# Modern Nutrition in Health and Disease

# Modern Nutrition in Health and Disease

SEVENTH EDITION

Edited by

## MAURICE E. SHILS, M.D., Sc.D.

*Professor Emeritus of Medicine*
*Cornell University Medical College*
*Consultant in Clinical Nutrition*
*Memorial Sloan-Kettering Cancer Center*
*New York City, New York*

## VERNON R. YOUNG, Ph.D.

*Professor of Nutritional Biochemistry*
*Department of Applied Biological Sciences*
*Massachusetts Institute of Technology*
*Cambridge, Massachusetts*

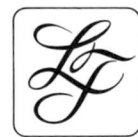

LEA & FEBIGER            *Philadelphia*            *1988*

Lea & Febiger
600 Washington Square
Philadelphia, PA   19106-4198
U.S.A.
(215) 922-1330

FIRST EDITION, 1955

SECOND EDITION, 1960

THIRD EDITION, 1964      *Reprinted February, 1966*

FOURTH EDITION, 1968     *Reprinted March, 1970*
                         *Reprinted July, 1971*

FIFTH EDITION, 1973      *Reprinted September, 1974*
                         *Reprinted April, 1975*
                         *Reprinted July, 1976*
                         *Reprinted January, 1978*
                         *Reprinted April, 1981*

SIXTH EDITION, 1980      *Reprinted April, 1984*

**Library of Congress Cataloging-in-Publication Data**

Modern nutrition in health and disease

   Includes bibliographies and index.
   1. Nutrition.  2. Diet therapy.
I. Shils, Maurice E. (Maurice Edward), 1914-
II. Young, Vernon R.
(Vernon Robert), 1937-
[DNLM: 1. Diet Therapy.  2. Nutrition.  WB 400 M689]
QP141.M64   1988        613.2       86-15314
ISBN 0-8121-0984-8

PRINTED IN THE UNITED STATES OF AMERICA

Print No.   4   3   2   1

To Cylia Shils–with affection and with appreciation for her critical support during the preparation of this book.

# Preface

The seventh edition of Modern Nutrition in Health and Disease continues the objectives of the previous editions in serving as a major textbook and reference source in basic and clinical nutrition for students and practitioners in the fields of biomedical research, medicine, dentistry, osteopathy, dietetics, nursing, pharmacy, and public health.

This volume considers the various aspects of the science and practice of nutrition in terms of the sources of calories and individual nutrients and their physiologic and metabolic interrelations, the adequacy and safety of diets and of the food supply, the assessment and therapy of malnutrition, nutritional needs during the life cycle and with work and exercise, modalities of nutrition support, and the role of diet and nutrition in the prevention and treatment of various diseases. Major revisions have been made and material updated to inform the reader of new information that we have gained rapidly in this vital and expanding field. The contributions to this volume emphasize the important role of nutrition in clinical medicine.

There are 20 new chapters or major subsections and 68 new authors compared to the previous edition. Additional space is devoted to trace elements, vitamin-like compounds, pseudovitamins, the role of intestinal flora, energetics, diet and drug interactions, nutrification of foods, nutrition assessment by various techniques, work and exercise, enteral feeding, diet and allergies, and nutrition and diet in relation to behavioral, neuro-logic, and rheumatic disorders. The Appendix with its various tables has been expanded.

This volume is the summary of current knowledge in the field by its distinguished contributors who, from seven countries, have made it an international edition. Our indebtedness to them is great. We extend appreciation to Kathleen Mannion, and also to Mr. Kenneth Bussy, Mr. Samuel Rondinelli, Ms. Amy Norwitz, and other members of the staff of Lea & Febiger who have been so helpful in the preparation of this volume.

This seventh edition of Modern Nutrition in Health and Disease is the first volume of its numerous editions which does not bear the name of Robert S. Goodhart, M.D., D.M.S. as an editor or author. Dr. Goodhart pioneered in vitamin research and clinical nutrition practice, headed the industrial feeding program of the U.S. Government in World War II, served as Director of the National Vitamin Foundation for many years, supporting basic and clinical research when funding from other sources was hard to come by, and was one of the founders of the American Society for Clinical Nutrition. The senior author has long been associated with Dr. Goodhart in many ways and acknowledges, with gratitude and respect, his indebtedness for having had the opportunity of learning from his agile, critical, and objective mind and for his friendship. We wish him and Mrs. Goodhart continued good health in their retirement.

*New York, NY*                     Maurice E. Shils
*Cambridge, MA*                    Vernon R. Young

# Contributors

Phyllis B. Acosta, Dr.P.H.
*Professor and Head, Nutritional Food Science*
*Department of Nutrition and Food Science*
*Florida State University*
*Tallahassee, Florida*

G. Harvey Anderson, Ph.D.
*Professor and Chairman*
*Department of Nutritional Sciences*
*Associate Dean, Research*
*University of Toronto*
*Toronto, Ontario*
*Canada*

James W. Anderson, M.D.
*Professor of Medicine and Clinical Nutrition*
*University of Kentucky*
*Chief, Endocrine-Metabolic Section*
*Veterans Administration Medical Center*
*Lexington, Kentucky*

Richard A. Anderson, Ph.D.
*Lead Scientist*
*U.S. Department of Agriculture*
*Human Nutrition Research Center*
*Beltsville, Maryland*

Louis V. Avioli, M.D.
*Shoenberg Professor of Medicine*
*Director, Division of Bone and Mineral Metabolism*
*Washington University School of Medicine*
*St. Louis, Missouri*

J. Christopher Bauernfeind, Ph.D.
*Formerly, Director of Agrochemistry and Nutrition*
*Research Coordinator*
*Hoffman-La Roche, Inc.*
*Gainseville, Florida*

George H. Beaton, Ph.D.
*Professor, Department of Nutritional Sciences*
*University of Toronto*
*Toronto, Ontario*
*Canada*

Ernest Beutler, M.D.
*Chairman, Department of Basic and Clinical Research*
*Research Institute of Scripps Clinic*
*Scripps Clinic and Research Foundation*
*Head, Division of Hematology/Oncology*
*Green Hospital of Scripps Clinic*
*La Jolla, California*

Edwin L. Bierman, M.D.
*Professor of Medicine*
*Chief, Division of Metabolism, Endocrinology, and*
*Nutrition*
*School of Medicine*
*University of Washington*
*Seattle, Washington*

Laurence M. Blendis, M.D.
*Professor of Medicine*
*Department of Medicine*
*University of Toronto*
*Senior Physician*
*Division of Internal Medicine and Gastroenterology*
*Toronto General Hospital*
*Toronto, Ontario*
*Canada*

Abby Stolper Bloch, M.S., R.D.
*Director, Clinical Nutrition Support Kitchen*
*Memorial Sloan-Kettering Cancer Center*
*New York, New York*

Alfred J. Bollet, M.D.
*Clinical Professor of Medicine*
*Yale University School of Medicine*
*New Haven, Connecticut*
*Adjunct Professor of Medicine*
*New York Medical College*
*Valhalla, New York*
*Chairman, Department of Medicine*
*Danbury Hospital*
*Danbury, Connecticut*

Benjamin Borenstein, Ph.D.
*Director, Product Development and Applications*
*Roche Vitamins and Fine Chemicals*
*A Division of Hoffmann-La Roche, Inc.*
*Nutley, New Jersey*

Harry P. Broquist, Ph.D.
*Division of Nutrition*
*Department of Biochemistry*
*Vanderbilt University*
*Nashville, Tennessee*

Alan Chait, M.B., M.D.
*Professor of Medicine*
*Head, Section of Clinical Nutrition*
*University of Washington*
*Seattle, Washington*

Ranjit Kumar Chandra, M.D.
*Professor of Pediatric Research, Medicine, and*
  *Biochemistry*
*Memorial University of Newfoundland*
*Director of Immunology*
*Janeway Child Health Center*
*St. John's, Newfoundland*
*Canada*

Ronni Chernoff, Ph.D., R.D.
*Associate Director, Geriatric Research, Education, and*
  *Clinical Center for Education and Evaluation*
*John L. McClellan Memorial Veterans Hospital*
*Little Rock, Arkansas*

Neville Colman, M.B., Ph.D.
*Professor of Medicine*
*Mt. Sinai School of Medicine*
*New York, New York*
*Hematology and Nutrition Laboratory*
*Bronx VA Medical Center*
*Bronx, New York*

Arthur Cooper, M.D.
*Assistant Professor of Surgery and of Pediatrics*
*Robert Wood Johnson Medical School*
*University of Medicine and Dentistry of New Jersey*
*Piscataway, New Jersey*
*Assistant Professor of Clinical Surgery (Adjunct)*
*College of Physicians and Surgeons*
*Columbia University*
*New York, New York*

Marilyn C. Crim, M.D., Ph.D.
*Medical Director*
*Eating Disorder Center*
*Marshall Hale Memorial Hospital*
*San Francisco, California*

Hector F. DeLuca, Ph.D.
*Steenbock Research Professor*
*Department of Biochemistry*
*University of Wisconsin-Madison*
*Madison, Wisconsin*

Mukesh B. Desai, M.B., B.S.
*Fellow*
*Division of Gastroenterology*
*Toronto General Hospital*
*Toronto, Ontario*
*Canada*

John T. Devlin, M.D.
*Assistant Professor of Medicine*
*University of Vermont*
*Burlington, Vermont*

Pierre M. Dreyfus, M.D.
*Professor of Neurology and Pediatrics*
*Department of Neurology*
*University of California School of Medicine-Davis*
*Davis, California*

Johanna T. Dwyer, D.Sc., R.D.
*Professor of Medicine (Nutrition) and Professor of*
  *Community Health*
*Tufts University School of Medicine*
*Director, Frances Stern Nutrition Center*
*New England Medical Center Hospital*
*Boston, Massachusetts*

Daniel Einhorn, M.D.
*Clinical Assistant Professor of Medicine*
*University of California—San Diego*
*Medical Director, Nutritional Disorders Program*
*San Diego Endocrine and Medical Clinic*
*Teaching Faculty*
*Mercy Hospital Medical Center*
*San Diego, California*

Louis J. Elsas, II, M.D.
*Professor of Pediatrics*
*Director of Division of Medical Genetics*
*Department of Pediatrics and Biochemistry*
*Emory University School of Medicine*
*Atlanta, Georgia*

Virgil F. Fairbanks, M.D.
*Professor*
*Laboratory Medicine and Internal Medicine*
  *(Hematology)*
*Mayo Medical School*
*Consultant in Hematology and Internal Medicine*
*Mayo Clinic and Mayo Foundation*
*Rochester, Minnesota*

Michael D. Fallon, M.D.
*Assistant Professor of Pathology*
*Department of Pathology and Laboratory Medicine*
*University of Pennsylvania School of Medicine*
*Attending Pathologist*
*Hospital of the University of Pennsylvania*
*Philadelphia, Pennsylvania*

Philip M. Farrell, M.D., Ph.D.
*Professor and Chairman*
*Department of Pediatrics*
*Affiliate Faculty Member*
*Department of Nutritional Sciences*
*University of Wisconsin*
*Chief of Pediatrics*
*University of Wisconsin Hospital and Clinics*
*Milwaukee, Wisconsin*

Gilbert B. Forbes, M.D.
*Professor of Pediatrics and Biophysics*
*University of Rochester School of Medicine and*
  *Dentistry*
*Pediatrician*
*Strong Memorial Hospital*
*Rochester, New York*

Beat E. Glatthaar, Ph.D.
*Department of Vitamin and Nutrition Research*
*Vitamin and Fine Chemicals Division*
*F. Hoffmann-La Roche and Co., Ltd.*
*Basel, Switzerland*

Barry R. Goldin, Ph.D.
*Associate Professor*
*Departments of Community Health and Medicine*
*Tufts University School of Medicine*
*Boston, Massachusetts*
*Adjunct Associate Professor*
*School of Nutrition*
*Tufts University*
*Medford, Massachusetts*

Elizabeth J. Gong, M.P.H., M.S., R.D.
*Instructor*
*Division of Adolescent Medicine*
*Department of Pediatrics*
*University of Maryland School of Medicine*
*Baltimore, Maryland*

Sherwood L. Gorbach, M.D.
*Professor of Medicine, Community Health, and*
   *Microbiology*
*Tufts University School of Medicine*
*New England Medical Center*
*Boston, Massachusetts*

Gordon R. Greenberg, M.D.
*Associate Professor of Medicine*
*University of Toronto*
*Staff Gastroenterologist*
*Department of Medicine*
*Toronto General Hospital*
*Toronto, Ontario*
*Canada*

Harry L. Greene, M.D.
*Professor of Pediatrics*
*Associate Professor of Biochemistry*
*Vanderbilt Medical School*
*Head, Division of Pediatric Gastroenterology*
*Director, Clinical Nutrition Research Unit*
*Vanderbilt University Medical Center*
*Nashville, Tennessee*

Herman Grossman, M.D.
*Professor of Radiology*
*Duke University Medical Center*
*Durham, North Carolina*

Roger C. Harris, Ph.D.
*Principal Biochemist*
*Physiology Unit*
*Equine Research Station*
*Suffolk, England*
*U.K.*

Kenneth C. Hayes, D.V.M., Ph.D.
*Director and Professor of Biology (Nutrition)*
*Foster Biomedical Research Laboratory*
*Brandeis University*
*Waltham, Massachusetts*

Felix P. Heald, M.D.
*Professor of Pediatrics*
*Director, Division of Adolescent Medicine*
*Department of Pediatrics*
*University of Maryland School of Medicine*
*Baltimore, Maryland*

William C. Heird, M.D.
*Associate Professor of Pediatrics*
*College of Physicians and Surgeons*
*Columbia University*
*Associate Attending Pediatrican*
*Babies Hospital*
*New York, New York*

Victor D. Herbert, M.D., J.D.
*Chief, Hematology and Nutrition Laboratory*
*Bronx VA Hospital*
*Bronx, New York*

Steven B. Heymsfield, M.D.
*Associate Professor of Medicine*
*College of Physicians and Surgeons*
*Columbia University*
*Director, Human Body Composition Laboratory*
*Director, Outpatient Obesity Research*
*Obesity Research Center*
*St. Luke's-Roosevelt Hospital Center*
*New York, New York*

L. John Hoffer, M.D., Ph.D.
*Assistant Professor of Medicine*
*Department of Medicine*
*McGill Nutrition and Food Science Center*
*McGill University*
*Attending Physician*
*Division of General Internal Medicine*
*Royal Victoria Hospital*
*Montreal, Quebec*
*Canada*

Dietrich H. Hornig, Ph.D.
*Department of Human Nutrition and Health*
*Vitamin and Fine Chemicals Division*
*F. Hoffman-La Roche and Co., Ltd.*
*Basel, Switzerland*

Edward S. Horton, M.D.
*Professor of Medicine*
*Director of Endocrinology and Metabolism*
*Department of Medicine*
*University of Vermont School of Medicine*
*Burlington, Vermont*

Eric Hultman, M.D.
*Professor, Karolinska Institute*
*Department of Clinical Chemistry II*
*Huddinge University Hospital*
*Huddinge, Sweden*

Diane M. Huse, M.S., R.D.
*Assistant Professor in Nutrition*
*Mayo Medical School*
*Nutritionist, Clinical Dietetics*
*Division of Endocrinology, Metabolism, and Internal*
   *Medicine*
*Mayo Clinic and Mayo Foundation*
*Rochester, Minnesota*

Khursheed N. Jeejeebhoy, M.B., Ph.D.
*Professor of Medicine*
*University of Toronto*
*Director, Division of Gastroenterology*
*Toronto General Hospital*
*Toronto, Ontario*
*Canada*

David J.A. Jenkins, M.D., Ph.D.
*Professor, Department of Nutritional Sciences and*
   *Department of Medicine*
*University of Toronto*
*Staff Physician*
*Division of Endocrinology and Metabolism*
*St. Michael's Hospital*
*Associate Physician*
*Division of Gastroenterology*
*Toronto General Hospital*
*Toronto, Ontario*
*Canada*

John M. Kinney, M.D.
*Visiting Professor*
*Rockefeller University*
*Senior Attending, Medical and Surgical Services*
*St. Luke's-Roosevelt Hospital Center*
*New York, New York*

Joel D. Kopple, M.D.
*Professor of Medicine and Public Health*
*University of California—Los Angeles*
*Los Angeles, California*
*Chief, Division of Nephrology and Hypertension*
*Harbor-UCLA Medical Center*
*Torrance, California*

Paul A. Lachance, Ph.D.
*Professor of Nutrition and Food Science*
*Department of Food Science*
*Rutgers University*
*New Brunswick, New Jersey*

Lewis Landsberg, M.D.
*Professor of Medicine*
*Harvard Medical School*
*Chief, Division of Endocrinology and Metabolism*
*Beth Israel Hospital*
*Boston, Massachusetts*

Orville A. Levander, Ph.D.
*Research Chemist*
*Vitamin and Mineral Nutrition Laboratory*
*Human Nutrition Research Center*
*U.S. Department of Agriculture*
*Beltsville, Maryland*

Alice H. Lichtenstein, D.Sc.
*Assistant Research Professor of Medicine and*
*    Biochemistry*
*Boston University School of Medicine*
*Boston, Massachusetts*
*Visiting Assistant Professor*
*School of Nutrition*
*Tufts University*
*Medford, Massachusetts*

Charles S. Lieber, M.D.
*Professor of Medicine*
*Mt. Sinai School of Medicine*
*City University of New York*
*New York, New York*
*Chief, Section of Liver Disease and Nutrition*
*Director, Alcohol Research and Treatment Center and*
*    GI-Liver Training Program*
*Bronx VA Medical Center*
*Bronx, New York*

Willem G. Linscheer, M.D., Ph.D.
*Professor of Medicine*
*State University of New York—Syracuse*
*Chief, Gastroenterology Section*
*VA Medical Center*
*Syracuse, New York*

David A. Lipschitz, M.D., Ph.D.
*Professor of Medicine*
*Head, Division on Aging*
*University of Arkansas for Medical Sciences*
*Director, Geriatric Research, Education, and Clinical*
*    Center for Education and Evaluation*
*John L. McClellan Memorial Veterans Hospital*
*Little Rock, Arkansas*

Alexander R. Lucas, M.D.
*Professor in Psychiatry*
*Mayo Medical School*
*Consultant, Section of Child and Adolescent*
*    Psychiatry*
*Mayo Clinic and Mayo Foundation*
*Rochester, Minnesota*

Ian MacDonald, M.D., D.Sc.
*Professor*
*Head, Division of Physiology*
*Guy's Hospital*
*London, England*
*U.K.*

Donald B. McCormick, Ph.D.
*Fuller E. Callaway Professor and Chairman*
*Department of Biochemistry*
*Executive Associate Dean for Science*
*Emory University School of Medicine*
*Atlanta, Georgia*

Donald S. McLaren, M.D., Ph.D.
*Reader in Clinical Nutrition*
*Department of Medicine*
*University of Edinburgh*
*Honorary Consultant Physician*
*The Royal Infirmary*
*Edinburgh, Scotland*
*U.K.*

Morton A. Meyers, M.D.
*Professor and Chairman of Radiology*
*State University of New York—Stony Brook*
*Stony Brook, New York*

Therese D. Mondeika, R.D.
*Assistant Director*
*Department of Personal Health*
*Division of Clinical Sciences*
*American Medical Association*
*Chicago, Illinois*

Ulrich Moser, Ph.D.
*Head, Vitamin C Research Laboratory*
*Department of Vitamin and Nutrition Research*
*Vitamin and Fine Chemicals Division*
*F. Hoffmann-La Roche and Co., Ltd.*
*Basel, Switzerland*

Hamish N. Munro, M.D., D.Sc.
*Professor of Medicine and Professor of Nutrition*
*Tufts University School of Medicine*
*Boston, Massachusetts*
*Adjunct Professor of Physiological Chemistry*
*Massachusetts Institute of Technology*
*Cambridge, Massachusetts*
*USDA Human Nutrition Research Center on Aging*
*Boston, Massachusetts*

Quentin N. Myrvik, Ph.D.
*Professor of Microbiology and Immunology*
*Bowman Gray School of Medicine*
*Winston-Salem, North Carolina*

Paul M. Newberne, D.V.M., M.Sc., Ph.D.
*Professor of Pathology*
*Boston University School of Medicine*
*Department of Pathology*
*Mallory Institute of Pathology*
*Boston, Massachusetts*

Forrest H. Nielsen, Ph.D.
*Research Chemist*
*Grand Forks Human Nutrition Research Center*
*USDA Agricultural Research Service*
*Grand Forks, North Dakota*

James A. Olson, Ph.D.
*Distinguished Professor of Sciences and Humanities*
*Professor of Biochemistry*
*Chairman, Department of Biochemistry and*
*    Biophysics*
*Iowa State University*
*Ames, Iowa*

Robert E. Olson, M.D., Ph.D.
*Professor of Medicine and Pharmacological Sciences*
*School of Medicine*
*Attending Physician*
*University Hospital*
*State University of New York–Stony Brook*
*Stony Brook, New York*

F. Xavier Pi-Sunyer, M.D.
*Professor of Clinical Medicine*
*College of Physicians and Surgeons*
*Columbia University*
*Chief, Division of Endocrinology and Diabetes*
*Associate Director, Obesity Research Center*
*St. Luke's-Roosevelt Hospital Center*
*New York, New York*

Henry T. Randall, M.D., D.M.Sc.
*Professor Emeritus of Medical Science*
*Brown University Program in Medicine*
*Consulting Surgeon, Former Surgeon-in-Chief*
*Rhode Island Hospital*
*Providence, Rhode Island*

Daphne A. Roe, M.D.
*Professor of Nutrition*
*Division of Nutritional Sciences*
*Cornell University*
*Ithaca, New York*
*Adjunct Professor of Nutrition*
*Upstate Medical Center*
*State University of New York—Syracuse*
*Syracuse, New York*

Irwin H. Rosenberg, M.D.
*Professor of Medicine*
*Tufts University*
*Director, USDA Human Nutrition Research Center on*
*    Aging*
*Boston, Massachusetts*

Robin I. Russell, M.D., Ph.D.
*Professor of Medicine*
*University of Glasgow*
*Consultant-in-Charge*
*Gastroenterology Unit*
*Royal Infirmary*
*Glasgow, Scotland*
*U.K.*

Frederic R. Senti, Ph.D.
*Senior Scientific Consultant*
*Life Sciences Research Consultant*
*Life Sciences Research Office*
*Federation of American Societies of Experimental*
*    Biology*
*Bethesda, Maryland*

James H. Shaw, Ph.D.
*Professor Emeritus of Nutrition*
*Harvard School of Dental Medicine*
*Boston, Massachusetts*

Spencer Shaw, M.D.
*Associate Professor of Medicine*
*Mt. Sinai School of Medicine*
*New York, New York*
*Assistant Chief, Section of Liver Disease and*
*    Nutrition*
*Bronx VA Medical Center*
*Bronx, New York*

Maurice E. Shils, M.D., Sc.D.
*Professor Emeritus of Medicine*
*Cornell University Medical College*
*Consultant in Clinical Nutrition*
*Memorial Sloan-Kettering Cancer Center*
*New York, New York*

Noel W. Solomons, M.D.
*Senior Scientist and Coordinator*
*Center for Studies of Sensory Impairment, Aging, and*
*    Metabolism (CeSSIAM)*
*Research Branch for the Committee for the Blind and*
*    Deaf of Guatemala*
*Guatemala City, Guatemala*
*Central America*

Wiley W. Souba, M.D., Sc.D.
*Assistant Professor of Surgery and Biochemistry*
*Chief, Surgical Metabolism*
*Director, Surgical Nutrition/Metabolism Laboratories*
*Department of Surgery*
*University of Florida School of Medicine*
*Gainseville, Florida*

John B. Stanbury, M.D.
*Professor Emeritus of Experimental Medicine*
*Senior Lecturer*
*Massachusetts Institute of Technology*
*Lecturer*
*Harvard Medical School*
*Senior Physician*
*Massachusetts General Hospital*
*Boston, Massachusetts*

Edward A. Sweeney, D.M.D.
*Clinical Associate Professor of Pediatric Dentistry*
*University of Pennsylvania School of Dental Medicine*
*Senior Dentist*
*Children's Hospital of Philadelphia*
*Philadelphia, Pennsylvania*

James A. Thomson, Ph.D.
*Associate Professor*
*Department of Kinesiology*
*University of Waterloo*
*Waterloo, Ontario*
*Canada*

Benjamín Torún, M.D., Ph.D.
*Senior Scientist and Head*
*Program of Clinical Nutrition and Metabolism*
*Institute de Nutrición de Centro América y Panamá*
  *(INCAP)*
*Professor of Basic and Human Nutrition*
*INCAP/Universidad de San Carlos de Guatemala*
*Visiting Scientist*
*Hospital Roosevelt*
*Guatemala City, Guatemala*

Antoine J. Vergroesen, M.D., Ph.D.
*Unilever Research Laboratory*
*Vlaardingen*
*Nederland*

Fernando E. Viteri, M.D., Sc.D.
*Professor of Nutrition*
*Department of Nutritional Sciences*
*University of California–Berkeley*
*Berkeley, California*
*Scientist, Bay Area Human Nutrition Center*
*San Francisco General Hospital*
*San Francisco, California*

Robin C. Watson, M.D.
*Professor of Radiology*
*Cornell University Medical College*
*Chairman, Department of Medical Imaging*
*Memorial Sloan-Kettering Cancer Center*
*New York, New York*

Philip L. White, Sc.D.
*Former Director, Division of Personal and Public*
  *Health*
*American Medical Association*
*Chicago, Illinois*

R.G. Whitehead, M.D.
*Director, MRC Nutrition Unit*
*University of Cambridge and Medical Research*
  *Council*
*Fellow, Darwin College*
*Cambridge, England*
*U.K.*

Elsie M. Widdowson, D.Sc., F.R.S.
*Department of Medicine*
*University of Cambridge, Clinical School*
*Adenbrooke's Hospital*
*Cambridge, England*
*U.K.*

Patricia J. Williams, B.S., R.D., M.M.Sc.
*Research Nutritionist*
*Department of Medicine*
*Emory University*
*Atlanta, Georgia*

Douglas W. Wilmore, M.D.
*Professor of Surgery*
*Harvard Medical School*
*Director, Nutrition/Metabolism Laboratory*
*Brigham and Women's Hospital*
*Boston, Massachusetts*

Peter C. Wilson, M.B.
*Associate in Gastroenterology and Medicine*
*Queen Elizabeth Hospital*
*Gastroenterologist*
*Repatriation General Hospital*
*Adelaide, S. Australia*
*Australia*

Stephen L. Wolman, M.D.
*Assistant Professor, Departments of Nutrition and*
  *Medicine*
*University of Toronto*
*Staff Physician*
*Division of Gastroenterology*
*Toronto General Hospital*
*Toronto, Ontario*
*Canada*

Steven H. Zeisel, M.D., Ph.D.
*Assistant Professor of Pathology and Pediatrics*
*Boston University School of Medicine*
*Assistant Visiting Physician, Pediatrics*
*Boston City Hospital*
*Boston, Massachusetts*

# Contents

**Part III**
*Adequacy and Safety of the Food Supply*

**Part IV**
*Malnutrition, Its Assessment and Therapy*

**Part V**
*Nutrition in Growth, Aging, and Physiologic Stress*

**Part VI**
*Techniques in Meeting Special Nutritional Needs*

**Part VII**
*Diet and Nutrition in the Prevention and Treatment of Disease*

# Part I
## *Nutrients, Minerals, Vitamins*

*Chapter* **1**

# THE PROTEINS AND AMINO ACIDS

## Hamish N. Munro and Marilyn C. Crim

Proteins are associated with all forms of life, an observation that dates back to the original identification of proteins as a class by Mulder in 1838, although earlier investigators had evidence of a less precise character for a similar group of compounds associated with living matter.[1] The proteins of living matter act as organic catalysts (enzymes), as structural features of the cell, as messengers (peptide hormones), and as antibodies. The accumulation of proteins during growth and development and the maintenance of tissue proteins in the adult represent important objectives in ensuring nutritional well-being. A knowledge of how dietary protein is optimally utilized by the body is important in determining how much protein is needed for health and for the restoration of body tissue in disease. For this reason, this chapter begins with the metabolism of amino acids, including their uses as a source of nitrogen for the biosynthesis of other major constituents of the body. The next section describes the roles of individual organs in the utilization of dietary protein, providing an integrated picture of protein metabolism and its responses to food intake. Estimates of the requirements of human sub-

jects for protein and for individual amino acids are then discussed, and changes in such needs as a result of disease are evaluated.

The importance of protein in the diet is primarily to act as a source of amino acids, some of which are *essential* (indispensable) dietary constituents because their carbon skeletons are not synthesized in the bodies of animals; others are *nonessential* (dispensable) because they can be made within the animal from carbon and nitrogen precursors. A survey of species ranging from single-celled animals (protozoa) to man shows that all animal species from single-celled organisms onward need some preformed amino acids in their diets.[2] In general, these essential amino acids include histidine, isoleucine, leucine, lysine, methionine, phenylalanine, threonine, tryptophan, and valine; in addition, cysteine and tyrosine are synthesized in the body from methionine and phenylalanine, respectively. All of these 11 amino acids occur in most proteins in the cells of the body. An additional nine amino acids (alanine, arginine, aspartic acid, asparagine, glutamic acid, glutamine, glycine, proline, and serine) are also present in proteins, but can be deleted from the diet because the body has the capacity to synthesize them from simple precursors. They are thus *nonessential* in the diet. Other amino acids occur in proteins, but these are made by modifying the side chains of one of the aforementioned after the protein has been synthesized. For example, hydroxyproline occurs in collagen by hydroxylation of certain proline residues in the collagen peptides as they are being made. Similarly, the contractile proteins actin and myosin of muscle contain 3-methylhistidine, made by methylation of certain histidine residues in these proteins. These derived amino acids are not used again for de novo protein synthesis. When proteins containing them are broken down within the body, they are either metabolized (hydroxyproline) or excreted quantitatively (3-methylhistidine).

Figure 1–1 shows the structural formulas of the 20 amino acids used for protein synthesis. All except glycine have an asymmetrical carbon atom, and thus can exist as optically active isomers that rotate the plane of polarized lights to the left (levorotatory) or to the right (dextrorotatory). Only one out of each amino acid isomer pair is used by the body for constructing its proteins. The amino acid isomers used for protein synthesis all have similar structural conformations around the asymmetric carbon atom, the amino group and the carboxyl group occupying the same relative spatial relationship to one another. These amino acids are

therefore designated as the L-series, whereas those never found in proteins are called the D-series, regardless of how they rotate the plane of polarized light. Many metabolic reactions, including those of protein synthesis and transport across cell walls, distinguish L- from D-forms. However, certain reactions (transaminations) can transform the D-form into the L-form and thus make it available to the body. The capacity to use dietary D-amino acids is limited to certain amino acids that vary from species to species.[2] In man, these are D-methionine and D-phenylalanine.[2] Studies with intravenous infusion of D-methionine indicate that it is utilized less efficiently than the L-form.

The structural features of the 20 amino acids show that some are dibasic (arginine, lysine, histidine) and some diacidic (aspartic acid, glutamic acid.) (see Fig. 1–1). These characteristics are important in determining the properties of proteins containing an abundance of dibasic or diacidic amino acids (e.g., diacidic amino acids are especially abundant in proteins forming parts of membranes). Most amino acids are, however, neutral with an aliphatic or aromatic side chain. The classification of amino acids into neutral, basic, and acidic has particular relevance to amino acid transport across membranes, since each amino acid class appears to be carried by a separate mechanism.

## METABOLISM OF AMINO ACIDS: INTRACELLULAR EVENTS

This section deals with free amino acid pools, their metabolic effects, the pathways of their degradation and some other pathways using amino acids.

### Free Amino Acid Pools and their Metabolic Effects

Protein consumed in the diet is enzymatically hydrolyzed in the alimentary tract and passes into the blood as free amino acids that mingle with amino acids coming from the tissues. Amino acids occur in the body in the free form and in the form of the body proteins. The concentration of protein-bound amino acids in the tissues averages 2 M, whereas the free amino acid pools are about 0.01 M,[3] that is, 0.5% of the concentration of protein-bound amino acids. Table 1–1 shows the distribution of individual amino acids between the body proteins and the free amino acid pools in the tissues of the young rat. The tissue concentrations of the free *essential* amino acids are very low, whereas the concentrations of four of the *nonessential* amino acids (alanine, glutamic acid, glutamine, and glycine) are higher. On the other hand, the concentrations of free amino acids in rat

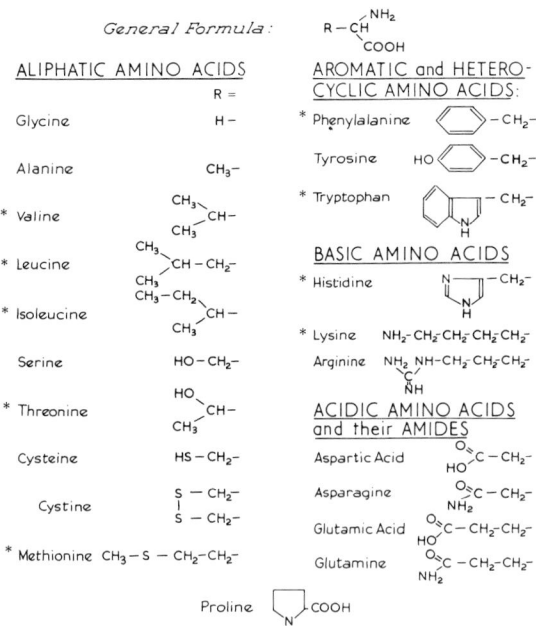

**Fig. 1–1.** Formulas of the 20 common amino acids found in proteins. Essential amino acids are marked with an asterisk(*).

**Table 1–1.    Amounts of Protein-Bound and Free Amino Acids in the Body of a 50-g Rat, and the Concentrations of Free Amino Acids in Rat Plasma***

| Amino Acid | Total Body Content of Amino Acids (μmoles/100-g rat) | | Free Amino Acids in Rat Plasma (μmoles/dl) | Daily Amino Acid Requirement (μmoles/100-g rat) |
|---|---|---|---|---|
| | Protein-bound | Free | | |
| *Essential* | | | | |
| Arginine | 8,400 | 7 | 16 | — |
| Histidine | 3,600 | 24 | 11 | 140 |
| Isoleucine | 8,400 | 10 | 8 | 400 |
| Leucine | 16,500 | 14 | 16 | 500 |
| Lysine | 8,900 | 15 | 41 | 600 |
| Methionine | 4,050 | 6 | 9 | 350 |
| Phenylalanine | 5,800 | 9 | 9 | 450 |
| Threonine | 7,550 | 20 | 24 | 400 |
| Tryptophan | 980 | 2 | — | 55 |
| Valine | 9,400 | 12 | 18 | 500 |
| *Nonessential* | | | | |
| Alanine | 13,500 | 100 | 32 | — |
| Aspartic acid | 11,300 | 19 | 1 | — |
| Glutamic acid | 17,700 | 132 | 15 | — |
| Glutamine | — | 223 | 55 | — |
| Glycine | 24,700 | 323 | 45 | — |
| Serine | 12,400 | 20 | 23 | — |
| Tyrosine | 3,550 | 8 | 9 | — |

*Adapted by Munro, H.N.,[4] from Herbert, J.D., et al.[5]

plasma all fall within a similar range (see Table 1–1). This occurs because the four nonessential amino acids present in most abundance in the tissues are extensively synthesized within the cells.

Comparison of the concentrations of free essential amino acids in the body with the essential amino acid requirements for the growing rat (see Table 1–1) demonstrates that the free amino acid pool must turn over several times daily through the flux from dietary sources. The magnitude of the flux of amino acids in the body is increased even further by recycling of amino acids coming from the breakdown of proteins in the tissues.

Transport of free amino acids across cell membranes has been extensively studied, and has been found to occur by several carrier mechanisms, each common to a number of amino acids.[3] In general, basic, acidic, and neutral amino acids each enter the tissues by different transport mediators. In each category, a degree of competition for the carrier can be demonstrated between any two amino acids of that class. Within the neutral class, Christensen described two groups of transport mechanisms.[3] One has high affinity for alanine and for alpha-aminoisobutyric acid, a synthetic nonprotein amino acid. This carrier is sensitive to respiratory inhibitors. On the other hand, the branched-chain neutral amino acids are taken up by a different mechanism that is relatively insensitive to respiratory inhibitors. This second form of uptake appears to depend for its driving force on exchange of intracellular neutral amino acids for extracellular amino acids. Finally, Meister has proposed a transport mechanism located in the cell membrane and involving glutathione for the actual movement of amino acids into the cells.[6]

There has been considerable dispute about whether free intracellular amino acids are the ultimate source for protein synthesis within cells, or whether extracellular amino acids charge transfer RNA (tRNA) for protein synthesis without entering the cell fluid.[7,8] This problem is important in studies of protein synthesis in whole animals because breakdown of tissue protein within cells contributes amino acids that dilute the intracellular free amino acid pool more than the plasma pool. In consequence, isotopically labeled amino acids undergo a greater reduction in specific activity within cells than in the blood,[9] so that the rate of synthesis of intracellular proteins computed from the specific activity of the free amino acids in each precursor pool can be quite different. Khairallah has measured the specific activity of liver amino-acyl-tRNA after giving labeled leucine to rats, and has found that the tRNA has an activity midway between that of free leucine in the plasma and in the liver cells.[10] He concludes that tRNA is charged with amino acids by a pool closely associated with the cell membrane and receiving amino acids from both the external and intracellular sources.

Amino acids are subjected within the body to

the series of metabolic reactions outlined in Figure 1–2. Although this diagram represents a complex series of pathways, we can group these reactions into three categories:

1. Part of the free amino acid pool is incorporated into tissue proteins. Because of protein breakdown, these amino acids return to the free pool after a variable length of time and thus become available for reutilization for protein synthesis or for catabolism.

2. Part of the free amino acid pool undergoes catabolic reactions. This process leads to loss of the carbon skeleton as $CO_2$ or its deposition as glycogen and fat, while the nitrogen is eliminated as urea. Individual pathways of amino acid catabolism are discussed later in this chapter.

3. Some free amino acids are used for synthesis of new N-containing compounds, such as purine bases, creatine, and epinephrine. These are subsequently generally degraded without return of end products to the free amino acid pool (e.g., purines are degraded to uric acid, creatine to creatinine, epinephrine to vanillylmandelic acid). In addition, the nonessential amino acids are made in the body using amino groups derived from other amino acids and carbon skeletons formed by reactions common to intermediary metabolism.

The relative magnitudes of these three pathways in the whole animal are represented by studies in which rats were fed by stomach tube with 1-mg doses of uniformly [14]C-labeled L-tyrosine, L-phenylalanine, or L-tryptophan.[12] The investigators measured the proportion of absorbed radioactivity excreted during the first four hours in the form of [14]$CO_2$ or recovered from the liver, gut, and total skeletal musculature in the form of protein-bound activity or nonprotein compounds. At 15 minutes after feeding, 20 to 40% of the absorbed radioactivity of the three amino acids was recovered as acid-soluble compounds in liver, gut, and muscle, most being in muscle. Considerable amounts of nonaromatic radioactive compounds were present at this time, indicating rapid breakdown of the free amino acids. Thereafter, acid-soluble [14]C activity decreased, whereas output as [14]$CO_2$ rose and eventually accounted for 19 to 40% of the absorbed dose. Protein-bound activity in the three tissues represented 34 to 51% of the absorbed activity at four hours after feeding. The relative magnitudes of these pathways depend, of course, on the nutritional state of the animal. In a later section, we shall see that the proportion of lysine degraded to $CO_2$ increases progressively as intake of lysine exceeds requirement, and that this is regulated by the liver.

### Pathways of Degradation

Each amino acid is degraded by undergoing a special sequence of chemical reactions. The details of these are not relevant in this volume, and can be obtained from texts on biochemistry. In Figure 1–3 the routes of degradation of the essential and nonessential amino acids are outlined to show how $NH_3$ and glutamic acid are made avail-

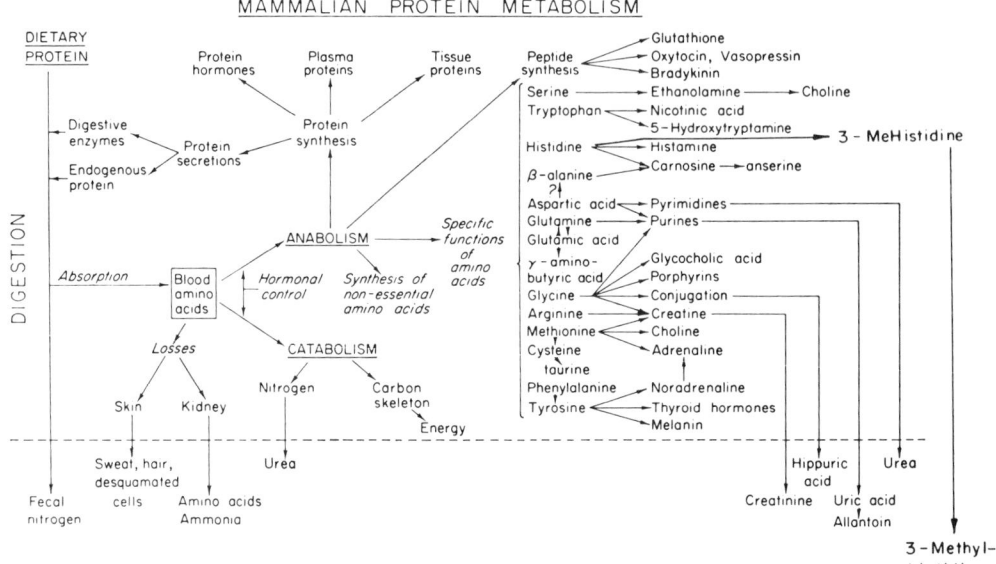

**Fig. 1–2.**　General features of mammalian protein metabolism. (From Munro, H.N.)[11]

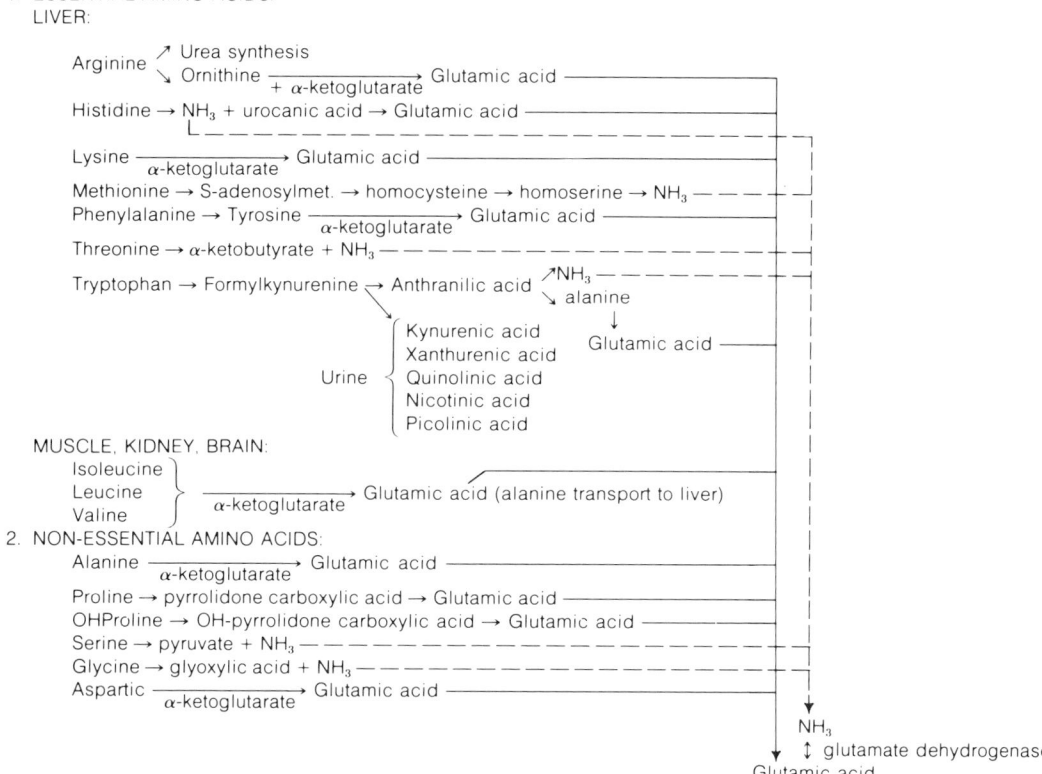

**Fig. 1–3.** Degradative pathways of amino acid metabolism.

able by these degradative reactions for eventual excretion as urea. The figure also shows that 7 of the 10 amino acids essential to the rat are primarily degraded in the liver, whereas the other 3 (the branched-chain amino acids isoleucine, leucine, and valine) are mostly catabolized in muscle, as well as in kidney and brain. Much of the amino group made available by transamination of the branched-chain amino acids in muscle is transferred to pyruvate and glutamate to produce, respectively, alanine and glutamine. In these forms they go by way of the blood to the liver (alanine) and the gut (glutamine). In the gut wall, alanine and glutamic acid are formed, and the alanine passes by way of the portal system to the liver. This process facilitates the transport of amino-N to the liver for urea formation, while the carbon of alanine becomes available for gluconeogenesis.

Urea synthesis is performed in the liver.[13] The process is summarized in Figure 1–4. Ammonia and $CO_2$ first form carbamyl phosphate. This reacts in turn with ornithine to give citrulline, which then acquires another N from aspartic acid to form argininosuccinate. This substance splits into arginine and fumarate, the latter going back to the tricarboxylic acid cycle while the arginine

is finally split by arginase into urea and ornithine. Ornithine is thus released to participate in another cycle. Note that glutamic acid contributes N through aspartic acid. The urea so formed is mostly secreted directly into the urine, but some passes into the lumen of the gut where urease in the bacteria causes release of ammonia. This ammonia returns via the portal vein to the liver, where urea is again formed. About 20% urea is recycled in this way through the gut flora.[14]

## Other Pathways Utilizing Amino Acids

**Synthesis of Nonessential Amino Acids.** The division of amino acids into essential and nonessential was originally defined by Rose on the basis of whether they were necessary in the diet for optimal growth of rats.[15] Nonessential amino acids could be deleted from the diet without impairing optimal growth. In the case of adults beyond the stage of growth, N balance was impaired by withdrawal of essential amino acids. It has since been shown with isotopic labels that nonessential amino acids are made from precursors such as glucose, whereas the carbon skeletons of the essential amino acids do not take up the labeled precursor.[2] The pathways of synthesis of the

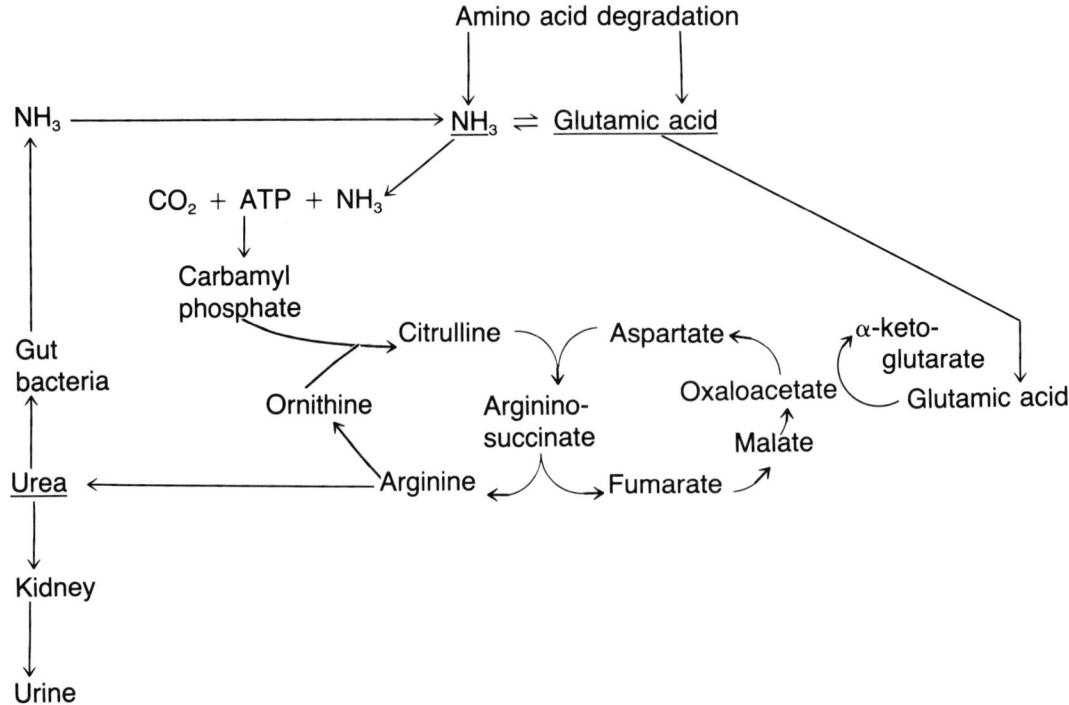

**Fig. 1–4.**   Mechanism of urea synthesis and recycling. (From Valgeirsdottir, K. and Munro, H.N.)[71]

nonessential amino acids are well established and are shown in Figure 1–5. These pathways are not always present in all tissues (e.g., tyrosine is formed by hydroxylation of phenylalanine only in the liver), and more than one biosynthetic route can exist (e.g., for serine).

**Purine and Pyrimidine Biosynthesis.** Purine and pyrimidine bases are synthesized in most cells of the body from simpler carbon and nitrogen precursors.[16] The major reactions are shown in Figures 1–6 and 1–7. These substances permit the formation of the ribonucleotides of adenine, guanine, uracil, and cytosine, which provide high-energy phosphate compounds (di- and triphosphates) in the cell, and also become polymerized to form RNA. The deoxyribonucleotides found in DNA are made by reduction of the ribose in the ribonucleotides.

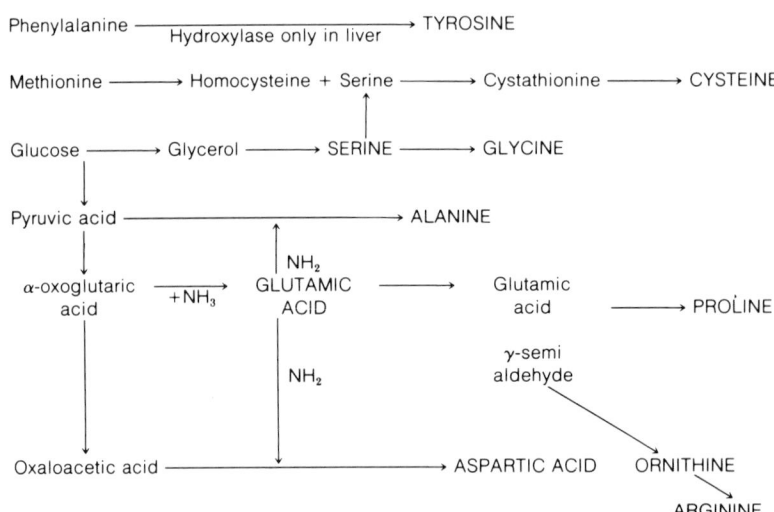

**Fig. 1–5.**   Pathways of synthesis of nonessential amino acid. (From Munro, H.N.)

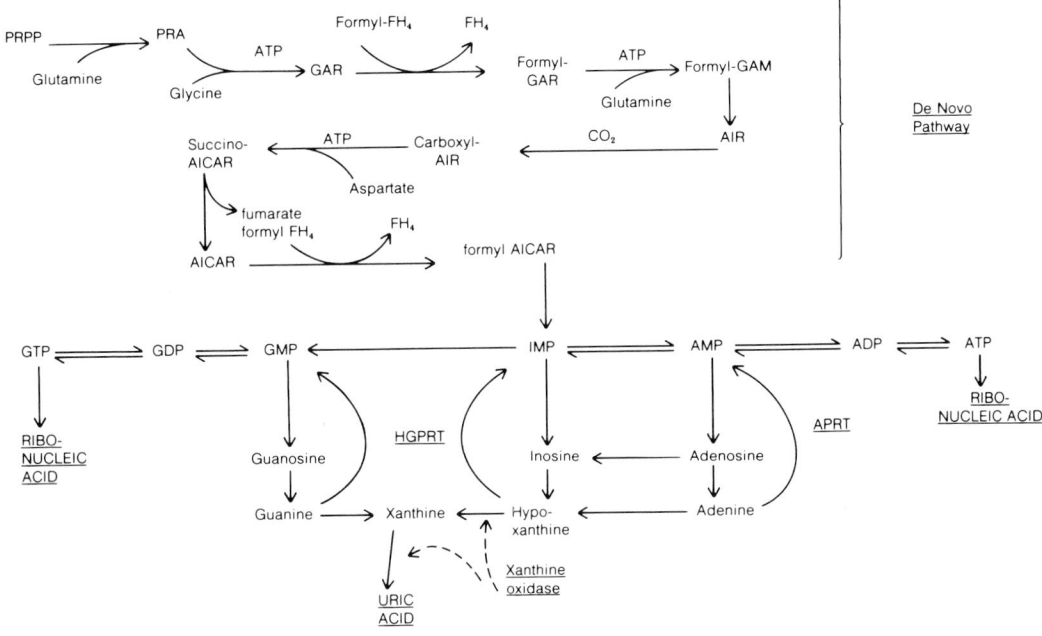

**Fig. 1–6.** De novo synthesis of purine nucleotides, nucleotide interchange, the salvage pathways, and purine degradation routes. *De novo pathway:* PRPP = phosphoribosylpyrophosphate; PRA = phosphoribosylamine; GAR = glycinamide ribonucleotide; formylGAM = N-formylglycinamidine ribonucleotide; AIR = amino-iminazole ribonucleotide; AICAR = amino-iminazole-carboxyamide ribonucleotide. *Nucleotide interchange:* IMP = inosinic acid (hypoxanthine ribonucleotide); AMP = adenylic acid; GMP = guanylic acid. *Salvage pathways:* APRT = adenine phosphoribosyltransferase; HGPRT = hypoxanthine-guanine phosphoribosyltransferase.

Biosynthesis of purine nucleotides can occur by two routes: de novo and salvage pathways. In de novo synthesis (see Fig. 1–6), glycine and phosphoribosylpyrophosphate (PRPP) initially react to form a series of products eventually providing the nucleotide inosine monophosphate (IMP) containing the base hypoxanthine. Adenylic acid (AMP) and guanylic acid (GMP) are then made from this nucleotide by altering substituents on certain carbon atoms of the purine ring (see Fig. 1–6). These mononucleotides can be phosphorylated to form the high-energy compounds ADP, ATP, GDP, and GTP. They can also undergo degradation to adenosine and adenine or guanosine and guanine. In turn, the free bases adenine and guanine can be deaminated to hypoxanthine and

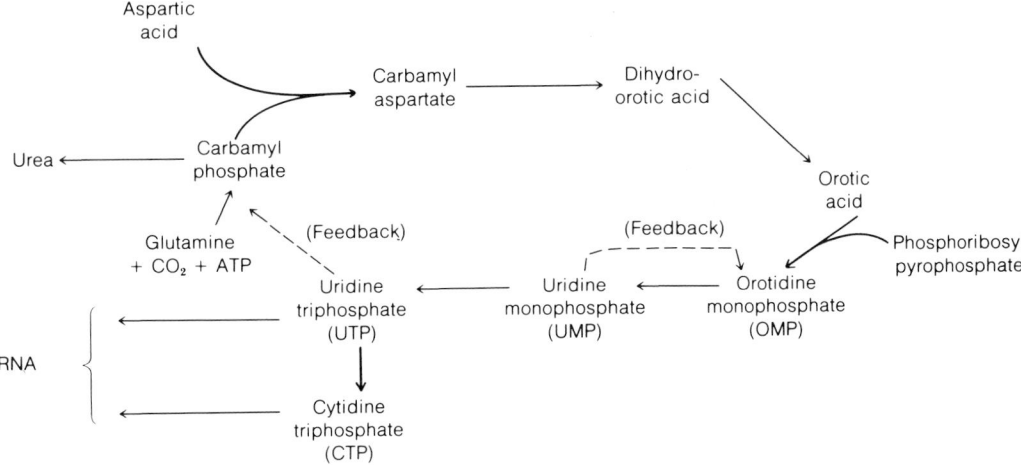

**Fig. 1–7.** Pyrimidine nucleotide synthesis.

xanthine, respectively. Finally, the hypoxanthine forms xanthine, which is irreversibly made into uric acid, the last two reactions being catalyzed by xanthine oxidase.

Figure 1–6 shows that de novo synthesis of AMP and GMP requires a considerable number of high-energy phosphate bonds. However, purine nucleotides can also be synthesized by means of the salvage pathways in which the free purine bases react with phosphoribosylpyrophosphate to form the monocleotides by a route involving only one molecule of ATP. Two enzymes, adenine-phosphoribosyl-transferase (APRT) and hypoxanthine-guanine phosphoribosyl-transferase (HGPRT), catalyze the reactions for reutilizing free adenine (APRT) and free guanine and hypoxanthine (HGPRT). The latter enzyme is defective in the Lesch-Nyhan syndrome,[17] leading to loss of salvage and consequent increased activity in the de novo pathway to compensate. The failure to salvage guanine leads to excessive formation of uric acid and is thus one cause of gout.

Finally, synthesis of the pyrimidine bases utilizes amino acid N, the initial reaction in the pathway requiring aspartic acid (see Fig. 1–7). In addition, the first step in this biosynthetic pathway requires carbamyl phosphate, which is also a substrate for urea synthesis. Lack of adequate amounts of dietary arginine to prime the urea synthesis cycle (see Fig. 1–4) can result in diversion of unutilized carbamyl phosphate to the pyrimidine biosynthetic pathway.[18] The consequent overload of the latter pathway results in accumulation of orotic acid and its excretion in the urine due to feedback regulation at this point in the pathway (see Fig. 1–7). Thus, arginine deficiency can be detected by excessive output of orotic acid in the urine.

**Creatine and Creatinine.** Most of the creatine of the body is found in skeletal muscle where it exists both as creatine and as creatine phosphate. In resting muscle the creatine is present largely in the high-energy phosphate form, whereas in fatigued muscle the concentration of creatine phosphate is insignificant.[19] This depletion is the result of the biochemical coupling of the conversion of creatine phosphate to creatine with synthesis of ATP, a reversible reaction mediated by the enzyme ATP-creatine transphosphorylase (also known as creatine phosphokinase). This reaction allows the muscle to generate an additional but limited amount of ATP from creatine phosphate under anaerobic conditions.

Creatine is synthesized extramuscularly in a two-reaction sequence, each step of which is enzymatically mediated (Fig. 1–8). The first is the transamidination reaction occurring in the kidney between the amino acids arginine and glycine, resulting in the formation of guanidinoacetic acid and ornithine. This reaction is followed by the methylation in the liver of the guanidinoacetic acid by S-adenosyl-methionine to form creatine. The creatine is then transported to the muscle and actively taken up by it. Both creatine phosphate and creatine undergo a nonenzymatic irreversible dehydration to form creatinine, the rate of reaction being twice as fast for creatine phosphate as for creatine. Unlike creatine, creatinine is not retained by muscle but is distributed in total body water and cleared from the body by the kidney. The daily rate of creatinine formation from its creatine precursors is remarkably constant and is estimated to be about 1.7% of the total creatine pool per day.

Daily urinary output of creatinine has been used as a measure of total muscle mass in the body, on the assumption that the creatine content of muscle is fairly constant. Indeed, population studies have shown a good correlation between creatinine output and lean body mass.[20] However, the creatine pool in the muscles of an individual represent a composite of the amount of creatine synthesized and the amount taken in the diet, notably from meat. Crim and collegues have shown that ingestion of creatine can increase the body pool of creatine appreciably.[21,22] Muscle creatine concentration can vary almost two-fold, from 0.3 to 0.5%. Thus the use of urinary creatinine excretion to assess the muscle mass could be associated with a considerable error if used for individuals or populations with different dietary patterns.

Clinically, the customary constancy of urinary creatinine output is also used to estimate the adequacy of 24-hour collections of urine. On a short-term basis, such as 1 to 2 weeks, this estimate is generally accurate, since the rate of degradation of creatine to creatinine is so small that large changes in the body pool of creatine would need to occur over a long period before a significant change in the 24-hour output of creatinine would occur. This use of creatinine output assumes, however, that during the collection period there are no significant sources of dietary creatinine, which, unlike creatine, is rapidly excreted in the urine.

**Ammonia Synthesis in the Kidney.** An important end product of protein metabolism is urinary ammonia, which increases in amount with acidosis occurring in conditions such as starvation or uncontrolled diabetes mellitus.[23] Urinary ammonia is derived from plasma glutamine (Fig. 1–9). In the cells of the proximal convoluted tubule of the kidney, glutaminase causes the amide N of glutamine to form ammonia and glutamate.[24]

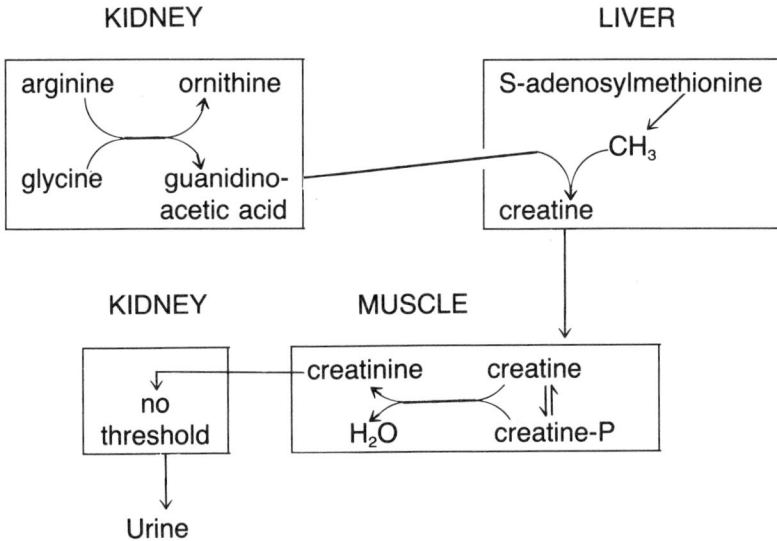

**Fig. 1–8.** Synthesis of creatine. (From Valgeirsdottir, K. and Munro, H.N.)[71]

The latter then yields another $NH_3$, leaving alpha-ketoglutarate as the other product of the reaction. This product is then available for gluconeogenesis, so that in acidosis the kidney becomes a source of glucose in tandem with $NH_3$ excretion. It has been suggested that the first response to acidosis is the production of glucose by the kidney, to which $NH_3$ formation is secondary.[25] Ammonia formation allows the body to conserve potassium and sodium ions, which would otherwise have to be used to neutralize the acid being excreted.

## UTILIZATION OF DIETARY PROTEIN

In the preceding section, the pathways of amino acid metabolism were examined individually. Proteins are intimately related to life processes, so that regulation of protein metabolism with its

20 amino acids in an integrated fashion is necessary to maintain bodily function. This concept will now be explored in a description of overall protein metabolism, especially as it responds to intake of a meal.

### Digestion and Absorption of Protein

Digestion of the protein of the diet begins with an attack by pepsin secreted in the gastric juice, followed by proteolytic enzymes from the pancreas and the mucosa of the small intestine.[27,28] These enzymes are mostly made in precursor (zymogen or proenzyme) form and become activated by loss of a small part of their peptide chains through "limited proteolysis." The pancreatic proenzymes become activated on meeting the intestinal juice where enterokinase is present and

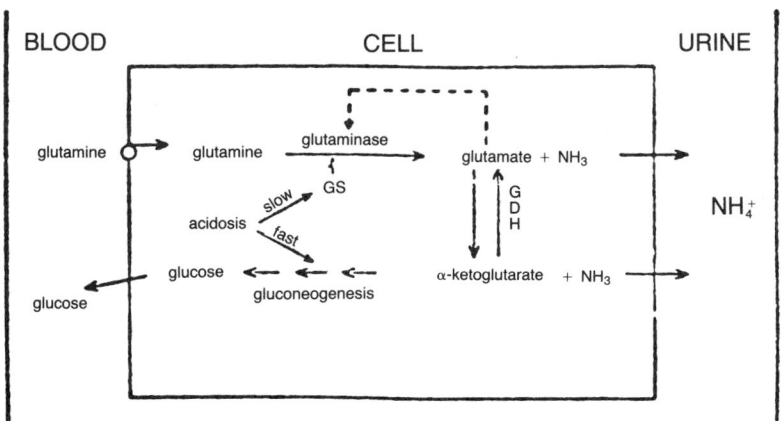

**Fig. 1–9.** Mechanism for control of ammonia production and gluconeogenesis by the kidney. GS = glutaminase synthesis; GDH = glutamate dehydrogenase. (From Goldstein, L. and Schooler, J.M.)[26]

activates trypsinogen. This process is followed by a cascade of activation of the other pancreatic proenzymes, again through selective proteolysis by the active trypsin (Fig. 1–10). Premature activation can occur within the pancreas in association with acute pancreatitis, resulting in autolysis of the pancreas.

Secretion of proteolytic enzymes by the pancreas appears to be regulated by the presence of dietary protein in the gut contents. In the case of trypsin, this enyzme binds to protein in the gut lumen until an excess is present.[29] This excess of free enzyme then operates a feedback regulation system to the pancreatic acinar cells which causes inhibition of synthesis of the precursor trypsinogen (Fig. 1–11). Some plants contain inhibitors of proteolytic enzymes, notably the trypsin inhibitor of the soybean. Feeding unheated soybean or its trypsin inhibitor to rats results in hypertrophy of the pancreas,[29] presumably because of tenacious binding of the free trypsin and the consequent overstimulation of enzyme formation in the pancreas. This control mechanism in pancreatic secretory activity does not appear as yet to have found an application in cases of acute and recurrent pancreatitis, where the giving of small peptides or free amino acid would be expected to reduce the secretory stimulus caused by whole protein.

The events occurring in the course of protein digestion are described in detail by Gitler.[27] Successive proteolytic enzymes attack peptide bonds selected on the basis of one of the amino acid residues adjacent to the bond (see Fig. 1–10). Thus

pepsin, with a relatively low specificity, preferentially hydrolyzes bonds adjacent to leucine or the aromatic amino acids, whereas the enzymes of the pancreatic juice show a greater specificity toward bonds adjacent to lysine or arginine (trypsin), to aromatic amino acids (chymotrypsin), or to neutral aliphatic amino acids (elastase). In addition, exopeptidases attack the free ends of the peptide chain. Thus the carboxyl terminal end loses one amino acid at a time through the action of two carboxypeptidases from the pancreas with different specificities, while the intestinal juice contributes aminopeptidases that perform a similar action at the N terminal end of the peptide.

The end products of digestion of protein are absorbed through the mucosal cells of the small intestine (see Fig. 1–11). Some of the protein in the gut lumen is finally hydrolyzed to free amino acids prior to absorption. Numerous studies confirm that transport of free amino acids into the mucosa involves energy-dependent carriers with some specificity for neutral, basic, and acidic classes of amino acids. However, the absorption of small peptides, notably dipeptides, plays a significant role in assimilation of dietary protein.[30] Because of the presence of peptide hydrolases in the brush border and cytosol of the mucosal cells, these small peptides of dietary origin undergo resolution to free amino acids on entering the mucosal cells so that virtually only free amino acids pass into the portal vein and to the liver (see Fig. 1–11). The transport mechanism for uptake of peptides by mucosal cells differs from the mechanism for free amino acid uptake, notably by ab-

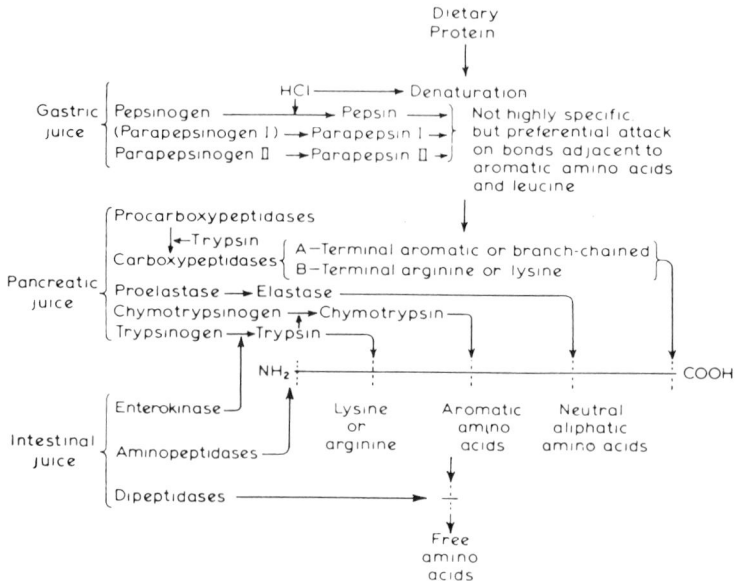

**Fig. 1–10.** Digestion of protein in the alimentary tract. (From Gitler, C.)[27]

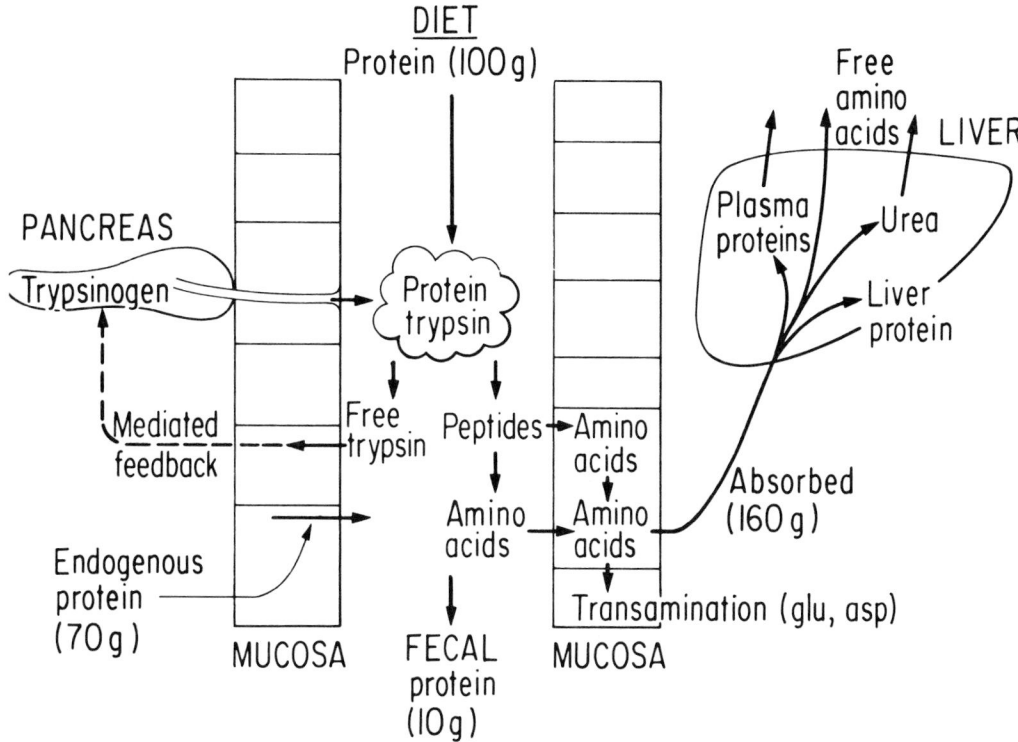

**Fig. 1–11.** Fate of dietary protein, secretion of endogenous protein, feedback control of pancreatic enzyme secretion, and absorption through the mucosa. (From Crim, M.C. and Munro, H.N.[31] Reprinted with permission from the American Medical Association.)

sence of competition for absorption between the two. The absorption of peptides is likely to represent a significant major route of amino acid uptake. Thus, although subjects with Hartnup's disease cannot transport free tryptophan into the mucosal cells, they nevertheless grow almost normally.[32] It must be assumed that their need for the essential amino acid tryptophan is adequately met by its absorption in peptide form.

It is significant that the mucosal cells can metabolize some incoming amino acids (see Fig. 1–11).[28] A notable pathway is the transamination of glutamic acid to yield alanine. Aspartic acid is also transaminated to alanine by the mucosal cells. The capacity of mucosal cells to transaminate dicarboxylic amino acids may play a significant role in reducing the toxicity of excessive intakes of these amino acids, which in enormous doses have been shown to cause damage to the hypothalamic regions of the brains of rats and mice[33] but not of primates.[34] The work of Windmueller[35] has demonstrated that glutamic acid and glutamine of dietary origin are extensively converted to alanine with a smaller yield of ornithine, citrulline, and proline by the pathways shown in Figure 1–5.[35] Glutamine perfused through the mesenteric vessels going to the gut

mucosa is also partly converted to alanine and thus participates in the transfer of amino groups from the peripheral tissues to the liver.

Finally, it is necessary to consider the fate of protein added to the gut contents in the form of digestive enzymes and the epithelial cells of the mucosa. These cells are continuously replaced by mitotic division in the crypts, followed by passage of each cohort of cells up the villus to be sloughed off from its tip. The extent of endogenous protein secretion is controversial, particularly estimates of the contribution of protein from mucosal sloughing. One intermediate estimate is that 70 g of protein (17 g as secreted juices and 50 g as sloughed mucosal cells) are added to the intestinal contents daily.[28] When this amount is added to the 100 g of protein consumed by the average person eating a Western type of diet, a total of 170 g in the gut lumen is available for absorption (see Fig. 1–11). Since fecal nitrogen output is equivalent to only 10 g of protein daily, the efficiency of digestion and absorption of both dietary and endogenous protein must be high. This turnover of protein in the gut wall is sensitive to dietary change. Protein deficiency[36] and starvation[37] both reduce the rate of cell division in the mucosa, which can be correlated with evidence in rats that protein deficiency leads to reduced secretion of endogenous protein into the gut.[38]

### Role of the Liver

The absorbed amino acids pass to the liver by way of the portal vein. After a meal of protein, there are changes in the amount and pattern of amino acids in the portal vein, but a less dramatic increase in amino acid levels in the general circulation. This change occurs because the liver is the main or only site of catabolism for seven of the essential amino acids, the remaining three, the branched-chain amino acids, being degraded mainly in muscle and kidney. This finding was demonstrated by Miller,[39] who compared the catabolism of individual labeled amino acids in the perfused liver and in the eviscerated liverless rat.[39] The liver monitors the absorbed amino acids and adjusts the rate of their metabolism according to bodily needs. Using dogs fed excessive amounts of meat, Elwyn demonstrated that much of this incoming amino acid load is immediately degraded to urea as it enters the liver cells, a small proportion is temporarily retained as liver protein presumably mostly as additional enzyme protein, another small portion is secreted as plasma protein, while only about a quarter of the absorbed amino acids pass into the general circulation (Fig. 1–12).[40]

The process of monitoring amino acid intake by the liver regulates the amounts of individual essential amino acids available to the rest of the body from the diet. When the dietary intake of an essential amino acid is progressively increased, induction of liver enzyme activity usually occurs when intake exceeds requirement.[41] This induction (e.g., threonine dehydratase in Figure 1–13) often shows a sudden increase at levels of intake beyond the needs of the body, indicating that the liver accurately monitors intake in relation to the needs of the body and destroys only essential amino acids extensively when their levels exceed that critical content in the diet. In the case of nonessential amino acids, the levels of enzymes (e.g., glutamic aminotransferase) responsible for their metabolism do not show this inflection, but increase progressively with rising intake (see Fig. 1–13). This conservation of essential amino acids is indicated also by studies in which different amounts of lysine were given to young growing rats.[42] At an intake of 100 mg of lysine, gain in body weight was maximal. At intakes beyond 100 mg daily, growth was not further stimulated, but [14]C-carbon dioxide production from injected [14]C-

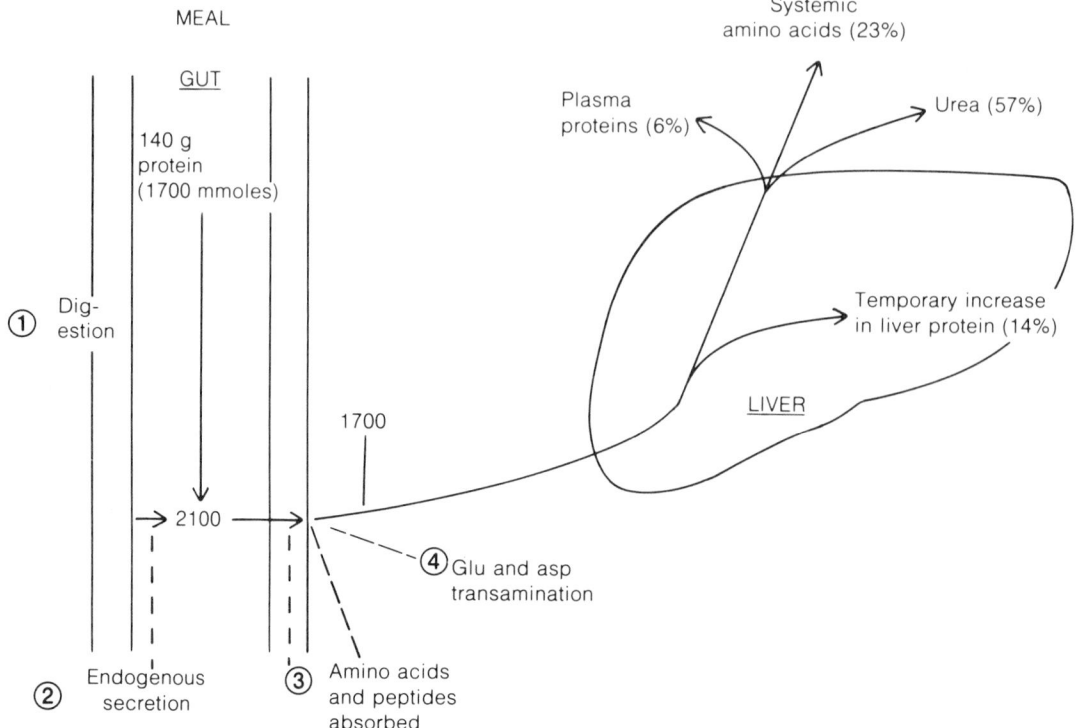

**Fig. 1–12.** Fate of a meal of meat fed to a dog: role of liver in monitoring incoming amino acids. The data are based on Elwyn's studies.[40]

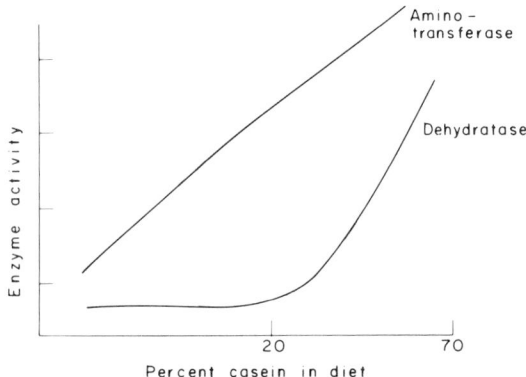

**Fig. 1–13.** Effect on liver enzymes of increasing the protein content of a diet fed to growing rats. The upper line shows the response of a liver enzyme metabolizing a nonessential amino acid (glutamic acid), while the lower line indicates the response of an enzyme for degradation of an essential amino acid (threonine). (Data from Harper, A.E.)[41]

lysine showed a rapid increase, indicating that the intake that gave maximal growth corresponded to the point at which the liver began to destroy excess lysine. In rats, the plasma levels of lysine show a response curve similar to that seen with $CO_2$ production,[43] the level of lysine rising steeply when more lysine is in the diet than is necessary for maximal growth. This finding suggests that increases in the peripheral blood levels of essential amino acids provide the signal for enzyme induction in the liver.

Finally, synthesis by the liver of degradative enzymes of amino acid metabolism and probably of other proteins is reflected in increased aggregation of polyribosomes during the absorptive period after a meal containing protein. In the rat, this process gives rise to diurnal variation in polyribosome aggregation related to the time of food intake.[44] Reduced breakdown of enzyme proteins also occurs,[45] presumably resulting from stabilization by their substrates derived from the incoming amino acids. Thus, degradative enzymes such as tyrosine aminotransferase[44] and tryptophan pyrolase[46] show diurnal variations related to meal consumption. In addition, other metabolic events in the liver cell are subject to diurnal variations related to protein intake from the diet. Synthesis of RNA accelerates while RNA breakdown decreases. This latter leads to changes in purine nucleotide pools, and consequent stimulation of de novo purine biosynthesis occurs after meals containing protein.[47] A scheme coordinating these various metabolic responses with changes in amino acid supply has been presented elsewhere.[48] Some secreted proteins, such as albumin, do not appear to undergo diurnal rhythms in syn-

thesis in normal animals, but their rate of synthesis increases when protein is given to protein-depleted animals. It has therefore been suggested that synthesis of albumin by the normal animal is regulated in relation to the plasma level, and responds to protein intake in the depleted animal because the serum albumin level has fallen below this critical control level and is not regulated in relation to amino acid supply.[48] Some secreted proteins, such as the alpha$_{2u}$-globulin (molecular weight 20,000) made by the liver of the mature male rat and excreted in the urine, show diurnal responses to protein intake even in well-nourished animals.[49]

## Regulation of Blood Amino Acid Levels

As indicated previously, the liver monitors the passage of amino acids into the peripheral circulation. However, this process does not completely eliminate excess amino acids beyond what the peripheral tissues are able to use or metabolize. Consequently, plasma levels of many essential amino acids increase when dietary supply exceeds the requirements of the tissues, as previously discussed for lysine. In some cases this increase in the level of an essential amino acid in the peripheral blood occurs abruptly when requirements are exceeded. For example, we examined the influence of the age of the rat on the response of its plasma tryptophan concentration to different levels of dietary tryptophan.[50] The rats used were either weanlings or mature adults. As the amount of tryptophan in the diet was increased from less than adequate to more than sufficient for maximal need, the tryptophan content of the plasma rose sharply beyond the point of requirement at each age. For the rapidly growing weanlings, the point of inflection was 0.1% tryptophan in the diet, above which growth was not stimulated and plasma tryptophan started to rise. For the mature rats, 0.03% dietary tryptophan was just sufficient to satisfy weight maintenance; above this level plasma tryptophan concentration rose. The findings are thus interesting in showing that the method is sensitive to age-related changes in requirements. This method has been used to determine the requirements of human subjects for essential amino acids, and indeed the point of inflection of tryptophan (3 mg/kg body weight) agrees with the amount required for N balance of young adults.[51] However, other essential amino acids such as lysine have given less clear-cut points of inflection, and the use of the inflection as a measure of optimal requirements has also been disputed.[52]

The plasma levels of amino acids are also affected by dietary carbohydrate through a mechanism involving insulin secretion. Shortly after an individual consumes carbohydrate, the concentrations of most plasma amino acids decrease because of deposition in muscle through insulin-mediated transport (Fig. 1–14).[53] The effect is maximal for branched-chain amino acids, which can fall as much as 40% after a dose of glucose, whereas some amino acids (e.g., tryptophan) are affected only minimally. The same mechanism is also the basis of a metabolic interaction between dietary protein or amino acids and carbohydrate consumed in the same meal.

The alterations in plasma-free amino acid patterns caused by the protein and carbohydrate components of a meal have significance for the availability of amino acids to the peripheral tissues. In particular, the free tryptophan content of the rat brain can be elevated by tryptophan administration, and this maneuver increases the serotonin content of the brain.[54] Entry of tryptophan into the cells of the brain is also determined by the plasma levels of other competing neutral amino acids, notably the branched-chain amino acids.[54] Consequently, following a meal of carbohydrate, the extensive reduction in plasma levels of branched-chain amino acids results in greater passage of tryptophan into the brain, and more serotonin is synthesized.

### Role of Skeletal Muscle in Protein Metabolism

Skeletal muscle is the largest tissue in the body.[2] Consequently, metabolism of amino acids in this tissue is of considerable significance for general protein metabolism. Muscle is also the main site of metabolism of the branched-chain amino acids (leucine, isoleucine, and valine). As described previously, muscle is a major target for the action of insulin, which promotes entry of amino acids

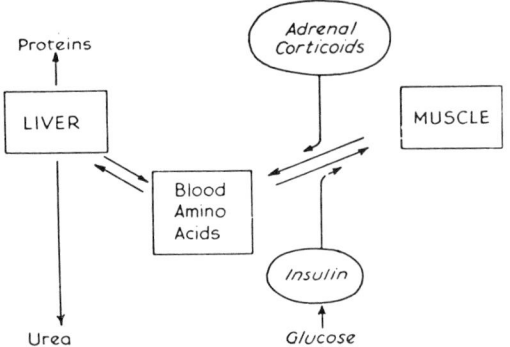

**Fig. 1–14.** Scheme showing the action of dietary carbohydrate on levels of blood amino acids. Adrenocortical hormones have the opposite action. (From Munro, H.N.)[53]

(especially the branched-chain amino acids). Insulin also promotes synthesis of muscle protein and reduces muscle protein breakdown. Corticosteroids have opposite effects (see Fig. 1–14).

The effects of hormones and of nutrient intake on muscle protein metabolism have been examined by various techniques, including use of radioactive amino acids. In man two main nonradioactive procedures have been used, namely, measurement of the differences in amino acid levels of blood entering and leaving muscle (arteriovenous differences) and measurement of 3-methylhistidine as a urinary compound proportional to the rate of myofibrillar protein breakdown. The measurement of uptake and release of amino acids indicates that fasting results in the release of large amounts equivalent to a loss of 50 g of protein daily from the muscles of a 70-kg man.[55] Most of this takes the form of alanine and glutamine. The alanine is formed by transamination between pyruvate derived from glucose and amino groups transferred from amino acids present in muscle. In consequence, alanine becomes a carrier of nitrogen from muscle to liver, where its carbon skeleton enters the gluconeogenic pathway while its amino group is converted into urea. The other carrier of nitrogen from muscle is glutamine, formed when glutamic acid accepts nitrogen as its amide group. This glutamine passes to the intestine where about half undergoes transamination to alanine, which now goes to the liver. By means of these reactions, muscle thus has a special mechanism that allows transport of nitrogen and carbon to the liver. Following gluconeogenesis in the liver, some of the carbon comes back to muscle as glucose, the overall exchange between liver and muscle being named the glucose-alanine cycle. Measurement of the arteriovenous differences across the forearm has demonstrated that, if a meal is given, the output of amino acids diminishes, and that after a meal containing protein, it is completely reversed so that muscle actually gains protein. Thus, fluctuations in the A-V loss occur in response to feeding and fasting throughout the day.[56,57] This mechanism implies that, from the body mass of muscle (45% of the body weight of the average adult), a considerable amount of carbon is available for metabolism during fasting or other emergency.

Interpretation of arteriovenous difference data is difficult, however, because of amino acid recycling within the muscle cell. For example, the diminution of arteriovenous difference after insulin administration[55] could be the result of retardation of muscle protein breakdown or increased synthesis of protein through the known stimulant action on muscle protein synthesis. In order to monitor muscle protein breakdown without reutilization, 3-methylhistidine output in urine has been exploited. Methylation of histidine in actin and myosin occurs only after these proteins have been synthesized in muscle. When the protein of the myofibril is eventually catabolized, 3-methylhistidine is not reused for protein synthesis but is excreted quantitatively in the urine and thus provides an index of muscle protein breakdown (Fig. 1–15). Several lines of evidence confirm that 3-methylhistidine in fact fulfills this purpose. First, tRNA and its charging enzymes were prepared from rat muscle and were shown not to charge with 3-methylhistidine.[58] This finding implies that it is not recycled for protein synthesis within the muscle cell. Second, analysis of various major tissues and organs of the rat for their content of 3-methylhistidine shows that skeletal muscle is the overwhelming reservoir of methylhistidine in body proteins. Third, by administering [14]CH$_3$-labeled 3-methylhistidine to rats[58] and to human subjects,[59] it was demonstrated that essentially all was excreted in the urine over a short period.

The output of 3-methylhistidine has been used to study dietary effects on muscle protein breakdown rate. Changes in methylhistidine excretion have been examined in young growing rats receiving either a normal diet or diets deficient in protein alone or protein and calories.[60] Protein depletion caused a rapid reduction in output of 3-methylhistidine, which declined steadily to 20% of initial output, while output again rose following repletion on a protein-rich diet. In the case of protein-calorie deficiency, however, an initial rise was followed by a gradual fall in 3-methylhistidine output. Thus, muscle is conserved in response to protein depletion by reducing breakdown. However, with semistarvation, breakdown at first increases and then diminishes. In similar fashion, malnourished children in India showed a low output of methylhistidine for weight, which rose during repletion.[61] We have also observed that grossly obese subjects undergoing prolonged fasting show a progressive reduction in 3-methylhistidine output.[62]

Finally, 3-methylhistidine output is affected by age and by hormonal status. Output per kg body weight is higher in the newborn than in the mature adult[63] and declines further in old age.[64] Output is increased by thyroxine secretion within the normal range of thyroid activity,[65] but by corticosterone secretion[66] only at plasma levels of this hormone equivalent to severe stress.

## Plasma Protein Metabolism

Most major proteins in the plasma are secreted from the liver. Furthermore, most are glycoproteins, a notable exception being serum albumin. The metabolism of plasma proteins is more readily studied than that of most other proteins, since plasma proteins can be more readily sampled in man. Pool size and turnover rate have been frequently reported for a variety of plasma proteins. These data are obtained by injecting samples of the plasma protein labeled with [131]I or [125]I and by measuring the kinetics of the disappearance of the label.[67] Synthesis of plasma proteins can be measured by administering radioactive [14]CO$_2$ or the stable isotope [13]CO$_2$, which labels liver arginine in the carbon of the guanido group (see Fig. 1–4). The specific activity of free arginine in liver can be measured from the arginine-derived carbon of urea excreted in the urine, and this value can be used to correct the specific activity of arginine in plasma protein made from the same free liver arginine pool. We have adapted this procedure for the use of [15]N-glycine, fed to human subjects every 3 hours over a 60-hour period, to label N in the guanido group of arginine.[68] This procedure allows the liver arginine to achieve a constant enrichment with N[15] that is reflected in the urinary urea, and thus permits analysis of the data using steady-state kinetics.

Table 1–2 shows the intravascular concentration, the percentage of total body content that is intravascular, the fractional turnover rate, and the mass synthesized per day for a variety of plasma proteins measured in human subjects. Nutritional status usually affects these parameters, which have therefore been used to recognize malnutrition. Rats fed a diet low in protein show a progressive reduction in plasma albumin level due to reduced synthesis of this plasma protein.[69] Addition of protein to the diet now stimulates protein

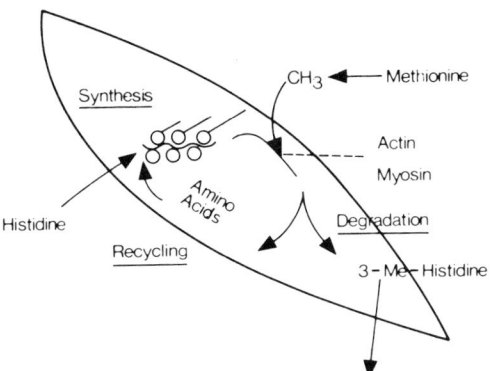

**Fig. 1–15.** Synthesis of 3-methylhistidine in muscle actin and myosin, and its release and quantitative excretion in the urine following breakdown of these muscle proteins. (From Munro, H.N.)[57a]

**Table 1–2.   Turnover of Plasma Proteins***

| Plasma Protein | Plasma Concentration (g/dl) | Intravascular Pool (% total) | Total per 70-kg Man (g) | Fractional Catabolic Rate (% total mass/day) | Amount Synthesized (g/day) |
|---|---|---|---|---|---|
| Albumin | 4.2 | 45 | 280 | 4 | 11 |
| Transferrin | 0.2 | 49 | 12 | 8 | 1.1 |
| IgG | 1.1 | 58 | 58 | 4 | 2.1 |
| IgM | 0.1 | 74 | 4.5 | 8 | 0.3 |
| Fibrinogen | 0.4 | 84 | 15 | 21 | 2.2 |
| Prealbumin | 0.03 | 40 | 2 | 27 | 0.5 |
| Retinol-binding protein | 0.006 | — | — | 120 | — |

*From Valgeirsdottir, K. and Munro, H.N.[71]

synthesis and is slowly followed by restoration of the level of albumin in the plasma. Serum albumin is thus too insensitive to serve as a reliable indicator of subclinical malnutrition. However, Shetty et al. have shown that plasma proteins with more rapid turnover rates than albumin can be more sensitive indicators of protein or calorie depletion and repletion.[70] For example, they showed that pre-albumin and retinol-binding proteins (which have high rates of turnover) provided suitable indicators of changed nutritional status when obese subjects were put on diets restricted in calories and/or protein.

## INTEGRATION OF BODY PROTEIN METABOLISM

From the preceding information, a composite picture of the daily flux of amino acids in various compartments of the body of an adult man can be assembled.[72] These estimates for a 70-kg man are shown in Figure 1–16. The customary daily pro-

tein intake in Western countries is about 100 g, augmented by addition of an estimated 70 g of protein secreted into the gastrointestinal tract; consequently, the total load available for absorption is estimated to be 170 g of protein of which 160 g is calculated to be absorbed (see Fig. 1–11). Experiments involving amino acids labeled with stable isotopes suggest that some 250 to 300 g of protein are synthesized daily in the body of the adult. The difference between the intake of 100 g of protein and the daily turnover of some 250 g indicates the extensive reutilization of amino acids involved in protein metabolism. Some major components in this daily protein turnover can be identified, namely, gut, muscle, plasma proteins, white blood cells, and hemoglobin. Note that the free amino acid pool of the body, estimated at 100 g, is primarily made up of nonessential amino acids, as shown earlier for the rat (Table 1–1).

Such data on the magnitude of protein metabolism in the whole body and its compartments continue to be refined using amino acids labeled with radioactive or stable isotopes of carbon, hydrogen, or nitrogen. The stable isotopes are preferred for human studies on grounds of safety. These experiments have been refined recently. Early studies of whole-body protein and amino acid metabolism were complicated by the use of single-pulse doses of labeled amino acid, followed by often complex kinetic analysis. To simplify it, Waterlow and his colleagues have developed the use of continuous administration of labeled amino acid orally or intravenously in order to achieve a steady state reflected by a constant concentration of isotopically labeled amino acid in the plasma.[73] Under these conditions, a simple model can be used to derive useful conclusions about the flux of the administered amino acid and the turnover of body protein, and can even be extended to the rate of synthesis of nonessential amino acids. Figure 1–17 shows such a model using 1-[13]C-leucine as the amino acid infused intravenously into the vein for a few hours. When a steady level of [13]C

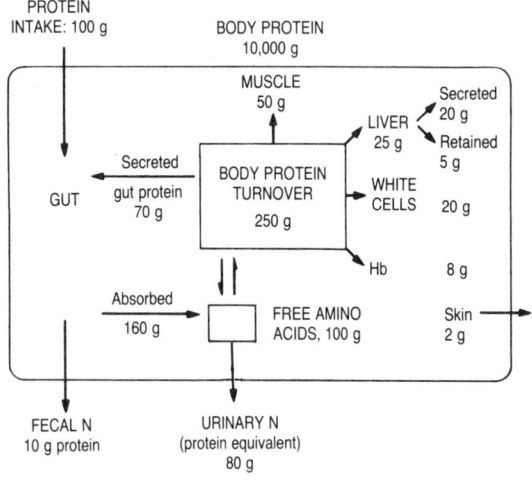

**Fig. 1–16.**   Estimated daily turnover of protein in the whole body and some organs of a 70-kg man. (From Munro, H.N., Raven Press, New York, 1982.)[72]

## MODEL OF WHOLE-BODY LEUCINE FLUX

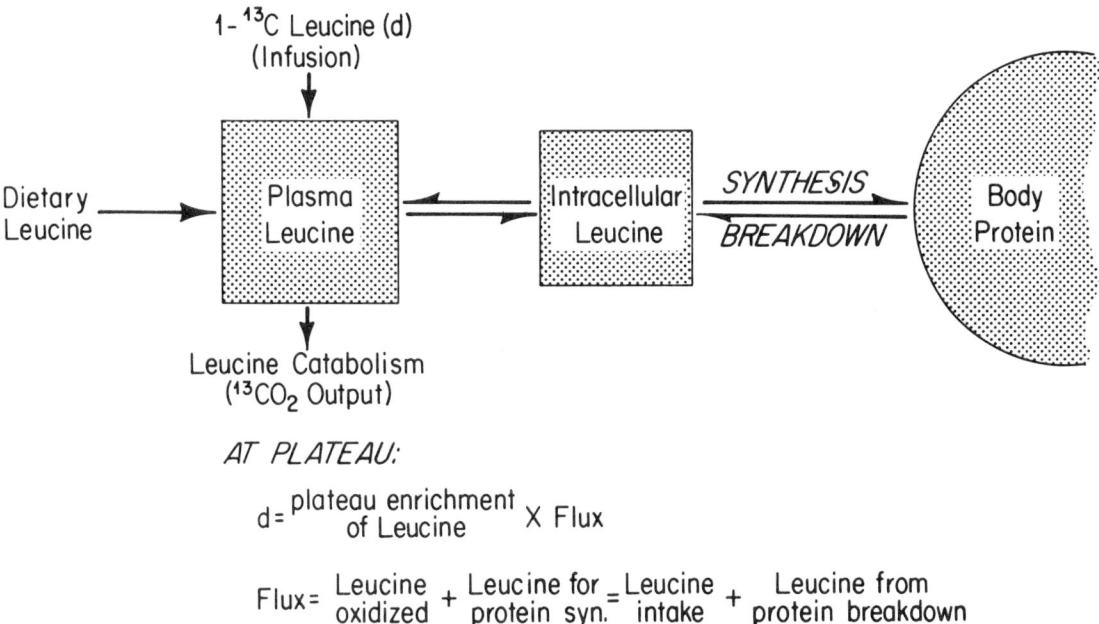

$$d = \frac{\text{plateau enrichment of Leucine}}{} \times \text{Flux}$$

$$\text{Flux} = \frac{\text{Leucine}}{\text{oxidized}} + \frac{\text{Leucine for}}{\text{protein syn.}} = \frac{\text{Leucine}}{\text{intake}} + \frac{\text{Leucine from}}{\text{protein breakdown}}$$

**Fig. 1–17.** Model of whole-body leucine flux.[74]

enrichment has been attained in the leucine of the plasma, it is considered to represent the level of labeling in the free leucine pools in most tissues. It is therefore accepted as a single metabolic pool from which label is withdrawn in two directions, namely for protein synthesis or for catabolism with release of $^{13}CO_2$. The flux of leucine through the metabolic pool can therefore be described by the equation:

$$Q = S + C = B + I$$

where Q is the rate of leucine flux, S represents rate of leucine utilization for protein synthesis throughout the body, C is the rate of catabolism to $CO_2$, B is the rate of leucine release from breakdown of body proteins, and I is leucine intake from the diet. Owing to the short time interval of the study, it is assumed that body proteins will not recycle isotope into the metabolic pool again. Motil et al. have used this technique to study the effect of level of protein intake on rate of protein synthesis and leucine oxidation in the fasting and in the fed states.[75] Table 1–3 shows that protein synthesis was increased in both the postabsorptive and the fed states when protein intake was raised from low through marginal to excess, whereas catabolism to $CO_2$ rose sharply only during the absorptive phase after the intake of excess dietary protein, including excess leucine. This meal-related increase in leucine breakdown is

compatible with other evidence discussed in the following section.

### Metabolic Integration of Organs

From the picture presented in preceding sections, it is apparent that certain organs play a major cooperative role in ensuring the utilization of free amino acids.[72,76] This process is seen most convincingly in the response to a meal containing protein, as illustrated in Figure 1–18 for three groups of amino acids: glutamate and glutamine, the aromatic amino acids, and the branched-chain amino acids. The intestinal mucosa responds to an influx of glutamine and glutamic acid from either the diet or the peripheral organs by transamination of a part to pyruvic acid to form alanine. Alanine then passes up the portal vein to the liver to yield glucose by gluconeogenesis, while the nitrogen becomes urea. In the liver, the rates of catabolism of most incoming amino acids are regulated according to the body's needs, as in the case of tryptophan (see earlier). Such regulation of rate of hepatic degradation is important because tryptophan is rate-limiting for synthesis of the neurotransmitter serotonin in the brain. If the level of plasma tryptophan is not kept within certain limits, the synthesis of serotonin would be uncontrolled (see later discussion of liver cirrhosis).

In contrast to tryptophan and most other essen-

**Table 1–3.    Metabolism in 1-¹³C-Leucine in Young Men*†**

| Protein Intake | Nitrogen Balance | Protein Synthesis | | | Leucine Oxidation | | |
|---|---|---|---|---|---|---|---|
| | | Post-absorptive | Fed | Difference | Post-absorptive | Fed | Difference |
| g/kg/day | mg/kg/day | | | μmoles/kg/hr‡ | | | |
| 0.1 | −42 | 76 | 64 | −8 | 13 | 12 | −1 |
| 0.6 | −21 | 89 | 102 | +13 | 22 | 22 | ±0 |
| 1.5 | +12 | 113 | 113 | ±0 | 18 | 46 | +28 |

*In the postabsorptive and absorptive states at low, marginal, and excess levels of protein intake.
†Adapted from Motil, K.J. et al.[75]
‡Expressed as μmoles leucine.

tial amino acids, the major site of branched-chain amino acid catabolism is not the liver but the peripheral tissues, notably muscle, adipose tissue, and kidney. Following a meal containing protein, dramatic changes occur in the exchange of branched-chain amino acids between the liver and the peripheral tissues. Thus DeFronzo and Felig describe experiments on human subjects in which the amino acid flux across the splanchnic area (gut and liver) and across the leg were measured by comparing the concentrations of each amino acid entering and leaving these body compartments.[77] The differences in amino acid concentrations, adjusted for the rates of blood flow through the splanchnic area and through the leg, provided quantitative measures of uptake or release by these organs. Figure 1–19 shows that, following a meal of 250 g of meat, 70% of the amino acids leaving the liver took the form of the branched-chain amino acid; this contrasts with their concentration in meat protein (about 20%), thus indicating the selective catabolism by the liver of other entering amino acids. Figure 1–19 also shows that a large percentage of the amino nitrogen taken up by the leg during the absorptive period is accounted for by branched-chain amino acids. Thus, following a protein meal, the branched-chain amino acids become the major

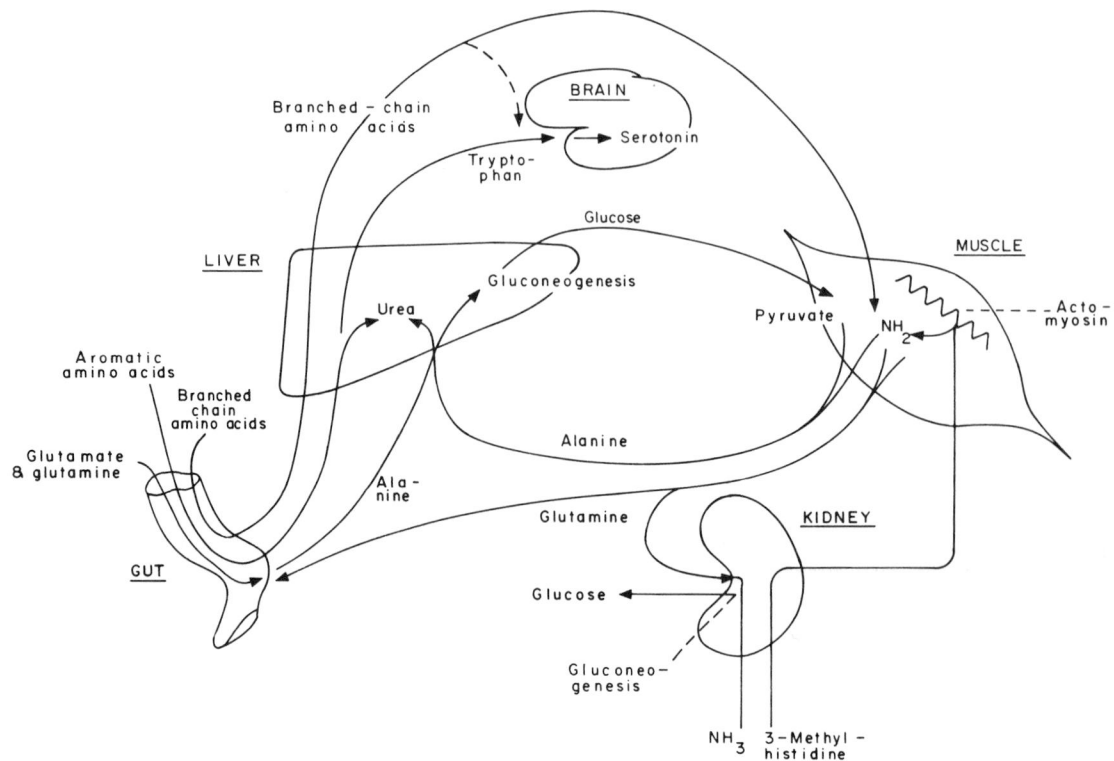

**Fig. 1–18.**   Interactions of organs in the metabolism of some major amino acids discussed in the text. (From Munro, H.N., Raven Press, New York, 1982.)[72]

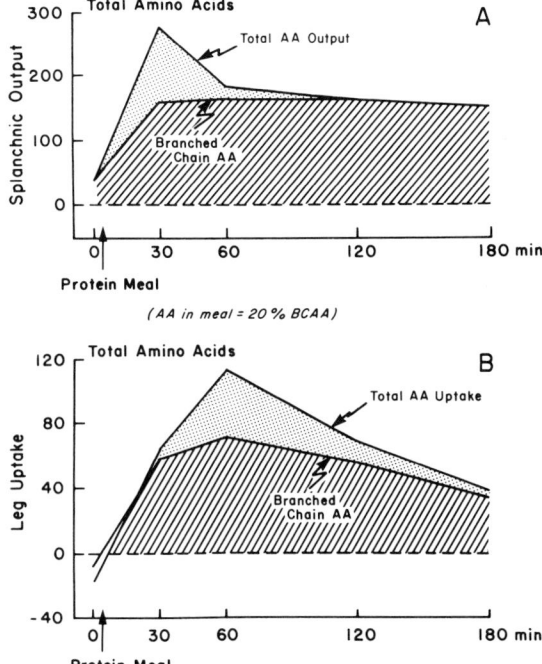

**Fig. 1–19.** Effect of a meal of protein on splanchnic amino acid release (A) and leg uptake of amino acids (B). The exchanges are expressed in μM/min. (Modified from DeFronzo, R.A. and Felig, P. ©Am. J. Clin. Nutr., American Society for Clinical Nutrition.)[77]

carriers of amino nitrogen between the viscera and the peripheral tissues, notably muscle.

There is also a selective release of amino acids from muscle into the blood.[78] Figure 1–20 shows arteriovenous differences across the leg and across the splanchnic area in fasting human subjects. Of the amino acids released from the tissues of the leg, glutamine and alanine each account for 30 to 40% of the total amino-N released. Calculation shows that only one third of these two released amino acids could come from muscle protein breakdown, the remaining two thirds being synthesized in the tissues of the leg. The arteriovenous difference across the splanchnic area in the same fasting subjects shows uptake of amino acids to be the inverse of the release of the leg (see Fig. 1–20); thus, most of the amino-N taken up during its passage across the splanchnic viscera represents removal of alanine and glutamine. As mentioned earlier, much of the glutamine is removed by the small intestinal mucosa, which transforms it to alanine for transfer to the liver. One might expect more to be released from muscle after a meal from the active absorption of amino acids and the transfer of large amounts of leucine to muscle. However, Elia and Livesey[57] have shown that glutamine release from a limb is unchanged

and alanine output actually decreases after a high-protein meal.[57]

Finally, glutamine is the source of nitrogen for ammonia synthesis by the kidney. The tissues contributing glutamine for this purpose have been elegantly documented in the acidotic rat by Schrock and Goldstein using amino acid exchange across the kidney compared with muscle, liver, and gut.[79] Acidosis caused by $NH_4Cl$ or HCl administration resulted in increased $NH_3$ output by the kidney, which could be accounted for by release of more glutamine from muscle and liver; the gut remained uninvolved.

In order to provide a reasonably complete picture of the interaction of metabolites within and between tissues in response to various physiologic conditions, it is necessary to add profiles of interorgan changes in carbohydrate and fat metabolites (Fig. 1–21). The interchange of these between liver, muscle, and adipose tissue is regulated by insulin and glucagon.[72] In the *fasting* state, insulin levels are low, which allows adipose tissue lipase to become active, releasing large amounts of free fatty acids and glycerol from the fat stores. Coincident with the fall in insulin levels, the plasma glucagon level rises and accelerates the loss of liver glycogen. The incoming free fatty acids entering the liver are diverted to ketone body formation, while in muscle the free fatty acids, and with more prolonged fasting, the ketone bodies, replace glucose as the major fuel. When the subject is now *fed*, the insulin level rises and favors glycogen deposition in liver and in muscle, so that carbohydrate becomes the main fuel in both tissues. Insulin also inhibits the action of lipase and thus shuts off the free fatty acids that are the alternative fuel. In muscle, the deposited tissue glycogen provides muscle energy, but under conditions of inadequate oxygen supply, lactate is released into the blood and passes to the liver for gluconeogenesis (Cori cycle).

The interactions of metabolites exchanged between organs are most clearly seen during progressive starvation. As pointed out by Cahill and Aoki, the brain uses large amounts of energy that must be supplied as water-soluble energy substrates, that is, glucose in well-nourished people and ketones during starvation.[80] Figure 1–22 shows metabolic profiles at four stages of the process of starvation. Between meals (interprandial state), blood glucose is maintained for the brain by release of sugar from glycogen stored in the liver, while the fall in insulin level allows free fatty acids to be released from the fat deposits and provides energy for muscle. At the next stage (overnight fast), liver glycogen is nearly exhausted and the maintenance of blood sugar now depends

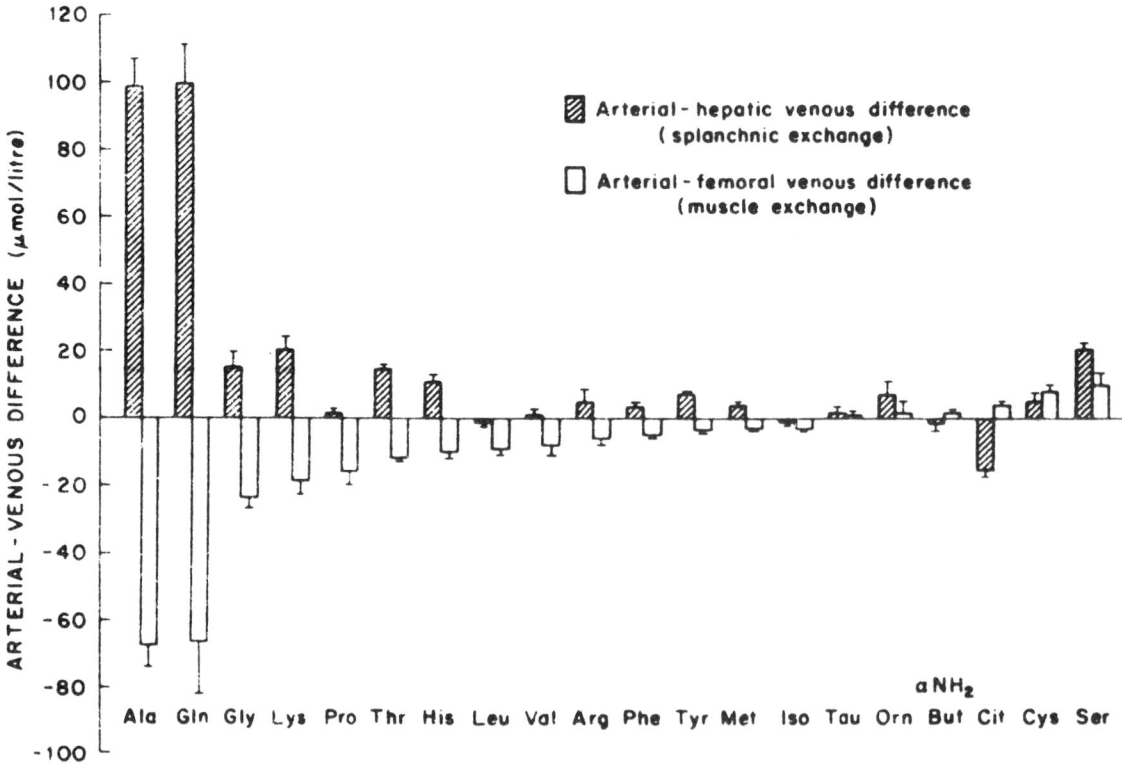

**Fig. 1–20.**　Splanchnic and leg exchange of amino acids in normal humans after an overnight fast, based on arterial-hepatic and arterial-femoral venous differences. Above the line, uptake; below, loss. (From Felig, P.)[78]

on gluconeogenesis from alanine released by muscle and intestine. At the same time, free fatty acids coming from the adipose tissue begin to form ketone bodies in the liver, this being encouraged by a rise in plasma glucagon level. At the next stage (early starvation), muscle becomes the major source of carbon for glucose released from the liver and utilized by the brain, while ketone bodies from the liver are the major energy source for muscle. Finally, in prolonged starvation, muscle protein breakdown diminishes, so that release of alanine and glutamine from muscle for use by the liver decreases. The brain then adapts to using ketone bodies as its major fuel, thus sparing glucose production in the liver.

### Metabolic Profiles in Disease

The preceding data present a picture of amino acid metabolism and energy metabolism that emphasizes cooperation between organs in regulating the flow and utilization of metabolites. One factor involved in the regulation of both amino acid and energy is insulin. The plasma level of insulin can determine tissue uptake of amino acids, especially into muscle, while it also regulates whether muscle and other peripheral tissues receive glucose or fatty acids and ketones as their

main energy source. Consequently, diseases involving changes in insulin secretion should cause changes in metabolite profiles in the blood and tissues. The five diseases discussed here show abnormalities of insulin regulation: in diabetes, lack of insulin secretion following a meal; in renal failure and in sepsis, resistance of tissues to the action of insulin; in liver failure, excessive levels of insulin entering the peripheral circulation; and in cancer, which is associated with low blood glucose and insulin. In Table 1–4, these altered patterns of insulin action are correlated with changes in metabolites of protein and energy. The following short account of these metabolic changes in disease can be supplemented by consulting more detailed reviews.[72,76]

One response of the normal person to carbohydrate administration is a fall in concentration of amino acids in the plasma, most extensive in the case of the branched-chain amino acids (see Fig. 1–14). This response does not occur in diabetic rats or in diabetic humans dependent on insulin, and in consequence, the concentrations of branched-chain amino acids increase in the plasma.[53] Since blood sugar is elevated in such diabetics, hepatic gluconeogenesis from alanine and lactate has to be increased. However, there is

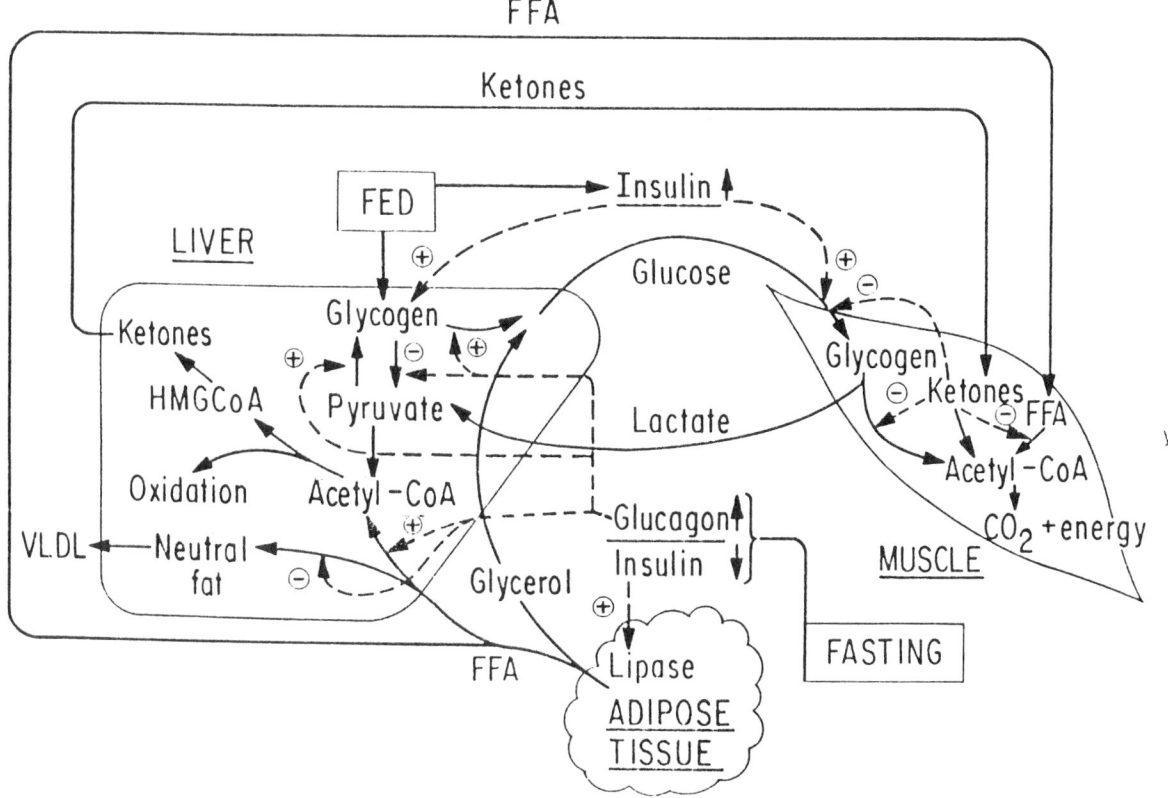

**Fig. 1–21.** Role of liver and muscle in the metabolism of carbohydrate and fat in the fed and fasted states. (From Munro, H.N., Raven Press, New York, 1982.)[72]

no corresponding increase in the release of alanine from muscle. Plasma alanine then falls because the liver extracts a higher percentage of alanine from the plasma. Finally, lack of insulin allows adipose tissue lipase to release excessive amounts of free fatty acids that raise the plasma level and contribute to ketone body formation by the liver.

In the case of kidney failure, the tissues show insulin resistance, so that administration of glucose to patients with uremia results in a higher blood sugar level than occurs in healthy people.[77] However, insulin resistance does not extend to amino acid entry into muscle. Unlike diabetics, these patients have plasma levels of branched-chain amino acids that are not elevated but are subnormal in uremia. This depression is caused by the elevated levels of insulin in the blood.

In cirrhosis of the liver, failure of several important liver functions contributes to the metabolic abnormalities.[81] As shown in Figure 1–23, amines and ammonia formed by bacterial action in the gut are no longer trapped by the liver but pass freely into the systemic blood and thence to the brain cells. For example, bacterial action pro-

duces phenethylamine from phenylalanine; this substance is transformed to octopamine in the brain where it may serve as a false neurotransmitter competing with the catecholamines. Amino acids for which metabolism is normally regulated in the liver (e.g., tryptophan and phenylalanine) are no longer subject to control, so that their plasma levels rise and are more available for entry into the brain. Finally, the liver normally inactivates a large part of the insulin secreted by the pancreas. In individuals with cirrhosis, this no longer occurs and plasma insulin levels rise extensively. This rise enhances transport of branched-chain amino acids into muscle in patients with cirrhosis. The consequent reduction in the plasma levels of the branched-chain amino acids allows a larger proportion of the already elevated tryptophan content of the plasma to pass into the brain, so that excessive levels of serotonin are generated and contribute to hepatic coma. This concept of the role of excess serotonin formation in hepatic coma has received some confirmation from studies showing reversal of the comatose state following administration of branched-chain amino acids to laboratory animals and patients

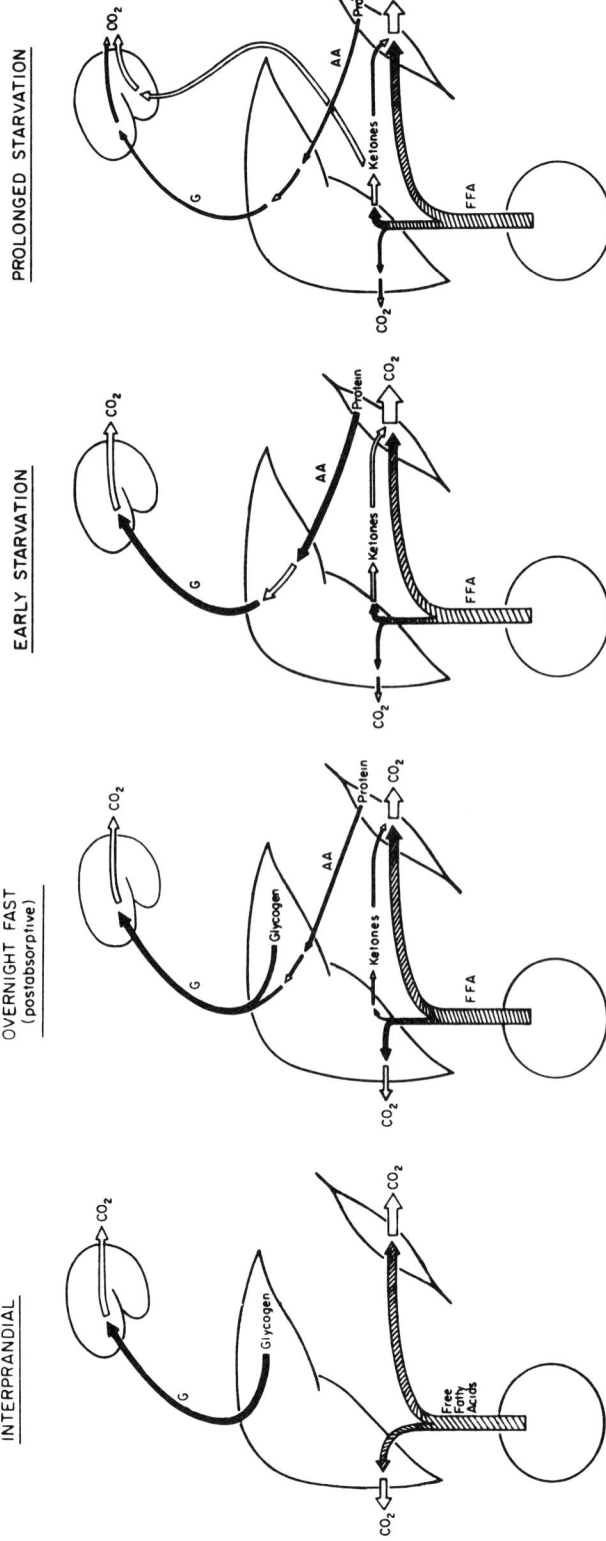

**Fig. 1–22.** Sequence of diagrams showing metabolic adaptation of man to starvation. (1) Man in the interprandial state, with hepatic glycogen providing glucose (G) for brain. (2) Overnight fasting state, with hepatic gluconeogenesis from muscle-derived amino acids (AA) providing glucose (G) for brain. The remainder of the body is using free fatty acids (FFA). (3) Early starvation, with muscle providing the major share of gluconeogenic precursor. (4) Prolonged starvation, with ketoacids being mainly rejected by muscle to elevate blood levels to permit their facilitated diffusion into brain. Thus brain glucose (G) utilization is diminished and, pari passu, muscle proteolysis. (Modified from Cahill, G.F., and Aoki, T.T. Reprinted with permission of Ross Laboratories, Columbus, OH 43216, ©1980 Ross Laboratories.)[80]

**Table 1–4.  Metabolic Profiles in Disease***

| Metabolite | Diabetes | Uremia | Cirrhosis | Sepsis | Cancer |
|---|---|---|---|---|---|
| Blood sugar | ↑ | ↑ |  | ↑ | ↓ |
| Insulin | ↓ | ↑ | ↑ | ↑ |  |
| Glucagon |  |  |  | ↑ |  |
| Free fatty acids |  |  |  | ↓ |  |
| Ketones | ↑ |  |  | ↓ |  |
| Plasma triglycerides | ↑ | ↑ |  | ↑ |  |
| Very low-density lipoprotein | ↑ | ↑ |  |  |  |
| Plasma branched-chain amino acids | ↑ | ↓ | ↓ |  |  |
| Branched-chain amino acid removal | ↓ | ↑ | ↑ | ↑ | ↑ |
| Glutamine release | ↑ |  |  | ↑ | ± |
| Alanine release (muscle) | ± | ± |  | ↑ | ↓ |
| Alanine uptake (liver) | ↑ | ± |  | ↑ |  |
| Plasma alanine | ↓ | ± |  |  | ↓ |

*From Munro, H.N.[76]

with hepatic coma,[82] but has also been challenged.[83]

Fever and sepsis cause metabolic and hormonal changes related to the increased energy output demanded by these conditions.[84] Several hormonal levels become elevated, notably insulin,

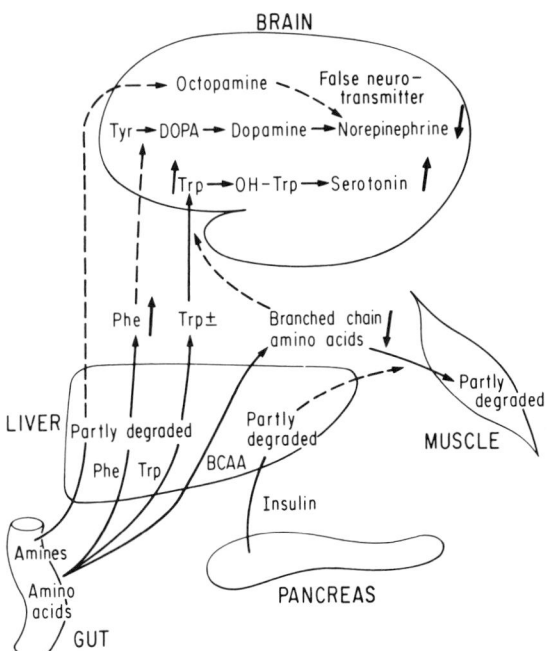

**Fig. 1–23.**  Role of branched-chain amino acids in hepatic coma. Owing to unrestricted passage of insulin into the general circulation in hepatic cirrhosis, branched-chain amino acids are removed excessively by muscle. In consequence of this lowering of plasma branched-chain amino acids, there is less competition with tryptophan and phenylalanine for entry into the brain and thus more serotonin and less norepinephrine are made. (From Crim, M.C., and Munro, H.N.[31] Reprinted with permission from the American Medical Association.)

which affects metabolism in the predicted ways. The rise in insulin results from the raised blood sugar levels in fever and sepsis; in response, the increased insulin level inhibits release of free fatty acids from the adipose tissue, and substrate for ketone formation is restricted even in the fasting state. The elevation of plasma insulin level also promotes entry of amino acids into muscle, which increases release of alanine and glutamine from muscle. Because of the increased output of the last two amino acids, gluconeogenesis is augmented, allowing more glucose to be passed into the blood and sustaining the elevated blood sugar.

Finally, as reviewed elsewhere, animal models are responsible for much of the evidence on metabolic changes in the body of cancer-bearing animals or humans.[85,86] The tumor itself takes up amino acids and glucose avidly and releases lactate, which can be used by the liver for gluconeogenesis. At the same time, loss of muscle mass is striking. It has been shown in vitro that muscle from the tumor-bearing rat oxidizes leucine more rapidly, less being available for muscle protein synthesis.[87] Less alanine is released in vitro from muscle taken from tumor-bearing rats, whereas glutamine output from muscle is not affected. The low alanine release can be corrected by adding glucose to the medium. These findings correlate with the low plasma alanine levels of patients with cancer.[88]

## Metabolic Body Size and Protein Metabolism

It has long been known that among mammals the intensity of energy metabolism decreases as mature body size increases. This general principle of metabolism affects the relative sizes of some organs intimately concerned with metabolic regulation, such as the liver.[2] Table 1–5 is based on

**Table 1–5.    The Influence of Body Size on the Relative Weights of Individual Organs and on Several Parameters of Metabolism***

| Measurement | Amount of Metabolic or Body Component/kg Body Weight | | |
| --- | --- | --- | --- |
| | At 200 g (rat) | At 70 kg (man) | Ratio $\frac{rat}{man}$ |
| Organ weights: | | | |
| Skeletal muscle (g) | 450 | 450 | 1.0 |
| Blood (g) | 52 | 48 | 1.1 |
| Heart (g) | 6.0 | 5.5 | 1.1 |
| Liver (g) | 41 | 19 | 2.1 |
| Kidney (g) | 9.4 | 3.8 | 2.5 |
| Pituitary (mg) | 360 | 80 | 4.5 |
| Adrenal (mg) | 380 | 120 | 3.2 |
| Thyroid (mg) | 150 | 90 | 1.7 |
| Metabolic Parameters: | | | |
| Basal energy metabolism (kcal/day) | 108 | 23 | 4.7 |
| Endogenous urinary N (mg N/day) | 230 | 45 | 5.1 |
| Threonine requirement (mg/day) | 28 | 7 | 4.2 |
| Methionine requirement (mg/day) | 56 | 16 | 3.5 |
| Total body protein synthesis (mg N/day) | 1010 | 218 | 4.6 |
| Creatinine in urine (mg N/day) | 14 | 8 | 1.8 |
| Total body albumin (g) | 4.0 | 4.6 | 0.9 |
| Albumin turnover (days$^{-1}$) | 0.24 | 0.04 | 6.0 |
| Ceruloplasmin turnover (days$^{-1}$) | 0.49 | 0.11 | 4.4 |

*Data abstracted from Munro, H.N.[2]

regression analysis of data from a wide range of mammals of varying mature size. It shows the results as organ weights or metabolic components per kg body weight for animals weighing 200 g (rat) and 70 kg (man), as predicted by these regression analyses. The proportion of skeletal muscle is constant at 45% of body weight. Blood and heart weights are also maintained at the same weight per kg body weight, but liver and kidney, two organs intimately concerned with metabolism of food, are relatively smaller in man than in the rat. The endocrine organs (pituitary, adrenal, and thyroid glands) are also smaller relative to body weight. In addition, most metabolic parameters (basal energy metabolism, endogenous urinary N output, requirements for the essential amino acids, total body protein synthesis, and turnover of albumin and ceruloplasmin) are about five times more intense per kg body weight in the rat than in man. However, the daily excretion of creatinine per kg body weight is less affected by body size of the species, reflecting its relationship to the amount of muscle in the bodies of rat and man.

### Nitrogen Excretion and Nitrogen Balance

The end products of nitrogen (N) metabolism within the body are excreted in the urine (see Fig. 1–2), whereas unabsorbed protein coming from the diet or protein secreted into the lumen of the intestines and not reabsorbed is voided in the

feces. In addition, some nitrogenous materials are lost from the skin both as soluble N (e.g., urea) and as shed epithelial cells. Finally, minor routes of N loss are represented by nasal secretions, hair cuttings, menstrual fluid, and semen.

The major N compounds in the urine are urea, ammonia, uric acid, and creatinine. These compounds respond differently to changes in protein intake (Table 1–6). On a diet of normal protein content, urea accounts for more than 80% of urinary N, but this proportion falls when a diet low in protein is consumed. During fasting, the absolute amount and percentage of ammonia N rise in response to the acidosis. On the other hand, creatinine output tends to be independent of diet because it reflects the pool of creatine in muscle when a creatine-free diet is taken.

The overall metabolism of protein in the body can be summarized by nitrogen balance. This represents the difference between N intake and N output, the difference being either positive (N retention, as in active growth), negative (N loss), or zero (N equilibrium). The determination of N balance (B) thus requires a careful estimate of intake (I) and of all routes of N loss, namely urine (U), feces (F), and dermal losses (S):

$$B = I - (U + F + S)$$

Thus, the balance is obtained by a usually small difference (10 to 15%) between two larger num-

**Table 1–6.   Partition of Urinary N Output Under Different Nutritional Conditions by Adult Human Subjects***

| | High-protein Diet | Low-protein Diet | During Fasting Day 1 | During Fasting Day 2 |
|---|---|---|---|---|
| Urinary N Source | Total daily output (g N) | | | |
| Total N | 16.80 | 3.60 | 10.51 | 8.77 |
| Urea N | 14.70 | 2.20 | 8.96 | 6.62 |
| Ammonia N | 0.49 | 0.42 | 0.40 | 1.05 |
| Uric acid N | 0.18 | 0.09 | 0.12 | 0.17 |
| Creatinine N | 0.58 | 0.60 | 0.44 | 0.39 |
| Undetermined N | 0.85 | 0.27 | 0.59 | 0.54 |
| | Percentage of total N output | | | |
| Urea N | 87.5 | 61.7 | 85.1 | 75.4 |
| Ammonia N | 3.0 | 11.3 | 3.8 | 12.0 |
| Uric acid N | 1.1 | 2.5 | 1.1 | 1.9 |
| Creatinine N | 3.6 | 17.2 | 4.2 | 4.4 |
| Undetermined N | 4.9 | 7.3 | 5.6 | 6.1 |

*From Allison, J.B. and Bird, J.C.[89]

bers and is subject to the combined errors of these estimates. Furthermore, Wallace has pointed out that N intake tends to be overestimated through unconsumed diet while output tends to be underestimated because of losses.[90] There is thus a built-in bias toward a positive balance. In addition, it is unusual to make direct measurements of dermal losses, the custom being to accept a constant (estimated) correction for dermal N, or to ignore this N loss. The contribution of such dermal N losses is discussed in the next section.

Nitrogen balance is also affected by energy intake.[74] Not only does N balance become progressively more negative as energy intake is reduced below the needs of the body, but it becomes more favorable when energy intake is increased above the subject's requirements for energy. There is accordingly a continuous relationship between energy intake and N balance from negative low-energy levels to positive at excessive intakes of energy, as shown by the upper line of Figure 1–24. The lower line in this diagram shows the consequence of limiting the amount of protein in the diet. Restriction of dietary protein prevents further improvement in N balance beyond a certain point. Note that the difference between the two lines results from increase in protein intake. The conclusions to be drawn from this figure are that N balance is the result of both protein intake and energy intake and that studies of factors affecting N balance, such as dietary protein, must be carried out under conditions where the subject's energy intake is carefully defined in relation to his requirements. The latter is not easy to accomplish.

Finally, N balance in influenced by hormones.[53] These can be divided into anabolic (growth hormone, testosterone) and catabolic (corticosteroids, thyroxine). These hormones are especially effec-

tive on protein metabolism in muscle. Because skeletal muscle is such a large tissue, anabolic and catabolic changes in muscle tend to determine alterations in N balance. This phenomenon can obscure effects of these hormones on protein metabolism in other tissues, such as liver.

## REQUIREMENTS OF MAN FOR PROTEIN AND AMINO ACIDS

In contrast to molecular biology, our knowledge of nutritional principles continues to evolve slowly. In the field of protein requirements, a

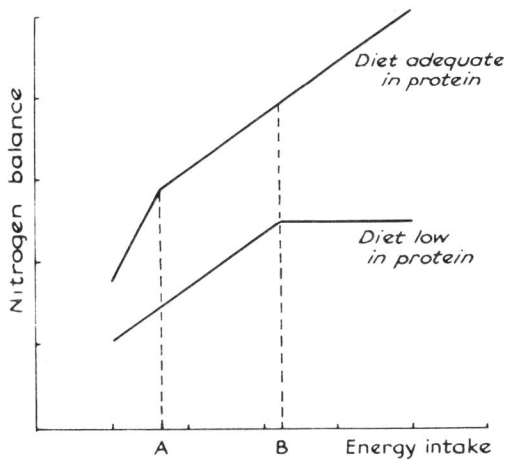

**Fig. 1–24.** Diagram showing the relationship of N balance and energy intake on diets of different protein content. *Upper line,* Diet adequate in protein; *lower line,* diet deficient in protein. An increase in energy intake evokes an improvement in N balance at both levels of protein intake, but at the lower protein intake increments in energy intake are not effective beyond point B. Presumably the upper slope will also eventually show a similar leveling off if sufficient energy is consumed. (From Munro, H.N.)[53]

major advance was achieved in 1946 by Block and Mitchell who showed that various biologic measures of the quality of dietary proteins could be correlated with their content of essential amino acids expressed as a "chemical score," i.e., the concentration of the essential amino acid in least abundance relative to requirements.[91] The emphasis on essential amino acids as an explanation for the need for dietary protein was further underlined in the period from 1950 to 1960 by a series of quantitative estimates of human requirements for individual amino acids. The protein and amino acid requirements of man have been frequently reviewed, and recommendations have been made in the publications of expert international committees[92–95] and also in recommended dietary allowances for the United States.[96] The requirements for protein and for individual essential amino acids will initially be considered separately.

### Protein Needs and Allowances

The requirement for protein in the diet can be estimated in two ways. One way is to measure all losses of nitrogenous compounds from the body when the diet is devoid of protein and then assume that sufficient nitrogen from high-quality dietary protein to replace these obligatory nitrogen losses will provide the adult human subject with his requirement. This is the so-called factorial method, since it is based on adding up a series of factors that represent obligatory nitrogen losses from the body. Enough protein to replace these losses should meet requirements. The second procedure for estimating protein requirements is to determine directly the minimum amount of dietary protein needed to keep the subject in nitrogen equilibrium. Ideally, the two methods should arrive at similar estimates of protein requirements. For infants and children, optimal growth, and not zero nitrogen balance, is the criterion used; similarly, the additional needs of pregnancy and lactation must be fulfilled.

The factorial method of measuring dietary protein needs depends on adding all the losses of organic nitrogen by a subject on a nitrogen-free diet. Two major questions thus arise: What are the routes of obligatory nitrogen loss, and what is the magnitude of N loss by each channel under these basal conditions on a protein-free diet? When a protein-free diet is fed to a human subject or to an animal such as a rat, urinary N output decreases rapidly for a few days, followed by a plateau (Fig. 1–25). Based on literature surveys by two successive WHO/FAO expert committees[93,94] and confirmed by a recent WHO/FAO/UNU panel,[95] this minimum output has been estimated to be 37 mg

N/kg body weight for adult men. Even on a diet without protein, there is also a loss of N in the feces, representing enzymes and desquamated intestinal cells that have not been fully digested and reabsorbed. This obligatory fecal N output of adults is about 12 mg N/kg body weight. Organic nitrogen is also lost from the skin in the form of desquamated cells, hair and nail clippings, and sweat. On the basis of direct studies of skin losses conducted under rigorous collection conditions involving minimal sweating,[98] the cutaneous N loss by adult men eating a normal diet in a temperate environment is about 5 to 8 mg/kg body weight; this amount decreases to 3 mg when a protein-free diet is consumed. In addition to these major routes of N loss, there are a series of minor routes of N excretion, such as ammonia in the breath, nasal secretions, menstrual flow in the female, and seminal fluid in the male.[98] For all these minor routes, an estimate of 2 mg N/kg body weight for men and 3 mg N/kg for women approximates the average daily loss.

The factorial approach predicts that protein requirements are the amounts needed in the diet to replace these combined obligatory losses of nitrogen. The sum of urinary, fecal, cutaneous, and minor routes of N loss given previously adds up to 54 mg N/kg body weight. These estimates of obligatory N loss can be expressed as amounts of body protein that have to be replaced daily from dietary sources, using the conversion factor of N × 6.25 to provide the weight of protein. Thus, the obligatory N losses would represent a net daily loss of 0.34 g of body protein/kg body weight, if not replaced from the diet. By this method, the daily protein requirement of the average adult would be 0.34 g/kg of a dietary protein that is fully utilized. The WHO/FAO reports suggest a coefficient of individual variation of 15% for the obligatory N losses in the urine and feces.[93,94] Consequently, Table 1–7 also includes a value reflecting the addition of 30% (twice the coefficient of variation of 15%) to cover the range of individual losses for 97.5% of the population. The upper limit of the amount of body protein to be replaced thus becomes 0.45 g/kg body weight, an estimate confirmed by re-examination of available data by the most recent international committee.[95]

It should be possible to test these predictions by feeding different amounts of protein and finding the minimum amount needed to restore N equilibrium. Several authors have added different levels of protein to a protein-free diet and have measured the improvement in N balance. In general, addition of increasing amounts of high-quality protein, such as whole-egg protein, has produced a nonlinear response (Fig. 1–26).[99] At lower

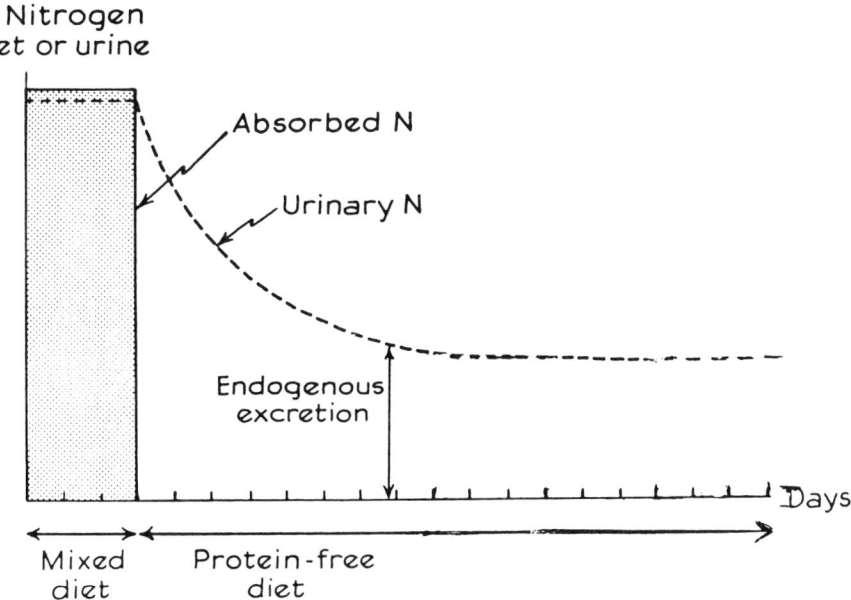

**Fig. 1–25.**   Effect of a protein-free diet on urinary N output. (Adapted from Munro, H.N.)[97]

intakes, the improvement in N balance is proportional to the amount of protein added to the diet, but as intake is further increased, the efficiency of utilization falls off. The amount then needed to achieve zero N equilibrium (i.e., output = intake) is much greater than predicted from the earlier part of the curve. This loss of efficiency as equilibrium is approached has been estimated to add 30% to the amount of whole egg protein needed for N equilibrium, and therefore the requirement for dietary protein is increased by this percentage, namely, from 0.45 to 0.57 g protein/kg body weight (see Table 1–7). If the protein of the diet is used less efficiently than egg protein, the amount needed to replace body protein will be correspondingly increased. Thus if the average

dietary protein has only 75% of the biologic quality of egg protein, the requirement should be increased to 0.8 g/kg body weight (0.57 × 100/75), that is, 56 g protein daily are needed to meet the requirements of a 70-kg man.

   These conclusions are less secure than such precise calculations would lead one to believe. Nitrogen balance is influenced by energy intake.[53] In the past not enough attention has been paid to ensuring energy equilibrium during N balance experiments; in general, the tendency has been to increase energy intake beyond requirements in order to prevent weight losses on low-protein diets. This approach confounds the N balance data by improving N retention from the surfeit of calories. This change has been well illustrated by

**Table 1–7.   Obligatory Nitrogen Losses by Adult Men on Protein-Free Diets and the Equivalent Loss of Body Protein**

|  | *Daily N Loss (mg/kg b wt)* | *Equivalent Amount of Protein (g/kg b wt)* |
|---|---|---|
| Obligatory Losses: | | |
| Urine | 37 | 0.23 |
| Feces | 12 | 0.08 |
| Cutaneous | 3 | 0.02 |
| Minor Routes | 2 | 0.01 |
| Total (Mean) | 54 | 0.34 |
| +2 S.D. above mean* | 70 | 0.45 |
| Amount of whole-egg protein needed for equilibrium† | | 0.57 |

*Additional 30% to cover upper level of individual requirements extending 2 S.D. above the mean.
†Loss of efficiency 30%.

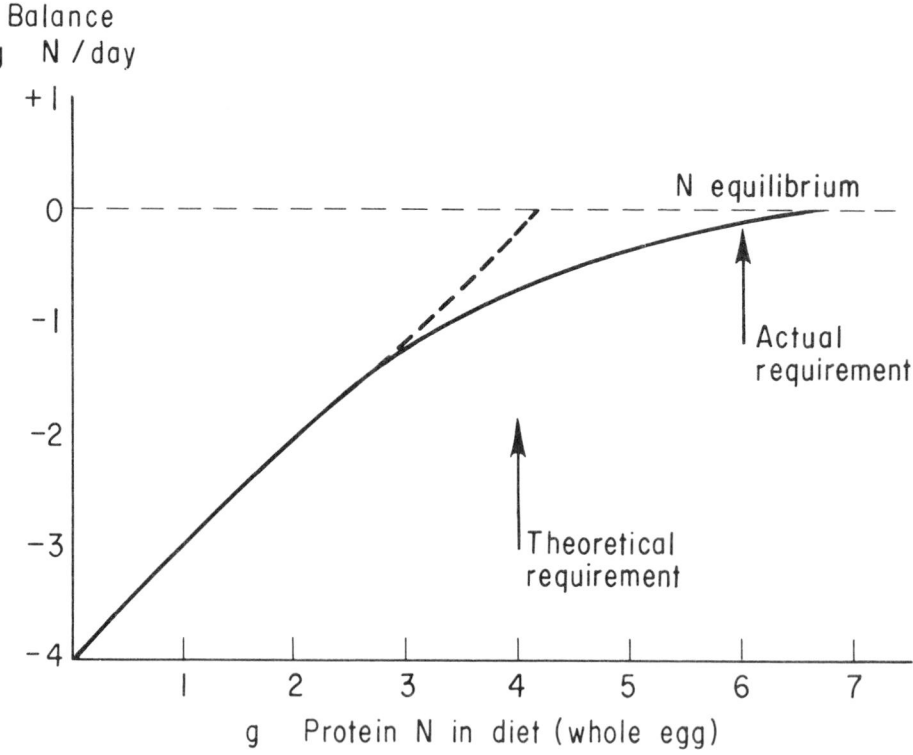

**Fig. 1–26.**   Response of N balance to increasing amounts of whole-egg protein added to a protein-free diet.

Inoue, who showed that the apparent requirement of young men for protein could be altered significantly by changing energy intake.[100] At an intake of energy just sufficient for maintenance (45 cal/kg), the average requirement of egg protein for N equilibrium was 0.65 g/kg body weight, whereas at a higher energy intake (57 cal/kg), the requirement fell to 0.45 g/kg. Similarly, the requirement for rice protein as the sole dietary protein changed from 0.87 g/kg at the lower caloric intake to 0.58 g/kg at the higher level of energy. Furthermore, it has been suggested that the use of a correction factor of 30% for loss of efficiency of utilization of egg protein (see Fig. 1–26) may not describe the reduction in utilization of other proteins such as wheat gluten. This correction of 30% has also been challenged by the most recent international committee, who considered that it should be much higher.[98] Garza et al. have also concluded that 0.57 g egg protein/kg body weight/day may not be sufficient to provide the optimum protein intake for young adult men receiving adequate but not excessive energy intakes.[101] At this level of intake, serum levels of certain liver enzymes (e.g., transaminases) rose, an effect that disappeared when protein intake was increased. In a more recent study, Garza et al. found that addition of non-essential amino acids to increase protein intake

from 0.57 to 0.8 g/kg allowed young adults to achieve N equilibrium,[102] thus pointing to a major requirement for more nonspecific nitrogen by the adult. This conclusion will also emerge in later comments on the essential amino requirements of adults.

In 1985, an international committee convened by the Food and Agricultural Organization, the World Health Organization, and the United Nations University issued a new report on protein and energy requirements.[95] On this occasion, the safe intake of protein for adults was based on published studies in which the least amount of good-quality dietary protein for maintaining zero nitrogen balance had been estimated directly. This literature survey led to the conclusion that the requirement for the *average* young adult was 0.6 g protein/kg body weight. When protein was increased by 25% to allow for individual variability (2 standard deviations), the safe intake to cover 97.5% of young adults rose to 0.75 g/kg body weight. Since adults are considered to have only small requirements for essential amino acids, no correction for biologic value was thought to be necessary, but digestibility was emphasized as a factor causing differences in availability varying from 95% for many animal proteins to only 80% for foods with a high content of fiber. Thus, the protein requirements of adults on mixed diets do not need correction, whereas those with low digestibility require an increase.

The needs of other age groups for protein have also been explored to various extents (Table 1–8). During its first year, the infant increases in weight by about 7 kg. The daily increment in body protein over this period is about 3.3 g. The estimates of daily protein requirements of infants are based on the amount of milk protein needed to sustain maximal growth, namely, 2.4 g/kg during the first month, declining to 1.75 g/kg by 6 months. After the first year, requirements are less well established but are believed to fall progressively from 1.2 g/kg at 1 to 2 years of age to the adult level of 0.75 g/kg (other WHO data in Appendix).

During pregnancy, about 1 kg of protein is deposited in the fetus and the maternal body, much of it during the later stages.[96] To meet this need, the pregnant woman should receive an average additional 6 g of protein daily. During early lactation, 17.5 g of protein should be added to the total daily amount recommended for nonpregnant women to offset the secretion of protein in the milk; beyond 6 months of lactation the extra dietary protein can be reduced. Studies of the protein requirements of elderly men and women are controversial. Two groups found no difference from the needs of young adults.[103,104] In one series, the elderly probably received more energy than they required,[103] whereas those in the second study were evaluated following a period of protein deficiency, which commonly improves the effi-

ciency of use of dietary protein.[104] An additional two studies performed at appropriate levels of energy intake suggest that half the elderly adults find it difficult to achieve zero N balance on 0.8 protein/kg.[105,106] These studies are evaluated elsewhere in more detail.[107]

## Factors Influencing Protein Requirements

While severe psychologic stress increases N output,[108] the ordinary stresses of living are allowed for in the estimates of protein allowances. Although high environmental temperatures cause excessive N loss through sweat, this loss is eventually compensated for by reduced urinary N output. Heavy work is also not thought to be a significant factor in protein requirements. However, athletes in training may temporarily need more protein during the period of increase in muscle mass.[109] The effect of the energy content of the diet on protein utilization has been well established, and the necessity for ensuring an adequate but not excessive calorie level during determinations of protein needs has already been emphasized.

## Essential Amino Acids and Their Needs by Man

For adult man, the essential amino acids are isoleucine, leucine, lysine, methionine, phenylalanine, threonine, tryptophan, and valine. Infants also require histidine, and small amounts are probably needed by adults. Our ideas on the amino acid needs of adults are based primarily on N balance studies, whereas requirements for infants and children are predicated on the least amounts compatible with maximal growth. Irwin and Hegsted have reviewed all studies of human amino acid needs published before 1971.[110] The conditions used for assaying amino acid requirements are discussed elsewhere in detail.[111] Published estimates obtained by nitrogen balance measurements show a wide range of estimated needs even within a single study

In order to extract useful figures from this literature, the middle of the range of values obtained by Rose and his colleagues has been accepted for men on the grounds that requirements for all the essential amino acids were studied by a single investigator under constant conditions.[111] These midrange values are shown in Table 1–9 expressed per kg body weight for adult men. They agree closely with data on Japanese men obtained by Inoue et al., who examined the requirement for each amino acid by plotting N balances at several levels of intake and interpolating to zero balance.[112] They also agree with the requirements of

**Table 1–8. WHO/FAO/UNU (1985) Safe Levels of Protein Intake***

| Age Group | | Males | Females |
|---|---|---|---|
| | | g protein/kg body weight† | |
| 3–6 | months | 1.85 | |
| 6–9 | " | 1.65 | |
| 9–12 | " | 1.50 | |
| 1–2 | years | 1.20 | |
| 2–3 | " | 1.15 | |
| 3–5 | " | 1.10 | |
| 5–7 | " | 1.00 | |
| 7–10 | " | 1.00 | |
| 10–12 | " | 1.00 | 1.00 |
| 12–14 | " | 1.00 | 0.95 |
| 14–16 | " | 0.95 | 0.90 |
| 16–18 | " | 0.90 | 0.80 |
| Adults | | 0.75 | 0.75 |
| Pregnancy | | | +6 g‡ |
| Lactation 0–6 months | | | +17.5 g‡ |
| 6 months + | | | +13 g‡ |

*Assembled from WHO/FAO/UNU Report.[95]
†Uncorrected for biologic values (amino acid scores) of mixed dietary proteins for infants and children and for digestibility for all groups.
‡Total added per subject.

**Table 1–9. Essential Amino Acid (EAA) Requirements in mg/kg Body Weight of Human Subjects of Various Ages***

| Requirement | Infant (Holt) | Child, 10–12 yr. (Nakagawa) | Adult Man (Rose) | Adult Man (Inoue) | Adult Woman (Hegsted) |
|---|---|---|---|---|---|
| Histidine | ( 25) | — | — | — | — |
| Isoleucine | 111 | 28 | 10 | 11 | 10 |
| Leucine | 153 | 49 | 11 | 14 | 13 |
| Lysine | 96 | 59 | 9 | 12 | 10 |
| Methionine and Cystine | 50 | 27 | 14 | 11 | 13 |
| Phenylalanine and Tyrosine | 90 | 27 | 14 | 14 | 13 |
| Threonine | 66 | 34 | 6 | 6 | 7 |
| Tryptophan | 19 | 4 | 3 | 3 | 3 |
| Valine | 95 | 33 | 14 | 14 | 11 |
| Total EAA (excluding histidine) | 680 | 261 | 81 | 87 | 80 |

*Adapted from Munro, H.N.[111]

women for essential amino acids per kg body weight estimated by Hegsted from regression equations obtained by recalculating all available published data on women.[113] It should be noted that these are average needs; in order to compare them with the allowances for protein, it would be necessary to increase the estimates by 30% in order to cover all but the top 2.5% of the population according to normal distribution. Even so, this adjustment would be based on the assumption that the variability of needs for individual essential amino acids follows that of protein.

Regarding amino acid requirements of the infants and children, Table 1–9 gives the estimates by Holt and Snyderman of the essential requirements of infants up to 6 months of age growing maximally.[114] Although the data were expressed as ranges, we have taken the midpoint of the range of values as the average need. Values of the same order have been obtained by Fomon and Filer from amino acid intakes of infants growing optimally on milk-formula diets.[115] The requirements of older children (10 to 12 years of age) have been estimated by Nakagawa et al.[116]

When expressed per kg body weight, the needs for protein and for each essential amino acid decline progressively with increasing age from infancy (Fig. 1–27). However, the requirements for essential amino acids decrease more extensively than do those for total protein. Consequently, the proportion of total protein needs represented by essential amino acids falls from 43% for infants to 36% for older children and to 19 to 20% for adults. On the basis of this information, it should be possible to dilute egg and other good-quality protein having an overabundance of essential amino acids with nonessential amino acids or with ammonium salts and still maintain N equilibrium. Indeed, some authors were able to achieve N equilibrium when adult subjects received only 13 to 15% of dietary N in the form of essential amino acids.[117,118] Scrimshaw and co-workers replaced a small part of the nitrogen of egg, beef, and milk with nonessential nitrogen from glycine and diammonium citrate without impairing nutritive value.[119] At a level of 0.4 g protein/kg body weight, N equilibrium could be maintained with dilution of these proteins up to 25 to 30%. The source of nonessential nitrogen may also be important. In contrast to these positive findings, Daniel et al. found that replacement of milk protein with nonessential nitrogen significantly

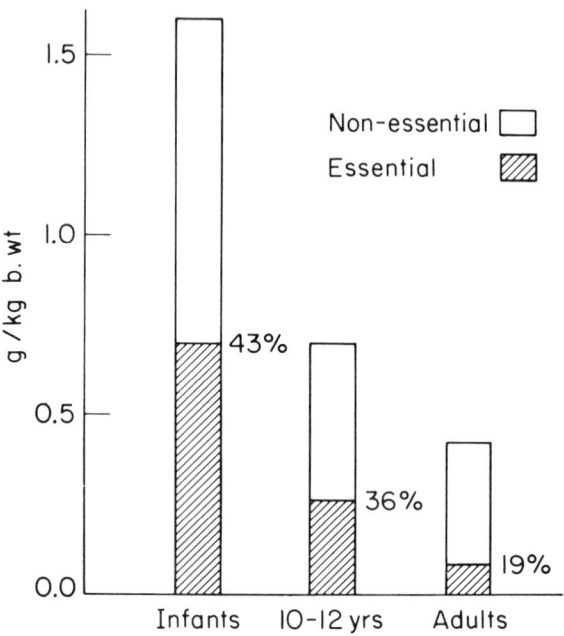

**Fig. 1–27.** Average requirements for protein and for the sum of eight essential amino acids at 6 months, 10 to 12 years, and in adulthood. (From Munro, H.N.)[111]

reduces the biologic value of the protein for 10- to 11-year-old girls,[120] suggesting that their essential amino acid needs are proportionately higher than those of adults. However, Snyderman et al. observed that nonessential nitrogen added to cow's milk protein to the extent of about 20% stimulated the growth of young infants.[121] The published data on dilution studies are thus too variable to indicate whether proteins can be diluted to a greater extent for adult use than for feeding infants.

## Protein and Essential Amino Acid Needs in Disease

There are two difficulties in deciding on protein requirements in disease: (1) Individual diseases affect protein needs to different extents and (2) each disease process varies in intensity. In a number of these conditions (fever, fracture, burns, and surgical trauma), body protein is lost extensively during the acute phase of the disease and should be regained during convalescence. Hence, we have two problems: the nutritional requirements during the acute phase and the requirements during recovery. Opinion about the desirability of high protein and energy intakes during the height of the metabolic response to a severe injury or illness varies. The loss of protein during such illness can be appreciable.[122] For example, simple disuse atrophy during bed rest can cause a loss of 0.3 kg body protein. To this can be added 0.4 kg body protein after a gastrectomy, 0.7 kg after fracture of a femur, and 1.2 kg after a 35% burn. Opinion is undivided about the need to replace such losses during convalescence. Studies on depleted adult rats indicate that during repletion the needs for essential amino acids increase to two to three times those for maintenance of the adult.[123] The repleting adult animal has the requirements of the growing rat. This is reflected in the recommendation of an essential amino acid pattern for the protein-depleted patient based on that of the rapidly growing child.[124]

In some diseases, protein intake must be restricted, e.g., acute liver failure, in which intake has to be restricted in order to avoid hepatic coma, and uremia, in which capacity to excrete nitrogenous end products is limited. The problem is to provide sufficient protein to avoid depletion of tissue protein without exceeding the capacity of the patient to deal with the amino acid load. Thus, in the dietary management of uremia, an intake of 0.5 g protein/kg body weight allows the patient to resist intercurrent infections better than an earlier recommendation of 0.25 g/kg. In order to reduce the amount of N to be excreted by uremic patients, recent attempts have used nitrogen-free

analogs of essential amino acids ("keto-analogues") to provide some of the dietary amino acid supply.[125] Finally, evidence suggests that wasting (cachexia) associated with the anorexia of malignant diseases reduces the capacity of the patient to withstand vigorous treatment. Nutritional rehabilitation allows the cancer patient to better withstand surgery, chemotherapy, and radiation therapy.[126] In judging the effectiveness of nutritional support, a useful observation is that many patients with cancer cachexia have lost the normal responses of cellular immunity. Responsiveness can often be restored by vigorous nutritional rehabilitation, and becomes an index of the repletion of the body.

## DIETARY SOURCES OF PROTEIN AND AMINO ACIDS

In performing nitrogen balance studies and similar nutritional experiments using normal diets, one usually assumes that almost all dietary nitrogen takes the form of protein, so that dietary N $\times$ 6.25 is accepted as a reasonable approximation of the amount of protein in the diet. This practice is based on two assumptions: first, that almost all the N in the diet is protein, and second, that the factor 6.25 represents the ratio of total weight to N for most proteins and protein mixtures. These propositions will now be examined.

### Forms of Dietary Nitrogen

Natural foods consist mostly of the tissues of plants and animals, so that the diet will reflect tissue constituents (see Munro[97] for details). Analysis of animal tissues such as liver and muscle confirms that indeed almost all the N is present in the form of protein, with only a small amount (1 to 2%) as free amino acids or peptides. An equally small amount is in the form of nucleic acids and phospholipid N and, in the case of muscle, as creatine and the dipeptides carnosine and anserine. However, the muscle of fish is richer in nonprotein N (20% or more), and contains a greater variety of N compounds. Similarly, about 20% of the N in human milk is nonprotein N, most of which is *not* free amino acids (e.g., urea).

In plant tissues, the proportion of nonprotein N is variable. Seeds contain mostly (95%) protein N. In roots, such as the potato and carrot, less than half the total N is protein, most of the N being present in the form of peptides and free amino acids with glutamine and asparagine especially abundant in the potato. In addition, plant tissues contain an abundance of amino acids that do not occur in proteins. Over 100 have been identified, some of which can be metabolized in the animal body, whereas many are excreted unchanged in the urine, and a few (e.g., hypoglycin A in the fruit of the West Indian Blighia and cyanoalanine in the grain of the East Indian *Lathyrus*) produce serious toxic effects.

In view of these findings, it is reasonable to accept the assumption that the N of Western mixed diets is essentially protein in nature. However, in the case of some root crops, such as cassava, the N content seriously overestimates the true protein content as obtained by hydrolysis followed by analysis of individual amino acids. Use of the conversion factor N × 6.25 implies that the average protein contains 16% N. However, the proteins of individual foods can vary from 15.7% N in milk to 19% in nuts. The use of varying conversion factors from N to protein has, in fact, been employed in calculating the protein content of foods assembled in some tables of food composition.

## Evaluation of Protein Quality

In a preceding section it was pointed out that proteins differ in their capacity to provide amino acids for utilization in the body. As discussed earlier, these differences in protein quality can sometimes be significant in computing the amount of protein needed to meet the needs of certain groups, notably infants. Measures for assessing protein quality have been surveyed in a publication that can be consulted for details.[127] Basically, the evaluation of a protein source begins with nitrogen and amino acid analysis and proceeds to biologic tests. Thus, we have to consider first the evidence obtained from amino acid analysis and then that obtained from evaluation based on biologic assays.

In 1946, Block and Mitchell introduced the concept of assessing the nutritional quality of a protein on the basis of its constituent amino acids.[91] They pointed out that all amino acids must be provided simultaneously at the sites of protein synthesis in the body and that intracellular deficits of any one could result in limitation of the rate of protein synthesis. Accordingly, they proposed that the biologic value of a dietary protein would be determined by the essential amino acid present in least concentration relative to the needs of the animal or human. This is therefore the "most limiting amino acid" from which a "chemical score" of protein quality could be calculated.

In practice, a protein with an ideal amino acid pattern is first established so that it provides all essential amino acids in optimal concentrations to meet requirements when it is fed at adequate levels. Then the concentrations of essential amino acids in 1 g of the dietary protein source are expressed as percentages of the amounts of each essential amino acid in 1 g of the ideal standard protein. The amino acid showing the lowest percentage is the "limiting amino acid," and its percentage determines the "chemical score" ("amino acid score") of the protein. A provisional amino acid pattern for scoring has been provided in the FAO/WHO report of Energy and Protein Requirements.[94] This pattern is based on the essential amino acid needs of the preschool child. The percentages of essential amino acids in this ideal pattern are: isoleucine 4%, leucine 7%, lysine 5.5%, methionine + cystine 3.5%, phenylalanine + tyrosine 6%, threonine 4%, tryptophan 1%, and valine 5%. Thus, as shown in Table 1–10, cereal protein in which lysine is the limiting amino acid at a concentration of 2.4% would have an amino acid score of

$$\frac{2.4}{5.5} \times 100 = 44.$$

Although amino acid analysis is thus a useful tool in establishing the nutritional potential of a dietary protein, there are some limitations to its use, including the finding that proteins totally lacking one essential amino acid can still have some biologic value in supporting slow growth. There is also a problem related to nonavailability of some essential amino acids present in the protein, as discussed later.

Further information about protein quality can be obtained from biologic tests. Many biologic assays of quality are based on growth of rats in which weight gain or nitrogen retention is the criterion of efficiency. In man, growth and N retention have been used for infants and N balance for adults. Relationships among various assays based on growth are illustrated diagrammatically in Figure 1–28.

The earliest assay to measure protein quality was the protein efficiency ratio (PER). In this test, young animals (usually rats) are fed the protein source at a standard level (e.g. 9%) for 10 or more days, and the weight gain per g protein eaten over this period provides the PER. For example, in one series of tests, the standard (casein) had a PER of 2.8, soy protein 2.4, and wheat gluten 0.4. This means that the young rat gained 2.8 g for every g of casein eaten, but only 0.4 g for every g of gluten eaten. However, this finding makes gluten appear to be of less value than it really is. If a protein-free diet is fed to young cats for 10 days, they will lose several g in weight. In most of the alternative assays to be described, this problem is recognized by including a control group on zero intake of protein.

The classic procedure for measuring protein quality by changes in body protein is biologic

**Table 1–10.** **Essential Amino Acid Composition of Ideal Reference Protein and of Cereal, Legume, and Milk Powder Proteins and of a Mixture of All Three\***

| Protein Source | Amino Acid Content of Protein | | | | Amino Acid Score (limiting amino acid) |
| | Lysine | Sulfur amino acids | Threonine | Tryptophan | |
|---|---|---|---|---|---|
| | % | % | % | % | |
| Ideal pattern | 5.5 | 3.5 | 4.0 | 1.0 | 100 |
| Cereal | 2.4 | 3.8 | 3.0 | 1.1 | 44 (lysine) |
| Legume | 7.2 | 2.4 | 4.2 | 1.4 | 68 (SAA)† |
| Milk powder | 8.0 | 2.9 | 3.7 | 1.3 | 83 (SAA)† |
| Mixture: cereal-legume-milk (67:22:11) | 5.1 | 3.2 | 3.5 | 1.2 | 88 (threonine) |

\*Data recalculated from Nutritional Evaluation of Protein Foods.[127]
†SAA = sulfur amino acids.

value (BV) (see Fig. 1–28). It can be applied to growing or adult animals and to man. As originally described, it involved measurement of N intake from the dietary protein and the output of N in the feces and in the urine. A group is also run on a protein-free diet to obtain values for excretion of N at zero protein intake. If the output of N in the feces is increased about this basal level, less than 100% of the dietary protein, is being absorbed. It is thus possible to calculate the amount of dietary N absorbed. The extent of utilization of this absorbed N is indicated by the proportion excreted in the urine above the basal N output

observed with animals or humans fed a protein-free diet. Biologic value thus is the fraction of absorbed N retained in the body for growth or maintenance.

A simpler procedure than measurement of BV by N balance is to assay the amount of protein N in the body of the animal at the end of the experiment. This amount is compared with the carcass N of a group fed a protein-free diet for the same length of time. The gain in N of the group receiving dietary protein is compared with their N intake, and the proportion retained in their bodies is computed to obtained net protein utilization

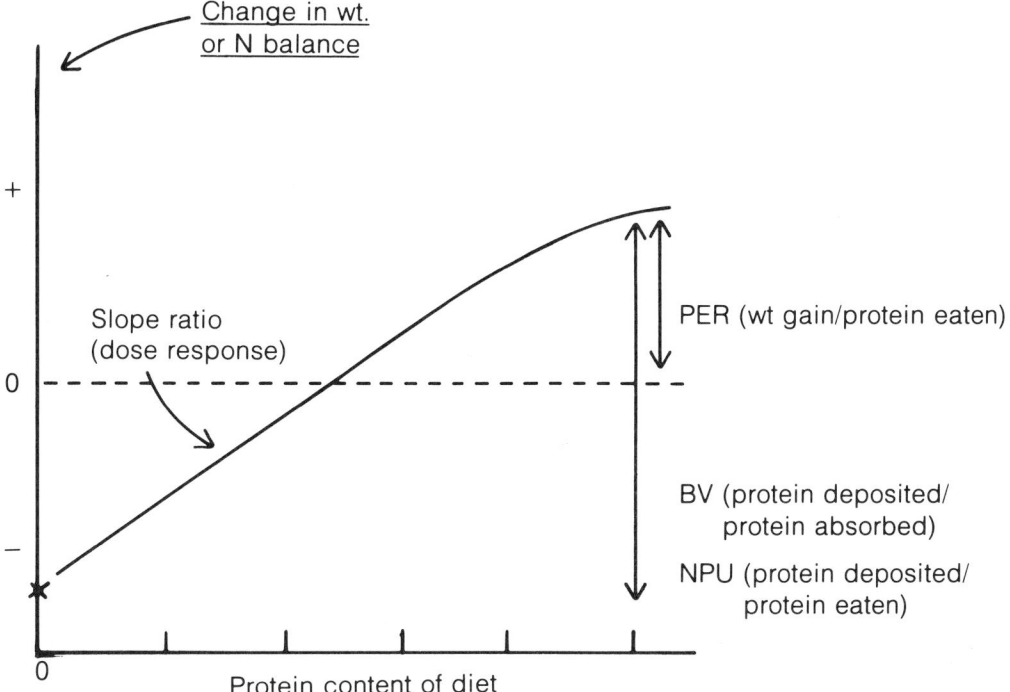

**Fig. 1–28.** Comparison of different indices of protein quality. N = nitrogen; PER = protein efficiency ratio; BV = biologic value; NPU = net protein utilization.

(NPU) (see Fig. 1–28). Because this index takes no account of digestibility, a poorly digested protein would be recorded as having a low value. The NPU procedure appeals because of its relative simplicity. It has been widely used with modifications in which the analysis of the carcass N content has been simplified by measuring dry weight or carcass water content. Said and Hegsted modified this procedure by measuring carcass N content at various levels of intake of dietary protein, from which they constructed a dose-response line, the slope of which is determined by the biologic quality of the dietary protein.[128] This procedure is representative of slope ratio assay methods. A problem associated with such dose-response assays is that the line relating protein consumed to growth rate may not be straight.

### Amino Acid Availability from the Diet

In general, the amino acid composition of the protein in a foodstuff is useful in predicting its nutritive value for growing animals and humans, using the chemical score as an index of quality. However, in certain circumstances, amino acid availability can be less than that indicated by chemical analysis. Some raw plants contain inhibitors of proteolytic digestion, the best known being the trypsin inhibitor of the soybean, which is inactivated by cooking.[129] Reduced biologic availability can also occur as a result of heat treatment or of storage under adverse conditions. This second type of underavailability has been extensively studied, because of its relevance to food processing procedures.[130]

Four types of damage to amino acids can occur as a result of food processings:

1. Loss of available lysine can occur from mild heat treatment in the presence of reducing sugars, e.g., during milk processing; in this instance, the sugar reacts with free side chains of lysine residues to render them unavailable.
2. Under severe heating conditions in the presence of either sugars or oxidized lipids or even without either of these, food proteins can become resistant to digestion so that availability of all amino acids is reduced.
3. When protein is exposed to severe treatment with alkali, lysine and cysteine residues can react together with formation of lysinoalanine, which may be toxic.
4. Conditions of oxidation, such as the use of $SO_2$, give rise to a loss of methionine in the protein.

In addition to the loss of essential amino acids from the diet by chemical reactions, their utilization by the recipient can be affected by the pres-

ence of excess of other essential or nonessential amino acids.[131] Such disproportionate amounts of amino acids can produce effects on the animal that are classified into toxicities, antagonisms, and imbalances. These effects have been demonstrated primarily with growing animals that respond with a reduction in growth rate and sometimes other changes. The term *amino acid toxicity* describes adverse effects from intake of large amounts of individual amino acids. Amino acids differ in the level at which such toxic effects occur; the most toxic are methionine and tyrosine, whereas threonine in large excess causes only a moderate reduction in growth rate. *Amino acid antagonism* is the term used when excess of one amino acid in the diet causes depression in growth rate that can be alleviated by the addition of a structurally similar amino acid. The best established example is the antagonism between the branched-chain amino acids leucine, isoleucine, and valine.

The term *amino acid imbalance* is used when a change in the proportion of amino acids causes a depression in growth rate that is alleviated by adding more of the most limiting essential amino acid in the diet. For example, when a mixture of amino acids lacking histidine is added to a diet containing 6% fibrin as the protein, young rats cease to grow. The addition of the amino acid mixture depresses growth, even though all the amino acids of the fibrin are still present. The most limiting amino acid in the diet is histidine, and growth can be restored by adding histidine to the diet imbalanced by the mixture of amino acids lacking it. Thus, utilization of the histidine in fibrin has been impaired by imbalancing the proportions of the essential amino acids through addition of the mixture lacking histidine. When the imbalance mixture is fed to rats, the level of histidine in the plasma falls sharply, and the animal reduces its food intake, presumably because of an effect of the low plasma amino acid level on appetite control by the brain. The extent to which the normal diet of man can be imbalanced without impairing utilization of essential amino acids is not known. The effects of imbalances are observed in growing animals under special circumstances in which suboptimal intakes of protein are fed. These effects are unlikely to occur in human subjects at normal levels of dietary protein.

### REFERENCES

1. Munro, H.N.: Historical introduction: The origin and growth of our present concepts of protein metabolism. *In* Mammalian Protein Metabolism, Vol. I (Munro, H.N., Allison, J.B., Eds.) New York, Academic Press, 1964, pp. 1–29.
2. Munro, H.N.: Evolution of protein metabolism in mammals. *In* Mammalian Protein Metabolism, Vol

III. (Munro, H.N., Ed.) New York, Academic Press, 1969, pp. 133–182.

3. Christensen, H.N.: Free amino acids and peptides in tissues. *In* Mammalian Protein Metabolism, Vol. I. (Munro, H.N., Allison, J.B., Eds.) New York, Academic Press, 1964, pp. 105–124.

4. Munro, H.N.: Free amino acid pools and their role in regulation. *In* Mammalian Protein Metabolism, Vol. IV. (Munro, H.N., Ed.) New York, Academic Press, 1970, pp. 299–386.

5. Herbert, J.D., Coulson, R.A., Hernandez, T.: Comp. Biochem. Physiol. *17*:583–598, 1966.

6. Meister, A.: Science *180*:33–39, 1973.

7. Hider, R.C., Fern, E.B., London, D.R.: Biochem. J. *114*:171–178, 1969.

8. Fern, E.B., Garlick, P.J.: Biochem. J. *142*:413–419, 1971.

9. Gan, J.C., Jeffay, H.: Biochim. Biophys. Acta *148*:448–458, 1967.

10. Airhart, J., Vidrich, A., Khairallah, E.A.: Biochem. J. *140*:539–548, 1974.

11. Munro, H.N.: An introduction to biochemical aspects of protein metabolism. *In* Mammalian Protein Metabolism, Vol. I. (Munro, H.N., Allison, J.B., Eds.) New York, Academic Press, 1964, pp. 31–34.

12. Dalgleish, C.E., Tabechian, H.: Biochem. J. *62*:625–631, 1956.

13. Krebs, H.A.: The metabolic fate of amino acids. *In* Mammalian Protein Metabolism, Vol. I. (Munro, H.N., Allison, J.B., Eds.) New York, Academic Press, 1964, pp. 125–176.

14. Walser, M.: Urea metabolism. *In* Nitrogen Metabolism in Man. (Waterlow, J.C., Stephen, J.M.L., Eds.) London, Applied Science Publishers, 1981, pp. 229–240.

15. Rose, W.C.: Physiol. Rev. *18*:109–136, 1938.

16. Lehninger, A.L.: Biochemistry, 2nd ed. New York, Worth, 1975, pp. 729–747.

17. Seegmiller, J.E.: Harvey Lect. *63*:28–51, 1971.

18. Milner, J.A., Visek, W.J.: Nature *145*:211–212, 1973.

19. Hultman, E., Bergstrom, J., Nilsson, L.H.: Acta Anaesthesiol. Scand. (Suppl.) *55*:28–49, 1974.

20. Forbes, G.B., Bruin, G.G.: Am. J. Clin. Nutr. *29*:1359–1366, 1976.

21. Crim, M.C., Calloway, D.H., Margen, S.: J. Nutr. *105*:428–438, 1974.

22. Crim, M.C., Calloway, D.H., Margen, S.: J. Nutr. *106*:371–381, 1975.

23. Cahill, G.F., Owen, O.E.: The role of the kidney in the regulation of protein metabolism. *In* Mammalian Protein Metabolism, Vol. IV. (Munro, H.N., Ed.) New York, Academic Press, 1970, pp. 539–584.

24. Curtoys, N.P., Lowry, O.H.: J. Biol. Chem. *248*:162–168, 1973.

25. Simpson, D.P.: J. Clin. Invest. *51*:1969–1978, 1972.

26. Goldstein, L., Schooler, J.M.: Adv. Enzyme Regul. *5*:71–86, 1967.

27. Gitler, C.: Protein digestion and absorption in nonruminants. *In* Mammalian Protein Metabolism, Vol. I. (Munro, H.N., Allison, J.B., Eds.) New York, Academic Press, 1964, pp. 35–69.

28. Fauconneau, G., Michel, M.C.: The role of the gastrointestinal tract in the regulation of protein metabolism. *In* Mammalian Protein Metabolism, Vol. IV. (Munro, H.N., Ed.) New York, Academic Press, 1970, pp. 481–522.

29. Green, G.M., Olds, B.A., Matthews, G., et al.: Proc. Soc. Exp. Biol. Med. *142*:1162–1167, 1973.

30. Kim, Y.S., Freeman, H.J.: The digestion and absorption of protein. *In* Clinical Nutrition Update: Amino Acids. (Greene, H.L., Holliday, M.A., Munro, H.N., Eds.) Chicago, American Medical Association, 1977, pp. 141–146.

31. Crim, M.C., Munro, H.N.: Protein and amino acid requirements and metabolism in relation to defined formula diets. *In* Defined Formula Diets for Medical Purposes. (Shils, M.E., Ed.) Chicago, American Medical Association, 1977, pp. 5–15.

32. Asatoor, A.M., Cheng, E., Edwards, K.D., et al.: Clin. Sci. *39*:1P, 1970.

33. Olney, J.N.: Toxic effects of glutamate and related amino acids on the developing central nervous system. *In* Heritable Disorders of Amino Acid Patterns. (Nyhan, W.L., Ed.) New York, John Wiley & Sons, 1974.

34. Filer, L.J.: Potential neurotoxic effects of amino acid imbalance. *In* Clinical Nutrition Update: Amino Acids. (Greene, H.L., Holliday, M.A., Munro, H.N., Eds.) Chicago, American Medical Association, 1977, pp. 97–101.

35. Windmueller, H.G.: Adv. Enzymol. *53*:202–237, 1982.

36. Munro, H.N., Goldberg, D.M.: The effect of protein intake on the protein and nucleic acid metabolism of the intestinal mucosal cell. *In* The Role of the Gastrointestinal Tract in Protein Metabolism. (Munro, H.N., Ed.) Oxford, Blackwell, 1964, pp. 189–196.

37. Ju, J.S., Nasset, E.S.: J. Nutr. *68*:633–645, 1959.

38. Twombley, J., Meyer, J.H.: J. Nutr. *74*:453–460, 1961.

39. Miller, L.L.: The role of the liver and the non-hepatic tissues in the regulation of free amino acid levels in the blood. *In* Amino Acid Pools. (Holden, J.T., Ed.) New York, Elsevier Science Publishing Co., 1962, pp. 708–721.

40. Elwyn, D.W.: The role of the liver in regulation of amino acid and protein metabolism. *In* Mammalian Protein Metabolism, Vol. IV. (Munro, H.N., Ed.) New York, Academic Press, 1970, pp. 523–557.

41. Harper, A.E.: Am. J. Clin. Nutr. *21*:358–366, 1968.

42. Brookes, I.M., Owens, F.N., Garrigus, U.S.: J. Nutr. *102*:27–36, 1972.

43. Pawlak, M., Pion, R.: Ann. Biol. Animal Biochim. Biophys. *8*:517–527, 1968.

44. Fishman, B., Wurtman, R.J., Munro, H.N.: Proc. Natl. Acad. Sci. USA *64*:667–683, 1969.

45. Schimke, R.T.: Regulation of protein degradation in mammalian tissues. *In* Mammalian Protein Metabolism, Vol. IV. (Munro, H.N., Ed.) New York, Academic Press, 1970, pp. 177–228.

46. Wurtman, R.J.: Diurnal rhythms in mammalian protein metabolism. *In* Mammalian Protein Metabolism, Vol. IV. (Munro, H.N., Ed.) New York, Academic Press, 1970, pp. 445–479.

47. Clifford, A.J., Riumallo, J.A., Baliga, B.S., et al.: Biochim. Biophys. Acta *277*:443–458, 1972.

48. Munro, H.N., Hubert, C., Baliga, B.S.: Regulation of protein synthesis in relation to amino acid supply. *In* Alcohol, Nutrition and Protein Synthesis. (Rothschild, M., Oratz, M., Schreiber, S.S., Eds.) New York, Pergamon Press, Inc., 1975, pp. 33–66.

49. Driscoll, H., Crim, M.C., Zahringer, J., et al.: J. Nutr. *108*:1691–1701, 1978.

50. Young, V.R., Munro, H.N.: J. Nutr. *103*:1756–1763, 1973.

51. Young, V.R., Hussein, M.A., Murray, E., et al.: J. Nutr. *101*:45–50, 1971.

52. Young, V.R., Tontisirin, R.K., Ozalp, I., et al.: J. Nutr. *102*:1159–1170, 1972.

53. Munro, H.N.: General aspects of the regulation of protein metabolism by diet and by hormones. *In* Mammalian Protein Metabolism, Vol. I. (Munro, H.N., Allison, J.B., Eds.) New York, Academic Press, 1964, pp. 381–481.

54. Fernstrom, J., Wurtman, R.J.: Science *178*:414–415, 1972.

55. Pozefsky, T., Felig, P., Tobin, J.D., et al.: J. Clin. Invest. *48*:2273–2282, 1969.

56. Wahren, J., Felig, P., Hagenfeldt, J.: J. Clin. Invest. *57*:970–999, 1978.

57. Elia, M., Livesey, G.: Branched-chain amino acid and oxo-acid metabolism in human and rat muscle. *In* Metabolism and Clinical Implications of Branched Chain Amino Acids and Keto Acids. (Walser, M., Williamson, D.R., Eds.) New York, Elsevier Science Publishing Co., 1981, pp. 257–262.

57a. Munro, H.N.: Control of plasma amino acid concentrations. *In* Aromatic Amino Acids in the Brain. Ciba Foundation Symposium 22. New York, North-Holland, 1974, pp. 5–18.

58. Young, V.R., Alexis, S.D., Baliga, B.S., et al.: J. Biol. Chem. *247*:3592–3600, 1972.

59. Long, C.L., Haverberg, L.N., Young, V.R., et al.: Metabolism *24*:929–935, 1975.

60. Haverberg, L., Deckelbaum, L., Bilmazes, C., et al.: Biochem. J. *152*:503–510, 1975.

61. Narasinga Rao, B.S., Nagabushan, V.S.: Life Sci. *12*:205–211, 1973.

62. Young, V.R., Haverberg, L., Bilmazes, C., et al.: Metabolism *22*:1929–1936, 1973.

63. Munro, H.N., Young, V.R.: Am. J. Clin. Nutr. *31*:1608–1614, 1978.

64. Munro, H.N.: Br. Med. Bull. *37*:83–88, 1981.

65. Burini, R., Santidrian, S., Moreyra, M., et al.: Metabolism *30*:679–687, 1981.

66. Tomas, F.M., Munro, H.N., Young, V.R.: Biochem. J. *178*:139–146, 1979.

67. McFarlane, A.S.: Metabolism of plasma proteins. *In* Mammalian Protein Metabolism, Vol. 1. (Munro, H.N., Allison, J.B., Eds.) New York, Academic Press, 1964, pp. 297–341.

68. Gersovitz, M., Munro, H.N., Udall, J., et al.: Metabolism *29*:1075–1086, 1980.

69. Kirsch, R., Firth, L., Black, E., et al.: Nature *217*:579, 1968.

70. Shetty, P.S., Jung, R.T., Wastrasiewicz, K.E., et al.: Lancet II: 230–232, 1979.

71. Valgeirsdottir, K., Munro, H.N.: Protein and amino acid metabolism. *In* Surgical Nutrition. (Fischer, J.E., Ed.) Boston, Little, Brown and Co., 1983, pp. 129–163.

72. Munro, H.N.: Interaction of liver and muscle in the regulation of metabolism in response to nutritional and other factors. *In* The Liver: Biology and Pathobiology. (Arias, I.M., Popper, H., Schachter, D., et al., Eds.) New York, Raven Press, 1982, pp. 677–691.

73. Waterlow, J.C., Garlick, P.J., Millward, D.J.: Protein Turnover in Mammalian Tissues and in the Whole Body. Amsterdam, North-Holland, 1978.

74. Young, V.R., Gersovitz, M., Munro, H.N.: Human aging: protein and amino acid metabolism and implications for protein and amino acid requirements. *In* Nutritional Approaches to Aging Research. (Moment, G.B., Ed.) Boca Raton, Fl. CRC Press, 1981, pp. 47–81.

75. Motil, K.J., Matthews, D.E., Bier, D.M., et al.: Am. J. Physiol. *240*:E712–E721, 1981.

76. Munro, H.N.: J. Parenter. Enteral. Nutr. *6*:271–279, 1982.

77. DeFronzo, R.A., Felig, P.: Am. J. Clin. Nutr. *33*:1378–1386, 1980.

78. Felig, P.: Annu. Rev. Biochem. *44*:933–954, 1975.

79. Schrock, H., Goldstein, L.: Am. J. Physiol. *240*:E519–E525, 1981.

80. Cahill, G.F., Aoki, T.T.: Conditions with abnormal energy balance: Partial and total starvation. *In* Assessment of Energy Metabolism in Health and Disease. (Kinney, J.M., Lense, E., Eds.) Columbus, Ross Laboratories, 1980, pp. 129–134.

81. Munro, H.N., Fernstrom, J., Wurtman, R.J.: Lancet I: 722–724, 1975.

82. Fischer, J.R., Rosen, H.M., Ebeid, A.M., et al.: Surgery *80*:77–82, 1976.

83. Conn, H.O.: Nutritional management of advanced liver disease. *In* Nutritional Support of the Seriously Ill Patient. (Winters, R.W., Greene, H.L., Eds.) New York, Academic Press, 1983, pp. 107–132.

84. Beisel, W.R., Wannemacher, R.W., Jr., Neufeld, H.A.: Relation of fever to energy expenditure. *In* Assessment of Energy Metabolism in Health and Disease. (Kinney, J.M., Lense, E., Eds.) Columbus, Ross Laboratories, 1980, pp. 144–150.

85. Goodlad, G.A.J.: Protein metabolism and tumor growth. *In* Mammalian Protein Metabolism. Vol. II. (Munro, H.N., Allison, J.B., Eds.) New York, Academic Press, 1964, pp. 415–555.

86. Munro, H.N.: J. Am. Diet. Assoc. *71*:380–384, 1977.

87. Goodlad, G.A.J., Clark, C.M.: Eur. J. Cancer Clin. Oncol. *16*:1153–1162, 1980.

88. Waterhouse, C., Jeanpetre, N., Keilson, J.: Cancer Res. *39*:1968–1972, 1972.

89. Allison, J.B., Bird, J.C.: Elimination of nitrogen from the body. *In* Mammalian Protein Metabolism, Vol. I. (Munro, H.N., Allison, J.B., Eds.) New York, Academic Press, 1964, pp. 483–512.

90. Wallace, W.M.: Fed. Proc. *18*:1125–1130, 1959.

91. Block, R.J., Mitchell, H.H.: Nutr. Abstr. Rev. *16*:249–278, 1946.

92. FAO Report: Protein Requirements. FAO Nutrition Studies No. 16. Rome, FAO, 1959.

93. WHO/FAO Report: Protein Requirements. FAO Technical Report Series No. 301. Geneva, WHO, 1965.

94. WHO/FAO Report: Energy and Protein Requirements. WHO Technical Report Series No. 522. Geneva, WHO, 1973.

95. WHO/FAO/UNU Report: Energy and Protein Requirements: WHO Technical Report Series No. 724, Geneva, WHO, 1985.

96. Food and Nutrition Board, National Academy of Sciences: Recommended Dietary Allowances, 8th Revision. Washington, DC, 1980.

97. Munro, H.N.: An introduction to nutritional aspects of protein metabolism. *In* Mammalian Protein Metabolism, Vol. II. (Munro, H.N., Allison, J.B., Eds.) New York, Academic Press, 1964, pp. 3–39.

98. Calloway, D.H., Odell, A.C., Margen, S.: J. Nutr. *101*:775–786, 1971.

99. Calloway, D.H., Margen, S.: J. Nutr. *101*:204–216, 1971.

100. Kishi, K., Mitayani, S., Inoue, G.: J. Nutr. *108*:658–669, 1978.
101. Garza, C., Scrimshaw, N.S., Young, V.R.: J. Nutr. *107*:335–352, 1977.
102. Garza, C., Scrimshaw, N.S., Young, V.R.: J. Nutr. *108*:90–96, 1978.
103. Cheng, A.H.R., Gomez, A., Gergan, J.G., et al.: Am. J. Clin. Nutr. *31*:12–22, 1978.
104. Zanni, E., Calloway, D.H., Zezulka, A.Y.: J. Nutr. *109*:513–524, 1979.
105. Uauy, R., Scrimshaw, N.S., Young, V.R.: Am. J. Clin. Nutr. *31*:779–785, 1978.
106. Gersovitz, M., Motil, K., Munro, H.N., et al.: Am J. Clin. Nutr. *35*:6–14, 1982.
107. Munro, H.N.: Protein nutriture and requirement in elderly people. *In* Nutritional Problems of the Elderly, No. 33. (Somogyi, J.C., and Fidanza, F., Eds.) Basel, Karger, Bibliotheca Nutr. Dieta., 1983, pp. 61–79.
108. Scrimshaw, N.S., Habicht, J.P., Piche, M.Z., et al.: Am. J. Clin. Nutr. *18*:321–324, 1966.
109. Torun, B., Scrimshaw, N.S., Young, V.R.: Am. J. Clin. Nutr. *30*:1983–1993, 1977.
110. Irwin, M.I., Hegsted, D.M.: J. Nutr. *101*:539–566, 1971.
111. Munro, H.N.: Amino acid requirements and metabolism and their relevance to parenteral nutrition. *In* Parenteral Nutrition. (Wilkinson, A.W., Ed.) London, Churchill-Livingstone, 1972, pp. 34–67.
112. Inoue, G., Komatsu, T., Kishi, K., et al: Amino acid requirements of Japanese young men. *In* Amino Acids: Metabolism and Medical Applications. Edited by G.L. Blackburn, J.F. Grant, and V.R. Young. Boston, John Wright, 1983, pp. 55–62.
113. Hegsted, D.M.: Fed. Proc. *22*:1424–1430, 1963.
114. Holt, L.E., Snyderman, S.E.: The amino acid requirements of children. *In* Amino Acid Metabolism and Genetic Variation. (Nyhan, W., Ed.) New York, McGraw-Hill Book Co., 1967, pp. 381–390.
115. Fomon, S., Filer, L.J.: Amino acid requirements for normal growth. *In* Amino Acid Metabolism and Genetic Variation. (Nyhan, W., Ed.) New York, McGraw-Hill Book Co., 1967, pp. 391–401.
116. Nakagawa, I., Takahashi, T., Suzuki, T., et al.: J. Nutr. *83*:115–118, 1964.
117. Kofranyi, E., Jekat, K.: Hoppe Seylers Z. Physiol. Chem. *338*:154–167, 1964.
118. Swendseid, M.E., Feeley, R.J., Harris, E.L., et al.: J. Nutr. *68*:203–211, 1959.
119. Scrimshaw, N.S., Young, V.R., Huang, P.C., et al.: J. Nutr. *98*:9–17, 1969.
120. Daniel, D.A., Doraiswamy, T.R., Swaminathan, M., et al.: Br. J. Nutr. *24*:741–747, 1970.
121. Snyderman, S.E., Holt, L.E., Dancis, J., et al.: J. Nutr. *78*:57–72, 1962.
122. Cuthbertson, D.P.: Protein requirements after injury—quality and quantity. *In* Parenteral Nutrition. (Wilkinson, A.W., Ed.) London, Churchill-Livingstone, 1972, pp. 4–23.
123. Steffee, C.H., Wissler, R.W., Humphreys, E.P., et al.: J. Nutr. *40*:483–497, 1950.
124. Winters, R.W., Hasselmeyer, E.: Intravenous Nutrition in the High-Risk Infant. New York, John Wiley & Sons, Inc., 1975.
125. Walser, M.: Keto-analogues of essential amino acids. *In* Clinical Nutrition Update—Amino Acids. (Greene, H.L., Holliday, M.A., Munro, H.N., Eds.) Chicago, American Medical Association, 1977, pp. 183–191.
126. Copeland, E.M.: The patient with malignancy. *In* Nutritional Support of the Seriously Ill Patient. (Winters, R.W., Greene, H.L., Eds.) New York, Academic Press, 1983, pp. 231–250.
127. Nutritional Evaluation of Protein Foods. Washington, National Academy of Sciences, 1978.
128. Said, A.K., Hegsted, D.M.: J. Nutr. *99*:474–480, 1969.
129. Kakade, M.L., Hoffer, D.E., Liener, I.E.: J. Nutr. *103*:1772–1778, 1973.
130. Carpenter, K.: Nutr. Abstr. Rev. *43*:424–451, 1973.
131. Harper, A.E., Benevenga, N.J., Wohlhueter, R.M.: Physiol. Rev. *50*:428–558, 1970.

*Chapter* 2

# CARBOHYDRATES

## (A) GENERAL

### Ian MacDonald

## HISTORY

The earliest record of a carbohydrate was 3000 B.C., in India, when an extraction process for sugar was described. From India sugarcane was brought to Europe by Alexander the Great, helped later by the returning Crusaders. In 1493 Columbus, in his second voyage, introduced sugarcane to the New World. It was not until 1812 that a Russian chemist named Kirchoff stated that starch, when boiled with dilute acid, was converted to a sugar identical with the sugar of grapes. Seven years later it was found that a similar acid treatment to sawdust, linen, rags, and straw also yielded grape sugar.[1] About this time carbohydrates, as they were to be called by Schmidt in 1844,[2] were found to be comprised of atoms of carbon, hydrogen, and oxygen. At the same time, Schmidt showed that sugar was present in blood, though the "honey urine" of the diabetic had been noticed by the Hindus in the sixth century. The presence of starch (glycogen) in the liver of a well-fed animal was discovered by the well-known physiologist Claude Bernard in 1856. He believed it to be formed from the protein of the food.

In more modern times carbohydrates tended to be dismissed as compounds whose sole role was the provision of energy, but in fact they play an important part in providing satisfactory organoleptic and preservative properties to food. Perhaps because of the desired taste, flavor, and texture of carbohydrates they have been accused in the causation of numerous diseases in man, including dental caries, obesity, cardiovascular disease, and diabetes.

## DEFINITIONS

Classically carbohydrates are substances having the empirical formula $C_n(H_2O)_n$ and would include under this definition such substances as glycerol. However, it is usual to consider only those in which $n>4$, and also to include the sugar alcohols when referring to dietary carbohydrates. This chapter restricts itself to the so-called "available" carbohydrates, those that can be digested and/or absorbed in the gut in man and metabolized by the body. The sugar alcohols, though not consumed in large quantities, do have clinical significance (Table 2A–1). The carbohydrates in foods are made up of polysaccharides and sugars, with most foods containing a mixture of both.

**Table 2A–1.  Summary of Principal Dietary Carbohydrates**

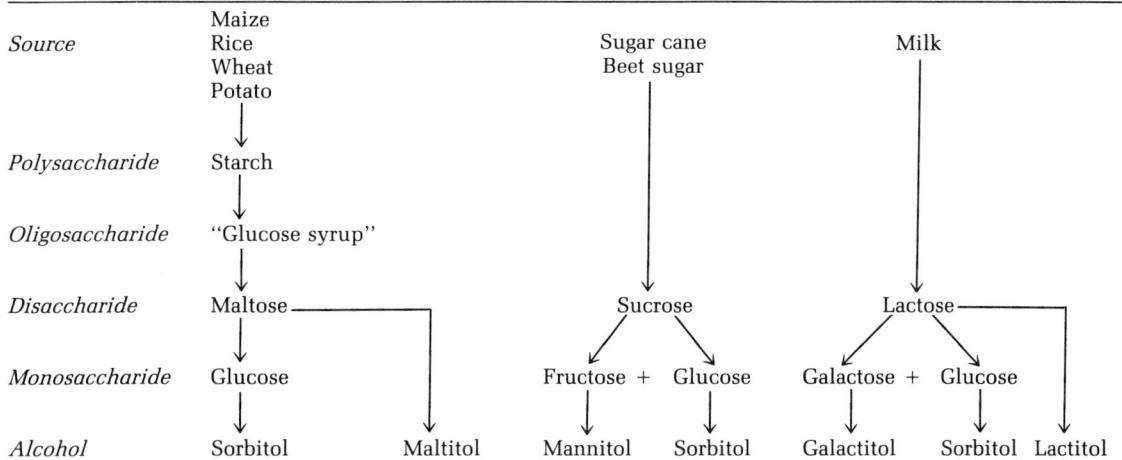

*Source* — Maize, Rice, Wheat, Potato; Sugar cane, Beet sugar; Milk

*Polysaccharide* — Starch

*Oligosaccharide* — "Glucose syrup"

*Disaccharide* — Maltose; Sucrose; Lactose

*Monosaccharide* — Glucose; Fructose + Glucose; Galactose + Glucose

*Alcohol* — Sorbitol; Maltitol; Mannitol; Sorbitol; Galactitol; Sorbitol; Lactitol

## Polysaccharides

The two main polysaccharides consumed by man are *starch* and *cellulose,* the latter having little metabolic role as it is largely indigestible. Starches, found in seeds and roots, are polymers of glucose, with the exception of *inulin* (found in artichokes), which is a polymer of fructose and is also indigestible. Raw starch is difficult to digest because the carbohydrate lies within thin-walled cells, and this makes it difficult for enzymatic attack. However, moist heat causes the starch to swell and burst the confining cell wall, thus becoming readily available for hydrolysis by amylolytic enzymes.

## Disaccharides

Perhaps the most common and best known disaccharide in the diet is *sucrose* (cane sugar, beet sugar) made up of a molecule of glucose and a molecule of fructose. Sucrose rotates polarized light to the right, but when hydrolyzed into its constituent molecules, the mixture is often referred to as "invert sugar" because polarized light is now rotated to the left.

*Lactose* is a disaccharide of glucose and galactose. Because it is only found in milk, it is unique to mammals.

*Maltose* consists of two glucose molecules and is formed from the breakdown of starch.

## Monosaccharides

*Glucose* (grape sugar, dextrose) is the main carbohydrate in the body although little is consumed in this form. It mainly arises from the hydrolysis of dietary starch. *Fructose* (fruit sugar, levulose) has the same formula as glucose, but the different spatial arrangement of the atoms makes polarized light rotate to the left. *Galactose* is also a hexose (six carbon atoms), but is rarely consumed as such.

The pentoses (five carbon atoms) *ribose* and *deoxyribose*, though not consumed in any quantity, are essential components of nucleic acids.

The alcohol of glucose, namely *sorbitol* (glucitol), had a therapeutic value as a replacement carbohydrate in the diet of diabetics and in parenteral feeding. Sorbitol is converted by the liver to fructose.

The alcohol of the pentose xylose is *xylitol,* which has also been used therapeutically as it has a sweetness similar to that of sucrose. It is reputed to be less cariogenic, and less insulinogenic.

## CONSUMPTION PATTERNS

In 1974 the supply of carbohydrates for human consumption was similar in both developed and developing countries (1,680 and 1,672 kcal/day, respectively).[3] Although the intake was almost identical, the nature of the carbohydrates eaten and the proportion they contributed to the energy intake were not similar. The carbohydrates from staple foods such as cereals and roots, and composed mainly of starch, represented 85% of the carbohydrate intake in developing countries, but only 62% in affluent ones. The difference was largely made up by carbohydrates from fruit and sugar. The proportion of carbohydrate taken as lactose was about 2%.

More recent surveys have shown that the consumption of sugar has varied, tending to fall in the more developed countries while rising in the others, and it has been suggested that the saturation point is approximately 160 g/day/person.[4] Starch consumption from cereals and roots, in developing regions seems to be related to income level, rising in 1965 to 1974 when personal income increased. In developed regions cereal consumption has fallen, especially in Japan and Eastern Europe, with little change in North America and Australasia. These changes perhaps reflect income, for at high income levels food choice is not limited to purchasing power. It has been shown that the proportion of energy obtained from carbohydrate falls as income rises.[5]

## CARBOHYDRATE AS AN ENERGY SOURCE

The intake of energy as carbohydrate can be calculated by two methods. In one, the amount of carbohydrate in a food is multiplied by its "apparent digestibility" to give a value to which the heat of combustion can be applied. "Apparent digestibility" is determined from human studies in which the food under consideration is added to a basal diet and the fecal excretion of carbohydrate is measured. As the heat of combustion (Table 2A–2) varies with the type of carbohydrate, this method could lead to some inaccuracy if the proportion of sugars to polysaccharides is not known. This method of assessing energy intake is used by the United States and by the Food and Agriculture Organization.

The other method assumes that all carbohydrates are completely digested and absorbed. Therefore, the energy available is calculated by applying the heat of combustion to monosaccharides. This method, used in the United Kingdom and other countries, implies that an assessment can be made of "available carbohydrates," that is, by measuring the amount of free sugars and starches. (See Chapter 2B for further discussion of these methods.)

The main function of dietary carbohydrate, then, is to provide energy. Carbohydrates not only contribute to the taste and texture of foods, but they also play a part in determining viscosity, in stabilizing emulsions, and in preserving food. Perhaps their most useful role, apart from nutritional energy, is as sweetening agents (Table 2A–3).

### Digestion

All carbohydrates have to be hydrolyzed to their constituent monosaccharide in order to cross the intestinal wall and be absorbed. After absorption,

**Table 2A–2. Heat of Combustion of Various Carbohydrates**

| Carbohydrate | k cal/g | kJ/g |
|---|---|---|
| Starch | 4.15 | 17.36 |
| Sucrose | 3.96 | 16.57 |
| Fructose | 3.76 | 15.73 |
| Glucose | 3.75 | 15.69 |

**Table 2A–3. Relative Sweetness of Various Carbohydrates**

| Sugar | Sweetness |
|---|---|
| Sucrose | 100 |
| Maltose | 40 |
| Lactose | 20 |
| Glucose | 70 |
| Fructose | 115–170 (sweeter when cooler) |
| Sorbitol | 70 |
| Mannitol | 70 |
| Xylitol | 90 |
| Glucose syrup | 30–60 |
| High-fructose corn syrup | 100–150 |

most of the monosaccharides pass in the portal circulation to the liver, but small quantities are used by the gut wall for maintaining its own viability. As most of the carbohydrates consumed are not monosaccharides, the alimentary tract has the responsibility to hydrolyze the starches and sugars to monosaccharides. This process commences in the mouth.

### Starch Hydrolysis

Plant starch, which occurs in granules, consists of amylose and amylopectin. Amylose is a straight-chain polymer of glucose linked by α–1, 4–glucosidic bonds, whereas amylopectin is a branched-chain polymer of glucose having not only the α–1, 4–glucosidic bonds but also branches of α–1, 6–glucosidic bonds approximately every 25 units. The proportion of amylose is approximately 25% and that of amylopectin about 75% in many native starches, with molecular weights of $10^5$ to $10^6$ and $10^7$ to $10^8$ respectively. The "waxy" cereal starches contain amylopectin only,[6] as does glycogen. The linkage between glucose molecules is important in view of the specificity of the hydrolyzing enzymes. For example, cellulose is a polysaccharide but has a β–linkage. Because no gut enzyme in man can hydrolyze this linkage,[7] cellulose can be considered a dietary fiber.

The enzyme that accelerates the hydrolysis of the one to four links is an α-amylase present in saliva and in pancreatic juice. The α-amylase splits the starch to maltose, maltotriose, and branched tri-, tetra-, and penta-polysaccharides with only small amounts of glucose. The pancreatic α–amylase, which is the major amylolytic enzyme, probably acts at two sites. One is obviously in the lumen of the jejunum and the other is on the outer surface of the intestinal brush border where pancreatic amylase can be absorbed. The digestion of starch by this membrane-bound α-amylase seems to be more efficient than by that in the lumen of the intestine.[8]

The α–1, 6 linkages of amylopectin are not affected by α-amylase, hence the branched remnants remain after hydrolysis with α-amylase. These remnants are further split by isomaltase (oligo-1, 6-glucosidase) present in the brush border of the small intestine.[9]

The saliva and pancreatic secretions contain α-amylase whose optimum pH is 6.9, and salivary α-amylase is destroyed at the low pH usually present in the stomach. Therefore the contribution of salivary α-amylase to starch digestion is small because the starch is not present for long in the mouth. Although some salivary amylase activity continues in the lumen of the stomach, this ceases as soon as the acid penetrates through the bolus. The low gastric pH also contributes to starch hydrolysis, though probably to only a minor extent overall. Among the physical factors that influence the rate of starch hydrolysis are obviously the extent of mixing of the digestive juice with the food helped, for example, by chewing. (It is of passing interest to note that dogs, which do not chew their food, have no α-amylase in the saliva.) As in the natural state starch granules are encased, failure to remove the outer covering delays starch hydrolysis. The intestinal discomfort that follows ingestion of large quantities of raw starch is evidence of this fact.

The remaining residues of dietary starch, namely the oligosaccharides such as maltotriose as well as the remnants of the branched starch (α-limit dextrins with 5 to 10 glucose residues), are hydrolyzed in the brush border of the intestine. Also hydrolyzed by enzymes in the brush border are the disaccharides lactose and sucrose. The main site of action of these enzymes is the upper and midjejunum. The α-dextrins or branch remnants are split by isomaltase (which removes the α 1–6 glucose stub), and the oligosaccharides are

hydrolyzed by maltases (glucosidases) of which there are three. Sucrose is cleaved by sucrase, an enzyme that is also active against maltose and maltotriose. The enzyme lactase (β-glucosidase) is specific for lactose (Tables 2A–4, 2A–5).

The efficiency of these surface enzymes is such that, with the exception of lactase, surface digestion is not rate-limiting for absorption and, in fact, a slight excess of monosaccharide is usually found on the luminal side. The splitting of lactase, on the other hand, is a comparatively slow process that releases insufficient glucose and galactose for maximal uptake.[10] If too great a quantity of monosaccharide is released into the gut lumen, the dangers of osmotic efflux of water with subsequent diarrhea and water loss would arise. This problem does not occur because the monosaccharides released probably cause inhibition of the enzymes.

Some vegetables, e.g., pulses, contain oligosaccharides of the raffinose family such as raffinose itself, stachyose, and verbascose. These oligosaccharides contain α-galactoside links. As these links cannot be hydrolyzed by the gut, the oligosaccharides will, if consumed in large quantities, give rise to flatulence and abdominal discomfort.

Starch should not be given to newborn infants because of the small amount of α-amylase produced by the pancreas. An increase in blood glucose following starch ingestion is absent at this age.[11] It is not until 3 to 4 years of age that the α-amylase output is maximal, though small amounts of starch can be hydrolyzed from 1 to 2 months of age.

The amylolytic enzyme present in the brush border can be influenced by the type of carbohydrate in the diet. When the diet contains large quantities of sucrose, the sucrase and maltase activities are significantly higher after 2 to 5 days than when glucose replaces sucrose, whereas

**Table 2A–4.   Hydrolysis of Dietary Carbohydrates to Monosaccharides**

| Starch | Saliva and Pancreatic Juice | Oligosaccharide | Brush Border | Monosaccharide |
|--------|------------------------------|-----------------|--------------|----------------|
| Amylose | Amylase → | Maltotriose Maltose | Maltase → Sucrase | Glucose |
| Amylopectin | Amylase → | α-Dextrin (branched) | Isomaltase → | Glucose |
| | | Sucrose | Sucrase → | Glucose and fructose |
| | | Lactose | Lactase → | Glucose and galactose |

**Table 2A–5.   Carbohydrate Hydrolyzing Enzymes in Human Brush Border**

| Substrate | Enzyme | Relative Importance For Substrate |
|---|---|---|
| Isomaltose (Limit dextrin) | Isomaltase (α-dextrinase) | 95 |
|  | Maltase | 5 |
| Maltose and Maltotriose | Isomaltase (α-dextrinase) | 50 |
|  | Sucrase | 25 |
|  | Maltase | 25 |
| Sucrose | Sucrase | 100 |
| Lactose | Lactase | 100 |

when lactose, maltose, or galactose replaces glucose no change in sucrase and maltase activity is seen.[12] The clinical interest in the failure of lactose to induce lactase activity lies in the inability to treat subjects with reduced lactase activity by gradually adding lactose to the diet. This finding that the enzyme regulation is not dependent on substrate is reinforced by the finding that fructose is the active principle in sucrose that leads to increased sucrase and maltase activity.

## ABSORPTION

Several methods are used, either singly or combined, to transport monosaccharides across the intestinal mucosa into the splanchnic capillaries. These transport systems include diffusion, facilitated (or carrier-mediated) diffusion, and active transport, the latter being distinguished by the need for energy input. Passive diffusion, which applies to the sugar alcohols and to the L-isomers of the monosaccharides glucose and galactose, prevents large quantities from being transported. The water withdrawal these compounds promote while in the gut lumen reduces the steepness of the concentration gradient. The amount that an adult can consume of these passively diffusing sugar and sugar alcohols before symptoms arise is about 50 g at any one time.

In man the only nutritionally significant monosaccharides that are actively absorbed are D-glucose and D-galactose. D-fructose, though not actively absorbed, has a rate of absorption greater than would be expected by passive diffusion, and its transfer from the lumen is by facilitated diffusion. Although glucose and galactose in the gut lumen can cross the mucosa down a diffusion gradient, the speed of this method is such that water would diffuse in the opposite direction leading to a lessening in the concentration gradient. When it is recalled that the efficiency of diffusion is inversely proportional to the distance, then the advantages of a rapid transport system for glucose and for galactose (in infancy) are obvious.

For active transport to occur, the monosaccharides involved must have certain structural requirements: at least six carbon atoms, a hydroxyl group at carbon -2, a D-pyranose ring structure, proper steric orientation, and substituent groups that are not too large.[13] In view of these limitations, it is not surprising that glucose and galactose share the same transport system and are competitive, so that one will inhibit the other when both are present. It is envisaged that the transport mechanism involves a mobile carrier and that the first step is the binding of the monosaccharide to the carrier at the luminal (brush border) side of the membrane. The sugar-carrier complex then moves across the cell and dissociates at the lateral side or the serosal surface of the cell. No carrier molecule has yet been identified, nor indeed is it certain that only one carrier is involved.[14]

Central to the mechanism of active transport of glucose and galactose is $Na+$. $Na+$ is essential for this process in the small intestine,[15] where it has been shown that the rate of glucose absorption is related to the flux of $Na+$ from mucosal to serosal surface.[16] When $Na+/K+$ ATPase is inhibited (as by ouabain), the active transport of sugar is inhibited,[17] and, perhaps unexpectedly, this inhibition is at the serosal surface of the cell. This process suggests that the $Na+$ is involved in the carrier mechanism as such, as well as in the system that provides the energy. These and other findings[18] led to the $Na+$ gradient hypothesis in which the carrier has a binding site for $Na+$ as well as for the particular sugar, with the suggestion that the carrier has a higher affinity for the sugar when the $Na+$ site is filled, as is normally found extracellularly. Inside the cell is an $Na+$ depleted environment. The $Na+$ leaves the carrier and hence releases the sugar, the free carrier then returning to the surface. The process continues resulting in a higher sugar concentration inside the cell, which then passes out into a capillary using facilitated diffusion[19] (Fig. 2A–1). Since the $Na+$ gradient hypothesis was first postulated it has become apparent that not enough energy is available to account for the sugar transport capability if only the chemical potential for $Na+$ is considered, based primarily on the fact that $K+$

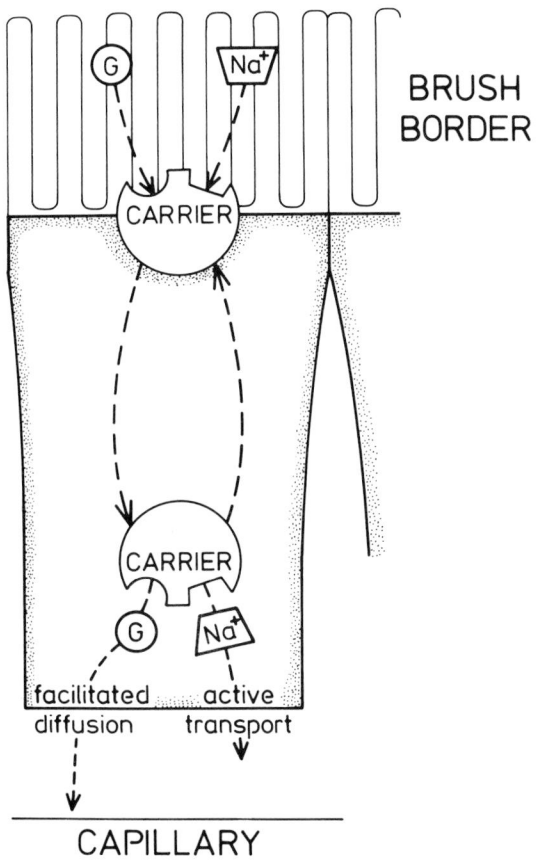

**BRUSH BORDER**

facilitated .......... active
diffusion　　transport

**CAPILLARY**

**Fig. 2A–1.** Diagrammatic representation of active absorption of glucose and galactose. G = glucose or galactose.

replacement of Na + on the carrier inhibits sugar transport.[20] This finding has led to more recent views suggesting that the potential difference across the brush border membrane of the cell may play an important role in the mechanism that concentrates sugar in the cell. Little seems to be known concerning factors that might modify the facilitated diffusion of sugar at the serosal surface.

Fructose, which is increasing in the human diet as a result of the advent of high-fructose syrups, comes from the disaccharide sucrose. It is not absorbed actively but by facilitated diffusion, and there does not appear to be any competition from other sugars. The rate of absorption may depend on the concentration of fructose at the brush border because higher plasma concentrations of fructose are found after ingestion of sucrose than after ingestion of equimolecular amounts of glucose and fructose.[21] This finding implies that, in man, only a limited amount of the fructose is converted to glucose in the intestinal wall.[22] Further, as sucrose hydrolysis occurs at the brush border, a greater concentration of fructose is present there than when fructose is in the gut lumen. Clinical confirmation is seen in the fact that in most adults 100 g of fructose by mouth will give rise to an osmotic diarrhea, whereas over 250 g of sucrose (which as a disaccharide contains over 100 g of fructose) does not produce any intestinal symptoms.

Earlier it was mentioned that the level of enzymes in the brush border can adapt to an increase in intake of sucrose and fructose but not lactose. It appears that intestinal transport can also respond to differences in intake of specific nutrients. Increase in fructose transport following a high-fructose diet has been observed in rats.[23] Similar observations have been noted after sucrose intake.[24] Findings have been similar in baboons.[25] The reverse has also been found in that glucose and galactose transport is decreased in rats fed carbohydrate-free diets.[26] Meal pattern may also influence carbohydrate absorption in that rats fed ad libitum showed less intestinal absorption of glucose than those given only one meal a day,[27] a change that could have survival value.

**INTOLERANCE**

The inability to hydrolyze or absorb dietary carbohydrate is well recognized, especially with reference to lactose. The signs and symptoms of carbohydrate intolerance include abdominal discomfort, borborygmi, flatulence, and diarrhea. Examination of the stools may reveal quantities of the undigested carbohydrate or, if the condition has been present for some time, increased quantities of lactate due to bacterial fermentation of the carbohydrate.

Oral tolerance tests using the carbohydrate under investigation are used in the diagnosis of carbohydrate intolerance. Measurements of the appropriate carbohydrate in blood are compared to normal values and, if necessary, an enzyme assay in a mucosal biopsy can be carried out as can a breath hydrogen examination.

Enzyme or carrier deficiency (and hence dietary carbohydrate intolerance) can be primary or secondary. In primary deficiency there is an enzyme or carrier defect; examples include lactase deficiency found in many adults and lactase or sucrase-isomaltase deficiency present at birth. Secondary deficiencies may arise due to a disease or disorder of the intestinal tract, and these defects disappear when the disease is resolved. Such disease could include protein deficiency, celiac disease, and intestinal infections.

Adult lactase deficiency is the most common of all enzyme deficiencies, with well over half the world's adults being lactose intolerant. Small quantities of lactose can be tolerated, however, and most individuals can tolerate up to 100 ml of milk (5 g lactose) without symptoms. Unlike other enzymes mentioned, intestinal lactase cannot be induced. Congenital lactase deficiency has been reported, but is rare and the infant would need to transfer to another carbohydrate soon after birth. A congenital defect of the glucose-galactose carrier has also been reported.

## METABOLISM

Glucose is the most common source of energy available to cells. Most cells are able to metabolize glucose to carbon dioxide and water with the release of energy. In this process the glucose is phosphorylated and converted to trioses before entering the tricarboxylic cycle. However, immediate breakdown to release energy is not the only intracellular fate for glucose. It may be converted to glycogen or to fat for future energy needs. (Although glucose can be converted to fat, it should be noted that fat cannot be converted to glucose.) The other monosaccharides in the diet, fructose and galactose, are metabolized in a comparable fashion.

Although glucose can be utilized by all cells, it is essential only in a few organs, including the brain and the red cells. Under normal circumstances the adult brain needs about 140 g glucose/day and the red cells about 40 g/day.[28] During pregnancy and growth, glucose is essential for the formation of cell constituents such as mucopolysaccharides and, of course, for lactose in lactation. Endogenous sources of glucose include some amino acids and the glycerol of glycerides. Glucose is thus ruled out as an essential nutrient in that the body is capable of gluconeogenesis to a limited extent.

In the absence of dietary carbohydrate, gluconeogenesis occurs from noncarbohydrate sources up to about 130 g/day. This amount would not meet the needs for glucose were it not for the fact that the brain adapts in such a situation and can oxidize ketone bodies.[29] Ketone bodies are formed during the breakdown of fatty acids for energy release and, in the absence of carbohydrate, the final steps in fat breakdown cannot be achieved. About 180 g glucose/day is needed to complete fat oxidation; thus, the diet should provide about 50 g glucose/day. The ketotic state has two possible disadvantages. One is that the judgment of the ketotic person may be impaired and the other is the ketone bodies, which contain utilizable energy, are excreted in breath and urine diminishing further the energy reserve of the body. Thus it is possible to state a minimum desirable intake of glucose (or its polymer equivalent), but there does

not appear to be an ideal level of intake. If dietary recommendations for protein and fat are met, the remainder of the energy needs of the body should be met by dietary carbohydrate.

## STORAGE

The only form of carbohydrate storage in the body is as the polymer of glucose, namely glycogen. The cost of storing glucose this way has been calculated as a loss of 5% compared to the direct oxidation of the glucose. When glucose is converted to fatty acid, the cost rises to approximately 28%, which makes it a less efficient way of storing energy originating as glucose.[30] Despite the efficiency of glycogen storage, however, the size of the store is small, limited, and negligible compared to the fat store. The size of the store in muscle is about 150 g and can increase about five-fold with training and dietary manipulations, but this amount is still relatively small. Added to this are the following disadvantages: glycogen is not as energy-dense as fat and, in addition, each gram of deposited glycogen needs 2.7 g of bound water,[31] making the store even less energy-dense compared with triglyceride. The glycogen store in adult liver is about 90 g.

The glycogen in muscle is probably almost entirely derived from circulating glucose because the absence of fructokinase in the muscle cell would prevent fructose metabolism there.[32] A regimen has been described and used by athletes in which the glycogen store in the muscle can be enlarged for the sporting occasion that is an endurance event[33] (see Chapter 53).

## CARBOHYDRATE AND ADIPOSE TISSUE

It was first noted in 1852 that dietary carbohydrate could be converted to fat,[34] and this fact is now recognized by all anxious overweight people. Using the respiratory quotient increases as an indication that the carbohydrate was being converted to fat, Benedict and Lee found that the Strasbourg goose force-fed corn had a respiratory quotient of 1.4.[35] It was not clear from this experiment where the fat was being formed or deposited, but the three main triglyceride pools are adipose tissue, liver, and plasma.

In the adipose tissue the adipocyte can convert glucose to fatty acid, a process whose rate is variable. Factors affecting the rate of this synthesis including fasting and a high-fat diet, which reduce it, and a high-carbohydrate diet and high-insulin level, which increase it. Little fructose enters the adipocyte because its transport into the cell is slow compared with that of glucose. Some findings suggest that not all dietary carbohydrates are equal in the extent to which they are converted to adipose tissue, though whether this is a direct or indirect effect is unclear.[36–38]

## CARBOHYDRATE AND LIVER METABOLISM

Until recently it was assumed that, in a first pass through the liver, much of the glucose that had just been absorbed from the gut would be converted by the liver cell to glycogen or to lipid. However, this simple concept may be incorrect, and therefore glucose may not be a substrate for liver metabolism. It appears that after absorption glucose is converted to liver glycogen and fat largely via a $C_3$ unit that is formed in tissues other than liver and then recycled to the liver.[39] In normal man it is reported that over two thirds of a glucose load escapes splanchnic removal and that the peripheral tissues quantitatively play the dominant role in glucose disposal.[40]

The presence of large quantities of fat in the liver is a feature of protein-calorie malnutrition where the calorie intake may approach normal, but where the protein intake is inadequate. The fat in the liver under these pathologic circumstances may represent an extension of the depot fat.[41] Its extent in experimental animals seems to be related to the type of carbohydrate accompanying the low protein intake, with sucrose leading to a greater accumulation than starch or glucose.[42]

In man most of the fructose absorbed reaches the liver,[22] little being converted by the intestinal mucosa to glucose, as occurs in rats.[43] Considerable amounts of fructose are removed by the liver because the plasma fructose levels do not rise greatly after fructose ingestion compared to intravenous infusion. The conversion of fructose by the liver can be to glucose, to lipid, or to lactate. The conversion to glucose requires glucose-6-phosphatase, the conversion to lipid can be via glucose, but as the amount of triglyceride formed seems to be greater with fructose than with glucose[44] another pathway is involved. It has been suggested that fructose, because its breakdown to trioses is not as rate-limiting as is that of glucose, forms quantities of glyceraldehyde -P which are then converted to glycerol. This glycerol then forms the basis for attachment of fatty acids.[45] Evidence to support this theory is seen in the increased levels of serum triglycerides following glycerol ingestion.[46] The formation of triglyercide glycerol is greater after fructose than after glucose.[47]

Fructose also increases the lactate levels[48,49] and the uric acid levels in blood, possibly owing to its unlimited rate of breakdown to the trioses.[50] Although these effects may not be important when fructose is given orally, intravenous administration would seem to be contraindicated. Another contraindication to intravenous infusion of fructose is the intense pain produced in the liver region if too much is given too rapidly.

Fructose, unlike glucose, accelerates the breakdown of ethanol whether it is given orally[51] or intravenously, though the extent of the increased rate of breakdown is probably not sufficient for any social advantage. Galatose metabolism is inhibited by ethanol, probably because of a decrease in the NAD+:NADH ratio in the liver.[52]

Galactose metabolism is mainly in the liver, although kidney and erythrocyte are to a minor extent involved. Galactose breakdown involves uridine diphosphoglucose and diphosphogalactose before it can be converted to glucose.[53] In milk as well as in gangliosides, cerebrosides, and some phospholipids, galactose is derived from glucose.[54] Galactose ingestion in fasted man increases the serum lactate and pyruvate levels,[55] whereas glucose has the reverse effect.[49] Glycogen may be less readily formed from galactose than from glucose.[56]

The control, in the liver, of carbohydrate metabolism is hormonal, whether after either acute or chronic ingestion. After chronic ingestion control is affected by enzyme induction, but in the short term the control is via alterations in inhibitory and/or facilitative factors. Insulin accelerates glycogen formation in keeping with its role as an anabolic hormone, but with long-term increased overall levels, it can induce enzyme activity and vice versa. Insulin thus differs from its more usual role of accelerating transfer of glucose into cells. Glucagon has the reverse effect on glycogen in that it accelerates its breakdown, as does circulating adrenaline. Glucagon stimulates insulin release, whereas adrenaline does not; glucagon does not accelerate muscle glycogen breakdown, whereas adrenaline does. Glucocorticoids aid gluconeogenesis.

## CARBOHYDRATE TOLERANCE TESTS

The tolerance test is used clinically to assess the subject's ability to metabolize a given compound or his ability to absorb it. The most common tolerance test is that in which glucose is given by mouth in water and blood glucose is measured before and at various intervals after ingestion. Any values found to be raised above normal indicate some inadequate handling of glucose. (Details are seen in Table 2A–6.) In view of the ability of insulin to keep blood glucose levels within limits, it is perhaps unwise to assess the extent of glucose absorption from the tolerance curve because varying doses of glucose give similar blood glucose

**Table 2A–6.  Glucose Concentrations\***

| Diabetes Mellitus | Venous Blood (mg/dl) | Capillary Blood (mg/dl) |
|---|---|---|
| Fasting | >120 | >120 |
| After 2 hours | >180 | >200 |
| *Impaired Glucose Tolerance* | | |
| Fasting | <120 | <120 |
| After 2 hours | 120–180 | 140–200 |

\*Before and two hours after 75 g glucose in 250 to 350 ml water.[57] Modified from W.H.O.: Tech. Rep. Ser. 646:10, 1980.

responses.[49] Of more value as an indicator of the extent of glucose absorption is the serum insulin response, which is directly related to the amount of glucose ingested.[49] Because insulin can induce liver enzymes, researchers have found that after a period on a reduced glucose intake the serum response to a glucose meal is much greater than if a higher intake of glucose (or its polymers) had preceded the tolerance test.[58] This effect does not appear to be as marked in animals.[59]

When a high-carbohydrate diet is consumed, the glucose and insulin levels in the blood over a 24-hour period are lower when the ingested carbohydrate is sucrose than when it is corn syrup. In one study, the mean 24-hour insulin level was 50% greater during the corn syrup diet than during the sucrose diet, this decrease being due to the fructose component of sucrose.[60]

Galactose tolerance curves are unlike glucose curves in that the maximum galactosemia and the time in which this is achieved are dose-related.[61] Because the liver is the major site of galactose uptake, galactose tolerance tests have been used to assess liver function.[62] The serum glucose level is raised after ingestion of galactose, but this increase is, as expected, not dose-related.[63] Galactose itself is not insulinogenic.[55]

When glucose accompanies ingested galactose, as in lactose, the serum galactose is markedly modified, in that the serum galactose response is decreased by the presence of glucose in the test meal, and this decrease is related to the dose of the glucose.[62] As glucose and galactose share the active absorption system, researchers have concluded that the explanation involved competition for absorption. This cannot be the entire explanation, however, since intravenous glucose given during a galactose tolerance test also reduces the serum galactose response.[64]

The lactose tolerance test may be used to assess lactase deficiency. It is accepted that after ingestion of 50 g of lactose an increase in the serum glucose concentration of 25 mg/dl or more indicates efficient hydrolysis and absorption of lactose.

The lactate and pyruvate levels in serum fall after glucose ingestion but rise after ingestion of fructose or sucrose, a fact that may have athletic consequence. In addition, uric acid in the serum tends to be raised after ingestion of fructose and sucrose.[49]

## CARBOHYDRATE AND SERUM LIPIDS

It has been known since 1961 that dietary carbohydrate can affect the level of lipids in the serum in both the long term[65] and the short term[66] Following the acute ingestion of carbohydrate, the level of serum triglyceride falls. Some consider this effect to be due to an increase in insulin output,[67] but others believe this explanation may not be entirely correct.[49]

The rise in the level of fasting serum triglyceride seen after the chronic ingestion of a high-carbohydrate diet seems to be short-lived. The undoubted increase in fasting serum triglyceride concentration on a raised intake of dietary carbohydrate appears, after several weeks, to fall.[68] Furthermore, many people in the world who subsist on a high-carbohydrate diet do not develop hypertriglyceridemia.[69] The increase in the serum triglyceride varies depending on the type of carbohydrate consumed, with fructose being more lipogenic than glucose.[70] All dietary carbohydrates seem to reduce the level of high-density lipoprotein (HDL) cholesterol in the serum,[71] and the HDL cholesterol:total cholesterol ratio in the serum is reduced to a greater extent by sucrose than by glucose.[72]

Any study of serum lipids and dietary carbohydrate can be confounded by the fact that triglyceride concentration falls after a meal of carbohydrate and rises after a meal containing fat. For this reason the triglycerides in the sample of serum taken after a 12-hour fast can be considered endogenous in origin.

## DIETARY CARBOHYDRATE INTERRELATIONSHIPS

**Consistency of Food.** The glucose and insulin responses to a carbohydrate are affected by the physical consistency in which it is consumed, as well as by the accompanying fat or "fiber." For example, the glucose and insulin response to potato are greater than the response to a similar carbohydrate intake given as rice,[73] and ingested ground rice also results in greater serum glucose and insulin response than whole rice.[74] Cooked starch results in a higher insulin response than raw starch but less than an equivalent amount of glucose.[75]

**Accompanying Carbohydrates.** As already mentioned, fructose seems to be absorbed more rapidly when ingested as sucrose compared to an isomolecular mixture of fructose and glucose. In addition, serum galactose levels following galactose ingestion are reduced when accompanied by glucose.

**Accompanying Protein.** When a reducing sugar is heated with protein, a Maillard reaction occurs that reduces the availibility of some amino acids, notably lysine.[76]

The monosaccharide in the intestinal lumen may influence the rate of uptake of certain amino acids, fructose seeming to accelerate this reaction.[77,78] Amino acid uptake across the blood-brain barrier is influenced indirectly by serum glucose in that the insulin concentration is directly related to the movement of tryptophan into the brain.[79]

**Accompanying Fat.** Apart from the important role of dietary carbohydrate in preventing ketosis, the type of fat accompanying ingested carbohydrate modifies the lipid response to carbohydrate. Polyunsaturated fat reduces the rise in fasting serum triglyceride levels seen after a sucrose diet.[80] In addition, a synergistic effect of sucrose and animal fat has been seen in the fasting serum triglyceride concentration when it is abnormally raised.[81]

**Minerals.** It is possible that lactose improves the absorption of calcium from the gut,[82] and carbohydrate intake is associated with sodium retention.[83]

**Ethanol.** As mentioned, fructose increases the rate of breakdown of ethanol.[51] In addition, the presence of ethanol slows the metabolism of galactose to carbon dioxide, whereas glucose is unaffected.[84]

**Sex of the Consumer.** Over 50 years ago a sex difference in carbohydrate metabolism was noted in that male rats had higher levels of liver glycogen than female animals on a similar diet.[85] More recently it has been found that after intravenous infusion in primates, males clear fructose more rapidly than females, a difference not seen with glucose.[86] In addition, the fall in plasma triglyceride after intravenous glucose is more marked in men than in women.[87] Apparently, the metabolism of fructose is affected by the sex of the consumer, and the premenopausal woman fails to show the rise in fasting serum triglycerides seen after ingestion of diets high in fructose (or sucrose).[88] This difference in response may be due to the fact that women clear serum triglycerides more rapidly than men.[89]

The glucose tolerance test varies with the phase of the menstrual cycle, with the blood glucose levels being highest at the time of ovulation.[90] Estrogens[91] but not progestogens[92] impair the glucose tolerance. Since these changes are not seen when glucose is given intravenously, they are probably mediated through changes in gastrointestinal motility.[92]

The estrogenic component of the oral contraceptive has been considered to impair the glucose tolerance,[93] whereas progesterone seems to have little effect.[94] A study in nonhuman primates on diets high in sucrose or glucose showed the level of fasting serum triglyceride to be significantly raised when the oral contraceptive was given.[95]

**"Sensitivity" of the Consumer.** If the influence of dietary carbohydrate on endogenous triglyceride as seen in the level of triglyceride in fasting serum is used as a marker, then there are some individuals whose triglyceride response is more striking than others. Their lipid level may show little change when they are placed on high-carbohydrate diets. Presumably the type IV hyperlipidemic individual is more reactive to dietary carbohydrate, with all its consequences in terms of ensuing disease. An attempt has been made to quantify this "sensitivity" (in the strictly nonallergic sense).[96] Hypertriglyceridemic individuals seem to be more sensitive to fructose than controls[97] as are patients with coronary artery disease.[98]

**Species.** The absorption of fructose in rats is different from that in man,[99] and the response to dietary carbohydrate can vary with the strain of rat.[100] The metabolism of galactose by the rat[101] and the mouse[102] is dissimilar to that reported in dogs,[103] rabbits,[104] and man.

## CARBOHYDRATE CONSUMPTION AND DISEASE

**Caries.** The role of carbohydrates in the etiology of dental caries varies with the particular carbohydrate as well as its mode and frequency of intake. There is no correlation between the amount of sucrose and the prevalence of caries,[105] nor is a correlation evident between solubility and caries incidence, although insoluble carbohydrates are noncariogenic. The acid production rates, by oral bacteria of various carbohydrates, are given in Table 2A–7.

**Obesity.** Although carbohydrates can be con-

**Table 2A–7. Acid Production Rate in Mouth of Various Carbohydrates[4]**

| Carbohydrate | Relative Acid Production Rate |
|---|---|
| Sucrose | 100 |
| Glucose syrups | 100 |
| Invert sugars | 100 |
| Fructose | 80–100 |
| Lactose | 40–60 |
| Sorbitol | 10–30 |
| Xylitol | 0 |

F.A.O./W.H.O.: Carbohydrates in Human Nutrition, Rep. 15:18, Rome 1980.

verted into adipose tissue, there is little evidence that they are markedly more efficient in this respect than protein or fat. In fact, with respect to fat, the reverse is true.[106] There are small differences in the effect on body weight of various carbohydrates. Sucrose and fructose in the diet seem to cause greater weight increase than glucose when rats[36] and baboons[37] are fed isoenergetically. Conversely, weight loss on a hypocaloric intake is greater with glucose than sucrose in rats[38] and in man,[108] thereby implying that the energy value of carbohydrates as measured on the bench may not be the same as the biologic energy value.

In diets for the treatment of the overweight, recommendations for intake of carbohydrates vary from a high intake (but reduced energy/day)[110] to a very low intake.[111] The metabolic response to a low-carbohydrate intake (less than 120 to 140 g/day for an adult) is ketosis. Although ketosis means the loss through breath and urine of products that have not completed their metabolic breakdown, the energy loss is negligible, amounting to no more than 2 g/day or 16 kcal/day.[112] Furthermore, ketosis is associated with feelings of fatigue and depression, although it may also reduce the feeling of hunger.

**Diabetes Mellitus.** Evidence associating and relating carbohydrate consumptions and sucrose consumption in particular, to diabetes mellitus is far from conclusive, largely owing to the inability to control variables other than the dietary carbohydrate intake.[113,114] There is no evidence that excessive sucrose consumption causes diabetes mellitus.[115]

In the treatment of maturity-onset diabetes (apart from the need to reduce body weight), there is a consensus that the amount of carbohydrate in the diet should increase,[116] a view diametrically opposed to that held for many years. When blood insulin levels are used to monitor the effect of dietary carbohydrate, fructose and sorbitol produce a minimal response, and sucrose produces an insulin response about half that of an equiva-

lent amount of glucose.[49] When these carbohydrates are taken as part of a meal, fructose produces a smaller increment in plasma glucose level than does sucrose, glucose, potato starch, or wheat starch. Sucrose, when consumed as part of a meal, does not aggravate postprandial hyperglycemia.[117] The glucose responses to complex carbohydrates are dissimilar and unpredictable, and the use of a glycemic response, which is based on the blood glucose response of a food to that of glucose, has been suggested.[118] The role of nondigestible carbohydrates on serum glucose is discussed in Chapter 2B.

**Cardiovascular Disease.** There is currently little evidence to suggest that dietary carbohydrates are involved in the etiology of cerebrovascular disorders, but they may have a role in ischemic heart disease. Type IV hyperlipidemia is associated with an increased incidence of coronary artery disease. Since in type IV, the serum lipid, notably the triglyceride levels, is dependent on the amount of dietary carbohydrate consumed,[119] then in certain individuals it may be deduced that dietary carbohydrate can be of etiologic significance. The type of dietary carbohydrate can alter the level of triglyceridemia in that the effect of dietary sucrose is greater than that of starch, with a fructose:glucose mixture being similar to sucrose.[120] This effect can be negated by the addition of polyunsaturated fat to the diet.[121]

Several epidemiologic studies and reviews have failed to find sufficient evidence that in the general population sucrose is associated with the development of coronary artery disease.[122–125] There is a reported correlation between coronary lesions at postmortem and dietary fructose.[126] With the other variables, such as blood pressure and smoking known to be associated with coronary artery disease, it is not possible to ascribe with any certainty an etiologic role for sucrose/fructose in this condition. The complex carbohydrate intake, however, does not seem to be associated with atherosclerosis in those individuals who subsist on large quantities.[127]

The role of dietary carbohydrate, and especially sucrose, in the causation of coronary disease is perhaps not a direct effect. It may act through a rise in blood pressure brought about by the dietary sucrose[128] working directly or through sodium retention.[129]

**Cataracts.** Galactose and glucose can give rise to cataracts because of the further metabolism of these monosaccharides in the lens and subsequent osmotic effects.[130] The glucose cataract is usually seen in diabetes where the blood glucose level is raised for a considerable time, whereas the galactose cataract is found in galactosemia[131] or im-

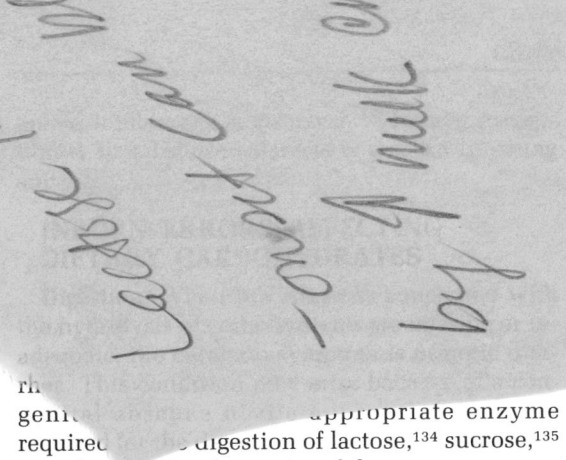

gen... ...appropriate enzyme required ...gestion of lactose,[134] sucrose,[135] or maltose.[136] Inadequacies of these enzymes may also be secondary to gut mucosal damage due to such conditions as celiac diesase or protein deficiency.[137]

Intolerance to dietary lactose due to inadequate lactase in the gut is common in the world except in individuals of Northern European origin. This intolerance appears after weaning. Its onset, which can be delayed by a high milk consumption,[138] is accompanied by symptoms of increase in intestinal fluid volume such as colic and diarrhea. The extent of the intolerance varies, but it is unusual to find complete lactase deficiency. Despite the low intake of galactose in those who are lactose-intolerant, the metabolic handling of galactose seems unimpaired.[139]

**Metabolism.** Genetic errors may occur in the conversion of fructose and galactose with important clinical effects. Absence of the enzyme fructokinase in the liver prevents fructose breakdown, and it is then excreted in the urine (fructosuria). Diminished activity of fructose-1-phosphate aldolase in the liver results in hypoglycemia and hypophosphatemia with associated vomiting (hereditary fructose intolerance). The hypoglycemia is the result of the inhibition by fructose-1-phosphate of glycogenolysis.[140] These two disorders are inherited as an autosomal recessive trait.[141]

Two clinical forms of galactosemia occur as inborn errors of metabolism and result from enzyme deficiencies. In one condition, the metabolism of galactose is halted at the galactose-1-P step with accumulation of galactose and galactose-1-P,[142] resulting in liver malfunction, cataracts, mental retardation, and failure to thrive. The other deficient enzyme is galactokinase in which galactose is not phosphorylated. This condition may lead to cataracts in an otherwise normal subject,[143] thus indicating that phosphorylated galactose is more toxic than galactose.

Certain metabolic errors in the handling of glucose by the body are, strictly speaking, not nutritional in origin. One of these is glucose-6-phosphate dehydrogenase (G6PD) deficiency, which possibly affects over 100 million persons,[144] males more frequently than females. G6PD deficiency manifests through the red cell and results in an inability to maintain glutathione in a reduced form during exposure to drugs such as sulfonamides or some antimalarials, leading to hemolysis and anemia. G6PD deficiency is prevalent in populations subject to malaria and with the sickle ... trait.[145]

...rer metabolic abnormalities affecting carbohydrate metabolism are concerned with gluconeogenesis (glucose-6-phosphate deficiency) or errors in glycogen synthesis and utilization. The latter are not common and fall into several distinct types.[146]

## REFERENCES

1. Braconnot, H.: Ann. de Chim. et de Phys. *12*:181, 1819.
2. Schmidt, C.: Liebig's Ann. *51*:30, 1844.
3. F.A.O.: Provisional Food Balance Sheets 1972/74 average. Rome, 1977.
4. F.A.O./W.H.O.: Carbohydrates in Human Nutrition, Rep. *15*:18, Rome 1980.
5. Perisse, J., Sizaret, F. Francois, P.: F.A.O. Newsletter 7, 1969.
6. Geddes, R.: Q. Rev. Chem. Soc. *23*:57–72, 1969.
7. Whelan, W.J.: Biochem. Soc. Symp. *11*:17–26, 1953.
8. Jesuitova, N.N., De Lacey, P., Ugolev, A.M.: Biochem. Biophys. Acta *86*:205–210, 1964.
9. Dahlqvist, A., Auricchio, A., Semenza, G., et al.: J. Clin. Invest. *42*:556–562, 1963.
10. Gray, G.M., Santiago, N.A.: Gastroenterology *51*:489–498, 1966.
11. Husband, J., Husband, P., Mallinson, C.N.: Lancet *2*:290–292, 1970.
12. Rosenweig, N.S.: *In* Sugars in Nutritional. (Sipple, H.L., McNutt, K.W., Eds.) New York, Academic Press, 1974, pp. 173–186.
13. Crane, R.K.: Physiol. Rev. *40*:789–825, 1960.
14. Honegger, P., Gershon, E.: Biochem. Biophys. Acta. *352*:127–134, 1974.
15. Riklis, E., Quastel, J.H.: Can. J. Biochem. Physiol. *36*:347–362, 1958.
16. Clarkson, T.W., Rothstein, A.: Am. J. Physiol. *199*:898–906, 1960.
17. Garrahan, P.J., Glynn, I.M.: J. Physiol. (Lond.) *192*:217–235, 1967.
18. Crane, R.K.: A.C.S.. Symp. Ser. *15*:2–19, 1975.
19. Kimmich, G.A.: *In* Physiology of the Gastrointestinal Tract, Vol. 2. (Johnson, L.R., Ed.) New York, Raven Press, 1981, pp. 1035–1062.
20. Crane, R.K., Forstner, G., Eicholz, A.: Biochem. Biophys. Acta *109*:467–477, 1965.
21. Macdonald, I., Turner, L.J.: Lancet *1*:841–843, 1968.
22. Cook, G.C.: Clin. Sci. *37*:675–687, 1969.
23. Mavrias, D.A., Mayer, R.J.: Biochem. Biophys. Acta *291*:531–537, 1973.
24. Reiser, S., Michaelis, D.E., Putney, J., et al.: J. Nutr. *105*:894–905, 1975.
25. Crossley, J.N., Macdonald, I.: Nutr. Metab. *12*:171–178, 1970.
26. Goldsmith, R.M., Munday, K.A., Turner, M.A.: Proc. Nutr. Soc. *30*:80A, 1971.

27. Leveille, G.A., Chakrabarty, K.: J. Nutr. *96*:69–75, 1968.
28. Cahill, G.F., Owen, O.E., Felig, P.: Physiologist *11*:97–102, 1968.
29. Owen, D.E., Morgan, A.P., Kemp, H.G.: et al.: J. Clin. Invest. *46*:1589–1595, 1967.
30. Horton, E.S.: Am. J. Clin. Nutr. *38*:972–977, 1983.
31. Karlsson, J., Saltin, B.: J. Appl. Physiol. *29*:598–602, 1970.
32. Axelrod, B.: *In* Metabolic Pathways 1. (Greenberg, D.M., Ed.) New York, Academic Press, 1967, pp. 112–145.
33. Astrand, P.O.: Fed. Proc. *26*:1772–1777, 1967.
34. Lawes, J.B., Gilbert, J.H.: Br. Assoc. Adv. Sci. Rep. 323, 1852.
35. Benedict, F.G., Lee, R.C.: Carnegie Instit. Wash Publ. No. 489, 1937.
36. Allen, R.J.L., Leahy, J.S.: Br. J. Nutr. *20*:339–347, 1966.
37. Brook, M., and Noel, P.: Nature (London) *222*:562–563, 1969.
38. Macdonald, I., Grenby, T.H., Fisher, M.A., et al.: J. Nutr. *111*:1543–1547, 1981.
39. Katz, J., McGarry, J.D.: J. Clin. Invest. *74*:1901–1909, 1984.
40. Katz, L.D., Guckman, G., Rapoport, S., et al.: Diabetes *32*:675–679, 1983.
41. Macdonald, I., Hansen, J.D.C., Bronte-Stewart, B.: Clin. Sci. *24*:55–61, 1963.
42. Macdonald, I.: J. Physiol. (Lond.) *162*:334–344, 1962.
43. Ginsberg, V., Hers, H.G.: Biochem. Biophys. Acta *38*:427–434, 1960.
44. Zakim, D.: Prog. Biochem. Pharmacol. *8*:161–188, 1973.
45. Kupe, I., Lamprecht, W.: Hoppe Seylers, Z. Physiol. Chem. *348*:929–935, 1967.
46. Macdonald, I.: Br. J. Nutr. *24*:537–543, 1970.
47. Maruhama, Y.: Metab. Clin. Exp. *19*:1085–1093, 1970.
48. Oppenheimer, S.: Biochem. Z. *45*:30–44, 1912.
49. Macdonald, I., Keyser, A., Pacy, D.: Am. J. Clin. Nutr. *31*:1305–1311, 1978.
50. Woods, H.F., Alberti, K.: Lancet *2*:1354–1357, 1972.
51. Brown, S.S., Forrest, J.A.N., Roscoe, P.: Lancet *2*:898–899, 1972.
52. Isselbacher, K.J., Krane, S.M.: J. Biol. Chem. *236*:2394–2398, 1961.
53. Leloir, L.F.: Arch. Biochem. Biophys. *33*:186–190, 1951.
54. Kalchar, H.M.: Science, *150*:305–313, 1965.
55. Royle, G., Kettlewell, M.G.W., Ilic, U., et al.: Clin. Sci. *54*:107–109, 1978.
56. Deuel, H.J.: Physiol. Rev. *16*:173–215, 1936.
57. W.H.O.: Tech. Rep. Ser. *646*:10, 1980.
58. Himsworth, H.P.: Clin. Sci. *1*:1–38, 1933.
59. Uram, J.A., Friedman, L., Kline, O.L.: Am. J. Physiol. *192*:521–524, 1958.
60. Thompson, R.G., Hayford, J.T., Danney, M.M.: Diabetes *27*:1020–1026, 1978.
61. Williams, C.A., Macdonald, I.: World Rev. Nutr. Diet *39*:23–52, 1982.
62. Tygstrup, N.: Acta. Med. Scand. *175*:281–289, 1964.
63. Stenstam, T.: Acta. Med. Scand. (Suppl.) *177*:1946.
64. Williams, C.A., Phillips, T., Macdonald, I.: Metabolism *32*:250–256, 1983.
65. Ahrens, E.H., Hirsch, S., Oettle, K., et al.: Trans. Assoc. Am. Physicians *74*:134–146, 1961.
66. Havel, R.J.: J. Clin. Invest. *36*:855–859, 1957.
67. Kessler, J.I.: J. Clin. Invest. *42*:362–367, 1963.
68. Antonis, A., Bersohn, I.: Lancet *1*:3–9, 1961.
69. Schwartz, M.J., Rosenweig, B., Toor, M., et al.: Am. J. Cardiol. *12*:157–168, 1963.
70. Macdonald, I.: Prog. Biochem. Pharmacol. *8*:216–241, 1973.
71. Schonfeld, G., Weidman, S.W., Witztum, J.L., et al.: Metabolism, *25*:261–275, 1976.
72. Macdonald, I.: Nutr. Rep. Internat. *17*:663–668, 1978.
73. Crapo, P.A., Reaven, G., Olefsky, J.: Diabetes *26*:1178–1183, 1977.
74. O'Dea, K., Nestel, P.J., Antonoff, L.: Am. J. Clin. Nutr. *33*:760–765, 1980.
75. Collings, P., Williams, C.A., Macdonald, I.: Br. Med. J. *282*:1032, 1981.
76. Landes, D.R., Miller, J.: Cereal Chem. *53*:678–682, 1976.
77. Cooke, G.C.: J. Physiol. (Lond.) *217*:61–70, 1971.
78. Reiser, S., Michaelis, D.E., Hallfrisch, J.: Proc. Soc. Exp. Biol. Med. *150*:110–114, 1975.
79. Fernstrom, J.D.: Metabolism *26*:207–223, 1977.
80. Macdonald, I.: Clin. Sci. *43*:265–274, 1972.
81. Antar, M.A., Little, J.A., Lucas, P., et al.: Atherosclerosis *11*:191–201, 1970.
82. Condon, J.R., Nassim, J.R., Millard, F.J.C.: et al.: Lancet. *1*:1027–1029, 1970.
83. Hoffman, R.S., Martino, J.A., Wahl, G., et al.: Metabolism *20*:1065–1073, 1971.
84. Segal, S., Blair, A.: J. Clin. Invest. *40*:2016–2025, 1961.
85. Greisheimer, E.M.: J. Nutr. *4*:411–418, 1931.
86. Jourdan, M.H.: J. Physiol. (Lond.) *201*:27P, 1969.
87. Perry, W.F., Corbett, B.N.: Can. J. Physiol. Pharmacol. *42*:353–356, 1964.
88. Macdonald, I.: Am. J. Clin. Nutr., *18*:369–372, 1966.
89. Kekki, M., Nikkila, E.A.: Metabolism *20*:878–889, 1971.
90. Macdonald, I., Crossley, J.N.: Diabetes *19*:450–452, 1970.
91. Buchler, D., Warren, J.C.: Am. J. Obstet. Gynecol. *95*:479–483, 1966.
92. Larsson-Cohn, U., Tengstrom, B., Wide, L.: Acta Endocrinol. *62*:242–250, 1969.
93. Ajabor, L.N.A., Tsai, C.C., Vela, P., et al.: Am. J. Obstet. Gynecol. *113*:383–387, 1972.
94. Adams, P.W., Wynn, V.: J. Obstet. Gynecol. Br. Comm. *79*:744–752, 1972.
95. Stovin, V., Macdonald, I.: Proc. Nutr. Soc. *34*:55A, 1975.
96. Hallfrisch, J., Reiser, S., Prather, E.S.: Am. J. Clin. Nutr. *37*:740–748, 1983.
97. Nikkila, E.A.: *In* Sugars in Nutrition. (Sipple, H., McNutt, K., Eds.) New York, Academic Press, 1974, pp. 439–448.
98. Palumbo, P.J., Briones, E.R., Nelson, R.A., et al.: Am. J. Clin. Nutr. *30*:394–401, 1977.
99. Dahlqvist, A., Thompson, D.L.: J. Physiol. (Lond.) *167*:193–209, 1963.
100. Durand, A.M., Fisher, N., Adams, M.: Arch. Pathol. *85*:318–324, 1968.
101. Newstead, G.C.: Proc. Nutr. Soc. *38*:38A, 1979.
102. Williams, C.A., Owens, A.M.: Proc. Nutr. Soc. *43*:58A, 1984.

103. Bollman, J.L., Mann, F.C., Power, M.H.: Am. J. Physiol. *111*:483–491, 1935.
104. Roe, J.H., Schwartzman, A.S.: J. Biol. Chem. *96*:717–735, 1932.
105. Rugg-Gunn, A.J.: *In* Prevention of Dental Disease. (Murray, J.J., Ed.) Oxford, Oxford Medical Publishers, 1983, pp. 3–82.
106. Wood, J.D., Reid, J.R.: Br. J. Nutr. *34*:15–24, 1975.
107. Reference deleted.
108. Macdonald, I., Taylor, J.: Guy's Hosp. Rep. *122*:155–159, 1973.
109. Reference deleted.
110. Dempner, W., Newborg, B.C., Peschel, R.L., et al.: Arch. Intern Med. *135*:1575–1584, 1975.
111. Flatt, J.P., Blackburn, G.L.: Am. J. Clin. Nutr. *27*:175–187, 1979.
112. Yang, M.U., Van-Italie, B.: J. Clin. Invest. *58*:722–730, 1976.
113. Stare, F.J.: Nutr. Metab. *18*(Suppl. 1): 133–142, 1975.
114. Khan, H.A., Herman, J.B., Medalie, J.H., et al.: J. Chronic Dis. *23*:617–629, 1971.
115. Bierman, E.L., Nelson, R.: World Rev. Nutr. Diet. *22*:280–287, 1975.
116. American Diabetes Association Report: Diabetes *20*:633–634, 1971.
117. Bantle, J.P., Laine, D.C., Castle, G.W., et al.: N. Engl. J. Med. *309*:7–12, 1983.
118. Jenkins, D.J.A., Wolever, T.M.S., Taylor, R.H.: Am. J. Clin. Nutr. *34*:362–366, 1981.
119. Nestel, P., Carroll, K.F., Havenstein, N., et al.: Metabolism *19*:1–18, 1970.
120. Blum, C.B., Levey, R.I., Eisenberg, S., et al.: J. Clin. Invest. *60*:795–807, 1977.
121. Nikkila, E.A., and Kekki, M.: Acta Med. Scand. (Suppl.) *542*:221–227, 1972.
122. M.R.C. Working Party: Lancet *2*:1265–1271, 1970.
123. Walker, A.R.P.: Atherosclerosis *14*:137–152, 1971.
124. Keys, A.: Atherosclerosis *14*:193–202, 1971.
125. Grande F.: *In* Sugars in Nutrition. (Sipple, H.L., McNutt, K.W., Eds.) New York, Academic Press, 1974, pp. 402–437.
126. Moore, M.C., Guzman, M.A., Schilling, P.E., et al.: J. Am. Diet. Assoc. *70*:602–606, 1977.
127. Higginson, J., Pepler, W.J.: J. Clin. Invest. *33*:1366, 1954.
128. Arhens, R.A.: Am. J. Clin. Nutr. *27*:403–422, 1974.
129. Hodges, R.E., Rebello, T.: Ann. Intern. Med. *98*:838–841, 1983.
130. Van Heyningen, R.: Nature (Lond.) *184*:194–195, 1959.
131. Rennert, O.M.: Ann. Clin. Lab. Sci. *7*:443–448, 1977.
132. Bhat, K.S., Gopolan, C.: Nutr. Metab. *17*:8, 1974.
133. Richter, C.P., Duke, J.R.: Science *168:*1372–1374, 1970.
134. Dahlqvist, A.: *In* Sugars in Nutrition. (Sipple, H.L., McNutt, K.W., Eds.) New York, Academic Press, 1974, pp. 187–214.
135. Prader, A., Auricchio, S., Murset, G.: Schweiz. Med. Wochenschr. *91*:465–476, 1961.
136. Semenza, G., Auricchio, S., Rubino, A.: Biochem. Biophys. Acta *96*:487–497, 1965.
137. Bayless, T.M., Christopher, N.L.: Am. J. Clin. Nutr. *22*:181–190, 1969.
138. Lebenthal, E., Antonowicz, I., Shwachman, H.: Am. J. Clin. Nutr. *28*:595–600, 1975.
139. Williams, C.A., Macdonald, I.: Hum. Nutr. *36C*:149–153, 1982.
140. Nisell, J., Linden, L.: Scand. J. Gastroenterol. *3*:80–82, 1968.
141. Gitzelmann, R., Steinmann, B., Van Der Berghe, G.: *In* Metabolic Basis of Inherited Disease. (Stanbury, J.B., et al., Ed.) New York, McGraw-Hill Book Co., 1983, pp. 118–140.
142. Anderson, E., Kalckar, H., Isselbacher, K.: Science *125*:113–114, 1957.
143. Gitzelmann, R.: Pediatr. Res. *1*:14–23, 1967.
144. Yoshida, A.: Science *179*:532–537, 1973.
145. Buetler, E., Johnson, C., Powars, D., et al.: N. Engl. J. Med. *290*:826–828, 1974.
146. Howell, R.R., Williams, J.C.: *In* Metabolic Basis of Inherited Disease. (Stanbury, J. B., et al., Ed.) New York, McGraw-Hill Book Co., 1983, pp. 141–166.

## SELECTED READINGS

1. Berdanier, C.D., (Ed.): Carbohydrate Metabolism. Hemisphere Publishing,1976.
2. F.A.O/W.H.O.: Carbohydrates in Human Nutrition. Rep. 15. Rome, 1980.
3. F.A.S.E.B.: Dietary Sugars in Health and Disease. I. Fructose. II. Xylitol. III. Sorbitol. Evaluation of the Health Aspect of Sucrose as a Food Ingredient, 1976. Evaluation of the Health Aspects of Starch and Modified Starches as Food Ingredients, 1979.
4. Lee, V.A.: The Nutritional Significance of Sucrose Consumption 1970–80. Critical Reviews in Food Science and Nutrition *14*:1, 1981.
5. Randle, P.J., Steiner, D.F., Whelan, W.J.: Carbohydrate Metabolism and its Disorders, Vols 1, 2, & 3. New York, Academic Press, 1981.
6. Sipple, H.L., McNutt, K.W. (Eds.): Sugars in Nutrition. New York, Academic Press, 1974.

*Chapter* **2**

# CARBOHYDRATES

## *(B) DIETARY FIBER*

### David J.A. Jenkins

The current interest in dietary fiber in terms of research and clinical application is in large measure attributable to the original observations and the hypothesis subsequently evolved by Denis Burkitt and Hugh Trowell.[1] Both practiced for 25 to 30 years following World War II as surgeon and physician, respectively, at Makareree University in Kampala, Uganda, before returning to Britain. They were struck by the great differences in the pattern and nature of diseases affecting the affluent West as opposed to more primitive communities. They were especially impressed with the differences in diet and bowel habit. In Uganda much bulky vegetable material was consumed and constipation was unknown. Their attention was therefore focused on the unabsorbable material in the diet, which they recognized as dietary fiber. They concluded that this was not only responsible for the increase in fecal bulk but was directly or indirectly related to the different pattern of diseases seen.[1]

## DIETARY FIBER HYPOTHESIS

As a result their "fiber hypothesis" was formulated in which they suggested that the consumption of unrefined, high fiber carbohydrate foods protected against many Western ailments including: colon cancer, diverticular disease, appendicitis, constipation, hemorrhoids, hiatus hernia, varicose veins, diabetes, heart disease, gallstones, obesity, and many others.[1] As presented, these claims appeared too extensive to be realistic. Detractors suggested that the incidence of these diseases related as well to food availability, exercise patterns, motor cars, televisions, and those variables that divide the more from the less developed communities throughout the world. However, with the passage of time, basic laboratory data and clinical evidence have been gathered to support much of the original hypothesis. The disorders where the hypothesis has had greatest clinical impact include constipation,[2,3] diverticular disease,[4,5] diabetes,[6–12] hyperlipidemia,[13–16] and, to some extent, obesity.[17] In addition, evidence has also been adduced to suggest a use for high fiber diets in the treatment of Crohn's disease,[18] gallstones,[19] and peptic ulcers.[20]

Nevertheless, in view of the many nutritional differences between Western and primitive communities, the exact importance of dietary fiber per se will be debated for some time to come. It may be that in the long term the greatest value of this hypothesis will be in increasing awareness of the possible differences between foods, their degree of processing, the form in which they are eaten, and the contents of their other non- or antinutrient components. All these factors may influence digestibility and subsequent metabolic events.

## DEFINITION

Hipsley in 1953 appears to have been the first to use the term *dietary fiber.*[21] Prior to this the term *crude fiber* had been developed to describe the material that reduced the energy value of animal feed. Crude fiber is largely cellulose and lignin and is still the fiber value given in food tables. The defectiveness of this term was seen in 1929 by McCance and Lawrence.[22] The problem that faced Lawrence, as a diabetologist, was how to assess the absorbable or "available" carbohydrate in the diets he wished to prescribe for his diabetic patients. Together with McCance he therefore constructed food tables that divided carbohydrate into both "available" and "unavailable."[22] It is this unavailable carbohydrate that together with lignin we currently term *dietary fiber.* These tables are currently the most comprehensive list of dietary fiber food values.[23] A reasonable working definition of dietary fiber has evolved: "The plant polysaccharides and lignin which are resistant to hydrolysis by the digestive enzymes of man."[24]

## CHEMISTRY AND STRUCTURE

Since fiber is not a single substance, its chemistry is both complex and diverse, with each plant species having both widely different fiber components and different proportions of the major classes: cellulose, lignin, and the noncellulosic polysaccharides. Histologically, dietary fiber is seen as forming the structural components of plant cell walls. The "crude" fiber, cellulose, and lignin forming the supportive skeleton and noncellulosic or what was previously termed the "hemicellulosic" water-soluble or gel-forming polysaccharides form the ground substance or matrix for this skeleton. In addition, **gums** may be secreted over the outer surface of the cell for protection (e.g., algal polysaccharides) or in response to injury, and mucilaginous polysaccharides may be found in the endosperm of the plant seed to prevent dehydration (e.g., guar gum). The dietary fiber composition of a given species of plant is not constant over the life span but changes as the plant ages. Notably the lignin content increases with time, imparting the fibrous texture to older plants.

The chief components of dietary fiber are therefore cellulose, lignins, and the noncellulosic polysaccharides (Table 2B–1).[25] Cellulose is a linear α-linked 1-4 glucose polymer of as many as 3,000 units or more and is the β-isomer of starch. It is resistant to salivary and pancreatic amylase. It is, however, capable of being degraded by the cellulases of colonic bacteria. Lignin is a complex cross-linked polymer of approximately 40 oxygenated phenylpropane units. This is the noncarbohydrate component of fiber and is very resistant to degradation, the greater proportion being recovered in the feces.[27] The noncellulosic polysaccharides include pectic substances, gums, mucilages, and algal polysaccharides. They are a diverse group, usually with less than 10% of the number of sugar residues compared to those in cellulose. The so-called hemicellulosic materials have been divided into A and B (Table 2B–1). Many are polymers of xylose with side chains of galactose, glucose, mannose, or arabinose. The so-called B hemicelluloses contain uronic acid linked to the sugars. Some investigators have classed pectins in this group, since they are polymers of galacturonic acid. The gums and mucilages are likewise branched carbohydrate polymers (e.g., guar gum, which is a linear mannan with galactose side chains). As mentioned, the proportions of these components and their chemical structure (whether mixed or single sugar main chain, the nature of the side chain residues and the frequency of side chains) will vary from plant to plant.

It is therefore not possible to think of fiber as a group of distinct entities or, far less, a single entity. Rather, there are an almost infinite number of plant fiber "complexes." However, an exact knowledge of the chemical components of fiber in a food may still not allow the physiologic effect of the dietary fiber component of that food to be predicted. It may depend very much on a tertiary chemical structure where one fiber component interacts with another.

## OCCURRENCE

The occurrence of dietary fiber is ubiquitous in all plant material[27,28] (see Appendix Table A–19).

**Table 2B–1. Chemical Components of Dietary Fiber***

| Class of Compound | Polymer | | Monomeric Units |
|---|---|---|---|
| Carbohydrate | Cellulose | | Glucose |
| | Noncellulosic polysaccharide ("hemicellulose A," gums, mucilaginous polysaccharides) | Hexose | Glucose Galactose Mannose |
| | | Pentose | Xylose Arabinose |
| | | Deoxyhexose | Rhamnose Fucose |
| | ("hemicellulose B," acidic polysaccharides, pectins, etc.) | Uronic acid | Galacturonic and glucuronic acids |
| Noncarbohydrate | Lignin | Ferulic Sinapic Coumaric | Alcohols and acids |

*Adapted from Cummings, J.H.[25]

As mentioned, the exact nature will differ from species to species and vary with stage of growth and growing conditions.

Some of the highest fiber foods are the unprocessed seeds and grains (legumes and cereals).[27,28] Nuts also are rich sources of fiber; however, these are often also high in calories. On a fiber/calorie basis the green leafy green vegetables, especially those of the *Brassica* family, are good sources, as are certain root vegetables such as parsnips and carrots.[27,28]

Although total fiber content of foods may differ, as already mentioned, the nature of the fiber may be equally important. Thus the fiber of rye and wheat is a relatively inert lignified fiber, whereas oats and barley contain mucilaginous β-glucans, and the fiber of legumes is largely noncellulosic, which in some instances may have great viscosity when hydrated (e.g., guar galactomannans). Thus, at present, in nutritional terms, knowledge of the physical rather than the chemical properties of fiber may be more rewarding.

## ANALYSIS

Perhaps the major barrier in preventing our understanding of the nutritional significance of fiber in the diet has been the problem associated with its analysis (Table 2B–2).[28–34]

### Crude Fiber

Originally all that was measured was *crude fiber,* which was simply the material (largely cellulose and lignin) remaining after extraction with dilute acid and alkali. The technique dates back to Einof in 1806 and has been in continuous use since then. Today it remains the measurement of fiber referred to in most food tables (with the notable exception of McCance and Widdowson's

"Composition of Foods").[23] This results in a gross underestimate of the fiber content of the food[27,28] and a corresponding overestimate of the available carbohydrate, since this is usually calculated as the difference by weight from the total of the sum of fat, protein, fiber, ash, and moisture. The crude fiber estimate may be as low as 10 to 20% of the dietary fiber estimate.

### Detergent Methods

To overcome these problems Van Soest developed two gravimetric techniques. One was an acid detergent method, which solubilized all constituents except cellulose and lignin, the weight of which gave a value comparable to crude fiber. The other was a neutral detergent extraction, which left a proportion of the hemicellulosic materials (Table 2B–2).[35] This technique more closely approximates to dietary fiber, but in its original form losses of the more soluble fibers, gums, mucilages, and pectic substances in the filtrate was large and the final value was likely to be an underestimate, especially if the fiber source was rich in soluble fiber. However, this approach is undergoing continuous development.

### Enzyme Techniques

Enzyme techniques provide the most complete assessment of fiber content. Perhaps the first technique to measure total dietary fiber was that of McCance and his co-workers who measured starch and protein in the food residue following alcohol extraction to remove fat; fiber or "unavailable carbohydrate" was then determined by difference.[30] This method has been refined by Southgate and now represents one of the most comprehensive methods of fiber analysis. The food is first extracted in alcohol and ether, and

**Table 2B–2.  Summary of Analytical Methods for Dietary Fiber and Fiber**

| Analytic Measurement | Outline of Method and Fraction Actually Measured | Nature of Fraction Measured |
|---|---|---|
| Dietary fiber (= Unavailable carbohydrates) | | |
| Total (McCance, Widdowson, and Shackleton, 1936)[30] | Preparation of residue insoluble in alcohol. Measurement of starch and protein and deduction of these from the residue | All components of dietary fiber in one fraction |
| As the components (Southgate, 1969)[31] | Sequential extraction and hydrolysis of residue insoluble in alcohol | Noncellulosic polysaccharides as component hexoses, pentoses, and uronic acids |
| | | Celluose as glucose |
| | | Lignin as the residue insoluble in 72% (W/W) $H_2SO_4$ |
| Total (Prosky, Asp, Furda, et al. 1984)[32] | Enzymatic digestion of defatted residue to remove protein and starch | All components of dietary fiber in one fraction (minus some soluble fiber) |
| Fiber | | |
| Crude (AOAC, 1970)[33] | Extraction of food with boiling acid and alkali. Measurement of organic matter in residue | Celluose plus lignin (incompletely in many foods) |
| Acid detergent (ADF) (Van Soest, 1963)[34] | Extraction of food with boiling acid detergent solution. Measurement of organic matter in residue | Cellulose plus lignin |
| Neutral detergent (NDF) (Van Soest, 1963)[34] | Extraction of food with boiling neutral detergent and weighing residue | Cell-wall materials less water-soluble components |

Adapted from Southgate, D.A.T., et al.[28]

the starch is removed by enzymatic hydrolysis. The residue is then subjected to a series of hydrolyses and extraction procedures specific for specific components (e.g., cellulose), and the sugars liberated are estimated.[31] This technique is, however, time consuming. Most recently, Prosky, Asp, Furda, et al.[32] have developed a technique to gelatinize starch in fat-extracted material by heating in a boiling water bath with termamyl (heat-stable α-amylase) and then enzymically digest it with protease and amyloglucosidase to remove protein and starch. Ethanol (95%) is added to precipitate the soluble dietary fiber, the total residue is filtered and washed with ethanol (71% and 95%) and acetone, and the residual protein content is measured on the dried material. The protein value is subtracted from the dried weight to give the dietary fiber (Table 2B–2). This technique has the advantage of being relatively quick, but some losses of the soluble fiber components (gums, mucilages, and pectic substances) are still experienced. In addition, analysis of the residual protein in the fiber precipitate is essential, especially in legumes where it may be considerable. Nevertheless, this is likely to be developed as a standard technique for routine analysis, comprising as it does elements of all the other techniques discussed.

## PHYSICAL AND PHYSICOCHEMICAL PROPERTIES AND PHYSIOLOGIC ACTIONS

The physical and physicochemical attributes of fiber that have attracted most interest are its water-holding capacity, viscosity, and cationic exchange properties. The relationship between these and other properties and the physiologic effects of fiber have been well summarized by Eastwood and Kay,[36] with emphasis on the changing form and role of fiber as it passes along the gastrointestinal tract. Table 2B–3[36,37] shows some of the physicochemical properties of fiber and the gastrointestinal events it may modify.

### Viscosity

Certain fibers, such as the gums and pectins, increase the viscosity of the intraluminal contents within the gastrointestinal tract so delaying gastric emptying,[38–41] increasing the mouth-to-cecum transit time,[32] and reducing the rate of small intestinal absorption,[38,42,43] in part probably through increasing the thickness of the unstirred water layer.[43] On the other hand, this is not the response to a particulate fiber such as wheat bran, which both in bread[44] or as a bran-glucose mixture[42] leaves the stomach and passes through the small intestine more rapidly than its low fiber or fiber-

**Table 2B–3.  Physicochemical, Physiologic and Clinical Aspects of Fiber**

| *Physicochemical Property* | *Type of Fiber* | *Physiologic Effect* | *Clinical Implication* |
|---|---|---|---|
| Viscosity | Gums, mucilages, pectins | ↓ Gastric emptying, ↑ mouth to cecum transit, ↓ rate of small intestinal absorption (e.g., of glucose, bile acids) | Dumping syndrome<br><br>Diabetes Hypercholesterolemia |
| Particle formation and water-holding capacity | e.g., Wheat bran, pentosan content, polysaccharide-lignin mixtures | ↑ Gastric emptying, ↓ mouth to cecum transit, ↓ total GI transit time, ↓ Colonic intraluminal pressure, ↑ fecal bulk | Peptic ulcer Constipation<br><br>Diverticular disease Dilute potential carcinogens |
| Adsorption and non-specific effects | Lignin, pectin mixed fibers | ↑ Fecal steroids output ↑ fecal fat and N losses (small) | Hypercholesterolemia Cholelithiasis |
| Cation exchange | Acidic polysaccharides (e.g., pectins) | ↑ Small intestinal losses of minerals (±), trace elements (±), heavy metals | Negative mineral balance, probably compensated for by colonic salvage, antitoxic effect |
| Antioxidant | Lignin (reducing phenolic groups) | ↓ Free radicals in digestive tract | Anticarcinogenesis? |
| Degradability (colonic bacteria) | Polysaccharides (free of lignin) | ↑ Gas and SCFAs production, ↓ cecal pH | Flatus, energy production |

Modified from Eastwood, M.A., Kay, R.M.,[36] and Kay, R.M., Strasberg, S.M.[37]

free equivalent. In the colon this property may have little relevance to many of the viscous fibers because of their complete degradation by colonic bacteria. Many particulate fibers, on the other hand, continue to reduce the transit time and increase fecal bulk, since they are relatively resistant to degradation.

## Water-Holding Capacity

The relevance of water-holding capacity in terms of small intestinal absorptive function is not clear. In the colon, however, water-holding capacity may be of importance in reducing colonic transit time and hence the overall transit time, since the colon contributes the major component. By the law of Laplace by increasing the intraluminal contents, and hence expanding the luminal diameter, the intraluminal pressure will tend to be reduced. In addition, fecal weight is increased. In this situation particulate fiber with low digestibility such as coarse wheat bran is very effective.[2,3] It has been suggested that the increase in fecal bulking effect is directly related to the pentosan content of the fiber[45] (Fig. 2B–1), which is very high in the case of wheat bran. It also appears to be related to the lignin content.[46] Although lignin in purified form is considered to be a constipating agent, through combination with pentosans it may limit their degradation by bacteria in the colon. In this way the fecal bulking effect is preserved. This illustrates an important point that the physiologic effects of combinations of fibers may

be very different from their individual effects given in purified form.

## Digestibility

The digestibility of fiber is a major factor determining fecal bulk. Perhaps because of their open or branched structure many of the noncellulosic polysaccharides readily undergo bacterial degradation contributing volatile fatty acids for uptake and utilization by colonic mucosa.[46] Some fibers such as the pectins are almost completely metabolized[47] and have no laxative effect, but other fiber sources such as cabbage encourage bacterial growth and contribute materially to the increase in fecal output.[48] Despite the different effects in both instances, the degradable material is noncellulosic polysaccharide. It may therefore be associated materials, for example, in cabbage fiber, that determine whether or not noncellulosic polysaccharides result in an increased fecal bulk.

## Cation Exchange Potential

Cationic exchange properties are possessed by acidic polysaccharides with free-COOH groups such as pectins and lignins. It has been suggested that most plant fibers appear to act as monofunctional ion-exchange resins, although fibers from cereals (oats, wheat, and maize) and certain tubers (e.g., potatoes) may be weakly polyfunctional.[37] The mechanism of binding is not clearly understood. However, extensive in vitro studies have been carried out by Reinhold and associates using

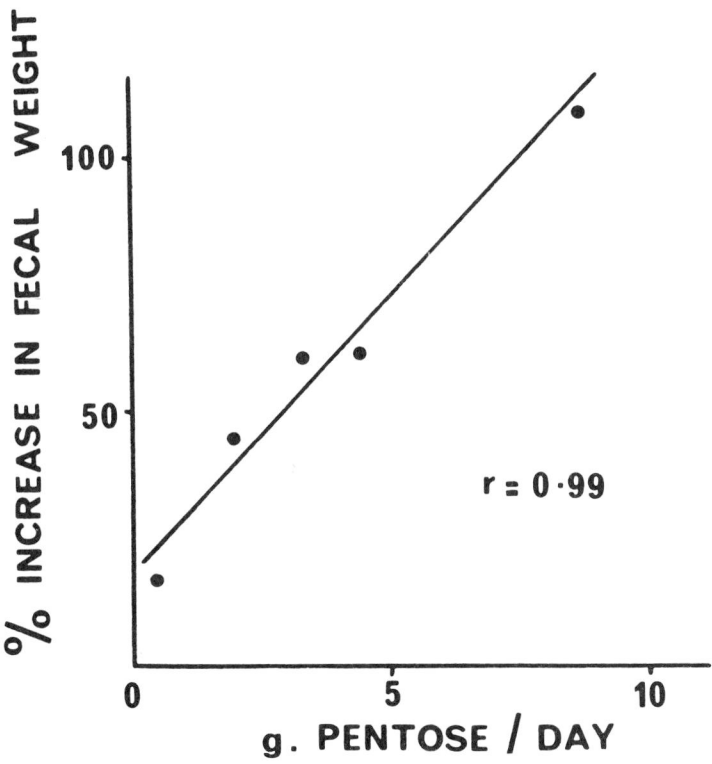

**Fig. 2B–1.** Mean percentage increase in fecal weight for each fiber (bran, cabbage, carrot, apple, and guar, in ascending order) plotted against daily intake of pentose sugars from noncellulosic polysaccharide fraction of each fiber preparation. (From Cummings, J.H., et al.,[45] with permission of Lancet.)

neutral detergent fiber prepared from maize and wheat.[49] It was found that binding for iron was pH dependent with a maximum binding capacity for maize fiber at pH 7.0 and no binding at pH 1.0.[49] This binding can be competitively inhibited by the presence of phytate, ascorbate, citrate, cysteine, and EDTA, which also bind iron. Since EDTA and ascorbate have been used as adjuvants to enhance iron absorption, it may be that they aid absorption because of their release of iron and other metals during metabolism in the gut. On the other hand, fiber that is not fermented may retain iron throughout the digestive tract.[49] This same principle may also apply to the binding of other metal ions by fiber. Binding has been shown to occur with a number of types of fiber, especially in respect of calcium, magnesium, iron, and zinc. The exact physiologic relevance, however, is not certain. James has suggested that calcium binding is in proportion to the uronic acid content of the fiber but that fermentation of these polysaccharides by colonic microflora will liberate calcium for colonic absorption, thus providing a mechanism for long-term adaptation on high fiber diets.[50] The possible deleterious effects of fiber on metal and trace element balance are discussed

later in the section on trace elements and minerals.

Fiber also has the property of adsorbing materials of biologic importance such as proteins, bile salts, certain toxic substances, and bacterial cells. Again the exact mechanisms have not been defined. Early on, lignin was shown to bind bile salts in vitro,[51] and extensive studies were carried out by Kritchevsky indicating that bile salt binding was a feature of a wide range of plant fibers[52–55] (Table 2B–4). No single physicochemical attribute appears responsible for this feature, and the binding of bile acids may be through different mechanisms for different fibers. The process appears to be enhanced in the presence of saponins.[56] The binding by lignin has been shown to be pH dependent, which would render it more effective in more acidic conditions[57] as, for example, in the cecum. On the other hand, viscous fibers such as guar[58] and pectin[59] may increase bile salt losses possibly by reducing the effectiveness of ileal absorption through increasing the thickness of the unstirred water layer. This mechanism would be analogous to their effect in limiting nutrient absorption higher in the small intestine.[37]

**Table 2B–4.  Binding in Vitro of Bile Acids and Salts to Fiber**

| Bile Acid or Salt | Fiber | | | |
|---|---|---|---|---|
| | Alfalfa* | Bran | Cellulose | Lignin |
| Cholic | 1.00 | 0.51 | 0.15 | 2.20 |
| Chenodeoxycholic | 1.25 | 0.91 | 0.10 | 1.17 |
| Deoxycholic | 0.52 | 0.27 | 0.01 | 0.87 |
| Taurocholic | 1.00 | 0.20 | 0.15 | 3.20 |
| Taurochenodeoxycholic | 2.18 | 1.42 | 0 | 3.68 |
| Taurodeoxycholic | 1.65 | 0.49 | 0.10 | 4.48 |
| Glycocholic | 1.00 | 0.33 | 0.10 | 1.96 |
| Glycochenodeoxycholic | 1.30 | 1.86 | 0.02 | 2.19 |
| Glycodeoxycholic | 2.42 | 0.68 | 0.41 | 4.57 |

From Story, J.A., Kritchevsky, D.[54] With permission of Journal of Nutrition.
*For each group alfalfa-cholic acid or salt is set as 1.00. Actual percentage binding to alfalfa-cholic, 19.9; taurocholic, 6.9; glycocholic, 11.5.

## Interaction with Proteins and Carbohydrates

Fiber, as cellulose or xylan, has also been shown to reduce the activity in vitro of human pancreatic trypsin in protein digestion.[61] The mechanism of this effect is not clear, but it may be responsible in part for the slightly increased fecal losses of nitrogen on high fiber diets. In addition, amylase and lipase activity was depressed,[6] with possible implications in carbohydrate and fat digestion.

Studies by Monoz and colleagues have indicated the importance of addition of protein to the diet in modifying the effects of fiber on minerals and trace elements such that the lower the protein the more positive the mineral balance.[62] These studies have further emphasized the importance of fiber-nutrient interactions. The diversity of sources of fiber manifesting the effect allowed no identification of specific mechanism. However, it may have been in part another adsorption effect of fiber. Equally difficult to explain is the abolition of the improved glucose tolerance seen on a high fiber diet when the level of dietary protein was doubled (120 to 140 g/day).[62]

Finally, bacteria may also be adsorbed onto fiber, possibly through interaction with the carbohydrate in the bacterial cell wall. In this way, theoretically, the colonic flora may be reduced or altered and possibly depleted of specific bacteria, an issue that has been raised with the use of microcrystalline cellulose.

## Free-Radical Scavenger

It has been suggested that the lignin component of fiber may act as a free-radical scavenger related to its reducing phenolic groups.[37] In this way fiber may be protective in reducing the risk of cancer development.[37] However, the association of lignin with other fibers may well modify this effect. Nevertheless, it is recognized in the food industry that the oil in high fiber wheat products is less prone to rancidity, and this feature supports an overall antioxidant property.

## Antitoxic Effects

In general, fiber preparations have been increasingly ascribed antitoxic properties, especially in the Japanese literature.[63–66] Again, no single property or chemical type of fiber has been identified as responsible. Fibers have been shown to prevent the toxic effects of detergents on the enterocyte,[63] to prevent adsorption of toxic metals such as cadmium by lignin, cellulose, and carbomethyl cellulose,[64] and to reduce toxicity of iron-chlorophyllin by cellulose, alfalfa, and yeast β-glucan (but not by other viscous or hemicellulosic fibers).[65] However, only delignified fiber from wheat, corn, and barley reduced the toxic effect of amaranth on rat growth.[66] This effect was not related to physical binding ability of the fibers but to their "settling" volume in water, suggesting that the bulking effect of the fiber and the physical factors involved may have been important.[66]

## Effect of Fiber on Structure of Small Intestine and Colon

Recent studies suggest that the nature of the fiber may alter the structure and turnover of cells lining the gastrointestinal tract. The blunted villous structure independent of tropical sprue seen in inhabitants of countries where diets are high in fiber[67] suggests an association with fiber intake. Studies with rats have indicated that pectin results in blunted villous appearance in the small intestine,[68] whereas cellulose and wheat bran have no effect in the small intestine.[68] However, wheat bran increased mucosal cell turnover in the colon.[69]

Such data suggest that viscous fibers that reduce the rate of small intestinal absorption may influence small intestinal structure and function. In this respect lower brushborder sucrase and lactase levels have also been reported after inclusion of viscous fiber in the diet.[70] On the other hand, the particulate fiber preparations with fecal bulking activity may alter colonic mucosal structure, function, and cell turnover.[69]

## Classification of Fiber on Structure-Function Basis

Studies of the physicochemical properties of fibers that determine the physiologic effects have yielded much useful data but much more is required to allow classification of fiber on a structure-function basis. One of the problems highlighted here is the difference between purified fiber sources and mixtures of dietary fibers in foods. Removal of the fiber component from a food deprives the fiber of its original intimate relationships with carbohydrates, proteins, and lipids and most certainly alters many of its properties. In addition, a number of fiber-associated substances, the so-called antinutrients, have marked physiologic effects. Their removal from the fiber will greatly alter its activity. Finally, progress in this area has been slow because of the difficulty of analysis both of total dietary fiber in foods and the components of fiber.

## Fiber-Associated Substances: Antinutrients

Many antinutrients are physically associated with dietary fiber or are found in high concentrations in high fiber foods, especially plant storage organs, seeds, and grains. They include lectins, saponins, phytates, tannins, and enzyme inhibitors. In the plant these substances may protect against attack by predators, parasites, and molds and inhibit autodigestion by the plant's own digestive enzymes. As with dietary fiber the level of these substances within a plant will vary with growing conditions (usually higher levels in unfavorable conditions) and the stage in the life cycle of the plant (e.g., lower concentrations in the seed after germination when digestion of the storage organ is actually required).

In general, lectins, phytates, and enzyme inhibitors are found in association with the plant protein fraction, and tannins are associated with carbohydrate and saponins with oils. Nevertheless, large amounts may also be present in the fiber fraction when separated physically (by milling and air classification). Lectins are glycoproteins,[71] which may bind stereospecifically to sugars on the surfaces of cells and induce lysis of the cell. This is important in the context of their ability to induce possible small intestinal damage or reduced intestinal absorption of nutrients.[72] They are heat labile. Saponins are triterpenoid mole-

cules with sugar residues.[73] These have the ability to alter surface characteristics of cell membranes and to stabilize lipid emulsions or foams[73] (hence the saponification property from which they derive their name). Their physiologic importance is that they may enhance the binding of bile acids to fiber,[56] reduce cholesterol absorption,[74] and so reduce serum cholesterol levels. They also enhance the immune response by acting as adjuvants.[75] Saponins are not normally absorbed from the gastrointestinal tract, but if they are, they may cause intravascular hemolysis and liver necrosis.

Phytate or myoinositol 1,2,3,4,5,6 hexakis dihydrogen phosphate has a marked ability to bind metal ions and proteins[76,77] and thus by direct interaction with digestive enzymes or the food components can limit the rate of digestion and enhance the loss of metal ions and trace elements in the stool. Tannins are polyphenolic compounds, which may also reduce the digestibility of the food by direct binding or binding to proteins[78] (hence "tanning"). Enzyme inhibitors are ubiquitous in the plant kingdom, but beans and cereal grains are particularly rich sources.[79] Inhibitors of lipase, amylase, trypsin, and proteases have been identified. The majority of enzyme inhibitors are heat labile,[80] but their degree of stability varies such that low levels may survive standard cooking procedures.[81]

It can be seen that the spectrum of effects ascribed to antinutrients in limiting the rate of absorption and enhancing elimination of bile acids and metal ions overlaps with the purported actions of dietary fiber. In view of this and the fact that in their active forms these substances are largely unabsorbed, it is difficult to interpret data on physiologic effects of fiber in whole foods. They should therefore probably be considered as part of the fiber complex of substances or at least as fiber-associated substances.

## METABOLISM OF FIBER

In man, by definition, the fiber that is digested within the body is degraded by colonic bacteria. There does, however, appear to be some limited breakdown of pectin within the human small intestine.[82] The degree to which different fibers are broken down in the colon varies from fiber to fiber. In general, the more lignified the fiber, the less it is metabolized by colonic bacteria, and the more water soluble its noncellulosic components, the greater is its breakdown.[46] Thus the noncellulosic polysaccharides, especially pectin and the gums, are largely broken down in the colon[25,47,83–88] (Table 2B–5). However, as already discussed, the combination of fibers with each other greatly influences the properties of the constituent fibers.

Thus, the presence of lignin in, for example, wheat bran may render it virtually inert in terms of potential for bacterial degradation. Similarly the source and physical state of the fiber may be crucial. Finely divided bran is degraded to a greater extent than coarse bran.[89] Cellulose is degraded about 5% in man (Table 2B–6). Highly crystalline cellulose from wood, however, is far less readily digested than that from root vegetables and fruit.[46] In addition, the length of time fiber remains in the colon determines its breakdown. Elderly people with slower transit times may degrade fiber more than their younger counterparts with an intrinsically more rapid transit time. It is difficult to determine whether this effect is due to altered motility of colonic musculature with age or to differences in bacterial populations.

In the colon the plant polysaccharides are metabolized by bacterial enzymes to short chain fatty acids (SCFA), including acetate, propionate, and butyrate in the percentage molar ratios of 60:24:16.[92] In addition, carbon dioxide, hydrogen, methane, and water are produced. Unless large amounts of carbohydrate are malabsorbed, lactate production is minimal.[92] The equation for fermentation in the human colon has been derived by Miller and Wolin,[93] based on the molar ratios of short chain fatty acids in feces and known production rates of carbon dioxide and methane:

$$34.4\ C_6H_{12}O_6 \rightarrow 64\ SCFA + 23.75\ CH_4$$
$$+ 34.23\ CO_2 + 10.5\ H_2O$$

It has been estimated that if 20 g of unavailable plant polysaccharide (fiber) is taken in daily then approximately 200 mmol SCFA will be produced.[92] If 70% of these are absorbed,[94] this amount would yield an additional 73 Cal/day. If on the other hand the SCFA produced is calculated as the amount required to support the observed colonic bacterial population, then three times the amount of SCFA are produced daily[92] (see Chapter 56 section D–1). With greater fiber intakes production of SCFA will increase. Since only small amounts are recovered in the feces, it is likely that metabolism of unavailable carbohydrate could contribute significantly to the energy intake of the individual when fiber intakes are high. Colonic bacteria may thus fulfill a function similar to those of the rumen of ruminant herbivores and in the cecum of monogastric herbivores. SCFAs are taken up by the enterocyte where butyrate may selectively be used for enterocyte metabolic processes,[95] leaving acetate and propionate to contribute to whole body metabolism after uptake by the liver. Studies of cecal infusion of labeled glucose in man confirm the considerable ability of the colon to salvage carbohydrate.[96] In addition, the SCFAs contribute to colonic bacterial metabolism and in the presence

**Table 2B–5. Noncellulose Polysaccharide Digestion in Man**

| Subjects (N) | Sources | Intake | % Digested | (range) | Reference |
|---|---|---|---|---|---|
| Young men (3) | Wheat bran | 14.3 | 35 | (32–39) | Williams and Olmsted (1936)[83] |
| | Carrot | 7.8 | 84 | (80–89) | |
| | Peas | 2.4 | 84 | (80–87) | |
| | Cabbage | 6.9 | 80 | (79–80) | |
| | Agar | 13.4 | 60 | (55–65) | |
| Young men (12) | Mixed diet | 13.5 | 72 | (69–78) | Southgate and Durnin (1970)[84] |
| Young women (14) | Mixed diet | 11.0 | 77 | (73–84) | |
| Elderly men (11) | Mixed diet | 20.4 | 84 | (80–87) | |
| Elderly women (12) | Mixed diet | 15.0 | 85 | (82–89) | |
| Adults (5) | Mixed diet | 9.2 | 76 | (60–90) | Southgate et al. (1976)[85] |
| | Mixed diet and bran biscuit | 19.5 | 72 | (66–78) | |
| Young men (8) | Wheat bran | | | | Heller (1977)[86] |
| | Coarse | 9.0 | 50 | | |
| | Fine | 9.0 | 54 | | |
| Young men | Cabbage | — | 53 | | Van Soest et al. (1978)[87] |
| Adults (14) | Mixed diet | 18.5 | 99 | | Farrell et al. (1978)[88] |
| | Mixed diet and bran | 21.4 | 42 | | |
| Adults (4) | Mixed diet | 8.8 | 81 | | Cummings et al. (1979)[47] |
| | Mixed diet and pectin | 39.6 | 93 | | |
| Adults (4) | Mixed diet | 14.7 | 73 | | |
| | Mixed diet and ispaghula | 37.4 | 87 | | |

From Cummings, J.H.,[46] with permission of Plenum Press.

**Table 2B–6. Cellulose Digestion in Man**

| Subjects (N) | Sources | Intake (g/day) | % Digested (range) | | Reference |
|---|---|---|---|---|---|
| Young men (3) | Wheat bran | 6.9 | 29 | (24–33) | Williams and Olmsted (1936)[83] |
| | Carrot | 8.7 | 67 | (62–72) | |
| | Peas | 9.6 | 45 | (40–49) | |
| | Cabbage | 9.1 | 55 | (43–61) | |
| | Celluflour | 10.1 | 7 | (0–11) | |
| Young men (16) | All bran | 10–19 | 0–6 | | Hoppert and Clark (1945)[90] |
| | Lettuce | 5.6 | 29 | | |
| | Cabbage | 4.1 | 42 | | |
| | Celery | 8.0 | 29 | | |
| | Oranges | 7.5 | 24 | | |
| | Apples | 10.4 | 57 | | |
| Young men (12) | Mixed diet | 8.0 | 15 | (−7–29) | Southgate and Durnin (1970)[84] |
| Young women (14) | Mixed diet | 5.2 | 26 | (6–40) | |
| Elderly men (11) | Mixed diet | 7.9 | 44 | (21–59) | |
| Elderly women (12) | Mixed diet | 5.9 | 26 | (−9–51) | |
| Adults (16) | Mixed diet | 8.5 | 43 | (15–87) | Milton-Thompson and Lewis (1971)[26] |
| Adults (5) | Mixed diet | 4.9 | 82 | (69–91) | Southgate et al. (1976)[85] |
| | Mixed diet and bran biscuit | 7.7 | 64 | (42–73) | |
| Young men (8) | Wheat bran | | | | Heller et al. (1977)[86] |
| | Coarse | 2.7 | 6 | | |
| | Fine | 2.7 | 23 | | |
| Young men | Solka floc | — | 20 | | Van Soest et al. (1978)[87] |
| | Cabbage | — | 81 | | |
| Adults (14) | Mixed diet | 10.5 | 74 | | Farrell et al. (1978)[88] |
| | Mixed diet and bran | 18.7 | 63 | | |
| Adults (4) | Mixed diet | 6.1 | 82 | | Cummings et al. (1979*)[47] |
| Adults (4) | Mixed diet | 4.9 | 73 | (62–81) | Prynne and Southgate (1979*)[91] |

*These studies were all performed as "blanks" in which cellulose intake and fecal excretion were measured in subjects on controlled or known diets.
From Cummings, J.H.,[46] with permission of Plenum Press.

of nitrogen sources will encourage bacterial cell multiplication.[97] At the same time alteration in bacterial pH may exert an inhibitory effect on bacterial types, numbers, and metabolism. Perman and colleagues found that acidification of colonic contents through fermentation of unavailable carbohydrate (lactulose) greatly reduced hydrogen production when the lactulose was taken daily for one week.[98]

A wide range of substances may be produced in the fermentation of fiber. In the anaerobic environment of the colon it is likely that significant amounts of alcohols will be produced. Of interest in this respect is the increased urinary excretion of formic acid in individuals consuming high methoxyl pectin.[99] Presumably methanol produced in the colon was metabolized to formaldehyde and formic acid, either in the colonic lumen or in the liver after absorption, and excreted. The effects are unlikely to have any relationship to those seen after consumption of methanol, since the rate of synthesis and hence absorption would be very slow. However, what other effects, if any, the chronic absorption of these and other fiber derived substances have in the long term,

either beneficial or detrimental, remain to be assessed.

## CLINICAL IMPLICATIONS

The fiber hypothesis suggested that dietary fiber might have a part to play in the prevention or treatment of a long list of diseases.[1] Those that are currently of greatest interest include constipation,[1,2] diverticular disease,[4,5] diabetes,[6–12] hyperlipidemia,[13–16] and, to some extent, obesity,[17] as well as Crohn's disease[18] and peptic ulcer.[20] Some of these areas are reviewed here and in Chapters 56 and 57.

### Carbohydrate Metabolism: Diabetes

The fiber hypothesis and its implications have contributed to significant changes in the approach to dietary therapy for persons with diabetes. The major English speaking diabetes associations are now in agreement that there may be definite benefits from increasing the consumption of high fiber carbohydrate foods.[100–102]

Studies in normal and diabetic volunteers with purified fiber indicated that the glucose and endocrine (insulin and GIP) responses to test meals could be reduced by addition of fibers and fiber analogues, especially viscous fibers such as guar, pectin, and tragacanth[9,42,103,104] (Fig. 2B–2). Longer term studies involving both metabolic and outpatient trials of fiber in diabetes confirmed the effects in reducing blood glucose levels, urinary glucose,[8,10,11,105–107] and ketone body losses.[108] Studies with the artificial pancreas indicated reduced insulin requirements.[109] The effect of wheat bran, although present, appeared to be smaller[110] and the acute effects on glycemic response more variable.[42] For the viscous fibers the mechanism appeared to relate to their ability to reduce the rate of gastric emptying[30–41] and to slow absorption in the small intestine.[42,43] More recently, the studies of Reed and his group have done much to define the actions of fiber within the gut.[110a,110b]

Intubation studies in man indicated slower absorption rates for glucose in the presence of guar and a lack of relationship between the glycemic peak and the gastric emptying rate for glucose loads taken with or without guar. Such evidence indicated that the slowing of small intestinal absorption rather than the gastric emptying may be of major importance. In addition, further in vitro studies and in vivo studies in man suggested that, for guar, the mechanism of action within the gut was due to reduced rates of diffusion in the bulk phase[110a,110b] rather than alteration in thickness of the unstirred water layer postulated for pectin.[110c] As judged by studies of breath $H_2$[111] and xylose,[42] increased malabsorption of available carbohydrate did appear to explain the phenomenon of

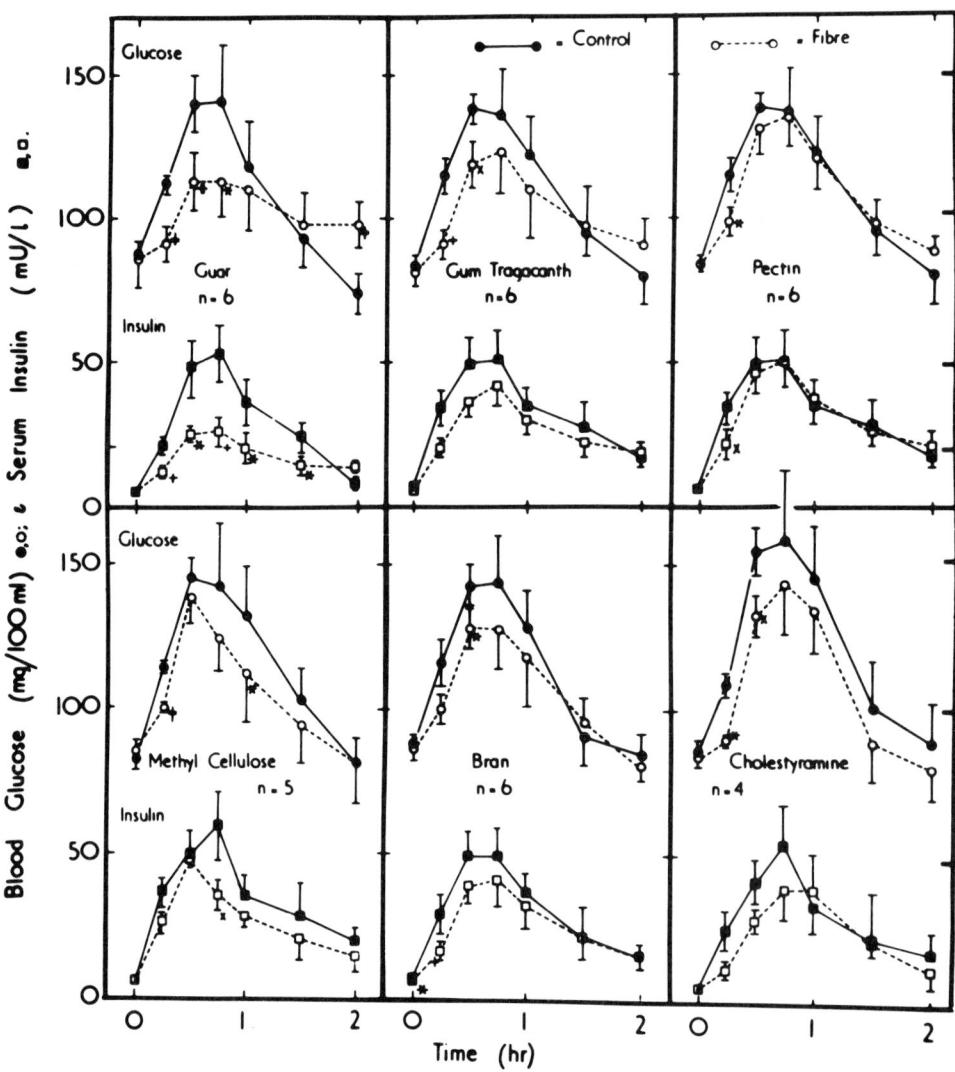

**Fig. 2B–2.** The mean blood glucose and serum insulin concentrations of volunteers after taking control and fiber-containing test meals. Conversion: S1 to traditional units—Glucose:1 mmol/1 ≈18 mg/100 ml. (From Jenkins, D.J.A., et al.,[42] with permission of British Medical Journal.)

flatter blood glucose responses to high fiber meals. It has been suggested that fiber may act by slowing the absorption of carbohydrate and so create what has been termed "lente" carbohydrate.[112] Failure to observe these effects has often resulted from inadequate mixing of the carbohydrate and fiber or the use of nonviscous forms of fiber.

Studies with fiber in unprocessed foods were pioneered by Anderson in therapeutic dietary trials, and other workers copied this model. These usually entailed increasing the available carbohydrate intake in addition to the fiber.[6,7,12,113,114] The studies indicated that, by raising both dietary fiber and carbohydrate levels in the diabetic diet, control of diabetes could be improved[6,7,12,113,114] and lower serum cholesterol levels could be achieved.[6,7,12,19] Criticism has been leveled at such work on the grounds that many studies were carried out on non-insulin-dependent diabetics whose control was improved simply by better adherence to a diabetic diet. In others it has been pointed out that weight loss, albeit small, had also been a feature. An alternative explanation, however, is that many of the diets contained low glycemic index foods (such as beans),[6,7,12,19] and the low glycemic response to these foods may have been a major reason for their success. (See Chapter 56, Section C6.) Nevertheless, it was on the basis of such studies that diabetic individuals have been advised to consume diets rich in carbohydrate fiber. In this area the impact of the fiber hypothesis has therefore been significant.

### Dumping Syndrome

As mentioned already, certain types of fiber (the gums, mucilages, and pectic substances) slow gastric emptying.[38–41] In patients with the late dumping syndrome, pectin has been found to reduce the high rises in blood glucose and insulin and so prevent the subsequent undershoot in blood glucose.[39–41] In addition, the hemoconcentration associated with the early dumping syndrome is minimized.[40] This effect was seen in pectin-supplemented test meals together with a more normalized gut endocrine response[41] (Fig. 2B–3) and diminished carbohydrate losses.[39] In the longer term, administration before meals of 5 g pectin 2 to 3 times daily has been shown to reduce the symptoms associated with dumping.[39] An explanation for this effect came from studies of healthy volunteers who ate 20 g apple pectin a day for 4 weeks.[115] These indicated, at the end of 4 weeks' supplementation, when no pectin remained in the gastrointestinal tract, that chronic administration of pectin had resulted in a chronically slower rate of gastric emptying. It may be that pectin and other similar fiber forms have a long-term therapeutic

role in the dumping syndrome through altering gastrointestinal motility patterns. Further work is required before specific advice can be given on the use of fiber in this condition. However, if appropriate, it will be the viscous forms that prove therapeutically useful.

### Duodenal Ulcer

Traditionally in the treatment of duodenal ulcer small bland low fiber meals have been advocated. This regimen has been challenged by Malhotra in India, who successfully used diets high in wheat and rice fiber to treat duodenal ulcer.[20] More recently, Norwegian workers using diets rich in fiber from unleavened wholemeal bread, oatmeal porridge, and a gruel of barley, oats, rye, and wheat recorded endoscopic freedom from relapse in 19 (55%) of 38 subjects in the high fiber group as opposed to only 7 (20%) in control groups.[116] Although high fiber diets have not been successful in ulcer treatment, this approach may be another area where, in addition to eliminating smoking and alcohol consumption and reducing coffee intake, a high fiber diet will be advocated for prophylaxis and to prevent relapse. The fiber recommended in this case is likely to be particulate fiber, such as bran, which encourages more rapid gastric emptying.[44]

### Lipid Metabolism: Hyperlipidemia

In terms of official recommendations or therapeutic measures in the management of hyperlipidemia, the fiber hypothesis has as yet made less impact than in diabetes, although it has stimulated much research and thought in this area. Nevertheless, an increase in fiber consumption has been recommended as part of a unitary dietary approach to the treatment of hyperlipidemia.[117]

In the 1960s, guar, pectin, and a wide range of unabsorbable viscous plant polysaccharides had all been shown to have hypocholesterolemic properties[54,118] with little fecal bulking action.[50,106] In this respect they differed from particulate fiber, which affected only transit time and fecal bulk[119,120] (Fig. 2B–4). Lignin was shown to increase fecal bile acid losses,[51] as was pectin.[59] The important studies of Kritchevsky and colleagues demonstrated that a range of indigestible plant materials was capable of binding bile salts in vitro.[13,51–55] This finding did much to provide a rationale for further work in allowing an analogy to be drawn between some of the actions of dietary fiber and those of synthetic hypocholesterolemic agents, the bile salt binding anion exchange resins, e.g., cholestyramine, used in clinical practice. The theory developed that fiber may reduce serum cholesterol at least in part by inducing increased

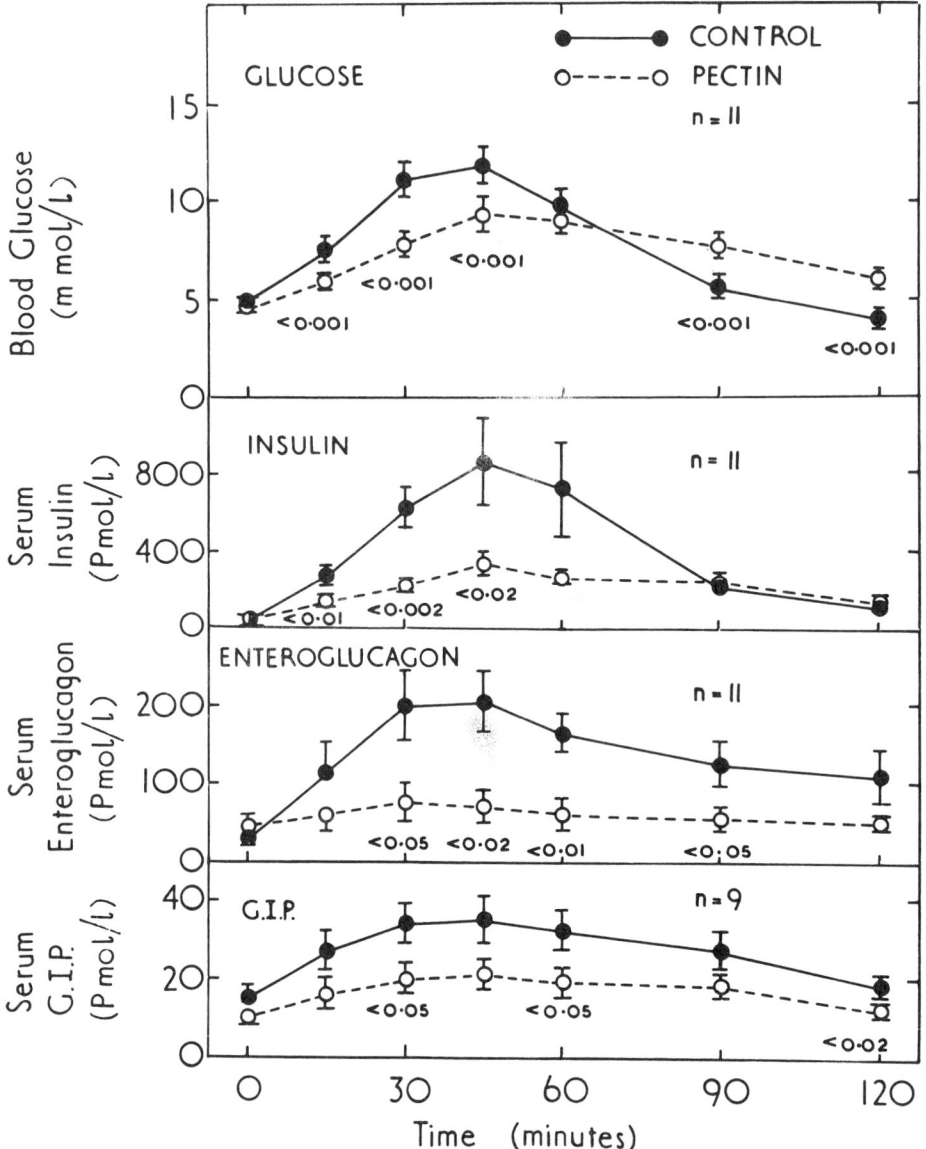

**Fig. 2B–3.** Mean levels over 2 hours of blood glucose, serum insulin, enteroglucagon, and gastric inhibitory polypeptide (GIP) in 11 postgastric surgery patients who took 50 g GTT on two occasions, to one of which was added 14.5 g pectin. (From Jenkins, D.J.A., et al.,[41] with permission of Gut.)

losses of bile acids or by altering the ratio of different bile acids in the bile salt pool. In addition, the more distal absorption of fat in high fiber diets may have a favorable influence on blood lipid and lipoprotein levels.[120a,120b] The successful use of cholestyramine in a major lipid research clinics (LRC) trial has emphasized the possible importance of this approach in the prevention of cardiovascular disease[121] and is likely to stimulate further interest in dietary fiber in this respect. However, extensive studies in patient groups have not yet been possible with fiber because fiber preparations acceptable for long-term use are not generally available.

## Purified Fiber and Hypolipidemic Effects

Guar,[15,122] pectin,[14] lignin,[16] oat bran,[123] and locust bean gum[124] have now all been used in trials involving type II and IV hyperlipidemic patients. The viscous materials, guar (10 to 25 g/day)[15,108] and pectin (40 g/day),[14] have been found to lower the serum cholesterol levels by 10 to 16%, the effect being more marked with guar. In studies involving diabetics, guar has also been shown to be hypocholesterolemic.[11] Reports on the effect of lignin have been conflicting.[125] Where measured, the falls on fiber have been in the LDL cholesterol[14,15] with no reduction in HDL cho-

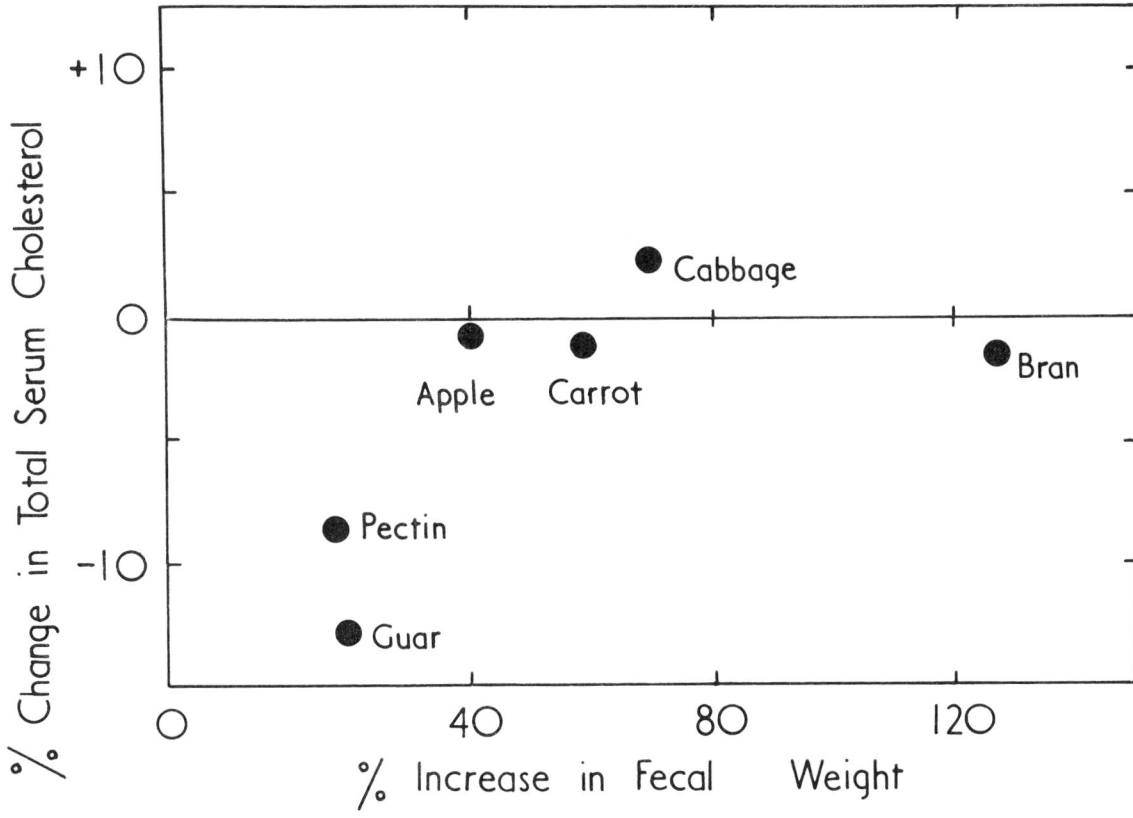

**Fig. 2B–4.** Relationship of percentage change in mean total serum cholesterol to percentage mean increase in fecal weight for six different fiber supplements. (From Jenkins, D.J.A., et al.,[120] with permission of Am. J. Clin. Nutr., American Society for Clinical Nutrition.)

lesterol[15] (Fig. 2B–5). Mean serum triglyceride levels have tended to fall in most studies; however, the falls have not usually reached significance. The modes of administration of these supplements have included the powders,[14,15,54,131] canned soups,[15] breads, and biscuits.[124] More recently, a guar crisp-bread and granulates that can be mixed with fruit drinks have become available. Mixing with the food did not seem to be as important for the hypocholesterolemic effect as it was to induce a flattening of postprandial glycemia in diabetes, and thus a granulate may be particularly suitable for long-term treatment.

### High Fiber Foods and Hypolipidemic Effects

The presence of other potentially hypocholesterolemic factors in high fiber foods make it difficult to assess the individual role played by fiber in unprocessed foods. The majority of studies using foods have been carried out on diabetics who for the most part were normolipidemic. In such studies falls in serum cholesterol have been produced,[6,7,12,113,114,126] but since these studies in-

volved both high fiber and high carbohydrate intakes, the reduced fat intake may have contributed to the lower cholesterol levels observed. These studies are remarkable, however, in that high carbohydrate diets, when they were high in fiber, failed to raise serum triglyceride levels. On the contrary, in hypertriglyceridemic individuals reductions in serum triglyceride levels were actually seen.[6,114] The fiber foods included cereals, starchy vegetables, and beans. More recently, studies of Trappist monks placed on diets where the fiber again came from legumes, cereals, and vegetables demonstrated significant reductions in serum cholesterol.[127] In addition, a recent prospective study suggested that increasing the fiber intake may usefully form part of dietary manipulation in preventing the development of cardiovascular disease.[128]

Only in a retrospective study by Morris and co-workers was there a suggestion that cereal fiber may be protective for cardiovascular disease.[129] However, cereal fiber, for the most part, has had little effect on blood lipids. The majority of studies have therefore emphasized the possible value of

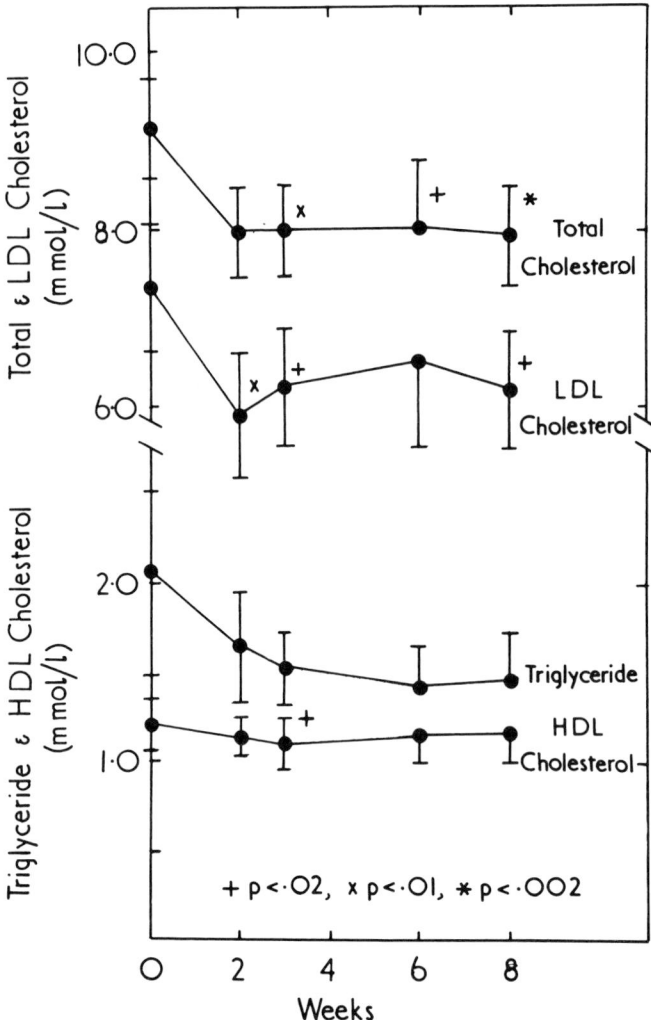

**Fig. 2B–5.** Mean levels of total LDL and HDL cholesterol and triglyceride in 7 patients on guar crispbread for 8 weeks. (From Jenkins, D.J.A., et al.,[15] with permission of Am. J. Clin. Nutr., American Society for Clinical Nutrition.)

legumes or legume fiber in studies where the lipid lowering effects have been observed.

Most recently a report of a study from a Szechwan province indicated that supplementing a Chinese diet with 30 g or more of dried beans daily resulted in a 10% fall in serum cholesterol in a large group of hyperlipidemic individuals over a 3-month period.[130] This is perhaps the first report of successful supplementation of a hyperlipidemic group with a high fiber food. No change was seen in serum triglyceride in this study, but a subsequent study demonstrated a 20% fall in a group of predominantly type IV hypertriglyceridemic patients who exchanged 30% of their carbohydrate from conventional sources for that in beans.[131] Since then, a number of studies have indicated that altering the amount of soluble fibers in the diet by the use of such foods as beans, oats,

and barley may result in reductions in blood lipids in hyperlipidemic individuals.[131a,131b,131c] Falls have been recorded in both LDL cholesterol and serum triglyceride levels with no consistent reductions in HDL cholesterol. In this respect it is also important to bear in mind that many of the effects in whole foods may be due to associated nutrients or antinutrients. This is especially true of possible effects of vegetable protein and perhaps saponins in diets that have been shown to reduce serum lipids. Further studies are therefore required before definitive advice can be given.

### Gallstones, Hiatus Hernia, Varicose Veins

Comparison of diet histories from test and control groups again suggested that not only patients with diverticular disease but also sufferers from the remaining two diseases of Saint's triad, gallstones and hiatus hernia, consumed significantly less fiber in their diets.[132] In the original fiber hypothesis it was suggested that both varicose veins and hiatus hernia may be the result of increased intraabdominal pressure in an attempt to pass constipated feces.[133] Fiber, by regularizing bowel habit, was considered to prevent this. The rationale for fiber in the prevention of gallstones was not clearly stated initially, but subsequent studies have indicated that bran supplements increase the proportion of chenodeoxycholic acid in the circulating bile salt pool. It was also shown that wheat bran reduced the lithogenic index of bile.[134] In addition, Falaiye showed that Africans consuming a high fiber diet had expanded bile salt pools, increased synthesis rates, and reduced cholesterol saturation of the bile.[135] The possible role of fiber has been further stressed by a case control study suggesting that patients with gallstones have lower fiber intakes than controls.[136] At present it is not possible to recommend specific types or amounts of fiber for gallstone prophylaxis.

### Weight Control

With the development of the "fiber hypothesis" it was pointed out that obesity was not seen in those parts of the world where large amounts of fiber were eaten. Again, however, the use of unprocessed foods is related to decreased total calorie intake relative to energy expenditure in many communities. Thus a causal relationship is difficult to define. Methylcellulose, cellulose, and other nonabsorbable materials have been used to induce satiety as noncalorific "fillers."[17] Small (1.5 to 2.5 kg) weight losses were seen in both diabetics[11] and hyperlipidemics[15] on long-term guar supplementation, and similar small weight losses have been reported in diabetics on high fiber-high carbohydrate diets.[12]

Increased fecal fat losses have been found in association with diets supplemented with bran,[3] guar,[58] or pectin,[58,59] but these have seldom been above 7 g/day more than the control diet.

It is possible that the weight loss with viscous fiber may be due to its ability to prolong absorption and so prevent large postprandial excursions both above and below the fasting blood glucose level. This, together with associated alterations in amino acid metabolism,[137] may enhance satiety. In addition, reduction in production of endogenous insulin or decreased requirement in diabetics for exogenous insulin may be another important factor favoring weight loss.[11,12]

Not only the type of fiber but also the effect it has on food form and food selection must be considered. This effect has been well shown in studies where rats became obese when fed human "junk" foods (biscuits and chocolate-coated pastries) as opposed to rat chow.[17] Recent studies have indicated that, in both obese and nonobese, reduction of the energy density of test meals reduced energy consumption by half despite comparable acceptability.[138] However, in a study conducted in a Swedish weight reducing club, weight loss was similar in ispaghula and bran-treated groups compared with controls despite a reduction in hunger ratings in the fiber supplemented groups.[139] Further studies must therefore be undertaken before the role of fiber per se in the prevention and treatment of obesity can be defined.

## POSSIBLE ADVERSE EFFECTS OF FIBER

### Minerals and Trace Elements

Consumption of certain high fiber diets have been associated with zinc deficiency, sigmoid volvulus, and esophageal cancer. Although the circumstances involved may have little relevance to increased fiber intake on a Western diet, the possible adverse effects of fiber must be considered.

At present there is no clear indication that dietary fiber per se compromises mineral and trace element status in the long term to produce clinical deficiency states in healthy individuals on a varied diet. However, zinc deficiency has been described in Iran where a major food item was a high fiber unleavened flat bread, and such flat breads have been shown to be associated with negative $Ca^{++}$, $Mg^{++}$, and $Zn^{++}$ balances.[140] In addition, a number of relatively short-term studies indicate that purified fiber preparations may induce negative $Ca^{++}$, $Mg^{++}$, and $Zn^{++}$ balance.[140–143] When whole foods have been used, fiber-associated substances such as phytate may also have been responsible for the metal binding.[144] However, in studies where leavened wholemeal bread was used, negative $Ca^{++}$ and $Mg^{++}$ balances were still seen despite the fact that a proportion of the phytate would normally be reduced by leavening.[140] Similarly, with wheat bran lower serum iron levels have been reported.[145,146] On the other hand, although a recent study using a mixed fiber source of fruit and vegetables demonstrated negative balances for $Ca^{++}$ or $Mg^{++}$,[146] the careful metabolic studies of Sandstead and collaborators showed no relationship between fiber content of the diet and $Zn^{++}$ and $Cu^{++}$ balance.[142] In addition, although serum levels may be misleading, long-term studies with guar given to diabetics for 6 months failed to show any reduction in serum $Ca^{++}$, $Zn^{++}$, or $Cu^{++}$ levels.[11] Similar results have been found using high fiber-high carbohydrate diets.[147] Further studies are therefore required to define the effects of fiber on mineral and trace element status.

In addition, the relevance of some of these findings with purified fiber or high phytate foods to fiber supplementation of a Western diet is not clear. In general, diets from mixed sources containing as much as 25 g NDF fiber daily (possibly equivalent to 35 g total dietary fiber) do not appear to have adverse effects on mineral metabolism.[141] Acutely higher levels may cause negative balances.[141] Information is lacking on longer-term deleterious effects of high fiber, although many communities appear to be well adapted to very high fiber intakes. Certain groups such as the malnourished and elderly may require special consideration, but evidence for general cautioning is lacking.

### Volvulus of the Colon

Volvulus is an acute form of intestinal obstruction produced when the colon, usually the sigmoid, twists on its mesentery and so obstructs the lumen. Unless relieved it may prove fatal. As a cause of death it remains rare even in high fiber eating areas of the world despite its undisputed relationship with fiber intake. Data have been gathered from Iran[148] and India.[149] It is of interest that diverticular disease is rare in those areas where volvulus is found.

### Esophageal Cancer

Although not directly related to fiber intake, the silica associated with certain cereal fibers, notably millet, has been implicated as a possible factor in the etiology of esophageal cancer.[150] Silica particles have been found in large amounts in esophageal tissue surrounding the tumors of patients from Northern China where such particles comprise almost 20% of the maize bran that is a staple part of their diet. The relationship between silica and esophageal cancer is further strengthened by the fact that high intakes of fiber-associated silica are also peculiar to the two other areas in the world, the Transkei in South Africa and Northeast Iran, where a high incidence of esophageal cancer is recorded.[150] There was no suggestion that cereal fiber was the cause, but such studies indicate the possible importance of fiber-associated materials such as silica. The silica was actually found in the tumors, a situation perhaps reminiscent of asbestosis.

### CONCLUSION

The study of dietary fiber has clearly indicated the physiologic importance of food form, that is, the interaction of digestible and indigestible elements in foods. It has further emphasized the diversity of physical and chemical attributes of the fiber components and the complexity of their relationships with each other. A purified preparation of a single fiber type may behave very differently from a mixture. This in turn may behave differently in the context of the whole unrefined food.

Studies have also indicated that the different physical and chemical attributes of different fibers result in diverse physiologic effects. These, in turn, may be relevant to the treatment or prophylaxis in an equally wide range of clinical states, but much remains speculation and subject to the results of further research. At present the major impact of the fiber hypothesis has been in stimulating nutritional research, especially in relation to the functions of the gut and in the nutritional management of constipation, diverticular disease, and diabetes.

### REFERENCES

1. Trowell, H.C., Burkitt, D.P.: *In* Refined Carbohydrate Foods and Disease. (Burkitt, D.P., Trowell, H.C., Eds.) London, Academic Press, 1975, pp. 333–345.
2. Eastwood, M.A., Kirkpatrick, J.R., Michell, W.D., et al.: Br. Med. J. *4*:392–394, 1973.
3. Cummings, J.H., Hill, M.J., Jenkins, D.J.A., et al.: Am. J. Clin. Nutr. *29*:1468–1473, 1976.
4. Brodribb, A.J.M., Humphreys, D.M.: Br. Med. J. *1*:424–430, 1976.
5. Painter, N.S., Almeida, A.Z., Colebourne, K.W.: Br. Med. J. *1*:137–140, 1972.
6. Anderson, J.W., Chen, W.J.: Am. J. Clin. Nutr. *32*:346–363, 1979.
7. Anderson, J.W., Ward, K.: Am. J. Clin. Nutr. *32*:2312–2321, 1979.
8. Doi, K., Matsuurama, M., Kawara, A., et al.: Lancet *1*:978–988, 1979.
9. Jenkins, D.J.A., Leeds, A.R., Gassull, M.A., et al.: Lancet *2*:172–174, 1977.
10. Jenkins, D.J.A., Wolever, T.M.S., Nineham, R., et al.: Br. Med. J. *2*:1744–1746, 1978.
11. Jenkins, D.J.A., Wolever, T.M.S., Taylor, R.H., et al.: Br. Med. J. *1*:1353–1354, 1980.
12. Kiehm, T.G., Anderson, J.W., Ward, K.: Am. J. Clin. Nutr. *29*:895–899, 1976.
13. Kritchevsky, D.: Am. J. Clin. Nutr. *31*:565–574.
14. Miettinen, T.A., Tarpila, S.: Clin. Chem. Acta. *79*:471–477, 1977.
15. Jenkins, D.J.A., Reynolds, D., Slavin, B., et al.: Am. J. Clin. Nutr. *33*:575–581, 1980.
16. Thiffault, C., Belanger, M., Pouliot, M.: Can. Med. Assoc. J. *103*:165–166, 1970.
17. Van Italie, T.B.: Am. J. Clin. Nutr. *31*:543–552, 1978.
18. Heaton, K.W., Thornton, J.R., Emmett, P.M.: Br. Med. J. *2*:764–766, 1979.
19. Pomare, E.W., Heaton, K.W., Low-Beer, T.S., et al.: Am. J. Dig. Dis. *21*:521–525, 1976.
20. Malhotra, S.L.: Postgrad. Med. J. *54*:6–9, 1978.
21. Hipsley, E.H.: Br. Med. J. *2*:420–422, 1953.

22. McCance, R.A., Lawrence, R.D.: MRC Special Report series No.135. HMSO, London pp. 22–73, 1929.
23. Paul, A.A., Southgate, D.A.T.: McCance and Widdowson's The Composition of Foods, 4th Ed. MRC Spec. Rep. Ser. 297. London, HMSO, 1978.
24. Trowel, H., Southgate, D.A.T., Wolever, T.M.S., et al.: Lancet *1*:967, 1976.
25. Cummings, J.H.: *In* Colon and Nutrition (Kasper, H., Goebell, H., Eds.) (Falk Symposium 32) MTP Press, pp. 91–103, 1982.
26. Milton-Thompson, E.J., Lewis, B.: Gut *12*:853–854, 1971.
27. Gordon, A.J.: *In* Topics in Dietary Fiber Research. (Spiller, G.A., Ed.) New York, Plenum Press, 1978, pp. 59–103.
28. Southgate, D.A.T., Bailey, B., Collinson, E., et al.: J. Hum. Nutr. *30*:303–313, 1976.
29. Watt, B.K., Merrill, A.L.: Handbook of the Nutritional Contents of Foods. USDA Handbook 8. New York, Dover Publications, 1975.
30. McCance, R.A., Widdowson, E.M., Shackleton, L.R.B.: Spec. Rep. Scr. Med. Res. Coun. Lond 213. London, HMSO, 1936.
31. Southgate, D.A.T.: J. Sci. Food Agric. *20*:331–335, 1969.
32. Prosky, L., Asp, N-G., Furda, I., et al.: *In* Determination of Total Dietary Fiber in Foods, Food Products and Ingredients: Collaborative Study. To be published.
33. AOAC: Official Methods of Analysis, 11th Ed. (Horwitz, W., Ed.) AOAC: Washington DC, Association of Official Analytical Chemists, 1970, p. 129.
34. Van Soest, P.J.: J. Assoc. Off. Agric. Chem. *46*:825, 829, 1963.
35. Van Soest, P.J., McQueen, R.W.: Proc. Nutr. Soc. *32*:123–130, 1973.
36. Eastwood, M.A.., Kay R.M.: Am. J. Clin. Nutr. *32*:364–367, 1979.
37. Kay, R.M., Strasberg, S.M.: Clin. Invest. Med. *1*:9–24, 1978.
38. Holt, S., Heading, R.L., Carter, D.L., et al.: Lancet *1*:636–639, 1979.
39. Jenkins, D.J.A., Gassull, M.A., Leeds, A.R., et al.: Gastroenterology *73*:215–217, 1977.
40. Leeds, A.R., Ralph, D.N.L., Ebied, F., et al.: Lancet *1*:1075–1078, 1981.
41. Jenkins, D.J.A., Bloom, S.R., Albuquerque, R.H., et al.: Gut *21*:574–579, 1980.
42. Jenkins, D.J.A., Wolever, T.M.S., Leeds, A.R., et al.: Br. Med. J. *1*:1392–1394, 1978.
43. Elsenhaus, B., Sufke, U., Blume, R., et al.: Clin. Sci. *59*:373–380, 1980.
44. McCance, R.A., Prior, K.M., Widdowson, E.M.: Br. J. Nutr. *7*:98–104, 1953.
45. Cummings, J.H., Branch, W., Jenkins, D.J.A., et al.: Lancet *1*:5–9, 1978.
46. Cummings, J.H.: *In* Dietary Fiber in Health and Disease (Vahouny, G.V., Kritchevsky, D., Eds.) New York, Plenum, 1982, pp. 9–21.
47. Cummings, J.H., Southgate, D.A.T., Branch, W.J., et al.: Br. J. Nutr. *41(3)*:477–485, 1979.
48. Stephen, A.M., Cummings, J.H.: Nature *284*:283–284, 1980.
49. Reinhold, J.G., Garcia-L, P.M., Arias-Amado, L., et al.: *In* Dietary Fiber in Health and Disease (Vahouny, G.V., Kritchevsky, D., Eds.) New York, Plenum, 1982, pp. 117–132.
50. James, W.P.T., Branch, W.J., Southgate, D.A.T., et al.: Lancet *1*:638–639, 1978.
51. Eastwood, M.A., Hamilton, D.: Biochem. Biophys. Acta *152*:165–173, 1968.
52. Kritchevsky, D., Story, J.A.: J. Nutr. *104*:458–462, 1974.
53. Kritchevsky, D., Story, J.A.: Am. J. Clin. Nutr. *28*:305–306, 1975.
54. Story, J.A., Kritchevsky, D.: J. Nutr. *106*:1292–1294, 1976.
55. Vahouny, G.V., Tombes, R., Cassidy, M.M., et al.: Lipids *15*:1012–1018, 1980.
56. Oakenfull, D.G., Fenwick, D.E.: Br. J. Nutr. *40*:299–309, 1978.
57. Eastwood, M.A., Mowbray, L.: Am. J. Clin. Nutr. *29*:1461–1467, 1976.
58. Jenkins, D.J.A., Leeds, A.R., Gassull, M.A., et al.: Clin. Sci. Mol. Med. *51*:8–09P, 1976.
59. Kay, R.M., Truswell, A.S.: Am. J. Clin. Nutr. *30*:171–175, 1977.
60. Fahrenbach, M.J., Riccardi, B.A., Saunders, J.L., et al.: Circulation *31/32* (Suppl. 2):1141, 1965.
61. Schneeman, B.O.: *In* Dietary Fiber in Health and Disease (Vahouny, G.V., Kritchevsky, D., Eds.) New York, Plenum, 1982, pp. 73–83.
62. Monoz, J.M.: *In* Dietary Fiber in Health and Disease. (Vahouny, G.V., Kritchevsky, D., Eds.) New York, Plenum, 1982, pp. 83–89.
63. Kimura, T., Imamura, H., Hasegawa, K., et al.: J. Nutr. Sci. Vitaminol. *28*(5):483–489, 1983.
64. Kiyozumi, M., Mishima, M., Noda, S., et al.: Clin. Pharm. Bull. *30*(12):4454–4459, 1982.
65. Ebihara, K., Kiryama, S.: J. Agric. Chem. Soc. Jpn. *56*:195–202, 1982.
66. Takeda, H., Tsuijta, J., Emoto, T., et al.: Nutr. Rep. Int. *25*(1):169–187, 1982.
67. Tasman-Jones, C.: *In* Medical Aspects of Dietary Fiber. (Spiller, G.A., Kay, R.M., Eds.) New York, Plenum, 1980, pp. 67–74.
68. Tasman-Jones, C., Owen, R.L., Jones, A.L.: Dig. Dis. Sci. *27*(6):519–524, 1982.
69. Jacobs, L.R., White, F.A.: Am. J. Clin. Nutr. *37*:945–953, 1983.
70. Thomsen, L.L., Tasman-Jones, C.: Digestion *23*(4):253–258, 1982.
71. Dean, F.M.: *In* Naturally Occurring Oxygen Ring Compound. London, Butterworths, 1962, pp. 485–548.
72. Purstai, A., Clarke, E.M.W., King, T.P.: Proc. Nutr. Soc. *38*:115–120, 1979.
73. Birk, Y., Peri, I.: *In* Toxic Constituents of Plant Food Stuffs. (Leiner, I.E., Ed.) New York, Academic Press, 1980.
74. Malinow, M.R., McLaughlin, P., Stafford, C., et al.: Am. J. Clin. Nutr. *32*:1810–1812, 1979.
75. Blomford, R.: Clin. Exp. Immunol. *39*:435–441, 1980.
76. Erdman, J.W.: J. Am. Oil Chem. Soc. *56*:736–740, 1979.
77. Cheryan, M.: CRC Crit. Rev. Food Sci. Nutr. *13*:297–335, 1980.
78. Tamir, M., Alumot, E.: J. Sci. Food Agric. *20*:199–202, 1969.
79. Salunkhe, D.K., Wu, M.T.: CRC Crit. Rev. Food Sci. Nutr. *9*:265–324, 1977.
80. Leiner, I.E.: Proc. Nutr. Soc. *38*:109–113, 1979.
81. Militzer, W., Ideka Kneen, E.: Arch. Biochem. *9*:30, 1946.

82. Holloway, W.D., Tasman-Jones, C., Maher, K.: Am. J. Clin. Nutr. *37*:253–255, 1983.
83. Willliams, T.D., Olmsted, W.H.: J. Nutr. *11*:433–449, 1936.
84. Southgate, D.A.T., Durnin, J.V.G.A.: Br. J. Nutr. *24*:517–535, 1970.
85. Southgate, D.A.T., Branch, W.J., Hill, M.J., et al.: Metabolism *25*:1129–1135, 1976.
86. Heller, S.N.: Ph.D Thesis, Cornell University, Ithaca, New York, 1977.
87. Van Soest, P.J., Robertson, J.D., Roe, D.A., et al.: Proceedings, 1978 Cornell Nutrition Conference for Feed Manufacturers, 1978.
88. Farrell, D.J., Girle, L., and Austher, J.: Aust. J. Exp. Biol. Med. Sci. *56*:469–479, 1978.
89. Heller, S.N., Hackler, L.R., Rivers, J.M., et al.: Am. J. Clin. Nutr. *33*:1734–1744, 1980.
90. Hoppert, C.A., Clark, A.J.: J. Am. Diet. Assoc. *21*:157–160, 1945.
91. Prynne, C.J., Southgate, D.A.T.: Br. J. Nutr. *41*:495–503, 1979.
92. Cummings, J.H.: Gut *22*:763–779, 1981.
93. Miller, T.L., Wolin, M.J.: Am. J. Clin. Nutr. *32*:164–172, 1979.
94. Smith, C.J., Bryant, M.P.: Am. J. Clin. Nutr. *32*:149–157, 1979.
95. Roediger, W.E.W.: Gut *21*:793–798, 1980.
96. Bond, J.H., Currier, B.E., Cuchwald, H., et al.: Gastroenterology *78*:444–447, 1980.
97. Stephen, A.M., Cummings, J.H.: Proc. Nutr. Soc. *38*:141A, 1979.
98. Perman, J., Modler, S., Olson, A.C.: J. Clin. Invest. *67*:643–650, 1981.
99. Werch, S.G., Ivy, A.C.: Am. J. Dis. Child. *62*:499–511, 1941.
100. Committee of the American Diabetes Association on Food and Nutrition. Diabetes Care *2*:520–523, 1979.
101. Special Report Committee on Guidelines for the Nutritional Management of Diabetes Mellitus. J. Can. Diet. Assoc. *42*:110–118, 1981.
102. The Nutrition Sub-Committee of the British Diabetic Association's Medical Advisory Committee. Hum. Nutr. Appl. Nutr. *36A*:378–394, 1982.
103. Morgan, L.M., Goulder, T.J., Tscoladis, D., et al.: Diabetologia *17*:85–89, 1979.
104. Jenkins, D.J.A., Wolever, T.M.S., Taylor, R.H., et al.: Br. Med. J. *281*:1248–1250, 1980.
105. Aro, A., Uusitupa, M., Voutilainen, E., et al.: Diabetologia *21*:29–33, 1981.
106. Smith, C.J., Rosman, M.S., Levitt, N.S., et al.: S. Afr. Med. J. *61*:196–198, 1982.
107. Smith, U., Holm, G.: Atherosclerosis *45*:1–10, 1982.
108. Jenkins, D.J.A., Wolever, T.M.S., Nineham, R., et al.: Br. Med. J. *2*:1555, 1979.
109. Christiansen, J.S., Bonnevie-Nielsen, V., Svendsen, P.A., et al.: Diabetes Care *3*:659–662, 1980.
110. Bosello, O., Ostuzzi, R., Armellini, F., et al.: Diabetes Care *3*:46–49, 1980.
110a.Reed, N.W.: *In* Dietary Fiber: Basic and Clinical Aspects. (Vahouny, G.V., Kritchevsky, D., Eds.) New York, Plenum Press, 1986, pp. 81–100.
110b.Blackburn, N.A., Redfern, J.S., Jayis, M., et al.: Clin. Sci. *66*:329–336, 1984.
110c.Flourie, B., Vidon, N., Florent, C.H., et al.: Gut *25*:936–941, 1984.
111. Jenkins, D.J.A., Leeds, A.R., Gassull, M.A., et al.: Ann. Intern. Med. *86*:20–23, 1977.
112. Jenkins, D.J.A.: Diabetes Care *5*:634–641, 1982.
113. Simpson, R.W., Mann, J.I., Eaton, J., et al.: Br. Med. J. *2*:523–525, 1979.
114. Simpson, H.C.R., Simpson, R.W., Lonsley, S., et al.: Lancet *1*:1–15, 1981.
115. Schwartz, S.E., Levin, R.A., Singh, A.: Gastroenterology *83*:812–817, 1982.
116. Rydring, A., Berstad, A., Asland, E.: Lancet *2*:736–739, 1982.
116a.Rydring, A., Berstad, A.: Scand. J. Gastroenterol. *20*:1078–1082, 1985.
117. Connor, W.E., Connor, S.L.: Med. Clin. N. Am. *66*(2):485–518, 1982.
118. Palmer, G.H., Dixon, D.G.: Am. J. Clin. Nutr. *18*:437–442, 1966.
119. Raymond, T.L., Connor, W.E., Lin, D.S., et al.: J. Clin. Invest. *60*:1429–1437, 1977.
120. Jenkins, D.J.A., Reynolds, D., Leeds, A.R., et al.: Am. J. Clin. Nutr. *31*:2430–2435, 1979.
120a.Story, J.A.: *In* Dietary Fiber: Basic and Clinical Aspects. (Vahouny, G.V., Kritchevsky, D., Eds.) New York, Plenum Press, 1986, pp. 253–264.
120b.Schneeman, B.O., Lefevre, M.: *In* Dietary Fiber: Basic and Clinic Aspects. (Vahouny, G.V., Kritchevsky, D.: Eds.) New York, Plenum Press, 1986, pp. 309–321.
121. The Lipid Research Clinics Coronary Primary Prevention Trial Results. JAMA *251*:351–364, 365–374, 1984.
122. Jenkins, D.J.A., Leeds, A.R., Slavin, B., et al.: Am. J. Clin. Nutr. *32*:16–18, 1979.
123. Kirby, R.W., Anderson, J.W., Sieling, B., et al.: Am. J. Clin. Nutr. *34*:824–829, 1981.
124. Zavoral, J.H., Smith, C.M., Hedlund, B.E., et al.: ACS Symposium Series. *214*:71–92, 1983.
125. Lindner, P., Moller, B.: Lancet *2*:1259–1260, 1973.
126. Rivellese, A., Riccardi, G., Giacco, A., et al.: Lancet *2*:447–450, 1980.
127. Lewis, B., Hammett, F., Katen, M., et al.: Lancet *2*:1310–1313, 1981.
128. Hjerman, I., Byre, K.V., Holme, I., et al.: Lancet *2*:1303–1310, 1981.
129. Morris, J.N., Marr, J.W., Clayton, D.G.: Br. Med. J. *2*:1307–1314, 1977.
130. Bingwen, L., Zhaofeny, W., Wanshen, L., et al.: Chin. Med. J. *94*:455–458, 1981.
131. Jenkins, D.J.A., Wong, G.S., Patten, R., et al.: Am. J. Clin. Nutr. *38*:567–573, 1983.
131a.Anderson, J.W., Story, L., Sieling, B., et al.: J. Can. Dietet. Assoc. *45*:140–149, 1984.
131b.Anderson, J.W., Story, L., Sieling, B., et al.: Am. J. Clin. Nutr. *4*:1146–1155, 1984.
131c.Jenkins, D.J.A., Wolever, T.M.S., Kalmusky, J., et al.: Am. J. Clin. Nutr. *42*:604–617, 1985.
132. Capson, J.P., Pajenneville, H., Dumont, M., et al.: Lancet *2*:329–331, 1978.
133. Burkitt, D.P., Meisuer, P.: Med. Rep. *24*:30–32, 1979.
134. Pomare, E.W., Heaton, K.W., Low-Beer, T.S., et al.: Am. J. Dig. Dis. *21*:521–526, 1976.
135. Falaiye, J.M.: Lancet *1*:1002, 1974.
136. Alessandrini, A., Fusco, M., Gatti, E., et al.: Ital. J. Gastroenterol. *14*(3):156–158, 1982.
137. Anderson, G.H.: Can. J. Physiol. Pharmacol. *57*:1043–1057, 1979.
138. Duncan, K.H., Bacon, J.A., Weinsier, R.L.: Am. J. Clin. Nutr. *37*:763–767, 1983.
139. Hylander, B., Rossner, S.: Acta Med. Scand. *213*:217–220, 1983.

140. Reinhold, J.G., Faradji, B., Abadi, P., et al.: J. Nutr. *106*:493–503, 1976.
141. Kelsay, J.: *In* Dietary Fiber: Basic and Clinical Aspects (Vahouny, G.V., Kritchevsky, D., Eds.) New York, Plenum, 1986, pp. 361–372.
142. Sandsted, H.H., Mong, J.M., Jacob, R.A., et al.: *In* Dietary Fibers Chemistry and Nutrition. (Inglett, G.E., Falkehag, S.I., Eds.) New York, Academic Press, 1979, pp. 147–156.
143. Ismail-beigi, F., Reinhold, J.G., Faraji, B., et al.: J. Nutr. *107*:510–518, 1977.
144. Widdowson, E.M., McCance, R.A.: Nature *148*:219–220, 1942.
145. Jenkins, D.J.A., Hill, M.J., Cummings, J.H.: Am. J. Clin. Nutr. *28*:1408–1411, 1975.
146. Kelsay, J.I., Behall, K.M., Prather, E.S.: Am. J. Clin. Nutr. *32*:1876–1880, 1979.
147. Anderson, J.W., Ferguson, S.K., Karounos, D., et al.: Diabetes Care *3*:38–40, 1980.
148. Ghavami, A., Saidi, F.: Dis. Colon Rectum *12*:462–466, 1969.
149. Gulati, S.M., Grover, N.K., Tagore, N.K., et al.: Dis. Colon Rectum *17*:219–225, 1974.
150. O'Neil, C., Pan, Q-Q., Clark, G., et al.: Lancet *1*:1202–1206, 1982.

*Chapter* **3**

# LIPIDS

Willem G. Linscheer and Antoine J. Vergroesen

Lipids are compounds soluble in organic solvents, e.g., acetone, ether, chloroform. Of nutritional interest are triglycerides, phospholipids, sphingolipids, and sterols present in food products of animal or plant origin. The fat-soluble vitamins A, D, E, and K are also lipids but will be discussed in chapters 12 to 15. Since many fatty acids and sterols have double bonds in the carbon chain and are prone to oxidation, the presence of natural antioxidants such as vitamin E and selenium (see Chapter 10) is important.

## CLASSIFICATION

Dietary lipids consist mainly of *triglycerides* (TG), a useful and concentrated source of energy. (1 g of TG provides approximately 9 kcal = 38 kjoule after absorption). Fat maldigestion and malabsorption lead to steatorrhea, an appreciable loss of energy. A fecal fat excretion of 40 g/day, which is not uncommon in the case of severe pancreatic insufficiency, represents an energy loss of >360 kcal (>1500 kJ). An adequate TG supply and absorption are especially important for infants[1] and also for adults with a high energy requirement, such as patients with major burns, malignant tumors, and surgical wounds. The alternative energy sources, proteins and carbohydrates, deliver per gram, 4 kcal = 17 kJ, less than half the energy density of fats, and require bulky meals to cover high energy requirements. In practice the energy density of common sources of proteins and carbohydrates is much less due to their fiber and water content.

Triglycerides consist of a molecule of glycerol esterified with 3 fatty acid (FA) molecules. The melting point of a TG is determined by the type of its FA (carbon chain length and the number and cis- or trans-configuration of its double bonds) and the position to which it is esterified with the glycerol molecule (1st, 2nd, or 3rd position). The melting point of a TG is important for intestinal absorption and for developments in modern food technology. By varying the chain length of fatty acids, reducing the number of natural cis double bonds, and/or increasing the number of trans double bonds, inter/trans esterification can produce a range of fats with a specific melting behavior. Fatty acids on the 2-position of TG are easily absorbed after digestion as monoglycerides even if they normally would be poorly absorbed if present as free FA, released by lipolysis in case they were bound to the 1- or 3-position. This holds true especially for saturated FA with a chain length of 18 or more and for monounsaturated FA (especially if the double bond is in the trans configuration) with more than 20 carbon atoms.

The foregoing observations demonstrate why the nutritional characterization of a TG requires more than a FA analysis limited to only chain length and number of double bonds and why too many nutritional studies on the role of fats can be interpreted incompletely.

Table 3–1 gives a review of the more important fatty acids and their natural sources.[1-3] Genetic and climatic differences are responsible for a rather wide variation in the compositions of vegetable oil; the composition of animal feed determines to a great extent animal fat composition, especially that of nonruminants. For this reason, a fat is insufficiently described by only its source

(e.g., safflower seed or lard). See Appendix Tables A–20a and b for lipid contents of selected foods and oils.

The vital importance of the essential fatty acids (EFA) to both man and animals in respect to the adequate composition of the biomembranes and as precursors of the prostaglandins (PGs), leukotrienes (LTs) and various hydroxy fatty acids will be discussed later in this chapter. As no animal, including man, can synthesize EFA, it is completely dependent on vegetable lipids (directly or indirectly via consumption of herbivores) to meet EFA requirements. Shifting the position of one of the double bonds of the EFA from the n-3, 6, 9 all

**Table 3–1. Average Triglyceride Fatty Acid Composition of Important Edible Fats**

| Food | Average Fat % | Saturated Total[a] | 16:0 | 18:0 | Mono- and Polyunsaturated 18:1 | 18:2 | 18:3 | 20:4 |
|---|---|---|---|---|---|---|---|---|
| milk (cow) | 3.5 | 65[a] | 25 | 11 | 26 | 1–3 | 2 | tr |
| butter | 80 | | | | identical to milk | | | |
| lard (pig) | 100 | 42 | 28 | 13 | 46 | 6–8 | 2 | 2 |
| pork | 35 | | | | approx. as lard | | | |
| tallow | 100 | 53 | 29 | 20 | 42 | 2 | tr | — |
| beef | 25 | | | | approx. as tallow | | | |
| chicken | 15 | 30 | 25 | 4 | 42 | 21 | — | — |
| egg | 11 | | | | identical to chicken | | | |
| turkey | 20 | | | | approx. as chicken | | | |
| groundnut oil | 100 | 19[b] | 11 | 3 | 40–55[b] | 20–43[b] | | |
| groundnut | 50 | | | | identical (variable, climate dependent) | | | |
| sesame oil | 100 | 15 | 9 | 5 | 39 | 40 | 1 | — |
| sesame seed | 53 | | | | identical to oil | | | |
| soybean oil | 100 | 15 | 11 | 4 | 23 | 51 | 7 | — |
| soybean | 18 | | | | identical to oil | | | |
| corn oil | 100 | 13 | 11 | 2 | 25 | 55 | tr | — |
| corn | 4 | | | | identical to oil | | | |
| sunflower seed oil | 100 | 12 | 6 | 4 | 24 | 60–70 | tr | — |
| olive oil | 100 | 17 | 14 | 3 | 71 | 10 | tr | — |
| olive | 14 | | | | identical to oil | | | |
| cottonseed oil | 100 | 30 | 25 | 3 | 18 | 51 | tr | |
| safflower seed oil | 100 | 10 | 7 | 3 | 15[c] | 75[c] | tr | |
| palm oil | 100 | 52 | 45 | 5 | 38 | 10 | — | |
| coconut oil | 100 | 88[a] | 8 | 3 | 6 | 2 | — | |
| palm kernel oil | 100 | 80[a] | 7 | 2 | 14 | 1 | — | |
| rapeseed oil (new) | 100 | 7 | 5 | 2 | 53 | 22 | 10 | |
| rapeseed oil (old) | 100 | 4 | 3 | 1 | 11 | 13 | 9+[d] | |
| mustard seed oil | 100 | 5 | 3 | 1 | 16 | 15 | 10+[d] | |
| cashew nut | 68 | 24 | 14 | 10 | 30 | 35 | tr | |
| walnut | 63 | 10 | 7 | 2 | 15 | 60 | 10 | |
| herring[e] (menhaden) | 16–25 | 30 | 19 | 4 | 13 | 1 | 1+[e] | |
| mackerel[f] | 25 | 25 | 17 | 5 | 18 | 1 | | [f] |

The figures given are approximations, as climate, species, fodder composition, etc. cause great variations. The data given are compiled from ref. 1,2,3.

[a]The balance of saturated fatty acids is formed by fatty acids with chain lengths < 12 (butter 14%) and 12 and 14 (butter 16%, coconut and palm kernel 65–70%).

[b]Circa 4% of C 20:0 and C 22:0, groundnuts from Argentina and Virginia (USA) have relatively low C 18:1 and high C 18:2 concentrations.

[c]Also safflower seed oil with the reverse C 18:1/18:2 composition is available.

[d]Contrary to new rapeseed varieties like Canbra and LEAR, old varieties of rapeseed oil and also mustard seed oil have 10% C 20:1 n-9 and 30–50% C 22:1 n-9.

[e]Menhaden herring oil has 11% C 20:5 n-3, 9% C 22:6 n-3, but Norwegian herring oil has 13% C 20:1 n-9, 21% C 22:1 n-11, 7% C 20:5 n-3, and 7% C 22:6 n-3.

[f]Dependent on fishing grounds mackerel oil is similar to Menhaden or to Norwegian/Northsea herring (see e).

cis or n-6, 9 all cis position (biologists prefer to count from the methyl end of the fatty acid) or changing the cis into the trans configuration, as will happen during hydrogenation (or by bacteria during fodder digestion in ruminants or catalytically by some types of oil processing), will result in a complete loss of EFA activity. Even worse is the fact that the polyunsaturated fatty acids without EFA activity may act as competitive inhibitors of EFA metabolism. For these reasons, careful application of sophisticated analytical methods is crucial in the study of the pathophysiologic effects of EFA and other (poly)unsaturated fatty acids.

Edible fats and oils also contain *sterols* and *phospholipids.* During the processing of vegetable oils, most of the sterols and phospholipids are removed for technological and taste reasons. However, other lipid-containing foods have varying amounts of these compounds, which are integral parts of all animal and plant biomembranes. Man can normally biosynthesize adequate amounts of cholesterol and phospholipids. As will be discussed later, dietary cholesterol, in contrast to most vegetable sterols, which are poorly absorbed, plays an important role in lipoprotein composition and metabolism (see also Chapter 63).

Figure 1 lists the more important sterols[4] and their main dietary sources and molecular differences. Since minor differences in structure are responsible for clear differences in absorption, complicated analytical methods are essential. Chemical characterization of sterols is important because plant sterols have long been known to diminish absorption of cholesterol in mammals and birds; this effect is presumably due to competition with cholesterol for incorporation into micelles or for transport across the intestinal cell wall. β-sitosterol has been used as a therapeutic agent for lowering plasma cholesterol, usually in doses of 10 to 20 g/day. However, it has been shown that maximal inhibition of cholesterol absorption—50% reduction—in man is achieved with 3 g of β-sitosterol per day and no further reduction occurs with higher intakes.[5]

Phospholipids from vegetable sources are absorbed as well as those from animal origin, but they normally have a different fatty acid composition. Recently, interest in the nutritional effects of phospholipids was renewed. Oral or intraduodenal administration of soya phosphatidylcholine will decrease markedly absorption of cholesterol and is in rats[6] and men[7] a more potent hypocholesterolemic agent than TG with a similar fatty acid composition. Furthermore, phosphati-

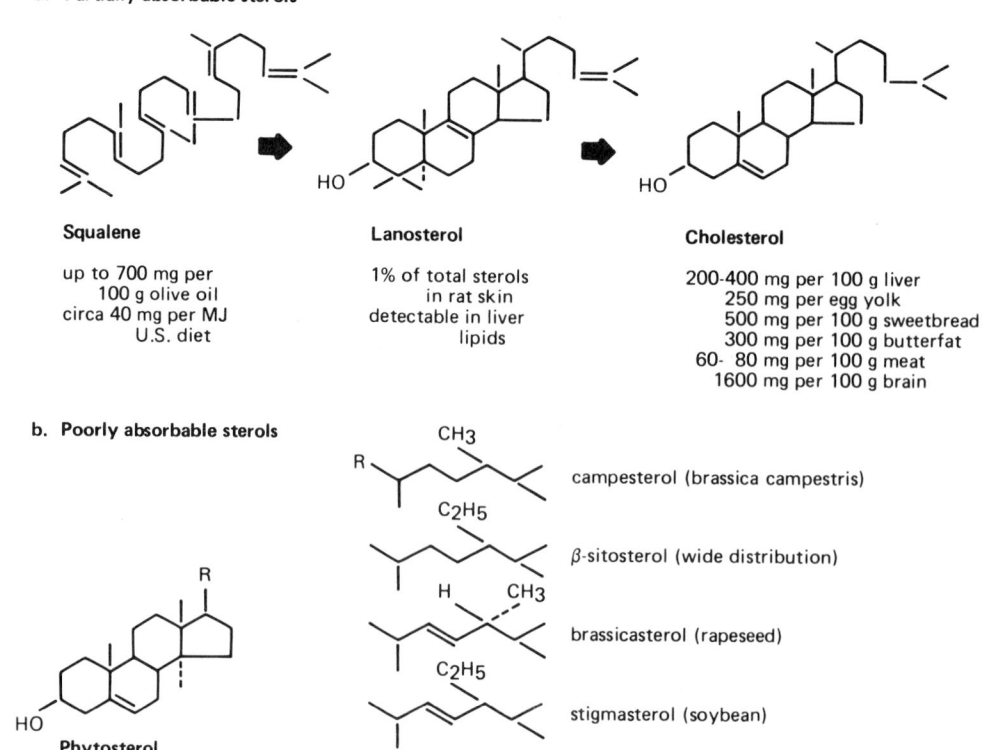

**Fig. 3–1.** Molecular structures and average concentrations of the more important sterols in various food components.

dylcholine given orally is much more efficient in raising blood choline levels than equimolar amounts of free choline,[8,9] which might have significant effects on biosynthesis of acetylcholine in the brain.[10] This is considered to have interesting therapeutic implications in diseases such as Alzheimer's (pre)senile dementia, tardive dyskinesia, and other conditions probably caused by a failing cholinergic activity.

A useful review of the sources of choline and lecithin in the diet has been published.[11] If the preliminary results can be confirmed, the demand for pure phosphatidylcholine (and sphingomyelin), instead of the crude lecithin preparations [mixtures of phosphatidylcholine (20 to 25%), -serine, -ethanolamine, -inositol, nonphosphorus-containing lipids (45 to 50%), and about 10% hydrophilic impurities (sugar, amino compounds)], which are now available, will increase. Again, accurate analytical data are necessary for a correct evaluation of data; for example, the hypocholesterolemic effects of soya phosphatidylcholine referred to above could not be confirmed in man by a study in which egg-phosphatidylcholine with a different fatty acid composition was used.[12]

Dietary triglycerides, along with carbohydrates, are the main *source of digestible energy* (consumption of proteins being rather constant between 10 and 15% of digestible energy (en%)). In most industrialized countries, fat intake is 40 to 45 en%, with a fatty acid composition predominantly high in saturated and mono-unsaturated fatty acids (about 50% and 40% of fat, respectively) and only 2 to 3 en% of EFA. Because this unbalanced fatty acid composition is considered to be a causal factor in atherogenesis, modern dietary recommendations emphasize a reduction of total fat intake and a 1 to 1 ratio between saturated fatty acids and EFA.[1,13] A reduction in fat intake will result in an increased carbohydrate consumption, accompanied by increased dietary levels of fiber, water-soluble vitamins, and trace elements if cereals, potatoes, etc. are the main carbohydrate source. However, prosperous population groups in general consider diets high in starch and fiber unattractive and prefer the sweetness of mono- and disaccharides (sucrose, but also, of course, fruits).

A healthy diet, however, becomes progressively more difficult when lowering dietary fat intakes because the "hidden" fat in meat and dairy products, bread, pastries, etc. is mainly saturated. Laymen will be inclined to limit fat intake by cutting down on "visible" fat intake (oils, spreads), which may be important sources of EFA. One should realize that any excess intake of digestible energy (sugar, alcohol, as well as protein) will be efficiently converted into palmitic and oleic acid and deposited as TG in adipose tissue. In this way, excess food intake contributes to an unphysiologic FA composition of human tissues.

This chapter reviews in greater detail (1) the digestion and absorption of triglycerides, sterols, and phospholipids; (2) the lipid transport and metabolism of various lipoproteins; (3) the functions of essential fatty acids of the n-3 and n-6 type; and (4) the role of dietary EFA as precursors for the biosynthesis of prostaglandins (PG), thromboxanes (TXA), leukotrienes (LT), and hydro(per)oxy FA such as hydroperoxypereicosatetraenoic acid (HPETE) and hydroxyeicosatetraenoic acid (HETE).

## ABSORPTION AND DIGESTION

### Triglycerides (TG)

Triglycerides represent the bulk of ingested fats; the second major group of fats contained in a normal diet, the phospholipids (PL), contribute only an estimated 2% to the total fat intake,[14] but an additional 12 g PL is secreted in the bile every 24 hours.[15] PL play an important role in the digestion and absorption of TG. Other lipids are either present in such minute quantities that they do not play a role in the absorptive process, or they are poorly absorbed (such as wax and wax-like compounds).

Although the proportion of vegetable fat in the diet has increased significantly over the past 40 years in the United States, only 41% of the daily intake is of vegetable origin.[16] Practically all PL in vegetable fat have been removed during preparation for consumption except for the addition of lecithin used as emulsifier. As mentioned in the introduction, the differences between two classes of lipids (animal vs. vegetable) in relation to composition, digestion, absorption, and in the composition and concentration of sterols incorporated in ingested fat affect metabolism and the composition of fat depots.[1-4]

Although digestion of TG consists of highly complicated digestive physicochemical reactions and numerous interactions between lipolytic products, PL, bile salts, proteins, and carbohydrates, certain major principles of lipid digestion have been elucidated. Since interactions with carbohydrates and proteins have not been clarified and are probably of minor importance, we will ignore these effects on the intraluminal phase of fat absorption and discuss the major principles of lipid digestion in the gastrointestinal tract, starting with digestion and absorption of TG.

The two initial steps in digestion of TG are to prepare for enzymatic hydrolysis by increasing the surface area of the TG and to make the TG surface accessible to lipase. These two steps are initiated in the mouth where chewing exposes the TG to lipase by disrupting cell walls and mechanically dispersing the fat into small droplets. Contrary to the teaching of some textbooks, TGs are exposed immediately to the lipolytic activity of a lipase that originates not from the salivary glands or stomach but from lingual serous glands (von Ebner) located on the back of the tongue in the region of the circumvallate papillae.[17-20] As a matter of fact, a small portion of TG is hydrolyzed prior to ingestion by exposure to lipases already present in food or added to sauces during preparation of food. Lipases are present in human milk (not in cow's milk),[21,22] meat, cheese, vegetables, salad dressings, and soy sauces. However, free FAs are reactive, unpleasant tasting molecules and are tolerated only at very low concentrations.

For a long time, acid treatment of food in the stomach was thought to delay lipid digestion. One of the main advantages of a low gastric pH is the sterilization of food prior to digestion, since continued multiplication of microorganisms (which are always present in food) while food is still in the upper gastrointestinal tract would interfere with the digestive process and, in addition, expose the host to all kinds of infections. TG digestion, however, is not inhibited by the low gastric pH, since lipases present in the stomach are active in an acid environment, and the lower pH in the proximal intestine is actually a favorable factor for the intraluminal digestion and uptake of lipids.

It has been shown that the lingual lipase is active at the gastric pH spectrum (pH 2 to 6), and it plays a very important role in TG digestion of the suckling infant.[23] It forms primarily diglycerides with a strong preference for hydrolysis of the Sn-3 position of long-chain TG (>C12). Like most lipases, it has a high activity for hydrolysis of medium (C6–C12) and short-chain (<C6) TG. In addition to lingual lipase, gastric esterase lyses the medium and short-chain TG (MCT and SCT), but it does not hydrolyze long-chain TG (LCT).[24,25] As a result of the buccoesophagogastric digestion, LCTs are partly emulsified and digested in the stomach. The medium and short chain FAs are also partly absorbed by the stomach before gastric chyme reaches the duodenum.

**Intestinal Digestion of TG.** Borgstrom's studies,[26] using a high fat liquid test meal (75 gm of fat) and an intubation technique, has demonstrated TG absorption to be practically completed in the first 120 cm of the small bowel in healthy human volunteers. Following a meal, small quantities of partly hydrolyzed TG (up to 30% depending on saturation and carbon chain length of

FA) are delivered to the duodenum by the gastric peristalsis and intermittent relaxation of the pyloric musculature. The combination of an acid pH, the presence of essential amino acids, and FA and monoglycerides in the gastric chyme strongly stimulate the release of cholecystokinin (CCK; identical to pancreozymin) and secretin from the duodenal mucosa into the circulation.[27-30] Secretin is the physiologic stimulant for release of most of the pancreatic electrolytes; CCK stimulates the synthesis and release of exocrine pancreatic enzymes and, to a lesser degree, the release of electrolytes.[31] The overlapping effect of CCK on excretion of pancreatic bicarbonate assures a more continuous pH adjustment in the duodenum because secretin release is primarily dependent on the short episodes of the pH lowering effect of freshly arrived gastric chyme in the proximal duodenum. CCK also induces sustained gallbladder contraction and synthesis and the release of hepatic bile, containing bile salts, PL, and cholesterol.

The obligatory steps in TG absorption are hydrolysis of TG and solubilization of the hydrolytic products. Based on physicochemical properties of lipids and lipid membranes (= luminal mucosal membranes), one can predict that (1) TG and diglycerides may not permeate the absorptive mucosal membrane and that (2) only 2-monoglycerides (2-MG) and primarily protonated (or nonionized) FA can pass through the membrane by diffusion as free monomers in the aqueous phase adjacent to the luminal membrane. It has been shown that 75 gm of LCT can be absorbed from the aqueous phase as monomers of 2-monoglycerides and protonated FA within 4 hours by 120 cm of small bowel.[26] This is a formidable accomplishment considering the fact that the maximum concentration of oleic acid in water is 80 $\mu$molar and the solubility of glyceryl 2-monooleate is only 5 $\mu$molar.[32]

As mentioned before, TG are partly hydrolyzed in the stomach, and hydrolysis of TG in chyme resumes immediately in the proximal duodenum following alkalinization of acid chyme and exposure to pancreatic lipase and intestinal esterase. Intraluminal digestion of lipids in the proximal small bowel is discussed in more detail.

*pH Changes.* Sodium bicarbonate released by the pancreas increases the duodenal pH to the activity level of pancreatic lipase (pH 5.5 to 6.5). Although this is still below the optimal pH for pancreatic lipase, such an excess of lipase is secreted (a 1,000 fold excess[33]) that, under optimal conditions, 100 kg of TG could be hydrolyzed in 24 hours instead of the ingested 100 g of fat in a normal diet.

*Hydrolysis of TG.* Pancreatic lipase, released simultaneously with the other exocrine enzymes of the pancreas, is inactivated by bile. The bile salts (BS) and PL present in bile would normally adhere to the surface of TG droplets, thereby displacing lipase from its substrate. However, as Borgstrom,[34] Desnuelle,[35] and Morgan and Hoffman[36] have elucidated, lipolysis does take place because procolipase (MW 10,000) is also released by the pancreas simultaneously with lipase (MW 50,000) in a 1:1 ratio. Procolipase is activated by pancreatic trypsin by the removal of a small group of less than 12 amino acids.[37] In the presence of TG (or FA), colipase then complexes firmly with lipase and also binds to the surface of TG droplets thereby supplanting BS and PL molecules. The mixed micelles present in bile, consisting of BS, PL, and cholesterol, participate in this complex.[38] Thus, colipase gives lipase access to its substrate, and micelles remove the products of lipolysis, thereby increasing the effectiveness of lipase (Fig. 3–2A and B).

In contrast to lingual lipase, pancreatic lipase hydrolyses long-chain fatty acids (LCFA) not only to a diglyceride but also to a 2-monoglyceride. The FA on the 2-position is resistant to pancreatic lipase; this resistance results in the release of FA and 2-monoglycerides. Lipolysis is greatly stimulated by the presence of the bile micelles, which facilitate lipolysis by removing the hydrophobic lipolytic end products of this enzymatic reaction (FA, monoglycerides) by micellar solubilization.

*Micellar Solubilization.* Pure bile salts are poor detergents. Bile micelles, however, are very efficient detergents due to the presence of PL, which are always secreted simultaneously with BS in relatively fixed molar ratios (3:1). Bile salts are the essential micelle-forming component of the mixed micelles because they are strong amphiphiles.[39] The strongly hydrophilic sites are located on one side of the molecule (OH, COOH, $NH_2$) with strongly hydrophobic groups ($CH_2$) on the other side. The low pKa (average = 3) renders the BS water soluble. The hydrophobic end of the molecule tends to adhere to any surface area and will form clusters of molecules when all available surface area is taken up. The hydrophobic part of the BS is directed towards the core of the aggregate, and the hydrophilic sites are located on the outside of the multimolecular sphere.

Micelle formation occurs when a certain concentration of BS has been reached; it is called the critical micellar concentration (CMC). The CMC is different for each bile salt. The average CMC for the mixture of BS is approximately 1 to 2 mmol. Physiologic concentrations of BS in intestinal chyme are about 12 mmol. The highly polar water soluble bile salts are poorly absorbed in the proximal small bowel and BS concentrations are therefore above the CMC during lipid digestion.

Solubilizing properties of bile micelles for FA and cholesterol are further enhanced by the incorporation of the exogenous 2-MG released from the TG by pancreatic lipase. Thus, the resistance to hydrolysis of the FA at the No. 2 position by pancreatic lipase facilitates micellar solubilization of the lipolytic products. Micellar aggregates, as present in bile, are in fact highly efficient in absorbing the 2-MG and FA released by the pancreatic lipase from the surface of the TG droplets. Because lipolysis is an extremely fast process (the turnover is approximately 400,000 mol/min/mol lipase,[40] formation of 2-MG and FA takes place at a higher rate than micellar solubilization, resulting in a new oil phase consisting of TG, DG, 2-MG, and FA. Lipid droplets are also emulsified during hydrolysis by the combination of released 2-MG and biliary PL. In short, the micelles surrounding the surface of the oil droplets incorporate immediately the 2-MG + FA, yet this expanded micelle is still a water-soluble macromolecule dispersed throughout the intestinal chyme.

Micelles consists of 2 to 40 molecules of BS and can incorporate 2 molecules of mono-olein (less for saturated MG) and 1 molecule of LCFA per molecule of BS.[32] MG is better solubilized in the micellar phase than FA, because swelling amphiphiles (like MG or PL) are much better incorporated in micelles than nonswelling amphiphiles. FA, with a lower melting point, is better incorporated than FA with a higher melting point, which is determined by the length of the carbon chain and degree of unsaturation. Therefore, the micellar solubility of FA is inversely related to the carbon chain length and degree of saturation; also, LCFA is better absorbed as 2-MG. Thus, in case of a poorly absorbable long chain saturated FA, the position of the FA in the TG molecule is important.

Ionized FA is better solubilized in micelles than protonated FA.[32] TG and diglycerides are poorly incorporated into the mixed micelles because they have a high partition in the oil phase. The mixed micellar aggregates in bile, consisting of cholesterol, PL, and bile salts, are in essence macromolecules with a loose, but organized structure determined by attracting and repulsing electromagnetic forces (v.d. Waals). As we have seen, these aggregates have the property to incorporate specifically the two end products of TG lipolysis by pancreatic lipase, the 2-MG, and the FA. Both lipid species are poorly water soluble; they are absorbed only as free monomers from the aqueous phase, which is in close contact with the luminal

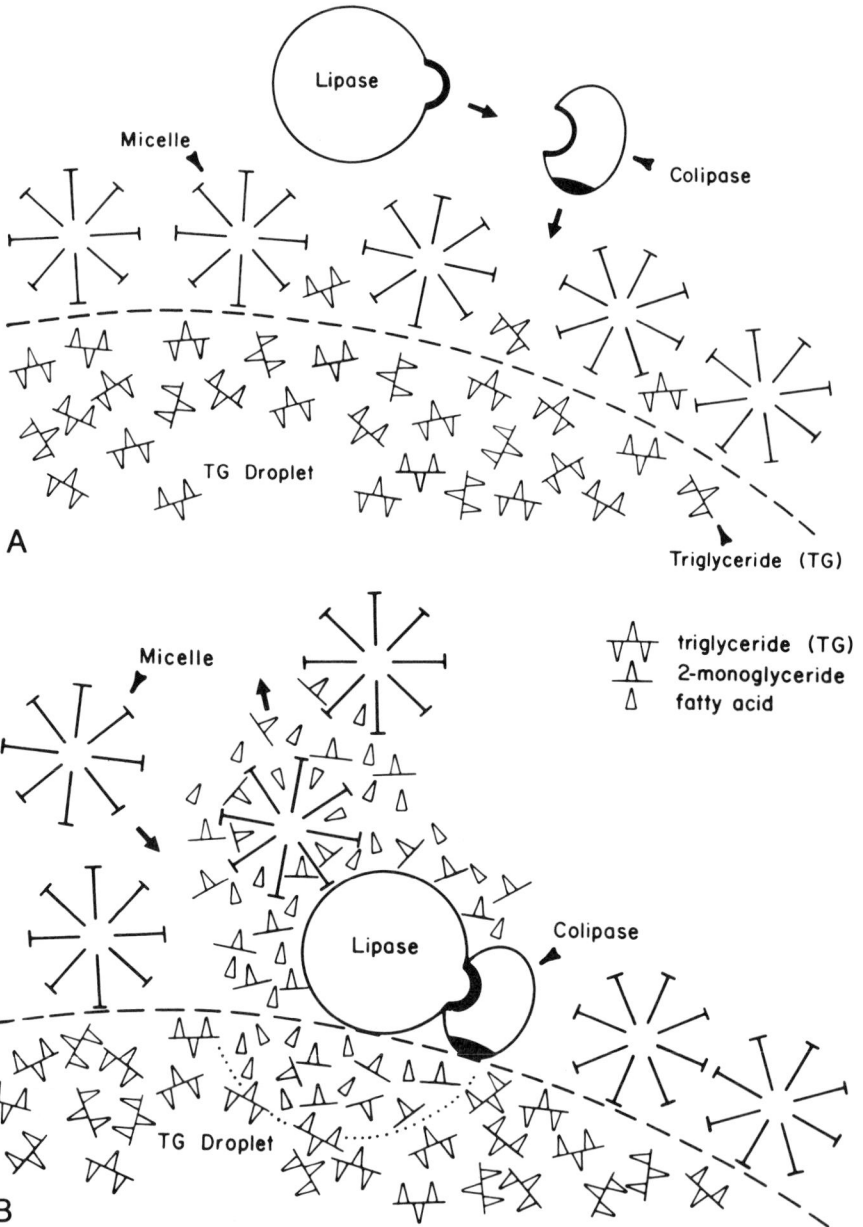

**Fig. 3–2.** *A*, Bile micelles and their components would prevent access of lipase to its substrate by adhering to the surface of TG droplets. ("Micelle" is the symbol for a bile micelle). *B*, Colipase with a high affinity to TG displaces the micelles and their components and at the same time complexes with the oil phase and the micelles.

membrane of the enterocytes. Uptake is dependent on passive diffusion gradients without an energy requiring facilitating mechanism.

*Passive Diffusion.* The final step in the digestive phase of absorption, namely, the uptake of free monomers of FA and 2-MG by passive diffusion from a water phase located between micelle and cell membrane, is a rate-limiting step; complicated mechanisms are involved in order to sustain monomer concentrations at the luminal cell sur-

face. In order to clarify some of these mechanisms, we will discuss in more detail properties and interactions of the micelles with the oil phase and the cell membrane.

Micelles are called flickering clusters because they are in constant movement (Brown's movements). Their constituents also exchange continuously between the micellar and aqueous phase, thereby sustaining the concentrations of lipid monomers in the intermicellar aqueous phase according to the partition coefficient between the two phases. Since there is an equilibrium between the constituents of the micelles and the surrounding aqueous phase, a fast exchange of these constituents between the micelles will take place when micelles move close to each other. This leads to an equalization of their composition. Due to their flickering random movements, in combination with the peristaltic movements of the bowel, the intermicellar aqueous phase of the intestinal chyme will be saturated with the newly formed FA and 2-MG.

The rate of lipolysis, as we have seen, exceeds the rate of micellar solubilization, and the presence of an emulsified oil phase of FA and MG keeps micelles in the bulk phase saturated. Conditions are different in the unstirred water layer (UWL) bordering the mucosal surface. Emulsified oil droplets, because of their large size (25,000 ± 20,000 A), diffuse very slowly compared to the much smaller micelles (30 to 100 A) and do not penetrate the UWL. Micelles, due to their small size and constant movements, migrate into the UWL (thickness 100 to 500 $\mu$m in vitro),[41] and, in addition, a constant exchange with the micelles in the bulk phase takes place. In contrast to the saturated intermicellar phase with FA and MG monomers because of the presence of an oil phase in the bulk phase of the proximal small bowel, there is no equilibrium phase in the UWL. Almost no oil phase is present, and monomers disappear continuously from the aqueous phase across the luminal membrane of the enterocytes. This is a unidirectional flow practically without back diffusion.[33]

As deduced from literature and our own observations, we propose the following mechanism for the transport of FA and 2-MG from the surface of their emulsified droplets to the cell membrane as illustrated by Figure 3–3. Micelles in the UWL, located close to the cell membrane, become partly unsaturated for FA and 2-MG. Monomer concentrations decrease in the aqueous phase surrounding the micelle and are partly replaced by monomers moving out of the micelle into the aqueous phase since the partition coefficient between micelle and the aqueous phase is constant. These partly depleted micelles by their constant movements come in contact with other (saturated) micelles and incorporate "lost" lipid monomers by the mechanism of fast exchange of their constituents. Thus, during absorption, micelles donate their lipid monomers to the cell membrane, and depleted micelles are replenished by contact with other micelles, creating a kind of chain reaction of monomers jumping from micelle to micelle and from micelle to membrane. As indicated in this figure the micelles in the bulk phase are saturated by the existence of FA and MG oil droplets.

To date, the rapid exchange of monomers between micelles has been shown,[32] but a chain reaction of monomers moving from the bulk phase through the UWL by jumping from micelle to micelle (from the more saturated to the less saturated micelle) has not yet been demonstrated. A somewhat similar process, however, has been proposed by Scholander for oxygen transport in hemoglobin solutions when a tension gradient is imposed.[42] He postulates that oxygen molecules are handed down from one hemoglobin molecule to another in a chain fashion. Because hemoglobin molecules are large molecules, delivery of oxygen via a shuttle system would be a much slower process than the jumping of oxygen molecules from one hemoglobin molecule to the next.

In addition to the transfer of monomers by jumping from micelle to micelle, there is also an exchange of micelles between the bulk phase and the UWL; this has led Dietschy to propose his so-called shuttle system as the major transport mechanism for lipid monomers.[43] The weakness of this hypothesis, however, is the fact that micelles move at random and there is, in our opinion, no driving force to move micelles from the bulk phase to the cell membrane or vice versa. Furthermore, the lifetime of a micelle is probably too short for completion of a shuttle roundtrip through the UWL. Dietschy later changed his concept, but was unable to express it in a mathematical model.

The most favorable condition for maximal TG absorption by the small bowel mucosa exists in the proximal small bowel when 2-MG and FA are present in the oil phase as well as in the micellar phase with an aqueous phase practically saturated with monomers. Phospholipids (PL), mainly lecithin (phosphatidylcholine), although contributing to micellar solubility by expansion of the micelle,[30] inhibit the exchange of monomers between the micellar and aqueous phase, resulting in decreased monomer activity[45] and FA absorption.[46] However, a phospholipase $A_2$, secreted by the pancreas, metabolizes most of the PL to lyso-PL. Lysolecithin does not inhibit the monomer activity (monomer activity is an expression for the total amount of protonated FA in solution available for absorption).[45]

Transfer of FA monomers from micelles via the aqueous interface to the cell membrane is optimal when micelles are saturated. Linscheer has demonstrated in the rat that the rate of absorption of oleic acid is proportionally related to the degree of saturation of micelles with FA (Fig. 3–4).[47] Chijiiwa and Linscheer have also demonstrated that the rate of oleic acid absorption from micellar so-

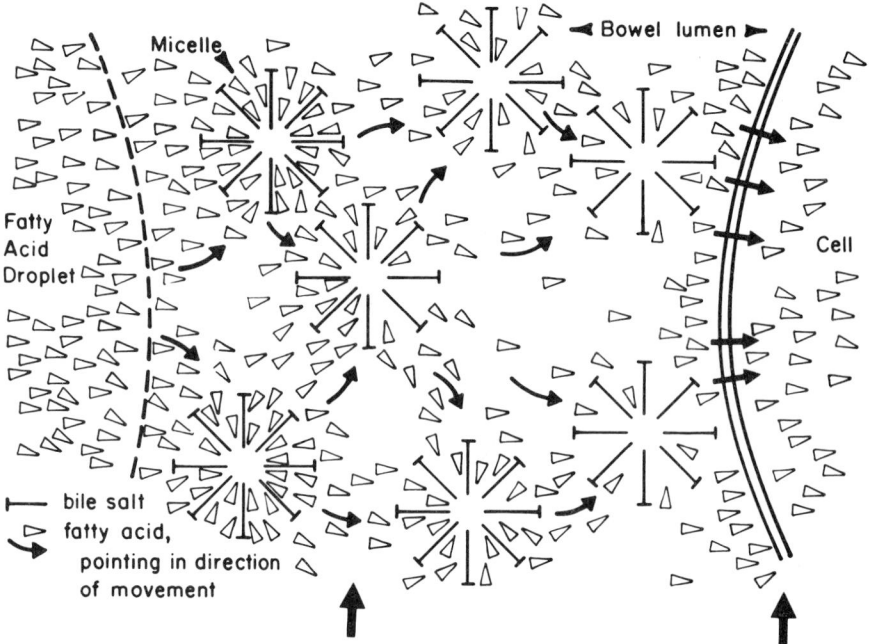

**Fig. 3–3.** Illustration of the transport hypothesis of FA and 2-MG from the oil droplets to micelles, from the more "saturated" micelles to the less saturated micelles, and from micelles to cell membrane. The arrows at the base of the figure indicate the unstirred water layer.

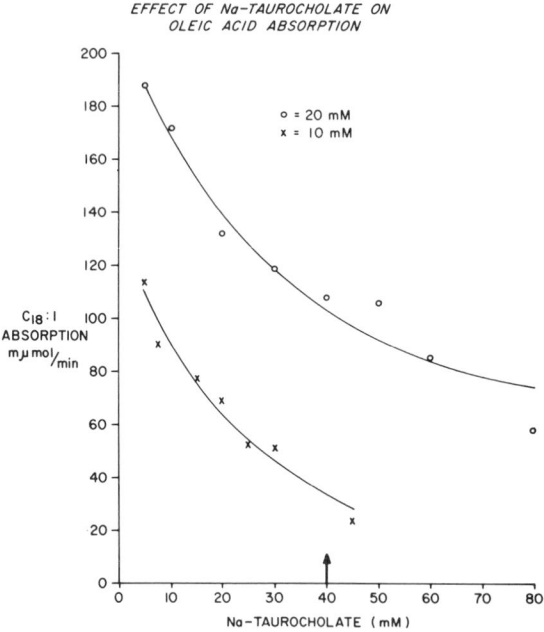

**Fig. 3–4.** Rates of absorption by the rat small bowel in vivo (see reference 48 for the technical procedure) at two concentrations of oleic acid (10 mmol (x) and 20 mmol (o) are plotted against increasing concentrations of Na-taurocholate. Micelles become more depleted for fatty acid with increasing concentrations of bile salt.

lutions was lower at a pH 6.5 as compared with pH 5.5. This was explained by the fact that more FA was solubilized at the higher pH, resulting in FA-depleted micelles and decreased monomer activity.[48] These experimental observations have clinical significance, since the pH in the duodenum is lower compared to that of the jejunum. The oil phase disappears more distally in the bowel, not only by absorption but also by increased micellar solubilization at the higher pH, and micelles become unsaturated for FA and 2-MG. Thus, intraluminal, as well as extraluminal factors, (more enterocytes/cm) are more favorable for lipid absorption in the proximal than in the distal small bowel.

An adult human being has a great reserve for fat absorption. Relatively independent of the composition of the ingested fat, the average daily stool fat excretion is 4 to 6 g, even when twice the normal amount has been consumed. The difference is that with an increasing load of fat, absorption is completed more distally in the small bowel. Newborns, however, have no reserve, and the source of fat is important. On mother's milk, fat excretion (6% of ingested fat) is similar to that in adults, but infants reared on cow's milk may have, for up to one year, a certain degree of fat malabsorption.[49]

In contrast to cow's milk, mother's milk contains a lipase that is resistant to gastric acid and pepsin.[21,22] Babies have a relative deficiency of BS, and the intestinal BS concentration is frequently below the critical micellar concentration (CMC).[50] It is interesting that human milk lipase can hydrolyze the FA from all three positions of the TG. It is known that 2-MG is practically not absorbed without prior micellar solubilization in contrast to FA whose absorption is less dependent on micelles.[32] This mechanism may compensate for the low BS concentrations in the infantile intestinal chyme.

The elderly have a limited capacity for lipid absorption,[51] but since their appetite also decreases, the fat intake has usually decreased also. Their mild fat malabsorption may be clinically manifested by malabsorption of vitamin D, as manifested by low serum concentrations of vitamin $D_2$ following oral administration of vitamin $D_2$.[52] In addition, the elderly have an increased incidence of achylia gastrica. This leads to a higher than normal pH in the proximal duodenum, which further limits the absorption of fat and sterols.[48] pH effect may also contribute to the mild steatorrhea after a partial gastric resection.

**Very Long Chain Fatty Acids (C 20 and more).** In some parts of the world, edible oils (rapeseed, mustard seed, and fish oil) with a high percentage of very long chain FA (C 20 and more) are produced and consumed as a natural oil or after (partial) hydrogenation. In addition to dihomo-γ-linolenic acid (C 20:3, n-6, 9, 12) and arachidonic acid (C 20:4, n-6, 9, 12, 15)—which occur in TG of animals only in limited amounts (<2%)—natural FA with 20 or more C-atoms with terminal cis double bond at either the n-3 or the n-9 position also can be present. Peanut oil has a relatively high amount (5 to 10%) of saturated FA with 20 to 24 C-atoms; these probably are responsible for the peculiar atherogenic effect of peanut oil.[53] The atherogenic effect disappears after re-esterification. This might be explained by the very poor absorption of free saturated FA with a carbon chain length ≥18, whereas those if present as a 2-MG are well absorbed.

Erucic acid (C 22:1, n-9) is present in many conventional varieties of rapeseed oil (Brassica napus and campestris) (20 to 50%) and in mustard seed oil (>50%). Genetic selection has led to varieties with less than 1% C 22:1, but in India, Pakistan, and China edible cruciferous oils high in C 20:1, n-9 and C 22:1, n-9 are still being produced.

Marine oils (Table 3–1) contain 27 to 50% FA with 20 and more C-atoms. Many of these have 4 to 6 cis double bonds starting at n-3 (except some species in tropical areas like North Australia) and are remarkably high in arachidonic acid C 20:4, n-6. Consumption of fish, seal, and whale can lead

to high intakes of especially C 20:5, n-3 and C 22:6, n-3. These are efficiently absorbed in contrast to saturated and monounsaturated FA of the same chain length and can be responsible for a series of interesting pathophysiologic effects (see "n-3 Polyunsaturated Fats, Thrombosis, and Atherosclerosis"). As a consequence of the fish meal industry, reasonably large quantities of fish oil are produced (>10^6 tons/year). Fish oil, after partial hydrogenation to improve preservation and melting ability, is used in some margarines, shortening, and bakery products.[1,3] Some types of herring, menhaden, and also eel have about 20% C 22:1, n-11, an isomer of C 22:1, n-9 (erucic acid). Due to hydrogenation, a whole range of cis- and trans-isomers with 1 or 2 double bonds is produced and, consequently, an extremely complicated FA composition.

As early as 1948, Deuel et al. related the poor growth performance of rats fed 10% rapeseed oil (high C 22:1, n-9 variety) to poor digestibility (circa 80%).[54] This was ascribed to the unusually slow rate of absorption of erucic acid, which occupies positions 1 and 3 in the TG of rapeseed oil. Seventy-five percent of the recovered fecal FA in rats fed rapeseed oil is erucic acid, which is excreted as free FA or diglycerides.[55] After interesterification, however, which randomly distributes the FA on the three positions of a TG, erucic acid was better absorbed by the rat.[56]

The slower and incomplete absorption of high erucic acid rapeseed oil has been found also in men and pigs,[57,58] lamb and poultry.[59] It is interesting that the relatively poor absorption of both tallow (mainly C 16:0 and C 18:0) and high erucic acid rapeseed oil is significantly improved when a mixture of both fats was fed.[59] This type of synergistic effect on digestibility of fat mixtures indicates the difficulty of interpretation of nutritional effects of extreme fat compositions and quantities. Intestinal absorption of other FA with a chain length of 20 or more C-atoms is not systematically studied, but, in general, it can be stated that rates of absorption decrease with increasing melting points. Melting points of FA depend on carbon chain length and the configuration and location of the double bonds.

Erucic acid containing TG is not only absorbed more slowly, but the absorbed, very long chain FA is also more slowly metabolized. Thus, it has a tendency to accumulate in tissues with a preferential metabolism for FA such as the heart muscle.[58] Following a certain adaptation phase, these lipid accumulations disappear, but scar tissue is observed in rats at the locations of previous lipid depots. These problems will be discussed later in more detail. In contrast to the very long chain FA, medium chain length FA (C6 to C12) are absorbed more quickly due to the essential differences in digestion, mucosal transport, and metabolism.

**Medium Chain Triglycerides (MCT).** MCT contain saturated FA with a carbon chain length of 6 to 12 carbon atoms. They occur in milk fat and especially in coconut and palm kernel oil. Some suppliers use coconut oil in commercially prepared baby formulas and in coffee whiteners. Furthermore, fractions rich in lauric and myristic acid (12:0, 14:0) are used in margarine manufacturing to improve melting. Because of this fractionation of coconut and palm kernel oil, fractions rich in MCT are formed as a by-product. The usefulness of MCT for human consumption was subsequently discovered in certain pathologic conditions,[60] based upon multiple differences in the digestion, absorption, transport, and metabolism of MCT vs. LCT.[61]

In summary, the principal difference from LCT is that MCT is much more water soluble; this solubility increases the effectiveness of lipase. MCFA are also more water soluble and require less BS for solubilization. They are not re-esterified by the enterocyte and transported as FA (bound to albumin) via the portal circulation, which has a much faster flow rate than the lymphatic system. Therefore, MCT are more quickly digested, they are relatively independent of pancreatic lipase, bile salts, and enterocytic metabolic transformations, and by being more water soluble, they still possess sufficient lipophylic properties for rapid passage through cell membranes. They are, therefore, transported and metabolized much faster than LCT, and they are not stored in fat depots.[62–65] It is not surprising that they can be successfully applied in most forms of fat malabsorption and in some forms of hyperlipidemia.[62–66]

Consumption of MCT may cause ketosis and, in the presence of portosystemic shunting (in liver cirrhosis), high blood levels of MCFA can saturate serum albumin, disturbing its carrier function for amino acids, vitamin E, and other compounds. Free nonalbumin bound MCFA crosses the blood/brain barrier and may induce coma.[66] However, the MCT have now been evaluated extensively in various disease entities, and their indications and contraindications are easily obtained. They are the preferred treatment in a number of fat malabsorption syndromes. It is regrettable that MCT in the United States is only commercially available either as MCT oil or as a formula feeding. Modern emulsifying techniques allow for production of a stable margarine that is commercially available in Europe.

### Common Causes of Fat Maldigestion

*Gastric Surgery.* Gastric resections interfere with the following physiologic conditions: (1) reservoir function for hydrolysis by lingual lipase and gastric esterase; (2) portionwise delivery of gastric chyme to the duodenum as regulated by pH adjustment in the duodenum; (3) lack of acidification of gastric chyme; (4) bypassing of the duodenum (Billroth II operation) preventing food-induced release of duodenal CCK and secretin. Patients with a partial gastric resection rarely regain their preoperative body weight and frequently have a mild fat malabsorption (approximately 15 g of stool fat/24 hr instead of 4 to 6 g).[67] Recently, it has been shown that loss of acidity is not only of significance in the inhibition of bacterial growth and gastric digestion, but also acid chyme leads normally to a mild acidity (pH 4.5 to 6.5) in the duodenum and proximal jejunum, which probably has a favorable effect on FA and cholesterol absorption. As discussed earlier, micellar solutions of FA and cholesterol have higher monomer activity and rate of absorption at a pH of 5.5 than at a pH of 6.5.[48]

*Lipase Deficiency.* Lack of lingual lipase activity causes malabsorption in rats;[68] however, it is unlikely to induce malabsorption in the adult human since pancreatic lipase is secreted in excessive amounts. Deficiency of pancreatic lipase is of clinical significance only when the secretion of pancreatic lipase is below 10% normal levels. At the same time, lipase activity is decreased by lack of chyme neutralization due to a concomitant $NaHCO_3$ deficiency. Triglycerides reaching the colon are partly split by bacterial lipases,[69] but LCFA are poorly absorbed by the colon.[70] Unsaturated hydroxy-FA change the permeability of the colonic mucosa, resulting in an influx of water into the bowel lumen causing diarrhea.

*Bile Salt Deficiency.* Bile salt deficiency caused by ileal dysfunction, iliectomy, or liver disease interferes with the transport mechanism of lipolytic products and inhibits lipase activity. Diarrhea caused by fat malabsorption is potentiated by concomitant bile salt malabsorption (iliectomy, nonfunctioning ileum). Dehydroxy bile salts have an effect similar to FA on the permeability of the colonic mucosa in man.[71]

*Disturbed Neutralization of Chyme in Duodenum.* Excessive release of gastric HCl (Zollinger-Ellison syndrome) prevents neutralization of gastric chyme in the duodenum. A low duodenal pH inactivating pancreatic lipase and impairing micelle formation results in deficient hydrolysis and micellar solubilization.[72]

### Phospholipids

Dietary PL plays only a minor role in the digestive process, since the average diet contains approximately only 2 g (mainly from legumes and egg yolk).[11] However, about 12 g are secreted in bile, which plays an essential role in the micellar solubilization of endogenous as well as exogenous cholesterol and which solubilizes FA and 2-MG. Current literature has paid little attention to the role of pancreatic phospholipase A on the absorption of TG. The PL, consisting primarily of lecithin, is so efficient in solubilizing 2-MG and FA in the mixed micelles that it inhibits the monomer activity of FA and MG and thereby the rates of absorption.[46] However, pancreatic phospholipase A hydrolyzes PL to lyso PL (mainly lysolecithin), which has no inhibitive effect on monomer activity or absorption.

In contrast to TG lipase, which hydrolyzes the No. 1 and 3 positions of TG, phospholipase $A_2$ hydrolyzes the FA at the No. 2 position. Lysolecithin is an active and potentially toxic molecule, particularly in combination with bile salts, and it may cause reflux gastritis and pancreatitis when refluxed into the pancreatic duct. Hydrolysis of lecithin is a slower process than hydrolysis of TG. In contrast to lecithin, lysolecithin is well absorbed and under physiologic conditions only very low concentrations of lysolecithin are present in the bowel lumen. It is partly re-esterified following uptake by the enterocyte and used by the cell for chylomicron formation and partly further hydrolyzed by phospholipase $A_1$ (Fig. 3–5).

PL is secreted in bile in a relatively stable ratio with BS (1:3), and isolated PL deficiencies as a cause of maldigestion are extremely rare. Its main functions in the absorptive process are (1) solubilizing of endogenous and exogenous cholesterol in mixed micelles (preventing gallstone formation and facilitating cholesterol absorption), (2) facilitating micellar solubilization of lipolytic products, steroids, and fat soluble vitamins; and (3) facilitating transport of TG in the intestinal mucosa. Since secretion of BS and PL by the hepatocyte are always coordinated, BS deficiency is always associated with biliary PL deficiency.

## Cholesterol

Since cholesterol is present in all tissues of vertebrates (and some invertebrates—crustacea (crab, shrimp) and higher molluscs (e.g., squid)—it follows that carnivores ingest appreciable quantities of cholesterol (Fig. 3–1). Not only food but also the bile and, to a small extent, the intestine itself (by de novo synthesis of cholesterol and by desquamation of mucosal cells) contribute to the cholesterol available for absorption. Experimental work suggests that the intestinal cholesterol pool is heterogeneous because biliary cholesterol is

more effectively absorbed than dietary cholesterol.[73]

In rats, biliary cholesterol is primarily absorbed in the proximal half of the small bowel, but dietary cholesterol is absorbed in the distal half.[74] Although these observations suggest much better absorption of endogenous cholesterol, actually only slightly more endogenous than exogenous cholesterol is absorbed. Several investigators using an isotopic-equilibrium method,[75,76] concluded that in normal human subjects the maximal capacity for absorbing dietary cholesterol is about 300 to 500 mg/day. Others,[77–80] using combined chemical and isotope balance methods, have shown that 30 to 40% of dietary cholesterol is absorbed in most men over an intake range of 40 mg/day to more than 2 g/day.

Although some disagree about the percentage of absorption, all investigators agree that only part of the cholesterol of both origins is absorbed. This in itself is a remarkable fact if one considers the different conditions for cholesterol absorption for the two sources of cholesterol. Bile cholesterol, for example, consists of unesterified cholesterol already solubilized in mixed (BS, PL) micelles. Exogenous cholesterol is partly esterified. Esterified cholesterol is not water soluble and is not absorbed as an FA ester.[75] Pancreatic cholesterol esterase, activated by BS, is capable of splitting cholesterol ester into the free sterol and FA, but this is a rather slow process compared to the hydrolysis of TG. Free cholesterol is dissolved in the oil phase and into micelles. When the oil phase disappears, cholesterol precipitates slowing down the rate of absorption.

The fact that cholesterol is only absorbed via micellar solubilization may explain the relatively poor absorption of exogenous cholesterol in healthy subjects, but it does not explain why endogenous cholesterol is poorly absorbed also. It is most likely that cholesterol absorption from micelles slows down considerably when MG, FA, and PL have disappeared from the micelle because their rate of absorption is much faster and BS micelles alone are poor detergents. Chijiiwa and Linscheer's observation that absorption rates of cholesterol are much higher at the lower pH of the duodenum and proximal jejunum than at the higher pH in the distal half of the small bowel suggests that this may be the contributing factor.[48]

The physiologic malabsorption of cholesterol (related to its very low solubility in water) is essential for the intestinal excretion mechanism of cholesterol. Cholesterol is also the substrate for BS synthesis, but reabsorption of BS is highly efficient and the amount of BS excreted in feces is not the main excretory pathway of cholesterol.

## Absorption of PL

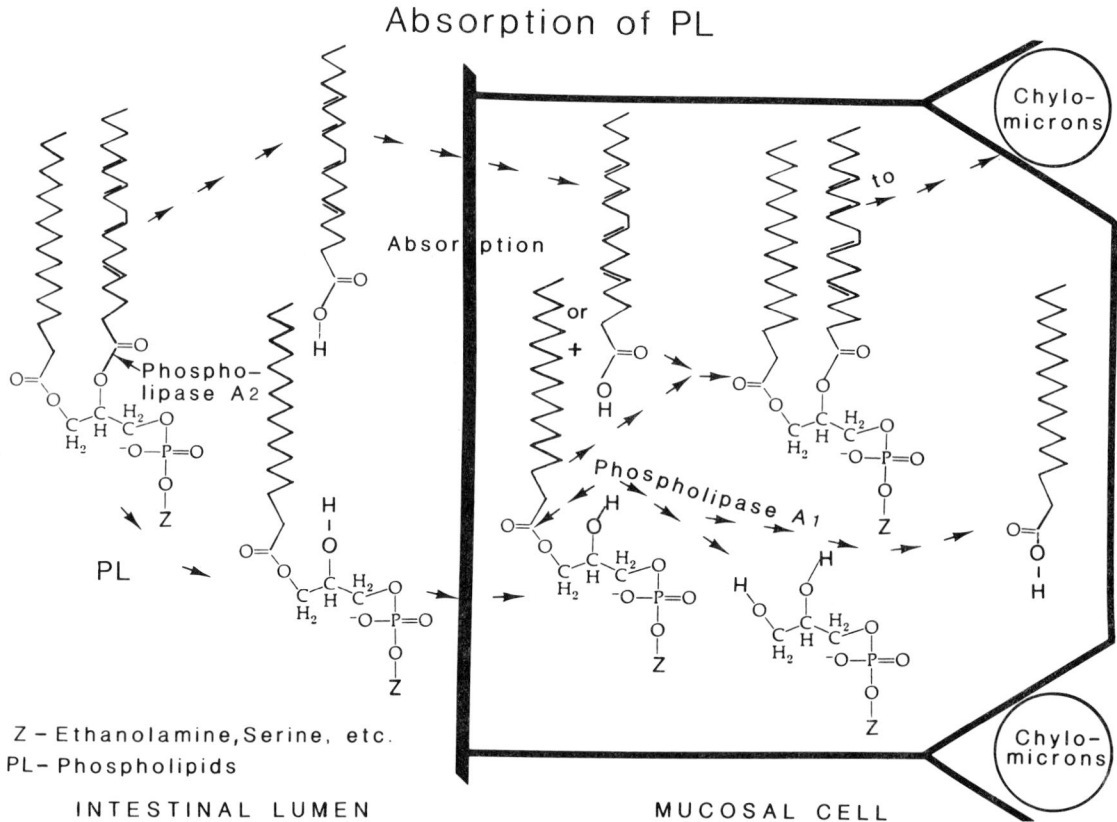

**Fig. 3–5.** Most of the phospholipids (PL) in the intestinal lumen consist of lecithin (Z-choline). Lecithin is poorly absorbed, but pancreatic phospholipase $A_2$ hydrolyzes the unsaturated fatty acid (FA) in the No. 2 position, and the hydrolytic products—lysolecithin and FA—are readily absorbed. Inside the enterocyte the lysolecithin is partly re-acetylated with an unsaturated FA by lysophosphatidyl cholin acyltransferase, the magnitude of which seems to be related to the need for phospholipid for the assembly and transport of chylomicrons. The rest of the absorbed lecithin is further metabolized by hydrolysis of the saturated FA in the No. 1 position by phospholipase $A_1$.

Since no evidence indicates that significant amounts of cholesterol are absorbed form an emulsified oil phase, it seems likely that one of the rate-limiting factors in the absorption of cholesterol is micellar solubilization. Cholesterol absorption is facilitated by the TG in the diet by the mechanism discussed above.

The normal intake of cholesterol (200 to 600 mg/day) accounts for only a small fraction of the total cholesterol transported, and because its contribution to the pool is small, no saturation will be apparent for the absorption of dietary cholesterol. Although individual responses of blood cholesterol show marked variations when animals and men are exposed to increased amounts of dietary cholesterol and some may even show no clear change,[77,81] the majority will react with an increase in concentrations of blood (and tissue) cholesterol.[73,76,83,84] Apparently no adequate compensatory mechanism exists for the augmented absorption by the reduction of endogenous cho-

lesterol synthesis and for the increased excretion via the bile.

Another consequence of the limited absorption of a high dietary cholesterol load is the increased concentration of excreted cholesterol, BS, and their bacterial degradation products in the colon and rectum; these are believed to have carcinogenic effects. High cholesterol diets are usually low in (vegetable) fibers and are associated with long intestinal transit times and reduced fecal bulk; these might be an additional explanation for the (epidemiologically) observed association between high saturated fat, high cholesterol, low fiber diets, and colon cancer.

As stated in the introduction of this chapter, plant sterols diminish the absorption of cholesterol in animals, presumably because of the competition with cholesterol for incorporation into micelles and for transport across the intestinal mucosa.[5] Absorption of β-sitosterol, a steroid similar in its molecular composition to cholesterol, is less than 5% of a single oral dose in vivo, but it is remarkably similar to cholesterol uptake in vitro (inverted sac experiments).[85] The enterocytes apparently have an effective selective ability for absorption of steroids in vivo. In some patients with β-sitosterolemia, absorption is increased to circa 30%.[86] This rare familial storage disease is characterzed by tendon xanthomas, tuberous lesions of the skin, and substantial amounts of plant sterols in plasma, adipose tissue, and erythrocytes even though plasma concentrations of cholesterol are normal. The accumulation of plant sterols is most likely caused by the loss of normal intestinal selectivity for the absorption of cholesterol.

Since animal tissue lacks the ability to alkylate the sterol side chain at the C-24 position, the β-sitosterol must be derived from vegetable matter in the diet;[4] a further study of this rare disease might give a better understanding of the development of the more common cholesterol-containing xanthomas at an early age despite near normal concentrations of plasma cholesterol. The intestinal absorption specificity for cholesterol is unlikely to be related to differences in incorporation in micelles, since β-sitosterol and cholesterol have the same partition coefficients between the oil and micellar phases.[80] It is not known whether the specificity is related to the transportation of the sterol into the mucosa, its intracellular esterification, or to its incorporation into TG-rich lipoproteins (VLDL and chylomicrons). The presence of BS in the bowel lumen seems to be essential for re-esterification and mucosal transport of cholesterol. The poor intestinal absorption of β-sitosterol is used to obtain a measurable degree of bacterial degradation of sterols in the intestinal tract, necessary in the combined chemical and isotopic balance studies performed to determine cholesterol absorption in man.[4,73]

In many of the studies reported so far, it is obvious that there are wide variations, intra- and interindividually, in respect to the amount of cholesterol that is degraded; figures of 10 to 500 mg of cholesterol/day have been published. One may summarize this discussion by stating that approximately half of the cholesterol in the bowel lumen is of endogenous origin. About 40 to 50% of the cholesterol is absorbed from the bowel lumen, thereby establishing a balance. A cholesterol-rich diet increases the cholesterol pool including higher blood cholesterol levels. Human beings can regulate their blood cholesterol with little variation, and although they increase blood cholesterol approximately 15% as a response to an increase of a dietary cholesterol load, most of the serum cholesterol is of endogenous origin, and its level is mainly regulated by endogenous synthesis.

However, it has now been well established that in the long run a diet low in cholesterol and saturated fats with limited amounts of animal protein leads to significantly lower serum cholesterol levels in a high percentage of the population.

## TRANSPORT AND METABOLISM

Absorbed lipids are transported in water-soluble form from the small intestine to other tissues. Fatty acids with chain lengths shorter than 12 carbon atoms are bound to albumin and preferentially transported directly to the liver via the portal vein. Only a small proportion of the medium-chain FA undergoes a conversion to long-chain FA and is esterified to TG.[87] A very small fraction of LCFA is transported via the portal route. This fraction increases when LCTs are fed in combinations with MCTs. The absorbed lipid fractions consist of FA, 2-MG, lyso PL, some PL, and small amounts of glycerol and cholesterol. Some of these lipid fractions (like FA and lysolecithin) are reactive molecules and may lyse cell membrane. The first step in mucosal transport is re-esterification, and the second step is synthesis of transport particles: the so-called lipoprotein particles.

### Re-esterification of TG and PL

Re-esterification of TG and PL is inter-related and discussed together.

**Re-esterification Pathway.** Most TGs are resynthesized in the enterocytes by the monoacylglycerol pathway. FAs are activated in the microsomes by CoA lipase to acyl-CoA and then reesterified with absorbed 2-monoglycerides. Diglyceride synthesis followed by TG formation takes place at the endoplasmic reticulum with mono- and diglyceride acyltransferases. Activity of these transacylases is high at the tip of the villi and relatively low in the crypt cells. The second pathway, accounting for 20% of enterocytic TG, is the α-glycerophosphate pathway. α-Glycerophosphate is synthesized de novo from triose phosphate and from absorbed free glycerol. Phosphatidic acid is formed and then dephosphorylated, resulting in 1,2-diglyceride which is then esterified to TG. Part of the phosphatidic acid is metabolized into phospholipids, which participate in chylomicron formation.

Another minor pathway for the formation of phosphatidic acid is the dihydroxyacetone phosphate pathway.[96] The ratio of TG formed from exogenous sources or esterification of endogenously formed diglycerides (an average ratio of 4:1) depends on the amount of exogenous TG. Following ingestion of a high-fat meal, more phosphatidic acid is used for PL synthesis because there is a maximum ratio between TG and PL in the chylomicron. The pathways of transportation of MCFA are different, and they have been discussed earlier.

**Esterification of Cholesterol.** Cholesterol is transported by the chylomicrons in two forms: as free cholesterol forming part of the hydrophylic outer layer of the chylomicron and as esterified cholesterol in the hydrophobic core of the chylomicron. Esterification of cholesterol takes place in the mucosa shortly before the chylomicron enters the lymph through the lateral leaky cell membrane of the enterocyte. Esterification is accomplished by incorporation of acyl-CoA into the cholesterol molecule by the microsomal acyl-CoA-cholesterol acyltransferase. In summary, the absorbed lipids are incorporated in the chylomicrons as TG, PL, free cholesterol, and cholesterol esters.

**Principles of Intravascular Transport.** Before comparing the changes and activities of the lipoprotein particles to vascular lipid transport, we would like to review schematically the principles of intravascular transport. Of the three main classes of lipids (TG, PL, and cholesterol), the TGs are used primarily as a fuel or are stored in fat depots. The PL and cholesterol are the principal constituents of plasma and biomembranes and also participate in intracellular transport as constituents of micelles and emulsified particles. As mentioned previously, they are also secreted with BS as mixed micelles into the canicular bile.

Since most of the energy for muscle contractions (including the heart muscle) in the fasting state is supplied by oxidation of FA released by adipose tissue, a continuous uptake of FA from the blood stream takes place. In the non-fasting state, FA are derived from chylomicrons and VLDL under the influence of lipoprotein lipase.

Like enterocytes, endothelial cells cannot take in TG, but MG and FA pass through the plasma membranes. TG, containing LDL, HDL, and remnants, however, can pass through the endothelial gaps and by pinocytosis. FA bound to albumin are rapidly taken up by the endothelium. The major source of FA is the TG present in the circulating lipoprotein particles. Although located in the lipid core of the lipoprotein particle, they are an accessible substrate for lipoprotein lipase present at the surface of the endothelial membrane and also to a hepatic lipase secreted by the liver.

## Chylomicrons and VLDL

The long chain nutritional TG are not transported from the intestinal mucosal cells until chylomicrons have been formed. These consist of about 86% TG, 8.5% PL, 3% cholesterol and cho-

lesteryl ester, and 2% protein. There is evidence that apo-B proteins in intestinal VLDL and chylomicrons are different from liver VLDL. Up to 20% of total VLDL is synthesized in the intestine and carries exogenous lipids, whereas liver VLDL contains only endogenous FA. The apoproteins of the two intestinal lipoproteins are different from liver VLDL and contain apo-B48 instead of apo-B100 and do not react with the apo-B100 receptors of peripheral cells. The intestinal VLDL and chylomicrons exchange components with HDL particles during lymphatic transport and blood circulation. The apo-C and E transferred from the HDL are essential for the metabolism of the intestinal chylomicron particles. This is because apo-C is the cofactor for lipoprotein lipase activation, and apo-E, remaining in the chylomicron remnants, is essential for uptake by the hepatocyte by binding to the apo-E receptors to initiate endocytosis. Lipoprotein lipase not only hydrolyzes TG but also the PL to lyso PL. As illustrated by Figure 3–6, hydrolysis affects particle size.

Thus, FA and MG in the circulation originate from exogenous and endogenous sources. Normal individuals have a large reserve of TG in their fat depots and can tolerate prolonged periods of fasting. The constant exchange of surface materials and apolipoproteins, donated by the HDL to chylomicrons and VLDL particles in exchange for PL, induce complicated changes in the properties of the lipoprotein particles and regulate binding to the specific apoprotein binding sites located on the membranes of various cell systems.[89] Transportation of cholesterol and the role of esterification by the lecithin-cholesterol acyltransferase (LCAT) system by transfer of FA from PL is discussed elsewhere.

In short, the principal vehicles for transport of TG from the gut to tissues via lymph and blood circulation to the liver, fat depots, and muscles are the chylomicrons and intestinal VLDL. Hepatic VLDL and LDL function primarily as an internal transport mechanism for TG, PL, and cholesterol; whereas, HDLs function primarily a reverse transport system of tissue cholesterol to the hepatocytes.

We will now discuss in more detail the interactions between the lipoproteins as affected by exchange or transfer of their constituents, hormones, and enzymes (Fig. 3–7). Alimentary lipemia starts 1 to 2 hours after ingestion of fat, reaches a maximum at 3 to 5 hours, and decreases to reach fasting levels usually by 8 to 10 hours.[90] Hydrolysis of chylomicrons and VLDL TG is catalysed by lipoprotein lipase, an enzyme situated in part at the luminal surface of the endothelium, but also present in fat cells. Liver also contains a

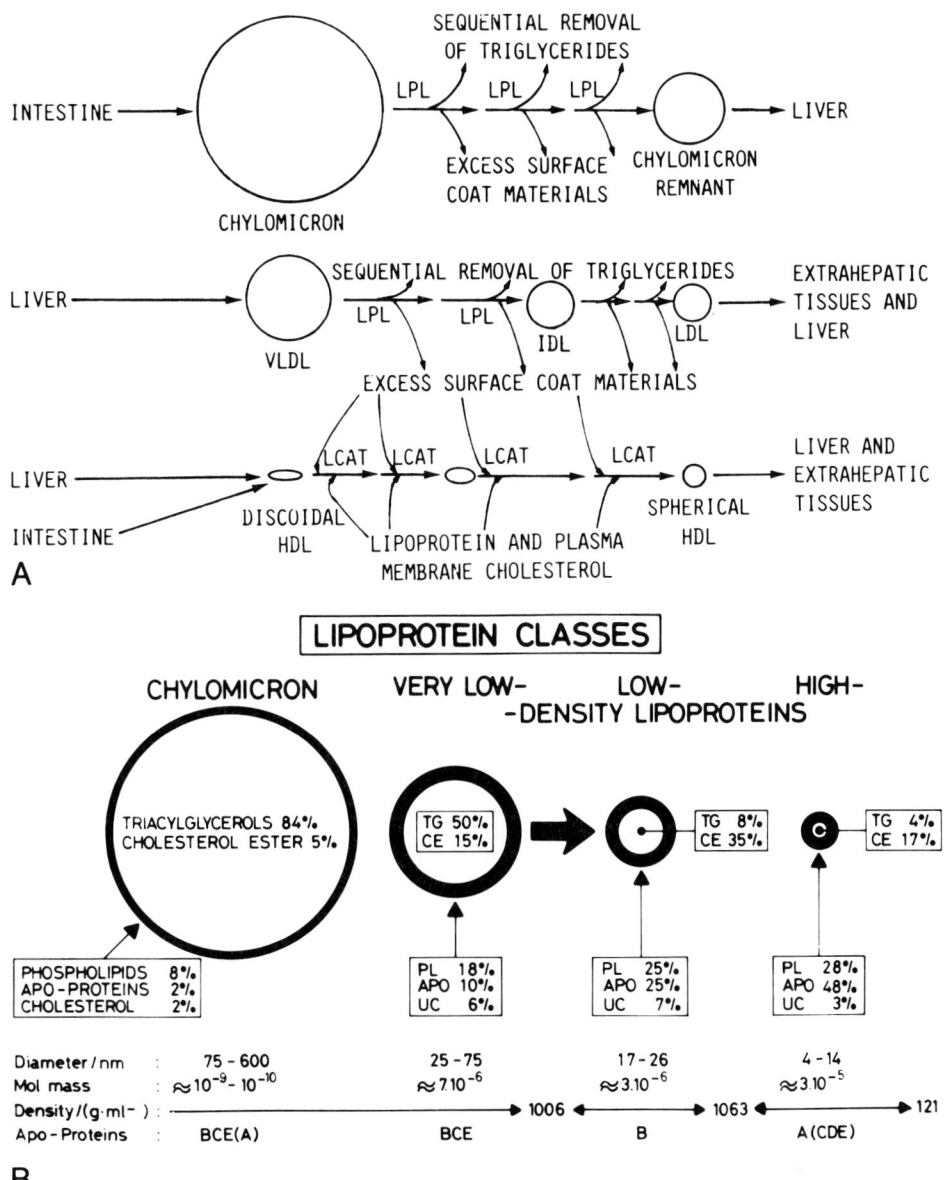

**Fig. 3–6.** *A*, Schematic representation of lipid transport processes. (Used with permission of publisher and author. Nishida, T.: *In* Dietary Fats and Health. Perkins, E.J., and Visek, W.J., Eds. Champaign, IL, American Oil Chemists' Society, 1983.) *B*, Composition of lipoprotein particles.

lipase that can hydrolyze lipoprotein TG, but it has different properties from lipoprotein lipase or endothelial and adipose tissue cells. Lipoprotein lipase activity in blood is affected by many circulating compounds.[91,92]

As stated before, apo-C2 activates lipoprotein lipase. Heparin in small doses releases lipoprotein lipase instantly into plasma, and it has been suggested that heparin of endogenous origin is an important regulating mechanism in the circulation of this enzyme. Furthermore, there is a definite stimulating effect of insulin on lipoprotein

lipase activity; this explains the high incidence of hypertriglyceridemia in diabetes mellitus. The earliest effect of insulin on adipose tissue lipoprotein lipase appears to be enhanced secretion of the enzyme by adipocytes;[93] this leads to increased extracellular activity. Nicotinic acid also activates lipoprotein lipase, but glucagon, ACTH, and TSH inhibit it. In general, its activity is decreased by several hormones with high activity in the fasting state.

The FA of chylomicron and VLDL TG are largely taken up by extra-hepatic tissues and used for: (1)

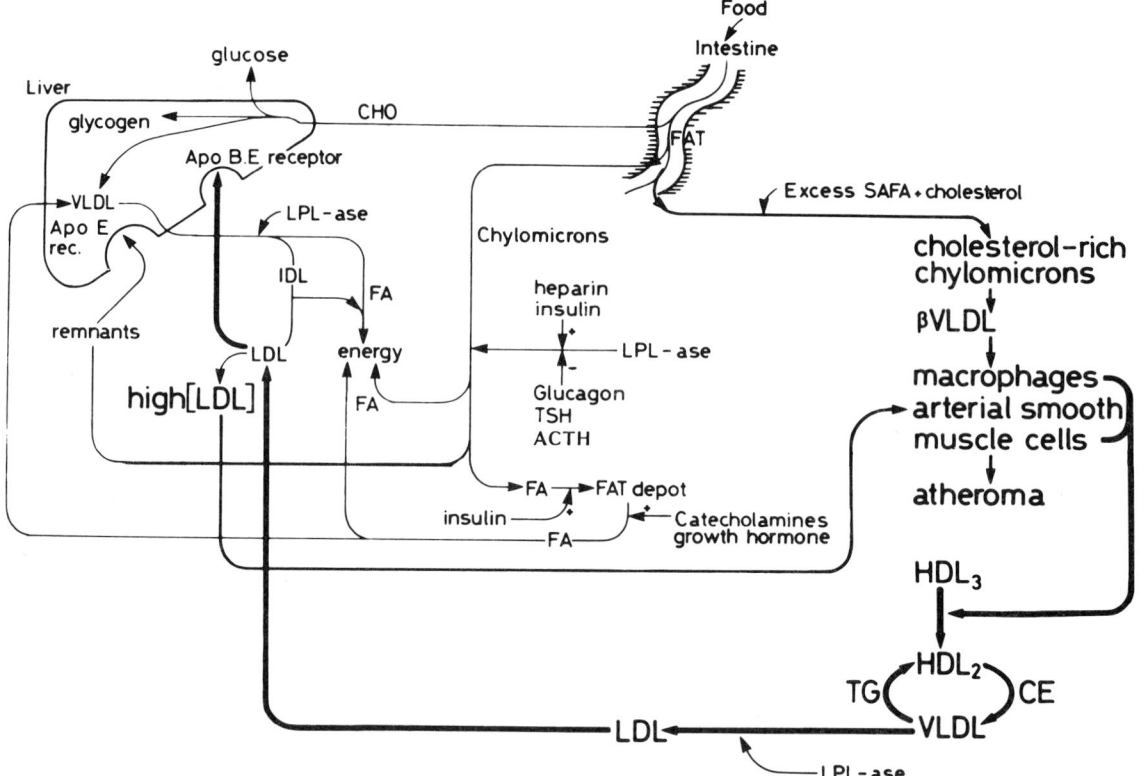

**Fig. 3–7.** Simplified scheme of the conversion of absorbed carbohydrates (CHO), fat and cholesterol to liver VLDL (with apo-B100), chylomicrons (with apo-B48) and β-VLDL. Lipoprotein lipase (LPL-ase) activity is stimulated by heparin and insulin and inhibited by glucagon, thyroid-stimulating hormone (TSH), and adrenocorticotrope hormone (ACTH). Insulin stimulates triglyceride formation in fat depots, and catecholamines and growth hormone stimulated adipose tissue lipase with fatty acid (FA) are released as a consequence. Excess VLDL formation in liver by excess dietary CHO or blood FA results in excess formation of LDL and atheroma. The same occurs at too high saturated fat (SAFA) and cholesterol consumption with the consequent formation of the atherogenic β-VLDL. HDL3 is within certain limits capable of removing excess cholesterol from macrophages. The resulting HDL2 particles transport the cholesterol to VLDL and are converted to LDL, which is taken up by liver and peripheral cells. The latter pathway is contributing also to atheroma formation, however. (Scheme is based on Ref. 98, 100, 101, 102, 103.)

energy production, especially by heart, red muscle fibers, smooth muscle cells, kidney, and platelets; (2) incorporation into phospholipids of all cellular biomembranes; the FA composition determines to a great extent biomembrane function and integrity, as well as biosynthesis of prostaglandins, thromboxanes, and leukotrienes; (3) a major source of stored energy by its deposition in adipose tissues as TG.

The types of dietary FA determine to a great extent whether they can be used for function 1, 2, or 3. Saturated and monounsaturated FA with chain lengths of 20 C or more cannot be used optimally for function 1[58] and MCFA not for 3. These specific effects were discussed earlier in this chapter. It is important to realize though that the FA composition of endogenous TG—transported mainly in VLDL—is affected indirectly by dietary composition because this determines adipose tissue composition and the degree of FA bio-

synthesis from carbohydrates by the liver. The latter mainly consists of C16:0, C18:0 and C18:1 n-9, contrary to the much greater variety of FA present in normal foods.

**Free Fatty Acids.** The tissue uptake of FA is proportional to its plasma concentration[90] and probably also is dependent upon FA binding within plasma. Free FA are transported largely in the form of firmly bound but rapidly reversible complexes with plasma albumin, which has two active binding sites for free FA and four to five weaker sites. Very low concentrations of free FA are present as monomers in solution, but they are transferred only as monomers into the cells. Most of the albumin-bound free FAs in blood are derived from lipolysis of TG in adipose tissue during fasting. In addition, they are released postprandially during hydrolysis of chylomicron and VLDL TG by lipoprotein lipase.

Lipolysis of adipose tissue TG increases during

fasting to meet the energy requirements of tissues (muscle especially) dependent on FA oxidation for ATP synthesis. The capacity of adipose tissue for stored energy is far greater than the available energy from muscle and liver glycogen. It is therefore useful that free FA mobilization increases as a result of stimulation by catecholamine during muscular activity and acute stress.[94,95] In man, plasma free FA are also increased by the growth hormone, glucagon, and thyroxine[90] (Fig. 3–7).

After the FA have entered the cells (particularly adipocyte and muscle cells), they are rapidly re-esterified to TG if not taken up by mitochondria for oxidation and ATP synthesis. The glycerol-3 phosphate, required for re-esterification of FA in extrahepatic tissue, is derived from glucose, and therefore TG accumulation is dependent upon insulin concentrations. During TG hydrolysis, glycerol is released. Plasma glycerol concentration is a reliable index of lipolysis because glycerol is not reutilized for esterification by adipocytes.

The release of free FA depends on the balance between lipolysis and re-esterification. Carbohydrate feeding reduces the concentration of plasma-free FA by augmenting insulin concentration. Insulin regulates primarily FA levels in plasma, since it has not only a potent stimulating effect upon re-esterification, thereby opposing the effects of catecholamines, growth hormone, and glucagon, but it also inhibits lipolysis.

These hormonal interactions are further complicated by locally synthesized prostaglandins $E_1$ and $E_2$, which also inhibit catecholamine-stimulated lipolysis in adipose tissue.[96] Because prostaglandin biosynthesis is stimulated by catecholamines, these observations are compatible with a physiologic role of prostaglandin E in the regulation of lipolysis, possibly by a feedback mechanism.

The intestine and particularly the liver take up about 40 to 50% of the free FA leaving plasma in man.[97] In the liver, FA are largely incorporated into TG, and some may be stored there to be utilized for energy production on subsequent hydrolysis. The major part, however, is incorporated into VLDL and secreted again in the plasma.[98] An increased peripheral lipolysis during prolonged starvation or diabetes will result in greater esterification to TG in the liver, thereby producing a fatty liver.[99] Increased synthesis of VLDL also leads to hypertriglyceridemia.[100]

The properties of the VLDL secreted by the liver are to some extent dependent upon the load of TG requiring transport; this is analogous to the situation occurring in the intestinal mucosa. High carbohydrate feeding in man results in increased production of VLDL having the characteristics of chylomicrons.[90] Diets high in saturated fat and cholesterol also cause major changes in the lipoproteins.[101] These changes include a reduction of typical HDL (without apo-E), an increase of HDL with apo-E (HDLc), and an increase of LDL and of a cholesterol-rich lipoprotein that floats at a density of less than 1.006 g/ml and has β-electrophoretic mobility (β-VLDL).

Important advances in our understanding of the function of apolipoprotein E in the metabolism of TG-rich lipoproteins has been derived from mutations of this protein. Three common isoforms of apo-E have now been identified. Two of those (E-3 and E-4) are associated with normal lipoprotein concentrations. However, E-2 is associated with accumulation of chylomicron and VLDL remnants in blood.[91] In rats, the apo-E, together with several C-apoproteins, are added to the surface of chylomicrons from HDL after their secretion from the intestine mainly in exchange for phospholipids. Until the apo-C is removed from chylomicrons during hydrolysis by lipoprotein lipase, the chylomicron remnants are not taken up by the liver because the liver has mainly apo-E receptor sites.

As already discussed, two apo-B proteins also play a role in selective hepatic uptake of remnants of VLDL and LDL.[92] HDLc (with apo-E) is formed in plasma or in extracellular space as a result of HDL (without apo-E) accepting cholesterol from peripheral tissue.[102] The free cholesterol is esterified by lecithin-cholesterol acyltransferase (LCAT). After the HDL enrichment with cholesteryl ester, the apo-E is redistributed from other plasma lipoproteins to HDLc.[101] HDLc with apo-E interacts with apo-B,E receptors. These receptors are only exposed when the cells lack the required amount of cholesterol for cholesterol homeostasis. HDL with apo-E will not only redistribute cholesterol to other cells that require cholesterol for cell growth and steroid synthesis (e.g., adrenals, testis, ovary) but it will redistribute cholesterol also to hepatocytes for biliary secretion or lipoprotein synthesis.

Recent studies have shown that apo-E may serve as the major determinant for lipoprotein recognition by hepatic receptors.[101] In immature dogs and pigs, the liver also possesses typical apo-B,E receptors in addition to the apo-E receptors. The apo-B,E receptor binds LDL and HDL without apo-E. In the liver of adult dogs, the apo-B,E receptor can be induced by treatment with cholestyramine (a drug binding intestinal cholesterol so that it is no longer available for reabsorption) or by prolonged fasting.[103] In the immature dog liver, the apo-B,E receptors are blocked by cholesterol feeding. This suggests that the apo-B,E receptors in the immature liver facilitate the increased cholesterol requirement in fast growing tissues in the absence of adequate endogenous cholesterol biosynthesis. Recently it has been found that a cholesteryl ester transfer protein can transfer cholesteryl esters from HDLc to VLDL and chylomicrons and subsequently transport it to the liver.[104] This pathway will be less effective if the VLDL and chylomicrons are already rich in cholesterol as is the case in hypercholesterolemia, including the diet-induced ones.

Diets high in saturated fats and cholesterol are atherogenic and are associated with a marked reduction in HDL without apo-E; apparently, the regulating role of HDL in cholesterol metabolism is stressed beyond its capacity in this situation. When there are sufficient other lipoproteins available for cholesterol transport, the excess cholesterol will be transported to other tissues than the liver and will cause atherosclerosis in the arterial walls by accumulation in macrophages and smooth muscle cells in the subendothelial tissue. Especially important in this respect are the β-VLDL that float at d <1.006 but have a β-electrophoretic mobility and are formed in diet-induced hypercholesterolemia. There are clear species-related differences in the origin of β-VLDL: in rabbits these arise as chylomicron remnants,[105] but in dogs and rats, species characterized by a high resistance to atherosclerosis, the β-VLDL appear to be of hepatic origin.[101,106]

Irrespective of their origin, β-VLDL are cholesterol-rich, contain apo-B,E, and interact with a specific high affinity apo-B,E receptor on the surface of macrophages. Unlike the apo-B,E receptor of fibroblasts or smooth muscle cells, the β-VLDL uptake is only partially suppressed as the macrophages accumulate cholesterol.[101] Actually β-VLDL seems to be the only naturally occurring lipoprotein that can cause a substantial (20- to 160-fold) increase in the cholesteryl-ester content of macrophages, converting these into foam cells.[107] Because production of β-VLDL can be induced in man by high cholesterol feeding[109,110] and is present in plasma of patients with hyperlipoproteinemia type III, one can assume that these lipoproteins play a role in atherogenesis in man in addition to the well-known atherogenic properties of LDL.[110]

In familial hypercholesterolemia (type II), patients are deficient in apo-B, and E receptors in all tissues; this deficiency produces corresponding high LDL levels in plasma. This does not explain, however, how the high LDL concentration can lead to accumulation of cholesteryl ester in subendothelial arterial tissue. Diets high in saturated fat (and cholesterol) cause, in most subjects, augmented LDL5 levels, with the size of these LDL

particles being greater than 5 times that of normal LDL.[101,111,112] In rhesus monkeys, the rise in cholesterol-induced high molecular weight LDL is correlated with the occurrence and the severity of coronary heart disease.[111] Furthermore, it has been found in several animal species that cholesterol feeding leads to a type of LDL containing a variable amount of apo-E next to the normally major apo-B moiety.[101] However, neither the apo-B LDL nor the apo-B,E LDL causes cholesteryl ester accumulation in macrophages. Recently[111] it has been shown that LDL can be modified to an unknown extent by, e.g., malondialdehyde released from platelets (malondialdehyde is one of the metabolic end products produced from thromboxane A released during platelet aggregation) or from lipid peroxidation at sites of damaged arterial tissue. This modified LDL appears to be capable of delivering cholesterol to macrophages and might explain the atherogenicity of raised concentrations of LDL. Individual genetically-based differences in β-VLDL formation, apo-B,E receptors, and LDL metabolism can at least partly explain the existence of hypo- and hyper-responders to dietary modification in many animal species, including man.[113,115,117,118] For a simplified scheme of these pathways see Figure 3–7.

## BIOSYNTHESIS

Given an adequate energy uptake, cholesterol and related sterols, phospholipids, sphingo- and glycolipids, and TG can be synthesized by many animal tissues if the requirements for essential minerals, vitamins, essential aminoacids, and the essential FA are met adequately.

### Phospholipids (PL)

PL and cholesterol are the principal components of all biomembranes, and they are both synthesized by the endoplasmic reticulum (ER) of many cell systems, particularly the liver and intestine. The ER itself consists of bilayers with PL being assembled from its components by the synthesizing enzymes located in the ER bilayer. The membranes, consisting of PL, cholesterol, and protein molecules, serve not only as boundaries between individual cells but also as a means to compartmentalize several major biochemical processes within the cell. The FA composition of the PL contributes significantly to the physical and biochemical properties of the membranes and is closely regulated by the proportion of saturated, mono-, and polyunsaturated FA.

The saturated and monounsaturated FA are derived from either diet or de novo synthesis by the condensation of acetate units, eventually followed by direct oxidative desaturation of long chain FA to, e.g., oleic acid. In contrast, essential FA with cis double bonds on the n-3 and/or n-6 position can be derived only from dietary sources (for further details see the section on essential FA). Under normal conditions, most tissues have phospholipids in cellular plasma membranes, which are characterized by having predominantly either linoleic or arachidonic acid esterified in the two position. On activation of phospholipase A-2, the released arachidonic acid is the preferred substrate for both lipoxygenase and cyclo-oxygenase; this leads to instantaneous biosynthesis of various leukotrienes, thromboxane $A_2$ or prostaglandins of the two-type. These are reviewed in the last section.

Continued feeding of an essential fat deficient diet leads to partial replacement of arachidonic acid by 20:3, n-9, 12, 15 all cis,[165] which is a substrate for lipoxygenase but not for cyclo-oxygenase.[188,191] Feeding a diet high in polyunsaturated fats of the n-3 type (linseed oil, fish oil) results in an enrichment of membrane PL with eicosapentaenoic acid (20:5, n-3, 6, 9, 12, 15, all cis) and docosahexaenoic acid (C22:6, n-3, 3, 6, 9, 12, 15, 18).[202]

*Phosphatidylcholine* (the preferred name for lecithin, a term also used for crude mixtures of various PL, oil, and carbohydrates produced during processing of edible oils is a prominent PL in the outer layer of the cell plasma membranes (in platelets 41%) and in lipoproteins. Recent research by Wurtman et al. has demonstrated that dietary phosphatidylcholine is an important contributor to blood and brain choline concentrations,[119] which codetermine the rate of acetylcholine biosynthesis, especially during rapid firing of cholinergic neurons.

Phosphatidylcholine is mainly responsible for the hydrophilic properties of the surface coat of chylomicrons and VLDL. When TG are mobilized from the hydrophobic core by lipoprotein lipase and the particle decreases in size, lecithin is exchanged for apoproteins of the HDL particles. Nascent HDL particles are excellent receptors of free cholesterol from other lipoprotein particles or endothelial membranes. Circulating LCAT, secreted by the liver and activated by apoprotein $A_1$ of the HDL surface, synthesizes cholesterol ester via transfer to free cholesterol by acyltransferase of the (poly) unsaturated FA located on the 2 position of the HDL PL. The HDL particles have then become spherical (mature) and are partly catabolized by the liver, fibroblasts, and elements of the vascular wall. Lysolecithin can be re-esterified by FA released by lipolysis of TG, of chylomicrons, or VLDL or LDL, and LCAT now has lysolecithin-acyltransferase activity.[120]

**Regulation of Biliary Phospholipids.** Synthesis and secretion of biliary PL depends on biliary BS secretion. BS output is regulated by hepatic uptake of BS from plasma. When plasma BS levels are very low during fasting, synthesis and secretion of BS are also at a very low level. Plasma concentrations of BS depend on absorption of BS from the intestinal lumen. CCK released from the gut mucosa stimulates BS synthesis and induces contraction of the gallbladder. Both actions of CCK result in increased BS levels in blood plasma by absorption from the gut lumen. The composition of the FA of biliary PL is different from that of lipoprotein PL. Secretion rates reach a plateau, and it is most likely that de novo synthesis has a maximum rate of 3 to 4 $\mu$mol/ml lecithin.[121] Synthesis of PL, which will be incorporated in the hepatic lipoprotein particles, takes place at a much slower rate and is independent of BS synthesis.

### Sterols

Outstanding reviews of the biosynthesis of cholesterol by several authors have been published in the last decade and will be summarized here only in respect to the main points.[4,73,90]

Cholesterol can be synthesized in all tissues from acetate. The rate of synthesis is high in the liver and the intestine but very low in the adult brain.[123] As early as the 18th week of gestation, the fetus is capable of synthesizing cholesterol from small molecules.[124] Incorporation of the carbon of acetate and glucose into cholesterol is much higher in the fetus than in the adult; however, it falls sharply at birth and rises again at weaning to a level higher than in adults. Eventually, though, it falls again to adult levels. The concentrations of $\beta$-hydroxy-$\beta$-methyl glutaryl (HMG)-CoA reductase per mg of protein in the liver follow a similar growth pattern. This fact suggests that the reduction of HMG-CoA by this enzyme is a rate-limiting step in the conversion of acetate into cholesterol in fetal and neonatal life as well as in the adult.[125]

The rate of synthesis is not only different in relation to the stage of development but varies widely in different tissues and in a given tissue under different conditions. However, the biosynthetic pathway beginning with acetate is similar and has been largely elucidated.[126–129]

Acetate can be converted into mevalonic acid by a sequence of reactions starting with acetate + ATP + CoA → acetyl-CoA + AMP + PP. However, most of the acetyl-CoA used for sterol synthesis is not derived from this reaction but is generated within the mitochondria by the $\beta$-oxidation of FA or, via oxidative decarboxylation, pyruvate is converted into citrate, which diffuses into the cytosol and is hydrolyzed to acetyl-CoA and oxaloacetate by citrate-ATP lyase:

$$\text{citrate} + \text{ATP} + \text{CoA} \longrightarrow$$
$$\text{acetyl-CoA} + \text{oxaloacetate} + \text{ADP} + \text{P} + \text{H}_2\text{O}$$

The citrate participating in this reaction acts as a carrier for transporting acetyl carbon across the mitochondrial membranes, which are impermeable to acetyl-CoA. Subsequently, in the cytosol, acetyl-CoA is converted into mevalonate via:

$$2 \text{ acetyl-CoA} \longrightarrow \text{acetoacetyl-CoA} + \text{CoA}$$

$$\text{Acetoacetyl-CoA} + \text{acetyl-CoA} + \text{H}_2\text{O} \longrightarrow$$
$$\text{HMG-CoA} + \text{CoA}$$

$$\text{HMG-CoA} + 2\text{NADPH} + 2\text{H}^+$$
$$\underline{\text{HMG-CoA reductase}} \longrightarrow \text{mevalonate}$$
$$+ 2\text{NADP}^+ + \text{CoA}$$

HMG-CoA reduction is suppressed by prolonged cholesterol feeding (probably by the increased flux of chylomicron remnants into the liver) and by fasting. A rise in cyclic-AMP concentration also appears to decrease the activity of HMG-CoA reductase.[90] This provides a plausible explanation for the effect of some hormones on HMG-CoA reductase activity, e.g., the stimulatory effect of insulin and the inhibitory effect of glucagon.[130]

Mevalonic acid is phosphorylated, isomerized, and converted via geranyl- and farnesyl-pyrophosphate into squalene (Table 3–2). Squalene is then oxidized and cyclized to a steroid ring—lanosterol. In the last steps, lanosterol is converted into cholesterol by the loss of 3 methyl groups, saturation of the side chain, and a shift of the double bond from $\Delta^8$ to $\Delta^5$. During the later stages of cholesterol biosynthesis, the intermediates are bound to a sterol carrier protein. Dietary manipulations—e.g., fat and cholesterol feeding—alter the concentration of this protein and its ability to stimulate later stages in cholesterogenesis in vitro.[131] A similar role in the intact living cell, however, has yet to be demonstrated conclusively.[90]

Suppression of cholesterol synthesis by cholesterol feeding—"feedback inhibition"—has been shown to occur in many animal species, including man.[132] In most mammals, the inhibitory effect is confined almost entirely to the liver, though prolonged feeding with cholesterol may cause some inhibition of sterol synthesis in the intestinal wall and the adrenals.

Interruption of the enterohepatic circulation by means of a bile fistula, an ileal bypass, diets high in β-sitosterol, or therapy with cholestyramine and similar drugs enhances the rate of synthesis of cholesterol in the liver. Part of this effect can

probably be explained by a depressing effect of bile salts, such as taurocholate, on the activity of HMG-CoA reductase in the liver.[133,134]

The effects of various hormones upon sterol synthesis in the liver are difficult to interpret because many conflicting data exist.[135] In vivo, the hormones will influence the liver not only directly but also indirectly via their actions on other tissues. Of these, adipose tissue plays an important role as a supplier of FA, which are used as a source for the production of acetyl-CoA in the liver. The nutritional state of the subject, for example, will influence insulin levels. Since insulin suppresses FA mobilization, the acetyl-CoA pool in the liver will be affected by insulin levels, especially in the diabetic state or by prolonged fasting. The regulation of cholesterol synthesis in the small intestine differs from that in the liver. Intestinal synthesis is inhibited only to a small extent by fasting and is uninfluenced by cholesterol feeding.[90] However, bile acids in the lumen of the gut do inhibit intestinal synthesis of cholesterol.[136] In rats, guinea pigs and monkeys, synthesis of cholesterol in other tissues was considerably lower than in the liver and intestinal wall and showed little response to the above mentioned factors influencing synthesis of cholesterol in the liver and intestine.

From these data, the view emerged that the regulation of the amount of cholesterol in the body as a whole is mainly centered in the liver. In several types of human cells an essential part of this regulatory system is the ability to develop cell-surface receptors with high affinity for a specific lipoprotein (LDL).[90] In the presence of LDL-receptors, the cell will bind LDL and internalize it; after cholesteryl ester is released from the LDL by hydrolysis, free cholesterol will be available for cell growth and maintenance without using the cellular capacity to synthesize its own cholesterol.

In the absence of LDL receptors as occurs in type IIA hypercholesterolemia, LDL is taken up by a low-affinity process and does not inhibit intracellular synthesis or esterification of cholesterol. The resulting continuous synthesis of cholesterol is responsible for the high levels of cholesterol in familial hypercholesterolemia (type IIA).

Although the lipoprotein particles synthesized by the liver contain mostly esterified cholesterol, the bile contains primarily free cholesterol. Biliary cholesterol is partly synthesized from the lipoprotein particles and partly synthesized de novo by the hepatocytes. Synthesis and release of this free cholesterol into the biliary system is regulated by a BS-dependent and a BS-independent mechanism, which are not yet defined. BS-dependent cholesterol secretion varies curvilinearly with BS secretion, but it reaches its maximum rate much earlier than PL. However, during fasting, when rates of secretion of BS are very low, cholesterol is still secreted by a BS-independent mechanism, resulting in a physiologic supersaturation of bile with cholesterol during fasting.

Cholesterol crystals and eventually cholesterol gallstones may form in patients. This formation is related to the duration of the existence of lithogenic bile in the gallbladder and the presence of a nucleating protein. This protein has been isolated, and analysis of its composition is in progress. Supersaturation of bile depends on the micellar solubilization of cholesterol and is primarily dependent on cholesterol output. As mentioned before, catabolism of sterols is very limited, and elimination of cholesterol depends largely on biliary secretion and, to a minor degree, on formation of BS (cholesterol is the substrate for synthesis of BS).

The populations of western countries have a diet relatively high in cholesterol, saturated fat, and animal protein. They have a high incidence of cholesterol gallstones (USA 15%, England 25%, Sweden >35%). Oriental countries (as documented well in Japan) and African populations on low cholesterol diets have a very low incidence of gallstones. The high incidence of cholesterol gallstones in the female American Indian population (>80%) is related to a genetic disorder resulting in a low output of BS and PL and high concentrations of biliary cholesterol.

Similarly for the PL, there are arguments for the existence of two hepatic cholesterol pools: one based on fast synthesis of biliary free cholesterol for biliary secretion and the other on the much slower synthesis of mostly esterified lipoprotein cholesterol secreted by the hepatocytes in the blood circulation. Both pools have access to cholesterol absorbed from the small bowel lumen and only a fraction of cholesterol secreted by the liver is de novo synthesis.

## Cholesteryl Ester

Tissue cholesterol is mainly in the free alcohol form, but in blood and adrenals about two thirds are esterified. In man, the esterification largely takes place in the plasma by transfer of the FA from the 2-position of plasma PL, under the influence of lecithin-cholesterol acyltransferase (LCAT), to the 3-β-OH group of cholesterol. Because the fatty acids in the 2-position of phospholipids are predominantly of the polyunsaturated type, there is a high percentage of linoleic acid and arachidonic acid in circulating choles-

teryl ester. LCAT is secreted by the liver bound to HDL and reacts preferentially with the free cholesterol of HDL.[138] As discussed before, the esterified cholesterol of HDL is transferred to VLDL subsequently.

Several other esterifying enzymes exist. In the small intestine mucosa, the absorbed free cholesterol is esterified largely with oleic acid before incorporation into chylomicrons. In the liver, acyl-CoA cholesterol:acyltransferase (ACAT), a microsomal enzyme, catalyzes the reaction:

long chain acyl-CoA

$$+ \text{ cholesterol} \rightarrow \text{cholesteryl ester} + \text{CoA}$$

ACAT has a marked specificity towards its fatty acid substrate. In the presence of CoA and ATP, C18:1 is the preferred substrate; in the livers of rats, the order of preference is C18:1 >16:0 >18:0 >18:2. ACAT has been demonstrated in many other tissues, and the activity of this enzyme is increased by a rise of free cholesterol in the cell as a consequence of the uptake of LDL from the medium by the specific LDL receptors as demonstrated in human skin fibroblasts and aortic smooth muscle cells. This increase in ACAT activity may have important consequences for the development of atherosclerotic lesions.

## Bile Acids

Cholesterol is metabolized mainly by conversion into bile acids and steroid hormones. The catabolism of cholesterol to bile acids accounts for 30 to 60% of the cholesterol lost from the human body, a much lower proportion than, for example, in rats (80 to 90% lost as bile acid).[4,90] The conversion takes place in the liver and is under negative feedback control by the bile acids reabsorbed from the intestine. The major known rate-limiting step in this pathway is the first oxidative step, catalyzed by 7-α-hydroxylase. Subsequently the 12α-position is hydroxylated, the 3β-OH is inverted to the 3α-position, the 4 double bond become saturated, and the three terminal carbon atoms of the side chain are removed by a process analogous to β-oxidation. Cholic acid is then formed as cholyl-CoA and is conjugated with glycine or taurine by the formation of a peptide bond between the carboxyl carbon of cholic acid and the amino group of the amino acid.[90]

The pathway for the formation of chenodeoxycholic acid is similar to the formation of cholic acid with the exception that there is no 12α-hydroxylation.[38] In man also, other pathways have been found.[90] After their secretion into the intestinal lumen, the conjugated primary bile acids are modified by bacteria in the lower ileum and large intestine; this process results in the formation of deoxycholate, lithocholate, allocholate, and some 20 other bile acid modifications. Some of these are reabsorbed; therefore, human bile contains also deoxycholic, lithocholic, and urosodeoxy-cholic acids.[90]

About 95% of bile salts participate in an enterohepatic circulation, which plays, as discussed before, an essential role in the absorption of lipids and the regulation of cholesterol metabolism in the liver. If the enterohepatic circulation is interrupted, the rate of synthesis of bile acids increases. This can occur in Crohn's disease of the distal ileum and after ilial resection or a bypass procedure formerly performed for treatment of morbid obesity. Bile acid synthesis increases too by the addition of cholesterol to the diet and by the amount of certain types of fiber added to the food. The latter may be mediated by binding, which inhibits the reabsorption of bile salts from the intestine.[140] This occurs also during therapy with cholestyramine and other anion exchangers that bind bile salts.

## Steroid Hormones

Cholesterol is an obligatory precursor of the adrenocortical hormones. The synthesis of steroids in the gonads and the placenta from cholesterol acts further as the precursor of vitamin D formed through ultraviolet (UV) irradiation of the skin. In man, the amount of cholesterol converted into steroid hormones is much less than that converted into bile acids but by no means negligible. Since the steroid hormone metabolites are excreted mainly in the urine, this loss may be a source of error in the estimation of the overall sterol balance.

## Fatty Acids (Fig. 3–8)

With the exception of the n-3 and n-6 polyunsaturated fatty acids or essential fatty acids (EFA), all other fatty acids can be synthesized by man from any excess of dietary energy. The rate of fatty acid synthesis is strongly linked to the availability of glucose and is marked depressed by fasting, dietary fat, and insulin deficiency. Glucagon also causes a rapid drop in hepatic lipogenesis, probably mediated by the effect of increased cAMP on a hormone-stimulated protein kinase.[141] The pathway for biosynthesis of saturated fatty acids is basically the same in all organisms examined to date. The universal substrate is acetyl-CoA. Citrate transported from the mitochondria is cleaved to acetyl-CoA and oxaloacetate. This reaction is of main importance in controlling the production of fatty acids.

The first step in the fatty acid biosynthetic pathway proper is the conversion of acetyl-CoA to malonyl-CoA. This reaction is catalyzed by acetyl-CoA carboxylase, which is rate-limiting for fatty acid synthesis.[142] Acetyl-CoA then combines sequentially with a series of malonyl-CoA as follows:

$$\text{Acetyl-CoA} + 7 \text{ malonyl-CoA} + 14 \text{ NADPH} + 14\text{H}$$
$$\longrightarrow \text{C16:0 (palmitic acid)} + 7CO_2 + 8CoASH$$
$$+ 14 \text{ NADP} + 6H_2O$$

The whole reaction is catalyzed by a group of enzymes known as fatty acid synthetases, which are localized in the cytosol of hepatocytes.

In man, synthesis of fatty acid takes place mainly in the liver; the adipose tissue apparently is much less active than in many other animal species such as the rat. In mammals, the product is mainly C16:0, which serves as a substrate for microsomal malonyl CoA dependent elongase. Subsequently $\Delta^9$-oxidative desaturation leads to C16:1 and C18:1 by microsomally bound desaturases with a broad chain length specificity—the $\Delta^9$-, $\Delta^6$-, $\Delta^5$- and $\Delta^4$-fatty acyl-CoA desaturases.[143] The monoenoic C16:1, n-7 cis and C18:1, n-9 cis and also linoleic acid (C18:2, n-6, 9 cis, cis) and α-linolenic acid (C18:3, n-3, 6, 9 all cis) are desaturated by the $\Delta^6$-desaturase, which is the regulatory enzyme in this sequence of reactions and which prerequires the presence of a n-9, cis double bond. Consequently, elaidic acid (C18:1, n-9 trans, formed by rumen bacteria or by chemical hydrogenation from the natural cis type of double bonds) cannot be converted by this enzyme. Newly inserted double bonds are always located between the existing ones and the carboxyl group.

In general, it may be stated that the enzymes display highest affinity for the highest unsaturated substrate,[144] the order of preference is:

α-linolenic acid family (n-3) > linoleic acid family (n-6) > oleic acid family (n-9) > palmitoleic acid family (n-7) > elaidic acid family (n-9, trans)[145]

This sequence of preferences has many implications. C20:3, n-9, 12, 15 (all cis) will be synthesized from carbohydrates via C18:1, n-9 cis only in the nearly complete absence of the EFA both of the n-3 and the n-6 types. The presence of C20:3, n-9, 12, 15 in phospholipids instead of C20:4, n-6, 9, 12, 15, C20:5, n-3, 6, 9, 12, 15 and C22:6, n-3, 6, 9, 12, 15, 18 is solid proof for the existence of EFA-deficiency.[146,166]

During the catalytic hydrogenation process of vegetable oils (primarily soy bean oil) and fish oils for the production of some margarines and shortenings, a variety of geometric (i.e., trans) and positional isomers of unsaturated fatty acids are formed in varying amounts. After absorption, these may compete with the EFA and endogenously synthesized fatty acids for desaturation and chain elongation. The biologic effects of trans fatty acids have been reviewed.[147] Long-term nu-

FATTY ACIDS MENTIONED IN THIS CHAPTER

| Name | Code | Formula |
|---|---|---|
| Short and medium-chain saturated fatty acids | C 4:0 – C10:0 | $CH_3 \cdot (CH_2)_{2-8} \cdot COOH$ |
| Lauric acid | C12:0 | $CH_3 \cdot (CH_2)_{10} \cdot COOH$ |
| Myristic acid | C14:0 | $CH_3 \cdot (CH_2)_{12} \cdot COOH$ |
| Palmitic acid | C16:0 | $CH_3 \cdot (CH_2)_{14} \cdot COOH$ |
| Stearic acid | C18:0 | $CH_3 \cdot (CH_2)_{16} \cdot COOH$ |
| Arachidic acid | C20:0 | $CH_3 \cdot (CH_2)_{18} \cdot COOH$ |
| Behenic acid | C22:0 | $CH_3 \cdot (CH_2)_{20} \cdot COOH$ |
| α - Linolenic acid | C18:3, n-3, 6, 9, all cis | $CH_3 \cdot CH_2 \cdot CH\overset{c}{=}CH \cdot CH_2 \cdot CH\overset{c}{=}CH \cdot CH_2 \cdot CH\overset{c}{=}CH \cdot (CH_2)_7 \cdot COOH$ |
| Timnodonic (eicosapentaenoic) acid | C20:5, n-3, 6, 9, 12, 15, all cis | $CH_3 \cdot CH_2 \cdot CH\overset{c}{=}CH \cdot CH_2 \cdot CH\overset{c}{=}CH \cdot CH_2 \cdot CH\overset{c}{=}CH \cdot CH_2 \cdot CH\overset{c}{=}CH \cdot CH_2 \cdot CH\overset{c}{=}CH \cdot (CH_2)_3 \cdot COOH$ |
| Clupanodonic (docosahexaenoic) acid | C22:6, n-3, 6, 9, 12, 15, 18, all cis | $CH_3 \cdot CH_2 \cdot CH\overset{c}{=}CH \cdot CH_2 \cdot CH\overset{c}{=}CH \cdot CH_2 \cdot CH\overset{c}{=}CH \cdot CH_2 \cdot CH\overset{c}{=}CH \cdot CH_2 \cdot CH\overset{c}{=}CH \cdot CH_2 \cdot CH\overset{c}{=}CH \cdot (CH_2)_2 \cdot COOH$ |
| Linoleic acid | C18:2, n-6, 9, all cis | $CH_3 \cdot (CH_2)_4 \cdot CH\overset{c}{=}CH \cdot CH_2 \cdot CH\overset{c}{=}CH \cdot (CH_2)_7 \cdot COOH$ |
| γ - Linolenic acid | C18:3, n-6, 9, 12, all cis | $CH_3 \cdot (CH_2)_4 \cdot CH\overset{c}{=}CH \cdot CH_2 \cdot CH\overset{c}{=}CH \cdot CH_2 \cdot CH\overset{c}{=}CH \cdot (CH_2)_4 \cdot COOH$ |
| Columbinic acid | C18:3, n-6, cis, 9, cis, 13, trans | $CH_3 \cdot (CH_2)_4 \cdot CH\overset{c}{=}CH \cdot CH_2 \cdot CH\overset{c}{=}CH \cdot (CH_2)_2 \cdot CH\overset{t}{=}CH \cdot (CH_2)_3 \cdot COOH$ |
| Dihomocolumbinic acid | C20:3, n-6, cis, 9, cis, 13, trans | $CH_3 \cdot (CH_2)_4 \cdot CH\overset{c}{=}CH \cdot CH_2 \cdot CH\overset{c}{=}CH \cdot (CH_2)_2 \cdot CH\overset{t}{=}CH \cdot (CH_2)_5 \cdot COOH$ |
| Dihomo - γ - linolenic acid | C20:3, n-6, 9, 12, all cis | $CH_3 \cdot (CH_2)_4 \cdot CH\overset{c}{=}CH \cdot CH_2 \cdot CH\overset{c}{=}CH \cdot CH_2 \cdot CH\overset{c}{=}CH \cdot (CH_2)_6 \cdot COOH$ |
| Arachidonic acid | C20:4, n-6, 9, 12, 15, all cis | $CH_3 \cdot (CH_2)_4 \cdot CH\overset{c}{=}CH \cdot CH_2 \cdot CH\overset{c}{=}CH \cdot CH_2 \cdot CH\overset{c}{=}CH \cdot CH_2 \cdot CH\overset{c}{=}CH \cdot (CH_2)_3 \cdot COOH$ |
| Palmitoleic acid | C16:1, n-7, cis | $CH_3 \cdot (CH_2)_5 \cdot CH\overset{c}{=}CH \cdot (CH_2)_7 \cdot COOH$ |
| Oleic acid | C18:1, n-9, cis | $CH_3 \cdot (CH_2)_7 \cdot CH\overset{c}{=}CH \cdot (CH_2)_7 \cdot COOH$ |
| Elaidic acid | C18:1, n-9, trans | $CH_3 \cdot (CH_2)_7 \cdot CH\overset{t}{=}CH \cdot (CH_2)_7 \cdot COOH$ |
| Eicosaenoic acid | C20:1, n-9, cis | $CH_3 \cdot (CH_2)_7 \cdot CH\overset{c}{=}CH \cdot (CH_2)_9 \cdot COOH$ |
| Eicosatrienoic acid | C20:3, n-9, 12, 15, all cis | $CH_3 \cdot (CH_2)_7 \cdot CH\overset{c}{=}CH \cdot CH_2 \cdot CH\overset{c}{=}CH \cdot CH_2 \cdot CH\overset{c}{=}CH \cdot (CH_2)_3 \cdot COOH$ |
| Erucic acid | C22:1, n-9, cis | $CH_3 \cdot (CH_2)_7 \cdot CH\overset{c}{=}CH \cdot (CH_2)_{11} \cdot COOH$ |
| Brassidic acid | C22:1, n-9, trans | $CH_3 \cdot (CH_2)_7 \cdot CH\overset{t}{=}CH \cdot (CH_2)_{11} \cdot COOH$ |
| Cetoleic acid | C22:1, n-11, cis | $CH_3 \cdot (CH_2)_9 \cdot CH\overset{c}{=}CH \cdot (CH_2)_9 \cdot COOH$ |

**Fig. 3–8.** Name, code, and formula of fatty acids mentioned in this chapter.

tritional evaluation of hydrogenated vegetable oils has shown that in mice, rats, and rabbits, no significant differences occur in respect of mortality, life span, growth, organ weights, or histopathology compared to palmitic, stearic, and oleic acid. Although it has been suggested that they may have unfavorable effects by interference with the necessary desaturation steps of linoleic acid to arachidonic acid, the main precursor acid for prostaglandin, thromboxane, and leukotriene biosynthesis, this does occur only at unrealistically high concentrations of n-6, n-9 trans, trans linoleic acid.[147]

Careful studies have found that conversion of C18:2 n-6, 9 (all cis) to C20:4 n-6, 9, 12, 15 (all cis) is affected only by excessive amounts of trans-9, trans-12 octadecadienoic acid (C18:2, n-6, 9 trans, trans)—a minor component of hydrogenated oils.[147] Furthermore, trans fatty acids or their derivatives are not incorporated in the 2-position of phospholipids when n-3 or n-6 polyunsaturated fatty acids are available. Interference of trans FA with the first phase of prostaglandin synthesis— hydrolysis of biomembrane phospholipids by phospholipase $A_2$, which releases the fatty acid on the 2-position—seems unlikely also for this reason.

Dietary polyunsaturated fatty acids play an important role in controlling the conversion of carbohydrate to storage triacylglycerols by selective inhibition of the lipogenic enzymes.[148,149] It is still not known why or how this should be and at what level dietary polyunsaturated FA exert this effect.

This phenomenon explains, at least partly, the very significant VLDL-lowering effect of linoleic acid-rich diets. As LDL is derived from VLDL, a lower VLDL synthesis contributers to the well-known LDL lowering effects of linoleic acid. Interesting in this context are the studies that suggest enhanced synthesis of VLDL-cholesterol by oleic acid (whether from dietary origin or from endogenous synthesis from excess carbohydrates).[150,151] Inhibition by linoleic acid of C18:0-CoA desaturase will limit the C18:1, n-9 synthesized and its control of cholesterol synthesis and so may limit VLDL secretion too.

The degradation of long-chain FA to acetyl-CoA by β-oxidation is important for ATP synthesis (energy production), but it is also potentially of great importance in regulating the composition of membrane lipids and cholesteryl esters. β-oxidation normally takes place in mitochondria, and it would seem capable of modulating not only the quantity but also, by selective degradation, the variety of FA available for structural lipid synthesis. Unfortunately, little is known regarding the specificity or regulation of β-oxidation. For mitochondrial β-oxidation, the FA have to be transported across the mitochondrial membrane in the form of acylcarnitine. Two types of carnitine acyltransferase are involved. These transferases are located on the inner and outer surface of the inner mitochondrial membrane,[152] which is considered a prime regulatory site for β-oxidation.

Rat liver cells have also a peroxisomal β-oxidation activity.[153] Although only low activity was found in normal livers, the livers of rats fed clofibrate and derivatives or oils rich in C20:5, n-3 and C22:6, n-3 contained greatly elevated levels of peroxisomal activity. Because peroxisomes can produce $H_2O_2$, which is potentially harmful for the cell, the cell needs defense mechanisms to protect itself from uncontrolled peroxidative reactions.[153] In the last section, some examples will demonstrate that the defense mechanism fails when diets high in n-3 polyunsaturated fatty acids (a linolenic acid family) are fed.

Feeding rapeseed oil (the high C22:1, n-9 cis variety) or partially hydrogenated marine oil, rich in trans or cis-trans mono- and di-unsaturated FA with 20, 22 and 24 carbon atoms, causes an acute accumulation of triacyl glycerols (high in C20:1 and C22:1 fatty acids) in the heart and red muscle fibres of many animal species.[58,154,155] The fat infiltration reaches a peak after approximately 5 days and decreases gradually, but incompletely, on prolonged feeding. This accumulation slowly leads to focal fibrotic changes in the heart. The acute lipidosis can be explained by an inhibition block of carnitine acyltransferase by C20:1 and C22:1, resulting in reesterification of the C20:1 and C22:1 to TG in the cytoplasm.[157] After a few days, increased lipase activity will induce fatty acid transport from the heart to the liver,[156] which, contrary to the heart muscle, can metabolize these very long chain FA, although more slowly than normal.

Another explanation can be found in the fact that C22:1 acylcarnitines are poorly oxidized by mitochondria.[154] In the liver an adaptive increase in peroxisomal β-oxidation seems to be the most important process explaining the partial adaptation to dietary C20:1 and C22:1.[158] As far as C22:1 FAs are concerned, brassidic (C22:1, n-9, trans), cetoleic (C22:1, n-11, cis) and erucic acid (C22:1 n-9, cis) are all oxidized by rat liver peroxisomes at similar rates, corresponding to approximately 20% of the rate obtained with palmitoyl-CoA.[154]

Although peroxisomal β-oxidation is not complete, the resulting short-chain fatty acids are good substrates for mitochondrial energy production. Although peroxisomal β-oxidation of the very long chain fatty acids is not very efficient, it is a process independent of carnitine. In this way, it plays an important role in converting C22:1 FA to short-chain fatty acids utilizable by the mitochondria. During peroxisomal, β-oxidation $H_2O_2$ is produced, thus increasing the requirements for antioxidant capacity of, for example, superoxide dysmutase and other glutathione- and tocopherol-dependent systems.

It is striking that diets with very long chain FA have many effects common with the action of drugs like clofibrate. A common feature may be the conversion to CoA esters, which are difficult to metabolize, thus triggering the previously discussed adaptation mechanisms. It is therefore not surprising that clofibrate has been found to give a partial protection (50%) against C22:1 induced myocardial lipidosis.[159] These data indicate that consumption of oil and fats rich in C20, C22 and C24 fatty acids creates some complicated biochemical adaptation processes, which explain the observed growth retardation in experimental animals and functional changes in the heart, adrenals, and the liver (for a complete review see ref. 154).

Oils derived from seeds of various Brassica species, e.g., rapeseed and mustard seed oil, are produced and consumed in many countries. In Canada and Northwest Europe, production of rapeseed oil has expanded rapidly since the 1940s. Because fat consumption is high in these areas, some national and international[1] recommendations suggest limiting the amount of C22:1, e.g., in the European Economic Community (EEC) the percentage of C22:1 n-9 and its isomers should be less than 5 of total fatty acid in oils and margarines. Because the modern varieties of rapeseed are very low in C22:1, n-9, this can be easily achieved. In the case of partially hydrogenated fish oils, the FAO/WHO recommends its blending with other oils in the production of food products.[1]

## FUNCTIONS OF ESSENTIAL FATTY ACIDS (EFA)

The Golden Jubilee International Congress on EFA and Prostaglandins convened in 1980 to commemorate the discovery of EFA by Burr and Burr[160] and of the prostaglandins (PG) by von Euler[161] fifty years ago. Quite remarkably, this was the first congress at which numerous scientists working in one of both fields met and reaffirmed, since its discovery in 1964, how closely related the metabolisms of EFA and PG are.[162–164]

This long history has created a confusing amount of literature. In studies on EFA, the main emphasis has been on C18:2, n-6, 9 all cis and C20:4, n-6, 9, 12, 15 all cis; studies have neglected, however, systematic research on the possible dietary essentiality of C18:3, n-3, 6, 9 all cis. Serious gaps in our knowledge also exist with regard to the PG because most of the research has been done on cyclo-oxygenase products of C20:4, n-6 and much less on those of C20:3, n-6 and C20:5, n-3. In respect to the lipoxygenase products of the various EFA, the data are even less complete, although the published results suggest important pathophysiologic functions, especially in inflammatory and thrombotic processes. For these reasons this review will be limited to a summary of the well-documented area of EFA deficiency, followed by a discussion of the pathophysiologic effects of dietary C18:2, n-6 and C20:5, n-3 as far as these are known to involve prostaglandins and leukotrienes metabolism.

## EFA Requirements

Because EFA are necessary for the normal function of all tissues, it is therefore not surprising that the list of symptoms of EFA deficiency is a long one.[165–167] Reduced growth rate, abnormal scaliness, increased loss of water by a change of skin permeability, and male and female infertility are the classic signs. To these can be added kidney abnormalities (papillary necrosis, hematuria, and renal hypertension), abnormal liver mitochondria (increased swelling, depressed ATP synthesis), decreased capillary resistance, increased fragility of erythrocytes, increased susceptibility to infections, decreased myocardial contractility, and decreased prostaglandin biosynthesis.[167] The most sensitive symptom is probably the increased triene (n-9)/tetraene (n-6) ratio ($>0.1$) in phospholipids.[165] Feeding linoleic acid C18:2, n-6 to decrease an abnormally high triene/tetraene ratio has been accepted in the past as curing EFA deficiency.[166] However, it is known now that for an optimal function of various tissues a higher en% of C18:2, n-6 is necessary for normalizing the triene/tetraene ratio.

With regard to growth rate, capillary resistance, fragility of erythrocytes, and mitochondrial function of liver and heart, linolenic acid C18:3, n-3 is similar to C18:2, n-6. On the other hand, with regard to skin condition, increased water consumption, and prostaglandin biosynthesis, dietary C18:3, n-3 and C20:5, n-3 are very much inferior to C18:2, n-6 and the other n-6 polyunsaturated fatty acids. For example, to a greater or lesser extent, a series of synthetic and natural polyunsaturated fatty acids of variable chain lengths and different degrees of unsaturation can normalize abnormal swelling properties of EFA-deficient rat liver mitochondria. For a proper structural function in liver mitochondria, the incorporated fatty acid should have at least 19, but preferably 20, carbon atoms and at least 4 double bonds, two of which are in the cis configuration and the n-6 and n-9 position; the remaining bonds should be methylene interrupted or farther away in respect to these double bonds.[168]

Other fatty acids (such as C20:5, n-3 and C22:6, n-3) had only a minor effect on growth rate and skin condition, although they reduced the C20:3, n-9 levels (increased in EFA deficiency) even

more efficiently than C18:2, n-6, thereby erroneously suggesting a return to normal EFA status. The scaliness of an EFA-deficient skin has been ascribed to insufficient synthesis of PGs,[169] which might be cured by local application of $PGE_2$ or EFA. The efficacy of $PGE_2$ in this respect could not be confirmed by other laboratories, but the efficacy of various EFA of the n-6 type has been confirmed at very low dose levels.[168,170,178,180]

Columbinic acid (C18:3, n-6, 9 cis, cis, 13 trans), present in the seed oil of the *Aquilegia vulgaris*—the columbine—and dihomocolumbinic acid (C20:3, n-6, 9 cis, cis, 13 trans), cannot be converted into PG and has been used as a biochemical tool to differentiate between the structural roles of EFA in various biomembranes and the role of EFA as PG precursor.[170] Columbinic acid, given to EFA-deficient rats either orally or by topical skin application, does restore very efficiently the growth rate of rats and normal skin function. Very interestingly, dihomocolumbinic acid (C20:3, n-6, 9 cis, cis, 13 trans) cured EFA-deficient skin completely, but is had disastrous effects on growth rate, liver and heart mitochondria, and kidney function and was not incorporated in membrane PL. The latter occurred only after shortening of the chain to columbinic acid. In severe EFA deficiency, hematuria is often observed; this is due to lesions in the papillary region. This condition was severely aggravated by dihomocolumbinic acid. There are indications that the abnormal kidney function in EFA deficiency (causing hematuria and hypertension) is caused by a deficiency of PG biosynthesis. Dihomocolumbinic acid, which cannot be converted in PGs, inhibits competitively the conversion of arachidonic acid into PGs. Since EFA deficiency results in low concentrations of arachidonic acid, the consequences of this deficiency are further aggravated. Columbinic acid can prevent the development of infertility in EFA deficiency, which apparently is not caused by low PG biosynthesis. However, when EFA-deficient rats treated with columbinic acid became pregnant, they died of inadequate labor during the parturition. Uterine labor is strongly dependent on normal PG biosynthesis, which was not improved by the addition of columbinic acid.[170]

Until recently, the development of human EFA deficiency was regarded as an extreme rarity. However, with the very sensitive triene/tetraene ratio as a criterion,[1,165] the existence of EFA deficiency has been demonstrated in elderly patients with peripheral vascular disease,[171] in fat malabsorption after major intestinal resection,[172,173] during prolonged fat-free intravenous feeding,[174,175] during low-fat, high-protein dietary supplementation for treatment of kwashiorkor,[176] and in patients after serious accidents and burns.[177] In all these conditions, oral or intravenous feeding of linoleic acid-containing TG easily cured not only the abnormal triene/tetraene ratio but also skin abnormalities. Although not tried, the use of polyunsaturated fatty acids of the n-3 family (e.g., fish oil) would have resulted in persistent dermal lesions that do not respond sufficiently to these fatty acids. It has been shown that a normally low dietary intake of n-6 EFA (in Northwest Europe, North America, Australia, and other countries where the average C18:2, n-6, 9 intake is only 2 to 4 en%) leads to EFA deficiency when a sudden increase of cell regeneration and rapid growth occurs.[176,177] For these reasons, it has been advised (1) that maternal EFA consumption during pregnancy and lactation should be increased from 3 en% to 4.5% and 5 to 7 en%, respectively, to compensate for losses via the placenta and milk. For example, in human milk, lipid provides 60% of the infant's dietary energy, and 10 to 12% of that is EFA. For the prevention of atherosclerosis, equal amounts of linoleic acid and of the various saturated fatty acids are generally recommended.[1] This amount results in 10 to 13 en% of linoleic acid in an American diet.

Lipids are significantly involved in brain development. Most of the EFAs in the brain are of the n-3 type, and it has been postulated that during pregnancy an increased intake of EFA of the n-3 type may be advantageous.[178]

Permanent learning defects and alterations in synaptic function, observed in EFA deficiency, can be prevented by feeding both n-6 or n-6 and n-3 EFA.[179] In rats, EFA deficiency cannot be prevented by feeding only n-3 polyunsaturated fatty acids, but brain development seems normal after feeding high n-6 EFA diets free of n-3 EFA; thus in mammals the n-3 EFAs are probably not absolutely essential.

The determination of human EFA requirements is further complicated from the interactions of EFA with other nutrients. Most investigations on interactions have been made on laboratory animals, but the phenomena observed are considered to operate also in humans.[166] Dietary saturated fatty acids, measured by growth, dermal symptoms, and the triene/tetraene ratio in tissue lipids, increase the EFA requirements. The magnitude of the effect is small, however, because relatively large changes in content of saturated fatty acids are necessary to induce small changes. Saturated fatty acids in human diets increase significantly the levels of VLDL and LDL cholesterol[180,181] and the thrombotic activity of platelets, which can be counteracted by dietary linoleic acid.[182,183] Cis monounsaturated fatty acids (mainly C18:1, n-9, oleic acid) substitute partially for EFA in the lipids of EFA-deficient animals and humans. At high dietary levels, however, the utilization of EFA is suppressed. For example, if the amount of C18:1, n-9 is 10 times higher than C18:2, n-6, 9, a triene/tetraene ratio of 1 was observed; this indicates a frank EFA deficiency.[184]

Trans monounsaturated fatty acids also have been found to increase EFA requirement in animals when fed at moderate levels. In man, C18:1, n-9 trans (elaidic acid) behaves in respect to blood lipids rather like palmitic acid if consumed in diets with a moderate cholesterol content.[2,147] Finally an increased serum cholesterol induced by cholesterol feeding has been found to accentuate EFA deficiency in various animal species.

In several other human diseases like cystic fibrosis,[184] acrodermatitis enteropathica,[184] and peripheral vascular disease,[171] signs of EFA deficiency have been found. Further research will be required before more definite conclusions about causality can be drawn.

## Synthesis of Prostaglandins (PG)

Since the discovery of the possibility of biosynthesis of the prostaglandins $E_2$ and $F_{2\alpha}$ ($PGE_2$ and $PGF_{2\alpha}$) from arachidonic acid (20:4, n-6, 9, 12, 15 all cis) nearly two decades ago,[162,163] our knowledge about the influence of polyunsaturated fatty acids (PUFA) on the biosynthesis of PGs, thromboxane (TXA), leukotrienes (LT) and hydroxy fatty acids has grown explosively. However, the physiologic significance of the various PGs, TXAs, LTs and hydroxy fatty acid pathways has not been clarified, mainly because of a lack of adequate analytical data. The short biologic half-lives, inter- and intraspecies differences, and the synergistic as well as antagonistic biologic activities of the various products synthesized by different tissues in the same individual from the same precursor fatty acid explain why reliable predictions about the influence of dietary PUFA cannot be made (Fig. 3–9 and 3–10). As explained earlier, neither linoleic acid (18:2, n-6, 9 all cis) nor α-linolenic acid (18:3, n-3,6, 9 all cis) can be produced by animal organisms. This means that, for an adequate PG biosynthesis via the cyclooxygenase (CO) pathway or the LT and hydroxy fatty acids biosynthesis by various lipoxygenases (LO), man is dependent on the presence of 18:2, n-6 and 18:3 in the diet. Chain elongation and desaturation of 18:2, n-6 to 20:3, n-6 and 20:4, n-6, which are good substrates for both CO and LO, have been well studied in several animal species[143,145] (Fig. 3–11).

The conversion of 18:3, n-3 to timnodonic acid (20:5, n-3) proceeds efficiently in the rat, but it is much less effective in man[190] (and even less so in rabbits). Several (nonhydrogenated) fish oils are relatively rich in 20:5, n-3 and 22:6, n-3 (cod liver, menhaden, mackerel) and are therefore to be pre-

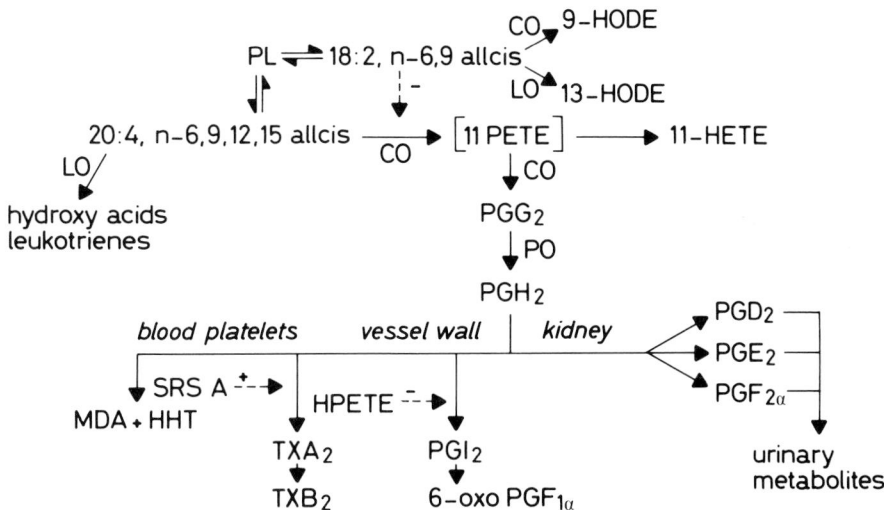

**Fig. 3–9.** Conversion of linoleic acid and arachidonic acid into prostaglandins and thromboxanes. PL = plasma membrane phospholipid; HODE = hydroxyoctadecadienoic acid; HPETE = hydroperoxyeicosatraenoic acid; HETE = hydroxyeicosatetraenoic acid; LO = lipoxygenase; CO = cyclooxygenase; PG = prostaglandin; TX = thromboxane; MDA = malondialdehyde; HHT = hydroxyheptadecatrienoic acid; SRS-A = slow reacting substance of anaphylaxis.

ferred in studies in man (and rabbits) if one is interested in the physiologic effects of dietary PUFA of the n-3 type in relation to PG and LT biosynthesis. 20:5, n-3 is a poor substrate for CO,[186,188] but a good one for LO.[191]

PUFA, especially of the n-3 type, are incorporated preferentially at the 2-position of most cell membrane phospholipids and are considered to play an important role in both cell membrane integrity and function. Cellular stimulation leads to activation of phospholipase A-2 followed by mobilization of the fatty acids on the 2-position of cell membrane phospholipids. The types of these fatty acids determine to a great extent the types of CO and LO products. Important in this respect is that 18:2, n-6, 18:3, n-3, 20:3, n-9 and various cis-trans isomers show competitive inhibition with 20:3, n-6, 20:4, n-6 and 20:5, n-3, the precursors for the known biologically active PG and LT.[170] Many of the other PUFA are substrates for LO, but insufficient data exist to determine whether these LO products are biologically significant.

For the preceding reasons, the best approach to evaluate the physiologic significance of dietary PUFA and their CO and LO products is by doing dietary studies in relation to specific organ functions. The existence of relatively specific inhibitors of CO and LO, such as acetylsalicylic acid, indomethacin, eicosatetraynoic acid, and others, facilitates the interpretation of functional changes. The following short review is limited to EFA of the n-6 or n-3 type, since these types are

involved in the prevention of atherosclerosis and its complications via the CO and LO pathways. This does not mean that essential and nonessential PUFA might not have other important effects on inflammatory and immunologic processes.

### n-6 Polyunsaturated Fatty Acids and Atherosclerosis

Causally related to the induction and progression of atherosclerosis are:

1. Abnormal lipoprotein metabolism leading to increased very low density (VLDL) and low density lipoprotein (LDL) levels. As reviewed earlier, this condition is normally associated with a decreased high-density lipoprotein (HDL) concentration in blood.
2. Increased tendency of blood platelets to form arterial thrombi; mural thrombi narrowing the lumen directly, while embolizing thrombi, are also held responsible for acute myocardial, cerebral, and renal infarcts. As aggregating platelets release also TXA$_2$, a potent vasoconstrictor, it is difficult to differentiate the role of vasospasm from the reduced blood flow due to the thrombus or embolus itself.
3. Increased arterial blood pressure.
4. Abnormal carbohydrate and insulin metabolism (both insulin-dependent and insulin-independent diabetes mellitus).

Available data support the concept that dietary composition—amount and type of fatty acids, cholesterol concentration, Na$^+$ content—in com-

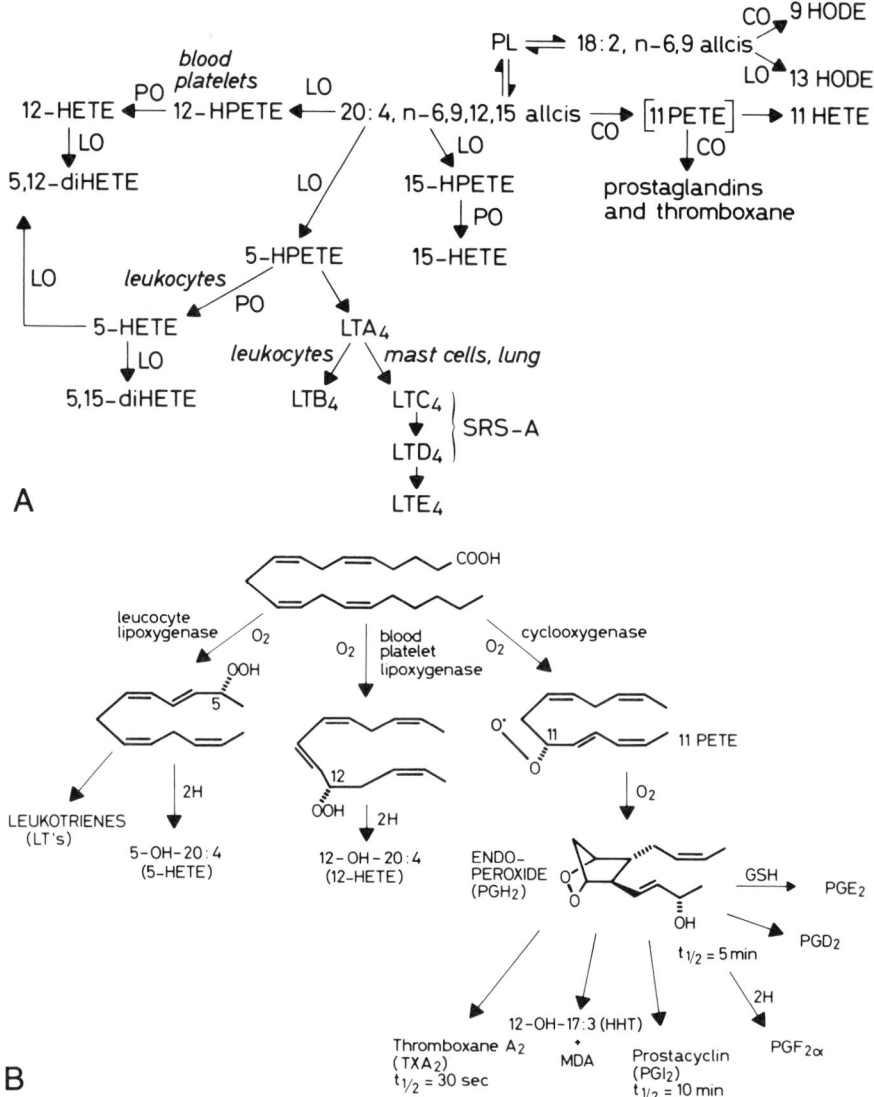

**Fig. 3–10.** *A,* Various prostaglandins synthesized by different organ systems. *B,* Prostaglandin endoperoxide (PGH₂).

bination with genetically determined predispositions determines to a great extent the risk of developing atherosclerosis and its complications. The effects of increased dietary intake of PUFA have been studied in respect to the four factors mentioned and in general have shown to be beneficial.

Measurements of urinary excretion of prostaglandin metabolites in rats and man showed clearly that an increase in linoleic acid consumption does lead to an augmented excretion of PG metabolites.[191,193]

It has been demonstrated convincingly that diets enriched in linoleic acid and reduced in saturated fatty acids do lower significantly LDL and VLDL cholesterol in man at both 30 and 40 en%

of fat levels.[180,181,194] In a series of studies by Iacono et al.,[194] similar diets also lowered moderate age-related hypertension to normal values. The latter results have been confirmed by several other groups[195,196] and are in agreement with epidemiologic data[197] and studies in salt-loaded rats.[198,199] Hornstra has reviewed his own studies and those of others in respect to the relationship between the type of dietary fat and the risk of arterial thrombosis.[183] These studies clearly show that saturated fats are prothrombotic and dietary PUFA antithrombotic in man,[182] as well as in rats.[183] Although it is generally accepted that atherosclerosis and arterial thrombosis are related phenomena, some conflicting data in this respect will have to be discussed later.

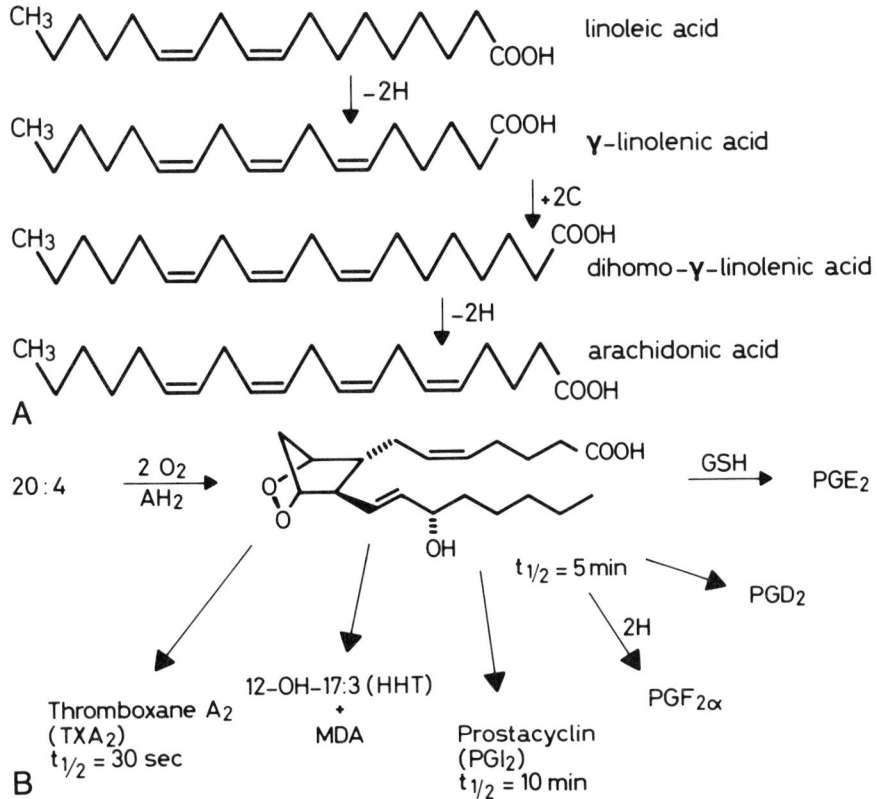

**Fig. 3–11.** *A*, Conversion of linoleic acid into arachidonic acid. *B*, Oxygenations of arachidonic acid.

The known pharmacologic effects of PG on kidney function (especially $PGE_2$), platelet aggregation and adhesion ($PGI_2$, $PGE_1$, $TXA_2$), and blood pressure ($PGE_1$, $E_2$, $D_2$), and the inhibitory effect of cycloxygenase inhibitors (aspirin, indomethacin) on the physiologic effects of dietary linoleic acid on blood pressuure[199] and platelet function[183] support the hypothesis that the atherosclerosis-inhibiting action of dietary PUFA is partially based on an improved PG biosynthesis. However, in the control of lipoprotein metabolism, no clear role for PG and LT has been identified.

The same holds for the observed beneficial effects of increased dietary linoleic acid (40 en% fat, P/S circa 1) in the prevention of retinopathy and macrovascular complications in 51 male and female type II diabetes mellitus patients when compared to 51 age-sex matched diabetic control patients treated with a "standard" diabetes diet (35 en% fat, P/S circa 0.3).[200] Some of these results have been confirmed.[200a] Especially interesting in this prospective (6 years) study is that, although serum cholesteryl linoleate concentration was increased significantly by the P/S 1 diet, total cholesterol levels during the whole period were similar to those of the controls on the P/S 0.3 diet.

Nevertheless, the incidence of diabetic retinopathy, myocardial infarctions, and mortality due to cardiac and cerebral complications was significantly lower at P/S 1. If this important study can be confirmed, the question can be raised whether changes in fatty acid composition of blood lipids (increased linoleic acid mainly) and cellular membranes might not be more important in diabetes mellitus than the present preoccupation with the possible effects of various lipoprotein concentrations.

### n-3 Polyunsaturated Fats, Thrombosis and Atherosclerosis

Dyerberg and Bang have concentrated attention on the epidemiologic data of Greenlanders who reportedly have a low incidence of myocardial infarction.[201] Although this could be expected because of the observed low levels of LDL and VLDL in these Eskimos combined with a high degree of physical activity compared to that of Danes, another explanation via a reduced platelet aggregatability in vivo, which fits the observed prolonged bleeding times typical of Greenlanders, has been stressed.[201,202] The diet of Greenlanders was (and to some extent still is) characterized by a high intake of eicosapentaenoic acid (timnodonic acid, 20:5, n-3). As already mentioned, 20:5, n-3 will be incorporated preferentially into plasma and biomembrane phospholipids at the expense of 18:2, n-6 and 20:4, n-6.[201] Hemostasis in Greenlanders was found to support the hypothesis that contrary to 20:4, n-6, which with CO leads to the formation of both the proaggregatory TXA$_2$ and antiaggregatory, PGI$_2$—20:5, n-3 is converted with CO into an inactive TXA$_3$ and platelet aggregation inhibiting PGI$_3$. A weak point in this hypothesis has always been that 20:5, n-3 is a very poor substrate for CO, and it is not surprising that no convincing data exist about the in vivo biosynthesis of significant amounts of PGI$_3$ and TXA$_3$.[188,189,191] On the other hand, it has been confirmed that feeding of 20:5, n-3 does reduce TXA$_2$ and PGI$_2$ biosynthesis from 20:4, n-6 (aspirin and similarly acting drugs have the same effect and also induce an increased bleeding time).

More important than the correctness of the hypothesis postulated by Dyerberg, Moncada, and Vane is whether increased intake of 20:5, n-3 really leads to a reduced incidence of arterial thrombosis and atherosclerosis. In order to contribute data to this discussion, in vivo studies have been performed on the role of 20:5, n-3 in arterial thrombosis (rat) and atherosclerosis (rabbit).[192,212]

Mural thrombus formation has been induced in aortae of rats fed diets deficient in EFA (5 en% hardened coconut oil), or with either 1.5 en% n-3 type PUFA (5 en% cod liver oil) or 3 en% 18:2, n-6 (5 en% sunflower seed oil), using Hornstra's method.[183] Because of the shortage of 20:4, n-6 and consequently a low production of TXA$_2$, thrombus formation is delayed in EFA deficiency. At 2.3 en% 18:2, n-6, biochemical conditions are such that the growth rate of mural thrombus is maximal; this decreases again (dose-effect related) at higher dietary 18:2, n-6 concentration.[183] Because it is claimed that PUFA of the n-3 type will reduce arterial thrombus formation due to a decreased production of TXA$_2$,[201,202,213] formation of thrombus should have been delayed by the cod liver oil-containing diet, especially since production of both TXA$_2$ and TXA$_3$ was negligible compared to the production in the diet containing 3 en% 18:2, n-6. However, thrombus formation in both groups was identical. This indicates that, at least in rats, TXA$_2$ production is not well-related to in vivo thrombus formation and that n-3 PUFA does not have a specific antithrombotic activity in comparison to n-6 PUFA. Also at a higher dietary intake (up to 40 en% of either sunflower seed oil or n-3 PUFA-rich fish oils) no significant differences have been observed with regard to the in vivo antithrombotic activities of these oils.[183]

In respect to the possible preventive effect of diets rich in fish oil on the development of atherosclerosis, a recently published 2-year study in rabbits is of great interest.[192]. The rabbits were fed cholesterol-free semisynthetic diets with soy protein instead of the more atherogenic casein as a source of protein and 32 en% of either palm, olive, sunflower seed, fish (menhaden), or linseed oil (Fig. 3–12). All diets contained 8 en% sunflower seed oil to prevent EFA deficiency. As could be expected, serum cholesterol levels were highest in the palm oil group and lowest in the 3 high-PUFA diets. The lowest incidence and degree of severity of atherosclerosis was observed in the group fed sunflower oil, as has been observed previously in rabbits and many other animal species (Fig. 3–12). Surprisingly, however, the most severe degree of atherosclerosis was observed in the rabbits fed fish oil, with a similar trend in the linseed oil group, rather than after feeding palm oil with its high concentration of palmitic and stearic acid.

These data certainly do not support the widely published assumption that n-3 fatty acids possess a specific retarding effect on atherogenesis.[201,202,213] On the contrary, in rabbits at least, they seem to stimulate atherosclerosis. Furthermore, in this study the rabbits fed fish oil showed dramatically increased levels of serum enzymes, indicative of liver damage (GOT, GPT, alkaline phosphatase). Histopathologic examination confirmed the macroscopically detected liver damage at autopsy. Periportal fibrosis, lipogranulomas filled with lipofuscin, and bile duct hyperplasia, were observed. Lipogranulomas were also present in the mesenteric lymph nodes.[192]

Other potentially harmful effects of 20:5, n-3 and 22:6, n-3 rich fish oils are neglected by the advocates of increased human consumption of fish oils. The pathologically increased bleeding times, as observed after aspirin ingestion, also occurs in Eskimos on a high fish oil diet.[201] Gudbjarnason has described a promoting role of 20:5, n-3 and 22:6, n-3 in the development of cardiac necrosis and an increased sensitivity to catecholamine stress.[203] Yellow fat disease, as a consequence of feeding n-3 PUFA, has been observed in cats,[204] swine,[205], wild rabbits,[206] Shetland ponies,[207] rats,[208] horses,[209] and minks.[210] Yellow fat disease is a result of tocopherol deficiency, which probably occurs only when oils rich in n-3 PUFA are present in the food. In piglets, even excess tocopherol from administering mackerel oil cannot prevent yellow fat disease.[211] For this reason, long-term studies involving humans ingesting large amounts of n-3 PUFA should be performed with care.

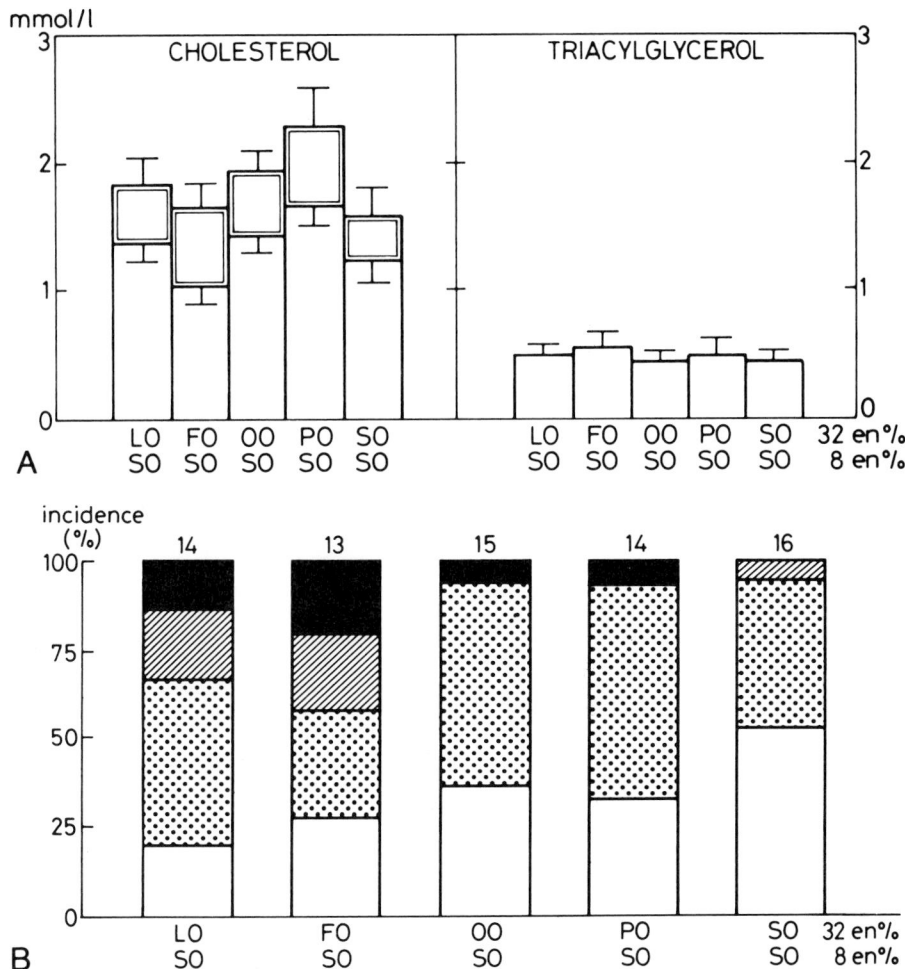

**Fig. 3–12.** *A,* Mean serum cholesterol (☐ free, ☐ ester) and triacylglycerol in rabbits fed for 90 weeks diets containing different oils. *B,* Effects of dietary fat mixtures on aorta atherosclerosis in rabbits after 93 to 95 weeks' feeding. Affected aorta area: ☐ 0%; ▦ 0–10%; ▨ 10–20%; ■ ≥ 20%

Up till now, no long-term studies in man have been published. Short-term studies consistently show the predictable effects of concentrates of cod liver oil, mackerel oil, and fish oil (e.g., Maxepa) on the increase in bleeding time and the reduction of blood triglyceride concentrations.[214,215]

On the other hand, the safety of long-term increased consumption of linoleic acid has been amply demonstrated in a great variety of animal species, including man.[1,2] As reviewed in the last section of this chapter, an increase of dietary linoleic acid intake over the minimal requirement of 3 en% will improve lipoprotein metabolism,[2,82,83,181] reduce the tendency to arterial thrombosis in vivo,[182,183] lower Na[+]-induced hypertension,[193–199] and reduce micro- and macrovascular complications in type II diabetes mellitus patients.[200] Some of these effects can be explained by an improved prostaglandin biosynthesis, but many other complicated biochemical pathways are also involved but not yet sufficiently understood to justify a definite explanation of the favorable effects of linoleic acid on the prevention of atherosclerosis.

## REFERENCES

1. FAO/WHO Expert Consultation: The Role of Dietary Fats and Oils in Human Nutrition. FAO Food and Nutrition Paper 3. Rome, FAO, 1978.
2. Vergroesen, A.J., Gottenbos, J.J.: The role of fats in human nutrition: An introduction. *In* The Role of Fats in Human Nutrition. (Vergroesen, A.J., Ed.) London, Academic Press, 1975.
3. Ackman, R.G.: Fatty acid composition in fish oils. *In* Nutritional Evaluation of Long-Chain Fatty Acids in Fish Oils. (Barlow, S.M., Stansby, M.E., Eds.) London, Academic Press, 1982.
4. Myant, N.B.: The Biology of Cholesterol and Related Steroids. 1st ed. London, William Heinemann Medical Books Ltd, 1981.

5. Grundy, S.M., Mok, H.Y.I.: J. Lipid Res. *18*:263–271, 1977.

6. O'Mullane, J.E., Hawthorne, J.N.: Atherosclerosis *45*:81–90, 1982.

7. Beil, F.U., Grundy, S.M.: J. Lipid Res. *21*:525–536, 1980.

8. Houtsmuller, U.M.T.: Metabolic fate of dietary lecithin. *In* Nutrition and the Brain, Vol. 5. (Barbeau, A., Growdon, J.H., Wurtman, R.J., Eds.) New York, Raven Press, 1979.

9. Zeisel, S.H., Growdon, J.H., Wurtman, R.J., et al.: Neurology *30*:1226–1229, 1980.

10. Cohen, E.L., Wurtman, R.J.: Science *191*:561–562, 1976.

11. Wurtman, J.J.: Sources of choline and lecithin in the diet. *In* Nutrition and the Brain, Vol. 5. (Barbeau, A., Growdon, J.H., Wurtman, R.J., Eds.) New York, Raven Press, 1979.

12. Simonsson, P., Nilsson, A., Akesson, B.: Am. J. Clin. Nutr. *35*:36–41, 1982.

13. WHO Expert Committee: Prevention of Coronary Heart Disease. WHO Technical Report Series 678, Geneva, WHO, 1974.

14. Borgstrom, B.: Phospholipid absorption. *In* Lipid Absorption: Biochemical and Clinical Aspects. (Rommell, K., Goebell, H., Bohmer, R., Eds.) Baltimore, University Park Press, 1976.

15. Northfield, T.C., Hofmann, A.F.: Gut *16*:1–11, 1975.

16. Rizek, R.L., Welsh, S.O., Marstron, R.M.: *In* Dietary Fats and Health. (Perkins, E.F., and Visek, W.J., Eds.) Am. Chemist. Soc., 1983.

17. Hamosh, M., Hand, A.R.: Dev. Biol. *65*:100–113, 1978.

18. Hamosh, M., Klaeveman, H.L., Wolf, R.O., et al.: J. Clin. Invest. *55*:908–913, 1975.

19. Hamosh, M., Scow, R.O.: J. Clin. Invest. *52*:88–95, 1973.

20. Hamosh, M., Burns, W.A.: Lab. Invest. *37*:603–608, 1977.

21. Olivecrona, T., Hernell, O.: Padiatr. Padol. *11*:600–604, 1976.

22. Fredrikzon, B., Hernell, O., Blacksberg, L., et al.: Pediatr. Res. *12*:1048–1052, 1978.

23. Hamosh, M.: Pediatr. Res. *13*:615–622, 1979.

24. Barrowman, J.A., Darnton, S.J.: Gastroenterology *59*:13–21, 1970.

25. Brockerhoff, H., Jensen, R.G.: Lipolytic Enzymes. New York, Academic Press, 1974.

26. Borgstrom, B., Dahlqvist, A., Lundh, G., et al.: J. Clin. Invest. *36*:1521–1536, 1957.

27. Meyer, J.H.: Release of secretion and cholecystokinin. *In* Gastrointestinal hormones. (Thompson, J.C., Ed.) Austin, University of Texas Press, 1975.

28. Moore, E.W., Verine, H.J., Grossman, M.I.: Acta Hepatogastroenterol. *26*:30–36, 1979.

29. Malagelada, J., Di Magno, E.P., Summerskill, W.H., et al.: J. Clin. Invest. *58*:493–499, 1976.

30. Ertan, A., Brooks, F.P., Ostrow, Y.D., et al.: Gastroenterology *61*:686–692, 1971.

31. Grossman, M.I.: Effect of gastrin, cholecystokinin and secretin on gastric and pancreatic secretion: a theory of interaction of hormones. *In* Origin, Chemistry, Physiology and Pathophysiology of Gastrointestinal Hormones. (Creutzfeldt, W., Ed.) Stuttgart, Verlag, Schattauer, 1970.

32. Hofmann, A.F., Mekhijian, H.S.: Bile acids and the intestinal absorption of fat and electrolytes in health and disease. *In* The Bile Acids, Vol. 2. (Nair, P.P., Kritchevsky, D., Eds.) New York, Plenum Press, 1973.

33. Patton, J.S.: Gastrointestinal lipid digestion. *In* Physiology of the Gastrointestinal Tract, Vol. 2. (Johnson, L.R., Ed.) New York, Raven Press, 1981.

34. Borgstrom, B.Y.: J. Lipid Res. *16*:411–417, 1975.

35. Desnuelle, P.: The lipases. *In* The Enzymes, Vol. 7. (Boyer, I.D., Ed.) New York, Academic Press, 1972.

36. Morgan, R.G., Hoffman, N.E.: Biochim. Biophys. Acta *248*:143–148, 1971.

37. Borgstrom, B., Weiloch, T., Erlanson-Albertsson, C.: FEBS Lett. *108*:407–410, 1979.

38. Lairon, D., Nalbone, G., Lafont, H., et al.: Biochemistry *17*:5263–5269, 1978.

39. Hofmann, A.F.: Fat digestion: the interaction of lipid digestion products with micellar bile acid solutions. *In* Lipid Absorption: Biochemical and Clinical Aspects. (Rommel, H.G., Guhmer, R., Eds.) Baltimore, University Park Press, 1976.

40. Vandermeers, A., Vandermeers-Piret, M.C., Rathe, J., et al.: Biochim. Biophys. Acta *370*:257–268, 1974.

41. Dietschy, J.M., Sallee, V.L., Wilson, F.A.: Gastroenterology *61*:932–934, 1971.

42. Scholander, P.F.: Science, *131*:585–590, 1960.

43. Dietschy, J.M.: Helv. Med. Acta *37*:89–102, 1973.

44. Mazer, N.A., Kwasnick, R.F., Carey, M.C., et al.: Quasi-elastic light scattering spectroscopic studies of aqueous bile salt, bile salt-lecithin, and bile salt-lecithin-cholesterol solutions. *In* Micellization, Solubilization and Microemulsions, Vol. 1. (Mittal, K.L., Ed.) New York, Plenum Press, 1977.

45. Sallee, V.L.: J. Lipid Res. *15*:56–64, 1974.

46. Saunders, D.R., Sillery, J.: Lipids *11*:830–832, 1976.

47. Linscheer, W.G.: Gastroenterology *62*:777, 1972.

48. Chijiiwa, K., Linscheer, W.G.: Am. J. Physiol. *246*:G492–G499, 1984.

49. Kamer, J.H., van de Weijers, H.A.: Fed. Proc. *20*(Suppl. 7):335–344, 1961.

50. Lavy, U., Silverberg, M., Davidson, M.: Pediatric Res. *5*:387, 1971.

51. Becker, G.H., Meyer, J., Necheles, H.: Gastroenterology *14*:80–92, 1950.

52. Corless, D., Boucher, B.J., Cohen, R.D., et al.: Lancet *1*:1404–1406, 1975.

53. Anonymous: Nutr. Rev. *41*:322–323, 1983.

54. Deuel, H.J. Jr., Cheng, A.L., Morehouse, M.G.: J. Nutr., *35*:295–300, 1948.

55. Rocquelin, G., Leclerc, J.: Ann. Biol. Anim. Bioch. Biophys. *9*:413–426, 1969.

56. Rocquelin, G.: Ann. Biol. Anim. Biochim. Biophys. *13*:51–154, 1973.

57. McDonald, B.E.: J. Am. Oil Chem. Soc. *49*:304A, 1972.

58. Vles, R.O.: Nutritional aspects of rapeseed oil. *In* The Role of Fats in Human Nutrition. (Vergroesen, A.J., Ed.) London, Academic Press, 1975.

59. Salmon, R.E., O'Neil, J.B.: Poultry Sci. *50*:1456–1467, 1971.

60. Greenberger, N.J., Ruppert, R.D., Tzagournis, M.: Ann. Intern. Med. *66*:727–734, 1967.

61. Greenberger, N.J., Rodgers, J.B., Isselbacher, K.J.: J. Clin. Invest. *45*:217–227, 1966.

62. Senior, J.R.: Introductory remarks by Chairman. *In* Medium Chain Triglycerides. (Senior, J.R., Ed.) Philadelphia, University of Pennsylvania Press, 1968.

63. Isselbacher, K.J.: Mechanisms of absorption of long and medium chain triglycerides. *In* Medium Chain Triglycerides. (Senior, J.R., Ed.) Philadelphia, University of Pennsylvania Press, 1968.

64. Scheig, R.: Hepatic metabolism of medium chain fatty acids. *In* Medium Chain Triglycerides. (Senior, J.R., Ed.) Philadelphia, University of Pennsylvania Press, 1968.

65. Hashim, S.A.: Studies of medium chain fatty acid transport in portal blood. *In* Medium Chain Triglycerides. (Senior, J.R., Ed.) Philadelphia, University of Pennsylvania Press, 1968.

66. Linscheer, W.G.: Replacement of dietary fat by medium chain triglycerides in cirrhotic patients. *In* Medium Chain Triglycerides. (Senior, J.R., Ed.) Philadelphia, University of Pennsylvania Press, 1968.

67. Gray, J.M.: Maldigestion and malabsorption. *In* Gastrointestinal Disease. (Sleisenger, M.H., Fordtran, J.S., Eds.) Philadelphia, W.B. Saunders Co., 1983.

68. Roy, C.C., Roulet, M., Lefebvre, D., et al.: Lipids *14*:811–815, 1979.

69. James, A.T., Webb, J.P., Kellock, T.D.: Biochem J. *78*:333–339, 1961.

70. Ammon, H.V., Thomas, P.J., Phillips, S.F.: J. Clin. Invest. *53*:374–379, 1974.

71. Mekhjian, H.S., Phillips, S.F., Hofmann, A.F.: Gastroenterology *62*:783, 1972.

72. Shimoda, S.S., Saunders, D.R., Rubin, C.E.: Gastroenterology *55*:705–723, 1968.

73. Boyd, G.S.: Cholesterol absorption. *In* The Role of Fats in Human Nutrition. (Vergroesen, A.J., Ed.) London, Academic Press, 1975.

74. Lutton, C., Brot-Laroche, E.: Lipids *14*:441–446, 1979.

75. Kaplan, J.A., Cox, G.E., Taylor, C.B.: Arch. Pathol. *76*:359–368, 1963.

76. Wilson, J.D., Lindsey, C.A.: J. Clin. Invest. *44*:1805–1814, 1965.

77. Quintao, E., Grundy, S.M., Ahrens, E.H.: J. Lipid Res. *12*:233–247, 1971.

78. Connor, W.E., Lin, D.S.: J. Clin. Invest. *53*:1062–1070, 1974.

79. Whyte, M., Nestel, P., MacGregor, A.: Eur. J. Clin. Invest. *7*:53–60, 1977.

80. Borgstrom, B.: J. Lipid Res. *10*:331–337, 1969.

81. Sodhi, H.S., Kudchodkar, B.J.: Lancet *1*:513–519, 1973.

82. Keys, A., Anderson, J.T., Grande, F.: Metabolism *14*:759–765, 1965.

83. Bronsgeest-Schoute, D.C., Hermus, R.J., Dallinga-Thie, G.M., et al.: Am. J. Clin. Nutr. *32*:2193–2197, 1979.

84. Katan, M.B., Beynen, A.C.: Lancet *1*:1213, 1983.

85. Treadwell, C.R., Vahouny, G.V.: Cholesterol absorption. *In* Handbook of Physiology, section 6, Vol. 3. (Cole, C.F., Ed.) Washington, American Physiological Society, 1968.

86. Bhattacharyya, A.K., Connor, W.E.: β-sitosterolemia and xanthomatosis. *In* The Metabolic Basis of Inherited Disease, 4th ed. (Stanbury, J.B., Wijngaarden, J.B., Fredrickson, D.S., Eds.) New York, McGraw-Hill, 1978.

87. Greenberger, N.J., Franks, J.J., Isselbacher, K.J.: Proc. Soc. Exp. Biol. Med. *120*:468–472, 1965.

88. Sabesin, S.M., Isselbacher, K.J.: Science *147*:1149–1151, 1965.

89. Osborne, J.C., Jr., Brewer, H.B., Jr.: Ann. N.Y. Acad. Sci. *348*:104–121, 1980.

90. Lewis, B.: The Hyperlipidaemias. Oxford, Blackwell Scientific Publications, 1976.

91. Mahley, R.W., Rall, S.C., Innerarity, T.L., et al.: Apolipoprotein E and cholesterol metabolism. *In* Atherosclerosis VI. (Schettler, G., Gotto, A.M., Middelhoff, G., Habenicht, A.J.R., Jurutka, K.R., Eds.) Berlin, Springer Verlag, 1983.

92. Havel, R.J.: Metabolism of triglyceride-rich lipoproteins. *In* Atherosclerosis VI. (Schettler, G., Gotto, A.M., Middelhoff, G., et al., Eds.) Berlin, Springer Verlag, 1983.

93. Garfinkel, A.S., Nilsson-Ehle, P., Schotz, M.C.: Biochim. Biophys. Acta *424*:264–273, 1976.

94. Steinberg, D., Vaughan, M.: In vitro and in vivo effects of prostaglandins on free fatty acid metabolism. *In* Nobel Symposium 2: Prostaglandins. (Bergström, S., Samuelsson, B., Eds.) Stockholm, Almqvist and Wiksell, 1967.

95. Carlson, L.A.: Metabolic and cardiovascular effects in vivo of prostaglandins. *In* Nobel Symposium 2: Prostaglandins. (Bergstrom, S., Samuelsson, B., Eds.) Stockholm, Almqvist and Wiksell, 1967.

96. Christ, E.J., Nugteren, D.H.: Biochim. Biophys. Acta *218*:296–307, 1970.

97. Boberg, J., Carlson, L.A., Freyschuss, U., et al.: Europ. J. Clin. Invest. *2*:454–466, 1972.

98. Havel, R.J.: Metabolism *10*:1031–1034, 1961.

99. Nestel, P.J., Steinberg, D.: Circulation *28*:667 (abstract), 1963.

100. Carlson, L.A., Boberg, J., Hogstedt, B.: Some physiological and clinical implications of lipid mobilization from adipose tissue *In* Handbook of Physiology, Vol. 5. (Renold, A.E., Cahill, G.F., Eds.) Washington, American Physiological Society, 1965.

101. Mahley, R.W.: Med. Clin. N.A., *66*:375–402, 1982.

102. Nestel, P.J., Miller, N.E.: Mobilization of adipose tissue cholesterol in high density lipoprotein during weight reduction in man. *In* High Density Lipoproteins and Atherosclerosis. (Gotto, A.M., Miller, N.E., Oliver, M.F., Eds.) New York, Elsevier/North Holland Biomedical Press, 1978.

103. Mahley, R.W., Hui, D.Y., Innerarity, T.L., et al.: J. Clin. Invest. *68*:1197–1206, 1981.

104. Fielding, P.E., Fielding, C.J.: Proc. Natl. Acad. Sci. USA *77*:3327–3330, 1980.

105. Ross, A.C., Zilversmit, D.B.: J. Lipid Res. *18*:169–181, 1977.

106. Swift, L.L., Manowitz, N.R., Dunn, G.D., et al.: J. Clin. Invest. *66*:415–425, 1980.

107. Goldstein, J.L., Ho, Y.K., Brown, M.S., et al.: J. Biol. Chem. *255*:1839–1848, 1980.

108. Mahley, R.W., Innerarity, T.L., Brown, M.S., et al.: J. Lipid Res. *21*:970–980, 1980.

109. Mistry, P., Nicoll, A., Niehaus, C., et al.: Circulation *54*(suppl. II):178, 1976.

110. Fredrickson, D.S., Goldstein, J.L., Brown, M.S.: The familial hyperlipoproteinemias. *In* The Metabolic Basis of Inherited Diseases, 4th ed. (Stanbury, J.B., Wijngaarden, J.B., Fredrickson, D.S., Eds.) New York, McGraw-Hill, 1978.

111. Rudel, L.L., Shah, R., Greene, D.C.: J. Lipid Res. *20*:55–65, 1979.

112. Tall, A.R., Small, D.M., Atkinson, D., et al.: J. Clin. Invest. *62*:1354–1363, 1978.

113. Lofland, H.B., Jr., Clarkson, T.B., St. Clair, R.W., et al.: J. Lipid Res. *13*:39–47, 1972.

114. Roberts, D.C., West, C.E., Redgrave, T.G., et al.: Atherosclerosis *19*:369–380, 1974.
115. Van Zutphen, L.F., Fox, R.R.: Atherosclerosis *28*:435–446, 1977.
116. Quintao, E., Grundy, S.M., Ahrens, E.H., Jr.: J. Lipid Res. *12*:233–247, 1971.
117. Mistry, P., Miller, N.E., Laker, M., et al.: J. Clin. Invest. *67*:493–502, 1981.
118. Katan, M.B., Beynen, A.C.: Lancet *1*:1213, 1983.
119. Wurtman, R.J.: Precursor control of transmitter synthesis. *In* Nutrition and the Bain, Vol. 5. (Barbeau, A., Growdon, J.H., Wurtman, R.J., Eds.) New York, Raven Press, 1979.
120. Subbaiah, P.V., Albers, J.J., Chen, C.H., et al.: J. Biol. Chem. *255*:9275–9280, 1980.
121. Kawamoto, T., Okano, G., Akino, T.: Biochim. Biophys. Acta *619*:20–34, 1980.
122. Young, D.L., Hanson, K.C.: J. Lipid Res. *13*:244–252, 1972.
123. Waelsch, H., Sperry, W.N., Stoyanoff, V.A.: J. Biol. Chem. *135*:297–302, 1940.
124. Solomon, S., Bird, C.E., Ling, W., et al.: Recent Progr. Hormone Res. *23*:297–347, 1967.
125. McNamara, D.J., Quackenbush, F.W., Rodwell, V.W.: J. Biol. Chem. *247*:5805–5810, 1972.
126. Bloch, K.: Science *150*:19–28, 1965.
127. Popjak, G.: J. Am. Oil Chem. Soc. *54*:647A–655A, 1977.
128. Lynen, F.: Pure Appl. Chem. *14*:137–167, 1967.
129. Conforth, J.W., Popjak, G.: Chemical synthesis of substrates of sterol biosynthesis. *In* Methods of Enzymology, Vol. 15. (Clayton, R.B., Ed.) New York, Academic Press, 1969.
130. Ingebritsen, T.S., Lee, H.-S., Parker, R.A., et al.: Biochem. Biophys. Res. Commun. *81*:1268–1277, 1978.
131. Frnka, J.V., Dempsey, M.E.: Circulation Suppl. *52* #4:82, 1975.
132. Siperstein, M.D.: Regulation of cholesterol biosynthesis in normal and malignant tissues. *In* Current Topics in Cellular Metabolism. Vol. 2. (Horecher, B.L., and Stadtman, E.R., Eds.) New York, Academic Press, 1970.
133. Mosbach, E.H.: Regulation of bile acid synthesis. *In* Bile Acids in Human Disease, II. (Back, P., Gerok, W., and Stuttgart, F.K., Eds.) Stuttgart Schattauer Verlag, 1972.
134. Barth, C.A., Hillmar, I.: Eur. J. Biochem. *110*:237–240, 1980.
135. Rodwell, V.W., Nordstrom, J.L., Mitschelen, J.J.: Adv. Lipid Res. *14*:1–74, 1976.
136. Wilson, J.D.: Arch. Internal Med. *130*:493–505, 1972.
137. Goldstein, J.L., Brown, M.S.: Annu. Rev. Biochem. *46*:879–930, 1977.
138. Glomset, J.A.: J. Lipid Res. *9*:155–167, 1968.
139. Bjorkhem, I., Danielsson, H., Einarsson, K., et al.: J. Clin. Inv. *47*:1573–1582, 1968.
140. Miettinen, T.A.: Clinical implications of bile acid metabolism in man. *In* The Bile Acids, Chemistry, Physiology and Metabolism, Vol. 2. Physiology and Metabolism. (Mair, P.C., Kritchevsky, D., Eds.) New York, Plenum Press, 1973.
141. Volpe, J.J., Vagelos, P.R.: Physiol. Rev. *56*:339–417, 1976.
142. Wakil, S.J.: J. Am. Chem. Soc. *80*:6465, 1958.
143. James, A.T.: Adv. Exp. Med. Biol. *83*:51–74, 1977.
144. Brenner, R.R., Peluffo, R.O.: J. Biol. Chem. *241*:5213–5219, 1966.

145. Houtsmuller, U.M.T.: Fette Seifen Anstrichm. *80*:162–180, 1978.
146. Holman, R.T.: J. Nutr. *70*:405–410, 1960.
147. Gottenbos, J.J.: Biological effects of trans fatty acids. *In* Dietary Fats and Health. (Perkins, E.G., Visek, W.J., Eds.) Champaign, American Oil Chemists Society, 1983.
148. Jeffcoat, R., James, A.T.: FEBS Lett. *85*:114–118, 1978.
149. Muto, Y., Gibson, D.M.: Biochem. Biophys. Res. Comm. *38*:9–15, 1970.
150. Goh, E.H., Heimberg, M.: Biochem. Biophys. Res. Commun. *55*:382–388, 1973.
151. Goh, E.H., Heimberg, M.: J. Biol. Chem. *252*:2822–2826, 1977.
152. Hoppel, C.L.: Carnitine palmitoyltransferase and transport of fatty acids. *In* The Enzymes of Biological Membranes, Vol. 2. (Martonosi, A., Ed.) New York, Plenum Press, 1976.
153. Lazarow, P.B.: J. Biol. Chem. *253*:1522–1528, 1978.
154. Christophersen, B.O., Norseth, J., Thomasson, M.S., et al.: Metabolism and metabolic effects of C 22:1 fatty acids with special reference to cardiac lipidosis. *In* Nutritional Evaluation of Long Chain Fatty Acids in Fish Oil. (Barlow, S.M., Stansby, M.E., Eds.) London, Academic Press, 1982.
155. Beare-Rogers, J.L.: Fortschr. Med. *95*:29–56, 1977.
156. Hülsmann, W.C., Stam, H.: Biochem. Biophys. Res. *82*:53–59, 1978.
157. Norseth, J.: Biochem. Biophys. Acta *575*:1–9, 1979.
158. Borrebaek, B., Osmundsen, H., Christiansen, E.N., et al.: FEBS Lett. *121*:23–24, 1980.
159. Christiansen, R.Z., Norseth, J., Christiansen, E.N.: Lipids *14*:614–618, 1979.
160. Burr, G.O., Burr, M.M.: J. Biol. Chem. *82*:345–367, 1929.
161. Euler, U.S. von: J. Physiol. *88*:213–234, 1936.
162. Dorp, D.A. van, Beerthuis, R.K., Nugteren, D.H., et al.: Biochim. Biophys. Acta *90*:204–207, 1964.
163. Bergström, S., Danielsson, H., Samuelsson, B.: Biochim. Biophys. Acta *90*:207–210, 1964.
164. Bergström, S.: Prog. Lipid Res. *20*:7–12, 1981.
165. Holman, R.T.: Essential fatty acid deficiency. *In* Progress in the Chemistry of Fats and Other Lipids, Vol. 9, part 2. (Holman, R.T., Ed.) New York, Pergamon Press, 1968.
166. Holman, R.T.: Biological activities of and requirement for polyunsaturated acids. *In* Progress in the Chemistry of Fats and Other Lipids, Vol. 9, part 5. (Holman, R.T., Ed.) New York, Pergamon Press, 1970.
167. Vergroesen, A.J.: Bibl. Nutr. Dieta *23*:19–26, 1976.
168. Houtsmuller, U.M.: Specific biological effects of polyunsaturated fatty acids. *In* The Role of Fats in Human Nutrition. (Vergroesen, A.J., Ed.) London, Academic Press, 1975.
169. Ziboh, V.A., Hsia, S.L.: J. Lipid Res. *13*:458–467, 1972.
170. Houtsmuller, U.M.: Prog. Lipid Res. *20*:889–896, 1981.
171. Kingsbury, K.J., Brett, C., Stovold, R., et al.: Postgrad. Med. J. *50*:425–440, 1974.
172. Collins, F.D., Sinclair, A.J., Royle, J.P., et al.: Nutr. Metab. *13*:150–167, 1971.
173. Shimoyama, T., Kikuchi, H., Press, M., et al.: Gut *14*:716–722, 1973.
174. Paulsrud, J.R., Pensler, L., Whitten, C.F., et al.: Am. J. Clin. Nutr. *25*:897–904, 1972.

175. Friedman, Z., Frolich, J.C.: Pediatr. Res. *13*:932–936, 1979.

176. Naismith, D.J.: Br. J. Nutr. *30*:567–576, 1973.

177. Wolfram, G., Eckart, J., Zollner, N.: Klin. Wochenschr. *58*:1327–1337, 1980.

178. Crawford, M.A., Hassam, A.G., Stevens, P.A.: Prog. Lipid Res. *20*:31–40, 1981.

179. Galli, C., Spagnuolo, C., Bosisio, E., et al.: Dietary essential fatty acids, polyunsaturated fatty acids and prostaglandins in the central nervous system. *In* Advances in Prostaglandin and Thromboxane Research, Vol. 4. (Coceani, F., Olley, P.M., Eds.) New York, Raven Press, 1978.

180. Brussaard, J.H., Dallinga-Thie, G., Groot, P.H., et al.: Atherosclerosis *36*:515–527, 1980.

181. Lewis, B., Hammett, F., Katan, M., et al.: Lancet *2*:1310–1313, 1981.

182. Hornstra, G., Chait, A., Karvonen, M.J., et al.: Lancet *1*:1155–1157, 1973.

183. Hornstra, G.: Dietary fats, prostanoids and arterial thrombosis. *In* Developments in Hematology and Immunology, Vol. 4. The Hague, Martinus Nijhoff Publishers, 1982.

184. Holman, R.T.: Essential fatty acid deficiency in humans. *In* Handbook of Nutrition and Foods. (Recheigl, M., Ed.) Cleveland, CRC Press, 1977.

185. Lloyd-Still, J.D., Johnson, S.B., Holman, R.T.: Am. J. Clin. Nutr. *34*:1–7, 1981.

186. Struijck, C.B., Beerthuis, R.K., Pabon, H.J.J. et al.: Recl. Trav. Chim. Pays Bas *85*:1233–1250, 1966.

187. Dyerberg, J., Bang, H.O., Hjorne, N.: Am. J. Clin. Nutr. *28*:958–966, 1975.

188. Lands, W.E.M., LeTellier, P.R., Rome, L.H., et al.: Inhibition of prostaglandin biosynthesis. *In* Advances in the Biosciences 9. (Bergstrom, S., Ed.) Oxford, Pergamon Press, 1972.

189. Needleman, P., Raz, A., Minkes, M.S., et al.: Proc. Natl. Acad. Sci. USA *76*:944–948, 1979.

190. Sanders, T.A.B., Roshanai, F.: Clin. Sci. *64*:91–99, 1983.

191. Vergroesen, A.J., Hoor, F., ten, Hornstra, G.: Effects of dietary essential fatty acids on prostaglandin synthesis. *In* Nutritional Factors: Modulating Effects on Metabolic Processes. (Beers, R.F., Bassett, E.G., Eds.) New York, Raven Press, 1981.

192. Kloeze, J., Haddeman, E., Hornstra, G. et al.: J.A.O.C.S., *60*:721, 1983.

193. Adam, O., Wolfram, G., Zollner, N.: Ann. Nutr. Metab. *26*:315–323, 1982.

194. Iacono, J.M., Judd, J.T., Marshall, M.W., et al.: Prog. Lipid Res. *20*:349–364, 1981.

195. Vergroesen, A.J., Fleischman, A.I., Comberg, H.-U., et al.: Acta Biol. Med. Ger. *37*:879–883, 1978.

196. Rao, R.H., Rao, U.B., Srikantia, S.G.: Clin. Exp. Hypertens. *3*:27–38, 1981.

197. Oster, P., Arab, L., Schellenberg, B., et al.: Ernahrungsumschau *27*:143–144, 1980.

198. Triebe, G., Block, H.U., Forster, W.: Acta Biol. Med. Ger. *35*:1223–1224, 1976.

199. Ten Hoor, F., van de Graaf, H.M.: Acta Biol. Med. Ger. *37*:875–877, 1978.

200. Houtsmuller, A.J., Hal-Ferwerda, J., Zahn, K.J., et al.: Prog. Lipid Res. *20*:377–386, 1981.

200a.Howard-Williams, J., Patel, P., Jelfs, R., et al.: Br. J. Ophthalmol. *69*:15–18, 1985.

201. Dyerberg, J., Bang, H.O.: Effects on hemostasis by feeding eicosapentaenoic acid. *In* Nutritional Factors: Modulating Effects on Metabolic Processes. (Beers, R.F., Bassett, E.G., Eds.) New York, Raven Press, 1981.

202. Dyerberg, J., Bang, H.O., Stoffersen, E., et al.: Lancet *2*:117–119, 1978.

203. Gudbjarnason, S.: Nutr. Metab. (Suppl. 1) *24*:142–146, 1980.

204. Editorial: *In* Merck Veterinary Manual. (Sigmund, O.H., McKae, J.W., Eds.) Rahway, N.J., Merck & Co., Inc., 1961.

205. Danse, L.H., Steenbergen-Botterweg, W.A.: Vet. Pathol. *11*:465–476, 1974.

206. Jones, D., Gresham, G.A., Lloyd, H.G., et al.: Nature *207*:205–206, 1965.

207. Kroneman, J., Wensvoort, P.: Neth. J. Vet. Sci. *1*:42–48, 1968.

208. Danse, L.H.J.C., Stolwijk, J., Verschuren, P.M.: Vet. Pathol. *16*:593–603, 1979.

209. Wensvoort, P.: Tijdschr. Diergeneesk. *99*:1060–1066, 1974.

210. Danse, L.H., Steenbergen-Botterweg, W.A.: Zentralbl. Veterinaermed. [A] *23*:645–660, 1976.

211. Ruiter, A., Jongbloed, A.W., van Gent, C.M., et al.: Am. J. Clin. Nutr. *31*:2159–2166, 1978.

212. Hornstra, G., Haddeman, E., Kloeze, J., et al.: Dietary-fat-induced changes in the formation of prostanoids of the 2 and 3 series in relation to arterial thrombosis (rat) and atherosclerosis (rabbit). *In* Advances in Prostaglandin, Thromboxane, and Leukotriene Research, Vol. 12. (Samuelsson, B., Paoletti, R., Ramwell, P., Eds.) New York, Raven Press, 1983.

213. Gryglewski, R.J., Salmon, J.A., Ubatuba, D.B., et al.: Prostaglandins *18*:453–478, 1979.

214. Phillipson, B.E., Rothrock, D.W., Connor, W.E., et al.: N. Engl. J. Med. *312*:1210–1216, 1985.

215. Singer, P., Wirth, M., Berger, I., et al.: Atherosclerosis *56*:111–118, 1985.

## SELECTED READINGS

FAO/WHO Expert Consultation: The Role of Dietary Fats and Oils in Human Nutrition. FAO Food and Nutrition Paper 3. Rome, FAO, 1978.

Holman, R.T.: Essential fatty acid deficiency in humans. *In* Handbook of Nutrition and Foods. (Rescheigl, M., Ed.) Cleveland, CRC Press, 1977.

Mahley, R.W.: Med. Clin. N.A. *66*:375–402, 1982.

Rommel, H.G., Gotzmer, R., Eds.: Lipid Absorption: Biological and Clinical Aspects. Baltimore, University Park Press, 1976.

Stanbury, J.B., Wÿngaarden, J.B., Fredrickson, D.S., et al. Eds.: The Metabolic Basis of Inherited Disease, 5th Ed. New York, McGraw-Hill, 1983.

Vergroesen, A.J., Ed.: The Role of Fats in Human Nutrition. London, Academic Press, 1975.

*Chapter* **4**

# WATER, ELECTROLYTES, AND ACID-BASE BALANCE

Henry T. Randall

Water is an essential and major component of all living things on earth. Far from being just a passive solvent for inorganic salts and gasses and a medium for solution or suspension of organic molecules, it is an enormously complex substance that is actively involved in a wide variety of biological processes. These processes include nutrient transport across cell membranes both in the gastrointestinal tract and from plasma and interstitial fluid to the body cells. Water is also an active agent in transporting waste materials out of cells and in carrying them through the circulation to the kidneys and lungs for excretion.

Electrolytes comprise a wide variety of substances, from simple inorganic salts (such as the chlorides, sulfates, and phosphates of sodium, potassium, and magnesium) to highly complex organic molecules. They share with water itself the ability to dissociate into positively and negatively charged ions. These ions variably affect the concentration of hydrogen ions in water, an effect depending both on individual ion characteristics, and on interaction with other ionized and partially ionized substances in the solution. Major differences in specific ion concentrations exist between intracellular fluid and extracellular, interstitial fluid. These concentration differences are maintained by complex energy-dependent structures in cell membranes that transport ions against chemical gradients and across electrical potential differences.

The concentration of hydrogen ions within cells and in the extracellular fluids in which they live is controlled within narrow limits by chemical systems that buffer potentially dangerous increases in hydrogen or hydroxyl ions so that minimal changes in acid-base balance occur.

Exogenous acid loads, such as those present in the usual diets of man, and the nonvolatile products of the metabolism of food including urea, inorganic salts, and water are excreted by the kidneys as urine. The oxidized carbon atoms of foods are excreted by the lungs as carbon dioxide.

The famous physiologist of the early twentieth century, Walter B. Cannon, suggested the word *homeostasis* to encompass all the multiple and highly complex physical, biochemical, and physiologic processes and controls by which highly evolved animals including man "preserve uniform and stable their internal economy."[1] This chapter reviews the water and electrolyte composition of the human body, and examines the mechanisms by which volume, electrolyte concentration, and acid-base balance are maintained. It then discusses the more common abnormalities of water, electrolyte, and acid-base disturbances, their diagnosis, and treatment.

A brief review of the history of understanding water and electrolyte disturbances in human disease and injury provides a background for current treatment.

## HISTORICAL PERSPECTIVES

Cholera is an acute infectious disease of man that is characterized by sudden onset of very high-volume diarrhea. Vomiting occurs after several hours, often preventing oral intake. Dehydration occurs rapidly and, in severe cases, may result in circulatory collapse and heart failure within hours of onset. Death occurred in 50% or more of severe cases during the nineteenth century in Western Europe and North America.

The disease probably existed for many centuries in the Indian subcontinent. It was first described by the Portuguese in the sixteenth century, but it did not affect the Western World until the early nineteenth century. The first epidemic of cholera appeared on the Miditerranean Coast as well as in China and Japan from 1817 to 1823.[2] The second epidemic, 1829 to 1835, spread through Persia, Russia, and Poland west to affect England, Ireland, and France. It came to the New World in 1832, spreading from Quebec and New York to the rest of the east coast of North America. As much as 10 to 15% of the population was affected, and mortality was high, particularly during the early stages of the epidemic.

The cholera epidemic of 1829 to 1835 was a major one in England, particularly in London and other crowded cities. Usual treatment included opiates, brandy, purgatives including castor oil and croton oil, and bleeding which was used to treat numerous illnesses at that time.

In this setting, there appeared in The Lancet in London, Volume 1 for 1831 to 1832, a letter dated 29 December, 1831 that William B. O'Shaughnessy, M.D., a physician and chemist who reported the results of his chemical analysis of the blood of cholera victims and of the diarrheal fluid.[3] The letter stated in part:

> Sir, - Having been enabled to complete the experimental inquires on which I have some time back been engaged in Newcastle upon-Tyne, I beg you will have the kindness to give insertion to the annexed outlines of the results I have obtained:
>
> 1. The blood drawn in the worst cases of the chol- is unchanged in its anatomical or globular structure.
> 2. It has lost a large proportion of its water, 1000 parts of cholera serum having but the average of 860 parts of water.
> 3. It has lost also a great proportion of its NEU- saline ingredients.
> 4. Of the free alkali contained in healthy serum, not a particle is present in some cholera cases, and barely a trace in others.
> 5. Urea exists in the cases where suppression of has been a marked symptom.
> 6. All the salts deficient in the blood, especially the carbonate of soda, are present in large quantities in the peculiar white dejected matters.

A summary of a detailed report filed by O'Shaughnessy with the Central Board of Health in London was published in The Lancet in March of 1832.[4] O'Shaughnessy stated that the normal constituents of blood consisted of water, fibrin, albumin, coloring matter (hemoglobin), extractive matter, and various saline substances including carbonate of soda, muriates (chlorides), phosphates and sulfates of sodium and potassium, carbonates and phosphates of lime or magnesia, and minute quantities of iron. Extractable substances consisted of oily and crystallizable matter and urea. The mineral elements were all expressed as salts because ionization of salts in water was not known at that time. Table 4–1 compares blood from healthy persons with O'Shaughnessy's findings in the blood of cholera patients.

O'Shaughnessy also observed that the blood of a patient who had been given a strong saline cathartic showed changes similar to those of cholera patients but much less in degree.

O'Shaughnessy stated that the objective of treatment of cholera patients should be "to restore the blood to normal specific gravity and to restore deficient saline matters." He recommended in mild cases of the disease the use of stringents (opiates), in more severe cases the use of copious quantities of enema fluid containing saline and carbonate of soda, and in desperate cases the use of "intravenous fluids containing the deficient matters."[4]

O'Shaughnessy's report in The Lancet was read with interest by a number of physicians in England. Thomas Latta, M.D. of Leith wrote to the

**Table 4–1. Comparison of Normal and Cholera Blood as Noted by O'Shaughnessy[4]**

|  | *Normal* | *Cholera* |
|---|---|---|
| Specific gravity of blood | 1.028 | 1.041 |
| Composition of blood, parts per 1,000 |  |  |
| Water | 906 | 854 |
| Albumin | 78 | 133 |
| Urea | 0 | 0.40 |
| Saline matters | 11 | 5.60 |
| Carbonate of soda with phosphate and sulfate | 2.10 | 0 |
| Ratio of serum of cells and fibrin clot (approximates hematocrit) | 43/57 | 57/43 |

Diarrhea of cholera patients contained: water, sodium carbonate, saline matters, fibrin, and traces of albumin in a highly alkaline solution.

Central Board of Health in London in May of 1832 stating that he had treated several patients using intravenous fluids as recommended by O'Shaughnessy.[5] He stated that as soon as he had read the results of Dr. O'Shaughnessy's analysis he attempted to restore the blood to its natural state by "injecting copiously in the large intestine warm water holding in solution the requisite salts and also administering quantities from time to time by mouth." He reported that he had little success with this method of treatment with no permanent benefit, and he felt increased vomiting and purging resulted. For a dying patient, he said, "I at length resolved to throw the fluid immediately into the circulation. In this, having no precedent to direct me, I proceeded with much caution." He inserted a tube into a basilic vein and, using a syringe, cautiously began to inject ounce after ounce of his solution.

> At first no visible changes were produced. Still persevering I thought that she began to breathe less laboriously, soon the sharpened features and sunken eyes and fallen jaw—began to glow with returning animation. The pulse, which had long ceased, returned to the wrist, first small and quick, by degrees became more and more distinct, fuller, slower and firmer and in the short space of a half an hour when six pints has been injected she expressed in a firm voice that she was free from all uneasiness, actually became jocular and fancied that she was in need of a little sleep.

He thought that he had cured the patient. After he had left, vomiting and diarrhea returned and within 5½ hours she sank into her former state of debility and died. Latta observed that were the remedy to have been repeated he had no doubt that she might have survived.

The solution that Dr. Latta used consisted of "2 or 3 drachms of muriate of soda and 2 scruples of the subcarbonate of soda in 6 pints of water, injected at a temperature of 112°F." This solution of sodium chloride and sodium bicarbonate is hypotonic to plasma containing approximately 80 meq Na, 70 meq Cl, and 10 meq $HCO_3$/L. The os-

molality is 160 mO, which is slightly more than 50% of the normal osmolality of plasma. It is, however, of sufficient concentration when mixed with some blood to protect red cells from hemolysis.

It is of particular interest that not only did Latta and other physicians endeavor to restore some of the missing chemical elements of the blood, but also that they were aware of the need for *substantial volumes* of fluids in patients who were in shock from dehydration. Latta recorded having given a total of 330 ounces (almost 10 liters) of his infusion fluid in 12 hours. He also reported that after an initial rapid injection, he slowed the infusion rate to two to three ounces a minute. These rates of infusion of electrolyte solutions are comparable to those used today in initial rapid resuscitation of hypovolemic patients where the solution commonly used is Ringer's lactate without glucose.

Dr. Latta and a Dr. Lewins succeeded in salvaging 5 of 15 patients. They went into great detail to describe that the patients were all in extremis and "within an hour or two of death."[6]

In a series of questions submitted to Lewins and Latta by the Central Board of Health in London,[6] the first was whether any of the patients had been *bled* prior to or following intravenous injections of fluid. Dr. Lewins noted that of the 15 patients he reported, one was bled to the amount of 12 ounces immediately after the first injection of fluid and none of the others had been bled.

Another question pertaining to proof of "absolute suppression of urine output" asked what happened when the injections were given. The reply was that all but two patients had complete suppression for several hours prior to treatment. "In all the successful cases and some of the unsuccessful ones the effect of the injection was to restore the secretion of urine."

Dr. James L. Gamble, a famous twentieth-century pioneer in the study of fluid and electrolyte balance, in an article reviewing the early history of fluid replacement therapy, noted that Dr. Latta and his followers had "inadvertently covered the all important requirements for adequate repair of dehydration. They were not aware of the relation of water loss to circulatory failure. Their concern was to supply enough of the curative sodium salts but their bedside observations guided them correctly. So that in the year 1832 both rationale and the effectiveness of fluid replacement therapy were roughly but adequately demonstrated."[7]

The O'Shaughnessy-Latta technique of intravenous infusion of water containing sodium chloride and sodium bicarbonate (or carbonate) was then frequently used in England for desperate patients with cholera. The Lancet gave strong editorial support. However, the cholera epidemic subsided by 1835, and intravenous infusion for treatment of acute dehydration was soon forgotten.

Gamble[7] and Moyer[8] have reviewed events that brought further understanding of the pathophysiology of diarrheal dehydration and its treatment. During the third cholera epidemic in 1850, Carl Schmidt confirmed and extended O'Shaughnessy's observations both on the normal constituents of blood, plasma, and serum, and on the profound changes that occurred in the blood in severe cholera. From Schmidt's data, Gamble calculated the bicarbonate deficit in the serum of cholera patients and demonstrated a severe metabolic acidosis. This finding was confirmed by Sellards in 1911 when the bicarbonate of the blood of patients with cholera was directly measured using Van Slyke's burette.[7]

The effectiveness of large volumes of alkaline fluids in treating the acute dehydration of cholera was also reported by Cantani of Naples in 1892[7] and by Sellards who treated cholera patients in the Philippines in 1910.[8] Large volumes of fluid containing 4 g of NaCl and 3 g of $NaHCO_3$/L were administered subcutaneously with dramatic results.

Not until the studies by Butler, Gamble, and Darrow in the 1930s of infants and young children with severe diarrhea was the tremendous loss of potassium that occurs with diarrhea appreciated. The use of potassium as well as sodium salts in rehydration of these infants began in 1936.[7] Cholera diarrhea also causes massive loss of potassium with resulting hypokalemia unless potassium as well as sodium salts are used in rehydration solutions. Oral hydration of cholera patients, using the World Health Organization formula of 3.5 g NaCl, 2.5 $NaHCO_3$, 1.5 g KCl, and 20 g of glucose per liter, volume for volume of diarrheal output, is now used throughout the world. The WHO intravenous solutions containing 4 g NaCl, 6.5 g Na acetate or lactate, 1 g KCl, and 8 g glucose per liter

is reserved for the most severe cases. Tetracycline shortens the period of intense diarrhea. As a result, mortality from cholera has dropped almost to zero except in remote areas, despite the fact that the disease is again pandemic in several parts of the world.[2]

The use of intravenous fluids for conditions other than dehydration due to diarrhea was slow to develop. Treatment of diabetic coma with intravenous saline was reported in 1874, with "partial success."[8]

George W. Crile in 1899 published a monograph on 138 carefully monitored experiments using dogs.[9] He assessed the contribution of hemorrhage, anesthesia, and the severity and duration of surgery to development of shock, which he attributed to loss of vasomotor tone. He was impressed with the effect of the infusion of warm saline noting that when a small amount was injected, the effect was not maintained. When, however, larger quantities up to 7.5% of body weight were injected, blood pressure was maintained unless the animal had been close to death before treatment was begun. He asked, "What has the saline done? It has increased the venous pressure, which in turn filled the heart; this in its turn beat strongly and sent out large quantities of saline blood, which in turn fed the exhausted and starving centers, and carried the overcharged blood to the lungs for the respiratory exchanges."

In 1923, Penfield and Teplitsky reported a method of control of intravenous infusions that incorporated a manometer for measuring venous pressure at frequent intervals during the infusion.[10] Infusions of glucose up to 10% and also of physiologic saline or Ringer's solution were given at rates of 800 to 1,500 ml/hour for 3 or 4 hours. In patients suffering from dehydration or shock, saline or Ringer's solution was used to avoid the diuresis produced by glucose when infused at high rates. A sharp rise in venous pressure was an indication to slow or stop the infusion.

Penfield and Teplitsky also attempted to find the cause of infusion reactions that occurred frequently with either glucose or saline. These reactions were characterized by a shaking chill, tachycardia, a rise in temperature to 103°F or more, and a rise in venous pressure all occurring within an hour after the start of the infusion. Where dogs were studied, they found that neither the temperature of infused fluid nor the hydrogen ion concentration of the infusate within a fairly wide range produced a chill or fever. They suspected that "particulate matter" in improperly cleaned rubber tubing was responsible for the chills seen in patients, and established an elaborate protocol for cleaning and sterilizing all apparatus using only distilled water for solutions.

Matas in 1924 referred to his review of the use of intravenous saline at Charity Hospital in New Orleans between 1881 and 1891, and recounted his own experience beginning in 1911 in which primary "massive" infusions of saline or glucose were used for treatment of "profoundly shocked, exhausted or starved surgical patients."[11] He noted that the immediate effect of "hot intravenous salt or glucose infusion is, for the time being, brilliant, but the effect is more often transitory." He felt that such solutions "ran out of the vessels into the tissues." He reported that a continuous infusion of 5% glucose by "drip" not only replaced lost fluid but also provided nutrition, particularly for patients without gastrointestinal function. He stated that hypodermoclysis, i.e., injection of fluid subcutaneously, was ineffective in patients in shock because of delayed absorption.

Matas advocated infusion of citrated whole blood as the most effective means of treating shock, but noted that blood was not always available in emergencies, and that it could not be used indefinitely. Next was "prompt intravenous infusion of a stimulating isotonic fluid (either saline or glucose) capable of replacing the lost or displaced blood." Then, if the patient relapsed, or showed evidence of failing circulation, he advocated his continuous drip of 5% dextrose at a rate of 6 ounces an hour, 140 to 150 ounces in 24 hours. (4,500 to 5,000 ml).

He was opposed to the use of the saline beyond acute resuscitation, stating that in his experience continuous infusion led to edema and excessive chloride retention. Neither did he favor solutions developed in physiology laboratories by Ringer, Locke, Straub, or a remarkable solution developed by Thiess in Germany that contained sodium, potassium, and calcium chlorides at normal plasma concentrations.

Matas also reported frequent occurrences of "infusion reaction" with chills and fever and sometimes hypotension, mottling of the skin, and peripheral cyanosis. He wondered why some patients had the reaction and others did not, even though the same apparatus and solutions were used. Such infusion reactions with intravenous fluids, glucose, or saline severely limited the use of infusions other than massive amounts of saline in treatment of shock until shortly before World War II. At that time, disposable plastic tubing, pyrogen-free distilled water, and purified glucose and sodium chloride were prepared commercially and became widely available. Before then, subcutaneous administration of glucose or saline, hypodermoclysis, or rectal infusion was used except when massive and rapid infusions of saline were needed to treat shock.

Matas in 1924 clearly recognized the nutritional value of glucose in "starved" patients, and stated that his continuous intravenous drip of 5% dextrose provided 750 to 1,000 kilocalories a day. It was not until 1939, however, that Elman in a seminal paper demonstrated that a combination of protein hydrolysate as a source of amino acid and glucose with electrolytes could provide not only water and salt, but also sufficient calories and amino acids to maintain a positive nitrogen balance in postoperative patients.[12] Ten years later, the importance of providing potassium intravenously to postoperative surgical patients was demonstrated to be as important as Darrow and Gamble had shown it to be in rehydration of infants and children dehydrated by diarrhea.[13]

The regulation of neutrality in the blood by the buffering action of weak acids and their sodium salts in solution was described by L. J. Henderson in 1908.[14] By studying the equilibrium among carbonic acid, sodium bicarbonate, and monosodium phosphate and disodium phosphate, he showed that acids whose ionization constants were nearly equal to the concentration of hydrogen ions in a neutral solution "possess, with the aid of their salts, a great capacity of preserving neutrality." He demonstrated the unusual capacity of the system $\dfrac{H_2CO_3}{NaHCO_3}$ to neutralize acid with minimal change in hydrogen ion concentration. He was aware of the abundance of carbon dioxide in the body, and the control of its concentration by the circulation and respiration. With his four-part equilibrium, he estimated that intracellular hydrogen ion concentration closely approximated $1 \times 10^{-7}$ at 38°C which is a pH 7.0.

In 1921, Van Slyke summarized research that he had undertaken with L. J. Henderson, Y. Henderson, Haldane, Hasselbalch, Peters, and others to determine normal and abnormal variations in the acid-base balance of blood in man.[15] He defined the average normal hydrogen ion concentration of plasma as $[H^+] = 4 \times 10^{-8}$ and the logarithm as $\log \dfrac{1}{[H^+]} = $ pH 7.4. Normal venous blood pH was only 0.02 below that of arterial blood. Extremes of pH with survival were defined as pH 7.0 in acidosis and pH 7.8 in alkalosis.

Henderson's equation, $H^+ = K_1 \dfrac{[H_2CO_3]}{[B\ HCO_3]}$, and its negative logarithmic equivalent as proposed by Hasselbalch, pH $= pK_1 + \log_{10} \dfrac{[B\ HCO_3]}{[H\ HCO_3]}$, were used to define normal limits of the total $CO_2$ content of plasma and its relationship to $CO_2$ tension and pH. The value PK for the dissociation constant for $H_2CO_3$ was stated to be 6.1, and the normal tension or partial pressure of $CO_2$ was stated as 40 mm Hg. A solubility coefficient for $CO_2$ in plasma at 37°C determined by Bohr was used in calculating the relationship between total $CO_2$ and pH. This step enabled Van Slyke to postulate nine possible acid-base states with high, low, or normal bicarbonate and high, low, or normal pH. Only one of these states was physiologically normal, when both pH and millimolar bicarbonates were within normal range. It was recognized that both alkali loading and loss of chloride from the stomach and uncompensated $CO_2$ deficit from hyperventilation could produce an elevated pH of the plasma, called "alkali excess." Similarly, these researchers recognized that abnormal retention of acid metabolites, as with renal insufficiency or diabetic ketoacidosis, and abnormal retention of $CO_2$ with respiratory obstruction or depression could result in a fall in pH and acidosis. Most significantly, compensation for both "alkali excess" and acidosis was defined, and both the respiratory and renal roles explained.

The clinical diagnosis of acid-base abnormalities at first depended on determining the "$CO_2$ combining power" of plasma equilibrated with $CO_2$ at 40 mm Hg partial pressure and measured in a Van Slyke burette. This process eliminated the respiratory causes and compensations for acid-base abnormalities and produced an incomplete and sometimes erroneous interpretation of the "alkali reserve." For example, a patient with a compensated respiratory acidosis would have a high bicarbonate and total $CO_2$ and a relatively normal pH. To assume that the patient was alkalotic because of the high bicarbonate would be in error. However, if the cause of $CO_2$ retention were suddenly removed, the patient would then indeed have an elevated plasma pH.

It was not until reliable and durable glass electrodes became available shortly before World War II that pH became widely available for clinical use, and $P_{CO_2}$ could be calculated from pH and total $CO_2$. Only recently have accurate devices for direct measurement of $P_{CO_2}$ become available but, as pointed out by Van Slyke, only two of the three determinations are necessary for assessment of acid-base status in blood.

## NORMAL BODY COMPOSITION

Knowledge of normal body composition is essential to understand the requirements of men, women, and children for water and the major electrolytes as a part of nutrition. For the purposes of this chapter, the data and terminology developed by F.D. Moore and his associates based on isotope dilution studies are used.[16] Additional information derived from whole body neutron irradiation and induced radioactivity analysis is also presented. Changes in body composition produced by intensive nutritional support have been assessed.

Total water, extracellular fluid, and intracellular water have been defined over a wide age span for both men and women. The range of normal values is substantial for both sexes and depends on body build and physical activity as well as sex and age.

Abnormalities of fluid and electrolyte balance are the result of alterations in *volume* of body compartments, or in *concentration* of electrolytes, or both. The importance of consideration of *volume* as well as *concentration* cannot be overemphasized.

### Total Body Water

The largest single component of the human body is water. It constitutes about 60% of body weight of young adult males and 50% of body weight in young adult females (Table 4–2). Water is in highest concentration intracellularly in metabolically active cells of muscle and viscera, and in lower concentration in relatively inert and inactive tissues such as the skin, dense fascia, and cortical bone of the skeleton. Water constitutes 93% of plasma and 97% of interstitial fluid—the "milieu interieur" of Claude Bernard in which body cells actually live. Intracellular water is the major component of cells, except fat cells, and constitutes 73% of the weight of metabolically active cells of muscle and viscera.

Water is capable of weak ionization into hydrogen and hydroxyl ions: $H_2O \rightleftarrows [H^+] + [OH^-]$. Its dissociation constant $[H^+] \times [OH^-] = Kw \times [H_2O]$ is very small: $Kw = 4.3 \times 10^{-16}$ at 37°C.[23]

The structure of water is substantially modified when substances that dissociate into ions in solution are introduced in small quantities, for example NaCl, which dissociates completely into $(Na^+)$ and $Cl^-$ at physiologic concentrations of 0.150 mol/L. Water molecules form hydration shells around each ion, separating them from each other. The process greatly enhances the passage of an electrical current through the solution, hence the term electrolyte to describe these solutions. Weak aqueous electrolyte solutions have been termed "the most important type of physical chemical system in our world."[24]

Water is also modified by proximity to solid surfaces, and to hydrophilic or hydrophobic membranes including cell membranes.[25] It participates actively metabolically with electrolytes, and with

**Table 4–2. Total Body Water (TBW) Related to Body Weight, Age, and Sex**

| Body Type | Age Group (yrs) | Subjects | Mean Body Wt. (Kg) | TBW (L) | % $\frac{TBW(L)}{Wt(kg)}$ | Ref. |
|---|---|---|---|---|---|---|
| **I. NORMAL** | | | | | | |
| Male | 16–30 | 63 | 71.75 | 42.96 ± 3.38 | 58.9 | |
| Male | 31–60 | 56 | 73.57 | 40.24 ± 3.42 | 54.7 | |
| Male | 61–90 | 13 | 69.42 | 35.82 ± 2.85 | 51.6 | |
| Female | 16–30 | 54 | 60.89 | 30.99 ± 2.41 | 50.9 | |
| Female | 31–90 | 34 | 62.62 | 28.36 ± 2.76 | 45.2 | (17) |
| Male | 17–52 | 223 | 72.23 | 44.5 ± 6.04 | 61.6 | |
| Female | N.S. | 36 | 61.75 | 31.5 ± 3.28 | 51.0 | (18) |
| Male | 21–56 x̄ 30.6 | 36 | 83.76 ± 18.7 | 46.3 ± 6.44 | 55.3 | (19) |
| **II. OBESE** | | | | | | |
| Male | 26–56 x̄ 34.2 | 10 | 110.72 ± 13.75 | 52.8 ± 4.41 | 47.7 | (19) |
| **III. MORBIDLY OBESE** (40 female; 5 male) | 20–57 x̄ 33 | 42 | 145.59 | 51.83 ± 2.38 | 35.6 | (20) |
| **IV. ATHLETES** Male | | | | | | |
| Football players | 20.3 ± 0.92 | 16 | 96.4 ± 10.4 | 60.46 ± 4.90 | 63.08 | |
| Basketball players | 20.8 ± 0.92 | 10 | 83.3 ± 11.4 | 51.3 ± 4.63 | 62.82 | |
| Swimmers | 20.6 ± 1.19 | 7 | 78.9 ± 7.2 | 55.2 ± 5.91 | 69.58 | |
| Runners | 21.3 ± 1.08 | 9 | 71.64 ± 12.7 | 50.04 ± 5.64 | 70.52 | |
| Gymnasts | 20.3 ± 0.86 | 7 | 69.22 ± 5.37 | 48.23 ± 2.46 | 69.82 | (21) |
| **V. CHILDREN** | | | | | | |
| Neonates | | | | | 75 | |
| 1 year | | | | | 58 | |
| 6–7 years | | | | | 62 | (22) |

cell membranes, membrane macromolecules, and enzymes in transport of ions across cell membranes. The physical state of ions and of water itself is probably different inside of cells, and perhaps in different parts of individual cells. These physical-chemical differences are intimately involved with many properties of cell structure and metabolism.[26]

In terms of molecular weight, 1 mol of water weighs 18.02 g. There are approximately 55.4 mol of water *per liter* of water at 37°C and therefore 2,327 ± 183 mol of water in a 70-kg man. Compare this total content of water to 3.40 mol K (48 meq/kg), 2.89 mol exchangeable Na (42 meq/kg), and 2.06 mol Cl (29.4 meq/kg). It shows that our body fluids are dilute solutions (0.15% or less) of specific electrolyte ions, with a total ionic concentration of about 0.3% in plasma and extracellular fluid water.

Water content of the human body varies by sex, age, and body habitus. Table 4–2 shows average water content of males in three age groups, and females in two groups from the work of Moore and his associates.[16,17] Note the descending percentage of body water with increasing age in both males and females. Two other series of normals are also shown.[18,19] It is important to note the wide variation within groups. Approximately 95% of the group populations are included in the mean figure for total body water by group ± 2 standard deviations. The range is large, from 15 to 25% of the mean.

In obese patients, the percentage of body water to weight declines, being 47.7% of body weight in a group of males 50% above ideal weight,[19] and 35.6% of body weight in a group of morbidly obese patients, largely female, who averaged 78.8 kg (172 lbs) in excess of ideal weight for sex and age.[20]

The reverse is true with body composition in young male athletes. As shown in Table 4–2, Novak[21] demonstrated that football and basketball players had only a slightly higher percentage of water than usual for young males. However, swimmers, track men, and gymnasts had such a high percentage of body weight as water that their bodies had to contain very little fat.

Total body water is substantially higher as a percentage of body weight in newborn babies. Body water ratio to weight in children resembles that of young adult males until adolescence, when an increase in the percentage of body weight that occurs as fat alters the female ratio.[22]

**Distribution of Body Water.** Total body water is distributed in two major compartments or spaces, based on differential concentration of the two major cations sodium and potassium and the volume represented by dilution of radioactive isotopes or other substances that appear to reach equilibrium in a portion of the total water pool.[16] The two major compartments are intracellular water (ICW) and extracellular water (ECW). Intracellular water is that portion of total body water (TBW) within cells. Body composition studies indicate that 50 to 58% (average 55%) of TBW is intracellular in normal healthy adults. Lean individuals with a relatively large skeletal muscle mass, such as trained young male athletes, have a higher percentage of TBW within cells, whereas females tend to have a more nearly equal distribution of TBW between ICW and ECW. Extracellular water consists of the water component of the extracellular fluids, plasma, interstitial fluid, and the water component of extracellular solids including tendon, fascia, dermis, collagen, elastin, and skeleton. Because there is no way of distinguishing in vivo among the various areas of distribution of ECW, except for measurement of plasma volume and total ECW, ECW is usually considered as a two-compartment distribution of interstitial fluid and plasma.

The size of the ECW compartment as a volume or space depends upon methods used for measurements. The size varies from 15 to 16% of body weight when inulin, sucrose, or mannitol is the indicator to as high as 27% of body weight if $^{24}Na$ is assumed to be distributed entirely extracellularly, which it is not. Measurement of other small ions, such as $^{35}SO_4$ and $^{82}Br$, gives equilibration values of distribution of 21 to 26% of body weight for ECW. These data suffer from the fact that these ions enter into cells to some degree with time as does $^{24}Na$.[27] As a practical matter, ECW can be considered as 23% of body weight in normal adults, or even as 20% of body weight as is commonly used clinically for extracellular fluid estimation in water and electrolyte balance problems.

### Total Body Potassium

This value in the healthy young adult male is stated to be 42 to 48 meq per kg body weight.[16] A 70-kg man contains 2,940 to 3,360 meq (115 to 131 g) of potassium. In trained athletes with larger than normal muscle mass, total body counting of $^{40}K$ gives values of 60 and 65 meq per kg body weight.[21] Virtually all body potassium appears to be exchangeable with $^{42}K$ in the normal adult in 24 hours. The exceptions are potassium in the erythrocytes, which is slowly exchanged, and that in the skeleton where the small amount present is not readily exchanged. In morbidly obese patients, as long as 38 hours may be required for equilibration of $^{42}K$; exchangeable K (Ke) may be underestimated with shorter equilibration periods.[20]

Ellis et al. measured the potassium content of 881 normal individuals at Brookhaven National Laboratory by [40]K whole body counting. The isotope [40]K is naturally occurring, and can be measured in man with a precision and accuracy of ± 3.3%.[28] They found total body potassium to be a function of age, weight, height, and sex. Subsequent evaluation of 1,714 children and another 808 adults ages 4 to 75 confirmed and expanded the Brookhaven studies. Formulas were developed for prediction of total K (Kp) in grams: $Kp = A W^{1/2} H^2$ where A is age in years, W is weight in kg, and H is height in meters. For males, $Kp = (5.52 - 0.014A) W^{1/2} H^2$ and for females $Kp = (4.58 - 0.010A) W^{1/2} H^2$. The ratio of measured total body K to predicted K was 1.000 ± 0.103 for males and 0.987 ± 0.102 for females.

A special and expensively equipped laboratory including a heavily shielded room is necessary for [40]K counting, but the normal values and the formula for predicting normal are important to compare with [42]K dilution studies of Ke.

Table 4–3 shows ranges of total body water by sex, weight, and age and total body potassium by sex, weight, and age from Moore.[16,17] Also listed are formulas for calculation of fat, lean body mass, fat-free solids, and body cell mass based on total body water and exchangeable potassium.

## BODY COMPOSITION BY NEUTRON ACTIVATION

Hill et al.[29] have reported body composition studies by whole body irradiation with 14 MeV neutrons, and whole body counting of the short-lived radiation from isotopes of nitrogen, potassium, sodium, chloride, phosphorus, and calcium that were produced.

The patients studies were 12 male and 13 female adults, all seriously ill with surgical diseases or postoperative complications[8] following major surgery. Seven were septic. All were studied by neutron activation, tritiated water for TBW, and muscle biopsy before and after 14 days of total parenteral nutrition (TPN). The average age was 52.2 years, the S.D. 14.8, and the age range 31 to 87 years. Mean body weight was 51.7 kg ± 10.9, which was 79.4% ± 10.5% of ideal weight for each patient. Weight gain on TPN was 2.62 ± 0.54 kg, with a gain of 2.33 ± 0.55 L water and 0.55 ± 0.17 kg fat. The only significant change by neutron activation and muscle biopsy analysis was in total body K, and in intracellular K concentration, both of which rose to normal.

Table 4–4 gives the data from the Hill study. Calculation of major components of body composition is derived from these data for comparison with Table 4–3 where isotope dilution techniques were used to determine body composition.

Of particular significance in the Hill study is the measurement of phosphorus and calcium, and of total nitrogen and total sodium. These data permit estimation of nonECF sodium and intra- and extracellular protein.

The TPN solution used by Hill et al. did not contain trace metal additives, particularly zinc, which may become significantly depleted on prolonged administration of TPN solutions with inadequate zinc or in patients with serious gastrointestinal losses prior to TPN.

Oxygen consumption and caloric expenditure are closely correlated with body cell mass (BCM). Kinney et al. measured oxygen consumption as 8 to 10 ml per minute per kg BCM, and caloric expenditure as 2.7 to 3.6 kcal per hour per kg BCM.[30] Novak et al. measured basal oxygen consumption of young athletes, which varied from 6.6 to 7.56 ml/kg BCM/min at rest to 100 to 125 ml/min/kg BCM at maximum exercise.[21] These observations are, of course, at extremes of energy production.

Moore has proposed that four biologic situations are basic for analysis of calories and nitrogen: fasting, established starvation, injury, and febrile illness. Each places a different demand on BCM and body fat stores, and each requires a different provision of calories and nitrogen, as well as of water and electrolytes.[17]

Figure 4–1 is a diagrammatic representation of the relationship of body cell mass to total body in *average* normal adult men and women. Based on body composition studies by Moore et al.,[16] the figure shows fat, body cell mass, extracellular fluid (including plasma, transcellular fluid, and bone and dense fascia), collagen, and cartilage as percent of total body weight. *Normal variation* of weight is approximately 20% ± the "ideal." Fat has the widest variation as percentage of body weight, ranging from as low as 3 to 4% in trained young male athletes[20,21] to 66.7% of body weight in morbidly obese patients averaging 172 pounds above ideal weight.[20]

Body cell mass varies with sex, age, physical activity, and nutritional status, from a high of 54% in young lean athletes[21] to 20% of body weight in the extremes of morbid obesity and cachectic malnutrition.

## ELECTROLYTE CONCENTRATION OF BODY FLUIDS

Figure 4–2, modified from the famous diagrams of Gamble,[31] illustrates the approximate composition of interstitial fluid and intracellular water in comparison with that of plasma with its more

**Table 4–3. Estimation of Body Composition by Methods of F.D. Moore[16,17]**

1. Total Body Water (TBW) by Age, Sex, and Body Weight (BWt) (Normal Adults)

| | Age (yrs.) | TBW (liters) | ± 2 Standard Deviations (%) |
|---|---|---|---|
| Males | 16–30 | TBW = 0.4 × BWt in kg + 13 | ±16 |
| Males | 31–60 | TBW = 0.4 × BWt in kg + 11 | ±17 |
| Males | 61–90 | TBW = 0.34 × BWt in kg + 12 | ±16 |
| Females | 16–30 | TBW = 0.31 × BWt in kg + 11.6 | ±13 |
| Females | 31–90 | TBW = 0.33 × BWt in kg + 8.84 | ±21 |

2. Estimation of:

   Body fat (BF) $= 1 \dfrac{\% \text{ TBW}}{0.732}$

   Lean body mass = BWt − B fat

   Fat-free solids (FFS) = Lean body mass − TBW

3. Total Exchangeable Potassium (Ke) by Age, Sex, and Body Weight[16,17]

| | Age (yrs.) | Total Ke (meq) | ± 2 Standard Deviations (%) | |
|---|---|---|---|---|
| Males | 16–30 | Ke = 38 × BWt + 735 | ±23 ) | |
| Males | 31–60 | Ke = 26 × BWt + 1,383 | ±20 ) | Average normal: 47 meq/kg |
| Males | 61–90 | Ke = 27 × BWt + 723 | ±16 ) | |
| Females | 16–30 | Ke = 18 × BWt + 1,250 | ±20 ) | |
| Females | 31–60 | Ke = 17 × BWt + 1,176 | ±23 ) | Average normal: 40 meq/kg |
| Females | 61–90 | Ke = 18 × BWt + 757 | ±29 ) | |

4. Estimation of Ke from Total Body Water

| Males and females | 20–60 | Ke = 97.4 × TBW − 409 |
|---|---|---|
| | 61–84 | Ke = 2 + 77 × TBW |

5. Calculation of Body Cell Mass

   Body cell mass, the sum of all living cells in the body, is calculated from TBW and total exchangeable potassium, assuming that potassium in intracellular water is 150 meq/L and that body cells are 73.2% water, the rest being protein and salts.

   Body Cell Mass (BCM) in kg $= \dfrac{Ke}{150} \times \dfrac{1,000}{0.732}$

   BCM = Ke × 9.10 where Ke is in mols

6. Calculation of Intracellular and Extracellular Water Compartments

   Intracellular Water (ICW) $= \dfrac{Ke \text{ (meq)}}{150}$

   Extracellular Water (ECW) = TBW − ICW

7. Ratios of Exchangeable Na and K

   $Na_e/Ke$ ratios: Normal male 0.87. Normal females 0.95.

8. Calculation of Amount of Wet Bone (B)[17]

   $B = \dfrac{\text{FFS} - 0.61}{1.61 + 0.0062\dfrac{(Ke)}{(FFS)}}$

precisely known values. Table 4–5 gives the range of normal and the analytic error of laboratory determinations for the major electrolytes of plasma as usually determined in serum. Values in this table are from the literature and from our laboratories. It should be remembered that a range of values is present in normal individuals and an error is present in any laboratory determination. The ranges shown take into consideration both the normal variation and the 95% confidence limits of the laboratory procedure in a well-run clinical laboratory. Repeating any laboratory test reduces the probability of error due to the test. *When laboratory reports do not help to confirm the clinical diagnosis or course, it is wise both to repeat the test and to reexamine and reevaluate the patient.*

Since the sum of the cations and the anions in any biologic system must be equal, and since sodium ion is the major cation of extracellular fluid and of serum or plasma most of the anions balance sodium. The anionic structure of serum or plasma is somewhat more complex than that of the cations because of the presence of a substantial amount of plasma protein, the molecules of which behave primarily as anions at the pH of plasma. The sum of bicarbonate (27 meq) and chloride (105 meq) equals all but 10 meq of the normal sodium concentration. The relationship between the sum of

**Table 4–4.   Body Composition From Neutron Activation and Isotope Counting***

(Initial average body weight 54 kg = 80% of ideal for 25 patients)
Neutron activation data after 2 weeks of TPN (see text):

| | *Total* | | *Per Kg* |
|---|---|---|---|
| K mmol | = 2,230 | ± 101 | 41.29 mmol |
| Na mmol | = 3,038 | ± 719 | 56.26 mmol |
| Cl mmol | = 1,828 | ± 74 | 33.85 mmol |
| P mmol | = 15,053 | ± 636 | 278.8 mmol = 8.6 g/kg |
| Ca mmol | = 19,152 | ± 1,213 | 354.63 mmol = 14.2 g/kg |
| N g | = 1,333 | ± 49 | g protein/kg = 154.3 |

Calculated Body Composition:

$$\text{Extracellular fluid} = \frac{\text{Total Cl}}{\text{Plasma Cl}/.93} = 15.57 \text{ L}$$

$$\text{Intracellular water} = \frac{\text{Total K}}{167.3} = 13.33 \text{ L}$$

Total body water = 28.4 L = 53.5% BWt

Body cell mass (BCM) = K × 9.10 = 20.29 kg = 37.6% BWt

$$\text{Body fat} = 1 - \frac{\% \text{ water}}{0.732} = 12.9 \text{ kg} = 23.9\% \text{ BWt}$$

Lean body mass = wt − fat = 41.08 kg

Total protein = N × 6.25 = 8.331 kg = 15.43% wt

$$\text{Intracellular protein} = \frac{\text{BCM}}{4} = 5.7 \text{ kg}$$

Extracellular protein = 2.63 kg

$$\text{Extracellular fluid Na} = \frac{137.6}{0.95} \times \text{ECF} = 2,255 \text{ mmol}$$

Bone and other nonECF Na = 782.8 mmol

Calcium     14.2   g/kg   Normal = 20–24 g/kg, 90% in bone†

Phosphorus   8.62 g/kg   Normal = 11–14 g/kg, 85% in bone†

Muscle Intracellular Fluid Before and After TPN for 14 Days:

| | *Na* mmol/L | *Cl* mmol/L | *K* mmol/L | *Nitrogen* g |
|---|---|---|---|---|
| PreTPN | 4.35 ± 1.3 | 3.36 ± 0.32 | 135.8 ± 5.2 | 58.8 ± 8.1 |
| PostTPN | 5.89 ± 3.6 | 4.22 ± 0.04 | 167.3 ± 9.4 | 60.0 ± 4.4 |
| Significance, P = | NS | NS | 0.005 | NS |

*Data from Hill, G.L., et al.[29]
†Data from Avioli, L.V.[39]

the two anions and the serum sodium concentration normally remains constant.

An approximation of the accuracy of determination of the sodium, chloride, and bicarbonate concentrations of the plasma or serum or the determination of the existence of a major electrolyte abnormality in the patient can be made by equating the serum sodium concentration (in meq) with the sum of the chloride and bicarbonate concentrations (in meq) plus 10 meq:

$$\text{meq Na} \pm 3 = \text{meq HCO}_3 + \text{meq Cl} + 10 \text{ meq}$$

If the sum of bicarbonate plus chloride plus 10 meq is *less* than 3 meq of the sodium concentration on repeated determinations, one of two conditions exists: either substantial amounts of another anion have been added or a major error in the laboratory determination of one or more of the three components has occurred. Conversely, if $HCO_3$ + Cl + 10 is greater than sodium by more than 4 to 5 meq, hypoproteinemia is the likely cause if laboratory error is ruled out.

The composition of intracellular electrolytes is less precisely known and more difficult to measure. Moore gives an *average* intracellular K concentration per liter of ICW as 149.7 meq.[16]

Bergström has analyzed skeletal muscle composition by neutron activation of needle biopsies.[32] Potassium concentration was 167.1 ± 11.9 meq/kg $H_2O$, phosphorus 109.8 ± 7.5 m/mol/kg $H_2O$, and intracellular sodium 4.4 ± 3.3 meq/kg $H_2O$. Water content was 77.45 ± 0.97% of weight of fresh fat-free muscle. Magnesium content of skeletal muscle averages 16 meq/kg wet weight[33] or 21.9 meq/L ICW.

Nitrogen averages 28.6 to 33 g/kg fresh fat-free

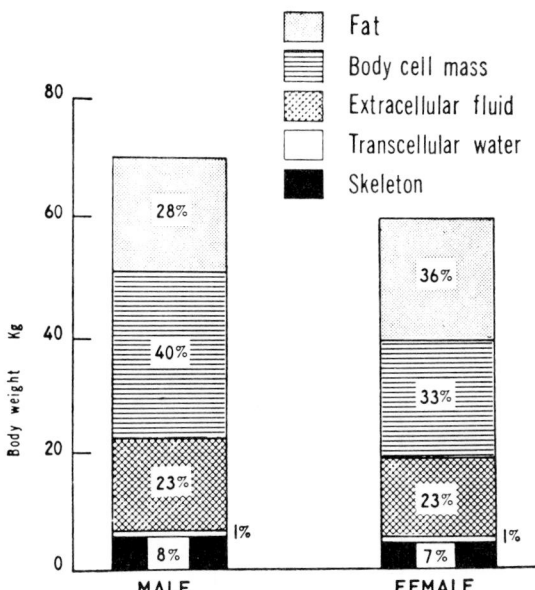

Fat
Body cell mass
Extracellular fluid
Transcellular water
Skeleton

**Fig. 4–1.** Body composition. Fat, body cell mass, extracellular fluid, transcellular water, and skeleton are shown as percent of body weight for average adult men and women. Extracellular fluid includes noncellular elements of connective tissue and tendons as well as interstitial fluid and plasma. Transcellular fluid is fluid in joints, cerebrospinal fluid, and fluid in the resting gastrointestinal tract. (Based on data from Moore, F.D., et al.[17])

muscle which, if N × 6.25 equals protein, would represent 17.9 to 20.6% protein by weight in normal young men.[17]

Hill showed a low intracellular K of 135.8 meq/L in ill patients prior to TPN, which rose to 167 meq/L after two weeks of TPN.[29] Very small amounts of intracellular Na and Cl did not change appreciably. Cell water was determined by drying, and intracellular electrolytes were determined from fat-free, dried specimens (see Table 4–4).

As shown in Figure 4–2, the major intracellular cations are potassium and magnesium, with small amounts of sodium. Anions include phosphate, sulfate, and protein, as well as about one half the plasma concentration of ($HCO_3^-$). As noted, the activity of both ions and water in cells is probably substantially modified by cell membranes, and by the gel-like properties of cytoplasmic proteins.

## OSMOLALITY AND OSMOTIC PRESSURE

A substance in solution in water on one side of a semipermeable membrane that is freely permeable to water but through which the solute cannot pass exerts an effect such that water molecules tend to diffuse in larger numbers toward the solution side where the water molecule concentra-

tion (or activity) is less. Osmotic pressure is the physical force necessary on the solution side of the membrane to prevent the net movement of water across the membrane toward the solution and to maintain equilibrium. One gram molecular weight (GMW) of a substance that does not dissociate into ions, such as glucose or urea, contains $6.06 \times 10^{23}$ molecules and is termed 1 mol. Dissolved in one liter of water, it becomes 1 osmole, which requires a pressure equal to 17,004 mm Hg on the solution side to maintain equilibrium across a membrane permeable only to water. One milliosmole (mOsm or mO) is one one-thousandth of an osmole and, when dissolved in one liter of water, has an osmotic pressure of 17 mm Hg.

Because the number of *particles* in a liter determines osmotic pressure, substances that ionize affect osmotic pressure according to the degree of dissociation. For example, sodium chloride dissociates into $Na^+$ and $Cl^-$ in such fashion that at 0.154 molar concentration (approximating extracellular fluid) there are about 1.85 particles for each original molecule. Hence, the activity of water molecules is altered by a ratio of $\frac{1.85}{2}$,[23,34] and a pressure of 286 mO, rather than 308 mO, is exerted.

Osmality of a solution can be determined on the basis that one osmole dissolved in one liter of water will depress the freezing point of water by 1.86°C. Normal plasma or serum freezes at −0.533°C, and osmolality is therefore 0.553/1.86 or 297 mO. Freezing point depression osmometers, widely available in clinical laboratories, are of great value in determining not only plasma osmolality but that of urine and other biologic fluids, thereby assisting the clinician in evaluation of fluid and electrolyte balance.

With such large forces present, and the fact that cell membranes, with limited exceptions, such as the distal nephron of the kidney, are freely permeable to water, osmolality must be nearly if not exactly equal within cells and in their surrounding extracellular fluids. Such is almost certainly the case despite substantial differences in individual ion content and in protein concentration between cells and ECF (see Fig. 4–2).

In order to permit such ionic discrepancies to exist, other forces must be at work and energy must be expended. The Gibbs-Donnan equilibrium rule provides that under equilibrium conditions the product of concentrations of any pair of diffusible cations and anions on one side of a membrane will equal the product of the same pair of ions on the other side. When a nondiffusible ion is present on one side of a membrane, the

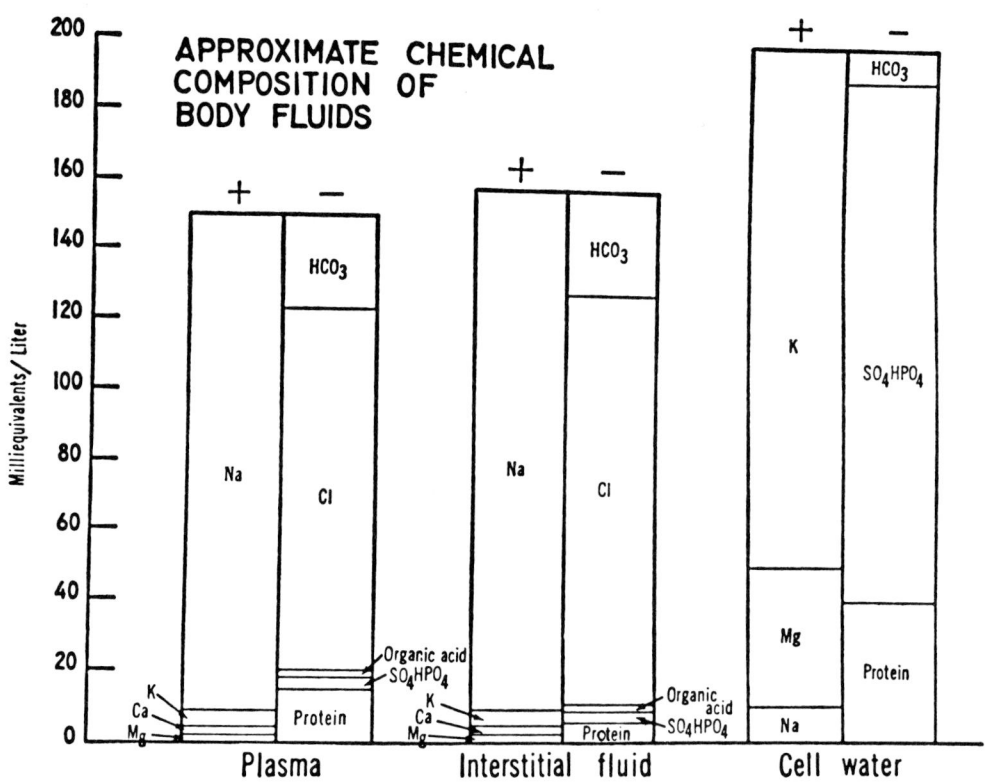

**Fig. 4–2.** The electrolyte concentrations of plasma and interstitial fluid are compared with an approximation of the electrolytes of intracellular water. (Modified from Gamble, J.L.[31])

**Table 4–5. Normal Electrolyte Concentration of Serum**

| Electrolytes | Range of Normal Including Laboratory-Method Variance | Reliability of Laboratory Test (95% Confidence Limits) |
|---|---|---|
| *Cations* | | |
| Sodium | 136–145 meq/L | ± 3 meq |
| Potassium | 3.5–5.0 meq/L | ± 0.2 meq |
| Calcium | 4.5–5.5 meq/L | ± 0.1 meq |
| | (9.0–11.0 mg/dl) | |
| Magnesium | 1.5–2.5 meq/L | ± 0.04 meq |
| | (1.8–3.0 mg/dl) | |
| *Anions* | | |
| Chloride | 96–106 meq/L | ± 2.0 meq |
| $CO_2$ (content) $TCO_2$ | 24–28.8 meq/L | ± 0.2 meq |
| Phosphorus (inorganic) | 3.0–4.5 mg/dl | Considerable variance due to |
| | (1.9 to 2.85 meq/L as $HPO_4^{2-}$) | analytic problem |
| Sulfate (as S) | 0.8–1.2 mg/dl | Method dependent |
| | (0.5–0.75 meq/L as $SO_2^{2-}$) | |
| Lactate | 0.7–1.8 meq/L | Method dependent |
| | (6 to 16 mg/dl) | |
| Protein | 6.0–7.6 g/dl | Method dependent |
| | (14–18 meq/L) | |
| | Depends on albumin | |

situation is altered: while the products of the concentration of the pairs of diffusible ions are equal, the concentrations on the two sides are unequal, and remain so. Within cells, organic phosphates and protein are nondiffusible and hold an excess of the cations K and Mg (see Fig. 4–2).[39] These forces are balanced by the remarkable property of living cells of keeping sodium out of the cell by continuous pumping. This counter-osmotic gradient, together with the probability that not all the ions and protein molecules are osmotically active (some being "bound" in large protein aggregates), provides the best current explanation of the ability of the body cell mass to maintain the transmembrane differences that are essential to life.

The extrusion of sodium from cells requires that sodium ions be pumped out against a chemical gradient (higher outside than inside) and an electrical potential that is more positive outside the cell by approximately 90 millivolts. At the same time, potassium must be moved against an even steeper chemical gradient from 4 meq/L in the extracellular fluid into a concentration of approximately 150 meq/L K in cell water. A remarkable enzyme, sodium- and potassium-dependent adenosinetriphosphatase (ATPase), is present in cell membranes and is responsible for active transport of both cations. The substantial energy required is provided by ATP, which is produced by the mitochondria in cells.[35,36]

All forms of this enzyme transport three sodium ions to two potassium ions, both against large chemical gradients. Other transport sites are also present in cell membranes that appear to use the energy of the sodium gradient created and maintained by the ATPase pump for transportation of nutrients into the cell. An example is the sodium-driven uptake of glucose and amino acids by the mucosal cells of the small bowel. Similarly, the sodium gradient energy is used to exchange sodium for intracellular calcium. The membrane potential created by Na- and K-dependent ATPase action are essential to polarization, depolarization, and repolarization of axons in the nervous system, and to intracellular concentration of calcium. This concentration is essential to and affects the strength and duration of contraction of myocardial muscle. The same pump is probably responsible for much of the net reabsorption of NaCl in the loop of Henle in the kidney.[36]

One of the effects of differing concentrations of potassium and other ions on opposite sides of a cell membrane is the development of an electrical potential across the membrane. A potential of −90 mV exists within muscle cells when compared to the ECF surrounding them. This negative potential may help to explain the rejection of Cl ion by most cells not involved in chloride transport.

Leaf has postulated that a balance of solutes stabilizes cell volume; extracellular sodium balances the effects of intracellular colloids, and a dynamic steady state results.[37] As much as one third of the total resting energy of skeletal muscle cells may be directed to the sodium pump. When metabolism of cells is interfered with by injury, hypoxia, or any other metabolic inhibitor, cells swell. The mechanism appears to be the entrance of Na and Cl ions into the cell, producing increased intracellular osmolality, which results in increased water content as water follows solute. At the same time, K is lost, but not equivalently to sodium, so that the result is a net gain in water. Figure 4–3 illustrates schematically the processes involved. If the cell survives, a new equilibrium appears to be established with time in which the intracellular Na concentration, and probably Cl, is higher than normal while the total water content of the tissue returns approximately to control levels.

Analysis of the potassium, sodium, chloride, water, and magnesium content by wet weight of fascia and gross fat-free abdominal rectus muscle of rats has been made following a standard surgical incision through the muscle compared to untraumatized muscle from the opposite side.[38] The injured muscle showed a rapid and significant increase in water, sodium, and chloride content by the time of completion of the operation. Water content reached its peak by day 2 and decreased slowly thereafter, reaching control level by day 20. Sodium content, however, continued to rise and potassium content to fall independent of change in total water content until day 10. A slow fall in sodium and chloride content of muscle matched by a progressive rise in potassium content then occurred over the next 50 days to the end of the experiment. Figures 4–4 and 4–5 show these changes. These observations suggest that a range of dynamic equilibria exists in skeletal muscle following trauma, with different ratios of intracellular and extracellular ions, that is compatible with survival. Repair by replacement of sodium by potassium within the cells proceeds slowly and is relatively independent of changes in water content.

Similar processes may occur in severe debilitating illness as well as with the hypoxia of hypoperfusion and acidosis of shock. Intracellular sodium may be higher than normal and intracellular potassium lower per unit of intracellular water in severe illness. In addition, a substantial expansion of the ECF and an increase in TBW with

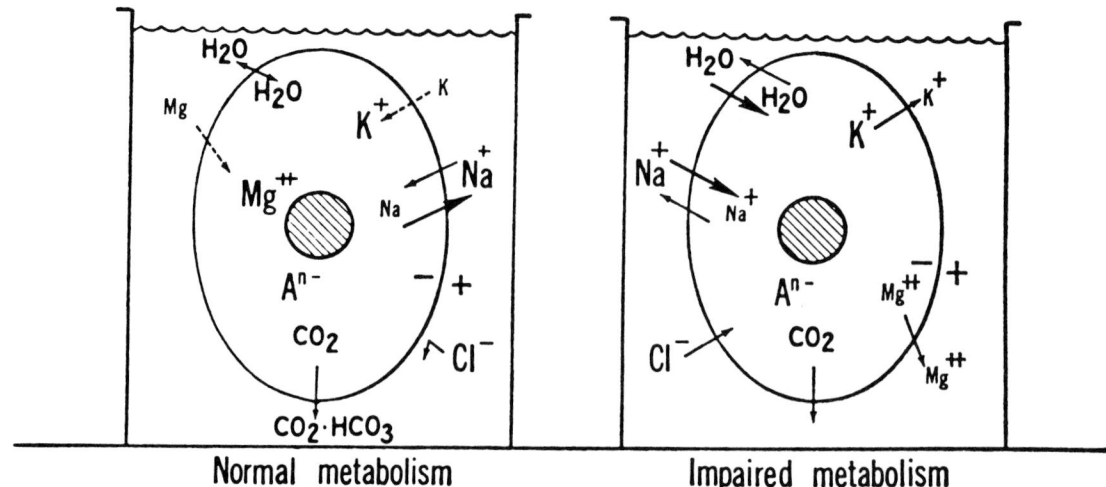

**Normal metabolism**      **Impaired metabolism**

**Fig. 4–3.** Schematic illustration of normal balance of water and electrolytes between cells and interstitial fluid compared with cell injury. Inhibition of normal metabolism results in depression of Na K-activated ATPase in cell membrane. Sodium and chloride enter the cell followed by water, while potassium and magnesium are lost. The injured cell increases in volume. (Modified from Leaf, A.[37])

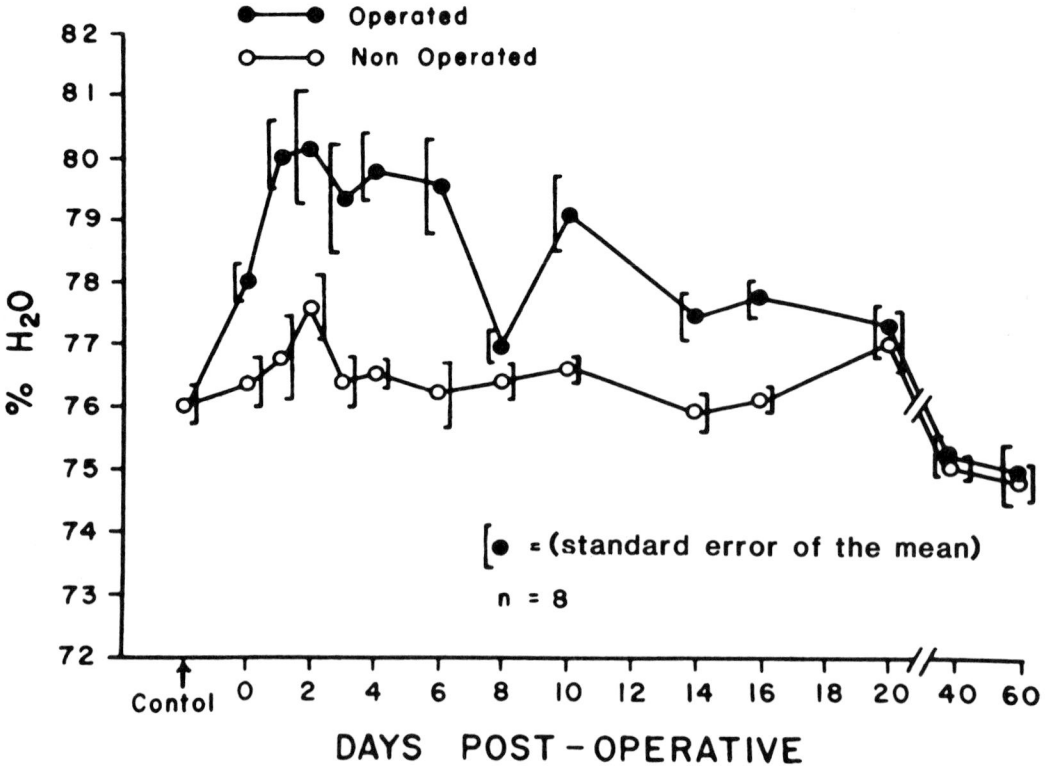

**Fig. 4–4.** Changes in the water content of incised rectus muscle of rats compared with the uninjured opposite rectus muscle of each rat. N = 8 rats for each time of sacrifice. Muscles were excised intact and dried to constant weight. (From Rocchio, M.A. and Randall, H.T.[38])

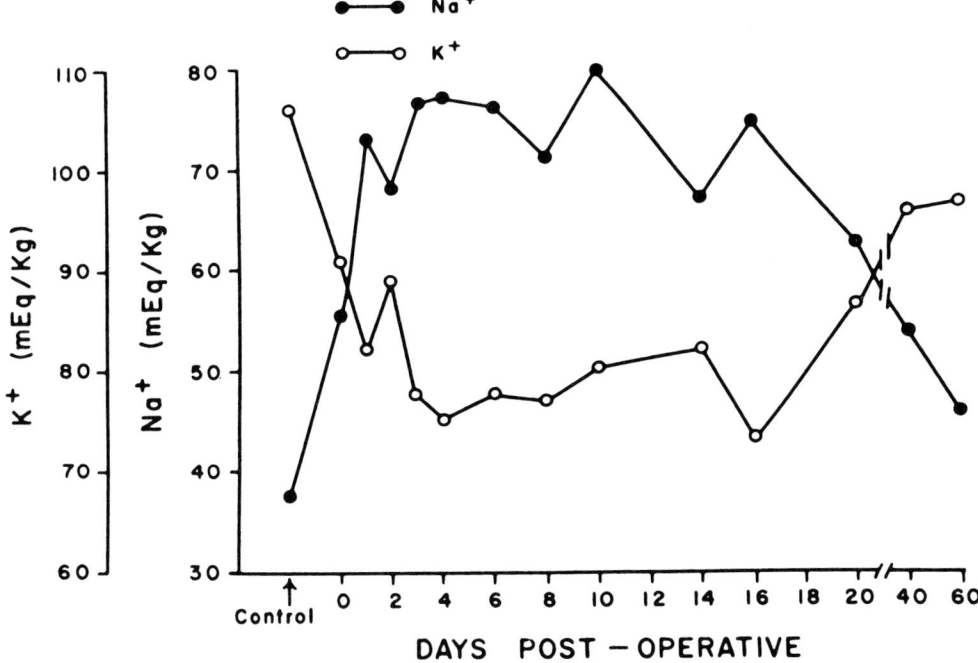

**Fig. 4–5.** Sodium and potassium content of incised rectus muscle of rats in meq/kg wet weight. N = 6 rats for each time interval. Note that the sodium concentration approximately doubled in 48 hours, while potassium concentration fell by 30%. This change occurred while the total water content of injured muscle increased only 5.5% (see Fig. 4–4), indicating intracellular sodium increase and potassium loss substantially in excess of water shift. Intracellular sodium excess and potassium deficit lasted longer than did increased water. (From Rocchio, M.A. and Randall, H.T.[38])

Na/K ratios substantially greater than 1.0 have been demonstrated.

## ACID BASE BALANCE (CONCENTRATION OF HYDROGEN ION AND ITS CONTROL IN BIOLOGIC SYSTEMS)

As noted in the historical introduction to this chapter, Henderson in 1908 described the role of weak acids and their sodium salts in resisting change in hydrogen ion [H$^+$] concentration in blood with the addition of strong acid or strong base (HCl or NaOH).[14] Van Slyke in 1921 developed volumetric apparatus for measuring the total $CO_2$, $H_2CO_3$ + $HCO_3^-$, in blood and serum, and demonstrated that the Gibbs-Donnan equilibrium theory also applied across cell membranes.[15] Peters and van Slyke introduced the terms *metabolic acidosis* and *metabolic alkalosis* and also *respiratory acidosis* and *respiratory alkalosis*, referring to conditions in the body that primarily affected plasma bicarbonate as "metabolic," and those that affected $CO_2$ tension as "respiratory."

Van Slyke noted the interdependence of both types of acid-base derangements and recorded the compensations in the alternate system that occurred to return [H$^+$] concentration toward or to a normal concentration. "A Summary of Acid Base History in Physiology and Medicine" by Van Slyke gives details of the evolution of understanding acid-base balance in man and is recommended.[40]

Some basic physical and chemical facts are needed to understand acid-base balance.

1. Water itself plays an active role in all biochemical processes. It dissociates into hydrogen [H$^+$] and hydroxyl ions [OH$^-$] to a very small degree: [H$^+$] + [OH$^-$] $\leftrightarrows$ H$_2$O and [H$^+$] × [OH$^-$] = K$_w$ H$_2$O. K$_w$, the dissociation constant of water, = 4.3 × 10$^{-16}$ eq/L at 37°C.[23]

2. The salts of strong acids dissociate completely or nearly so in physiologic concentrations in water. NaCl in solution → [Na$^+$] + [Cl$^-$]. Similarly, strong acids are almost completely dissociated HCl → [H$^+$] + [Cl$^-$].

3. Weak acids (HA) are usually those with organic acid ions; these dissociate only in a small amount so that as equilibrium is achieved between [H$^+$] + [A$^-$] and HA:

$$[H^+] \times [A^-] = K_A HA, \text{ or } [H^+] = K_A \frac{HA}{A^-}.$$

K$_A$ and pK, the negative logarithm of K$_A$

for some representative acids, are listed in Table 4–6.

4. Weak acids and their salts with strong cations (e.g., Na or K) have the ability to resist change in [$H^+$] concentration from addition of strong acid or strong base. They "buffer" the change in [$H^+$] by forming a neutral salt and increased weak acid with a small dissociation constant. For example, as noted by Henderson in 1908,[14] the complex $\frac{H_2CO_3}{NaHCO_3}$ is uniquely capable of buffering changes in plasma ($H^+$) because of two reactions:

    1. $HCl + NaHCO_3 \rightleftarrows Na^+ + Cl^- + H_2CO_3$
    2. $H_2CO_3 = P_{CO_2} \times 0.0306$. $CO_2$ in solution and $P_{CO_2}$ are regulated by respiration. Bicarbonate represents more than one half of extracellular fluid buffers, which include hemoglobin and plasma proteins. Phosphate and protein constitute major intracellular buffers.

5. The *strong* ions (sodium, potassium, magnesium, calcium) and the strong anions (chloride and sulfate) *do not function as buffers, and are neither acids nor bases.* Their charges, either + or −, however, are highly significant. Electroneutrality (+ = −) must exist in all solutions. Therefore, the strong ion difference (SID), the sum of strong cations *minus* strong anions, plays an important role in acid-base balance.

According to Stewart, only three *independent* variables control acid-base.[23] They are SID, $P_{CO_2}$, and the total of weak acid buffers (HA) + (A−) = (A total).

The magnitude of SID is approximately 31 meq/L in interstitial fluid and 42 meq/L in plasma. A total is about 20 meq/L in plasma.

Stewart calculates SID to be very large in intracellular fluid, as large as 130 meq/L. A total is approximately 200 meq/L ICW.

6. In clinical practice, *pH*, the negative logarithm of (H⁺), $\log_{10} \frac{1}{H^+}$ or − log [H⁺], is commonly used to denote hydrogen ion concentration in biologic fluids. If hydrogen ion is expressed in nanomoles per liter, $10^{-9}$ mol, at pH values of whole blood compatible with survival, the concentration of hydrogen ion at 37°C is:

| pH | 7.0 | 7.1 | 7.2 | 7.3 | 7.4 | 7.5 | 7.6 | 7.7 |
|---|---|---|---|---|---|---|---|---|
| [H] (nmol/L) | 100 | 80 | 63 | 50 | 40 | 32 | 25 | 20 |

It is essential to record temperature and whether whole blood or plasma is examined in reporting both pH and hydrogen ion content or activity.

## Carbon Dioxide System

Total carbon dioxide concentration ($T_{CO_2}$) is the total carbon dioxide extractable from a biologic fluid with strong acid. This amount includes dissolved carbon dioxide, carbonic acid, bicarbonate ion, and carbamino compounds. This is the usual value reported by clinical laboratories as total $CO_2$ or $CO_2$ content of plasma.

The partial pressure of carbon dioxide in gas phase ($P_{CO_2}$) in equilibrium with a biologic fluid is usually reported in mm Hg or torr. Although $P_{CO_2}$ can be directly measured by diffusion through a specially prepared Teflon membrane standardized with gas of known $CO_2$ concentration, the value is often calculated from pH and $T_{CO_2}$ by use of a nomogram based on the Henderson-Hasselbalch equation.

Carbonic acid concentration [$H_2CO_3$] in biologic fluids is small in comparison to dissolved carbon dioxide concentration. The usual units are nmol/L or meq/L.

Dissolved carbon dioxide concentration is the quantity of dissolved carbon dioxide gas in a specified volume; however, usually $H_2CO_3$ is included also. The sum of the two is designated as S × $P_{CO_2}$ where S is the solubility coefficient relating the sum of the concentrations of dissolved $CO_2$ and $H_2CO_3$ in nmol/L to $P_{CO_2}$ in mm Hg. This value is temperature dependent; at 37°C for blood or plasma, S = 0.0306.

## Table 4–6. Acid Dissociation Constants

| Substance | $K_A^1$* | $pK_A$* |
|---|---|---|
| Acetic acid | $2.0 \times 10^{-5}$ | 4.7 |
| Acetoacetic acid | $1.6 \times 10^{-4}$ | 3.8 |
| Carbonic acid | $7.95 \times 10^{-7}$ | 6.1 |
| Hydroxybutyric acid | $1.6 \times 10^{-5}$ | 4.8 |
| Lactic acid | $1.3 \times 10^{-4}$ | 3.9 |
| Phosphoric acid A²* | $3.0 \times 10^{-7}$ | 6.8 |

*$K_A^1$ is the dissociation constant for the first hydrogen of each weak acid; $pK_A^1$ is $\frac{1}{\log K_A^1}$. When a second dissociation occurs, as with phosphoric acid, the constant for the second dissociation is designated $K_A^2$.

Bicarbonate ion concentration $[HCO_3^-]$ is chemically defined as the concentration of $HCO_3^-$ in biologic fluids. In physiologic studies and clinical use, however, it is calculated as total $CO_2 - S \times P_{CO_2}$. This value includes carbamino compounds and carbonate ion in addition to bicarbonate ion. Their inclusion makes little difference in plasma or interstitial fluid, but introduces large errors for intracellular fluid:

$$[HCO_3^-] = T_{CO_2} - S \times P_{CO_2}$$

## Henderson-Hasselbalch Equation

This equation describes the relationships in serum or plasma among total $CO_2$ ($T_{CO_2}$), bicarbonate $[HCO_3^-]$, partial pressure of $CO_2$, and pH. Two constants are involved in the equation: $pK$, the $\log_{10}$ of $\dfrac{1}{K1}$ for $HHCO_3$, which is 6.1, and $S$, the solubility coefficient of $CO_2$ in plasma at $37°C$. $[HCO_3^-]$ is a derived figure, $T_{CO_2} - S \times P_{CO_2} = (HCO_3)$

$$pH = pK_1 + \log_{10} \frac{(T_{CO_2} - S \times P_{CO_2})}{S \times P_{CO_2}}$$

or

$$pH = pK_1 + \log_{10} \frac{[HCO_3^-]}{S \times P_{CO_2}}$$

The relationships among total $CO_2$ ($T_{CO_2}$), $P_{CO_2}$, and pH can be expressed graphically, as shown in Figure 4–6. The pH scale has been expanded so that the $P_{CO_2}$ isobars are linear. Clinical laboratories often use a nomogram or table to predict the third value when two of the three (pH, $T_{CO_2}$, and $P_{CO_2}$) have been measured.

In general, plasma bicarbonate, calculated from the Henderson-Hasselbalch equation, is used as a measure of the *metabolic* derangements of acid-base balance, recognizing that alterations in plasma bicarbonate also reflect compensatory changes secondary to a respiratory $P_{CO_2}$ derangement.

Similarly, $P_{CO_2}$ regarded as a measure of the *respiratory component* of acid-base disequilibria, recognizing that such changes may either represent a primary disorder or result from secondary compensatory changes.

Mixed primary derangements are also possible; one example, is the simultaneous existence of respiratory and metabolic acidosis in severe injury, or sepsis complicating chronic obstructive pulmonary disease. Another example is metabolic alkalosis due to gastric chloride loss or potassium deficiency, occurring with either respiratory acidosis or alkalosis, particularly in patients on ventilators.

The *usual* findings in changes of $T_{CO_2}$, $P_{CO_2}$, and pH with a primary metabolic or respiratory disturbance with a change in pH are shown in the designated areas in Figure 4–6. Partial but incomplete compensation is included. Values that fall in between the designated areas are often the product of *two simultaneous* derangements. Note that pH may be in the normal range.

Figure 4–7 indicates the primary defect produced by metabolic and respiratory acidosis and alkalosis and the early secondary compensation that will occur. Both renal and respiratory compensations are indicated. These compensations *should not* be considered as acidosis or alkalosis, but should be reported as "metabolic acidosis with compensatory fall in $P_{CO_2}$" or "respiratory acidosis with compensatory fall in plasma chloride and increase in bicarbonate." When possible, independent measurements of pH, $T_{CO_2}$, and $P_{CO_2}$ should be made for seriously ill patients. Arterial blood provides greater accuracy in assessing pulmonary function and $P_{CO_2}$. In addition, it permits measurement of the partial pressure of oxygen, oxygen content, and hemoglobin saturation of arterial blood. These determinations are called blood gases.

Mixed venous blood, preferably drawn from a large vein without a tourniquet, or a minute or two after tourniquet removal, has a pH averaging 0.02 pH units lower than arterial blood, and a $P_{CO_2}$ 3 to 5 mm higher than arterial blood. When cardiac output is significantly reduced, peripheral venous blood becomes inaccurate in assessing acid-base status, and arterial blood is required.

## Whole Blood Base Excess, or $\Delta$ Buffer Base Method

This system, based on the work of Siggaard-Andersen,[42,43] holds that the metabolic component of acid-base equilibrium can be most precisely determined by titrating to pH 7.40 with strong acid or alkali whole blood that is equilibrated with $P_{CO_2}$ at 40 mm Hg at $37°C$. The determination of the number of meq of base lost or gained by 1 L of whole blood under these circumstances is independent of respiratory function and represents nonvolatile acid or base accumulation. It is stated that the two most valuable parameters for clinical evalution of acid-base metabolism are $P_{CO_2}$ and the accumulation of nonvolatile acids or bases.

Values that are determined include: whole blood base excess or $\Delta$ Bb, blood or plasma $P_{CO_2}$, plasma pH. These are usually reported as "base excess" or -base excess (deficit) in meq/L. Base excess is not independent of $P_{CO_2}$ in vivo. The titration curve of blood in vivo is slightly different

# ···ACID-BASE PATTERN-ANALYSIS DIAGRAM···

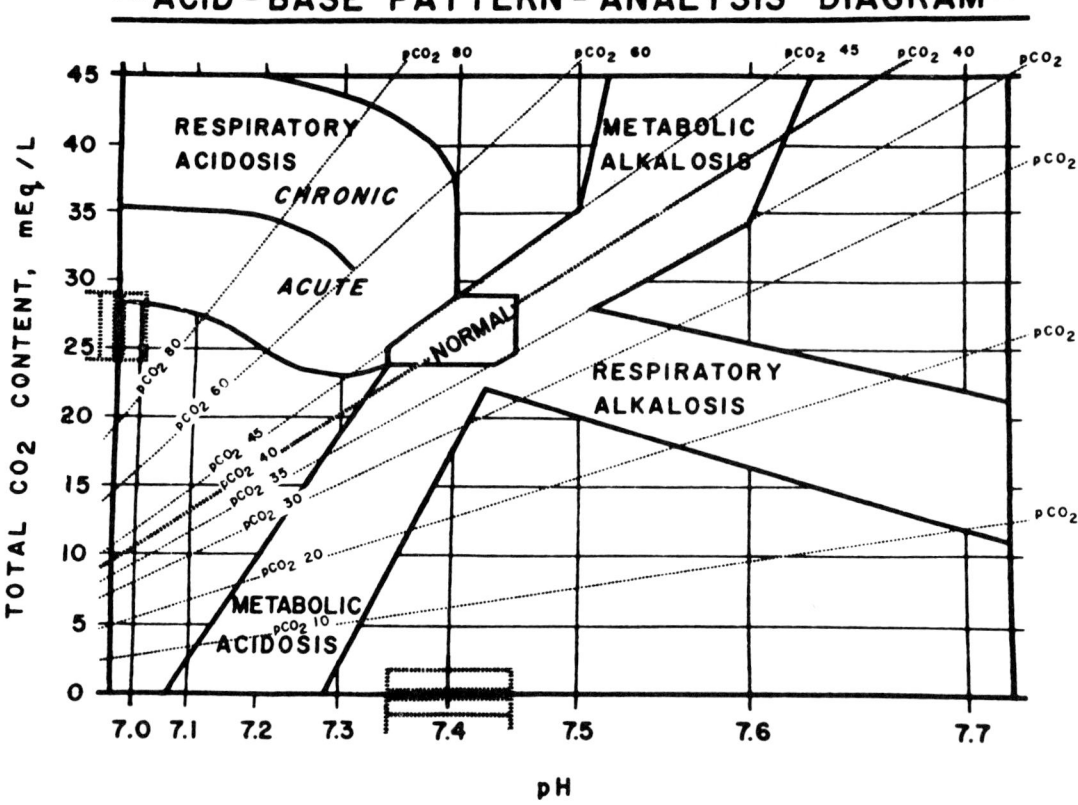

**Fig. 4–6.**   Acid base analysis diagram developed by R.V. Stephens, M.D. in our laboratory. The pH scale is inverted $(\frac{1}{pH})$ so that the $P_{CO_2}$ isobars are straight lines. Designated areas for metabolic acidosis and alkalosis and respiratory acidosis and alkalosis represent findings with a *single primary derangement with compensation.* Normal ranges for $T_{CO_2}$ and pH are shown as heavy bars. When plotted on the diagram two coexisting derangements will fall between the areas indicated for a single primary change and the usual compensation. See also Figure 4–7. (From Randall, H.T. Surg. Clin. North Am. *56*:1019–1058, 1976. Reprinted with permission from W.B. Saunders Co.[44])

than in vitro. As with any system of analysis of acid-base status, a careful assessment of the patient is essential for clinical interpretation and for determination of therapy.[44]

## METABOLISM OF WATER AND ELECTROLYTES

### Water Intake and Losses

Man requires free water to maintain water balance. Even with maximum concentration of urine solutes, the water contained in the foods of a normal diet and the water produced by oxidation of food are inadequate to provide for urinary excretion of the end products of metabolism, for losses of water from the bowel, and for losses by evaporation from the respiratory tract and skin.

Water contained in food averages from 1,000 to 1,500 ml per day. Water of oxidation of fat provides 1.07 g water/g of fat, that from starch 0.6 g/g, and that from protein approximately 0.41 g.

Thus, water of oxidation from a 2,500-kcal diet, containing 15% protein, 50% carbohydrate, and 35% fat, is approximately 330 ml per day.

The volume of ingested free water and dilute fluids varies greatly with environment, being largest in warm humid areas. Habit also plays a significant role in the volume of intake. Adults in a temperate climate drink 1,000 to 2,000 ml or more of water and dilute fluids a day. Thus, total available water ranges from 2,000 to 3,500 ml or more per day, or about 10% of total body water of 30 to 40 L.

Loss takes place by four different routes: by urinary output and the water content of stool, both of which are measurable, and by evaporation from the respiratory tract and the skin. The latter two, measured only with great difficulty, are termed "insensible losses." In the normal individual, water intake and loss balance closely, and daily body weight fluctuates less than 1% if determined

| STATE | $\Delta$pH | $\Delta$PCo$_2$ | $\Delta$TCo$_2$ | EARLY SECONDARY COMPENSATION |
|---|---|---|---|---|
| Metabolic Alkalosis | ↑ | ± TO ↑ | ↑ * | Variable $\Delta$PCo$_2$ within O$_2$ limits, Renal excretion HCo$_3$] |
| Respiratory Alkalosis | ↑ | ↓ * | ± TO ↓ | Renal ? [HCo$_3$]⁻ excretion ↑Organic acid c̄ Hypoxia |
| Metabolic Acidosis | ↓ | ↓ | ↓ * | Hyperventilation, Renal [H]⁺ excretion |
| Respiratory Acidosis | ↓ | ↑ * | ↑ | Renal excretion of Cl⁻ and [H] |

\* INITIAL AND PRIMARY CHANGE

**Fig. 4–7.** Primary changes in Pco$_2$ and Tco$_2$ are shown for metabolic alkalosis, respiratory alkalosis, metabolic acidosis, and respiratory acidosis. Early secondary compensation that produces a tendency to return pH toward 7.40 is also shown. The renal compensation for metabolic alkalosis is limited by volume depletion of the ECF, and is largely blocked by significant total body potassium deficiency.

at the same time of day. Insensible losses depend on body size, on degree of physical exertion, and on environmental temperature and humidity. In an environment of moderate temperature and humidity, losses are substantially less than in a warm humid environment where sweat loss becomes large. Respiratory insensible loss averages 300 to 500 ml per day in females and up to 750 ml per day in large males. Surface evaporation and sweat together average 400 to 600 ml a day. Total insensible water loss is between 300 and 500 ml per m² of body surface area per day, with minimal activity in a temperate environment.[45–47] Sweat volume is small in a temperate climate except with vigorous activity. It may reach several liters a day, with serious losses of both water and sodium chloride, in warm humid environments with exposure to the sun.

Gump et al. have found total insensible loss in afebrile surgical patients to average 23 ml/m²/hour. Insensible losses increase with fever, but the standard deviations are so large that prediction of increased loss for a particular individual is not possible.[48] Markedly obese patients have an increased insensible water loss. Brill measured losses of 2.4 to 2.9 L a day in a group of markedly obese patients compared to an average loss of 0.9 L per day in normal individuals.[49]

Daily or more frequent determination of body *weight* is the only reliable method of estimating insensible losses, and it must be combined with an accurate intake and output record to achieve useful clinical data.

Urine volume represents the difference between total water intake plus water of oxidation and the sum of insensible losses plus the water in stool (normally 100 to 200 ml per day). Normal adults excrete 1,000 to 2,500 ml of urine a day. Minimal urine volume in a young adult with normal renal function is about 600 ml per day. This volume requires the ability to concentrate the urine to a specific gravity above 1.030 and with an osmolality of 1,000 to 1,200 mO. Urea represents more than one half the total solutes from a normal diet. Urea excretion is increased by a high-protein intake and by trauma or sepsis, which produces increased catabolism of body protein. A large protein intake or acute illness may substantially increase minimal urine volume. Renal disease increases the minimal urine volume required to clear a given solute load, since the ability to concentrate the urine is diminished or lost. Renal efficiency progressively decreases with age.

Concentration of the urine beyond the osmolality of plasma (290 mO) and excretion of very dilute urine both require increased renal work. Unless there are compelling medical or surgical reasons to alter fluid intake, sufficient water should be ingested or provided in intravenous solutions so that the urine osmolality is less than 600 mO and more than 150 mO/kg $H_2O$. In the absence of glucose, mannitol, intravenous radiographic contrast media, xylose, or other substances that increase urine specific gravity abnormally, this range of osmolality usually corresponds to a specific gravity between 1.006 and 1.020. Depending on the size, sex, and age of the individual and assuming reasonably normal renal function, these limits can be maintained with a urine volume of 800 to 1500 ml in 24 hours.

With starvation, and particularly in patients who suffer from sepsis or major trauma, intracellular water is mobilized and transferred to the extracellular fluid space where it may cause overexpansion and dilution of the normal extracellular electrolytes, particularly sodium and chloride. This endogenous water reflects excessive catabolism of intracellular protein. It is accompanied by transfer of potassium to the extracellular fluid from which it is excreted by the kidneys. As much as 500 ml of intracellular water and 75 meq of potassium per day may be added to the extracellular fluid in a sick septic patient.[49a]

### Electrolyte Intake and Excretion

This section discusses the metabolism of sodium, potassium, and chloride. Calcium, magnesium, phosphate, iron, iodine, and other trace elements are considered in other chapters.

**Sodium Balance and Intake.** The value of salt, sodium chloride in relatively pure state, has been recognized since early recorded history as not only a pleasurable but also an essential component of man's diet. In most of the world today, intake of sodium salts is regulated more by taste, custom, and habit than by need. Careful planning of diets is necessary to reduce sodium intake below 1 g (43 meq) a day, which is approximately the minimal requirement for an active normal adult in a temperate climate. Diets containing less than 0.3 g of sodium are unpalatable and not well tolerated by most patients.

Normal sodium intake varies from 2 g to as much as 10 a day. A group of 28 adults who volunteered to undergo metabolic balance studies for 2 weeks prior to elective surgery for gallbladder disease or inguinal hernia were permitted to select their own diets and seasoning. The only limitation was moderate fat restriction for those with gallstones and a total caloric intake of 30 to 40 calories per kg body weight a day. Thirty-five diet weeks yielded an average sodium intake in food and added salt of 98.9 meq (2.28 g) a day, with two thirds of the group selecting an intake of 76 to 120 meq (1.75 to 2.75 g). Potassium intake ranged from

65 to 88 meq (2.5 to 3.4 g) and chloride from 85 to 145 meq (2.4 to 4.1 g).[50] All but 6 to 10 meq of the ingested sodium and 4 to 6 meq of potassium were recovered from urine and stool of these patients. Since the patients neither gained nor lost significant weight and were in nitrogen balance, the missing sodium and potassium were interpreted as "insensible loss," probably losses from skin cells shed, and as sweat. Streeten and Rapoport found a mean surface loss of 3.3 meq of sodium a day in normal volunteers bathed in distilled water whose clothes were also analyzed for sodium loss.[51]

*Plasma Sodium Concentration.* Sodium is the major cation of the extracellular fluid. It is normally maintained within narrow limits at a concentration of 140 ± 3 meq/L of plasma or 147 ± 3 meq/L in extracellular fluid. It is the major determinant of the osmolar strength of the ECF and, in turn, of intracellular osmolality as well. Plasma osmolality can be closely approximated from data or plasma sodium (meq/L) and the concentrations of urea and glucose:

$$\text{Plasma osmolality (mO)} = 2 \times \text{Na (meq)/L} + \frac{\text{BUN (mg/dl)}}{3} + \frac{\text{glucose (mg/dl)}}{18}$$

*ECF Volume and Total Sodium.* The volume of ECF is also closely related to the *total* sodium in the ECF. Regulation of the volume of interstitial fluid and plasma is controlled by volume sensors, which are pressure and distention sensitive and are located in the cardiac atria, the right ventricle, and the pulmonary capillaries. Arterial pressure sensors also exist in the carotid arteries and the aortic arch.[52,53] Signals from these receptors proceed to the medulla and hypothalamus where they invoke multiple responses. With a *decrease* in ECF or blood volume, sympathetic inhibition is released, and sympathetic activity increases. Renin release is increased, leading to an increase in angiotensin II. Adrenal medullary secretion of epinephrine and norepinephrine is increased, as is the secretion of glucagon by the pancreas. ACTH is released by the pituitary in response to acute volume change, as is seen in hemorrhage. This ACTH and angiotensin II result in an increased adrenal secretion of aldosterone and cortisol. These factors promote sodium retention by the kidneys and usually lead to increased potassium loss.

Central nervous signals also increase the secretion of antidiuretic hormone (ADH), which promotes increased absorption of water and, acting together with aldosterone, increases sodium reabsorption from the distal collecting ducts of the kidneys.[53]

*Thirst* is a prominent symptom resulting from reduction in the volume of the ECF without a change in osmolality, or from an increase in osmolality, or both. A 1 to 2% decrease in total body water is the usual stimulus, and represents a change of 350 to 700 ml in the normal adult. A decrease in intravascular volume, as seen with acute hemorrhage, and the infusion or ingestion of hypertonic solutions are also effective stimuli to the sensation of thirst. The centers for control of thirst, located in the ventromedial and anterior hypothalamus, are in close relationship to or overlap the centers of the neurohypophysis that regulate ADH.[54]

Thirst may occur in spite of a normal or even overexpanded total body water if *intracellular* fluid is decreased by infusion of hypertonic extracellular fluids. Thirst may also occur if effective interstitial and intravascular fluid volumes are decreased by rapid sequestration of a part of the volumes into an area of injury, such as a burn, a crush injury, or an infection, or by rapid accumulation of ascitic fluid or peripheral edema. Thirst is inhibited by expansion of total body water, by reduction of osmolality, or by isotonic expansion of body fluids.

*Fasting and Sodium Homeostasis.* ECF volume and total ECF sodium are also affected by caloric intake. Total fasting is accompanied by a substantial loss of water and sodium by renal excretion with an initial rapid weight loss. After several days, renal conservation of sodium becomes evident. Boulter et al. have shown that the water and sodium losses occur even if 50 meq of Na and 87 meq of K a day are provided with water during fasting.[55] The critical nutrient appears to be carbohydrate. When dietary carbohydrate was restricted to 50 g a day or less in obese adults by isocaloric substitution with fat, the same pattern of sodium and water excretion occurred as with total fasting. Following six days of sodium loss, sodium conservation and positive balance resulted with 50 meq/day intake.

Blood volume has been shown to decrease by an average of 770 ml or 14% during 10 days of fasting. This change was markedly reduced by the oral administration of 90 meq Na per day. However, the negative water and sodium balance of the first seven days of fasting was not prevented.[56]

Analysis of the urine of fasting patients showed a large increase in ammonia, particularly during the second week of fasting. $NH_4$ permits release of $[H^+]$ as an organic cation, e.g., $NH_3 + [H^+] \rightarrow [NH_4^+]$, accompanied by decreased sodium and potassium secretion. Urine pH rose steadily as urine phosphate declined and organic anions increased. Creatinine clearance diminished as did urea output and clearance.[57,58]

A sudden reduction in the intake of sodium and carbohydrate in a diet will also result in initial weight loss with urinary sodium and potassium losses. After, the first week, to 10 days on a subcaloric diet with lower than usual carbohydrate intake, however, weight loss becomes related to the amount of metabolized fat and is much slower. High protein supplements and diuretics potentiate potassium loss, and without careful monitoring are potentially dangerous with serious food restriction.

*Hyponatremia and Hypernatremia.* To this point, changes in ECF *volume* and total body water have been discussed in situations in which the *concentration* of plasma sodium remains relatively constant and within normal range. *Total body sodium is decreased* with volume loss of the ECF, whether due to starvation or semistarvation, acute losses from the gastrointestinal tract as in vomiting or diarrhea, excessive sweating in a hot humid environment, or renal losses due to diuretics, or as the result of renal excretion of sodium as the primary compensation for metabolic alkalosis (see Fig. 4–7). Restitution of ECF volume and concentration to normal requires both water and sodium salts.

In some clinical situations, an imbalance between ECF volume and plasma sodium exists. Because sodium is the dominant determinant of osmolality, significant hyponatremia determines a hypo-osmolar ECF and also changes intracellular ion concentrations. A sudden drop in plasma sodium concentration (as for example with large volumes of infusion of dextrose in water, or oral intake of water without salt to replace severe diarrhea) results in entry of water into cells and cell swelling.

Inappropriate secretion of antidiuretic hormone (ADH) results in major alteration of body fluid balance through water retention. The clinical findings are (1) hyponatremia with hypo-osmolality of the plasma, (2) continued renal excretion of $Na^+$ despite hyponatremia, (3) absence of clinical evidence of volume depletion, (4) urine less than maximally dilute, and (5) normal renal and adrenal function.[59] The primary causes of the syndrome of inappropriate secretion of ADH include tumors (particularly cancer of the lung or pancreas, which may synthesize ectopic ADH), trauma, tumors of the brain or its meninges, severe pulmonary infection, the postoperative state following anesthesia, sepsis,[60] and certain drugs, such as vincristine.

Symptoms appear to be related to the *rate of*

*change* of the sodium concentration and osmolality of the plasma. If these fall slowly, over several days or weeks, essentially no complaints occur until the sodium concentration falls to approximately 120 meq/L. With a rapid dilution by water ingestion or infusion, or when the serum sodium is below 120 meq/L, the chief complaints are loss of appetite, nausea, vomiting, and weakness. Patients become drowsy, irritable, confused, and sometimes hostile. Muscle weakness is pronounced, deep tendon reflexes are diminished or absent, and neurologic signs resembling bulbar palsy may be seen. Coma, convulsions, and death may occur. Edema is rare except with water overloading in excess of 3 to 4 L.

Plasma sodium and chloride concentrations tend to fall together in patients with inappropriate ADH release. Bicarbonate concentration of the plasma remains nearly normal, as does blood pH. The urine volume is not increased, and a relative oliguria may exist. The characteristic finding of substantial amounts of sodium in the urine (30 to 50 meq/L or more) in the presence of hyponatremia is seen only with inappropriate ADH, adrenal insufficiency, or severe renal disease.

Treatment consists of water restriction. A maximum intake of 500 to 700 ml a day in the adult, with 150 g of carbohydrate either orally or as 25% dextrose given slowly intravenously into the superior vena cava, results in a progressive rise in the serum sodium and often in a brisk diuresis with diminished urine sodium. Unless sodium deficit is known to exist concurrently, sodium salts should probably not be administered. If there is a sodium deficit, 100 to 150 meq of NaCl as 3% or 5% saline may be given slowly I.V., *followed by strict restriction of total fluid intake.*

Table 4–7 lists common causes of hyponatremia and hypernatremia.

**Chloride Balance.** Normal chloride intake in diet was 85 to 145 meq a day in a series of patients on an ad libitum diet intake.[50] Intake varied with types of food and added NaCl.

Normal plasma chloride concentration is 100 to 106 meq/L, a value that, like that of plasma sodium, is subject to little normal variation. Dietary intake of chloride is usually in excess of sodium. Virtually all the intake is excreted in the urine in conjunction with sodium and potassium ions. The *strong ion* difference (SID) in plasma and ECF between $Na^+ + K^+ + Mg^{++} + Ca^{++}$ and $Cl^- + HPO_4^{2-} + SO_4^{2-}$ is maintained.

The 40 to 60 meq of $H^+$ excreted in the urine daily with an "acid ash" diet is buffered by the $\dfrac{Na_2HPO_4}{NaH_2PO_4}$ buffer system and, to a small degree,

normally by the weak base $NH^+_4$ so that urine pH seldom falls below pH 5.0.

Changes in chloride ion concentration in the plasma follow those of sodium in dilutional hypotonicity and in desiccation dehydration. Deviation from the normal plasma sodium/chloride ratio of slightly less than 3:2 is usually due to excessive chloride loss from the gastrointestinal tract or kidneys or to chloride retention with renal disease or ureterointestinal anastomoses. Table 4–8 shows the common causes of hypochloremia and hyperchloremia.

**Potassium Balance.** As noted earlier, more than 95% of body potassium is intracellular. Daily dietary intake of potassium of 60 to 100 meq equals or exceeds the total ECF potassium. Plasma and interstitial fluid potassium concentrations are held within narrow limits of concentration by a combination of prompt renal excretion of excess K and some intracellular transfer induced by glucose and insulin. A small amount of potassium is excreted normally in feces; however, losses may become marked with large volumes of diarrhea or loss of fluid from small bowel.

Immediately following trauma, including surgical operations, potassium is lost substantially in excess of the usual intracellular ratio of 3 meq/g nitrogen, and appears in high concentration in the urine. This response may be accentuated in debilitated hyponatremic patients. On the other hand, potassium plasma concentration may rise to dangerously high levels if significant dehydration also exists.

Potassium balance becomes positive before nitrogen balance does in convalescence., often by two or more days.

*Plasma or Serum Potassium Concentration.* This concentration is *not* a reliable index of total body potassium, nor is it per se an indication for the administration or withholding of potassium. Only the extremes of high and low concentration are important of themselves. Potassium concentration in excess of 6 meq/L with no hemolysis in the specimen requires an explanation and appropriate treatment. Levels of potassium of 7 meq/L or higher constitute an emergency requiring immediate action to prevent cardiac arrest.

Plasma potassium concentrations of 3 meq/L or less usually represent significant loss of total body potassium, and levels of 2.5 meq/L or less present additional serious complication of cardiac arrhythmias and skeletal and smooth muscle paralysis.

*Hypokalemia.* The ingestion of carbohydrate without potassium or the infusion of glucose solutions will reduce the resting plasma K concentrations in many patients by as much as 0.5 meq/

**Table 4–7.  Causes of Hyponatremia and Hypernatremia**

*Hyponatremia* = plasma sodium concentration less than 135 meq/L
1. In chronic wasting illnesses: e.g., cancer, chronic infection, liver disease, semistarvation, ulcerative colitis, congestive heart failure, ascites, and edema.
2. Following major surgical treatment or extensive trauma: e.g., extensive soft tissue injury, burns, major fractures, severe infection, fluid sequestration in a third space of tissue injury, transcellular pooling, anesthesia, or treatment with morphine and meperidine.
3. With excessive water intake, usually iatrogenic: e.g., antidiuresis of trauma or chronic debility, excessive intravenous glucose and water, retained water from irrigations or hypotonic wet dressings, excessive oral intake, acute renal insufficiency without adequate water restriction, or inappropriate ADH syndrome.
4. As the result of abnormal external loss of sodium with inadequate replacement: e.g., gastrointestinal losses through diarrhea, vomiting, or intestinal intubation; bowel, biliary, or pancreatic fistulas; decompression of incompletely obstructed distal urinary tract; osmotic diuresis from glucose, mannitol, or urea; excessive sweating; or adrenal insufficiency.
5. As the result of dietary restriction or drugs: e.g., chlorothiazide, mercurial diuretics, ethacrynic acid or furosemide diuresis, low sodium diets for prolonged periods, particularly in chronic heart, liver, or kidney disease, or for hypertension.
6. Factitious: e.g., laboratory error or sampling error with dilution by glucose infusion or other sodium-free sources of water. In addition, the presence of very high levels of plasma lipid or protein, which decrease plasma water concentration.

*Hypernatremia* = plasma sodium more than 150 meq/L
1. Dehydration by loss of hypotonic fluid (desiccation) without adequate water replacement: e.g., respiratory loss with fever, dry oxygen, tracheotomy, hyperventilation of dyspnea, or metabolic acidosis; skin losses with burns; or prolonged exposure to dry heat.
2. Excessive solute loading: e.g., concentrated tube feedings of all types high in protein and salts without adequate supplemental water intake or isotonic electrolyte solutions as the total source of water intake.
3. Large volume of dilute urine: e.g., ineffective antidiuretic hormone level, diabetes insipidus, brain stem injury, and the posthypophysectomy state.

L. This occurrence is partially due to the incorporation of potassium with glucose in the intermediate stages of glycogen formation. In addition, insulin stimulates sodium- potassium-dependent ATPase to enhance intracellular transfer of potassium.[61,62] Alkalosis, either metabolic or respiratory, enhances both intracellular potassium transfer and renal excretion of potassium.

Most patients with hypokalemia have *decreased total body potassium* caused by renal excretion, losses in gastrointestinal tract fluids, and wounds. In surgical patients, these sources of loss often exist concurrently.

Undesirable effects of hypokalemia and reduced total body K include:[62]

1. Impaired glucose tolerance, with impaired insulin secretion.
2. Impaired protein anabolism.
3. Cardiac effects: reduced amplitude of T waves; development of U waves; atrial and ventricular PVC, possibly worse with digitalis; heart failure with salt and water retention, and myocardiolysis with severe and prolonged low $K^+$.
4. Smooth and striated muscle effects: weakness and paralysis due to increased resting membrane potential, ileus, urinary retention, and respiratory and vocal cord muscle weakness.
5. Renal effects: impairment of renal concentration of urine, enhanced $HCO_3^-$ reabsorption by proximal tubules, increased $NH_4^+$ excretion, vacuolization of proximal convoluted tubular cells and interstitial nephritis.
6. Metabolic alkalosis with hypochloremia refrac-

tory to NaCl administration, with paradoxical aciduria.

Common causes of hypokalemia are shown in Table 4–9.

The treatment of hypokalemia consists of the administration of potassium chloride. Intravenous solutions should not exceed 40 meq/L of potassium ion per liter except in certain instances, and the salt must therefore be given in 5% glucose in water or other isotonic solutions. The rate of intravenous administration of potassium salts should not normally exceed 15 to 20 meq per hour in the average-sized adult, except in emergency situations such as digitalis toxicity or skeletal muscle paralysis when constant electrocardiogram monitoring is essential. Therapeutic doses of potassium chloride are 50 to 150 meq per day, and 40 meq per day is indicated in baseline parenteral fluids. Potassium can be given by mouth either in the form of citrus or tomato juices, or as flavored solutions containing 5 to 10% KCl. Slowly dissolving oral capsules or tablets are also available.

Infusion of KCl in small volumes with concentration exceeding 40 meq/L is sometimes used to treat cardiac arrhythmias in patients with plasma levels of 3.0 meq/L or less or those with chronic renal tubular losses secondary to nephrotoxic drugs. *The greatest care must be used* to assure that the small volume of concentrated KCl is administered *slowly* and *uniformly* at a rate not to

### Table 4–8.  Common Causes of Hypochloremia and Hyperchloremia

*Hypochloremia* = plasma chloride level less than 95 meq/L

1. Dilutional, with hyponatremia, in an expanded extracellular fluid following trauma, with wasting diseases, in water retention with overloading, or with sequestration of extracellular fluid in a third space of injury.
2. Chloride loss from the gastrointestinal tract, particularly from vomiting or gastric suction, but common with salt loss from all levels without adequate replacement.
3. Diuretics, with a loss of chloride in excess of sodium and with high loss of potassium in urine.
4. Adrenal steroid administration with sodium retention and potassium and chloride loss in urine.
5. Compensating mechanism in chronic respiratory acidosis, with high plasma $PCO_2$, total $CO_2$ and $HCO_3^-$ levels, and normal or low pH.
6. Elevated plasma carbon dioxide level and pH and low plasma potassium level in hypokalemic hypochloremic alkalosis.
7. Chronic renal disease and acute renal failure.

*Hyperchloremia* = plasma chloride level above 110 meq/L.

1. Hypernatremia in desiccation dehydration, excess solute loading, diabetes insipidus, or brain stem injury.
2. Ureterointestinal anastomoses due to reabsorption of chloride by the bowel, potentiated by renal insufficiency and by prolonged exposure of bowel mucosa to urine.
3. Iatrogenic with excessive administration of ammonium chloride, hydrochloric acid, or NaCl.
4. Carbonic anhydrase inhibitors, such as mafenide (Sulfamylon), absorbed from burn wounds.

### Table 4–9.  Common Causes of Hypokalemia*

*Hypokalemia* = plasma $K^+$ less than 3.5 meq/L

1. Intracellular potassium shifts
   Increased pH of blood, e.g., respiratory alkalosis
   Increased plasma $HCO_3$, primary or compensatory, metabolic alkalosis
   Glucose and insulin
2. Decreased potassium intake
   Decreased dietary intake
   Infusion of potassium-free intravenous fluids
   Underestimation of sum of gastrointestinal tract and renal losses
3. Gastrointestinal tract losses
   Diarrhea, 20 to 30 meq K/L
   Small bowel fistulae
   Long tube drainage of small bowel
   Prolonged vomiting or gastric suction
   Villous adenoma of the colon
   Saline cathartics
4. Renal losses
   Dehydration and K shift from cells
   Either acidosis or alkalosis when prolonged
   Excessive intake of sodium
   Following trauma, anesthesia, surgery
   Administration of diuretics
   Chronic renal disease
   Antibiotics or other drugs affecting tubular function, e.g., amphotericin
5. Metabolic alterations with secondary K loss usually renal in origin
   Starvation
   Reduced carbohydrate intake
   Surgical trauma, sepsis, burns, with K loss greater than nitrogen loss
   Antidiuresis following acute ECF volume depletion, with sodium and water retention and increased K loss, aldosterone
   Intracellular sodium shifts and potassium loss due to tissue injury, with initial K loss followed by increased demand for K, $HPO_4$, and amino acids with recovery
   Alteration in pH due to change in strong ion difference, commonly chloride loss from vomiting or gastric suction, metabolic alkalosis with excessive K loss
   Exogenous steroid administration
   Endogenous endocrine abnormalities: hyperaldosteronism, excess cortisol, adrenal hyperplasia, and adenoma
   Effect of circulating epinephrine in reducing plasma K level
   Magnesium deficiency

*Compiled from the literature[13,16,17,33,62–67] and personal experience.

exceed 20 meq/hour. Monitoring by EKG and by frequent plasma potassium levels is essential if acute treatment of hypokalemia is necessary.[62] When chronic large administration is necessary, frequent plasma determinations are also necessary.

*Hyperkalemia.* Plasma levels of potassium above 6 meq/L must be considered abnormally elevated and potentially dangerous, and levels of 7 meq/L or higher are emergencies. The biochemistry laboratory should notify the floor staff and the responsible physician *at once* when plasma potassium levels of 6.5 meq/L or more are found. The electrocardiogram changes include peaking of T waves and widening of the QRS complex. Various arrhythmias may develop. The chief danger is death from cardiac arrest. Causes of this condition are listed in Table 4–10. The most common cause is renal insufficiency. Some degree of renal failure exists together with hypovolemia in most patients with hyperkalemia, except that caused by acute hypoxia.

Immediate treatment of hyperkalemia consists

of measures to decrease the plasma concentration rapidly, including:

1. The administration of sodium bicarbonate intravenously to combat acidosis and to shift potassium intracellularly; 44 meq in 200 ml of 5% glucose in water can be used as a test dose, with electrocardiogram monitoring. Decreases in the amplitude and spiking of T waves are favorable signs.
2. The administration of glucose and insulin

**Table 4–10.   Common Causes of Hyperkalemia**

*Hyperkalemia* = plasma potassium 6.0 meq/L or more; emergency level 7.0 meq/L or higher

1. As the result of decreased renal excretion of K
   Acute or chronic oliguric renal failure, ATN (acute tubular necrosis)
   Hypovolemia, with decreased perfusion due to hemorrhage, sepsis, burns
   Acute dehydration
   Adrenal insufficiency, hypoaldosteronism
2. Due to massive release of K from cells
   Crush injury, major surgical operations
   Severe metabolic or respiratory acidosis
   Shock, whether cardiogenic or hypovolemic
   Gastrointestinal hemorrhage with rapid absorption of K from red blood cells
   Major infection, particularly gram-negative bacterial septicemia
3. Due to high K intake in the presence of some renal insufficiency
   Rapid intravenous infusion of K salts
   Oral administration of K supplements
   Potassium penicillin in large doses
4. Major osmotic shifts with ECF hyperosmolality
   Hyperglycemia—nutritional with total parenteral nutrition (TPN) or diabetic
   Mannitol, roentgenogram contrast media I.V., excess saline

intravenously. One unit of regular insulin for each 5 g of glucose, given together, is usually safe. Careful mixing is essential.

3. The administration of intravenous calcium gluconate, which temporarily alleviates the effect of elevated plasma potassium on the heart. An exception is when serum phosphate is also markedly elevated (e.g., when marked tumor lysis occurs in association with renal failure). In this situation, dialysis is essential.

Further treatment includes immediate elimination of exogenous sources of potassium in food and in infusions. Peritoneal dialysis or hemodialysis is necessary if the cause is renal, particularly if the plasma potassium level tends to rise after emergency treatment. Hydration with potassium-free fluids is essential if the cause is hypovolemia.

Sodium-charged polystyrene sulfonate resins (Kayexalate), given orally or as an enema, will absorb about 1 meq K per gram of resin.

## A GUIDE TO CLINICAL PARENTERAL FLUID THERAPY

### Water, Electrolytes, and Baseline Glucose Requirements

This section provides an outline for clinical management of water, sodium, potassium, and chloride requirements of patients who must be maintained wholly or partially by parenteral infusion. The principles described must be integrated with total parenteral nutrition (TPN) and enteral nutrition by tube feeding, both of which are described in Chapter 54.

The purpose of administering parenteral fluids and electrolytes is to prevent deficiencies that otherwise result from inability of the patient's gastrointestinal tract to fulfill its normal functions. In addition, when a substantial loss of water and electrolytes from the body has occurred without adequate oral replacement, parenteral fluid therapy is required to restore a normal distribution of body fluids and concentration of electrolytes.

The requirements for parenteral therapy can conveniently be considered in three categories:

1. *Baseline requirements:* What does the patient require in water, electrolytes, basic calories, and micronutrients to minimize the effects of dehydration and of starvation due to cessation or reduction of oral intake? The calculation of baseline requirements disregards any preexisting dehydration or any abnormal losses, but baseline volumes may require modification in patients with extracellular fluid excess or dilutional hyponatremia.

2. *Abnormal losses:* What does the patient require in order to replace ongoing abnormal fluid and electrolyte losses or internal fluid derangements resulting from the disease or its treatment, or both?

3. *Deficits or excesses:* What deficits (or excesses) does the patient have in volume of water, concentration of electrolytes, blood volume, and plasma protein concentration? What should be done to correct these abnormalities, and at what *rate* should reconstitution be effected?

   The daily or more frequent orders, in the case of the seriously ill patient, that are written for parenteral fluid and electrolyte therapy should take into consideration all three of these major categories. The parenteral fluids needed are the sum of baseline requirements and abnormal losses plus (or when an excess exists, minus) a part or all of the deficits existing at the time treatment is begun.

### Estimation of Baseline Requirements

Normal baseline parenteral water requirements in the adult vary from 1,250 to 3,000 ml per day depending on total body size, body cell mass size, age, and sex. Table 4–11 illustrates methods for estimating the baseline parenteral or combined

**Table 4–11.  Baseline Fluid Requirements in Temperate Climate**

| | Age (yrs.) | Average Water Requirements (ml per kg per day) |
|---|---|---|
| I. *Adults:* Based on "Ideal" Weight for Height and Age ± 20% of Ideal Weight | | |
| Average | 20 to 55 | 35 |
| Young active | 16 to 30 | 40 |
| Older | 55 to 75 ± | 30 |
| Elderly | 75 | 25 |
| II. *Children:* Over 5 kg Body Weight to Age 18* | | |
| First 10 kg of body weight | | 100 |
| Second 10 kg of body weight | | 50 |
| Weight above 20 kg | | 25 |

*For fluid requirements of infants and young children, see Filston, H.C., et al.:[68]

parenteral and oral fluid requirements for patients on parenteral fluids.

### Body Weight

Body weight is the most practical index of the state of hydration and of water balance. Several different types of scales are available on which the patient may be weighed in the supine position; one of these should be on every floor in a modern hospital. Daily weights of patients on routine parenteral fluid therapy, with the usual accompanying caloric insufficiency, should *decrease* with a weight loss of approximately 0.3 to 0.5% of body weight per day until adequate oral or parenteral nutrition is instituted. Exceptions occur with blood transfusions, with deliberate changes in hydration, and during the first 24 to 48 hours following trauma or operation with local sequestration of fluid and increased parenteral therapy to compensate for it. The patient who gains weight in circumstances other than these while on routine parenteral therapy is almost certainly being overhydrated. The patient who rapidly loses weight, except during the normal post-traumatic diuresis, has usually had an abnormal loss that has been inadequately replaced.

*Daily or more frequent body weight measurements are the single most important method of controlling water balance.*

### Factors that Modify Baseline

Factors that increase baseline requirements are essentially those that increase the insensible loss.

**Fever.** Fever increases the baseline water requirements largely through hyperventilation with increased water evaporation. A patient with a fever of 103°F requires about 500 ml of additional baseline water per day. Endogenous water production is also increased.

**Excessive Sweating.** A general guideline with respect to sweat loss is to increase the average adult baseline water requirement by 500 ml per day for each 5° above 85°F of ambient temperature in the absence of air conditioning. High humidity increases the need. Sweat is about one-third isotonic sodium chloride or less in the summertime with adaptation in temperate climates. Sweat may be nearly two thirds isotonic in winter, so that additional salt must be provided in baseline therapy to compensate. When the environmental temperature approaches body temperature, the environment of the seriously ill patient should be cooled, preferably by air conditioning, because insensible loss of water becomes very large when the ambient temperature exceeds body temperature. Grossly obese patients have substantially increased water loss through sweating and will require additional free water.

**Increased Metabolism.** Hyperthyroidism increases the baseline water turnover and caloric requirements substantially. Hyperthyroid patients in the semistarving state tend to consume massive amounts of lean body tissue and body fat, producing unusual amounts of endogenous water. Simultaneously they lose water both by respiratory evaporation and skin sublimation as well as by sweating.

### Factors that Reduce Baseline Water Requirements

These factors include reduced metabolic activity, as seen in hypothyroidism, in the elderly, and in situations having an excessive amount of body water with overexpanded extracellular fluid space, as in cardiac edema, in hypoproteinemia with starvation, in prolonged infection, and in carcinoma of the gastrointestinal tract. In the special circumstances of acute oliguric renal failure, fluid replacement should be restricted to insensible loss plus measured urine volume and gastrointestinal losses.

## Sodium and Potassium Requirements in Baseline

In the absence of abnormal losses, or of dehydration and salt losses preexisting, the sodium requirements of the average adult are easily met by 75 meq of sodium a day. One liter of 0.45% NaCl with 5% dextrose provides this amount. The remainder of water requirements should be given as sodium-free glucose solutions.

Potassium is also required in baseline and should be administered *unless* plasma $K^+$ levels are elevated or oliguric renal insufficiency is evident. Forty meq of $K^+$ a day as KCl provides about one half of normal potassium intake. KCl can be added to glucose and saline, and to glucose solutions. Concentrations of 20 meq/L are suggested to avoid the pain caused by higher concentrations. With *normal* renal function, infusion rates should not exceed 15 meq of $K^+$/hour.

Magnesium is indicated in baseline infusions, particularly when deficiency is likely or when drugs affecting renal tubular reabsorption are being given.

Glucose should not be administered at a rate in excess of *0.5 g per kg per hour to avoid hyperglycemia* and probable osmotic diuresis with dehydration. Hence, three hours should be a minimum time required for infusion of a liter of 5% dextrose. More usual infusion rates are 100 to 200 ml per hour. If more rapid rates of infusion are required, glucose should be reduced to 2.5% or omitted.

It is unphysiologic to provide 2,500 ml of fluid containing 125 g of glucose, 4.5 g of sodium chloride, and 3.0 g of potassium chloride in an infusion beginning at seven in the morning and completed by noon, and then to expect the patient to "coast" the remaining 19 hours of the day on nothing. By evening the patient will have disposed of most of the excess water load and will have metabolized the glucose. By midnight, the patient will be dehydrated, and some degree of starvation acidosis will be developing in most instances. Either a continuous infusion at a rate calculated to give the required volume in 24 hours, or two infusions spaced 12 hours apart, each taking 4 to 6 hours, is recommended. Patients should be out of bed, and walking when possible, at least part of the day.

Needles or small catheters used for infusion should be *changed* and a new site started at least every 48 hours to avoid risk of infection at the site of infusion.

Vitamins and trace elements may be indicated, particularly in debilitated patients. See individual chapters on these important substances and Chapter 54 for details.

## Nutritional Considerations

Baseline requirements of the adult for carbohydrate are met by the administration of 1.5 to 2 g of glucose per kg body weight per day. Administration of 100 to 150 g of glucose a day reduces the demand for amino acids mobilized from skeletal muscle for gluconeogenesis in starvation by about one half. This is a significant saving. For surgical patients undergoing moderately stressful operations who are unable to eat for a few days to a week, and who were well nourished with normal skeletal muscle mass preoperatively, this amount is usually all the caloric nutritional support required.

However, in patients who are debilitated by chronic illness, or who have suffered loss of 10% of body weight or more in the immediate past, and in those suffering from major trauma, sepsis, or burns or having surgery that will result in gastrointestinal dysfunction for a prolonged period, a nutritional regimen must be carefully planned to provide the energy requirements of the patient until he is able to eat, digest, and absorb enough normal foods to survive and convalesce. Total parenteral nutrition and defined formula diets (elemental diets) both play a significant and vital role in accomplishing these objectives. Details of methodology are presented in Chapter 54. Important to this discussion is that water and electrolyte requirements and acid-base abnormalities must receive constant attention with *nutritional formulas being adjusted in volume and content* to maintain fluid-electrolyte and acid-base balance. It is short-sighted to assume that all is well once a patient is on 2 to 3 liters a day of a standard TPN preparation, or on an equivalent amount of a defined formula or polymeric diet.

### Abnormal Loss

This is the second major category for consideration in determining fluid and electrolyte requirements. It includes both external abnormal losses of water, electrolytes, and plasma protein, and internal fluid shifts with functional loss of fluids by sequestration within the body.

External abnormal loss may be in the form of excessive loss of water and electrolytes by normal routes of excretion or secretion, or losses that occur from nasogastric or long small intestinal tubes, drains, fistulae, or wounds. The most common source of external abnormal losses in surgical patients is the gastrointestinal tract; next in frequency are losses from surgical wounds, increased evaporation from the skin and respiratory tract, and burns. Sequestration of extracellular fluids into areas of traumatized or infected tissue produces a decrease in the usual distribution of extracellular fluid *without external loss or change in body weight.*

### Losses From the Gastrointestinal Tract

The normal daily volume of secretions into the gastrointestinal tract is not precisely known, but has been estimated to be 8,000 to 10,000 ml, of which saliva constitutes 1 to 2 liters; gastric juice, including both acid and mucoid secretions, about 2,500 ml; bile, 500 to 750 ml; and pancreatic juice, more than 1,000 ml. In addition, secretion of the upper small bowel contributes between 2,000 and 3,000 ml. All but 100 to 200 ml is normally reabsorbed by the small bowel and the colon.

Abnormal losses from the gastrointestinal tract include water, electrolytes, and varying amounts of protein. The electrolyte content of fluid from the gastrointestinal tract varies significantly with the level from which the bulk of the fluid is derived. Table 4–12 summarizes the average and the range of variation of sodium, potassium, chloride, and bicarbonate in fluid from different levels of the intestine in patients with various causes for drainage. Of all the secretions of the gastrointestinal tract, only bile and pancreatic juice are isotonic in their electrolyte content. The average calculated osmolarity of saliva is about 160 mO; of fasting gastric juice, in patients without duodenal ulcer, about 180 mO; of upper small bowel content, 220 mO; and of fluid from the distal ileum, about 240 mO. Other substances, including mucoproteins, other polysaccharides, urea, calcium, and phosphate, increased the total osmolality beyond these approximations.

The average values shown may be used for semiquantitative replacement of gastrointestinal tract losses. When volumes exceed 2,000 ml in 24 hours or when substantial losses (1 L or more per day) continue for more than two days, it is wise to send an aliquot of the 24-hour drainage to the laboratory for analysis for electrolytes and protein and to determine the pH of a freshly obtained specimen. With this information, more precise replacement can be made.

It is important to note that replacement of abnormal losses is *in addition to* baseline requirements.

### Internal Fluid Shifts

If the intracellular and extracellular fluid spaces are considered as the two major body fluid compartments, an abnormal "third" fluid space is created when interstitial fluid, plasma, and sometimes red blood cells are sequestered in large amounts in an area of tissue injury. Although this sequestered fluid is in continuity with the remaining extracellular fluid from which it was derived, it is unavailable for restoring diminished interstitial fluid and plasma volumes. It is apparent as wound edema in patients with burns; it also occurs in crush injuries, in peritonitis, in pulmonary infection, in soft tissue and wound infection, and in areas distal to obstructed venous flow. Sequestered fluid, which is accumulated to some degree postoperatively in all surgical wounds, is substantial with retroperitoneal dissection or with visceral or muscle trauma.

A special type of internal fluid shift is seen with the development of transcellular pooling such as occurs within the gastrointestinal tract with intestinal obstruction or adynamic ileus; the volume of fluid involved may be quite large. These collections of transcellular fluid may become abnormal external losses if they are vomited or drained by intestinal intubation. They may resolve by reabsorption as the patient recovers gastrointestinal function. If the volume of sequestered fluid is significantly large, it must be replaced exactly

**Table 4–12.   Electrolyte Concentration of Gastrointestinal Secretions[†]**

| Source of Fluid | NA (meq/L) | K (meq/L) | Cl (meq/L) | Effective $HCO_3^-$ (meq/L) |
|---|---|---|---|---|
| Saliva, average of 3 pt (based on 1 ml/min) | 60 | 30 | 16 | 50 |
| Gastric, average | 59 | 9.3 | 89 | 0–1 |
| Range* | 30–90 | 4.3–12 | 52–155 | |
| Upper small bowel, average | 105 | 5.1 | 99 | 10 |
| Range | 72–128 | 3.5–6.8 | 69–127 | |
| Ileum, average | 117 | 5.0 | 106 | 15–20 |
| Range | 91–140 | 3.0–7.5 | 82–125 | |
| Bile, average | 145 | 5.2 | 100 | 50 |
| Range | 134–156 | 3.9–6.3 | 83–110 | |
| Pancreatic fistula, average of 3 pt | 141.6 | 4.6 | 76.6 | 70 |

*Patients under major stress, or with peptic ulcer disease, usually have highly acid gastric juice, with a large difference between $Cl^-$ and $Na^+$ concentration. Pharmacologic modification by $H_2$ blocking is usually indicated.
†From Randall, H.T.[50] With permission of Surg. Clin. North Am.

as if an external loss had occurred. Isotonic electrolyte solutions, such as Ringer's lactate without glucose, are given in sufficient volume and rate to support the circulation and to provide adequate urine output.

The major difference between development of a third space of sequestered fluid and an abnormal external fluid loss is that sequestered fluid remains within the body, so that there is no loss of weight. A *gain* in weight results from the necessary replacement of diminished plasma and interstitial fluid volumes of the rest of the body. In addition, unlike an external loss, the sequestered fluid eventually returns to the circulation as normal capillary function returns to the affected area, presenting a potential problem in water and electrolyte overloading.

It is usually necessary to reduce fluid and electrolyte administration when a third space begins to resolve. A diuresis of water and sodium indicates mobilization of sequestered fluid. *The excess urine output should not be replaced* because the patient is unloading excess fluid and electrolytes given earlier to maintain circulation and urine output when the third space was being formed.

### Deficits or Excesses

The administration of water, electrolytes, calories, and vitamins as baseline therapy, the replacement of abnormal external losses, and the provision of internal fluid shifts are intended to help the patient to maintain normal functional volumes of body fluids, normal concentrations of electrolytes, and a normal pH of plasma and interstitial fluid. However, patients may have deficits or excesses of some or all of the component body fluids at the time when they are first seen and treatment is begun. In other patients, significant abnormalities of volume, concentration, and pH may develop while the patient is under treatment. The replacement of deficits of water and electrolytes and the recognition and treatment of excessive fluid volumes or electrolyte concentrations constitute the third major category for clinical consideration in fluid and electrolyte therapy. The reader is referred to Narins et al.[69] for detailed diagnostic strategies useful when causes of derangements are not apparent.

### Acute Dehydration

Acute change in the *volume* of total body water can occur as the result of either failure of intake, or abnormal external loss, or both simultaneously. The comparable change in body weight, if known, greatly assists in diagnosis. Rapid weight loss due to dehydration is almost entirely extracellular

fluid. A loss of 2% of body weight produces thirst and some oliguria. A loss of 4% of body weight (20% of extracellular fluid) causes oliguria, tachycardia, and often postural hypotension. An acute extracellular fluid loss of 6% of body weight is a life-threatening event, reducing interstitial fluid and plasma volumes by about 30% and compromising both blood pressure and renal function.

**Treatment.** Replacement of acute loss of extracellular fluid or its functional loss by sequestration or transcellular pooling is best accomplished by infusion of water containing the electrolytes of extracellular fluid. Balanced salt solutions, such as Ringer's lactate, *without* glucose are effective. If blood loss has occurred, three to four times the volume of blood lost will be required to maintain cardiac output if replaced by electrolyte solutions.

Losses by vomiting or nasogastric suction usually result in excess chloride loss, and produce a metabolic alkalosis. Ringer's lactate solution *should never be used* to replace vomiting or gastric suction unless plasma electrolyte determinations show a low $TCO_2$ and nearly normal plasma chloride concentration. *Isotonic sodium chloride,* 0,9% without glucose, is the best solution for replacement when dehydration is due to vomiting. Ringer's lactate solution is preferred to replace diarrhea or small bowel losses.

Urine volume and concentration, hematocrit, pulse, and blood pressure are clinical guides to replacement of fluids, which initially should be quite rapid in the absence of increased venous pressure. A urine volume of 50 ml/hour, with a falling specific gravity and osmolality, and a falling hematocrit in the absence of blood loss are clinical indications of improvement. Diminishing thirst in an alert patient is a useful symptom.

Plasma potassium concentration should be monitored, and potassium chloride should be added when plasma levels fall within normal range and urine volume is sufficient to permit excretion of any excess K. Substantial potassium losses occur with severe dehydration and the metabolic acidosis that usually accompanies dehydration.

### Chronic Dehydration

A patient who has become chronically dehydrated over several days to a week or more, as a result of inadequate intake of water and food, may lose 10% or more of body weight. The loss of body water in such instances is more evenly distributed between intracellular and extracellular fluids. The effects of slow combined fluid depletion are less severe than those with acute extracellular fluid dehydration; hypotension and hemoconcentration are less marked, and the degree of oliguria is less.

**Treatment.** Rehydration in such a patient requires replacement of the extracellular fluid deficit in sufficient volume to raise urine volume to 25 to 50 ml per hour and to reduce the hematocrit to normal levels. A period of days rather than hours is desirable for repletion of the intracellular water and potassium deficits. Emergency surgical measures, if required, can be performed after repletion of the extracellular fluid component. Complete rehydration should not result in return to predehydration weight because of the loss of protein and fat during the period of underhydration and semistarvation.

Substantial total body potassium deficit is common in this condition and requires replacement once hydration is satisfactorily under way.

## Hypertonicity Due to Solute Loading

This condition is usually the result of inadequate water intake in patients who are receiving tube feedings of mixtures that are high in protein and salt in relation to water content. It can also occur with TPN. The syndrome is likely to develop in patients who have had head and neck surgical treatment, those on gastrostomy feedings, unconscious patients being tube-fed, and patients with brain stem injury. Hypertonicity due to solute loading can result from the exclusive use of an isotonic balanced salt solution, such as Ringer's lactate, given with the mistaken idea that such a solution will meet baseline requirements for patients on parenteral fluids. Unless renal function permits excretion of urine of very high specific gravity with elimination of excessive electrolyte, urea, and other solutes in a volume of water smaller than that administered, both hypernatremia and azotemia will result.

Laboratory findings demonstrate an increased concentration of all plasma solutes, both electrolytes and crystalloids, which is out of proportion to changes in hematocrit. An elevated plasma sodium level in the presence of a moderate to large urine output is the key to diagnosis differentiating these patients from those with desiccation dehydration. The serum sodium may reach levels of 170 meq/L or more in severe cases.

**Treatment.** Treatment consists of the administration of large volumes of water orally or via a tube, or parenterally as 5% glucose in water, while at the same time eliminating, or at least reducing, the osmolar load. Insulin may be required if blood glucose is high. *Caution must be exercised to reduce the osmolarity relatively slowly.* The entire body, including the cerebrospinal fluid and brain, becomes hypertonic during the solute loading pe-

riod; cerebral edema, convulsions, or coma may result if the extracellular fluid osmolality is reduced too rapidly. Large volumes of urine persist for several days during solute release, and the hematocrit does not change greatly unless significant dehydration has also been present.

## Chronic Overexpansion of Extracellular Fluid

With chronic illnesses such as cancer, liver disease, infection, starvation, or cardiac decompensation, the patient often presents with an overexpansion of the extracellular fluid space with an *excess of total body sodium despite hyponatremia.* Such a patient has a decrease in the normal total intracellular water because of a diminished volume of body cell mass. With the fall in body cell mass, as percent of body weight, there is a relative expansion of the extracellular fluid space. Such patients are usually hyponatremic, with serum sodium concentrations in the low 130 meq/L range. Usually, total body potassium is markedly depleted, although the plasma concentrations of potassium may be normal or even a little high. In addition, hypoproteinemia is usually considerable and the normal osmolality of the plasma is reduced with the osmolality in the range of 260 to 270 mO.

Water and sodium retention are exaggerated with superimposed acute illness or surgery in such patients. More marked hyponatremia and hyperkalemia often occur. These individuals have a poor tolerance for the administration of large volumes of extracellular fluid expander such as Ringer's lactate solution or saline solution. They also tolerate free water, as glucose in water, poorly, holding on to excessive water intake with further dilution. An expanded extracellular fluid space with hyponatremia is the most common pattern of water and electrolyte abnormality seen in debilitated patients, and it is one of the most difficult to treat once it becomes established.

**Treatment.** Treatment of this dilutional hyponatremia must *not* be by the administration of salt solutions on some formula based on unit deficit multiplied by a theoretical volume for extracellular fluid. Rather, it must be based on a combination of restriction of water intake to less than that required by the normally hydrated individual and the restoration of the red cell mass and plasma volume to normal by the transfusion of blood or the infusion of albumin, or both. Because a large intracellular potassium deficit is usually present in such patients, the major electrolyte need is usually for potassium rather than for sodium. These patients frequently benefit from TPN, with high-caloric-density, low-volume, and low-sodium solutions.

## Overhydration, Hypotonicity, and Water Intoxication

Water intoxication is an acute form of hypotonic dilution. Drowsiness, weakness, and a *fall* in urine volume are early symptoms, followed by convulsions and coma. A rapid weight gain always occurs. Peripheral and pulmonary edema may appear but are not always present. Water intoxication may result from excessive administration of parenteral glucose and water, from absorption of water from the colon as the result of enemas or colon irrigations given for distention, or from water absorption from wounds and burns treated with hypotonic wet dressings. Water intoxication is a particular hazard of the dilute silver nitrate treatment of burns. It is particularly likely to occur in patients with inappropriate antidiuretic hormone release. (See previous sections on body water and ADH.)

Laboratory findings include a low concentration of serum sodium, usually less than 120 meq/L and often less than 110 meq/L. The urine may contain a substantial concentration of sodium, 30 meq/L or more despite the extremely low plasma value, owing to an inappropriate sodium release in the presence of a large extracellular fluid volume. Adrenal insufficiency and primary renal tubular disease must be excluded. The rapidity of fall of the plasma sodium concentration is apparently of greater significance than the absolute values. Cerebral edema from a shift of water into the cerebrospinal fluid due to the difference in osmolality is the probable cause of convulsions and coma.

**Treatment.** Either total water restriction for a time or the slow administration of a small volume of water as hypertonic glucose (20%)—not more than 500 ml over 24 hours—is required. If the patient has good cardiovascular function and central venous pressure is within normal limits, small volumes (300 ml or less) of hypertonic sodium chloride solution (5%) can be given slowly with monitoring of central venous pressure. This regimen will begin restoration of extracellular fluid osmotic pressure and promote renal excretion of water. No attempt should be made to administer salt with a "formula" based on extracellular fluid deficit because severe overloading can result. Time and patience will result in a rising urine volume and an increase in serum sodium concentration with recovery in most cases. In an emergency, hemodialysis with ultrafiltration to remove water may be necessary.

## SUMMARY OF CLINICAL APPLICATION: FLUID AND ELECTROLYTE BALANCE

Fluid and electrolyte requirements of patients on intravenous fluids may be considered in three categories:

1. Baseline requirements include the amount of water, sodium, potassium, and chloride needed to meet normal requirements of a patient deprived of oral intake. This category also consists of minimal carbohydrate requirements to reduce protein catabolism in starvation.

2. Abnormal losses include the semiquantitative replacement with respect to volume and electrolyte content of losses from the gastrointestinal tract and wounds. Also included is provision for the formation of a third space of sequestered extracellular fluid, and sometimes blood, in areas of trauma, sepsis, and burns, using volumes sufficient to restore or maintain cardiovascular and renal function.

3. Deficit includes estimation of and provision for water and electrolyte needs in dehydration, or restriction of water and sodium intake in patients with overexpansion of extracellular fluid.

Adjustment of the ionic composition of infusions to assist in correction of metabolic acidosis or metabolic alkalosis, together with careful attention to abnormalities of ventilation and pulmonary alveolar perfusion, compensates for or corrects the respiratory causes of acidosis or alkalosis, and hypoxia.

## REFERENCES

1. Cannon, W.B.: The Wisdom of the Body. New York, W. W. Norton & Company, Inc., 1932.
2. Benenson, A.S.: Cholera. *In* Bacterial Infections of Humans—Epidemiology and Control. (Evans, A.S., and Feldman, H.A., Eds.) New York, Plenum Publishing Corp., 1982.
3. O'Shaughnessy, W.B.: Lancet *1*:490, 1831–1832.
4. O'Shaughnessy, W.B.: Lancet *1*:929–936, 1831–1832.
5. Latta, T.: Lancet *2*:274–277, 1831–32.
6. Lewins, R.: Lancet *2*:279–280, 1831–32.
7. Gamble, J.L.: Pediatrics *11*:554–567, 1953.
8. Moyer, C.A.: Fluid Balance—A Clinical Manual. Chicago, Year Book Medical Publishers, 1952.
9. Crile, G.W.: An Experimental Research into Surgical Shock. Philadelphia, J. B. Lippincott Co., 1899.
10. Penfield, W.G., Teplitsky, D.: Arch. Surg. *7*:111–124, 1923.
11. Matas, R.: Ann. Surg. *79*:643–661, 1924.
12. Elman, R., Weiner, D.O.: J.A.M.A. *112*:796–802, 1939.
13. Randall, H.T., Habif, D.V., Lockwood, J.J., et al.: Surgery *26*:341–363, 1949.
14. Henderson, L.J.: Am. J. Physiol. *21*:427–448, 1908.
15. Van Slyke, D.D.: J. Biol. Chem. *48*:153–176, 1921.

16. Moore, F.D., Olesen, K.H., McMurrey, J.D., et al.: The Body Cell Mass and Its Supporting Environment—Body Composition in Health and Disease. Philadelphia, W. B. Saunders Co., 1963.

17. Moore, F.D.: J. Parenter. Enter. Nutr. 4:228–260, 1980.

18. Krzywicki, H.J., Ward, G.M., Rahman, D.P.: Am. J. Clin. Nutr. 27:1380–1385, 1974.

19. Boling, E.A., Taylor, W.L., Entenman, C.: J. Clin. Invest. 41:1840–1849, 1962.

20. Golberger, J.H., Cha, C-J., Hazard, W.L., et al.: Surgery 80:493–497, 1976.

21. Novak, L.P., Hyatt, R.E., Alexander, J.F.: J.A.M.A. 205:764–770, 1968.

22. Widdowson, E.M.: Growth and composition of the fetus and newborn. In Biology of Gestation. Vol. II. (Assali, N.S., Ed.) New York, Academic Press, 1968.

23. Stewart, P.A.: How to Understand Acid-Base. A Quantitative Acid-Base Primer for Biology and Medicine. New York, Elsevier Science Publishing Co., Inc., 1981.

24. Horne, R.A.: Introduction. In Water and Aqueous Solutions. Structure, Thermodynamics, and Transport Processes. (Horne, R.A., Ed.) New York, John Wiley & Sons, Inc., 1972.

25. Peschel, G., Belouschek, P.: The problem of water structure in biological systems. In Cell-Associated Water. (Drost-Hansen, W., Clegg, J.S., Eds.) New York, Academic Press, 1979.

26. Hazlewood, C.F.: A view of the significance of understanding of the physical properties of cell-associated water. In Cell-Associated Water. (Drost-Hansen, W., and Clegg, J.S., Eds.) New York, Academic Press, 1979.

27. Ikkos, D.: Metabolism 4:19–28, 1955.

28. Ellis, K.J., Shukla, K.K., Cohn, S.H., et al.: J. Lab. Clin. Med. 83:716–727, 1974.

29. Hill, G.L., King, R.F.G.J., Smith, R.C.: Br. J. Surg. 66:868–872, 1979.

30. Kinney, J.M., Lister, J., Moore, F.D.: Ann. N.Y. Acad. Sci. 110:711–722, 1963.

31. Gamble, J.L.: Chemical Anatomy. Physiology and Pathology of Extracellular Fluid. Cambridge, Harvard University Press, 1964.

32. Bergström, J.: Scand. J. Clin. Lab. Invest. (Suppl.) 14:1–110, 1962.

33. Shils, M.E.: Magnesium. In Modern Nutrition in Health and Disease. 7th ed. (Shils, M.E., and Young, V., Eds.) Philadelphia, Lea & Febiger, 1986.

34. Gennari, F.J.: N. Engl. J. Med., 310:102–105, 1984.

35. Katz, A.I., Epstein, F.H.: N. Engl. J. Med., 278:253–261, 1968.

36. Sweadner, K.J., Goldin, S.M.: N. Engl. J. Med. 302:777–783, 1980.

37. Leaf, A.: Am. J. Med. 49:291–295, 1970.

38. Rocchio, M.A., Randall, H.T.: Am. J. Surg. 121:460–466, 1971.

39. Avioli, L.V.: Calcium and phosphorus. In Modern Nutrition in Health and Disease. 7th ed. (Shils, M.E., and Young, V. Eds.) Philadelphia, Lea & Febiger, 1986.

40. Van Slyke, D.D.: Ann. N. Y. Acad. Sci. 133:5–14, 1966.

41. Pitts, R.F.: Physiology of the Kidney and Body Fluids. Chicago, Year Book Medical Publishers, 1963.

42. Siggaard-Andersen, O.: Scand. J. Clin. Lab. Invest. 12:311–314, 1960.

43. Siggaard-Andersen, O.: The Acid-Base Status of the Blood. 3rd ed. Baltimore, Williams & Wilkins, 1965.

44. Randall, H.T.: Surg. Clin. North Am. 56:1019–1058, 1976.

45. Bland, J.H.: Basic physiologic considerations of body water and electrolytes. In Clinical Metabolism of Body Water and Electrolytes. (Bland, J.H., Ed.) Philadelphia, W.B. Saunders Co., 1963.

46. Shires, G.T.: Fluid and electrolyte therapy. In Manual of Preoperative and Postoperative Care. 2nd ed. (Kinney, J.M., Chairman, and Egdahl, R.H., and Zuidema, G.D., Eds.) Philadelpha, W. B. Saunders Co., 1971.

47. Share, L., Claybaugh, J.R.: Ann. Rev. Physiol. 34:235–260, 1972.

48. Gump, F.E.: Fluid and electrolyte management. In Manual of Surgical Intensive Care. (Kinney, J.M., Chairman, and Bendixen, H.H., and Powers, S.R., Jr., Eds.) Philadelphia, W. B. Saunders Co., 1977.

49. Brill, A.B., Sandstead, H.H., Price, R., et al.: Am. J. Surg. 123:49–56, 1972.

49a. Moore, F.D.: Metabolic Care of the Surgical Patient. Philadelphia, W.B. Saunders Co., 1959, pp. 287, 288.

50. Randall, H.T.: Surg. Clin. North Am. 32:445–469, 1952.

51. Streeten, D.H.P., Rapoport, A.: J. Clin. Endocrinol. Metab. 23:928–937, 1963.

52. Skorecki, K.L., Brenner, B.M.: Am. J. Med., 70:77–88, 1981.

53. Gann, D.S.: Response to injury. In The Scientific Management of Surgical Patients. (Peters, R.M., Peacock, E.E., and Benfield, J.R., Eds.) Boston, Little, Brown & Co. 1983.

54. Kleeman, C.R., Fichman, M.P.: N. Engl. J. Med. 277:1300–1307, 1967.

55. Boulter, P.R., Hoffman, R.S., Arky, R.A.: Metabolism, 22:675–683, 1973.

56. Maage, H.: Metabolism 17:133–138, 1968.

57. Rapoport, A., From, G.L.A., Husdan, H.: Metabolism 14:31–46, 1965.

58. Sigler, M.H.: J. Clin. Invest. 55:377–387, 1975.

59. Bartter, F.C., Schwartz, W.B.: Am. J. Med. 42:790–806, 1967.

60. Cooke, C.R., Turin D.D., W.D., Walker, W.G.: Medicine 58:240–251, 1979.

61. Cox, M., Sterns, R.H., Singer, I.: N. Engl. J. Med., 299:525–532, 1978.

62. Schultze, R.G., Nissensen, A.R.: Potassium: physiology and pathophysiology. In Clinical Disorders of Fluid and Electrolyte Metabolism. 3rd ed. (Maxwell, M.H., Kleeman, C.R., Eds.) New York, McGraw-Hill Book Co., 1979.

63. Cox, M.: Med. Clin. North Am. 65:363–383, 1981.

64. Lawson, D.H., Henry, D.A., Lowe, J.M., et al.: Arch. Intern. Med. 139:978–980, 1979.

65. Thomas, T.H., Morgan, D.B.: Br. J. Surg., 66:540–542, 1979.

66. Brown, M.J., Brown, D.C., Murphy, M.B.: N. Engl. J. Med. 309:1414–1419, 1983.

67. Moore-Ede, M.C., Meguid, M.M., Fitzpatrick, G.F., et al.: Clin. Pharmacol. Ther. 23:218–227, 1978.

68. Filston, H.C., Edwards, C.H., III, Chitwood, W.R., Jr., et al.: Ann. Surg. 196:76–81, 1982.

69. Narins, R.G., Jones, E.R., Stom, M.C.: Am. J. Med. 72:496–520, 1982.

## SELECTED READINGS

Drost-Hansen, W., Clegg, J. (Eds.): Cell Associated Water. New York, Academic Press, Inc., 1979. A comprehensive review of problems of water structure in biologic systems.

Dudrick, S.J., Baue, A.E., Eiseman, B., et al. (Eds.): Manual of Preoperative and Postoperative Care, 3rd ed. Philadelphia, W. B. Saunders Co., 1983. Includes chapters on parenteral and enteral nutrition as well as a surgical view of fluid and electrolyte balance, and pulmonary and renal function.

Maxwell, M.H., Kleeman, C.R. (Eds.): Clinical Disorders of Fluid an Electrolyte Metabolism. 3rd ed. New York, McGraw-Hill Book Co., 1979. A major and authoritative medically oriented text that includes unusual as well as ordinary causes of disorders of fluid, electrolyte, and acid-base metabolism and how to diagnose and treat them.

Moore, F.D.: J. Parenter. Enter. Nutr. *4*:228–260, 1980, The 1980 Jonathan E. Rhoads Lecture. A major monograph by this world-renowned authority integrates body composition and energy needs over a wide spectrum of normal and pathologic states.

Starling, E.H.: The Fluids of the Body. Chicago, W.T. Keener and Company, 1909. For lovers of the history of medicine, and modern users of Starling hypotheses, this is a true classic.

Stewart, P.A.: How to Understand Acid-Base. A Quantitative Acid-Base Primer for Biology and Medicine. New York, Elsevier Science Publishing Co., Inc., 1981. A highly mathematical approach to acid-base balance in man. Excellent reading for computer experts and those who want to know more about aqueous solutions.

*Chapter* **5**

# CALCIUM AND PHOSPHORUS

## Louis V. Avioli

Calcium and phosphorus are considered together because they constitute the major part of the mineral content of the skeleton. Over 99% of the total-body calcium and approximately 85% of the phosphorus are in the bones. The ratio of calcium to phosphorus in the bone is slightly over 2:1 and is approximately constant. Thus, marked changes in the body content of one of these minerals will be reflected in changes in the other.

Many phosphorus compounds are present in the body, and phosphorylated compounds are involved in several metabolic pathways. No attempt is made in this chapter to discuss these functions of phosphorus, since they are considered in standard textbooks of biochemistry. Attention is directed primarily toward the nutritional requirement of calcium and phosphorus. Since phosphorus is ordinarily considered to occur in adequate amounts in most diets consumed by man, primary discussion is given to calcium requirements. It is remarkable that, in spite of the prominence given to calcium in the nutrition literature, there is much argument as to its nutritional significance in most diets. Increasing knowledge has served primarily to emphasize how little is known of calcium requirements and how great the need is for additional criteria to estimate requirements and adequacy of calcium intake.

## CALCIUM

Calcium is the most abundant cation and the fifth most common inorganic element of the human body. It not only serves as the principal component of skeletal tissue, imparting to it the structural integrity essential to support the increasing body size of the individual during growth, but also plays a vital role in various essential physiologic and biochemical processes. The functions of the calcium ion include its influence on blood coagulation, neuromuscular excitability, cellular adhesiveness, transmission of nerve impulses, maintenance and function of cell membranes, and activation of enzyme reactions and hormone secretion. The skeleton, a huge reservoir of insoluble complexes of calcium, is in dynamic equilibrium with physicochemically soluble forms of circulating calcium that are maintained at a remarkably constant level, with a diurnal plasma variation of ± 3%. This fluctuation in circulating calcium is comparable to that of plasma sodium (± 3%) and is lower than the range of variation for the potassium (± 12%) or the hydrogen ion (± 10%). Although the primary homeostatic mechanism that controls the plasma calcium concentration in adults is a function of the parathyroid and thyroid glands and the biologically active vitamin D metabolite $(1,25(OH)_2D_3)$, various other hormones, vitamins, inhibitors of biologic calcification (such as inorganic pyrophosphate), and other less well understood factors prevent the fluctuation of calcium over a wide range, despite the enormous insoluble skeletal reservoir and wide variations in intake and output.[1] Disruption of this exquisite control system leads ultimately to derangements in skeletal and extraosseous calcium metabolism. These changes, in turn, often result in characteristic clinical manifestations and alterations in both chemical and roentgenographic findings, which serve to define the pathologic state.

## Calcium in Bone

The average adult human contains 1,000 to 1,200 g of calcium or 20.7 to 24.8 g per kg of fat-free body tissue. Whereas, quantitatively, 30% of body sodium and 50% of body magnesium are stored in bone, over 99% of the body calcium resides in the skeleton. Calcium in the solid mineral phase of bone is usually considered to be a variant of poorly crystalline hydroxyapatite, $Ca_{10}(PO_4)_6$ $(OH)_2$, the unit cell of the crystal lattice containing all 18 ions of the formula. It has been suggested, from studies on synthetic and biologic hydroxyapatites, that the apatite portion of bone mineral does not have the ideal stoichiometry $(Ca_{10}(PO_4)_6(OH)_2$, but is approximately 10% deficient in calcium, with the structure remaining generally intact.[2]

There appear to be two distinct phases other than hydroxyapatite: brushite and a β-tricalcium phosphate.[3] No temporal relationship has been established between the nonapatitic and apatitic phases of bone, nor is there presently any evidence that nonapatitic phases are precursors of a final apatitic phase in bone.[3]

The hydroxyapatite crystals are tubular hexagons with average dimensions of $40 \times 50 \times 600$ nm. Although calcium and phosphate are the principal ions in hydroxyapatite, the crystal contains significant amounts of $Na^+$, $Mg^{++}$, $CO_3^{2-}$, and citrate$^{3-}$ ions[4] which, with the exception of $Mg^{++}$, can substitute for either calcium or phosphate in the apatite lattice and can be absorbed on its surface or incorporated into its hydration shell.

Trace elements[5] and bone-seeking ions, such as strontium (Sr), radium (Ra), plutonium, lead, and fluorine, are also incorporated into or adsorbed onto the crystal. This process assumes importance when their radioactive isotopes (e.g., $^{90}Sr$ from fallout or Ra from luminous paints) are ingested, because their accumulation may lead to radiation damage and malignant degeneration of bone cells. The release of mineral from bone during resorption buffers hydrogen ions, whereas the formation of bone mineral generates hydrogen ions—8 $H^+$ released per unit cell of the crystalline lattice. This may assume significant proportions in the growing skeleton wherein, during the process of skeletal mineralization and hydroxyapatite synthesis, approximately 20 meq of $H^+$ are released by the deposition of 1 g of calcium.[6] Bone, therefore, not only represents a calcium depot for the miscible

calcium pool, but also assumes an important role as a reservoir for electrolytes and buffers.

Bone affords an enormous depot of calcium which, when appropriately stimulated by various hormones and metabolic agents, serves as the guardian of the circulating calcium pool.[7] Unlike the mineral of tooth enamel, which is relatively inert,[8] bone undergoes constant remodeling and turnover. The dynamic process of the bone turnover in the adult normally releases into blood and then reaccumulates from 250 mg to 1 g of calcium per day. Little calcium is deposited in the fetus during the first trimester of pregnancy, but the concentration rises rapidly subsequently until a body weight of 0.5 kg is attained.[9] Gradual increments are observed thereafter until term. During the final trimester, when maternal levels of circulating parathyroid hormone[10] and intestinal calcium absorption[11] are increased, the human fetus acquires approximately 20 g of calcium from maternal sources. The total calcium content of a full-term neonate weighing 3,500 g approaches 30 g, or about 1% of the body weight.

The turnover of skeletal calcium varies with age. It has been estimated to be 100% per annum in infants up to 1 year and decreases with age to a turnover rate of 10% in older children. The skeleton weighs approximately 100 g at birth and actually doubles in weight during the first year of life. Skeletal growth during childhood involves calcium retention of not more than 150 mg per day until after the first decade. During peak adolescent growth, bone development is at its maximum, and calcium retained as bone may range between 275 and 500 mg per day. The rate of turnover is higher in cancellous or trabecular bones (e.g., vertebrae and ribs) than in compact bones (i.e., long bones of the limbs). In adults, after epiphyseal closure and longitudinal growth have ceased, the turnover rate is approximately 2 to 4% per annum.

During adult life skeletal growth does not entirely cease. Both subperiosteal bone formation and the later adolescent shift to endosteal bone formation, or apposition, continue to some extent. At this time, skeletal maintenance requires the deposition of approximately 180 g of calcium per annum, or 18% of the total skeletal content. The skeleton is in a relatively steady state because bone formation equals bone resorption, with no net change in skeletal mass. Between the third and fourth decades this equilibrium shifts in cancellous bone (vertebrae), primarily in women, and vertebral bone mass begins to decline (Fig. 5–1).[12]

Appendicular or cortical bone loss begins between the fourth and fifth decades in women and much later in men (Fig. 5–2).[12] Since in the past

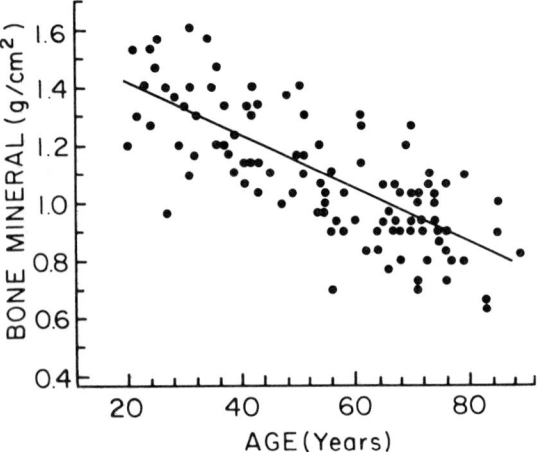

**Fig. 5–1.** Regression of lumbar spine density in 105 normal women as determined by dual-photon absorptiometry. Equation for regression is $y = 1.59 - 0.0092$ age. (From H.J. Riggs, et al. J. Clin. Invest. 67:330, 1981.)

changes in cortical and appendicular bone mass observed in postmenopausal women were observed to be minimized by estrogen replacement therapy, and because oophorectomy resulted in rapid bone loss, osteoporosis and fracture were attributed to a decrease in circulating estrogen levels. No cause for the early loss of trabecular or cancellous bone in ovulating females has been established, although subclinical estrogen deficiency[13] and inadequate calcium intake[14] may prove important in this regard. The significant features of the skeletal changes that occur throughout

life are: (1) among young adults, the skeletal mass is greater in males than in females and greater in blacks than in whites; (2) the bone loss begins earlier in females than in males; and (3) although the onset of loss in the females antedates the menopause, the rate of skeletal loss in some females is distinctly accelerated after the menopause. Thus, since the maximum skeletal mass at maturity is less for the white female than for the white male or the black individual of either sex, and because the loss begins earlier in the female and proceeds at a more rapid rate after the menopause, net skeletal mass is lowest in the menopausal white female, a fact that increases the predisposition to skeletal fracture.

The exchange of calcium between bone and circulating fluids is still ill-defined and poorly understood. It appears to be divisible into the slow processes of bone formation and resorption and the far more rapid processes of ion exchange with accessible crystal surfaces. The osteon surface, or haversian units, of compact bone plus the surfaces afforded by trabecular bone provide an enormous surface area for interchange between extracellular fluids and bone mineral. Normally, less than 1% of the skeletal calcium is available for free ionic exchange with the extracellular fluid. The calcium in blood, extracellular fluid, and extraosseous cellular compartments accounts for 1% of whole-body calcium and, together with the exchangeable calcium of bone, comprises the miscible, or readily exchangeable, calcium pool. Since most of the skeletal calcium is not in a form that is readily

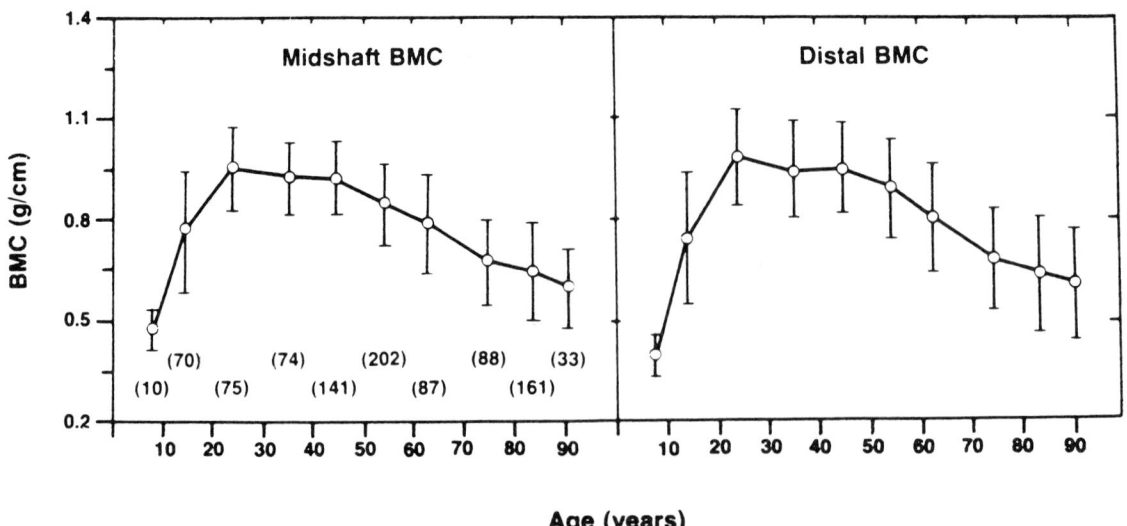

**Fig. 5–2.** Age-related changes in appendicular (radius) bone mass (BMC) content in 941 white women using single-photon absorptiometry. The population was divided into decades of life. Mean values ± SD are plotted at the mean age of each group. Number of subjects in each group is shown in parentheses. (Reprinted from Geriatrics, Vol. 33, No. 11, pp. 67–76, November 1978. Copyright 1978 by Harcourt Brace Jovanovich, Inc.)

diffusible to combat hypocalcemia and maintain homeostasis, calcium must be mobilized by active resorptive processes.

Bone lability is maintained by the concurrent activities of bone formation and resorption. Osseous tissue is continually being deposited and resorbed, primarily as a result of the activity of the connective tissue cells covering its surfaces. Changes in bone resorption are not simply consequent to changes in the activity of existing cell machinery but depend on the continuous transformation of resting undifferentiated cells to osteocytic cells, osteoblasts, and osteoclasts. Osteoclastic and osteocytic responses to parathyroid hormone represent one of the most singularly effective control mechanisms available to facilitate the resorption of bone. The regulating action of parathyroid hormone is normally accomplished through continuous secretion, which is inversely related to the extracellular fluid calcium ion concentration.

In contrast to the action of parathyroid hormone on bone, the inhibition of bone resorption is the principal, if not sole, function of the hormone calcitonin.[1,15] It is noteworthy that the resorptive activity of osteoclasts decreases in response to calcitonin, the action of which is rapid and short-lived, relative to that of parathyroid hormone. Calcitonin is elaborated by the parafollicular cells of the thyroid in response to elevations in circulating ionized calcium concentration. Together with parathyroid hormone, calcitonin constitutes the dual proportional control system that effectively maintains a constant extracellular calcium concentration.[15] In addition, vitamin D, through its biologically active $1,25(OH)_2D_3$ metabolite, controls the intestinal absorption of calcium in order to maximize the utilization of dietary calcium and minimize the use of skeletal reservoir for the maintenance of calcium homeostasis.[16]

Although the roles of parathyroid hormone, calcitonin, and $1,25(OH)_2D_3$ in maintaining calcium homeostasis are of paramount importance, insulin, growth hormone, thyroxine, androgens, estrogens, adrenal corticosteroids, and inorganic phosphate also contribute in this regard.[1]

## Calcium in Plasma

The total calcium concentration of blood plasma or serum of man is remarkably constant, ranging between 2.25 and 2.75 mmol, with 2.5 mmol (10 mg/dl or 5.0 meq/L) the average value.[17] In men, the serum calcium decreases with age, paralleling a decrease in both total serum protein and albumin, whereas in women, despite similar decrements in total serum protein, serum calcium remains rather constant with advancing years.

Serum total calcium also decreases 5 to 10% during pregnancy until the end of the third trimester, when it tends to rise. The values begin to fall in the second or third month, attaining the lowest values in the seventh or eighth month. Because the "free" ionized calcium concentration is not significantly altered during pregnancy, the reduction in total calcium can best be explained by the lower amount of protein-bound calcium. The latter may reflect the 20 to 30% fall in circulatory albumin that normally obtains during the third trimester.

Calcium exists in three forms in the blood and body fluids: (1) protein-bound calcium; (2) ionized calcium; and (3) diffusible calcium complexed with organic acids such as citrate or inorganic acids such as sulfate or phosphate.[17] The free and complexed calciums are often referred to as the nonprotein-bound or ultrafilterable fraction. The physiologic properties of calcium are all functions of the free ionic calcium. Because of the compartmentalization of plasma calcium, total calcium may often fail to reflect the free ionic calcium levels, particularly in subjects with acidosis, alkalosis, or abnormal plasma protein concentration. In normal plasma, the protein-bound calcium accounts for about 46% of the total (Fig. 5–3). Albumins and globulins are the principal plasma proteins to which calcium is bound, with the prealbumin fraction accounting for the highest degree of binding affinity. About 81% of the protein-bound calcium is bound to albumin, the globulins accounting for the remainder.

For the protein-poor fluids of the body, such as the cerebrospinal and extracellular fluids, the calcium concentration is generally about 1.25 mm/L (5 g/dl) and is virtually all in the ultrafilterable form. A small fraction of this amount is also in the form of nonionized diffusible complexes. The ionized calcium fraction is the physiologically active form; alterations in its concentration are critical for the regulation of neuromuscular excitability. Plasma ionized calcium concentrations normally range between 0.94 and 1.33 mmol/L (mean 1.14 mmol/L). When this plasma concentration is reduced, as in hypoparathyroidism or vitamin-D-deficient rachitic states (Table 5–1), increased neuromuscular irritability results. Other signs of hypocalcemia include seizures, cardiac cramps, and choreiform movements. More chronic and less severe forms of hypocalcemia often result in cataract formation, intermittent paresthesias of the extremities, and loss of cognitive function. The protective effect of acidosis against hypocalcemic tetany (i.e., as may occur in patients with chronic renal insufficiency) may not result entirely from an increased concentration of

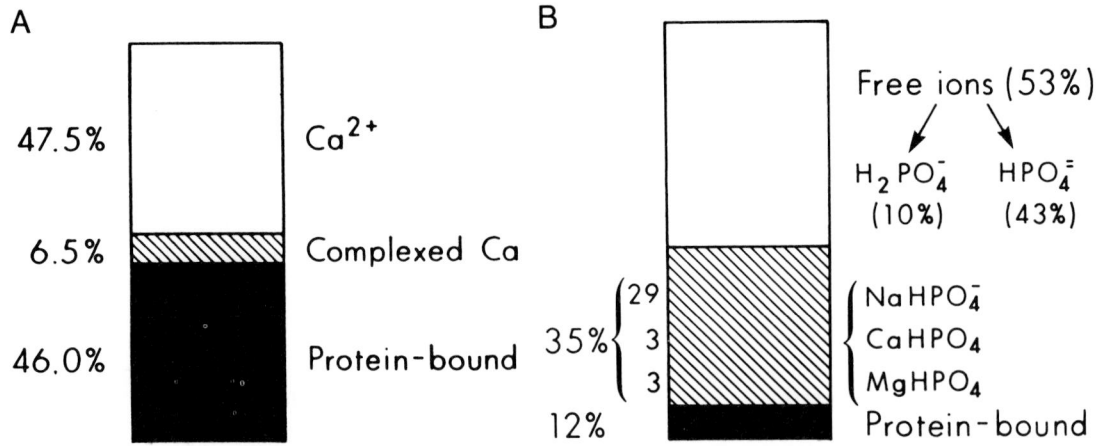

Fig. 5–3. *A*, Calcium distribution in normal human plasma. *B*, Phosphate distribution in normal human plasma. (Modified from M. Walser.[16])

ionized calcium. The hydrogen (or hydroxyl) ion exerts a depressive effect on neuromuscular irritability, even though it does not affect the inotropic response of the heart to calcium ions.

Hypercalcemia, which occurs in various clinical disorders (Table 5–2), may result in nausea, vomiting, generalized fatigue, constipation, nocturia, vomiting, hypertension, polyuria, subjective proximal muscular weakness, myopathy, and renal calculi. Unlike most symptoms attributable to hypercalcemia, the degree of elevation of the serum calcium does not appear to correlate with the severity of the observed myopathy. Mental disturbances have also been noted in hypercalcemic patients.[18] They range from simple functional behavioral disorders, confusion, and depression to severe neurasthenic personality changes, organic

psychosis, and catatonic stupor. A definite quantitative correlation is apparent between the degree of psychosocial disturbance and serum calcium; the higher the serum calcium, the more severe the mental disturbance. Moreover, the disturbed behavioral patterns are completely reversible when the serum calcium is returned to normal.[18] Hypercalcemia is attended by a depression of cere-

**Table 5–1.  Causes of Hypocalcemia**

Hypoparathyroidism
    Post-thyroidectomy
    Postparathyroidectomy
    Idiopathic causes
    Pseudohypoparathyroidism
Hypomagnesemia
Chronic renal failure
Malabsorption syndromes
Acute pancreatitis
Osteoblastic metastasis
Chemotherapy of acute leukemia
Chronic anticonvulsant therapy
Phosphate enemas or infusions
Neonatal hypocalcemia
Osteomalacia or rickets due to:
    Vitamin D-deficient states
    Poor sunlight exposure
    Inadequate vitamin D intakes
Transfusion of citrated blood
Tumors producing vitamin D "antagonists"*

*Specifically tumors that produce substance(s) that interfere with the biologic activation of vitamin D.

**Table 5–2.  Causes of Hypercalcemia**

Solid tumors: breast, ovarian, lung, renal
Hematologic malignancies: myeloma, leukemia, lymphoma
Primary hyperparathyroidism
Hyperthyroidism
Familial benign hypercalcemia (with hypocalciuria)
Pheochromocytoma
Acute adrenal insufficiency (glucocorticoid treated)
Myxedema
Acromegaly
"Pancreatic cholera" often associated with islet cell tumor
Immobilization (children, Paget's disease, and paraplegics)
Hypophosphatasia
Sarcoidosis
Coccidioidomycosis
Histoplasmosis
Tuberculosis
Berylliosis
Lymphogranuloma venereum
Vitamin D toxicity
Vitamin A toxicity
Thiazide diuretics
Chlorthalidone
Lithium
Tamoxifen (antiestrogen)
Vasomotor nephropathy (diuretic phase)
Acute renal failure
Idiopathic hypercalcemia of infancy
Generalized periostitis
Idiopathic hypertrophic subaortic stenosis
Benign breast dysplasia

bral function and nonspecific EEG patterns, characterized by a diffusely slow record with paroxysms of frontal dominant and 2 to 4 c/s bursts of modulality high voltage. Reversal of the hypercalcemia also leads to a gradual disappearance of the abnormal EEG patterns.

Oral calcium supplementation is the treatment of choice for most of the hypocalcemic disorders listed in Table 5–1. In prescribing oral calcium supplements, which usually range from 1.5 to 2.5 g of elemental calcium per day, the physician must recognize that various forms of calcium differ in the content of *elemental* calcium. Tablets of calcium gluconate (9% calcium), calcium lactate (13% calcium), and calcium carbonate (40% calcium) are all considered appropriate supplemental agents. In order to ensure the maximal intake of calcium with adequate patient compliance, calcium carbonate should be considered the supplement of choice. Calcium chloride should not be prescribed because it often causes gastrointestinal irritation. When oral calcium supplementation fails to reverse the hypocalcemia, treatment with pharmacologic quantities of either vitamin $D_3$ or $D_2$, dihydrotachysterol (Hytakerol), $25OHD_3$ (calcidiol), or $1,25(OH)_2D_3$ (calcitriol) is recommended. Maximal response to each of these agents can only be assumed with concomitant oral calcium therapy in a range of 1.5 to 2.5 g of elemental calcium per day. Unlike hypocalcemic states where adjustments in calcium intake may prove therapeutic, changes in dietary calcium usually have insignificant effects on serum calcium in hypercalcemic patients. Primary exceptions to this rule are patients with vitamin D intoxication syndromes and sarcoidosis.[19]

In normal subjects, a relation exists between plasma calcium and inorganic phosphate. When expressed in terms of total calcium (mg per dl) and inorganic phosphate (mg per dl), the "ion product" or Ca × P solubility product normally averages 35. This calculated circulating ion product has no theoretical significance, and its values are extremely variable in normal man. In molar units, the ion product calculated by this method is 0.2 to 0.3 times the actual plasma ion product, $(Ca^{+2}) \times (HPO_4^{2-})$, which in human plasma averages $0.72 \times 10^{-6}$ mmol. A "solubility product constant" can be defined as the ion product at concentrations of the ions at which the rates of solution and precipitation of the salt are equal. A solubility product constant thus physicochemically defines conditions present at equilibrium.

Despite many uncertainties concerning the mineralizing propensity of plasma and the exact chemical nature of either the earliest form of bone mineral or of the fluids in direct contact with bone mineral in vivo, it has been suggested that ionic interchange between bone and tissue fluids exhibits a solubility relationship. The ion product of hydroxyapatite ($1 \times 10^{-25}$ mmol) is considerably lower than that of $(Ca^{+2}) \times (HPO_4^{2-})$ in extracellular fluid. At normal plasma pH, the body fluids are, in effect, supersaturated with respect to the final mineral bone phase. This finding has been interpreted to mean that mineral can be extracted from the surrounding fluids with great efficiency during bone formation. Moreover, it has been suggested that a fall in the Ca × P ion product in the extracellular fluid leads to a dissolution of the exchangeable bone mineral and, conversely, an increase leads to increased deposition of these elements into bone.

It seems likely that the formation of inorganic crystals in bone occurs by a process of heterogeneous phase transformation, which does not occur within the lumen of blood vessels and in soft tissue. This implies that calcium and phosphate from the fluids bathing bone are rendered mineralizable by the interaction of ions in the bathing fluids with a unique "nucleating center" in bone (probably collagen fibrils). In order for heterogeneous nucleation to occur, the tissue fluid in contact with the nucleation center in bone must be in metastable equilibrium. To date, this hypothesis has not been verified because it cannot be determined a priori from the chemical composition and properties of the fluids bathing bone whether they are in metastable equilibrium with the mineral phase of bone. Therefore, until the determination of the plasma Ca × P ion product can be correlated in vivo with the mineralizing propensity of plasma and until the effective ion product that governs mineralization in vivo is known, it appears unwise to consider the plasma Ca × P ion product a precise physiologic determinant of new bone formation and skeletal turnover.

### Calcium Absorption

The homeostasis of calcium in blood and extracellular fluid represents an exquisite biologic control system in man. The level of circulating calcium depends on a balance between the amount added by the resorption of bone, intestinal absorption, and renal tubular reabsorption on one hand, and the calcium lost by skeletal formation, or "accretion," and renal and intestinal excretion on the other.

Measurements of "calcium balance" in man are likely to be poor estimates of actual calcium absorption or retention.[20] Since the "balance" is, in essence, the calculated difference between a large intake and a large excretion, the difference between these is inherently inaccurate. The usual errors, namely, failure of the subject to consume all of the diet and failure to collect all of the excreta, often lead to false-positive balances. The extent to which such errors have influenced prevailing concepts of calcium homeostasis in health and disease is unknown. The absorptive efficiency of the intestine for calcium is dependent on amount of exposure to ultraviolet light[16] and vitamin D intake, the sex and age of the individual, the food source, the total calcium content of the source, and the bioavailability of calcium. Whereas during periods of active skeletal growth children may absorb up to 75% of ingested calcium, normal adults, with daily intakes of 400 to 1,000 mg, absorb 30 to 60%.[21] Dietary factors that increase calcium absorption include certain amino acids, such as lysine and arginine, vitamin D, and lactose. Cocoa, soybeans, kale, spinach (or other foods high in oxalate), and foods with high phosphate content, such as unpolished rice or hexaphosphinositol in bran or wheat meal, decrease the intestinal absorptive efficiency for calcium.[22-24] Other factors that decrease calcium absorption include the ingestion of alkali, increased gastrointestinal transit time, stress, immobilization, anticonvulsant medications, thyroid hormone, and cortisol or any of its synthetic analogues. Antibiotics such as penicillin, neomycin, and chloramphenicol may actually enhance the absorption of calcium.

The localization of the actual intestinal site(s) of calcium absorption in man and animals has preoccupied a host of investigators for considerable time. It seems well established that absorption occurs primarily in the upper portion of the small intestine of most species tested thus far (rat, rabbit, horse, mouse, and chick) and that the most efficient mechanism of absorption resides in the duodenum. In vitro experiments with everted intestinal loops, as well as in vivo intestinal perfusion studies in the rat and dog, have demonstrated that the rate of calcium ion absorption per unit segment (in terms of the amount of calcium transferred per unit time) is maximal in the duodenum.[25,26] However, when one also considers the transit time of calcium through the intestinal tract, it becomes obvious that more distal intestinal segments contain the major effective sites of calcium absorption in both rat and dog. Studies in man have suggested that similar dictates apply.[27,28] These latter studies demonstrated that, although the calculated rate of calcium absorption by the human duodenum was three times that of the rest of the intestine, the intestinal segment distal to the duodenum was more sensitive to factors controlling calcium absorption under normal physi-

ologic conditions. The studies also showed that in man, the calcium flux from lumen to blood was independent of intraluminal calcium concentration and was maximal in the more proximal intestinal segments. More recent studies in healthy normal subjects reveal that in the basal state, calcium absorption is significantly higher in the jejunum than in the ileum. Administration of the active vitamin $D_3$ metabolite, $1,25(OH)_2D_3$, results in an increase in calcium absorption in both jejunum and ileum of similar magnitudes.[29] Changes in net calcium absorption are due primarily to an increase in lumen-to-plasma calcium flux.[29] Observations in the rat suggest that the large intestine may also play a role in calcium homeostasis, particularly when dietary calcium is restricted.[30] It is evident from these animal studies that the large intestine must also be considered potentially significant in regulating calcium homeostasis in man, particularly during calcium deprivation or as a consequence of the loss of ileal absorptive function.

The effect of inorganic phosphate on calcium absorption is controversial. Earlier reports of an inhibition of calcium absorption induced by supplemented phosphate feeding[31] conflict with later studies demonstrating no effect of dietary phosphorus increments on calcium absorption.[32] Calcium absorption is more efficient in males than in females. This finding may be related to reports of stimulated calcium absorption when androgens are administered to females.[33] Absorption decreases as individuals age[34,35] (Fig. 5–4). The adaptive efficiency of the intestine to fluctuations in calcium intake is one whereby, with decreasing calcium intake, the percent absorbed increases.[35,36] This intestinal adaptive efficiency appears to be also blunted by the aging process[35] (see Fig. 5–4). Despite the recognized inverse relation between calcium absorption and intake, prolonged fasting paradoxically results in decreased absorption,[37] and absorption may actually increase as calcium intake rises, with absorptive capacities of more than 1.0 g per day documented at intakes of 7.5 g.[38] Although it has been reported that calcium is significantly better absorbed when given to human subjects as the lactate than as the gluconate salt,[39] it has also been observed that no difference exists in the utilization of calcium from milk, gluconate, lactate, carbonate, or sulfate salts.[40,41]

Fecal calcium consists not only of unabsorbed ingested calcium but also of the endogenous calcium secreted into the gastrointestinal tract and not absorbed. About 85% of the calcium entering the intestine in this manner is secreted proximal to the site of absorption. It is thus presented to

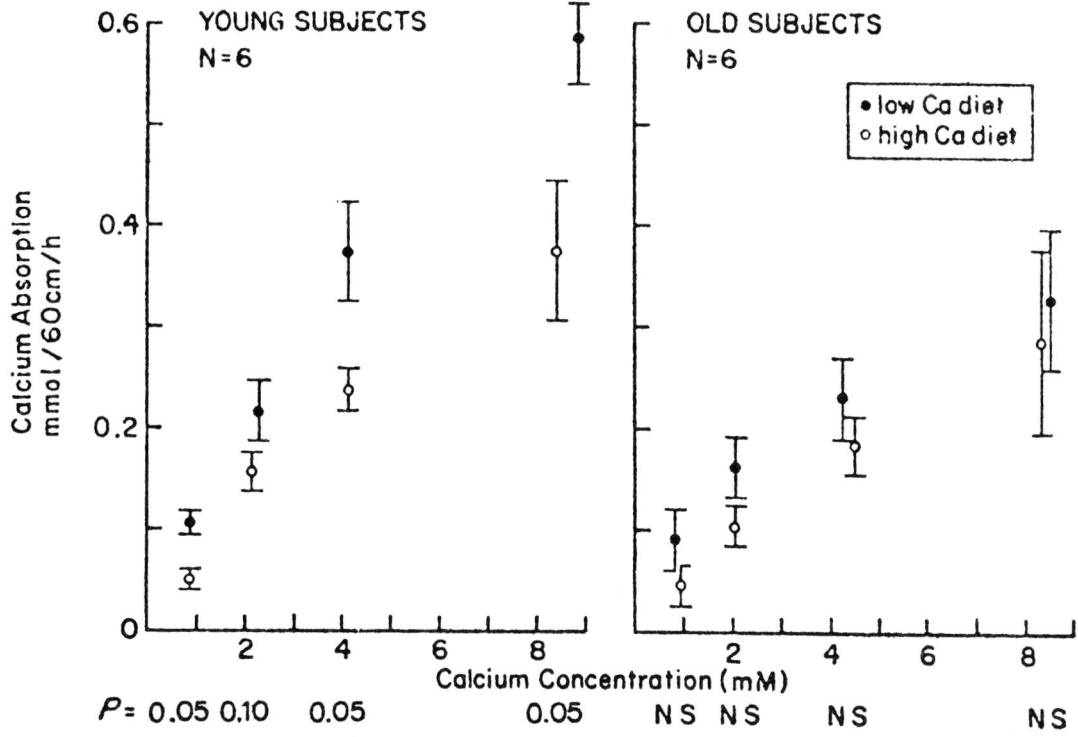

**Fig. 5–4.** Effect of calcium intake on calcium absorption rates in young and old subjects. Each subject was studied on a high- and low-calcium diet. The rate of calcium absorption in old subjects was significantly less than that observed in younger individuals. Note that the intestinal response of old subjects to calcium deprivation (i.e., compare values obtained on low- *vs.* high-calcium diet) was blunted. NS = no significant difference. In this study, urinary calcium was higher in the older subjects despite the fact that they absorbed less calcium. (From Ireland and Fordtran.[35])

the absorptive sites and is assumed to be handled with the same efficiency as the calcium of dietary origin. Approximately 15% of the total intestinal calcium secretion is assumed to be nonabsorbable, even under conditions when dietary calcium is completely absorbed. Total intestinal calcium excretion in man averages 0.194 ± 0.073 g per day; the secreted calcium that is not absorbed, endogenous fecal calcium, averages 130 mg per day. This endogenous fecal fraction, like the daily losses of calcium in sweat, exerts little effect on the day-to-day regulation of calcium balance. In certain clinical situations, such as overt hyperthyroidism, however, the calcium losses in sweat, which normally range between 20 and 350 mg per day,[20] may be considerable because of the increased concentrations of calcium in the sweat, as well as the increased volume of sweat. Calcium losses in sweat may also be as large as 1 g per day in individuals working in high temperatures.

## Calcium Excretion

Once absorbed, calcium enters the extracellular fluid and rapidly exchanges with the calcium in the exchangeable moiety of bone mineral and that

in the glomerular filtrate. The daily urinary excretion of calcium in normal human subjects on diets containing 600 to 1,000 mg of calcium per day ranges between 80 and 250 g.[42] An exponential relationship exists between dietary and urinary calcium, so that wide variations in intake are accompanied by parallel but only slight alterations in excretion.[43] The urinary excretion of calcium is determined more by the absorption of calcium from the intestine than by the dietary intake. The more efficient the intestinal absorption of calcium, the greater the absolute change in urinary calcium for a given change in calcium intake. In young adults, urinary calcium increases by approximately 6% for any given change in dietary calcium intake.[43] Since the efficiency of absorption decreases in man with advancing age,[34,35] the variation in urinary calcium with changes in calcium intake is greater in young than in older individuals. Variations in urinary calcium excretion normally play an insignificant role in modifying the effect of wide swings in calcium intake on calcium homeostasis. There is also a diurnal variation in the rate of calcium excretion, with the greatest excretion occurring during the day and a nadir observed during the evening hours.[42]

The amount of nonprotein-bound calcium filtered by the glomeruli in man averages 10,000 mg per 24 hours. Normally, approximately 99% of the filtered load is reabsorbed by the renal tubules, so that, on the average, 100 to 150 mg of calcium are excreted per day. In hypocalcemic states (i.e., serum calcium concentration below 7.5 mg per dl), renal tubular reabsorption of calcium is so complete that calcium virtually disappears from the urine. The major part of calcium reabsorption, like that of sodium, occurs in the proximal convoluted tubule and in the ascending limb of Henle's loop; presumably the remainder is absorbed in more distal parts of the nephron. Whereas the distal tubular reabsorption of calcium appears independent of sodium, calcium and sodium ions appear to share a common pathway of active transport in the proximal tubule. To this extent, excretion is dependent upon simultaneous sodium excretion, the latter governing the excretion of the free calcium ion. Calcium excretion is increased not only by saline diuresis but also by carbohydrate and sodium ingestion, phosphate deprivation,[44] metabolic acidosis, cortisol or any of the synthetic glucocorticoids, thyroid and growth hormones,[42,45] and diets rich in protein and magnesium. In fact, urinary calcium appears to be more dependent on protein and salt intake than on calcium intake.[46] The reasons for all of these seemingly unrelated causes of hypercalciuria are still not well delineated.

Carbohydrate-induced increments in urinary calcium have been attributed to an inhibition of calcium reabsorption in the distal tubules (or collecting ducts) by enhanced glucose uptake and glycolysis.[47–49] The hypercalciuria observed during phosphate deprivation or in patients ingesting large amounts of phosphate-binding gels[50] results from an increased intestinal absorption of calcium, the latter due primarily to hypophosphatemic-stimulated increments in circulating $1,25(OH)_2D_3$.[50]

At present, there is no conclusive evidence for a direct action of glucocorticoids on transepithelial calcium transport in the kidney. All available data are compatible with an extrarenal effect of glucocorticoids. The elevation in urinary calcium can be accounted for by an increase in skeletal resorption, and an increase in the filtered load of ionized calcium. The calcium effect of high-protein diets has been attributed to increments in glomerular filtration rates,[51,52] to sulfur-containing amino acids of dietary protein that inhibit the tubular reabsorption of filtered calcium,[53,54] and to the stimulation of insulin secretion.[55] An evaluation of these many and diverse observations must be attempted with caution with full recognition that high-protein diets rich in phosphate cause a *decrease* in urinary calcium,[56] a phenomenon that results from a direct effect of parathyroid hormone on increasing the renal tubular reabsorption of the filtered calcium load.

Clinical disorders characterized by hypercalciuria include hyperthyroidism, sarcoidosis, acromegaly, hyperparathyroidism, Cushing's disease, metastatic bone disease, the chronic ingestion of phosphate-binding gels such as $Al(OH)_3$, and either the "absorptive" or "renal" hypercalciuric syndromes of stone-forming patients.[57] In "absorptive" hypercalciuria, the basic abnormality is an acquired (or inherited) intestinal hyperabsorption of calcium. Increased calcium absorption results in a suppression of parathyroid hormone release and hypercalciuria. In "renal" hypercalciuria, the primary abnormality is a defect in the renal tubular reabsorption of calcium. The constant "renal calcium leak" stimulates parathyroid function resulting in elevation in blood levels of the hormone. In some patients with the renal hypercalciuric syndrome, parathyroid "autonomy" may be anticipated if untreated. The "hyperparathyroid" syndrome in these patients may prove to respond to calcium therapy with 1,000 mg of elemental calcium per day. Finally, it should be noted that the renal tubular reabsorption of calcium is increased by benzothiadiazine diuretics. Thiazide diuretics augment calcium reabsorption in the distal tubules and stimulate proximal tubular resorption of calcium, the latter resulting from extracellular volume contraction. Although short-term administration of thiazides may prove beneficial to maintaining calcium homeostasis, chronic administration results in a progressive fall in blood parathyroid hormone, the latter causing a decrease in the production of $1,25(OH)_2D_3$ and a decrease in the intestinal absorption of calcium.

## Calcium Requirements

Several dietary surveys reveal that among Western populations the mean adult calcium intake ranges between 400 and 1,300 mg calcium per day.[50–60] At all ages, men consume more calcium than women (Fig. 5–5), and at all ages some individual men and women ingest two to four times the recommended allowances of calcium.

The full-term infant contains about 25 to 35 g of calcium, about half of which is deposited during the last lunar month of pregnancy at a rate of approximately 300 mg per day. It has been demonstrated that the reproductive process is not impaired when the calcium intake of pregnant

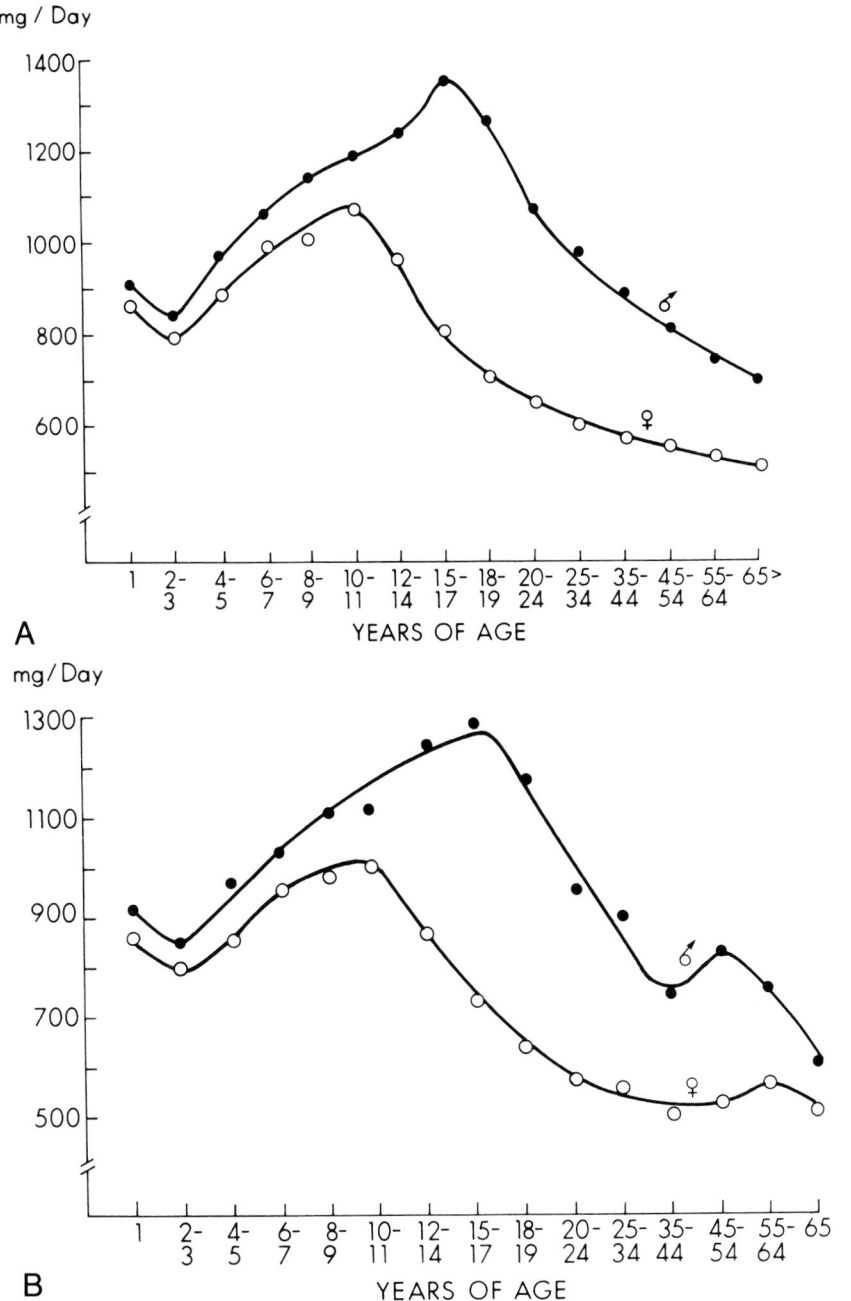

**Fig. 5–5.** Mean *(A)* and median *(B)* calcium intakes of men and women in the United States from 1971 to 1974. (Adapted from DHEW Publication No. (HRA) 77–1647, July, 1977.)

women ranges between 700 mg and 1.2 g per day.[61,62] More recent estimates place the calcium requirement of pregnant women at 2 g per day,[63] although this has been contested.[64] A young baby receives about 200 mg calcium per day while ingesting 650 ml of breast milk during early lactation, and by 8 months of age the infant's daily calcium intake has increased to 350 mg.[65] Assuming a maintenance calcium requirement of 3 mg per kg body weight and an efficiency of utilization of 30%, it has been estimated that a lactating mother requires 1 to 2 g of calcium per day in order to ensure adequate calcium supply in breast-feedings and skeletal balance.[66] The needs for the third trimester of pregnancy and normal lactation, as recommended by the Joint FAO/WHO Expert Group on Calcium Requirements, has been set at 1,200 mg per day,[67] although it is recognized that many women have lactated adequately on low intakes.

A premature infant needs about 90 to 120 g calcium per kg body weight and 60 to 90 mg phosphorus per kg daily, amounts that are easily provided by 100 g of whole cow's milk per kg of body weight.[68] An average 1-month-old infant weighing 4 kg obtains 235 mg of calcium daily from breast milk, and at 3 months approximately 300 mg calcium per day—amounts sufficient to meet his skeletal demands. Maternal bone loss during this period approximates 2 to 3%.[69] Formula-fed children up to 1 year of age require no more than 600 mg of calcium per day for adequate skeletal development and growth.[20] For children 1 to 10 years of age with adequate vitamin D intakes, 800 mg per day appears to be sufficient to ensure normal skeletal growth.

Preadolescent growing children, however, may need 2 to 4 times as much calcium as does an adult. Higher intakes of calcium of 1 to 1.5 g daily are recommended during preadolescence and puberty because of the demands of rapid skeletal growth. Intakes greater than this need not be advocated because maximal calcium retention obtains in children and young adults at this level of intake.

The nutritional status of the aged in the United States has been evaluated on innumerable occasions and found to be relatively inadequate when judged by Recommended Daily Allowance (RDA) standards[58–60] (see Fig. 5–5). An increasing volume of data implicates calcium deficiency in tooth and mandibular bone loss[70,71] and the osteopenic postmenopausal fracture syndrome.[72–83] Although dietary sources should provide sufficient calcium to maintain a positive calcium balance in the average U.S. woman, it has been well documented that the intake of the average woman is consistently below the RDA.[58–60] Moreover, there is increasing concern that the U.S. RDA of calcium, which had been established earlier at 800 mg/day, may prove to be inadequate to maintain the integrity of bone[76] (Fig. 5–6). It should be emphasized that as early as 1955 the Household Food Consumption Survey of the USDA cited that calcium was one of three nutrients most often to be ingested at levels below the RDA.[60] Subsequent dietary surveys not only revealed that at any age men ingest more calcium than women, but also that during the period of life when bone mass is approaching its peak value, more than two thirds of all U.S. females ingest calcium below the RDA. This observation becomes significant in view of the fact that those women who fail to generate their full adolescent bone complement are destined to develop symptomatic osteoporosis at an earlier age. An additional insult to the integrity of bone occurs after the age of 35 when more than 75% of all females ingest less than the RDA in any given day.

On calcium intakes of 450 to 500 mg/day, normal perimenopausal and postmenopausal women develop a negative calcium balance greater than 40 mg/day; this degree of calcium loss results in a bone loss of approximately 1.5% per year.[75] As cited earlier, elderly postmenopausal women do not absorb oral or dietary calcium as well as younger menstruating women (Fig. 5–4). Estrogen loss at menopause also results in a decrease in renal calcium conservation. The intestinal adaptability to changes in calcium intake is blunted by age, and is inadequate to maintain the homeostatic equilibrium between bone and circulating calcium that characterizes the adolescent and young-adult periods of life. Consequently, it is naive to assume that the efficiency of calcium absorption necessarily "adapts" to low-calcium diets, and that the total amount of consumed calcium is relatively unimportant.[73] Defective renal adaptation to low calcium intakes (see Fig. 5–4) with mild (but persistent) hypercalciuria probably also contributes to the negative calcium balance seen in the fracture-prone osteoporotic individual.[75] Probable causes are relative degrees of immobilization that necessarily attend senescence and peculiar diets containing excessive amounts of sodium carbohydrate and proteins with low phosphate and high sulfate content (vide supra).

Until more definitive prospective studies become available, the beneficial effects of dietary calcium supplements on either retarding the rate of bone loss or decreasing bone resorption in peri- and postmenopausal women must be acknowledged (Fig. 5–7).[72,75,77,79,80,83,84] Diets should be programmed to include foods rich in elemental calcium and/or supplemented with calcium salts in order to ensure a total intake of 1.0 to 1.5 g per day. For those individuals with lactose intolerance, yogurt may prove to be an excellent dietary source of calcium.[85] Although a variety of foods are rich in calcium (i.e., dark green leafy vegetables), they also contain oxalic acid, which binds calcium and interferes with its absorption. Similarly, diets high in bran or whole grain are also poor sources of elemental calcium because of either high-fiber content or the presence of phytates which, like oxalic acid, interfere with calcium absorption. When anticipating the use of dietary supplements in patients who are either intolerant to milk or who refuse to adjust their diet to ensure adequate calcium intake, one must always consider patient compliance. Thus, one can anticipate more consistent adherence to a rou-

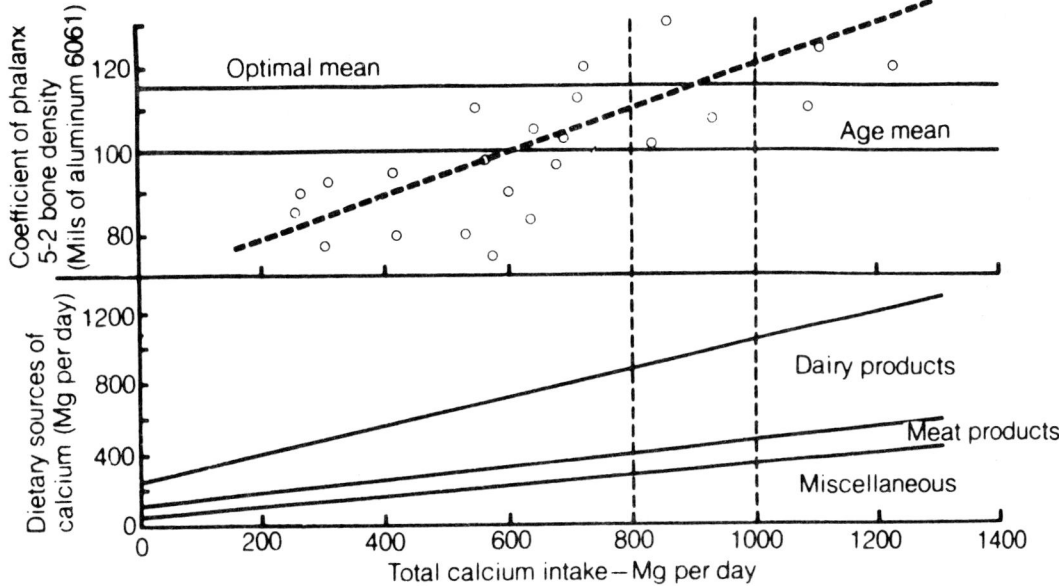

**Fig. 5–6.** Relationship between bone density (upper panel) and calcium intake (lower panel) from various sources in 23 postmenopausal women 53 to 60 years of age. (From Postgrad. Med. 63(3):171, 1978.)

tine program that requires only one to two tablets per day rather than one that would necessitate five to six tablets per day for adequate calcium supplementation. In this regard, the physician is well advised to become familiar with the elemental calcium content of commercially available calcium supplements and be reminded that *elemental calcium content is the important ingredient in the calcium preparation in question and not the total weight of the preparation.*

Modern diets, which are characteristically rich in animal proteins and phosphorus with low Ca/P ratios, may prove deleterious to bone because they may promote hypercalciuria and stimulate the release of parathyroid hormone with a resultant progressive decrease in bone mass. Immobilization, or the relative inactivity that often attends the infirmities of age, promotes skeletal demineralization. Peculiar dietary habits may also lead to increased urinary calcium loss and a negative

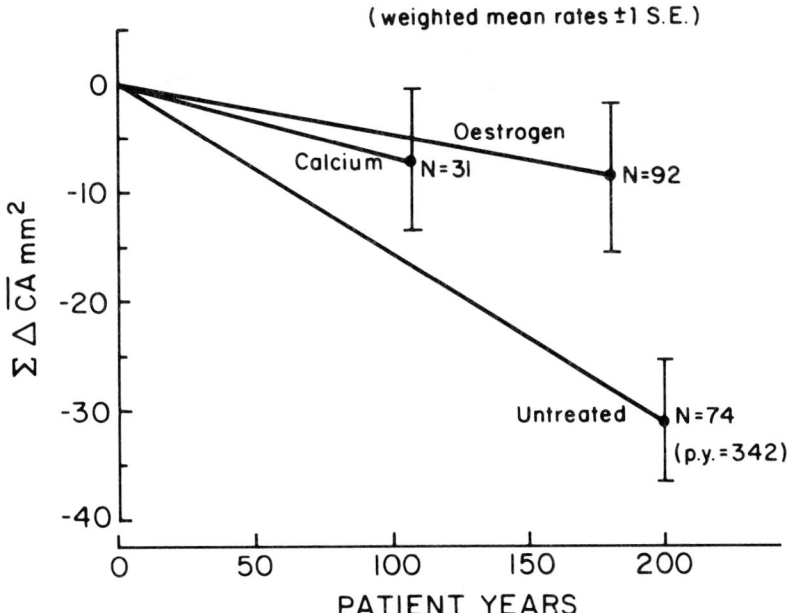

**Fig. 5–7.** Cumulative plots of the change in mean metacarpal cortical area (CA) in untreated postmenopausal women and others treated with either calcium or estrogens. (From Geriatric Medicine Today, 2:66, 1983.)

calcium balance, despite an adequate intake. Not only may calcium intakes be inadequate in geriatric populations, but vitamin D deficiency and inadequate sunlight exposure may also prevent maximal absorption of the ingested calcium.[16]

Calcium intakes ranging from 1,000 to 2,500 mg per day do not result in hypercalcemia or significant hypercalciuria in normal individuals.[42,43] Ingestion of larger amounts, as may occur with ulcer patients consuming large amounts of milk and antacid (alkali) products for patients with sarcoidosis[19] may result in hypercalciuria, hypercalcemia, and a rapid deterioration in renal function.[86–89] An acquired or inherited vitamin D-sensitive hyperabsorption of calcium occurs in patients with sarcoidosis and in certain hypercalciuric individuals with renal calculi. In these subjects, hypercalcemia and/or hypercalciuria result from only modest increments in dietary vitamin D supplementation of diets containing 800 to 1,500 mg calcium per day.[90–92]

## PHOSPHORUS

Of the 11 to 14 g of phosphorus per kg fat-free tissue in the normal adult, 85% is in the skeleton. The remainder is distributed between tissue and membrane components of skeletal muscle, skin, nervous tissue, and other organs. Whereas most of the phosphorus in soft tissue and cell membranes is in the form of organic esters, almost all the phosphorus in bone is contained in the mineral phase as inorganic orthophosphate and small amounts of inorganic phosphate. The regulation of plasma phosphate is not as readily explained as that of plasma calcium. The circulating phosphate is in equilibrium not only with skeletal and cellular inorganic phospate but also with a large number of organic compounds resulting from cellular metabolism. The phosphate ion is essential for the metabolism of carbohydrate, lipids, and protein, functioning as a cofactor in a multitude of enzyme systems and contributing to the metabolic potential in the form of "high-energy-phosphate" compounds. Phosphate functions to modify acid-base equilibrium in plasma and within cells and plays fundamental roles in modifying the development and maturation of bone, in governing renal excretion of hydrogen ions, and in modifying the effects of the B vitamins.

Although the sequence of events that obtains during the nucleation of bone collagen is still imperfectly understood, collagen fibrils exhibit a remarkable faculty to form covalent bonds with phosphate. The phosphorylation of collagen has been considered the initiating event in the nucleation of bone. Phosphate, in addition to its conditioning role in the formation of the apatitic structure, also affects bone resorption, mineralization, and collagen synthesis and thus plays an integral role in calcium homeostasis. The available evidence is consistent with the interpretation that these are direct effects of phosphate upon the metabolic functions of bone cells.[1]

### Phosphate in Plasma

In the human adult, plasma inorganic phosphate ranges between 2.5 and 4.4 mg/dl, with a mean of 3.5 mg/dl. Dietary phosphate, stage of growth and age, time of day, hormonal interplay, and renal function all contribute to the variability of the fasting serum phosphate concentration. Eighty-eight percent of the plasma phosphate is ultrafilterable (Fig. 5–3); some of this is complexed with mono or divalent cations such as $Na^+$, $Ca^{++}$, and $Mg^{++}$. At normal blood pH, 85% of the ultrafilterable phosphate is in the form of $HPO_4^{-2}$, the remainder existing mainly as $H_2PO_4$.

As noted earlier for calcium, the concentration of plasma phosphate varies with age. In prepubertal children, the mean value for circulating phosphate approximates 5 mg/dl with an upper normal limit approaching 6 mg/dl. Normal adult values are gradually approached by the third decade, after which, in men, plasma phosphate decreases progressively with advancing age.[93] The trend of values for plasma phosphate in females represents a unique cicrcumstance: they decline gradually between ages 20 and 35 and rise after age 40. The higher levels of phosphate in the female over 40 years of age seem to be related to the menopause. This finding assumes more significance because not only are postmenopausal females deficient in estrogen, but a positive correlation reportedly exists between serum inorganic phosphate and the extent of bone resorption in middle-aged and elderly women.[94]

Total serum phosphate may also normally fluctuate by as much as 1 to 2 mg per dl. These variations generally reflect abrupt shifts of inorganic phosphate between extracellular fluid and intracellular compartments, rather than a net gain or loss of phosphate from the body. The administration of hormones such as insulin, glucagon, or epinephrine results in a reduction in serum phosphate, presumably by stimulating the cellular utilization of glucose and accelerating the formation of intracellular phosphate esters.[95,96] A systemic alkalosis has been associated with a fall in circulating phosphate and has been attributed to a shift of phosphate out of the extracellular fluid compartment. The fall in plasma phosphate concentration is apparently greater in respiratory than in comparable levels of metabolic alkalosis. Thus, the evaluation of hypophosphatemia should always include measurements of the pH and total $CO_2$ content of plasma.

Phosphate depletion syndromes in humans are often the result of inappropriate ingestion of nonabsorbable antacids such as $Al(OH)_3$ gels.[44,50] The syndrome is readily reversed when the medication is discontinued and sufficient amounts of dietary phosphate are consumed. Recognition and appropriate therapy require medical supervision, particularly when adjustments in drug therapy for peptic ulcer are involved.[44,50]

Whereas starvation is occasionally associated with a decrease in plasma inorganic phosphate, acidosis and excessive catabolism of body tissue associated with starvation or lysis of neoplastic lymphoid cells during therapy may lead to cellular release of phosphate, hyperphosphatemia, and reciprocal hypocalcemia.[97]

Severe hypophosphatemia has been reported in total parenteral nutrition, alcoholism,[98] and other hypokalemia states, independent of the attendant metabolic alkalosis. Complications ascribed to hypophosphatemia include hemolytic anemia, osteomalacia, congestive heart failure, kidney stones, renal glycosuria, and proximal tubular dysfunction, central nervous system abnormalities, myopathy, rhabdomyolysis, and acute respiratory failure.[99–103] Because a large amount of phosphorus may shift rapidly between extracellular and intracellular or bone compartments, the total body deficit in hypophosphatemic subjects cannot be estimated from the serum phosphate level. Concrete recommendations for correcting the serum phosphate by the infusion of phosphate are not readily available, especially for situations wherein serum phosphate levels are less than 0.32 mmol/L (1 mg/dl) because it is difficult to estimate the extent of the total body deficit. Therapeutic guidelines must be empiric with serum phosphate levels monitored continuously in order to prevent hyperphosphatemia and hypocalcemia.[104] The latter, observed during therapy with intravenous phosphate solutions, may cause hypotension and acute renal failure.

Variations in the plasma level of inorganic phosphate probably contribute to the regulation of bone turnover and to bioactivation of the vitamin D metabolite $25OHD_3$ to $1,25(OH)_2D_3$.[16,44,105–107] It is noteworthy that severe dietary phosphate deprivation results in hypophosphatemia and increased circulating $1,25(OH)_2D_3$ in women, whereas insignificant changes in the plasma levels of either substance obtain in phosphate-depleted males.[44]

## Phosphate Absorption

Most if not all of the dietary phosphorus is absorbed as free phosphate. The efficiency of phosphate absorption is a function of both the dietary intake and food source.[108] On a normal intake, 60 to 70% is absorbed, and maximal absorption (up to 90%) is achieved on very low intakes.[109] Various dietary forms of organic phosphate esters, such as the phytic acid of cereals and seeds, are not readily available to man, since the human intestine is relatively deficient in the enzyme phytase, essential for hydrolysis of the organic esters. Organic phosphate ester compounds may also interfere with calcium absorption because they form insoluble calcium salts within the intestinal lumen. In animals and man, unsaturated fatty acids, iron, magnesium, and aluminum interfere with intestinal phosphate absorption.[110–112]

Although vitamin D increases intestinal phosphate absorption in certain animal species,[106] a direct effect of vitamin D (or its biologically active metabolites) on phosphate absorption in man is still to be adequately demonstrated. There is no known effective physiologic mechanism regulating the intestinal absorption of phosphate in man; the control of the phosphate economy is achieved primarily by variations in dietary intake and renal excretion.[42] Fecal phosphorus represents both unabsorbed phosphate and that secreted into the gastrointestinal tract.[109] In man, with phosphorus intakes of approximately 1 to 1.5 g per day, the secretion of endogenous phosphate into the intestinal lumen averages 3 mg/kg per day.[109] Dietary phosphorus is absorbed to a greater extent than is calcium and, consequently, the renal excretion of phosphate is much greater than that of calcium.[42]

## Phosphate Excretion

Urinary phosphorus is largely inorganic phosphate, the amount depending primarily upon how much is absorbed from the intestinal tract. Phosphate exists in the forms of $HPO_4^{2-}/H_2PO_4$ in the glomerular filtrate in a ratio of 4 to 1. With normal renal function, urinary phosphorus usually amounts to approximately two thirds of the dietary phosphorus. Normally, a diurnal variation in phosphate clearance occurs with the usual pattern, that of a matitudinal increase in urinary phosphorus/creatinine ratios. This circadian rhythm is related to physical activity, with the nadir appearing a few hours after the end of sleep. The loss of diurnal variation in adrenal-insufficient states and the documented inverse correlation between phosphate excretion and plasma cortisol levels suggest that this rhythm is controlled by the adrenal glands.[42]

In man, the tubular reabsorption of phosphate cleared by the glomeruli is normally 85 to 95%.[42] This is an age-related and rate-limited process, with a maximum tubular reabsorptive capacity in adults of 4 to 8 mg per min. The tubular reabsorption of phosphate is increased by short-term cortisol therapy and growth hormone, and is decreased by digoxin, estrogen, thyroid hormone, parathyroid hormone, long-term cortisol therapy, and elevations in circulating calcium.[42]

## Phosphorus Requirements

The average daily phosphorus requirement of adults is estimated to be 0.8 to 1.5 g per day.[31,108,113] Dietary surveys reveal that the level of phosphorus in the diet of the average American is approximately 45 to 62 mg phosphorus per 100 calories consumed, 15 mg phosphorus per gram protein, or 1.5 to 1.6 mg phosphorus per mg calcium. National food consumption surveys show that males generally consume more phosphorus daily, the difference resulting primarily from difference in total energy intake. Phosphorus intakes (as expressed as mg per 100 K cal) also vary with age with values for infants and young children greater than the average values of adolescents and adults.[114] The average diet of blacks, who have greater bone mass than nonblacks, contains considerably less phosphorus than the diet of nonblacks. Approximately four fifths of the dietary phosphorus in all age groups is contained in milk products, grains, and meat products. Obviously, milk and milk products are the primary source of phosphorus for infants, the latter accounting for two thirds of the phosphorus consumed. Only one fifth of the phosphorus consumed by adults is from milk and milk products. Food additives also contribute a considerable amount of phosphorus. These phosphorus-containing additives are used primarily in baked goods, cheeses, and other dairy products; phosphoric acid is also used in cola and carbonated beverages. It has been estimated that food additives may contribute as much as 30% of the phosphorus of an average adult diet in the U.S.[114] These estimates can only increase in the future because the segment of older adults who consume processed foods containing food additives is increasing annually as America is "graying," and also because processed foods are being used with increasing frequency by families in which both adults are employed.[114]

The relative greater availability of phosphate-containing foodstuffs has resulted in a calcium/phosphate dietary ratio in Western diets much lower than that deemed essential to maintain the integrity of skeletal tissue. This matter is of some concern, since diets with a low Ca/P ratio have led to progressive bone loss in rats,[115] dogs,[115–117] and horses[118] owing to excessive parathyroid stimulation. Similar effects may occur in humans on high-phosphate diets for prolonged periods because excessive phosphate ingestion does result in a stimulated release of parathyroid hormone.[119]

Short-term dietary habits that include relatively high (1.5 to 2.5 g phosphorus per day) levels of phosphorus and P/Ca ratios of less than 3/1 have not been associated with abnormalities in calcium and bone metabolism in humans.[32] Although many agree that the daily consumption of 2.0 g of phosphorus does not affect bone adversely when sufficient calcium is ingested, the "adequacy" of calcium intake essential to protect skeletal resources, and hence prevent bone loss, is still a contestable issue.[14]

With the exception of young infants, the recommended allowance of phosphorus per day is the same as that of calcium, although the Ca/P ratio of diets ingested throughout the world today is reported to be less than 0.75.[120,121] The Ca/P ratio of cow's milk of 1.3/1, compared with a Ca/P ratio of 2/1 in breast milk,[120] may contribute to the syndrome of "idiopathic hypocalcemia" and tetany of infants on formula feedings.

Since the kidney is capable of excreting 600 to 900 mg of phosphorus daily, hyperphosphatemia is rare in the absence of chronic renal disease and then only occurs when the glomerular filtration rate falls below 20 mg per min.[42] Hyperphosphatemia is also characteristic of disorders of parathyroid secretion and metabolism, such as hypoparathyroidism[122–124] and pseudohypoparathyroidism,[124,125] and can be accentuated by phosphate feeding. There are no specific signs or symptoms of hyperphosphatemia per se, although the hypocalcemia often associated with the hyperphosphatemia in these syndromes (and exacerbated by phosphate feeding) can result in enhanced neuroexcitability, tetany, and convulsions.[122]

## REFERENCES

1. Raisz, L.: Bone Metabolism and Calcium Regulation. *In* Metabolic Bone Disease, Vol. 1 (Avioli, L.V., and Krane, Eds.) New York, Academic Press, 1977, pp 1–42.
2. Robinson, R.A.: Clin. Orthop. *112*:263–315, 1975.
3. Lee, D.D., Lander, W.J., and Glimcher, M.J.: J. Bone Min. Res. *1*:425–432, 1986.
4. Termine, J.D.: Clin. Orthop. *85*:207–241, 1972.
5. Becker, R.D., Spadaro, M.S., Berg, W.: J. Bone Joint Surg. *50A*:326–334, 1968.
6. Kildeberg, P., Engel, K., Winters, R.W.: Acta Paediatr. Scand. *58*:321–329, 1969.
7. Centrella, M., Canalis, E.: Endoc. Rev. *6*:544–551, 1985.
8. Daniell, H.W.: Arch. Int. Med. *143*:1678–1682, 1983.
9. Pitkin, R.M.: Am. J. Obstet. Gynecol. *121*:724–737, 1975.
10. Cushard, N.G. Jr., Creditor, M.A., Canterbury, J.M., et al.: J. Clin. Endocrinol. Metab. *34*:767–771, 1972.

11. Heaney, R.P., Shillman, T.G.: J. Clin. Endocrinol. Metab. *53*:661–670, 1971.

12. Riggs, B.L., Wahner, H.W., Dunn, W.L., et al.: J. Clin. Invest. *67*:328–335, 1981.

13. Johnston, C.C., Jr., Hui, S.L., Witt, R.M., et al.: J. Clin. Endocrinol. Metab. *61*:905–911, 1985.

14. Avioli, L.V.: Calcium and osteoporosis. Ann. Rev. Nutrition *4*:471–491, 1984.

15. Avioli, L.V.: Calcitonin. *In* The Year in Endocrinology. (Ingbar, Ed.) New York, Plenum Press, 1976, pp 233–248.

16. Miller, S.M.: Am. J. Med. Tech. *49*:27–37, 1983.

17. Walser, M.: J. Clin. Invest. *40*:723–730, 1961.

18. Avioli, L.V.: Geriatrics *41*:30–37, 1986.

19. Bell, N.H.: J. Clin. Invest. *76*:1–6, 1985.

20. Isaksson, B., Lindholm, B., Sjogren, B.: Metabolism *16*:303–313, 1967.

21. Mautalen, C.A., Cabrejas, M.L., Soto, R.J.: Metabolism *18*:395–405, 1969.

22. Irwin, M.J., Kienholz, E.W.: J. Nutr. *103*:1019–1095, 1973.

23. McCance, R.A., Widdowson, E.M.: J. Physiol. *101*:44–85, 1942.

24. Reinhold, J.G., Faradji, B., Abadi, P., et al.: J. Nutr. *106*:493–503, 1976.

25. Urban, E., Schedl, H.P.: Am. J. Physiol. *217*:126–130, 1969.

26. Cramer, C.F.: Qualitative studies on absorption of calcium from intestinal loops in dogs. *In* The Transfer of Calcium and Strontium Across Biological Membranes. (Wasserman, Ed.) New York, Academic Press, 1963.

27. Birge, S.J., Peck, W.A., Berman, M.: J. Clin. Invest. *48*:1705–1713, 1969.

28. Wensel, R.H., Rich, C., Brown, A.C.: J. Clin. Invest. *48*:1768–1775, 1969.

29. Krejs, G.J., Nicar, M.J., Zerwekh, J.E., et al.: Am. J. Med. *75*:973–976, 1983.

30. Petith, M.M., Scheal, H.P.: Gastroenterology *71*:1039–1042, 1976.

31. Leichsenring, J.M., Norris, L.M., Lamison, S.A., et al.: Br. J. Nutr. *45*:477–485, 1951.

32. Spencer, H., Menczel, J., Lewin, I., et al.: J. Nutr. *86*:125–132, 1965.

33. Jaworski, Z.F., Brown, E.M., Fedoruk, M.A., et al.: N. Engl. J. Med. *269*:1103–1111, 1963.

34. Avioli, L.V., McDonald, J.E., Lee, S.W.: J. Clin. Invest. *44*:1960–1967, 1965.

35. Ireland, P., Fordtran, J.S.: J. Clin. Invest. *52*:2672–2681, 1973.

36. Spencer, H., Lewin, I., Fowler, J., et al.: Am. J. Med. *46*:197–205, 1969.

37. Fromm, G.A., Litvak, J., Degrossi, O.J.: Lancet *1*:616–617, 1970.

38. Heaney, R.P., Saville, P.D., Recker, R.R.: J. Lab. Clin. Med. *85*:881–890, 1975.

39. Spencer, H., Scheck, J., Lewin, I., et al.: J. Nutr. *89*:283–292, 1966.

40. Bronner, F., Harris, E., Moor, L., et al.: MIT Report A-81C, 1960.

41. Patton, M.B., Sutton, T.S.: J. Nutr. *48*:443–452, 1952.

42. Massry, S.G., Friedler, R.M., Coburn, J.W.: Arch Intern. Med. *131*:828–859, 1973.

43. Lemann, J. Jr., Adams, N.D., Gray, R.W.: N. Engl. J. Med. *301*:535–541, 1979.

44. Gray, R.W., Wilz, D.R., Caldas, A.E., et al.: J. Clin. Endocrinol. Metab. *45*:299–306, 1977.

45. Fallon, M.D., Perry, H.M., Bergfeld, M., et al.: Arch. Intern. Med. *143*:442–444, 1983.

46. Linkswiler, H.M., Joyce, C.L., Anand, C.R.: Trans. N.Y. Acad. Sci. *36*:333–340, 1974.

47. Lemann, Lennon, Piering, et al.: J. Lab. Clin. Med. *75*:578, 1970.

48. Lemann, J. Jr., Piering, W.F., Lennon, E.J.: N. Engl. J. Med. *280*:232–237, 1969.

49. Lindeman, R.D., Adler, S., Yiengst, M.J., et al.: J. Lab. Clin. Med. *70*:236–245, 1967.

50. Cooke, N., Teitelbaum, S., Avioli, L.V.: Arch. Intern. Med. *138*:1007–1009, 1978.

51. Hegsted, M., Linkswiler, H.M.: J. Nutr. *111*:244–251, 1981.

52. Kim, S., Linkswiler, H.M.: J. Nutr. *109–112*: 1399, 1980.

53. Schuette, S.A., Zemel, M.B., Linkswiler, S.M.: J. Nutr. *110*:305–315, 1980.

54. Zemel, M.B., Schuette, S.A., Hegsted, M.: J. Nutr. *111*:545–552, 1981.

55. Allen, L.H., Block, G.D., Wood, R.J.: Fed. Proc. *39*:1043, 1980. (abstract)

56. Hegsted, M., Linkswiler, H.M.: J. Nutr. *111*:120–125, 1981.

57. Pak, C.Y.C.: Am. J. Physiol. *237*:F415–F423, 1979.

58. National Health Survey, Vital and Health Statistic Series 11, No. 202, Pub. (HRA) 77–1647. Washington, D.C., U.S. Dept. HEW PHS, 1977.

59. U.S. Dept. Agriculture: Nationwide Food Consumption Survey, 1977–1978. Report #2, USDA, 1980.

60. U.S. Dept. Agriculture: Household Food Consumption Survey Report #6. Agricultural Res. Sec., 1955.

61. Thomson, P.: Br. J. Nutr. *13*:190–193, 1959.

62. Thomson, P.: Br. J. Nutr. *13*:509–511, 1959.

63. Duggin, G.G., et al.: Lancet *2*:926–927, 1974.

64. Walker, A.R.P.: Lancet *1*:107, 1975.

65. Sterns, M.S.: Physiol. Rev. *19*:415–431, 1939.

66. Nordin, B.E.C., J. Food and Nutr. *42*:67–82, 1986.

67. Food and Agriculture Organization. Rome, Series No. 30, 1962.

68. Hovels, O., Stephan, U.: Ernahrung *2*:178–180, 1961.

69. Atkinson, P.J., West, R.R.: J. Obst. Gyn of Brit. Commonwealth *77*:555–560, 1970.

70. Daniell, H.W.: Arch. Intern. Med. *143*:1678–1682, 1983.

71. Krook, L., Lutwak, L., Whalen, J.P., et al.: Cornell Veterinarian *62*:32–53, 1972.

72. Albanese, A.A., Edelson, A.H., Lorenze, E.J. Jr., et al.: N.Y. State J. Med. *75*:326–336, 1975.

73. Allen L.H.: Am. J. Clin. Nutr. *35*:783–808, 1982.

74. Avioli, L.V.: Fed. Proc. *40*:82–84, 1965.

75. Heaney, R.P., Recker, R.R., Saville, P.D.: J. Lab. Clin. Med. *92*:953–963, 1978.

76. Heaney, R.P., Gallagher, J.C., Johnston, C.C., et al.: Am. J. Clin. Nutr. *36*:986–1013, 1982.

77. Horsman, A., Marshall, D.H., Nordin, B.E.C., et al.: Clin. Sci. *59*:137–145, 1980.

78. Hurxthal, L.M., Vose, G.P.: Calcif. Tissue Res. *4*:245–256, 1969.

79. Riggs, B.L., Kelly, P.J., and Kenney, V.R.: J. Bone Joint Surg. *49A*:915–924, 1967.

80. Seeman, E., Riggs, B.L.: Geriatrics *36*:71–79, 1981.

81. Smith, D.A., Nordin, B.E.: Proc. R. Soc. Med. *57*:868–870, 1964.

82. Smith, D.A., Nordin, B.E.C. Effect of calcium supplements in spinal density in osteoporosis. *In* Bone

and Tooth. (Backwood, Ed.) New York, MacMillan Publishing Co. Inc., 1964.

83. Thallasinos, N.C., Gutteridge, G., Joplin, G.F., et al.: Clin. Sci. *62*:221–224, 1982.
84. Horsman, A., Gallagher, J.C., Simpson, M., et al.: Br. Med. J. *2*:789–792, 1977.
85. Kolars, J.C., Levitt, M.D., Aouji, D.A.G., et al.: N. Engl. J. Med. *310*:1–9, 1984.
86. Ivanovich, P., Fellows, H., Rich, C.: Ann. Intern. Med. *66*:917–923, 1967.
87. Henneman, P.: Fed. Proc. *18*:1093–1095, 1959.
88. McMillan, D.E., Freeman, R.B.: Medicine *44*:485–501, 1965.
89. Hoth, E.J. (editorial): Ann. Intern. Med. *66*:1021–1022, 1967.
90. Jackson, W.P., Dancaster, C.D.: J. Clin. Endocrinol. Metab. *19*:658–682, 1959.
91. Bell, N.H., Gill, J.R. Jr., Bartter, F.C.: Am. J. Med. *36*:500–513, 1964.
92. Sandler, L.M., Winearls, C.G. Fraher, L.J., et al.: Quart. J. Med. *210*:165–180, 1984.
93. Keating, F.R., Jones, J.B., Elveback, L.R., et al.: J. Lab. Clin. Med. *73*:825–834, 1969.
94. Kelly, P.J., Jowsey, J., Riggs, B.L., et al.: J. Lab. Clin. Med. *69*:110–115, 1967.
95. Ditzel, J.: Horm. Metab. Res. *5*:471–472, 1973.
96. Riley, M.S., Schade, D.S., Eaton, R.P.: Metabolism *28*:191–197, 1979.
97. Clarkson, D.R., Blondin, J., Cryer, P.E.: Metabolism *22*:611–616, 1973.
98. Knochel, J.P.: Arch. Intern. Med. *140*:613–615, 1980.
99. Newman, J.H., Neff, T.A., Ziporin: P.N.: N. Engl. J. Med. *296*:1101–1103, 1978.
100. Darsee, J.H., Nutter, D.O.: Ann. Intern. Med. *89*:867–870, 1978.
101. Knochel, J.P., Barcenas, C., Cotton, J.R., et al.: J. Clin. Invest. *62*:1240, 1978.
102. O'Connor, L.R., Wheeler, W.S., Bethune: J.E.: N. Engl. J. Med. *297*:901–903, 1977.
103. Juan, D., Elrazak, M.A.: JAMA *242*:163–164, 1979.
104. Lentz, R.D.: Ann. Intern. Med. *89*:941–944, 1978.
105. Haddad, J.G. Jr., Avioli, L.V.: Endocrinology *87*:1245–1250, 1970.
106. DeLuca, H.F.: Fed. Proc. *32*:2211–2217, 1974.
107. Hughes, M.R., Haussler, M.R., Brumbaugh, D.F., et al.: Science *190*:578–579, 1975.
108. Moon, W.H., Malzer, J.L., Clark, H.E.: J. Am. Diet. Assoc. *64*:386, 1974.
109. Wilkinson, R.: Absorption of calcium, phosphorus and magnesium. *In* "Calcium, Phosphorus and Magnesium Metabolism." Ed. B.E.C. Nordin, 36–113, Churchill-Livingstone, 1976.
110. Guillot, A.P., Hood, V.L., Runge, C.F., et al.: Nephron *30*:114–117, 1982.
111. Street, H.R.: J. Nutr. *24*:111–119, 1942.
112. Cox, G.J., Dodds, M.L., Wigman, H.B., et al.: J. Biol. Chem. *92*:11–12, 1931.
113. Recommended Dietary Allowances: Washington, National Academy of Sciences, 1958.
114. Greger, J.L., Krystofiak, M.: Food Technology, January, 78–84, 1982.
115. Draper, H.H., Sie, T.L., Bergan, J.G.: J. Nutr. *102*:1133–1141, 1972.
116. Krook, R., Lutwak, L., Henrikson, R., et al.: J. Nutr. *101*:233–238, 1971.
117. LaFlamme, G.H., Jowsey, J.: J. Clin. Invest. *51*:2834–2840, 1972.
118. Argenzio, R.A., Lowe, J.E., Hintz, H.F., et al.: J. Nutr. *104*:18–27, 1974.
119. Reiss, E., Canterbury, J.A., Bercovitz, M.A., et al.: J. Clin. Invest. *49*:2146–2149, 1970.
120. Beal, V.A.: J. Am. Diet. Assoc. *53*:450–455, 1968.
121. Lorenz, R., Burr, I.M.: J. Pediatr. *85*:522–525, 1974.
122. Avioli, L.V.,: Am. J. Med. *57*:34–42, 1974.
123. Peden, V.H.: Am. J. Hum. Genet. *12*:323–327, 1960.
124. Parfitt, A.M.: J. Clin. Endocrinol. Metab. *34*:152–158, 1972.
125. Farriaux, J.P.: Am. J. Dis. Child. *130*:780, 1976.

*Chapter* **6**

# MAGNESIUM

## Maurice E. Shils

The first systematic observations on the effects of magnesium deficiency in laboratory animals were performed by McCollum and associates in the early 1930s.[1] The resulting changes in rats were particularly striking and led to the association of magnesium deficiency with neuromuscular abnormalities. Since that time a very large number of species, including man, have been investigated experimentally.[2]

The first description of clinical depletion in man in a small number of patients with various underlying diseases was published in 1934.[3] Flink and associates in the early 1950s documented depletion of this ion in alcoholics and in patients on magnesium-free I.V. solutions and described the clinical consequences of this deficiency.[4a,b] A series of clinical case reports in the early 1960s helped focus attention on the occurrence of hypomagnesemia in various malabsorptive states and stimulated efforts to study magnesium deple-

tion and its consequences under controlled conditions. Increasing numbers of clinical disorders associated with magnesium depletion have been recognized, as have the effects of certain drugs in inducing renal losses of this nutrient. The increasing use in clinical chemistry laboratories of atomic absorption spectrophotometry for magnesium analysis has shown that human depletion occurs more commonly than was previously assumed. Experimental and clinical observations have revealed fascinating interrelations of this ion with other electrolytes, second messengers, hormone receptors, parathyroid hormone secretion and action, vitamin D metabolism, bone function, and other changes that are not unexpected, given the major role that this ion plays in cellular functions in all organs.

## BODY PARTITION

Magnesium is the fourth most abundant cation in the body and is second only to potassium in its intracellular concentration. Like calcium, it undergoes limited intestinal absorption and is stored primarily in bone, with only a small proportion present in extracellular fluid. It is similar to potassium and phosphate as an important intracellular constituent and resembles sodium in its efficient retention by the normal kidney. It is now apparent that a deficiency of magnesium affects the homeostatic control of calcium, potassium, and sodium ions.

The adult human weighing 70 kg contains approximately 20 to 28 g of magnesium, equalling 1667 to 2400 meq (1 meq = 0.5 mmol = 12 mg).[5-7] About 60 to 65% of the total is present in bone, about 27% is in muscle, another 6 to 7% is in other cells, and only about 1% is in extracellular fluid. Muscle, liver, heart, and other soft tissues contain about the same amount (approximately 14 to 20 meq/kg wet weight, i.e., 7 to 10 mmol).[5,7,8-14] Erythrocyte content varies from 4.3 to 6.2 meq/L, depending on the age of the cells and the analytic measurement used.[5] As the red cells age, the magnesium content slowly drops.[9] This age difference possibly explains the increased concentrations of red cell magnesium in certain pathologic conditions associated with shortened erythrocyte survival time such as chronic renal failure, thalassemia, and sickle cell anemia.

Normal serum levels vary somewhat depending on analytic methods. With atomic absorption spectrophotometry, the usual range for neonates, older children, and adults is 1.5 to 2.1 meq/L.[10] Magnesium ion in erythrocytes and plasma exists as free, complexed (with citrate, phosphate, and other ions), and protein-bound forms; in plasma the approximate percentages are 55% free, 13% complexed, and 32% of protein bound. Cerebrospinal fluid magnesium is approximately 2.5 meq/L, with 55% free and the remainder in complexed form.[5] Magnesium in sweat averages 0.6 meq/L in man in a hot environment.[11] Its concentration is relatively small (0.6 to 1.4 meq/L) in saliva and in gastric, biliary, and pancreatic secretions.

Of bone magnesium, 30% is in a surface-limited pool present either within the hydration shell or on the crystal surface. In adult men, the large fraction of bone magnesium does not appear to be associated with bone matrix but, rather, is an integral part of the bone crystal. Both magnesium pools are increased in patients with chronic renal failure.[12] In vitro studies suggest that bone surface magnesium rapidly reflects changes in the serum levels; the deeper pool is probably deposited at the time of bone formation, with mobilization dependent on resorptive processes.

Magnesium as well as calcium forms complexes with phospholipids of various cell membranes (e.g., plasma, endoplasmic, and mitochondrial) and with nucleic acids.[13] Total intracellular magnesium concentration varies from about 6 to 10 mmol/kg wet weight, depending on the tissue, with the exception of the erythrocyte, which has less.[14] Expressed on the basis of water, values are higher (e.g., 16.4 mmol in guinea pig hearts). Measured by 31 phosphorus nuclear magnetic resonance (NMR), the ratio of cytosolic magnesium to total heart magnesium was 0.85.[15a] One example of the distribution of magnesium is reported in the frog muscle cells, where free $Mg^{2+}$* was 0.6 mmol, while ATP Mg was 5.8, phosphocreatine Mg was 1.7, and myosin Mg was 0.3 mmol.[15b] The range often given for free $Mg^{2+}$ in many cells is 0.3 to 0.6 mmol.[14] However, the selection of stability constants for Mg ATP and the conditions for calculation of free $Mg^{2+}$ concentration are critical; Wu et al., for example, have found free $Mg^{2+}$ to be 2.5 to 7 mmol in guinea pig hearts, an amount four times that reported for frog skeletal muscle by 31 P NMR under different conditions.[15c]

## Analytic Procedures

A review of the development of methods for determining total magnesium in biologic fluids, cells and isolates of cells, foods, and other materials has been given by Alcock.[16a] Atomic absorption spectrophotometry is currently the procedure usually employed in clinical chemistry laboratories.[16b] Indirect procedures have been used for estimating free and bound magnesium in living cells.[15,17,18]

Isotopes of magnesium have been used as biologic tracers in analyzing absorption and distribution of this ion. The radioisotope $^{28}$Mg with a short half-life (21.3 hours), first described in 1953, has been used in human subjects. It disappears from the circulation rapidly after injection and is initially concentrated in the soft tissues; however, over 80% of the $^{28}$Mg in the body appears to be in slowly exchanging components.[19] Naturally occurring magnesium contains 78.99 atom percent $^{24}$Mg, 10.0 percent $^{25}$Mg, and 11.01 percent $^{26}$Mg. $^{26}$Mg has been used as a tracer in biomedical research, including absorption studies in man.[20]

## HOMEOSTATIC CONTROLS

The homeostasis of the individual with respect to magnesium balance—as with all mineral substances—is dependent on intake, absorption, and excretion (Fig. 6–1).

---

*Ionized magnesium is referred to as $Mg^{2+}$.

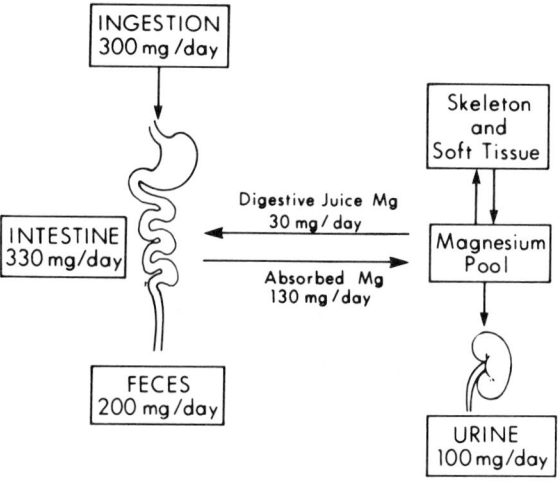

INGESTION
300 mg/day

Skeleton
and
Soft Tissue

Digestive Juice Mg
30 mg/day

INTESTINE
330 mg/day

Magnesium
Pool

Absorbed Mg
130 mg/day

FECES
200 mg/day

URINE
100 mg/day

**Fig. 6–1.** Magnesium homeostasis in man. A schematic representation of its metabolic economy indicating a) its relatively poor absorption from the alimentary tract, b) its distribution into a number of tissue pools with a major distribution into bone, and c) its dependence on the kidney for excretion. Homeostasis depends upon the integrity of intestinal and renal absorptive processes. (From Slatapolsky, E.: Pathophysiology of Calcium, Magnesium and Phosphorus Metabolism in the Kidney and Body Fluids, (Edited by S. Klahr) New York, Plenum Publishing Corp, 1984, with permission.)

## Intake

Magnesium is widely distributed in foods. (See Appendix Table A–25a). Because magnesium is the mineral ion of chlorophyll, green vegetables are an important source. Similarly, ingestion of animal products, legumes, and cereals helps assure a good intake. The daily intake of healthy individuals in the United States and Western Europe has been estimated at between 15 and 40 meq (180 to 480 mg).

As has been noted in the recently published summary of a 1977 United States survey of food consumption, the analytic data for magnesium in foods in this and earlier surveys have been less reliable than those for other nutrients.[21a] With this disclaimer, the 1977–78 Nationwide Food Consumption Survey found that diary products contributed 21% of the nation's magnesium intake; vegetables, 17%; dairy products, 16%; meat, fish, and fowl, 15%; other protein foods, 10%; fruits, 7%; and various beverages and "foods of little nutritional value," 11%.[21a] Magnesium in the United States food supply in 1982 was estimated to be 18% lower than at the beginning of this century, primarily because of decreased consumption of grain products. Intakes in this survey for adult males averaged approximately 310 mg/day, and for adult females, approximately 230 mg/day.

Data on magnesium intake have been collected

on 16 men and 18 women ages 20 to 53. These individuals subsisted on their customary diets. At the beginning and every 3 months over a year, duplicate food and beverage samples, urine, and stools were collected for a period and analyzed. Daily intakes among individuals varied greatly (e.g., from 132 to 350 mg for women, mean 234; and from 157 to 595 mg for males, mean 323 mg).[21b]

## Absorption

Magnesium is absorbed primarily in the small intestine. Perfusion of the jejunum and ileum of normal human subjects indicated that both segments absorb this ion equally well up to concentrations of about 10 mmol; however, the ileal absorption process became saturated above that concentration, while that in the jejunum increased.[22] In these experiments water movement was near zero. In usual enteric conditions, contraction or expansion of luminal volume would tend to increase or decrease luminal magnesium concentration, and absorption would be influenced significantly by water movement (i.e., solvent drag).[23]

Individuals subsisting for 4 to 8 weeks on a high-calcium diet (1900 mg/day) had significantly less absorption in the ileum (but not the jejunum) of a standard amount of magnesium perfused in a 30-cm segment compared to the same subjects previously maintained on a low-calcium intake (200 mg/day)[24]; however, the intersubject variations were great. Furthermore, as is discussed in the section on human requirements, many metabolic balance studies suggest that calcium in a fairly broad range of intake has relatively little influence on magnesium absorption, although there are some conflicting claims about calcium as well as phosphate.[2,25,26]

Comparison of intestinal transport of magnesium has been made in normal children and in a child with the rare, genetically determined disorder designated as primary (or idiopathic) hypomagnesemia.[27] The data suggest that two separate transport systems participate in the absorption of this ion from the proximal small intestine. One appears to be a carrier-mediated system that saturates at low intraluminal concentrations (2 and 4 meq/L); this system appears to be defective in primary hypomagnesemia. The other system appears to be that of simple diffusion and occurs at higher concentrations—for example, 20 meq/L.

Overall, magnesium is not absorbed efficiently. Data from earlier studies averaged from 50[28] to 60 or 70%[5,29] on usual diets. More recent studies indicate a greater range. For example, with a magnesium intake of 189 to 342 mg/day, healthy adult males excreted 35 to 68% in stool on a diet containing 200 mg of calcium/day.[26a] In free-living adults evaluated periodically over the course of a year, absorption averaged 21% for males and 27% for females[21b] (Table 6–1, study 8). In other metabolic studies, the average absorption was appreciably higher; in most of these studies the diet was not self-selected (Table 6–1).

When [28]Mg was used as a tracer, the absorption varied from 75% on a very low intake (23 mg/day) to 44.3% on a more usual intake (240 mg/day) and to only 23.7% on a very high daily intake (1764 mg/day).[28] In studies in which subjects were fed [26]Mg incorporated into leafy vegetables, absorption varied from 39 to 50% in adult males in diets containing 331 to 447 mg of magnesium/day.[20b] The absorption of the labeled greens varied between 57.5 and 62%.

Much literature accumulated over four or so decades reports the effects of the interactions of various nutrients and magnesium on magnesium's absorption, requirement, and overall balance. Reports have been contradictory concerning the effect of dietary calcium and phosphate on magnesium absorption in various species.[2,25] Spencer et al. have briefly reviewed some of the human data, which are also conflicting.[26a–26c] Many of these studies were performed before precise methods for determining magnesium were available; this imprecision was particularly true of methods in which magnesium was analyzed in the presence of significant amounts of calcium and phosphate (e.g., in fecal specimens or certain foods). It was not until the mid and late 1960s that measurement by atomic absorption spectrophotometry began to be used widely. Another issue involves the duration of human feeding experiments. Spencer et al. have pointed out that the transition period required for equilibrium to be established following changes in calcium or magnesium intake ranges from 6 to 18 days, depending on the individual.[26b] Hence, absorption studies require a significant adaptation period before valid data can be collected.

Spencer et al. conducted many studies in healthy adults under rigorous metabolic ward conditions showing long-term adaptation to specific diets of various compositions. On an average, with usual magnesium intakes absorption was 50% (Table 6–1).[26b,c] The percentages of absorption did not change when the daily calcium intake was increased from 200 to 800 to 2000 mg. Regardless of calcium intake, an increase of magnesium in the basal diet (251 to 342 mg/day) by about 575 mg as MgO reduced absorption from

about 50% to 35% with some increase in net absorption.[26b]

Increasing the daily phosphate content of the basal diet from 800 mg to 2000 mg (as glycerophosphate) did not affect the absorption of magnesium on a 250-mg/day diet, regardless of calcium intake; however, on a magnesium intake of 850 mg (increased with MgO), the higher phosphate intake was associated with a drop in absorption from about 55% to 40%.[26d]

**Vitamin D and Magnesium Absorption.** In contrast to the demonstrated effect of vitamin D and its active metabolites on improving the reabsorption of calcium and phosphate in the intestine, the influence of vitamin D on magnesium absorption is uncertain because of contradictory evidence. The magnesium–vitamin D relationship involves two factors, one having to do with eumagnesemic individuals, the other with hypomagnesemic individuals. (The latter aspect is discussed in the section on Clinical Interrelations.) 1-α-OH vitamin D did not increase magnesium absorption in short-term studies in animals or in balance studies in several patients with chronic renal failure despite increases in calcium retention.[33] Moderate amounts of vitamin D given to patients with various disorders of calcium metabolism and/or bone disease had only a small incremental effect on magnesium absorption.[34] Significant absorption of this ion (and phosphate) has been noted in individuals having no detectable plasma $1,25(OH)_2$ vitamin D (calcitriol).[35] There was no significant correlation between plasma levels of calcitriol and magnesium absorption.[34,35] Despite a claim that 1-α-OH vitamin D was associated with a major rise in serum magnesium, this report shows that the rise was associated with an intake of magnesium antacids; when these were eliminated, serum magnesium fell despite continuation of the vitamin D metabolite.[36]

Conversely, the claim has been made that a supplement of calcitriol (2 μg/day for 1 week) to healthy subjects resulted in a significant increase in absorption of magnesium in the jejunal segment, but not in the ileal segment as measured by steady-state perfusion studies in 30-cm segments.[37] Calcium absorption improved in both jejunal and ileal segments with calcitriol. The markedly lower basal absorption in the jejunal segment in this study is not in accord with other data from the same laboratory, which indicate that the absorption rate of magnesium at the same 5-mmol concentration is very similar in jejunal and ileal segments in healthy individuals.[22,24] In a similar experiment with patients with chronic renal disease, 2 μg calcitriol resulted in a significant in-

**Table 6–1.  Summary of Recent Magnesium Balance Studies**

| Study No. | Subjects N | Sex | Age (yrs) | FL/MU | Adaptation Period (d) | Collection Period (d) | Diet Magnesium (mg) Total/d | /per kg | Balance (mg) | Absorption Percent | Ref |
|---|---|---|---|---|---|---|---|---|---|---|---|
| 1) | 14 | F | 12½–14½ | FL* | 6 | 18 | 190±26[a] | — | −1.8±2.2 | 50 | 30a |
|  |  |  |  |  |  |  | 95±29[b] |  | −6.8±10.4 | 43 |  |
|  |  |  |  |  |  |  | 95±29[c] |  | −5.6±16.5 | 47 |  |
| 2) | 12 | M | 37–38 | FL* | 19 | 7 | 356±10[d] | — | 28±17 | 40 | 31a |
|  |  |  |  |  |  |  | 322±12[e] |  | 32±10 | 29 |  |
| 3) | 7 | F | 20–39 | FL* | 5 | 25 | 276[f] | 4.5 | 14±24 | 58 | 31b |
|  |  |  |  |  |  |  | 300[g] |  | −15±16 | 52 |  |
| 4) | 10 | M | 50–67 | MU‡ | 14 | 40 | 263±17 (Ca = 220 mg) | 4.6 | −16±12.5 | 48.5 | 26a |
| 5) | 15 | M | — | MU‡ | ? | ? | 250 (Ca = 210 mg) |  | 44 | 55 | 26b |
|  | 12 | M | — |  |  |  | 250 (Ca = 1270 mg) |  | 40 | 54 |  |
| 6) | 8 | M | 22–29 | FL* | 6 | 12 | 371 |  | −10±13 | 40 | 30b |
| 7) | 10 | M | 19–64 | MU‡ | 16 | 12 | 229±24[h] | 3.0 | 13±30 | 52 | 32 |
|  |  |  |  |  |  |  | 258±24[i] | 3.4 | 17±36 | 53 |  |
| 8) | 16 | M | 20–53 | FL† | + + | 7 | 323 | — | −32 | 21 | 21b |
|  | 18 | F | 20–53 | FL† |  | 7 | 234 | — | −25 | 27 |  |

FL* = free living with controlled diets
FL† = free living with self-selected diets over one year
MU‡ = on metabolic unit with controlled diets
a = control diet with meat; added zinc
b = soy replacing 30% meat; extra zinc
c = b− no extra zinc
d = low fiber diet
e = high fiber diet
f = control diet
g = added cellulose
h = protein at 65 g/d
i = protein at 94 g/d
+ + = subjects on study one year; diets, stool, urine collected for 7 days quarterly
　　7/11 males in equilibrium or positive balance
　　6/18 females in equilibrium or positive balance

crease in magnesium absorption, but this increase was appreciably less than the increase noted for calcium absorption.[38] Further support for the concept that magnesium and calcium have different intestinal transport processes is the observation that patients with absorptive hypercalciuria with increased calcium absorption have normal magnesium absorption.[22]

Intestinal absorption of magnesium is reduced in a variety of malabsorption syndromes, in particular those associated with steatorrhea (Table 6–2). Chronic renal disease of varying severity has been reported to either reduce intestinal absorption of this ion to a major degree,[22,26c,38] or have little or no effect.[39,40]

### Renal Regulation

Absorbed magnesium is retained either for tissue growth (including bone growth) or for turnover replacement; the remainder is excreted in the urine (Fig. 6–1). Following glomerular filtration, tubular reabsorptive processes are the key to magnesium homeostasis. Micropuncture and in vitro microperfusion studies in the rat, rabbit, and dog have revealed information on magnesium reabsorption along the nephron.[41] Although claims have been made for a secretory process,[42] it seems

that secretion, if it actually occurs, must be a minor factor.[41,43]

Of serum magnesium, 80% is ultrafilterable. In the proximal convoluted tubule, the magnesium concentration in the tubular fluid was increased to about 1.5 times that of the plasma ultrafiltrate (TF/UF = 1.5) because of the relatively low permeability of magnesium in this segment.[44] This increase was in marked contrast to sodium and calcium. *Hyper*magnesemia reduced fractional reabsorption to a modest degree as the result of its osmotic inhibitory effect on net sodium and water reabsorption.[45a] With *hypo*magnesemia, filtered load and luminal concentration decreased with a major reduction in net absorption but with the fractional reabsorption remaining normal.[45b]

As magnesium progressed into the descending limb of the loop of Henle (LH), its concentration became greater than that of other ions (TF/UF = 3 to 4). The thick ascending limb (TAL) of the loop was the major site of magnesium reabsorption and the major site of control of excretion. Of filtered magnesium, 50 to 60% was resorbed between the thin descending limb and the early distal tubule (DT) (Fig. 6–2).[41,44]

When the *intraluminal* concentration of mag-

### Table 6–2. Clinical Conditions Associated with Magnesium Depletion

Gastrointestinal Disorders
  Malabsorption
    Inflammatory bowel disease
    Gluten enteropathy; sprue
    Intestinal fistulas or bypass
    Ileal dysfunction with steatorrhea
    Immune diseases with villous atrophy
    Short-bowel syndrome
    Radiation enteritis

Renal Tubular Dysfunction
  Metabolic—See Table 6–3
  Hormonal—See Table 6–3
  Drugs—See Table 6–3

Endocrine Disorders (See Table 6–3)
  Hyperaldosteronism
  Hyperparathyroidism with hypercalcemia
  Postparathyroidectomy period
  Hyperthyroidism

Genetic and Familial Disorders
  Primary idiopathic hypomagnesemia
  Renal wasting syndromes
  Bartter's syndrome
  Infants born of diabetic or hyperparathyroid
    mothers

Inadequate Intake or Provision of Magnesium
  Alcoholism
  Protein-calorie malnutrition (usually with infection)
  Prolonged infusion of magnesium-low nutrient
    solutions
  Hypercatabolic states (burns, trauma)
  Excessive lactation

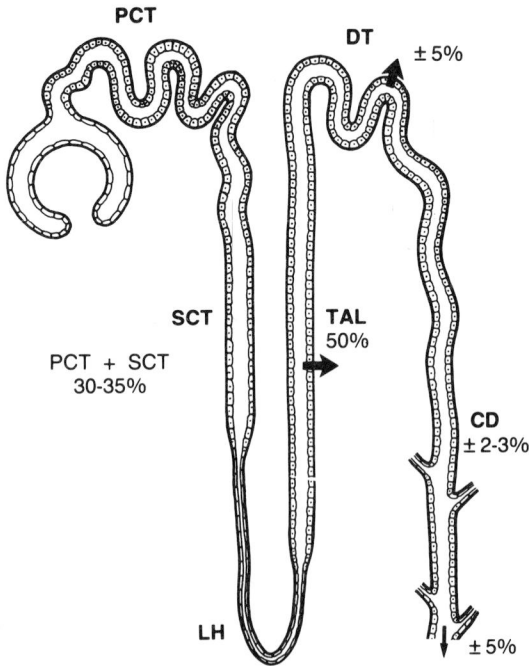

**Fig. 6–2.** Magnesium reabsorption in various segments of the nephron. While a significant proportion of filtered magnesium is reabsorbed in the convoluted tubule (CT), the major site of reabsorption is the thick ascending limb of the loop of Henle. Reabsorption is influenced by various metabolic, hormonal, and drug factors. PCT is partial convoluted tubule; SCT is straight convoluted tubule.

nesium was elevated progressively, this segment absorbed more, maintaining a fractional reabsorption rate of 80% of the delivered load.[45a] On the other hand, when the *plasma* magnesium was raised by I.V. infusion of magnesium salts, the reabsorption ability of this segment was progressively blunted, presumably because of raised peritubular capillary magnesium concentrations; hence, as plasma magnesium rose, increasing amounts of this ion entered the urine. In addition, as plasma magnesium levels increased, resorption of calcium declined but that of sodium remained normal until the magnesium concentration was very high.

In magnesium-depleted rats the reabsorption in the loop of Henle was more complete than it was in normally fed animals; by the time the urine reached the early distal tubule, concentrations were very low (TF/UF = 0.4).[41,45b] The amount reabsorbed by this time was more than 95% of the amount filtered, and fractional excretion was approximately 3%, as compared to the normal 15%. With rapid I.V. magnesium repletion, there appeared to be some delay in the ability of the loop of Henle to reabsorb magnesium as efficiently as expected; it was suggested that this inability might reflect a mild cellular dysfunction secondary to the preceding depletion. Whether this observation holds for less severe depletion is not known. In deficient human beings who were repleted with moderate amounts of intramuscular or oral magnesium, the kidney retained magnesium tenaciously until significant amounts had been given and the serum level rose to an apparent threshold level.[46,47]

The distal convoluted tubule was found to have a limited reabsorptive ability (<5% of the filtered load) while the collecting tubules and collecting ducts (CD) normally absorbed little (Fig. 6–2).[45b]

Studies of renal reabsorption of magnesium in dogs suggested a maximal transport rate (Tm) for this ion.[48] Observations of segmental reabsorption by micropuncture technique in dogs who underwent thyroparathyroidectomy (TPTX) indicated increased reabsorption of filtered magnesium up to 3.5 meq/L of plasma magnesium.[49] While these data fitted the pattern characteristic of a Tm, the segmental studies also revealed that the urinary excretory pattern was a summation of the distinct transport properties of the proximal tubule and the loop of Henle,[49] so that a true Tm is not operative. However, the summation results in an *apparent* Tm of 1.25 to 1.30 meq/L of serum in my experience.

**Metabolic and Drug Influences on Renal Regulation.** Magnesium reabsorption in the nephron is influenced by a number of physiologic and metabolic factors as well as by drugs and disease states (Table 6–3). Of particular clinical significance with respect to renal losses are the loop diuretics such as furosemide and ethacrynic acid and nephrotoxic drugs. Relatively short term use of thiazide diuretics causes relatively little or no effect on magnesium status[41]; reports on the effect of long-term ingestion are conflicting.[56a–56d] Hypomagnesemia is likely to occur in a setting of poor dietary intake and hypokalemia associated with concomitant usage of diuretics and other drugs for patients with heart failure, cirrhosis, hypertension, and other fluid-retaining states (see Disease State and Magnesium Correlates). The diuretics triamterene and amiloride exert a magnesium-sparing effect, as they do for potassium.[68]

The persistent long-term renal wasting secondary to the cancer chemotherapeutic drug cisplatin is of particular concern in affected patients, as are

**Table 6–3. Metabolic, Hormonal, and Drug Influences on Magnesium Excretion**

*Increased Excretion*
Hypermagnesemia*
Hypercalciuria[41,45a]
Hyperaldosteronism[50]
Hyperparathyroidism†[51]
Familial renal wasting syndromes
  Primary,[52a,b,d] Bartter's, and related
    syndromes[52c;207–209]
Potassium depletion[53]
Alcoholism[4,54]
Increased extracellular fluid volume[41]
Phosphate depletion[64]
Diuresis
  Osmotic (diabetes, glucose, mannitol)[55,65c]
  Postrenal obstruction[57]
  Postrenal transplantation[57]
Nephrotoxic drugs
  Amphotericin[58]; cisplatin[59–61]
  Aminoglycosides[62]; cyclosporin[63]
Acidosis
  Fasting[65a]; ketoacidosis[65b]; NH$_4$Cl[65c]
Mineralocorticosids‡[67]
Hyperthyroidism[66]

*Decreased Excretion*
Hypomagnesemia[41,46,47,73,74]
Parathyroid hormone[51,71]
Hypocalcemia[67]
Alkalosis[65d,75]
Hypothyroidism[72]
Contracted extracellular fluid volume[41]
Antidiuretic hormone[70]
Calcitonin[67,70]
Glucagon[70]
K$^+$, Mg$^{2+}$ sparing diuretics[68]

*When associated with magnesium infusion/injection
†Secondary to hypercalcemia; transient negative balance
‡Secondary to increased extracellular fluid volume

the similar effects of the antibiotics amphotericin B, ticarcillin, carbenicillin, and gentamicin. The renal tubular effects of cisplatin may develop rapidly with serious losses; furthermore, renal wasting may persist for many months after the drug is discontinued.

A number of hormones affect magnesium absorption by the kidney (Table 6–2); the effects of most are usually minimal and may be indirect. Calcitonin can reduce magnesium excretion by increasing loop reabsorption provided there is a fall in absolute plasma calcium.[67] Mineralocorticoids cause urinary magnesium excretion largely through extracellular volume expansion. Excess parathyroid hormone (PTH) may result in increased urinary excretion, as has been documented frequently in primary hyperparathyroidism.[51] The resulting hypercalcemia in the intact organism may in itself inhibit tubular reabsorption of magnesium. Control of calcium levels by acute TPTX in rats indicated that cyclic AMP had no effect.[69,70] Similarly, in perfusion studies of the loop of Henle in magnesium-deficient TPTX rats, PTH did not overcome the defect in absorption associated with deficiency.[71] Chronic (12-day) I.V. infusion of b (1-34) PTH into normal human subjects resulted in the expected hypercalcemia, hypercalciuria, and negative calcium balance. Plasma magnesium, however, did not change. Hypermagnesuria (30% above that of controls) occurred but negative magnesium balance was transient because of an increase in intestinal magnesium absorption.[51] In TPTX Brattleboro rats infused with somatostatin, both PTH and glucagon increased fractional reabsorption of magnesium, primarily in the loop of Henle, as did ADH and calcitonin. There was some increase also in the distal tubule.[70]

Thyroid-deficient rats conserved magnesium much more efficiently than did euthyroid or hyperthyroid animals; however, the thyroid-deficient rats had sodium and calcium wasting. Prior administration of thyroid hormone to thyroid-deficient or euthyroid rats was without effect.[72]

When magnesium intake is severely restricted in human subjects with normal kidney function, output becomes very small in a matter of days (Fig. 6–3).[47,73] Supplementing normal intake increases urinary excretion without altering normal serum levels, providing renal function is normal and the amounts given are not excessive.[74] The intestinal and renal conservation and excretory mechanisms in normal individuals permit homeostasis over a wide range of intake of dietary magnesium. Unlike with sodium, there does not appear to be a hormonal homeostatic mechanism for regulating serum magnesium. The normal range

is the result of a balance between the gastrointestinal and renal absorption and the excretion processes reviewed above.

## REQUIREMENTS FOR HEALTHY INDIVIDUALS

A large number of balance studies have been performed over the years in an effort to obtain quantitative data on magnesium requirements.[21b,26b–d,29a,29b] Much of the older data is unreliable because of analytic and procedural problems, as noted earlier. Spencer et al. have pointed out that, of the 22 balance studies cited by Seelig, only 4 had been carried out longer than 15 days in any individual and only 2 had been performed in adults maintaining a constant dietary intake in a hospital metabolic ward.[26a,29a]

Table 6–1 summarizes balance data in some recent studies, including observations on the possible influences of varying intake of protein, soy protein, fiber, and calcium. Results of studies on the effects of varying the levels of calcium or phosphate, protein or fiber on magnesium balance are contradictory.[21b,26b–d]

The variance in the reports of magnesium needs based on classic balance studies is noteworthy. The fact that clinically significant hypomagnesemia is uncommon and the lack of verified reports of symptomatic magnesium deficiency in a healthy population raise the question about the reliability of the current recommended dietary allowances (RDA) for magnesium.

The RDA for magnesium are given in Appendix Table A–1b. They are based on consumption data, old balance studies, and human milk content. These allowances recommended 40 to 70 mg/day for infants, rising to 250 mg/day as children mature to 10 years. Adolescent and adult males and nonpregnant and nonlactating females have recommendations in the range of 300 to 400 mg (5 to 6 mg/kg and 14 to 15 mg/100 kcal of recommended energy intake), with 450 mg during pregnancy and lactation.

The figures for male and female adolescents and adults are 5 to 6 mg/kg and 14 to 15 mg/100 kcal of recommended energy intake. Utilizing the data of Spencer et al., which indicate that equilibrium or positive balance is attained on 200 mg of magnesium/day,[26a–c] and assuming that average adult male weights and expenditures were 65 kg and 2000 kcal, respectively, the need for magnesium is about 3.1 mg/kg or 10 mg/100 kcal. Such data suggest a very large "safety" factor for stable adults in the RDA.

The RDA may be inadequate for those with serious intestinal and renal absorptive defects and for patients being nutritionally repleted after a se-

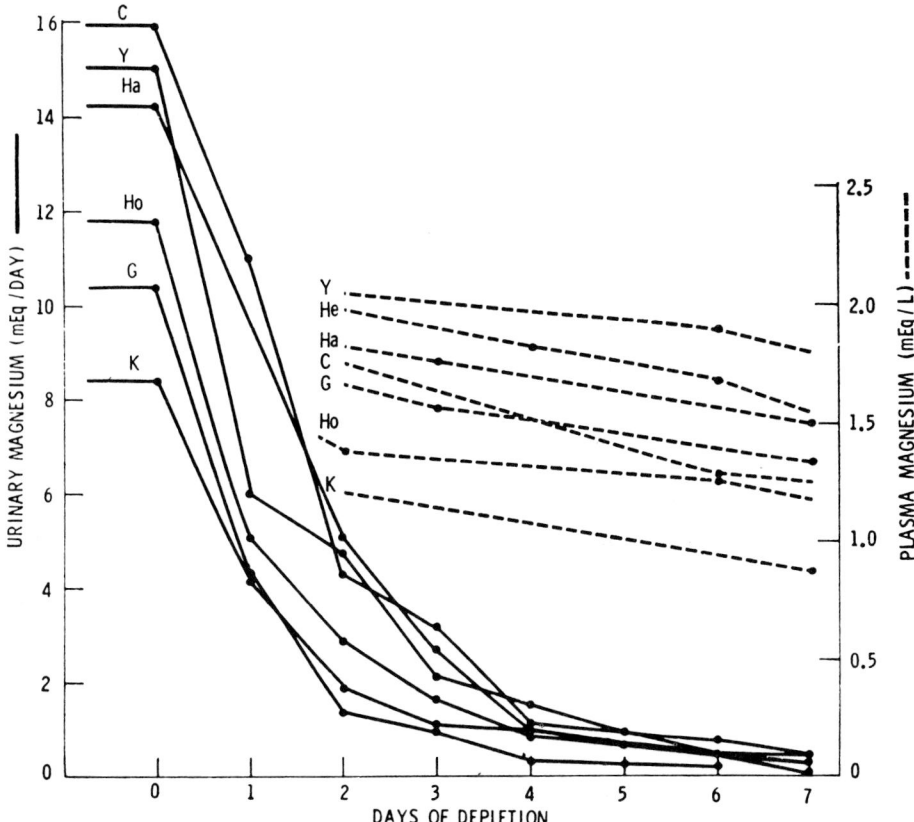

**Fig. 6–3.** Plasma and urine magnesium in the week following omission of magnesium from the diet. The rapid decrease in excretion is depicted for 6 subjects. By the tenth day, all plasma values except that of Y were more than 2 standard deviations below the normal mean for the method used. (From Shils, M.E.,[47] with permission.)

rious hypercatabolic disease; such patients need careful serial analyses of serum, stool, and urine magnesium to permit adequate replacement.

Based on the 1980 RDA for magnesium, 25% of those surveyed in 1977–78 Nationwide Food Consumption Survey had intakes equal to or greater than the RDA. Among children 8 years of age or younger, 89% achieved the RDA levels. Mean intake was 83% of RDA.[21a] As noted earlier, however, analytic data for magnesium in foods are not considered highly reliable.

The currently "suppressed" 1985 report of The National Research Council Food and Nutrition Board Committee on the RDA tentatively recommended that the RDA for magnesium be made "provisional"; most of the 1980 figures were retained with this proviso but allowances for infants were reduced somewhat (i.e., from 50 to 70 mg/day to 30 to 50 mg/day), and extra amounts for pregnancy and lactation were reduced from 150 mg/day to 20 mg/day during pregnancy and to 60 mg/day during lactation.[76] This position is of interest in view of the recent statement of the Food and Nutrition Board of the National Research Council/National Academy of Science (NCR/NAS) which asks, "Since few studies have been devoted exclusively to magnesium requirements and the reliability of many of the resultant data is questionable, should there be an RDA or should only a provisional intake be established for magnesium," and "Since there is no apparent evidence of magnesium deficiency in the general population, are data on the magnesium content of the average diet reliable enough to justify lowering the RDA?"[77]

The need for more quantitative data on various age groups using adequate analytic and more precise and prolonged balance techniques under strictly controlled conditions in conjunction with bone biopsy analyses is obvious.

## SOME BIOCHEMICAL AND PHYSIOLOGIC FUNCTIONS

Merely to list some of the reactions and functions of this divalent cation is to emphasize its importance. Magnesium plays a key role as an essential prosthetic group in at least 300 enzymatic reactions in intermediary metabolism.

These enzymes include those involved in (1) hydrolysis and transfer of phosphate groups (phosphokinases); for example, magnesium is involved in the phosphorylation of glucose in glucose's anaerobic metabolism and in its oxidative decarboxylations in the citric acid cycle requiring thiamin pyrophosphate, (2) initiation by thiokinases of fatty acid degradation; (3) activities of alkaline phosphatase and of pyrophosphatase; (4) activation of amino acids, protein synthesis through magnesium's action on ribosomal aggregation, and its role in binding messenger RNA to 70S ribosomes; (5) the synthesis and degradation of DNA; (6) contractibility of cardiac and smooth muscles per se and magnesium's relation to calcium ion transport and utilization; and (7) the adenylate cyclase system. Some of these reactions are noted here. These and others are reviewed in some detail elsewhere.[78–86]

The activation of enzymes by magnesium is thought to occur according to the following mechanisms as stated by Ebel and Gunther.[13]:

1.  $Mg + S \rightleftharpoons MgS$
    $MgS + E \rightleftharpoons MgES \rightleftharpoons MgP + E$

Where E = enzyme, S = substrate, P = reaction product

In this sequence, magnesium is reacting with the substrate. It reduces the high negative charge of the substrate which is normally $ATP^{4-}$. As a consequence, MgS, as the true substrate, reacts with the enzyme. This type of reaction also occurs with hexokinase and phosphoglycerate kinase.

2.  $Mg + E \rightleftharpoons MgE$
    $MgE + S \rightleftharpoons MgSE \rightleftharpoons MgE + P$

In this reaction sequence, magnesium first reacts with the enzyme. A conformational change of the enzyme follows resulting in the enzyme's activation. Thereafter, the substrate is bound to the enzyme. Results of this type of reaction include enolase, pyruvate kinase, and pyrophosphatase. The binding of S to MgE can also be accomplished with participation of magnesium. In both types of reaction, magnesium facilitates the reaction by polarization. Also, a combination of both types of reaction is possible. Another effect of magnesium is to change the equilibrium of a reaction; this change occurs when magnesium forms complexes with the substrate and the reaction product, which have different stabilities; alternatively, the free substrate and its magnesium complex may have different affinities for the enzyme.

A role for magnesium was noted in the formation of adenyl cyclase when cyclic adenosine monophosphate (cAMP) was identified as the "second messenger" for glucagon and epinephrine in the liver. Subsequent research has revealed that numerous other hormones in various tissues are mediated by cAMP.[87,88] Various pharmacologic agents including hormones function through cAMP by either increasing or decreasing its production.

Cyclic AMP is now known to be part of a cascade—the adenylate cyclase system. The membrane-bound enzyme system is composed of a number of interdependent functional components (Fig. 6–4). These include cell-surface specific hormone receptors—either stimulatory (e.g., the beta adrenergic receptor for catecholamines) or inhibitory (e.g., alpha$_2$ adrenergic agonists); stimulatory or inhibitory guanine nucleotide proteins ("G proteins"); a catalytic site for the conversion of magnesium ATP to cAMP (the latter two are located at the intracellular membrane surface); and a regulatory site for divalent cations such as $Mg^{2+}$.[89]

Free $Mg^{2+}$ (in excess of substrate ATP) enhanced enzyme catalytic activity in hormone-adenylate cyclate systems.[90–92] In one study the divalent cations $Mg^{2+}$, $Mn^{2+}$, and $Ca^{2+}$ caused a fivefold increase in the binding of a proterenol compound to the beta adrenergic receptors in frog erythrocyte membranes; $Mg^{2+}$ was the most potent ion at 0.4 mm. $Mg^{2+}$ caused a fivefold increase in the binding of PGE$_1$ to prostaglandin receptors[91] and appeared to participate in the formation of a

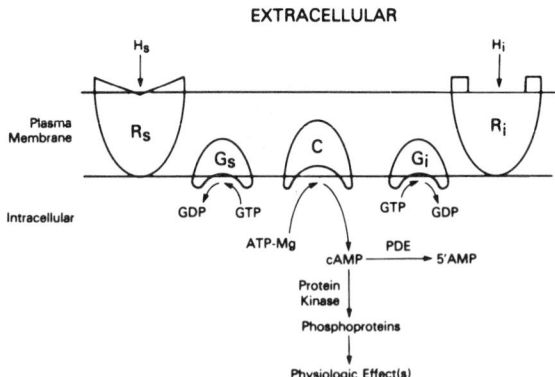

**Fig. 6–4.** Schematic outline of the adenylate cyclase–cyclic AMP system that involves magnesium. The adenylate cyclase system is a membrane-bound enzyme complex found in virtually every cell; it seems to modulate cAMP through a wide variety of hormones and metabolic agents. Magnesium plays a key role as indicated. H$_s$ and H$_i$ denote stimulatory and inhibitory agents, respectively; R$_s$ and R$_i$ stimulatory and inhibitory receptors; and G$_s$ and G$_i$, the stimulatory and inhibitory guanine nucleotide-binding proteins. C denotes the catalytic unit of adenylate cyclase; PDE indicates phosphodiesterase; cAMP indicates cyclic AMP. (From Speigel, et al.[89] Reprinted, by permission of the New England Journal of Medicine *312*:26–33, 1985.)

high-affinity complex between agonist and adenylate-coupled receptors, with resultant catalytic activity. Subsequent work has extended the role of free $Mg^{2+}$, particularly in a number of hormone-receptor adenylate cyclase–coupled receptor systems.[93,94]

In addition to the roles of Mg ATP and of free $Mg^{2+}$ with the receptor-cyclase complex, there is evidence of hormonal transport of $Mg^{2+}$ across the plasma membrane. This inhibition is not mediated by cyclic AMP but rather appears to be a property of the complex or of a possible $Mg^{2+}$ transport protein associated with the hormone receptor.[92] It has been further suggested that $Mg^{2+}$ may serve as an intracellular messenger for integration of opposing physiologic signals.[92]

**Effects on Muscle.** The concentration of myoplasmic free $Ca^{++}$ ions regulates contractile activity in vertebrate skeletal and cardiac muscle by binding to $Ca^{2+}$-specific sites on troponin as well as to paralbumins, myosin, and calmodulin. Some of these sites have a high affinity for $Ca^{2+}$ and bind $Mg^{2+}$ competitively ($Ca^{2+}$-$Mg^{2+}$ sites); the other sites have a lower affinity for $Ca^{2+}$ and are essentially specific for $Mg^{2+}$ with a rapid off rate. The $Ca^{2+}$-$Mg^{2+}$ sites appear not to be directly involved in the rapid switching mechanisms.[95]

The sarcoplasmic reticulum of muscle cells has an ATP-driven calcium pump, and the $Ca^{2+}$ transport system depends on $Mg^{2+}$ as well as $Ca^{2+}$. At a given $Ca^{2+}$ concentration, increasing the $Mg^{2+}$ enhances both $Ca^{2+}$ transport and $Ca^{2+}$-stimulated ATP cleavage. $Mg^{2+}$ enters the reaction chain chelated with ATP when the system operates as an ATP-driven $Ca^{2+}$ pump; it is a component of the ADP-sensitive phosphoprotein species involved in the ATP-ADP exchange reaction. In the reverse mode when the system operates as a $Ca^{2+}$ efflux-driven ATP synthetase, $Mg^{2+}$ together with inorganic phosphate rapidly forms the initial phosphorylated intermediate.[96]

Actin and myosin filaments of cardiac muscle attach by cross-bridges containing myofibrillar ATPase activity. Hydrolysis of magnesium ATP by this enzyme yields energy for the contractile process. The relations of $Mg^{2+}$, $Ca^{2+}$, $K^+$, $Na^+$, and cardiac contractile proteins have been reviewed,[80,99] as has the action of $Mg^{2+}$ in cardiac functions among various species.[80]

The $Mg^{2+}$-$Ca^{2+}$ interactions of skeletal muscle pertain also to smooth muscle (e.g., uterine and vascular).[97] The concentrations of free $Mg^{2+}$ and $Ca^{2+}$ in the extracellular fluid have pronounced effects on the activity of vascular smooth muscle. In general, increased $Mg^{2+}$ concentration or decreased $Ca^{2+}$ concentration caused relaxation, whereas increased $Ca^{2+}$ concentration or decreased $Mg^{2+}$ concentration caused vasoconstriction.[84,98a,98b] Increasing the levels of extracellular $Mg^{2+}$ (i.e., > 1.2 mmol) was reported in many species to depress the reactivity of isolated and perfused blood vessels to certain contractile agonists (i.e., $K^+$, ouabain, and certain neurohumoral agents); conversely, removal of $Mg^{2+}$ enhances reactivity of arterial, arteriolar, and venous vessels to several hormonal agents (catecholamines, angiotensin, acetylcholine, and serotonin). In these studies, magnesium was either very low, normal, or high. No other divalent cation acted as substitute for $Mg^{2+}$ in its effects on these smooth muscles' reactivity reactions and on the uptake and distribution of cellular $Ca^{2+}$.[98b]

Contradictory evidence has been obtained by in vitro measurements of the tone of perfused cattle coronary arteries when exposed to varying concentrations of $Mg^{2+}$.[99] It was concluded that $Mg^{2+}$ concentration must be very low (0.2 mm or less) to induce even moderate tone increases in the vessels or to sensitize them to agonists such as potassium or 5-hydroxytryptamine; there was no increase in response to acetylcholine and norepinephrine.

Seelig et al. studied the $Mg^{2+}$ relaxation effects on cerebral arteriolar smooth muscle in vivo in cats. They found that the dilator effect of an eightfold increase in cerebrospinal fluid (CSF) $Mg^{2+}$ (from 1.2 to 9.6 meq/L) was modest (i.e., 15 to 20%).[84] The authors pointed out that the blood-brain barrier is relatively impermeable to $Mg^{2+}$ and CSF $Mg^{2+}$ is closely regulated.

## Magnesium, Calcium, and Parathyroid Hormone (PTH) Interactions

While the concentration of extracellular $Ca^{2+}$ is the principal physiologic regulator of PTH secretion,[100] for two decades it has been recognized that, when $Mg^{2+}$ is present in increased concentrations, it uniformly suppresses PTH release both in vivo and in vitro.[101,102] However, reports differ as to the relative effectiveness of extracellular $Ca^{2+}$ and $Mg^{2+}$ as inhibitors of PTH secretion. In vitro studies utilizing bovine parathyroid gland cultures indicated equimolar potency while varying the concentration of each in opposite directions and while maintaining the total equivalent ion concentration. There was an exception; at very low $Mg^{2+}$ concentration, PTH secretion fell.[103] On the other hand, in vitro studies have indicated that $Ca^{2+}$ was approximately $2\frac{1}{2}$ to 3 times more potent than $Mg^{2+}$ on a molar basis[101,104]; an exception was noted when $Ca^{2+}$ was very low, at which time $Mg^{2+}$ was markedly less effective on the 3:1 basis.[101,106] In vivo studies in calves also indicated that $Ca^{2+}$ was 2 to 3 times more effective than $Mg^{2+}$.[105]

The influence of variations in the extracellular concentrations of $Ca^{2+}$ and $Mg^{2+}$ on the cytosolic $Ca^{2+}$ concentration in dispersed bovine parathyroid cells was determined in relation to PTH secretion[102]; the cytosolic $Ca^{2+}$ was measured using a $Ca^{2+}$-sensitive fluorescent dye taken up intracellularly. As expected, raising either extracellular $Ca^{2+}$ or $Mg^{2+}$ suppressed hormone production. The noteworthy finding was that an increase of either of these two ions was associated with an increase in cytosolic $Ca^{2+}$. This intracellular free $Ca^{2+}$ increase correlated inversely with the PTH production.[102] These studies, together with previous studies, implicate cytosolic $Ca^{2+}$ as an intracellular mediator of hormonal secretion in parathyroid cells; that is, cytosolic $Ca^{2+}$ may act as a second messenger mediating the effect of extracellular $Ca^{2+}$, $Mg^{2+}$, and other divalent cations. Hence, these ions do not act independently.[102]

Cyclic AMP mediates the response of the parathyroid gland to various agonists (e.g., dopamine, catecholamines, prostaglandins, and polypeptide hormones) as well as to divalent cations. PTH secretion and cAMP production are influenced by $Ca^{2+}$ and $Mg^{2+}$ concentrations.[106] The action of adenylate cyclase (derived from rat parathyroid membranes) was inhibited directly by $Ca^{2+}$ and stimulated by $Mg^{2+}$ with the enzyme sensitivity to $Ca^{2+}$ being dependent upon $Mg^{2+}$ concentration.[106] Oldham et al. noted two $Ca^{2+}$ inhibition sites on porcine parathyroid adenylate cyclase[107] and found that $Mg^{2+}$ concentration influences the relative contribution on these sites to $Ca^{2+}$ inhibition.[108] These authors point out that the concentration of intracellular $Ca^{2+}$ in parathyroid cells is reportedly at a level that could inhibit adenylate cyclase activity; consequently, the $Ca^{2+}$ inhibitable activity involving competition with $Mg^{2+}$ would be particularly significant at low intracellular $Mg^{2+}$ concentrations.

The interdependent effects of $Ca^{2+}$ and $Mg^{2+}$ on parathyroid hormone levels is further evident in many studies in which magnesium was present at levels above the physiologic levels in in vitro studies, experimental animals, and human subjects. In one such study, pregnant women were given continuous I.V. magnesium sulfate over 3 hours to suppress premature labor.[109] Serum magnesium remained elevated while total and ionized calcium fell gradually into the hypocalcemic range at 3 hours (Fig. 6–5). PTH decrease preceded the decline in calcium, which stayed below baseline levels even after 2 hours of hypocalcemia. In contrast to this study, in pre-eclamptic pregnant women the hypocalcemia associated

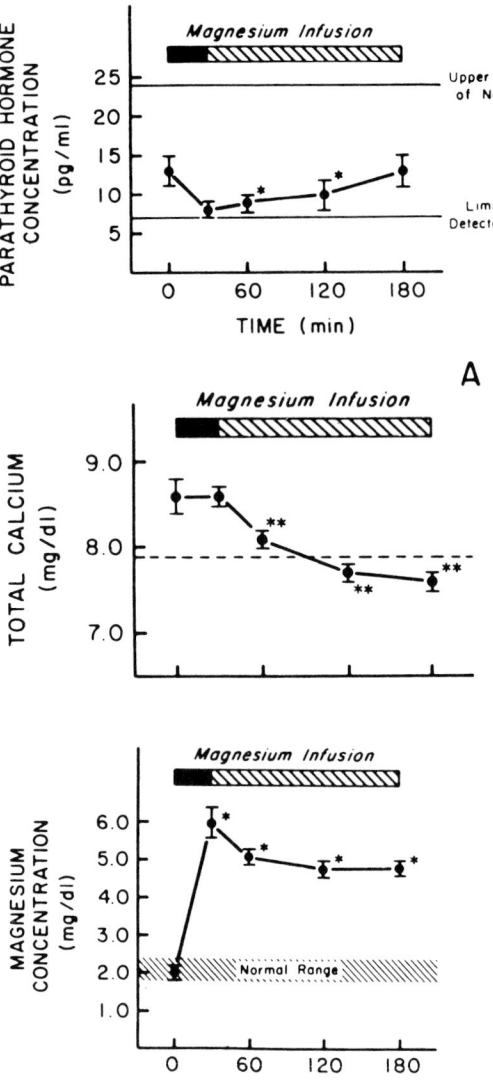

**A**

Fig. 6–5.  Effect of hypermagnesemia on parathyroid hormone and serum levels. Loading and maintenance intravenous infusion of magnesium for the suppression of premature labor increased serum magnesium to approximately twice the upper normal range (lower panel) with an associated decline in parathyroid hormone levels (top panel) and a gradual fall in total and ionized calcium (middle panel). (From Cholst et al.,[109] with permission of the New England Journal of Medicine.)

with induced hypermagnesemia was associated with either unchanged or slightly elevated PTH levels.[110,111] The maternal and fetal magnesium levels at delivery were at approximately similar levels. Fetal blood total and ionized calcium levels were lower than those in controls; serum PTH was undetectable in many of the fetuses from the magnesium-treated women.[110] In the second study, the differences from controls were slight or absent.[111]

Increased calcium excretion occurs in hypermagnesemia.[41] If a state of relative hypoparathyroidism also occurs, excretion of magnesium ion should decrease as serum calcium falls. Hypermagnesemia may also suppress peripheral PTH action.[112] The doubling of magnesium concentration in hemodialysis fluid resulted in a rise in plasma magnesium in the dialyzed uremic patient from 1.25 to 1.70 mmol/L (i.e., 2.5 to 3.40 meq/L). This rise was associated with a 23% decline in mean plasma iPTH. Plasma calcium, phosphate, and 25-OH vitamin D declined, but not significantly.[113]

It is apparent from this brief survey that there are multiple magnesium interactions. Magnesium interaction with calcium is variable from cell type to cell type and even among species. In some cells, e.g., muscle contractile proteins, $Ca^{2+}$ is stimulatory and $Mg^{2+}$ is competitively inhibitory, whereas with parathyroid adenylate cyclase, $Ca^{2+}$ is inhibitory and $Mg^{2+}$ competitively stimulatory. Extracellular $Mg^{2+}$ may increase cytosolic $Ca^{2+}$ through cellular depolarization either by influencing calcium channels or by affecting phospholipid metabolism resulting in an increase in plasma membrane permeability for calcium.[101b] The presynaptic neuron $Mg^{2+}$ can compete with $Ca^{2+}$ for sites at which calcium binding leads to acetylcholine release. Competitive $Mg^{2+}$ binding, however, does not cause acetylcholine release with consequent relaxation of smooth muscle.[81]

These and other $Mg^{2+}$-$Ca^{2+}$ interactions have led to designation of magnesium as a "mimic weak $Ca^{2+}$ antagonist" and "the mimic/antagonist of calcium."[98,114] These designations identify an association that, while apparently correct in many instances, is not a universal concept since magnesium also has independent attributes.

## MAGNESIUM DEFICIENCY

### Laboratory Animals

Although the rat has been by far the most widely used animal, many other species have been studied, including various fowl, guinea pigs, mice, pigs, sheep, cattle, dogs, and monkeys.[2] The acutely depleted young rat develops rapid signs in what is probably the most dramatic of all deficiency syndromes. After 3 to 5 days rats developed peripheral vasodilatation with intense erythema that increased for approximately 1 week and then gradually subsided.[1] This hyperemia occurred in association with a rise and fall in the number of mast cells and associated histamine release.[115,116] Concomitantly, the animals became progressively hyperkinetic and suddenly developed tonic-clonic convulsions—usually associated with a sudden noise—which were often fatal.[1] These early observations in the rat were the basis for the association of magnesium depletion with neuromuscular changes. Other signs of deficiency noted in rats include reduced growth, alopecia, and skin lesions.

With more chronic deficiency, edema and hypertrophic gums occurred with leukocytosis, splenomegaly, and thymic changes. The thymic abnormalities in deficient rats have been described as a malignant lymphosarcoma[117,118] or as disseminated lymphoblastic leukemia.[119] Other investigators, however, have noted two very different changes; the thymus in some magnesium-deficient animals was atrophic, whereas it was markedly enlarged in 18 to 52% of deficient rats that survived more than 6 weeks.[120] In the enlarged gland the normal structure was replaced by cells morphologically resembling transformed lymphocytes. There were no metastases. One of the diets utilized by Alcock et al. had the same composition as that which others associated with lymphosarcoma[118]; this malignancy was not observed, however.

Immunologic changes (with depressed IgG and 7S antibody) and certain other antibody titers occurred in rats.[121,122] Profound changes in the immune functions would be expected to occur in magnesium deficiency on the basis of its essentiality for protein synthesis—a situation resembling that of zinc.

Studies of calcium absorption in magnesium-deficient rats have yielded conflicting results, with reports of an increase,[123a] a decrease,[123b] or no change[123c,d] from controls.

Crystalluria, calcification, and degenerative changes in various organs, especially in the kidney, are prominent in deficient rats and certain other species maintained on low-magnesium diets,[124–125] particularly with the diets containing calcium in relatively high percentage concentrations compared to human diets.[2] Renal changes may occur rapidly[125]; within 12 hours of initiating the low-magnesium diet in the rat, the brush border of the proximal tubules contained electron dense material.[125a] These changes coincided with virtual disappearance of magnesium from the urine; however, at this time renal cellular magnesium was normal. Within 36 hours concretions were present in the lumen of the proximal tubules; by the fifth day much larger crystalline masses were present and disruption of the epithelium was noted in some areas. The pathologic changes in the kidney, heart, and muscles have been described in detail.[124a,124b]

The rat is not representative of other species with respect to certain deficiency signs, e.g., the hyperemia, the repetitive and usual fatal tonic-clonic convulsions, and serum calcium changes. Mice on the same diet developed no hyperemia, became hypocalcemic, and often died with a single abrupt and massive convulsion.[126] Deficient dogs and monkeys on diets of the same composition developed spasticity, tremors, and convulsions with hypocalcemia; increasing the oral calcium in the diet did not increase the serum calcium or prevent the neuromuscular changes.[127]

## Experimental Human Studies

Symptomatic human deficiency observed in patients usually develops in a setting of predisposing and complicating disease states (Table 6–2) that often reduce intestinal absorption or are associated with impaired renal reabsorption (Table 6–3). Decreased intake or failure to provide adequate amounts of parenteral magnesium may be a complicating factor. Often, associated complex and uncontrolled variables are present because the individuals are often quite ill. In the early days of clinical interest in magnesium depletion, many nutritional inadequacies, metabolic abnormalities, electrolyte and fluid imbalances, manifestations of basic disease, infection, and administration of various medications occurred in conjunction with magnesium therapy and often created a situation in which it was difficult to ascribe certain clincial manifestations specifically to magnesium deficiency.

Experimental studies and additional case reports have helped clarify the clinical, biochemical, and physiologic aspects and interrelationships of this deficiency.

Four groups of investigators have recorded their efforts to induce magnesium deficiency experimentally in human volunteers.[46,47,128–130] In the study that produced symptomatic depletion, the experimental diet provided somewhat less than 0.8 meq of magnesium/day.[46,47] Plasma magnesium fell progressively to levels that were 10 to 30% those of control periods (Fig. 6–6). Erythrocyte magnesium declined more slowly and to a lesser degree. Urine (Fig. 6–3) and fecal magnesium decreased to extremely low levels within 7 days. Hypomagnesemia, hypocalcemia, and hypokalemia were present in all of the consistently symptomatic patients (Fig. 6–7). These effects were associated with good intestinal calcium absorption and hypocalciuria so that the patients had positive calcium balance. Serum phosphate values were variable among the subjects (Fig. 6–6). Most deficient subjects developed hypokalemia with negative potassium balance as the re-

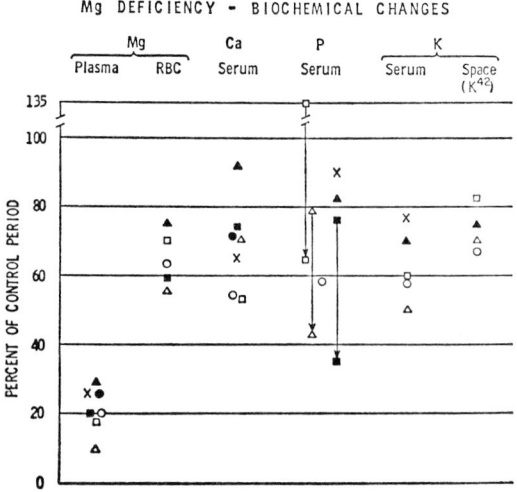

**Fig. 6–6.** Biochemical changes observed in the course of experimental human magnesium depletion. The maximum deviation observed in the course of the depletion is indicated as a percentage of the average control levels for each subject for magnesium, calcium, inorganic phosphate, and potassium. $K^{42}$ space indicated the estimate of exchangeable body potassium using $^{42}K$. The transient decrease in serum inorganic phosphate noted in 3 individuals immediately following magnesium repletion is indicated by a line connecting values observed in the late depletion period with those observed in early repletion. (From Shils, M.E.,[47] with permission.)

sult of increased urinary losses. Serum sodium remained normal and the subjects were in positive sodium balance. Neuromuscular signs (positive Trousseau's signs, tremors, fasciculations, and gross muscle spasms) occurred in five of the seven subjects after deficiency periods ranging from 25 to 110 days. Marked personality changes occurred in several patients.

Despite the hypocalcemia, deep tendon reflexes were either normal or decreased. The electromyogram revealed rapid-firing high-pitched potentials during the deficiency period in the five patients tested. The electroencephalograms were normal. Anorexia, nausea, and apathy occurred frequently and heralded exacerbation of the neurologic changes. When electrocardiographic changes occurred, they were compatible with coexisting hypocalcemia and/or hypokalemia.

All symptoms and signs (including personality changes) reverted to normal with reinstitution of magnesium. A characteristic finding (which has been repeatedly confirmed in cases of clinical magnesium depletion) was the delayed rise in serum calcium despite the rapid return to normal of serum magnesium upon repletion with this ion; a week or even longer intervened before calcium returned to baseline levels (Fig. 6–7). Potassium balances became strongly positive as sodium bal-

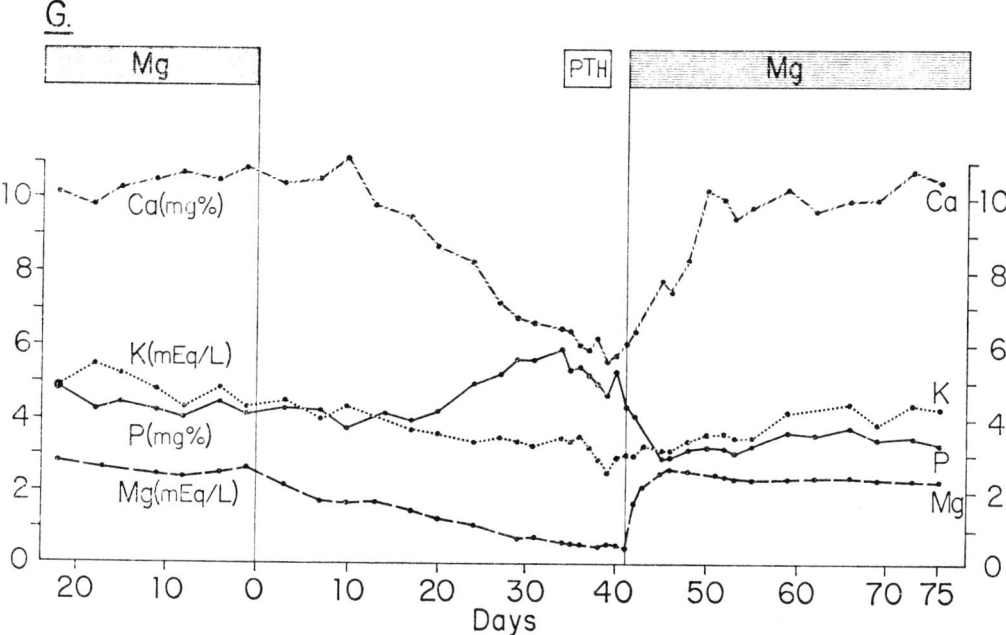

**Fig. 6–7.** Blood chemistries in subject on experimental magnesium (Mg) depletion. Mg was omitted after the patient was one month on the control diet. The rise in serum inorganic phosphate (P) with Mg depletion in this patient was unique among the depleted subjects. On depletion day 25, Trousseau's and Chvostek's signs first occurred, and the former became progressively stronger as plasma calcium (Ca), Mg, and potassium (K) continued to decline. On depletion day 35, parathyroid hormone (PTH) was given I.M. at 50 units t.i.d. for 5 days; this had no effect on plasma Ca but appeared to decrease P. On day 41, anorexia, nausea, paresthesias, and generalized muscle spasticity developed; 17 meq of Mg I.V. was then given with rapid improvement. This was followed by similar amounts of Mg I.M. 12 and 15 hours later. Dietary Mg (40 meq daily) was resumed on the third repletion day. (From Shils, M.E.,[47] with permission.)

ances became negative and as serum potassium returned to normal, over a matter of days (Fig. 6–7). Urine magnesium and calcium rose.

This study led to the conclusion that magnesium is essential for the normal metabolism of potassium and calcium in adult man, that it is essential for the mobilization of calcium from bone, and that the signs and symptoms secondary to magnesium deficiency are associated with complex electrolyte changes. The extent of alterations in concentrations of the various electrolytes in blood and tissues, their relative intakes and losses, and the accompanying alkalosis influence the manifestations of the deficiency in a given individual.

Hypomagnesemia occurred with hypocalciuria but without hypocalcemia and without clinical symptoms or signs of deficiency in two subjects ingesting 2 to 5 meq of magnesium/day in another study.[130] The four subjects in the other two experimental studies did not become hypomagnesemic within the 20 to 38 days of the experimental diet.[128,129] The numerous differences in types of subjects, diet composition, and experimental conditions in these investigations have been reviewed.[47]

The signs and symptoms noted above in experimental deficiency have been described separately or in various combinations in clinical cases of hypomagnesemia. They included Trousseau's and Chvostek's signs, muscle fasciculations, tremor, muscle spasm, personality changes, anorexia, nausea, and vomiting. Frank tetany, myoclonic jerks, athetoid movements, convulsions, and coma have been reported. Convulsions with or without coma seem to occur much more frequently in acutely deficient infants than in adults.

**Blood and Tissue Electrolyte Changes**

Hypomagnesemia occurs uniformly in all species on low-magnesium diets. Magnesium levels are significantly lower than those of controls within a day or two of onset of deficiency in rats[131] and within 5 to 7 days in human volunteers with severe magnesium restriction.[46,47]

The condition most closely related to "pure" experimental human magnesium deficiency is familial hypomagnesemia—a congenital primary hypomagnesemia occurring in males[132,133] and related to a specific defect in intestinal absorption of magnesium ion, as mentioned earlier.[27] There were 18 cases verified by 1981, with the usual age of onset being 2 to 4 weeks. Hypomagnesemia and hypocalcemia with tetany and often with convulsions were corrected with magnesium supplements. Calcium and vitamin D supplements were ineffective. Serum potassium was low and sodium and phosphate elevated.[132] During relatively short periods of depletion under controlled conditions, serum iPTH, calcitonin, and 25-OH vitamin D remained normal despite the hypomagnesemia.

Three children with this disease were treated from 3 to 4 weeks of age with oral magnesium supplements for 9 to 12 years with normal somatic and intellectual development. Optimal daily dosages were 0.5 to 0.75 mmol (1.0 to 1.5 meq/kg).[132]

Table 6–4 summarizes findings on serum/plasma calcium levels in various species, as culled from a review of publications of different research groups. Many groups had multiple reports on this topic. The findings from individual laboratories were usually consistent when the species and diets were the same. In the rat, which has been most widely used, most groups have observed consistent hypercalcemia when the usual diets are employed. There is only one report of hypocalcemia; I found the diet used in that study to be associated with marked azotemia in rats, which may have been the responsible factor. In contrast to the rat, other species have been reported to be either normocalcemic or hypocalcemic.

Factors that affect serum calcium levels in deficient rats are age and the calcium content of the diet. Young animals are more likely to develop hypercalcemia than are older animals when both subsist on the same diet. The usual calcium content of the diet has varied among investigators

from 400 to 1500 mg/dl (usually 600 to 700 mg/dl). On such diets hypercalcemia is usual. When rats are fed a diet more closely reflecting the daily human calcium intake (140 mg/dl in a purified diet), serum calcium was either normal or elevated.[126,127] Reduction of calcium to 70 mg/dl resulted in normocalcemia in all. When the dietary calcium was reduced further, hypocalcemia occurred in the magnesium-depleted rats but not in controls.[134,135]

Hypocalcemia occurred consistently in mice, dogs, monkeys, and human volunteers on the same magnesium-deficient diet with 140 mg/dl of calcium.[126,127] A diet with 1200 mg/dl calcium fed to mice resulted in normocalcemia[136]; when mice of the same strain were fed a diet with 140 mg/dl calcium, they were hypocalcemic.[126]

The variability reported in dogs also appears to reflect age and calcium content of the deficient diet. For example, significant hypocalcemia was noted in a study with 340 mg/dl of calcium in mature dogs[137] and in puppies with 600 mg/dl dietary calcium.[135] There was mild hypocalcemia on a diet with 950 mg/dl calcium[138] and normocalcemia on a diet with 1680 mg/dl.[139] There is also evidence that the severity of magnesium deficiency is increased as dietary calcium is increased. Differences in dietary calcium content may also be reflected in differences in bone calcium and histology.

**Serum Potassium.** In the two experimental human deficiency studies in which hypomagnesemia was observed, hypokalemia also occurred.[47,130] Teenagers with familial hypomagnesemia had low potassium levels.[132] In case reports of adult clinical magnesium deficiency of various causes, hypokalemia has been frequently reported.[4,140–144] In malnourished children with magnesium depletion, hypokalemia is often pres-

**Table 6–4.** The Influence of Experimental Mg Depletion on Serum Calcium Levels in Various Species (Analysis of Published Reports from 14 Different Laboratories)*†

| Species | Serum Calcium | | |
| | Increased | Normal | Decreased |
| --- | --- | --- | --- |
| Rat | Numerous References | Numerous References | 1‡ |
| Mouse | — | 1 | 1 |
| Guinea pig | — | 1 | 1 |
| Chick | — | — | 2 |
| Dog | — | 5 | 6 |
| Pig | — | — | 1 |
| Sheep | — | — | 2 |
| Cow | — | 1 | 5 |
| Monkey | — | — | 3 |
| Man | — | 1‡ | 1 |

*Modified slightly from ref 2. Number of laboratories reporting data. Individual references in ref 2.
†Diets were variable in composition including Mg, Ca, and other minerals.
‡See text

ent.[145,146] However, the majority of cases of neonatal tetany associated with hypomagnesemia and hypocalcemia showed normal serum.[127] Hypokalemia may or may not occur in deficient laboratory animals.

**Serum Phosphate.** During experimental human depletion, serum inorganic phosphate was variable ranging from slightly elevated to low[47]; following treatment with magnesium, three of the six patients had an abrupt fall in phosphate (Fig. 6–6). Children with familial hypomagnesemia often have elevated serum phosphate; in a closely supervised study, two of three such patients had a "spontaneous" fall in phosphate following repletion.[132] In mature dogs on experimental diets, inorganic phosphate may remain unchanged[137,139] or fall modestly[138]; in puppies it may be elevated.[147,148] Hypophosphatemia associated with phosphaturia and hypercalcemia in the rat, noted early by MacIntyre et al., has been noted frequently in that species.[149] Mice became hyperphosphatemic and hypocalcemic on the same magnesium-deficient diet that induces hypophosphatemia and hypercalcemia in rats.[126]

**Skeletal Muscle Changes.** Magnesium in cells is bound to ligands, especially to ATP. Since only a small amount is free $Mg^{2+}$, only a relatively small amount is freely exchangeable (probably less than 15%). In adult rats on a magnesium-deficient diet with the usual high calcium and phosphate intake there were no significant changes in skeletal muscle magnesium, calcium, sodium, or potassium after 2 weeks of depletion.[150] There was a significant lowering of Mg-ATPase activity but not of Na-K-ATPase or of Ca-ATPase. Resting soleus muscle potentials were lower but not significantly so from controls.

In the adult magnesium-deficient dog fed a very high calcium diet, muscle magnesium was transiently decreased at 7 weeks but equal to baseline value at 11 weeks; sodium was consistently and markedly elevated, and chloride and calcium were also significantly increased; potassium was unaltered and phosphate was decreased.[139] Resting membrane potential was significantly elevated by 10 weeks and in some dogs was greater than 100 mV (hyperpolarization). Rhabdomyolysis and focal necrosis occurred in some subjects, while 4 others had normal histology. Despite marked hypomagnesemia, plasma calcium, phosphate, and potassium were unchanged.[139]

## Bone Metabolism and Morphology

A major proportion of magnesium in bone is complexed with apatite crystal. Alfrey et al. showed that the surface-limited magnesium bone pool is rapidly utilized to replace other tissue deficits during deficiency.[153] In contrast to muscle magnesium, the magnesium present in bone correlates well with serum magnesium in normal, depleted, and overloaded laboratory animals and human subjects.[154] The availability of magnesium in bone deposits during a period of deficient intake depends on the age of the animal. A large percentage is lost, compared to the initial control value in young depleted rats (varying from 30 to 40% in one study)[151] and to 60 to 67% in others.[131b,152]

Studies of bone mineralization patterns and histology in deficient animals have resulted in very different findings, perhaps resulting partly from differences in the calcium content of diets, age of subjects, and duration of observation. In a 21-day study by Jones et al., magnesium in the femurs of young control rats increased from 1.935 $mg/cm^3$ to 2.349 $mg/cm^3$, while the magnesium in the bones of deficient rats fell from the initial control values to 0.647 $mg/cm^3$, a difference of 72%.[131b] In this study utilizing a moderately high calcium dietary level (0.6 g%), the animals became hypomagnesemic and hypercalcemic. The femurs of the deficient animals had more calcium and total ash than the controls; radiographs revealed greater density, with many abnormalities including much unmineralized osteoid tissue. When slightly older rats were observed for longer periods while subsisting on either a control or a magnesium-deficient diet with a calcium content similar in percentage to a human diet (0.140 g%), Mirra et al. obtained very different results.[152] The markedly deficient animals were only slightly (but significantly) hypercalcemic as compared to controls; femur magnesium was only 40% of controls and bone calcium was 3% less at 40 days and 11% less at 80 days, with diminished bone growth; histologically, cortical bone in the deficient group was normal but decreased in thickness. Bony trabeculae were strikingly diminished and there was no osteoid. Plasma alkaline phosphatase activity in deficient rats was markedly depressed.[150,152] The addition of magnesium to the medium did not restore activity to control values, suggesting decreased apoenzyme concentration.[152]

The femurs of magnesium-deficient chicks on a diet with 1.2% calcium appeared similar to those of the rats studied by Jones et al. in that thickening of the cortex was marked and osteoid was increased.[152a]

Adult dogs with chronic magnesium depletion for 4 to 6 months on a very high calcium diet had a 27% decrease in serum magnesium, a 23% decrease in phosphorus, and an 8% decrease in calcium—all significant changes from controls.[138] The magnesium content of rib bone at the end of the study was decreased 31%, while the calcium and phosphorus concentrations were similar to those of controls. Histologically there was a marked decrease in osteoid, expressed as percent relative osteoid volume and percent total osteoid surface.

## Comparison of Human Experimental and Clinical Depletion

Reports are conflicting of serum, muscle, and bone levels of magnesium in sick patients who were claimed to be magnesium deficient. The number of patients studied in most reports is small. The findings include (1) decreased serum and muscle magnesium with normal bone level,[155] (2) decreased serum, variable muscle, and low bone magnesium levels,[156] (3) normal serum and erythrocyte magnesium levels with decreased muscle magnesium and potassium,[157] (4) reduced serum level with normal muscle content,[157a] (5) reduced muscle level in association with normal serum, erythrocyte, and bone magnesium levels and variable muscle potassium,[158] (6) consistently reduced serum concentrations with variable muscle levels,[159] and (7) low serum magnesium with variable muscle magnesium concentration but with a highly significant correlation between serum and bone magnesium levels.[154]

During magnesium deficiency, muscle magnesium varies directly with muscle potassium in man,[4,143,154,160] rats,[161] and guinea pigs.[162] It is noteworthy that the development of potassium depletion with depressed muscle potassium is associated with decreased muscle magnesium in man.[143,154,160,163]

The rather bewildering variations noted in ill patients with respect to their blood and tissue magnesium and other electrolytes emphasize a point made earlier, namely, the difficulty in ascribing cause and effect to a specific nutrient deficiency in uncontrolled situations in sick individuals. Normal cellular metabolism and homeostasis of cellular composition are critically dependent on an adequate supply of energy and the many essential nutrients. Significant deficiency of one or more nutrients has an impact on retention of other nutrients; for example, magnesium depletes potassium while potassium depletion reduces the magnesium content of cells.

Starvation caused protein catabolism, acidosis, and loss of cellular constituents including magnesium, even though serum magnesium remained normal or near normal. In a 2-month period of total starvation, magnesium was lost from tissue in two ways, firstly, by depletion of lean body mass; in four of six obese subjects a loss of 400 g of nitrogen was calculated to be associated with

a loss of approximately 700 meq of magnesium. Secondly, magnesium was lost by an additional renal loss that appeared to be related, at least in good part, to the degree of acidosis.[164] When 50 to 150 g of glucose were given, urinary magnesium decreased by 55%. Muscle magnesium decreased, but the electrolyte excretion patterns indicated that very significant amounts came from bone. Presumably, serum magnesium was maintained by a fairly constant input of magnesium into the blood. In the blood, serum magnesium was presented to the glomerulus for filtration and to the renal tubular cells, in which some reabsorption occurred, affected by the presence of organic acids.

Whatever the explanation for the relatively normal serum magnesium, we have here a model that is very different from that of primary or experimental magnesium depletion, which is always associated with hypomagnesemia. The same pattern seen in the starving individual could occur in the patient with significantly decreased glomerular filtration resulting from renal disease, who is eating poorly, is in negative nitrogen balance, and has acidosis; it could occur also in any patient with serious cellular catabolism (i.e., trauma, burns, sepsis) with little or no nutritional support who is releasing into the circulation magnesium that for some reason is not being normally excreted by the kidneys because of prerenal factors (i.e., hypotension and/or dehydration).

It may be useful clinically to distinguish three types of magnesium depletion: (1) that caused by a failure to ingest, absorb, or retain sufficient magnesium in an individual with normal glomerular function which is associated with the characteristic hypomagnesemia and sequelae noted in experimental deficiency; (2) that of depressed magnesium intake associated with other deficiencies (including energy deficiency) that induce serious cellular catabolism, potassium depletion, and/or acidosis associated with tissue (including bone) loss of magnesium in an individual in whom tissue-derived magnesium, together with some oral intake, maintains a normal to near normal serum level. The normal sequelae of experimental deficiency except for tissue depletion are absent in this type. The serum level will depend on the oral intake and extent of tissue loss; and (3) either of the first two types but of less severity, associated with glomerular dysfunction of varying degrees with resultant normal or high serum magnesium levels.

It is recommended that clinical reports attempting to correlate serum magnesium with tissue levels (muscle, bone, or white or red cells) should provide sufficient clinical and metabolic data to allow the reader to evaluate the situation in the light of the three situations listed above.

## MAGNESIUM DEFICIENCY: PHYSIOLOGIC AND BIOCHEMICAL CORRELATES

### Response to PTH

Studies have shown that magnesium-deficient rats often develop hypercalcemia, hypophosphatemia, hypocalciuria, and hyperphosphaturia suggestive of a hyperparathyroid state.[149,165,166] Parathyroidectomy eliminated the relative hypercalcemia, further strengthening the relationship between magnesium deficiency and increased activity of the parathyroid gland in this species.[42,165–167] However, despite the hypercalcemia, histologic studies in intact magnesium-deficient rats have indicated that the parathyroid glands were actually smaller than those of controls.[131,145] The hypocalcemia found in most other deficient species (including those maintained on a diet identical to that of the rat[2]) suggests a secondary hypoparathyroid state.

Numerous observations have been made as to the degree of responsiveness of magnesium-deficient laboratory animals and patients to injected parathyroid extract (PTE).[2] With the exception of the chick, other species including the rat, dog, and monkey respond to PTE with an elevation of serum calcium despite magnesium deficiency. Deficient dogs appeared to have varying degrees of resistance to PTE, suggesting a refractory state of bone responsiveness to the hormone. In deficient adults and children, responses in terms of serum calcium and renal excretion of phosphate and cAMP have been variable, but in general the expected rise has been blunted. In most subjects in whom the PTE response was retested following institution of magnesium, the calcemic response was appreciably greater than during the deficiency period but still appeared to be blunted. Interpretation of the results in a number of these studies is complicated by the variable degrees of deficiency and treatments and by the calcium rise, which, although attributed to PTE, was occurring at a time when the calcemic effect of magnesium repletion may have been occurring as well. Despite variability and unresolved differences, however, a significant percentage of deficient patients did appear to have some end-organ resistance to PTE.[2]

### PTH Levels in Humans

The advent of immunologic assays for circulating PTH has contributed importantly to our understanding of the effect of magnesium depletion on calcium metabolism and afforded further insight on species differences in response to this depletion. The first reported depleted patient on whom immunoparathyroid hormone (iPTH) assays were performed had a genetically related hypomagnesemia with undetectable iPTH.[168] When magnesium was given, iPTH levels rose markedly, followed by a good calcemic response. These results indicated that magnesium depletion was associated with a failure of the parathyroid gland to either manufacture or secrete the hormone. Over the next few years, as more cases with iPTH measurements were reported, it became apparent that the situation was more complex. For example, a survey of data on 36 hypomagnesemic patients by me and others from the literature revealed that 10 had iPTH levels that were low or undetectable, 18 had values in the "normal" range (which were, however, inappropriately low for the degree of hypocalcemia present), and 8 had elevated levels.[2] These data indicated a complex situation involving both iPTH secretions and bone reactivity.

Many patients with very low or normal iPTH concentrations had developed significant increases in hormone levels following magnesium administration, with the rise in iPTH occurring appreciably earlier than the rise in serum calcium. When iPTH measurements were done serially before and at very short intervals after a rapid bolus I.V. injection of magnesium, serum iPTH rose within 1 minute to very high levels in association with very rapid elevations of serum magnesium but without any detectable rise in serum calcium over the next 30 to 360 minutes.[169,170] It is apparent that the magnesium-depleted parathyroid gland is capable of producing PTH and that magnesium induces rapid secretion (Fig. 6–8). The differences in baseline iPTH appear to reflect the severity of the magnesium depletion.[170] Eumagnesemic subjects given magnesium had the expected rise in magnesium with a fall in iPTH.

### Bone Resistance

Bone resistance to PTH was predicted from the finding of normal or elevated iPTH levels in hypomagnesemic/hypocalcemic patients and relative refractoriness of deficient animals and humans to PTE. Resistance has been confirmed by observation in chronic magnesium depletion in dogs. Isolated tibias were perfused with a synthetic bovine PTH (syn b-PTH 1-34).[138] The uptake (i.e., the arteriovenous difference for iPTH across the bones) of control dogs was 37.5% as compared to 10.1% in the depleted animals. This correlated with a significant depression in cAMP production by the deficient dogs. The deficient bones had a histologic picture of skeletal inactivity.

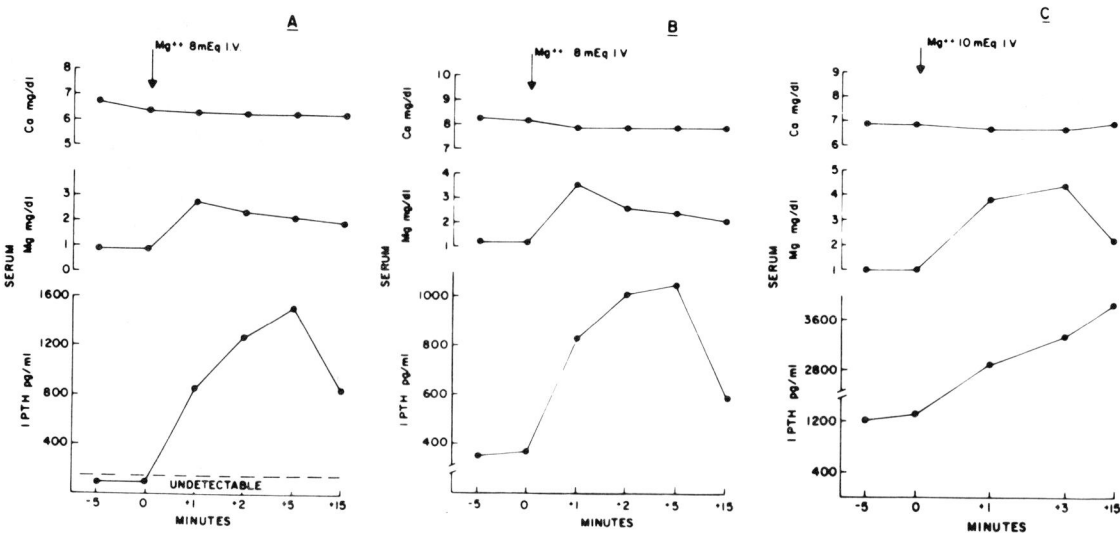

**Fig. 6–8.** Effect of rapid intravenous injection of magnesium (Mg) on the serum concentrations of Mg, immuno-reactive parathyroid hormone (iPTH), and calcium in hypomagnesemic hypocalcemic patients with undetectable iPTH (A), normal iPTH (B), and elevated iPTH (C) levels prior to Mg injection. Level of iPTH detectability 150 pg/ml. The PTH level reflects in part the severity the magnesium depletion and its effect on bone resistance to PTH and on suppression of PTH secretion. Despite the normal (B) or high (C) iPTH levels, serum calcium remained low. In response to the rapid rise in Mg, the iPTH rose in all instances within the first minute. (From Rude, et al.,[70] with permission of The Endocrine Society.)

### Sequence of Effects of Deficiency and Repletion in Humans

1. The initiation of hypocalcemia: When an intake of calcium is adequate, calcium balance is positive; consequently, calcium depletion can be ruled out as an etiologic factor in the development of hypocalcemia. The initiating factor appears to be failure of the normal heterionic exchange of bone calcium for magnesium in the bathing medium at the labile bone mineral surface.[171–174] As magnesium depletion progresses, a more important influence is impairment of osteoclast receptor responsiveness to PTH with reduction of active bone resorption. At this stage hypocalcemia develops in a setting of progressive increase in the level of circulating PTH.

2. The perpetuation of hypocalcemia: As depletion progresses further, secretion of PTH diminishes to very low levels despite adequate intraparathyroid gland hormonal reserves. The hallmarks of severe magnesium depletion are present at this stage; namely, very low circulating PTH, unresponsive bone, hypocalcemia, hypokalemia, sodium retention, and neuromuscular and other clinical signs and symptoms.

3. The regression of hypocalcemia: With adequate magnesium administration, serum magnesium rises rapidly; this rise is followed closely by an increase in serum PTH, which also may be rapid. Following a lag period of some days, serum calcium and potassium begin to rise. In this interval magnesium ions are entering the hydration shell of bone, permitting heterionic calcium exchange to begin. This early exchange may explain the rapid improvement that occurs subjectively and with some decrease in neuromuscular signs with litle or no detectable change in circulating calcium. The delayed rise in serum calcium reflects the failure of resorptive calcium release associated with continuing osteoclast end-organ insensitivity. During this interval, however, receptors to PTH on the osteoclasts are renewing their responsiveness. As end-organ resistance recedes and elevated PTH levels continue, serum calcium rises. With normalization of serum calcium, the hormone level declines and the electrolyte abnormalities and clinical signs and symptoms disappear.

### PTH in the Magnesium-Deficient Rat

The enigmatic behavior of serum calcium in the magnesium-deficient rat has been noted above. Rayssiguier et al. and Anast and Forte measured iPTH sequentially as magnesium depletion progressed in young rats.[175a,175b] The changes observed in iPTH were different in the two studies although the experimental conditions appeared rather similar. In the report of Rayssiguier et al., plasma iPTH levels were significantly above those of controls by day 7 and increased further by day 14; they then fell to control levels by day 20, at which time plasma calcium in the different rats continued to *increase* over that of controls while the plasma magnesium remained at the same low level.[175a] In the study of Anast and Forte, serum magnesium fell during the first 4 days of depletion associated with a modest increase in serum calcium; at the fourth day serum iPTH was at levels twice those of controls (Fig. 6–9A). The iPTH rise was transient; thereafter, as serum magnesium continued to fall (<0.6 mg/dl) and serum total and ionized calcium progressively rose, iPTH fell to values below those of the controls (Fig. 6–9B). Further experiments indicated that the parathyroid glands of the severely magnesium depleted rats were capable of secreting large amounts of iPTH when they were made hypocalcemic by depletion of either calcium or vitamin D.[175b] It was concluded that the cause of the reduced iPTH in hypomagnesemic rats was the hypercalcemia.

Thus, the parathyroid glands of the magnesium-depleted rat, in contrast to those of other species, responded appropriately to the calcium level induced by the deficiency. Although these two studies have somewhat different findings, their data question prior statements that the hypercalcemia of magnesium deficiency in the rat is the result of increased PTH secretion.[149,163] The decreased

iPTH output with the marked rise in calcium is consistent with the observations, mentioned earlier, of histologic evidence of reduced parathyroid gland activity.[131b,145] We are left without a clear-cut explanation of the etiology of the hypercalcemia. More data are needed on calcium absorption and calcium release from bone in relation to iPTH levels as deficiency progresses.

## Vitamin D Resistance

The role of vitamin D metabolites in the absorption of magnesium was mentioned above briefly with the evidence of a stimulatory effect being inconclusive and rather unlikely. There is another area of interaction between these two nutrients, namely, the resistance to vitamin D reported to occur as the result of magnesium depletion. A series of clinical reports, originally following a report in rats,[176] suggested that the calcemic effect of vitamin D—often in a high dose—is blunted in the presence of magnesium depletion.[177–180] Low levels of magnesium (0.25 mmol) in the culture medium of live fetal rat bone and killed fetal rat bones in vitro inhibited the PTH- or calcitriol-stimulated release of labeled calcium from bone, in contrast to the effectiveness

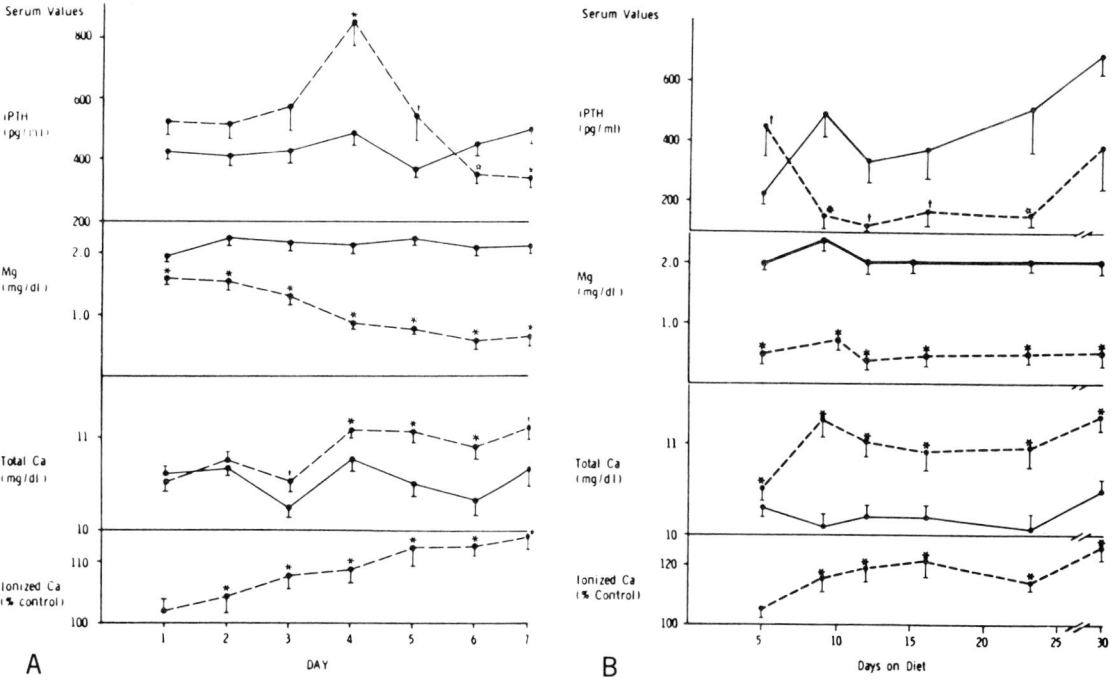

**Fig. 6–9.** Effect of magnesium deficiency (Mg) in the rat on serum magnesium, calcium, and immunoreactive parathyroid hormone (iPTH). Mg deficient rats •- - - -•, control rats •——• A, iPTH and calcium (total and ionized) rose significantly in first 4 days of deficiency as serum Mg declined. iPTH then fell progressively with further deficiency as calcium rose over the succeeding 20 days (B). Statistical differences between controls and deficient rats: *p<0.05; †p<0.02; *p<0.01. (From Anast, et al.,[175b] with permission of the Endocrine Society.)

of calcitriol in the presence of magnesium at 0.8 mmol.[174]

PTH is necessary for the formation of calcitriol,[181] and calcitriol is necessary for PTH to exert its effect on calcium mobilization from bone[182] (see Chap. 13). A patient who underwent thyroparathyroidectomy and who became magnesium depleted was reportedly resistant to calcitriol until repleted with magnesium, after which there was a good calcemic response.[180] There are conflicting data on the levels of serum/plasma calcitriol in cases of human magnesium deficiency. In one case it was high prior to treatment.[183] In another, it was in the normal range but doubled following magnesium treatment.[184] This increase was associated with a rather abrupt fall in plasma phosphate as serum magnesium rose, a situation that may stimulate calcitriol formation.

### Magnesium, Vitamin D, and Citrate

It has been known for 50 years or more that there is a relationship between vitamin D status and citrate levels in blood and urine.[185] Treatment of rickets with the vitamin increased citrate excretion in children[185] and rats.[186] It is well known that urinary citrate is increased with bicarbonate loading[186,187]; nevertheless, vitamin D supplementation of rachitic rats increased citrate excretion far more than did bicarbonate, and despite a fall in urine pH.[186] A combined calcium-magnesium-vitamin D–deficient diet fed to rats resulted in a low urinary citrate and increased intestinal wall citrate.[188] Giving vitamin D did not appreciably increase citrate excretion or decrease gut citrate until magnesium and calcium were present in the diet. Rats deficient in magnesium, but with adequate calcium and vitamin D intake had elevated serum citrate levels and decreased urinary citrate. A combined vitamin D deficiency and magnesium deficiency decreased serum citrate and reduced urinary citrate further.[189]

Individuals either chronically depleted of magnesium as the result of intestinal malabsorption or acutely depleted by the reduction of the magnesium content of their total parenteral nutrition solutions were found to have a markedly decreased content of citrate in urine secondary to increased renal tubular citrate reabsorption.[190]

### DISEASE STATES AND MAGNESIUM CORRELATES

The list of causes of magnesium depletion (Table 6–3) emphasizes that this condition is not likely to be rare in hospitals with both acutely and chronically ill patients. In a survey of 2300 patients in a Veterans Administration hospital, 6.9% were hypomagnesemic.[191] Another study found

11% of patients in routine magnesium determination to have hypomagnesemia.[192]

Earlier discussion in this chapter of the metabolic effects of magnesium depletion emphasized the associated multiple electrolyte abnormalities. Because serum magnesium determinations are not done routinely whereas serum potassium, sodium, phosphate, and calcium often are, Whang et al. investigated the incidence of hypomagnesemia when the other electrolytes were below normal.[193] Hypomagnesemia (<1.25 meq/L) occurred in 42% of patients with hypokalemia (<3.5 meq/L), 29% of those with hypophosphatemia (<2 mg/dl), 27% of those with hyponatremia (<130 meq/L), and 22% of those with hypocalcemia (<8.0 mg/dl). The distribution of the depressed values in the population was not given. In a retrospective study of 421 hospitalized patients in whom plasma magnesium and potassium had been measured concurrently, Boyd et al. found the incidence of hypokalemia (<3.5 meq/L) to be 12%, while hypomagnesemia (<1.4 meq/L) was 26%.[193b] Hypomagnesemia was present in 38% in the hypokalemic samples; hypomagnesemia was present in 25% of normokalemic samples. Data on drug ingestion or disease were not reported. The frequent association suggested that magnesium determinations should be performed routinely.

### Alcoholism

Thirty percent of all alcoholics and 86 percent of those with delirium tremens had hypomagnesemia during the first 24 to 48 hours after admission.[194] In 27 patients admitted with severe diabetic ketoacidosis, 7% had hypomagnesemia initially; after 12 hours of insulin and fluid therapy, hypomagnesmia was present in 55% as the result of continued urinary loss and/or shift into cells or bone.[195] It is noteworthy that 68% of these patients had elevated serum magnesium initially. In the survey of Whang et al., of 2300 hospitalized patients, 5.6% were hypermagnesemic.[191]

### Diabetes

Losses of magnesium in diabetic ketosis have been appreciated for many years.[65b] Of infants born to diabetic mothers, 37% were found to be hypomagnesemic during the first 3 days of life; the degree of decline was related to the severity of maternal diabetes and prematurity.[196] Children ages 5 to 18 with well-controlled type 1 diabetes tended to have lower serum magnesium values than controls; iron, copper, and zinc values were similar to those of controls.[197]

### Malabsorption

Serum magnesium is often subnormal in patients with malabsorption syndromes.[199–201] In one series, 15 of 42 patients with various types of malabsorption had low values; 9 of 63 patients with Crohn's disease were hypomagnesemic, as were 10 of 24 patients with idiopathic steatorrhea.[156] In another series of 17 patients with Crohn's disease severe enough to require hospitalization, 6 had low serum magnesium and 15 had low urine magnesium.[199] Increased amounts of fatty acids in the intestinal lumen form insoluble soaps with $Mg^{2+}$ and $Ca^{2+}$, leading to loss of these ions from dietary and endogenous sources; hence, their losses will bear some direct relation to fat intake.

### Nephrotoxic Drugs

Certain antibiotics may impair the renal conserving ability of magnesium (Table 6–3). In an early report on the use of cisplatin, 23 of 44 treated patients developed hypomagnesemia[59]; the renal defect may occur shortly after the drug is initiated and it may persist for months or even for years after it is discontinued. Administration of cisplatin in hypertonic saline together with extensive hydration provides some protection against the nephrotoxic action of the drug.[60]

### Protein-Energy Malnutrition

Magnesium depletion occurs in children with inadequate intake for various reasons in combination with malabsorption, persistent vomiting and/or diarrhea, and infection. It has been documented frequently in protein-energy malnutrition. Serum or plasma magnesium was noted to be low in various studies in Africa, i.e., in 19 of 28 children,[145] 39 of 100,[200] and 10 of 13 having serum values below the lower limit of normal and with all having very low urinary magnesium.[201] In a study in Central America, 50% of serum magnesium values were below 1.3 meq/L on admission to the hospital and during recovery in unsupplemented children and an equal percent had low muscle magnesium.[202] The authors noted that some children had elevated serum and muscle magnesium and speculated that such findings were related to reduced renal function, which was known to occur.

### Kidney Disease

Earlier discussion in this chapter and the data in Table 6–3 emphasize the number of factors that may modify adversely the critical role of the kidney in magnesium homeostasis. In addition to nephrotoxic drugs, increased excretion is associated with various metabolic changes such as acidosis, phosphate depletion, and tissue wasting and with diseases such as postobstructive nephropathy, chronic glomerulonephritis, postrenal transplantation, and familial urinary magnesium wasting syndromes.[52a,b,d]

The risk of stone formation and nephrocalcinosis in magnesium-depleted rats is well documented. Presumably, long-term unrecognized chronic magnesium depletion in humans with a good calcium intake could lead to soft-tissue calcification. A more common risk is associated with the hypocitraturia that occurs within a matter of days in magnesium-depleted patients.[190] Since both citrate and magnesium tend to keep calcium from precipitating in urine, the value of maintaining adequate urine concentrations of both is obvious.

A relatively uncommon situation is reported in which magnesium deficiency occurs in a setting of impaired glomerular filtration.[203] In this setting (which usually induces hypermagnesemia), the hypomagnesemia must occur because of associated clinical problems, such as tubular dysfunction with depressed reabsorption, prolonged infusion of magnesium-free I.V. fluids as the major nutritional input into the patient, reversal of severe acidosis with magnesium-poor I.V. fluids, or concomitant serious intestinal malabsorption.[204]

Hypermagnesemia and its potential toxicity in patients with renal failure ingesting magnesium-containing antacids are discussed below.

Reference has been made earlier to the depression of PTH in obstetric patients made hypermagnesemic.[109] Related observations have been made in patients with chronic renal failure on hemodialysis. Because of secondary hyperparathyroidism and bone disease in patients on long-term hemodialysis, the dialysate magnesium was increased from 1.5 to 2.5 meq/L, and in some it was reduced from the usual 1.5 to 0.5 meq/L. Raising magnesium reduced serum PTH, calcium, and phosphate, while its reduction caused a marked rise in the PTH without a concomitant increase in calcium and phosphate.[205]

### Familial Disorders

Mention has been made in various sections of this chapter of primary hypomagnesemia involving impairment of the normal reabsorptive mechanism for magnesium of the small bowel.[2,132,133,147,168] Daily oral magnesium supplements of 1.0 to 1.5 meq/kg resulted in serum magnesium levels of about 1.2 meq/L, serum calcium of about 9.4 mg/dl, and small but definite amounts of magnesium in the urine. These dosages avoided diarrhea and permitted normal development for many years of children with this abnormality.[132]

A familial disorder of impaired renal conservation of magnesium and potassium was described by Gitelman et al. with hypomagnesemia, hypokalemia, and alkalosis. In some cases magnesium restriction was associated with hypercalcemia.[52a] A familial disorder with renal magnesium wasting was noted in a mother and son with associated hypomagnesemia; the mother also had calcium pyrophosphate synovitis and chondrocalcinosis.[52b,52d]

Bartter's syndrome, a rare condition, is characterized by hypokalemic alkalosis with hyperplasia of the juxtaglomerular apparatus, hyperreninemia, normal or high plasma aldosterone levels, increased sympathoadrenal activity, high urinary prostaglandin levels, normal blood pressure, and hyporesponsiveness of the pressure to pressor agents such as angiotensin II and norepinephrine. Hypomagnesemia may occur but is not a common finding.[52c] An infant with a severe type of this disorder made a dramatic and sustained improvement when magnesium was added following failure to improve with potassium and other supplements.[206] A normal serum magnesium level was associated with a low muscle magnesium (as well as low potassium and high sodium) content with significant renal dysfunction.[206] In another case, prolonged magnesium infusion corrected the renal potassium wasting.[207]

A new syndrome similar to that of Bartter's syndrome has been described with characteristics of the latter but with normal juxtaglomerular apparatus. The kidneys were abnormal with hypertrophy of the proximal tubular basement membranes and characteristic changes of the tubular cells on electron microscopy.[208] Serum magnesium was normal as was serum creatinine, but hypokalemia was severe. Supplementation with magnesium chloride (40 to 60 meq/day) was associated with decreased potassium excretion, positive potassium balance, elevation of serum potassium, and an increase in supine and upright plasma aldosterone.[209]

## Postparathyroidectomy Hypomagnesemia

Cases have been described of symptomatic hypomagnesemia following parathyroidectomy for primary hyperparathyroidism in association with the expected hypocalcemia. Symptoms of muscle weakness, tremor, and mental changes were reversed by magnesium despite continuing low calcium.[210] This appears to be a manifestation of the "hungry bone" syndrome, in which not only calcium but also magnesium is deposited into bone at a rate exceeding absorption following removal of the parathyroid adenoma.

## Antiepileptic Drugs

Early claims were made that serum magnesium levels are lower than controls in epileptic patients treated with antiepileptic medications.[211] More recent evidence, however, indicates that epileptic patients on such drugs, e.g., diphenylhydantoin,[212,214] with or without phenothiazines, had serum or CSF magnesium levels similar to those of matched untreated controls.[213,214]

## Coronary Artery Disease

It has been suggested that there is an inverse relationship between magnesium intake and coronary artery disease and its sequelae.[29b,215,216] The prevalence, morbidity, and mortality of this disease are such that these claims merit examination. The arguments advanced rest in large part on interpretations of analytic data in epidemiologic reports of decreased prevalence of deaths from coronary artery disease in areas where the water is "hard" (i.e., higher in calcium and magnesium than "soft" water).[29b,217–219]

In these and other reports the prevalence of coronary artery disease (as evidenced by deaths or survived acute myocardial infarction) was evaluated in populations living in areas with different amounts of magnesium, calcium, or fluoride in the drinking water. Marier summarized data on magnesium and calcium contents of different waters and the ratios of these divalent ions; he noted the wide variations encountered in water of different "hardness".[29b] In a complex case-controlled study by Luoma et al. with a relatively small number of men, the relative risk for the association between low magnesium in the water ($\leq$ 1.2 ppm) and myocardial infarction was 2.0 in a group of surgical patients matched for age and community, and 4.7 in a group similarly matched but drawn from a population registry. Nevertheless, there was no significant difference between the *mean* content of magnesium or calcium in the drinking waters of the two groups.[219] The authors point out that the average daily dietary intake of magnesium of Finns is about 440 mg; the intake of this ion from 2 L of water containing 3 ppm would provide 6 mg; hence, water-derived magnesium made a relatively small contribution. Others have found much greater contributions to the total intake of magnesium from water.[29b]

Elwood et al. in their study in England and Wales found no association between the myocardial content of magnesium or calcium and their levels in domestic tap water.[220] Hammer and Heyden summarized briefly a series of studies that failed to implicate a causal relationship between water hardness and heart disease, particularly mortality from cardiovascular disease.[221a] More recently, Leoni et al. recorded negative correlations for cardiovascular diseases and water hardness in 12 Italian locales during the period 1968-

1978.[221b] Hence, consensus regarding the role of hard water is lacking.

The observation that both the intake of magnesium of the American people and the age-adjusted death rate from ischemic heart disease in the United States have declined from earlier in the century[21a] suggests to me that the level of magnesium intake is not likely to be a significant etiologic factor in this disease. This view is supported by serum data studies.

**Serum Values of Magnesium of Patients with Acute Myocardial Infarction.** Although the data in various reports conflict, the majority noted that the patients' serum or plasma values decreased "soon after" or "upon admission" to the hospital. As indicated below, the time of drawing the sample is critical. Table 6–5 reviews some of the more recent data bearing on this issue. In the first three studies, magnesium values in the patients with acute myocardial infarction on day 1 were significantly less than controls, but only when there were complications[223] or when severe coronary artery disease was detected by angiography.[225] Patients in the coronary care unit (CCU) with or without infarction had similar magnesium values.[224] In the patients with coronary artery surgery, serum magnesium declined significantly postoperatively both in those suffering acute infarction and in those who did not. There was no significant difference between the two groups.[226]

In only two of these reports (Table 6–5) was there any mention of medications being used by the patients prior to the studies. Manthey et al. noted that the serum magnesium levels were significantly lower in the patients on either digitalis drugs or diuretics.[225] Dyckner noted that a significant minority of CCU patients with or without infarction had been on either digitalis or diuretic drugs.[224]

The study of Rector et al. revealed that by the third day postinfarction, serum magnesium levels had returned to normal in those with complications.[223] Urinary excretion of magnesium diminished on days 1 and 2 but was not significantly different from controls until the third day in those patients eating at least 85% of the daily diet. Because the infarcted myocardium loses magnesium and because there were decreases in both the serum and the urine of the infarcted patients, the data imply temporary redistribution of the magnesium within the body following acute infarction with complications.

It has been known for many years that lipolysis occurs soon after the onset of symptoms of acute myocardial infarction; similar changes have been noted with ethanol withdrawal, epinephrine administration, surgery, cold stress, and severe exercise.[227] Flink et al. found a mean rise of free fatty acids (FFA) of 0.56 meq/L (to about 3 times baseline) in 16 patients shortly after infarction,

**Table 6–5. Serum Magnesium in Patients with Advanced Coronary Artery Disease***

| Mg Units | Controls | Acute Infection or Ischemia AMI† | ACI† | Ref |
|---|---|---|---|---|
| mg/dl | 1.91 ± 0.03 (80) | 1.70 ± 0.04 (42)☆ | 1.61 ± 0.08 (9)‡ | 222 |
| mg/dl | 1.95 ± 0.23 | 1.97 ± 0.16‖ (27) 1.75 ± 0.19# (11)‡ 1.70 ± 0.26¶ (6)§ | 1.92 ± 0.23‖ (15) 1.92 ± 0.15 (7) (CHF) | 223 |
| mmol/L | Non-CCU 0.86 ± 0.11 (167) | CCU—AMI 0.82 ± 0.11 (392) | CCU—No AMI 0.82 ± 0.10 (563) | 224 |
| | | Coronary Lesions by Angiography | | |
| meq/L | None 1.78 ± 0.16 (31) | Moderate 1.72 ± 0.15 (31) | Severe 1.63 ± 0.16 (39) | 225 |
| | | Post-Operative Coronary By-Pass Surgery | | |
| | Post-Op: No AMI (20) | Post-Op: AMI (10) | Medical AMI (8) | |
| | Pre-op / Post-op | Pre-op / Post-op | | |
| mg/dl | 1.84 ± 0.2 / 1.43 ± 0.19 | 1.91 ± 0.14 / 1.48 ± 0.25 | 1.76 ± 0.15 | 226 |

*Analyses performed on blood drawn on day of admission or on occurrence of AMI
†AMI = Acute myocardial infarction
 ACI = Acute coronary ischemia
 CCU = Coronary care unit
 CHF = Congestive heart failure
☆P < 0.001 relative to control
‡P <0.01 relative to controls
§P <0.05 relative to controls
‖No complications
#Congestive failure with arrhythmias
¶Ventricular fibrillation
(  ) = Number of subjects; value X ± S.D.

this increase was associated with a decrease in magnesium level of 0.22 meq/L.[227] The rapid fall in FFA in the ensuing 48 to 72 hours was associated with a rise in serum magnesium to normal levels in 48 hours. It was suggested that FFA bind magnesium ions; this binding may result in decreased free $Mg^{2+}$ concentration, especially in patients depleted of magnesium by poor intake or diuretic treatments.

Despite the significant reduction noted in some patients with infarction or ischemia—especially in conjunction with complications or severe artery involvement—the reduced levels were not in the range that would be a cause for concern in terms of clinical magnesium depletion (i.e., <1.2 meq/L). The biochemical significance of these changes and their possible relation to arrhythmias are discussed below.

No association has been noted between the levels of serum magnesium and the presence or absence of clinically apparent chronic coronary artery disease.[228] On the other hand, there is some reduction—small but significant—in patients with painful conditions requiring acute surgery, in medical patients with painful disease states, and in women in labor; surgical, medical, or obstetric patients without pain had normal magnesium levels.[229]

**Magnesium in the Myocardium.** A moderate number of reports from 1969-1980 noted decreased magnesium in the myocardium of patients dying with ischemic heart disease.[29b]

When acute myocardial damage was induced in rats with isoprenaline, serum magnesium rose approximately 30 to 40% over predamage values in 30 to 60 minutes and then returned to normal, whereas heart magnesium declined by 40% in the same period and then made a partial recovery by 6 to 24 hours.[229] Measurement of intracellular free $Mg^{2+}$ in perfused beating guinea pig hearts by 31P NMR spectra of ATP revealed no difference between control hearts and those with ischemic arrest.[15c]

In human hearts obtained at necropsy, the left ventricles from individuals without infarction who died following acute trauma (controls) contained approximately 11% more magnesium than the right ventricles. Both ventricles (noninfarcted areas) from patients dying of acute myocardial infarction had 20 to 28% less magnesium than in the respective control ventricles. Magnesium in the infarcted areas of left ventricles was only one half that found in control left ventricles. Potassium, calcium, and sodium concentrations were also lower in the noninfarcted portions of the heart compared to those of controls. As the result of cytolysis and anoxia in the infarcted areas the

magnesium-calcium ratios were significantly inverted and the potassium-sodium ratios were significantly smaller.[230] No data were given about the medication history of the patients with infarction.

The causes and significance of the decreased magnesium content in ischemic hearts are not clear because there are many complicating factors and such information is not included in most of the published reports. These complicating factors include duration of the heart disease; prior medications and dietary therapies; elapsed time between the infarction, death, and tissue sampling; areas of sampling; and variability in sampling. Some of these factors have been noted, e.g., prior drugs[224] and sampling area.[230] The relation of the reported changes in tissue magnesium content on the overall state of magnesium nutrition is also uncertain.

### Cardiac Arrhythmias

Salts of magnesium (chloride or sulfate) have been used for 50 years in the treatment of atrial, junctional, and ventricular tachyarrhythmias occurring in patients with myocardial ischemia, alcoholism, digitalis toxicity, diuretic therapy, and other conditions.[80,231]

In recent years, interest and concern have been stimulated by reports of increased in vitro coronary artery tone ("spasms") and its possible relationship to sudden death in ischemic heart disease.[98] However, a contradictory report indicates that the concentration of $Mg^{2+}$ in the bath must be very low to induce even a moderate increase in tone.[99] (See section on Biochemistry and Physiologic Function; effect on muscle.)

These interventions have been based on physiologic considerations of electrolytes (including magnesium), membrane interactions, and calcium-magnesium antagonism,[80] as well as a report that magnesium-deficient monkeys and dogs had increased susceptibility to toxic arrhythmias from acetylstrophanthidin.[232] Iseri and French postulated that the beneficial effects of magnesium reside in its action as a calcium blocker and that magnesium depletion leads to loss of cellular potassium and to an increase in calcium, failure of membrane Ca-ATPase to extrude calcium from the cell, and influx of calcium into mitochondria.[233]

As noted earlier, digitalis drugs and diuretics are commonly prescribed for patients with cardiac disease.[224] Analysis of abnormal potassium and magnesium levels in 103 consecutive patients admitted to a CCU indicated that hypokalemia (< 3.5 meq/L) occurred in 18% and hypomagnesemia (<1.4 meq/L) was present in 24%.[234] Wester and Dyckner found hypokalemia in 30% of their magnesemic patients.[56c] Boyd et al. found the mean plasma concentrations of potassium and magnesium were lower in the group of patients treated with diuretic drugs compared with the nontreated group.[234]

Dyckner noted that the incidence of serious ventricular ectopic beats, ventricular tachycardia, and ventricular fibrillation on admission of patients to the CCU was higher in hypomagnesemic patients with acute myocardial infarction, as was the incidence of atrial fibrillation and supraventricular tachycardia[224]; on the other hand, atrioventricular block and supraventricular bradycardia were higher in the hypermagnesemic patients. In a series of 136 serum samples sent to the laboratory for digitalis estimation, hyponatremia was found in 21%, hypomagnesemia in 19%, and hypokalemia in 9%.[235]

An increase in sudden death was noted in the Multiple Risk Factor Intervention Trial (MRFIT) in a subgroup of patients with baseline electrocardiographic abnormalities who were part of the special intervention group of hypertensives who had received a higher dose of diuretics and who had developed a greater degree of hypokalemia; the latter was not uniformly corrected at the time the study was initiated because hypokalemia secondary to diuretic therapy was not believed to lead to ventricular ectopic activity in hypertensive patients without overt cardiac disease.[236] More recent studies provided evidence to the contrary.[237–239] Because hypokalemia and hypomagnesemia can be induced by the same mechanisms and are often clinically correlated with one another, magnesium as well as potassium should be routinely measured in patients given chronic diuretic therapy in which hypokalemia and hypomagnesemia may occur.[240] Electrolyte balance should be maintained. Alternatively, the choice of diuretic agents in patients with cardiac disorders should be to avoid those agents that induce hypokalemia and hypomagnesemia.

**Magnesium in Cardioplegic Solutions.** Such solutions are designed to induce rapid diastolic ischemic arrest, minimize the extent of ischemic injury, and prevent myocardial damage during reperfusion after aortocoronary bypass. The addition of magnesium to cardioplegic potassium solutions has been reported to mitigate the deleterious effects of excess calcium.[233] Experiments with rat and rabbit hearts suggest that the protective action of high magnesium content depends on its having a negative inotropic effect before the onset of ischemia. High magnesium content is effective with rat hearts but not with rabbit hearts and perhaps not with other species.[247a] Reduction of magnesium from 9 to 4

mmol/L improved post-ischemic recovery in dog models.[241b]

In a prospective randomized study of 76 patients undergoing coronary bypass grafting with varying concentrations of magnesium (0 or 0.25 meq/kg) in the solution during bypass with the aorta clamped or with 0.375 meq/kg before bypass, magnesium administration did not affect resumption of a cardiac rhythm or spontaneous defibrillation during reperfusion.[242] However, the number of shocks to initial and to sustained defibrillation and the energy required for the last direct-current shock were greatest in the patients who received magnesium before bypass and in those whose plasma magnesium was greater than 2.26 mg/dl (1.88 meq/L).

### Hypertension

Older studies have noted lower mean serum magnesium levels in hypertensive patients as compared to normal individuals (e.g., 1.4 vs 1.6 meq/L)[243] or lower values in hypertensive men but not women.[244] In an intervention study, hypertensive patients on diuretic therapy were given 365 mg of magnesium as the aspartate·HCl with a subsequent drop in blood pressure over 6 months with no change in plasma magnesium or other electrolytes.[245] One of a limited number of reports on magnesium intake in relation to the presence of hypertension indicated no difference from normotensives,[246] another indicated lower intake by hypertensives.[247]

Serum ionized calcium, total magnesium, and plasma renin activity were determined in 102 normotensive patients and 98 patients with essential hypertension; the latter had not been taking medications for at least 2 weeks and had essentially normal serum BUN and creatinine values.[248] Patients with low-renin hypertension had serum magnesium of $2.07 \pm 0.03$ meq/L, those with normal renin had $1.94 \pm 0.02$ meq/L, and those with high renin had $1.83 \pm 0.02$ meq/L. Each group was significantly different from the other, and the high- and low-renin groups differed significantly from the normotensive group, which had a magnesium value of $1.91 \pm 0.02$ meq/L. Opposite relationships were noted for serum ionized calcium; hypertensive patients with low renin had the lowest levels of ionized calcium ($2.09 \pm 0.03$ meq/L), which were significantly lower than those with normal-renin hypertension ($2.24 \pm 0.03$ meq/L) or patients with high-renin hypertension ($2.34 \pm 0.03$ meq/L). Again, the high- and low-renin groups were significantly different from the control group, which had values of $2.20 \pm 0.04$ meq/L. The range of variability within all groups covered essentially the normal clinical range.[248,249] Resnick

et al. also found a close inverse correlation between intracellular red-cell free $Mg^{2+}$ concentration, systolic blood pressure, and ionized extracellular $Ca^{2+}$ pressures. Untreated hypertensives
had the lowest values ($192 \pm 8$ $\mu M$); treated hypertensives were higher ($237 \pm 7.8$ $\mu M$), and normotensives highest ($261 \pm 9.8$ $\mu M$). The physiologic and biochemical relevance of these relatively
small but apparently statistically significant
changes is still unclear but may be related to
changes in intracellular $Ca^{2+}$, which could act by
affecting renin, parathyroid secretion, and vascular tone.

## HYPERMAGNESEMIA AND MAGNESIUM TOXICITY

Magnesium salts as cathartics have a long history and are still in use, with the sulfate, hydroxide, and citrate forms being commonly used. Their
slow and incomplete absorption from the digestive tract is used to explain water retention in the
lumen on the basis of osmotic forces.[251] Since 20%
or more of $Mg^{2+}$ may be absorbed, magnesium
salts may have a systemic effect and must be given
in reduced amounts or, better, avoided in the presence of renal insufficiency.

$Mg^{2+}$ may have a more direct effect on ion transport. In in vitro studies with short-circuited rabbit
terminal ileum, an increase in $Mg^{2+}$ as the chloride from 0.3 mmol/L (low basal) to 10.3 abolished
net sodium absorption and converted net chloride
absorption into net secretion.[252] These data suggest that at least part of the cathartic effect of magnesium salts is the result of the marked changes
in ileal ion transport.

The normal kidney is capable of excreting absorbed or injected magnesium ion so rapidly that
serum levels do not rise to clinically significant
levels. In the treatment of preeclampsia, eclampsia, and premature labor with magnesium salts,
relatively massive doses have been given as a loading dose followed by maintenance doses with the
objective of maintaining the serum level at 5 to 8
meq/L.[109–111] Patients with normal kidneys were
able to excrete 40 to 60 g of magnesium sulfate/
day.[253] Hypermagnesemia may develop in other
clinical situations in which magnesium-containing drugs, usually antacids or cathartics are given
to individuals with renal insufficiency or in
which large amounts of the ion are given inadvertently by the parenteral routes.[86] In acute renal
failure with oliguria, especially in the presence of
acidosis, tissue release in association with the
usual intake of magnesium will result in some
degree of hypermagnesemia.

Mordes and Wacker have reviewed in great detail the many and potentially lethal effects of mag-

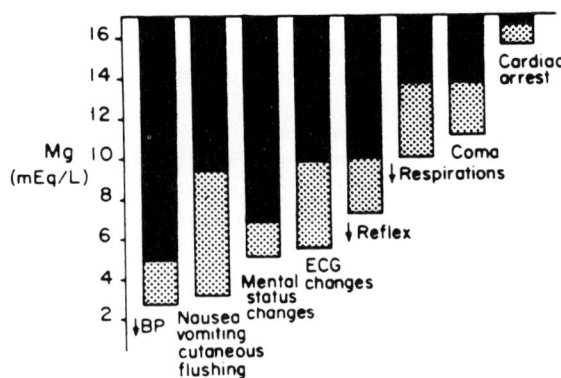

**Fig. 6–10.** The toxic effects of elevated serum magnesium progress in severity with increasing concentration. Nausea, vomiting and hypotension may occur in
the range of 3 to 9 meq/L; bradycardia and urinary retention also occur in this range. Electrocardiogram
changes, hyporeflexia, and secondary central nervous
system depression may appear in the 5- to 10-meq/L
range followed at higher concentrations by life-threatening respiratory depression, coma, and asystolic cardiac arrest. (From Mordes and Wacker,[86] with permission of the American Society of Pharmacology and
Experimental Therapeutics.)

nesium excess (Fig. 6–10).[86] As Mordes and
Wacker emphasize and as others had pointed out,
the widely held belief that magnesium is an anesthetic and a major central nervous system depressant is not correct unless magnesium is given
intrathecally or intraventricularly or is applied directly to nervous tissue. Uptake of magnesium
from the blood into the central nervous system is
quite limited. Calcium infusion counteracts magnesium toxicity.[86]

Avoidance of magnesium-containing medications in patients with significant renal disease is
recommended unless otherwise indicated and unless serum levels are closely monitored. Serum
magnesium determinations should be made in all
instances of acute renal failure at suitable intervals and monitored in chronic renal insufficiency.
Hypermagnesemia should be suspected in instances of low anion gap in stable patients and
normal anion gap in severely ill acidotic patients.[86]

## MAGNESIUM THERAPY IN DEPLETION

This review has noted the very large number of
clinical conditions and factors that can cause hypomagnesemia. Ideally the physician should
apply knowledge about predisposing conditions
and factors in order to anticipate hypomagnesemia and institute early therapeutic regimens to
prevent its occurrence. Such preventive measures
include instituting treatment of underlying dis-

ease, minimizing therapeutic insult, and initiating nutritional and dietary intervention to minimize or overcome magnesium losses in stool and urine.

When the patient presents for the first time with hypomagnesemia, it is essential to determine the etiology of the magnesium depletion. Usually this can be determined by a careful history to delineate intestinal and/or renal causes. If the cause is uncertain, a combination of serum and urine determinations is indicated. If the serum magnesium has fallen below the apparent threshold of the normal kidney (1.2–1.3 meq/L) for several days, renal excretion falls and only small amounts of magnesium (i.e., < 2 meq/day) should be present. If the renal tubular insufficiency is present, urinary magnesium will be appreciably higher, to the point of equalling or exceeding the magnesium absorbed from the intestine or that given parenterally.

The amount and route of magnesium administration will depend on the severity of depletion, its etiology, and the kidney function. Symptomatic deficiency is best treated by the intravenous or intramuscular route in conjunction with any indicated therapy for the underlying condition and with correction of other electrolyte and acid-base abnormalities. It is our practice to initiate treatment in symptomatic adolescents and adults with good renal function with 3 g (25 meq) of 50% magnesium sulfate given intravenously over 2 or 3 hours in saline or dextrose solutions, with other nutrients as required. Another 3 to 4 g are then given by continuous infusion over the remaining 24 hours or by periodic intramuscular injections. This administration is given daily for 2 or more days and the situation reassessed. An estimate of the degree of depletion may be obtained by measuring daily urinary magnesium levels during repletion. When a sudden increase in urine levels occurs, serum magnesium levels usually have become normal and the first goal of repletion has been achieved.

Intravenous calcium administration in the treatment of hypocalcemia secondary to magnesium deficiency is usually unnecessary unless overt or latent tetany is apparent; in this case, the calcium infusion is usually necessary only for several days as magnesium replacement takes effect.

The return to the normal range of serum magnesium with the above or higher dosage schedule is relatively rapid. Repletion of magnesium lost from bone and other tissues, however, requires a more prolonged period of magnesium therapy. This treatment should be combined—although at smaller doses or different routes if desirable— with periodic evaluation of serum and/or urine magnesium levels as the dosage is reduced until

a stable and adequate state is achieved with normal serum magnesium.

For the asymptomatic patient with serum levels below 1.0 meq/L, the dosage prescribed above is indicated; when the level is higher, half the dosage parenterally or orally should be sufficient unless renal losses are very high.

Where indicated and feasible, supplementary magnesium may be given as tablets of milk of magnesia (MgO) or as gelatin capsules packed with powdered magnesium sulfate (Epsom salts), magnesium chloride, or magnesium oxide; one capsule is given 3 to 6 times/day. Improvement of existing steatorrhea will decrease fecal magnesium losses. Treatment of other underlying disease and replacement of chronic potassium deficits are essential.

The need for prolonged magnesium therapy that cannot be met adequately by increased oral intake presents a practical problem. Intramuscular injection of magnesium salts is painful and often induces a fibrotic reaction. The alternative is intravenous infusion or the old-fashioned but useful hypodermic clysis. In the latter procedure a dilute solution of 50% magnesium sulfate (e.g., 2 g) in 250 ml of 0.45% saline is infused slowly through a small needle inserted under the skin over the abdomen as frequently as is necessary to meet the patient's magnesium requirement. The intravenous route may be through a peripheral line, through percutaneous catheter into the subclavian vein, or, for very prolonged infusion, via a tunneled central venous catheter or subcutaneously implanted reservoir (e.g., Mediport). For the patient with serious persistent renal wasting from cisplatin toxicity, for example, the tunneled catheter or reservoir is very useful. Using this catheter, the daily requirement for magnesium (together with any other electrolytes that are needed) may be given at home in a matter of 2 to 4 hours nightly or, less frequently, if so indicated. Periodic assessment of serum magnesium levels prior to periodic infusion allows an estimate of stable or changing needs.

Alternative programs of magnesium replacement in deficient adults have been utilized, usually with higher doses than advocated here. Flink, for example, recommended 112 to 128 meq intramuscularly or intravenously over the first day, with smaller doses subsequently.[253] The larger the dose and the faster the rate of administration, the higher the serum level achieved and the greater the amount excreted by the normal kidney. Flink reported that 50 meq of I.V. magnesium given over 12 hours raised serum levels to 2.0 to 3.3 meq/L, while 100 meq in 12 hours raised the levels to 3 to 3 meq, with some subjects having serum values up to 5.5 meq/L with continued infusion.[253]

Experience in the treatment of symptomatic magnesium depletion in infants is unanimous concerning the rapid efficacy of relatively small amounts of intravenous or intramuscular magnesium in controlling neurologic signs and restoring serum levels.[254–256] Parenteral administration is recommended at 0.3 to 0.5 meq (3.6–6 mg)/kg body weight as 50% magnesium sulfate over the first several hours, followed by an equal amount either I.M. or I.V. over the remainder of the day. If the child is symptomatic, calcium should also be infused, with potassium and other electrolytes, as indicated. Duration, route of administration, and dosage will depend on the severity and cause of the depletion.

Where malabsorption is serious, as in primary magnesium depletion in children, 1.0 to 1.5 meq/kg in multiple divided oral doses should be tested; experience has indicated that this dosage schedule raises serum levels to near normal without inducing diarrhea.[132]

## REFERENCES

1. Kruse, H.D., Orent, E.R., McCollum, E.V.: J Biol Chem *96*:519–539, 1932.
2. Shils, M.E.: Ann NY Acad Sci *355*:165–180, 1980.
3. Hirschfelder, A.D., Haury, V.G.: JAMA *102*:1138–1141, 1934.
4a. Flink, E.B., Stutzman, F., Anderson, A.R., et al.: J Lab Clin Med *43*:169–183, 1954.
4b. Flink, E.B.: J Am Coll Nutr *4*:17–31, 1985.
5. Walser, M.: Erg Physiol *59*:185–196, 1967.
6. Widdowson, E.M., McCance, R.A., Spray, C.M.: Clin Sci *10*:113–125, 1951.
7. Schroeder, H.A., Nason, A.P., Tipton, I.H.: J Chron Dis *21*:815–841, 1969.
8. Iyengar, G.V., Kollmer, W.E., Bowen, H.J.M.: The Elemental Composition of Human Tissues and Body Fluids. New York, Verlag, 1978.
9. Watson, W.S., Lyon, T.D.B., Hilditch, T.E.: Metab Clin Exp *29*:397–399, 1980.
10a. Tsang, R.C.: Am J Dis Child *124*:282–294, 1972.
10b. Wacker, W.E.C., Parisi, A.F.: N Engl J Med *278*:712–717, 1968.
11. Consolazio, C.F., Matoush, L.O., Nelson, R.A., et al.: J Nutr *79*:407–415, 1963.
12. Alfrey, A.C., Miller, N.L.: J Clin Invest *52*:3019–3027, 1973.
13. Ebel, H., Gunther, T.: J Clin Chem Clin Biochem *18*:257–270, 1980.
14. Erdos, J.J., Vauquelin, G., Cech, S.Y., et al.: Adv Cycl Nucleot Res *14*:69–81, 1981.
15a. Shulman, R.G., Brown, T.R., Urgubil, K., et al.: Science *205*:160–166, 1979.
15b. Gupta, R.K., Moore, R.D.: J Biol Chem *255*:3987–3993, 1980.
15c. Wu, S.T., Pieper, G.M., Salhany, J.M., et al.: Biochemistry *22*:7399–7403, 1981.
16a. Alcock, N.W.: Ann NY Acad Sci *162*:707–716, 1969.
16b. Willis, J.B.: Clin Chem *11*(Suppl):251–258, 1965.

17. Scarpa, A., Brinkley, J.: Fed Proc *40*:2646–2652, 1981.
18. Altura, B.M., Altura, B.T.: Magnesium *4*:245–271, 1985.
19a. Aikawa, J.K., Gordon, G.S., Rhoades, E.L.: J Appl Physiol *15*:503–507, 1960.
19b. Avioli, L.V., Berman, M.: J Appl Physiol *21*:1688–1694, 1960.
20a. Schwartz, R.: Fed Proc *41*:2709–2713, 1982.
20b. Schwartz, R., Spencer, H., Welsh, J.J.: Am J Clin Nutr *39*:571–576, 1984.
21a. U.S. Dept Health and Human Svcs., Dept of Agriculture: Nutrition Monitoring in the U.S. DHHS Publ #86-1255. Pub. Health Svce U.S. Gov't Printing Office Washington D.C., July 1986.
21b. Lakshmanan, F.L., Rao, R.B., Kim, W.W., et al.: Am J Clin Nutr *40*:1380–1389, 1984.
22. Brannan, P.G., Vergne-Marini, P., Pak, C.Y.C.: J Clin Invest *57*:1412–1418, 1976.
23. Behar, J.: Am J Physiol *227*:334–340, 1974.
24. Norman, D.A., Fordtran, J.S., Brinkley, L.J., et al.: J Clin Invest *67*:1599–1603, 1981.
25. O'Dell, B.L.: Fed Proc *19*:648–654, 1960.
26a. Spencer, H., Lesniak, M., Gatza, L.A., et al.: Gastroenterology *79*:26–34, 1980.
26b. Spencer, H., Lesniak, M., Kramer, L., et al.: Studies of magnesium metabolism in man. *In* Magnesium in Health and Disease. Edited by M.S. Seelig. New York, Spectrum Publishers, 1980, pp 911–919.
26c. Spencer, H.: J Am Diet Assoc *86*:864–867, 1986.
26d. Spencer, H., Kramer, L., Gatza, C., et al.: Magnesium-phosphorus interactions in man. *In* Trace Substances in Environmental Health-XIII. Editd by D.D. Hemphill. Columbia, Univ. Missouri, 1979.
27. Milla, P.J., Agett, P.J., Wolff, O.H., et al.: Gut *20*:1028–1033, 1979.
28. Graham, L.A., Ceasar, J.J., Burgen, A.S.U.: Metab Clin Exper *9*:646–659, 1960.
29a. Seelig, M.S.: Am J Clin Nutr *14*:342–390, 1964.
29b. Marier, J.R.: Magnesium *1*:3–15, 1982.
30a. Greger, J.L., Baligar, R.P., Abernathy, O.A., et al.: Am J Clin Nutr *31*:117–121, 1978.
30b. Johnson, M.A., Baier, M.J., Greger, J.L.: Am J Clin Nutr *35*:1332–1338, 1982.
31a. Kelsay, J.L., Behall, K.M., Prather, E.S.: Am J Clin Nutr *32*:1876–1880, 1979.
31b. Slavin, J.L., Marlett, J.A.: Am J Clin Nutr *33*:1932–1939, 1980.
32. Mahalko, J.R., Sandstead, H.H., Johnson, L.K.: Am J Clin Nutr *37*:8–14, 1983.
33. Fox J., Care A.D.: *In* Calcified Tissues. Copenhagen, FADL's Forlag, 1976, p 147.
34. Hodgkinson, A., Marshall, D.H., Nordin, B.E.E.: Clin Sci *57*:121–123, 1979.
35. Wilz, D.R., Gary, R.W., Dominquez, J.H., et al.: Am J Clin Nutr *32*:2052–2060, 1979.
36. Sorensen, E., Tougaard, L., Brochner-Mortensen, J.: Br Med J *2*:215, 1979.
37. Krejs, G.J., Nicar, M.J., Zewekh, J.E., et al.: Am J Med *75*:973–976, 1983.
38. Schmulen, A.C., Lerman, M., Pak, C.Y.C., et al.: Am J Physiol *238*:G349–G352, 1980.
39. Clarkson, E.M., McDonald, S.J., DeWardener, E., et al.: Clin Sci *28*:107–115, 1965.
40. Kopple, J.D., Coburn, J.W.: Medicine *52*:597–607, 1973.
41. Dinks, J.H.: Kidney Intl *23*:771–777, 1983.
42. Heaton, F.W.: Ann NY Acad Sci *162*:775–785, 1969.

43. Quamme, G.A., Dirks, J.H.: Am J Physiol *238*:F393–F401, 1980.
44. LeGrimellec, C., Roinel, N., Morel, F.: Pfluegers Arch *340*:181–196, 1973.
45a.Quamme, G.A., Dirks, J.H.: Am J Physiol *238*:F187–F198, 1980.
45b.Carney, S.L., Wong, N.L.M., Quamme, G.A., et al.: J Clin Invest *65*:180–188, 1980.
46. Shils, M.E.: Am J Clin Nutr *15*:133–143, 1964.
47. Shils, M.E.: Medicine *48*:61–85, 1969.
48. Massry, S.G., Coburn, J.W., Kleeman, C.R.: Am J Physiol *216*:1460–1467, 1969.
49. Wong, N.L., Dirks, J.H., Quamme, G.A.: Am J Physiol *244*:F78–F83, 1983.
50. Horton, R., Biglieri, E.G.: J Clin Endocrinol Metab *22*:1187–1192, 1962.
51. Hulter, H.N., Paterson, J.C.: Metabolism *33*:662–666, 1984.
52a.Gitelman, H.J., Graham, J.B., Welt, L.G.: Ann NY Acad Sci *162*:856–864, 1969.
52b.Evans, R.A., Carter, J.N., George, C.R.P., et al.: Quart J Med Ser L No: *197*:39–52, 1981.
52c.Bardgette, J.J., Stein, J.H.: Pathophysiology of Bartter's syndrome. *In* Acid-Base and Potassium Homeostasis. Edited by B.M. Brenner and J.H. Stein. New York, Churchill-Livingstone, 1978, p 272.
52d.Milazzo, S.C., Ahern, M.J., Cleland, L.G.: J Rheumatol *8*:767–771, 1981.
53. Old, C.W., Siedlecki, M., Duarte, C.G., et al.: Magnesium *3*:95–106, 1984.
54. McCallister, R.J., Flink, E.B., Lewis, M.D.: Am J Clin Nutr *12*:415–420, 1963.
55. Wong, N.L., Quamme, G.A., Sutton, R.A., et al.: J Lab Clin Med *94*:683–692, 1979.
56a.Duarte, C.G.: Metabolism *17*:867–876, 1968.
56b.Sheehan, J., White, A.: Br Med J *285*:1157–1159, 1982.
56c.Wester, P.O., Dyckner, T.: Acta Pharmacol Toxicol (Copenh) *54*:(Suppl) 59–65, 1984.
56d.Wong, N.L.M., Quamme, G.A., Dirks, J.H.: Can J Physiol Pharmacol *60*:1160–1165, 1982.
57. Davis, B.B., Preuss, H.G., Murdaugh, H.V., Jr.: Nephron *14*:275–280, 1975.
58. Burges, A.L., Birchall, R.: Am J Med *53*:77–84, 1972.
59. Schilsky, R.L., Anderson, T.: Ann Intern Med *90*:929–931, 1979.
60. Blachley, J.D., Hill, J.B.: Ann Intern Med *95*:628–632, 1981.
61. Ozols, R.F., Corden, B.J., Jacob, J., et al.: Ann Intern Med *100*:19–24, 1984.
62a.Bar, R.G., Wilson, H.E., Mazzaferri, E.C.: Ann Intern Med *82*:646–649, 1975.
62b.Kelnar, C.J.H., Taor, W.S., Reynolds, D.J.: Arch Dis Child *53*:817–820, 1978.
63. Thompson, C.B., June, C.H., Sullivan, K.M., et al.: Lancet *2*:1116–1120, 1984.
64a.Dominquez, J.H., Gray, R.W., Lemann, J., Jr.: J Clin Endocrinol Metab *43*:1056–1068, 1976.
64b.Kreusser, W., Kurakawa, K., Azner, E., et al.: J Clin Invest *61*:573–581, 1978.
64c.Wong, N.L., Quamme, G.E., O'Callaghan, T., et al.: Canad J Physiol Pharmacol *58*:1063–1071, 1980.
65a.Drenick, E.J., Hunt, I.F., Swendseid, M.E.: J Clin Endocrinol *29*:1341–1348, 1969.
65b.Butler, A.M.: N Engl J Med *234*:648–656, 1950.
65c.Lennon, E.J., Piering, W.F.: J Clin Invest *49*:1458–1468, 1970.
65d.Wong, N.L.M., Quamme, G.A., Dirks, J.H.: J Clin Invest Med *5*:44B, 1982.
66. Jones, J.E., Desper, P.C., Shane, S.R., et al.: J Clin Invest *45*:891–900, 1966.
67. Quamme, G.A.: Am J Physiol *283*:E573–E578, 1980.
68. Ryan M.P., Devane, J., Ryan, M.F., et al.: Drugs *28*(Suppl 1):167–181, 1984.
69. Kantziger, H., Amiel, C., Roinel, N., et al.: Am J Physiol *227*:905–911, 1974.
70a.Sharego, G.R., Agus, Z.S.: J Clin Invest *69*:759–769, 1982.
70b.Bailly, C., Roinel, H., Amiel, C.: Am J Physiol *246*:Pt2, F205–F212, 1984; Pflueger's Arch *403*:28–34, 1985.
71. Quamme, G.A., Carney, S.L., Wong, N.L.M., et al.: Pfluger's Archiv *386*:59–65, 1980.
72. McCaffrey, C., Quamme, G.A.: Can J Comp Med *48*:51–57, 1984.
73. Barnes, B.A., Cope, O., Gordon, E.B.: Ann Surg *152*:518–533, 1960.
74. Heaton, F.W.: Ann NY Acad Sci *162*:775–785, 1969.
75. Marone, C.C., Sutton, R.A.: Metabolism *32*:1033–1037, 1983.
76. Dr. M.L. Brown: Personal communication.
77. Food Nutrition Bd NRC-NAS: J Nutrition *116*:482–488, 1986.
78. Wacker, W.E.C.: Ann NY Acad Sci *162*:717–726, 1969.
79. Gunther, T.: Artery *9*:167–181, 1981.
80. Shine, K.L.: Am J Physiol *237*:H413–H423, 1979.
81. Anast, C.S., Gardner, D.W.: Magnesium metabolism. *In* Disorders of Mineral Metabolism: Pathophysiology of Calcium, Phosphorus and Magnesium. (Edited by F. Bronner and J.W. Coburn.) New York, Academic Press, 1981, pp 423–522.
82. Altura, B.M., et al.: Symposium: Role of magnesium ions in regulation of muscle contraction. Fed Proc *40*:2645–2679, 1981.
83. Betz, E., Heuser, D.: Adv Neurol *20*:71–76, 1978.
84. Seelig, J.M., Wei, E.P., Kontos, H.A., et al.: Am J Physiol *245*:H22–H26, 1983.
85. Cronin, R.E., Knochel, J.P.: Adv Intern Med 509–533, 1983.
86. Mordes, J.P., Wacker, W.E.C.: Pharmacological Rev *29*:274–300, 1978.
87. Robison, G.A., Butcher, R.W., Sutherland, E.W.: Cyclic AMP. New York, Academic Press, 1971.
88. Lefkowitz, R.J., Caron, M.G., Stiles, G.L.: New Engl J of Med *310*:1569–1579, 1984.
89. Spiegel, A.M., Gierschik, P., Levine, M.A., et al.: N Engl J Med *312*:26–33, 1985.
90. Severson, D.L., Drummond, G.I., Sulakhe, P.V.: J Biol Chem *247*:2949–2958, 1972.
91. Williams, L.T., Mullikin, D., Lefkowitz, R.J.: J Biol Chem *253*:2984–2989, 1978.
92. Cech, S.Y., Broadus, W.C., Maguire, M.E.: Mol Cell Biochem *33*:67–92, 1980.
93. Abramowitz, J., Iyengar, R., Birnbaumer, L.: Endocrinology *110*:330–346, 1982.
94. Burrows, G.H., Barnes, A.J.: Neurochem *38*:569–573, 1982.
95. Potter, J.D., Robertson, S.P., Johnson, J.D.: Fed Proc *40*:2653–2656, 1981.
96. Hasselbalch, W., Fassold, E., Migala, A., et al.: Fed Proc *40*:2657–2661, 1981.
97. Somylo, A.P., Somylo, A.V.: Fed Proc *40*:2667–2671, 1981.

98a.Altura, B.M., Altura, B.T.: Fed Proc *40*:2672–2679, 1981.

98b.Altura, B.M., Altura, B.T.: Magnesium *4*:245–271, 1985.

99. Kalsner, S.: Br J Pharmacol *78*:629–638, 1983.

100a.McLean, F.C., Hastings, A.B.: Am J Med Sci *189*:601–613, 1935.

100b.Copp, D.H., Davidson, A.G.F.: Proc Soc Exp Biol Med *107*:342–344, 1961.

100c.Sherwood, L.M., Potts, Jr., J.T., Care, A.D., et al.: Nature (London) *209*:52–55, 1966.

101a.Buckle, R.M., Care, A.D., Copper, C.W., et al.: J Endocrinol *42*:529–534, 1968.

101b.Brown, E.M., Thatcher, J.G., Watson, E.J., et al.: Metabolism *33*:171–176, 1984.

102. Shoback, D.M., Thatcher, J.G., Brown, E.M.: Mol Cell Endocrinol *38*:179–186, 1984.

103. Targovnik, J.H., Rodman, J.S., Sherwood, L.M., Endocrinology *88*:1477–1482, 1971.

104. Habener, J.F., Potts, Jr., J.T.: Endocrinology *98*:197–202, 1976.

105. Mayer, G.D., Hurst, J.G.: Endocrinology *102*:1803–1807, 1978.

106. Mahaffee, D.D., Cooper, C.W., Ramp, W.K., et al.: Endocrinology *110*:487–495, 1982.

107. Oldham, S.B., Molloy, C.T., Lipson, L.G.: Endocrinology *114*:207–214, 1984.

108. Oldham, S.B., Rude, R.K., Molloy, C.T., et al.: Endocrinology *115*:1883–1890, 1984.

109. Cholst, I.N., Steinberg, S.F., Tropper, P.J., et al.: N Engl J Med *310*:1221–1225, 1984.

110. Donovan, E.F., Tsang, R.C., Steichen, J.J., et al.: J Pediat *96*:305–310, 1980.

111. Cruikshank, D.P., Pitkin, R.M., Reynolds, W.A., et al.: Am J Obstet Gynecol *134*:243–249, 1979.

112. Slatopolsky, E., Mercado, A., Morrison, J.A., et al.: J Clin Invest *58*:1273–1279, 1976.

113. McGonigle, R.J., Weston, M.J., Keenan, J., et al.: Magnesium *3*:1–7, 1984.

114. Levine, B.S., Coburn, J.W.: N Engl J Med *310*:1253–1254, 1984.

115. Belanger, L.F., Van Erkel, G.A., Jakerow, A.: Science *126*:29–30, 1957.

116. Kraeuter, S.L., Schwartz, R.: J Nutrition *110*:851–858, 1980.

117. Jasmin, G.: Rev Cancer Biol *22*:383–390, 1963.

118. Bois, P., Sanborn, E.B., Messier, P.E.: Cancer Res *29*:763–775, 1969.

119. Hass, G., Laing, G., Galt, R., et al.: Magnesium Bull *1*:217–228, 1981.

120. Alcock, N.W., Shils, M.E., Lieberman, P.H., et al.: Cancer Res *33*:2196–2204, 1973.

121. Alcock, N.W., Shils, M.E.: Proc Soc Exp Biol Med *145*:855–858, 1974.

122. McCoy, J.H., Kenney, M.A.: J Nutrition *105*:791–797, 1975.

123a.Kessner, D., Epstein, F.: Proc Soc Exp Biol Med *122*:721–725, 1966.

123b.Chou, H., Wasserman, R., Schwartz, R.: Proc Soc Exp Biol Med *159*:171–175, 1978.

123c.Krawitt, E.L.: Proc Soc Exp Biol Med *141*:569–572, 1972.

123d.Rayssiguier, Y., Carre, M., Ayigbede, O., et al.: C R Acad Sci Paris Ser D *281*:731–734, 1975.

124a.Whang, R., Oliver, J., Welt, L.G., et al.: Ann NY Acad Sci *162*:766–774, 1969.

124b.Heggtveit, H.A.: Ann NY Acad Sci *162*:758–765, 1969.

125a.Bunce, G.E., Saacke, R.G., Mullins, J.: Exp Mol Pathol *33*:203–210, 1980.

125b.Rushton, H.G., Spector, M.: J Urology *127*:598–604, 1982.

126. Alcock, N.W., Shils, M.E.: Proc Soc Exp Biol Med *146*:137–141, 1974.

127. Shils, M.E.: Magnesium deficiency and calcium and parathyroid hormone interrelation. *In* Trace Elements in Human Health and Disease. Vol. 2 (Edited by A. Prasad) New York, Academic Press, 1976.

128. Fitzgerald, M.G., Fourman, P.: Clin Sci *15*:635–647, 1956.

129. Barnes, B.A., Cope, O., Gorden, E.B.: Ann Surg *152*:518–533, 1960.

130. Dunn, M.J., Walser, M.: Metabolism *15*:884–895, 1966.

131a.Orent, E.R., Kruse, H.D., McCollum, E.V.: J Biol Chem *106*:573–593, 1934.

131b.Jones, J.E., Schwartz, R., Krook, L.: Calc Tissue Int *31*:231–238, 1980.

132. Strømme, J.H., Steen-Johnsen, J., Harnaes, K., et al.: Pediatr Res *15*:1134–1139, 1981.

133. Garty, R., Arkalay, A., Bernheim, J.L.: Isr J Med Sci *19*:345–348, 1983.

134. McManus, J., Heaton, F.W.: Clin Sci *36*:297–306, 1969.

135. Suh, S.M., Csima, A., Fraser, D.: J Clin Invest *50*:2668–2678, 1971.

136. Goldman, R.H., Kleiger, R.E., Schweizer, E., et al.: Proc Soc Exp Biol Med *136*:747–749, 1971.

137. Levi, J., Massy, S.G., Coburn, J.N., et al.: Metabolism *23*:323–335, 1974.

138. Freitag, J.J., Martin, K.J., Conrades, E., et al.: J Clin Invest *64*:1238–1244, 1979.

139. Cronin, R.E., Ferguson, E.R., Shannon, Jr., W.A., et al.: Am J Physiol *243*:F113–F120, 1982.

140. Webb, S., Chade, D.S.: JAMA *233*:23–24, 1975.

141. Medalle, R., Waterhouse, C.: Ann Intern Med *79*:76–79, 1973.

142. Whang, R., Oei, T.O., Aikawa, J.K., et al.: Arch Intern Med *144*:1794–1796, 1984.

143. Jones, J.E., Shane, S.R., Jacobs, W.H., et al.: Ann NY Acad Sci *162*:934–946, 1969.

144. Gerlach, K., Morowitz, D.A., Kirsner, J.B.: Gastroenterology *59*:567–574, 1970.

145. Caddell, J.L., Goddard, D.R.: N Engl J Med *276*:535–540, 1967.

146. Back, E.H., Montgomery, R.D., Ward, E.E.: Arch Dis Child *37*:106–109, 1962.

147. Suh, S.M., Tashjian, A.H., Jr., Matsuo, N.: J Clin Invest *52*:153–160, 1973.

148. Bunce, G.E., Jenkins, K.J., Phillips, P.H.: J Nutr *76*:17–22, 1962.

149. MacIntyre, I., Boss, I., Troughton, V.A.: Nature *198*:1058–1060, 1963.

150. Robeson, B.C., Maddox, T.L., Martin, W.G.: J Nutr *109*:1383–1389, 1979.

151. Breibart, S., Lee, G.S., McCoord, A., et al.: Proc Soc Exp Biol Med *105*:361–363, 1960.

152. Mirra, J.M., Alcock, N.W., Shils, M.E., et al.: Magnesium *1*:16–33, 1982.

152a.Reddy, C.R., Coburn, J.W., Hartenbower, D.L., et al.: J Clin Invest *52*:3000–3010, 1973.

153. Alfrey, A.C., Miller, N., Trow, R.: J Clin Invest *54*:1074–1081, 1974.

154. Alfrey, A.C., Miller, N., Butkus, D.: J Lab Clin Med *84*:153–162, 1974.

155. MacIntyre, I., Hanna, S.S., Booth, C.C., et al.: Clin Sci 20:297–305, 1961.
156. Booth, C.C., Barbouris, N., Hanna, S., et al.: Br Med J 2:141–144, 1963.
157. Montgomery, R.D.: Lancet 2:74–75, 1960.
157a. Muldowney, F.P., McKenna, T.J., Kyle, L.H., et al.: N Engl J Med 281:61–68, 1970.
158. Lim, P., Jacobs, E.: J Lab Clin Med 80:313–321, 1972.
159. Stendig-Lindberg, G., Bergstrom, J., Hultman, E.: Acta Med Scand 201:273–280, 1977.
160. Baldwin, D., Robinson, P.K., Zierler, K.L., et al.: J Clin Invest 31:850–858, 1952.
161. Whang, R., Welt, L.G.: J Clin Invest 42:305–313, 1963.
162. Grace, N.D., O'Dell, B.L.: J Nutr 100:45–50, 1970.
163. Alleyne, G.A.O., Millward, D.J., Scullard, G.H.: J Pediatr 76:75–81, 1970.
164. Drenick, E.G., Hunt, J.F., Swendseid, M.E.: J Clin Endocrinology 29:1341–1348, 1969.
165. Gitelman, H.J., Kukolj, S., Welt, L.G.: J Clin Invest 47:118–126, 1968.
166. MacManus, J., Heaton, F.W., Lucas, P.W.: J Endocrinol 49:253–258, 1971.
167. Hahn, T.J., Chase, L.R., Avioli, L.V.: J Clin Invest 51:886–891, 1972.
168. Anast, C.S., Mohs, J.M., Kaplan, et al.: Science 177:606–609, 1972.
169. Anast, C.S., Winnacker, J.L., Forte, L.R., et al.: J Clin Endocrinol Metab 42:707–717, 1976.
170. Rude, R.K., Oldham, S.B., Sharp, C.F., Jr., et al.: J Clin Endocrinol Metab 47:800–806, 1978.
171. Raisz, L.G., Niemann, J.: Endocrinology 85:446–452, 1969.
172. MacManus, J., Heaton, F.W.: Biochem Biophys Acta 215:360–367, 1970.
173. Pak, C.Y.C., Diller, E.C.: Calc Tissue Res 4:69–77, 1969.
174. Johannesson, A.J., Raisz, L.G.: Endocrinol 113:2294–2298, 1983.
175a. Rayssiguier, Y., Thomasset, M., Garel, J.M., et al.: Horm Metab Res 14:379–382, 1982.
175b. Anast, C.S., Forte, L.F.: Endocrinology 113:184–189, 1983.
176. Lifshitz, F., Harrison, H.C., Harrison, H.E.: Endocrinology 81:849–853, 1967.
177. Petersen, V.P.: Acta Med Scand 173:285–298, 1973.
178. Rosler, A., Rabinowitz, D.: Lancet 1:803–804, 1973.
179. Medalle, R., Waterhouse, C., Hahn, T.J.: Am J Clin Nutr 29:854–858, 1976.
180. Graber, M.L., Schulman, G.: Ann Intern Med 104:804–805, 1986.
181. Tanaka, Y., DeLuca, H.F.: Proc Natl Acad Sci USA 78:196–199, 1981.
182. Garabedian, M., Tanaka, Y., Holick, M.F., et al.: Endocrinology 94:1022–1027, 1974.
183. Jacobs, A.L., Pennell, J.P., Lambert, P.W., et al.: Min Elect Metab 6:316–322, 1981.
184. Ralston, S., Boyle, I.T., Cowan, R.A., et al.: Acta Endocrinologica 103:535–538, 1983.
185. Harrison, H.E., Harrison, H.C.: Yale J Biol Med 24:273–283, 1952.
186. Bellin, S.A., Herting, D.C., Cramer, J.W., et al.: Arch Biochem Biophys 50:18–24, 1954.
187. Simpson, D.P.: Am J Physiol 244:F223–F234, 1983.
188. Hanna, S., Alcock, N., Lazarus, B., et al.: J Lab Clin Med 61:220–229, 1963.

189. Lifschitz, F., Harrison, H.C., Bull, E.C., et al.: Metabolism 16:345–357, 1967.
190. Rudman, D., Didonis, J.L., Fountain, M.T., et al.: N Engl J Med 303:657–661, 1980.
191. Whang, R., Aikawa, J.K., Oei, T.O., et al.: Routine serum magnesium determinations—an unrecognized need. In Magnesium in Health and Disease. Edited by M. Cantin and M.S. Seelig. New York, Spectrum Publishers, 1980, pp 1–5.
192. Wong, E.T., Rude, R.K., Singer, F.R., et al.: Am J Clin Pathol 79:348–352, 1983.
193a. Whang, R., Oei, T., Aikawa, J.K., et al.: Arch Intern Med 144:1794–1796, 1984.
193b. Boyd, J.C., Bruns, D.E., Wills, M.R.: Clinical Chem 29:178–179, 1983.
194. Sullivan, J.F., Wolpert, P.N., Williams, R., et al.: Ann NY Acad Sci 162:947–962, 1969.
195. Martin, H.E.: Ann NY Acad Sci 162:891–900, 1969.
196. Tsang, R.C., Strub, R., Brown, D.R., et al.: J Pediatr 89:115–119, 1976.
197. Ewald, U., Gebre-Medhin, M., Tuvemo, T.: Acta Paediatr Scand 72:367–371, 1983.
198. Gerlach, K., Morowitz, D.A., Kirsner, J.B.: Gastroenterology 59:567–574, 1970.
199. Main, A.N.H., Morgan, R.J., Russell, R.I., et al.: J Parenteral Enteral Nutr 5:15–19, 1981.
200. Rosen, E.U., Campbell, P.G., Moosa, G.M.: J Pediatr 72:709–714, 1970.
201. Linder, G.C., Hansen, J.D.L., Karabus, C.D.: Pediatr 31:552–568, 1963.
202. Nichols, B.L., Alvarado, J., Hazlewood, C.F., et al.: Am J Clin Nutr 31:176–188, 1978.
203. Meunes, P., Rosenbaum, R., Martin, K., et al.: Ann Intern Med 88:206–209, 1978.
204. Krebs, R.A., Neal, B.J., et al.: JAMA 241:722–723, 1979.
205. Petka, P., Bernstein, D.S., Hampers, C.L., et al.: Lancet 2:462–463, 1961; Metabolism 23:619–630, 1974.
206. Mace, J.W., Hambidge, M., Gotlin, R.W., et al.: Arch Dis Childh 48:485–487, 1973.
207. Baehler, R.W., Work, J., Kotchen, T.A., et al.: Am J Med 69:933–938, 1980.
208. Güllner, H.-G., Bartter, F.C., Gill, J.R., Jr., et al.: Arch Intern Med 143:1534–1540, 1983.
209. Güllner, H.-G., Gill, J.R., Jr., Bartter, F.C.: Am J Med 71:578–582, 1981.
210. Jones, C.T.A., Sellwood, R.A., Evanson, J.M.: Br Med J 3:391–392, 1973.
211. Christiansen, C., Nielson, S.P., Rodero, P.: Br Med J 1:98–99, 1974.
212. Katz, S.H., Gerstman, J., Lautenbacher, H.W., et al.: Br Med J 1:341, 1976.
213. Heipertz, R., Eickhoff, K., Karstens, K.H.: J Neurol Sci 41:55–60, 1979.
214. Yassa, R., Schwartz, G.: NY State J Med 84:114–115, 1984.
215. Seelig, M.S., Heggtviet, H.A.: Am J Clin Nutr 27:59–79, 1974.
216. Altura, B.M., Altura, B.T.: Magnesium 4:226–244, 1985.
217. Crawford, T., Crawford, M.D.: Lancet 1:229–232, 1967.
218. Anderson, T.W., Neri, L.C., Schreiber, G., et al.: Canad Med Assoc J 113:199–203, 1975.
219. Luoma, H., Aromaa, A., Helminen, S., et al.: Acta Med Scand 213:171–176, 1983.
220. Elwood, P.C., Sweetnam, P.M., Beasley, W.H., et al.: Lancet 2:720–722, 1980.

221a.Hammer, D.I., Heyden, S.: JAMA *243*:2399–2400, 1980.

221b.Leoni, V., Fabiani, L., Tichiarelli, L.: Arch Environ Health *40*:274–278, 1985.

222. Abraham, A.S., Eylath, V., Weinstein, M., et al.: N Engl J Med *296*:862, 1977.

223. Rector, W.G., Jr., DeWood, M.A., Williams, R.V., et al.: Am J Med Sci *281*:25–29, 1981.

224. Dyckner, T.: Acta Med Scand *207*:59–66, 1980.

225. Manthey, J., Stoeppler, M., Morgenstern, W., et al.: Circulation *64*:722–729, 1981.

226. Forster, A., Stalder, R., Bloch, A., et al.: J Cardiovasc Surg *22*:163–165, 1981.

227. Flink, E.B., Brick, J.E., Sliane, S.R.: Arch Intern Med *141*:441–443, 1981.

228. Abraham, A.S., Weinstein, M., Eylath, V., et al.: Am J Clin Nutr *31*:1400–1402, 1978.

229. Abraham, A.S., Shaoul, R., Shimonovitz, S., et al.: Biochem Med *24*:21–26, 1980.

230. Speich, M., Bousquet, B., Nicolas, G.: Clin Chem *26*:1662–1665, 1980.

231. Eisenberg, M.J.: NY State J Med *86*:133–136, 1986.

232. Kleiger, R.E., Seta, K., Vitale, J.J., et al.: Am J Cardiol *17*:520–527, 1966.

233. Iseri, L.T., French, J.H.: Am Heart J *108*:188–193, 1984.

234. Boyd, J.C., Bruns, D.E., Dimarco, J.P., et al.: Clinical Chem *30*:754–757, 1984.

235. Whang R, Oei, TO, Watanable, A.: Arch Intern Med *145*:655–656, 1985.

236. Sherwin, R.: Drugs *28*(Suppl 1):46–53, 1984.

237. Holland, O.B.: Drugs *31*(Suppl 4):78–84, 1986.

238. Caralis, P.V., Perez-Stable, E.: Drugs *31*(Suppl 4):85–100, 1986.

239. Ikram, H., Espener, E.A., Nicholls, M.G.: Drugs *31*(Suppl 4):101–108, 1986.

240. Wills, M.R.: Drugs *31*(Suppl 4):121–131, 1986.

241a.Bersohn, M.M., Shine, K.I., Sterman, W.D.: Am J Physiol *242*:H89–H93, 1982.

241b.Gebhard, M.M., Preusse, C.J., Schnabel, P.A., et al.: Thorac Cardiovasc Surg *32*:271–276, 1984.

242. Hecker, B.R., Lake, C.L., Kron, I.L., et al.: Am J Cardiol *55*:61–64, 1985.

243. Albert, D.G., Morita, Y., Iseri, L.T.: Circulation *17*:761–763, 1958.

244. Bauer, F., Martin, H.E., Mickey, M.R.: Proc Soc Exper Biol Med *120*:466–468, 1965.

245. Dyckner, T., Wester, P.O.: Br J Med *286*:1847–1849, 1983.

246. Thulin, T., Abdulla, M., Dencker, I., et al.: Acta Med Scand *208*:367–373, 1980.

247. McCarron, D.A., Morris, C.D., Cole, C.: Science *217*:267–269, 1982.

248. Resnick, L.M., Laragh, J.H., Sealy, J.E., et al.: N Engl J Med *309*:888–891, 1983.

249. Resnick, L.M., Miller, F.B., Laragh, J.H., et al.: N Engl J Med *311*:605–606, 1984.

250. Resnick, L.M., Gupta, R.K., Laragh, J.H.: Proc Natl Acad Sci USA *81*:6511–6515, 1984.

251. Fingl, E.: Laxative and cathartics. *In* Pharmacological Basis of Therapeutics. 5th Ed. Edited by L.S. Goodman, and A. Gilman. New York, MacMillan, 1975, p 980.

252. Booth, I.W., Milla, P.J., Harries, J.T.: Clin Sci *66*:465–471, 1984.

253. Flink, E.B.: Ann NY Acad Sci *162*:901–905, 1969.

254. Davis, J.D., Harvey, D.R., Yu, J.S.: Arch Dis Child *40*:286–290, 1965.

255. Clarke, P.C.N., Carre, I.J.: J Pediatr *70*:806–809, 1967.

256. Wong, H.B., Teh, Y.F.: Lancet *2*:8–21, 1968.

*Chapter* **7**

# IRON

## Virgil F. Fairbanks and Ernest Beutler

## HISTORY OF IRON IN MEDICINE

Iron was a familiar metal in most of the ancient civilizations of the Mediterranen littoral, and was used in numerous tools and weapons. This familiarity with iron may also have led to its early medicinal use. In the earliest extant manuscript, the Ebers papyrus of Egypt, rust was prescribed in an ointment to prevent baldness. In early Greece, a solution of iron in wine was esteemed as a means of restoring male potency. It was not until the seventeenth century, however, that the most important clinical application of iron was discovered: the treatment of chlorosis, a disorder now regarded as having been due to iron deficiency. Yet, such was the role of dogma in medicine, that for nearly three centuries the use of iron in chlorosis was controversial, until unassailable scientific proof of the value of iron in this disorder was published in 1932. Even before then, however, investigations of iron metabolism had begun to bear fruit, and thousands of careful studies have now largely elucidated the complex and fascinating roles of this extraordinary element in human nutrition, metabolism, and disease.*

## BIOLOGIC IMPORTANCE

Iron is one of the most abundant metals in the universe and in the earth's crust. It is also one of the most useful, both in technology and in biology, for iron compounds are involved in numerous oxidation-reduction reactions, beginning with the reduction of hydrogen and its incorporation into carbohydrates during photosynthesis in the pres-

---

*It is of historical interest that one of the principal players in this unfolding drama was Dr. Carl Moore, of Washington University, St. Louis, Missouri, who was also the author of the iron chapter in the first edition of this book. The authors consider it a privilege to have known Dr. Moore and an honor to succeed him in authorship of this chapter.

ence of ferredoxins. Aerobic metabolism is dependent on iron because of its role in the functional groups of most of the enzymes of the Krebs cycle and as an electron carrier in cytochromes.

Iron is essential to vertebrate forms of life because its central role in the heme molecule permits oxygen and electron transport. The total quantity of body iron varies with weight, hemoglobin concentration, sex, and size of the storage compartment. A broad range of individual values exists (Table 7–1), with an average level of about 50 mg/kg of body weight in adult men and 35 mg/kg in adult women.[1,2]

The amount of iron that must be absorbed from food in order to maintain body iron levels is determined by the amount excreted, the loss in menstrual flow or from hemorrhage, the demands of pregnancy and, in children, the needs related to growth.

Two functional compartments of body iron are recognized: (1) an essential component, comprising about 70% of the total, which is contained in hemoglobin, myoglobin, heme enzymes, cofactor, and transport iron and (2) the remainder nonessential storage iron, found predominantly in liver, spleen, and bone marrow as ferritin and hemosiderin. Quantitative distribution of the essential fraction is approximately as follows: 85% in hemoglobin, 5% in myoglobin, 10% in the ubiquitous intracellular heme enzymes (e.g., cytochromes, cytochrome oxidase, peroxidase, catalase) or serving as a cofactor in other enzyme systems, and less than 0.1% (about 3 mg) as transport iron bound to transferrin in the plasma.[1–3]

When iron deficiency is well developed, insufficient iron is available to sustain normal hemoglobin production. An anemia results that is characterized, in its severe form, by hypochromic, microcytic erythrocytes. Reduced synthesis of the other heme complexes and iron-containing metalloenzymes may be responsible for the fatigue, epithelial changes, and other associated clinical manifestations. Iron-deficiency anemia is a medical and public health problem of prime impor-

tance, causing few deaths but contributing seriously to the weakness, ill health, and substandard performance of millions of people. Iron deficiency too mild to produce anemia appears to have a relatively high incidence among children and young women; whether it impairs performance or causes symptoms is still uncertain. Such latent iron deficiency is reliably detected by assay of serum ferritin except in patients who have other concurrent disorders, especially inflammatory disease (e.g., rheumatoid arthritis or infection) or cancer. Iron excess or overload is also a serious and often lethal disorder that is more prevalent than formerly recognized. It occurs as a genetic disorder or inborn error of metabolism. Iron excess also occurs in patients with refractory anemia or thalassemia, or in those who have been given numerous blood transfusions.

The main metabolic pathways of iron[4,5] are summarized in Figure 7–1.

## INTAKE

Information concerning dietary iron intake is still fragmentary. Most published figures, obtained from dietary surveys rather than from actual analysis, indicate that the average daily intake is between 10 and 30 mg.[6] The diets of people who live in western countries contain about 5 to 7 mg of iron per 1,000 calories.[1] A weight-conscious young women who limits her intake to 1,000 to 1,500 calories per day will therefore consume only 6 to 9 mg of food iron. These estimates, however, ignore the iron content of beverages and that added or lost during food preparation. Exogenous iron is of particular significance in the iron-rich diets of some African peoples; the iron is derived largely from the iron pots used for cooking and for the preparation of fermented beverges.[4]

The iron content of meals served to military personnel in five countries, shown in Figure 7–2, reveals that (1) the *calculated* iron intake was comparatively high (20 to 30 mg per day), and (2) in every instance, the chemically analyzed iron content of the food was even higher.[7] The food

**Table 7–1.  Estimates of Total Body Iron in Adults to Emphasize the Wide Variations Produced by Body Size and Normal Range of Hemoglobin Values**

|  | Male, 70 kg<br>Hb 16 g/dl | Male, 100 kg<br>Hb 18 g/dl | Female, 45 kg<br>Hb 12 g/dl |
|---|---|---|---|
| "Essential" iron |  |  |  |
| Hb Fe | 2.67 g | 4.2 g | 1.26 g |
| Functional tissue iron* | ~.45 | ~.64 | ~.29 |
| Transport iron | ~.005 | ~.007 | ~.003 |
| Storage iron | 0.5–1.5 | 0.5–1.5 | 0.3–1.0 |
| Total: as low as |  |  | <2 g |
| as high as |  | >6 g |  |

*Myoglobin, metalloenzymes.

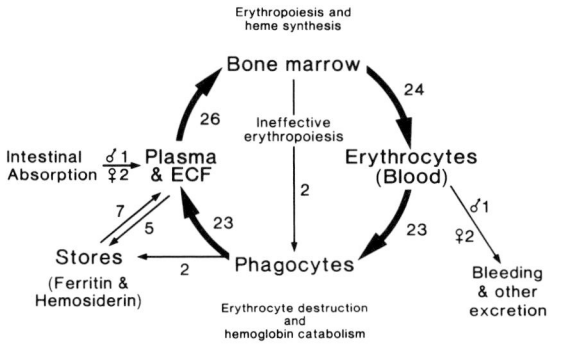

**Fig. 7–1.** Pathways of iron metabolism. Iron is tightly conserved in a nearly closed system in which each iron atom cycles repeatedly from plasma and extracellular fluid (ECF) to the bone marrow where it is incorporated into hemoglobin. Then it travels to the peripheral blood where within erythrocytes it circulates in the blood for 4 months. It then travels to phagocytes of the reticuloendothelial system, where senescent erythrocytes are engulfed and destroyed, hemoglobin is digested, and iron is released to plasma where the cycle continues. With each cycle, a small proportion of iron is transferred to storage sites where it is incorporated into ferritin or hemosiderin, a small proportion of storage iron is released to plasma, a small proportion is lost in urine, sweat, feces, or blood, and an equivalent small amount of iron is absorbed from the intestinal tract. In addition, a small proportion (about 10%) of newly formed erythrocytes normally is destroyed within the bone marrow and its iron released, bypassing the circulating blood part of the cycle (ineffective erythropoiesis). The numbers indicate the approximate amount of iron (in mg) that enters and leaves each of these iron compartments every day in healthy adults who do not have bleeding or other blood disorders. (From Fairbanks, V.F. Klee, G.G.: Biochemical aspects of hematology. *In* Textbook of Clinical Chemistry. Tietz, N.W., Ed.) Philadelphia, W.B. Saunders Co., 1986.)

had been prepared in iron cooking utensils. The diets of military personnel doubtless are nutritionally better and contain more meat, and thus more iron, than the diets of most of the populations of these countries. Other studies have shown that iron utensils contribute significantly to the iron content of cooked foods.[8] The substitution of aluminum, stainless steel, or plastic-coated pots and pans has almost certainly had an adverse effect on dietary iron intake. The iron content of canned food may increase significantly when the cans are stored for a few months.

Failure to consider the iron content of drinking fluids introduces into dietary surveys another source of error that is of varying significance in different areas. Some ciders and wines may contain as much as 2 to 16 mg of iron or more per liter. However, the iron content of American wines and other alcoholic beverages is believed to be negligible. The iron content of city water supplies is usually low, but more than 5 mg/L may be found in the water from some deep wells or bore holes.[9]

## ABSORPTION

### Mechanism and Regulating Factors

Since iron loss is limited, normal iron balance is maintained largely by regulation of the iron absorbed. Ingested inorganic iron is solubilized and ionized largely by the acid gastric juice, reduced to the ferrous state, and chelated. Substances that form low molecular weight chelates, such as ascorbic acid, sugars, and amino acids, tend to promote absorption (see Fig. 7–1). The concept that only ferrous forms of iron traverse the brush border of intestinal mucosal cells may be an oversimplification. The much greater solubility of ferrous than of ferric hydroxide at the neutral to alkaline pH of the duodenum may be of great importance. Normal gastric secretions contain a chemically unidentified stabilizing factor, probably an endogenous chelate, which helps slow the precipitation of ingested iron at the alkaline pH of the small intestine.[10] Impaired iron absorption in achlorhydria and in gastrectomized subjects is presumably related to decreased solubilization and chelation of the ferric iron in food.[11]

Absorption may occur at any level of the small intestine, but it is most efficient in the upper portion or duodenum. The chemical form of iron that enters mucosal cells, the nature of receptor sites, and the transmucosal transport system are unknown. Iron-binding compounds that have been purified may play a role in iron transport by the gastrointestinal system.[12] Ferritin was once believed to impede iron transport across the mucosa, but it seems doubtful that it plays such a role.[2,5] Apotransferrin of the epithelial cytosol may accelerate iron absorption. The increased cellular apotransferrin in iron deficiency may play a regulatory role by facilitating iron absorption when the body's need for iron is augmented. It has even been proposed that transferrin is secreted by mucosal cells into the lumen, where it binds iron, and that the iron-tranferrin complex then binds to mucosal epithelial cells and is absorbed.[13] Other iron-binding proteins of the cytosol have also been described, but their role in iron metabolism is still to be elucidated. Mucosal xanthine oxidase has been proposed as a ferroxidase that oxidizes Fe(II) to Fe(III), thus promoting absorption of iron and its uptake by transferrin of the mucosal cell cytosol.[14] Most of the iron absorbed into the blood passes rapidly through the mucosal cells in the form of small molecules; that portion exceeding the rapid transport capacity combines with apoferritin to form ferritin. Some of the fer-

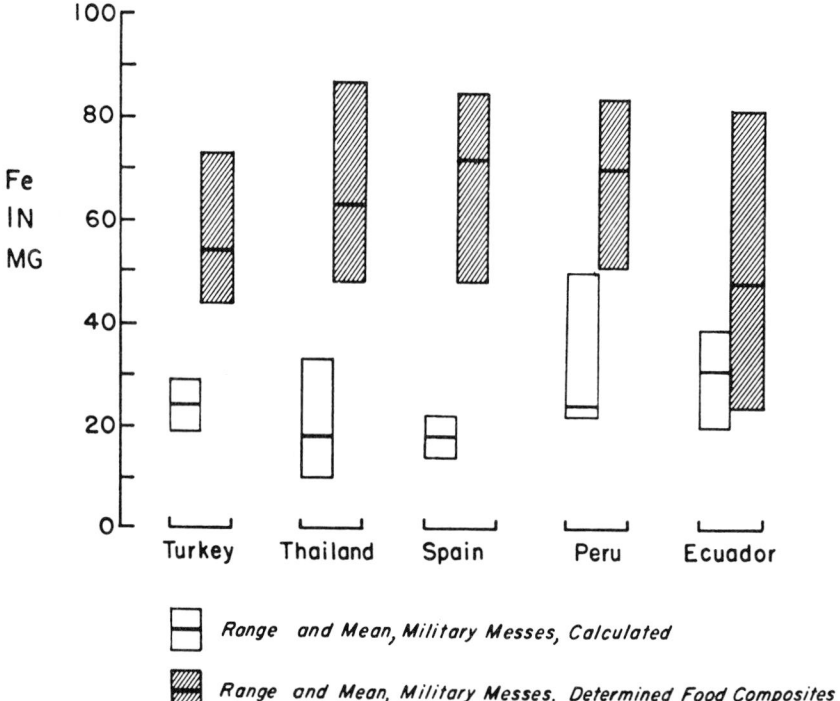

**Fig. 7–2.** Iron intake (mg) per man per day in military messes. In each case the values are much higher when determined on food composite than when calculated from food composition tables. (Data from U.S. Interdepartmental Committee for National Defense Nutrition Survey.[7])

ritin iron may later be released for uptake into the blood, but most of it seems to remain in the mucosal cells until they are desquamated at the end of their two- to three-day life span. Direct entry into lymphatic channels is insignificant.

### Intraluminal Factors

Intraluminal factors that decrease absorption include: rapid transit time, achylia, malabsorption syndromes, precipitation by alkalinization, phosphates, phytates, and ingested alkaline clays[15] or antacid preparations. Tea and coffee both reduce iron absorption substantially, in proportion to the amount of tea or coffee ingested. Iron absorption is reduced about 60% by tea and about 40% by coffee.[16] Phytates are polyphenols that normally occur in wheat, refined flour, bran and maize. They chelate iron, reducing its absorption. Although the effect of phytates in retarding food iron absorption has long been recognized, some doubt has been cast on the importance of this effect because both rats and anemic pigs seem to absorb iron equally well from phytate-rich and phytate-poor diets.[17] A high-molecular-weight substance ("gastroferrin") has been described in gastric juice, and its function was said to be the chelation of iron to prevent its absorption.[18,19] However, the role and even the existence of "gastroferrin" are

in doubt.[5,20] As the intraluminal concentration of iron is increased, the percentage absorbed decreases but the total amount retained by the body rises steadily. When the logarithm of iron dosage is plotted against the logarithm of iron absorbed, a straight line is obtained.[21] The following equation describes the relationship between the amount of iron absorbed (A) and iron dosage (D)[22]:

$$A = 0.022 \times D^{0.676} \text{ for males and}$$

$$A = 0.025 \times D^{0.668} \text{ for females}$$

This relationship indicates that for each two-fold increment in iron dosage a 1.6-fold increment in absorption can be anticipated. Uptake is increased by ascorbic acid, by certain weak chelating agents (e.g., ascorbic acid, succinic acid, sugars, sulfur-containing amino acids), and possibly by the stabilizing gastric factor previously mentioned.[10] The effects of ethanol ingestion and of deficiency of pancreatic exocrine function on iron absorption are disputed. Whether ingested or administered parenterally, ethanol has little, if any, direct effect on iron absorption,[23] and may even retard it.[24]

### Systemic Regulation

The systemic regulatory mechanisms that influence iron absorption have never been identified in spite of intensive search.[2,4,5,25,26] They operate: (1) to increase absorption in iron deficiency and in hemochromatosis, during the latter half of pregnancy, and when erythropoiesis is stimulated (including ineffective erythropoiesis) and (2) to decrease absorption in iron overload, and when erythropoiesis is depressed.

Various possible mechanisms have been investigated, including decreased saturation of plasma transferrin, local hypoxia, humoral factors, and mucosal iron concentration. For several decades, the concept of a "mucosal block" of iron absorption dominated the literature. Ferritin was regarded as the mediator of absorption; uptake was thought to continue until the intracellular concentration of ferritin blocked further assimilation. Compelling reasons for rejecting the theory have been documented.[2,5] The signal that determines whether iron is to be absorbed may reside within the mucosal cells modulating iron absorption in this manner: (1) The columnar mucosal cells formed in crypts at the base of villi contain a variable amount of transferrin-derived iron, (2) the size of its intracellular deposit regulates, within limits, the quantity of intraluminal iron that enters cells, and (3) the cellular iron may enter the body according to need or may remain within the cells to limit absorption and be lost when the cells are sloughed from the tips of villi at the end of their brief life spans. According to this concept, little iron is incorporated from transferrin into mucosal cells of iron-deficient subjects, and absorption is enhanced. Conversely, in iron-loaded subjects, the mucosal cells formed are well endowed with iron, absorption is limited, and the cellular iron is excreted when desquamation occurs.

Heme iron, an important dietary form of iron, is absorbed by a mechanism different from that described for inorganic and nonheme forms of food iron. Some investigators believe that heme is taken up by mucosal cells after it has been released from its globin combination by proteolytic duodenal enzymes, whereas others believe that the protein portion is removed largely within the mucosal epithelium.[11,27] In either case, iron is liberated by a heme-splitting substance, probably the enzyme heme-oxygenase,[28] and is transferred to plasma in a form that can be bound by transferrin. Only a small portion of the heme absorbed by mucosal cells is delivered to the portal blood as the iron-porphyrin complex.[24] Absorption of heme iron is increased in iron deficiency, but less so than is the ferrous ion. Unlike nonheme forms of iron, absorption of heme is not increased by ascorbic acid nor is it depressed by such substances as phytates and desferrioxamine. Its absorption is inhibited less by simultaneous administration of inorganic iron than is that of nonheme forms,[29–32] and it has a slower rate of appearance in plasma.

## Absorption from Foods

Healthy persons absorb about 5 to 10% of dietary iron, and those who are iron-deficient absorb about 10 to 20%. The maximum amount of iron absorption expected from an average diet in the United States is about 1 to 2 mg in normal adults and 3 to 6 mg in iron-deficient patients.

The earliest measurements of iron absorption were made with nonisotopic balance techniques.[33] The small difference between oral intake and fecal loss is difficult to measure with precision. Furthermore, differentiation between excreted and unabsorbed iron is not possible by these methods. The studies have merit because they were done on mixed diets fed over several weeks, so that the effect of daily variation on results was minimized. Absorption, calculated on the basis of positive balance, ranged from 7.3 to 21%.[2,32]

Since 1950, most data have been obtained by measuring the absorption of iron from single foods prepared or grown to contain radioactive iron. Isotopic methods can be used to measure absorption from these foods after they are prepared and fed as in a normal diet. Figure 7–3 presents typical results.[32] The overall absorption in 219 normal subjects approximated 10% and that in 148 iron-deficient patients 20%. Absorption from any given food varies widely, and is greater from liver, muscle, hemoglobin, and soybeans than from eggs, milk, and cereals. It is generally greater in children than in adults.

Figure 7–4 summarizes results obtained in 520 subjects using 7 foods of vegetable origin and 5 of animal origin.[34] Absorption exceeded 10% from animal foods, was poor from rice and spinach, and was somewhat better from soybeans than from other vegetable sources. Contradictory results have been reported as to the effect of soybeans and soy protein on iron absorption; further data to resolve this issue would be welcome. Since radioiron-tagged foods were given as a single test dose, daily variations in absorption were not measured, nor was the effect of possible interaction of foods on iron absorption. For example, ascorbic acid increased,[2] while eggs decreased[35] the uptake of iron from some foods.

Reference has already been made to the effects of polyphenols on retarding absorption of food iron. The effect of organic acid phytates and other polyphenols on absorption of dietary iron was studied by the external tag method in which $^{59}FeSO_4$ is mixed with food prior to ingestion by

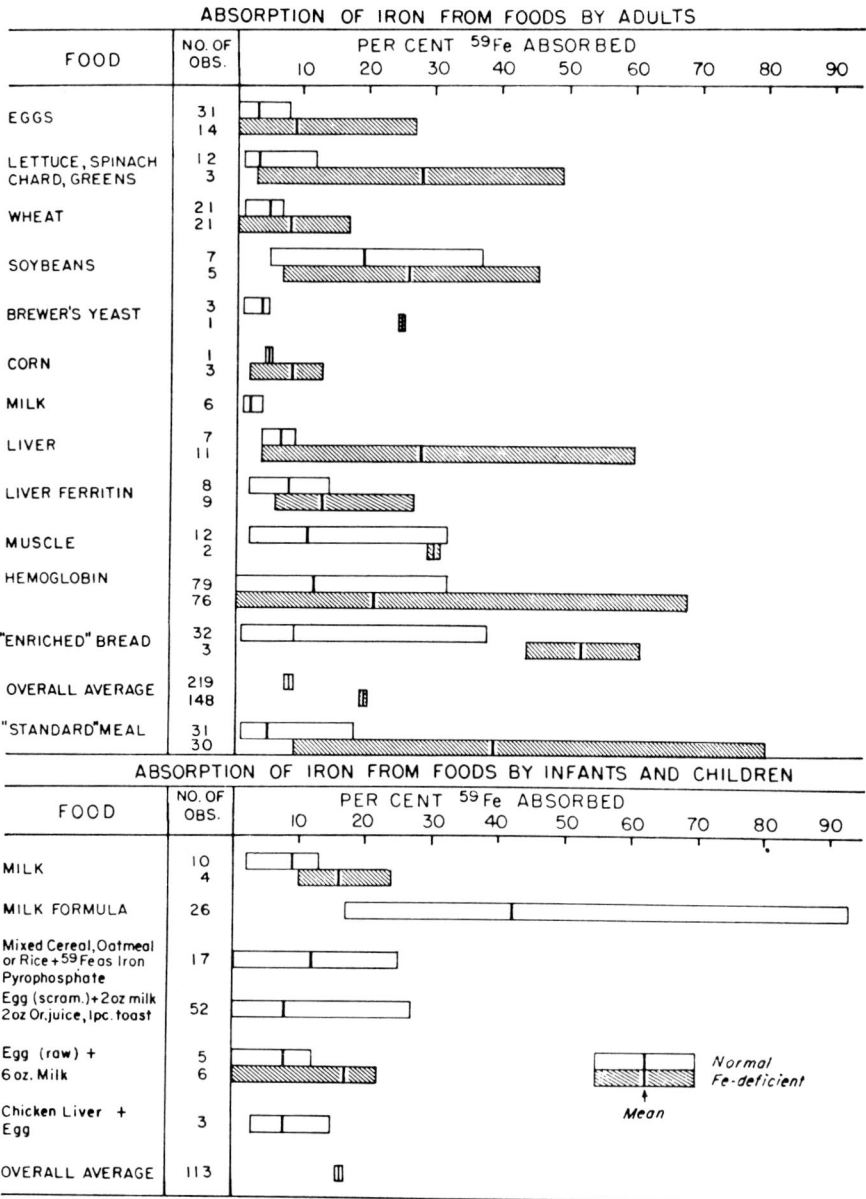

**Fig. 7–3.** Radioiron measurements of the absorption of iron from foods by adults, infants, and children. The length of the bars indicates the variation among different subjects for each food; the heavy vertical lines across each bar indicates the average value. The amount of iron in each feeding varied from 1 to 17 mg. Clear bars = normal subjects; crosshatched bars = iron-deficient patients. (From Moore, C.V.[32] Reprinted by permission of the Swedish Nutrition Foundation.)

human subjects. Iron was poorly absorbed from wheat germ, butter beans, spinach, lentils, and beetroot greens—all foods with high phytate content. In contrast, good-to-moderate iron absorption resulted when carrots, potatoes, beetroots, pumpkin, broccoli, tomatoes, cauliflower, cabbage, turnips, or sauerkraut were eaten—all vegetables that contain substantial amounts of malic, citric, or ascorbic acids.[36] Studies of bioavailability or iron from western-type whole meals indi-

cated that either meat, fish, or ascorbic acid enhanced iron absorption. Meals that included principally pizza, hamburger, or spaghetti and cheese resulted in poor iron absorption, whereas those containing cod, beef, shrimp, or chicken yielded good iron absorption. (It is not clear why iron absorption from the hamburger-based meal was poor; perhaps phytates in the bun or the milk in the milkshake inhibited iron absorption.) In this study the best iron absorption resulted from

| | Food of vegetable origin | | | | | | | Food of animal origin | | | | | |
| | Rice | Spinach | Black beans | Corn | Lettuce | Wheat | Soybean | Ferritin | Veal liver | Fish muscle | Hemo-globin | Veal muscle | Total |
| Dose of food Fe | 2 mg | 2 mg | 3-4 mg | 2-4 mg | 1-17 mg | 2-4 mg | 3-4 mg | 3 mg | 3 mg | 1-2 mg | 3-4 mg | 3-4 mg | |
| N° cases | 11 | 9 | 137 | 73 | 13 | 42 | 38 | 17 | 11 | 34 | 39 | 96 | 520 |

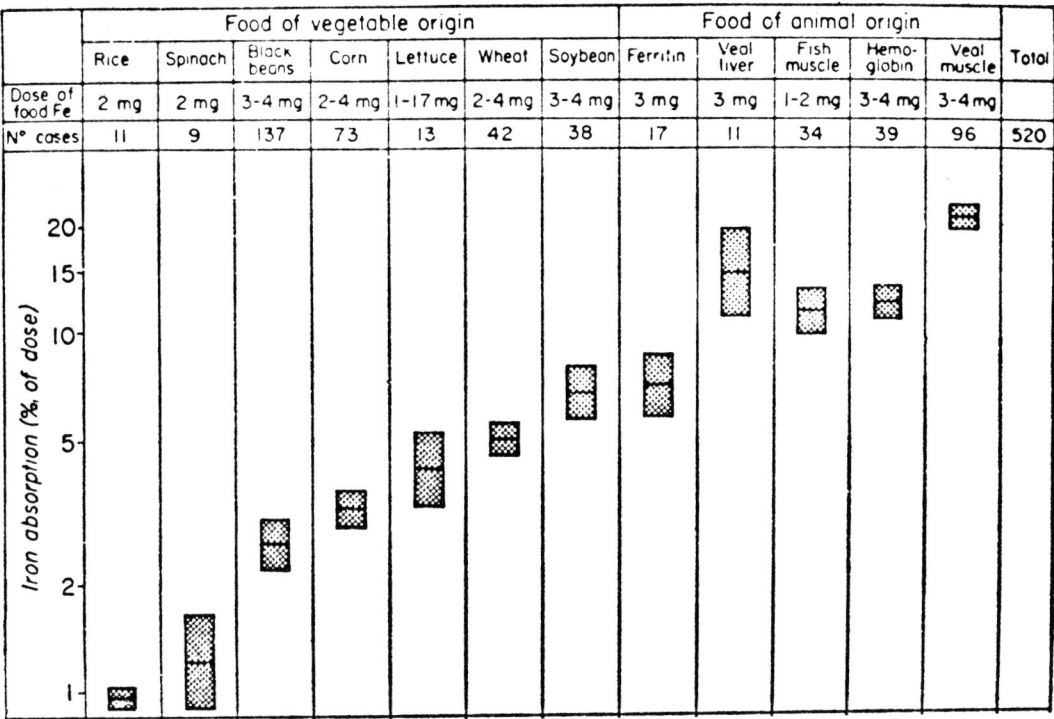

**Fig. 7–4.** Absorption of iron from foods. (From Layrisse, M., Martinez-Torres, C.[34] Reprinted by permission of Grune and Stratton.)

an Italian meal of antipasti misti, spaghetti, meat, bread, oranges, and wine.[37] In addition to the aforementioned dietary factors, soybean products are believed also to retard iron absorption.[38] This finding may pose a problem for vegetarian meals in which soy protein is a meat substitute.

The effect on absorption of certain foods has also been investigated.[39–41] One vegetable (maize or black beans) and one animal food (fish or veal muscle) tagged with different isotopes ($^{55}$Fe and $^{59}$Fe) were fed to the same subjects separately and mixed in the same meal. Veal iron absorption was diminished about 20% when veal was combined with vegetable foods; iron absorption from either maize or black beans was almost doubled when these foods were mixed with animal food. Furthermore, the enhancing effect could be duplicated by substituting amino acids in the same composition as those found in fish muscle. Cysteine seemed to be the amino acid primarily responsible for the enhancing effect.

These results indicate that overall iron absorption from a meal that contains a number of components cannot be estimated from what is known of the iron absorption that would occur if these component were taken separately. Therefore, there has been interest in the use of composite data on absorption or iron from a complete diet, and stimulated interest in the use of "standard"

or mixed meals[32,42] to which a tracer dose of inorganic radioiron is added as an external tag. Nonheme iron in food appears to be converted into a common pool during cooking and digestion, and absorption of the external tag provides a measure of the iron absorbed from this pool.[34,43] In this way, the laborious isotopic labeling of individual foods can be circumvented and the effect of interaction of different foods on absorption more easily studied. Radioiron-labeled hemoglobin may be added to food as a means of measuring the absorption of dietary heme iron. Absorption of iron from a complete diet can, therefore, be determined by adding to food both ionic radioiron and hemoglobin-bound radioiron.

### TRANSPORT

Iron is transported in plasma bound to transferrin, a $\beta_1$ globulin with a molecular weight of approximately 80,000 and a plasma half-life of 8 to 10.5 days.[44] Transferrin is synthesized in the liver. The plasma transferrin concentration is about 200 mg/dl. The total amount of transferrin present in the normal adult is equally distributed between the intra-and extravascular spaces. Transferrin serves a dual function in the transport of iron. It accepts iron from the intestinal tract or from sites of storage or hemoglobin destruction. It then delivers this iron to the bone marrow for hemoglobin synthesis, to reticuloendothelial cells for storage, to the placenta for fetal needs, and to all cells for iron-containing enzymes.

Transferrin has two separate binding sites, each capable of binding one atom of ferric iron.[45,46] Data regarding the identity of the two binding sites are contradictory. Fletcher and Huehns suggested that the sites were different, one having a greater affinity for iron than the other.[46] These observations have sparked much controversy. Clearly there are species differences in the functional heterogeneity or homogeneity of the two iron-binding sites of transferrin.[47–55] However, from the practical standpoint, in humans, the small difference in function between the two sites seems to be of little consequence. In the presence of bicarbonate, Fe(III) binds to transferrin at physiologic pH. Exchange occurs at specific cellular receptor sites. The best studied are the receptor sites on developing red blood cells (normoblasts). The normoblast membrane surface receptors for Fe(III) transferrin gradually diminish in number as the cells mature.[56] The transferrin-iron complex binds to receptors on the normoblast or reticulocyte and then is internalized, as by pinocytosis, into the cytosol. There the iron is released and the apotransferrin returned to the plasma.[56–66] However, the mechanisms of entry of iron into the normoblast remain controversial.[67]

Little attention has been paid to iron transport to cells other than erythrocytes, probably because of technical difficulties. Cultured skin fibroblasts represent a suitable system for such studies, however, and transferrin may also play a role in iron delivery to these cells. When cultured fibroblasts are incubated with increasing concentrations of iron tagged with $^{59}$Fe, rapid incorporation of iron occurs. The amount of iron incorporated into fibroblasts increases more rapidly than the concentrations of iron itself. This finding is the opposite of that which would be expected if carrier mechanisms were involved, and is compatible with the concept of membrane damage by ionized iron. On the other hand, if the iron is first complexed to transferrin, the relationship between the concentration of iron and the amount of iron incorporated into fibroblasts follows saturation kinetics. These findings strongly suggest that fibroblasts, like reticulocytes, contain specific binding sites for transferrin.

At least 19 genetic variants of transferrin have been recognized;[68] all seem functionally identical. The average transferrin content of normal plasma varies from 215 to 350 mg/dl, but concentration is ordinarily expressed in physiologic terms as total iron-binding capacity (TIBC): roughly 300 to 450 µg/dl. The amount of iron in plasma (90 to 180 µg/dl in men and 70 to 150 µg/dl in women) is sufficient to saturate only about one third of the available iron-binding sites. The remaining two thirds represent a latent or unsaturated iron-binding capacity (UIBC). The plasma iron concentration exhibits diurnal variation, with morning values being about 30% higher than those in the evening. The plasma iron concentration is not influenced by season, exercise, or normal meals.

Although only 3 or 4 mg of iron circulates bound to transferrin, the iron turnover rate is rapid.[3,69] About 70 to 90% of the total is transported to the bone marrow where it is transferred to developing red blood cells to support hemoglobin synthesis. Except for a small fraction, which is used for myoglobin and cellular metalloenzymes, the remainder is exchanged largely with reticuloendothelial and hepatic parenchymal cells. The plasma iron turnover rate (PITR) can be determined with reasonable accuracy. After the intravenous injection of trace amounts of radioiron, the disappearance of radioactivity is followed for 2 or 3 hours and plotted semilogarithmically (Fig. 7–5). The time required for the activity to reach half that initially present ($T_{1/2}$) varies in normal subjects from 60 to 120 minutes. More rapid clearance rates are found in patients with iron deficiency or accelerated erythropoiesis; slower rates occur in those with erythroid hypoplasia. Using the $T_{1/2}$ and plasma iron values, one can calculate the PITR from the following formula:

$$\text{PITR (mg/day)} = \frac{\begin{array}{c}0.693 \times \text{Fe (mg/ml plasma)} \\ \times \text{ plasma volume (ml)} \times 24\end{array}}{^{59}\text{Fe } T_{1/2}\text{(hr)}}$$

Normal PITR values range from 25 to 40 mg per day. The PITR is increased when erythropoiesis is stimulated and decreased when erythropoiesis is depressed. In iron deficiency, the $T_{1/2}$ is rapid, the plasma iron value is low, and the PITR is usually normal or increased. If the disappearance of plasma iron is followed for many hours, a second and even a third component of the clearance curve can be measured. This finding suggests that the iron cleared from the plasma is not simply being incorporated into stable compounds but that some is entering other compartments, e.g., "the labile iron pool" from which iron is fed back into the plasma. Complex mathematical models have been constructed to describe the movement of iron among different compartments in the body.[70,71] Such models are of little clinical value.

Changes in the TIBC and plasma iron levels are useful diagnostic indicators of various diseases (Fig. 7–6). The plasma TIBC is often increased in iron deficiency, in the third trimester of pregnancy, and in response to hypoxia. It is decreased

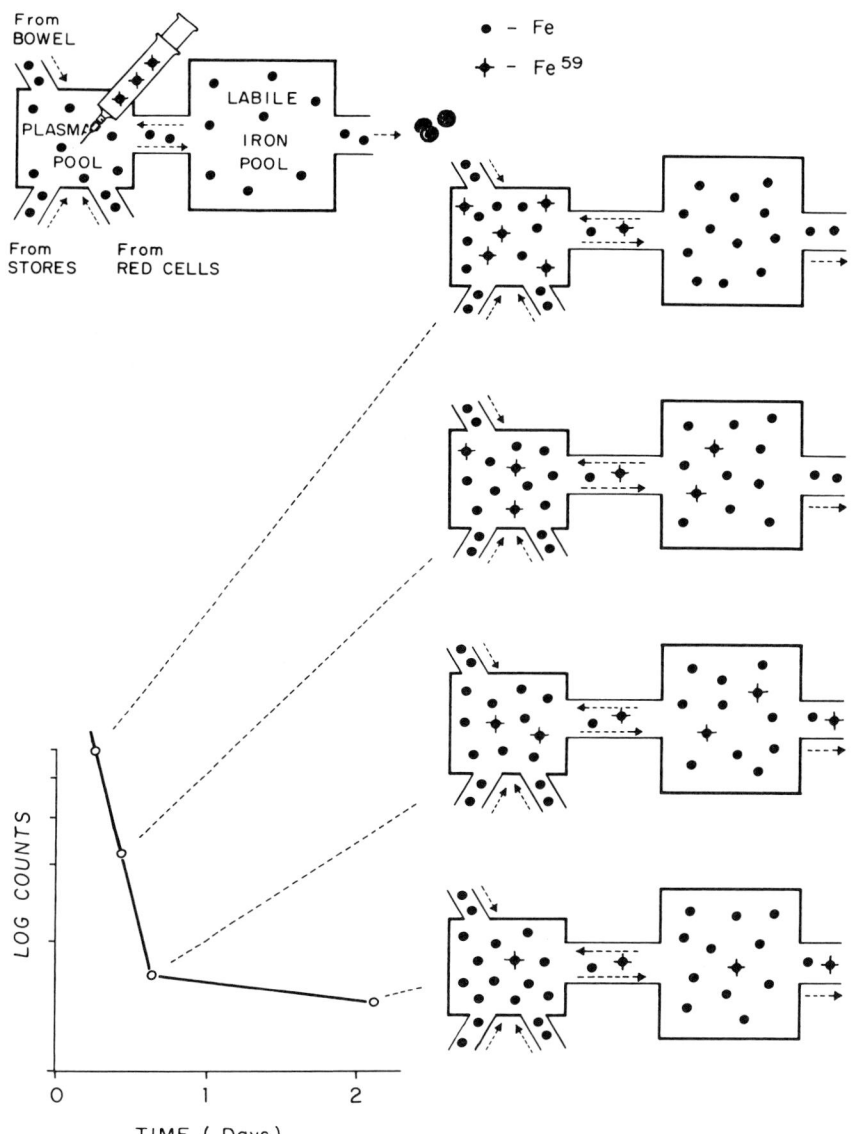

**Fig. 7–5.** The mechanism by which two-component iron clearance curves may be produced. $^{59}$Fe is injected into the plasma iron pool and the first rapid clearance component represents dilution of the radioactive iron by nonradioactive iron coming from iron stores, bowel, red cells, and a labile iron pool. However, the radioactive iron mixes with the iron in the labile iron pool until the specific activity of both pools has become equal. The second, slower slope now results form the dilution of the larger, combined pool by iron from the stores, bowel, and red cells. The fractional loss from this much larger pool is less, and therefore the slope is not as steep. (Modified from Fairbanks, V.F., Fahey, J.L., Beutler, E.[5])

in patients with infections or cancer, in protein-calorie malnutrition (kwashiorkor), in many types of iron overload, and in conditions in which protein is lost, such as nephrosis or protein-losing enteropathies. The plasma iron concentration represents the balance between iron extracted from the blood by organs of utilization or storage and that delivered to the blood by absorption, hemolysis, or release from storage sites. Consequently, it is often low in patients with iron deficiency,

accelerated eythropoiesis, or inflammatory states (infections or cancer) in which release from reticuloendothelial cells is impaired. The plasma iron concentration is generally high in people with iron overload, hemolysis, or depressed rates of red blood cell formation.

Ferritin may also be detected in plasma or serum, normally in minute concentration. The normal range of the serum ferritin concentration depends in part on the method of assay, but 20 to

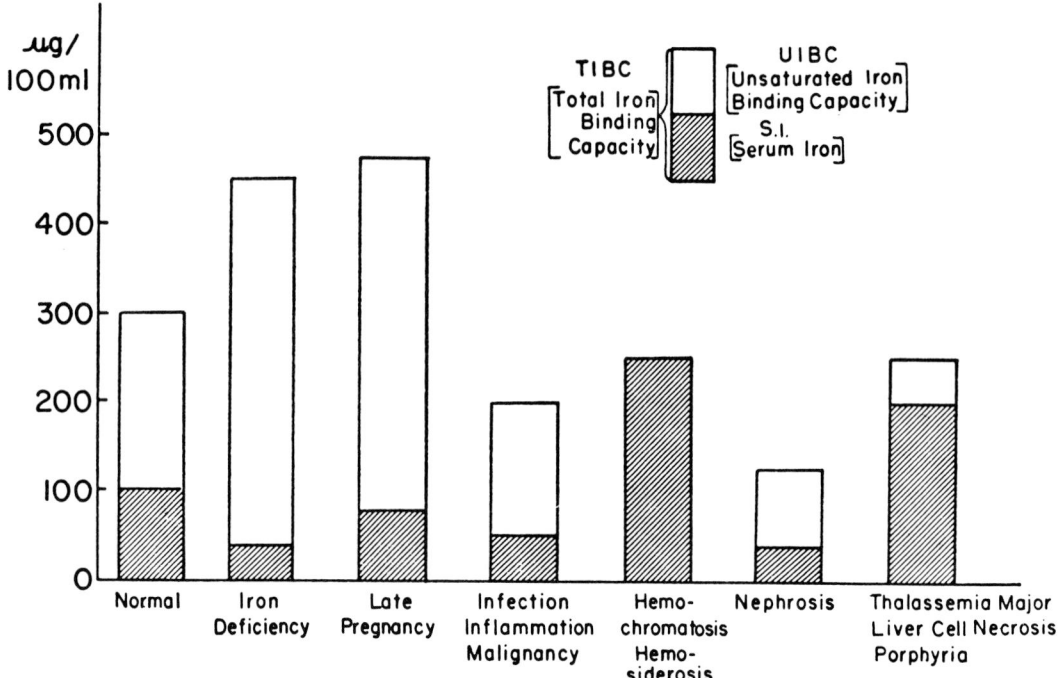

**Fig. 7–6.** Representative values for serum iron concentration, unsaturated iron-binding capacity, and total iron-binding capacity in various clinical conditions. (Modified from Laurell, C.-B.[45] and Moore, C.V.[2])

300 μg/L is a typical normal range for males and 10 to 300 μg/L for healthy adult women. The serum ferritin concentration is increased moderately in persons with inflammatory disorders or cancer and markedly in those with acute liver injury, as in hepatitis. In the latter disorder, hyperferritinemia may exceed 10,000 μg/L as a consequence of the release of ferritin from hepatic cells into plasma. It is also very high in patients with Gaucher's disease. Plasma ferritin does not appear to function as a means of transport of iron to cells.

## UTILIZATION

The amount of iron utilized for hemoglobin synthesis in a normal adult is approximtely 20 to 25 mg per day. These values can be calculated as follows:

> A man with a blood volume of 5,000 ml and a hemoglobin level of 15 g/dl has 750 g of circulating hemoglobin or 2.55 g of circulating hemoglobin iron (total hemoglobin multiplied by 0.34%). Since the normal life span of the red cell is about 120 days, 2.55 g ÷ 120, or 21 mg of iron, would be required daily to replace the catabolized hemoglobin. Iron utilization can also be determined after a tracer dose of radioiron is given intravenously. The amount of injected radioactive iron that is utilized for hemoglobin synthesis and delivered to the peripheral blood in newly formed erythrocytes is then measured. Normally, erythrocyte radioactivity rises for 7 to 14 days and then levels off at 75 to 90% of the injected amount. The PITR in mg per 24 hours is multiplied by the maximum percentage of the dose of radioactivity injected that appears in circulating blood. This calculation gives the amount of iron used daily for hemoglobin formation. For example,

> if the PITR is 35 mg/day and if 80% of the injected dose appears in the circulating blood, then (35 mg × 80% =) 28 mg Fe is used for hemoglobin synthesis each day.

For a detailed discussion of these ferrokinetic considerations, the reader is referred to Bothwell and Finch,[4] Finch et al.,[70] Fairbanks et al.,[5] or Cook et al.[72]

A normally functioning bone marrow can effect a six-fold increase in its production of red blood cells and of hemoglobin. Under maximal stimulation, therefore, as much as 100 to 150 mg of iron could be used for hemoglobin synthesis per day.

## STORAGE AND TISSUE IRON

Iron in excess of need is stored intracellulary as ferritin and hemosiderin, principally in the macrophage ("reticuloendothelial") system of liver, spleen, bone marrow, and other organs. Ferritin is the basic storage iron molecule. Hemosiderin appears to be aggregated ferritin partially stripped of its protein component, or apoferritin. A complete ferritin molecule consists of an apoferritin protein shell that is 13 nm in outer diameter and has an internal cavity of 7 nm in diameter.[73,74]

Within the internal cavity are one or more crystals of ferric oxyhydroxide, FeOOH, together with trace amounts of phosphate that may occur at imperfections or cleavage planes in the FeOOH crystals. The cavity of each ferritin molecule has the capacity to hold at maximum 4,300 iron atoms in the FeOOH crystals, although most ferritin molecules contain 2,000 iron atoms.

The apoferritin protein shell is composed of 24 monomers, each of approximately 20,000 molecular weight, and each formed, in turn, by four long nearly parallel helical chains of amino acids, two short helical segments, and connecting nonhelical segments of amino acids.[73,74] The monomers are so arranged as to form a nearly spherical structure that is the apoferritin shell, with groups of four monomers so aligned that their short helices form pores, altogether six in number, that permit ingress and egress of small molecules in the interior of the apoferritin shell. The pores are approximately 0.7 nm in diameter, just large enough to permit monosaccharides, flavin mononucleotide, ascorbic acid, and desferrioxamine to enter the interior cavity (Fig. 7–7).[74] Furthermore, the pores appear to function as catalytic sites for the binding of Fe(II), its oxidation to FeOOH, and the facilitated passage of the FeOOH so formed to the interior, where it is added to the growing core crystal (Fig. 7–8).[75] Thus the apoferritin shell is not only an efficient iron trap, but it also functions enzymatically.

The oxidation and uptake of iron by apoferritin are very rapid. Similarly, the release of iron is rapid. Iron release from ferritin may be mediated by reduced flavin mononucleotide, although an enzymatic mechanism has not been excluded.[75] The complete amino acid sequence of horse spleen ferritin has been determined.[76] Human ferritins may exist in multiple isomeric states.[77] H and L monomers have been described that differ in molecular weights, the former being about 20,000 and the latter about 18,000. It has been proposed that 25 isoferritins exist, depending on the proportion of H and L monomers.[77,78] Ferritin that contains mostly H monomers is relatively acidic, contains relatively more iron, and is found predominantly in heart. Ferritin that contains mostly L monomers is relatively basic, contains little iron, and is characteristically found in liver. Ferritin predominantly of the H type is said to be increased in the serum, especially in patients with carcinoma of the breast, embryonal carcinomas, and lymphomas.[79,80] Some studies have suggested that the isoferritins may only represent laboratory artefacts, or at most may merely reflect the amount of sialic acid associated with ferritin monomers.[81] Other studies indicate that acidic (predominantly H chain) isoferritins are derived from basic isoferritins by post-translational modification, and that the proportion of basic isoferritin may be increased by iron loading.[82,83]

Hemosiderin is traditionally differentiated from ferritin by the solubility of the latter in aqueous media, and the insolubility of hemosiderin. Chemically they differ in that hemosiderin contains slightly more iron (about 30% by weight) than does ferritin. Immunologically they appear to be identical. On electron microscopy, the apoferritin shell of ferritin is not seen, but the electron-dense FeOOH crystalline core appears as a tetrad, owing to its octahedral shape. By electron microscopy, hemosiderin is seen to contain great numbers of ferritin core crystal tetrads.[84,85] From these considerations, it may be seen that a molecular weight cannot be given for hemosiderin. The molecular weight of ferritin is partly dependent on its iron content, but is usually stated as 620,000.

The immediate source of most iron in the reticuloendothelial system is hemoglobin iron released from erythrocytes phagocytosed at the end of their life spans. Hepatic parenchymal iron probably comes primarily from plasma transferrin. The

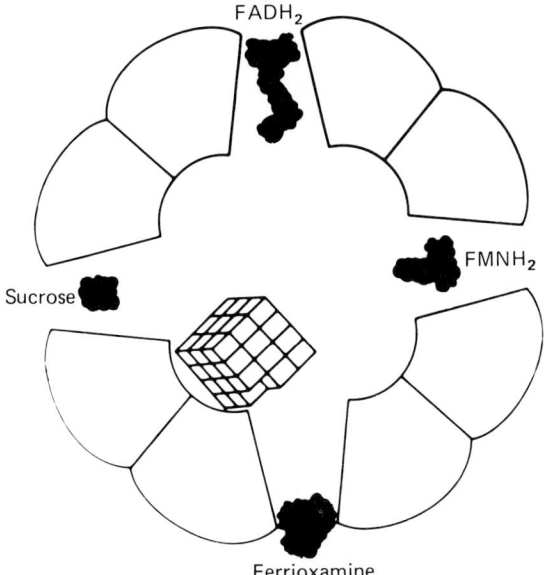

**Fig. 7–7.** Relationship of molecular size to diameter of intermonomeric pores of apoferritin. Small molecules such as sucrose, ascorbate, or flavin adenine nucleotides appear to be capable of diffusing passively through the intermonomeric pores to the internal cavity of ferritin. Desferrioxamine-B may be small enough to enter the internal cavity, but ferrioxamine may be hindered in this passage. $FADH_2$ = reduced flavin adenine dinucleotide; $FMNH_2$ = reduced flavin mononucleotide. (From Harrison, P.M.: Semin. Hematol. *14*:55–70, 1977. Reprinted by permission of Grune and Stratton.)

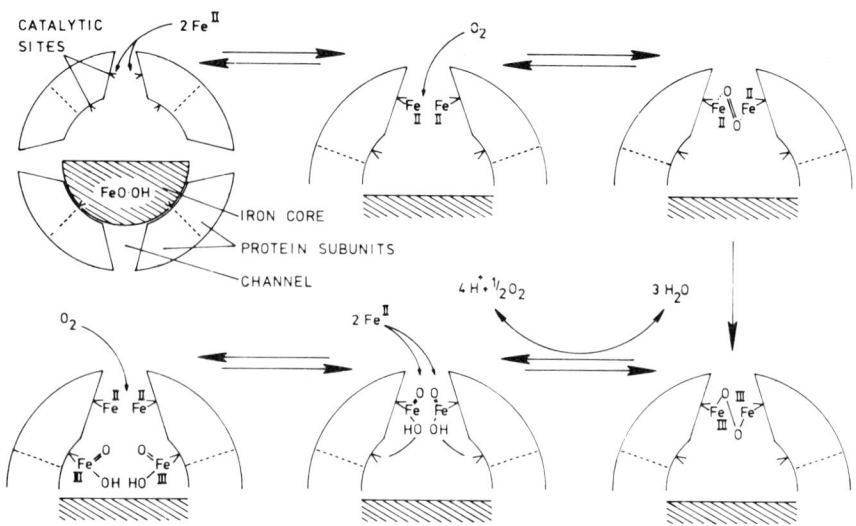

**Fig. 7–8.** Scheme for uptake and deposition of iron by ferritin. Two pairs of iron-binding sites are envisioned in this scheme, and these are located close to the intermonomeric pores of the apoferritin shell. See text for a more complete explanation of this interesting model. (From Crichton, R.R., Roman, F.: J. Mol. Catalysis 4:75–82, 1978.) (Reprinted with permission.)

liver and spleen of normal animals have a slight preponderance of ferritin over hemosiderin iron. With increasing concentrations of tissue iron, this ratio is reversed, and at high levels the additional storage iron is deposited as hemosiderin.[85] Both forms are capable of being mobilized for hemoglobin synthesis when the need for iron exists. The mechanism by which ferritin iron is released to the plasma is obscure.[86] However, such reducing substances as ascorbate, dithionite, and reduced flavin mononucleotide (FMNH$_2$) cause rapid release of iron from ferritin. Thus FMNH$_2$ might serve as the physiologic mediator of iron release.[87]

Quantitative measurement of normal iron stores has proved difficult, but reasonable estimates derived from available data are 300 to 1,000 mg for adult women and 500 to 1,500 mg for adult men. More individuals appear to fall into the lower half of these ranges than into the upper half, and many healthy women have virtually no iron reserves.[88]

The amount of stored iron may increase as a result of a shift of iron from the red cell mass to the stores. This process occurs in all anemias except those due to iron deficiency. A true increase in total body iron is found in patients with hemochromatosis, transfusion hemosiderosis or, rarely, after excessive and prolonged iron therapy. The total body burden of storage iron may exceed 30 g. Whether iron stores are deficient or excessive may be estimated from the serum iron, TIBC, serum ferritin,[88–91] and stainable iron in bone marrow aspirates.[4,5,92–96]

At one time it was believed that iron enzymes

were "inviolate" in iron-deficiency anemia.[97] Extensive studies in experimental animals have shown that iron enzymes are, in fact, quite sensitive to depletion of iron. The degree of loss varies from enzyme to enzyme and from tissue to tissue. Cytochrome $c$[98] and aconitase[99] are readily depleted, whereas cytochrome oxidase appears to be less susceptible[100] and catalase [101] most resistant of all to depletion. It has been relatively difficult to extend such studies to human subjects because most of the iron-containing enzymes are not readily accessible. However, investigations of human leukocytes[102] and buccal mucosa[103] have shown depletion of cytochrome oxidase, even in relatively mild iron defiency.

Iron deficiency in rats is associated with marked (approximately 70%) reduction in activity of the iron-sulfur enzymes succinate-ubiquinone oxidoreductase and NADH-ubiquinone oxidoreductase in rat skeletal muscle mitochondria. The reduction in activities of these important enzymes of the respiratory chain is due to a quantitative change rather than to altered function because the peptide components as well as the flavin prosthetic groups were reduced in studies.[104] Iron-deficient rats also have hyperphenylalaninemia that is directly proportional to the severity of anemia. The mechanism is uncertain, as the hepatic activity of the iron-containing enzyme phenylalanine hydroxylase is not reduced. Iron deficiency may result in metabolism of phenylalanine by an alternative pathway that might generate increased quantities of phenylpyruvic acid and thereby disturb brain function. Treatment of iron deficiency with iron dextran resulted in normal serum concentrations of phenylalanine within one week.[105]

Poor work performance in iron-deficient rats has been attributed to reduced activity of muscle $\alpha$-glycerophosphatase dehydrogenase, as noted in the section on Clinical Manifestations. Mitochondrial $\alpha$-glycerophosphate dehydrogenase is a flavoprotein that contains nonheme iron. It plays an important electron transport role in aerobic metabolism.

That iron deficiency results in impairment of activities of cytochromes and the aforementioned iron-containing enzymes is understandable since iron plays an important role in the function of these enzymes. However, iron deficiency is also associated with reduced activity of many enzymes that do not contain iron. The activity of monoamine oxidase (MAO), a copper-containing enzyme important in the synthesis of neurotransmitters, is diminished in the liver and in platelets of iron-deficient humans.[106–108] However, MAO was normal in the brains of iron-deficient rats.[107]

Some reduction in the activities of other enzymes has also been reported in association with iron deficiency in rats. These enzymes include hepatic glucose-6-phosphate dehydrogenase,[109] 6-phosphogluconic dehydrogenase,[110] and various transaminases.[111] Diminution inactivity of these enzymes is minor and of no physiologic import. It is puzzling that activities of these enzymes should be affected, as none of them contains iron or requires iron as a cofactor.

### Conservation

The avid manner in which the body conserves and reutilizes iron is an important characteristic of iron metabolism. A normal adult catabolizes enough hemoglobin each day to release 20 to 25 mg of iron. If this amount were excreted, the iron requirement would be enormously increased and would far exceed the dietary iron absorbed. Actually, more than 90% is conserved so that it can be reutilized repeatedly. Iron released from cells that die anywhere in the body is presumably conserved in a similar manner.

### Iron Transfer to the Fetus

The fetus has a highly effective acceptor system for assimilating iron. Iron from the maternal transferrin is transferred to the placental tissue, to the plasma transferrin of the fetus, and then to the fetal tissues via a unidirectional pathway that operates against increased maternal requirements for iron despite maternal iron deficiency. During the last trimester of pregnancy 3 to 4 mg of iron are transferred to the fetus each day.[112,113]

### EXCRETION

The body has a limited capacity to excrete iron. Daily iron loss in adult men is between 0.90 and 1.05 mg or approximately 13 $\mu$g per kg of body weight irrespective of climate-dependent variation in perspiration.[114,115] The external loss is distributed roughly as follows: gastrointestinal (blood 0.35 mg, mucosal 0.10 mg, biliary 0.20 mg), urinary 0.08 mg, and skin 0.20 mg.

As shown in Figure 7–9, a slight increase in iron excretion, principally fecal, and not greater than about 4 mg per day, may occur in persons with iron overload, in partial compensation for increased iron stores. Urinary iron excretion may be increased significantly in patients with proteinuria, hematuria, hemoglobinuria, and hemosiderinuria. The etiologic role of hemosiderinuria in the iron deficiency associated with cardiac anemia (e.g., implanted artificial heart valves, calcific aortic stenosis) is of considerable clinical importance. The iron excreted in feces is derived from blood lost into the alimentary canal (1.2 ± 0.5 ml whole blood per day),[118] from unabsorbed biliary iron, and from desquamated intestinal mucosal cells.

It is difficult to quantitate the "normal" iron loss due to menstruation or pregnancy, because of the wide variation that is encountered. Although the menstrual blood loss for any individual normal woman tends to be constant from month to month, the difference among women is considerable.[119] In an extensive study of Swedish women, the mean menstrual loss was found to be 43 ml, equivalent to an average of about 0.6 to 0.7 mg of iron per day.[120,121] No great difference was found between the various age groups except that the smallest mean value occurred among the 15-year-old girls and the largest among women in the 50-year group. The upper normal limit of menstrual loss was between 60 and 80 ml per period. In 95% of women, loss was found to average less than 1.4 mg Fe per day. Women who consider their menses normal may lose more than 100 ml and occasionally more than 200 ml per period. Menstrual blood losses are influenced by intrauterine devices, which increase menstrual bleeding,[122] and by contraceptive pills, which decrease it.[123]

The iron "cost" of pregnancy is high.[1,124] The external loss in urine, feces, and sweat continues and amounts to about 170 mg for the gestational period. About 270 mg (200 to 370 mg) are contributed to the fetus, and another 90 mg (30 to 170 mg) are contained in the placenta and cord. The amount of iron lost in hemorrhage at delivery has been underestimated in the past, and is now believed to average about 150 mg (90 to 300 mg).

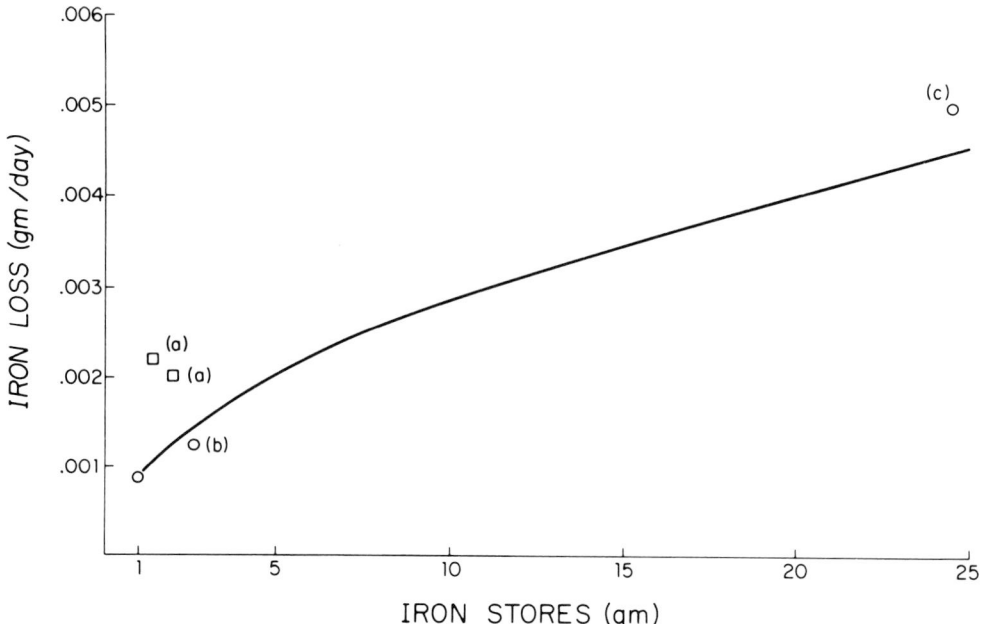

**Fig. 7–9.** The relationship between iron stores and iron loss. The curve fits the equation $L = .0009 \sqrt{F}$, where L is the iron loss in g per day and F represents the iron stores in g. The points designated (a) are based on the data of Bothwell et al., [112,115] the point labeled (b) is from the data of Finch,[116] while point (c) is from Crosby et al.[117]

Iron is required for the expansion of the red blood cell mass that occurs during the last half of pregnancy, but this amount is largely recovered when the circulating red blood cell volume is returned to normal after delivery. Lactation causes an additional drain of approximately 0.5 to 1 mg of iron per day. If one ignores both the external loss, since it represents an amount roughly equal to a year's menstrual loss, and the iron needed for the expanded blood volume and the enlarging uterus, since it is largely conserved, then the total iron "cost" of a normal pregnancy can be estimated to vary from about 420 to 1,030 mg (Table 7–2), or 1 to 2.5 mg per day spread over the 15-month period of pregnancy and lactation.

Pathologic bleeding from any site constitutes an important form of iron loss: 1 ml of blood with a hemoglobin concentration of 15 g/dl contains 0.5 mg of iron. A rule-of-thumb is that 1 ml of packed red cells contains about 1 mg of iron. The chronic loss of only a small volume of blood, therefore, may significantly increase iron requirements. Rec-

ognition must also be given to the fact that each 500 ml of blood removed for transfusion removes between 200 and 250 mg of iron from the donor. Spread equally over a year, that amounts to roughly 0.6 to 0.7 mg per day. A donor who gives blood every two months will have an increase in the average daily iron loss of 4 mg, and will require at least a four-fold increase in iron intake in order to avoid becoming anemic. This is especially a problem for women who are blood donors. If they do not receive iron supplementation, many cease being blood donors because of anemia. In a double-blind randomized study of the effects of iron alone, iron with vitamin C, and vitamin C alone as supplement for women blood donors, the dropout rate due to anemia was 32% for those not receiving iron supplements and only 4.5% for those given regular oral iron supplement. As little as 39 mg of iron daily (120 mg of ferrous sulfate) in a single dose was sufficient to prevent anemia and to allow 96% of adult women to donate blood at 8- to 12-week intervals.[125]

## IRON REQUIREMENTS

### Growth

The iron required for growth and its attendant increase in circulating hemoglobin mass is obviously influenced by the rate of growth, i.e., the rapid growth during infancy and the growth spurt of adolescent males. The calculations in Table 7–3

**Table 7–2.   Iron "Cost" of a Normal Pregnancy**

| | |
|---|---|
| Iron contributed to fetus | 200–370 mg |
| In placenta and cord | 30–170 |
| In blood loss at delivery | 90–310 |
| In milk, lactation 6 months | 100–180 |
| | 420–1030 mg |
| Average per day (pregnancy 9 mo, lactation 6 mo) | 1–2.5 |

**Table 7–3. Estimates of Average Daily Iron Requirements for Growth**

|  | Boys | Girls |
|---|---|---|
| Adult wt greater than birth wt by | 50–100 kg | 45–70 kg |
| Normal body iron per kg | 50 mg | 35 mg |
| Iron in total wt gained | 2,500–5,000 mg | 1,575–2,450 mg |
| Years of growth | 20 yr | 15 yr |
| Estimated iron required for growth: Av per year | 125–250 mg | 100–163 mg |
| Av per day | 0.35–0.70 mg | 0.3–0.45 mg |

provide a rough estimate of an average iron requirement of 0.35 to 0.7 mg per day for boys and 0.3 to 0.45 mg for girls.

## Nutritional Allowances

The foregoing discussion has emphasized the limitations of our information about iron loss, the dietary intake of iron, and the efficiency of iron absorption from the gastrointestinal tract. In addition, the variations from person to person are relatively large. Enough data are available, however, to permit reasonable estimates of the amount of iron required to maintain a positive balance at various age levels of the population. These approximations suffice to guide physicians and health organizations in their attempts to reduce the prevalence of iron deficiency. The estimated requirements are summarized in Table 7–4. Calculations of the daily food iron requirement are based on an average absorption of 10%—an assumption that seems reasonable since assimilation tends to become more efficient as need increases. It is evident that men and nonmenstruating women, in the absence of pathologic bleeding, should have little difficulty obtaining the iron they need from diets customary in the United States (12 to 18 mg Fe per day). The balance may be precarious, however, in many menstruating women and adolescent girls who, because of concern about weight, restrict their diets and frequently have low iron intakes of 10 mg or less per day. The requirements during pregnancy are frequently so large that they are greater than the amount available from diet alone. Particularly in women with depleted iron stores, supplemental iron therapy is necessary during the latter half of pregnancy if iron deficiency is to be prevented.

## IRON DEFICIENCY AND IRON-DEFICIENCY ANEMIA

Iron deficiency is without a doubt the most common nutrient deficiency. Indeed, it seems likely that it is the most common organic disease of man, excluding such nearly universal maladies as chickenpox, dental caries, constipation, and acne vulgaris.

Iron deficiency is common in infants, and nearly always affects the premature unless iron supplements are administered.[126] In children over the age of 4, anemia has been reported to occur in 0.6 to 7.7%.[127] Relatively advanced iron-deficiency anemia was found in 5.5% of poor children

**Table 7–4. Estimated Iron Requirements in Mg/Day**

|  | External Loss* | Menses | Pregnancy "Cost" | Growth | Fe Requirement | Daily Food Intake Requirement‡ |
|---|---|---|---|---|---|---|
| Adult males (50–100 kg) | 0.65–1.3 |  |  |  | 0.65–1.3 | 6.5–13 |
| Nonmenstruating women (45–70 kg) | 0.6–0.9 |  |  |  | 0.6–0.9 | 6–9 |
| Menstruating women (45–70 kg) | 0.6–0.9 | 0.1–1.4 |  |  | 0.7–2.3 | 7–23 |
| Pregnancy (50–80 kg) | 0.65–1.0 |  | 1.0–2.5 |  | 1.65–3.5 | 16.5–35 |
| Adolescent boys (50–100 kg) | 0.65–1.3 |  |  | 0.35–0.7 | 1–2 | 10–20 |
| Adolescent girls (45–70 kg) | 0.6–0.9 | 0.1–1.4 |  | 0.3–0.45 | 1–2.7 | 10–27 |
| Children† |  |  |  |  | 0.4–1.0 | 4–10 |
| Infants† |  |  |  |  | 0.5–1.5 | 5–15 |

*0.013 mg/kg
†Estimates by the Committee on Iron Deficiency[1]
‡Assuming 10% absorption. The figures given in this column assume that the daily iron needs of healthy persons vary depending on age, body size, the nature of the dietary iron sources, and other factors. Thus, they differ from the Recommended Daily Allowance, which is arbitrarily selected on the basis of average needs.

aged 5 to 8.[128] Some degree of iron deficiency occurs in 35 to 58% of young, healthy women.[80–82] During pregnancy, the incidence is even higher.[129–132] In areas where intestinal helminthiasis exists in a large proportion of the population, iron deficiency anemia is nearly universal.

Studies of the paleopathology of the ancient inhabitants of the southwestern United States indicate that severe iron deficiency may have been prevalent among sedentary agricultural people of the canyon bottomlands, who depended upon maize as their nearly sole dietary resource. Maize is poor in iron an also contains phytates that chelate iron, further reducing iron availability. Skeletons excavated in such areas reveal marked bony deformities and spongy porosity of the skull (porotic hyperostosis), attributed to extreme iron impoverishment.[133,134] Nomadic highland peoples, who were hunters, appear not to have suffered this deformity. Similarly, the peoples of the Aztec and Maya cultures of meso-America, where maize was the major food, do not appear to have been afflicted with this disorder, perhaps because they also consumed beans rich in iron.

In earlier studies of nutritional status of the people of the United States, it appeared that iron deficiency had a high prevalence, especially among the poor and among black people. The methods used for ascertainment of iron deficiency were not very sensitive or specific. Microcytosis and low blood hemoglobin concentration have been used as criteria for the prevalence of iron deficiency, on the assumption that other causes are rare. However, since (1) 3% of black Americans have only two rather than four α-globin loci[135,136] a form of α-thalassemia characterized by microcytosis, (2) about 1% are β-thalassemia heterozygotes, and (3) the mean hemoglobin concentration of healthy, non-iron-deficient black people is slightly lower than that of whites,[137,138] earlier interpretations of the prevalence of iron deficiency in blacks are probably overstated. In tropical regions where helminthiasis is nearly universal and nutrition poor, and among impoverished people, multiparous women, and premature babies or those breast-fed too long, iron deficiency is a prevalent disorder with adverse consequences.

## Pathogenesis

Iron deficiency results from one or a combination of the following: inadequate diet, impaired absorption, blood loss, or repeated pregnancies. An iron-poor diet is *very rarely* the primary cause of iron deficiency in adults. This is because the normal excretory loss of iron is so small that once a person has attained adulthood with normal body iron stores, a subsequent iron-poor diet and poor iron absorption deplete iron reserves and lead to anemia only after many years. Thus, the two most common causes of iron deficiency among adults are increased menstrual bleeding and hemorrhage from the alimentary tract.[139] The development of iron deficiency in an adult man or a postmenopausal woman should be assumed to be due to blood loss until proved otherwise.

*Defective absorption* can be caused by diets that are grossly iron-deficient or high in cereal content and low in animal protein. Geophagia interferes in the absorption of iron, probably because the ingested clay chelates or precipitates iron as insoluble compounds in the lumen of the intestine.[12] Clay-eating is practiced particularly by children and adult women. Among the poor its prevalence is probably much greater than generally realized. Inadequate uptake of iron occurs in malabsorption syndromes and in chronic diarrhea from any cause. After partial or total gastrectomy two defects in iron absorption are observed: absorption of food iron is subnormal,[140] and the increase in absorption that usually accompanies iron deficiency does not take place.[141,142] When patients with atrophic gastritis and achlorhydria become iron-deficient, they also are not able to increase the uptake of iron as much as are comparable individuals with normal gastric function.

Except for pregnancy, large losses of iron are most commonly caused by bleeding. Hemorrhage from wounds, the nose or mouth, genitourinary tract, and hemorrhoids is obvious. Bleeding from the gastrointestinal tract is often occult, and adults may lose as much as 30 ml of blood from esophagus, stomach, or small bowel without stools being discolored or positive for occult blood by the guaiac test. Hemorrhoidal bleeding is usually obvious, if the patient is observant, but in some instances even marked hemorrhoidal bleeding may pass unnoticed. Occult gastrointestinal bleeding is most commonly due to peptic ulcer, large hiatal hernia, esophageal varices, salicylate ingestion, intestinal diverticula, benign or malignant tumors, intestinal helminthiasis (particularly hookworm disease), regional enteritis, or ulcerative colitis. Occult gastrointestinal blood loss may be detected in nearly 50% of iron-deficient infants.[143] Usually no anatomic lesions can be identified. Meckel's diverticulum may be particularly difficult to identify as a cause of occult bleeding in infants or children.

The effect of normal menstrual blood loss on iron requirements has been discussed. Women frequently, however, fail to recognize an abnormal flow. Menstrual volume may be excessive if: double pads must be worn because one soaks through, duration of periods is greater than five days, large clots are passed, and more than 12 pads per period are needed. The use of intrauterine devices increases menstrual bleeding.

The admirable and necessary donation of blood for transfusions and the collection of large amounts of blood for diagnostic study are forms of hemorrhage. Iron deficiency as a result of transferrin loss through a nephrotic kidney has been reported,[144] but must be rare.

Iron-deficiency anemia is common after subtotal gastric resection, particularly when the anastomosis between remaining stomach and small bowel is end-to-side respectively (e.g., Billroth II). Approximately 45% of patients who have had such surgery ultimately become iron-deficient.[145,146] Sometimes they have combined iron and vitamin $B_{12}$ or folate deficiency. A small proportion of such patients experience low-grade chronic blood loss from lesions around the anastomosis site, not amounting to more than 5 or 10 ml per day.[147] However, most such patients appear to have an impaired ability to absorb heme iron.[148] They respond well to administration of medicinal iron orally, as their absorption of inorganic iron is unimpaired.

Sometimes the cause for iron deficiency is not found during the course of careful clinical evaluation: the diet seems adequate, no absorptive defect can be recognized, no blood loss can be detected. In a study of iron-deficient patients seen at the Radcliffe Infirmary of Oxford, England, bleeding could not be demonstrated in 17% of 371 patients.[139] No other distinctive features characterized this group. In all probability, blood loss in such patients goes unrecognized because it is intermittent or very small in amount.

Hereditary hemorrhagic telangiectasia has long been recognized as a cause of chronic bleeding and iron-deficiency anemia. The diagnosis is usually made early, especially if there is a family history or the presence of typical cutaneous lesions on palms, soles, face, and elsewhere. The telangiectatic lesions may be widespread in the gastrointestinal tract. A similar vascular anomaly that is not hereditary, does not have a cutaneous counterpart, and usually is not manifested until middle age is angiodysplasia of the gastrointestinal tract, also called vascular ectasia or arteriovenous anomaly. These tiny telangiectasis-like lesions are most common in the cecum or ascending colon, but may occur at any level of the alimentary canal. They seem to be a relatively frequent cause of occult gastrointestinal blood loss that cannot be diagnosed by traditional roentgenographic examinations or sigmoidoscopy. Mesenteric angiography, gastroscopy, or colonoscopy is usually required.[149,150]

Mild anemia is commonly encountered in elite long-distance runners.[151–153] The anemia has been characterized as microcytic; plasma hemoglobin concentration has been increased, serum iron and ferritin concentrations decreased. The anemia responds to iron therapy.[151] The mechanism might be iron loss from hemoglobinuria that results from mechanical trauma to erythrocytes, as has long been recognized in march hemoglobinuria sometimes experienced by soldiers on forced marches. Significant gastrointestinal blood loss was demonstrated in 20 of 24 long-distance runners, and postulated as the probable cause of anemia in runners.[152] However, other studies have cast doubt on iron deficiency as the mechanism of "runner's anemia."[153]

Iron-deficiency anemia is a frequent long-term complication of gastric bypass surgery for refractory obesity. In this setting, iron deficiency may be accompanied by vitamin $B_{12}$ deficiency, folate deficiency, or both.[154]

In four conditions, the availability of iron for hemoglobin synthesis is reduced although body iron is normal or greater than normal. These conditions are: (1) idiopathic pulmonary hemosiderosis; (2) paroxysmal nocturnal hemobloginuria; (3) inflammation, with inability to mobilize iron from reticuloendothelial cell depots; and (4) the extremely rare (only seven cases known worldwide) disorder congenital atransferrinemia.[155–159] In these four disorders, increased amounts of iron are found in (1) lungs, (2) kidneys, and (3 and 4) liver and reticuloendothelial systems, respectively, but the amount of iron transported to normoblasts of the bone marrow is markedly reduced. Despite this reduced availability of iron from sequestered stores, patients with idiopathic pulmonary hemosiderosis and those with paroxysmal nocturnal hemoglobinuria usually respond to iron therapy with a rise in blood hemoglobin concentration.

## Diagnosis

In most disorders, the fully developed disease state is easy to detect, but when its expression is mild it may be difficult to diagnose. Iron deficiency is no exception. *Severe iron-deficiency anemia* is characterized by hypochromia and microcytosis of the red blood cells.[160] Erythrocytes are not only small and pale when observed on the blood smear, but they vary greatly in size and shape. The serum iron concentration is diminished, and the TIBC may be increased.[92,93] In consequence, the saturation of the iron-binding protein is reduced; generally, less than 16% of the available iron-binding sites are saturated. The free protoporphyrin level of the erythrocytes is increased,[161–163] and the serum ferritin concentration is diminished.[88–91,164,165] Examination of the bone marrow generally reveals a decrease in the amount of storage iron in macrophages.[86,96,166,167] Exceptions to this rule are patients who have been transfused within the previous few months or who have been given parenteral iron preparations. In such persons, storage iron may be present in bone marrow despite hypochromic, microcytic erythrocytes in blood, low serum iron concentration, and low serum ferritin. Such cases are puzzling unless it is recalled that some patients utilize iron dextran poorly.[5,168,169] The number of sideroblasts (the normoblasts that contain cytoplasmic granules (that stain for iron) is also markedly diminished in the bone marrows of patients with iron-deficiency anemia.[93,94]

The diagnosis of *mild iron-deficiency anemia,* or *iron deficiency without anemia,* is more difficult to establish than that of the severe form. Mildly anemic patients do not manifest the microcytic hypochromic cells that are characteristic of the severe iron-deficiency state.[160] Neither is the serum iron concentration invariably diminished nor the TIBC increased. The transferrin may be normally saturated with iron.[93] However, the serum ferritin concentration is usually diminished even in mild iron deficiency,[88–90,100,164,170–172] and even following recent administration of exogenous iron such as iron dextran.[171] The free erythrocyte protoporphyrin concentration is increased.[160–162] With the exception of patients who have been given blood transfusions or parenteral iron therapy, the bone marrow iron stores are depleted, even in the mildest degree of iron deficiency.[5,96,165,167]

It is important to differentiate iron-deficiency anemia from other anemias, particularly hypochromic anemias that may simulate it. Thalassemias and certain hemoglobinopathies are also characterized by hypochromia and microcytosis of erythrocytes, and are easily misdiagnosed as iron deficiency, sometimes with serious consequences. These disorders are prevalent in North America. Alpha-thalassemia, which is particularly common, is often overlooked. Approximately 28% of American blacks lack one of the four normal α-globin loci, and about 3% lack two of these genes.[135–136] Characteristically, erythrocytes of individuals with only two α-globin loci are slightly smaller than normal with mild hypochromia and slight target cell formation. Those with three normal α-globin loci do not usually exhibit any major blood abnormalities, but for such persons the median hemoglobin concentration and median value for the mean erythrocyte volume (MCV) are slightly less than the corresponding median values of persons who have four functional α gene loci.

More than 25% of the Indochinese refugees now living in North America also have forms of α-thalassemia.[173] This population contains persons who lack three of the normal loci. With only one functioning α gene, they have hemoglobin H disease, a moderately severe hemolytic anemia characterized by jaundice, enlargement of the spleen, moderate anemia (blood hemoglobin concentration of 8 to 10 g/dl), increase in reticulocytes in the blood, microcytosis, hypochromia, and target erythrocytes. Approximately 10% of the Indochinese refugees have hemoglobin E trait, which is also characterized by mild microcytosis and hypochromia, and may be mistaken for iron deficiency.[173–175] Indeed, the presence of smaller than normal erythrocytes in the blood of persons from Southeast Asia now residing in North America is far more often due to hemoglobin E trait or a thalassemia than to iron deficiency. Beta-thalassemia minor occurs in about 5% of people of Mediterranean, Southern Chinese, or Southeast Asian origin, and in about 1% of American blacks. Thus, it is prevalent in North America, and must not be mistaken for iron deficiency, which it may resemble from examination of the blood or blood film. It is characterized by an increase in the hemoglobin $A_2$ content of blood, usually to 4 to 9%. When iron deficiency and β-thalassemia minor coexist, however, the hemoglobin $A_2$ content is often normal, and the correct diagnosis may be overlooked.

Delta-beta-thalassemia is less common than β-thalassemia. It is characterized by small erythrocytes, hypochromia, target erythrocytes, and an increase in the hemoglobin F content of blood to 5 to 15% of total hemoglobin. Hemoglobin Lepore trait, once believed rare, is in fact quite common, with a prevalence about one-fortieth that of β-thalassemia minor. It is associated with blood changes like those of β-thalassemia minor, but not with anemia or splenomegaly. Of these disorders, all but the minor α-thalassemias are easily identified by hemoglobin electrophoresis and the measurement of hemoglobins $A_2$ and F. Identification of the α-thalassemias requires measurement of globin chain synthesis or restriction mapping of the globin genes. At present these are tedious and costly tests that are not practical for routine use. Therefore, the diagnosis of α-thalassemias (except hemoglobin H disease) is based on exclusion of other known causes of microcytosis: iron deficiency, β-thalassemia, δβ-thalassemia, chronic disease (e.g., infection or cancer), and sideroblastic anemias. Sometimes a family history of anemia or microcytosis is a useful clue. Knowledge of the patient's ethnic origin is often helpful, since thalassemias have high prevalence in certain ethnic groups.

Measurement of the serum iron concentration, TIBC, and transferrin saturation and assay of serum ferritin concentration are useful in distinguishing iron deficiency from most other disorders that produce microcytic anemias. Except when these conditions coexist with iron deficiency (a not uncommon problem), the serum iron concentration, total iron-binding capacity, transferrin saturation (serum iron × 100 ÷ TIBC), and serum ferritin concentration are normal in all except inflammatory disorders or cancer (chronic disease). In early iron deficiency, the serum iron, TIBC, and transferrin saturation are often normal, but the serum ferritin concentration is diminished. In more advanced iron deficiency, the serum iron concentration, transferrin saturation, and ferritin concentration are usually low and the TIBC may be increased. In chronic disease, on the other hand, the serum iron concentration and TIBC are usually both diminished, the transferrin saturation normal, and the ferritin concentration increased. Unfortunately, exceptions to these generalizations are not infrequent.

A particular problem is the interpretation of serum ferritin concentration as a test for iron deficiency in patients who have such disorders as rheumatoid arthritis, chronic renal disease, malignant lymphomas, leukemias, or other cancers or inflammatory disorders. The problem stems from the fact that serum ferritin concentration is typically increased in these conditions, and may reflect the severity of the disease.[79,80,176–180] Thus, an elevated or abnormal serum ferritin concentration in patients with these disorders may mislead the physician into assuming erroneously that iron deficiency does not coexist. In such cases, diagnosis requires bone marrow examination with iron stain.

Differentiation of iron-deficiency anemia from the sideroblastic anemias is particularly important, since patients with sideroblastic anemia tend to accumulate excess amounts of iron in the tissues. As a result, they frequently develop iron storage disease. In such circumstances, iron therapy not only fails to benefit the patient but hastens the appearance of complications of iron storage disease and may cause earlier death.

Studies of patients with iron-deficiency anemia are never complete until the cause for the deficiency is recognized. The source of any blood loss that may underlie the deficiency state must be identified. Carcinomas of the gastrointestinal tract may occasionally be detected in this search long before other manifestations would have appeared. At times it is helpful to tag a sample of the patient's red blood cells with radioactive chromium, readminister the blood, and then measure the radioactivity of feces: it will be greater than normal if blood is oozing from a gastrointestinal lesion.[118] The same technique may be used to measure menstrual loss.

## Clinical Manifestations

It is often assumed that the manifestations of iron-deficiency anemia result from reduction of the hemoglobin concentration of the blood. Certain clinical observations suggest that this is not the case: (1) The severity of symptoms is not closely correlated with the degree of anemia. (2) Response to treatment often seems to precede rise in the hemoglobin concentration of the blood. (3) Certain clinical manifestations such as koilonychia and esophageal webs cannot be accounted for on the basis of anemia alone.

For these reasons, it was suggested long ago that symptoms in iron-deficient individuals may arise from alterations in tissue metabolism.[10,181,182] Indeed, it was proposed that iron deficiency might produce symptoms in the absence of any anemia at all; a double-blind study in nonanemic, chronically fatigued women suggested that those who were iron-depleted responded better symptomatically to iron than to placebo.[183] The concept that iron deficiency might produce symptoms through mechanisms distinct from its effect on the hemoglobin of the blood should not be surprising. In pernicious anemia, it is quite clear that the neurologic symptoms are related to the metabolic effects of vitamin $B_{12}$ deficiency on nonhematopoietic tissues; there is no reason why iron deficiency could not produce symptoms through an analogous mechanism.

Nonetheless, the concept that iron deficiency is a systemic disorder in which symptoms do not arise from the anemia alone has received increasing support only in the past few years. Iron deficiency may contribute to scholastic underachievement and behavioral disturbances in children,[184–191] possibly through defects in the metabolism of monoamines involved in neurotransmission.[106,185–192]

Iron-deficient rats cannot exercise maximally even if transfused to a normal hemoglobin level. This impaired exercise tolerance is associated with lactic acidosis and has been attributed to reduction in α-glycerophosphate dehydrogenase activity of the skeletal muscle of affected rats.[193] Subsequent studies in guinea pigs indicate that iron deficiency results in reduction of $O_2$ consumption by skeletal muscle mitochondria and lower than normal amounts of cytochromes C + $C_1$ and flavoproteins, but no reduction in α-glycerophosphate dehydrogenase activity.[194] In humans, many studies have shown that work tolerance is impaired as a consequence of iron deficiency,[195–207] and blood lactate concentration rises more rapidly during work in iron-deficient humans.[206] However, some contradictory results have been reported, as reviewed elsewhere.[207]

Many studies have considered the relationship between iron deficiency and resistance to infectious diseases.[208–213] Although some disturbances of leukocyte function have been documented, it is still unclear whether iron-deficient persons are more or less susceptible to infection than normal persons. (As noted in the section on iron overload, persons with hemochromatosis may be unusually susceptible to serious infection with certain microorganisms.)

Some patients with iron-deficiency anemia are unaware of being in ill health. Even these individual, however, often experience an unaccustomed feeling of well-being once iron therapy is initiated.[181] Apparently they considered their reduced level of function as normal, since it had existed for a long time. Often the vague symptoms of iron-deficient women have been ascribed to tension, boredom, psychoneurosis, or some other form of complex psychopathology. In symptomatic patients with moderately severe to severe degrees of anemia, most of the complaints are common to all anemias: weakness, fatigability, pallor, dyspnea on exertion, palpitation, and a sense of being very tired. When standardized exercise is carried out on a bicycle ergometer, the time needed to restore cardiorespiratory functions to preexercise resting values is markedly prolonged.[196] Coldness and paresthesias of the hands and feet are not infrequent. Only a minority of iron-deficient patients complain of the abnormality causing the anemia, e.g., hiatal hernia, peptic ulcer, hemorrhoids. Symptoms are usually so insidious in onset that their duration cannot be dated with accuracy.

Manifestations related to the oral cavity and the gastrointestinal tract have attracted attention both because of their frequency and because of uncertainty as to their pathogenesis. Vague gastrointestinal complaints—capricious appetite, flatulence, epigastric distress with eructation, constipation or diarrhea, and nausea—are fairly common. Pica in the form of geophagia, starch-eating, and pagophagia, is practiced by some patients with iron deficiency.[214] Geophagia is often but not always corrected by iron therapy.[215] Severe degrees of iron deficiency may cause secondary malabsorption phenomena, possibly related to a decrease in iron-containing or iron-dependent enzymes in intestinal mucosal cells.[216] Glossitis, characterized by

varying degrees of papillary atrophy and soreness, is found more often in patients over the age of 40 years and with greater frequency in women than in men. Angular stomatitis occurs in 10 to 15% of patients, particularly among those who are edentulous. Dysphagia, iron-deficiency anemia, and postcricoid esophageal stricture, often accompanied by a web at this site, constitute an interesting triad (the Paterson-Kelly or Plummer-Vinson syndrome) found particularly but not exclusively in middle-aged women. It has been regarded as a precancerous lesion, but the relationship has been questioned.[217] Gastroscopic examination with gastric biopsy in northern Europeans with iron deficiency has demonstrated gastritis with varying degrees of glandular damage in about 80% of patients and atrophic gastritis in a few.

The relationship of these oral and gastrointestinal manifestations to iron deficiency is still a matter of dispute. For instance, the incidence of glossitis, angular stomatitis, and dysphagia varies greatly among patients in different population groups and seems to be decreasing in communities where iron deficiency remains prevalent. The varying incidence of these epithelial changes plus their greater frequency in "low-input" (decreased absorption) than "high-output" (blood loss) iron deficiency suggest that they may be caused by associated deficiencies. Hypochlorhydria and achlorhydria occur more commonly in populations with high prevalence of iron deficiency than in similar population groups that have low prevalence of iron-deficiency. The frequency of these abnormalities depends on the methods used for stimulating gastric secretion, on the age of the patients, and on the cause of iron deficiency. For instance, achlorhydria is unusual in chronic iron deficiency and hookworm disease.[218] In the Oxford series, the frequency of achlorhydria was about 40% if the single-dose histamine test was used, but only 16% with the augmented histamine test.[139] Particularly in younger patients with achlorhydria, the secretion of acid may return after treatment with iron. However, usually it does not.[219] The histologic appearance of the gastric mucosa has only rarely been observed to improve.[139] That impairment of iron absorption itself might be the *result* of iron deficiency as well as its *cause* was first suggested many years ago.[220] More recent data also show diminution of the expected increase in serum iron after oral iron loading,[221] but such cannot be interpreted as unequivocally indicating impaired absorption.[95,221]

The fingernails, and sometimes the toenails as well, may become lusterless, thin, brittle, flattened, and then spoon-shaped (koilonychia).

When the hemoglobin falls below 6 g/dl, the heart may become dilated and "hemic" murmurs may be heard. Infrequently, the spleen is palpable at the costal margin. Mild degrees of vitiligo and of dependent edema are not infrequent. Neurologic examination is normal in spite of paresthesias. Rarely, papilledema, visual disturbances, and elevated cerebrospinal fluid pressure, which simulates intracranial tumors, may be found in iron-deficient patients; these unusual manifestations are corrected by iron therapy.[5] Another interesting syndrome consisting of dwarfism, iron-deficiency anemia, hepatosplenomegaly, hypogonadism, and geophagia occurs among young males in Iran.[222] A similar syndrome without geophagia has been observed in Egypt. Coexistent zinc deficiency may be responsible.

As noted previously, several groups of investigators have repeatedly documented behavioral and cognitive abnormalities in iron-deficient infants. In a study of iron deficiency induced by phlebotomy in seven adult men, disturbance in cognitive function could not be demonstrated with confidence. However, subtle changes in mental function may require a much larger series in order to attain statistical significance. Asymmetries of electroencephalograph recordings in the occipital area were observed and were positively correlated with severity of iron deficiency.[223]

Significant depressions of the ST segments of electrocardiograms were observed during treadmill tests in 14 of 55 patients with iron-deficiency anemia and in only 1 of 55 age- and sex-matched controls. Total-dose iron dextran infusion resulted in abolition of the electrocardiographic abnormality in 10 ot 11 patients so treated. The electrocardiographic effect of iron replacement was observed before any rise in blood hemoglobin concentration, thus suggesting that the observed electrocardiogram abnormality was probably the result of impairment of cytochrome or enzyme function within the cells of the conducting system.[224]

Severe iron-deficiency anemia in pregnant rats results in excess embryonic and fetal mortality and increased frequency of microphthalmia or anophthalmia.[225] We know of no comparable study of the effect of severe iron-deficiency anemia on the outcome of human pregnancy. Iron-deficient rats also have decreased cold tolerance due to failure to increase the blood levels of thyroid hormones, the normal adaptive response of rats to cold.[226] Whether a similar failure of thermal homeostasis affects iron-deficient humans is unknown at present.

The leukocyte count in severely iron-deficient patients is usually normal, but in about 10% of cases may be as low as $2.5 \times 10^9/L$. Platelet counts may be elevated, but thrombocytopenia also occurs[227–229] and may be quite severe.[230]

## Treatment

Adequate therapy must not only correct the deficiency but also treat its cause. Increased menstrual flow, occult loss of blood from the urinary or gastrointestinal tracts, or defective absorption must be detected and corrected if possible. Appropriate selection of a therapeutic agent requires understanding the maximum expected hematologic response, the amount of iron required to produce this maximum effect, and the absorption that can be expected from a given iron compound. The physician should observe the patient to make certain that a response is obtained. A satisfactory rise in the hemoglobin level attributable to the iron therapy constitutes final proof of the correctness of the diagnosis.

### Hematologic Response and Amount of Iron Required for Maximum Effect

About 7 to 10 days after therapy is initiated, the reticulocyte count begins to rise. It reaches a peak between 12 and 16 days and then falls to normal levels during the next two weeks. The height of the reticulocyte peak is inversely proportional to the original hemoglobin value, sometimes exceeding 20% in severely anemic patients. The blood hemoglobin concentration begins to increase after 10 to 14 days; it rises at a rate of 0.2 to 0.3 g/dl per day when the anemia is severe and 0.1 to 0.2 g/dl when the initial hemoglobin level is greater than 7.5 g/dl. As the hemoglobin concentration approaches normal, the rate of increase slows; 4 to 8 weeks are required before normal values are attained. The response in children is somewhat more rapid than that of adults, and some data suggest that after intravenous infusion of iron dextran a substantial change in the hemoglobin concentration may be observed even after one week.[231]

The *daily* dose of iron ideally should be sufficient to support a maximum hemoglobin increase: 0.3 g/dl per day or 15 g of new circulating hemoglobin in a patient with a blood volume of 5 L. This amount requires absorption of 50 mg of iron. The exact amount obviously varies with the blood volume and with other factors, but 50 mg of absorbed iron is a reasonable average quantity to provide for adults. The comparable figure for children varies with body weight and can be calculated by estimating the blood volume to be 70 ml/kg body weight.

The *total* amount of iron that must be absorbed

or injected to correct the deficiency can also be estimated. If, for example, a woman with severe iron-deficiency anemia has a hematocrit of only 15%, each 1,000 ml of blood is deficient in approximately 300 ml of packed red cells. If the patient's blood volume is 4 L, enough iron must be supplied to provide four times as many red cells, i.e., 1,200 ml. Since each ml of red cells contains about 1 mg of iron, 1.2 g of iron are needed to restore the red cell mass to normal. In addition, 0.5 to 1 g of iron should be provided in replete the stores. The total amount needed to correct the deficiency in this instance, therefore, would be 1.7 to 2.2 g.

## Oral Therapy

The ideal iron preparation for oral therapy should be well absorbed, well tolerated by the gastrointestinal tract in therapeutic doses, and inexpensive. Since ferrous iron is more efficiently absorbed than the ferric form, simple highly soluble ferrous salts come closest to approaching the ideal. Ferrous sulfate is generally recognized as the standard against which all other compounds must be evaluated. An elegant comparison of absorption from different iron compounds used a double isotope iron tracer technique.[232] Thirty mg of iron as ferrous sulfate and 30 mg as the preparation under study were given on alternate days for a total of 10 days. The two preparations were labeled with two different isotopes of iron so that absorption from the preparation under study could be compared with that from ferrous sulfate (Fig. 7–10). Several compounds were absorbed about as well as ferrous sulfate: ferrous succinate, ferrous lactate, ferrous fumarate, ferrous glycine sulfate, ferrous glutamate, and ferrous gluconate; none was clearly superior. Relatively large amounts of ascorbic acid given with ferrous sulfate increased absorption of iron.

Each of the preparations listed in Table 7–5 is acceptable. An iron-deficient patient will absorb approximately 20% of the iron in these tablets. Since the recommended daily dose provides 200 to 240 mg of iron, the desired 40 or 50 mg should be absorbed. Much has been made of the supposed gastrointestinal irritating qualities of medicinal iron salts. In fact, iron preparations are much better tolerated by patients than is generally believed. In a double-bind study in which iron was given at a slightly lower dosage than that usually employed, no difference could be observed between the effects of placebo and those of iron.[233] On the other hand, a few patients did encounter difficulty in tolerating iron medication given in full therapeutic dosage. In those patients who complain of severe epigastric distress, tolerance can frequently

be induced by reducing the dose to one tablet per day and then gradually adding one tablet per day until the full therapeutic dose is reached. Alternatively, other preparations may be tried until one is found that can be tolerated. Children tend to have less gastrointestinal distress from iron therapy than do adults. A satisfactory schedule is to give half the adult dose to children who weigh 15 to 35 kg, and the full dose to those heavier than 35 kg. For smaller children, and those unable to take tablets, liquid preparations are available.

A common error is to discontinue iron therapy after the two or three months required for correction of the anemia. Replacement of iron stores occurs slowly when iron is given orally because absorption falls off as the hemoglobin rises toward normal. Consequently, oral therapy must be continued for 6 to 12 months if stores are to be repleted. If the chronic bleeding responsible for iron deficiency cannot be corrected or controlled, continuous iron therapy is required.

Iron preparations that contain molybdenum, copper, cobalt, ascorbic acid, and various other vitamins such as folic acid and vitamin $B_{12}$ liver, or bone marrow extracts are more expensive, are no more effective in correcting iron deficiency and, in some instances, have more serious disadvantages. Injections of folic acid and of vitamin $B_{12}$ do not increase the response to iron. Also to be deplored is the prevalent practice of packaging ferrous sulfate in enteric-coated tablets or in capsules containing delayed-release granules. The fraction of iron absorbed from some of these preparations is distinctly less because iron is released more distally in the small intestine where absorption is less efficient. As a result, the expected response to treatment does not occur or is suboptimal.[234,235] In our experience, this is one of the more common explanations for "refractory iron-deficiency anemia" in the United States. Although adequate responses may be observed with some so-called delayed-release iron preparations, such capsules presumably release iron quite rapidly.[236] However, the most widely used preparation of this type, Feosol Spansule capsules, is often ineffective.[235,237]

Oral iron therapy may fail in patients with malabsorption syndromes or diarrhea, or in those who have had a gastrectomy. In the latter two instances, iron tablets may move so quickly through the small intestine that they reach the cecum before disintegrating; roentgenographic films of the abdomen may demonstrate the radiopaque pellets in the large bowel.

## Parenteral Therapy

Parenteral administration of iron should be reserved for those subjects who are unable to tol-

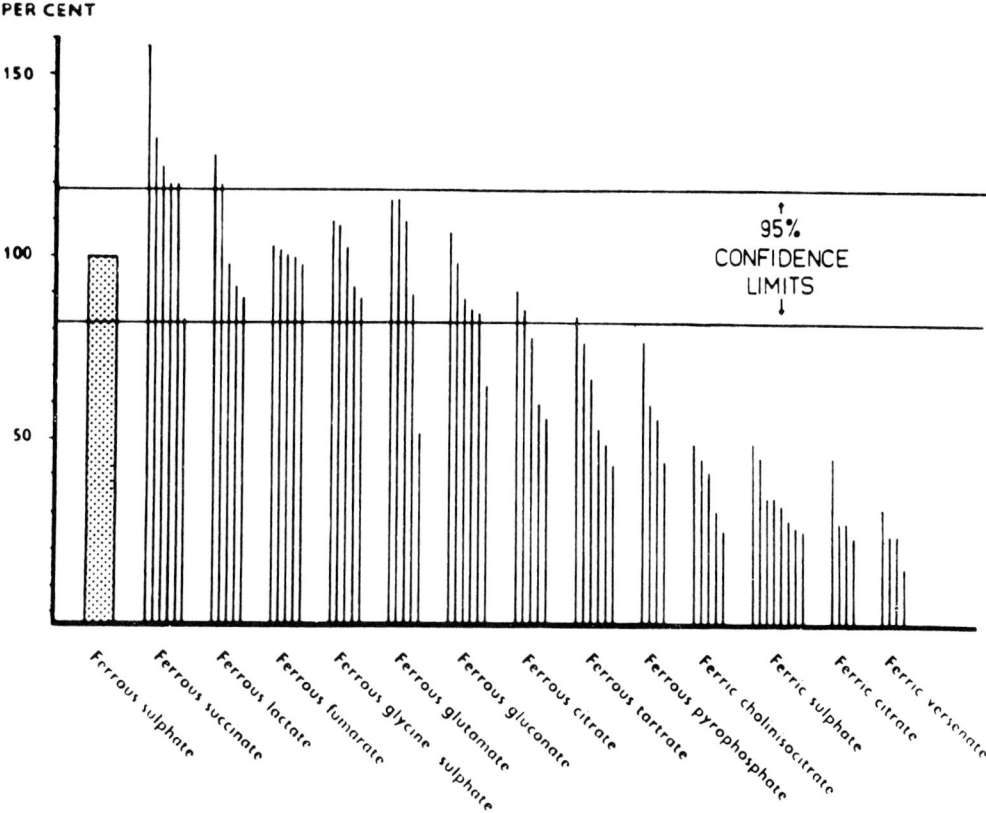

**Fig. 7–10.** Comparison of the absorption of iron from ferrous sulfate and from various iron compounds. Daily dose is equivalent to 30 mg elemental iron. Ferrous sulfate and the other compounds under study were tagged with different isotopes of iron and given on alternate days for 10 days. (From Brise, H., Hallberg, L.[232] Reprinted by permission of Acta Med. Scand.)

erate or absorb orally administered iron: (1) patients with ulcerative colitis, regional enteritis, intestinal shunts, colostomy, or ileostomy, (2) patients with malabsorption syndromes, (3) the rare person who is unable or unwilling to cooperate or who has severe intolerance ro oral therapy, and (4) patients in whom the rate of blood loss is so rapid that it is desirable both to introduce large amounts of iron into the body quickly and to reestablish iron stores.

The most widely used and most satisfactory parenteral iron preparation is iron dextran (Imferon). This preparation may be given either intramus-

cularly or intravenously. The possibility of an anaphylactoid response may be slightly greater when iron dextran is given by the intravenous route. Intramuscular administration of iron produces staining of the skin and may also result in local discomfort. Because iron dextran in very large doses has the capacity to induce sarcomas in experimental animals, its possible carcinogenesis in man is of some concern. However, after more than 30 years of extensive use, there are only scattered reports of the appearance of such tumors.[238] Indeed, so few cases of sarcomas at or near the site of iron dextran injection have been

**Table 7–5.  Recommended Oral Iron Preparations**

| Preparation | g/tablet | Iron Content % | mg Fe/tablet | Acceptable Adult Dose tablets/day |
|---|---|---|---|---|
| Ferrous sulfate·7H$_2$O | 0.32 | 20 | 60 | 4 |
| Ferrous sulfate, exsiccated | 0.20 | 29 | 60 | 4 |
| Ferrous gluconate | 0.32 | 12 | 40 | 4 or 5 |
| Ferrous fumarate | 0.20 | 33 | 66 | 4 |
|  | 0.32 | 33 | 105 | 2 or 3 |
| Ferroglycine sulfate | 0.25 | 16 | 40 | 5 |

observed that a cause-and-effect relationship cannot be considered to be established in man. The total dose should be calculated to correct the hemoglobin deficit and to provide at least an additional 1,000 mg for storage. An easily remembered formula for estimation of mg Fe needed is: venous blood hemoglobin deficit (in g/dl) times body weight in pounds. To this amount one adds 1,000 mg to provide an adequate storage iron reserve.

Intramuscular injections should be given using a "Z-track" technique in which the skin is pulled to one side during the injection. This technique helps to minimize unsightly staining of the skin. According to the manufacturer, not more than 2 ml (100 mg) should be injected on any day, whether intramuscularly or intravenously. Systemic reactions are unusual but may be severe: headache, fever, arthralgia, generalized lymphadenopathy, splenomegaly, back pain and, rarely, peripheral vascular collapse and death. Marked neutrophilic leukocytosis of peripheral blood has been reported as has pleocytosis of the cerebrospinal fluid.[5] Whenever iron dextran is injected, by either parenteral route, a physician should be prepared to treat anaphylactic shock, if it occurs, with epinephrine and other supportive measures. There is no evidence that doses 2 ml or less are any less likely to cause severe adverse reactions than are much larger doses such as total dose infusion by intravenous route. Rates of hemoglobin increase do not differ significantly from those produced by proper oral iron therapy.

*Blood transfusions* are rarely needed in the treatment of iron-deficiency anemia and should generally be reserved for patients who have serious complications (angina, congestive heart failure, or severe pneumonia) that demand immediate correction of anemia. For patients with cardiac failure, transfusions must be given slowly and cautiously. Healthy young adults are able to tolerate levels of hemoglobin as low as 2.5 or 3 g/dl with remarkably little discomfort or danger. The patient's clinical status, not the numerical value of the blood hemoglobin concentration, should be given primary consideration in reaching a decision regarding the advisability of blood transfusion. Patients with bleeding who are iron-deficient must sometimes be transfused. In these instances, however, the purpose of the transfusion is not primarily to correct the anemia but rather to restore a falling blood volume to normal, thus avoiding the development of hemorrhagic shock.

## Prognosis

Recurrence of iron-deficiency anemia is common because the precipitating cause is not rec-

ognized, continues, or recurs.[139] Patients with chronic severe epithelial changes in the oral cavity have a somewhat higher attack rate of carcinoma of the upper gastrointestinal tract. In affected children whose growth and development are retarded, iron therapy frequently produces at least partial correction of the defect.[184–191,239]

## Supplements to Prevent Development of Iron Deficiency

In the United States and several other countries, the cereal most commonly eaten, usually wheat flour or rice, is usually fortified with iron. In the United States, flour is enriched with 12 mg of iron per pound (460 g). Bread baked under commercial conditions contains about 0.022 to 0.037 mg Fe per g of wet weight. That the iron can be absorbed was proved in experiments in which people ate bread fortified with radio-labeled iron. Normal subjects absorbed 1 to 12%, whereas iron-deficient subjects assimilated several times as much.[240] Soluble inorganic iron added to food is absorbed to the same extent as is iron intrinsic to that food.[43] However, the usual method for iron fortification of flour in the United States is addition of finely powdered metallic iron. The absorption of iron in this form is poor, and it has been suggested that the principal effect of such iron fortification of flour is in public relations: millers are able to list a high percentage of the recommended daily allowance for iron. Concern has also been expressed regarding the potential risk of iron fortification of cereal to persons with unrecognized hemochromatosis. Although this potential hazard may be small in comparison to the potential benefit to large numbers of persons with marginal iron reserves, it could be more substantial than previously believed if, as now believed, two or three persons per thousand are at risk.

Since iron in rice and corn is poorly absorbed,[34] these cereals are poor vehicles for fortification. Approximately 10% of the iron is absorbed from iron-fortified cereals prepared for infants.[241] The exact amounts may differ considerably, however, varying not only with the iron compound used but also with the particle size and presumably with the method of preparation of the food. Although wheat flour has received the most emphasis as a vehicle for iron supplementation, other foodstuffs may be equally or more suitable, particularly in certain countries. Thus, sugar,[242] fish sauce,[243] and salt[244] may be suitable vehicles for iron supplementation. Their effectiveness, however, has been vigorously challenged.[35,245]

There are two times in life when iron supplementation is recommended: during infancy and pregnancy. A daily dietary allowance of 1.0 to 1.5

mg dietary iron per kg per day achieves optimal iron nutrition for a majority of the infant population.[126,163,246] In an infant of average weight, an intake of 6 to 9 mg/day at 3 months of age, gradually increasing to 8 to 12 mg/day at 6 months, and to 10 to 15 mg/day by 12 months will satisfy this requirement. Supplementation by iron-enriched cereals or by iron salts is usually required if an intake of 15 mg per day is to be achieved. In pregnant women, it has been found that 78 mg of ferrous iron per day for 24 weeks is sufficient to achieve optimal hemoglobin mass and maintain normal iron stores, but 39 mg daily is not.[247] Pregnant women who receive adequate iron supplementation have continually normal values for serum iron concentration, total iron-binding capacity, transferrin saturation, ferritin concentration, and free erythrocyte protoporphyrin, although their blood hemoglobin concentration may decline to between 10 and 11 g/dl, owing to expanded plasma volume.[248]

The prevalence of iron deficiency is also correlated with age in both sexes. Persons 60 years of age are more likely to be iron-deficient than are younger persons. In males over the age of 60 there is a greater frequency of those whose hemoglobin concentrations are less than 14 g/dl and whose serum iron and ferritin concentrations are below normal limits.[249] In healthy elderly persons of New Mexico, only a small proportion had hemoglobin, serum iron, or ferritin values below the generally accepted normal ranges for their sex.[250] Very likely the low values documented in these studies of the elderly reflect a higher frequency of occult blood loss or chronic disease in the elderly. Iron supplementation is not justified for healthy elderly persons who are not iron-deficient.

## OVERLOAD

An excessive body burden of iron can be produced by greater-than-normal absorption from the alimentary canal, by parenteral injection, or by a combination of both mechanisms. The excess iron is deposited largely as hemosiderin in reticuloendothelial cells, or in the parenchymal cells of certain tissues. The site of deposition is in part dependent on the portal of entry. When excess iron is derived from intestinal absorption, it is carried to tissues bound by plasma transferrin and transferred to parenchymal and reticuloendothelial cells as well as to developing erythroblasts. On the other hand, parenterally administered iron, given usually as transfused blood, accumulates largely in reticuloendothelial cells where the transfused erythrocytes are eventually destroyed and their hemoglobin degraded. In iron overload, the serum iron concentration and transferrin saturation are usually increased, and the TIBC may be depressed (see Fig. 7–6). A simple classification based on mechanism of production is:

1. Excessive absorption of iron
   A. Hereditary hemochromatosis
   B. Excessive intake (African or "Bantu" siderosis; prolonged therapeutic administration of iron to subjects not iron-deficient)
   C. Chronic alcoholism or chronic liver disease (usually alcoholic cirrhosis) and possibly pancreatic insufficiency
   D. "Shunt hemochromatosis"
   E. Certain types of refractory anemia, usually associated with ineffective erythropoiesis, and increased hemolysis
2. Transfusional hemosiderosis

The term *hemosiderosis* denotes an increase in iron storage without associated tissue damage. *Hemochromatosis* indicates that such damage is present, particularly in the liver, that the iron overload is generalized, and that the amount of iron is greatly increased (usually 20 to 40 g).[4,251] The classic "triad" of hemochromatosis—cirrhosis, diabetes, and hyperpigmentation of the skin—summarizes the most striking clinical features of this disorder. The other major clinical features of hemochromatosis are cardiac arrhythmias, restrictive cardiomyopathy (due to iron deposition in heart muscle cells), cardiac failure, arthropathy that may mimic rheumatoid arthritis, gonadal failure secondary to marked reduction in pituitary hormone secretion, and testicular atrophy.[251–253] The diabetes, arthropathy, and sterility are usually irreversible, but cardiac function and hepatic function commonly improve following treatment by removal of 50 L or more of blood over the period of one or two years. Patients with hemochromatosis have a substantially increased risk of hepatocellular carcinoma. The frequency of hepatoma is as high as 29% of cases in some series,[252] but overall about one out of every seven hemochromatosis patients dies of hepatoma. The frequency of this lethal complication is probably greater than the frequency of its occurrence in alcoholic cirrhosis and certainly much greater than in noncirrhotic subjects. The incidence and progression of hepatoma are not affected by phlebotomy therapy. Aberrations in mental function may be observed in about a third of patients with hemochromatosis. These aberrations include marked lethargy, somnolence, confusion, and disorientation.[252]

Patients with hereditary hemochromatosis manifest increased susceptibility to infection. Sudden onset of overwhelming sepsis and shock was once a common cause of death in patients with this disorder. Persons with iron overload of any cause are especially susceptible to septicemia from the marine bacterium *vibrio vulnificus,* a microorganism that grows rapidly when iron is readily available.[255–257] The infection is usually acquired by handling or eating raw shellfish such as oysters. Septicemia is rapidly progressive and commonly fatal. Cases have also been reported of peritonitis and of septicemia due to *Yersinia enterocolitica* in patients with hereditary hemochromatosis, thalassemia major, or oral iron overdosing.[258–262] However, since this microorganism appears to be an "opportunistic pathogen," causing severe or fatal infections in persons debilitated from a variety of disorders, the relationship of *Y. enterocolitica* infections to iron overload seems doubtful.

## Hereditary Hemochromatosis

Hereditary ("idiopathic") hemochromatosis is a relatively common inborn error of metabolism, in which the increased intestinal absorption of iron results in slow progressive accumulation of the metal throughout life. It is caused by a single recessive gene that is closely linked to the HLA histocompatibility locus on chromosome 6.[263–265] We and others[266] have been unable to demonstrate a defect in iron uptake from transferrin by fibroblasts, and the molecular basis of hemochromatosis is still unknown. Earlier studies based on postmortem examinations suggested a prevalence for the fully expressed clinical disorder of about 1/10,000.[251–254] More recent studies seem to indicate a much higher prevalence of about 2 to 3/1,000 in Sweden, France, Scotland, Canada (Ontario), the United States (Utah), and Australia.[263,264,267–273]* This higher prevalence rate implies a gene frequency of about 0.04 to 0.09 and a carrier rate of about 10% of Caucasians of northern European derivation. Furthermore, it implies that most cases of hemochromatosis are not correctly diagnosed during life. Very likely many such cases are diagnosed as diabetes mellitus, rheumatoid arthritis, or idiopathic cardiomyopathy, without the underlying iron storage disease being recognized. Many experienced clinicians, including many who are expert in the field of iron metabolism, are uncomfortable with these newer

---

*In an unpublished review of 511 Mayo Clinic cases of hepatic cirrhosis, Dr. Juergen Ludwig found that 7.6% had hemochromatosis and that 0.1% of 33,465 consecutive Mayo Clinic autopsy cases had hepatic cirrhosis with hemochromatosis. These results are nearly identical with those reported from Glasgow, Scotland.[268] Since patients with precirrhotic hemochromatosis were excluded from both of these studies, these autopsy data are consistent with the predicted homozygote prevalence rate of 2 to 4/1,000.

estimates and question whether hemochromatosis is so common a disorder as the gene frequency estimates imply. A careful reappraisal of the prevalence data is greatly needed. The previous problem of occasional apparent autosomal dominant inheritance of hemochromatosis now appears to be the result of homozygote-heterozygote matings, as has been demonstrated in several kindreds.[271–273]

The homozygous state may be manifest any time after puberty in men, but usually not prior to menopause in women, since menstruation functions as a "safety valve."

For some time there was controversy as to whether "idiopathic" hemochromatosis ought to be regarded as a truly separate nosologic entity or merely as a manifestation of alcoholic cirrhosis. However, careful genetic studies have eliminated the latter hypothesis. In this regard, the close linkage to the HLA locus has been extremely useful. The frequency of the HLA-A3 phenotype in patients with hemochromatosis is about 70%, whereas in the general population the HLA-A3 phenotype has a 28% prevalence.[274] Were hemochromatosis merely an epiphenomenon of alcoholic cirrhosis, the HLA-A3 frequency should also be 70% in the latter group. In fact, it is 28%, as in the general population. These and extensive genetic studies prove that hereditary hemochromatosis and alcoholic cirrhosis are distinct and separate disease entities, although they share some clinical manifestations.

Some physicians may be tempted to use HLA typing as a screening test for hemochromatosis or in the attempt to differentiate it from alcoholic cirrhosis. Either application is illogical, wasteful of resources, and meaningless, since any patient with alcoholic cirrhosis has nearly a 30% likelihood of having the HLA-A3 antigen (and the same proportion of patients with hemochromatosis do not have HLA-A3), and since the test is time-consuming and costly. The procedure has some merit, however, for examining the siblings of a person who is a known case of hemochromatosis, since those who are genotypically identical with their affected sibling may be presumed also to be homozygous for hereditary hemochromatosis; those who are not genotypically identical may be reassured. In this application, it does not matter whether the HLA type is A3 or any other type.

Screening tests for hemochromatosis should include assay of serum iron concentration, TIBC, percent transferrin saturation, and ferritin concentration. Taken together, these tests provide a high level of confidence for identification of persons likely to have hemochromatosis, although a few cases may still be missed.[275] Persons with serum iron concentrations greater than 180 $\mu$g/dl and transferrin saturation greater than 55% must be assumed to be at risk of hemochromatosis until proven otherwise. Such proof usually requires liver biopsy.

In African (Bantu) siderosis, a positive correlation exists between the concentration of iron in the liver and the incidence of portal cirrhosis: with concentrations greater than 2 g/100 g dry weight, most of the patients have portal cirrhosis.[276] The large amount of intracellular iron may cause progressive destruction of parenchymal cells and replacement by fibrous tissue.[277] The relationship between diabetes mellitus and cardiomyopathy on the one hand and deposition of hemosiderin in the pancreas and myocardium on the other has also been cited as evidence favoring toxicity of the iron. The improvement reported in patients with idiopathic hemochromatosis after removal of most of their excess iron by therapeutic phlebotomy argues strongly for a noxious effect of iron when present in great excess.

Of particular nutritional interest are the secondary forms of iron overload that are caused by increased alimentary intake, such as "Bantu siderosis" and that resulting from inappropriate and prolonged iron therapy.

## African ("Bantu") Siderosis

Iron overload in blacks of South Africa (first recognized in those of the Bantu linguistic stock, although not limited or predetermined by language) results from long-continued exposure to diets containing too much iron, derived largely from cooking pots and from the steel barrels used in the preparation of fermented alcoholic beverages.[278,279] In adult males, the intake may exceed 100 mg iron per day. The condition frequently becomes manifest in late adolescence, reaches its greatest severity between the ages of 40 and 60 years, and is usually more severe in males because their alcoholic consumption tends to be greater. The pathologic pattern of the iron overload is one of hepatic and reticuloendothelial involvement. Portal cirrhosis becomes evident in most (but not all) patients when the hepatic concentration of iron reaches 2 g or more per 100 g of dry weight.[276] Redistribution of iron takes place so that parenchymal deposits of hemosiderin are found in the epithelial cells of many organs, particularly in the pancreas and the myocardium. Approximately 20% of these subjects develop clinical diabetes, but myocardial failure has not been described. To what extent these changes are caused by iron alone, by chronic alcoholism, or by the associated nutritional disturbances is unknown.

## Alcoholic Cirrhosis, Chronic Alcoholism, and Pancreatic Insufficiency

Patients with alcoholic or nutritional portal cirrhosis of the liver frequently have increased amounts of stainable iron in their livers, although the total amount present is rarely greater than 1 g.[254,274,280] With the larger amounts, hemosiderin deposits are found in parenchymal cells of the liver, pancreas, heart, and adrenal glands. Clinical similarity to hemochromatosis is accentuated by the occurrence also in alcoholic cirrhosis of increased skin pigmentation, a higher incidence of diabetes mellitus than can be ascribed to coincidence, testicular atrophy, and an increased risk of hepatoma. Cardiac failure, when it occurs, can usually be accounted for on other grounds. More males than females are affected and clinical manifestations are most prominent in late middle life.

A number of possible explanations for the iron overload have been cited. Patients with portal cirrhosis are frequently wine drinkers, and may consume several liters daily. European wines may contain significant quantities of iron (although American wines do not), and several mg per day may be derived from that source alone.[8] Patients with chronic liver disease or chronic pancreatitis absorb iron excessively from the intestine.[281,282]

Although the controversy over the genetic basis of "idiopathic" hemochromatosis has been resolved, there remains the issue whether alcoholic cirrhosis per se can lead to serious iron overload. Seventy percent of cirrhotic patients with marked iron overload have the HLA-A3 allele, a frequency identical with that in hereditary hemochromatosis, whereas the frequency of HLA-A3 is 30% in cirrhotics without iron overload, a frequency identical within the general population.[274] These data suggest that all or most of the alcoholic cirrhosis patients with iron overload probably have hereditary hemochromatosis, and that ethanol abuse is additive but not the primary cause. However, the issue is still not fully resolved.

### Shunt Hemochromatosis

Many cases have been observed of "shunt hemochromatosis" that appears within a few years of the establishment of a shunt between the portal and systemic venous systems. The shunt has usually been created surgically to relieve pressure in esophageal varices, and in most instances the iron loading has followed end-to-side anastomoses.[283-285] However, the disorder has also developed spontaneously, presumably from formation of collateral channels between portal and systemic veins. The rate of iron accumulation seems rapid. The mechanism is unknown. The manifestations are the same as those of hemochromatosis from other causes.

## Chronic Renal Disease

During the 1970s and early 1980s iron dextran was commonly given prophylactically to patients who were subjected to frequent hemodialysis for severe chronic renal disease. The objective was to prevent iron deficiency that often resulted from blood loss during the dialysis procedure. Subsequently, many of these patients have manifested marked iron overload, and some nephrologists have instituted chelation therapy with desferrioxamine.[286-288] It seems too early to judge the efficacy of this treatment. The need for iron chelation therapy has been questioned by the observation that hepatic dysfunction was not observed in a series of such patients during as much as 7 years.[289] Clearly, however, parenteral iron therapy should not be given indiscriminately to long-term hemodialysis patients.

## Prolonged Iron Therapy

In rare instances, the prolonged administration of iron to patients who did not need it has been responsible for iron overload.[290-293] Manifestations indistinguishable from hemochromatosis may have been secondary to increased iron intake. Since iron preparations are advertised widely in the United States, are available without prescription, and are consumed in large quantities, it is of interest that more examples of overload have not been reported. For this reason, the potential of iron preparations for the production of iron storage disease deserves special attention. On the basis of present-day knowledge of iron metabolism, it is possible to make some rough estimates of the amount of iron that might accumulate in the body of normal persons when different amounts of medicinal iron are administered over long periods. The rate of increase ($\Delta F$) is the difference between the amount of iron absorbed (A) and the amount of iron lost from the body (L): $\Delta F = A - L$. Both of these functions depend upon the amount of stored iron already present in the body; storage iron decreases iron absorption and increases iron loss.

Scant data are present to define either of these parameters, but on the basis of those data that are available[115-117,294] L may be approximated as .0009 $\sqrt{F}$ for males or .0009 $\sqrt{F}$ + .0005 for menstruating females, where F is the body iron store in g (Fig. 7–11). We have already pointed out that the amount of iron absorbed from a given dose is:

$$A = 0.022\ D^{0.676} \text{ for males and}$$

$$A = 0.025\ D^{0.668} \text{ for females.}$$

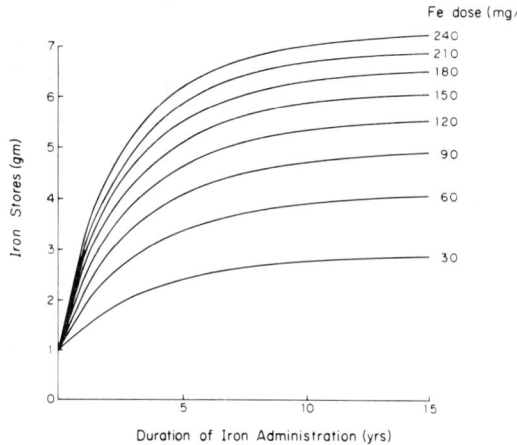

ACCUMULATION OF IRON STORES AT DIFFERENT SINGLE DAILY DOSAGES IN WOMEN

**Fig. 7–11.** The expected accumulation of iron in menstruating women receiving single daily doses that ranged from 30 to 240 mg. These data are based on the assumptions that iron absorption in females is .025 × $D^{0.668}$, where D is the dose of iron in g, that iron absorption is modified by stores to the extent of $e^{-0.196(F-1)}$, and that excretion is .0009 $\sqrt{F}$ + .0005, where F is the iron stores in g.

This amount seems to be modified by the amount of storage iron by a factor of approximately $e^{0.196(F-1)}$, based on modification of iron absorption in man with different levels of iron burden.[65,66,295] As the fraction of iron absorbed decreases and the amount excreted increases, an equilibrium is established at a level of body iron that depends upon the dose given. The results of calculations of the expected body iron burden at different doses of medicinal iron taken over long periods of time are shown in Figure 7–11. Finally, in view of the high prevalence of idiopathic hemochromatosis, and the relatively low frequency of hemochromatosis ascribed to chronic ingestion of iron, it is plausible that many of the latter cases also are homozygous for hereditary hemochromatosis.

Clearly there is some hazard from prolonged administration of large doses or iron to persons who are not iron-deficient. This is particularly a problem for patients with thalassemia major and other chronic anemias, for whom the ultimate development of hemochromatosis is a serious complication of treatment. For premenopausal women who have normal menses and do not have thalassemia or other chronic anemia, the hazard of serious iron overload resulting from exogenous iron is slight. However, the inappropriate and prolonged administration of iron, by oral or parenteral route, to other adults who are not bleeding and not iron-deficient needlessly exposes them to the risk of hemochromatosis with all its serious complications. This hazard has, of course, long been recognized. The demonstration that 2 or 3 Americans/1,000 are homozygous for the hereditary hemochromatosis gene emphasizes the high prevalence of vulnerability to development of this serious disease, and should lead physicians not to prescribe iron medications indiscriminately for prolonged periods.

## Refractory Anemia

The amount of iron found in the tissues of patients with refractory anemia,[4,5] particularly those with hypercellular marrows and ineffective erythropoiesis, is occasionally greater than can be accounted for by the tranfusions they have received. In some cases, little blood was given during the course of the illness, yet excess iron was present. Not all these subjects have been inappropriately treated with iron, although that has happened in some instances. Excessive absorption of dietary iron must have occurred, supposedly because of the accelerated but ineffective erythropoiesis. Bothwell and Finch found 31 such patients reported in the literature: the anemias included refractory anemia (now called sideroblastic anemia), thalassemia major, and paroxysmal nocturnal hemoglobinuria; all had erythroid hyperplasia of their bone marrows.[4] Portal cirrhosis occurred in 26, and an additional 4 had increased portal tract fibrosis; 5 had diabetes and 6 more had impaired glucose tolerance; at least 15 showed increased pigmentation of the skin. Indeed, the cardiac and hepatic complications of hemochromatosis are common causes of death in patients with sideroblastic anemias or thalassemias.

We and others have encountered severe iron overload in patients with congenital dyserythropoietic anemia. Hereditary spherocytosis and thalassemia minor apparently are not usually associated with iron overload except in those patients misdiagnosed as having iron deficiency and given copious amounts of iron over many years. However, some cases have been reported in which these disorders coexisted with hereditary hemochromatosis. In view of the high prevalence of the latter disorder in persons of European ancestry, the concurrence of these disorders is hardly surprising. In patients such as these, large amounts of hemosiderin are found in parenchymal as well as in reticuloendothelial cells. Why they develop the changes of hemochromatosis, whereas transfusional hemosiderosis without parenchymal damage is found in most multitransfused subjects with similar loads of body iron, remains a mystery. Nutritional differences between the two groups

cannot clearly be identified. Factors of possible significance include cirrhosis resulting from serum hepatitis and the possibility that primarily parenchymal (hepatocyte) distribution of iron may be related to the gastrointestinal portal of entry of a significant portion of the excess body iron. Parenterally administered iron accumulates predominantly in the Kupffer cells of the macrophage system, where it may do much less harm.

## REFERENCES

1. Committee on Iron Deficiency: J.A.M.A. *203*:407–412, 1968.
2. Moore, C.V.: Harvey Lecture *55*:67–101, 1960.
3. Moore, C.V. and Dubach, R.: Iron. *In* Mineral Metabolism: An Advanced Treatise, Vol. 2. (Comar, L., Bronner, F., Eds.) New York, Academic Press, 1962.
4. Bothwell, T.H., Finch, C.A. (Eds.): Iron Metabolism. Boston, Little, Brown and Company, 1962.
5. Fairbanks, V.F., Fahey, J.L., Beutler, E.: Clinical Disorders of Iron Metabolism. 2nd ed. New York, Grune and Stratton, 1971.
6. Moore, C.V.: Ser. Haematol. *6*:1–14, 1965.
7. U.S. Interdepartmental Committee for National Defense Nutrition Survey of the Armed Forces: Iran, 1956. Turkey, 1958. Spain, 1958. Ethiopia, 1959. Peru, 1959. Ecuador, 1960. The Kingdom of Thailand, 1961.
8. MacDonald, R.A.: Arch. Intern. Med. *112*:184–190, 1963.
9. Taylor, E.W.: The Examination of Water and Water Supplies. 7th ed. London, Churchill, 1958.
10. Beutler, E., Fairbanks, V.F., Fahey, J.L.: Clinical Disorders of Iron Metabolism. New York, Grune and Stratton, 1963.
11. Conrad, M: Iron Deficiency: Pathogenesis, Clinical Aspects, Therapy. (Hallberg L., Harwerth, H.-G., Vannotti, A., Eds.) New York, Academic Press, 1970.
12. Pollack, S., Lasky, F.D.: J. Lab. Clin. Med. *87*:670–679, 1976.
13. Huebers, H.A., Huebers, E., Csiba, E., et al.: Blood *61*:283–290, 1983.
14. Topham, R.W., Walker, M.C., Calisch, M.P., et al.: Biochemistry *21*:4529–4535, 1982.
15. Minnich, V., Okcuoglu, A., Tarcon, Y., et al.: Am. J. Clin. Nutr. *21*:78–86, 1968.
16. Morck, T.A., Lynch S.R., Cook, J.D.: Am. J. Clin. Nutr. *37*:416–420, 1983.
17. Frölich, W., Lysø, A.: Am. J. Clin. Nutr. *37*:31–36, 1983.
18. Murray, M.J.: J. Lab. Clin. Med. *70*:866, 1967. (Abstract)
19. Luke, C.G., Davis, P.S., Deller, D.J.: Lancet *2*:844–846, 1968.
20. Wynter, C.V.A., Williams, R. Lancet *2*:534–537, 1968.
21. Beutler, E., Kelly, B.M., Beutler, F.: Am. J. Clin. Nutr. *11*:559–567, 1962.
22. Heinrich, H.C.: Iron Deficiency. (Hallberg, L., Harwerth, H.-G., Vannotti, A., Eds.) New York, Academic Press, 1970.
23. Chapman, R.W., Morgan M.Y., Boss, A.M., et al.: Dig. Dis. Sci. *28*:321–327, 1983.
24. Celada, A., Rudolf, H., Donath, A.: Am. J. Hematol. *5*:225–237, 1978.

25. Morgan, E.H.: Q. J. Exp. Physiol. *65*:239–252, 1980.
26. Huebers, H.A., Huebers, E., Csiba, E., et al.: Blood *61*:283–290, 1983.
27. Weintraub, L.R., Weinstein, M.B., Huser, H.-J., et al.: J. Clin. Invest. *47*:531–539, 1968.
28. Raffin, S.B., Woo, C.H., Roost, K.T., et al.: J. Clin. Invest. *54*:1344–1352, 1974.
29. Brown, E.B., Hwang, Y.-F., Nicol, S., et al.: J. Lab. Clin. Med. *72*:58–64, 1968.
30. Turnbull, A., Cleton, F., Finch, C.A.: J. Clin. Invest. *41*:1897–1907, 1962.
31. Hallberg, L., Sölvell, L.: Acta Med. Scand. *181*:335–354, 1967.
32. Moore, C.V.: Symposium on Occurrence, causes and prevention of nutritional anaemias. Swedish Nutrition Foundation, Tylösand, 1967. Symposia 6. (Blix, G., Ed.) Uppsala, Almqvist and Wiksells, 1968.
33. Josephs, H.W.: Blood *13*:1–54, 1958.
34. Layrisse, M., Martinez-Torres, C.: Prog. Hematol. *7*:137–160, 1971.
35. Elwood, P.C.: Lancet *2*:516, 1968. (Letter to editor)
36. Gillooly, M., Bothwell, T.H., Torrance, J.D., et al.: Br. J. Nutr. *49*:331–342, 1983.
37. Hallberg, L., Rossander, L.: Scand. J. Gastroenterol. *17*:151–160, 1982.
38. Cook, J.D., Morck, T.A., Lynch, S.R.: Am. J. Clin. Nutr. *34*:2622–2629, 1981.
39. Layrisse, M., Cook, J.D., Martinez, C., et al.: Blood *33*:430–443, 1969.
40. Martinez-Torres, C., Layrisse, M.: Blood *35*:669–682, 1970.
41. Layrisse, M., Martinez-Torres, C., Cook, J.D., et al.: Blood *41*:333–352, 1973.
42. Pirzio-Biroli, G., Bothwell, T.H., Finch, C.A.: J. Lab. Clin. Med. *51*:37–48, 1958.
43. Cook, J.D., Layrisse, M., Martinez-Torres, C., et al.: J. Clin. Invest. *51*:805–815, 1972.
44. Awai, M., Brown, E.B.: J. Lab. Clin. Med. *61*:363–396, 1963.
45. Laurell, C.-B.: Pharmacol. Rev. *4*:371–395, 1952.
46. Fletcher, J., Huehns, E.R.: Nature *218*:1211–1214, 1968.
47. Huebers, H.A., Csiba, E., Huebers, E., et al.: Proc. Natl. Acad. Sci. USA *80*:300–304, 1983.
48. Morgan, E.H., Huebers, H., Finch, C.A. Blood *52*:1219–1228, 1978.
49. Awai, M., Chipman, B., Brown, E.B.: J. Lab. Clin. Med. *85*:769–784, 1975.
50. Princiotto, J.V., Zapolski, E.J.: Nature *255*:87–88, 1975.
51. Harris, D.C., Aisen, P.: Nature *257*:821–823, 1975.
52. Schlabach, M.R., Bates, G.W.: J. Biol. Chem. *250*:2182–2188, 1975.
53. Delaney, T.A., Morgan, W.H., Morgan, E.H.: Biochim. Biophys. Acta *701*:295–304, 1982.
54. Marx, J.J.M., Klein Gebbink, J.A.G., Nishisato, T., et al.: Br. J. Haematol. *52*:105–110, 1982.
55. van Bockxmeer, F.M., Morgan, E.H.: Comp. Biochem. Physiol. [A] *71*:211–218, 1982.
56. Jandl, J.H., Katz, J.H.: J. Clin. Invest. *42*:314–326, 1963.
57. Iacopetta, B.J., Morgan, E.H., Yeoh, G.C.T.: Biochim. Biophys. Acta *687*:204–210, 1982.
58. Octave, J.-N., Schneider, Y.-J., Hoffmann, P., et al.: Eur. J. Biochem. *123*:235–240, 1982.
59. Iacopetta, B.J., Morgan, E.H., Yeoh, G.C.T.: J. Histochem. Cytochem. *31*:336–344, 1983.
60. Schneider, Y.-J., Limet, J.N., Octave, J.-N., et al.: Prog. Clin. Biol. Res. *91*:495–521, 1982.
61. van Bockxmeer, F.M., Yates, G.K., Morgan, E.H.: Eur. J. Biochem. *92*:147–154, 1978.
62. van Bockxmeer, F.M., Morgan, E.H.: Biochim. Biophys. Acta *584*:76–83, 1979.
63. Light, A., Morgan, E.H.: Scand. J. Haematol. *28*:205–214, 1982.
64. Armstrong, N.J., Morgan, E.H.: Biochim. Biophys. Acta *762*:175–186, 1983.
65. Rao, K., van Renswoude, J., Kempf, C., et al.: FEBS Lett *160*:213–216, 1983.
66. Lim, B.C., Morgan, E.H.: Comp. Biochem. Physiol. [A] *79*:317–323, 1984.
67. Nunez, M.-T., Cole, E.S., Glass, J.: J. Biol. Chem. *258*:1146–1151, 1983.
68. Giblett, E.R.: Genetic Markers in Human Blood. Philadelphia, F.A. Davis Co., 1969.
69. Conrad, M.E., Jr., Crosby, W.H.: Blood *22*:406–415, 1963.
70. Finch, C.A., Deubelbeiss, K., Cook, J.D., et al.: Medicine (Baltimore) *49*:17–53, 1970.
71. Colli Franzone, P., Paganuzzi, A., Stefanelli, M.: J. Math. Biol. *15*:173–201, 1982.
72. Cook, J.D.: Meth. Hematol. *1*:1–172, 1980.
73. Harrison, P.M., Clegg, G.A., May, K.: Iron in Biochemistry and Medicine, II. (Jacobs, A., Worwood, M., Eds.) New York, Academic Press, 1980. pp. 131–171.
74. Clegg, G.A., Stansfield, R.F.D., Bourne, P.E., et al.: Nature *288*:298–300, 1980.
75. Crichton, R.R., Roman, F.: J. Mol. Catalysis *4*:75–82, 1978.
76. Heusterpreute, M., Wustefeld, C., Mathijs, J.M., et al.: Proc. Peptides Biol. Fluids Colloq. *28*:91, 1980.
77. Bjork, I., Fish, W.W.: Biochemistry *10*:2844–2848, 1971.
78. Arosio, P., Adelman, T.G., Drysdale, J.W.: J. Biol. Chem. *253*:4451–4458, 1978.
79. Worwood, M., Summers, M., Miller, F., et al.: Br. J. Haematol. *28*:27–35, 1974.
80. Jacobs, A., Jones, B., Ricketts, C., et al.: Br. J. Cancer *34*:286–290, 1976.
81. Jacobs, A., Slater, A., Whittaker, J.A., et al.: Br. J. Cancer *34*:162–166, 1976.
82. Treffry, A., Harrison, P.M.: Biochim. Biophys. Acta *610*:421–424, 1980.
83. Treffry, A., Harrison, P.M.: Biochem. Soc. Trans. *8*:656–657, 1980.
84. Fischbach, F.A., Gregory, D.W., Harrison, P.M., et al.: J. Ultrastruct. Res. *37*:495–503, 1971.
85. General Discussion I: Haemosiderin. CIBA Found. Symp. *51*:69–78, 1977.
86. Crichton, R.R.: N. Engl. J. Med. *284*:1413–1422, 1971.
87. Hoy, T.G., Harrison, P.M., Shabbir, M.: Biochem. J. *139*:603–607, 1974.
88. Jacobs, A., Miller, F., Worwood, M., et al.: Br. Med. J. *4*:206–208, 1972.
89. Lipschitz, D.A., Cook, J.D., Finch, C.A.: N. Engl. J. Med. *290*:1213–1216, 1974.
90. Siimes, M.A., Addiego, J.E., Jr., Dallman, P.R.: Blood *43*:581–590, 1974.
91. Jacobs, A., Worwood, M.: Br. J. Haematol. *31*:1–3, 1975. (Annotation)
92. Bainton, D.F., Finch, C.A.: Am. J. Med. *37*:62–70, 1964.
93. Beutler, E., Robson, M.J., Buttenweiser, E.: Ann. Intern. Med. *48*:60–82, 1958.

94. Weinfeld, A.: Acta Med. Scand. [Suppl.] *427*:1–155, 1964.

95. Beutler, E.: N. Engl. J. Med. *256*:692–697, 1957.

96. Beutler, E., Drennan, W., Block, M.: J. Lab. Clin. Med. *43*:427–439, 1954.

97. Hahn, P.F., Whipple, G.H.: Am. J. Med. Sci. *191*:24–42, 1936.

98. Beutler, E.: Am. J. Med. Sci. *234*:517–527, 1957.

99. Beutler, E.: J. Clin. Invest. *38*:1605–1616, 1959.

100. Beutler, E.: Acta Haematol. (Basel) *21*:371–377, 1959.

101. Beutler, E., Blaisdell, R.K.: J. Clin. Invest. *37*:833–835, 1958.

102. Beutler, E.: Ill. Med. J. *116*:16, 1959.

103. Jacobs, A.: Lancet *2*:1331–1333, 1961.

104. Ackrell, B.A.C., Maguire J.J., Dallman, P.R., et al.: J. Biol. Chem. *259*:10053–10059, 1984.

105. Mackler, B., Person, R., Miller L.R., et al.: Pediatr. Res. *13*:1010–1011, 1979.

106. Symes, A.L., Sowkes, T.L., Youdim, M.B.H., et al.: Can. J. Biochem. *47*:999–1002, 1969.

107. Youdim, M.B.H., Green, A.R.: CIBA Found. Symp. *51*:201–221, 1977.

108. Youdim, M.B.H., Green, A.R.: Proc. Nutr. Soc. *37*:173–179, 1978.

109. Srivastava, S.K., Zaheer, N., Krishnan, P.S.: Arch. Biochem. Biophys. *105*:446–447, 1964. (Letter to editor)

110. Bailey-Wood, R., Blayney, L.M., Muir, J.R., et al.: Br. J. Exp. Pathol. *56*:193–198, 1975.

111. Kyaw, A., Win, T., Pe, U.H.: Biochem. Med. *11*:194–197, 1974.

112. Bothwell, T.H., Pribilla, W.F., Mebust, W., et al.: Am. J. Physiol. *193*:615–622, 1958.

113. Davies, J., Brown, E.B., Jr., Stewart, D., et al.: Am. J. Physiol. *197*:87–92, 1959.

114. Green, R., Charlton, R., Seftel, H., et al.: Am. J. Med. *45*:336–353, 1968.

115. Bothwell, T.H., Seftel, H., Jacobs, P., et al.: Am. J. Clin. Nutr. *14*:47–51, 1964.

116. Finch, C.A.: Physiopathologic mechanisms of iron excretion. *In* Iron Metabolism: An International Symposium. (Gross, F., Ed.) Berlin, Springer-Verlag, 1964.

117. Crosby, W.H., Conrad, M.E., Jr., Wheby, M.S.: Blood *22*:429–440, 1963.

118. Ebaugh, F.G., Jr., Clemens, T., Jr., Rodnan, G., et al.: Am. J. Med. *25*:169–181, 1958.

119. Hallberg, L., Nilsson, L.: Acta Obstet. Gynecol. Scand. *43*:352–359, 1964.

120. Hallberg, L., Högdahl, A.-M., Nilsson, L., et al.: Acta Obstet. Gynecol. Scand. *45*:320–351, 1966.

121. Rybo, G.: Iron Deficiency: Pathogenesis, Clinical Aspects, Therapy. (Hallberg, L., Harwerth, H.-G., Vannotti, A., Eds.) New York, Academic Press, 1970.

122. Guillebaud, J., Bonnar, J., Morehead, J., et al.: Lancet *1*:387–390, 1976.

123. Mears, E., Grant, E.C.G.: Br. Med. J. *2*:75–79, 1962.

124. Moore, C.V.: Iron nutrition. *In* Iron Metabolism: An International Symposium. (Gross, F., Ed.) Berlin, Springer-Verlag, 1964, pp. 241–255.

125. Simon, T.L., Hunt, W.C., Garry, P.J.: Transfusion *24*:469–472, 1984.

126. Sturgeon, P.: Studies or iron requirements in infants and children. *In* Iron in Clinical Medicine. (Wallerstein, R.O., Mettier, S.R., Eds.) Berkeley, University of California Press, 1958, pp. 183–203.

127. Pearson, H.A., Abrams, I., Fernbach, D.J., et al.; Pediatr. Res. *1*:169–172, 1967.

128. Karp, R.J., Haaz, W.S., Starko, K., et al.: Am. J. Dis. Child. *128*:18–20, 1974.

129. Fielding, J., O'Shaughnessy, M.C., Brunström, G.M.: Lancet *2*:9–12, 1965.

130. Monsen, E.R., Kuhn, I.N., Finch, C.A.: Am. J. Clin. Nutr. *20*:842–849, 1967.

131. Scott, D.E., Pritchard, J.A.: J.A.M.A. *199*:897–900, 1967.

132. Pritchard, J.A., Hunt, C.F.: Surg. Gynecol. Obstet. *106*:516–518, 1958.

133. El-Najjar, M.Y., Robertson, A.L., Jr.: Science *193*:141–143, 1976.

134. El-Najjar, M.Y., Lozoff, B., Ryan, D.J.: A. J. R., *125*:918–924, 1975.

135. Dozy, A.M., Kan, Y.W., Embury, S.H., et al.: Nature *280*:605–607, 1979.

136. Johnson, C.S., Tegos, C., Beutler, E.: Arch. Intern. Med. *142*:1280–1282, 1982.

137. Garn, S.M., Ryan, A.S., Owen, G.M., et al.: Am. J. Clin. Nutr. *34*:1645–1647, 1981.

138. Liebman, M., Kenney, M.A., Billon, W., et al.: Am. J. Clin. Nutr. *38*:109–114, 1983.

139. Beveridge, B.R., Bannerman, R.M., Evanson, J.M., et al.: Q. J. Med. *34*:145–161, 1965.

140. Magnusson, B.E.O.: Scand.J. Haematol. [Suppl.] *26*:7–111, 1976.

141. Baird, I.M., Wilson, G.M.: Q. J. Med. *28*:35–41, 1959.

142. Stevens, A.R., Jr., Pirzio-Biroli, G., Harkins, H.N., et al.: Ann. Surg. *149*:534–538, 1959.

143. Hoag, M.S., Wallerstein, R.O., Pollycove, M.: Pediatrics *27*:199–203, 1961.

144. Hancock, D.E., Onstad, J.W., Wolf, P.L.: Am. J. Clin. Pathol. *65*:73–78, 1976.

145. Adams, J.F.: Scand. J. Gastroenterol. *3*:145–151, 1968.

146. Hines, J.D., Hoffbrand, A.V., Mollin, D.L.: Am. J. Med. *43*:555–569, 1967.

147. Kimber, C., Patterson, J.F., Weintraub, L.R.: J.A.M.A. *202*:935–938, 1967.

148. Hallberg, L., Sölvell, L., Zederfeldt, B.: Acta Med. Scand. [Suppl. 179] *445*:269–275, 1966.

149. Meyer, C.T., Troncale, F.J., Galloway, S., et al.: Medicine (Baltimore) *60*:36–48, 1981.

150. Clouse, R.E., Costigan, D.J., Mills, B.A., et al.: Arch. Intern. Med. *145*:458–461, 1985.

151. Hunding, A., Jordal, R., Paulev, P.-E.: Acta Med. Scand. *209*:315–318, 1981.

152. Stewart, J.G., Ahlquist, D.A., McGill, D.B., et al.: Ann. Intern. Med. *100*:843–845, 1984.

153. Magnusson, B., Hallberg, L., Rossander, L., et al.: Acta Med. Scand. *216*:149–164, 1984.

154. Crowley, L.V., Seay, J., Mullin, G.: Am. J. Gastroenterol. *79*:850–860, 1984.

155. Heilmeyer, L., Keller, W., Vivell, O., et al.: Schweiz. Med. Wochenschr. *91*:1203, 1961.

156. Cap, J., Lehotska, V., Mayerova, A.: Cesk. Pediatr. *23*:1010–1025, 1968.

157. Loperena, L., Dorantes, S., Medrano, E., et al.: Bol. Med. Hosp. Infant. Mex. *31*:519–535, 1974.

158. Goya, N., Miyazaki, S., Kodate, S., et al.: Blood *40*:239–245, 1972.

159. Fairbanks, V.F., Beutler, E.: Congenital atransferrinemia and idiopathic pulmonary hemosiderosis. *In* Hematology. 3rd ed. (Williams, W.J., Beutler, E., Erslev, A.J., et al., Eds.) New York, McGraw-Hill Book Company, 1983, pp. 300–310.

160. Beutler, E.: Ann. Intern. Med. *50*:313–322, 1959.
161. Lund, C.J.: Am. J. Obstet. Gynecol. *62*:947–961, 1951.
162. Piomelli, S., Brickman, A., Carlos, E.: Pediatrics *57*:136–141, 1976.
163. Sturgeon, P.: Pediatrics *17*:341–348, 1956.
164. Burks, J.M., Siimes, M.A., Mentzer, W.C., et al.: J. Pediatr. *88*:224–228, 1976.
165. Rios, E., Lipschitz, D.A., Cook, J.D., et al.: Pediatrics *55*:694–699, 1975.
166. Hutchinson, H.E.: Blood *8*:236–248, 1953.
167. Rath, C.E., Finch C.A.: J. Lab. Clin. Med. *33*:81–86, 1948.
168. Beutler, E.: J. Lab. Clin. Med. *51*:415–419, 1958.
169. Olsson, K.S., Weinfeld, A.: Acta Med. Scand. *192*:543–549, 1972.
170. Sies, H., Grosskopf, M.: Eur. J. Biochem. *57*:513–520, 1975.
171. Jacobs, P., Dommissee, J.: J. Med. *13*:309–321, 1982.
172. Harju, E., Pakarinen, A., Larmi, T.: Scand. J. Clin. Lab. Invest. *44*:555–556, 1984.
173. Monzon, C.M., Fairbanks, V.F., Burgert, E.O., Jr., et al.: Am. J. Hematol. *19*:27–36, 1985.
174. Fairbanks, V.F., Gilchrist, G.S., Brimhall, B., et al.: Blood *53*:109–115, 1979.
175. Fairbanks, V.F., Oliveros, R., Brandabur, J.H., et al.: Am. J. Hematol. *8*:109–121, 1980.
176. Ali, M.A.M., Luxton, A.W., Walker, W.H.C.: Can. Med. Assoc. J. *118*:945–946, 1978.
177. Luxton, A.W., Walker W.H.C., Gauldie, J., et al.: Clin. Chem. *23*:683–689, 1977.
178. Siimes, M.A., Dallman, P.B.: Br. J. Haematol. *28*:7–18, 1974.
179. Smith, R.J., Davis, P., Thomson, A.B.R., et al.: J. Rheumatol. *4*:389–392, 1974.
180. Fairbanks, V.F., Klee, G.G.: Prog. Clin. Pathol. *8*:175–203, 1981.
181. Heilmeyer, L., Ploetner, K.: Das Serumeisen und die Eisenmangelkrankheit. Jena, Gustav Fischer, 1937.
182. Jasinski, B., Roth, O.: Larvierte Eisenmangelkrankheit. Basel, Schwabe, 1954.
183. Beutler, E., Larsh, S.E., Gurney, C.W.: Ann. Intern. Med. *52*:378–394, 1960.
184. Webb, T.E., Oski, F.A.: J. Pediatr. *82*:827–829, 1973.
185. Pollitt, E., Leibel, R.L.: J. Pediatr. *88*:372–381, 1976.
186. Voorhess, M.L., Stuart, M.J., Stockman, J.A., et al.: J. Pediatr. *86*:542–547, 1975.
187. Lozoff, B., Brittenham, G.M., Viteri, F.E., et al.: J. Pediatr. *101*:948–952, 1982.
188. Oski, F.A., Honig, A.S., Helu, B., et al.: Pediatrics *71*:877–880, 1983.
189. Walter, T., Kovalskys, J., Stekel, A.: J. Pediatr. *102*:519–522, 1983.
190. Lozoff, B., Brittenham, G., Viteri, F.E., et al.: Behavioral abnormalities in infants with iron deficiency anemia. *In* Iron Deficiency: Brain Biochemistry and Behavior (Pollitt, E., Leibel, R.L., Eds.) New York, Raven Press, 1982, pp. 183–194.
191. Pollitt, E., Viteri, F., Saco-Pollitt, C., et al.: Behavioral effects of iron deficiency anemia in children. *In* Iron Deficiency: Brain Biochemistry and Behavior (Pollit, E., Leibel, R.L., Eds.) New York, Raven Press, 1982, pp. 195–208.
192. Youdim, M.B.H., Yehuda, S., Ben-Shachar, D., et al.: Behavioral and brain biochemical changes in iron deficient rats: the involvement of iron in dopamine receptor function. *In* Iron Deficiency: Brain Biochemistry and Behavior (Pollitt, E., Leibel, R.L., Eds.) New York, Raven Press, 1982, pp. 39–56.
193. Finch, C.A., Gollnick, P.D., Hlastala, M.P., et al.: J. Clin. Invest. *64*:129–137, 1979.
194. MacDonald, V.W., Charache, S., Hathaway, P.J.: J. Lab. Clin. Med. *105*:11–18, 1985.
195. Vellar, O.D., Hermansen, L.: Acta Med. Scand. [Suppl.] *522*:1–62, 1971.
196. Anderson, H.T., Barkve, H.: Scand J. Clin. Lab. Invest. [Suppl.] *25*:1–62, 1970.
197. Andersen, H.T., Stavem, P.: Nutr. Metab. *14*:129–135, 1972.
198. Viteri, F.E., Torun, B.: Clin. Haematol. *3*:609–626, 1974.
199. Lieden, G., Adolfsson, L.: Scand. J. Clin. Lab. Invest. *34*:37–42, 1974.
200. Davies, C.T.: Acta Paediatr. Belg. [Suppl.] *28*:253–256, 1974.
201. Gardner, G.W., Edgerton, V.R., Senewiratne, B., et al.: Am. J. Clin. Nutr. *30*:910–917, 1977.
202. Charlton, R.W., Derman, D., Skikne, B., et al.: Clin. Sci. Mol. Med. *53*:537–541, 1977.
203. Beutler, E., Larsh, S., Tanzi, F.: Am. J. Med. Sci. *239*:759–765, 1960.
204. Beutler, E., Larsh, S.E., Gurney, C.W.: Ann. Intern. Med. *52*:378–394, 1960.
205. Edgerton, V.R., Ohira, Y., Gardner, G.W., et al.: Effects of iron deficiency anemia on voluntary activities in rats and humans. *In* Iron Deficiency: Brain Biochemistry and Behavior (Pollitt, E., Leiber, R.L., Eds.) New York, Raven Press, 1982, pp. 141–160.
206. Ohira, Y., Edgerton, V.R., Gardner, G.W., et al.: J. Nutr. Sci. Vitaminol. (Tokyo) *27*:87–96, 1981.
207. Beutler, E., Fairbanks, V.F.: The effects of iron deficiency. *In* Iron in Biochemistry and Medicine, II (Jacobs, A., Worwood, M., Eds.) New York, Academic Press, 1980, pp. 393–425.
208. Buckley, R.H.: J. Pediatr. *86*:993–995, 1975.
209. Chandra, R.K., Saraya, A.K.: Pediatrics *86*:899–902, 1975.
210. Macdougall, L.G., Anderson, R., McNab, G.M., et al.: J. Pediatr. *86*:833–843, 1975.
211. Masawe, A.E.J., Swai, G.: Lancet *1*:1241, 1975. (Letter to editor)
212. Chandra, R.K.: Nutr. Rev. *34*:129–132, 1976.
213. van Asbeck, B.S., Verhoef, J.: Eur. J. Clin. Microbiol. *2*:6–10, 1983.
214. Coltman, C.A., Jr.: J.A.M.A. *207*:513–516, 1969.
215. Lanzkowsky, P.: Arch. Dis. Child. *34*:140–148, 1959.
216. Kimber, C., Weintraub, L.R.: N. Engl. J. Med. *279*:453–459, 1968.
217. Jacobs, A.: Br. J. Cancer *15*:736–744, 1961.
218. Foy, H., Kondi, A.: Trans. R. Soc. Trop. Med. Hyg. *54*:419–433, 1960.
219. Lees, F., Rosenthal, F.D.: Q. J. Med. *27*:19–26, 1958.
220. Jasinski, B.: Schweiz. Med. Wochenschr. *79*:291–293, 1949.
221. Gross, S.J., Stuart, M.J., Swender, P.T., et al.: Pediatrics *88*:795–799, 1976.
222. Halsted, J.A., Prasad, A.S., Nadimi, M.: Arch. Intern. Med. *116*:253–256, 1965.
223. Tucker, D.M., Sandstead, H.H., Swenson, R.A., et al.: Physiol. Behav. *29*:737–740, 1982.
224. Mehta, B.C., Panjwani, D.D., Jhala, D.A.: Acta Haematol. *70*:189–193, 1983.
225. Shepard, T.H., Mackler, B., Finch, C.A.: Teratology *22*:329–334, 1980.

226. Beard, J., Finch, C.A., Green, W.L.: Life Sci *30*:691–697, 1982.

227. Marchasin, S., Wallerstein, R.O., Aggeler, P.M.: Calif. Med. *101*:95–100, 1964.

228. Kasper, C.K., Whissel, D.Y.E., Wallerstein, R.D.: J.A.M.A. *191*:359–363, 1965.

229. Sahud, M.A., Olsen, H., Pedemont, L.: Ann. Intern. Med. *81*:132–133, 1974. (Letter to editor)

230. Scher, H., Silber, R.: Ann. Intern. Med. *84*:571–572, 1976. (Letter to editor)

231. Mehta, B.C., Lotliker, K.S., Patel, J.C.: Indian J. Med. Res. *61*:1818–1823, 1973.

232. Brise, H., Hallberg, L.: Acta Med. Scand. [Suppl.] *376*:1–73, 1962.

233. Kerr, D.N.S., Davidson, S.: Lancet *2*:489–492, 1958.

234. Beutler, E.: Clin. Med. *71*:1889–1901, 1964.

235. Beutler, E., Meerkreebs, G.: N. Engl. J. Med. *274*:1152–1153, 1966. (Letter to editor)

236. Baird, I.M., Walters, R.L., Sutton, D.R.: Br. Med. J. *4*:505–508, 1974.

237. Beutler, E.: Blood *15*:288–290, 1960.

238. MacKinnon, A.E., Bancewicz, J.: Br. Med. J. *2*:277–279, 1973.

239. Seshadri, S., Hirode, K., Naik, P., et al.: Br. J. Nutr. *48*:233–240, 1982.

240. Steinkamp, R., Dubach, R., Moore, C.V.: Arch. Intern. Med. *95*:181–193, 1955.

241. Schulz, J., Smith, N.J.: Am. J. Dis. Child. *93*:30, 1957. (Abstract)

242. Layrisse, M., Martinez-Torres, C., Renzi, M., et al.: Am. J. Clin. Nutr. *29*:8–18, 1976.

243. Garby, L.: Unpublished data, 1976.

244. Sayers, M.H., Lynch, S.R., Charlton, R.W., et al.: Br. J. Haematol. *28*:483–495, 1974.

245. Elwood, P.C., Benjamin, I.T., Fry, F.A., et al.: Am. J. Clin. Nutr. *23*:1267–1271, 1970.

246. Moe, P.J.: Acta Paediatr. Scand. [Suppl.] *150*:1–67, 1963.

247. De Leeuw, N.K.M., Lowenstein, L., Hsieh, Y.-S.: Medicine (Baltimore) *45*:291–315, 1966.

248. Romslo, I., Haram, K., Sagen, N., et al.: Br. J. Obstet. Gynaecol. *90*:101–107, 1983.

249. National Center for Health Statistics, Singer, J.D., Granahan, P., Goodrich, N.N., et al.: Diet and iron status, a study of relationships: United States, 1971–74. Vital and Health Statistics. Series 11, No. 229. DHHS Pub. No. (PHS) 83–1679. Public Health Service. Washington, D.C., U.S. Government Printing Office, December, 1982.

250. Garry, P.J., Goodwin, J.S., Hunt, W.C.: J. Am. Geriatr. Soc. *31*:389–399, 1983.

251. Finch, S.C., Finch, C.A.: Medicine (Baltimore) *34*:381–430, 1955.

252. Milder, M.S., Cook, J.D., Stray, S., et al.: Medicine (Baltimore) *59*:34–49, 1980.

253. Powell, L.W.: Ann. N.Y. Acad. Sci. *252*:124–134, 1975.

254. Powell, L.W., Halliday, J.W.: Idiopathic haemochromatosis. *In* Iron in Biochemistry and Medicine, II. (Jacobs, A., Worwood, M., Eds.) New York, Academic Press, 1980, pp. 461–498.

255. Blake, P.A., Merson, M.H., Weaver, R.E., et al.: N. Engl. J. Med. *300*:1–5, 1979.

256. Wright, A.C., Simpson, L.M., Oliver, J.D.: Infect. Immun. *34*:503–507, 1981.

257. National Institutes of Health: J.A.M.A. *251*:323–325, 1984.

258. Kruijs, F.J., Tan T.G.: Ned. Tijdschr. Geneeskd. *128*:2036–2038, 1984.

259. Capron, J.P., Capron-Chivrac, D., Tossou, H., et al.: Gastroenterology *87*:1372–1375, 1984.

260. Robins-Browne, R.M., Rabson, A.R., Koornhof, H.J.: Contrib. Microbiol. Immunol. *5*:277—282, 1979.

261. Roche, G., Leheup, B., Gerard, A., et al.: Rev. Med. Interne *3*:65–74, 1982.

262. Melby, K., Slørdahl, S., Gutteberg, T.J., et al.: Br. Med. J. *285*:467–468, 1982.

263. Simon, M., Alexandre, J.-L., Fauchet, R., et al.: Prog. Med. Genet. *4*:135–168, 1980.

264. Simon, M., Bourel, M., Fauchet, R., et al.: Gut *17*:332–334, 1976.

265. Simon, M., Bourel, M., Genetet, B., et al.: N. Engl. J. Med. *297*:1017–1021, 1977.

266. Ward, J.H., Kushner, J.P., Ray, F.A., et al.: J. Lab. Clin. Med., *103*:246–254, 1984.

267. Olsson, K.S., Ritter, B., Rosen, U., et al.: Acta Med. Scand. *213*:145–150, 1983.

268. MacSween, R.N.M., Scott, A.R.: J. Clin. Pathol. *26*:936–942, 1973.

269. Cartwright, G.E., Edwards, C.Q., Kravitz, K., et al.: N. Engl. J. Med. *301*:175–179, 1979.

270. Dadone, M.M., Kishner, J.P., Edwards, C.Q., et al.: Am. J. Clin. Pathol. *78*:196–207, 1982.

271. Edwards, C.Q., Skolnick, M.H., Kushner, J.P.: Prog. Hematol. *12*:43–71, 1981.

272. Borwein, S.T., Ghent, C.N., Flanagan, P.R., et al.: Clin. Invest. Med. *6*:171–179, 1983.

273. Bassett, M.L., Doran, T.J., Halliday, J.W., et al.: Hum. Genet. *60*:352–356, 1982.

274. LeSage, G.D., Baldus, W.P., Fairbanks, V.F., et al.: Gastroenterology *84*:1471–1477, 1983.

275. Bassett, M.L., Halliday, J.W., Ferris, R.A., et al.: Gastroenterology *87*:628–633, 1984.

276. Isaacson, C., Seftel, H.C., Keeley, K.J., et al.: J. Lab. Clin. Med. *58*:845–853, 1961.

277. Block, M., Moore, G., Wasi, P., et al.: Am. J. Pathol. *47*:89–123, 1965.

278. Charlton, R.W., Bothwell, T.H.: Prog. Hematol. *5*:298–323, 1966.

279. Bothwell, T.H.: Ser. Haematol. *6*:56–65, 1965.

280. MacDonald, R.A., Pechet, G.S.: Arch. Intern. Med. *116*:381–391, 1965.

281. Callender, S.T., Malpas, J.S.: Br. Med. J. *2*:1516–1518, 1963.

282. Davis, A.E., Badenoch, J.: Lancet *2*:6–8, 1962.

283. Tuttle, S.G., Figueroa, W.G., Grossman, M.I.: Am. J. Med. *26*:655–658, 1959.

284. Grace, N.D., Balint, J.A.: Am. J. Dig. Dis. *11*:351–358, 1966.

285. Nixon, D.D.: Am. J. Dig. Dis. *11*:359–366, 1966.

286. Ali, M., Fayemi, A.O., Rigolosi, R., et al.: J.A.M.A. *244*:343–345, 1980.

287. Krumlovsky, F.A.: Int. J. Artif. Organs *5*:223–225, 1982.

288. Hilfenhaus, M., Koch, K.-M., Bechstein, P.B., et al.: Contrib. Nephrol. *38*:167–173, 1984.

289. Kothari, T., Swamy, A.P., Lee, J.C.K., et al.: Dig. Dis. Sci. *25*:363–368, 1980.

290. Castleman, B., Towne, V.W.: N. Engl. J. Med. *247*:986–995, 1952.

291. Castleman, B., Kibbee, B.U.: N. Engl. J. Med. *258*:652–661, 1958.

292. Wallerstein, R.O., Robbins, S.L.: Am. J. Med. *14*:256–260, 1953.
293. Turnberg, L.A.: Br. Med. J. *1*:1360, 1965.
294. Pollycove, M.: Iron Kinetics. *In* Iron Metabolism: An International Symposium. (Gross, F., Ed.) Berlin, Springer-Verlag, 1964, pp. 148–170.
295. Pirzio-Biroli, G., Finch, C.A.: J. Lab. Clin. Med. *55*:216–220, 1960.

*Chapter* **8**

# IODINE

## John B. Stanbury

The necessity for a dietary supply of iodine arises from its role as a component of the two hormones of the thyroid gland, thyroxine ($T_4$) (Fig. 8–1), containing 4 atoms of iodine per molecule and triiodothyronine ($T_3$) (Fig. 8–1), containing 3 atoms of iodine. These hormones are required for normal growth and development and for maintenance of a normal metabolic state. Iodine is thinly and unevenly distributed in the earth's crust and the biosphere, and deficiency of this element may be the most prevalent of all deficiency states encountered in man. Although iodine deficiency is one of the simplest and least expensive of deficiencies to remedy, vast populations in the developing countries continue to manifest the effects of the deficiency state by reason of inaction on the part of governments and agencies charged with protecting the public health.[1]

## HISTORICAL OVERVIEW

Iodine was discovered by Courtois in 1811, and the discovery was announced in 1813. Courtois had observed a violet vapor arising from heated vats in a factory producing gunpowder.[2] Part of the process employed seaweed ash (varek or wrack), a source of sodium carbonate. The seaweed also, of course, was impure and contained iodine, which was vaporized in the process. Proof that the substance was an element came from Gay-Lussac.[3] Although seaweed had been a Chinese remedy for goiter for centuries, iodine was first employed for the treatment of goiter in 1816 by Prout[4] and later by Coindet.[5] In 1895 the element was discovered in the thyroid gland by Baumann.[6] The first hormone of the thyroid, thyroxine, which was crystalized from the gland by Kendall,[7] was synthesized by Harington and Barger.[8] The second thyroid hormone, triiodothyronine, was identified by Gross and Pitt-Rivers in 1953.[9] The first indication that dietary components might influence the metabolism of iodine and modify dietary requirements was the observation of Chesney et al. in 1928 that goiter occurred in rabbits fed cabbage.[10] Since then, substances that impede uptake or utilization of iodine by the thyroid have been identified in various foods and water.[11–13] The role these substances may play in naturally occurring human disease is not fully established, but a cyanogenic glycoside clearly has a contributory role in the iodine deficiency disease of Zaire, and Gaitan has strong evidence for a waterborne factor in addition to iodine deficiency in the endemic goiter of Colombia.[14]

A landmark event in the history of iodine nutriture was the demonstration in 1917 by Marine and Kimball in Akron, Ohio[15] that endemic goiter can be prevented by administration of small

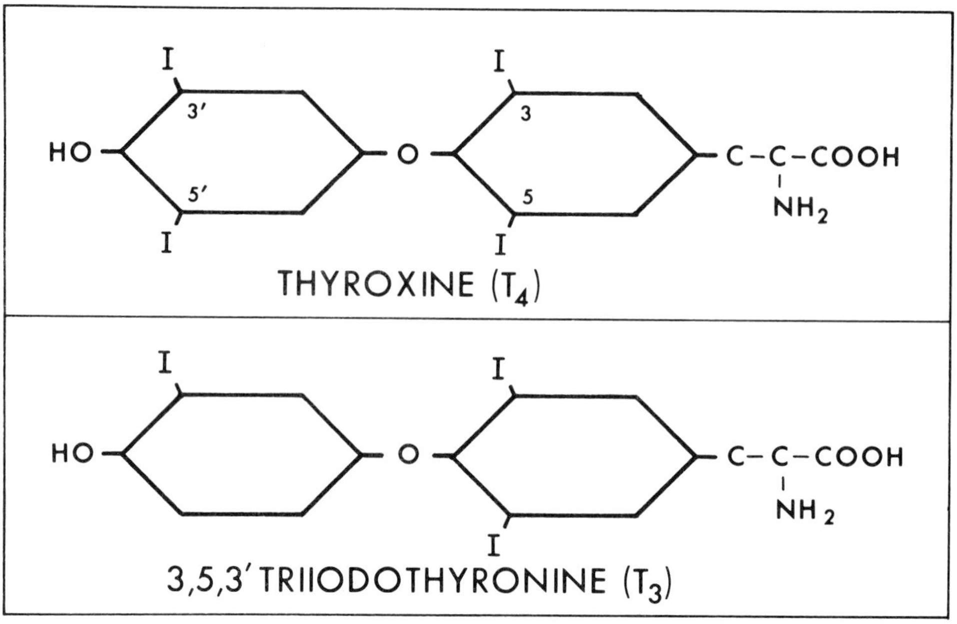

**Fig. 8–1.** Structural chemical formulas of the thyroid hormones, thyroid ($T_4$) and 3,5,3'-triiodothyronine ($T_3$). The numerals within the aromatic rings are used to designate the position of the iodine-substituents. When not occupied by an iodine atom, the "corners" of each aromatic ring are occupied by a hydrogen atom (not shown). The alanine side chain of each hormone is the L-isomer.

amounts of iodine to children at risk. A second highly significant and practical contribution was that of McCullagh (at the suggestion of Dr. John Gunther), who first used iodized poppy seed oil in the prevention of endemic goiter in Papua New Guinea.[16]

## OCCURRENCE AND CHEMISTRY

Iodine occupies the sixty-first place in order of abundance of the elements in the earth's crust. It is one of the rarest of nonmetallic elements and occurs in free form only rarely in sea mists or above iodine-rich mineral springs. It never occurs in rich deposits, veins, or lodes.[17] Relatively high concentrations are found in certain marine plants and animals such as corals, sponges, and sea-weeds, in the thyroid glands of vertebrates, in fossil fuels, in some natural mineral waters, in sedimentary phosphate rock, in soils that are usually richer in iodine than the parent rocks from which they were formed, and in the nitrate deposits of northern Chile. The last may contain as much as 2% iodine, but the range of concentrations is wide. Metamorphic and sedimentary rocks contain more iodine than igneous rocks, but soil derived from the last is richer in iodine, presumably because it is less subject to leaching.

Plants extract iodine from the soil and return it to the soil unless they are cropped, thereby enriching the soil as it is produced from the under-lying rocks. Iodine is added to the atmosphere by photo-oxidation of the iodide in seawater and falls to the earth with rain and sea mists where it is retained by the soil and plants. Thus there is a gradual incremental increase in the iodine of soils. Glaciation, by removal of topsoil, depleted vast areas that are now poor in iodine. Leaching by rain and periodic flooding have also created great plains areas that are poor in iodine, as in the central plains of the United States, the lowlands of central Africa, and the plains south of the Himalayas, such as the Indian Terai. The concept that iodine deficiency is found only in the mountainous regions of the world is a myth: the most severely depleted regions of the world are not mountainous.

Iodine is found in plants, and the amount is a function of the type of plant and the soil in which it grows. Some plants are more efficient in extracting iodine from the soil than others.[18] The role of iodine in the economy of plants is unknown, but is said to be a growth factor for some plants. The average content of foods varies widely both between and within types and depending on origin (Table 8–1).[19]

The iodine content of dairy products is dependent largely on the iodine available to the cow. Thus the iodine content of milk varies widely. The introduction of iodophors (iodine-containing sterilizing agents) for cleaning udders and milk con-

**Table 8–1.  Average Iodine Content of Foods (Values are in μg/kg)**

| | Fresh Basis | | Dry Basis | |
|---|---|---|---|---|
| | *Mean* | *Range* | *Mean* | *Range* |
| Fish (freshwater) | 30 | 17–40 | 116 | 68–194 |
| Fish (marine) | 832 | 163–3,180 | 3,715 | 471–1,591 |
| Shellfish | 798 | 308–1,300 | 3,866 | 1,292–4,987 |
| Meat | 50 | 27–97 | | |
| Eggs | 93 | | | |
| Cereal grains | 47 | 22–72 | 65 | 34–92 |
| Fruits | 18 | 10–29 | 154 | 62–277 |
| Legumes | 30 | 23–36 | 234 | 223–245 |
| Vegetables | 29 | 12–201 | 385 | 204–1,636 |

Compiled by the Chilean Iodine Educational Bureau.[19]

tainers has caused a sharp increase in the iodine content of milk products. The estimated range of iodine intake in this country has been slowly rising since the early 1950's also because of the use of iodine-containing dough conditioners in the baking industry, as dietary supplements for stock, and in many medications. It appears to be leveling off now. Recent figures place the mean intake between 400 and 800 μg/day. This contrasts with the minimal daily need of about 50 μg.

Certain algae concentrate iodine to a remarkable degree. Among these are the common seaweeds *Laminaria*, *Fucus*, *Ecklonia*, and *Nereocystis*. Concentrations may reach nearly 1% of dry weight. The metabolism of *Nereocystis* has been studied by Tong and Chaikoff,[20] who found that the iodide was actively concentrated by the organism and appeared primarily as iodide, monoiodotyrosine, and diiodotyrosine. The iodoamino acids were protein-bound. An iodide peroxidase was found on the cell surface. The role of the iodine in algae is unknown. Iodine is also concentrated in the exoskeleton of sponges and corals.[21] The marine iguana of the Galapagos Islands has been found to have a high concentration of protein-bound iodine in its blood, but this is not thyroxine.[22] It presumably is derived from absorption of protein-bound iodine from the algae on which the iguana feed. The marine algae have replaced Chilean nitrate as the major source of commercial iodine.

## ABSORPTION AND METABOLISM

Iodine is rapidly reduced in the gut to iodide and, like iodide, is unusually rapidly absorbed by the stomach and upper small bowel. Iodate is either reduced in the gut to iodide or is reduced immediately after absorption. Most organically bound iodine is first reduced to iodide prior to absorption, but not all. Certain iodinated dyes are absorbed unchanged and can be used in contrast roentgenography because of their concentration in the gallbladder. Thyroxine and triiodothyronine

are largely absorbed without degradation, but not entirely. Malabsorption of iodine appears not to be a feature of malabsorption syndromes because of its ready transfer in the upper bowel. The metabolic circuit of iodine is illustrated in simplified form in Figure 8–2.[23]

The volume of distribution of iodide is approximately that of the extracellular fluid. It is rapidly cleared from the plasma with a halflife of about 7 hours by the thyroid gland and the kidneys. The ratios of these two clearances determines the value of the familiar radioiodine uptake test of thyroid function. The clearance rate by the thyroid is determined by recent and past availability of iodine and the need for thyroid hormone. Under conditions of iodide supply prevailing in most western countries at the present time, approximately 5 to 10 ml/min of plasma are cleared of iodide by the thyroid gland. Clearance by the kidney is not determined by iodine need or supply and is approximately 30 ml/min. Renal clearance in man does not contribute to the adaptation to iodide deficiency or excess. Renal clearance is the result of glomerular filtration and tubular reabsorption.

Iodide is also actively cleared from the plasma by the salivary glands, the gastric mucosa, the secreting mammary gland, and the choroid plexus. These structures, like the thyroid, pump iodide against an electrochemical gradient and expend energy in the process. Certain anions compete with iodide for transport. Among these are bromide, perchlorate, thiocyanate, and other anions of approximately the same charge and molecular size, but these are concentrated selectively very little if at all.

No function has been assigned to iodine in the body except as a component of the thyroid hormones. The possibility has been entertained that iodide may have a direct role in early fetal development, but proof is lacking.

Iodide transported into the thyroid fills the so-called iodide space of the gland and is oxidized

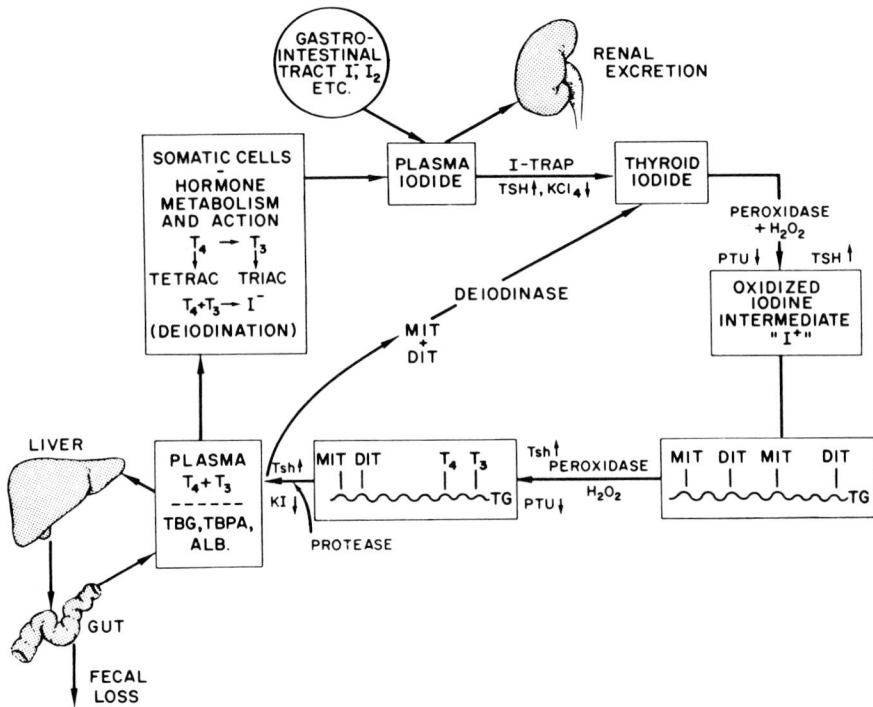

**Fig. 8–2.** A simplified diagram designed to represent the flow of iodine related metabolites through the body. The rectangles represent body compartments. $T_4 + T_3$/TBG represent iodothyronines, the essential hormones, in non-covalent linkage with thyroxine binding globulin in the plasma. Iodine from the gut is absorbed, usually in the reduced state, is actively transported into the thyroid, and iodinates mono- and diiodotyrosine (MIT, DIT), which are then coupled to form the thyroid hormones. These are stored in the thyroglobulin (TG), and the hormones, thyroxine ($T_4$) and $T_3$, are released to circulate in blood to their characteristic action on target cells. PTU = pro-pylthiouracil. TBG = thyroxine binding globulin. TBPA = thyroxine binding prealbumin. Tetrac = tetraiodothy-roacetic acid. Triac = triiodothyroacetic acid. TBPA, the thyroxine binding prealbumin, is a blood component. Albumin is also a hormone carrier protein of much lower affinity than TBG or TBPA.

by a thyroid-specific peroxidase which has a flavin nucleotide as cofactor and requires a per-oxide generating system (Fig. 8–2). It then dis-places a proton in the 3 and 5 positions on tyrosyl residues of thyroglobulin (TG) (mw = 680,000). Mono- and diiodotyrosyl (MIT and DIT) residues are formed, and these, through another oxidative step within the matrix of the thyroglobulin mole-cule, are coupled through an oxygen bridge, an alanine side chain is lost, and an iodothyronine residue is formed. Under normal conditions of iodine supply the DIT to MIT ratio in thyroglob-ulin is about 2, the ratio of $T_4$ to $T_3$ is about 5, and the ratio of iodotyrosine to iodothyronine is about 5. Under conditions of iodine deficiency these ra-tios shift toward the less well-iodinated forms, favoring production of the physiologically more active hormone, $T_3$.

Iodine in the form of the iodoamino acids of thyroglobulin is stored in the colloid of the thy-roid follicles. Secretion of hormone follows pro-teolytic degradation of the thyroglobulin. The re-leased MIT and DIT are deiodinated within the

thyroid and the iodide enters the iodide pools of the body. The hormones $T_3$ and $T_4$ are transported in the plasma largely bound to carrier proteins. Most of the $T_3$ that appears in the plasma is de-rived from peripheral deiodination of $T_4$.

The thyroid hormones enter the cells of the pe-ripheral tissues and bind to the nuclear chroma-tin, where they presumably have their effects in controlling cellular metabolism. Most, but per-haps not all, of these effects are due to $T_3$. The pathways of degradation of the thyroid hormones are complex and include deiodination, rupture of the ether bridge, and formation of glucuronic and sulfate conjugates and other derivatives.

Iodine metabolism is controlled primarily by a biofeedback system, which includes the thyroid itself and the pituitary through secretion of thy-rotropic hormone (TSH). This system is modu-lated by a hypothalamic hormone, thyrotropin re-leasing hormone. TSH is not thought to exert any effect on organs other than the thyroid either for uptake, release, secretion, or degradation of iodine or iodine-containing substances. The set point of the system is governed by iodine in the diet. If supplies are abundant, thyroid hormone can be produced in normal amounts at a low level of TSH secretion. If supplies are limited, the system responds by increasing TSH secretion, which promotes iodine uptake by the thyroid and, if of sufficient degree, hyperplasia and hypertrophy of the gland. The system is well protected against rapid fluctuations in dietary iodine. The gland stores enough hormone normally to meet needs for several months in the absence of dietary iodine and stores iodine when supplies increase. The seasonal changes in dietary iodine may have no effect on hormone secretion unless they fluctuate about a mean that is barely adequate or worse. The physiology and biochemistry of the thyroid system have been extensively reviewed elsewhere.[24,25]

In chronic illness and with semistarvation there is customarily initially a fall in $T_3$ content of the plasma and later a fall in $T_4$. The reasons are complex but are primarily a result of decreased peripheral deiodination of $T_4$. A fall in concentration of the plasma carrier proteins may also contribute to the fall. This does not imply that there is hypothyroidism. Nothing appears to be gained by treating these changes with hormone replacement.

## MINIMUM DAILY REQUIREMENTS

Since iodine has no established physiologic function other than in the thyroid system, one must use the thyroid system as an indicator of iodine nutritional state. This is complicated by the fact that many disorders of the system are unrelated to iodine nutrition. Accordingly, the minimum daily requirement must be established on statistical grounds against a background of thyroid disease that is unrelated. A further complication is what value to accept as "normal." Is the doubling of thyroid size that occurs in many adolescent females abnormal?

Most investigators at present would agree that a 10% prevalence of distinctly enlarged thyroid glands–a gland that is enlarged to the size of the distal phalanx of the subject's thumb–of school children between the ages of 8 and 14 years indicates iodine deficiency. This level of thyroid disease will occur if the mean daily excretion of iodine in the urine falls below 50 μg or below 50 μg/g creatinine. Many observations support an inverse relationship between iodine excretion and activity of the thyroid as measured by radioiodine uptake by the thyroid.[26] This value of 50 μg may be accepted as a rather fuzzy minimal daily requirement. It may be insufficient if goitrogens are present in the diet. When the mean values of iodine excretion fall below 20 to 30 μg/24 hours or 1 g creatinine, then one may expect to find severe goiter and appearance in the community of individuals with mental deficiency with or without deaf-mutism and neurologic signs and with or without other characteristic features. They are called cretins, and their numbers vary with the degree of iodine deficiency. They may be accompanied by a larger group of more modestly retarded persons with lesser neurologic disorders.

It is not known whether subtle changes in neuromotor function occur with increased frequency in communities with mean urinary iodine excretion values between 20 and 50 μg daily. One might expect this in families subsisting for long periods at the lower end of this range, but proof has not been obtained.

## CONSEQUENCES OF IODINE DEFICIENCY: IODINE DEFICIENCY DISEASE

### Endemic Goiter

Endemic goiter is an exceedingly common disorder in many of the developing countries. Its clinical spectrum extends from modest enlargement of the thyroid affecting the periadolescent females, as in Colombia and parts of Panama, to regions where most of the population have thyroids that are several times normal in size, are frequently nodular, and, as in the Indian Terai, are oftentimes huge (Fig. 8–3) and clearly evident in children (Fig. 8–4). Severity varies with the degree of iodine deficiency. In severe endemics, such as in rural mountainous Nepal, most schoolboys have nodular goiter, and pregnant and nursing women, as in some communities of the Ubangi region of Zaire, may nearly all have very large nodular goiters.

Endemic goiter is not entirely confined to the underdeveloped countries. It may still be found in parts of Europe.[26a,26b]

When not severe, endemic goiter per se is not a major medical problem. In females the goiter frequently diminishes in size or ceases to grow, and in males it disappears with maturity. Larger and nodular goiters may cause obstructive symptoms from compression of the trachea or esophagus and may impinge on the recurrent laryngeal nerve. Acute symptoms may arise from hemorrhage into a nodule. Tracheomalacia may be a serious complication following surgery for large goiters of long standing. Whether endemic goiter increases the risk of malignant neoplasms of the thyroid is unsettled at present but is certainly not a strong factor. Introduction of iodine prophylactically as iodized salt, iodized oil, or through other media will precipitate thyrotoxicosis in a small number of subjects (Jod-Basedow). The dis-

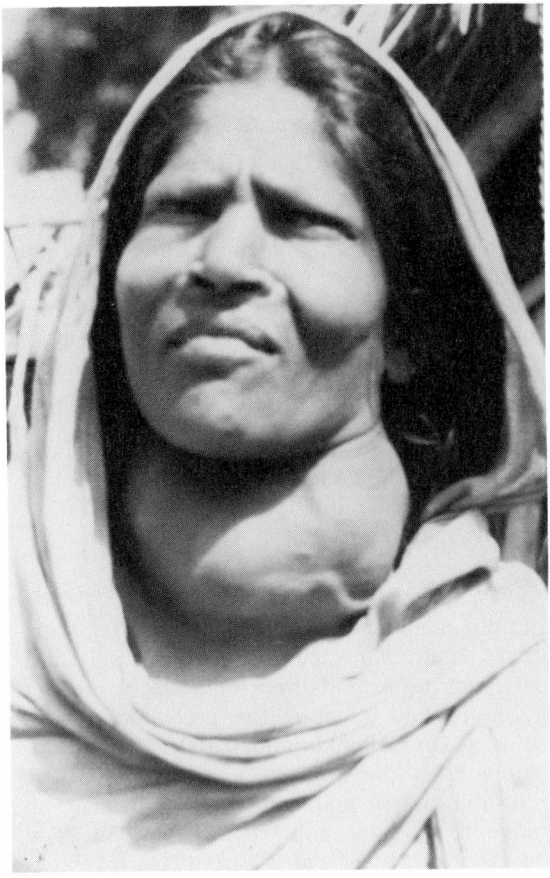

Fig. 8–3. Adult woman from the Indian Terai with a huge goiter.

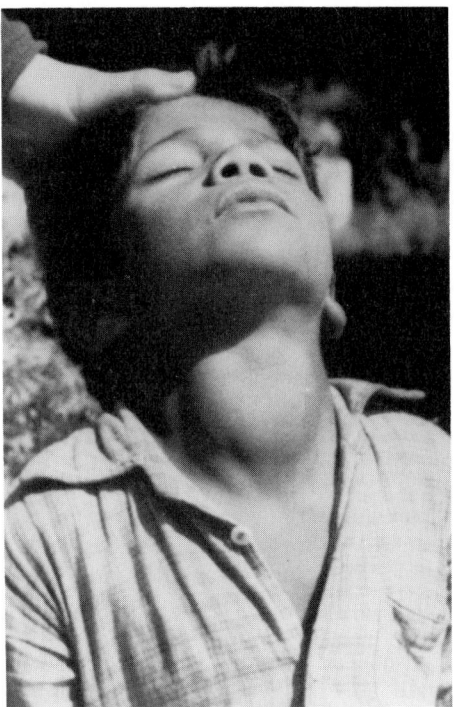

Fig. 8–4. Schoolboy from the Indian Terai with goiter.

order is generally mild, self-limited, and easily controlled. Its precise incidence has not been established, and available figures vary widely.

### Endemic Cretinism

Accompanying endemic goiter of severe degree is the syndrome of endemic cretinism. The sine qua non of this syndrome is mental deficiency. In addition, one may find in various combinations spastic diplegia or quadriplegia affecting primarily the proximal muscle groups, deaf-mutism or dysarthria, a characteristic shuffling gait, sometimes squint, shortened stature, and clinical evidence of hypothyroidism. Some isolated communities have been described in which 8 to 12% of the inhabitants conform to this syndrome. The true incidence of cretinism is only beginning to emerge as screening tests for neonatal hypothyroidism are being introduced into endemic regions. Prevalence rates, though interesting, do not indicate the incidence, since mortality rates among these subjects are high, on the one hand, and prevalence does not necessarily accord with

incidence, since iodine available to the pregnant women and infants may have changed since the cretins in the community were conceived.

The finding of endemic cretins in a community is a reason for concern and an indication of need for immediate investigation of current iodine nutriture and usually for a crash program of iodine prophylaxis. In countries where endemic goiter does not exist congenital hypothyroidism may be expected in 0.025% of live births. A diagnosis of endemic cretinism in 0.25% of a goitrous population would certainly be sufficient to trigger a prophylaxis campaign. Querido et al. find that reduced hearing is an excellent objective marker for neurologic impairment resulting from iodine deficiency.[27]

The pathogenesis of endemic cretinism is not entirely clear. Although there is ample evidence that development is dependent on thyroid hormone at the right time during fetal and postnatal growth, there are unexplained geographical differences in clinical manifestations. Thus, in Zaire most of the cretins are severely hypothyroid, do not have goiter, have very short stature, are often not deaf, and have few other neurologic defects, whereas, generally, the endemic cretin has major neurologic defects, more moderate growth retardation, and goiter and is often severely affected in hearing and speech (Fig. 8–5). Some hypotheses to explain these differences have been offered.[28]

## Endemic Deaf-Mutism

It is said that endemic deaf-mutism may be a consequence of iodine deficiency without other defects or manifestations of cretinism. Experimentally the development of the ear is dependent on the presence of thyroid hormone.[29,30] In underdeveloped regions where endemic goiter is found, assessment of intellectual function may be difficult and misleading. Until formal pyschologic testing designed for the local cultural setting is applied to these noncretinous deaf-mutes, one might be cautious in accepting deaf-mutism as a sole sequela of iodine deficiency.

## Endemic Neuropsychic Retardation

From the socioeconomic point of view endemic neuropsychic retardation may be the most important of the iodine deficiency disorders. One is often struck by the numbers of superficially normal-appearing persons in endemic goiter regions who on closer inspection appear to be subnormal mentally or to have mild motor defects or both (Fig. 8–6). A multitude of factors influences development in socially and economically deprived regions. Parenting may be deficient, as may be general nutrition and schooling. The investigator must work across cultural and often language barriers with test instruments not necessarily compatible with the local experience or ethos. Cooperation may be difficult or deceptive. Nevertheless, a number of attempts have been

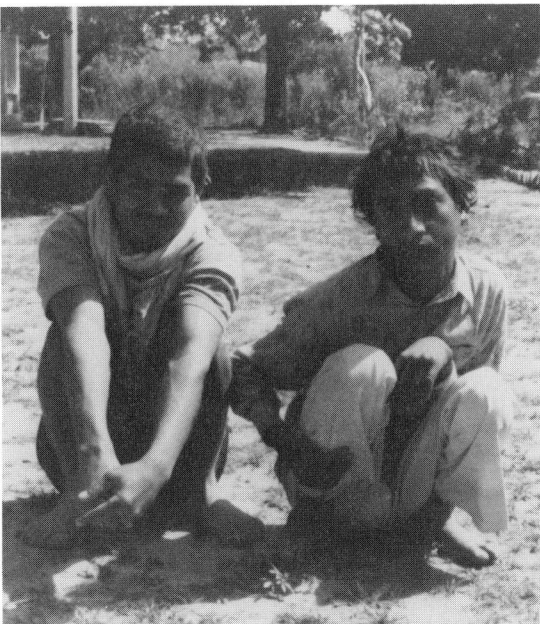

**Fig. 8–6.** Two retarded males from the highly endemic Indian Terai.

made, and with surprising uniformity the results have favored the existence of large numbers of mild or moderate retardation in intellectual, motivational, or neuromotor maturation in conjunction with endemic goiter.[31–36] In a recent study of subjects a decade or so after iodized oil was introduced into a community, school and work performance and results of testing were compared between those whose mothers received the iodized oil during pregnancy or before, or who received it at a young age, and a group who received no iodized oil.[37] Test results strongly favored the group that received the iodine. The number of obviously retarded persons who are not typical cretins in the severely goitrous villages of the Indian Terai is striking.

In the Terai and in a village in rural Ecuador 4 to 5% of newborns have had high TSH or low $T_4$ values or both,[38,39] and the figure is reported as being much higher in the Ubangi.[40] It is possible that not only the most severely deprived of these would be permanently and irreversibly damaged, but that less severely deprived individuals might find access to iodine at some date postnatally, grow, and appear relatively normal but with mental deficiency and perhaps mild motor incoordination, without the stigmata of typical cretinism. Large numbers of such retarded persons could severely impede social progress and negate programs designed to improve the quality of life in such communities.

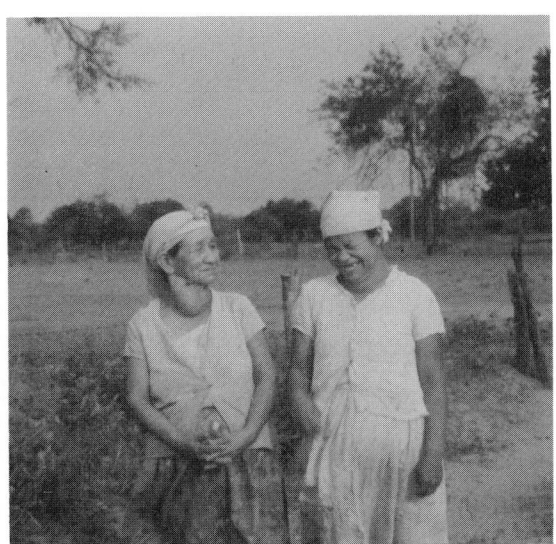

**Fig. 8–5.** Two cretinous adult women from rural Bolivia.

## DISORDERS OF IODIDE EXCESS

As has been described, ingestion of 100 to 200 μg of iodine daily is sufficient to prevent iodine deficiency disease, except in those rare subjects with inborn errors of thyroid metabolism that can be corrected by administration of very large daily dietary supplements.[24] What are the consequences of administration of iodine far in excess of daily needs?[41] Organification of iodine in the normal thyroid is blocked if the plasma iodide concentration exceeds 15 to 25 μg/ml. This is the Wolff-Chaikoff effect.[42] The block is usually temporary and is lifted after 24 to 48 hours, when hormone synthesis resumes. Discharge of iodide from the thyroids of such subjects by perchlorate suggests that the block is at a point beyond iodide transport and before organification. Occasional subjects will have a persistent block under the same conditions, and a goiter may develop. Goiters large enough to cause dystocia appeared in fetuses whose mothers were given iodide as medication.

An entirely satisfactory explanation for the Wolff-Chaikoff effect has not been forthcoming, nor do we know why the block fails to be lifted in some subjects. In this regard it is interesting that patients successfully treated for Graves' disease by surgery or with radioiodine or those with lymphocytic thyroiditis may be unusually and persistently sensitive to increased daily intake of iodine and may become fully hypothyroid.

Administration of iodine well beyond that to which the subject is accustomed in iodine-deficient areas occasionally precipitates thyrotoxicosis (Jod-Basedow) as it may in some with long-standing nodular goiter. Thus, there was a sharp and well-studied epidemic of thyrotoxicosis in Tasmania when iodide was introduced in the bread baking industry,[43] and there was much anecdotal evidence for this in the United States and in Europe following iodization of salt as prophylaxis against endemic goiter. Thyrotoxicosis has appeared in a small fraction of subjects given iodized oil prophylactically, either intramuscularly or orally, but in other large preventive programs the phenomenon has not been observed.

The precise mechanism of Jod-Basedow is uncertain. It may be that administration of iodine unmasks Graves' disease that has been held in check by the prevailing iodine deficiency, or it may be that thyroid nodules of the iodine-deficient glands become autonomous of normal control; when iodine becomes more available these produce an excess of hormone. It may be that long-term iodine deficiency alters upward the set point of the thyroid feedback control system.

Goiter from an unusually abundant supply of iodine may be endemic. This has been described in the northern island of Japan[44] and in China in regions where seaweeds are a dietary staple. Since some seaweeds may contain nearly 1% iodine, the daily consumption can be huge if seaweed is a principal component of the diet. Withdrawal of iodine from such persons is said to result in rapid reduction in thyroid size. The pathophysiology of endemic goiter due to iodide excess is presumably the same as that of sporadic iodide goiter, but it is puzzling that it should be so frequent in some localities.

Acute necrosis of the thyroid of the dog has been produced by administration of pharmacologic doses of iodide.[45] Analogous lesions have not been described in man. Lymphocytic infiltrates in the thyroids of man have been attributed to intake of large quantities of iodine, and an apparent rise in the incidence of chronic lymphocytic thyroiditis during the past two decades has been related to the rise in iodine consumption in the United States during the corresponding time. A cause and effect relationship remains unproven.

## EVALUATION OF IODINE NUTRITURE

Iodine deficiency disease can be prevented by readily available and relatively inexpensive methods, as described in the section on prevention, but an assessment of need is required before a prophylactic program is implemented. Several complementary techniques are available.

### Goiter Surveys

A goiter survey is the time-tested method of establishing need for a preventive program. Standards have been developed for use by the survey team in order that inter-team results may be comparable and that the severity of the endemia can be estimated (Table 8–2). Much confusion has arisen in the past, either because differing criteria for gland size were used or because prevalence data were published without regard to any standards. In the future, surveys should adhere strictly to World Health Organization criteria.[46]

Sample size, source, and composition are important in any survey. Military recruits have often been used and are a biased sample that ignores sex differences and the obviously unfit, such as the retarded. School pupils have often been chosen, but may also be a biased sample. House-to-house surveys may exclude the more fit and males who are working, but is probably the fairest method if all family members can be counted. There has been too much emphasis in the past on having large numbers of subjects. In general, a smaller but well-selected random sampling is probably best. Careful training of the members of

**Table 8–2. Criteria for Definition of Goiter by Stages**

| Grade 0 | 0a: | Thyroid not palpable or, if palpable, not larger than normal. |
| | 0b: | Thyroid distinctly palpable but usually not visible with the head in a normal or raised position, considered to be definitely larger than normal, at least as large as the distal phalanx of the subject's thumb. |
| Grade I | | Thyroid easily palpable and visible with the head in either a normal or a raised position. The presence of a discrete nodule qualifies a patient for inclusion in this grade. |
| Grade II | | Thyroid easily visible with the head in a normal position. |
| Grade III | | Goiter visible at a distance. |
| Grade IV | | Monstrous goiters. |

From Tilly, C.H., et al.[46]

the survey team to a set of uniform criteria, and pretesting team members against each other and against a small but varied set of subjects is important in ensuring comparability of results.

### Iodine Excretion

A widely used and reliable indicator of iodine nutriture is the daily excretion of iodine in the urine. This is based on the assumption that the daily excretion is a close reflection of iodine intake and that for the surveyed group as a whole excretion rates are a fair sample of iodine intake over an extended period of time. Seasonal swings in iodine intake with seasonal shifts in diet surely occur but have not been documented in any endemic region. A small fraction of iodine is excreted in the feces, but this is neglected for survey purposes, and the assumption is made that most members of the surveyed community are in a state of equilibrium, i.e., are neither storing iodine nor losing iodine from their thyroids.

In order to be useful the analyses must be done with reference to a time unit. Many investigators report excretion rates relative to creatinine excretion, assuming that creatinine excretion is constant over time. This may be refined to creatinine excreted per square meter body surface derived from height, weight, and sex tables. Although there are inaccuracies in this method, it seems to be a practical and useful base. Other investigators report their analyses on a first morning specimen, assuming that, on average, urine volumes are sufficiently close within the community that quantity of iodine excreted in the morning specimen per unit volume is sufficient for all practical purposes. Some observers have been able to obtain successive 24-hour collections. The difficulties with this method are obvious, but if accurate collections can be assured, then it provides the best denominator for calculating a 24-hour excretion rate.

### Other Criteria

Various laboratory tests have been used in surveys, but for the most part they are not applicable for routine assessment of the degree of need for prophylaxis. These include measurements of $T_3$ or $T_4$ or both and TSH. These are more applicable for identifying need through detection of neonatal hypothyroidism. As such, they reach the core of the problem. For routine survey work these methods are relatively expensive and are difficult or impossible in many settings in the developing countries at the present time. Measurement of plasma iodide is difficult because of the low concentration and has not yet been proven to be a measurement of any clinical usefulness.

### PREVENTION OF IODINE DEFICIENCY DISEASE

Iodine deficiency disease is prevented by ensuring an adequate intake of iodine. This was first demonstrated by Marine and Kimball among school children in Akron, Ohio, in 1917.[15] Fortification of table salt with iodine quickly became widespread in the United States and Europe. It was rapidly followed by a rapid and sharp decline in the prevalence of goiter and the disappearance of new cases of endemic cretinism.[47] Other methods of dispensing iodine to populations at risk have also been used.

### Iodized Salt

Iodide added to table salt as the sodium or potassium salt remains stable under dry conditions and if packed in impervious containers. Impure salt, when allowed to become warm and moist and if packed in bulk, may lose much of its iodine with time. Salts of iodate are considerably more stable. Other salts of iodine have been used with no noteworthy advantage.

The levels of concentration of iodine in salt have varied from country to country. In the United States it is 0.01%, which is well above minimal daily needs if average table salt intake is 5 g daily. Other countries employ 0.002 to 0.005%. The salt is iodized at the plant usually by a spray method, but at times by a dry mixing method. Agencies concerned with health monitoring should ascertain the concentration of iodine in "iodized" salt at the consumer level.

In some localities in need of wide distribution of iodide prophylactically, programs have failed for many reasons, including government inattention or lack of concern, Laocoön-like bureaucracy, the modest extra expense involved in salt iodization, consumer resistance or indifference, the unavailability of refined salt for logistical or economic reasons, or the availability of salt from nearby noncommercial or cottage industry sources.

## Iodized Oil

Iodized poppy seed oil has been used for many years in contrast roentgenography. It was introduced as an agent for long-term delivery of iodine in 1959 in Papua New Guinea and has been successfully used there and elsewhere in large programs.[16] It is effective, a single 2 ml dose given intramuscularly providing protection for 2 to 4 years. The only significant complication is the rare appearance of thyrotoxicosis. It is suitable for those foci of endemic goiter where there is no hope of early introduction of iodized salt to the general population. Iodized oil may also be given orally, but it probably has a shorter period of effectiveness. There has been much less experience with iodized oil given orally than by the intramuscular route. Iodized soya oil and walnut oil have also been used.

## Iodized Bread

Various iodine-containing food additives are used in the baking industry to improve the quality of the product by catalyzing the cross-linking of gluten. Iodide has also been added to bread expressly for prevention of goiter. In Tasmania use of the additive was followed by an increase in the incidence of thyrotoxicosis.[43] As a technique for prevention of goiter it has not become widely used, perhaps in part because of the great variation in consumption patterns.

## Other Methods

Iodide has been distributed in candies to school children, as drops or tablets at intervals, and in the drinking water. The last method is said to be cost effective and to have the additional advantage of improving the bacterial purity of the water, but it can be employed only when there is a central supply.[48]

## REFERENCES

1. Stanbury, J.B., Hetzel, B.S. (Eds.): Endemic Goiter and Endemic Cretinism. New York, John Wiley & Sons, 1980.
2. Courtois, B.: Ann. Chim. *88*:304, 1813.
3. Gay-Lussac, J.L.: Ann. Chim. *91*:5, 1814.
4. Prout, W.: Chemistry, Meteorology and the Function of Digestion Considered with Reference to Natural Theology. London, Wm. Pickering, 1834, p. 100.
5. Coindet, J-F.: Ann. Chim. *15*:49, 1820.
6. Baumann, E.: Z. Physiol. Chem. *21*:319, 1895.
7. Kendall, E.C.: J.A.M.A. *64*:204, 1915.
8. Harington, C.R., Barger, G.: Bioch. J. *22*:1429, 1927.
9. Gross, J., Pitt-Rivers, R.: Lancet *1*:439, 1952.
10. Chesney, A.M., Clawson, T.A., Webster, B.: Bull. Johns Hopkins Hosp. *43*:261, 1928.
11. Greer, M.A.: Physiol. Rev. *30*:513, 1950.
12. Delange, F., Ermans, A.M.: Am. J. Clin. Nutr. *24*:1354, 1971.
13. Gaitan, E., Wahner, J.W., Correa, R., et al.: J. Clin. Endocrinol. Metab. *28*:1730, 1968.
14. Gaitan, E.: World Rev. Nutr. Diet. *17*:53, 1973.
15. Marine, D., Kimball, O.P.: J. Lab. Clin. Med. *3*:40, 1917.
16. McCullagh, S.F.: Papua New Guinea Med. J. *3*:43, 1959.
17. Chilean Iodine Educational Bureau: Geochemistry of Iodine. London, 1956.
18. Chilean Iodine Educational Bureau: Iodine Content of Plants. London, 1950.
19. Chilean Iodine Educational Bureau: Iodine Content of Foods. London, 1952.
20. Tong, W., Chaikoff, I.L.: J. Biol. Chem. *215*:473, 1955.
21. Saenko, G.N., Kravtsova, Y.Y., Ivanenka, V.V., et al.: Marine Biol. *47*:243, 1978.
22. Fierro-Benitez, R., Chapman, E.M., and Stanbury, J.B.: Rev. Ecuatoriano de Med. *18*:135, 1981.
23. DeGroot, L., Stanbury, J.B.: The Thyroid and its Diseases. New York, John Wiley & Sons, 1973.
24. Stanbury, J.B., Wyngaarden, J.B., Fredrickson, D.S., et al. (eds.): The Metabolic Basis of Inherited Diseases, New York, McGraw-Hill, 1983. Ch. 11.
25. DeGroot, L., Larsen, P.R., Refetoff, S., Stanbury, J.B.: The Thyroid and Its Diseases. New York, John Wiley & Sons, 1984.
26. Stanbury, J.B., Brownell, G., Riggs, D.S. et al.: Endemic Goiter: The Adaptation of Man to Iodine Deficiency. Cambridge, Harvard University Press, 1954.
26a. Scriba, P.C.: Goitre and Iodine Deficiency in Europe–A Review. *In* Treatment of Endemic and Sporadic Goitre. (Reinwein, D., Scriba, P.C., Eds.) Stuttgart, Schattauer, 1985. p. 19.
26b. Subcommittee Study Endemic Goitre and Iodine Deficiency. Europ. Thyroid Assoc. Lancet *1*:1289, 1985.
27. Querido, A., Delange, F., Dunn, J.G., et al.: *In* Dunn, J.T. and Medeiros-Neto, G.A., Eds.: Endemic Goiter and Cretinism: Continuing Threats to World Health. PAHO, Washington, 1974, Page 267.
28. Stanbury, J.B.: The pathogenesis of endemic retardation associated with endemic goiter. *In* Diminished Thyroid Hormone Formation. (Reinwein, D., Klein, E., eds.) Stuttgart, Schattauer Verlag, 1982, p. 8.
29. Deol, M.: J. Med. Genet. *10*:235, 1973.
30. Bargman, G.J., Gardner, L.I.: *In* The Thyroid Gland: Relation to Endemic Cretinism. (Stanbury, J.B., Kroc, R.L., Eds.) New York, Plenum, 1972, p. 305.
31. Fierro-Benitez, R., Ramirez, I., Suarez, J.: *In* Human Development and the Thyroid Gland. (Stanbury, J.B., Kroc, R.L., Eds.) New York, Plenum Press, 1972, p. 239.
32. Bautista, A., Barker, P.A., Dunn, J.T., et al.: Am. J. Clin. Nutr. *35*:127, 1982.
33. Thilly, C.H.: *In* Psychomotor Development in Fetal Brain Disorders–Recent Approaches to the Problem of Mental Deficiency. (Hetzel, B.S., Smith, R.M., Eds.) Amsterdam, Elsevier North-Holland, 1981.
34. Bleichrodt, N., Drenth, P.J.D., Querido, A.: Am. J. Phys. Anthropol. *53*:55, 1980.

35. Bleichrodt, N.: Presented at a meeting of the International Council for the Control of Iodine Deficiency Disorders held in Kathmandu, Nepal, March, 1986. To be published.

36. Hetzel, B.S., and Potter, B.J.: Iodine deficiency and the role of thyroid hormones in brain development. *In* Neurobiology of the Trace Elements. Vol. 1. (I.E. Dreosti and R.M. Smith, Eds.) New Jersey, Humana Press, 1983, p. 45.

37. Fierro-Benitez, R.: Presented at the second meeting of the Latin American Thyroid Association, Lima, Peru, 1984. In Press.

38. Kochupillai, N., Godbole, M.M., Pandav, C.S., Karmarkar, M.G., and Ahuja, M.M.S.: Neonatal thyroid status in the iodide deficient environment of the Sub-Himalayan region of India. *In* Thyroid Disorders Associated with Iodine Deficiency and Excess. R. Hall and J. Kobberling, eds. Raven Press, New York, 1985, p. 61.

39. Fierro-Benitez, R.: Personal communication.

40. Thilly, C.H., Bourdoux, P., Vanderpas, J., Mafuta, M., Berquist, H., Due, D. Le My, Delange, F. and Ermans, A.M. *In* Epidemiology and prophylaxis of endemic goiter in developing countries. *In* Thyroid Disorders Associated with Iodine Deficiency and Excess. R. Hall and J. Kobberling, eds. Raven Press, New York, 1985.

41. Hall, R. and Kobberling, J., eds.: Thyroid Disorders Associated with Iodine Deficiency and Excess. Raven Press, New York, 1985.

42. Wolff, J. and Chaikoff, I.L.: J. Biol. Chem. *174*:555, 1948.

43. Vidor, G.I., Stewart, J.C., Wall, J.R., Wangel, A., and Hetzel, B.S.: Pathogenesis of iodine-induced thyrotoxicosis: Studies in Northern Tasmania. J. Clin. Endocrinol. Metab. *37*:901, 1973.

44. Suzuki, H., Higuchi, T., Sawa, K., Ohtaki, S., Horuchi, Y.: Endemic coast goitre in Hokkaido, Japan. Acta Endocrinol. *50*:161, 1965.

45. Belshaw, B.E. and Beckers, D.V.: J. Clin. Endocrinol. Metab. *36*:466, 1973.

46. Thilly, C.H., Delange, F., and Stanbury, J.B.: Epidemiologic surveys in endemic goiter and cretinism. *In* Endemic Goiter and Endemic Cretinism. (J.B. Stanbury and B.S. Hetzel, Eds.) John Wiley & Sons, New York, 1980, p. 157.

*Chapter* **9**

# ZINC AND COPPER

## Noel W. Solomons

## ZINC

### History of Zinc as a Nutrient

Zinc was recognized as a distinct element in 1509. Todd et al. in 1934 showed the essentiality of zinc in the rat.[1] Swine parakeratosis was shown to be a zinc-deficiency disease in 1955.[2]

Malnourished Chinese patients in wartime were found to have low concentrations of zinc in the circulation in 1940,[3] and in 1956, a conditioned zinc-deficiency syndrome in man was demonstrated.[4] Since 1961, when the endemic hypogonadism and dwarfism of rural Iran was suggested to derive from zinc deficiency,[5] a wide appreciation of the magnitude of both the clinical and the public health significance of episodic and endemic zinc deficiency states has developed.

### Chemistry

Zinc bears atomic number 30, and an atomic weight of 65.37. It has five naturally occurring stable isotopes: $^{64}Zn$, $^{66}Zn$, $^{67}Zn$, $^{68}Zn$, and $^{70}Zn$. Three radioisotopes—$^{65}Zn$ ($t_{1/2}$ = 245 days), $^{69m}Zn$ ($t_{1/2}$ = 13.8 h), and $^{63}Zn$ ($t_{1/2}$ = 38.1 min)—have been applied as tracers in biologic experiments. Zinc can exist in several valence states, but is almost universally found as the divalent ion $Zn(II)$. The zinc ion can be chelated and precip-

itated by a number of chelating agents including some natural constituents of the diet.

### Metabolism

#### *Zinc in the Human Body*

The neonate contains up to 140 mg of zinc at birth, most of which was transferred from mother to fetus during the third trimester of pregnancy.[5] It has been estimated that the adult body contains 2 to 3 g of zinc.

The distribution of zinc within the body has not been established. Two important studies,[6,7] and several lesser sources provide data on zinc concentrations in various tissues and organs. The World Health Organization expert committee cites a figure of 30 µg/g of wet weight as the *average* zinc concentration in fat-free tissue, with bone having 200 µg/g and muscle 50 µg/g.[8] Prostatic fluids and ocular tissues have the highest zinc levels, 600 to 800 µg/g. Muscle, bone, skin, and liver combined contain most of the zinc in humans.

#### *Zinc Uptake*

**Site of Absorption.** The site of predilection for zinc absorption is uncertain. A series of in vitro studies suggested that the efficiency of transfer of zinc was greatest in the duodenum,[9,10] whereas in vivo studies suggested that the more distal intestinal segment has the greater uptake capacity for zinc.[11,12] In vivo perfusion studies in man showed that the human intestine was capable of extracting 3.3 to 5.0 mg of zinc from the intestinal lumen through the first 90 cm of the jejunum.[13] At what level of the gastrointestinal tract the majority of meal zinc is absorbed remains to be settled.

**Intraluminal Factors.** In the process of the gastrointestinal passage and digestion of a meal, Zn(II) is presumably liberated from the original food matrices. As such, it is free to form coordination complexes with both exogenous and endogenous ligands. There is evidence that zinc can be bound by histidine and absorbed as a zinc-histidine complex,[14] and that glutathione enhances zinc absorption.[15] Various substances, most notably citric acid and picolinic acid (a metabolite in the tryptophan to niacin pathway,[16,17] have been suggested as endogenous zinc-binding ligands (ZBL).

Unlike iron, the intestinal pH does not appear to influence zinc uptake, and ascorbic acid plays little or no role.[18] The concentration of other metal ions such as calcium[19] and iron[20,21] may antagonize the uptake of zinc. Intraluminal prostaglandins may exert an influence on zinc absorption, $PGE_2$ being enhancing, and $PGF_{2\alpha}$ being inhibitory.[22] It is doubtful that they act as ZBLs, however.

**Cellular Factors.** Zinc demonstrates a prominent *bidirectional* (mucosa-to-serosa and serosa-to-mucosa) flux. Thus, a constant pool of zinc within the cell is capable of being displaced from the cell in either direction.[23] The absorption of zinc from the intestinal lumen displays saturation kinetics at lower concentrations of zinc.[24,25] Similar results were shown with isolated brush-border membrane vesicles.[26] Because metabolic inhibitors do not influence zinc entry into intestinal cells and zinc transport by brush-border vesicles is not an active process,[27] the sum total of the observations suggests that the initial uptake of zinc across the mucosal membrane is a carrier-mediated process. Specific receptor proteins have not been identified.

The disposition of zinc within the intestinal cell is complex. It can be used locally for nutritional purposes of the cell, or it can continue its passage through the cell or displace another ion in the zinc pool resulting in a net transfer of zinc in one or another direction, or it can be captured and held within the cell firmly bound to metallothionein.[28] Zinc so trapped is then lost into the fecal stream in the normal course of cell turnover of the intestinal villus. The overall process of mucosa-to-serosa transport of zinc would appear to be en-

ergy-dependent, as the transfer of zinc across the basolateral membrane into the blood is an active transport process.[29]

**Portal Transport.** The zinc released by the intestinal cells at the basolateral-serosal surface into the mesenteric capillary is carried in the portal blood to the liver. Albumin acts as the major portal transport protein in pig, human,[30] and rat.[31]

**Homeostatic Regulation.** The body content of zinc can be controlled by re-excretion and by homeostatic regulation of intestinal uptake.[32] The fractional absorption of zinc decreases as the intraluminal concentration of the ion increases.[23,25,33] Administration of both parenteral and enteral zinc reduces zinc absorption in laboratory animals and in human subjects.[33,34] Induction of metallothionein is a component of the down-regulation of zinc absorption.[28] Experimental zinc deficiency also enhances zinc uptake,[35] and zinc absorption in humans can also be up-regulated by relative zinc restriction in the diet.[36] Certain hormonal influences associated with stress (corticosteroids and leukocytic endogenous mediators) also increase the efficiency of zinc absorption.[37]

### Zinc Excretion

The major route for excretion of endogenous zinc from the body is back into the fecal stream. It has long been thought that this process occurs mainly via the pancreatic secretions; however, the demonstration of a two-way transepithelial flux of zinc in the intestine permits a role for a contribution by intestinal secretion. Perfusion studies have showed an increment of 2.5 to 4.8 mg of zinc in the content of a meal as it passed through the duodenum, presumably as a consequence of the addition of pancreatic zinc to the lumen from the meal-stimulated pancreatic secretion.[13] Unlike copper, the re-excreted zinc can be absorbed and returned to the body. Thus, there is an important *enteropancreatic* circulation of zinc, and the intactness of this circulation contributes to the conservation of this mineral by the body.

The kidney also contributes to zinc excretion. Normally, about 400 to 600 µg of zinc are excreted daily in the urine. Surface losses through desquamation of skin, outgrowth of hair, and sweat can also contribute up to 1 mg of the zinc lost daily from the body. An ejaculum of semen can contain up to 1 mg of zinc.[38]

### Zinc Turnover and Transport

Sophisticated compartmental models using [65]Zn have begun to reveal information about zinc pools and their turnover.[39,40] Total-body biologic half-time for zinc is normally over 360 days, but it is shortened to 235 days by daily loading with 100 mg of zinc.

About 3.5 mg of zinc are normally circulating in the plasma at any given moment. This zinc is partitioned into various species. Forty percent is firmly bound to alpha-2 macroglobulin.[41] This fraction does not participate in nutritionally relevant transport of the mineral. The remaining zinc is loosely bound, either to albumin (55%) or to amino acids (5%). This loosely bound fraction of circulating zinc provides the transport and delivery of the nutrient to the tissues. The amino acid-bound fraction determines the amount that is filtered by the kidneys. Figure 9–1 illustrates the metabolism of zinc in mammals in a schematic fashion.[42]

### Zinc in the Acute-Phase Response

The acute-phase response (APR) to injury is an immunologic response occurring primarily in the liver (with the synthesis of acute-phase proteins), and mediated by bacterial endotoxin or by circulating polypeptides derived from activated white cells (leukocytic endogenous mediators, endogenous pyrogen, interleukin I). One of the characteristic features of the APR is a rapid and dramatic fall in plasma zinc levels to less than 50% of the premorbid level.[43] The mechanism appears to be the sequestering of circulating zinc by the liver, probably after the hormonal induction of

thionein synthesis.[44] A transient fall in zinc levels occurs commonly in the severe illnesses of hospitalized patients,[45] and corticosteroids may be the dominant hormonal mediators of this form of zinc depression. The teleologic significance of this APR-related zinc depression may be directed at making zinc available for the increased protein synthetic duties of the liver in the APR.[44] Sugarman et al. have also shown that zinc ions enhance bacterial adherence to HeLa cells.[46] They speculate that free zinc might be a virulence factor in certain bacterial infections and that the zinc depression response is a protective adaptation.

### Biochemical and Physiologic Function and Mode of Action

Considerable scientific effort has been expended in recent years to further our understanding of the biology of zinc.

### Biochemistry

Zinc appears to have four distinct roles in mammalian metabolism: (1) as a component of zinc-containing metalloenzymes; (2) in the conformation of polysomes; (3) in the stabilization of membranes; and (4) in assorted functions as a free ion within the cell. The biochemistry of zinc has been reviewed extensively.[47,48]

The most important function of zinc is as a constituent of metalloenzymes. To qualify as a me-

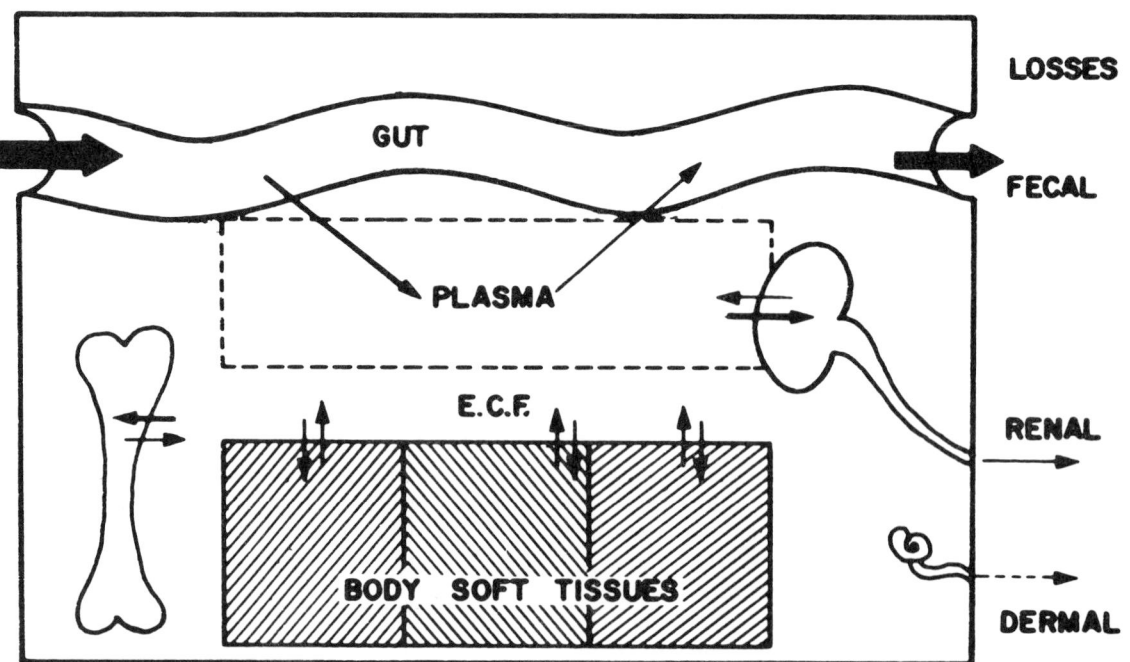

**Fig. 9–1.** Schematic representation of the metabolism of zinc in mammals. From Beisel, W.R., et al.,[42] with permission of Academic Press.

talloenzyme, three criteria must be met: (1) a stoichiometric relationship between metal and protein must be established; (2) the ion must be tightly bound to the protein; and (3) removal or chelation of the metal must impair the catalytic function of the enzyme. The metal can have a conformational role and/or participate at the active site. Many metalloenzymes have more than one metal species (e.g., Zn-Cu superoxide dismutase). The first enzyme confirmed as a zinc metalloenzyme was carbonic anhydrase in 1940. Since then, more than 120 zinc enzymes have been identified in plant and animal species[47] embracing all six I.U.B. classes. Selected zinc metalloenzymes are listed in Table 9–1. Not all have been shown to occur in mammalian tissues.

Certain additional enzymes are classified as "zinc-dependent." Their zinc content has not been confirmed chemically, but *nutritional* experiments have shown them to be uniquely sensitive to dietary zinc deprivation. An important example is thymidine kinase. It is reduced in experimental zinc deficiency in rats and humans.[49]

The intracellular role of zinc ions in the confirmation of polysomes during protein synthesis has been demonstrated.[50] Protein synthesis is not uniformly sensitive to zinc restriction. As pointed out by Chesters:[48]

> DNA synthesis and cell replication are impaired by Zn deficiency to a greater extent than protein synthesis and cell hypertrophy....In normal cells, lack of zinc seems to prevent individual cells from acquiring the groups of proteins that must be synthesized during each cell cycle before the onset of DNA synthesis in the S phase.

Much of the action of zinc, specifically on circulating cells (red cells, white cells, platelets), can be explained by its role in stabilizing membranes.[51]

There are emerging indications that ionic zinc may play a sundry of intracellular roles beyond polysomal conformation, i.e., in the polymeriza-tion and regulation of tubulin synthesis,[52,53] in activating serum thymic factors,[54] and as a soluble cofactor analogous to Mg(II) and Ca(II) by the enzyme fructose-1,6-bisphosphate.[55]

## Physiology

Ideally, our detailed understanding of the biochemistry of zinc would allow the prediction and description of its physiology. This is not the case. In fact, most of what is known about the role of zinc in physiology comes from experiments in zinc-restricted animals or clinical observations in zinc-deficient humans. Although we have a catalogue of zinc metalloenzymes (see Table 9–1), it is important to remember that only in those biochemical pathways in which the metalloenzyme governs the rate-limiting or determinant step will the biochemical defect be manifest as a pathophysiologic lesion. Moreover, the nonenzymatic role of zinc could determine the functional lesion. Table 9–2 lists the physiologic functions dependent on adequate zinc nutriture.

The most important consequence of zinc deficiency is growth failure. Part of this phenomenon might be explained by the anorexia and inanition of the animal; the remainder appears to have a cellular explanation. Protein synthesis impairment is ascribed to the role of zinc in RNA polymerases, in polysomes, and perhaps also to the catabolic effect of an elevation in RNase in zinc deficiency.[56] A complex participation of zinc in cell replication has been postulated.[47] Impaired nuclear division would result from deficiencies of DNA polymerase, deoxynucleotidyl transferases, and thymidine kinase. In addition, an enzyme in the pathway for purine degradation, nucleoside phosphorylase, is zinc-dependent[57] and zinc-containing.[58] This finding has further implications for a role for zinc in the regulation of cell proliferation.[59]

The interaction of zinc and vitamin A metabolism has been recognized.[60,61] It is here that a pure example of a deficiency of a rate-limiting enzyme might be illustrated. The dehydrogenase for vitamin A alcohol (retinol dehydrogenase), like most mammalian alcohol dehydrogenases, would logically be a zinc enzyme. The night blind-

**Table 9–1.  Selected Zinc Metalloenzymes**

α-mannosidase
Alcohol dehydrogenase
Alkaline phosphatase
Carbonic anhydrase
Carboxypeptidase
Deoxynucleotidyl transferase
DNA polymerase
Glutamic acid dehydrogenase
Malic acid dehydrogenase
Nucleoside phosphorylase
Reverse transcriptase
RNA polymerase
Thermolysin
Zn-Cu superoxide dismutase

**Table 9–2.  Physiologic Functions of Zinc in Mammals**

Cell growth
Cell replication
Sexual maturation
Fertility and reproduction
Night vision
Immune defenses
Taste and appetite

ness of zinc deficiency has been ascribed to depletion of retinal and retinol dehydrogenases.[62] Even this may not be the unique explanation because zinc deficiency has also been shown to influence the integrity of the retina itself.[63]

An enormous amount of information on zinc and immune function has been published in the past decade. Zinc deficiency impairs phagocytic function, cellular immunity, humoral immunity, and their intercommunication.[64,65] It may also impair the acute-phase response as well. The molecular basis for the taste impairment and appetite suppression of zinc deficiency remains an enigma.

## Zinc Deficiency

**Clinical Manifestations.** The list of manifestations of zinc deficiency in humans is growing. The original observations in the Persian and Egyptian dwarfs included growth retardation, hypogonadism, and delayed sexual maturation.[66,67] Diverse forms of skin lesions, including papular, pustular, eczematous, seborrheic, and acneiform rashes, have been described in zinc deficiency, in addition to the classic scaly rash on the acral surfaces.[68] A chemotactic defect of phagocytes[69] and cellular immune deficiencies[70] are often seen in zinc-depleted patients. Zinc-responsive night blindness has been documented in patients with alcoholic cirrhosis,[71] sickle cell disease,[72] and Crohn's disease.[73] Not all taste impairment is due to nutritional causes, but in experimental zinc depletion, a clear reversible hypogeusia developed in volunteers.[74] A list of the clinical manifestations, confirmed by their resolution with zinc supplementation, is given in Table 9–3.

**Biochemical and Laboratory Abnormalities.** A number of biochemical and laboratory abnormalities are recognized in zinc deficiency (Table 9–4). Some of these alterations have been known for many years, but a large number have been recognized only since the last edition of this book. Some of the abnormalities became evident in the context of spontaneous or experimental human zinc deficiency, but most have been revealed in laboratory animals or livestock.

### Table 9–3. Clinical Manifestations of Human Zinc Deficiency

Growth retardation
Delayed sexual maturation
Hypogonadism and hypospermia
Alopecia
Skin lesions
Immune deficiencies
Behavioral disturbances
Night blindness
Impaired taste (hypogeusia)
Impaired wound healing

### Table 9–4. Biochemical and Laboratory Abnormalities in Zinc Deficiency

Decreased circulating zinc
Decreased albumin synthesis
Decreased alkaline phosphatase activity (serum)
Decreased carboxypeptidase activity (intraduodenal)
Decreased alcohol dehydrogenase activity (retina, testis)
RNA polymerase activity (liver)
Decreased nucleoside phosphorylase activity (lymphocyte)[a]
Elevated RNase activity (serum)
Increased serum ammonia[b]
Impaired glucose metabolism[c]
Decreased insulin response
Disordered prostaglandin sensitivity[d]
Decreased testosterone levels[e]
Decreased white cell chemotaxis
Impaired T-lymphocyte function
Decreased serum thymic factor[f]
Decreased resistance to experimental infections[g]
Increased resistance to autoimmune disease[h]
Decreased intestinal disaccharidase activity[i]
Elevated 3-hydroxy-3-methylglutamyl coenzyme A reductase[i]
Abnormalities of retinal pigment[j]
Decreased collagen synthesis
Decreased platelet aggregation[k]

[a]Pilz, R.B., et al.: J. Biol. Chem., *257*:13544, 1982.
[b]Rabbani, P., Prasad, A.S.: Am. J. Physiol. *235*:E203. 1978.
[c]Reeves, P.G., O'Dell, B.L.: Br. J. Nutr. *41*:441, 1983.
[d]Gordon, P.R., et al.: J. Nutr. *113*:755, 760, 766, 1983.
[e]Abbasi, A.A., et al.: Lab. Clin. Med., *96*: 544, 1980.
[f]Dardenne, M., et al.: Proc. Natl. Acad. Sci. USA *19*:5370, 1982.
[g]Fraker, P.J., et al.: J. Nutr. *112*:1224, 1982.
[h]Beach, R.S., et al.: J. Immunol. *129*:2686, 1982.
[i]Gebhardt, R.L., et al.: J. Nutr. *113*:855, 1983.
[j]Leure-du Pree, A.E., McClain, C.J.: Invest. Ophthalmol. Vis. Sci. *23*:425, 1982.
[k]Gordon, P.R., et al.: Am. J. Clin. Nutr. *35*:113, 1982.

It is important to understand the conventional model used to investigate the effects of zinc deficiency in animal experiments. Zinc-deficient diets rapidly produce anorexia, causing animals to grow poorly or even lose weight. Thus, in addition to the control and deficient groups, a third group of pair-fed or pair-weighted animals is often included to control for the inanition produced by the anorexia in the zinc-deficient experimental group. Hence, most of the abnormalities listed in Table 9–4 refer to differential changes in zinc-restricted and pair-fed animals.

Although taste dysfunction and reduced appetite may be present in human zinc deficiency, the amount of feed restriction is not analogous to that of animals. Zinc-depleted humans usually maintain reasonable total energy intake. This factor of normal weight maintenance is crucial to the interpretation of experimental data and the extrapolation to the human situation. Although human zinc deficiency is characterized by elevated RNase activity, increased serum ammonia, and depressed testosterone, many of the abnormalities in Table 9–4 may not apply to the human deficiency state. A major experimental and conceptual breakthrough in the induction of zinc deficiency in animals has been made by the tube feeding of rats with a ration of low zinc density while achieving energy intakes of animals fed ad libitum.[75,76] The animals gained weight. Appropriate controls were animals tube-fed with zinc-adequate diets. The preliminary findings are interesting because RNase activity did not increase in this form of zinc deficiency.[75]

## Zinc Toxicity

Zinc toxicity can result from oral or parenteral exposure, and can be either acute or chronic. The different forms produce different manifestations.

**Acute Toxicity.** With oral zinc, doses above 25 mg can produce a metallic taste, nausea, and epigastric distress. Doses in excess of 225 to 450 mg are frankly emetic. Several outbreaks of food poisoning have resulted from preparing fruit drinks in galvanized containers. In the most recent incidence, the illness was characterized by nausea, abdominal cramps, metallic taste, headache, dizziness, vomiting, and chills.[77] Treatment of a premature infant with a daily dose of 3 mg of zinc per kg produced irritability, tremor, seizures, and tachycardia, and serum zinc rose to 224 $\mu$g/dl.[78]

Overly rapid infusion of zinc in TPN solutions can produce symptoms. Bos et al. observed transient flushing, blurred vision, and sweating when 10 mg of zinc was perfused within a brief period.[79] A fatality resulted from a massive inadvertent infusion of 1.6 g of zinc over a three-day period in a woman on home dialysis.[80]

**Chronic Toxicity.** The major consequence of the chronic ingestion of zinc for medicinal purposes is copper deficiency and anemia as a result of the intestinal interaction of zinc and copper. These conditions developed rapidly in a patient given 5 g of zinc daily.[81] Long-term administration of a 150-mg daily dose produced the same result. Gastric erosion is another complication of daily dosage of zinc in the 150-mg range.[84]

A 10-fold error in formulation of a TPN solution, providing 23 mg of zinc daily instead of the prescribed 2.3 mg, resulted in asymptomatic hyperamylasemia in 7 patients.[85]

## Conditions Predisposing to Zinc Depletion

Not only is decreased intake a potential cause of zinc depletion, but also decreased absorption, decreased utilization, increased loss, and increased requirements can lead to the manifestations of a zinc deficiency state. Table 9–5 outlines clinical and environmental situations that might predispose to human zinc deficiency.

### Primary and Dietary-Induced Deficiency

Primary zinc depletion is most commonly seen in patients on total parenteral nutrition when insufficient care has been taken to supply adequate zinc intravenously. Virtually all the manifestations listed in Table 9–3 have been observed in patients on TPN with iatrogenic zinc deficiency. This is of more than academic interest because nitrogen retention and insulin secretion are improved when patients on TPN are maintained in positive zinc balance.[86] Deficient intakes of zinc are found in association with anorexia nervosa,[87] anorexia of cancer,[88] and protein-energy malnutrition (PEM),[89] but multiple nutrient deficiencies are also seen in these conditions. Specific *experimental* zinc deficiency in volunteers has provided important insights into the biology of human zinc depletion.[90,91]

In a public health context, primary zinc deficiency is relatively rare. Shrimpton, however, has provided convincing evidence that zinc is the limiting nutrient in the river fish and rice diet of the population of the upper Amazon basin of Brazil.[92] Since the zinc content of plants is largely determined by the zinc content of soil,[93,93a] this type of endemic deficiency may become common as the mineral content of the world's topsoil becomes depleted.

The more common scenario for dietary-induced deficiency of zinc, however, is not an absolute intake restriction, but rather consumption of a staple diet with a high content of inhibitors of zinc absorption. The classic example is the nutritional dwarfs of Egypt and Iran. High-fiber, high-phytate diets of this region are primarily responsible for limiting the zinc nutriture of the population.[94] A subsegment of the children develops overt signs of deficiency. Vegetarian diets in the United States appear to be less detrimental to zinc nutriture.[95] Some concern had been raised that increasing the amount of texturized soy protein in the diet might have an adverse impact on zinc nutrition, but not all observers share this concern.[95a]

Mineral imbalances in the diet may be the more relevant dietary factor influencing zinc nutriture in Western populations. The antagonism of iron and zinc had been cited.[19,20] Analyses of infant formulas show that some preparations have an iron:zinc ratio as high as 50:1.[96] The delayed infant growth with iron-fortified diet formulas not supplemented with zinc reported by Walravens

**Table 9–5. Clinical Situations Predisposing to Zinc Depletion**

*Decreased Intake*
  Anorexia nervosa
  Anorexia of malignant disease
  Protein-energy malnutrition
  Chronic uremia
  Abnormal food selection pattern
  Experimental depletion
  Total parenteral nutrition without added zinc
*Decreased Absorption*
  High-phytate diet
  High-fiber diet
  High dietary iron/zinc ratio
  Geophagia
  Acrodermatitis enteropathica
  Hyposucrasia
  Celiac disease
  Inflammatory bowel diseases
  Short-bowel syndrome
  Jejunoileal bypass
  Alcoholic cirrhosis
  Pancreatic insufficiency
  Chronic uremia
*Decreased Utilization*
  Protein-energy malnutrition
  Alcoholic cirrhosis
  Phenylketonuria (?)
  Anticonvulsant therapy (?)
*Increased Loss*
  Diarrheal fluid loss
  Ileostomy fluid loss
  Celiac disease
  Inflammatory bowel diseases
  Intestinal parasitosis (giardiasis)
  Pancreaticocutaneous fistula
  Pancreaticocolic fistula
  Nephrotic syndrome
  Thiazide diuretics
  Parenteral ethylenediamine tetra-acetate therapy
  Oral ethylenediamine penta-acetate therapy
  Oral D(-)penicillamine therapy
  Alcoholism
  Acute alcoholic pancreatitis
  Alcoholic cirrhosis
  Viral hepatitis
  Infantile biliary cirrhosis
  Hemolytic anemias (thalassemia, sickle cell)
  Post-surgery/post-trauma/post-infection periods
  Extracorporeal dialysis
  Thermal burn exudation
  Exfoliative dermatitis
  Psoriasis
*Increased Requirement*
  Neoplastic diseases
  Post-burn re-epithelialization
  Infantile and adolescent growth spurts
  Pregnancy
  Lactation
  Psoriasis (?)

(?) = Speculation as to mechanism of observed zinc deficiency.

and Hambidge[97] is likely to have been influenced by the 6:1 iron:zinc ratio. High-dose iron supplementation during pregnancy may influence plasma zinc levels.[98,99] The high concentration of calcium in the hard water of Guelph (330 ppm in Ontario versus 33 ppm of Nova Scotia) may interfere with zinc absorption.[100]

### Inborn Errors of Zinc Metabolism

**Acrodermatitis Enteropathica.** The autosomal recessive disease, acrodermatitis enteropathica (AE), is an inherited abnormality of zinc absorption. The hyperpigmented skin lesions over the acral surfaces of elbows and knees (often also involving the face, buttocks, and other surfaces and frequently superinfected with suppurative and nonsuppurative organisms) are characteristic. Intestinal disturbances and growth failure are also prominent. The phenotypic expression of AE is totally related to manifestations of zinc deficiency per se.[101] The efficiency of zinc absorption in AE is reduced, with abnormalities of secretory factors and mucosal membrane factors having been identified.

Barnes and Moynahan determined that oral therapy could produce complete and long-lasting clinical remissions.[102] The association of zinc therapy with clinical improvement has been conclusively correlated in balance studies. The intestinal barrier to zinc absorption in this disease is not absolute; increments in oral intake of only 100 to 200% of the RDA of zinc salts are therapeutically effective.[103] As women with AE survived to childbearing age, concern for safety during pregnancy arose. However, with adequate attention to zinc prophylaxis and the maintenance of normal plasma zinc levels during gestation, women with treated AE have been successfully delivered of healthy infants.[104]

An animal model for understanding the pathophysiology of AE can be found in the Friesian cattle who have a malabsorption of zinc leading to zinc deficiency signs.[105] They respond to dietary supplementation with zinc. Figure 9–2 shows the clinical features of human AE, and a calf with Adema disease.

**Familial Hyperzincemia.** Persistent elevation of plasma zinc to levels >300 μg/dl has been identified in a black kinship in Washington D.C.[106] No pathologic consequences are yet identified. The excess circulating zinc is associated with the albumin fraction.[107]

### Secondary Acquired Zinc Deficiency

Aside from AE, the two secondary zinc deficiency conditions best characterized are sickle cell anemia and chronic uremia.[108–111] There is

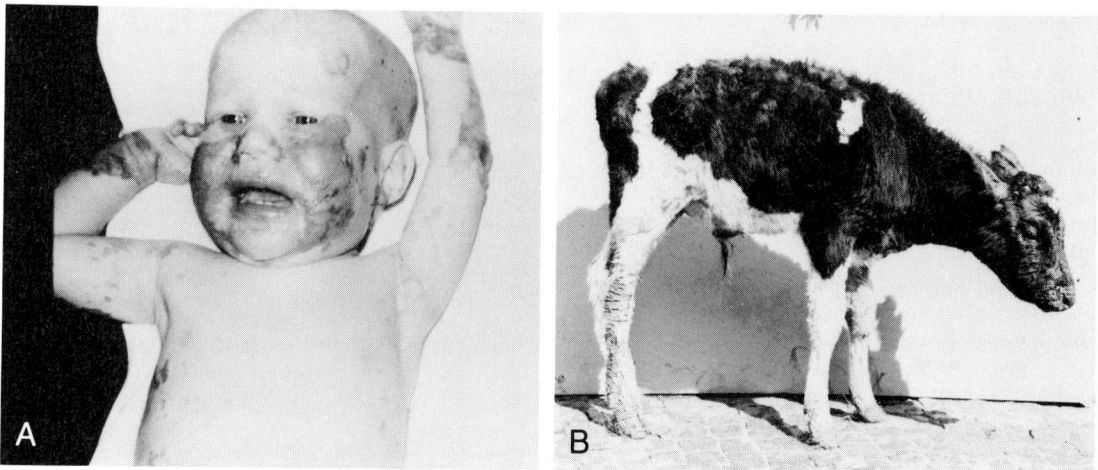

**Fig. 9–2.** *A,* Typical clinical features of a patient with acrodermatitis enteropathica. (Courtesy of Dr. Kenneth Neldner.) *B,* A calf with Adema disease. (Courtesy of Dr. Thor Flagstad.)

evidence for zinc deficiency in childhood protein-energy malnutrition; delayed cutaneous hypersensitivity, thymus size, and the composition of weight regained during recovery are all influenced by the level of zinc intake.[112]

The major pathophysiologic abnormalities contributing to secondary zinc depletion are zinc malabsorption and excessive urinary zinc excretion (see Table 9–5). In many diseases, multiple causative factors contribute to zinc deficiency. The most important example is alcoholism in which intestinal malabsorption, pancreatic insufficiency, decreased albumin affinity, and excessive urinary excretion all contribute to abnormal zinc metabolism. Zinc deficiency commonly occurs in Crohn's disease and celiac disease, and both malabsorption and wastage from the gastrointestinal tract occur with protein-losing enteropathy and diarrhea. Zinc malabsorption is even a factor in the zinc deficiency of chronic uremia. A role for vitamin D nutriture in the efficient absorption of zinc by uremic patients has been suggested.[113] Finally, the substantial amount of zinc that can be lost with diarrheal episodes has only recently been appreciated.[86,114] The plasma zinc levels within a group of psoriasis patients correlated with the extent of skin surface involved with the rash.[115]

Rapid turnover of tissue is the basis for increased zinc requirements. This process is seen in neoplastic diseases, during re-epithelialization after burns, and during the newborn and adolescent growth spurts. The most important examples of increased zinc requirements, however, are lactation and pregnancy. However, in lactating women in Maryland, there were no changes observed in plasma or red cell zinc as compared to

nonlactating postpartum women.[116] Both groups consumed only 42% of their respective RDAs for zinc. Pregnancy would potentially stress zinc reserves even more than lactation. Two inquiries have evaluated the prevalence of zinc deficiency in terms of responses to intragestational supplementation, one in 213 pregnant Hispanic women in Los Angeles,[117] the other in 46 pregnant middle-income women in Denver.[99] The natural history of circulating zinc in both groups was a decline throughout gestation. A daily supplement of 20 mg of zinc in the Los Angeles subjects reduced significantly the number of women with abnormally low zinc levels at parturition; 15 mg of supplementary zinc in 10 of the Denver mothers produced a higher alkaline phosphorylase activity in serum. These studies have cautiously been interpreted to imply a prevalence of subadequate zinc status in pregnancy. Moreover, the outcome of pregnancy may be related to maternal zinc status.[118–121] Experimental zinc deficiency in pregnant animals produces teratogenesis in the offspring.[122] A prospective/retrospective study of mothers delivering babies with congenital abnormalities revealed a significantly lower blood zinc as compared to mothers of infants without malformations.[123] Mean cord blood in 20 congenitally abnormal babies was also lower than that for normal babies. Abnormalities of zinc metabolism in both experimental and human fetal alcohol syndrome have led to strong speculation that fetal zinc deprivation is an etiologic factor.[124]

## Dietary Considerations

Species differ with respect to their requirements for zinc. The amount of zinc per kg of ration for a select group of vertebrates is shown in Table 9–6.

### Human Dietary Allowances

The Recommended Dietary Allowance Committee has specified an RDA for zinc for healthy individuals consuming a mixed North American diet[125] (Appendix Table A1b). There is, however, both little certainty and little agreement on the values for allowances. The Canadian recommendations for zinc intake (Appendix Table A2c) are considerably lower than those for the United States. For instance, adult men and women in Canada have allowances of 9 and 8 mg, respectively, whereas for lactating women in Canada, the daily recommendation for zinc is 14 mg.[126] On the other hand, the 1973 Expert Committee of the World Health Organization based a series of zinc intake recommendations on a factorial estimate for daily zinc losses and retentions, and on assumptions about the average bioavailability of the diet.[8] They estimated that a lactating woman would need to absorb 5.5 mg of zinc daily. If her diet provided a 40% fraction absorption for its zinc content, the recommended intake in lactation would be 13.6 mg, similar to the Canadian figure; if dietary zinc were 10% absorbable, the daily intake requirement would be 54.6 mg.

### Food Sources

Foods differ widely in their intrinsic zinc content[126a] (Table 9–7. See also Appendix Table A37 for detailed data). Oysters are the richest sources of zinc among food whereas sweets, fats and oils, fish, and pastries are relatively low in zinc. Depending on the traditional constituents of regional diets, a population might receive an extraordinarily high total zinc intake or a subadequate amount. Drinking water usually makes a negligible contribution to zinc intake; under certain environmental circumstances, however, tap water can provide up to 10% of the daily requirement.[127] Exclusively breast-fed children in the

### Table 9–6. Comparative Zinc Requirement in Several Mammalian Species

| Species | Zinc Requirement (mg/kg of Ration) |
|---|---|
| Mouse | 30 |
| Rat | 12 |
| Cat | 30 |
| Dog | 50 |
| Pig | 50 |
| Sheep | 35–50 |
| Squirrel monkey | 15 |
| Human | 15* |

*Assumes that an adult human consumes about 1 kg of food daily.

### Table 9–7. Food Sources of Zinc*

| Zinc Category (mg/1,000 kcal) | Foods |
|---|---|
| Very poor 0–2 | Fats, oils, butter, cream cheese, sweets, chocolates, soft drinks, alcoholic drinks, sugars, jams, and preserves |
| Poor 1–5 | Fish, fruits, refined cereal products, pastries, biscuits, cakes, puddings, tubers, plantains, sausages, chips |
| Rich 4–12 | Whole grains, pork, poultry, milk, low-fat cheese, yogurt, eggs, nuts |
| Very rich 12–882 | Lamb, leafy and root vegetables, crustacea, beef, kidney, liver, heart, mollusks |

*Classification of dietary zinc sources based on nutrient-energy density.
From Solomons, N.W., Shrimpton, R.,[126a] with permission of McGraw-Hill Book Co.

United States will receive an average of 0.5 mg zinc/kg body weight with normal suckling.[128]

### Factors Affecting Zinc Bioavailability

The intake of zinc from the diet, however, is not the only factor influencing the satisfaction of zinc requirements. For instance, in one study, children in rural Iran near Shiraz consumed an average of 12 mg of zinc,[129] but deficiency was common in this population. Similarly, breast-fed children generally ingest between 1 and 2 mg of zinc daily,[130] less than the RDA allowance of 3 mg, yet their zinc status is superior to that of bottle-fed infants consuming a milk-based formula with 5.8 mg of zinc daily.[131] The *biologic availability* of zinc is an important consideration.[8] The nature of the food in the meal influences the absorbability of zinc by inhibiting, or occasionally enhancing, the uptake of dietary zinc. Factors affecting zinc bioavailability are listed in Table 9–8. This topic has been discussed in detail elsewhere.[130,132]

The absorbability of zinc appears to be largely a function of the presence or absence of inhibitory substances in the food or meal in which it is consumed. Meats are considered to be sources of highly available zinc because of the relative absence of chemical constituents that inhibit zinc. Unlike iron, zinc does not gain absorptive efficiency by being consumed with flesh.[133]

Some foods and drugs appear to enhance zinc absorption, notably zinfandel wine, breast milk, and certain drugs. The factor(s) in human milk that increase the absorption of zinc have been a matter of considerable speculation, with picolinic acid and citric acid mentioned prominently, but no functional role for either organic acid has been confirmed. Recent evidence suggests that excess

**Table 9–8. Factors Affecting Zinc Bioavailability**

INHIBITORY FACTORS

*Specific Foods/Beverages*
Soy protein
Whole wheat
Tea
Coffee
Celery
Cow milk
Cheese
Corn tortillas
Beans
Hamburger

*Chemical Constituents of the Diet*
Dietary fiber
Phytic acid
Oxalate
Iron
Ethanol
"Tannins" (polyphenols)
Ethylenediamine tetra-acetic acid
Calcium
Tin

ENHANCING FACTORS

*Specific Foods/Beverages*
Human breast milk
Zinfandel wine

*Chemical Constituents of the Diet*
? Citric acid
? Picolinic acid

*Drugs*
Iodoquinol (Diodoquin)
Phenytoin
D(-)penicillamine

consumption of alcohol can reduce intestinal zinc absorption.

Net delivery of zinc, or any nutrient, to the organism is a function of the bioavailability (fractional absorption) *and* the total amount of zinc in the meal. For instance, whole grains have a low bioavailability of zinc, but they contain substantially more zinc than milled flour. On a meal-for-meal basis, one might actually absorb more zinc from wheat as whole-grain items than from the same foods prepared from refined flour.[134]

## Assessment of Zinc Nutriture

Despite our knowledge about the biology of zinc and about factors promoting or predisposing to depletion, the management of clinical problems of zinc nutrition is complicated by the difficulties in assessing the zinc status of an individual. Clinical assessment of zinc nutriture remains highly problematic. Approaches to assessing nutritional status in the laboratory involve the measurement of *static* indices (e.g., concentration of the nutrient in tissues or fluids, or measurement of surrogates for the nutrient, such as metal-containing enzymes and proteins), or *functional* indices (i.e.,

performance on nutrient-dependent physiologic functions).[135] The problem is that many measures do not accurately reflect either total-body zinc or the pool of nutritionally available zinc in the body.

**Static Indices.** The development of atomic absorption spectrophotometry (AAS) has made the determination of serum and plasma zinc levels a routine procedure; it is fairly simple and reliable for determination of the zinc content of hair or the concentration in urine. However, emission spectrophotometry, x-ray fluorescence, proton- and electron-induced x-ray emission spectrometry, and neutron activation analysis all have the capacity to measure zinc. In an attempt to characterize human zinc status, zinc has been measured in human plasma, serum, saliva, sweat, cerumen, red cells, white cells, platelets, skin, hair, nails, and urine. Normal values for commonly used static indices are shown in Table 9–9. The most common index, by far, has been circulating zinc measured by AAS. Extreme caution must be exercised to avoid pitfalls in the quantification or interpretation of serum or plasma zinc in terms of human zinc nutriture. These pitfalls are enumerated in Table 9–10.

**Functional Indices.** Table 9–11 lists the in vitro and in vivo tests of physiologic function (functional indices) that have been used to assess the adequacy of zinc nutriture. The most definitive index would be isotope turnover tests from which the size of various body pools could be determined.[39,40] This test and the others are quite limited to varying degrees in their routine application in nutritional assessment. The other indices listed have each been shown to respond to zinc repletion. Wound healing and nitrogen retention are cumbersome measures to be reserved for extraordinary and specific circumstances. Other procedures among the functional indices of zinc nutriture are dark adaptometry, taste, olfactory acuity, and the in vitro tests of white cell function.

**Diagnostic Approach to Suspected Impairment of Zinc Nutriture.** The role of signs and symptoms

**Table 9–9. Normal Range of Value for Selected Static Indices of Zinc**

| Areas of Zinc Content | Reported Ranges of Normal |
|---|---|
| Serum | 140–65 μg/dl |
| Red cell | 44–40 μg/g Hgb |
| White cell | 130–80 μg/$10^{10}$ cells |
| Saliva (parotid) | 79–23 ng/g |
| Sweat | 1.75–0.55 mg/L |
| Skin | 80–10 μg/g |
| Nails | 400–100 μg/g |
| Hair | 250–100 μg/g |
| 24-hr urine | 600–230 μg/g |

**Table 9–10.  Pitfalls and Limitations of Use of Circulating Levels of Zinc to Assess Nutritional Status**

| Condition | Direction of Change Relative to "True" Zinc Level |
|---|---|
| External contamination | increased |
| Hemolysis | increased |
| Venous occlusion | increased |
| Prolonged fasting | increased |
| Estrogens, oral contraceptives | decreased |
| Corticosteroids | decreased |
| Inflammation/infection | decreased |
| Post-prandial sampling | decreased |
| Albumin concentration | either direction* |
| Protein-binding affinity | either direction† |

*Hypoalbuminemia caused *decrease,* relative.
†Decreased binding affinity in alcoholic cirrhosis and pregnancy; increased binding affinity in familiar hyperzincemia.

**Table 9–11.  Functional Indices of Zinc Nurinture**

*In Vitro Tests*
  Leukocyte chemotaxis
  Lymphocyte blastogenesis
  Platelet aggregation
  $^{65}$Zn uptake by red cells

*In Vivo Tests*
  Dark adaptation
  Taste acuity
  Olfactory acuity
  Rate of healing of experimental wound
  Collagen accumulation in subcutaneous sponge implant
  Sperm production
  Nitrogen retention
  Glucose tolerance and insulin production
  Intestinal zinc uptake
  Zinc retention
  Isotopic turnover (radiozinc or stable isotope)

in the diagnosis of zinc deficiency is similar to that for any other nutrient deficiency syndrome. That is, they are (by definition) useless for pinpointing a specific marginal or *sub*clinical deficiency. If a patient has a disease commonly predisposing to zinc depletion, a systematic search for the classic signs and symptoms of zinc deficiency (see Table 9–3) should be made. When one or more compatible clinical manifestations are discovered on a routine examination and/or a disease state is associated with an increased likelihood of deficiency (e.g., malabsorption with chronic diarrhea), a differential diagnosis including zinc deficiency should be constructed, and a concerted search for other zinc deficiency signs and symptoms should be conducted. Laboratory and functional indices should be measured.

It is important to recognize that, in a malnour-

ished patient, the manifestations of zinc deficiency are usually not specific for this nutrient. However, the skin lesions (palmar bullae and dermatitis around the mouth and at pressure points) are quite suggestive. Thus, as in the diagnosis of subclinical deficiency states, the confirmation of zinc deficiency by collateral laboratory indices should be attempted prior to the institution of a therapeutic trial with zinc. The same principle of using some static and functional indices applies equally to the patient with clinical manifestations compatible with zinc deficiency as it does to the person thought to be at risk for a marginal subclinical deficiency state.

**Therapeutic Use**

When a presumptive diagnosis of zinc deficiency or of a zinc-responsive condition has been made, zinc supplementation is indicated. Various zinc compounds are available for oral administration, including the sulfate, gluconate, acetate, and oxide. Dosages of elemental zinc per tablet or capsule range from 5 to 50 mg. Various claims for superiority in bioavailability, therapeutic efficacy, or tolerance have been made for one or another compound, but these are largely unsubstantiated. Studies in our laboratory showed no differences in the availability of zinc from the inorganic sulfate salt and the organic gluconate compound. Although gastrointestinal irritation may be lessened by taking zinc with meals, the absorption of therapeutic zinc is markedly reduced by food.[136] Administration of zinc preparations should be displaced from mealtime.

Traditionally, treatment of zinc deficiency has involved daily oral dosages of 150 mg of zinc in three divided doses. Given the risk of inducing copper deficiency on this regimen, Sandstead has recommended that therapeutic doses of oral zinc to treat zinc deficiency be limited to 40 mg per day.[137] In some conditions, such as acrodermatitis enteropathica, lesser amounts of medicinal zinc will produce the desired therapeutic effect.

A new class of conditions is being described in which oral zinc in *therapeutic levels* is claimed to be effective even in the absence of preexisting zinc deficiency. These are so-called "zinc-responsive" conditions, with claims for daily doses in excess of 40 mg. There are claims for beneficial effects on immune responses by supplementing elderly subjects (>60 years) with 150 mg of zinc daily.[138,139] The long-term benefits of this immunoreconstitution have not been evaluated in terms of its ultimate influence on carcinogenesis or infection susceptibility. Maintenance of the "decoppered" state in Wilson's disease, after initial treatment with D-penicillamine, by high levels of oral zinc, represents another zinc-responsive condition.[140] The amount of zinc required to suppress absorption of dietary and endogenous copper is 150 mg daily. With a similar rationale, attempts to control the excess liver copper in primary biliary cirrhosis are far less successful.[141]

When individuals are unable to consume nutrients orally, total parenteral nutrition (TPN) may be instituted. If TPN is continued for more than a few days, zinc must be added to the regimen unless evidence for prior depletion indicates immediate parenteral therapy. Recommendations have been made for the administration of daily maintenance levels of intravenous zinc for patients on TPN[142] (see Chapter 54).

## COPPER

### History of Copper as a Nutrient

The element copper has been known since antiquity, the bronze of the "Bronze Age" being an alloy of copper and tin. Copper compounds were used in folk medicine to treat arthritic conditions. Aberhalden in 1900 first showed that laboratory animals fed a whole-milk diet developed an iron-resistant anemia. In 1928, Hart et al. found that the anemia of a milk or milk-rice ration would respond to iron therapy only after copper had also been added to the diet.[143] A clear-cut, copper-responsive syndrome of copper deficiency in humans was reported in 1966.[144] Since the advent of total parenteral nutrition, the frequency of reported cases of human copper deficiency has increased. More detailed historical notes on copper as a nutrient have appeared.[145,146]

### Chemistry

Copper has atomic number 29, and an atomic weight of 63.54. It has two naturally occurring isotopes: $^{63}Cu$ (69.1%) and $^{65}Cu$ (30.9%). Two radioisotopes—$^{64}Cu$ ($t_{1/2}$ = 12.7 hours) and $^{67}Cu$ ($t_{1/2}$ = 61.9 hours)—have been used as biologic tracers. Copper ions exist in two oxidation states: Cu(I), which is *cuprous*, and Cu(II), which is *cupric*. The cupric ion is a potent oxidizing agent. Copper ions complex with greater or lesser affinity to many of the same chelating agents known to bind zinc.

### Metabolism

#### Copper in the Human Body

Estimates for total-body copper for an adult man range from 70 to 80 mg.[145] Others make a factorial estimate of 99.4 mg.[147] Copper is distributed among organs as follows: skeletal muscle (24.7%), skin (15.3%), bone marrow (14.8%), skeleton (19.0%), liver (8.0 to 15.0%), and brain (8.0%). The full-term infant is born with 15 to 17 mg of copper.[148] Copper concentration per gram of wet weight of tissue is highest in the brain (6.3 µg/g) and liver (5.1 µg/g). Skin, bone, kidney, and heart all have concentrations in excess of 2.0 µg/g wet tissue. The concentration of copper in skeletal muscle is 0.9 µg/g.[147]

### Copper Uptake

**Site of Absorption.** The human stomach and upper duodenum are capable of absorbing copper in soluble form as attested to by the rapid appearance of copper in the circulation and the quantitative removal of copper from the upper lumen. Copper in foods is in bound form and requires digestion of the food for its dissociation into a free, ionic form, which is less rapidly absorbed. The exposure of copper to bile may influence its bioavailability. Thus, the majority of dietary copper that is absorbed is probably taken up at a site distal to the duodenum.

**Intraluminal Factors.** Copper complexes tend to dissociate at low pH. It has been calculated that the salivary and gastric secretions have sufficient capacity to bind all the dietary copper in a meal.[149] The interplay of the luminal pH, endogenous macroligands, and smaller binding species probably influences the absorption of dietary copper. Histidine may play a role in copper absorption under physiologic conditions. Copper complexed to histidine presumably shares the absorption kinetics of its amino acid carrier. Whether the putative endogenous ligands or small binding ligands from breast milk that act on zinc also influence copper absorption has received some speculation, but no conclusions are forthcoming.[150] There is some evidence of increased copper absorption in patients with pancreatic insufficiency, interpreted to indicate that pancreatic secretions at mealtime serve normally to moderate the uptake of copper.[151]

A direct intraluminal mineral:mineral competition of copper and an antagonistic ion may be operative with some dietary metals. Nutritional studies suggest such a competition for iron and copper. Zinc inhibits the uptake of copper at Zn/Cu ratios of >500:1, ratios that rarely occur in normal foods or animal feeds.[152]

**Cellular Factors.** Two mechanisms for the cellular uptake of copper are available. The minor route is active transport in association with amino acid complexes. The major route is diffusional and, being saturable, has the characteristics of carrier-mediated diffusion. It is not glucose-dependent. The transport of copper across the cell and into the blood is the point of maximum control. Evidence from a number of sources suggests that mucosal metallothionein plays a regulatory role, impeding the passage of copper from mucosa to serosa. The induction of intestinal metallothionein by oral zinc decreases copper uptake in proportion to the zinc supplied.[153] Intramucosal transferrin may also be involved in copper transfer, but more in a facilitating role.[154]

**Portal Factors.** Newly absorbed copper is initially bound to albumin for transport to the liver.[155] Incorporation of copper into ceruloplasmin is an elaborate process that takes place exclusively in the liver.

**Homeostatic Regulation.** The efficiency of copper absorption is increased in copper-deficient rats and humans, suggesting homeostatic regulation at the level of gastrointestinal absorption.[156] The efficiency of absorption, furthermore, decreases as the amount of copper in the lumen increases.[157] Intestinal senescence does not influence the absorption of copper in elderly men. Whether pregnancy or lactation enhances the efficiency of absorption in women remains to be determined.

### Copper Excretion

The major route of excretion of copper is via the bile. An in vivo perfusion technique revealed human biliary copper excretion to be 1.7 ± 0.8 mg daily.[149] Biliary copper excretion is the major homeostatic regulator of body copper balance as well, responding to changes in copper absorption and to parenteral administration of copper.[149,151,157]

The precise chemical form of copper in bile is debated; it is reportedly bile associated with a high-molecular-weight (protein) fraction[158] or complexed with conjugated bilirubin.[159] Whatever the nature of biliary copper, it appears to be poorly absorbed by the mammalian intestine.[160] Hence, the enterohepatic recirculation of endogenous copper is minimal. Copper in salivary, gastric, and intestinal juices makes a contribution to fecal copper excretion. This copper may be more available for reabsorption than biliary copper.

Urine represents a minor route of excretion. Daily output of copper in the urine is 30 to 50 μg, with only a limited capacity to increase excretion with biliary obstruction. Small amounts of copper are also lost in sweat, with the outgrowth of hair and nails, and with desquamation of skin.

### Copper Turnover and Transport

Although it contains only 8 to 15% of total-body copper, the liver is the dominant terminal for the turnover of copper. It is also the organ most susceptible to toxic accumulation of copper when the mechanisms to excrete copper from the body are impaired. The biologic half-life of an intravenous dose of $^{67}Cu$ in a normal, healthy individual was computed to be 27.1 days.[161]

The primary transport protein in copper, providing the copper to nourish the peripheral tissues of the body, is ceruloplasmin.[162] Each mole of ceruloplasmin contains 6 gram atoms of copper[162,163] attached post-translationally within the liver. The synthesis of apoceruloplasmin appears to be somewhat independent of copper availability.[164] It was previously a consensus that 92 to 94% of circulating copper was in the form of ceruloplasmin. Linder et al. have reported that 5% of serum copper is associated with a protein fraction (fraction II) of greater molecular weight than ceruloplasmin.[165] The concentration of ceruloplasmin does not appear to be rate-limiting for the nurture of peripheral tissues, since patients with Wilson's disease have minute serum levels of this protein but show no evidence of copper deficiency.

A number of physiologic and hormonal influences affect the synthesis and release of ceruloplasmin. Acutely, high doses of corticosteroids increase serum copper but, administered chronically, steroids may reduce serum copper levels. Pregnancy[166] and the use of oral estrogen-containing contraceptives[167] produce a two- to three-fold increase in ceruloplasmin levels. Cigarette smokers[168] and individuals taking anticonvulsant drugs[169] have increased ceruloplasmin concentrations. Various malignant conditions, such as leukemia,[170] lymphoma,[171] and assorted solid tumors,[172] produce chronic elevation of ceruloplasmin.

In the perinatal period, developmental changes in the liver govern the ability of the fetal and newborn liver to accumulate and release copper.[173] A specific degree of hepatic maturation is required before copper can be released to the tissues. Thus, premature infants have lower copper concentrations than full-term infants,[174] and copper supplementation of premature infants does not produce normal ceruloplasmin levels until appropriate liver maturation occurs.[175] A schematic illustration of copper metabolism in mammals is shown in Figure 9–3.

### Copper and the Acute-Phase Response (APR)

The APR also affects circulating copper, although in a manner quite distinct from that for zinc. Ceruloplasmin is not only a major transport protein for copper, it is also an acute-phase protein. Circulating concentrations of copper can become significantly elevated in 18 hours following the onset of infection, and the total ceruloplasmin levels, and hence circulating copper, can rise

COPPER

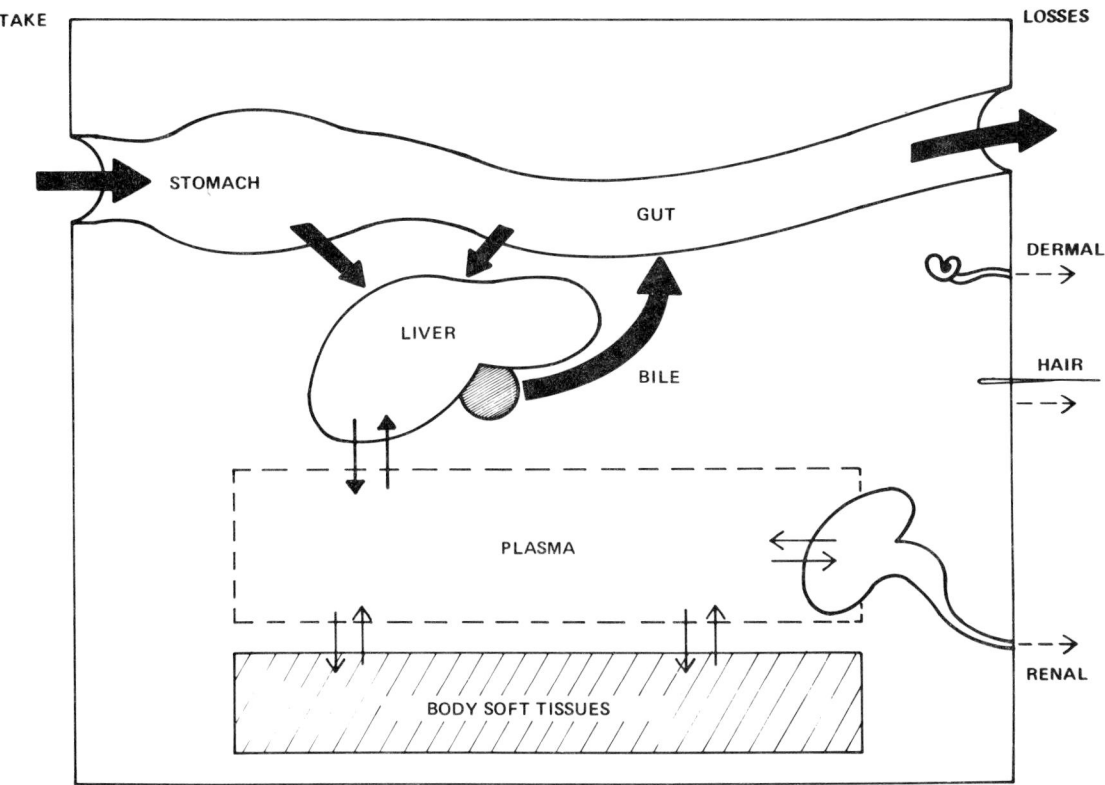

**Fig. 9–3.** Schematic representation of the metabolism of copper in mammals.

threefold during the course of an infection.[176] Tuberculosis, leprosy, schistosomiasis, advanced cystic fibrosis, and drug rashes are all associated with acute-phase elevations of copper.[177] There appears to be a potential teleologic significance to this outpouring of ceruloplasmin. Ceruloplasmin apparently exerts a physiologically important superoxide dismutase activity in the plasma to neutralize superoxide radicals released by activated white cells phagocytosing invading organisms.[178]

## Biochemical and Physiologic Function and Mode of Action

Reviews of the biochemistry of copper have appeared.[179,180] The primary role of copper is as a component of copper metalloenzymes. A list of common cuproenzymes is presented in Table 9–12. Although the substrates, reactions, and metabolic roles are vastly different, *all* cuproenzymes, mammalian and nonmammalian alike, share a common biochemical principle: They all involve reactions in which molecular oxygen or a related species (e.g., superoxide radicals) is consumed. Water or hydrogen peroxide are commonly

formed. A typical example is the reaction catalyzed by superoxide dismutase:

$$2O_2^- + 2\,H^+ \rightarrow H_2O_2 + O_2$$

The nature of the reactions makes the cuproenzyme step the thermodynamically determinant step in a given metabolic pathway. Thus, copper deficiency induces physiologic lesions that can often be attributed to a specific enzymatic defect.[179]

**Table 9–12. Metalloenzymes of Copper**

| |
|---|
| *Mammalian* |
| Ceruloplasmin (ferroxidase I) |
| Ferroxidase II |
| Tyrosinase |
| Monoamine oxidase |
| Diamine oxidase |
| Lysyl oxidase |
| Cytochrome *c* oxidase |
| Dopamine-beta-hydroxylase |
| Zn-Cu superoxide dismutase |
| |
| *Nonmammalian* |
| Ascorbate oxidase |
| Galactose oxidase |
| Laccase |

Tyrosinase is important in the formation of melanin. Cytochrome *c* oxidase governs the terminal reaction in mitochondrial oxidative phosphorylation. The amine oxidases catalyze the oxidative deamination of amines. An amine oxidase of specific importance is lysyl oxidase, key enzyme for the cross-linking reactions for collagen and elastin supportive connective tissues. Both ferroxidase I (ceruloplasmin) and ferroxidase II are capable of catalyzing the oxidation of *ferrous* ions to *ferric* ions. Although one might suppose that ferroxidation plays a role in supporting the erythron, the biochemical basis for copper-deficiency anemia is still not clearly delineated.[181] In fact, other substrates such as ascorbic acid and circulating free superoxide radicals may be physiologically relevant to the catalytic function of ceruloplasmin.

As with zinc, a number of enzymes are considered to be "copper-dependent" even though no confirmation of their metalloenzyme status has been produced. O'Dell and Prohaska have published a superb review of the enzymatic functions that respond to copper restriction in laboratory animals.[180] Activity of 2'3'-cyclonucleotide-3'-phosphodiesterase is reduced in the copper-deficient rat and mouse. Because this enzyme is an index of myelination in developing nervous tissue, its deficient activity may explain the documented hypomyelination lesion. Additionally, tyrosine hydroxylase, which is involved in the pathway from tyrosine to DOPA, UDP-galactose:HFA-ceramide galactosyl transferase, which is involved in the formation of cerebrosides in the brain, and latent hexokinase in synaptic membranes of the cerebellum are all reduced with nutritional deprivation of copper in experimental animals. None is yet known to *contain* copper.

The enzymatic reactions and physiologic functions for copper correspond more closely than those for zinc, but many of the functions that have been assigned to this metal are based on nutritional (copper restriction) experiments in animals and do not have any molecular basis in copper biochemistry. Indeed, an impressive list of physiologic roles for copper in mammals can now be compiled (Table 9–13). The ensuing discussion of copper deficiency will clarify the reason for ascribing dependence of the various functions on adequate copper nutriture.

## Copper Deficiency

**Clinical Manifestations.** Clinical manifestations of copper deficiency can be seen with acquired copper deficiency or with the inborn error of metabolism, Menkes' syndrome, which is de facto a copper deficiency condition despite elevated copper concentrations in some organs. The

**Table 9–13. Physiologic Functions of Copper in Mammals**

Erythropoiesis
Leukopoiesis
Skeletal mineralization
Connective tissue synthesis
Myelin formation
Melanin pigment synthesis
Catecholamine metabolism
Oxidative phosphorylation
Thermal regulation
Antioxidant protection
Cholesterol metabolism
Immune function
Cardiac function
Glucose metabolic regulation

**Table 9–14. Clinical Manifestations of Human Copper Deficiency\***

Microcytic hypochromic anemia
Neutropenia
Skeletal demineralization
Subperiosteal hemorrhages
Depigmentation of hair and skin
Defective elastin formation with:
   arterial aneurysms
   decreased tensile strength of skin
Cerebral and cerebellar degeneration
Hypotonia
Hypothermia

\**Pili torti* or kinky hair is only observed in patients with kinky hair syndrome, not in acquired deficiency.

manifestations are listed in Table 9–14. The twisted, brittle, "steel wool" hair of Menkes' disease has not been seen in acquired copper deficiency in humans, but all the other manifestations have been observed in primary copper deficiency in children.[182,183] The most recently described sign is leg swelling due to subperiosteal hemorrhages.[183] In adult patients, however, *only* the microcytic anemia and neutropenia have been observed.

Most of the lesions can be ascribed to deficiencies of one or another pathway governed by a documented cuproenzyme. The depigmentation of integumentary tissues can be ascribed to insufficient tyrosinase activity, defective elastin, and collagen formation is attributed to lysyl oxidase deficiency. The hypothermia and hypotonia are likely to be due to cytochrome *c* oxidase deficiency causing the failure of oxidative phosphorylation. Cerebral and cerebellar degeneration could be due, in part, to defects in cytochrome *c* oxidase and dopamine-beta-hydroxylase. Another factor is demyelination, the biochemical basis of which is not yet clear. The skeletal demineralization and subperiosteal hemorrhage are reminiscent of scurvy. In plants, ascorbate oxidase is a cuproenzyme. Although no mammalian ascorbate oxidase is known, one of the other cuproproteins with oxidase activity, such as ceruloplasmin, may act on ascorbic acid; such a role could explain the scorbutic lesion of copper deficiency.[184] The bone lesion of copper depletion is only seen in *growing* bone.

The biochemical bases of the anemia and neutropenia are not resolved. Copper appears to play several roles in iron metabolism,[181] but none is clearly limiting of iron availability to the erythron. The neutropenia of copper deficiency is only relative. With infection, a normal leukocytosis response can be seen.[185] Because the superoxide dismutase of white cells is a cuproenzyme, and superoxide radical generation is an important component of the bactericidal mechanism of the white cell,[186] one could speculate on an "auto-oxidation" lesion in white cells with an imbalance between superoxide generation and its normal dismutation to hydrogen peroxide.

**Biochemical and Laboratory Abnormalities.** The biochemical and laboratory abnormalities of mammalian copper deficiency are listed in Table 9–15. Since the publication of the last edition of this book, several new abnormalities have been catalogued, primarily from research in experimental animals, but also in the human context (see Table 9–15 b,c,h). A number of noncuproenzymes have their activity reduced by dietary copper restriction. This phenomenon has been found for lecithin:cholesterol acyltransferase activity (Table 9–15 f), which may explain a failure of cholesterol clearance in copper deficiency, and may add new insights into the long observed effect of copper depletion on hypercholesterolemia. This finding, in turn, combines with several specific new cardiac lesions of copper deficiency—altered muscle metabolism (Table 9–15 k) and electrocardiographic abnormalities (Table 9–15 l)—providing experimental bases for the zinc/copper hypothesis of the origin of ischemic heart disease. Another enzymatic abnormality produced by experimental copper deficiency in rats was reduced activity of the *seleno*enzyme, glutathione peroxidase (Table 9–15 e). This reduction in concert with the decline in the cuproenzyme, Zn-Cu superoxide dismutase, might produce a double impairment of cellular antioxidant protection.

Abnormalities of carbohydrate metabolism are produced by copper deficiency. The most important is impaired glucose tolerance. Others have noted interactions of copper deficiency with the metabolism of diverse carbohydrates (Table 9–15 h). Finally, with copper, as with zinc, a wide range of immune defects of lymphocytic function has been described (Table 9–15 i,f). Their implica-

**Table 9–15. Biochemical and Laboratory Abnormalities in Copper Deficiency**

Decreased circulating copper
Decreased ceruloplasmin concentration
Decreased red cell counts
Decreased neutrophils
Decreased red cell life span in vivo[a]
Decreased liver copper
Elevated liver iron
Decreased red cell superoxide dismutase activity[b]
Decreased lysyl oxidase activity in tissue culture[c]
Decreased 2′, 3′ cyclic nucleotide 3′ phosphodiesterase activity in brain[d]
Decreased glutathione peroxidase activity in liver[e]
Decreased lecithin:cholesterol acyltransferase activity[f]
Elevated serum cholesterol
Decreased brain catecholamines[g]
Elevated brain dopamine-beta-hydroxylase activity[g]
Decreased glucose tolerance[h]
Decreased serum thymic factor activity[i]
Decreased plaque-forming splenocytes in vitro[j]
Decreased T-cell blastogenesis in vitro[i]
Elevated cardiac oxygen consumption[k]
Altered electrocardiogram[l]

[a]Russanov, E.M., et al.: Int. J. Biochem. *14*:321, 1982.
[b]Castillo-Duran, C., et al.: Am. J. Clin. Nutr. *37*:898, 1983.
[c]Kivirikko, K.I., Peltonen, L.: Med. Biol. *60*:45,1982.
[d]Prohaska, J.R., Wells, W.W.: J. Neurochem. *25*:221, 1975.
[e]Jenkinson, S.G., et al.: J. Nutr. *112*:197, 1982.
[f]Harvey, P.W., Allen, K.G.: J. Nutr. *111*:1855, 1981.
[g]Prohaska, J.R., Smith, T.L.: J. Nutr. *112*:1706, 1982.
[h]Klevay, L.M., et al.: Am. J. Clin. Nutr. *37*:717, 1983; Fields, M., et al.: Proc. Soc. Exp. Biol. Med. *173*:137, 1983 and J. Nutr. *113*:1335, 1983.
[i]Lukasewycz, O.A., Prohaska, J.R.: Nutr. Res. *3*:335, 1983.
[j]Vyas, D., Chandra, R.K.: Nutr. Res. *3*:343, 1983.
[k]Prohaska, J.R., Heller, L.J.: J. Nutr. *112*:2142, 1982.
[l]Klevay, L.M., Vienstenz, K.E.: Am. J. Physiol. *240*:H185, 1981.

tions for host resistance to infection have yet to be defined.

## Copper Toxicity

**Acute Toxicity.** Oral copper is an emetic, with dosages of copper sulfate in excess of 250 mg (64 mg of copper) producing vomiting.[187] As little as 10 mg of oral copper, however, can produce nausea, with the lethal dose of copper compounds in humans thought to be 3.5 to 35 g.[187] Poisoning with gram amounts of copper causes jaundice due to both hepatic necrosis and intravascular hemolysis. Gastric hemorrhage is also seen. Cases of attempted suicide in which the circulating level of copper exceeded 265 µg/dl were universally fatal in one series.[188]

Fatal hemolytic anemia has also occurred as a result of systemic absorption of copper nitrate salves applied to burn patients. Even the acute release of copper from the liver into the blood of

Wilson's disease patients, due to sudden massive hepatic necrosis, can lead to fatal intravascular hemolysis.[189]

**Chronic Toxicity.** As reviewed by Klevay,[190] the tolerance for high levels of dietary copper in monogastric animals is considerable, ranging from 200 to 800 mg/kg of ration. Underwood estimated that healthy humans could tolerate a dietary intake of copper of 200 mg/kg ration (about 200 mg daily) for a prolonged period.[191] Daily consumption of 10 to 35 mg of copper would probably be safe indefinitely.[190]

A theoretical danger of chronic copper toxicity arises with long-term home parenteral nutrition. Amounts of intravenous copper in excess of 0.5 mg/day have been retained.[192] This amount could be deposited in liver tissue over long periods and lead to hepatic overload and scarring.

## Conditions Predisposing to Copper Depletion

The clinical situations that predispose to copper depletion can be classified by presumptive cause (Table 9–16).

### *Primary and Dietary-Induced Deficiency*

Copper deficiency was not recognized in humans until 1964.[193] The setting was in children

**Table 9–16. Clinical Situations Predisposing to Copper Deficiency**

*Decreased Intake*
  Low-copper infant formulas
  Total parenteral nutrition without added copper
*Decreased Absorption*
  Megadose and high therapeutic zinc intakes
  High dietary intakes of ascorbic acid
  Chronic oral alkali therapy
  Chronic infantile diarrhea
  Short-bowel syndrome
  Celiac disease
  Jejunoileal bypass
  Menkes' kinky-hair syndrome
*Decreased Utilization*
  Menkes' kinky-hair syndrome
  Phenylketonuria (?)
  Protein-energy malnutrition
*Increased Loss*
  Tropical sprue
  Celiac disease
  Crohn's disease
  Nephrotic syndrome
  Parenteral chelation therapy
  Burns and scalds
  Primary hyperparathyroidism
  High amino acid total parenteral nutrition
*Increased Requirement*
  Prematurity
  Pregnancy
  Lactation

with PEM and antecedent diarrhea fed milk-based diets reconstituted with water flowing through new, noncopper pipes at a nutritional research center in Lima, Peru. Subsequently, copper deficiency has been seen repeatedly in PEM.[194] In addition to dietary factors, malabsorption and malutilization may contribute to the copper deficiency manifestation in children with PEM.

The advent of total parenteral nutrition, an alimentary situation with no oral intake and total dependency on the nutrients in intravenous solutions, led to copper deficiency among TPN patients, especially in the early years of widespread use of this technique.[195–198] This *primary* copper deficiency resulted from the failure to supply sufficient parenteral copper. The continued significant use of blood products, e.g., packed cells or fresh frozen plasma, with the TPN solution can prevent copper deficiency.[199] This is an expensive and potentially dangerous procedure, however, particularly when copper solutions are available and inexpensive.

Human copper deficiency related to diet has been seen in infants fed primarily milk-based or other low-copper formulas. Premature infants are especially sensitive to insufficient copper intakes and manifest frank symptoms.[182,200,201] Cordano estimated the oral requirements for premature infants to be 100 μg/kg body weight.[202] Copper deficiency has also developed in full-term infants fed milk-based diets.[203]

Two oral medications are notable for their contribution to impaired copper absorption, which can lead to copper depletion. One such medication is antacid that alkalinizes the gastrointestinal lumen, presumably reducing copper bioavailability. The second and more important medication, mentioned previously, is high-dose oral zinc. The mechanism is intestinal blockade with zinc-induced metallothionein.[153] Indeed, copper-deficiency anemia is a principal manifestation of chronic oral zinc toxicity.[82,83]

It has long been known that ascorbic acid interferes with copper absorption in rodents and other monogastric mammals. Milne et al. showed an impairment of copper uptake with high doses of vitamin C in nonhuman primates,[204] and Finley and Cerklewski provided preliminary data that megadose intakes of vitamin C (1.5 mg) decrease copper availability in man.[205] Whether frank copper depletion can result in humans remains to be determined.

### *Inborn Errors of Copper Metabolism*

**Menkes' Disease.** Kinky-hair syndrome is an X-linked disease of male infants with an onset in early infancy described by Menkes and colleagues in 1962.[206] It is characterized by growth retardation, uncontrollable seizures with progressive cerebral degeneration and mental retardation, depigmentation of hair and skin, diffuse arterial aneurysms, bone demineralization, hypotonia, and hypothermia. The characteristic sign is a brittle, kinky hair texture resembling steel wool. The neurologic condition usually evolves to coma, and death by inanition and infection is the common fate. Survival beyond the second year of life is rare.

Because of the similarities of the phenotypic expression of Menkes' disease to copper deficiency in livestock (sheep) in Australia, Danks et al. proposed that the disease involved abnormal copper metabolism.[207] It has subsequently been demonstrated that transintestinal uptake of radiocopper is impaired, although mucosal copper levels of the intestine are elevated. Liver copper levels are extremely low, while kidney copper content is elevated.[208] The failure to absorb copper is not the only abnormality. Within cells, copper cannot gain access to the usual functional cuproproteins. Thus, *malutilization* of copper, in addition to malabsorption, operates in the pathogenesis of Menkes' syndrome. Unlike acquired copper deficiency, hematologic indices are normal. Variant presentations of Menkes' disease have been identified: Milder cases, representing a *form fruste* or incomplete penetrance of the gene, have been described in which patients survive beyond infancy and have relatively normal health.[209]

The abnormal distribution of copper in Menkes' kinky hair syndrome was originally suspected to be due to an abnormal form of metallothionein, but physiologic studies suggested that it was the *amount,* not the type, of thionein that was disordered.[210] Since the syndrome of Menkes is X-linked, the mapping of the thionein genes to an autosomal location strongly indicates that pathologic regulation of synthesis, rather than an abnormal protein itself, is the defect.[211]

An animal model for Menkes' syndrome has been discovered in the brindled variety of the mottled mutant of the house mouse. The mottled locus is on the X chromosome, and the most severely affected animals are brindled males, $Mo^{br/y}$. They have decreased pigmentation of hair, low brain and liver copper levels with elevated intestinal and kidney copper concentrations, reduced lysyl oxidase levels, similar neurologic abnormalities, and brain biochemical defects. Unlike animals with nutritional copper deficiency, the mutant mice do not have anemia. A treatise comparing Menkes' disease and the mottled mouse mutants has been published.[212] Figure 9–4 shows a brin-

dled male mouse and a child who depicts the typical features of Menkes' syndrome.

**Wilson's Disease (Hepatolenticular Degeneration).** Wilson's disease is characterized by excessive copper retention and specific toxic accumulation of copper in the liver and basal ganglia of the brain leading to cirrhosis and ataxia, respectively.[213] The hepatic concentration of copper ranges from 750 to 980 µg/dl (dry weight)[214] or 184 µg/g wet weight.[215] Kidney and cornea (Kayser-Fleischer rings) also accumulate copper. Crippling neurologic disease and lethal cirrhosis result in the untreated patient with Wilson's disease.

The outstanding biochemical abnormality is low ceruloplasmin concentrations.[216] The underlying biochemical abnormality remains a mystery. The excess body burden of copper can be removed by therapy with D-penicillamine that chelates copper, normalizing hepatic copper levels.[217] Penicillamine treatment, however, is not without side effects. The antagonism of zinc and copper has been used in the maintenance of normal copper balance in patients with Wilson's disease.[140] A daily intake of 150 µg of zinc proved adequate to maintain copper balance in the "decoppered" patient, presumably by inducing mucosal thionein and blocking the transfer of dietary and endogenous copper into the body.

**Atypical Ehlers-Danlos Syndrome.** A variant form of a hereditary connective tissue disorder, Ehlers-Danlos syndrome, characterized by generalized integumentary laxity and hyperelasticity, has been identified in which lysyl oxidase activity, a cuproenzyme, is deficient.[218] In this case, a cross-linking defect due to abnormal copper metabolism may be the basis for the connective tissue lesion.

### Secondary Acquired Copper Deficiency

In addition to food and dietary factors, a number of disease states, including short-gut celiac sprue, jejunoileal bypass, and chronic diarrhea, can interfere with efficient absorption of copper, contributing to copper depletion.

Malutilization of copper may account for the manifestations of copper deficiency in situations besides Menkes' syndrome. For instance, it may contribute to copper deficiency in PEM. Abnormalities of copper metabolism have been found in phenylketonuria patients ingesting adequate amounts of dietary copper.[219] Malutilization may play a role.

Secondary copper deficiency can also result from excessive wastage of copper. Protein enteropathy states with gastrointestinal seepage of ceruloplasmin, such as sprue or Crohn's disease, are one route. Excessive renal excretion in nephrotic

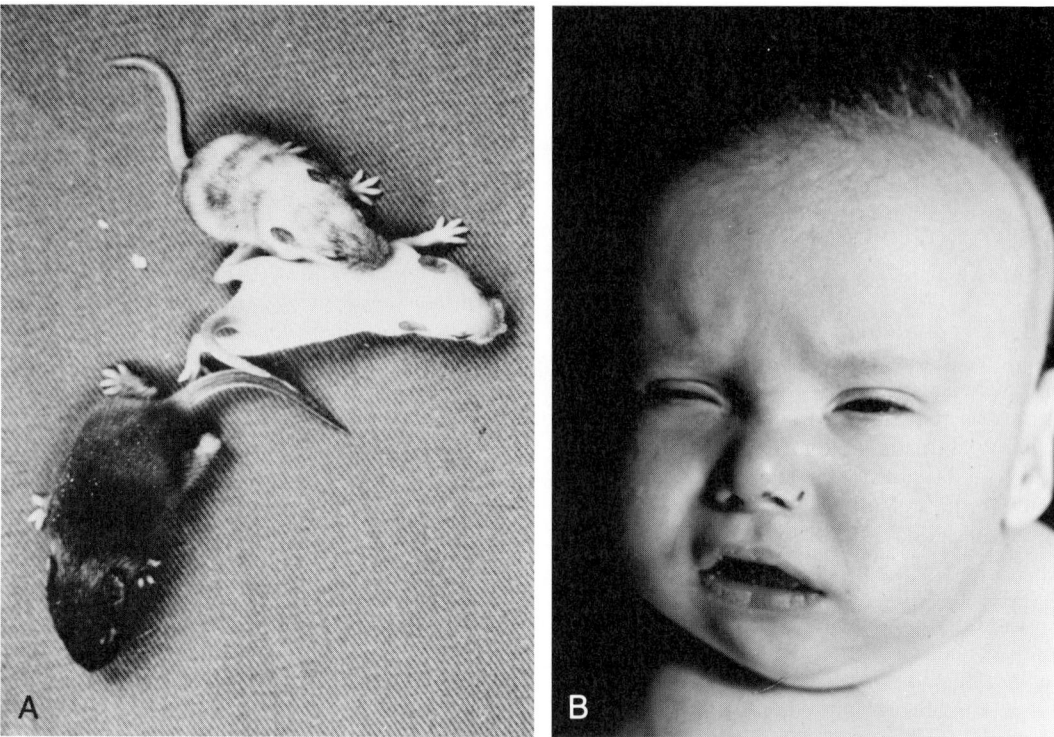

**Fig. 9–4.** *A,* Genetic consequences of disordered metabolism in a rodent model, the house mouse, with the brindled allele at the mottled locus of the X chromosome. At the bottom is a normal male ($Mo^{+/y}$); at the top is a heterozygous female ($Mo^{br/+}$) showing intermediate discoloration of fur; in the center is a homozygous male ($Mo^{br/y}$), showing less vitality, stunted growth, and marked pallor. *B,* A male infant with Menkes' kinky-hair syndrome. Note the depigmented, dystrophic, and sparse hair. The child also has severe nervous retardation. Photographs courtesy of Professor David Danks.

syndromes, with chelation therapy and in various other conditions that increase filterable copper, is another route for excess copper loss. When D-penicillamine is used for the treatment of rheumatoid arthritis, clinical copper depletion is a concomitant risk.[220]

Prematurity, pregnancy, and lactation all increase copper requirements. A significant correlation has been found between neonatal head circumference and maternal serum copper, and between birth weight and maternal hair copper content.[221]

**Copper Status and Cardiovascular Disease.** Lysyl oxidase activity is essential for the cross-linking of collagen and elastin. Tilson has suggested that diminished hepatic copper may be a marker for the pathogenesis of aortic aneurysms in man.[222]

A more elaborate theory relating copper status to ischemic (coronary) heart disease has been promulgated by Klevay in several reviews.[223] It is known as the "zinc/copper hypothesis" and, simply stated, it postulates: "Either a relative or absolute deficiency of copper characterized by a high ratio of zinc to copper results in hypercholesterolemia, myocardial and arterial damage and increased mortality" from ischemic heart disease.[223] This theory derives from the original observation of Klevay that increasing the zinc/copper ratio in rat diets produced hypercholesterolemia. Either an absolute deficiency of copper intake or an aggravation of copper bioavailability by a high zinc uptake should effectively produce a reduced copper delivery. Young men given 160 mg of zinc daily[224] and young women fed 100 mg of zinc per day[225] had a decline in high-density lipoprotein (HDL), possibly due to a zinc:copper interaction at the intestinal level.

### Dietary Considerations

Understanding of the specific human requirements and bioavailibility for dietary copper is incomplete.

#### Comparative Requirements

Shown in Table 9–17 are the requirements for copper in the rations of different vertebrate spe-

**Table 9–17.  Comparative Copper Requirements in Several Mammalian Species**

| Species | Copper Requirements (mg/kg of ration) |
|---------|----------------------------------------|
| Mouse | 4.5 |
| Rat | 5 |
| Rabbit | 3 |
| Cat | 5 |
| Dog | 7.3 |
| Pig | 5 |
| Sheep | 5 |
| Human | 2–3 |

cies. As with zinc, a wide variability exists among species.

### Human Dietary Allowances

There are as yet no RDAs for copper. Recognizing that insufficient bases for a formal allowance for copper were available, the RDA Committee in 1980 established "Safe and Adequate Daily Dietary Intakes" (SADDI) for human consumption of copper[125] (Appendix Table A1). This guideline represents a *range* of intake above which one would risk possible toxic accumulation and below which the copper intake from the diet might be considered inadequate. Since the preparation of the copper SADDIs, metabolic balance data in a large number of healthy adult volunteers from the USDA Grand Forks Human Nutrition Research Laboratory have been published, providing an empirical estimate of a daily intake from a mixed diet of 1.24 to 1.35 mg of copper for adult men as the level that achieves copper equilibrium.[226] The upper limits for safe copper intake provided in the SADDI are at variance with the much larger tolerable doses proposed by Underwood[191] and Klevay.[190]

### Food Sources

Copper is widely distributed in foods, although the concentration varies (Appendix Table A37). Rice and milk, two foods often used alone or in combination for infant feeding, are notoriously low in copper. The richest sources of copper are oysters, other shellfish, and legumes. In an earlier era, the copper in pipe tubing and water tanks would leach into the drinking water supply and increase human copper intakes. Copper alloys were also used in cooking pots and table utensils. Modern materials, such as aluminum and Teflon, have eliminated these contaminant sources of copper from the diet of western industrialized countries.

### Factors Affecting Copper Availability

The factors affecting copper bioavailability in the human diet are generally less well understood than those for zinc. Our present state of understanding is summarized in Table 9–18. Of the factors listed, ascorbic acid is notable for the observations on high vitamin C intakes in primates.[204] High zinc intakes induce intestinal metallothionein, which traps dietary copper within the intestinal cell as well. Important antagonistic interactions of zinc and copper have been demonstrated in human nutrition.[81–83] In ruminant animals, molybdenum can reduce copper utilization and produce copper deficiency.[227] The operation of this interaction in *monogastric* species such as primates has not been shown.

Several dietary constituents can enhance copper uptake. One such beverage appears to be breast milk,[228] although the specific factors in human milk that promote copper absorption have yet to be defined. It is known that, like zinc, ionic copper is bound by low-molecular-weight ligands in milk. Their role in copper bioavailability is unknown. Free amino acids, notably histidine, can complex with copper and promote its uptake. Whether this process makes an important positive contribution to the intestinal uptake of dietary copper has not been determined.

### Assessment of Copper Nutriture

The clinical assessment of human copper nutriture, like that of zinc, remains problematical. An unequivocal, indirect laboratory index that reflects the total-body or nutritionally available copper reserves has yet to be identified. The options for nutritional assessment include measuring copper or a surrogate (e.g., copper protein) in fluids and tissue, or measuring a physiologic function dependent on adequate copper nutriture.

**Table 9–18.  Factors Affecting Copper Bioavailability**

INHIBITORY FACTORS
*Specific Foods/Beverages*
  Uncooked meat
*Chemical Constituents of the Diet*
  Cellulose
  Ascorbic acid
  Zinc
  Iron
  ? Molybdenum
  Phosphorus

ENHANCING FACTORS
*Specific Foods/Beverages*
  Breast milk
*Chemical Constituents of the Diet*
  Histidine
  ? Other amino acids

## Static Indices

The advent of atomic absorption spectrophotometry (AAS) has opened the way for accurate determination of copper in body fluids and tissues. The other more sophisticated techniques mentioned for zinc can also be applied to the analysis of copper. Copper has been measured in serum, red cells, nails, hair, and urine in efforts to assess human nutriture. As with zinc, circulating (plasma or serum) levels of copper are the most commonly used index of nutritional status and, as with zinc, a number of pitfalls and limitations in the application and interpretation of this index are inherent (Table 9–19). Although animal studies demonstrate a good correspondence between hair copper and hepatic copper in rats,[229] practical experience with human hair shows that the adsorption of environmental copper from air, soaps, shampoos, and rinses contributes to an increasing hair copper content with increasing distance from the scalp.[230] Furthermore, the rate of growth of hair affects copper content. The technical capacity for measuring copper in white cells has been demonstrated.[231] Measurement of several cuproenzymes in serum or in circulating cells has been reported, including cytochrome *c* oxidase in white cells,[232] superoxide dismutase in red cells,[233] and serum amine oxidase,[232] but such analyses are not yet routinely available in the average clinical laboratory.

### Table 9–19. Pitfalls and Limitations of Use of Circulating Levels of Copper to Assess Nutritional Status

| Condition | Direction of Change Relative to "True" Zinc Level |
|---|---|
| External contamination | increased |
| Hemolysis | minimal change |
| Estrogens, oral contraceptives | increased |
| Cigarette smoking | increased |
| Infection/inflammation | increased |
| Corticosteroids, acute | increased |
| Corticosteroids, chronic | decreased |
| Impaired synthesis or release of ceruloplasmin | decreased |

### Table 9–20. Functional Indices of Copper Nutriture

Bone mineralization
Arterial angiography
Skin elastin morphology
Tissue culture or cell culture; lysyl oxidase production
Glucose tolerance
Cellular immunity
Copper retention
Isotopic turnover of radiocopper ($^{67}$Cu; $^{64}$Cu)

## Functional Indices

Table 9–20 provides a list of functional indices of copper nutriture. The first three indices listed actually represent the pathologic consequences of copper deficiency on tissue integrity, but have been included here as functional tests. Bone demineralization and arterial wall defects are likely only to present in young children with chronically severe copper depletion. Impaired glucose tolerance, reduced cellular immunity, and lysyl oxidase activity in cell culture in vitro, however, are all tests with minimal exploration for the evaluation of marginal copper deficiency.

An individual with *primary* copper deficiency (e.g., a patient on TPN with inadequate copper) should have a greater avidity to retain the nutrient where administered and would be in more positive copper balance than a well-nourished individual. However, in *secondary* copper depletion, copper balance is negative as a result of the disease process itself, and copper retention becomes less useful as an index of nutriture. Theoretically, *pool-size* data from formal isotopic turnover studies should allow a precise estimate of total-body copper status in most clinical situations. Radiation exposure, cost, and short radioactive half-life, however, all impose serious limitations on the use of isotopic studies to assess human copper status.

### Diagnostic Decision-Making

To assess human copper status, one must compile indications from one or more static indices (e.g., serum or plasma copper concentration and/ or 24-hour copper excretion) with as many appropriate functional indices as are practical and accessible. Attention to the clinical setting is critical. A low serum copper is not as great a *nutritional* concern in a patient with Wilson's disease as in one receiving TPN. An individual might be copper-deficient and still have *normal* hair copper levels with exogenous contamination of hair contributing to the false-negative result. If a clear deficiency of a tissue cuproenzyme or definite impairment of a functional test can be documented, and unique supplementation with copper restores activity or function in a disease state or condition predisposing to copper depletion, then a definitive, albeit *retrospective,* diagnosis of human copper deficiency can be made with assurance.

### Therapeutic Use

When a presumptive diagnosis of copper deficiency has been made, copper supplementation is indicated. The most commonly used salt for oral copper supplementation is cupric sulfate. It is important to recognize that oral copper is a potent emetic, with as little as 5 to 10 mg producing nausea. The conventional dose of oral copper for therapeutic use to treat copper deficiency is 2 mg, which can be taken three to four times daily. To date, no "copper-responsive" conditions, other than primary or secondary copper deficiency, have been reported.

Copper can be delivered by a parenteral route as well as by mouth. Patients on TPN are susceptible to copper deficiency, and require routine maintenance supplementation of their alimentation regimen with this mineral. The AMA panel has recommended intravenous copper administration in TPN[142] (see Chapter 54). Balance studies by Shike et al. in TPN patients, however, have shown that copper balance was achieved in stable adults in an intake of about 0.25 mg per day.[234] Copper delivered in excess of this level was retained by the patients, presumably accumulating in the liver. Obviously, individuals with cholestasis or biliary compromise on TPN should receive much lower maintenance doses. Alternatively, TPN patients with gastric fistula or gastric suction may require slightly more copper to maintain nutritional balance.

A variety of parenteral routes, including subcutaneous, intramuscular, and intravenous, have been used for the administration of copper to patients with Menkes' syndrome. In general, the therapeutic results of parenteral or oral supplementation of patients with Menkes' disease have been disappointing with all routes of administration.

# REFERENCES

1. Todd, W.R., Elvehjem, C.A., Hart, E.B.: Am. J. Physiol. *107*:146–156, 1934.
2. Tucker, H.F., Salmon, W.D.: Proc. Soc. Exp. Biol. Med. *88*:613–616, 1955.
3. Eggleton, W.G.E.: Biochem. J. *34*:991–997, 1940.
4. Vallee, B.L., Wacker, W.E.C., Bartholomay, A.F., et al.: N. Engl. J. Med. *255*:403–408, 1956.
5. Prasad, A.S., Halsted, J.A., Nadimi, M.: Amer. J. Med. *31*:532–546, 1961.
6. Perry, H.M., Jr., Tipton, I.H., Schroeder, H.A., et al.: J. Lab. Clin. Med. *60*:245–253, 1962.
7. Tipton, I.H., Schroeder, H.A., Perry, H.M., Jr.: Health Phys. *11*:403–451, 1965.
8. Trace Elements in Human Nutrition. Tech Rept Series #532. Geneva, World Health Organization, 1973.
9. Methfessel, A.H., Spencer, H.: J. Appl. Physiol. *34*:58–62, 1973.
10. Davies, N.T.: Br. J. Nutr. *43*:189–203, 1980.
11. Emes, J.H., Arthur, D.: Proc. Soc. Exp. Biol. Med. *148*:86–88, 1975.
12. Antonson, D.L., Barak, A.J., Vanderhoof, J.A.: J. Nutr. *109*:142–147, 1974.
13. Matseche, J.W., Phillips, S.F., Malagelada, J-R, et al.: Am. J. Clin. Nutr. *33*:1946–1953, 1980.
14. Suso, F.A., Edwards, H.M.: Nature *236*:230–232, 1972.
15. Ostereich, P., Cousins, R.J.: J. Nutr. *112*:1978–1982, 1982.
16. Lönnerdal, D., Schneeman, B.O., Keen, C.L., et al.: Biol. Trace Elem. Res. *2*:149–161, 1980.
17. Evans, G.W.: Nutr. Rev. *38*:137–141, 1980.
18. Solomons, N.W., Jacob, R.A., Pineda, O., et al.: Am. J. Clin. Nutr. *32*:2495–2499, 1979.
19. Erdmann, J.W., Forbes, R.M., Kondo, H.: Zinc bioavailability from processed soybean products. *In* Nutritional Bioavailability of Zinc. (Inglett, G.E., Ed.) Washington, D.C., American Chemical Society Press, 1983.
20. Solomons, N.W., Jacob, R.A.: Am. J. Clin. Nutr. *34*:475–482, 1981.
21. Solomons, N.W., Pineda, O., Viteri, F., et al.: J. Nutr. *113*:337–349, 1983.
22. Cunnane, S.C.: Pediatr. Res. *16*:559–603, 1982.
23. Smith, K.T., Cousins, R.J.: J. Nutr. *108*:1849–1857, 1978.
24. Davies, N.T.: Br. J. Nutr. *43*:189–302, 1980.
25. Steel, L., Cousins, R.J.: Fed. Proc. *43*:2592, 1984.
26. Menard, M.P., Cousins, R.J.: J. Nutr. *113*:1434–1442, 1983.
27. Menard, M.P., Oestereicher, P., Cousins, R.J.: Zinc transport by isolated vascular perfused rat intestine and brush border vesicles. *In* Nutritional Bioavailability of Zinc. (Inglett, G.E., Ed.) Washington, D.C., American Chemical Society Press, 1983.
28. Cousins, R.J.: Nutr. Rev. *37*:97–103, 1979.
29. Kowarski, S., Blair-Stanek, C.S., Schachter, D.: Am. J. Physiol. *226*:401–407, 1974.
30. Chester, J.K., Will, M.: Br. J. Nutr. *46*:111–118, 1981.
31. Smith, K.T., Cousins, R.J.: J. Nutr. *110*:316–323, 1980.
32. Evans, G.W., Grace, C.I., Hahn, C.: Proc. Soc. Exp. Biol. Med. *143*:723–725, 1973.
33. Solomons, N.W., Guerrero, A-M., Torun, B., et al.: Fed. Proc. *42*:823, 1983.
34. Richards, M.P., Cousins, R.J.: Proc. Soc. Exp. Biol. Med. *153*:52–56, 1976.
35. Flanagan, P.R., Haist, J., Valberg, L.S.: J. Nutr. *113*:962–972, 1983.
36. Freeland-Graves, J.H., Ebangit, M.L., Hendriksen, P.J.: Am. J. Clin. Nutr. *33*:1757–1766, 1980.
37. Bonewitz, R.F., Jr., Foulkes, E.C., O'Flaherty, E.J., et al.: Am. J. Physiol. *244*:G314–G320, 1983.
38. Baer, M.T., King, J.C.: Am. J. Clin. Nutr. *39*:566–571, 1984.
39. Aamodt, R.L., Rumble, W.F., Babcock, A.K., et al.: Metabolism *31*:326–334, 1982.
40. Babcock, A.K., Henkin, R.I., Aamodt, R.L., et al.: Metabolism *31*:335–347, 1982.
41. Parisi, A.F., Vallee, B.L.: Biochemistry *9*:2421–2426, 1970.
42. Beisel, W.R., Pekarek, R.S., Wannemacher, R.W., Jr.: Homeostatic mechanisms affecting plasma zinc levels in acute stress. *In* Trace Elements in Human Health and Disease, Vol. I. Zinc and Copper. New York, Academic Press, 1976.
43. Pekarek, R.S., Wannemacher, R.W., Jr., Chapple, F.E., III, et al.: Proc. Soc. Exp. Biol. Med. *141*:643–648, 1972.
44. Sobocinski, P.Z., Canterbury, W.J., Jr., Mapes, C.A., et al.: Am. J. Physiol. *234*:E399–E406, 1978.
45. Falchuk, K.H.: N. Engl. J. Med. *296*:1129–1134, 1977.
46. Sugarman, B., Epps, L.R., Stenbeck, W.A.: Infect. Immun. *37*:1191–1199, 1982.

47. Vallee, B.L., Falchuk, K.H.: Phil. Trans. R. Soc. (Lond.) *B294*:185–197, 1981.
48. Chesters, J.K.: Metabolism and biochemistry of zinc. *In* Clinical, Biochemical, and Nutrition Aspects of Trace Elements. (Prasad, A.S., Ed.) New York, Alan R. Liss, 1982.
49. Prasad, A.S., Fernandez-Madrid, F., Ryan, J.F.: Am. J. Physiol. *236*:E272–E275, 1979.
50. Fosmire, G.J., Fosmire, M.A., Sandstead, H.H.: J. Nutr. *106*:1152–1158, 1976.
51. Bettger, W.J., O'Dell, B.L.: Life Sci. *28*:1425–1438, 1981.
52. Hesketh, J.F.: Int. J. Biochem. *14*:983–990, 1982.
53. Eagle, G.R., Zomnola, R.R., Hines, R.H.: Biochemistry *22*:221–228, 1983.
54. Cunningham-Rundles, C., Cunningham-Rundles, S., Iwata, T.: Clin. Immunol. Immunopathol. *21*:387–396, 1981.
55. Cowen, L.A., Cousins, R.J.: Fed. Proc. *41*:285, 1982.
56. Prasad, A.S., Oberleas, D.: J. Lab. Clin. Med. *82*:461–466, 1973.
57. Prasad, A.S., Rabbani, P.: Trans. Assoc. Am. Physicians *94*:314–321, 1981.
58. Pilz, R.B., Willis, R.C., Seegmiller, J.E.: J. Biol. Chem. *257*:13544–13549, 1982.
59. Anonymous: Nutr. Rev. *42*:279–281, 1984.
60. Solomons, N.W., Russell, R.M.: Am. J. Clin. Nutr. *33*:2031–2040, 1980.
61. Russell, R.M., Cox, M.E., Solomons, N.W.: Ann. Intern. Med. *99*:227–239, 1983.
62. Morrison, S.A., Russell, R.M., Carney, E.A., et al.: Am. J. Clin. Nutr. *31*:276–281, 1978.
63. Leure-du Pree, A.E., McClain, C.J.: Invest. Ophthalmol. Vis. Sci. *23*:425–434, 1982.
64. Keusch, G.T., Wilson, C.S., Waksal, S.D.: Nutrition, host defenses, and the lymphoid system. *In* Advances in Host Defense Mechanisms, Vol. 2. (Gallin, J.I., Fauci, A.S., Eds.) New York, Raven Press, 1983.
65. Fraker, P.: Surv. Immunol. Res. *2*:155–163, 1983.
66. Prasad, A.S., Miale, A., Farid, Z., et al.: J. Lab. Clin. Med. *61*:537–549, 1963.
67. Ronaghy, H.A., Halsted, J.A.: Am. J. Clin. Nutr. *28*:831–836, 1975.
68. Weston, W.L., Huff, J.C., Humbert, J.R., et al.: Arch. Dermatol. *113*:422–425, 1977.
69. Briggs, W.A., Pedersen, M.M., Mahajan, S.K.: Kidney Int. *21*:827–832, 1982.
70. Allen, J.I., Korchik, W., Kay, N.E.: Am. J. Clin. Nutr. *36*:410–415, 1982.
71. Keeling, P.W., O'Day, J., Ruse, W., et al.: Clin. Sci. *62*:109–111, 1982.
72. Warth, J.A., Prasad, A.S., Zwas, F., et al.: J. Lab. Clin. Med. *98*:189–194, 1981.
73. McClain, C.J., Le-Chu, S., Gilbert, H., et al.: Dig. Dis. Sci. *28*:85–87, 1983.
74. Wright, A.L., King, J.C., Baer, M.T., et al.: Am. J. Clin. Nutr. *34*:848–852, 1981.
75. Faraji, B., Swenseid, M.E.: J. Nutr. *113*:447–455, 1983.
76. Flanagan, P.R.: J. Nutr. *114*:493–502, 1984.
77. Anonymous: M.M.W.R. *32*:257–258, 1983.
78. Tasic, V., Gordova, A., Delidzhakova, M., et al.: Pediatrics *70*:660–661, 1982.
79. Bos, L.P., van Vloten, W.A., Smit, A.F., et al.: Neth. J. Med. *20*:263–266, 1977.
80. Brocks, A., Ried, H., Glazer, G.: Br. Med. J. *1*:1390–1391, 1977.
81. Pfeiffer, C.C., Jenny, E.H.: Fed. Proc. *37*:324, 1978.
82. Porter, K.G., McMaster, D., Elmes, M.E.: Lancet *2*:774, 1977.
83. Prasad, A.S., Brewer, G.J., Schoomaker, E.B., et al.: JAMA *240*:2166–2168, 1978.
84. Moore, R.: Br. Med. J. *1*:754–755, 1978.
85. Faintuch, J., Faintuch, J.J., Toledo, M., et al.: J. Parenter. Enter. Nutr. *2*:640–645, 1978.
86. Wolman, S.L., Anderson, G.H., Marliss, E.B., et al.: Gastroenterology *76*:458–467, 1978.
87. Casper, R.C., Kirschner, B., Sandstead, H.H., et al.: Am. J. Clin. Nutr. *33*:1801–1808, 1980.
88. Askari, A., Long, C.L., Blakemore, W.S.: J. Parenter. Enter. Nutr. *4*:561–571, 1980.
89. Golden, B.E., Golden, M.H.N.: Am. J. Clin. Nutr. *32*:2490–2494, 1979.
90. Hess, F.M., King, J.C., Margen, S.: J. Nutr. *107*:2219–2227, 1977.
91. Prasad, A.S., Rabbani, P., Abbasi, A., et al.: Ann. Intern. Med. *89*:483–490, 1978.
92. Shrimpton, R.: Studies on zinc nutrition in the Amazon Valley. Thesis, University of London, 1980.
93. Lorenz, K., Loewe, R.: Agric. Food Chem. *25*:806–809, 1977.
93a. Davis, K.R., Peters, L.J., Cain, R.F., et al.: Cereal Foods World *29*:246–248, 1984.
94. Reinhold, J.G., Faradji, B., Abadi, P., et al.: Binding of zinc to fiber and other solids of wholemeal bread. *In* Trace Elements in Human Health and Disease, Vol. 1. Zinc and Copper (Prasad, A.S., Ed.) New York, Academic Press, 1976.
95. Abdulla, M., Aly, K-O., Andersson, I., et al.: Am. J. Clin. Nutr. *34*:2464–2477, 1981.
95a. Hogarth, F.W.: J. Hum. Nutr. *35*:379–382, 1981.
96. Lönnerdal, B., Keen, C.L., Ohtake, M., et al.: Am. J. Dis. Child. *137*:433–437, 1983.
97. Walravens, P.A., Hambidge, K.M.: Am. J. Clin. Nutr. *29*:1114–1121, 1976.
98. Breskin, M.W., Worthington-Roberts, B.S., Knopp, R.H., et al.: Am. J. Clin. Nutr. *38*:943–953, 1983.
99. Hambidge, K.M., Krebs, N.F., Jacobs, M.A., et al.: Am. J. Clin. Nutr. *37*:429–442, 1983.
100. Gibson, R.S., Anderson, B.M., Scythes, C.A.: Am. J. Clin. Nutr. *37*:37–42, 1983.
101. Hambidge, K.M.: Int. J. Dermatol. *15*:38–39, 1976.
102. Barnes, P.M., Moynahan, E.J.: Proc. R. Soc. Med. *66*:327–329, 1973.
103. Krieger, I.: Nutr. Rev. *38*:148–149, 1980.
104. Jackson, M.J.: J. Clin. Pathol. *30*:284–287, 1977.
105. Brummerstedt, E., Basse, A., Flagstad, T., et al.: Am. J. Pathol. *87*:725–728, 1977.
106. Smith, J.C., Jr., Zeller, J.A., Brown, E.D., et al.: Science *193*:496–498, 1976.
107. Failla, M.L., van de Veerdonk, M., Morgan, W.T., et al.: J. Lab. Clin. Med. *100*:943–952, 1982.
108. Prasad, A.S., Cossack, Z.T.: Trans. Assoc. Am. Physicians *95*:165–176, 1982.
109. Ballester, O.F., Prasad, A.S.: Ann. Intern. Med. *98*:180–182, 1983.
110. Prasad, A.S., Cossack, Z.T.: Am. J. Clin. Nutr. *37*:720, 1983.
111. Mahajan, S.K., Prasad, A.S., Rabbani, P., et al.: Am. J. Clin. Nutr. *36*:1177–1183, 1982.
112. Golden, M.H.N., Golden, B.E.: Am. J. Clin. Nutr. *34*:900–908, 1981.
113. Antoniou, L.D., Shalhoub, R.J., Elliot, S.: Clin. Nephrol. *16*:181–187, 1981.
114. Naveh, Y., Lightman, A., Zinder, O.: J. Pediatr. *101*:730–732, 1982.

115. McMillan, E.M., Rowe, D.: Br. J. Dermatol. *108*:301–305, 1983.
116. Moser, P.B., Reynolds, R.D.: Am. J. Clin. Nutr. *38*:101–108, 1983.
117. Hunt, I.F., Murphy, N.J., Cleaver, A.E., et al.: Am. J. Clin. Nutr. *37*:572–582, 1983.
118. Meadows, N.J., Smith, M.F., Keeling, P.W.N., et al.: Lancet *2*:1135–1137, 1982.
119. Patrick, J., Dervish, C., Gillieson, M.: Lancet *1*:169–170, 1982.
120. McMichael, A.J., Dreosti, I.E., Gibson, G.T.: Early Hum. Dev. *7*:59–69, 1982.
121. Jameson, S.: Zinc status and pregnancy outcome in humans. *In* Clinical Application of Recent Advances in Zinc Metabolism. (Prasad, A.S., Dreosti, I.E., Hetzel, B.S., Eds.) New York, Alan R. Liss, 1982.
122. Hurley, L.S., Shrader, R.E.: Proc. Soc. Exp. Biol. Med. *123*:692–696, 1966.
123. Soltan, M.H., Jenkins, D.M.: Br. J. Obstet. Gynaecol. *89*:56–58, 1982.
124. Anonymous: Nutr. Rev. *40*:43–45, 1982.
125. Recommended Dietary Allowances. 9th Ed. Washington, D.C., National Research Council, 1980.
126. Recommended Nutrient Intakes for Canadians. Ottawa, Canadian Government Publishing Centre, 1983.
126a. Solomons, N.W., Shrimpton, R.: Zinc. *In* Tropical and Geographic Medicine. (Mahmoud, A.F., Warren, K.W., Eds.) New York, McGraw-Hill Book Co., 1984.
127. Gillies, M.E., Paulin, H.V.: Hum. Nutr. Appl. Nutr. *36*:287–292, 1982.
128. Feeley, R.M., Eitenmiller, R.R., Jones, J.B., Jr., et al.: Am. J. Clin. Nutr. *37*:443–448, 1983.
129. Ronaghy, H., Spivey-Fox, M.R., Garn, S.M., et al.: Am. J. Clin. Nutr. *22*:1279–1289, 1969.
130. Solomons, N.W.: Biological availability of zinc in humans. Am. J. Clin. Nutr. *35*:1048–1075, 1982.
131. Hambidge, K.M., Walravens, P.A., Casey, C.E., et al.: J. Pediatr. *94*:607–608, 1979.
132. Sandstead, H.H.: J. Am. Coll. Nutr. *4*:73–82, 1985.
133. Shah, B.G., Belonje, B.: Nutr. Res. *4*:71–77, 1984.
134. Frolich, W., Sandström, B.: Zinc absorption from composite meals. *In* Nutritional Bioavailability of Zinc. (Inglett, G.E., Ed.) Washington, D.C., American Chemical Society Press, 1983.
135. Solomons, N.W., Allen, L.H.: Nutr. Rev. *41*:33–50, 1983.
136. Brewer, G.B., Ellis, F., Bjork, L.: Pharmacology *23*:254–263, 1981.
137. Sandstead, H.H.: JAMA *240*:2188–2189, 1979.
138. Duchateau, J., Delespesse, G., Vereecke, P.: Am. J. Clin. Nutr. *34*:88–93, 1981.
139. Wagner, P.A., Jernigan, J.A., Bailey, L.B., et al.: Int. J. Vitam. Nutr. Res. *53*:94–101, 1983.
140. Brewer, G.B., Hill, G., Prasad, A.S., et al.: Ann. Intern. Med. *99*:314–319, 1983.
141. Olsson, R.: Acta Med. Scand. *212*:191–192, 1982.
142. American Medical Association: JAMA *241*:2051–2054, 1979.
143. Hart, E.B., Steenbock, H., Waddell, J., et al.: J. Biol. Chem. *77*:797–812, 1928.
144. Cordano, A., Baertl, J.M., Graham, G.G.: Pediatrics *38*:596–604, 1966.
145. Mason, K.E.: J. Nutr. *109*:1979–2066, 1979.
146. O'Dell, B.L.: Copper. *In* Present Knowledge of Nutrition. 5th ed. Washington, D.C., Nutrition Foundation, 1984.
147. Bloomer, L.C., Lee, G.R.: Normal hepatic copper metabolism. *In* Metals and the Liver. (Powell, L.W., Ed.) New York, Marcel Dekker, Inc., 1978.
148. Shaw, J.C.L.: Am. J. Dis. Child, *134*:74–81, 1980.
149. Van Berge Henegouwen, G.P., Tangedahl, T.N., Hofmann, A.F.: Gastroenterology *72*:1228–1231, 1977.
150. Sandstead, H.H.: Am. J. Clin. Nutr. *35*:809–814, 1982.
151. Braganza, J.M., Klass, H.J., Bell, M., et al.: Clin. Sci. *60*:303–310, 1981.
152. Evans, G.W., Grace, C.I., Hahn, C.: Bioinorg. Chem. *3*:115–120, 1974.
153. Fischer, P.W.F., Giroux, A., L'Abbe, M.R.: J. Nutr. *113*:462–469, 1983.
154. El-Shobaki, F.A., Rummel, W.: Res. Exp. Med. (Berlin) 197:187–195, 1979.
155. Peters, T., Jr., Hawn, C.: J. Biol. Chem. *242*:1566–1573, 1967.
156. Strickland, G.T., Beckner, W.M., Leu, M-L, et al.: Clin. Sci. *43*:605–615, 1972.
157. Owen, C.A., Jr.: Am. J. Physiol. *207*:1203–1206, 1964.
158. Terao, T., Owen, C.A.: Am. J. Physiol. *224*:682–686, 1973.
159. McCullars, G.M., O'Reilly, S.O., Brennan, M.: Clin. Chim. Acta *74*:33–38, 1977.
160. Gollan, J.L.: Clin. Sci. Mol. Med. *49*:237–245, 1975.
161. Dekaban, A.S., O'Reilly, S., Aamodt, R., et al.: Trans. Am. Neurol. Assoc. *99*:106–109, 1974.
162. Marceau, N., Aspin, N.: Biochim. Biophys. Acta *328*:351–358, 1973.
163. Ryden, L., Deutsch, H.F.: Biochemistry *15*:3411–3417, 1976.
164. Matsuda, I., Pearson, T., Holtzman, N.A.: Pediatr. Res. *8*:821–825, 1974.
165. Linder, M.C., Hixon, T., Gonzalez, R.: Fed. Proc. *42*:670, 1983.
166. Scheinberg, I.H., Cook, C.D., Murphy, J.A.: J. Clin. Invest. *33*:963, 1954.
167. Johnson, N.C., Kheim, T., Kountz, W.B.: Proc. Soc. Exp. Biol. Med. *102*:98–99, 1959.
168. Davidoff, G.N., Votaw, M.L., Coon, W.W., et al.: Am. J. Clin. Pathol. *70*:790–792, 1978.
169. Tutor, J.C., Paz, J.M., Fernandez, M.P.: Clin. Chem. *28*:1367–1370, 1982.
170. Hrgovcic, M., Te-smer, C.F., Mincler, T.N., et al.: Cancer *21*:743–755, 1968.
171. Asbjörnsen, G.: Scand. J. Haematol. *22*:193–196, 1979.
172. Capel, I.D., Pinnock, M.H., Williams, D.I., et al.: Oncology *39*:38–41, 1982.
173. Keen, C.L., Hurley, L.S.: Mech. Ageing Dev. *13*:161–176, 1980.
174. Hillman, L.S.: J. Pediatr. *98*:305–308, 1981.
175. Manser, J.L., Tran, N.N., Kotwal, M., et al.: J. Pediatr. *100*:511, 1982.
176. Pekarek, R.S., Powanda, M.C., Wannemacher, R.W., Jr.: Proc. Soc. Exp. Biol. Med. *141*:1029–1031, 1972.
177. Solomons, M.W.: J. Am. Coll. Nutr. *4*:83–105, 1985.
178. Goldstein, I., Kaplan, H.B., Edelson, H.S., et al.: J. Biol. Chem. *254*:4040–4045, 1979.
179. O'Dell, B.L.: Biochemical basis of the clinical effects of copper deficiency. *In* Clinical, Biochemical and Nutritional Aspects of Trace Elements. New York, Alan R. Liss, Inc., 1982.
180. O'Dell, B.L., Prohaska, J.R.: Biochemical aspects of copper deficiency in the nervous system. *In* Neu-

robiology of the Trace Elements, Vol. 1. Trace Element Neurobiology and Deficiencies. (Dreosti, I.E., Smith, E.M., Eds.) Clifton, N.J., Humana Press, 1983.

181. Lee, G.R., Williams, D.M., Cartwright, G.E.: Role of copper in iron metabolism and heme biosynthesis. *In* Trace Elements in Human Health and Disease, Vol 1. Zinc and Copper. (Prasad, A.S., Ed.) New York, Academic Press, 1976.

182. Griscom, N.T., Craig, J.N., Newhowser, E.B.D.: Pediatrics *48*:883–895, 1971.

183. McGill, L.C., Boas, R.N., Zerella, J.T.: J. Pediatr. Surg. *15*:740–747, 1980.

184. Fleming, C.R., Hodges, R.E., Hurley, L.S.: Am. J. Clin. Nutr. *29*:70–77, 1976.

185. Graham, G.G., Cordano, A.: Copper deficiency in human subjects. *In* Trace Elements in Human Health and Disease, Vol. 1. Zinc and Copper. (Prasad, A.S., Ed.) New York, Academic Press, 1976.

186. Johnston, R.B., Jr., Lehmeyer, J.E.: J. Clin. Invest. *57*:836–841, 1976.

187. Gosselin, R.E., Hodges, H.C., Smith, R.P., et al.: Clinical Toxicology of Commercial Products. 4th ed. Baltimore, Williams & Wilkins, 1977.

188. Wahal, P.K., Mehrotra, M.P., Kishore, B., et al.: J. Assoc. Physicians India *24*:153–158, 1976.

189. Roche-Sicot, J., Benhamou, J.P.: Ann. Intern. Med. *86*:301–303, 1977.

190. Klevay, L.M.: The role of copper, zinc, and other chemical elements in ischemic heart disease. *In* Metabolism of Trace Metals in Man, Vol. 1. (Rennert, O.W., Chan, W.-Y., Eds.) Boca Raton, C.R.C. Press, 1984.

191. Underwood, E.J.: Trace elements. *In* Toxicants Occurring Naturally in Foods. 2nd ed. Washington, D.C., National Academy of Sciences, 1973.

192. Shike, M., Jeejeebhoy, J.N.: Clin. Nutr. Suppl. *2*:5–7, 1983.

193. Cordano, A., Baertl, J.M., Graham, G.G.: Pediatrics *34*:324–326, 1964.

194. Fisberg, M., Castillo, C., Uauy, R.: Rev. Chil. Pediatr. *52*:410–414, 1981.

195. Karpel, J.T., Peden, V.H.: J. Pediatr. *80*:32–36, 1972.

196. Vilter R.W., Bozian, R.C., Hess, E.V., et al.: N. Engl. J. Med. *291*:188–191, 1974.

197. Zidar, B.L., Shadduck, R.K., Ziegler, Z., et al.: Am. J. Hematol. *3*:177–185, 1977.

198. Allen, T.M., Manoli, A., La Mont, R.L.: Clin. Orthop. *168*:206–210, 1982.

199. Askari, A., Long, C.L., Blakemore, W.S.: Metabolism *31*:1185–1193, 1982.

200. Seely, J.R., Humphrey, G.B., Matter, B.J.: N. Engl. J. Med. *286*:109–110, 1972.

201. Blumenthal, I., Lealman, G.T., Franklyn, P.P.: Arch. Dis. Child. *55*:224–231, 1980.

202. Cordano, A.: Pediatrics *54*:524, 1974.

203. Naveh, Y., Hanzani, A., Beranti, M.: Pediatrics *68*:397–400, 1981.

204. Milne, D.B., Omaje, S.T., Amos, W.H.: Am. J. Clin. Nutr. *34*:2389–2393, 1981.

205. Finley, E.B., Cerklewski, F.L.: Am. J. Clin. Nutr. *37*:553–556, 1983.

206. Menkes, J.H., Alter, M., Steiglede, G.K., et al.: Pediatrics *29*:764–779, 1982.

207. Danks, D.M., Campbell, P.E., Stevens, B.J., et al.: Pediatrics *50*:188–201, 1972.

208. Williams, D.M., Atkins, C.L.: Am. J. Dis. Child. *135*:375–376, 1981.

209. Dinno, N.D., Yacoub, U., Holmes, W., et al.: J. Pediatr. *99*:325, 1981.

210. Labadie, G.U., Hirschhorn, K., Katz, S., et al.: Pediatr. Res. *15*:257–261, 1981.

211. Schmidt, C.J., Hamer, D.H., McBride, O.W.: Science *224*:1104–1106, 1984.

212. Prohaska, J.R., Wells, W.W.: J. Neuro Chem. *23*:91–98, 1974.

213. Scheinberg, I.H.: Med. Clin. North Am. *60*:705–712, 1976.

214. Sternlieb, I., Scheinberg, I.H.: N. Engl. J. Med. *278*:352–359, 1968.

215. Lefkowitch, J.H.: N. Engl. J. Med. *307*:271–277, 1982.

216. Matsuda, I., Pearson, T., Holtzman, N.A.: Pediatr. Res. *8*:821–825, 1974.

217. Grand, R.J., Vawter, G.F.: J. Pediatr. *87*:1161–1170, 1975.

218. Kuivanieni, H., Peltonen, L., Palotie, A., et al.: J. Clin. Invest. *61*:730–733, 1982.

219. Acosta, P.B., Fernhoff, P.M., Warshaw, H.S., et al.: J. Parenter. Enter. Nutr. *5*:406–409, 1981.

220. Cutolo, M., Accardo, S., Cimmino, M.A., et al.: Arthritis Rheum. *25*:119–120, 1982.

221. Vir, S.C., Love, A.H., Thompson, W.: Am. J. Clin. Nutr. *34*:2382–2388, 1981.

222. Tilson, M.D.: Arch. Surg. *117*:1212–1213, 1982.

223. Klevay, L.M.: Biol. Trace Elem. Res. *5*:245–255, 1983.

224. Hooper, P.L., Visconti, L., Garry, P.J., et al.: JAMA *244*:1960–1961, 1980.

225. Freeland-Graves, J.H., Friedman, B.J., Han, W.-H., et al.: Am. J. Clin. Nutr. *35*:988–992, 1982.

226. Klevay, L.M., Reck, S.J., Jacob, R.A., et al.: Am. J. Clin. Nutr. *33*:45–50, 1980.

227. Dick, A.T., Dewey, D.W., Gawthorne, G.M.: J. Arg. Sci. *85*:567–568, 1975.

228. Fransson, G.B., Lönnerdal, B.: J. Pediatr. *101*:504–508, 1982.

229. Jacob, R.A., Klevay, L.M., Logan, G.M., Jr.: Am. J. Clin. Nutr. *31*:477–480, 1978.

230. Hambidge, K.M.: Am. J. Clin. Nutr. *26*:1212–1215, 1973.

231. Hinks, L.J.: Analyst *107*:815–823, 1982.

232. Garnica, A.D., Friad, J.L., Rennert, O.M.: Clin. Genet. *11*:159–161, 1977.

233. Alexander, N.M., Benson, G.D.: Life Sci. *16*:1025–1032, 1975.

234. Shike, M., Roulet, M., Kurian, R., et al.: Gastroenterology *81*:290–297, 1981.

*Chapter* **10**

# SELENIUM, CHROMIUM, AND MANGANESE

## (A) SELENIUM

### Orville A. Levander

Selenium first attracted practical biologic interest in the 1930's when it was found to cause alkali disease, a chronic poisoning of livestock resulting from the consumption of plants that grow on high-selenium soils.[1] Then in 1957, Schwarz discovered that traces of selenium prevented liver necrosis in vitamin E-deficient rats.[2] Soon thereafter selenium was shown to play a beneficial role in several economically important nutritional diseases in cattle, sheep, swine, and poultry,[3] but the first reports of possible significance in human nutrition did not appear until 1979.[4,5]

## CHEMISTRY AND MODE OF ACTION

The biologically important oxidation states of selenium are $+6$ (selenic acid, $H_2SeO_4$; selenates), $+4$ (selenous acid, $H_2SeO_3$; selenites), and $-2$ (seleno-amino acids; selenides). Like sulfur, selenium is a member of the Group VIa elements, and many of its compounds are analogous to sulfur compounds (e.g., selenomethionine, selenocystine).[6] Sodium selenate, sodium selenite, and selenomethionine are of similar potency for preventing liver necrosis in rats, whereas elemental selenium is inert nutritionally because of its insolubility.[7]

Although several microbial enzymes containing selenium have been described,[8] the only well-characterized mammalian selenoenzyme is glutathione peroxidase.[9] The primary metabolic role of this enzyme is thought to be the destruction of intracellular $H_2O_2$ and other hydroperoxides.[9]

This biochemical function of selenium explains its long-known nutritional relationship with the fat-soluble antioxidant vitamin E[10] (Fig. 10A–1). Glutathione peroxidase is inactive against fatty acid hydroperoxides esterified in phospholipids,[11] so the mechanism by which selenium acts in vivo as an antioxidant is still uncertain. Moreover, studies on the metabolism of phenobarbital in rats suggest that selenium is needed for the normal functioning of the hepatic microsomal P–450 system by a mechanism independent of glutathione peroxidase, thereby suggesting additional functions for the element.[9]

## METABOLISM

Values reported for total body selenium content range from 3 to 6 mg in New Zealanders[12] to about 15 mg in North Americans[13] and are thought to reflect differences in dietary intake.[14] The highest concentrations of selenium occur in the kidneys and liver and the lowest in the lung and brain.[13] Intestinal absorption of selenium compounds generally is 80% or more.[15] Little is known about selenium transport in the body, and no human selenium transport protein has been identified. About 60% of the total selenium excreted appears in the urine.[16] No effective homeostatic control over selenium absorption is apparent, and homeostasis is achieved mainly by the kidney.[17] Selenium compounds tend to be reduced in vivo to the selenide level that contrasts with the tendency of sulfur compounds to be oxidized and excreted as sulfate.[6] Selenium as selenide is methylated to

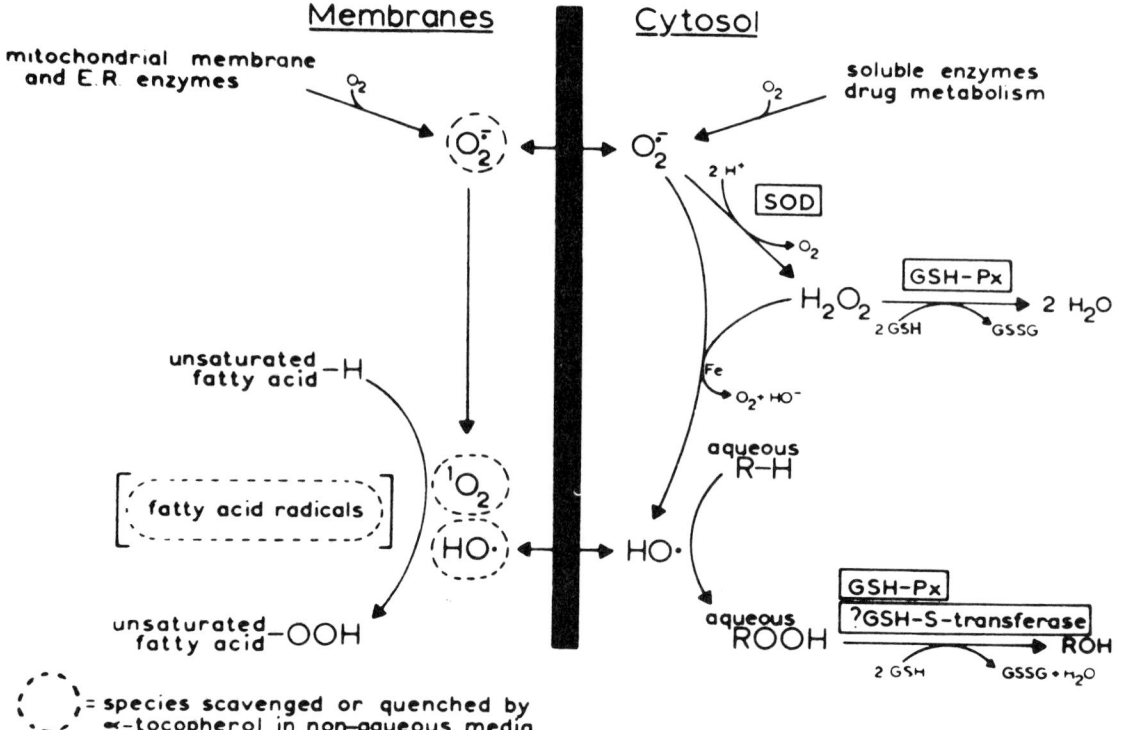

**Fig. 10A–1.** Functional interrelationships of glutathione peroxidase (GSH–Px), α-tocopherol (vitamin E), superoxide dismutase (SOD), and GSH-S-transferase (so-called selenium-independent glutathione peroxidase) in a liver cell. The compartmentalization between aqueous (cytosolic) and nonaqueous (membrane) domains of the cell are shown. (From Sunde, R.A., and Hoekstra, W.G.: Nutr. Rev. *38*: 269, 1980).

form trimethylselenonium ion, which is excreted in the urine.[17] Selenium overexposure leads to the production of dimethyl selenide, a volatile compound excreted via the lungs that is responsible for the "garlicky breath" characteristic of selenium poisoning.[17]

## EFFECTS OF DEFICIENCY AND EXCESS

A combined deficiency of both selenium and vitamin E causes liver necrosis in rats and swine, exudative diathesis in chickens, and white muscle disease in sheep and cattle.[3] The first descriptions of a specific selenium deficiency in animals fed nutritionally adequate levels of vitamin E did not appear until 1969. The symptoms included hair loss, growth retardation, and reproductive failure in rats fed a deficient diet for two generations and pancreatic degeneration in the chick.[18,19] Later work, however, showed that the pancreatic atrophy in the chick can be prevented by feeding high levels of vitamin E or other antioxidants.[20] Adult squirrel monkeys fed a low-selenium diet for nine months lost weight and developed alopecia, myopathy, nephrosis, and hepatic degeneration,[21] but attempts to produce selenium deficiency in

rhesus monkeys by feeding a selenium-deficient diet for four years were unsuccessful.[22] This difference between squirrel and rhesus monkeys may be a result of differences in the metabolism of selenium.[23]

Evidence that selenium is essential for humans is based upon the response of a total parenteral nutrition (TPN) patient in New Zealand and upon experience with Keshan disease in China. The New Zealand patient complained of increasing bilateral discomfort in her quadriceps and hamstring muscles that disappeared after about one week of daily supplementation with 100 μg of selenium as selenomethionine.[4] Keshan disease is an endemic cardiomyopathy affecting children and young women that occurs in a long belt running from northeastern to southwestern China.[24] The acute form is characterized by sudden onset of insufficient heart function, whereas individuals with chronic cases exhibit moderate or severe heart enlargement with varying degrees of heart insufficiency. The histopathologic features include multifocal necrosis, fibrous replacement of the myocardium, and myocytolysis. Keshan disease is related to a low dietary selenium intake and low blood and hair selenium levels.[25] An intervention trial demonstrated protection by selenium supplements.[5] Because certain features of the disease could not be explained solely on the basis of selenium status (e.g., seasonal variation), a cardiotoxic agent, such as a virus, might also be necessary for the disease to occur.[24]

The level of dietary selenium needed to cause chronic selenium toxicity in animals is 5 µg/g. In livestock, chronic selenosis (alkali disease) is characterized in liver cirrhosis, lameness, hoof malformations, hair loss, and emaciation.[3] Laboratory rats chronically poisoned with selenium exhibit growth depression, liver cirrhosis, and splenomegaly. The mechanism of selenium toxicity is not known,[26] and the toxic effects of selenium may be modified by adaptation and certain dietary factors.[3]

Two public health surveys carried out in seleniferous areas of the United States in the late 1930's failed to establish any symptom specific for selenium poisoning.[27,28] Field studies conducted in Venezuela showed that the incidence of dermatitis, loose hair, and pathologic nails was greater in children from a seleniferous area than in those from Caracas,[29] but no differences were seen in the various biochemical tests performed. A report from China described an outbreak of endemic selenium poisoning in humans.[30] The most common sign of intoxication was loss of hair and nails. In high-incidence areas, lesions of the skin, nervous system, and possibly teeth were observed.

## CLINICAL SITUATIONS INDUCING DEFICIENCY

Low selenium status in TPN patients has been associated with cardiomyopathy, elevation of serum enzymes, muscle pain, and abnormal nail beds.[4,31–33] Very little selenium exists in purified TPN solutions,[34] but the diversity of signs and symptoms observed suggests that other factors may also be operating. More research is needed to clarify the role of selenium in TPN and to determine the most appropriate form for intravenous administration.[34]

Children with inborn errors of amino acid metabolism have been fed therapeutic diets that were very low in selenium. Such children had serum selenium levels much less than normal but no evidence of hematologic, electrocardiographic, or electromyographic abnormalities.[35] Declines in plasma and red cell selenium levels and red cell glutathione peroxidase activity may contribute to hemolytic events in premature infants during the first few months of life.[36]

## DIETARY CONSIDERATIONS

**Requirements.** In 1980, the National Research Council established a safe and adequate daily selenium intake for adults of 50 to 200 µg.[37] Healthy North American men and women need 57 to 80 µg/day to replace fecal and urinary losses,[16] whereas only 20 µg/day were needed to achieve balance in healthy New Zealand women.[12] This difference, thought to be due to differences in the total body selenium pools of North Americans vs. New Zealanders,[12,13] suggests that the amount of selenium needed to attain balance is a function of previous dietary intake. Keshan disease did not occur in any areas of China where the dietary selenium intake was 30 µg/day or more,[38] and no health problems could be ascribed to the habitual consumption of 28 to 32 µg/day in New Zealand.[39] Therefore, an intake of about 30 µg/day seems sufficient to prevent selenium deficiency in adults. Some workers advocate much higher intakes of selenium (250 to 300 µg/day) as a way of preventing certain human diseases such as cancer.[40] However, the National Research Council has advised that firm conclusions regarding any protective effect of selenium against the risk cancer cannot be drawn on the basis of the present limited evidence.[41] The 200-µg limit of the safe and adequate range is meant to warn persons against consuming megadoses of selenium. The intake at which selenium becomes harmful to people is not known, but a tentative maximum acceptable daily intake of 500 µg has been proposed.[42] This figure, however, is based on Japanese consumption of large quantities of fish. If the toxicologic potency of the selenium in fish is as low as its nutritional bioavailability, then this number would have to be lowered accordingly.

**Food Sources.** Adults consuming self-selected diets in Maryland, an area with marginal soil selenium levels, ingested an average of 81 µg of selenium per day.[16] Other estimates of selenium intakes in North America ranged from 62 to 224 µg/day,[43] but any estimate of more than 150 µg/day was derived from high-calorie diets, idealized diets, or diets sampled in high-selenium areas. Seafoods, kidney, liver, and muscle meats are high in selenium, whereas fruits and vegetables are, with some exceptions, low in selenium.[43] Grains are variable depending upon where they are grown. Drinking water contributes negligible selenium to the North American diet.[44] Animal studies have shown that the availability of selenium in wheat and beef kidney is high, whereas that in tuna is low.[45] A human bioavailability trial carried out in Finland, a country with selenium-poor soils, showed significant differences in various forms of selenium tested (e.g., selenate, wheat, yeast) depending upon the criterion of availability used (increase in platelet glutathione peroxidase activity, elevation of plasma or red cell selenium level, retention of selenium).[46] The advantages of using a functional test of selenium bioavailability, such as glutathione peroxidase, are discussed elsewhere.[15]

**Interrelationships with Other Nutrients.** Because of its role in glutathione peroxidase, selenium probably interacts with any nutrient that affects the antioxidant/pro-oxidant balance of the cell.[47] For example, the selenium requirement of chicks is inversely proportional to the dietary vitamin E intake.[19] Selenium also protects against the toxicity of mercury, cadmium, and silver,[47] and a physiologic role for selenium in counteracting heavy metal pollutants has been proposed.[48] The low bioavailability of the selenium in tuna may be due to complexation with mercury, but this issue needs further investigation.[15]

## EVALUATION OF NUTRIENT STATUS

**Analytical Evaluation.** Random urine samples are of little use in assessing selenium status since they are affected by dilution and the previous meal.[39] Blood selenium levels vary widely in different countries and are thought to reflect dietary intakes[14] (Fig. 10A–2), although a direct relation to muscle or total body selenium levels has yet to be established.[39] Average blood selenium levels reported in different areas of the U.S. range between 160 and 260 ng/ml,[49] whereas extreme values of 8 and 7,500 ng/ml have been reported in Keshan disease and endemic selenosis areas of China, respectively.[30] Plasma selenium levels, which respond to selenium supplementation more rapidly than whole blood levels, are an index of short-term status.[39] Average plasma selenium levels observed in areas with marginally adequate (Maryland) or low (Ohio) levels of soil selenium in the U.S. were 134 and 119 ng/ml, respectively.[16,50] Levels less than 50 ng/ml are

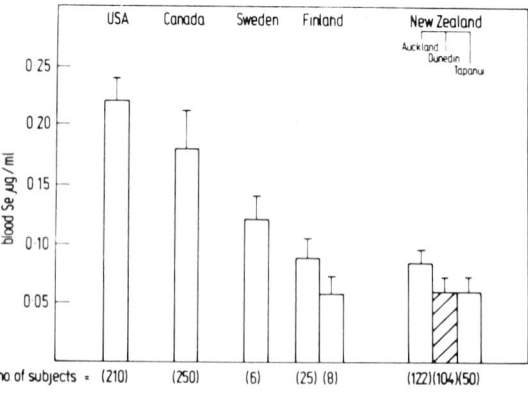

**Fig. 10A–2.** Blood selenium levels reported in healthy adults in various countries. (From Thomson, C.D., Robinson, M.F.[39])

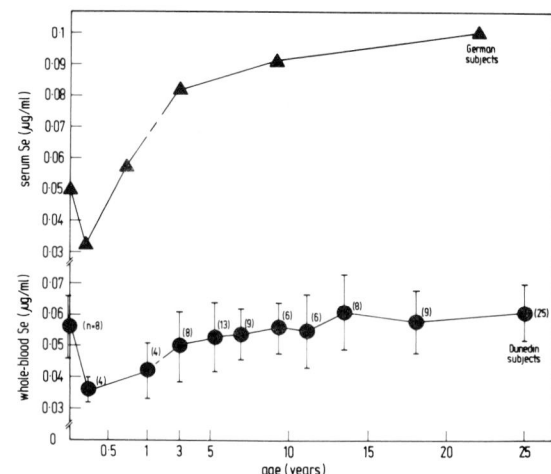

**Fig. 10A–3.** Serum selenium concentrations in healthy German children and young adults in comparison with whole-blood selenium concentrations in healthy New Zealand children and young adults. (From Thomson, C.D., Robinson, M.F.[39])

often seen in healthy residents of the south island of New Zealand.[51] Serum selenium concentrations fall soon after birth and then gradually increase to adult values (Fig. 10A–3). Response to selenium supplementation was observed in a New Zealand TPN patient who had a plasma level of 9 ng/ml.[4] Hair selenium was utilized in China to evaluate status,[38] but may not be valid in Western countries where shampoos containing selenium are used.

**Biochemical and Clinical Evaluation.** A direct relationship exists between blood glutathione peroxidase activity and blood selenium level up to 100 ng/ml.[52] Beyond that point the activity of the enzyme plateaus and cannot be used to evaluate selenium nutriture. Moreover, numerous other factors can affect glutathione peroxidase activity.[53] Some workers have shown that hemoglobin interferes with assay of the enzyme in human erythrocytes.[23] Others have taken advantage of the relatively short life span of platelets to avoid this problem and have measured changes in platelet glutathione peroxidase activity to monitor the bioavailability of various forms of dietary selenium in humans.[46] At present, there are no suitable clinical parameters for evaluating selenium status.

## REFERENCES

1. Moxon, A.L., Rhian, M.A.: Physiol. Rev. *23*: 305–337, 1943.
2. Schwarz, K., Foltz, C.M.: J. Am. Chem. Soc. *79*: 3292–3293, 1957.
3. National Research Council: Selenium in Nutrition, revised ed. Washington, National Academy of Sciences, 1983.

4. van Rij, A.M., Thomson, C.D., McKenzie, J.M., et al.: Am. J. Clin. Nutr. *32*:2076–2085, 1979.

5. Keshan Disease Research Group: Chin. Med. J. *92*: 471–476, 1979.

6. Levander, O.A.: Selected aspects of the comparative metabolism and biochemistry of selenium and sulfur. *In* Trace Elements in Human Health and Disease, Vol. 2: Essential and Toxic Elements. (Prasad, A.S., Ed.) New York, Academic Press, 1976.

7. Schwarz, K., Folz, C.M.: J. Biol. Chem. *233*: 245–251, 1958.

8. Stadtman, T.C.: Annu. Rev. Biochem. *49*:93–110, 1980.

9. Burk, R.F.: Annu. Rev. Nutr. *3*:53–70, 1983.

10. Hoekstra, W.G.: Fed. Proc. *34*:2083–2089, 1975.

11. Grossman, A., Wendel, A.: Eur. J. Biochem. *135*: 549–552, 1983.

12. Stewart, R.D.H., Griffiths, N.M., Thomson, C.D., et al.: Br. J. Nutr. *40*:45–54, 1978.

13. Schroeder, H.A., Frost, D.V., Balassa, J.J.: J. Chron. Dis.*23*:227–243, 1970.

14. Levander, O.A.: Ann. N.Y. Acad. Sci. *393*: 70–82, 1982.

15. Levander, O.A.: Fed. Proc. *42*:1723–1727, 1983.

16. Levander, O.A., Morris, V.C.: Am. J. Clin. Nutr. *39*: 809–815, 1984.

17. Burk, R.F.: World Rev. Nutr. Diet. *30*:88–106, 1978.

18. McCoy, K.E.M., Weswig, P.H.: J. Nutr. *98*: 383–389, 1969.

19. Thompson, J.N., Scott, M.L.: J. Nutr. *97*: 335–342, 1969.

20. Whitacre, M.E., Combs, G.F., Parker, R.S.: Fed. Proc. *42*:928, 1983.

21. Muth, O.H., Weswig, P.H., Whanger, P.D., et al.: Am. J. Vet. Res. *32*:1603–1605, 1971.

22. Butler, J.A., Whanger, P.D., Patton, N.M., et al.: Fed. Proc. *40*:943, 1981.

23. Beilstein, M.A., Whanger, P.D.: J. Nutr. *113*: 2138–2146, 1983.

24. Ge, K., Xue, A., Bai, J., et al.: Virchows Arch. *401*: 1–15, 1983.

25. Keshan Disease Research Group: Chin. Med. J. *92*: 477–482, 1979.

26. Levander, O.A.: Selenium: Biochemical actions, interactions, and some human health implications. *In* Clinical, Biochemical, and Nutritional Aspects of Trace Elements. (Prasad, A.S., Ed.) New York, Alan R. Liss, 1982.

27. Smith, M.I., Franke, K.W., Westfall, B.B.: U.S. Public Health Rep. *51*:1496–1505, 1936.

28. Smith, M.I., Westfall, B.B.: U.S. Public Health Rep. *52*:1375–1384, 1937.

29. Jaffe, W.G.: Effect of selenium intake in humans and in rats. *In* Proc. Symp. Selenium-Tellurium in the Environment. Pittsburgh, Industrial Health Foundation, 1976.

30. Yang, G.Q., Wang, S., Zhou, R., et al.: Am. J. Clin. Nutr. *37*:872–881, 1983.

31. Johnson, R.A., Baker, S.S., Fallon, J.T., et al.: N. Engl. J. Med. *304*:1210–1212, 1981.

32. Fleming, C.R., Lie, J.T., McCall, J.T., et al.: Gastroenterology, *83*:689–693, 1982.

33. Kien, C.L., Ganther, H.E.: Am. J. Clin. Nutr. *37*: 319–328, 1983.

34. Levander, O.A.: Bull. N.Y. Acad. Med. *60*: 144–155, 1984.

35. Lombeck, I., Kasperek, K., Feinendegen, L.E., et al.: Low selenium state in children. *In* Selenium in Biology and Medicine. (Spallholz, J.E., Martin, J.L., Ganther, H.E., Eds.) Westport, CT AVI Publ. Co., 1981.

36. Gross, S.: Semin. Hematol. *13*:187–199, 1976.

37. National Research Council: Recommended Dietary Allowances. 9th Ed. Washington, National Academy of Sciences, 1980.

38. Chen, X., Yang, G.Q., Chen, J., et al.: Biol. Trace Element Res. *2*:91–107, 1980.

39. Thomson, C.D., Robinson, M.F.: Am. J. Clin. Nutr. *33*:303–323, 1980.

40. Schrauzer, G.N., White, D.A.: Bioinorg. Chem. *8*: 303–318, 1978.

41. National Research Council: Diet, Nutrition, and Cancer. Washington National Academy of Sciences, 1982.

42. Sakurai, H., Tsuchiya, K.: Environ. Physiol. Biochem. *5*:107–118, 1975.

43. Levander, O.A.: Selenium in foods. *In* Proc. Symp. Selenium-Tellurium in the Environment. Pittsburgh, Industrial Health Foundation, 1976.

44. National Research Council: The contribution of drinking water to mineral nutrition in humans. *In* Drinking Water and Health, Vol. 3. Washington, National Academy of Sciences, 1980.

45. Douglass, J.S., Morris, V.C., Soares, J.H., et al.: J. Nutr. *111*:2180–2187, 1981.

46. Levander, O.A., Alfthan, G., Arvilommi, H., et al.: Am. J. Clin. Nutr. *37*:887–897, 1983.

47. Levander, O.A., Cheng, L.: Ann. N.Y. Acad. Sci. *355*: 1–372, 1980.

48. Parizek, J., Ostadalova, I., Kalouskova, A.: The detoxifying effects of selenium: Interelations between compounds of selenium and certain metals. *In* Newer Trace Elements in Nutrition. (Mertz, W., Cornatzer, W.E., Eds.) New York, Marcel Dekker, Inc., 1971.

49. Allaway, W.H., Kubota, J., Losee, F., et al.: Arch Environ. Health 16: 342–348, 1968.

50. Snook, J.T., Palmquist, O.L., Moxon, A.L., et al.: Am. J. Clin. Nutr. *38*:620–630, 1983.

51. Thomson, C.D., Robinson, M.F., Campbell, D.R., et al.: Am. J. Clin. Nutr. *36*:24–31, 1982.

52. Thomson, C.D., Rea, H.M., Doesburg, V.M., et al.: Br. J. Nutr. *37*:457–460, 1977.

53. Ganther, H.E., Hafeman, D.G., Lawrence, R.A., et al.: Selenium and gultathione peroxidase in health and disease—A review. *In* Trace Elements in Human Health and Disease, Vol. 2: Essential and Toxic Elements. (Prasad, A.S., Ed.) New York, Academic Press, 1976.

*Chapter* # 10

# SELENIUM, CHROMIUM, AND MANGANESE

## *(B) CHROMIUM*

### Richard A. Anderson

Chromium (Cr) entered into mammalian nutrition in the late 1950's when Schwarz and Mertz reported that rats fed Cr-deficient diets exhibited glucose intolerance.[1,2] They subsequently isolated fractions containing chromium from brewers' yeast and pork kidney powders that restored glucose removal rates to normal when fed to rats raised on low-Cr diets. Marginal dietary intakes of Cr lead to signs and symptoms similar to those associated with diabetes and cardiovascular disease. Cr is involved in carbohydrate, lipid, and nucleic acid metabolism. Chromium functions in carbohydrate and lipid metabolism as a potentiator of insulin action. In nucleic acid metabolism, it is postulated to be involved in maintaining the structural integrity of the nuclear strands and regulation of gene expression.

## EFFECTS OF DEFICIENCY AND EXCESS IN LABORATORY ANIMALS AND MAN

Glucose intolerance is usually one of the first signs of Cr deficiency, followed by additional abnormalities in glucose and lipid metabolism and nerve disorders (Table 10B–1). Most of the signs of Cr deficiency listed in this table have been observed in both experimental animals and man. Signs that have not been conclusively demonstrated in man include those that are not readily differentiated using human subjects, such as impaired growth and decreased longevity. Although it may be a factor, Cr also has not been demonstrated to affect sperm count and fertility in man.

Reduction of aortic intimal plaque area and aortic total cholesterol content were observed in rabbits that were fed a diet containing 1% cholesterol for 30 days and then administered potassium chromate for an additional 30 days.[4] In rats supplemented with 5 μg of Cr per ml in drinking water for 24 to 26 months, Schroeder and Balassa also observed a reduction in serum cholesterol from 108 mg/dl in the controls to 77 mg/dl in the Cr-supplemented rats.[5]

Glucose removal rates for weanling rats are usually between 4 and 5%/min and decrease slightly with age to 3.5 to 3.8%; removal rates of rats raised on a low-Cr diet are decreased to approximately 2.7%/min. Growth of animals with those decreased glucose removal rates is not affected by Cr supplementation. However, more severe Cr deficiency observed when rats are raised in a strictly controlled low-Cr environment results in glucose removal rates of less than 1% per min. Under those conditions, growth rate and longevity have been reported to be improved with supplemental Cr.[6] The median age of male mice at death was 99 days longer for the animals receiving Cr in the drinking water than for the nonsupplemented controls.[7]

Exposure of weanling mice raised on a moderately low Cr diet (0.112 μg/g) to 4% glucose in the drinking water for 7 weeks caused a drop in food energy utilization of approximately 33%. An addition of 5 ng of Cr per ml to the drinking water containing glucose prevented this decreased food energy utilization and also protected against glu-

**Table 10B–1.  Signs and Symptoms of Chromium Deficiency***

| Function | Animal |
|---|---|
| Impaired glucose tolerance | Human, rat, mouse, squirrel, monkey |
| Elevated circulating insulin | Human, rat |
| Glycosuria | Human, rat |
| Fasting hyperglycemia | Human, rat, mouse |
| Impaired growth | Rat, mouse, turkey |
| Decreased longevity | Rat, mouse |
| Elevated serum cholesterol and triglycerides | Human, rat, mouse |
| Increased incidence of aortic plaques | Rabbit, rat, mouse |
| Neuropathy | Human |
| Encephalopathy | Human |
| Reduction in aortic intimal plaque areas | Rabbit |
| Corneal lesions | Rat, squirrel, monkey |
| Decreased fertility and sperm count | Rat |

*Adapted from ref. 3.

cose-induced losses of chromium, zinc, iron, copper, and manganese in the liver and heart.[7a]

Toxicity of chromium is limited almost exclusively to hexavalent forms of Cr which may be absorbed by ingestion through the skin and by inhalation. From the toxicologic data available, the only group at special risk from exposure to ambient levels of chromium are workers in industries that use or manufacture products containing hexavalent Cr. Chronic exposure to hexavalent chromate dust has been correlated with increased risk of respiratory diseases, especially lung cancer. Exposure to hexavalent Cr and, to a lesser extent, trivalent Cr compounds may also induce dermatitis and related symptoms in some Cr-sensitive individuals.[8] No toxicity has been reported for the oral administration of trivalent Cr, the form found in foods.

## CLINICAL SITUATIONS INDUCING DEFICIENCY

Overt signs of chromium deficiency, such as neuropathy and encephalopathy, have been observed only in patients receiving total parenteral nutrition (TPN).[9,10] The first reported case of a severe Cr deficiency was observed in a subject receiving TPN for 3.5 years who developed impaired glucose tolerance, inability to utilize glucose for energy, neuropathy with normal insulin levels, high fatty acid levels, low respiratory quotient, and abnormalities of nitrogen metabolism. Daily infusion of 45 units of insulin did not improve glucose tolerance or respiratory quotient. However, addition of 250 µg daily of Cr as chromic chloride for 2 weeks restored intravenous glucose tolerance and respiratory quotient to normal. The individual was then placed on a daily maintenance dose of 20 µg of Cr. Over the next 5 months, exogenous insulin was not needed, glucose intake had to be reduced to avoid excess weight, and nerve conduction and well-being returned to nor-

mal. Similar results were reported for a woman who had been receiving total parenteral nutrition for 5 months following complete bowel resection. This patient displayed severe glucose intolerance, weight loss, and a confusional state similar to metabolic encephalopathy. Within 3 to 4 days of supplementation of 150 µg of Cr per day, the patient was able to maintain normal glucose levels with no added insulin. Chromium supplementation restored the glucose tolerance to normal, reduced insulin requirements, improved weight gain, and eliminated the encephalopathy.[10]

Not all total parenteral solutions are low in Cr.[11,12] Mean daily Cr intake from TPN solutions for 8 subjects was 18.1 ± 0.9 µg. Chromium was not added to these solutions but was present as a contaminant; therefore, Cr intake should be monitored during long-term TPN to ensure proper Cr nutriture.

Various other forms of stress may also lead to altered Cr metabolism. For example, serum and urinary Cr concentrations are affected by sandfly fever,[13] glucose loading,[14] pregnancy,[15] and protein calorie malnutrition.[16] Urinary losses of Cr are also elevated markedly following physical injury[11] and strenuous exercise.[17] Various forms of stress that affect glucose metabolism often also influence Cr metabolism.

## FUNCTIONS AND METABOLISM

The biologically active form of Cr that functions in carbohydrate and lipid metabolism is postulated to be comprised of Cr, nicotinic acid, and glutathione or its constituent amino acids.[18–24] A method to synthesize biologically active chromium complexes has been developed[20] and, based upon chromatographic evidence and maximal insulin potentiating activity, the products appear similar to those isolated from brewers' yeast, the richest known source of biologically active Cr.

Insulin potentiation is measured by determining the increase in insulin activity as a response to biologically active Cr complexes in the breakdown of glucose to carbon dioxide by adipose tissue[22] or adipocytes.[23] Insulin potentiation, due to organic Cr complexes, is relatively specific because inorganic Cr complexes, most organic Cr complexes, and individual or combined constituents of biologically active Cr complexes are inactive (Table 10B–2). Only trivalent organic Cr complexes have been shown to yield insulin-potentiating activity. Activity of insulin alone in Table 10B–2 is listed as 1.0 and is the basis of calculating insulin-potentiating activity of the other complexes. Insulin potentiation due to biologically active Cr complexes at pH 7.0, instead of 7.4 as shown in Table 10B–2, is often 7 to 10 times as great.[24] In the presence of biologically active Cr complexes, much lower levels of insulin are required to yield the same apparent insulin activity.[22–24]

Chromium also functions in nucleic acid metabolism. Chromium, found primarily in cell nuclei, binds tightly to DNA, RNA, and nuclear proteins. Chromium stimulates RNA synthesis in vitro when incubated with DNA or chromatin, whereas other metals tested inhibited synthesis, suggesting that Cr may be involved in the regulation of gene expressions.[25]

The structures of the chromium complexes functioning in carbohydrate, lipid, and nucleic acid metabolism are not known. Simple inorganic chromium compounds appear to affect in vitro nucleic acid metabolism but inhibit or have no effect on in vitro carbohydrate and lipid metabolism.

The mechanism of action of chromium in carbohydrate and lipid metabolism remains to be elucidated. Chromium potentiates the action of insulin, but whether it binds directly with insulin in vivo or exerts its primary effects through increased receptor number or affinity needs to be documented. The binding of biologically active chromium to insulin in vitro but not in vivo has been established.[18] Mertz et al.[22] proposed the catalysis of the disulfide interchange between insulin and sulfhydryl membrane receptor sites as one possible mechanism whereby chromium may potentiate insulin action.[22]

Numerous chromium compounds are present in biologic systems. Anderson et al prepared ethanol and ammonia extracts from yeast grown with radioactive chromium added to the growth medium and found that less than 5% of the total chromium was associated with insulin-potentiating activity.[21] Haylock et al also found numerous chromium-containing fractions from brewers' yeast.[26] The uniqueness or interconversions of these compounds remains to be established. Biologically active chromium compounds isolated from different sources are also significantly different based upon their elution profiles using size exclusion chromatography.[20,21,24,26,27] Reported apparent molecular weights of naturally occurring insulin-potentiating Cr compounds range from 400 to 2,000 daltons or more. Biologically active chromium appears to encompass a number of complexes that may or may not be related and/or interconverted.

## DIETARY CONSIDERATIONS

In 1980, the suggested safe and adequate intake for chromium was established at 50 to 200 μg per day for adolescents and adults, and 10 to 120 μg

**Table 10B–2.  Biological Activity of Synthetic Cr Complexes and Their Components§**

| Samples* | Insulin Potentiation† |
|---|---|
| Control (no additions) | 1.0 |
| Control + $CrCl_3$ | $1.0 \pm 0.05$ |
| Control + $Cr(C_2H_3O_2)_3$ | $0.9 \pm 0.10$ |
| Control + nicotinic acid | $1.1 \pm 0.05$ |
| Control + glutathione | $1.2 \pm 0.14$ |
| Control + glycine | $1.1 \pm 0.05$ |
| Control + $CrCl_3$ + nicotinic acid | $1.1 \pm 0.10$ |
| Control + $CrCl_3$ + glutathione | $1.3 \pm 0.14$ |
| Control + $CrCl_3$ + glutathione + nicotinic acid | $1.3 \pm 0.11$ |
| Control + Cr, nicotinic acid, glutathione complex | $3.2 \pm 0.23$‡ |
| Control + Cr, nicotinic acid, glycine complex | $2.7 \pm 0.15$‡ |
| Control + yeast isolate | $3.3 \pm 0.11$‡ |

*One hundred micrograms of all samples were added. For more than one addition, 100 μg of each were added.
†Potentiation of insulin activity when 2 μunits of insulin were added to the fat cell bioassay. Insulin potentiation was calculated by dividing the radioactive $CO_2$ released in the presence of insulin plus component added by that released in response to insulin alone, e.g., an insulin potentiation of 1 indicates that the components tested had no measurable effect on insulin action. All numbers are mean ± standard deviation of four or more separate determinations.
‡Significantly greater than lines 1–9 at $P < 0.001$.
§Adapted from ref. 23.

for infants and children.[28] This recommended range is for total chromium and not for specific organic forms. Chromium intake in the United States appears to be near the lower end of the suggested range and may be less. Levine et al reported a daily intake of 5 to 115 μg for elderly institutionalized subjects.[29] One third of the diets, designed by a nutritionist to be well-balanced and to contain the recommended daily intake of vitamins and minerals (except Cr) contained less than the minimum safe and adequate intake of 50 μg of chromium.[30] Kozlovsky et al recently completed a study involving the daily and weekly Cr intake of 32 male and female adult subjects consuming self-selected diets.[31] Chromium daily intake ranged from 8 to 89 μg, with a mean of 27 ± 1 μg, and weekly intake ranged from 91 to 273 μg. Approximately 90% of the daily diets contained less than the minimum suggested safe and adequate intake for Cr.

Reported Cr content of foods and diets seems to vary depending upon the method of homogenizing samples. For example, stainless steel blenders and/or stainless steel blender blades are usually used for homogenizing foods. When they are used, the apparent Cr content of foods depends more upon duration of blending than upon the endogenous Cr content. Methods of food preparation may also affect Cr intake since Cr tends to leach from stainless steel cookware.[32] Heating 10% lemon juice in a stainless steel container for 5 minutes at 98 to 100° increases the Cr concentration of the lemon juice more than 30-fold. Chromium that is incorporated into foods during preparation may be utilized. For example, Cr in beer, some of which originates from contamination during preparation, is absorbed and therefore presumably utilized.[33] The long-term consequences of food preparation using Teflon-coated and other types of cookware need to be evaluated.

No comprehensive studies have been undertaken to determine the Cr content of individual foods eaten in the United States. Finnish workers, however, determined Cr content of numerous foods from each of the basic food groups.[34] Foods high in Cr include mushrooms, brewers' yeast, prunes, nuts, asparagus, wine, and beer. The relative Cr distribution among the food groups is similar for fruits and vegetables, dairy products, beverages, and meat with lesser amounts from cereal products, and negligible dietary Cr from most seafoods and drinking water.

## SUPPLEMENTATION STUDIES IN HUMANS

Several studies have reported significant improvements in glucose tolerance and/or serum lipids following Cr supplementation of humans. In a controlled clinical trial, three of six patients with mild diabetes displayed significant improvements in glucose tolerance following oral supplementation with chromium as $CrCl_3.6H_2O$. Two more patients showed some improvement, and in one the glucose tolerance was not altered by Cr supplementation. Decreases in 120-min glucose (100-g glucose load), due to Cr supplementation, were approximately 40 to 50 mg/dl with the presupplementation 120-min values ranging from 154 to 179 mg/dl.[35] In a study of impaired glucose tolerance of older subjects (74 to 96 years of age), 10 subjects with abnormal glucose tolerance curves were supplemented with 150 μg of Cr for 2 to 30 months.[29] Glucose tolerance curves of four of the subjects improved to normal, and glucose tolerance of the remaining six subjects was unchanged. The group that responded to Cr had a milder impairment than the nonresponders. Hopkins et al treated six malnourished infants from Jordan and six from Nigeria with 250 μg Cr as $CrCl_3$.[36] Within 18 hr after supplementation, glucose removal rates of the Jordanian infants improved from an average glucose removal rate of 0.6% per min to 2.9% per min, and those of the Nigerian infants improved from 1.2 to 2.9% per min. Glucose tolerance of malnourished Jordanian infants, from a valley with three times higher levels of Cr in the drinking water, was not improved by Cr supplementation.

Riales and Albrink gave 200 μg chromic chloride or placebo to 23 healthy adult men 21 to 60 years of age.[37] After 12 weeks, high-density lipoprotein cholesterol increased significantly in the chromium group from 35 to 39 mg/dl and did not change in the control group. The largest increases in high-density lipoprotein cholesterol and decreases in insulin and blood glucose were found in those subjects having normal glucose levels together with elevated basal insulin levels. Mossop supplemented 13 diabetic patients with 2 mg chromium chloride for three months and 13 with placebo.[38] Initial mean fasting blood glucose for the 13 patients receiving Cr was 259 mg/dl and decreased to 119 mg/dl after two to four months of Cr supplementation. Initial mean fasting blood glucose for the control patients was 259 mg/dl and was 221 mg/dl at the conclusion of the study. Insulin doses in five of the patients taking Cr were reduced during the study, and four of the controls required higher doses of insulin. High-density lipoprotein cholesterol of Cr-supplemented subjects also increased 38%.

Anderson el al[39] reported significant improvements in glucose tolerance following two and three months of Cr supplementation (200 μg Cr daily as chromium chloride) in 18 of 20 subjects with marginally elevated blood glucose (90-min glucose greater than 100 mg/dl). The study design was double-blind crossover with each test period lasting three months. Mean 90-min glucose decreased from 135 mg/dl to 116 mg/dl following Cr supplementation. This report has been verified by Canadian workers.[40] In the study of Anderson et al, glucose tolerance of subjects with near optimal glucose tolerance was nearly identical following Cr supplementation. Serum glucose of subjects with 90-min glucose less than fasting was elevated following Cr supplementation. In a follow-up study involving eight hypoglycemic patients, using the same double-blind crossover study design, hypoglycemic response was improved in seven of eight patients, insulin binding and insulin receptor number also improved following supplementation, and immunoreactive insulin decreased in five patients following Cr supplementation.[41]

Numerous studies have attributed improvements in glucose and lipid metabolism of human subjects, following brewers' yeast supplementation, to the Cr present in the yeast. Brewers' yeast is the richest known source of biologically active Cr. Because yeast contains several other nutrients, however, and improvements may not be due solely to Cr, this supplementation is not discussed here.

Not all studies have reported significant improvements in glucose tolerance and/or serum lipids.[42] However, not all subjects would be expected to be improved by Cr supplementation, and response to Cr should depend upon the Cr status of the individual. Chromium supplementation can only correct that part of the problem due to insufficient dietary Cr. Chromium functions as a nutrient and not as a therapeutic agent.

## EVALUATION OF NUTRIENT STATUS

Evaluation of reported values pertaining to the Cr content of biological materials and their relation to status is difficult because of problems associated with total Cr analysis. Literature values for the Cr concentration of biological fluids have decreased precipitously in the past two decades. For example, reported values for serum Cr range from several hundred parts per billion (ppb) to the presently accepted values of less than 0.5 ppb (0.5 ng per ml or per g) for normal individuals. Similar decreases have been observed in reported values for urinary Cr concentration. Mean Cr values greater than 0.5 ppb for normal human urine, serum, and milk samples may be in error and, unless verified by independent means, should not be considered accurate. Values for the Cr concentration of human tissues should be viewed with

caution since most studies have not incorporated appropriate collection techniques excluding stainless steel, or the samples have not been analyzed using improved laboratory techniques and instrumentation. Studies validating the correlation of Cr concentration of physiologic fluids and/or tissues with Cr status need to be completed. Preliminary results, especially those involving Cr concentrations of urine and serum, indicate that, except in extreme cases, Cr content of these physiologic fluids may not be indicative of status.

The Cr status of infants, adolescents, adults, and the elderly cannot be readily evaluated at present because no known enzymes or abnormal metabolic products of Cr can be measured as indicators of status. However, relative Cr status can be evaluated retrospectively following daily Cr supplementation of approximately 200 μg to adult subjects for one to three months. Studies should be placebo-controlled double-blind crossover studies. Subjects who showed improvements in glucose and/or lipid parameters following Cr supplementation appear to have been in marginally low Cr status.

## REFERENCES

1. Schwarz, K., Mertz, W.: Arch. Biochem. Biophys. *72*:515–518, 1957.
2. Schwarz, K., Mertz, W.: Arch. Biochem. Biophys. *85*:292–295, 1959.
3. Anderson, R.A.: Sci. Total Environ. *17*:13–29, 1981.
4. Abraham, A.S., Sonnenblick, M., Eini, M.: Atherosclerosis *41*:371–379, 1982.
5. Schroeder, H.A. and Balassa, J.J.: Am. J. Physiol. *209*:433–437, 1965.
6. Mertz, W., Roginski, E.E., Schroeder, H.A.: J. Nutr. *86*:107–112, 1965.
7. Schroeder, H.A., Vinton, W.H. Jr., and Balassa, J.J.: J. Nutr. *80*:39–45, 1963.
7a. Schrauzer, G.N., Shrestha, K.P., Molenaar, T.B., and Mead, S.: J. Biol. Trace Element Res. *9*:79–87, 1986.
8. Environmental Protection Agency: Health Effects Assessment Document for Chromium, Research Triangle Park, NC, 1983.
9. Jejeebhoy, K.N., Chu, R.C., Marliss, E.B., et al.: Am. J. Clin. Nutr. *30*:531–538, 1977.
10. Freund, H., Atamian, S., Fischer, J.E.: J.A.M.A. *241*:496–498, 1979.
11. Borel, J.S., Majerus, T.C., Polansky, M.M., et al.: Biol. Trace Element Res. *6*:317–325, 1985.
12. Borel, J.S.: Urinary chromium excretion of trauma patients and chromium supplementation of trauma patients receiving total parenteral nutrition: Effect on chromium and glucose metabolism. Thesis, Univ. of Maryland, College Park, 1983.
13. Pekarek, R.S., Hauer, E.C., Rayfield, E.J., et al.: Diabetes *24*:350–353, 1975.
14. Anderson, R.A., Polansky, M.M., Roginski, E.E., et al.: Am. J. Clin. Nutr. *36*:1184–1193, 1982.
15. Hambidge, K.M., Rodgerson, D.O.: Am. J. Obstet. Gynecol. *103*:320–321, 1969.
16. Gurson, C.T., Saner, G.: Am. J. Clin. Nutr. *26*:988–991, 1973.

17. Anderson, R.A., Polansky, M.M., Bryden, N.A., et al.: Diabetes *31*:212–216, 1982.
18. Anderson, R.A., Polansky, M.M., Brantner, J.H., et al.: Chemical and biological properties of biologically active chromium. *In* Trace Element Metabolism in Man and Animals, Vol. II. (Kirchgessner, M., Ed.) Freising-Weihenstephan, West Germany, Arbeitskreis für Tierernährungsforschung, 1978.
19. Mertz, W., Toepfer, E.W., Roginski, E.E., et al.: Fed. Proc. Am. Soc. Exp. Biol. *33*:2278–2280, 1974.
20. Toepfer, E.W., Mertz, W., Polansky, M.M., et al.: J. Agric. Food Chem. *25*:162–166, 1977.
21. Anderson, R.A., Polansky, M.M., Roginski, E.E., et al.: J. Agric. Food Chem. *26*:858–861, 1978.
22. Mertz, W., Roginski, E.E.: Chromium metabolism: The glucose tolerance factor. *In* Newer Trace Elements in Nutrition. (Mertz, W., Cornatzer, W.E., Eds.) New York, Marcel Dekker, Inc., 1971.
23. Anderson, R.A., Brantner, J.H., Polansky, M.M.: J. Agric. Food Chem. *26*:1219–1221, 1978.
24. Anderson, R.A., Polansky, M.M., Brantner, J.H.: Assay and study of biologically active chromium utilizing adipocytes. *In* Chromium in Nutrition and Metabolism. (Shapcott, D., Hubert, J., Eds.) New York, Elsevier Science Publishing Co., Inc., 1979.
25. Okada, S., Ohba, H., Taniyama, M.: J. Inorg. Biochem. *15*:223–231, 1981.
26. Haylock, S.J., Buckley, P.D., Blackwell, L.F.: J. Inorg. Biochem. *18*:195–211, 1983.
27. Mirsky, N., Weiss, A., Dori, Z.: J. Inorg. Biochem. *13*:11–21, 1980.
28. National Research Council: Recommended Dietary Allowances. Washington, D.C., National Academy of Sciences, 1980.
29. Levine, R.A., Streeten, D.H.P., Doisy, R.J.: Metabolism *17*:114–125, 1968.
30. Kumpulainen, J.T., Wolf, W.R., Veillon, C., et al.: J. Agric. Food Chem. *27*:490–494, 1979.
31. Kozlovsky, A.S., Hallfrisch, J., Anderson, R.A.: Fed. Proc. *43*:471, 1984.
32. Offenbacher, E.G., Pi-Sunyer, F.X.: J. Agric. Food Chem. *31*:39–42, 1983.
33. Anderson, R.A., Bryden, N.A.: J. Agric. Food Chem. *31*:308–311, 1983.
34. Koivistoinen, P.: Acta Agric. Scand. Suppl. 22, 1980.
35. Glinsmann, W.H., Mertz, W.: Metab. Clin. Exp. *15*:510–520, 1966.
36. Hopkins, L.L., Jr., Ransome-Kuti, O., Majaj, A.S.: Am. J. Clin. Nutr. *21*:203–211, 1968.
37. Riales, R., Albrink, M.J.: Am. J. Clin. Nutr. *34*:2670–2678, 1981.
38. Mossop, R.T.: Cent. Afr. J. Med. *29*:80–82, 1983.
39. Anderson, R.A., Polansky, M.M., Bryden, N.A., et al.: Metabolism *32*:894–899, 1983.
40. Martinez, O.B., MacDonald, C.A., Gibson, R.S.: Western Hemisphere Nutrition Congress VII, Miami Beach, 1983.
41. Anderson, R.A., Polansky, M.M., Bryden, N.A., et al.: Metabolism (in press).
42. Borel, J.S., Anderson, R.A.: Biochemistry of chromium. *In* Biochemistry of the Elements. (Frieden, E., Ed.) New York, Plenum Publishing Corp., 1984.

*Chapter* **10**

# SELENIUM, CHROMIUM, AND MANGANESE

## (C) MANGANESE

Orville A. Levander

The essentiality of manganese to mammals was discovered in 1931 when it was shown to be necessary for growth in mice[1] and reproduction in rats.[2] A nutritional role for the element has subsequently been demonstrated in several animal species,[3] but evidence for its essentiality to humans is limited to one report.[4,5] Human manganese poisoning was first described in 1837 as a condition in workers that resembled paralysis agitans.[6] Chronic manganese intoxication was considered rare until World War II when increased mining led to an increased incidence of chronic manganism among the miners.[6]

## CHEMISTRY AND MODE OF ACTION

Manganese occurs in many oxidation states, but the manganous ($+2$) and manganic ($+3$) forms are of the greatest biologic interest. In vitro, $Mn^{+2}$ ion can act as a nonspecific divalent metal activator for several enzymes,[7] particularly by substituting for $Mg^{+2}$. The discrepancy between the relatively complete interchangeability of $Mn^{+2}$ and $Mg^{+2}$ in vitro and the great differences in the metabolism of these cations in vivo was resolved by concluding that manganese assumes valences higher than $+2$ in vivo while magnesium does not.[8] Even in vitro, however, $Mn^{+2}$ does not fully replace $Mg^{+2}$ since, for example, manganese decreases the fidelity of DNA synthesis in cell-free assays of DNA polymerases that require the presence of a divalent cation.[9]

The two manganese-containing mammalian metalloenyzmes, pyruvate carboxylase and su-

peroxide dismutase, are both located in the mitochondria, the cellular organelle that contains the highest level of manganese. The former catalyzes an adenosine triphosphate-dependent $CO_2$ fixation to form oxaloacetate, whereas the latter catalyzes the breakdown of superoxide free radicals to hydrogen peroxide and water thereby protecting the cell against peroxidative damage.[7] Manganese can also activate several enzymes known as the glycosyltransferases that catalyze the synthesis of glycosaminoglycans and glycoproteins.[10]

## METABOLISM

A normal 70-kg person contains 12 to 20 mg of manganese.[3] In mammals, the highest concentrations occur in the bones, liver, and pituitary gland (2.5 to 3.3 µg/g) and the lowest in muscle (0.04 to 0.18 µg/g). Manganese levels in human plasma are very low, ranging from 0.4 to 1.0 ng/ml.[11] In the general population, tissue levels remain remarkably constant over most of the life cycle,[12] which suggests adequate dietary intake coupled with effective homeostasis. Manganese is poorly absorbed from the gastrointestinal tract; only about 3% is absorbed in healthy humans.[13] Once absorbed, $Mn^{+2}$ is transported to the liver where a small proportion is oxidized to $Mn^{+3}$, becomes bound to transferrin, and is transported to the tissues.[10] The primary route of excretion is the bile, and little appears in the urine. Although regulation of biliary excretion is considered to be the primary means of manganese homeostasis, it has been suggested that changes in absorption may also play a homeostatic role.[14]

## EFFECTS OF DEFICIENCY AND EXCESS

Several signs of manganese deficiency have been reported in various species of experimental animals. The skeletal defects observed include shortening and thickening or bowing of the long bones, malformation of the skull, enlarged joints, and slipping of the gastrocnemius tendon from its condyles.[3] These bone abnormalities are not caused by impaired calcification but rather by defective synthesis of the mucopolysaccharide organic matrix of cartilage. This failure in mucopolysaccharide biosynthesis is explained biochemically by a decreased activity of glycosyltransferase enzymes important in polysaccharide and glycoprotein synthesis.

The neonatal ataxia of manganese deficiency also appears to result from faulty mucopolysaccharide metabolism.[3] The newborn of manganese-deficient mothers displays incoordination and head retraction owing to poor fetal development of otoliths, the structure of the inner ear responsible for balance. The positive stain for mucopolysaccharides characteristic of normal otoliths is missing in otoliths from deficient animals.[15] This depressed mucopolysaccharide synthesis again is thought to be related to the decreased activity of certain glycosyltransferases. Mice with the mutant gene *pallid* have both a congenital ataxia and abnormal otoliths indistinguishable from those seen in prenatal manganese deficiency.[16] The otolith abnormality of the pallid mice can be prevented by supplementing the diet of the mother with high levels of dietary manganese (1,000 ppm) during gestation.[15]

The deleterious effects of manganese deficiency on reproductive function may be caused by interference with the synthesis of sex hormones.[3] Manganese deficiency also leads to an impaired glucose tolerance in guinea pigs, but the biochemical mechanism of this impairment is unknown.[3] Several ultrastructural abnormalities have been observed in manganese-deficient animals, including enlargement of the Golgi apparatus and disorganization of mitochondrial cristae.[16]

Although manganese deficiency has been produced in every animal species studied,[16] evidence for its essentiality in humans is limited to the experience of one male subject who was fed a chemically defined diet as part of an investigation of vitamin K requirements in people.[4,5] In the course of that study, manganese was inadvertently omitted from the purified diet, which then furnished only about 0.35 mg of manganese per day

over a 17-week period. The subject developed mild dermatitis, reddening of his black hair and beard, slowed growth of hair, nails, and beard, occasional nausea and vomiting, decreased serum phospholipids and triglycerides, and moderate weight loss. During this period, his serum and stool manganese levels decreased 55 and 85%, respectively, as determined by retrospective analysis.

Dietary manganese is of low toxicity to animals, and levels greater than 1,000 µg/g are needed to produce toxic signs.[3] Feeding 3,000 to 5,000 µg of manganese per g diet as various inorganic salts resulted in only a slight growth depression and mild anemia in young chicks.[17] Because hepatic iron levels were depressed in the manganese-treated birds, it was postulated that manganese produced the anemia by blocking iron absorption. In man, manganese toxicity has not been observed as a consequence of dietary intake and is known primarily in miners or workers occupationally exposed to high concentrations of airborne manganese dust or fumes.[6] The clinical features of manganism resemble those of parkinsonism, suggesting that both conditions may have common biochemical abnormalities in the extrapyramidal system of the brain. The successful therapeutic use of L-dopa for both of these diseases indicates that this shared abnormality may be a defect in the metabolism of dopamine.[6] The study of manganese neurotoxicity has been hampered by the lack of a suitable animal model. Recent work, however, suggests that the chronic, extrapyramidal stage of manganism may occur when excess $Mn^{+2}$ is oxidized to higher valences that can potentiate the auto-oxidation of catecholamines, particularly dopamine.[18]

## CLINICAL SITUATIONS INDUCING DEFICIENCY

Manganese deficiency has never been reported in free-living humans. No instance of manganese deficiency has been noted in patients undergoing total parenteral nutrition, but guidelines exist for its parenteral use.[19] Human breast milk is low in manganese.[20] Even though no mechanism for storage of the element during fetal development has been established,[21] no cases of manganese deficiency have been documented in human infants.[22] Low blood manganese levels were reported in children with convulsive disorders and adults with epilepsy,[16] but the clinical significance, if any, of these observations is at present unknown.

## DIETARY CONSIDERATIONS

**Requirements.** Manganese requirements have been estimated by short-term metabolic balance studies. Positive balances were observed in persons receiving 2.5 to 3.0 mg of manganese or more per day.[23,24] Slight negative balances were reported in men given about 2.1 mg per day.[25] The safe and adequate daily dietary intake for adults is 2.5 to 5.0 mg as established by the National Research Council.[26] This range also protects against overexposure to manganese since no evidence of poisoning has been seen in adults habitually consuming 8 to 9 mg per day in their diet.[27] The manganese requirement of the human infant is uncertain. Human breast milk has been reported to contain 4 to 15 $\mu$g/L.[20] Breast-fed infants are in negative manganese balance[28] but, as discussed previously, manganese deficiency has not been recognized in human infants. Increased manganese needs during pregnancy or lactation are likely to be low, and animal studies indicate increased absorption during such physiologic states.[29]

**Food Sources.** Adults consuming self-selected diets in the United States ingested an average of 2.9 mg of manganese per day.[30] Grains, cereals, fruits, and vegetables contain much manganese, whereas dairy products, meat, fish, and poultry contain little. Tea has high levels of manganese,[31] but usual drinking water sources contribute little to the dietary intake.[32] Extrinsically added radiomanganese bound to different ligands in human milk, cow's milk and infant formulas,[33] but little is known regarding the chemical form or nutritional availability of the manganese in foods.

**Interrelationships with Other Nutrients.** Animal studies have shown that manganese has several interrelationships with other nutrients, but its interaction with iron is potentially the most important in terms of possible effects on human health. Hemoglobin repletion in anemic lambs and pigs is impaired by relatively modest dietary levels of manganese, possibly by interference of manganese with iron absorption.[34,35] On the other hand, iron deficiency leads to increased manganese absorption in humans.[13] Thus, iron deficiency could make an individual more vulnerable to manganese toxicity, whereas manganese overexposure might induce anemia by blocking iron absorption.

## EVALUATION OF NUTRIENT STATUS

**Analytical Evaluation.** Whole-blood manganese level was evaluated as an index of total body manganese in rats fed either deficient or adequate dietary manganese.[36] Because the blood levels tended to reflect liver levels, this finding may be a useful means of assessing manganese status. Further work is indicated to determine whether this promising approach is valid in hu-

mans. From the toxicologic point of view, the use of blood as a means of evaluating occupational exposure to manganese has been disappointing.[6]

As analytical techniques have improved over the past 20 years, the concentrations of manganese reported in human plasma or serum have declined by almost two orders of magnitude. It is now generally agreed that a typical concentration of manganese in plasma from healthy subjects is 0.5 to 0.6 ng/ml with an upper limit of about 1.0 to 1.2 ng/ml.[11] Values in the older literature that exceed this limit must be interpreted with caution.

**Biochemical and Clinical Evaluation.** Mitochondrial superoxide dismutase appears to be a promising indicator of manganese status because it responds to dietary manganese intake in rats, mice, and chicks.[37,38] However, its mitochondrial location severely limits its usefulness as a tool for nutritional assessment. Pyruvate carboxylase is not sensitive to manganese deficiency because magnesium replaces manganese in the enzyme with only minor changes in its catalytic properties.[39] Since human manganese deficiency has been described in only one unconfirmed report that was also complicated by concurrent vitamin K deficiency, it is not possible to describe any clinical parameters that can be used to evaluate manganese status.

## REFERENCES

1. Kemmerer, A.R., Elvehjem, C.A., Hart, E.B.: J. Biol. Chem. *92*:623–630, 1931.
2. Orent, E.R., McCollum, E.V.: J. Biol. Chem. *92*:651–678, 1931.
3. Underwood, E.J.: Trace Elements in Human and Animal Nutrition. 4th ed. New York, Academic Press, 1977.
4. Doisy, E.A., Jr.: Micronutrient controls on biosynthesis of clotting proteins and cholesterol. *In* Trace Substances in Environmental Health—VI. (Hemphill, D.D., Ed.) Columbia, University of Missouri Press, 1973.
5. Doisy, E.A., Jr.: Effects of deficiency in manganese upon plasma levels of clotting proteins and cholesterol in man. *In* Trace Element Metabolism in Animals—2. (Hoekstra, W.G., Suttie, J.W., Ganther, H.E., et al., Eds.) Baltimore, University Park Press, 1974.
6. National Research Council: Manganese. Washington, National Academy of Sciences, 1973.
7. Utter, M.F.: Med. Clin. North Am. *60*:713–727, 1976.
8. Cotzias, G.C.: Fed. Proc. *20* (Suppl. 10):98–103, 1961.
9. Goodman, M.F., Keener, S., Guidotti, S., et al.: J. Biol. Chem. *258*:3469–3475, 1983.
10. Leach, R.M., Lilburn, M.S.: World Rev. Nutr. Diet. *32*:123–134, 1978.
11. Versieck, J., Cornelis, R.: Anal. Chim. Acta. *116*:217–254, 1980.
12. Schroeder, H.A., Balassa, J.J., Tipton, I.H.: J. Chronic Dis. *19*:545–571, 1966.

13. Mena, I., Horiuchi, K., Burke, K., et al.: Neurology *19*:1000–1006, 1969.
14. Abrams, E., Lassiter, J.W., Miller, W.J., et al.: J. Anim. Sci. *45*:1108–1113, 1977.
15. Leach, R.M., Jr.: Fed. Proc. *30*:991–994, 1971.
16. Hurley, L.S.: Clinical and experimental aspects of manganese in nutrition. *In* Clinical, Biochemical, and Nutritional Aspects of Trace Elements. (Prasad, A.S., Ed.) New York, Alan R. Liss, 1982.
17. Southern, L.L., Baker, D.H.: Poult. Sci. *62*: 642–646, 1983.
18. Donaldson, J., McGregor, D., LaBella, F.: Can. J. Physiol. Pharmacol. *60*:1398–1405, 1982.
19. AMA Department of Foods and Nutrition: J.A.M.A. *19*:2051–2054, 1979.
20. Lonnerdal, B., Keen, C.L., Hurley, L.S.: Annu. Rev. Nutr. *1*:149–174, 1981.
21. Widdowson, E.M., Dauncey, J., Shaw, J.C.L.: Proc. Nutr. Soc. *33*:275–284, 1974.
22. Lonnerdal, B., Keen, C.L., Ohtake, M., et al.: Am. J. Dis. Child. *137*:433–437, 1983.
23. McLeod, B.E., Robinson, M.F.: Br. J. Nutr. *27*:221–227, 1972.
24. Greger, J.L., Snedeker, S.M.: J. Nutr. *110*:2243–2253, 1980.
25. Spencer, H., Asmussen, C.R., Holtzman, R.B., et al.: Am. J. Clin. Nutr. *32*:1867–1875, 1979.
26. National Research Council: Recommended Dietary Allowances. 9th ed. Washington, National Academy of Sciences, 1980.
27. W.H.O. Expert Committee: Trace Elements in Human Nutrition. W.H.O. Techn. Rep. Ser. No. 532. Geneva, World Health Organization, 1973.
28. Widdowson, E.M.: Trace elements in human development. *In* Mineral Metabolism in Paediatrics. (Barltrop, D., Ed.) Oxford, Blackwell, 1969.
29. Kirchgessner, M., Sherif, Y.S., Schwarz, F.J.: Ann. Nutr. Metab. *26*:83–89, 1982.
30. Wolf, W.R.: Assessment of inorganic nutrient intake from self-selected diets. *In* Human Nutrition Research, Beltsville Symposia in Agricultural Research—4. (Beecher, G.R., Ed.) Totowa, Allanheld, Osmun, 1981.
31. Gillies, M.E., Birkbeck, J.A.: Am. J. Clin. Nutr. *38*:936–942, 1983.
32. National Research Council: The contribution of drinking water to mineral nutrition in humans. *In* Drinking Water and Health, Vol. 3. Washington, National Academy of Sciences, 1980.
33. Chan, W.Y., Bates, J.M., Jr., Rennert, O.M.: J. Nutr. *112*:642–651, 1982.
34. Hartman, R.H., Matrone, G., Wise, G.H.: J. Nutr. *57*:429–439, 1955.
35. Matrone, G., Hartman, R.H., Clawson, A.J.: J. Nutr. *67*:309–317, 1959.
36. Keen, C.L., Clegg, M.S., Lonnerdal, B., et al.: N. Engl. J. Med. *308*:1230, 1983.
37. Paynter, D.I.: J. Nutr. *110*:437–447, 1980.
38. DeRosa, G., Keen, C.L., Leach, R.M., et al.: J. Nutr. *110*:795–804, 1980.
39. Scrutton, M.C., Griminger, P., Wallace, J.C.: J. Biol. Chem. *247*:3305–3313, 1972.

*Chapter* **11**

# ULTRATRACE MINERALS

### Forrest H. Nielsen

Ultratrace minerals are those elements with estimated dietary requirements usually less than 1 μg/g, and often less than 50 ng/g of diets for laboratory animals.[1] At least 14 elements have been suggested to fit in the ultratrace mineral category: arsenic, boron, bromine, cadmium, chromium, fluorine, lead, lithium, molybdenum, nickel, selenium, silicon, tin, and vanadium. The quality of the evidence supporting nutritional essentiality varies widely among the ultratrace elements. In this chapter, an element is considered essential if a dietary deficiency of the element consistently results in a suboptimal biologic function that is preventable or reversible by intake of physiologic amounts of that element. The evidence for the essentiality (initially appearing in the 1950s) of chromium and selenium is substantial and noncontroversial. Their nutritional importance in health and disease is discussed in Chapters 10A and 10B. A critical review of the experimental evidence supporting the suggestion of nutritional essentiality of the other 12 ultratrace elements indicated that only arsenic, molybdenum, nickel, and silicon meet the definition of essentiality.[1] Since that review, substantial evidence has accumulated to indicate that boron is an essential nutrient. These five elements are emphasized in this chapter. In addition, vanadium is discussed because it may have some pharmacologic importance. Only weak evidence supports the nutritional essentiality of bromine, cadmium, fluorine, lead, lithium, tin, and vanadium. However, certain benefits of fluorine are well known. Table 11–1 is a classification summary of the ultratrace elements.

Deficiency in humans has not been described for any of the 12 ultratrace elements, except possibly for molybdenum. Thus, their importance in human nutrition can be inferred only from the results of animal studies. Generally, extrapolation of experimental findings from animals to humans must be done with caution. For the major trace elements (e.g., iron, zinc) that are clearly required by humans, however, signs of deficiency often correspond closely with signs observed in animals. Possibly, therefore, most of the ultratrace elements that are essential for other animals are also essential for humans. Furthermore, some of the deficiency signs and requirements of animals might have counterparts in humans.

The extremely low amounts of ultratrace elements needed to satisfy the requirements of laboratory animals suggest that finding a pure deficiency of any ultratrace element outside the experimental laboratory is unlikely. However, factors other than a simple acute deficiency (Table 11–2) may make these elements of nutritional significance for humans. Persons concerned with human nutrition should be cognizant of this possibility and, therefore, should not consider the ultratrace elements as esoteric when considering the adequacy of diets for health maintenance.

## ARSENIC

**Historic Overview.** Since ancient times, arsenicals have been associated with actions benevolent and malevolent. Very early in the history of arsenic, people found that some arsenic compounds were convenient, scentless, and tasteless instruments for homicide. Thus, for about 1,100

**Table 11–1.  Classification Summary of the Ultratrace Elements**

| Element | Evaluation of Essentiality* | Selected Major or Reported Deficiency Sign† | Possible Need in Normal Function Of/In |
|---|---|---|---|
| Arsenic | E | depressed growth (C,R,P,G) myocardial damage (G) | taurine or sulfate production from methionine |
| Boron | E | depressed growth (C) | major mineral (Ca, P, Mg) metabolism via parathormone |
| Bromine | NE | insomnia? (H) | ? |
| Cadmium | NE | depressed growth? (G,R) | ? |
| Chromium | E | insulin resistance (R) altered lipid metabolism (R,H) | insulin potentiation |
| Fluorine | NE‡ | depressed growth? (M,R) depressed hematopoiesis? (M) | calcified tissue structure |
| Lead | NE | hypochromic microcytic anemia? (R) disturbed iron metabolism? (R) | iron absorption |
| Lithium | PE | depressed growth (G) depressed fertility (R,G) | endocrine regulation |
| Molybdenum | E | depressed growth (C,R,G,P) depressed molybdoenzyme activity (C,R) | xanthine, aldehyde, sulfite oxidase§ |
| Nickel | E | depressed growth (G,P,R,S,B) depressed hematopoiesis (C,R,S,G) | iron absorption; some metalloenzyme |
| Selenium | E | muscle degeneration (B,C,S.) | glutathione peroxidase§ |
| Silicon | E | bone abnormalities (C,R) depressed bone collagen (C) | cross-linking of connective tissue |
| Tin | NE | depressed growth? (R) | ? |
| Vanadium | PE | many reported (C,R), but not one consistently | phosphoryl-transfer enzyme regulation |

*E = essential; PE = probably essential, but further study required to establish essentiality; NE = should not be considered essential at present because evidence for essentiality is weak, has shortcomings, or is questionable.
†Letter in parentheses indicates species: B = bovine-cow; C = chicken; G = goat; H = human; M = mice; P = minipig; R = rat; S = sheep. For citations to original reports describing signs of deficiency, refer to other sources.[1,3]
‡Fluorine should be recognized as an element with beneficial pharmacologic properties (i.e., anticariogenic property).
§Enzyme cofactor function established.

**Table 11–2.  Factors that Influence the Appearance of Trace Element Deficiencies**

1. Amount ingested or given parenterally
2. Biologic effectiveness of form ingested
3. Interactions with other dietary components affecting absorption, transport, retention (utilization, storage), or excretion.
4. Elevated requirements caused by inborn errors of metabolism affecting absorption, retention, or excretion; alterations to metabolism and/or biochemistry as a secondary consequence to malnutrition, disease, injury, or stress; nutrient imbalance; or anabolic demand (growth, pregnancy, lactation).

years, through the nineteenth century, arsenic reigned as the king of poisons. Although arsenic was considered synonymous with "poison," its bad reputation did not prevent it from becoming an important pharmaceutic agent. By 1937, the pharmacologic actions of 8,000 arsenicals had been recorded. Arsenicals were considered at various times to be specific remedies for the treatment of anorexia, other nutritional disturbances,

syphilis, neuralgia, rheumatism, asthma, chorea, malaria, tuberculosis, diabetes, various skin diseases, and numerous hematologic abnormalities. The use of arsenicals for these disorders has either fallen into disrepute or been replaced by more effective alternatives.

The first conclusive evidence for arsenic essentiality was published in 1975 to 1976. Arsenic deprivation signs were described for rats, minipigs, and goats. Subsequently, signs also were described for chickens and hamsters.

For citations to original reports that are the basis for the discussion on arsenic, see reviews.[1–5]

**Chemistry.** Probably the most biochemically important organic arsenic compounds are those that contain methyl groups. Those compounds include arsenocholine, arsenobetaine, and trimethylarsoniumlactate, all of which are relatively nontoxic. Also included are dimethylarsinic acid and methylarsonic acid, which are products of metabolism of various organisms, including humans. Other arsenic compounds of interest are those formed when arsenate esterifies with biologically important molecules. Examples of those compounds are glucose-6-arsenate and ADP-arsenate, which are counterparts of biologically important phosphate esters. Phosphoryl compounds are usually more stable than arsenyl compounds. Under certain conditions, however, arsenate esters are quite stable and might be the form of arsenic that performs an essential function.

**Metabolism.** Orally ingested inorganic arsenate and arsenite are well absorbed. The form of organic arsenic determines whether it is well absorbed. For example, eight days after ingesting flounder containing arsenic, humans excreted in urine more than 75% of the arsenic. In contrast, more than 90% of a dose of sodium-p-N-glycolyl-arsanilate was recovered in the feces within three days. Urinary excretion accounted for only 4 to 5% of the dose.

Only a limited number of studies have examined the mechanisms involved in the intestinal absorption of arsenic. Arsenic as arsenate apparently is absorbed in a manner similar to that of phosphorus as phosphate. In rats, some forms of organic arsenic are absorbed at rates directly proportional to their intestinal concentration over a 100-fold range. This finding suggests that organic arsenicals are absorbed mainly by simple diffusion through lipoid regions of the intestinal boundary.

The excretion of ingested arsenic is quite rapid with both urine and feces serving as major routes of elimination. Organic arsenic that is absorbed apparently undergoes little or no chemical change. Ingested inorganic arsenic appears in urine in both the inorganic and methylated forms. One analysis found the proportions of the forms of arsenic in human urine to be 51% dimethylarsinic acid, 21% monomethylarsonic compound, and 27% inorganic arsenic after an oral dose of inorganic arsenic.

Arsenic retention in persons given [74]As orally as arsenic acid was found to be represented best by a three-component exponential function whose coefficients were 65.9% with a half-life of 2.09 days, 30.4% with a half-life of 9.5 days, and 3.7% with a half-life of 38.4 days. The finding of little retained arsenic after 10 days is similar to findings in some experimental animals. Thus, homeostatic mechanisms, probably involving biomethylation, are present in most higher animals. Under usual circumstances, these mechanisms prevent arsenic accumulation, or retention, in amounts greater than required.

The mechanism whereby mammals methylate arsenic is incompletely understood. Rat liver apparently methylates arsenic in vitro through two different enzymes because monomethylarsonic acid is formed in all subcellular fractions, whereas dimethylarsinic acid is formed primarily in the supernatant fraction of the liver. Both the liver and kidney have been suggested as the major sites of biomethylation.

**Functions and Mode of Action.** The metabolic function, or mode of action, of arsenic is not clearly defined. Recent findings suggest that arsenic might have a role that affects taurine or sulfate production from methionine. Such a role seems reasonable because arsenic affects, or is affected by methyl, and thus methionine, metabolism. Perhaps the effect is through a function in some enzyme system because arsenic has been shown to activate and inhibit enzymes in vitro. It has not been shown, however, to be a specific activator or inhibitor of any enzyme. As an activator, arsenic, as arsenate, probably replaces phosphate in phosphorylation reactions. As an inhibitor, arsenic, as arsenite, apparently exerts its effects on enzymes by reacting with sulfhydryl groups. The presence of arsenocholine, arsenobetaine, and the novel membrane phospholipid O-phosphatidyltrimethylarsoniumlactic acid in marine organisms supports the suggestion that arsenic might have a role related, or similar, to that of lipid phosphorus in biological systems. Further support for this idea is that in higher animals arsenocholine can replace choline in some of its functions. Arsenocholine has an antiperotic and growth-promoting effect in the choline-deficient fowl.

**Deficiency Signs.** Arsenic deprivation has been induced in chickens, hamsters, goats, minipigs, and rats. Studies with goats, minipigs, and rats were done with growing, pregnant, and lactating animals, and with their first- and second-generation offspring. The first signs of arsenic deprivation were seen in $F_1$ offspring and also, for goats, in lactating dams. The most consistent signs of arsenic deprivation were depressed growth and abnormal reproduction characterized by impaired fertility and elevated perinatal mortality. Other notable signs in goats were depressed serum triglycerides and maternal death during lactation. Myocardial damage was present in lactating goats. The organelle of the myocardium most markedly affected was the mitochondria at the membrane level. In advanced stages, the membrane actually ruptured, allowing mitochondrial materials to lie free in the cytoplasm. Other signs of arsenic deprivation have been reported. Listing the signs must be done with care, however, because studies with chicks indicate that the extent, severity, and direction of the signs of arsenic deprivation are affected by the arginine, methionine, and zinc status of the animal.

**Toxicology.** The toxicity of a given arsenical depends upon its rate of excretion from the body and, thus, the degree to which it accumulates in tissues. Arsenicals that are excreted the slowest are the most toxic. The general pattern of toxicity is:

$$AsH_3 > As^{3+} > As^{5+} > R - As - X > As^\circ$$

However, the physical state of the arsenic compound influences its toxicity. For example, with $As^{3+}$, the oral $LD_{50}$ of sodium arsenite and arsenic trioxide in rats was reported to be 24 and 293 mg/kg body weight, respectively. In addition, arsenic trioxide given orally in the solid form is less toxic than compounds given in solution. The estimated fatal acute dose of arsenic trioxide for humans is 70 to 180 mg (about 0.76 to 1.95 mg As/kg body weight of a 70-kg human). This amount is much less than that required to kill rats. A major clinical consequence of chronic excess oral arsenic is hyperkeratosis.

The toxicity of arsenite and trivalent organoarsenicals stems from their ability to react with sulfhydryl groups. The formation of an arylbis (organylthio) arsine inhibits normal tissue protein and enzyme function. Toxicity of arsenate apparently stems from its ability to substitute competitively for inorganic phosphate in phosphorylation reactions, forming unstable arsenyl esters that then spontaneously decompose. Pentavalent organoarsenicals are nontoxic. Elemental arsenic, being insoluble, is for practical purposes nontoxic.

**Dietary Considerations.** Although a specific biochemical function for arsenic is unknown, evidence is strong that arsenic is an essential nutrient. Only data from animal studies are available for estimating the needs of humans. An arsenic requirement of less than 50 ng/g of diet and probably near 25 ng/g was suggested for chickens and rats fed an experimental diet containing 20% protein, 9% fat, 60% carbohydrate, and 11% fiber, minerals, and vitamins. Thus, the arsenic requirement is apparently between 6.25 and 12.5 μg/1,000 kcal. Based on these data, a possible arsenic requirement for humans eating 2,000 kcal would be about 12 to 25 μg daily.

Tabulations of the arsenic content of a number of foods show that most diets provide adequate arsenic if the requirements of humans are similar to those suggested for chickens. Recent surveys indicate that dietary intakes are 20 to 130 μg/day. Diets rich in fish and seafood contain much more arsenic than diets high in dairy products, certain vegetables, and fruits.

The ability of a diet to provide the postulated requirement for arsenic may be influenced by other factors (see Table 11–2). Other nutrients with which arsenic interacts include arginine, methionine, and zinc. In addition, arsenic is an antagonist of selenium and, perhaps, vice versa. Since 1938, when arsenic was found to protect against selenium toxicity, the protective effect has been demonstrated for many animal species under various conditions. The finding that arsenic and selenium each increase the biliary excretion of the other has led to the suggestion that these two elements react in the liver to form a detoxication conjugate that is excreted in bile. If dietary selenium is high, the formation of this conjugate could possibly increase the need for arsenic.

**Clinical Considerations.** Until more is known about the physiologic function of arsenic, it would be inappropriate to associate specific disorders with deficient arsenic nutriture. At present, what is important is to recognize the likelihood that arsenic is essential for humans. Furthermore, although arsenic has been synonymous with poison for centuries and has been associated with the occurrence of some forms of cancer, arsenic is much less toxic than selenium, a trace element with a well-established nutritional value. Thus, the belief that any form or amount of arsenic is unnecessary, toxic, or carcinogenic is unrealistic if not potentially harmful.

## BORON

**Historic Overview.** Between 1939 and 1944, several attempts to induce a boron (B) deficiency in rats were unsuccessful, although the diets used apparently contained only 155 to 163 ng of B/g. In 1945 a report indicated that supplemental dietary boron enhanced survival and maintenance of body fat and elevated liver glycogen in potassium-deficient rats. Those findings were not confirmed in a subsequent study in which rats were fed a different diet with an unknown boron content and different levels of boron supplementation. After those reports, boron was generally accepted as being essential for plants (discovered in 1910, confirmed in 1923), but not for animals. Between 1981 and 1985, however, evidence was accumulated that indicated boron might be an essential nutrient.

For citations to original reports that are the basis for the discussion on boron, the reader is referred to other reviews.[1,6]

**Chemistry.** Boron complexes with organic compounds containing hydroxyl groups; this complexing is best when the groups are adjacent and *cis*. Compounds with more than two hydroxyl groups react more strongly, and the intensity of the reaction increases with the increase in the number of adjacent hydroxyl groups. Thus, boron complexes with many substances of biological interest, including sugars and polysaccharides, adenosine-5-phosphate, pyridoxine, riboflavin, dehydroascorbic acid, and pyridine nucleotides. To date, two naturally occurring organoboron compounds have been identified. They contain boron bound to four oxy groups. These compounds are aplasmomycin, a novel ionophoric macrolide antibiotic that was isolated from strain SS–20 of *Streptomyces griseus,* and boromycin, an antibiotic synthesized by *Streptomyces antibioticus.*

**Metabolism.** Food boron, sodium borate, and boric acid are rapidly absorbed and excreted largely in the urine. Because of variations in the boron dose and length of the study, reported recoveries of ingested boron from the urine ranged from 30 to 92%. For example, in human balance studies in which a 352-mg dose of boron as boric acid was ingested on day one, over 90% of the boron was recovered from the urine at the end of one week. On the other hand, only 40% of a dose of boron ingested by dogs was found in a 24-hour urine collection. Very little is known about the mechanism by which boron is absorbed from the gastrointestinal tract.

**Functions and Mode of Action.** Although conclusive proof has not been presented, many findings support the hypothesis that boron has an essential function that somehow influences parathormone action, and therefore indirectly influences the metabolism of calcium, phosphorus, magnesium, and cholecalciferol. Boron seems to be beneficial in nutritional disorders characterized by secondary hyperparathyroidism, i.e., magnesium deficiency in rats and fluoride toxicity in rabbits.

Boron also may be directly involved in maintaining the functional efficiency of membranes. Most of the evidence for this possible role has come from studies on the function of boron in plants. In one animal study, however, the binding of palytoxin to membranes was potentiated by borate. Palytoxin, an extremely poisonous animal toxin from coral, raises the permeability of excitable and nonexcitable membranes of animals. In addition, aplasmomycin, a novel ionophoric (thus affecting membranes) macrolide antibiotic, is an organoboron compound.

The possibility that boron has a role in some enzymatic reactions cannot be dismissed because boron has been shown to affect the activity of enzymes in vitro and in plants. Borate competitively inhibits two classes of enzymes. One class is the pyridine or flavin nucleotide-requiring oxidoreductases such as aldehyde dehydrogenase, xanthine dehydrogenase, and cytochrome $b_5$ reductase. Borate apparently competes with the enzyme for NAD or flavin because of its great affinity for *cis*-hydroxyl groups. The other class of borate-inhibited enzymes are those in which borate and boronic acid derivatives bind to the active enzyme site. These enzymes include chymotrypsin, subtilisin, and glyceraldehyde-3-phosphate dehydrogenase.

**Deficiency Signs.** Studies defining the signs of boron deprivation are not complete. Therefore, definitively stating deficiency signs is difficult. The most consistent sign of deficiency is depressed growth. Most other reported signs vary in extent, severity, and direction as the diet is varied in content of calcium, phosphorus, magnesium, cholecalciferol, aluminum, and methionine. For example, in one study, dietary boron markedly affected the response of rats to treatments that supposedly cause changes in parathormone activity. Magnesium deficiency, which causes an apparent hyperparathyroid state in rats, depressed growth and elevated the spleen weight/body weight, liver weight/body weight, and kidney weight/body weight ratios. The changes were more marked in boron-deprived than in boron-supplemented rats. Furthermore, the differences due to dietary boron were the greatest when dietary methionine was marginal or possibly deficient.

**Toxicology.** Boron has a low order of toxicity when administered orally. Toxicity signs generally occur only after dietary boron concentration exceeds 100 μg/g. In studies, when boron exceeded 150 mg/L in drinking water, rats exhibited depressed growth, continued prepubescent fur, lack of incisor pigmentation, aspermia, and impaired ovarian development. When the boron content of drinking water was 300 mg/L, rats also exhibited depressed plasma triglycerides, protein and alkaline phosphatase, and depressed bone fat and calcium. In humans, the signs of acute toxicity are well known and include nausea, vomiting, diarrhea, dermatitis, and lethargy, In addition, high boron ingestion induces riboflavinuria. The association between riboflavin status and boron toxicity is not unusual because, in chick enbryos, boron-induced teratogenic abnormalities, including several types of skeletal abnormalities, were reduced by the administration of riboflavin. Other polyhydroxy compounds (D-ribose, pyridoxine•HCl, D-sorbitol hydrate) also reduced or abolished the teratogenic effects of boric acid on chick embryos.

**Dietary Considerations.** The minimum amounts of boron required by animals to maintain health, based on the addition of graded increments to a known deficient diet in the conventional manner, have not been determined. However, based on the finding that rats and chicks sometimes have altered mineral metabolism when fed diets containing 0.3 to 0.4 µg B/g, diets probably should contain more than this level of boron.

The daily intake of boron by humans can vary widely depending upon the proportions of various food groups in the diet. Foods of plant origin, especially fruits, vegetables, and nuts, are rich sources of boron. Wine, cider, and beer are also high in boron content. Meat or fish apparently are poor sources of boron. Recent surveys indicate dietary intakes of 1.7 to 7 mg B/day are average.

**Clinical Considerations.** It is too early to suggest specific disorders in which subnormal boron nutrition is a contributing factor; more information is needed about its physiologic function. However, boron is apparently a dynamic ultratrace element that affects major mineral metabolism in higher animals. Thus, boron nutrition might have a role in some disorders of unknown etiology that exhibit disturbed major mineral metabolism (e.g., osteoporosis).

## MOLYBDENUM

**Historic Overview.** Evidence for the essentiality of molybdenum first appeared in 1953 when xanthine oxidase was identified as a molybdenum metalloenzyme. Subsequently, attempts to produce molybdenum deficiency signs in rats and chickens were successful only when the diet contained massive levels of tungsten, an antagonist of molybdenum metabolism. These studies showed that the dietary requirement to maintain normal growth of animals was less than 1 µg molybdenum/g diet, a level substantially lower than requirements for other trace elements recognized as essential at the time. Thus, molybdenum was not considered to be of much practical importance in animal and human nutrition. Consequently, over the past 30 years, relatively little effort was devoted to studying the metabolic and pathologic consequences of molybdenum deficiency in monogastric animals or humans.

For citations to original reports that are the basis for most of the discussion of molybdenum, the reader is referred to other sources.[7–9]

**Chemistry.** Molybdenum is a transition element that readily changes its oxidation state and can thus act as an electron transfer agent in oxidation-reduction reactions. Animal enzymes known to contain molybdenum are shown in Table 11–3. In the oxidized form of those enzymes, molybdenum is probably present as the 6 + state. Although the enzymes during electron transfer are probably first reduced to the 5 + state, the oxidation state of the completely reduced enzyme is uncertain. Evidence suggests that one or more of the enzymes,

**Table 11–3. Animal Molybdenum Enzymes**

| Enzyme | Substrate | Electron Donor or Acceptor |
|---|---|---|
| Aldehyde oxidase | Aldehydes | $O_2$ |
| Sulfite oxidase | $SO_3^{2-}$ | $O_2$ |
| Xanthine dehydrogenase | Purines | NAD |
| Xanthine dehydrogenase | Purines | Ferredoxin |
| Xanthine oxidase | Purines | $O_2$ |

in the presence of excess substrate, can have molybdenum present in either the 4 + or 3 + state. The molybdenum apparently is present at the active site of the enzyme in a small nonprotein cofactor containing a pterin nucleus. Findings indicate that over 50% of the nonenzymatic form of molybdenum in the liver exists as this cofactor that is bound to the mitochondrial outer membrane. This form can be transferred to an apoenzyme of xanthine oxidase or sulfite oxidase, transforming it into an active enzyme molecule.

In addition to the molybdenum cofactor and/or enzymatic molybdenum, the other important form of molybdenum is molybdate. In herbage, molybdenum is present as sodium, calcium, and ammonium molybdate. Plants also contain some molybdenum sulfide and molybdenum oxide. Evidence suggests that molybdenum in blood and urine exists mainly as the molybdate ion ($MoO_4^{2-}$). Thus, molybdate in food and water apparently is not radically changed by absorption and transport in the blood.

**Metabolism.** Molybdenum (except as $MoS_2$) in foods and in the form of soluble complexes is readily absorbed. In humans, between 25% and 80% of ingested molybdenum is absorbed. Studies with rats indicate that molybdenum absorption occurs in the stomach and small intestine, the rate of absorption being higher in the proximal than in the distal parts of the small intestine. No absorption of molybdenum takes place in the large intestine. Whether an active or a passive mechanism is most important in the absorption of molybdenum is uncertain. One study indicated that at low concentrations of molybdenum its absorption was carrier-mediated and active. Another study showed that in vivo absorption rates were essentially the same over a 10-fold range of molybdenum concentrations. This finding and the finding that the rate of absorption in both stomach and the small intestine was high suggest that the molybdate was absorbed via diffusion only. The possibility exists that molybdate is moved both by diffusion and by active transport, but that at high concentrations the relative intensity of the latter is small. After absorption, molybdenum is rapidly turned over and eliminated as molybdate via the kidney, thus indicating that this, rather than regulated absorption, is the major homeostatic mechanism for this element.

**Functions and Mode of Action.** Molybdenum functions as an enzyme cofactor. Animal molybdoenzymes identified to date are shown in Table 11–3. These enzymes catalyze the transfer of an oxygen atom from water to various compounds. Aldehyde oxidase oxidizes and detoxifies various pyrimidines, purines, pteridines, and related compounds. Xanthine oxidase/dehydrogenase catalyzes the transformation of hypoxanthine to xanthine, and xanthine to uric acid. Sulfite oxidase catalyzes the transformation of sulfite to sulfate.

**Deficiency Signs.** In rats and chickens, molybdenum deficiency, aggravated by excessive dietary tungsten, results in depression of the molybdenum enzymes (xanthine oxidase, aldehyde oxidase, and sulfite oxidase), disturbances of uric acid metabolism, and increased susceptibility to sulfite toxicity. Deficiency uncomplicated by tungsten has been produced in goats and minipigs fed diets containing less than 60 ng molybdenum/g. Deficiency signs were depressed feed consumption and growth, impaired reproduction characterized by elevated mortality in both mothers and offspring, and elevated copper concentrations in liver and brain.

Under field conditions, a molybdenum-responsive syndrome was found in hatching chicks. This syndrome was characterized by a high incidence of late embryonic mortality, mandibular distortion, anophthalmia, and defects in leg bone development and feathering. Skeletal lesions, subsequently detected in older birds, included separation of the proximal epiphysis of the femur, osteolytic changes in the femoral shaft, and lesions in the overlying skin that were ultimately attributed to intense irritation in these areas. The incidence of this syndrome was particularly high in commercial flocks reared on diets containing high concentrations of copper (a molybdenum antagonist) as a growth stimulant. These apparent dissimilar pathologic changes could possibly be explained by a defect in sulfur metabolism. Recognition of the role of molybdenum as a component of sulfite oxidase and evidence that sulfite oxidase deficiency markedly deranges cysteine metabolism suggest that the metabolic consequences of molybdenum deprivation should be reappraised.

The need for this reappraisal is further supported by two recent human studies.[10] A lethal inborn error in metabolism that markedly deranged cysteine metabolism in a patient was determined to be a sulfite oxidase deficiency. Another patient on prolonged total parenteral nutrition (TPN) therapy acquired a syndrome described as acquired molybdenum deficiency.[10] This syndrome, exacerbated by methionine administration, was characterized by hypermethioninemia, hypouricemia, hyperoxypurinemia, hypouricosuria, and very low urinary sulfate excretion. In addition, the patient suffered mental disturbances that progressed to coma. The symptoms were indicative of a defect in sulfur amino acid metabolism at the level of sulfite transformation to sulfate (sulfite oxidase deficiency) and a defect in uric acid production at the level of xanthine and hypoxanthine transformation to uric acid (xanthine oxidase deficiency). Supplementation of the patient with ammonium molybdate improved the clinical condition, reversed the sulfur handling defect, and normalized uric acid production.

**Toxicology.** Large oral doses are necessary to overcome the homeostatic control of molybdenum. Thus, molybdenum is a relatively nontoxic element; in nonruminants, an intake of 100 to 5,000 mg/kg of food or water is required to produce clinical symptoms. Ruminants are more susceptible to elevated dietary molybdenum. The mechanisms of molybdenum toxicity are uncertain. Most toxicity signs are similar or identical to those of copper deficiency (i.e., growth depression, anemia). Signs obviously due to a direct action of molybdenum are not known. However, both occupational and high-level dietary exposures to molybdenum have been linked through epidemiologic methods to elevated uric acid levels in blood and an increased incidence of gout.

**Dietary Considerations.** Minimum dietary requirements for molybdenum in animals and humans are unknown. Thus, human requirements can be estimated only on the basis of balance studies. The National Academy of Sciences has estimated that an adequate and safe intake of molybdenum is 0.15 to 0.5 mg/day.[11] This amount is easily furnished by most diets consumed in the United States. One review estimated that the daily intake of molybdenum from food and water was 0.08 to 0.35 mg, with an average near 0.18 mg/day.[7] Foods highest in molybdenum are milk and milk products, dried legumes, organ meats (liver, kidney), and grain products (cereals, baked goods). Foods lowest in molybdenum are pork, fish, nuts, fats, sweets, and citrus fruits.

Other nutrients and substances that affect molybdenum, and therefore molybdenum requirement and toxicity, include copper, sulfate, manganese, zinc, iron, lead, tungstate, ascorbic acid, methionine, cystine, and protein. The bases for many of these interactions are as yet unexplained. The most important interaction, which is between molybdenum and copper, can be modified by dietary sulfur. The formation of copper tetrathiomolybdates in the gastrointestinal tract apparently is the basis for this interaction. In this compound, copper and molybdenum are unavailable for biologic action.

Another important interaction is between molybdenum and sulfate. Inorganic sulfate inhibits the intestinal absorption of molybdate in the chicken, rat, and sheep. Other findings indicate that elevated dietary sulfate enhances the excretion of molybdenum. Thus, the possibility that high dietary sulfate might induce a molybdenum-responsive syndrome in humans cannot be ignored.

**Clinical Considerations.** Except for the molybdenum-responsive patient with TPN "acquired molybdenum deficiency," there is no indication that molybdenum deficiency is of clinical importance. The existence of this patient, however, suggests that further studies examining for possible molybdenum-responsive syndromes in humans are warranted. These studies also might reveal if some basis exists for the epidemiologic finding that molybdenum levels in foods and water were lower in areas with high incidence of esophageal cancer than in areas with normal incidence.[12]

## NICKEL

**Historical Overview.** The first study of the biologic action of nickel was reported in 1826 when the oral nickel toxicity signs exhibited by rabbits and dogs were described. The first reports on the presence of nickel in plant and animal tissues appeared in 1925. Although nickel was first suggested to be an essential element in 1936, conclusive evidence for essentiality did not appear until 1970 to 1975. Thus, most of the studies on the biochemical, nutritional, and physiologic roles of nickel were done after 1970.

For citations to original reports that are the basis for the discussion on nickel, the reader is referred to other sources.[1,3,13]

**Chemistry.** Both divalent and trivalent nickel forms apparently are important in biochemistry. Divalent nickel forms a large number of complexes encompassing coordination numbers 4, 5, and 6 and all main structural types, which include square planar, square pyramidal, tetrahedral, octahedral, and trigonal pyramidal. Therefore, it is not surprising that nickel complexes, chelates, or binds with many substances of biologic interest and is ubiquitous in all biologic material. The binding of divalent nickel by various ligands probably is important in the extracellular transport and intracellular binding of nickel, and in the excretion of nickel in urine and bile. In some recently identified nickel metalloenzymes from microorganisms, a substantial amount of trivalent nickel was found. Therefore, redox-sensitive nickel may be an important catalytic component, and may represent the binding site for the substrate in some nickel metalloenzymes.

**Metabolism.** Most ingested nickel remains unabsorbed by the gastrointestinal tract and is excreted in the feces. Limited studies indicate that less than 10% of ingested nickel is normally absorbed. A higher percentage, however, may be absorbed in an iron-deficient, gravid, or lactating state. Nickel is apparently absorbed via the iron transport system located in the proximal part of the small intestine and is an energy-driven, rather than a simple diffusion, process. Nickel is transported in blood by serum albumin and by ultrafilterable serum amino acid ligands. No tissue, except possibly fetal tissue and amniotic fluid, significantly accumulates orally administered physiologic doses of nickel. Although fecal nickel excretion (mostly unabsorbed nickel) is 10 to 100 times as great as urinary excretion, the small fraction of nickel absorbed from the intestine and transported to the plasma is excreted primarily via the kidney as urinary low-molecular-weight complexes believed to include histidine and aspartic acid. Urine also contains a nickel-binding glycoprotein that is present in the kidney. The glycoprotein, with a molecular weight of about 15,000 to 16,000, contains 10% carbohydrate (high mannose), and a protein moiety high in glycine and low in cysteine and tyrosine. Only large oral doses of nickel salts can overcome the excellent homeostatic control of nickel.

**Functions and Mode of Action.** No evidence clearly defines the metabolic function or mode of action of nickel in higher animals. Some recent findings, however, indicate that nickel functions as a cofactor or structural component in specific metalloenzymes. This hypothesis was stimulated by the discovery of several nickel-containing enzymes in plants and microorganisms. These enzymes include: (1) urease, which converts urea to carbon dioxide and ammonia, (2) hydrogenases involved in the conversion of hydrogen to methane or water, (3) component C of methyl coenzyme M methylreductase, which reduces $CH_3$-S-CoM to methane and HS-CoM, and (4) a moiety exhibiting carbon monoxide dehydrogenase activity and forming part of a multienzyme complex that catalyzes the reductive carboxylation of methyltetrahydrofolate to acetate. Nickel can activate many enzymes in vitro, but a role as a specific cofactor for any animal enzyme has not been shown.

**Deficiency Signs.** Signs of nickel deprivation have been described for six animal species:

chicken, cow, goat, minipig, rat, and sheep. The most prominent and consistent of these signs include depressed growth and hematopoiesis, and changes in the levels of iron, copper, and zinc in liver. Numerous other signs exhibited by one or more of the six species have been listed. Many of these signs, however, were obtained with animals that apparently were marginally iron-deficient. Further study is needed to establish which of those signs are true indications of nickel deficiency, and which suggest that nickel acted through pharmacologic mechanisms to overcome a limited iron deficiency.

**Toxicology.** Life-threatening toxicity of nickel through oral intake is unlikely. Because of excellent homeostatic regulation, nickel salts exert their toxic action mainly by gastrointestinal irritation and not by inherent toxicity. Generally, 250 μg or more of nickel/g of diet are required to produce signs of nickel toxicity (such as depressed growth) in rats, mice, chickens, rabbits, and monkeys. If animal data can be extrapolated to humans, a daily dose of 250 mg of soluble nickel would produce toxic symptoms in humans.

Some findings, however, suggest that oral intake of nickel in moderate doses could adversely affect health under certain conditions. Moderate levels of dietary nickel exacerbate signs of copper deficiency and severe iron deficiency in rats. Nickel may act similarly in humans. The tendency of the fetus to retain nickel suggests that elevated levels of nickel in blood should be avoided during pregnancy. Finally, evidence suggests that the ingestion of small amounts of nickel may be of greater importance than external contacts in maintaining eczema caused by nickel allergy. An oral dose of nickel (as nickel sulfate) as low as 0.6 mg produced a positive reaction in some nickel-sensitive individuals. That dose is only 12 times as high as the human daily requirement postulated from animal studies (vide infra).

**Dietary Considerations.** Because nickel is essential for several animals, a reasonable hypothesis is that nickel is required by humans also. Moreover, the nickel requirement of animals should suggest the amount of nickel possibly required by humans. For rats and chickens, the nickel requirement apparently is about 50 μg/kg of diet, or 16 μg/1,000 kcal; thus, a suggested dietary nickel requirement for humans would be near 35 μg daily. Limited studies indicate that the oral intake of nickel by humans ranges between 170 and 700 μg/day, an intake that would be ample to meet the hypothetical nickel requirement. Diets based on foods of animal origin and fats may be low in nickel. Rich sources of nickel include chocolate, nuts, dried beans and peas, and grains.

In animals, plants, and microorganisms, nickel interacts directly or indirectly with at least 13 essential minerals. Of the dietary interactions, the one with iron probably is the most significant. An antagonistic interaction occurs between nickel and ferrous iron, perhaps during absorption because they apparently use the same transport system. It seems likely, therefore, that iron nutriture influences nickel metabolism and requirement. That is, high intakes of iron increase and low intakes decrease the nickel requirement.

In rats, copper deficiency signs are exacerbated by nickel. This process presumably occurs through an isomorphous replacement of copper by nickel at various functional sites and not by interference with intestinal absorption of copper. This antagonistic interaction between copper and nickel suggests that high dietary copper might also elevate nickel requirement.

**Clinical Considerations.** Until more is known about the physiologic function of and requirement for nickel, it is inappropriate to suggest specific disorders other than nickel dermatitis as wholly or partially attributable to abnormal nickel nutrition. Imaginative research is needed on the role of nickel in human nutrition. The findings that nickel affects the absorption and metabolism of iron and copper, and that iron and possibly copper influence nickel metabolism, should be helpful in defining situations in which nickel nutriture is of clinical significance.

## SILICON

**Historic Overview.** Silicon was first found in the ash of animals in 1848. In 1901, it was reported that high concentrations of silicon were present in tendons, aponeuroses, and eye tissues. As early as 1911, researchers suggested that silicon might have an anti-atheroma action. Until 1972, however, silicon was generally considered to be nonessential except in some lower classes of organisms (diatoms, radiolarians, and sponges), in which silica serves a structural role. In that year, the first substantial evidence was published that indicated silicon is an essential element for chickens and rats. Most of the limited studies on the biochemical, nutritional, and physiologic roles of silicon have been published since 1974.

For citations to original reports that are the basis for most of the discussion on silicon, the reader is referred to other sources.[1,3,14–19]

**Chemistry.** The chemistry of silicon is similar to that of carbon, its sister element. Silicon forms silicon-silicon, silicon-hydrogen, silicon-oxygen, silicon-nitrogen, and silicon-carbon bonds. Thus, organosilicon compounds are analogues of organocarbon compounds. However, the substitution of silicon for carbon, or vice versa, in organocompounds results in molecules with different properties because silicon is larger and less electronegative than carbon.

In animals, silicon is found both in the free and bound forms. Silicic acid probably is the free form. The bound form has never been rigorously identified. Silicon may be present in biologic material as a silanolate—an ether (or ester-like) derivative of silicic acid. $R_1$-O-Si-O-$R_2$ or $R_1$-O-Si-O-Si-O-$R_2$ bridges may play a role in the structural organization of some mucopolysaccharides.

**Metabolism.** Little is known about the metabolism of silicon. Increasing the intake of silicon increases urinary silicon output up to fairly well-defined limits in humans, rats, and guinea pigs. However, the upper limits of urinary silicon excretion apparently are not set by the excretory ability of the kidney because urinary excretion can be elevated above these upper limits by peritoneal injections of silicon. Thus, the limits apparently are set by the rate and extent of silicon absorption from the gastrointestinal tract. The form of dietary silicon determines whether it is well absorbed. In one study, humans absorbed only about 1% of a large single dose of an alumino-silicate compound, but absorbed over 70% of a single dose of methylsilanetriol salicylate, a drug used in the treatment of circulatory ischemias and osteoporosis. Further evidence that some forms of silicon are well absorbed is the fact that in rats and humans, daily urinary silicon excretion can be a high percentage (close to 50%) of daily silicon intake.[20] Silicon absorption has been found to be affected in rats by age, sex, and the activity of various endocrine glands. The mechanisms involved in intestinal absorption and in blood transport of silicon are unknown.

**Functions and Mode of Action.** Both the distribution of silicon in animals and the effect of silicon deficiency on the form and composition of connective tissue support the view that silicon functions as a biologic cross-linking agent that contributes to the architecture and resilience of connective tissue. The connective tissue components in which silicon apparently plays a fundamental role in the cross-linking mechanism are collagen, elastin, and mucopolysaccharide. Silicon is required for maximal bone prolylhydroxylase activity.[18] This function suggests that silicon is required for bone and cartilage collagen biosynthesis.

Silicon apparently is involved in bone calcification; however, the mechanism of involvement remains unclear. Some findings suggest a catalytic function for silicon. The marked influence of silicon on collagen and mucopolysaccharide formation and structure may result in its indirect influence on bone calcification. In support of this latter view is the finding, in silicon-deficient animals, that the formation of organic matrix, whether cartilage or bone, is apparently more impaired than the mineralization process.

**Deficiency Signs.** Most of the signs of silicon deficiency in chickens and rats indicate aberrant metabolism of connective tissue and bone. Chicks fed a semisynthetic, silicon-deficient diet exhibit skull structure abnormalities associated with depressed collagen content in bone and long-bone abnormalities characterized by small, poorly formed joints and defective endochondral bone growth. Tibias of silicon-deficient chicks exhibit depressed contents of articular cartilage, water, hexosamine, and collagen. In optimally growing chickens, growth is not significantly retarded by silicon deficiency.

**Toxicology.** Silicon is essentially nontoxic when taken orally. Evidence for its nontoxicity is the observation that magnesium trisilicate, an over-the-counter antacid, has been used by humans for more than 40 years without obvious deleterious effects. Other silicates are food additives used as anticaking or antifoaming agents. However, ruminants consuming plants with a high silicon content may develop siliceous renal calculi. Renal calculi in humans may also contain silicates.

**Dietary Considerations.** Although the essentiality of silicon was suggested more than 10 years ago, the form of silicon needed and the minimum requirement for it have not been ascertained for any animal. Therefore, nothing is known about possible human requirements. The estimated requirement of chickens for silicon, as sodium silicate, is in the range of 100 to 200 $\mu$g/g diet, or about 26 to 52 mg/1,000 kcal of an experimental diet. However, other silicon compounds might be 5 to 10 times as effective, per atom of silicon, in preventing nutritional deficiency. Thus, the absolute requirement for chickens (and humans) is probably much lower than 26 to 52 mg/1,000 kcal.

Silicon is ubiquitous and is supplied by many foods, especially unrefined grains of high fiber content, cereal products, and root vegetables. Foods of animal origin, except skin (e.g., chicken), are relatively low in silicon. A human balance study indicated that oral intake of silicon could be about 21 to 46 mg/day.[21]

Several nutrients can affect the absorption or metabolism and, perhaps, the dietary requirement of silicon. These nutrients include fiber, molybdenum, magnesium, and fluoride. In chickens, plasma and tissue silicon levels were markedly and inversely affected by molybdenum intake and vice versa. In young chickens, a severe leg weakness caused by the addition of magnesium and fluoride to the purified diet was associated with large changes in blood and bone silicon concentrations. In humans, silicon balance was significantly lower on a high-fiber than on a low-fiber diet. Apparently, all these nutrients elevate the silicon requirement.

**Clinical Considerations.** Ample evidence indicates that silicon can be accepted as an essential nutrient, but more work is needed to clarify the consequences of silicon deficiency in humans. This need has not prevented speculation that silicon lack is involved in the causation of several human disorders, including atherosclerosis, osteoarthritis, and hypertension, as well as the aging process. Those speculations demonstrate the critical need for studying the importance of silicon nutrition, especially in aging humans.

## VANADIUM

**Historic Overview.** In 1876, Priestley reported on the toxicity of sodium vanadate. It was not until 1912, however, that the first classical paper on the pharmacologic and toxicologic actions of vanadium appeared. At this time, high vanadium concentrations were discovered in the blood of ascidian worms. The hypothesis that vanadium may play a physiologic role in higher animals has had a long and inconclusive history. In the 1940s it was stated that "we are completely ignorant of the physiological role of vanadium in animals, where its presence is constant." In 1963, Schroeder et al. reviewed the early studies on vanadium essentiality and concluded that, although vanadium behaves like an essential trace metal, final proof of essentiality for mammals was still lacking.[22] Between 1971 and 1974, a number of findings reported by four different research groups led many to conclude that vanadium is an essential nutrient. Recently, however, a convincing argument indicates that most evidence presented as proof for the essentiality of vanadium is nothing more than evidence that vanadium has very active in vitro and pharmacologic actions. Because of these actions, interest in the biochemical, nutritional, and pharmacologic roles of vanadium has been stimulated.

For citations to original reports that are the basis for most of the discussion on vanadium, see reviews.[1,3,22–27]

**Chemistry.** The chemistry of vanadium is complex because the element can exist in oxidation states from $-1$ to $+5$ and can form polymers. In biologic systems, the tetravalent and pentavalent valence states are the most important forms of vanadium. The tetravalent state appears most simply as $VO^{2+}$, or the vanadyl cation, and easily complexes with other substances such as transferrin or hemoglobin, which stabilizes it against oxidation. The pentavalent state of vanadium is known as vanadate ($H_2VO_4^-$ or more simply $VO_3^-$). Vanadate forms complexes with other biologic substances, in particular, those with *cis* diols. Vanadate is easily reduced by ascorbate, glutathione, or NADH.

Kustin and Macara stated that three types of behavior could be predicted for vanadium in biologic systems.[24] First, as vanadate, the element competes at the active sites of phosphate-transport proteins, phosphohydrolases, and phosphotransferases. Second, as vanadyl, the element competes with other transition metal ions for binding sites on metalloproteins and for small ligands such as ATP. Third, vanadium participates in redox reactions within the cell, particularly with relatively small molecules that can reduce vanadate nonenzymatically, such as glutathione.

**Metabolism.** Limited information exists about vanadium metabolism at physiologic levels in animals. Nonetheless, it is apparent that most ingested vanadium is unabsorbed and is excreted via the feces. Urine is the major excretory route for absorbed vanadium. Based on the very low concentrations of vanadium normally in urine (0.2 to 0.8 μg/L), in comparison with the estimated daily intake and fecal level of vanadium, $\leq 1\%$ of vanadium ingested is absorbed. However, more evidence is needed to confirm this finding because two studies with rats indicated much greater vanadium absorption ($>30\%$) from the intestine. Dietary composition and vanadium species probably affect the percentage of ingested vanadium absorbed from the intestine. Regardless, the rat studies suggest caution in assuming that ingested vanadium will always be poorly absorbed from the gastrointestinal tract.

Evidence suggests that the binding of the vanadyl ion to iron-containing proteins is important in vanadium metabolism. Regardless of the oxidation state administered to animals, vanadium apparently is converted into vanadyl-transferrin and vanadyl-ferritin complexes in plasma and body fluids. However, it remains to be determined whether ferritin is a storage vehicle for vanadium as well as for iron in the liver and whether vanadyl-transferrin can transfer vanadium through the transferrin receptor.

**Functions and Mode of Action.** To date, no demonstration that vanadium deficiency reproducibly and consistently impairs a biologic function has been shown in any animal. Nonetheless, because vanadium is so active in vitro and pharmacologically, possible biochemical and physiologic functions for the element have been suggested. These functions include:

1. *Regulation of (Na,K)-ATPase and the sodium pump.* In vitro vanadate inhibits (Na,K)-ATPase activity, and reduction of vanadate to vanadyl reverses that inhibition. Because of this action, it was hypothesized that in vivo vanadium might function as a physiologic regulator of sodium pump activity. (Na,K)-ATPase plays a key role in the maintenance of membrane potential and sodium-gradient across the plasma membrane. Such a role would be a more acceptable possibility if an in vivo mechanism, whereby vanadium in tissue is converted from vanadyl to vanadate, could be demonstrated.

2. *Regulation of an ATPase.* A number of ATPases are inhibited by physiologic concentrations of vanadium in vitro. These include $Ca^{2+}$-ATPase, gastric mucosa and colon epithelium $H^+$, $K^+$-ATPase, and myosin ATPase. However, like (Na,K)-ATPase, a regulatory role for an ATPase would seem more likely if an in vivo mechanism whereby vanadium in tissue is converted from vanadyl to vanadate could be demonstrated.

3. *Regulation of phosphoryl transfer enzymes.* Phosphohydrolases and phosphotransferases are inhibited by physiologic concentrations of vanadate in vitro. These types of enzymes include glucose-6-phosphatase, alkaline phosphatase, acid phosphatase, and phosphoglucomutase. The inhibitory action of vanadium on phosphoryl transfer enzymes is quite selective. This selectivity prompts the belief that vanadium has a regulatory role in vivo. However, the vanadate ion, which is inhibitory, is not prevalent in tissue.

4. *Regulation of adenylate cyclase.* Vanadium stimulates the synthesis of cyclic AMP in various cell membranes through the activation of adenylate cyclase. Vanadium apparently activates the adenylate complex by promoting its association with an otherwise inactive guanine nucleotide regulatory protein. However, a physiologic role played by vanadium in regulating adenylate cyclase activity is questionable because the effective concentration needed to affect the enzyme is relatively high—much higher than that normally found in tissue or required for ATPase inhibition.

5. *Vanadyl as an enzyme cofactor.* Other than a possible regulatory role through vanadate and redox mechanisms, vanadium as the vanadyl cation might have a catalytic function or might be a cofactor for some enzyme. When vanadyl replaces other metals in metalloproteins, the metals replaced include $Zn^{2+}$, $Cu^{2+}$, and $Fe^{3+}$; thus it is possible that vanadyl has a role similar to that of these cations.

6. *Role in glucose metabolism.* In vitro studies have shown that vanadium might affect glucose metabolism by altering or mimicking the action of insulin, or by altering the activity of the multifunctional enzyme glucose-6-phosphatase. Insulin-mimetic actions of vanadium contribute to an increased utilization of glucose. Vanadium stimulates glucose oxidation and transport in adipocytes and glycogen synthesis in liver and diaphragm, and inhibits hepatic gluconeogenesis and intestinal glucose transport. Vanadium seems to act like insulin by altering membrane function for ion transport processes. However, whether vanadyl or vanadate is more important in this action is controversial. Insulin stimulatory actions of vanadium are exemplified by the finding that it enhances the stimulatory effect of insulin on DNA synthesis in cultured cells. Vanadate is a potent inhibitor of glucose-6-phosphatase. Because of such a range of in vitro actions on glucose metabolism, it is not surprising that pharmacologic levels of dietary vanadium improved oral glucose tolerance in studies on guinea pigs. Pharmacologic levels of dietary vanadium also prevented an increase in glucose, despite low insulin, in blood, and prevented the decline in cardiac performance of rats made diabetic with streptozocin.[28]

7. *Role in lipid metabolism.* Vanadium at pharmacologic levels has been shown to inhibit cholesterol biosynthesis in human and animal organs. This inhibition was accompanied by decreased plasma phospholipid and cholesterol levels and reduced aortic cholesterol concentrations. In older individuals and in patients with hypercholesterolemia and ischemic heart disease, no such effect from vanadium was apparent, whereas in older rats the inhibition was demonstrated in vitro but not in vivo. The site of the inhibition by vanadium apparently was the microsomal enzyme system referred to as squalene synthetase. In contrast, another study showed that 100 μg V/g diet fed to young chicks increased liver and plasma total lipid and cholesterol levels and plasma cholesterol turnover rate. Thus, de-

pending upon the dose, pharmacologic, toxicologic, or in vitro studies show that vanadium depresses, enhances, or has no effect on the biosynthesis or metabolism of various lipids. Deprivation studies also provide a similar array of findings. These confusing results suggest a role for vanadium that influences lipid metabolism.

8. *Role in bone and tooth metabolism.* Radiovanadium injected into mice or rats is concentrated in the areas of rapid mineralization of bones and tooth dentine. Aqueous solutions of $V_2O_5$ (0.1 mg/kg) given intraperitoneally to rabbits with holes drilled in their mandibles accelerated reparative regeneration of bone by stimulation of ossification. The function of vanadium in developing bone and tooth, if any, is unknown.

**Deficiency Signs.** To date, no sign of vanadium deprivation has been reproducibly or consistently induced in any animal. One of the most recent attempts to establish a reproducible set of signs of vanadium deprivation was a failure. In several experiments with rats fed diets of different composition, vanadium "deprivation" adversely affected perinatal survival, growth, physical appearance, hematocrit, plasma cholesterol, and lipids and phospholipids in liver. Unfortunately, no sign of deficiency was found consistently throughout all experiments. Findings from chick studies were similarly inconsistent. Recent studies suggest that the reported differences between vanadium-deprived and vanadium-supplemented animals in these and other earlier studies were the consequence of high vanadium supplements (10 to 100 times the amount normally found in the diet) that resulted in pharmacologic changes in suboptimally performing animals fed imbalanced diets. The diets used in the early studies had widely varying contents of protein, sulfur amino acids, ascorbic acid, iron, copper, and perhaps other nutrients that affect, or can be affected by, vanadium. In conclusion, no sign of vanadium deficiency can be confidently listed here.

**Toxicology.** Vanadium can be a relatively toxic element to some animal species. However, the concentration of dietary vanadium that is toxic can be affected by dietary composition. A number of substances can ameliorate vanadium toxicity, including ascorbic acid, EDTA, chromium, protein, ferrous iron, chloride, and perhaps aluminum hydroxide. Age and animal species also influence vanadium toxicity. From their in-depth study of vanadium toxicity, Proescher et al. concluded that vanadium was a neurotoxic and a hemorrhagic-endotheliotoxic poison with a nephrotoxic, hepatotoxic, and probably a leukocyto-

tactic and hematotoxic component.[29] Thus, it is not surprising that a variety of signs of vanadium toxicity exist and that they can vary among species and with dosage. Some of the more consistent signs include depressed growth, elevated organ vanadium, diarrhea, depressed food intake, and death. Excessive in vivo vanadium has been suggested to be a factor in manic-depressive illness.

**Dietary Considerations.** Failure to define the conditions that induce reproducible deficiency in animals or that establish an essential function for vanadium prevents any suggestion of a vanadium requirement. However, any human requirement for vanadium would be very small. Diets containing 4 to 25 ng V/g apparently adversely affected chicks and rats only under certain conditions. Since foods contain very little vanadium, the metabolism of which apparently is affected profoundly by other dietary components, vanadium intake may not always be optimal. The daily dietary intake of vanadium is approximately a few tens of μg and may vary widely. One study found that nine institutional diets supplied 12.4 to 30.1 μg of vanadium daily, with intake averaging 20 μg. Foods rich in vanadium include shellfish, mushrooms, parsley, dill seed, black pepper, and some prepared foods.

**Clinical Considerations.** Although vanadium is a pharmacologically and in vitro active element, no primary beneficial pharmaceutical or nutritional role for vanadium has been developed. Perhaps the right questions have yet to be addressed. It would not be surprising to find in the future that vanadium is an element of some clinical or nutritional importance.

## OTHER ULTRATRACE ELEMENTS

The other elements listed in Table 11–1 but not discussed in this chapter need further research to establish essentiality.[1,3] Thus, a complete description of any possible biologic function, nutritional requirement, and clinical consideration seems inappropriate at this time. Nonetheless, the possible deficiency of some yet-to-be-established essential ultratrace element affecting optimal health in humans merits some consideration. Individuals concerned with human nutrition should be cognizant of the possibility. Fortunately, the consumption of a varied diet increases the probability of an adequate supply of all essential micronutrients, including any not yet identified.

## REFERENCES

*1. Nielsen, F.H.: Ann. Rev. Nutr. *4:*21–41, 1984.
*2. Nielsen, F.H., Uthus, E.O.: Arsenic. *In* Biochemistry of the Essential Ultratrace Elements. (Frieden, E., Ed.) New York, Plenum Publishing Corp., 1984, p. 319.

*3. Nielsen, F.H.: Ultratrace elements: Current status. *In* Nutrition Update, Vol. 2. (Weininger, J., Briggs, G., Eds.) New York, John Wiley & Sons, Inc., 1985, p. 107.

*4. Nielsen, F.H., Uthus, E.O., Cornatzer, W.E.: Biol. Trace Element Res. *5*:389–397, 1983.

*5. Anke, M., Schmidt, A., Groppel, B., et al.: Further evidence for the essentiality of arsenic. *In* 4. Spurenelement-Symposium. (Anke, M., Baumann, W., Braunlich, H., Bruckner, C., Eds.) Jena, Friedrich-Schiller-Univ., 1983, p. 97.

*6. Nielsen, F.H.: Other elements: Ba, B, Br, Cs, Ge, Rb, Ag, Sr, Sn, Ti, Zr, Be, Bi, Ga, Au, In, Nb, Sc, Te, Tl, W. *In* Trace Elements in Human and Animal Nutrition, Vol. 2. (Mertz, W., Ed.) New York, Academic Press, 1986, p. 415.

*7. Winston, P.W.: Molybdenum. *In* Disorders of Mineral Metabolism, Vol. 1. (Bronner, F., Coburn, J.W., Eds.) New York, Academic Press, 1981, p. 295.

*8. Mills, C.F., Bremner, I.: Nutritional aspects of molybdenum in animals. *In* Molybdenum and Molybdenum-Containing Enzymes. (Coughlan, M.P., Ed.) Oxford, Pergamon Press, 1980, p. 519.

*9. Spence, J.T.: Reactions of molybdenum coordination compounds: Models for biological systems. *In* Metal Ions in Biological Systems, Vol. 5. Reactivity of Coordination Compounds. (Sigel, H., Ed.) New York, Marcel Dekker, 1976, p. 279.

*10. Abumrad, N.N., Schneider, A.J., Steel, D., et al.: Am. J. Clin. Nutr. *34*:2551–2559, 1981.

*11. National Academy of Sciences: Recommended Dietary Allowances. 9th Ed. Washington, D.C., Food and Nutrition Board, National Academy of Sciences, 1980.

12. Luo, X.-M., Wei, H.-J., Yang, S.P.: J. Natl. Cancer Inst. *71*:65–70, 1983.

*13. Nielsen, F.H.: Nickel. *In* Biochemistry of the Essential Ultratrace Elements. (Frieden, E., Ed.) New York, Plenum Publishing Corp., 1984, p. 293.

*14. Wannagat, U.: Nobel Symposium *40*:447–472, 1978.

*15. Safe Drinking Water Committee: Drinking Water and Health, Vol. 3. Washington, D.C., National Academy of Science, 1980, p. 355.

*16. Carlisle, E.M.: Fed. Proc., Fed. Am. Soc. Exp. Biol. *33*:1758–1766, 1974.

*17. Schwarz, K.: Fed. Proc., Fed. Am. Soc. Exp. Biol. *33*:1748–1757, 1974.

*18. Carlisle, E.M.: Nutr. Rev. *40*:193–198, 1982.

*19. Carlisle, E.M.: Silicon. *In* Biochemistry of the Essential Ultratrace Elements. (Frieden, E., Ed.) New York, Plenum Publishing Corp., 1984, p. 257.

20. Benke, G.M., Osborn, T.W.: Fd. Cosmet. Toxicol. *17*:123–127, 1979.

21. Kelsay, J.L., Behall, K.M., Prather, E.S.: Am. J. Clin. Nutr. *32*:1876–1880, 1979.

*22. Schroeder, H.A., Balassa, J.J., Tipton, I.H.: J. Chron. Dis. *16*:1047–1071, 1963.

*23. Nechay, B.R.: Annu. Rev. Pharmacol. Toxicol. *24*:501–524, 1984.

*24. Kustin, K., Macara, I.G.: Comments Inorg. Chem. *2*:1–22, 1982.

*25. Stoecker, B.J., Hopkins, L.L.: Vanadium. *In* Biochemistry of the Essential Ultratrace Elements. (Frieden, E., Ed.) New York, Plenum Publishing Corp., 1984, p. 239.

*26. Nechay, B.R., Nanninga, L.B., Nechay, P.S.E., et al.: Role of vanadium in biology—symposium summary. Fed. Proc., Fed. Am. Soc. Exp. Biol. *45*:123–132, 1986.

*27. Nielsen, F.H.: Vanadium. *In* Trace Elements in Human and Animal Nutrition. Vol. 2*. (Mertz, W., Ed.) New York, Academic Press, 1986, in press.

28. Heyliger, C.E., Tahiliani, A.G., McNeill, J.H.: Science *227*:1474–1477, 1985.

*29. Proescher, F., Harvey, H.A., Stillians, A.W.: Am. J. Syph. *1*:347–405, 1917.

*Review article.

*Chapter* **12**

# VITAMIN A, RETINOIDS, AND CAROTENOIDS

## James A. Olson

## HISTORICAL OVERVIEW

Night blindness was a well-recognized disease in ancient Egypt. The cure, as expressed in the Papyrus Ebers and the London Medical Papyrus, was to apply topically to the eyes juice squeezed from cooked liver. The ancient Greeks, who were familiar with Egyptian medical practice, recommended the ingestion of cooked liver as well as its topical application.[1] Interestingly, this tradition of applying cooked liver oil or juice topically to the eye has persisted in many societies to this day. The active principle of liver oil or juice, of course, is vitamin A.

In the early part of this century, Frederick Gowland Hopkins in England found that a growth-stimulating principle in milk was present in the alcoholic extract rather than in the ash, and soon thereafter Stepp in Germany identified one of these so-called "minimal qualitative factors" as a lipid. In 1915 E. V. McCollum and Marguerite Davis in Wisconsin showed that butter or egg yolk, but not lard, contained an essential growth factor

for rats. They termed this factor "fat-soluble A." Concomitantly Osborn and Mendel in New Haven found a similar fat-soluble growth factor in cod liver oil and butter. Thus, 1915 marks the beginning of the modern nutritional history of vitamin A.

The fact that active fractions from plant tissues were often colored, whereas those from liver and animal tissues were not, puzzled many investigators during the following decade. This problem finally was resolved when Moore in England showed that β-carotene was converted biologically to a color-less form of vitamin A, which was then stored in liver tissue. In 1930 Karrer and his colleagues in Switzerland determined the structures of both vitamin A and β-carotene. Five years later Wald identified the chromophore of visual pigments as retinene, now termed retinal, thereby defining one of the primary functions of the vitamin. During the 1920s the marked effects of vitamin A deficiency on appetite, growth, and tissue differentiation were also well noted. These early studies on vitamin A are well reviewed in Moore's elegant treatise.[2]

## CHEMISTRY

Vitamin A and over 400 carotenoids have been crystallized and fully characterized by a variety of chemical and physical methods. Furthermore, both vitamin A and many of its analogues, as well as selected carotenoids, have been synthesized chemically from simple, readily available precursors. Mainly because of the structure of conjugated double bonds that are characteristic of both vitamin A and carotenoids, these substances are sensitive to oxidation.

### Nomenclature

The nomenclature of vitamin A and related substances has been revised.[3,4] Vitamin A is now considered chemically as a subgroup of the retinoids, which are defined as a class of compounds consisting of four isoprenoid units joined in a head-to-tail manner and customarily containing five conjugated double bonds. The term vitamin A is used as a generic descriptor for retinoids exhibiting qualitatively the biologic activity of retinol. The numbering system for all-*trans* retinol is depicted in Figure 12–1*A*. Other naturally occurring retinoids of biologic interest, mainly in the all-*trans* form, include retinal (also termed retinaldehyde), retinoic acid, 3-dehydroretinol (vitamin A$_2$), 11-*cis* retinal, 4-oxoretinoic acid, retinyl palmitate, retinyl phosphate, retinoyl β-glucuronide, and retinotaurine (Fig. 12–1*B* to *J*).

The nomenclature of carotenoids primarily is based on β-carotene, or more formally, on β,β-carotene.[4,5] The formulas and numbering system for β-carotene and α-carotene are given in Figure 12–1 *M, N*. The term provitamin A carotenoids is used as a generic descriptor for all carotenoids exhibiting qualitatively the biologic activity of β-carotene.

### Isolation and Synthesis

Vitamin A, mainly in the form of esters, was initially prepared commercially by molecular distillation from extracts of fish liver oils.[2] As early as 1937, however, vitamin A was synthesized from β-ionone, although in poor yield. In 1947 a commercially feasible process was developed by Otto Isler in Switzerland, and later another excellent commercial process, employing the Wittig reaction, was devised by Pommer.[6] Simple compounds, such as acetone, formaldehyde, isobutylene, acetylene, methanol, hydrogen gas, and acetic acid anhydride, are now used as precursors in the complete synthesis of retinol.

Carotenoids, which contain 40 carbon atoms, are commercially synthesized in the presence of suitable catalysts either from two molecules of retinal, a C-20 compound, or from two molecules of a C-19 aldehyde and acetylene.[6] Most, if not all, of the vitamin A and β-carotene available commercially, whether in concentrated solution, stabilized beadlets, or crystalline form, is of synthetic origin. These synthetic compounds are identical in every way, both chemically and biologically, with the same substances isolated from natural sources. Commercially available preparations of vitamin A are almost invariably in the form of fatty acyl esters, i.e., retinyl acetate, propionate, or palmitate, which are more stable than retinol. Stabilized dry forms of vitamin A, which contain an antioxidant in a matrix of gelatin and carbohydrates, are commonly used as supplements in animal feed and can be used as well with humans.

In view of the intense current interest in analogues of vitamin A for the treatment of skin disorders and as possible anticancer agents, many additional retinoids have been synthesized.[7] The formulas of two highly active synthetic retinoids that are *not* found in nature are depicted in Figure 12–1*K, L*.

### Properties

Vitamin A and carotenoids are soluble in most organic solvents but not in water. In their extraction from plasma and tissues, therefore, the cell structure must be disrupted, the proteins denatured, and the lipid fraction dissolved in some solvent, such as hexane or dichloromethane, which is immiscible with water. In crystalline form or when dissolved in oil containing an antioxidant, vitamin A is stable for long periods, providing it is kept in a sealed container under a dry nitrogen or argon atmosphere in the dark. Carotenoids, although somewhat less stable than retinol, are also preserved well under similar conditions.

Vitamin A and the carotenoids are sensitive to oxidation, isomerization, and/or polymerization when dissolved in dilute solution under light in the presence of oxygen, particularly at elevated temperatures. The destruction of these compounds is particularly rapid when they are absorbed as a thin surface film in the presence of light and oxygen.

Vitamin A is stable when stored in frozen liver tissue in the dark below −20°C, and in frozen serum stored in sealed vials under ideal conditions. Carotenoids present in stored frozen serum or tissues tend to be more sensitive than vitamin A to destruction.

Vitamin A has several physical properties that have been used often in its analysis: (1) a char-

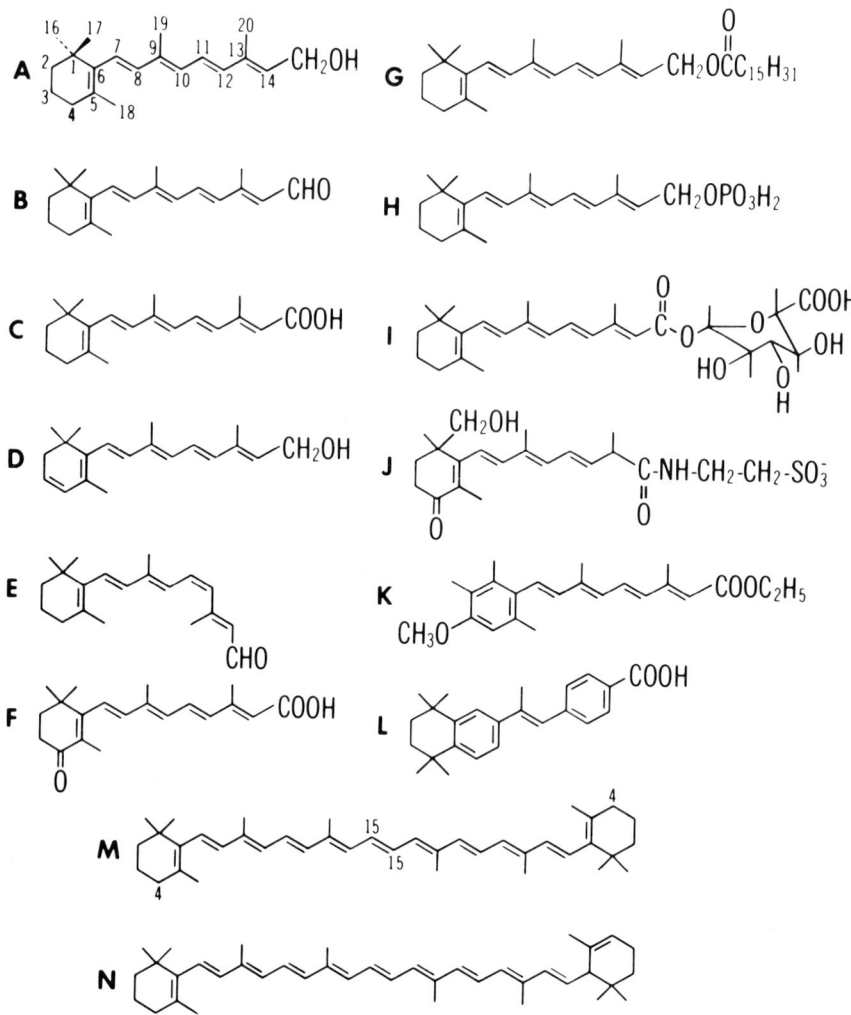

**Fig. 12–1.** Formulas and numbering systems for retinoids and carotenoids. *A,* all-*trans* retinol; *B,* all-*trans* retinal; *C,* all-*trans* retinoic acid; *D,* 3-dehydroretinol (vitamin $A_2$); *E,* 11-*cis* retinal; *F,* 4-oxoretinoic acid; *G,* retinyl palmitate; *H,* retinyl phosphate; *I,* retinoyl β-glucuronide; *J,* retinotaurine; *K,* trimethyl-methoxy-phenyl analogue of ethyl retinoate; *L,* tetrahydro, tetramethyl naphthyl-isopropenyl-benzoic acid; *M,* all-*trans* β-carotene; *N,* α-carotene.

acteristic UV absorption spectrum with a λmax of 325 nm and a molecular extinction coefficient of 53,000 $cm^{-2}M^{-1}$ ($E_{1cm}^{1\%}$ of 1850) in hexane, (2) a greenish fluorescence at 470 nm when excited at 325 nm, and (3) the capability to form a brilliant blue chromophore, albeit transient, at 620 mm when exposed to various Lewis acids, e.g., antimony trichloride, trifluoroacetic acid, and trichloroacetic acid, in anhydrous chloroform.

Carotenoids also show characteristic absorption spectra; β-carotene, for example, has a λmax of 450 nm in hexane with a molecular extinction coefficient of 136,900 $cm^{-2}M^{-1}$ ($E_{1cm}^{1\%}$ of 2550). Under normal laboratory conditions, carotenoids do not fluoresce to any significant extent. Although carotenoids will form colored complexes

with Lewis acids, the intensity is much less than those formed with vitamin A.

Most pure retinoids and many individual carotenoids have been well characterized by UV/VIS absorption spectroscopy, infrared spectroscopy, nuclear magnetic resonance spectroscopy, mass spectrometry, and other physical methods.[7,8]

## BIOLOGIC ACTIVITY

The primary unit of biologic activity for vitamin A is 1 μg of all-*trans* retinol, whether present as the free alcohol or as one of several natural or synthetic fatty acyl esters. Although retinyl esters are more common than retinol in foodstuffs and are almost exclusively present in synthetic preparations of vitamin A, the biologic activity is still calculated in terms of the amount of all-*trans* retinol present.

A unit of historical value, which is still extensively used in food composition tables and in labeling of vitamin A supplements, is the International Unit, or IU. One IU equals 0.300 μg of all-*trans* retinol, or a corresponding amount of retinol in ester linkage. Thus, whether the vitamin A in a given solution is present as free retinol, retinyl acetate, or retinyl palmitate, the number of IU will be the same.

A growing, but still minor, practice is the use of the Système International (SI) units. In such units, retinol is expressed in molar terms, e.g., moles, μM/L, μM/g. Thus, 1 μg retinol is equal to 0.003491 μmoles or, conversely, 1 μmole of retinol equals 286.46 μg of retinol.

Among the 400 or more carotenoids that exist in nature, only about 50 show provitamin A activity. The most active, and often major, provitamin A carotenoid in food is all-*trans* β-carotene. In stimulating the growth of vitamin A-depleted animals, most other provitamin A carotenoids, such as α- and γ-carotene, show biologic activities between 20 and 60%. On the average, other provitamin A carotenoids in foods possess approximately 50% of the growth-promoting action of β-carotene. To express all provitamin A carotenoids as a single unit, the β-carotene equivalent was defined, where 1 β-carotene equivalent equals 1 μg of all-*trans* β-carotene or 2 μg of other, largely all-*trans*, provitamin A carotenoids in foods.

To express *both* preformed vitamin A *and* β-carotene equivalents as a single nutritive value, the retinol equivalent (RE) was created.[9] One RE is equal to 1 μg of all-*trans* retinol in food, or to 6 μg of all-*trans* β-carotene in food, or to 12 μm of other provitamin A carotenoids in foods. Although the ratios are somewhat arbitrary, the logic is as follows: In the biologic conversion of β-carotene to vitamin A, one molecule of the former yields two of the latter, i.e., a weight ratio of precursor to product of approximate unity. Not all ingested β-carotene is converted to vitamin A, however, and the absorption efficiency of synthetic β-carotene is somewhat poorer than that of vitamin A. Thus, a low dose of ingested vitamin A, on a weight basis, is approximately two to four times as efficacious as a low dose of ingested pure β-carotene.[2,10] Carotenoids in foods are less bioavailable, however, than is preformed vitamin A, and the absorption efficiency of carotenoids, unlike vitamin A, falls markedly with increasing doses or dietary amounts. If the bioavailability of vitamin A in food is presumed to be 1.5 to 3 times greater than that of β-carotene, 1 μg of retinol in food would be equivalent to 6 μg β-carotene. In the absence of carefully controlled studies of this conversion ratio in man under normal dietary conditions, the ratio of one to six is an acceptable, albeit arbitrary, value.

However, some confounding factors exist. On the basis of carefully conducted but older experiments in animals, one IU of vitamin A added to a diet was found to be equivalent to approximately 0.6 μg of added β-carotene under optimal conditions of absorption and conversion.[2] Thus, one IU of β-carotene was defined as 0.6 μg and presumed to be equal to one IU of retinol (0.3 μg). Food composition tables have been compiled in large part by simply adding IU from preformed vitamin A and from β-carotene equivalents, although the revision of Handbook 8 expresses values both as total IU and as RE. Confusion exists because the equivalency is different in the two systems: in the RE system one μg retinol equals six μg β-carotene, whereas in the IU system, one μg retinol equals two μg β-carotene. If an IU of retinol is denoted as $IU_a$ and an IU of β-carotene as $IU_c$, where one $IU_a$ equals three $IU_c$, this impasse might be resolved.[11]

The resolution of this issue is of key importance in food labeling and in assessing the vitamin A status of a population.

There is another aspect of relative biologic activity. In vitamin A and all known provitamin A carotenoids, ingested all-*trans* forms are significantly more active than any of the *cis* isomers. All-*trans* retinal is almost as active as all-*trans* retinol, whereas 3-dehydroretinol shows about 40% as much activity. Retinoic acid is active in growth but ineffective in vision and, depending on the species, in reproduction. Interestingly, the synthetic aromatic retinoid depicted in Figure 12–1L is active in growth, but also is highly toxic at somewhat elevated doses.[12]

All provitamin A carotenoids possess at least one unsubstituted β-ionone ring, a structure convertible to it, or a 3-dehydro β-ionone moiety. Reports that β-carotene may play a direct role in enhancing fertility in cattle, independent of the intake of preformed vitamin A, are interesting, but thus far are highly controversial.[13]

## METABOLISM

The metabolism of vitamin A and carotenoids consists of several aspects, namely their digestion and absorption, transport as chylomicra, uptake and storage by the liver, release as holo-retinol-binding protein, intracellular binding, biologic transformation, and excretion. These aspects are considered in the following sections.

## Digestion, Absorption, and Carotenoid Cleavage

In the presence of adequate amounts of fat and protein in the diet, preformed vitamin A and carotenoids are largely released from protein during proteolysis in the stomach. Vitamin A and carotenoids tend to aggregate with lipids into globules, which then pass into the small intestine. The upper intestine is the major site of lipid hydrolysis. Dietary fat, protein, and their hydrolytic products stimulate, via cholecystokinin, the secretion of bile, which first emulsifies lipids and then forms micelles. Bile salts also stimulate both pancreatic lipase, which hydrolyzes triglycerides, and other esterases that hydrolyze retinyl esters and cholesteryl esters. Hydrolysis is an important factor in the bioavailability of vitamin A, inasmuch as retinol in a bile salt-containing micelle is well absorbed (70 to 90%) from the small intestine, whereas retinyl esters are poorly utilized. As already mentioned, carotenoids are not as well absorbed as vitamin A, perhaps in part because of their more fastidious requirements for a suitable micellar suspension.[14,15] Vitamin A seems to be absorbed by a carrier-mediated process at low concentrations, but mainly by diffusion from the micellar phase at high doses.[16]

β-Carotene and most other provitamin A carotenoids are cleaved by a carotenoid 15,15′-dioxygenase in the cytosol of mucosal cells. β-Carotene is cleaved to two molecules of retinal,[17,18] which are in large part reduced and esterified to retinyl ester.[19] The cleavage enzyme requires molecular oxygen and apparently contains a metal, possibly iron, at its catalytic site. Some carotenoids may be cleaved asymmetrically to yield a β-apocarotenal that in turn is converted to retinal. Carotenoid 15,15′-dioxygenase is also present in the liver, the corpus luteum, and possibly in other tissues. At the level of retinal, therefore, which is reversibly reduced to retinol by alcohol dehydrogenases in many tissues, the metabolism of carotenoids and that of preformed vitamin A coincide. Retinol of whatever origin may well be transported through the cytosol of intestinal mucosal cells by a special retinol-binding protein, tentatively termed intestinal CRBP-II.[20]

## Transport in Chylomicra

Within intestinal cells, newly formed chylomicra contain retinyl ester, cholesteryl ester, some retinol, phospholipids, much triglyeride, and apolipoproteins A–1, A–4, B, and several others. In the complex conversion of the secreted chylomicra into chyiomicron remnants in the plasma, the triglyceride content is markedly reduced by the hydrolytic action of lipoprotein lipase, the predominant apolipoproteins on the chylomicron remnant become B and E, and the relative concentration of retinyl ester increases.[21,22]

## Uptake and Storage by the Liver

By interaction with cell surface receptors on liver parenchymal cells for apolipoprotein E, and possibly for apolipoprotein B, chylomicron remnants are internalized by receptor-mediated endocytosis. Retinyl esters are hydrolyzed, combined with cellular retinol-binding protein (CRBP) in the cytosol of the hepatocyte, and then subjected to several possible metabolic routes. In regard to storage, retinol may be directly esterified primarily to retinyl palmitate, which is stored in vitamin A-containing lipid globules in the hepatocyte. Alternatively, retinol may be transferred, probably by means of a specific protein carrier, to stellate cells,[23] where retinol is also esterified and stored in vitamin A-containing globules. Stellate cells have also been termed lipocytes, Ito cells, and fat-storing cells.[24] Under normal physiologic conditions, stellate cells contain 80 to 90% of the stored vitamin A, hepatocytes 10 to 20% and other liver cells only a few percent.[25,25a–c] The retinyl ester stored in lipocytes and hepatocytes can be readily and completely mobilized and utilized by the organism.

## Transport of Retinol on Retinol-Binding Protein (RBP)

Within the hepatocyte, a precursor of RBP, pre-apo-RBP is first formed, which is then proteolytically cleaved, with the loss of a peptide, to apo-RBP.[26] All-*trans* retinol combines with apo-RBP in a specific 1:1 molecular complex to form holo-RBP. The latter is transported through the Golgi apparatus and then is secreted into the plasma. Human RBP is a single polypeptide chain with 182 amino acids in a known sequence[27] and shows a molecular weight of 21,230. Within the plasma, holo-RBP combines in large part with transthyretin (prealbumin), which specifically binds one thyroxine molecule per tetramer.[26]

In adults the total RBP concentration is 40 to 50 μg/ml, 80 to 90% of which exists as holo-RBP.[26] In children up to the age of puberty, the total RBP concentration is approximately 50% of the adult level.[28]

Holo-RBP interacts with cell surface receptors for RBP on target tissue cells, which are mainly epithelial. Retinol is internalized, whereas apo-RBP is modified in conformation and released. This modified apo-RBP no longer binds retinol, no longer interacts with transthyretin, and ultimately is catabolized primarily by the kidney.

Holo-RBP can also be taken up by liver stellate and parenchymal cells.[28a]

## Intracellular and Interstitial Binding Proteins

Cells of most tissues contain a specific binding protein for all-*trans* retinol (CRBP).[29] Most fetal tissues and many adult tissues contain a binding protein for all-*trans* retinoic acid (CRABP).[29] Müller cells of the retina and pigment epithelial cells of the eye possess a fairly specific binding protein for 11-*cis* retinal (CRALBP).[30] Fetal and adult intestine contains a distinct binding protein for all-*trans* retinol (intestinal CRBP–II).[20] Cells of regenerating liver also transiently contain a special binding protein for retinol and retinoic acid, termed CRBP–F.[31] An intercellular binding protein for retinol in the eye, termed interstitial (or interphotoreceptor) binding protein (IRBP), has been identified[32-34] and characterized.[35] Yet a different retinol-binding protein (RBP–S) is secreted from an established cell line (TM–4) of Sertoli cells.[36] The properties of these retinoid-binding proteins are given in Table 12–1. These binding proteins may play a role in the function of vitamin A in differentiation, may serve as intracellular (or intercellular) transport agents for vitamin A, may protect vitamin A from destruction within cells, or may protect cellular structures from the surface-active properties of retinoids. These possible roles, of course, are not mutually exclusive.

## Metabolic Transformations and Excretion

Quite apart from its interaction with specific binding proteins, vitamin A is extensively metabolized in the body. The major reactions, which are summarized in Figure 12–2, are esterification, oxidation at C–15, oxidation at C–4, conjugation, phosphorylation, isomerization, other miscellaneous oxidative reactions, and chain cleavage. Retinol and retinal, as well as other metabolites reversibly converted to them, all possess significant biologic activity. Retinoic acid and its glucuronide are active in growth but not in vision or, in most species, in reproduction. More oxidized products, e.g., 4–hydroxyretinoic acid, 5,6-epoxyretinoic acid, and C–19 metabolites, are largely devoid of biologic activity. Retinoyl β-glucuronide, retinyl β-glucuronide, and retinoic acid are normally present in small amounts (1 to 10 µg/ml) in human plasma.[36a]

Approximately 5 to 20% of ingested vitamin A and a larger percentage of carotenoids, depending on their nature, bioavailability, and amount, are not absorbed from the intestinal tract and consequently are excreted in the feces. A significant portion (10 to 40%) of the *absorbed* vitamin A is oxidized and/or conjugated in the liver and then is secreted into the bile. Although some of these biliary metabolites, such as retinoyl β-glucuronide, are reabsorbed in the intestine and transported back to the liver, most of the biliary metabolites are excreted in the feces. Vitamin A that is oxidized and chain-shortened in various tissues ultimately is excreted in the urine. Finally, carbon dioxide that is released in the oxidation and cleavage of the side chain in vitamin A is excreted in the respired air. In quantitative terms, of the dietary intake of vitamin A, an average of 10% is not absorbed, 20% appears in the feces via the bile, 17% is excreted in the urine, 3% is released as $CO_2$, and 50% is stored, primarily in the liver. Much less is known about the metabolism and excretion of carotenoids.[36b]

## FUNCTIONS

Physiologic fuctions involving vitamin A might be considered from two different perspectives: (1) those processes in which vitamin A shows specific effects, and (2) those processes that are adversely affected by vitamin A deficiency. In the

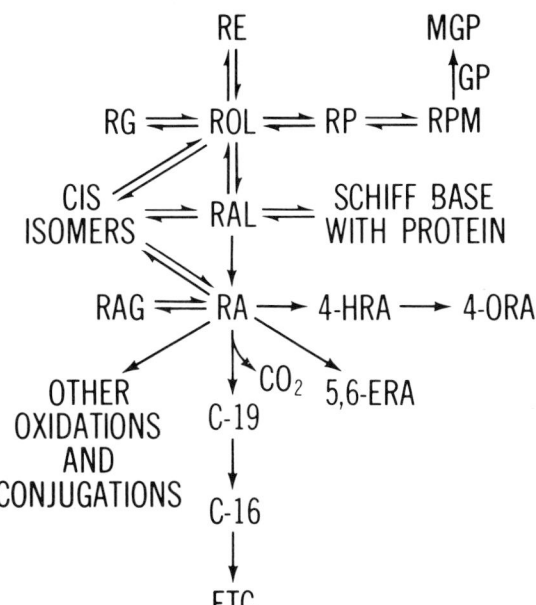

**Fig. 12–2.** Major metabolic transformations of vitamin A. ROL = retinol; RE-retinyl ester; RAL = retinal; RA = retinoic acid; RG = retinyl β-glucuronide; RAG = retinoyl β-glucuronide; RP = retinyl phosphate; RPM = retinyl phosphomannose; GP = glycoprotein acceptor; MGP = mannosylated glycoprotein; 4-HRA = 4-hydroxyretinoic acid; 4-ORA = 4-oxoretinoic acid; 5,6 ERA = 5,6-epoxyretinoic acid; C-19, C-16 = chain shortened, oxidized products with the indicated number of carbon atoms. Double arrows indicate reversible reactions; single arrows denote irreversible changes.

**Table 12–1.  Properties of Retinoid-Binding Proteins**

| Binding Protein | Molecular Weight | Major Ligand | Major Tissue |
| --- | --- | --- | --- |
| RBP | 21,230 | all-*trans* retinol | Synthesized in hepatocytes Circulates in plasma |
| CRBP | 14,600 | all-*trans* retinol | Most tissues |
| CRBP-II (intestinal) | 16,000 | all-*trans* retinol | Many fetal tissues Adult intestine |
| CRBP-F | ~15,000 | all-*trans* retinol and all-*trans* retinoic acid | Regenerating liver |
| CRABP | 14,600 | all-*trans* retinoic acid | Most fetal tissues Many adult tissues |
| CRALBP | 33,000 | 11-*cis* retinal | Müller cells, pigment epithelia |
| IRBP | 249,000 | all-*trans* retinol | Matrix between pigment epithelia and photoreceptor cells |
| RBP-S | ≥70,000 | all-*trans* retinol | Secreted by Sertoli cells (TM-4) |

former category are vision, the proton-pumping capability of *Halobacterium halobium,* and the differentiation of some types of cells. In the latter category are food intake, amino acid metabolism, the differentiation of mucus-secreting cells as well as many other types of epithelial cells, the immunologic system, reproduction, and ultimately the structure and function of most cells and organs of the body. In the latter case, of course, a primary deficiency of vitamin A may give rise to secondary effects that ultimately produce the observed signs of deficiency. Sorting out those abnormalities that are primarily caused by a lack of vitamin A from those that are secondary has not been easy. Consequently, well-defined functions will first be considered, followed by those in which vitamin A has been implicated.

## Vision

The role of vitamin A in vision is well defined.[37,38] In the outer segment of rod cells in the retina, 11–*cis* retinal forms a protonated Schiff base with a specific lysine residue of the membrane-bound protein, opsin, to yield rhodopsin, with an absorption maximum of 498 nm. Similar complexes exist in human cone cells to give three specific iodopsins that absorb maximally at 420 nm (blue cones), 534 nm (green cones), and 563 nm (red cones).[39] When a photon of light strikes the dark-adapted retina, the 11–*cis* bond of retinal in rhodopsin is isomerized to the all-*trans* form. This isomerization destabilizes rhodopsin, which passes through a series of different conformational states and ultimately dissociates into all-*trans* retinal and opsin (Fig. 12–3). Metarhodopsin II and probably other like conformers, but not rhodopsin, may also be phosphorylated by rhodopsin kinase.

All-*trans* retinal may be isomerized back to the 11-*cis* form, either by light in the presence of cer-

tain phospholipids, or in the dark by a yet undefined mechanism. As depicted in Figure 12–3, the isomerization pathway may also involve 11-*cis* retinol as an intermediate. During extensive bleaching, all-*trans* retinal, although possibly oxidized in part to retinoic acid, is largely reduced to retinol, which is transported to the pigment epithelial cell, presumably in a complex with IRBP. Thereafter, retinol can be esterified, mainly to retinyl palmitate, and stored in vitamin A-containing lipid globules similar to those found in liver cells.

Vitamin A in the pigment epithelial cells may also arise from the phagocytosis of rhodopsin-containing discs shed from the rod outer segment, a process subject to a diurnal rhythm,[40] or by receptor-mediated uptake from holo-RBP of the plasma.[41]

During the regeneration of rhodopsin in the dark, the sequence of changes is reversed, i.e., retinyl palmitate is hydrolyzed to retinol, which is transported to the rod outer segment. There it is oxidized and isomerized to 11-*cis* retinal, which then reacts with opsin to form rhodopsin.

The light-activated transformation of rhodopsin ultimately results in a reduction in the sodium ion current into the rod outer segment, which induces hyperpolarization of the membrane. The probable sequence of steps in this amplification cascade[42,43] is summarized in Figure 12–4. In essence, light converts rhodopsin to an active intermediate, probably metarhodopsin II. The latter induces the exchange of GDP for GTP on a disc protein termed transducin. The complex of GTP with transducin activates phosphodiesterase, which in turn hydroylzes cGMP to GMP. As the concentration of cGMP falls, more ionic calcium appears in the cytosol, which blocks the sodium channel and leads to membrane hyperpolarization. The cascade is turned off by the time-

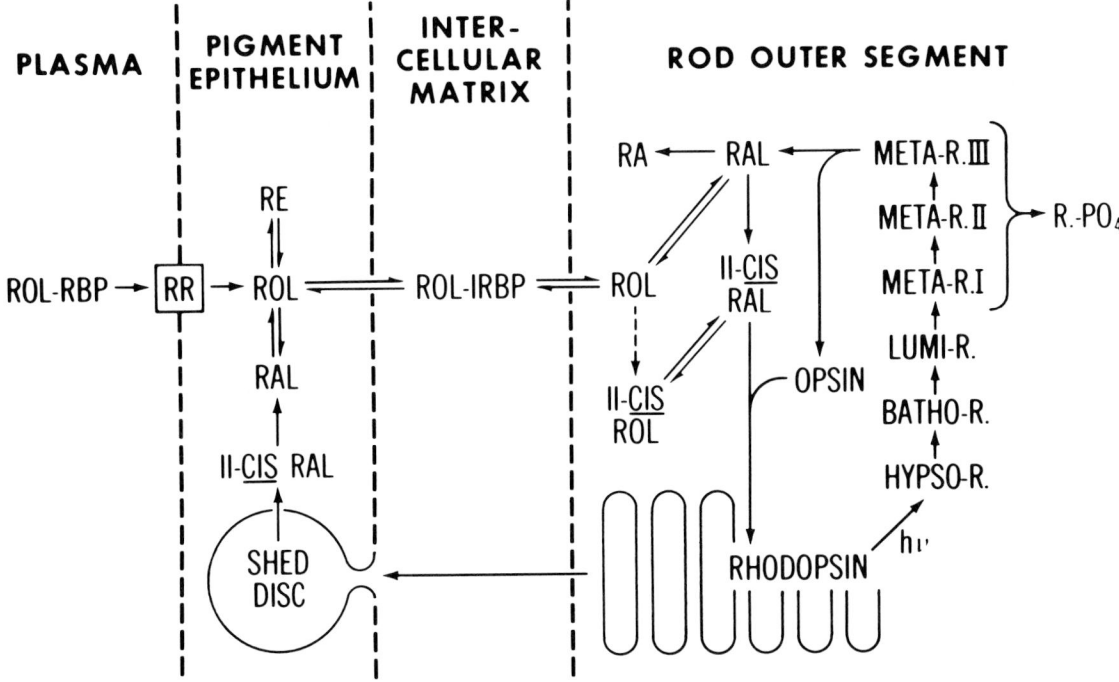

**Fig. 12–3.** Vitamin A metabolism and the visual cycle in the eye. ROL-RBP = holo-RBP; RR = cell surface receptor for holo-RBP on the pigment epithelial cell; ROL = retinol; RE-retinyl ester; RAL = retinal, ROL-IRBP = holo-interstitial RBP; RA = retinoic acid; HYPSO-R = hypsorhodopsin; BATHO-R = bathorhodopsin; R.-PO4 = phosphorylated rhodopsin. All isomers are *trans* unless otherwise noted. Double and single arrows denote reversible and irreversible reactions, respectively.

dependent decay of metarhodopsin II to opsin, by the conversion of metarhodopsin II to an inactive phosphorylated form, and by the hydrolysis of bound GTP by the inherent GTPase activity of transducin.

Bacteriorhodopsin, a light-sensitive, retinal-containing protein similar to rhodopsin, is found in the purple patches on membranes of *Halobacterium halobium*.[44] In response to light, this protein also undergoes a series of conformational changes that are ultimately linked to the transfer of a proton from the cytosol to the external medium.[44] During this cycle, the 13-*cis* and all-*trans* isomers of retinal are involved, however, rather than the 11-*cis* and all-*trans* forms.

### Differentiation

In vitamin A deficiency, mucus-secreting cells are replaced by keratin-producing cells in many tissues of the body.[2,45] Conversely, the addition of

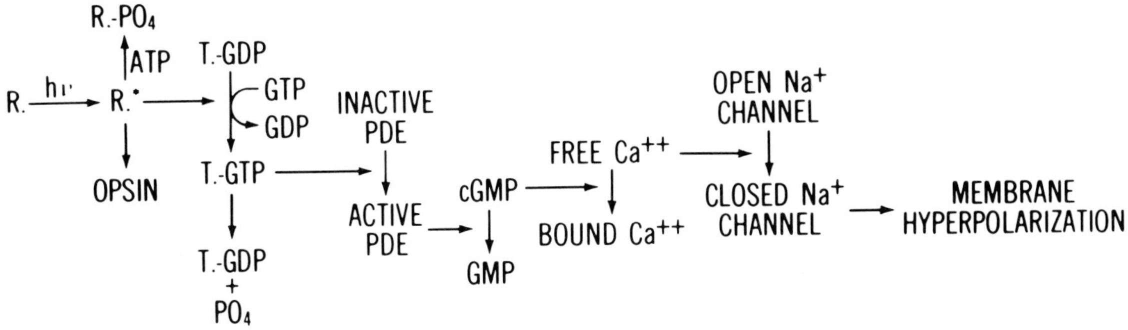

**Fig. 12–4.** A possible sequence of steps between the light-induced activation of rhodopsin and hyperpolarization of the rod cell membrane. R = rhodopsin; R* = light-activated rhodopsin, possibly metarhodopsin II; R-PO4 = phosphorylated rhodopsin; ATP = adenosine triphosphate; GTP = guanosine triphosphate; GDP = guanosine diphosphate; cGMP = cyclic 3′, 5′-guanosine monophosphate; GMP = guanosine monophosphate; T = transducin; T-GDP = a complex of transducin with GDP; T-GTP = a complex of transducin with GTP; PDE = phosphodiesterase.

vitamin A to vitamin A-deficient keratinizing cells in tissue culture induces a shift to mucus-producing cells.[46,47] Retinoids also rapidly induce F–9 teratocarcinoma cells, as well as many other cell lines, to differentiate.[48] In this process, many new proteins appear in the newly differentiated cells. Thus, vitamin A and its analogues, both in vivo and in vitro, markedly influence the way in which cells differentiate.[49,50]

The mechanism by which retinoids produce these changes is far from clear. One attractive hypothesis, defined by Chytil and Ong, is that vitamin A directly affects gene expression.[50,51] In their view, the cellular binding proteins for retinol and retinoic acid play a key role in this process. Their hypothesis is summarized in Figure 12–5. Cytosolic retinol derived from plasma holo-RBP is in part oxidized through retinal to retinoic acid. Then retinol and retinoic acid, in combination with their respective intracellular binding proteins, enter the nucleus and interact with specific sites on chromatin. In this process, the retinoids are bound to chromatin, and the binding proteins are released. These interactions specifically affect the process of transcription, giving rise to a different set of mRNA molecules, which then code for a new group of cellular proteins. Although individual steps in this process are well supported by experimental evidence, it is still unclear whether this is the major or sole way that vitamin A affects cellular differentiation. In this regard, the nucleus clearly is not essential for *all* effects of vitamin A on cells. For example, retinoic acid inhibits the phorbol ester-dependent release of fibronectin both in normal and in enucleated 3T3 cells.[52] Nonetheless, further developments in this hypothesis will be of great interest.

Both in vitamin A deficiency and in tissue culture cells exposed to retinoids, glycoprotein patterns markedly change.[53,54] Of particular interest is the change in cell surface glycoproteins, which are involved in cellular adhesion, interaction with hormones, and intercellular communication. In this regard, retinoids enhance the binding of epidermal growth factor to several cell lines.[55] A molecular mechanism to account for the marked effects of retinol on glycoprotein patterns has been proposed by DeLuca and Wolf.[53,54] The suggested mechanism, already outlined in Figure 12–2, is as follows: Retinol is phosphorylated to retinyl phosphate, which reacts with GDP–mannose to yield retinyl phosphomannose. The latter compound then transfers mannose to an acceptor glycoprotein to produce a specific mannosylated glycoprotein. Some other sugars, such as galactose, may undergo similar reactions, but mannose is clearly preferred. Although the individual steps of the reaction sequence have been well demonstrated, some unresolved issues still remain: (1) that retinoic acid and some aromatic retinoids normalize glycoprotein patterns without directly forming a phosphomannose complex,[49] (2) that the dolichol-dependent glycosylation system is similar to that postulated for retinol, and (3) that the mannosylated glycoproteins formed have not been shown to exert specific effects in differentiation that are in harmony with those produced by vitamin A. Nonetheless, the hypothesis has rightfully drawn

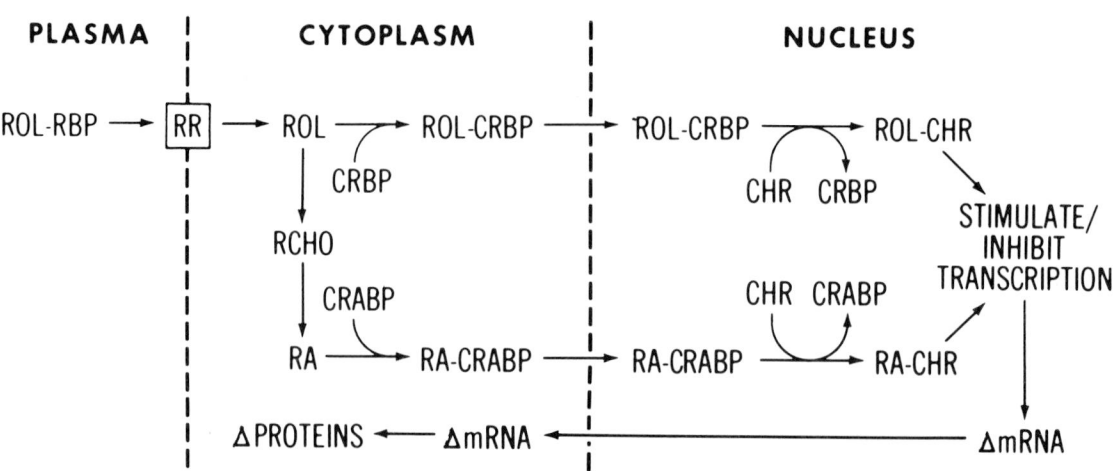

**Fig. 12–5.** The direct interaction genome hypothesis of Chytil and Ong.[50] ROL-RBP = holo-RBP; RR = cell surface receptor for holo-RBP on the target cell membrane; ROL = retinol; RCHO = retinal; RA = retinoic acid; CRBP = cellular retinol-binding protein; CRABP = cellular retinoic acid–binding protein; ROL-CRBP = a complex of ROL with CRBP; RA-CRABP = a complex of RA with CRABP; CHR = chromatin; ROL-CHR = a complex between ROL and a specific site on CHR; RA-CHR = a complex between RA and a specific site on CHR; Δ mRNA = new mRNA molecules produced as a result of ROL and RA interactions with CHR; Δ PROTEINS = new proteins produced from the new mRNA.

much attention to the marked effects of vitamin A on glycoprotein patterns, and currently is the only specific molecular hypothesis of vitamin A action.

All aspects of vitamin A action are not fully explained by either of the two major aforementioned hypotheses. Some other possibilities are that vitamin A may trigger differentiation by creating specific metabolic imbalances, possibly in ions, amino acids, or other essential metabolic intermediates. Vitamin A might also modulate the action of hormones,[56] and it certainly influences the process of embryogenesis.[57] Retinoids may predominantly act at the plasmalemma of cells, inasmuch as HL–60 cells that do not contain detectable amounts of CRABP still differentiate in response to retinoic acid.[57a] Retinoids markedly affect pattern formation in tissues,[58,59] and can be teratogenic.[60,61] Thus, the molecular way or ways that vitamin A affects cellular differentiation and tissue development may still be largely undefined.

### Other Processes

Vitamin A is essential, either directly or indirectly, for the proper functioning of most organs of the body. For example, reproductive processes in both males and females are particularly dependent on adequate vitamin A status. Whether these complex physiologic processes have unique needs for vitamin A or are primarily dependent on the action of vitamin A in cellular differentiation is not clear. Several aspects of the immune system are also affected by vitamin A status, namely, cell-mediated immunity and the complement system.[62] Splenic T-lymphocytes of mice injected with retinoic acid, for example, show enhanced antitumor cytotoxic activity, and augmented allograft responses induced by feeding mice with large doses of retinyl acetate can be passively transferred in Lyt–1 lymphocytes.[63] The possibility that the anticancer effect of retinoids are expressed through their enhancement of the immune system has stimulated much interest in probing the underlying mechanisms of their actions.

### DEFICIENCY

Most vertebrate species, including man, experimental and farm animals, birds, and fish, suffer from vitamin A deficiency. Crustacea and insects also employ retinal as a chromophore in their photosensitive pigments. The signs of vitamin A deficiency in most species are similar.

### Humans

Vitamin A deficiency is a practical nutritional problem among preschool children in southern and southeastern Asia and in parts of Africa and South America.[64–66] It has been estimated that 250,000 preschool children go blind each year in Asia alone.[65] The major signs of vitamin A deficiency in preschool childen are a history of night blindness, low serum vitamin A values, and a sequence of abnormalities of increasing severity in the conjunctiva and cornea of the eye, generically termed xerophthalmia. Severe irreversible changes in the cornea, which ultimately perforates with loss of the aqueous humor, is called keratomalacia. Another corneal abnormality, punctate keratopathy, is often found, even during the early stages of corneal involvement.[65] These pathologic changes in the conjunctiva and cornea have been well documented.[64–67] Use of these eye signs in the diagnosis of vitamin A deficiency is discussed later in the section on the evaluation of vitamin A status.

Why does vitamin A deficiency have such selective and disastrous effects on the cornea? The best explanation, given by Pirie,[68,69] is as follows: In vitamin A deficiency, the plasma vitamin A values fall, and as a consequence the amount of holo-RBP diffusing into the cornea decreases.[70] Mucus-secreting cells of the cornea and conjunctiva tend to disappear,[67] and the first eye signs become evident. Leukocytes that contain acidic and neutral proteases as well as elastase infiltrate into the corneal stroma, which concomitantly becomes edematous and shows peripheral vascularization. Proteases released from invading leukocytes hydrolyze collagen and other structural proteins in the cornea, with an increase in hydroxyproline release and a decrease in the strength of the fiber network supporting the cornea. At a certain point, the latter perforates and collapses.

Other factors contribute to corneal destruction. Human tears contain a discrete amount of glycoprotein as well as approximately 2 μg retinol/dl,[71] both of which fall markedly in vitamin A deficiency. The lack of glycoprotein in the tear fluid lowers the break-up time of the liquid layer bathing the cornea and allows dry areas (xerosis) to appear. The cells in such areas consequently are prone to attack by both bacteria and viruses. Finally, a general state of malnutrition, although not necessary for the eye changes caused by vitamin A deficiency, must certainly exacerbate the condition.

The night blindness resulting from vitamin A deficiency can be readily explained. As plasma vitamin A values fall to low levels, the amount of vitamin A in the pigment epithelium and in the retina declines. As a consequence, less rhodopsin is formed. Because the sensitivity of the dark adaptation response is directly proportional to the amount of rhodopsin in the rod outer segment, night blindness results. Protein-calorie malnutrition and zinc deficiency, which also lowers the rhodopsin content of the eye,[72] exacerbate the condition.

Vitamin A deficiency also produces skin changes in humans, namely follicular hyperkeratosis and phrynoderma. Because other nutritional deficiencies produce similar skin disorders, these changes are not useful as unique indicators of vitamin A deficiency. Nonetheless, vitamin A is necessary for the maintenance of skin. Normally, vitamin A in the form of holo-RBP diffuses into the dermis and epidermis from capillaries in the skin.[73] Upon entering cells of the skin, retinol and its oxidation product, retinoic acid, are bound by CRBP and CRABP, respectively. Under normal conditions, human keratinocytes synthesize keratins with molecular weights of 40,000 and 52,000, as well as many others.[74] When vitamin A is absent, these "small" keratins are replaced by larger keratins (molecular weight ≥67,000) characteristic of the stratum corneum.[74] Hair follicles, particularly sensitive to vitamin A, become obstructed and enlarged in the deficient condition. In all likelihood, vitamin A deficiency sets in motion a large number of changes in skin structure and metabolism that ultimately lead to the observed pathologic signs.

## Other Species

The albino rat has been most extensively studied as a model for vitamin A deficiency. To differentiate between direct effects of vitamin A deficiency and secondary changes resulting from generalized malnutrition, rats have been cycled on retinol-free diets containing retinoic acid for 18 days followed by diets free of both retinol and retinoic acid for 10 days.[75,76] After five or six cycles, the animals became exquisitely sensitive to removal of retinoic acid from the diet. Retinoic acid was used because, unlike retinol, it is not stored in the liver and other tissues but is completely metabolized and excreted within a day. In such animals, the sequence in which deficiency signs appear[77,78] is listed in Table 12–2. Three major phases are noted: (1) the early period, characterized by reduced food intake and some histologic defects, (2) the mid-period, in which many abnormalities in cellular differentiation, responsiveness to drugs, and metabolism appear, and (3) the late phase, in which neuromuscular defects and other physiologic abnormalities in many tissues and processes become evident. By use of this technique, these signs can be directly attributed to vitamin A deficiency, which clearly can affect

**Table 12–2.** Sequence in the Appearance of Signs of Vitamin A Deficiency in Rats Cycled on Retinoic Acid

| Sign | Day of Onset |
|---|---|
| Lowered food intake | 1–2 |
| Plateau in weight | 2–3 |
| Decreased intestinal goblet cells | 2–3 |
| Marked weight loss | 6–8 |
| Enhanced taurine excretion | 6–8 |
| Reduced sensitivity to pilocarpine | 6–8 |
| Augmented tracheal metaplasia | 6–8 |
| Periocular porphyrin deposits | 6–8 |
| Decreased salivary secretion | 9–10 |
| Inadequate stomach emptying | 12 |
| Neuromuscular defects | 12 |
| Increased susceptibility to infection | 12 |

nearly all tissues of the body. Similar signs of vitamin A deficiency have been noted in most other affected species by conventional dietary procedures.[2]

## EXCESS

In amounts several times higher than the recommended dietary allowances (RDA), preformed vitamin A causes toxicity in man and animals.[79,80] Two toxic syndromes exist: acute and chronic. Acute toxicity is produced by a single very large dose of vitamin A, or several doses taken during a short period, whereas chronic toxicity is caused by the recurrent ingestion of smaller, but still large, doses. Teratogenic effects, leading to spontaneous abortion, birth defects, and permanent learning disabilities, occur from lower doses, particularly when taken in early pregnancy. The excessive dietary intake of carotenoids does not produce hypervitaminosis A, but rather a benign, albeit sometimes preoccupying, condition known as hypercarotenosis. Large daily therapeutic doses of some carotenoids can cause retinopathies when taken chronically.

## Humans

When a single dose of ≥ 200 mg of vitamin A (≥660,000 IU) is ingested by adults or of ≥ 100 mg (≥ 330,000 IU) by children, nausea, vomiting, headache, increased cerebrospinal pressure, vertigo, blurred (double) vision, muscular incoordination, and (in infants) bulging of the fontanelle may occur. These signs are generally transient and subside within one to two days.[79–81] When the dose is very large, drowsiness, malaise, inappetence, reduced physical activity, skin exfoliation, itching, particularly around the eyes, and recurrent vomiting soon follow. Finally, when lethal doses are given to young monkeys, which incidently are an excellent model for vitamin A toxicity in the human, deepening coma, convulsions, respiratory irregularities, and finally death from either respiratory failure or convulsions finally ensue.[81] The $LD_{50}$ value of vitamin A injected intramuscularly in a water-miscible form in the young monkey is 168 mg retinol/kg body weight.[81] Extrapolated to a 3-kg child and a 70-kg adult, the total $LD_{50}$ dose would be 0.5 and 11.8 g, respectively. Because a newborn child receiving 25 mg daily (8 mg/kg) for 11 days died of apparent vitamin A toxicity,[81a] monkeys seem to be more tolerant of vitamin A than are humans. Such enormous amounts of vitamin A are present only in high-potency preparations of vitamin A or in large amounts (~1 kg) of livers particularly rich in vitamin A ($\geq$10 mg/g).

Chronic toxicity is induced by the recurrent in-

**Table 12–3. Toxic Signs Attributed to Chronic Vitamin A Toxicity**

Alopecia
Anemia
Anorexia
Ataxia
Bone pain
Brittle nails
Cheilitis
Conjunctivitis
Dermatitis
Diarrhea
Diplopia
Dysuria
Edema
Elevated CSF pressure
Epistaxis
Exanthema
Fatigue
Fever
Fontanelle bulging
Headache
Hepatomegaly
Hepatotoxicity
Hypercalcemia
Hyperlipemia
Hyperostosis
Insomnia
Irritability
Membrane dryness
Menstrual irregularities
Muscular pain
Nausea
Negative N balance
Nervous ailments
Papilledema
Petechiae
Polydipsia
Premature epiphyseal closure
Pruritus
Pseudotumor cerebri
Skin desquamation
Skin erythema
Skin rash
Skin scaliness
Vomiting
Weight loss

take of vitamin A in amounts at least 10 times the RDA, i.e., 4.2 mg retinol (14,000 IU) for an infant or 10 mg retinol (33,300 IU) for an adult. A health food enthusiast who ingested daily 25,000 IU of vitamin A as a supplement plus 25,000 IU in food showed severe signs of toxicity.[81b] Signs of chronic toxicity, reported in over 200 patients,[79] are summarized in Table 12–3. Clearly all symptoms do not appear in all patients, and the relative severity of the signs varies widely in different individuals. Upon elimination of the supplemental intake of vitamin A, these signs also disappear over a period of weeks to months.

In chronic hypervitaminosis A, holo-RBP in the plasma is not elevated, whereas retinyl esters are increased often markedly.[26,81c] Retinyl esters, being transported by plasma lipoproteins, can react more randomly with the membranes of cells than the physiologically sequestered retinol bound in holo-RBP. Thus, circulating retinyl esters, by disrupting membrane functions, may well be a major toxic form of vitamin A. Administered retinoic acid and other acidic retinoids, however, although not forming similar esters, are nonetheless equally, if not more, toxic than vitamin A. The toxicity of retinoids is probably caused by their interaction at several cellular loci. Physiologic conditions or disease that enhance the plasma levels of lipoprotein-bound retinyl ester, therefore, may well increase the risk of vitamin A toxicity.

Vitamin A and other retinoids are powerful teratogens, both in experimental animals[82] and in women.[83,83a–83d] A single very large dose, exposure for as short as a week on high daily doses (30 to 90 mg), or chronic daily intakes of 25,000 IU (7,500 RE) during early pregnancy can induce spontaneous abortions or major fetal malformations. Common defects are craniofacial abnormalities, including microcephaly, microtia and harelip, congenital heart disease, kidney defects, thymic abnormalities, and central nervous system disorders. Permanent learning disabilities have been noted in otherwise normal rat pups whose dams received nonteratogenic doses of vitamin A.[83e,83f,83g] Synergism between vitamin A and other teratogens, such as alcohol and drugs, at nonteratogenic doses of each is probable. A safe daily intake of vitamin A during pregnancy has not been defined.[83h] Thus women who are pregnant, or who might become so, should carefully control their intake of vitamin A, both in regard to rich food sources, such as liver, and vitamin A supplements.

The International Vitamin A Consultative Group has formally taken the position that the diet of healthy, well-nourished pregnant women should supply the recommended dietary intake of 9.3 RE/kg body weight + 100 RE or a total of 675 RE (2,250 IU) daily for a 62–kg woman.[83i] Only in populations in which the vitamin A status is demonstrably poor should daily supplements of vitamin A not exceeding 3,000 RE (10,000 IU) be considered for pregnant women.[83i] Vitamin A deficiency, just like its excess, interferes with the reproductive process.

Because of the widespread and increasing use of large doses of retinoids, including vitamin A, for the treatment of various skin disorders and some types of cancer, retinoid toxicity will increasingly be encountered. Doses of vitamin A that have been tolerated by most patients undergoing these treatments are 1.3 to 1.6 mg retinol/kg/day, or approximately 200,000 IU/m$^2$/day.[84,85] Other retinoids, such as etretinate and isoretinoin, show toxic signs at similar doses.[80] The major toxic signs observed in these patients are cheilitis, conjunctivitis, and dryness of the mucous membranes. Upon lowering the treatment dose, the discomfort lessens. Because of the teratogenic action of retinoids, fertile women treated with large doses of retinoids should employ rigorous contraceptive practices during treatment and for several months and perhaps as long as two years after the termination of therapy.[85a]

### Other Species

Hypervitaminosis A has been described in many domestic animals, including chickens, pigs, and calves.[2] The signs of toxicity are similar to those described previously for primates. Although adult rats are particularly resistant to hypervitaminosis A, large doses of retinoids given to the pregnant dam induce many congenital malformations in rat fetuses.

### Hypercarotenosis

Individuals who routinely ingest large amounts of carotenoids, such as are found in carrot juice, tomato juice, and red palm oil, may be affected by hypercarotenosis. The condition is characterized by hypercarotenemia and carotenodermia, a yellow jaundice-like coloration of the skin that is particularly evident in the nasolabial folds, the fat pads of the palms of the hands, and the fatty areas on the soles of the feet. The sclerae of the eyes are clear in hypercarotenosis, unlike jaundice. Insofar as is known, the condition is completely benign and slowly disappears upon removing the carotenoid-rich foods from the diet. Patients with erythropoietic protoporphyria and related disorders who ingest large daily therapeutic doses of canthaxanthin (50 to 100 mg) for long periods, however, often show a mild retinopathy.[85b] Hyper-

vitaminosis A does *not* result from the excessive intake of carotenoids, primarily because of the relatively slow rate of conversion of carotenoids into vitamin A. It should be stressed, however, that this conversion rate is fully adequate to meet nutritional needs.

## HIGH-RISK CLINICAL SITUATIONS

Newborn infants contain low reserves of vitamin A in the liver, e.g., median values of 11 µg retinol/g in one American study[25] and 24 µg/g in a Brazilian study.[86] When appropriately nourished, essentially all infants show adequate liver reserves ($\geq$ 20 µg retinol/g) by one year of age.[25] Premature infants, although showing at birth the same median value of liver reserves as term infants, seem to deteriorate in vitamin A status over the first two months of life.[25,87] Because orally administered vitamin A may not be utilized well in premature infants, this group seems to be at special risk.

Fat malabsorption syndromes, such as cholestasis, cystic fibrosis, sprue, chronic diarrhea, pancreatic insufficiency, and biliary cirrhosis, markedly reduce the digestion and absorption of vitamin A and carotenoids, and ultimately lead to a state of vitamin A depletion. The effects of these disorders are more marked in young children, who possess limited vitamin A reserves and need vitamin A for growth, than in adults. Nonetheless, adults with chronic malabsorption problems of long duration can also be affected, particularly if their diets are low in vitamin A and carotenoids.

Subjects nourished for long periods by means of total parenteral nutrition conventionally receive vitamin A in the infusion fluid. Because variable amounts of the vitamin A present can be adsorbed on the plastic delivery tubing, the vitamin A status of these individuals should receive careful attention.

The liver clearly is of primary importance in the storage and utilization of vitamin A. The chronic ingestion of alcohol, even in relatively small amounts, tends to reduce vitamin A storage.[88] In clinical cases of alcoholism, both the storage of vitamin A and the structure of the liver are markedly affected.[89] In this condition, stellate cells tend to disappear, and fibroblasts increase in number. Thus, it is not surprising that the abnormal dark adaptation response found in many alcoholic subjects is usually ameliorated by administration of vitamin A.[90] Other liver poisons, such as halogenated hydrocarbons, and some drugs, such as phenobarbital, also lower liver reserves of vitamin A.[91] Cadmium and other heavy metals, which predominantly affect tubular reabsorption in the kidney, cause a marked excretion of holo-

RBP in the urine.[92] Other kidney disorders with decreased glomerular and tubular functions give rise to *increased* plasma levels of holo-RBP because of reduced metabolism of RBP in the kidney.[26,92a]

Although estrogens and estrogen-containing contraceptives cause a significant increase in the steady-state concentration of holo-RBP in the plasma,[93] the rate of mobilization of vitamin A from liver reserves is only slightly affected.[94] Thus, in otherwise well-nourished women, the routine use of contraceptive agents does not significantly affect their vitamin A requirement.

No serious genetic defects in the metabolism and utilization of vitamin A and carotenoids have ever been identified. Some young children do seem to metabolize carotenoids rather slowly, however, which produces mild hypercarotenosis on relatively normal intakes of carotenoids. With increasing age, this condition tends to disappear. Some individuals also seem to be particularly susceptible to hypervitaminosis A at generous but not excessive intakes of the vitamin. In one case, for example, a reported daily supplement of 1.5 mg (5,000 IU) of retinol, given regularly for five years in addition to vitamin A in the food, induced toxic signs and a serum vitamin A value of 1,500 $\mu$g/retinol/dl in a 10-year-old boy.[95] The author presumed that the clearance of vitamin A from the plasma was defective, thereby giving rise to toxicity at only a slightly elevated intake. Such reports, however, are rare.

As discussed previously, the significant teratogenic risk of increased vitamin A intakes during early pregnancy, and particularly of supplements of vitamin A and of other retinoids, should be carefully noted.

## DIETARY CONSIDERATIONS

The average daily intake of vitamin A by adults in the United States has been estimated to be approximately 5,400 IU in a national food consumption survey conducted in 1977,[96] and approximately 4,750 IU in a national survey carried out from 1971 to 1972.[97] The most recent national nutrition survey conducted between 1976 and 1980 reported mean and median intakes of 5,150 IU and 3,320 IU, respectively.[98] Based on an analysis of 50 foods that contributed most to vitamin A intake in this survey, researchers concluded that 44% of the total IU was derived from preformed vitamin A and 56% from provitamin A carotenoids.[98a] Thus, the mean and median intakes of vitamin A in the United States are approximately 1,000 RE and 620 RE, respectively, of which carotenoids and preformed vitamin A contribute approximately 25% and 75%, respec-

tively, of the total. During the decade from 1970 to 1980, the mean and median intakes of vitamin A in the United States have not appreciably changed.

### Human

Table 12–4 summarizes the recommended daily dietary allowances (RDA) for selected age groups for vitamin A, determined in 1980 by the Food and Nutrition Board (FNB) of the United States Academy of Science,[99] and the recommended dietary intakes (RDI) for vitamin A, set by joint expert committees of the Food and Agriculture Organization (FAO) and of the World Health Organization (WHO) in 1967, republished in 1974,[9] and in 1986.[99a]

Recommended dietary allowances (or intakes) are usually defined as the amount of nutrient, expressed as the average daily intake over a period of several weeks, that meets the nutritional needs and is consistent with the good health of most persons in the selected population group.[99,100] Ideally, the recommended dietary allowance would indicate the amount of a given nutrient that would meet the needs of over 97% of the population considered, i.e., a mean value plus two standard deviations.

For most nutrients, including vitamin A, the standard deviation for humans falls in the range of 12 to 25% of the mean requirement. Thus, a safety factor of 25 to 50% is conventionally used. The mean requirement can be defined operationally in several ways, namely, as the average daily amount needed: (1) to prevent the appearance of signs of vitamin A deficiency; (2) to maintain normal growth in children; (3) to cure the signs of vitamin A deficiency in depleted subjects over a specified period; (4) to provide a specified total body reserve of the vitamin in order to minimize the effects of occasional periods of low intake, infections, and other stresses; and (5) to ensure maximal body reserves, but without producing signs of toxicity. The amounts required clearly will increase from criterion 1 to 5, and any definition might be selected as the basis for the RDA (RDI).

Because of the multiplicity of possible definitions, the most recent FAO/WHO recommendations include a "two-tier" system of values: the basal dietary requirement (BDR), which meets criteria 1 and 2 in children and 1 to 3 in adults, and the RDI, which additionally meets criterion 4.[99a] Criterion 5 has not been used for vitamin A, although it has been considered for some other nutrients. The *curative* dose (criterion 3) will certainly be greater than the *preventive* dose (criterion 1), largely because the former must be

**Table 12–4.** **Recommended Daily Dietary Allowances (or Intakes) of Vitamin A in Retinol Equivalents\***

| Category | Age | FNB[†] 1980 | FAO/WHO 1967 | FAO/WHO 1986[‡] BDR[†] | RDI | BW[†] |
|---|---|---|---|---|---|---|
| Infants | 0–½ | 420 | 300 | 120–170 | 350 | 5.5 |
| | ½–1 | 400 | 300 | 180 | 320 | 9 |
| Males | 15–75 + | 1000 | 750 | 325 | 605 | 65 |
| Females | 15–75 + | 800 | 750 | 275 | 510 | 55 |
|   Pregnant | | + 200 | 0 | | + 100 | |
|   Lactating | | + 400 | + 450 | | + 350 | |

\*One retinol equivalent equals 1 μg retinol, 6 μg β-carotene, or 12 μg other provitamin A carotenoids in foods.
†FNB = Food and Nutrition Board RDA
‡BDR denotes a basal dietary requirement, RDI a recommended dietary intake with a storage reserve, and BW the midperiod body weights of reference individuals in kg.

used to rebuild tissues and to restore processes in addition to preventing their deterioration. The mean curative dosage in adult humans is approximately 5 μg/kg/day,[99a,100] whereas the preventive dose, although not yet quantitatively determined, may well be half or even less of that amount.

The recommendations given in Table 12–4 clearly differ considerably, primarily because different criteria were used in setting them. The FAO/WHO value for adults in 1967 was primarily based on the daily amount of retinol required to cure signs of vitamin A deficiency and to raise plasma vitamin A levels in vitamin A-depleted human volunteers.[101] Because 440 μg retinol given daily for 60 days did not induce further improvement, 750 μg was selected as a suitable recommended intake, i.e., by use of a generous safety factor of 70%.[101]

The 1980 (and 1974) RDA values of the FNB were based on the observations that 600 μg retinol given daily for 11 to 15 days cured all signs of deficiency in adult male subjects and raised their plasma values to approximately 20 μg/dl. To raise plasma retinol values closer to 30 μg/dl, however, 1,200 μg were required daily for 9 to 14 days.[10] Although mean plasma vitamin A values in healthy American adults are homeostatically controlled from 40 to 65 μg retinol/dl,[101b] restoration of the complex control process after severe vitamin A depletion is both slow and often unresponsive to low levels of intake.[11] Thus, the *curative* doses of 300 μg retinol for most clinical signs of deficiency and of 600 μg retinol for all signs, including the raising of the plasma retinol level close to 20 μg/dl, seem to be more appropriate dosage levels for recovery than the higher doses needed to reactivate the homeostatic control system. A safety factor is not specifically cited in those recommendations.

A new and different approach was used by FAO/WHO in 1986,[99a] namely the selection of an adequate body reserve of 20 μg/g liver, calculation of the amount of dietary vitamin A required to maintain that reserve, and the use of a safety factor of 1.40. The resultant RDI was 9.3 μg dietary retinol/kg/day. For the representative adult male (76 kg) and female (62 kg) in the United States, the RDI values would be approximately 700 RE and 600 RE, respectively. These values accord well with the median dietary intake values previously noted.

The relationship between the RDA and the actual intake of total vitamin A in a population is rendered somewhat uncertain, unfortunately, by the somewhat arbitrary ratio of 6:1 set for the relative biologic activities of β-carotene and retinol in foods, a point discussed earlier in this chapter.

For infants, the RDA of the FNB is based on a presumed mean breast milk volume of 840 ml and a mean milk concentration of 50 μg retinol/dl.[99] If a more realistic mean breast milk volume of 750 ml is assumed, the RDA would be 375 RE.[11] A safety factor is not included in the calculation, inasmuch as no signs of inadequate vitamin A status have been observed in breast-fed infants ingesting this quantity of vitamin A.

## Other Species

The requirements and recommended intakes of vitamin A have been defined for a large number of experimental and domestic animals. In general, the requirement for maintenance and growth of young animals, regardless of size, is approximately 15 RE (50 IU)/kg/day.[2] Maintenance requirements alone, based both on preventive and on curative studies, are 3 to 6 RE/kg/day.[101a] To induce storage and to ensure maximal fertility and longevity, higher amounts must be given. In the United States, the mean recommended levels of vitamin A in the feed of various animals, expressed as RE/kg feed are: cats (3,000), poultry (2,400), horses (2,000), swine (1,500), cattle, sheep, dogs, foxes, and fish (1,300), and rats and mice (1,200). In Europe, the recommended levels of vitamin A in feeds are approximately twice as high.

## Food Sources

Good food sources of vitamin A and carotenoids are listed in Table 12–5. A particularly rich source of carotenoids, although ingested primarily only in parts of Western Africa and Brazil, is red palm oil, which contains 0.2 to 0.8 mg of α- and β-carotene/ml.[2] In regard to vitamin A, liver oils of marine mammals and of fish may contain up to 300 mg retinol/g oil.[2] Although cod liver oil was once given as a vitamin A supplement, this practice has largely been replaced by the use of pills containing either multivitamins or vitamin A alone. Perhaps up to 30% of selected groups in the American population use such supplements.

In one American survey, major ingested food sources of all forms of vitamin A, expressed in RE, were milk and dairy products (31%), vegetables and fruits (22%), the meat group (16%), fats, oils, and fortified margarines (10%), grain (9%), eggs (8%), and miscellaneous foods (4%).[96] The vitamin in the grain group is present largely as preformed vitamin A added to grain products. In contrast, carotenoid-containing foods are by far the major source of ingested vitamin A in much of the less industrialized world.[65]

## Nutrient Interrelationships

The efficient absorption of vitamin A and carotenoids is dependent on the presence of fat in the diet, both in its stimulation of bile flow and in the formation of micelles suitable for absorption. Dietary protein is also necessary for the normal metabolism and transport of vitamin A. In protein-calorie malnutrition, for example, both carotenoid cleavage activity in the intestine and the synthesis and release of plasma RBP are depressed.[102] Thus, the addition of protein alone to the diet of protein-deficient but vitamin A-sufficient children can markedly increase plasma vitamin A levels.[100] A deficiency of iron, as expressed in anemia, and vitamin A deficiency are associated epidemiologically. In physiologic terms, vitamin A may affect the release of stored iron from the liver.[102] The clinical signs of zinc deficiency and of vitamin A deficiency are similar in many ways, e.g., hyper-

keratosis, reduced food intake, and night blindness. At a molecular level, zinc seems to be necessary for the formation of proteins essential for vitamin A function, such as plasma RBP and opsin.[72,102] Protein synthesis seems to be generally affected, however, rather than only those proteins involved in the metabolism and binding of vitamin A.[102] In vitamin E deficiency, vitamin A is poorly absorbed from the intestinal tract and is poorly stored in the liver. Vitamin E is known to stabilize lipid-containing membranes, particularly those with high concentrations of unsaturated fatty acids, such as the disc membranes of the rod outer segment. Thus, vitamin E is probably acting as an antioxidant in protecting vitamin A, both in the intestinal lumen and within cells.[102] Vitamin E also enhances the esterification of vitamin A in the liver and inhibits the hydrolysis of retinyl esters.[102a]

## EVALUATION OF VITAMIN A STATUS

Vitamin A status can be evaluated by biochemical, physiologic, and clinical procedures. Various criteria will first be considered, followed by discussion of the biochemical methods used.

### Criteria

Vitamin A status can be classified into four categories: poor, marginal, acceptable, and excessive.[100] As shown in Table 12–6, which primarily relates to preschool children, each category can be assessed by different criteria.[103] Outside of clinical eye signs, which will be considered later, night blindness is often present in young children suffering from vitamin A deficiency. Because quantitative measurement of the dark adaptation threshold in young children is not feasible, a history of night blindness, obtained by interviewing the mother, has been found in Indonesia to correlate well both with low plasma vitamin A values and with clinical eye signs.[65] Plasma vitamin A values are diagnostic of vitamin A deficiency when very low (<10 μg/dl) and of hypervitaminosis A when high (>100 μg/dl). In the latter case the presence of significant amounts (>50%) of circulating retinyl ester in fasting plasma is confirmatory of a hypervitaminotic state. In regard to

**Table 12–5. Good Common Food Sources of Preformed Vitamin A and Provitamin A Carotenoids**

| *Preformed Vitamin A* | *Provitamin A Carotenoids* | |
| --- | --- | --- |
| Liver | Carrots | Tomatoes |
|  |  | Yellow maize |
| Whole eggs | Spinach | Papayas |
| Whole milk | Yams | Ripe mangoes |
| Chicken meat | Dark green leaf lettuce | Oranges |

**Table 12–6.  Indicators of Vitamin A Status in Preschool Children**

| | | | Vitamin A | | | | |
|---|---|---|---|---|---|---|---|
| Status | Eye Signs | Night Blindness | Plasma μg/dl | Breast Milk* μg/dl | Liver μg/g | Diet RE/day | RDR† % |
| Poor | Present | Present | <10 | <10 | <5 | <100 | ≥50 |
| Marginal | Absent | Absent | 10–20 | 10–20 | 5–20 | 100–300 | >20 |
| Adequate | Absent | Absent | 20–100 | 20–100 | 20–300 | 300–2,000 | <20 |
| Excessive | Some‡ | Absent | >100 | — | High | >5,000 | — |

*Nursing infants only.
†Relative dose response.
‡Conjunctivitis; different from signs of deficiency.

breast milk, a suggested minimally adequate concentration of vitamin A for nursing infants is 20 μg/dl.[103] In this regard, when lactating women in Guatemala ingested sugar fortified with vitamin A, the percentage with milk vitamin A values below 20 μg/dl fell from 39 to 11%.[103]

Because the liver is the major repository of vitamin A in the body, direct measurement of liver stores indicates vitamin A status. Median values of liver vitamin A concentrations in well-nourished adult individuals in many countries are approximately 100 μg retinol/g.[86] A suggested adequate reserve, both for adults and children, is 20 μg of retinol/g.[86,103,104] Lower liver stores are associated with increased risk of deficiency. The amount of dietary vitamin A required for preschool children is a function of their age, size, and rate of growth. Certainly intakes of <100 RE/day are inadequate for all preschool children, and intakes of 100 to 300 RD/day may prevent the appearance of clinical signs but would not lead to increased reserves. For adequate intakes, a presumed safe range (300 to 2,000 RE) is given in Table 12–6, but the upper limit is admittedly arbitrary. Toxicity may well appear at intakes ≥5,000 RE (≥16,700 IU) in this age group. This value is also arbitrary, in that toxic signs may not appear at much higher daily intakes in many in-

dividuals, but may be found at lower intakes in some persons.[95]

The relative dose response (RDR), a technique developed by Underwood and co-workers,[105] is a useful indicator of marginal vitamin A status. The principle of the method is as follows: When vitamin A stores in the liver are low, apo-RBP accumulates in the hepatocyte.[106] After the oral administration of a small dose (450 μg) of vitamin A in oil, the holo-RBP concentration of the plasma rapidly rises to a plateau at approximately 5 hours. The increment in plasma retinol levels betwen 0 and 5 hours divided by the retinol value at 5 hours, and then multiplied by 100, yields the RDR value as a percentage. Values above 50% have been noted in vitamin A-depleted children[107] as well as in vitamin A-deficient rats, whereas values above 14 to 20% have been found in adult subjects with night blindness correctable with vitamin A[108] or with liver reserves below 20 μg/g.[109]

The most frequently used indicators of vitamin A deficiency in children are the clinical eye signs. The classification scheme of such signs, adopted by the World Health Organization,[110] is given in Table 12–7. In the same table, the diagnostic usefulness of each sign is indicated, and the prevalence values of selected indicators in a preschool age population that should arouse public health

**Table 12–7.  Classification of Clinical Eye Signs and Associated Changes Characteristic of Vitamin A Deficiency**

| Code | Condition | Diagnostic Use | Prevalence Limits (%) |
|---|---|---|---|
| X1A | Conjunctival xerosis | Nonspecific | |
| X1B | Bitot's spot with conjunctival xerosis | Useful in very young children | 0.5 |
| X2 | Corneal xerosis | Useful | |
| X3A | Corneal ulceration/keratomalacia (<⅓ of corneal surface) | Useful | 0.01 |
| X3B | Corneal ulceration/keratomalacia (≥⅓ of corneal surface) | Useful | |
| XN | Night blindness | Qualitative use | |
| XF | Xerophthalmia fundus | Not employed | |
| XS | Corneal scars | Uncertain specificity | 0.05 |

concern are noted.[66,110] A prevalence of $\geq$ 5% of preschool children with plasma values <10 μg retinol/dl is also an approved WHO criterion for public health concern.[66,110] Suggested prevalence values of public health concern for the other indicators listed in Table 12–6 are night blindness (1%), breast milk values <20 μg/dl (15%), liver vitamin A concentrations <5 μg/g (3%), and liver vitamin A concentrations <20 μg/g (15%).[103] The disappearance of goblet cells from the conjunctiva of the eye, which is dramatic in the vitamin A-deficient rabbit, may also prove to be useful in diagnosing vitamin A deficiency in children.[110a]

Vitamin A deficiency in adults is rare, except when associated with some genetic disease, such as cystic fibrosis, with severe defects in lipid absorption, as in cholestasis, severe intestinal disease, or resection, or with liver malfunction, as in alcoholic cirrhosis. The percentile distribution of total vitamin A values in plasma as a function of age and sex in apparently healthy individuals in the United States[101b] is set forth in Table 12–8. Clearly, few values in children are below 20 μg/dl. In adult American patients suffering from liver cirrhosis, however, impaired dark adaptation has been associated with plasma values below 40 μg/dl.[110b] Because the mean plasma retinol values of healthy adults in many countries fall below 40 μg/dl, a cutoff vaue of universal utility cannot be set. Nonetheless, within the United States, an expert panel on vitamin A nutriture has suggested that plasma total vitamin A values of 30 μg/dl or higher are generally consistent with good health. They have also presented some guidelines, summarized in Table 12–9, for interpreting lower plasma values in the United States.[101b] It must be stressed that these suggested guidelines, particularly those for adolescents and adults, are based primarily on the frequency distribution of serum vitamin A values, that the population studied was healthy and well-nourished, and that these American guidelines may or may not be generally relevant to other countries or to specific sociocultural groups.

## Methods

Methods used for the analysis of vitamin A in plasma, milk, tissues, and foods include high-pressure liquid chromatography (HPLC) linked to a UV detector, UV spectrophotometry with ultraviolet inactivation, colorimetry using one of several Lewis acids, and fluorescence assay. These methods have been reviewed, both as survey[103] and as research[111] techniques. Although all methods can give valid results under proper conditions, the HPLC procedure for the analysis of retinol in serum by using a reverse-phase column[112] is preferred at present. A reverse-phase gradient HPLC system is of particular use as well in analyzing retinol and the pattern of retinyl esters in liver samples.[113,113a]

Results obtained by using different methods can be influenced, sometimes markedly, by the following: (1) UV spectrophotometry, by the absorption of other unsaturated compounds at 325 nm; (2) colorimetry, by the formation of colored complexes with carotenoids and other unsaturated compounds, particularly in frozen samples; and (3) fluorescence, by the presence of other highly fluorescent substances, and particularly of phytofluene, in the samples. The conditions of storage of samples over long periods can also markedly affect the values obtained.[111] Thus, if aberrant results are obtained with any selected method, possible sources of error must be carefully assessed.

Carotenoids have conventionally been analyzed in serum and foods by their absorption at 450 nm in an organic solvent after the chromatographic separation of major carotenoid classes, e.g., hydrocarbons or oxygenated analogues.[114] This procedure, although valuable, clearly does not allow suitable estimates to be made of individual provitamin A carotenoids in foods.[103,115] The use of HPLC is at present providing new and more accurate information about the carotenoid content of foods.[115–117] Food composition tables that are revised by employing these new values will be

**Table 12–8. Percentile Distribution of Total Vitamin A Values in the Serum of Apparently Healthy Individuals in the United States***

| Age in Years | Males | | | Females | | |
|---|---|---|---|---|---|---|
| | *3rd* | *50th* | *97th* | *3rd* | *50th* | *97th* |
| 3–5 | 20 (19) | 35 (31) | 64 (63) | 20 (17) | 35 (29) | 60 (54) |
| 6–11 | 23 (20) | 36 (33) | 61 (52) | 24 (20) | 37 (33) | 60 (51) |
| 12–17 | 29 | 45 | 68 | 27 | 43 | 68 |
| 18–44 | 37 | 58 | 92 | 29 | 49 | 85 |
| 45–74 | 37 | 64 | 108 | 34 | 57 | 104 |

*Expressed as μg retinol/dl.
Values not in parentheses are from NHANES I, 1971–1974; those in parentheses are from NHANES II, 1976–1980.
Data fron Pilch, S.M.[101b]

**Table 12–9.  Suggested Relationships between Total Vitamin A Levels in the Serum and the Vitamin A Status of Apparently Healthy Individuals in the United States[101b]**

|  | *Age in Years* | | |
|---|---|---|---|
| *Serum Vitamin A* | *3–11* | *12–17* | *18–74* |
| μg/dl | | | |
| Less than 10 | SSS†,FF‡ | SSS,FF | SSS,FF |
| 10–19 | SS | SS,F | SSS,FF |
| 20–29 | S* | S | S,F |

*In some individuals.
†S: With increased intakes of vitamin A, vitamin A status may improve (S), is likely to improve (SS), or is very likely to improve (SSS).
‡F: Impairment of vitamin A function may be present (F), or is likely to be present (FF).

more reliable in estimating carotenoid intakes than those currently available.

## REFERENCES

1. Wolf, G.: Am. J. Clin. Nutr. *31*:290–292, 1978.
2. Moore, T.: Vitamin A. Amsterdam, Elsevier, 1957.
3. IUPAC–IUB Joint Commission on Biochemical Nomenclature: Eur. J. Biochem. *129*:1–5, 1982.
4. Nomenclature Policy: J. Nutr. *114*:643–644, 1984.
5. IUPAC–IUB Commission on Biochemical Nomenclature: Biochemistry *10*:4827–4837, 1971.
6. Mayer, H., Isler, O.: Total synthesis. *In* Carotenoids. (Isler, O. Ed.) Basel, Birhauser Verlag, 1971, pp. 325–575.
7. Mayer, H., Bollag, W., Hanni, R., et al.: Experientia *34*:1105–1119, 1978.
8. Frickel, F.: Chemistry and physical properties of retinoids. *In* The Retinoids, Vol. 1. (Sporn, M.B., Roberts, A.B., Goodman, D.S., Eds.) New York, Academic Press, 1984, pp. 7–145.
9. WHO: Handbook on human nutritional requirements. Monograph No. 61. Geneva, World Health Organization, 1974.
10. Sauberlich, H.E., Hodges, R.E., Wallace, D.L., et al.: Vitam. Horm. *32*:251–275, 1974.
11. Olson, J.A.: Am. J. Clin. Nutr., In press, 1986.
12. Stephens-Jarnigan, A., Miller, D., DeLuca, H.F.: Fed. Proc. *43*:789, 1984.
13. Lotthammer, K.H., Ahlswede, L., Meyer, H.: Deutsche Tierarztl. Wochenschr. *83*:353–359, 1976.
14. Olson, J.A.: Am. J. Clin. Nutr. *9*:1–11, 1961.
15. El-Gorab, M.I., Underwood, B.A., Loerch, J.D.: Biochim. Biophys. Acta *401*:265–277, 1975.
16. Hollander, D.: J. Lab. Clin. Med. *97*:449–462, 1981.
17. Goodman, D.S., Huang, H.S.: Science *149*:879–880, 1965.
18. Olson, J.A., Hayaishi, O.: Proc. Natl. Acad. Sci. USA *54*:1364–1370, 1965.
19. Olson, J.A.: Formation and function of vitamin A. *In* Biosynthesis of Isoprenoid compounds, Vol. 2. (Porter, J.W., and Spurgeon, S.L., Eds.) New York, Wiley-Interscience, 1983, pp. 371–412.
20. Ong, D.E.: J. Biol. Chem. *259*:1476–1482, 1984.
21. Green, P.H.R., Glickman, R.M.: J. Lipid Res. *22*:1153–1173, 1981.
22. Goodman, D.S.: Biosynthesis, Absorption and Hepatic Metabolism of Retinol. *In* The Retinoids, Vol. 2. (Sporn, M.B., Roberts, A.B., Goodman, D.S., Eds.) New York, Academic Press, 1984, pp. 1–39.
23. Blomhoff, R., Helgerud, P., Rasmussen, M., et al.: Proc. Natl. Acad. Sci. USA *79*:7326–7330, 1982.
24. Wake, K.: Int. Rev. Cytol. *66*:303–353, 1980.
25. Olson, J.A., Gunning, D.: J. Nutr. *113*:2184–2191, 1983.
25a. Hendriks, H.F.J., Verhoofstad, W.A.M.M., Brouwer, A., et al.: Exp. Cell. Res. *160*:138–149, 1985.
25b. Blomhoff, R., Rasmussen, M., Nilsson, A., et al.: J. Biol. Chem. *260*:13560–13565, 1985.
25c. Batres, R.O., Gunning, D., Olson, J.A.: Fed. Proc. *45*:832, 1986.
26. Goodman, D.S.: Plasma retinol-binding protein. *In* The Retinoids, Vol. 2. (Sporn, M.B., Roberts, A.B., Goodman, D.S., Eds.) New York, Academic Press, 1984, pp. 41–88.
27. Rask, L., Anundi, H., Peterson, P.A.: FEBS Lett. *104*:55–58, 1979.
28. Vahlquist, A., Rask, L., Peterson, P.A., et al.: Scand. J. Lab. Clin. Invest. *35*:569–574, 1975.
28a. Blomhoff, R., Norum, K.R., Berg, T.: J. Biol. Chem. *260*:13571–13575, 1985.
29. Chytil, F., Ong, D.E.: Adv. Nutr. Res. *5*:13–29, 1983.
30. Bunt-Milam, A.H., Saari, J.C.: J. Cell Biol. *97*:703–712, 1983.
31. Omori, M., Muto, Y., Nagao, T.: J. Lipid Res. *22*:899–904, 1981.
32. Adler, A.J., Martin, K.J.: Biochem. Biophys. Res. Commun. *108*:1601–1608, 1982.
33. Lai, V.L., Wiggert, B., Liu, Y.P., et al.: Nature (London) *298*:848–849, 1982.
34. Liou, G.I., Bridges, C.D.B., Fong, S-L.: Vision Res. *22*:1457–1468, 1982.
35. Fong, S-L., Liou, G.I., Landers, R.A., et al.: J. Biol. Chem. *259*:6534–6542, 1984.
36. Carson, D.D., Rosenberg, L.I., Blaner, W.S., et al.: J. Biol. Chem. *259*:3117–3123, 1984.
36a. Barua, A.B., Olson, J.A.: Am. J. Clin. Nutr. *43*:481–485, 1986.
36b. Davies, B.H.: Pure Appl. Chem. *57*:679–684, 1985.
37. Chader, G.J.: Retinoids in ocular tissue: Binding proteins, transport and mechanism of action. *In* Cell Biology of the Eye. (McDevitt, D.S., Ed.) New York, Academic Press, 1982, pp. 377–433.
38. Bridges, C.D.B.: Retinoids in photosensitive systems. *In* The Retinoids, Vol. 2. (Sporn, M.B., Roberts, A.B., Goodman, D.S., Eds.) New York, Academic Press, 1984, pp. 125–176.
39. Bowmaker, J.K., Dartnall, H.J.A.: J. Physiol. *298*:501–511, 1980.
40. Young, K.W.: Invest. Ophthalmol. *17*:105–116, 1978.
41. Heller, J.: J. Biol. Chem. *250*:3613–3619, 1975.
42. Fung, B. K-K.: J. Biol. Chem. *258*:10495–10502, 1983.

43. Miller, W.H.: Adv. Cyclic Nucleotide Res. *15*:495–511, 1983.
44. Oesterhelt, D., Stoeckenius, W.: Nature (London) *233*:149–152, 1971.
45. Wolbach, S.B., Howe, P.R.: J. Exp. Med. *42*:753–757, 1925.
46. Sporn, M.B., Newton, D.L.: Fed. Proc. *38*:2528–2534, 1979.
47. Sietsema, W.K., DeLuca, H.F.: J. Nutr. *112*:1481–1489, 1982.
48. Strickland, S., Sawey, M.J.: Dev. Biol. *78*:76–85, 1980.
49. Sporn, M.B., Roberts, A.B.: Cancer Res. *43*:3034–3040, 1983.
50. Chytil, F., Ong, D.E.: Fed. Proc. *38*:2510–2514, 1979.
51. Omori, M., Chytil, F.: J. Biol. Chem. *257*:14370–14374, 1982.
52. Bolmer, S.D., Wolf, G.: Proc. Natl. Acad. Sci. USA *79*:6541–6545, 1982.
53. DeLuca, L.M.: Vitam. Horm. *35*:1–57, 1977.
54. DeLuca, L.M., Bhat, P.V., Sasak, W., et al.: Fed. Proc. *38*:2535–2539, 1979.
55. Jetten, A.M.: Fed. Proc. *43*:134–139, 1984.
56. Ganguly, J., Rao, M.N., Murphy, S., et al.: Vitam. Horm. *38*:1–54. 1980.
57. Thompson, J.N.: The role of vitamin A in reproduction. *In* The Fat-Soluble Vitamins. (DeLuca, H.F., Suttie, J.W., Eds.) Madison, University Wisconsin Press, 1969, pp. 267–281.
57a. Johnson, J.D., Davies, P.J.A.: Fed. Proc. *44*:544, 1985.
58. Olson, J.A.: Isr. J. Med. Sci. *8*:1170–1178, 1972.
59. Maden, M.: J. Embryol. Exp. Morphol. *77*:273–295, 1983.
60. Kochhar, D.M.: Teratology *1*:299–305, 1968.
61. Willhite, C.C., Dawson, M.I., Williams, K.J.: Toxicol. Appl. Pharmacol. *83*:563–575, 1986.
62. Dennert, G.: Retinoids and the immune system. *In* The Retinoids, Vol. 2. (Sporn, M.B., Roberts, A.B., Goodman, D.S., Eds.) New York, Academic Press, pp. 373–390.
63. Malkovsky, M., Edwards, A.J., Hunt, R., et al.: Nature (London) *302*:338–440, 1983.
64. McLaren, D.S., Ballintine, E.J., ten Doesschate, J., et al.: The Symptoms and Signs of Vitamin A Deficiency and Their Relationship to Applied Nutrition. International Vitamin A Consultative Group, Washington, D.C., The Nutrition Foundation, 1981, p. 20.
65. Sommer, A.: Nutritional Blindness. Oxford, Oxford University Press, 1982. p. 282.
66. McLaren, D.S.: Vitamin A deficiency and toxicity. *In* Present Knowledge of Nutrition. 5th ed. Washington, D.C., The Nutrition Foundation, 1984, pp. 192–208.
67. Sommer, A.: Ophthalmology *90*:592–600, 1983.
68. Pirie, A., Werb, Z., Burleigh, M.C.: Br. J. Nutr. *34*:297–309, 1975.
69. Pirie, A.: Trans. Ophthalmol. Soc. U.K. *98*:357–360, 1978.
70. Rask, L., Geijer, C., Bill, A., et al.: Exp. Eye Res. *31*:210–211, 1980.
71. Ubels, J.L., MacRae, S.M.: Curr. Eye Res. *3*:815–822, 1984.
72. Dorea, J.G., Olson, J.A.: J. Nutr. *116*:121–127, 1986.
73. Törmä, H., Vahlquist, A.: Arch. Dermatol. Res. *275*:324–328, 1983.
74. Fuchs, E., Green, H.: Cell *25*:617–625, 1981.
75. Lamb, A.J., Apiwatanaporn, P., Olson, J.A.: J. Nutr. *104*:1140–1148, 1974.
76. Moore, T., Holmes, P.D.: Lab. Anim. *5*:239–250, 1971.
77. Rojanapo, W., Olson, J.A., Lamb, A.J.: Biochim. Biophys. Acta *633*:386–399, 1980.
78. Anzano, M.A., Lamb, A.J., Olson, J.A.: J. Nutr. *11*:496–504, 1981.
79. Bauernfeind, J.C.: The Safe Use of Vitamin A. International Vitamin A Consultative Group, Washington, D.C., The Nutrition Foundation, 1980, p. 44.
80. Olson, J.A.: Semin. Oncol. *10*:290–293, 1983.
81. Macapinlac, M.P., Olson, J.A.: Int. J. Vitam. Nutr. Res. *51*:331–341, 1981.
81a. Bush, M.E., Dahms, B.B.: Arch. Pathol. Lab. Med. *108*:838–842, 1984.
81b. Herbert, V.: Am. J. Clin. Nutr. *36*:185–186, 1982.
81c. Smith, F.R., Goodman, D.S.: N. Engl. J. Med. *249*:805–808, 1976.
82. Shenefelt, R.E.: Am. J. Pathol. *66*:589–592, 1972.
83. Stänge, L., Carlstrom, K., Erickson, M.: Acta Obstet. Gynecol. Scand. *57*:289–295, 1978.
83a. Pilotti, G., Scorta, A.: Minerva Ginecol. *17*:1103–1108, 1965.
83b. Bernhardt, I.B., Dorsey, D.J.: Obstet. Gynecol. *43*:750–755, 1974.
83c. Rosa, F.W.: Lancet *2*:513, 1983.
83d. Lammer, E.J., Chen, D.T., Hoar, R.M., et al.: N. Engl. J. Med. *313*:837–841, 1985.
83e. Butcher, R.E., Brunner, R.L., Roth, T., et al.: Life Sci. *11*:141–145, 1972.
83f. Hutchings, D.E., Gibbon, J., Kaufman, M.A.: Dev. Psychobiol. *6*:445–457, 1973.
83g. Vorhees, C.V.: Teratology *10*:269–273, 1974.
83h. Editorial: Vitamin A and teratogenesis. Lancet *1*:319–320, 1985.
83i. Underwood, B.A.: IVACG Recommendations for Safely Improving the Vitamin A Status of Pregnant and Lactating Women and the Nursing Infant. International Vitamin A Consultative Group, Washington D.C., The Nutrition Foundation, 1986.
84. Goodman, G.E., Alberts, D.S., Ernest, D.L., et al.: J. Clin. Oncol. *1*:394–399, 1983.
85. Kligman, A.M., Leyden, J.J., Mills, Jr. O.: Oral vitamin A (retinol) in acne vulgaris. *In* Retinoids: Advances in Basic Research and Therapy. (Orfanos, C.E., Braun-Falco, O., Farber, E.M., et al., Eds.) Berlin, Springer-Verlag, 1981, pp. 245–253.
85a. Kietzmann, H., Schwarze, I., Grote, W., et al.: Dtsch. Med. Wochenschr. *111*:60–62, 1986.
85b. Weber, U., Goerz, G., Hennekes, R.: Klin. Monatsbl. Augenheilkd. *186*:351–354, 1985.
86. Olson, J.A.: Latino-Am. Arch. Nutr. *29*:521–545, 1979.
87. Latham, C.B., Woodruff, C.W.: Fed. Proc. *43*:468, 1984.
88. Leo, M.A., Lieber, C.S.: Hepatology *3*:1–11, 1983.
89. Leo, M.A., Lieber, C.S.: Alcoholism, Clin. Exp. Res. *7*:15–21, 1983.
90. Russell, R.M.: Retina *2*:303–304, 1982.
91. Olson, J.A.: Vitamin A. *In* Handbook of Vitamins. (Machlin, L.J., Ed.) New York, Marcel Dekker, Inc., 1984, pp. 1–43.
92. Kanai, M., Iwanaga, T., Hagino, N., et al.: World Rev. Nutr. Diet. *31*:31–42, 1978.
92a. Shils, M.E., Baker, H., Frank, O.: J. Parenter. Enter. Nutr. *9*:179–188, 1985.

93. Briggs, M., Briggs, M., Bennum, M.: Contraception *67*:275–279, 1972.
94. Supopark, W., Olson, J.A.: Int. J. Vitam. Nutr. Res. *45*:113–123, 1975.
95. Schurr, D., Herbert, J., Habibi, E., et al.: J. Pediatr. Gastroenterol. Nutr. *2*:705–707, 1983.
96. U.S. Public Health Service: Dietary Source Data, United States 1976–1980. DHHS Publ. No. PHS 83–1681, Hyattsville, Md., 1983.
97. First National Health and Nutrition Examination Survey, United States, 1971–1972. Health Resources Administration, U.S. Dept. of Health, Education and Welfare, Rockville, Md., 1974, p. 183.
98. McDowell, M.A., Sempos, C.T., Yetley, E.A., et al.: Fed. Proc. *43*:665, 1984.
98a. Block, G., Dresser, C.M., Hartman, A.M., et al.: Am. J. Epidemiol. *122*:13–26, 1985.
99. Food and Nutrition Board: Recommended Dietary Allowances, 9th ed. U.S. National Academy Science, Washington, D.C., 1980, p. 185.
99a. FAO/WHO: Requirements of Vitamin A, Iron, Folate, and Vitamin $B_{12}$. World Health Organization, Geneva, and Food and Agriculture Organization, Rome, 1986. In press.
100. Underwood, B.A.: Vitamin A in animal and human nutrition. *In* The Retinoids, Vol. 1. (Sporn, M.B., Roberts, A.B., Goodman, D.S., Eds.) New York, Academic Press, 1984, pp. 281–392.
101. Hume, E.M., Krebs, H.A. (compilers): Vitamin A Requirement of Human Adults. Medical Research Council, Special Report No. 264. London, H.M. Stationery Office, 1949, p. 145.
101a. Rubin, S.H., DeRitter, E.: Vitam. Horm. *12*:101–135, 1954.
101b. Pilch, S.M. (Ed.) Assessment of the Vitamin A Nutritional Status of the U.S. Population Based on Data Collected in Health and Nutrition Examination Surveys. Life Science Research Office, Federation of American Societies for Experimental Biology, Bethesda, Md., 1985.
102. DeLuca, L.M., Glover, J., Heller, J., et al.: Recent Advances in the Metabolism and Function of Vitamin A and their Relationship to Applied Nutrition. International Vitamin A Consultative Group, Washington, D.C., The Nutrition Foundation, 1979, p. 44.
102a. Napoli, J.L., McCormick, A.M., O'Meara, B., et al.: Arch. Biochem. Biophys. *230*:194–202, 1984.
103. Arroyave, G., Chichester, C.O., Flores, H., et al.: Biochemical Methodology for the Assessment of Vitamin A Status. International Vitamin A Consultative Group, Washington, D.C., The Nutrition Foundation, 1982, p. 88.
104. Suthutvoravoot, S., Olson, J.A.: Am. J. Clin. Nutr. *27*:883–891, 1974.
105. Loerch, J.D., Underwood, B.A., Lewis, K.C.: J. Nutr. *109*:778–786, 1979.
106. Muto, Y., Smith, J.E., Milch, P.O., et al.: J. Biol. Chem. *247*:2542–2550, 1972.
107. Flores, H., Araujo, C.R.C., Campos, F.A.C.S., et al.: Int. J. Vitam. Nutr. Res. *24* (Suppl.):23–24, 1983.
108. Mobarhan, S., Russell, R.M., Underwood, B.A., et al.: Am. J. Clin. Nutr. *34*:2264–2270, 1981.

109. Amédéé-Manesme, O., Anderson, D., Olson, J.A.: Am. J. Clin. Nutr. *39*:898–902, 1984.
110. Control of Vitamin A Deficiency and Xerophthalmia. Technical Report No. 672. Geneva, World Health Organization, 1982, p. 70.
110a. Hatchell, D.L., Sommer, A., Hatchell, M.C.: Proceedings, Tenth Conference of the International Vitamin A Consultative Group, Hyderabad, India, 1985.
110b. Russell, R.M., Morrison, S.A., Smith, F.R., et al.: Ann. Intern. Med. *88*:622–626, 1978.
111. Frolik, C.A., Olson, J.A.: Extraction, separation and chemical analysis of retinoids. *In* The Retinoids, Vol. 1. (Sporn, M.B., Roberts, A.B., Goodman, D.S., Eds.) New York, Academic Press, 1984, pp. 181–233.
112. Catignani, G.L., Bieri, J.G.: Clin. Chem. *29*:708–712, 1983.
113. Furr, H.C., Amédéé-Manesme, O., Olson, J.A.: J. Chromatogr. *309*:299–307, 1984.
113a. Furr, H.C., Cooper, D.A., Olson, J.A.: J. Chromatogr. *378*:45–53, 1986.
114. Official Methods of Analysis, 12th ed. Washington, D.C., Assoc. of Off. Analyt. Chem., 1980.
115. Simpson, K.L.: Proc. Nutr. Soc. *42*:7–17, 1983.
116. Simpson, K.L., Chichester, C.O.: Annu. Rev. Nutr. *1*:351–374, 1981.
117. Taylor, R.F.: Adv. Chromatogr. *22*:157–213, 1983.

## SELECTED READINGS

Arroyave, G., Chichester, C.O., Flores, H., et al.: Biochemical Methodology for the Assessment of Vitamin A Status. International Vitamin A Consultative Group, Washington, D.C, The Nutrition Foundation, 1982.
Britton, G.: Carotenoids and Polyterpenoids. Natural Product Depts. *2*:349–387, 1985.
Chytil, F., Ong, D.E.: Cellular retinol- and retinoic acid-binding proteins in vitamin A action. Fed. Proc. *38*:2510–2514, 1979.
DeLuca, L.M., Shapiro, S.S. (Eds.): Modulation of Cellular Interactions by Vitamin A and Derivatives (Retinoids). New York, New York Academy of Science, (Annals Vol. 359), 1981.
Goodman, D.S.: Vitamin A and retinoids in health and disease. N. Engl. J. Med. *310*:1023–1031, 1984.
Goodwin, T.W.: Biochemistry of the Carotenoids, Vol. 2. Animals, London, Chapman and Hall, 1984.
McLaren, D.S.: Vitamin A deficiency and toxicity. *In* Present Knowledge in Nutrition. 5th ed. (Olson, R.E., Ed.) Washington, D.C., The Nutrition Foundation, 1984, pp. 192–208.
Miller, W.H.: Physiological effects of cyclic GMP in the vertebrate retinal rod outer segment. Adv. Cyclic Nucleotide Res. *15*:495–511, 1983.
Olson, J.A.: Vitamin A. *In* Handbook of Vitamins. (Machlin, L.J., Ed.) New York, Marcel Dekker, Inc., 1984, pp. 1–43.
Sommer, A.: Nutritional Blindness: Xerophthalmia and Keratomalacia. Oxford, Oxford University Press, 1982.
Sporn, M.B., Roberts, A.B., Goodman, D.S., (Eds.): The Retinoids, Vol. 1 and 2. New York, Academic Press, 1984.

*Chapter* 13

# VITAMIN D AND ITS METABOLITES

### Hector F. DeLuca

Rickets apparently was evident even in ancient times, possibly resulting indirectly from advances in urbanization.[1] Bardsley, in 1807, wrote about the effective use of cod liver oil in the treatment of osteomalacia,[2] and Palm, in 1890, suggested that sunlight possessed antirachitic action.[3] In 1919 Sir Edward Mellanby succeeded in producing rickets in experimental animals and found it could be prevented by the administration of cod liver oil.[4] McCollum and associates demonstrated that the antirachitic factor in cod liver oil is relatively stable to heat and aeration,[5] thereby differing from the previously discovered vitamin A. McCollum named the factor vitamin D.[6] Also in 1919, Huldshinsky demonstrated clearly that ultraviolet light from either sunlight or ultraviolet lamps could cure rickets.[7] The elegant work of Steenbock and associates established that antirachitic activity could be produced in food and other biologic materials by ultraviolet irradiation.[8,9] This discovery provided the basic information needed for the isolation and identification of vitamin $D_2$[10,11] and the elimination of rickets as a major medical problem because food could be easily fortified with the antirachitic vitamin.

A distinct time lag exists between administration of vitamin D to deficient animals and detection of a physiologic response[12] (e.g., enhanced intestinal calcium absorption). It is now known that the conversion of vitamin D to active metabolites and the stimulation of protein synthesis and/or assembly constitute the main events occurring during this time.

By current definitions, vitamin D can be considered both a vitamin and a hormone. Vitamin D is an organic compound that acts as a micronutrient; its ingestion is required by most urban populations (i.e., it acts as a vitamin). However, vitamin D supplementation is unnecessary in people who are able to meet their vitamin D requirement through the sunlight activation of 7-dehydrocholesterol in the skin. The vitamin D thus produced is metabolized to an active form that then acts on distinct target tissue with feedback control occurring at the site of active metabolite synthesis. Thus the active metabolite 1,25-dihydroxyvitamin $D_3$ (1,25-$(OH)_2D_3$), which is produced exclusively in the kidney and functions in intestine and bone, is considered a hormone and vitamin D a prohormone.[12,13]

## CHEMISTRY

The D vitamins are characteristically found in the sterol fraction of biologic extracts. Vitamins $D_2$ and $D_3$, the more common forms of the vitamin, are derived from ergosterol and 7-dehydrocholes-

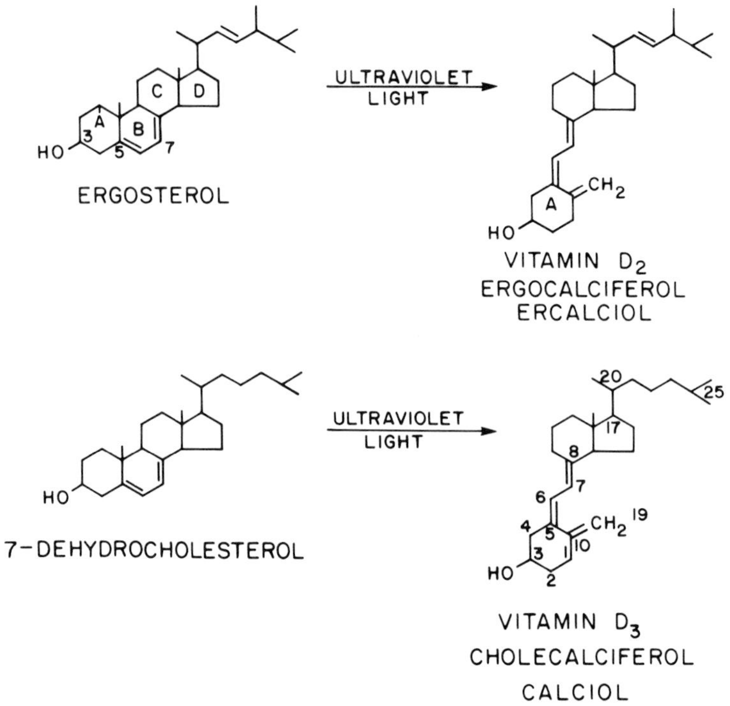

**Fig. 13–1.** The precursors and the medically important forms of vitamin D. The new terminology for vitamin $D_2$ is ercalciol and for vitamin $D_3$, calciol (see Table 13–1).

terol, respectively, and are therefore named ergocalciferol and cholecalciferol or, by modern nomenclature, ercalciol and calciol (Fig. 13–1). Table 13–1 provides both old and new nomenclature for the vitamin D compounds.

The triene structure of vitamin D gives a characteristic absorption band at 265 nm with an absorption minimum at 228 nm and a molar extinction coefficient of 18,200 at 265 cm. Vitamin D is fairly stable and is soluble in a wide range of organic solvents. Care should be taken, however, to store solutions of the vitamin under nitrogen in the absence of light and acid and at cold temperatures if possible. The main problem is the ease of oxidation of the triene system, its sensitivity to acid, and light-catalyzed isomerization. Often an antioxidant such as α-tocopherol or butylated hydroxytoluene can be used to help prevent oxidation. Aqueous suspensions are particularly unstable because of dissolved oxygen. Oil or propylene glycol solutions of the vitamin with an antioxidant, however, are stable.

Chemical alteration of existing functional groups or double bonds results in a product with decreased antirachitic activity. Vitamin $D_4$ is produced by the reduction of the 22,23 double bond in vitamin $D_2$ and is only one half to three fourths as active as vitamin $D_2$ in rats. Substitution of a Cl,Br[14] or a mercaptan[15] group for the 3-OH function results in loss of activity. Reduction of the methylene group on ring A and rotation of the ring 180 degrees result in dihydrotachysterol (present in solutions of AT-10), a compound that is less active than the vitamin at low doses but is of therapeutic value when given at a pharmacologic level[16] because it acts as an analogue of 1,25-$(OH)_2D_3$.[17]

## MEASUREMENT

Only a small amount of vitamin D is required (e.g., 1 I.U. in the rat, where 1 mg = 40,000 I.U.)

**Table 13–1. Names of Vitamin D Compounds**

| | | |
|---|---|---|
| Vitamin $D_3$ | Cholecalciferol | Calciol |
| 25-Hydroxyvitamin $D_3$ | 25-Hydroxycholecalciferol | Calcidiol |
| 1,25-Dihydroxyvitamin $D_3$ | 1,25-Dihydroxycholecalciferol | Calcitriol |
| 24R,25-Dihydroxyvitamin $D_3$ | 24R,25-Dihydroxycholecalciferol | 24-Hydroxycalcidiol |
| Vitamin $D_2$ | Ergocalciferol | Ercalciol |
| 25-Hydroxyvitamin $D_2$ | 25-Hydroxyergocalciferol | Ercalcidiol |
| 1,25-Dihydroxyvitamin $D_2$ | 1,25-Dihydroxyergocalciferol | Ercalcitriol |

to elicit a physiologic response. Thus the amounts of vitamin D that must be measured in biologic materials are extremely small. High-performance liquid chromatography (HPLC) coupled to a sensitive ultraviolet absorbance detector is now used for measurement, and will largely replace the biologic assays for concentrated samples; however, biologic assays represent the only reliable method for analyses of foods and feeds.[18]

The rat-line test or calcification test[19] remains the biologic method of choice. A single dose of standard vitamin D promotes calcification in the epiphyseal plate of the rachitic rat. Silver nitrate (1.5% w/v) staining of sectioned bone is used for visual detection of new calcification, which increases as a function of the dose of vitamin D.

Percent bone ash is also used in chicks and rats as an assay for vitamin D. The bone ash content of tibia is determined after feeding chicks a rachitogenic diet and standard doses of vitamin D for 21 days.[20] Increase in percent bone ash is correlated to the dose of vitamin D. The chick bone ash method is the primary method used for vitamin $D_3$. To differentiate between vitamins $D_2$ and $D_3$, an efficacy ratio of rat to chick response is used. Chicks give a response to vitamin $D_3$ tenfold greater than to vitamin $D_2$, whereas rats respond equally well to both compounds. HPLC can be used for vitamin D determination but is largely inaccurate on any samples but concentrates.[21]

## ABSORPTION AND EXCRETION

Vitamin D is generally absorbed with food fats; therefore, inhibition of normal fat absorption (steatorrhea) results in a diminished absorption of ingested vitamin D. Patients with chronic pancreatitis, celiac disease, and biliary obstruction malabsorb vitamin $D_3$.[22] Absorption occurs in the jejunum and/or ileum, and bile is essential.[23,24] Most of an absorbed dose of vitamin D is present in the chylomicrons of the lymphatic system.[22] Vitamin D concentrates rapidly in the liver where it is hydroxylated to 25-hydroxyvitamin $D_3$ (25-OH-$D_3$).[25,26] The movement of vitamin D from the plasma chlyomicrons and lipoproteins appears to occur in the liver by transfer to an $\alpha$-globulin with a molecular weight of 52,000 that acts as a carrier for the vitamin and all its metabolites.[27–29] Although enterohepatic circulation has been reported for vitamin D metabolites, its extent is small and not believed to be significant.[30,31]

Bile appears to be the major pathway of vitamin D metabolite excretion. Patients having biliary fistulas excrete little radioactivity from a dose of $^3H$-vitamin $D_3$.[32] A significant amount (i.e., 3%) of $^3H$-vitamin $D_3$ is also detectable in the urine during the 48- to 72-hour period following an intravenous dose.[32]

## PHOTOBIOGENESIS

For the most part, vitamin D is derived from the photobiogenesis process occurring in skin. 7-Dehydrocholesterol was first discovered by Windaus and colleagues as a chemical entity. Upon irradiation, it yielded vitamin $D_3$. 7-Dehydrocholesterol later became known in relation to the process of cholesterol biosynthesis. Its presence in skin was clearly demonstrated to be in the preputial glands and in the malpighian layer of the epidermis. Thus, animals and man on a vitamin D-deficient diet will not become vitamin D deficient if exposed to sufficient amounts of ultraviolet light. 7-Dehydrocholesterol absorbs 282 nm ultraviolet light; in a strictly chemical photolysis reaction, rupture of the 9-10 double bond is followed by a 5,7-sigmatropic shift of the double bonds to yield an intermediate previtamin D as shown in Figure 13–2. Previtamin D is in itself biologically inert and undergoes a chemical isomerization to become vitamin $D_3$. The aforementioned vitamin D transport protein recognizes the vitamin D compounds but does not recognize the previtamin D.[33,34] Thus, previtamin D becomes converted to vitamin D and is transported by the vitamin D transport protein to the liver where it begins its metabolic activation. Equilibration at body temperatures between vitamin D and previtamin D requires approximately 36 hours for completion and is 96% in the form of vitamin $D_3$ and approximately 4% in the form of previtamin D.

The entire process of conversion of 7-dehydrocholesterol to vitamin $D_3$ is a strictly chemical reaction, not involving proteins or enzymes. It is not regulated; however, under circumstances of high plasma 1,25-$(OH)_2D_3$ levels the amount of 7-dehydrocholesterol found in skin appears to be increased.[35] The photolysis system is efficient. It has been estimated that approximately 10 to 15 minutes of summer sun exposure of hands and face will produce 10 $\mu$g of vitamin $D_3$, sufficient to meet the recommended daily allowance.[36] Pigmented skin is less efficient in production of vitamin D.[37] Tanning also reduces the efficiency of vitamin D production. Although increased blood levels of 25-OH-D can be achieved by ultraviolet light exposure, it is of considerable interest that vitamin D intoxication has not resulted from excessive sunlight exposure.[38] A possible explanation is that the damaging effects of excessive ultraviolet light may be more critical on systems other than the vitamin D system.

Intravenously administered vitamin D and its

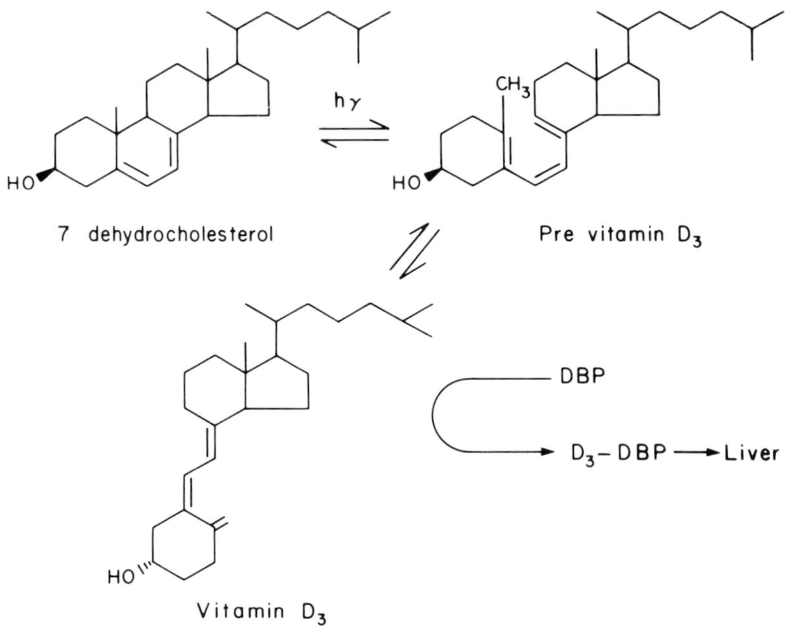

**Fig. 13–2.** The conversion of 7-dehydrocholesterol to vitamin $D_3$ in skin and its subsequent transport to the liver. Ultraviolet light is absorbed by the B-ring of 7-dehydrocholesterol bringing about a rupture of the 9,10 bond and a subsequent shift of the double bonds to form previtamin $D_3$. Previtamin $D_3$ is biologically inert and remains in the skin. It slowly equilibrates to form vitamin $D_3$. Vitamin $D_3$ is recognized by the vitamin D plasma transport protein (DBP) that transports it to the liver to begin its metabolic activation. DBP does not recognize previtamin $D_3$.

metabolites are efficiently utilized resulting in the highest biologic responses in animals.[39,40] Although it has been suggested that vitamin D given intravenously causes osteomalacia in patients fed intravenously,[41] this conclusion is not warranted from the data provided and appears unlikely.

For unexplained reasons, fish accumulate large quantities of vitamin D in their livers.[42] Cod liver oil and tuna liver oil have high concentrations of this substance. It can be argued that this accumulation is a result of the position of these fish in the food chain. On the other hand, fish may possess a nonphotochemical process for production of vitamin D.[43] This possibility has not, however, been sufficiently documented and remains an unsolved biologic problem.

## DIETARY IMPLICATIONS

Because of food fortification with vitamin D, the daily vitamin D requirement (200 to 400 I.U. or 5 to 10 μg vitamin $D_3$) can be achieved without vitamin supplementation.[44] However, rickets can occur in breast-fed infants and in those fed unfortified milk,[45] in which case a vitamin D supplement is recommended (e.g., 400 I.U. daily). It is currently suggested that prophylactic doses of vitamin D in excess of 1,000 I.U. daily are inadvisable.[46] Fomon and associates showed, however, that moderate overdoses of vitamin D (i.e., 1,380 to 2,370 I.U. daily), common in a substantial

number of children in the United States, had no detrimental effect on growth.[47] A high frequency of a mild form of idiopathic hypercalcemia in Great Britain has been associated with a vitamin intake of 4,000 I.U. daily, mainly from fortified infant foods.[48] Of course, an excessive intake of vitamin D (i.e., 50,000 to 100,000 I.U. daily) is potentially dangerous to both normal children[49] and to adults[50] and must be avoided. As a precaution, intakes of vitamin D in excess of 1,000 I.U. per day should be taken only if prescribed by a physician and provided that serum calcium concentration or fasting 24-hour urinary calcium levels are routinely monitored once every month and remain in the normal range.

Improper dietary intake of calcium and/or phosphorus can impair growth and cause bone disease. Infants require 400 to 600 mg of calcium daily, children (1 to 10 years of age) and adults (over 18 years of age) require 800 mg daily, and adolescents (10 to 18 years of age) and pregnant women need 1,300 mg daily.[45] Phosphorus should be consumed at a level equivalent to that of calcium with the dietary ratio of the two ions approximately 1:1. A high-phosphorus diet, as afforded by cow's milk, may result in hypocalcemia tetany during early infancy.[51] The high phosphate intake in the United States afforded through soft drinks and meat is also of interest concerning possible long-term effects in children and adults. High-phosphate diets may cause a secondary hyperparathyroidism that causes bone loss. Phytate in bread and certain cereals forms insoluble calcium phytate, which interferes with intestinal calcium absorption.[52]

One result of low blood calcium and phosphorus is the softening and deformity of the maxillary bones. Mellanby and Mellanby reported that, in London between 1945 and 1947, children (up to 5 years of age) who had increased availability of calcium and vitamin D possessed markedly improved dental status.[53]

## METABOLITES: FORMATION AND ACTIVITIES

As a result of work carried out during the past 20 years, it is now clear that vitamin D must be metabolized before it can function[54,55] (Fig. 13–3). There is little doubt that the first event in the metabolism of vitamin D is 25-hydroxylation, which occurs primarily in the liver and in the endoplasmic reticulum of the hepatocytes.[56] The product, 25-OH-D, is the major circulating form of vitamin D and is the form measured when physicians assess the vitamin D status of a patient

suffering from metabolic bone disease. In the United States, this level is approximately 30 ng/ml[21,41] whereas in Europe, where vitamin D intakes are lower, the levels have been reported to be approximately 20 ng/ml.[57] 25-Hydroxylase found in the endoplasmic reticulum is a cytochrome P-450-dependent two-component mixed function mono-oxygenase.[58] It does not appear to be regulated to any degree, although the hydroxylase level is approximately two-fold higher in vitamin D deficiency than in animals given a source of vitamin D.[59] 25-OH-$D_3$ is delivered to the kidney where it undergoes its next obligatory conversion to the final vitamin D hormone, 1,25-$(OH)_2D_3$. This conversion takes place in the mitochondria and involves a three-component mixed function mono-oxygenase, including a flavoprotein, an iron sulfur protein, and a cytochrome P-450.[60] It is this system that is tightly regulated and that constitutes a major regulatory position of the vitamin D endocrine system as will be described in the section on calcium homeostasis.

In the nonpregnant mammal, the kidney re-

PHYSIOLOGIC   METABOLISM  OF  VITAMIN $D_3$

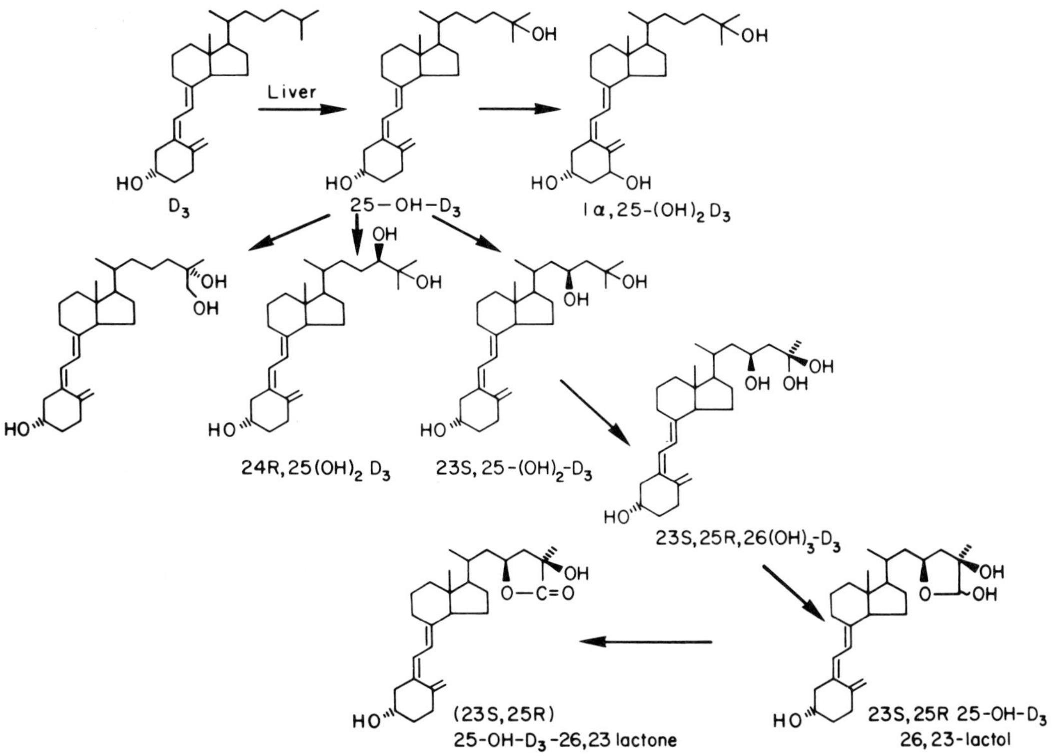

**Fig. 13–3.** The physiologic metabolism of vitamin $D_3$. Only metabolites that have been identified as being physiologically relevant are illustrated. Other metabolites have been isolated and identified following pharmacologic doses of vitamin D or following incubation with large amounts of vitamin D. These metabolites have not been listed because it is unclear whether they have relevance in vivo.

mains the exclusive site of synthesis of 1,25-$(OH)_2D_3$.[61,62] This hormonal form of the vitamin is transported on the vitamin D transport protein to target organs such as intestine or bone and elsewhere in the kidney where it exerts its biologic effects (to be described in subsequent sections).

The placenta is a normal site of 1α-hydroxylation of 25-OH-$D_3$.[63] The major concentration of this enzyme is in the yolk sac, although some activity is also found in the chorioallantoic membrane.[63a] Why it is found in the placenta and what is the function of the resultant 1,25-$(OH)_2D_3$ remain unknown. Certainly fetal kidney is a site of 1α-hydroxylation as well as a provider of any fetal needs for this hormone.[64] Thus, the placental 1α-hydroxylase may provide additional 1,25-$(OH)_2D_3$ needed during pregnancy.

There have been reports of other extrarenal sites of 1,25-$(OH)_2D_3$ synthesis.[65,66] Some of these sites are found only in tissue culture and not in vivo (e.g., bone and intestinal cells).[61,62] On the other hand, macrophages have been reported to synthesize 1,25-$(OH)_2D_3$. Because high concentrations of 1,25-$(OH)_2D_3$ are found in the absence of kidneys in patients with sarcoidosis,[67] and this potent hormone may be the cause of hypercalcemia, it is possible that under this disease state extrarenal synthesis of 1,25-$(OH)_2D_3$ is a major consideration. In other disease states in which hypercalcemia is found, such as neoplastic diseases and lymphomas, it is possible that 1,25-$(OH)_2D_3$ synthesis may occur ectopically.[68]

Besides the activation pathway just described, 25-OH-$D_3$ undergoes other important metabolic conversions. The most important is 24R-hydroxylation to form 24R,25-$(OH)_2D_3$, a major circulating metabolite of the vitamin. Despite many efforts to delineate an active role, it is now clear that 24R,25-$(OH)_2D_3$ possesses no biologic function and represents an alternative hydroxylation likely needed for removal of 25-OH-$D_3$. Alternatively, the 24R-hydroxylation may be meant as an initial event in the inactivation of 1,25-$(OH)_2D_3$ because 24R-hydroxylation of that compound occurs to produce 1,24,25-$(OH)_3D_3$, a metabolite with much lower biologic activity.[69] This substance may be the first intermediate in the metabolic degradation of 1,25-$(OH)_2D_3$ ultimately to its side chain cleavage product, calcitroic acid.[70] Whether this is in fact the case remains to be determined. Experiments with 24,24-$F_2$-25-OH-$D_3$ have largely excluded any biologic function of 24R,25-$(OH)_2D_3$.[71–73] 26-Hydroxylation can also occur, resulting in an epimeric mixture of 25,26-$(OH)_2D_3$.[74] This compound is biologically less active than 25-OH-$D_3$ and does not represent an activation pathway.[75]

The most recent series of reactions discovered involves side chain oxidation. 23S-Hydroxylation occurs on 25-OH-$D_3$ to bring about the synthesis of an important intermediate of a major metabolite, 25-OH-$D_3$-26,23-lactone.[76,77] Again the fluoro derivative, 26,26,26,27,27,27-$F_6$-25-OH-$D_3$, has been used to demonstrate that both the lactone formation and 26-oxidation are not involved in the functions of vitamin D.[78] Thus from a functional point of view, these pathways can be largely ignored.

Vitamin $D_2$ is metabolized functionally in identical fashion with vitamin $D_3$ producing 25-OH-$D_2$ and 1,25-$(OH)_2D_2$.[79] 24R,25-$(OH)_2D_2$ has also been isolated and identified.[80] However, much work remains to be done on vitamin $D_2$ metabolism because it is unlikely that the lactone pathway is followed in this case. In birds and New World monkeys, vitamin $D_2$ and its metabolites are less active than vitamin $D_3$.[81,82] Vitamin $D_2$ compounds are more rapidly metabolized and excreted in the case of the chicken.[83] Furthermore, in New World monkeys, the vitamin D-binding proteins, including the transport protein as well as the receptor protein, appear to have less affinity for the vitamin $D_2$ series.[84] A major contributor to discrimination against vitamin $D_2$ in birds is the vitamin D transport protein.[85] This protein does not bind the vitamin $D_2$ derivatives, whereas it does bind vitamin $D_3$ derivatives as well as the mammalian transport proteins. In contrast, the mammalian transport protein binds vitamin $D_2$ and vitamin $D_3$ compounds equally well.

It appears that 1,25-$(OH)_2D_3$ carries out all the known functions of vitamin D. Furthermore, when delivered by an osmotic minipump to animals for two generations, this compound brings about normal animals in every respect,[72] thus eliminating the necessity for postulating other pathways of functional metabolism of vitamin D.

Measurement of vitamin D metabolites, especially 25-OH-$D_3$, 25-OH-$D_2$, and 1,25-$(OH)_2D$, has become useful in the diagnosis of metabolic bone diseases. Table 13–2 provides normal levels of these metabolites in human plasma along with

**Table 13–2. Approximate Levels of Vitamin D Metabolites and Their Half Lives in Man**

| Metabolite | Blood Level | Half Life in Blood |
|---|---|---|
| Vitamin $D_3$ | 2.3 ± 1.6 ng/ml | 36 days |
| Vitamin $D_2$ | 1.2 ± 1.4 ng/ml | ? |
| 25-OH-$D_3$ | 27.6 ± 9.2 ng/ml | 28 days |
| 25-OH-$D_2$ | 3.9 ± 3 ng/ml | — |
| 1,25-$(OH)_2D_3$ | 31 ± 9 pg/ml | 2–4 hours |
| 24,25-$(OH)_2D_3$ | 3.5 ± 1.4 ng/ml | ? |

their approximate half lives. Measurements of $24,25\text{-}(OH)_2D_3$ are of no diagnostic value.

Vitamins $D_2$ and $D_3$ are now measured with high-performance liquid chromatography (HPLC), using absorbance at 254 or 265 nm. 25-OH-D metabolites are measured best by HPLC and absorption at 254 or 265 nmol or by competitive binding assay, whereas $1,25\text{-}(OH)_2D_3$ is measured by chromatographic purification followed by binding assay using the receptor for $1,25\text{-}(OH)_2D_3$ or an antibody for that metabolite.[86–89] A cellular uptake assay has also been devised but has not received significant popularity.

The biologic activity of the metabolites has also been determined in animals and approximated in man. The relative activities in mammals for the important metabolites and analogues are:

$$\text{vitamin } D_3 = 1$$
$$\text{vitamin } D_2 = 1$$
$$25\text{-OH-}D_3 = 2 \text{ to } 5$$
$$25\text{-OH-}D_2 = 2 \text{ to } 5$$
$$1,25\text{-}(OH)_2D_3 = 10$$
$$1,25\text{-}(OH)_2D_2 = 10$$
$$1\alpha\text{-OH-}D_3 = 5$$

These activities are based on results obtained with vitamin D-deficient animals that were otherwise normal.

Vitamin D deficiency is best diagnosed using measurements of 25-OH-D. When levels below 7 to 10 ng/ml are observed, vitamin D deficiency can be expected even if $1,25\text{-}(OH)_2D$ levels are 35 pg/ml. Under conditions of osteomalacia treated with physiologic levels of vitamin D, levels of $1,25\text{-}(OH)_2D_3$ rise to the 200 to 300 pg/ml level during the healing process. Thus, a normal level of $1,25\text{-}(OH)_2D$ under this circumstance is higher than 35 pg/ml. It is clear, therefore, that the 25-OH-D level is the best diagnostic test of vitamin D deficiency.

## FUNCTIONS

Vitamin D brings about normal bone and endochondral calcification, preventing rickets in the young and osteomalacia in the adult.[90] It also plays an important role in the prevention of hypocalcemic tetany, a function it shares with the parathyroid hormone.[91] Because the vitamin is essential for calcium absorption, it may also function in the prevention of osteoporosis by ensuring adequate calcium from the environment, thus preventing reliance on the skeleton to support normal serum calcium concentration.[92] To prevent hypocalcemic tetany and to provide for normal mineralization of bone and cartilage, vitamin D is re-

sponsible for the elevation of plasma calcium and phosphorus concentration to supersaturation.[12,13] Although it has been suggested that some form of vitamin D is required for matrix synthesis and the calcification process, recent studies have excluded this possibility.[92,93] To elevate plasma calcium and phosphorus, vitamin D activates active transport of calcium[94] and phosphorus[95] in the intestine, improves renal reabsorption of calcium,[96] and stimulates the mobilization of calcium from the bone fluid compartment.[97] All these mechanisms then result in the elevation of plasma calcium and phosphorus concentrations to normal levels required for normal mineralization of bone. Vitamin D stimulates bone resorption in culture[98] and bone remodeling in vivo.[99] Thus, this function must be recognized as an important one distinct from the bone calcium mobilization system. Bone remodeling is required to maintain a healthy skeleton, whereas modeling is required for shaping the skeleton during growth and development.[99]

There is evidence that vitamin D functions to improve muscle strength,[90] but the nature of this function is not known.

### $1,25\text{-}(OH)_2D_3$ as a Hormone

Vitamin D is converted in the liver to 25-OH-$D_3$ and subsequently in the kidney to $1,25\text{-}(OH)_2D_3$ before it exercises its metabolic functions. Nephrectomized animals do not synthesize $1,25\text{-}(OH)_2D_3$.[100] The target organs of intestine[101] and bone[102] thus do not respond to physiologic doses of 25-OH-$D_3$ and vitamin $D_3$, but do respond normally to $1,25\text{-}(OH)_2D_3$. Because $1,25\text{-}(OH)_2D_3$ is made exclusively in kidney and functions in bone and intestine, it is considered a hormone.[12,13] As a hormone, its biosynthesis is stimulated by hypocalcemia, hypophosphatemia, and certain hormones.[54,55] It is the major calcium-regulating hormone and serves as an important phosphate-regulating hormone.

Figure 13–4 illustrates the role of serum calcium and phosphorus in the regulation of vitamin D metabolism. Low blood calcium indirectly stimulates $1\alpha$-hydroxylation of 25-OH-$D_3$ by the kidney system via the parathyroid gland.[103] Hypocalcemia itself may directly stimulate the $1\alpha$-hydroxylase, but this possibility has not yet been proven. Low blood phosphorus also stimulates $1\alpha$-hydroxylase,[104–105] whereas $1,25\text{-}(OH)_2D_3$ suppresses that system. Suppression of the $1\alpha$-hydroxylase is usually associated with a stimulation of 25-OH-$D_3$-24-hydroxylase. This system 24-hydroxylates not only 25-OH-$D_3$ but also 1,25-

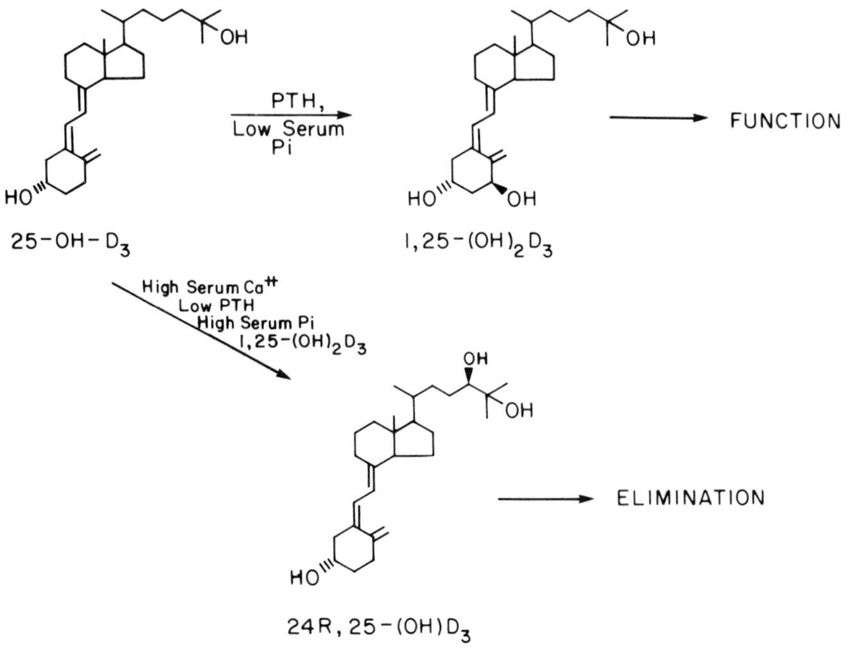

**Fig. 13–4.** Regulation of 25-OH-D$_3$ metabolism by serum calcium, phosphorus, and parathyroid hormone (PTH).

(OH)$_2$D$_3$ as well. 24-Hydroxylation is viewed as an inactivation system and does not play a role in the functions of vitamin D.[106]

### Calcium Homeostasis

A fall in serum calcium concentration stimulates secretion of the parathyroid hormone. This peptide hormone stimulates biosynthesis of 1,25-(OH)$_2$D$_3$.[103] The 1,25-(OH)$_2$D$_3$ stimulates intestinal calcium absorption and, together with the parathyroid hormone, stimulates renal reabsorption of calcium and mobilization of calcium from bone.[107] The resultant rise in serum calcium suppresses parathyroid hormone secretion, thus shutting down 1,25-(OH)$_2$D$_3$ biosynthesis and calcium mobilization. When calcium rises above normal, the C cells of the thyroid secrete the hormone calcitonin, which blocks mobilization of calcium from bone and perhaps stimulates calcium and phosphorus excretion in the kidney, thus restoring calcium to normal.[55]

Parathyroid hormone does not bind to intestine and thus does not directly influence calcium absorption.[108] Rather it stimulates calcium absorption by stimulating 1,25-(OH)$_2$D$_3$ synthesis.[109] In the bone and kidney, however, both parathyroid hormone and 1,25-(OH)$_2$D$_3$ must be present to stimulate the mobilization and retention of calcium.[107] The parathyroid hormone is rapid-acting, and its actions are spent in minutes. On the other hand, the stimulation of 1,25-(OH)$_2$D$_3$ and its actions require many hours.[110] Thus, short-term con-

trol of serum calcium is by parathyroid hormone acting on kidney and bone with existing 1,25-(OH)$_2$D$_3$, whereas prolonged hypocalcemia causes 1,25-(OH)$_2$D$_3$ to increase, stimulating the intestine to absorb calcium. Thus the ability to adjust calcium absorption to the needs of the organism is by parathyroid hormone-1,25-(OH)$_2$D$_3$ stimulation.[109-111] Exogenous parathyroid hormone or 1,25-(OH)$_2$D$_3$ eliminates the ability of the intestine to adapt.[110,111] Thus, Nicolaysen's "endogenous factor" is the parathyroid hormone-vitamin D endocrine complex.[112]

### Differentiation of Marrow Stem Cells in Response to Vitamin D Hormone

Suda and his colleagues have provided an interesting new development in the field of vitamin D function.[113] The addition of the vitamin D hormone to cultures of human promyelocyte HL-60 cells causes them to differentiate into monocytes or macrophages. Concentrations required for this differentiation are near physiologic. These findings suggest that the vitamin D compounds may be utilized in the treatment of acute myelocytic-type leukemic diseases. A major problem is that the vitamin D compounds in such instances would cause a hypercalcemia because of their calcemic actions, and thus might prevent the achievement of sufficient concentrations to be of therapeutic value in the treatment of acute myeloid leukemias.

The other interesting implication of this development is that the macrophages are natural precursors of osteoclasts. Thus it is enticing to consider that the vitamin D may have an important role in the formation of bone resorbing cells, the osteoclasts. Osteoclasts, however, are certainly found in vitamin D deficiency, both in young animals and in lactating mothers.[93,114] Although the vitamin D hormone may be involved in the formation of osteoclasts, this cannot represent the sole pathway because of the existence of osteoclasts in frank vitamin D deficiency.

Vitamin D compounds have also been used to inhibit growth of several neoplastic cell lines, including a melanoma cell line, a T47D human breast carcinoma cell line, and certain types of lymphomas. Whether this approach will be fruitful in the anticancer field remains undetermined.

## MECHANISM OF ACTION OF 1,25-(OH)$_2$D$_3$

1,25-(OH)$_2$D$_3$ is believed to bind to a 3.2-3.7 receptor[115,116] located in the nucleus[117] to initiate transcription of genes[118] that code for calcium and phosphate transport proteins. Indeed, 1,25-(OH)$_2$D$_3$ is located in the nucleus in the functioning intestine consistent with the steroid hormone receptor mechanism.[119] Further, receptor proteins have been identified and shown to bind to nuclei.

The nature of the calcium-phosphorus transport remains unknown. Wasserman and co-workers identified a calcim-binding protein in chicks and mammalian species that may play a role in calcium transport.[120] Although this possibility is likely to be true, it is also clear that additional proteins must function in this process. Thus there is a current search for the vitamin D-induced proteins in target cells that carry out the function of this hormone. Another possibility is that a nonnuclear mechanism may supplement the nuclear mechanism in terms of expression of vitamin D action.[121] In any case, the ultimate effect is that the vitamin D hormone alters the intestinal epithelial cells to permit calcium to enter the cell to be transferred across the cell and to be expelled in the serosal medium by a sodium-dependent process.[122] Much remains to be learned about the molecular mechanism of action of this steroid hormone in inducing expression of specific genes.

Little is known concerning the phosphate transport system of intestine except that it requires sodium and is active.[123,124]

In the bone, 1,25-(OH)$_2$D$_3$ binds to a 3.2S receptor and ultimately appears in the nuclei of osteoblasts and/or osteocytes. It initiates calcium mobilization by a transcriptive event because this action is blocked by actinomycin D.[110]

## VITAMIN D DEFICIENCY AND DISEASE STATES

### Deficiency

Many biochemical and physiologic imbalances occur in the deficient state, which, if not corrected, result in rickets in growing children and osteomalacia in adults.[125] Characteristic biochemical changes include low plasma calcium and inorganic phosphorus levels with a concomitant high plasma alkaline phosphatase. Early in deficiency a defect in calcium absorption occurs. This condition often leads to secondary hyperparathyroidism, in which parathyroid hormone is secreted in response to a low plasma calcium concentration. With remaining 1,25-(OH)$_2$D$_3$, bone calcium is mobilized, restoring serum calcium to normal, but parathyroid hormone also causes phosphaturia leading to hypophosphatemia, which results in a failure of mineralization and bone disease. Rickets occurs when the newly synthesized organic matrix, osteoid, fails to mineralize, resulting in soft bones. Most striking is the failure of endochondral calcification, resulting in widening of the epiphyseal plate and the buildup of osteoid tissue.

Vitamin D affects citrate metabolism; for example, in one study the serum citrate in 10 rachitic infants was 1.5 mg/dl compared to 2.5 mg/dl in normal infants.[126] Vitamin D treatment (i.e., 600,000 I.U.) resulted in elevation of the serum citrate; however, it is now clear that the citrate response is a consequence of, rather than a participant in, the vitamin-induced changes in mineral metabolism.[127]

Diagnosis of rickets is usually made from the characteristic bony deformities seen on radiographs (see Chapter 48) and from the plasma calcium, phosphorus, and alkaline phosphatase values. The noncalcified epiphyseal plate becomes more apparent, and broadening and irregularity occur in the adjacent regions of the epiphysis and metaphysis (see Chapter 46 for a discussion of changes seen on bone biopsy).

Although vitamin D-deficiency rickets is now rare in the western world, several disorders still exist in which the action of the vitamin is apparently lacking within the calcium homeostatic system. It is now clear that vitamin D is converted to an active hormone that acts on the target tissue, resulting in appropriate responses. Thus some diseases of bone are probably the result of a defective vitamin D metabolism, regulation, or target organ response.

## Refractory or Vitamin D-Resistant Rickets (Familial Hypophosphatemia)

This disease is usually manifest during childhood and during the rapid phase of growth before puberty. It is characterized by hypophosphatemia and an X-linked dominant inheritance.[128] Although the exact resulting molecular defect that causes the disease is not clearly known, the most characteristic dysfunction is a renal loss of phosphate. In addition, intestinal calcium absorption is below normal. Abnormal vitamin D metabolism has been reported in this disease,[129] but the phosphate defect is not corrected by the administration of $1,25\text{-}(OH)_2D_3$ or $25\text{-}OH\text{-}D_3$.[130] It is likely that a generalized defect in phosphate transport mechanisms is not related to abnormal vitamin D metabolism. The low calcium absorption is the result of inadequate $1,25\text{-}(OH)_2D_3$ levels in blood.[131] Furthermore, the defective absorption of calcium in the disease is corrected by administration of $1,25\text{-}(OH)_2D_2$ or $1\alpha\text{-}OH\text{-}D_3$.[132] Treatment with massive doses of vitamin D (e.g., 50,000 to 100,000 I.U. daily) gives variable results.[133] Some investigators have reported better success by using lower amounts of vitamin D (e.g., 15,000 to 50,000 I.U. daily) in conjunction with oral phosphate supplements.[134]

More recently, $1,25\text{-}(OH)_2D_3$ has been used in the treatment of the disease, together with oral phosphate, with good success.[132] The oral phosphate replaces the renal loss of phosphate while the $1,25\text{-}(OH)_2D_3$ repairs the calcium transport mechanism and prevents secondary hyperparathyroidism.

## Hypoparathyroidism

Hypoparathyroidism usually occurs as a result of surgical removal of the parathyroid glands. Idiopathic hypoparathyroidism is uncommon. This rare disease frequently persists with major convulsive seizures in addition to tetanic spasms. Such patients often have years of anticonvulsant therapy before the underlying pathologic condition is detected. In this context it is interesting that the long-term use of anticonvulsant drugs apparently accelerates the metabolic breakdown of vitamin D.[135,136]

Hypoparathyroidism has been treated with high doses of dihydrotachysterol or vitamin $D_2$. Dihydrotachysterol is reported to be the more active compound on a weight basis.[137] Occasionally, hypoparathyroid patients develop a resistance to treatment with vitamin D and dihydrotachysterol, necessitating the search for derivatives that may be more active. $25\text{-}OH\text{-}D_3$ is more effective than vitamin $D_3$ or dihydrotachysterol.[138] Of great importance is the fact that parathyroid hormone stimulates $1,25\text{-}(OH)_2D_3$ synthesis; thus, hypoparathyroid patients produce inadequate $1,25\text{-}(OH)_2D_3$ in response to hypocalcemia. Exogenous $1,25\text{-}(OH)_2D_3$ and its analogue $1\alpha\text{-}OH\text{-}D_3$ are effective at physiologic doses in management of this disease, provided dietary calcium is adequate.[139,140]

## Vitamin D-Dependency Rickets Types I and II

Prader and his associates have described a vitamin D-resistant rickets in children that is completely curable with doses of vitamin D ranging from 50,000 to 100,000 I.U. daily.[141] Vitamin D-dependency rickets differs from familial hypophosphatemia in that the latter does not respond completely to vitamin D, and the former is an autosomal recessive trait. Several children suffering from this disease have responded to 30 to 500 µg $25\text{-}OH\text{-}D_3$ daily.[142] Because pharmacologic amounts of this form of the vitamin are required for treatment, the disease is not the result of a block in 25-hydroxylation of vitamin D. However, it is probably a specific genetic block in 1-hydroxylation of $25\text{-}OH\text{-}D_3$ because physiologic amounts (0.05 µg/kg) of $1,25\text{-}(OH)_2D_3$ will cure the disease, and low blood levels of $1,25\text{-}(OH)_2D_3$ have been found.[142] Cure with $25\text{-}OH\text{-}D_3$ probably results from excess $25\text{-}OH\text{-}D_3$ substituting for small amounts of $1,25\text{-}(OH)_2D_3$ in the receptor mechanisms.[143]

By means of new methods for determining $1,25\text{-}(OH)_2D_3$ levels, a new type of vitamin D-resistant rickets has been discovered that is named vitamin D-dependency rickets type II.[144,145] Although not clearly established, the genetics are likely to be autosomal recessive, and the affected subjects present with severe rickets, alopecia, and high plasma levels of $1,25\text{-}(OH)_2D_3$. These patients are resistant to levels of $1,25\text{-}(OH)_2D_3$ as high as 32 µg/subject/day, with the normal production rate of this hormonal form of vitamin D being about 1 µg/day. At least one subset of this disease is a defect in the receptor mechanism for $1,25\text{-}(OH)_2D_3$ in the target organs.[146] In any case, treatment of the affected subjects is by administration of large amounts of $1,25\text{-}(OH)_2D_3$ and large amounts of dietary calcium and phosphorus with only limited success.

## Osteoporosis and Possible Involvement of Vitamin D System

In normal subjects, a need for calcium is reflected in slightly low plasma calcium concentration that stimulates the parathyroid glands to secrete parathyroid hormone. This process in turn stimulates production of the vitamin D hormone that then stimulates intestinal calcium absorption. Thus under circumstances where calcium is required, the normal response brings about an elevated efficiency of calcium absorption to provide the needed calcium. If this mechanism fails, the organism will continue to secrete parathyroid hormone and will mobilize calcium from the skeleton to provide for its presence at the neuromuscular junction. This mechanism, although preventing the serious disorder of hypocalcemia tetany, causes a loss of the skeleton. If loss of skeleton continues daily to provide for plasma calcium concentration required by the soft tissues, trabecular bone is sacrificed resulting in thin bones that are prone to fractures. In this concept, a defect in vitamin D metabolism might contribute to some of the osteoporotic syndromes. Furthermore since $1,25\text{-}(OH)_2D_3$ is involved in the initial event in bone modeling and remodeling, i.e., stimulation of osteoclastic resorption, this process of bone is also compromised under these circumstances.

Deficiency of the vitamin D hormone can result as either a primary event or a secondary event in osteoporosis. In the case of the postmenopausal woman, loss of estrogen somehow brings about the release of bone calcium that suppresses parathyroid secretion that in turn suppresses $1,25\text{-}(OH)_2D_3$ production.[147] A failure of calcium absorption results, and the organism shifts its dependency from dietary sources to skeletal calcium with a continuous loss of skeletal calcium regardless of dietary calcium levels. In fact, increased calcium intake of postmenopausal women suffering from osteoporosis does not prevent their bone loss, a fact that is consistent with a low circulating level of $1,25\text{-}(OH)_2D_3$.[148]

In addition, as a function of age, plasma level of $1,25\text{-}(OH)_2D_3$ is inadequate regardless of sex.[147] In the case of aging subjects, the capacity to produce $1,25\text{-}(OH)_2D_3$ is markedly reduced in response to a parathyroid hormone challenge.[149] Thus the thinning of bones as a result of aging itself could be a primary defect in the production of $1,25\text{-}(OH)_2D_3$ to provide for adequate intestinal calcium absorption and for adequate bone remodeling.

Another possible mechanism is that which is induced by high levels of glucocorticoids. The glucocorticoids inhibit directly intestinal calcium absorption, thereby limiting environment calcium and shifting the dependence of the organism to bone calcium. All these circumstances bring about a loss of bone mass resulting ultimately in the disappearance of trabecular bone. This condition gives rise to vertebral crush fractures initially and ultimately to fractures elsewhere.

Promising results have been obtained by treat-ing postmenopausal women with osteoporosis with $1,25\text{-}(OH)_2D_3$.[148] Doses of approximately 0.5 µg/day improve intestinal absorption of calcium to increase calcium balance, to increase the amount of trabecular bone and, most importantly, to reduce the fraction rate. Probably $1,25\text{-}(OH)_2D_3$ does more than merely increase calcium absorption; it likely increases bone remodeling, giving rise to a stronger skeleton. This important new development will be widely explored in the future to provide for a major treatment for the most widespread of the metabolic bone diseases.

## Azotemic Chronic Renal Failure

Patients suffering from chronic renal failure often exhibit abnormally low intestinal calcium absorption, low plasma calcium, secondary hyperparathyroidism, and osteodystrophy.[150,151] Such patients have features of both osteitis fibrosa and/or osteomalacia.[152] They are resistant to vitamin D and show abnormal vitamin D metabolism.[153] These patients respond satisfactorily to 50 to 100 µg/day of $25\text{-}OH\text{-}D_3$ as compared to much larger doses of vitamin D.[99] Because renal tissue is responsible for the metabolism of $25\text{-}OH\text{-}D_3$ to $1,25\text{-}(OH)_2D_3$, which is the metabolically active form of vitamin D, it is likely that, in chronic renal disease, $1,25\text{-}(OH)_2D_3$ is not made in sufficient amounts. Thus a "vitamin D"-deficient intestine and, ultimately, bone result. The resulting hypocalcemia brings about secondary hyperparathyroidism and osteitis fibrosa (see Chapter 46). Another abnormal feature of this disease is a rise in serum phosphorus because of failure of excretion. The rise in serum phosphorus also suppresses remaining renal $1\alpha$-hydroxylase, contributing to the failure of calcium absorption and suppression of parathyroid secretion.[154] Osteomalacia results from aluminum intoxication.[155] Aluminum was found to be a contaminant of dialysis fluids until this was recognized and corrected. Aluminum hydroxide is used as oral phosphate binder to control plasma phosphorus, and some aluminum is also absorbed. To heal osteomalacia, removal of aluminum is required as well as correction of the hypocalcemia. The $1,25\text{-}(OH)_2D_3$ satisfactorily restores calcium absorption to normal in nephrectomized rats.[101] Furthermore, $1,25\text{-}(OH)_2D_3$ and $1\alpha\text{-}OH\text{-}D_3$ are used in the successful treatment of a high proportion of renal osteodystrophy patients.[156–159] Pharmacologic amounts of $25\text{-}OH\text{-}D_3$ are also successfully employed in the treatment.[153]

Other bone diseases may also be of interest with regard to vitamin D metabolism. The vitamin D resistance of such diseases as hepatic rickets and Fanconi syndrome makes the investigation into the use of vitamin D metabolites for the treatment of such illnesses an exciting area of clinical investigation.

## HYPERVITAMINOSIS D (VITAMIN D TOXICITY)

Care should be taken to detect any hypercalcemia or hypercalciuria when one is using large doses of vitamin D. Either condition could be indicative of intoxication. Irreversible renal, heart, and aortic damage results from prolonged hypercalcemia. Serum calcium should not be permitted to rise above 12 mg/dl.[160]

Treatment in mild cases consists of withdrawing vitamin D until serum calcium falls, necessitating the readministration of vitamin D, usually at a reduced level. More severe cases may require the use of glucocorticoids to reduce serum calcium concentration.[161] Calcitonin may also occasionally be used in the treatment of hypervitaminosis D.[162] Toxicity of vitamin D is believed to be the result of high circulating 25-OH-D levels that substitute for $1,25\text{-}(OH)_2D_3$ on the receptor when at excessive concentrations.[143] Thus calcium transport and bone resorption continue at high and unchecked rates, causing hypercalcemia and nephrocalcinosis.

## IMPORTANT ANALOGUES OF $1,25\text{-}(OH)_2D_3$

A synthetic analogue of importance is $1\alpha\text{-}OH\text{-}D_3$, which is not naturally occurring.[163] It is converted in the liver to the active hormone $1,25\text{-}(OH)_2D_3$ before it acts.[164] It is relatively easy to synthesize and is used therapeutically as a substitute for $1,25\text{-}(OH)_2D_3$.

Dihydrotachysterol$_2$ is a reduction product of vitamin $D_3$ or the photoisomer tachysterol$_2$. The 9,10 double bond is reduced, and the A ring is rotated about the 5,6 double bond.[17] Thus the 3-OH group is in the spatial position of the 1-OH of $1,25\text{-}(OH)_2D_3$. It therefore acts without undergoing 1-hydroxylation. Similarly, the 5,6-*trans* vitamin $D_3$ acts without 1-hydroxylation. They are, however, poor substitutes for $1,25\text{-}(OH)_2D_3$.[164]

## SUMMARY

In summary, the mode of action for vitamin D is becoming increasingly clear; as evidenced by the discovery of the kidney-based vitamin D endocrine system and the hydroxylated vitamin D metabolites, especially $1,25\text{-}(OH)_2D_3$. Vitamin D is first hydroxylated in the liver to $25\text{-}OH\text{-}D_3$, which represents the major circulating form of the vitamin in blood. Further hydroxylation of $25\text{-}OH\text{-}D_3$ to $1,25\text{-}(OH)_2D_3$ occurs in the kidney. It is the latter compound that acts directly to carry out the functions of vitamin D.

The realization that vitamin D serves only as a precursor for the synthesis of a hormone suggests that some vitamin D-related diseases may involve a block in the production of the active form of the vitamin. It is already apparent that renal osteodystrophy, vitamin D dependency, and hypoparathyroidism are such diseases. These and several other diseases are managed with the active metabolites of vitamin D and their analogues.

## REFERENCES

1. Griffenhagen, G.: Bull. Natl. Inst. Nutr. *2*:8, 1952.
2. Bennett, J.H.: Treatise on the Oleum Jecoris Aselli or Cod-liver Oil. Edinburgh, 1848.
3. Palm, T.A.: Practitioner *45*:270, 1890.
4. Mellanby, E.: J. Physiol. *52*:Liii, 1919.
5. McCollum, E.V., Simonds, N., Becker, J.E., et al.: J. Biol. Chem. *53*:293, 1922.
6. McCollum, E.V., Simonds, N., Becker, J.E., et al.: Bull. Johns Hopkins Hosp. *33*:229, 1922.
7. Huldshinsky, K.: Dtsch. Med. Wochenschr. *45*:712–713, 1919.
8. Steenbock, H., Black, A.: J. Biol. Chem. *61*:405–422, 1924.
9. Steenbock, H.: Science *60*:224–225, 1924.
10. Askew, F.A., Bourdillon, R.B., Bruce, H.M., et al.: Proc. R. Soc. *B107*:76, 1931.
11. Windaus, A., Schenck, F., von Werder, F.: Hoppe Seylers Z. Physiol. Chem. *241*:100–103, 1936.
12. DeLuca, H.F.: Vitam. Horm. *25*:315–367, 1967.
13. DeLuca, H.F.: Fed. Proc. *33*:2211–2219, 1974.
14. Bernstein, S., Oleson, J.J., Ritter, H.B., et al.: J. Am. Chem. Soc. *71*:2576–2577, 1949.
15. Bernstein, S., Sax, K.J.: J. Org. Chem. *16*:685–693, 1951.
16. Parfitt: Aust. Ann. Med. *16*:114, 1967.
17. Hallick, R.B., DeLuca, H.F.: J. Biol. Chem. *246*:5733–5738, 1971.
18. Jones, G.: In Vitamin D: Biochemical, Chemical and Clinical Aspects Related to Calcium Metabolism. (Norman, A.W., Schaefer, K., Coburn, J., et al., Eds.) Berlin, Walter de Gruyter, Inc., 1977.
19. U.S. Pharmacopoeia, 15th Revision, U.S.P. XV. Easton, Mack Publishing, 1955.
20. Association of Official Analytical Chemists, (E. Horwitz, Ed.) Box 540, Benjamin Franklin Station, Washington, D.C.
21. Shepard, R.M., Horst, R.L., Hamstra, A.J., et al.: Biochem. J. *182*:55–69, 1979.
22. Thompson, G.R., Lewis, B., Booth, C.C.: J. Clin. Invest. *45*:94–96, 1966.
23. Schachter, D., Finkelstein, J.D., Kowarski, S.: J. Clin. Invest. *43*:787–796, 1964.
24. Greaves, J.D., Schmidt, C.L.A.: J. Biol. Chem. *102*:101–112, 1933.
25. Ponchon, G., DeLuca, H.F.: J. Clin. Invest. *48*:1273–1279, 1969.
26. Bhattacharyya, M., DeLuca, H.F.: Arch. Biochem. Biophys. *160*:58–62, 1974.
27. Botham, K.M., Ghazarian, J.G., Kream, B.E., et al.: Biochemistry *15*:2130–2135, 1976.
28. Imawari, M., Goodman, D.S.: J. Clin. Invest. *59*:432–442, 1977.
29. Haddad, J.G., Walgate, J.: J. Biol. Chem. *251*:4803–4809, 1976.
30. Kumar, R., Nagubandi, S., Mattox, V.R., et al.: J. Clin. Invest. *65*:277–284, 1980.

31. Kumar, R., Nagubandi, S., Londowski, J.M.: J. Lab. Clin. Med. *96*:278–284, 1980.
32. Avioli, L.V., Williams, T.F., Lund, et al.: J. Clin. Invest. *46*:1907–1915, 1967.
33. Esvelt, R.P., Schnoes, H.K., DeLuca, H.F.: Arch. Biochem. Biophys. *188*:282–286, 1978.
34. Holick, M.F.: J. Invest. Dermatol. *76*:51–58, 1981.
35. Esvelt, R.P., DeLuca, H.F., Wichmann, J.K., et al.: Biochemistry *19*:6158–6161, 1980.
36. MacLaughlin, J.A., Anderson, R.R., Holick, M.F.: Science *216*:1001–1003, 1982.
37. Clemens, T.L., Henderson, S.L., Adams, J.S., et al.: Lancet *9*:74–76, 1982.
38. Eisman, J.A., Shepard, R.M., DeLuca, H.F.: Anal. Biochem. *80*:298–305, 1982.
39. Tanaka, Y., Frank, H., DeLuca, H.F.: Endocrinology *92*:417–422, 1973.
40. Tanaka, Y., Frank, H., DeLuca, H.F.: J. Nutr. *102*:1569–1577, 1972.
41. Shike, M., Sturtridge, W.C., Tam, C.S., et al.: Ann. Intern. Med. *95*:560–567, 1981.
42. Bills, C.E.: Vitamin D group (Sections II-V). *In* The Vitamins. Vol. II (Sebrell, W.H., Jr., Harris, R.S., Eds.) New York, Academic Press, 1954.
43. Blondin, G.A., Kulkarni, B.D., Nes, W.R.: Comp. Biochem. Physiol. *20*:379–390, 1967.
44. Recommended Dietary Allowances. 9th ed. Washington, National Academy of Sciences, National Research Council, 1980.
45. Maternal Nutrition and Child Health, Bull. 123. Washington, National Research Council, Food and Nutrition Board, 1950 (reprinted 1957).
46. Fraser, D., Salter, R.B.: Pediatr. Clin. North Am. May, 417–441, 1958.
47. Fomon, S.J., Younozai, K., Thomas, L.N.: J. Nutr. *88*:345–350, 1966.
48. Fellers, F., Schwartz, R.: N. Engl. J. Med. *259*:1050–1058, 1958.
49. Paterson, C.R., Path, M.R.C.: Lancet *1*:1164–1166, 1980.
50. Hess, A.F., Lewis, J.M.: JAMA *91*:783–788, 1928.
51. Gardner, L.I.: Pediatrics *9*:534–543, 1952.
52. Bruce, H.M., Callow, R.K.: Biochem. J. *28*:517–528, 1934.
53. Mellanby, M., Mellanby, H.: Br. Med. J. *2*:409–413, 1948.
54. DeLuca, H.F., Schnoes, H.K.: Annu. Rev. Biochem. *52*:411–439, 1983.
55. DeLuca, H.F.: The vitamin D-calcium axis—1983. *In* Calcium in Biological Systems. (Rubin, R.P., Weiss, G.B., Putney, J.W., Jr., Eds.) New York, Plenum Publishing Corp., 1985, pp. 491–511.
56. Dueland, S., Holmberg, I., Berg, T., et al.: J. Biol. Chem. *256*:10430–10434, 1981.
57. Haddad, J.G., Jr., Hahn, T.J.: Nature *244*:515–517, 1973.
58. Yoon, P.S., DeLuca, H.F.: Arch. Biochem. Biophys. *203*:529–541, 1980.
59. Madhok, T.C., DeLuca, H.F.: Biochem. J. *184*:491–499, 1979.
60. Ghazarian, J.G., Jefcoate, C.R., Knutson, J.C., et al.: J. Biol. Chem. *249*:3026–3033, 1974.
61. Reeve, L., Tanaka, Y., DeLuca, H.F.: J. Biol. Chem. *258*:3615–3617, 1983.
62. Shultz, T.D., Fox, J., Heath, H., III, et al.: Proc. Natl. Acad. Sci. USA *80*:1746–1750, 1983.
63. Tanaka, Y., Halloran, B., Schnoes, H.K., et al.: Proc. Natl. Acad. Sci. USA *76*:5033–5035, 1979.
63a. Paulson S., DeLuca, H.F.: Unpublished data, 1986.
64. Weisman, Y., Sapir, R., Harell, A., et al.: Biochim. Biophys. Acta *428*:388–395.
65. Howard, G.A., Turner, R.T., Sherrard, D.J., et al.: J. Biol. Chem. *256*:7738–7740, 1981.
66. Turner, R.T., Puzas, J.E., Forte, M.D., et al.: Proc. Natl. Acad. Sci. USA *77*:5720–5724, 1980.
67. Barbour, G.L., Coburn, J.W., Slatopolsky, E., et al.: N. Engl. J. Med. *305*:440–443, 1981.
68. Epstein, S., Stern, P.M., Bell, N.H., et al.: Calcif. Tissue Int. *36*:541–544, 1984.
69. Kleiner-Bossaller, A., DeLuca, H.F.: Biochim. Biophys. Acta *338*:489–495, 1974.
70. Esvelt, R.P., Schnoes, H.K., DeLuca, H.F.: Biochemistry *18*:3977–3983, 1979.
71. Tanaka, Y., DeLuca, H.F., Kobayashi, Y., et al.: J. Biol. Chem. *254*:7163–7167, 1979.
72. Brommage, R., Jarnagin, K., DeLuca, H.F., et al.: Am. J. Physiol. *244*:E298–E304, 1983.
73. Parfitt, A.M., Mathews, C.H.E., Brommage, R., et al.: J. Clin. Invest. *73*:576–586, 1984.
74. Ikekawa, N., Koizumi, N., Ohshima, E., et al.: Proc. Natl. Acad. Sci. USA *80*:5286–5288, 1983.
75. Lam, H-Y., Schnoes, H.K., DeLuca, H.F.: Steroids *25*:247–256, 1975.
76. Wichmann, J.K., DeLuca, H.F., Schnoes, H.K., et al.: Biochemistry *18*:4775–4780, 1979.
77. Tanaka, Y., Wichmann, J.K., Schnoes, H.K., et al.: Biochemistry *20*:3875–3879, 1981.
78. Tanaka, Y., Pahuja, D.N., Wichmann, J.K., et al.: Arch. Biochem. Biophys. *218*:134–141, 1982.
79. Jones, G., Schnoes, H.K., DeLuca, H.F.: J. Biol. Chem. *251*:24–28, 1976.
80. Jones, G., Schnoes, H.K., LeVan, L., et al.: Arch. Biochem. Biophys. *202*:450–457, 1980.
81. Jones, G., Baxter, L.A., DeLuca, H.F., et al.: Biochemistry *15*:713–716, 1976.
82. Hunt, R.D., Garcia, F.C., Hegsted, D.M.: Lab. Anim. Care *17*:222–234, 1967.
83. Imrie, M.H., Neville, P.F., Snellgrove, A.W.: Arch. Biochem. Biophys. *120*:525–532, 1967.
84. Takahashi, N., Suda, S., Shinki, T., et al.: Biochem. J. *227*:555–563, 1985.
85. Belsey, R.E., DeLuca, H.F., Potts, J.T., Jr.: Nature *247*:208–209, 1974.
86. Shepard, R.M., Horst, R.L., Hamstra, A.J., et al.: Biochem. J. *182*:55–69, 1979.
87. Eisman, J.A., Hamstra, A.J., Kream, B.E., et al.: Arch. Biochem. Biophys. *176*:235–243, 1976.
88. Clemens, T.L., Hendy, G.N., Graham, R.F., et al.: Clin. Sci. Mol. Med. *54*:329–332, 1978.
89. Clemens, T.L., Hendy, G.N., Papapoulos, S.E., et al.: Endocrinology *11*:225–234, 1979.
90. Hess, A. (Ed.): *In* Rickets, Including Osteomalacia and Tetany. Philadelphia, Lea & Febiger, 1929, pp. 22–37.
91. DeLuca, H.F.: Proceedings of the Annual Meeting of the Royal College of Physicians and Surgeons of Canada. January 29, 1977. Toronto, 1977, pp. 216–225.
92. Underwood, J.L., DeLuca, H.F.: Am. J. Physiol. *246*:E493–E498, 1984.
93. Weinstein, R.S., Underwood, J.L., Hutson, M.S., et al.: Am. J. Physiol. *246*:E499–E505, 1984.
94. DeLuca, H.F., Franceschi, R.T., Halloran, B.P., et al.: Fed. Proc. *41*:66–71, 1982.
95. Chen, T.C., Castillo, L., Korycka-Dahl, M., et al.: J. Nutr. *104*:1056–1060, 1974.
96. Sutton, R.A.L., Dirks, J.H.: Fed. Proc. *37*:2112–2119, 1978.

97. Carlsson, A.: Acta Physiol. Scand. *26*:212–220, 1952.
98. Raisz, L.G., Trummel, C.L., Holick, M.F., et al.: Science *175*:768–769, 1972.
99. Frost, H.M.: Bone dynamics in osteoporosis and osteomalacia. *In* Henry Ford Hospital Surgical Monograph Series. Springfield, Charles C Thomas Co., 1966.
100. Gray, R., Boyle, I., DeLuca, H.F.: Science *172*:1232–1234, 1971.
101. Boyle, I.T., Miravet, L., Gray, R.W., et al.: Endocrinology *90*:605–608, 1972.
102. Holick, M.F., Garabedian, M., DeLuca, H.F.: Science *176*:1146–1147, 1972.
103. Tanaka, Y., DeLuca, H.F.: Proc. Natl. Acad. Sci. USA *78*:196–199, 1981.
104. Baxter, L.A., DeLuca, H.F.: J. Biol. Chem. *251*:3158–3161, 1976.
105. Tanaka, Y., DeLuca, H.F.: Am. J. Physiol. *246*:E168–E173, 1984.
106. Garabedian, M., Holick, M.F., DeLuca, H.F., et al.: Proc. Natl. Acad. Sci. USA *69*:1673–1676, 1972.
107. Garabedian, M., Tanaka, Y., Holick, M.F., et al.: Endocrinology *94*:1022–1027, 1974.
108. Zull, J.E., Repke, D.W.: J. Biol. Chem. *247*:2195–2199, 1972.
109. Ribovich, M.L., DeLuca, H.F.: Arch. Biochem. Biophys. *175*:256–261, 1976.
110. Tanaka, Y., DeLuca, H.F.: Arch. Biochem. Biophys. *146*:574–578, 1971.
111. Ribovich, M.L., DeLuca, H.F.: Arch. Biochem. Biophys. *170*:529–535, 1975.
112. Boyle, I.T., Gray, R.W., Omdahl, J.L., et al.: *In* Endocrinology 1971. (Taylor, Ed.) London, Wm. Heinemann Medical Books, 1972, pp. 468–476.
113. Abe, E., Miyaura, C., Sakagami, H., et al.: Proc. Natl. Acad. Sci. USA *78*:4990–4994, 1981.
114. Miller, S.C., Halloran, B.P., DeLuca, H.F., et al.: Calcif. Tissue Int. *34*:245–252, 1982.
115. Kream, B.C., Reynolds, R.H., Knutson, J.M., et al.: Arch. Biochem. Biophys. *176*:779, 1976.
116. Brumbaugh, P.F., Haussler, M.R.: Life Sci. *16*:353–362, 1975.
117. Brumbaugh, P.F., Haussler, M.R.: J. Biol. Chem. *249*:1258–1262, 1974.
118. Emtage, J.S., Lawson, D.E.M., Kodicek, E.: Nature *246*:100–101, 1973.
119. Chen, T.C., DeLuca, H.F.: J. Biol. Chem. *248*:4890–4895, 1973.
120. Wasserman, R.H., Feher, J.J.: Vitamin D-dependent calcium-binding proteins. *In* Calcium Binding Proteins and Calcium Function. (Wasserman, R.H., Corradino, R.A., Carafoli, E., et al., Eds.) New York, Elsevier Science Publishing Co., Inc., 1977, pp. 292–302.
121. Rasmussen, H., Matsumoto, T., Fontaine, O., et al.: Fed. Proc. *41*:72–77, 1982.
122. Martin, D.L., DeLuca, H.F.: Am. J. Physiol. *216*:1351–1359, 1969.
123. Taylor, A.N.: J. Nutr. *104*:489–494, 1974.
124. Walling, M.W.: Effects of 1α,25-dihydroxyvitamin D$_3$ on active intestinal inorganic phosphate absorption. *In* Vitamin D: Biochemical, Chemical, and Clinical Aspects Related to Calcium Metabolism. (Norman, A.W., Schaefer, K., Coburn, J.W., et al., Eds.) Berlin, Walter de Gruyter, 1977, pp. 321–330.
125. Fraser, D., Kooh, S.W., Scriver, C.R.: Pediatr. Res. *1*:425–435, 1967.
126. Harrison, H.E., Harrison, H.C.: Yale J. Biol. Med. *24*:273–283, 1952.
127. Harrison, H.E., Harrison, H.C.: Am. J. Physiol. *199*:265–271, 1960.
128. Williams, T.F., Winter, R.W., Burnett, C.H.: *In* The Metabolic Basis of Inherited Disease. (W. Stanbury, H. Wyngaarden, J. Fredrickson, Eds.) New York, McGraw-Hill Book Co., 1966, pp. 1179–1204.
129. Avioli, L.V., Williams, T.F., Lund, J., et al.: J. Clin. Invest. *46*:1907–1915, 1967.
130. Glorieux, F.H., Scriver, C.R., Holick, M.F., et al.: Lancet *2*:287–289, 1973.
131. Scriver, C.R., Reade, T.M., DeLuca, H.F., et al.: N. Engl. J. Med. *299*:976–979, 1978.
132. Glorieux, F.H., Marie, P.J., Pettifor, J.M., et al.: N. Engl. J. Med. *303*:1023–1031, 1980.
133. Harrison, H.E.: J. Pediatr. *64*:618–620, 1964.
134. Wilson, D.R., York, S.E., Jaworski, Z.R., et al.: Medicine *44*:99–134, 1965.
135. Hahn, T.J., Halstead, L.R.: Calcif. Tissue Int. *27*:13–18, 1979.
136. Richens, A., Rowe, D.J.F.: Br. Med. J. *4*:73–76, 1970.
137. Harrison, H.E., Lifshitz, F., Blizzard, R.M.: N. Engl. J. Med. *276*:894–900, 1967.
138. Pak, C., DeLuca, H.F., Chavez de los Rios, J.M., et al.: Arch. Intern. Med. *126*:239–247, 1970.
139. Kooh, S.W., Fraser, D., DeLuca, H.F., et al.: N. Engl. J. Med. *293*:840–844, 1975.
140. Neer, R.M., Holick, M.F., DeLuca, H.F., et al.: Metabolism *24*:1403–1413, 1975.
141. Prader, A., Illig, R., Heierli, E.: Helv. Paediatr. Acta *16*:452–468, 1961.
142. Fraser, D., Kooh, S.W., Kind, H.P., et al.: N. Engl. J. Med. *289*:817–822, 1973.
143. Eisman, J.A., DeLuca, H.F.: Steroids *30*:245–257, 1977.
144. Bell, N.H., Hamstra, A.J., DeLuca, H.F.: N. Engl. J. Med. *298*:997–999, 1978.
145. Rosen, J.F., Fleischman, A.R., Finberg, L., et al.: J. Pediatr. *94*:729–735, 1979.
146. Eil, C., Liberman, U.A., Rosen, J.F., et al.: N. Engl. J. Med. *304*:1588–1591, 1981.
147. Gallagher, J.C., Riggs, B.L., Eisman, J., et al.: J. Clin. Invest. *64*:729–736, 1979.
148. Gallagher, J.C., Jerpbak, C.M., Jee, W.S.S., et al.: Proc. Natl. Acad. Sci. USA *79*:3325–3329, 1982.
149. Slovik, D.M., Adams, J.S., Neer, R.M., et al.: N. Engl. J. Med. *305*:372–375, 1981.
150. Stanbury, S.W., Lumb, G.A.: Medicine *41*:1–32, 1962.
151. Kimberg, D.V., Baerg, R.D., Gershon, E.: Arch. Intern. Med. *126*:891–895, 1970.
152. Avioli, L.V., Birge, S., Lee, S.W., et al.: J. Clin. Invest. *47*:2239–2252, 1968.
153. Teitelbaum, S.L., Bone, J.M., Stein, P.W., et al.: JAMA *235*:164–167, 1976.
154. Brommage, R., DeLuca, H.F.: Endocr. Rev. *6*:491–511, 1985.
155. Ott, S.M., Maloney, N.A., Coburn, J.W., et al.: N. Engl. J. Med. *307*:709–711, 1982.
156. Silverberg, D.S., Bettcher, K.B., Dosetor, J.B., et al.: Can. Med. Assoc. J. *112*:190–195, 1975.
157. Brickman, A.S., Sherrard, D.J., Jowsey, J., et al.: Arch. Intern. Med. *134*:883–888, 1974.
158. Pierides, A.M., Kerr, D.N.S., Ellis, H.A., et al.: Clin. Nephrol. *5*:189–196, 1976.
159. Chan, J.C.M., Oldham, S.B., Holick, M.F., et al.: JAMA *234*:47–52, 1975.
160. Yendt, E.R., DeLuca, H.F., Garcia, D.A., et al.: *In*

The Fat Soluble Vitamins. (H.F. DeLuca, J.W. Suttie, Eds.) Madison, University of Wisconsin Press, 1970, pp. 125–158.

161. Connor, T.B., Hopkins, T.R., Thomas, W.C., et al.: J. Clin. Endocrinol. *16*:945, 1956.

162. Milhaud: *In* Parathyroid Hormone and Thyrocalcitonin (Calcitonin). (R.V. Talmage, L.F. Belanger, Eds.) New York, Excerpta Medica, 1968.

163. Holick, M.F., Semmler, E.J., Schnoes, H.K., et al.: Science *180*:190–191, 1973.

164. Holick, M.F., Tavela, T.E., Holick, S.A., et al.: J. Biol. Chem. *251*:1020–1024, 1976.

*Chapter* # 14

# VITAMIN K

Robert E. Olson

While studying cholesterol biosynthesis in chicks fed a fat-free diet, Dam in 1929 observed subcutaneous and intraperitoneal hemorrhages in these chicks after a few days and demonstrated that this disease was caused by a deficiency of a previously unrecognized fat-soluble substance in the diet.[1] The absence of this factor caused delayed coagulation of the blood, which was traced to the absence of prothrombin activity. This factor was not identical with any known lipid or the then known fat-soluble vitamins A, D, and E, and was found to be broadly distributed in the plant kingdom, particularly in green leafy vegetables. Dam christened the new substance "vitamin K" for the "koagulation" vitamin. McFarland et al. in 1931 confirmed Dam's finding and they and others reported that fish meal was a source of the new vitamin K.[2,3]

In 1939, Doisy and his colleagues[4] and Dam and his colleagues[5] announced the isolation of a vitamin K from alfalfa. In addition, Doisy's group reported the isolation of a related but not identical vitamin K from putrified fish meal.[6] They named these compounds vitamins $K_1$ and $K_2$.

## CHEMISTRY OF THE K VITAMINS

Vitamin $K_1$, now known as phylloquinone, was identified by Doisy's group as 2-methyl-3-phytyl-1,4-naphthoquinone[7] (Fig. 14–1). It is the only homologue of vitamin K synthesized by plants. Vitamin $K_2$, isolated from fish meal, was originally believed to be 2-methyl-3-difarnesyl-1,4-naphthoquinone.[8] Because it has since been shown to have seven isoprene units in the side chain instead of six, however, it is now called menaqui-

none-7.[9] Traces of MK-6 were also found. The menaquinone family of $K_2$ homologues is a large series of vitamins containing unsaturated side chains, which differ in the number of isoprenyl units. Menaquinone-4 is synthesized in animals and birds from the provitamin menadione (2-methyl-1,4-naphthoquinone),[10] formerly known as vitamin $K_3$, by enzymatic alkylation with digeranyl pyrophosphate. The enzyme has been partially purified and characterized from chick and rat liver microsomes.[11,12] The other menaquinones are products of bacterial biosynthesis and range from menaquinone-7 to menaquinone-13.[13,14] Partially saturated menaquinones, menaquinone-9-H[15] and menaquinone-8-H,[16] are known.

## ESTIMATION OF VITAMIN K

Except for selected vitamin K-rich foods, vitamin K is present in animal and plant tissues in

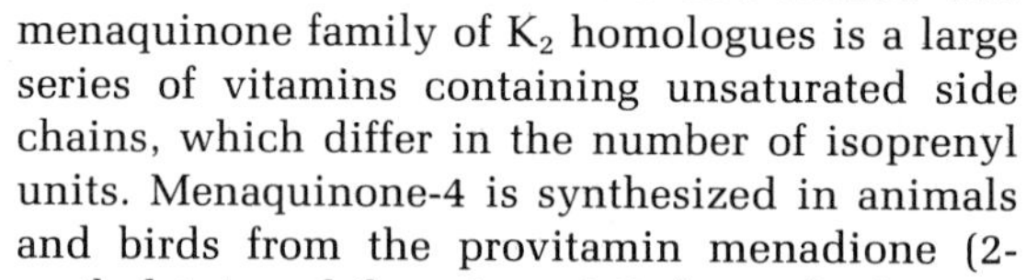

Phylloquinone (Vitamin $K_1$)

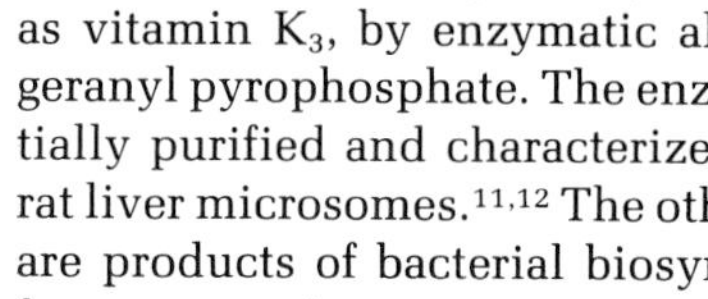

Menaquinone-n (MK-n, Vitamins $K_2$)

**Fig. 14–1.** Structures of phylloquinone (vitamin $K_1$) and menaquinone (vitamin $K_2$)

concentrations less than 1 µg/g of fresh weight. The concentration of phylloquinone in liver is about 50 ng/g fresh weight and in plasma about 1 ng/ml. Such low concentrations make chemical determinations difficult, particularly because all the vitamin K homologues are labile to alkali and light.

## Physiochemical Methods

Extraction of desiccated tissue with neutral solvents, followed by column and thin-layer chromatography and, more recently, high-pressure liquid chromatography (HPLC),[17] has resulted in the isolation of several vitamin K homologues from various tissues.[16,18] When purified in sufficient quantity, the vitamin Ks can be identified by mass and absorption spectrometry. The molecular extinction coefficient at 248 mµ is 19,000. With animal tissues and blood plasma, the analytical method of choice is multiple preparation TLC and HPLC followed by analytical reverse-phase HPLC using an ultraviolet or electrochemical detector.[19]

## Biologic Methods

Methods based upon measurement of prothrombin times in vitamin K-deficient animals or birds can be used for determination of the vitamin K activity of pure compounds and tissue extracts. Usually, the assay is curative, i.e., deficient chicks are given a supplement containing the food for seven days. The prothrombin level obtained with the unknown preparation is compared to that obtained with known amounts of phylloquinone.[20,21] The sensitivity of the chick bioassay is 0.1 µg of phylloquinone/g food or a total of 2 to 3 µg per day. Such assays, however, do not yield information about the form of vitamin K present in the material.[21] In a study of homologues, Matschiner and Doisy found that menaquinone-1 had only 1% of the activity of phylloquinone per os, whereas MK-4, MK-5, MK-6, and MK-7 were identical to phylloquinone in biologic activity.[21] MK-2 and MK-10 gave 20 to 29% of the activity of phylloquinone and showed that the very-short-chain and the very-long-chain homologues were less active by mouth than the medium-chain derivatives. Similar findings were made by Wiss and coworkers.[22]

The vitamin K content of common foods as determined by bioassay and HPLC methods is presented in Table 14–1. In general, green leafy vegetables are high, fruits and cereals are low, and meats and dairy products are intermediate. Some of these bioassays were done on an "as-is" basis, without extraction which, in the instances of green vegetables, gave less than the actual content of vitamin $K_1$. In fact, the intestinal absorption of

vitamin K from plant sources ranges from 30 to 70% of the actual content determined by extraction. It appears that tobacco is one of the richest sources of phylloquinone known. It contains about 5 mg/100 g, a small percentage of which is volatilized in smoking and absorbed through the mucous membranes of the nasopharynx and bronchi.[23]

## ABSORPTION, DISTRIBUTION, AND METABOLISM

The absorption of phylloquinone and the menaquinones requires bile and pancreatic juice for maximum effectiveness.[24] Dietary vitamin K is absorbed in the small bowel, is incorporated into chylomicrons, and appears in the lymph.[25] Efficiency of absorption has been measured from 40 to 80%, depending upon the vehicle in which the vitamin is administered and the extent of the enterohepatic circulation generally characteristic of isoprenoid lipids. When isotopically labeled phylloquinone was administered to animals[26] and man[27] by mouth in doses ranging from the physiologic to the pharmacologic, the vitamin appeared in the plasma within 20 minutes, peaked at two hours, and then declined exponentially to low values over 48 to 72 hours, reaching fasting levels of 1 to 3 ng/ml. During this period, it appeared to be transferred from the chylomicrons to the β-lipoproteins. No specific carrier protein for vitamin K in plasma has been identified. Between 8 and 30% of the administered radioactivity was recovered in polar metabolites in the urine over a three-day period in both animals and man, whereas total fecal radioactivity accounted for 45 to 60% of the administered dose over a five-day period. About one third of this fecal radioactivity was unchanged vitamin $K_1$. The administration of nonabsorbable lipids, such as mineral oil or squalene, greatly reduced the absorption of vitamin K in animals.[28]

Wiss et al.[26] observed that the principal excretory form of vitamin K in rat urine is a metabolite resembling the lactone of vitamin E first described by Simon, Gross, and Milhorant.[29] It was identified as a chain-shorted and oxidized derivative of vitamin K, which forms a gamma lactone and is probably excreted as a glucuronide. Vitamin K-2,3-epoxide has also been identified as a metabolite of vitamin K in rats.[30]

As much as 50% of a parenterally administered dose of vitamin $K_1$ may appear in the liver within one hour. After oral administration, the liver may contain as much as 20% of the administered dose in two hours; this amount then declines to low values after 24 hours. In one study, the relative concentration of vitamin K in kidney, heart, skin,

**Table 14–1.  Average Vitamin K Content of Ordinary Foods***

| Food | Vitamin K $\mu g/100\ g$ | Food | Vitamin K $\mu g/100\ g$ | Food | Vitamin K $\mu g/100\ g$ | Food | Vitamin K $\mu g/100\ g$ |
|---|---|---|---|---|---|---|---|
| Milk and Milk Products | | Fats | | Vegetables | | Fruits | |
| butter | 30 | beef fat | 15 | asparagus | 57 | applesauce | 2 |
| cheese | 35 | corn oil | 0 | beans, green | 40 | banana | 2 |
| milk (cows) | 1 | safflower oil | 10 | broccoli | 175 | orange | 1 |
| milk (human) | 0.2 | | | cabbage | 125 | peach | 8 |
| Eggs | | Cereals and Grain Products | | kale | 729 | raisin | 6 |
| hens (whole) | 11 | bread | 4 | lettuce | 129 | strawberry | 10 |
| | | maize | 5 | peas, green | 29 | | |
| Meat and Meat Products | | oats | 10 | potato | 1 | Beverages | |
| bacon | 46 | rice | 3 | pumpkin | 2 | coffee | 38 |
| beef liver | 92 | wheat flour | 4 | spinach | 415 | cola | 2 |
| chicken liver | 7 | whole wheat | 17 | tomato | 10 | tea, black | — |
| ground beef | 7 | | | turnip greens | 650 | tea, green | 712 |
| ham | 15 | | | watercress | 80 | | |
| pork liver | 25 | | | | | Tobacco | |
| pork tenderloin | 11 | | | | | cigarettes | 5,000† |

*Data from Shearer, M.J., et al.,[17] Dam, H., et al.,[20] Matschiner, J.T., et al.,[21] Richardson, L.R., et al.,[140] Doisy, E.A.[141]
†Only a small percentage is volatilized and absorbed by mucous membranes.

and muscle increased to maximum values over a 24-hour period, and then declined. The principal sites of uptake, after liver, were skin and muscle. Fractionation of liver tissue, after the administration of $^3$H-phylloquinone to rats, showed the following relative distribution of radioactivity: nuclei, 13%; mitochondria, 9%; microsomes, 63% and cytosol, 14%.[31] In omnivorous animals, such as man, both phylloquinone and the higher-molecular-weight menaquinones (MK-7 to MK-13), of bacterial origin and probably derived from intestinal flora, are found in the liver.[32,33]

The turnover of vitamin K in the animal body is rapid, and the total body pool size is surprisingly small. Bjornsson et al. infused 300 $\mu$g of $^3$H-phylloquinone into human volunteers with or without previous drug loading with warfarin or clofibrate.[34] The initial half-time ($T_{1/2\alpha}$) for the first exponential phase was 26 ± 8 min, and the average terminal half-time was 166 ± 9 min under all conditions. Shearer et al. found similar results with a 1-mg intravenous dose of $^3$H-phylloquinone, namely $T_{1/2\alpha}$ = 20 to 24 min and $T_{1/2\alpha}$ = 120 to 150 min.[35] From data on the volume of distribution and clearance rate, Bjornsson et al. calculated the fractional turnover rate to be 0.4/hr, suggesting the body pool was turning once every 2.5 hours,[36] although more recent studies by Olson et al., employing 0.3 $\mu$g of $^3$H-phylloquinone and longer periods of observation, have suggested the metabolic turnover time for vitamin $K_1$ is about once per day.[37] From approximate daily intakes of vitamin K, body pool sizes were estimated to be 50 to 100 $\mu$g, which is less than the body pool size for vitamin $B_{12}$, and extraordinarily low for a fat-soluble vitamin.

When menadione (2-methyl-1,4-naphthoqui-none) is administered to animals or man, only a small amount (0.05 to 1.0%) is converted to an active vitamin, menaquinone-4.[38–40] The principal metabolites of menadione are the sulfate and glucuronide of dihydromenadione.[41] Menadione also reacts with free sulfhydryl groups in proteins to form a thioether linkage, first described by Fieser,[42] which may account for some of its reported toxicity.[43]

## PHYSIOLOGIC FUNCTION

### Regulation of Clotting Protein Synthesis

Shortly after the discovery of vitamin K, Dam and others[44] demonstrated that the hemorrhagic diathesis caused by vitamin K deficiency in the chick was caused by a reduction in plasma prothrombin activity. Over the next 10 years, researchers learned that three other procoagulant proteins, factors VII,[45] IX,[46] and X,[47] are also regulated by vitamin K. Prothrombin has a molecular weight of 72,000 and is present in plasma at a concentration of 100 $\mu$g/ml. The other vitamin K-dependent proenzymes have molecular weights between 45,000 and 55,000 and are present in plasma at levels of 1 to 20 $\mu$g/ml.

More recently, four new vitamin K-dependent proteins containing $\gamma$-carboxyglutamate (Gla) have been isolated, namely proteins C,[48] S,[49] M,[50] and Z.[51] All require Ca$^{++}$ for activity and contain areas of amino acid homology with the established vitamin K-dependent factors. Factors C and S are anticoagulants. Activated protein C rapidly and selectively inactivates factors V and VIII, which are respectively the cofactors for the activation of factors X and II (prothrombin). Factor S enhances the inactivation of factor V in the presence of phospholipid. Factors Z and M appear to stimulate platelet activity in coagulation. An abbreviated clotting scheme showing the proteolytic cascade hypothesis proposed by Biggs and McFarlane[52] and by Davie and Ratnoff,[53] which shows the role of the vitamin K-dependent factors, is shown in Figure 14–2.

### Discovery of γ-Carboxyglutamate (Gla)

Since 1935, several hypotheses have been proposed to account for the action of vitamin K. These theories suggested a role in: (1) mammalian electron transport;[54] (2) specific mRNA synthesis and uptake by ribosomes;[55] and (3) the post-translational modification of a precursor peptide by addition of a prosthetic group.[56] The discovery of γ-carboxyglutamate (Gla) was the first specific clue to the action of the vitamin (Fig. 14–3). Gla was discovered in a tetrapeptide (Leu-Gla-Gla-Val) isolated from bovine prothrombin representing residues 6 to 9 by Stenflo and his colleagues,[57] followed by independent reports of similar findings by Nelsestuen et al.[58] and Magnusson et al.[59] This new amino acid was absent from the corresponding peptide derived from the abnormal inactive prothrombin present in the plasma of cows that had been fed dicumarol. These findings strengthened the view that vitamin K was involved in the post-translational carboxylation of an inactive precursor peptide. Magnusson et al. observed that not only were residues 7 and 8 γ-carboxyglutamate, but also that in the first 40 amino acids from the N terminus all glutamic acids (at positions 7, 8, 15, 17, 20, 21, 26, 27, 30, and 33) were γ-carboxylated.[59]

The discovery of γ-carboxyglutamate in prothrombin stimulated numerous studies of $CO_2$ fixation into prothrombin under various conditions. Girardot and others dosed vitamin K-deficient rats with $H^{14}CO_3$ and reported that a $^{14}C$-tryptic peptide derived from plasma prothrombin contained a labeled acidic amino acid resembling γ-carboxyglutamate.[60] The first vitamin K-dependent in vitro system that produced prothrombin was that described by Shah and Suttie.[61] Postmitochondrial supernatants from vitamin K-deficient rats responded to the addition of vitamin K by producing a significant amount of biologically active prothrombin in the presence of cycloheximide. Esmon and associates then demonstrated that the same postmitochondrial supernatant would catalyze a vitamin K-dependent incorporation of

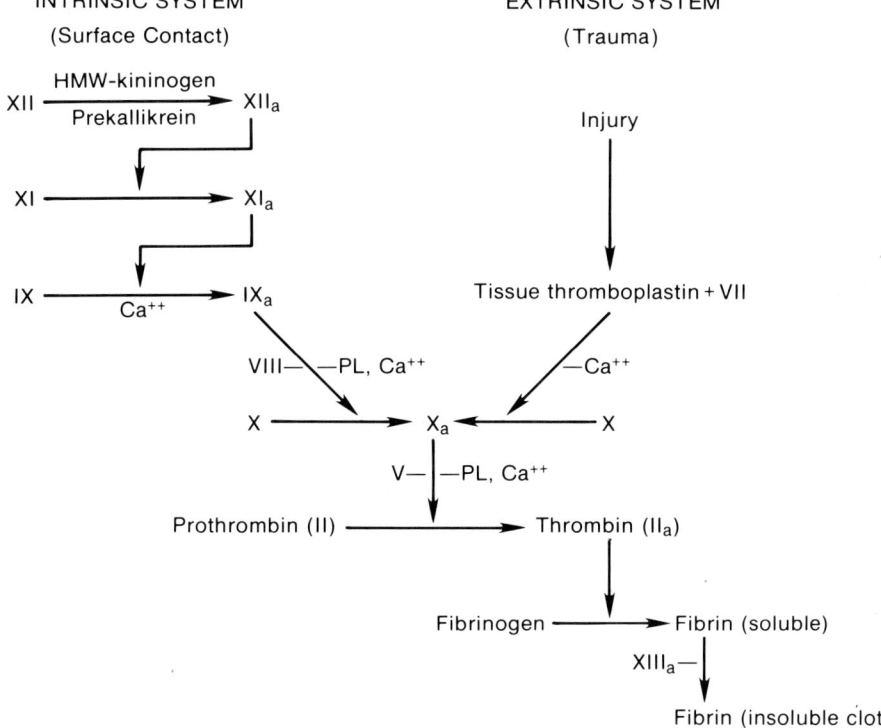

**Fig. 14–2.** Clotting factor cascade. Factors II (prothrombin), VII (proconvention), IX (Christmas factor), and X (Stuart-Prower factor) are vitamin K-dependent, contain γ-carboxyglutamate, and occupy the core of the clotting scheme. Activation of these factors requires calcium ions leading to an active protease (factor). Factor V is accelerated globulin and factor VIII is antihemophilic globulin, both cofactors for specified reactions. Factor X is fibrin-stabilizing factor, a transpeptidase, and PL is phospholipid.

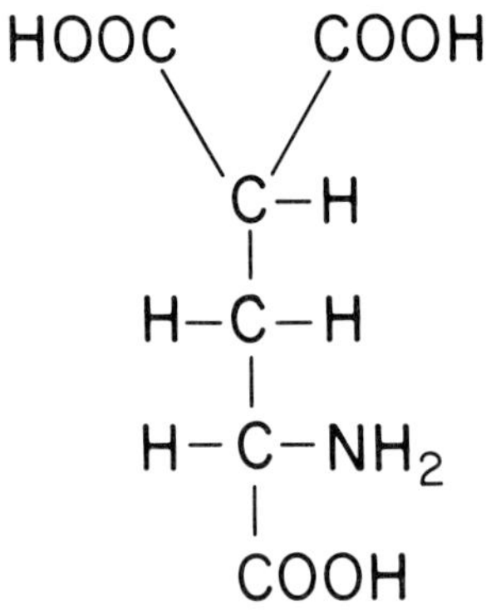

$$HOOC \quad COOH$$

(Structure diagram of γ-carboxyglutamic acid)

**Fig. 14–3.** Structure of γ-carboxyglutamic acid.

H[14]CO$_3$ into the endogenous microsomal precursor protein, which is heterogeneous and consists of a group of proteins in isoelectric points ranging from 5.8 to 7.7.[62] Radioactive prothrombin formed in this in vitro system was isolated, and essentially all the radioactivity was shown to be present as γ-carboxyglutamic acid residues in the N-terminal portion of prothrombin. These observations offered final proof that vitamin K was concerned with the post-translational carboxylation of glutamate residues in a prothrombin precursor. The vitamin K-dependent synthesis and modification of precursor prothrombin have also been demonstrated in H-35 hepatoma cells in culture.[63]

The vitamin K-dependent carboxylase system is a membrane-bound component of microsomes. It has been solubilized[64–66] and, in the soluble form, retains most of the properties of the microsomal system. The system requires a peptide substrate, O$_2$, CO$_2$, and either vitamin K plus NADH or vitamin K hydroquinone; ATP is not required. The active form of the vitamin is the hydroquinone (the reduced form) and constitutes the electron donor for a microsomal electron transport system for which oxygen is the terminal acceptor. This electron transport system is coupled to a CO$_2$-fixation reaction converting peptide-bound glutamate (Glu$_p$) to γ-carboxyglutamate. Artificial substrates initiating partial sequences of prothrombin precursor such as Phe-Leu-Glu-Glu-Leu[67,68] have proved to be active in this system.

The mechanism of the vitamin K-dependent carboxylation is still obscure. Jones and colleagues investigated the species of "CO$_2$" utilized by the microsomal system and discovered that it was CO$_2$ and not bicarbonate.[68] Biotin is clearly not involved in this CO$_2$ fixation. Chemically synthesized carbonates for vitamin K hydroquinone are inactive. Vitamin K is thus not a CO$_2$ carrier, but may be an oxygen carrier, particularly since vitamin K-2,3-epoxide is a product of the reaction.

A reaction mechanism proposed by Larson et al. is shown as follows:[69]

$$KH_2 + O_2 \xrightarrow[Mg^{2+}]{carboxylase} KHOO^{(-)} + H^+$$

$$KHOO^{(-)} + Glu_p \rightleftharpoons KHOOH + Glu_p{}^{(-)}$$

$$Glu_p{}^{(-)} + CO_2 + H^+ \rightarrow Gla_p$$

$$KHOOH \rightarrow KO + H_2O$$

*Sum:* vitamin KH$_2$ + O$_2$ + CO$_2$ + Glu$_p$

$$\rightarrow \text{vitamin KO} + Gla_p + H_2O$$

Arguments for and against this sequence of reactions have been advanced.[70–72] Larson and Suttie proposed that a hypothetical vitamin K-hydroperoxy anion might be sufficiently basic to remove the γ-methylene proton from peptide-bound glutamate.[65] Olson et al., however, argued that the organic hydroperoxy anion was insufficiently basic to remove a proton from the γ-methylene group and suggested an induction mechanism for the labilization of the γ-methylene proton.[66] Vitamin K hydroperoxide is thus a hypothetical intermediate that has never been isolated or identified. Further studies are needed to clarify the nature of the oxygen derivative of vitamin K and the mechanism of γ-glutamyl-peptide activation.

**Vitamin K Cycle**

The vitamin K cycle is shown in Figure 14–4. In essence, this cycle is a salvage pathway for vitamin K, which is present in only nanomolar quantities in liver and other tissues. It postulates that the vitamin K epoxidase (which is linked to the carboxylase) converts vitamin K to its 2,3-epoxide, usually in excess of the carboxylation rate. The epoxide is then reduced to the quinone by a dithiol-dependent epoxide reductase. The regenerated vitamin K is now reduced to the vitamin K hydroquinone by one of several possible enzymes, at least one driven by a dithiol and several by NAD(P)H. The dithiol-dependent epoxide reductase and quinone reductase are strongly inhibited by warfarin, whereas the NAD(P)H-dependent dehydrogenase is relatively insensitive.[73] The net effect of the cycle is the salvage of the vitamin K-2,3-epoxide formed in association with the carboxylation reaction by reducing it in two steps to vitamin K hydroquinone, which is the active form of the vitamin for carboxylation.

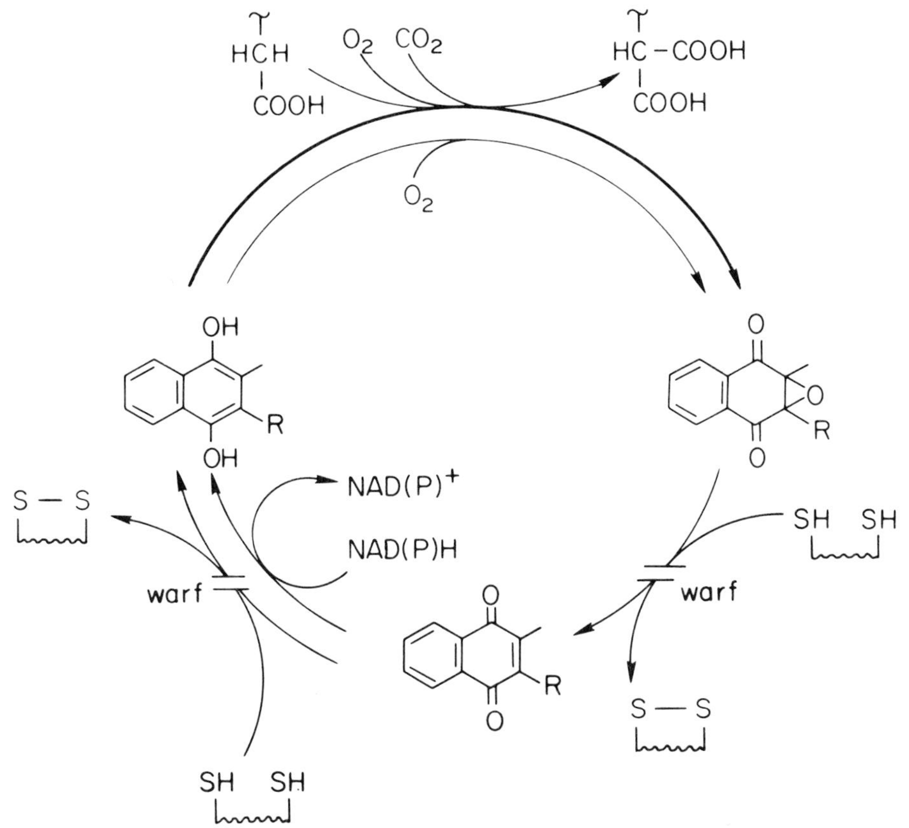

**Fig. 14–4.** The vitamin K-vitamin K oxide cycle. Vitamin K hydroquinone is the substrate for the carboxylase-epoxidase enzyme system shown at the top. The product of this reaction, the vitamin K-2,3-epoxide, is reduced to vitamin K by a dithiol-driven epoxide reductase to form vitamin K. The vitamin is then reduced to regenerate the hydroquinone by several reductases. Warfarin inhibits both the dithiol-driven vitamin K epoxide reductase and the dithiol-driven vitamin K reductase, but not the NAD(P)H-driven vitamin K reductase.

## Bone and Kidney Proteins Containing γ-Carboxyglutamate

A bone Gla-protein (BGP) was discovered independently by Hauschka et el.[74] and Price et al.[75] This matrix protein is extractable from bone with EDTA, makes up 20% of EDTA extractable protein, and represents 1% of total bone protein. The Harvard group has called this protein osteocalcin. The amino acid composition and sequence have been determined by Price in calf, swordfish, and man.[76] The BGP for calf and human bone has a molecular weight of 5,700, contains 49 residues of which residues 17, 21, and 24, clustered around a disulfide bridge, are Gla. The swordfish protein is homologous with 47 residues. None of these proteins is homologous with the coagulation factors, but all bind $Ca^{++}$ and particularly hydroxyapatite. Its precise function in bone metabolism is not known.

Microsomes from embryonic chick bone contain a vitamin K-dependent γ-glutamyl carbox-ylase that can carboxylate endogenous bone protein and Gla-containing pentapeptides.[77] The synthesis of BGP in embryonic chick and calf bones is inhibited by warfarin.[78,79] Several cases have been reported of the Conradi-Hunermann type of chondrodysplasia punctata in infants born of mothers taking warfarin during the first trimester. These findings suggest that warfarin may be a teratogen because of its inhibition of osteocalcin synthesis and perhaps the synthesis of other vitamin K-dependent proteins concerned with the maturation of bony tissue.[73–75,80–88]

The synthesis of BGP, furthermore, is regulated by 1,25-dihyroxy-vitamin $D_3$ in cultured osteosarcoma cells.[89] This process suggests that BGP may mediate some action of vitamin D on bone. Although the present data show that a deficiency of BGP does not affect bone structure or fracture repair, plasma BGP is elevated in metabolic bone disease[90] and may stimulate bone modeling and mobilization of calcium. A protein closely related to BGP has been found in calcified atherosclerotic plaques (athero-calcin)[75,91] and in calcified aortic valves.[92]

In 1976, Lian and Prien reported the presence of another Gla-containing protein in the matrix of calcium-containing renal stones in man.[93] It was reported to have a molecular weight of 18,000 and to contain three to four residues of Gla. It may function to solubilize calcium salts in urine. In 1976 Hauschka et al. demonstrated that mena-quinone-3 stimulated the synthesis of $^{14}C$-Gla from $^{14}CO_2$ in kidney microsomes from dicou-marol-treated animals.[94] Friedman et al. have localized this synthesis to the tubular cells.[95] Gla biosynthesis has also been demonstrated in a mouse renal adenocarcinoma in tissue culture.[96]

## COUMARIN ANTICOAGULANT DRUGS

A hemorrhagic disease in cattle that have consumed spoiled clover was described by Schofield in 1922[97] and was attributed to a depressed pro-thrombin level by Roderick in 1931.[98] In 1941, Campbell and Link reported that the active agent in spoiled clover was bishydroxycoumarin (di-cumarol).[99] A variety of related compounds, derivatives of either 4-hydroxycoumarin or phen-indandione, have been synthesized and tested for anticoagulant activity in animals and man. One of the more popular ones in the Unites States is warfarin (3-[α-acetonylbenzyl]-4-hydroxycou-marin), a more soluble compound than dicumarol (Fig. 14–5).

The oral anticoagulant agents regulate the biosynthesis of prothrombin (factor II) and other vitamin K-dependent factors in the liver. They also induce hypoprothrombinemia and other factor deficiencies at specific rates when given in saturating doses, even though the half-life of various drugs varies from hours to days in different animals and man. As soon as there is an effective concentration of the drug, vitamin K-dependent factor biosynthesis by liver is shut off and the factors then decay in plasma at their specific half-lives.[100] Hydroxylated products of these drugs, generated by the enzymes in the liver microsomes, are inactive.

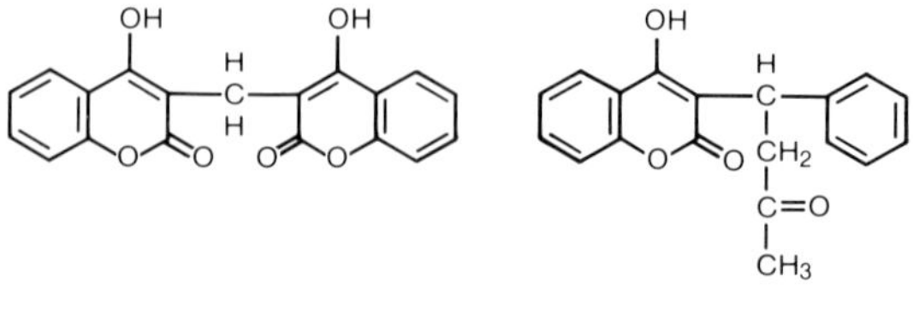

DICUMAROL                          WARFARIN

**Fig. 14–5.** Structure of dicumarol and warfarin.

The mechanism of action of the 4-hydroxycou-marin drugs is still under investigation, although it seems fairly clear now that these agents do not directly block the vitamin K-dependent carboxylase. As noted earlier, Bell and Matschiner proposed that the primary action of warfarin was to inhibit vitamin K-2,3-epoxide reductase and prevent the recycling of the epoxide to vitamin K, thus reducing the concentration of $KH_2$ in vivo to ineffective levels.[101] This view has been strongly supported by others.[102] More recently, Fasco et al. have shown that the dithiothreitol (DTT)-driven vitamin K reductase is more sensitive to warfarin than the vitamin K-epoxide reductase in both normal and warfarin-resistant rats and that the vitamin K-KO cycle is blocked at both reduction steps by warfarin.[103,104]

The apparent $K_m$ for vitamin K carboxylation by intact microsomes is about 100 pmoles/g and corresponds to the amount actually present in mammalian liver.[105,106] It is possible that the DTT-driven vitamin K reductase has a very low $K_m$ when compared to the NAD(P)H-dependent vitamin K reductase. Hence, under physiologic conditions, the DTT-powered warfarin-sensitive enzyme is the pathway used. In order to overcome a warfarin block, large amounts of vitamin K are necessary. At these high levels, the NAD(P)H reductases, which are relatively insensitive to warfarin, are used.[107] These enzymes restore carboxylation as long as $KH_2$ can be formed. Warfarin-binding studies have also shown that normal microsomes bind warfarin more tightly and in larger amounts than those from warfarin-resistant rats.[108–110]

When overdosage with coumarin drugs occurs in patients who have received anticoagulant agents to prevent thrombosis (coronary artery disease, pulmonary embolic disease), the intravenous administration of pharmacologic doses of vitamin $K_1$ in the milligram range reinitiates prothrombin synthesis within minutes, gives protective levels of prothrombin within hours, and gives normal values for prothrombin and other vitamin-K dependent factors in 24 hours. Water-soluble derivatives of menadione (e.g., Synkay-vite) are largely ineffective against the coumarin anticoagulant drugs because, as previously mentioned, the rate of conversion to menaquinone-4 is so slow that pharmacologically effective levels of the alkylated vitamin are not attained.[111,112]

## VITAMIN K DEFICIENCY

Primary vitamin K deficiency is uncommon in healthy persons. This fact is due to widespread distribution of vitamin K in plant and animal tissues and to the microbiologic flora of the normal gut, which synthesizes the menaquinones in amounts that may supply a significant part of the requirement for vitamin K. The causes of deficiencies in the vitamin K-dependent coagulation factors are thus largely secondary to disease or drug therapy and are presented in Table 14–2. These causes are considered in order.

## Hemorrhagic Disease of the Newborn

Newborn infants represent a special case of vitamin K nutrition because (1) the placenta is a relatively poor organ for the transmission of lipids and (2) the gut is sterile during the first few days. In normal infants, the plasma prothrombin concentration and that of the other vitamin K-dependent factors may decrease to a level as low as 30% in the second and third days of life. As food is taken, the levels gradually climb to normal adult values over a period of weeks. If prothrombin values fall below 10%, hemorrhagic disease of the newborn appears.[113] Premature infants are even more susceptible to vitamin K deficiency than are full-term ones.[114]

High-pressure liquid chromatographic studies of the vitamin K content of human and cow's milk have shown that human milk contains only 1 to 2 μg/L, whereas cow's milk contains 5 to 17 μg/L.[17] Since the requirement for vitamin K in the newborn is estimated to be 5 μg/day, the very low content of vitamin K in human milk accounts for the greater predisposition of breast-fed infants to develop the hemorrhagic syndrome. Since breast milk is sterile and delays colonization of the gut with bacteria, Seeler recommends that babies who are to be breast-fed receive 1 mg phylloquinone (Aquamephyton) intramuscularly at birth.[115]

Infants of mothers on hydantoin anticonvulsants should have prophylactic vitamin K because diphenylhydantoin is an antagonist to vitamin K.[116] Neonatal complications such as diarrhea, malabsorption, cystic fibrosis, idiopathic cholestasis, atresia of the bile duct, and prolonged par-

**Table 14–2. Causes of Deficiencies of Vitamin K-Dependent Coagulation Factors**

Hemorrhagic disease of the newborn
Dietary inadequacy (low-fat diets, protein-calorie malnutrition)
Total parenteral nutrition deficient in the vitamin
Biliary obstruction (gallstones, stricture, fistulas)
Malabsorption syndromes (cystic fibrosis, sprue, celiac disease, ulcerative colitis, regional ileitis, short-bowel syndrome)
Liver disease
Drug therapy
    Coumarin anticoagulants and related drugs (warfarin, indanediones, phenprocoumon, hydantoins, salicylates)
    Antibiotics including cephalosporins
    Megadoses of vitamin E

enteral nutrition are all indications for intramuscular or intravenous vitamin K administration.

## Dietary Inadequacy

Healthy adult subjects fed low-vitamin-K diets (10 μg/day) for several weeks show minimal signs of vitamin K deficiency (i.e., plasma prothrombin values of 60 to 90%) unless they are also given bowel-sterilizing antibiotics such as neomycin.[117,118] In one study of apoplectic patients, intravenous nutrition plus neomycin was required to lower the vitamin-K-dependent clotting factors to below 20% of normal in four weeks.[118] The intravenous administration of vitamin K in various doses (0.03 to 1.5 μg/kg) to these patients caused a proportional rise in the concentration of these depressed values to normal levels. In unusual cases, self-imposed dietary restriction induces hypoprothrombinemia with hemorrhage responsive to oral vitamin K.[119,120] Dietary deficiency of vitamin K becomes manifest more quickly in debilitated patients with or without antibiotics.[121,122]

In protein-calorie malnutrition, amino acid deprivation may cause a hypoprothrombinemia that is not responsive to vitamin K but does respond to protein feeding.[123]

## Total Parenteral Nutrition

With the advent of subclavian-vein catheterization in 1968 for long-term total parenteral nutrition of both surgical and medical patients unable to eat, new nutritional deficiency syndromes have been reported,[124] among which is hemorrhage due to vitamin K deficiency.[125] It is advisable to give doses of 1 mg phylloquinone per week (equivalent to about 150 μg vitamin K per day).

## Biliary Obstruction

Prior to the discovery of vitamin K and recognition of its deficiency in obstructive jaundice, bleeding commonly occurred after surgical correction of biliary obstruction.[126] Because the secretion of bile salts is essential for the absorption of fats and fat-soluble vitamins, it is not surprising that biliary obstruction was early identified as a cause of vitamin K deficiency. All patients with obstructive jaundice should receive parenteral vitamin $K_1$ (5 mg/day) for three days prior to surgery.

## Malabsorption Syndrome

Depression of the vitamin K-dependent coagulation factors is frequently found in the malabsorption syndromes and in other gastrointestinal disorders (e.g., cystic fibrosis, sprue, celiac disease, ulcerative colitis, regional ileitis, ascaris infection, and short-bowel syndrome).

Severe abnormalities of coagulation with extensive bleeding are not as common in these disorders as in biliary obstruction, but they do occur with sufficient frequency to be a concern of physicians caring for these patients. One of the complications of ileojejunostomy for morbid obesity is hemorrhage due to vitamin K deficiency. Such patients should be treated with all the fat-soluble vitamins, including vitamin K, in doses that are 1 to 2 mg/day, some 20 times the usual requirement.

### Liver Disease

Patients with parenchymal liver disease may have hypoprothrombinemia and an elevation in plasma $\gamma$-carboxyprothrombin. They are unable to utilize vitamin K in the biosynthesis of vitamin K-dependent clotting factors, usually as a result of destruction of the rough reticulum in the hepatocyte. Patients with liver disease, however, should be challenged with vitamin K to determine the extent of the organic disorder preventing biosynthesis of prothrombin.

### Drug Therapy

Various drugs, including the 4-hydroxy coumarins, salicylates, certain broad-spectrum antibiotics, and vitamin K in pharmacologic doses will antagonize the action of vitamin K.

**Coumarin- and Salicylate-Induced Hemorrhagic Disease.** The coumarin anticoagulant drugs can induce serious hypoprothrombinemia by blocking the vitamin K epoxide and vitamin K reductases. Some of the contributory causes are reduction in dietary intake of vitamin K, ingestion of interfering drugs, and the inadvertent alteration of the anticoagulant dosage schedule. Coumarin drugs, in rare cases, may cause coumarin skin necrosis. This condition probably occurs because coumarin drugs inhibit the biosynthesis of the anticoagulant protein C before they affect the levels of the procoagulant factors II, VII, IX, and X. The temporary imbalance may, in fact, stimulate local coagulation in venules with resulting thrombosis.[127] Salicylates in large doses may also depress vitamin K-dependent factors. When mild overdosage unaccompanied by bleeding occurs, the anticoagulant should be discontinued, 2 mg of vitamin $K_1$ should be given parenterally, and prothrombin times should be monitored over the next 24 hours. If more severe hypoprothrombinemia with hemorrhage occurs, 25 to 50 mg of vitamin $K_1$ should be administered intravenously. When the patient's bleeding is under control (usually achieved within 48 hours), vitamin K should then be discontinued and coumarin drugs reinstituted until a proper prothrombin level is obtained.

**Broad-Spectrum Antibiotics.** An important source of vitamin K in humans is their own intestinal bacteria. As has been mentioned, the gastrointestinal flora may supply an individual's entire requirement. Vitamin K, however, is not well absorbed from the colon. Udall showed that large amounts of vitamin K (approximately 500 mg/day) instilled into the cecum did not elevate depressed coagulation factors in anticoagulated patients, whereas the same dose given orally gave a prompt response.[117] The microorganisms synthesizing vitamin K in the intestine probably reside in the ileum, where absorption of vitamin K is possible.

Sulfa drugs, neomycin, and other broad-spectrum antibiotics are capable of sterilizing the bowel. The classic occurrence is that of a patient who has undergone gastrointestinal surgery, preceded by a limited intake of food, and who has been given large doses of antibiotics preoperatively and postoperatively. The sudden appearance of melena, perhaps along with hematemesis, is the first clue. Prophylactic vitamin K is effective.

Certain broad-spectrum cephalosporin antibiotics (moxalactam, cefamandole) cause vitamin K-reversible hemorrhage in man.[128] Lipsky reported that the N-methylthiotetrazole moiety of these antibiotics blocks vitamin K-dependent peptide carboxylation in triton-solubilized rat liver microsomes in a dose-dependent manner.[129] Uotila and Suttie verified the effect of these antibiotics on the vitamin K-dependent carboxylase in vitro.[130]

**Vitamin E.** Large amounts of vitamin E may also antagonize the action of vitamin K. March et al. observed that when diets containing 2,200 I.U. vitamin E per kg were fed to chicks, prothrombin times were lengthened.[131] This prothrombin deficiency was responsive to vitamin K. Prolongation of prothrombin times as a result of megavitamin E therapy has also been reported in man.[132] This conditioned vitamin K deficiency in human subjects taking megadoses of vitamin E has also been expressed as a hypersensitivity to the coumarin anticoagulant drugs. Corrigan and Marcus reported clinical evidence of vitamin K deficiency in a patient taking 5 mg warfarin, 2.0 clofibrate, and 1,200 I.U. of vitamin E each day.[133] Upon discontinuation of megavitamin E therapy, the bleeding tendency and prolonged prothrombin time normalized. Lesser doses of vitamin E in man (42 I.U./day for 30 days) do not potentiate the anticoagulant effects of warfarin.[134]

## NUTRITIONAL REQUIREMENTS

The vitamin K requirements of mammals is met by a combination of dietary intake and microbiologic biosynthesis in the intestine. In conventional rats, the vitamin K requirement is about 10 μg/kg body weight per day, whereas, in germ-free rats, the requirement is more than doubled to about 25 μg/kg per day.[135] Genetic factors no doubt influence the vitamin K requirement in both animals and man.

In human subjects, 50% of the vitamin K in liver has been found to be vitamin $K_1$ and the remainder a mixture of menaquinone-7, menaquinone-8, menaquinone-9, menaguinone-10, and menaquinone-11.[32,136] If both phylloquinone and menaquinone are mobilized with equal ease, on the average 50% of the requirement is probably met by phylloquinone and 50% by bacterial synthesis. However, the fact that plasma vitamin K is principally phylloquinone[137] makes that conclusion questionable.

If it is assumed that the intravenous dose of vitamin K required to raise depressed vitamin K-dependent factors to normal for one day is 0.2 μg/kg[118] and that 50% of the vitamin K appearing in the lumen of the intestine each day *is absorbed,* the total daily requirement for the vitamin would be 0.4 μg/kg/day. If the assumption is that 50% of the requirement is derived from intestinal microorganisms, then the *dietary* requirement would fall back to 0.2 μg/kg/day. With the information at hand, this is a rough estimate, particularly since the relative activity of phylloquinone and the menaquinones in stimulating prothrombin synthesis is controversial.[138,139] Studies of healthy young volunteers on elemental diets containing 10 μg of phylloquinone per day show no change in coagulation factors over an eight-week period.[37]

Certainly 30 μg of phylloquinone per day would protect all healthy adults from a dietary deficiency of vitamin K.

From the dietary information presented in Table 14–2, it can be calculated that a "normal mixed diet" in the United States will contain 300 to 500 μg of vitamin K per day, an amount more than adequate to supply the dietary requirement.

## REFERENCES

1. Dam, H.: Biochem. Z. *215*:475–492, 1929.
2. McFarland, W.D., Graham, W.R., Richardson, F.: Biochem. J. *25*:358–366, 1931.
3. Almquist, H.J., Stokstad, E.L.R.: J. Nutr. *12*:329–335, 1936.
4. Binkley, S.B., MacCorquodale, D., Thayer, S.A., Doisy, E.A.: J. Biol. Chem. *130*:219–234, 1939.
5. Dam, H., Geiger, A., Glavind, J., et al.: Helv. Chim. Acta *22*:310, 1939.
6. McKee, R.W., Binkley, S., Thayer, S.A., et al.: J. Biol. Chem., *131*:327, 1939.
7. Binkley, S., Cheney, H., et al.: J. Am. Chem. Soc. *61*:2558, 1939.
8. Binkley, S., McKee, R.W., Thayer, S.A., et al.: J. Biol. Chem. *133*:721–729, 1940.
9. Isler, O., Ruegg, R., Chopard-dit-Jean, et al.: Helv. Chim. Acta *41*:786–807, 1958.
10. Martius, C., Esser, H.O.: Biochem. Z. *331*:1–9, 1958.
11. Dialameh, G.H., Yekundi, K.G., Olson, R.E.: Biochim. Biophys. Acta *223*:332–338, 1970.
12. Lee, F.C., Olson, R.E.: Biochim Biophys. Acta *799*:166–170, 1984.
13. Matschiner, J.T., Taggart, W.V., Amelotti, J.M.: Biochemistry *6*:1243–1248, 1967.
14. Pennock, J.F.: Vitam. Horm. *24*:307–329, 1966.
15. Gale, P.H., Arison, B.H., Trenner, N.R., et al.: Biochemistry *2*:196–200, 1963.
16. Scholes, P.B., King, H.K.: Biochem. J. *97*:766–768, 1965.
17. Shearer, M.J., Allan, V., Haroon, Y., et al.: Nutritional aspects of vitamin K in the human. *In* Vitamin K Metabolism and Vitamin K-Dependent Proteins. (J.W. Suttie, Ed.) Baltimore, University Park Press, 1980, pp. 317–327.
18. Martius, C.: Am. J. Clin. Nutr. *9*:97, 1961.
19. Haroon, Y., Hauschka, V.: J. Lipid Res. *24*:481–484, 1983.
20. Dam, H., Glavind, J.: Biochem. J. *32*:485, 1938.
21. Matschiner, J.T., Doisy, E.A., Jr.: J. Nutr. *90*:97–100, 1966.
22. Wiss, O., Weber, F., Ruegg, R., et al.: Z. Physiol. Chemie *314*:245–249, 1959.
23. Doisy, E.A., Jr.: Unpublished work.
24. Mann, J.D., Mann, F.D., Bollman, J.L.: Am. J. Physiol. *158*:311–314, 1949.
25. Blomstrand, R., Forsgren, L.: Int. Z. Vitaminforsch *38*:328–344, 1968.
26. Wiss, O., Gloor, H.: Vitam. Horm. *24*:575–586, 1966.
27. Shearer, M.J., Barkhan, P., Webster, G.R.: Br. J. Haematol. *18*: 297–308, 1970.
28. Matschiner, J.T., Hsia, S.L., Doisy, E.A., Jr.: J. Nutr. *91*:299–306, 1967.
29. Simon, E.J., Gross, C.S., Milhorat, A.T.: J. Biol. Chem. *221*:797–805, 1956.
30. Matschiner, J.T., Bell, R.G., Amelotti, J.M., et al.: Biochim. Biophys. Acta *201*:309–315, 1970.
31. Bell, R.G., Matschiner, J.T.: Biochim. Biophys. Acta *184*:597–603, 1969.
32. Matschiner, J.T., Amelotti, J.M.: J. Lipid Res. *9*:176–179, 1968.
33. Rietz, P., Gloor, U., Wiss, O.: Int. Z. Vitamforsch *40*:351–362, 1970.
34. Bjornsson, T.D., Meffin, P.J., Swezey, S.E., et al.: Disposition and turnover of vitamin $K_1$ in man. *In* Vitamin K Metabolism and Vitamin K-Dependent Proteins. (J.W. Suttie, Ed.) Baltimore, University Park Press, 1980, pp. 328–332.
35. Shearer, M.J., McBurney, A., Barkhan, P.: Vitam. Horm. *32*:513–542, 1974.
36. Bjornsson, T.D., Meffin, P.J., Swezey, S.E., et al.: Pharmacol. Exp. Ther. *210*:322–326, 1979.
37. Olson, R.E., Meyer, R.G., Chao, J., et al.: Circulation *70* (Part II):97, 1984.
38. Billeter, M., Bolliger, W., Martius, C.: Biochem. Z. *340*:290–303, 1964.
39. Taggart, W.V., Matschiner, J.T.: Biochem. J. *8*:1141–1146, 1969.
40. Dialameh, G.H., Taggart, W.V., Matschiner, J.T., et al.: Int. J. Vitam. Nutr. Res. *41*:391–400, 1971.
41. Losito, R., Owen, C.A., Jr., Flock, E.V.: Biochemistry *6*:62–68, 1967.

42. Fieser, L.F., Turner, R.B.: J. Am. Chem. Soc. *69*:2335–2338, 1947.
43. Mezick, J.A., Cornwell, D.G.: Biochim. Biophys. Acta *219*:361, 1970.
44. Dam, H., Schonheyder, F., Tage-Hansen, E.: Biochem. J. *30*:1075–1079, 1936.
45. Owen, C.A.: Bull. Am. Coll. Surg. *32*:256, 1947.
46. Naeye, R.L.: Proc. Soc. Exp. Biol. Med. *91*:101–104, 1956.
47. Hougie, C., Barrow, E.M., Graham, J.B.: J. Clin. Invest. *36*:485–496, 1957.
48. Stenflo, J.: J. Biol. Chem. *251*:355–363, 1976.
49. DiScipio, R.G., Hermodson, M.A., Yates, S.G., et al.: Biochemistry *16*:698–706, 1977.
50. Seegers, W.H., Ghosh, A., Wu, V-Y.: Function of previously unrecognized plasma protein M in thrombin generation. *In* Vitamin K Metabolism and Vitamin K-Dependent Proteins. (J.W. Suttie, Ed.) Baltimore, University Park Press, 1980, pp. 96–101.
51. Prowse, C.V., Esnouf, M.P.: Biochem. Soc. Trans. *5*:255–256, 1977.
52. Biggs, R.P., McFarlane, R.G.: Human Blood Coagulation and Its Disorders. Philadelphia, F.A. Davis Co., 1962.
53. Davie, E.W., Ratnoff, O.D.: Science *145*:1310–1312, 1964.
54. Martius, C.: Vitam. Horm. *24*:441–445, 1966.
55. Olson, R.E.: Vitam. Horm. *32*:483–511, 1974.
56. Suttie, J.W.: Vitam. Horm. *32*:463–481, 1974.
57. Stenflo, J., Fernlund, P., Egan, W., et al.: Proc. Natl. Acad. Sci. U.S.A. *71*:2730–2733, 1974.
58. Nelsestuen, G.L., Zytokovicz, T.H., Howard, J.B.: J. Biol. Chem. *249*:6347–6350, 1974.
59. Magnusson, S., Sottrup-Jensen, L., Petersen, T.E., et al.: FEBS Lett. *44*:189–193, 1974.
60. Girardot, J.M., Delaney, R., Johnson, B.C.: Biochem. Biophys. Res. Commun. *59*:1197–1203, 1974.
61. Shah, D.V., Suttie, J.W.: Biochem. Biophys. Res. Commun. *60*:1397–1402, 1974.
62. Esmon, C.T., Sadowski, J.A., Suttie, J.W.: J. Biol. Chem. *250*:4744–4748, 1975.
63. Munns, T.W., Johnston, M.F.M., Liszewski, M.K., et al.: Proc. Natl. Acad. Sci. U.S.A. *73*:2803–2807, 1976.
64. Willingham, A.K., Laliberte, R.E., Bell, R.G., et al.: Biochem. Pharmacol. *25*:1063–1066, 1976.
65. Larson, A.E., Suttie, J.W.: Proc. Natl. Acad. Sci. U.S.A. *75*:5413–5416, 1978.
66. Olson, R.E., Hall, A.L., Lee, F.C., et al.: Vitamin K-dependent carboxylase: A heme protein? *In* Post-translational Covalent Modifications of Proteins. (Johnson, B.C., Ed.) New York, Academic Press, 1983, pp. 295–319.
67. Suttie, J.W., Hagemen, J.M., Lehrman, S.R., et al.: J. Biol. Chem. *251*:5827–5830, 1976.
68. Jones, J.P., Gardner, E.J., Cooper, T.G., et al.: J. Biol. Chem. *252*:7738–7742, 1977.
69. Larson, A.E., Friedman, P.A., Suttie, J.W.: J. Biol. Chem. *256*:11032–11035, 1981.
70. Hall, A.L., Kloepper, R., Zee-Cheng, R. K-Y., et al.: Arch. Biochem. Biophys. *214*:45–50, 1982.
71. DeMetz, M., Soute, B.A., Hemker, H.C., et al.: J. Biol. Chem. *257*:5326–5329, 1982.
72. Meyer, R.G., Lee, F.C., Olson, R.E.: Fed. Proc. *43*:1862, 1984.
73. Wallin, R., Hutson, S.: J. Biol. Chem. *257*:1583–1586, 1982.
74. Hauschka, P.V., Lian, J.B., Gallop, P.M.: Proc. Natl. Acad. Sci. U.S.A. *72*:3925–3929, 1975.
75. Price, P.A., Otsuka, A.S., Poser, J.W., et al.: Proc. Natl. Acad. Sci. U.S.A. *73*:1447–1451, 1976.
76. Price, P.A., Poser, J.W., Raman, N.: Proc. Natl. Acad. Sci. U.S.A. *73*:3374–3375, 1976.
77. Lian, J.B., Friedman, P.A.: J. Biol. Chem. *253*:6623–6626, 1978.
78. Gallop, P.M., Lian, J.B., Hauschka, P.V.: N. Engl. J. Med. *302*:1460–1466, 1980.
79. Nishimoto, S.K., Price, P.A.: J. Biol. Chem. *254*:437–441, 1979.
80. Friedman, P.A., Shia, M.A.: Biochem. J. *163*:39–43, 1977.
81. Wood, H.G. and Utter, M.F.: Essays in Biochemistry. New York, Academic Press, 1965.
82. Olson, R.E., Suttie, J.W.: Vitam. Horm. *35*:59–108, 1977.
83. Sadowski, J.A., Schnoes, H.K., Suttie, J.W.: Biochemistry *16*:3856–3863, 1977.
84. Hauschka, P.V.: Biochem. Biophys. Res. Commun. *71*:1207, 1976.
85. Pettifor, J.M., Benson, R.: J. Pediatr. *86*:459–462, 1975.
86. Warkany, J.: Am. J. Dis. Child. *129*:287–288, 1975.
87. Fourie, D.T., Hay, I.T.: S. Afr. Med. J. *49*:2081–2083, 1975.
88. Shaul, W.L., Emery, H., Hall, J.G.: Am. J. Dis. Child. *129*:360–362, 1975.
89. Price, P.A., Baukol, S.A.: J. Biol. Chem. *255*:11660–11663, 1980.
90. Price, P.A., Parthemore, J.G., Deftos, L.J.: J. Clin. Invest. *66*:878–883, 1980.
91. Levy, R.J., Lian, J.B., Gallop, P.: Biochem. Biophys. Res. Commun. *91*:41–49, 1979.
92. Levy, R.J., Zenker, J.A., Lian, J.B.: J. Clin. Invest. *65*:563–566, 1980.
93. Lian, J.B., Prien, E.L., Jr.: Fed. Proc. *35*:1763, 1976.
94. Hauschka, P.V., Friedman, P.A., Traverso, H.P., et al.: Biochem. Biophys. Res. Commun. *71*:1207–1213, 1976.
95. Friedman, P.A., Mitch, W.E., Silva, P.: J. Biol. Chem. *257*:11037–11040, 1982.
96. Traverso, H.P., Hauschka, P.V., Gallup, P.M.: Calcif. Tissue Int. *30*:73–76, 1980.
97. Schofield, F.W.: Can. Vet. Rec. *3*:74–79, 1922.
98. Roderick, L.M.: Am. J. Physiol. *96*:413–425, 1931.
99. Campbell, H.A., Link, K.P.: J. Biol. Chem. *138*:21–33, 1941.
100. O'Reilly, R.A., Aggeler, P.M.: Pharmacol. Rev. *22*:35–96, 1970.
101. Bell, R.G., Matschiner, J.T.: Arch. Biochem. Biophys. *141*:473–476, 1970.
102. Suttie, J.W.: CRC Crit. Rev. Biochem. *8*:191–223, 1980.
103. Fasco, M.J., Hildebrandt, E.F., Suttie, J.W.: J. Biol. Chem. *257*:11210–11212, 1982.
104. Fasco, M.J., Principe, L.M., Walsh, N.A., et al.: Biochemistry *22*:5655–5660, 1983.
105. Jones, J.P., Fausto, A., Houser, R.M., et al.: Biochem. Biophys. Res. Commun. *72*:589–597, 1976.
106. Whitlon, D.S., Sadowski, J.A., Suttie, J.W.: Biochemistry *17*:1371–1379, 1978.
107. Wallin, R., Hutson, S.: J. Biol. Chem. *257*:1583–1586, 1982.
108. Lorusso, D.J., Suttie, J.W.: Mol. Pharmacol. *8*:197–203, 1972.

109. Thierry, M.J., Hermodson, M.A., Suttie, J.W.: Am. J. Physiol. *219*:854–859, 1970.
110. Searcey, M.T., Graves, C.B., Olson, R.E.: J. Biol. Chem. *252*:6260–6267, 1977.
111. Douglas, A.S., Brown, A.: Br. Med. J. *1*:412–415, 1952.
112. Dam, H.: Vitam. Horm. *24*:295–306, 1966.
113. Brinkhous, K.M., Smith, H.P., Warner, E.D.: Am. J. Med. Sci. *193*:475–480, 1937.
114. Sutherland, J.M., Glueck, H.I., Gleser, G.: Am. J. Dis Child. *113*:524–533, 1967.
115. Seeler, R.A.: Ill. Med. J. *147*:59–61, 1975.
116. Evans, A.R., Forrester, R.M., Discombe, C.: Lancet *1*:517–518, 1970.
117. Udall, J.A.: J.A.M.A. *194*:107–109, 1965.
118. Frick, P.G., Riedler, G., Brogli, H.: J. Appl. Physiol. *23*:387–389, 1967.
119. Kark, R., Lozner, E.L.: Lancet *2*:1162–1164, 1939.
120. Aggeler, P.M., Lucia, S.P., Fishbon, H.M.: Am. J. Dig. Dis. *9*:227–229, 1942.
121. Ansell, J.E., Kumar, R., Deykin, D.: J.A.M.A. *238*:40–42, 1977.
122. Pineo, G.F., Gallus, A.S., Hirsh, J.: Can. Med. Assoc. J. *109*:880–883, 1973.
123. Damrongsak, D.: The fat-soluble vitamins and protein-calorie malnutrition. *In* Protein-Calorie Malnutrition. (Olson, R.E., Ed.) New York, Academic Press, 1975, pp. 195–197.
124. Dudrick, S.J., Wilmore, D.W., Vars, H.M., et al.: Surgery *64*:134–142, 1968.
125. Ryan, J.A., Jr. : Complication of total parenteral nutrition. *In* Total Parenteral Nutrition. (Fischer, E., Ed.) Boston, Little, Brown and Co., 1976, pp. 55–100.
126. Boland, E.W.: Proc. Staff Meet. Mayo Clinic *13*:70–72, 1938.
127. McGehee, W.G., Klotz, T.A., Epstein, D.J., et al.: Ann. Intern. Med. *100*:59–60, 1984.
128. Hooper, C.A., Harvey, B.B., Stone, H.H.: Lancet *1*:39–40, 1980.
129. Lipsky, J.J.: Lancet *2*:192–193, 1983.
130. Uotila, L., Suttie, J.W.: J. Infect. Dis. *148*:571–578, 1983.
131. March, B.E., Wong, E., Seier, L., et al.: J. Nutr. *103*:371–377, 1973.
132. Korsan-Bengsten, K., Elmfeldt, D., Holm, T.: Thromb. Diath. Haemorr. *31*:505–512, 1974.
133. Corrigan, J.J., Marcus, F.I.: J.A.M.A. *230*:1300–1301, 1974.
134. Schrogie, J.J.: J.A.M.A. *232*:19, 1975.
135. Gustafsson, B.E., Daft, F.S., McDaniel, E.G., et al.: J. Nutr. *78*:461–468, 1962.
136. Duello, T.J., Matschiner, J.T.: J. Nutr. *102*:331–335, 1972.
137. Chiu, Y.J.D., Zee-Cheng, R.K.-Y, Olson, R.E.: Fed. Proc. *40*:873, 1981.
138. Matschiner, J.T., Taggart, W.V.: J. Nutr. *94*:57–59, 1968.
139. Isler, O., Wiss, O.: Vitam. Horm. *17*:53–90, 1959.

## SELECTED READINGS

Olson, R.E.: The function and metabolism of vitamin K. Ann. Rev. Nutr. *4*:281–337, 1984.

Suttie, J.W., Olson, R.E.: Vitamin K. *In* Present Knowledge in Nutrition. 5th ed. 1984, pp. 241–259.

Suttie, J.W.: Vitamin K-dependent carboxylase. Ann. Rev. Bioch. *54*:459–477, 1985.

*Chapter* **15**

# VITAMIN E

## Philip M. Farrell

In the interval since Horwitt's review,[1] there have been many developments relating to nutritional and clinical aspects of vitamin E. Methods for assessment of nutritional status have been re-examined critically and improved, particularly with the advent of high performance liquid chromatography (HPLC) to separate the major vitamin E isomers of the tocopherol family.[2,3] Populations of vitamin E deficient patients have been identified and studied with respect to pathologic alterations that might be attributed to the deficiency state.[4] Yet, the vitamin remains an enigma and a continued challenge to both nutritional and clinical scientists. The subcellular role of vitamin E has been particularly difficult to establish, although it clearly functions as a biologic antioxidant. Partly as a result of this gap in knowledge, confusion also persists among medical scientists as to the indications for vitamin E therapy. Although medical benefits of tocopherol pharmacotherapy have been claimed when large doses of dietary supplements were taken by individuals not deficient in vitamin E, the evidence for favorable responses is generally unconvincing.[4–6]

Nevertheless, the essentiality of this vitamin for humans has been well established during the past two decades, and many challenging new concepts have emerged from relevant basic research. The search for clinical disturbances in the human deficiency state has been aided by extensive investigation of the pathobiology of vitamin E deficiency in lower animals. Provocative experimental results in free radical biology have stimulated ever increasing interest during recent years in the antioxidant capability of vitamin E. Thus, review of vitamin E requires comprehensive discussion of current multidisciplinary research, including information on free radical biology and lipid peroxidation.

## HISTORICAL PERSPECTIVE

The early history of vitamin E was reviewed in detail by Mason.[7] Its discovery can be traced to the observation that reproductive failure often occurred in rats fed semipurified diets that contained adequate amounts of vitamins A, B, C, and D and supported good growth and general health. The existence of vitamin E was recognized in 1922 when it became clear that this fat-soluble factor prevented fetal death in animals fed a diet containing rancid lard. By 1925, the term *vitamin E* was accepted as the fifth serial alphabetical designation for vitamins. Subsequently, Evans proposed the word *tocopherol* from the Greek "tos" for childbirth and "phero" meaning to bring forth and "ol" for the alcohol portion of the molecule.

The early years of research were characterized by descriptions of the structural and functional changes of vitamin E deficiency in various animals. Degeneration of the germinal epithelium in the male rat was noted as the underlying problem in testicular atrophy, whereas fetal resorption was identified as the major problem of pregnant females. Paralysis associated with dystrophic muscle and occurrence of encephalomalacia were described in rodents and fowl as reviewed by Nelson.[8] Also, "exudative diathesis" (subcutaneous edema with lipid peroxidation) was described in vitamin E deficient chicks, and an early clue to the nutritional interrelationship with selenium was recognized. In the 1930s, the ferric chloride-dipyridyl method of tocopherol analysis developed by Emmerie and Engel[9] allowed determination of the vitamin E content of foods. Lipids with vitamin E activity were isolated from wheat germ oil, and their chemical synthesis was achieved in 1938 by Karrer et al.[10] Similar methods of chemical synthesis were reported soon thereafter by Smith et al.[11] Nutritional surveys in the 1940s and 1950s revealed that premature infants and patients with malabsorption had low levels of blood tocopherol and abnormal hemolysis of erythrocytes incubated in the presence of hydrogen peroxide.[12,13] Finally, in 1968, vitamin E was recognized formally as an essential nutrient for humans by inclusion in the Recommended Dietary Allowances table of the United States Food and Nutrition Board (National Academy of Sciences).

It is somewhat surprising that during the first two decades of vitamin E research the pathologic conditions of the dietary deficiency state in animals were well defined, the chemical nature and biologic properties of the tocopherols were established, and chemical synthesis was achieved, whereas definitive information on subcellular function(s) and the precise role of this vitamin in human health remain to be elucidated. This paradox adds to the challenge of vitamin E research and has stimulated ever increasing scientific interest in tocopherol around the world.

## CHEMISTRY AND NOMENCLATURE

In comparison to the other fat-soluble vitamins, the chemistry of vitamin E is rather complex because there are eight naturally occurring compounds with the characteristic biologic activity. Four vitamers are members of the tocopherol family and four are tocotrienols. Moreover, the stereochemistry of commercially synthesized tocopherols further complicates structural considerations because there are three asymmetric carbon atoms and therefore numerous stereoisomers.

The most abundant and active isomer is alpha-tocopherol, the structure of which is shown in Figure 15–1. The compound is also referred to as 5,7,8-trimethyl tocol, the latter being 2-methyl-2-(4,8,12-trimethyl-tridecyl)-6-chromanol IX). Natural alpha-tocopherol as found in foods is [d]-alpha-tocopherol, whereas chemical synthesis produces a mixture of eight epimers.

In addition to the alpha vitamer, three other tocopherols with biologic activity are present in foods: β-, γ-, and δ-tocopherols. As illustrated in Figure 15–2, they differ from alpha-tocopherol only in regard to methyl substitutions on the benzene ring. In particular, β-tocopherol is 5,8-dimethyl-tocol, γ-tocopherol is 7,8-dimethyl tocol, and δ-tocopherol is 8-methyl tocol. The tocotrienols consist of four compounds similar to the corresponding tocopherols but with unsaturated side chains as shown in Figure 15–2. These unsaturated isomers have not been well studied, and only α-tocotrienol appears to have significant vitamin E activity.

Detailed information on the nomenclature of vitamin E compounds has been published by Kasparek[14] and Bieri and McKenna.[15] In addition, the January issue of the *Journal of Nutrition* publishes a policy statement on terminology each year. Although common usage has dictated that certain terms be retained, the systemization of biochemical nomenclature by the International Union of Biochemistry (IUB) has specified that the prefixes *d*- and *l*- are not appropriate for indicating stereoisomers of tocopherols. Instead, it was proposed that modification of the RS system be used in accordance with the approach commonly accepted for other organic compounds with asymmetric carbon atoms.[15] Because of the three asymmetric carbon atoms, however, the nomenclature for the tocopherol family is complicated. In brief, [d]-α-tocopherol is now designated RRR-α-tocopherol, and the commercially synthesized all racemic compound formerly referred to as [dl]-α-tocopherol is now known as all-*rac*-α-tocopherol. The RS system is essential for presentation of chemical data, for discussing synthetic processes, and describing structural formulas with stereochemical accuracy. On the other hand, it is an awkward system and has not yet been used widely in clinical nutrition, nor does it seem necessary for communications among nutritionists and clinicians, particularly since analytical methods used commonly do not distinguish the stereoisomers. Therefore, in this article, the term *vitamin E* is employed as the generic descriptor for tocol and tocotrienol derivatives with the characteristic biologic activity. In general, α-, β-, δ-, and γ-tocopherol have been used in an unqualified fashion herein to indicate the various vitamers being assessed in human nutrition, and the prefixes *d*- and *l*- have been largely avoided.

Methods for the chemical production of tocopherols have been reviewed by Kasparek.[14] In general, two approaches have been employed, involving either partial synthesis from naturally available compounds or total synthesis. The usual method of complete chemical synthesis depends upon construction of the heterocyclic ring of tocopherols along with the isoprenoid side chain at C-2 using methylated hydroquinones and an ali-

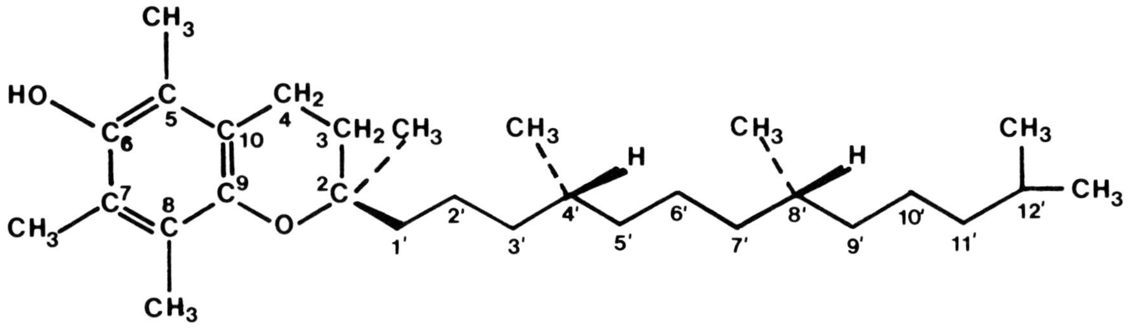

**CHEMICAL NAME:** 2, 5, 7, 8-Tetramethyl-2-(4', 8', 12'-trimethyl tridecyl)-6 chromanol

**IUPAC NAME:** 2R, 4'R, 8'R-Alpha Tocopherol

**TRIVIAL NAME:** RRR-Alpha Tocopherol

**COMMON NAMES:** Natural Vitamin E
Alpha Tocopherol

**Fig. 15–1.** Structure and nomenclature of the most active vitamin E isomer. See text for details of nomenclature.

phatic reactant. Originally, natural phytol was used as the starting material to yield 2RS,4'R,8'R-alpha-tocopherol. This product contained approximately equimolar amounts of the 2R and 2S stereoisomers and was, therefore, marketed commercially under the designation [dl]-alpha-tocopherol and referred to as 2-ambo-alpha-tocopherol (Table 15–1). Currently, synthetic phytol or isophytol is used to yield a mixture of four racemates or eight stereoisomers which is correctly designated all-*rac*-α-tocopherol. In partial synthetic procedures, methyl groups are introduced into the benzene ring of the lower methyl homolog of 5,7,8-trimethyl tocol. This method yields α-tocopherol from the 5,8-dimethyl, 7,8-dimethyl, and 8-methyl tocol compounds which are naturally present in many sources. In essence, this allows conversion of biologically less active vitamers into the most active RRR-α-tocopherol.

## BIOLOGIC ACTIVITY

There is widespread agreement that vitamin E can function in general as a biologic antioxidant to protect cellular membranes from oxidative destruction. Most of the evidence for this function has been obtained from in vitro experiments, but there are also data from studies of various tissues that tocopherols have antioxidant potential in vivo.[19] Moreover, it has been well established that

some manifestations of vitamin E deficiency in chicks and rats can be prevented completely by feeding antioxidants such as ethoxyquin. Many enzyme activities in plasma are altered during severe vitamin E deficiency because tissue necrosis causes release of cellular enzymes.[5,16] Partly as a result of these enzymatic alterations, other functions have been proposed for vitamin E but have not been established. These include regulation of nucleic acid synthesis and gene expression and control of the growth cycle in certain protozoa.[16]

McCay and King have reviewed the evidence indicating that α-tocopherol functions as a free radical scavenger in membranes.[18] As illustrated in Figure 15–3, phospholipids in cellular and subcellular membranes contain polyunsaturated fatty acids (PUFA) that are susceptible to peroxidation. Vitamin E is the fat-soluble antioxidant capable of protecting these fatty acids by interrupting free radical reactions that otherwise can cause membrane damage in subcellular organelles. Other antioxidant systems involving enzymes (e.g., glutathione peroxidase and superoxide dismutase) can also function in helping the cell control free radical attacks on peroxidizable fatty acids. Thus, the well-known interrelationship between α-tocopherol and selenium has been explained by the fact that glutathione peroxidase is a selenoenzyme.[17]

| COMMON NAME | STRUCTURE | RELATIVE BIOLOGIC ACTIVITY |
|---|---|---|
| Alpha-Tocopherol | | 1 |
| Beta-Tocopherol | | 0.4 |
| Gamma-Tocopherol | | 0.1 - 0.3 |
| Delta-Tocopherol | | 0.01 |
| Alpha-Tocotrienol | | 0.3 |

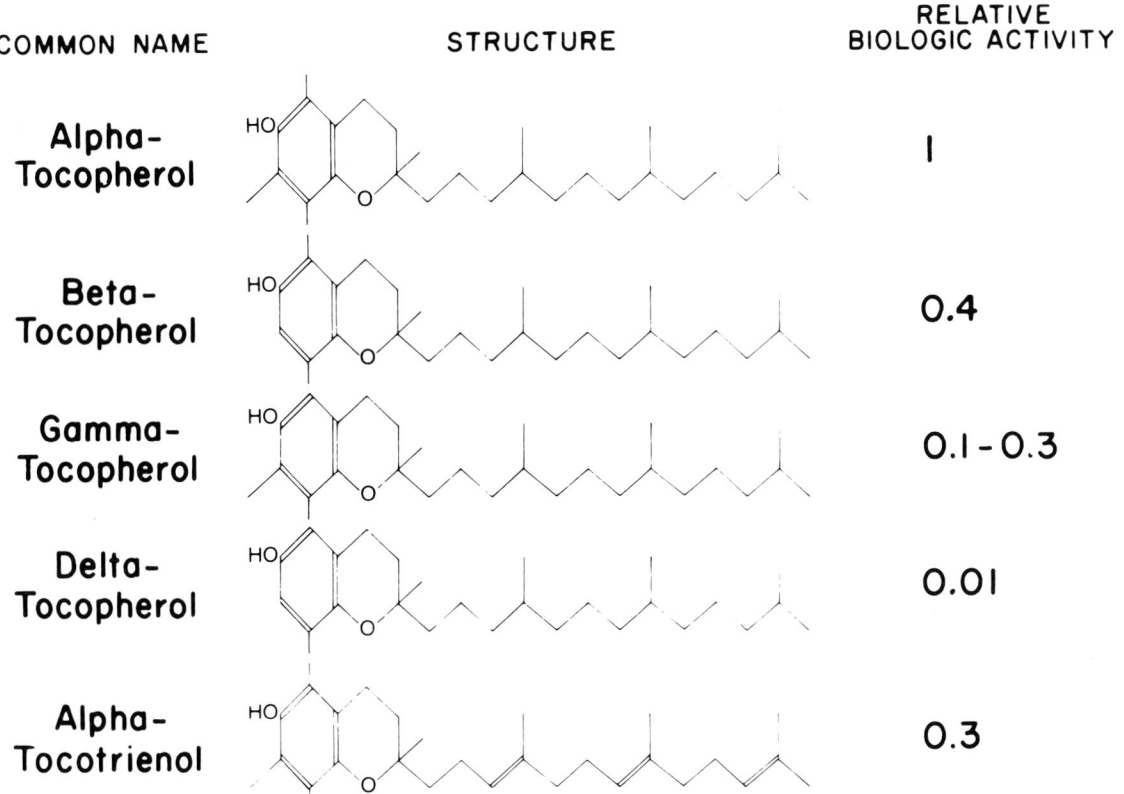

**Fig. 15–2.** Naturally occurring vitamin E compounds and their biologic activities relative to RRR-α-tocopherol, which is designated officially as having 1.49 IU/mg.

The importance of free radicals in cellular metabolism has become apparent because of concurrent investigations in several fields, including studies on the generation of lipid hydroperoxides, on oxidoreductase systems, and on the subcellular role of superoxide dismutase.[18,19] Also, considerable interest has been stimulated in recent years because of concern that adverse effects of environmental toxins are mediated through free radicals, that aging is associated with inadequately controlled free radical reactions, and that carcinogenesis can be triggered by peroxidation.[20]

There are several mechanisms for formation of free radicals in biologic systems: (1) cleavage of covalent bonds in organic compounds in which each of the two new molecules retain one electron from the original bonding pair after the splitting; (2) capture of an electron by a receptor molecule such as in the production of the superoxide anion radical when molecular oxygen captures an electron; and (3) self-generation of additional free radicals when reaction occurs with certain compounds such as PUFA molecules. Endogenous production of free radicals can be catalyzed by iron and can also be promoted by inhaled atmospheric pollutants and ingested toxins like carbon tetrachloride.[20] Cellular generation of superoxide and hydrogen peroxide can initiate free radical-mediated lipid peroxidation in exposed membranes. As illustrated in Figure 15–3, a chain reaction can occur during the formation of free radicals because of methylene group reactions of PUFA molecules. It appears that fatty acid radicals formed in this fashion can react spontaneously with oxygen to form a fatty acid peroxy radical; this may propagate the peroxidation of more fatty acid molecules by abstracting hydrogen atoms to form hydroperoxides and new fatty acid radicals. Thus, the self-propagating reaction may lead to oxidation of many fatty acid molecules from production of a single fatty acid radical as the initiating event. As a result of peroxidation of fatty acids, malondialdehyde is produced in tissues subjected to peroxidation of PUFA within phospholipid membranes.[18] Lipid peroxidation can also be detected by analysis of exhaled ethane and pentane.[21]

As envisioned, the major role of vitamin E as an antioxidant is to "neutralize" free radicals, which could otherwise initiate the change reac-

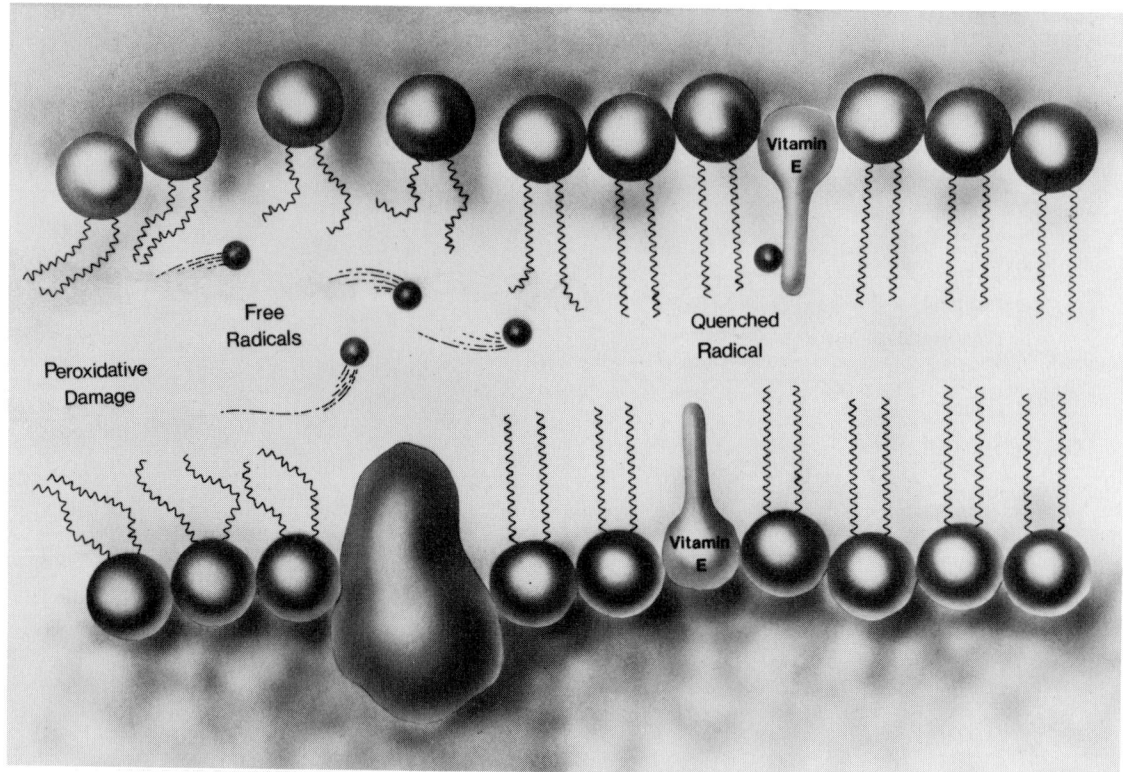

**Fig. 15–3.** Proposed antioxidant role of vitamin E as a free radical scavenger in biologic membranes halting the chain reaction of polyunsaturated fatty acid peroxidation.

tion, especially in membranes that contain a large proportion of highly unsaturated fatty acids. To be effective, α-tocopherol must be localized in membrane sites that contain free radicals. Oxidation of vitamin E caused by reaction with free radicals leads to the formation of α-tocopherol semiquinone, which is rapidly converted to other products such as α-tocopherol quinone and hydroquinone. In view of the relationship between vitamin E and unsaturated fatty acids, it is not surprising that the requirement for α-tocopherol is somewhat dependent upon the amount of PUFA consumed, which can alter membrane fatty acid composition.[5] This relationship appears to be particularly important in young growing animals in which formation of normal membrane structures and maintenance of their integrity are very active biochemical processes.

Cellular enzyme antioxidant systems can play a potentially important role in preventing free radical initiation of chain reactions. For instance, glutathione peroxidase is an effective scavenger of hydrogen peroxide because of its high affinity for this substrate. On the other hand, catalase is relatively ineffective at low hydrogen peroxide concentrations.[18] In selenium deficiency, lower glutathione peroxidase activity probably is associated with greater levels of hydrogen peroxide in certain cells; as a result, α-tocopherol might be consumed more rapidly by free radical attacks on unsaturated lipids in the membranes. The enzyme superoxide dismutase appears also to be highly effective in removing superoxide radicals formed by a number of oxido-reductase systems such as microsomal NADPH oxidase.[18] Despite the presence of these antioxidant enzyme systems, tocopherol deficiency in membranes will lead to insufficient protection against hydroxy-radical-induced damage from superoxide formation and hydrogen peroxide in the cell.

## STRUCTURAL-FUNCTIONAL RELATIONSHIPS

The biologic antioxidant activity of tocopherol isomers has been measured by using both in vitro and in vivo techniques. It must be recognized that the vitamin E of a given isomer will depend not only on the compound's structure, but also on its relative absorption, uptake by target tissues, and turnover rate. Consequently, results of in vitro assay systems do not give the same data as in vivo bioassays. This has lead to controversy over the assignment of relative potencies, an important consideration with respect to dietary allowances. The in vivo bioassay systems used most commonly are based on assessing pathologic changes in rats, chicks, and hamsters. In these bioassays, fetal resorption, production of muscular dystrophy, and occurrence of encephalomalacia may be used to detect relative biologic activity. More recently, quantitative measures of in vivo lipid peroxidation have been used, particularly in rats.[21] Unfortunately, the relative potencies of the vitamers determined by these various in vivo methods can differ substantially, and this fact adds to the controversy.

Table 15–1 summarizes the relative biologic activities of vitamin E compounds according to current consensus.[5,15] The original international standard of vitamin E, synthesized from natural phytol and initially designated [dl]-α-tocopheryl acetate, was defined as having 1 IU/mg; however, this product is no longer available. The replacement compound (all-rac-α-tocopheryl acetate) is currently being investigated to determine if it has the same biologic activity as the original standard.[22] On the basis of in vivo bioassays, the approximate relative potencies of the other tocopherol isomers compared to α are: β = 40 to 50%; γ = 10 to 30%; δ = about 1%. Thus, the presence and location of methyl groups in the benzene ring is of great importance in determining biologic activity among the tocopherol isomers. As for the stereoisomers, it appears from some data that only the 2-position is significant in influencing biologic antioxidant activity, with the 2R configuration being essential to account for the potency of natural vitamin E.[14,22]

Assessment of γ-tocopherol's relative activity is of special interest because of the high content of this vitamer in the American diet.[24,25] Although 10% of the activity of α-tocopherol has been accepted,[15] recent comparative assessment of lipid peroxidation in vivo by determination of pentane production in iron-loaded rats suggests that γ-tocopherol is 31% as effective as α-tocopherol.[21] In contrast to the in vivo bioassays, the usual in vitro tests indicate that gamma-tocopherol in the red blood cell membrane shows 30 to 67% the activity of the alpha vitamer.[5] Also, measurement of biochemical antioxidant potential in vitro has yielded values as high 68 to 100% for γ-tocopherol.[23] The difference in γ-tocopherol's level of vitamin E activity has been attributed to a faster turnover rate (compared to that for α-tocopherol) and lesser amounts in the phospholipid membranes where the antioxidant function is needed.[5,24] Because of its uncertain bioavailability, therefore, γ-tocopherol in foods was assigned only 10% the activity of α-tocopherol by the Food and Nutrition Board in the 9th Edition of *Recommended Dietary Allowances.*

Very little information is available on the vitamin E activity of the tocotrienols, but there is evidence that the effects of methyl substitution are similar to those observed with the tocopherol family. Thus, only α-tocotrienol has biologically significant vitamin E activity, approximating 30% that of α-tocopherol.[26]

## DIETARY CONSIDERATIONS

Most of the information on the vitamin E activity in foods has been derived from analysis of tocopherols, rather than tocotrienols. Bauernfeind has presented a list of tocopherol concentrations including the distribution of isomers in various foods.[25] The tocopherol content of diets shows great variation depending upon harvesting, proc-

**Table 15–1. Vitamin E. Activities of Tocopherol Isomers as Originally Designated[15]**

| Compound | Vitamin E Activity |
|---|---|
| [d]-alpha-tocopherol (RRR-alpha-tocopherol) | 1.49 IU/mg |
| [d]-alpha-tocopheryl acetate (RRR-alpha-tocopheryl-acetate) | 1.36 IU/mg |
| [dl]-alpha-tocopherol (originally 2-ambo-alpha-tocopherol, now all *rac*-alpha-tocopherol) | 1.1 IU/mg |
| [dl]-alpha-tocopheryl acetate (originally 2-ambo-alpha-tocopheryl acetate, now all *rac*-alpha-tocopheryl acetate) | 1.0 IU/mg* |
| [d]-beta-tocopherol | 0.60 IU/mg† |
| [d]-gamma-tocopherol | 0.15–0.45 IU/mg† |
| [d]-delta-tocopherol | 0.015† |

*The original international standard is no longer available, and the activity of the current replacement compound is being investigated to determine if its specific biologic activity is less than 1 IU/mg.[15,22]
†Derived by calculation, since only alpha vitamers are officially recognized by assigned international units of biologic activity.

essing, storage, and final food preparation procedures.[25] The major sources of vitamin E consumed by Americans are the vegetable and seed
oils, such as corn oil, soybean oil, and safflower
oil. Although these common oils, and the less
commonly consumed wheat germ, are rich
sources of tocopherols, the actual concentration
and distribution of vitamin E isomers are quite
variable. As shown in Table 15–2, animal products are not good sources. Although butter provides very little α-tocopherol, American margarine contains a range from 3.2 to 32.7 mg/100 g
and, therefore, can supply a significant amount of
vitamin E in the diet.

The proportion of non-α isomers provided by
fats and oils has become a topic of great nutritional
interest since corn oil and soybean oil have become major components of the American diet, [5,24]
rather than animal fat. Soybean oil has become
particularly prevalent and accounted for 74% of
oils and fats used in edible United States products
according to a USDA survey in 1982/83.[27] Soybeans contain predominantly γ-tocopherol with
lesser amounts of δ-tocopherol and only a relatively small amount of α-tocopherol (see Table
15–2). As a result of the rather high content of
non-α vitamers, soybean oil provides a disproportionately low amount of vitamin E activity in
comparison to its concentration of total tocopherols. Other dietary lipid sources such as coconut
and fish oils are low in tocopherols. Except for

fish oil, however, the concentration of tocopherols
increases in proportion to the amount of PUFA
present.

In calculating the vitamin E activity of mixed
diets, the traditional approach has been to adjust
the amount of β-tocopherol by a factor of 0.5, γ-
tocopherol by 0.1, and alpha-tocotrienol by 0.3.
For instance, the γ-tocopherol content of soybean
oil (59.3 mg/100 g) would be multiplied by 0.1 to
yield a value of 5.93 mg/100 g and, similarly, the
contribution of delta-tocopherol would be reduced from 26 to 0.26 mg/100 g; these concentrations would be added to the 10.1 mg/100 g of
α-tocopherol to yield a total "α-tocopherol equivalent" value of 16.29 mg/100 g. For studies of
mixed diets in which only RRR-α-tocopherol is
reported, the value in milligrams can be increased
by 20% to allow for the presence of other vitamin
E compounds and thereby estimate "α-tocopherol
equivalents."[15]

## INTESTINAL ABSORPTION, TRANSPORT, AND STORAGE

A variety of methods have been used to measure
vitamin E absorption and transport as discussed
by Bieri and Farrell.[5] Although the data have been
obtained almost exclusively in studies of α-
tocopherol, it appears that transport processes are
similar for the other tocopherol vitamers.[24] On the
other hand, tissue storage and turnover are considerably different. The absorption of tocopherols

**Table 15–2.  Tocopherol Content of Representative Dietary Components[25]**

| | Tocopherols Measured by Various Techniques (mg/100g) | | | |
|---|---|---|---|---|
| Dietary Component | α | β | γ | δ |
| Milk | 0.04 | – | – | – |
| Bread—white | 0.04 | 0.02 | 0.24 | 0.1 |
| —whole wheat | 0.16 | 0.15 | 0.38 | 0.2 |
| Beef—steak† | 0.30 | – | – | – |
| —liver† | 0.63 | – | – | – |
| Fish (haddock)† | 0.60 | – | – | – |
| Butter | 1.68 | – | 0.14 | – |
| Lard | 1.20 | – | 0.70 | – |
| Margarine | 11.70* | – | 29.00 | 8.1 |
| Seeds and Nuts | | | | |
| Peanuts | 9.7 | – | 6.60 | – |
| Almonds | 27.4 | 0.30 | 0.90 | – |
| Sunflower seeds | 49.5 | 2.73 | – | – |
| Oils | | | | |
| Corn | 11.2 | 5.00 | 60.20 | 1.8 |
| Cottonseed | 38.9 | – | 38.70 | – |
| Peanut | 13.0 | – | 21.60 | 2.1 |
| Safflower | 38.7 | – | 17.40 | 24.0 |
| Soybean | 10.1 | – | 59.30 | 26.4 |
| Sunflower | 48.7 | – | 5.10 | 0.8 |
| Wheat germ | 133.0 | 71.00 | 26.00 | 27.1 |

*α-tocopherol content varies from 3.2 to 32.7 mg/100 g depending on multiple factors (oil source, processing methods);
  the average for 27 brands listed by Bauernfeind was 12.0 mg/100 g.[25]
†Values listed are prepared food (e.g., cooked meat).

depends upon factors generally important in lipid digestion and intestinal uptake, as discussed elsewhere in the book. Bile salts and pancreatic enzymes are known to be important in the absorption process.[4] In general, the degree of absorption of tocopherols will vary depending upon total lipid absorption.[5] The efficiency of the absorption, however, decreases as large amounts of tocopherol are consumed.[28] Most of the quantitative information has been obtained by administering radioactive α-tocopherol and measuring fecal excretion of radioactivity. The percentage absorption in rats observed by Losowsky et al.[28] decreased from about 60% when 0.04 mg of α-tocopherol was administered (in either arachis oil, a Tween emulsion, or alcohol) to 30% when 20 mg were given. Vitamin E-deficient rats also absorbed about 60% of 0.04 mg of α-tocopherol. In normal humans, an average absorption of at least 50% and perhaps as high as 70% can be assumed for dietary levels of α-tocopherol consumption (e.g., 0.4 to 1 mg);[5,28] however, the efficiency falls to less than 10% with pharmacologic doses such as 200 mg.

The malabsorption of fat seen in patients with various forms of steatorrhea results in a parallel loss of tocopherols. As shown in **Figure 15–4**, the fecal excretion of radiolabeled tocopherol correlates with the extent of steatorrhea in patients with pancreatic disease, biliary obstruction, celiac disease, postgastrectomy malabsorption, and lymphangiectasia.[29] Children with pancreatic achylia due to cystic fibrosis have been studied extensively with respect to vitamin E status, and their levels of circulating tocopherol have been found to correlate closely with various indices of malabsorption.[30]

Once absorbed, vitamin E isomers are transported with fat predominately by lymphatic vessels to the venous system. Tocopherols are distributed in plasma in association with lipoproteins, but no specific carrier protein has been identified. In general, the concentrations of tocopherol in plasma subfractions vary depending upon the amount of lipid present. A rapid exchange of plasma tocopherol and erythrocyte tocopherol occurs at the red blood cell membrane.[31] α-tocopherol is taken up by most tissues, including liver, lung, heart, skeletal muscle, and adipose tissue.[32] Contrary to the other tissues, fat

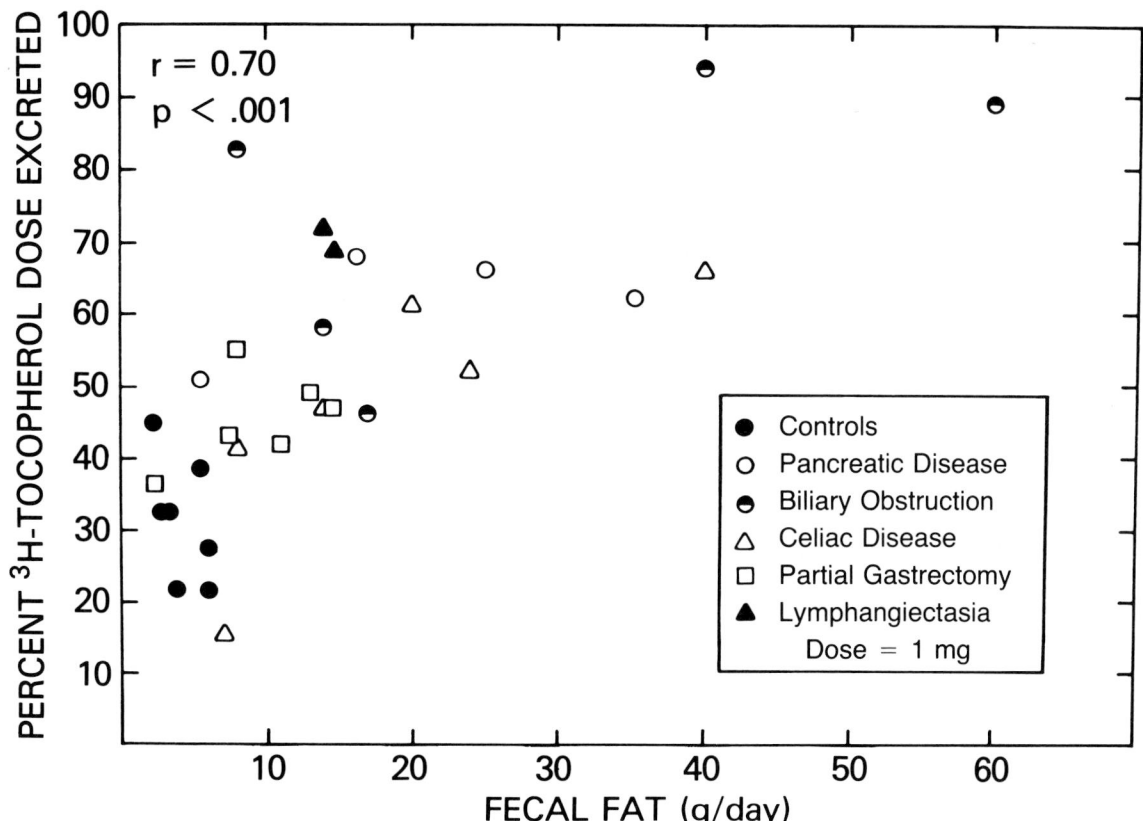

**Fig. 15–4.** Degree of tocopherol malabsorption in patients with various gastrointestinal disorders as determined by MacMahon and Neal,[29] using 1 mg doses of labeled α-tocopherol. (Reproduced from Farrell, P.M., Machlin, L.J.,[4] with permission of Marcel Dekker, Inc.)

accumulates α-tocopherol continuously and can sequester the vitamin.[5,32,33] In general, vitamin E compounds are apparently concentrated wherever there is abundant fatty acid, especially in structures of the cell containing phospholipid membranes, such as mitochondria, microsomes, and plasma membranes. When the intake of vitamin E is high, the liver is a major repository, but the total body pool in adipose tissue is much higher. Although adipose tissue is sometimes considered a "store" of vitamin E, it should be recognized that the tocopherol present in adipocytes is not readily available to other tissues.[32]

The concentration of tocopherol present in tissues is related to the amount of vitamin E consumed,[32,34] and the lipid content of the organ in question. The amount of α-tocopherol present in the liver is considered to be an index of dietary intake. Tissues with greater lipid content tend to have more vitamin E. In blood, the amount of lipid present also has a major influence, if not a determining role, on the level of circulating plasma tocopherols.[35] Therefore, vitamin E concentrations in biologic specimens should be expressed both in terms of mg/unit volume or weight and as mg/g lipid.

The metabolism and turnover of α-tocopherol have been investigated only to a limited extent in humans and have not been adequately quantitated in any species. According to the scheme proposed by Gallo-Torres,[36] the chromane ring is hydrolyzed to α-tocopheryl quinone, which may be reduced to the hydroquinone. Further metabolism leads to oxidation of the terminal methyl group in the side chain; the resulting carboxylate may be then be shortened, giving rise to tocopheronic acid, which can subsequently be converted to tocopheronolactone. Small amounts of tocopherol metabolites such as tocopheryl quinone and tocopheryl hydroquinone have been found in various tissues. Only traces of tocopherol metabolites are found in urine. Tocopheronolactone has been detected in urine of animals given free tocopherol, but the amount excreted is quite low. The major route of excretion of tocopherol metabolites appears to be fecal elimination, possibly in association with bile secretion.

When a vitamin E-deficient diet is fed to animals, plasma and liver levels of α-tocopherol decrease rapidly. There seem to be two pools present, at least in rats, a rapidly metabolized pool and a component that is retained for longer periods.[32] Depletion of tocopherol from adipose tissue and skeletal muscle is a slow process. Thus, these organs should not be considered physiologic storage sites for vitamin E.

Using both short-term labeling techniques and longer feeding studies, Bieri and Poukka Evarts have assessed γ-tocopherol metabolism in rats in comparison to α-tocopherol.[24] γ-tocopherol showed similar absorption and initial distribution in plasma lipoproteins. Within two hours, however, there was a twofold enrichment of the α vitamer and by 24 hours a threefold relative increase of α- relative to γ-tocopherol in both chylomicrons and lipoproteins. Tissue deposition was similar for the two isomers at two hours, but at 24 hours there was only about half as much labeled γ-tocopherol in liver and spleen. When partially depleted animals were fed for two weeks with a diet providing γ- and α-tocopherols in a 2:1 ratio, an average of only 23% as much γ was deposited in seven tissues. With greater proportions of γ-tocopherol fed longer, relatively more of this isomer was deposited, but never to a level approaching α-tocopherol except in adipose tissue. The results of Bieri and Poukka Evarts indicate that γ-tocopherol disappears from the circulation and tissues much faster than the α vitamer, implying a more rapid turnover rate.[24] Whether this is due simply to the one methyl group difference in structure or to a specific cellular receptor helping to retain α-tocopherol or to some other mechanism remains to be determined.

Quantitative information on γ-tocopherol turnover in humans is lacking. Nevertheless, it is reasonable to conclude that the same faster turnover phenomenon applies to children and adults in view of the low proportion of γ-tocopherol in blood despite higher consumption than that of α-tocopherol. Because depletion of γ-tocopherol from tissues is relatively rapid, one must be careful not to overestimate its contribution to total vitamin E activity in the American diet.

## EVALUATION OF VITAMIN E STATUS

In nutritional surveys and clinical diagnostic studies, assessment of vitamin E status has depended upon biochemical analyses of plasma or serum, erythrocytes, adipose tissue biopsies, and organs obtained at autopsy. In common practice, serum has generally been used for measurement of total tocopherol concentrations. A better assessment, however, is provided by measuring tocopherol isomers either by thin layer chromatography[37] or, preferably, by HPLC.[2,3] The latter will provide precise determination of α-tocopherol concentrations, as well as data on the other isomers. Separation of the β and γ isomers, however, is extremely difficult using either method. As a result, these two vitamers are generally reported together as the β + γ fraction. Although 90% or more of the circulating vitamin E is normally α-tocopherol, large amounts of β +

γ-tocopherol and δ-tocopherol can be found in some circumstances. For instance, Gutcher et al. showed that infants on formulas containing corn oil had high levels of circulating γ-tocopherol,[3] and Farrell et al. commented that infants receiving Intralipid (intravenous fat emulsion) had high levels of γ-tocopherol.[38] Also, Horwitt et al. have detected unusually high proportions of β + γ tocopherol in adults on diets containing a predominance of γ tocopherol (i.e., corn oil supplemented subjects).[39]

In addition to measuring tocopherol concentrations in blood, one finds that the peroxide hemolysis test is helpful in providing an index of antioxidant potential. Although this test is not entirely specific, a normal result [less than 5% hemolysis during 3 hours incubation in 2% $H_2O_2$[30]] can be assumed to rule out vitamin E deficiency. In performing peroxide hemolysis tests, one must be very careful with technical details to avoid artifacts as discussed elsewhere.[30]

Because of the marked influence of plasma lipids on tocopherol concentrations, tocopherol/lipid ratios have been used in some studies as recommended by Horwitt et al.[35] These more recent investigations have demonstrated that although children have significantly lower levels of plasma vitamin E than adults, a tocopherol/total lipid ratio of 0.6 or 0.8 mg/g of total plasma lipids indicates adequate nutritional status.[40] Without the concurrent assessment of circulating lipids, it is possible that some individuals with low lipids will be misclassified as vitamin E deficient when they are actually normal. Conversely, some hyperlipidemic subjects can have normal tocopherol concentrations per unit volume of plasma or serum, but in reality may be low in vitamin E.[41]

Most of the previous investigations have utilized colorimetric determination of total plasma or serum tocopherols and have shown that a level above 0.5 mg/dl indicates adequate nutritional status.[5] Although many infants and children have levels less than 0.5 mg/dl because of lower lipid concentrations, they usually do not show other evidence of vitamin E deficiency. This conclusion is based on the finding of normal resistance of erythrocytes to hemolysis in the presence of hydrogen peroxide promoted membrane peroxidation.[40]

The ideal approach to assessing vitamin E nutritional status, therefore, involves a combination of methods including determination of tocopherol isomers in plasma or serum, measurement of circulating lipids such as the total lipid fraction or cholesterol esters, determination or erythrocyte hemolysis in the presence of 2% hydrogen peroxide, and (if warranted) determination of the tocopherol content of a tissue biopsy.

## PATHOLOGY OF VITAMIN E DEFICIENCY

Table 15–3 summarizes the abnormalities present in animals raised on vitamin E-deficient diets. Perhaps the most notable aspect of vitamin E deficiency in animals is the marked degree of species specificity. Also, there is a great diversity of tissue and organ functions affected by low tocopherol levels. Nelson has reviewed the histopathology of the reproductive organs, skeletal muscles, and nervous system in vitamin E-deficient animals.[8] In general, tissue necrosis is a major feature and is accompanied by accumulation of lipopigments thought to represent peroxidized lipid. In some instances, especially in rapidly growing animals, disorders such as muscular degeneration and encephalomalacia occur over a matter of several days to a few weeks. It must be recognized, however, that young animals that are studied with respect to vitamin E deficiency are typically placed on diets that are virtually devoid of all antioxidants and sometimes contain large amounts of PUFA to further stress vital tissues. It is conceivable that this experimental approach may cause an isolated, severe vitamin E deficiency state in circumstances where other mechanisms involving antioxidants cannot become compensatory.

The search for a clinical correlate of vitamin E deficiency in humans has been based largely on our understanding of the pathologic disturbances in animals on synthetic diets. In humans, rapid development of vitamin E deficiency apparently does not occur except in unusual clinical circumstances. Because of the marked differences in nutritional status between animals investigated comprehensively and human subjects available for clinical investigations, it has become necessary to probe for insidious pathologic processes in humans, possibly leading only to biochemical abnormalities. Yet, extensive research to uncover specific clinical signs of human tocopherol deficiency has met with frustration in many instances. This is quite in contrast, of course, to observations on the other fat-soluble vitamins where prominent manifestations of the deficiency state generally develop (e.g., hemorrhage with vitamin K, rickets with vitamin D, and night blindness with vitamin A). It was largely for this reason that vitamin E was not added to the nutrients included on the list of those with a Recommended Dietary Allowance until 1968.

Human vitamin E deficiency can be defined for

**Table 15–3. Vitamin E Deficiency***

| Condition | Tissue Affected | Species |
|---|---|---|
| Hemolysis and possible anemia | Erythrocyte | Rat, chick, monkey, premature human, human with malabsorption |
| Neuronal degeneration | Axons† | Rat, monkey, probably human |
| Nutritional "muscular dystrophy" | Skeletal muscle | Rabbit, fowl, guinea pig, sheep, others |
| Myocardial necrosis and fibrosis | Cardiac muscle | Calf, rat, hamster |
| Reproductive failure | | Rat,‡ mouse,‡ guinea pig,‡ dog, monkey |
|   (Fetal death in females)‡ | ?Placenta | |
|   (Testicular degeneration in males) | Testicle | |

*Also, encephalomalacia and exudative diathesis in fowl, ceroid pigment deposition in smooth muscle of various species, and possible "disappearance" of mitochondrial and microsomal membranes in ducks and human jejunum.
†Axons of the spinal cord and peripheral nerves degenerate and may accumulate lipopigment.
‡During pregnancy fetal death and resorption have been observed in rats, mice, and guinea pigs.

practical purposes as a low plasma (or serum) tocopherol level (below at least 0.5 mg/dl), accompanied by a low ratio of tocopherol to lipid and/or hemolysis of erythrocytes incubated in 2% hydrogen peroxide. The term *subclinical* or biochemical deficiency may be used to indicate that laboratory evidence of low tocopherol levels in humans is not necessarily equivalent to biologically or clinically evident deficiency. With the exception of the Elgin project described by Horwitt and associates,[42] in which adult male volunteers were placed on special diets low in α-tocopherol, the occurrence of vitamin E deficiency of pure dietary origin is rare in developed countries. On the other hand, there are three categories of patients who have been well established as susceptible to vitamin E deficiency: (1) premature infants, (2) patients with gastrointestinal diseases leading to malabsorption, and (3) individuals with abetalipoproteinemia. Also, children with protein-calorie malnutrition have sometimes been noted to show abnormally low levels of circulating tocopherol. Because the three categories of patients who commonly are low in vitamin E have reviewed in detail previously,[4] only a brief account has been included herein.

Newborn infants delivered prematurely show evidence of vitamin E deficiency due to several factors, including limited tissue storage at birth, intestinal malabsorption for as long as 8 to 12 weeks,[43] and rapid growth rates that increase nutrient requirements in general. Also, some infant formula preparations have been marginal to low in α-tocopherol content relative to the amount of PUFA and iron present. Although pregnancy is associated with high maternal levels of circulating vitamin E proportional to rising plasma lipids,[35] transplacental delivery of tocopherols to the fetus is limited, resulting in low circulating concentrations in the premature infant. Furthermore, neonatal tissue concentrations are not only low, but a paucity of adipose tissue in premature infants limits their total body vitamin E pool even further.

The possible adverse consequences of vitamin E deficiency in premature infants were first suggested by Owens and Owens in relationship to retrolental fibroplasia (RLF), a tragic disease that nearly caused an epidemic of blindness in premature neonates.[44] This disorder was eventually attributed to oxygen toxicity when hyperoxemia was found to lead to degeneration of retinal arteries. Although the importance of vitamin E deficiency in RLF has been disputed, recent investigations support the benefits of correcting the deficiency state early in these patients with parenteral or enteral α-tocopheryl acetate.[45,46] Convincing evidence, therefore, continues to be published indicating that vitamin E therapy in high doses can ameliorate the retinal artery abnormality.[47]

Hemolytic anemia is another abnormality of premature infants associated with vitamin E deficiency. Oski and Barness were the first to report data indicating that vitamin E deficiency plays a role in the exaggerated anemia that occurs in some premature infants.[48] Although subsequent changes in the composition of infant formula and less use of supplemental iron during the neonatal period have reduced the impact of vitamin E deficiency and raised questions about the reproducibility of the original data,[49] Gross and Melhorn confirmed and extended the original observations with respect to: (1) the pattern of fall in erythrocyte indices, (2) the poor intestinal absorption of vitamin E in premature infants, and (3) the beneficial effects of tocopherol supplementation on hematologic status.[43] In particular, Gross and Melhorn found significantly improved hemoglobin and reticulocyte values in a vitamin E-treated group compared to premature controls (as shown in Figure 15–5).[43] Data on red cell turnover ob-

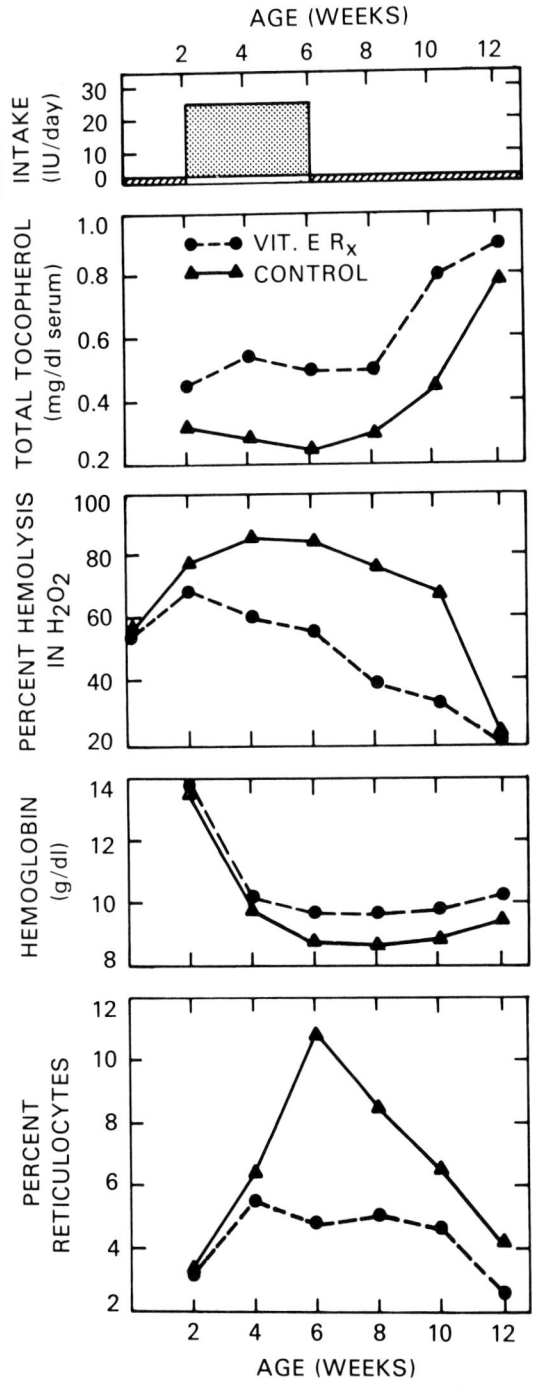

**Fig. 15–5.** Vitamin E and hematologic status of 28- to 32-week-gestation infants studied by Gross and Melhorn.[43] (Reproduced from Farrell, P.M., Machlin, L.J.,[4] with permission of Marcel Dekker, Inc.)

tained before and after correction of vitamin E deficiency would be helpful in establishing the conclusion concerning hemolysis in vivo. Unfortunately, erythrocyte survival studies involving radioisotope-tagged cells are hazardous to perform in newborns and yield data that are difficult to interpret. Thus, little information is available on erythrocyte kinetics to confirm the clinical observations.

In addition to RLF and hemolytic anemia, one report suggests that a hemorrhagic tendency might develop in vitamin E-deficient premature infants.[50] Another case report suggests that encephalomalacia might also be present when large amounts of PUFA are given.[51]

The second category of human subjects who manifest vitamin deficiency includes a variety of patients with intestinal malabsorption. This is a very heterogeneous group with a common clinical feature, namely steatorrhea. Vitamin E deficiency has been associated with disturbances affecting nearly every component of the gastrointestinal tract, including the stomach (postgastrectomy syndrome), liver (biliary atresia and cirrhosis), pancreas (cystic fibrosis, chronic pancreatitis, and pancreatic carcinoma), and intestinal mucosa (gluten enteropathy and regional enteritis). Although the degree of tocopherol malabsorption varies in these conditions and in individual patients (see Figure 15–4), it may be concluded in general that if steatorrhea is of sufficient duration and magnitude, vitamin E deficiency is likely to ensue as a consequence of tocopherol malabsorption.

Of those patients with enteropathies leading to chronic steatorrhea, children with cystic fibrosis (CF) have been of particular interest, since they represent a relatively large group of human subjects (1 of 2000 children in the United States) that are readily available for research, and since they manifest a prolonged, permanent digestive defect that cannot be completely corrected by oral pancreatic enzyme replacement therapy. The first report describing vitamin E deficiency in CF patients appeared in 1949 and resulted from a survey of 200 hospitalized patients by Darby et al.[12] Subsequently, Nitowsky, and associates showed that low serum tocopherol levels were common in these patients and associated with in vitro hemolysis.[52,53] Farrell et al. later found that vitamin E deficiency occurred invariably in CF patients with long-term fat malabsorption and that the severity of tocopherol deficiency was proportional to the degree of steatorrhea.[30] Underwood and Denning found that tissue α-tocopherol concentrations were also low,[54] and this was confirmed by others.[30]

Studies on the possible consequences of vitamin E deficiency in patients with cystic fibrosis and other malabsorption syndromes have focused on erythrocyte stability and the neuromuscular system. Although severe anemia is unlikely to occur in patients with malabsorption, significant decreases in the survival of [51]Cr-labeled erythrocytes have been described in CF patients and shown to respond favorably to tocopherol therapy.[4] The average [51]Cr-RBC half-life values observed by Farrell el al. increased significantly in CF patients from 19.0 days to 27.6 days (normal range = 25 to 35 days) before and after supplementation with 100 to 200 IU/day.[30] In a similar experimental design, Leonard and Losowsky found that adults with tocopherol malnutrition due to malabsorption or alcoholism were found to show a similar reduction in the [51]Cr-RBC survival to 19.3 days and an increase to 24.9 days following treatment with vitamin E.[55] Erythrocyte survival was also found to be significantly decreased in the volunteers fed diets low in vitamin E by Horwitt et al.[56] It should be noted, however, that the average degree of shortening of erythrocyte survival in tocopherol-deficient patients with malabsorption is not sufficient to produce clinically evident hemolytic anemia. Nevertheless, on the basis of the above studies it is clear that human vitamin E deficiency is associated not only with in vitro hemolysis but also with decreased erythrocyte survival in vivo from diminished antioxidant activity.

Investigation of the neuromuscular system in vitamin E-deficient children with malabsorption has been of interest because of the alterations in lower animals.[8] Some evidence of a primary myopathy has been reported, but the data are unconvincing and not supported by histologic examination of skeletal muscle biopsies.[41] On the other hand, recent investigations of children with chronic cholestasis due to biliary atresia and other etiologies, as well as evaluation of patients with abetalipoproteinemia, suggest that a neurologic disease can develop that is similar to that found in animals.[57,58] Histologic abnormalities are especially prominent in the spinal cord where axonal dystrophy leads to degeneration of the posterior column. Furthermore, preliminary data suggest that the characteristic neurologic symptoms improve with vitamin E treatment and perhaps can be prevented with such therapy in patients with abetalipoproteinemia.[57,58]

Several reports suggest that destruction of cellular membranes can occur in patients with vitamin E deficiency such as those with abetalipoproteinemia.[59] Many investigations also indicate that lipopigment (ceroid) will be deposited in human tissues such as small instestine, just as in animals.[8] This deposit is thought to represent accumulation of peroxidized lipid and reflects altered PUFA metabolism.

## NUTRITIONAL REQUIREMENTS

Because of the adequacy of vitamin E nutrition in healthy Americans consuming balanced diets, the recommended daily allowance for this nutrient has been based largely upon dietary analyses. According to a study by Bieri and Evarts in 1972, daily intakes of RRR-α-tocopherol in adults averaged 9 mg (13.5 IU) and ranged from 4.4 to 12.7 mg (6.6 to 19 IU).[60] Witting and Lee found similar values.[61] Because of the dietary contribution of the gamma vitamers, total tocopherol ingestion is generally twofold to threefold higher. Thus, the level of "alpha-tocopherol equivalents" consumed may range from 6 to 15 mg/day for adults, corresponding to 9 to 22.5 IU/day.[15] Although this is a relatively low level compared to the amounts ingested by young growing animals, there is no indication of deficiency when this amount is ingested. The minimum daily requirement is not known, but the Elgin project revealed that for adult men the level is above 2 mg/day of dietary α-tocopherol.[62]

It has been demonstrated that the requirement for vitamin E in animals is elevated when the intake of PUFA is increased substantially. Horwitt showed that the same applies to humans.[62] Alteration of the fat source in diets consumed by volunteers in the Elgin project elevated the concentration of linoleic acid in adipose tissue markedly and increased the need for dietary tocopherol. Although the consumption of certain oils raises the intake of PUFA, a corresponding increase in vitamin E intake occurs, except in the case of fish oils. When the primary unsaturated fatty acid in the diet is linoleic acid, a ratio of 0.4 mg RRR-α-tocopherol/g of polyunsaturated fatty acid is more than adequate to maintain normal vitamin E status. Bieri and Evarts found that the average α-tocopherol/PUFA ratio in representative American diets was 0.42 mg/g.[60]

In the United States the current recommendations concerning vitamin E allowances reflect the usual dietary intake of Americans. In reaching a conclusion about vitamin E, the committee appointed to develop the tenth edition of *Recommended Dietary Allowances* agreed that 10 mg of α-tocopherol equivalents are satisfactory for young adults.[63] This recommendation is based on assigning γ-tocopherol a vitamin E activity of 0.1 relative to α-tocopherol. The value recommended by the Committee for infants from birth to 3 months of age is 2 mg of α-tocopherol equivalents.[63]

## PHARMACOLOGIC APPLICATIONS AND TOXICITY

The medical uses of vitamin E have been described in detail elsewhere.[4-6] Management of patients with vitamin E deficiency due to malabsorption can generally be achieved by supplementing the diet with water-miscible α-tocopheryl acetate preparations. Although the dose has not been firmly established, experience with CF patients indicates that the following dosages will either correct or prevent vitamin E deficiency: 25 IU/day for infants; 50 to 100 IU/day for 1 to 10-year-old children; 100 IU/day for 10 to 18-year-olds; and 200 IU/day for those above 18 years of age.[64] Presumably, these same dosages will be effective for other patients with steatorrhea due to pancreatic insufficiency.

On the other hand, patients with biliary atresia and abetalipoproteinemia are extremely difficult to treat and may require parenteral (usually intramuscular) supplementation. An injectable vitamin E preparation has been described and investigated in both infants and adults.[65] Further research, as well as approval of the United States Food and Drug Administration, will be needed before routine intramuscular therapy can be recommended for these two categories of patients.

Premature infants are also difficult to treat adequately using the oral supplementation approach because of the necessity of delayed feedings in sick babies, the frequent occurrence of early gastrointestinal intolerance, and the presence of prolonged tocopherol malabsorption. Thus, intramuscular vitamin E is under investigation,[45] and multivitamin mixtures can be given intravenously to provide α-tocopheryl acetate, which seems to be hydrolyzed in vivo to α-tocopherol. Gutcher et al. have shown that 1 to 5 IU/day rapidly normalizes plasma tocopherol levels and peroxide hemolysis test results.[66] After a few days, 1 IU/kg/day given intravenously will maintain vitamin E adequacy. When enteral feedings are established, the usual oral dose of water-miscible α-tocopheryl acetate is 25 IU/day.

Pharmacologic use of vitamin E has been recommended in certain disease states that are not accompanied by vitamin E deficiency. This usage constitutes megavitamin therapy and has been reviewed in detail elsewhere.[4] Most of the disorders that have been reported as being responsive to vitamin E supplements, such as ischemic heart disease, intermittent claudication, and pulmonary oxygen toxicity, have not been adequately investigated. Although the most favorable results have been obtained with intermittent claudication, only one controlled study is convincing. This is an ongoing investigation by Haeger that includes objective data on beneficial responses in 158 patients given 300 mg/day.[67]

Because of claims that vitamin E supplementation will lead to great benefits in the quality of one's life, it is not surprising that a large proportion of the American population appears to take vitamin E supplements. The usual doses range from 100 to 800 mg/day, but the amount absorbed is far less. Observational experience over many years and limited studies have indicated no convincing evidence of toxicity.[68] It is not appropriate, however, to conclude that long term self-treatment with large amounts of vitamin E is without risk. Further research is needed in this area, especially in view of the toxicity recently noted in premature infants given parenteral vitamin E[69] and the observation that tocopherol can accumulate continuously in adipose tissue.

## REFERENCES

1. Horwitt, M.K.: Vitamin E. *In* Modern Nutrition in Health and Disease. 6th ed. (Goodhart, R.S., Shils, M.E., Eds.) Philadelphia, Lea & Febiger, 1980.
2. Bieri, J.G., Tolliver, L.J., Catignani, G.L.: Am. J. Clin. Nutr. *32*:2143, 1979
3. Gutcher, G.R., Lax, A.A., Farrell, P.M.: J.P.E.N. *8*:269, 1984
4. Farrell, P.M., Machlin, L.J.: *In* Vitamin E, A Comprehensive Treatise. (Machlin, L.J., Ed.) New York, Marcel Dekker, 1980.
5. Bieri, J.G., Farrell, P.M.: Vitam. Horm. *34*:31, 1976
6. Bieri, J.G., Corash, L., Hubbard, V.S.: N. Engl. J. Med. *308*:1063, 1983.
7. Mason, K.E.: The first two decades of vitamin E history. *In* Vitamin E. A Comprehensive Treatise. (Machlin, L.J., Ed.) New York, Marcel Dekker, 1980.
8. Nelson, J.S.: Pathology of vitamin E deficiency. *In* Vitamin E. A Comprehensive Treatise. (Machlin, L.J., Ed.) New York, Marcel Dekker, 1980.
9. Emmerie, A., Engel, C.: Rec. Trav. Chim. *57*:1351, 1938.
10. Karrer, P., Fritzche, H., Ringier, B.H., et al.: Helv. Chim. Acta *21*:520, 1938.
11. Smith, L.I., Ungnada, H.E., Pritchard, W.W.: Science *88*:37, 1938.
12. Darby, C.W., Davidson, A.G.F., Fosbrooke, A.S.: Arch. Dis. Child. *48*:72, 1973.
13. Mackenzie, J.B.: Pediatrics *13*:346, 1954.
14. Kasparek, S.: Chemistry of tocopherols and tocotrienols. *In* Vitamin E. A Comprehensive Treatise, (Machlin, L.J., Ed.) New York, Marcel Dekker, 1980.
15. Bieri, J.G., McKenna, M.C.: Am. J. Clin. Nutr. *34*:289, 1981.
16. Catignani, G.L.: Role in nucleic acid and protein metabolism. *In* Vitamin E. A Comprehensive Treatise. (Machlin, L.J., Ed.) New York, Marcel Dekker, 1980.
17. Hoekstra, W.G.: Fed. Proc. *34*:2083, 1975.
18. McCay, P.B., King, M.: Biochemical Function. *In* Vitamin E. A Comprehensive Treatise. (Machlin, L.J., Ed.) New York, Marcel Dekker, 1980

19. McCay, P.B., King, M.M., Poyer, J.L., et al.: Ann. N.Y. Acad. Sci. *393*:23, 1982.
20. Pryor, W.A.: Free radical biology: Xenobiotics, cancer, and aging. *In* Vitamin E: Biochemical, Hematological, and Clinical Aspects. (Lubin, B., Machlin, L.J., Eds.) New York, New York Academy of Sciences. 1982.
21. Dillard, C.J., Gavino, V.C., Tappel, A.L.: J. Nutr. *113*:2266, 1983.
22. Machlin, L.J., Gabriel E., Brin, M.: J. Nutr. *112*:1437, 1982.
23. Burton, G.W., Ingold, K.U.: J. Am. Chem. Soc. *103*:6472, 1981.
24. Bieri, J.G., Poukka Evarts, R.: J. Clin. Nutr. *27*:980, 1974.
25. Bauernfeind, J.: Tocopherols in food. *In* Vitamin E. A Comprehensive Treatise. (Machlin, L.J., Ed.) New York, Marcel Dekker, 1980.
26. Bunyan, J., McHale, D., Green, J., Marcinkiewicz, S.: Br. J. Nutr.*15*:253, 1961.
27. USDA, Oil Crops—Outlook and Situation Report. May, 1983.
28. Losowsky, M.S., Kelleher, J., Walker, B.E.: Ann. N.Y. Acad. Sci. *203*:212, 1972.
29. MacMahon, M.T., Neale, G.: Clin. Sci. *38*:197, 1970.
30. Farrell, P.M., Bieri, J.G., Fratantoni, J.F., et al.: J. Clin. Invest. *6*:233, 1977.
31. Poukka, R.K.H., Bieri, J.G.: Lipids *5*:757, 1970.
32. Bieri, J.G.: Ann. N.Y. Acad. Sci. *203*:181, 1972.
33. Bieri, J.G., Evarts, R.P.: Proc. Soc. Exp. Biol. Med. *34*:913, 1975.
34. Wiss, O., Bunnell, R.H., Gloor, U.: Vitam. Horm. *20*:441, 1962.
35. Horwitt, M.K., Harvey, C.C., Dahm, C.H., et al.: Ann. N.Y. Acad. Sci. *203*:223, 1972.
36. Gallo-Torres, H.E.: Transport and metabolism. *In* Vitamin E. A Comprehensive Treatise. (Machlin, L.J., Ed.) New York, Marcel Dekker, 1980.
37. Bieri, J.G.: Chromatography of tocopherols. *In* Lipid Chromatographic Analysis. Vol. 2. (Marinetti, G.V., Ed.) New York, Marcel Dekker, Inc., 1969.
38. Farrell, P.M.: J. Pediatr. *95*:869, 1979.
39. Horwitt, M.K., Harvey, C.C., Harmon, E.M.: Vitam. Horm. *26*:487, 1968.
40. Farrell, P.M., Levine, S.L., Murphey, M.D., et al.: Am. J. Clin. Nutr. *31*:1720, 1978.
41. Sokol, R.J., Heubi, J.E., Iannaccone, S.T., Bove, K.E., et al.: N. Eng. J. Med. *310*:1209, 1984.
42. Horwitt, M.K.: Vitam. Horm. *20*:541, 1962.
43. Gross, S., Melhorn, D.K.: Ann. N.Y. Acad. Sci. *203*:141, 1972.
44. Owens, W.C., Owens, E.U.: Am. J. Ophthalmol. *32*:1, 1949.
45. Johnson, L., Schaffer, D., Boggs, T.R.: Am. J. Clin. Nutr. *27*:1158, 1974.
46. Hittner, H.M., Godio, L.B., Rudolph, A.J., et al.: N. Engl. J. Med. *305*:1365, 1981.
47. Hittner, H.M., Godio, L.B., Speer, M.E., et al.: Pediatrics *71*:423, 1983.
48. Oski, F.A., Barness, L.A.: J. Pediatr. *70*:211, 1967.
49. Goldbloom, R.B., Cameron, D.: Pediatrics *32*:36, 1963.
50. Nitowsky, H.M., Jus, M.J., Gordon, H.H.: Vitam. Horm. *20*:559, 1962.
51. Horwitt, M.K., Bailey, P.: Arch. Neurol. Psychiatr. *1*:312, 1959.
52. Nitowsky, H.M., Cornblath, M., Gordon, H.H.: AMA. J. Dis. Child. *92*:164, 1956.
53. Nitowsky, H.M., Tildon, J.T., Levin, S., et al.: Am. J. Clin. Nutr. *10*:368, 1962.
54. Underwood, B.A., Denning, C.R.: Pediatr. Res. *6*:26, 1972.
55. Leonard, P.J., Losowsky, M.S.: Am. J. Clin. Nutr. *24*:388, 1971.
56. Horwitt, M.K., Century, B., Zeman, A.A.: Am. J. Clin. Nutr. *28*:706, 1963.
57. Guggenheim. M.A., Ringel, S.P., Silverman, A., et al.: Ann. N.Y. Acad. Sci. *393*:84, 1982.
58. Muller, D.P.R., Lloyd, J.K.: Ann. N.Y. Acad. Sci. *393*:133, 1982.
59. Molenaar, I., Hommes, F.A., Braams, W.G., et al.: Proc. Nat. Acad. Sci. *61*:982, 1968.
60. Bieri, J.G., Evarts. R.P.: J. Am. Diet. Assoc. *62*:147, 1973.
61. Witting, L.A., Lee, L.: Am. J. Clin. Nutr. *28*:571, 1975.
62. Horwitt, M.K.: Am. J. Clin. Nutr. *8*:451, 1960.
63. Food and Nutrition Board: Recommended Dietary Allowances, 10th ed. Washington, D.C., National Academy of Sciences, National Research Council, in press.
64. Farrell, P.M., Mischler, E.H., Gutcher, G.R.: Ann. N.Y. Acad. Sci. *393*:96, 1982.
65. Newmark, H.L., Pool, W., Bauernfeind, J.C., et al.: J. Pharmacol. Sci. *64*:655, 1975.
66. Gutcher, G.R., Farrell, P.M., Lax, A.: J. Pediatr. Gastroenterol. Nutr. *4*:604, 1985.
67. Haeger, K.: Ann. N.Y. Acad. Sci. *393*:369, 1982.
68. Farrell, P.M., Bieri, J.G.: Am. J. Clin. Nutr. *28*:1381, 1975.
69. Phelps, D.L.: Pediatrics *74*:1114, 1984.

*Chapter* # 16

# THIAMIN

## Donald B. McCormick

Though the role of thiamin (vitamin $B_1$) in the cure of human beriberi has been recognized for more than a generation, the disorder itself was clearly described as long ago as 7th century China. Apparently, it took a thousand years for the spread of the disease to Japan, seemingly causally related to the introduction of polished rice into the diet. Takaki (1884–1887) may have been the first to publish that beriberi seemed to be a nutritional deficiency; this was based on his ability to decrease its incidence in Japanese sailors by giving a diet that included dry milk and additional meat.[1] Eijkman (1890–1897), working in Batavia, found that fowls fed a diet consisting mainly of polished rice developed polyneuritic symptoms similar to those common in beriberi;[2] addition of rice polishings to the avian diet effected a cure. His associate Grijns noted that addition of green peas, green beans, and meat could also prevent beriberi in fowl and correctly deduced, about the turn of the century, that such natural foodstuffs contained a factor needed for the prevention of beriberi.[3] About ten years later, Funk, at the Lister Institute in London, isolated a material from rice polishings, which he believed would cure beriberi;[4] for such trace vital nutrients, he coined the term *vitamine*.[5] By 1926, Jansen and Donath, working in the laboratory where Eijkman and Grijns had experimented, actually succeeded in obtaining the crystalline antiberiberi vitamin.[6] Jansen suggested the name *aneurine*, which has since been replaced by thiamin.

A coenzymic role as part of the heat-stable co-carboxylase (thiamin pyrophosphate, TPP) asso-ciated with "carboxylase" (pyruvate decarboxylase) was reported by Auhagen in 1932.[7] R. R. Williams and his colleagues isolated a sufficient quantity of the vitamin in 1934[8] and by 1936 had elucidated its structure.[9] In 1937, Lohmann and Schuster isolated crystalline cocarboxylase, determined its structure, and synthesized it.[10] The coenzymic role of TPP with transketolase was firmly established by Horecker and his associates in 1953.[11] Following studies by Breslow in the latter 1950s on the chemical reactivity of the thiazole moiety of thiamin and its pyrophosphate,[12] work in the early 1960s, notably by Holzer and his colleagues in Germany and by Krampitz in the United States, led to identity of the active intermediates formed during α-ketoacid decarboxylations and ketolations catalyzed by TPP-dependent enzymes.

## CHEMISTRY, INCLUDING PRINCIPAL ANALOGUES

Thiamin is a pyrimidyl-substituted thiazole, which can be systematically named as 3-(2'-methyl-4'-amino-5'-pyrimidylmethyl)-4-methyl-5- (β-hydroxyethyl) thiazole. The free vitamin is a base, which is isolated or synthesized and handled as a solid thiazolium salt, e.g., thiamin chloride hydrochloride. The principal, if not sole, coenzymic form is the pyrophosphate ester (TPP) formed at the β-hydroxyethyl substituent (Fig. 16–1).

Chemical synthesis of thiamin has been accomplished along two routes. In one developed by Williams et al.,[9] the pyrimidine and thiazole

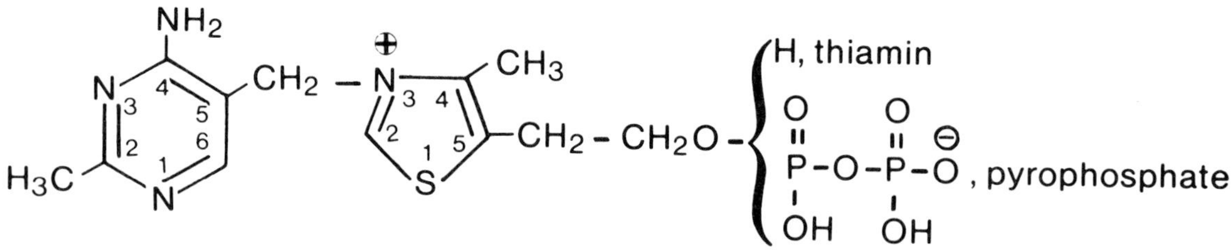

**Fig. 16–1.** Thiamin and the pyrophosphate coenzyme.

moieties are separately synthesized and then joined to form the vitamin. In another method developed by Todd and Bergel,[13] a pyrimidine is synthesized to contain a side chain suitable for reaction to form the thiazole. A variation of this is the thiothiamin method developed by Matsukawa et al.[14]

Numerous analogues of thiamin have been made, including those used as experimental antithiamins, e.g., oxythiamin first produced by Bergel and Todd[15] and pyrithiamin synthesized by Tracy and Elderfield.[16] Amprolium is a commercially useful poultry coccidiostat.[17] (See Fig. 16–2.)

Usually salts of thiamin are very water soluble; 1 g of thiamin chloride hydrochloride can be dissolved in 1 ml of water. Such polar salts are poorly soluble in common organic solvents. Colorless solutions at pH 7 exhibit absorption maxima at 235 and 267 nm corresponding to the pyrimidine and thiazole moieties, respectively.

Thiamin is generally stable to heating in aqueous solutions that are somewhat acidic, but sulfite ion even at room temperature causes cleavage at the methylene bridge to produce 2-methyl-4-amino-5-methyl-pyrimidylsulfonate and 4-methyl-5-(2-hydroxyethyl)thiazole.[18] In alkaline solution, thiamin rapidly loses its biologic activity because the thiazole ring is subject to base attack at carbon 2. The base can be a hydroxyl ion leading to a pseudobase, ring opening and some thiamin disulfide under mild oxidizing, e.g., $O_2$, conditions.[19,20] Also, the 4-amino on the pyrimidyl portion can attack as an intramolecular base to form the tricyclic amino adduct, which can be oxidized, e.g., with potassium ferricyanide, to yield

thiochrome, which is fluorescent ($\lambda$ excit = 385 nm; $\lambda$ emit = 440 nm) (Fig. 16–3).

The chemical synthesis of TPP by pyrophosphorylation of thiamin and the separation from contaminating mono- and triphosphates provide commercial quantities of the coenzyme.[14]

## BIOLOGIC ACTIVITY RELATING TO STRUCTURE

From testing of diverse analogues of thiamin, usually administered to birds or rodents, the relationship of molecular structure to vitaminic activity has been circumscribed.[20] In summary, both pyrimidine and thiazole portions are needed and are optimal with only one methylene group bridging the moieties and are inactive with greater than two. A primary alcohol is required at position 5 of the thiazole, but some activity is found with three-carbon as well as the natural two-carbon length. The quaternary nitrogen in the thiazole is essential as is the amino at carbon 4 in the pyrimidine. The methyl functions at 2′ and 4′ positions can be replaced to some extent with other short alkyl chains.

## ABSORPTION, TRANSPORT, METABOLISM, AND EXCRETION

Thiamin is readily absorbed in the small intestine by an active transport process that is probably carrier-mediated so long as intakes are less than 5 mg/d; at higher intakes, passive diffusion increasingly contributes to absorption.[21–23] Phosphorylation takes place in the jejunal mucosa to yield thiamin pyrophosphate. Thiamin is carried by the portal blood to the liver. The free vitamin occurs in the plasma, but the coenzyme, TPP, predominates in the cellular components. Approxi-

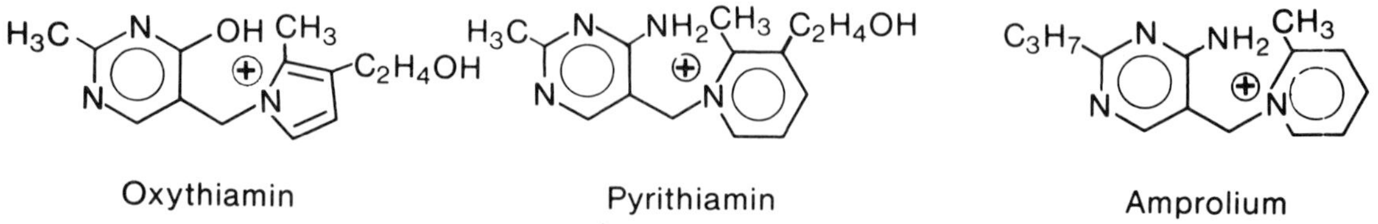

Oxythiamin          Pyrithiamin          Amprolium

**Fig. 16–2.** Thiamin antagonists.

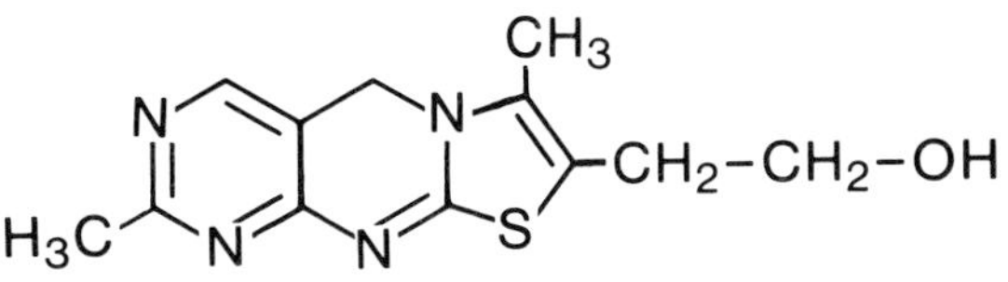

**Fig. 16–3.** Thiochrome.

mately 30 mg are stored in the body with 80% as the pyrophosphate, 10% as triphosphate, and the rest as thiamin and its monophosphate. About half of the body stores are found in skeletal muscles with much of the remainder in heart, liver, kidneys, and nervous tissue, including brain, which contains most of the triphosphate. The three tissue enzymes known to participate in formation of the phosphate esters are thiaminokinase (a pyrophosphorylase), which catalyzes formation of TPP and AMP from thiamin and ATP; TPP-ATP phosphoryl-transferase, which forms the triphosphate and ADP from TPP and ATP; and thiamin triphosphatase, which hydrolyzes TTP to the monophosphate. Though thiaminokinase is widespread, the phosphoryl transferase and membrane-associated triphosphatase are mainly in nervous tissue.

In addition to urinary excretion of excess thiamin (by renal tubules), several catabolites have been identified[21,24] (Fig. 16–4).

As a thiamin deficiency develops, there is a rather rapid loss of the vitamin from all tissues except the brain. The decrease of TPP in the erythrocyte roughly parallels the decrease of this coenzyme in other tissues. During this time, the thiamin in urine falls to near zero; the urinary metabolites remain high for some time before decreasing.

Very little thiamin is excreted in the bile. Early milk contains low levels, but administration of the vitamin to the mother causes some increase in the level in milk. Though coliforms in the bowel synthesize considerable thiamin, little, if any, is available to the host.

## BIOCHEMICAL AND PHYSIOLOGIC FUNCTIONS

There are two general types of reactions in the human where TPP functions as the $Mg^{2+}$-coordinated coenzyme for so-called active aldehyde transfers. These are the oxidative decarboxylation of $\alpha$-keto acids catalyzed by dehydrogenase complexes and the formation of $\alpha$-ketols (ketoses) as catalyzed by transketolase.[25] There are several pathways where coenzymic TPP cycles in such reactions (Fig. 16–5).

The multienzymic dehydrogenase complexes that effect decarboxylative conversion of $\alpha$-keto

acids to acyl-CoA derivatives, for example, pyruvate dehydrogenase, are localized in the mitochondria where efficient utilization in the Krebs tricarboxylic acid (citric acid) cycle follows. Three types of subunit proteins comprise such dehydrogenase complexes: a TPP-dependent decarboxylase, which converts the $\alpha$-keto acid to an $\alpha$-hydroxyalkyl-TPP complex (e.g., $\alpha$-hydroxyethyl-TPP from pyruvate or $\alpha$-hydroxy-$\gamma$-carboxypropyl-TPP from $\alpha$-ketoglutarate); a transacylase core, which contains lipoyl residues that are acylated by the $\alpha$-hydroxyalkyl-TTP; and an FAD-dependent dihydrolipoyl dehydrogenase, which reoxidizes the reduced lipoyl residues produced after transfer of their acyl functions to reduce CoA. In addition to energy and ultimate ATP supply derived from reactions in the Krebs cycle, the initial pyruvate dehydrogenase-catalyzed step importantly provides acetyl-CoA as a biosynthetic precursor to other essential compounds such as lipids and acetylcholine of the parasympathetic nervous system.

Transketolase is a TPP-dependent enzyme found in the cytosol of many tissues, especially liver and blood cells, where principal carbohydrate pathways exist. This enzyme catalyzes the reversible transfer of a glycolaldehyde moiety ($\alpha,\beta$-dihydroxyethyl-TPP) from the first two carbons of a donor ketose phosphate to the aldehyde carbon of an aldose phosphate of the pentose phosphate pathway, which additionally supplies NADPH needed for biosynthetic reactions.

Though thiamin as its pyrophosphate contributes to nervous system composition and function by such essential reactions as energy production and biosyntheses of lipids and acetylcholine, it appears that there is another incompletely understood role, particularly for the triphosphate. Thiamin and its phosphate esters are located in axonal membranes of nerves; electrical stimulation leads to hydrolysis and release of both the di- and triphosphate.[21] As noted before, enzymes involved in formation and cleavage of thiamin triphosphate are in nervous tissue. Moreover, a subacute necrotizing encephalomyelopathy in patients with Leigh's syndrome results from the presence of an inhibitor of TPP-ATP phosphoryl transferase.[21,25]

## DEFICIENCY AND EXCESS

Opisthotonus, a characteristic noise-elicited head retraction in birds, was one of the first recorded signs of thiamin deficiency in experimental animals.[26] Deficient pigeons also have ataxia and leg weakness, tachycardia with cardiac failure, and ultimate necrosis of the heart muscle. Rodents also develop both neuromuscular and cardiac symptoms during thiamin deficiency.

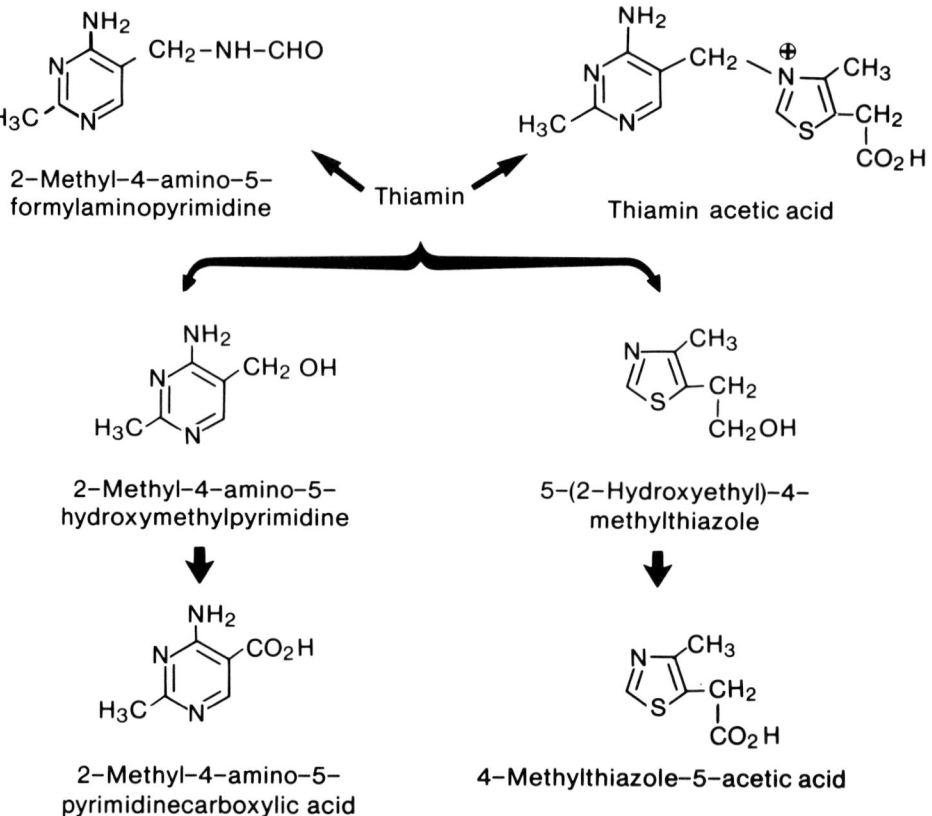

**Fig. 16–4.** Principal urinary catabolites of thiamin.

Major occurrences in rats are anorexia with weight loss, convulsions, bradycardia, and a decrease in body temperature.

Beriberi is the disease resulting from thiamin deficiency in the human. Clinical signs primarily involve the nervous and cardiovascular systems.[27] In the adult, symptoms most frequently observed are mental confusion, anorexia, muscle weakness, ataxia, peripheral paralysis, ophthalmoplegia, edema (wet beriberi), muscle wasting (dry beriberi), tachycardia, and an enlarged heart. In infants, symptoms appear suddenly and severely, often involving cardiac failure and cyanosis. Commonly, the distinction between wet (cardiovascular) and dry (neuritic) manifestations of beriberi relate to duration and severity of the deficiency, the degree of physical exertion, and caloric intake.[22] The wet or edematous condition results from severe physical exertion and high carbohydrate intake, whereas the dry or polyneuritic form stems from relative inactivity with caloric restriction during the chronic deficiency. The three major physiologic derangements that involve the cardiovascular system are peripheral vasodilatation leading to a high output state, biventricular

myocardial failure, and retention of sodium and water leading to edema. Nervous system involvement includes peripheral neuropathy, Wernicke's encephalopathy, and the amnesic psychosis of Korsakoff syndrome.[28]

Normally, excess ingested thiamin, as with most water-soluble vitamins, is readily excreted and is not a potential hazard. Rats have been maintained for three generations on doses up to 100 times above the requirement level without harmful effects.[18] Thiamin is also harmless administered orally to humans.[29]

Death in animals after intravenous injection of sufficient thiamin is caused by depression of the respiratory center.[30] The lethal dose in mg/kg body weight is for mice, 125; rats, 250; rabbits, 300; and dogs, 350. Monkeys tolerate even higher levels.[31]

Pharmacologic effects in humans are similarly found only with parenterally administered doses hundreds of times larger than required for optimal nutrition.[29,32] Prolonged injections of high amounts can lead to a sensitized anaphylactoid reaction. Parenteral doses greater than 400 mg of thiamin cause nausea, anorexia, lethargy, solemness, mild ataxia, heaviness in the limbs, and a diminution of gut tone.

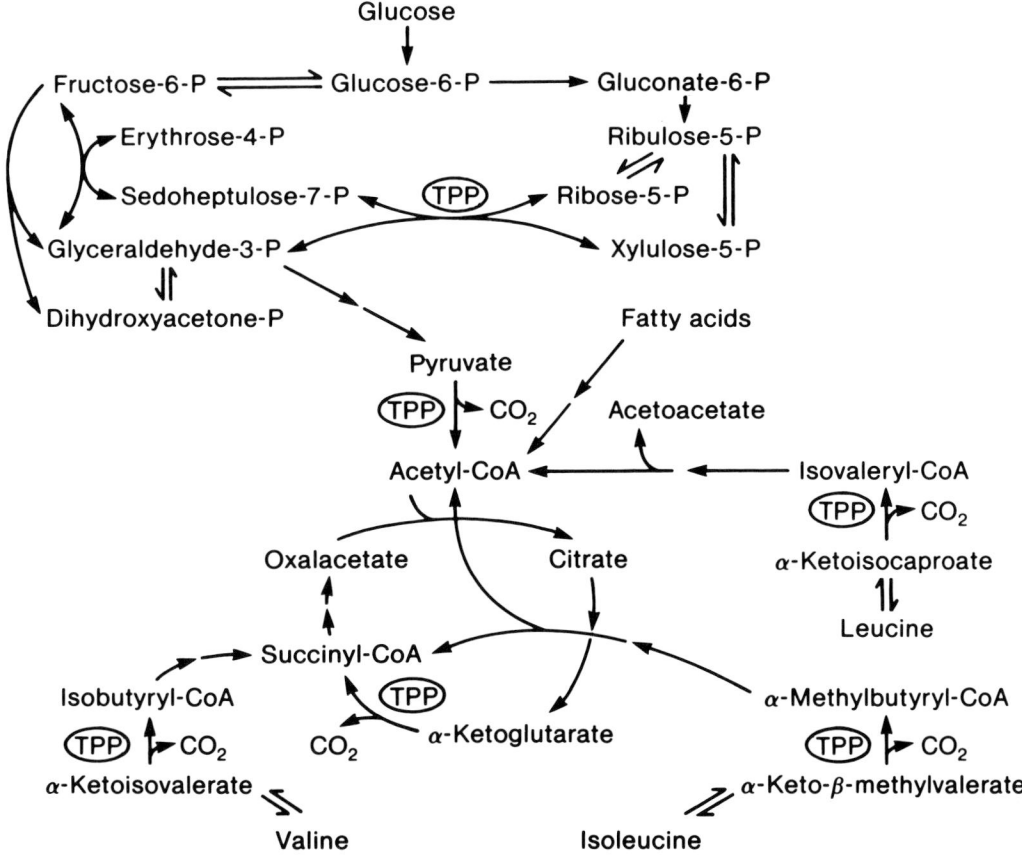

**Fig. 16–5.** Pathways dependent upon coenzyme forms of thiamin.

## CAUSES OF DEFICIENCY

The causes for deficiency are several and include inadequate intake due to diets largely dependent on milled, nonenriched grains such as rice and wheat,[21,27] or the ingestion of raw fish containing microbial thiaminases,[33] which hydrolytically destroy the vitamin in the gastrointestinal tract. Tea may contain antithiamin factors that have been detected in certain other plant extracts, though the presumption is often based on thiochrome assays, which may be interfered with by other compounds affecting its fluorescence. Chronic alcoholism is a common contributor to deficiency in that there is not only a low intake of thiamin (and other B vitamins) but also impaired absorption and storage. There are several thiamin-responsive inborn errors of metabolism;[34,35] these include a megaloblastic anemia of unknown mechanism, lactic acidosis due to low or defective pyruvate decarboxylase, branched-chain ketoaciduria with poor activity of the keto acid dehydrogenase system, and subacute necrotizing encephalomyelopathy where there is lack of thiamin triphosphate in neural tissues. Therapeutic doses of 5 to 20 mg of thiamin daily have proved beneficial in some cases.[28] Finally, other at-risk patients are those undergoing long-term renal dialysis or intravenous feeding and even those with chronic febrile infections.[27]

## DIETARY CONSIDERATIONS

The requirement levels for thiamin vary considerably, since there is a direct correlation of need with amount of metabolizable carbohydrate intake. There is a generally increased requirement under numerous situations where metabolism is heightened, for example, in the normal conditions of increased muscular activity, pregnancy, and lactation or in the abnormal cases of protracted fever and hyperthyroidism.[36] Clinical signs of deficiency in adults can be prevented with intakes of thiamin above 0.15 to 0.2 mg/1000 kcal, but 0.35 to 0.4 mg/1000 kcal may be closer to the level necessary to maintain urinary excretion and TPP-dependent erythrocyte transketolase activity within normal ranges.[27] On the basis of these considerations, an adult allowance of 0.5 mg/1000 kcal has been recommended. With further considerations of average caloric intakes and activities in different age groups, the RDAs, expressed as mg, range from 1.0 for older women to 1.5 for young men. The requirement for pregnant women increases early in pregnancy and then remains constant; an additional allowance of 0.4 mg/d is recommended. Because the lactating woman secretes 0.1 to 0.2 mg of thiamin per day in milk, an additional 0.5 mg/d allowance is suggested. Based on thiamin content of human milk and with an increment considered to provide a margin of safety, 0.3 mg/d is the allowance for young infants. Increases above this are suggested for growing children.

Small amounts of thiamin and its phosphates are present in most plant and animal tissue, but more abundant sources are unrefined cereal grains, liver, heart, kidney, and lean cuts of pork. The enrichment of flour and derived food products has increased considerably the availability of this vitamin.

## METHODS FOR ASSAY AND STATUS DETERMINATION

Microbiologic methods including use of *Ochromonas danica,*[37] and the chemical conversion (by ferricyanide in alkaline solution) of thiamin to fluorometrically determined thiochrome were the principal means to determine the vitamin in various biologic fluids and still are in use. There are now several useful modifications for chemical determination of the free vitamin as well as phosphate esters, which can be separated by electrophoresis, ion-exchange, or HPLC techniques.[37–39] Determination of the urinary excretion of thiamin in a 4-hour period, especially with comparison of excretion before and after a test load, is helpful in differentiating between extremes of thiamin status, but as is the case in most assessments based on amount of water-soluble vitamins in urine, excretion can be influenced considerably by dietary intake, absorption, and other factors. Excretion of <27 μg thiamin/g creatinine usually reflects deficiency in the adult, whereas ≥66 μg/g is acceptable.[40] Certain urinary metabolites, notably thiamin acetic acid, have also been suggested as reflective of status.[41]

Biochemical tests based on the functional level of TPP may reflect more adequately the immediate status of an individual. One such diagnostic test is the measurement of the ratio of lactic to pyruvic acid in the blood after administration of glucose. Blood and urinary levels of these metabolites are characteristically elevated in deficiency, as would be expected when the TPP-dependent pyruvate dehydrogenase is decreased. One disadvantage of this test is the potential of provoking lactic acidosis in a severely deficient patient given a glucose load.[36] Other catabolites elevated as a consequence of thiamin deficiency include α-ketoglutarate, glyoxylate, and urinary methylglyoxal.[4]

The most useful and reliable method presently used is a measurement of whole blood or erythrocyte transketolase, particularly if the assay is performed before and after addition of TPP to the incubation sample. A discussion of this reaction and the interpretation of values and the TPP effect have been given previously,[42] as has a detailed description of the Brin method.[38,39] Typically, deficiency is reflected by TPP stimulation of >20%, whereas acceptable ranges are considered to be 0 to 15%.

## REFERENCES

1. Takaki: Lancet *2*:189, 1887.
2. Eijkman, C.: Geneesk. Tijdschr. Nederland-Indie *30*:295, 1890.
3. Grijns, G.: J. Noorduyn. Gorinchem. *37*:38, 1935.
4. Funk, C.: J. Physiol. (London) *43*:395, 1911.
5. Funk, C.: J. State Med. *20*:341, 1912.
6. Jansen, B.C.P., Donath, W.F.: Koninkl. Ned. Akad. Wetenschap. Proc. *29*:1390, 1926.
7. Auhagen, E.: Z. Physiol. Chem. *204*:149, 1932.
8. Williams, R.R., Waterman, R.E., Keresztesy, J.C.: J. Am. Chem. Soc. *56*:1187, 1934.
9. Williams, R.R., Cline, J.K., Finkelstein, J.: J. Am. Chem. Soc. *58*:1504, 1936.
10. Lohmann, K., Schuster, P.: Biochem. Z. *294*:188, 1937.
11. Horecker, B.L., Smyrniotis, P.Z., Klenow, H.: J. Biol. Chem. *205*:661, 1953.
12. Breslow, R.: J. Am. Chem. Soc. *80*:3719, 1958.
13. Todd, A.R., Bergel, F.: J. Chem. Soc. 364: 1937.
14. Matsukawa, T., Hirano, H., Yurugi, S.: Preparation of thiamine derivatives and analogs. *In* Vitamins and Coenzymes. Methods in Enzymology, Vol. 18, Part A. (McCormick, D.B., Wright, L.D., Eds.) New York, Academic Press, 1970.
15. Bergel, F., Todd, A.R.: J. Chem. Soc. 1504, 1937.
16. Tracy, A.H., Elderfield, R.C.: J. Org. Chem. *6*:54, 1941.
17. Rogers, E.F., Clark, R.L., Pessolano, A.A., et al.: J. Am. Chem. Soc. *82*:2974, 1960.
18. Williams, R.R., Spies, T.D.: Vitamin B. New York, Macmillan, 1938.
19. Maier, G.D., Metzler, D.E.: J. Am. Chem. Soc. *79*:4386, 1957.
20. Isamu, U., Harada, K., Kohno, K., et al.: Oxidation products of thiamine derivatives. *In* Vitamins and Coenzymes. Methods in Enzymology, Vol. 18, Part A (McCormick, D.B., Wright, L.D., Eds.) New York, Academic Press, 1970.
21. Tanpaichitr, V.: Thiamin. *In* Present Knowledge in Nutrition, 4th ed. (Hegsted, D.M., et al., Eds.) Washington, The Nutrition Foundation, 1976.
22. Wilson, J.A.: Disorders of vitamins-deficiency, excess and errors of metabolism. *In* Harrison's Principles of Internal Medicine, 10th ed. (Petersdorf, R.G., et al., Eds.) New York, McGraw-Hill, 1982.
23. Hoyumpa, A.M., Jr.: Fed. Proc. 42: Minisymposium, 1983.

24. Nutr. Rev. *29*:120, 1971.
25. White, A., Handler, P., Smith, E.L., et al.: Principles of Biochemistry. New York, McGraw-Hill, 1978.
26. Suzuki, U., Shamimura, T., Okade,S.: Biochem. Z. *43*:89, 1912.
27. Recommended Dietary Allowances, 9th ed. Committee on Dietary Allowances and Food and Nutrition Board, National Research Council, National Academy of Science, Washington, D.C., 1980.
28. Blass, J.P.: Thiamin and the Wernicke-Korsakoff syndrome. *In* Vitamins in Human Biology and Medicine (Briggs, M.H., Ed.) Boca Raton, CRC Press, 1981.
29. Cumming, F., Briggs, M., Briggs, M.: Chemical toxicology of vitamin supplements. *In* Vitamins in Human Biology and Medicine (Briggs, M.H., Ed.) Boca Raton, CRC Press, 1981.
30. Haley, T.J.: Proc. Soc. Exp. Biol. Med. *68*:153, 1948.
31. Mouriquand, G., Coisnard, J.: Presse Med. *53*:369, 1945.
32. Campbell, T.C., Allison, R.G., Carr, C.J.: Feasibility of Identifying Adverse Health Effects of Vitamins and Essential Minerals in Man. Life Sciences Research Office, F.A.S.E.B., Bethesda, 1980.
33. Evans, W.C.: Thiaminases and their effects on animals. *In* Vitamins and Hormones, Vol. 33 (Munson, P.E., et al., Eds.) New York, Academic Press, 1975.
34. Scriver, C.R.: Metabolism *22*:1319, 1973.
35. Rosenberg, L.E.: Vitamin-responsive inherited diseases affecting the nervous system. *In* Res. Publ. Assoc. Nerv. Ment. Dis., Vol. 53 (Plum, F., Ed.) New York, Raven Press, 1974.
36. Harper, H.A., Rodwell, V.A., Mayes, P.A.: Review of Physiological Chemistry, Chpt. 13. Los Altos, CA, Lange Medical Publications, 1979.
37. Baker, H., Frank, O., Fennelly, J.J., et al.: Am. J. Clin. Nutr. *14*:197, 1964.
38. McCormick, D.B., Wright, L.D. (Eds.): Vitamins and Coenzymes. Methods in Enzymology. Vol. 18, Part A. New York, Academic Press, 1970.
39. McCormick, D.B., Wright, L.D. (Eds.): Vitamins and Coenzymes. Methods in Enzymology. Vol. 62, Part D. New York, Academic Press, 1979.
40. Sauberlich, H.E., Dowdy, R.P., Skala, J.H.: Laboratory tests for the assessment of nutritional status. Boca Raton, CRC Press, 1974.
41. Neal, R.A.: Vitamin deficiencies: thiamin. *In* Workshop on Problems of Assessment and Alleviation of Malnutrition in the U.S. (Hansen, R.G., Munro, H.N., Eds.) Nashville, GSMHA and NIH, 1970.
42. McCormick, D.B.: Vitamins. *In* Textbook of Clinical Chemistry. (Tietz, N.W., Ed.) Philadelphia, W.B. Saunders, 1986.

*Chapter* **17**

# RIBOFLAVIN

## Donald B. McCormick

The "water-soluble B" fraction, reported by McCollum and Kennedy in 1916 to contain an antiberiberi substance,[1] was subsequently shown by Emmett and Luros (1920)[2] and Smith and Hendrick (1926)[3] to contain at least a second more heat-stable antipellagra factor, which was termed $B_2$. It soon became apparent that this $B_2$ fraction was a complex containing a yellow growth factor called riboflavin in England and vitamin G in the United States, as well as the subsequently identified pellagra-preventive factor (niacin) and the rat antidermatitis factor (vitamin $B_6$). Although a water-soluble, yellow, fluorescent compound was known in the latter part of the 19th century (Blyth, 1879)[4] to occur in such natural materials as whey, association of the pigment with vitaminic properties was not secured until its isolation in 1933 by several groups.[5–7] Terms applied to riboflavin indicated the origin, e.g., lactoflavin (milk), ovoflavin (egg), hepatoflavin (liver), and uroflavin (urine). Warburg and Christian in Germany had meanwhile isolated by 1932 a yellow respiratory ferment (now called "Old Yellow Enzyme") from yeast.[8] This flavoprotein was soon dissociated into a protein apoenzyme and a yellow prosthetic coenzyme that was clearly similar to riboflavin.[9] Stern and Holiday (1934) found the coenzyme was an alloxazine derivative,[10] and Theorell (1934) demonstrated it was a phosphate ester.[11]

By 1935, the groups of Kuhn[12,13] at Heidelburg and Karrer[14,15] in Zurich had achieved synthesis of the vitamin. Theorell, in 1937, secured the structure of the simpler coenzyme as riboflavin 5'-phosphate (flavin mononucleotide, FMN).[16] By 1938 Warburg and Christian had isolated and characterized the more abundant but complex prosthetic group, flavin-adenine dinucleotide (FAD), and showed its participation as the coenzyme of D-amino oxidase.[17–20] In more recent years, it has become known that there are diverse natural flavins that have alterations in side chain or ring system of the basic flavin structures.[21] No less than four 8α-modified forms of FAD occur covalently attached to important flavoproteins in the mammal, viz., the N(3)-histidyl-linked cases of succinate and sarcosine dehydrogenases of the inner mitochondrial membrane, S-cysteinyl-linked monoamine oxidase of the outer mitochondrial membrane, and the N(1)-histidyl-linked L-gluconolactone oxidase of the liver microsomal fraction.

## CHEMISTRY, INCLUDING PRINCIPAL ANALOGUES

Riboflavin (vitamin $B_2$) was chemically specified as 6,7-dimethyl-9-(1'-D-ribityl)isoalloxazine, but with evolution of systematic nomenclature is now correctly given as 7,8-dimethyl-10-(1'-D-ribityl) isoalloxazine. The free vitamin is a weak base normally isolated or synthesized as a yellowish orange amorphous solid. The 5'-hydroxymethyl terminus of the ribityl side chain in the vitamin is reacted to become an orthophosphate ester in the simpler coenzyme, flavin mononucleotide (FMN), which can be further enlarged to the more complex and frequently encountered FAD with a pyrophosphate-bridged adenylate moiety (Fig. 17–1).

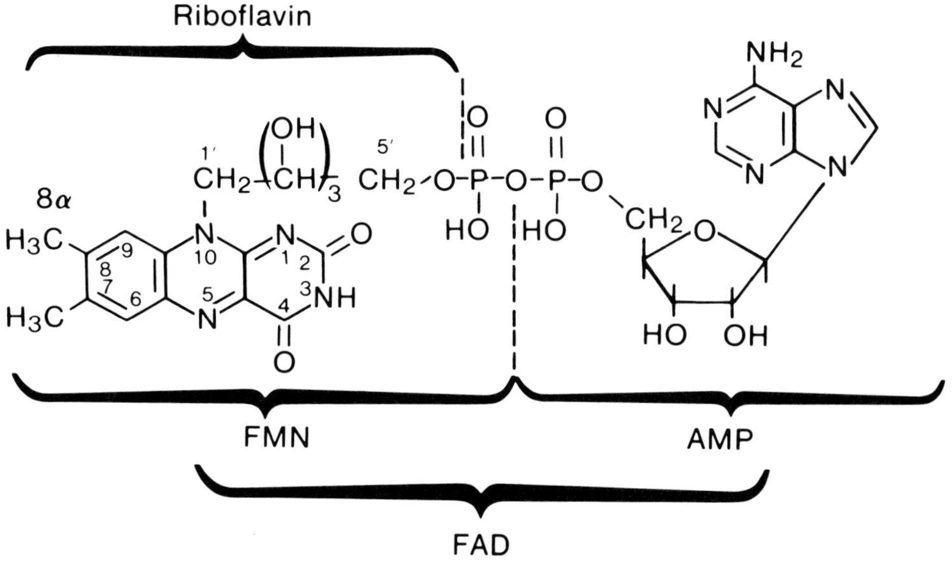

**Fig. 17–1.** Riboflavin and FMN as components of FAD.

There are some biosynthetic variations on the parent vitaminic structure, e.g., the 8-dimethylamino group of roseoflavin produced by *Streptomycetes davawensis*[22] and 5'-glycosides of riboflavin, which can be formed by plant and fungal species.[23] In addition, several natural variants of the coenzyme forms are listed in Table 17–1.

Chemical syntheses of riboflavin and similar isoalloxazines have been accomplished by several routes,[24] most adapted from the earlier procedures of Kuhn and Karrer and more recently from modifications introduced by Tishler and his associates.[25]

Riboflavin is only modestly soluble in aqueous solutions, though strong acid flavinium salts formed at low pH (<1) and flavin anion formed at alkaline pH (>10) are considerably more soluble. Neutral and slightly alkaline solutions are yellow with a long-wavelength absorption band near 450 nm. Strongly acidic flavin solutions are paler, since their primary absorbance shifts with intensification to about 385 nm. Solutions of the neutral oxidized (quinoid) form of the vitamin are strongly fluorescent with an emission wavelength at 525 nm. Riboflavin also has phosphorescent character reflecting triplet state reactivity following light excitation. One consequence of flavin photochemistry is the photolability of the side chain. Riboflavin is photodegraded ultimately to yield vitaminically inactive lumiflavin (7,8,10-trimethylisoalloxazine) under alkaline conditions and lumichrome (7,8-dimethylalloxazine) at all pH values, especially in neutral to acidic solutions (Fig. 17–2). Flavins are chemically and biologically reduced, often through the radical (semiquinone) forms, to the nearly colorless, nonfluorescent 1,5-dihydro forms that rapidly reoxidize upon exposure to air (oxygen).

Chemical syntheses of flavocoenzymes involve phosphorylation of riboflavin,[26] commonly with chlorophosphoric acid, to form crude FMN, which is purified chromatographically. Conversion of FMN to FAD usually involves condensation of activated AMP, such as adenosine 5'-phosphoromorpholidate, with an FMN salt.[27,28] Extension of these techniques has been useful to form coenzyme analogues.[29]

## BIOLOGIC ACTIVITY RELATING TO STRUCTURE

Numerous analogues of riboflavin and the coenzyme derivatives have been tested in whole organisms[30] and with apoflavoproteins,[21,31] respectively. In general, the full D-ribityl side chain is needed, though weak vitaminic activity has been found with the D-arabo configuration. D-galactoflavin is an antagonist. In addition to a normal pyrimidinoid portion, both 7- and 8-methyl substituents are required for optimal vitaminic activity, though sparing with corresponding monoethyl analogues has been reported. The 7,8-dihaloflavins are inhibitors as is isoriboflavin with a 6,7-dimethyl structure. The 5'-phosphate, commonly as the dianionic ester, is needed for binding in FMN-dependent systems and an additional 5'-AMP moiety with FAD-dependent enzymes.

## ABSORPTION, TRANSPORT, METABOLISM, AND EXCRETION

The processes by which riboflavin and lesser amounts of natural derivatives are released by

**Table 17–1.  Naturally Occurring Variants of FMN and FAD[21]**

| Name | Sources |
|---|---|
| 6-Hydroxy-FMN | Glycolate oxidase (pig liver) |
| 6-S-Cysteinyl (peptide)-FMN | Trimethylamine dehydrogenase (bacterium W3A1) |
| 6-Hydroxy-FAD | Electron-transferring flavoprotein (*Megasphaera elsdenii*) |
| 8α-S-Cysteinyl(peptide)-FAD | Monoamine oxidase (outer mitochondrial membrane) Cytochrome $C_{533}$ (*Chlorobium*) |
| 8α-O-Tyrosyl(peptide)-FAD | *p*-Cresol methylhydroxylase (*Pseudomonas*) |
| 8α-N(1)-Histidyl(peptide)-FAD | L-Glucono-γ-lactone oxidase (rat liver) L-Galactono-γ-lactone oxidase (yeast) Cholesterol oxidase (*Schizophyllum*) β-Cyclopiazonate oxidocyclase (*Penicillium cycloplum*) |
| 8α-N(3)-Histidyl(peptide)-FAD | Succinate dehydrogenase (inner mitochondrial membrane) Sarcosine dehydrogenase (*Pseudomonas*, mitochondria) D-6-Hydroxynicotine oxidase (*Arthrobacter oxidans*) Fumarate reductase Chlorine oxidase |
| Coenzyme $F_{420}$ (5-deaza-5-carba-7,8-didemethyl-8-hydroxy; 5'-phospholactyldiglutamyl) | Methane synthetase (*Methanobacterium*) |

digestion of complexes with food proteins and then absorbed, transported, and metabolically altered has been reviewed in a fairly comprehensive manner.[21] Salient features are that coenzyme forms of the vitamin (mainly FAD and less FMN) are released from noncovalent attachment to proteins as a consequence of gastric acidification. Nonspecific action of pyrophosphatase and phosphatase on the coenzyme forms occurs in the upper gut. Several percent of 8α-(amino acid)riboflavins originally in covalent attachment to certain enzymes, *e.g.,* mitochondrial succinate dehydrogenase or monoamine oxidase, and traces of other ring and side-chain substituted flavins are also released by these actions following proteolysis. The vitamin is primarily absorbed in the human in the proximal small intestine by a saturable transport system that is rapid and proportional to dose before leveling off at 25 mg of riboflavin. Bile salts appear to facilitate the uptake, and a modest amount of the vitamin circulates via the enterohepatic system. Active transport at lower levels of intake may be Na$^+$-dependent and involve phosphorylation. An active transport process dependent on Na$^+$ has been indicated from studies on riboflavin uptake in rat intestine in vivo[32] and in vitro.[33,34] In the human, some of the riboflavin circulating in blood plasma is

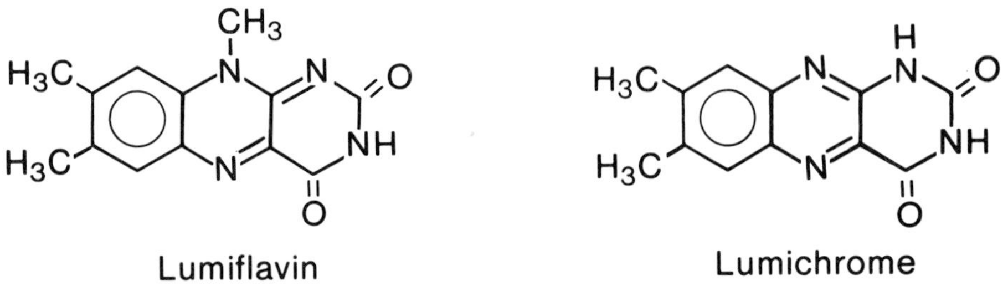

Lumiflavin          Lumichrome

**Fig. 17–2.**  Photodegradation products from riboflavin.

loosely associated with albumin, though significant amounts complex with other proteins. A subfraction of IgG has been found to bind avidly a small portion of the total free flavin in blood,[35] and several immunoglobulins contribute significantly to the circulatory transport of the vitamin. Uptake of riboflavin by hepatocytes from rat liver has been shown to involve metabolic trapping dependent upon flavokinase, but not $Na^+$ as with enterocytes.[37] Metabolic interconversions of flavins at the cellular level are outlined in Figure 17–3.

Conversion of riboflavin to coenzymes occurs within the cellular cytoplasm of most tissues, but particularly in the small intestine, liver, heart, and kidney.[21,38] The obligatory first step is the ATP-dependent phosphorylation of the vitamin catalyzed by flavokinase. The FMN product can be complexed with specific apoenzymes to form several functional flavoproteins, but the larger quantity is further converted to FAD in a second ATP-dependent reaction catalyzed by FAD synthetase (pyrophosphorylase). It seems likely that the biosynthesis of flavocoenzymes, particularly at the flavokinase step, is tightly regulated and dependent upon riboflavin status.[39] Thyroxine and triiodothyroxine stimulate FMN and FAD synthesis in mammalian systems.[40,41] This seems to involve a hormone-mediated increase in an active form of flavokinase.[42] FAD is the predominant flavocoenzyme present in tissues where it is mainly complexed with numerous flavoprotein dehydrogenases and oxidases. Less than 10% of the FAD can also become covalently attached to specific amino acid residues of a few important apoenzymes. Examples include the 8α-N(3)-histidyl FAD within succinate dehydrogenase and 8α-S-cysteinyl FAD within monoamine oxidase, both of mitochondrial localization. Turnover of covalently attached flavocoenzymes requires intracellular proteolysis, and further degradation of the coenzymes involves nonspecific pyrophosphatase cleavage of FAD to AMP and FMN and action by nonspecific phosphatases on the latter.

Since there is little storage of riboflavin as such, the urinary excretion reflects dietary intake. Both 7- and 8-hydroxymethylflavins appear in urine from the human and rat and are the result of microsomal mixed-function oxidases.[43] Smaller amounts of side-chain degradation products, such as lumichrone, 10-formylmethylflavin, and 10-(2'-hydroxyethyl)-flavin, are also excreted and may largely result from intestinal microorganisms.[21,44] Traces of 8α-flavin peptides and catabolites are found in urine and feces.[45] Cow's milk contains reasonable quantities of the vitamin and lesser amounts of coenzyme, principally FMN, whereas human milk contains relatively more of the coenzymes.

## BIOCHEMICAL AND PHYSIOLOGIC FUNCTIONS

In bound coenzymic form, riboflavin participates in oxidation-reduction reactions in numerous metabolic pathways and in energy production via the respiratory chain. A variety of chemical reactions are catalyzed by flavoproteins.[21,38,40,46] The redox functions of a flavocoenzyme, illustrated in Figure 17–4, include one-electron transfers, during which the biologically encountered, neutral, oxidized quinone level of flavin is half reduced to the radical semiquinone, which can exist within natural pH ranges as neutral or anionic species. A further electron transfer can lead to a fully reduced hydroquinone. Additionally, a single-step two-electron transfer from substrate to flavin can occur with hydride ion transfer, e.g., from reduced pyridine nucleotide or by base abstraction of a substrate proton together with carbanion addition.[21]

There are flavoprotein-catalyzed dehydrogenations that are both pyridine nucleotide-dependent and independent, reactions with sulfur-containing compounds, hydroxylations, oxidative decar-

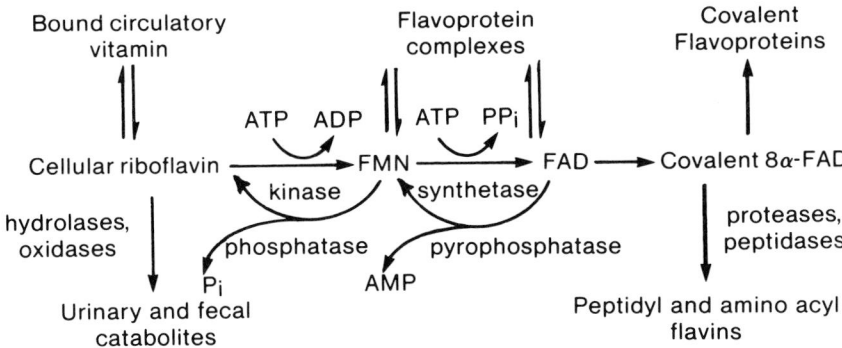

**Fig. 17–3.** Cellular interconversions of flavins.

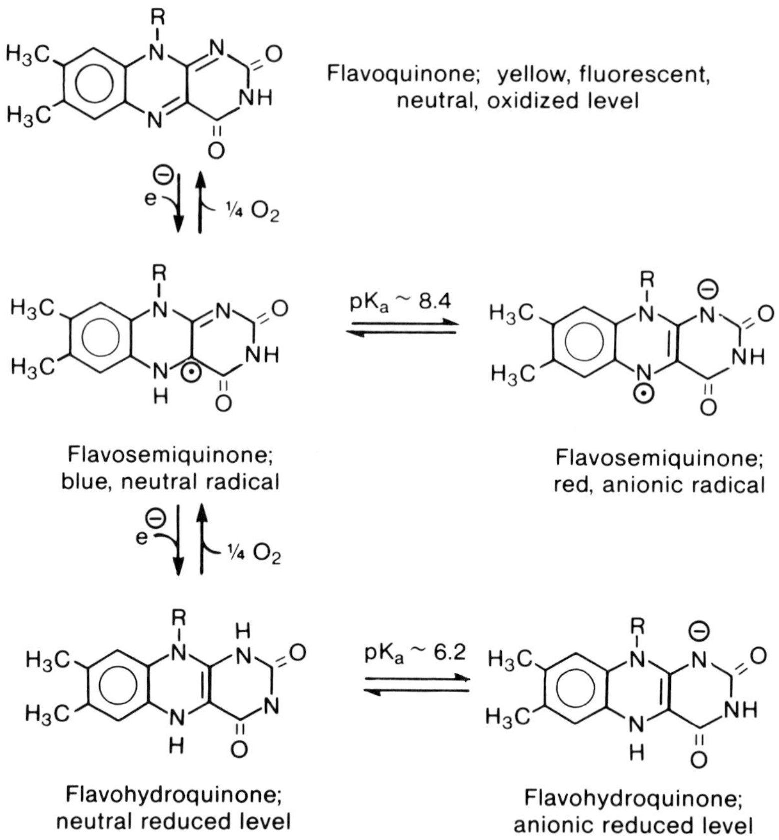

**Fig. 17–4.** Physiologically relevant redox states of flavocoenzymes.

boxylations, dioxygenations, and reduction of $O_2$ to hydrogen peroxide. The intrinsic abilities of flavins to be varyingly potentiated as redox carriers upon differential binding to proteins, to participate in both one- and two-electron transfers, and in reduced (1,5-dihydro) form to react rapidly with oxygen permits wide scope in their operation.

## DEFICIENCY AND EXCESS

Though riboflavin has a wide distribution in foodstuffs, many people live for long periods on low intakes and, consequently, minor signs of deficiency are common in many parts of the world.[47] Moreover, such deficiency as is encountered almost invariably occurs in combination with deficiency of other water-soluble vitamins. Clinical deficiency of riboflavin has been induced by feeding a riboflavin-deficient diet and/or by the administration of an antagonist such as galactoflavin. The deficiency syndrome is characterized by sore throat, hyperemia and edema of the pharyngeal and oral mucous membranes, cheilosis, angular stomatitis, glossitis (magenta tongue), seborrheic dermatitis, and normochromic, normo-

cytic anemia associated with pure red cell cytoplasia of the bone marrow.[48] As noted above, though, some of these symptoms, e.g., glossitis and dermatitis, when encountered in the field, may have resulted from other complicating deficiencies. Severe riboflavin deficiency can also affect the conversion of vitamin $B_6$ to its coenzyme[49] and even curtail conversion of tryptophan to niacin.[50]

No cases of toxicity from ingestion of excess riboflavin by experimental animals or humans have been reported.[51] The capacity of the human gastrointestinal tract to absorb orally administered riboflavin may be less than 20 mg in a single dose.[52,53] The limited solubility and absorptivity of this vitamin as encountered in multivitamin preparations and natural foodstuffs and its ready excretion as typical of water-soluble vitamins precludes a health risk even with megavitamin fads.

## CAUSES OF DEFICIENCY

Pure, uncomplicated riboflavin deficiency is probably never encountered in patients, but is accompanied by multiple nutrient deficiencies. Ariboflavinosis can result from such primary and secondary factors as commonly affect supply or utilization of other nutrients as well.[54] Inadequate dietary intake most commonly related to limited availability of food, but sometimes exacerbated by poor storage or processing, remains the major cause. Additionally, anorexic persons rarely ingest adequate amounts of riboflavin and other nutrients.

Decreased assimilation results from abnormal digestion, absorption, or both. Lactose intolerance as a result of lactase insufficiency, mostly encountered among blacks and Asians, argues against such afflicted people's consuming milk, which is a good source of the vitamin. Malabsorption can occur as a result of tropical sprue, celiac disease, malignancy and resection of the small bowel, and gastrointestinal and biliary obstruction. Poor absorption also results from disorders that increase motility and decrease gastrointestinal passage time, such as diarrhea, infectious enteritis, and irritable bowel syndrome.

Defective utilization can result from disturbances in hormonal production, certainly as relates to thyroid hormone,[40,41] but less likely as may be affected by oral contraceptives.[55] Phenothiazine derivatives appear to impair use of riboflavin.[56]

Increased destruction of riboflavin occurs during treatment of neonatal jaundice with phototherapy.[57,58] In this case, the side chain of the vitamin is photochemically destroyed, as it is involved in the photosensitized oxidation of bilirubin to more polar excretable compounds.

The recent finding that phenobarbital induced microsomal oxidation of the 7-methyl function of the vitamin[43] lends credence to the belief that long-time use of barbiturates may jeopardize flavin status.

Enhanced excretion of riboflavin occurs in catabolic patients undergoing nitrogen loss. The relationship of the vitamin to protein status has long been recognized. Also, certain antibiotics and phenothiazine drugs increase excretion of riboflavin.[59,60]

Increased requirements can, of course, be the consequence of one or more of the above-mentioned factors. For example, protein-calorie malnutrition commonly accompanies a diminution in both absorption and utilization of riboflavin. Systemic infections even without gastrointestinal involvement sometimes lead to increased requirements that can result from decreased intake, defective absorption, poor utilization, and increased excretion.

## DIETARY CONSIDERATIONS

The requirement levels for riboflavin, in contrast to those for thiamin, are not raised when energy utilization is increased.[51] Because of the interdependence of protein, energy intake, and metabolic body size, however, allowances calculated on these three bases do not differ significantly. Clinical signs of deficiency in adults can be prevented with intakes of riboflavin above 0.4 mg/1000 kcal, but over 0.5 mg/1000 kcal may be required to maintain tissue reserves in adults and children as reflected in urinary excretion, red cell riboflavin, and erythrocyte glutathione reductase. From these considerations, the riboflavin allowances are now computed as 0.6 mg/1000 kcal for people of all ages. This leads to RDAs ranging from 0.4 mg/day for early infants to 1.7 mg/day for young adult males. However, for elderly people and others whose daily calorie intake may be less than 2000 kcal, a minimum of 1.2 mg/day is recommended. Since pregnancy imposes extra demands, reflected by decreased excretion and an elevated FAD stimulation of erythrocyte glutathione activity, an additional 0.3 mg/day is recommended. The lactating woman secretes approximately 40 μg/100 ml of milk for an output of about 0.34 mg/day. Since the utilization of the additional riboflavin for milk production is assumed to be 70%, an additional intake of 0.5 mg is recommended.

Small amounts of riboflavin, largely as digestible coenzymes, are present in most plant and animal tissue. Especially good sources are eggs, lean meats, milk, broccoli, and enriched breads and cereals.[62] Such losses as occur during cooking are largely attributable to leaching of the heat-stable but light-sensitive flavins into water.

When supplementation or therapy with riboflavin is warranted, oral administration of 5 to 10 times the RDA usually is satisfactory.[59]

## METHODS FOR ASSAY AND STATUS DETERMINATION

Numerous biochemical methods are aimed at the separation and quantitation of the diverse natural flavins.[62,63] Among the more sensitive are those that invoke specific binding, e.g., riboflavin with egg white riboflavin-binding protein, FMN with apoflavodoxin, and FAD with apoproteins for D-amino acid oxidase or glucose oxidase. However, nutritional status is commonly assessed by measuring urinary excretion of the vitamin in fasting, random, or 24-hour specimens; or by load return tests, measurement of erythrocyte riboflavin concentration, and determination of the erythrocyte glutathione reductase activity coefficient.[54,64]

Urinary riboflavin can be measured by fluorometric as well as by microbiologic procedures. Under conditions of adequate intake, the amount excreted per day is more than 120 μg, or at least 80 μg are excreted per gram of creatinine. The rate of excretion expressed as μg/g creatinine is greater for children than for adults who normally have ≤80 but fall to <27 μg when deficient. Conditions causing negative nitrogen balance and the administration of antibiotics and certain psychotropic (phenothiazine) drugs increase urinary riboflavin as a consequence of tissue depletion and displacement, respectively. A load return test augments the applicability to a given case.

Erythrocyte riboflavin can also be determined by either fluorometric or microbiologic means. Since changes observed are rather small, there is some problem with sensitivity and interpretation of results. Nevertheless, it is clear that values below 10 μg/dl cells should be considered as reflecting a deficient status, as compared to ≤ 15 μg/dl for an acceptable status.

The most commonly used current method for assessing riboflavin status utilizes the determination of FAD-dependent glutathione reductase activity in freshly lysed red cells as detailed for routine clinical use[65] from the procedure described by Sauberlich et al.[66] Activities of holo and apo forms of glutathione reductase in erythrocyte hemolysates are measured before and after addition of FAD, respectively, by spectrophotometric determinations of NADPH oxidation. Values obtained are expressed in terms of "activity coefficients" (AC = $\Delta A_{340}$ with FAD/$\Delta A_{340}$ without FAD), which represent the degree of stimulation of apoenzyme resulting from addition in vitro of FAD. An AC of 1.0 would indicate no stimulation and only the presence of holoenzyme as a result of excess FAD (and riboflavin) in the original erythrocytes. Guidelines suggested for such coefficients are: <1.2, acceptable; 1.2 to 1.4 low; >1.4, deficient. Though presently the biochemical method of choice for assessing riboflavin status, the erythrocyte glutathione reductase assay has some drawbacks.[54] The test cannot be used in persons with glucose 6-phosphate deficiency because of an increased avidity in the reductase for FAD in this disease, which is about 10% among American Blacks.

## REFERENCES

1. McCollum, E.V., Kennedy, C.: J. Biol. Chem. *24*:491, 1916.
2. Emmett, A.D., Luros, G.O.: J. Biol. Chem. *43*:265, 1920.
3. Smith, M.I., Hendrick, E.G.: Public Health Rep. *41*:201, 1926.
4. Blyth, A.W.: J. Chem. Soc. *35*:530, 1879.
5. Kuhn, R., Gyorgy, P., Wagner-Jauregg, T.: Ber. *66*:317, 576, 1034, 1933.
6. Ellinger, P., Koschara, W.: Ber. *66*:315, 1933.
7. Booker, L.E.: J. Biol. Chem. *102*:39, 1933.
8. Warburg, O., Christian, W.: Biochem. Z. *254*:438, 1932.
9. Warburg, O., Christian, W.: Biochem. Z. *266*:377, 1933.
10. Stern, K.G., Holiday, E.R.: Chem. Ber. *67*:1104, 1442, 1934.
11. Theorell, H.: Biochem. Z. *272*:155, 1934.
12. Kuhn, R., Reinemund, K., Kaltschmitt, H., et al.: Naturwissenschaften *23*:260, 1935.
13. Kuhn, R., Reinemund, K., Weygand, F., et al.: Chem. Ber. *68*:1765, 1935.
14. Karrer, P., Schöpp, K., Benz, F.: Helv. Chim. Acta. *18*:426, 1935.
15. Karrer, P., Salomon, H., Schopp, K., et al.: Helv. Chim. Acta. *18*:1143, 1935.
16. Theorell, H.: Biochem. Z. *290*:293, 1937.
17. Warburg, O., Christian, W.: Biochem. Z. *294*:261, 1938.
18. Warburg, O., Christian, W.: Biochem. Z. *296*:294, 1938.
19. Warburg, O., Christian, W.: Biochem. Z. *297*:417, 1938.
20. Warburg, O., Christian, W.: Biochem. Z. *298*:150, 1938.
*21. Merrill, A.H., Jr., Lambeth, J.D., Edmondson, D.E., McCormick, D.B.: Formation and mode of action of flavoproteins. *In* Ann. Rev. Nutr. (Darby, W.J., Broquist, H.P., Olson, R.E., Eds.) Palo Alto, Annual Reviews, 1982.
22. Otani, S.: Studies on roseoflavin: isolation, physical, chemical, and biological properties. *In* Flavins and Flavoproteins (Singer, T.P., Ed.) Amsterdam, Elsevier, 1976.
23. Whitby, L.G.: Glycosides of riboflavin. *In* Vitamins and Coenzymes. Methods in Enzymology, Vol. 18, part B (McCormick, D.B., Wright, L.D., Eds.) New York, Academic Press, 1971.
24. Lambooy, J.P.: The alloxazines and isoalloxazines. *In* Heterocyclic Compounds, Vol. 9 (Elderfield, R.C., Ed.) New York, Wiley, 1967.
25. Tishler, M., Pfister, K., Babson, R.D., et al.: J. Am. Chem. Soc. *69*:1487, 1947.
26. Flexer, L.A., Farkas, W.G.: XIIth Internat. Congr. Pure Appl. Chem., New York, Sept. 1951, Abstracts p. 71.
27. Moffatt, J.G., Khorana, H.G.: J. Am. Chem. Soc. *80*:3756, 1958.
28. Moffatt, J.G., Khorana, H.G.: J. Am. Chem. Soc. *83*:649, 1961.
29. Föry, W., McCormick, D.B.: Chemical synthesis of flavin coenzymes. *In* Vitamins and Coenzymes. Methods in Enzymology, Vol. 18, Part B (McCormick, D.B., Wright, L.D., Eds.) New York, Academic Press, 1971.
*30. McCormick, D.B., N.Y. State J. Med. *62*:2842, 1962.
*31. McCormick, D.B.: Metabolism of riboflavin. *In* Riboflavin (Rivlin, R.S., Ed.) New York, Plenum Press, 1975.
32. Rivier, D.A.: Experientia *29*:1443, 1973.
33. Meinen, M., Aeppli, R., Rehner, G.: Nutr. Metab. *21 (Suppl. 1)*:264, 1977.
34. Daniel, H., Wille, U., Rehner, G.: J. Nutr. *113*:636, 1982.
35. Merrill, A.H., Jr., Froehlich, J.A., McCormick, D.B.: Biochem. Med. *25*:198, 1981.
36. Innis, W.S.A., McCormick, D.B., Merrill, A.H., Jr.: Biochem. Med. *34*:151, 1985.
37. Aw, T.-Y., Jones, D.P., McCormick, D.B.: J. Nutr. *113*:1249, 1983.

*38. McCormick, D.B.: Riboflavin. *In* Present Knowledge in Nutrition, 4th ed. (Hegsted, D.M., et al., Eds.) Washington, D.C., The Nutrition Foundation, 1976.

39. Lee, S.S., McCormick, D.B.: J. Nutr. *113*:2274, 1983.

*40. Rivlin, R.S., (Ed): Riboflavin. New York, Plenum Press, 1975.

*41. Rivlin, R.S.: Hormones, Drugs, and Riboflavin. Nutr. Rev. *37*:241, 1979.

42. Lee, S.S., McCormick, D.B.: Arch. Biochem. Biophys. *237*:197, 1985.

43. Ohkawa, H., Ohishi, N., Yagi, K.: J. Biol. Chem. *258*:5623, 5629, 1983.

44. Oka, M., McCormick, D.B.: J. Nutr. *115*:496, 1985.

45. Chia, C.P., Addison, R., McCormick, D.B.: J. Nutr. *108*:373, 1978.

46. Bray, R.C., Engel, P.C., Mayhew, S.G. (Eds.): Flavins and Flavoproteins. New York, de Gruyter, 1984.

47. Winick, M.: Nutrition in Health and Disease. New York, Wiley, 1980.

*48. Wilson, J.A.: Disorders of vitamins-deficiency, excess and errors of metabolism. *In* Harrison's Principles of Internal Medicine, 10th ed. (R.G. Petersdorf, et al., Eds.) New York, McGraw-Hill, 1982.

*49. Nutr. Rev. *39*:331, 1981.

50. White, A., Handler, P., Smith, E.L., et al.: Principles of Biochemistry. New York, McGraw-Hill, 1978.

*51. Recommended Dietary Allowances, 9th revised ed., Committee on Dietary Allowances and Food and Nutrition Board, National Research council, National Academy of Science, Washington, D.C., 1980.

52. Stripp, B.: Acta Pharmacol. Toxicol. *22*:353, 1965.

53. Mayersohn, M., Feldman, S., Gibaldi, M.: J. Nutr. *98*:288, 1969.

*54. Nichoalds, G.E.: Riboflavin. Symposium in laboratory medicine. *In* Clinics in Laboratory Medicine, Philadelphia, W.B. Saunders, Vol. 1, No. 4, 1981.

55. Roe, D.A., Boguzz, S., Sheu, J., et al.: Am. J. Clin. Nutr. *35*:495, 1982.

56. Horvath, C., Szonyi, L., Mold, K.: Teratology *14*:167, 1976.

57. Rubatelli, F.F., Allegri, G., Costa, et al.: J. Pediatr. *85*:865, 1974.

58. Gromisch, D.S., Lopez, R., Cole, H.S., et al.: J. Pediatr. *90*:118, 1977.

59. Goldsmith, G.A.: Prog. Food Nutr. Sci. *1*:559, 1975.

60. Pinto, J., Huang, Y.P., Rivlin, R.S.: Clin. Res. *27*:444A, 1979.

61. Watt, B.K., Merrill, A.L.: Composition of food: raw processed, prepared. *In* Agriculture Handbook No. 8. U.S. Department of Agriculture, 1963.

62. McCormick, D.B., Wright, L.D. (Eds.): Vitamins and Coenzymes. Methods in Enzymology, Vol. 18, Part B. New York Academic Press, 1971.

63. McCormick, D.B., Wright, L.D. (Eds.): Vitamins and Coenzymes. Methods in Enzymology, Vol. 66, Part E. New York, Academic Press, 1980.

*64. Briggs, M., (Ed.): Vitamins in Human Biology and Medicine. Boca Raton, CRC Press, 1981.

*65. McCormick, D.B.: Vitamins. *In* Textbook of Clinical Chemistry. (Tietz, N.W., Ed.) Philadelphia, W.B. Saunders, 1986.

66. Sauberlich, H.E., Judd, J.H., Jr., Nichoalds, G.E., et al.: Am. J. Clin. Nutr. *25*:756, 1972.

* A review.

*Chapter* **18**

# NIACIN

## Donald B. McCormick

The present knowledge of niacin derived from the need to understand the cause and prevention of a disease, pellagra, which as recently as this century ravaged large numbers of the population, especially among rural and poor. Pellagra is a classic deficiency disease that has been most often found among those who subsist chiefly on corn (maize).[1] After the Spanish introduced to Europe, about 1720, the planting of corn, a longtime food crop in Central America, the poorer classes who subsisted largely on this stable began to evidence a disease described by physician Casal in 1735 as "Mal de la Rosa" (sickness of the rose) after the redness of the skin. The peasantry in Italy began to use the term *pellagra* (for rough skin), which was the name passed on in a description published in 1771 by Frapolli. Although the British epidemiologist Sandwith, working in Egypt, suggested in 1913 that pellagra was a deficiency disease probably resulting from lack of tryptophan,[2] the certainty that it was a dietary deficiency of some factor was secured in the 1920s by the classic studies of Goldberger in the southeast United States.[3]

Tanner, an associate of Goldberger, described (quoted by Sebrell[4]) in 1921 the cure of a pellagrous patient by the administration of tryptophan. Since some foodstuffs other than those known to be good tryptophan sources were also varyingly effective in curing pellagra, it remained likely that another factor was needed. It was not until 1937 that Elvehjem et al. demonstrated that nicotinic acid, known chemically since 1867, could cure the pellagrous black tongue condition in a dog.[5]

Correlation between human pellagra and deficiency of nicotinic acid was then rapidly secured.[6–10] By 1946, the biologic transformation of tryptophan to the equivalent of niacin was finally understood.[11] It is now known that we have the ability to metabolize tryptophan to an altered form of the vitamin (nicotinic acid mononucleotide), which is a common intermediate in conversion of nicotinic acid to essential coenzymes.[12] Warburg and Christian in 1934 had isolated nicotinamide from a coenzyme, triphosphopyridine nucleotide (TPN),[13] now commonly known as NADP, shorthand for nicotinamide adenine dinucleotide phosphate. In 1935, Von Euler et al. isolated nicotinamide from DPN (diphosphopyridine nucleotide[14] now commonly known as NAD from nicotinamide adenine dinucleotide). Hence, the biochemical function of the vitamin uniquely preceded the discovery of its nutritional significance.

## CHEMISTRY, INCLUDING PRINCIPAL ANALOGUES

Though the term *niacin* is chemically synonymous with nicotinic (pyridine-3-carboxylic) acid, it is now used as the generic descriptor for the specific compound as well as for derivatives exhibiting qualitatively the biologic activity of nicinamide (nicotinamide, nicotinic acid amide). Thus "niacin activity" and "niacin deficiency" carry this broader meaning in nutritional literature.[15] A distinction between the two primary vitamin forms needs to be borne in mind, however, when dealing with some aspects of their metabolism and especially their different pharmacologic actions at high doses. Structures of both vitamers and the two coenzyme forms containing the nicotinamide moiety are given in Figure 18–1.

Free forms of the vitamin are white, stable solids that are quite soluble in water. The acid sublimes without decomposition at 230°C. The oxidized coenzymes are labile to alkali, whereas the reduced (1,4-dihydro) coenzymes are labile to acid. Reduction of the oxidized coenzymes commonly occurs by addition of a hydride ion to the *para* (4) position of the nicotinamide ring with simultaneous formation of a solvated proton. NADH and NADPH (but not NAD and NADP) absorb light in the near ultraviolet (340 nm).

Significant steps toward the elucidation of structure and synthesis of nicotine, a natural alkyl β-substituted pyridine, were begun by Pinner in 1893.[16] Ladenburg then showed that oxidation of such β-alkyl pyridines yielded nicotinic acid.[17] Various other approaches have provided means for obtaining niacin.[18–20] The amide is achieved via the nitrile or by such conventional procedures as converting nicotinic acid to the acid chloride and then treating the latter with ammonia.

Numerous analogues of niacin have been synthesized, but most vitaminically active are those *meta*-substituted pyridines with R-(CO)-functions which include esters as well as N-substituted amides. Among antivitamin analogues that have been employed are those depicted in Figure 18–2. Synthesis of the natural pyridine nucleotide coenzymes has been accomplished by various methods.[21–24] Analogues of NAD and NADP are usually made by direct modification of the natural coenzymes or by the pyridine base exchange reaction catalyzed by NADases.[25]

## BIOLOGIC ACTIVITY RELATING TO STRUCTURE

From the testing of many analogues of niacin and niacinamide, it is clear that some, e.g., pyridine-3-sulfonate, are more effective as an inhibitor in vitro than in vivo, whereas others, e.g., 6-aminonicotinamide, can be converted biologically to NAD(P) analogues, which become good competitive inhibitors in vivo as well. For coenzymic activity, the analogue must not only bind suitably to a pyridine nucleotide-dependent enzyme, which requires an appropriate meta substituent on the pyridine ring, but also have an unsubstituted *para(4)*-position in the pyridine ring capable of allowing hydride ion transfers to and from substrate/product. There is considerable variation in activity caused by replacement of the natural *meta(3)*-carboxamido substituent with other related functions.[26] For example, an isopropyl ketone group is more active in an NAD analogue with liver alcohol dehydrogenase than is the natural NAD; yet such an analogue is much less active than NAD with muscle glyceraldehyde phosphate dehydrogenase. In no instance has an analogue been found more reactive than the natural coenzymes for all of their known oxidation-reduction roles with enzymes, and in most cases the analogue serves less well. When the *para* position is substituted, as through keto product carbanion attack on the natural coenzyme in concentrated so-

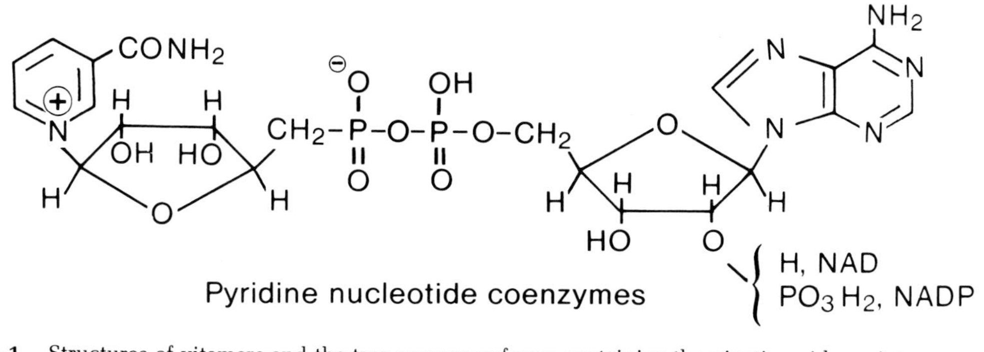

Nicotinic acid (niacin)          Nicotinamide (niacinamide)

Pyridine nucleotide coenzymes

H, NAD
PO₃H₂, NADP

**Fig. 18–1.** Structures of vitamers and the two coenzyme forms containing the nicotinamide moiety.

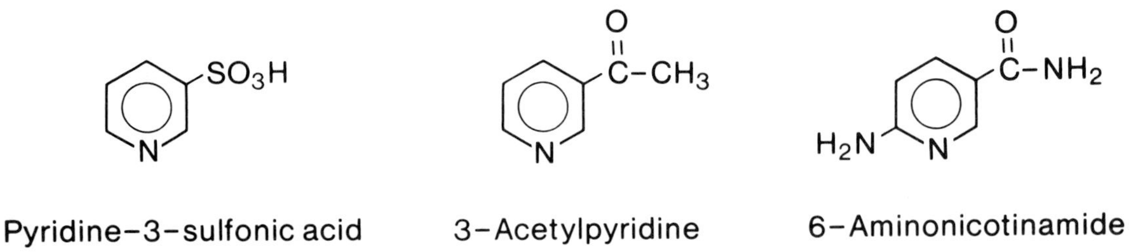

Pyridine-3-sulfonic acid　　　　3-Acetylpyridine　　　　6-Aminonicotinamide

**Fig. 18–2.** Antivitamin analogues.

lution of a dehydrogenase, turnover stops because the *para* adduct disallows normal redox function.[27]

## ABSORPTION, TRANSPORT, METABOLISM, AND EXCRETION

A recent review has served to bring together much of the material on mammalian metabolism of niacin.[28] The coenzymes are hydrolyzed in the intestinal tract to such fragments as nicotinamide mononucleotide (NMN), nicotinamide riboside (NMR) and nicotinamide.[29] Nicotinic acid is absorbed from the stomach,[30] and both acid and amide forms of the vitamin are readily absorbed from the small intestine as is some quantity of NMN.[31] Nicotinic acid and nicotinamide are both present in blood plasma. There may be a facilitated diffusion between blood and cerebrospinal fluid.[32]

The vitaminic forms are converted to coenzymes in blood cells, kidney, brain, and liver. The principal aspects of niacin metabolism in the human are summarized in Figure 18–3. The first step involves the cytosolic pyrophosphorylase (phosphoribosyltransferase)-catalyzed reaction of nicotinate or nicotinamide with 5-phosphoribosyl-1-pyrophosphate to form pyrophosphate and nicotinic acid mononucleotide (NaMN) or nicotin-

amide mononucleotide (NMN), respectively.[12] Additionally in liver, quinolinate from metabolism of tryptophan is similarly converted with concomitant decarboxylation to NaMN. A nuclear mononucleotide adenyltransferase catalyzes attachment of the AMP moiety from ATP to form pyrophosphate plus deamido-NAD from NaMN. The deamido compound subsequently reacts with glutamine in a cytosolic ATP-dependent synthetase step to yield NAD, glutamate AMP, and pyrophosphate. NMN is directly converted by the adenyltransferase to NAD. NADP is formed by a kinase-catalyzed phosphorylation of NAD. In the tissues, most of the vitamin is present as nicotinamide in NAD and NADP, although liver may contain a significant fraction of the free vitamin. There is little storage of niacin as such.

Although nicotinamide can be converted to nicotinic acid by a rather widespread microsomal deamidase, there is no direct reamidation of the nicotinic acid. Rather a glycohydrolase (NADase) catalyzes hydrolysis of NAD to nicotinamide plus adenosine 5'-pyrophospho-5-ribose (ADPR). A considerable number of catabolites of vitaminic forms have been identified from several animal species. These include conjugation of the acid with glucuronic acid or glycine, methylation of nicotinamide with some further oxidation of 1-methylnicotinamide to the 4- and 6-pyridones,

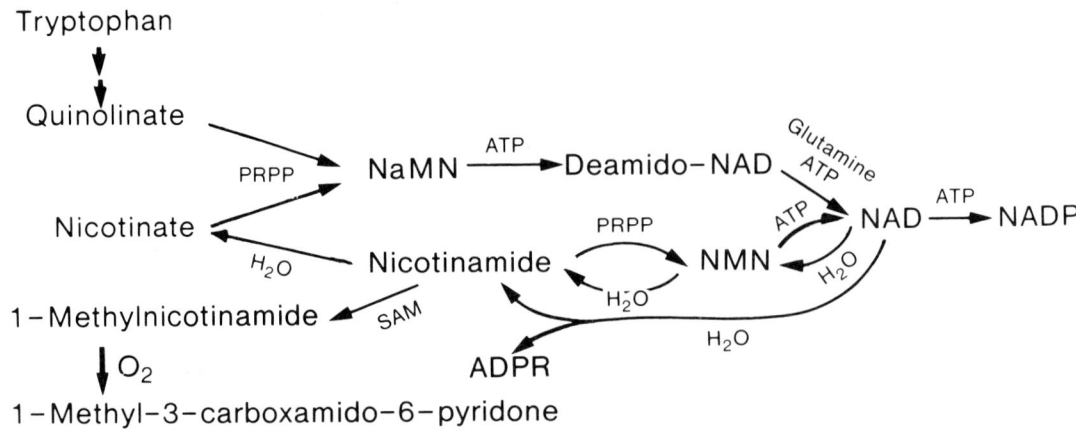

**Fig. 18–3.** Principal aspects of niacin metabolism in the human body.

and nicotinamide $N^1$-oxide. The human excretes normally 1-methylnicotinamide and 1-methyl-3-carboxamido-6-pyridone (or 1-methyl-2-pyridone-5-carboxamide) which are primary urinary metabolites.[12,15,28,33] With abnormally high intake of nicotinic acid (>1 g), increasing amounts of the methylnicotinamide and nicotinuric acid (the glycine conjugate) appear; with nicotinamide, a considerable amount of the free amide is excreted. Some 4-pyridone is also found but at a lower, constant ratio compared to the 6-pyridone. Nicotinamide $N^1$-oxide is a minor product from both acid and amide.

## BIOCHEMICAL AND PHYSIOLOGIC FUNCTIONS

Hundreds of enzymes require the nicotinamide moiety within either NAD or NADP. Most of these oxidoreductases function as dehydrogenases and catalyze such diverse reactions as the conversion of alcohols (often sugars and polyols) to aldehydes or ketones, hemiacetals to lactones, aldehydes to acids, and certain amino acids to keto acids. The common mechanism of operation, as generalized in Figure 18–4, involves the stereospecific abstraction of a hydride ion from substrate, with *para* addition to one or the other side of carbon 4 in the pyridine ring of the nucleotide coenzyme. The second hydrogen of the substrate group oxidized is concomitantly removed as a proton and ultimately exchanges as hydronium ion.

Most dehydrogenases utilizing NAD or NADP function reversibly. Glutamate dehydrogenase, for example, favors the oxidative direction, whereas others, like glutathione reductase, catalyze preferential reduction. A further generality is that most NAD-dependent enzymes are involved in catabolic reactions, whereas NADP systems are more common to biosynthetic reactions. As has been reviewed,[28] the discovery that some NAD glycohydrolases have the ability to transglycosidate, i.e., transfer the ADPR moiety of NAD to macromolecules, led to recognition of non-redox functions of the coenzyme. ADP-ribosyl transferases catalyze the transfer of ADPR to such prokaryote macromolecules as elongation factor 2,

thereby blocking translocation on ribosomes.[34] Poly-(ADPR)synthetases (polymerases) of eukaryotes catalyze n NAD + acceptor → (ADPR)n – M + n nicotinamide + n $H^+$. This activity is found in mitochondria and bound to ribosomes as well as in nuclei where it affects operation of DNA.[35] This non-redox function of NAD probably accounts for the rapid turnover of NAD in human cells.

## DEFICIENCY AND EXCESS

The diagnostic symptoms of pellagra were not clearly recognized until about 1908, and the early manifestations—weakness, lassitude, anorexia, and indigestion—were more recently appreciated as indicators for insufficient intake of niacin as well as other B-complex vitamins.[36] The typical presentation of pellagra is that of a chronic wasting disease associated with dermatitis, dementia, and diarrhea.[37] The characteristic erythematous dermatitis is bilateral and symmetrical. It occurs especially on skin areas exposed to sunlight, but may be additionally aggravated by heat and trauma. Mental changes include fatigue, insomnia, and apathy, which precede an encephalopathy characterized by confusion, disorientation, hallucination, loss of memory, and eventually frank organic psychoses. The diarrhea, when it occurs, reflects a widespread inflammation of the intestinal mucous surfaces; it may be accompanied by vomiting and dysphagia. Other gastrointestinal manifestations include achlorhydria, glossitis, stomatitis, and vaginitis.

While relatively large daily intakes of niacin (40 to 200 mg) may be required in treatment of Hartnup disease and carcinoid syndrome,[37] the use of pharmacologic doses is of doubtful value for other dysfunctions, e.g., poor glucose tolerance and atherosclerosis,[28] and may even prove harmful.[15,33,38] Massive (gram) doses of nicotinic acid (but not the amide) produce vascular dilation or "flushing" with an accompanying sensation of burning or stinging of the face and hands. Pruritus, nausea, vomiting, and diarrhea have been commonly reported but often abate with continued therapy. Varying degrees of hyperpigmentation and acan-

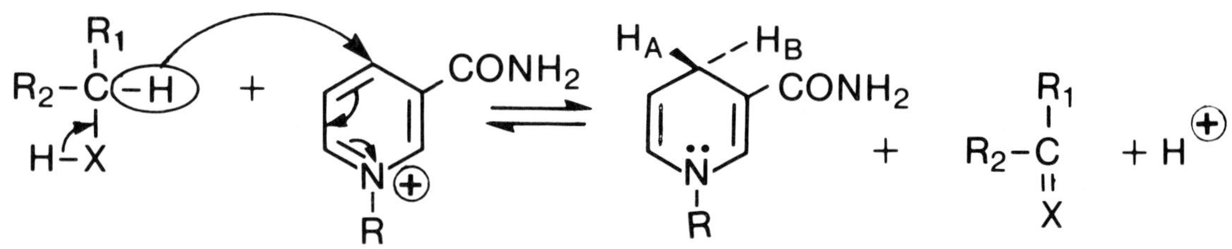

**Fig. 18–4.** The common mechanism of operation for niacin.

thosis nigricans occur in rare cases. Additional effects are abnormal glucose tolerance, hyperuricemia, peptic ulcer, hepatomegaly, jaundice, and increased serum transaminases. Hence, high chronic doses of nicotinic acid appear hepatotoxic.

## CAUSES OF DEFICIENCY

Though the pathogenesis of pellagra has been attributed to a deficiency of niacin (and tryptophan), other associated complicating factors may be an imbalance of amino acid intake, particularly the ingestion of high levels of leucine,[33,37] and the presence of mycotoxins elaborated by mold infestations, mainly by *Fusarium*.[37] Pellagra is also an occasional secondary manifestation of two disorders that profoundly affect tryptophan metabolism:[37] carcinoid syndrome in which up to 60% of tryptophan is catabolized by what is ordinarily a minor pathway of metabolism, and Hartnup disease, an autosomal recessive disorder in which several amino acids, including tryptophan, are poorly absorbed.

## DIETARY CONSIDERATIONS

Estimations of niacin requirements take into account the contribution of protein-tryptophan. A dietary intake of 60 mg of this amino acid is considered equivalent to 1 mg of niacin.[15] Average diets in the United States supply 0.5 to 1 g of tryptophan plus 8 to 17 mg of niacin for a total of 16 to 34 mg of niacin equivalents (NE).[15] Moreover, utilization of niacin within pyridine nucleotide coenzymes can be generally related to energy expenditure. Hence, the niacin equivalents have been related to caloric intake. The allowance recommended is 6.6 during childhood; for adults the recommended range is 9 to 19 NE/d. An increase of 2 NE/d during pregnancy is based on the recommended daily increase in energy intake of 300 kcal/d. Similarly, 5 equivalents daily for lactation relates to an increased energy intake of 500 kcal/d and will offset the 1.6 mg of preformed niacin lost in 850 ml of milk. Human milk contains approximately 0.17 mg of niacin and 22 mg of tryptophan per 100 ml or 70 kcal, and these amounts are adequate to meet niacin needs of the infant. RDAs are set at 6 NE/d for infants up to six months and 8 for the period of six months to a year.

The pyridine nucleotides, NAD(H) and NADP(H) represent most of the niacin activity found in good food sources such as yeast, lean meats, liver, and poultry.[39] Milk, canned salmon, and several leafy green vegetables contribute lesser amounts, but sufficient to prevent deficiency. Additionally, some plant foodstuffs, especially cereals such as corn and wheat, contain niacin bound in forms nutritionally not readily available.[15,33] Among these are niacinogens and niacytin. At least part of such material appears to be constituted by nicotinic acid that is amide linked to the ε-amino lysyl groups of peptides. Also there is evidence for esterification of nicotinic acid with glucose imbedded in a glycopeptide.[28] Protein provides a considerable portion of niacin equivalents because of the tryptophan content. As much as two thirds of niacin required by adults can be derived from tryptophan metabolism via nicotinic acid ribonucleotide to NAD and NADP. The "equivalence" of 60 mg of this amino acid to 1 mg niacin varies somewhat among individuals. Most notable is the report that women in the third trimester of pregnancy excrete considerably more metabolites of tryptophan and of niacin following a tryptophan load test than is the case during the fourth postpartum month.[40] From such evidence and other studies involving use of contraceptive steroids or steroid hormones, it appears that estrogens stimulate tryptophan oxygenase, which is rate-limiting in the pathway for conversion of tryptophan to NMN.[41,42]

## METHODS FOR ASSAY AND STATUS DETERMINATION

Microbiologic methods that utilize bacteria *(Lactobacilli)* and protozoa *(Tetrahymena)* have been used to estimate the quantities of niacin in biologic fluids and tissue extracts; however, these and other methods applied to blood or urine do not adequately reflect nutritional status. Since the urinary excretion of metabolites of niacin and tryptophan is lower than average in patients with generalized malnutrition, the measurement of these analytes is not entirely satisfactory as diagnostic indices for niacin deficiency.[33,37,43] However, the excretion of 1-methylnicotinamide and 1-methyl-3-carboxamide-6-pyridone has received continued use in the biochemical assessment of niacin nutriture. Normally, adults excrete 20 to 30% of their niacin in the form of methylnicotinamide and 40 to 60% as the pyridone.[43] An excretion ratio of pyridone to methylnicotinamide of 1.3 to 4.0 is acceptable, but latent niacin deficiency is indicated by a value below 1.0. As depletion occurs, the pyridone is absent for weeks before clinical signs are noted, and the methylnicotinamide excretion falls to a minimum about the time clinical signs are evident.

Although assays for coenzymes derived from niacin have not yet been adapted well to assess nutritional status, there are several efficient means to separate and sensitively quantitate both vitaminic and coenzymic forms.[44,45] Some of these rely on the absorbance of reduced pyridine nucleotides at 340 nm, especially in coupled enzyme systems: others utilize fluorescent properties of addition products, e.g., with methyl ethyl ketone.

## REFERENCES

1. Roe, D.A.: A Plague of Corn. Ithaca, Cornell University Press, 1973.
2. Sandwith, F.M.: Trans. Soc. Trop. Med. Hyg. *6*:143, 1913.
3. Goldberger, J.: J.A.M.A. *78*:1676, 1922.
4. Sebrell, W.H.: J. Nutr. *55*:3, 1955.
5. Elvehjem, C.A., Madden R.J., Strong, F.M., et al.: J. Am. Chem. Soc. *59*:1767, 1937.
6. Fouts, P.J., Helmer, O.M., Lepkovosky, S., et al.: Proc. Soc. Exp. Biol. Med. *37*:405, 1937.
7. Smith, D.T., Ruffin, J.M., Smith, S.G.: J.A.M.A. *109*:2054, 1937.
8. Spies, T.D., Cooper, C., Blankenhorn, M.A.: J.A.M.A. *110*:622, 1938.
9. Spies, T.D., Bean, W.B., Stone, R.E.: J.A.M.A. *111*:584, 1938.
10. Schmidt, Jr., H.L., Sydenstricker, V.P.: J.A.M.A. *110*:2065, 1938.
11. Krehl, W.A., Sarma, P.S., Teply, L.J., Elvehjem, C.A.: J. Nutr. *31*:85, 1946.
12. White, A., Handler, P., Smith, E.L. et al.: Principles of Biochemistry. New York, McGraw-Hill, 1978.
13. Warburg, O., Christian, H.: Biochem. Z. *274*:112, 1934.
14. von Euler, H., Albers, H., Schlenk, F.: Z. Physiol. Chem. *237*:180 I, 1935.
15. Recommended Dietary Allowances, 9th ed. Committee on Dietary Allowances and Food and Nutrition Board, National Research Council, National Academy of Science, Washington, D.C., 1980.
16. Pinner, A.: Ber. *26*:292, 1893.
17. Ladenburg, A.: Ann. *301*:152, 1898.
18. McElvain, S.M.: Org, Syn. *4*:49, 1925.
19. Woodward, C.F., Badgett, C.O., Williaman, J.J.: Ind. Eng. Chem. *36*:540, 1944.
20. McElvain, S.M., Goese, M.A.: J. Am. Chem. Soc. *63*:2283, 1941.
21. Shuster, L., Kaplan, N.O., Stolzenbach, F.E.: J. Biol. Chem. *215*:195, 1955.
22. Hughes, N.A., Kenner, G.W., Todd, A.R.: J. Chem. Soc. 3733, 1957.
23. Woenckhaus, C.: Top. Curr. Chem. *52*:209, 1974.
24. Fisher, T.L., Vercellotti, S.V., Anderson, B.M.: J. Biol. Chem. *248*:4293, 1973.
25. Zatman, L.J., Kaplan, N.O., Colowick, S.P.: J. Biol. Chem. *200*:197, 1953.
26. Kaplan, N.O.: The Pyridine Coenzymes. *In* The Enzymes. 2nd ed. Vol. 5. (Boyer, P., Lardy, H., Myrback, K., Eds.) New York, Academic Press, 1960.
27. Everse, J., Kaplan, N.O.: Adv. Enzymol. *37*:61, 1973.
28. Henderson, L.M.: Niacin. *In* Ann. Rev. Nutr. Vol. 3. (Darby, W.J., Broquist, H.P., Olson, R.E., Eds.) Palo Alto, CA, Annual Reviews, 1983.
29. Baum, C.L., Selhub, J., Rosenberg, I.H.: Biochem. J. *204*:203, 1982.
30. Bechgaard, H., Jespersen, S.: J. Pharm. Sci. *66*:871, 1977.
31. Baum, C.L., Selhub, J., Rosenberg, I.H.: Fed. Abst. *42*:1319, 1983.
32. Spector, R.: J. Neurochem. *33*:895, 1979.
33. Narasinga Rao, B.S., Gopalan, C.: Niacin. *In* Present Knowledge in Nutrition. 5th ed. (Olson, R.E., et al., Eds.) Washington, The Nutrition Foundation, 1984.
34. Honjo, T., Nishizuka, Y., Hayaishi, O.: J. Biol. Chem. *243*:3553, 1968.
35. Ogata, N., Ueda, K., Kawaichi, M., et al.: J. Biol. Chem. *256*:4135, 1981.
36. Elvehjem, C.A.: Physiol. Rev. *20*:249, 1940.
37. Wilson, J.A.: Disorders of vitamins—Deficiency, excess and errors of metabolism. *In* Harrison's Principles of Internal Medicine. 10th ed. (Petersdorf, R.G., et al., Eds.) New York, McGraw-Hill, 1982.
38. Campbell, T.C., Allison, R.G., Carr, C.J.: Feasibility of identifying adverse health effects of vitamins and essential minerals in man. Bethesda, Life Sciences Research Office, F.A.S.E.B., 1980.
39. Harper, H.A., Rodwell, V.A., Mayes, P.A.: Review of Physiological Chemistry, Chpt. 13. Los Altos, CA, Lange Medical Publications, 1979.
40. Wertz, A.W., Lojkin, M.E., Bouchard, B.S., et al.: J. Nutr. *64*:339, 1958.
41. Rose, D.P., Braidman, I.P.: Am. J. Clin. Nutr. *24*:673, 1971.
42. Brin, M.: An. J. Clin. Nutr. *24*:704, 1960.
43. Sauberlich, H.E., Skala, J.H., Dowdy, R.P.: Laboratory Tests for the Assessment of Nutritional Status. Boca Raton, FL, CRC press, 1974.
44. McCormick, D.B., Wright, L.D. (Eds.): Vitamins and Coenzymes. Methods in Enzymology. Vol. 18, Part B. New York, Academic Press, 1971.
45. McCormick, D.B., Wright, L.D. (Eds.): Vitamins and Coenzymes. Methods in Enzymology. Vol. 66, Part E. New York, Academic Press, 1980.

*Chapter* **19**

# VITAMIN B$_6$

## Donald B. McCormick

As with some other members of the vitamin B complex, recognition of the vitamin B$_6$ group came only after adequate distinction of its activity could be made with sufficiently enriched material. For a time, it was believed that a dermatitic condition in rats (rat acrodynia) was an experimental model for pellagra in humans. Following the separation of a heat-labile, antiberiberi vitamin B$_1$ (thiamin) from a crude vitamin B$_2$, it became apparent that the latter comprised a mixture of activities. Since riboflavin was the first factor characterized from such a mixture, it has remained synonymous with vitamin B$_2$. By 1934, when György could show that vitamin B$_2$ was not a rat pellagra-preventive factor, he proposed the name *vitamin B$_6$* to cover such activity.[1] Later György and his associates secured the fact that rat acrodynia was not cured by the real pellagra-preventive factor (vitamin B$_3$ or niacin), and vitamin B$_6$ became an entirely new entity.[2,3]

The isolation of a crystalline vitamin B$_6$ from extracts of rice bran[4–7] and yeast[8] was reported by five groups of investigators in 1938. The structure of this form of vitamin B$_6$ was determined in 1939 and led to the name *pyridoxine.*[9–11] In the same year, synthesis of pyridoxine was accomplished by Harris and Folkers.[12] When the effect of vitamin B$_6$ in natural materials was compared in microorganisms and animals, it became evident to Snell and associates that at least another form, then called pseudopyridoxine,[13] must be present to account for the greater growth activities found with some bacteria. Their proposed structures were then synthesized by the Merck group. Pyridoxal

and pyridoxamine proved to be the active compounds.[14] The coenzymic activity of a natural derivative of vitamin B$_6$ was recognized with the discovery and identification of pyridoxal 5'-phosphate (PLP).[15–18] The similar phosphorylated form of pyridoxamine, interchangeable with pyridoxal phosphate during transaminations, was also shown to occur naturally.[19]

## CHEMISTRY, INCLUDING PRINCIPAL ANALOGUES

The vitamin B$_6$ group is comprised of three natural forms—pyridoxine (pyridoxol), pyridoxamine, and pyridoxal—all of which are 4-substituted 2-methyl-3-hydroxyl-5-hydroxymethyl pyridines. The free vitamin forms are bases normally provided as the white crystalline hydrochloride salts; pyridoxine hydrochloride is the common commercial form. The 5'-phosphate esters of all three forms are also found in nature. Pyridoxal 5'-phosphate is the predominant coenzyme form, though pyridoxamine 5'-phosphate interconverts as coenzyme during transaminations (Fig. 19–1). Chemical syntheses of pyridoxine have been developed by several routes.

The hydrochloride salts of vitamin B$_6$ are quite water soluble and give colorless solutions with absorption maxima near 290 nm characteristic of the protonated pyridinium compounds. B$_6$ compounds are somewhat fluorescent and in general are sensitive to light, particularly at alkaline pH.

A large number of vitamin B$_6$ analogues have been synthesized,[20,21] several other compounds have been found to interfere with specific or gen-

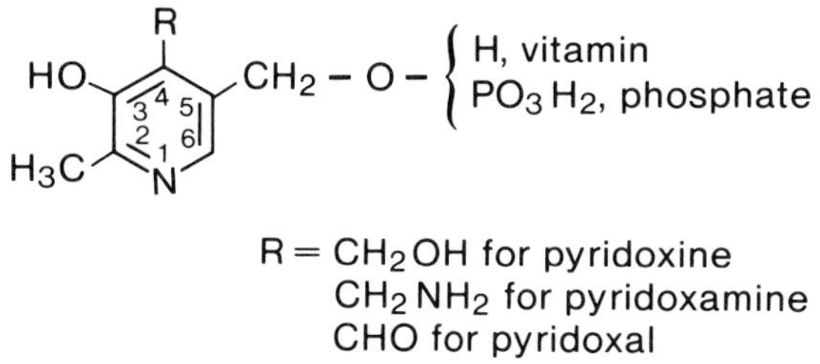

R = CH$_2$OH for pyridoxine
CH$_2$NH$_2$ for pyridoxamine
CHO for pyridoxal

**Fig. 19–1.** Free and phosphorylated forms of vitamin B$_6$.

eral function of B$_6$, and there are known to be a number of naturally occurring B$_6$ antagonists.[22] Among generally useful synthetic antagonists is 4′-deoxypyridoxine;[23] this can be phosphorylated by the pyridoxal kinase system[24] to form the 5′-phosphate, which competes for binding to PLP-dependent enzymes but cannot function as a coenzyme. Toxopyrimidine, the alcohol derived from the pyrimidine portion of thiamin, is a structural analogue of vitamin B$_6$ and causes running fits in rats and mice; these symptoms of B$_6$ antagonism are stopped by administration of the vitamin.[25] Among pharmacologically used compounds that inhibit by virtue of reacting with and depleting pyridoxal and its phosphate are penicillamine, otherwise useful as a chelator to work against heavy metal poisoning and to remove excess copper in Wilson's disease, and isoniazid (isonicotinic acid hydrazide), which is a tuberculostatic drug.[26] More generally, such carbonyl reagents, which include β-thiolamines, hydrazines, semicarbazides, and hydroxylamines, also form substrate inhibitors of pyridoxal kinase: thiazolidines, hydrazones, semicarbazones, and oximes, of pyridoxal.[24] All the vitamin B$_6$ antagonists of natural origin are of the carbonyl reagent type and therefore act on the pyridoxal form of the vitamin or its coenzymic derivate, PLP. A list of these natural anti-B$_6$ compounds is given in Table 19–1.

Chemical phosphorylation of vitamin B$_6$ and numerous analogues has been used to produce coenzyme and analogue forms.[20,21] Most commonly the vitamin form can be dissolved in and reacted with a polyphosphoric acid mixture (P$_2$O$_5$ with H$_3$PO$_4$) followed by chromatographic purification. In some instances, yield and purity of product are enhanced by selective blocking or protection of functions other than the 5-hydroxymethyl, which bears the natural phosphate.

## BIOLOGIC ACTIVITY RELATING TO STRUCTURE

Some alterations in the structure of vitamin B$_6$ decrease biologic activity, and most lead to inactive or inhibitory compounds.[27,28] Because coenzymic function depends on the dianionic 5′-phosphate for optimal binding to apoenzymes, the phosphorylatable vitaminic 5-hydroxymethyl is needed. Participation of the formyl group (or the aminomethyl in transaminations) is obligatory in the 4-position of a 3-hydroxypyridine, since this permits condensation with amines (or ketones) to form reactive intermediates. Though the 4-hydroxymethyl of pyridoxine and 4-aminomethyl of pyridoxamine can be biologically oxidized to the requisite 4-formyl function, a 4-methyl cannot. Hence 4′-deoxypyridoxine can be phosphorylated but cannot function as coenzyme. 5′-Deoxypyridoxal, on the other hand, could conceivably function, but does not bind well enough to apoenzymes.

## ABSORPTION, TRANSPORT, METABOLISM, AND EXCRETION

The processes by which vitamin B$_6$ is taken in and utilized in numerous biochemical reactions has been treated in a fairly recent textbook.[27] The three B$_6$ vitamers, mostly released from their 5′-phosphate esters by intraluminal action of intestinal alkaline phosphatase, are readily absorbed by the mucosal cells, which contain cytoplasmic pyridoxal kinase responsible for

**Table 19–1. Naturally Occurring Antagonists of Vitamin B$_6$[29]**

| *Reagent* | *Precursor* | *Source* |
|---|---|---|
| Substituted hydrazines: | | |
| 1-Amino-D-proline | Linatine | *Linus usitatissimus* |
| Methylhydrazine | Giromitrin | *Gyromitra esculenta* |
| 2-(1-Methylhydrazino)-acetic acid | Negamycin | *Streptomyces purpeofuscus* |
| 3-(1,3,5-Hexatrienyl)-phenylhydrazine | Spinamycin | *Streptomyces albinospinus* |
| 4-Hydroxymethyl-phenylhydrazine | Agaritine | *Agaricus* spp. |
| Substituted hydroxylamines: | | |
| L-Canaline | Canavanine | *Lotoidae* spp. |
| D-Cycloserine | | *Actinomyces* spp. |
| O-Amino-D-serine | D-Cycloserine | Rat urine |

catalyzing the ATP-dependent phosphorylation of all three vitamin forms. As shown in Figure 19–2, it is probable that other cells utilizing $B_6$ allow entry of free vitamin into the cell followed by "metabolic trapping" as the phosphates. Clearly, this is the case with isolated liver cells.[28] Most cells contain a cytosolic FMN-dependent, pyridoxine (pyridoxamine)-5'-phosphate oxidase responsible for catalyzing the $O_2$-dependent conversion of pyridoxine phosphate and pyridoxamine phosphate to pyridoxal phosphate (PLP) (and $H_2O_2$). The coenzyme can enter directly into subcellular organelles, such as hepatocyte mitochondria.[29] PLP binds for catalytic function with numerous specific apoenzymes throughout the cell. The erythrocyte, in addition, traps PLP as a conjugate Schiff base with hemoglobin.[30] Glycogen phosphorylase contains most of the PLP in skeletal muscle.[31] The adult body pool of $B_6$ compounds has been estimated to be at least 25 mg.

Release of free vitamin, mainly pyridoxal when physiological nonsaturating levels of vitamin are absorbed, occurs when the phosphates are hydrolyzed by nonspecific alkaline phosphatase located in the plasma membrane of cells. However, some PLP is also released into circulation by the liver.[27] Since the reactive aldehyde is capable of forming Schiff bases with amino groups, PLP in plasma is more tightly complexed to proteins, mostly albumin, than is pyridoxal, which forms an intramolecular hemiacetal between the 4-formyl and 5-hydroxymethyl functions. All forms of $B_6$, specifically PLP, cross the placenta readily and are concentrated in fetal blood.[32] Although PLP is the principal tissue form of $B_6$ and pyridoxal constitutes much of the circulating vitamin, the main catabolite excreted in urine is 4-pyridoxic acid, which is formed by the action of the FAD-dependent general liver aldehyde oxidase and especially by NAD-specific aldehyde dehydrogenase found in most tissues.

The concentration of vitamin $B_6$, mainly pyridoxal, in human milk is approximately 10 to 20 μg/L during the first days of lactation and thereafter gradually increases to 100 to 250 μg/L, reflecting nutritional status of the mother.[32] The $B_6$ content of cow's milk is considerably higher.

## BIOCHEMICAL AND PHYSIOLOGIC FUNCTIONS

As coenzyme PLP, vitamin $B_6$ functions in numerous reactions that embrace the metabolism of macronutrients, i.e., proteins, carbohydrates, and lipids.[25,33] Especially diverse are PLP-dependent enzymes that are involved in amino acid metabolism. By virtue of the ability of PLP to condense its 4-formyl substituent with an amine, usually the α-amino group of an amino acid, to form an azomethine (Schiff base) linkage, a conjugated double bond system extending from the α-carbon of the amine (amino acid) to the pyridinium nitrogen in PLP results in reduced electron density about the α-carbon. This potentially weakens each of the bonds from the amine (amino acid) carbon to the adjoined functions (hydrogen, carboxyl, or side chain). A given apoenzyme then locks in a particular configuration of the coenzyme-substrate compound such that maximal overlap of the

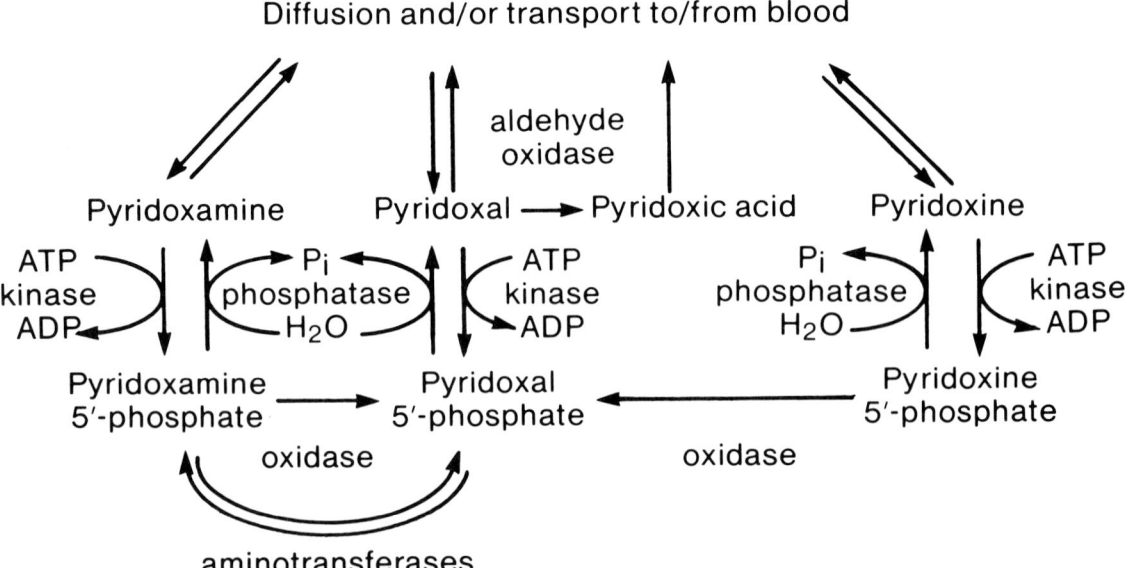

**Fig. 19–2.** Mammalian metabolism of vitamin $B_6$.

bond to be broken will occur with the resonant, coplanar, electron-withdrawing system of the coenzyme complex (Fig. 19–3).

Aminotransferases effect rupture of the α-hydrogen bond of an amino acid with ultimate formation of an α-keto acid and pyridoxamine 5′-phosphate; this reversible reaction provides an interface between amino acid metabolism and that for ketogenic and glucogenic reactions. Amino acid decarboxylases catalyze breakage of the α-carboxyl bond and lead to irreversible formation of amines, including several that are functional in nervous tissue, e.g., epinephrine, norepinephrine, serotonin, and γ-aminobutyrate. The biosynthesis of heme depends upon the early formation of δ-aminolevulinate from PLP-dependent condensation of glycine and succinyl-CoA followed by decarboxylation. There are many examples of enzymes, such as cysteine desulfhydrase and serine hydroxymethyltransferase, which effect the loss or transfer of amino acid side chains. PLP is the essential coenzyme for phosphorylase that catalyzes phosphorolysis of the α-1, 4-linkages of glycogen. An important role in lipid metabolism is the PLP-dependent condensations of L-serine with palmitoyl-CoA to form 3-dehydrosphinganine, a precursor of sphingolipids.

As with other water-soluble vitamins that function as coenzymes, the relative affinity of the coenzyme for a given apoenzyme and the extent to which a particular holoenzyme-catalyzed reaction is essential is reflected in the progressive symptomatology of deficiency in the vitamin.

## DEFICIENCY AND EXCESS

Recognition of deficiency symptoms ultimately attributed to lack of vitamin B$_6$ was gained through use of experimental animals, (e.g., that of rat acrodynia) before the sequelae of events that occur in the human were appreciated. Investigations of the consequences of vitamin B$_6$ deficiency in the human have utilized diets deficient in the vitamin and/or diets containing an antagonist, usually 4′-deoxypyridoxine.[30] Otherwise, a deficiency of B$_6$ alone is uncommon, and it is more usual to expect the problem to occur in association with deficits in other vitamins of the B-complex. Biochemical changes occur early and become more marked as deficiency of B$_6$ progresses.[26,34,35] Plasma levels of PLP and urinary output of B$_6$ and 4-pyridoxic acid decrease within a week of removal of the vitamin from the diet. There is increased xanthurenic acid in urine, since liver kynureninase activity is decreased. Transaminases in serum and red cells also decrease. Electroencephalographic abnormalities appear within three weeks. Epileptiform convulsions, probably the result of insufficient activity of PLP-dependent L-glutamate decarboxylase responsible for production of the inhibitory neurotransmitter γ-aminobutyrate, are a common finding in young subjects deficient in B$_6$. In addition, skin changes include a dermatitis with cheilosis and glossitis. Hematologic manifestations may include a decrease in circulating lymphocytes and possibly a normocytic, microcytic, or sideroblastic anemia.

Ingestion of moderate excesses of vitamin B$_6$ appears to be without ill effect, although it has been reported that a B$_6$ dependency is induced in normal human adults given a supplement of 200 mg of pyridoxine for each of 33 consecutive days.[36] Acute toxicity of pyridoxine, however, is low.[37,38] Doses up to 1 g/kg of body weight seem to be tolerated by rats, rabbits, and dogs. The toxicity of pyridoxamine and pyridoxal is also low, although pyridoxal was found about twice as toxic as pyridoxine or pyridoxamine for animals.[39,40] As with a number of other micronutrients, however,

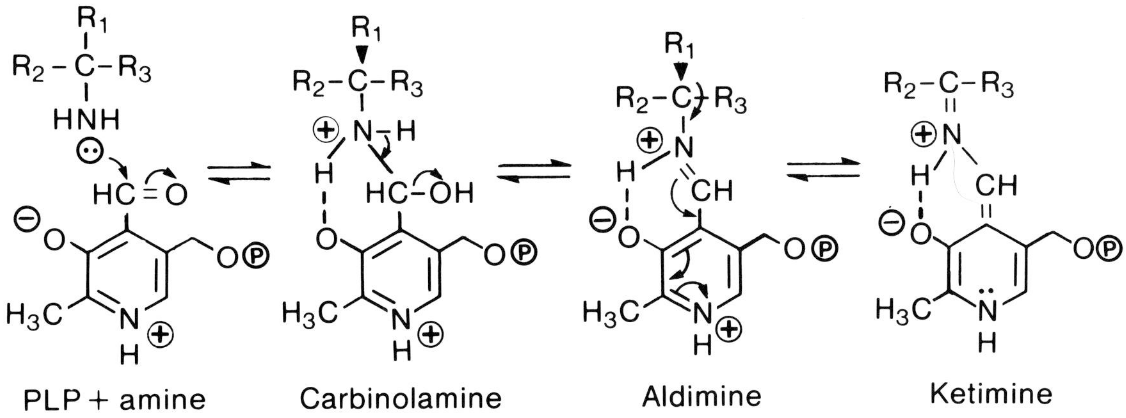

**Fig. 19–3.** Generalized operation of pyridoxal phosphate with an amine.

the use of megadoses of vitamin $B_6$ is fraught with real danger. The toxic outcome of the chronic use of 1000 to 2700 times the RDA (2 to 6 g/d) of pyridoxine in the human, generally for the putative treatment of carpal tunnel syndrome or pre-eclampsic edema, has now been documented.[41] Interestingly, a peripheral neuropathy develops with such excesses, similar to the peripheral nervous system involvement and convulsions that occur in deficiency.

## CAUSES OF DEFICIENCY

Uncomplicated primary deficiency of vitamin $B_6$ in the adult human is rarely encountered, since ingestion of diets so poor as to be insufficient in this vitamin group would likely lack adequate amounts of some other B-complex vitamins. Infrequent reports of improperly constituted infant formulas, viz., those singularly inadequate in $B_6$, have been made. There is also evidence that inadequate intake of vitamin $B_6$, as well as other nutrients, can be a problem for the elderly and certainly is in chronic alcoholics.[32]

There are instances where chemotherapeutic use or fortuitous ingestion of antagonists has led to hypovitaminosis $B_6$.[26,34] These include the tuberculostatic drug isoniazid which, as mentioned earlier, can form hydrazones with pyridoxal and PLP. As with other "carbonyl reagents," such compounds not only cause loss by displacement and urinary excretion, but the Schiff bases formed with pyridoxal inhibit pyridoxal kinase,[24,42] and the PLP Schiff bases may additionally inhibit some PLP-dependent enzymes.[27] There are known to be several naturally occurring substituted hydrazines and hydroxylamines that pose such risk (Table 19–1).[22]

Abnormalities in the function of $B_6$ occur in several genetic conditions. Pyridoxine-responsive genetic diseases include the following: (1) cases of infantile convulsions where the apoenzyme for glutamate decarboxylase has a poor affinity for the coenzyme; (2) a type of chronic anemia where the number but not the morphologic abnormality of erythrocytes is improved by pyridoxine supplementation; (3) xanthurenic aciduria where affinity of the mutant kynureninase for PLP is decreased; (4) primary cystathioninuria due to similarly defective cystathionase; (5) homocystinuria where there is less of the normal cystathionine synthetase. Usually these inborn errors of metabolism respond to increased levels (5 to 50 mg/d) of administered vitamin $B_6$.[43]

## DIETARY CONSIDERATIONS

Requirements for vitamin $B_6$ are complicated by differences in protein intake, the probable avail-

ability of a fraction of the quantity needed through bacterial synthesis in the intestinal tract, the use of alcohol and oral contraceptives, and less frequently, cases when extra needs are apparent.[26,32,35] Estimates of requirements with some margin of safety have been based on production and cure of clinical signs of deficiency and, more often, on biochemical parameters. The latter include the determination of urinary excretion of vitamin $B_6$ and 4-pyridoxic acid or xanthurenic acid after a tryptophan load test and the plasma levels of PLP and red cell transaminase activity.[32] A ratio of 0.02 mg of $B_6$/g of protein intake has been suggested for normal adults and may be extrapolated to children and adolescents. For adult males ingesting 100 g of protein per day, the RDA is 2.2 mg; for females ingesting 100 g per day, it is 2.0 mg. An addition of 0.6 mg $B_6$ per day is suggested for the pregnant woman to match the increased protein allowance during gestation. During lactation, an addition of 0.5 mg/d is recommended to accommodate for extra protein intake and provide a level of the vitamin in milk (0.10 to 0.25 mg/L) adequate for the breast-fed infant.

Vitamin $B_6$ is widely distributed in animal and plant tissues where mainly the phosphorylated forms, and particularly PLP, predominate. Meats, poultry, and fish are good sources, as are yeast, certain seeds, and bran; somewhat more limited are milk, eggs, and green leafy vegetables.[26,32,35,44] The common commercial form of the vitamin is pyridoxine hydrochloride, which is a water-soluble, white, crystalline solid. Solutions of the $B_6$ vitamers are decomposed by light, especially in the ultraviolet region at neutral to alkaline pH. The reactive aldehyde function of PLP leads to significant loss during thermal processing of foods.[45]

## METHODS FOR ASSAY AND STATUS DETERMINATION

Several methods have proved useful for assays of $B_6$ and PLP, PLP-dependent enzymes, and metabolites of $B_6$ and those amino acids that reflect vitamin $B_6$ status in the human.[27,34,46–48] There are a number of reliable modifications that are adapted for diverse biologic samples.

Direct assessment of all or separate vitaminic forms of $B_6$ in urine and blood have utilized microbiologic assays with specific strains of *Saccharomyces carlsbergensis (S. uvarum)* for all three natural vitamers, *Streptococcus faecium* for pyridoxal and pyridoxamine, and *Lactobacillus casei* for pyridoxal. Levels of 20 μg $B_6$/g creatinine in human urine are considered indicative of marginal or inadequate dietary intake of the vitamin.

Fluorometric assays of urinary 4'-pyridoxic acid and blood PLP after conversion of the latter to the cyanide complex or condensation with a fluorophore such as methyl anthranilate followed by reduction have also found application. During deficiency, the level of 4-pyridoxic acid will drop well below the normal of at least 0.8 mg/d in urine. The PLP concentration in human plasma, usually measured by using radioactive tyrosine and the apodecarboxylase, has been judged the most reliable indicator of $B_6$ status. The reference range is 5 to 23 ng/ml of plasma.

Activities of blood transaminases have been frequently used as a reflection of $B_6$ status. Though the enzyme activity in serum is depressed in $B_6$ deficiency, a considerable variability results because release of these enzymes reflects cell death and breakdown in various tissues. Erythrocyte levels of aspartate and alanine aminotransferases provide a better reflection of $B_6$ status. Enzymatic assays are best run after and before addition of PLP in vitro to yield an activity coefficient ratio. Values less than about 1.5 are considered normal, but may depend somewhat on the assay method used.[46]

Measurement of urinary tryptophan metabolites, particularly xanthurenic acid, following an oral load (2 to 5 g) of L-tryptophan, is one of the most common indices used in studies of $B_6$ nutriture, because changes can be recognized early and measurements are relatively easy. Amounts of xanthurenate well above the normal (near 25 mg/d) are seen in $B_6$ deficiency. Levels of other metabolites such as kynurenic acid and 3-hydroxykynurenine are also increased. The methionine load test has also been utilized.[34,46] The ratio of cystathionine to cysteine sulfinic acid is elevated in a 24-hour urine sample from $B_6$ deficient patients who have received a 3-g methionine load. This method, however, requires an amino acid analyzer.

## REFERENCES

1. György, P.: Nature *133*:498, 1934.
2. Birch, T.W., György, P., Harris, L.J.: Biochem. J. *29*:2830, 1935.
3. Birch, T.W., György, P.: Biochem. J. *30*:304, 1936.
4. György, P.: J. Am. Chem. Soc. *60*:983, 1938.
5. Lepkovsky, S.: J. Biol. Chem. *124*:125, 1938.
6. Keresztesy, J.C., Stevens, J.R.: J. Am. Chem. Soc. *60*:1267, 1938.
7. Ichiba, A., Michi, K.: Sci. Papers Inst. Phys. Chem. Res. (Tokyo) *34*:623, 1938.
8. Kuhn, R., Wendt, G.: Ber. *71*:780, 1938.
9. Stiller, E.T., Keresztesy, J.C., Stephens, J.R.: J. Am. Chem. Soc. *61*:1237, 1939.
10. Kuhn, R., Wendt, G., Westphal, K.: Chem. Ber. *72B*:310, 1939.
11. Harris, S.A., Stiller, E.T., Folkers, K.: J. Am. Chem. Soc. *61*:1242, 1939.
12. Harris, S.A., Folkers, K.: Science *89*:347, 1939.
13. Snell, E.E., Guirard, B.M., Williams, R.J.: J. Biol. Chem. *143*:519, 1942.
14. Harris, S.A., Heyl, D., Folkers, K.: J. Biol. Chem. *154*:315, 1944.
15. Gunsalus, I.C., Bellamy, W.D., Umbreit, W.W.: J. Biol. Chem. *155*:685, 1944.
16. Heyl, D., Luz, E., Harris, S.A., et al.: J. Am. Chem. Soc. *73*:3430, 1951.
17. Baddiley, J., Mathias, A.P.: J. Chem. Soc. 2583, 1952.
18. Schlenk, F., Snell, E.E.: J. Biol. Chem. *157*:425, 1945.
19. Rabinowitz, J.C., Snell, E.E.: J. Biol. Chem. *169*:643, 1947.
20. Korytnyk, W., Ikawa, M.: Synthesis of vitamin $B_6$ analogs. *In* Vitamins and Coenzymes. Methods in Enzymology, Vol. 18, Part A. (McCormick, D.B., Wright, L.D., Eds.) New York, Academic Press, 1970.
21. Korytnyk, W.: Synthesis and biological activity of vitamin $B_6$ analogs. *In* Vitamins and Coenzymes. Methods in Enzymology, Vol. 62, Part D (McCormick, D.B., Wright, L.D., Eds.) New York, Academic Press, 1979.
22. Klosterman, H.J.: Vitamin $B_6$ antagonists of natural origin. *In* Vitamins and Coenzymes. Methods in Enzymology, Vol. 62, Part D (McCormick, D.B., Wright, L.D., Eds.) New York, Academic Press, 1979.
23. Coburn, S.P.: The Chemistry and Metabolism of the Vitamin $B_6$ Antagonist, 4'-Deoxypyridoxine. Boca Raton, CRC Press, 1981.
24. McCormick, D.B., Snell, E.E.: J. Biol. Chem. *236*:2085, 1961.
25. Metzler, D.E.: Biochemistry. The Chemical Reactions of Living Cells, Chpt. 8. New York, Academic Press, 1977.
26. Wilson, J.A.: Disorders of vitamins: Deficiency, excess and errors of metabolism *In* Harrison's Principles of Internal Medicine. 10th ed. (Petersdorf, R.G., et al., Eds.) New York, McGraw-Hill, 1982.
27. Tryfiates, G.P. (Ed.): Vitamin $B_6$ Metabolism and Role in Growth. Westport, CT, Food and Nutrition Press, 1980.
28. Kozik, A., McCormick, D.B.: Arch. Biochem. Biophys. *229*:187, 1984.
29. Lui, A., Lumeng, L., Li, T.-K.: J. Biol. Chem. *256*:6041, 1981.
30. Mehansho, H., Henderson, L.M.: J. Biol. Chem. *255*:11901, 1980.
31. Black, A.L., Guirard, B.M., Snell, E.E.: J. Nutr. *108*:670, 1978.
32. Recommended Dietary Allowances, 9th revised ed. Committee on Dietary Allowances and Food and Nutrition Board, National Research Council, National Academy of Science, Washington, DC, 1980.
33. White, A., Handler, P., Smith, E.L., et al.: Principles of Biochemistry. New York, McGraw-Hill, 1978.
34. Gershoff, S.N.: Vitamin $B_6$. *In* Present Knowledge in Nutrition, 4th ed. (Hegsted, D.M., et al., Eds.) Washington, DC, The Nutrition Foundation, 1976.
35. Harper, H.A., Rodwell, V.A., Mayes, P.A.: Review of Physiological Chemistry, Chpt. 13. Los Altos, CA, Lange Medical Publications, 1979.
36. Canham, J.E., Nunes, W.T., Eberlin, E.W.: Electroencephalographic and central nervous system manifestations of $B_6$ deficiency and induced $B_6$ dependency in normal human adults. *In* Proceedings VI International Congress on Nutrition. Edinburgh, E. and S. Livingstone, Ltd., 1964.
37. Bauernfeind, J.C., Miller, O.N.: Vitamin $B_6$ nutri-

tional and pharmaceutical usage, stability, bioa-vailability, antagonists, and safety. *In* Human Vitamin B₆ Requirements. Washington, DC, National Academy of Sciences, 1978.

38. Brin, M.: Vitamin B₆: chemistry, absorption, metabolism, catabolism and toxicity. *In* Human Vitamin B₆ Requirements. Washington, DC, National Academy of Sciences, 1978.

39. Sebrell, W.H., Jr., Harris, R.S. (Eds.): The Vitamins, Vol. II. New York, Academic Press. 1968.

40. Kraft, H.-G., Fiebig, L., Hotovy, R.: Arzneim. Forsch. *11*:922, 1961.

41. Schaumburg, H., Kaplan, J., Windebank, A., et al.: N. Engl. J. Med. *309*:445, 1983.

42. McCormick, D.B., Snell, E.E.: Proc. Natl. Acad. Sci. U.S. *45*:1371, 1959.

43. Rosenberg, L.E.: Vitamin-responsive inherited diseases affecting the nervous system. *In* Res. Publ. Assoc. Nerv. Ment., Vol. 53 (Plum, F., Ed.) New York, Raven Press, 1974.

44. Winick, M.: Nutrition in Health and Disease. Chpt. 9. New York, Wiley, 1980.

45. Gregory, J.F., Kirk, J.R.: Vitamin B₆ in foods: assessment of stability and bioavailability. *In* Human Vitamin B₆ Requirements. Washington, DC, National Academy of Sciences, 1978.

46. Briggs, M. (Ed.): Vitamins in Human Biology and Medicine. Boca Raton, CRC Press, 1981.

47. Sauberlich, H.E.: Vitamin B₆. *In* The Vitamins, 2nd ed., Vol. VII (Gyorgy, P., Pearson, W.N., Eds.) New York, Academic Press, 1967.

48. McCormick, D.B.: Vitamins. *In* Textbook of Clinical Chemistry. (Tietz, N.W., Ed.) Philadelphia, W.B. Saunders, 1986.

*Chapter* # 20

# PANTOTHENIC ACID

## Donald B. McCormick

Among the components of "bios," a term coined by Wildiers[1] for the yeast growth factor(s) in natural extracts, R.J. Williams and his associates described in 1933 a particular acidic compound, pantothenic acid, which seemed to have widespread occurrence.[2] Highly active concentrates of this substance were described in 1939.[3,4] Somewhat parallel to this work was the use of fuller's earth to separate "eluate factor," which contained a substance (pyridoxine) that was a rat antidermatitis factor, and "filtrate factor," which Elvehjem et al.[5,6] and Jukes and associates[7,8] showed could cure the chick dermatitis first described by Norris and Ringrose.[9] By 1939, Wooley et al. had isolated the pure hydroxy acid[10] and obtained β-alanine[6] from alkaline degradation of the chick antidermatitis factor, and Weinstock et al. had found it was not only a cleavage product of pantothenic acid, but could replace the vitamin in some microorganisms.[11] In 1940 Mitchell et al. reported that an α-hydroxy-γ-lactone was also released from hydrolysis of pantothenic acid.[12] The pure lactone was identified as α-hydroxy-β, β-dimethyl-γ-butyrolactone by Williams and Major,[13] who also demonstrated that racemic pantothenic acid was formed when the lactone (racemized during isolation) was coupled to β-alanine. The lactone became known as pantoic lactone (pantolactone) and the acid as pantoic acid.[14,15] The first clear identification of a biochemical function for the vitamin was made in 1947, when Lipmann et al. reported that the coenzyme required for the acetylation of sulfanilamide contained 10% pantothenic acid in a bound form.[16]

The full structure was elucidated by Baddiley et al. in 1953.[17] The name *coenzyme A* was given to indicate this was a coenzyme of acetylation, now in a broader sense for acylations. The second known coenzyme-like substance with a pantothenyl moiety is acyl carrier protein which contains a 4'-phosphopantetheine residue.[18,19]

## CHEMISTRY, INCLUDING PRINCIPAL ANALOGUES

Pantothenic acid, as noted in the preceding section, is composed of pantoic acid and β-alanine. These are conjoined via amide linkage with the natural dextrarotatory isomer to form D-N-(2,4-dihydroxy-3,3-dimethyl-butyryl)-β-alanine. The acid is a viscous oil (syrup) which is hygroscopic and fairly labile to acids, bases, and heat. The vitamin is an integral part of 4'-phosphopantetheine, which serves as a covalently attached prosthetic group of acyl carrier protein and as a component within the structure of coenzyme A (CoA) (Fig. 20–1).

Modifications in one or the other portion of pantothenate have led to analogues, some of which have significant antivitamin activity. Replacements of the β-alanine portion with taurine in pantoyltaurine and with a β-aminoethylphenyl ketone in phenylpantothenone produce antipantothenates for bacteria, whereas ω-methylpantothenate, in which the hydroxymethyl is replaced by a methyl group, is antivitaminic for animals and bacteria (Fig. 20–2).

Pantothenic acid is soluble in water, but nearly insoluble in such organic solvents as benzene or

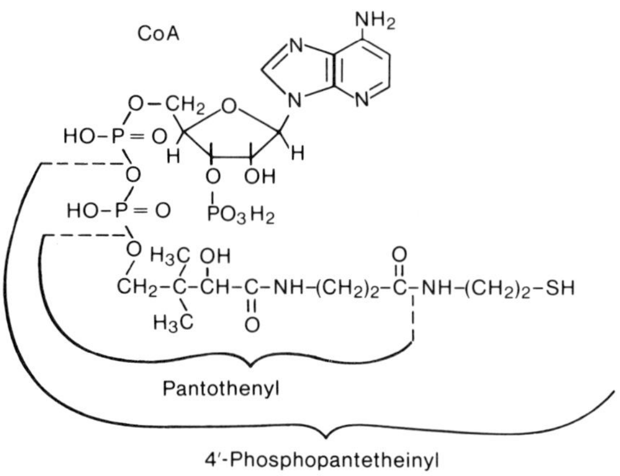

**Fig. 20–1.** Pantothenate and 4'-phosphopantetheine as components of CoA.

chloroform. The usual and common salt form of the vitamin is calcium pantothenate, which is soluble at the level of 1 g/2.8 ml of water. Such solutions are most stable between pH 5 and 7 but, even so, are not stable to autoclaving; sterilization by ultrafiltration is necessary.[20]

The total synthesis of coenzyme A was reported by Moffatt and Khorana,[21] Michelson,[22] and Shimizu et al.[23] Analogues of CoA, including those made via thiazoline intermediates[24] and those in which the sulfur is replaced,[25] have been synthesized.

Since the isolation of a *Leuconostoc oenos* growth factor from tomato juice[26] and its characterization as 4'-O-(β-D-glucopyranosyl)-D-pantothenic acid,[27] a number of glycosyl derivatives of pantothenic acid and pantetheine also have been synthesized.[28]

## BIOLOGIC ACTIVITY RELATING TO STRUCTURE

With regard to the vitamin level of activity, removal of the terminal hydroxy group of the pantoyl moiety produces an inhibitor, since the ω-methyl compound interferes with phosphorylation of the hydroxymethyl function during ultimate formation of CoA. Removal of the methyl functions destroys activity, and replacing one with an ethyl group decreases activity. The β-alanyl moiety cannot be replaced by α-alanine or other amino acids, but esters can be hydrolyzed

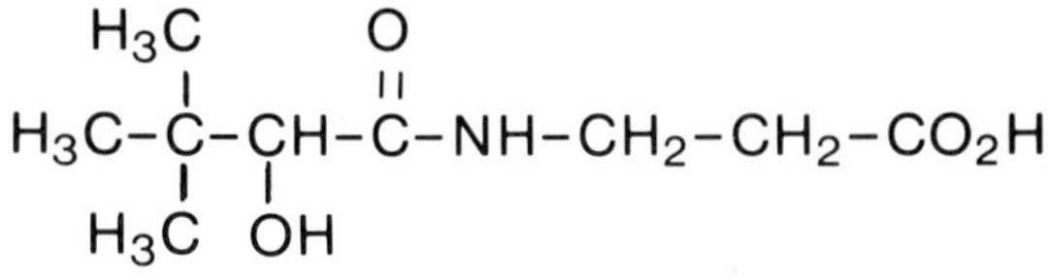

**Fig. 20–2.** ω-Methyl pantothenate.

to the active vitamin salt and even pantothenol (produced by replacing the carboxyl with —$CH_2OH$) has activity in the animal where some oxidation of the hydroxymethyl to natural carboxyl terminus can occur. At the CoA level, most molecular alterations also decrease activity and generally lead to competitive inhibitors or partial antagonists.[24,25] Clearly, the sulfur of the functional mercapto terminus is needed, as its replacement by a hydrogen or hydroxyl group in desulfo (dethio) and oxy analogues leads to potent antagonists. Even seleno-CoA is only poorly active in such systems as acetyl-CoA synthetase.

## ABSORPTION, TRANSPORT, METABOLISM, AND EXCRETION

Coenzyme A, the form in which much of the pantothenic acid is ingested, is hydrolyzed by intestinal pyrophosphatase and phosphatase to pantetheine (pantothenyl cysteamine), which together with pantothenate is absorbed into the portal circulation.[29] Within cells resynthesis of coenzyme level compounds occurs via successive conversions of pantothenate as shown in the biosynthetic scheme[30,31] (Fig. 20–3).

Formation of acyl carrier protein (ACP) occurs by transfer of the 4'-phosphopantetheinyl moiety of CoA, which binds via a phosphodiester link to apo-ACP in a reaction catalyzed by ACP holoprotein synthase.[31] About 80% of the vitamin in animal tissues is in CoA form, and the rest exists mainly as phosphopantetheine and phosphopantothenate. Cleavage enzymes catalyzing hydrolysis of the phosphate moieties (CoA→dephospho CoA→4'-phosphopantetheine→pantetheine) and release of β-mercaptoethylamine (cysteamine) and pantothenate from pantetheine operate during turnover and release of the vitamin, which is excreted in the urine. Only a small fraction of pantothenate is secreted into milk and even less into colostrum.

## BIOCHEMICAL AND PHYSIOLOGIC FUNCTIONS

The myriad acyl thiol esters of CoA, of which pantothenic acid is a constituent, are central to the metabolism of numerous compounds, especially lipids and the ultimate catabolic disposition of carbohydrates and ketogenic amino acids.[30,31] The chemical properties of the thiol ester, which has a high group-transfer potential, permits facile acylations and hydrolysis; the ready formation of enolate ions and the carbanion-like property of the carbon α to the carbonyl facilitate condensation reactions. For example, acetyl-CoA, which is formed during metabolism of carbohydrates, fats, and amino acids, can acetylate compounds, such

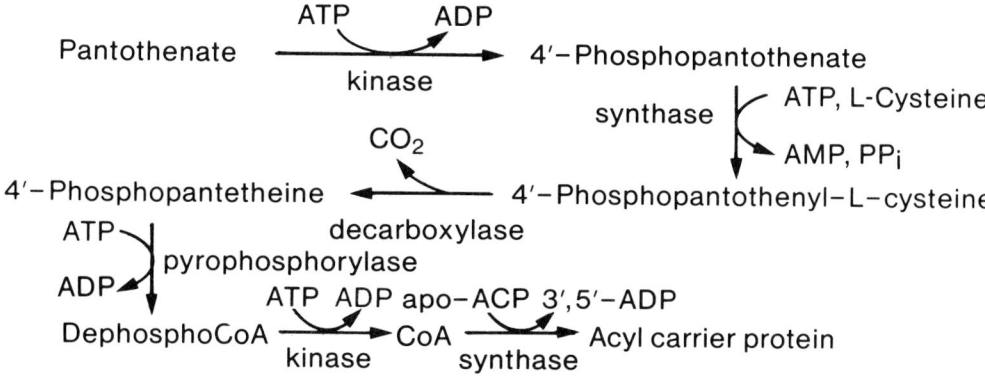

**Fig. 20–3.** Biosynthesis of CoA and the 4′-phosphopantetheine of ACP.

as choline and hexosamines, to produce essential biochemicals; it can also condense with other metabolites, such as oxalacetate, to supply citrate and can lead to cholesterol.

Another essential role of pantothenic acid is its participation in the 4′-phosphopantetheine moiety of acyl carrier protein (ACP) where the phosphodiester-linked prosthetic group utilizes the sulfhydryl terminus to exchange with malonyl-CoA to form an ACP-S-malonyl thioester, which can chain elongate during fatty acid biosynthesis.

Though the reactive thiol function of CoA and ACP is not an immediate part of the pantothenyl structure within these compounds, the steric and chemical properties conferred by the vitamin structure is important for enzymic recognition.

## DEFICIENCY AND EXCESS

The widespread occurrence of pantothenic acid in foods is commensurate with its many roles and makes an uncomplicated dietary deficiency of pantothenate unlikely. The use of experimental animals, which can be more rigorously controlled, permitted recognition of the requirement for this vitamin and established the bases of symptomatology, some of which extend to the human. In poultry, pantothenate deficiency results in a classic dermatitis around the beak, feet, and eyes; feathering is poor; there is a myelin degeneration of the spinal cord leading to incoordination and paralysis; involution of the thymus and fatty degeneration of the liver occur.[32–34] Ducks additionally develop anemia and show an impaired ability to develop antibodies.[35,36] Deficiency in rats results in a scaling and erythematous dermatitis; achromotrichia (loss of hair color); spectacle alopecia (circumocular loss of hair); chromodacryorrhea ("bloody" whiskers due to protoporphyrin release by the Harderian glands via the nasolacrimal duct); hemorrhagic necrosis of the adrenals with altered synthesis of corticosterone, duodenal ulcer, spastic gait, anemia, leukopenia, impaired antibody production; and gonadal atrophy with infertility.[37–39] There is also a lower CoA level when a high-fat diet is fed[40] and there is decreased urinary excretion of the vitamin.[41]

Dogs develop hair changes, irritability, gastrointestinal disturbances, fatty livers, hemorrhagic adrenals, hypoglycemia, convulsions, and coma. Swine develop dermatitis and hair loss; excessive lachrymation; impaired sodium, potassium, and glucose absorption with diarrhea, ulcerative colitis, degenerative lesions of the spinal cord, and peripheral nerves; and a spastic gait described as "goose-stepping."[42] Induction of deficiency in other animals, such as the guinea pig and cat, has also been reported.[43] Overall, it is clear that growth impairment[44] and dermatitic involvement, common to deficits of other vitamins, result not only from a pantothenate deficiency but also from adrenal cortical insufficiency and its attendant sequelae.

With the human, the best-defined signs and symptoms were enumerated after deficiency had been produced in a few volunteers who had received ω-methylpantothenic acid as an antagonist,[45] and more recently in persons fed semisynthetic diets virtually free of pantothenate.[46] Subjects became irascible, developed postural hypotension and rapid heart rate on exertion, and evidenced epigastric distress with anorexia and constipation, numbness and tingling of the hands and feet ("burning feet" syndrome), hyperactive deep tendon reflexes, and weakness of finger extensor muscles. The eosinopenic response to ACTH was also impaired.

There is no evidence that therapeutic doses (10 to 100 mg range) of pantothenate chronically administered cause any harmful effects. Even with oral amounts as high as 10 to 20 g of the calcium salt, the only reported problem was occasional diarrhea.[47,48]

## DIETARY CONSIDERATIONS

An intake of pantothenic acid of 4 to 7 mg/d seems sufficient for adults, since consumption averages 7 mg/d when supplied with a range of ordinary foods, and even 4 mg/d was consumed by low-income women who were deemed at least marginally adequate in other vitamins.[49] Urinary excretion, which generally correlates with dietary intake, is 2 to 7 mg/d in adults consuming 5 to 7 mg/d; another 1 to 2 mg/d is lost in feces. A slightly higher intake may be warranted for pregnant or lactating women. Human milk contains approximately 2 mg/L. Adequate intakes for younger age groups are based on proportional energy needs and range from a suggested 2 mg/d for young infants to 4 to 5 mg/d for adolescents.

Pantothenic acid occurs ubiquitously in nature where it is synthesized by most microorganisms and plants from pantoic acid derived from L-valine, and β-alanine derived from L-aspartate. The vitamin is widely distributed in foods, mostly within CoA-containing compounds, and is particularly abundant in animal sources, legumes, and whole grain cereals.[30,49] Excellent food sources (100 to 200 μg/g dry weight) include egg yolk, kidney, liver, and yeast. Fair sources (35 to 100 μg/g) include broccoli, lean beef, skimmed milk, sweet potatoes, and molasses. Over half the pantothenate in wheat may be lost during manufacture of flour and up to a third is lost during cooking of meat.

## METHODS FOR ASSAY AND STATUS DETERMINATION

Since urinary output of pantothenate is directly proportional to dietary intake, present assessment relies mainly on this index.[50–52] Urinary excretion of <1 mg/d is considered abnormally low with a mean of 4 (1 to 15 mg range).[52] Suspicion of inadequate intake is further supported if whole blood values are <100 μg/dl, since 103 to 183 are normal values.[52] Functional tests based on acetylation of sulfanilamide by red cells[53] and urinary excretion of acetylated *p*-aminobenzoic acid after a load test of the acid[54] have been suggested, but their value is not yet established.

Pantothenic acid is usually measured by microbiologic procedures, often using *Lactobacillus plantarum*[51,52,55] but also *Lactobacillus casei, Tetrahymena pyriformis,* or *Saccharomyces uvarum. Pedioccus acidilactici* NCIB 6990 has been found to be especially sensitive as an assay organism. A radioimmunoassay is also being used.[56]

Gas chromatographic methods are employed for pharmaceutical preparations. Enzymatic assays can be used determining the quantity of CoA and ACP.[57,58]

## REFERENCES

1. Wildiers, E.: La Cellule *18*:313, 1901.
2. Williams, R.J., Lyman, C.M., Goodyear, G.H., et al.: J. Am. Chem. Soc. *55*:2912, 1933.
3. Williams, R.J.: Science *89*:486, 1939.
4. Williams, R.J., Weinstock, Jr., H.H., Rohrmann, E., et al.: J. Am. Chem. Soc. *61*:454, 1939.
5. Elvehjem, C.A., Koehn, Jr., C.J.: J. Biol. Chem. *108*:709, 1935.
6. Wooley, D.W., Waisman, H.A., Elvehjem, C.A.: J. Am. Chem. Soc. *61*:977, 1939.
7. Lepkovsky, S., Jukes, T.H.: J. Biol. Chem. *114*:109, 1936.
8. Jukes, T.H.: J. Am. Chem. Soc. *61*:975, 1939.
9. Norris, L.C., Ringrose A.T.: Science *71*:643, 1930.
10. Wooley, D.W., Waisman, H.A., Michelson, O., et al.: J. Biol. Chem. *125*:715, 1938.
11. Weinstock, Jr., H.H., Mitchell, H.K., Pratt, E.F., et al.: J. Am. Chem. Soc. *61*:1421, 1939.
12. Mitchell, H.K., Weinstock, Jr., H.H., Snell, E.E., et al.: J. Am. Chem. Soc. *62*:1776, 1940.
13. Williams, R.J., Major, R.T.: Science *91*:246, 1940.
14. Stiller, E.T., Harris, S.A., Finkelstein, J., et al.: J. Am. Chem. Soc. *62*:1779, 1785, 1940.
15. Kuhn, R., Wieland, T.: Chem. Ber. *73*:971, 1134, 1940.
16. Lipmann, F., Kaplan, N.O., Novelli, G.D., et al.: J. Biol. Chem. *167*:869, 1947.
17. Baddiley, J., Thain, E.M., Novelli, G.D., et al.: Nature *171*:76, 1953.
18. Vagelos, P.R., Larrabee, A.R.: J. Biol. Chem. *242*:1776, 1967.
19. Vanaman, T.C., Wakil, S.J., Hill, R.L.: J. Biol. Chem. *243*:6420, 1968.
20. Frost, D.V., McIntire, F.C.: J. Am. Chem. Soc. *66*:425, 1944.
21. Moffatt, J.G., Khorana, H.G.: J. Am. Chem. Soc. *81*:1265, 1959, *83*:663, 1961.
22. Michelson, A.M.: Biochim. Biophys. Acta *50*:605, 1961.
23. Shimizu, M., Nagase O., Okada, S., et al.: Chem. Pharm. Bull. *13*:1142, 1965.
24. Shimazu, M.: Pantothenic acid and coenzyme A: Preparation of CoA analogs. *In* Vitamins and Coenzymes. Methods in Enzymology, Vol. 18, Part A (McCormick, D.B., and Wright, L.D. Eds.) New York, Academic Press, 1970.
25. Mautner, H.G.: Synthesis of coenzyme A analogs. *In* Vitamins and Coenzymes. Methods in Enzymology, Vol. 18, Part A (McCormick, D.B., and Wright, L.D., Eds.) New York, Academic Press, 1970.
26. Amachi, T., Yoshizumi, H.: Agric. Biol. Chem. *33*:139, 1969.
27. Amachi, T., Imamoto, S., Yoshizumi, H.: Agric. Biol. Chem. *35*:1222, 1971.
28. Imamoto, S., Amachi, T., Yoshizumi H.: Syntheses of glycosyl derivatives of pantothenic acid and pantetheine. *In* Vitamins and Coenzymes. Methods in Enzymology, Vol. 62, Part D (McCormick, D.B., Wright, L.D., Eds.) New York, Academic Press, 1979.
29. Rose, R.C., Hoyumpa, A.M., Jr., Allen, R.H., et al.: Transport and metabolism of water-soluble vita-

mins in intestine and kidney. Symposium Report. Fed. Proc. *43*:2423, 1984.

30. Harper, H.A., Rodwell, V.A., Mayes, P.A.: Review of Physiological Chemistry, Ch. 13. Los Altos, CA, Lange Medical Publications, 1979.

31. White, A., Handler, P., Smith, E.L., et al.: Principles of Biochemistry. New York, McGraw-Hill, 1978.

32. Kratzer, F.H., Williams, D.E.: Poul. Sci. *27*:518, 1948.

33. Milligan, J.L., Briggs, Jr., G.M.; Poul. Sci. *28*:202, 1949.

34. Gries, C.L., Scott, M.L.: J. Nutr. *102*:1269, 1972.

35. Schulman, M.P., Reichert, D.A.: J. Biol. Chem. *226*:181, 1957.

36. Axelrod, A.E., Hopper, S.: J. Nutr. *72*:325, 1960.

37. Eida, K., Kubato, N., Nishigaki, T., et al.: Chem. Pharm. Bull. *23*:1, 1975.

38. Axelrod, A.E.: Am. J. Clin. Nutr. *24*:265, 1971.

39. Pietrzik, K., Hesse, C., Hötzel, D.: Int. J. Vitam. Nutr. Res. *45*:251, 1975.

40. Williams, M.A., Chu, L.-C., McIntosh, D.J., et al.: J. Nutr. *94*:377, 1968.

41. Pietrzik, K., Hesse, C., Wiesch, E.S.Z., et al.: Int. J. Vitam. Nutr. Res. *45*:153, 1975.

42. Nelson, R.A.: Am. J. Clin. Nutr. *21*:495, 1968.

43. Gershoff, S.N., Gottlieb, L.S.: J. Nutr. *82*:135, 1964.

44. Follis, R.H.: Pantothenic acid. *In* Deficiency Disease. Springfield, IL, Charles C Thomas, 1958.

45. Hodges, R.E., Bean, W.B., Ohlson, M.A., et al.: J. Clin. Invest. *38*:1421, 1959.

46. Fry, P.C., Fox, H.M., Tao, H.G.: J. Nutr. Sci. Vitaminol. *22*:339, 1976.

47. Ralli, E.P., Dumm, M.E.: Relation of pantothenic acid to adrenal cortical function. *In* Vitamins and Hormones, Vol. 11. (Harris, R.S., Marrian, G.F., Thimann, K.V., Eds.) New York, Academic Press, 1953.

48. Harris, R.S., Lepkovsky, S.: Pantothenic acid. *In* The Vitamins: Chemistry, Physiology, Pathology, Vol. 2. (Sebrell, Jr., W.H., Harris, R.S., Eds.) New York, Academic Press, 1954.

49. Recommended Dietary Allowances, 9th ed.: Committee on Dietary Allowances and Food and Nutrition Board, National Research Council, National Academy of Science, Washington, DC, 1980.

50. Briggs, M. (Ed.): Vitamins in Human Biology and Medicine. Boca Raton, FL, CRC Press, 1981.

51. Sauberlich, H.E., Skala, J.H., Dowdy, R.P.: Laboratory Tests for the Assessment of Nutritional Status. Boca Raton, FL, CRC Press, 1974.

52. Sauberlich, H.E., Logan, N.M.: Vitamins. *In* Clinical Guide to Laboratory Tests (Tietz, N.W., Ed.) Philadelphia, W.B. Saunders, 1983.

53. Ellestad, J.J., Nelson, R.A., Adson, M.A., et al.: Fed. Proc. *29*:820, 1970.

54. Sarma, P.S., Menon, P.S., Venkatachalan, P.S.: Curr. Sci. *18*:367, 1949.

55. Wright, L.D.: Pantothenic acid. *In* Present Knowledge in Nutrition, 4th ed. (Hegsted, D.M., et al., Eds.) Washington, DC, The Nutrition Foundation, 1976.

56. Wyse, B.W., Wittmer, C., Hansen, R.G.: Clin. Chem. *25*:108, 1979.

57. McCormick, D.B., Wright, L.D. (Eds.): Vitamins and Coenzymes. Methods in Enzymology, Vol. 18, Part A. New York, Academic Press, 1970.

58. McCormick, D.B., Wright, L.D. (Eds.): Vitamins and Coenzymes. Methods in Enzymology, Vol. 62, Part D. New York, Academic Press, 1979.

*Chapter* **21**

# FOLIC ACID AND VITAMIN B$_{12}$

## Victor D. Herbert and Neville Colman

## HISTORY

The unraveling of the relation of vitamin B$_{12}$ and folic acid to anemia traces back almost two centuries.[1–3] In 1822, physician Combe reported to the Royal Medical and Surgical Society of Edinburgh on the "history of a case of anemia" which he surmised was due to "some disorder of the digestive and assimilative organs."[4] Thus was launched the study of pernicious anemia in particular and megaloblastic anemia in general, after restimulation by physician Thomas Addison's description, in 1849 and 1855,[5] of what his contemporaries evidently recognized as pernicious anemia, even though he did not mention the characteristic glossitis, jaundice, or nerve damage. He did mention "the disease having uniformly occurred in fat people," which would imply deficiency of vitamin B$_{12}$ rather than of folate; deficiency of the latter tends to be associated with wasting.

The nutritional basis of pernicious anemia was suspected by the American physician Austin Flint in 1860, when he stated that "in these cases there exists degenerative disease of the glandular tubuli of the stomach."[6] Another two thirds of a century had passed when the classic work of physician William Castle and his associates demonstrated that normal human gastric juice contains an "intrinsic factor" (i.e., within the body) that combines with an "extrinsic factor" (i.e., outside the body—in food) contained in animal protein to result in absorption of the "antipernicious anemia principle."[7] Vitamin B$_{12}$ was finally reported as isolated in 1948 in the United States,[8] and three weeks later, entirely independently in England,[9] Berk and his associates[10] showed that this vitamin was "extrinsic factor" and "antipernicious anemia principle."

Early reports of disease now recognizable as probable folate deficiency include those of Channing[11] and Barclay,[12] who reported a severe form of anemia in pregnancy and the puerperium, which was often fatal when it resulted from the nutritional drains of several pregnancies superimposed on a nutritionally inadequate diet. Osler postulated that megaloblastic anemia of pregnancy and the puerperium was "caused by an agent which differs from that which causes the anemia of Addison."[13] Support for this hypothesis emerged a decade later when Wills and her associates described a macrocytic anemia in Hindu women in Bombay, usually associated with pregnancy,[14] that responded to therapy with a commercial preparation of autolyzed yeast called marmite (still a favored home remedy in Commonwealth countries). By feeding the same type of diet ingested by their patients to monkeys, they produced in them a similar macrocytic anemia that responded to a "Wills factor" present in crude but not purified liver extracts.

We now know that the more purified extract consisted of a fairly pure solution of vitamin $B_{12}$, and that the Wills factor removed from the crude liver extract in the process of purification is folic acid. This fact gradually became clear after the purification of pteroylglutamic acid in 1943 by Stokstad,[15] its crystallization from liver in the same year by Pfiffner and associates,[16] its synthesis and structural identification by Angier and his co-workers,[17] and the 1948 isolation of crystalline vitamin $B_{12}$. The rapid isolation of vitamin $B_{12}$ by the American workers was greatly aided by a microbiologic assay based on Shorb's[18] discovery that "LLD factor," a growth factor required by *Lactobacillus lactis Dorner*, was not only the "animal protein factor" necessary for proper growth and function in animals fed an all-vegetable diet. It was also present in liver extracts in amounts that closely paralleled their potency in the treatment of pernicious anemia.

Folic acid proved to be not only the Wills factor but also the vitamin M contained in dried brewer's yeast that corrected the deficiency anemia, leukopenia, diarrhea, and gingivitis of monkeys studied by Day and associates.[19] It also proved to be the vitamin $B_c$ contained in yeast that corrected the deficiency syndrome in chicks characterized by anemia and growth failure. Furthermore, folic acid proved to be the norite eluate factor (i.e., it could be adsorbed on and eluted from charcoal) of liver, described by Snell and Peterson[20] as essential to the growth of *Lactobacillus casei* (and therefore also called the "*L. casei* factor"). The term *folic acid* was coined by Mitchell and co-workers[21] because they found this material in a leafy vegetable (spinach). At that time, it was not recognized that vitamin $B_{12}$, and not folic acid, was the active ingredient in the oral liver therapy that Minot and Murphy reported in 1926 as successful in treating pernicious anemia[22] (for which work they received the Nobel Prize in Medicine in 1934).

# CHEMISTRY[3,23,23a,23b,23c,24,24a,24b,24c,24d]

Neither cyanocobalamin nor pteroylglutamic acid, the common pharmaceutical forms of vitamin $B_{12}$ and folic acid, is present as such in significant quantity in either the human body or the various foods from which these agents were isolated. In the body and in foods, they are present in various reduced metabolically active coenzyme forms, often conjugated (in the case of vitamin $B_{12}$ to peptide and in the case of folate to one or more glutamates) in peptide linkage. During the extraction procedure, these labile active forms are either destroyed by oxidation (particularly folates) or oxidized and converted to cyanocobalamin or pteroylglutamic acid, which are the stable forms of the respective vitamins. These stable forms are partially oxidized and not known to be metabolically active; not until they are reduced by metabolic systems present within gut and other tissue cells do they become metabolically active cobalamins or folates.

## Vitamin $B_{12}$[3,23,23a,23b,23c,25–27]

Figure 21–1 shows the structural formula of vitamin $B_{12}$ (cyanocobalamin): Delineation of this structure, using x-ray crystallography, by Hodgkin and her co-workers was partly responsible for her winning the 1964 Nobel Prize in Chemistry. The chemistry of the vitamin has been repeatedly reviewed.[23,23a,23b,23c] The two major portions of the molecule are the corrin nucleus (a planar group) and a "nucleotide" lying in a plane nearly at right angles to the corrin nucleus and linked to it by D-1-amino-2-propanol. The "nucleotide" (5-6-dimethylbenzimidazole) is attached to ribose by an alpha-glycoside linkage. A second bond between the two major parts of the molecule is the coordinate linkage of the cobalt atom to one of the nitrogen atoms of the "nucleotide."

In cyanocobalamin, the anionic (–R) group in coordinate linkage with the cobalt is cyanide. Fortunately, the original isolation of $B_{12}$ from liver yielded a stable product, cyanocobalamin, because the unstable linkage of the 5'-deoxyadenosyl anionic group to the rest of the molecule in coenzyme $B_{12}$ (the form naturally dominant in liver) was ruptured and replaced by cyanide, which leached from the charcoal columns used in the isolation procedure.

Cyanocobalamin crystals are dark red and the substance absorbs water. The official product in the USP contains 12% absorbed moisture. Cobalamins are destroyed by heavy metals and strong oxidizing or reducing agents, but not by autoclaving for short periods at 121°C. Ascorbate and other nutrients that are strong reducing agents, when placed in solution with cobalamins, destroy co-

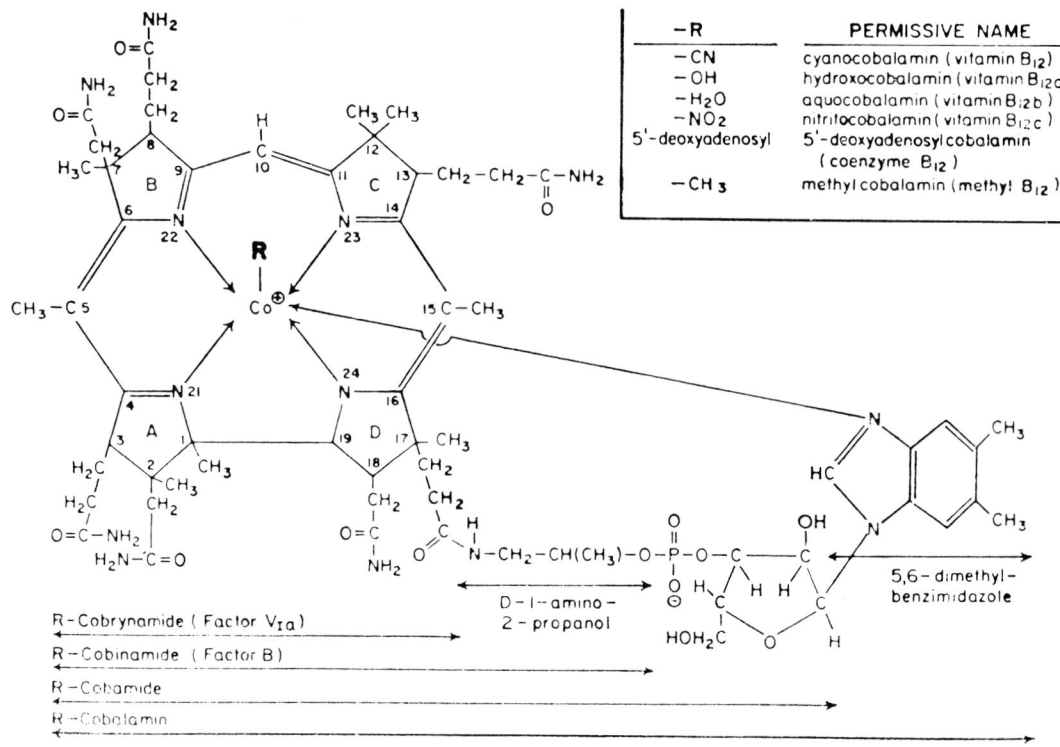

**Fig. 21–1.** Structural formula of vitamin $B_{12}$ (cyanocobalamin). The numbering system for the corrin nucleus is made to correspond to that of the porphin nucleus by omitting the number 20. (Modified from Brown and Reynolds: Annu. Rev. Biochem. *32*:419, 1963.)

balamins by converting them to various analogues,[27a] some of which may actually block cobalamin metabolism (i.e., function as antimetabolites).[27b] Cyanocobalamin is soluble 1:80 in water, and stable in solution. Aqueous solutions are neutral; maximal stability is at pH 4.5 to 5, making this the favored pH for extracting the vitamin from foods and tissues.

Coenzyme $B_{12}$ (5-deoxyadenosylcobalamin) and methylcobalamin (methyl-$B_{12}$) are the two vitamin $B_{12}$ coenzymes known to be metabolically active in mammalian tissues. Both should be extracted in the dark[27c] because they are unstable in light and undergo photolysis with formation of aquocobalamin or, in the presence of potassium cyanide, cyanocobalamin. Under the rules of the International Union of Pure and Applied Chemistry (IUPAC) Commission on Biochemical Nomenclature,[28] cyanocobalamin is a permissive (semisystematic) name for vitamin $B_{12}$, and the term vitamin $B_{12}$ without qualification means cyanocobalamin exclusively. However, the term is also entrenched in the literature as a generic term for all the cobalamins active in man. The permissive term cobalamin (or vitamin $B_{12}$) is used to describe the vitamin $B_{12}$ molecule minus the cyanide group, and is prefixed by the desig-

nation of the anionic R group (Fig. 21–1) attached to the cobalt. The terms coenzyme $B_{12}$ and vitamin $B_{12}$ coenzyme are not interchangeable; the former means 5'-deoxyadenosylcobalamin exclusively, and the latter applies to any coenzyme form of $B_{12}$.

Figure 21–1 delineates some of the family of natural and semisynthetic cobalamins; others include dicyanocobalamin, thiocyanatocobalamin, chlorocobalamin, and sulfitocobalamin. The alphabetic congeners of vitamin $B_{12}$ ($B_{12a}$, $B_{12b}$, $B_{12c}$) listed on this figure are believed to be equipotent in treatment of vitamin $B_{12}$ deficiency (unless that deficiency is due to a congenital or acquired defect in enzymes involved in converting one $B_{12}$ form to another). However, minimal dose therapy (0.1 µg daily) suggests[29] that coenzyme $B_{12}$ is more potent therapeutically than cyanocobalamin. Therapy with doses greater than minimal is always used clinically, and all forms of $B_{12}$ appear equipotent when used in greater than minimal doses.

## Folic Acid[3,24,24a,24b,24c,24d,30]

Figure 21–2 presents the structural formula of folic acid (pteroylglutamic acid [PteGlu or PteGlu₁]), the reference compound of the folate vi-

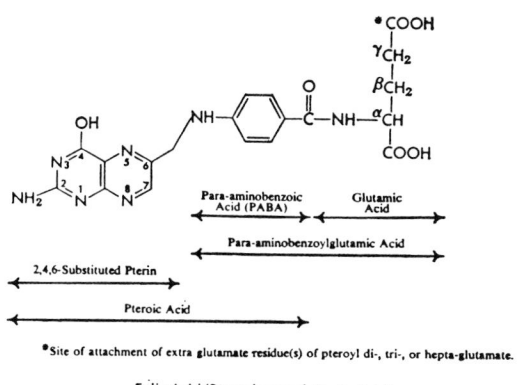

Fig. 21–2. Structural formula of folic acid (pteroylglutamic acid). (From Herbert,[3] with permission of Macmillan Publishing Co., Inc.)

tamin forms. Because it is an oxidized and therefore more stable form, it is the pharmaceutical form usually used therapeutically. Oxidized forms of folate cannot function in one-carbon metabolism in humans until converted by tissue enzymes to reduced forms. Reduced forms are the ones normally found in food and tissues. The major subunits of the molecule are the pteridine moiety linked by a methylene bridge to para-aminobenzoic acid, which is joined by peptide linkage to glutamic acid.

Crystalline folic acid is yellow. The free acid is almost insoluble in cold water, but the disodium salt is more soluble (about 1.5 g/dl). Injectable solutions are prepared by dissolving folic acid in isotonic sodium bicarbonate solution, or by using the disodium salt. Folic acid is destroyed at pH below 4, but is relatively stable above pH 5, with no destruction in one hour at 100°C. The molecule usually splits into pteridine and para-aminobenzoyl glutamate.

The nomenclature of folic acid and its derivatives is currently undergoing revision. Recommendations of an advisory panel to Commissions on Nomenclature of the International Union of Biochemistry (IUB) and the International Union of Pure and Applied Chemistry (IUPAC)[28] are that

> "Folate and folic acid are the preferred synonyms for pteroylglutamte and pteroylglutamic acid, respectively...The term folates may also be used in a generic sense to designate any member of the family of pteroylglutamates, or mixtures of them, having various levels of reduction of the pteridine ring, one-carbon substitutions, and numbers of glutamate residues."

The term "folacin" is no longer to be used.

Pteroylglutamic acid, an oxidized compound, is not normally found as such in foods or in the human body in significant concentrations. The

forms that are found in such sources are the reduced forms indicated in Figure 21–3. They differ from the parent compound by virtue of one to three structural modifications. First, all are reduced folates and, except for 7,8-dihydrofolate, all are 5,6,7,8-tetrahydrofolates (THF). Second, as indicated in Figure 21–3, various 1-carbon adducts may be linked to THF at the N-5, N-10, or 5,10 position, conferring on folates their role as 1-carbon carriers. It has been suggested that only five natural 1-carbon substitutions are on THF, and that N[5] formyl THF (folinic acid, citrovorum factor) represents nonenzymatic conversion of folate during processing of natural materials.[30] Third, the number of glutamate residues may vary from one to seven, and sometimes up to 11, each linked by peptide bonds between its amino group and the gamma-carboxyl group of the preceding glutamate (see Fig. 21–2).

## UNITS OF MEASUREMENT AND METHODS OF ASSAY

### Vitamin B$_{12}$[3,23,23a,23b,23c,32–35]

Human serum levels of vitamin B$_{12}$ are measured in picograms (pg: 10$^{-12}$ grams, also called μμg [micromicrograms]) per ml of serum. Normal values range from 200 to 900 pg/ml; below 80 pg/ml represents unequivocal B$_{12}$ deficiency according to the WHO Scientific Group on Nutritional Anemias.[31,31a,31b] However, the level below which one can state there is unequivocal deficiency actually varies from laboratory to laboratory depending on microbiologic or radioassay methodology used; there is no "gold standard" method for assay.[31,31a,31b,32a,35h] In fact, as vitamin B$_{12}$ deficiency develops, B$_{12}$ *analogue* levels may rise,[32b] making assays that measure total corrinoids instead of cobalamins alone unreliable.[32c] The tiny quantity of vitamin B$_{12}$ activity in human serum may be measured only microbiologically or by radioassay. Many microoganisms require vitamin B$_{12}$ in order to grow, and therefore there are many microbiologic assays for vitamin B$_{12}$. Radioassay has the advantage over microbiologic assay that false low results do not occur if serum contains antibiotics or other substances that inhibit growth of microorganisms, causing the microbiologic assays to yield false low results. Additionally, one can perform differential radioassay to separate cobalamins from other corrinoids,[32c,32d] which cannot be adequately done by differential microbiologic assay.[32e,32f,32g] Radioassay for vitamin B$_{12}$ was first described by Herbert in 1958.[33] The most widely employed assay uses coated charcoal[34,35] to separate free from bound vitamin B$_{12}$, but many

| | R | OXIDATION STATE |
|---|---|---|
| $N^5$ formyl THFA | —CHO | formate |
| $N^{10}$ formyl THFA | —CHO | formate |
| $N^5$ formimino THFA | —CH=NH | formate |
| $N^{5,10}$ methenyl THFA | >CH | formate |
| $N^{5,10}$ methylene THFA | >CH₂ | formaldehyde |
| $N^5$ methyl THFA | —CH₃ | methanol |

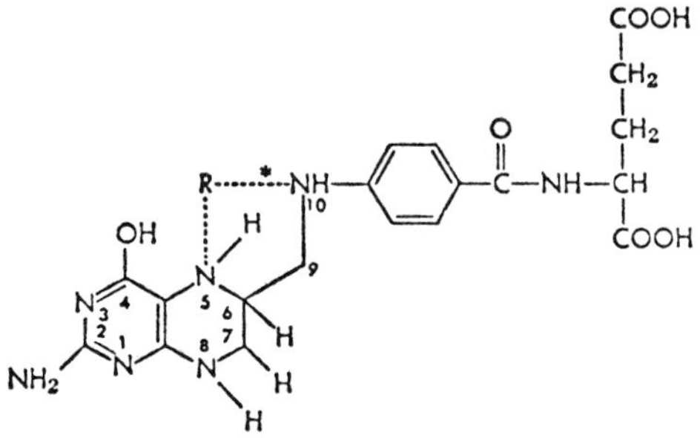

*Broken lines indicate the $N^5$ and/or $N^{10}$ site of attachment of various 1-carbon units for which THFA acts as a carrier.

5,6,7,8-Tetrahydrofolic Acid (THFA)(FH₄)(R==—H)

**Fig. 21–3.** Structures and nomenclature in the folate field. The table above the formula lists some of the possible 1-carbon adducts formed with THFA. (From Herbert[3] with permission of Macmillan Publishing Co., Inc.)

other satisfactory separation methods exist.[23,23a,23b,23c,31,31a,31b,32a]

Human serum and tissues contain not only biologically active "true B₁₂" (i.e., cobalamins), but also analogues (i.e., noncobalamin corrinoids) of varying to no activity; some may even be antimetabolites.[32a–g,35b–g] Radioassays that do not use pure intrinsic factor or impure intrinsic factor with its nonintrinsic factor blocked by an analogue (which binds only "true B₁₂," i.e., "true cobalamins")[35a] measure "total B₁₂" ("total corrinoids," i.e., cobalamins plus noncobalamin analogues) rather than "true B₁₂." Thus they may not pick up early vitamin B₁₂ deficiency, since in early deficiency only that portion of "total B₁₂" that is "true B₁₂" may fall, and analogues may still be in the normal range[32c,35b,35c] or may even rise.[32b] In addition, heat plus the presence of large amounts of vitamin C or other nutrients with strong reducing activity may destroy vitamin B₁₂ unless the B₁₂ is protected by cyanide, –S, or another protective mechanism.[27a,27b,35d]

Differential radioassay is necessary to distinguish cobalamin from noncobalamin corrinoids in human serum,[32c] erythrocytes,[35e] liver,[35e] nervous system,[35e] and bile.[35f] Differential microbiologic assays are incapable of doing so. Workers unaware

of this fact represented that the early data of Herbert et al. on B₁₂ destruction by vitamin C was incorrect. In fact, the vitamin C converted the vitamin B₁₂ to noncobalamin corrinoids that nondifferential microbiologic assays and radioassays were unable to distinguish from true B₁₂.[35d–f]

Larger quantities of vitamin B₁₂ than those present in human serum may be assayed colorimetrically, spectroscopically, fluorometrically, or chemically. A serum standard was proposed.[35h]

The USP assay for vitamin B₁₂ in pharmaceutical preparations is spectrophotometric. Although liver extract for injection was deleted from the USP in 1960, such largely obsolete often allergenic products are still being used, assayed by a nondifferential microbiologic method for their "vitamin B₁₂" content, despite the fact that some of this "B₁₂" is noncobalamin analogues.[35e,f] Differential radioassay demonstrates that 10 to 30% of "B₁₂" in multivitamin-mineral pills may be such analogues.[32g]

## Folic Acid[3,35–37]

Normal human serum contains 5 to 16 nanograms (ng: $10^{-9}$ grams; mμg [millimicrograms]) of folic acid activity (i.e., PteGlu equivalents) per ml. These tiny quantities could be measured only microbiologically, as originally described in 1959,[38–42] until a radioisotopic assay was described in 1970.[43,43a] The dominant folate in serum and red cells is 5-methyltetrahydrofolate, and folate assays must therefore be capable of measuring this derivative. Because *Lactobacillus casei* is the only microorganism known to grow well on this folate, the only microbiologic assay that adequately measures serum and red cell folate uses *L. casei*. Similarly, the only radioassays that accurately measure serum folate are those that measure 5-methyltetrahydrofolate; these are mainly done at pH 9.3, where folic acid (used as a stable standard) and serum folate have similar reactivity.[44]

Simultaneous radioisotope determinations of serum vitamin $B_{12}$ and folate can be done in the same test tube. The results correlate well with those of other radioassays. This procedure considerably simplifies assay of the two vitamins.[45,46] It may be the method of choice for use in most laboratories.

Because serum folate is labile, false low values for serum folate activity occur if the serum has not been protected against oxidative destruction before assay. Such protection is brought about by storing the serum frozen, storing it in the presence of a reducing agent such as ascorbate, or both. It must be remembered that ascorbate may destroy $B_{12}$ in storage.[35d]

Larger quantities of folate activity than those normally present in human serum may be measured chemically, fluorometrically, by paper and thin-layer chromatography, enzymatically, or by animal assay.[35a]

## CAUSES OF NUTRITIONAL DEFICIENCY

In the final analysis, nutritional deficiency means there is inadequate usage of a nutrient in one or more intracellular systems to sustain normal biochemical functions. Such inadequate usage falls in one or more of six basic categories: inadequate ingestion, inadequate absorption, inadequate utilization, increased requirement, increased excretion, and increased destruction. Any one or combination of these three inadequacies and three excesses may result in nutritional deficiency. Table 21–1 presents the currently known possible etiologic factors in each of these six categories that may produce nutritional deficiency of vitamin $B_{12}$ or folic acid. The ensuing sections will discuss in more detail mechanisms of inadequate absorption and utilization of these two vitamins.

## ABSORPTION

### Vitamin $B_{12}$[3,23,23a,23b,23c,47–51a–e]

There are two separate and distinct mechanisms for the absorption of vitamin $B_{12}$. The *physiologic* mechanism, the derangement of which accounts for much human vitamin $B_{12}$ deficiency, is capable of handling a maximum of 1.5 to 3 μg of free vitamin $B_{12}$ at any one time. This mechanism operates as follows: (1) Ingested vitamin $B_{12}$ is freed from its polypeptide linkages to food by gastric acid and gastric and intestinal enzymes. (2) The free vitamin $B_{12}$ attaches to salivary R binder in preference to the gastric intrinsic factor (IF) of Castle (a glycoprotein of molecular weight in the range of 50,000, produced by normal gastric parietal cells, which dimerizes on combination with vitamin $B_{12}$ so that a complex is formed containing two molecules of vitamin $B_{12}$). (3) The salivary R binder is destroyed by pancreatic trypsin, releasing $B_{12}$ onto IF to create the $B_{12}$-IF complex, which is carried down to the ileum, where it attaches to receptors for $B_{12}$-IF on the brush border of the ileal mucosal cells in the presence of ionic calcium and a pH above 6. (4) Via a currently uncertain mechanism, the vitamin $B_{12}$ is released from the $B_{12}$-IF complex probably at (but possibly within) the ileal enterocyte (epithelial cell). (5) The vitamin then finds its way across the enterocyte into the portal venous blood, at which point it is attached to serum vitamin $B_{12}$-binding proteins, perhaps having attached to transcobalamin (TC) II in the enterocyte.[93b] Bicarbonate and trypsin from the pancreas facilitate this mechanism by selectively destroying R binders.[51b,51c,78c] Pancreatic enzymes similarly effect transfer of biliary cobalamin from R binder to intrinsic factor, creating much of the enterohepatic cobalamin circulation[78b–d] so important to the vitamin $B_{12}$ economy of the vegetarian. R binder (particularly TC III) delivers $B_{12}$ and analogues to the liver but not to other tissues. TC II preferentially binds cobalamins and delivers them to all tissues that need them. TC II is to cobalamin economy what transferrin is to iron economy. Holo-TC III is more a reflection of cobalamin stores.

The other, or *pharmacologic*, mechanism of vitamin $B_{12}$ absorption appears to be diffusion.[48,48a] It accounts for the absorption along the entire length of the small intestine of approximately 1% of *any* quantity of *free* vitamin $B_{12}$ in the small bowel. This mechanism makes possible oral (rather than parenteral) therapy for vitamin $B_{12}$ deficiency caused by vitamin $B_{12}$ malabsorption. However, such therapy is less reliable than parenteral therapy.[3]

**Table 21–1.   Etiologic Classification of Megaloblastic Anemias: A Tabular Lexicon**

*I. Vitamin B₁₂ deficiency* (normal $B_{12}$ body stores last 3 to 6 years after cessation of $B_{12}$ absorption, but 20 to 30 years after cessation of only $B_{12}$ ingestion, because of continuation of reabsorption of the 3 to 6 μg of $B_{12}$ excreted daily in bile)

A. Inadequate ingestion
1. Poor diet (lacking microorganisms and animal foods, which are the sole $B_{12}$ sources)
   a. Strict vegetarianism (eating no meat, fowl, seafood, eggs, milk, or any products thereof)
   b. Chronic alcoholism (no $B_{12}$ or folate in hard liquor; folate deficiency occurs first, and is more common, partly because body stores of $B_{12}$ last much longer than those of folate)
   c. Poverty, religious tenets (Hinduism, Seventh-Day Adventism,* certain Catholic orders), dietary faddism
B. Inadequate absorption
1. Gastric disorder, producing inadequate or absent secretion by gastric parietal cells of intrinsic factor
   a. Addisonian pernicious anemia (PA—that form of $B_{12}$ deficiency disease due to inadequate intrinsic factor secretion of uncertain etiology)
      (1) Hereditary absence of normal intrinsic factor secretion; absent secretion at birth (circulating antibody to intrinsic factor never present; supports theory that antibody only occurs when antigenic stimulus is produced by intrinsic factor, which enters blood from damaged parietal cells and is recognized as foreign by the immunologic surveillance system); rare
      (2) Congenital production of defective intrinsic factor molecule (three published cases)
      (3) Autoimmunity-associated gastric atrophy. These patients usually have nondiagnostic-for-PA circulating parietal cell antibody which is index only of past or present gastric damage and *not* of amount of intrinsic factor secretion (circulating diagnostic-for-PA antibody to intrinsic factor is always present under age 21; there is a gradual decrease in measurable antibody, so that by age 65 only two thirds of patients present with measurable circulating antibody to intrinsic factor)
         (a) Juvenile pernicious anemia (usually presents between ages 3 and 14)
         (b) Hereditarily determined degenerative gastric atrophy (gradually progressing with increasing age; almost half of all adult PA cases fall in this category)

           (c) Acquired gastric atrophy as the end result of superficial inflammatory gastritis; superficial gastritis with atrophy (almost half of all adult PA cases fall in this category, which includes acquired gastric damage related to iron deficiency or alcohol)
           (d) Endocrine disorders (hypothyroidism, polyendocrinopathy) associated with gastric damage
   b. Gastrectomy
      (1) Total
      (2) Subtotal (approximately 20% develop PA within 10 years after surgery, associated with atrophy of remaining parietal cells)
         (a) Proximal
         (b) Distal
   c. Lesions that destroy the gastric mucosa (ingested corrosives, linitis plastica)
   d. Intrinsic factor inhibitor in gastric secretion
      (1) Antibody to intrinsic factor (in saliva or gastric juice)
         (a) "Blocking" antibody (attaches to intrinsic factor to block ability of intrinsic factor to take up $B_{12}$)
         (b) "Binding" antibody (attaches to intrinsic factor at site distal to site of $B_{12}$ attachment)
2. Small intestinal disorder (affecting ileum, which is the main site of $B_{12}$ absorption)
   a. Gluten-induced enteropathy (childhood and adult celiac disease); idiopathic steatorrhea; nontropical sprue
   b. Tropical sprue ($B_{12}$ is often the first nutrient to be subnormally absorbed and the last to return to normal absorption)
   c. Regional enteritis
   d. Strictures or anastomoses of the small bowel, other "stagnant bowel" syndromes
   e. Intestinal resection
   f. Cancers and granulomatous lesions involving the small intestine
   g. Other conditions characterized by chronically disturbed intestinal function
   h. Drugs damaging $B_{12}$ absorption
      (1) Para-aminosalicylic acid (PAS) (therapy of tuberculosis)
      (2) Colchicine (therapy of gout)
      (3) Neomycin (antimicrobial)
      (4) Ethanol (societal)
      (5) Metformin (and other biguanide oral antidiabetic agents?)
      (6) Oral contraceptive agents?
   i. Specific malabsorption for vitamin $B_{12}$
      (1) Due to long-term ingestion of calcium-chelating agents (ionic calcium required for $B_{12}$ absorption)

*Only 1–2% of Seventh-Day Adventists eat no animal foods.

**Table 21–1.  *Continued***

(2) Due to inadequately alkaline pH in ileum (Zollinger-Ellison syndrome, pancreatic disease) (pH >6 required for B$_{12}$ absorption)

(3) Unknown causes (lack of intestinal receptors for B$_{12}$-intrinsic factor complex? absence of "releasing factor"?)

(a) Congenital (Imerslund-Gräsbeck syndrome; receptors probably functioning)

(b) Acquired (forme fruste of sprue; receptors absent or nonfunctioning?)

3. Competition for vitamin B$_{12}$ by intestinal parasites or bacteria
   a. Fish tapeworm (*Diphyllobothrium latum;* decreasing in Finland because of pollution)
   b. Bacteria: The blind loop syndrome (B$_{12}$ adsorbing bacteria)

4. Pancreatic disease (normal pancreatic exocrine secretion of trypsin and bicarbonate required for normal B$_{12}$ absorption)

C. Inadequate utilization
   1. Vitamin B$_{12}$ antagonists
      a. Substituted B$_{12}$ amides and anilides (experimental agents)
      b. Cobaloximes (experimental agents)
      c. Anti-B$_{12}$ analogues?
   2. Congenital or acquired enzyme deficiency or deletion
      a. Methylmalonyl-CoA mutase
      b. Methyltetrahydrofolate-homocysteine methyltransferase
      c. B$_{12a}$ reductase
      d. B$_{12r}$ reductase
      e. Deoxyadenosyltransferase
      f. Other enzyme reduction or deletion
   3. Abnormal B$_{12}$-binding protein in serum, irreversibly binding B$_{12}$ and making it unavailable to tissues
      a. Increased TC I or TC III glycoprotein (myeloproliferative disorders—"granulocyte-related" B$_{12}$ binders)
      b. Increased TC II protein (liver disease; "liver-related" B$_{12}$ binders)
      c. Other abnormal B$_{12}$ binding (a glycoprotein in some hepatoma cases)
   4. Inadequate serum B$_{12}$-binding protein (congenital or acquired)
      a. TC II protein (lack produces megaloblastic anemia; it delivers B$_{12}$ to blood cells, as transferrin delivers iron)
      b. TC I glycoprotein (lack not known to produce megaloblastic anemia; it is mainly a storage protein for B$_{12}$, somewhat akin to ceruloplasmin for copper)
      c. TC III (larger amounts produced in vitro by granulocytes)
   5. Protein malnutrition?
   6. Cancer?
   7. Liver disease?
   8. Renal disease?
   9. Thiocyanate intoxication?

D. Increased requirement (normal adult daily requirement for exogenous sources is 0.1 μg)
   1. Hyperthyroidism
   2. Increased hematopoiesis?
   3. Infancy (increased requirement for growth)
   4. Parasitization
      a. By fetus
      b. By malignant tissue?
E. Increased excretion
   1. Inadequate B$_{12}$-binding protein in serum (inadequate TC II particularly?)
   2. Liver disease (inadequate storage capacity for B$_{12}$)
   3. Renal disease?
F. Increased destruction by antioxidants
   1. By pharmacologic doses of ascorbic acid

II. *Folic acid deficiency* (normal folate body stores will last only 3 to 6 months after cessation of folate ingestion or absorption)
   A. Inadequate ingestion
      1. Poor diet (lacking unprocessed fresh, uncooked, or slightly cooked food or fruit juices—folates are heat-labile)
         a. Nutritional megaloblastic anemia
            (1) Tropical
            (2) Nontropical
            (3) Scurvy (diets poor in vitamin C are also poor in folate)
         b. Chronic alcoholism with or without cirrhosis
   B. Inadequate absorption (affecting upper third of small intestine, which is the main site of folate absorption; since most food folates are in polyglutamate forms, biliary and intestinal gamma glutamyl conjugases are necessary to split off excess glutamates to make folates absorbable)
      1. Malabsorption syndromes
         a. Gluten-induced enteropathy (childhood and adult celiac disease; idiopathic steatorrhea, nontropical sprue; coincident B$_{12}$ malabsorption rare)
         b. Any other chronic functional or structural disorder involving the upper small intestine
            (1) Tropical sprue (coincident B$_{12}$ malabsorption almost invariably present)
            (2) Associated with herpetic and other skin disorders
         c. Drugs
            (1) Diphenylhydantoin (Dilantin—anticonvulsant)
            (2) Primidone (anticonvulsant)
            (3) Barbiturates
            (4) Oral contraceptive agents (?)
            (5) Cycloserine (tuberculosis)
            (6) Ethanol (societal)
            (7) Metformin (diabetes therapy)
            (8) Dietary amino acid excess of glycine or methionine
            (9) Nitrofurantoin? (antimicrobial)
            (10) Glutethimide? (sedative)
            (11) Cholestyramine
            (12) Salicylazosulfapyridine (Azulfidine)

**Table 21–1.** *Continued*

2. Specific malabsorption for folate
   a. Congenital nonconjugase defects (four cases published)
   b. Acquired nonconjugase defects
   c. Inadequate biliary or intestinal conjugase
   d. Conjugase inhibitors (such as contained in some beans)
3. Blind loop syndrome (folate-greedy bacteria; more commonly, bacteria make folate and actually raise serum folate level of host)

C. Inadequate utilization (metabolic block)
1. Folic acid antagonists (dihydrofolate reductase inhibitors)
   a. 4-amino-4-deoxyfolates (i.e., methotrexate)    (Chemotherapy, immunosuppression, psoriasis)
   b. 2,4-Diaminopyrimidine
      Pyrimethamine    (Malaria, toxoplasmosis)
      Trimethoprim    (Antibacterial)
   c. Triamterene    (Diuretic)
   d. Diamidine compounds (i.e., pentamidine isothionate)    (*Pneumocystis carinii,* protozoacidal)
2. Diphenylhydantoin and possibly other anticonvulsants (possibly block cell uptake or use of folate)
3. Enzyme deficiency
   a. Congenital
      (1) Formiminotranferase
      (2) Dihydrofolate reductase
      (3) Methyltetrahydrofolate transmethylase
      (4) Other enzymes (some secondarily affect folate)
   b. Acquired
      (1) Liver disease
         (a) Formiminotransferase
         (b) Other enzymes
4. Vitamin B₁₂ deficiency (reduces folate uptake and retention by cells)
5. Alcohol (both specific and nonspecific damage to folate metabolism)
6. Ascorbic acid deficiency (increased hematopoiesis associated with bleeding reduces folate stores; may also decrease ability of body to retain folates in their metabolically active reduced state)
7. Dietary amino acid excess (glycine, methionine)

D. Increased requirement (normal adult daily requirement from exogenous sources is 50 µg)
1. Parasitization
   a. By fetus (especially in multiple and twin pregnancies)
   b. By malignant tissue (especially lymphoproliferative disorders)
   c. By breast-fed infant
2. Infancy (increased requirement for growth)
3. Increased hematopoiesis (hemolytic anemias; chronic blood loss, including scurvy)
4. Increased metabolic activity (hyperthyroidism, chronic temperature elevations)
5. Lesch-Nyhan syndrome
6. Drugs (L-Dopa?)

E. Increased excretion
1. Vitamin B₁₂ deficiency? (? of obligatory excretion of folate in urine and bile; possible inability to reabsorb methylfolate excreted in bile because B₁₂ required for it)
2. Liver disease?
3. Kidney dialysis
4. Chronic exfoliative dermatitis

F. Increased destruction
1. Oxidant in diet?

III. *Interference with purine ring synthesis and interconversion of purine bases*
A. Purine antagonists
1. 6-Mercaptopurine (6-MP)    Chemotherapy, immunosuppression
2. Thioguanine    Chemotherapy, immunosuppression
3. Azathioprine    Immunosuppression

B. Enzymatic defects in ability to make purine nucleotide from preformed bases
1. Lesch-Nyhan syndrome (there is an associated increased requirement for folate, which is needed at two steps in the increased de novo biosynthesis of purine)

IV. *Interference with pyrimidine synthesis*
A. Pyrimidine antagonists
1. 5-Fluorouracil (5-FU) (blocks thymidylate synthetase)    Chemotherapy
2. 6-Azauridine    Chemotherapy, psoriasis

B. Enzymatic defects in ability to make pyrimidine
1. Hereditary oroticaciduria (not responsive to therapy with vitamin B₁₂ or folic acid, but responsive to yeast extract or its active ingredients, uridine or the pyrimidine nucleotides, cytidylic, and uridylic acids)

V. *Inhibition of ribonucleotide reductase (cytidylic to deoxycytidylic acid)*
A. Cytosine arabinoside (inhibits DNA polymerase also)    Chemotherapy, antiviral
B. Hydroxyurea    Chemotherapy, psoriasis
C. Iron deficiency: Iron is required for ribonucleotide reductase, but it is not yet established that lack of iron can produce megaloblastosis; some workers have reported hypersegmented polys in iron deficiency that disappear with iron therapy, but coincident folate deficiency has not been excluded fully
D. Procarbazine (depolymerizes DNA)

VI. *Inhibition of protein synthesis*
A. L-Asparaginase    Chemotherapy

**Table 21–1.** *Continued*

| | |
|---|---|
| *VII. Mechanism unknown*<br>   A. Benzene       Solvent<br>   B. Azulfidine     Ulcerative colitis<br>   C. Arsenic        Poison<br>   D. Pyridoxine-responsive megaloblastic anemia (only about 10% of patients with pyridoxine-responsive sideroblastic anemia have megaloblastic morphology)<br>   E. Thiamin-responsive megaloblastic anemia (one case reported)<br>   F. Megaloblastoid anemias (differentiated from megaloblastic anemias by bizarre morphology, including marked polyploidy, few to no orthochromatic megaloblasts, tendency to hyposegmentation, and sometimes karyorrhexis in nucleated red cells) | 1. DiGuglielmo syndrome (erythremic myelosis—a myeloproliferative disorder usually presenting as refractory anemia and eventuating in death from "erythroleukemia" or myelogenous leukemia); preleukemia<br>2. Occasional cases of polycythemia vera and other myeloproliferative disorders<br>3. Occasional cases of aplastic anemia (which may subsequently develop myeloproliferative disorders)<br>4. Occasional cases of miliary tuberculosis (in such cases, the megaloblastoid marrow is often accompanied by monocytosis and leukopenia or leukocytosis) |

## Folate[3,24,24a,24b,24c,24d,48,48a,52,53]

Current evidence suggests that food folate is absorbed primarily from the proximal third of the small intestine, although it is capable of being absorbed from the entire length of the small bowel. Folate in food is present primarily in polyglutamate form. Before absorption, the "excess" glutamates must be split off the side chain of the vitamin molecule by conjugases (pteroylpolyglutamate hydrolase). The products of conjugase action are detectable in the intestinal lumen before absorption,[54] and preliminary evidence suggests that this occurrence may be due to a surface-active brush border conjugase functionally and chromatographically distinguishable from intracellular conjugase.[55] Conjugase action may be specifically inhibited by food factors described in yeast and beans[56] and may be nonspecifically impaired at acid pH.[57]

However, impaired mucosal transport of monoglutamyl folates after deconjugation probably accounts for most instances of folate malabsorption. Active mucosal transport is accelerated by glucose[58] and galactose and impaired by unidentified factors present in many foods.[59,60] However, studies using milk folate binder suggest that folate uptake in the gut is facilitated by prior binding.[60a]

It is probable that a small but relatively unchanging percentage of ingested folate is absorbed by passive diffusion after deconjugation,[61] as is the case with vitamin B₁₂.

## TRANSPORT, DISTRIBUTION, STORAGE, FATE, AND EXCRETION

### Vitamin B₁₂ (Fig. 21–4A)[3,25,49,49a,62,62a,62b,63]

Vitamin B₁₂ in human serum is bound to three different vitamin B₁₂-binding proteins: transcobalamins I, II, and III (TC I, TC II, TC III). The normal total vitamin B₁₂-binding capacity (TBBC)

of serum ranges from about 1000 to 1800 pg/ml, and the unsaturated vitamin B₁₂-binding capacity (UBBC) ranges from 600 to 1400 pg/ml, normally largely (450 to 1000 pg/ml) due to TC II.[64] TC I and TC III are glycoproteins that are synthesized largely in granulocytes,[63,63a,63b,63c] but possibly also in salivary glands, gastric mucosa, and some hepatomas.[65,65a,65b] They have a molecular weight of about 60,000, and appear to have largely a storage function, although TC III may be involved in redelivery of vitamin B₁₂ to the liver, to which TC III may attach via a terminal galactose.[63,63a,63b,63c,65a,65b] The amounts of unsaturated TC I and TC III in serum range from 30 to 110 and 120 to 300 pg/ml respectively.[64] These glycoproteins are referred to by some as cobalophilins (R proteins). They are microheterogeneous mixtures of various isoproteins in different proportions.[65,65a,65b,65c]

TBBC, UBBC, and serum vitamin B₁₂ levels all tend to be elevated in any situation in which the total body neutrophil pool is increased (as in myeloproliferative disorders). This elevation is caused by an increase in the amounts of unsaturated TC I and TC III.[66] These glycoproteins, however, do not deliver vitamin B₁₂ to the bone marrow, as illustrated by the following: one patient with chronic myelogenous leukemia and pernicious anemia had a normal serum vitamin B₁₂ level because of these glycoproteins and yet the tissues were starved of the vitamin to the point where biochemical deficiency was severe.[67]

Further evidence that TC I and TC III do not participate in transport of the vitamin to bone marrow and nervous tissue is provided by the report of two brothers with congenital lack of these proteins who had low serum vitamin B₁₂ levels but no hematologic or other manifestations of tissue B₁₂ deficiency.[63,63b,63c]

Unlike the cobalophilins (TC 1 and TC III), which are glycoproteins, TC II is a pure protein.

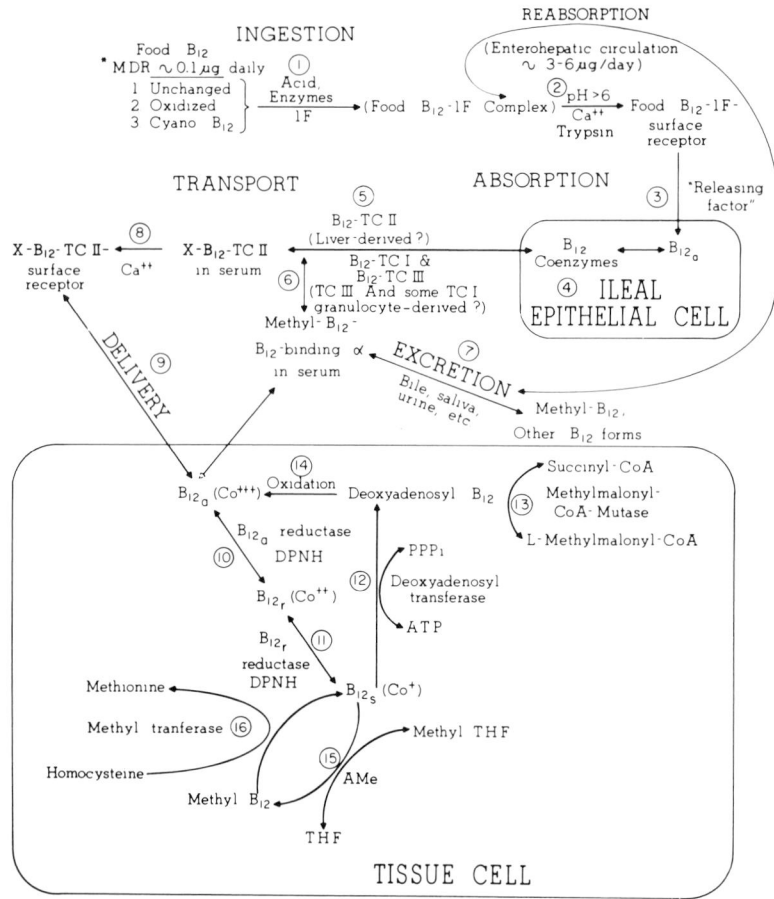

**Fig. 21–4.** *A*, Cobalamin (B$_{12}$) metabolism in man. (From Herbert[149] with permission of W.B. Saunders Co.)

It has an apparent molecular weight of 38,000,[65,65a,65b] is synthesized largely in the liver,[68-70] is a betaglobulin, and is chiefly responsible for transport and delivery of the vitamin. Relatively little vitamin B$_{12}$ is attached to it in vivo because of the rapidity with which it is degraded as it delivers B$_{12}$ to tissues. When a sample of blood is drawn, only 10 to 20% of plasma vitamin B$_{12}$ (which is mainly methyl-B$_{12}$) is bound to TC II; the rest is bound to cobalophilin, largely TC I (which is 80 to 100% saturated with B$_{12}$). The plasma survival time of TC III is very short (minutes) compared to TC II, which in turn is short (hours) compared to TC I (days) and the cobalophilins in chronic myelogenous leukemia and hepatoma.[65,65a,65b]

When it enters the blood, vitamin B$_{12}$ is bound by TCs in proportion to their binding capacity and delivered by TC II to liver, bone marrow cells, reticulocytes, lymphoblasts, fibroblasts, and tumor cells via a mechanism similar to that by which intrinsic factor delivers the vitamin to ileal

mucosal cells. Bone marrow cells, reticulocytes, and many other cells contain on their surfaces "receptor sites" for the TC II-B$_{12}$ complex. These sites will take up the complex only in the presence of ionic calcium and a pH greater than 6[71]; liver cells may contain receptor sites for TC III.[63,63a,63b,63c,65,65a,65b] Thus, delivery of B$_{12}$ to the gut enterocyte and the immature erythrocytes both require (1) a transport protein, (2) pH above 6, (3) ionic calcium, and (4) a receptor site for the protein-vitamin B$_{12}$ complex on the surface of the cell.

The importance of TC II in the absorption, transport, and delivery of vitamin B$_{12}$ to the tissues is emphasized by the finding of individuals with congenital absence of TC II who have defective vitamin B$_{12}$ delivery and therefore require treatment with large frequent parenteral doses of the vitamin.[72,73] The possible "acute phase reactant" status of TC II may be important,[73a] including elevated TC II in autoimmune disease.[73b]

"Normal" stores of vitamin B$_{12}$ range between 1 and 10 mg,[32,74,75] with the liver containing 50 to

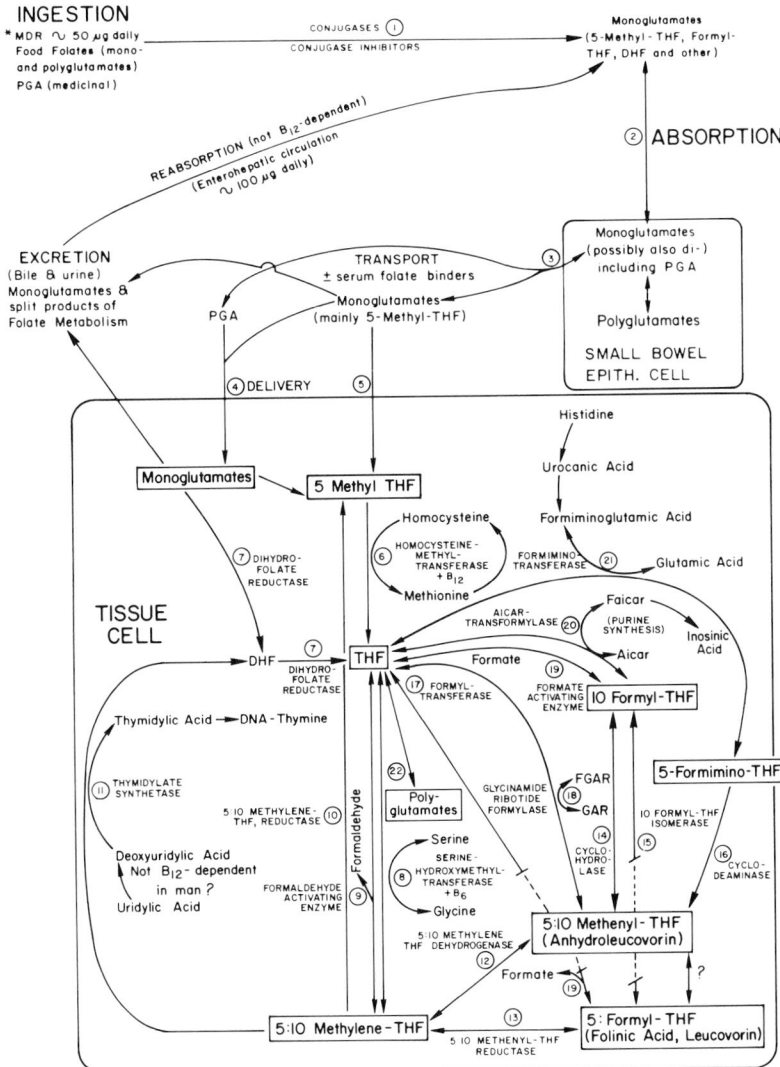

**Fig. 21–4.** *B,* Flow chart of folate metabolism in man. Circled numbers identify individual steps in folate metabolism. In mammals, the same enzyme catalyzes reactions 12, 14, and 19,[147] and another single enzyme catalyzes both steps 16 and 21.[148] THF = tetrahydrofolate, DHF = dihydrofolate. (From Herbert[149] with permission of W.B. Saunders Co.)

90% of the total stored vitamin (averaging 1 μg B$_{12}$/g of liver). Some of the stores are not cobalamins but rather noncobalamin analogues.[35e] Average vitamin B$_{12}$ stores range between 2 and 5 mg. There is little evidence for significant catabolism of vitamin B$_{12}$ by man, and it is probable that loss occurs only by excretion, mainly in the bile. The noncobalamin analogues do not appear to derive mainly by catabolism, but seem to be absorbed across the ileum.[35g] The whole-body turnover of vitamin B$_{12}$ is between 0.1 and 0.2% daily, regardless of whether body stores are normal or reduced. Coenzyme B$_{12}$ appears to be the main storage form, and methyl-B$_{12}$ appears to be the main serum transport form.[23,23a,23b,23c,25]

The normal enterohepatic circulation of vitamin B$_{12}$ may account for approximately 0.6 to 6 μg of the vitamin excreted daily in the bile and reabsorbed in the ileum.[3,76–78] This almost total conservation of vitamin B$_{12}$ explains why pure vegetarians, who eat almost no vitamin B$_{12}$, take decades to develop deficiency of the vitamin. It is only when the reabsorption phase of the enterohepatic circulation of the vitamin is damaged, by damage to the stomach, ileum, or pancreas, that vitamin B$_{12}$ deficiency disease develops more rapidly (i.e., in 3 to 6 years).[91a]

The effect of the enterohepatic circulation is to remove noncobalamin vitamin B$_{12}$ analogues from the body, because about 60% of the corrinoids excreted in bile are analogues,[78a,b] and cobalamin is normally preferentially reabsorbed over analogues.[78c] The role of noncobalamin vitamin B$_{12}$ analogues in human vitamin B$_{12}$ economy is unknown, but some may act as antivitamins and could prove harmful.[27a,b,32d] Although some have suggested that all noncobalamin corrinoids in humans derive from vitamin supplements fed to livestock and taken by humans, we found analogue levels of Americans similar to those in Kalahari Bushmen never exposed to supplements.[35f]

## Folate (Fig. 21–4*B*)[3,30,79–82]

Plasma transport of folate remains far less clearly elucidated than that of vitamin B$_{12}$. Folate in plasma appears to be distributed in three fractions. Free folate and that loosely bound to low-affinity binders are similar in magnitude, whereas much less is bound to high-affinity binders.

Low-affinity binding is a nonspecific property of many different plasma proteins and is similar to nonspecific binding of bilirubin and various drugs. It was detected many years ago using ultrafiltration (which overestimates the amount bound), equilibrium dialysis, and gel filtration. The potential binding capacity is several hundred times greater than the amount of folate in serum. Early data showing failure to half-saturate these binders at high concentrations of free folate indicate that the affinity constant of the system is less than 10$^4$ liters per mole, which is less than the 10$^6$ liters per mole affinity constant of the carrier-mediated cell transport systems for folate.[82]

Study of the high-affinity serum folate binders was initiated by Rothenberg's serendipitous discovery of such binders in chronic myeloid leukemia cells,[83] and subsequently in the serum of the same patients. They are demonstrable in granulocytes of a proportion of nonleukemic subjects, and are released into the serum by these cells.[84] Although their release has not yet been detected in most normal subjects, all human (and animal) serum contains these binders,[80] which more often than not are largely saturated.

Current data suggest that there is only one class of high-affinity serum folate binders—glycoproteins with a molecular weight of about 40,000 probably granulocyte-derived but modified in liver and perhaps kidney.[80] They have binding constants (K$_d$) of approximately 10$^{-10}$ M folic acid and of the order of 10$^{-8}$ M 5-methyltet-

rahydrofolate, the main folate present in serum. Although these affinities indicate that binder would only be half saturated at usual serum methyltetrahydrofolate concentrations, they normally average 67% saturation. This phenomenon may be due to the presence of small quantities of nonmethyl unsubstituted folates on binders. These binders carry less than 5% of serum folate. Their physiologic function has not yet been demonstrated, but at least three lines of inquiry are currently being pursued: (1) The binders may play a role in folate delivery to liver similar to the role of transcobalamin I in vitamin B$_{12}$ transport. (2) They may be important in controlling folate distribution, breakdown, and excretion in deficient states. (3) Their presence in cerebrospinal fluid,[85,85a] their increased affinity for oxidized folate, and the active transport of oxidized folates out of cerebrospinal fluid[86] all suggest that they may function as carriers important in transporting oxidized folates from cerebrospinal fluid to blood. As discussed earlier, they are also present in milk, where they may enhance folate absorption from gut, and they may be related to a membrane protein-mediated uptake of folate.

Folate is delivered to bone marrow cells, reticulocytes, liver, cerebrospinal fluid, and renal tubular cells against a concentration gradient in a manner that suggests energy-dependent carrier-mediated transport.[82] The transport constant of these systems is about 10$^{-6}$ M. Methyltetrahydrofolate, which accounts for almost all serum folate, appears to be transported more efficiently than folic acid across the intestinal cell and into the cells of the body. A red cell membrane protein that binds folates (including methyltetrahydrofolate) and is immunologically cross-reactive with folate binders in placenta, milk, and serum,[82a] increases in quantity when cells are grown in low-folate medium.[82b] This phenomenon suggests that it may be important in cellular folate transport.

Normal total-body folate stores range from 5 to 10 mg, of which approximately half is in the liver.[31] It has been suggested that the enterohepatic circulation, which transports about 0.1 mg of biologically active folate daily,[3] is important in the maintenance of serum folate levels.[87]

Most stored folate is present as polyglutamates,[30] which have far greater molecular size and charge than monoglutamates. Transport across cell walls probably requires hydrolysis to monoglutamates, and the enzymes responsible for polyglutamate synthesis and hydrolysis are thus thought to play a major role in folate storage. These enzymes, which have been incompletely characterized, are known respectively as polyglutamate synthetase and conjugase (pteroylpolyglu-tamate hydrolase; gamma-glutamylcarboxypepti-dase). Conjugase, which has been more fully studied than the synthetase, is present in almost all mammalian tissue and is under partial hor-mone control. Some of the folate-dependent re-actions shown in Figure 21–4B are altered by varying glutamyl chain lengths, and it is thus probable that conjugase and polyglutamate syn-thetase effect the metabolism role of folate as well as its storage.

Folate is excreted in urine and bile in metabol-ically active and inactive forms. Urinary excretion of the biologically active material occurs after glo-merular filtration of the free fraction and reab-sorption of some filtered folate by active transport across the tubular cell wall. The principal break-down product of folate in urine, acetamidoben-zoylglutamate, suggests that the principal route of folate catabolism occurs through oxidative cleav-age of the folate molecule at the 9-10 bond, with acetylation of the para-aminobenzoyl moiety in the liver before excretion.[81] Some workers believe that scorbutic patients may lose large amounts of folate through irreversible oxidation of 10-for-myltetrahydrofolate to 10-formylfolate and excre-tion of the latter in the urine.[88]

As mentioned previously, about 100 μg of bi-ologically active folate is excreted in the bile daily. In addition, studies with radioactive tracer folates[89] indicate that a large proportion of in-jected radioactivity is excreted in the bile as a biologically inactive compound that is not a prod-uct of 9-10 cleavage, but that has not been well characterized. Alcohol interferes with the folate enterohepatic cycle.[87]

## NUTRITIONAL REQUIREMENTS AND NATURAL SOURCES

The term *minimal daily requirement* (MDR), as used in this chapter, means the minimum *from exogenous sources* required to sustain normality, with normality defined as the absence of any bio-chemical hypofunction that is correctable by ad-dition of greater quantities of the vitamin. By this definition, the minimal daily requirement for vi-tamin $B_{12}$ of a normal subject would be only 0.1 μg, since this quantity will sustain normality in a normal subject.[90,91] The minimum daily require-ment for vitamin $B_{12}$ of a patient with gastric or ileal structural or functional damage would be greater because such damage eliminates not only the normal absorption of vitamin $B_{12}$ from exog-enous (food) sources, but also the normal daily reabsorption from the ileum of almost all the vi-tamin $B_{12}$ normally excreted each day in bile.

The minimal daily requirements can be reduced

to a formula[92] applicable generally to essential (i.e., required from exogeneous sources) nutrient deficiency, as follows:

$$MDR \text{ (units/day)} = \frac{UBS \text{ (units)}}{D \text{ (days)}}$$

where MDR = minimal daily requirement of nu-trient from exogenous sources, UBS = utilizable body stores of nutrient, and D = number of days required to develop tissue deficiency after ces-sation of absorption from exogenous sources of nutrient (with appropriate correction for *incom-plete* cessation of absorption).

This formula may also be written as:

$$D = UBS/MDR$$

or

$$UBS = D \times MDR$$

As suggested previously, one can predict the time it would take any given nutrient deficiency to de-velop in any given person after reduction or ces-sation of absorption of the nutrient if one knows (or can reasonably estimate) the MDR for the nu-trient and the utilizable body stores thereof.

The Recommended Dietary Allowance (RDA) "are the levels of intake of essential nutrients con-sidered, in the judgment of the Food and Nutrition Board (of the National Academy of Sciences of the US) on the basis of available scientific knowledge, to be adequate to meet the known nutritional needs of practically all healthy persons."[91] The RDA for each nutrient is intentionally substan-tially greater than the MDR in order to produce some measurable amount of body stores to allow for normal variation in utilization and transient increased requirements. There is a tendency to err on the side of larger body stores when information is incomplete. Small storage surpluses of nutrients are rarely detrimental, whereas small deficits may result in deficiency over a long period of subtle negative balance. Other countries often use the term "RDI" (recommended dietary intake) to de-scribe the concept termed "RDA" in the United States.[91a]

### Vitamin $B_{12}$

**Nutritional Requirements.**[3,29–31,74,90,91,91a–b] Vi-tamin $B_{12}$ requirements have been estimated from three different types of study:[31] (1) those designed to determine the minimal amount needed to pre-vent or to cure megaloblastic anemia resulting from vitamin $B_{12}$ deficiency, (2) those correlating the relationship between the levels of vitamin B$_{12}$ in serum and in liver in deficient and healthy subjects, and (3) those correlating body stores and turnover rates of vitamin B$_{12}$.

The results of such studies[30] demonstrated that: (1) The minimum quantity of vitamin B$_{12}$ that would produce a hematologic response in patients with uncomplicated vitamin B$_{12}$ deficiency was approximately 0.1 μg daily, and 0.5 to 1 μg of the vitamin daily produced maximum hematologic responses, with similar amounts maintaining a normal picture. (2) Patients with moderate vitamin B$_{12}$ deficiency resulting from B$_{12}$ malabsorption had an average liver vitamin B$_{12}$ content of 0.16 μg/g wet weight of liver, associated with serum vitamin B$_{12}$ levels ranging from 80 to 130 pg/ml and an average total body B$_{12}$ of approximately 250 μg. (A second group of individuals who were also suffering from vitamin B$_{12}$ malabsorption, but who had not yet developed morphologic evidence of blood damage due to vitamin B$_{12}$ deficiency, all had serum levels between 130 and 200 pg/ml, associated with approximately 0.28 μg of vitamin B$_{12}$/g wet weight of liver and an average total body vitamin B$_{12}$ content of approximately 525 μg.) (3) The daily whole-body turnover of vitamin B$_{12}$ measured with tracer doses of radioactive vitamin indicates a radioactivity turnover of between 0.1 and 0.2% daily, regardless of whether the body vitamin B$_{12}$ stores are normal or reduced.

Loss of 0.1 to 0.2% of radioactive vitamin B$_{12}$ daily means less than that quantity of vitamin is lost from the body stores daily because the radioactive B$_{12}$ excreted in the bile mixes with nonradioactive B$_{12}$ in the diet, and some of the radioactive B$_{12}$ that would otherwise be reabsorbed in the ileum is replaced by absorbed nonradioactive vitamin. The net result is a gradual reduction in the radioactivity of the body vitamin B$_{12}$ stores, but a much lesser reduction in the actual vitamin B$_{12}$ content of those stores.

The Food and Nutrition Board of the National Academy of Sciences (NAS) set the RDA for vitamin B$_{12}$ in 1980 at 3 μg/day for adolescents and normal adults.[91] This amount is much higher than the intake of millions of healthy vegetarians, is associated with gradually increasing body stores each decade of life and, for this and other reasons, it was reduced to 2 μg/day by the 1980-1985 RDA Committee.[91a] The Joint FAO/WHO Expert Group recommended in 1987 a daily intake of 1 μg of vitamin B$_{12}$ for the normal adult and 2 μg for those with achlorhydria.[31b] The 1980 recommendation of the NAS group was based almost entirely on studies of the body turnover of radioactive vitamin B$_{12}$—studies that seem to have no relation to

minimal daily requirements, since such turnover tends to be a fixed percentage of body stores regardless of their size. On the other hand, the 1 μg daily intake recommended in 1987 for adults by the FAO/WHO group[31b] is based not only on the same radioactivity turnover studies on which the NAS relied almost exclusively, but also on studies of minimal amounts needed to prevent or to cure megaloblastic anemia resulting from vitamin B$_{12}$ deficiency, and on studies of the relationship between the levels of vitamin B$_{12}$ in serum and in liver in deficient and in healthy subjects. The daily allowance of 2 μg of vitamin B$_{12}$ for adults recommended by the 1980–1985 RDA Committee[91a] carries a greater margin above normal physiologic requirements for absorption of the vitamin by the nonachlorhydric adult than does the FAO/WHO recommendation, resulting in larger tissue stores. There is no clear evidence that these larger stores constitute a benefit (or a harm).

Vitamin B$_{12}$ deficiency does not occur in breast-fed infants unless their mothers are deficient in the vitamin. Infants showing such deficiency respond hematologically to 0.1 μg of vitamin B$_{12}$ orally.[93] In the economically advanced countries, breast milk with a content of about 0.4 μg/L supplies about 0.3 μg of vitamin B$_{12}$ daily, which is clearly adequate as manifested by lack of evidence of any deficiency in the infant. Available evidence suggests that the milk from mothers whose serum contains vitamin B$_{12}$ concentrations close to the lower limit of normality (i.e., 200 pg/ml) is also adequate, but that of vegetarian mothers with lower serum levels is not adequate when it falls to 0.07 μg/L of breast milk or less.[31] The Joint FAO/WHO Expert Group in 1987[31b] therefore recommended a daily intake of 0.1 μg of vitamin B$_{12}$ in breast milk as adequate for infants. The 1980-1985 RDA Committee recommended for those on artificial feeding 0.3 μg at age 0 to 2.9 months, 0.4 μg at 3 to 5.9 months, 0.5 μg at 6 to 11.9 months, 0.7 μg at 1 to 1.9 years, 1 μg at 2 to 5.9 years, 1.5 μg at 6 to 9.9 years, and 2.0 μg thereafter.[91a]

Vitamin B$_{12}$ deficiency does not occur in normal children on adequate calorie and animal protein intakes. The Joint FAO/WHO Expert Group in 1987 calculated desirable intakes of vitamin B$_{12}$ for children as 0.04 μg/kg body weight/day to a maximum of 1 μg/day.[31b]

Pregnancy produces an increased requirement for vitamin B$_{12}$ owing to the fetal drain on maternal stores. The fetus removes approximately 0.2 μg of vitamin B$_{12}$ daily from the maternal stores in the latter half of pregnancy. The Joint FAO/WHO Expert Group in 1987 calculated the desirable daily intake of vitamin B$_{12}$ in pregnancy to be the adult 1 μg plus an additional 0.4 μg, and in lactation an additional 0.3 μg on top of the adult 1 μg.[31d]

Total recommended intake during lactation is 2.5 μg/day (4 μg RDA) based on the recommended daily intake of 2 μg for the normal adult (3 μg RDA) plus an additional 0.5 μg to accommodate the approximately 0.3 μg lost in the milk of nursing mothers.[91a]

The sequence of events in developing vitamin $B_{12}$ deficiency[74,74a,74b] is delineated in Figure 21–5 and involves the concept of four stages of depletion for vitamins using vitamin $B_{12}$ and folate as models.[93a,101b] The first stage, negative vitamin $B_{12}$ balance, begins when vitamin $B_{12}$ absorption falls low enough to deplete the amount of vitamin $B_{12}$ on its primary delivery protein, transcobalamin II (TC II), resulting in a low holo-TC II level.[93b,93c] For any laboratory test, because of individual variability, deviation from the value normal for the

individual often precedes deviation from the range of normal for the laboratory,[93d] i.e., the individual's low holo-TC II may be low for him and may indicate that he is in negative vitamin $B_{12}$ balance before his holo-TC level falls below the *laboratory* range of normal. The same is true for other tests, such as the granulocyte nuclear lobe average, which can be high enough to indicate slowed DNA synthesis in granulocytes of the individual owing to vitamin $B_{12}$ or folate deficiency even when the lobe average is still within the laboratory normal range.[93d]

When one understands this normal sequence of events, it is not surprising to learn that about 10% of Hindu Indian vegetarians with early cobalamin deficiency did not yet have an elevated mean corpuscular volume (MCV) (particularly with their frequent iron deficiency) or anemia.[93e]

**Natural Sources.**[2,3,23,23a,23b,23c,25–27,32,74,91,94] The

| Stage: | Normal $B_{12}$ Balance | Negative $B_{12}$ Balance | $B_{12}$ Depletion | $B_{12}$-Deficient Erythropoiesis | $B_{12}$-Deficiency Anemia |
|---|---|---|---|---|---|
| Liver $B_{12}$ / HoloTC II / RBC+WBC $B_{12}$ | | | | | |
| HoloTC II | >30 pg/ml | <20 pg/ml | <20pg/ml | <12 pg/ml | <12 pg/ml |
| TC II % sat. | >5% | <5% | < 2% | < 1% | < 1% |
| Holohap | >150 pg/ml | >150pg/ml | <150 pg/ml | <100 pg/ml | <100 pg/ml |
| dU suppression | Normal | Normal | Normal | Abnormal | Abnormal |
| Hypersegmentation | No | No | No | Yes | Yes |
| TBBC*% sat. | >15% | >15% | >15% | <15% | <10% |
| Hap % sat. | >20% | >20% | >20% | <20% | <10% |
| RBC Folate | >160 ng/ml | >160 | >160 | <140 | <140 |
| Erythrocytes | Normal | Normal | Normal | Normal | Macroovalocytic |
| MCV | Normal | Normal | Normal | Normal | Elevated |
| Hemoglobin | Normal | Normal | Normal | Normal | Low |
| TC II | Normal | Normal | Normal | Elevated | Elevated |
| Methylmalonate | No | No | No | ? | Yes |
| Myelin damage | No | No | No | ? | ? |

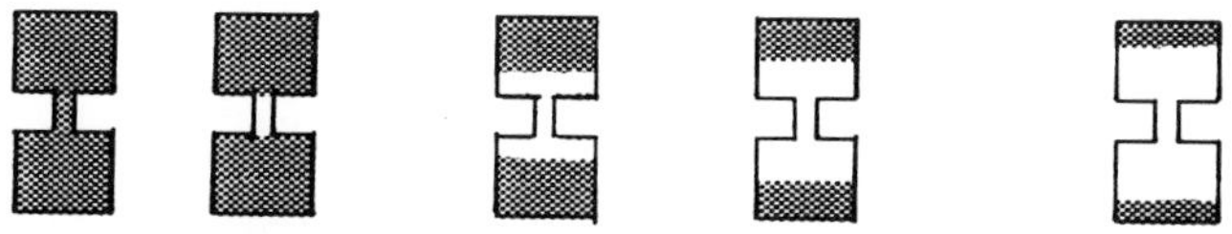

**Fig. 21–5.** Sequential stages in the development of vitamin $B_{12}$ deficiency. Biochemical and hematologic sequence of events as negative vitamin $B_{12}$ balance progresses. Holo TC II = holotranscobalamin II (i.e., transcobalamin II with cobalamin on it). Without cobalamin, it is apotranscobalamin II. TC II % sat = % of total TC II that has cobalamin on it. Holohap = holohapatocorrin (i.e., haptocorrin with cobalamin on it). Synonyms for haptocorrin are cobalaphilin and transcobalamin (I and II).

dU suppression = diagnostic test of ability of cells (bone marrow cells, peripheral blood lymphocytes) to make DNA. Hypersegmentation = increase in number of lobes in granulocytic white cell nuclei.

TBBC % sat = % of total $B_{12}$ binding capacity of plasma that has $B_{12}$ on it.

RBC = red blood cell.

MCV = mean corpuscular volume of red cells.

sole source of vitamin B$_{12}$ in nature is synthesis by microorganisms. The vitamin is not found in plants except when they are contaminated by microorganisms. Fruits, vegetables, and grains and grain products are usually devoid of vitamin B$_{12}$. However, the root nodules of certain legumes contain microorganisms that make vitamin B$_{12}$, and unwashed vegetable products may also contain vitamin B$_{12}$ because of contamination by soil or fecal matter. These small amounts of vitamin B$_{12}$ in legumes and in contaminated food may provide the only dietary source of vitamin B$_{12}$ for strict vegetarians. The usual dietary sources of vitamin B$_{12}$ are meat and meat products (including shellfish, fish, and poultry) and, to a lesser extent, milk and milk products. Rich sources of vitamin B$_{12}$ (greater than 10 μg/100 g of wet weight) are organ meats such as lamb and beef liver, kidney, and heart and bivalves (clams, oysters) that siphon large quantities of vitamin B$_{12}$-synthesizing microorganisms from the sea. Moderately high amounts (3 to 10 μg/100 g of wet weight) are present in nonfat dry milk, some seafood (crabs, rock fish, salmon, sardines), and egg yolk. Moderate amounts (1 to 3 μg/100 g of wet weight) are found in fluid milk products, cream, cheddar cheese, and cottage cheese. Bacteria in the knobby growth of some seaweeds make the vitamin,[94a,94b] and some manufacturers add the vitamin to breakfast cereals.

The vitamin B$_{12}$ molecule is resistant to heat unless exposed in an alkaline medium to temperatures in excess of 100°C; the molecule splits at 250°C. Thus, hamburgers cooked on a hot griddle may lose some of their B$_{12}$ from the surface flat against the hot griddle, but the vitamin B$_{12}$ deep within the patty is preserved. Of the vitamin B$_{12}$ in liver, 8% is lost by boiling at 100°C for five minutes. Boiling muscle meat at 170°C for 45 minutes results in a loss of 30% of the vitamin from the meat. Milk pasteurized for two to three seconds losses 7% of its available vitamin B$_{12}$; when boiled for two to five minutes, it loses 30%. Sterilization in a bottle for 13 minutes at 119 to 120°C causes a loss of 77%; rapid sterilization (3 to 4 seconds) with superheated steam at 143°C destroys only about 10% of the vitamin.[74] In the presence of ascorbic acid, vitamin B$_{12}$ is less heat-stable, and substantial amounts in food may be destroyed by 0.5 g of ascorbic acid.[35c,93,95,96,97] In light of this, if ascorbic acid is added to food, as has been suggested in some schemes of iron fortification,[88,98] vitamin B$_{12}$ intake may be significantly reduced. In some circumstances, large doses of ascorbic acid may reduce vitamin B$_{12}$ absorption.[99a]

The enzymatically active forms of vitamin B$_{12}$

(coenzyme B$_{12}$ and methylcobalamin) are the dominant forms in foodstuffs, in which they are generally attached to polypeptides. Cyanocobalamin per se is probably not present to a significant extent in any natural source. This stable form of vitamin B$_{12}$ results from the action of cyanide on natural vitamin B$_{12}$ coenzymes. Thiocyanate ingestion and absorption of cyanide from tobacco smoke may convert a small amount of enzymatically active cobalamins in blood and tissue to cyanocobalamin.

## Folic Acid

**Nutritional Requirements.**[3,30,31,74,90,91,91a,100,100a,100b] The minimal daily requirement (MDR) for folate is approximately 50 μg for adults. The FAO/WHO Expert Group in 1987 recommended a daily dietary intake for adults of 3.1 μg/kg of body weight, to equal a daily intake of 200 μg for a 65-kg man and 170 μg for a 55-kg woman.[31e] This amount will provide stores sufficient to prevent deficiency for 3 to 4 months of zero intake. Because of the possibility of an acute drain on stores from acute blood loss or pregnancy, a smaller daily intake is not recommended. To meet the added needs of pregnant women, WHO/FAO recommends a supplement of 200 to 300 μg daily, so that the daily folate intake is no less than 350 μg (or 7 μg/kg body weight), and a supplement of 100 μg/day during lactation (i.e., a total of 5 μg/kg body weight). The 1980 RDA of the Food and Nutrition Board of the NAS ranged from 50 μg for infants (under 1 year) through 100 μg (1 to 3 years), 200 μg (4 to 6 years), and 300 μg (7 to 10 years) to 600 μg for lactating women and 800 μg in pregnancy.[91]

The 1980-1985 NRC RDA Committee for folate, based on considerably more data correlating food folate intake with red cell and liver folate stores, proposed a daily intake of 16 μg for ages 0 to 2.9 months, 24 μg for ages 3 to 5.9 months, 32 μg for ages 6 to 11.9 months, 3.3 μg/kg body weight for ages 1 to 9.9 years, and 3 μg/kg body weight thereafter, with a total of 500 μg/day during pregnancy and 3 μg/kg plus 100 μg/day during lactation.[91a]

Because the daily folate requirement is hinged to the daily metabolic and cell turnover rates, it is increased by anything that increases metabolic rate (such as infection and hyperthyroidism), and anything that increases cell turnover (such as hemolytic anemia and rapid tissue growth in the fetus and malignant tumors). Folate consumption by individual cells is proportional to their rate of one-carbon-unit transfer. Alcohol interferes with folate utilization, and thereby increases folate requirement.[101]

The sequence of events[74,101a,101b] in developing

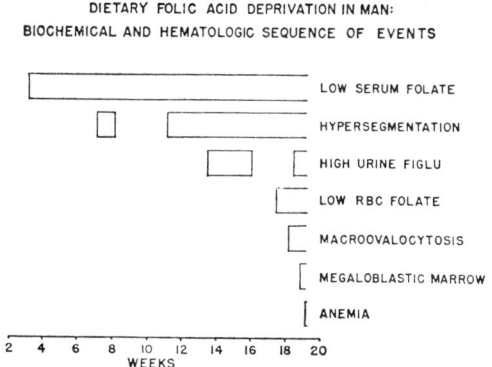

DIETARY FOLIC ACID DEPRIVATION IN MAN:
BIOCHEMICAL AND HEMATOLOGIC SEQUENCE OF EVENTS

**Fig. 21–6.** Biochemical and hematologic sequence of events in developing dietary folate deficiency in man. (From Herbert, V.: Trans. Assoc. Am. Physicians *75*:307, 1962.)

folate deficiency in man is depicted in Figures 21–6 and 21–7.* The concept in Figure 21–7 was first presented in slightly different form at the 1985 International Congress of Nutrition.[93a,101b,101c,101d] As Figure 21–7 depicts, the stages are: negative folate balance (characterized by a fall in erythrocyte folate to below 3 ng/ml); tissue folate depletion (characterized by a fall in erythrocyte folate to below 160 ng/ml (and a pari passu fall in hepatic folate); defective DNA synthesis (characterized by an abnormal diagnostic dU suppression test and by granulocyte nuclear hypersegmentation); and finally, gross macroovalocytosis, elevated mean corpuscular volume (MCV), and anemia. More than half of folate-depleted individuals have not yet reached the stage of anemia and will be missed by screening tests that do not recognize that folate depletion may precede anemia by months.

**Natural Sources.**[24,91,102–105] Unlike vitamin $B_{12}$, which is present only in animal protein, folates are ubiquitous in nature, being present in nearly all natural foods. Unlike vitamin $B_{12}$, folate is highly susceptible to oxidative destruction; 50 to 95% of the folate content of foods may be destroyed by protracted cooking or other processing, such as canning, and all folate is lost from refined foods such as hard liquor and hard candies. Foods with the highest folate content per unit of dry weight include yeast, liver and other organ meats, fresh green vegetables, and some fresh fruits.

The naturally occurring folates are active metabolic forms, usually in polyglutamate linkage[30] (with pteroylheptaglutamates dominant in yeast). Conjugases present in vegetable and mammalian

tissues[106] (including human intestine) liberate pteroyldiglutamates and pteroylmonoglutamates from the conjugates, thereby making the folate available for absorption. About 90% of monoglutamate is absorbed by humans when ingested on its own, but this proportion is markedly decreased in the presence of many foods, irrespective of whether the folate was derived from or added to the food.[59,60] Prior data suggested that polyglutamate was poorly absorbed compared with monoglutamate; however such data were probably affected by other factors in the foods from which polyglutamate was derived. The efficiency of polyglutamate hydrolysis in intestine[53,54] appears to rule out this process as a rate-limiting step in folate absorption unless conjugase inhibitors are present.

The pharmaceutic product pteroylglutamic acid (PGA), like the pharmaceutic product cyanocobalamin, is not usually found as such in natural sources. Its isolation from natural sources, like the isolation of cyanocobalamin, was the result of oxidation and deconjugation of the naturally occurring conjugated forms to a stable form.

## METABOLIC FUNCTIONS AND INTERRELATIONSHIPS[2,3,25,107–109]

### DNA Synthesis

As illustrated in Figure 21–8, both vitamin $B_{12}$ and folic acid are required for synthesis of thymidylate and, therefore, of DNA. A vitamin $B_{12}$-containing enzyme removes a methyl group from methyl folate and delivers it to homocysteine, thereby converting homocysteine to methionine (methyl-homocysteine) and regenerating tetrahydrofolic acid (THFA) from which the 5,10-methylene THFA involved in thymidylate synthesis is made. Methyl folate is the dominant form of folate in human serum and liver, and probably also in other body storage depots for folate. Because methyl folate may only return to the body's folate pool via a vitamin $B_{12}$-dependent step, a patient with vitamin $B_{12}$ deficiency has much of his folate "trapped" as methyl folate, which is metabolically useless. This "folate trap" hypothesis[32d,107–110] may provide much of the explanation for the hematologic damage of vitamin $B_{12}$ deficiency that is not clinically distinguishable from that of folate deficiency. In both instances, the hematologic defect results from lack of adequate 5,10-methylene THFA, which delivers its methyl group to deoxyuridylate to convert that substance to thymidylate, and thus makes DNA during the S (synthesis) phase. In either deficiency, lack of adequate DNA synthesis causes many hematopoietic cells to die in the bone marrow, possibly without ever com-

---

*Note: Herbert has introduced a stage of negative nutrient balance between the stages of normality and tissue nutrient depletion.[93a,101b,150]

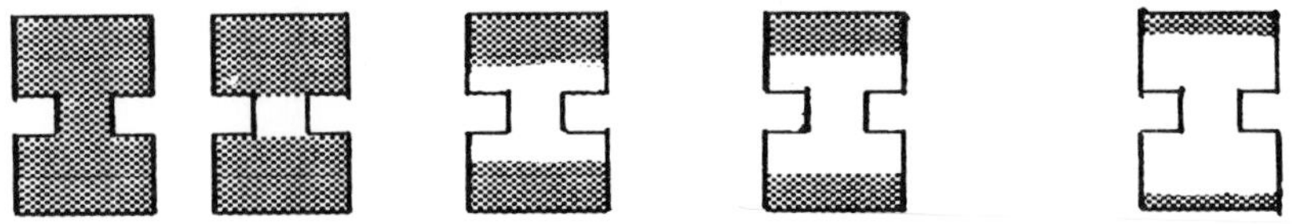

| | Normal | Negative Folate Balance | Folate Depletion | Folate Deficient Erythropoiesis | Folate Deficiency Anemia |
|---|---|---|---|---|---|
| Liver folate | | | | | |
| Plasma folate | | | | | |
| Erythron folate | | | | | |
| Serum folate | >5 ng/ml | <3 ng/ml | <3 ng/ml | <3 ng/ml | <3 ng/ml |
| RBC folate | >200 ng/ml | >200 ng/ml | <160 ng/ml | <120 ng/ml | <100 ng/ml |
| Diagnostic dU suppression | Normal | Normal | Normal | Abnormal* | Abnormal* |
| Lobe average§ | < 3.5 | < 3.5 | < 3.5 | > 3.5 | > 3.5 |
| Liver folate | >3 μg/g | >3 μg/g | <1.6 μg/g | <1.2 μg/g | <1 μg/g |
| Erythrocytes | Normal | Normal | Normal | Normal | Macroovalocytic |
| MCV | Normal | Normal | Normal | Normal | Elevated |
| Hemoglobin | > 12 g/dL | > 12 g/dL | > 12 g/dL | > 12 g/dL | < 12 g/dL |
| Plasma clearance of intravenous folate | Normal | Normal | Normal | Increased | Increased |

**Fig. 21–7.** Sequential stages in the development of folate deficiency. In the first three lines, the area of the shaded boxes in the normal individual shows the relative quantities of folate in each compartment. The sequentially increasingly unshaded areas show its proportional disappearance during successive stages of folate deficiency development. In our laboratory, in 100 normal adults, arithmetic mean serum folate = 8.125 ± 5.06 ng/ml, and geometric mean serum folate = 6.92 with range (± 2 s.d.) = 1.89 to 21.8. In the same 100, arithmetic mean red cell folate = 359.5 ± 158.2 ng/ml, and geometric mean red cell folate = 329.7 with range (± 2 s.d.) = 129.8 to 773.3. Boxes enclose laboratory abnormalities which characterize onset of the stage indicated in the column heading.

    RBC = red blood cell.

    Diagnostic dU suppression = the test of DNA synthesis normality described in other references.[32d,108,128a,128b,128d]

    MCV = mean corpuscular volume of erythrocytes.

    *Abnormal in bone marrow first and subsequently in lymphocytes, except with concomitant iron deficiency, when the reverse occurs.

    §Normal lobe average = 3.2 ± 0.15.[93d,128b]

pleting the S phase of cell replication (i.e., a form of "ineffective erythropoiesis").

Megaloblastosis (the presence of giant germ cells) is the end product of deranged DNA synthesis of any cause. It is most easily understood as an arrest in the S phase of cell replication, usually because of inadequate availability of vitamin B$_{12}$ or folate, with most replicating cells in the body, instead of being in a resting phase, in the process of attempting (with poor success) to double their DNA in order to divide. The underlying biochemical defect that translates poor thymidylate synthesis (due to folate and/or vitamin B$_{12}$ deficiency) into morphologic megaloblastosis may be failure to elongate DNA chains in the presence of a relatively normal capacity to initiate DNA synthesis. This process occurs, presumably, because the lowered thymidylate concentrations remain adequate to serve as substrate for "initiat-

ing" but not for "elongating" DNA polymerase.[111] Alternatively, the mechanism of the defect may be "illicit" incorporation of thymidylate precursors (such as deoxyuridylate) into DNA, with subsequent cleavage of the DNA containing the "illicit" nucleotide.[111a]

Morphologic changes are most striking in bone marrow cells, with the "ineffective hematopoiesis" resulting in peripheral blood pancytopenia (anemia, leukopenia, and thrombopenia). However, megaloblastosis is also present in all other duplicating cells of the body[3,112] and may be strikingly noted in the epithelial cells of the entire alimentary tract, producing glossitis and variable degrees of megaloblastosis along the entire alimentary tract epithelium. It is not yet clear why gut changes associated with vitamin B$_{12}$ deficiency are often related to constipation whereas those associated with folate deficiency are more

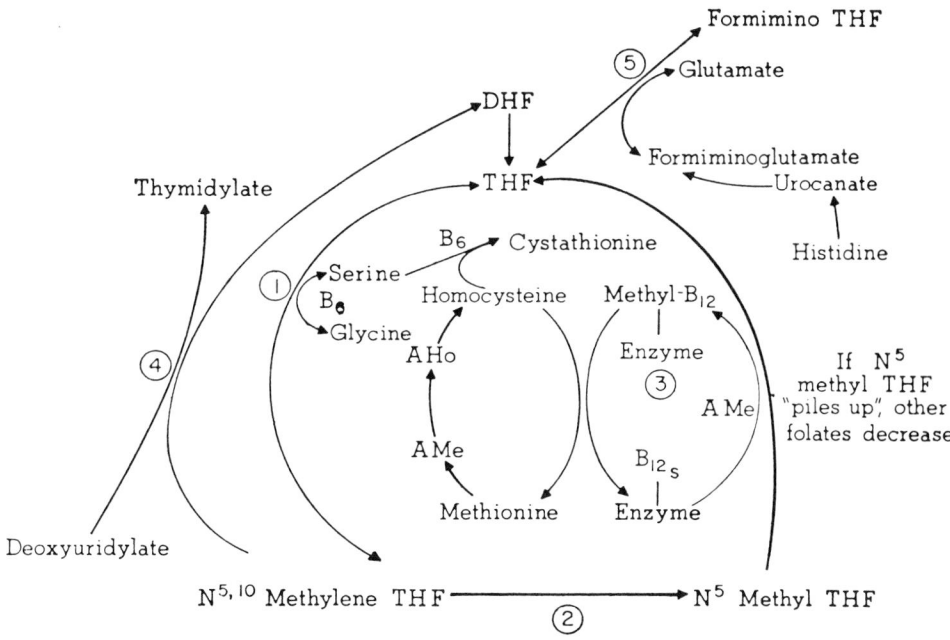

**Fig. 21–8.** Interrelationships of vitamin B$_{12}$, B$_6$, and folate. (From Herbert[25] with permission of J. & A. Churchill.)

commonly related to diarrhea. These differences may be connected to phenomena other than the nutrient deficiency per se.

Because growth is dependent on cell replication, and cell replication is dependent on DNA synthesis, both vitamin B$_{12}$ and folic acid are required for growth.

### "Packaging" Folate in Cells

Another important interrelationship of these two vitamins is the involvement of vitamin B$_{12}$ in the transport and storage of folate in cells.[113–118] In vitamin B$_{12}$ deficiency, transport of methyltetrahydrofolate into bone marrow cells and into transformed lymphocytes[116] is impaired with correction of the defect after addition of vitamin B$_{12}$.[116] Similarly, humans and experimental animals with vitamin B$_{12}$ deficiency have low erythrocyte folate and decreased liver folate stores. These defects are probably attributable to failure of vitamin B$_{12}$-dependent homocysteine: methionine transmethylation. Failure to remove the methyl group from folate, which causes an intracellular "methyl trap,"[3,112] may interfere with dissociation of the carrier-folate complex at the inner cell wall and may impair transport into the cell.[32] It does impair folate storage because tetrahydrofolate is preferred over methyltetrahydrofolate as a substrate for polyglutamate synthetase.[117,118]

### Nerve Damage

Inadequate myelin synthesis with resultant neurologic damage results from vitamin B$_{12}$ de-

ficiency but not from folate deficiency.[3,112] The biochemical basis for this defective myelin synthesis is unknown. Because myelin is lipoprotein, vitamin B$_{12}$ must have some as yet undetermined role in synthesis of either the lipid or the protein component of myelin. It has been proposed that the neurologic damage relates to the B$_{12}$ requirement for the propionate-methylmalonate conversion. This hypothesis is probably not correct, however, because infants born lacking the apoenzyme for this conversion do not have damaged myelin, and the abnormalities reported in fatty acids in myelin of vitamin B$_{12}$-deficient subjects[119] may well relate to plasmalogen[120] rather than to B$_{12}$ deficiency. The nervous system damage caused by vitamin B$_{12}$ deficiency involves, in addition to myelinated peripheral nerves, the myelinated posterior and lateral cords of the spinal column.[112] Therefore, nervous system damage from this deficiency has been variously termed subacute combined degeneration, combined system disease, posterolateral sclerosis, and funicular degeneration. However, the disease usually starts insidiously and not subacutely. Combined lesions are often absent, and lesions of the peripheral nerves occur more frequently and earlier than lesions of the central nervous system. For these reasons, the nervous system changes are more accurately described by direct reference to the actual involvement (i.e., peripheral nerve, spinal cord, or cerebral damage).

The various neurologic symptoms and signs resulting from the inadequate myelin synthesis caused by vitamin B$_{12}$ deficiency include paresthesia, especially numbness and tingling in the hands and feet, diminution of vibration sense and/or position sense (usually but not always occurring first in the ankles and feet), unsteadiness, poor muscular coordination with ataxia, moodiness, mental slowness, poor memory, confusion, agitation, depression, and central scotomata (sometimes with dim vision due to optic atrophy and tobacco amblyopia). Delusions, hallucinations, and even overt psychosis (usually with paranoid ideas) may occur. The wide variety of sensory and motor changes tend to be symmetrical, especially if present for weeks or months.

Early subtle nerve damage (inability to sense position in index toes, inability to perceive the vibrations of a 256-vps tuning fork) precedes by months grosser nerve damage (inability to sense position in great toes, inability to perceive the vibrations of a 128-vps tuning fork).[112] Correction by vitamin B$_{12}$ therapy confirms that the damage is due to vitamin B$_{12}$ deficiency rather than to the normal process of aging.

Comparing "private" with "ward" patients in large hospital populations, we observed that economically advantaged people with vitamin B$_{12}$ deficiency tend to have relatively severe neurologic damage and relatively mild hematologic damage, whereas economically deprived people with vitamin B$_{12}$ deficiency tend to have relatively equal severity of neurologic and hematologic damage.[112] A major explanation for the variable degree of hematologic damage with fixed amount of neurologic damage in vitamin B$_{12}$ deficiency is the quantity of folate in the diet. Well-to-do people tend to eat better diets, richer in high-folate foods such as fresh fruits, vegetables, and meats. The folate retards development of hematologic damage while allowing neurologic damage to progress.

Folate deficiency does not damage myelin, but it is associated with a high frequency of irritability, forgetfulness and, often, hostility and paranoid behavior. These phenomena often strikingly improve within 24 hours of the start of therapy with folic acid. Other neurologic sequelae attributed by some to folate deficiency have been reviewed elsewhere,[121] but the association has not been convincingly demonstrated.[85]

Cerebration may improve rapidly when vitamin B$_{12}$ deficiency is appropriately treated, but the neurologic damage resulting from inadequate myelin synthesis heals slowly. Because the nerve damage is related to deterioration of the axon underneath the deteriorated myelin, healing is related to the speed of regeneration of damaged axons; this regeneration creeps peripherally from the nerve head at the rate of 0.1 mm/day.

## B$_{12}$ in Fat and Carbohydrate Metabolism[3,23,23a,23b,23c,25,27,30,122]

Because coenzyme B$_{12}$ is required for the hydrogen transfer and isomerization whereby methylmalonate is converted to succinate,[23,25] B$_{12}$ is involved in both fat and carbohydrate metabolism. As indicated previously, although it is an attractive speculation that the neurologic damage of patients with vitamin B$_{12}$ deficiency is caused by inability to make the lipid portion of the lipoprotein myelin sheath (due to inadequate propionic acid utilization related to inadequate interconversion of methylmalonate and succinate), there is not yet evidence to associate this with the neurologic damage of vitamin B$_{12}$ deficiency in man.

More recently, researchers have shown that rat glial cells in vitamin B$_{12}$-deficient media produce two odd-chain fatty acids that are not found when the cells are grown in the presence of vitamin B$_{12}$.[123] Further, nerve biopsies from subjects with vitamin B$_{12}$ deficiency incubated in $^{14}$C-labeled propionate produced labeled $^{15}$C and $^{14}$C fatty acids.[124] The explanation for this finding and its relationship to the functional and histologic changes have not yet been elucidated.

## B$_{12}$ in Protein and Fat Metabolism[23,23a,23b,23c,25,27,30]

Vitamin B$_{12}$ is involved in protein synthesis through its role in the synthesis of the amino acid methionine, and possibly in other ways as well. Because methionine is involved in making available more of the lipotropic substances choline and betaine, this is another area where cobalamin may play a role in lipid metabolism.

## B$_{12}$ as a Reducing Agent[3,23,23a,23b,23c,125]

Vitamin B$_{12}$ appears to be involved in maintenance of sulfhydryl (SH) groups in the reduced form necessary for function of many SH-activated enzyme systems. Vitamin B$_{12}$ deficiency is characterized by a decrease in reduced glutathione (which is changed from reduced glutathione [GSH] to oxidized glutathione [GSSG]) of erythrocytes and liver. This condition may be corrected by administration of vitamin B$_{12}$. In vitro, vitamin B$_{12}$ derivatives catalyze the nonenzymatic oxidation of sulfhydryl derivatives.

## Folate in One-Carbon Unit Transfers[24,30,126]

Folate coenzymes are concerned with mammalian metabolic systems involving transfer of a one-carbon unit. These reactions include (1) de novo purine synthesis (formylation of glycinamide ribonucleotide [GAR] and 5-amino-4-imidazole carboxamide ribonucleotide [AICAR]), (2) pyrimidine nucleotide biosynthesis (methylation of deoxyuridylic acid to thymidylic acid), (3) three amino acid conversions: the interconversion of serine and glycine (which also requires vitamin B$_6$), catabolism of histidine to glutamic acid, conversion of homocysteine to methionine (which also requires vitamin B$_6$), (4) generation of formate into the formate pool (and utilization of formate), and (5) methylation of small amounts of transfer RNA. The suggestion that folate may be involved in physiologic methylation of biogenic amines[127] has been refuted.[128]

## Role of Ascorbic Acid

It is possible that ascorbate in vivo may aid in the protection against oxidative destruction of reduced folates in the body. There is no evidence that ascorbate plays any role in the reduction of pteroylglutamic acid to tetrahydrofolic acid, a reaction mediated by folate reductases. The original such evidence proved to be protection by ascorbate of the end product against oxidative destruction.

## Selective Nutrient Deficiency

An important area of nutrition research is selective nutrient deficiency in one cell line or one tissue and not another in the same patient. This condition can result from one tissue obtaining food folate first, as do intestine cells when food folate is decreased.[101a] Another cause may be the presence of more machinery and/or more efficient machinery for folate uptake and less for folate rejection and loss in relation to one cell line as compared to another. Selective folate deficiency can occur, for example, in white cells but not in red cells.[128a,128b] Therefore, lymphocytes (which in their resting form in the human blood appear impervious to the vitamins B$_{12}$ and folic acid, and also other nutrients, such as nicotinamide[128c]) can be used to measure past nutrient deficiency up to two months after therapy,[128a] and also to measure covert folate deficiency in patients who lack macro-ovalocytosis because of coincident iron-deficiency or hemoglobinopathy.[128d,128e,128f] Only when lymphocytes are making DNA do they appear to be pervious to nutrients.[128a,128b,128c]

## THERAPY

The only established therapeutic use of vitamin B$_{12}$ or folic acid is in treating deficiency of the respective vitamins. Claims made for nutritional value of either of these vitamins in clinical situations in which deficiency of the vitamin does not exist are without foundation in fact.

When the deficiency is of vitamin B$_{12}$, only this vitamin should be used for therapy; conversely, when the deficiency is of folate, only that vitamin should be used for therapy. The use of folic acid in the treatment of a patient whose deficiency is of vitamin B$_{12}$ often produces temporary hematologic improvement, but allows the neurologic damage of the underlying vitamin B$_{12}$ deficiency to progress, often to an irreversible state.

Although liver extract for injection was deleted from the USP in 1960, such products are still being used by some practitioners and appear in the National Formulary. For clinical purposes, the injectable unit is approximately the equivalent of 1.33 μg of vitamin B$_{12}$. Because preparations of liver extract contain hematopoietic materials other than vitamin B$_{12}$ (e.g., folic acid, folinic acid), they constitute "shotgun therapy," like many other multi-ingredient therapies, and such use is to be avoided.

The signs and symptoms of deficiency of vitamin B$_{12}$ or folate in humans[1–3,111,129–131] are listed in Table 21–2.

### Therapy of Critically Ill Patients

It is rarely necessary to institute immediate therapy before determining the cause of megaloblastic anemia. Major indications for emergency therapy include severe thrombocytopenia (platelet count less than 50,000/mm$^3$) associated with bleeding, severe leukopenia (white cell count less than 3,000/mm$^3$) associated with infection, infection itself, coma, severe disorientation, marked neurologic damage, severe hepatic disease, uremia, or other debilitating illness complicating the anemia. The anemia itself is not a problem because the dyspnea and occasional angina that may accompany a hematocrit of less than 15 volumes % are relieved by a transfusion of one to two units of packed erythrocytes. Transfusion is unwarranted in the absence of symptoms of anemia. When venous pressure is elevated, transfusion of packed erythrocytes should be accompanied by withdrawal of equivalent or slightly smaller quantities of whole blood, which will reduce rather than raise the venous pressure. Transfusion of whole blood without withdrawal of blood has been responsible for acute rises in venous pressure with resultant irreversible congestive failure in elderly patients with megaloblastic anemia and unrecognized elevated venous pressure. Ideally, venous pressure should be determined before transfusion and monitored during both the transfusion of packed cells and the simultaneous withdrawal of whole blood. An alternate to exchange transfusion

**Table 21–2.   Clinical Picture of the Megaloblastic Anemias**

1. Symptoms
   Weakness, tiredness
   Dyspnea
   Sore tongue
   Paresthesia (B$_{12}$ deficiency only)
   Diarrhea (especially folate deficiency)
   Constipation (especially B$_{12}$ deficiency)
   Irritability and forgetfulness (especially folate deficiency)
   Anorexia
   Syncope
   Headache
   Palpitation
2. Signs
   Megaloblastic bone marrow (orthochromatic megaloblasts, giant metamyelocytes)
   Anemia, leukopenia, thrombocytopenia, with macro-ovalocytes (normal MVC = $87 \pm 5$ cu $\mu$) and "hyper-segmented polys" (normal Arneth count 2 lobes = 20 to 40%, 3 lobes = 40 to 50%, 4 lobes = 15 to 25%, 5 lobes = 0 to 5%, 6 lobes = 0 to 0.1%, more than 6 lobes = 0) (normal "lobe average" = $3.17 \pm 0.25$). (Rule of fives: When 100 neutrophils are counted, the presence of more than 5% containing 5 or more lobes means hypersegmentation.)
   Morphologic red herrings: congenital hypersegmentation (approximately 1% of population), hypersegmentation with renal disease; twinning deformities; macrocytes of pyruvate kinase deficiency, aplastic anemia, reticulocytosis, hypothyroidism, neoplasia.
   Fever
   Icterus plus pallor (lemon-yellow skin)
   Glossitis
      Acute
      Chronic atrophic
   Neurologic damage (only proven in B$_{12}$ deficiency, which damages myelin)
      Vibration sense diminished
      Position sense diminished, ataxia, "combined systems disease"
      Impaired mentation, paranoid ideation (seen in both deficiencies)
   Malabsorption
   Achylia gastrica (primary with B$_{12}$ deficiency, secondary with folate deficiency) (reduced intrinsic factor)
   Splenomegaly (in approximately one third of cases, if looked for radiologically)
   Weight loss (especially folate deficiency)
   Pigmentation; vitiligo
   Postural hypotension (especially B$_{12}$ deficiency)
   Low serum vitamin B$_{12}$ or folate level
   Elevated serum lactic dehydrogenase (LDH)
   Elevated urine formiminoglutamate
   Methylmalonic aciduria (B$_{12}$ deficiency only)
   High serum iron, increased saturation of iron-binding capacity of serum, increased bone marrow iron stores, normal free erythrocyte protoporphyrin (findings that may obscure occult Fe deficiency)
   Low red cell folate is present in either deficiency
   Circulating antibody to intrinsic factor in two thirds of pernicious anemia patients
   Circulating antibody to gastric parietal cells in most patients with gastric damage, regardless of cause
   Abnormal "dU suppression test" (corrected by adding vitamin in vitro)
   Abnormal liver function tests
   Subnormal intestinal absorption
   Low red cell B$_{12}$ or folate level; low lymphocyte B$_{12}$ or folate

is to precede the administration of blood by the parenteral injection of a diuretic.

When, for one of the reasons discussed previously, immediate vitamin therapy is necessary before etiologic diagnosis, 100 µg of cyanocobalamin and 15 mg of folic acid are given intramuscularly, followed by 5 mg of folic acid by mouth and 100 µg of vitamin B$_{12}$ intramuscularly daily, for a week. Such treatment produces excellent hematologic response except in patients in whom hematopoiesis is suppressed by infection, uremia, chloramphenicol administration, or some other factor.

## Vitamin B$_{12}$ Therapy

Vitamin B$_{12}$ deficiency in man is nearly always the result of inadequate ingestion and/or inadequate absorption, and therapy is guided by adequate etiologic diagnosis (see Table 21–1).

Inadequate ingestion of vitamin B$_{12}$ is corrected by adding to the daily diet any food containing vitamin B$_{12}$ (i.e., animal products, including meat, milk, fish, shellfish, or poultry). If the patient, because of poverty, cannot afford animal products or, for religious or other reasons, is a strict vegetarian, adequate treatment consists of 1 µg of vitamin $B_{12}$ orally supplied daily as a liquid or tablet or $B_{12}$-containing food supplement.

When the vitamin $B_{12}$ deficiency is the result of inadequate absorption, 1 μg of vitamin $B_{12}$ parenterally (subcutaneously or intramuscularly) daily constitutes adequate therapy. A single injection of 100 μg or more of vitamin $B_{12}$ produces a complete therapeutic remission in any patient whose deficiency is not complicated by unrelated systemic disease or other factors. The remission is sustained for life by monthly injections of 100 μg of vitamin $B_{12}$. It is important to inform the patient who has permanent gastric or ileal damage that he must receive monthly injections of vitamin $B_{12}$ for life.

For simultaneous differential diagnosis and therapy, patients should be treated with an injection of 1 μg of vitamin $B_{12}$ daily for 10 days, after a control period of a few days to establish the constancy of the reticulocyte level, and the elimination of dietary sources of vitamin $B_{12}$ and folic acid (by provision of a diet consisting exclusively of well-cooked finely particulate grains or vegetables, such as rice and beans, and beverages devoid of vitamin $B_{12}$ and folate, such as tea, coffee, and soft drinks).[129]

Initial therapy with doses of vitamin $B_{12}$ greater than 1 μg daily is desirable when the vitamin $B_{12}$ deficiency is complicated by other debilitating illness such as infection, hepatic disease, uremia, coma, severe disorientation, or marked neurologic damage. In such patients, 30 μg or more of vitamin $B_{12}$ is given daily parenterally for 5 to 10 days. Daily parenteral doses larger than 30 μg have no proven therapeutic advantage, and much of the excess is rapidly excreted in the urine.[130]

Vitamin $B_{12}$ can also be administered in a nasal gel, facilitating self-administration. Preliminary data indicate that nasal $B_{12}$ is more effectively absorbed than oral $B_{12}$ in normal individuals, that it is effective in $B_{12}$ malabsorption, and that it can be used to treat $B_{12}$-deficient patients.[130a,b]

Hydroxocobalamin and other depot preparations of vitamin $B_{12}$ may be retained longer at the site of injection and in serum, but this possible slight therapeutic advantage over cyanocobalamin does not warrant their greater cost; they also may have undesirable side effects. More detailed discussion of vitamin $B_{12}$ preparations, routes of administration, dosage, and therapeutic responses may be found in *The Pharmacological Basis of Therapeutics*.[3]

## Folic Acid Therapy

For combined differential diagnosis and therapy, the patient is treated with 100 μg of folic acid orally daily (if the suspected diagnosis is folate malabsorption). This dosage produces a maximal hematologic response in patients with folate deficiency, but does not produce hematologic response in patients with vitamin $B_{12}$ deficiency.[129] As in treated vitamin $B_{12}$ deficiency, treatment of folate deficiency returns subnormal leukocyte and platelet levels to normal within a week after the start of therapy, at approximately the time of the reticulocyte peak.

Therapy with doses of folic acid larger than 0.1 mg daily is desirable when the folate deficiency state is complicated by conditions that may suppress hematopoiesis (such as unrelated systemic disease), conditions that increase folate requirement (pregancy, hypermetabolic states, alcoholism, hemolytic anemia), and conditions that reduce folate absorption. Therapy should then consist of 0.5 to 1 mg daily. There is no evidence that doses greater than 1 mg daily have any greater efficacy; additionally, loss of folate in the urine becomes roughly logarithmic as the amount administered exceeds 1 mg.

Maintenance therapy is normally 0.1 mg of folic acid daily for one to four months, and then should be discontinued only if the diet contains at least one fresh fruit or fresh vegetable daily. If the daily folate requirement is increased owing to an increased metabolic or cell-turnover rate, the maintenance dose should be 0.2 to 0.5 mg daily.

Ideal nutritional therapy for dietary folate deficiency is the ingestion of one fresh fruit or one fresh vegetable daily. Such a diet would probably eliminate nutritional folate deficiency from the earth.[130–132] At present, nutritional folate deficiency probably encompasses approximately a third of all the pregnant women in the world.[74]

## PREVENTION OF FOLATE DEFICIENCY

It is the consensus that pregnant women should receive folate supplements,[3] and they have been recommended in clinical disorders that increase the risk of folate deficiency. Major problems have been encountered in the delivery of such supplements to patients. Significant numbers of pregnant women do not ingest iron tablets given to them.[133] This problem may not be as severe when tablets containing both iron and folate are given, because a separate report suggests that the adverse gastrointestinal effects of iron ingestion may be decreased when folic acid is simultaneously ingested.[134] However, the iron in the supplement should not exceed the 30-mg iron daily pregnancy supplement recommended by the 1980–1985 RDA Committee.[133a] Tablets containing 100 mg iron and 350 μg folate significantly interfere with the absorption of needed zinc.[133b] The largest component of the problem is that antenatal care is not available to, or taken advantage of, by large numbers of pregnant women, particularly in populations in which folate deficiency is common.[135] This phenomenon has again been highlighted by the observation that of 110 consecutive women seeking prenatal care in New York City, 61 were in the second trimester and 26 already in the third trimester of pregnancy.[136,136a]

As an alternative approach to the alleviation of the problem, a series of studies was devised to determine the feasibility of fortifying staple foods with folic acid.[60,135,137–140] When the data generated in these studies are judged against criteria delineated by an Expert Committee of the World Health Organization (WHO) and Food and Agricultural Organization (FAO),[141] such fortification appears feasible, inexpensive, effective, and safe in populations with a demonstrable need for increased dietary levels of folic acid. It has been suggested that such elevations may increase the incidence and/or severity of neurologic damage in subjects with pernicious anemia, but the literature contains little data to support this view. This reservation thus seems minor when weighed against the primary object of food fortifications, namely, the elevation of dietary folate levels in large undernourished populations to amounts present in the diet of more affluent people who rarely suffer folate deficiency, i.e., to levels approaching the RDA. A joint meeting of the WHO and other bodies has recommended that authorities concerned with populations in which folate deficiency is common should initiate trials to determine the feasibility and effectiveness of food fortification with folate in those populations.[142]

## TOXICITY

There is no evidence that either vitamin B$_{12}$ or folic acid, in the human-active forms necessary for life, is toxic to humans in quantities close to minimal daily requirements. These substances in their human-active forms are nontoxic in man not only in small doses but also in doses that exceed the minimal daily adult human requirement by 10,000 times for vitamin B$_{12}$ and several hundred times for folic acid. Being water-soluble, excesses of these vitamins tend to be excreted in the urine rather than, like fat-soluble vitamins, being stored in tissues. Vitamin B$_{12}$ and folic acid both appear to require binding to polypeptides as a precondition of storage; excesses above the limited serum- and tissue-available-binding capacity tend to be excreted rather than retained.

A rare allergic reaction has been reported, possibly due to impurities in a rare preparation of crystalline cyanocobalamin.[25] Hydroxocobalamin

injections and injections of various depot preparations of cyanocobalamin have been associated with the appearance of antibody to plasma vitamin B$_{12}$-binding protein.[127] Although the significance of this antibody is not yet clear, such preparations offer no clear advantage over cyanocobalamin to warrant their use, especially in view of their greater cost and the pain on injection of some of the depot preparations. The pharmaceutical preparation, cyanocobalamin, is not metabolically active in humans. Tissue enzymes remove the cyanide to make the cobalamin active. The rare infant who is born with a congenital lack of this cyanide-removing mechanism can, of course, be harmed by cyanocobalamin, because for him it is an antimetabolite of vitamin B$_{12}$.[142a]

The efficacy and safety of the vitamin B$_{12}$ analogues created by nutrient-nutrient interaction in vitamin-mineral supplements is unknown.[32g]

One questionable instance of an allergic reaction to folic acid has been reported in man.[2] Daily doses of up to 15 mg in healthy humans without convulsive disorders are without known toxic effects; this daily dose is well below that which could lead to precipitation of crystalline folic acid in the kidneys (such precipitation produces renal toxicity in rats given massive doses of folic acid). Very large amounts of folic acid in its pharmaceutical oxidized form (pteroylglutamic acid) may be noxious to the nervous system and can reverse the antiepileptic effects of phenobarbital, diphenylhydantoin, and primidone, and have provoked seizures in patients otherwise under control on anticonvulsant therapy.[121,144,144a,144b,144c]

Although no such effect has been observed in controlled studies using oral doses of 15 mg folic acid daily, experimental and clinical evidence suggests that very high concentrations of folic acid can have a convulsant effect.[121] The convulsant dose in normal rats was 45 to 125 mg if administered intravenously and 15 to 30 mg if preceded by the induction of a focal cortical lesion.[145] Convulsions have been reported in one of eight epileptics given parenteral folic acid under electroencephalographic monitoring.[146] This reaction occurred after the rapid intravenous infusion of 14.4 mg folic acid, which presumably elevated serum folate concentration in the cerebral vessels several times higher than would be the case after folic acid ingestion.[85,121] Anticonvulsants and folic acid compete with each other for absorption across the intestinal epithelial cells,[146a] and probably also compete at the brain cell wall.[107,144,14a,144b,144c] However, at present, despite evidence in uncontrolled studies suggesting increased fit frequency in epileptics given oral therapeutic doses of folic acid, no such effect of oral folic acid has so far been demonstrated in carefully conducted controlled trials.

Oral folic acid supplements of 350 μg daily reduce zinc absorption and may be a problem where maternal zinc depletion and intrauterine growth retardation are common.[91a,133b]

## REFERENCES

1. Castle, W.B.: Trans. Am. Clin. Climatol. Assoc. *73*:53, 1961.

1a. Kass, L.: Pernicious Anemia. Philadelphia, W.B. Saunders Co., 1976.

2. Chanarin, I.: The Megaloblastic Anemias. Oxford, Blackwell Scientific Publications, 1979.

3. Herbert, V.: *In* The Pharmacological Basis of Therapeutics, 5th ed. (Goodman, L.S., Gilman, A., Eds.) New York, Macmillan Publishing Co., Inc., 1975.

4. Combe, J.S.: Trans R. Med. Chir. Soc. Edinb. *7*:194, 1824.

5. Addison, T.: On the Constitutional and Local Effects of Disease of the Suprarenal Capsules. London, S. Highley, 1855.

6. Flint, A.: Am. Med. Times *7*:181, 1960.

7. Castle, W.B.: Am. J. Med. Sci. *178*:748, 1929.

8. Rickes, E.L., Brink, N.G., Koniuszy, F.R., et al.: Science *107*:396, 1948.

9. Smith, E.L., Parker, L.F.J.: Biochem. J. *43*:viii, 1948.

10. Berk, L., Castle, W.B., Welch, A.D., et al.: N. Engl. J. Med. *39*:911, 1948.

11. Channing, W.: N. Engl. Q. J. Med. Surg. *I*:157, 1824.

12. Barclay, A.W.: Quoted by Castle.[1]

13. Osler, W.: Br. Med. J. *I*:1, 1919.

14. Wills, L., Clutterbuck, P., Evans, B.D.F.: Biochem. J. *31*:2136, 1937.

15. Stokstad, E.L.R.: J. Biol. Chem. *149*:573, 1943.

16. Pfiffner, J.J., Binkley, S.B., Bloom, E.S., et al.: Science *97*:404, 1943.

17. Angier, R.B., Boothe, J.H., Hutchings, B.L., et al.: J. Am. Chem. Soc. *103*:667, 1946.

18. Shorb, M.S.: Science *107*:397, 1948.

19. Day, P.L., Mims, V., Totter, J.R., et al.: J. Biol. Chem. *157*:423, 1945.

20. Snell, E.E., Peterson, W.H.: J. Bacteriol. *39*:273, 1940.

21. Mitchell, H.K., Snell, E.E., Williams, R.J.: J. Am. Chem. Soc. *63*:2284, 1941.

22. Minot, E.R., Murphy, W.P.: JAMA *87*:470, 1926.

23. Smith, E.L.: Vitamin B₁₂, 3rd ed. New York, John Wiley & Sons, 1965.

23a. Babior, B.M. (Ed.): Cobalamin. New York, John Wiley & Sons, 1975.

23b. Pratt, J.M.: Inorganic Chemistry of Vitamin B₁₂. London, Academic Press, 1972.

23c. Dolphin, D. (Ed.): B₁₂, Vols. 1 and 2. New York, John Wiley & Sons, 1982.

24. Blakley, R.L.: The Biochemistry of Folic Acid and Related Pteridines. New York, American Elsevier, 1969.

24a. Food and Nutrition Board: Folic Acid. Washington, National Academy of Sciences, 1977.

24b. Kisliuk, R.L., Brown, G.M. (Eds.): Chemistry and Biology of Pteridines, Vol. IV. New York, Elsevier/North Holland, 1979.

24c. Blakley, R.L. (Ed.): Folates and Pterines, Vol 3. New York, John Wiley & Sons, 1986.

24d. Cooper, B.A., Whitehead, V.M. (Eds.): Chemistry and Biology of Pteridines. Berlin and New York, Walter de Gruyter, 1986.

25. Arnstein, H.R.V., Wrighton, R.J. (Eds.): The Cobalamins. London, Churchill-Livingstone, 1971.

26. Heinrich, H.C. (Ed.): Vitamin B₁₂ and Intrinsic Factor, Second European Symposium. Stuttgart, Ferdinand Enke Verlag, 1962.

27. Perlman, D. (Ed.): Ann. N.Y. Acad. Sci. *112*:547, 1964.

27a. Herbert, V., Drivas, G., Foscaldi, R., et al.: N. Engl. J. Med. *307*:255, 1982.

27b. Kondo, H., Binder, M.J., Kolhouse, J.F., et al.: J. Clin. Invest. *70*:889, 1982.

27c. Jacobsen, D.W., Green, R.: Blood *68*(Suppl. 1):247a, 1986.

28. IUPAC-IUB Commission on Biochemical Nomenclature: Nomenclature of vitamins, coenzymes and related compounds. Tentative rules. *In* Folates and Pterins, Vol. I: Chemistry and Biochemistry of Folates. (Nomenclature pp. xi-xiv). (Blakley, R.L., Benkovic, S.J. Eds.) New York, John Wiley & Sons, 1984, p. 29.

29. Sullivan, L.W., Herbert, V.: N. Engl. J. Med. *272*:340, 1965.

30. Herbert, V.: Am. J. Clin. Nutr. *21*:743, 1968.

30a. Scott, Weir: Clin. Haematol. *5*:547, 1976.

31. WHO Scientific Group: WHO Tech. Rep. Ser. #450, 1968.

31a. FAO/WHO Expert Group: Requirements of ascorbic acid, vitamin B₁₂, folate and iron. WHO Tech. Rep. Ser. #452, 1970.

31b. FAO/WHO Expert Group: Requirements of vitamin A, iron, folate and vitamin B₁₂. (In press), 1987.

31c. Herbert, V., Bierfass, M., Wasserman, L.R., et al.: Am. J. Clin. Nutr. *7*:325–327, 1959.

32. Skeggs, H.R.: Vitamin B₁₂. *In* The Vitamins: Chemistry, Physiology, Pathology, Methods, 2nd ed., Vol. VII. (Gyorgy, P., Pearson, W.N., Eds.) New York, Academic Press, 1967.

32a. Herbert, V., Colman, N., Palat, D., et al.: J. Lab. Clin. Med. *104*:824–841, 1984.

32b. Herbert, V., Memoli, D., March, R., et al.: Blood *68*(5)(Suppl. 1):46a, 1986.

32c. Kolhouse, J.F., Kondo, H., Allen, R.H., et al.: N. Engl. J. Med. *299*:785, 1978.

32d. Herbert, V.: Lab. Invest. *52*:3, 1985.

32e. Herbert, V., Drivas, G., Chu, M., et al.: Blood *62*(Suppl. 1): 37A, 1983.

32f. Herbert, V., Drivas, G., Manusselis, C., et al.: Trans. Assoc. Am. Physicians *97*:161, 1984.

32g. Herbert, V., Drivas, G., Foscaldi, R., et al.: N. Engl. J. Med. *307*:255, 1982.

33. Herbert, V.: Am. J. Clin. Nutr. *7*:433, 1959.

34. Lau, K.S., Gottlieb, C., Wasserman, L.R., et al.: Blood *26*:202, 1965.

35. Herbert, V.: *In* B₁₂ and Folate Analysis with Radionuclides in Hematopoietic and Gastrointestinal Investigations with Radionuclides. (Gilson, A.J., Smoak, W.M., Weinstein, M.B., Eds.) Springfield, Charles C Thomas, 1972.

35a. Herbert, V., Colman, C.: *In* Methods of Vitamin Assay, 4th ed. (Augustin, J., Klein, B.P., Becker, D., et al., Eds.) New York, John Wiley & Sons, 1985.

35a. Gottlieb, C., Retief, F.P., Herbert, V.: Biochem. Biophys. Acta *141*:560, 1967.

35b. Cooper, B.A., Whitehead, V.M.: N. Engl. J. Med. *299*:816, 1978.

35c. Donaldson, R.M.: N. Engl. J. Med. *299*:827, 1978.

35d.Herbert, V., Jacob, E., Wong, K-T.J., et al.: Am. J. Clin. Nutr. *31*:253, 1978.

35e.Kanazawa, S., Herbert, V.: Am. J. Clin. Nutr. *37*:774, 1983.

35f.Kanazawa, S., Herbert, V., Herzlich, B., et al.: Lancet *i*:707, 1983.

35g.Shaw, S., Meyers, S., Colman, N., et al.: Fed. Proc. *46*:1004, 1987 (abstract).

35h.Internat. Comm. Stds Haematol. (ICSH): Br. J. Haematol. *64*:809, 1986.

36. Herbert, V., Bertino, J.R.: *In* The Vitamins: Chemistry, Physiology, Pathology, Methods, 2nd ed, Vol. VII. (Gyorgy, P., Pearson, W.N., Eds.) New York, Academic Press, 1967.

37. Herbert, V.: *In* Clinical Biochemistry. (Curtius, H-Ch., Roth, M., Eds.) Berlin and New York, Verlag Walter DeGruyter, 1974.

38. Herbert, V., Wasserman, L.R., Frank, O., et al.: Fed. Proc. *18*:246, 1959.

39. Baker, H., Herbert, V., Frank, O.: Clin. Chem. *5*:275, 1969.

40. Herbert, V., Baker, Frank, O., et al.: Blood *15*:228, 1960.

41. Herbert, V.: J. Clin. Invest. *40*:81, 1961.

42. Herbert, V.: J. Clin. Pathol. *19*:12, 1966.

43. Waxman, S., Schreiber, C., Herbert, V.: Blood *36*:858, 1970; *38*:219, 1971.

43a.Rothenberg, S.P., da Costa, M., Rosenberg, Z.: N. Engl. J. Med. *286*:1335, 1972.

44. Longo, D.L., Herbert, V.: J. Lab. Clin. Med. *87*:138, 1976.

45. Gutcho, S., Mansbach, L.: Clin. Chem. *23*:1609, 1977.

46. Jacob, E., Colman, N., Herbert, V.: Clin. Res. *25*:537A, 1977.

47. Glass, G.B.J., Physiol. Rev. *43*:529, 1963.

48. Herbert, V.: Gastroenterology *54*:110, 1968.

48a.Herbert, V.: Semin. Nucl. Med. *2*:220, 1972.

49. Gräsbeck, R.: Intrinsic Factor and Other Vitamin B$_{12}$ Transport Proteins. *In* Progress in Hematology, Vol. VI. (Brown, E., Moore, C., Eds.) New York, Grune & Stratton, 1969.

49a.Nexø, E., Oleson, H.: *In B$_{12}$*, Vol. 2., (Dolphin, D., Ed.) New York, John Wiley & Sons, 1982.

50. Carmel, R., Rosenberg, A.H., Lau, K-S., et al.: Gastroenterology *56*:548, 1969.

51. Corcino, J., Waxman, S., Herbert, V.: Am. J. Med. *48*:562, 1970.

51a.Chanarin, I.: J. Clin. Pathol. *24*(Suppl.):60, 1971.

51b.Bernstein, L., Herbert, V.: Am. J. Clin. Nutr. *26*:340, 1973.

51c.Allen, R.H., Seetharam, B., Allen, N.C., et al.: J. Clin. Invest. *61*:1628, 1978.

52. Butterworth, C.E., Jr., Krumdieck, C.L.: Br. J. Haematol. *31*(Suppl.):111, 1975.

53. Rosenberg, I.H.: Clin. Haematol. *5*:589, 1976.

54. Halsted, C.H., Baugh, C.M., Butterworth, C.E., Jr.: Gastroenterology *68*:261, 1975.

55. Reisenauer, A.M., Krumdieck, C.L., Halsted, C.H.: Fed. Proc. *36*:1120, 1977.

56. Butterworth, C.E. Jr., Newman, J.H., Krumdieck, C.L.: Trans. Am. Clin. Climatol. Assoc. *86*:11, 1974.

57. Tamura, T., Shin, Y.S., Buehring, K.U., et al.: Br. J. Haematol. *32*:123, 1976.

58. Gerson, C.D., Cohen, N., Hepner, G.W., et al.: Gastroenterology *61*:224, 1971.

59. Tamura, T., Stokstad, E.L.R.: Br. J. Haematol. *25*:513, 1973.

60. Colman, N., Green, R., Metz, J.: Am. J. Clin. Nutr. *28*:459, 1975.

60a.Colman, N., Hettiarachchy, N., Herbert, V.: Science *211*:1427, 1981.

61. Smith, M.E., Matty, A.J., Blair, J.A.: Biochim, Biophys. Acta *219*:37, 1970.

62. Hall, C.A.: Ann. Intern. Med. *75*:297, 1971.

62a.Stenman: Scand. J. Haematol. *14*:91, 1975.

62b.Allen, R.H.: Br. J. Haematol. *33*:161, 1976.

63. Herbert, V.: Am. J. Clin. Nutr. *7*:433, 1959.

63a.Castro, Z., Herbert, V., Wasserman, L.R., et al.: J. Clin. Invest. *40*:66, 1961.

63b.Herbert, V.: Blood *32*:305, 1968.

63c.Carmel, Herbert: Blood *40*:542, 1972.

64. Jacob, E., Wong, K-T.J., Herbert, V.: J. Lab. Clin. Med. *89*:1145, 1977.

65. Allen, R.H.: Prog. Hematol. *9*:57, 1975.

65a.Stenman, U-H.: Scand. J. Clin. Lab. Invest. *35*:157, 1975.

65b.Gräsbeck, R.: Br. J. Haematol *31*(Suppl.):103, 1975.

65c.Jacob, E., Baker, S.J., Herbert V.: Physiol. Rev. *60*:918, 1980.

66. Begley, J.A., Hall, C.A.: Blood *45*:287, 1975.

67. Corcino, J., Zalusky, R., Greenberg, M., et al.: Br. J. Haematol. *20*:511, 1971.

68. Tan, C.H., Hansen, H.J.: Proc. Soc. Exp. Biol. Med. *127*:740, 1968.

69. Cooksley, W.G.E., England, J.M., Louis, L., et al.: Clin. Sci. Mol. Med. *47*:531, 1974.

70. Savage, C.R., Jr., Green, P.D.: Fed. Proc. *34*:905, 1975.

71. Retief, F.P., Gottlieb, C., Herbert, V.: J. Clin. Invest. *45*:1907, 1966.

72. Hakami, N., Neiman, P.E., Cannellos, G.P., et al.: N. Engl. J. Med. *285*:1163, 1971.

73. Scott, C.R., Hakami, N., Teng, C.C., et al.: J. Pediatr. *81*:1106, 1972.

73a.Fleming, A.F., Ogunfunmilade, V.A., Carmel, R.: Am. J. Clin. Nutr. *31*:1732, 1978.

73b.Fräter-Schröder, M., Hitzig, W.H., et al.: Lancet *2*:238, 1978.

74. Herbert, V.: *In* Food and Agricultural Research Opportunities to Improve Human Nutrition for the 21st Century. (Doberenz, A.R., Milner, J.A., Schweigert, B.S., Eds.) University of Delaware, Newark, DE, College of Human Resources Press, 1986.

74a.Herbert, V., Herzlich, B.: Blood *66*(Suppl. 1): 45a, 1985.

74b.Herbert, V.: B$_{12}$ deficiency. *In* Book of Abstracts, XXIst Congress, International Soc. Haematol. Sydney, Australia, 1986.

75. Rappazzo, M.E., Salmi, H.A., Hall, C.A.: Br. J. Haematol. *18*:427, 1970.

76. Okuda, K., Gräsbeck, R., Chow, B.F.: J. Lab. Clin. Med. *51*:17, 1958.

77. Gräsbeck, R., Nyberg, W., Reizenstein, P.: Proc. Soc. Exp. Biol. Med. *97*:780, 1958.

78. Heinrich, H.C.: Semin. Hematol. *1*:199, 1964.

78a.Kanazawa, S., Herbert, V., Herzlich, B., et al.: Lancet *i*:707, 1983.

78b.Kanazawa, S., Herbert, V.: Trans. Assoc. Am. Physicians *96*:336–344, 1983.

78c.Herzlich, B., Herbert, V.: Am. J. Gastroenterol. *79*:489–493, 1984.

78d.Kanazawa, S. Herzlich, B., Herbert, V.: Am. J. Gastroenterology *80*:964–969, 1985.

79. Colman, N., Herbert, V.: *In* Topics in Hematology.

(Seno, S., Takaku, F., Irino, S., Eds.) Amsterdam, Excerpta Medica, 1977.

80. Colman, N., Herbert, V.: Blood *48*:911, 1976.
81. Murphy, M., Keating, M., Boyle, P., et al.: Biochem. Biophys. Res. Commun. *71*:1017, 1976.
82. Goldman, I.D.: Ann. N.Y. Acad. Sci. *186*:400, 1971.
82a.Antony, A., Utley, C., Kolhouse, J.F.: J. Biol. Chem. *257*:10081, 1982.
82b.Kane, M.A., Portillo, R.M., Elwood, P.E., et al.: J. Biol. Chem. *261*:44–49, 1985.
82c.Antony, A.C., Kane, M.A., Kolhouse, J.F.: J. Biol. Chem. *260*:14911–14917, 1985.
83. Rothenberg, S.P.: Proc. Soc. Exp. Biol. Med. *133*:428, 1970.
84. Colman, N., Herbert, V.: Program, 17th Annual Meeting of American Society of Hematology, 1974, p. 155.
85. Colman, N., Herbert, V.: Clin. Res. *25*:336A, 1977.
85a.Herbert, V., and Colman, N.: *In* Folic Acid and the Nervous System. (Botez, Reynolds, Eds.) New York, Raven Press, 1979.
86. Spector, R., Lorenzo, A.V.: Am. J. Physiol. *229*:777, 1975.
87. Hillman, R.S., McGuffin, R., Campbell, C.: Trans. Assoc. Am. Physicians *90*:145, 1977.
88. Stokes, J.B., Melikian, V., Leeming, R.J., et al.: Am. J. Clin. Nutr. *28*:126, 1975.
89. Lavoie, A., Cooper, B.A.: Clin. Sci. Mol. Med. *46*:729, 1974.
90. Herbert, V.: Am. J. Clin. Nutr. *27*:743, 1968.
91. Food and Nutrition Board, National Research Council: Recommended Dietary Allowances, 9th ed. Washington, National Academy of Sciences, 1980.
91a.Herbert, V.: Am. J. Clin. Nutr. *45*:661, 671, 1987.
91b.Herbert V: *In* Present Knowledge in Human Nutrition. 5th ed. (Olson, R.E., Ed.) New York, The Nutrition Foundation, 1984.
92. Herbert, V.: N. Engl. J. Med. *284*:976, 1971.
93. Jadhav, M., Webb, J.K.G., Vaishava, S., et al.: Lancet *2*:903, 1962.
93a.Truswell, A.: *In* Proceedings of the XIII International Congress of Nutrition. (Taylor, Jenkins, Eds.) London, John Libbey & Co., 1986.
93b.Herzlich, B., Drivas, G., Herbert, V.: Clin. Res. *33*:605A, 1986.
93c.Herzlich, B., Herbert, V.: Am. J. Hematol. In press, 1987.
93d.Herbert, V., Memoli, D., McAleer, E., et al.: Clin. Res. *34*:718A, 1986.
93e.Chanarin, I., Malkowska, O'Hea, et al.: Lancet *2*:1168, 1985.
94. Lichtenstein, H., Beloian, A., Murphy, E.W.: Vitamin B₁₂ Microbiological Assay Methods and Distribution in Selected Foods. Home Econ. Res. Rep. #13. Washington, U.S. Department of Agriculture, 1961.
94a.Ericson, Banhidi: Acta Chem. Scand. *7*:167, 1953.
94b.Lindenbaum, J.: Personal communication.
95. Herbert, V., Jacob, E.: JAMA *230*:241, 1974.
96. Newmark, H.L., Scheiner, J., Marcus, M., et al.: Am. J. Clin. Nutr. *29*:645, 1976.
97. Herbert, V., Jacob, E., Wong, K-T.J.: Am. J. Clin. Nutr. *30*:297, 1977.
98. Sayers, M., Lynch, S., Jacobs, P., et al.: Br. J. Haematol. *24*:209, 1973.
99. Sayers, M., Lynch, S., Charlton, R., et al.: Br. J. Haematol. *28*:483, 1974.
99a.Herbert, V., Landau, L., Shang, C., et al.: Blood *52*:(Suppl. 1): November, 1978.
100. Colman, N.: *In* Advances in Nutritional Research. (Draper, H.H., Ed.) New York, Plenum Press, 1977.
100a.Rodriguez: *In* Nutritional Requirements of Man. (Irwin, Ed.) New York, The Nutrition Foundation, 1980.
100b.Wagner, C.: *In* Present Knowledge in Nutrition, 5th Ed. (Olson, R.E. Ed.) New York, The Nutrition Foundation, 1984.
101. Sullivan, L.W., Herbert, V.: J. Clin. Invest. *43*:2048, 1964.
101a.Herbert, V.: Trans. Assoc. Am. Physicians *75*:307, 1962.
101b.Herbert, V.: *In* Proceedings of the XIII International Congress Nutrition. (Taylor, Jenkins, Eds.) London, John Libbey & Co., 1986.
101c.Herbert, V., Colman, N., Drivas, G.: Blood *66* (Suppl. 1):45a, 1985.
101d.Herbert, V.: *In* Book of Abstracts, XXI Congress, International Soc. Haematol, Sydney, Australia, 1986.
102. Herbert, V.: Am. J. Clin. Nutr. *12*:17, 1963.
103. Hurdle, A.D.F., Barton, D., Searles, I.H.: Am. J. Clin. Nutr. *21*:1202, 1968.
104. Hoppner, K., Lampi, B., Perrin, D.E.: J. Inst. Cancer Sci. Tech. Aliment. *5*:60, 1972.
105. Perloff, Butrum, R.R.: J. Am. Diet. Assoc. *70*:161, 1977.
106. Reed, B., Weir, D.G., Scott, J.M.: Am. J. Clin. Nutr. *29*:1393, 1976.
107. Herbert, V., Zalusky, R.: J. Clin. Invest. *41*:1263, 1962.
108. Metz, J., Kelly, A., Swett, V.C., et al.: Br. J. Haematol. *4*:575, 1968.
109. Das, K.C., Herbert, V.: Clin. Haematol. *5*:697, 1976.
110. Noronha, J.M., Silverman, M.: *In* Vitamin B₁₂ and Intrinsic Factor, 2nd European Symposium. (Heinrich, H., Ed.) Stuttgart, Ferdinand Enke Verlag, 1962.
111. Hoffbrand, A.V., Ganeshaguru, K., Hooton, J.W.L., et al.: Clin. Haematol. *5*:727, 1976.
111a.Luzzatto, L., Falusi, A.O., and Joju, E.A.: N. Engl. J. Med. *299*:1156, 1981.
112. Herbert, V.: The Megaloblastic Anemias. New York, Grune and Stratton, 1959.
113. Herbert, V.: Proc. R. Soc. Med. *57*:377, 1964.
114. Cooper, B.A., Lowenstein, L.: Blood *24*:502, 1964.
115. Das, K.C., Hoffbrand, A.V.: Br. J. Haematol. *19*:203, 1970.
116. Tisman, G., Herbert, V.: Blood *41*:465, 1973.
117. Spronk, A.M.: Fed. Proc. *32*:471A, 1974.
118. Shane, B., Brody, T., Stokstad, E.L.R.: Fed. Proc. *36*:1120, 1977.
119. Frenkel, E.P.: J. Clin. Invest. *50*:33a, 1971.
120. Marcus, A., Ullman, H.L., Safier, L.B., et al.: J. Clin. Invest. *41*:2198, 1962.
121. Colman, N., Herbert, V.: *In* Biochemistry of Brain. (Kumar, Ed.) Oxford, Pergamon Press, 1979, pp. 127–142.
122. Weissbach, H., Taylor, R.T.: Vitam. Horm. *28*:395, 1968.
123. Barley, F.W., Sato, G.H., Abeles, R.H.: J. Biol. Chem. *247*:4270, 1972.
124. Frenkel, E.P.: J. Clin. Invest. *52*:1237, 1973.
125. Ellenbogen, L.: *In* Newer Methods of Nutritional Biochemistry, Vol. 1. (Albanese, Ed.) New York, Academic Press, 1963.
126. Herbert, V., Das, K.C.: Vitam. Horm. *34*:1, 1976.

127. Pearson, A.G.M., Turner, A.J.: Nature *258*:173, 1975.
128. Meller, E., Rosengarten, H., Friedhoff, A., et al.: Science *187*:171, 1975.
128a.Das, K.C., Herbert, V.: Br. J. Haematol. *38*:219, 1978.
128b.Das, K.C., Herbert, V., Colman, N., et al.: Br. J. Haematol. *39*:357, 1978.
128c.Colman, N., Herbert, V.: Blood *52*(Suppl. 1): 132, 1978.
128d.Herbert, V.: Med. Grand Rounds, *1*:320, 1982.
128e.Green, R., Kuhl, W., Jacobsen, R., et al.: N. Engl. J. Med. *307*:1322, 1982.
128f.Spivack, J.L.: Arch. Intern. Med. *142*:2111, 1982.
129. Herbert, V.: N. Engl. J. Med. *268*:201, 368, 1963.
130. Herbert, V.: Semin. Hematol. *7*:2, 1970.
130a.Colman N., Demartino, L., McAleer, E.: Blood *68*:45A, 1986.
130b.Herbert, V., Huebscher, T., Stopler, T.: Unpublished data.
131. Herbert, V.: *In* Disease-A-Month. Chicago, Year Book Medical Publishers, 1965.
132. Zalusky, R., Herbert, V.: N. Engl. J. Med. *265*:1033, 1961.
133. Bonnar, Goldberg, Smith: Lancet *1*:451, 1969.
133a.Herbert, V.: Am. J. Clin. Nutr. *45*:679, 1987.
133b.Simmer, K., Iles, C.A., James, N., et al.: Am. J. Clin. Nutr. *45*:122, 1987.
134. Sood, Ramachandran, Mathur, et al.: Q. J. Med. *44*:241, 1975.
135. Colman, N., Barker, M., Green, R., et al.: Am. J. Clin. Nutr. *27*:339, 1974.
136. Herbert, V., Colman, N., Spivack, M., et al.: Am. J. Obstet. Gynecol. *123*:175, 1975.
136a.Herbert, V.: *In* Nutritional Disorders of American Women. (Winick, Ed.) New York, John Wiley & Sons, 1977.
137. Colman, N., Larsen, J.V., Barker, M., et al.: Am. J. Clin. Nutr. *28*:465, 1975.
138. Colman, N., Barker, E.A., Barker, M., et al.: Am. J. Clin. Nutr. *28*:471, 1975.
139. Colman, N., Larsen, J.V., Barker, M., et al.: S. Afr. Med. J. *48*:1763, 1974.
140. Colman, N., Green, R., Stevens, K., et al.: S. Afr. Med. J. *48*:1795, 1974.
141. FAO/WHO: WHO Tech. Rep. Ser. #477, 1971.
142. WHO: WHO Tech. Rep. Ser. #580, 1975.
142a.Rosenberg, L.: *In* Metabolic Basis of Inherited Disease, 5th Ed. (Stanbury, Wyngaarden, Fredrickson, et al., Eds.) New York, McGraw-Hill Book Co., 1983.
143. Hom, B.L., Olsen, H., Schwartz, M.: Scand. J. Haematol. *5*:107, 1968.
144. Reynolds, E.H.: Brain *91*:197, 1968.
144a.Herbert, V., Tisman, G.: *In* Biology of Brain Dysfunction (Gaull, Ed.) New York, Plenum Press, 1973.
144b.Herbert, V., Colman, N.: *In* Folic Acid in Neurology, Psychiatry, and Internal Medicine. (Botez, M.I., Reynolds, E.H., Eds.) New York, Raven Press, 1979.
144c.Colman, N., Herbert, V.: *In* Folates and Pterins, Vol 3. (Blakley, R.L., Ed.) New York, John Wiley & Sons, 1986, pp. 340–357.
145. Hommes, O.R., Obbens, E.A.M.T., et al.: J. Neurol. Sci. *19*:63, 1973.
146. Chi'en, L.T., Krumdieck, C.L., Scott, C.W., Jr., et al.: Am. J. Clin. Nutr. *28*:51, 1975.
146a.Gerson, C.D., Hepner, G.W., Brown, N., et al.: Gastroenterology *63*:363, 1972.
147. Paukert, J.L., Straus, L.D., Rabinowitz, J.C.: J. Biol. Chem. *251*:5104, 1976.
148. Drury, E.J., Bazar, L.S., MacKenzie, R.E.: Arch. Biochem. Biophys. *169*:662, 1975.
149. Herbert, V.: *In* Textbook of Medicine, 14th ed. (Beeson, P.B., McDermott, W., Eds.) Philadelphia, W.B. Saunders, Co., 1975.
150. Herbert, V.: Am. J. Clin. Nutr. *45*:661, 1987.

*Chapter* **22**

# ASCORBIC ACID

## Dietrich H. Hornig, Ulrich Moser, and Beat E. Glatthaar

## HISTORY

The ancient disease known as scurvy, and later recognized as vitamin C deficiency disease, accompanied mankind through history. It affected many people in ancient Egypt, Greece, and Rome. Scurvy influenced the course of history because rations during military campaigns and long ocean voyages seldom contained adequate amounts of vitamin C.[1] Between 1556 and 1857, 114 scurvy epidemics were reported from several countries, most occurring during winter and spring when fresh fruits and vegetables were not available.[2] Equally large were the number of reports from sea voyages during which scurvy proved to be devastating on long journeys.[3]

This large number of accounts of scurvy led to the first clues to the treatment of the disease. In 1536, Jacques Cartier, on advice from Newfoundland Indians, took an extract from spruce tree needles to cure an epidemic among his crew. Subsequently, in several other incidences, the use of oranges, lemons, all kinds of berries, fruits, and fresh vegetables proved to be an effective treatment. In 1720, Kramer prescribed fresh herbs or lemons to the Austrian soldiers fighting the Turks. Although numerous indications began to appear that scurvy was associated with diet, this knowledge had to be rediscovered many times until the nineteenth century.[4]

As a consequence of the disastrous voyage around the world from 1740 to 1744, when Admiral George A. Anson lost most of his men, most due to scurvy, James Lind in 1742 performed his famous experiment, which may have been the first controlled clinical trial. He published his findings in his "Treatise of the Scurvy," described the disease as a dietary deficiency, and demonstrated that patients given lemon juice recovered.[5] Captain Cook succeeded in avoiding scurvy altogether on his three voyages between 1768 and 1779. Only in 1804, however, did the British Navy adopt the use of lime juice rations for all crews. Still, scurvy incidents continued to occur periodically even though prevention had been demonstrated. Particularly during wars poor nutrition caused the disease.

The history of scurvy research leading to the discovery of vitamin C only began in 1907 when Holst and Frölich found the guinea pig to be as susceptible to scurvy as man.[6] The findings that the disease could be experimentally produced led to the development of an assay for the biologic determination of the antiscorbutic potency of foodstuffs. Between 1910 and 1921 Zilva and his associates extracted the elusive substance from lemons and discovered that the antiscorbutic activity was probably associated with a capacity for reducing phenolindophenol.[7] In 1922, Drummond's proposal to name the antiscorbutic factor vitamin C was accepted.[8]

The characterization of vitamin C was first accomplished by Szent-Györgyi in 1928. He isolated a reducing agent in crystalline form from orange juice, cabbage juice, and adrenal glands that he called "hexuronic acid." In 1932, Svirbely and Szent-Györgyi[9] and independently King and Waugh[10] demonstrated hexuronic acid to be identical with vitamin C. In 1933, Hirst and Haworth determined the structure of vitamin C,[11] and Reichstein worked out a synthesis[12] that 50 years later still forms the basis for large-scale industrial production. The name L-ascorbic acid was coined by Haworth and Szent-Györgyi in 1933 to point out the antiscorbutic properties of vitamin C. It was proved unambiguously that the synthetic product has the same biologic activity as the product isolated from natural tissues.

## CHEMISTRY AND ANALYTICAL DETERMINATION

Ascorbic acid is a white, odorless, crystalline solid with a sharp acidic taste. Its chemical composition is $C_6H_8O_6$, resulting in a molecular weight of 176.13. At 190 to 192°C decomposition takes place. One gram of ascorbic acid dissolves in 3 ml water, but it is insoluble in most organic solvents.

The original structure determination of L-ascorbic acid was confirmed by the synthesis from L-xylose, assigning it to the L series. Biosynthesis of ascorbic acid in animals and plants begins from either D-glucose or D-galactose. Chemical synthesis starts from glucose, but follows different steps. In addition to vitamin C and L-ascorbic acid, there exist the chemical names L-xyloascorbic acid and L-threo-hex-2-uronic acid γ-lactone.[13-15] Among the chemical properties of ascorbic acid, the reversible oxidation-reduction with dehydro-L-ascorbic acid is the most important and is probably the basis for most of its known physiologic functions. Although ascorbic acid is stable when dry, it tends to undergo rapid oxidation by atmospheric oxygen in an aqueous solution (Fig. 22–1). No dehydroascorbic acid could be found in these solutions kept at room temperature. Ascorbic acid in tap water becomes more stable with increasing concentrations, and it is rapidly oxidized below a concentration of 10 mg/dl. In aqueous solutions, it is more sensitive to alkalies than to acids; it is most stable at pH 4 to pH 6. Ascorbic acid is sensitive to heat. Most metals, especially copper, catalyze its oxidation. Degradation products of ascorbate are dehydroascorbic acid, 2,3-diketo-L-gulonic acid, oxalic acid, and L-threonic acid. In acidic solution, the degradation process furnishes a number of additional products.

In liquid vitamin preparations, the degradation of ascorbic acid depends on the composition of the mixture; preaddition of this vitamin to TPN solutions must be avoided.[16] Of the various derivatives and analogues prepared, only salts and C-6 substituted esters have biologic activity. They are readily converted to ascorbic acid in the body.[17]

A large number of spectroscopic, electrochemical, enzymatic, and chromatographic methods for the analysis of ascorbic acid in food products, pharmaceuticals, and biologic samples have been described.[18-20a] Colorimetric reactions with metal ions, which are unspecific and subject to interference by a large number of substances contained in foods and other natural products, can be combined with enzymatic techniques in order to increase specificity without losing the advantage of a simple and fast method.[18] The application of gas chromatography dramatically improves the sensitivity and selectivity of the analysis, but ascorbic acid has to be transformed into a derivative.[20b]

The separation of ascorbic acid from other compounds with high-performance liquid chromatography (HPLC) allows the detection of an isomer, erythorbic acid, together with ascorbic acid using electrochemical detection. The determination of ascorbic acid together with its oxidized form (dehydroascorbic acid) is only possible after transformation into a derivative. HPLC allows the highly selective and sensitive detection of ascorbic acid in tissues and plasma. However, the appropriate method must be chosen according to the nature of the sample and the lab facilities.[20a] To assess the biologic activity of ascorbic acid, a test system is required that is dependent on ascorbic acid. For practical reasons, the guinea pig is virtually the only suitable model, although monkeys may also be used.

## SOURCES OF VITAMIN C

Ascorbic acid occurs in all living tissues, which is not surprising in view of its redox function in cell metabolism. Important sources of vitamin C are fresh fruits and vegetables (Table 22–1).[21]

## ABSORPTION, DISTRIBUTION, ELIMINATION

Vitamin C has been demonstrated in guinea pigs and in man to be absorbed in the intestine by an active $Na^+$-dependent, energy-requiring, electroneutral, carrier-mediated transport mechanism. The apparent $K_m$ values for transport of ascorbate into brush border membrane vesicles from guinea pig small intestine were determined to be approximately 0.3 mmol; in model experiments with human material, $K_m$ was found to be 0.5 mmol.[22-25] Absorption in the rat and in all species that are not prone to scurvy follows a passive diffusion mechanism.[25,26]

Because an active transport mechanism is a saturable process, the relative absorption capacity is

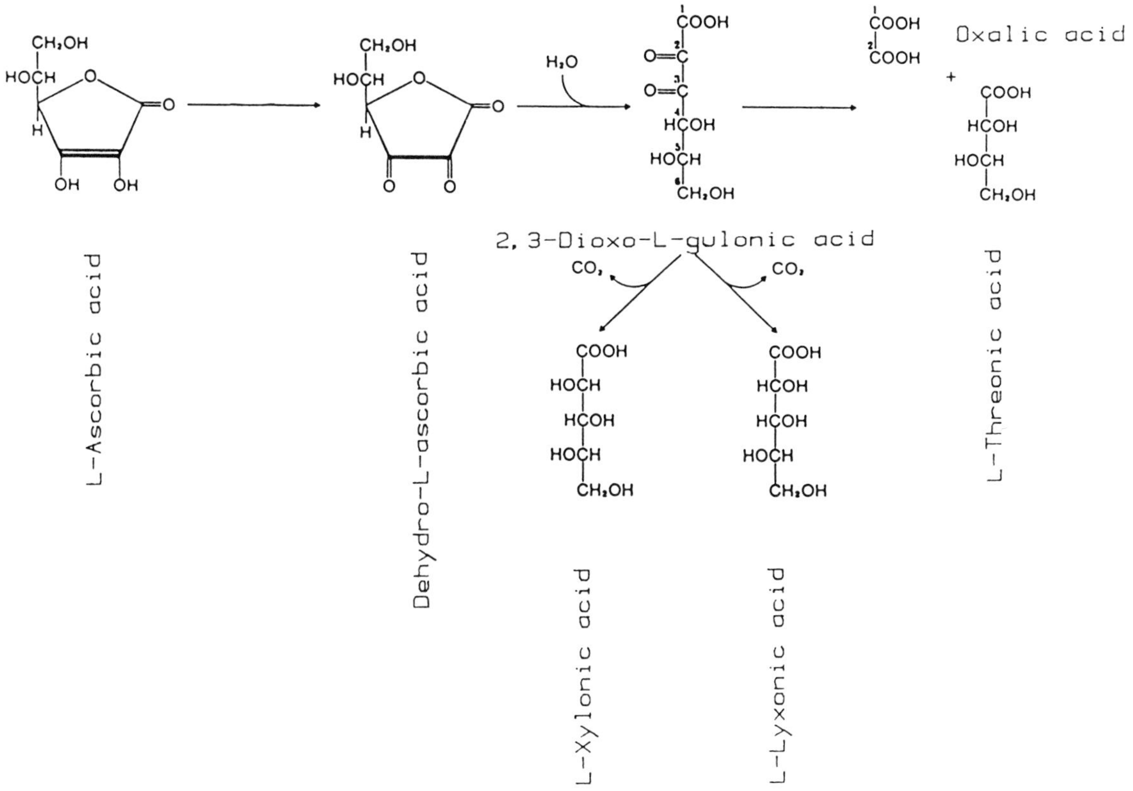

**Fig. 22–1.** Degradation products of ascorbic acid.

reduced with increasing intakes of the compound. In volunteers, saturation kinetics of absorption were demonstrated with a $K_m$ of 5.44 mmol at different vitamin C concentrations. The transport was studied by intestinal perfusion of vitamin C using the triple lumen technique.[27] With a pharmacokinetic approach, at oral intakes increasing from 1.5 to 12 g, the relative absorption decreased from approximately 50% to only 16%. An average absorption of 70% was extrapolated for intakes of up to 180 mg.[28] Estimation of the absorption of ascorbic acid in volunteers using (1-[14]C) ascorbic acid yielded a mean absorption of 84% of the dose (up to 180 mg) as estimated from the urinary elimination of ([14]C) radioactivity.[29] Similar results were found in smokers (mean 76%).[30] These results indicate losses of up to 20% during the absorption process of physiologic doses. This conclusion can be made because the appearance of label in the feces is negligible.[31,32]

The absorption capacity of the intestine for vitamin C in man was found to be saturated at oral intakes of 3 g. By using urinary ascorbate excretion as a parameter, researchers determined an absorption of 75% with an intake of 1 g as a *single* dose, of 44% with 2 g, of 39% with 3 g, of 28% with 4 g, and of 20% with 5 g of the ingested dose. A maximum absorption capacity of approximately 1,200 mg was calculated, which is reached with a single intake of 3 g.[33,34] The absorption capacity can only be increased by administration of graded intakes. Following loading with 5 × 1 g ascorbic acid daily, the urinary excretion within 24 hours resulted in 1,600 to 1,800 mg, whereas with intakes of 5 × 2 g of ascorbic acid, the excretion rose to approximately 2,500 mg, indicating an absorption of 30% and 25% of the dose.[35] Increasing intakes of ascorbic acid resulted in an increase of urinary excretion of unaltered ascorbic acid, since in man the mechanism of elimination involves a saturable $Na^+$-dependent and potentially sensitive reabsorption process.[36] Studies on the kinetic

**Table 22–1.  Content of Ascorbic Acid in Selected Foods**

| Food | mg/100 g |
|------|----------|
| fruits of *Terminalia ferdinandiana* (Australia) | 3,000 |
| acerola | 2,000 |
| hips | 1,000 |
| black currants | 200 |
| broccoli | 70–160 |
| brussels sprouts | 90–150 |
| cauliflower | 50–90 |
| strawberries | 40–90 |
| lemons | 50–80 |
| cabbage | 50–80 |
| oranges | 40–60 |
| grapefruit | 35–45 |
| pineapples | 20–40 |
| turnips | 15–40 |
| liver, kidney | 10–40 |
| tomatoes | 10–30 |
| peaches | 5–25 |
| potatoes | 10–20 |
| beans | 10–20 |
| peas | 10–15 |
| apples | 5–10 |
| bananas | 5–10 |
| cow's milk | 1–2 |
| meat, beef, and pork | up to 2 |

**Table 22–2.  Unchanged Ascorbate Recovered from Urine***

| Dosage (mg/day) | Number of Subjects Studied | 14C-Ascorbate (%) |
|-----------------|----------------------------|-------------------|
| 1 × 30 | 4 | 6.6 |
| 2 × 30 | 4 | 20.3 |
| 2 × 45 | 3 | 34.1 |
| 4 × 45 | 4 | 61.7 |
| 4 × 250 | 4 | 82.4 |
| 4 × 500 | 3 | 87.9 |
| 2 × 1,000 | 8 | 87.0 |

*In relation to total amounts of radioactivity in urine, at various levels of oral intake.
From Kallner, A., et al.,[37] with permission of Am. J. Clin. Nutr., American Society for Clinical Nutrition.

behavior of (1-14C) ascorbic acid demonstrated that the steep increase in renal turnover of unmetabolized ascorbic acid observed at plasma concentrations of 0.8 to 0.9 mg/dl is the consequence of the saturability of the reabsorption process.[37] This value indicates the threshold.

The investigation by Kallner et al. using (1-14C) ascorbic acid as tracer (15 to 25 μCi per subject) demonstrated that the percentage of total urinary radioactivity excreted as unmetabolized (1-14C) ascorbic acid increases with intakes of unlabeled ascorbic acid (Table 22–2).[37] In addition, with low intakes (30 mg/day), a substantial amount was excreted unaltered in urine (6.6%). Thus, with large intakes only 10 to 15% of the total urinary excre-

tion derived from ascorbate can be represented by metabolites. With the limited absorption capacity of the intestine with high intakes, then, the total amount of metabolites that may be formed from ascorbic acid will not be higher than 100 to 150 mg/day, even with very high intakes.[37]

The distribution of ascorbic acid has been reported for mice,[38] rats,[39] and guinea pigs.[40,41] Ascorbic acid is widely distributed throughout the tissues. In man, the highest concentrations were found, by analyses of postmortem specimens, in the adrenal and pituitary glands (30 to 50 mg/100 g wet tissue). High levels were also found in liver, spleen, and brain (10 to 15 mg/100 g wet tissue), but their contribution to the total body pool was by far larger than that from glands and secretory organs (Table 22–3).[40] At present, no information is available on tissue concentrations of ascorbate in man following continuous high intakes. Studies have documented that the body pool of ascorbic acid approaches "saturation" at approximately 20 mg/kg of body weight, but it has been claimed that the pool may be further enlarged with intakes far higher than the physiologic range.[42]

## METABOLISM

A number of review papers on the metabolism of ascorbic acid have been published in the past decade.[13,16,33,40,43–47] In animals such as guinea pigs and rats there is a considerable conversion of carboxy-group labeled ascorbic acid to carbon dioxide. In guinea pigs, respiratory exhalation of (14C) carbon dioxide after administration of (1-14C) ascorbic acid is the major route of catabolism. Urinary and fecal excretion contribute only to a minor part.[41] Of the approximately 8 to 10% of label recovered in urine, unchanged ascorbic acid, de-

**Table 22–3.  Ascorbic Acid Levels of Adult Human Tissues**

| Tissue | Ascorbic Acid (mg/100 g wet tissue) |
|--------|-------------------------------------|
| Adrenal glands | 30–40 |
| Pituitary gland | 40–50 |
| Liver | 10–16 |
| Spleen | 10–15 |
| Lungs | 7 |
| Kidneys | 5–15 |
| Testes | 3 |
| Thyroid | 2 |
| Heart muscle | 5–15 |
| Skeletal muscle | 3–4 |
| Brain | 13–15 |
| Pancreas | 10–15 |
| Eye lens | 25–31 |
| Plasma | 0.4–1.0 |
| Saliva | 0.07–0.09 |

From Hornig, D.,[40] with permission of Ann. N.Y. Acad. Sci.

hydroascorbic acid, and 2,3-diketo-L-gulonic acid accounted for approximately 2 to 3% of the given dose. Most of the excreted label was incorporated in oxalate (7% of the given dose). Other metabolites were isolated and identified in rat and/or guinea pig urine: 2-0-methyl ascorbate, ascorbic acid 2-sulfate, and saccharoascorbic acid, all of which are excreted in small amounts.[44]

The metabolism of ascorbic acid in the trained monkey is similar to that in man. The monkey is therefore an excellent study model. In studies, the size of the body pool varied with the level of dietary intake. With an intake of 1 mg/kg body weight, a pool size of 24 mg/kg could be maintained. The turnover rate was calculated to be 2.5 mg/day, and the half-life was estimated to be approximately 15 days. Half-lives were substantially prolonged when lower amounts of ascorbic acid were ingested. The percentage of unmetabolized ascorbic acid excreted in urine increased with the dietary intake; feces contained only negligible amounts. Following ingestion of (1-[14]C) ascorbic acid, two main fractions of the urinary radioactivity were identified as unmetabolized (1-[14]C) ascorbate and ([14]C) oxalate. With low ascorbate intake, unmetabolized ascorbate accounted for 10 to 20% and oxalate for 25 to 48% of the urinary radioactivity. With increasing intakes of ascorbate (larger than 10 mg/kg body weight), however, unmetabolized ascorbate (about 75%) was identified as the major fraction. Oxalate contributed only 7%, suggesting the metabolic conversion of ascorbate to oxalate to be limited.[48] The conversion of ascorbate into 5-keto metabolites suggests that there may be other metabolites of ascorbic acid of functional importance.[44,45] As in the trained monkey,[46] ascorbic acid is not converted to carbon dioxide in man. Less than 5% of (1-[14]C) ascorbic acid was exhaled during a 10-day period following intravenous injection of labeled ascorbate.[37,49,50]

In humans the principal route of elimination of metabolic products of ascorbate is urinary excretion. Dehydroascorbate, 2,3-diketo-L-gulonate, ascorbate 2-sulfate, and oxalate are the main metabolites.[32] Under physiologic intakes of vitamin C, oxalate contributes on average about half of the daily oxalate excretion of approximately 40 to 50 mg. However, more recent evidence has clearly demonstrated that the conversion rate of ascorbate to oxalate is limited. In healthy volunteers, intakes of 10 g ascorbic acid per day (5 × 2 g) enhanced the mean urinary oxalate excretion only slightly from about 50 to 90 mg per day. The average increase in oxalate excretion was only small, especially when compared with the large amount of vitamin C available for a possible conversion to oxalate.[35,51] Hyperoxaluria has been attributed to ascorbic acid administration of 1 to 1.5 g/day during parenteral nutrition in one patient.[51a] However, ascorbic acid may be oxidized to oxalate in urine at room temperature.[51b] Special care must be taken for the oxalate determination because ascorbic acid may also be degraded to oxalate during the analytical procedure, leading to false positive results.[51c]

In summary, it is concluded that ascorbic acid, even at large intakes, is not a risk factor in the multifactorial process of oxalate stone formation. Patients suffering from oxaluria and people with a history of oxalate stones, however, should avoid any source of additional oxalate.

One investigation found that man produced and exhaled carbon dioxide from oral (1-[14]C) ascorbic acid if the amount of unlabeled carrier of ascorbic acid was larger than at least 300 mg.[52] Perorally administered ascorbate is perhaps metabolized presystematically, that is, by gastrointestinal microflora, to compounds that may be further catabolized to carbon dioxide. The finding that low doses of ascorbate given with tracer doses of (1-[14]C) ascorbate do not give rise to carbon dioxide is explained by the rapid and almost complete absorption of the compound in the proximal part of the duodenum.

## BIOCHEMICAL AND PHYSIOLOGIC FUNCTIONS

L-Ascorbic acid is a cofactor of hydroxylating enzymes, either as part of the active site[53] or as a protective reducing agent.[54] However, these enzymatic reactions cannot be used as early signs of vitamin C depletion at this time because the relationship between enzymatic activity and vitamin concentration is not well documented. Owing to its reducing properties and its reaction with free radicals, however, it plays important roles in many biochemical reactions. Although actual reaction mechanisms are not fully understood at the molecular level, there is evidence that ascorbic acid may be critical in reactions depending on reduced iron or copper. The only role of ascorbic acid that is categorically established is its function in the prevention and cure of clinical scurvy.

**Collagen Synthesis.** Hydroxylation of proline is essential for the formation and stabilization of the triple helical structure of collagen. Hydroxylation of lysine is essential for glycosylation and therefore for the formation of hydroxylysine-derived cross-links.[55] These reactions are catalyzed by prolylhydroxylase (EC 1.14.11.2) or lysyl hydroxylase (EC 1.14.11.4), both of which require iron in the ferrous form.[56] Oxygen and 2-oxoglutarate inactivate prolylhydroxylase unless ascorbic acid is present, which presumably prevents S-S bridge formation in the enzyme.[56a] Although compounds such as tetrahydropterin, tetrahydrofolate, cysteine, and dithiothreitol can function as reducing agents, ascorbic acid is the most efficient agent and the physiologic cofactor.[57] Lack of ascorbic acid results in under-hydroxylated proline in tropocollagen, which leads to a reduced stability of connective tissue.[58] In guinea pigs, skin, bone, and tendon are sensitive to ascorbate deficiency, whereas internal organs such as skeletal muscle, lung, heart, and kidney exhibit only small effects.[59]

Beneficial effects have been claimed for ascorbic acid in doses of 1 to 4 g daily in humans suffering from pressure sores, ulcers, and Ehlers-Danlos syndrome type VI (lysyl hydroxylase deficiency). In a double-blind controlled clinical trial in a group of 20 surgical patients suffering from pressure sores, the treatment with 1 g ascorbic acid daily was followed by an 84% reduction of the ulcers, whereas the corresponding reduction in the placebo group was 43%.[60] Seven patients given 1 g ascorbic acid daily showed an increased collagen synthesis at the site of pressure sores compared with other patients given a placebo.[61] A higher rate of complete or partial healing of leg ulcers could be observed in individuals with β-thalassemia given 3 g ascorbic acid daily in a double-blind cross-over trial.[62] In one patient with Ehlers-Danlos syndrome type IV, the application of 4 g ascorbic acid daily led to an improvement of wound healing, corneal growth, bleeding time, muscle strength, and pulmonary residual volume.[63]

**Carnitine Synthesis.** L-Carnitine is essential for carrying long-chain fatty acids into mitochondria for β-oxidation, providing energy to cells, especially to myocardium and to skeletal muscle. The distribution of enzymes involved in carnitine metabolism, e.g., short-chain and medium-chain carnitine acyltransferases, has led to the conclusion that carnitine has multiple roles in mammalian metabolism.[64] The highest concentration of carnitine is found in the epididymis (60 mmol). Therefore, carnitine may play an important role in the maturation and maintenance of spermatozoa.[65] Carnitine can be either obtained via the diet or synthesized from lysine and methionine. Two dioxygenases in this pathway (EC 1.14.11.8 and EC 1.14.11.1) are dependent on ferrous iron and L-ascorbic acid similar to prolyl and lysyl hydroxylases.[66] Studies in guinea pigs have shown that ascorbic acid depletion results in a significant reduction in skeletal and heart muscle carnitine well before any classic signs of scurvy can be observed,[67] whereas brain and serum contents remain unchanged.[67a] Experiments with perfused guinea pig livers demonstrated that the γ-butyrobetaine, 2-oxoglutarate-dioxygenase, but not the trimethyl-lysine, 2-oxoglutarate-dioxygenase, becomes the rate-limiting enzyme in ascorbate-deficient animals.[67a] Muscle carnitine may therefore be a highly sensitive indicator of ascorbate status. Furthermore, symptoms such as fatigue and lassitude seen in vitamin C-depleted human volunteers may be the result of poor energy production due to decreased carnitine biosynthesis.[68]

**Noradrenaline Synthesis.** One of the enzymes of the biosynthesis of noradrenaline and also of adrenaline from tyrosine, the copper-containing dopamine-β-mono-oxygenase (EC 1.14.17.1), necessitates stoichiometric amounts of ascorbic acid (Fig. 22–2). This enzyme catalyzes the incorporation of oxygen into the side chain of dopamine, forming the end-products noradrenaline and water.[69] Thus, the function of ascorbic acid in this reaction is clearly different from its role in collagen and carnitine synthesis. Noradrenaline is synthesized in neural tissues and in the adrenal medulla. Experiments with guinea pigs deficient in ascorbic acid suggest that the synthesis of biogenic amines is dependent on the ascorbic acid status.[70] Ascorbic acid consumed during the biosynthesis of noradrenaline in adrenal chromaffin granules must be regenerated in order to maintain intragranular reduced ascorbic acid. Cytosolic ascorbate serves as a source of reducing equivalents, and cytochrome $b_{561}$ may act as an electron shuttle between the ascorbate pools.[70a,70b] Furthermore, the injection of ascorbate into the brain affects dopamine function by increasing its metabolism to noradrenaline.[71] Therefore, vitamin C therapy is claimed by some to be of advantage in conditions of dopamine excess such as schizophrenia, chorea, and dyskinesia.

**Peptide α-Amidation.** Many of the bioactive peptides, such as α-melanocyte-stimulating hormone and adrenocorticotropic hormone, isolated from neural and endocrine tissues have an α-amide moiety at their carboxyl terminus. The α-amidation is catalyzed by the enzyme peptidylglycine α-amidating mono-oxygenase, which is dependent on copper, oxygen, and ascorbic acid as cofactors. This enzymatic activity is associated with secretory granules and secreted along with amidated product peptides.[71a,71b] In one study of guinea pigs deprived of ascorbic acid, only two thirds of the gastrin isolated from the antrum was amidated compared to 100% in animals receiving ascorbic acid.[71c]

**Degradation of Cholesterol.** The first and rate-limiting step in the conversion of cholesterol to bile acids is the hydroxylation in liver micro-

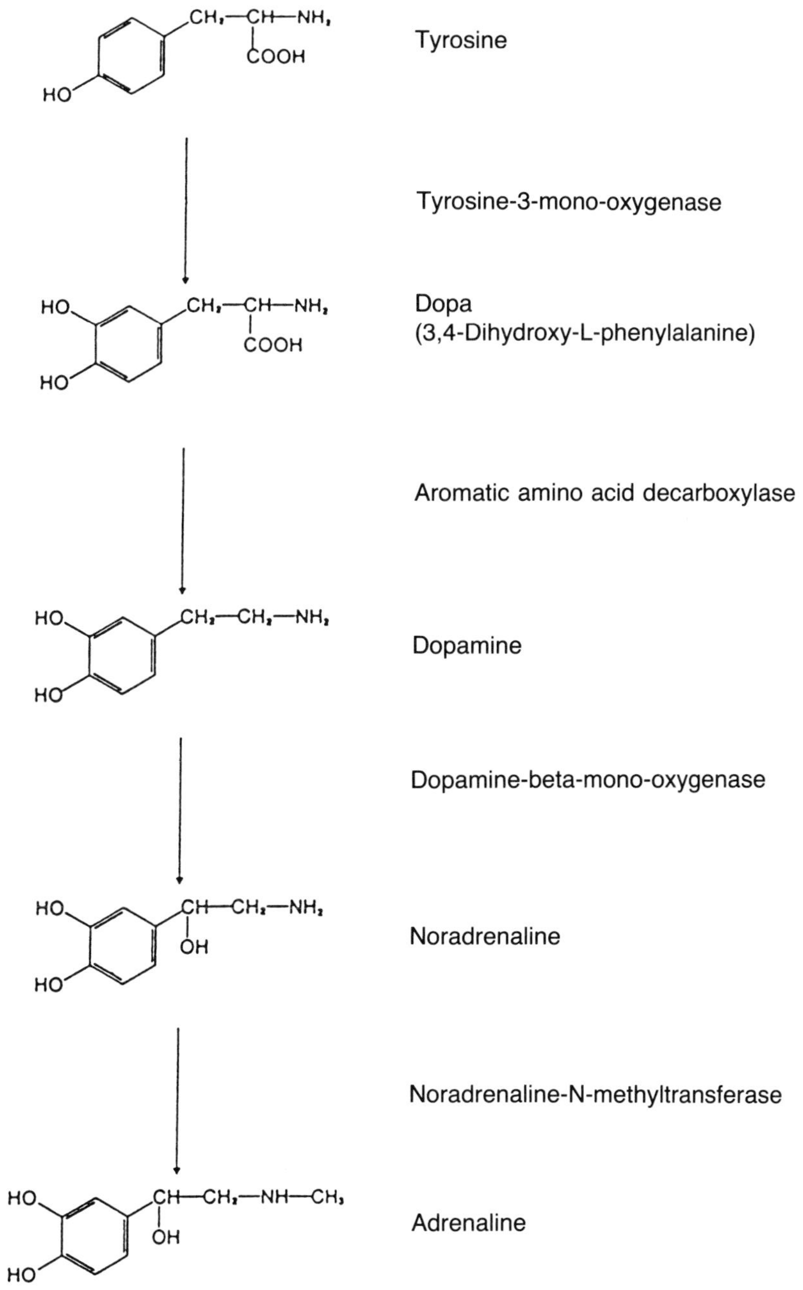

**Fig. 22–2.** Biosynthesis of catecholamines. Ascorbic acid acts as a cofactor of dopamine-β-mono-oxygenase.

somes catalyzed by the cytochrome P450-dependent cholesterol-7α-mono-oxygenase (EC 1.14.13.17). The enzyme activity is depressed by 46% in the liver of guinea pigs with chronic marginal vitamin C deficiency leading to an accumulation of cholesterol in tissues and plasma.[72–74] Thus, hypovitaminosis C may be implicated as an etiologic risk factor in the pathogenesis of hypercholesterolemia and coronary artery disease.[73,74]

**Degradation of Tyrosine.** In the main pathway,

tyrosine is metabolized to fumarate and acetoacetate. The enzyme 4-hydroxyphenylpyruvate dioxygenase (EC 1.13.11.27) is protected by ascorbic acid from substrate inhibition under tyrosine loading. In case of ascorbate deficiency, p-hydroxypyruvic, p-hydroxylactic, and homogentisic acids are excreted in urine.[75]

**Recycling of 5,6,7,8-Tetrahydrobiopterin.** The hydrogen donor of several mono-oxygenases, such as phenylalanine-4-mono-oxygenase (EC

1.14.16.1), tyrosine-3-mono-oxygenase (EC 1.14.16.2), and tryptophan-5-mono-oxgenase (EC 1.14.16.4), is 5,6,7,8-tetrahydrobiopterin. The formed 6,7-dihydroxybiopterin is recycled by dihydropteridinereductase (EC 1.6.99.7) using NADPH. Two studies have indicated that ascorbic acid may enhance the recycling of tetrahydrobiopterin.[76,77]

**Steroid Synthesis.** Ascorbic acid is released from the adrenal glands upon stimulation by adrenocorticotropic hormone.[78] Although some of the metabolic steps of steroid hormone synthesis are hydroxylations, no direct function of ascorbic acid is known. Only the steroid-21-mono-oxygenase (EC 1.14.99.10) has been shown to be inhibited by ascorbate in vitro.[79]

**Drug Metabolism.** Many drugs and toxic agents produced by the body must be modified before excretion. Hydroxylation and other reactions occur in liver microsomes and reticuloendothelial tissues by the mixed-function oxygenase system, which requires a number of components: hydroxylating and demethylating enzymes, flavoproteins, cytochrome P450, oxygen, and reducing agents in the form of NADP or NAD. This mixed-function oxidase is depressed by 50% in ascorbic acid-deficient guinea pigs if the liver ascorbate drops to 40% of normal.[80–82] However, extrahepatic detoxification systems and some hepatic drug metabolizing enzyme systems are less dependent or even independent of ascorbic acid status.[83,84]

**Ascorbic Acid in Iron Nutrition.** Iron is an essential nutrient that plays a vital role in oxygen transport as well as in many other metabolic processes. Ascorbic acid is a powerful promoter of non-heme iron absorption from food and acts by reducing the ferric iron in the stomach and by forming complexes with iron ions that remain in solution at the alkaline pH in the duodenum. To be most effective, ascorbic acid should be ingested together with food. The effect of ascorbic acid is dose-dependent, and the iron absorption is increased manifold. Because even small increases in the content of ascorbic acid in food enhance iron absorption, ascorbic acid is the most suitable compound to stimulate iron absorption and to improve iron nutrition.[85] The effect on iron absorption together with the action on carnitine biosynthesis may explain why the working capacity is impaired in vitamin C inadequacy.

Of a population of approximately 200 schoolchildren aged 12 to 15 years, 30% exhibited a vitamin C level below 2.0 mg/L, as well as deficiencies of riboflavin (33%) and pyridoxine (17%). Supplementation with 70 mg ascorbic acid, 2 mg riboflavin, and 2 mg pyridoxine daily for three months resulted in a significantly increased working capacity, serum iron, transferrin saturation, and vitamin C plasma level.[86]

## EXTRASCORBUTIC AND PHARMACODYNAMIC FUNCTIONS

Apart from the basic antiscorbutic role, ascorbic acid has prophylactic and therapeutic effects in pathologic conditions. These conditions include infectious diseases, immune deficiency disorders, atherosclerosis, malignant disease, nitrosamine formation, and toxicity of heavy metals. These functions emerged from clinical and experimental studies that used ascorbic acid in doses of up to 1 g daily or more.

**Ascorbic Acid and Immunity.** The immune response consists of cellular and humoral immune functions. Ascorbic acid has been shown to increase some cellular immune functions in vitro and in vivo, and to influence humoral immune reactions. The migration of human neutrophils toward leukoattractants can be stimulated by ascorbic acid in vitro and in vivo. An oxidative environment, such as the myeloperoxidase/$H_2O_2$/halide system, completely blocks the chemotaxis of granulocytes. This process can be reversed by ascorbic acid.[87] The importance of the action of ascorbic acid can best be demonstrated in diseases in which leukocyte functions are impaired, such as chronic granulomatous disease, an inherited disorder of neutrophil function. The defect in the killing of microorganisms leads to repeated bacterial infections. In patients, addition of 1 g ascorbic acid daily or 50 mg/kg/day to standard therapy improved the chemotaxis of neutrophils, leading to a dramatic reduction of infectious attacks.[88,89] Ascorbate has also been reported to restore partially or completely the antimicrobial activity impaired in the Chédiak-Higashi syndrome.[90]

Data indicate that ascorbic acid modulates cyclic nucleotide levels in B as well as in T cells, a process that may mediate immune reactions.[91] Humoral factors involved in the immune response include histamine and prostaglandins. Oral administration of ascorbate to 11 volunteers resulted in a reduction of blood histamine levels.[92] On the other hand, intracellular ascorbic acid is essential for the release of small quantities of histamine. How ascorbic acid regulates the histamine level is not clear.[93] Furthermore, ascorbic acid may also be involved in the release of prostaglandins of the E and F types[94] as well as in the synthesis of prostacyclin.[95]

**Ascorbic Acid and Lipid Metabolism.** The function of ascorbic acid on the cholesterol-7-mono-oxygenase has been discussed previously. The plasma triglyceride concentration increases in vitamin C-deficient guinea pigs, which results in an accumulation of triglycerides in liver and arteries.[73] Vitamin C administration in gram amounts to hyperlipidemic subjects and to two patients with hypertriglyceridemias led to a massive decrease in circulating triglycerides.[96–98] Ascorbic acid may also be effective in reducing the incidence of thrombotic episodes. A clinical trial with surgical patients who received 1 g vitamin C daily or a placebo showed that the incidence of thrombosis was reduced by 50% in the supplemented group.[99] Circumstantial and indirect evidence has indicated that hypovitaminosis C may be a risk factor in arterial diseases. However, additional trials must substantiate the still controversial role of ascorbate in lipid metabolism.

**Ascorbic Acid and Cancer.** The debate about a possible role of ascorbic acid in cancer therapy started when data from a trial with 100 terminal cancer patients were published. Ten g ascorbic acid daily was claimed to increase the survival time fourfold as compared with 1,000 claimed matched historical controls.[100] The authors concluded that supplemental ascorbate can offer some degree of benefit to all advanced cancer patients. A controlled clinical trial did not confirm these results, but these patients had received chemotherapy that impairs immunologic functions.[101] To overcome this problem, the study was repeated, with the same negative results, in a controlled double-blind clinical trial with 100 patients suffering from colorectal cancer. These patients had not received chemotherapy or irradiation, as opposed to the former study.[101a] An exchange of views about this controversy has been published.[101b]

Observations of terminal cancer patients in two hospitals who were receiving either low-dose ascorbate (4 g daily or less) or high-dose ascorbate (5 g daily or more) showed a significantly higher median survival of 105 days in the high-dose group compared with 35 days in the low-dose group. The administration of ascorbic acid seemed to improve the well-being of many cancer patients, as measured by decreased requirement for pain-controlling drugs, improved appetite, and increased mental alertness.[102] However, these studies were poorly controlled, and the classification of "low dose" and "high dose" was arbitrary. Furthermore, the site of primary tumor seems to be important for the effectiveness of ascorbic acid; uterus and stomach are the most promising. In vitro, an inhibitory effect of ascorbic acid on the growth of human melanoma cells was demonstrated.[103] In 1 mmol ascorbate no melanoma colonies were observed, and in 0.6 mmol ascorbate

the ability of melanoma cells to form colonies was 10 to 20 times less than for normal human amniotic cells.[103] Again, additional controlled studies are needed to eventually establish a role for vitamin C in cancer.

**Blockage of Nitrosamine Formation.** Nitrosamines, formed by a reaction of nitrate with either amines or amides, occur in food, cosmetics, tobacco, and body fluids such as blood, gastric juice, and urine. Many of the nitrosamines have been identified in animal experiments as carcinogenic. Nitrosamines can be formed in vivo in animals as well as in humans.[104–106] Ascorbic acid, present in a molar ratio of 2:1 (ascorbate to nitrite), blocks the nitrosamine formation.[107] Oral ingestion of nitrate, the precursor of nitrite, from beet root juice and proline leads to the formation of the noncarcinogenic N-nitrosoproline, which is excreted unchanged and can be analyzed in urine. Simultaneous administration of ascorbate completely inhibits N-nitrosoproline formation in rats and man.[108] Formation of nitrosamines in gastric juice of patients with atrophic conditions was significantly reduced following therapy with ascorbate (4 × 1 g daily).[109] Supplementation of the diet with 400 mg ascorbic acid and 400 mg α-tocopherol resulted in a significant reduction of mutagenic compounds excreted with human feces.[110] These studies suggest that ascorbic acid may have a direct inhibitory effect on carcinogenic N-nitrosamine formation and may help reduce the probability of malignant tumor formation.

**Interaction with Heavy Metal Ions.** There is evidence that ascorbic acid has a protective effect against the toxicity of heavy metals. Ascorbic acid is capable of reducing the toxic hexavalent chromium to the trivalent form known to cause no major adverse effects.[111] Ascorbic acid together with ferrous iron prevents the absorption of cadmium. This effect is not dependent on the ascorbate status, which suggests that ascorbic acid must be present at the site of absorption at the same time as the ions in order to be effective.[112,113] The deleterious effects of nickel, lead, and vanadium can also be alleviated by simultaneous administration of ascorbic acid.[114] Forty lead-burdened mothers were treated during pregnancy with a combined therapy of calcium phosphate and vitamin C (1 g/day). The urinary excretion of 5-amino levulinic acid, a parameter of lead intoxication, was decreased by 65%, the lead content of placenta by 90%, and the lead content of mother's milk by 15%. In addition, the cadmium content of the placenta was reduced to 40% of that found in untreated mothers.[115] Investigations into the possible effect of ascorbate on mercury are inconclusive. A study of vitamin C in guinea pigs demonstrated that administration of vitamin C prior to $HgCl_2$ poisoning is essential to protect this animal from any fetal consequences.[116]

It has also been suggested that ascorbic acid interferes with the intestinal absorption of copper and its distribution in tissues.[117] Copper absorption and utilization as demonstrated by copper serum levels and ceruloplasmin activity were increased in ascorbate deficiency states and decreased during high-ascorbate treatment in guinea pigs. This finding is consistent with results from studies in other species in which high vitamin C supplements together with low copper intakes increased the severity of copper deficiency.[118,119] The role of vitamin C in the detoxification of heavy metals in man has to be elucidated further.

## MARGINAL VITAMIN C DEFICIENCY

Marginal deficiency of nutrients is associated with reduced biochemical functions without the appearance of clinical symptoms. Depending on the duration of undernourishment, various phases of vitamin C depletion can be observed.

The *preliminary stage* of depletion is caused by an inadequate availability of vitamin C owing to either dietary changes, malabsorption, or increased requirements (e.g., pregnancy, lactation, smoking). Plasma concentration of vitamin C remains normal or is slightly reduced.

In the *biochemical deficiency stage,* a reduction in plasma and leukocyte concentrations and in urinary excretion of ascorbic acid and metabolites occurs. Only a limited amount of vitamin C is ingested, which is not sufficient to maintain the body pool. First correlations with certain enzyme activities or certain physiologic parameters, such as the proline/hydroxyproline ratio, serum carnitine, or histamine concentrations, may be noted.

The *physiologic deficiency stage* is accompanied by the concurrent appearance of unspecific symptoms such as loss of appetite, physical fatigue or weakness, reduced working capacity, impaired immune response, retarded wound healing, and poor iron absorption. This stage may be maintained over months by a limited intake of vitamin C without the appearance of manifest clinical deficiency symptoms, but may also be a transient situation in the case of extreme physiologic or pathologic conditions. It is only in the *clinically manifest vitamin deficiency stage* that clinical symptoms related to overt scurvy are noted.

The first three stages can be understood as a definition of *latent vitamin C deficiency,* and they can be considered as *marginal vitamin C deficiency.* There are two possibilities: The supply of vitamin C may be so small that after a short time

(80 to 100 days) the vitamin C body pool is depleted.[126,127] This situation causes the rapid appearance of clinically manifest vitamin C deficiency. On the other hand, when only a limited amount of vitamin C may be ingested daily for a long time, no clinical signs are observed. As a result, such a person remains in a long-lasting stationary marginal vitamin C deficiency state.

What factors might cause or initiate this marginality of vitamin C and to what extent it is prevalent in certain population segments have been considered in several investigations.[128] Two types of factors will be highlighted: those affecting the intake of vitamin C, such as season, age, institutionalization, hospitalization, and chronic disease; and those affecting metabolism or daily requirement, such as pregnancy, lactation, long-term drug therapy or alcohol abuse, smoking, and acute disease.

Reports are available demonstrating seasonal differences in vitamin C reserves.[121] The lowest levels occur at the end of winter, and the highest levels during summer months. This finding was also documented in an epidemiologic study.[129] Healthy and hospitalized persons showed a fall in vitamin C reserves in late winter and early spring. Whereas the healthy individuals remained adequately supplied despite insufficient intakes, a large percentage of those with marginal intakes in hospital became depleted.[130] The impact of seasonal variation in vitamin C intake was seen in the risk that higher requirements, caused by infection or any other disease, will further deplete the body pool and result in a marginal vitamin C deficiency.

Numerous reports have shown low plasma and leukocyte ascorbate levels in the elderly.[121] This finding is also reflected by the concentrations in tissues analyzed in postmortem samples. As an example, brain ascorbate concentration fell in one study to as little as 25% of that found in children.[131] In elderly persons living at home or in nursing homes, vitamin C deficits were more prevalent when compared with the profile in young healthy subjects. Vitamin C levels were strikingly depressed in the noninstitutionalized elderly as compared with the institutionalized population or the controls (healthy volunteers).[132,133] In another study on nutrition in the elderly[134] involving 48 subjects, 63% had plasma vitamin C levels below 0.2 mg/dl and were at a high risk of vitamin C deficiency. All of the men and 68% of the women showed plasma levels below 0.4 mg/dl. Elderly men required a higher daily intake of vitamin C to maintain the same plasma level as the elderly women. In a longitudinal study on the nutritional and health status of a large elderly population, daily intakes needed to maintain a plasma vitamin C level of 1.0 mg/dl were estimated to be 75 mg for women and 150 mg for men.[135] In evaluating the relationship between nutritional status and mental function (cognitive functioning) in the same elderly population, the authors stated that subclinical malnutrition may play a role in the depression of cognitive function observed in some of the elderly individuals, or that depressed cognitive function may result in reduced nutrient intake.[136] These data document the importance of normalizing the vitamin status in the elderly by adequate intakes.

Evaluation of the nutritional status of patients upon consecutive admissions to a general medical service revealed 5 of 108 patients with serum vitamin C levels within the scorbutic range of less than 0.2 mg/dl. Of the patients hospitalized 2 weeks or longer, approximately 25% showed a deterioration of their vitamin C status.[137] Estimation of several vitamins in 656 hospital inpatients by means of dietary interview, biochemical studies, and a clinical evaluation showed that a vitamin C deficiency state occurred more frequently in elderly, obese, or sedentary subjects, and more frequently in male than in female patients.[138]

Subclinical vitamin C deficiency is often seen in chronic or acute disease states. In chronic disease, however, anorexia is considered to be the major cause for the lowered vitamin C status. In acute disease it is unlikely that the cause is dietary restriction only because the vitamin C concentration falls rapidly. The prevalence of marginal vitamin C deficiency in various disease states is summarized in Table 22–4.[139] The vitamin C status in one study was marginally deficient in gastrointestinal disorders such as peptic ulcers and duodenal ulcers, and in intestinal malabsorption.[140] Malnutrition is common in malabsorption. Of the patients with steatorrhea, about 40 to 50% had low serum vitamin C levels. Subnormal leukocyte ascorbate levels were noted in about 15%

of patients with nonalcoholic chronic liver disease. A highly significant reduction was also seen in chronic alcoholics without any liver disease.[141] Ethanol caused a significant attenuation of the increase in plasma vitamin C after ingestion of vitamin C. This finding was interpreted as an adverse effect of alcohol on the absorption of ascorbate.[142]

Of rheumatoid patients 85% were deficient in vitamin C. Because their dietary intake of ascorbate did not differ from that of controls and absorption was found to be normal, rheumatoid subjects may utilize ascorbic acid at a faster rate, possibly owing to drug-vitamin interaction.[143] Nutritional depletion is a common accompanying phenomenon in patients with cancer. Low vitamin C levels were found in 71% of 120 cancer patients.[144,145] A rapid decrease in leukocyte vitamin C levels occurred in the first 24 hours following myocardial infarction. Within 12 hours the mean level in ascorbate had fallen to 8.5 $\mu$g/$10^8$ leukocytes, and the serum ascorbate level to 0.32 mg/dl, indicating a marginal vitamin C deficiency status. This lowering of ascorbate concentrations may be a general effect in states of stress, that is, the body's response to physical infective or traumatic insult.[146]

Numerous reports demonstrate a negative effect of long-term cigarette smoking on plasma and leukocyte vitamin C levels.[147] These levels were reduced by up to 43%[147a] (Table 22–5). This phenomenon is caused by a higher metabolic turnover in smokers, 70.0 ± 20.2 (17) mg/day, compared with 35.7 ± 9.3 (14) mg/day in nonsmokers.[30] Therefore, it would appear that, for reasons yet unknown, smokers require a 40% higher intake than nonsmokers to maintain comparable vitamin C plasma levels. Because the half-life of ascorbic acid in smokers is shorter at lower plasma con-

**Table 22–4.  Prevalence of Marginal Vitamin C Deficiency in Disease States**

| Disease State | Percentage with Low Vitamin C Status* |
|---|---|
| Malnutrition-Steatorrhea | 40–50 |
| Nonalcoholic liver disease | 35 |
| Alcoholic liver disease | 57 |
| Rheumatoid disease | 85 |
| Cancer | 71 |
| Malignant disease | 65 |

*Assessed by plasma, serum, or leukocyte vitamin C concentrations.

From Kelleher, J.,[139] with permission of MTP Press.

**Table 22–5.  Plasma Vitamin C Levels in Smokers and Nonsmokers**

| *Vitamin C Plasma Concentration (mg/L)* | | |
|---|---|---|
| *Nonsmokers* | *Smokers* | *P* |
| 9.1 ± 3.8 (91)*† | 5.2 ± 3.9 (31) | <0.00001 |
| 6.2 ± 4.0 (32)† | 4.4 ± 2.8 (22) | 0.037 |
| 1.8 ± 0.1 (34)† | 1.3 ± 0.2 (18) | <0.00001 |
| 7.4 ± 3.8 (80)† | 5.1 ± 3.7 (96) | <0.00001 |
| 9.6† | 8.3 | |
| 5.9† | 5.3 | |
| 8.8 ± 2.7 (10)† | 6.9 ± 2.6 (12) | 0.0545 |
| 6.0 ± 1.9 (14)† | 4.2 ± 2.2 (14) | 0.0143 |
| 13.2 ± 2.4 (12)† | 13.2 ± 2.4 (7) | 0.5 |
| 6.6 ± 2.1 (100)‡ | 3.9 ± 1.3 (96) | <0.00001 |

*Mean ± SD (N).

†Data modified from Hornig, D.H., Glatthaar, B.E.,[147] with permission of Huber Verlag.

‡Data from Murata, A.[147a]

centrations than in nonsmokers, smokers have a higher risk of becoming deficient in vitamin C than nonsmokers, should there be a restriction in the normal vitamin C intake.[30]

The increased need for vitamin C during pregnancy and lactation is also well documented, and most official recommendations for the intake of this vitamin have considered this fact.[148] A marginal vitamin C deficiency state is only seen when a woman has a low vitamin C status before pregnancy, since during pregnancy the vitamin C levels fall progressively. During prolonged lactation, exclusively breast-fed infants were found to be well protected against vitamin C undernutrition.[149] They maintained their vitamin C status independently of the maternal vitamin C status and the milk vitamin C concentration, but marginal vitamin C nutrition of lactating mothers was more common than assumed.[149] Significantly decreased plasma vitamin C levels are consistently noted in hemodialysis patients who therefore have an increased requirement for this vitamin.[150]

## IMPACT OF MARGINAL VITAMIN C DEFICIENCY ON HEALTH

The most important aspect is the extent to which a marginal vitamin C deficiency status may compromise health. Are there any symptoms, specific or unspecific, that could clearly be attributed to the lack of ascorbic acid, and will health improve when the marginal vitamin C status is normalized either by an improved diet or by supplementary vitamin C? This question can only be answered with adequately controlled, double-blind trials with the aim to alleviate or even prevent symptoms related to a marginal vitamin C deficiency state. Because degenerative alterations caused by a continuous hypovitaminosis may take many months or even years to manifest themselves, and may even be irreversible, such investigations are long-term.

It has been suggested that changes in capillary fragility are associated with marginal leukocyte ascorbate concentrations.[152] However, this is a subject with considerable negative data and controversy. Greco et al. investigated a group of 100 subjects, 45 of them apparently healthy, and the remainder with hemorrhagic ocular diseases (hemorrhagic clouding of the vitreous body, central vein thrombosis, apoplectic glaucoma).[153] In all patients the blood vitamin C levels were insufficient. Daily supplementation with vitamin C caused a progressive amelioration of the eye state and a clear regression of the hemorrhagic spots.

In experimentally induced vitamin C deficiency in man, a decreased ability in physical performance was reported at low levels of plasma ascorbate (0.17 mg/dl).[154] Seventy milligrams vitamin C daily, together with riboflavin and vitamin $B_6$, improved working capacity as measured by oxygen consumption.[86] Working capacity was significantly reduced when several vitamins ($B_1$, $B_2$, $B_6$, and C) were supplied in the amount of only one third of the Dutch recommended dietary allowances (RDA) for eight weeks. It was not fully restored when twice the RDA of these vitamins was given for two weeks.[155] In young adolescents, the optimum aerobic capacity was associated with a daily intake of 80 to 100 mg of vitamin C or a plasma vitamin C level of 0.8 to 0.9 mg/dl. This relationship was more pronounced in subjects having low or deficient plasma vitamin C concentrations. The increase in plasma vitamin C was accompanied by an increase in aerobic capacity, but only up to a concentration of 0.8 to 0.9 mg/dl.[156]

A relation between histamine and ascorbate concentrations in blood has been shown in pregnant women, adult males, and nonpregnant females. Blood histamine increased gradually when ascorbate dropped below 1.0 mg/dl. The increase in histamine was highly significant at vitamin C concentrations below 0.7 mg/dl.[92]

In general, more research is needed to substantiate the impact of a marginal vitamin C deficiency state on physiologic parameters.

## VITAMIN C DEFICIENCY IN MAN

Evans described the medical history of infantile scurvy or Barlow's disease.[157] In his Bradshaw Lecture in 1894, Sir Thomas Barlow mentioned the following symptoms: pallor, inadequate subcutaneous fat, screaming when the legs were handled, pseudoparalysis, swelling of limbs, crepitus due to fracture in or near the epiphyses, occasional proptosis, spongy gums with fetor and bleeding, deformities of the ribs, osseous sheaths surrounding bones, and albumin and blood in the urine.

In the adult, the onset of scurvy may be detected after 60 to 90 days on a vitamin C-deficient diet[126,127] (Fig. 22–3). The earliest manifestations consist of a few petechial spots and small ecchymoses that fade within a few days, but are replaced by others. They first appear when the plasma ascorbic acid ranges from 0.13 to 0.24 mg/dl. Larger ecchymoses may be accompanied by petechiae that become perifollicular in location. At the same time, follicular hyperkeratosis develops, especially on the buttocks, thighs, and calves. Many hyperkeratotic lesions contain fragmented or coiled hairs, and some demonstrate the classic lesion of scurvy: the hyperkeratotic follicle with a red hemorrhagic halo. Gums become swollen

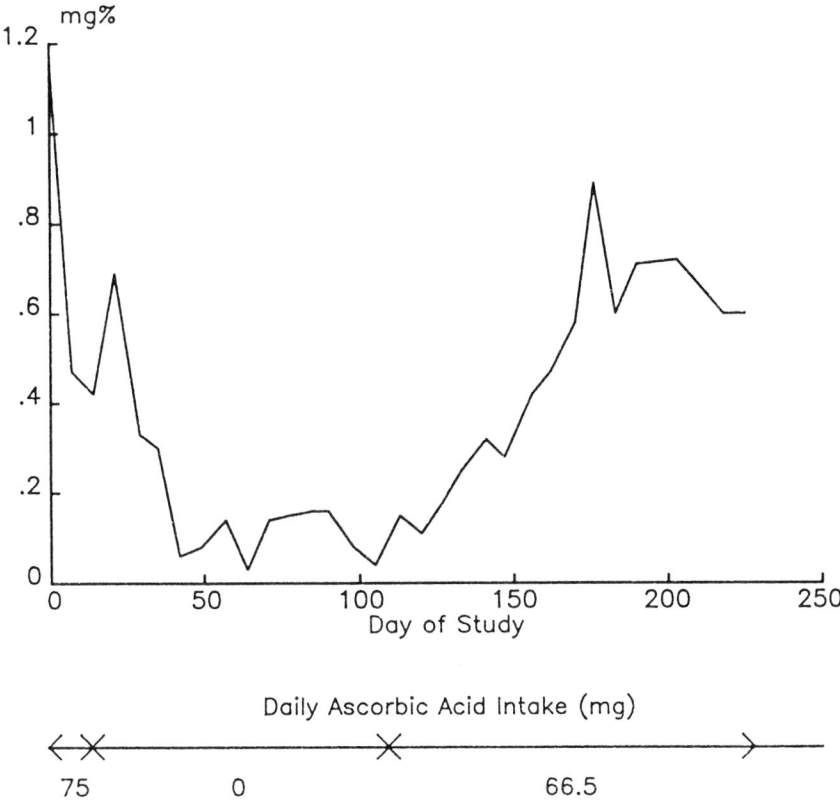

**Fig. 22–3.** Plasma ascorbate values in scurvy. Average plasma ascorbate values of two men during depletion and repletion. (From Hodges, R.E., et al.[127], with permission of Am. J. Clin. Nutr., American Society for Clinical Nutrition.)

and bleed easily. It is noteworthy that the gums do not become involved if the patient has no teeth, and gum lesions are seldom severe in subjects who practice good dental hygiene. A unique characteristic of scurvy is the development of Sjögren's (sicca) syndrome: dryness of the mouth and eyes, loss of hair, dry itchy skin, and loosening of teeth and dental fillings. Scurvy may be characterized by weakness and lethargy, followed by aching of the legs, arthralgia, and joint effusions. A peculiar form of vasomotor instability may be observed and accompanied by pitting edema of the feet and ankles. Oliguria is also observed in severe scurvy. Psychologic changes, common in this condition, are characterized as the "neurotic triad," which consists of hysteria, depression, and hypochondriasis. Peripheral neuropathy was observed in one scorbutic subject who developed hemorrhages into the femoral nerve sheaths of both legs. The description of scurvy symptoms by Hodges[3] confirms the observations made during the ex-

periments of the British Medical Research Council.[120]

Treatment of scorbutic patients must not be delayed because sudden death can result. After several doses of 100 mg ascorbic acid either orally or intravenously, improvement of the severe condition is rapid. Continuous daily administration of vitamin C rapidly repletes the body pool. Whereas the first signs of scurvy are observed at a pool size of 300 to 400 mg, the last signs upon repletion (hyperkeratosis) only disappear at a pool size of about 1,000 mg (healthy adults have a body pool size of approximately 20 mg/kg body weight or about 1,500 mg).[31,32]

## DAILY REQUIREMENTS

Man is dependent on exogenous sources of vitamin C because he is unable to synthesize it endogenously. The supply of vitamin C necessary to offer protection against scurvy is about 10 mg daily.[120] However, ascorbic acid exerts many physiologic as well as extra-antiscorbutic functions for which tissue concentrations greater than those to prevent the emergence of the deficiency disease appear desirable. How much is required to attain optimum health is a matter of controversy, although more evidence is being accumulated, not only for vitamin C, but for all essential nutrients, to allow researchers to establish daily requirements. Therefore, it is not surprising that different recommended dietary allowances (RDA) exist for the various countries, ranging between 30 mg and 120 mg including groups with increased needs (e.g., pregnant and lactating women, smokers). These differences reflect the various definitions of the RDAs: either to be adequate to meet the needs of practically all healthy persons, or to be merely sufficient to prevent scurvy. Figure 22–4 shows the relationship between plasma vitamin C levels and intake of the vitamin, taking into account the 95% range for the mean values in reports published during the last 40 years.[121]

In the National Survey of Canada of 1973, three risk categories were introduced.[122] A high risk was postulated to exist for all age groups having a plasma level below 0.2 mg/dl. Conversely, a low risk of vitamin deficiency was expected above 0.4 mg/dl for the age group over 19 years, and above 0.6 mg/dl for those younger than 19 years. A mod-

erate risk was defined to exist at the plasma levels in between. These conclusions were translated into necessary daily vitamin C intakes of 60 mg and 80 mg, respectively, to maintain a low-risk vitamin C nutritional status.[121]

Newton et al. studied the relation between intake and plasma concentration of vitamin C in elderly women.[123] They found a sigmoidal relation demonstrating a rapid change in plasma concentration as the intake increased from 30 to 60 mg daily. This finding suggested saturation of a pathway of metabolic utilization. To protect against impairment of health, the authors of this study suggested maintaining the intake of vitamin C above 60 mg daily.

The most comprehensive survey assessing the overall health status and nutritional status of the population probably is the Nationwide Health and Nutrition Examination Survey conducted by the U.S. Department of Health and Human Services between 1976 and 1980 (NHANES II).[125] It included 21,000 people from 6 months to 74 years of age and provided a representative sample of the civilian noninstitutionalized population. First evaluations regarding vitamin C nutritional status revealed a close correlation between critical vitamin C serum levels of less than 0.3 mg/dl and intakes corresponding to low percentages of the vitamin C RDA.

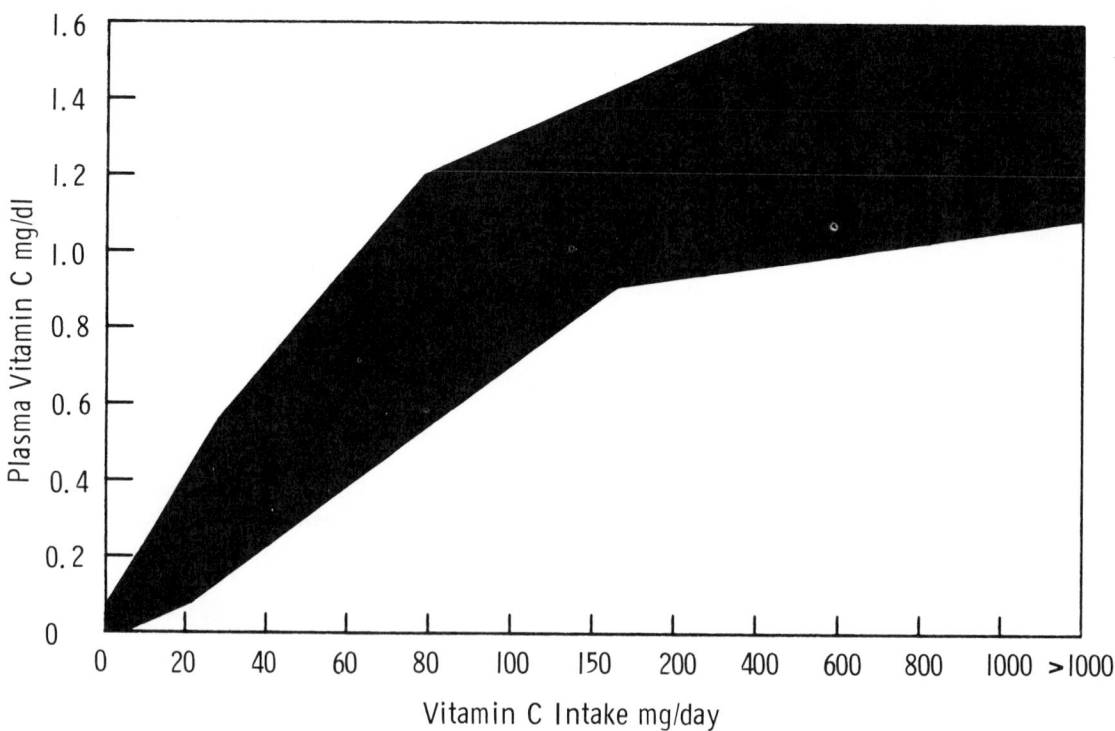

**Fig. 22–4.** The relationship between plasma levels and intake of vitamin C. (From Basu, T.K., Schorah, C.J.,[174] with permission of The Avi Publishing Company, Inc.)

A comprehensive review of research on vitamin C requirement of man was compiled by Irwin and Hutchins[158] and more recently by Hornig.[159] Conclusions were derived mostly from blood or plasma levels, from urinary excretion of ascorbic acid, or from investigations of the minimum intake of ascorbic acid to prevent the appearance of scorbutic symptoms. Other approaches have been the saturation of the body ascorbic acid and the estimation of the requirement by urinary response to large intakes of this vitamin. As a result of the different methods employed for assessing the vitamin C status, the published estimates of the daily requirement vary considerably. For example, the estimates of the necessary daily intake for children range between 60 and 125 mg.

The studies with $(1-^{14}C)$ labeled or $(^3H)$ labeled ascorbic acid[66,67] have contributed to the elucidation of body pool sizes and turnover of vitamin C in man.[30-32,37,47,50,126,127] There are several limitations to the studies by Baker et al.[31,32,50,126,127] First, these studies were performed in depleted and hence physiologically abnormal subjects, suggesting that the turnover of only a "deep" compartment was determined. Second, the use of urinary excretion data alone normally results in an overestimate of the pool size, although this fact does not seem to be crucial in the case of vitamin C. Third, after oral administration, the absorbed amount of ascorbic acid was considered to be equal to the ingested amount. Based on these studies, the National Research Council recommended in 1980 a daily intake of 60 mg for adults of both sexes, taking into consideration an average absorption efficiency of 85%.[148] In their reinvestigation using plasma and urinary data, Kallner et al.[30,37,47] presented evidence that with intakes of up to 180 mg the absorption is incomplete.[29] In addition, at a total turnover of about 60 mg ascorbic acid daily, the metabolic turnover (turnover of metabolites derived from ascorbate) levels off at about 40 to 50 mg/day. This total daily turnover of 60 mg/day corresponds to a plasma concentration of 0.8 to 0.9 mg/dl and a total body pool size of 20 mg/kg body weight. Consequently, owing to the incomplete absorption (80 to 90%), the daily intake for healthy nonsmoking males necessary to reach this defined total turnover of 60 mg is approximately 70 to 75 mg/day. The statistical variation observed (SD = 14 mg/day) indicates that a daily intake of approximately 100 mg should be appropriate to cover the physiologic requirement of 95% of this population[37,59] in order to achieve ascorbate tissue saturation. Because pharmacokinetic studies with radiolabeled material have not been done in children, appropriate recommendations would need to be extrapolated from studies with adults. Similar investigations with smokers have shown an increase in the metabolic turnover. To match the increased requirement, a daily intake of approximately 140 mg of vitamin C per day should be attained for smokers.[30]

The enhanced requirements of vitamin C during pregnancy and lactation have generally been accepted.[148]

## SAFETY OF VITAMIN C

Reviews on the safety and tolerance of vitamin C have been published along with reports about adverse effects of high doses.[16,160,161] The most frequently cited adverse effect of high intakes of ascorbic acid concerns the production of oxalate. However, as outlined in the section on metabolism, vitamin C cannot be considered as a risk factor in oxalate stone formation.[51] Observations on the occurrence of ascorbic acid deficiencies upon the termination of a high-dose regimen due to a faster turnover are poorly documented or even anecdotal.[162] Long-term administration of massive doses of ascorbic acid to guinea pigs has caused no induction on the metabolizing enzyme system.[163] High doses of vitamin C were reported to destroy vitamin $B_{12}$ in an in vitro system.[164] This statement, however, had to be revised because of analytical inadequacies.[165,166]

Ascorbic acid may interfere with laboratory tests involving nonspecific color reactions caused by redox mechanisms. Such interactions were reported for the analyses of glucose, uric acid, creatinine, and inorganic phosphate.[167] Ascorbic acid ingested in amounts higher than 1 g/day may appear in feces and may interfere with the detection of occult blood.[168] These unfavorable effects can easily be avoided by using appropriate laboratory methods.

A study in women seemed to confirm earlier findings in animals that high doses of vitamin C caused reduced fertility and fetotoxicity.[169] In humans high doses of vitamin C up to 10 g daily for several years neither reduced the fertility in 3,000 women nor affected the newborn. However, these conclusions have been drawn from occasional observations and not from a controlled study.[170] Furthermore, vitamin C has been used as therapy in nonspecific sperm agglutination where it was reported to increase seminal levels of zinc, magnesium, calcium, and potassium,[171,172] and has also been used to induce ovulation in anovulatory women.[173] Other adverse effects frequently cited are occasional diarrhea, deep vein thrombosis, and hemolysis in glucose-6-phosphate dehydrogenase deficiency. These allegations were based on anecdotal and uncontrolled studies.[16]

# REFERENCES

1. Hess, A.F.: Scurvy, Past and Present. Philadelphia, J.B. Lippincott Co., 1920.
2. Hirsch, A.: Handb. d. histor. geograph. Vol. I. Pathologie, Erlangen, pp. 537–551, 1860.
3. Hodges, R.E.: Ascorbic acid. *In* Modern Nutrition in Health and Disease. 6th ed. (Goodhart, R.S., Shils, M.E., Eds.) Philadelphia, Lea & Febiger, 1980.
4. Wintermeyer, U., Lahann, H., Vogel, R.: Vitamin C. Stuttgart, Deutscher Apotheker Verlag, 1981.
5. Lind, J.: A Treatise on the Scurvy. London, A. Millar, 1753. (Republished Edinburgh, Edinburgh University Press, 1953.)
6. Holst, A., Frölich, T.: J. Hyg. (Lond.) *7*:634–669, 1907.
7. Zilva, S.S.: Lancet *1*:478, 1921.
8. Drummond, J.C.: Biochem. J. *13*:77–80, 1919; *14*:660, 1920.
9. Svirbely, J.L., Szent-Györgyi, A.: Biochem. J. *26*:865–870, 1932.
10. King, C.G., Waugh, W.A.: Science *75*:357–358, 1932.
11. Haworth, W.N., Hirst, E.L.: J. Soc. Chem. Ind. *52*:645–646, 1933.
12. Reichstein, T., Grüssner, A., Oppenhauer, R.: Helv. Chir. Acta *16*:561–565, 1933.
13. Tolbert, B.M., Downing, M., Carlson, R.W.: Ann. N.Y. Acad. Sci. *258*:48–69, 1975.
14. Crawford, T.C.: Synthesis of L-ascorbic acid. *In* Ascorbic Acid: Chemistry, Metabolism, and Uses. (Seib, P.A., Tolbert, B.M., Eds.) Advances in Chemistry Series, No. 200. Washington, D.C., American Chemical Society, 1982, pp. 1–36.
15. Jaffe, G.: Vitamin C. *In* Handbook on Vitamins: Nutritional, Biochemical and Clinical Aspects. (L.J. Machlin, Ed.) New York, Marcel Dekker, Inc., 1984, pp. 199–244.
16. Nordfjeld, K., Lang-Pedersen, J., Rasmussen, M., et al.: J. Clin. Hosp. Pharm. *9*:293–301, 1984.
17. Mohn, G.: Vitamin C, L-(+)-Ascorbinsäure. *In* Fermente, Hormone, Vitamine. 3rd ed. (Ammon, R., Dirschel, W., Eds.) Stuttgart, Thieme Verlag, 1974, pp. 873–961.
18. Beutler, H.O., Beinstingl, G.: Dtsch. Lebensm. Rdsch. *76*:69–75, 1980.
19. Cooke, J.R.R., Moxon, R.E.D.: The detection and measurement of vitamin C. *In* Vitamin C (Ascorbic Acid). (Counsell, J.N., Hornig, D.H., Eds.) London, Applied Science Publications, 1981, pp. 167–198.
20. Sauberlich, H.E., Green, M.D., Omaye, S.T.: Determination of ascorbic acid and dehydroascorbic acid. *In* Ascorbic Acid: Chemistry, Metabolism, and Uses. (Seib, P.A., Tolbert, B.M., Eds.) Advances in Chemistry Series, No. 200. Washington, D.C., American Chemical Society, 1982, pp. 199–221.
20a. Pachla, L.A., Reynolds, D.L., Kissinger, P.T.: J. Assoc. Off. Anal. Chem. *68*:1–12, 1985.
20b. Vecchi, M., Kaiser, K.: J. Chromatogr. *26*:22–29, 1967.
21. Paul, A.A., Southgate, D.A.T.: McCance and Widdowson's The Composition of Foods. 4th ed. (Medical Research Council's Special Report No. 297) London, HMSO, 1978.
22. Stevenson, N.R.: Gastroenterology *67*:952–956, 1974.
23. Siliprandi, L., Vanni, P., Kessler, M., et al.: Biochim. Biophys. Acta *552*:129–142, 1979.

24. Toggenburger, G., Landolt, M., Semenza, G.: FEBS Lett. *108*:473–476, 1979.
25. Stevenson, N.R., Brush, M.K.: Am. J. Clin. Nutr. *22*:318–326, 1969.
26. Spencer, R.P., Purdy, S., Hoeldtke, R., et al.: Gastroenterology *44*:768–773, 1963.
27. Nelson, E.W., Lane, H., Fabri, J., et al.: J. Clin. Pharmacol. *18*:325–335, 1978.
28. Kübler, W., Gehler, J.: Int. J. Vitam. Nutr. Res. *40*:443–453, 1970.
29. Kallner, A., Hartmann, D., Hornig, D.: Int. J. Vitam. Nutr. Res. *47*:383–388, 1977.
30. Kallner, A., Hartman, D., Hornig, D.: Am. J. Clin. Nutr. *34*:1347–1355, 1981.
31. Baker, E.M., Hodges, R.E., Hood, J., et al.: Am. J. Clin. Nutr. *22*:549–558, 1969.
32. Baker, E.M., Hodges, R.E., Hood, J., et al.: Am. J. Clin. Nutr. *24*:444–454, 1971.
33. Hornig, D., Vuilleumier, J.P., Hartmann, D.: Int. J. Vitam. Nutr. Res. *50*:309–314, 1980.
34. Angel, J., Alfred, B., Leichter, J., et al.: Int. J. Vitam. Nutr. Res. *45*:237–243, 1975.
35. Schmidt, K.H., Hagmaier, V., Hornig, D., et al.: Am. J. Clin. Nutr. *34*:305–311, 1981.
36. Toggenburger, G., Häussermann, M., Mütsch, B., et al.: Biochim. Biophys. Acta *646*:433–443, 1981.
37. Kallner, A., Hartmann, D., Hornig, D.: Am. J. Clin. Nutr. *32*:530–539, 1979.
38. Hammarstroem, L.: Acta Physiol. Scand. *70*(Suppl. 289):1–83, 1966.
39. Martin, G.R., Mecca, C.E.: Arch. Biochem. Biophys. *93*:110–114, 1961.
40. Hornig, D.: Ann. N.Y. Acad. Sci. *258*:103–118, 1975.
41. Hornig, D., Hartmann, D.: Kinetic behavior of ascorbic acid in guinea pigs. *In* Ascorbic Acid: Chemistry, Metabolism, and Uses. (Seib, P.A., Tolbert, B.M., Eds.) Advances in Chemistry Series, No. 200. Washington, D.C., American Chemical Society, 1982, pp. 293–316.
42. Ginter, E.: Am. J. Clin. Nutr. *33*:538–539, 1980.
43. Hornig, D.: World Rev. Nutr. Diet. *23*:225–258, 1975.
44. Tolbert, B.M., Ward, J.B.: Dehydroascorbic acid. *In* Ascorbic Acid: Chemistry, Metabolism, and Uses. (Seib, P.A., Tolbert, B.M., Eds.) Advances in Chemistry Series, No. 200. Washington, D.C., American Chemical Society, 1982, pp. 101–123.
45. Tolbert, B.M.: Metabolism and function of ascorbic acid and its metabolites. *In* Vitamins in Nutrition and Therapy. (Hornig, D.H., Hanck, A.G., Eds.) Berne, Huber Verlag, 1985, pp. 121–138.
46. Omaye, S.T., Tillotson, J.A., Sauberlich, H.E.: Metabolism of L-ascorbic acid in the monkey. *In* Ascorbic Acid: Chemistry, Metabolism, and Uses. (Seib, P.A., Tolbert, B.M., Eds.) Advances in Chemistry Series, No. 200. Washington, D.C., American Chemical Society, 1982, pp. 317–334.
47. Kallner, A., Hartmann, D., Hornig, D.: Kinetics of ascorbic acid in humans. *In* Ascorbic Acid: Chemistry, Metabolism, and Uses. (Seib, P.A., Tolbert, B.M., Eds.) Advances in Chemistry Series, No. 200. Washington, D.C., American Chemical Society, 1982, pp. 335–348.
48. Tillotson, J.A., O'Connor, R.J.: Am. J. Clin. Nutr. *34*:2397–2404, 1981.
49. Hellman, L., Burns, J.J.: J. Biol. Chem. *230*:923–930, 1958.

50. Baker, E.M., Halver, J.E., Johnsen, D.O., et al.: Ann. N.Y. Acad. Sci. *258*:72–80, 1975.

51. Moser, U., Hornig, D.: Trends Pharmacol. Sci. *3*:480–483, 1982.

51a. Swartz, R.D., Wesley, J.R., Somermeyer, M.G., et al.: Ann. Intern. Med. *100*:530–531, 1984.

51b. Chalmers, A.H., Cowley, D.M., McWhinney, B.C.: Clin. Chem. *31*:1703–1705, 1985.

51c. Conyers, R.A.J., Bais, R., Rofe, A.M., et al.: Aust. N.Z. J. Med. *15*:353–355, 1985.

52. Kallner, A., Hornig, D., Pallita, R.: Am. J. Clin. Nutr. *41*:609–613, 1985.

53. Visser, C.M.: Bioorganic Chemistry *9*:261–271, 1980.

54. Levene, C.I., Bates, C.J.: Ann. N.Y. Acad. Sci. *258*:288–306, 1975.

55. Bates, C.J.: The function of vitamin C in man. *In* Vitamin C (Ascorbic Acid). (Counsell, J.N., Hornig, D.H., Eds.) London, Applied Science Publishers, 1981, pp. 1–22.

56. Myllylä, R., Kuutti-Savolainen, E.R., Kivirikko, K.I.: Biochem. Biophys. Res. Commun. *83*:441–448, 1978.

56a. Nietfeld, J.J., Kemp, A.: Biochem. Biophys. Acta *657*:159–167, 1981.

57. Peterkovsky, B., Kalwinsky, D., Assad, R.: Arch. Biochem. Biophys. *199*:362–373, 1980.

58. Barnes, M.J., Kodicek, E.: Vitam. Horm. *30*:1–43, 1972.

59. Bates, C.J.: Int. J. Vitam. Nutr. Res. *49*:77–86, 1979.

60. Taylor, T.V., Rimmer, S., Day, B., et al.: Lancet *2*:544, 1974.

61. Burr, R.G., Rajan, K.T.: Br. J. Nutr. *28*:275–281, 1972.

62. Afifi, A.M., Ellis, L., Huntsman, R.G., et al.: Br. J. Dermatol. *92*:339–341, 1975.

63. Elsas, L.J., Miller, R.L., Pinnell, S.R.: J. Pediatr. *92*:378–384, 1978.

64. Bieber, L.L., Emaus, R., Valknor, K., et al.: Fed. Proc. *41*:2858–2862, 1982.

65. James, M.J., Brooks, D.E., Snoswell, A.M.: FEBS Lett. *126*:53–56, 1981.

66. Broquist, H.P.: Fed. Proc. *41*:2840–2842, 1982.

67. Nelson, P.J., Pruitt, R.E., Henderson, L.L., et al.: Biochim. Biophys. Acta *672*:123–127, 1981.

67a. Dunn, W.A., Rettura, G., Seifter, E., et al.: J. Biol. Chem. *259*:10764–10770, 1984.

68. Hughes, R.E.: Recommended daily amounts and biochemical roles—the vitamin C, carnitine, fatigue relationship. *In* Vitamin C (Ascorbic Acid). (Counsell, J.N., Hornig, D.H., Eds.) London, Applied Science Publishers, 1981, pp. 75–86.

69. Ullrich, R., Duppel, W.: Iron- and copper-containing monooxygenases. *In* Enzymes. 3rd ed., Vol. XII. (Boyer, P.D., Ed.) New York, Academic Press, 1975.

70. Deana, R., Bharaj, B.S., Verjee, Z.H., et al.: Int. J. Vitam. Nutr. Res. *45*:175–182, 1975.

70a. Beers, M.F., Johnson, R.G., Scarpa, A.: J. Biol. Chem. *261*:2529–2535, 1986.

70b. Levine, M., Morita, K.: Vitam. Horm. *42*:1–64, 1985.

71. Tolbert, L.C., Thomas, T.W., Middaugh, L.D., et al.: Life Sci. *25*:2189–2195, 1979.

71a. Eipper, B.A., Mains, R.E., Glembotski, Ch.C.: Proc. Natl. Acad. Sci. USA *80*:5144–5148, 1983.

71b. Murthy, A.S.N., Mains, R.E., Eipper, B.A.: J. Biol. Chem. *261*:1815–1822, 1986.

71c. Hilsted, L., Rehfeld, J.F., Schwartz, T.W.: FEBS Lett. *196*:151–154, 1986.

72. Björkhem, I., Kallner, A.: J. Lipid Res. *17*:360–365, 1976.

73. Ginter, E., Bobek, P.: The influence of vitamin C in lipid metabolism. *In* Vitamin C (Ascorbic Acid). (Counsell, J.N., Hornig, D.H., Eds.) London, Applied Science Publishers, 1981, pp. 299–347.

74. Hornig, D., Weiser, H.: Experientia *32*:687–689, 1976.

75. LaDu, B.N., Zannoni, V.G.: Ann. N.Y. Acad. Sci. *92*:175–191, 1961.

76. Lerner, P., Hartman, P., Ames, M.M., et al.: Arch. Biochem. Biophys. *182*:164–170, 1977.

77. Stone, K.J., Townsley, B.H.: Biochem. J. *131*:611–613, 1973.

78. Sayers, G., Sayers, M.A., Liang, T.Y., et al.: Endocrinology *38*:1–9, 1946.

79. Greenfield, N., Ponticorvo, L., Chasalow, F., et al.: Arch. Biochem. Biophys. *200*:232–244, 1980.

80. Zannoni, V.G., Sato, P.H., Rikans, L.E.: Ascorbic acid and drug metabolism. *In* Nutrition and Drug Interrelationships. (Hathcook, J.H., Coon, J., Eds.) New York, Academic Press, 1978.

81. Degkwitz, E., Walsch, S., Dubberstein, M., et al.: Ann. N.Y. Acad. Sci. *258*:201–208, 1975.

82. Weis, W.: Ann. N.Y. Acad. Sci. *258*:190–200, 1975.

83. Omaye, S.T., Green, M.D., Turnbull, J.D., et al.: J. Clin. Pharmacol. *18*:325–335, 1980.

84. Sikic, B.I., Mimnaugh, E.G., Litterst, C.L., et al.: Arch. Biochem. Biophys. *179*:663–671, 1977.

85. Hallberg, L.: Annu. Rev. Nutr. *1*:123–147, 1981.

86. Buzina, R., Grgic, Z., Jusic, J., et al.: Hum. Nutr. Clin. Nutr. *36*:429–438, 1982.

87. Anderson, R., Jones, P.T.: Clin. Exp. Immunol. *47*:487–496, 1982.

88. Anderson, R.: Int. J. Vitam. Nutr. Res. Suppl. *23*:23–34, 1982.

89. Patrone, R., Dallegri, F., Bonvini, E., et al.: Acta Vitaminol. Enzymol. *4*:163–168, 1982.

90. Boxer, L.A., Watanabe, A.M., Lister, M., et al.: N. Engl. J. Med. *295*:1041–1045, 1976.

91. Panush, R.S., Katz, P., Powell, G., et al.: Int. J. Vitam. Nutr. Res. *53*:61–67, 1982.

92. Clemetson, C.A.: J. Nutr. *110*:662–668, 1980.

93. Sharma, S.C., Molloy, A., Walzman, M., et al.: Int. J. Vitam. Nutr. Res. *51*:266–273, 1981.

94. Sharma, S.C.: Interactions of ascorbic acid with prostaglandins. *In* Vitamin C. New Clinical Applications in Immunology, Lipid Metabolism and Cancer. (Hanck, A., Ed.) Berne, Huber Verlag, 1982, pp. 239–256.

95. Beetens, J.R., van den Bossche, R., Herman, A.G.: Arch. Int. Pharmacodyn. Ther. *256*:151–152, 1982.

96. Sokoloff, B., Hori, M., Saelhof, C.C., et al.: J. Am. Geriatr. Soc. *14*:1239–1260, 1966.

97. Ginter, E.: N. Engl. J. Med. *294*:559–560, 1976.

98. Geoly, K.L., Diamond, L.H.: Ann. Intern. Med. *93*:511, 1980.

99. Spittle, C.R.: Lancet *2*:199–201, 1973.

100. Cameron, E., Pauling, L., Leibovitz, B.: Cancer Res. *39*:633–681, 1979.

101. Creagan, E.T., Moertel, C.G., O'Fallon, J.R., et al.: N. Engl. J. Med. *301*:687–690, 1979.

101a. Moertel, Ch.G., Fleming, T.R., Creagan, E.T., et al.: N. Engl. J. Med. *312*:137–141, 1985.

101b. Pauling, L., Moertel, Ch.G.: Nutr. Rev. *44*:28–32, 1986.

102. Murata, A., Morishige, F., Yamaguchi, H.: Prolongation of survival times of terminal cancer patients by administration of large doses of ascorbate. *In*

Vitamin C. New Clinical Applications in Immunology, Lipid Metabolism and Cancer. (Hanck, A., Ed.) Berne, Huber Verlag, 1982, pp. 103–114.

103. Bram, S.: Nature *284*:629–631, 1980.

104. Sander, J., Burkle, G.: Z. Krebsforsch. *73*:54–66, 1969.

105. Mirvish, S.S.: Toxicol. Appl. Pharmacol. *31*:325–351, 1975.

106. Walters, C.L.: The influence of ascorbic acid on the formation of N-nitrosamines in foods, drugs, cosmetics and tobacco. *In* Vitamin C (Ascorbic Acid). (Counsell, J.N., Hornig, D.H., Eds.) London, Applied Science Publishers, 1981, pp. 199–213.

107. Mirvish, S.S., Wallcave, L., Eagan, M., et al.: Science *177*:65–68, 1972.

108. Ohshima, H., Bartsch, H.: The influence of vitamin C on the in vivo formation of nitrosamines. *In* Vitamin C (Ascorbic Acid). (Counsell, J.N., Hornig, D.H., Eds.) London, Applied Science Publishers, 1981, pp. 215–224.

109. Reed, P.I., Summers, K., Smith, P.L.R., et al.: Scand. J. Gastroenterol. *17*(Suppl. 78):239, 1982.

110. Dion, P.W., Bright-See, E.B., Smith, C.C., et al.: Mutat. Res. *102*:27–37, 1982.

111. Samitz, M.H., Scheiner, P.H., Katz, S.A.: Arch. Environ. Health *17*:44–45, 1968.

112. Fox, M.R.S., Jacobs, R.M., Jones, A.O.L., et al.: Ann. N.Y. Acad. Sci. *355*:249–261, 1980.

113. Lyall, V., Chauhan, V.P.S., Sarkar, A.K., et al.: Toxicol. Lett. *9*:403–407, 1981.

114. Suzuki, T., Yoshida, A.: J. Nutr. *109*:1974–1978, 1979.

115. Altman, P., Maruna, R.F.L., Maruna, H., et al.: Wien. Med. Wochenschr. *131*:311–314, 1981.

116. Mokranjac, M., Petrovic, C., Fabre, H.R.: C.R. Acad. Sci. (Paris) *258*:1341–1342, 1964.

117. Disilvestro, R.A., Harris, E.D.: J. Nutr. *111*:1964–1968, 1981.

118. Milne, D.B., Omaye, S.T.: Int. J. Vitam. Nutr. Res. *50*:301–308, 1980.

119. Smith, C.H., Bidlack, W.R.: J. Nutr. *110*:1398–1408, 1980.

120. Bartley, W., Krebs, H.A., O'Brien, J.R.P.: Vitamin C Requirement of Human Adults. A Report by the Vitamin C Subcommittee of the Accessory Food Factors Committee. Med. Res. Council Spec. Rep.Ser. No. 280. London, Her Majesty's Stationery Office, 1953.

121. Schorah, C.J.: Vitamin C status in population groups. *In* Vitamin C (Ascorbic Acid). (Counsell, J.N., Hornig, D.H., Eds.) London, Applied Science Publishers, 1981, pp. 23–47.

122. Nutrition Canada National Survey: Information Canada. Ontario, 1973.

123. Newton, H.M.V., Morgan, D.B., Schorah, C.J., et al.: Br. Med. J. *287*:1429, 1983.

124. Reference deleted.

125. Dallman, P.R., Yip, R., Johnson, C.: Methods for estimating the prevalence of iron deficiency and iron deficiency anemia in industrialized countries. *In* Groupes à Risque de Carence en Fer dans les Pays Industrialisés. (Dupin, H., Herzberg, S., Eds.) Paris, I.S.T.A. CNAM, 1983, pp. 21–31.

126. Hodges, R.E., Baker, E.M., Hood, J., et al.: Am. J. Clin. Nutr. *22*:535–548, 1969.

127. Hodges, R.E., Hood, J., Canham, J.E., et al.: Am. J. Clin. Nutr. *24*:432–443, 1971.

128. Hornig, D.: J. Jap. Soc. Clin. Nutr. *3*:91–105, 1984.

129. Ritzel, G.: Evaluation von Ernährungserhebungen im Rahmen der Basler Studie III. In Zur Ernährungssituation der Schweizer Bevölkerung. (Brubacher, G., Ritzel, G., Eds.) Berne, Huber Verlag, 1975, pp. 57–82.

130. Schorah, C.J.: Inappropriate vitamin C reserves: Their frequency and significance in an urban population. *In* Importance of Vitamins to Human Health. (Taylor, T.G., Ed.) Lancaster, MTP Press, 1979, pp. 61–72.

131. Kirk, J.E.: Vitam. Horm. *20*:83–92, 1962.

132. Baker, H., Frank, O., Thind, I.S., et al.: J. Am. Geriatr. Soc. *27*:444–450, 1979.

133. Bates, C.J., Rutishauser, I.H.E., Black, A.E., et al.: Br. J. Nutr. *42*:43–56, 1979.

134. Silink, S.J., Nobile, S., Woodhill, J.M., et al.: J. Geriatrics. *3*:29–36, 1972.

135. Garry, P.J., Goodwin, J.S., Hunt, W.C., et al.: Am. J. Clin. Nutr. *36*:332–339, 1982.

136. Goodwin, J.S., Goodwin, J.M., Garry, P.J.: J.A.M.A. *249*:2917–2921, 1983.

137. Weinsier, R.L., Hunker, E.M., Krumdieck, C.L., et al.: Am. J. Clin. Nutr. *32*:418–426, 1979.

138. Lemoine, A., Le Devehat, C., Codaccioni, J.L., et al.: Am. J. Clin. Nutr. *33*:2595–2600, 1980.

139. Kelleher, J.: Vitamin deficiencies in disease states. *In* Importance of Vitamins to Human Health. (Taylor, T.G., Ed.) Lancaster, MTP Press, 1979, pp. 139–149.

140. Wilson, C.W.M.: Practitioner *212*:481–492, 1974.

141. Bonjour, J.P.: Int. J. Vitam. Nutr. Res. *49*:434–441, 1979.

142. Fazio, V., Flint, D.M., Wahlqvist, M.L.: Am. J. Clin. Nutr. *34*:2394–2396, 1981.

143. Basu, T.K.: The influence of drugs with particular reference to aspirin on the bioavailability of vitamin C. *In* Vitamin C (Ascorbic Acid). (Counsell, J.N., Hornig, D.H., Eds.) London, Applied Science Publishers, 1981, pp. 273–281.

144. Calman, K.C.: Proc. Nutr. Soc. *37*:87, 1978.

145. Moriartry, M., Murphy, C., Keogh, R., et al.: Ir. Med. J. *74*:43–45, 1981.

146. Hume, R., Vallance, B., Weyers, E.: Ascorbic acid and stress. *In* Re-evaluation of Vitamin C. (Hanck, A., Ritzel, G., Eds.) Berne, Huber Verlag, 1977, pp. 89–98.

147. Hornig, D.H., Glatthaar, B.E.: Vitamin C and smoking: Increased requirement of smokers. *In* Vitamins: Nutrients and Therapeutic Agents. (Hornig, D.H., Hanck, A.B., Eds.) (Supplement 3, No. 27 of International Journal for Vitamin and Nutrition Research)—Hans Huber Publishers, Bern Stuttgart Toronto, 1985, pp. 139–155.

147a. Murata, A., Morinage, N., Kato, F., et al.: Vitamins *58*:61–69, 1984.

148. The National Research Council: Recommended Dietary Allowances, 9th ed. Washington, D.C., National Academy of Sciences, 1980.

149. Salmenperä, L.: Am. J. Clin. Nutr. *40*:1050–1056, 1984.

150. Pönkä, A., Kuhlbäck, B.: Acta Med. Scand. *213*:305–307, 1983.

151. Reference deleted.

152. Eddy, T.P.: Br. J. Nutr. *27*:537–542, 1972.

153. Greco, A.M., Fioretti, F., Rimo, A.: Acta Vitaminol. Enzymol. *2*:21–25, 1980.

154. Kinsman, R.A., Hood, J.: Am. J. Clin. Nutr. *24*:455–464, 1971.

155. Van der Beek, E.J., van Dokkum, W., Schrijver, J., et al.: Int. J. Sports Med. *5*, Suppl.:28–31, 1984.

156. Buzina, R., Suboticanec, K.: Vitamin C and physical working capacity. *In* Vitamins in Nutrition and Therapy. (Hornig, D.H., Hanck, A.B., Eds.) Berne, Huber Verlag, 1985, pp. 157–166.

157. Evans, P.R.: Br. Med. J. *287*:1862–1863, 1983.

158. Irwin, M.I., Hutchins, B.K.: J. Nutr. *106*:821–879, 1976.

159. Hornig, D.: Trends Pharmacol. Sci. *3*:294–296, 1982.

160. Barness, L.A.: Ann. N.Y. Acad. Sci. *258*:523–528, 1975.

161. Hanck, A.: Tolerance and effects of high doses of ascorbic acid. *In* Vitamin C. New Clinical Applications in Immunology, Lipid Metabolism and Cancer. (Hanck, A., Ed.) Berne, Huber Verlag, 1982, pp. 221–238.

162. Schrauzer, G.N., Rhead, W.J.: Int. J. Vitam. Nutr. Res. *43*:201–211, 1973.

163. Hornig, D., Weiser, H., Weber, F., et al.: Int. J. Vitam. Nutr. Res. *43*:28–33, 1973.

164. Herbert, V., Jakob, E.: J.A.M.A. *230*:241–242, 1974.

165. Newmark, H.L., Schreiner, J., Marcus, M., et al.: Am. J. Clin. Nutr. *29*:645–649, 1976.

166. Marcus, M., Prabhudesai, M., Wosseft, S.: Am. J. Clin. Nutr. *33*:137–144, 1980.

167. Siest, G., Appel, W.: J. Clin. Chem. Clin. Biochem. *16*:103–110, 1978.

168. Ganick, D.P., Close, J.R.: Lancet *2*:820–821, 1977.

169. Samborskaya, E.P., Ferdman, T.D.: Byull. Éksp. Biol. Med. *62*:934–935, 1967.

170. Hoffer, A.: Lancet *2*:1146, 1973.

171. Harris, W.A., Harden, T.E., Dawson, E.B.: Fertil. Steril. *32*:455–459, 1979.

172. Dawson, E.B., Harris, W.A., McGanity, W.J.: Clin. Res. *31*:616A, 1983.

173. Igarashi, M.: Int. J. Fertil. *22*:168–173, 1977.

174. Basu, T.K., Schorah, C.J.: Vitamin C in Health and Disease. Westport, Connecticut, The Avi Publishing Company, Inc., 1982.

*Chapter* **23**

# BIOTIN

## Donald B. McCormick

The ultimate recognition that the vitamin biotin was the unique factor common to apparently different functions in diverse species required the efforts of a number of laboratories spanning approximately 40 years. In early studies with microorganisms, Wildiers reported in 1901 on a substance "bios," present in extracts of natural materials, which was a growth factor for yeasts.[1] This was later found composed of Bios I, determined to be inositol, and Bios II, which turned out to be a mixture containing biotin. It was not until 1936 that Kögl and Tönnis succeeded in isolating from the Bios II fraction of egg yolk a crystalline compound, which they named biotin.[2] Before this, Allison et al. had reported on a factor called coenzyme R, which was found to stimulate respiration in legume nodule bacteria.[3] Among notable studies with animals, Boas reported in 1927 that a toxic condition observed upon feeding raw (uncooked) egg white could be prevented by providing foods containing an "X factor."[4] György described in detail the histologic changes that occur in skin due to egg white injury, and he called the protective factor, vitamin H (Haut-skin).[5] In 1940, du Vigneaud and his associates proved that the Bios II component, coenzyme R, and vitamin H were identical to biotin,[6] and by 1942 they reported the structure. The Merck group led by Harris et al. announced the synthesis of biotin in 1943.[8] Traub elucidated the absolute configuration by x-ray crystallographic analysis.[9]

The manner in which biotin functions took longer to ascertain, though the suggestion that it might be particularly involved in the process of

$CO_2$ fixation was first advanced by Burk and Winzler in 1943.[10] Participation of biotin in a carboxylation reaction involving β-methylcrotonyl-CoA, a catabolite of leucine, was demonstrated in experiments of Lardy and Peanasky in 1953.[11] These workers demonstrated a decrease in the carboxylase from biotin-deficient animals. Lynen et al. reported in 1959 that specific activity of the carboxylase purified from mycobacteria was directly proportional to its biotin content.[12] The importance of biotin in fatty acid biosynthesis was underscored by its occurrence as a functional component in acetyl-CoA carboxylase.[13] Through the work of Lynen,[14] Knappe,[15] and their colleagues during the 1960s, the involvement of biotin, covalently attached as an amide through the ε-amino lysyl residues of carboxylating enzymes, was largely elucidated. The way in which biotin as the 5'-adenylate becomes covalently appended to an apoenzyme also has been elucidated for several systems.[16]

## CHEMISTRY, INCLUDING PRINCIPAL ANALOGUES

Natural *d*-biotin is chemically specified as *cis*-tetrahydro - 2 - oxothieno[3,4 - *d*] - imidazoline - 4 - valeric acid (or *cis*-hexahydro-2-oxo-1H-thieno[3,4] imidazole-4-valeric acid (Fig. 23–1). The free vitamin is an acid ($pK_a = 4.51$),[17] which crystallizes as fine, white needles.

Though the acid form of the vitamin is only modestly soluble at room temperature (25°C), in water (22 mg/dl), or 95% ethanol (80 mg/dl) and essentially insoluble in other common organic

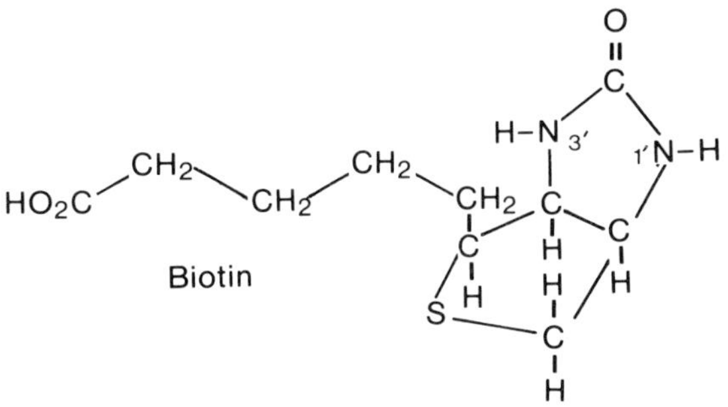

**Fig. 23–1.** Biotin. Natural derivatives include the dethio compound in which 2 H's replace the divalent S, the sulfoxides in which an SO function replaces S, and biocytin with an ε-lysyl attachment.

solvents, the anionic salts are significantly more water soluble. The colorless, pure compound in neutral, aqueous solution is quite stable, but alkaline solutions decompose with heating. Moreover, oxidizing reagents rapidly form sulfoxides.[22] Stronger oxidants lead to biotin sulfone.

Compounds related to biotin continue to be synthesized often starting with the parent vitaminic structure.[18] A number of such analogues, e.g., certain side chain-shortened compounds and the sulfoxides and sulfone, have since been found to be catabolites; others, e.g., dethiobiotin, are biosynthetic precursors of the vitamin. Biocytin (ε-N-biotinyl-L-lysine) is a natural fragment derived by degradation of biotinyl enzymes. An unnatural synthetic analogue of biotin, which is weakly active in microorganisms and animals, is oxybiotin where O has replaced S in the ring system. Synthetic homologues of biotin, e.g., homobiotin with five methylenes in the side chain and norbiotin with three, are antagonists,[20,21] yet they are subject to partial β-oxidative cleavage of the acid side chains.[22]

## BIOLOGIC ACTIVITY RELATING TO STRUCTURE

Since there are four asymmetric carbons in biotin, there are eight chemical stereoisomers; however, only the natural d-biotin has been found vitaminically active.[18] The imidazole ring (ureido carbonyl) is required for activity including binding to avidin. Replacement of sulfur in the thiolane ring by oxygen leads to oxybiotin, which has decreased activity. Dethiobiotin has no activity. The latter appears to have vitamin-like activity in those organisms, e.g., *Aspergillus niger,* that can convert dethiobiotin to biotin,[23] but not in mammals that lack the biosynthetic pathway. Oxidation of the sulfur impairs vitaminic activity: the d-sulfoxide can be metabolically slowly reduced to biotin,[24] but not the l-sulfoxide;[25] the sulfone

is not significantly metabolized by microorganisms where it can serve as an antagonist.[18]

## ABSORPTION, TRANSPORT, METABOLISM, AND EXCRETION

The salient features of biotin uptake and turnover in organisms have been reviewed earlier[26] and updated in chapters on the subject.[27] The main points, especially with regard to the human,[28] are summarized in the following.

Digestion of dietary proteins containing bound biotin yields considerable biocytin (ε-N-biotinyl-L-lysine). Biocytin is resistant to hydrolysis by proteolytic enzymes in the intestinal tract as is the biotin-avidin complex. Biocytin and biotin are readily absorbed. An enzyme called biocytinase (biotin amidohydrolase) is in plasma and erythrocytes and catalyzes the hydrolysis of biocytin to yield free biotin. Biotin is cleared from the circulating blood more rapidly in deficient than in normal mammals, taken up by such tissues as liver, muscle, and kidney, and localized in cytosolic and mitochondrial carboxylases. Covalent attachment of biotin to apoenzymes involves ATP-dependent conversion of the vitamin to biotinyl-5'-adenylate followed by condensation of the biotinyl moiety with ε-amino groups of specific lysyl residues in apoenzymes preformed from subunits. The enzymes responsible for catalyzing the formation on the ε-N-biotinyl-L-lysyl (biocytinyl) moiety of proteins are holoenzyme synthetases.

Details on the biosynthesis and metabolism of biotin have been elucidated and summarized.[27] Although a soil bacterium isolated to grow on the vitamin as a sole source of C, H, O, N, and S can extensively degrade biotin in the ways outlined in Figure 23–2, the catabolic machinery of animals is more limited. Following turnover and during fractional catabolism of biotin, the mammal is able to effect some oxidation of the thioether function; both d- and l-sulfoxides are formed. Partial cleavage of the valeric acid side chain is effected by β-oxidation. Trace amounts of biotin sulfoxides and bisnorbiotin are excreted in the urine with larger (but still μg) amounts of free vitamin. Careful balance studies in man, where perhaps only 1 mg is the total body content, showed that urinary excretion of biotin often exceeded dietary intake, and that in all cases fecal excretion was as much as 3 to 6 times greater than dietary intake because of microfloral biosynthesis.[29,30]

## BIOCHEMICAL AND PHYSIOLOGIC FUNCTIONS

At present, nine biotin-dependent enzymes are known: 6 carboxylases, 2 decarboxylases, and a transcarboxylase.[27,31,32] Four carboxylases are

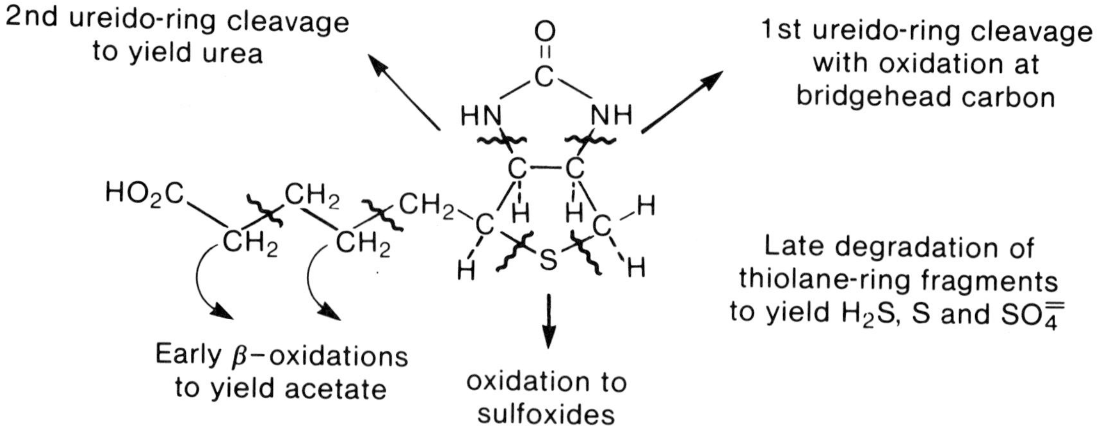

**2nd ureido-ring cleavage to yield urea**

**1st ureido-ring cleavage with oxidation at bridgehead carbon**

**Late degradation of thiolane-ring fragments to yield $H_2S$, S and $SO_4^=$**

**Early $\beta$-oxidations to yield acetate**

**oxidation to sulfoxides**

**Fig. 23–2.** Degradation of biotin and catabolites.

found in human tissues. These are carboxylases for acetyl-CoA, proprionyl-CoA, β-methylcrotonyl-CoA, and pyruvate, which catalyze formation of malonyl-CoA, methylmalonyl-CoA, β-methylglutaconyl-CoA, and oxalacetate, respectively. The biotin-dependent carboxylases operate via a common mechanism, which involves phosphorylation of bicarbonate by ATP to form carbonyl phosphate, followed by transfer of the carboxyl group to the sterically less hindered nitrogen of the biotin moiety (Fig. 23–3). The resulting $N(1)$-carboxybiotinyl enzyme can then exchange the carboxylate function with a reactive center in a substrate. With cytosolic acetyl-CoA carboxylase, the product is malonyl-CoA utilized for fatty acid biosynthesis. This carboxylase is allosterically regulated by citrate and coenzyme A as positive modulators and by long-chain fatty acyl-CoAs, which are negative effectors. Hence, the consumption of excess carbohydrates can lead to higher concentrations of citrate, which turn on acetyl-CoA carboxylase to make more fat. As the production of fatty acyl-CoAs increases, there is somewhat of a braking effect to slow down the carboxylase. In mitochondria, pyruvate carboxylase catalyzes formation of oxalacetate, which together with acetyl-CoA forms citrate. Acetyl-

CoA is a positive modulator of this carboxylase. Hence, as more acetyl-CoA is produced by pyruvate breakdown, another fraction of pyruvate is carboxylated to supply coordinately the other substrate needed for citrate formation. The other carboxylases are involved in the metabolism of odd-numbered and branched-chain fatty acids, some of which derive from metabolism of certain amino acids.

## DEFICIENCY AND EXCESS

Dietary deficiency of biotin is infrequently seen and has been produced in the adult usually only after ingestion of diets that have included large amounts of raw egg white (containing avidin).[27–29] With the advent of total parenteral nutrition and the use by some physicians of vitamin preparations devoid in biotin, deficiency of this micronutrient has been reported in children[33] and adults.[34] Symptoms include anorexia, nausea, vomiting, glossitis, pallor, depression, and a dry scaly dermatitis. A seborrheic dermatitis in infants under six months of age can also be caused by inadequate biotin, but the condition responds promptly to biotin therapy. Significantly lowered urinary excretion or circulating blood levels have also been found in pregnant women, alcoholics,

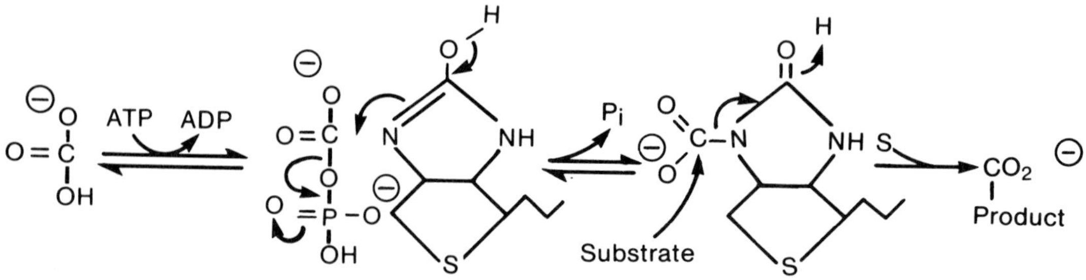

**Fig. 23–3.** Mechanisms of biotin-catalyzed carboxylations.

patients with achlorhydria, and among the elderly and some athletes.[28] Finally, there are rather rare genetic defects such as in holoenzyme synthetase (reflected in inadequate conversion of apo- to holocarboxylases) or a defect in an enzyme such as propionyl-CoA carboxylase (reflected in a distinguishing acidemia).[27]

Though no direct studies on toxicity of biotin given to humans appear to have been published, the injection of 5 to 10 mg daily in infants less than six months old produced no ill effect. Because of the modest solubility of the vitamin, it is not likely that a large amount could even be absorbed in a single passage through the gut.

## DIETARY CONSIDERATIONS

Intestinal microflora make a significant contribution to the body pool of available biotin so that the dietary requirement is uncertain.[29] Mean urinary excretion, reflective of dietary intake, ranges from 18 to 46 $\mu$g/d for adults who ingest 50 to 200 $\mu$g/d. It is felt that an intake of 100 to 200 $\mu$g/d is quite adequate. Since urinary concentration of biotin in infants after the age of six months is comparable with that of adults, the requirement for older infants and children is probably proportional to body weight and energy consumption. A ratio of 50 $\mu$g/1000 kcal has been suggested, and adequate intakes are increased from 50 $\mu$g/d for the half-year old up to the adult level. The suggested intake of 35 $\mu$g/d for young infants is more than adequate when compared to the low biotin content of human milk at 10 $\mu$g/1000 kcal or 0.16 $\mu$g/dl.

Good sources of biotin include yeast, liver, kidney, and pancreas; moderate sources are eggs, milk, fish, and nuts; poorer sources are muscle meats, cereal grains, and fruits.

## METHODS FOR ASSAY AND STATUS DETERMINATION

At the trace concentrations present in biologic samples, biotin can be quantitated using microbiologic assays.[35] Bound biotin is first liberated by proteolytic digestion of the sample using, for example, papain with whole blood. Then aliquots are added to a biotin-deficient medium inoculated with a test organism such as *Lactobacillus plantarum*. Standard curves are derived from growth in controls containing known amounts of biotin. Other methods include isotopic dilution assays that are generally applicable and even a colorimetric determination with acidic *p*-dimethylaminocinnamaldehyde, which forms a red Schiff base;[36] this is suitable only when quantity and purity of specimens are adequate.

## REFERENCES

1. Wildiers, E.: La Cellule *18*:313, 1901.
2. Kögl, F., Tönnis, B.: Z. physiol. Chem. *242*:43, 1936.
3. Allison, F.E., Hoover, S.R., Burk, D.: Science *78*:217, 1933.
4. Boas, M.A.: Biochem. J. *21*:712, 1927.
5. György, P.: J. Biol. Chem. *131*:733, 1939.
6. du Vigneaud, V., Melville, D.B., György, P., et al.: Science *92*:62, 1940.
7. du Vigneaud, V.: Science *96*:455, 1942.
8. Harris, S.A., Wolf, D.E., Mozingo, R., et al.: Science *97*:447, 1943.
9. Traub, W.: Nature *178*:649, 1956.
10. Burk, D., Winzler, R.G.: Science *97*:59, 1943.
11. Lardy, H.A., Peanasky, R.: Physiol. Rev. *33*:560, 1953.
12. Lynen, F. Knappe, J., Lorch, E., et al.: Angew. Chem. *71*:481, 1959.
13. Wakil, S., Gibson, D.M.: Biochim. Biophys. Acta *41*:122, 1960.
14. Lynen, F.: Biochem. J. *102*:381, 1967.
15. Knappe, J.: Ann. Rev. Biochem. *39*:757, 1970.
16. Achuta Murthy, P.N., Mistry, S.P.: Biochem. Rev. *XLIII*:1, 1972.
17. Sigel, H., McCormick, D.B., Griesser, R., et al.: Biochemistry *8*:2687, 1969.
18. Sternbach, L.H.: Biotin. *In* Comprehensive Biochemistry, Vol. II (Florkin, M., Stotz, E.H., Eds.) New York, Elsevier, 1963.
19. Melville, D.B.: J. Biol. Chem. *208*:495, 1954.
20. Rubin, S.H., Scheiner, J.: Arch. Biochem. Biophys. *23*:400, 1949.
21. Goldberg, M.W., Sternbach, L.H., Kaiser, S., et al.: Arch. Biochem. *14*:480, 1947.
22. Ruis, H., Brady, R.N., McCormick, D.B., et al.: J. Biol. Chem. *243*:547, 1968.
23. Li, H.-C., McCormick, D.B., Wright, L.D.: J. Biol. Chem. *243*:6442, 1968.
24. Im, W.B., Roth, J.A., McCormick, D.B., et al.: J. Biol. Chem. *245*:6269, 1970.
25. Roth, J.A., McCormick, D.B., Wright, L.D.: J. Biol. Chem. *245*:6264, 1970.
26. Mistry, S.P., Dakshinamurti, K.: Biotin. *In* Vitamins and Hormones, Vol. 22 (Harris, R.S., Wool, I.G., and Loraine, J.A., Eds.). New York, Academic Press, 1965.
27. McCormick, D.B., Olson, R.E.: Biotin. *In* Present Knowledge in Nutrition, 5th edit. (Olson, R.E., Ed.). Washington, DC, The Nutrition Foundations, 1984.
28. Bonjour, J.P.: Int. J. Vit. Nutr. Res. *47*:107, 1977.
29. Recommended Dietary Allowances, 9th ed.: Committee on Dietary Allowances and Food and Nutrition Board, National Research Council, National Academy of Science, Washington, DC, 1980.
30. Harper, H.A., Rodwell, V.A., Mayes, P.A.: Review of Physiological Chemistry, Ch. 13. Los Altos, CA, Lange Medical Publications, 1979.
31. Moss, J., Lane, M.D.: Adv. Enzymol. *35*:321, 1971.
32. Wood, H.G., Barden, R.E.: Ann. Rev. Biochem. *46*:385, 1977.
33. Mock, D.M., Boswell, D.C., Baker, H., et al.: J. Pediatr. *106*:762, 1985.
34. McClain, C.J., Baker, H., Onstad, G.R.: J.A.M.A. *247*:3116, 1982.
35. Sauberlich, H.E., Skala, J.H., Dowdy, R.P.: Laboratory Tests for the Assessment of Nutritional Status. Boca Raton, FL, CRC Press, 1974.
36. McCormick, D.B., Roth, J.A.: Anal. Biochem. *34*:2265, 1970.

*Chapter* **24**

# "VITAMIN-LIKE" MOLECULES

## (A) CHOLINE*

### Steven H. Zeisel

Choline (trimethyl-beta-hydroxyethylammonium) is widely distributed in plant and animal tissues. It is a precursor for the biosynthesis of the neurotransmitter acetylcholine (ACh), a source of labile-methyl groups, and a precursor of phospholipids, important constituents of membranes.

Choline, first discovered by Strecker in 1862, was chemically synthesized in 1866.[1,2] It was known to be a component of phospholipids, but the pathway for its biosynthesis was first described in 1941 by duVigneaud.[3] The route for its incorporation into phosphatidylcholine (lecithin) was not elucidated until 1956.[4] The importance of choline as a nutrient was first appreciated during the pioneering work on insulin.[5,6] Depancreatized dogs, maintained on insulin, developed fatty infiltration of the liver and died. Administration of raw pancreas prevented hepatic damage; the active component was the choline moiety of pancreatic phosphatidylcholine.[5,6] In 1935 the association between a low-choline diet and fatty infiltration of the liver in rats was recognized.[7] The term "lipotropic" was coined to describe choline and other substances that prevented deposition of fat in the liver. Subsequently researchers suggested that the liver disease associated with alcoholism might respond to choline therapy.[8] However, little data supported this hypothesis. The assays for choline available at the time were not particularly sensitive or specific, and the therapy did not prove to be very effective. In 1975, Wurtman and colleagues and Haubrich and associates reported that administration of choline accelerated the synthesis and release of the ACh by neurons.[9–12] At the same time, technical breakthroughs in the assay of choline made it possible to accurately detect picomoles of the substance.[13,14] A revival of interest in choline ensued, resulting in a plethora of publications characterizing the metabolism, physiologic effects, and pharmacology of choline.

## BIOCHEMISTRY AND METABOLISM OF CHOLINE

Table 24A–1 presents the structures of choline and the major choline metabolites.

### Pathways Utilizing Choline

In mammalian tissue four enzyme-catalyzed pathways utilize choline: it can be oxidized, ace-

*Some of the work described in this chapter was supported by grants from the National Institutes of Health (AM33163, HD16727, CA26731), the United States Department of Agriculture (CRCR-1-1828), and the International Life Sciences Institute-Nutrition Foundation.

**Table 24A–1. Structures of Choline and Major Choline Metabolites**

| | |
|---|---|
| Choline | $(CH_3)_3-N^+-CH_2-CH_2OH$ |
| Phosphorylcholine | $(CH_3)_3-N^+-CH_2-CH_2O-PO_3$ |
| Acetylcholine | $(CH_3)_3-N^+-CH_2-CH_2-COO-CH_3$ |
| Betaine | $(CH_3)_3-N^+-CH_2-COO$ |
| Phosphatidylcholine (Lecithin) | $CH_2-O-CO-$ *Fatty Acid* |
| | \| |
| | $CH-O-CO-$ *Fatty Acid* |
| | \| |
| | $CH_2-O-PO_2-OCH_2-CH_2-N^+-(CH_3)_3$ |
| Lysophosphatidylcholine (Lysolecithin) | $CH_2-O-CO-$ *Fatty Acid* |
| | \| |
| | $CH-OH$ |
| | \| |
| | $CH_2-O-PO_2-OCH_2-CH_2-N^+-(CH_3)_3$ |
| Sphingomyelin | $CH=CH-(CH_2)_{12}-CH_3$ |
| | \| |
| | $CH-NH-CO-(CH_2)_{14}-CH_3$ |
| | \| |
| | $CH_2-O-PO_2-OCH_2-CH_2-N^+-(CH_3)_3$ |

tylated, transferred by "base" exchange, and phosphorylated. Betaine formation is probably the predominant fate of most excess choline presented to the liver.[15] Choline is oxidized to betaine aldehyde, which is then converted to betaine in reactions catalyzed by choline dehydrogenase and betaine aldehyde dehydrogenase (collectively called choline oxidase). These enzymes are present in several mammalian tissues including liver and kidney, but are not present in blood, brain, or muscle.[16–21] Once betaine is formed it cannot be reduced to reform choline; however, it can donate a methyl group to homocysteine, thereby producing dimethylglycine and methionine (see section on Interrelationships). Dimethylglycine is converted to sarcosine and then to glycine, producing a 1-carbon fragment.[22] Thus, the oxidation pathway acts to remove free choline from tissues while scavenging methyl groups. Figure 24A–1 summarizes the metabolic pathways of choline.

The activity of choline acetyltransferase (ChAT) is of interest because of the role that ACh plays as a neurotransmitter. However, only a small fraction of ingested choline is acetylated.[23] ChAT is highly concentrated in the terminals of cholinergic neurons, but it is also present in such nonnervous tissues as the placenta.[24–26] The availability of choline and acetyl-CoA influences in vivo ChAT activity.[27] In brain it is unlikely that ChAT is saturated with either of its substrates, so that choline (and possibly acetyl-CoA) availability determines the rate of ACh synthesis.[9–11,27] A carrier mechanism, within the blood-brain barrier, transports free choline into the brain against a concentration and charge gradient.[28] This carrier has a low affinity for choline (km = 0.44 mmol). Thus at physiologic concentrations of choline in serum (10 μM), this carrier is unsaturated and is able to carry choline into the brain at a rate that is proportional to serum choline concentration.[28] When large doses of choline and phosphatidylcholine are ingested, blood choline concentrations increase,[29] thereby accelerating the entry of choline into, and inhibiting its efflux out of, the brain. Some choline molecules may also be transported into the brain as part of phospholipids such a phosphatidylcholine or lysophosphatidylcholine.[30]

Some investigators report that administration of choline or phosphatidylcholine results in the accumulation of ACh within brain neurons,[9–12] whereas others observe that such acceleration of ACh synthesis by choline administration can only be detected after pretreatments with agents that cause cholinergic neurons to fire rapidly.[31] The increase in brain ACh synthesis is associated with an augmented release into the synapse of this neu-

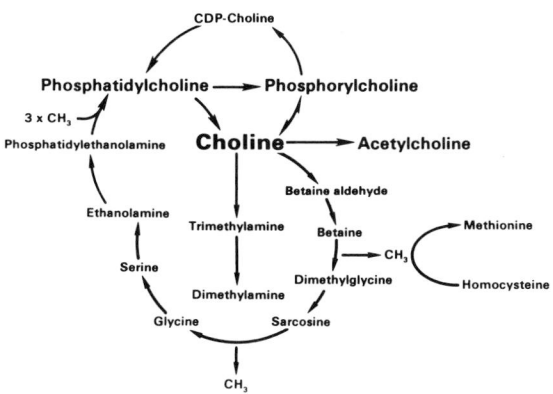

**Fig. 24A–1.** Metabolic pathways of choline.

rotransmitter. Choline itself is a weak cholinergic receptor agonist.[32] It has been possible to actually measure an increase in the number of ACh molecules released by certain in vitro preparations of heart and nerves exposed to higher than normal levels of choline in their perfusion media.[33,34] A temporal dissociation between choline administration and effects on brain ACh synthesis and release has been observed.[35] Choline taken up by brain may first enter a storage pool (perhaps the phosphatidylcholine in membranes) before being converted to ACh.[36]

A base-exchange pathway has been described in several tissues including liver and brain.[37–39] It involves the substitution of choline for serine, inositol, or ethanolamine head groups on endogenous phospholipids. The reaction is reversible and requires the presence of calcium. In most tissues this is probably a minor pathway for choline utilization.

Choline kinase catalyzes the phosphorylation of the hydroxyl group of choline, using ATP as the phosphate donor.[40] It is widely distributed in mammalian tissues including the liver, brain, kidney, and lung.[40–44] Phosphorylation of choline is the first step in the CDP pathway for phosphatidylcholine synthesis.[4] In this pathway cytidine triphosphate and phosphorylcholine are combined, generating cytidine diphosphocholine (CDP-choline). The CDP-choline is then combined with diacylglycerol, forming phosphatidylcholine (Fig. 24A–2).

## Pathways Forming Choline De Novo

Three enzymatic pathways catalyze phosphatidylcholine biosynthesis, yet only one generates new choline molecules. The cytidine diphosphocholine (CDP) and base exchange pathways do not cause a net synthesis of choline, but only redistribute preexisting molecules.[4,37,39] The methylation pathway, catalyzed by the enzyme(s) phosphatidylethanolamine-N-methyltransferase (PEMT), makes new choline molecules by sequentially methylating phosphatidylethanolamine, using S-adenosylmethionine (SAM) as the methyl donor.[45–49] This enzyme has its highest activity in the liver, but it is also found in kidney, testes, heart, adrenal gland, lung, erythrocyte, brain, and spleen.[45–51] PEMT is probably composed of several enzyme activities.[49,50] The first of these activities has a high affinity for SAM and is located on the inner (cytoplasmic) side of the plasma membrane. In the membrane of the endoplasmic reticulum this enzyme is also on the cytoplasmic surface.[52] As monomethyl-phosphatidylethanolamine is formed it flips into the middle of the phospholipid bilayer of the membrane

where it is methylated by the second PEMT enzyme.[49,50] This enzyme has a low affinity for SAM. A third methyl group is then added (either by the second enzyme or, possibly, by a third enzyme), and the newly formed phosphatidylcholine flips into the outer (extracellular) leaflet of the phospholipid bilayer. This pathway is one of the major mechanisms whereby the asymmetry of the membrane bilayer is maintained (i.e., more phosphatidylethanolamine on the cytoplasmic side, more phosphatidylcholine on the extracellular side).[53,54a]

The methylation pathway may be especially important in brain, where it provides choline for acetylcholine synthesis.[54a] PEMT (first methylation) catalyzes the rate-limiting step in phosphatidylcholine synthesis in brain, and phosphatidylcholine formation via this pathway is greatest during the neonatal period.[55]

There are no accurate estimates of the activity of PEMT in vivo. Investigators have attempted to assess PEMT activity by measuring excretion of labile methyl groups in humans eating diets devoid of choline.[54b] These studies have assumed that choline can only be derived from the diet or from PEMT activity, but such assumptions are not valid, as choline can also, at least temporarily, be withdrawn from storage pools such as the phosphatidylcholine in membranes. In vitro data suggest that 15 to 40% of the phosphatidylcholine present in liver is synthesized via the PEMT pathway, with the remainder coming from the CDP pathway.[46,56] Choline deficiency and exposure to ethanol increase the in vitro activity of the methylation pathway in liver.[57–59] Female rats have more hepatic PEMT activity than do males.[45,48] In brain and red blood cells, stimulation of noradrenergic receptors acts to increase the rate of phosphatidylethanolamine methylation.[60,61] The accumulation of the methylated products may alter membrane fluidity and thereby modulate the activity of enzymes that are embedded within the membrane.[62] The methylation pathway makes new free choline molecules because the phosphatidylcholines produced are hydrolyzed.[63]

## Absorption of Choline by Tissues

Some ingested choline is metabolized before it can be absorbed from the gut. Enterocytes degrade it to form betaine, and gut bacteria use it to make methylamines (see section on Toxicity).[64–66] Free choline that survives these fates is absorbed all along the small intestine.[66–69] We have identified two mechanisms for choline transport by rat small intestine, one involving mediated transport (saturation-type kinetics) and one involving diffusion.[67] Choline is absorbed from colon only via

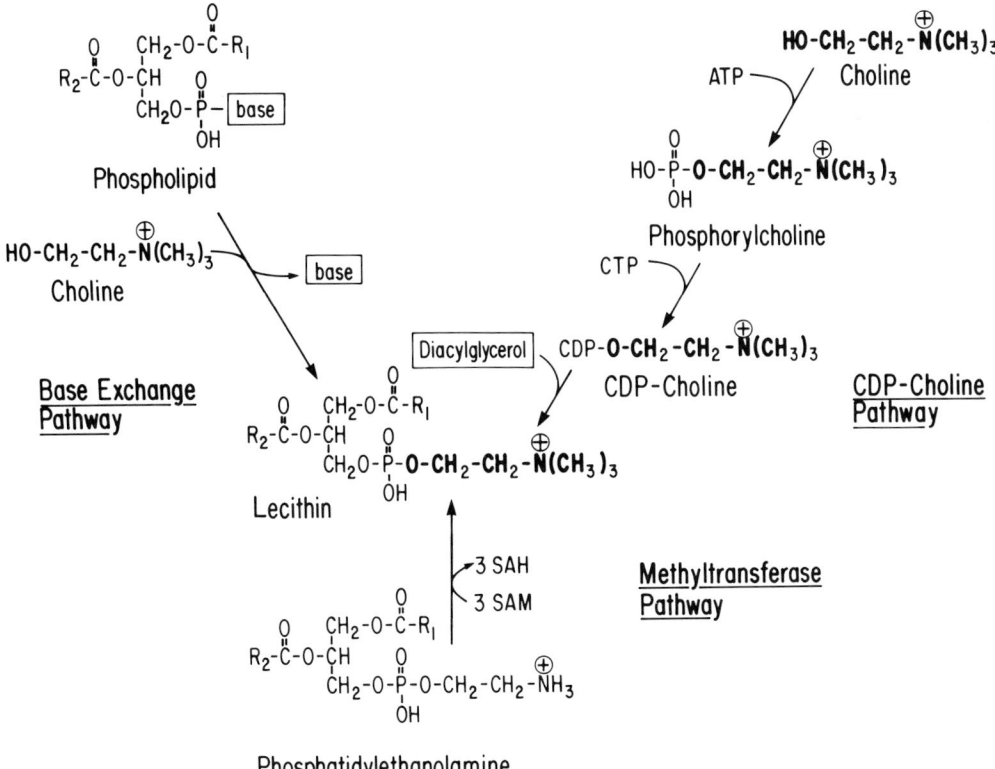

**Fig. 24A–2.** Biosynthesis of phosphatidylcholine.

diffusion. In the guinea pig, choline absorption is not sodium- or energy-dependent, whereas in the hamster energy is required.[66,69] At this time no other component of the diet has been identified that competes with choline for transport by this carrier.

Most foods contain choline in the form of phosphatidylcholine[70–72] (Table 24A–2). Both pancreatic secretions and intestinal mucosal cells contain enzymes capable of hydrolyzing this phospholipid. Phospholipase A2 (which cleaves the beta-fatty acid moiety) is found in pancreatic juice and in the intestinal brush border.[73–79] It is secreted as a zymogen, which is activated in the gut by trypsin, calcium and bile salts.[73,74] Within the gut mucosal cell, phospholipase A1 cleaves the alpha-fatty acid, and phospholipase B cleaves both fatty acids.[80] These enzymes degrade much less phosphatidylcholine than the pancreatic lipase does. The net result is that most ingested phosphatidylcholine is absorbed as lysophosphatidylcholine (deacylated in the beta position).[77] Within the enterocyte, lysophosphatidylcholine can be deacylated to form glycerophosphorylcholine (GPC), or it can be acylated to re-

form phosphatidylcholine.[77,80] The latter reaction is catalyzed by a dismutase found in both the microsomal and soluble fractions of the mucosal cell.[80] It uses a second lysophosphatidylcholine molecule as the fatty acid donor. Thus two lysophosphatidylcholine molecules are converted to a phosphatidylcholine and a GPC molecule. For this reason, approximately twice as many phosphatidylcholine molecules are absorbed from the gut as are reconstituted and secreted from the mucosal cell into the lymphatic circulation.[76,77]

GPC is present in small quantities in the diet and, as discussed previously, is formed from ingested phosphatidylcholine. Within the gut mucosal cell, GPC diesterase (L-3-glycerophosphorylcholine glycerophosphohydrolase, EC 3.1.4.2) catalyzes the conversion of GPC to glycerophosphate and free choline. This free choline enters the portal circulation of the liver.[75–77] Phosphorylcholine is also present in small amounts in the diet. It is rapidly degraded by intestinal alkaline phosphatases, liberating free choline, and inorganic phosphate.[81]

The phosphatidylcholine formed within gut mucosal cells enters the lymphatic circulation,

Table 24A–2.  Choline Content of Foods*

| Food | Choline Chloride (mg/100 g food) | Phosphatidylcholine |
|---|---|---|
| Peanuts | — | 1,113 |
| Pecans | — | 333 |
| Peanut butter | — | 966 |
| Wheat germ | — | 2,820 |
| Wheat | — | 613 |
| White flour | — | 346 |
| Polished rice | — | 586 |
| Corn meal | — | 280 |
| Spinach | 10 | 10 |
| Cauliflower | 78 | 2 |
| Kale | 89 | 2 |
| Potatoes | 40 | 1 |
| Lettuce | 18 | 0.2 |
| Carrots | 10 | 7 |
| Brussels sprouts | 43 | 2 |
| Calf liver | 650 | 850 |
| Lamb chops | — | 753 |
| Beef round | — | 453 |
| Ham | — | 800 |
| Trout | — | 580 |
| Cheese | — | 50–100 |
| Eggs | 0.4 | 394 |
| Milk | 5 | 10 |

*Data from Wood, J.L., Allison, R.G.[157]

and then enters the blood. Many tissues possess enzymes that are capable of degrading phosphatidylcholines and lysophosphatidylcholines. Phospholipases A1 and A2 remove fatty acid moieties from phosphatidylcholine.[82] Lysophospholipase performs the same function for lysophosphatidylcholine. GPC diesterase then acts to release free choline and glycerol phosphate.[83,84] Phosphatidylcholines can also be degraded by phospholipase C activity, which produces diacylglycerol and phosphorylcholine.[85] Phospholipase D activity has been identified in mammalian tissues where it forms free choline and diacylglycerolphosphate from phosphatidylcholine.[86] Lysophospholipase D acts in a similar manner upon lysophosphatidylcholine.[87] Although we are sure that blood choline concentration increases after humans eat phosphatidylcholine,[29] we do not know which organ or which enzyme activity is responsible for the liberation of most of the free choline seen.

As discussed earlier, the liver actively phosphorylates and oxidizes choline. All ingested choline, and free choline liberated from phosphatidylcholine, enters the hepatic circulation after absorption from the gut.[75–77] Choline is accumulated by liver, and much of it is converted to betaine.[15,88,89] Hepatectomy increases the half-life of choline and results in an increase in blood choline concentration.[89] The rate at which liver takes up

choline is sufficient to explain the rapid disappearance of choline injected systemically.

The kidney also accumulates choline.[89] Some of this choline appears in the urine unchanged, but most is oxidized within kidney to form betaine.[90] Nephrectomized dogs show a decreased rate of choline disappearance from the plasma.[89] Mean free choline in the plasma of azotemic humans is several times greater than in normal controls.[91] Hemodialysis rapidly removes choline from the plasma.[91]

## EFFECTS OF CHOLINE DEFICIENCY

Chronic ingestion of a diet deficient in choline has major consequences that include hepatic, renal, memory, and growth disorders. In the rat, hamster, pig, dog, and chicken, choline deficiency results in fatty infiltration of the liver.[5–7,92–102] This process is probably due to a disturbance in the synthesis of phosphatidylcholine, which is needed to export triglycerides as part of lipoproteins. Fatty infiltration of the liver begins in the central area of the lobule and spreads peripherally. This process is different than what occurs in kwashiorkor or essential amino acid deficiency, where fatty infiltration usually begins in the portal area of the lobule.[102a] Choline deficiency in adult rats causes a decrease in plasma choline, cholesterol, and phospholipid, a reduction in high-density lipoproteins, and a marked decrease in low-density betalipoproteins[103] (Fig. 24A–3). Induction of he-

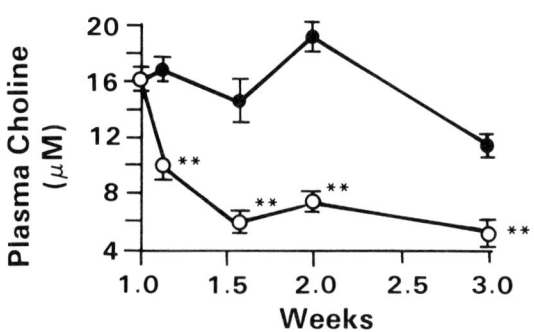

**Fig. 24A–3.** Plasma choline concentration in rats fed a choline-deficient diet. Rats were fed on a choline-supplemented, semisynthetic diet (0.7 mg choline/g wet weight diet) for one week. They were then randomly assigned to one of two groups: five rats were fed on a choline-deficient diet, and five rats were continued on the choline-supplemented diet. Animals were pair-fed, with calculations made on a daily basis. Data are expressed as mean ± SEM. ● = control group; ○ = choline-deficient group; ** = p <0.01. (From Zeisel, S.H., DaCosta, K-A., Fox, J.G., The Biochemical Society, London.[159a])

patocarcinoma by chemical carcinogens is enhanced in animals fed choline-deficient diets.[104] Renal function is also compromised, with abnormal concentrating ability, free water reabsorption, sodium excretion, glomerular filtration rate, renal plasma flow, and gross renal hemorrhage.[105–109] Infertility, growth impairment, bony abnormalities, decreased hematopoiesis, and hypertension have also been reported to be associated with diets low in choline content.[110–114] In mice choline deficiency is associated with memory impairment.[115]

## Clinical Situations Likely to Induce Choline Deficiency

Choline and phosphatidylcholine are so ubiquitous in the food supply that a deficiency syndrome in humans has not yet been identified. Only in clinical populations denied access to normal foods could choline deficiency be identified.

Hepatic complications associated with total parenteral nutrition (TPN), which include fatty infiltration of the liver and hepatocellular damage, have been reported by many clinical groups.[116–127] Frequently TPN must be terminated because of the severity of the associated liver disease. Although no definitive studies have tested the hypothesis, it is possible that some of the liver disease associated with TPN is related to choline deficiency. When rats were fed intravenously with choline-free TPN solutions (4.25% FreAmine II in 25% glucose), they developed fatty infiltration of

the liver, and had elevated serum levels of conjugated bilirubin and transaminases.[117] In these animals, oral or intravenous supplements of choline were effective in reversing hepatic lipid accumulation. This finding suggests that these rats were choline-deficient and that the methyl groups supplied by methionine within the TPN solution were not available in adequate amounts or were not utilized to spare choline requirements. Other investigators, however, have observed that I.V.-administered choline did not prevent fatty liver in rats on TPN.[117a] The rat requires cystine for hair formation. This requirement may increase the demand for methionine and the methyl groups of choline. Thus, data about choline requirements in rats may not necessarily be transferable to humans.

Amino acid-glucose solutions used in TPN of humans contain no choline. Lipid emulsions contain choline in the form of phosphatidylcholine (20% emulsion contains 13.2 μmol/ml.)[127a] Burt et al. reported that plasma choline concentrations were decreased in TPN patients at the same time that liver dysfunction was present.[128] We have found that malnourished humans, at the time they were referred for TPN therapy, had significantly lower plasma choline concentrations than did well-fed control subjects[127a] (Fig. 24A–4). Plasma choline concentrations in these patients declined further when they were treated with an amino acid-glucose solution lacking choline during the first week of therapy. However, when patients were treated with lipid emulsion as well as an amino acid-glucose solution, their plasma choline concentrations rose slightly. Neither group received sufficient choline to restore plasma choline concentrations to normal. We calculated that humans treated with TPN required 1,000 to 1,700 μmol of choline-containing phospholipid per day during the first week of TPN therapy to maintain plasma choline levels.[127a] Enteral food supplements, which contained choline, contributed to the rising plasma choline that we observed after the first week of TPN therapy.

Conditions that enhance hepatic triglyceride synthesis (such as carbohydrate loading) increase the requirement for choline-containing lipoprotein envelope.[128a] Thus, treatment of malnourished patients with high-calorie TPN solutions, at a time when choline stores are depleted, might cause hepatic dysfunction. The definitive experiment, in which supplemental choline is administered and found to decrease the incidence of hepatic dysfunction during TPN, has not yet been performed. Until such data are available, it is impossible to state that humans require choline dur-

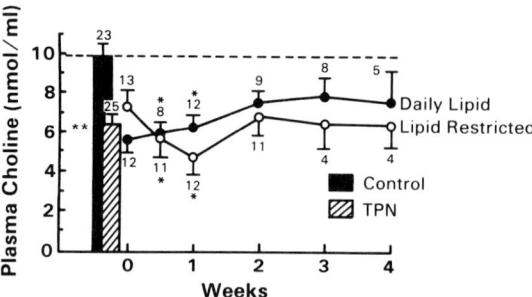

**Fig. 24A–4.** Plasma choline concentration during TPN therapy. Plasma samples were obtained by venepuncture from well-fed hospitalized controls (n = 23;■) and from malnourished patients treated with total parenteral nutrition therapy. (n = 25;■). Choline was measured using a radioenzymatic assay. The TPN patients were prospectively divided into two groups. Group 1 (Daily Lipid;●) was treated with amino acid, glucose, vitamin, and trace mineral parenteral nutrition solutions with a daily supplement of intravenous lipid emulsion. Group 2 (Lipid-Restricted;○) was treated with same TPN solutions, but received no supplemental lipid during the first week of therapy. After this period, both groups were supplemented with daily lipid infusion, and with oral or enteral feedings. Data are expressed as mean ± SEM; n for each point is indicated.** = p <0.001 different from control group.* = p <0.05 different from baseline value. (From Sheard, N.F., Tayek, J.A., Bistrian, B.R., et al.[127a])

ing TPN. The information available to date only suggests that this may be so.

## EFFECTS OF CHOLINE EXCESS

### Therapeutic Effects of Choline and Phosphatidylcholine

The use of foods as "drugs" is not a new idea. Many individuals ingest coffee, tea, or soft drinks because of the pharmacologic effects of their constituents. The isolation and purification of choline and phosphatidylcholine from foods have made possible the use of these compounds as treatments for human illnesses.

**Nervous System.** The data accrued from studies in animals suggest that choline could be used to augment cholinergic neurotransmission in humans. A large number of clinical studies using choline or phosphatidylcholine therapy for neurologic diseases have already been undertaken. Administration of choline-containing compounds may augment acetylcholine synthesis and release in humans, but usually the effect is modest. Most recently, clinical trials have focused on treatments that combine pharmacologic agents (which augment cholinergic transmission) with choline-containing compounds.[129] Lecithin (95% phosphati-

dylcholine) administration (20 to 30 g/day in adults) seems the preferred mode of delivering choline, as the effect on blood choline is more sustained, and patients do not smell like rotten fish.[29]

Choline and phosphatidylcholine therapy benefits patients with tardive dyskinesia, a syndrome thought to involve deficient cholinergic neurotransmission.[130–134] This disorder is characterized by involuntary choreic movements of the tongue, lips, and jaw. It is thought to be a side effect of many of the antipsychotic drugs currently being marketed in the United States.

Cholinergic neurons are vital for normal memory in rats and humans.[135] Choline administration improves the memory of humans who are poor initial learners in serial-learning and selective-reminding tasks.[136,137] Mice exhibit an age-related diminution of memory that is exacerbated by a diet low in choline and alleviated by a diet high in choline.[115] Such diets are also associated with anatomic differences in the brains of these mice.[138] Diminished memory in old age is not peculiar to mice. Benign senescent forgetfulness is a problem in humans as well. Some humans are afflicted with rapid loss of memory at a relatively young age, a syndrome called Alzheimer's disease. This disease is characterized by the loss of acetylcholine neurons in brain.[139,140] A number of reports have described memory function in Alzheimer's disease patients treated with choline or phosphatidylcholine. Most have described open-label studies, but several have been double-blind.[141–142] In most studies some of the subjects improve while others are not helped at all.

Serious problems face investigators who wish to study memory in humans. There is little agreement as to what constitutes an objective memory test, and clinicians are not able to identify a homogenous population to study. It may be that multidrug pharmacy is required. Preliminary reports indicate that choline or phosphatidylcholine plus piracetam (a drug thought to increase the firing rate of acetylcholine neurons) has more effect than precursor alone.[129] Definitive evidence of the efficacy of choline or phosphatidylcholine treatment in patients with Alzheimer's disease awaits further investigation.

It has been proposed that mania is the result of increased activation of adrenergic receptors in brain, whereas depression is the result of increased cholinergic stimulation.[143] Physostigmine, a cholinergic agonist, induces depression, and it decreases symptoms in patients with mania.[144] When phosphatidylcholine was administered along with lithium, the improvement in patients' behavior was greater than after lithium treatment alone.[145] The erythrocyte accumulates choline from the plasma via a specific transport mechanism. This mechanism is irreversibly inhibited by lithium.[146] In humans with mania or depression, red blood cell choline levels are extremely high. This finding is true even in those patients with no history of treatment with lithium.[147,148] An abnormality in choline transport may be involved in the pathophysiology of these diseases.

**Cardiovascular System.** In both humans and animals intravenous choline administration lowers blood pressure slightly.[149–152] Because this effect is prevented by pretreatment with hemicholinium-3, choline must be transported via a carrier into some cell, possibly a neuron, to lower blood pressure.[152] Oral administration of choline has a slight hypotensive effect in humans.[153] Choline could be acting by increasing vagal tone to the heart, or by dilating arterioles. Although choline administration increases acetylcholine release in in vitro preparations of heart,[34] changes in cardiac rate have not been observed in healthy humans treated with choline. Rats exposed to transient periods of dietary choline deficiency develop irreversible hypertension.[105,154] These changes may be related to changes in renal as well as cardiovascular function.

## Toxicity of Choline-Containing Compounds

Much of the clinical use of choline and phosphatidylcholine has occurred recently. Little attention has been given to the pharmacology and side effects of these compounds. The LD50 of choline iodide in rats is 1.7 mmol/kg i.p. and 28.7 mmole/kg orally.[32] The growth rate of rats is slowed when they are fed high-choline diets (depressed 100% on a 10% choline intake).[155] Dogs develop a macrocytic, hypochromic anemia after ingesting 10 mg/kg/day choline chloride for 25 days.[156] Neither choline nor phosphatidylcholine is teratogenic by the Ames test.[157]

In the treatment of neurologic diseases large doses (20 to 30 mmoles/70 kg body weight) of choline and phosphatidylcholine have been used on humans. High doses of choline have been associated with "fishy" body odor, vomiting, salivation, sweating, and gastrointestinal distress.[157] These side effects are probably dose-dependent, and all but the fishy body odor can be prevented by prior administration of a muscarinic receptor blocker such as methscopolamine.[158] Rarely, humans have become depressed after ingesting large amounts of choline.[159] Fishy body odor occurs because methylamines are formed from ingested choline by the action of gut bacteria.[64] This prob-

lem does not occur when choline is injected intravenously, or when it is fed to germ-free or antibiotic-treated animals.[65,159a,160–162]

Some dimethylamine is formed from endogenous sources even when the diet is completely devoid of choline.[159a] Methylamine, dimethylamine, and trimethylamine produced from choline could be substrates for the formation of nitrosamines.[64] Nitrosamines have marked carcinogenic activity in a wide variety of animal species.[163] Gastric fluid is a likely site for endogenous biosynthesis of nitrosamine because the precursors of nitrosamines are efficiently delivered to gastric fluid, and nitrosation of dimethylamine is most likely to occur in an acidic medium.[164] Nitrosamine formation has been shown to occur in the stomach of humans and experimental animals.[164a,164b] The formation of nitrosamines is a theoretical risk of choline ingestion; no investigators have tried to measure nitrosamines in body fluids of humans treated with choline or phosphatidylcholine.

Large doses of phosphatidylcholine are also associated with "cholinergic" side effects (sweating, gastrointestinal distress, vomiting, and diarrhea).[157] Again, these side effects are dose-dependent: most humans tolerate 20 g/day of phosphatidylcholine and many experience no problems with 30 g/day. When phosphatidylcholine is consumed as a component of common foods, as much as 35 g/day have been ingested for several days without difficulty.[165]

## SOURCES OF CHOLINE IN THE DIET

Free choline concentration in blood and other tissues depends upon dietary intake of choline[12,29,165] (Fig. 24A–5). In the adult human, serum choline concentration fluctuates between narrow limits when common foods are ingested.[29] Administration of choline chloride (2 g/70 kg body weight) elevates plasma choline concentration three- to fourfold, with peak concentrations being attained three hours post dose and lasting for several hours.[12] Free choline is found in some foods such as liver, oatmeal, soybeans, cauliflower, kale, and cabbage.[70–72] Because phosphatidylcholine is a part of almost all biologic membranes, we consume a great deal of this choline-containing phospholipid as part of our diet.[70–72] Foods such as eggs, liver, soybeans, and peanuts are rich in phosphatidylcholine.[70–72] It is often added to processed foods because it acts as an emulsifying agent or as an antioxidant. Healthy humans in the United States probably ingest about 6 g of phosphatidylcholine/day (100 mg/day of this amount is added to foods during processing).[29] Total choline intake (as free choline and the choline in phosphatidyl-

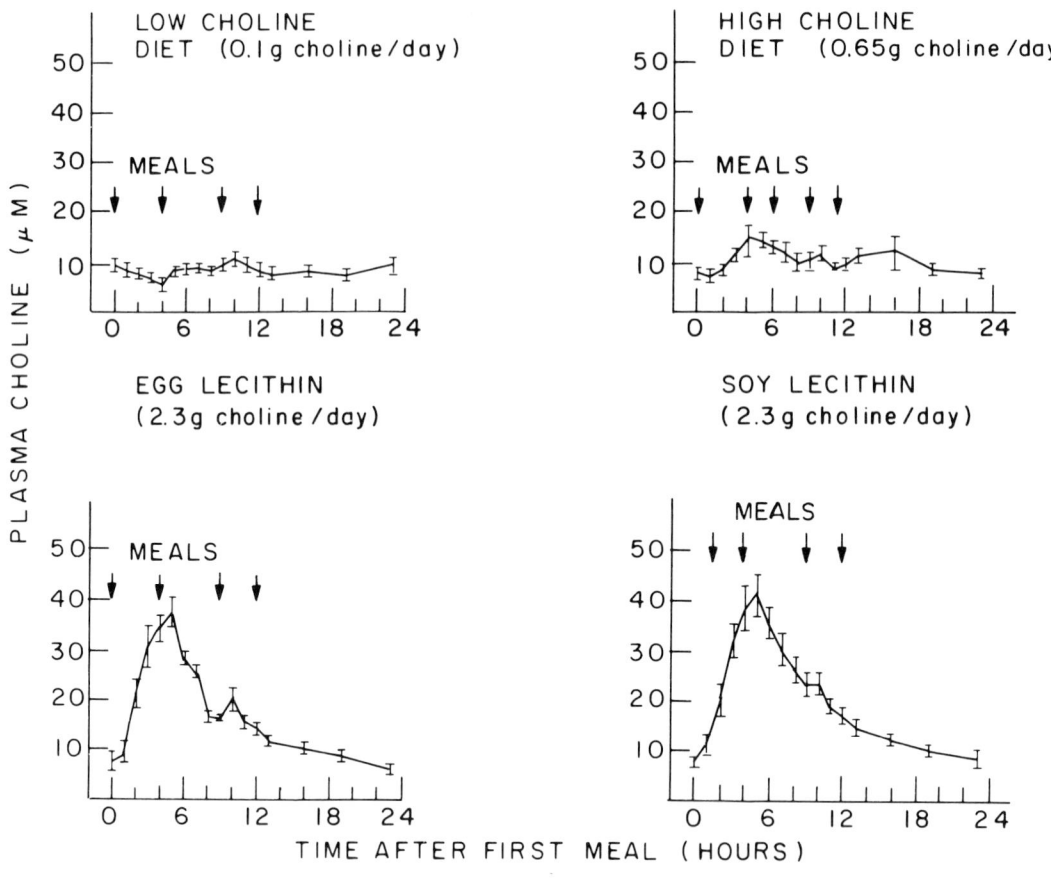

**Fig. 24A–5.** Plasma choline response to ingested choline and lecithin. Six adult human subjects ingested each of four diets (common foods high in choline, common foods low in choline, low-choline diet plus breakfast supplement of 25 g 80% pure egg lecithin, and low-choline diet plus breakfast supplement of 25 g 80% pure soy lecithin). Plasma samples were obtained at regular intervals and assayed for choline. Meal times are indicated by arrows. Data are expressed as mean ± SD. (From Zeisel, S.H., Growdon, J.H., Wurtman, R.J., et al.[29])

choline) amounts to 600 to 1,000 mg/day in the adult.[29] Phosphatidylcholine (called lecithin) is also available to the public as a dietary supplement sold in retail stores. The capsules or granules sold in this manner are usually impure (35% phosphatidylcholine).

## Interrelationships with Other Nutrients

In view of all the disease associated with choline-deficient diets, why are we not able to definitively say that humans must eat some choline-containing compounds in their diet? It is because we are unsure to what extent methionine and other labile methyl donors can spare choline requirements. Methionine or vitamin B[12] deficiency exacerbates the hepatic and renal damage associated with choline deficiency.[93,96,100] Choline is an intermediate in a labile methylgroup cycle. Vitamin B[12] and folic acid catalyze the de novo synthesis of methyl groups from 1-carbon fragments

via formation of 5-methyltetrahydrofolate[55] (see Chap. 21). These methyl groups can be incorporated into choline via the PEMT pathway. Choline can be degraded to betaine, which can donate a methyl group to homocysteine, forming methionine. Methionine can be utilized for protein synthesis, creatine synthesis, or formation of S-adenosylmethionine (SAM). This methyl donor can then be involved in one of several pathways (e.g., the formation of phosphatidylcholine).[55] These transmethylation reactions allow methionine, vitamin B[12], folate, and betaine in the diet to substitute, in part, for choline. This makes it difficult to establish an RDA for choline, as several other dietary constituents must be taken into consideration. It is possible that exogenous choline is only needed during periods of rapid tissue growth (i.e., during infancy), for it is at these times that the sequelae of choline deficiency are the easiest to elicit.

Carnitine is a cofactor for long-chain acetylCoA carnitine transferase; human deficiency syndromes have been identified.[166] Rats fed a choline-deficient diet had reduced levels of carnitine in liver, heart, and skeletal muscle.[167] This finding has been attributed to a methyl-group deficiency, i.e., carnitine is derived from trimethyl-lysine. However, a single injection of choline (but not of methionine, betaine, or sarcosine) was able to raise the concentration of hepatic carnitine in these animals to control values within 1.5 hours.[167] This suggests that choline was capable of facilitating carnitine release from some storage pool, as de novo synthesis of carnitine would have taken much more time. Paradoxically, plasma carnitine was higher in choline-deficient rats.[167]

## EVALUATION OF STATUS OF CHOLINE NUTRITURE

No definitive studies have been done to suggest a clinical approach to the evaluation of choline nutriture in humans theoretically at risk for choline deficiency (e.g., TPN patients). If humans were to become choline-deficient, what biochemical markers could be used to detect this? It appears that we may expect plasma choline concentrations to be lower than in well-fed persons.[12,127a,128] Red blood cells accumulate choline actively, and may reflect changes in the availabilty of choline more accurately than plasma choline levels.[168] Plasma and urinary betaine is formed from choline within the liver. In the rat, exclusion of choline from a carbohydrate-rich diet results in a fivefold decrease in hepatic betaine concentrations.[169] In these studies, the levels of free choline and phosphorylcholine in liver were also significantly decreased (two- to three-fold).[169,170] Choline stores (in the form of phosphatidylcholine) are probably used up to maintain tissue-free choline levels; therefore, it is possible that the phosphatidylcholine content of liver membranes might decrease.

## METHODS FOR CHOLINE ANALYSIS

Sensitive and specific chemical methods for the quantification of choline have superseded bioassay procedures. These include a radioenzymatic method, in which choline is isolated by liquid cation exchange and converted to choline-$^{32}$P in a reaction catalyzed by choline kinase.[13] A gas chromatograph method requires that choline be volatilized by pyrolysis or by chemical methods, and that it can be detected with a flame ionization detector or a mass spectrometer.[14] One method isolates choline using high-pressure liquid chromatography and quantitates it after a post-column reaction, converting the choline to betaine and

then forming hydrogen peroxide.[171] Each of these methods is capable of detecting 100 pmoles or less of choline, and is not subject to major interference from other biologic quaternary amines (such as carnitine). The radioenzymatic method has the advantage of allowing analysis of 100 samples in two days.

## REFERENCES

1. Strecker, A.: Ann. Chem. Pharmacie *123*:353–360, 1862.
2. Baeyer, A.: Ueber Neurin Ann. Chem. Liebigs *140*:306–313, 1866.
3. duVigneaud, V., Cohn, M., Chandler, J.P., et al.: J. Biol. Chem. *140*:625–641, 1941.
4. Kennedy, E.P., Weiss, S.B.: J. Biol. Chem. *222*:193–214, 1956.
5. Hershey, J.M.: Am. J. Physiol. *93*:657–658, 1930.
6. Best, C.H., Huntsman, M.E.: J. Physiol. *75*:405–412, 1932.
7. Best, C.H., Huntsman, M.E., Ridout, J.: Nature *135*:821, 1935.
8. Gabuzda, G.J.: Am. J. Clin. Nutr. *6*:280, 1958.
9. Cohen, E.L., Wurtman, R.J.: Life Sci. *17*:1095–1102, 1975.
10. Cohen, E.L., Wurtman, R.J.: Science *19*:561–562, 1976.
11. Haubrich, D.R., Wang, P.F.L., Clody, D.E., et al.: Life Sci. *17*:975–980, 1975.
12. Haubrich, D.R., Wedeking, P.W., Wang, P.F.L.: Life Sci. *14*:921–929, 1974.
13. Goldberg, A.M., McCaman, R.E.: J. Neurochem. *20*:1–8, 1973.
14. Hanin, I., Skinner, R.F.: Anal. Biochem. *66*:568–583, 1975.
15. Zeisel, S.H., Story, D.L., Wurtman, R.J., et al.: Proc. Natl. Acad. Sci. USA *77*:4417–4419, 1980.
16. Haubrich, D.R., Gerber, N.H.: Biochem. Pharmacol. *30*:2993–3000, 1981.
17. Bernheim, F., Bernheim, M.L.C.: Am. J. Physiol. *104*:438–440, 1933.
18. Bernheim, F., Bernheim, M.L.C.: Am. J. Physiol. *121*:55–60, 1938.
19. Hatefi, Y., Stiggall, D.: Choline dehydrogenase. *In* The Enzymes, Vol. 13. (Boyer, P., Ed.) New York, Academic Press, 1976, pp. 261–263.
20. Mann, P.J., Quastel, J.H.: Biochem. J. *31*:869–878, 1937.
21. Wilken, D.R.: Anal. Biochem. *36*:323–331, 1979.
22. MacKenzie, C.G., Frisell, W.R.: J. Biol. Chem. *232*:417–427, 1958.
23. Haubrich, D.R., Wang, P.F.L., Wedeking, P.W.: J. Pharmacol. Exp. Ther. *193*:246–255, 1975.
24. Fonnum, F.: Brain Res. *62*:497–507, 1973.
25. Wajda, I.J., Manigault, I., Hudick, J.P., et al.: J. Neurochem. *21*:1385–1390, 1973.
26. Rama Sastry, B.V., Olubadewo, J., Harbison, R.D., et al.: Biochem. Pharmacol. *25*:425–431, 1976.
27. White, H.L., Wu, J.C.: J. Neurochem. *20*:297–307, 1973.
28. Cornford, E.M., Braun, L., Oldendorf, W.: J. Neurochem. *30*:299–308, 1978.
29. Zeisel, S.H., Growdon, J.H., Wurtman, R.J., et al.: Neurology *30*:1226–1229, 1980.
30. Illingsworth, D.R., Portman, O.W.: Biochem. J. *130*:557–567, 1972.
31. Wecker, L., Dettbarn, W.: Neurochem. J. *32*:961–967, 1979.

32. Ladinsky, H., Consolo, S., Pugnetti, P.: *In* Nutrition and the Brain, Vol. 5. (Barbeau, A., Growdon, J., Wurtman, R., Eds.) New York, Raven Press, 1979, pp. 95–108.

33. Bierkamper, G.G., Goldberg, A.M.: Brain Res. *202*:234–237, 1980.

34. Loffelholz, K., Lindmar, R., Weide, W.: Relationship between choline and acetylcholine release in the autonomic nervous system. *In* Nutrition and the Brain, Vol. 5. (Barbeau, A., Growdon, J., Wurtman, R., Eds.) New York, Raven Press, 1979, pp. 233–241.

35. Trommer, B.A., Schmidt, D.E., Wecker, L.: J. Neurochem. *39*:1704–1709, 1982.

36. Wecker, L.: Abstract, Conference on Dynamics of Cholinergic Function, West Virginia, 1983.

37. Orlando, P., Arienti, G., Cerrito, F., et al.: Neurochem. Res. *2*:191–201, 1977.

38. Salerno D.M., Beeler, D.A.: Biochim. Biophys. Acta *326*:325–338, 1973.

39. Porcellati, G., Arienti, G., Pirotta, M., et al.: J. Neurochem. *18*:1395–1417, 1971.

40. Brophy, P., Choy, P., Toone, J., et al.: Eur. J. Biochem. *78*:491–496, 1977.

41. Sundler, R., Arvidson, G., Akesson, B.: Biochim. Biophys. Acta *280*:559–568, 1972.

42. Haubrich, D.R.: J. Neurochem. *21*:315–328, 1973.

43. McCaman, R.E.: J. Biol. Chem. *237*:672–676, 1962.

44. Farrell, P.M., Epstein, M.F. Fleischman, A.R., et al.: Biol. Neonate *29*:238–246, 1976.

45. Bjornstad, P., Bremer, J.: J. Lipid Res. *7*:38–45, 1966.

46. Bremer, J., Figard, P., Greenberg, D.: Biochim. Biophys. Acta *43*:477–488, 1960.

47. Bremer, J., Greenberg, D.: Biochim. Biophys. Acta *46*:205–216, 1961.

48. Linblad, L., Schersten, T.: Scand. J. Gastroenterol. *11*:587–591, 1976.

49. Blusztajn, J.K., Zeisel, S.H., Wurtman, R.J.: Brain Res. *179*:319–327, 1979.

50. Hirata, F., Axelrod, J.: Proc. Natl. Acad. Sci. USA *75*:2348–2352, 1978.

51. Hirata, F., Viveros, O.H., Dilberto, E.J., et al.: Proc. Natl. Acad. Sci. USA *75*:1718–1721, 1978.

52. Higgins, J.A.: Biochim. Biophys. Acta *640*:1–15, 1981.

53. Crews, F.T., Hirata, F., Axelrod, J.: Neurochem. Res. *5*:983–991, 1980.

54. Rothman, J.E., Kennedy, E.P.: Proc. Natl. Acad. Sci. USA *74*:1821–1825, 1977.

54a. Blusztajn, J.K., Wurtman, R.J.: Nature (London) *290*:417–418, 1981.

54b. Mudd, H.S., Ebert, M.H., Scriver, C.R.: Metabolism *29*:707–720, 1980.

55. Blusztajn, J.K., Zeisel, S.H., Wurtman, R.J.: Biochem. J. *232*:505–511, 1985.

56. Sundler, R., Akesson, B.: J. Biol. Chem. *250*:3359–3367, 1975.

57. Fallon, H.J., Gertman, P.M., Kemp, E.L.: Biochim. Biophys. Acta *187*:94–104, 1969.

58. Hoffman, D.R., Uthus, E.O., Cornatzer, W.E.: Lipids *15*:439–446, 1980.

59. Uthus, E.O., Skurdal, D.H., Cornatzer, W.E.: Lipids *11*:641–644, 1976.

60. Hirata, F., Strittmatter, W.J., Axelrod, J.: Proc. Natl. Acad. Sci. USA *76*:368–372, 1979.

61. Strittmatter, W.J., Hirata, F., Axelrod, J., et al.: Nature *282*:857–859, 1979.

62. Hirata, F., Axelrod, J.: Nature *275*:219–220, 1978.

63. Blusztajn, J.K., Wurtman, R.J.: Nature *290*:417–418, 1981.

64. Zeisel, S.H., Wishnok, J., Blusztajn, J.K.: J. Pharmacol. Exp. Ther. *225*:320–324, 1983.

65. De La Huerga, J., Popper, H.: J. Clin. Invest. *31*:598–603, 1952.

66. Flower, R.J., Pollitt, R.J., Sanford, P.A., et al.: J. Physiol. *226*:473–489, 1972.

67. Sheard, N.F.S., Zeisel, S.H.: Pediatr. Res. *20*:768–772, 1986.

68. Kuczler, F.J., Nahrwold, D.L., Rose, R.C.: Biochim. Biophys. Acta *465*:131–137, 1977.

69. Sanford, P.A., Smyth D.H.: J. Physiol. *215*:769–788, 1971.

70. Engel, R.W.: J. Nutr. *25*:441–446, 1943.

71. Food and Nutrition Board, National Academy of Sciences USA: Comprehensive GRAS survey, usage levels reported for NAS appendix A substances (group 1) used in regular foods. Washington, D.C., 1973.

72. McIntire, M., Schweigert, B.S., Elvehiem, C.A.: J. Nutr. Rev. *28*:219–223, 1944.

73. DeHaas, G.H., Postema, N.M., Nieuwenhuizen, W., et al.: Biochim. Biophys. Acta *159*:103–117, 1968.

74. DeHaas, G.H., Postema, N.M., Nieuwenhuizen, W., et al.: Biochim. Biophys. Acta *159*:118–129, 1968.

75. Fox, J.M., Betzing, H., Lekim, D.: Pharmacokinetics of orally ingested phosphatidylcholine. *In* Nutrition and the Brain, Vol. 5. (Barbeau, A., Growdon, J., Wurtman, R., Eds.). New York, Raven Press, 1979.

76. Houtsmuller, U.M.T.: Metabolic fate of dietary lecithin. *In* Nutrition and the Brain, Vol. 5. (Barbeau, A., Growdon, J., Wurtman, R., Eds.). New York, Raven Press, 1979, pp. 83–93.

77. Lekim, D., Betzing, H.: Hoppe Seylers Z. Physiol. Chem. *357*:1321–1331, 1976.

78. Parthasarathy, S., Subbaiah, P.V., Ganguly, J.: Biochem. J. *140*:503–508, 1974.

79. Subbaiah, P.V., Ganguly, J.: Biochem. J. *118*:233–239, 1970.

80. Subbaiah, P.V., Ganguly, J.: Indian. J. Biochem. Biophys. *8*:197–203, 1971.

81. McFarlane, M.G., Petterson, L.M.B., Robison, R.: Biochem. J. *28*:720–724, 1934.

82. Goracci, G., Porcellati, G., Woelk, H.: Adv. Prostaglandin Thromboxane Res. *3*:55–67, 1978.

83. Webster, G.R., Marples, E.A., Thompson, R.H.S.: Biochem. J. *65*:374–377, 1957.

84. Baldwin, J.J., Cornatzer, W.E.: Biochim. Biophys. Acta *176*:193–195, 1969.

85. Hostetler, K.Y., Hall, L.B.: Biochim. Biophys. Res. Commun. *96*:388–393, 1980.

86. Taki, T., Kanfer, J.N.: Methods Enzymol. *71*:746–750, 1981.

87. Wykle, R.L., Schremmer, J.M.: J. Biol. Chem. *249*:1742–1746, 1974.

88. Haubrich, D.R., Wang, P.F.L., Wedeking, P.W.: J. Pharmacol. Exp. Ther. *193*:246–255, 1975.

89. Bligh, J.: J. Physiol. *120*:53–62, 1953.

90. Rennick, B., Acara, M., Glor, M.: Am. J. Physiol. *232*:F443–447, 1977.

91. Rennick, B., Acara, M., Hysert, P., et al.: Kidney Int. *10*:329–335, 1976.

92. Allan, F.N., Bowie, D.J., Macleod, J.J.R., et al.: Br. J. Exp. Pathol. *5*:75–83, 1934.

93. Ketola, H.G., Nesheim, M.C.: J. Nutr. *104*:1484–1486, 1974.

94. Deeb, S.S., Thornton, P.A.: Poult. Sci. *38*:1198–1202, 1959.

95. Fairbanks, B.W., Krider, J.L.: N. Am. Vet. *26*:18–23, 1945.

96. Lombardi, B.: Fed. Proc. *30*:139–142, 1971.

97. Dutra, F.R., McKibben J.M.: J. Lab. Clin. Med. *30*:301–307, 1945.

98. Fouts, P.F.: J. Nutr. *24*:217–224, 1943.

99. Handler, P., Bernheim, F.: Proc. Soc. Exp. Med. Biol. *72*:569–571, 1949.

100. Aoyama, H.J., Yasui, H., Ashida, K.: J. Nutr. *101*:730–734, 1971.

101. Assushi, I., Hellerstein, E.E., Hegsted, D.M.: J. Nutr. *79*:488–492, 1963.

102. Daft, F.S., Sebrell, W.H., Lillie, R.D.: Proc. Soc. Exp. Biol. Med. *48*:288–293, 1941.

102a. Rogers, A., Fox, J., Gottlieb, L.: *In* Frontiers of Science and the Liver. (Burke, P.D., Ed.) New York, Thieme-Stratton, 1981.

103. Olson, R.E., Jablonski, J.R., Edmund, T.: Am. J. Clin. Nutr. *6*:111–118, 1958.

104. Rogers, A.E., Newberne, P.M.: Nutr. Cancer *2*:104–112, 1980.

105. Michael, U.F., Cookson, S.L., Chavez, R., et al.: Proc. Soc. Exp. Biol. Med. *150*:672–676, 1975.

106. Baxter, J.H.: J. Nutr. *34*:333–337, 1947.

107. Best, C.H., Hartroft, W.S.: Fed. Proc. *8*:610–622, 1949.

108. Griffith, W.H., Wade, N.J.: J. Biol. Chem. *131*:567–573, 1939.

109. Patterson, J.M., McHenry, E.W.: J. Biol. Chem. *156*:265, 1944.

110. Chang, C.H., Jensen, L.S.: Poult. Sci. *54*:1718, 1975.

111. Ensminger, M.E., Colby, R.W., Canha, T.J.: Wash. Agr. Exp. Sta. Circ. *134*:1–35, 1951.

112. Jukes, T.H.: J. Biol. Chem. *134*:789–792, 1940.

113. Caniggia, A.: Haematologica *34*:625–627, 1950.

114. Kratzing, C.C., Perry, J.J.: J. Nutr. *101*:1657–1662, 1971.

115. Bartus, R.T., Dean, R.L., Goas, A.J., et al.: Science *209*:301–303, 1980.

116. Poley, J.R.: *In* Textbook of Gastroenterology and Nutrition in Infancy. (Lebenthal, E., Ed.) New York, Raven Press, 1981, pp. 743–763.

117. Kaminski, D.J., et al.: Surgery *88*:93–100, 1980.

117a. Hall, R.I., Ross, L.H., Bozovic, M.G., et al.: J. Parenter. Enteral Nutr. *9*:597–599, 1985.

118. Broviac, J.W., Scribner, B.H.: Gastroenterology *62*:727, 1972.

119. Grant, J.P., et al.: Surg. Gynecol. Obstet. *145*:573, 1977.

120. Lindor, D., et al.: J.A.M.A. *241*:2398, 1979.

121. Sheldon, G.F., et al.: Arch. Surg. *113*:504, 1978.

122. McDonald, A.T.J., et al.: Gastroenterology *64*:885, 1973.

123. Rager, R., Finegold, M.J.: J. Pediat. *86*:264, 1975.

124. Touloukian, R.J., Downing, S.E.: Arch. Surg. *106*:58, 1973.

125. Rodgers, et al.: Amer. J. Surg. *131*:149, 1976.

126. Postuma, R., Trevenen : Pediatr. *63*:110, 1979.

127. Beale, C.J., et al.: Pediatrics *64*:342, 1979.

127a. Sheard, N.F., Tayek, J.A., Bistrian, B.R., et al.: Am. J. Clin. Nutr. *43*:219–224, 1986.

128. Burt, M.E., Hanin, I., Brennan, M.F.: Lancet *2*:638–639, 1980.

128a. Carroll, C., Williams, L.: Nutr. Reports. Internat. *25*:773–782, 1982.

129. Growdon, J.H., Corkin, S., Huff, F.J.: *In* Alzheimer's Disease: Advances in Basic Research and Therapies (Wurtman, R., Corkin, S., Growdon, J., Eds.) Cambridge, Center For Brain Sciences and Metabolism, 1984, pp. 375–389.

130. Davis, K.L., Berger, P.A., Hollister, L.E.: N. Engl. J. Med. *293*:152, 1975.

131. Growdon, J.H., Hirsch, M.J., Wurtman, R.J., et al.: N. Engl. J. Med *297*:524, 1977.

132. Gelenberg, A.J., Doller-Wojick, J.C., Growdon, J.H.: Am. J. Psychiatry *136*:772–776, 1979.

133. Tamminga, C.A., Smith, R.C., Ericksen, S.E., et al.: Am. J. Psychiatry *134*:769–776, 1977.

134. Jackson, I.V., Nuttall, E.A., Ibe, I.O., et al.: Am. J. Psychiatry *136*:1458–1460, 1979.

135. Drachman, D.A.: Neurology *27*:783–790, 1977.

136. Sitaram, N., Weingartner, H., Caine, E.D., et al.: Life Sci. *22*:1555–1560, 1978.

137. Sitaram, N., Weingartner, H., Gillin, J.C.: Science *201*:274–276, 1978.

138. Mervis, R., Meyer, D.R., Wallace, L.J., et al.: Abstract, Conference on Dynamics of Cholinergic Function, West Virginia, 1983.

139. Davies, P., Maloney, A.J.F.: Lancet *2*:1903, 1976.

140. Perry, E.K., Perry, R.H., Blesses, G., et al.: Lancet *1*:189, 1977.

141. Zeisel, S.H., Reinstein, D., Corkin, S., et al.: Nature *293*:187–188, 1981.

142. Fisman, M., Merskey, H., Helmes, E., et al.: Can. J. Psychiatry *26*:426–428, 1981.

143. Janowsky, D.S., El-Yousef, M.K., Davis, J.M., et al.: Lancet *2*:632–635, 1972.

144. Janowsky, D.S., El-Yousef, M.K., Davis, J.M., et al.: Arch. Gen. Psychiatry *28*:542–547, 1973.

145. Cohen, B.M., Miller, A.L., Lipinski, J.F., et al.: Am. J. Psychiatry *137*:242–243, 1980.

146. Jenden, D.J., Jope, R.S., Fraser, S.L.: Commun. Psychopharmacol. *4*:339–344, 1980.

147. Hanin, I., Kopp, U., Spiker, G., et al.: Psychiatry. Res. *3*:345–355, 1980.

148. Jope, R.S., Jenden, D.J., Erlich, B.E.: Proc. Natl. Acad. Sci. USA *77*:6144–6146, 1980.

149. Anton, V.: Rev. Esp. Fisiol. *10*:179–188, 1954.

150. Kapp, J., Mahaley, M.S., Odom, G.L.: J. Neurosurg. *32*:468–472, 1970.

151. Steigmann, F., Firestein, R., De La Huerga, J.: Fed. Proc. *11*:393, 1952.

152. Singh, G.S.: Indian J. Physiol. Pharmacol. *17*:125–131, 1973.

153. Boyd, W.D., Graham-White, J., Blackwood, G., et al.: Lancet *2*:711, 1977.

154. Kratzing, C.C., Perry, J.J.: J. Nutr. *101*:1657–1662, 1971.

155. Hodge, H.C.: Proc. Exp. Biol. Med. *58*:212–215, 1945.

156. Davis, J.E.: Am. J. Physiol. *142*:65–67, 1944.

157. Wood, J.L., Allison, R.G.: Effects of consumption of choline and lecithin on neurologic and cardiovascular systems. Life Sciences Research Office of the Federation of American Societies for Experimental Biology. Technical Report to the Bureau of Foods, Food and Drug Administration, Washington, D.C., 1981, pp. 1–105.

158. Jenden, D.J.: The neurochemical basis of acetylcholine precursor loading as a therapeutic strategy. *In* Brain Acetylcholine and Neuropsychiatric Disease. (Davis, K., Berger, P., Eds.) New York, Plenum Press, 1979, pp. 483–513.

159. Tamminga, C.A., Smith, R.C., Chang, S., et al.: Lancet *2*:905, 1976.

159a. Zeisel, S.H., DaCosta, K-A., Fox, J.G.: Biochem. J *232*:403–408, 1985.

160. Asatoor, A., Simenhoff, M.: Biochim. Biophys. Acta *111*:384–392, 1965.
161. De La Huerga, J., Popper, H., Stiegmann, F.: J. Lab. Clin. Med. *38*:904–920, 1951.
162. Prentiss, P.G., Rosen, H., Brown, N., et al.: Arch. Biochem. Biophys. *94*:424–429, 1961.
163. Lijinsky, W., Epstein, S.S.: Nature *225*:21–23, 1970.
164. Zeisel, S.H., DaCosta, K-A., Edrise, B., et al.: Carcinogenesis *7*:775–778, 1986.
164a.Lane, R.P., Bailey, M.E.: Food Cosmet. Toxicol. *11*:851–854, 1973.
164b.Lintas, C., Clark, A., Fox, J.G., et al.: Carcinogenesis *3*:161–165, 1982.
165. Hirsch, M.J., Growdon, J.H., Wurtman, R.J.: Metabolism *27*:953–960, 1978.
166. Borum, P.: Annu. Rev. Nutr. *3*:233–259, 1983.
167. Carter, A.L., Frenkel, R.: J. Nutr. *108*:1748–1754, 1978.
168. Martin, K.: J. Gen. Physiol. *51*:497, 1968.
169. Arvidson, A.S.P.: Ann. Nutr. Metab. *26*:12, 1982.
170. Barak, A.J., Tuma, D.J.: Lipids *14*:304, 1979.
171. Buchanan, D.N., Fucek, F.R., Domino, E.F.: J. Chromatogr. *181*:329–335, 1980.

# Chapter 24

# "VITAMIN-LIKE" MOLECULES

## (B) CARNITINE

### Harry P. Broquist

Carnitine was discovered as a minor nitrogenous compound in muscle tissue in 1905, and its structure subsequently was shown to be β-hydroxy-γ-trimethyl-ammonium butyrate. It received little further attention until 1952 when Carter el al. established that carnitine was required for growth of the meal worm, *Tennebrio molitor,* thus implying that carnitine had an important physiologic function.[1] What that function might be was suggested by experiments of Fritz and Yue, who showed that carnitine stimulated the oxidation of long chain fatty acids by heart muscle preparations.[2] Ultimately this observation led to a role for carnitine in the intramitochondrial transport of fatty acids, a process essential for subsequent fatty acid oxidation and energy release. In general, animal foods are rich in carnitine in contrast to plant-derived foods. Man obtains carnitine from both dietary sources and via de novo synthesis. The biosynthesis of carnitine from lysine and methionine is now well understood.[3,4] Considerable current nutritional and clinical interest is centered on defining carnitine deficiency in man resulting from (1) dietary insufficiency of carnitine, e.g., as in protein malnutrition and/or (2) an impairment in carnitine biosynthesis, e.g., arising from nutritional, pathologic, iatrogenic, or genetic causes. A number of reviews emphasize nutritional,[5,6,7] physiologic,[8,9] and biochemical[3,4] aspects of carnitine.

## CHEMISTRY AND METABOLISM

The structure of free carnitine is shown in Figure 24B–1 and as a functional fatty acyl ester. There are thought to be three separate carnitine fatty acyl transferases: long-chain, middle-chain, and short-chain transferases; examples of respective substrates are: R = palmitate or oleate or acetate (Fig. 24B–1.) The structural relationship of carnitine to choline is evident, since the β and γ carbon atoms of carnitine bear the respective substituents of choline. Yet choline is not a structural precursor of carnitine, though a functional relationship may exist between these two similar compounds.

The biogenesis of carnitine from lysine and methionine is shown in Figure 24B–2; carbon atoms 3, 4, 5, and 6 and the 6-amino group of lysine form the backbone of carnitine, and the N-methyl groups derive from methionine S-methyl. The biosynthetic pathway involves methylation, hydroxylation, an aldolase type cleavage, an oxidation, and a second hydroxylation. Several vitamins and iron are involved in these transformations, which have been discussed in detail elsewhere.[3,4] In animals ε-N-trimethyl-lysine covalently bound in proteins such as actin, myosin, and histones is released via lysosomal hydrolases and then may enter the carnitine pathway (Fig. 24B–2). A unique feature of carnitine enzymology is the presence of two distinct α-ketoglutarate depend-

$$(CH_3)_3 \overset{\oplus}{N}CH_2 \underset{\underset{OH}{|}}{CHCH_2}COO^{\ominus}$$

## CARNITINE

$$(CH_3)_3 \overset{\oplus}{N}CH_2 \underset{\underset{OCOR}{|}}{CHCH_2}COO^{\ominus}$$

## ACYL CARNITINE

**Fig. 24B–1.** Structure of carnitine, β-hydroxy-γ-trimethylammonium butyrate and a generalized structure for an acylcarnitine.

ent dioxygenases, one mitochondrial and the other cytosolic (hydroxylases 2 and 5, respectively, Fig. 24B–2). The enzymes of carnitine biogenesis show species variation in tissue distribution. In general, the liver of all mammals studied carry out reactions 2 to 5 (Fig. 24B–2); these reactions also occur in the kidney of certain higher animals, including the rhesus monkey and man. In man carnitine is largely excreted unchanged in the urine; some minor degradation products, such as methyl choline, have been identified but are likely due to the action of intestinal microflora.

## BIOCHEMICAL AND PHYSICAL FUNCTION AND MODE OF ACTION

**Long-Chain Fatty Acyl Transfer.** At present the carnitine-dependent acyl group transfer system of mitochondria is believed to consist of an "outer" and an "inner" carnitine acyltransferase connected by a carnitine translocase (enzymes 2, 4, 3, respectively, Fig. 24B–3).[9] Palmitic acid, for example, following activation to palmitoyl CoA (enzyme 1, Fig. 24B–3) has only a limited ability to cross the mitochondrial membrane, but its entry is facilitated by enzyme 2 (Fig. 24B–3) catalyzing a transesterification reaction forming palmitoylcarnitine. The latter ester is then thought to cross the inner mitochondrial membrane via translocase (enzyme 3, Fig. 24B–3). A second transesterification reaction then occurs via enzyme 4, regenerating palmitoyl CoA in the mitochondria for subsequent β-oxidation. Carnitine is also released to function repeatedly in this transport system, which constitutes the initial events mandatory for the subsequent oxidation of long-chain fatty acids. Recent studies show reciprocal control for fatty acid oxidation and synthesis in liver.[10] A regulatory site for hepatic acid fatty acid oxidation appears to be "outer" carnitine palmitoyl transferase (enzyme 2, Fig. 24B–3). Fatty acid synthesis depends on the level of malonyl CoA, and as fatty acid needs are met, excess malonyl CoA now inhibits the activity of enzyme 2.

**Medium- and Short-chain Acyl Transfer.** The role of medium- and short-chain carnitine acyltransferases is less clear, since the medium- and short-chain acyl CoA syntheses are localized in the mitochondria.[9] In this regard, a β-oxidation system for fatty acids has been demonstrated in peroxisomes.[11] Interestingly enough, this organelle contains the medium- and short-chain car-

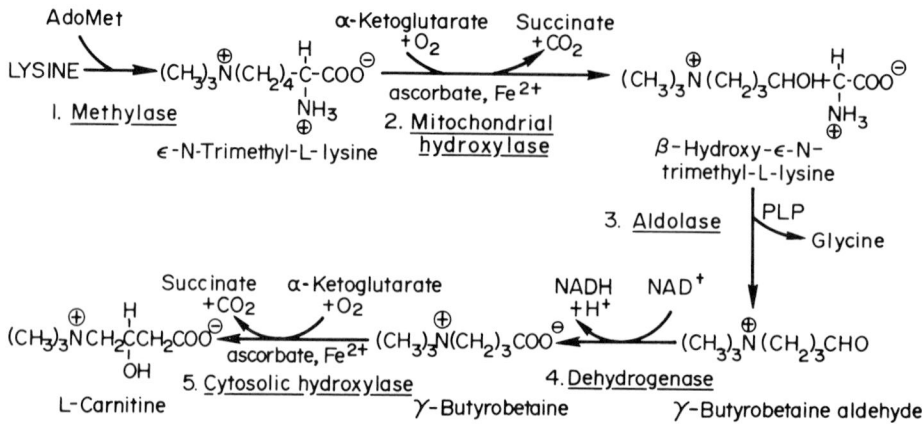

**Fig. 24B–2.** The biogenesis of carnitine from lysine and methionine.

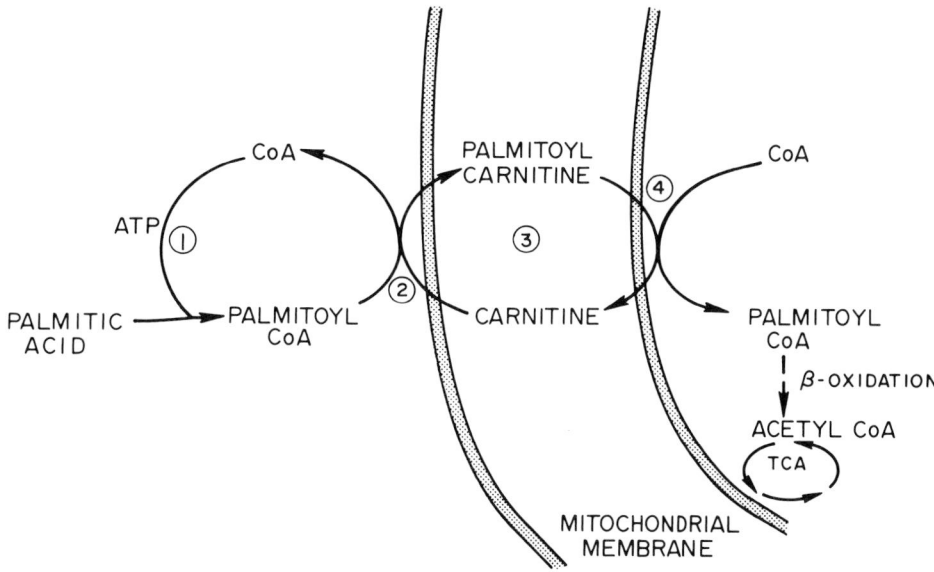

**Fig. 24B–3.** Carnitine and intramitochondrial transport of long-chain fatty acids.

nitine acyltransferases, but not the long-chain carnitine transferase. Acetyl CoA synthase is found both intra- and extramitochondrially, especially in lipogenic tissues; but there is no general agreement on whether carnitine is active in the oxidation of extramitochondrial acetyl CoA. A long-standing view is that carnitine acts mainly as a sink for mitochondrial acetyl CoA allowing a shift of the "acetyl pressure" from the mitochondria to the cytoplasm.[9]

**Branched Chain Amino Acid (BCAA) Metabolism.** BCAA metabolism in muscle initially proceeds as follows:

BCAA→BC β-ketoacid→
$$\text{BC aliphatic acyl CoA } + CO_2$$

Many observations suggest that carnitine then functions in such metabolism by involvement in the intramitochondrial transport of the respective BC aliphatic acyl esters (analogous to the events of Fig. 24B–3) as a prerequisite for subsequent entry into the individual pathways of BCAA metabolism.

## BIOCHEMICAL, PHYSIOLOGIC, AND PATHOLOGIC EFFECTS OF CARNITINE DEFICIENCY AND EXCESS IN LABORATORY ANIMALS AND MAN

Many attempts have been made to induce a nutritional carnitine deficiency in animals by feeding diets limited in nutrients concerned in carnitine biogenesis. In general, weanling rats fed cereal grain diets limiting in lysine exhibited somewhat lower carnitine levels in the heart and skeletal muscle, epididymis, and plasma,[12,13] a significant fatty liver,[14,15] and an impairment in palmitic acid oxidation by heart homogenates.[15] These latter aberrations in lipid metabolism could be significantly counteracted by dietary carnitine. Khairallah and Wolf reported that carnitine gave a growth response in the methionine-deficient rat,[16] but this observation has not been confirmed.[17] It is relevant to point out that lysine-ketoglutarate reductase, the first enzyme of lysine catabolism, is repressed,[18] and homocysteine methyltransferase concerned in methionine synthesis de novo, is activated[19] when lysine and methyl groups are respectively limiting in the diet. Such regulatory mechanisms would act to conserve the penultimate precursors of carnitine and may explain the inability to call forth severe carnitine deficiency in diets low in lysine and methionine.

Scorbutic young male guinea pigs had 50% less carnitine in heart and skeletal muscle than control animals and in vivo hydroxylation of trimethyllysine (reaction 2, Fig. 24B–2) was decreased in scorbutic animals.[20] Possibly muscle carnitine deficiency seen in these scorbutic animals reflects the lassitude and fatigue preceding the emergence of frank scurvy in man. (See Chapter 22, Ascorbic Acid.) When rat liver was perfused in the presence of a vitamin $B_6$ antagonist, 1-amino-D-proline, conversion of protein-bound trimethyllysine to carnitine and related metabolites was markedly depressed and β-hydroxytrimethyllysine accumulated concomitantly (reaction 3, Fig. 24B–2).[21]

Taken together, these animal experiments indicate how generalized malnutrition could significantly retard carnitine biosynthesis as a consequence of limiting dietary amino acid precursors and/or cofactors (vitamins) required for the transformations shown in Figure 24B–2.

Several studies (Egypt,[22] India,[23] and Thailand[24]) have shown significantly lowered blood levels of carnitine in patients suffering from severe protein malnutrition. To what degree such depressed carnitine levels have significant clinical implications needs further study. In the newborn a switch from carbohydrate to fatty acid oxidation for energy takes place, and carnitine palmitoyltransferase activity increases immediately after birth. Infants fed soybean formulas (which contain no detectable carnitine[25]) had plasma carnitine levels lower than breast-fed, or milk-based-formula-fed infants. Borum has summarized several lines of evidence indicating that carnitine may be an essential nutrient for the newborn.[26] Fatty acid oxidation is a major source of energy for cardiac tissue and would be expected to be seriously affected by a carnitine deficiency. The relation of carnitine to aspects of cardiac disease and liver disease in man are active areas of clinical nutrition investigation (see 27 and 6 for discussion and references).

The β-carbon atom of carnitine (Fig. 24B–1) is asymmetric. Many differences in biologic activity have been shown between L and D carnitine, the natural and unnatural forms, respectively. Recent clinical evidence indicates that the L isomer and not the DL racemic mixture should be administered to humans.[28,29]

## CLINICAL SITUATIONS LIKELY TO INDUCE CARNITINE DEFICIENCY

The most obvious examples of carnitine deficiency described to date in man arise from inborn errors of metabolism resulting in lipid storage myopathies associated with muscle fatigue and low carnitine content of the skeletal muscle.[6] Some 50 cases have now been described; these have been partially summarized in Table IV of reference 5. The response to treatment with supplemental carnitine in these instances has been variable; however, this might be anticipated if the genetic lesion has resulted, for example, in (1) defective intestinal absorption of carnitine, (2) alterations in cellular mechanisms for carnitine transport, (3) abnormal renal handling of carnitine, or (4) excessive degradation of carnitine.[29a] The severity of the disease varies and can be fatal.

A carnitine deficiency may also advertently be of iatrogenic origin. For example, patients maintained for long periods on enteral or parenteral solutions lacking carnitine also exhibit lower plasma carnitine levels and may be candidates for carnitine deficiency (see Borum's article[6] and its references). In kidney disease also a sharp decline in serum carnitine has been observed during hemodialysis.[30] A study of carnitine nutriture in cirrhosis revealed that 20 of 60 cirrhotic patients had low serum and urinary levels of carnitine.[31] They exhibited severe hepatocellular disease and advanced protein calorie undernutrition. Their intakes of preformed carnitine and of lysine and methionine were only 30% of the intakes of normal individuals. It is difficult to know to what degree a "lower than normal" serum or tissue carnitine level signals carnitine deficiency and pending pathologic consequences. In this regard it might again be noted that in the studies mentioned earlier of low serum carnitine levels in kwashiorkor[23] and schistosomiasis[22] that such diseases are accompanied by severe disturbances in lipid metabolism. The study of Rudman et al. with cirrhotic patients indicated an association between low serum carnitine levels and severe fatty liver.[31] Primary muscle carnitine deficiency has as one of its major clinical features variable excesses of lipid in the skeletal muscle fibers.[31a] It is attractive to view these examples in terms of cause and affect.

It can be appreciated then from the foregoing how a carnitine deficiency could arise insidiously in man by a confounding of (1) malnutrition limiting intake of dietary carnitine, carnitine precursors, and/or cofactors concerned in carnitine biogenesis, coupled with (2) a pathologic state that could impair, for example, protein synthesis, thus concomitantly limiting formation of carnitine biosynthetic and functional enzymes.

## DIETARY CONSIDERATIONS

**Food Sources.** Data on the carnitine content of foodstuffs are limited, but information on some foodstuffs has been tabulated by Mitchell.[7] Considering these data together with an analysis of several hundred foodstuffs in ready-to-eat form that have been analyzed by Borum,[32] it is clear that meat and dairy products are the major sources of carnitine in the diet, whereas cereals, fruit, and vegetables frequently contain little if any carnitine. For example, one meat serving per day may furnish 50 mg of carnitine, 1 g lysine, and ½ g methionine. On the other hand, cereal grains such as wheat, oats, corn, and rice, consumed by much of the world's population as the major source of protein, are not only lacking in carnitine, but may be low in its amino acid precursors, lysine and methionine, as well. Hence, the chance for a dietary carnitine deficiency is much greater in poplations where little meat and dairy products are consumed, and herein lies the relevancy of human nutritional studies alluded to earlier.[22–24] Borum determined the carnitine content of 14 different United States hospital diets and calculated the carnitine intake from a large number of patients consuming the test diets as varying between 2 to 100 mg carnitine per day, although certain intakes reached 300 mg.[32] It is not known if carnitine biosynthesis is repressed in individuals consuming diets high in carnitine, although in *Neurospora crassa* 33933 (lys⁻), which can synthesize carnitine from lysine, both carnitine and trimethyllysine repress the synthesis of carnitine.[32a]

Carnitine of dietary origin and/or arising from de novo biosynthesis in the tissues (principally liver and kidney) is transported via the blood to the relevant tissues (e.g., muscle and heart) where it carries out its function(s). The epididymis has the highest concentration of carnitine found in any tissue in the adult animal[33] and may imply it has a role in reproduction. Most tissues have a carnitine concentration >10-fold higher than that of the blood plasma implying active uptake mechanisms. A number of studies have appeared on the uptake and exchange of carnitine in different tissues (see Bremer[9] for discussion and references). Cantrell and Borum have extracted a carnitine-binding protein from heart with properties agreeing closely with the carnitine-uptake characteristics of the heart.[34]

**Requirements.** It might be stated somewhat facetiously that carnitine is an essential biocatalyst in search of a requirement. Nutritionists have not seen the need, in the classic sense, to consider a dietary requirement in man for carnitine. It should be clear, from the foregoing, however, that varying degrees of carnitine deficiency, as indicated, for example, by decreased tissue or blood levels of carnitine, can be induced via consumption of diets limiting in carnitine and nutrients concerned in its biogenesis, and/or clinical situations that impact on carnitine biogenesis or function. As Borum concludes in her review: "Carnitine nutriture can no longer be ignored."[6]

## EVALUATION OF NUTRIENT STATUS

Present methods for the determination of carnitine are based on the carnitine acetyltransferase (CAT) reaction:

$$\text{L-carnitine + acetyl CoA} \xrightarrow{\text{CAT}} \text{acetyl-L-carnitine + CoASH}$$

In a spectrophotometric method carnitine extracts are incubated with freshly prepared acetyl CoA and CAT (a stable, commercially available enzyme preparation).[35] The carnitine-dependent appearance of CoASH is determined spectrophotometrically with Ellman's reagent, dithiobisnitrobenzoic acid. In a radioisotope assay, which is at least 10 times as sensitive,[36] [1-¹⁴C] acetyl CoA is employed; radioactive acetylcarnitine formed is separated from residual [1-¹⁴C] acetyl CoA by cation exchange filtration and radioactivity is counted. In these methods a mild alkaline hydrolysis is employed such that free carnitine is measured; if acyl carnitine forms are to be measured, more selective procedures must be followed. Recent developments in methodology for carnitine assays have been reviewed.[37]

## REFERENCES

1. Carter, H.E., Bhattacharyya, P.K., Weidman, K.R., et al.: Arch. Biochem. Biophys. *38*:405–416, 1952.
2. Fritz, I.B., Yue, K.T.N.: J. Lipid Res. *4*:279–288, 1963.
3. Frenkel, R.A., McGarry, J.D.: Carnitine Biosynthesis, Metabolism, and Functions. New York, Academic Press, 1980.
4. Broquist, H.P.: Fed. Proc. *41*:2840–2842, 1982.
5. Broquist, H.P., Borum, P.R.: Adv. Nutr. Res. *4*:181–204, 1982.
6. Borum, P.R.: Ann. Rev. Nutr. *3*:233–259, 1983.
7. Mitchell, M.E.: Am. J. Clin. Nutr. *31*:293–306, 1978.
8. Mitchell, M.E.: Am. J. Clin. Nutr. *31*:481–491, 1978.
9. Bremer, J.: Physiol. Rev. *63*:1420–1480, 1983.
10. McGarry, J.D., Foster, D.W.: J. Biol. Chem. *254*:8163–8168, 1979.
11. Lazarow, P.B.: J. Biol. Chem. *253*:1522–1528, 1978.
12. Tanpaichitr, V., Broquist, H.P.: J. Nutr. *103*:80–87, 1973.
13. Borum, P.R., Broquist, H.P.: J. Nutr. *107*:1209–1214, 1977.
14. Tanpaichitr, V., Zaklama, M.S., Broquist, H.P.: J. Nutr. *106*:111–117, 1976.
15. Khan, L., Bamji, M.S.: J. Nutr. *109*:24–31, 1979.
16. Khairallah, E.A., Wolf, G.: J. Nutr. *87*:469–476, 1965.
17. Felice, J., Mason, P., Broquist, H.P.: Unpublished observations.
18. Chu, S.W., Hegsted, D.M.: J. Nutr. *106*:1089–1096, 1976.
19. Mudd, S.H., Poole, J.R.: Metabolism *24*:721–734, 1975.
20. Nelson, P.J., Pruitt, R.E., Henderson, L.L., et al.: Biochim. Biophys. Acta *672*:123–127, 1981.
21. Dunn, W.A., Aronson, N.N. Jr., England, S.: J. Biol. Chem. *257*:7948–7951, 1982.
22. Mikhail, M.M., Mansour, M.M.: Clin. Chim. Acta *71*:207–214, 1976.
23. Khan, L., Bamji, M.S.: Clin. Chim. Acta *75*:163–166, 1977.
24. Tanpaichitr, V., Lerdvuthisopon, N., Dhanamitta, S., et al.: Am. J. Clin. Nutr. *33*:876–880, 1980.
25. Borum, P.R., York, C., Broquist, H.P.: Am. J. Clin. Nutr. *32*:2272–2276, 1979.
26. Borum, P.R.: Nutr. Rev. *39*:385–390, 1981.
27. Mitchell, M.E.: Am. J. Clin. Nutr. *31*:645–659, 1978.
28. Bazzato, G., Mezzina, C., Ciman, M., et al.: Lancet *1*:1041–1042, 1979.
29. DeGrandis, D., Mezzina, C., Fiaschi, A., et al.: J. Neurol. Sci. *46*:365–371, 1980.
29a.Rebouche, C.J., Engel, A.G.: Mayo Clin. Proc. *58*:533–540, 1983.

30. Bartel, L.L., Hussey, J.L., Shrago, F.: Am. J. Clin. Nutr. *34*:1314–1320, 1981.
31. Rudman, D., Sewell, C.W., Ansley, J.D.: J. Clin. Invest. *60*:716–723, 1977.
31a.Engel, A.G., Angelini, C.: Science *179*:899–902, 1973.
32. Borum, P.R.: Unpublished observations.
32a.Rebouche, E.J., Broquist, H.P.: J. Bacteriol. *126*:1207–1214, 1976.
33. Casillas, E.R.: Biochim. Biophys. Acta *280*:545–551, 1972.
34. Cantrell, C.R., Borum, P.R.: J. Biol. Chem. *257*:10599–10604, 1982.

35. Marquis, N.R., Fritz, I.B.: J. Lipid Res. *5*:184–187, 1964.
36. Cederblad, G., Lindstedt, S.: Clin. Chim. Acta *37*:235–243, 1972.
37. Anonymous: Nutrit. Rev. *38*:338–340, 1980.

## SELECTED READINGS

Broquist, H.P., Borum, P.R.: Carnitine Biosynthesis: Nutritional Implications in Advances in Nutritional Research, Vol. 4 (Draper, H.H., Ed.). New York. Plenum Press, 1982.
Bremer, J.: Carnitine Metabolism and Functions: Physiol. Rev. *63*:1420–1480, 1983.

*Chapter* **24**

# "VITAMIN-LIKE" MOLECULES

## (C) INOSITOL

### Harry P. Broquist

Inositol has long been recognized as a constituent of animal tissue and of higher and lower plant tissues, but its status as an essential nutrient has been somewhat of an enigma. Nutritionists first became interested in inositol following the pioneer work of Woolley describing a dietary inositol deficiency in mice, characterized by decreased rate of growth and occurrence of alopecia.[1] Doubt soon arose, however, over the status of inositol as a dietary essential, and it gradually became apparent that an inositol deficiency may be manifested more readily in some animal species than others, depending upon a variety of circumstances including the purity of the diet, biosynthesis by intestinal flora, endogenous synthesis by various tissues, and by physiologic or metabolic stress. Exogenous inositol is required as an essential growth factor for some 18 normal and malignant human cell lines in tissue culture,[2] attesting to a vital metabolic role of inositol at the cellular levels.

A major impetus was the discovery of Gavin and McHenry that dietary inositol, like choline, is a lipotropic agent, which reduces the amount of fat in the liver of rats fed under certain dietary conditions.[3] This observation has received renewed research emphasis, particularly in relation to the effect of various dietary fats on the lipotropic function of inositol. That inositol, like choline, also exists in cells as a phosphatide points to a metabolic role for it in membrane and lipoprotein function. Current research indicates that inositol lipids appear to be intimately involved in $Ca^{++}$-mediated control of cell functions by hormones and other ligands, in cell proliferation, and in the attachment of enzymes to the plasma membrane.[4]

Several exceedingly useful reviews give in-depth coverage of research on inositol,[4–7] as well as a complete text, *Cyclitols and Phosphoinositides.*[8]

## CHEMISTRY

Of the nine possible isomers of hexahydrocyclohexane, *myo*-inositol is the sole isomer of nutritional and metabolic consequence. Its structure and stereochemical relationship to D-glucose is shown in Figure 24C–1. Such free inositol, phosphates of inositol, and inositol phospholipid(s) are the principal forms of inositol in nature. Phosphatidylinositol is shown in a general form with the acyl groups in the glyceride unspecified and consists of a hydrophylic head group, *myo*-inositol, linked via a phosphodiester to diacylglycerol, the hydrophobic moiety of the phosphatide. In animal cells about 10% or less of the membrane phospholipids are composed of phosphatidylinositol. The phosphatide may be further phosphorylated (Fig. 24C–1) via ATP-dependent ki-

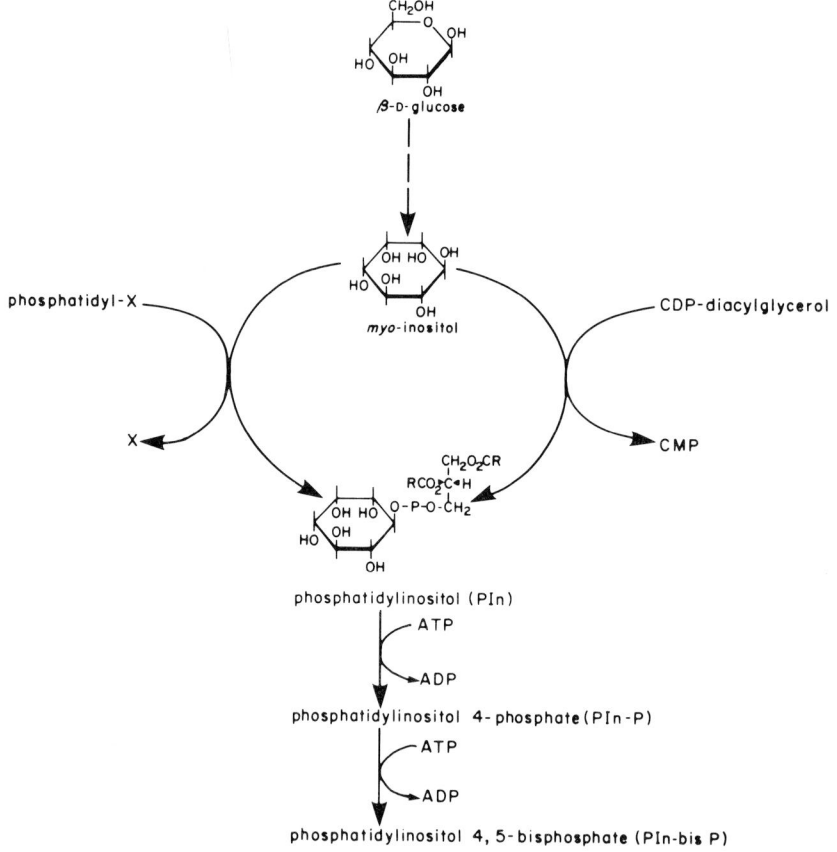

**Fig. 24C–1.** Inositol and phosphatidylinositol: structures and biosynthesis. The predominant route of phosphatidylinositol (1,2-diacyl-sn-glycero-3-phosphoryl-inositol, PIn) biosynthesis is via a transferase reaction of myo-inositol with the liponucleotide, cytidine diphosphodiacylglycerol (CDP-diacylglycerol), giving PIn and cytidine monophosphate (CMP). Some free inositol may also react in an exchange reaction with the base moiety (expressed in the general form, X) of endogenous microsomal phospholipid to give PIn and X.

nases, and such phosphates (PIn-P, and PIn-bis P) may also be degraded via specific monophosphomonoesterases or phosphodiesterases. The acyl groups in inositol phosphatide(s) vary as a consequence of enzymic transformations involving deacylation of the phosphatide and reacylation by differing R groups. Stearic and arachidonic acid esterified in the 1 and 2 positions, respectively, of the sn-glycero-3-phosphorylinositol backbone, represent the major fatty acids in the phosphatidylinositol of rat liver and other mammalian tissues.[9]

## BIOLOGIC ACTIVITY

In many instances the underlying requirement of cells for *myo*-inositol resides in its phosphatide(s), but current research indicates that each form of inositol may have distinct, unique biologic activity in a particular species or tissue or physical process. Phytic acid or inositol hexaphosphate, the predominant form of inositol in plants, has long been known to readily bind divalent cations such as $Ca^{++}$, $Zn^{++}$, and $Fe^{++}$, thus decreasing gastrointestinal absorption of these minerals. This, of course, has serious nutritional implications; zinc deficiency in humans, for example, was first recognized in young Iranian men consuming cereal grain diets high in phytate.[10]

## METABOLISM

Free *myo*-inositol arises in animal cells both from dietary sources and from biosynthesis from D-glucose (Fig. 24C–1). The enzymatic biosynthesis of inositol has been studied extensively, and relevant enzymes have been purified, e.g., in rat testis, rat mammary gland *Neurospora*, and yeast. The overall reactions, stemming particularly from work in Eisenberg's laboratory involve an internal cyclization of glucose-6-phosphate yielding inositol-1-phosphate with subsequent hydrolysis to inositol.[11] The absolute requirement for $NAD^+$ but with no net gain of NADH suggests a tightly coupled oxidation reduction mechanism; 5-ketoglucose-6-phosphate and inosose 2,1-phosphate have been suggested as reaction intermediates.[12]

**glucose-6-phosphate**
  NAD$^+$ ↓ L-*myo*-inositol-1-phosphate synthase
**inositol-1-phosphate**
  Mg$^{++}$ ↓ L-*myo*-inositol-1-phosphatase
  **inositol**

The kidney appears to be the principal organ concerned with the turnover of inositol in mammalian systems.[13] Excretion per se appears to be minor; instead inositol is catabolized in the kidney via the glucuronic acid and pentose phosphate pathways to give such products as glucose, glucuronolactone, and ultimately $CO_2$ and water.[13,14]

Of prime importance is the conversion of inositol to its phosphatide(s), a process occurring in all animal organs studied to date. The major route is the CDP pathway (Fig. 24C–1), wherein inositol reacts with CDP-diacylglycerol in the presence of a transferase enzyme to yield phosphatidylinositol.[15] A minor alternate synthesis involves an exchange of free inositol with the base moiety of endogenous phospholipid in a Mn$^{++}$ activated enzyme exchange reaction (X, Fig. 24C–1) to yield phosphatidylinositol.[15]

## BIOCHEMICAL AND PHYSIOLOGIC FUNCTIONS AND MODE OF ACTION

The predominance of free inositol in concentration over the inositol-containing phospholipids in most tissues may imply a cellular function. The high concentration of inositol in the epididymis versus the testis, for example is suggestive of a role in spermatogenesis.[16] Another hypothesis is that inositol may in some manner control the functional state of microtubules, which together with inositol are enriched in nervous and secretory tissues.[17] Several disparate functions for various inositol phosphates are claimed. For example, inositol hexaphosphate can act as an allosteric effector in interacting with human adult hemoglobin to shift the quaternary equilibrium from the R (relaxed) state toward the T (tensed) state.[18]

The predominant physiologically active form of inositol is as the phosphatide, which functions primarily at the membrane level. It is now clear that membrane phosphatidylinositol has a special function in the response of various cells to external stimuli such as certain hormones and neurotransmitters. An impressive list of stimuli that produce enhanced phosphatidylinositol metabolism in appropriate target tissues has been summarized by Michell.[4] Stimuli whose major effects are to produce rapid physiologic responses include muscarinic cholinergic, α-adrenergic, 5-hydroxytryptamine, histamine (H$_1$) receptors, angiotensin, vasopressin, or those that bring about longer-term stimulation of cell proliferation, e.g., phytohaemagglutinins and other mitogens and high serum concentrations. Such events appear to involve degradation of membrane phosphatidylinositol,[4,19] as postulated in Figure 24C–2, and may control cell surface Ca$^{++}$ permeability giving rise to an elevation in intracellular Ca$^{++}$ concentration.[19a] Some evidence for the scheme of Figure 24C–2 was the discovery that Li$^+$ is a potent inhibitor of inositol-1-phosphatase, which permitted a demonstration of the accumulation of inositol-1-phosphate released concomitantly by appropriate receptor activity from phosphatidylinositol in the presence of Li$^+$ (see discussion in Michell[20]).

## BIOCHEMICAL, PHYSIOLOGIC, AND PATHOLOGIC EFFECTS OF DEFICIENCY AND EXCESS IN LABORATORY ANIMALS AND MAN

The most dramatic example of inositol deficiency described to date in experimental animals is in female gerbils.[21,22] Female animals (and castrated males) fed semipurified diets lacking inositol had hypocholesteremia, excessive fat deposition in the intestinal mucosa (lipodystrophy), and eventually dermatitis, weight loss, and death. The intestinal lipodystrophy could be reversed by inositol; saturated fat caused a greater accumulation of intestinal lipid compared to unsaturated fat. A similar interaction between saturated fat and inositol deficiency has been described by Hayashi et al. in the rat,[23] but Anderson and Holub reported that lipid accumulation in inositol-deficient rat livers is independent of dietary fat saturation.[24] The latter group of investigators has developed a nutritionally acceptable diet,[25] which may standardize experimental conditions for studying inositol "syndrome(s)." In this regard it is also apparent that such factors as age of animals and physiologic stress must also be considered. One mechanism suggested for lipid accumulation in the liver during inositol deficiency is that the transport of lipoproteins from liver into plasma is impeded.[26,27] Inositol appears to be relatively nontoxic in normal subjects, but when inositol catabolism is impaired, there may be a problem (see next section).

## CLINICAL SITUATIONS LIKELY TO INDUCE DEFICIENCY

There is growing evidence of altered metabolism of inositol in patients with diabetes mellitus,

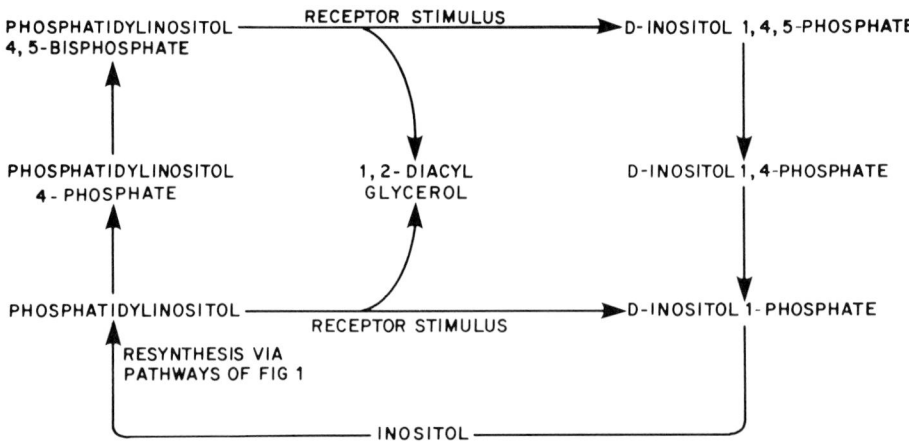

**Fig. 24C–2.**   Postulated mechanism of receptor stimuli and concomitant breakdown of phosphatidylinositol (or the 4,5-bisphosphate) and subsequent reformation of phosphatidylinositol. See Michell[20] for references and discussion.

chronic renal failure, galactosemia, and multiple sclerosis.[5] Diabetics are known to exhibit decreased peripheral motor and sensory nerve conduction velocities with or without evidence of polyneuropathy. In this regard, diabetic rats given streptozotocin show an impaired ability to maintain normal concentrations of free inositol in peripheral nerves that is related to a decreased velocity in motor nerve conduction.[29] Such effects were negated either by insulin or by dietary supplementation with inositol (1%). There is some evidence for an impaired synthesis of inositol phosphatides and of inositol transport in nerve tissue from diabetic rats. It has been hypothesized that the hyperglycemia associated with untreated human diabetes may impair inositol transport,[30] presumably by an unfavorable competition with glucose for a common transport mechanism, thus resulting in a gross intracellular inositol deficiency. Partial support for this view derives from studies of Salway et al., who found an improvement in neurophysiologic measurements in diabetic patients given inositol orally (500 mg twice daily for two weeks).[31]

The catabolism of inositol via the kidney inositol oxygenase system is markedly decreased in experimental diabetes, as evidenced by elevated levels of inositol in the kidney and by an inositoluria, and there is a dramatic elevation of serum inositol in human subjects with chronic renal failure. Such findings raise concerns of potential inositol toxicity. Animal experiments support the possibility that hyperinositolemia may contribute to the pathogenesis of polyneuropathy in subjects with chronic renal failure.

## DIETARY CONSIDERATIONS

**Requirements.** Holub notes that, although the National Research Council does not list inositol

as a required nutrient for the rat, animal nutritionists found it expedient in 71% of 184 studies reported in the *Journal of Nutrition* to include inositol in their experimental diets.[5] The female gerbil has an absolute requirement for inositol (70 to 120 mg/kg diet) under conditions described by Hegsted et al.[21] There is no demonstrable requirement for inositol in man, though various pathologic states and consumption of refined diets (e.g., parenteral solutions presently devoid of inositol) could reveal a partial requirement for inositol. In this regard, it is of interest that the Committee on Nutrition of the American Academy of Pediatrics has recommended that inositol be included in infant formulas at or above the amounts found in milk-based formulas.[32]

**Food Sources.** Inositol is present mainly as phytic acid in plant tissues and is hydrolyzed in varying degree in the gut of monogastric animals by the enzyme phytase. In animal tissues it is present principally in the free form and as the phosphatide. There is much analytic data on the content of inositol and related forms in food and plant and animal tissues.[7,33] It has been estimated that a six-month-old breast-fed infant weighing 7.5 kg may ingest 130 mg inositol per day. An adult eating a mixed North American diet may consume approximately a gram of inositol per day. Based on experiments with segments of hamster small intestine,[34] inositol appears to be absorbed by an active transport process requiring energy and $Na^+$. The absorption of phosphatidylinositol might parallel that for lecithin, although this is not known with certainty.

## EVALUATION OF NUTRIENT STATUS

Detailed methods for the extraction of the inositol lipids and their separation by appropriate chromatographic methods are available.[7] Inositol levels in biologic materials can be measured by microbiologic, titrimetric, enzymatic, and various chromatographic procedures.[35] A yeast microbiologic cup-plate assay[36] and a qualitative paper chromatographic assay method[35] describe simple, economical procedures adaptable for the assay of many samples, though with limited sensitivity. A more elegant procedure for the determination of polyols in general, based on acetylation of the polyols and subsequent analysis by gas liquid chromatography, has been described[37] and appears to have useful clinical application.

## REFERENCES

1. Woolley, D.W.: J. Biol. Chem. *139*:29–34, 1941.
2. Eagle, H., Oyama, V.I., Levy, M., et al.: J. Biol. Chem. *226*:191–205, 1057.
3. Gavin, G., McHenry, E.W.: J. Biol. Chem. *139*:485, 1941.
*4. Michell, R.H.: Trends Biol. Sci. *4*:128–131, 1979.
*5. Holub, B.J.: Adv. Nutr. Res. *4*:107–141, 1982.
*6. Kuksis, A., Mookerjea, S.: Nutr. Rev. *36*:233–238, 1978.
*7. Hawthorne, J.N., White, D.A.: Vitam. Horm. *33*:529–573, 1975.
*8. Wells, W., Eisenberg, F., Jr.: Cyclitols and Phosphoinositides. New York, Academic Press, 1978.
9. Holub, B.J.: Studies on the metabolic heterogeneity of different molecular species of phosphatidylinositols. *In* Cyclitols and Phosphoinositides (Wells, W., Eisenberg, F., Jr., Eds.), New York, Academic Press, 1978.
10. Prasad, A.S.: Fed. Proc. *26*:172–185, 1967.
11. Eisenberg, F., Jr.: J. Biol. Chem. *242*:1375–1382, 1967.
12. Chen, C.H., Eisenberg, F., Jr.: J. Biol. Chem. *250*:2963–2967, 1975.
13. Howard, C.F., Jr., Anderson, L.: Arch. Biochem. Biophys. *118*:332–339, 1967.
14. Lewin, L.M., Yannai, Y., Sulimovici, S., et al.: Biochem. J. *156*:375–380, 1976.
15. Paulus, H., Kennedy, E.P.: J. Biol. Chem. *235*:1103–1311, 1960.
16. Morris, R.N., Collins, A.C.: J. Reprod. Fertil. *27*:201–210, 1971.
17. Kirazov, E.P., Lagnado, J.R.: FEBS Lett. *81*:173–178, 1977.
18. Neya, S., Morishima, I.: J. Biol. Chem. *256*:793–798, 1981.
19. Hokin-Neaverson, M., Sadeghian, K., Harris, D.W., Merrin, J.S.: The mechanism of stimulated phosphatidylinositol breakdown. *In* Cyclitols and Phosphoinositides (W.W. Wells, Eisenberg, F., Jr., Eds.) New York, Academic Press, 1978.
19a. Holub, B.J.: Ann. Rev. Nutr. *6*, 1986 (in press).
20. Michell, R.H.: Trends Biol. Sci. *7*:387–388, 1982.
21. Hegsted, D.M., Gallagher, A., Hanford, H.: J. Nutr. *104*:588–592, 1974.
22. Hoover, G.A., Nicolosi, R.J., Corey, J.E., et al.: J. Nutr. *108*:1588–1594, 1978.
23. Hayashi, E., Maeda, T., Tomita, T.: Biochim. Biophys. Acta *360*:134–145, 1974.
24. Anderson, D.B., Holub, B.J.: J. Nutr. *106*:529–536, 1976.
25. Anderson, D.B., Holub, B.J.: J. Nutr. *110*:488–495, 1980.
26. Hasan, S.H., Kotaki, A., Yagi, K.: J. Vitaminol. *16*:144–148, 1970.
27. Hasan, S.H., Nakagawa, Y., Nishigaki, I., et al.: J. Vitaminol. *17*:159–162, 1971.
28. Daughaday, W.H., Larner, J., Hartnett, C.: J. Biol. Chem. *212*:869–875, 1955.
29. Greene, D.A., De Jesus, P.V., Winegrad, A.I.: J. Clin. Invest. *55*:1326–1336, 1975.
30. Clements, R.S., Jr., Reynertson, R.: Diabetes *26*:215–221, 1977.
31. Salway, J.G., Finnegan, J.A., Barnett, D., et al.: Lancet *2*:1282–1284, 1978.
32. American Academy of Pediatrics Committee on Nutrition: Pediatrics, *57*:278–285, 1976.
33. Sebrell, W.H., Jr., Harris, R.S.: The Vitamins, Vol. III. New York, Academic Press, 1967.
34. Caspary, W.F., Crane, R.K.: Biochem. Biophys. Acta *203*:308–316, 1970.
35. Lewin, L.M., Melmed, S., Bank, H.: Clin. Chim. Acta *54*:377–379, 1974.
36. Yamada, M., Tsukahara, T.: J. Nutr. Sci. Vitaminol. (Tokyo) *19*:205–214, 1973.
37. Pitkanen, E.: Clin. Chim. Acta *38*:221–230, 1972.

## SELECTED READING

Holub, B.J.: Adv. Nutr. Res. *4*:107–141, 1982.

*Review article.

Although taurine has been recognized as a component of living organisms since 1827[1] and has long been considered an end product of sulfur amino acid metabolism, its potential importance in biologic functions other than bile acid conjugation has only recently been emphasized.[2-4] Originally isolated from ox bile, from which it acquired its name, taurine has since attained nutrient status in its own right and is currently discussed as a possible essential nutrient for human infants, largely from evidence obtained in kittens and infant monkeys that demonstrated the essentiality of taurine for normal retinal function and growth.[4] Because of its unique failure to be incorporated into proteins, coupled with the minimal amount (500 ppm) needed in the diet to assure vision and growth in kittens, it is often referred to as a vitamin-like compound. The focus of current interest has centered on its recent addition to human infant formulas and pending inclusion in solutions for parenteral nutrition.

### CHEMISTRY

Taurine, β-aminoethanesulfonic acid, is unique among the amino acids because of its sulfonic acid group, which replaces the carboxyl group of what would normally be glycine. It takes part in few biochemical reactions and is not incorporated into proteins, but is found instead as the free amino acid in most animal tissues and biologic fluids, often as the mostly highly concentrated free amino acid (e.g., in muscle, platelets, developing CNS).[2] A notable exception to its nonreactivity is its con-

jugation with bile acids and with the powerful oxidant, hypochlorous acid, generated in leukocytes, to form the relatively stable taurchloramine.[5] Although taurine has been described as a component of a peptide, glutaurine, isolated from the thyroid gland, this observation awaits confirmation and more specific elucidation of its physiologic relevance.[6]

Taurine is synthesized from cysteine by certain mammalian cells, but not usually by plant cells, which means that it is essentially absent from the plant kingdom. Its sulfur moiety can be oxidized to sulfate by intestinal bacterial flora, but not by mammalian cells. A colorless compound with a MW of 125, taurine is soluble in water up to 0.84 M solution, but essentially insoluble in ethanol or ether. Since it is a free amino acid without dissociable side groups, it exists in zwitter ion form with a pKa of 1.5 (sulfonic acid group) and pKb of 8.7 (amino group) and is presumably neutral at physiologic pH:

$$\begin{matrix} & O & \\ & | & \\ HO\text{-}S\text{-}CH_2\text{-}CH_2 & \\ & | & | \\ & O & NH_2 \end{matrix}$$

Taurine (β-aminoethanesulfonic acid)

### BIOSYNTHESIS AND METABOLISM

In lower vertebrates and mammals taurine derives from the metabolism of the sulfur amino acids, methionine and cysteine, through decarboxylation of cysteine sulfinic acid to hypotaurine with subsequent oxidation to taurine (Fig. 24D–1). Although other pathways have been suggested, such as the fixation of sulfate with serine to form cysteamine and eventually taurine, little evidence exists that this represents a metabolically significant pathway; and it is generally agreed that enzymatic activity of cysteine sulfinic acid decarboxylase (CSAD) reflects the synthetic capacity of different organs (tissues) for taurine biosynthesis. Whereas the enzymatic involvement of CSAD is well characterized, other enzymes and biochemical conversions, such as hypotaurine to taurine, have not been carefully delineated. Enzymes in the transulfuration pathway to taurine are heavily dependent upon vitamin $B_6$ as a cofactor (cystathione synthase, cystathionase, and CSAD). This pathway has been documented in the liver and brain of many species and is most likely age-dependent, i.e., it may be poorly developed in the preterm and newborn infant, making the synthesis of taurine even more restricted in the neonate.[3]

On the basis of CSAD activity, various tissues from a number of species have been compared for their taurine synthetic capacity (Table 24D–1). It is apparent that humans (and primates in general) represent species with poor synthetic ability, worse even than cats, in contrast to species such as the rat and the dog where hepatic synthesis is extremely high. It is noteworthy that the CNS, including the retina, has moderate taurine synthetic capacity in most species, even while hepatic synthesis varies among species. In the frog chronic light exposure depresses retinal taurine biosynthesis. In terms of available taurine it is not clear that the hepatic taurine pool is readily circulated as a donor pool for other tissues, since bile acids constitute the primary demand for liver taurine. For this reason and because most tissues appear to concentrate taurine against a concentration gradient, low plasma concentration of taurine may not be a good indicator of individual tissue pools and very likely reflects dietary intake most closely.

Taurine is relatively inactive because of its sulfonyl group, the notable exception being the rather stable taurine conjugate of bile acids. Although most species conjugate bile acids with glycine in addition to taurine, all seem to prefer taurine con-

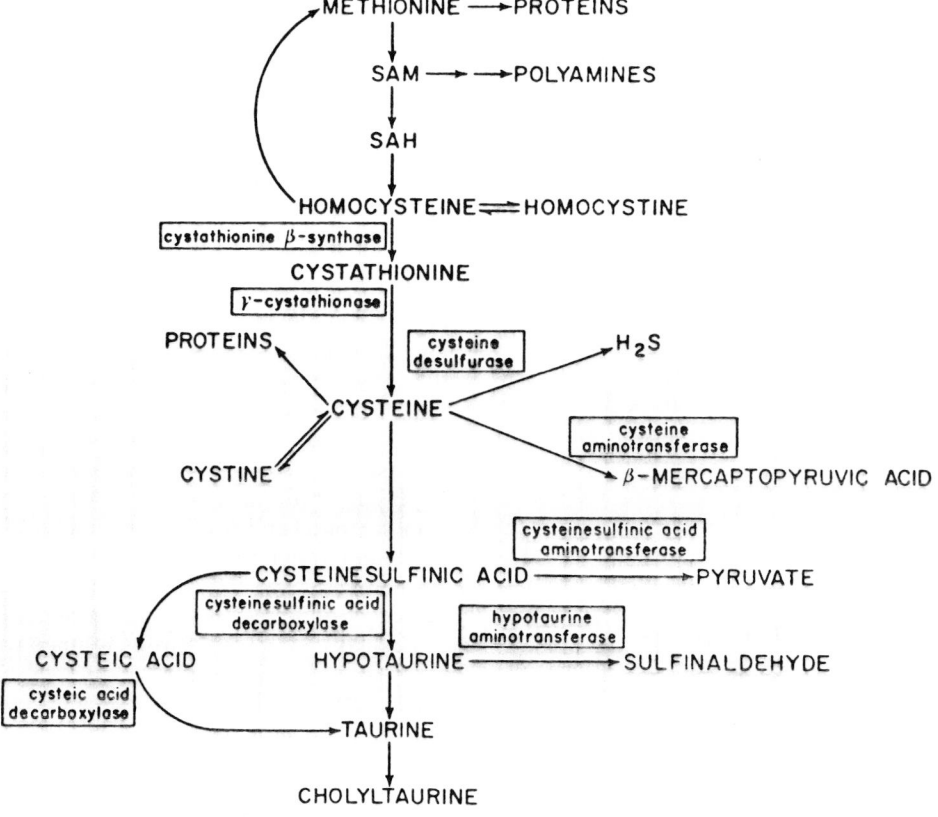

**Fig. 24D–1.** Taurine biosynthesis derives from the transulfuration pathway involving methionine and cysteine. The three key enzymes depicted along this route require vitamin $B_6$ as cofactor.

**Table 24D–1. Cysteinesulfinic Acid Decarboxylase Activity in Liver and Brain of Various Species***

| Species | Liver | | Brain | |
|---|---|---|---|---|
| | Adult | Fetus | Adult | Fetus |
| | mmol $CO_2$ produced/mg protein/hr | | | |
| Man | <1 | <1 | 5 | — |
| Rhesus | 5 | 4 | 5 | trace |
| Rat | 468 | 9 | 63 | 1 |
| Cat | 4 | 7 | 59 | 6 |
| Rabbit | 14 | 16 | 25 | 8 |
| Guinea pig | 3 | 2 | 6 | 4 |

*Adapted from Sturman, J.A., Hayes, K.C.[3]

jugation when supplemented with taurine. Noteworthy is the fact that cats conjugate exclusively with taurine and secrete free bile acids rather than reverting to glycine when hepatic taurine is exhausted. In primates depleted of taurine, chenodeoxycholic acid seems to have preferential access to the remaining taurine, and cholic acid conjugates readily with glycine. This preference depends on the species of primate,[4] suggesting that bile acid conjugation with taurine is more complex than the simple hepatic concentration of this amino acid.

Studies with $S^{35}$-taurine in man have suggested a multicompartmental model for taurine metabolism with a total body pool of 100 to 150 mmol (12 to 18 g).[7] Turnover is best described by two exchangeable pools, a small (2-mmol), rapidly miscible pool. ($T_{1/2}$ = 0.1 hr) and a larger (100-mmol) pool with a slow turnover rate ($T_{1/2}$ = 70 hr).[7] Excretion occurs from the rapidly miscible plasma pool into the urine, resulting in loss of 0.5 to 2.0 mmol/day. Subcompartments of the actively exchangeable pool would include bile acids, the central nervous system and "other" tissues, most of which actively take up taurine against a concentration gradient.

Under normal circumstances plasma taurine ranges from 50 to 220 μmol/L in humans with any excess being readily excreted via the kidney in the urine. Both urine and plasma concentrations are reduced when the combined dietary and synthetic contributions are inadequate.[2]

**Table 24D–2. Biologic Functions That Are Affected by Taurine**

Retinal photoreceptor activity
Bile acid conjugation
WBC antioxidant activity
CNS neuromodulation (depressant)
Platelet aggregation (reduces)
Cardiac contractility (enhances)
Sperm motility (enhances)
Growth (enhances)
Insulin activity (enhances)

## PHYSIOLOGIC MODE OF ACTION

Although the mode of action for taurine is not adequately delineated, its ubiquitous presence (in most cells) and varied biologic activity (Table 24D–2) suggest a prominent role for taurine in cell function. The high concentration in the developing nervous system, muscle, and platelets, along with its association with calcium, has fueled speculation that it functions as a modulator of cation flux, especially for calcium. In this capacity it may stabilize or sequester membrane calcium during depletion of electrolytes.[8] In platelets taurine has the effect of decreasing aggregation sensitivity, presumably by increasing calcium ion concentration, which, in turn, is enhanced by increasing alkalinity.[9]

In heart muscle, taurine increases the calcium available for contractions at low calcium concentrations, yet protects against intracellular calcium overload when calcium is abundant. This regulation is thought to be modulated by the sarcolemma, possibly by interacting with specific phospholipids, such a phosphatidylinositol, or alternatively by taurine binding to specific high- and low-affinity protein receptors in the membrane.[8] The inotropic effect of taurine in cardiac muscle mediates contractility and work load to the extent that taurine has been considered effective therapy in congestive heart failure and is thought to exert a hypotensive action on the cardiovascular system. A summary of cardiac effects is presented in Table 24D–3.

In the retina and CNS taurine may serve a structural and functional role in stabilizing neural membranes, especially those situated in the lamellae of photoreceptor outersegments.[3,4]

Mollusks and other marine animals existing in

**Table 24D–3. Taurine Influence on the Heart***

Antiarrhythmic agent
Inotropic in regard to calcium ion
Enhancer of digitalis inotropy
Osmotic agent
Hypotensive agent

*After Huxtable and Sebring.[8]

environments with varying alkalinity presumably utilize taurine in an osmoregulatory function, a role it does not seem to have in similar freshwater species, but which may exist in the mammalian CNS.[2,10]

Van Gelder has postulated that a centralized mechanism for taurine function involves the basic regulation of the excitation threshold.[10] In this model taurine would stabilize membranes by controlling mobilization of calcium ions during depolarization. Control is influenced by pH, bicarbonate ion availability, and a zinc-taurine membrane-associated complex that would interact with $CO_2$ and $NH_3$ to regulate glutamate generation, the latter then acting in its role as neurotransmitter. In this capacity taurine would function as a neuromodulator indirectly depressing neuroexcitation through its control over glutamate metabolism. Several aspects of the hypothesis remain to be tested.

## DEFICIENCY

Taurine is not known to be a dietary essential for humans, but interest has been kindled by the fact that plasma and urinary taurine decreased in preterm and full-term infants fed synthetic formulas without taurine[11] and in infants maintained by parenteral nutrition.[12] Interestingly, taurine concentration is exceedingly high in colostrum and milk of early lactation, including breast milk.[3] Cow's milk, on the other hand, is generally not a rich source of taurine, presumably because most such milk is obtained during prolonged lactation when taurine secretion has waned.

The strongest evidence for the biologic importance of taurine has been obtained in kittens,[4] a species in which taurine biosynthesis is limited and demand is relatively high because cat bile acids are conjugated exclusively with taurine. This requirement places an unusual demand on the body taurine pool, depleting most tissues to 10% or less of their normal concentration when kittens are fed a taurine-free diet. In kittens, bile acids, retina, and olfactory bulb maintain their taurine concentration most avidly. However, when the retina has depleted to approximately 50% normal concentration, electrical and morphologic changes are demonstrable in the photoreceptor cells. If allowed to persist, continued depletion of taurine results in extensive, irreparable degeneration of the retina. Repletion with taurine in less advanced stages of degeneration allows restoration of photoreceptor outer segments and restored vision, although cone-timing delays and distorted cone morphology remain for up to 2 years. Similar, less clinically noticeable changes

have been reported in monkeys raised on human infant formulas lacking taurine.[13]

Additional responses to taurine depletion include depressed body weight gain and a decrease in the taurine/glycine ratio of bile acid conjugates, both of which were observed in infant monkeys fed soy-based, human infant formula.[4] Weight depression was apparently not noted in a similar study with a larger species of infant monkey.[13]

Whether these observations are relevant to humans is unclear because of difficulty in documenting physiologic evidence of human taurine deficiency, particularly in the premature infant, in whom the problem is most apt to occur. Preterm and full-term neonates develop reduced plasma and urinary concentrations of taurine when fed infant formulas without taurine compared to infants fed human breast milk or infant formula containing a normal taurine concentration.[11] However, in premature infants weighing about 2300 g following 3 weeks of taurine supplementation at 30 μmol/dl, neither bile acid synthesis nor primary or total bile acid pools were affected by taurine, even though the taurine/glycine bile acid ratio was increased.[14] In what were described as "sicker" premature infants weighing between 1400 and 2100 g who were fed 25 μmol/dl of formula supplemented with taurine, low plasma taurine values failed to increase, whereas urine values increased significantly but remained low (2.7 vs 12.4 μmol/dl). The concentration of duodenal bile salts was higher and that of cholesterol lower in the taurine-supplemented infants.[15] The implications of the latter observations are not clear except to indicate that the smallest premature infants (unlike larger infants) may be subject to taurine manipulation of their bile metabolism.[14,16] In another study a 10-day intravenous supplementation of taurine failed to improve cholestasis induced by parenteral nutrition in premature infants weighing <1500 g.[17]

By contrast, adult human males fed 3.0 g/day of taurine revealed a modest, but significant, decrease (11%) in their bile acid pool size. The relative biliary lipid composition, i.e., biliary saturation index, and the distribution of primary bile acids were unaffected.[18]

Taurine supplementation of infant formula (30 μmol/dl) also failed to have an impact on infant growth, serum cholesterol, BUN, serum proteins, blood acid-base balance,[19] or fat absorption,[20] all of which tend to suggest that the dietary taurine requirement is minimal in humans. More sophisticated measures of taurine function on the central nervous system must be utilized if an exogenous (dietary) requirement is to be identified. The likelihood of demonstrating such a requirement would seem to be greatest during parenteral nutrition.

Geggel et al.[21] expanded their original description of taurine depletion in humans receiving parenteral nutrition, again emphasizing that children, as compared to adults, are at high risk of taurine depletion under these circumstances. It has been noted[22] that the infused parenteral solutions lacked cysteine, the sulfur amino acid that stimulates the enzyme (cysteine sulfinic acid decarboxylase) leading to formation of taurine. Furthermore, the flux through the transsulfuration pathway is thought to be diminished in very young patients because of the low activity of cystathionase needed to convert methionine to cysteine. Thus, more definitive data are needed in neonates and young children receiving adequate cysteine before the dietary essentiality of taurine for infants can be ascertained.

## INDIVIDUALS AT RISK OF TAURINE DEPLETION

Based on the above information, and if we can extrapolate from kittens and monkeys, one might predict that taurine depletion depends upon an inability to synthesize appreciable taurine (low CSAD activity) in the face of extreme demand (Fig. 24D–2). A rationale for taurine depletion suggests that an organism is susceptible to depletion if taurine biosynthesis is inadequate when dietary supply is minimal and the demand (requirement) by tissues is high.[23] For instance, the carnivorous cat normally eats meat to assure a dietary intake of taurine that compensates for poor hepatic synthesis. However, the bile acid pool in cats is extremely demanding (obligate taurine conjugator), such that most endogenous taurine becomes sequestered by bile to the detriment of other tissues when the dietary supply fails. The whole-body demand for taurine is further exacerbated by the extremely rapid growth rate in kittens and a rapidly expanding muscle mass that requires taurine.

| INPUT | = | DEMAND |
|---|---|---|
| biosynthesis (CSAD) | | muscle growth |
| diet | | bile acid conjugation |
| | | CNS development |
| | | (retina) |
| | | (brain) |
| | | other cell functions |
| | | WBC |
| | | platelets |
| | | endocrine glands |

**Fig. 24D–2.** Requirements for whole-body taurine balance.

Thus depletion occurs. Most species that grow rapidly, like the rat and dog, synthesize taurine avidly. Other species, such as man and most monkeys that experience poor synthesis, grow slowly or are able to conjugate bile acids with glycine and thereby relieve the demand for taurine considerably so that minimal synthesis is adequate.

In human infants the supply/demand balance might conceivably be compromised when already limited sythesis is impaired by prematurity or hepatic dysfunction when growth rate is maximal and an exogenous supply is nonexistent (infant formulas, parenteral nutrition). Once growth has been completed, it is difficult to imagine a situation in which taurine would become limiting in normal circumstances. Excessive taurine loss in association with bile acids (as in chronic malabsorption) or impaired synthesis (as in chronic hepatic disease where synthesis is precluded) might provide clinical situations where concern for taurine depletion would be real.

That dietary taurine might be most critical to the neonate is further suggested by numerous studies of placental and milk transfer of taurine in utero and during the suckling period, respectively, in rhesus monkeys and rats. These results suggest an importance for taurine during development, underscored by the high concentration in fetal brain. These transfers are critical because the synthetic pathway (via CSAD) is limited in its capacity for taurine biosynthesis during development.[3]

## DIETARY CONSIDERATIONS

The noteworthy relationship between taurine and diet is its relative absence from vegetable sources and abundance in muscle, particularly that of shellfish (Table 24D–4). Thus, vegetarians should be at a disadvantage in terms of taurine status if it were an essential nutrient for humans. Since there are no reports that vegetarians suffer unduly from lack of taurine and their plasma taurine concentrations are presumably normal, adults probably do not require a dietary supply of taurine under normal physiologic conditions.

As mentioned earlier, a concern for the dietary taurine requirement in humans has arisen in infants fed substitute milk formulas or maintained by parenteral nutrition where plasma and urinary taurine are known to decline.[11,12,21] Whether an actual dietary requirement exists under these circumstances is under consideration and awaits further corroborating evidence of physiologic dysfunction.

The situation is quite different for cats fed commercial diets based on vegetable protein that have resulted in retinal degeneration.[4] In the cat the

**Table 24D–4.  Dietary Sources of Taurine***

|  | Fresh | Boiled | Cooking Fluid |
|---|---|---|---|
|  | *mg/100g net wt* | | |
| Beef (lean round) | 36–46 | 6 | 20 |
| Beef steak | 7 | | |
| Pork liver | 16 | 4 | 16 |
| Pork chop | 8 | | |
| Chicken | 34 | | |
| Lamb kidney | 13 | 5 | 2 |
| Sheep mutton | 6 | | |
| Cod | 31 | | |
| Clams | 240 | | |
| Oysters | 93 | 13 | 120 |
| Several plants & vegetables | 0 | | |
| Milk | | *mol/100 ml* | |
|    Human (1–12 wk) | | 20–48 | |
|    Cow's (marked drop after 1 wk) | | 1–30 | |

*adapted from refs.[27–31]

dietary requirement is thought to be 500 to 750 ppm for the growing kitten and lactating queen. Based on the urinary excretion rate in the adult human, a dietary intake of 125 to 500 ppm should suffice if diet were the exclusive source of taurine. For the cat the dietary requirement is at least 2 or more orders of magnitude above most vitamins and an order of magnitude less than the typical essential amino acid requirement. The fact that taurine is synthesized to some extent by most tissues precludes its being a true vitamin and renders its dietary essentiality conditionally dependent upon metabolic peculiarities of individual species, particularly reflecting age and growth status. The actual daily intake of taurine in humans is estimated to range between 40 and 400 mg or approxiately 100 to 1,000 ppm on a dietary basis.

To date no interrelationships have been described linking the requirement for taurine with that of other nutrients per se. However, since taurine synthesis depends on sulfur amino acid metabolism, limited intake of methionine or cysteine can increase the dietary requirement for taurine, at least in cats, and a high taurine intake may spare the requirement for cysteine or methionine. Because the transulfuration pathway also requires vitamin $B_6$, inadequate supply of this vitamin could theoretically increase the dependency on dietary taurine. In actual fact evidence of vitamin $B_6$ deficiency has been found to precede any evidence of taurine depletion in cebus monkeys.[24]

## EVALUATION OF TAURINE STATUS

The most acceptable and convenient assessment of taurine status is based on plasma and urinary taurine concentrations. The plasma concentration of taurine normally varies widely between 25 and 150 $\mu$mol/L, although it is not really known what constitutes a "low" or deficient plasma concentration in humans. Infants and children thought to be depleting their taurine pools still maintained plasma values in the 30 to 40 $\mu$mol/L range.[11,12,21] Values of 1 to 10 $\mu$mol/L are common in depleted cats.

A recurring problem is the spuriously high plasma concentration that derives from platelets or white blood cells if care is not taken to prevent contamination from these highly concentrated sources of taurine. Ironically, some of the highest plasma taurine values (>200 $\mu$mol/L) have been reported during the first 2 weeks of life,[2] presumably because of the high concentration transferred in early breast milk or the lack of taurine conversion to sulfate, the latter attributed to bacterial flora in the more mature intestine.

Urinary taurine values are usually high, 200 to 2,000 $\mu$mol/day, or roughly 2 to 10 times the plasma taurine concentration. Normal urinary values are difficult to ascertain, since variation within and between individuals is appreciable, with variation being dependent upon dietary intake. Normally renal tubular reabsorption of taurine is extremely low, leading to constant loss of circulating taurine and reducing the efficacy of the plasma as an interorgan transport system.

A number of methods have been utilized for taurine analysis, including paper chromatography and direct taurine quantitation following separation from other amino acids by ion-exchange chromatography. More recently, techniques have been described for ion-change separation and subsequent quantitation of fluorescent derivatives utilizing conventional spectrofluorometry[25] or fluorescence detection by HPLC.[26] The latter is probably the most sensitive and allows detection in the $\mu$mole range on minimal amounts of tissue or fluid.

## REFERENCES

1. Tiedemann, F., Gmalin, L.: Ann. Physik. Chem. *9*:326, 1827.
2. Jacobsen, J.G., Smith, L.H.: Physiol. Rev. *48*:424, 1968.
3. Sturman, J.A., Hayes, K.C.: Adv. Nutr. Res. *3*:231, 1980.
4. Hayes, K.C., Sturman, J.A.: Ann. Rev. Nutr. *1*:401, 1981.
5. Weiss, S.J., Klein, R., Slivka, A., Wei, M.: J. Clin. Invest. *70*:598, 1982.
6. Feuer, L., Torok, L.J., Kapa, E., Csaba, G.: Comp. Biochem. Physiol. *61C*:67, 1978.
7. Sturman, J.A., Hepner, G.W., Hofmann, A.F., Thomas, P.J.: J. Nutr. *105*:1206, 1975.
8. Huxtable, R.J., Sebring, L.A.: Prog. Clin. Biol. Res. *125*:5, 1983.
9. Raghu, C.N., Manikeri, S.R., Sheth, U.K.: Indian J. Exp. Biol. *20*:481, 1982.
10. van Gelder, N.: J. Neurochem. Res. 8:687, 1983.
11. Gaull, G.E., Rassin, D.K., Raiha, N.C.R. Heinonen, K.: J. Pediatr. *90*:348, 1977.
12. Geggel, H.S., Heckentively, J.R., Martin, D.A., Doc: Ophthalmology *31*:199, 1982.
13. Sturman, J.A., Wen, G.Y., Wisniewski, H.M., Neuringer, M.: Int. J. Dev. Neurosci. *2*:121, 1984.
14. Watkins, J.B., Jarvenpaa, A-L., Szczepanik-Van Leeuwen, P., et al.: Gastroenterology *85*:793, 1983.
15. Okamoto, E., Rassin, D.K., Zucker, C.L., et al.: J. Pediatr. *104*:936, 1984.
16. Jarvenpaa, A-L, Rassin, D.K., Kuitunen, G.E., et al.: Pediatrics *72*:677, 1983.
17. Cooke, R.J., Whitington, P.F., Kelts, D.: J. Pediatr. Gastro. Nutr. *3*:234, 1984.
18. Hardison, W.G.M., Grundy, S.M.: Gastroenterology *84*:617, 1983.
19. Jarvenpaa, A-L, Raiha, N.C.R., Rassin, D.K., Gaull, G.E.: Pediatrics *71*:171, 1983.
20. Jarvenpaa, A-L: Pediatrics *72*:684, 1983.
21. Geggel, H.S., Ament, M.E., Heckenlively, J.R., et al.: N. Engl. J. Med. *312*:142, 185.
22. Vandewonde, M.F.J., De Leeuw, I.H.: N. Engl. J. Med. *313*:121, 1985.
23. Hayes, K.C., Sturman, J.A.: Adv. Exptl. Med. Biol. *139*:79, 1982.
24. Stephan, Z.F., Sturman, J.A., Hayes, K.C.: Nutr. Res. *4*:421, 1984.
25. Baskin, S.I., Klekotka, S.J., Kendrick, Z.V., Bartuska, D.G.: J. Endo. Invest. *2*:245, 1979.
26. Stabler, T.V., Siegel, A.L.: Clin. Chem. *27*:1771, 1981.
27. Roe, D.A., Weston, M.O.: Nature *205*:287, 1965.
28. Awapara, J.: J. Biol. Chem. *218*:571, 1956.
29. Armstrong, M.D., Yates, K.N.: Proc. Soc. Exp. Biol. Med. *113*:680–683, 1963.
30. Mansford, K., Raper, R.: Nature *174*:314, 1954.
31. Rassin, D.K., Sturman, J.A., Gaull, G.E.: Early Human Dev. *2*:1, 1978.

*Chapter* **25**

# PSEUDOVITAMINS

## Victor D. Herbert

## CATEGORIES OF PSEUDOVITAMINS

The word "vitamin" describes those organic accessory food factors left in food after removal of the basic food factors (carbohydrates, fats, proteins, minerals, and water) that meet two specific requirements: (1) they are necessary in trace amounts for health (i.e., daily intake measured in micrograms to milligrams), and (2) they are essential in the diet because the body either does make them at all or does not make them in adequate quantities. The trace amounts necessary for health are measured by the two criteria of the Hopkins-Funk vitamin theory of deficiency disease: withdrawing the substance from the diet produces deficiency disease, and supplying the substance corrects the disease.[1]

Over the years, a number of organic substances that do not meet the necessary criteria have been alleged to be vitamins for humans.[2,2a] These pseudovitamins continue to be represented as vitamins by those who profit thereby, to a total of more than a billion dollars yearly. According to Cody, "misuse of the term vitamin to describe these compounds is a health fraud, since it is an implicit promise for a "natural curative" that has no scientific basis."[2a] The pseudovitamins fall into three categories:

(1) Metabolites: These include mislabeled intermediary metabolites like orotic acid ("vitamin B_{13}")[2a]; substances whose metabolism requires B vitamins, like inositol, choline, and methionine; and substances that are B vitamins for bacteria, worms, or other nonvertebrate forms of life, but not for humans. Two examples are para-amino-

benzoic acid (PABA) (mislabeled "vitamins B_x")[2a] a B vitamin for certain bacteria (that make folic acid from it), but not for humans (who must have preformed folic acid),[3] and "vitamin B_T," which is carnitine, a B vitamin for the mealworm (*Tenebrio molitor*) but not for humans.[4] Sulfonamides are structural antagonists to certain bacteria requiring PABA. Hence, people being treated with sulfonamides who take food supplements containing PABA are actually feeding their infecting bacteria the antidote to the sulfa drug, and risk overwhelming sepsis.[3] Entrepreneurs represent PABA as "a member of the B complex family," omitting the words "for bacteria," so that they can sell it as a food supplement.[2,3] PABA is a sunscreen when applied to the skin, but one should not drink one's suntan lotion.

(2) Pharmacologics: These are pharmacologic substances that are alleged to affect favorably certain metabolic process or processes in humans but that have not been objectively demonstrated to be necessary or even desirable for the normal physiologic functioning of that process or processes.[2,3] Bioflavonoids are typical such substances.

(3) Frauds: Snake oil nutrition remedies[2,3,6,7,7a] were created by what has been described in testimony before the United States Congress as "the quackery mafia."[5] These are pharmacologic substances, called "vitamins" by hucksters, that are of no objectively ascertained value in normal human physiology and that meet the legal definition of fraud (i.e., deceit for profit).[7] The deceit includes false representations of efficacy[6,7] and concealment of harms,[6,7] and it is accompanied by

**471**

remorseless smearing of responsible health professionals who point out the facts.[5,8] Two classic examples are vitamin $B_{15}$ (pangamate, pangamic acid)[9,10] and vitamin $B_{17}$ (Laetrile).[11,12] Gerovital "vitamin $H_3$" also falls in this category.[2a,3]

## FLAVONOIDS ("BIOFLAVONOIDS," "VITAMIN P")

In his original work on vitamin C, Szent-Gyorgyi thought an extract of Hungarian peppers, rich in vitamin C, was more effective than vitamin C alone in treating the fragile blood vessels of scurvy. He believed another vitamin was present, which he called "P" (for "permeability" of the blood capillaries, and for paprika).[13,14] Extraction of the peppers showed that they contained several chemically related substances—the flavonoids— derived from phenol. The flavone fraction (citron) of lemon was also alleged to decrease tissue hemorrhages and prolong the life of scorbutic guinea pigs.

Subsequent work by the same and other authors failed to establish that these substances were necessary, and in 1950 the Joint Committee on Biochemical Nomenclature of the American Society of Biological Chemists (ASBC) and the American Institute of Nutrition (AIN) recommended that the term "vitamin P" be discontinued.[15] The word bioflavonoids—designating flavonoids having biologic (i.e., pharmacologic) activity—was introduced to replace the erroneous designation vitamin P.[16]

### Chemistry and Occurrence in Foods

The flavonoids are a large group of generally insoluble phenolic compounds widely distributed in plants.[17] The basic flavone structure consists of a 1,4-benzopyrone with a phenyl substitution at the 2 position (Fig. 25–1). Hydroxyl group substitutions enable naturally occurring flavonoids to combine with sugars to form glycosides. Flavonoids can also form chelates with metals. The chemistry and biochemistry of the major classes are discussed systematically in the comprehensive text The Flavonoids.[18] The structures

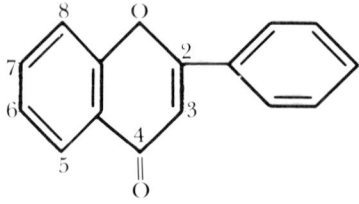

**Fig. 25–1.** Basic flavone structure.

of some common bioflavonoids are given in Figure 25–2.

As pigments that produce the colors of many flowers, fruits, and vegetables, flavonoid compounds range from the pale yellow and colorless flavanones in citrus fruit to the red and blue anthocyanins in berries.[17,19,20] Most flavonoids are concentrated in the skin, peel, and outer layers of fruits and vegetables, the areas most accessible to light. Beverages such as tea, coffee, wine, and beer also contain significant amounts. The amounts of different flavonoids in various foodstuffs are presented in two reviews.[17,19]

There is no bioflavonoid deficiency condition. Because an average daily intake of about 1000 mg of flavonoids occurs in a typical mixed diet,[17] health-food store tablets of 20 to 30 mg hardly make a difference. Bioflavonoids are among the many chemicals in food with pharmacologic activity. About one half of the amount ingested is absorbed in a pharmacologically active form, the rest being degraded by intestinal bacteria. Certain bioflavonoids may inhibit an enzyme involved in the formation of cataracts in diabetes mellitus and galactosemia, but there is no evidence that they interfere with cataract formation.[21,22] By pharmacologic action,[23] bioflavonoids may reduce red blood cell aggregation[24] or decrease bleeding associated with capillary fragility.[16]

Some of the observed effects may be explained by bioflavonoids' ability to chelate metals or by their ascorbate-protecting antioxidant effects.[18] Some of the inconsistent findings may be results of variable actions of different flavonoids as well as of different study designs.

Despite claims of usefulness,[17,23,24] bioflavonoids have no accepted preventive or therapeutic role in vascular purpura, hypertension, degenerative vascular disease, rheumatic fever, arthritis, cancer, or any other condition nor do they have any role in human nutrition.[2,7a]

Pills containing bioflavonoids may be unsafe, because quercetin (Fig. 25–2), a common bioflavonoid, is a mutagen.[2a] Whereas in food there are many mutagens and antimutagens (as well as carcinogens and anticarcinogens) that balance each other out,[7] such is not the case in pills, in which ingredients by definition are unbalanced, i.e., not in the same relationships as they are in the diet.

## PANGAMATE ("VITAMIN $B_{15}$")[6,7,9,10]

In 1943, Ernst Krebs, Sr. and Jr., applied for a patent, granted in 1949, for an uncharacterized remedy. The senior Krebs died in 1970 at age 93 pending a California antiquackery action against him, and the junior Krebs was jailed in San Francisco in 1983 for promoting the pseudovitamins

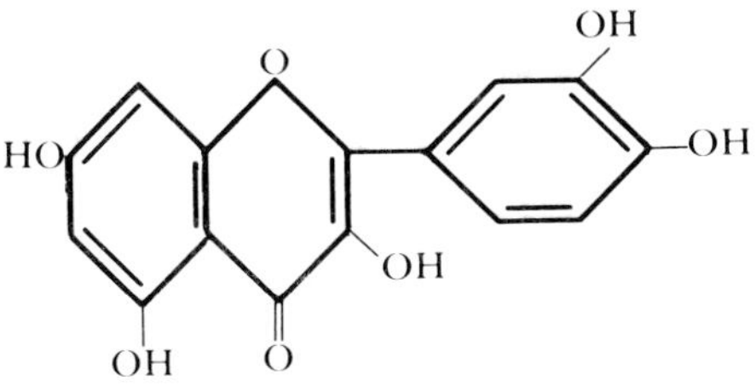

Quercetin

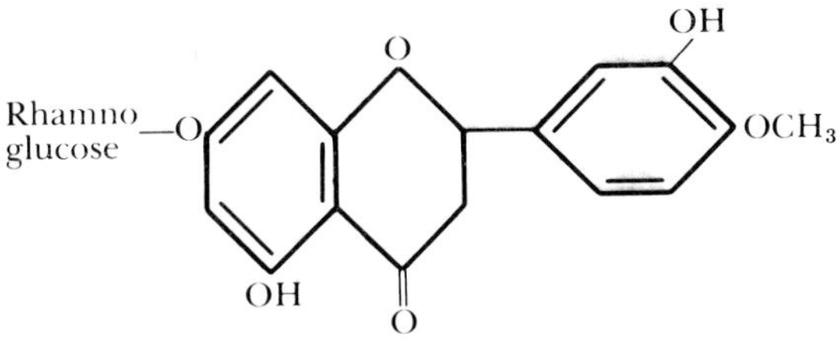

Hesperidin

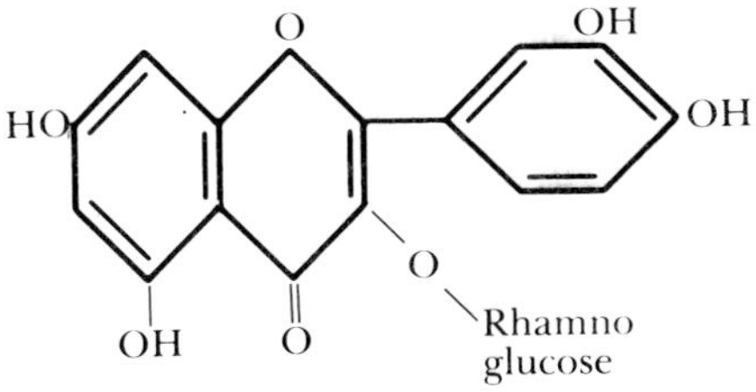

Rutin

**Fig. 25–2.** Structures of some common bioflavonoids.

$B_{15}$ and $B_{17}$ in violation of the terms of his probation, following a 1973 conviction.[6,7,12] The patented remedy was an uncharacterized extract "from seeds ... of the *Prunus* family and seeds of rice and barley." Presenting no supporting data, they claimed the extract as "a preparation for the immunization of toxic products present in the human or animal system" to produce "relief and immunity to persons afflicted with asthma and allied disease ... eczema ... arthritis, neuritis ... affections of the skin, respiratory tract, painful nerve and joint affections, and even cell proliferation ..."[9,10] The United States Patent Office will legally issue a patent on anything that claims novelty and usefulness, whether or not it works, is what it claims to be, actually exists, or does what it claims to do.[10]

The Krebs named their extract "pangamic acid" (pan = universal; gam = seed) and "vitamin $B_{15}$"[25] and alleged it conformed to the structural formula $C_{10}H_{19}O_8N$, molecular weight 281, for an ester of dimethylglycine (DMG) and gluconic acid (Fig. 25–3), an ester so unstable as to be unmeasurable in any reproducible manner.[26–28] To achieve a stable ester with DMG, a ring sugar is needed, such as $\alpha$-glucose.[26,28]

They alleged synthesis of a "family of compounds ... characterized by the presence of one or more labile methyl groups" with the common formula A-G, where A was any amino acid with one or more methyl groups and G was any glycone, sugar, or other carbohydrate. Any mixture of A and G that combined when mixed was designated

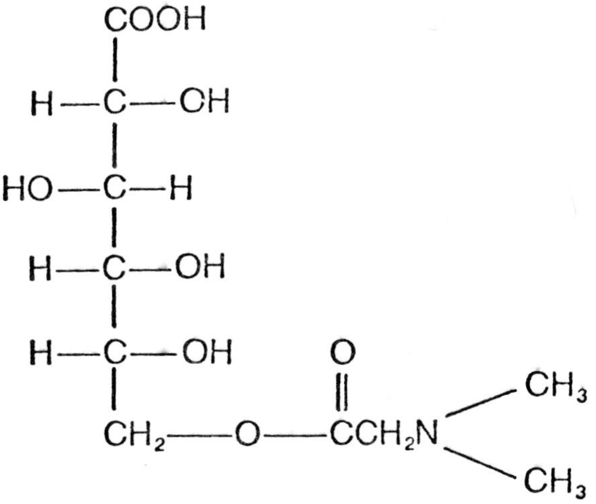

**Fig. 25–3.** Pangamic acid ("vitamin $\bar{B}_{15}$"), $C_{10}H_{19}O_8N$, an ester of dimethylglycine (DMG) and gluconic acid. The claims that this substance exists as a stable compound are as elusive as the claims it or its DMG component is a magic potion. Nitrosated DMG is mutagenic by Ames test. DMG is a waste product of choline breakdown, and is a "natural food" in the same sense any other waste product in stool or urine is a natural food. Failure of alleged esterification explains presence of DMG and gluconic acid separately in tablets of pangamate ("$B_{15}$"). DMG is not found in urine except as a drug catabolite.

a pangamate or $B_{15}$ analogue, and even compounds consisting only of A (amino acid with one or more methyl groups), preferably of DMG, or only of G (glycone; carbohydrate), preferably halogenated carbohydrates like dichloroacetate (DCA), were "sister compounds of $B_{15}$."[9,10] DCA was a bizzare preference in view of the mutagenicity of halogenated hydrocarbons.

Beard, a co-author of the paper that created the trade names pangamic acid and vitamin $B_{15}$,[25] subsequently claimed that it was a sugary compound formed by the union of gluconic acid with glycine in its methylated state, or it was the dimethylaminoacetate of gluconic acid.[10] In 1953 he sent capsules of $B_{15}$ to William Darby, who was unable to find any transmethylating activity in them and eventually sent those left over to me. Evaluation by nuclear magnetic resonance (NMR) in a Food and Drug Administration (FDA) laboratory showed an NMR spectrum of pure lactose, with no trace of either DMG or gluconic acid.[10]

Among the compounds mentioned as a major $B_{15}$ form in a follow-up 1955 Krebs patent[9,10] was a condensation product of diisopropylamine with dichloroacetate, the drug diisopropylamine dichloroacetate[4,22] (Fig. 25–4). The Merck Index lists diisopropylamine dichloroacetate (trade named DIPA; more accurately DIPA-DCA) as a vasodilator and hypotensive,[29] which explains why those who take it believe they "can feel it working" and that "this must be a powerful vitamin." Its pharmacologic properties were summarized by a stepson of Krebs.[30] The diisopropylamine (DIPA) component is a strongly alkaline liquid for which the Merck Index issues the warning, "Caution: Irritating to skin, mucous membranes."[29] The dichloroacetate (DCA) component is a strongly acid liquid, which the Merck Index describes as "escharotic' topical keratolytic; topical astringent."[29] When mixed together in equimolar concentrations, these two liquids become a solid crystalline salt with no loss of water.[29] The salt

dissociates easily in water into its component parts, DIPA and DCA.

In 1978, Stacpoole et al.[31] used DCA in the treatment of lactic acidosis. After we noted its mutagenicity,[32,33] they terminated all oral use because of its severe toxicity to nerves, gonads, and eyes of rats and dogs, and its generation of polyneuropathy in at least one human.[34]

In 1980, in a Federal Court, DIPA-DCA was found to be "an unsafe food additive" (USA vs. GNC).[9,10] DIPA-DCA is mutagenic by Ames test.[35]

Some $B_{15}$ products contain DMG (N-methylsarcosine, a tertiary amine) in doses of 20 to 50 mg/tablet. Such large amounts of DMG are not found in food or human tissues, nor do they play any known salutary physiologic role.[9,10] DMG is transiently present in trace amounts during choline catabolism.[10]

DIPA cannot be a methyl donor because its methyl groups are on carbon, and only methyl groups on a nitrogen or a sulfur can serve as methylating agents, and then only when there is no need for an added energy source. DMG methyl groups, like those of sarcosine, are not labile and so must be removed by oxidation and only then can enter the 1-carbon unit pool.[36,37] DIPA is not lipotropic.[37] DMG enters 1-carbon metabolism at the oxidation level of formaldehyde. It worsens methyl depletion of rats given nicotinamide supplements and on diets creating methyl deficiency, resulting in renal cortical necrosis in mature females and damaged growth and development of fetal rats.[38] DMG consumes oxygen; it does not supply it.

DMG reacts with nitrites (which are formed de novo in saliva, the stomach, and the intestine)[39] to form both the potent carcinogen, dimethylnitrosamine, and the weaker carcinogen, nitrososarcosine,[40] which induces cancer of the oral pharyngeal cavity and esophagus in the rat.[41] DMG ingested in concentrated, multimilligram freeform as a tablet is therefore much more likely carcinogenic than when ingested in the trace amount present in 100 g of meat. Additionally, pills sold as pangamate $B_{15}$ are not DMG, but DMG-HCl, of greater reactivity. The mixture of DMG-HCl and nitrite is mutagenic by Ames test.[42]

In 1981, DMG was ruled in a Federal Court to be an unsafe food additive (U.S.A. vs. Food-Science).[10] The FDA considers the sale of pangamate ($B_{15}$) illegal[43] because the terms are meaningless as descriptions of the contents of bottles so labeled and because no substantial evidence was submitted to the FDA that products so labeled have therapeutic efficacy or are safe for human consumption.[9] None of the studies published through 1986 claiming health value of DMG pills

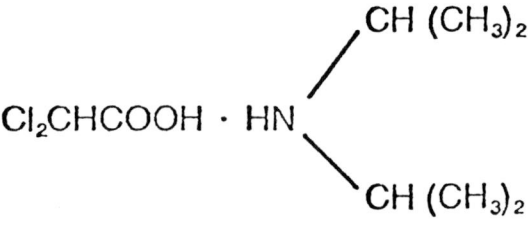

**Fig. 25–4.** Diisopropylamine dichloroacetate (DIPA-DCA, registered as the drug DIPA), the "active ingredient of vitamin $B_{15}$." It is a vasodilator and hypotensive drug (1976 Merck Index #3181). The DCA portion is mutagenic by Ames test, as is DIPA-DCA.

have been confirmed as showing any efficacy for humans, and its safety remains questionable.

## LAETRILE ("VITAMIN B$_{17}$")[6,11,12]

### Chemistry: A Source of Cyanide

Laetrile and vitamin B$_{17}$ are 20th century trade names created by Krebs[6,12] for a 19th-century product, amygdalin, a cyanogenetic glycoside[44] isolated in 1830[11] in France from almonds (hence the designation "amygdalin"). Cyanogenetic glycosides are naturally present as toxicants (poisons) in many species of plants including the kernels of apricot pits, a number of other stone fruits in members of the Malaceae and Amygdalaceae (formerly Rosaceae) families (apples, cherries, peaches, pears, plums), and nuts (almonds, macadamia nuts, etc.)[44,45] Laetrile was first erroneously represented as a cancer cure in 1840 in Presse Medicale by a French country doctor, who gave it to six cancer patients and reported it cured cancer because all were still alive 2 months later. The evidence has been equally bad since.[6,7,11,12]

### Toxicity

Cyanogenetic glycosides (trade named "Laetrile," "Nitrilosides," and "vitamin B$_{17}$" by Krebs) are chemical substances made up of cyanide, aldehyde or ketone, and sugar.[44] Laetrile is 6% cyanide by weight, consisting of two parts glucose, one part benzaldehyde (itself mildly poisonous), one part cyanide, and no parts vitamin[45,46] (Fig. 25–5). The cyanide in Laetrile is released as hydrogen cyanide (prussic acid) by hydrolysis in the presence of the enzyme β-glucosidase (which is present in a wide variety of vegetables and other plant products),[44,47–51] by heat, mineral acids, or megadoses of ascorbic acid, especially in the presence of blood.[52] The released hydrogen cyanide (hydrocyanic acid, HCN) is so penetrating a poison that victims have died within 2 minutes after ingestion of 300 mg hydrocyanic acid in aqueous solution,[53] an amount released by 2½ ounces of some varieties of bitter apricot kernels mixed with saliva, or a sixth of an ounce of Laetrile mixed with saliva and vegetables.

The claim that cyanide from Laetrile is immediately detoxified to thiocyanate by rhodanese (mitochondrial sulfur transferase) and sulfur in the body is disproved by the undetoxified cyanide measureable in the blood of persons poisoned by Laetrile or apricot kernels[6,12,47,53] and by the fact that thiocyanate is itself toxic.[53]

Cyanide prevents respiration in normal cells and, to a lesser extent, in cancer cells.[46,47,54] by inhibiting cytochrome oxidase at a concentration of $10^{-8}$M cyanide.[53] For humans, the lethal dose

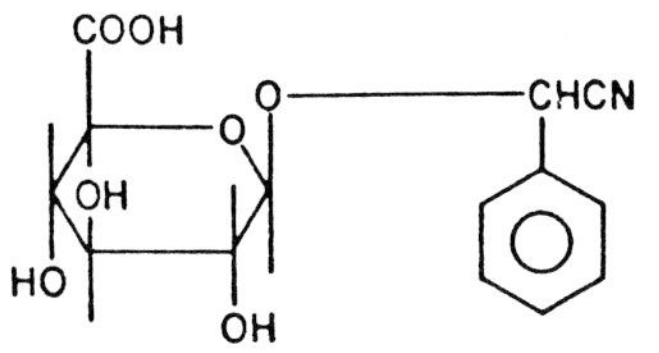

**LAETRILE ®**

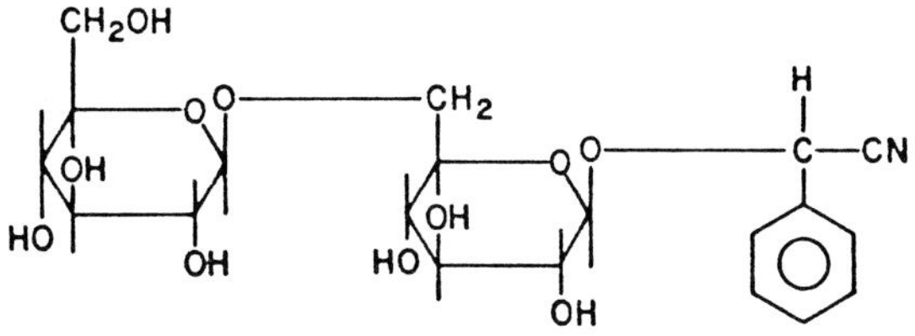

**AMYGDALIN (laetrile)**

**Fig. 25–5.** Laetrile with a capital "L" is a synthetic substance that has never been marketed, and the claimed method of synthesis of it by Krebs was never reproduced. The "natural" substance closest to it is prunasin, which differs only in having a "-CH$_2$OH" replacing "-COOH". Laetrile with a lower case "l" is amygdalin, the product marketed by laetrile promoters. The popular term "laetriles" is a synonym for "cyanogenetic glycosides."

of cyanide taken orally is between ½ and 3½ millionths of a pound per pound of body weight.[47] About 10 of some varieties of bitter apricot kernels can be eaten without acute toxicity by adults, but 25 kernels of other varieties can be lethal eaten at once.[55] Twenty-five to 35 average-variety bitter apricot kernels eaten over 1 or 2 hours may produce nonfatal symptoms of cyanide toxicity such as headache, dizziness, nausea, drowsiness, a sharp fall in blood pressure, difficulty breathing, damage to heart action, and possibly convulsions or coma.[47] The average fatal dose of cyanide is 50-60 mg[45]; the entire 60-mg cyanide content of 1 g Laetrile taken at once can be lethal. Deaths were reported in an infant who ingested approximately five 500-mg tablets[6,12,53] and in a 17½-year-old girl who drank 3½ ampules (10½ g) of Laetrile.[56,57]

Chronic cyanide intoxification from laetriles in the diet (manioc—bitter cassava) has produced thousands of cases of slowly progressing neurologic damage with blindness (bilateral optic atrophy), nerve deafness, myelopathy, and muscle weakness in a demyelinating syndrome of toxic ataxic neuropathy and its variants.[44,58–65] Small amounts of cyanide may be oxidized to $CO_2$ via cyanate,[56] which is neurotoxic.[66,67] Cyanate toxicity in man includes not only hypoxia-like damage to the nervous system (drowsiness, diminished vision, severe debilitating peripheral neuropathy with muscle weakness, gait disturbance, footdrop, electroencephalogram changes, possible diffuse encephalopathy, demyelination, and paresthesia), but also marked weight loss and cataracts (which may appear months or years after exposure).[62]

A recent epidemic of spastic paraparesis neuropathy in Mozambique children was traced[63] to cyanide from laetriles in cassava and the low-sulfur amino acid vegetarian intake. (Vegetarian intakes are favored by Laetrile proponents.[6]) Congenital malformations induced in animals by laetriles continue to be reported,[64] and Laetrile promoters are now being sued for wrongful death from cyanide poisoning (1983, Las Vegas, Clark County, Nevada).

Laetriles in the diet may produce goiters from the inhibition of iodine uptake by the thyroid caused by the thiocyanate produced from cyanide.[57,59,65] About half a million Zaire nationals developed cretinism and mental[59,65] retardation from laetriles.[55,62,66]

The human toxic reactions to cyanide, all of which have been seen with Laetrile and which may be erroneously ascribed to the patient's cancer, include, from high doses, tachypnea, dyspnea, paralysis, unconsciousness, convulsions, respiratory arrest, and death; from lesser doses, headache, vertigo, nausea, and vomiting; and from chronic exposure over long periods, fatigue and weakness. Lassitude, insomnia, cardiac discomfort, anemia, skin eruption, and ocular and auditory disturbances also occur.[67-70] Low concentrations of Laetrile may produce insidious loss of appetite, weight loss, cachexia, and mental deterioration. Thiocyanate can produce weakness, nausea, vomiting, diarrhea, skin eruptions, arthralgia, palpitations, precordial pain, muscle cramps, facial edema, depressed thyroid function, irritability, blurred vision, tinnitus, motor aphasia, hallucinations, and delirium.[58,71] There may be bizzare behavior. A 3½-year-old girl who ate about 15 apricot kernels exhibited "disorientation and confusion, vertigo and restlessness.[55]

As a poison, Laetrile is much more toxic when taken by mouth than when injected, because gastric juice may release some cyanide from Laetrile. Also, the enzymes that split off the 6% cyanide from the rest of the Laetrile molecule are found not only in plant foods, but in intestinal bacteria and possibly in intestine epithelial cells.[46-48] Because enzymes are not absorbed from the intestine into the blood stream, the releasing of cyanide from Laetrile occurs largely in the intestine,[46-48] including the colon.[74] Human feces hydrolyze

enough Laetrile that children (and possibly adults) have died from Laetrile enemas.[6,72]

## Ineffectiveness as an Anticancer Agent

In over a century of studies, Laetrile has never been objectively demonstrated to be more effective for cancer treatment than doing nothing, or as safe as doing nothing. In fact, patients treated with Laetrile deteriorate faster and die faster than those treated with nothing.[2,2a,6,7,11,12] The combined effects of lack of proper medical care and chronic cyanide poisoning have reduced by half the life span of cancer patients taking Laetrile.[73]

A number of studies in the first half of this century testing cyanide as a cancer chemotherapy agent always proved the levels harmful to tumors to be too harmful to the host as well to be of clinical value.[74] While cyanide clearly can kill cancer cells, it does so only in doses that kill the patient.[6,12] Although a major 1982 multi-institution study reconfirmed the worthlessness of Laetrile against cancer[75] the lucrative Laetrile industry continues.[3,6,7,12]

Five lines of evidence suggest Laetrile may actually promote cancer: Laetrile is goitrogenic[65,66] and such goiters are precancerous lesions[54]; it is mutagenic[47,76]; and it gives a positive Ames test.[77] Also, one patient with cancer developed a second cancer while being "treated" with Laetrile;[78] and cyanate, an oxidation product of cyanide, reduces the ability of mice to reject tumor inocula.[62] The myth that natives of Hunza (Hunzakuts) do not get cancer because they eat apricot kernels was long ago shattered by autopsy findings of cancer in Hunzas.[79,80]

## REFERENCES

1. Herbert: Vitamin. *In* World Book Encyclopedia. Chicago, World Book—Childcraft International Inc., 1979, pp. 333–336.
1a. Herbert: Arch. Int. Med. *140*:173, 1980.
2. Marshall: Vitamins and Minerals: Help or Harm? Philadelphia, Stickley Co., 1983.
2a. Cody: Food Sci. Technol. *13*:571, 1984.
3. Herbert, Barrett: Vitamins and "Health" Foods: The Great American Hustle. Philadelphia, Stickley Co., 1981.
4. Borum: Ann. Rev. Nutr. *3*:233, 1983.
5. Herbert: Testimony, Select Committee on Aging, House of Representatives. Comm. Pub. 98-463 "Quackery: A $10-Billion Scandal." Washington, DC, U.S. Government Printing Office, May 31, 1984.
6. Herbert: Nutrition Cultism: Facts and Fictions. Philadelphia, Stickley Co., 1981.
7. Herbert: Cancer *58*:1930–1941, 1986.
7a. Bender: Health or Hoax? The Truth about Health Foods and Diets. Buffalo, Prometheus Books, 1986.
8. Herbert: Testimony, Health Fraud and the Elderly, Dec. 3, 1985. Available free from Assembly Republican Task Force on Health Fraud and the Elderly, 99 Washington Avenue, Room 1010, Albany, NY 11210.
9. Herbert: Am. J. Clin. Nutr. *32*:1534, 1979.

10. Herbert, Herbert: Pangamate ("Vitamin B$_{15}$"). *In* Controversies in Nutrition (Edited by Ellenbogen). New York, Churchill Livingstone, 1981, pp. 159–170.
11. Dorr, Paxinos: Ann. Int. Med. *89*:389, 1978.
12. Herbert: Am. J. Clin. Nutr. *32*:1121, 1979.
13. Rusznyak, Szent-Gyorgyi: Nature *138*:27, 1936.
14. Bentsath, Rusznyak, Szent-Gyorgyi: Nature *138*:798, 1936.
15. Joint Committee on Nomenclature: Science *112*:628,1950.
16. Miner: Bioflavonoids and the capillary. Ann. NY Acad. Sci. *61*:637, 1955.
17. Kuhnau: World Rev. Nutr. Diet. *24*:117, 1976.
18. Harborne, Mabry, Mabry (Eds.): *The Flavonoids*, Part I and Part 2. New York, Academic Press, 1975.
19. Herrmann: J. Food Technol. *11*:433, 1976.
20. Hughes: J. Hum. Nutr. *32*:47, 1978.
21. Varma, Mikuni, Kinoshita: Science *188*:1215, 1975.
22. Varma and Kinoshita: Biochem. Pharmacol. *25*:2505, 1976.
23. Pearson, JAMA. *164*:1675, 1957.
24. Robbins: Int. J. Vitam. Nutr. Res. *47*:373, 1977.
25. Krebs, Krebs, Jr., Beard, et al.: Int. Rec. Med. *164*:19–24, 1951.
26. Yurkevich, Verenikina, Dolgikh, et al.: Zh. Ob. Khim. *37*:1267, 1967.
27. Skupin, Giec: Chemia. Analityczna *15*:1127–1133, 1970.
28. Micheau, Lattes, Podesta, et al.: Chim. Ther. *7*:103–121, 1972.
29. Windholz, Budavari, Stroumtsos, Fertig (Eds.): The Merck Index. 9th Ed. Rahway, NJ, Merck and Co., Inc., 1976. Entries #3021 (Dichloroacetic acid); #3180 (Diisopropylamine) #3181 (Diisopropylamine dichloroacetate); #9676 (Vitamin B$_{15}$, Pangamic acid). Dimethylglycine is not listed.
30. Stacpoole: J. Clin. Pharm. *9*:282–291, 1969.
31. Stacpoole, Moore, Kornhauser: N. Engl. J. Med. *298*:526–530, 1978.
32. Herbert, Gardner, Colman: Clin. Res. *27*:551a, 1979.
33. Herbert, Gardner, Colman: Am. J. Clin. Nutr. *33*:1179–1182, 1980.
34. Stacpoole, Moore, Kornhauser: N. Engl. J. Med. *300*:372, 1979.
35. Gelernt, Herbert: Nutr. Cancer *3*:129–133, 1982.
36. White, Handler, Smith: Principles of Biochemistry. New York, McGraw-Hill, 1973.
37. Jukes: Nutr. Notes *14*:13, 1978.
38. Woodard: J. Nutr. *100*:125, 1970.
39. Tannenbaum, Fett, Young, et al.: Science *200*:1487–1489, 1978.
40. Friedman: Bull. Environ. Contam. Toxicol. *13*:226–232, 1975.
41. Hartman: Science *200*:260, 1978.
42. Colman, Herbert, Gardner, et al.: Proc. Soc. Exper. Biol. Med. *164*:9–12, 1980.
43. Check: JAMA *243*:2473–2480, 1980.
44. Conn: *In* Toxicants Occurring Naturally in Foods 2nd Ed. Washington, DC, National Academy of Science, 1973, pp. 299–308.
45. Windholz Budavari, Stroumtsos. (Eds.) The Merck Index. 9th Ed. Rahway, NJ, Merck and Co., Inc., 1976. Entries #630 (Amygdalin); #1057 (Benzaldehyde); #4688 (Hydrogen Cyanide); #5197 (Laetrile).
46. Greenberg: West. J. Med. *122*:345, 1975.
47. Lewis: West. J. Med. *127*:55, 1977.
48. Schmidt, Newton, Sanders, et al.: JAMA *239*:943, 1978.
49. Herbert: JAMA *240*:1139, 1978.
50. Herbert: Am. J. Clin. Nutr. *32*:96, 1979.
51. Conn: *In* Effects of Poisonous Plants on Livestock. Edited by Keefer, Kampen, James. New York, Academic Press, 1978, pp. 301–310.
52. Backer, Herbert: JAMA *241*:1891, 1979.
53. Humbert, Tress Braico: JAMA *238*:482, 1977; Braico, Humbert, Terplan, Lehotay: N. Engl. J. Med. *300*:238, 1979.
54. Jukes: JAMA *236*:1984, 1976.
55. Gunders, Abrahamov, Weisenberg, et al.: J. Israel Med. Assoc. *76*:535, 1969.
56. Sandoff, Fuchs, Hollander: JAMA *239*:1532, 1978.
57. Anonymous. Med. World News. Jan. 9, 1978, pp. 16, 21.
58. Dreisbach: Cyanides, sulfides and carbon monoxide. *In* Handbook of Poisoning: Diagnosis and Treatment. Los Altos, CA, Lange Medical Publishers, 1977, pp. 241–245.
59. Osuntokun: Bull. Schweiz. Akad. Med. Wiss. *31*:353, 1975.
60. Shaw, Papyannopoulou, Stamatoyannopoulous. Pharmacology *12*:166, 1974.
61. Peterson, Tsairis, Onishi, et al.: Ann. Intern. Med. *81*:152, 1974.
62. Harkness, Roth: Prog. Hematol. *9*:157, 1975.
63. Cliff, Lundqvist, Mårtensson, et al.: Lancet *ii*, 1211, 1985.
64. Willhite: Science *215*:1513, 1982.
65. Ermans: *In* The Thyroid. 4th Ed. Edited by Werner and Ingbar. Hagerstown, MD, Harper & Row, 1978, pp. 537–553.
66. Dorozynski: Nature *272*:121, 1978.
67. Anonymous: Emergency Med. *10*:155, 1978.
68. Hamilton, Hardy: Industrial Toxicology. 3rd Ed. Acton, MA, Publishing Sciences Group, Inc., 1974, pp. 221–228.
69. Gettler, St. George: Am. J. Clin. Pathol. *4*:429, 1934.
70. Smith, Butler, Cohan, Schein: JAMA *238*:1351, 1977; Cancer Treatment Rept. *62*:169, 1978.
71. Nickerson, Reundy: Antihypertensive agents and drug therapy of hypertension. *In* The Pharmacologic Basis of Therapeutics, Edited by Goodman and Gilman. New York, Macmillan, 1975, p. 717.
72. Klassen and Stavric: 91st Ann. Meet., AOAC, 1977, p. 18.
73. Young: On the harmful effects of laetrile. IV. Clinical experience with laetrile. Joint Hearing, Florida State Board of Medical Examiners and Osteopathic Board of Medical Examiners. Orlando, FL, Feb. 25, 1978.
74. Brown, Wood, Smith: Am. J. Obstet. Gynecol. *80*:907, 1960.
75. Moertel, Fleming, Rubin, et al.: N. Engl. J. Med. *306*:201, 1982.
76. Selby, Menges, Houser, et al.: Arch. Environ. Health *22*:496, 1971.
77. Fenselau, Pallante, Batziner, et al.: Science *198*:625, 1977.
78. Dainer, Long: N. Engl. J. Med. *297*:220, 1977.
79. Subcommittee on Health and Scientific Resources, United States Senate. Proceedings of the July 12, 1977 Hearings on Banning of the Drug Laetrile from Interstate Commerce by F.D.A. Washington, DC, Government Printing Office, 1977.
80. Harada, Myoshi: Results of the Kyoto University Scientific Expedition to the Karakoram and Hindukush, 1955, vol. V, pp. 1–14, 1963.

Supported in part by USPHS Grant DK37509 and by the Medical Research Service of the United States Veterans Administration, NY.

# Part II
## *Physiologic and Metabolic Interrelations*

*Chapter* **26**

# THE GASTROINTESTINAL TRACT: PORTAL TO NUTRIENT UTILIZATION

Peter C. Wilson and Harry L. Greene

This chapter provides an overview of gastrointestinal function as it relates to nutrient intake, digestion, absorption, and expulsion of unextracted substances; a detailed explanation of physiology and pathophysiology is beyond its scope. Particulars of intestinal handling of most major and minor nutrients are discussed in more detail in other chapters.

The gastrointestinal tract is a complex organ system whose primary functions are to carry out digestion and absorption of ingested nutrients and simultaneously to protect the body from ingested microorganisms and noxious substances. After ingestion, food is mechanically divided, mixed with digestive enzymes, and cleaved into readily absorbable particles. Nutrients are then absorbed through specialized mucosa and nonabsorbed substances are expelled. More than 95% of ingested carbohydrate, fat, and protein is usually absorbed during passage through a normally functioning gastrointestinal tract, although absorption of vitamins, minerals, and trace elements may be less efficient.[1]

Protection against harmful, non-nutritive substances is provided first by the practice of food selection and preparation before ingestion, and to some extent by sensory discrimination at the time of ingestion. The chemical action of saliva and production of mucus, gastric acid, and digestive enzymes further alter potentially harmful substances.[2] A complex immune system that involves the production of luminal antibodies to neutralize many ingested parasites, bacteria, and viruses adds further protection. Additional protective mechanisms include vomiting, which is coordinated by the brain stem vomiting center sensitive both to the influence of central chemoreceptors and to afferent impulses from the gastrointestinal tract,[3] and diarrhea. Prostaglandins also appear to aid this protective action by modulating the motor and secretory activity of the intestine.[4] Inhibition of prostaglandin synthesis by agents, such as nonsteroid anti-inflammatory drugs, appears to disrupt the functional integrity of the gastric and duodenal mucosa creating the potential for ulcer formation.

## INTEGRATION OF THE GASTROINTESTINAL TRACT WITH OTHER ORGANS

The gastrointestinal tract is an extremely active metabolic organ. Although it contains most of the enzymes that are present in the liver, the metabolic pathways are generally less active than those of the liver. Its metabolic functions are therefore directed primarily toward supporting digestion and delivery of ingested nutrients to the liver for further processing. This function demands substantial quantities of energy in the postabsorptive state. In order to meet these energy demands, the gastrointestinal tract consumes 30% of the cardiac output from two major arteries.[2] Together they carry more blood than any other branch of the aorta; the blood flow may increase even further with eating. In fact, postprandial increases in blood flow may produce cardiac and mesenteric angina in susceptible subjects.

**Liver.** The liver is the organ most responsible for metabolic homeostasis of ingested nutrients. The liver participates directly in intestinal function through secretion of bile, which is required for lipid absorption. Other hepatic functions include detoxification of drugs and noxious chemicals, modulation of certain circulating hormones, and elimination of pathogenic organisms.

Venous blood from the gastrointestinal tract is carried to the liver via the portal vein. With the exception of intestinal chylomicrons that enter the lymphatics, all absorbed products pass initially through the liver and, in most instances, are extracted or modified before passage into the systemic circulation. Many nutrients and some drugs are subject to an enterohepatic circulation through their excretion in bile and subsequent reabsorption by the small intestine. Interruption of this cycle by biliary diversion or failure of reabsorption accounts for a more rapid onset of specific deficiencies than might otherwise be anticipated. Examples of substances with enterohepatic circulation include bile salts, vitamin D, vitamin $B_{12}$, folate, cholesterol, and drugs such as methotrexate. The enterohepatic circulation of methotrexate increases the liver and intestinal exposure to the drug and contributes to its tendency toward hepatic and intestinal toxicity.[5]

**Pancreas.** The endocrine and exocrine activity of the pancreas is integrally related to gastrointestinal and hepatic handling of nutrients. Insulin is released from beta cells in response to a rise in plasma amino acids or glucose, vagal stimulation, or a rise in circulating gastrin, cholecystokinin (CCK), or secretin. All such postprandial signals appear to originate in the intestine. The anabolic actions of insulin facilitate intracellular transfer of glucose, amino acids, and fatty acids and increase glucose oxidation, glycogenesis, lipogenesis, and protein synthesis. Glucagon, which is secreted by alpha islet cells in response to rises in circulating alanine, ketones, and CCK, or a fall in blood glucose, balances in part the many actions of insulin. Pancreatic exocrine function, which is stimulated by hormones released from the small

bowel mucosa in response to luminal nutrients, aids in the digestion and absorption of food. The exocrine pancreas also produces somatostatin and possibly other hormones that may further modulate metabolic and functional activities of the intestine by as yet unidentified mechanisms.

**Brain.** The relationship between the brain and the gastrointestinal tract is more complex than initially supposed. More than 15 peptides with dual distribution in brain and intestine have now been described.[6] Apart from hormonal and neurotransmitter functions in the intestine, several of these peptides show paracrine activity between adjacent cells. Many of these same peptides also appear to act as neurotransmitters at central nerve ganglia. A new term has therefore evolved to describe this system of common transmission in brain in gastrointestinal tract—the "peptidergic nervous system."[7] Peptide transmitters include vasoactive intestinal peptide (VIP), motilin, cholecystokinin, and somatostatin. In addition, many opiate peptides or endorphins are also found in both the brain and the intestinal mucosa. In the brain, these transmitters may modulate pain; in the gut, they appear to inhibit gastrointestinal motility and secretion. Although the integrated function of these peptides in the control of intestinal function is unclear at present, a number of the peptides have been individually studied. Some of the peptides common to brain and gut are shown in Table 26–1.

Appetite plays a major role in food-seeking behavior, and although it is incompletely understood, it is apparently regulated by the central nervous system, particularly the hypothalmus.[6,8]

**Immune System.** The gut is an important interface between the internal and external environment. In protecting the body from potentially harmful foreign substances, the immune system may favorably influence nutrient absorption, but conversely, malnutrition or certain dietary toxins adversely affect immune function. The intestinal immune system acts to reduce the amount of antigen absorbed by the intestine and, by humoral communication, may prevent undesirable immune reactions from otherwise harmless antigenic substances that have managed to cross the intestinal mucosa. Impairment of the intestinal immune system is implicated in the genesis of several diseases that affect gut function and nutritional status.[9] These diseases include gluten-sensitive enteropathy, food allergies, immunodeficiency syndromes, and possibly inflammatory bowel disease. The role of the immune system is discussed in detail in Chapter 33.

**Table 26–1. Polypeptides Common to Brain and Gastrointestinal Tract**

| Peptide | Location | Main Function in Gut |
|---|---|---|
| CCK* | Upper small intestine | Stimulation of pancreatic enzyme release and gallbladder contraction |
| Substance P; neuromedin K | Small intestine. In both neuronal and endocrine cells | Atropine-resistant contractions in peristalsis |
| Neurotensin | Lower small intestine | Unknown |
| Somatostatin | Throughout small intestine | Paracrine inhibitory effects |
| VIP-PHI* | Small intestine | Receptive relaxation, reflex vasodilation with descending inhibition |
| Secretin | Upper small intestine | Stimulation of pancreatic $HCO_3$ |
| Glucagon-like | Lower small intestine, colon | Unknown |
| Enkephalins | Throughout small intestine | Inhibition of acetylcholine release |
| Endorphins | Small bowel endocrine cells | Unknown |
| Bombesin | Upper small intestine, neuronal origin | Release of gastrin |
| Motilin | Upper small intestine | Initiation of mean migratory complex |

*CCK = cholecystokinin; VIP = vasoactive intestinal peptide; PHI = peptide with histidine at the N-terminus and isoleucineamide at the C-terminus.

## STRUCTURE AND DEVELOPMENT OF THE GASTROINTESTINAL TRACT

### Embryology

The primitive gut forms during the fourth week of gestation from the foregut, midgut, and hindgut. The foregut gives rise to the pharynx, esophagus, stomach, duodenum (proximal to the ampulla of Vater), liver and biliary apparatus, and pancreas. With the exception of the pharynx and esophagus, the blood supply for these organs derives from the celiac artery. Because the trachea and esophagus have a common origin, incomplete partitioning may lead to stenoses, atresias, and fistulas. Duodenal atresia occurs when vacuolization between the foregut and the midgut fails to occur.

The derivatives of the midgut are the small intestine (below the opening of the common bile duct), the cecum, the appendix, the ascending colon, and the proximal part of the transverse colon. Blood is supplied to these structures by the superior mesenteric artery. Omphaloceles, malrotations, and abnormalities of fixation occur when the midgut fails to return from the umbilical cord or fails to rotate appropriately.

The hindgut begins at the distal part of the transverse colon and extends through the descending and sigmoid colon, the rectum, and the superior portion of the anal canal. Hindgut derivatives are supplied by the inferior mesenteric artery.

### Anatomy and Growth

The gastrointestinal tract is a musculomembranous tube that stretches from the mouth to the anus. Accessory organs include the salivary glands, liver, and pancreas (Fig. 26–1).

The wall of the gastrointestinal tract contains a series of cellular layers. These layers are the epithelium (including glands), lamina propria, muscularis mucosae, submucosa (containing blood

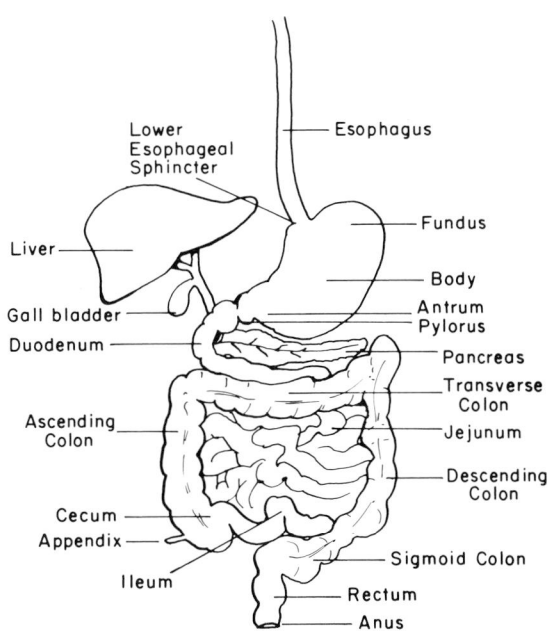

THE GASTROINTESTINAL TRACT

**Fig. 26–1.** Diagram of the major parts of the gastrointestinal tract.

vessels, nerves, lymphatics), muscularis externa, and serosa. The two nerve plexuses of the enteric nervous system lie within the submucosa and between the two muscle layers of the bowel, the circular and longitudinal layers of the muscularis externa.

The stomach is a food reservoir where digestion begins. Although its capacity is normally 1,000 to 1,500 ml, under unusual circumstances as much as 6,000 ml may be present. The area just below the lower esophageal sphincter is designated the cardia; the fundus is that portion of the stomach that continues lateral to and above the cardia, and the body extends from the cardia to the antrum, which stretches from the angulus to the pylorus. The antrum, which differs markedly from the remainder of the stomach in function, may be distinguished grossly by the absence of rugae as well as by its histologic appearance. The pylorus, a muscular sphincter between the stomach and the duodenum, controls gastric emptying and limits reflux of bile.

Gastric epithelium contains numerous glands lined by mucous cells, parietal (acid-producing) cells, and chief (pepsinogen-producing) cells. In the cardia and antrum, these glands contain predominantly mucous cells. Gastrin cells are located in the antral epithelium and have surface microvilli that monitor the intragastric pH. These cells secrete gastrin into the blood in response to rises in intragastric pH. Adjacent to gastrin-producing cells are D cells, which produce somatostatin and may modulate gastrin production.[10]

The pancreas is a triangular compound racemose gland lying deeply between the duodenum, bile duct, stomach, colon, and spleen. Pancreatic acini produce exocrine secretions that drain into a branching duct system and eventually into the duodenum to aid in primary digestion of food. Scattered throughout the pancreas are islets of Langerhans, which produce insulin, glucagon, somatostatin, and possibly other peptide hormones.

The liver is a large bilobular organ in the right upper abdomen. It receives 30% of its blood supply from the hepatic artery and the remainder from the portal vein that carries blood from the stomach, intestines, pancreas, and spleen. The liver is composed of microscopic lobules. In each lobule the blood flows from the hepatic artery and portal vein through sinusoids lined with cords of liver cells (hepatocytes) to central veins and eventually to hepatic veins that drain into the vena cava. The difference in oxygen and nutrient content in blood at the periportal areas versus that at the central vein areas accounts for certain differences in metabolic activity between the periportal and central lobular cells. Bile flows from the he-

patocyte through microscopic bile canaliculi to bile ductules and then along the biliary system to the duodenum.

The adult small intestine measures about 22 feet long at post mortem, though it may appear less than half that length at surgery. The jejunum is arbitrarily defined as the upper 40% and the ileum as the remainder. The epithelial lining of the small bowel has a far greater surface area than the muscle coat to which it is attached. This is the result of many invaginations (crypts) and projections (villi) as shown in Figure 26–2. Each villus has its own microscopic projections (microvilli), which in turn are covered by a fuzzy coat or glycocalyx containing many digestive enzymes. Several cell types have been identified within the intestinal mucosa, but their functions are incompletely established. The villus epithelial cells have digestive as well as absorptive function. Rapidly dividing cells at the base of the crypts are responsible for secretion, but as they migrate to the villus they mature into absorptive cells and are eventually extruded from the villus tip. Small intestinal cell turnover time (48 to 72 hours) is one of the most rapid of any tissue. Consequently, malnutrition and compounds (such as methotrexate[7]) that interfere with protein sythesis or cell replication may adversely affect intestinal function.

The colon is a large-diameter muscular organ that frames the small intestine. The vermiform appendix, which is attached to the cecum, contains specialized lymphatic structures. The epithelial surface of the normal colon is composed of absorptive cells that predominantly absorb water and electrolytes. Goblet (mucus-producing) cells line the glandular crypts. Endocrine cells are also present, but hormonal function as related to the colon is not well understood. The turnover time of colonic mucosa is three to eight days, substantially longer than that of the small intestine.

The gastrointestinal tract grows in length and caliber until somatic growth ceases after puberty. This visceral growth appears to be dependent upon the same general factors as somatic growth (nutritional adequacy, insulin, growth hormone, thyroid hormone, cortisol, androgens, and estrogens) as well as specified factors such as the direct effect of ingested nutrients, gastrointestinal hormones, and secretions.[11] The principal factors affecting the growth of the gastrointestinal mucosa are shown in Figure 26–3. Several of the hormones affecting growth, secretion, and contractility are shown in Table 26–2.

## Intestinal Immune System

Elements of the intestinal immune system include (1) lymphocytes scattered between the cells

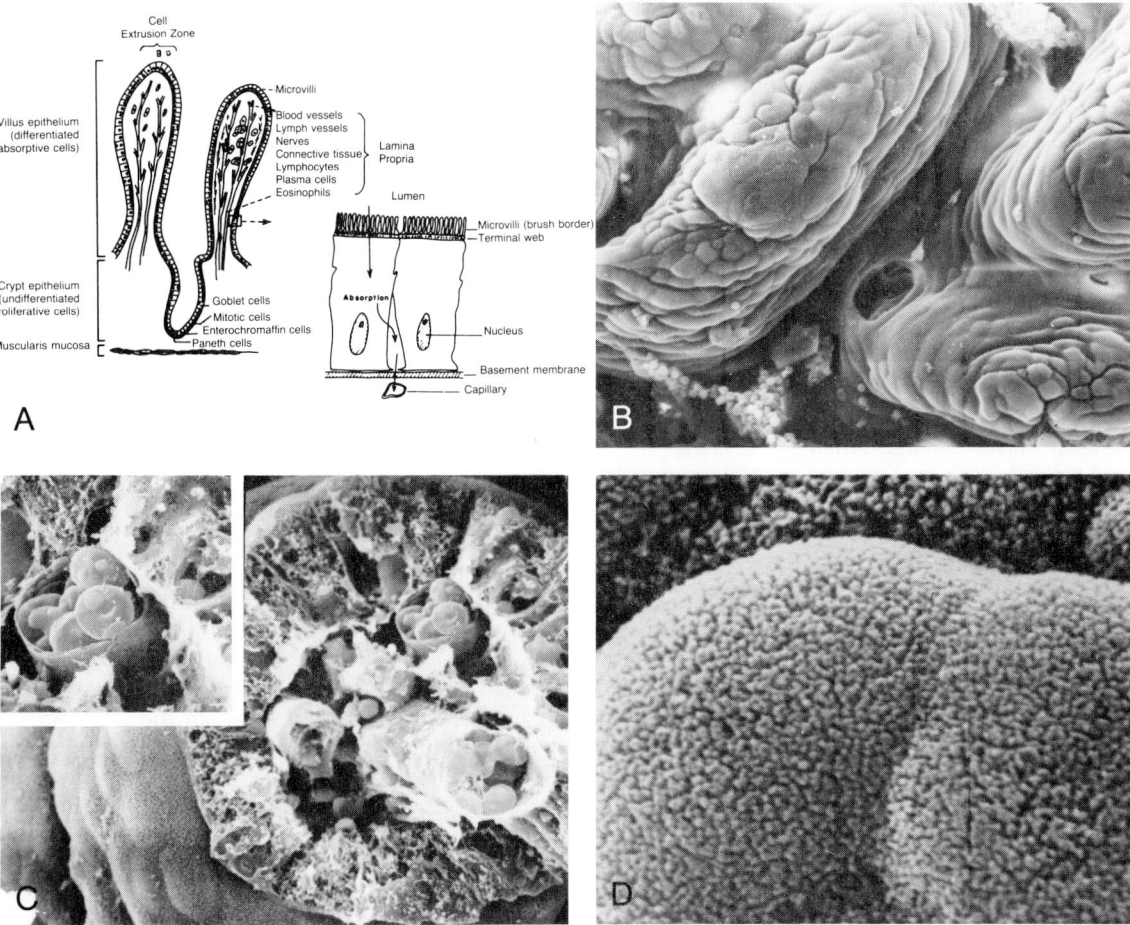

**Fig. 26–2.** *A*, Diagram of the functional units of the intestine (magnified about 1,000 ×) and two epithelial cells showing the brush border and primary direction of nutrient transport through the cell into the capillary. *B*, Scanning electron micrograph of jejunal villi with crypts (magnified about 1,000 ×) apparent between and at the base of the villi. *C*, Scanning electron micrograph of a jejunal villus tip fractured in a single plane to illustrate the structures of the lamina propria (magnified about 3,000 ×). The diagrams of the two epithelial cells shown in *A* are similar in size to the columnar cells viewed in *C*. The basolateral space demonstrated in *A* is apparent between several cells in *C*. Inside the villus, the lamina propria contains three tubular-appearing capillaries that can be identified because of the concave red cells within. The insert is a higher magnification (about 10,000 ×) of one capillary (containing red cells), showing the proximity of the adjacent basement membrane and intracellular space between two epithelial cells where the cellular nutrients are expelled en route to the adjacent capillary. *D*, Scanning electron micrograph of epithelial cell microvilli (magnified about 30,000 ×). (Reprinted with permission of Ross Laboratories, Columbus, OH 43216, from Developmental Nutrition.)

of the gastrointestinal epithelium, (2) lymphocytes and macrophages scattered diffusely in the lamina propria of the stomach and intestine, and (3) differentiated lymphoid structures located along the course of the gastrointestinal tract. The latter, which include the tonsils, the Peyer's patches, and the lymphoid structures of the appendix, are the initial site of interaction between many antigens and the immune system. The overlying epithelial surface contains T-lymphocytes, which appear to facilitate the binding and entry of antigens. Memory cells produced in response to antigens migrate to other parts of the body and the intestine via the general circulation. Re-ex-

posure to antigens leads to differentiation of these memory cells into plasma cells that produce type-specific IgA or IgE.[12]

Plasma cells in the lamina propria of the gut synthesize and secrete immunoglobulins including antibodies directed against antigens present in the gut lumen. Plasma cells produce IgA in contrast to other lymphoid tissues where IgG is the predominant immunoglobulin produced. IgA enters the intestinal lumen with two additional peptide chains: one of these, the secretory component, protects the IgA from luminal digestion; the second facilitates polymerization. Secretory IgA may prevent bacterial adherence to the mu-

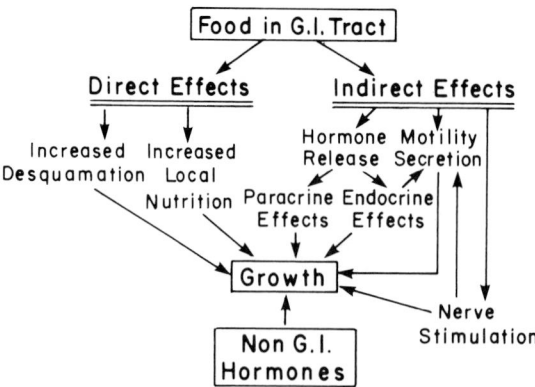

**Fig. 26–3.** Factors influencing growth of the gastrointestinal mucosa. (Redrawn from Johnson, L.R.[69])

cosal surfaces, but it does not appear to fix complement. Details of the immune system are discussed in Chapter 33.

## FUNCTIONS OF THE GASTROINTESTINAL TRACT

After ingestion, food is chewed and swallowed. Integrated motility and secretion subsequently enhance digestion and mucosal contact for ultimate absorption. Secretion and motility are subject to exogenous influences but are organized by primary autonomous intrinsic neurologic and hormonal systems.

### Neural and Hormonal Control of Intestinal Activity

The functions of eating and evacuation are controlled by the central nervous system through its somatic division and modulated by numerous hormonal interactions.

Autonomic innervation of the gastrointestinal tract (efferent sympathetic fibers arising from the ganglia of the sympathetic trunk and parasympathetic fibers in the vagus, pelvic, and splanch-

nic nerves) modifies motility and secretions but is not essential for coordinated function. The usual autonomic neurotransmitters appear to have only a limited role in the intrinsic nervous system of the gut, which is maintained primarily by a different set of transmitters described subsequently.

The enteric nervous system (ENS) contains over 108 neurons in humans (roughly equivalent to all the neurons in the spinal cord).[13,14] The physiologic independence of the enteric nervous system was described with considerable precision by Bayliss and Starling in 1899.[15] The ENS contains sensory receptors, primary afferent neurons, interneurons to carry reflexes, and motor neurons to relax or excite smooth muscle. Loss of certain intrinsic components of the enteric nervous system, as is seen in Hirschsprung's or Chagas' diseases, is associated with functional obstruction and proximal dilatation. Propulsive movement of the bowel thus depends on local reflex activity mediated by ganglia of the ENS.

The ENS is composed of two interconnected ganglionated plexuses (neuroglial sheaths) lying in the submucosa and between the longitudinal and circular muscle layers. Nerve endings and muscle fibers are widely separate with consequent nondiscrete control—the gut does not twitch but shows broad regional responses. Putative neurotransmitters (in addition to catecholamines and acetylcholine) include serotonin,[16] purines,[17] VIP,[18] substance P,[19] somatostatin,[20] encephalins,[21] bombesin,[22] pancreatic polypeptide, and neurotensin.[23] Acetylcholine appears to act as an excitatory transmitter between vagal fibers and enteric neurons, between enteric interneurons, and between enteric neurons and intestinal smooth muscle. Intestinal motility is thus vulnerable to interruption by ganglion-blocking agents such as hexamethonium and by muscarinic antagonists such as atropine. Noradrenergic in-

**Table 26–2.    Principal Peptide Hormones From Gut**

| | | Main Function | | |
|---|---|---|---|---|
| Peptide | Location | Hypertrophy-Hyperplasia | Secretion | Contractility |
| Gastrin | Pyloric antrum | ↑ | ↑ gastric acid | 0 |
| Secretin | Upper small intestine | ↓ | ↑ bicarbonate | 0 |
| Enteroglucagon | Lower small intestine, colon | ↑ (?) | 0 | ↓ |
| VIP* | Pancreas | 0 | ↑ | 0 |
| GIP* | Upper small intestine | ↑ (?) | ↓ | 0 |
| Motilin | Upper small intestine | 0 | 0 | ↑ |
| Somatostatin | Throughout | 0 | ↓ | 0 |
| PP* | Pancreas | 0 | ↓ (?) | 0 |
| Bombesin | Throughout | 0 | ↑ (?) | ↑ (?) |
| Neurotensin | Lower small intestine | ? | ? | ? |
| CCK | Upper small intestine | ↑ (?) | ↑ | 0 |

*VIP = vasoactive intestinal peptide; GIP = gastrone; PP = pancreatic polypeptide; CCK = cholecystokinin nervation is concentrated at the periphery of the myenteric and submucosal plexuses, although sympathetic axons may directly activate neuroendocrine cells and affect absorption. Norepinephrine inhibits gastrointestinal motility by direct beta and indirect alpha actions. More powerful than sympathetic inhibition of gastrointestinal motility is the inhibition mediated by the ENS. This inhibition is unrelated to norepinephrine, but a specific ENS neurotransmitter has not yet been identified. Candidates include adenosine triphosphate (ATP) and VIP, both of which cause gut relaxation.

Many different types of endocrine cells are found in the epithelial lining of the gastrointestinal tract.[24] These cells characteristically have villi on the luminal surface, and contain secretory granules that can be released and cross the basolateral membrane. Their contents may then act locally or be transported to targets by the systemic circulation (see Table 26–1).

### Integration of Control of Motility

As described previously, many potential agents are involved in the control of intestinal motility. These mechanisms appear to act in concert to produce the various patterns of contractility seen in intact humans. Figure 26–4 illustrates the integration of the controlling influences on intestinal motility.

The primary unit of contractile activity is the smooth muscle cell. This unit can contract on its own and in a regular fashion. At least two other factors can modulate these intrinsic contractions, namely, circulating and locally released chemicals or "hormones," and neurotransmitters from either intrinsic or extrinsic neural fibers. Each system is capable of either excitatory or inhibitory influences to produce various patterns of contractions. Thus, the classification of motility into only two distinct types, segmental and propulsive, does not cover the wide spectrum of motility patterns of which the intestine is capable. On the other hand, the complexities of this system and its overall control are so poorly understood that the simplistic classification continues to serve as

a practical approach to evaluation of clinical problems relating to gastrointestinal motility.

Esophageal motor contractions begin at the upper end of the esophagus with each conscious swallow and travel toward the lower esophageal sphincter. A second wave of spontaneous peristalsis usually follows if the primary wave fails to empty the esophagus. The lower esophageal sphincter (LES) relaxes to allow the bolus of food to pass.

Although the resting pressure in the body of the esophagus is lower than that of the stomach, reflux of gastric contents, even in the head-down position, is prevented by the higher resting pressure of the LES, which only relaxes to allow a food bolus to pass. The LES appears to be subject to the influence of the vagus nerve, neurohormonal agents (gastrin, secretin, and other gastrointestinal hormones), and prostaglandins, although their exact physiologic roles are uncertain.

Gastric motility is coordinated by the enteric nervous system but is sensitive to vagal and hormonal factors. Gastric emptying depends upon antral motility, proximal gastric tone, pyloric resistance, and the consistency of the gastric contents. These factors are further modified by duodenal feedback (to protect against volume, tonicity, irritant, or pH overload) and gastric distention. The stomach normally empties exponentially at around 3%/min. Gastric emptying of fluid can be influenced by several conditions, some of which are listed in Table 26–3. In the fasting state, infrequent migrating motor complexes (peristaltic waves) originate in the gastric antrum or upper small intestine and travel down the small intestine, clearing secretions and sloughed cells. This activity aborts in the fed state (but not with total parenteral nutrition) and is replaced by irregular bursts of contractions (segmentation and peristalsis) interspersed with transient quiescence.

In the small intestine, rhythmic segmentation is weaker than peristalsis, but it occurs more frequently. Segments become ballooned between contraction rings, facilitating mixing and increasing lymph flow. These segmentations occur 10 to 12 times/min in the duodenum with a progressive

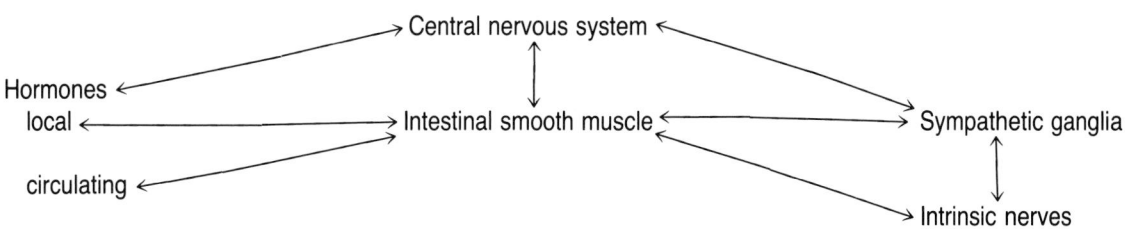

**Fig. 26–4.** Control of intestinal motility.

**Table 26–3.    Factors Determining the Rate of Gastric Emptying**

| Decrease Emptying | Increase Emptying |
|---|---|
| Foods | Foods |
| Fats > protein > carbohydrate | In Stomach |
| Thicker consistency (solids > liquids) |    Liquids |
| High osmolality > 800 mosm/L |      Change in temperature |
| | In Duodenum |
| |    High osmolality |
| |    High volume |
| |    Low pH |
| |    Irritant |
| Drugs | Drugs |
| Anticholinergics | Cholinergics |
| Ganglion blockers | Metoclopramide |
| GI Hormones | GI Hormones |
| Secretin | Gastrin |
| Cholecystokinin | Motilin |
| Glucagon | |
| Diseases or Surgery | Diseases or Surgery |
| Vagotomy | "Irritable colon" |
| Pseudo-obstruction | Pyloroplasty |
| Diabetic neuropathy | Partial gastrectomy |
| Autonomic neuropathy | |
| Scleroderma | |
| Mechanical | Mechanical |
| Peptic ulcer | Gravity |
| Extrinsic pressure | Gastric distention |

decrease in rate to 6 to 8/min in the terminal ileum. These segmental contractions are mediated by the myenteric plexus. Peristaltic contraction waves (which may be preceded by a relaxation wave) travel aborally for only a few centimeters. Their speed is faster in the proximal than in the terminal intestine. Peristalsis is dependent on the myenteric plexus and is abolished by atropine, removal of the mucosa, or plexus degeneration.

Motor activity (both peristalsis and segmentation) increases with entry of chyme into the duodenum, gastric distention, mucosal irritation, and intestinal distention. The latter produces powerful peristaltic rushes.

Colonic contractions are either mixing or propulsive. Mixing movements are segmental contractions of 10 to 60 seconds duration found in the cecum, colon, and rectum. Propulsive contractions are most frequent in the midtransverse colon, and their net effect is to move colonic contents toward the rectum. Propulsion, which occurs several times daily, especially postprandially, is preceded by loss of segmental contractions. Eating produces an increase in the amplitude and frequency of colonic propulsive movement. Colonic movements are coordinated by intrinsic enteric nerves, but are subject to autonomic modulation, which can be blocked by anticholinergic drugs and increased by opiates.

Anal continence is maintained by cortical suppression of the urge to defecate that comes with rectal stimulation. When colonic contents pass into the rectum, cortical perception of rectal distention produces contraction of the external anal sphincter to counteract reflex relaxation of the internal sphincter. If defecation is convenient, the external anal sphincter relaxes, the glottis closes, the diaphragm and abdominal muscles contract, and the increased intra-abdominal pressure leads to evacuation of feces.

## Membrane Transport

Substances are transported across the epithelial membranes by either passive (through electrochemical gradients) or active transport (energy-dependent mechanisms). The rate of diffusional transport depends on both size and fat solubility of the substrate. Carrier mediation increases the transport capabilities of some substrates.[25]

**Passive Transport.** The permeability of the gastrointestinal mucosa primarily governs passive transport. The principal force driving this passive transport of solutes, as well as water, is the electrochemical or concentration gradient across the gastrointestinal mucosa.[26] Because the membranes are composed of a lipid layer sandwiched between two protein layers, lipid solubility also plays a facilitative role in passive solute transport.

Movement of electrically charged particles through membranes presents special problems. These charged particles are generally fat-insoluble and can permeate the membrane only through aqueous channels. The passive distribution of charged particles across the membrane depends on the prevailing chemical and electrical difference.[27] The rate of passive solute transport depends on the size as well as the charge of the aqueous channels. The size of the channels ranges from about 15 nm in the jejunum to only 4 nm in the less permeable colon. The net charge in the channels depends on the ratio of carboxyl to amino groups. For example, the anionic carboxyl groups outnumber the cationic amino groups in the gallbladder, giving the channels a net negative charge. This makes the gallbladder more permeable to cations because opposite charges attract one another. In the stomach the reverse is true.

Another characteristic of the gastrointestinal tract is the variability of the microenvironment immediately adjacent to the luminal membrane. This fluid layer is not identical to the fluid in the middle of the lumen. Since no amount of peristaltic movement can affect this layer, it has been termed the "unstirred layer." Its presence has two important consequences: (1) Since it is aqueous, it comprises the principal diffusion barrier for lipid absorption. (2) Owing to the acidic groups in the glycocalyx, the lower pH of the layer influences absorption of weak electrolytes, including many drugs.[28]

Finally, in considering passive transport in the gastrointestinal tract, permeability paths between the epithelial cells must be discussed. These intercellular or paracellular "shunt" pathways are mainly of importance to small electrolytes and water. The protein cement of cellular junctions serves as an alternate channel for passive diffusion. In the ileum, about four times as much water and electrolytes traverse the paracellular pathways as cross the cellular membranes, and the gallbladder is an even looser epithelium, having a paracellular shunt 20 times that of the transcellular pathway.

In summary, many factors influence the permeability and therefore passive transport of water and substrate across the gastrointestinal epithelium. These factors are illustrated in Figure 26–5.

**Active Transport.** Active transport is distinguished by the interaction of the permeating substance with one of the protein components of the membrane. This interaction has all the characteristics of the interaction between an enzyme and substrate: i.e., the reaction is saturable, shows competition between structurally similar substrates, has specificity to stereoisomers of substrates, and is inhibited by metabolic poisons. Thus, the "carrier" protein that shuttles substrate from one side of the membrane to another may be considered a specialized membrane enzyme. This class of transport is termed "carrier-mediated" transport.

Carrier-mediated transport serves the needs of the gastrointestinal cell by allowing larger, water-soluble substances to cross the membrane. It can allow essential substrates to move against the prevailing diffusional forces of chemical and electrical differences.[27]

If mediated transport utilizes energy and operates the uphill shuttle across the membrane, it is termed "active" transport. The metabolic energy for this active movement of substances across the membrane is adenosine triphosphate (ATP). The release of energy is provided by an ATPase that hydrolyzes the terminal phosphate from ATP to form adenosine diphosphate (ADP). Thus, each active transport process is driven by the activity of membrane ATPase.[28] The ATPases are not necessarily specific for that substance being transported. For example, the active transport of sugars and amino acids lacks specific ATPases, and their active transfer comes about by specific coupling to the active transport of Na+. Thus, the carrier protein for sugars and amino acids has specific sites for glucose (or amino acids) and also for Na+. The binding of both Na+ and sugars or Na+ and amino acids occurs on the luminal side of the membrane where they then diffuse to the intracellular side for release.[29,30] This process does not require energy and is termed facilitated diffusion.

The requirements for metabolic energy mentioned previously occur at the opposite side of the cell at the basolateral membrane. Here, another

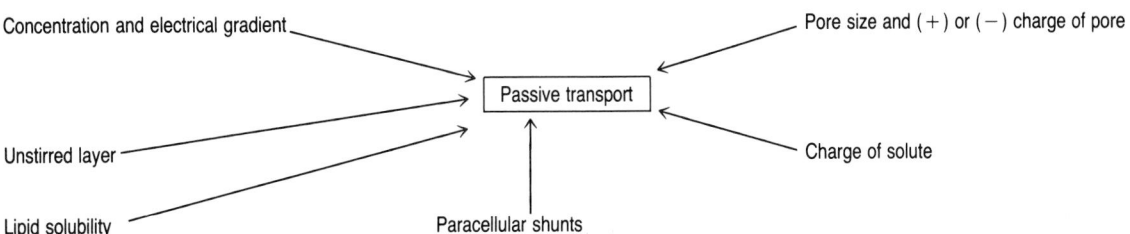

**Fig. 26–5.** Factors that influence the permeability and passive transport of water and substrate across the gastrointestinal epithelium.

carrier protein with a binding site for Na +, but not for sugar or amino acid, binds to the Na +. After binding Na +, this carrier protein is acted upon by ATPase, releasing metabolic energy so that Na + transfer out of the cell occurs against a concentration gradient (Figure 26–6).

Virtually all substances enter or leave the cells of the gastrointestinal tract partly or wholly by simple passive transport. Most classes of substances are transported in the absence of sodium coupling, and several are transported in more than one way. The various types of transport utilized in transfer across the intestinal membranes are listed in Table 26–4.

This table demonstrates that whole proteins may be transported by pinocytosis. This process may be important in the absorption of small amounts of immunoglobulins from breast milk. This process requires energy and is classified as active.

## Secretion

Secretions entering the gastrointestinal tract contain electrolytes, bile salts, digestive enzymes, antibodies, and other organic molecules. Table 26–5 lists mean concentrations of major electrolytes in these secretions. Normal adults ingest about 1 to 2 L of fluid and secrete an additional 6 to 10 L of fluid into the gastrointestinal tract daily. Since only about 1 L leaves the small intestine for the colon, the small intestine absorbs 200 to 400 ml of water per hour with a maximum rate of about 700 ml per hour. With a normal meal of 645 ml of food, the volume increases to about 1,500 ml by midduodenum, decreases to 750 ml by midjejunum, and is only 250 ml in the lower small bowel. The colon absorbs additional fluid

so that only about 75 ml, or 10% of the original intake, is excreted.

Saliva functions to moisten the mouth, maintaining oral hygiene. It contains thiocyanate and lysozyme, both of which are strongly bactericidal. Saliva is an effective buffer that contains calcium to minimize calcium loss from teeth. It also contains an amylase and hormones such as epidermal growth factor, nerve growth factor, and somatostatin. Secretion of saliva is controlled by conditioned cortical reflexes (made famous by Pavlov) and nonconditioned oral and gastrointestinal reflexes.

Gastric secretions contain acid, pepsins (proteolytic enzymes), mucus, and intrinsic factor. The parietal cell is responsible for secretion of hydrogen ion at concentrations of about 4 million times that of plasma (the highest ion gradient known in physiology). Three substances in the body are capable of acting directly on the parietal cell to increase acid secretion. These substances are acetylcholine (from the vagus nerve), histamine, and gastrin.[31] Histamine is abundant in mast-like cells of the lamina propria of the oxyntic gastric mucosa and, after release, diffuses into adjacent parietal cells. Its role in physiologic control of acid secretion is uncertain, although the introduction of an H2 antagonist, such as cimetidine, suggests it may play an important physiologic role in acid secretion. Cimetidine also inhibits the response to gastrin,[32] as do the cholinomimetics.[33] Table 26–6 summarizes several modulating effects of agents affecting gastric acid secretion. Secretin, cholecystokinin, and motilin may also play a modulating role in acid secretion.

Pepsins are principally secreted by cells in the acid-secreting part of the stomach. Somatostatin and glucose-dependent insulin-releasing peptide (GIP) reduce pepsin secretion. Mucoproteins pro-

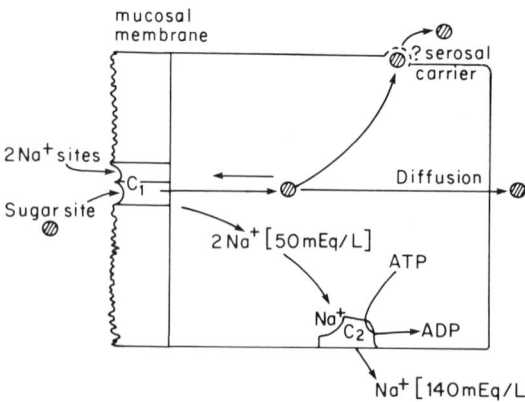

**Fig. 26–6.** Diagram of the proposed mechanism of sodium-coupled, active transport mechanism. C1 = carrier 1 for coupled transport into the cell; C2 = carrier 2 for transport of sodium out of the cell.

**Table 26–4. Types of Transport Used in Transfer Across Intestinal Membranes**

| Passive Transport | Active Transport |
|---|---|
| *Simple* | *Active* |
| Water | Electrolytes |
| Fats | Sugars |
| Drugs | Amino acids |
| Electrolytes | Dipeptides |
| Sugars | Vitamins |
| Amino acids | Bile acids |
| Vitamins | *Coupled Active* |
| Sterols | Electrolytes |
| *Facilitated* | Sugars |
| Sugars | Amino acids |
| Amino acids | Vitamins |
| Electrolytes | *Pinocytosis* |
| | Proteins |

**Table 26–5.  Electrolyte Characteristics of Enteric Secretions**

| Organ | Volume* ml/24h | H+ meq/hr | Fluid Na+ meq/L | K+ meq/L | Ca++ meq/L | Cl- meq/L | HCO3- meq/L |
|---|---|---|---|---|---|---|---|
| Saliva | 1,200 | — | 10 | 26 | 2 | 10 | 8 |
| Stomach† | 1,500 | 2 (basal)<br>17 (peak) | 150 | 15 | 2 | 130 | — |
| Pancreas† | 1,500 | — | 157 | 7.0 | 4 | 50 | 110 |
| Bile§ | 1,000 | — | 146 | 5.0 | 4 | 110 | 46 |
| Duodenum and small bowel‖ | 4,000 | — | 140# | 6.3 | 3 | 100 | 17 |
| Stool | 125 | — | 25 | 60 | 1 | 20 | 3 |

*Unstimulated volume. Total volume of GI secretions may be as little as 200 ml in the nonfed state or as high as 1,700 ml with hormonal stimulation.
†Stimulated by histamine. Data from Hunt, J.N.: Physiol. Rev. *491,* 1959 and Trudeau, W.L., McGuigan, J.E.: New Engl. J. Med. *284*:408, 1971.
‡Data from Swanson, C.H., Soloman, A.K.: J. Gen. Physiol. *62*:407, 1973.
§Data from Erlinger, S.: *In* The Liver Biopsy and Pathobiology. New York, Raven Press, 1982, p. 407.
‖Data from Krejs, G.J., Fortran, J.S.: *In* Gastrointestinal Disease. Philadelphia, W.B. Saunders Co., 1978, p. 297.
#This value for Na+ is higher than that generally given by others (see Chap. 4).

duced by the neck cells of the gastric glands provide a lubricant and mucosal buffer. Mucus secretion is increased by food, acid, and ethanol in the stomach and by vagal and sympathetic stimulation.

Intragastric food, especially protein breakdown products, promotes secretion of gastric juice. This effect is partly mediated by the local intrinsic plexus but predominantly through the dorsal motor nucleus of the vagus. Gastrin is the major factor stimulating gastric acid release; its release in response to food is not blocked by atropine or vagotomy. In response to intragastric food, acid secretion occurs at a rate of approximately 200 ml/hour for 2 to 3 hours.

Within the small intestine, the crypts of Lieberkühn produce small intestinal juice that contains electrolytes, bicarbonate, mucus, traces of brush border enzymes, and other contents of shed cells. Secretion of water and electrolytes is mediated by cyclic AMP. Cholera enterotoxin, by stimulating production of cyclic AMP, increases sodium and water excretion through its action on the NaCl pump at the cell-lumen interface. Other hormones that increase intestinal secretions are prostaglandins, calcitonin, and ADH, as well as the intestinal hormones listed in Table 26–2.

Bile is an isotonic fluid that is concentrated in the gallbladder and is released after stimulation by cholecystokinin (CCK). It contains bile salts, lecithin, cholesterol, and electrolytes.

Pancreatic secretions contain enzymes, bicarbonate, and electrolytes. The enzymes are responsible for digestion of protein, carbohydrate, lipids, and nucleic acids. They are secreted in an inactive form and activated in the duodenum, mostly by trypsin. Enterokinase from intestinal brush border activates trypsinogen to its active enzyme, trypsin. Trypsin inhibitors present in acinar cells and ducts adsorb and inactivate free trypsin.

A cephalic phase of pancreatic secretion (prior to the ingestion of food) results in direct vagal stimulation of pancreatic enzyme secretion without increased flow. This process fills the duct system with a viscous enzyme-rich fluid. As gastric juice enters the duodenum, acidity stimulates the release of secretin from the intestinal mucosa. This process promotes an increase in volume and bicarbonate output. Intraduodenal protein (or protein components), fat, carbohydrate, and luminal distention all stimulate release of CCK, which stimulates further secretion of enzymes. Pancreatic secretions are suppressed by intravenous administration of amino acids and dextrose. Less stimulation occurs with intraduodenal free amino acids than with peptides or intact protein. Thus,

**Table 26–6.  Factors Modulating the Primary Agents Increasing Gastric Secretion**

| Modulator | Acetylcholine (Vagal Stimulus) | Histamine | Gastrin |
|---|---|---|---|
| Atropine | decrease | 0 | 0 |
| Calcium | increase | 0 | 0 |
| Lanthanum | decrease | 0 | 0 |
| Cimetidine | mild decrease[33] | decrease | mild decrease[32] |
| PGE2 | 0 | decrease | 0 |

parenteral nutrition or the administration of a formula containing low fat, high carbohydrate, and amino acids may provide less stimulus to pancreatic secretion than food or a defined formula with intact or hydrolyzed protein and fat. This finding may be important in management of patients with pancreatitis. Intragastric feeding provokes acid secretion and, through secretin, increases the volume and bicarbonate output. Small bowel distention also activates the pancreas by vagovagal reflex.

### Digestion of Carbohydrates, Proteins, and Lipids

Secretions from the mouth, stomach, small intestine, liver, and pancreas are mixed with food. Complex molecules are consequently hydrolyzed to simple components that can then be absorbed.

**Carbohydrate.** The chief dietary forms of carbohydrate are polysaccharides (starches and components of dietary fiber), disaccharides (sucrose and lactose), and monosaccharides (glucose and fructose). Digestion and absorption of carbohydrate occur in the mouth, stomach, and small intestine[34-38] as illustrated in Figure 26–7A. In addition, carbohydrates not absorbed in the small bowel may be degraded by colonic bacteria. Although this process may provide substantial calories to some animal species, bacterial fermentation appears to provide an insignificant energy source for humans.

Simple sugars (glucose, fructose, galactose) are absorbed by carrier-mediated saturable processes.[36,37] Deficiency of the brush-border enzymes may result in carbohydrate malabsorption. The resulting diarrhea is often accompanied by flatulence due to bacterial fermentation of unabsorbed disaccharides in the cecum, producing gas and osmotically active particles.[39] Dietary fiber, which is predominantly composed of carbohydrate, is resistant to human digestive enzymes but is broken down by bacteria, resulting in increased stool volume and stool water. If fiber is consumed in excess, diarrhea with flatulence results.

**Protein.** Digestion of protein occurs in the stomach and small intestine, and the final products are amino acids and di- and tripeptides (Fig. 26–7B). In the stomach, activated pepsins hydrolyze protein to polypeptides of diverse size. Within the small intestine, pancreatic endopeptidases (trypsin, chymotrypsin, and elastase) split peptide bonds within the protein to produce smaller peptides. Exopeptidases (carboxypeptidase A and B) cleave the terminal bonds of large peptides to produce single amino acids and peptide fragments. These enzymes have an optimum pH of 8.0, and hypersecretion of gastric acid (as with the Zollin-

ger-Ellison syndrome) may impair their function. Brush-border and cytosolic peptidases hydrolyze small peptides to produce amino acids.

**Lipids.** The chief forms of dietary lipid are triglycerides, phospholipids, cholesterol, and cholesterol esters (Fig. 26–7C). Pharyngeal lipase hydrolyzes some triglyceride intragastrically to fatty acids and diglycerides. Within the small intestine, pancreatic lipase continues this hydrolysis to produce free fatty acids and glycerol. Co-lipase is a pancreatic polypeptide that acts as cofactor for pancreatic lipase, improving its activity in the presence of bile salts. An intestinal lipase has also been identified, but its precise function is uncertain. Bile salts, which have both hydrophilic and hydrophobic ends, form micelles, which have an external hydrophilic layer and are water-soluble. This process facilitates the absorption of their fat-soluble contents (fatty acids, cholesterol, fat-soluble vitamins). Triglycerides containing fatty acids of less than 12 carbons can be absorbed directly without undergoing hydrolysis, although this may not be quantitatively important since infants with lipase–co-lipase deficiency respond less well to medium-chain triglyceride formulas than to pancreatic enzyme extracts.

### Absorptive Function of the Gastrointestinal Tract

Glucose, ethanol, aspirin, and water can be absorbed from the oral and gastric mucosa. However, absorption of nutrients and most drugs occurs primarily in the small intestine. The colon absorbs principally water and electrolytes. A descending gradient of absorption exists for most nutrients, with most absorption occurring in the first four feet of intestine in normal adult humans. Substances actively transported are absorbed mainly in the jejunum.

**Absorption of Carbohydrate.** As discussed earlier, sodium entering from the luminal side of the cell provides the driving force for carbohydrate transfer.[34-38] Glucose is thus cotransported into the cell against a concentration gradient (see Fig. 26–6). Glucose freed from the carrier complex accumulates in the cell and establishes a concentration gradient for facilitated diffusion across the basolateral membrane into the intracellular spaces and ultimately the blood. Other water-soluble organic substrates that are transported by similar $Na^+$-dependent gradient coupling include amino acids, di- and tripeptides, ascorbic acid, sulfate and phosphate, bile salts, bilirubin, and riboflavin.[40-43] This transport mechanism appears to be ubiquitous throughout the animal and plant kingdoms. Amino acids and glucose reciprocally inhibit absorption of one another by competing

# CARBOHYDRATE DIGESTION

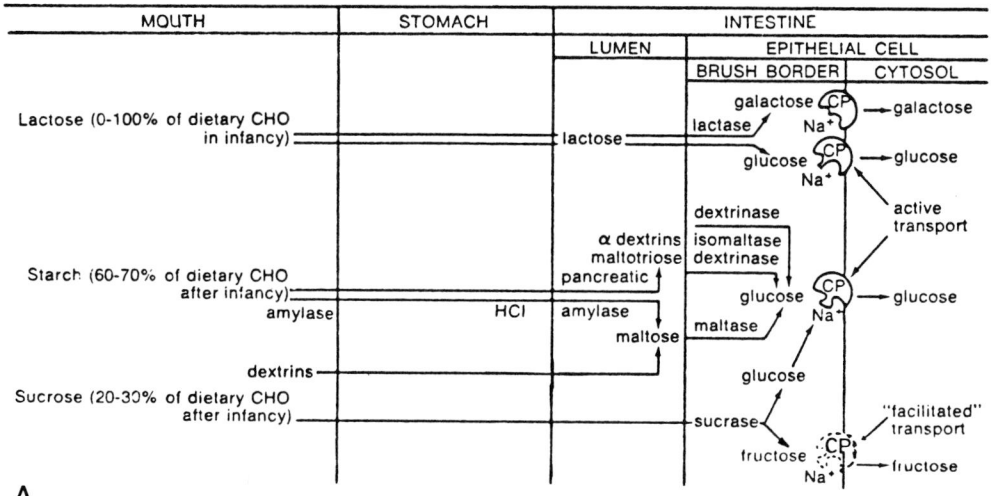

A

# PROTEIN DIGESTION

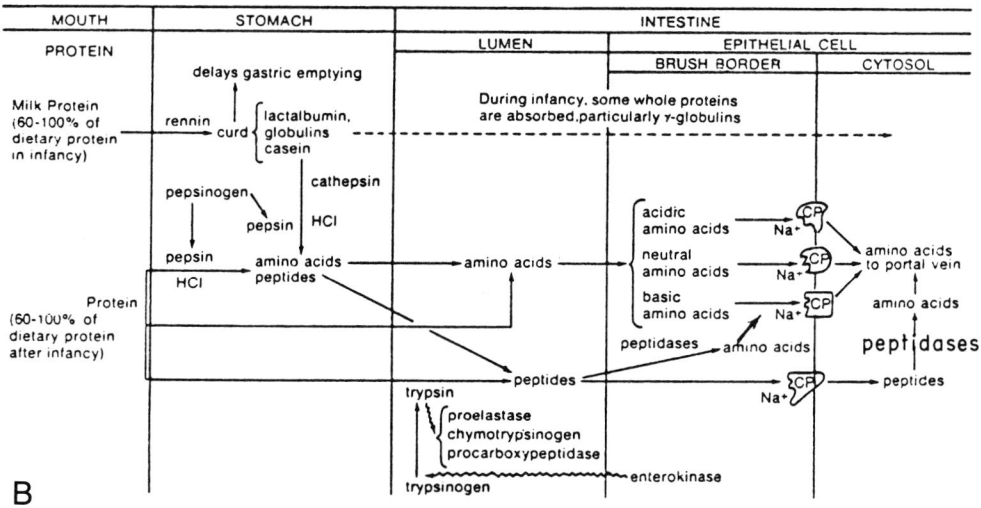

B

# LIPID DIGESTION

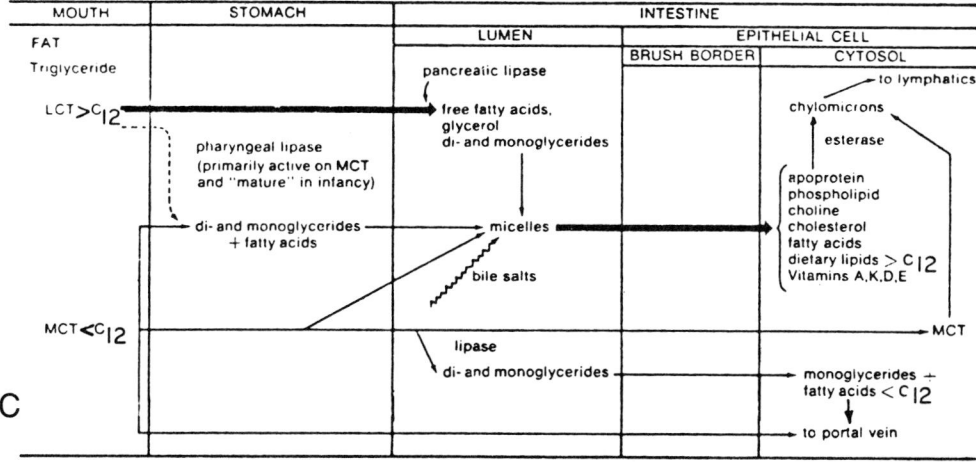

C

**Fig. 26–7.**  Schema of carbohydrate, protein, and lipid digestion. (CP = carrier protein.) (Reprinted with permission of Ross Laboratories, Columbus, OH 43216, from Developmental Nutrition.)

for a limited supply of energy from this electro-chemical gradient. An increase in the luminal concentration of $Na^+$ results in improved absorption of glucose and amino acids and vice versa. Knowledge of this phenomenon has led to the use of sodium-glucose solutions to aid in the management of patients with cholera or acute diarrheal syndromes.

**Absorption of Peptides and Amino Acids.** As described with absorption of glucose, amino acid absorption is a sodium-dependent, carrier-mediated, and saturable process. Di- and, to some extent, tripeptides may be absorbed intact. Cytoplasmic peptidases hydrolyze the di- and tripeptides and limit the amount of dietary protein reaching the liver as anything but amino acids. Single amino acids are transported across the basolateral membrane by both simple passive diffusion and carrier-mediated diffusion (see Fig. 26–6).

**Absorption of Fat.** Fat absorption is generally a passive process,[43–46] although fatty acids or triglycerides with less than 12 carbon atoms (short- and medium-chain triglycerides) can pass directly into the portal blood. Long-chain fat (more than 12 carbon atoms) requires digestion to fatty acids and monoglycerides for micellar solubilization and efficient absorption. Bile and pancreatic enzymes greatly facilitate fat absorption, but brush-border lipase and simple diffusion in a healthy intestine allow absorption of a considerable proportion of ingested fat. This absorptive fraction is relatively unaffected by the total amount ingested; under usual circumstances, the more fat ingested, the more will be absorbed. Unsaturated fats are more readily absorbed than saturated fats. Within the enterocyte, fatty acids and other lipid particles from within the micelle are packaged and released into lymphatics as chylomicrons.[47,48]

**Absorption of Water and Ions.** The $Na^+$ -$K^+$ ATPase-dependent pump located on the basolateral membrane extrudes $Na^+$ and thus maintains intracellular electronegativity.[49] Sodium is absorbed passively by diffusion from luminal chyme into enterocytes along an electrochemical gradient, and chloride follows passively. A small amount of $Cl^-$ is actively reabsorbed in exchange for excreted $HCO_3^-$.[50] This process occurs mainly in the lower ileum and large intestine. Intracellular sodium is actively transported into the extracellular space. Water moves passively according to the prevailing osmotic gradient and follows sodium into the extracellular space. Chyme remains isotonic during its passage through the small and large intestine. Sudden delivery of large volumes of hypertonic fluids into the small intestine results in a rapid water flux *into* the lumen,

which may produce circulating hypovolemia and the dumping syndrome. As the water and sodium move into the extracellular space, the hydrostatic pressure increases and flow occurs into the lymphatics and capillaries of the villi.[51]

Calcium is most actively absorbed in the duodenum. The low relative efficiency of this process (30%) is increased by 1,25-dihydroxycholecalciferol (calcitriol). Passive absorption also occurs in the jejunum and ileum. Absorption is impaired by multiple luminal factors and by high levels of circulating cortisol, thyroxine, and estrogen. Absorption is facilitated by parathormone, hypocalcemia, and increased duodenal acidity. See Chapters 5 and 13 for details of calcium metabolism.

**Absorption of Water-Soluble Vitamins.** Water-soluble vitamins are predominantly absorbed passively and are carrier-mediated at physiologic intakes. Some studies suggest that ascorbate,[52,53] riboflavin,[54] and thiamine[55] are absorbed by sodium-dependent mechanisms. Folate polyglutamate is hydrolyzed by zinc-dependent intestinal brush-border conjugase from dietary polyglutamates to monoglutamate before absorption. Absorption proceeds by a pH-dependent, active-carrier mediated process, predominantly in the jejunum.[56,57] Absorption is reduced during intestinal damage, folate deficiency, or vitamin $B_{12}$ deficiency by ethanol, sulfasalazine, and phenytoin.[58,59]

Vitamin $B_{12}$ is absorbed with approximately 10% efficiency. It initially binds to R protein (present in saliva and gastric juice) from which it is separated by pancreatic enzymes in the duodenum.[57] Free $B_{12}$ then binds to intrinsic factor (IF) released from gastric mucosa.[60] Intrinsic factor facilitates active $B_{12}$ absorption at specific sites on the brush border of cells in the distal ileum. Approximately 99% of B12-IF absorption occurs in the distal ileum, and passive absorption in the jejunum and proximal ileum accounts for only 1% of absorption. Impaired absorption and clinical deficiency may occur following gastric resection or atrophy (resulting in loss of intrinsic factor), small intestinal bacterial or parasitic overgrowth (resulting in consumption of the ingested $B_{12}$), pancreatic exocrine failure, or terminal ileal disease (regional enteritis, ileal resection, or congenital absence of ileal $B_{12}$ and IF receptors). Large oral doses of vitamin $B_{12}$ may allow adequate absorption in the absence of intrinsic factor or in the presence of terminal ileal disease, although parenteral therapy is usually preferred. Selective familial vitamin $B_{12}$ malabsorption has been described, but the specific defect has not been clearly defined.[61]

**Absorption of Fat-Soluble Vitamins.** The absorption of fat-soluble vitamins parallels the absorption of fat, although only about 50% of the ingested dose is generally retained.[62] These lipid-soluble molecules are absorbed in micelles and leave the intestine in chylomicrons. Vitamin K absorption is facilitated by a bile salt–dependent luminal esterase of pancreatic origin, making vitamin K deficiency common in bile salt deficiency syndromes such as biliary atresia.[63,64] Absorption of fat-soluble vitamins is impaired in any disease producing fat malabsorption such as pancreatic insufficiency, cholestasis, or nonspecific malabsorption, as seen with bacterial overgrowth or gluten-sensitive enteropathy.

**Absorption of Trace Elements.** Absorption of iron occurs predominantly in the duodenum. Absorption is passive and relatively inefficient with only 5 to 15% of ingested iron absorbed. Absorption is subject to modification by luminal agents and to mucosal influences, including reduced iron stores, active erythropoiesis, and idiopathic hemochromatosis. Iron is best absorbed as heme (organic) iron, although the inorganic ferrous ion is also well absorbed.

Zinc is absorbed by facilitated diffusion throughout the small intestine with an efficiency of 20 to 40%. Organic zinc is better absorbed than inorganic zinc, and the latter is more sensitive to interference by luminal factors such as phytates, dietary fiber, phosphate, other cations, and products of the Maillard reactions.[65] The absorption of zinc is facilitated by zinc-binding ligands found in human milk and in pancreatic secretions.[66] Although 1 to 2 mg of zinc may be secreted via the pancreas each day, it is reabsorbed by the small bowel. Patients with malabsorptive diseases are prone to zinc deficiency. If the malabsorption is due to exocrine pancreatic failure, however, clinical signs of zinc deficiency are uncommon. This phenomenon is possibly due to simultaneous decrease in zinc output by the pancreas. During zinc absorption, the intestinal cell retains a large amount of the absorbed zinc, which is bound to an intracellular protein, metallothioneine. This bound zinc is eventually sloughed with the cell and lost in the feces. Metallothioneine may, therefore, contribute to the regulation of absorption or retention of zinc, as well as other cations such as copper.[67]

Little is known about absorption of other trace elements such as iodine, chromium, manganese, selenium, and molybdenum. Each appears to be passively absorbed with varying degrees of efficiency. Except in geographic areas where the soil is severely deficient in iodine or selenium, deficiency of these minerals is extremely uncommon and is generally associated with severe bowel disease and/or the use of prolonged total parenteral nutrition.

**Absorption by the Colon.** The colon has a large absorptive capacity, particularly for water. It absorbs about 850 ml of the average 1,000 ml that daily crosses the ileocecal valve. Indiscriminate use of enemas over a few hours may lead to water intoxication. There is minor colonic absorption of glucose, amino acids, and vitamins but ready absorption of short-chain fatty acids (the products of colonic bacterial metabolism of unabsorbed carbohydrate). The rectal mucosa also provides a route for administration of certain drugs including antiemetics, sedatives, antipyretics, and steroids.

## FACTORS AFFECTING GASTROINTESTINAL FUNCTION

### Physiologic Factors

**Maturation.** The newborn gastrointestinal tract undergoes many maturational changes during the first months of life. Several of these changes are illustrated in Tables 26–7 and 26–8. During the first three to four months sucking reflexes are present, while extrusion reflexes protect against introduction of potentially indigestible solids. Esophageal motility is present at birth, but coordination of propulsive waves does not develop until after four months of postnatal life. Lower esophageal sphincter (LES) pressure remains low, and the intragastric pressure often exceeds the esophageal and LES pressure. This results in a high incidence of "spitting" of gastric contents for the first three to six months of life. Gastric motility is poorly coordinated for three to four months, which leads to poor antral mixing and therefore less digestion of solid foods than after four months of age. Usually at 12 weeks, intestinal peristalsis of a type seen in older children and adults develops, but it is approximately one third slower. The slower transit may serve to increase exposure time to the intestinal mucosa and thereby improve nutrient digestion and absorption. The motor function in the large intestine appears to be fully mature at birth.

Intestinal mucosal permeability is greatest during the neonatal period, and many large molecules, including proteins such as immunoglobulins, tend to be absorbed intact. This process provides a mechanism for passive transfer of antibodies from mother's milk but also permits the passage of whole proteins with a potential to provoke allergic responses. The relationship between ingestion of whole cow's milk and anemia from chronic intestinal blood loss during the first few months of life appears to result from this mechanism. Other nonhuman protein foods may also

**Table 26–7.  Gastric Analysis**

| Age | HCl Production* (meq/L:meq/hr/kg of wt—mean) | Volume Gastric Juice* (ml/hr—mean) | Pepsin* (ng/hr/kg of wt—mean) | IF† (mean) | Serum Gastrin‡ (pg/ml— mean ± SEM) |
|---|---|---|---|---|---|
| Birth | 8.1:0.01 | 3.3 | 0.40 | 8 | 64 ± 125 |
| 3–8 days | 14.4:0.02 | 3.7 | 0.06 | 17.8 | 151 ± 15.8 |
| 10–17 days | 34.4:0.12 | 4.0 | 0.15 | 29.2 | — |
| 25–32 days | 26.4:0.02 | 6.4 | 0.24 | 27.9 | 193 ± 28 |
| 60–90 days | 34.8:0.01 | 13.4 | 0.28 | 34.4 | — |
| 4–9 years | 114.2: −0.1 | 42.5 | — | 79.5 | 215 ± 37 |
| Adult | 91.2:0.19 | 143.2 | 0.60 | 78.7 | <90 |

*Tritratable acid obtained during one hour of intermittent suction after 1.0 mg/kg body weight of histalog. Data from Agunod, M., et al.: Am. J. Dig. Dis. *14*:400, 1969.
†IF = intrinsic factor.
‡Data from Rogers, I.M., et al.: Arch Dis. Child. *49*:796, 1974 and Rogers, I.M., et al.: Arch. Dis. Child. *50*:467, 1975.

cause similar changes in the first six months of life.

Secretory and absorptive functions of the intestine mature during the first two years of life (see Tables 26–7 and 26–8). In general, animal fat is less well digested and absorbed than vegetable oils by infants. The intestinal mucosal alpha-glucosidases (sucrase, maltase, isomaltase) are well developed by 32 weeks of gestation and are present at near adult levels at the time of the term delivery. By contrast, the beta-galactosidase, lactase, develops late in fetal life and does not reach maximal activity until feeding begins. In spite of the relatively low lactase activity, formulas containing lactose are well tolerated by term infants and many infants over 34 weeks gestation. For extremely premature infants (27 to 32 weeks gestation), formulas with less than 60% of total carbohydrate calories as lactose are generally best tolerated.

**Senescence.** Age-related changes in intestinal function occur simultaneously with loss of lean body mass.[68] Impaired glucose homeostasis, decreased clearance of drugs, variability in temperature control, and deterioration in immunologic function also occur with the alteration in gastrointestinal function.[69] Other changes include loss of dentition, reduced taste and smell acuity, esophageal dysmotility and delayed gastric emptying, hypochlorhydria, a tendency to ischemia, and intestinal amyloidosis. These factors and the frequent use of medication in the elderly may all contribute to impaired gastrointestinal tract function and an increased tendency toward malnutrition. Many of the physiologic changes observed with aging (immune senescence, reduction in visceral protein levels, decreased lean body mass) are similar to those observed in malnutrition in younger subjects,[20] although normal aging alone does not appear to impair protein-energy absorption substantially. Gastric emptying and intestinal transit are slowed, and the efficiency of absorption, particularly of vitamin A, may be improved as a result. On the other hand, absorption of vitamin $B_{12}$,[70] calcium,[71] and zinc seems to be impaired in the elderly.

**Adaptation.** The gastrointestinal tract is capable of extensive adaptation, particularly in children. Where intestinal function is marginal (as may occur after extensive resection), the residual intestine is capable of considerable dilation, increase

**Table 26–8.  Duodenal Fluid Analysis in 36 Premature Infants and in Children**

| Age | Volume* (ml) | αAmylase*‡ (U) | Trypsin*‡ (mg) | Lipase* (IU) |
|---|---|---|---|---|
| Premature (wt 2.0–2.4 kg) birth, before feeding | 44(4.3–152) | 0.88(0–3.6) | 60(0–482) | 77(3–343) |
| 24 hrs after first feeding | 55(16–98) | 0.62(0.2–1.4) | 43(1.6–148) | 66(2–209) |
| 1 wk | 82(17–168) | 2.07(0.2–8.2) | 233(5–660) | 329(7–1,249) |
| 4 wks | 90(34–187) | 1.67(0–4.6) | 196(0.9–660) | 284(11–730) |
| Children (9 mos–13 yrs)† | 390(180–810) | 665(160–2,150) | 765(215–2,000) | 1,465(350–5,000) |

*Data from Zoppi, G., et al.: Pediatr. Res. *6*:880, 1972. Values expressed on basis of body weights (kg) and represent mean and (range), during 50 min after injections of pancreozymin (2 units/kg) and secretin (2 units/kg).
†Data from Zoppi, G., et al.: Acta Paediatr. Scand. *59*:692, 1970.
‡Term infants had slightly lower enzyme activities one week after birth.

in rugosity, and hypertrophy of villi and micro-villi. Increased surface area and absorptive capacity result. Cell turnover and enzyme activities increase. These adaptive changes can be maximized by mucosal exposure to nutrients, pancreatic and biliary secretions, and by certain hormonal factors that remain unidentified. The search for trophic hormones has important therapeutic implications, but no candidates have shown conclusive growth-stimulating activity in the small intestine. Gastrin's trophic action affects primarily the esophagus, stomach, colon, and pancreas and may play some role in adaptation of the small intestine. Cholecystokinin and secretion are mildly trophic to the small intestine, but this reaction may be due to their stimulation of bile and pancreatic secretions.[72] Factors that limit intestinal adaptation include inadequate blood supply, poor nutritional status, and the presence of residual disease. The ileum is better able to adapt than the jejunum, which cannot assume certain specialized functions of the ileum such as active absorption of vitamin $B_{12}$ and bile salts. Slower transit in the ileum may improve absorptive capacity, but conversely provides a better milieu for bacterial overgrowth.

**Nutrition.** Inadequate nutrient intake over several days or weeks results in malnutrition and impaired intestinal function. With severe malnutrition, steatorrhea is characteristic even with a low fat intake.[73] Moderate degrees of protein calorie malnutrition may be associated with a reduction in gastric, biliary, pancreatic, and intestinal secretions and mucosal enzyme content, but minimal degrees of malabsorption. Severe protein deficiency also predisposes to immune dysfunction, leading to diarrhea from bacterial or parasite infections. Bacterial overgrowth of the small intestine may be the primary cause for a progressive decline in intestinal function due to impaired motility and depressed mucosal enzyme activity. Specific deficiencies of protein, vitamin $B_{12}$, folate, niacin, or minerals (calcium, potassium, magnesium, or zinc) may further impair intestinal function. Dietary fiber decreases absorption of some trace elements by as much as 20%. Whether such effects from dietary fiber are capable of producing specific trace-mineral deficiencies remains uncertain.

Total parenteral feeding is associated with atrophic changes in the muscular as well as the mucosal layers of the bowel.[74] Similar changes are also present in segments of the bowel that have been surgically bypassed.[75] Thus, exposure to food and upper gastrointestinal secretions is necessary to maintain mucosal vigor (see Chap. 54).

## Disease and Iatrogenic Factors

**Disease Factors.** Abnormalities of gastrointestinal function may produce manifestations that vary in nutritional importance from the mild discomfort of colonic spasm or heartburn to the debilitating or fatal consequences of regional enteritis or cancer. Many disorders affect more than one facet of gut activity, but in assessing the nutritional significance of any disorder, it is beneficial to consider its impact on each stage of assimilation (ingestion, luminal digestion, motility, brush border activity, transport, and intestinal vascular supply).

Congenital anomalies are usually manifested during infancy or early childhood and are composed primarily of atresias, abnormalities of rotation, duplications, and anorectal anomalies. Congenital enzyme deficiencies (disaccharidase, enterokinase, or lipase deficiencies and transport disorders) may also cause malabsorption. Reduction in biliary and pancreatic secretions produces severe fat malabsorption and less severe malabsorption of other nutrients. Immune deficiency syndromes frequently are associated with malabsorption, pernicious anemia, and increased gastrointestinal infections.[76] Enteropathy caused by sensitivity to cow's milk protein or soy protein and eosinophilic gastroenteritis are examples of abnormal responses of the intestinal epithelium to whole-food proteins.[76] Abnormalities of motility that prevent appropriate delivery of food (achalasia, pyloric stenosis) or affect intestinal transit, producing bacterial overgrowth (pseudo-obstruction, diabetic neuropathy), may result in bacterial deconjugation of bile salts and associated steatorrhea with severe nutrient deficiencies. Peptide-secreting endocrine tumors may result in watery diarrhea and malabsorption. Diseases involving the bowel wall (Whipple's disease, inflammatory bowel disease, scleroderma) may cause abnormalities of motility, secretion, digestion, and absorption with attendant malabsorption and diarrhea. In addition, vascular insufficiency, endocrine disorders (hypopituitarism, thyrotoxicosis), malignant tumors, and other remote conditions frequently compromise gut function.

**Surgery.** The surgical procedures that most commonly have impact on nutritional status are those performed for peptic ulcer disease and those involving small bowel resection. Approximately 10 to 25% of postgastrectomy patients have disabling symptoms of nausea, vomiting, or diarrhea. Weight loss of 10 to 15 pounds and mild steatorrhea are almost universal after partial gastrectomy, as is lactose intolerance. Malabsorption of vitamin

$B_{12}$, iron, and calcium may produce symptoms but usually responds to supplementation. The bacterial overgrowth that is common to some degree often responds to broad-spectrum antibiotics. Symptoms due to dumping can usually be handled with dietary restriction of foods with high osmolarity (i.e., reduction of simple carbohydrate load, juices, and certain soups). Although resection of up to 50% of the small bowel is well tolerated, adverse prognostic factors include loss of ileum, rather than jejunum, loss of the ileocecal valve, residual disease of the intestine, liver, or pancreas, advanced age, and massive resection.

**Radiation.** The severity of radiotherapy-induced damage to the gastrointestinal tract depends upon the total dose given and the time elapsed between exposures. Intestinal fibrosis due to small vessel ischemia results in mucosal dysfunction, disordered motility with bacterial overgrowth and, at times, severe malabsorption.

**Medications.** Many medications interact luminally with specific nutrients to alter availability for absorption or to affect their actions or metabolism. Some directly affect gut function and impair nutrient absorption. Examples of commonly used drugs that affect nutrition are neomycin, colchicine, sulfasalazine, diphenylhydantoin, alcohol, and cytotoxic agents.

With dietary guidance, nutrient supplementation, and adequate treatment of the primary disease, the gastrointestinal tract can withstand considerable insult and yet maintain acceptable nutritional status and activity. In cases of failure of the gastrointestinal tract, a temporary period of total parenteral nutrition can enable some patients to recover gastrointestinal function. If no functional return is possible, permanent home parenteral nutrition may be provided. Nutritional management of gastrointestinal tract disease is discussed in Chapter 59.

## REFERENCES

1. Robert, A., Nezamis, J.E., Lancaster, C., et al.: Gastroenterology *77*:433–443, 1979.
2. Donaldson, R.M.: The relation of enteric bacterial populations to gastrointestinal function and disease. *In* Gastrointestinal Disease. 3rd ed. (Sleisenger, M.H., Fordtran, J.S., Eds.) Philadelphia, W.B. Saunders Co., 1983, p. 79.
3. Bukhave, K., Rask-Madsen, J.: Gastroenterology *78*:32–42, 1980.
4. Tarnawski, A., Stachura, J., Ivey, K.T., et al.: Prostaglandins (Suppl.) *21*:147–159, 1980.
5. Trier, J.S.: Gastroenterology *42*:295–305, 1962.
6. Smith, G.P.: Lancet *2*:88–89, 1983.
7. Wood, J.D.: Physiology of the enteric nervous system. *In* Physiology of the Gastrointestinal Tract. (Johnson, L.R., Ed.) New York, Raven Press, 1981.
8. Morley, J.E., Levine, A.S.: Lancet *1*:398–401, 1983.
9. Kagnoff, M.F.: Immunology and allergic responses of the bowel. *In* The Role of the Gastrointestinal Tract in Nutrient Delivery. (Green, M., Greene, H.L., Eds.) New York, Academic Press, 1984.
10. Pearse, A.G.E., Polak, J.M., Bloom, S.R.: Gastroenterology *72*:746–761, 1977.
11. Johnson, L.R.: Regulation of intestinal growth. *In* Physiology of the Gastrointestinal Tract. (Johnson, L.R., Ed.) New York, Raven Press, 1981.
12. Doe, W.F., Hapel, A.J.: Clin. Gastroenterol. *12*:415–436, 1983.
13. Gershon, M.D., Erde, S.M.: Gastroenterology *80*:1571–1594, 1981.
14. Furness, J.B., Costa, M.: Neuroscience *5*:1–20, 1980.
15. Bayliss, W.M., Starling, E.H.: J. Physiol. (Lond.) *24*:99–143, 1899.
16. Gershon, M.D., Robinson, R.G., Ross, L.L.: J. Pharmacol. Exp. Ther. *198*:548–561, 1976.
17. Burnstock, G., Campbell, G., Satchell, D., et al.: Br. J. Pharmacol. *40*:668–688, 1970.
18. Said, S.I., Mutt, V.: Science *169*:1217–1218, 1970.
19. von Euler, U.S., Gaddum, J.H.: J. Physiol. *72*:74–87, 1931.
20. Costa, M., Patel, Y., Furness, J.B., et al.: Neurosci. Lett. *6*:215–222, 1977.
21. Hughes, J., Kosterlitz, H.W., Smith, T.W.: Br. J. Pharmacol. *61*:639–647, 1977.
22. Bloom, S.R., Ghatei, M., Warton, J.W., et al.: Gastroenterology *76*:1103–1107, 1979.
23. Polak, J.M., Sullivan, S.N., Bloom, S.R., et al.: Nature *270*:183–186, 1977.
24. Tatemoto, K.: Chemical assay for natural peptides: Application to the isolation of candidate hormones. *In* Gastrointestinal Hormones. (Glass, G.B.J., Ed.) New York, Raven Press, 1980.
25. Sernka, T., Jacobson, E.: Gastrointestinal Physiology. Baltimore, Williams & Wilkins, 1979.
26. Schultz, S.G., Zalusky, R.: J. Gen. Physiol. *47*:567–584, 1964.
27. Schultz, S.G., Zalusky, R.: J. Gen. Physiol. *47*:1043–1059, 1964.
28. Wilson, F.A., Dietchy, J.M.: Biochem. Biophys. Acta *363*:112–117, 1974.
29. Kimmich, G.A., Cater-Su, C.: Am. J. Physiol. *235*:C78, 1978.
30. Kimmich, G.A., Randles, J.: Biochem. Biophys. Acta *596*:439–444, 1980.
31. Gardner, J.D., Jackson, M.J., Batzvi, S., et al.: Gastroenterology *74*:348–354, 1978.
32. Grossman, M.I., Konturek, S.G.: Gastroenterology *66*:517–521, 1974.
33. Grossman, M.I.: Vagal stimulation and inhibition of acid secretion and gastrin released: Which aspects are cholinergic? *In* Gastrins and the Vagus. (Rehfeld, J.F., Andrup, E., Eds.) New York, Academic Press, 1979.
34. Cezard, J-P., Conklin, K.A., Das, B.C., et al.: J. Biol. Chem. *254*:8969–8975, 1979.
35. Conklin, K.A., Yamashiro, K.M., Gray, G.M.: J. Biol. Chem. *250*:5735–5741, 1975.
36. Crane, R.K.: Fed. Proc. *24*:1000–1006, 1965.
37. Crane, R.K., Malathi, P., Preiser, H.: Biochem. Biophys. Res. Commun. *71*:1010, 1976.
38. Fogel, M.R., Gray, G.M.: J. Appl. Physiol. *35*:262–267, 1973.
39. Gray, G.M.: Intestinal disaccharidase deficiencies and glucose-galactose malabsorption. *In* Metabolic Basis of Inherited Disease. 4th ed. (Stanbury, J.B., Wyngaarden, J.B., Fredrickson, D.S., Eds.) New York, McGraw-Hill Book Co., 1982.

40. Adibi, S.A.: J. Clin. Invest. *50*:2266–2275, 1971.
41. Rivier, D.: Experientia *29*:1443–1446, 1973.
42. Reichen, J., Baumgartner, G.: Am. J. Physiol. *231*:734–742, 1976.
43. Wilson, F.A., Dietschy, J.M.: J. Clin. Invest. *51*:3015–3025, 1972.
44. Wilson, F.A., Treanor, L.L.: J. Memb. Biol. *33*:213–230, 1977.
45. Sallee, V.L., Dietschy, J.M.: J. Lipid Res. *14*:475–484, 1973.
46. Chow, S.L., Hollander, D.: Lipids *13*:239–245, 1978.
47. Vodovar, H., Flanzy, J., Francois, A.C.: Ann. Biol. Anim. *9*:219–232, 1968.
48. Norum, K.R., Lilljeqvist, A.C., Helgerud, P., et al.: J. Clin. Invest. *9*:55–62, 1979.
49. Stirling, C.E.: J. Cell Biol. *53*:704–714, 1972.
50. Liedke, C.M., Hopfer, U.: Biochem. Biophys. Res. Commun. *76*:579–585, 1977.
51. Diamond, J.M., Bossert, W.H.: J. Gen. Physiol. *50*:2061–2083, 1967.
52. Rose, R., Nahrwold, D.: Int. J. Vitam. Nutr. Res. *48*:382–386, 1978.
53. Siliprandi, L., Vanni, P., Kessler, M., et al.: Biochem. Biophys. Acta *552*:129–142, 1979.
54. Rivier, D.: Experientia *29*:1443–1446, 1973.
55. Rindi, G., Ferrari, G.: Experientia *33*:211–213, 1977.
56. Said, H.M., Strum, W.B.: J. Pharmacol. Exp. Ther. *226*:95–99, 1983.
57. Said, H.M., Ghishan, F.K, Redha, R.: Gastroenterology *90*:1612, 1986 (abst).
58. Said, H.M., Strum, W.B.: Digestion *34*:350–355, 1986.
59. Rosenberg, I.H.: Intestinal absorption of folate. *In* Physiology of the Gastrointestinal Tract. (Johnson, L.R., Ed.) New York, Raven Press, 1981, pp. 1221–1230.
60. Allen, R.H., Seetharam, B., Podell, E., et al.: J. Clin. Invest. *61*:47–54, 1978.
61. Mackenzie, I.L., Donaldson, R.M., Trier, J.S., et al.: N. Engl. J. Med. *286*:1021–1025, 1972.
62. Thompson, G.R.: J. Clin. Pathol. *24*: Suppl. R. Coll. Pathol. *5*:85–89, 1971.
63. Gallo-Torres, H.E.: Lipids *5*:379–384, 1970.
64. Thompson, G.R., Scott, M.L.: J. Nutr. *100*:797–809, 1970.
65. Reinhold, J.G., Faradji, B., Abadi, P., et al.: Effects of cellulose consumption on zinc, calcium and phosphorus in man. *In* Trace Elements in Human Health and Disease. (Prasad, A.S., Ed.), New York, Academic Press, 1976.
66. Duncan, J.R., Hurley, L.S.: Am. J. Physiol. *235*:556–559, 1978.
67. Hunt, D.M.: Nature *249*:852–854, 1974.
68. Bowman, B.B., Rosenberg, I.H.: Am. J. Clin. Nutr. *37C*:75–78, 1983.
69. Shock, N.: Sci. Am. *206*:110–116, 1962.
70. King, C.E., Liebach, J., Toskes, P.P.: Dig. Dis. Sci. *24*:397–402, 1979.
71. Gallagher, J.C., Riggs, B.L., Eisman, J., et al.: J. Clin. Invest. *64*:729–732, 1979.
72. Johnson, L.R.: Regulation of gastrointestinal growth. *In* Physiology of the Gastrointestinal Tract. (Johnson, L.R., Ed.) New York, Raven Press, 1981.
73. Greene, H.L., McCabe, D.R., Merenstein, G.B.: J. Pediatr. *87*:695–704, 1975.
74. Johnson, L.R., Copeland, E.M., Dudrick, S.J.: Gastroenterology *68*:1177–1183, 1975.
75. Gronqvist, B., Engstrom, B., Grimelius, L.: Acta Chir. Scand. *141*:208–217, 1975.
76. Walker, A.: Intestinal transport of macromolecules. *In* Physiology of the Gastrointestinal Tract. (Johnson, L.R., Ed.) New York, Raven Press, 1981.

## SELECTED READINGS

Bloom, S.R., Polak, J.M.: Gut Hormones. Edinburgh, Churchill Livingstone, 1981.
Johnson, L.R.: Physiology of the Gastrointestinal Tract. New York, Raven Press, 1981.
Lebenthal, E.: Textbook of Gastroenterology and Nutrition in Infancy. New York, Raven Press, 1981.
McCaughan, G., Basten, A.: Immune system of the gastrointestinal tract. *In* Gastrointestinal Physiology IV, International Review of Physiology 28. (Young, J.A., Ed.) Baltimore, University Park Press, 1983.
Mutt, V.: Scand. J. Gastroenterol. (Suppl. 77) *17*:133–152, 1982.
Sleisenger, M.H., Fordtran, J.S.: Gastrointestinal Disease. 3rd ed. Philadelphia, W.B. Saunders Co., 1983.
Spiro, H.M.: Clinical Gastroenterology. 3rd ed. New York, Macmillan Publishing Co., Inc., 1983.
Thomas, H.C., Jewell, D.P.: Clinical Gastrointestinal Immunology. Oxford, Blackwell Scientific Publications, 1979.

*Chapter* **27**

# THE ROLES OF THE INTESTINAL FLORA

Barry R. Goldin, Alice H. Lichtenstein, and Sherwood L. Gorbach

In recent years there has been renewed interest in defining the capacity of the intestinal microflora to alter a wide variety of chemical compounds. This chapter reviews the current knowledge of the relationship between the intestinal microflora and the physiology and biochemistry of the host in health and disease.

## COMPOSITION AND DISTRIBUTION OF MICROFLORA

The bacterial inhabitants of the human gastrointestinal tract constitute a complex ecosystem. More than 400 bacterial species have been identified in feces of a single subject.[1,2] Anaerobic bacteria are the predominant microorganisms in the gastrointestinal tract, outnumbering aerobes by a factor of $10^2$ to $10^4$. The most prevalent anaerobic bacteria are *Bacteroides, Bifidobacterium, Fusobacterium, Clostridium, Eubacterium, Peptococcus,* and *Peptostreptococcus.* Numerous species are present in varying but lesser degrees.

In healthy humans the upper gastrointestinal tract is sparsely populated with microorganisms. Bacteria from the oral cavity are washed along with saliva into the stomach where most microorganisms are destroyed by gastric juice.[3] The most commonly isolated bacteria in the stomach are gram-positive facultative forms such as *Streptococcus, Staphylococcus,* and *Lactobacillus* (Table 27–1).

The small intestine constitutes a zone of transition between the sparsely populated stomach and the luxuriant bacterial flora of the distal ileum and colon. The microflora of the proximal small bowel is similar to that of the stomach. Here the concentration of bacteria increases to between $10^3$ and $10^4$ colony-forming units (CFU) per ml of intestinal contents. The most common organisms are gram-positive aerobes, although coliform and anaerobic bacteria can be isolated in low concentrations. In the distal ileum the concentration of bacteria increases to between $10^6$ and $10^7$ CFU per ml, and gram-negative bacteria outnumber gram-positive organisms. Coliforms are consistently present, and anaerobic bacteria, such as *Bacteroides, Bifidobacterium, Fusobacterium,* and *Clostridium,* are found in substantial concentrations.[4]

**Table 27–1.  Distribution and Composition of the Intestinal Flora**

| Site | Composition* | Total Number of Organisms/ ml Contents |
|---|---|---|
| Stomach | *Streptococcus* *Lactobacillus* | $10^1 – 10^2$ |
| Duodenum and jejunum | Similar to stomach | $10^2 – 10^4$ |
| Ileal-cecal | *Bacteroides* *Clostridium* *Streptococci* *Lactobacilli* | $10^6 – 10^8$ |
| Colon | *Bacteroides* *Clostridium* $(10^{10})$ *Eubacterium* $(10^{10})$ *Peptococcus* $(10^{10})$ *Bifidobacterium* $(10^9 – 10^{10})$ *Streptococcus* $(10^{10})$ *Fusobacterium* $(10^9 – 10^{10})$ | $10^{11.5} – 10^{12}$ |

*Organisms listed represent only the major species isolated from the different sites.

Distal to the ileocecal sphincter, bacterial concentrations increase sharply. Within the colon the bacterial concentration is between $10^{11}$ and $10^{12}$ CFU per ml of fecal material. One third of the fecal dry weight consists of viable bacteria. A summary of the distribution and composition of the gastrointestinal flora is presented in Table 27–1.

## COLONIZATION OF THE GASTROINTESTINAL TRACT

Colonization of the gastrointestinal tract of newborn infants occurs within a few days of birth.[5] The type of delivery, dietary constituents, and gestational age influence the colonization pattern. In one study, within 4 to 6 days of birth almost 100% of the full-term infants delivered vaginally had an anaerobic flora and 61% harbored *Bacteroides fragilis* in the gastrointestinal tract.[6] In contrast, 59% of infants delivered by cesarean section had anaerobes and only 9% had *B. fragilis,* suggesting that contamination occurred during passage through the birth canal. Prematurity and breast-feeding reduced the rate at which the infant's gastrointestinal tract was colonized with anaerobes.

## EFFECT OF DIET ON COMPOSITION OF MICROFLORA

Numerous animal and human studies have investigated the effect of diet on the composition of the intestinal microflora. In this section some of the human studies are summarized; subsequent sections will also discuss relevant examples.

The data are conflicting regarding the ability of diet to alter specific microbial components of the human adult flora. Moore et al. reported no change in the predominant organisms in the fecal flora of individuals shifted from an omnivorous to a vegetarian diet.[7] In another study Maier et al. investigated four subjects fed a meatless diet for four weeks, and then a high-meat diet for four weeks.[8] Increased fecal counts of *Bacteroides* and lower counts of coliforms were noted when subjects were eating the high-meat diet. However, a statistical analysis was not performed and the changes were not great. Reddy et al. reported a similar study in which eight volunteers, initially consuming a high-meat diet, were shifted for four weeks to a non-meat diet.[9] The shift resulted in a lower number of total anaerobic bacteria, including decreased counts of *Bacteroides, Bifidobacterium,* and *Peptococcus,* when the non-meat diet was consumed.

Intercountry studies performed in the early 1970s showed that people living in Britain or the United States eating a Western diet had more *Bacteroides* and fewer enterococci and other aerobic organisms than people eating a largely vegetarian diet in Uganda, India, and Japan.[10] In such large cross-cultural studies, however, it is difficult to eliminate factors other than diet that may influence the microflora.

The most detailed studies of the human microflora have been performed in the laboratory of Finegold. Subjects eating a Western diet were compared with subjects eating a Japanese diet, and with vegetarian and nonvegetarian Seventh-Day Adventists.[1,11] The subjects eating a Japanese diet had significantly higher fecal counts of *Streptococcus faecalis, Eubacterium lentum,* and *E. contortum;* they also had a lower counts of *Bacteroides,* although the values were not significantly different. The data were also evaluated in terms of populations at low and high risk for colon cancer.[11] The low-risk group included subjects eating a Japanese diet and the vegetarian and nonvegetarian Seventh-Day Adventists; the high-risk group included people eating a Western diet and patients with colonic polyps. The low-risk group had higher counts in their feces of *Klebsiella pneumoniae* and various *Lactobacillus* species, whereas the high-risk group had greater numbers of *Bifidobacterium, Peptococcus,* and *Clostridium.*

Drasar et al. studied the effect of fiber on the fecal flora of four volunteers.[12] Crude wheat fiber was increased from 3.6 to 11.7 g/day by adding wheat bran to the diet. These investigators reported no change in the microbial composition of the fecal flora as a result of this dietary modification.

In summary, studies of dietary influence on specific bacteria in intestinal flora indicate that people eating low-meat, high-complex-carbohydrate diets have higher fecal counts of aerobic bacteria and lower numbers of certain anaerobic bacteria. The overall shifts in the composition of the flora are hardly dramatic, and in some studies, no alterations are seen.

These studies of fecal microflora are based on classic principles of bacterial taxonomy, by which bacteria are named for their morphologic characteristics and their ability to perform certain biochemical reactions, usually having no relation to the physiology of the host. Since the flora is so complex (consisting of over 400 species), based on standard taxonomy, with a concentration of $10^{11}$ bacteria/g, it is difficult to show changes in any specific bacterium. Another approach, outlined in subsequent sections, deals with the metabolic activity of the microflora as a whole in relation to specific substrates. By this criterion diet can, indeed, alter the metabolic activity of the flora. These changes may be more relevant to the host than the Latin or Greek name of the microorganisms.

## EFFECT OF DIET ON BACTERIAL REACTIONS

Variations in bacterial metabolic activity can result from a variety of environmental factors.[13] Hill reported that feces from United States and English subjects contained higher levels of steroid nuclear dehydrogenating *Clostridium* than feces from African and Asian subjects.[14] The incriminated enzyme is involved in the production of unsaturated steroids from saturated steroids such as androgens and bile acids.

The microbial metabolism of bile acids and neutral steroids, as well as microbial β-glucuronidase, has been measured in the feces of various groups of people in the United States consuming diets of different compositions in order to assess the degree of microbial activity.[15] These measurements were performed among Americans consuming a mixed Western diet, and among American vege-

tarians and Seventh-Day Adventists (lacto-ovo vegetarians). When compared to the vegetarians, the Americans consuming a mixed Western diet had fecal microflora with a greater ability to hydrolyze glucuronide conjugates, to metabolize bile acids to lithocholic and deoxycholic acids, and to reduce cholesterol.

MacDonald et al. studied in Seventh-Day Adventists and subjects consuming a mixed Western diet the fecal NAD and NADP-dependent 7-α-hydroxysteroid dehydroxylase that converts hydroxy steroids to ketosteroids.[16] The activity of fecal 7-α-hydroxysteroid dehydroxylase was lower in the Seventh-Day Adventists.

Goldin and Gorbach reported that rats fed a high-fat (meat) diet for one month had higher levels of the fecal bacterial enzymes, β-glucuronidase, nitroreductase, and azoreductase, than rats on a low-fat (no meat) diet.[17] These results were confirmed and extended in a subsequent study that found that a high-fat diet, independent of the meat content, elevated the activity of these fecal bacterial enzymes.[18] Goldin et al. also studied these fecal bacterial enzymes, as well as 7-α-steroid dehydroxylase, in humans eating a Western diet and in lacto-ovo vegetarians and vegans.[19] All four bacterial enzymes were lower in the non-meat-eating vegetarian subjects. These studies confirm that the metabolic activity of the intestinal microflora can be altered by the nature of the diet. More detailed studies are required to determine the relationship of specific dietary components to the activity of different bacterial reactions.

Lindop et al. have compared intestinal bacterial β-glucuronidase activities in rats given a fiber-free diet or a diet containing pectin or cellulose.[19a] They found pectin and cellulose significantly reduced β-glucuronidase activity of cecal contents. Cellulose also lowered the β-glucuronidase activity of the jejunal and ileal contents while pectin reduced the activity in the ileum. Dietary fiber components had no effect on jejunal or ileal mucosal β-glucuronidase activity.

## METABOLIC ACTIVITIES OF MICROFLORA

The metabolic capacity of the gut bacteria is extremely diverse. Any compound taken orally or any substance entering the intestine via the biliary tract, via the blood, or by secretion directly into the lumen is a potential substrate for bacterial transformation. Table 27–2 contains a partial list of reactions that can be performed by the intestinal bacteria as well as examples of substrates for these reactions.

**Table 27–2.  Biochemical Reactions by Intestinal Bacteria**

| Reaction | Representative Substrate |
|---|---|
| Hydrolysis: | |
| Glucuronides | Estradiol-3-glucuronide |
| Glycosides | Cycasin |
| Sulfamates | Cyclamate, Amygdalin |
| Amides | Methotrexate |
| Esters | Acetyldigoxin |
| Nitrates | Pentaerythritol trinitrate |
| Dehydroxylation: | |
| C-hydroxy groups | Bile acids |
| N-hydroxyl groups | N-Hydroxyfluorenylacetamide |
| Decarboxylation | Amino acids |
| D-demethylation | Biochanin A |
| Deamination | Amino acids |
| Dehydrogenase | Cholesterol, bile acids |
| Dehalogenation | DDT |
| Reduction: | |
| Nitro groups | P-nitrobenzoic acid |
| Double bonds | Unsaturated fatty acids |
| Azo groups | Food dyes |
| Aldehydes | Benzaldehydes |
| Alcohols | Benzyl alcohols |
| N-oxides | 4-Nitroquinoline-1-oxide |
| Nitrosamine formation | Dimethylnitrosamine |
| Aromatization | Quinic acid |
| Acetylation | Histamine |
| Esterification | Galic acid |

## Glycosides

Hydrolysis of glycosidic bonds is one of the best-known examples of bacterial metabolism. Glycosides are compounds consisting of a non-sugar moiety (aglycone) bound to a sugar by either an $\alpha$ or $\beta$ glycosidic linkage. Glycosides enter the gut from two major sources: diet or the liver (via the bile). The diet contains a large number of plant glycosides, comprised predominantly of flavonoids. Glycosides coming from the liver include compounds that are detoxified by glucuronide formation and subsequently secreted into the bowel via the bile. The intestinal flora can then hydrolyze the $\beta$-glucuronide bond leading to the release of the biologically active aglycones, some of which are potentially toxic or carcinogenic.

The principal glycosidases produced by the intestinal flora are $\beta$-glucosidase, $\beta$-galactosidase, and $\beta$-glucuronidase.[3] On the basis of studying 50 strains each of 4 bacterial species commonly found in the bowel, Hawksworth et al. concluded that, on a per-cell basis, *Escherichia coli* and *Clostridium* had the highest $\beta$-glucuronidase activity and *Lactobacillus* and *Bifidobacterium* had the lowest activity.[20] The relative activities were different for $\beta$-glucosidase, where *Escherichia coli* had the lowest activity, and *Bacteroides* and *Streptococcus faecalis* the highest activity.

There are a number of interesting examples of the role of bacteria in the metabolism of glyco-sides. Cycasin methylazoxymethanol-$\beta$-D-glucoside is a naturally occurring compound that is a constituent of cycad plants, also known as tropical ferns. Much of the interest in cycasin stems from the finding that the aglycone, methylazoxymethanol, caused tumors in conventional but not in germfree rats. These results suggested that the hydrolysis was a result of the intestinal microorganisms. This hypothesis was confirmed by mono-contaminating germfree rats with bacteria having different levels of $\beta$-glucosidase activity. Toxicity after feeding cycasin was positively correlated with the $\beta$-glucosidase levels of the particular bacterial strain implanted.[21] A more detailed discussion of the interaction of the bacterial flora with cycasin is presented in a later section.

Rutin is a plant glycoside that is not mutagenic in tests such as the *Salmonella* test. Upon hydrolysis of the glycosidic linkages, however, the hydrolysate becomes mutagenic. Several studies have reported that mixed fecal cultures[21a] or fecal isolates, such as *Streptococcus faecalis*,[21b] can convert rutin (quercetin-3-0-B-D-glucose-$\gamma$-L-rhamnose) to quercetin, a compound that is mutagenic in the *Salmonella* liver homogenate test. Beverages such as red wine and tea contain glycosides of quercetin. In addition, cell-free extracts from fecal cultures grown in the presence of bile acids have increased ability to form quercetin from rutin.[21c]

The cathartic agent, cascara sagrada, is a mixture of glycosides. The glycosides themselves have no pharmacologic action; however, upon bacterial hydrolysis, the active aglycone is released. Hawksworth et al. found that the β-glucosidase of *S. faecalis* can hydrolyze cascara sagrada.[20]

The metabolism of the cardiac glycoside digoxin has been studied by Lindenbaum et al.[22] In order to produce pharmacologic effects, the bacterial flora must remove a trisaccharide from the parent compound, releasing digoxigenin. The intestinal flora of approximately 10% of patients given digoxin further metabolizes the drug by reducing the double bond in the lactone ring resulting in the formation of dihydrodigoxigenin. This compound is pharmacologically inactive. Therefore, about 10% of people receiving digoxin will not achieve predicted serum levels as a result of bacterial inactivation. The microorganism *Eubacterium lentum* is exclusively responsible for this reduction.[23]

The bacterial hydrolysis of disaccharides is another example of a hydrolytic glycosidic reaction. The dietary disaccharides, sucrose, lactose, and maltose, are normally hydrolyzed by mammalian enzymes in the intestinal mucosal brush border in the upper small bowel. This arrangement minimizes contact of the disaccharides with the high bacterial populations in the lower intestine. Those individuals who, either by genetic design or by an acquired disorder, lack mucosal disaccharidases have resultant insufficient absorption of related sugars in the upper small intestine. The sugars are transported to the ileum and large bowel where the bacterial enzymes lactase (β-galactosidase), maltase (α-glucosidase), and sucrose (α-glycosidase) hydrolyze the disaccharides. The monosaccharides produced from this hydrolysis are further metabolized by bacteria to short-chain acids in a classic fermentation reaction. The production of these acids leads to an osmotic imbalance, and water flows into the bowel lumen causing diarrhea. The acid production also lowers the pH of the fecal stream causing irritation of the colonic wall. The most common disaccharidase disorder is lactase deficiency leading to the well-known disorder of lactose intolerance. Deficiencies in sucrase or isomaltase, which produce similar symptoms, also occur, but are much rarer.

## Amines

Bacteria can deaminate or remove amino groups from amines by four direct pathways. There is also an indirect route of removal of amino groups via the Strickland reaction. These deamination reactions are discussed in greater detail with respect to amino acid metabolism in a later section.

The contribution of ammonia from bacterial deamination of amino acids is small, relative to the total intestinal pool. The major source of ammonia production in the intestine is deamination of primary amine, urea. Bacterial urease catalyzes the production of carbon dioxide and ammonia from urea. Urease is present in a wide range of organisms found in the intestinal tract including both aerobes and anaerobes.[24] Intestinal bacteria hydrolyze approximately 40% of the urea synthesized by the liver.[3]

Intestinal bacteria can esterify primary amino groups to a variety of compounds. This reaction is an important mechanism by which bacteria can inactivate sulfonamides and certain aminoglycoside antibiotics. The bacterial esterification of histamine is the major source for N-acetyl histamine in human urine. Additionally, the gut microflora can hydrolyze the N-acetyl linkage of secondary amines. An example of this reaction is the deesterification of the antibiotic chloramphenicol, with release of the dichloracetyl group.

The intestinal flora can also remove alkyl groups from secondary amines. The demethylation of methylamphetamine to produce amphetamine is an example of this reaction.

The bacterial flora can also add a nitroso group to secondary amines, producing nitrosamines, an addition known as N-nitrosation. Bacteria can use nitrate as the nitrosating agent. Aerobes such as *Streptococcus faecalis* and the common anaerobes, *Clostridium, Bacteroides,* and *Bifidobacterium,* can catalyze the N-nitrosation of diphenylamine. (The implication of this reaction to human health is discussed later.)

## Azocompounds

Most artificial coloring additives used in foods and in the textile industry are dyes containing a single azo bond (mono azo dyes). American consumption of azo dyes has been increasing steadily during the past 20 years. During that time more than a dozen dyes have been taken off the market following laboratory indications that they may be toxic and carcinogenic. The water-soluble dyes are not well absorbed from the intestine and are subject to bacterial action in the large bowel, which contributes to their detrimental effects. A number of studies have shown that the bacterial flora can reductively hydrolyze the azo bond, resulting in the formation of substituted aromatic amines.[25] This class of bacterially generated compounds contains a number of well-established carcinogens.[26] For example, orange II can be reductively cleaved leading to the formation of the bladder carcinogen 1-amino-2-naphthol.[27] Ponceau 3R,[28] methyl yellow, and methyl orange, formerly used as food colorants, can be transformed by intestinal anaerobes into mutagens.[29]

The bacterial reduction of an azocompound is not always harmful. Salicylazosulfapyridine (Azulfidine) is used for the treatment of ulcerative colitis. The drug was designed for therapeutic efficacy by combining the antimicrobial action of sulfapyridine with the anti-inflammatory action of aminosalicylate via an azo bond linkage. Peppercorn and Goldman demonstrated that salicylazosulfapyridine is cleaved in the bowel by the bacterial flora.[30] Germfree animals were incapable of reducing this azocompound and it passed unchanged into the feces. Conventional animals completely reduced the compound, but the reaction was blocked by feeding neomycin, a nonabsorbed antibiotic. The end result of this bacterial action is the release of the therapeutically active moieties at the site of the diseased tissue in the colon rather than the absorption of the compounds in the upper intestine, which would occur had they been administered separately. Additionally, because the larger azocompound is not well absorbed, slow release of the active halves of the molecule occurs in the large bowel. It has subsequently been found that only the aminosalicylate has therapeutic efficacy in ulcerative colitis; however, the delivery system is still a useful concept.

## Nitrocompounds

The reduction of nitro groups by the intestinal microorganisms can be another source for the production of aromatic amines. Germfree rats reduce the nitro group of p-nitrobenzoic acid at a much lower rate than conventional animals.[31] Goldin and Gorbach have found that diet and oral antibiotics can influence the level of fecal nitroreductase activity.[32]

Reduction of aromatic nitro groups is a complex reaction involving the addition of six electrons. The intermediates in this reaction include a nitrofree radical, a nitroso group, and an N-hydroxy group; all three of these functional groups have been associated with potentially deleterious genotoxic events.

## Sulfates

There have been several reports of bacterial sulfatase activity in the intestine.[33] The intestinal flora can hydrolyze C-sulfonates, O-sulfates, and N-sulfonates. An example of the significance of these reactions is the bacterial hydrolysis of cyclamate. Cyclamate (cyclohexylamine N-sulfonate) was used as an artificial sweetening agent until it was banned in 1969. Initially, researchers believed that cyclamate could not be metabolized

in the body. It was subsequently shown that cyclamate could be converted to the bladder carcinogen cyclohexylamine via an N-sulfate ester hydrolysis by the bacterial flora.[34,35] Cyclohexylamine was absorbed and excreted in the urine. Prolonged feeding of cyclamate to rats increased the amount of metabolite; removal of cyclamate from the diet led to a loss of hydrolytic activity of the flora within five days.[36] Other examples of bacterial sulfatase reactions have been reported.[33]

## Steroids

The bacterial deconjugation and dehydroxylation of bile acids are examples of the importance of the intestinal flora in the metabolism of endogenous compounds. Bile acids are synthesized in the liver and excreted via the bile into the small intestine. Prior to entering the small intestine they are conjugated to the amino acids taurine or glycine. The intestinal bacteria hydrolyze the conjugates releasing the free bile acids. Most bile acids have a hydroxyl group at the 7 position of the steroid nucleus. The bacterial enzyme 7-$\alpha$-steroid dehydrogenase can remove this hydroxyl group. It has been estimated that 80% of the cholic and chenodeoxycholic primary bile acids undergo 7-dehydroxylation to yield deoxycholic and lithocholic acid, respectively. The implications of this reaction in relation to the etiology of large bowel cancer are discussed later.

The nuclear dehydrogenation of steroids by intestinal microorganisms represents another class of bacterial intestinal reaction. In this case, double bonds are introduced into the steroid structure. When androgens are substrates for this reaction, the double bonds are introduced in the 1 and 4 position giving rise to 1,4 androgens.

## DOPA

Metabolism by the intestinal microflora is a complicating factor in the treatment of patients with Parkinson's disease with 3,4-dihydroxyphenylalanine (DOPA). The bacterial modification involves a dehydroxylation at the para position, leading to the formation of meta-hydroxyphenylacetic acid.[37] For this reason, high doses of DOPA have to be administered orally in order to deliver relatively small quantities to the brain. In addition, DOPA can be decarboxylated by *S. faecalis* in the same way as tyrosine and other amino acids. This reaction causes an increase in urinary excretion of amines.

## Aromatization

Quinic acid is present in a number of food products, including coffee, tea, vegetables, and fruits. The compound has an aliphatic cyclic structure.

Quinic acid is aromatized when taken orally and excreted in urine as hippuric acid. The aromatization does not occur when quinic acid is given parenterally, and the reaction is inhibited by the action of the antibiotic neomycin in the rat and man.[38] These data suggest the aromatization is a bacterially catalyzed event in the bowel.

### Glycoproteins

**Mucins.** Throughout the gastrointestinal tract goblet cells secrete mucins, which are glycoproteins. The function of the mucins apparently is to protect the epithelial cells against harmful agents in the luminal contents. In contrast to conventional rats, germfree animals accumulate large amounts of mucous material, as shown by Hoskins and Zamcheck.[39] They found the rate of excretion of nonhydrolyzed carbohydrate moieties to be 6 to 10 times higher in the feces of germfree rats. The blood group ABO antigens, which are also glycoproteins, were detected only in the feces of germfree animals. Feces from conventional, but not from germfree, animals contain enzymes capable of degrading ABO antigens.

For a more complete discussion of intestinal bacterial metabolism, the review articles by Scheline are recommended.[33,40]

## ENTEROHEPATIC CIRCULATION

A substance is said to undergo an enterohepatic circulation when it is metabolized in the liver, excreted into the bile, passed into the lumen of the intestine, reabsorbed through the intestinal wall, and then returned to the liver via the portal circulation. Many endogenous compounds have an enterohepatic circulation, including estrogens, folic acid, vitamin $B_{12}$, bile acids, cholesterol, protoporphyrin, and the metabolites of vitamin D.[41,42] Enterohepatic circulation has also been demonstrated for drugs and chemicals, including ouabain, promazine, morphine, colchicine, diethylstilbestrol, digoxin, rifampin, and iopanoic acid.[41]

Several factors determine whether a compound will be secreted from the liver into the bile. The compound generally is conjugated to a polar group such as glucuronic acid, sulfate, taurine, glycine, or glutathione prior to secretion into bile. In addition, a compound that undergoes an enterohepatic circulation tends to have a molecular mass in excess of 200 daltons. Once secreted into the small intestine, the microflora plays an important role in the next phase of the enterohepatic circulation. The conjugated compounds themselves are not well absorbed; they cannot undergo an enterohepatic circulation unless hydrolyzed by the enzymes of the bacterial flora. These bacterial enzymes include β-glucuronidase, sulfatase, and various glycosidases. These enzymes can hydrolyze a variety of conjugates resulting in the release of the nonconjugated compounds in the intestine with subsequent reabsorption.

There are several ways to interrupt the enterohepatic circulation. In one study, the absorption of diethylstilbestrol, which is excreted as a monoglucuronide in bile,[43] was inhibited 90% by glucuro-1-4-lactone, an inhibitor of bacterial β-glucuronidase.[44] Similarly, rats pretreated with the antibiotics neomycin or kanamycin also had decreased intestinal reabsorption of the diethylstilbestrol-monoglucuronide. Adlercreutz et al. showed that administration of ampicillin to pregnant women caused an increased fecal excretion of estrogens[45] and decreased urinary excretion.[46] The types of estrogens in the feces were also drastically altered. Prior to the administration of the antibiotic, conjugated estrogens made up only 1.8% of the total fecal estrogens, whereas after antibiotic administration, the conjugates made up 25 to 30% of the total fecal estrogens.

An example of the physiologic implications of diet-mediated alteration of the enterohepatic circulation has been reported by Goldin et al.[47] These investigators found that American vegetarian women excreted between two and three times more estrogen in their feces and had between 20 and 40% lower plasma levels of estrogen than American omnivores eating a Western diet. There was an inverse correlation between fecal excretion of estrogen and plasma estrogen levels.

In summary, the enterohepatic circulation contributes to an increased half-life and elevated plasma levels for these substances, which is advantageous for certain compounds but not for others. The composition of the diet can alter the enterohepatic circulation by affecting bacterial deconjugating enzymes.

## VITAMINS

The conversion of vitamin K, a member of the naphthoquinone family, is a classic example of the involvement by the bacterial flora in the metabolism of a vitamin. The prothrombin complex, a blood-clotting factor, is synthesized by the liver. The peptides that become the glycoproteins of the prothrombin complex cannot be synthesized on the appropriate mRNA unless the liver contains menaquinone, a substituted naphthoquinone. Since animals cannot synthesize the substituted naphthoquinone ring, they depend on vegetables in the diet for their supply.

Bacteria found in the intestinal tract also synthesize homologues of vitamin $K_2$ (menaquinone-7). These homologues range from menaquinone-6 (6 isoprene units in the side chain) to menaquinone-13.[47a,47b] The bacterial metabolism apparently occurs, at least in part, in the ileum where the menaquinone can be absorbed.

The importance of bacterial synthesis of vitamin K has been demonstrated in studies in which healthy adult subjects were given low vitamin K diets for several weeks without causing a deficiency. Treatment of subjects on low vitamin K diets with bowel sterilizing antibiotics, such as neomycin, caused a significant decrease in plasma prothrombin levels.[47c,47d]

In contrast, vitamin $B_{12}$ (cyanocobalamin) is synthesized solely by microorganisms. Vitamin $B_{12}$ is synthesized by the microflora of ruminants, and is absorbed in the small intestine of these animals. The meat and milk from these animals are a major dietary source of vitamin $B_{12}$ for humans. The human microflora also synthesizes significant amounts of vitamin $B_{12}$, and approximately 5 μg are excreted in the feces daily. However, the primary site for the synthesis of vitamin $B_{12}$ in humans is the large bowel. Absorption from this site is poor or nonexistent because of a lack of receptors in the mucosa. The ileum is the major location of vitamin $B_{12}$ absorption in humans. Albert et al. have reported the synthesis of vitamin $B_{12}$ in the jejunum and ileum of healthy Southern Indian subjects.[48] At least two organisms, *Pseudomonas* and *Klebsiella,* were shown to synthesize significant amounts of vitamin $B_{12}$ in the small intestine.

Biotin is synthesized to a major extent by the intestinal flora of animals and humans.[49] Large doses of antibiotics can cause biotin deficiency in experimental animals. Administration of antibiotics also lowers urinary biotin levels in humans. Germfree rats require biotin in their diet, whereas conventional rats appear to have sufficient bacterial synthesis to satisfy systemic requirements for biotin.

Several other B complex vitamins, such as folic acid and thiamine, are synthesized by bacteria in the gastrointestinal tract,[50] although this pathway does not provide adequate absorbable amounts to eliminate the requirement for a dietary source for these vitamins.

## AMINO ACIDS AND PROTEINS

In monogastric animals the microflora of the lower intestine hydrolyzes incompletely digested food proteins. Similarly, proteins from shed epithelial cells and digestive secretions such as enzymes and glycoproteins (mucins), secreted too far down in the gastrointestinal tract to be acted upon by intestinal protease, are metabolized by intestinal bacteria. The ability of the flora to destroy ABO blood antigens in the gut could be a measure of mucin degradation.[51] In addition, intestinal bacteria can ferment most amino acids. The initial reactions involve either deamination or decarboxylation. Many amines derived from amino acid metabolism by the gut flora are found in the urine, indicating subsequent resorption of the metabolites. Piperidine and pyrrolidine are examples of cyclic secondary amines that are formed from lysine and arginine via cadaverine and putrescine.

Five mechanisms of bacterial deamination have been described. Nonoxidative deamination by aspartate ammonia-lyase catalyzes the conversion of aspartate to fumarate; histidine ammonia-lyase produces urocanic acid from histidine, and cystathione-γ-lyase forms pyruvate from cysteine. Oxidative deamination is a minor pathway in bacteria. Only a few organisms utilize this pathway on a restricted range of amino acids such as glycine, alanine, and glutamic acid. Reductive deamination, producing a saturated fatty acid from an amino acid, is a major bacterial pathway. By this mechanism aspartic acid is deaminated to succinic acid, and tryptophan to indopropionic acid. Bacterial hydrolysis of amino acids is exemplified by the deamination of aspartic acid to yield malic acid. This route of metabolism generates α-hydroxy acids from amino acids. Another mechanism of deamination is the indirect removal of ammonia by the mixed amino acid, or Strickland reaction. Clostridia primarily catalyze this reaction in which two amino acids react to yield a keto-acid and a saturated fatty acid.

The bacterial degradation of proteins and metabolism of the resulting amino acids cause the formation of a wide range of different amines and short-chain organic acids.

## LIPIDS

In monogastric animals most of the fatty acids from dietary lipids are absorbed in the small intestine. Some unsaturated fatty acids do reach the lower small intestine and colon. The cecum of the rabbit has the capacity to hydrogenate these unsaturated fatty acids.[49] There is evidence in humans that anaerobic bacteria, in addition to hydrogenating, can also hydrate unsaturated fatty acids.[52] Small amounts of 10-hydroxystearic acid have been identified in human feces. In general, lipid metabolism by intestinal bacteria is important in ruminants, but has only minor significance in humans.

## CARBOHYDRATES

The anaerobic intestinal flora is capable of fermenting carbohydrate to short-chain fatty acids. Acetate, propionate, and butyrate are the major end products in the feces of humans. Carbon dioxide, hydrogen, methane, and water are also end products of the fermentation process. Acetate is usually formed by the oxidative decarboxylation of pyruvate and butyrate, and by reduction of acetoacetate from acetate. The production of propionate is by two pathways, involving either fixation of carbon dioxide to form succinate, which is subsequently decarboxylated, or formation of lactate and acrylate (the "acrylate pathway"). Lactate may also be formed from pyruvate by anaerobic bacteria, but lactate is not a key intermediate in fermentation, and significant amounts are rarely found in the human colon.

The major source of fermentable carbohydrates in the human colon is plant cell-wall polysaccharides such as cellulose, pectins, and hemicellulose, the major components of dietary fiber. Starch, intestinal mucus, and mono- and disaccharides can also be fermented in significant quantities. It is estimated that between 20 and 70 g of carbohydrate are fermented per day, depending on the fiber content of the diet. The plant cellwall polysaccharides are composed of glucose, galactose, xylose, arabinose, and uronic acid monomers, which are fermented by bacteria along various anaerobic pathways. Hexose breakdown is mainly via the Embden-Myerhof-Parnas glycolytic pathway to pyruvate. Alternatively, hexose is converted to 6-phosphogluconate and then metabolized by the pentose monophosphate shunt.

The short-chain fatty acids produced as a result of bacterial fermentation of carbohydrate can be absorbed by the colonic mucosa.[52] The rate of absorption is between 6 and 12 mol/cm²/hr and is more rapid than sodium transport.[53] Substantial amounts of these absorbed fatty acids are metabolized within the colonic epithelial cells. In isolated epithelial cells from human colon, butyrate is an important energy source for colonic mucosa, accounting for the major part of energy needs even in the presence of glucose.[52]

## BILE ACIDS

The bile acids synthesized in the liver and secreted in bile are substituted C-24 cholanic acids conjugated to glycine or taurine. In Table 27–3, the principal bile acids, and the various sidechain substitutions, are presented. The free bile acids are absorbed either by active transport from the terminal ileum or, to a lesser extent, by passive diffusion from the small or large intestine. The absorbed bile acids return to the liver via the portal circulation and are reconjugated and resecreted in the bile. Approximately 5% of the bile acids are lost in the feces in each cycle.[41] The bile acids found in the feces are deconjugated. Primary bile

acids are synthesized by the liver, and they are converted to secondary bile acids by intestinal bacteria. Studies with germfree animals show an absence of secondary bile acids in the feces.

The principal bacterial reactions involved in the conversion of bile acids include three separate classes: the hydrolysis of the amide bond to release the free bile acid from its glycine or taurine conjugates; an oxido-reduction reaction of the hydroxyl groups at C-3, C-7, and C-12 to give either oxo-bile acids (hydroxyl to keto group) or β-hydroxyl groups after the reduction of the keto group (inversion products); and dehydroxylation at C-7, and to a smaller extent at the C-3 and C-12 positions. The hydroxyl groups of the primary bile acids are in the α-configuration. The formation of a keto group and subsequent reduction of this group can lead to the formation of a β-hydroxyl group. The source and properties of these bacterial enzymes are discussed in detail by Drasar and Hill.[3]

## CHOLESTEROL

Cholesterol, the precursor of bile acids, is a substituted neutral (e.g., no charged groups) C-27 cholestene. There are two principal fecal metabolites of cholesterol, coprostanone and coprostanol, and one minor product, cholestenone. The production of coprostanol involves a steroid nuclear hydrogenation of the 5,6 double bond. The conversion of cholesterol to coprostanone results from the reduction of the 4,5 bond and a C-3 oxido-reductase converting the hydroxyl group to a keto group. The sequence of these reactions has not been fully elucidated. Coprostanone may be synthesized via cholestenone (4-cholesten-3-one). In general, coprostanol accounts for 50% of the total fecal neutral sterols, coprostanone 10 to 15%, and unmetabolized cholesterol makes up most of the remainder. In germfree rats, cholesterol is the only neutral sterol in the feces, indicating that the intestinal flora is solely responsible for the metabolism of cholesterol in the intestine. The percentage conversion of intestinal cholesterol to its metabolites varies from 70 to 85% in Americans and Western Europeans to 55 to 65% in Africans and Asians.[15]

## ESTROGENS AND ANDROGENS

Estrogens and androgens are a third class of steroids (C-18 and C-19) that undergo extensive modification by bacteria in the intestinal tract. The three principal estrogens (estrone, estradiol, and estriol) are excreted in the bile, mainly conjugated to glucuronic acid or sulfate. Fecal extracts can hydrolyze these conjugates releasing the free estrogens, and all subsequent reactions involve ox-

**Table 27–3. Major Fecal Bile Acids in Humans**

| Nature of Substituent at Position | | | |
|---|---|---|---|
| 3 | 7 | 12 | Trivial Name* |
| OH | OH | OH | Cholic acid |
| OH | OH | — | Chenodeoxycholic acid |
| OH | — | OH | Deoxycholic acid |
| OH | — | — | Lithocholic acid |
| β-OH | — | — | Isolithocholic acid |

*All are substituted 5 β-cholanic acids.

idoreduction of the C-17 position. Once deconjugated, intestinal bacteria can convert estrone to estradiol under anaerobic conditions.[54] The reverse reaction, estrone from estradiol, may be catalyzed by the fecal flora via an aerobic reaction. In vitro, this reaction only occurs when the oxygen concentration is high and the number of fecal bacteria is low. Since these conditions do not occur under normal physiologic circumstances, the significance of this oxidative reaction is unclear. The fecal flora is also capable of converting 16 α-hydroxyestrone to estriol. Although the significance of these steroid interconversions is not defined, there is evidence that the intestinal flora can influence the serum estrogen levels.[47]

Several bacterial conversions of androgens have been described.[54] The fecal flora is capable of reversibly oxidizing and reducing the 3-hydroxy group (C-3 oxidoreductase) and reducing steroid nuclear double bonds at the 1 and 4 positions,[54] leading to a complex set of interconversions of androgens. The introduction of double bonds into the androgen nucleus has also been described in vitro,[55] but this reaction requires oxidizing agents and low numbers of fecal bacteria. Because of these requirements, it is unlikely the reaction occurs in the colon.

## BILE PIGMENTS

Bile pigments, the end products of the breakdown of hemoglobin and heme-containing enzymes, are normal constituents of bile. Between 200 and 300 mg of bilirubin, the product derived from heme, are excreted daily in the bile. Approximately 90% of the bilirubin is conjugated as a glucuronide and 10% to sulfate in the liver prior to excretion into the bile. The glucuronide conjugate of bilirubin is hydrolyzed by the gut flora, releasing the free compound, which can be reabsorbed in the intestine. Alternately, bilirubin can be reduced by intestinal bacteria to urobilinogen. Approximately 20% of the urobilinogen is reabsorbed from the intestine of humans. Further nonenzymatic oxidation of urobilinogens results in the formation of pigmented urobilins that can also be resorbed from the small intestine. Urobilins

and bilirubin are the principal pigments of urine, bile, and feces.

Another component of bile, the phospholipid lecithin (phosphatidylcholine), is mostly degraded by pancreatic phosphatases to free fatty acids and phosphatidic acid. Residual lecithin can be hydrolyzed by phosphatases produced by *Clostridium* and *Escherichia coli*. Phospholipase A and C have been found in bacteria normally residing in the gastrointestinal tract.[3]

The four major components of bile (cholesterol, bile acids, bile pigments, and lecithin) as well as androgens and estrogens, which also are excreted by this route, are subject to bacterial action in the intestine. The physiologic importance of these reactions constitutes an area of ongoing research.

## BACTERIAL OVERGROWTH ("BLIND LOOP") SYNDROME

Anatomic and physiologic derangements of the gastrointestinal tract can lead to proliferation of bacterial growth in the upper small intestine. This condition, known as "bacterial overgrowth," may cause a variety of metabolic disorders, including steatorrhea, vitamin deficiencies, and carbohydrate malabsorption.[56]

One cause of bacterial overgrowth in the upper small bowel relates to gastric acid production. Gastric acid normally limits bacterial growth in the stomach and upper small intestine. However, a number of situations, such as atrophic gastritis, pernicious anemia, surgical resections, and therapy with drugs (e.g., cimetidine), can cause hypochlorhydria. These conditions are usually accompanied by overgrowth of bacterial populations in the stomach and upper small intestine.

Small-bowel bacterial overgrowth also can result from inadequate clearance of microorganisms due to disordered peristalsis. This situation can be caused by anatomic disorders such as small-bowel diverticula, surgically created blind loops, or strictures with partial small-bowel obstruction. Scleroderma and diabetic autonomic neuropathy are associated with ineffective peristalsis and bacterial overgrowth.

A complex flora is present in the upper small bowel of patients with bacterial overgrowth. More than 20 different species of bacteria have been identified, at concentrations ranging from $10^7$ to $10^9$ CFU/ml. Counts as high as $10^{11}$ CFU/ml have been reported,[57] which are considerably greater than the $10^2$ to $10^4$ CFU/ml in the normal state.

The most common clinical manifestation of small-bowel overgrowth is malabsorption of fat, along with the related malabsorption of fat-soluble vitamins. The major cause of fat malabsorption involves deconjugation of bile salts. Normally, the conjugated bile salts, which contain a hydrophilic and hydrophobic region (conferring detergent-like properties), solubilize fatty acids and monoglycerides by forming mixed micelles. In the setting of bacterial overgrowth, particularly with anaerobic bacteria, the concentration of conjugated bile acids in the upper small bowel is reduced by bacterial hydrolysis. This process results in impaired micelle formation, fat malabsorption, and steatorrhea.

In addition to the low concentration of conjugated bile salts associated with small-bowel overgrowth, there is a corresponding increase in free bile acids. Free bile acids can cause intestinal tissue damage and dysplasia.[57a,57b] Free bile acids, particularly deoxycholic acid, can also inhibit the esterification of fatty acids by the intestinal tissue during absorption. The combination of impaired micelle formation, altered intestinal cell structure and kinetics, and decreased intestinal esterification contributes to a malabsorption syndrome.

Small-bowel bacterial overgrowth is also associated with megaloblastic anemia due to vitamin $B_{12}$ deficiency. Reduced vitamin $B_{12}$ absorption is related to binding of the vitamin to the bacteria present in the proximal small bowel, thereby preventing vitamin $B_{12}$ absorption in the distal ileum.[58] Vitamin $B_{12}$ malabsorption in rats with surgically created blind loops was corrected by administration of metronidazole,[59] an antibiotic that acts exclusively against anaerobic bacteria. In vitro studies have demonstrated that *Bacteroides* binds the intrinsic factor-cobalamin complex. Patients with bacterial overgrowth syndrome have high levels of vitamin $B_{12}$ in the small intestine lumen, not only from nonabsorbed dietary sources but from local bacterial synthesis as well. Yet they still suffer from vitamin $B_{12}$ deficiency because there is no vitamin available for intestinal absorption.

Amino acid and carbohydrate absorption is impaired in patients with small-bowel bacterial overgrowth. There is increased fecal nitrogen, low serum proteins and, on occasion, a clinical picture of protein-calorie malnutrition.[60] These patients also have abnormally low D-xylose absorption resulting from bacterial metabolism of this pentose sugar and from impaired mucosal transport. Elevated levels of volatile fatty acids, degradation products of bacterial carbohydrate metabolism, have been demonstrated in the jejunal aspirates from patients with small-bowel bacterial overgrowth, suggesting bacterial utilization of ingested carbohydrates.[61]

## COLON CANCER: ASSOCIATION WITH MICROFLORA

More than 130,000 cases of large-bowel cancer are diagnosed annually in the United States. It has become the most frequently diagnosed cancer of internal organs in the United States, surpassing even lung and breast cancers. Epidemiologic studies have shown that the incidence of colon cancer is higher among North Americans and Western Europeans than among Africans, Asians, and South Americans. The critical factor that may account for these differences is the characteristic "Western" diet, which is high in beef, fat, and protein, and low in dietary fiber. Armstrong and Doll,[62] Howell,[63] and Drasar and Irving[64] have demonstrated, by using intercountry comparisons, positive correlation between the consumption of beef, total fat, animal fat, and animal protein and the incidence of colon cancer.

Studies of migrant populations indicate that their cancer incidence approximates the prevailing rates in the place of *residence,* rather than the place of *birth*. Dunn has compared the incidence of cancer in Japan with that among Japanese in California.[65] The incidence of stomach cancer, which is high in Japan, has undergone a stepwise reduction, with intermediate rates in immigrant Japanese, to lower rates in American-born Japanese. In contrast, cancer of the colon has shown the opposite trend; among American-born Japanese, the incidence of colon tumors is approaching that observed in native Caucasians.

In the past 10 years a number of investigators have proposed that the effect of diet on cancer development is indirect, primarily by affecting the ability of the host to metabolize procarcinogens to proximate carcinogens. In the case of colon cancer, however, activation of carcinogens may be mediated by the bacterial flora in the large bowel. Several bacterial enzymes have been implicated in generating mutagens, carcinogens, and various tumor promoters: β-glucuronidase, β-glucosidase, β-galactosidase, nitroreductase, azoreductase, 7-α-steroid dehydrogenase, and 7-α-hydroxy-steroid dehydroxylase.[17,18,21,66]

The carcinogenic potential of bacterial enzymes in the intestinal microflora has been illustrated in a series of studies involving experimental colon cancer induced by cycasin. This substance is a naturally occurring β-glucoside of the methylazoxymethanol, extractable from the seeds and roots of cycad plants. Laqueur et al. discovered that feeding cycasin to infant rats caused hepatomas, renal sarcomas, squamous cell carcinomas of the ear duct and, in greatest frequency, intestinal adenocarcinomas that were almost exclusively located in the large bowel.[21] The genetic strain of rat had little influence on the carcinogenic effect of cycasin; similar tumors were induced in Osborne-Mendel, Sprague-Dawley, Fischer, and Wistar rats.[21] The intestinal flora was required for the carcinogenic activity of cycasin because the compound was completely inactive when given orally to germfree rats.

The age of the animal was a critical factor. Cycasin was inactive when given parenterally to *adult* conventional animals. Newborn conventional and newborn germfree rats, however, developed tumors after subcutaneous or intraperitoneal injection of cycasin. A tissue (host) or bacterial (microflora) β-glucosidase is required to hydrolyze the glycolytic bond in cycasin in order to release the active aglycone, methylazoxymethanol. The observation that subcutaneous or intraperitoneal injections of cycasin caused tumors in infant rats, but not in older rats, supported the view that young animals have a tissue β-glucosidase that disappears by the third week of life. An additional supposition was that cycasin did not enter the bile in significant quantities since older animals did not develop intestinal adenocarcinomas when given cycasin by the subcutaneous route.

The discovery of the carcinogenicity of cycasin led Druckery et al. to test the precursors, azoxymethane, azomethane, and dimethylhydrazine.[67] These compounds were carcinogenic in conventional and germfree animals.[68] The route of administration was not critical since tumors developed after oral or subcutaneous administration.[21]

## Bacterial Enzymes

Bacterial β-glucuronidase seems to play an important role in colon carcinogenesis. This substance has a wide substrate specificity and, consequently, can hydrolyze a large number of different glucuronides. These reactions are potentially important in the generation of carcinogenic and toxic substances, inasmuch as many compounds are detoxified by glucuronide formation in the liver and subsequently enter the bowel via bile. Deconjugation in the intestine then regenerates the carcinogenic or toxic compound. Several studies have shown that intestinal β-glucuronidase can alter or amplify the biologic activity of exogenous and endogenous compounds. For example, toxic aglycones can be regenerated in situ in the bowel by bacterial β-glucuronidase. Fisher et al. have investigated the metabolic fate of diethylstilbestrol-β-D-glucuronide.[43] When given orally to germfree rats, the compound was rapidly recovered in the feces as a result of poor absorption of the glucuronide in the intestine. In contrast, when this compound was fed to conventional animals, both the rate and the amount of compound recovered in the feces decreased. These changes were accounted for by intestinal absorption of free diethylstilbestrol. In animals with a conventional microflora, diethylstilbestrol makes approximately 1.5 passes through the enterohepatic circulation. This increased exposure can amplify the biologic activity of this compound, which is believed to be a carcinogen for vaginal and mammary tissue.

Weisburger et al. have studied the metabolism of the carcinogen N-hydroxyfluorenylacetamide, administered parenterally to conventional and germfree rats.[69] Germ-free rats excreted appreciably larger amounts of the glucuronide of N-hydroxyfluorenylacetamide in their feces than did conventional animals. The cecal and fecal metabolites in conventional rats were mostly free, unconjugated compounds, whereas the major fraction in germfree animals was conjugated with glucuronic or sulfuric acid.

Morotomi et al. reported that cell-free extracts of some strains of intestinal bacteria, including *Bacteroides fragilis, B. vulgatus, B. thetaiotaomicron, Eubacterium lentum, Peptostreptococcus,* and *Escherichia coli*, enhanced the mutagenicity of bile from rats given 1-nitropyrene via stomach tube.[69a] These bacterial cell-free extracts hydrolyzed the synthetic β-D-glucuronides of phenolphthalein and/or p-nitrophenol. Cell-free extracts of bacteria not capable of increasing mutagenicity did not hydrolyze the glucuronides. These data indicate that the glucuronides of 1-nitropyrene metabolites secreted into the bile can be hydrolyzed in the intestine by bacterial β-glucuronidases to potent mutagenic aglycones.

Nitroreductase and azoreductase are responsible for reducing nitro and azo compounds, respectively, to aromatic amines. The highly reactive intermediates and end products are known mutagens and carcinogens with animals. These enzymes are mostly confined to bacteria residing in the bowel. Azo dyes are widely used in the textile, printing, and food dye industries and in laboratories. Water-soluble azo dyes are degraded by intestinal microorganisms in the gastrointestinal tract.[69b] Large-bowel cancer occurs more commonly in highly industrialized countries, and the extent of the use of azo dyes is related to the degree of industrialization of the country. A possible connection may exist between the number of cancer cases and the use of azo dyes.[69c]

There is a 90% correlation between carcinogenicity and mutagenicity for aromatic amines and azo dyes tested with the *Salmonella*/microsomal mutagenicity test. The transformation of azo dyes by intestinal bacteria may be a necessary prerequisite of carcinogenicity.

The reduction of azocompounds by azoreductase is believed to be mediated through a free radical mechanism, which produces intermediates that react with proteins and nucleic acids. Azoreductase also can reduce food dyes, releasing phenyl- and naphthyl-substituted amines. These compounds have been implicated as chemical carcinogens.[70] The amines generated in the bowel via the azoreductase reaction are probably further oxidized by microsomal enzymes in the intestinal mucosa to proximal carcinogens.

The role of bacteria in the generation of mutagens from a number of azo dyes is noteworthy. Trypan blue is widely used as a biologic stain and is not mutagenic, but reduction by a cell-free extract of *Fusobacterium* produces a mutagen, O-tolidine,[70a] which is mutagenic in the Ames assay and also carcinogenic.[70b] Ponceau 3R, another biologic stain, is reduced in vitro by *Fusobacterium* to a 2,4,5-trimethylaniline, which has been determined to be mutagenic.[70c] Incubation of methyl orange or methyl yellow with intestinal anaerobes and testing with a *Salmonella* TA 1538 in the presence of a microsomal activating system have proved positive for mutagenicity. Both dyes are reductively cleaved to the mutagen N,N-dimethyl-p-phenylene diamine.[70d] Other azo dyes that have been shown to undergo bacterial reduction to mutagenic or carcinogenic products are direct black 38, direct red 2, and direct blue 15. These dyes are converted to benzidine, 3-3-dimethylbenzidine, and 3,3 dimethoxybenzidine respectively. Congo red is also reduced by rat cecal bacteria to benzidine.[70e] In the absence of a bacterial reductase system, congo red is not mutagenic toward *Salmonella* TA 1538 in the presence of a liver activating system. However, preincubation of congo red with cecal bacteria has resulted in a positive mutagenic response.

Nitroreductase causes the formation of reactive nitroso and N-hydroxy intermediates in the course of converting aromatic nitro compounds to aromatic amines. The precursor aromatic nitro compounds are commonly found in factory effluents as industrial chemical pollutants. Wheeler et al. studied a similar reaction, the reduction of p-nitrobenzoic acid, in conventional and germfree rats.[31] Conventional animals rapidly converted p-nitrobenzoic acid, whereas germfree rats reduced little of the *nitrocompound*.

The nitrated polynuclear aromatic hydrocarbon called 1-nitropyrene is readily formed by reaction of nitrogen oxides with the combustion product pyrene. Its presence in diesel engine exhaust represents a potential health hazard because of its high mutagenicity in bacterial test systems and its carcinogenicity in rats. When 1-nitropyrene was administered orally to conventional rats, 5 to 6% of the dose was detected in the feces as 1-aminopyrene.[70f] When a similar experiment was performed on germfree rats, no 1-aminopyrene appeared in the feces. Since reduction of 1-nitropyrene to 1-aminopyrene is an activation process, the results indicate that intestinal microfloras are important in the metabolic activation of 1-nitropyrene.

Miller and Miller[71] and Weisburger and Weisburger,[70] after reviewing the evidence, have suggested that the products of these reactions are extremely important in chemical carcinogenesis.

The effect of diet on fecal bacterial nitroreductase and azoreductase activity has been studied in rats.[17] Rats initially maintained on a grain diet, then shifted after several weeks to a meat diet, showed a twofold rise in fecal nitroreductase activity on the meat diet. This increase started within 6 days, although the total effect required 12 to 17 days. Fecal azoreductase also increased approximately twofold when rats were shifted to the meat diet. An increase in specific activity of this enzyme was noted between 4 and 10 days after the dietary change.

Studies on human populations have revealed that American vegetarians have lower levels of fecal nitroreductase than Americans eating a Western diet.[19] Fiber supplements to the Western diet do not affect the levels of fecal azoreductase or nitroreductase.

## Bile Acids, Beef, and Bacteria

Bile acids have been studied extensively as candidate carcinogens because of their structural similarity to the carcinogenic polycyclic aromatic hydrocarbons. The concentration of fecal bile acids is increased in people eating a beef (high-fat) diet. This concentration induces colonic bacteria to produce larger amounts of 7-$\alpha$-dehydroxylase, the enzyme involved in conversion of primary to secondary bile acids.[72] White et al. showed that the addition of the chenodeoxycholic acid to a growing culture of *Eubacterium* resulted in a striking increase in 7-$\alpha$-dehydroxylase activity.[73] Salvioli and co-workers found increased fecal concentrations of cholic and chenodeoxycholic acid, and decreased fecal concentrations of secondary bile acids after daily administration of lyophilized *Streptococcus faecalis* to normal volunteers.[74]

Demographic studies have demonstrated a correlation between high fecal concentrations of secondary bile acids and the Western high-beef diet.[15] Hill et al. noted that the fecal microflora of North Americans and Western Europeans contained more bacterial strains capable of 7-α-dehydroxylation than did those from Ugandans or Indians.[10] In studies by Mower et al. involving Japanese living in Akita, Japan, and Japanese living in Hawaii who adopted a Western-style diet, the latter group had higher levels of fecal deoxycholic acid; however, little difference was noted in the other fecal bile acids.[75] In contrast to these studies, fecal concentrations of coprostanol and coprostanone, degradation products of cholesterol, are higher in people eating a Western-style diet. Mastromarino and co-workers studied patients with colon cancer and found elevated levels of both 7-α-dehydroxylase and cholesterol dehydrogenase compared with normal controls.[66] Elevations of both enzymes also were noted in patients with nonhereditary colonic polyps.[76]

MacDonald et al. studied in vegetarian Seventh-Day Adventists and subjects consuming a mixed Western diet the fecal NAD- and NADP-dependent 7-α-hydroxysteroid dehydrogenase, which converts hydroxy-bile acids to keto-bile acids.[16] The activity was lower in the vegetarian group, suggesting that increased fecal NAD- and NADP-dependent 7-α-hydroxysteroid dehydrogenase is associated with risk of large-bowel cancer.

## Nitrosamines

It has been 30 years since Magee and Barnes reported the induction of liver cancer in rats by feeding dimethylnitrosamine.[77] Since this first report, at least 80 different N-nitroso compounds have been found to produce tumors at different organ sites. Nitrosamines form readily by the reaction of the secondary amines with nitrite in an acidic medium. Nitrosation can occur in the mammalian stomach if both nitrites and amines are present.[78] The potential danger of this reaction is somewhat reduced by the relatively short residence time of these compounds in the stomach. Nitrite is added to cured meat and fish, and nitroso compounds have been found in these and other food sources.[79]

Bacteria have also been implicated in the formation of N-nitroso compounds. Nitrite is produced through the reduction of nitrate by many common microbial species. Certain leafy vegetables may accumulate high concentrations of ni-

trate that can then be converted to nitrite by bacteria during storage. Tannenbaum et al. reported that the oral microbial flora of humans can reduce nitrate to nitrite, producing levels in saliva as high as 6 to 10 ppm.[80]

Klubes et al. reported that dimethylamine and sodium nitrite, when incubated together with rat intestinal bacteria under anaerobic conditions at pH 7.0, gave rise to dimethylnitrosamine.[81] The formation was enhanced by the presence of riboflavin. The major implication of these findings lies in the possibility of generating nitrosamines in the intestine, where the pH is nearly neutral and where the reaction could be expected to occur nonenzymatically at a very slow rate. Potentially, this reaction could be important since secondary amines can come from many dietary sources and nitrites are present as food additives. Although rapid transit in the stomach may prevent to some extent nonenzymatic nitrosamine formation, the bacterially catalyzed reaction in the large bowel could lead to significant N-nitroso formation.

## Fecal Mutagens

Bruce et al. first reported the presence of a substance in the feces from healthy humans that caused mutagenesis in the Ames test using *Salmonella typhimurium*.[82] A high correlation exists between mutagenesis in this bacterial test system and the induction of tumors in various animal models.[83] Subsequent studies have shown that in a population at high risk of developing colon cancer, 17% of the individuals had mutagens in their feces, whereas in a population at low risk, only 5% of the individuals excreted mutagens.[84]

A number of studies have investigated the influence of specific dietary components for their effect on fecal mutagenic activity. Reddy et al. have investigated fat, protein, and fiber,[84a] and Land and Bruce have investigated ascorbic acid.[84b] The latter study showed that ascorbic acid given orally to volunteers decreased their levels of fecal mutagens. In general, persons consuming vegetarian diets with low levels of animal fat and protein, and relatively high levels of fruits, vegetables, and dietary fiber have less fecal mutagenic activity than those consuming typical meat-containing diets.[84c,84d]

Van Tassel et al. reported that the concentration of the mutagen increased dramatically when the feces was incubated anaerobically for several days at 37°C.[85] This observation indicates that the fecal flora, probably the anaerobic component, produces the mutagenic substance. In vitro production of the mutagen was enhanced by the addition of bile or bile acids. The addition of any one of five different strains of *Bacteroides,* a common component of the normal intestinal flora, to a broth containing feces from a person who excreted the mutagen resulted in a five- to eight-fold increase in mutagen production. The chemical structure of the mutagen has been identified as C-12 (dodeca) vinyl ether of glycerol.[86] The C-12 side chain has five double bonds. The chemical name of the mutagen is (S)-3-(1,3,5,7,9-dodecapentaenyloxy)-1,2-propanediol.

## Bacterial Reactions as Protection against Tumors

Most reports dealing with the relationship between the intestinal flora and cancer have emphasized the generation of carcinogens. There is evidence, however, that the opposite, an inactivation of carcinogenic compounds, also occurs. For example, Rowland and Grasso have shown that *E. coli, Lactobacillus, Bifidobacterium,* and *Bacteroides* can degrade the carcinogens dimethylnitrosamine and diphenylnitrosamine to nitrite and the corresponding amine.[87] The reaction could counteract the generation of N-nitroso compounds formed nonenzymatically in the stomach or by bacterial action in the lower intestine.

Williams et al. indicated that bacteria in the cecum of the rat have the ability to dehydroxylate N-hydroxyfluorenylacetamide, thereby generating fluorenylacetamide.[88] The dehydroxylation of N-hydroxyamines may reverse the activation of amines to proximal carcinogens.

Other studies by Wheeler et al. demonstrated that the intestinal flora can dehydroxylate N-hydroxyl-4-acetylaminobiphenyl to acetylaminobiphenyl.[89] The reversal of the metabolic activation of the parent carcinogen can be demonstrated in cultures of some bacteria that are indigenous to the intestinal tract. The flora of the cecum is particularly active in this reduction. These experiments may explain the observation that rats fed this compound develop tumors in the forestomach, but not in the cecum.

## SUMMARY

This chapter has reviewed the role of the intestinal flora in the metabolism and synthesis of exogenous and endogenous compounds. The ability of the flora to synthesize and activate nutrients as well as to metabolize hormones, bile acids, cholesterol, and various dietary components has been presented. The involvement of the intestinal flora in various diseases has also been discussed. It is clear that there are positive and negative metabolic effects of these organisms, and the balance of these forces has profound implications for the physiologic state of the host.

## REFERENCES

1. Finegold, S.M., Attebery, H.R., Sutter, V.L.: Am. J. Clin. Nutr. *27*:1456, 1974.
2. Moore, W.E.C., Holderman, L.V.: Appl. Micro. *27*:961, 1974.
3. Drasar, B.S., Hill, M.J.: Human Intestinal Flora. New York, Academic Press, 1974.
4. Drasar, B.S., Skinner, M., McLeod, G.M.: Gastroenterology *56*:71, 1969.
5. Haenel, H.: Am. J. Clin. Nutr. *23*:1433, 1970.
6. Long, S.S., Swenson, R.M.: J. Pediatr. *91*:298, 1977.
7. Moore, W.E.C., Holderman, L.V.: Cancer Res. *35*:3418, 1975.
8. Maier, B.R., et al.: Am. J. Clin. Nutr. *27*:1470, 1974.
9. Reddy, B.S., Weisburger, J.H., Wynder, E.L.: Science *183*:416, 1974.
10. Hill, M.J., et al.: Lancet *1*:95, 1971.
11. Finegold, S.M., et al.: Am. J. Clin. Nutr. *30*:1781, 1977.
12. Drasar, B.S., Jenkins, D.J.A., Cummings, J.H.: J. Med. Microbiol. *9*:423, 1976.
13. Goldin, B.R., Gorbach, S.L.: Microbial factors and nutrition in carcinogenesis. *In* Advances in Nutritional Research. (Draper, H.H., Ed.) New York, Plenum Press, 1979.
14. Hill, M.J.: Cancer Res. *35*:3398, 1975.
15. Reddy, B.S., Wynder, E.L.: J. Natl. Cancer Inst. *52*:1437, 1973.
16. MacDonald, I.A., Webb, G.R., Mahoney, D.C.: Am. J. Clin. Nutr. *31*:5233–5238, 1978.
17. Goldin, B.R., Gorbach, S.L.: J. Natl. Cancer Inst. *57*:371, 1976.
18. Goldin, B.R., Sullivan, C.E., Gorbach, S.L.: Etiologic factors in the development of colonic cancer: Bacteria, beef and animal fat. *In* Nutrition in Gastrointestinal Diseases. (Kurtz, R.C., Ed.) New York, Churchill Livingstone, Inc., 1981.
19. Goldin, B.R., et al.: J. Natl. Cancer Inst. *64*:255, 1980.
19a. Lindop, R., Tasman-Jones, C., Thomsen, L.L., et al.: Br. J. Nutr. *54*:21, 1985.
20. Hawksworth, G., Drasar, B.S., Hill, M.J.: J. Med. Microbiol. *4*:451, 1971.
21. Laqueur, G.L., Spatz, M.: Cancer Res. *28*:2262, 1968.
21a. Tamura, G., Gold, C., Ferro-Luzze, A., et al.: Proc. Natl. Acad. Sci. *77*:4961, 1980.
21b. Macdonald, I.A., Bassard, R.G., Hutchison, D.M., et al.: Appl. Environ. Microbiol. *47*:350, 1984.
21c. Moder, J.A., Macdonald, I.A.: Mutat. Res. *155*:99, 1985.
22. Lindenbaum, J., et al.: N. Engl. J. Med. *305*:789, 1981.
23. Lindenbaum, J.: Bacterial inactivation of digoxin. 8th International Symposium on Intestinal Microecology, Boston, 1983.
24. Suzuksi, K., et al.: Appl. Environ. Microbiol. *37*:379, 1979.
25. Parkinson, T.M., Brown, J.P.: Annu. Rev. Nutr. *1*:175, 1981.
26. Combes, R.D., Haveland-Smith, R.B.: Mutat. Res. *98*:101, 1982.
27. Bonser, G.M., Bradshaw, L., Clayson, D.B., et al.: Br. J. Cancer *10*:539, 1956.
28. Hartman, C.P., Andrews, A.W., Chung, K.T.: Infect. Immun. *23*:686, 1979.
29. Chung, K.T., Fulk, G.E., Andrews, A.W.: Mutat. Res. *58*:375, 1978.
30. Peppercorn, M.A., Goldman, P.: J. Pharmacol. Exp. Ther. *181*:555, 1972.

31. Wheeler, L.A., Soderberg, F.B., Goldman, P.: J. Pharmacol. Exp. Ther. *194*:135, 1975.
32. Goldin, B.R., Gorbach, S.L.: J. Natl. Cancer Inst. *73*:689, 1984.
33. Scheline, R.R.: Pharmacol. Rev.. *25*:454, 1973.
34. Kajima, S., Ichibagose, H.: Chem. Pharm. Bull. (Tokyo) *14*:1971, 1966.
35. Renwick, A.G., Williams, R.T.: Biochem. J. *129*:869, 1972.
36. Wallace, W.C., Lethco, E.T., Brouwer, E.A.: J. Pharmacol. Exp. Ther. *175*:325, 1970.
37. Goldin, B.R., Peppercorn, M.A., Goldman, P.: J. Pharmacol. Exp. Ther. *186*:160, 1973.
38. Asatoor, A.M.: Biochem. Biophys. Acta *199*:200, 1965.
39. Hoskins, L.C., Zamcheck, N.: Gastroenterology *54*:210, 1968.
40. Scheline, R.R.: Monogr. Pharmacol. Physiol. *5*:551, 1980.
41. Plaa, G.L.: The enterohepatic circulation. *In* Handbook of Experimental Pharmacology. (Gillette, J.R., Ed.) New York, Springer-Verlag, 1975.
42. Kumar, R., Nagubandi, S., Mattox, V.R., et al.: J. Clin. Invest. *65*:277, 1980.
43. Fisher, L.J., Millburn, P., Smith, R.L.: Biochem. J. *100*:69, 1966.
44. Clark, A.G., et al.: Biochem. J. *112*:17, 1969.
45. Adlercreutz, H., et al.: J. Clin. Endocrinol. Metab. *43*:497, 1976.
46. Adlercruetz, H., Martin, F., Tikkanen, J.M., et al.: Acta Endocrinol. (Kbh) *80*:551, 1975.
47. Goldin, B.R., et al.: N. Engl. J. Med. *307*:1542, 1982.
47a. Matschiner, J.T., Taggart, W.V., Amelotti, J.M.: Biochemistry *6*:1243, 1967.
47b. Pennock, J.F.: Vitam. Horm. *24*:307, 1966.
47c. Udall, J.A.: JAMA *194*:127, 1965.
47d. Frick, P.G., Riedler, G., Brogli, H.J.: Appl. Physiol. *23*:387, 1967.
48. Albert, M.J., Mathan, V.I., Baker, S.J.: Nature *283*:781, 1980.
49. Coates, M.E., Fuller, R.: *In* Microbial Ecology of the Gut Flora. (Clarke, R.T.J., Bauchop, T.) New York, Academic Press, 1977.
50. Wostman, B.S.: Annu. Rev. Nutr. *1*:257, 1981.
51. Hoskins, L.C., Boulding, E.T.: J. Clin. Invest. *57*:63, 1976.
52. Cummings, J.H.: Gut *22*:763, 1981.
53. McNeil, N.I., Cummings, J.H., James, W.P.T.: Gut *19*:819, 1978.
54. Lombardi, P., Goldin, B., Boutin, E., et al.: J. Steroid Biochem. *9*:795, 1978.
55. Goddard, P., Hill, M.J.: Biochem. Biophys. Acta *280*:336, 1972.
56. Simon, G.L., Gorbach, S.L.: Gastroenterology *86*:174, 1984.
57. Tabagchali, S., Booth, C.C.: Lancet *2*:12, 1966.
57a. Fry, R.J.M.: Nature *203*:1396, 1964.
57b. Raicht, R.F.F., Deschner, E., Salem, G.: Gastroenterology *68*:979, 1975.
58. King, C.E., Toskes, P.P.: Gastroenterology *76*:1035, 1979.
59. Welkos, S., Toskes, P., Baker, H.: Gastoenterology *80*:313, 1981.
60. Grocey, M.: Am. J. Clin. Nutr. *32*:234, 1979.
61. Prizont, R., Whitehead, J.S., Kim, Y.S.: Gastroenterology *69*:1254, 1975.
62. Armstrong, B., Doll, R.: Int. J. Cancer *15*:617, 1975.
63. Howell, M.A.: J. Chronic Dis. *28*:67, 1975.
64. Drasar, B.S., Irving, D.: Br. J. Cancer *27*:167, 1973.
65. Dunn, J.E.: Cancer Res. *35*:3240, 1975.
66. Mastromarino, A., Reddy, B.S., Wynder, E.L.: Am. J. Clin. Nutr. *29*:1455, 1976.
67. Druckery, H., Preussman, R., Matzbies, F., et al.: Naturwissenschaften *54*:285, 1967.
68. Laqueur, G.L., McDaniel, E.G., Matsumoto, H.: J. Natl. Cancer Inst. *39*:355, 1967.
69. Weisburger, J.H., Grantham, P.H., Horton, R.E.: Biochem. Pharmacol. *19*:151, 1970.
69a. Morotomi, M., Nanno, M., Watanrobe, T., et al.: Mutat. Res. *149*:171, 1985.
69b. Chung, K.T.: Mutat. Res. *114*:269, 1983.
69c. Wolff, A.W., Oehme, F.W.J.: Am. Vet. Med. Assoc. *164*:623, 1974.
70. Weisburger, J.H., Weisburger, E.K.: Pharmacol. Rev. *25*:1, 1973.
70a. Harman, C.P., Falk, C.E., Andrews, A.W.: Mutat. Res. *58*:125, 1978.
70b. Weisburger, J.J., Weisburger, E.K.: Chem. Eng. News *44*:124, 1966.
70c. Hartman, C.P., Andres, A.W., Chung, K.T.: Infect. Immun. *23*:686, 1979.
70d. Chung, K.T., Fulk, C.E., Andrews, A.W.: Mutat. Res. *58*:375, 1978.
70e. Reid, T.M., Morton, K.C., Wang, C.Y., et al.: Mutat. Res. *117*:105, 1983.
70f. El-Bayoumy, K., Fharma, C., Louis, Y.M., et al.: Cancer Lett. *19*:311, 1983.
71. Miller, J.A., Miller, E.C.: Prog. Exp. Tumor Res. *11*:273, 1969.
72. Weisburger, J.H.: Cancer *28*:60, 1971.
73. White, B.A., Lipsky, R.L., Prieke, R.J., et al.: Steroids *35*:103, 1980.
74. Salvioli, G., et al.: Digestion *23*:80, 1981.
75. Mower, H.F., et al.: Cancer Res. *39*:328, 1979.
76. Mastromarino, A.J., Reddy, B.S., Wynder, F.L.: Cancer Res. *38*:4458, 1978.
77. Magee, P.H., Barnes, J.M.: Br. J. Cancer *10*:114, 1956.
78. Mirvish, S.S.: J. Natl. Cancer Inst. *44*:633, 1970.
79. Ender, F., Ceh, L.: Food Cosmet. Toxicol. *6*:569, 1968.
80. Tannenbaum, S.R., Sinsky, A.J., Weisman, M., et al.: J. Natl. Cancer Inst. *53*:79, 1974.
81. Klubes, P., Cerna, I., Robinowitz, A.D., et al.: Food Cosmet. Toxicol. *10*:757, 1972.
82. Bruce, W.R., Varghese, A.J., Furrer, R., et al.: Cold Spring Harbor Conf. Cell Proliferation *4*:1641, 1977.
83. Ames, B.N., McCann, J., Yamasaki, E.: Mutat. Res. *31*:347, 1975.
84. Ehrich, M., Aswell, J.E., Van Tassell, R.L., et al.: Mutat. Res. *64*:231, 1979.
84a. Reddy, B.S., Sharma, C., Wynder, E.: Cancer Lett. *10*:123, 1980.
84b. Land, P.C., Bruce, W.R.: Proc. Am. Assoc. Cancer Res. *19*:167, 1978.
84c. Kuhnlein, H.V., Kuhnlein, V.: Nutr. Cancer *2*:119, 1981.
84d. Nader, C.J., Potter, J.D., Weller, R.A.: Nutr. Rep. Int. *23*:113, 1981.
85. Van Tassel, R.L., MacDonald, D.K., Wilkins, T.D.: Infect. Immun. *37*:975, 1982.
86. Hirai, N., Kingston, G.I., Van Tassell, R.L., et al.: J. Am. Chem. Soc. *104*:6150, 1982.
87. Rowland, I.R., Grasso, P.: Appl. Microbiol. *29*:7, 1975.
88. Williams, J.R., et al.: Biochem. Pharmacol. *19*:173, 1970.
89. Wheeler, L.A., Soderberg, F.B., Goldman, P.: Cancer Res. *35*:2962, 1975.

*Chapter* **28**

# FOOD AS FUEL: THE DEVELOPMENT OF CONCEPTS

John M. Kinney

Food has been considered to be fuel since the time of primitive man. Yet, the need for food was originally linked to general ideals of health and well-being. A central aspect of man's concern has been maintaining a comfortable body temperature closely associated with satisfying a sense of hunger. To the earliest physicians, the healthy body felt warm, whereas at the time of death the body became cool. Therefore, it is not surprising that some mechanism of heat production, or "vital heat," came to be synonymous with life. This vitalistic approach to life embraced all sorts of supernatural beliefs not subject to experimental study and delayed attempts to measure and to analyze biologic and medical observations.

By the time of Hippocrates, the Greeks had developed a hypothetical system that explained the mechanisms of health and illness in terms of four basic humors in the body. The four basic elements of Greek metaphysics (water, air, fire, and earth) had each a specific quality (moist, dry, hot, and cold) and were related to the visible secretions of the body (blood, phlegm, yellow bile, and black bile). It was believed that the body was in health when these humors were in balance, whereas an excess, or deficiency, in any of the humors caused illness. The use of specific drugs or nutrients was meant to restore the proper balance of these humors. The physician, Galen, linked the four humors with four basic temperaments: sanguine, phlegmatic, choleric, and melancholic. Aristotle had said, "Nature does nothing without a purpose," and Aristotle sought the explanation for the purpose. Galen felt that he knew the purpose. His writings remained the unimpeachable authority on medicine for nearly 1,500 years.

Fuel was understood as burning to produce heat or power, but the concept of the importance of air in supporting combustion and respiration had to await the work of Boyle and his contemporaries in the late 1600s. When the burning of fuel in combustion was recognized in the late 1700s as the combining of fuel with oxygen and the giving off of carbon dioxide and heat, the respiration of animals and man was quickly recognized as a special case of combustion.

The quantitative relationship between individual foods and their use in the body to produce a predictable amount of heat developed slowly over the nineteenth century. The new information regarding gas exchange was opposed by those who continued to believe in vitalistic concepts. Furthermore, the chemical composition of the main foodstuffs could only be clarified with the growth of organic chemistry, which led to the application of metabolic balance studies in animals and later in man.

Understanding the relationship of chemical energy to heat was greatly assisted by physical scientists who laid the groundwork for the field of thermodynamics. The quantitative relationship of respiration and heat production depended upon advances in nutritional chemistry, which allowed a pure foodstuff to have the heat output measured in a bomb calorimeter and then measured in the human body by indirect calorimetry. These studies demonstrated that the human body obeyed the law of conservation of energy.

The field of calorimetry from 1900 to 1940 was

**516**

mainly devoted to examining the abnormalities in energy expenditure associated with starvation and various diseases, in particular thyroid disease, diabetes, and the more common fevers. Interest in calorimetry then waned, to be followed by a resurgence of interest during the past 15 years as a result of the growing interest in adjusting food intake to energy expenditure to promote health and to treat hospital malnutrition.

The basic factors in measuring energy expenditure in man were considered to be understood early in the twentieth century. However, modern investigators are presenting new evidence suggesting that our ability to measure, or predict, the energy requirements for any given individual are not as precise as had been formerly thought. In addition, the knowledge of how food is utilized for energy in acute disease and injury, as well as in problems of starvation, suggests that we still have more to learn about the role of food and "vital heat."

## FROM VITAL HEAT TO EXPERIMENTAL MEDICINE

The title of this chapter will immediately suggest to the reader that food is fuel for cells and tissues working to support life processes. However, from the perspective of the past 2,000 years, it is important to remember that food as fuel had commonly been considered in terms of providing heat. Even today, in general references to food, the first thought of the lay person relates to the calorie content of the food. When a person is over- or underweight, it is usually assumed that he is consuming too many or too few calories.

The concept of innate heat was first proposed by early Greek writers. An innate body heat was thought to be intimately linked with or synonymous with all life processes. The theory was strengthened by postulating a source for this heat and by making it indistinguishable from life itself. Mendelsohn has pointed out that a generalization as powerful as innate heat made possible the unification and explanation of otherwise diverse natural phenomena.[1] Plato believed that this vital heat was an important factor in the digestion of food and drink. The principal seat of this internal fire was the heart and, therefore, the heart must be continually cooled. According to Plato, the lung was placed "around" the heart as a sort of buffer, so that respiratory movement could be a factor to continuously cool the heart.[2] Thus, the action of the heart, the structure of the heart, and the function of respiration were all considered to accommodate this vital heat. Plato felt that vital heat had an importance for life and death and many natural functions, such as growth.

Aristotle treated the concept of vital heat as a source of life and all of its powers—"of nutrition, of sensation, of movement, and of thought."[3] In fact, Aristotle wrote that "the soul is, as it were, set aglow with fire." In locating the vital heat in the heart, Aristotle made the heart preeminent in body functions and then designed much of his thinking about physiology to be consistent with this idea. In addition, Aristotle believed that nature had developed the brain as a counterbalance to the heart and its heat content. Hence, the human brain had to be large to offset the volume of heat and blood in the human heart. The innate heat was thought to control growth through the concoction and transformation of the fluid and solid matter of food. The mode of animal reproduction was also thought to be determined by the vital heat. The warmer an animal, the more perfect would be the state in which its young were generated. Thus, Aristotle found in the concept of innate heat a way of explaining the myriad functions of the living organism, from its generation to its death. While he thought that vital heat was like fire, however, it was not quite like fire; it needed to be moderated and cooled to keep it from burning to exhaustion. These details of Aristotle's view, together with the later contributions of Galen, formed part of the doctrine of the most influential and longest lived biologic and medical tradition that man has known. During the 1,500 years prior to the seventeenth century, the vital heat, as defined by Aristotle, was utilized in explanations by both physiologists and physicians. An important and powerful generalization that was useful for Aristotle became a rigid doctrine in later years and tended to prevent the further search for causal explanations into the mechanisms of life.

Galen, perhaps the greatest of the Greek men of medicine, practiced in Rome in the second century A.D. His doctrines provided a synthesis of the ideas from many previous philosophers. He believed that innate heat of the body was of paramount importance. Food clearly emerged as a fuel for the body, much in the manner that had been suggested by the Hippocratic authors. Galen even wrote that the fatty part of the blood acted as a kind of fuel for the heat of warm-blooded animals, whereas it was stored in that of cold-blooded animals. The very word "nutriment" implied an increase in the heat of the body and, conversely, the lack of nourishment, a cooling of the body. Galen wrote that food "is used up by our heat as oil is by a flame." Aristotle was hesitant to draw an analogy between fire and innate heat and sought to distinguish between the two. Galen seemed to find a complete identity between the flame and animal heat. Not only were both phenomena nourished by fuel, but they both utilized air in a process similar to that of respiration, and they both produced waste products of combustion that he referred to as ash, smoke, and soot. Respiration was then thought to provide not only cooling for the heart, but also an outflow of what Galen referred to as "smoky mist." The heart was considered to be the source of the heat and from that organ the pulse distributed warmth to various parts of the body. The substance of the air breathed in the lungs was thought by some to be involved in the formation of a "vital spirit" and not particularly related to heat production, a view in contrast to that of Hippocrates, who believed that respiration was useful for "nutrition" as well as for "refreshing cooling."[3]

Christian philosophers writing on the nature of man described the important role of innate heat. They represented Galen's views on the heart as the source of heat and the importance of respiration for maintenance of internal warmth at the proper level. Avicenna provided a codification of Muslim medical knowledge, and his views were, again, strongly influenced by the attitude of Galen toward vital heat.[5] Thus, a group of ideas concerning air, respiration, heat, blood, and heartbeat have been the focus of philosophic speculation since the dawn of man. Such preoccupations, whether in religion, myth, or science, long preceded "physiology" as an independent science.

William Harvey is credited with the single most important discovery in the history of the physiologic sciences: the circulation of the blood.[6,7] Harvey's dissections identified the heart's motion and led to the observation of the pulmonary transit and the arterial pulse. Such findings were not in themselves new. His innovation lay in noting that to keep the veins from being emptied of blood and the arteries from being choked with blood, the circulation in the periphery needed to pass from the arteries into the veins and, thence, to return to the heart in a circular motion. This concept required an understanding of the capillary circulation, which was not defined until the availability of the microscope.

When Harvey began his work, the anatomists commonly believed that the body was divided into three parts.[8] The abdomen was thought to serve the natural functions of nutrition, excretion, and procreation. Its principal organ was the liver, which was the seat of these natural functions and the origin of the abdominal venous circulation. Food, having passed through the stomach and the intestines, was absorbed and drawn off by the mesentery veins to pass through the substance of the liver. The second portion of the body, the thorax, served the vital functions of maintaining and distributing heat and life throughout the body. Its principal organ was the heart, which was the hottest part of the body, containing a vital heat that was distributed from the heart to the rest of the body and was moderated by the cool air from the lungs. Air that had passed through the pulmonary circulation was thought to serve as the raw material for the creation of vital spirits that were somehow linked to arterial blood. The third great center of the body was the head, with the principal part being the brain. The head was a source of all animal functions such as motion, sense, and reason, which it carried out through its effector vessels, the nerves. Some believed that the lungs were mainly involved in bringing air to the blood, which was somehow necessary for the production of vital heat. Others believed that the respiration also removed waste products in the expired air.

The concept of heat was obviously central to the explanatory framework of traditional physiology. Several kinds were distinguished. Every part of the body had its own innate heat proper to it as a living being. This heat in the extremities was continuously being dissipated into the surrounding environment. It therefore had to be replenished from some origin and source in the body, which was obviously the heart. This heat, together with the heartbeat, fabricated the vital spirit out of air and blood. The vital spirit was in turn carried by an activated arterial blood. What was the vital spirit? The animal faculty had animal spirits distributed through the nerves. Similarly, the vital faculty seated in the heart was heated and vivified through the vital spirits in arterial blood. The natural faculty in the liver, it was thought, needed no such natural spirit in the blood, since venous blood was in itself the natural material of nutrition. Because both nutrition and vivification were equally necessary for all organs, every part of the body had its own venous and arterial provision. Such were the kinds of physiologic opinions that Harvey found when he turned to the textbooks at the beginning of the seventeenth century. They contained a collection of explanations whose cardinal virtue was system. Every organ had its function and every function had its organ.

That system had to be replaced with one compatible with the newly discovered facts regarding the circulation. Harvey's methodology of dissection and experiment became for his students the model procedure for the solution of physiologic problems.[7] This was combined with the values of chemical experimentation and the stimulus of Bacon's writings, all of which provided the dominant theme in the construction of physiology at that time. By the early 1650s, Harvey found an English scientific world different from the one into which he had introduced his announcement of the circulation 25 years earlier. He had by then developed some implications of his announcement and had centralized the physiologic functions of the circulation strongly in the blood. Harvey was convinced that it was there, and not in the heart, that the innate heat of the body was to be found. The blood acted through its vital properties, not through some kind of spirit generated by the beating of the heart.

Harvey gathered around him a remarkable group of men who were interested in the investigation of medical and biologic problems, and this group became known as the "Oxford School of Physiology."[9] In the process of searching for the origin of body heat, these investigators tried to decide whether the process of the beating of the heart somehow was involved with producing the heat, or whether the motion of the blood produced friction and therefore heat as it passed through the vessels of the body. The lungs were considered by Harvey to represent an important heat dissipation mechanism that prevented the cardiac generation of heat from exceeding the body's tolerance. This group of physiologists included Robert Boyle, who is credited with discovering basic facts about the movement of air in and out of the airway. Until that time, air had been considered as a single substance that was somehow associated with life, but the relationship remained obscure. Boyle and his co-workers developed a pneumatic pump in which they were able to evacuate glass containers to show that a bird could not live in an evacuated container for more than a brief period, and to demonstrate that a flame was rapidly extinguished in the same circumstances.[10] However, they were unable to show a sufficiently close correlation between the combustion of a flame and the respiration of an animal to recognize that they were closely related processes.

Robert Hooke, who had served as Boyle's laboratory assistant in the work with the air pump, continued to be interested in problems of respiration.[11] In 1667 he performed an experiment before the Royal Society to prove that the motion of the lungs was not essential to life. He did this by keeping a dog with an open chest alive by blowing air through the lungs with a bellows. A review of the writings of the Oxford Physiologists calls attention to the number of important conclusions that they partially grasped, but that were not clearly stated until approximately a century later. One of the biggest differences between their work and the work that was possible in the second half of the 1700s was the improvement in thermometry and in the methods used by investigators to study gases and ultimately the composition of air.

During the seventeenth century, biologic concepts clearly began to move away from the old idea of circulating humors as governing body functions. The improved understanding of anatomy that followed the work of Vesalius stimulated explanations for digestion and absorption, together with a growing interest in other areas of physiology. There was widespread agreement that all functions in body tissues were based on biochemical processes. However, further efforts to explain such processes depended upon the tendency of the physician (or biologist) to become more interested in chemistry or in physics.

Van Helmont was a Belgian physician who devoted much of his life to chemical experiments.[12] His attitude toward human biology was a mixture of chemical science based in part on experiments and in part on religious mysticism. He obtained gases from a number of different sources and recognized that different gases had different properties. He rejected Aristotle because he believed that fire and earth could not be classified as elements and rejected the view that a living being was composed of mixtures of general qualities common to all things. Instead, he believed that organisms were composed of seeds which were active principles responsible for specific form and function. Water, which was at first an inert element, received the seeds of various materials such as metals or plants. As matter gradually took on special characteristics, it acquired a characteristic gas of its own. He believed that every substance in nature contained its own gas, a spirit that contained the essential specificity characteristic of nature. Van Helmont distinguished six separate kinds of digestion that were thought to take place before the food could become a specific tissue. The final digestion after these six phases was specific in each organ; that is, each had at its base a "kitchen" that directed the solution of the food material brought by the blood and its conversion to the material of that tissue. He concluded that the various solutions were the result of the specific action of individual ferments in various organs and tissues. He believed that, if the ferments acted properly, then solution of the food was complete and the organ was healthy. This was in contrast to the possibility that an "alien ferment" might enter the tissue from the outside and a residue would be left that could lead to disturbances in either the anatomy or the physiology of that tissue. Disease viewed this way involved an external cause that required the old humoral theories of disease to be abandoned. Specific medicines with their own particular forces were then required for treatment.

The view of the Greek philosophers regarding the soul was often expressed as some form of vitalism; however, by the seventeenth century this expression had acquired a different significance. Vital spirits were used to express some form of mechanism by which the living body operated, but with many different detailed interpretations. Sometimes the spirit was a mystic expression of a vital life force, whereas at other times it was a physical entity that obeyed the laws of mechanics and produced specific effects in accord with these laws.

A strong influence at the same time was that of Rene Descartes, who believed that everything in biology had to be accounted for in terms of motion and heat.[13] He stressed the distinction between mind and matter, but denied the existence of mind to all organisms except man. The body of man was a machine powered by the heat of the heart and fed by the food carried in the blood. This process led to the production of animal spirits made of extremely fine particles that obeyed the physical laws of fluids. The essential difference between animals and man was that, in addition to the animal spirits that operated in his body, man also possessed a rational soul, which was distinct from the matter that resided in the pineal gland.

During the second half of the seventeenth century, new anatomic discoveries were made at an increasing rate, and the growing custom of investigating organ function in living animals made possible the development of the new theories of physiologic mechanisms. This environment provided freedom for speculation and led to a great variety of theories that laid the groundwork for a more scientific approach to many biologic problems.

The development of physiologic concepts and their application to medicine received great impetus during the period from 1700 to 1750. Perhaps the most influential medical teacher of the early eighteenth century was Boerhaave, Professor of Medicine, Botany, and Chemistry at Leyden whose teachings were spread over much of Europe from Vienna to Edinburgh.[14] He not only ran a large clinic, but was also one of the most competent chemists of his day and carried out prolonged experiments with biologic fluids. He believed that motion was the distinguishing mark of life and that bodily heat came from the motion of body fluids. Boerhaave believed that air was an elastic element that could not enter into chemical reactions, although he did admit that it might have a certain occult virtue somehow related to the secret fuel of life. One of Boerhaave's students was

the Swiss anatomist, physiologist, and botanist von Haller.[15] Like Boerhaave, he carefully and critically reviewed the work of all his predecessors and was instrumental in eliminating a profusion of earlier theories that lacked sound experimental support. He then reviewed his experimental work in an eight-volume text on the physiology of the human body. Later physiologists and chemists were thus able to base their work on a more unified set of principles established by these medical leaders. Haller recognized that atmospheric air contained a "subtle element" that could penetrate the blood and, by the action of respiration, this air could be vitiated and rendered unfit either for inflating the lungs or for supporting a flame. He believed, however, that the reason was that such air had lost its elasticity.

During the second half of the eighteenth century, the division between vitalistic and nonvitalistic physiology became pronounced. During this time, physiologists observed the phenomena occurring in the animal body and tried to account for them by mechanisms analogous to those known, or observed, in similar cases. When they needed to fit some material substance into their general theory, they simply assumed that it must exist and must possess the desired properties. This method was the opposite from that usually employed by chemists who would isolate and characterize the specific compounds they found in mixtures and then would try to find a mechanism for their function in terms of the properties of the substances that had been found. During most of the eighteenth century, chemists had not prepared enough substances to permit them to frequently utilize this procedure, whereas physiologists had advanced their science to a point at which they could employ their method freely. Therefore, physiology prospered in the early years of the eighteenth century, but lost its prominence to chemistry in the latter part of the century. By 1800, chemists had developed analytical methods and preparative procedures to a point at which they could begin to determine the ultimate constituents of body fluids and tissues. Physiologists and chemists continued to pursue their disciplines separately, but by combining their results, a true science of physiologic chemistry began to emerge.

## EMERGENCE OF ENERGY METABOLISM (1750–1850)

The major chemical development from 1750 to 1800 was the discovery of a whole new class of substances, the gaseous elements and their compounds. The fundamental basis for the new chemistry was established by Joseph Black, a professor of medicine in Glasgow, who studied the carbonates of magnesium and calcium.[16] He demonstrated that these materials could be converted to their oxides with the loss of a gas that was termed "fixed air" and was later recognized as carbon dioxide. Black demonstrated by the use of a balance that his fixed air combined in definite proportions with the metallic element. He used the precipitation of calcium carbonate when fixed air was blown into lime water to demonstrate that air exhaled in respiration contained fixed air.

Discovery of new gases followed quickly. Oxygen and nitrogen were prepared by Scheele, the famous Swedish apothecary. The isolation of oxygen is generally credited to Priestley and Scheele.[17] As early as 1767, Priestley demonstrated by experiment that "a candle would not burn in air that had passed through a charcoal fire or through the lungs of an animal." When Priestley discovered oxygen, he found that mice lived in it longer and that it combined with more nitrous oxide than was the case with "common air." He then concluded that oxygen was "between four and five times as good as common air in supporting life." However, he was a firm believer in the phlogiston theory, which was one of the first great generalizations in chemistry, introduced by the German investigator Stahl.[18] This theory held that a material escaped from any substance when it was burned. Stahl believed that when oxygen joined another substance phlogiston left it, and that plants could absorb phlogiston. Therefore, Priestely accounted for respiration by assuming that the organism took a large amount of phlogiston into itself with its food and that this phlogiston became a waste product that had to be eliminated. In this way blood would carry phlogiston to the lungs where fresh air would remove it by exhalation.

The crowning achievement of the pneumatic chemists was the discovery not only of oxygen but also of the role of oxidation in many branches of chemistry and biology as demonstrated by Lavoisier.[19] Lavoisier also recognized that carbon dioxide was a compound of carbon and oxygen. From studies on the respiration of a bird, he proved that fixed air was given off by animal respiration and that only one fourth of the volume of fresh air could regenerate the original air, while the remaining air in fresh air was purely a passive medium that seemed to enter and leave the lungs unchanged. Lavoisier believed that combustion occurred in the lungs and that the resultant heat was carried by the pulmonary blood flow to the rest of the body. He also believed that gaseous oxygen was a compound of oxygen itself and heat, or "caloric," which was liberated during the process of oxygen combining with the material undergoing combustion. In 1783, Lavoisier worked with the mathematician Laplace to utilize an ice calorimeter similar to one used by Black and laid the foundations for the science of thermal chemistry.[20] From his studies on respiration, he calculated the amount of gas exchange of an animal and showed that predicted heat agreed well with the actual heat production measured directly in the calorimeter. Therefore, he wrote:

> Respiration is thus a combustion, very slow, but perfectly similar to that of carbon; it occurs in the interior of the lungs, without disengagement of visible light since the matter of fire which becomes free is at once absorbed by the humidity of these organs. The heat developed in this combustion communicates itself to the blood which traverses the lungs and from there it spreads over all the animal system.

After the composition of water was established by Cavendish, Lavoisier recognized in 1785 that some of the oxygen taken into the body must be used to form water. From 1785 until the end of his life nine years later, Lavoisier conducted a series of experiments with Seguin to measure the amount of oxygen absorbed by both animals and man under various conditions.[21] In one of these experiments, he showed that more oxygen was absorbed when the temperature outside the body was low, or when food was being ingested, or particularly when physical work was being performed.

Another biologic advance at the end of the eighteenth century was the recognition of photosynthesis. Priestley noticed in 1771 that a sprig of mint growing in water gave off an air in which candles could burn.[22] He then put the mint in a vessel containing air in which a candle had been extinguished. Ten days later a candle once more burned in this air. Lavoisier suggested in 1786 that since oxidation converted vegetable matter into carbonic acid and water that the reverse reaction must occur in plants.[23] The carbon cycle in nature that had been envisioned in reverse by the proponents of phlogiston could now be understood by the recognition of plants as the primary source of animal life. Important development of nutritional chemistry occurred during the period from 1800 to 1850. The source of animal heat had been one of the great biologic problems since the time of the Greeks, but a rational understanding of it was not possible until the discovery of oxygen and carbon dioxide. After the recognition by Lavoisier of the close relationship between respiration and combustion, the basis for animal calorimetry was established. It became apparent that the total amount of heat produced in a chemical reaction was the same no matter what intermediate pathway the reaction followed. The erroneous theory of heat as a material substance, termed "caloric" by Lavoisier, did not prevent valuable laboratory progress.

Boussingault, a French chemist, designed a series of experiments on his Alsatian farm in 1839, using a milk cow to prove that the nitrogen in the air was not used for nutritional purposes.[24] He compared the quantity and nature of the elementary material taken in as food with the quantity and nature of the elementary material eliminated in urinary and digestive products and milk. He then calculated by difference the amount of food eliminated in respiratory products. This was the first introduction of balance experiments in animals and demonstration of the existence of the nitrogen cycle. A few years later Carl Voit found that all the nitrogen in the body came from foods and that a condition of nitrogen equilibrium could be established when the level of nitrogen intake was kept constant.[25]

In the early years of the nineteenth century, the Industrial Revolution was reaching its height, and men were favoring mechanical explanations of natural phenomena. Watt had successfully demonstrated a new and efficient steam engine that emphasized that heat could produce work.[26] Physicists began to think in terms of "force" or "energy." The principle of the conservation of energy, upon which both physical and biologic science would become dependent, was developed during the midportion of this century.

A unique clinical observation was made by Mayer in 1840 when, as a ship's physician in Java, he was bleeding a seaman and observed that the venous blood that he drew in this tropical climate was a brighter red than was usual in Europe.[27] He suggested that in a tropical climate less heat was required for metabolic actvity and work and that the redder blood probably meant more unused oxygen and so less combustion. Thus, a certain amount of heat corresponded to a certain amount of work. Mayer tried unsuccessfully to understand this phenomenon by comparisons with a steam engine. However, 25 years later Voit and Pettenkofer, discussing the biologic utilization of energy, remarked, "As coal, burned under a boiler, moves a steam engine, so do fats and carbohydrates by their oxidation in the body to carbon dioxide and water yield the power for our mechanical performance.[28]

The period from 1790 to 1840 was characterized by many confrontations between chemistry and physiology. The rapid development of methods for identifying and analyzing organic compounds made it essential to investigate such vital phenomena as respiration, digestion, and nutrition in light of this new chemical knowledge. There were, however, divergent opinions concerning the most fruitful ways to pursue these investigations. Those who were trained primarily as chemists often sought to treat biologic problems by extensions of the methods they found successful in their own discipline. This approach was in contrast to that of researchers who were accustomed to dealing with organisms by anatomic studies or vivesection. In addition, results of the chemists' discoveries were rationalized in light of the physiologic observations. The chemical school was defined most distinctively in the efforts of Lavoisier and his followers who sought to extend the theory of respiration he had propounded at the end of the eighteenth century. Parisian chemists of the early nineteenth century were engaged in experiments to determine whether the heat actually produced by an animal matched the heat theoretically created by the chemical reactions of respiration.[29] They also attempted to determine whether the site of the reactions was in the lungs, or throughout the body, to measure the proportion between the oxygen inspired and the carbonic acid exhaled and also to detect whether nitrogen was absorbed or released. It was common for the investigator to place an intact animal in a chamber, arranged so that he could measure the net results of its chemical exchanges with the surrounding atmosphere, but without delving into the complications of the processes within the organism.

Two outstanding physiologists of the time, Johannes Muller of Germany and Francoise Magendie of France, both doubted the adequacy of Lavoisier's theories. Many biologists of this period questioned the adequacy of a given chemical process to account for animal heat and even questioned any chemical explanation of similar biologic phenomena. Investigators such as Muller did not deny that chemical combustion was a source of a portion of animal heat, but they felt that there was insufficient experimental evidence to state that chemical processes were the only conceivable source of heat. When Claude Bernard began his physiologic training, he was exposed to both the prominence and the doubts concerning the chemical theory of respiration and animal heat production. Holmes has carefully traced the growing conviction of Bernard that chemical theories were only useful when they were coupled with direct animal experimentation.[30]

In approximately 1840, a Parisian chemist named Dumas was actively engaged in the study of the exchanges of matter and force between organisms and their environment. A brilliant German contemporary, Justus Liebig, was pursuing a path of nutritional chemistry that was extremely similar to that of Dumas.[29] Liebig thought that by utilizing the ready-made constituents of animal blood, transformations of a synthetic nature were possible that might involve reduction or oxidation. Both of these functions Dumas ascribed exclusively to plants. Various differences developed into bitter acrimony between these two leaders in European chemistry. In a well-known lecture, Dumas repeated that "plants alone have the privilege of fabricating these products, which animals secure from them either to assimilate them or to destroy them." Slowly an extended confrontation developed over the principal issue between Dumas and Liebig, namely the source of animal fat.[31] Liebig maintained that formation of fat from sugar was possible in the animal body, whereas the French chemists maintained that preformed fat existing even in maize could provide for fat in the animal body.

Despite preliminary evidence that carbohydrate could indeed be transformed into fat in the animal body, Boussingault set out in the spring of 1844 in a massive effort to establish the French view of the source of animal fat. By the end of 1845 this investigator had proved both in the goose and in the pig that animals could form fat from other classes of food.[24]

Liebig has often been considered the father of the modern methods of organic analysis.[32] He copied the principle of Boussingault's balance method in order to account for the fate of carbon compounds in the animal economy. Liebig applied to the problems of biology the advantages of the new organic chemistry that he himself was creating. This method gradually produced a knowledge of the constitution of foods, urine, feces, and even of certain tissues that Lavoisier and his contemporaries had not possessed.

The word "energy" had its roots in the Greek language, but its emergence as a significant scientific concept dates from the early nineteenth century. At that time, it was a technical term limited to mechanical, or kinetic, energy. The use of the word "energy" was closely related to an individual's concept of the nature of heat. Two theories of the nature of heat were in vogue. One was a mechanical theory that heat was synonymous with motion. The physician, Boerhaave, had a theory that a heated body was like a struck bell in that it vibrated rapidly. This image influenced Benjamin Thompson, (Count Rumford); his observation on the heat generated when cannons were being bored represented a cornerstone in the belief that heat was the result of motion.[33]

However, the physicists and chemists of that day were not totally satisfied with the concept that heat was a mode of motion.[34] They were searching for a theory that would apply to the expansion on heating, to changes of state, and to the rapidly accumulating information on chemical compounds and reactions. Stahl's phlogiston theory was falling in disrepute. On the other hand, there was the caloric theory that had been proposed by Lavoisier together with the theory of latent heat proposed by Black. For most of the eighteenth century the theories of heat as motion and as material or caloric enjoyed equal popularity. Black and Lavoisier developed the material theory of heat into a quantitative science and made a serious attempt to explain all phenomena of heat in terms of an elastic fluid or, as it was termed, an "igneous fluid." Lavoisier used the word "caloric," which was later adopted as the official term for the matter of heat in the chemical usage. This "caloric" was considered a fluid, the particles of which were self-repulsive. This idea could provide an obvious explanation for the expansion of a material on heating and the contraction on cooling. Joseph Black carefully examined the contemporary theories of heat and decided to reject the Boerhaave version in which "the motion in which heat consists is not a vibration of the hot body itself but of the particles of some sort of subtle, highly elastic fluid matter which is contained in the pores of the hot body." It is thus evident that the caloric theory has enormous explanatory power covering most of the known phenomena of that day. Despite its popularity with the chemists at that time, however, it did not explain the "excitement" of heat on friction.

The central person in this subject area was Herman von Helmholtz, who was a towering scientific personality whose work left its marks on all branches of nineteenth-century science from theoretical mechanics to applied physiology.[35] German education at this time was characterized by a belief in the general conservation principles in nature and the cross-fertilization between the physical and physiologic sciences. Helmholtz was a physician who spent several years in the laboratory of the famous physiologist Johannes Müller. When he encountered the problem of "vital forces" and especially that of vital heat, he argued that vital forces were like other forces conserved in nature; since all phenomena are reducible to mechanics, vital forces could be considered as mechanical forces. The mathematical treatment of this argument led to his famous paper of 1847, "On the Conservation of Force." In the nineteenth century there was a strong realization that the intuitive primitive idea was one of "force" and that this concept was as ancient as human consciousness and therefore naturally vague in definition.

However, historians have noted that the concept of force undoubtedly owes its origin to the muscular effort that human beings experience when they attempt to set bodies in motion. The principle of conservation of force is that vaguely formulated principle to which Helmholtz was committed. Together with other influences this principle led him to a generalization of the conservation law, which resulted in the creation of the concept of energy.

## A CENTURY OF CALORIMETRY (1850–1950)

The tremendous contributions in metabolism and nutrition that came from Germany in the second half of the 1800s are often credited to the school of Carl von Voit. However, much of the interest of Voit was stimulated by his teacher, Max von Pettenkofer.[36] Pettenkofer was a student at the University of Munich were he qualified in both chemistry and medicine. Subsequently, he did postgraduate work with Justin von Liebig at Geissen, where he discovered creatine. In 1847, he was called to Munich as Professor of Medical Chemistry, a newly created position. One of his first students was Voit whose name is associated with that of his teacher in the Pettenkofer-Voit respiration apparatus. Voit continued to study the physiology and metabolism related to nutrition, whereas Pettenkofer moved by gradual stages into experimental hygiene, which included not only diet but also handling of food, sanitary regulations, and sewage disposal.[37]

One of the early contributions of Voit was a demonstration in 1857 that an animal could be brought into what he called "nitrogenous equilibrium."[38] The difference between the amount of nitrogen ingested and that recovered in the excreta of a dog over 58 days was only $3/_{10}$ of 1%. It therefore seemed probable that the excretion of protein nitrogen was in the urine and feces and that other sources of loss were negligible. However, the question remained whether nitrogen of the air had any exchange with organic compounds in the body. Lavoisier had said that nitrogen gas had nothing to do with respiratory metabolism. Voit and others produced additional evidence in the animal that urinary urea was not an incidental product, but one normally proportional to the protein destruction.

Lusk, a student of Voit's stated that the discovery of the method of calculating protein metabolism led Voit to suggest to Pettenkofer that he construct an apparatus with which the total carbon excretion might be measured, including that of the respiration, as well as that of the urine and feces. Voit saw that such data would make it possible to determine how much of each foodstuff was ac-

tually burned in the human body. He described the delight that he and Pettenkofer experienced when their wonderful machine began to explain life processes. Upon the death of Pettenkofer, Voit wrote:

> Imagine our sensations as the picture of the remarkable process of the metabolism unrolled before our eyes, and a mass of new facts became known to us! We found that in starvation protein and fat alone were burned, that during work more fat was burned, and that less fat was consumed during rest, especially during sleep; that the carnivorous dog could maintain himself on an exclusive protein diet, and if to such a protein diet fat were added, the fat was almost entirely deposited in the body; that carbohydrates, on the contrary, were burned no matter how much was given, and that they, like the fat of the food, protected the body from fat loss, although more carbohydrates than fat had to be given to effect this purpose; that the metabolism in the body was not proportional to the combustibility of the substances outside the body, but that protein, which burns with difficulty outside, metabolizes with the greatest ease, then carbohydrates, while fat, which readily burns outside, is the most difficult combustible in the organism.[39]

The best known of the investigators trained in the laboratories of Voit was Max Rubner. The apparatus for quantitative evaluation provided extensive opportunity for quantitative measurement of the metabolism of the principal foodstuffs in animals and man. Rubner built a self-registering calorimeter that combined measurements of expired carbon dioxide with the nitrogen excreted in the urine and feces. This work was the background for the law of constant heat sums expressed by Hess, namely, that in a chemical reaction the heat produced or absorbed is the same, irrespective of the pathway providing the end product. Rubner measured the varying influence of foods on energy production and found that a difference existed between carbohydrates, fats, and proteins that he termed "specific dynamic action." His standard caloric values for the major foodstuffs are still in use today.[40] He also introduced the "law of surface area," which states that the energy metabolism of any animal is proportional to the size and the surface area of the animal.[41] This seemed logical at the time, and many decades passed before it was seriously challenged. Rubner also presented evidence that the three groups of food are interchangeable in the body in relation to their caloric equivalents, which became known as the "isodynamic law." He classified temperature regulation into physical (heat loss) and chemical (heat production) factors.

Rubner was the recognized leader in the investigation of the metabolism of foodstuffs well into the current century. He prepared several monographs on food and energy metabolism and, as late as 1928, contributed a review on metabolism and energy exchange. One of the last experiments of Rubner used an animal calorimeter that could accurately measure the amount of heat produced by a dog over 24 hours. From data on gas exchange the heat production could be calculated. When this heat production was compared with the direct measurement of heat loss, the results were a dramatic demonstration that the animal body followed the law of the conseration of energy.[42]

Many investigators who had received their early training in the laboratories of Voit set up their own laboratories in Europe and in the United States and continued the study of calorimetry in animals and in man. W.O. Atwater, an American nutritionist who had studied under Voit, together with E.B. Rosa, a physicist, constructed a large calorimeter capable of measuring precisely the amount of heat given off by a man living in it.[43] This apparatus confirmed Rubner's experiments and demonstrated that the energy expended by a man in doing any work, such as bicycle riding, is equal to the heat released by the metabolism of food in the body. The physiologist Francis G. Benedict extended Atwater's work by constructing special equipment in the nutrition laboratory of the Carnegie Institute in Boston for the simultaneous measurement of gaseous metabolism and heat production. Such research was extended by the construction of the physiologic laboratory at the Cornell University Medical College in New York City under the direction of Graham Lusk. This laboratory had a small respiration calorimeter suitable for animals and babies. In addition, the Russell Sage Institute of Pathology constructed a respiration calorimeter in Bellevue Hospital for the determination of energy metabolism in various disease conditions. These elaborate and costly devices allowed the establishment and confirmation of general principles of energy metabolism in animals and in man.

Graham Lusk received a Ph.D. in 1891 from the University of Munich; his thesis discussed the influence of carbohydrate on protein metabolism with particular reference to diabetes mellitus. The clinical problem of diabetes remained of special interest to him, and he combined calorimetry for estimating fat metabolism with careful measurements of the glucose and nitrogen in the urine when insulin secretion from the pancreas was suppressed by phlorhizin. While still at the Bellevue Medical College in 1906, Lusk published the first edition of his famous monograph, *The Elements of the Science of Nutrition*, dedicated to Voit. This was a standard text on the subject for

a quarter of a century. Lusk's unique contribution was his ability to synthesize and to interpret data from both European centers and American investigators, while establishing an American school that trained many important investigators of its own.[44]

The Russell Sage calorimeter for the determination of energy metabolism in disease conditions was under the management of Eugene F. DuBois. He was a student and colleague of Lusk and a close friend of Max Rubner. The classic volume entitled *Basal Metabolism in Health and Disease*, authored by DuBois in 1924, presents data on 11 different conditions of particular interest to the field of internal medicine. This work demonstrated the relationship between increased energy metabolism and fever. It is best remembered for confirmation of the usefulness of measuring basal metabolism in the diagnosis and treatment of diseases of the thyroid gland.

Lusk's classic textbook first appeared in 1906 and had its fourth and final edition in 1931. Another outstanding book was written by E.V. McCollum entitled *Newer Knowledge of Nutrition* and first appeared in 1918.[45] These two books provided dramatic evidence of the shift away from energy metabolism during the 1920s. Lusk's book contained extensive material on energy metabolism, whereas McCollum's book contained essentially nothing on energy metabolism, emphasizing instead the biologic method of evaluating foods for their nutrient adequacy and the importance of vitamins.

Interest in calorimetry became relegated to the hospital measurement of the basal metabolic rate (BMR) as an indicator of thyroid function. This was a standard available measurement in hospital laboratories until approximately 1950.[46] At that time, new chemical methods for measuring materials in the urine and the blood related to thyroid metabolism caused hospitals to abandon the measurement and, therefore, to terminate the last remaining quantitative approach to energy metabolism in patients.

Research on the energy expenditure of surgical patients was undertaken by Kinney and co-workers utilizing a noninvasive head canopy system.[47] This system was acceptable to acutely ill, hyperventilating patients while still allowing medical care as required. However, the utilization of this type of measurement became more widespread only when specialized hospital nutrition became an accepted part of hospital care.

The addendum to this chapter outlines the principles of indirect calorimetry and gives examples of the calculations that provide information on the utilization of substrates and energy exchange.

## REEXAMINATION OF ENERGY REQUIREMENTS

The development of indirect calorimetry and the concept of the BMR have often been considered to be firmly established, and the normal range for large populations was thought to be relatively narrow. Therefore, at the beginning of this century, whenever there appeared to be much variation in the BMR of supposedly normal individuals, this phenomenon was often considered to be the result of carelessly conducted measurements or inadequacies in the measuring equipment.

The energy requirement of any individual can be determined by the following equation:

energy requirements = BMR + DIT + physical activity

The BMR is thought to represent the minimal energy expenditure of an awake individual. Diet-induced thermogenesis (DIT) is the current and more popular term for what was formerly called "the specific dynamic action" (SDA), meaning the heat increment that follows digestion of a meal. These factors, together with the energy requirements for physical activity, have led to conclusions such as "individuals of the same size, living in the same environment, and with the same mode of life have a similar energy requirement, whatever their ethnic origin."[48] However, during the past 15 years, many inquiries and new information have suggested that the three variables used to calculate energy requirements are neither as uniform nor as well understood as previously thought.[49]

**BMR in Relation to Body Size.** The convenience of using body weight was offset by the early recognition that energy metabolism did not vary as a linear function of body weight. A French physiologist, J.F. Rameaux, working with P.F. Sarrus, a mathematician, realized in 1830 that an animal loses heat through the surface of its body, while its capacity for heat production is related to its volume. They reasoned that the larger the animal, the greater its heat production relative to its heat loss.[50]

Rubner noticed that the ratio of metabolic rate to body weight was not constant, even within a series of dogs of different sizes. However, when the metabolic rate was expressed per square meter of body surface area, the effect of body size disappeared. From this and similar observations, Rubner deduced his simple rule that fasting homeotherms produce daily 1,000 kilocalories of heat per square meter of body surface area. He published a famous paper in 1883 proposing that the metabolic rate was somehow limited by body

surface area and citing the fact that oxygen comes in and heat goes out through surfaces that are proportional to the total body surface area. Voit published further observations supporting the surface area law.[41]

Problems and arguments remained about how to determine the surface area for animals and for man. DuBois and DuBois developed a formula in 1916 that allowed the calculation of the surface area of stout and slim human beings more accurately than did previous formulas by using body weight and body length.[51] This formula was:

$$S = 71.84W^{0.425} \times L^{0.725}$$

where S equals surface area in square centimeters, W equals body weight in kilograms, and L equals body length in centimeters.

Kleiber pointed out in 1932 that the various efforts to refine measurements of surface area did not clarify the underlying issue of whether metabolic rate was in fact determined by surface area. He carefully studied the various kinds of information used to support the surface law of animal metabolism, and he presented a careful critique of each.[52] He found strong evidence against the surface area being the determining factor of basal metabolism. Kleiber then proposed that metabolism should be considered as a power function of body weight. Lacking a better definition of the metabolic body size, he proposed a three-fourths power of the body weight as the best correlation between body size and resting metabolism.

**Relation to Lean Body Mass.** Grande emphasized the fact that the body composition is not homogeneous as far as energy expenditure is concerned and, therefore, the proper reference for energy expenditure should be neither body weight nor body surface area, but rather the lean tissue of the body or the fat-free mass (FFM).[53] He presented data indicating that sex and age differences could be corrected for if one used the FFM as the metabolic body size. Behnke, while working in the Navy submarine school, popularized the concept of underwater weighing as a way of determining the proportion of the body that was fat; he then arrived at what he called the "lean body mass."[54] This was similar to the concept of fat-free mass, usually arrived at by applying the Pace and Rathbun formula[55] for the hydration of lean tissue.

Moore and his co-workers extended the concept further to approach the metabolizing body cell mass by measuring total exchangeable potassium.[56] Kinney and Moore published preliminary data indicating the curvilinear relationship between the resting energy expenditure and total body potassium.[57]

Shizgal and co-workers divided the lean tissues of the body into the extracellular and intracellular portions by examining the ratio of total exchangeable sodium to total exchangeable potassium.[58] This method has a particular advantage: under various pathologic conditions, the extracellular phase tends to undergo relative or absolute expansion as represented by increases in exchangeable sodium, while the body cell mass tends to shrink; therefore, the ratio of exchangeable sodium to exchangeable potassium increases as a result of both changes.

Cohn,[59] Hill,[60] and McNeil[61] have all worked on methods utilizing neutron activation to try to determine body nitrogen content. Cohn has analyzed the relationship between exchangeable potassium and body nitrogen to try to separate the muscle mass from the remainder of the lean tissue. Such approaches may in the future separate the resting energy expenditure between the proportions associated with muscle and those of viscera.

Rubner emphasized that the resting energy expenditure of both animals and man increased following the ingestion of a meal. His studies revealed that most of this thermic effect of food concerned the administration of protein or amino acids. The administration of fat and carbohydrate was reported to be so small as to be insignificant. Studies of an average meal of mixed composition are usually reported to increase the resting energy expenditure by approximately 10% above the pre-meal level. Krebs suggested that the energy losses following administration of protein were somehow linked to urea production.[62] However, studies by Garrow and Hawes did not demonstrate such an association.[63] Attention to the thermic effect of food has shifted from the SDA of protein to DIT, which often involves mixed diets.

The thermic responses to food and to cold were formerly thought to be independent. However, in animals in which brown adipose tissue is the main organ responsible for non-shivering thermogenesis, thermogenic activity can be stimulated by feeding. Stock and Rothwell proposed that brown adipose tissue may perform a regulatory function in response to overfeeding.[64] This concept was based on the demonstration that rats could become obese on a palatable "snack food" diet, but that the animals maintain normal body weights when given rat chow. The brown adipose tissue of the rats with the abnormal weight gain was markedly increased on the former, suggesting that overfeeding may have led to a substantial increase in dietary-induced thermogenesis. Certain strains of genetically obese rodents, in contrast, possess a deficient diet-induced thermogenic response.

Brown adipose tissue has been reviewed in detail by Girardier.[65] Its presence in the rodent and in the human infant is well established, but its presence and functional significance in adult man remain controversial.

**Diet-induced Thermogenesis.** The thermic effect of food, can be divided into obligatory and adaptive components.[64] Obligatory DIT, formerly known as "specific dynamic action," is the energy cost of digestion, absorption, and the inner conversion of food substrates and is thought to be due largely to the synthesis of protein and fat from carbohydrate. Adaptive DIT (originally named Luxuskonsumption) represents the dissipation of energy over and above that associated with basal metabolism activity and the obligatory DIT. It is stimulated by the ingestion of a meal, a part of which is oxidized to produce adaptive DIT.

The existence of adaptive DIT in both man and other mammals is a controversial subject today. The concept that the body is able to control its weight and energy content by disposing of the excess consumed energy (hence, the term Luxus Konsumption) comes partly from studies in which individuals have maintained a constant body weight despite different levels of energy intake. The evidence for adaptive DIT from these studies relies upon the demonstration of an apparent discrepancy between estimates of energy intake as food, energy expenditure, and the energy storage or change in body fat. Unfortunately, most of these studies have not had actual measurements of energy balance. Since errors in the calculation of energy intake and expenditure in man may be of greater magnitude than those of diet-induced thermogenesis, the precise measurement of this aspect of human thermogenesis is difficult. The problem is not as great in animals because of the ability to do carcass analysis. When rats were offered palatable human foods, they increased their energy intake by as much as 150% of that observed when ingesting a normal chow diet.[66] The authors calculated that this extra energy intake could be accounted for as increases in the energy costs of digestion, absorption, metabolism, fat synthesis, and activity and that there is no evidence of energy imbalance attributable to adaptive DIT.

Early research on the specific dynamic action of foodstuffs indicated that this effect was small for carbohydrate. However, now that carbohydrate is being given for total parenteral nutrition (TPN) in amounts that may equal or exceed the daily energy expenditure, there is new evidence that the thermogenic response to carbohydrate loads is larger than formerly appreciated. King and co-workers utilized (TPN) in surgical patients in whom glucose was used as the only nonprotein calorie source.[67] They administered glucose at different rates with a fixed nitrogen intake. They found a progressive rise in oxygen consumption and $CO_2$ production, which accounted for a total of 31% of the additional glucose administered. The net rate of fat synthesis from glucose reached a maximum of 147 g/day at an energy supply of 14,500 kJ/(3,460 kcal) day. These data suggest that both fat synthesis and the associated obligatory thermogenesis are the main components of diet-induced thermogenesis in response to these large glucose intakes. If the energy cost of fat synthesis is taken to be 22% of the total energy of the increase in glucose supply, then roughly 9% of the glucose can be accounted for by adaptive thermogenesis.[67]

An important area for future investigation is to understand the role of the neuroendocrine system, particularly the sympathetic nervous system, in responding to a glucose load. When high-carbohydrate TPN was administered to depleted surgical patients and to acutely injured patients, the depleted patients had no thermogenic response, in contrast to a marked thermogenic response in the acutely injured patients.[68] The urinary norepinephrine excretion was three times the normal daily levels in the acutely injured patients before TPN was started and reached essentially a three-fold increase following a week of TPN administration. The contribution of the amino acids, compared to that of the carbohydrate, remains to be defined.

**Efficiency of Energy Utilization.** Body weight is the measurement most commonly thought of in assessing the nutritional status of human beings. Weight loss is an obvious manifestation of energy undernutrition, whereas weight gain is expected whenever there is a positive balance of energy. Because adipose tissue represents the main storage form of energy in the body and because the human body obeys the law of the conservation of energy, it is reasonable to expect that a positive energy balance will cause a corresponding increase in fat content of the body, whereas a negative energy balance must decrease the content of body fat. A kilogram of fat is thought to contain approximately 9,000 kcal, whereas adipose tissue contains sufficient fat to provide between 6,000 and 7,000 kcal/kg. Therefore, a reduction in daily energy intake of approximately 100 kcal below energy equilibrium each day should result in a weight loss of approximately 1 kg over 60 to 70 days, or twice that amount if the energy intake is reduced by twice as much.

Experimental studies do not agree with such calculations. Keys and co-workers performed detailed studies of partial starvation on previously healthy, young adult males.[69] During a 24-week period the subjects received a reduced intake, resulting in a calorie deficit of approximately 200 kcal/day. This reduction should have produced a minimum of 200 g weight loss/day if only fat was lost and a larger amount if some lean tissue was also lost. In fact, the men lost only about 100 g/day.

A number of overfeeding studies have been tabulated by Webb in which 1,000 kcal/day were fed in excess of energy equilibrium for 20 days or more.[70] If all the weight gain were adipose tissue, one would expect a gain of approximately 150 g/day. Only about 67 g were gained per day. The weight gain of the individuals in the study varied from 16 to 135 g/day, indicating a response that varied from near zero up to approximately theoretical levels. Such data strongly suggest that the common factors considered in calculating energy requirements are not sufficient to predict weight gain or weight loss in any given individual by simply knowing the energy intake.

Voit and Rubner published data on the energy requirements of various forms of physical activity, and these were later refined by Benedict, Lusk, and others.[71] However, it is extremely difficult to determine the actual energy expenditure of individuals throughout their normal daily life. Reports by Edmundson have challenged the ability to predict the energy utilization with various forms of work.[72,73] He monitored the work output and energy intake of 54 adult men on six days spread throughout the year.[72] Energy intakes varied from 1,450 to 3,800 kcal/day. This wide variation in intake appears to have no association with the work output. This finding led Edmundson to suggest that some "compensatory mechanisms" might allow greater work efficiency of those who are accustomed to low energy intakes than those with relatively high intakes. These findings prompted a second study in which he measured the total food intake, the basal metabolic rate, and the energy expenditure of men pedaling a bicycle ergometer at standard rates. These men were accustomed to receiving either a relatively high or a relatively low energy intake per day.[73] The two groups were similar in body size although the skinfold thickness of the habitual high-energy consumers seemed to be about twice that of the low-energy consumers. The BMR of the latter group was about 50% of that of the high-energy consumers. While performing medium work output on the ergometer, the low-energy consumers expended only 70% as many calories as did the high-energy consumers. This finding led Edmundson to state that: "In East Java many people who were small in stature and low in body weight seemed to live productive lives and work long hours with energy intakes that are only 60 to 80% of presently accepted energy requirements and recommendations."

Durnin and co-workers conducted energy balance studies in an identical fashion on a coastal and a highland group of people in New Guinea who were maintaining stable adult weights.[74] There was close agreement between the measured total daily energy expenditure and the energy intake of both men and women in the highland area. In contrast, both the men and women in the coastal area maintained a stable weight despite a measured energy intake that was about 500 kcal/day less than the measured energy expenditure.

Difficulties in the measurement of energy expenditure in normal man led Durnin and co-workers to publish a letter under the title "How Much Food Does Man Require?"[75] The letter stressed the importance of improved calorimetry studies in man and noted the efforts that had been put into calorimeters for domestic animals at a time when no comparable instruments existed for human studies. The authors believed that apparently comparable individuals may have widely differing energy intakes. Some individuals appear to be healthy, physically well built, and active on intakes that would, by current standards, be regarded as inadequate, whereas some obese people fail to lose expected weight when placed on low dietary intake. Apparently, variation in human metabolic efficiency is much greater than had formerly been appreciated. Hegsted has proposed that the requirement for energy should be related to the requirement for the formation of ATP and other high-energy compounds needed for chemical and physical work.[49] He has noted that, contrary to classic views (which maintain that the proportion of total energy converted to high-energy compounds is constant in different individuals and does not change in the same individual under varying conditions), there may be in fact many mechanisms, such as the uncoupling of phosphorylation, futile cycles or the direct hydrolysis of ATP via unregulated ATPases, that may modify the efficiency of energy utilization in a given individual.

## SUMMARY

The measurement of energy expenditure by indirect calorimetry was considered well established by 1920, and its use in medical practice over the next 30 years was largely limited to thyroid disease. The field seemed largely of historical interest until a resurgence of interest occurred in the 1970s. This new interest in energy metabolism was spurred by three special factors: efforts to treat obesity, awareness of hospital malnutrition, and the introduction of commercial instruments for measuring energy expenditure at the bedside with greater accuracy than before. This new attention to calculating energy intake in relation to a measured energy expenditure represents a major advance in patient care. However, important additional information is needed and is currently being sought in order to provide a better understanding of each of the major factors (BMR, DIT, and physical activity) that enter into the total energy expenditure each day.

## ADDENDUM: PRINCIPLES OF CALORIMETRY

Direct calorimetry is the direct measurement of the actual heat production of an individual or an animal. It is performed in a specialized chamber in which the walls of the chamber are able to measure the heat loss by the gradient layer principle or by transfer to a surrounding water jacket. Not only is such equipment expensive and time-consuming to operate, it also has the problems associated with the isolation of the subject or patient. Simultaneous measurements of direct calorimetry and gas exchange have demonstrated that measuring gas exchange alone could provide an accurate estimate of the heat production. Atwater and Benedict showed that 40-day determinations on three subjects revealed only 0.2% difference between the two methods of arriving at the total daily caloric output.[43]

The caloric value of any combustible substance, including food, is readily determined in an apparatus such as a bomb calorimeter. This device is a heavy metal cylinder in which the test sample of food is *completely* oxidized in an oxygen atmosphere, and the heat is transferred to surrounding water where the heat production is calculated in terms of calories.

In the living organism, the oxidation of carbohydrate and fat to $CO_2$ and water is complete, whereas the oxidation of protein is incomplete because of the urinary end products of protein excreted in the urine.

One can write an equation for the complete oxidation of glucose as follows:[76]

$$C_6H_{12}O_6 + 6O_2 \rightarrow 6CO_2 + 6H_2O + 673 \text{ kcal}$$

From this equation the respiratory quotient (RQ) or $CO_2/O_2 = 1.0$. Furthermore, since 1 mole of glucose utilizes 134.4 liters of $O_2$ upon yielding 673 kcal, each liter of $O_2$ involved in oxidizing carbohydrate will yield 5.01 kcal.

A similar equation can be written for mixed fat as follows:

$$2(C_{55}H_{106}O_6) + 157\ O_2 \rightarrow 110\ CO_2$$
$$+\ 106\ H_2O + 16{,}353\ kcal$$

In the case of fat, the RQ is 0.701 (or 0.71 for pure triolein). Upon complete oxidation of the 2 moles of fat, 16,353 Cal would be produced with a utilization of 3,516.8 liters of $O_2$; hence, each liter of $O_2$ used for oxidizing fat would equal 4.65 kcal.

The RQ for protein oxidation is not as clearcut because protein composition varies and the completeness of oxidation may also vary. However, the RQ of protein oxidation is between 0.80 and 0.82. Because food protein contains an average of 16% nitrogen, it follows that every gram of urinary nitrogen represents 6.25 g of protein metabolized in the body. The metabolism of an amount of protein sufficient to yield 1 g of urinary nitrogen results in the production of 26.51 kcal and 4.745 liters of $CO_2$ while 5.923 liters of oxygen are utilized.

An example of the calculation of indirect calorimetry may be taken from the data of a subject having complete measurements of $O_2$ consumption and $CO_2$ production for 60 minutes. During the study the individual consumed 20 liters of $O_2$, exhaled 16 liters of $CO_2$, and excreted 0.5 g of urinary nitrogen.

From the urinary nitrogen excretion:

0.5 × 26.51 = 13.25 kcal from protein oxidation
0.5 × 6.25 g = 3.13 g protein metabolized
0.5 × 5.923 L = 2.961 L $O_2$ used from protein oxidation
0.5 × 4.754 L = 2.377 L $CO_2$ produced by protein oxidation

The $O_2$ for oxidation of carbohydrate and fat = 20 − 2.961 or 17.041 L $O_2$.

0.5 × 4.754 L = 2.377 L $CO_2$ produced by protein oxidation

The $CO_2$ for oxidation from fat and carbohydrate is 16 − 2.377 = 13.623 liters.
The nonprotein RQ due solely to fat plus carbohydrate oxidation is:

$$\frac{13.62\ L}{17.04\ L} = 0.80$$

A nonprotein RQ of 0.80 can be found in Table 28–1 relating equivalence of carbohydrate and fat to 4.801 calories per liter of $O_2$ used. Thus, 17.04 × 4.80 = 81.79 kcal. The nonprotein RQ indicates that 31.7% of the calories came from carbohydrate and the remainder from fat. Therefore:

0.317 × 81.79 = 25.93 kcal from carbohydrate
0.683 × 81.79 = 55.89 kcal from fat
                13.25 kcal from protein
                ─────
                95.04 kcal per hour

**Table 28–1. Caloric Equivalents of Oxygen and Carbon Dioxide for Nonprotein Respiratory Quotients***

| Nonprotein Respiratory Quotient | kcal/liter | |
|---|---|---|
| | Oxygen | Carbon Dioxide |
| 0.70 | 4.686 | 6.694 |
| 0.72 | 4.702 | 6.531 |
| 0.74 | 4.727 | 6.388 |
| 0.76 | 4.732 | 6.253 |
| 0.78 | 4.776 | 6.123 |
| 0.80 | 4.801 | 6.001 |
| 0.82 | 4.825 | 5.884 |
| 0.84 | 4.850 | 5.774 |
| 0.86 | 4.875 | 5.669 |
| 0.88 | 4.900 | 5.568 |
| 0.90 | 4.928 | 5.471 |
| 0.92 | 4.948 | 5.378 |
| 0.94 | 4.973 | 5.290 |
| 0.96 | 4.997 | 5.205 |
| 0.98 | 5.022 | 5.124 |
| 1.00 | 5.047 | 5.047 |

*From Carpenter, T.M.: Tables, Factors, and Formulas for Computing Respiratory Exchange and Biological Transformation of Energy. 3rd ed. Washington, Carnegie Institute of Washington, 1939 Reprinted from Consolazio, C.F.[77]

The basal metabolic rate (BMR) is an abbreviated version of indirect calorimetry. A 6- to 12-minute measurement of $O_2$ consumption is made when the subject is postabsorptive (no food during the previous 12 hours), having rested quietly during the previous 30 minutes in a thermoneutral environment. The $CO_2$ production is not measured under traditional circumstances, but an assumption is made that the normal RQ under basal conditions is 0.82 and thus the calorie value of 1 liter of $O_2$ at this RQ is 4.825 kcal.

Standard tables for comparison of the measured BMR with a given body size often are based upon equations for calculation of the body surface area. Kleiber has developed extensive evidence that the metabolic body size is approximately the body weight to the three fourth power.[50] This value happens to be surprisingly close to estimates of body surface area from a knowledge of weight and height. Thus standard tables and nomograms continue to be expressed in calories per square meter per hour for males and females of various ages.[3]

In an example taken from Consolazio et al., a young adult male is found to consume 1.5 liter of $O_2$ in a six-minute BMR measurement.[77] This would amount to 15 liters of $O_2$ in one hour. Since the caloric value of 1 liter of $O_2$ under basal conditions is 4.825, then the hourly heat production would be 72.4 kcal. If the man's height were 150 cm and his weight 60 kg, a standard table or nomogram would indicate a body surface area of 1.54 M², which would yield a basal energy expenditure of 72.4/1.54 = 47.0 kcal/M²/hour. Utilizing the Mayo Clinic standards of Boothby and co-workers, one could determine that a man of this age should have a normal BMR of 41 kcal/M²/hour; hence, the subject would be ⁶/₄₁ or 15% elevation above the normal BMR.

## REFERENCES

1. Mendelsohn, E.: Heat and Life: The Development of the Theory of Animal Heat. Cambridge, Harvard University Press, 1964, pp. 1–7.
2. Mendelsohn, E.: Heat and Life: The Development of the Theory of Animal Heat. Cambridge, Harvard University Press, 1964, pp. 8–26.
3. Leicester, H.M.: Development of Biochemical Concepts from Ancient to Modern Times. Cambridge, Harvard University Press, 1974, pp. 5–24.
4. Lyons, A.S., Petrucelli, R.J.: Medicine: An Illustrated History. New York, Harry N. Abrams, Inc., 1978, p. 251.
5. Lyons, A.S., Petrucelli, R.J.: Medicine: An Illustrated History. New York, Harry N. Abrams, Inc., 1978, p. 310.
6. Harvey, W.: De Motu Cordis, 1628.
7. Frank, R.G., Jr.: Harvey and the Oxford Physiologists. Berkeley, University of California Press, 1980.
8. Frank, R.G., Jr.: Harvey and the Oxford Physiologists. Berkeley, University of California Press, 1980, pp. 1–9.
9. Frank, R.G.,Jr.: Harvey and the Oxford Physiologists. Berkeley, University of California, 1980, pp. 22–45.
10. Frank, R.G., JR.: Harvey and the Oxford Physiologists. Berkeley, University of California Press, 1980, pp. 128–134.
11. Frank, R.G., Jr.: Harvey and the Oxford Physiologists. Berkeley, University of California Press, 1980, pp. 142–148.
12. Lyons, A.S., Petrocelli, R.J., Medicine: An illustrated History. New York, Harry N. Abrams, Inc., 1978, p. 429.
13. Elkana, Y.: The Discovery of the Conservation of Energy. Cambridge, Harvard University Press, 1974, pp. 1–3.
14. Leicester, H.M.: Development of Biochemical Concepts from Ancient to Modern Times. Cambridge, Harvard University Press, 1964, pp. 116–120.
15. Leicester, H.M.: Development of Biochemical Concepts from Ancient to Modern Times. Cambridge, Harvard University Press, 1964, pp. 121–126.
16. Kent, A. (Ed.): An Eighteenth Century Lectureship in Chemistry. Glasgow, Jackson, Son & Company, 1950, pp. 99–106.
17. Leicester, H.M.: Development of Biochemical Concepts from Ancient to Modern Times. Cambridge, Harvard University Press, 1964, pp. 128–137.
18. Leicester, H.M.: Development of Biochemical Concepts from Ancient to Modern Times. Cambridge, Harvard University Press, 1964, p. 112.
19. Holmes, F.L.: Lavoisier and Chemistry of Life. Madison, University, of Wisconsin Press, 1985, pp. 3–128.
20. Holmes, F.L.: Lavoisier and the Chemistry of Life. Madison, University of Wisconsin Press, 1985, pp. 151–262.
21. Holmes, F.L.: Lavoisier and the Chemistry of Life. Madison, University of Wisconsin Press, 1985, pp. 411–468.
22. Leicester, H.M.: Development of Biochemical Concepts from Ancient to Modern Times. Cambridge, Harvard University Press, 1974, p. 135.
23. Holmes, F.L.: Lavoisier and the Chemistry of Life. Madison, University of Wisconsin Press, pp. 385–412.
24. Holmes, F.L.: Claude Bernard and Animal Chemistry. Cambridge, Harvard University Press, 1974, pp. 96–117.
25. Cathcart, E.P.: The early development of the science of nutrition. In Biochemistry and Physiology of Nutrition, Vol 1. (Bourne, G.H., Kidder, G.W., Ed.) New York, Academic Press, 1953, p. 1.
26. Robinson, E., McKie, D. (Eds.): Partners in Science (Watt to Black, July 24, 1778). Cambridge, Harvard University Press, 1970, p. 65.
27. Leicester, H.M.: Development of Biochemical Concepts from Ancient to Modern Times. Cambridge, Harvard University Press, 1974, p. 190.
28. Leicester, H.M.: Development of Biochemical Concepts from Ancient to Modern Times. Cambridge, Harvard University Press, 1974, p. 191.
29. Holmes, F.L.: Claude Bernard and Animal Chemistry. Cambridge, Harvard University Press, 1974, pp. 1–33.
30. Holmes, F.L.: Claude Bernard and Animal Chemistry. Cambridge, Harvard University Press, 1974, pp. 118–140.
31. Holmes, F.L.: Claude Bernard and Animal Chemistry. Cambridge, Harvard University Press, 1974, pp. 48–76.
32. Leicester, H.M.: Development of Biochemical Concepts from Ancient to Modern Times. Cambridge, Harvard University Press, 1974, pp. 170–175.
33. Elkana, Y.: The Discovery of the Conservation of Energy. Cambridge, Harvard University Press, 1974, pp. 66–71.
34. Elkana, Y.: The Discovery of the Conservation of Energy. Cambridge, Harvard University Press, 1974, pp. 61–65.
35. Lyons, A.S., Petrucelli, R.J.: Medicine: An Illustrated History. New York, Harry N. Abrams, Inc., 1978, p. 521.
36. Hume, E.E.: Max von Pettenkofer. New York, R.B. Hoeber, Inc., 1927.
37. Lusk, G.: Ann. Med. Hist. 3:583–594, 1931.
38. Leicester, H.M.: Development of Biochemical Concepts from Ancient to Modern Times. Cambridge, Harvard University Press, 1974, p. 192.
39. Leicester, H.M.: Development of Biochemical Concepts from Ancient to Modern Times. Cambridge, Harvard University Press, 1974, p. 193.
40. Rubner, M.: Z. Biol. 19:313–396, 1883.
41. Rubner, M.: Z. Biol. 19:535–562, 1883.
42. Leicester, H.M.: Development of Biochemical Concepts from Ancient to Modern Times. Cambridge, Harvard University Pess, 1974, p. 194.
43. Lusk, G.: The Elements of the Science of Nutrition. 4th ed. Philadelphia, W.B. Saunders Co., 1931, pp. 17–45.
44. "Graham Lusk." Editorial, JAMA 210:2385, 1969.
45. McCollum, E.V.: The Newer Knowledge of Nutrition. 1st ed. New York, McMillan Company, 1918, p. 199.
46. DuBois, E.F.: Basal Metabolism in Health and Disease. Philadelphia, Lea & Febiger, 1924, pp. 237–288.

47. Kinney, J.M.: The application of indirect calorimetry to clinical studies. *In* Assessment of Energy Metabolism in Health and Disease, Report of the First Ross Conference on Medical Research. (Kinney, J.M., Ed.) Columbus, Ross Laboratories, 1980, p. 42.

48. Energy and Protein Requirements, FAO Nutrition Meeting Report. Series No. 52, Rome, 1973.

49. Hegsted, D.M.: Energy needs and energy utilization. *In* Present Knowledge in Nutrition. 4th ed. (Hegsted, D.M., Ed.) Washington, DC, The Nutrition Foundation, 1976, p. 1.

50. Kleiber, M.: The Fire of Life, an Introduction to Animal Energetics. 2nd ed. Huntington, NY, Robert E. Krieger, 1975, p. 182.

51. DuBois, D., Dubois, E.F.: Arch. Intern. Med. *17*:863–871, 1916.

52. Kleiber, M.: The Fire of Life, an Introduction to Animal Energetics. 2nd ed. Huntington, NY, Robert E. Kreiger, 1975, pp. 179–221.

53. Grande, F.: Body weight, composition and energy balance. Present Knowledge in Nutrition. 5th ed. (Olson, R.E., Ed.) Washington, DC, The Nutrition Foundation, 1984, p. 7.

54. Behnke, A.R.: Comment on the determination of whole body density and a resume of body composition data. *In* Techniques for Measuring Body Composition. (Brozek, J., Henschel, A., Eds.) Washington, DC, National Academy of Sciences & National Research Council, 1961, p. 118.

55. Pace, H., Rathbun, E.N.: J. Biol. Chem. *158*:685, 1945.

56. Moore, F.D., et al.: The Body Cell Mass and Its Supporting Environment. Philadelphia, W.B. Saunders Co., 1963.

57. Kinney, J.M., Lister, J., Moore, F.D.: Ann. NY Acad. Sci. *110*:711–722, 1963.

58. Shizgal, H.M.: Nutritional failure. *In* Care of the Critically Ill Patient. (Tinker, J., Rapin, M. Eds.) Berlin, Springer-Verlag, 1983, p. 483.

59. Cohn, S.H., Vartsky, D., Yasumura, S., et al.: Am. J. Physiol. 239 (Endocrinol. Metab. 2):E524–E530, 1980.

60. Hill, G.L.,King, R.F.G.J., Smith, R.C., et al.: Br. J. Surg. *66*:868–872, 1979.

61. McNeill, K.G., Harrison, J.E., Mernagh, J.R., et al.: J. Parenter. Enter. Nutr. *6*:106–108, 1982.

62. Krebs, H.A.: The metabolic fate of amino acids. *In* Mammalian Protein Metabolism. (Munro, H.N., Allison, J.B., Eds.) New York, Academic Press, 1964, p. 125.

63. Garrow, J.S., Hawes, S.F.: Br. J. Nutr. *27*:211–219, 1972.

64. Rothwell, N.J., Stock, M.J.: Diet-induced thermogenesis. *In* Mammalian Thermogenesis. (Girardier, L., Stock, M.J., Eds.) New York, Chapman and Hall, 1983, p. 208.

65. Girardier, L.: Brown fat: An energy dissipating tissue. *In* Mammalian Thermogenesis. (Girardier, L., Stock, M.J., Eds.) London, Chapman and Hall, 1983, p. 50.

66. Armitage, G., Hervey, G.R., Tobin, G.: J. Physiol. *312*:58P, 1981.

67. King, R.F.G.J., McMahon, M.J., Almond, D.J.: Clin. Sci. *71*:31–39, 1986.

68. Askanazi, J., Carpentier, Y.A., Elwyn, D.H., et al.: Ann. Surg. *191*:40–46, 1980.

69. Keys, A., Brozek, J., Henschel, A., et al.: The Biology of Human Starvation. Minneapolis, University of Minnesota Press, 1950, p. 84.

70. Webb, P.: Am. J. Clin. Nutr. *33*:1299–1310, 1980.

71. Lusk, G., The Elements of the Science of Nutrition. 4th ed. Philadelphia, W.B. Saunders Co., 1931, pp. 400–446.

72. Edmundson, W.: Individual variations in work output per unit energy intake in East Java. Ecol. Food Nutr. *6*:147–151, 1977.

73. Edmundson, W.: Individual variations in basal metabolic rate and mechanical mark efficiency in East Java. Ecol. Food Nutr. *8*:189–195, 1979.

74. Durnin, J.V.G.A.: Proc. Nutr. Soc. *37*:5–12, 1978.

75. Durnin, J.V.G.A., Edholm, O.G., Miller, D.S., et al.: Nature London *242*:418, 1973.

76. West, E.S., Todd, W.R., Mason, H.S., et al.: Energy metabolism. *In* West, E.S., Todd, W.R., Mason, H.S., et al. (eds.): Textbook of Biochemistry. 4th ed. New York, Macmillan Publishing Co., Inc., 1966, pp. 970–984.

77. Consolazio, C.F., Johnson, R.E., Pecora, L.J.: Respiratory metabolism. *In* Consolazio, C.F., Johnson, R.E., Pecora, L.J. (eds.). Physiological Measurements of Metabolic Functions in Man. New York, McGraw-Hill Book Co., 1963, pp. 1–59.

*Chapter* **29**

# BODY COMPOSITION: INFLUENCE OF NUTRITION, DISEASE, GROWTH, AND AGING

Gilbert B. Forbes

> *"Der sehr fettarme Muskel eines verhungerten Tiers kann nicht ohne weiteres dem fettreichen bei normaler Ernährung gegenübergestellt werden. Zulässig ist nur der Vergleich fettfrei berechneter Organe." Adolph Magnus-Levy[1]* *

The promulgation of the concept of fat-free tissue at the turn of the century paved the way for the development of techniques for estimating body composition in vivo. Voit and Rubner spoke of the existence of an "active protoplasmic mass," to which various metabolic phenomena could be related.[2,3] The labors of the nineteenth century Continental chemists had established with some precision the composition of blood and tissue; now the twentieth century investigators were to supply the concept of volume, first with blood[4] and later with other body fluid compartments, and to conceive the idea of metabolic balance. Soon after the discovery of deuterium George von Hevesy used this isotope to estimate total body water,[5] and later Francis Moore introduced the concept of total exchangeable potassium and sodium.[6] By applying Archimedes' principle, Albert Behnke showed us how to estimate the relative proportions of lean and fat in the human body.[7] Rudolph Sievert found that the human body contained enough $^{40}K$ to be easily detectable,[8] and thus opened the way for the use of this technique to estimate lean and fat in a noninvasive manner.[9] More recent years have seen the use of neutron activation,[10,11] of special roentgenographic procedures (the latest being the CT scan), and of electrical conductivity; tomorrow may well see the use of nuclear magnetic resonance. Conceptualization and technical development both have played a role in this historical development, the one powerless without the other, to the point where we now possess a great deal of information on certain aspects of body composition throughout the age span of man. The composition of the "reference man" can now be found in textbooks, and those of the "reference infant" and "reference child"[12] will soon be at his side.

## BODY WEIGHT AND HEIGHT

Measurements of body weight and height are easily done and are of great use in assessing growth and nutritional status. For the infant and child, growth velocity is truly a bioassay for energy balance and for certain hormonal functions; in the adult a change in weight suggests an abnormal process, nutritional or otherwise.

---

*"The fat-poor muscle of a starved animal cannot be compared directly to one normally nourished and rich in fat. It is permitted only to compare organs on a fat-free basis."

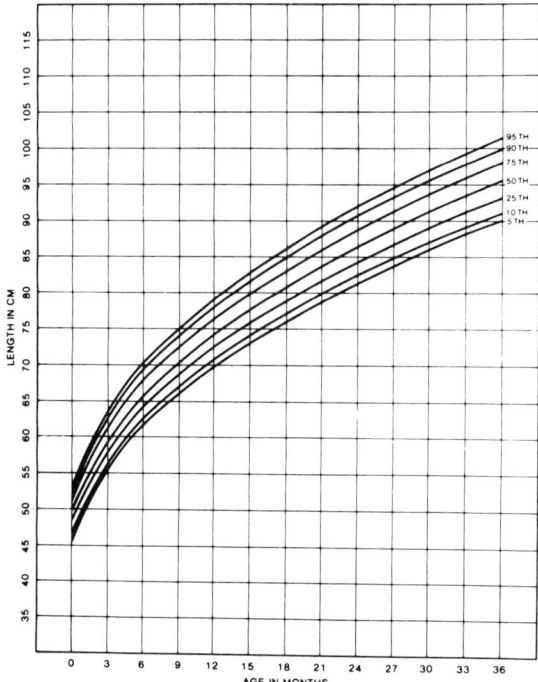

**Fig. 29–1.** Length for age, girls birth to 3 years. (From Hamill, P.V.V., et al.,[13] © Am. J. Clin. Nutr., with permission of the authors and the American Society for Clinical Nutrition.)

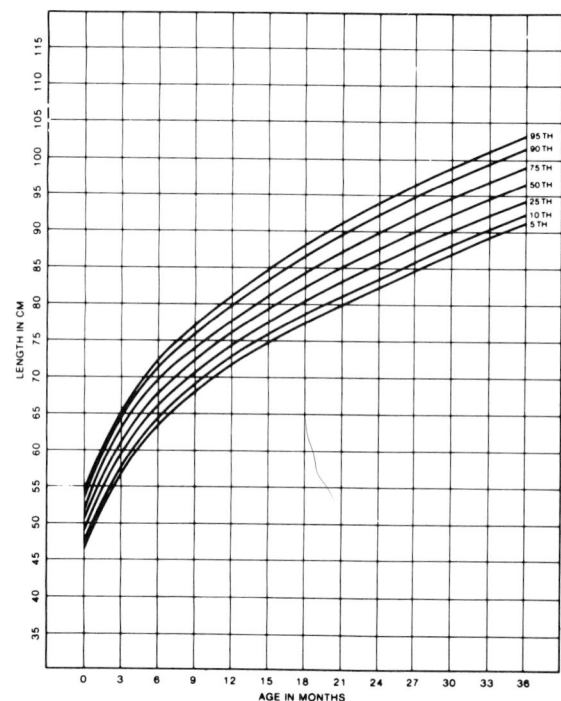

**Fig. 29–2.** Length for age, boys birth to 3 years. (From Hamill, P.V.V., et al.,[13] © Am. J. Clin. Nutr., with permission of the authors and the American Society for Clinical Nutrition.)

Due to the activities of the National Center for Health Statistics, we now have normative data for United States citizens, from the midgestation fetus to the adult. These values are shown in Figures 29–1 to 29–10. Since weight is related to height at all ages, stature must be taken into account, as well as age and sex, in evaluating weight. It should be remembered that norms for citizens of other countries may differ somewhat from those of the United States of America.

Normative values, despite what the adjective implies, cannot necessarily be construed as optimum. This is particularly apt to be true for a country such as ours where there is an abundant supply of high quality food, where a sizeable fraction of the population is clearly overweight, and where it is the usual practice for adults to gain weight after they reach their maximum stature at 18 to 20 years for women and 21 to 25 years for men. In an attempt to define optimum, tables of "desirable weight" for height have been developed from actuarial data gathered by the Metropolitan Life Insurance Company. Appendix Table A–5 lists such "desirable weights" for adults 25 years of age and older.[15] Although no provision is made for age, adults are categorized by body frame size, which is determined by inspection; and the

lack of precision in defining what is "desirable" is manifested by the range of values given for each frame and height category. These ranges vary progressively from 2.7 kg for the shortest "small frame" category to 11.8 kg for the tallest "large frame" category of persons. Of interest is the fact that the values in this table differ somewhat from those published in former decades.

**Body Mass Index (BMI).** This is body weight divided by a power of height, usually (height)$^2$, which is said to be independent of stature, at least in the adult.[16] Calculations based on values for ideal body weight (Appendix Table A–5) suggest that BMI for normal men and women should be in the range 19 to 27 kg/m$^2$. Indeed, this range roughly corresponds to 25th to 75th percentile values recorded from adult individuals who participated in the 1971–1974 National Health and Nutrition Survey.[17] In the case of infants and children, average BMI values change with age,[18,19] beginning at 13 at birth, reaching a peak of 18 at about 1 year, and then a nadir of 15 at about age 6 years, to be followed by a rise to adult values during adolescence. Individuals with high indices are classified as overweight, even obese, and those with subnormal indices as undernourished. Although such classifications cannot be applied, for

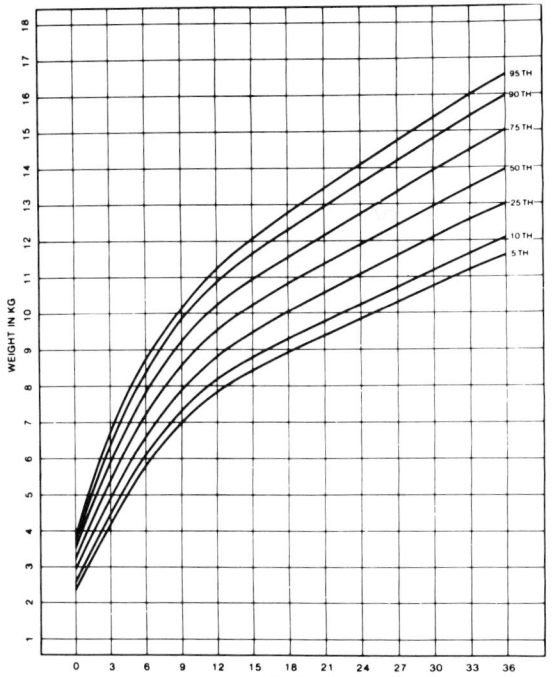

**Fig. 29–3.** Weight for age, girls birth to 3 years. (From Hamill, P.V.V., et al.,[13] © Am. J. Clin. Nutr., with permission of the authors and the American Society for Clinical Nutrition.)

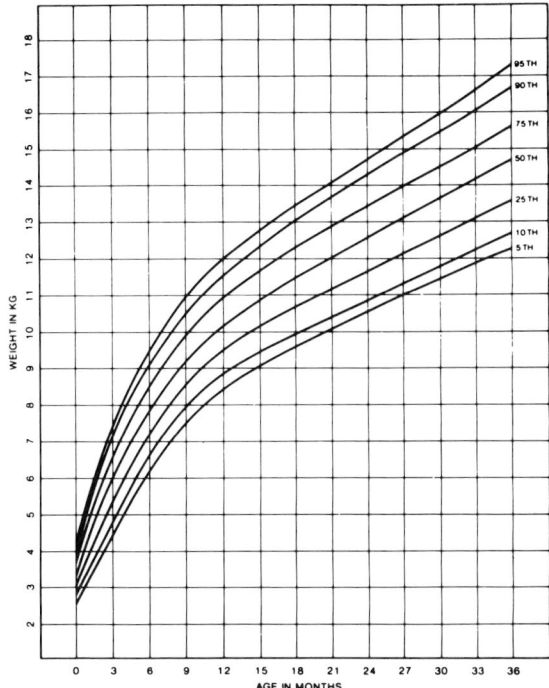

**Fig. 29–4.** Weight for age, boys birth to 3 years. (From Hamill, P.V.V., et al.,[13] © Am. J. Clin. Nutr., with permission of the authors and the American Society for Clinical Nutrition.)

instance, to short muscular men, or to tall asthenic women, the BMI has found usefulness in evaluating groups of individuals.

However, the BMI is not always an accurate index of body composition. This is evident from the fact that despite the difference in body fat the average index is about the same for both sexes during the adolescent and young adult years.[17,19]

**Constancy of Body Weight.** Support for the hypothesis that body weight is homeostatically controlled comes from the observation that many adults maintain their weight within narrow limits over long periods of time and that many children maintain their relative weight status as they grow. This is true of some overweight and underweight adults as well as those in the normal range. The coefficients of variation for successive daily weights in adults is 0.4 to 0.8%.[20] Short-term fluctuations in weight can result from changes in water balance or possibly changes in liver and muscle glycogen induced by diet and/or physical activity. Episodes of infection, serious trauma, enforced bed rest, malignancy, and nutritional inadequacy and surfeit lead to weight change; and many women state that they gain weight towards the end of the menstrual cycle.

The fluctuations noted above indicate that ho-

meostatic control is not perfect; nevertheless, the absence of long-term change in healthy individuals suggests that energy balance oscillates around a mean of zero and that appetite (which controls intake) is geared in some mysterious manner to metabolic rate (which determines expenditure). When these homeostatic mechanisms fail, body weight will change significantly, and the result is obesity or anorexia nervosa.

**Influence of Heredity.** Garn,[21] Tanner et al.,[22] and Wingerd et al.[23] have offered charts and tables showing the effect of parental stature on the height of children, and there can be no doubt that a significant influence on children's heights is the height of their parents. Family resemblances in relative weight and in body build are readily appreciated, as is the tendency towards obesity. Monozygotic twins are more concordant for body size, even if reared apart, than are dizygotic twins.[24] A genetic influence on metacarpal cortex thickness[25] and on skinfold thickness[26] has been demonstrated. Although family life-style and feeding practices may modulate the amount of body fat, studies of adopted children, as well as animal models, provide additional evidence for the role of heredity.[24,27,27a]

Racial differences in stature are well known:

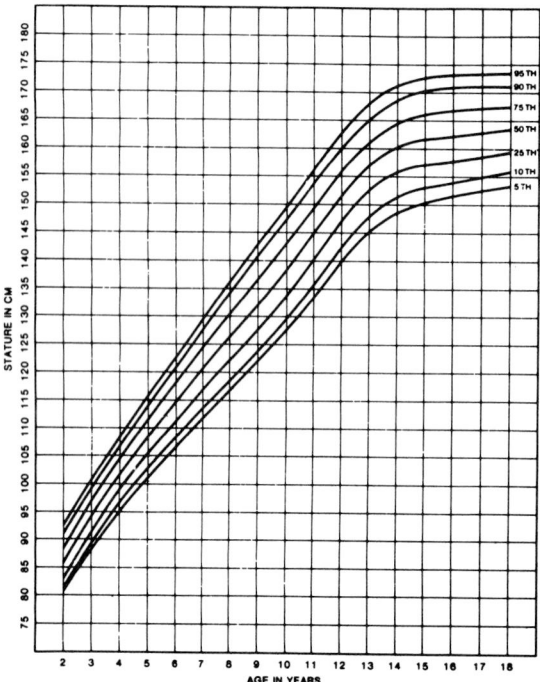

**Fig. 29–5.** Stature for age, girls 2 to 18 years. (From Hamill, P.V.V., et al.,[13] © Am. J. Clin. Nutr., with permission of the authors and the American Society for Clinical Nutrition.)

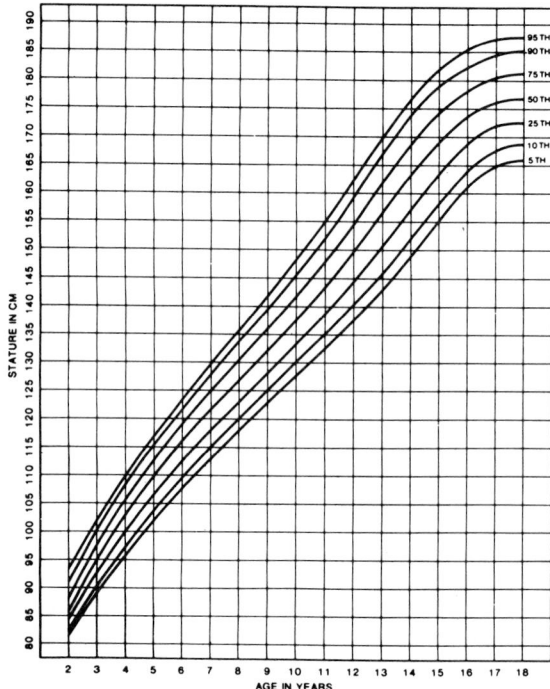

**Fig. 29–6.** Stature for age, boys 2 to 18 years. (From Hamill, P.V.V., et al.,[13] © Am. J. Clin. Nutr. with permission of the authors and the American Society for Clinical Nutrition.)

generally speaking, Oriental adults are shorter than Caucasians, and southern Europeans are shorter than northern Europeans. The average Pygmy male is 144 cm tall, the female 137 cm; and average birth weight is 2,600 g.[28]

**Secular Changes.** Today's children are taller and heavier than those of previous generations,[29,18] a phenomenon that has occurred in all countries in which it has been studied. Although the reason for this change is not known, it is likely that improved nutrition is a prime factor. However, the weight/height ratios have not changed appreciably.[18]

**Aging.** Once middle age is reached, there is a progressive decline in stature; the rate gradually increases to 0.9 to 1.4 cm per decade late in life.[30,31] This change is the result of thoracic kyphosis, compression of intervertebral discs, and change in angulation of the femoral neck. Borkan et al. report a loss of 7.3 cm in males between ages 22 and 82 years; and they estimate that 3.0 cm (41%) of the total is secular in origin, and 4.3 cm is due to aging.[30] As will be shown later, aging is also accompanied by a decline in LBM and in skeletal mass.

## BODY COMPOSITION

Body weight is the sum total of its parts. Modern techniques have made it possible to partition the body into several components, to carry out a "bloodless dissection."

**Body Fluid Volumes.** The various techniques used for this purpose are all based on the dilution principle: a known amount of material is injected intravenously, or in certain instances is given by mouth, and after an interval for equilibration, a sample of blood or urine or saliva is obtained for analysis (in the case of metabolizable substances, several such samples are required, with subsequent extrapolation to time zero). When urinary losses are appreciable, a correction is made for these; however, losses into the lumen of the gastrointestinal tract are usually neglected.

The general equation, V being volume and C concentration, is:

$$V_2 = \frac{C_1 V_1}{C_2}$$

where $C_1 V_1$ is the quantity of material administered, $C_2$ is the concentration in body fluid at equilibrium, and $V_2$ is body fluid volume.

Since the body is not a static system, true equilibrium may never be achieved, particularly in the

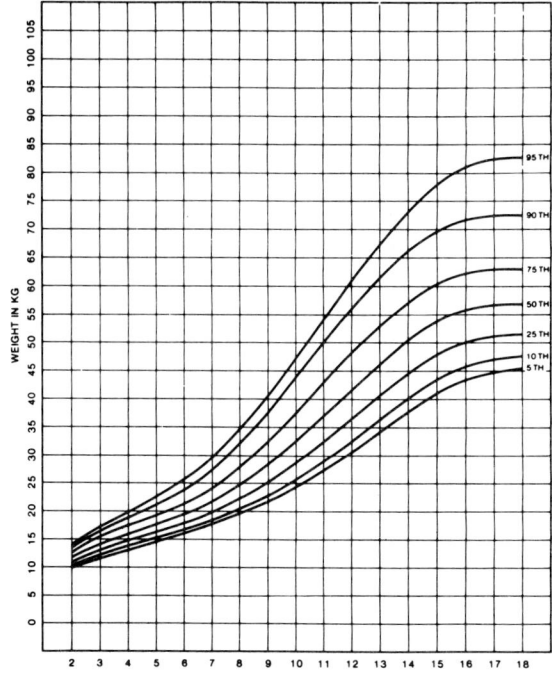

**Fig. 29–7.** Weight for age, girls 2 to 18 years. (From Hamill, P.V.V., et al.,[13] © Am. J. Clin. Nutr., with permission of the authors and the American Society for Clinical Nutrition.)

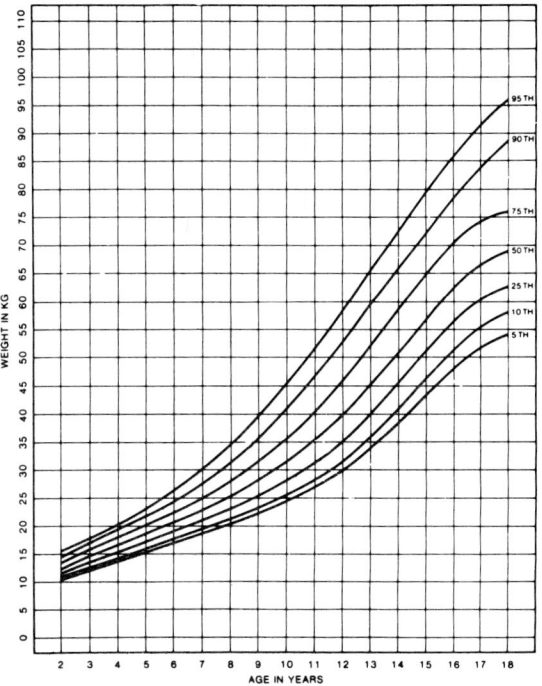

**Fig. 29–8.** Weight for age, boys 2 to 18 years (From Hamill, P.V.V., et al.,[13] © Am. J. Clin. Nutr., with permission of the authors and the American Society for Clinical Nutrition.)

central nervous system and in bone, and there is always some question as to whether the apparent volume of distribution of the administered material coincides with that of the compartment in question. Intracellular fluid volume cannot be determined directly, but only by the difference between total body water and extracellular fluid (ECF) volume, and the value for the latter varies with the material used for its determination.

Plasma volume can be estimated with Evans blue dye (T-1824) or $^{131}$I-labeled albumin, and erythrocyte volume with RBCs tagged with $^{32}$P, $^{51}$Cr, $^{55}$Fe, $^{59}$Fe, or $^{99m}$Tc or by CO uptake. Materials for extracellular fluid volume are inulin, $^{35}S_2O_3^-$, $^{35}SO_4^{2-}$, $SCN^-$, $Br^-$, and $^{82}Br^-$. Cohn et al. have used the ratio of total body Cl (by neutron activation) to serum Cl for this purpose.[32]* The first two materials in this list yield smaller values for ECF volume than the others. Appropriate corrections for serum water must be made, and in the case of

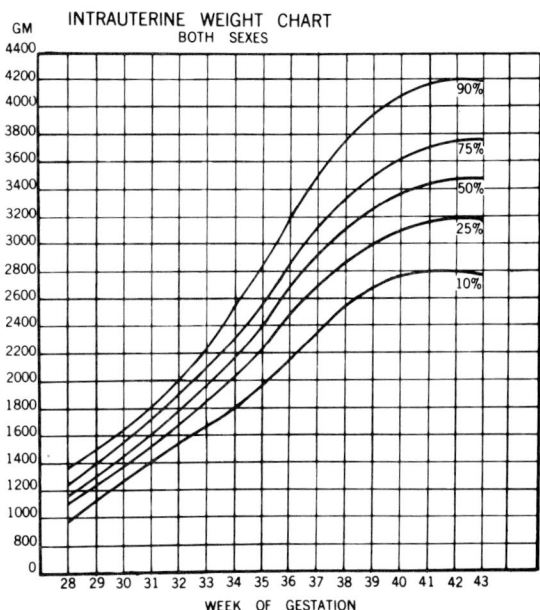

**Fig. 29–9.** Fetal weight for gestational age. (From Naeye, R.L., Dixon, J.B.,[14] with permission of the authors and Pediatric Research.)

---

*New methods for analysis of small amounts of stable Br are fluorescent excitation[33] and high-performance liquid chromatography (HPLC);[34] the detection limit for the latter method is 60 μgm Br/L serum. Preinjection samples are required.

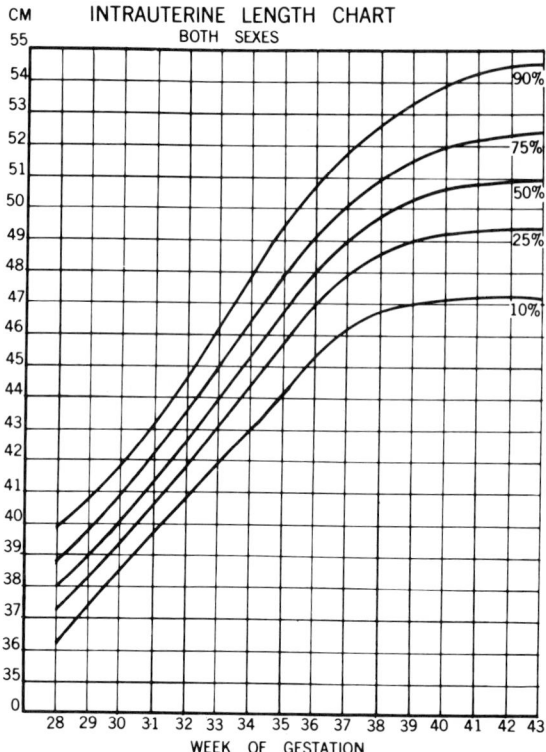

**Fig. 29–10.** Fetal length for gestational age. (From Naeye, R.L., Dixon, J.B.,[14] with permission of the authors and Pediatric Research.)

ionized injectates, corrections for the Donnan equilibrium.

Total body water is estimated by deuterium or tritium labeled water ($D_2O$ or THO) dilution, or by dilution of urea, alcohol, or N-acetyl-4-amino-pyrine. Deuterium can be assayed by infrared spectrometry. Water labeled with oxygen-18 is now being used to estimate total body water.[35] Administered deuterium and tritium undergo some exchange with nonaqueous hydrogen, and hence overestimate total body water by a few percentage points. Bromide and $SCN^-$ both overestimate extracellular fluid volume by about 10% because of penetration of erythrocytes.

Some of these materials can be given by mouth; others must be given intravenously; some readily penetrate the cerebrospinal fluid; others do so very slowly; however, all appear in gastrointestinal secretions. This latter phenomenon poses a problem in animals with a large gastrointestinal tract.

Repeat determinations in normal subjects show that the total error (i.e., biologic variation plus technical error) ranges from 2 to 9% for the various assay methods.[36-39] It should be remembered that body weight, which can be measured quite ac-

curately, varies by at least 1% during the course of a 24-hour day and that individuals tend to be 1 to 2 cm shorter in the evening than in the morning.

**Total Body Content.** The body content of a number of elements can now be assayed by several methods. The technique of isotopic dilution can be applied to Na, K, and Cl, as well as water, by using the following equation:

$$Q = \frac{Q^* \text{ admin.} - Q^* \text{ excreted}}{Q^*/Q \text{ (serum, urine)}}$$

where Q is body content (g, meq) and $Q^*$ is the isotope ($^{24}Na$, $^{22}Na$, $^{42}K$, $^{43}K$, $^{82}Br$, stable Br). Br is used since there is no convenient isotope of Cl. The result is expressed as total exchangeable content ($Na_e$, $K_e$, $Cl_e$), since this procedure underestimates total body content of both K and Na. Total exchangeable K is 90 to 95% of total body K because of incomplete exchange with erythrocytes and brain. Total exchangeable Na is only 70 to 80% of total body Na because of incomplete exchange with bone. However, Br dilution appears to be a good reflection of total body Cl.[40]

Shizgal et al. have devised a method for estimating total exchangeable K ($K_e$) without the need to use the short-lived and inconvenient $^{42}K$ ($t_{1/2}$ 12 hr).[41] Total body water and total exchangeable Na ($Na_e$) are measured together with Na, K, and $H_2O$ in a sample of whole blood. Then

$$K_e = \left[ \frac{Na + K}{H_2O} \text{ (blood)} \times \text{ body } H_2O \right] - Na_e$$

The correlation between measured $K_e$ and $K_e$ as estimated by this method is high. Since $Na_e$ is measured with long-lived $^{22}Na$, this method may not be suitable for children.

Neutron activation has been used to estimate total body Na, Cl, N, Ca, and P.[10,11,32] The subject is irradiated with neutrons, and the induced radioactivity is determined (some investigators do not include the head or lower legs in the radiation field). Table 29–1 lists the nuclear reactions involved. The dose of radiation to the subject is about 30 millirad. However, because the facilities

**Table 29–1.   Nuclear Reactions**

| Substance | | Activation Product Half-life |
|---|---|---|
| $^{48}Ca$ (0.18%)* | (n, γ)† $^{49}Ca$ | 8.8 min |
| $^{23}Na$ (100%) | (n, γ)$^{24}Na$ | 15 hr |
| $^{37}Cl$ (25%) | (n, γ)$^{38}Cl$ | 37 min |
| $^{31}P$ (100%) | (n, α)$^{28}Al$ | 2.3 min |
| $^{14}N$ (99.6%) | (n, 2n)‡ $^{13}N$ | 10 min |

*Isotopic abundance.
†Nuclear reaction.
‡Also prompt gamma emission (n, γ).

required are very expensive and sophisticated, only a very few are in existence.

The possibility exists of determining total body Mg, H, C, and O and individual organ content of I and Cd. Details can be found in reviews by Cohn.[42,43]

**⁴⁰K Counting.** The body contains enough of this naturally occurring isotope ($t_{1/2}$ $1.3 \times 10^9$ years, body content 0.1 μCi) to permit its detection and quantitation by low background scintillation counters. From the known abundance of $^{40}K$ (0.012%) one can then calculate total body K content. This technique has the advantage of being noninvasive and requiring little cooperation by the subject.

There are two types of detectors: one or more sodium iodide crystals activated with thallium, and large plastic or liquid scintillation chambers, both in heavily shielded rooms. The former provides excellent resolution so that contaminating radioisotopes can be detected, but low efficiency; the latter have poor resolution, but high efficiency, because the detector can be made large enough to completely surround the subject.* The former has a low background rate, of the order of one-third the net $^{40}K$ activity in adults, whereas the latter has, by virtue of its large size, a high background rate, amounting to 3 to 4 times the net $^{40}K$ activity. Two factors demand careful calibration of each instrument: the inverse square law of radiation and the attenuation of $^{40}K$ gamma rays by body tissues, especially the subcutaneous fat layer, which has a low K content.

**Body Density.** Archimedes is credited with the discovery that one can estimate the relative proportions of a two-component mixture, each of known density, by measuring the density of the whole system. Hence from a measurement of body density the relative proportions of lean (D = 1.100 g/cm³) and fat (D = 0.900 g/cm³) can be calculated. Let Wf represent weight of fat, Wl weight of lean, and Wb weight of body, and Vf, Vl, and Vb their respective volumes. Since density (D) = W/V, the relationship Vb = Vf + Vl can be written as

$$\frac{Wb}{Db} = \frac{Wf}{Df} + \frac{Wl}{Dl}$$

and since Wl = Wb − Wf, it follows that

$$\frac{Wb}{Db} - \frac{Wb}{Dl} = \frac{Wf}{Df} - \frac{Wf}{Dl}$$

whence

$$Wb \left( \frac{1}{Db} - \frac{1}{Dl} \right) = Wf \left( \frac{1}{Df} - \frac{1}{Dl} \right)$$

Dividing Wf by Wb yields the following (letting $\frac{1}{Df} - \frac{1}{Dl} = \frac{1}{a}$):

$$\frac{Wf}{Wb} = \frac{a}{Db} - \frac{a}{Dl}$$

Since Dl is known (letting $\frac{a}{Dl} = a'$),

$$\text{fraction fat} \left( \frac{Wf}{Wb} \right) = \frac{a}{Db} - a', \text{ and}$$

$$\text{fraction lean} = 1 - \frac{Wf}{Wb}$$

Using the values for Df and Dl noted above, $a = 4.95$ and $a' = 4.50$. Brozek et al. suggest values of 4.570 and 4.142, respectively, based on calculations derived from induced weight losses and gains and compositional differences between lean and obese young men.[44] Actually, these two sets of coefficients yield almost the same values for percentage of body fat. Body density can be measured by underwater weighing:

$$Db = \frac{W \text{ (air)}}{W \text{ (air)} - W \text{ (water)}}$$

with appropriate corrections for the densities of water and air and for the volume of air in the lungs (gastrointestinal air is either neglected or assumed to be 100 ml). Body volume can also be estimated by water displacement, by helium dilution, application of Boyle's law, and even by special photographic and acoustic techniques, whence density is simply W/V. The underwater weighing technique is the only one in common use.

**Other Techniques.** These include anthropometry (skinfold thickness—really a double layer of skin and subcutaneous tissue—and various body circumferences), radiographic assessment of widths of extremity muscles, subcutaneous fat, and bone cortex; photon densitometry of bone; ultrasound determination of subcutaneous fat and of individual organ size; uptake of fat soluble gases such as cyclopropane, xenon, and radiokrypton[45,46]; CT scan for subcutaneous and internal fat, individual organ size, and muscle widths; urinary excretion of creatinine and 3-methylhistidine as indices of total muscle mass. Metabolic balance can, of course, provide information on change in body content of a number of elements.

Various combinations of skinfold thickness and body circumferences have been used to estimate body density and/or body fat content.[47–54] Cross-sectional area of the muscle-bone component of the arm can be calculated from arm circumference

---

*During the 1960s the body burden of $^{137}Cs$ (a fallout product) was sufficient to cause interference with $^{40}K$ counts in low resolution counters; however, at the present time this is much less of a problem.

and skinfold thickness at the midpoint, as follows (T is triceps skinfold, B is biceps):

$$M + B \text{ area} = \frac{1}{4\pi} \left[ \text{circ.} - \frac{\pi}{2} (T + B \text{ SF}) \right]^2$$

and by subtraction, arm fat area. Data on arm M + B area and arm fat area for 6- to 17-year-old children have been published by the National Center for Health Statistics (1974).* Extensive studies by many investigators have established relationships between various anthropometric measurements and LBM or body fat, and although the correlations are not very high ($r^2$ in the range of 0.4 to 0.8), the simplicity of the techniques means that they can be readily applied to large numbers of individuals in the field. It is obvious that such measurements as skinfold thickness and abdominal and buttocks circumferences will bear some relationship to body fat and that biacromial, wrist, and knee diameters will vary with LBM. The quantitative relationships between anthropometric measurements and body composition varies somewhat by age and sex and, indeed, among various investigators; furthermore, there have been problems in applying the results to individuals other than those from whom the observations were made. In a recent review Johnston came to the conclusion that "accurate estimates of whole body composition from anthropometry are not possible."[56]

However, Slaughter et al. found that the inclusion of body weight with skinfold thickness and body circumferences in a multiple regression formula produced a good correlation with LBM ($r^2$ = 0.91) in adolescent boys.[57] Hume found that LBM could be estimated just as well from height and weight ($r^2$ = 0.92 male, 0.69 female adults) as from skinfold thickness.[58] Earlier, Allen et al. had found a good relationship between adiposity and a weight-height[3] function, though it produced spurious results in professional football players.[39]

Since LBM comprises 70 to 90% of body weight in normal children and adults, it is obvious that LBM and weight will be related; and in subjects of widely varying fat content one can anticipate that body fat and weight will also be related. As will be noted later, LBM is a function of stature at all ages. It was the failure of weight-height functions for individuals whose excess weight con-

sisted of muscle that led Behnke to develop the specific gravity technique.[7]

Some newer techniques now undergoing trials are the EMME (or TOBEC) instrument, which estimates lean weight by electrical conductivity,[59,60] and the measurement of electric impedance.[61,61a] Takunaga et al. did CT scans of several regions of the body;[62] by assuming cylindrical shapes for these regions they were able to estimate both internal (viscera) and subcutaneous fat volumes. The radiation dose was 0.6 to 0.9 rad. Nuclear magnetic resonance can identify both internal and external fat depots and even thin layers of fat between muscle bundles.

**Precision of Various Techniques.** Two factors must be considered: technical error per se, and biologic variability. The former includes such phenomena as the random nature of radioactive isotope emissions, the measurement of quantity of injectate, and flame photometer errors. For isotope dilution procedures, for instance, four measurements are necessary, each subject to error: composition of the injectate and its volume and assay of the equilibrium sample of body fluid for tracer and stable isotope; and in some instances there is a fifth measurement, urinary excretion of tracer. For $^{40}$K counting, the subject must be properly situated in the counting chamber. Underwater weighing entails measurement of residual pulmonary air volume as well as body weight both in air and submerged. Neutron activation requires that the neutron dose must be known as well as the amount of induced radioactivity. In the case of urinary creatinine excretion, creatinine concentration and 24-hour urine volume are both required; an error of 15 minutes in collection time represents 1% of a 24-hour period. The latter is in reality a component of technical error.

Biologic variability must also be considered in assessing the significance of observed changes in body composition. Earlier mention was made of the inconstancy of body weight and stature, and it is only reasonable to expect fluctuations in body composition. Once considered a "constant," 24-hour urine creatinine excretion is now known to have a coefficient of variation of several percentage points under controlled conditions. It is the *total* error—technical plus biologic—that must be taken into account, and this can be evaluated only by replicate assays on individuals, a procedure not always feasible with assays involving radiation exposure.

The magnitude of the observed error will depend on the method used to express the results. When LBM is measured, fat is gotten by subtraction; so in subjects where LBM exceeds 50% of

---

*These values were calculated from arm circumference and triceps skinfold only, whence the formula becomes

$$M + B \text{ area} = \frac{1}{4\pi} \left[ \text{circ.} - \pi \, T \, SF \right]^2$$

body weight, the relative error for fat will be greater than that for LBM; the same is true for densitometry.

Published data show coefficients of variation (cv) of 2 to 4% for $^{40}$K counting,[63–65] 2.5 to 6.1% for total exchangeable K,[36,37,66,67] a 7 to 8% "uncertainty" for cyclopropane and $^{85}$Kr uptake;[45] a cv of 5.5% for body Ca,[68,69] and one of ±3.5% for total body N.[70] Densitometry appears to be the most reproducible technique (cv 1.2%[71]); skinfold thickness is the worst, with recorded cvs of 6 to 24%.[55]

The existence on rare occasions of individuals with estimated body fat contents of 1% or less, or even a negative value, is proof that error can occur. Unlikely situations, such as a calculated increase in total body N during weight reduction in some subjects,[72] and a clearly aberrant value for total body water,[73] provide additional evidence.

**Cell Size and Number.** Methods are available for estimating the average size of skeletal muscle cells and of adipocytes and their total number in living subjects. A biopsy is taken of muscle, and the DNA and protein contents are determined; total muscle mass is estimated from urinary creatinine excretion. By using the value of 6.2 pg DNA per muscle cell, the average cell size can be estimated and then total muscle cell number.[74]

Adipocytes obtained by biopsy are sized by histologic techniques, and their average lipid content is assayed chemically; then cell number is calculated from assays of total body fat.[75] These values vary somewhat depending on the site of the biopsy.

**Urinary Creatinine Excretion.** The assumption that this is an index of muscle mass is supported by the work of Schutte et al. in dogs.[76] They found not only a good correlation between urinary creatinine excretion and dissectable muscle mass in this species but also a good correlation between creatinine excretion and total plasma creatinine (plasma Cr concentration times plasma volume). Urine collections must be timed accurately, and the excretion rate can be affected by diet. Studies of subjects of widely varying body size have also shown a good relationship between creatinine excretion and lean weight.[77] For subjects on ad libitum intake, this relationship is

$$\text{LBM (kg)} = 0.0291 \text{ Cr (mg/d)} + 7.38 \quad r^2 = 0.97[77]$$

and for those on meat-free diets it is

$$\text{LBM (kg)} = 0.0241 \text{ Cr (mg/d)} + 20.7 \quad r^2 = 0.91[78]$$

Based on both human and animal data, fat-free skeletal muscle, on average, makes up 49% of total fat-free weight.[77] Hence one can use these equations to estimate the ratio of muscle mass (MM) to urinary creatinine excretion (gm/d):

$$\text{MM/Cr} = 15.7 + 4/\text{Cr} \quad \text{(ad libitum diet)}$$

$$\text{MM/Cr} = 13.0 + 11/\text{Cr} \quad \text{(meat-free diet)}$$

This ratio will vary with the amount of creatinine excreted, from 19.7 kg muscle/g Cr at an excretion rate of one g Cr/d to 17.7 at 2 g Cr/d on ad libitum diet; the respective ratios are 24 and 18.5 for the meat-free diet. These values are close to those reported by Schutte (17.9 kg/g),[76] Cheek (20 kg/g),[74] and Talbot (17.9 kg/g);[79] however, none of these authors considered the possibility that the ratios were not invariant. Cheek suggests that the ratio is different for infants,[74] but it is not possible to derive a definite value from his data. The urinary excretion of 3-methylhistidine has also been proposed as an index of muscle mass.[80] A meat-free diet for at least two days is a prerequisite.

The result of this array of techniques is that the investigator is now in a position to undertake estimates of a number of body components in the living subjects: the amounts of lean and fat, skeletal size, body content of a number of elements, muscle mass, and body fluid volumes.

Table 29–2 lists the various techniques now available, together with the advantages and disadvantages of each. In selecting a technique the purpose of the study to be performed is a paramount consideration, as is the availability of equipment and facilities. Some require considerable cooperation on the part of the subject, some require elaborate and expensive instrumentation or the administration of a radioactive isotope, and some involve measurements of only portions of the body.

The metabolic balance technique, which antedated the others listed, can detect small changes in body content and body composition. For example, a change in body N content of 16 g, equivalent to 0.5 kg LBM, is easily detected, whereas such a change is well within the error of body composition techniques. However, it cannot provide data on actual body content, and it is actually rather expensive when one adds up the cost of running a metabolic ward and supporting laboratory facilities.

The usual procedure is to subtract urine and fecal excretions from intake and to neglect cutaneous losses, since these are difficult to measure. If balance is strongly positive or negative, the error is small, but it becomes appreciable as balance approaches zero. Cutaneous losses of N and K increase as their respective intakes rise.[86,87] Many authors automatically subtract 5 or 8 mg N/kg/day. Another problem is the nonrandom nature of the

**Table 29–2. Techniques to Determine Body Composition**

| | Advantages | Disadvantages |
|---|---|---|
| Density | Apparatus inexpensive<br>Estimates LBM and fat simultaneously<br>Nonhazardous<br>Can be repeated frequently | Subject cooperation necessary for underwater weighing technique<br>Unsuitable for young children, elderly<br>Error from intestinal gas |
| $^{40}$K counting | No hazard<br>Minimal subject cooperation<br>Can be repeated frequently | Instrument expensive<br>Proper calibration necessary<br>Problem in interpretation in subjects with K deficiency |
| Metabolic balance | No hazard<br>Suitable for many elements<br>Can detect small changes in body content (<1%) | Measures only *change* in body composition<br>Meticulous subject cooperation<br>Metabolic ward expensive<br>Error from unmeasured skin losses<br>Many laboratory analyses needed |
| Neutron activation | Minimal subject cooperation<br>Body content Ca, P, N, Na, Cl | Apparatus very expensive<br>Calibration very difficult<br>Radiation exposure |
| Creatinine excretion | No hazard<br>Estimate of muscle mass | Meticulous subject cooperation<br>Influenced by diet, collection time critical<br>Day-to-day variation (c.v. 5–10%) |
| Fat-soluble gases | Direct estimate of body fat | Cyclopropane, xenon, $^{85}$Kr<br>Apparatus expensive<br>Long equilibration time |
| Dilution methods | Estimate body fluid volumes<br>Inexpensive<br>Great variety: Na, K, Cl(Br), $H_2O$ | Radiation exposure (some materials)<br>Blood samples needed (some materials) (some require several samples)<br>Incomplete equilibration Na, K; overestimation by $D_2O$, THO; value for ECF depends on method used; $^{18}$O assay requires elaborate equipment |
| Anthropometry | Cheap<br>Direct estimate of body fat, muscle mass | Poor precision in obese subjects, and in those with firm s.c. tissue<br>Regional variation in subcutaneous fat layer; uncertainty ratio s.c. fat/total fat* |
| Radiography, photon densitometry | Bone density, volume, muscle widths | Limited regions<br>Radiation exposure |
| CT scan† | Organ size, configuration; s.c. fat; intraperitoneal, pericardial fat, bone | Instrument expensive<br>Radiation exposure |
| Ultrasound | Organ size<br>No hazard | Poor definition subcutaneous fat layer |
| 3-Methylhistidine excretion | Estimate of muscle mass | Meat-free diet 2 days prior to collection<br>Subject cooperation<br>? Variable contribution from gastrointestinal tissue<br>? Day-to-day variability |

*This ratio varies from 0.04 to 0.43 among various mammals.[81] There are only two reports for humans: in one newborn infant the ratio was 0.42,[82] and in one adult it was 0.32.[83] Recent observations by CT scan suggest that the ratio of intra-abdominal fat to subcutaneous fat varies considerably in adults.[84]

†See, for example, the analysis of the constituents of the human forearm by Maughan et al.[85]

intake and excretion variables; the result is that positive balances tend to be overestimated and negative balances underestimated, never the reverse. Corrections must be made for element content of blood samples and for menstrual losses. For those elements, such as Ca, Fe, and Pb, whose main route of excretion is fecal the balance periods must be long enough to account for day-to-day variations and to include intestinal transit time.

Garrow has put forth an ingenious method for estimating the composition of the tissue lost during weight reduction.[88] Energy balance is estimated, and from the energy equivalents of fat and lean (taken as 9 and one kcal/g, respectively*), the amount of fat lost is given as follows:

$$\Delta \text{ fat (kg)} = \frac{\Delta E \text{ (Mcal)} - \Delta W \text{ (kg)}}{8}$$

The problem is the measurement of energy expenditure, a tedious and time-consuming job requiring meticulous cooperation by the subject. Nor can the possession of a direct colorimeter provide a solution except for the rare subject willing to be confined in such an apparatus for several days. Nevertheless, Garrow and co-workers were able to show a reasonable correlation between this method and nitrogen balance for estimating body fat loss in a group of obese women kept on low energy diets for about three weeks.[88]

The calculation of lean weight from density, total body N, K, and $H_2O$ (Table 29-3) carries the assumption that the composition of the lean body mass does not vary among normal adult individuals. Sheng and Huggins have shown that the water content of the LBM does vary somewhat as determined by various investigators.[91] Bone has a low water and a low K content but a high density in comparison to soft tissue; hence one must assume that bone:soft tissue ratios do not vary greatly among individuals. In their neutron activation studies Ellis and Cohn do find that whole body Ca/K ratio is related to stature, and so is a little lower in men than in women;[92,93] nonetheless, the limited variability of this ratio indicates that the bone:soft tissue ratio does not vary a great deal among normal individuals.

Assessment of individuals with massive obesity presents a problem. They are unable to cooperate with the underwater weighing procedure; proper calibration of $^{40}K$ counters is difficult; skinfold measurements are imprecise, and the thickness may exceed the maximum jaw width of the usual calipers. Some patients have mild to moderate edema. Dilution methods and urinary creatinine excretion, however, should be satisfactory.

The ultimate precision of most techniques is limited by biologic variability; body weight exhibits diurnal and day-to-day variations, and it is safe to assume that certain features of body composition also exhibit some variability. An instructive exercise is to calculate the effect of adding or subtracting 500 ml $H_2O$ from an adult subject: this will change the density and the K, and N, and $H_2O$ contents of the LBM slightly, as well as the ratio of element balance to weight change.

Another consideration stems from the fact that the ratio ECF/total water varies somewhat with age, being higher in neonates than in young adults and then rising again in the elderly. Hence, neither the K, N, nor $H_2O$ contents of the LBM, nor its density can be considered to be constant throughout the age span of man (vide infra). In dealing with diseased subjects or those who are losing or gaining weight, it must be remembered that the K/N ratio varies among body tissues, from a high of 24 meq K/gN in erythrocytes, to 5.0 in brain, 2.8 in skeletal muscle, about 2.5 in viscera, to a low of 0.45 in plasma and skin.[94] Hence, the ratio of change in body K to change in body N resulting from a change in weight will depend on the particular tissue components involved. In states of under- or overhydration the density of the LBM will be altered from its usual value of 1.100 g/ml, and in states of K deficiency the K content of the LBM will be subnormal.

A number of investigators have used two or more techniques in the same subjects. Some report a reasonable correspondence between densitometric, body water, and $^{40}K$ techniques;[95,42] and Cohn et al. found rather small coefficients of variation for body N/K and body $K/H_2O$ ratios in normal adults.[96] A recalculation of the data published by Womersley et al. shows a good correspondence between LBM values derived from density and $^{40}K$ counts in both men and women;[97] and in a subsequent publication the same was true for muscular and obese individuals.[98] Krzywicki et al. found a good correspondence between density and $^{40}K$ and for density and body water for women, but not for men.[95] The results of $^{40}K$ and densitometric assays were comparable in a series of women with varying degrees of obesity;[99] and body K was closely related to body N in a group of adult men and women.[100] In a group of adult males Lukaski et al. found a good correspondence among all three techniques.[80,101]

The values for K, $H_2O$, and N contents of the LBM listed in Table 29-3 are based on cadaver analyses,[82] with the K/LBM ratio being altered for females on the basis of the reported sex difference in the $K_e/H_2O$ ratio.[102,64] Some investigators prefer to derive values for LBM composition from a comparison of in vivo assays. Cohn et al. have chosen values of 64.5 and 58 meq K/kg LBM for males and females, respectively,[96] but Womersley et al. suggest that these should be 66.4 and 59.7.[97] Lukaski et al. derived a value of 62.6 meqK/kg LBM for males.[80] They also offer one of 746 ml $H_2O$/kg LBM; however, their values of 32.1 gN[80] and 32.7

---

*Others have assigned slightly different values to these two body components: fat 9.4 and lean 1.16 kcal/g, the latter derived from the energy value of protein (5.65 kcal/g $\cong$ 1.16 kcal/g LBM.[89] Based on the data reported by Spady et al. a gain of 1 g fat requires 12 kcal, and a gain of 1 g protein requires 8.65 kcal ($\cong$ 1.78 kcal/g LBM).[90]

**Table 29–3.    Calculation of Lean Body Mass, Fat in Adults (Wt = LBM + Fat)**

| Method | Formula | Remarks |
|---|---|---|
| Density | $\text{Fraction fat} = \dfrac{4.570}{D} - 4.142$ | Brozek et al.[44] |
| | $\text{Fraction fat} = \dfrac{4.95}{D} - 4.50$ | Siri[103] |
| Total body water | $\text{LBM} = H_2O\ (l)/0.73$ | Multiply by 0.95 to correct for $^2H$ and $^3H$ exchange with nonaqueous hydrogen |
| $^{40}K$ counting | $\text{LBM} = \text{total K (meq)}/68.1\ (M),\ 64.2\ (F)$<br>$\text{BCM}^* = \text{total K (meq)} \times 0.00833$ | Multiply by 1.1 when $^{42}K$ dilution is used |
| Creatinine excretion | $\text{LBM} = 0.029\ \text{Cr (mg/ld)} + 7.38$<br>$\text{LBM} = 0.024\ \text{Cr (mg/d)} + 20.7$ | Ordinary diet[77]<br>Meat-free diet[78] |
| Neutron activation† | $\text{LBM} = \text{total N (g)}/33$ | Change in LBM can be estimated from N balance |
| Anthropometry (skinfold thickness, body circumferences) | Numerous formulae | Those of Steinkamp et al.[49] and Durnin and Womersley[50] are frequently used; many have less than adequate precision. |
| Density—total water | $\text{Fraction fat}$<br>$= \dfrac{2.1366}{D} - 0.78\,\dfrac{H_2O}{Wt} - 1.374$ | Siri[103] |
| Neutron activation—body water—$^{40}K$ | $\text{LBM} = 6.25\ N + H_2O + \dfrac{Ca}{0.34}$ | Cohn et al.[32] |
| | $\text{LBM} = \text{BCM} + \text{ECF} + \dfrac{Ca}{0.117}$ | Cohn et al.[96] |

*Francis Moore and co-workers put forth the concept of body cell mass (BCM), namely, that component of the body which contains 120 meq K/kg, which is stated to be the concentration of K in body cells.[104] In discussing this concept the authors admit that the factor of 0.00833 is not precise and that it could be as high as 0.010 or as low as 0.007.

†At the suggestion of L. Burkinshaw, Cohn and his associates have used measured body N and K to make estimates of the relative amounts of muscle (striated) and non-muscle components of the LBM in adults.[96] These calculations depend on the difference in K/N ratio for these two components. However, the various tissues that make up the non-muscle component have widely varying K/N ratios (see text), and the validity of this novel approach remains in doubt.

**Table 29–4.    LBM Composition**

| Age | Male $H_2O$ (%) | ECF/$H_2O$ | K (meq/kg) | N (%) | Density (g/ml) | Female $H_2O$ (%) | ECF/$H_2O$ | K (meq/kg) | N (%) | Density (g/ml) |
|---|---|---|---|---|---|---|---|---|---|---|
| Fetus 24 week | 89* | | 40* | | | | | | | |
| Fetus 32 week | 86* | | 46* | | | | | | | |
| Birth | 81 | 0.61 | 49 | 2.4 | 1.063 | 81 | 0.61 | 49 | 2.4 | 1.064 |
| 5 year | 77 | 0.46 | 64 | 2.96 | 1.078 | 78 | 0.48 | 62 | 2.88 | 1.073 |
| 10 year | 75 | 0.43 | 67 | 3.1 | 1.085 | 77 | 0.45 | 64 | 2.99 | 1.075 |
| 18.5 year | 73.6 | 0.38 | | 3.24 | 1.093 | | | | | |
| Young adult | 73 | | 68.1 | | 1.10 | 73 | | 64.2 | | 1.10 |
| | | | K/N (meq/g) | | | | | K/N (meq/g) | | |
| Young adult† | | 0.44<br>0.42‡ | 1.88 | | | | 0.48 | 1.73 | | |
| Old adult† | | 0.50<br>0.48‡ | 1.78 | | | | 0.52 | 1.65 | | |

*Combined sexes;[106] birth to 18.5 years.[12,107]
†Cohn et al.[32]
‡Borkan, Norris.[108]

gN/kg LBM[101] are close to the one derived from cadaver analysis.

A number of values for total body K/N ratios (meq/g) have been reported: 1.92,[96] 1.88,[105] 1.95[80] for males; 1.67,[96] 1.73,[105] 1.78[100] for females, although these latter authors derive a value of 1.81 meqK/gN for both sexes by regression analysis. Total body K/N ratios tend to be lower in older adults.[96] The average value from cadaver analysis is 2 meqK/gN.[82]

The variations noted above reflect the criteria used to assess LBM, possible differences in analytical technique, or even biologic variability. There is a distinct tendency among investigators to use the densitometric technique as the "standard" to which the results of other techniques should be compared. While densitometry has the advantage of being subject to less technical error than the other techniques, it is obviously impossible to determine its accuracy for living subjects, and it is likely that the density of the LBM (upon which the test implicitly depends) varies with age (it does change with growth) and perhaps with sex. There would seem to be no a priori reason for choosing any one technique as the standard to which others must be compared. Given the likelihood of interindividual variations in organ size, the goal of developing a highly precise method for estimating body composition may never be achieved.

**Effect of Age on Composition of LBM.** The values listed in Table 29–4 pertain to young and middle-aged adults. Composition is quite different for the fetus and newborn, and changes occur with aging. Some of those changes are given in condensed form in this table. Water content falls progressively during early life, as does the ratio of extracellular fluid volume to total body water; this ratio rises again in old age. Potassium and nitrogen contents rise, as does calculated density. With aging, total body K declines a little faster than total body N, and the K/N ratio falls.

## CHANGES IN BODY COMPOSITION WITH GROWTH, AGING

The "reference man" has been defined as indicated in Tables 29–5 and 29–6. Relative organ size is somewhat different in the neonate, with muscle accounting for 22% of body weight, brain for 10%, and liver for 4%, compared to 40%, 2%, and 2.6%, respectively, in the adult. A large fraction of the newborn skeleton consists of cartilage.

Table 29–7 lists average values for weight, LBM, and % body fat for the newborn, the ten-year-old, and the adult. As mentioned earlier, human beings rank among the fattest of mammals.[81] Newborn infants contain less K per unit fat-free weight than do adults (53 meq/kg versus 68), and less N (23 g/kg versus 33).[82,94] Calculated density of the fat-free mass increases, from 1.063 g/ml in the newborn[12] to 1.100 in the adult, and water content decreases from 81 to 73%. As mentioned earlier, K and N contents of the LBM decline somewhat with aging.

The ratio of extracellular fluid (ECF) volume to total body water also changes with age. This ratio is 0.61 in the newborn,[12] 0.42 to 0.44 in young adults, and 0.48 to 0.50 in the elderly.[32,109]

**LBM and Weight Variability Compared.** Among individuals of the same age and sex body fat ex-

**Table 29–5.  Reference Man: Gross Organ Size\* (g)**

| | | |
|---|---|---|
| Weight | 70,000 | |
| Skeletal muscle | 28,000 | |
| Adipose tissue | 15,000 | (fat 12,000) |
| Skeleton | 10,000 | (cortical bone 4,000; trabecular bone 1,000; marrow 3,000; cartilage 1,100; periarticular tissue 900) |
| Skin | 4,900 | |
| Liver | 1,800 | |
| Brain | 1,400 | |
| Heart | 330 | |
| Kidneys | 310 | |

\*From International Committee on Radiation Protection.[109]

**Table 29–6.  Reference Man: Total Body Content of Some Elements\***

| Element | Amount (g) | |
|---|---|---|
| Oxygen | 43,000 | (1,340 mol) |
| Carbon | 16,000 | (1,333 mol) |
| Hydrogen | 7,000 | (3,500 mol) |
| Nitrogen | 1,800 | (64 mol) |
| Calcium | 1,000† | (25 mol) |
| Phosphorus | 780† | (25 mol) |
| Sulfur | 140 | (4,370 mmol) |
| Potassium | 140 | (3,600 mmol) |
| Sodium | 100 | (4,170 mmol) |
| Chlorine | 95 | (2,680 mmol) |
| Magnesium | 19 | (780 mmol) |
| Silicon | 18 | |
| Iron | 4.2 | |
| Fluorine | 2.6 | |
| Zinc | 2.3 | |
| Copper | 0.07 | |
| Manganese | 0.01 | |
| Iodine | 0.01 | |
| Radium | $3 \times 10^{-11}$ | |

\*From International Committee on Radiation Protection.[109] Seventeen additional trace elements (all less than 330 mg) are listed in this reference. Values are lower in women.

†Newer data derived from neutron activation analyses show that Ca/P ratio is about 2:1 and that the content of both elements varies with stature, age, and sex.

**Table 29–7.    The Reference Person***

|  | Newborn | Ten-year-old Boy | Ten-year-old Girl | Adult Man | Adult Woman |
|---|---|---|---|---|---|
| Weight | 3.4 | 31 | 32 | 72 | 58 |
| LBM | 2.9 | 27 | 26 | 61 | 42 |
| % Fat | 14 | 13 | 19 | 15 | 28 |

*From references 12, 96, 98, 110, 111, 112.

hibits much more variability than LBM. This is shown in Figure 29–11, which is based on the author's $^{40}$K assays of 164 women aged 14 to 50 years and 156 to 170 cm in stature.[105a] It is evident that body fat accounts for most of the variability in body weight. In women the maximum LBM is about 70 kg; in men about 100 kg. Perhaps there is a limit to LBM size in humans, as there is for stature.

**Age and Sex.** Figures 29–12 and 29–13 show average values for LBM and fat from midgestation through the eighth decade, as compiled from several sources.[105a] Note that the abscissa scale for Figure 29–12 is in postconception years. The fetus does not acquire appreciable amounts of body fat until the last trimester of gestation, and it turns out that the human neonate has a larger percentage of body fat (14%) than other mammals at birth.[114] Relative body fat continues to increase during the first six months of postnatal life to a maximum of 25%, and then falls to a nadir of about 13% in boys and 16% in girls in late childhood.

It is of interest that sexual dimorphism in body composition is present in early life, well in advance of mature gonadal function. Once adoles-

cence is under way, the sex difference becomes pronounced, the male spurt in LBM being much more rapid and females acquiring more fat. Between the ages of 10 and 20 years the average increment in LBM is 33 kg in boys but only 16 kg in girls, and by age 20 years the male:female ratio is 1.45. This can be compared to a weight ratio of 1.25 and a height ratio of 1.08 at age 20. During the male adolescent spurt, the peak velocity for LBM coincides with peak height velocity.[48] It is likely that the sex difference in the magnitude of the adolescent spurt in LBM is due to the fact that the testosterone production rate in males is about 6 times that of females.

The adult years are characterized by a slow fall in LBM; this fall takes place somewhat more rapidly in males, and from the data at hand it would appear that female LBM is preserved until the age of menopause. By age 75 years, LBM in males is roughly equivalent to that of the average 14-year-old, and in females to that of the average 13-year-old. It appears that much of the LBM increment acquired during the adolescent growth spurt is dissipated by the aging process.

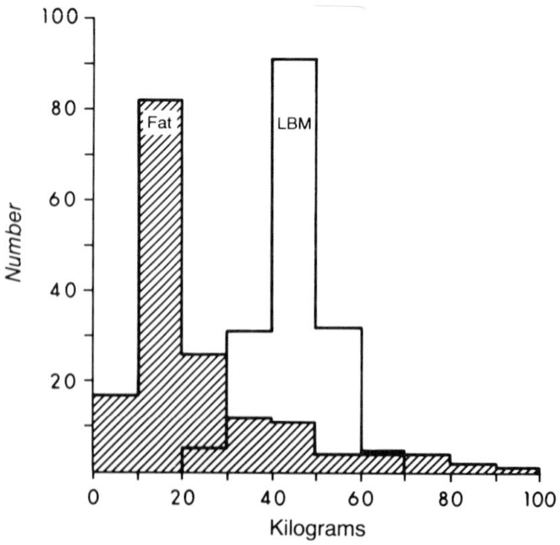

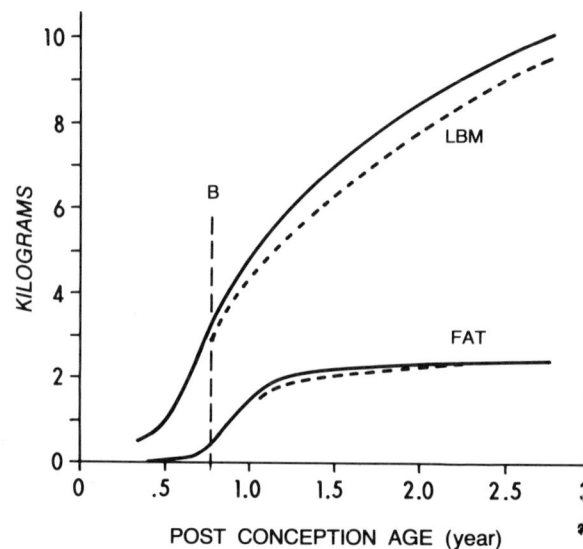

**Fig. 29–11.** Frequency distribution of lean body mass and body fat for 164 women and girls aged 14 to 50 years and 156 to 170 cm in height. Included are patients with anorexia nervosa and obesity, as well as normal subjects.

**Fig. 29–12.** Average values for LBM and fat in fetus and infant. Age in postconception years. Boys —; girls ---. (From Forbes, G.B.,[105a] with permission of Springer-Verlag.)

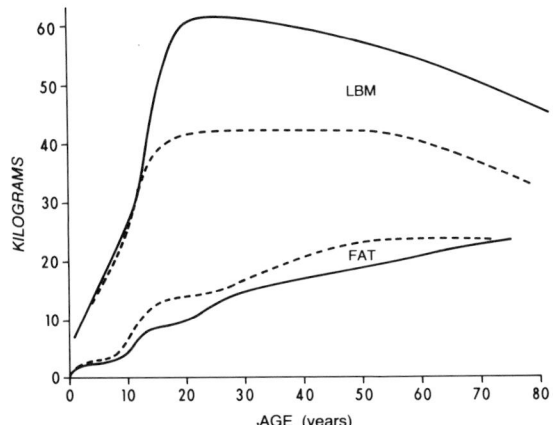

**Fig. 29–13.** Average values for LBM and fat in child and adult. Males —, females ---. Compiled from data in references 12, 96, 107, 110, 111, 112, 113.)

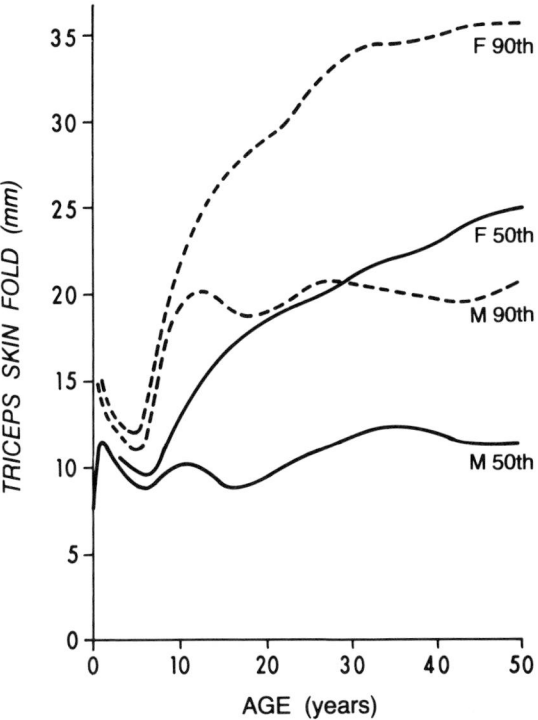

**Fig. 29–14.** 50th and 90th percentiles for triceps skinfold thickness. Infants and children less than 6 years from Tanner and Whitehouse;[117] individuals 6 to 50 years from Cronk and Roche.[17]

The studies of Cohn and associates show that there is a progressive decline in total body K, N, and Ca during the adult years.[32] Between ages 25 and 75 years body K declines by about 4.5% per decade and body N by about 3.5% per decade in both sexes; however, the decline in body Ca is 5.4% per decade in women compared to 2% per decade in men. A number of observers have confirmed the adult decline in LBM as derived from cross-sectional data.[113,115,116]

As shown in Figure 29–13, girls have slightly more body fat than boys from an early age; once adolescence is under way, girls acquire much more body fat than boys, and this sex difference persists throughout the adult years. These changes are reflected in triceps skinfold thickness (Fig. 29–14). The great variability in body fat is evident from Figures 29–11 and 29–14.

**Stature.** At all ages studied LBM is a function of height. On average the regression slope is 0.69 kg/cm in adult males and 0.29 kg/cm in adult females.[118] When the sexes are considered together, it turns out that LBM is related to the cube of height. Skeletal size is also a function of height;[119] and Ellis and Cohn's data show that the same is true for total body Ca, the regression slope being 20 g Ca/cm.[92,120] Based on these findings a 186 cm male would be expected to have about 1,370 g Ca in his body, a 154 cm woman only 730 g Ca. McNeill and Harrison found truncal Ca content to be proportional to height to the 3.1 power in adults and to the 2.9 power in children.[121] Allen et al. related blood volume to the cube of height.[39]

Data such as these mean that comparisons of LBM and total body Ca among individuals are valid only if height, age, and sex are controlled. Many athletes are taller than average, which is one reason they tend to have a larger LBM.[122] Indeed, Khosla found that the winners of a number of Olympic events were taller than the average of all participants in those events.[124] An analysis of the data compiled by Wilmore on male and female athletes showed that for most groups the relationship between LBM and height was steeper than others have found for nonathletes; for such individuals LBM is a function of height to the 4.4 power.[105a] Exceptions were basketball players who have a lower LBM:height ratio, and the weight lifters and body builders who have a higher ratio than the others.

**Pregnancy.** Of the total weight gain during pregnancy, some 12 to 13 kg on average, the fetus, placenta, and amniotic fluid together comprise about 4.2 kg. The remaining 8 kg is maternal tissue. All components of body water increase—plasma volume, extra- and intracellular fluid volume—and since the ratio of body water:body K increases, the increase in ECF volume is proportionately greater than that of ICF volume, which is in keeping with the observation that many pregnant women have mild edema. A portion of the weight gain—variously estimated at 2 to 4 kg—consists of fat.[125,126]

**Some Correlates of Body Composition.** Since the adult female has on average only about 70% the amount of LBM possessed by the average male, it is obvious that the requirements for energy and protein are correspondingly less. The Recommended Dietary Allowances of the National Research Council reflect this sex difference. Basal metabolic rate is more closely related to LBM than to body weight;[127–130] so it is to be expected that BMR per kg body weight would be lower in the obese than in the nonobese.

It would seem prudent to adjust the dose of various drugs on the basis of LBM rather than body weight. Women achieve higher blood alcohol concentrations than men when the amount ingested is based on body weight.[131] Some of the adult decline in such metabolic parameters as glucose tolerance, adrenocorticoid hormone excretion, and maximal oxygen consumption may possibly reflect the age-associated decline in LBM.

In considering studies done on individuals consuming "essentially" protein-free diets,[132–134] a linear relationship is seen between endogenous urinary nitrogen excretion and body cell mass (r = 0.85) over a range for the latter of 14 to 42 kg.

Some years ago Frisch and co-workers proposed the hypothesis that sexual maturity in females was related to the acquisition of a certain amount of body fat, namely 17% at menarche and 22% for continued menstruation, and a "critical" body weight of 47 kg.[135,136] This hypothesis generated widespread interest in the possible role of body fat as a determinant of mature sexual function. What was overlooked by many was the fact that Frisch derived values for body fat content not from body composition measurements but from height and weight. After a thorough review Scott and Johnston concluded that the Frisch hypothesis is invalid.[137] Loucks et al. reported that amenorrheic women athletes have the same degree of body fatness (by densitometry) as those who menstruate normally and that the height-weight equation used by Frisch yields erroneous values for body fat.[138]

Body fat stores serve an important function in times of caloric deprivation. Obese individuals who fast lose less nitrogen per unit weight loss than do the nonobese,[139] and it is well known that the obese can tolerate much longer fasts than those who are thin. The protective effect of body fatness is also seen in situations involving less severe caloric restriction. In relatively long-term studies of individuals given 1,400 to 1,900 kcal diets, LBM accounted for about 50% of the total weight loss in those who were thin, but only 15 to 26% in the obese.[48,140–143]

## INFLUENCE OF NUTRITION

**Energy Deficit.** Maintenance of body weight in the adult and satisfactory growth rate in the child depend on an adequate supply of energy. Subnormal intakes lead to a decline in growth velocity, and in the adult to a fall in body weight. Generally speaking, the rate of weight loss is a function of the magnitude of the energy deficit. After the first few days, fasting results in a loss of about 0.5 kg/day in the obese[144] and about 0.35 kg/day in the nonobese.[145] Mathematical analysis shows that the weight loss during fasting is exponential,[146] which suggests that the loss rate is proportional to weight itself and so tends to diminish with time. The fractional loss rate is less in the obese than in the nonobese (0.34%/day vs. 0.56%/day).

Smaller energy deficits produce slower rates of weight loss. Using data obtained during controlled observations on adults over periods of at least five weeks, it appears that 1,400 to 1,900 kcal diets produce a loss of 0.13 to 0.15 kg/day in nonobese males,[140,147] 0.16 to 0.20 kg/day in obese males, and 0.08 to 0.12 kg/day in obese females.[141–143] On intakes of 500 to 750 kcal/day the obese lose 0.25 to 0.39 kg/day.[148,149]

**Energy Excess.** Consumption of energy in excess of maintenance needs produces an increase in body weight. When subjects are under close observation, it turns out that the increase is roughly proportional to the total excess energy consumed during the overfeeding period.[150] Indeed, a re-evaluation of Neumann's and Gulick's classic studies on themselves showed that they always gained weight when they took excess food (and that they always lost when they ate less).[151]

The energy cost of the weight gain has been computed for several types of human subjects. On average this turns out to be 5.0 kcal/g gain for infants recovering from malnutrition,[90] 4.0 kcal/g gain for growing prematurely born infants,[152] 4.7 kcal/g for adolescent girls recovering from anorexia nervosa,[153] and 8.0 kcal/g for normal adults who are deliberately overfed.[153a] The energy cost of weight gain is about the same for women as it is for men.[153a] Based on estimates of the additional energy requirement for pregnancy,[126] and the average weight gain, the cost is 80,000 kcal ÷ 12,500 g = 6.4 kcal/g gain. As will be shown later, the energy cost varies according to the composition of the tissue gained.

**Effect on Body Composition.** Nutrition can affect lean weight as well as body fat. When compared to normal individuals of the same stature, age, and sex, undernourished subjects have a reduced LBM as well as less fat,[122,154,155] and the obese have an increase in both.[150] Indeed, Keys and Brozek spoke of "obesity tissue" as consisting of protein and body fluid as well as fat.[156]

Careful studies of underfed subjects, employing either nitrogen balance or body composition techniques, have shown that significant weight reduction involves a loss of both LBM and fat. The relative contribution of each of these components to the total weight loss depends on two principal factors: the initial body fat content and the magnitude of the energy deficit.

During a fast, thin individuals lose twice as much body N per unit weight loss as obese individuals lose,[139] and thin individuals consuming diets of 1400–1900 kcal have a greater loss of LBM ($\Delta$LBM/$\Delta$W ratio) than obese individuals.[140–143] When only those experiments lasting 4 weeks or longer are considered, the contribution of LBM to the total weight loss is an inverse function of initial body fat content. Obese individuals preferentially burn fat and so tend to conserve lean tissue.

The second factor is equally important: for all categories of initial body fat content studied to date, the $\Delta$LBM/$\Delta$W loss ratio is directly related to the energy deficit. As Benedict et al. showed many years ago,[147] even modest energy deficits lead to some loss of body N,[160] and densitometric techniques have confirmed the loss of LBM.[161] There are no well-controlled studies showing that body N and LBM can be preserved on low-energy diets, a conclusion reached some 30 years ago by Calloway and Spector.[162] Nitrogen losses do tend to diminish with time, however, as do calculated LBM losses,[140,149,158,163] both with low energy diets and during fasting.[164] Indeed, during fasting the N loss is exponential, and the fractional N loss is greater in nonobese than in obese individuals.[139] This phenomenon may partly account for the greater tolerance of obese individuals for fasting.

The combined influence of initial body fat content and energy deficit on the composition of the weight loss during weight reduction is shown in Table 29–8. Included are data on 70 men and 179 women who had body composition assays (total body water or densitometry or $^{40}$K counting) both

prior to and after at least 4 weeks on a weight-reduction diet. Except for those given 300 kcal or less daily, all had adequate protein intakes. The values for the proportion of weight loss represented by LBM ($\Delta$LBM/$\Delta$W ratio) are grouped in categories according to initial body fat content and energy intake. The $\Delta$LBM/$\Delta$W ratio is seen to fall progressively for all energy intake categories as initial body fat increases; and for any given value for body fat, the ratio progressively falls with increasing energy intakes (and hence decreasing energy deficits).

It is obvious that the amount of weight lost in response to a given energy deficit will vary with the composition of the weight loss. The energy value of fat is 9.4 kcal/g, and that of lean tissue is about 1.1 kcal/g (protein has a value of 5.6 kcal/g, and LBM is 20% protein). Hence, in general, the obese individual will lose less weight for a given energy deficit than the nonobese individual because the obese individual loses proportionately more fat. However, because the entire process is confounded by the associated fall in BMR, variability in physical activity, and lack of information on the actual energy deficit, precise estimates are very difficult to make.

Attempts to forestall the loss of LBM by using low-energy diets composed mainly, or entirely, of protein have not been successful in this respect. The careful studies by Fisler et al. showed that some body N was lost by obese subjects given a 400-kcal (100-g protein) diet, though the loss was less (8.2 gm N/kg weight loss) than during fasting (11.8 g N/kg).[158] In this connection it should be mentioned that a number of deaths have occurred in patients given such diets, and among the findings at autopsy have been a reduction in the size of the heart.[159]

Obese patients subjected to intestinal bypass or gastric stapling operations also lose LBM as they lose weight. In various studies, 15 to 40% of the weight lost by these patients has consisted of LBM.[165–168]

The only animal known to preserve LBM during weight reduction is the hibernating bear,[169] though migrating birds come close.[170] In the ab-

**Table 29–8.  Effect of Energy Deficit on $\Delta$LBM/$\Delta$W ratio***

| Intake kcal/day | Initial Body Fat (kg) | | | | | | |
|---|---|---|---|---|---|---|---|
| | *5–10* | *11–20* | *21–30* | *31–40* | *41–50* | *51–60* | *60+* |
| 0–300 | | | | .56(4) | .53(3) | | .40(7) |
| 450–900 | | | .51(7) | .38(35) | .31(17) | .26(10) | .21(17) |
| 1100–1400 | | | .26(21) | .13(31) | .14(17) | | |
| 1600–1900 | .69(18) | .49(14) | .21(45) | | | .15(3) | |

*Compilation of data from 19 reports (see reference 105a). Values represent means; unfortunately, many of the data were presented in such a way as to preclude calculation of a standard deviation or a range. Number of subjects in parentheses.

sence of food and water the bear has been observed to lose 17 kg (13% of initial weight) during 60 days of hibernation without a change in LBM. However, when bears are fasted (but not thirsted) in summer, they, like other mammals, lose LBM as well as fat.

When undernourished individuals are induced to gain weight, both LBM and fat increase[90,122,155,171]; the same is true for growing infants and children. There is also an increase in both components when normal adults are deliberately overfed.[150] For such subjects the energy cost of the weight gain averages 8 kcal/g, and 38% of the gain consists of LBM.[153a] Using the factors for LBM and fat reported by Spady et al.,[90] the recorded energy cost is almost exactly that predicted by theory, namely $(0.38 \times 1.78) + (0.62 \times 12) = 8.1$ kcal/g. On the other hand, in patients recovering from anorexia nervosa, 64% of the gain consists of LBM, so the energy cost is less, only 4.7 kcal/g.[153] In experiments involving rather modest degrees of overfeeding, Butterfield and Calloway found that 1 to 2 mg N was retained per kcal of added energy ($\sim$45 mg LBM/kcal).[172]

These data were collected from experiments lasting only a few weeks, the longest being 83 days. With no controlled studies of longer duration in man, the long-term situation is unknown. However, it is known that obese individuals who continue to gain weight accumulate additional lean tissue as well as fat.[78,105a]

The importance of adequate protein intake cannot be overemphasized. While undernourished men can gain weight on low protein diets,[171] some LBM is lost at the same time that body fat is gained. When adequate protein was given to these subjects without a change in energy intake, they gained LBM as well as fat. When Miller and Mumford gave excess food low in protein to normal individuals, they lost LBM as they gained weight, whereas excess food high in protein produced a gain in LBM and a greater total gain per excess calorie consumed.[173] Hence, low-protein diets are inefficient.

**Body Composition in Obesity.** Human obesity can occur only in the face of positive energy balance, and in this sense it is a nutritional disease. Studies of obese children, adolescents, and young adults show that a portion (10 to 30%) of their excess weight consists of LBM, although a few have normal values.[150*] Such data can be interpreted to mean only that most obese individuals

are overnourished. Autopsy data show that the obese have larger hearts, kidneys, and livers.[176] Basal metabolic rate is also increased.[177] However, Shizgal et al. found that the ratio of ECF/Total Body Water was much the same in the obese (average weight 137 kg) and the nonobese (70 kg).[178]

A great deal of attention has been paid to the cellular composition of adipose tissue in recent years. Adipocyte cell size can be determined on biopsy specimens of subcutaneous tissue and at surgery from internal sites. Then total adipocyte cell number is simply cell size per gram adipose tissue times total body fat. While some investigators have suggested that there are two types of obesity—the hypertrophic and the hyperplastic—extensive studies reveal a gradual increase in both cell size and number as total body fat increases. Adipocytes contain about 0.3 µg lipid in thin adults and 1.1 µg in the very obese; cell number averages $2.5 \times 10^{10}$ in the former and $7.5 \times 10^{10}$ in the latter.[75]

**Body Composition in Undernutrition.** Examples to be considered in undernutrition are individuals with more or less chronic energy deficits uncomplicated by significant infection or disease. They usually have normal or only slightly reduced serum protein levels and are not incapacitated.

Patients with anorexia nervosa have thin subcutaneous tissue, small heart volumes, a reduced blood volume, and even some reduction in renal function.[179] There is a reduction in both LBM and body fat.[122,155] The same is true of undernourished male laborers; however, ECF volume is not reduced, and the ratio of ECF/ICF volume is supranormal.[154]

The situation in severe, complicated undernutrition will be described in a section, "Influence of Disease."

## PHYSICAL ACTIVITY

**Exercise.** The phenomenon of work hypertrophy is well known; and this is nicely illustrated by the fact that the dominant arm of professional tennis players has larger muscles and thicker bones. However, the subcutaneous tissue thickness is about the same.[181,182]

Generally speaking, athletes of both sexes have a larger LBM than their nonathletic peers, and many have less body fat.[51,123] The enlarged LBM is particularly true of weight lifters, "body builders," discus throwers, shot putters, and football players. As is the case for others, LBM in athletes is related to stature.[122,183]

The question is whether the larger LBM is the result of training and exercise, or is merely an inherent feature of the athletic individual. A number of studies have been done on individuals who

---

*The situation is quite different in animals rendered obese by experimentally induced hypothalamic lesions, for they tend to have a smaller LBM than controls.[174,175]

have engaged in training and exercise programs of various types and who have presumably not taken androgenic-anabolic steroids. Although these studies show a tendency for LBM to rise and for body fat to fall, the documented changes have not been very great.[183] Wilmore's review of 55 such studies shows that LBM increased more than 1 kg in 22 (maximum 3.1 kg), LBM decreased in 7, and was unchanged in 26.[123] Parizkova studied gymnasts in training for the Olympics.[194] LBM increased by an average of 1.8 kg in the males and 1.2 kg in the females, and there was an equivalent loss of body fat. Once the contests were finished, body composition reverted in time to its pretraining status.

A number of reports describe exercise programs that are not very strenuous and of relatively brief duration, and many of the studies have been conducted on physically active individuals who may already have achieved their maximum LBM. The experiments described by Oscai et al. are of interest in this regard:[185] when rats are forced to swim daily for many weeks (about 20% of their life span) they acquire more LBM and less fat than their paired-weight sedentary controls; skeletal muscle accounts for one-third of the LBM increase. However, that they had less LBM and less fat than the control animals who were fed ad libitum suggests that the strenuous exercise blunted their appetite.

**Immobilization, Space Travel.** The decrease in muscle mass and bone density in immobilized or paralyzed limbs is a well-known phenomenon. Healthy young men placed in plaster spicas from the waist down for several weeks lost some nitrogen, calcium, and phosphorus and had a reduction in blood volume although body weight did not change.[186] Ordinary bed rest also results in negative balance of Ca, K, and P;[187] and these authors found that exercise in the supine position was of no help in this respect. Studies of astronauts have included estimates of LBM. The loss of LBM during the 84-day flight varied according to the method used: 3.4 kg by $^{42}$K dilution, 1.2 kg by densitometry, 2.6 kg by nitrogen balance, and 1.1 kg by total body water. The average is 2.1 kg LBM loss in the face of a 2.8 kg weight loss.[188] Blood volume declined by 10%.[189] The interpretation of these results is difficult because of the occurrence of mild hyponatremia, suggesting a change in body fluid osmolality, the strong positive N balance prior to the flight, and the fact that body weight was rapidly regained on returning to earth. Pitts and co-workers found an 8% drop in the fat-free weight, a drop in total body Ca, and an increase in body fat in rats who had spent 18 days in space.[190] Thus the maintenance of normal body composition is dependent on gravity and normal physical activity as well as muscle innervation.

## INFLUENCE OF HORMONES

Large doses of adrenal corticosteroids act to decrease muscle and bone mass; hence individuals with Cushing's syndrome have subnormal total body K and Ca and an increased Na/K ratio,[191] and total body K increases with treatment. Excessive amounts of parathyroid and thyroid hormones result in negative Ca balance, and the latter in loss of body N as well. On the other hand, administration of progesterone and estrogen causes retention of N,[192] as does administration of growth hormone.[193] Treatment of children with hypopituitarism is associated with an increase in LBM and a decrease in body fat.[194] Individuals with acromegaly have increased body K, N, Na, and Ca,[195] as well as ECF volume.[196] Cattle treated with stilbestrol gain more weight, and the tissue gained contains more lean and less fat than in controls.[197]

Striking effects are produced by the androgenic-anabolic steroids: nitrogen balance becomes positive, and animal studies have shown an increase in amino acid uptake in muscle and an increase in muscle size.[198] Large doses produce a significant increase in LBM and a fall in body fat in man.[199] These effects are apparently perceived by athletes, among whom the use of such steroids is said to be widespread.

It is likely that the sex difference in testosterone production rate (male:female ratio is about 6:1) is responsible in large part for the sex difference in LBM and body fat that develops during normal adolescence. Individuals with Klinefelter's syndrome (XXY karyotype) tend to have a smaller LBM than normal males,[200] possibly the result of lower serum testosterone levels.

Insulin has both anabolic and lipotropic activity, and deficiency of this hormone leads to negative nitrogen balance and fat dissolution. Normal pregnancy is associated with an increase in maternal LBM and fat, changes that are facilitated by the increased levels of testosterone, prolactin, progesterone, estrogen, and insulin that are known to occur.

## INFLUENCE OF DISEASE

Many years ago Cuthbertson showed that severe trauma to the limbs was accompanied by a significant loss of body nitrogen; the negative balance in his patients was as high as 137 g, equivalent to a loss of 4 kg LBM.[201] Earlier, Shaffer and Coleman had found that N losses occurred during the course of typhoid fever and further that the addition of energy in the form of carbohydrate could minimize the N loss in such patients.[202] Beisel et al. recorded significant N losses in other types of infections and showed that these losses exceeded those due to the decreased food intake that often accompanies infection.[203] They also recorded losses of K, Na, P, and Mg in their subjects. It is now common practice to provide extra nutrients—often by the parenteral route—to patients with severe trauma or infection or after major surgical procedures. Another feature of the metabolic response to surgery is an increase in the $Na_e/K_e$ ratio.[104]

Neuromuscular disease has a profound effect. Serial studies of boys with the Duchenne type of muscular dystrophy show a progressive departure from the normal total body K as they get older.[204] Female carriers of this trait are normal in this respect.[205]

There are conflicting reports of individuals with hypertension. Some report no abnormalities in the $Na_e/K_e$ ratio,[206,207] but others find an increase in $Na_e$ and show a relationship between total body Na and the $Na_e/K_e$ ratio and blood pressure.[208]

Individuals with cirrhosis,[209] as well as those with cardiac failure,[104] have an increase in the ratio of Na space to total body water. As expected, individuals with osteoporosis have a reduced total body Ca.[92]

Severe malnutrition is associated with an increase in the ECF/ICF ratio,[210] an increase in the $Na_e/K_e$ ratio,[211,212] an increase in intracellular Na in muscle and a decrease in K.[213] Waterlow and co-workers have reviewed these effects on body water distribution and the decrease in tissue K and Mg,[214] and Garrow et al. confirmed the relative increase in body water and the decrease in body K by carcass analysis.[215] In such states it appears that ECF volume is better preserved than cell mass, the shrunken cells retaining their fluid covering. Picou and co-workers evaluated the relative amounts of collagen and noncollagen protein in the bodies of malnourished infants.[216] Although the latter was reduced to about one half the expected value, the former had not changed significantly. Skin and bone account for about 70% of the total body collagen.

The observations of Picou et al. help to explain the difference in calculated changes in body composition recorded by different techniques.[216] Because tendon has a higher density[217] and a lower K concentration[94] than muscle, an increase in the ratio of collagen to noncollagen protein during weight loss would be expected to increase the density and to decrease the K content of the LBM. Hence the use of standard values for each will result in a slight underestimation of the LBM con-

tribution to the weight loss by densitometry and an overestimation by $^{40}K$ counting. The finding of a smaller contribution of LBM to total weight loss by density than by $^{40}K$ counting during weight reduction by Garrow[88] and during space flight by Leonard et al.[188] is in keeping with this hypothesis. Such inconsistencies serve as a reminder that body composition techniques may not always yield precise results.

## CONCLUSION

Modern techniques for assessing body composition have provided the human biologist with a new set of tools. He is no longer dependent on drawing analogies from the results of animal experiments; indeed, inferences derived from work on animals can now be tested in man; and the biologist is freed from the constraints of the metabolic balance technique in now being able to assess body content at any point in time as well as changes that occur over long periods. To mention one lesson that has been learned, it appears that the lean and fat components of the body are not independent of each other, for a change in one is often accompanied by a change in the other.

A new dimension has been added to the phenomena of growth and aging. One awaits with interest the application of computerized tomography and of nuclear magnetic resonance to the body composition in man.

## REFERENCES

1. Magnus-Levy, A.: Physiologie des Stoffwechsels. *In* Handbuch der Pathologie des Stoffwechsels. (von Noorden, C., Ed.) Berlin, Hirschwald, 1906, p. 446.
2. Voit, E.: Z. Biol. *41*:113–154, 1901.
3. Rubner, M.: Die Gesetze des Energieverbrauchs bei der Ernährung. Leipzig and Vienna, Deutsche, 1902.
4. Keith, N.M., Rowntree, L.G., Gerachty, J.T.: Arch. Intern. Med. *16*:547–576, 1915.
5. von Hevesy, G., Hofer, E.: Klin. Wochenschr. *13*:1524–1526, 1934.
6. Moore, F.D.: Science *104*:157–160, 1946.
7. Behnke, A.R., Jr., Feen, B.G., Welham, S.C.: JAMA *118*:495–498, 1942; Welham, W.C., Behnke, A.R., Jr.: Idem, p. 498.
8. Sievert, R.M.: Arch. Fysik. *3*:337–346, 1951.
9. Forbes, G.B., Gallup, J., Hursh, J.B.: Science *133*:101–102, 1961.
10. Anderson, J., Osborn, S.B., Tomlinson, R.W.S., et al.: Lancet *2*:1201–1205, 1964.
11. Cohn, S.H., Dombrowski, C.S.: J. Nucl. Med. *12*:499–505, 1971.
12. Fomon, S.J., Haschke, F., Ziegler, E.E., et al.: Am. J. Clin. Nutr. *35*:1169–1175, 1982.
13. Hamill, P.V.V., Drizd, T.A., Johnson, C.L., et al.: Am. J. Clin. Nutr. *32*:607–629, 1979.
14. Naeye, R.L., Dixon, J.B.: Pediatr. Res. *12*:987–991, 1978.
15. Metropolitan Life Insurance Co.: 1983.

16. Keys, A., Fidanza, F., Karvonen, M.J., et al.: J. Chronic Dis. *25*:329–343, 1972.
17. Cronk, C.E., Roche, A.F.: Am. J. Clin. Nutr. *35*:351–354, 1982.
18. van Wieringen, J.C.: Secular Changes in Growth. Leiden, Netherlands, Institute of Preventive Medicine, 1972.
19. Rolland-Cachera, M.F., Sempé, M., Guillond-Bataille, M., et al.: Am. J. Clin. Nutr. *36*:178–184, 1982.
20. Khosla, T., Billewicz, W.Z.: Br. J. Nutr. *18*:227–239, 1964.
21. Garn, S.M., Rohmann, C.C.: Pediatr. Clin. North Am. *13*:353–379, 1966.
22. Tanner, J.M., Goldstein, H., Whitehouse, R.H.: Arch. Dis. Child. *45*:755–762, 1970.
23. Wingerd, J., Salomon, I.L., Schoen, E.J.: Pediatrics *52*:555–566, 1973.
24. Foch, T.T., McClearn, G.E.: Genetics, body weight, and obesity. *In* Obesity (Stunkard, A.J., Ed.) Philadelphia, W.B. Saunders, 1980, pp. 48–71.
25. Smith, D.M., Nance, W.E., Kang, K.W., et al.: J. Clin. Invest. *52*:2800–2808, 1973.
26. Brook, C.G.D., Huntley, R.M.C., Slack, J.: Br. Med. J. *2*:719–721, 1975.
27. Biron, P., Mongeau, J.-G., Bertrand, D.: J. Pediatr. *91*:555–558, 1977.
27a.Stunkard, A.J., Sorensen, T.I.A., Hanis, C., et al.: N. Engl. J. Med. *314*:193–198, 1986.
28. Vincent, M., Jans, C., Ghesquiere, J.: Am. J. Phys. Anthropol. *20*:237–247, 1962.
29. Roche, A.F.: Monograph Society for Research in Child Development, Serial No. 179, 1979, p. 120.
30. Borkan, G.A., Hults, D.E., Glynn, R.J.: Hum. Biol. *55*:629–641, 1983.
31. Parizkova, J., Eiselt, E.: Hum. Biol. *52*:803–809, 1980.
32. Cohn, S.H., Vaswani, A.N., Yasumura, S., et al.: Am. J. Clin. Nutr. *40*:255–259, 1984.
33. Kaufman, L., Wilson, C.J.: J. Nucl. Med. *14*:812–815, 1973.
34. Miller, M.E., Cappon, C.J.: Clin. Chem. *30*:781–783, 1984.
35. Schoeller, D.A., Van Sauten, D.W., Dietz, W., et al.: Am. J. Clin. Nutr. *33*:2686–2693, 1980.
36. Price, W.F., Hazelrig, J.B., Kreisberg, R.A., et al.: J. Lab. Clin. Med. *74*:557–563, 1969.
37. Haxhe, J.J.: La Composition Corporelle Normale. Paris, Librairie Maloine S.A., 1963.
38. Greenway, R.M., Littell, A.S., Houser, H.B., et al.: Proc. Soc. Exp. Biol. Med. *120*:487, 1965.
39. Allen, T.H., Peng, M.T., Chen, K.P., et al.: Metabolism *5*:328–345, 1956.
40. Cheek, D.B., West, C.D.: J. Clin. Invest. *34*:1744–1755, 1955.
41. Shizgal, H.M., Spanier, A.H., Humes, J., et al.: Am. J. Physiol. *233*:F253–259, 1977.
42. Cohn, S.H. (Ed.): Non-invasive Measurements of Bone Mass and Their Clinical Application. Boca Raton, FL, CRC Press, 1981.
43. Cohn, S.H.: Med. Phys. *8*:145–154, 1981.
44. Brozek, J., Grande, F., Anderson, T., et al.: Ann. N.Y. Acad. Sci. *110*:113–140, 1963.
45. Lesser, G.T., Deutsch, S., Markofsky, J.: Metabolism *20*:792–804, 1971.
46. Mettau, J.W., Degenhart, H.J., Visser, H.K.A., et al.: Pediatr. Res. *11*:1097–1101, 1977.
47. Brozek, J., Keys, A.: Br. J. Nutr. *5*:194–206, 1951.
48. Pařizková, J.: Body Fat and Physical Fitness. The Hague, Martinus Nijhoff b.v., Publishers, 1977.
49. Steinkamp, R., Cohen, N.L., Gaffry, W.R., et al.: J. Chron. Dis. *18*:1291–1307, 1965.
50. Durnin, J.V.G.A., Womersley, J.: Br. J. Nutr. *32*:77–97, 1974.
51. Behnke, A.R., Wilmore, J.H.: Evaluation and Regulation of Body Build and Composition. Englewood Cliffs, NJ, Prentice-Hall, 1974, pp. 236.
52. Pollock, M.L., Wilmore, J.H., Fox, S.M. III: Exercise in Health and Disease. Philadelphia, W.B. Saunders, 1984.
53. Lohman, T.G.: Hum. Biol. *53*:181–225, 1981.
54. Gurr, M.I., Jung, R.T., Robinson, M.P., et al.: Int. J. Obes. *6*:419–436, 1982.
55. National Center for Health Statistics: DHEW Pub. No. (HRA) 74–614, Series 11, #132, 1974.
56. Johnston, F.E.: Hum. Biol. *54*:221–245, 1982.
57. Slaughter, M.H., Lohman, T.G., Boileau, R.A.: Ann. Hum. Biol. *5*:469–482, 1978.
58. Hume, R.: J. Clin. Pathol. *19*:389–391, 1966.
59. Klish, W.J., Forbes, G.B., Gordon, A., et al.: J. Pediatr. Gastroenterol. Nutr. *3*:349–350, 1984.
60. Presta, E., Wang, J., Harrison, G.G., et al.: Am. J. Clin. Nutr. *37*:735–739, 1983.
61. Hoffer, E.C., Meader, C.K., Simpson, D.C.: J. Appl. Physiol. *27*:531–534, 1969.
61a.Segal, K.R., Gutin, B., Presta, E., et al.: J. Appl. Physiol. *58*:1565–1571, 1985.
62. Tokunaga, K., Matsuzawa, Y., Ishikawa, K., et al.: Int. J. Obes. *7*:437–446, 1983.
63. Shukla, K.K., Ellis, K.J., Dombrowski, C.S., et al.: Am. J. Physiol. *224*:271–274, 1973.
64. Forbes, G.B., Schultz, F., Cafarelli, C., et al.: Health Phys. *15*:435–442, 1968.
65. Johny, K.V., Worthey, B.W., Lawrence, J.R., et al.: Clin. Sci. *39*:319–326, 1970.
66. Davies, D.L., Robertson, J.W.K.: Metabolism *22*:133–137, 1973.
67. James, A.H., Brooks, L., Edelman, I.S., et al.: Metabolism *3*:313–323, 1954.
68. McNeill, K.G., Harrison, J.E.: Partial body neutron activation-truncal. *In* Non-invasive Measurements of Bone Mass and Their Clinical Application. (Cohn, S.H., Ed.) Boca Raton, FL, CRC Press, 1981, pp. 165–190.
69. Nelp, W.B., Denney, J.D., Murano, R., et al.: J. Lab. Clin. Med. *79*:430–438, 1972.
70. Ellis, K.J., Yasumura, S., Vartsky, D., et al.: J. Lab. Clin. Med. *99*:917–926, 1982.
71. Durnin, J.V.G.A., Taylor, A.: J. Appl. Physiol. *15*:142–144, 1960.
72. Archibald, E.H., Harrison, J.E., Pencharz, P.B.: Am. J. Dis. Child. *137*:658–662, 1983.
73. Kyle, L.H., Werdein, E.J., Canary, J.J.: Ann. N.Y. Acad. Sci. *110*:55–61, 1963.
74. Cheek, D.B.: Human Growth. Philadelphia, Lea & Febiger, 1968.
75. Sjöström, L.: Fat cells and body weight. *In* Obesity (Stunkard, A.J., Ed.). Philadelphia, W.B. Saunders, 1980, pp. 86–100.
76. Schutte, J.E., Longhurst, J.C., Gaffney, F.A., et al.: J. Appl. Physiol. *51*:762–766, 1981.
77. Forbes, G.B., Bruining, G.J.: Am. J. Clin. Nutr. *29*:1359–1366, 1976.
78. Forbes, G.B., Brown, M.R.: Unpublished data.
79. Talbot, N.B.: Am. J. Dis. Child. *55*:42, 1938.
80. Lukaski, H.C., Mendez, J., Buskirk, E.R., et al.: Am. J. Physiol. *240*:E302–307, 1981.

81. Pitts, G.C., Bullard, T.R.: Some interspecific aspects of body composition in mammals. *In* Body Composition in Animals and Man. Washington, D.C., National Academy of Science, Pub. #1598, 1968, pp. 45–70.

82. Forbes, G.B.: Pediatrics *29*:477–494, 1962.

83. Moore, F.D., Lister, J., Boyden, C.M., et al.: Hum. Biol. *40*:135–188, 1968.

84. Borkan, G.A., Gerzof, S.G., Robbins, A.H., et al.: Am. J. Clin. Nutr. *36*:172–177, 1982.

85. Maughan, R.J., Watson, J.S., Weir, J.: Clin. Sci. *66*:683–689, 1984.

86. Calloway, D.H., Odell, A.C.F., Margen, S.: J. Nutr. *101*:775–786, 1971.

87. Forbes, G.B.: Am. J. Clin. Nutr. *38*:347–348, 1983.

88. Garrow, J.S.: Treat Obesity Seriously. London, Churchill Livingstone, 1981.

89. Pike, R., Brown, M.: Nutrition: An Integrated Approach. 2nd ed. New York, John Wiley & Sons, 1975.

90. Spady, D.W., Payne, P.R., Picou, D., et al.: Am. J. Clin. Nutr. *29*:1073–1088, 1976.

91. Sheng, H.-P., Huggins, R.A.: Am. J. Clin. Nutr. *32*:630–647, 1979.

92. Ellis, K.J., Cohn, S.H.: J. Appl. Physiol. *38*:455–460, 1975.

93. Cohn, S.H.: Personal communication.

94. Widdowson, E.M., Dickerson, J.W.T.: Chemical composition of the body. *In* Mineral Metabolism (Comar, C.L., Bronner, F., Ed.), Vol. 2, Part A. New York, Academic Press, 1964, pp. 2–247.

95. Krzywicki, H.J., Ward, G.M., Rahman, D.P., et al.: Am. J. Clin. Nutr. *27*:1380–1385, 1974.

96. Cohn, S.H., Vartsky, D., Yasumura, S., et al.: Am. J. Physiol. *239*:E524–530, 1980.

97. Womersley, J., Boddy, K., King, P.C., et al.: Clin. Sci. *43*:469–475, 1972.

98. Womersley, J., Durnin, J.V.G.A., Boddy, K., et al.: J. Appl. Physiol. *41*:223–229, 1976.

99. Halliday, D., Hesp, R., Stalley, S.F., et al.: Int. J. Obes. *3*:1–6, 1979.

100. Morgan, D.B., Burkinshaw, L.: Clin. Sci. *65*:407–414, 1983.

101. Lukaski, H.C., Mendez, J., Buskirk, E.R., et al.: Metabolism *30*:777–782, 1981.

102. Forbes, G.B., Amirhakimi, G.H.: Hum. Biol. *42*:401–418, 1970.

103. Siri, W.E.: Body composition from fluid spaces and density: analysis of methods. *In* Techniques for Measuring Body Composition (Brozek, J., Henschel, A., Eds.). Washington, D.C., National Academy of Sciences, 1961, pp. 223–244.

104. Moore, F.D., Olesin, K.H., McMurray, J.D., et al.: The Body Cell Mass and Its Supporting Environment. Philadelphia, W.B. Saunders, 1963.

105. Cohn, S.H., Vartsky, D., Yasumura, S., et al.: Am. J. Physiol. *244*:E305–E310, 1983.

105a.Forbes, G.B.: Human Body Composition. New York, Springer-Verlag, 1987.

106. Ziegler, E.E., O'Donnell, A.M., Nelson, S.E., et al.: Growth *40*:329–341, 1976.

107. Haschke, F.: Acta Paediatr. Scand. [Suppl.] *307*:1–23, 1983.

108. Borkan, G.A., Norris, A.H.: Hum. Biol. *49*:495–514, 1977.

109. International Committee on Radiation Protection: Report of the Task Group on Reference Man for Purposes of Radiation Protection. Oxford, Pergamon Press, 1975.

110. Burmeister, W., Bingert, A.: Klin. Wochenschr. *45*:409–416, 1967.

111. Forbes, G.B.: Body composition in adolescence. *In* Human Growth: An Advanced Treatise (Falkner, F., Tanner, J., Eds.), Vol. II. New York, Plenum, 1978, pp. 239–272.

112. Forbes, G.B.: Growth *36*:325–338, 1972.

113. Forbes, G.B.: Hum. Biol. *48*:161–173, 1976.

114. Widdowson, E.M.: Nature *166*:626–631, 1950.

115. Brozek, J.: Fed. Proc. *11*:784–793, 1952.

116. Noppa, H., Andersson, M., Bengtsson, C., et al.: Am. J. Clin. Nutr. *32*:1388–1395, 1979.

117. Tanner, J.M., Whitehouse, R.H.: Arch. Dis. Child. *50*:142–145, 1975.

118. Forbes, G.B.: Am. J. Clin. Nutr. *27*:595–602, 1974.

119. Borisov, B.K., Marei, A.N.: Health Phys. *27*:224–229, 1974.

120. Cohn, S.H.: Personal communication.

121. McNeill, K.G., Harrison, J.E.: Partial body neutron activation—truncal. *In* Non-Invasive Measurements of Bone Mass and Their Clinical Application (Cohn, S.H., Ed.). Boca Raton, FL, CRC Press, 1981, pp. 165–190.

122. Forbes, G.B.: Fed. Proc. *44*:343–47, 1985.

123. Wilmore, J.H.: Med. Sci. Sports Exerc. *15*:21–31, 1983.

124. Khosla, T.: Br. Med. J. *4*:111–113, 1968.

125. Pipe, N.G.J., Smith, T., Halliday, D., et al.: Br. J. Obstet. Gynaecol. *86*:929–940, 1979.

126. Hytten, F.E., Leitch, I.: The Physiology of Human Pregnancy. 2nd Ed. Oxford, Blackwell Scientific, 1971.

127. von Dobeln, W.: Acta Physiol. Scand. [Suppl.] *37*:126, 1956.

128. Halliday, D., Hesp, R., Stalley, S.F., et al.: Int. J. Obes. *3*:1–6, 1979.

129. MacMillan, M.G.: Lancet *1*:728–729, 1965.

130. Baker, S.P., Shock, N.W., Norris, A.H.: Influence of age and obesity in women on basal oxygen consumption expressed in terms of total body water and extracellular water. *In* Biological Aspects of Ageing (Shock, N.W., Ed.). New York, Columbia University, 1962.

131. Marshall, A.W., Kingstone, D., Boss, M., et al.: Hepatology *3*:701–706, 1983.

132. Rand, W.M., Young, V.R., Scrimshaw, N.S.: Am. J. Clin. Nutr. *29*:639–644, 1976.

133. Uauy, R., Scrimshaw, N.S., Rand, W.M., et al.: J. Nutr. *108*:97–103, 1978.

134. Huang, P.C., Chong, H.E., Rand, W.M.: J. Nutr. *102*:1605–1614, 1972.

135. Frisch, R.E., Revelle, R., Cook, S.: Hum. Biol. *45*:469–483, 1973.

136. Frisch, R.E., McArthur, J.: Science *185*:949–951, 1974.

137. Scott, E.C., Johnston, F.E.: J. Adolesc. Health Care *2*:249–260, 1982.

138. Loucks, A.B., Horvath, S.M., Freedson, P.S.: Hum. Biol. *56*:383–392, 1984.

139. Forbes, G.B., Drenick, E.J.: Am. J. Clin. Nutr. *32*:1570–1574, 1979.

140. Keys, A., Brozek, J., Heuschel, A., et al.: The Biology of Human Starvation. Minneapolis, University of Minnesota, 1950.

141. Young, C.M., Scanlon, S.S., Im, H.S., et al.: Am. J. Clin. Nutr. *24*:290–296, 1971.

142. Young, C.M., DiGiacomo, M.M.: Metabolism *14*:1084–1094, 1965.

143. Woo, R., Garrow, J.S., Pi-Sunyer, F.X.: Am. J. Clin. Nutr. *36*:478–484, 1982.

144. Drenick, E.J., Swendseid, M.E., Blahd, W.H., et al.: JAMA *187*:100–105, 1964.

145. Benedict, F.G.: A Study of Prolonged Fasting. Washington, D.C., Carnegie Institute of Washington, 1915.

146. Forbes, G.B.: Am. J. Clin. Nutr. *23*:1212–1219, 1970.

147. Benedict, F.G., Miles, W.R., Roth, P., et al.: Human Vitality and Efficiency under Prolonged Restricted Diet. Washington, D.C., Carnegie Institute of Washington, 1919, p. 701.

148. Phinney, S.D., Horton, E.S., Sims, E.A.H., et al.: J. Clin. Invest. *66*:1152–1161, 1980.

149. Brown, M.R., Klish, W.J., Hollander, J., et al.: Am. J. Clin. Nutr. *38*:20–31, 1983.

150. Forbes, G.B., Welle, S.L.: Int. J. Obes. *7*:99–108, 1983.

151. Forbes, G.B.: Am. J. Clin. Nutr. *39*:349–350, 1984.

152. Reichman, B., Cheessex, P., Putet, G., et al.: N. Engl. J. Med. J. Med. *305*:1495–1500, 1981.

153. Forbes, G.B., Kreipe, R.E., Lipinski, B.: Hum. Nutr.: Clin. Nutr. *36C*:485–487, 1982.

153a. Forbes, G.B., Brown, M.R., Welle, S.L., et al.: Br. J. Nutr. *56*:1–9, 1986.

154. Barac-Nieto, M., Spurr, G.B., Lotero, H., et al.: Am. J. Clin. Nutr. *31*:23–40, 1978.

155. Russell, D.McR., Prendergast, P.J., Darby, P.L., et al.: Am. J. Clin. Nutr. *38*:229–237, 1983.

156. Keys, A., Brozek, J.: Physiol. Rev. *33*:245–345, 1953.

157. Durrant, M.L., Garrow, J.S., Royston, P., et al.: Br. J. Nutr. *44*:275–286, 1980.

158. Fisler, J.S., Drenick, E.J., Blumfield, D.E., et al.: Am. J. Clin. Nutr. *35*:471–486, 1982.

159. Isner, J.M., Sours, H.E., Paris, A.L., et al.: Circulation *60*:1401–1412, 1979.

160. Young, V.R., Garza, C., Steinke, F.H., et al.: Am. J. Clin. Nutr. *39*:8–15, 1984.

161. Garrel, D.R., Todd, K.S., Calloway, D.H.: Am. J. Clin. Nutr. *39*:716–721, 1984.

162. Calloway, D.H., Spector, H.: Am. J. Clin. Nutr. *2*:405–412, 1954.

163. Bistrian, B.R., Winterer, J., Blackburn, G.L., et al.: J. Lab. Clin. Med. *89*:1030–1035, 1977.

164. Owen, O.E., Felig, G., Morgan, A.P., et al.: J. Clin. Invest. *48*:574–583, 1969.

165. Scott, H.W., Jr., Brill, A.B., Price, R.R.: Ann. Surg. *182*:395–404, 1975.

166. Spanier, A.H., Kurtz, R.S., Shibata, H.R., et al.: Surgery *80*:171–177, 1976.

167. Kral, J.G., Bjorntorp, P., Schersten, T., et al.: Eur. J. Clin. Invest. *7*:413–419, 1977.

168. Forbes, G.B.: Unpublished data.

169. Nelson, R.A., Jones, J.D., Wahner, H.W., et al.: Mayo Clin. Proc. *50*:141–146, 1975.

170. Odum, E.P., Connell, C.E.: Science *123*:892–894, 1956.

171. Barac-Nieto, M., Spurr, G.B., Lotero, H., et al.: Am. J. Clin. Nutr. *32*:981–991, 1979.

172. Butterfield, G.E., Calloway, D.H.: Br. J. Nutr. *51*:171–184, 1984.

173. Miller, D.S., Mumford, P.: Am. J. Clin. Nutr. *20*:1212–1222, 1223–1229, 1967.

174. Han, P.-W., Lin, C.-H., Chu, K.-C., et al.: Am. J. Physiol. *209*:627–631, 1965.

175. Goldman, J.K., Bernardis, L.L., Frohman, L.A.: Am. J. Physiol. *227*:88–91, 1974.

176. Naeye, R.L., Roode, P.: Am. J. Clin. Pathol. *54*:251–253, 1970.

177. James, W.P.T., Bailes, J., Davies, H.L., et al.: Lancet *1*:1122–1125, 1978.

178. Shizgal. H.M., Forse, R.A., Spanier, A.H., et al.: Surgery *86*:60–68, 1979.

179. Fohlin, L.: Acta Paediatr. Scand. [Suppl.] 268, 1977.

180. Jones, H.H., Priest, J.D., Hayes, W.C., Nagel, D.A.: J. Bone Joint Surg. *59A*:204–208, 1977.

181. Buskirk, E.R., Anderson, K.L., Brozek, J.: Res. Quart. *27*:127–131, 1956.

182. Gwinup, G., Chelvam, R., Steinberg, T.: Ann. Intern. Med. *74*:408–411, 1971.

183. Forbes, G.B.: Some influences on lean body mass: exercise, androgens, pregnancy, and food. *In* Diet and Exercise: Synergism in Health Maintenance (White, P.L., Mondeika, T., Eds). Chicago, A.M.A., 1982, pp. 75–91.

184. Parizkova, J.: Ann. N.Y. Acad. Sci. *110*:661–674, 1963.

185. Oscai, L.B., Mole, P.A., Krusack, L.M., Halloszy, J.O.: J. Nutr. *103*:412–418, 1973.

186. Deitrick, J.E., Whedon, G.D., Shorr, E.: Am. J. Med. *4*:3–36, 1948.

187. Greenleaf, J.E., Bernauer, E.M., Juhos, L.T., et al.: J. Appl. Physiol. *43*:126–132, 1977.

188. Leonard, J.I., Leach, C.S., Rambaut, P.C.: Am. J. Clin. Nutr. *38*:667–679, 1983.

189. Rambaut, P.C., Smith, M.C., Jr., Leach, C.S., et al.: Fed. Proc. *36*:1678–1682, 1977.

190. Pitts, G.C., Ushakov, A.S., Pace, N., et al.: Am. J. Physiol. *244*:R332–R337, 1983.

191. Aloia, J.F., Roginsky, M., Ellis, K., et al.: J. Clin. Endocrinol. Metab. *39*:981–985, 1974.

192. Landau, R.L.: The metabolic effects of anabolic steroids in man. In Anabolic-Androgenic Steroids (R.O. Greep, Ed.); Handbook of Physiology. Washington, D.C., Am. Physiological Society, pp. 573–589, 1973.

193. Ikkos, D., Luft, R., Gemzell, C.A.: Acta Endocrinol. (Kbh) *32*:341–361, 1959.

194. Collipp, P.J., Curti, V., Thomas, J., et al.: Metabolism *22*:589–595, 1973.

195. Aloia, J.F., Roginsky, M.S., Jowsey, Jr., et al.: J. Clin. Endocrinol. Metab. *35*:543–551, 1972.

196. Ikkos, D., Luft, R., Gemzell, C.A.: J. Clin. Invest. *33*:989–994, 1954.

197. Trenkle, A., Willham, R.L.: Science *198*:1009–1015, 1977.

198. Kochakian, C.D. (Ed.): Anabolic-Androgenic Steroids. New York, Springer-Verlag, 1976.

199. Forbes, G.B.: Metabolism, *34*:571–73, 1985.

200. East, B.W., Boddy, K., Price, W.H.: Clin. Endocrinol. *5*:43–52, 1976.

201. Cuthbertson, D.P.: Q.J. Med. N.S. *1*:233–246, 1932.

202. Shaffer, P.A., Coleman, W.: Arch. Intern. Med. *4*:538–600, 1909.

203. Beisel, W.R., Sawyer, W.D., Ryll, E.D., Crozier, D.: Ann. Intern. Med. *67*:744–779, 1967.

204. Griggs, R.C., Forbes, G.B., Moxley, R.T., Herr, B.E.: Neurology *33*:158–165, 1983.

205. Borgstedt, A., Forbes, G.B., Reina, J.C.: Neuropädiatrie *1*:447–451, 1970.

206. Rajagopalan, B., Thomas, G.W., Beilin, L.J., Ledingham, J.G.G.: Clin. Sci. *59*(Suppl. 6):427s–429s, 1980.

207. Hollander, W., Chobanian, A.V., Burrows, B.G.: J. Clin. Invest. *40*:408, 416, 1961.

208. Beretta-Piccali, C., Davies, D.L., Boddy, K., et al.: Clin. Sci. *63*:257–270, 1982.
209. Gilder, H., Redo, S.F., Barr, D., Child, C.G., III: J. Clin. Invest. *33*:555–564, 1954.
210. McConkey, B.: Clin. Sci. *18*:95–102, 1959.
211. Shizgal, H.M.: Surg. Gynecol. Obstet. *152*:22–26, 1981.
212. Moore, F.D., Edelman, I.S., Olney, J.M., et al.: Metabolism *3*:334–350, 1954.
213. Metcoff, J., Frenk, S., Antonowicz, I., et al.: Pediatrics *26*:960–972, 1960.
214. Waterlow, J.C., Cravioto, J., Stephen, J.M.L.: Protein Chem. *15*:163–238, 1960.
215. Garrow, J.S., Fletcher, K. Halliday, D.: J. Clin. Invest. *44*:417–425, 1965.
216. Picou, D., Halliday, D., Garrow, J.S.: Clin. Sci. *30*:345–351, 1966.
217. Allen, T.H., Krzywicki, H.J., Roberts, J.E.: J. Appl. Physiol. *14*:1005–1008, 1959.

## SELECTED READINGS

Brozek, J., Henschel, A.: Techniques for Measuring Body Composition. Washington, D.C., NAS-NRC, 1961.

Cheek, D.B.: Human Growth. Philadelphia, Lea & Febiger, 1968.

Cohn, S.H.: Measurement of total body calcium, sodium, chlorine, nitrogen and phosphorus in man by in vivo neutron activation analysis. Med. Phys. *8*:145–154, 1981.

Cohn, S.H. (Ed.): Non-invasive Measurements of Bone Mass and Their Clinical Application. Boca Raton, FL, CRC Press, 1981.

Forbes, G.B.: Human Body Composition. New York, Springer-Verlag, 1987.

Keys, A., Brozek, J.: Body fat in adult man. Physiol. Rev. *33*:245–345, 1953.

Moore, F.D., Olesin, K.H., McMurray, J.D., et al.: The Body Cell Mass and Its Supporting Environment. Philadelphia, W.B. Saunders, 1963.

Parizkova, J.: Body Fat and Physical Fitness. The Hague, Martinus Nijhoff b.v., 1977.

Whipple, H.E., Silverzweig, S., Brozek, J. (Eds): Body Composition. Ann. N.Y. Acad. Sci. *110*:1–1018, 1963.

Widdowson, E.M., Dickerson, J.W.T.: Chemical composition of the body. *In* Mineral Metabolism (Comar, C.L., Bronner, F., Eds.), Vol. 2, Part A. New York, Academic Press, 1964, p. 2–247.

*Chapter* **30**

# METABOLIC REGULATION OF FOOD INTAKE

## G. Harvey Anderson

The initiation and termination of feeding are complex processes that involve a large number of signals to the central nervous system (Fig. 30–1). In man, cultural and social conventions are significant modifiers of the impact of metabolic and physiologic signals. However, the focus of this chapter is restricted to the metabolic and physiologic cues that arise from the perception, ingestion, digestion, absorption, or metabolism of food and nutrients. The brain serves as the organizer and integrator of these signals with the goal of balancing output and storage of nutrients and energy with input (food intake). The purpose of this chapter is to illustrate the role of metabolism in mechanisms regulating food intake and to show that, in the past twenty years, concepts have changed with respect to the relevant metabolic signals and mechanisms.

Because the earlier theories of the regulation of total food intake and energy balance centered on the metabolism of glucose, fat, and amino acids, these theories and current views of their application will be examined first. Then the following sections will describe two relatively recent advances in our understanding of appetite regulation. First, it is now realized that regulation of food intake involves not only the quantitative or energy content of food but also its composition. Therefore, evidence for the regulation of nutrient intake and of food selection, with specific reference to the control of fat, protein, and carbohydrate will be examined.

A second important recent advance has occurred from development in the understanding of brain neurotransmitters and their function. Therefore, in the final sections of this chapter current views of the involvement of brain centers and the role of brain neurotransmitters in control pathways determining energy balance and food selection are described.

## REGULATION OF TOTAL FOOD INTAKE AND ENERGY BALANCE: METABOLIC REGULATORS

Historically, the focus of research on the regulation of energy intake has been motivated by ob-

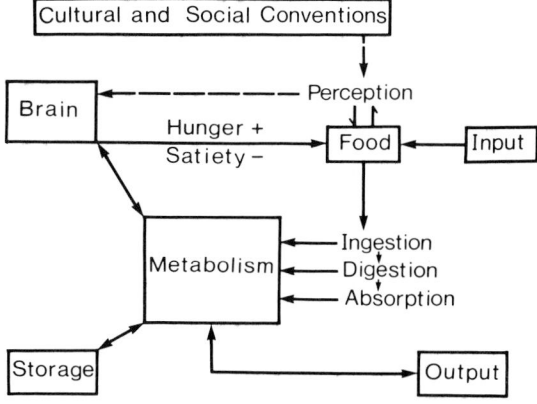

**Fig. 30–1.** An overview of sources of signals used by the brain in the regulation of body energy intake, output, and storage.

servations on the physiologic constancy of adult body weight and concern with deviations from this that occur in obesity and anorexia nervosa in the human.[1] It is clear that when energy requirements are changed, food intake is rapidly and appropriately adjusted. For example, both cold exposure[2] and exercise[3] bring about a quantitative increase in food intake of rats. Also, after food deprivation, rats show compensatory overeating during the first few days of refeeding.[4] Thus, maintenance of energy balance appears to be a primary goal of the mechanism controlling feeding behavior.[5,6] It should not be surprising, therefore, that considerable scientific inquiry has been dedicated to elucidating the feeding control mechanisms regulating this easily defined motivation for feeding.

Because metabolic energy is ultimately derived from the three macronutrients—carbohydrate, fat, and protein—each has been investigated for a putative role in control mechanisms. Each of these nutrients, in addition to providing energy, has other properties that may also provide signals to the central nervous system.

### Glucose

The enthusiasm for glucose as a primary metabolic substrate regulating food intake is related to its role as a ready source of cellular energy. Glucose is readily converted to energy (ATP), $CO_2$, and $H_2O$ in all cells of the body. Not all cells require glucose as the energy substrate, but the brain and presumably the appetite regulatory centers are dependent on glucose under normal day-to-day conditions of feeding. Thus, fluctuations in blood glucose levels, seen as an indication of availability of glucose to nervous tissue and glucose utilization by brain cells, have been suggested as primary signals leading to regulation of food intake. This is known as the glucostatic theory of food intake.

The role of blood glucose concentration in providing signals either indirectly or directly to the brain is uncertain, however. While it has been reported that a 7% decrease in blood glucose concentration occurs prior to the initiation of meals in the rat,[7] and that with food consumption, blood glucose increases,[8] it is also clear that hypoglycemia does not consistently elicit eating. For example, infusion of fructose, a sugar that does not cross the blood-brain barrier,[9] to insulin-treated rats terminated feeding despite the presence of hypoglycemia.[10] This observation suggests that feeding after insulin treatments may not be purely a consequence of hypoglycemia but due to other effects of insulin. These effects may include a reduction in the concentration of plasma free fatty

acids, ketone bodies, and amino acids, any one of which may influence, directly or indirectly, signals to the brain.[11] Conversely, hyperglycemia does not necessarily suppress feeding. Intravenous infusion of glucose sufficient to raise blood glucose by a constant 20 to 30 mg/dl did not affect either frequency of eating or the amount consumed by rats.[12]

Uncertainty with respect to the role of blood glucose concentrations in controlling feeding probably arises from the fact that blood concentration does not necessarily indicate the rate of glucose utilization by tissues. Therefore, it is encouraging for the subscribers to the glucostatic hypothesis of feeding to find that glucose utilization in brain cells appears to be more closely related to feeding. A high rate of cellular glucose utilization after a meal corresponds with a state of satiation in animals,[13] but the converse is associated with eating.[14]

In addition to energy utilization by brain cells serving as an indicator of glucose availability, it has been proposed that glucose in the liver influences glucoreceptors, which provide signals to the brain via the vagus nerve.[15] This would explain the observation that blocking of glucose utilization in the liver by infusion of 2-deoxy-D-glucose, an antimetabolite of glucose, into the portal vein of rabbits, elicits eating. Systemic infusions are much less effective.[16] Further evidence that there is a relationship between the liver's metabolism of glucose and satiety has been provided from studies of the effects of hepatic-portal glucose functions. A decrease in food intake after glucose infusion into the portal vein occurs in food deprived but not fed rabbits,[16] suggesting that liver energy reserve (glycogen) modifies the sensitivity of the hepatic glucoreceptors.

A link between glucoreceptors in the liver and the brain's control of feeding probably involves messages transmitted via the vagus nerve. Subdiaphragmatic vagotomy blocks suppression of food intake caused by duodenal glucose infusion.[17] The dependence of long-term energy balance or even meal size on hepatic glucoreceptors seems unlikely, however, because denervation of liver in dogs and rats does not affect food consumption.[18] Thus, while glucose concentrations in plasma and tissues and glucose utilization appear to influence feeding under certain conditions, it is also clear that glucose metabolism does not offer as much of an explanation of the mechanisms for regulation of food intake as originally expected.[19]

### Lipid

The lipostatic theory for regulation of food intake is based on the observation that depot fat in animals serves as an energy reservoir, suggesting that variations in total energy storage (adiposity) should provide signals that cause animals to alter their energy intake.[20] Whether there is any direct link, neural or otherwise, between body fat stores and the feeding control mechanism in the brain has not been established. Similarly, the significance of fat mass and its regulation is uncertain because it is clear that obese animals consume excess food.[21] It is probable, however, that circulating substrates derived from fat metabolism influence food consumption.

The mobilization of body fat, with the release of free fatty acids and glycerol and the interaction with glucose metabolism, provides a possible explanation of circadian fluctuation of food intake in the rat, as well some evidence of a link between brain function and lipid metabolism. On a day-to-day basis, lipid metabolism is synchronized with the circadian fluctuation in food intake and appears to be under the influence of the ventromedial hypothalamus (VMH), a brain region involved in feeding control and frequently called the "satiety" center.[22] Stimulation of the VMH enhanced lipolysis in white adipose tissue,[23,24] which in turn was associated with decreased feeding. Furthermore, electrical activity in the VMH, but not in the lateral hypothalamus (the "feeding" center) of rats, is enhanced during the light period when they do not eat and when lipolysis is occurring, but is suppressed during the dark hours when they do eat.[25] Consistent with the link between lipid metabolism and feeding is the observation that a daytime feeding pattern can be induced during the dark hours by stimulating lipid breakdown with adrenaline infusion.[26] Conversely, if lipid synthesis is stimulated during the light period by insulin infusions, rats develop hyperphagia and increase meal frequency similar to that normally observed at night.[27]

Mobilization of body fat during the light hours has been suggested as the reason that rats ingest only two or three meals, representing less than 25% of their daily intake, throughout the light period of a 24-hour light-dark cycle.[28] Those investigators who emphasize a role for glucose in the initiation and termination of feeding suggest that the expected initiation of a meal by a fall in blood glucose is delayed during the light portion of the day because there is an endogenous supply of energy from lipolysis.[29] In contrast, during the dark hours, the rat's insulin response to a glucose load is enhanced, as is lipogenesis and glucose utilization. This increase results in a rapid fall in blood glucose after each eating episode, reduced levels of substrates from fat breakdown, and more meals initiated at night. In this way it is proposed

that metabolism of glucose and lipid interact in signaling the brain's regulation of feeding.[22,29] Clearly, however, neither body lipid stores nor plasma lipid content independently controls feeding behavior.

No readily apparent product of lipid metabolism can be used to explain feeding behavior.[23,30,31] Plasma levels of the products of lipid metabolism, including free fatty acids, glycerol, triglycerides, and ketone bodies (β-hydroxybutyrate, acetoacetate) fluctuate with feeding and fasting. During and immediately after a meal triglycerides predominate and are the primary vehicle of transport of fat from the gut and liver to adipose tissue. Because of concurrent insulin release, concentrations of free fatty acids, glycerol, and ketone bodies are very low. Gradually, however, as availability of the products of digestion is depleted, adipose tissue switches from taking up fat to releasing it. This release results in an increase in plasma free fatty acids, glycerol, and ketone bodies. As pointed out earlier, it is thought that in the rat the presence of these energy substrates reduces frequency of eating during the day.[22] Similarly, it has been proposed that the loss of acute hunger associated with fasting or very restricted food intake of greater than two or three days in man is specifically due to the presence of ketone bodies in plasma.[30] Advocates of the lipostatic theory have also suggested that an increase in plasma free fatty acids, such as that which occurs when adipose tissue is mobilized, signals that food consumption should begin.[31] This hypothesis obviously contradicts the view that the presence of free fatty acids explains the rat's lack of eating during the light hours.

Possibly the mechanism of fat storage and mobilization is in itself a signal to the brain, although, as pointed out earlier, a direct link has not been found between adipose tissue and the brain. The activity of adipose tissue lipoprotein lipase (LPL), the enzyme that breaks down triglycerides for ultimate storage in adipose tissue, appears to correlate with food intake. For example, ovariectomy, which decreases LPL activity, decreases fat storage and food intake.[32] Because an increase in LPL activity precedes the increased food intake in genetically obese rats, the possibility exists that capacity for fuel storage has some effect on food consumption.[33] Overall, however, one can conclude only that the roles of fat metabolites, fat stores, and fat synthesis as components of food intake control mechanisms merit considerable further investigation.

### Amino Acids

Amino acids, like fat and glucose, provide energy to body cells. In addition, however, their primary role is in the formation of body proteins and in the provision of substrates for the synthesis of several important regulators of metabolism, including creatine, carnitine, polyamines, purine, pyrimidine, and neurotransmitters. Studies of the role of amino acids in regulating feeding behavior illustrate clearly that the production of energy is not the only aspect of macronutrient metabolism significant to appetite control.

The concept that plasma amino acids influence feeding behavior was introduced in the early 1950s.[34] Mellinkoff et al. observed an inverse relationship between concentration of serum amino acid and appetite in man, and proposed that the brain is sensitive to amino acids through mechanisms independent of their energy-producing property.[34] This postulate is known as the aminostatic theory of feeding control. In the following years, considerable work has been undertaken to identify the shifts in plasma and brain amino acids that may influence the brain's regulation of feeding.

High protein or imbalanced diets inhibit food intake in association with shifts in the plasma[35] and brain[36] amino acid patterns in rats. For example, rats fed high protein diets display a marked and sustained increase in plasma branched-chain amino acids,[37,38] which may be of significance to appetite control. Branched-chain amino acids could influence feeding behavior, either directly due to their elevation in brain-free amino acid pools or indirectly by blocking brain uptake of other large neutral amino acids that share a common system for uptake across the blood-brain barrier.[39] As will be seen later, some of the amino acids occurring in decreased concentrations in the brain serve as precursors for the synthesis of neurotransmitters involved in control mechanisms of feeding.[39] Thus, amino acid deficits may signal the brain through their effect on neurotransmitter synthesis,[40] but this is not necessarily the only mechanism by which appetite regulating centers are signaled by amino acids, as is illustrated by the effect of feeding imbalanced diets.

The decreased feeding induced by imbalanced diets appears to be due to decreased availability of a growth-limiting amino acid to the brain rather than to excesses of amino acids.[41] Imbalanced diets are created by adding to a low protein diet, usually 6% casein, an equal quantity of an amino acid mixture that does not contain one of the essential amino acids.[35] Feeding activity can be restored if the supply of the growth-limiting amino acid is increased by injecting it into the carotid artery. In contrast, the same quantity of amino acid injected into the jugular vein, and hence distrib-

uted to other tissues as well as to the brain, has no effect on food intake.[41]

Depression of food intake also occurs in response to individual amino acids. Most of the studies have been conducted with individual amino acids added in excess (1 to 10% of the diet) to a low-protein diet fed to rats.[35] However, there is now an indication that relatively small amounts of amino acids affect feeding behavior in man and experimental animals. For example, in man a mixture of four amino acids (phenylalanine 3 g; valine 2 g; methionine, 2 g; tryptophan 1 g) taken by overweight subjects one-half hour before a midday meal reduced their food intake by 22.5%.[42] Tryptophan alone, in amounts of 2 or 3 g also reduced lunchtime intake of normal weight young men and women.[43] Very small quantities of tryptophan (15 mg added to a 1-g meal of carbohydrate) fed to rats affected their food selection in a subsequent meal.[44] Similarly, tyrosine, fed by intubation to a slow-growing strain of chickens, caused an increased food intake in a subsequent meal.[45]

Brain regions sensitive to alterations in plasma amino acid patterns or concentrations appear to lie outside the hypothalamus, the center traditionally recognized in the regulation of food intake. Lesions of the VMH have little effect on the food intake depression observed following consumption of imbalanced diets.[46] Rather, it appears that the amygdala and prepyriform cortex may be involved in mediating the response to diets imbalanced and deficient in amino acids. Rats with lesions of the prepyriform cortex do not decrease their intake of imbalanced or deficient diets, whereas rats with lesions of the amygdala failed to respond to imbalanced diets.[41] These are not the only brain regions sensitive to plasma amino acids, however, since both groups showed depressed food intake after consumption of high protein diets.

In summary, a variety of mechanisms based on glucostatic, lipostatic, or aminostatic signals have been proposed as the metabolic basis for regulation of energy intake. Animals, however, can regulate energy balance on diets of widely differing macronutrient content and density if the conditions are such that protein and other nutrient requirements can be met. For example, animals fed high protein diets will initially show a food intake depression, but will quickly increase their metabolic capacity to catabolize amino acids, and as a result food intake returns to normal.[35,39] Hence, it would seem that the ingestion of sufficient food to achieve energy balance is a priority within appetite regulatory systems and that the system must be able to detect total energy flow and storage. It is reasonable, therefore, to ask why metabolites derived from each of the macronutrients appear to be involved in control mechanisms regulating food intake, but yet can be so easily ignored in the achievement of energy balance. An answer to this question may be found in the fact that animals have the ability to regulate quality in addition to quantity of food intake.

## REGULATION OF NUTRIENT INTAKE AND FOOD SELECTION

Animals survive and reproduce in a variety of nutritional environments. This fact suggests that they are able to choose from their environment foods that maximize their chance of survival by being adequate in essential nutrients and free of poisonous or harmful substances. It is clear that animals have adapted to their environments by a variety of anatomic and physiologic developments, so that, for example, some animals are principally herbivores and others carnivores. In addition, food selection is consistent with good nutritional health, suggesting that mechanisms have been developed to link internal metabolic processes to need and to consequences of eating.[47]

Despite the situation existing in nature, most scientists have chosen to feed their test animals diets of fixed composition. Thus, most of the literature on appetite regulation is comprised of reports describing whether the animal eats the one diet chosen by the investigators. Because only one diet is fed, it is easy to translate the feeding response into one indicating that the role of control mechanisms relates solely to the goal of achieving energy balance.

Yet, the early literature has also provided a clear indication of nutrient-specific appetites in animals. In 1918, Osborne and Mendel observed that rats ate little of a protein-free diet when also provided an 18% casein diet.[48] They wrote, "It is therefore interesting to have this evidence that the desire of a young animal for food is something more than a satisfaction of its caloric needs."

The concept of nutrient-specific appetites was more extensively investigated in the 1940s. Curt Richter demonstrated that rats offered a wide choice of foods survived and grew as well as rats fed a standard laboratory chow.[49] He suggested that rats were able to maintain relatively constant daily intakes of most nutrients by adjusting their food choices according to nutrient requirements and nutrient availability.

### Specific Appetites for Vitamins and Minerals

For some vitamins and minerals, specific appetites have been illustrated in a food choice situation and under circumstances where nutrient deficiencies or abnormal metabolisms occur. One of the best known examples of this is presented by adrenalectomized rats. These animals experience high sodium loss but compensate for deficits in body sodium by choosing to drink a salt solution rather than water.[50] Similarly, rats that are parathyroidectomized and unable to maintain plasma calcium levels by mobilization of stores show a preference for a dietary source of calcium.[51]

Vitamin deficiencies also can be detected and appropriate diets chosen, as illustrated in the case of thiamin. Thiamin-deficient rats quickly learn to detect a thiamin-containing diet and ignore the deficient one. If the rats have been maintained on a thiamin adequate diet, however, they do not illustrate a strong preference.[52] Although these examples illustrate that specific appetites for vitamins and minerals can be demonstrated under certain conditions of metabolic deficiencies, they do not show that there is a quantitative regulation of micronutrient intake. That is, the fact that animals fed deficient diets make appropriate choices, perhaps on the basis of gross metabolic disturbances, and learn to choose a food that alleviates the disturbances does not necessarily indicate that in normal rats metabolism guides their choice.

To date the best demonstration of a quantitative regulation of a micronutrient intake by well-nourished, healthy rats is that for phosphorus.[53,54] When given a choice of high and low phosphorus diets, growing or adult rats selected a remarkably constant 0.23 to 0.24% or 0.64 to 0.69%, respectively, of their diet as phosphorus.[54] Why phosphorus should be so precisely regulated on a day-to-day basis, whereas calcium is not, is presently unexplained. Whether intake of other micronutrients can be regulated in accordance with physiologic needs remains to be determined.

In contrast to current information on regulation of micronutrient intake, the better defined regulation of macronutrient consumption has offered some direction toward a definition of metabolically based control mechanisms regulating food intake. In particular, the fact that the animal is able to regulate intakes of protein, carbohydrate, or fat if offered dietary choices shows the benefit of metabolic signals arising from each of these food constituents.

### Regulation of Macronutrient Intake

Despite earlier investigations, the presence of macronutrient-specific appetites was not clearly established until the past decade. The early efforts by Richter[49] and others[55] were likely confounded because of the then existing lack of knowledge of the nutrient needs of the rat. As a result, although the rats were given food choices, the dietary circumstances were often such that it was impossible for the rat to obtain a nutritionally complete diet. It would be predicted then that metabolic signals arising in the brain from the micronutrient deficiencies would not allow the rat to provide the investigators with evidence for macronutrient-specific appetites. In the past ten years, however, macronutrient-specific appetites have been reinvestigated, and their presence has been firmly established.

**Protein Intake.** As pointed out earlier, the concept for regulation of protein intake is not new, and the first investigation of the rat's ability to regulate this component of the diet can be dated back to 1918.[48] Since then, studies designed to examine this aspect of regulation of food intake have used the approach of allowing the rats an opportunity to select for protein as well as for energy.[39] As a result, evidence has emerged showing that protein intake is regulated not only on a day-to-day basis,[56] but also within the day,[28] and even within a meal.[44,57]

A systematic investigation of the rat's ability to regulate protein intake on a day-to-day basis was reported in 1974 by Musten et al.[56] In their studies, young rats were simultaneously presented with two diets differing only in protein and carbohydrate content. One diet was low in protein and high in carbohydrate, whereas the other was high in protein and low in carbohydrate. By substituting carbohydrate for protein (or vice versa) the diets formed were kept isocaloric. Both diets were complete with respect to vitamins and minerals and contained identical nutrient to energy ratios because the fat content of both diets was the same.

From a number of dietary choices (e.g., 0 and 50%, 15 and 55%, 25 and 65% protein), rats regulated their protein intake at a constant proportion of their food consumed, averaging 33 to 35% of the dietary energy. Furthermore, this regulation was almost as precise as the regulation of total energy intake.[56] Other studies have shown that a constant energy density of the diets is not essential, since the rat seeks a constant protein intake under a variety of circumstances. When diets containing the protein sources were diluted with noncaloric materials such as water or agar, methyl cellulose and water, or nonnutritive fiber, both adult and weanling rats compensated by adjusting their intake of the protein-containing diet so that protein consumption remained relatively constant.[58]

Since the amount of protein selected is usually at or above the required level of 13 to 15% of dietary energy,[59] the existence of a protein intake regulatory mechanism in the rat might serve to ensure an intake of protein adequate to provide for its needs. In general, the quantity of protein consumed is a characteristic of the particular protein fed and the animal's usual intake.[58,59] By adding certain amino acids to the protein, the quantity consumed can be manipulated while energy intake remains unaffected. For example, adding lysine to gluten, tryptophan to casein and to zein, or methionine to casein causes the rat to select a lower proportion of food energy as protein, but energy intake is usually unaffected.[60,61] Whether this decrease in protein intake caused by amino acid additions is due to an improvement of protein quality or is the specific effect of the amino acids added awaits future investigation.

A dissociation between the control mechanisms that regulate protein and energy intake also occurs. When adjustment in energy intake is necessary, the rat's protein intake is usually unaffected. For example, animals selectively increase their energy intake while maintaining a constant intake of protein when their energy requirement is increased by either cold exposure[56] or increased activity.[3] Similarly, hyperphagia in rats with lesions of the ventromedial hypothalamus and in the genetically obese Zucker rats is characterized by overconsumption of total food energy as carbohydrate and fat, whereas protein intake is similar to that of appropriate control animals.[62] Although these findings indicate a functional separation of the controls of protein and energy intake, it is reasonable to assume that both mechanisms must interact to determine food intake.

An ability to quantitatively regulate protein intake has been demonstrated for species other than the rat, including mice,[63] dogs,[64] and chickens.[65] Furthermore, a protein intake regulatory mechanism might exist in humans. Whenever a diverse and adequate food supply is available, humans consume 14 to 16% of the dietary calories as protein, even though food varies in protein concentration from 0 to 96%, and the proportions of fat and carbohydrate calories consumed vary widely.[66] More direct evidence comes from a recent study of the dietary patterns of monozygotic versus dizygotic twins. Dietary records obtained from each of twin pairs raised in separate home environments showed that dietary protein concentration selected by monozygotic identical twin pairs was similar. In contrast, the diets of dizygotic twins raised in different home environments were quite dissimilar, suggesting that a primitive, genetically determined control mechanism may underlie protein intake in humans.[67]

Protein intake by the rat is regulated not only on a day-to-day but also on a meal-to-meal basis.

Evidence for meal-to-meal regulation emerged from studies in which selection of protein and of total food energy was monitored throughout the day. Rats given simultaneous access to a high protein and a protein-free diet showed different circadian patterns of protein and energy intake.[28] Energy intake, mainly from the protein-free, primarily carbohydrate diet, showed large circadian fluctuations, with the largest intake occurring in meals consumed during the dark period. In contrast, average protein intake at a meal is relatively constant throughout the day. However, variations in protein consumed within a meal occur, and, although small, appear to be of significance in determining both size and time of onset of the subsequent meal.[28] That is, a positive correlation is present between the quantity of protein in a meal and the postprandial interval. Also, the calories derived from the nonprotein components of a meal are directly related to the length of the interval immediately preceding that meal. Taken together, this information shows that after a low protein meal the rat will take a shorter than average time to start another meal and, consequently, this meal will be selected so that it contains relatively more protein and fewer carbohydrate calories than average.

The effect of recently ingested food composition on subsequent food choice and macronutrient preference has been more precisely defined by providing rats a choice of diets after they were fed either carbohydrate or protein meals. High protein meals not only suppressed total food intake as occurs in the absence of food choice[35] but also, in the presence of a food choice, led to decreased preference for protein (or a relatively increased preference for carbohydrate) in a subsequent meal.[44]

**Carbohydrate Intake.** The notion of a regulated carbohydrate appetite has also been with us for some time. By using a variation of the self-selection method of feeding, Soulairac attempted to quantitate the rat's ability to regulate carbohydrate intake.[68] He allowed rats access to carbohydrate-containing fluids, as well as to food. His observations had the benefit of showing that modification of carbohydrate metabolism can affect appetite for carbohydrate. Unfortunately, he did not report data on either total energy or carbohydrate intake, but only on amount of carbohydrate solution consumed.

More recent evidence, however, shows that rats regulate carbohydrate intake if offered dietary choices.[69] Again, as with the protein regulation studies, two diets have been presented to the animals. In this instance, however, the isocaloric diets contained different amounts of carbohydrate, but were identical in protein. When daily food and carbohydrate intakes were measured for 3 weeks it was found that rats consumed about 60 to 65% of their dietary calories as carbohydrate. This level of selection is achieved whether the rats were given a choice of 25 and 75% carbohydrate diets or of 50 and 75% carbohydrate diets. Of particular interest to the metabolic basis of food intake regulation are the studies showing that sweetness of the test diets did not influence the proportion of diet consumed as carbohydrate. When the two diet choices varying in carbohydrate content were comprised of sucrose, dextrose, or dextrin the rats consumed the same total carbohydrate.[69]

As is the situation for protein consumption, carbohydrate consumption has immediate effects on food selection. Food choice has been examined in fasting animals allowed to consume a small (6 kcal) premeal containing either carbohydrate or carbohydrate and protein. Ninety minutes later the rats were allowed access to a pair of isocaloric, isoprotein 25 and 75% carbohydrate diets. Those eating the carbohydrate premeal chose to eat less of the high-carbohydrate diet, even though they ate the same number of calories as those eating the mixed premeal.[70]

**Fat Intake.** There is little information on regulation of fat intake. Again, however, in a given set of circumstances, relative constancy of fat selection has been described.[71,72] For example, when the protein concentration of a high fat and a high carbohydrate diet choice was kept at 32% protein-energy, rats selected approximately 60% of the daily intake as fat. However, if the protein provided only 10% of the protein energy in both diets, the rats switched to the high carbohydrate diet and consumed only 20% of the diet as fat energy.[71] This switch to carbohydrate from fat energy when protein is limiting may offer further proof that protein intake is regulated closely to requirements. Carbohydrate, compared to fat, is known to be protein-sparing, and hence its consumption when protein is limiting would be an obvious advantage to the rat.

An examination of the literature will lead the reviewer to conclude that the absolute intake of protein, carbohydrate, and fat selected by rats varies considerably among reports. This variation cannot be readily explained and is in contrast to energy intake, which is found to be relatively constant, when expressed relative to body size, for animals fed different diets in different locations. Overall, however, it is clear that within a constant set of experimental conditions the selection of macronutrients by the rat is remarkably consistent. As a result, control mechanisms regulating each of these appetites can be examined. Studies to date have established the principle that control mechanisms previously thought to be involved only in regulating energy intake are also possible regulators of nutrient-specific appetites.

## BRAIN MECHANISMS AND THE REGULATION OF FOOD INTAKE

For metabolic events to affect feeding behavior, they must first be detected by the nervous system. Thus, the role of various brain regions in the control of feeding behavior has been extensively studied. From this work, the central role of the hypothalamus in the control of feeding has been identified. Originally, on the basis of lesion studies, the ventromedial hypothalamus (VMH) was identified as the satiety center because its destruction resulted in overeating and increased body weight. The lateral hypothalamus (LH) was identified as the feeding center because its destruction caused starvation. Although oversimplified, this concept of the hypothalamus having two control centers has served as a useful working model in the study of feeding mechanisms.[73] At this time, however, it is more appropriate to recognize the hypothalamus as an integrative unit functioning in the brain's reception and organization of the many signals arising from food ingestion.[73a]

How the brain receives and organizes the many signals arising from the metabolism of foods is unknown. Furthermore, the signals may arise preabsorptively as well as postabsorptively and reach the brain through neuronal input (via the vagus nerve) or through changes in plasma concentration of nutrients, of their metabolites, and of hormones released in the metabolism of these nutrients.

With the ingestion and digestion of food the resulting releases of fat, amino acids, and glucose have the potential to provide preabsorptive information to the brain via the vagus nerve. Evidence has been obtained for the presence of gastrointestinal chemoreceptors for glucose[76] and amino acids.[74] Glucose, amino acids, and fat also signal the release of gastrointestinal hormones, ten of which have been shown to inhibit feeding, including cholecystokinin, bombesin, gastrin, secretin, glucagon, insulin, somatostatin, neurotensin, substance P, and pancreatic polypeptide.[75]

Of the gut hormones, cholecystokinin (CCK) is the most studied modulator of food intake. The satiety effect of intravenous CCK has been demonstrated in mice, rats, rabbits, rhesus monkeys, and humans. CCK is released from the small intestine by fat and amino acids. It has a rapid onset of action and shortens the duration of eating without affecting the rate of eating. The peripheral action of the hormone appears to depend upon the vagus nerve, specifically the afferent branch arising from the stomach. If this branch of the vagus nerve is cut, CCK injections do not bring about reductions in food intake.[75a,75b]

After entry into the portal vein and passage to the liver, nutrients may also provide, via the vagus nerve, information to the brain. For example, as reviewed earlier, glucose entry into the liver and its storage are known to influence feeding behavior.[16]

Plasma fluctuations in nutrients are clearly useful to the brain in monitoring the milieu intérieur. These fluctuations create changes in brain concentrations due to the activity of many blood-brain-barrier transport systems.[76] Neurons sense changes in availability of nutrients by a variety of mechanisms, including direct interaction with receptors (e.g., glucose[77] and amino acids[78]), recognition of a change in rate of nutrient utilization for energy production (e.g., glucose[6]), recognition of altered neurotransmitter activity because of precursor (e.g., tyrosine or tryptophan) or cofactor (e.g., $B_6$, iron) roles of nutrients in neurotransmitters (e.g., glycine[79]). With altered neuronal activity, a large number of neuronal systems become involved and may utilize many monoamine and neuropeptide neurotransmitters. Eventually, the information provided becomes integrated, and feeding behavior is regulated to maintain the nutritional homeostasis of the organism.[80]

To fully understand the brain's regulation of feeding behavior, a determination of what brain signals initiate a meal, as well as those that terminate a meal, is of fundamental importance. Classic theories of feeding behavior have suggested that the lateral hypothalamus is always providing a tonic signal for the rat to eat, and appetite regulation is primarily an inhibition of this signal. However, both endogenous and exogenous opioid peptides have been shown to stimulate food intake, and it has been proposed that stress-induced eating in both human beings and experimental animals may be stimulated by opiate release.[80] While the attractive hypothesis has been stated that obesity may result from an autoaddiction to endogenous opioid peptides, it remains to be proven. Nevertheless, this information raises the possibility that eating is initiated by specific signals, rather than by a decreased presence of appetite suppressive signals.

The large number of signals already identified that influence feeding suggests that there is redundancy in feeding control mechanisms. Alternatively, it has been proposed that all of these factors may in some way be involved, such as in a cascade of events analogous to that occurring during blood clotting.[80] If so, many of the appetite signals identified to date may not be of independent significance, but may be interdependent components of a complex system.

## BRAIN MECHANISMS AND THE REGULATION OF MACRONUTRIENT INTAKE

Confusion with respect to the importance of each of the putative signals influencing feeding may also arise from the experimental design of the majority of feeding studies. As indicated previously, most studies of control mechanisms have utilized energy balance and total food intake, without regard to meal composition, as measures of feeding behavior. However, the determination of nutrient-specific appetites has indicated that some control mechanisms that were previously proposed as being involved in the determination of energy balance may also be nutrient-specific. For example, the hypothalamus and many neuronal systems are involved in the regulation of macronutrient intake.

The hypothalamus plays a role in the regulation of macronutrient selection,[81,82] in addition to its established role in the regulation of energy balance. Ventromedial hypothalamic lesions and parasagittal knife cuts through the medial hypothalamus cause hyperphagia. However, when the rat is allowed access to separate sources of protein, carbohydrate, and fat, the hyperphagia is expressed by a preferred consumption of carbohydrate.[82] This increase in carbohydrate appetite could be due to hyperinsulinemia, which also occurs with these lesions.[83] However, rats with paraventricular hypothalamic (PVH) lesions are not hyperinsulinemic,[84] but also have increased carbohydrate appetites, suggesting that the hypothalamic neuronal circuitry is directly involved in the regulation of carbohydrate intake.

Of the neurotransmitters now known to influence food choice, which include serotonin (5-HT), norepinephrine, and the opiates, the role of serotonin is perhaps best understood. Based on studies in which rats were allowed access to single diets while serotonergic systems were pharmacologically manipulated, its action has been described as inhibitory.[85] More recent research, however, suggests that another role of 5-HT may be to regulate the composition of food consumed in such a way as to achieve an adequate intake and balance of protein and carbohydrate. This role of 5-HT may be predicted for two reasons. First, brain 5-HT synthesis is under control by the availability of its tryptophan precursor. The rate-limiting enzyme in the pathway of conversion of tryptophan to serotonin is tryptophan hydroxylase.

Because this enzyme, which converts tryptophan to 5-hydroxytryptophan, the first product in the pathway to serotonin, is not fully saturated by normal brain tryptophan concentrations, fluctuations in tryptophan availability influence serotonin synthesis.[39,40,79] Thus, events that influence plasma tryptophan concentration and brain uptake can be expected to modify brain serotonin synthesis. A second reason for predicting that 5-HT may be involved in the regulation of food selection arises from the fact that brain tryptophan availability is modulated in opposite directions by carbohydrate and protein consumption.[39]

Tryptophan, a dietary essential amino acid, appears in the blood as a result of protein ingestion and body protein breakdown. It is transported across the blood brain barrier via a carrier mechanism specific for the large neutral amino acids (NAA), which include tryptophan (TRP), tyrosine, phenylalanine, valine, isoleucine, and methionine.[86] Because of the competitive nature of amino acid uptake, the effect of food ingestion on brain tryptophan is not simply related to its tryptophan content. Because tryptophan is present in protein in relatively small amounts, a meal of protein causes a greater increase in plasma concentrations of large neutral amino acids relative to tryptophan, decreasing the ratio of plasma TRP/NAA and therefore brain tryptophan uptake. Conversely, a carbohydrate meal increases the plasma TRP/NAA ratio.[87,88] This is due to carbohydrate-induced insulin release, which increases the uptake of all amino acids into tissues; but, insulin has a lesser effect on tryptophan, which is carried in plasma both in free form and bound to albumin.[89] Insulin reduces the free fatty acid content of plasma, and consequently the amount available to bind with albumin is decreased. Because tryptophan and fatty acids have the same binding site on albumin, tryptophan binding increases after a carbohydrate meal and tends to be retained in plasma. Tryptophan is released, however, as albumin transverses the brain capillaries, and because of tryptophan's increased concentration relative to other large neutral amino acids in the blood and hence its competitive advantage at the blood-brain barrier, tryptophan uptake is favored after a carbohydrate meal. Thus, protein ingestion decreases the level of serotonin in the brain by limiting uptake of tryptophan, whereas tryptophan administration and carbohydrate ingestion increase the concentration of tryptophan and serotonin in the brain.

The suggestion that brain 5-HT may regulate nutrient selection was supported by studies in which rats were given dietary choices after consuming meals of either carbohydrate or protein.

When the meal was rich in carbohydrate, the rats emphasized protein in the next meal,[70] and vice versa.[57]

A role for brain 5-HT in carbohydrate and protein selection has been explored by using both dietary and pharmacologic treatments. For example, increases in rat brain 5-HT are found after a carbohydrate meal with or without added tryptophan (15 mg). These increases in brain 5-HT synthesis are consistent with the behavior of rats fed carbohydrate. If the rats are given a choice of a high carbohydrate and a high protein diet after a carbohydrate meal, they will show a distinct preference for the protein diet.[44] Tryptophan additions to the carbohydrate meal increased brain 5-HT turnover by a further 30 to 50% and caused rats to further increase their preference for protein over that induced by the carbohydrate meal alone. Finally, because these feeding preferences did not occur when the diet-induced increases in 5-HT synthesis were blocked by para-chlorophenylalanine (p-CPA), an inhibitor of tryptophan hydroxylase,[44] further evidence was provided for a central role for 5-HT in the regulation of food selection.

Further support for the hypothesis that 5-HT plays a role in macronutrient selective appetites is provided by studies in which activity in serotonergic neurons was manipulated by specific drugs. Fenfluramine, injected at 1 to 2 mg/kg, caused rats to select more protein relative to carbohydrate in the subsequent hour of feeding.[44,90] However, in the next 3 to 8 hours the rats reversed their feeding preference and showed greater relative preference for carbohydrate.[44] These feeding responses can be explained by the action of fenfluramine, which causes an initial release of 5-HT into the synaptic cleft and hence increased activity in serotonergic neurons,[91] followed by depletion of 5-HT and decreased activity in the neurons.[92]

In addition to modulating the relative amount of protein and carbohydrate consumed from meal to meal, 5-HT also appears to be involved in regulating the absolute intake of these macronutrients over a longer term. When considered over the full day, fenfluramine reduced the absolute intake of protein but not of carbohydrate,[44] which is consistent with its long-term effect of depleting brain 5-HT. Similarly, long-term depletion of brain 5-HT induced by *para*-chlorophenylalanine, a tryptophan hydroxylase inhibitor, or by 5,7-dihydroxytryptamine, a neurotoxin, which destroys 5-HT nerve endings, or by lesion of the raphe nuclei of serotonin nerve cells, resulted in chronic suppression of protein intake relative to carbo-

hydrate intake but had no effect on total energy intake.[93]

In summary, an involvement of brain 5-HT in the regulation of protein and carbohydrate consumption can be described. Ingestion of a food (i.e., one high in carbohydrate) that raises brain 5-HT will cause the animal to seek a food (i.e., one high in protein) that decreases brain 5-HT (Fig. 30–2), and vice versa.

The role of other neurotransmitters, which are known to be involved in feeding control mechanisms, might also be elucidated by experiments in which the food choice paradigm is utilized. For example, the catecholamines and opioid peptides, primarily through a neuronal system coordinated by the hypothalamus, also influence food choice and meal composition. Rats selectively increased carbohydrate intake after microinjection of norepinephrine into the paraventricular nucleus of the hypothalamus (PVH).[94] Carbohydrate, however, is not the only nutrient whose selection is modified by activity of catecholaminergic neurons. When catecholaminergic tone was suppressed by clonidine, a presynaptic α-receptor agonist, rats increased their intakes of both protein and total food.[95] Conversely, amphetamine, a central catecholaminergic agonist, decreased total food intake, with a greater effect on protein intake.[96]

At the present time it is not possible to state that food selection is regulated in normal feeding situations as a result of signals to the central nervous system by precursor effects of tyrosine. The synthesis of the catecholamines is influenced by tyrosine availability, but there are no reports of the effect of diet-induced variations in brain tyrosine on food choice. One might speculate, however, that the elevated synthesis of norepinephrine that occurs after protein consumption might

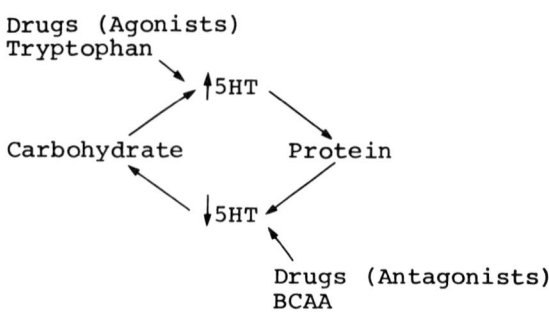

**Fig. 30–2.** Brain serotonin (5-HT) as a regulator of macronutrient preference. Foods or drugs that increase brain 5-HT cause the animal to prefer protein relative to carbohydrate. Conversely, when brain 5-HT is decreased, a preference for carbohydrate relative to protein occurs.

direct the animal to prefer carbohydrate in the next meal.[97]

In addition to norepinephrine and serotonin, the opiates also influence macronutrient choice. A selective preference for fat can be induced also by morphine[98] and decreased by naloxone, an opiate antagonist.[99] The site of action of the opiates appears to be in the hypothalamus with the feeding response involving norepinephrine-containing neurons.

Many, if not all, of the gut hormones are present in the brain. At the present time the view is that their presence in the brain is due to endogenous synthesis rather than active transport from the circulation and that they function in some way as neuromodulators. Despite the strong effect on food intake of systemic injections of some of these peptides, preliminary reports suggest that at least cholecystokinin (CCK) does not influence macronutrient choice.[75b]

## SUMMARY

An integrative view of the concepts presented in this review is provided in Figure 30–3. Feeding results in the ingestion of food containing energy and nutrients. The presence of macronutrient breakdown products in the gastrointestinal tract, particularly amino acids and fat, may directly or indirectly, via hormone release, stimulate vagal receptors and hence provide impulses directly to the brain. The products of digestion and hormones released from the gut and entering the liver also affect the brain through stimulation of the vagus nerve. Nutrients and hormones passing the liver result in changes in plasma concentrations, which in turn may signal the brain in some indirect man-

ner without uptake across the blood-brain barrier, or more directly as a result of brain uptake and changes in brain nutrient concentration and availability. Both energy utilization and storage in tissues also provide signals to the brain, although their mechanism is unknown. Through a complex system of neurotransmitters the brain organizes the information arising from the metabolism of food and directs feeding so that the animal's intake of both energy and macronutrients is quantitatively regulated.

In summary, it is clear that many metabolic factors are involved in the central regulation of appetite. The evolutionary process would appear to have generated a complex control system. As a result, it seems unlikely that appetite control will be understood within the near future. Indeed we seem further away from a unifying answer than three decades ago when hunger and satiety centers in the hypothalamus and the glucostatic theory were being explored. Given the complexity of the mechanism of regulation of food intake and its responsiveness to so many signals, however, one can only be amazed that in most animals and man it works as effectively as it does.

## REFERENCES

1. Durnin, J.G.V.A.: J. Physiol. *156*:294-299, 1961.
2. Sellers, E.A., You, R.W., Moffat, N.W.: Am. J. Physiol. *177*:367-371, 1954.
3. Collier, G., Leshner, A.I., Squibbs, R.L.: Physiol. Behav. 4:79-82, 1969.
4. Adolph, E.F.: Am. J. Physiol. *151*:1110-1125, 1947.
5. Hamilton, C.L.: J. Am. Diet. Assoc. *62*:35-40, 1973.
6. Mayer, J.: Physiology of hunger and satiety. *In* Modern Nutrition in Health and Disease, 6th ed. (Goodhart, R.S., Shils, M.E., Eds.) Philadelphia, Lea & Febiger, 1980.
7. Louis-Sylvestre, J., Le Magnen J.: Neurosci. Biobehav. Rev. *4*(Suppl. 1):13-15, 1980.
8. Strubbe, J.H., Steffens, A.B.: Physiol. Behav. *19*:303-308, 1977.
9. Rapoport, S.I.: Blood-brain barrier. *In* Physiology and Medicine. New York, Raven Press, 1976.
10. Stricker, E.M., Rowland, N., Saller, C.F.: Science *196*:78-81, 1977.
11. Friedman, M.I., Ramirez, I., Wade, G.N., et al.: Physiol. Behav. *29*:515-518, 1982.
12. Rezek, M., Havlicek, V., Novin, D.: Am. J. Physiol. *299*:545-548, 1975.
13. Glick, Z., Mayer, J.: Nature (Lond.) *219*:1374, 1968.
14. Muller, E.E., Paneri, A., Cocchi, D., et al.: Experientia *29*:874-875, 1973.
15. Russek, M.: Neurosci. Res. *4*:213-282, 1971.
16. Novin, D.: Visceral mechanisms in the control of food intake. *In* Hunger: Basic Mechanism and Clinical Implications. (Novin, D., Wyrwicka, W., Bray, G., Eds.) New York, Raven Press, 1976.
17. Novin, D., Sanderson, J.D., Vanderweele, D.A.: Physiol. Behav. *13*:3-8, 1974.
18. Bellinger, L.L., Williams, F.E.: Physiol. Behav. *26*:663-673, 1981.
19. Mayer, J.: N. Engl. J. Med. *249*:13-16, 1953.
20. Faust, I.M.: Signals from adipose tissue. *In* The Body

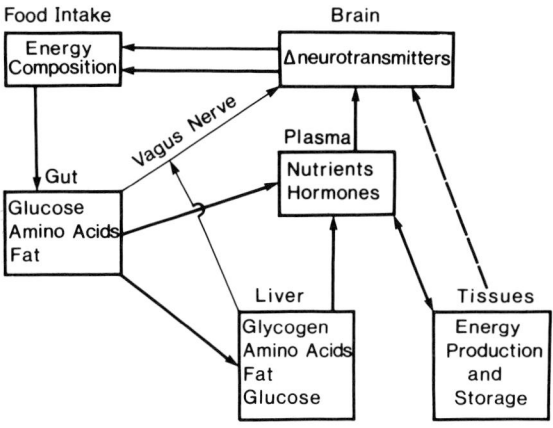

**Fig. 30–3.** An integrative view of the regulation of intake of food quantity (energy) and of composition. Signals arrive in the brain via many sources and are integrated in a manner that leads to food selection as well as to quantitative intake.

Weight Regulatory System: Normal and Disturbed Mechanisms (Cioffi, L., James, W.P.T., Van Italie, T.B., Eds.) New York, Raven Press, 1981.

21. Mrosovsky, N., Powley, T.L.: Behav. Biol. *20*:205-223, 1977.

22. Le Magnen, J., Devos, M.: Physiol. Behav. *5*:805-814, 1970.

23. Shimazu, T.: Diabetologia *20*(suppl):343-356, 1981.

24. Takahashi, A., Shimazu, T.: J. Auton. Nerv. Syst. *4*:195-205, 1981.

25. Schmitt, M.: Am. J. Physiol. *225*:1096-1101, 1973.

26. Danquir, J., Nicolaidis, S.: Am. J. Physiol. *228*:E223-E228, 1980.

27. Larue-Achagiotis, C., Le Magnen, J.: Physiol. Behav. *22*:435-440, 1979.

28. Johnson, D.J., Li, E.T.S., Coscina, D.V., et al.: Physiol. Behav. *22*:777-782, 1979.

29. Le Magnen, J.: Physiol. Rev. *63*:314-386, 1983.

30. Cahill, G.F. Jr.: New Engl. J. Med. *1282*:668-675, 1970.

31. Harris, R.B.S., Martin, R.J.: Nutr. Behav. *1*:253-275, 1984.

32. Wade, G.N., Gray, J.M.: Physiol. Behav. *22*:583-593, 1979.

33. Greenwood, M.R.C., Cleary, M., Steingrimsdotter, L., et al: *In* Recent Advances in Obesity Research III. (Bjorntorp, P., Cairella, M., Howard, A.N., Eds.) London, John Libbey, 1981.

34. Mellinkoff, S.M., Franklin, M., Boyle, D., et al.: J. Appl. Physiol. *8*:535-538, 1956.

35. Harper, A.E., Benevenga, N.J., Wohlhueter, R.M.: Physiol. Rev. *50*:428-558, 1970.

36. Peng. Y., Tews, J.K., Harper, A.E.: Am. J. Physiol. *222*:314-321, 1972.

37. Anderson, H.L., Benevenga, N.J., Harper, A.E.: Am. J. Physiol *214*:1008-1013, 1968.

38. Johnson, D.J., Anderson, G.H.: Am. J. Physiol. *243*:R99-R103, 1982.

39. Anderson, G.H., Li, E.T.S., Glanville, N.T.: Brain Res. Bull. *12*:167-173, 1984.

40. Anderson, G.H.: Br. Med. Bull *37*:95-100, 1981.

41. Rogers, Q.R., Leung, P.M.B.: Fed. Proc. Fed. Am. Soc. Exp. Biol. *32*:1709-1719, 1973.

42. Butler, R.M., Davis, M., Gehling, N.J., et al.: Am. J. Clin. Nutr. *34*:2045-2047, 1981.

43. Hrboticky, N., Leiter, L., Anderson, G.H.: Nutr. Res. *5*:595-607, 1985.

44. Li, E.T.S., Anderson, G.H.: Life Sci. *34*:2453-2460, 1984.

45. Lacy, M.P., Van Krey, H.P., Denbow, D.M., et al.: Nutr. Behav. *1*:65-74, 1982.

46. Scharrer, E., Baile, C.A., Mayer, J.: Am. J. Physiol. *218*:400-404, 1970.

47. Mugford, R.A.: External influences on the feeding of carnivores. *In* The Clinical Senses and Nutrition. (Kare, M.R., Maller, O., Eds.) New York, Academic Press, 1977.

48. Osborne, T.B., Mendel, L.B.: J. Biol. Chem. *35*:19-27, 1918.

49. Richter, C.P.: Harvey Lect. *38*:63-103, 1943.

50. Richter, C.P.: Am. J. Physiol. *115*:155-161, 1936.

51. Richter, C.P., Eckert, J.: Am. J. Med. Sci. *198*:9-16, 1939.

52. Harris, L.J., Clay, J., Hargreaves, F.J., et al.: Proc. R. Soc. London, Ser. B *113*:161-190, 1933.

53. Siu, G.M., Hadley, M., Draper, H.H.: J. Nutr. *111*:1681-1685, 1981.

54. Siu, G.M., Hadley, M., Agwu, D.E., et al.: J. Nutr. *114*:1059-1105, 1984.

55. Lát, J.: Handbook of Physiology, Section 6 Vol. 1, Chapter 27, Washington, DC, American Physiology Society, 1967.

56. Musten, B., Peace, D., Anderson, G.H.: J. Nutr. *104*:563-572, 1974.

57. Li, E.T.S., Anderson, G.H.: Physiol. Behav. *29*:779-783, 1982.

58. Li, E.T.S., Anderson, G.H.: Nutr. Abstr. Rev. Clin. Nutr. Series A *53*:169-181, 1983.

59. Anderson, G.H., Ashley, D.V.M.: Plasma amino acids, brain mechanisms and the control of protein intake. *In* Nutrition in Transition; Proceedings Western Hemisphere Nutrition Congress V, Vol. 67. (White, P.L., Selvey, N., Eds.) Chicago, Alan Liss, 1981.

60. Ashley, D.V.M., Anderson, G.H.: J. Nutr. *105*:1405-1411, 1975.

61. Ashley, D.V.M., Anderson, G.H.: Life Sci. *21*:1235-1244, 1977.

62. Anderson, G.H., Leprohon, C.E., Chambers, J.H., et al.: Physiol. Behav. *22*:777-780, 1979.

63. Chee, K.M., Romsos, D.R., Bergen, W.G.: J. Nutr. *111*:668-677, 1981.

64. Romsos, D.R., Ferguson, D.: J. Am. Vet. Assoc. *182*:41-43, 1983.

65. Summers, J.D., Leeson, S.: Br. Poult. Sci. *19*:425-430, 1978.

66. FAO/WHO: Joint Expert Committee on Energy and Protein Requirement. World Health Organization Technical Report Series, No. 522, Geneva, 1973.

67. Wade, J., Milner, J., Krondl, M.: Am. J. Clin. Nutr. *34*:143-147, 1981.

68. Soulairac, A.: Bull. Biol. Fr. Belg. *81*:273-432, 1947.

69. Wurtman, J.J., Wurtman, R.J.: J. Psychiat. Res. *17*:213-221, 1982/83.

70. Wurtman, J.J., Moses, P.L., Wurtman, R.J.: J. Nutr. *113*:70-78, 1983.

71. Ashley, D.V.M., Leathwood, P.D.: Nestlé Research News 1982/83, La Tour-De-Peilz, Switzerland, Nestlé Products Technical Assistance Co. Ltd. pp. 59-69. 1984.

72. Kanarek, R.B., Ho, L., Meade, R.G.: Pharmacol. Biochem. Behav. *14*:539-542, 1981.

73. Hoebel, B.G.: Neurotransmitters in the control of feeding and its rewards: monoamines, opiates and brain-gut peptides. *In* Eating and Its Disorders (Stunkard, A.J., Stellar, I., Eds.) New York, Raven Press, 1983.

73a.Sullivan, A.C., Gruen, R.K.: Fed. Proc. *44*:139-144, 1985.

74. Jeanningros, R.: Physiol. Behav. *28*:9-21, 1982.

75. Smith, G.P., Gibbs, J.: Brain-gut peptides and the control of food intake. *In* Neurosecretion and Brain Peptides (Martin, J.B., Rechlin, S., Bick, K.L., Eds.) New York, Raven Press, 1981.

75a.Smith, G.P., Jerome, C., Cushin, B.J., et al.: Science *213*:1036-1037, 1981.

75b.Li, E.T.S., Anderson, G.H.: Am. J. Physiol. *247* (Endocrinol. Metab. 10):E815-E821, 1984.

76. Pardridge, W.M., Oldendorf, W.H.: J. Neurochem. *28*:5-12, 1977.

77. Oomura, Y.: Significance of glucose, insulin and free fatty acids in the hypothalamic feeding and satiety neurons. *In* Hunger: Basic Mechanism and Clinical Implications (Novin, D., Wyrwicka, W., Bray, G., Eds.) New York, Raven Press, 1976.

78. Wayner, M.J., Ono, T., Young De, A., et al.: Pharmacol. Biochem. Behav. *3*(suppl. 1):85-90, 1975.

79. Anderson, G.H., Johnston, J.L.: Can. J. Physiol. Pharmacol. *61*:271-281, 1983.
80. Morley, J.E., Levine, A.S.: Lancet *8321*:398-401, 1983.
81. Kanarek, R.B., Feldman, P.G., Hanes, C.: Physiol. Behav. *27*:337-343, 1981.
82. Sclafani, A., Aravich, P.F.: Am. J. Physiol. *244*:R686-R694, 1983.
83. Kanarek, R.B., Marks-Kaufman, R., Lipeles, B.J.: Physiol. Behav. *25*:779-782, 1980.
84. Leibowitz, S.F., Hammer, N.J., Chang, K.: Physiol. Behav. *27*:1031-1040, 1981.
85. Blundell, J.E.: Int. J. Obes. *1*:15-42, 1977.
86. Pardridge, W.M.: Regulation of amino acid availability to the brain. *In*: Nutrition and the Brain. Vol. 1 (Wurtman, R.J., Wurtman, J.J., Eds.) New York, Raven Press, 1977.
87. Fernstrom, J.D., Wurtman, R.J.: Science *173*:149-152, 1971.
88. Wurtman, R.J., Fernstrom, J.D.: Biochem. Pharmacol. 25:1692-1696, 1976.
89. McMenamy, R.H., Oncley, J.L.: J. Biol. Chem. *233*:1436-1447, 1978.
90. Wurtman, J.J., Wurtman, R.J.: Science *198*:1178-1180, 1978.
91. Fuxe, K., Farnebo, L.O., Hamberger, B., et al.: Postgrad. Med. J. *51*(Suppl. 1):35-45, 1975.
92. Garattini, S., Buczko, W., Jori, A., et al.: Postgrad. Med. J. *51*(Suppl. 1):27-35, 1975.
93. Ashley, D.V.M., Coscina, D.V., Anderson, G.H.: Life Sci. *24*:973-984, 1979.
94. Leibowitz, S.F.: Neurochemical systems of the hypothalamus in control of feeding and drinking behavior and water-electrolyte excretion. *In* Handbook of the Hypothalamus, Vol. 3A. (Morgane, P.J., Panksepp, J., Eds.) New York, Marcel Dekker, 1980.
95. Mauron, C., Wurtman, J.J., Wurtman, R.J.: Life Sci. 27:781-791, 1980.
96. Blundell, J.E., McArthur, R.A.: Br. J. Pharmacol. *67*:436-438, 1979.
97. Gibson, C.J., Wurtman, R.J.: Life Sci. *22*:1399-1406, 1978.
98. Marks-Kaufman, R.M., Kanarek, R.B.: Pharmacol. Biochem. Behav. *12*:427-430, 1980.
99. Marks-Kaufman, R.M., Kanarek, R.B.: Psychopharmacology (Berlin) *74*:321-324, 1981.

*Chapter* **31**

# HORMONE AND NUTRIENT INTERACTIONS

John T. Devlin and Edward S. Horton

This chapter examines the interrelations of plasma hormone concentrations with the metabolism of various nutrients.

## PANCREATIC HORMONES: INSULIN, GLUCAGON, AND SOMATOSTATIN

Carbohydrate metabolism is finely regulated by interactions between insulin, the hormone promoting fuel storage, and the counterregulatory hormones, such as glucagon, epinephrine, cortisol, and growth hormone. Insulin's influences may be anabolic or may oppose the catabolic action of other hormones, thus acting in an anticatabolic manner (Table 31–1). Glucose homeostasis is maintained in the presence of widely varying quantities and compositions of food intake. Because the brain requires a constant supply of glucose even in the absence of available carbohydrate, the importance of these homeostatic mechanisms is apparent.

## Carbohydrate Metabolism

Insulin's central role in regulating glucose metabolism has long been recognized. Insulin, like other peptide hormones, initiates its metabolic effects by binding to a cell-surface receptor. Insulin's effects depend on the activation of a tyrosine-specific protein kinase, which is contained in the beta subunit of the receptor.[1,2] After binding to its cell-surface receptor, insulin accelerates the membrane transport of sugars, which increases 4 times in normal hearts and 6 to 7 times in diabetics.[3] This effect is mediated by glucose transporter units, which have been characterized in adipose

**Table 31–1. Insulin Action**

|  | Liver | Adipose Tissue | Muscle |
|---|---|---|---|
| Anticatabolic effects | ↓ Glycogenolysis<br>↓ Gluconeogenesis<br>↓ Ketogenesis | ↓ Lipolysis | ↓ Protein catabolism<br>↓ Amino acid output |
| Anabolic effects | ↑ Glycogen synthesis<br>↑ Fatty acid synthesis | ↑ Glycerol synthesis<br>↑ Fatty acid synthesis | ↑ Amino acid uptake<br>↑ Protein synthesis<br>↑ Glycogen synthesis |

(From Felig, P.: *In* Felig, P., Baxter, J.D., Broadus, A.E., Frohman, L.A., (eds.): Endocrinology and Metabolism. New York, McGraw-Hill, 1981.)

tissue, as well as in heart and diaphragm muscle tissues.[4,5] Insulin rapidly increases membrane glucose transport, within 1 to 2 minutes, with a maximal effect in 15 to 20 min. Whereas insulin is known to increase glucose transport into skeletal and heart muscle, adipocytes, fibroblasts, and other tissues, the uptake of glucose by hepatic cells is not insulin dependent. Although the use of glucose by the brain has been thought to be insulin independent,[6] a requirement for insulin does appear to exist for glucose use by the hypothalamus.[7]

In addition to increasing glucose transport, insulin has major effects on intracellular glucose metabolism (Fig. 31–1). In experimental diabetes, one sees decreased activities of enzymes for glycolysis and glucose oxidation, such as glucokinase, phosphofructokinase, and pyruvate kinase, and increased activities of gluconeogenic enzymes, such as glucose 6-phosphatase, fructose 1,6-diphosphatase, phosphoenolpyruvate (PEP) carboxykinase, and pyruvate carboxylase. These abnormalities are corrected by insulin replacement. Insulin also promotes glycogen synthesis, by promoting the conversion of glycogen synthase to its active, glucose 6-phosphate independent

("I") form and by decreasing the activity of phosphorylase. Insulin causes rapid decreases in phosphorylase activity and more gradual increases in synthase I activity, although the hormonal effect is of brief duration in vivo.[8] Recent data suggest that elevations in concentrations of plasma glucose, rather than serum insulin, may play a more important role in activation of glycogen synthase and glycogen deposition in the liver, whereas insulin has a key role in the regulation of glycogen metabolism in skeletal muscle.[9] Insulin is also able to stimulate glycolysis and lipogenesis in fat and both glycolysis and glycogen synthesis in muscle tissue and to inhibit gluconeogenesis in the renal cortex.[10] Although most tissues have the enzyme systems required to synthesize and to hydrolyze glycogen, only the liver and kidneys contain glucose 6-phosphatase, the enzyme necessary for the release of glucose into the circulation. The liver and kidneys also contain the enzymes necessary for gluconeogenesis (pyruvate carboxylase, PEP carboxykinase, and fructose 1,6-bisphosphatase). Except after prolonged starvation—when renal gluconeogenesis becomes important—the liver is the sole source of endogenous glucose production (EGP).

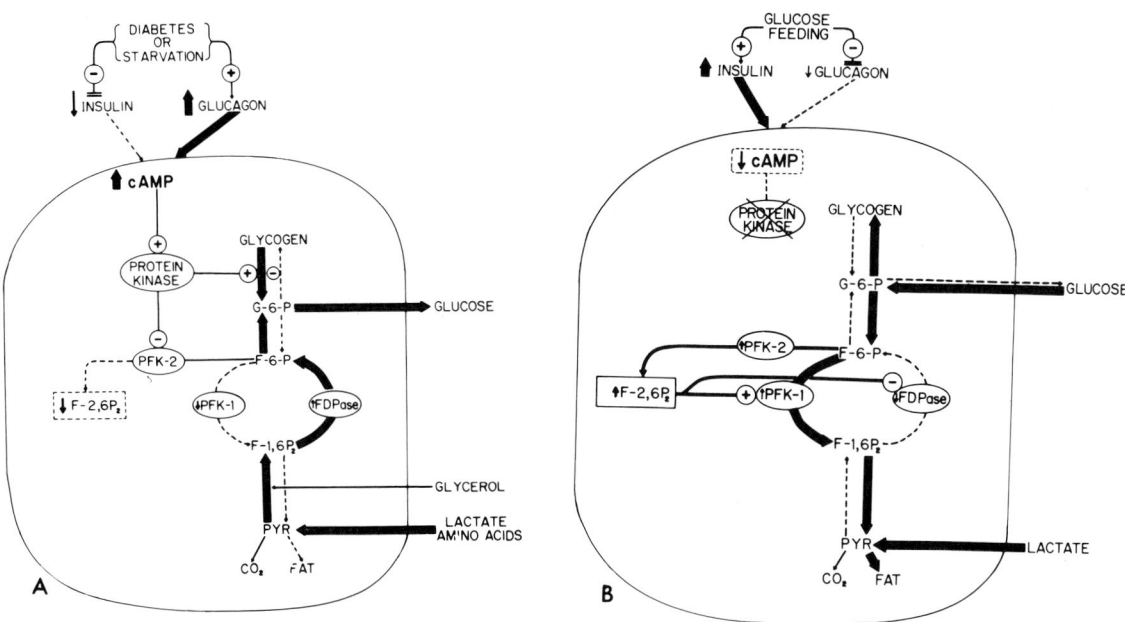

**Fig. 31–1.** *A*, Enhancement of gluconeogenesis and glycogenolysis by glucagon in diabetes and starvation. Both processes are activated by increases in cyclic AMP in the hepatocyte. Phosphofructokinase 1 (PFK-1) catalyzes formation of fructose 1,6-bisphosphate in the glycolytic pathway, while PFK-2 synthesizes fructose 2,6-bisphosphate, a regulator of PFK-1 activity. Cyclic AMP-induced phosphorylation of the enzyme decreases the former and increases the latter. Decreased F-2, 6-$P_2$ decreases glycolysis and increases gluconeogenesis. *B*, Inhibition of gluconeogenesis and activation of glycogen synthesis, and lipogenesis by insulin. Insulin decreases cyclic AMP, deactivates protein kinase, and reverses changes in F-2, 6-$P_2$ and substrate flux over the glycolytic-gluconeogenic pathway produced by glucagon. Glycogen synthesis and lipogenesis are also increased. (From Unger, R.H., Foster, D.W.: *In* Wilson, J.D., Foster, D.W. (eds.): William's Textbook of Endocrinology. 7th ed. Philadelphia, W.B. Saunders, 1985.)

During periods of starvation, the maintenance of euglycemia is critically important to the organism because in the nonketotic state, the energy needs of the brain can only be met by glucose, and the absence of glucose results in the death of central nervous system tissues. Starvation is associated with a decline in insulin and a rise in glucagon concentrations,[11] which result in increased rates of gluconeogenesis (Fig. 31–1). Decreased plasma insulin concentrations allow for a decrease in glucose use by peripheral tissues, as well as for enhanced lipolysis for the provision of increased lipid oxidation during starvation. These changes in serum insulin and glucagon concentrations also result in increased conversion of free fatty acids (FFA) to the ketone bodies, acetoacetate and beta-hydroxybutyrate, which can substitute for glucose as an energy supply for the brain.[12] Because the glucose pool can provide only 15 to 20 g in the adult, and because the amount of glycogen that can be mobilized to provide circulating glucose (that is, hepatic glycogen) averages 70 g, preformed glucose can provide less than an 8-hour supply of glucose on the average. Thus, gluconeogenesis is important for the maintenance of postabsorptive plasma glucose concentrations, and it becomes the sole source of glucose production after a 24- to 48-hour fast. Clearly, the change from a glucose-based to a lipid-based (FFA and ketone bodies) energy supply in prolonged starvation helps to minimize protein catabolism in skeletal muscle by reducing the need for amino-acid-derived gluconeogenesis.[13]

The ingestion of carbohydrate produces a prompt increase in plasma insulin and a decrease in glucagon concentrations.[14] The rise in insulin occurs before the rise in arterial glucose concentrations via the so-called "enteroinsular axis" and cephalic-phase insulin release, which are believed to be mediated through hormonal[15] and parasympathetic[16] mechanisms. This early insulin release allows for increased glucose use during the absorption of glucose and helps to minimize the extent of hyperglycemia following a meal. As glucose is absorbed, the hepatic production of glucose is decreased because of the foregoing hormonal changes, and glucose uptake by the liver, muscle, and adipose tissues accelerates.

When a carbohydrate-free protein meal is ingested, insulin concentrations increase slightly and promote protein synthesis in skeletal muscle, with a parallel rise in glucagon,[14] which prevents hypoglycemia.[17]

The effects of insulin deficiency are exemplified by type I, or insulin-dependent, diabetes mellitus (IDDM). As stated previously, this disorder is associated with increased activities of enzymes of gluconeogenesis and decreased activities of glycolytic and oxidative enzymes. In addition, IDDM is always associated with relative or absolute hyperglucagonemia,[18,19] resulting from loss of the restraining influence of insulin on the secretion of glucagon by the pancreatic alpha cell.[20,21] A rise in glucose concentrations also fails to inhibit glucagon secretion,[22,23] as it normally does, and it may paradoxically increase glucagon release.[24] Glucagon responses to protein are also excessive in IDDM[14]; they are not blunted by hyperglycemia.[25] Control of the plasma glucose to near-normal levels with insulin therapy corrects the basal hyperglucagonemia,[26] as well as the exaggerated response to protein ingestion.[25]

Inappropriate hyperinsulinemia, as seen in insulin-producing islet cell adenomas or hyperplasia, results in postabsorptive hypoglycemia. Insulin secretion is not normally decreased as the plasma glucose declines in the postabsorptive state. The result is a low rate of endogenous glucose production, with rates of glucose uptake that are not high in the absolute sense but are inappropriately high relative to the plasma glucose level. Insulin's hypoglycemic effect is potent, and when present in sufficient quantity, insulin can cause hypoglycemia despite the actions of all known counterregulatory factors. Postabsorptive hypoglycemia may also occur when both glucagon and epinephrine are deficient and insulin is present.[27] This phenomenon occurs in some patients with IDDM,[28,29] but it has not been convincingly demonstrated in other conditions.

Glucagon is secreted by the alpha cells of the pancreatic islets into the hepatic portal circulation, and it is thought to act exclusively on the liver under physiologic conditions. Glucagon exerts its effects through activation of adenyl cyclase.[30] Cyclic adenosine monophosphate (cAMP) concentrations in liver rise within seconds after the administration of glucagon. Glucagon is a potent activator of glycogenolysis and gluconeogenesis and is able to increase EGP within minutes, although the effect is transient. Glucagon decreases levels of fructose 2,6-bisphosphate, a key regulator of gluconeogenesis and glycolysis. Despite ongoing hyperglucagonemia, EGP decreases toward basal levels within 90 minutes. Glucagon-induced hyperglycemia is transient because the increase in glycogenolysis does not persist. This transient response is not the result of glycogen depletion, but more likely is caused by glucagon-induced insulin secretion coupled with an autoregulatory effect of hyperglycemia to inhibit EGP.

During fasting in humans, about 75% of EGP is mediated by glucagon,[31] whereas only about 40% of glucose use occurs in insulin-sensitive tissues.

Therefore, if both insulin and glucagon were deficient, EGP would decline by 75%, but glucose use would decrease by only 40%, and plasma glucose concentrations would remain constant or would even fall, at least initially. The major action of insulin on the liver is to oppose the effect of glucagon.[32] Insulin deficiency has a minimal influence on hepatic glucose and ketone metabolism in the absence of glucagon, and significant overproduction of glucose and ketones by the liver does not occur without glucagon.[33]

Glucagon deficiency, produced experimentally by infusion of somatostatin with partial insulin replacement, reduces nadir glucose concentrations after glucose ingestion by approximately 30%. Prolonged hypoglycemia does not occur because of epinephrine secretion, however. As noted previously, combined glucagon and epinephrine deficiency, as seen in some subjects with longstanding IDDM, totally disrupts the counterregulatory process and results in hypoglycemia late after glucose ingestion.

Glucagon excess, as seen in islet-cell glucagonoma, is associated with glucose intolerance, hypoaminoacidemia, and a characteristic skin rash, "necrolytic migratory erythema," thought to be the result of either the hyperglucagonemia or the decreased plasma levels of amino acids.[34,35] The glycogenolytic and gluconeogenic actions of glucagon result in mild hyperglycemia that can usually be controlled by dietary therapy.

In the somatostatinoma syndrome,[36] seen in somatostatin-producing islet cell adenomas, suppression of both insulin and glucagon causes mild diabetes mellitus. Neither the hyperglycemia nor the hyperketonemia is severe. Other features include cholelithiasis, steatorrhea, dyspepsia, and hypochlorhydria.

## Lipid Metabolism

Insulin and glucagon also play important roles in lipid metabolism; increased insulin concentrations stimulate lipogenesis and lipid storage, and the decreased insulin and increased glucagon levels seen in fasting promote lipolysis and lipid oxidation.[37] The major function of stored triglyceride in adipose tissue is as an efficient energy reserve. Triglyceride stores can serve as fuel to support many weeks of fasting, whereas stored carbohydrate is able to support a fast lasting only several hours. Stored triglyceride yields over twice as many calories per gram as either carbohydrate or protein and requires less than half the intracellular water for storage.

In the fed state, insulin and glucose are required for lipogenesis. Glucose use is needed for FFA synthesis and esterification and supplies the following: (1) acetyl coenzyme A (acetyl-COA) as a precursor of long-chain fatty acids; (2) α-glycerophosphate for esterification to fatty acids to form triglycerides; and (3) nicotinamide adenine dinucleotide phosphate (NADPH). Insulin stimulates carrier-mediated glucose transport and, in addition, is involved in the following steps: (1) activation of pyruvate dehydrogenase for conversion of glucose to acetyl-COA;[38] and (2) inhibition of lipolysis, thereby reducing palmityl-COA, an inhibitor of lipogenesis.[39]

Fatty acids stored in adipose tissue as triglyceride are derived from either dietary (chylomicrons) or endogenous (hepatic very low density lipoproteins (VLDL)) sources. Preformed triglycerides are transported from the gastrointestinal tract and liver to adipose tissue, where they are hydrolyzed by the enzyme lipoprotein lipase on the cell surface of the capillary endothelium. Insulin has an important role in maintaining and stimulating the activity of lipoprotein lipase.[40] In addition, insulin has a direct stimulatory effect on FFA uptake by adipose tissue. During insulin deficiency, lipoprotein lipase activity is reduced, and uptake of FFA by adipose tissue is diminished.[41]

In humans, liver as well as adipose tissue is a major site of lipid synthesis, occurring when dietary fat is replaced by carbohydrate. The liver removes a large proportion of circulating FFA delivered from adipose tissue, in a concentration-dependent manner. Lipogenesis depends on the availability of both glucose and insulin. During insulin deficiency, hexose monophosphate shunt activity is impaired, and NADPH is not provided for fatty acid synthesis.[42] In addition, decreased glucose use reduces the availability of acetyl-COA and citrate and thereby retards lipogenesis. Fatty acids synthesized in the liver are converted mainly to VLDL, are secreted into plasma, and are then cleared from the circulation minutes to hours later, by mechanisms similar to those involved in the removal of chylomicron triglycerides.

Lipolysis, with a net release of FFA and glycerol from adipose tissue, occurs during periods of fasting, exercise, stress, and uncontrolled diabetes mellitus. Low levels of insulin and increased glucagon concentrations enhance this mobilization of lipid from adipose tissue.[37] Several hormones, including glucagon, catecholamines, thyroid-stimulating hormone (TSH), and adrenocorticotropic hormone (ACTH), play important roles in lipolysis, through cAMP-mediated stimulation of "hormone-sensitive lipase." Insulin reduces catecholamine-stimulated cAMP concentrations in adipose tissue,[43] either by decreasing adenylate cyclase or by increasing phosphodiesterase activity.[44] During lipolysis, glycerol diffuses from the adipocyte because adipose tissue lacks the enzyme glycerolkinase and cannot reuse glycerol. FFA can either be released into the circulation or be reesterified into triglycerides in adipose tissue. Part of insulin's antilipolytic action is to stimulate reesterification of fatty acids.

On their release from adipose tissue, the glycerol and FFA circulate briefly in the plasma. Glycerol is metabolized primarily in the liver and kidney, where it is phosphorylated and either reesterified to triglyceride or used for gluconeogenesis. FFA are taken up by tissues in proportion to local blood flow and plasma concentrations. The potential fate of FFA taken up by the liver includes reesterification to triglyceride, oxidation, or conversion to ketone bodies, depending on the hormonal milieu. In the absence of either glucose or insulin, and in the presence of glucagon, only a small proportion of FFA taken up by the liver is reesterified to triglyceride and released as VLDL. The insulin-glucagon ratio appears to be critical in regulating the hepatic metabolism of FFA.[45] Activated fatty acids must be transported into the mitochondria for oxidation or conversion to ketone bodies, and neither FFA nor their COA derivatives can penetrate the inner mitochondrial membrane. Carnitine palmitoyl transferase I is an enzyme present on the inner mitochondrial membrane that reversibly transfers fatty acyl groups from COA to carnitine and allows entry into the mitochondria. A second enzyme, carnitine palmitoyl transferase II, irreversibly transfers the fatty acyl groups to mitochondrial COA and allows them to undergo either beta-oxidation or conversion to the ketone bodies, acetoacetate and beta-hydroxybutyrate. The activity of the key enzyme, carnitine palmitoyl transferase I, is regulated through the effects of insulin and glucagon on malonyl-COA concentrations.[46] In addition to their effects on carnitine palmitoyl transferase I activity, low insulin and high glucagon concentrations also contribute to increased lipid oxidation and ketogenesis by increasing adipose tissue lipolysis and FFA delivery. Ketone bodies circulate in plasma and are metabolized in skeletal muscle, heart, and brain tissues.

Alterations in lipid metabolism are common in subjects with diabetes mellitus; hypertriglyceridemia occurs in approximately one third of patients. This disorder is related to insulin's key role both in hepatic triglyceride production and in removal of triglyceride-rich lipoproteins.[47] Insulin is essential for the normal function of lipoprotein lipase, and with severe insulin deficiency hypertriglyceridemia is secondary to an acquired deficiency of this enzyme. "Diabetic lipemia," with milky plasma and eruptive xanthoma, may be the result of coexistent, poorly controlled IDDM and a familial form of hypertriglyceridemia.[48] This defect is promptly reversed with appropriate insulin replacement. Withdrawal of insulin from subjects with IDDM can decrease lipoprotein lipase activity and can produce hypertriglyceridemia within 48 hours.

Excess insulin, as most often encountered in obesity, leads to hypertriglyceridemia through a different mechanism. Elevated insulin concentrations act on the liver to increase VLDL production.[49] Obese subjects, both with and without diabetes, have higher-than-normal rates of VLDL triglyceride production.[50,51] This form of hypertriglyceridemia responds dramatically to weight reduction.

Increases in plasma low-density lipoproteins (LDL) may also be seen in diabetes mellitus. Insulin enhances LDL receptor-mediated catabolism,[52] and intensive insulin therapy in IDDM lowers both LDL and VLDL levels.[53] It is possible that glycosylation of LDL contributes to decreased rates of catabolism in diabetes. In noninsulin-dependent diabetes mellitus, increased LDL levels may result from increased rates of synthesis.[54,55]

## Protein Metabolism

Insulin and other hormones play an important role in *protein metabolism*. In as little as several hours of starvation, protein catabolism is increased to provide amino acids for gluconeogenesis. During more prolonged starvation, metabolic adjustments are made to spare muscle protein, such as increased reliance by the central nervous system on ketone bodies as an oxidative fuel. When fuel supplies are plentiful, protein synthesis occurs.

Insulin lowers blood concentrations of several amino acids in normal as well as in diabetic subjects, in a time pattern similar to that for glucose. The serum insulin concentrations required to produce half-maximal suppression of plasma amino acid concentrations are similar to those required for half-maximal stimulation of peripheral glucose disposal.[56] The lowering of plasma levels of the essential amino acids occurs in a pattern that corresponds to their relative concentrations in muscle protein. Isolated preparations incubated in vitro liberate amino acids, the rate of release of which is depressed by the addition of insulin. The presence of glucose may be, in part, necessary for insulin-mediated inhibition of heart muscle proteolysis.[57] Insulin also inhibits intracellular protein degradation in isolated hepatocytes, an effect that depends on internalization of insulin by the cells.[57] In addition to inhibiting release, insulin stimulates accumulation of amino acids in skeletal muscle. Of the six identified amino acid transport systems, insulin stimulates two, the A and the X systems.[58] Prior exercise may potentiate insulin's ability to increase amino acid uptake by muscle tissues.[59] When added to isolated muscle preparations, insulin promotes incorporation of labeled amino acids into tissue protein.[60] Glucose appears capable of lowering plasma amino acid levels through a mechanism independent of its effect on insulin secretion;[61] this finding suggests that glucose directly or indirectly affects amino acid metabolism in peripheral tissues. Recently, glucose infusions have been shown to increase de novo alanine synthesis, an important factor in interorgan nitrogen transfer.[62]

Insulin stimulates the incorporation of amino acids into protein tissues of normal animals, except in the liver, in which action of the hormone is evident only in diabetic preparations. Amino acid incorporation into diaphragm protein is stimulated by insulin,[63] and one also sees increased conversion of amino acids synthesized in muscle into tissue protein. Thus, insulin stimulates protein synthesis as well as amino acid uptake. Insulin stimulates the incorporation of labeled precursors into nucleic acid.[64] Although insulin increases RNA synthesis in muscle, the increase does not appear to be a requisite for hormone-mediated stimulation of protein synthesis, as shown by the observation that actinomycin, an inhibitor of RNA synthesis, did not impair the ability of insulin to increase protein synthesis.[65]

The importance of insulin in the regulation of protein balance has been most clearly demonstrated in subjects with type I diabetes (IDDM), who rapidly develop negative nitrogen balance when insulin therapy is discontinued. In the heart and most skeletal muscles studied, the absolute protein content, that is, the quantity of protein per tissue or organ, was much less in diabetic animals than in control animals. In contrast, the protein content of liver was unaffected in diabetic animals.[66] The most significant loss of protein in vivo, as the result of insulin deficiency, occurs in muscle. Studies using stable isotopes of amino acids to examine rates of whole-body protein turnover and oxidation have demonstrated increased rates of protein degradation and leucine oxidation in insulin-deprived subjects with IDDM; these rates could be decreased by insulin infusions.[67] In vitro and animal studies have shown decreased rates of protein synthesis in diabetes.[68,69] In contrast, increased rates of protein synthesis were found in insulin-deprived human subjects with IDDM, although protein breakdown was even more markedly accelerated.[70] The postulated

mechanism for this increase in protein synthesis in vivo is that accelerated protein degradation provides increased intracellular free amino acid concentrations as precursors for protein synthesis. Several studies have reported resistance to insulin-mediated suppression of branched-chain amino acid (BCAA) plasma concentrations,[71] as well as rates of BCAA turnover and oxidation,[72] in IDDM. Thus, it appears that diabetics are insulin resistant with respect to amino acid, as well as glucose, metabolism.

Glucagon's actions on amino acid metabolism are threefold: (1) to increase membrane transport of amino acids; (2) to decrease protein synthesis and increase catabolism; and (3) to increase amino acid conversion into glucose (gluconeogenesis).[73]

Glucagon increases gluconeogenesis in perfused liver, an effect that can be reproduced by perfusion with cAMP. Glucagon increases hepatic use of glycine, alanine, glutamate, and phenylalanine for gluconeogenesis. In addition to increasing gluconeogenesis, glucagon increases the rates of ureagenesis.

In fasted human subjects, during early starvation one sees an increase in plasma glucagon, and a decrease in insulin, concentrations, associated with increased rates of gluconeogenesis and ureagenesis. Splanchnic extraction of alanine is increased from 43% in the postabsorptive state to 71% after 3 days of fasting, but it decreases to 53% after 6 weeks of fasting.[74] During prolonged starvation, the brain adapts by developing the capacity to use ketone bodies as an energy source and thereby decreases the need for increased rates of gluconeogenesis.

Glucagon is able to increase liver protein catabolism in the intact animal. Liver protein content is decreased and BCAA release from the liver is increased by glucagon. This increased protein catabolism can be suppressed by the administration of insulin or a mixture of amino acids.

As mentioned previously, a common feature of patients with glucagonoma syndrome is hypoaminoacidemia. When similar degrees of hyperglucagonemia are produced by infusions of glucagon in normal volunteers, reductions in blood amino acid concentrations are similar.[75] High-protein diets can normalize the plasma amino acid profile and may cause a positive nitrogen balance in glucagonoma syndrome.[76] When glucagon deficiency is produced by infusions of somatostatin with insulin replacement, amino acid concentrations are increased.[76a] That urinary urea nitrogen and total nitrogen excretion rates are lower during glucagon deficiency than during glucagon excess suggests that alterations in the rate of gluconeogenesis are one mechanism by which glucagon controls blood amino acid levels.

## THYROID HORMONES

These hormones influence the metabolism of carbohydrates, lipids, and proteins.

### Carbohydrate Metabolism

Thyroid hormones exert multiple effects on carbohydrate metabolism. Patients with hyperthyroidism frequently (30 to 50%) display mild-to-moderate degrees of glucose intolerance.[77–79] Part of this abnormality is attributable to more rapid gastric emptying and intestinal absorption of glucose in hyperthyroidism,[80] whereas glucose absorption is delayed in hypothyroidism.

Rates of hepatic glucose production are increased by 20% in the basal state, and the liver is less sensitive to insulin infusions in hyperthyroid human subjects.[81] Hepatic glycogen stores are reduced in states of thyroid hormone excess. Thyroid hormones appear to modulate the magnitude of the glycogenolytic and hyperglycemic actions of epinephrine and norepinephrine, possibly by enhancing the responsiveness of the adenylate cyclase-cAMP system. In rats, thyroid hormone exerts a biphasic effect on liver glycogen. Small doses of thyroid hormone increase glycogen synthesis in the presence of insulin, whereas large doses augment hepatic glycogenolysis. Small doses of thyroid hormone enhance, and large doses depress, the glycogenolytic response to epinephrine.[82] That the glycogen content of liver and muscle tissues is decreased in hypothyroidism possibly reflects a new balance between simultaneously decreased rates of glycogen synthesis and degradation.[83]

Rates of gluconeogenesis are also increased in hyperthyroidism, in part because of an increase in substrate supply from protein breakdown and lipolysis. The splanchnic uptake of gluconeogenic precursors is also increased by 20 to 120% in hyperthyroidism.[81] Gluconeogenesis is suppressed in hypothyroidism. The in vitro addition of $T_3$ to hypothyroid hepatocytes stimulates hepatic gluconeogenesis by approximately 80 to 90% within 30 to 40 min.[83]

Rates of total glucose disposal during euglycemic, hyperinsulinemic clamp studies have been shown to be normal; this finding suggests that skeletal muscle is not insulin resistant in hyperthyroidism.[84] Rates of glucose oxidation are increased twofold, however.

Total body glucose turnover rates are increased in thyrotoxicosis. A major fraction of the increased glucose turnover is accounted for by increases in glucose recycling. Recycling, through both the Cori (glucose-lactate) and the glucose-alanine cycles, is increased in hyperthyroidism and is decreased in hypothyroidism.[83]

### Lipid Metabolism

Thyroid hormones also have an impact on multiple aspects of lipid metabolism, including lipid synthesis, mobilization, and degradation. Degradation is affected more than synthesis, so the net effect of excess thyroid hormone is a decrease in total body lipid stores and plasma concentrations. Thyroid hormones increase lipolysis in adipose tissue, both by directly stimulating cAMP production and by increasing the sensitivity to other lipolytic agents, such as catecholamines, TSH, ACTH, growth hormone, glucocorticoids, and glucagon. Conversely, lipolysis is impaired in hypothyroidism.

The delivery of FFA to peripheral tissues and to the liver is increased in hyperthyroidism. FFA turnover rates are increased approximately twofold in thyrotoxicosis.[85] That lipid oxidation rates are also increased in thyrotoxicosis may contribute to the calorigenic action of thyroid hormones.

Hepatic triglyceride synthesis is increased in hyperthyroidism, in large part because of the increased delivery of FFA and glycerol to the liver. The synthesis and clearance of cholesterol and triglyceride are accelerated in hyperthyroidism; the clearance effect predominates. Modest reductions in serum cholesterol and triglyceride levels are usually present.[86] Conversely, serum lipid levels may be increased in hypothyroidism because of impaired clearance. Lipoprotein lipase activity in both hepatic and adipose tissue has been reported to be low in hypothyroidism.[87,88]

### Protein Metabolism

With regard to protein metabolism, the short-term administration of thyroid hormones increases liver protein and RNA content, with a concomitant decrease in muscle protein. During more prolonged administration of these hormones, both liver and peripheral tissues decrease in size.[89] Thyroid hormone increases both amino acid uptake by the liver and incorporation of amino acids into protein by isolated liver microsomes and mitochondria.[90] That this second effect does not occur in the presence of actinomycin suggests that these effects of thyroid hormone are mediated by DNA transcription and RNA translation.[91]

Clinically, a great excess of thyroid hormone appears to have the opposite effect, with suppressed rates of protein synthesis,[92] increased catabolism of collagen,[93] and increased forearm amino acid release in human subjects.[94] Nitrogen excretion is increased in thyrotoxicosis, and nitrogen balance may be normal or negative, depending on whether intake is sufficient to meet the increased demand.

In hypothyroidism, rates of protein synthesis and degradation are both decreased. Patients are usually in positive nitrogen balance. Treatment of myxedema is accompanied by mobilization of extracellular protein and a marked temporary negative nitrogen balance. Total serum protein concentrations are usually normal in hypothyroidism.

## GLUCOCORTICOIDS

Corticosteroids in excess are known to produce increases in plasma insulin and glucose concentrations, that is, a state of insulin resistance. This insulin resistance is out of proportion to the degree of obesity seen in Cushing's syndrome.[95] Glucose intolerance in Cushing's syndrome has been reported to be present in 80 to 90% of patients, although overt diabetes occurs in only 15 to 20% of subjects.[96,97]

### Glucose and Glycogen Metabolism

Glucocorticoids counteract the effects of insulin at numerous steps in glucose homeostasis. Rates of gluconeogenesis are augmented by several mechanisms: (1) increased release of gluconeogenic precursors, that is, amino acids and lactate,[98,99] from peripheral tissues; and (2) increased activity of key gluconeogenic enzymes,[100] including pyruvate carboxylase and PEP carboxykinase. PEP carboxykinase is important in this regard because it is the unidirectional rate-limiting enzyme in the initiation of the gluconeogenic cascade from pyruvate. In addition, conditions of glucocorticoid excess result in stimulation of glucagon secretion by pancreatic alpha cells.[98,101] This effect may be the result of increased proteolysis and hyperaminoacidemia. Corticosteroids act in conjunction with glucagon to increase rates of gluconeogenesis in perfused rat liver.[102]

Glucocorticoids stimulate hepatic glycogen deposition and, in this regard, resemble the action of insulin. The carbon source for this new liver glycogen is derived from breakdown of muscle protein with release of amino acids. The activity of glycogen synthase, the rate-limiting enzyme for glycogen synthesis, is decreased in rats that have undergone adrenalectomy and is restored to normal by corticosteroid treatment.

In addition to increasing glucose production from amino acids and lactate, an excess of corticosteroids also results in diminished glucose use by muscle and adipose tissues, by multiple mechanisms.[103–105] These mechanisms include: (1) decreased activity of the plasma membrane glucose transport system;[106] (2) decreased insulin binding to its receptor through decreases in receptor affinity and number;[107,108] and (3) a defect at the postreceptor level.[105,109] The hyperglycemic action of glucocorticoids is amplified if levels of glucagon, catecholamines, or growth hormone are also increased.[110,111]

### Lipid Metabolism

Glucocorticoids appear to exert a permissive effect on lipolysis through activation of cAMP-dependent, hormone-sensitive lipase in the adipocyte. Epinephrine-induced lipolysis is prompted by cortisol,[112] which appears necessary for the full stimulation of lipolysis by catecholamines.[113] Glucocorticoids are similarly required for the maximal lipolytic action of growth hormone. Cortisol's lipolytic action is prevented by inhibitors of protein synthesis.[114]

Prolonged treatment with glucocorticoids may result in increased plasma triglyceride concentrations,[115] but this effect is most often seen in the presence of diabetes mellitus and reflects impaired triglyceride removal. LDL uptake and degradation by cultured fibroblasts and smooth muscle cells are also impaired by high doses of glucocorticoids.[116] Long-term glucocorticoid treatment may result in a "fatty liver," owing to increased lipolysis and FFA delivery associated with enhanced hepatic uptake of FFA.

Long-term administration of excess corticosteroids also produces increases in total body fat in humans and in experimental animals. Pair-feeding experiments suggest that increased food intake is the major factor producing obesity in steroid-treated rats.[117] Changes in body fat distribution are also characteristic of Cushing's syndrome, with accumulations of fat in the supraclavicular, truncal, and facial areas.[118] The reason for this regional fat deposition in states of glucocorticoid excess is unknown.

ACTH administration stimulates lipolysis through cAMP-mediated activation of hormone-sensitive lipase in adipose tissue. This effect is demonstrable in animals that have undergone adrenalectomy,[119] and therefore it does not depend on corticosteroid secretion.

### Protein Metabolism

One of the major metabolic effects of glucocorticoids is stimulation of skeletal muscle protein breakdown. Many of the clinical features of Cushing's syndrome, such as the loss of bone density, increased capillary fragility and dermal atrophy, muscle wasting, and growth retardation in children, are at least in part due to this augmented proteolysis. It has recently been shown that 5 days of physical training were able to reverse the muscle wasting present in patients taking low-to-moderate doses of prednisone.[120] In addition to increasing protein breakdown, corticosteroids appear to inhibit incorporation of amino acids into muscle protein.[121,122] Elevations of cortisol within the physiologic range have been shown to augment muscle proteolysis, with increased de novo alanine synthesis and muscle glutamine release.[123,124] Together, alanine and glutamine account for 60 to 65% of amino acid nitrogen exported from skeletal muscle during conditions of stress or following glucocorticoid treatment.[125] Alanine is transported to the liver, where it serves as a substrate for gluconeogenesis. Recent studies have shown that the major organ removing glutamine in the dexamethasone-treated dog is the gastrointestinal tract,[126] but glutamine may also be used by the kidney for gluconeogenesis.

In contrast to these effects on muscle tissues, corticosteroids have been shown to increase liver protein content. Administration of glucocorticoids increases the protein and RNA contents of liver and other viscera.[127] Amino acids delivered as a result of enhanced muscle proteolysis are transported to the liver, where they can be used for protein synthesis. Administration of cortisol to rats enhances hepatic uptake of alpha-amino-isobutyric acid,[122] as well as of increased free amino nitrogen concentrations in the liver.[128] These effects of glucocorticoids depend on the diet; increased protein synthesis occurs when the caloric and protein contents of the diet are adequate.

## GROWTH HORMONE AND SOMATOMEDIN-C (IGF I)

When discussing the metabolic effects of growth hormone, it is important to distinguish the direct effects of growth hormone from those of somatomedin-C. Somatomedin-C is synthesized by liver and other tissues in response to stimulation by growth hormone, although nutritional uptake appears to have a direct effect on somatomedin-C production. In normal human volunteers, somatomedin-C levels declined 60 to 70% during a 5-day fast.[129] Studies in the rat have shown that both adequate dietary protein and total energy contents are necessary for maintenance of somatomedin concentrations.[130] The "somatomedin hypothesis" states that many of the anabolic, growth-promoting effects of growth hormone are mediated by somatomedin-C, whereas growth hormone has direct catabolic effects on glucose and lipid metabolism.

## Metabolic Effects

A biphasic response to the short-term administration of growth hormone is seen. During the initial 2 hours after administration, growth hormone exhibits an insulin-like effect; it lowers plasma glucose levels by directly stimulating beta-cell insulin secretion,[131] as well as by stimulating glucose use in peripheral tissues. Whereas this effect has been demonstrated in animals that have undergone hypophysectomy,[132] growth hormone does not produce hypoglycemia in normal subjects. From 2 to 12 hours after short-term administration, growth hormone has anti-insulin effects. This state of insulin resistance is due to a postreceptor defect in peripheral glucose use, coupled with slight impairment in hepatic sensitivity to insulin.[133]

During long-term administration in animals and humans, growth hormone produces an insulin-resistant state. Glucose intolerance in acromegaly has been reported in 60 to 70% of patients, although elevations in fasting plasma glucose concentrations are reported to occur in only 6 to 25% of those with acromegaly.[134–137] Even more striking than glucose intolerance is the hyperinsulinemia and resistance to insulin that occur in acromegaly.[137] In most patients, increased insulin secretion compensates for the insulin-resistant state. Long-term administration of excess growth hormone increases the rates of hepatic glucose production and decreases glucose use by peripheral tissues.[138,139] Decreased peripheral glucose use is likely the result of defects in insulin action at both receptor and postreceptor sites.[140] Elevations in plasma FFA and ketone bodies inhibit glucose use by muscle tissue and may, in part, explain the postreceptor defect seen in acromegaly.[141] Successful treatment of acromegaly results in improved glucose tolerance and reductions in serum insulin concentrations in most patients.[135,142,143]

Whereas chronic elevations in growth hormone concentrations produce anti-insulin effects, many of the actions of somatomedin-C (IGF I) mimic those of insulin. This finding is not surprising when one considers the structural similarities in tertiary configuration between somatomedin-C and proinsulin.[144] IGF I has been shown to increase glucose transport,[145] as well as rates of glycolysis and glycogen synthesis,[146] in heart and skeletal muscle tissues.

In contrast to acromegaly, chronic growth hormone deficiency produces increased insulin sensitivity. This sensitivity is not usually associated with hypoglycemia, although occasionally, the adaptations in pancreatic islet cell secretion are inadequate to prevent fasting hypoglycemia. Such hypoglycemia is more often seen when deficiencies of growth hormone and cortisol coexist.

The effects of short-term growth hormone administration on lipid metabolism are similar to those described previously for glucose. Within the first few hours after growth hormone is given, reductions in plasma FFA concentrations are seen. In addition, reduced rates of epinephrine-stimulated lipolysis have been described in rats that have undergone hypophysectomy during this early period following administration of growth hormone.[147] Thereafter, increased rates of lipolysis are seen, associated with enhanced rates of FFA oxidation by muscle and ketogenesis in the liver.[148] In addition to increasing FFA delivery to the liver, growth hormone also appears to exert a direct hepatic effect to increase ketogenesis.[149] Studies in humans have shown that growth hormone produces significant increases in lipolysis and ketogenesis only in the presence of insulin deficiency, either induced by somatostatin administration or in subjects with IDDM.[150–153] Growth-hormone-mediated lipolysis is similar to that induced by glucocorticoids, in that a lag time of at least an hour is required before the effect can be observed, and the lipolytic effects can be blocked by inhibitors of protein synthesis.[154]

In contrast to the effects of growth hormone on lipid metabolism, somatomedin-C has been shown to increase lipogenesis and to inhibit epinephrine-stimulated lipolysis in adipose tissue.[155]

One of the major effects of growth hormone is the promotion of linear growth and skeletal maturation. Somatomedin-C is responsible for these effects and increases synthesis of DNA, RNA, and protein in fibroblasts and chondrocytes.[156] Extraskeletal effects include increased rates of protein synthesis and cell proliferation. Animals made deficient in growth hormone by hypophysectomy develop a negative nitrogen balance and decreased protein and RNA contents in various tissues. Growth hormone administration is able to stimulate amino acid uptake and incorporation into protein in both liver and skeletal muscle tissues.[157] This process involves translation of existing RNA, rather than new RNA synthesis, although the new RNA synthesis is also stimulated.

## CATECHOLAMINES: EPINEPHRINE, NOREPINEPHRINE

The catecholamines are epinephrine, norepinephrine, and dopamine. Norepinephrine is secreted from the sympathetic neurons throughout the body and, to a limited extent, from the adrenal medulla. The principal secretory product of the adrenal medulla is epinephrine. Both epinephrine

and norepinephrine have alpha- and beta-agonist activities, although norepinephrine predominantly produces alpha-adrenergic effects. The major stimuli to sympathetic nervous system stimulation and adrenomedullary secretion are physical exercise, trauma, cold exposure, emotional stress, and hypoglycemia. Although combined increases in epinephrine and norepinephrine secretion occur with most stresses, hypoglycemia predominantly augments epinephrine secretion.[158] Epinephrine appears to be critical for recovery from hypoglycemia only in the absence of glucagon, however.[159]

### Carbohydrate Metabolism

Catecholamines have multiple effects on carbohydrate metabolism (Fig. 31–2). Alpha-adrenergic stimulation inhibits insulin secretion, whereas beta-stimulation augments insulin release. The alpha-adrenergic inhibitory effects on pancreatic beta-cell function generally prevail under conditions of stress or sympathetic nerve stimulation. Both alpha- and beta-adrenergic stimulation appear to augment pancreatic glucagon secretion.[160,161]

Catecholamines increase glycogen breakdown in liver and muscle tissues. Beta-adrenergic stimulation activates phosphorylase and inhibits glycogen synthase, through a cAMP-dependent mechanism. In addition, the alpha-adrenergic system is able to activate phosphorylase and to inhibit glycogen synthase, through a cAMP-independent mechanism involving membrane calcium transport.[162–165] Liver glycogenolysis appears to be mediated predominantly through alpha-adrenergic, cAMP-dependent, mechanisms. This suggestion is derived from in vitro data showing inhibition of catecholamine-mediated hepatic glycogenolysis (and gluconeogenesis) by alpha-adrenergic, but not beta-adrenergic, blocking drugs.[164–166] A recent study in conscious dogs reports contradictory findings, however.[167] In contrast, skeletal muscle glycogenolysis is mediated by beta-adrenergic stimulation of adenylate cyclase,[168] and it does not appear to be affected by alpha-adrenergic mechanisms.[162,169] The effects of catecholamines on muscle glycogen metabolism are antagonized by insulin and are dependent on glucocorticoids.[170–172]

As mentioned, catecholamines also stimulate hepatic gluconeogenesis through alpha-adrenergic mechanisms. Catecholamines increase the delivery of gluconeogenic precursors to the liver through the lipolytic (glycerol) and muscle glycogenolytic (lactate and pyruvate) actions. In addition, alpha-adrenergic agonists increase hepatic uptake of amino acids and possibly of lac-

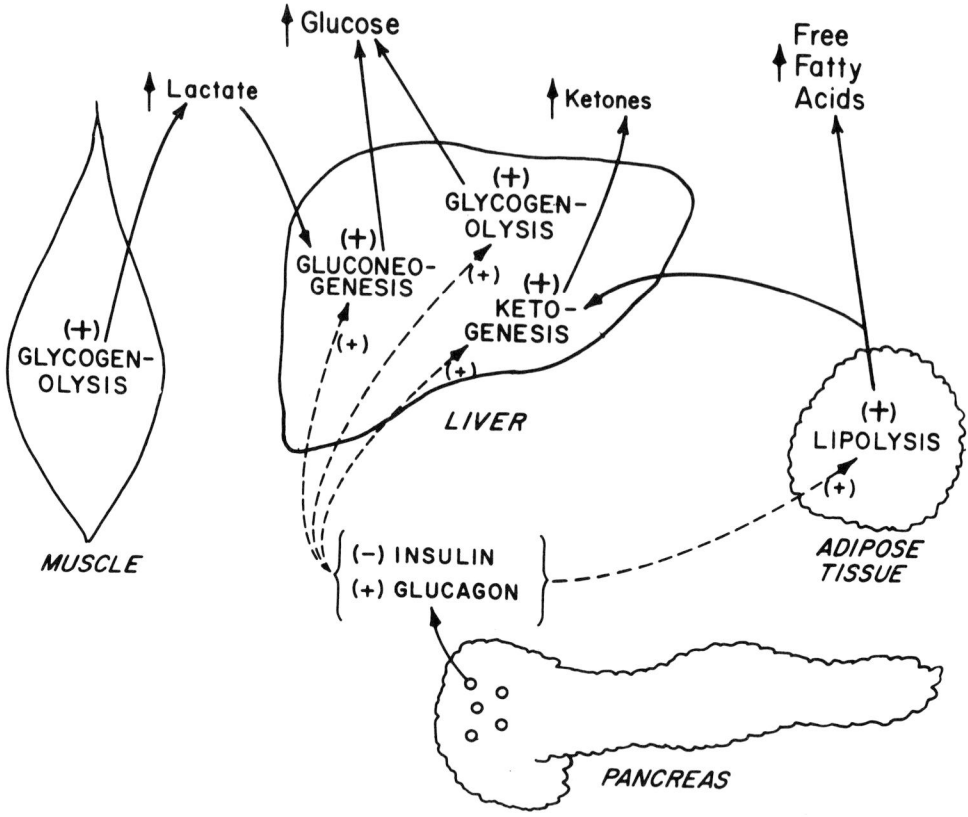

**Fig. 31–2.** Catecholamine effects on fuel mobilization in liver, adipose tissue, and muscle. Direct effects are reinforced by (but do not require) catecholamine-mediated suppression of insulin and stimulation of glucagon. (+ = stimulation; − = inhibition) (From Bondy, P.K., Rosenberg, L.E.: Metabolic Control and Disease. 8th Ed. Philadelphia, W.B. Saunders, 1980.)

tate.[173,174] The decreases in circulating insulin, and increases in glucagon, concentrations following sympathetic stimulation also promote glycogenolysis and gluconeogenesis.

Infusions of epinephrine resulting in physiologic elevations of plasma concentrations inhibit insulin-stimulated glucose uptake by peripheral tissues, even when plasma glucose and insulin concentrations are controlled by the insulin clamp technique.[175,176] In contrast to these short-term responses, long-term administration of terbutaline, a beta-adrenergic agonist, has resulted in significant increases in peripheral insulin sensitivity during insulin clamp studies.[177]

### Lipid Metabolism

The major effect of catecholamines on lipid metabolism is augmentation of lipolysis. Both epinephrine and norepinephrine activate hormone-sensitive lipase in adipose tissue, liver, heart, and skeletal muscle. Stimulation of lipolysis is dependent on cAMP and is mediated through beta-1-adrenergic stimulation of adenylate cy-

clase.[178,179] Alpha-2-adrenergic stimulation has an antilipolytic effect,[178] although this action may not be of physiologic importance. Many other hormonal factors affect catecholamine-induced lipolysis; insulin plays a major opposing role. Thus, catecholamine inhibition of insulin secretion is important in promoting lipolysis.

In addition to promoting lipolysis, catecholamines also increase lipogenesis and ketogenesis. Hepatic triglyceride synthesis is increased by adrenergic stimulation, although this effect is predominantly due to increased FFA delivery resulting from enhanced lipolysis.[168] Augmented ketogenesis is also partly the result of increased FFA delivery to the liver, although other mechanism(s) coexist. Norepinephrine produces dose-dependent increases in ketogenesis in isolated rat hepatocytes, without increasing FFA uptake.[180] In the postabsorptive dog, norepinephrine augments ketogenesis, whereas epinephrine has antiketogenic effects.[181]

Catecholamines also produce increases in plasma lipid levels. Cholesterol synthesis is increased following epinephrine administration, through activation of 3-hydroxy-3-methylglutaryl-COA reductase.[182-184] Triglyceride levels increase acutely during catecholamine infusions,[185] but they are not elevated after long-term administration.

## Protein Metabolism

Catecholamines have insulin-like effects on plasma amino acid levels. Infusions of epinephrine that produce plasma concentrations similar to those seen during acute stress decrease total amino acid levels, although alanine concentrations are unchanged.[186] This effect occurs in the absence of insulin secretion (in type I diabetics) and can be prevented by beta-adrenergic blockade with propranolol.

## SEX STEROIDS AND PROLACTIN

Disturbed fuel metabolism is seen in several conditions of altered sex steroid and prolactin secretion.

### Testosterone and Estrogen

Testosterone administration to hypogonadal or castrated men decreases urinary nitrogen excretion and results in weight gain.[187] A major component of this weight gain is augmentation of skeletal muscle mass, most prominently in the pectoral and shoulder girdle areas. In normal men, pharmacologic doses of androgens produce only about half the nitrogen retention seen in hypogonadal men, and the effect is short lived. Attempts to improve the rate of nitrogen repletion using androgens in patients suffering from catabolic illness have had minimal or no therapeutic benefit.[188] The increases in weight from androgens in such individuals are probably due to stimulation of appetite and increased food intake.

Estrogen therapy, as used in oral contraceptive preparations, has been reported to exacerbate mild diabetes mellitus. The recent literature suggests that it is the progestogen component, specifically the 19-nortestosterone derivatives, of oral contraceptives that alters glucose tolerance, however. Newer, low-dose compounds do not appear to affect carbohydrate metabolism adversely.[189]

Pharmacologic doses of estrogens influence the production and removal rates of plasma lipoproteins. Plasma concentrations of VLDL cholesterol are increased by enhanced hepatic production rates.[190] In contrast, the clearance of LDL is enhanced by estrogens. This effect has led to the therapeutic use of estrogens in some types of familial hypercholesterolemia; the most striking results have been seen in women with familial dysbetalipoproteinemia (type II) and in some postmenopausal women with heterozygous familial hypercholesterolemia (type II).[191] Whereas estrogens produce significant increases in plasma high-density lipoprotein (HDL) cholesterol levels, the progestogens of the 19-nortestosterone series lower HDL concentrations.[192]

In pharmacologic doses, estrogens inhibit somatic growth. This effect may be mediated by the suppression of somatomedin-C generation, as demonstrated in hypopituitary subjects treated with growth hormone.[193]

### Prolactin

Prolactin has a weak stimulatory effect on somatomedin-C generation in patients with prolactin-secreting pituitary tumors.[194] Prolactin administration to growth-hormone-deficient human subjects mimics many of the actions of growth hormone and produces nitrogen retention, lipid mobilization, glucose intolerance, and modest skeletal growth.

## REFERENCES

1. Kahn, C.R.: Clin. Res. *31*:326–335, 1983.
2. Kasuga, M., Zick, Y., Blithe, D.L., et al.: Nature *298*:667–669, 1982.
3. Park, C.R., Morgan, H.E., Henderson, M.J., et al.: Recent Prog. Horm. Res. *17*:493–538, 1961.
4. Wardzala, L.J., Cushman, S.W., Salans, L.B.: J. Biol. Chem. *253*:8,002–8,005, 1978.
5. Wardzala, L.J., Jeanrenaud, B.: J. Biol. Chem. *256*:7,090–7,093, 1981.
6. Hertz, M.M., Paulson, O.B., Barry, D.I., et al.: J. Clin. Invest. *67*:597–604, 1981.
7. Debons, A.F., Krimsky, I., From, A., et al.: Am. J. Physiol. *217*:1,114–1,118, 1969.
8. Curnow, R.T., Rayfield, E.J., George, D.T., et al.: Am. J. Physiol. *228*:80–87, 1975.
9. Parkes, J.L., Grieninger, G.: J. Biol. Chem. *260*:8,090–8,097, 1985.
10. Taunton, O.D., Stifel, F.B., Greene, H.L., et al.: J. Biol. Chem. *249*:7,228–7,239, 1974.
11. Aguilar-Parada, E., Eisentraut, A.M., Unger, R.H.: Diabetes *18*:717–723, 1969.
12. Owen, O.E., Morgan, A.P., Kemp, H.G., et al.: J. Clin. Invest. *46*:1,589–1,595, 1967.
13. Cahill, G.F., Herrera, M.G., Morgan, A.P., et al.: J. Clin. Invest. *45*:1,751–1,769, 1966.
14. Muller, W.A., Faloona, G.R., Aguilar-Parada, E., et al.: N. Engl. J. Med. *283*:109–115, 1970.
15. Unger, R.H., Ketterer, H., Dupre, J., et al.: J. Clin. Invest. *46*:630–645, 1967.
16. Bloom, S.R., Vaughan, N.J.A., Russell, R.C.G.: Lancet *2*:546–549, 1974.
17. Unger, R.H., Ohneda, A., Aguilar-Parada, E., et al.: J. Clin. Invest. *48*:810–822, 1969.
18. Aguilar-Parada, E., Eisentraut, A.M., Unger, R.H.: Am. J. Med. Sci. *257*:415–419, 1969.
19. Unger, R.H., Aguilar-Parada, E., Muller, W.A., et al.: J. Clin. Invest. *49*:837–848, 1970.
20. Samols, E., Tyler, J.M., Marks, V.: Glucagon-insulin interrelationships. *In* Glucagon: Molecular Physiology, Clinical and Therapeutic Implications. Edited by P.J. Lefebvre and R.H. Unger. New York, Pergamon Press, 1972, pp. 151–173.

21. Samols, E., Weir, G.C., Bonner-Weir, S.: Intraislet insulin-glucagon-somatostatin relationships. *In* Glucagon. Vol. 2. Edited by P.J. Lefebvre. Berlin, Springer, 1983, pp. 133–173.
22. Unger, R.H.: Diabetologia *20*:1–11, 1981.
23. Unger, R.H., Madison, L.L., Muller, W.A.: Diabetes *21*:301–307, 1972.
24. Buchanan, K.D., McCarroll, A.M.: Lancet *2*:1,394–1,395, 1972.
25. Raskin, P., Aydin, I., Yamamoto, T., et al.: Am. J. Med. *64*:988–997, 1978.
26. Raskin, P., Pietri, A., Unger, R.H.: Diabetes *28*:1,033–1,035, 1979.
27. Rosen, S.G., Clutter, W.E., Berk, M.A.: J. Clin. Invest. *73*:405–411, 1984.
28. White, N.H., Skor, D., Cryer, P.E., et al.: N. Engl. J. Med. *308*:485–491, 1983.
29. Santiago, J.V., White, N.H., Skor, D.A., et al.: Am. J. Physiol. *247*:E215–E220, 1984.
30. Rodbell, M.: The actions of glucagon at its receptor: regulation of adenylate cyclase. *In* Glucagon. Vol. 1. Edited by P.J. Lefebvre. Berlin, Springer, 1983, pp. 263–290.
31. Liljenquist, J.E., Mueller, G.L., Cherrington, A.D., et al.: J. Clin. Invest. *59*:369–374, 1977.
32. Boyd, M.E., Albright, E.B., Foster, D.W., et al.: J. Clin. Invest. *68*:142–152, 1981.
33. Dobbs, S., Sakurai, H., Sasaki, H., et al.: Science *187*:544–547, 1975.
34. Mallinson, C.N., Bloom, S.R., Warin, A.P., et al.: Lancet *2*:1–5, 1974.
35. Wood, S.M., Polak, J.M., Bloom, S.R.: Glucagonoma syndrome. *In* Glucagon. Vol. 2. Edited by P.J. Lefebvre. Berlin, Springer, 1983, pp. 411–430.
36. Krejs, G.J., Orci, L., Conlon, J.M., et al.: N. Engl. J. Med. *301*:285–292, 1979.
37. Felig, P.: N. Engl. J. Med. *283*:149–150, 1970.
38. Taylor, S.I., Mukherjee, C., Jungas, R.L.: J. Biol. Chem. *248*:73–81, 1973.
39. Weber, G., Lea, M.A., Stamm, N.B.: Lipids *4*:388–396, 1969.
40. Bagdade, J.D., Porte, D., Bierman, E.L.: N. Engl. J. Med. *276*:427–433, 1967.
41. Kessler, J.I.: J. Clin. Invest. *42*:362–367, 1963.
42. Siperstein, M.D., Fagan, V.M.: J. Clin. Invest. *37*:1,185–1,195, 1958.
43. Butcher, R.W., Baird, C.E., Sutherland, E.W.: J. Biol. Chem. *243*:1,705–1,712, 1968.
44. Keirns, J.J., Freeman, J., Bitensky, M.W.: Am. J. Med. Sci. *268*:62–91, 1964.
45. Unger, R.H.: Diabetes *20*:834–838, 1971.
46. McGarry, J.D., Wright, P.H., Foster, D.W.: J. Clin. Invest. *55*:1,202–1,209, 1975.
47. Bierman, E.L.: Isr. J. Med. Sci. *8*:303–308, 1972.
48. Chait, A., Brunzell, J.D.: Metabolism *32*:209–214, 1983.
49. Tobey, T.A., Greenfield, M., Kraemer, F., et al.: Metabolism *30*:165–171, 1981.
50. Grundy, S.M., Mok, H.Y.I., Zech, L., et al.: J. Clin. Invest. *63*:1,274–1,283, 1979.
51. Kissebah, A.H., Alfarsi, S., Evans, D.J., et al.: Diabetes *31*:217–225, 1982.
52. Chait, A., Bierman, E.L., Albers, J.J.: J. Clin. Invest. *64*:1,309–1,319, 1979.
53. Pietri, A., Dunn, F.L., Raskin, P.: Diabetes *29*:1,001–1,005, 1980.
54. Kesaniemi, Y.A., Grundy, S.M.: Arteriosclerosis *3*:170–177, 1983.
55. Kissebah, A., Alfarsi, S., Evans, D.J., et al.: J. Clin. Invest. *71*:655–667, 1983.
56. Fukagawa, N.K., Minaker, K.L., Young, V.R., et al.: Am. J. Physiol. *250*:E13–E17, 1986.
57. Sugden, P.H., Smith, D.M.: Biochem. J. *206*:467–472, 1982.
58. Longo, N., Franchi-Gazzola, R., Bussolati, O., et al.: Biochim. Biophys. Acta *844*:216–223, 1985.
59. Zorzano, A., Balon, T.W., Garetto, L.P., et al.: Am. J. Physiol. *248*:E546–E552, 1985.
60. Jefferson, L.S., Robertson, J.W.: Diabetes *21 (Suppl. 1)*:341, 1972.
61. Adibi, S.A., Morse, E.L., Amin, P.M.: J. Lab. Clin. Med. *86*:395–409, 1975.
62. Robert, J.-J., Bier, D.M., Zhao, X.H., et al.: Metabolism *31*:1,210–1,218, 1982.
63. Wool, I.G., Krahl, M.E.: Nature *183*:1,399–1,400, 1959.
64. Wool, I.G.: Am. J. Physiol. *199*:719–721, 1960.
65. Davidson, M.B., Goodner, C.J.: Diabetes *15*:835–838, 1966.
66. Manchester, K.L.: Sites of hormonal regulation of protein metabolism. *In* Mammalian Protein Metabolism. Vol. 4. Edited by H.N. Munro. New York, Academic Press, 1970, pp. 229–298.
67. Umpleby, A.M., Boroujerdi, M.A., Brown, P.M., et al.: Diabetologia *29*:131–141, 1986.
68. Jefferson, L.J., Rannels, D.E., Munger, B.L., et al.: Fed. Proc. *33*:1,098–1,104, 1974.
69. Sloan, G.M., Norton, J.A., Brennan, M.F.: J. Surg. Res. *28*:442–448, 1980.
70. Nair, K.S., Garrow, J.S., Ford, C., et al.: Diabetologia *25*:400–403, 1983.
71. Trevisan, R., Nosadini, R., Avogaro, A., et al.: J. Clin. Endocrinol. Metab. *62*:1,155–1,162, 1986.
72. Tessari, P., Nosadini, R., Trevisan, R., et al.: J. Clin. Invest. *77*:1,797–1,804, 1986.
73. Marliss, E.B., Aoki, T.T., Cahill, G.F.: *In* Glucagon: Molecular Physiology, Clinical and Therapeutic Implications. Edited by P.J. Lefebvre and R.H. Unger. New York, Pergamon Press, 1972.
74. Felig, P., Owen, O.E., Wahren, J., et al.: J. Clin. Invest. *48*:584–594, 1969.
75. Liljenquist, J.E., Lewis, S.B., Cherrington, A.D., et al.: Metabolism *30*:1,195–1,199, 1981.
76. Abraira, C., DeBartolo, M., Katzen, R., et al.: Am. J. Clin. Nutr. *39*:351–355, 1984.
76a. Boden, G., Rezvani, I., Owen, O.E.: J. Clin. Invest. *73*:785–793, 1984.
77. Kreines, K., Jett, M., Knowles, H.C.: Diabetes *14*:740–744, 1965.
78. Doar, J.W.H., Stamp, T.C.B., Wynn, V., et al.: Diabetes *18*:633–639, 1984.
79. Maxon, H.R., Kreines, K.W., Goldsmith, R.E., et al.: Arch. Intern. Med. *135*:1,477–1,480, 1975.
80. Holdsworth, C.D., Besser, G.M.: Lancet *2*:700–702, 1908.
81. Wennlund, A., Felig, P., Hagenfeldt, L., et al.: J. Clin. Endocrinol. Metab. *62*:174–180, 1986.
82. Ingbar, S.H.: The thyroid gland. *In* Textbook of Endocrinology. Edited by J.D. Wilson and D.W. Foster. Philadelphia, W.B. Saunders, 1985, 682–815.
83. Muller, M.J., Seitz, H.J.: Klin. Wochenschr. *62*:11–18, 1984.
84. Randin, J.-P., Tappy, L., Scazziga, B., et al.: Diabetes *35*:178–181, 1986.
85. Saunders, J., Hall, S.E.H., Sonksen, P.H.: Clin. Endocrinol. *13*:33–44, 1980.

86. Agdeppa, D., Macaron, C., Mallik, T., et al.: J. Clin. Endocrinol. Metab. *49*:726–729, 1979.

87. Krauss, R.M., Levy, R.I., Fredrickson, D.S.: J. Clin. Invest. *54*:1,107–1,124, 1974.

88. Pykalisto, O., Goldbert, A.P., Brunzell, J.D.: J. Clin. Endocrinol. Metab. *43*:591–600, 1976.

89. Munro, H.N.: General aspects of the regulation of protein metabolism by diet and by hormones. *In* Mammalian Protein Metabolism. Vol. 1. Edited by H.N. Munro. New York, Academic Press, 1964, pp. 381–481.

90. Roche, J., Dumazert, C., Emond, Y., et al.: Compt. Rend. Soc. de Biol. *136*:326, 1942.

91. Sokoloff, L., Kaufman, S., Gelboin, H.V.: Biochim. Biophys. Acta *52*:410–412, 1961.

92. Crispell, K.R., Parson, W., Hollifield, G.: J. Clin. Invest. *35*:164–169, 1956.

93. Kivirikko, K.I., Laitinen, O., Aer, J., et al.: Endocrinology *80*:1,051–1,061, 1967.

94. Foley, T.H., London, D.R., Prenton, M.A.: J. Clin. Endocrinol. Metab. *26*:781–785, 1966.

95. Wajchenberg, B.L., Leme, C.E., Lerario, A.C., et al.: Diabetes *33*:455–459, 1984.

96. Plotz, C.M., Knowlton, A.J., Ragan, C.: Am. J. Med. *13*:597–614, 1952.

97. Pupo, A.A., Wajchenberg, B.L., Schnaider, J.: Diabetes *15*:24–29, 1966.

98. Wise, J.K., Hendler, R., Felig, P.: J. Clin. Invest. *52*:2,774–2,782, 1973.

99. Issekutz, B., Allen, M.: Metabolism *21*:48–59, 1972.

100. Wicks, W.D., Barnett, C.A., McKibbin, J.B.: Fed. Proc. *33*:1,105–1,111, 1974.

101. Marco, J., Calle, C., Roman, D., et al.: N. Engl. J. Med. *288*:128–132, 1973.

102. Eisenstein, A.B., Strack, I.: Endocrinology *83*:1,337–1,348, 1968.

103. Cahill, G.F.: *In* The Human Adrenal Cortex. Edited by N.P. Christy. New York, Harper and Row, 1971, pp. 205–238.

104. Livingston, I.N., Lockwood, D.H.: J. Biol. Chem. *250*:8,353–8,360, 1975.

105. Olefsky, J.M.: J. Clin. Invest. *56*:1,499–1,508, 1975.

106. Munck, A.: Perspect. Biol. Med. *14*: 265–289, 1971.

107. Olefsky, J.M., Johnson, J., Liu, F., et al.: Metabolism *24*:517–527, 1975.

108. Kahn, C.R., Goldfine, I.D., Neville, D.M., et al.: Endocrinology *103*:1,054–1,066, 1978.

109. Nosadini, R., DelPrato, S., Tiengo, A., et al.: J. Clin. Endocrinol. Metab. *57*:529–536, 1983.

110. Shamoon, H., Hendler, R., Sherwin, R.S.: J. Clin. Endocrinol. Metab. *52*:1,235–1,241, 1983.

111. Eigler, N., Sacca, L., Sherwin, R.S.: J. Clin. Invest. *63*:114–123, 1979.

112. Nayak, R.V., Feldman, E.B., Carter, A.C.: Proc. Soc. Exp. Biol. Med. *111*:682–686, 1962.

113. Shafrir, E., Steinberg, D.: J. Clin. Invest. *39*:310–319, 1960.

114. Fain, J.N.: Science *157*:1,062–1,064, 1967.

115. Bagdade, J.D., Porte, D., Bierman, E.L.: Arch. Intern. Med. *125*:129–134, 1970.

116. Henze, K., Chait, A., Albers, J.J., et al.: Eur. J. Clin. Invest. *13*:171–177, 1983.

117. Krotiewski, M., Bjorntorp, P.: Acta Endocrinol. *80*:667–675, 1975.

118. Lamberts, S.W.J., Birkenhager, J.C.: J. Clin. Endocrinol. Metab. *42*:864–868, 1976.

119. Engel, F.L.: Vitam. Horm. *19*:189–227, 1961.

120. Horber, F.F., Scheidegger, J.R., Grunig, B.E., et al.: J. Clin. Endocrinol. Metab. *61*:83–88, 1985.

121. Kostyo, J.L.: Endocrinology *76*:604–613, 1965.

122. Noall, M.W., Riggs, T.R., Walker, L.M., et al.: Science *126*:1,002–1,005, 1957.

123. Simmons, P.S., Miles, J.M., Gerich, J.E., et al.: J. Clin. Invest. *73*:412–420, 1984.

124. Muhlbacher, F., Kapadia, C.R., Colpoys, M.F., et al.: Am. J. Physiol. *247*:E75–E83, 1984.

125. Kapadia, C.R., Smith, R.J., Wilmore, D.W.: Surg. Forum. *33*:19–21, 1982.

126. Souba, W.W., Smith, R.J., Wilmore, D.W.: Metabolism *34*:450–456, 1985.

127. Clark, I.: J. Biol. Chem. *200*:69–76, 1953.

128. Weber, G., Srivastava, S.K., Singhal, R.L.: J. Biol. Chem. *240*:750–756, 1965.

129. Isley, W.L., Underwood, L.E., Clemmons, D.R.: J. Clin. Invest. *71*:175–182, 1983.

130. Phillips, L.S., Orawski, A.T., Belosky, D.C.: Endocrinology *103*:121–127, 1978.

131. Frohman, L.A., MacGillivray, M.H., Aceto, T.: J. Clin. Endocrinol. Metab. *27*:561–567, 1967.

132. Kostyo, J.L., Reagan, C.R.: Pharmacol. Ther. (B) *2*:591–604, 1976.

133. Bratusch-Marrain, P.R., Smith, D., DeFronzo, R.A.: J. Clin. Endocrinol. Metab. *55*:973–982, 1982.

134. Beck, P., Schalch, D.S., Parker, M.L., et al.: J. Lab. Clin. Med. *66*:366–379, 1965.

135. Sonksen, P.H., Greenwood, F.C., Ellis, J.P., et al.: J. Clin. Endocrinol. Metab. *27*:1,418–1,430, 1967.

136. Boden, G., Soeldner, J.S., Steinke, J., et al.: Metabolism *17*:1–9, 1968.

137. Emmer, M., Gorden, P., Roth, J.: Med. Clin. North Am. *55*:1,057–1,064, 1971.

138. Weil, R.: Acta Endocrinol. *(Suppl. 98)*:7–92, 1965.

139. Kipnis, D.M.: *In* The Nature and Treatment of Diabetes. Edited by B.S. Leibel and G.A. Wrenshall. New York, Excerpta Medica, 1965, p. 258.

140. Muggeo, M., Bar, R.S., Roth, J., et al.: J. Clin. Endocrinol. Metab. *48*:17–25, 1979.

141. Randle, P.J., Garland, P.B., Hales, C.N., et al.: Lancet *1*:785–789, 1963.

142. Luft, R., Cerasi, E., Hamberger, C.A.: Acta Endocrinol. *56*:593–607, 1967.

143. Eastman, R.C., Gordon, P., Roth, J.: J. Clin. Endocrinol. Metab. *48*:931–940, 1979.

144. Blundell, T.L., Bedarkar, S., Rinderknecht, E., et al.: Proc. Natl. Acad. Sci. U.S.A. *75*:180–184, 1978.

145. Meuli, C., Froesch, E.R.: Eur. J. Clin. Invest. *5*:93–99, 1975.

146. Froesch, E.R., Muller, W.A., Burgi, H., et al.: Biochem. Biophys. Acta *121*:360–374, 1966.

147. Goodman, H.M.: Metabolism *19*:849–855, 1970.

148. Goodman, H.M., Schwartz, J.: *In* The Pituitary Gland and Its Neuroendocrine Control. Part 2. Edited by R.O. Greep and E.B. Astwood. Washington, D.C., American Physiological Society, 1974.

149. Villar-Palasi, C., Larner, J.: Annu. Rev. Biochem. *39*:639–672, 1970.

150. Gerich, J.R., Lorenzi, M., Bier, D.M., et al.: J. Clin. Invest. *57*:875–884, 1976.

151. Metcalfe, P., Johnston, D.G., Nosadini, R., et al.: Diabetologia *20*:123–128, 1981.

152. Schade, D.S., Eaton, R.P., Peake, G.T.: Diabetes *27*:916–924, 1978.

153. Luft, R., Ikkos, D., Gemzell, C.A., et al.: Lancet *1*:721, 1958.

154. Fain, J.N., Dodd, A., Novak, L.: Metabolism *20*:109–118, 1971.

155. Zapf, J., Schoenle, E., Waldvogel, M., et al.: Eur. J. Biochem. *113*:605–609, 1981.
156. Zapf, J., Schoenle, E., Froesch, E.R.: Eur. J. Biochem. *87*:285–296, 1978.
157. Nutting, D.F.: Endocrinology *98*:1,273–1,283, 1976.
158. Garber, A.J., Cryer, P.E., Santiago, J.V., et al.: J. Clin. Invest. *58*:7–15, 1976.
159. Clarke, W.L., Santiago, J.V., Thomas, L., et al.: Am. J. Physiol. *236*:E147–E152, 1979.
160. Smith, P.H., Madson, K.L.: Diabetologia *20*:314–322, 1981.
161. Smith, P.H., Porte, D.: Annu. Rev. Pharmacol. Toxicol. *16*:269–285, 1976.
162. Exton, J.H.: Am. J. Physiol. *238*:E3–E12, 1980.
163. Kneer, N.M., Bosch, A.L., Clark, M.G., et al.: Proc. Natl. Acad. Sci. U.S.A. *71*:4,523–4,527, 1974.
164. Hutson, N.J., Brumley, F.T., Assimacopoulos, F.D., et al.: J. Biol. Chem. *251*:5,200–5,208, 1976.
165. Cherrington, A.D., Assimacopoulos, F.D., Harper, S.C., et al.: J. Biol. Chem. *251*:5,209–5,218, 1976.
166. Tolbert, M.E.M., Butcher, F.R., Fain, J.N.: J. Biol. Chem. *248*:5,686–5,692, 1973.
167. Steiner, K.E., Stevenson, R.W., Green, D.R., et al.: Metabolism *34*:1,020–1,023, 1985.
168. Himms-Hagen, J.: Effects of catecholamines on metabolism. *In* Catecholamines: Handbook of Experimental Pharmacology. Vol. 33. Edited by H. Blaschko and E. Muscholl. Berlin, Springer, 1972, pp. 363–462.
169. Dietz, M.R., Chiasson, J.-L., Soderling, T.R., et al.: J. Biol. Chem. *255*:2,301–2,307, 1980.
170. Shikama, H., Chiasson, J.-L., Exton, J.H.: J. Biol. Chem. *256*:4,450–4,454, 1981.
171. Foulkes, J.G., Cohen, P., Strada, S.J.: J. Biol. Chem. *257*:12,493–12,496, 1982.
172. Green, G.A., Chenoweth, M., Dunn, A.: Proc. Natl. Acad. Sci. U.S.A. *77*:5,711–5,715, 1980.
173. Exton, J.H., Park, C.R.: J. Biol. Chem. *243*:4,189–4,196, 1968.
174. Le Cam, A., Freychet, P.: Endocrinology *102*:379–385, 1978.
175. Abramson, E.A., Arky, R.A.: Diabetes *17*:141–146, 1968.
176. Chiasson, J.-L., Shikama, H., Chu, D.T.W., et al.: J. Clin. Invest. *68*:706–713, 1981.
177. Scheidegger, K., Robbins, D.C., Danforth, E.: Diabetes *33*:1,144–1,149, 1984.
178. Fain, J.N., Garcia-Sainz, J.A.: J. Lipid Res. *24*:945–966, 1983.
179. Belfrage, P., Fredrickson, G., Olsson, H., et al.: Control of adipose tissue lipolysis by phosphorylation/dephosphorylation of hormone-sensitive lipase. *In* The Adipocyte and Obesity: Cellular and Molecular Mechanisms. Edited by A. Angel, C.H. Holleberg, and D.A.K. Ronicari. New York, Raven Press, 1983, pp. 217–224.
180. Oberhaensli, R.D., Schwendimann, R., Keller, U.: Diabetes *34*:774–779, 1985.
181. Steiner, K.E., Fuchs, H., Williams, P.E., et al.: Diabetes *34*:425–432, 1985.
182. Edwards, P.A.: Arch. Biochem. Biophys. *170*:188–203, 1975.
183. Edwards, P., Lemongello, D., Fogelman, A.M.: J. Lipid Res. *20*:2–7, 1979.
184. George, R., Ramasarma, T.: Biochem. J. *162*:493–499, 1977.
185. Miller, H.I.: Metabolism *16*:1,096–1,105, 1967.
186. Shamoon, H., Jacob, R., Sherwin, R.S.: Diabetes *29*:875–881, 1980.
187. Wilson, J.D., Griffin, J.E.: Metabolism *29*:1,278–1,295, 1980.
188. Tweedle, D., Walton, C., Johnston, I.D.A.: Br. J. Clin. Pract. *27*:130–132, 1972.
189. Brooks, P.G.: J. Reproduct. Med. *29 (Suppl.)*:539–546, 1984.
190. Glueck, C.J., Fallat, R.W., Scheel, D.: Metabolism *24*:537–545, 1975.
191. Tikkanen, M.J., Nikkila, E.A., Vartiainen, E.: Lancet *2*:490–491, 1978.
192. Wahl, P., Walden, C., Knopp, R., et al.: N. Engl. J. Med. *308*:862–867, 1983.
193. Wiedemann, E., Schwartz, E.: J. Clin. Endocrinol. Metab. *34*:51–58, 1972.
194. Clemmons, D.R., Underwood, L.E., Ridgway, E.C., et al.: J. Clin. Endocrinol. Metab. *52*:731–735, 1981.

*Chapter* **32**

# NUTRITION AND IMMUNOLOGY

## Quentin N. Myrvik

Immunology, as a biologic subject, can be defined as a study of the immunity of living organisms to harmful agents. Early in the development of immunology it was recognized that specifically reacting glycoproteins were produced against foreign substances. These protective glycoproteins were called *antibodies* because they reacted and neutralized the "foreign bodies," which induced the production of the specific antibodies. The foreign proteins capable of inducing the formation of antibodies were called *antigens* because they *gen*erated *anti*body in the host.

Since serum antibodies are special glycoproteins called globulins and are concerned with immunity they are called *immunoglobulins*. Five classes of immunoglobulins are recognized,

namely, IgG, IgM, IgA, IgE, and IgD. The production of antibodies is commonly referred to as the humoral immune response.

The early development of immunology took place within the discipline of microbiology because of the numerous observations that individuals who recovered from infectious disease were specifically resistant to subsequent infections by the same microorganism.

Before the turn of the century it was observed that the serum of animals that had recovered from experimental diphtheritic infection contained specific glycoprotein molecules that neutralized the potent toxin produced by *Corynebacterium diphtheriae,* the etiologic agent of diphtheria.

It is well established that B-lymphocytes are the

cells responsible for antibody formation. In addition, another class of lymphocytes designated T-lymphocytes can mediate cell-mediated immunity directly as cytotoxic immune cells (tissue graft and tumor immunity) or through macrophages that are mobilized and activated by T-lymphocyte products (lymphokines). This latter system is primarily involved in antimicrobial immunity.

The scope of immunology has extended to essentially every aspect of biology and medicine. Subdisciplines now include immunochemistry, immunogenetics, immunopathology, immunopharmacology, and immunohematology.

Since the immune system is a complex interplay of many cell types, which results in cell proliferation and synthesis of a wide variety of chemical moieties, it is not surprising that malnutrition can influence the immune response. One can safely predict that studies on the effects of nutrition on the immune response will spawn a new subdiscipline.

## EVOLUTION OF THE IMMUNE SYSTEM

The biologic world comprises a multitude of plant and animal species. Although some species benefit from association with other species, each competes with and may be harmed by other species as well. Every individual is endowed with attributes for self-preservation and preservation of the species to which it belongs. It is almost axiomatic that every multicellular animal possesses mechanisms to distinguish between components of self and foreign substances and to oppose invasion of its body by potentially harmful foreign agents. In mammals the ability to distinguish between foreign antigens and antigens of self is vested in the lymphocyte and is one of many of the important expressions whereby cells can recognize foreign substances.

Cell recognition rests primarily on molecular cell surface configurations called receptors. Receptors represent discrete and intrinsic components imbedded within the fluid matrix of the cell membrane that can move independently within the membrane. Receptors endow cells with the ability to respond to various stimuli and mediate such diverse events as hormone stimulation, phagocytosis, organogenesis, and the immunologic activities of cells.

Early in evolution the multicellular animals developed a primitive circulation called the hemolymph system which included phagocytic cells capable of recognizing, engulfing, and often destroying foreign particles. Cells that carry out the specialized function of phagocytosis are some-

times termed professional phagocytes to distinguish them from certain other cells that under special circumstances can engage in phagocytosis. Ultimately, in the course of evolution, the lower animals developed the ability to synthesize nonspecific humoral factors of defense, especially antimicrobial factors. Certain invertebrates, however, including the annelids and the truncates, evolved with the ability to mount a form of specific cellular immunity mediated by the coelomocyte, a cell similar to the mammalian macrophage. There is no evidence that this immune response has been retained by invertebrates; however, vertebrates have expanded and modified the basic invertebrate system and have developed their own specific immune system.

Concomitant with the development of higher animals, complex lymphoreticular organs and specialized cells called lymphocytes emerged that were capable of mounting specific immune responses to foreign agents. This ability also included the unique capacity to respond specifically with accelerated and enhanced responsiveness upon re-exposure to the same agent (anamnesis or memory). Anamnesis is mediated by special lymphocytes that are generated during the immune response and are referred to as memory cells.

The manner by which higher animals exercise such an astounding ability to mount a specific immune response to a nearly infinite number of different antigens remains a central unsolved problem in immunology. It is known, however, that large numbers of clones of lymphocytes exist and that the cells of each clone can possess surface receptors of unique configuration that bind specifically to a complementary structure on the antigen molecule called the antigen determinant or epitope. Accordingly, specific binding of antigen molecules to specifically immunocompetent lymphocytes that possess complementary surface receptors can trigger the lymphocyte to replicate, expand the number of cells in the specific clone, and induce differentiation to an antibody-secreting cell. In the case of T cells, the cells multiply and expand the clones in the same way; although the receptor responsible for specific responsiveness is intrinsic to the membrane of the T cell, it is not an immunoglobulin.

It is convenient to view the total immune response as consisting of three phases. The first is the afferent phase during which the antigen is bound to the immunocompetent cell; during the central phase the stimulated cell differentiates and proliferates; and during the efferent or effector phase immune T cells and/or antibodies are generated by B cells and react with residual antigen or reintroduced antigen.

*Total immunity* represents the sum of innate immunity, which is mediated by constitutive non-specific humoral and cellular mechanisms and specific acquired or adaptive immunity. Acquired immunity is dependent principally on the specific activities of antibodies and immune T cells.

The terms *antimicrobial immunity* and *antitissue immunity* are often used. The former designates immunity against microorganisms, and the latter designates immunity against cells of foreign grafts or autochthonous (of self) tumors. In some instances individuals can mount a specific immune response against their own tissues and destroy them (autoimmunity).

## CELLS OF THE IMMUNE SYSTEM

Conceptually the mammalian immune system is divided into the central lymphoid system and the peripheral lymphoid system. The terms lymphoid and lymphatic are used synonymously. The central lymphoid system comprises the bone marrow, thymus, and the theoretic bursa equivalent, whereas the peripheral lymphoid system comprises the spleen, lymph nodes, tonsils, mucous membrane-associated lymphoid tissue, and other diffuse lymphoid tissues of the body. It should be emphasized that the differentiation and proliferation of lymphocytes within the central system do not involve antigen-sensitive stem cells and are not antigen driven; however, differentiation and proliferation of lymphocytes in the peripheral lymphoid system are antigen-driven events.

It is well established that the immune responses are mediated by numerous cell types and complex cell interactions. These cells include lymphocytes, macrophages, granulocytes, mast cells, and dendritic cells (accessory cells for antigen presentation). As noted later, these cell interactions usually take place within the specialized microenvironment of the various organ systems involved in the immune response. The following cells have various important functions with respect to the affector and effector mechanisms of total immunity.

### Granulocytes

Blood granulocytes, which are comprised of basophils, eosinophils, and neutrophils, are found in the blood as fully differentiated and short-lived cells 12 to 15 μm in diameter. They originate from a common progenitor in the bone marrow. Neutrophils are usually multilobed and are commonly referred to as polymorphonuclear leukocytes, whereas eosinophils and basophils tend to possess bilobed nuclei.

*Neutrophils* comprise about 70% of the circu-

lating blood leukocytes. They are short-lived cells that persist in circulation for only a few days at most and constantly leave vessels in small numbers to migrate into the tissues. They have a number of functions including the liberation of the fever-producing agent endogenous pyrogen and are active in the digestion of foreign material and dead tissue. Neutrophils provide the first line of phagocytic defense against many microorganisms as will be noted later. Neutrophils, as well as eosinophils, are attracted by immune complexes, particularly when the complement factor C5a is generated. Neutrophils and eosinophils engulf immune complexes mainly because they possess receptors for the Fc segment of the IgG molecule and a receptor for the C3b component of complement.

The human adult produces about 126 billion neutrophils every day. The body reserve is staggering. Possibly 25 billion neutrophils circulate in the blood and equal numbers are attached to the endothelium of the blood vessels in the process of moving out to the extravascular tissues. For every circulating neutrophil there are 100 more in the bone marrow. Within an hour 20 times the number of neutrophils in the blood can be mobilized from the bone marrow reserve.

*Eosinophils* comprise about 2 to 6% of the circulating leukocytes. They are characterized by coarse membrane-invested cytoplasmic granules that stain with the acid dye eosin. Granules are rich in hydrolytic enzymes, peroxidase, and major basic protein as well as eosinophilic cationic protein. Although their ability to inhibit or kill ingested microbes is limited, they can be an important effector cell in immunity against several animal parasitic infections.

The *basophil* normally comprises about 0.05 to 1% of the circulating leukocytes. It possesses receptors that bind to the Fc segment of the IgE molecule. Cytoplasm of the basophil is characterized by coarse basophilic cytoplasmic granules containing stores of various biologically active molecules. The *mast cell,* which is the functional counterpart of the basophil in tissues, is abundant in perivascular and peribronchiolar connective tissue adjacent to smooth muscle. Basophils and mast cells become activated and release mediators when IgE molecules are bound to their Fc receptors and are cross-linked by reacting with specific antigen. Mast cell rupture resulting from tissue trauma can also result in the release of mediators that can cause marked inflammation.

### Macrophages

Macrophages are large long-lived mononuclear phagocytic cells that range in diameter from about

12 to 25 μm. They arise from radiosensitive promonocytes in the bone marrow. Macrophage precursors (promonocytes and monocytes) pass continually from the bone marrow to the blood as small (12- to 15-μm) nonactivated cells. They comprise about 5% of the blood leukocytes. Many of the monocytes in the blood become fixed to vessel walls within organs such as the liver and the spleen, where they engage in phagocytic and pinocytic activity, which in turn induces their activation and maturation. Some monocytes migrate through vessel walls to reach extravascular sites and tissues such as body cavities, lung alveoli, lymphoid organs, and even the brain. Macrophages possess various surface receptors including Fc receptors that bind antibodies of the human subclasses IgG1, IgG3, as well as C3b from complement. Bound antibodies are important in specifically trapping and promoting phagocytosis of antigen in lymphoid structures. Bound antibodies to macrophages also enable the macrophage to adhere and attack the membranes of foreign mammalian cells containing the corresponding antigens. Macrophages play a major role in acquired cell-mediated immunity. In this case immune T cells secrete lymphokines that can mobilize and activate macrophages to the site of infection. Lymphokine-activated macrophages have an enhanced capability to kill microorganisms. In addition, they also have elevated levels of hydrolytic enzymes packaged in lysosomes. These enzymes include plasminogen activator, collagenase, elastase, proteases, and lysozyme. Macrophages can also function in processing and presenting antigens to lymphocytes.

### Lymphocytes

Lymphocytes play the central role in mediating specific acquired immunity. A normal human adult possesses approximately $10^{12}$ lymphocytes, most of which reside in the lymphoid organ systems. The source of the stem cell progenitor of all lymphocytes resides in the bone marrow.

The three major groups of lymphocytes known are B cells, T cells, and null cells. The latter group lacks most of the surface characteristics of either B or T cells. Null cells appear to play an important role as killer cells in antitissue immunity.

The overall specific immune response is divided into two major types of responses: the humoral and the cell-mediated immune response. The immune cell responsible for the humoral response is the B cell, whereas the T cell is responsible for mediating cell-mediated immune responses.

It is well established that B cells are responsible for the production of all the immunoglobulins.

However, it is also established that certain antigens, referred to as thymus-dependent (TD) antigens, can induce antibody formation by B cells only if T helper cells (T4) are present. Accordingly, T helper cells can react with the antigen determinants of the antigen that is also stimulating the B cells. In contrast, when thymus-independent antigens are introduced to the host, B cells can be activated without the need of T helper cells. Null cells have been demonstrated to contain two subsets, one referred to as killer (K) cells, which can destroy mammalian cells when specific antibodies are bound to the surface antigens of the target cell. The second subset is natural killer (NK) cells, which are capable of killing tumor cells directly in the absence of any immunoglobulin.

Plasma cells are the end cells of antigen-stimulated B cells. These are the highly specialized fully differentiated cells derived from B cells that produce and secrete immunoglobulin. Plasma cells are found only in extravascular sites and do not circulate in the vascular compartment. The plasma cells are characteristic because of the enormous amounts of dilated endoplasmic reticulum that can be found in the cytoplasm.

## TISSUES AND ORGANS OF THE IMMUNE SYSTEM

**Reticular Tissue and Associated Cells.** Reticular cells possess dendrite-like cytoplasmic processes and are commonly found in lymphoreticular organs. These cells are particularly important in the presentation of antigens to immunocompetent lymphoid cells. There are three cell types: dendritic cells, interdigitating reticular cells, and Langerhans' cells. It is of special interest that dendritic cells appear to be associated with the B-dependent areas of lymphoid tissue, whereas interdigitating reticular cells are usually associated with T-dependent areas. Langerhans' cells are located abundantly in the thymus, eye, and epidermis. They have also been observed in the T-dependent areas of lymph nodes. These cells as a group are important in antigen presentation and the induction of humoral or cell-mediated immunity.

**Thymus and T Cell Differentiation.** The thymus originates as an epithelial outgrowth of an embryonic structure, the bronchial pouch, and is the principal lymphoid organ of the early embryo. The major function of the thymus is to provide the environment in which precursor lymphoid cells undergo differentiation and become T cells. Several hormones are produced by the thymus, including thymopoietin, thymosin, and thymulin. The thymic hormones presumably promote differentiation of precursor cells into T cells.

The thymus is well developed at birth and begins to diminish in size or involute after puberty. During early embryonic life and thereafter the thymus seeds the peripheral lymphoid system with differentiated T cells that express a high degree of clone diversity with respect to antigen recognition. In adulthood the organ seems to play a lesser role because adult thymectomy depresses T cell function only after a delay of weeks to months. This delay is probably due to the extensive seeding of T cells in peripheral lymphoid organs and the long life of certain T cell subsets.

**Potential Sites of B Cell Maturation.** It is well established that the bursa of Fabricius, the central lymphoid organ in birds, is involved in the early nonantigen-driven differentiation of B cells. Accordingly, the term of bursa cell is the origin of the term B cell or B-lymphocyte. In the case of the mammal, a bursa equivalent has not been precisely defined. Mammalian B cell maturation may occur at multifocal sites in the peripheral lymphoid system.

**Lymph Nodes.** The lymph node is an encapsulated lymphoreticular ovoid organ traversed by supporting trabeculae, connective tissue, and a radial arrangement of lymph sinuses that lead from the subcapsular marginal sinus to the medulla. The cells in the node are principally lymphocytes with lesser numbers of macrophages, plasma cells, and a few granulocytes. The paracortical area is populated largely by aggregates of T cells that emigrate from the thymus. Interdigitating reticular cells and a few Langerhans' cells are also present in the paracortex. The other portions of the node represent B-dependent areas (Fig. 32–1). Lymph nodes contribute to systemic as well as local defense by serving as important sites for production of antibodies and immune T cells. The slow percolation of lymph through the intricate network of lymphatic sinuses provides ample opportunity for soluble antigens, antigen-antibody complexes, and foreign particulates to come in contact with the surfaces of macrophages, dendritic cells, and lymphocytes. It is of special importance that over 99% of a soluble antigen can be trapped in the draining lymph nodes of an unprimed animal. Lymph nodes have both efferent and afferent lymph vessels. The lymph circulation is complex and allows for an orderly return of extravascular fluid, proteins, and lymphoid cells to the blood compartment via the thoracic duct.

**Lymphoid Follicles.** Lymphoid follicles occur in lymphoreticular structures including lymph nodes and comprise collections of B cell clones. Primary follicles that characterize the newborn consist of uniform clusters of small lymphocytes. Secondary follicles develop as a consequence of exposure to foreign antigens. Germinal centers arising from progenitor B cells derived from the bone marrow are commonly associated with the evolution of secondary follicles. Events that occur in germinal centers include trapping and presentation of antigen to lymphocytes, expansion of specifically reactive clones of antibody-forming cells, and production of memory B cells; however, most of the plasma cells that are generated in the humoral response develop outside the germinal centers.

**Spleen.** The spleen is a large lymphoreticular organ located within the circulation of the vascular compartment, where it serves as a filter for blood (Fig. 32–2). The spleen is pervaded by a reticular network whose organization varies in different segments of the organ. The capsule and trabeculae are rich in flexible tissue that lends elasticity to the organ. The small central arteries are surrounded by a cylindric collar of lymphatic tissue called the white pulp. The structural function of the white pulp resembles that of the lymph node. The white pulp contains lymphoid follicles rich in B cells, whereas the nonfollicular area is a T-dependent area. The red pulp is a large matrix rich in red cells and thin-walled vena sinuses. Lymphocytes leave the spleen via afferent lymphatics as well as via the vena sinuses. The spleen is a storehouse for blood and is a major site for the destruction of effete red blood cells. It can compensate for blood loss by contracting and expelling enormous numbers of red blood cells in the circulation.

**The Mucous Membrane Associated Lymphoid Tissue (MALT).** This highly specialized lymphoid system comprises lymphoid tissue directly associated with the mucosal surfaces of the body. The MALT possesses efferent but not afferent lymph vessels. It comprises both diffuse and organized lymphoid tissues containing essentially all the types of cells and fine structure that characterize major lymphoid organs. The effectors of specific immunity in the MALT include immune T cells, secretory IgA antibody, and lesser amounts of antibody of the other classes. Secretory IgA, which is uniquely resistant to digestive enzymes, is formed chiefly by plasma cells in the lamina propria of the mucosa of the gastrointestinal and bronchial tracts as well as the mammary gland. There is little doubt that the secretory IgA found at all mucosal surfaces plays an important part in protecting the mucosal surfaces against microbial agents.

**Circulation of Lymphocytes.** It is well established that certain populations of lymphocytes, especially virgin cells and memory cells, continually recirculate from the blood to lymph and back

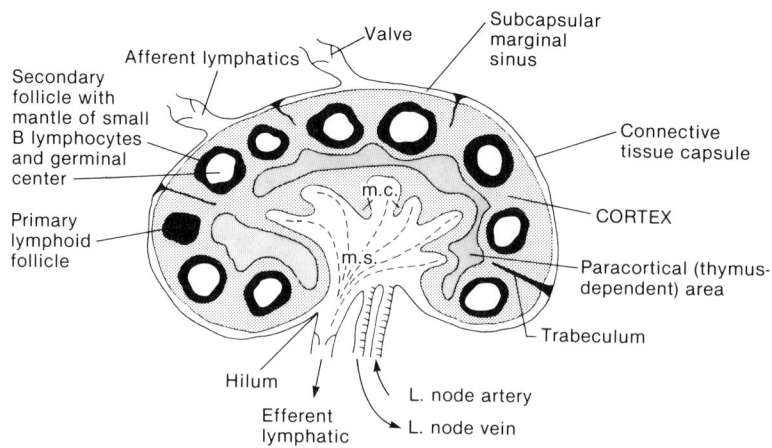

m.c. Medullary cords
m.s. Medullary sinuses

**Fig. 32–1.**   Diagrammatic representation of a typical lymph mode. Note B-dependent and T-dependent areas. (From Myrvik, Q.N., Weiser, R.S.: Fundamentals of Immunology. 2nd ed. Philadelphia, Lea & Febiger, 1984.)

again to the blood. The recirculating interval of T cells is about 30 hours; for B cells it is probably somewhat less. Most lymphocytes in the thoracic duct lymph and in the blood of normal adults are long-lived recirculating T cells.

Lymphocyte recirculation is of obvious importance because (1) it permits the rapid mobilization of specifically competent lymphocytes to the site of antigen deposition; (2) it ensures that committed cells can leave the organ and distribute the efferent specific immune response systemically to distant lymphoid tissues; and (3) it maintains in the immune cell population a large number of

mobile memory cells that can be readily deployed to mount either an afferent or an efferent response at any site where antigen may reappear.

**Immunologic Aspects of Phagocytosis.** Steps that lead to phagocytosis include directional movement of the phagocyte toward the particle (chemotaxis), recognition of the particle, adherence to the phagocyte, and finally engulfment. It is well established that some microorganisms resist phagocytosis and that specific antibody is necessary for the phagocytic event to take place. As a rule, phagocytosis of pathogenic bacteria is Fc and C3b receptor-dependent.

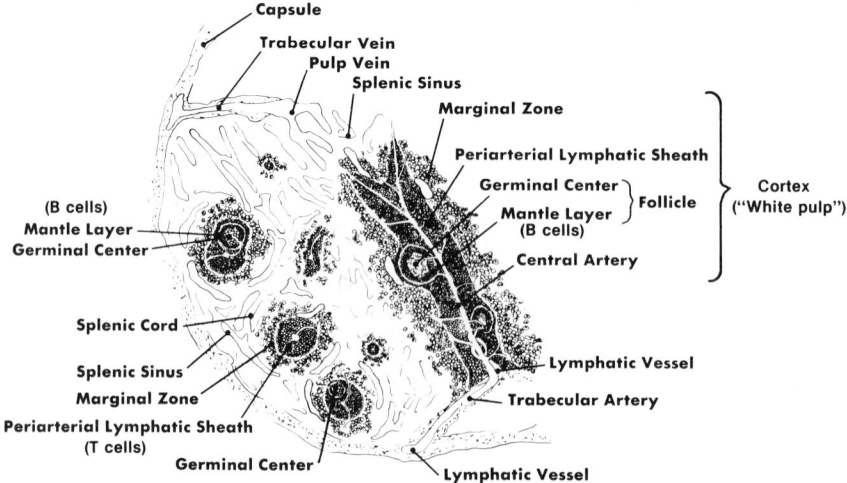

**Fig. 32–2.**   Diagrammatic representation of the spleen. Note T cell and B cell areas. (From Myrvik, Q.N., Weiser, R.S.: Fundamentals of Immunology. 2nd ed. Philadelphia, Lea & Febiger, 1984.)

## STRUCTURAL AND FUNCTIONAL CHARACTERISTICS OF HUMAN IMMUNOGLOBULINS

The gammaglobulins were first recognized and designated as a distinct group of serum proteins by Tiselius in 1937. He termed these proteins gammaglobulins because they migrated more slowly in an electric field than globulins of two other groups called alpha and beta. Five classes of immunoglobulins are recognized: IgG, IgM, IgA, IgD, and IgE (Fig. 32–3). The IgG molecule has been studied intensively and serves as a model of the basic structural unit of all immunoglobulins. It is a Y-shaped monomeric four-chain polypeptide complex containing two identical light chains and two identical heavy chains (either kappa or lambda) held together by noncovalent and covalent disulfide bonds. Extensive studies have been made on the amino acid sequence of various immunoglobulins. Each chain has a constant region and a variable region. The variable regions represent the site of the antibody molecule that reacts with the antigen determinants. Domains also have been identified on the respective chains. For example, in the case of the IgG molecule, each heavy chain has one V region domain referred to as the $V_H$ domain and three heavy chain domains called $C_H1$, $C_H2$, and $C_H3$. The $C_H2$ and $C_H3$ domains have a number of biologic activities including complement activation, transplacental transfer of IgG, and binding of the molecule to phagocytic cells and certain lymphoid cells possessing Fc receptors. Whereas the $C_H2$ domain is the site where complement components first interact to initiate the complement cascade, the $C_H3$ domain possesses sites that bind the molecule to Fc receptors on macrophages, granulocytes, and certain lymphocytes. A summary of the classification and structural properties of human immunoglobulins can be found in Table 32–1. The properties of human immunoglobulins can also be found in Tables 32–2 and 32–3. The following summary describes the various classes of immunoglobulins.

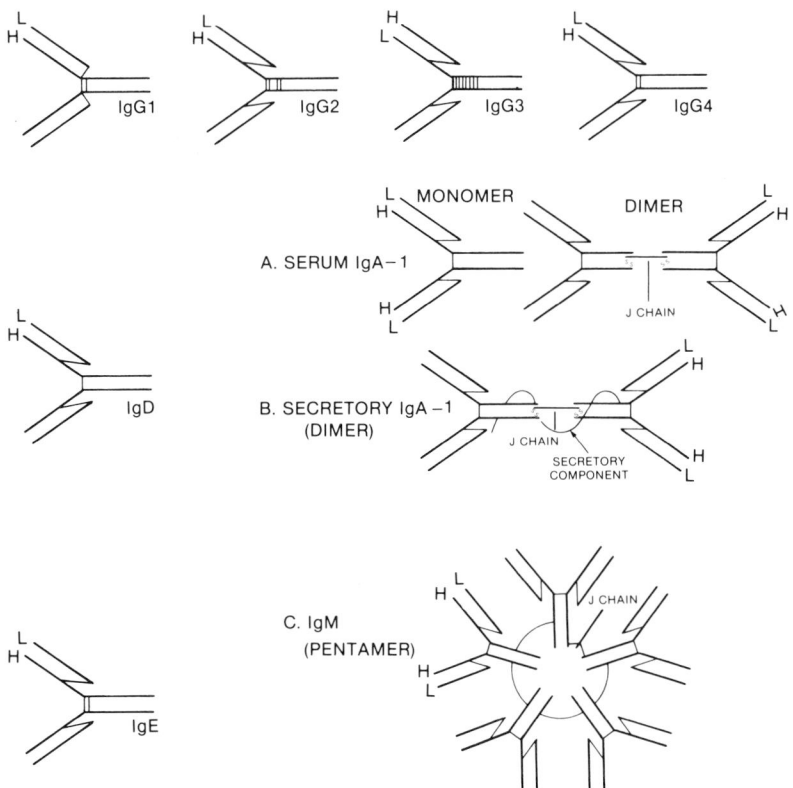

**Fig. 32–3.** Diagram illustrating human immunoglobulins. Human immunoglobulins belong to five classes: IgG, IgA, IgM, IgD, and IgE. Basic monomers of all immunoglobulin molecules are comprised of two L and two H chains. All immunoglobulins have either identical kappa (κ) or lambda (λ) chains. Heavy chains of each immunoglobulin class are designated by Greek letters corresponding to the capital letter identifying the class. (From Fudenberg, H.H., Stites, D.P., Caldwell, J.L., et al. (Eds.): Basic and Clinical Immunology. 3rd ed. Los Altos, CA, Lange Medical Publications, 1980.)

**Table 32–1.  Classification and Structural Properties of Human Immunoglobulins**

| Class | H Chain Ag Determinant | L Chain Ag Determinant | Molecular Formulae | Sedimentation Constant | Approximate Mol. Weight |
|---|---|---|---|---|---|
| IgG1 | $\gamma1$ | $\kappa$ or $\lambda$ | $\gamma1_2\kappa_2$ or $\gamma1_2\lambda_2$ | 7S | 160,000 |
| IgG2 | $\gamma2$ | $\kappa$ or $\lambda$ | $\gamma2_2\kappa_2$ or $\gamma2_2\lambda_2$ | 7S | 160,000 |
| IgG3 | $\gamma3$ | $\kappa$ or $\lambda$ | $\gamma3_2\kappa_2$ or $\gamma3_2\lambda_2$ | 7S | 160,000 |
| IgG4 | $\gamma4$ | $\kappa$ or $\lambda$ | $\gamma4_2\kappa_2$ or $\gamma4_2\lambda_2$ | 7S | 160,000 |
| IgA (serum) | $\alpha$ | $\kappa$ or $\lambda$ | $(\alpha_2\kappa_2)1{-}3$ or $(\alpha_2\lambda_2)1{-}3$ | 7S,11S,18S | 170,000 600,000 |
| IgA (secretory) | $\alpha$ | $\kappa$ or $\lambda$ | $(\alpha_2\kappa_2)_2+P*$ or $(\alpha_2\lambda_2)_2+P*$ | 11S | 390,000 |
| IgM | $\mu$ | $\kappa$ or $\lambda$ | $(\mu_2\kappa_2)_5$ or $(\mu_2\lambda_2)_5$ | 19S | 900,000 |
| IgD | $\delta$ | $\kappa$ or $\lambda$ | $\delta_2\kappa_2$ or $\delta_2\lambda_2$ | 7S | 160,000 |
| IgE | $\epsilon$ | $\kappa$ or $\lambda$ | $\epsilon_2\kappa_2$ or $\epsilon_2\lambda_2$ | 8S | 180,000 |

*P = Secretory piece produced by epithelial cells.
From Myrvik, Q.N., Weiser, R.S.: Fundamentals of Immunology. 2nd ed. Philadelphia, Lea & Febiger, 1984.

**Table 32–2.  Properties of Human Immunoglobulins**

| Class | Half-life (Days) | Serum Concentration (mg/dl)* | Distribution (% of Total in Intravascular Space) | Synthetic Rate (mg/kg/day) | Total Immuno-globulin (%) |
|---|---|---|---|---|---|
| IgG | 23 | 1000 | 45 | 33 | 80 |
| IgA (serum) | 6 | 200 | 42 | 24 | 16 |
| IgM | 5 | 120 | 76 | 6–7 | 4 |
| IgD | 3 | 3 | 75 | 0.4 | 0.001 |
| IgE | 3 | 0.05 | 51 | 0.02 | 0.00003 |

*dl = Deciliter.
From Myrvik, Q.N., Weiser, R.S.: Fundamentals of Immunology. 2nd ed. Philadelphia, Lea & Febiger, 1984.

**Table 32–3.  Properties of Human Immunoglobulins**

| Class | Immunologic Activities | Opsonic Activity | Placental Passage | Order of Appearance of Synthetic Ability in Infants | Functional Valence |
|---|---|---|---|---|---|
| IgG | Late response to Ag; antibacterial; antitoxic; antiviral; blood group Abs | + | Yes (all subclasses) | late | 2 |
| IgA (serum) | Block bacterial adherence; viral defense | – | No | intermediate | 2 (monomer) |
| IgA (secretory) | Activity in mucous secretions; block bacterial adherence; viral defense | – | No | intermediate | 2–4 (dimer) |
| IgM | Early response to Ag; antibacterial; antiviral; blood group Abs | + | No | early | 5 (10)* |
| IgD | Present on lymphocyte surface | + | No | | 2 |
| IgE | Allergic (anaphylactic) reactions; possible respiratory tract defense; mast cell fixation; raised in parasitic infections; cytophilic, for basophils and mast cells | + | No | | 2 |

*A valence of 10 is the theoretic maximum and could only be achieved with low-molecular-weight hapten.
From Myrvik, Q.N., and Weiser, R.S.: Fundamentals of Immunology. 2nd ed. Philadelphia, Lea & Febiger, 1984.

**Immunoglobulin G.** Human IgG can be subdivided into four subclasses, IgG1, IgG2, IgG3, and IgG4. They comprise 66%, 23%, 7%, and 4%, respectively, of the IgG in the blood. Whereas IgG3, IgG1, and IgG2 can fix complement in that order, the IgG4 subclass cannot activate the classic complement pathway.

**Immunoglobulin A.** Immunoglobulin A comprises two subclasses, IgA1 and IgA2, which occur in the serum in the ratio of 40 to 1. There are two basic molecular forms of IgA: serum IgA and secretory IgA. Serum IgA is, for the most part, a monomeric four-chain polypeptide unit, whereas secretory IgA consists of a J chain coupled dimer to which secretory component, a product of epithelial cells, is added.

**Immunoglobulin M.** The IgM molecule is a 19S star-shaped polymer composed of five basic monomers held together by disulfide bonds and a J chain. Each H chain carries four domains on the constant segment. Although the molecule has ten potential antigen-binding sites, only five can be readily demonstrated to bind high-molecular–weight antigens. Because of its multivalence, IgM possesses high avidity for antigens carrying repeating (identical) antigen determinants such as polysaccharides. It is an efficient agglutinin as well as efficient complement activating antibody.

**Immunoglobulin D.** This immunoglobulin class comprises only about 0.2% of the total immunoglobulins in serum. Although its role in acquired immunity is unknown, immunoglobulin D is commonly found on the surface of precursor immature lymphocytes in conjunction with monomeric IgM.

**Immunoglobulin E.** This immunoglobulin is found in very low concentrations in human serum; it is a potent antibody in terms of mediating anaphylactic hypersensitivity reactions such as hay fever, allergic asthma, and food allergies. This is largely based on its affinity for mast cells and basophils through its Fc segment. When specific antigen reacts with IgE bound to mast cells, they undergo degranulation releasing potent mediators such as histamine, serotonin, bradykinin, and the leukotrienes.

## THEORIES TO EXPLAIN ANTIBODY DIVERSITY

The specificity of an antibody molecule is due to the amino acid sequences of the variable regions of the L and H chains. Accordingly, the germ line theory has emerged as a major mechanism responsible for antibody diversity in terms of specificity for antigenic determinants. Since it has been shown that somatic mutation of these genes is frequent, this mechanism probably contributes importantly to the fine tuning of antibody specificity through a clonal selection process.

The heavy-chain V (variable) genes in man comprise at least four subgroups, and the gene products of any one of these genes can combine with the products of the constant-region gene. In addition, some four to six respective V-region gene subgroups have been tentatively identified for human light chains. Individually, these gene products also can combine with the constant-region genes through recombination events.

With respect to the L chain, this recombination takes place between a germ-line V-region gene and a distinct segment of DNA on the same chromosome referred to as a joining (J) gene, which encodes a 13 amino acid sequence. The J gene is responsible for at least two important signals, one for DNA recombination and one for RNA splicing. Ribonucleic acid splicing is required even after DNA transcription because the L and H chain genes remain at different discrete coding segments separated by intervening sequences of DNA (introns).

Whereas L chains are encoded by three genes (V, J, and C genes), the encoding of H chains involves an additional gene D for diversity. Thus the functional H chain gene complex represents a combination of V, D, J, and C genes in that order. Multiple different D genes exist, but the exact numbers are unknown. The combinatorial possibilities of the genes for L and H chains can account for the large number of specificities expressed in the immune responses to the large number of antigen determinants that are foreign to the host.

## THE COMPLEMENT SYSTEM

The complement system consists of 17 different plasma proteins. Nine major components comprise the classic pathway of complement activation and cell lysis initiated by certain antigen-antibody interactions on the cell surfaces. The nine major components of the classic pathway are designated C1 through C9 in the order of their discovery, which is not the order of their reaction sequence. C1 consists of three subunits: C1q, C1r, and C1s. A second pathway of complement activation, called the alternative pathway, is initiated nonspecifically by extrinsic agents other than antigen-antibody complexes such as bacterial endotoxin and high-MW polysaccharides. Serum factors unique to the alternative pathway are designated by the capital letters B, D, and P (properdin). Two other components of the complement system are (1) C3bINA, which inactivates C3b and (2) BIH, which enhances the activity of C3bINA. A summary of the classic and alternative pathway reactions is presented in Figure 32–4.

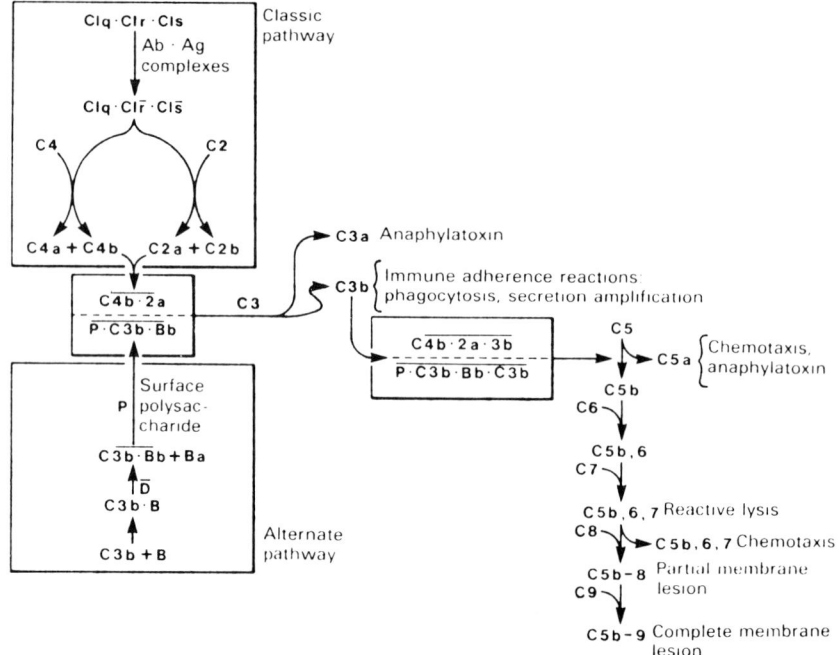

**Fig. 32–4.** Reaction sequence of the classic and alternative complement system. Note that C4b2a and PC3bBb are the C3 convertases for the classic and alternative C pathways, respectively. (From Eisen, H.N.: Immunology. 2nd ed. Hagerstown, MD, Harper & Row Publishers, Inc., 1980.)

The classic pathway as well as the alternative pathway can generate the chemotactic factor C5a and the opsonic factor C3b. In addition, if the factor sequences C5b through 9 are activated by either pathway, the lysis of cells can result. The alternative pathway is initiated with the C3 moiety of complement. Accordingly, C1, C2, and C4 are not involved in the alternative pathway.

The C3b component of complement, in conjunction with the C3b receptor and Fc receptor on phagocytes, produces a synergistic action in terms of stimulating opsonin-mediated phagocytosis of bacteria. Complement can also aid in the clearance of circulating immune complexes by way of the C3b and Fc receptors on phagocytes.

Individuals genetically deficient in C2 exhibit increased susceptibility to infection. Since C2 is not involved in the alternative pathway, this finding suggests that the alternative pathway alone is not sufficient for normal function of antimicrobial mechanisms of defense. In particular, patients with C3 deficiencies are highly susceptible to infections, particularly pulmonary infections. This finding indicates the importance of C3b in complement-mediated opsonic action.

## INTERACTIONS OF ANTIGENS AND ANTIBODIES IN VITRO

Antibodies of all the major immunoglobulin classes and subclasses can participate in various types of antigen-antibody interactions in vitro. Numerous studies have utilized haptens as monovalent determinants on proteins to study antigen-antibody interactions in vitro. An antigen determinant will react with the antibody-reacting site in a highly specific way. The typical antibody-reacting site on an antibody molecule is a three-dimensional cavity comprising approximately 500 to 700 $A^2$ in area. Antigen-antibody bonds are generally weak and range from 7 to 20 kilocalories/mole; however, the reactions can be highly specific.

If antigens and antibodies react in soluble state, a precipitate is usually formed upon their interaction. The antibody in this case is referred to as a *precipitin*. If the antigen is particulate or if it is on the cell surface of a cell, the specific antibody can produce agglutination or aggregation. Such antibodies are commonly referred to as *agglutinins*. A large array of gel precipitation tests utilize the reactions of soluble antigens and antibodies. In addition, immunoelectrophoresis is commonly used as a mechanism to separate antigen preparations in mixtures followed by developing precipitin arcs with appropriate antibodies. Discrete antigen-antibody systems can be visualized with this technique. Other immunologic techniques involve radioimmunoassays, immunofluorescence, immobilization tests, complement fixation tests, and virus neutralization tests. Enzyme immunoassays, as well as crossed immunoelectrophoresis, are other techniques that have been developed and utilize in vitro interactions of antigens and antibodies. Descriptions of these techniques are readily available in standard immunologic textbooks.

## CELLULAR BASIS OF AFFERENT IMMUNE RESPONSES

### Ontogeny of B-Lymphocytes

The early development and differentiation of B cells are not antigen-driven events. Differentiation proceeds from a pluripotential bone marrow stem cell that is unable to form immunoglobulin to a family of line progenitor cells called pre-B cells. These cells synthesize but do not secrete IgM. Two types of pre-B cells exist, a rapidly dividing large cell type and a slowly dividing small cell type. In the adult bone marrow, the large pre-B cell differentiates into a small pre-B cell. Both cell types contain a small amount of cytoplasmic IgM (monomeric) but little or no surface IgM. The small pre-B cell continues to differentiate to become an immature B cell possessing intrinsic surface monomeric IgM but no cytoplasmic IgM. Immature B cells leave the bone marrow and move to peripheral lymphoid tissues where they rapidly differentiate to become mature immunocompetent cells carrying both surface IgM and surface IgD but no cytoplasmic Ig. Prior to their experience with antigens, the mature cells are commonly called virgin B cells. Most peripheral B cells carry surface Ig. Upon encountering antigen, a virgin B cell can differentiate to become a memory cell, an antibody-secreting end cell (plasma cell), or a tolerized cell. A summary of ontogeny of B cells is presented in Figure 32–5.

### Ontogeny of T-Lymphocytes

Progenitor T cells migrate from the bone marrow to the thymus to differentiate and proliferate in the thymus cortex and pass to the medulla. Human T-lymphocyte antigens that characterize human T cells first appear at the pre-T cell stage together with the receptor for peanut agglutinin. Changes in the enzyme patterns of human thymocytes occur during maturation. For example, terminal deoxynucleotide transferase is only present in progenitor hematopoietic cells and immature thymocytes, whereas α-naphthol acetate esterase is present in mature T cells. One human T cell subset, the Tμ cell, which possesses receptors for the Fc segment of IgM, is a precursor of the T helper cell. Another T cell subset that possesses receptors for the Fc segment of IgG (T cells) is the

precursor of the T suppressor cell. Additional subsets of T cells possess Fc receptors for IgA (T cells) and IgE (T cells). A summary of the ontogeny of T cells is presented in Figure 32–6. The functions of human T cell subsets are presented in Table 32–4. A third group of lymphoid cells is referred to as null cells because they lack the characteristic B- and T-lymphocyte markers. One subset of this group possesses Fc receptors for both IgG and IgG-containing immune complexes and is referred to as killer (K) cells. A second set is referred to as natural killer (NK) cells. The K cells can act as killer cells against tumor cells in cooperation with specific antibody, whereas the NK cells can act as killer cells without immunoglobulin utilizing some undefined primitive recognition system.

It should be stressed that the immune responses in the fetus and neonate are relatively feeble and tolerance is easily induced. During fetal life excess suppressor T cells apparently exist which down regulate the maternal immune response. It has been suggested that this process prevents the mother from rejecting the fetus.

### B Cell Activation and the Humoral Response

The nonantigen-driven events in B cell maturation result in a marked randomization of a large number of clones that can fortuitously react with antigens encountered by the host. The genetic repertoire of specificities resides within the genome of the responding cell. When an antigen determinant reacts with a specifically reacting surface IgM molecule on a mature immunocompetent B cell, the B cell replicates and a clone is generated that subsequently synthesizes IgM antibodies with that single specificity. It is likely that subsets of specifically reacting T helper cells are responsible for the switch to other Ig classes. Switching occurs as follows: IgM to IgG, IgM to IgA, and IgM to IgE. As a rule switching only occurs with thymus-dependent antigens. As previously stated, thymus-independent antigens only stimulate production of IgM and do not require T helper cells.

### Role of T Cells in the Cell-Mediated Immune Response

The cell-mediated immune (CMI) response can only be induced by thymus-dependent antigens. Intracellular parasites like *Mycobacterium tuberculosis* and *Histoplasma capsulatum* develop good CMI responses because their antigens persist and are slowly released from the parasitized macrophages. Water-insoluble antigen complexes are apparently more effective in producing a CMI response than water-soluble proteins. Effector CMI responses in humans are mediated by at least two

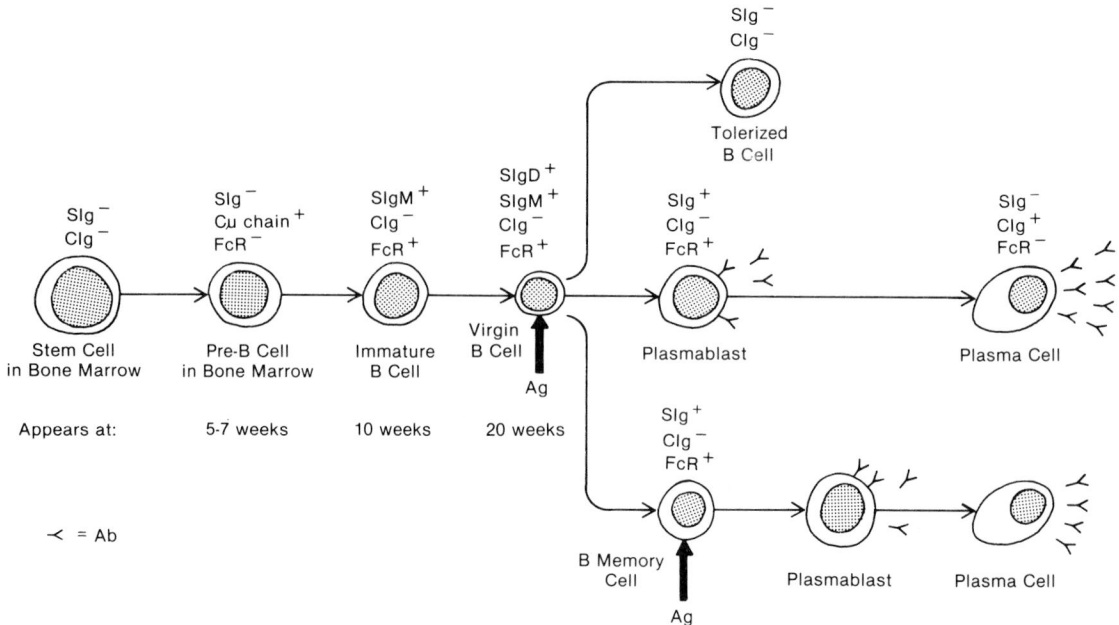

**Fig. 32–5.** Ontogeny of B cells. Note that surface IgM (SIgM) first appears on the immature B cell with loss of cytoplasmic Ig (CIg). The virgin B cell possesses SIgD and SIgM. Fc receptors (FcR) appear at the immature B cell stage. (From Myrvik, Q.N., Weiser, R.S.: Fundamentals of Immunology. 2nd ed. Philadelphia, Lea & Febiger, 1984.)

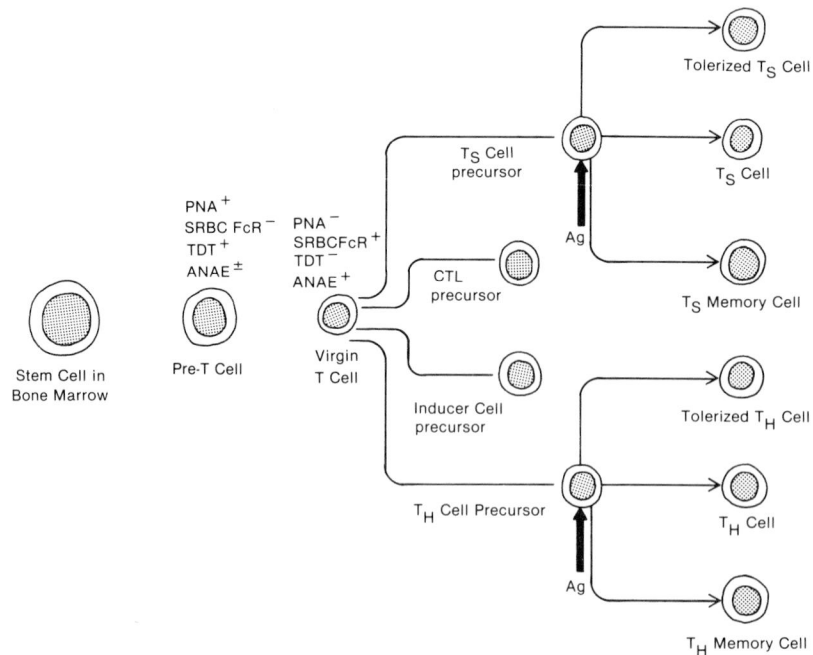

**Fig. 32–6.** Ontogeny of T cells. Note that pre-T cells are peanut agglutinin (PNA) positive and positive for terminal deoxynucleotidyltransferase (TDT). Virgin T cells, however, are negative for PNA and TDT but carry Fc receptors (FcRs) for sheep red blood cells and are positive for α-naphthol acetate esterase (ANAE). (From Myrvik, Q.N., Weiser, R.S.: Fundamentals of Immunology, 2nd ed. Philadelphia, Lea & Febiger, 1984.)

**Table 32–4. Immunologic Functions of Human T Cell Subsets**

| *Function* | *Helper/Inducer* | *Cytotoxic/Suppressor* |
|---|---|---|
| | OKT4, Leu 3a | OKT8, Leu 2a |
| Cytotoxic-effector function | − | + |
| Cell-mediated antimicrobial immunity | + | − |
| Delayed hypersensitivity | + | − |
| Regulatory events | | |
| Help (induction) | | |
| T–T | + | − |
| T–B | + | − |
| T-macrophage | + | − |
| Suppression | | |
| T–T | − | + |
| T–B | − | + |

From Reinherz, E.L., Schlossman, S.F.: N. Engl. J. Med. 303:370, 1980. Reprinted from Chandra, R.K.[143]

subsets of T cells: (1) Human T-lymphocytes expressing the T4 surface antigen and mediating antimicrobial CMI response through lymphokine-mediated macrophage deployment and activation and (2) precursor T-lymphocytes expressing T8 surface antigen and antitissue CMI. The T8-lymphocyte subset is commonly referred to as a cytotoxic T-lymphocyte (CTL).

## Activation of Suppressor T Cells

As indicated previously there are two prominent T-lymphocyte subsets: one comprised of T helper/inducer cells (T4) and a second subset of T suppressor/cytotoxic cells (T8). The intravenous injection of antigen tends to favor the development of T suppressor cells that are abundant in the spleen. Suppressor cells can be involved in suppressing the B cell response as well as the T cell response. It is obvious that suppressor cells play an important role in the regulation of the immune response.

## Contributions of Accessory Cells to Lymphocyte Activation

It is well recognized that macrophages play an important role as accessory cells and are effective in processing and presenting antigens to immunocompetent lymphocytes. Macrophages are also important in the production of interleukin 1, which activates T cells and induces them to replicate.

Macrophages contribute to the humoral response to thymus dependent (TD) antigens by processing antigen and presenting it to specifically competent T helper cells and virgin B cells. In accord with these events, interleukin 1, which is produced by macrophages, stimulates the activation and replication of T cells. In turn, T cells secrete interleukin 2, which plays an important role in the activation and replication of additional

T cells during an immune response. As mentioned previously, other cells also can function as accessory cells. In particular, the Langerhans' cells and the interdigitating reticular cells play an important role in the induction of the CMI response, whereas dendritic cells appear to play an important role in the activation of the humoral immune response. These accessory cells, as well as macrophages, always contain Ia antigens (mouse system) on their surface when functioning as accessory cells. The Ia equivalent in the human system is HLA-DR, which is involved in antigen presentation to immunocompetent lymphocytes.

## Genetic Basis for Afferent Immune Responses

Specific immune responses are controlled by two genetic systems in mammals. Genes of the first system, which encode for immunoglobulin structure, are present in three distinct unlinked loci on three respective chromosomes. Genes of the second system, which regulate the immune response to TD antigens, are associated with the major histocompatibility complex (MHC), so named because it contains genes encoding antigens concerned with allograft rejection. In the case of the mouse, the MHC is a major region on chromosome 17 comprising nine discrete loci grouped between five associated minor regions (K, I, S, G, and D). The analogue in man is the HLA complex or system. In the mouse the genes that determine the immune responses to TD antigens are located in the I region situated between the K and D regions and are called immune response (Ir) genes. It is of interest that no genes controlling the specific immune responses to T-independent antigens have been found in the MHC.

Following the identification of Ir genes, researchers observed that serologically distinct Ir gene products are present in various types of cells, particularly the cells of the immune system. They are low-molecular-weight polymorphic glycoproteins that can be identified with alloantisera. Because these gene products are antigenic they were called I region-associated antigens (Ia antigens). The I region has been divided into five subregions, including I-A, I-B, I-C, and I-E based on the mapping of Ir genes, most of which are present in the I-A subregion. The fifth subregion, I-J, is based on the serologic identification of a distinct gene product on T suppressor cells called Ia 4. Both macrophages and certain B cells carry Ia antigens encoded by I-A and I-C subregion genes. I-A genes also code for Ia antigens in certain T cell subsets and are present in the helper factor complexes shed by T helper cells.

An animal that is a nonresponder to a given T-dependent antigen may (1) lack T cells that bear that specific antigen receptor, (2) have defects in handling and presentation of antigens by accessory cells, (3) lack certain Ia antigens on T cells, or (4) have B cells that lack a receptor for the specific helper factor produced by T helper cells. In addition, excess suppressor cell function can dampen the immune response to the point where it may appear to be partially defective. This is particularly true during the fetal and neonatal period. On the other hand, old animals tend to have a lack of normal suppressor cell function. This in turn appears to lead to the development of autoimmune diseases in which the immune system begins reacting to antigens of self.

### Anamnestic (Memory) Response

One of the most important responses with respect to the function of the immune system is the secondary antibody response or anamnestic response to TD antigens. The secondary response is readily distinguished from the primary response by a shortened induction phase, an earlier appearance of antibodies in serum, a more rapid rate of antibody synthesis, particularly IgG antibody, a higher peak of total serum antibody, and a more prolonged phase of decline in the serum levels of IgG. These characteristics of the secondary response are attributable to increased numbers of B cells and T helper memory cells that play a major role in the secondary response. It is likely that virgin B cells play only a minor role in the secondary antibody response because of feedback suppression by IgG antibody (Fig. 32–7).

If antibody is still present in serum when the second dose of antigen is given, such serum antibody declines or disappears rapidly (negative phase) owing to its almost immediate reaction with antigen to form immune complexes that are removed by the reticuloendothelial system. If the

dose of antigen is adequate but low enough to allow its full incorporation into antigen antibody complexes, antigen is rapidly cleared from the blood and the titer of antibody formed later rises to levels of 10 to 100 times the serum level attained in the normal primary response. If the secondary dose of antigen is in sub-pg quantities, an antibody response may not occur, presumably because antigen-antibody complexes formed would be meager and would be rapidly reduced by phagocytic destruction to substimulatory levels. Serum antibodies generated during the secondary antibody response are for the most part high-affinity IgG antibodies because most of the antibody-forming cells participating in the response are the progeny of memory cells that have been selected to have high-affinity antigen receptors. Low doses of antigen will preferentially activate those lymphocytes that have receptors with the highest affinity. The ability of an animal to rapidly mount a secondary response yielding high-affinity antibodies is of great practical importance because it can result in the elimination of a viral or bacterial infection before clinical manifestations develop.

### Abnormalities of the Immune System

Immunodeficiencies can be characterized by decreased or abnormal function in one or more components of the immune system, which usually results in increased susceptibility to infection. As a rule, the primary immune deficiencies are hereditary or congenital and are considered to result from defects in the development of the immune system. In contrast, secondary immune deficiencies are the consequence of some other systemic disorder that indirectly causes a defect in the response of the immune system. A third category of immunodeficiency diseases can be referred to as "physiologic" and affects all individuals, although to different degrees. Such deficiencies could be age-dependent because of increased susceptibility to infection in the first few months of life as well as certain defects in the immune system that occur with old age. A physiologic immunodeficiency could also be the result of malnutrition at any age. This topic is discussed in more depth later in this chapter.

**Immunodeficiencies of the T Cell System.** These abnormalities are characterized by the classic DiGeorge syndrome, which is the prototype of a selective T cell deficiency. This immunodeficiency is manifested by increased susceptibility to infections of microorganisms of low virulence, such as *Pneumocystis carinii* and *Candida albicans*. Although the levels of immunoglobulins and the number of B cells can approach normal levels, secondary responses are generally de-

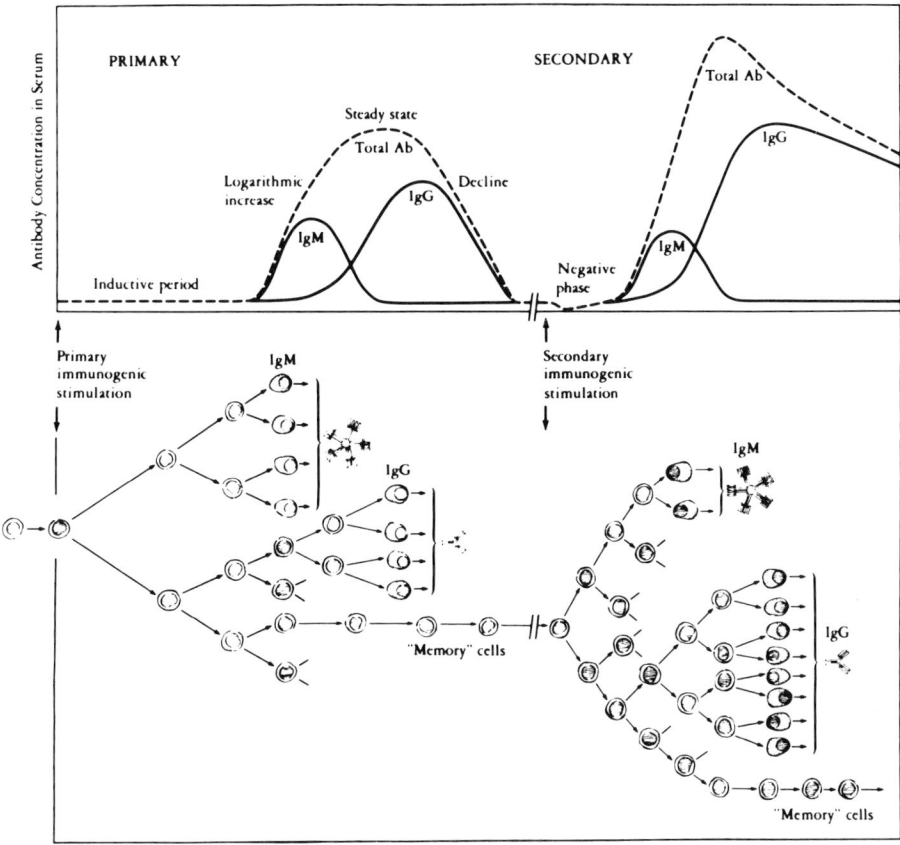

**Fig. 32–7.** Primary and secondary antibody responses. Note the kinetics of IgM and IgG responses. (From Bellanti, J.A.: Immunology III. Philadelphia, W.B. Saunders Company, 1985.)

pressed because of the lack of adequate numbers of T helper cells. A nucleoside phosphorylase deficiency has also been associated with T cell deficiency and, in this case, the enzyme nucleoside phosphorylase is missing. As a consequence, patients accumulate inosine, guanosine, and the respective deoxy compound. These metabolites exert inhibitory effects on normal T cell function in vitro.

**Immunodeficiencies of the B Cell System.** These can include panhypogammaglobulinemia (Bruton's agammaglobulinemia) and several dysgammaglobulinemias. In the case of the dysgammaglobulinemias, patients can have selective IgA deficiency, selective IgM deficiency, deficiencies of IgG and IgA with increased IgM, and selective deficiencies of any of the IgG subclasses. In the case of panhypogammaglobulinemia, the almost total lack of B cells suggests a developmental defect in B cell precursors. Inherited hypogammaglobulinemia is characterized by recurring sinus and pulmonary infections with *Hemophilus influenzae* and *Streptococcus pneumoniae*. The B-dependent areas of lymphoid tissue are usually depleted of lymphocytes with germinal centers and lymphoid follicles lacking in the lymph nodes. The lamina propria of the intestinal mucosa is also devoid of plasma cells.

**Combined Immunodeficiencies.** Combined immunodeficiencies are associated with syndromes such as reticular dysgenesis, ataxia-telangiectasia, Wiskott-Aldrich syndrome, and short-limbed dwarfism. Combined immunodeficiency disease has also been associated with adenosine deaminase deficiency. In this case, the patients suffer from an inborn error in purine metabolism. This disorder is inherited in an autosomal recessive manner. Lack of adenosine deaminase, which metabolizes adenosine and deoxyadenosine, results in accumulation of metabolites, such as cAMP and deoxy-ATP, which can depress lymphocyte function in vitro.

**Combined Immunodeficiencies Without Associated Adenosine Deaminase Deficiency or Specific Clinical Syndromes.** Patients with Nezelof's syndrome reveal severe T-lymphocyte depletion, although immunoglobulin levels may be close to normal. The antibody response to immunization is usually poor, and the serum antibodies frequently have restricted heterogeneity. This immunodeficiency may result from developmental arrest at the level of the stem cell or at early stages of lymphocyte differentiation.

**Immunodeficiencies of the Complement (C) System.** Primary deficiencies of C1q, C1r, C1s, C2, and C4 are frequently associated with autoimmune diseases. In addition, C2 and C4 deficiencies are also associated with increased frequency of certain histocompatibility antigens. Deficiencies of C3 and C5 are associated with increased susceptibility to infection that usually can be corrected by replacement therapy. Deficiency of C5, which commonly involves the presence of nonfunctional C molecules, has also been reported to be associated with autoimmune diseases. The generation of C3b and C5a is apparently an important component in opsonization and chemotactic functions. A host deficient in the production of these components will show increased susceptibility to infections.

**Acquired Immune Deficiency Syndrome (AIDS).** This disease surfaced in the United States about 1980. It is caused by a retrovirus that is designated as human immunodeficiency virus (HIV). It infects T cells and monocytes/macrophages and results in severe depression of immune functions with devastating consequences for the affected individuals. At this writing, no effective treatment is available, but experimental drugs to ameliorate the disease are under study.

## PRINCIPLES OF INNATE AND ACQUIRED IMMUNITY TO PARASITES

Immunity to a given agent may be complete or partial depending largely on two variables, the virulence of the parasite and the resistance of the host. It is useful to outline host immunity as set forth in Table 32–5.

**Innate Immunity.** Defined as immunity that is constitutive for the species, innate immunity is expressed in the early stages of primary infection before acquired immunity develops. The major factors responsible for innate immunity include anatomic barriers, phagocytes, special antimicro-

bial substances, and the basic response of inflammation.

**Acquired Immunity.** This immunity may be nonspecific as well as specific. For example, immunity naturally acquired by infection by one parasite may be nonspecifically operative concomitantly against another antigenically unrelated parasite.

**Artificial Active Immunity.** This form results from purposeful vaccination with immunogenic antigens derived from or associated with a specific or related microorganism.

**Artificial Passive Immunity.** Artificial passive immunity is usually accomplished by injection of an immune serum that contains antibodies capable of conveying specific immunity against the microbe to the recipient.

**Natural Passive Immunity.** For the most part this immunity is largely mediated by specific antibodies of the class IgG in humans because immunity is transferred almost exclusively to the human fetus by way of the placenta. Artificial passive immunity may be mediated by IgM and IgA, as well as IgG antibodies, all of which are present in injectable commercial human Ig preparations. However, IgG is the dominant and most important Ig.

## Internal Cellular Organ Systems of Defense

_Inflammation_ is important in antimicrobial defense largely because it creates a fibrin network to trap microorganisms and promotes the escape of fluid and leukocytes into the area of inflammation.

_Phagocytosis,_ a major mechanism of internal defense against invading microbes, can function in both innate and specific acquired immunity. The neutrophil or polymorphonuclear neutrophil leukocyte (PMN) represents the first line of defense against many microbes. Certain microorganisms, particularly encapsulated strains, can resist phagocytosis unless opsonized with specific antibody. Polymorphonuclear cells possess high levels of acid hydrolases as they emerge from the bone marrow to populate the blood. Hydrolases

**Table 32–5.  Host Immunity**

| | Type of Immunity | | | Example of Immunity Exhibited |
|---|---|---|---|---|
| | Innate or Constitutive | | | During early stages of primary infection |
| | Acquired naturally | | Active | Following a case of whooping cough |
| | | | Passive | Result of placental transfer of immunity from mother to fetus, e.g., immunity to diphtheria |
| Acquired | | | | |
| | Acquired artificially | | Active | Result of tetanus toxoid vaccination |
| | | | Passive | Result of injection of tetanus antitoxin |

are packaged in membrane-bound structures called lysosomes. There are two classes of antimicrobial systems, oxygen-dependent and oxygen-independent, expressed by polymorphonuclear cells. The toxic oxygen-derived radicals generated by a burst in the hexose monophosphate shunt upon phagocytosis are particularly important bactericidal agents in the course of phagocytosis.

The *mononuclear phagocyte system* involves large circulating mononuclear cells of the blood (monocytes) and tissue phagocytes (macrophages) such as alveolar macrophages of the lung, pleural macrophages, peritoneal macrophages, Kupffer's cells of the liver, and microglial cells in the brain. The macrophage is a highly adaptive cell that differentiates according to need. Because the macrophage can undergo limited mitosis in the local lesion, it is not wholly dependent on blood-borne cells. In the case of CMI, macrophages are mobilized and activated by T-lymphocyte products referred to as lymphokines. Once macrophages are immunologically activated, they possess a markedly increased capacity to inhibit and kill bacteria in a nonspecific manner. Oxygen-derived metabolites such as superoxide ion and hydrogen peroxide probably play major roles in microbial killing within macrophages.

## Nonantibody Biochemical Agents in Systems

The host can exert many nonspecific systems in the defense against microorganisms. The following substances illustrate this point.

*Lysozyme* hydrolyzes the muramic acid from the mucopeptide in the cell walls of gram-positive bacteria. It can also act synergistically with antibody and complement in the lysis of gram-negative bacteria because a thin mucopeptide layer is present. Lysozyme is normally present in most of the body fluids as well as neutrophils and macrophages.

*Beta-lysin (serum bactericidin)* system is activated by the clotting mechanism and is potent against several gram-positive organisms.

*Basic polypeptides,* which have been isolated from PMN lysosomes, can inhibit or kill several microorganisms.

*Spermine* is a polyamine that is found in renal tissue and semen. It is particularly inhibitory and lethal for tubercle bacilli and staphylococci.

*Lactoferrin* and *transferrin* are iron-binding compounds that can deprive bacteria of adequate supplies of iron and consequently exert bacteriostasis.

*Organic acids* can be bacteriostatic and are particularly toxic at low pH when they are in the nonionized state.

*Hematin* and *mesohematin* are iron porphyrins that have antibacterial properties owing largely to their ability to compete with other porphyrins in bacterial metabolism.

*The peroxidase-thiocyanate-hydrogen peroxide antimicrobial system.* Peroxidase, thiocyanate, and $H_2O_2$ form an antimicrobial system that inhibits the growth of a number of species of microorganisms. Lactoperoxidase, which is present in bovine milk, and myeloperoxidase, which is present in PMNs, can participate in this system. Thiocyanate is a constituent of extracellular fluids including serum, saliva, and milk. Microorganisms that accumulate $H_2O_2$ (and lack catalase) are inhibited by the addition of thiocyanate and peroxidase, whereas microorganisms that possess catalase are inhibited only if a $H_2O_2$ generating system is present. Accordingly, when leukocytes generate $H_2O_2$ during phagocytosis, the peroxidase thiocyanate system can be activated.

## Acquired Immunity to Bacteria

Classes of bacterial pathogens comprise (1) extracellular parasites such as *Staphylococcus aureus, Streptococcus pyogenes,* and *Klebsiella pneumoniae,* (2) facultative intracellular parasites such as *Mycobacterium tuberculosis, Francisella tularensis,* and *Brucella abortus,* and (3) obligate intracellular parasites such as *Rickettsia rickettsii, Rickettsia typhi,* and *Coxiella burnetii.* As a rule, pathogenic extracellular bacteria are resistant to humoral antimicrobial factors but are fully susceptible to killing by phagocytes. Accordingly, they usually express virulence factors that subvert and block phagocytosis. However, specific antibodies of acquired immunity can reverse the virulent effects by neutralizing toxins (IgG, IgA, and IgM) and functioning as opsonins (IgG, IgM).

On the other hand, facultative intracellular parasites characteristically are resistant to intracellular killing by both PMN and macrophages. As a consequence, the CMI system evolved to provide special phagocytes with superior killing powers. This system involves T helper cells that synthesize lymphokines that attract and activate macrophages to a level of antibacterial activity far above that expressed by normal macrophages. Obligate intracellular bacterial pathogens are also handled by activated macrophages and, in some instances, by an interplay with the humoral mechanisms.

**Humoral Mechanisms of Antibacterial Defense.** Antibodies of various classes play important and fundamental roles in acquired immunity against many bacterial pathogens.

*Chemotaxis.* The major factors of chemotaxis are derived from complement in which C5a and the complex C5b67 are formed. Oxidation products from arachidonic acid can also serve as important chemotaxins as well as certain chemotactic polypeptides that are liberated during inflammation.

*Opsonic Action.* Antibodies of the classes IgM and IgG play the major role in promoting phagocytosis of bacteria; human PMN and macrophages have Fc receptors for IgG1 and IgG3. Accordingly, IgG can function even in the absence of complement in the system. However, complement augments opsonization via the C3b receptor.

*Antibacterial Action of Antibody plus Complement.* Specific antibody, particularly IgM plus complement, can be highly bactericidal against some gram-negative organisms, especially *Escherichia coli,* a member of the gut flora. However, gram-positive bacteria are totally resistant to this mechanism. It is of special interest that lysozyme can act synergistically with this mechanism against gram-negative organisms.

*Neutralization of Toxin.* One of the major roles of specific antibody in acquired immunity is to neutralize bacterial toxins. Specific IgG, IgA, or IgM can contribute to toxin neutralization in toxigenic diseases such as diphtheria and tetanus.

*Blocking of Bacterial Colonization.* Certain bacteria must adhere to host cells to produce disease. This is the case with *Vibrio cholerae* organisms that colonize the surfaces of intestinal epithelial cells. If specific IgA antibodies are present in the gut and can react with surface antigens of the *V. cholerae,* colonization of this organism is blocked and the disease is prevented.

**Acquired Antibacterial Cell-Mediated Immunity.** In the development of CMI, the host produces an enormous expansion of clones of specifically reactive T memory cells. These circulating immune memory cells can be activated by specific antigen(s) in the course of a subsequent infection with the corresponding intracellular parasite. They then stimulate lymphokine mobilization and activation of macrophages. As mentioned earlier, the macrophages that are immunologically activated are far superior to the normal macrophage in terms of killing intracellular parasites. Immunologically activated macrophages can exhibit a 10- to 20-fold burst in the production of hydrogen peroxide in the course of phagocytosing intracellular parasites. T memory cells can migrate to interstitial tissues and probably remain there for extended periods without recirculating. Accordingly, if microorganisms invade and infect tissue, interstitial T memory cells (immune) can activate the whole process of CMI.

**Examples of Interplay of Specific and Nonspecific Mechanisms.** Total immunity depends on interplay between the factors of specific acquired immunity and those of innate immunity, as exemplified by the following:

1. Antibody, complement, and lysozyme can act synergistically against gram-negative bacteria. The opsonic action of antibody interplays with the bactericidal action of phagocytes. Opsonic action can also interplay with the bactericidal activity of complement and lysozyme.

2. Synergism also can exist between humoral immune and cell-mediated immune mechanisms. For example, opsonization can interact and interplay with immunologically activated macrophages that are destined to engulf facultative intracellular parasites.

## Acquired Immunity to Fungi

Cell-mediated immunity appears to be the major mechanism of acquired immunity against fungi, a finding that reflects the chronic nature of most fungi infection. In addition, odd-numbered fatty acids in skin, as well as the integuments, can be natural barriers to infection. The mononuclear phagocyte system and immune T cells play major roles in intracellular infections caused by fungi such as *Histoplasma capsulatum, Candida albicans,* and *Coccidioides immitis.*

One of the potential problems of chronic fungal infections is the generation of T suppressor cells that can negate acquired CMI.

## Acquired Immunity to Viruses

The major elements that participate in nonspecific internal defense against viral infections include interferon, NK cells, and macrophages. During virus replication, the virus induces the production of interferon, which can passively cause neighboring cells to become resistant. Macrophages can destroy virus if they are nonpermissive. Natural killer cells can destroy virus-infected cells.

Antibody-mediated immunity involves specific antibodies (IgG, IgA, and IgM) that neutralize extracellular virus and block infection; complement can enhance viral neutralization in the case of IgG and IgM. Specific IgG and IgM plus complement can also destroy viral-infected cells because, with some viruses, viral antigen is inserted in the membrane of the infected cell before virus maturation is completed. Hence the infection is aborted.

Cell-mediated immunity is mediated by specific cytotoxic T cells (T8) that can also react with viral antigen in the cell membrane and abort the infection before mature virus is made. Other CMI mechanisms can involve NK cells, K cells, and macrophages. The latter two cell types can participate in an antibody-dependent cell cytotoxic reaction.

## LABORATORY TESTS TO QUANTIFY IMMUNOLOGIC RESPONSES

**Plaque-Forming Assay.** This assay is useful experimentally to quantify the number of B-lymphocytes present in the spleen of laboratory animals, such as mice, that produce IgM or IgG antibody following administration of sheep red blood cells (SRBC). For example, IgM-producing B cells are dispersed in agar containing a lawn of SRBC to which complement is added. IgM specific for SRBC will lyse the surrounding SRBC in the presence of complement, forming a "clear plaque" around the lymphocyte (Fig. 32–8). The plaque-forming cells can be counted, and the kinetics of the number of specific IgM-producing cells can be plotted.

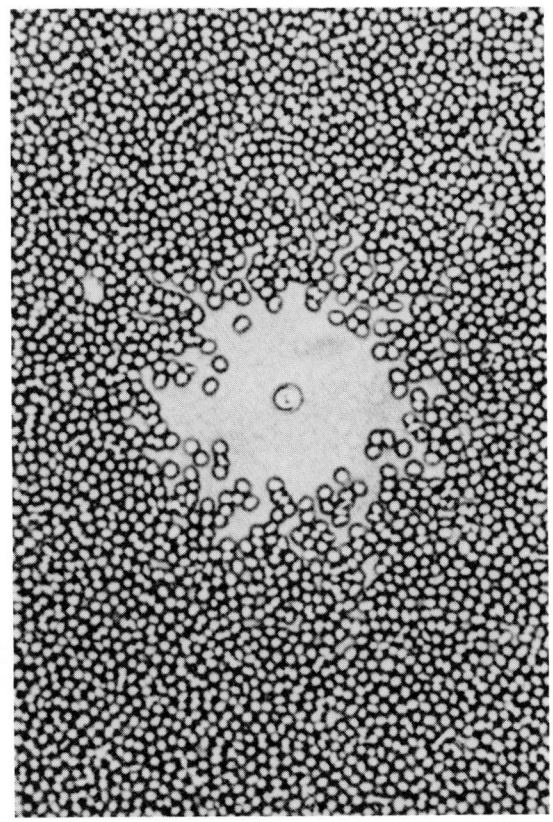

**Fig. 32–8.** Plaque-forming cell embedded in a layer of sheep red blood cells. Antibody secreted by the cell combines with the surrounding red cells. Addition of complement reacting with the antibody-red cell complex caused lysis of the red cells. (From Garvey, J.S., Cremer, N.E., Sussdorf, D.H.: Methods in Immunology. 3rd ed. Reading, MA, W.A. Benjamin, Inc., 1977.)

The quantitation of the IgG-producing B cells requires an overlay of IgM specific for the IgG (anti-SRBC) molecules made by the individual B cells. This step is required because the IgG-complement lysis of SRBC is much less efficient than that of IgM. Accordingly, the addition of IgM specific for IgG plus complement provides an amplification of SRBC lysis. The resulting plaques can be scored as the number of B cells producing IgG after subtracting the number of plaques that are formed by IgM antibodies specific for SRBC.

**Blastogenic Responses of Lymphocytes to Mitogens.** Both B- and T-lymphocytes can proliferate when incubated with certain mitogens. For example, phytohemagglutinin (PHA) and concanavilin A (Con A) cause T cells to proliferate, whereas lipopolysaccharide (LPS) causes B cells to proliferate. These proliferative responses are polyclonal responses with respect to antigenic specificity.

Proliferation is usually quantified by measuring the incorporation of tritiated thymidine, which reflects DNA synthesis. These tests measure important functional characteristics of lymphocytes, including the relative number of immunocompetent cells. The same principle is applied if one wishes to measure the specific proliferative response to antigens, except that the uptake of tritiated thymidine is less with antigens than with polyclonal mitogens because responses in this case are specific and clonal.

**Cell-Mediated Hypersensitivity (Delayed Hypersensitivity).** This immune effector response is commonly monitored by a skin test. Skin test antigens can include candidin, tuberculin, SK-SD, and so forth. A positive skin test response is characterized by an infiltration of lymphocytes and macrophages that peaks at 24 to 30 hours. Another approach involves the production of migration inhibition factor (MIF) when immune T cells (peripheral blood) are incubated with their specific antigen. This lymphocyte product(s) or lymphokine(s) causes activation and migration inhibition of macrophages. As one might expect, incubation of T cells with the polyclonal mitogens Con A or PHA also induces production of MIF. These tests are useful in obtaining relative data on changes in immunocompetence with respect to cell-mediated immune mechanisms.

**T Cytotoxic (Killer) Cell Activity.** Specific cytotoxic T cells are induced as a consequence of allogeneic tissue transplants, transplantable tumors, and certain viral infections. This arm of the CMI response can be readily evaluated in vitro using a chromium-51 release test. The target cells are first incubated with chromium-51 to allow endocytosis of the isotope and then incubated with immune cytotoxic T cells. Release of chromium-51 indicates lysis of target cells.

**Cytotoxic Antibodies.** These antibodies can lyse or destroy allogeneic target cells, viral-infected cells, or certain tumor cells when complement is present. The antibodies are specific and usually of the class IgM or IgG.

**Blocking Antibodies.** These antibodies do not activate complement and have no demonstrable effect on target cells. They can block the activity of cytotoxic antibodies or cytotoxic T cells due to steric effects.

**Enumeration T Helper and T Suppressor Lymphocytes.** It is common practice to quantify the numbers of T helper and T suppressor cells. This is readily accomplished using specific fluoresceinated monoclonal antibodies that are specific for T4 (helper) or T8 (suppressor) antigens (human) or Ly1 (helper) or Ly2,3 (suppressor) (mouse). Fluoresceinated cells can be counted by fluorescence microscopy or by a cytofluorograph (laser cell sorter).

**Quantitation of Serum Immunoglobulins.** The levels of serum Ig can be quantified by the use of radial immunodiffusion plates. These plates contain specific antibodies against IgG, IgM, or IgA. Sera are added to the wells and a precipitin ring is formed that relates to the amount of the respective Ig present in the serum (Fig. 32–9). Since IgE is in very low levels, a radioimmunoassay is required that is based on allowing an immobilized anti-IgE (IgG) to react with the total IgE present in the serum. After washing, a radiolabeled anti-IgG is added that specifically reacts with the complex. The bound radioactive counts relate to the amount of IgE present in the serum.

## EFFECT OF MALNUTRITION ON IMMUNE RESPONSES

Up to 1955 it was generally agreed that severe protein deficiencies suppressed antibody formation.[1] In addition, deficiencies of pyridoxine, pantothenic acid, and pteroylglutamic acid resulted in suppressed antibody responses. Deficiencies of components of the vitamin B complex also caused some depression in antibody formation.

Other questions pertained to whether malnutrition involved defective release of antibody or increased destruction, thus resulting in subnormal values. Although not proved at that time, the experimental data did not support impaired release or enhanced destruction.

Since 1955 the number of papers on this topic has increased. However, many questions remain unanswered or only partially answered. In particular, there has been a strong emerging interest in the effect of zinc deficiency on the immune response. This section summarizes the current state of knowledge on the role of malnutrition on the immune response.

### Complexities in Interpreting Data

Naturally occurring states of malnutrition are difficult to interpret largely because deficiencies usually involve multiple dietary factors. This problem is further compounded by infection, anorexia, debilitation, and severe negative nitrogen balances. For example, a marked reduction in food intake is commonly associated with vitamin and mineral deficiencies, thus contributing to the effects of protein-calorie undernutrition.

It is obvious that single nutrients can only be analyzed in defined and controlled animal experiments. Even in this context a word of caution is in order because there may be synergism between two or more required nutrients. Another issue is concerned with the degree of suppression of immunologic functions that reflect significant immunodeficiencies. Accordingly, caution must be exercised in the analysis of data from all nutritional experiments. Emphasis must be placed on proper controls, appropriate evaluation of immunologic assays, and careful scrutiny of perturbing influences such as infection and proper housing.

### Effect of Protein and Protein-Calorie Malnutrition

The studies by Cooper et al. revealed that the number of plaque-forming lymphocytes that became activated and the corresponding amount of antibody synthesized were directly correlated with protein or protein-calorie intake when three levels of dietary protein were given (6%, 12%, or 27%).[2] In contrast, under conditions of chronic protein or protein-calorie deprivation, some T cell-mediated immunologic functions were increased.[2,3] These functions included proliferative responses to the mitogens, concanavilin A, and phytohemagglutinin, development of delayed hypersensitivity, and formation of migration inhibition factor (MIF).[4]

Studies of tumor immunity further illustrated the depression of the B cell system and sparing of the T cell system when moderate protein-calorie restriction occurred. For example, T killer cell activity was normal or heightened in nutritionally deprived mice and rats using experimental tumor systems, whereas the formation of cytotoxic and blocking antibodies was reduced. However, with only a 3% protein intake, tumor cell killing was markedly reduced in mice. Similar results were noted with guinea pigs.[4]

Wunder et al. carried out a malnutrition study

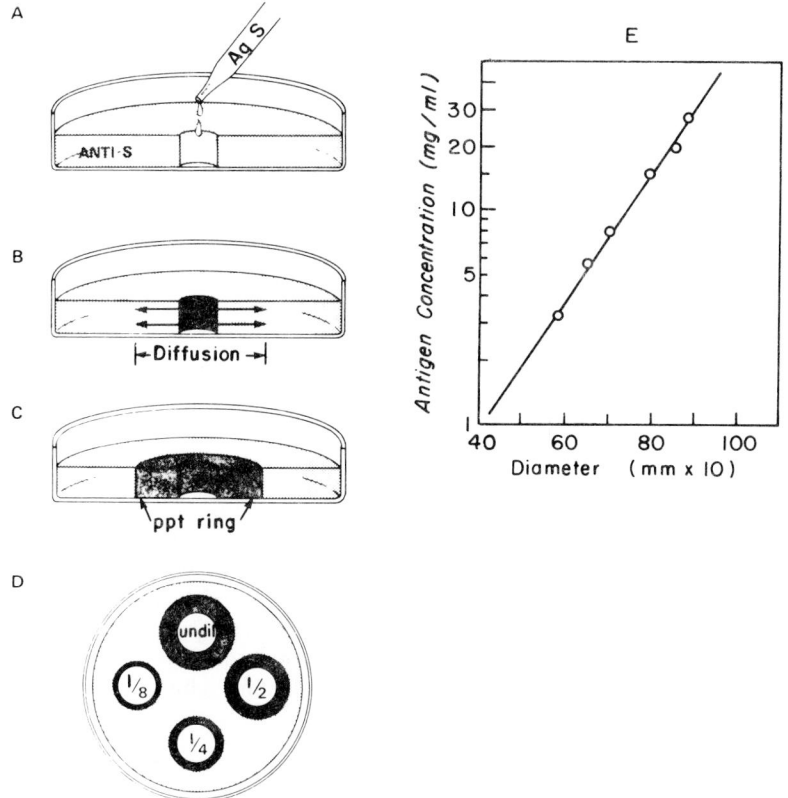

**Fig. 32–9.** Radial immunodiffusion in agar. *A,* Petri dish is filled with semisolid agar solution containing antibody (Ab) to antigen (Ag) S. The center well is filled with a precisely measured concentration of Ag S. *B,* Antigen S is allowed to diffuse radially from the center well. *C,* After reaction proceeds to completion, a sharp ring is formed. *D,* By serial dilution of a known standard quantity of Ag S in a defined measure of time (24 hours), rings of progressively decreasing size are formed. The amount of Ag S in unknown specimens can be calculated and compared with a standard Ag (24 hours) (1/1, 1/4, 1/8). *E,* Relationship of the log of Ag concentration to the diameter of immune precipitate. (From Fudenberg, H.H., Stites, D.P., Caldwell, J.L., et al. (Eds.): Basic and Clinical Immunology. Los Altos, CA, Lange Medical Publications, 1976.)

in guinea pigs using two different protocols.[5] In the first one, test animals started on a normal diet that was reduced by 25% weekly for a 4-week period. In the second protocol, groups of animals were given 5%, 30%, and 60% casein; other dietary components were constant. In the first experiment and in the group that received 5% casein, comparable declines in phagocytic function occurred by the third week. A depression of opsonization was also evident. Serum C3 was significantly lower, and mitogenic responses to phytohemagglutinin were 85% lower in these malnourished animals.

Sakamoto et al. reported that complement components C1, C4, C2, and C3 were lower in the 0.5% protein rat group compared to the 18% protein group.[6] In addition, the $CH_{50}$ titers were also lower in the 0.5% protein group. Sakamoto et al. also found that rats maintained on 0.5% protein diet for 4 weeks exhibited reduced tuberculin skin reactivity.[7] Tuberculin reactivity disappeared

completely in all rats after they were on a 0.5% protein diet for 8 weeks.

It is generally acknowledged that severe protein-calorie malnutrition in humans affects many systems and is usually complicated by multiple simultaneous nutrient deficiencies that also can be aggravated by infection. Nevertheless, the significant body of knowledge available can be helpful in the dissection of this complex problem. In this regard, the weight of evidence now indicates that severe protein or calorie malnutrition in humans results in marked impairment of both humoral and cell-mediated immune functions.[8–11] Severe thymic atrophy and associated T cell deficiencies are particularly common in undernourished children.[12] A depression of T helper cells and possibly an increase in T suppressor cells also can occur in protein-calorie malnutrition.[13] Salimonu et al.[14] and Schlesinger et al.[15] reported decreased killer cell activity and decreased production of interferon in children with protein calorie malnutrition and patients with marasmus, respectively. Several investigators have observed reduced levels of sIgA in pharyngeal secretions, tears, and saliva that could be responsible for the compromised resistance to organisms that cause respiratory infections.[25–28] Impairment of sIgA is thought to represent depression of IgA synthesis in the submucosa or impaired synthesis of secretory component or both.[12] These observations are compatible with the findings in protein-calorie malnutrition of the loss of intestinal epithelium, mucosal thinning, and atrophy of gut-associated lymphoid tissue.[29] A summary of the reported changes in the immune system resulting from protein-calorie malnutrition is presented in Table 32–6.[24]

### Single-Nutrient Deficiencies

Most clinical studies of nutrition-related immunodeficiencies in humans involve multiple-deficiency states commonly complicated by infection. Although data on animals are probably more reliable, selected clinical data have been helpful in arriving at a consensus of how single nutrients affect the immune system. A summary of the effects of single nutrients is presented in Table 32–7.[30]

**Amino Acids.** Aschkenasy noted that isoleucine and valine deficiencies impaired the recovery of both thymus and peripheral lymphoid populations after acute protein deficiency.[31] In addition, deficiencies of methionine and cysteine-cystine also resulted in delayed effects on the recovery of the thymus, lymph nodes, and spleen. The aforementioned amino acids, when deficient, also caused severe lymphocyte depletion of gut-associated lymphoid tissue similar to that seen in total protein deficiency.

Tryptophan is vital in the maintenance of normal antibody production.[31–33] Although methionine appears to be essential in lymphopoiesis, the requirement for antibody synthesis is low.[31]

Jose and Good fed rats diets deficient in single amino acids.[33,34] Diets were given at 50%, 25%, or 10% of normal levels. At 50% dietary level, leucine deficiency resulted in a reduction in the tumor cytotoxic response, whereas serum blocking and hemagglutinating antibody levels were in-

**Table 32–6.   Summary of Effects of Protein-Calorie Malnutrition on Immune Functions**

|  | *Human* | *Animal* |
|---|---|---|
| Lymphoid anatomy[12] | | |
|   Thymus | ↓ | ↓ |
|   Spleen | ↓ | ↓ |
|   Lymph nodes | ↓ | ↓ |
|   Other lymphoid tissue | ↓ | ↓ |
|   Total circulating lymphocytes | ↓ | ↓ |
| Humoral immunity[16] | | |
|   Circulating B-lymphocytes | ↓ or N* | |
|   Serum Ig levels | ↑ or N | |
|   Serum Ab, response to Ag | ↓ | ↓ |
|   Secretory IgA | ↓ | |
|   Splenic plaque-forming cell responses | | ↓ |
| Cellular immunity[9–11] | | |
|   Circulating T-lymphocytes[13,17] | ↓ | |
|   Delayed cutaneous hypersensitivity[9,11,18] | ↓ | ↓ |
|   Allograft rejection | | N or ↑ or ↓ |
|   Tumor cytotoxicity | | ↑ |
|   Immunity to intracellular organisms | ↓ | |
|   Lymphocyte proliferation[9,10,19,20,21] | | |
|     (a) Concanavilin A | ↓ or N | |
|     (b) PHA | ↓ or N | N or ↑ or ↓ |
|     (c) PWM | ↑ or N | |
|   Lymphokine production[15] | ↓ | |
| Phagocytic function[22] | | |
|   Monocyte chemotaxis | ↓ | ↓ |
|   PMN* chemotaxis | N | ↑ |
|   PMN phagocytosis | N | |
|   RES* function | | ↑ or ↓ |
|   Intracellular killing | ↓ or N | N |
| Complement[23] | ↓ | ↓ |

*PMN = polymorphonuclear leukocyte; RES = reticuloendothelial system; N = normal; ↓ = depressed; ↑ = increased.
From Dowd, P.S., Heatley, R.V.,[24] with permission of Clin. Sci., The Biochemical Society, London.

## Table 32–7. Single-Nutrient Effects on Immunologic Functions

| | Lymphocytes | | | | | Immunoglobulins | | | | | Other Immune Functions | | | | | | | | |
|---|---|---|---|---|---|---|---|---|---|---|---|---|---|---|---|---|---|---|---|
| | Lymphoid Anatomy | Total Lymphs in Blood | T and B Cell Differential | Proliferative Response | Splenic PFC Response | Serum Ig Values | Primary Response | Secondary Response | Secretory IgA | Blocking Ig | Delayed Skin Sensitivity | Graft Rejection | PMN Phagocytosis | PMN Bactericidal | Monocyte Function | RES Function | Complement | Inflammatory Response | Host Resistance |
| **Vitamins** | | | | | | | | | | | | | | | | | | | |
| A, Excess | ⇧ | | | ⇧ | | N⇧N | ⇧ | | | | N⇧ | ⇧ | | | ⇧N | ⇧ | ⇧ | | ⇧ |
| A, Deficit | ⇩ | N⇧↓⇩N⇩ | | ⇩ | | ⇩ | ⇩↓ | | | | ↓ | | ⇧ | | ⇧ | ⇩↓⇩ | | | |
| Thiamine | ⇧ | ⇧ | | ⇧ | | ⇧ | | | | | ⇧ | | | | | | | ↓ | |
| Riboflavin | ⇩ | ⇧ | | ⇧ | | ⇧ | | | | | | | | | | | | | |
| Pantothenic acid | ⇩ | N ⇩ | ⇩ | | ↓ ↓⇩ | ⇧ | | | | | | | | | | | | | |
| Pyridoxine | ↓⇩↓⇩ | ⇩ | ⇩ | ⇩ | ↓ ↓⇩ | ⇩ | | | | ↓⇩ | ⇩ | | | | N | ⇩ | | |
| B₁₂ | | ↓ | | | N | ↓ | | | | ⇧ ↓ | | | | | | | | |
| Folic acid | ⇩ | ↓⇩↓⇩ | ⇧ | | ⇩ | ⇩ | | | | ↓⇩ | N ⇩N | | | | ⇩⇩⇩ | | |
| C, Excess | ⇧ | N | ↓ | ⇧ | | | | | ↓ ⇧ | ⇧ | ↓ | | | | | ↓ | ↓⇧ | |
| C, Deficit | ⇩ | N ⇩ | | N⇩N | | ⇩ | ⇩ | ⇩ | ⇩ | N ⇧ | | | ↓⇩ | |
| E, Excess | ⇧ | ↓⇧ | ⇧ | | ⇧ ⇧ ⇧ | ⇧ | | | | ⇧ | ⇧↓ | | ⇧ | | ⇧ |
| E, Deficit | ⇧ | N | ⇩ | ⇧ | | ⇧ | | | | | | | ⇩ | | ⇧ | ⇩ |
| **Minerals** | | | | | | | | | | | | | | | | | | | |
| Iron, Excess | | | | | | | | | | | ⇩ | | | | | | | ⇩⇧ |
| Iron, Deficit | ↓⇩↓↓⇩↓⇧ | | N | N⇩ | ↓ | ↓ | N⇩⇩↓ | ⇩ | ↓ | ↓ ↓⇩↓⇩ |
| Zinc, Excess | | | | | | | | | | ↓⇩ | ⇩ | ⇩ | ⇩ | | |
| Zinc, Deficit | ↓↓⇩⇩↓⇩ | | ⇧ ⇧ | ⇧ | ↓↓ | ⇧↓⇧ | ↓⇩ | ↓ | ↓ |
| Magnesium, Deficit | ⇧ | ⇩ | | ⇩⇩ | ⇧ | | ⇩ ↓ | ⇧ | | ⇧ |
| Selenium, Excess | ⇧ | | ⇧ | | | | | | | | |
| **Amino Acids** | | | | | | | | | | | | | | | | | | | |
| Branch chain | ⇩ | ⇩ | ⇩ | ⇩ | | ⇩ | | | | | | | | | | | | |
| Aromatic | ⇩ | | | | | ⇩ | ⇩ | | ⇩ | | | | | | | ⇩ | | |
| Other | ⇩ | | | | | ⇩ | | ⇩ | | | | | | | | ⇩ | | |
| **Lipids** | | | | | | | | | | | | | | | | | | | |
| Cholesterol, Excess | | | ⇧ | | | ↓⇧ | | | | | ⇩ | ⇩ ⇧ | ⇩ | | ⇩ |
| Fatty Acids, Excess | | ⇩ | ⇩ | | ⇩ | ⇩ | | | ⇩ | ⇧ | | ⇩ |
| Fatty Acids, Deficit | ⇧ | | | ↓ ↓ | | | ↓ | ⇧ | | ⇧ |
| Polyunsaturated fatty acids, Excess | ⇧ | ↓⇩↓⇩ ⇩ | | ⇩ ⇩ | ↓⇩↓ ↓ | ↓⇧ | ↓ | ⇩ |

Any reported change in immune function (top) associated with nutritional variable (left) is indicated by direction and length of arrows. Solid arrows indicate human studies; open arrows, animal findings. N = normal findings; PMN = polymorphonuclear leukocyte; PFC = plaque-forming colonies; RES = reticuloendothelial system.

From Beisel, W.R., et al.: J.A.M.A. 245: 53–58, 1981.

tact. Tryptophan deficiency resulted in depressed cytotoxic function with further reduction with leucine deficiency at the 25% dietary level. However, marked depression of serum blocking and hemagglutinating antibody levels was noted with single deficiencies of methionine-cystine, valine, tryptophan, threonine, and phenylalanine-tyrosine at the 25% dietary level.

Most amino acid deficiencies apparently result in more severe suppression of humoral antibody synthesis than cell-mediated immunity.[34,35] When dietary protein was reduced to 4% in the diet or phenylalanine was reduced to 0.2% of the diet, the reticuloendothelial (RE) system of mice exhibited impaired clearance of labeled polyvinylpyrrolidone.[36,37] Tryptophan deficiency produced similar results.

**Zinc.** Zinc deficiency causes atrophy of lymphoid tissue and produces abnormalities in both cellular and humoral immunity.[38-40]

Zinc deficiency may be one of the most prevalent nutritional problems worldwide. The average adult must obtain about 15 mg of zinc per day from the diet. Since the body stores of this element are limited, a constant steady-state intake of zinc is required. Zinc deficiencies can be due to inadequate diet, disease, or unknown factors that interfere with intestinal absorption.

It now appears that zinc deficiency is primarily caused by diets that contain large amounts of grains, cereals, and unleavened bread. Because these foods contain high amounts of the zinc chelator phytic acid, zinc becomes unavailable for absorption.

Clinically, zinc-deficient children present with lymphopenia, retarded wound healing, thymic atrophy, reduced capacity to exhibit delayed hypersensitivity, and increased susceptibility to disease. A similar pattern of immune defects has been observed in children with acrodermatitis enteropathica, which is an inherited defect in intestinal absorption of zinc. This clinical entity was described in 1942.[41] A zinc supplement was found to be a cure for this disease.[42] Children with this disease tend to be plagued with severe skin disturbances, CNS disorders, GI malfunction, and recurrent infections, particularly with fungi. A similar disease has been found in the A-46 mutant of black, pied Danish cattle, a variant of the Holstein-Friesian line.[43] Calves born with this trait have alopecia, hyperkeratosis, and severely involuted thymus and usually die of infections. Administration of zinc totally cures this syndrome.

Fraker et al.[44,45] observed that young adult mice maintained on a zinc-deficient diet (1 μg zinc/g/day) for 30 days exhibited only 10 to 30% as many IgM and IgG plaque-forming cells per spleen in response to sheep red blood cells (SRBC) when compared to mice receiving 25 μg zinc/g/day. Zinc-deficient mice also experienced severe thymic atrophy. In addition, they responded poorly to T-independent antigens. Secondary responses were also markedly reduced even if the primary immunization was given prior to zinc deprivation.[44] Taste activity and appetite were gradually lost, which resulted in anorexia. This is a serious problem in such experiments because it always raises the potential complicating problem of superimposed protein-calorie malnutrition. To control this potential problem, the investigators included a group of mice that were given a diet containing adequate amounts of zinc, but were given a restricted total diet limited to the average amount consumed by the mice receiving the zinc-deficient diet. The diet-restricted mice experi-enced no suppression of their immune capacity compared to controls for a 30-day period. However, inanition became evident, and the immune response deteriorated when the animals were monitored for an additional 10 days.[46]

In this regard, in vitro studies reveal that splenocytes from zinc-deficient mice gave depressed responses to concanavilin A but exhibited enhanced responses to lipopolysaccharide. These observations suggest a reduced response of T cells with an enhanced response by B cells. Furthermore, the responses of lymphocytes of zinc-deficient mice to allogeneic cells (mixed lymphocyte reaction) were enhanced 100% compared to control or diet-restricted mice. These results indicate that greater numbers of immature T cells occur in the spleens of zinc-deficient mice, a finding that suggests an arrest of T cell maturation.[47]

Hildebrandt et al. reported that the avidities of antibodies in plaques produced by deficient 17-day-old neonates in response to trinitrophenol conjugated to lipopolysaccharide were much lower than those of the normal controls.[48] These data suggest that there is an interference with differentiation and expansion of nonantigen-driven B cell clones. Accordingly, zinc deficiency also may suppress and delay ontogeny of lymphoid cells.

DePasquale-Jardieu and Fraker noted that splenocytes from zinc-deficient mice gave suboptimal secondary responses.[49] Their data suggest that zinc deficiency appears to destroy or block the development of memory cells. Other studies by the same authors revealed that plasma levels of corticosterone were elevated in zinc-deficient mice (115 μg/dl compared to 30 μg/dl for controls).[50-53] Furthermore they noted that in adrenalectomized zinc-deficient mice the thymus did not involute and appeared to contain normal numbers of thymocytes. However, these mice had only marginally better responses to SRBC than intact zinc-deficient mice. Again, the idea emerges that zinc deficiency results in an arrest of T cell maturation. Thymus involution appears to be stress-induced under conditions of zinc malnutrition.

In view of the large number of zinc-dependent enzymes, it is readily understandable how zinc deficiency affects the immune response. Zinc is a cofactor for at least 90 metalloenzymes, including enzymes required for transcription and translation. Because cells of the immune system are under continuous proliferation and differentiation and require numerous enzymes that utilize zinc as a cofactor, it is apparent how this deficiency can affect both the affector and effector responses. T cell maturation and replication in this case are absolute requirements for normal function. A summary of the potential roles of zinc as a cofactor in immune-related enzymes is presented in Table 32–8.[53]

In this regard, it is important that the thymic hormone facteur thymique serique (FTS) exists in two forms. The first form has no zinc and is biologically inactive, whereas the second form contains zinc and is biologically active; this latter form is termed thymulin.[55] At least two laboratories have reported that FTS levels drop sharply after the onset of zinc deficiencies.[55,56]

Studies to date indicate that restoration of zinc to a zinc-deficient diet results in a return of normal immune function within two weeks or less.[57] However, it is puzzling that the kinetics of repair demonstrate a period of augmentation. For example, Zwickl and Fraker observed that previously zinc-deficient mice immunized 4 days after beginning a normal diet produced 2.5 times more PFC/spleen following immunization with SRBC than did controls.[58]

It appears to be well established that zinc deficiency can lead to breakdown in cell-mediated immunity, particularly killer T cell function[59] and helper T cell function.[60] In addition, plaque-forming cell responses also drop dramatically. Because terminal deoxyribonucleotidyltransferase is a zinc-containing DNA polymerase required by immature T cells for replication and function, the unique sensitivity of the T cell system to zinc deficiency can be explained in part.[61]

**Iron.** Human subjects with iron deficiency exhibit impaired delayed hypersensitivity reactions as well as defective neutrophil and macrophage killing functions.[62] It is noteworthy that severely malnourished patients with coexisting deficiencies of protein and iron exhibit very low concentrations of iron-binding proteins in plasma. Such patients may experience a clinical activation of intracellular infections (malaria, tuberculosis, or brucellosis) during iron repletion therapy because iron is freely available to the infective organisms, stimulating their growth in the face of impaired cell-mediated immunity.[63]

Antia et al.[64] reported that the mean level of serum transferrin in patients with kwashiorkor was only 34% of control levels, whereas patients with marasmus had mean transferrin levels that were 71% of those of controls.[64] McFarlane et al. noted that transferrin levels correlated with subsequent survival of children with kwashiorkor.[65] Survivors had transferrin levels about four-fold higher than the levels for those who did not survive. Because low levels of transferrin might make iron more available to bacteria, a low transferrin level might impede the natural antibacterial properties of transferrin if adequate free iron were available. Researchers have suggested that, since transferrin levels are depressed in patients with severe protein-calorie malnutrition, this nutritional deficit must be corrected before iron is administered.[66] Accordingly, hyperferremia or hypotransferrinemia are conditions that result in increased susceptibility to infection.[67]

Iron deficiency in the presence of normal transferrin levels results in atrophy of lymphoid tissues and depletion of lymphocytes with a subsequent decrease in antibody production.[68,69] There is evidence that infants receiving adequate iron and vitamins experienced only one half the incidence of respiratory infections compared to controls who were iron-deficient but received vitamins only.[70]

The effects of iron deficiency on the immune system are controversial.[71–73] Some have suggested that any effect of iron must be via an indirect mechanism that involves perturbation of folate metabolism.[74,75] The role of iron in increased susceptibility to infection as well as its role in lymphocyte and phagocyte function is still partially unresolved largely because of problems relating to coexisting nutrient deficiencies.

**Copper.** Deficiencies of copper appear to prevent the RE system from reacting normally to infection. For example, control spleens increased from 0.21 to 0.92% of body weight during the course of infection, whereas in copper-deficient animals the increase was from 0.17 to 0.22%.[76,77] In summary, these limited studies suggest that a copper deficiency produced a more depressed re-

**Table 32–8. Biochemical Roles of Zinc**

| | *Examples* |
|---|---|
| Cofactor for Enzymes | DNA polymerase |
| | RNA polymerase |
| | Thymidine kinase |
| | Reverse transcriptase |
| | Terminal deoxynucleotidyl- transferase |
| | Alkaline phosphatase |
| | Alcohol dehydrogenase |
| | Carbonic anhydrase |
| | Carboxypeptidase A |
| | Pyruvate carboxylase |
| | Superoxide dismutase |
| | (~ 60 other metalloenzymes) |
| Cofactor of Hormones | Insulin |
| | Facteur thymique serique |
| Membranes | Stabilizer of plasma and lysosomal membranes |
| Cell Replication | Essential to DNA synthesis |
| Mitogen | Weak mitogen at high concentrations |

From Fraker, P.J.[53] with permission of Surv. Immunol. Res.

sponse to infection than either a vitamin $B_{12}$ or protein deficiency.

**Magnesium.** Limited studies reveal that rats depleted of magnesium for 6 to 12 weeks exhibited thymic hyperplasia.[78] In addition, serum IgG levels were 40 to 50% of control levels.[79] Subsequent studies suggested that peak serum hemagglutinin and hemolysin responses were depressed in magnesium-deficient rats (45% of control titers).

**Selenium.** The role of selenium in the immune response is not clear. It has been reported that a moderate increased intake of selenium appears to enhance the immune response in animals.[30] On the other hand, a selenium deficiency that results in a suppressed antibody response can be reversed by giving vitamin E.[80] Other studies reveal that a selenium deficiency leads to a depressed killing of yeast cells by leukocytes.[81,82] A recent report indicates that selenium deficiency affects the secondary antibody response to T cell-dependent antigens.[171]

### Vitamin Deficiencies

Because vitamins have critical roles as coenzymes, it is not unexpected that they play important roles in the immune response.

**Pyridoxine ($B_6$).** As early as 1946, Stoerk and Eisen convincingly demonstrated that pyridoxine-deficient animals produced less antibody than controls.[83] Pruzansky and Axelrod noted that pyridoxine deficiency had the greatest impairment on the anamnestic response.[84] In a clinical study, Hodges et al. observed that experimental pyridoxine deficiency resulted in only slight impairment of antibody formation against tetanus toxoid and typhoid vaccine.[85] However, when human volunteers were deficient in both pyridoxine and pantothenic acid the impairment of the antibody response was substantial, resulting in hypogammaglobulinemia.[86]

Pyridoxine deficiency markedly affects cell-mediated immunity.[87] For example, pyridoxine deficiency increases allogeneic graft survival.[88–90] Pyridoxine-deficient guinea pigs expressed a profound depression of delayed hypersensitivity to purified protein derivative (PPD).[91,92] The afferent limb of the immune response apparently remains intact because restoration of pyridoxine to deficient animals results in a normal response.[91]

**Vitamin C.** An early observation revealed that vitamin C deficiency abolished tuberculin hypersensitivity.[93] In particular, a deficiency during the induction period of immunization severely impaired the responsiveness to tuberculin. Impaired allograft rejection has also been described in guinea pigs deficient in vitamin C.[94] Other studies suggest that vitamin C plays an important role in the development and maintenance of lymphoid tissue.[95] The idea has emerged that vitamin C is involved as a cofactor in the production of thymic humoral factors.[95,96]

Evidence also indicates that vitamin C plays an important role in phagocytic function. In this regard, Shilotri observed that leukocytes from guinea pigs deficient in vitamin C had severely impaired bactericidal activity.[97,98] He also demonstrated that phagocytosis-induced stimulation of NADPH oxidase activity was reduced in leukocytes from ascorbate-deficient animals. In contrast, other investigators found that peritoneal exudate macrophages from guinea pigs deficient in vitamin C were normal except for yield and migratory ability.[99,100]

The effect of megadoses of vitamin C remains controversial. However, no substantial body of data supports the concept that megadoses are beneficial. The weight of evidence supports the concept that physiologic levels are required for proper maintenance of phagocyte function.

**Vitamin A.** Vitamin A is important in the maintenance of epithelial and mucosal surfaces and secretions as a form of primary defense.[101,102] Vitamin A deficiency apparently results in decreased antibody production as well as significant reduction of T cell levels and function.[84,103–106] In contrast, other investigators report an adjuvant-like effect of vitamin A for both antibody and cell-mediated immune response.[107–110] It appears certain that adequate levels of vitamin A are required for optimal humoral and cell-mediated responses.

A recent study is of special significance because it reports that more severe experimental herpes keratitis occurred in rats deficient in vitamin A than in control animals.[172] Other recent studies indicate that rats deficient in vitamin A had reduced blood clearance of bacteria as well as phagocytic activity. The conclusion was that the RE system and PMN functions were impaired.[173]

**Vitamin $B_{12}$.** Deficiencies of vitamin $B_{12}$ result in megaloblastic changes, particularly in the bone marrow. Das and Hoffbrand noted that the lymphocytes from subjects deficient in $B_{12}$ were more "megaloblastoid" than normal cells.[111] They found the lesion to involve methylation of deoxyuridylate to thymidylate. MacCuish found significant depression of lymphocyte transformation to PHA in patients with pernicious anemia.[112] However, T and B cell levels were normal in peripheral blood.

**Folic Acid.** In folic acid deficiency, synthesis of thymidylate stops, which also results in megaloblastic changes of replicating cells. Because body stores of folic acid are depleted rapidly in the face of insufficient intake, megaloblastic changes are evident in a few weeks.[113] One of the most common conditions that leads to folate deficiency is pregnancy.[114,115] The effect on the fetus is yet to be elucidated. There appears little doubt that a folic acid deficiency can lead to decreased responses of T cells to PHA as well as to cytotoxic T cell function.[96,116] Changes are evident in a few weeks.[113]

**Pantothenic Acid.** Axelrod and associates reported that the primary antibody response to SRBC was markedly decreased in rats deficient in pantothenic acid.[117–119] Cells in pantothenic-deficient animals may be incapable of secreting newly synthesized proteins into the extracellular compartment.

**Riboflavin.** Deficiencies of riboflavin in dogs resulted in increases in PMN but a decrease in peripheral lymphocytes.[120] Other reports indicate that riboflavin-deficient rats and swine had impaired agglutinin responses to human RBC. In addition, riboflavin-deficient mice were more susceptible than control animals to *Salmonella typhimurium*.[105,121]

**Biotin.** Deficiency of biotin results in impairment of primary and secondary antibody responses.[105,119]

## Fatty Acids

Di Luzio reported that administration of methyl palmitate impaired reticuloendothelial system (RES) clearance of colloidal carbon.[122] In addition, primary and secondary antibody responses to SRBC were markedly suppressed.[123]

Other investigations indicate that the administration of cholesterol oleate and ethyl palmitate reduces the antibody response when given before immunization.[124] Although mice on a high-fat diet had prolonged graft survival, the effect of excessive lipid intake on delayed hypersensitivity appeared to be negligible.[125,126]

With respect to polyunsaturated fatty acids, other studies indicate an increased inhibition of the in vitro responses to PHA and PPD by the addition of C18:1 to C20:4 fatty acids.[127] Incorporation of [³H] thymidine was inhibited to a greater degree than [³H] uridine incorporation, which suggested that DNA synthesis was more susceptible than RNA synthesis. Curiously, palmitate is effective in reversing the inhibitory effects of arachidonate, linoleate, and oleate.[128]

It has also been reported that rats raised on diets deficient in polyunsaturated fatty acids had increased susceptibility to experimental encephalomyelitis.[129,130]

Of particular interest are the observations that administration of polyunsaturated fatty acids prolonged allograft survival.[131–134] Conversely, animals fed diets deficient in polyunsaturated fatty acids rejected allografts sooner than did controls.[133] It has been suggested that polyunsaturated fatty acids induce splenomegaly with a possible overproduction of spleen suppressor cells. Another possibility is that unsaturated fatty acids serve as precursors of prostaglandins, a theory that is based on the inhibitory effect of PGE, on PHA-induced lymphocyte transformation, as well as on cytotoxic T cell destruction of allogeneic target cells.[135,136]

## Prenatal and Postnatal Malnutrition

The developing thymolymphatic system of the fetus is highly sensitive to malnutrition involving deficiencies of protein, calories, lipotropic factors, vitamins, and iron. In utero malnutrition can result in profound defects of immunologic functions in the face of only a slightly reduced birth weight.

Experimental maternal protein deficiency resulted in decreased thymus weights, as well as cellularity, DNA, RNA, and protein in the thymuses of rat offspring even when the postnatal diet was normal.[137] Thymus weights remained suppressed for four months even though an adequate postnatal diet was given.[138]

Although the data are somewhat uncertain, it is potentially important that humans can suffer apparent long-term immunologic defects as a consequence of in utero or early postnatal malnutrition.[139] For example, maternal malnutrition during the third trimester had marked effects on fetal body weight and organ development. In particular, low-birth-weight infants from nutritionally deficient mothers had impressive reductions in spleen and thymus weights.[140] Immunologic defects that result from intrauterine malnutrition may be fully as severe as those seen in postnatal protein-calorie malnutrition.[141–144] Because of the low cord blood levels of IgG in newborn infants having experienced intrauterine malnutrition, placental transfer of maternal IgG may be impaired.[143]

Long-term studies on effects of intrauterine malnutrition have revealed decreased T cell levels as well as marked impairment of delayed hypersensitivity.[144] Collectively, the results indicate that immunologic defects resulting from intrauterine malnutrition may be more refractory to reversal than the defects that accrue following only postnatal undernutrition.

Infants with only slight fetal growth retardation due to malnutrition have exhibited minimal immunologic impairment, whereas those infants who suffered from severely retarded intrauterine growth have exhibited marked impairment of delayed hypersensitivity. Deficiency of protein or calories usually results in chronic suppression of both humoral and cell-mediated immunity.

## Immunologic Sequelae in Malnourished Children

One of early changes that has been noted in severely malnourished children is thymic atrophy.[145] Decreased cellularity was evident in certain areas of the spleen and lymph nodes usually populated by T-lymphocytes. Postmortem studies on African children with marasmus and kwashiorkor revealed markedly reduced weights of thymuses, spleens, Peyer's patches, and appendices. In particular paracortical areas were depleted and germinal centers were absent. The histopathologic picture correlated well with the reduced level of responsiveness to dinitrochlorobenzene (DNCB) and lowered blastogenic activity of their lymphocytes to PHA.[146]

Neumann et al. examined the immune status of Ghanaian children with moderate or severe malnutrition.[147] Marked depression of CMI responses was noted in all severely malnourished children with either marasmus or kwashiorkor. The authors found close correlations between delayed hypersensitivity to SKSD and candidin and levels of serum albumin, carotene, vitamin C, and total serum protein. Whereas relatively rapid recovery of normal CMI responses has been observed upon nutritional rehabilitation, in some instances impairment of CMI responses has persisted for several years.[148] For example, Dutz et al. reported that orphans who had been severely malnourished with infection during early infancy exhibited depression of CMI responses for at least five years even though they were free of intercurrent disease and well nourished.[149] McMurray et al. demonstrated that severely protein-malnourished children did not exhibit normal CMI responses even after nutritional rehabilitation.[150] Moderately malnourished children have responded with significantly less delayed hypersensitivity to PPD following BCG vaccination.[151] Most CMI parameters are impaired in malnourished children, whereas some of the same parameters are normal or enhanced in moderately malnourished experimental animals.

It has been conclusively demonstrated that serum complement levels are reduced in children with protein-calorie malnutrition followed by an increase during nutritional rehabilitation.[150,152,153] Children suffering from moderate and severe protein malnutrition experience significant suppression (50%) of lysozyme secretion into tears.[154] In addition, the synthesis and secretion of secretory IgA are also reduced. Severely protein-malnourished Thai,[155] Indian,[156] and Colombian[157] children had 35 to 50% reduction of secretory IgA in secretions. However, levels of IgG or albumin were not reduced. A summary of secretory IgA levels in malnourished children in found in Table 32–9.

Numerous pressing questions remain unanswered as to the duration of immunologic impairment of a neonate who experiences intrauterine malnutrition as well as the degree and reversibility in terms of timing and qualitative nature of the deficiency.

## Overnutrition

Definitive studies that elucidate the effects of obesity or overnutrition on the immune system are lacking. It appears that excess intake of saturated and unsaturated fatty acids interferes with normal RE system functions. Excess intake of polyunsaturated fatty acids causes suppression of cell-mediated immune functions. In contrast, low intake causes some potentiation of the immune response.

A moderate excess of vitamin A and vitamin E seems to exert an adjuvant-like effect on humoral and cell-mediated immunity. Excess sugar intake or hyperglycemia, as in diabetes, has been reported to impair phagocyte function.

In general, the incidence of lower respiratory tract infections is higher in obese infants than in infants of normal weight.[158,159]

## Interaction of Nutrition and Infection

The effect of infection on an existing state of malnutrition is poorly understood.[12] Infection causes negative balances of nitrogen, zinc, iron, potassium, phosphates, magnesium, and sulfates as well as plasma amino acids.[160] For example, bacterial diarrhea is associated with malabsorption and possible nutrient deficiencies.[161] Infection also can cause anorexia, which can result in undernutrition or, in some instances, an unexplainable temporary resistance to infection.[162,163] Gopalan theorized that marasmus is an extreme degree of adaptation to malnutrition in which organs and body functions are protected at the expense of muscle tissue, whereas kwashiorkor develops when this adaptation breaks down.[164] Beisel has suggested that infection may be a common factor that triggers the breakdown.[160]

Malnourished populations have impaired resistance to certain infections. Accordingly, it is readily understandable how anorexia and a negative nitrogen balance brought on by infection could aggravate even a moderate state of malnutrition.[165–167] Subclinical infections produced with living vaccines can induce measurable deficits in the nutritional status of apparently healthy

**Table 32–9.  Secretory Immunoglobulin A (SIgA) and Antibody Titers in Malnourished Children**

| | Well Nourished | Malnourished |
|---|---|---|
| Indian children[25] | | |
| SIgA in nasopharyngeal secretions | 2.8 mg/dl[20]* | 1.56 mg/dl[20]† |
| Neut. measles antibody titer | 1:64 titer[20] | 1:4 titer[20]† |
| Neut. poliovirus antibody titer | 1:64 titer[20] | 1:4 titer[20]† |
| Thai children[155] | | |
| SIgA in nasal washings | 28.5 ± 3.4 mg/dl[23] | 11.5 ± 7.8 mg/dl[24]† |
| Indian children[169] | 42 ± 4 mg/dl[12] | 7 ± 2 mg/dl[16]† |
| SIgA in duodenal fluid | 120 ± 17 mg/g protein | 25 ± 9 mg/g protein† |
| SIgA in saliva | 24 ± 7 mg/dl[12] | 4 ± 2 mg/dl[160]† |
| | 60 ± 14 mg/g protein | 13 ± 8 mg/g protein† |
| SIgA in tears | 31 ± 14 mg/dl[12] | 10 ± 2 mg/dl[16]† |
| | 91 ± 15 mg/g protein | 32 ± 8 mg/g protein† |
| Indonesian children[170] | 15.1 ± 2.5 mg/dl[6] | 42.7 ± 6[29] |
| SIgA in duodenal fluids | | |

*Number studied
†Significantly reduced
From Stiehm, E.R.,[16] with permission of Fed. Proc.

children, a finding that is also reflected in subnormal weight gain.[168]

## SUMMARY

It can be concluded that protein-calorie malnutrition has a greater effect on cell-mediated immunity than humoral immunity, although it is recognized that this point is somewhat controversial. Some of this controversy may be the result of simultaneous uneven multicomponent nutritional deficiencies. For example, a concurrent zinc deficiency could cause an exaggerated impairment of the cell-mediated immune response. Single amino acid deficiencies such as tryptophan also could exaggerate a marginal protein-calorie deficiency.

Aside from an impairment of the B- and T-lymphocyte network and resultant defective afferent responses, it is likely that impaired phagocyte function also becomes a sequela of malnutrition. This alone could explain increased incidence of infection in malnourished children. Phagocyte defects in protein-calorie malnutrition can include impaired chemotaxis, phagocytosis, bactericidal action, and metabolic responses, including the monophosphate shunt.

There is little doubt that single vitamin deficiencies can impair the immune response. This issue takes on great importance when one considers that 88% of a United States hospital population had at least one deficiency based on the results of a recent survey.

Of the so-called trace elements, zinc undoubtedly plays an essential role in the lymphocyte and mononuclear phagocyte systems. It is plausible that this deficiency is more common than realized, particularly in the aging population. The need for iron is well recognized.

An important area for future research involves the quantitative and qualitative nature of the effects of intrauterine malnutrition. The suggestion that impaired immune function in this case may be irreversible at least in part calls for extensive research of this problem.

Immunologists and nutritionists must not draw major conclusions concerning nutrient effects based on small shifts in Ig levels, T and B cell counts, and phagocytic functional assays. It is always tempting to generalize from significant deviations of normal values. More research is needed to determine what degree of shifts of immunologic parameters is required to place a subject at risk of infection or disease. Furthermore, infections can aggravate an already nutrition-compromised host and exacerbate immunologic functional impairment. In this regard, "hospital malnutrition" is an established phenomenon that is undoubtedly the result of synergism between marginal nutrition and an already existing disease complicated by physician-induced disease.

Future research needs to examine carefully why the incidence of infection is not more extensive in severe undernutrition considering the gross alterations of immunologic parameters that have been observed. Questions that remain unanswered include the following: (1) Are infectious organisms less aggressive or virulent in a host that provides a poor nutritional environment? This theory would support the old adage, "starve the patient and starve the disease." (2) Is there compensatory nonspecific activation of the mononuclear phagocyte system when acquired immune mechanisms are compromised by undernutrition? Research in nutrition and immunology will have many unresolved topics for future investigation.

# REFERENCES

1. Axelrod, A.E., Pruzansky, J.: Vitam. Horm. *13*:1, 1955.
2. Cooper, W.C., Good, R.A., Mariani, T.: Am. J. Clin. Nutr. *27*:647, 1974.
3. Jose, D.G., Good, R.A.: Nature *231*:323, 1971.
4. Kramer, T.R., Good, R.A.: Clin. Immunol. Immunopathol. *11*:212, 1978.
5. Wunder, J.A., Stinnett, J.D., Alexander, J.W.: Surgery *84*:542, 1978.
6. Sakamoto, M., Ishii, S., Nishioka, K., et al.: Infect. Immun. *32*:553, 1981.
7. Sakamoto, M., Nishioka, K., Shimada, K.: Immunology *38*:413, 1979.
8. Watson, R.R., Petro, T.M.: CRC Crit. Rev. Microbiol. *10*:297, 1984.
9. Neumann, C.G., Lawlor, G.J., Stiehm, E.R., et al.: Am. J. Clin. Nutr. *28*:89, 1975.
10. McMurray, D.N., Loomis, S.A., Casazza, L.J., et al.: Am. J. Clin. Nutr. *34*:68, 1981.
11. Bistrian, B.R., Blackburn, G.L., Scrimshaw, N.S., et al.: Am. J. Clin. Nutr. *28*:1148, 1975.
12. Chandra, R.K., Newberne, P.M.: Nutrition, Immunity and Infection: Mechanism of Interactions. New York, Plenum Publishing Corp., 1977.
13. Chandra, R.K.: Pediatrics *59*:423, 1977.
14. Salimonu, L.S., Ojo-Amaize, E., Williams, A.I.O., et al.: Clin. Immunol. Immunopathol. *24*:1, 1982.
15. Schlesinger, L., Ohlbaum, A., Grez, L., et al.: Am. J. Clin. Nutr. *29*:758, 1976.
16. Stiehm, E.R.: Fed. Proc. *39*:3093, 1980.
17. Salimonu, L.S., Johnson, A.O.K., Williams, A.I.O., et al.: Br. J. Nutr. *48*:7, 1982.
18. Schlesinger, L., Stekel, A.: Am. J. Clin. Nutr. *27*:615, 1974.
19. Rafii, M., Hashemi, S., Nahani, J., et al.: Clin. Immunol. Immunopathol. *8*:1, 1977.
20. Beatty, D.W., Dowdle, E.B.: Clin. Exp. Immunol. *35*:433, 1979.
21. Messer, H.H., Murray, E.J., Goebel, N.K.: J. Nutr. *112*:652, 1982.
22. Strauss, R.G.: Am. J. Clin. Nutr. *31*:660, 1978.
23. Haller, L., Zubler, R.H., Lambert, P.H.: Clin. Exp. Immunol. *34*:248, 1978.
24. Dowd, P.S., Heatley, R.V.: Clin. Sci. *66*:241, 1984.
25. Chandra, R.K.: Br. Med. J. *2*:583, 1975.
26. McMurray, D.N., Rey, H., Casazza, L.J., et al.: Am. J. Clin. Nutr. *30*:1944, 1977.
27. Shilotri, P.G., Bhat, K.S.: Am. J. Clin. Nutr. *30*:1077, 1977.
28. Suskind, R.M., Shrisinha, S., Edelman, R., et al.: Immunoglobulins and antibody response in Thai children with protein-calorie malnutrition. *In* Malnutrition and the Immune Response. (Suskind, R.M., Ed.) New York, Raven Press, 1977.
29. Smythe, P.M., Brereton-Stiles, G.G., Grace, H.J., et al.: Lancet *2*:939, 1971.
30. Beisel, W.R., Edelman, R., Nauss, K., et al.: J.A.M.A. *245*:53, 1981.
31. Aschkenasy, A.: World Rev. Nutr. Diet. *21*:152, 1975.
32. Gershoff, S.N., Gill, T.J., Simonian, S.J.: J. Nutr. *95*:184, 1968.
33. Jose, D.G., Good, R.A.: J. Exp. Med. *137*:1, 1973.
34. Jose, D.G., Good, R.A.: Cancer Res. *33*:807, 1973.
35. Jose, D.G., Good, R.A.: Nature (London) *231*:323, 1971.
36. Coovadia, H.M., Soothill, J.F.: Clin. Exp. Immunol. *23*:373, 1976.
37. Coovadia, H.M., Soothill, J.F.: Clin. Exp. Immunol. *23*:562, 1976.
38. Dreizen, S.: Int. J. Vitam. Nutr. Res. *49*:220, 1978.
39. Beisel, W.R.: Malnutrition and the immune response. *In* Biochemistry of Nutrition I. (Neuberger, A., Jukes, T.H., Eds.) Baltimore, University Park Press, 1979.
40. Edelman, R.: Cell-mediated immune response in protein-calorie malnutrition—a review. *In* Malnutrition and the Immune Response. (Suskind, R.M., Ed.) New York, Raven Press, 1977.
41. Danbolt, N., Closs, K.: Acta Derm. Venereol. *23*:127, 1942.
42. Moynahan, E.J., Barnes, P.M.: Lancet *1*:676, 1973.
43. Khalid, M., Kabiel, A., El-Khateeb, S., et al.: Am. J. Clin. Nutr. *27*:260, 1974.
44. Fraker, P.J., Haas, S.M., Luecke, R.W.: J. Nutr. *107*:1889, 1977.
45. Fraker, P.J., DePasquale-Jardieu, P., Zwickl, C.M., et al.: Proc. Natl. Acad. Sci. USA *75*:5660, 1978.
46. Luecke, R.W., Simonel, C.E., Fraker, P.J.: J. Nutr. *108*:881, 1978.
47. Nash, L., Iwata, T., Fernandes, G., et al.: Cell. Immunol. *48*:238, 1979.
48. Hildebrandt, K.J., Luecke, R.W., Fraker, P.J.: Fed. Proc. *41*:84a, 1982.
49. DePasquale-Jardieu, P., Fraker, P.: J. Nutr. *114*:1762, 1984.
50. Jardieu, P., Fraker, P.J.: Fed. Proc. *41*:218a, 1982.
51. DePasquale-Jardieu, P., Fraker, P.J.: J. Nutr. *109*:1847, 1979.
52. DePasquale-Jardieu, P., Fraker, P.J : J. Immunol. *124*:2650, 1980.
53. Fraker, P.J.: Surv. Immunol. Res. *2*:155, 1983.
54. Dardenne, M., Pleau, J., Lefrancier, P., et al.: C. Hebd. Seanc. Acad. Sci. Paris *292*:793, 1981.
55. Iwata, T., Incefy, G.S., Tanaka, T., et al.: Cell. Immunol. *47*:100, 1979.
56. Chandra, R.K., Heresi, G., Au, B.: Clin. Exp. Immunol. *42*:332, 1980.
57. Fraker, P.J., Zwickl, C.M., Luecke, R.W.: J. Nutr. *112*:309, 1982.
58. Zwickl, C.M., Fraker, P.J.: Immunol. Commun. *9*:a611, 1980.
59. Fernandes, G., Nair, M., Onoe, K., et al.: Proc. Natl. Acad. Sci. USA *76*:457, 1979.
60. Fraker, P.J., Haas, S.M., Luecke, R.W.: J. Nutr. *107*:1889, 1977.
61. McCaffrey, R., Smoler, D.F.: Proc. Natl. Acad. Sci. USA *70*:521, 1973.
62. Chandra, R.K., Au, B., Woodford, G., et al.: Iron status, immune response and susceptibility to infection. *In* Iron Metabolism. (Kies, H., Ed.) Ciba Foundation Symposium 51. Amsterdam, Elsevier/Excerpta Medica/North Holland, 1977.
63. Murray, M.J., Murray, A.B., Murray, M.B., et al.: Br. Med. J. *2*:1113, 1978.
64. Antia, A.U., McFarlane, H., Soothill, J.F.: Arch. Dis. Child. *43*:459, 1968.
65. McFarlane, H., Reddy, S., Adcock, K.J., et al.: Br. Med. J. *4*:268, 1970.
66. Weinberg, E.: Am. J. Clin. Nutr. *30*:1485, 1977.
67. Powanda, M.C.: Am. J. Clin. Nutr. *30*:1254, 1977.
68. Chandra, R.K.: Nutr. Rev. *34*:129, 1976.
69. Nalder, B.N., Mahoney, A.W., Makrishnan, R., et al.: J. Nutr. *102*:535, 1972.
70. Andelman, M.G., Sered, B.R.: Am. J. Dis. Child. *111*:45, 1966.

71. Gross, R.L., Reid, J.V.O., Newberne, P.M., et al.: Am. J. Clin. Nutr. *28*:225, 1975.

72. Kulapongs, P., Suskind, R.M., Vithayasai, V., et al.: Lancet *2*:689, 1974.

73. Suskind, R.M., Kulapongs, P., Vithayasai, V., et al.: Iron deficiency anemia and the immune response. *In* Malnutrition and the Immune Response. (Suskind, R.M., Ed.) New York, Raven Press, 1977.

74. Hershko, C., Karasi, A., Eylon, L., et al.: Blood *36*:321, 1970.

75. Toskes, P.P., Smith, G.W., Bensinger, T.A., et al.: Am. J. Clin. Nutr. *27*:355, 1974.

76. Newberne, P.M., Gebhardt, B.M.: Nutr. Rep. Int. *7*:407, 1973.

77. Newberne, P.M., Hunt, C.E., Young, V.R.: Br. J. Exp. Pathol. *49*:448, 1968.

78. Alcock, N.W., Shils, M.E., Lieberman, P.H., et al.: Cancer Res. *33*:2196, 1973.

79. Alcock, N.W., Shils, M.E.: Proc. Soc. Exp. Biol. Med. *145*:855, 1974.

80. Chandra, R.K.: Can. J. Physiol. Pharmacol. *61*:290, 1983.

81. Serfass, R.E., Ganther, H.E.: Nature *255*:640, 1975.

82. Boyne, R., Arthur, J.R.: Proc. Nutr. Soc. *38*:14a, 1978.

83. Stoerk, H.C., Eisen, H.N.: Proc. Soc. Exp. Biol. Med. *62*:88, 1946.

84. Pruzansky, J., Axelrod, A.E.: Proc. Soc. Exp. Biol. Med. *89*:323, 1955.

85. Hodges, R.E., Bean, W.B., Ohlson, M.A., et al.: Am. J. Clin. Nutr. *11*:180, 1962.

86. Hodges, R.E., Bean, W.B., Ohlson, M.A., et al.: Am. J. Clin. Nutr. *11*:187, 1962.

87. Axelrod, A.E., Trakatellis, A.C.: Vitam. Horm. *22*:591, 1964.

88. Parkes, A.S.: Nature (London) *184*:699, 1959.

89. Axelrod, A.E., Fisher, E.B., Fisher, E., et al.: Science *127*:152, 1975.

90. Herr, N.G., Coursin, D.B.: J. Nutr. *88*:273, 1966.

91. Axelrod, A.E., Trakatellis, A.C., Bloch, H., et al.: J. Nutr. *79*:161, 1963.

92. Stinebring, W.R., Trakatellis, A.C., Axelrod, A.E., et al.: J. Immunol. *91*:39, 1963.

93. Mueller, P.S., Kies, M.W.: Nature (London) *195*:813, 1962.

94. Kalden, J.R., Guthy, E.A.: Eur. Surg. Res. *4*:114, 1972.

95. Dieter, M.P.: Proc. Soc. Exp. Biol. Med. *132*:1147, 1969.

96. Gross, R.L., Newberne, P.M.: Malnutrition, the thymolymphatic system, and immunocompetence. *In* The Reticuloendothelial System in Health and Disease, Vol. B. (Friedman, H., Escobar, M.R., Reichard, S.M., Eds.) New York, Plenum Press, 1976.

97. Shilotri, P.G.: J. Nutr. *107*:1507, 1977.

98. Shilotri, P.G.: J. Nutr. *107*:1513, 1977.

99. Ganguly, R., Durieux, M.F., Waldman, R.H.: Am. J. Clin. Nutr. *29*:762, 1976.

100. Stankova, L., Gebhardt, N.B., Nagel, L., et al.: Infect. Immun. *12*:252, 1975.

101. Beisel, W.R.: Nonspecific host factors—a review. *In* Malnutrition and the Immune Response. (Suskind, R.M., Ed.) New York, Raven Press, 1977.

102. Neumann, C.G.: Nonspecific host factors and infection in malnutrition. *In* Malnutrition and the Immune Response. (Suskind, R.M., Ed.) New York, Raven Press, 1977.

103. Krishnan, S., Bhuyan, U.N., Talwar, G.P., et al.: Immunology *27*:383, 1974.

104. Nauss, K.M., Mark, D.A., Suskind, R.M.: J. Nutr. *109*:1815, 1979.

105. Ludovici, P.P., Axelrod, A.E.: Proc. Soc. Exp. Biol. Med. *77*:526, 1951.

106. Harmon, B.G., Miller, E.R., Hoeffer, J.A., et al.: J. Nutr. *79*:263, 1963.

107. Cohen, B.E., Cohen, I.K.: J. Immunol. *111*:1376, 1973.

108. Jurin, M., Tannock, I.F.: Immunology *23*:283, 1972.

109. Floersheim, G.I., Bollag, W.: Transplantation *15*:564, 1972.

110. Levis, W.R., Emden, R.G.: Proc. Am. Assoc. Cancer Res. *17*:112, 1976.

111. Das, K.C., Hoffbrand, A.V.: Br. J. Haematol. *19*:459, 1970.

112. MacCuish, A.C., Urbaniak, S.J., Goldstone, A.H., et al.: Blood *44*:849, 1974.

113. Chanarin, I.: The Megaloblastic Anaemias. Oxford, Blackwell, 1969.

114. Chanarin, I., Rothman, D., Ward, A., et al.: Br. Med. J. *2*:390, 1968.

115. Lowenstein, L., Cantile, G., Ramos, O., et al.: Can. Med. Assoc. J. *95*:797, 1966.

116. Hollingsworth, J.W., Carr, J.: Cell. Immunol. *8*:270, 1973.

117. Axelrod, A.E.: Nutrition in relation to acquired immunity. *In* Modern Nutrition in Health and Disease. 6th ed. (Goodhart, R.S., Shils, M.E., Eds.) Philadelphia, Lea & Febiger, 1980, p. 578.

118. Lederer, W.H., Kumar, M., Axelrod, A.E.: J. Nutr. *105*:17, 1975.

119. Axelrod, A.E.: Am. J. Clin. Nutr. *24*:265, 1971.

120. Morgan, A.F., Groody, M., Axelrod, A.E.: Am. J. Physiol. *146*:723, 1946.

121. Harmon, B.G., Miller, E.R., Hoefer, J.A., et al.: J. Nutr. *79*:269, 1963.

122. Di Luzio, N.R.: Adv. Lipid Res. *10*:43, 1972.

123. Di Luzio, N.R., Wooles, W.R.: Am. J. Physiol. *206*:939, 1961.

124. Stuart, A.E., Davidson, A.E.: J. Pathol. Bacteriol. *87*:305, 1964.

125. Santiago-Delpin, E.A., Szepsenwol, J.: J. Natl. Cancer Inst. *59*:459, 1977.

126. Fiser, R.H., Denniston, J.C., McGann, V.G., et al.: Infect. Immun. *8*:105, 1973.

127. Mertin, J., Huges, D.: Int. Arch. Allergy Appl. Immunol. *48*:203, 1975.

128. Weyman, C., Belin, J., Smith, A.D., et al.: Lancet *2*:33, 1975.

129. Clausen, J., Moller, J.: Int. Arch. Allergy Appl. Immunol. *36*:224, 1969.

130. Selivonchick, D.P., Johnston, P.V.: J. Nutr. *105*:288, 1975.

131. Meade, C.J., Mertin, J.: Int. Arch. Allergy Appl. Immunol. *48*:203, 1975.

132. Mertin, J.: Transplantation *21*:1, 1976.

133. Mertin, J., Hunt, R.: Proc. Natl. Acad. Sci. USA *73*:928, 1976.

134. Mertin, J., Meade, C.J., Hunt, R., et al.: Int. Arch. Allergy Appl. Immunol. *53*:469, 1977.

135. Smith, J.W., Steiner, A.L., Parker, C.W.: J. Clin. Invest. *50*:442, 1971.

136. Henney, C.S., Bourne, H.R., Lichtenstein, L.M.: J. Immunol. *108*:1526, 1972.

137. Zeman, F.J., Stanbrough, E.C., Shrader, R.E.: Fed. Proc. *28*:1288a, 1969.

138. Olusi, S.O., McFarlane, H.: Pediatr. Res. *10*:707, 1976.

139. Naeye, R.L., Blanc, W.B., Paul, C.: Pediatrics *52*:491, 1973.
140. Jelliffe, D.B.: J. Trop. Pediatr. *20*:232, 1974.
141. Chandra, R.K.: Lancet *2*:1393, 1974.
142. Chandra, R.K.: Am. J. Dis. Child. *129*:450, 1975.
143. Chandra, R.K.: Cell-mediated immunity in fetally and postnatally malnourished children from India and Newfoundland. *In* Malnutrition and the Immune Response. (Suskind, R.M., Ed.) New York, Raven Press, 1977.
144. Chandra, R.K., Ali, S.K., Kutty, K.M., et al.: Biol. Neonate *31*:15, 1977.
145. Watts, T.: J. Trop. Pediatr. *15*:155, 1969.
146. Smythe, P.M., Schonlan, M., Brereton-Stiles, G.G., et al.: Lancet *2*:1939, 1971.
147. Neumann, C.G., Lawlor, G.J., Stiehm, E.R., et al.: Am. J. Clin. Nutr. *28*:89, 1975.
148. Watson, R.R., McMurray, D.N.: CRC Crit. Rev. Food Sci. Nutr. *12*:113, 1979.
149. Dutz, W., Rossipal, E., Ghavami, H., et al.: Eur. J. Pediatr. *122*:117, 1976.
150. McMurray, D.N., Watson, R.R., Reyes, M.A.: Am. J. Clin. Nutr. *34*:2117, 1981.
151. Ziegler, H.D., Ziegler, P.B.: Johns Hopkins Med. J. *137*:59, 1975.
152. Sirisinha, S., Suskind, R.M., Edelman, R., et al.: The complement system in protein-calorie malnutrition. *In* Malnutrition and the Immune Response. (Suskind, R.M., Ed.) New York, Raven Press, 1977.
153. McMurray, D.N., Reyes, M.A., Watson, R.R.: Fed. Proc. *36*:1171, 1977.
154. McMurray, D.N., Rey, H., Casazza, L.J., et al.: Am. J. Clin. Nutr. *30*:1944, 1977.
155. Sirisinha, E., Edelman, R., Asvapaka, C., et al.: Pediatrics, *55*:166, 1975.
156. Chandra, R.K.: Br. Med. J. *2*:583, 1975.
157. McMurray, D.N., Rey, H., Casazza, L.J., et al.: Fed. Proc. *35*:588, 1976.
158. Hutchinson-Smith, B.: Med. Off. *123*:257, 1970.
159. Leonard, P.J., MacWilliam, K.M.: J. Endocrinol. *29*:273–279, 1964.
160. Beisel, W.R.: Adv. Nutr. Res. *1*:125, 1977.
161. Ghadimi, H., Kamar, S., Abaci, F.: Pediatr. Res. *7*:161, 1973.
162. Wing, E.J., Young, J.B.: Infect. Immun. *28*:771, 1973.
163. Murray, J., Murray, A.: Prospect. Biol. Med. *20*:471, 1977.
164. Gopalan, C.: Am. J. Clin. Nutr. *23*:35, 1970.
165. Beisel, W.R.: Am. J. Clin. Nutr. *30*:1236, 1977.
166. Scrimshaw, N.S.: Bibl. Nutr. Dieta. *18*:153, 1973.
167. Arbeter, A., Echeverri, L., Franco, D., et al.: Fed. Proc. *30*:1421, 1971.
168. Kielmann, A.A.: Am. J. Clin. Nutr. *30*:592, 1977.
169. Reddy, V., Raghuramulu, N., Bhaskaram, C.: Arch. Dis. Child. *51*:871, 1976.
170. Bell, R.G., Turner, K.J., Gracey, M., et al.: Am. J. Clin. Nutr. *29*:392, 1976.
171. Mulhern, S.A., Taylor, G.L., Magruder, L.E., et al.: Nutr. Res. *5*:201, 1985.
172. Nauss, K.M., Anderson, C.A., Conner, M.W., et al.: J. Nutr. *115*:1300, 1985.
173. Ongsakul, M., Sirisinha, S., Lamb, A.J : Proc. Soc. Exp. Biol. Med. *178*:204, 1985.

## SELECTED READINGS

Diet, Nutrition, and Cancer. National Academy Press, 1982.

Eisen, H.N.: Immunology. 2nd edition. Harper & Row, 1980.

Golub, E.S.: The Cellular Basis of the Immune Response, An Approach to Immunobiology. 2nd edition. Sunderland, MA, Sinauer Associates, 1981.

Hood, L.E., et al.: Immunology. 2nd edition. Menlo Park, CA, The Benjamin/Cummings Publishing Company, 1984.

McMurray, D.N.: Cell-mediated immunity in nutritional deficiency. Prog. Food Nutr. Sci. *8*:193–228, 1984.

Myrvik, Q.N., Weiser, R.S.: Fundamentals of Immunology. 2nd edition. Philadelphia, Lea & Febiger, 1984.

Nisonoff, A.: Introduction to Molecular Immunology. Sunderland, MA, Sinauer Associates, 1982.

Panush, R.S., Delafuente, J.C.: Vitamins and immunocompetence. World Rev. Nutr. Diet. *45*:97–132, 1985.

Megadose zinc intakes impair immune responses. Nutr. Rev. *43*:141–143, 1985.

Johnston, D.V., Marshall, L.A.: Dietary fat, prostaglandins and the immune response. Prog. Food Nutr. Sci *8*:3–25, 1984.

*Chapter* **33**

# NUTRITION AND CELL AND ORGAN GROWTH

## Elsie M. Widdowson

All mammals start life as a single cell, the fertilized ovum. During the early part of gestation this cell divides and redivides many times, and different kinds of cell develop during the process of differentiation and arrange themselves to form part of the various organs of the body. No two types of cell and no two organs are the same and, moreover, within any one organ there are often several kinds of cell. Some cells have a single nucleus, those of the kidney for example; others like muscle fibers have many nuclei, and others again such as the red blood cells have no nuclei at all. Some cells, such as the neuronal and glial cells of the brain, are relatively stable, but others, like the cells of the intestinal mucosa, are continually being removed and new cells take their place. Thus cell growth and organ growth are complex processes, and broad generalizations may be misleading. However, certain principles apply to all cells, whatever their situation and function. Cells are the metabolically active part of the body, and they are surrounded by extracellular fluid. All transport of nutrients and waste products to and from the cell must take place through the extracellular fluid, for there is no direct exchange between one cell and another. Mechanisms are necessary to replenish the nutrients by absorption from the digestive tract and to remove the waste products through the kidneys if the extracellular fluid is to remain constant in volume and composition. Since all exchanges between cell and extracellular fluid have to take place through the surface of the cell, there must be a limit to the

volume a cell can attain if its more slowly expanding surface is to fulfill the demands made upon it by the metabolism of the inclusions within it.

The fluid inside and outside the cells is in osmotic equilibrium, but the composition of the two fluids is very different: potassium is the cation of the cells and sodium of the fluid surrounding them (Table 33–1). Within the past 10 to 15 years it has gradually been realized, however, that the relatively minute amounts of calcium within the cells and their mitochondria are of vital importance to function. Phosphorus is the main cellular anion, and chloride is the extracellular one. A large part of the protein in the body is inside the cells.

The composition of the intra- and extracellular fluid remains remarkably constant in many re-

**Table 33–1. Composition of Plasma and Intracellular Fluid***

| | Plasma meq/L water | Intracellular Fluid meq/L water |
|---|---|---|
| Na | 169 | 8 |
| K | 6 | 151 |
| Ca | 6 | 2 |
| Mg | 6 | 28 |
| Cl | 123 | — |
| HCO$_3$ | 32 | 10 |
| PO$_4$ | 2 | 100 |
| SO$_4$ | 1 | 10 |

*From Black, D.A.K.,[1] with permission of Blackwell Scientific Publications.

spects, not only from age to age, but also from species to species. However, the relative amounts of the two fluids within the body vary greatly from one age and one organ to another and may alter in malnutrition and disease. The immature organism is characterized by having a large volume of extracellular fluid in all its organs and tissues in relation to the cell mass. As development proceeds and the cells increase in number and size, the proportion of the tissue taken up by the cells increases, and the percentage of extracellular material decreases. This is true of all the separate parts of the body and of the body as a whole. However, some organs develop earlier in this respect than others, the fetal heart and kidney, for example, being nearer their adult composition than skeletal muscle at the time of birth.

## CELL AND ORGAN GROWTH

Growth in the early stages of gestation is brought about entirely by cell division. Because the first divisions of the ovum are not preceded by any increase in size, the individual cells become successively smaller. By the time the blastocyst is implanted in the wall of the uterus, the cells begin to enlarge before they divide. There is a change too in the timing of the divisions. The first few occur almost simultaneously, but after a few days cell division becomes staggered so that only a small proportion of the cells is dividing at the same time. Cell division goes on more rapidly in the first weeks after conception in some species than in others. It has been estimated that the rat increases from a single cell to 3,000 million during its first 3 weeks of development,[2] whereas the human fetus increases only to 1.3 thousand million after 8 weeks' gestation.[3] These are rough figures, but they are confirmed by body weight. The rat emerges from the uterus at 3 weeks weighing 5 g, whereas the human fetus takes 8 weeks to reach a weight of 1 g. The rate of cell division just after conception sets the pace for growth later and is genetically determined; nutrition plays little part at this stage of development. There comes a time, however, when cells begin to increase in size and Winick and Noble described three phases of cellular growth: first, increase in number without any increase in average size; then, increase in size and number; finally, increase only in size of cells.[4] This concept has been criticized by Sands, Dobbing, and Gratrix,[5] and it will be discussed in more detail later. It is obvious that the description of the last stage could not be strictly true, for we know that some organs like the liver, pancreas, and adrenal cortex are capable of almost unlimited cellular division when occasion demands, for example, after surgical removal of part of the

organ. Further, as already explained, cells cannot go on increasing in size in an unlimited way, so once the maximum size has been attained further growth of the organ can only be by increase in number of cells.

## Measurement of Number and Size of Cells

Up to the 1940s the only method of measuring the number and size of cells in a tissue was to count them in a section of tissue in a field of known dimensions under a microscope. This technique had been in use for many years for red blood cells, and it remained the only method until the introduction of the Coulter counter. For nucleated cells, however, another method became available with the description by Schneider[6] and Burton[7] of chemical methods for the determination of DNA. These involved smashing up the cells so that all the cell walls were broken down and the chemical reagents could get at the contents of the nuclei, including the DNA, and react with it so that it could be measured. It was proposed by Boivin, Vendrely, and Vendrely that all the diploid nuclei of a given animal species contain the same amount of DNA,[8] and this is 6 pg for man and 6.2 pg for the rat. Davidson and Leslie suggested that if the total amount of DNA was measured in an organ or tissue, which has mononuclear cells with only diploid nuclei within them, the number of nuclei and hence of cells in an organ could be calculated.[9] The constancy of DNA may not be strictly true,[10] but in view of all the other inaccuracies of this kind of work minor variations in the amount of DNA within the nucleus are probably not important.

Since most of the protein within soft tissues, except skin, is in the cells, a measurement of protein gives an index of the amount of cytoplasm, so the ratio of protein to DNA, or of protein per nucleus, gives an index of the average size of the cell. Intracellular protein is sometimes measured, and this is in theory more accurate, but in practice does not make much difference, especially when comparisons are being made. Some investigators have measured RNA, which is responsible for protein synthesis within the cell, and this method gives a more dynamic approach to cellular growth than the measurement of the protein that is already there. However, although the total RNA in an organ increases during growth, it increases in parallel with the DNA, that is, with the number of nuclei and so gives no indication of the amount of cytoplasm associated with each nucleus.

The speed with which determinations of DNA, RNA, and protein can be made has enabled us to learn a great deal about the quantitative side of cellular growth and multiplication, which we should never have been able to get with a microscope. But the method has its limitations. Perhaps the most important of these is related to the fact that the cells within an organ or tissue are rarely homogenous. The cells of the liver, kidney, and pancreas, for example, and above all of the brain, are functionally highly differentiated, but a measurement of DNA gives no clue about this or to the way the different structures within the organ develop and begin to function. Further, the cells may or may not represent the functional units within an organ. In the kidney the number of cells goes on increasing long after the number of nephrons is complete. Even among the same type of cell within an organ there is often a wide range in the size of the cells. Other difficulties arise because some tissues have many nuclei within a cell, the most obvious being the skeletal muscle fiber. In this case DNA gives a measure of the number of nuclei, but not the number of muscle fibers, which must still be determined by histologic methods.

Adipose tissue presents other problems. Adipoctyes are nucleated and are specialized connective tissue cells localized mostly in the subcutaneous tissue and around the internal organs. Adipose tissue contains other nucleated cells, fibroblasts, some but not all of which are designated preadipocytes, which will become adipocytes when they start to fill with fat. A measurement of DNA, therefore, gives a falsely high number of adipose cells. In fact, this is no different from the problem encountered in other tissues, for example, the brain, where a measurement of DNA gives no indication of the number of nuclei present in the different types of cell. However, investigators concerned with the cellular development of adipose tissue have generally been interested in one type of cell, that containing lipid, and other methods that detect only lipid-containing cells were therefore devised. These depend on the measurement of the size of the actual cells. The size of the adipocytes depends in turn on the amount lipid within them. In one method the fat in a known weight of adipose tissue is fixed with osmium tetroxide. The little balls of fixed lipid are then freed from connective tissue, suspended in glycerin and saline, and counted in a Coulter counter. In the other method frozen sections are cut, and the mean volume of cells in the adipose tissue is determined from their diameter measured under the microscope. Volume of lipid is converted to weight, and the number of cells in a known weight of tissue is determined chemically so that the number of adipocytes containing that lipid can be calculated. Then, if it is desired to know the total number of fat cells in the whole body, the amount of fat in the body is determined, either by calculation from the body density determined by weighing in air and under water, or from skinfold measurements, using a formula such as that suggested by Durnin and Womersley for relating skinfold measurements at four sites to total body fat.[11] Alternatively, lean body mass is calculated from a measurement of the amount of water or of potassium in the body and the amount of fat is obtained by difference. By extrapolation from the number of cells in, say, 20 mg of adipose tissue obtained by biopsy from one site, the number of adipocytes in the adipose tissue of the whole body is calculated. The adipose tissue in an obese person may weigh 100 kg.

The assumptions and inaccuracies in calculating the number of fat cells in an individual from the measurements just described are now accepted as so great that the whole concept of relating obesity to number and size of fat cells in childhood or in later life has largely been abandoned. However, it was pursued with great enthusiasm in the early 1970s and, even if only for historical reasons, the more important of the difficulties will be briefly described. Quite apart from all the inaccuracies involved in measuring total body fat, we now know that the mean fat cell size is not the same all over the body, so a biopsy from one site will not be representative of all the adipose tissue in the body. In the full term infant, for example, cells in the gluteal region averaged 68 μm in diameter, and those in the anterior abdominal wall 50 μm.[12] Because of the relation between the diameter of a sphere and its volume, the amount of fat in a cell differs much more than its diameter. The average cell in these two sites contained 0.17 and 0.06 μg of fat, respectively. Thus the number of fat cells calculated to be present in the body might vary by a factor of 3, depending on which site was chosen for a biopsy.

The other serious problem arises because, if the Coulter counter is used to measure the number of fat cells in a sample of adipose tissue, then the cell must contain a minimum of 0.01 μg of lipid in order to register on the machine. The average lipid content of the adipocyte in the human adult is 0.5 to 0.8 μg, with a maximum of about 1.2 μg. However, a lean individual may well have millions of potential fat cells that contain less than 0.01 μg lipid, and these would never appear in an adipose cell count, but are ready to be filled if the intake of energy becomes greater than the expenditure and the capacity of storage of energy in cells already containing fat is exhausted.

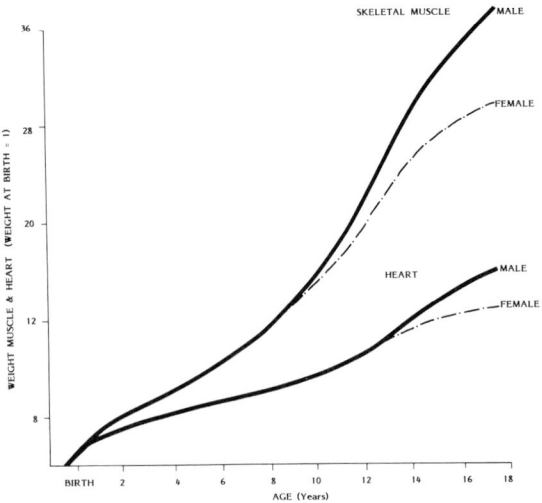

**Fig. 33–1.** Weight of skeletal muscle and heart. Weight at birth = 1. Documenta Geigy Scientific Tables. 7th ed. (Diem, K., Lentner, C., Eds.) Basel, J.R. Geigy, S.A., 1970.

## Growth of the Body and its Tissues

Figures 33–1 to 33–3 show the weight of skeletal muscle, heart, liver, brain, and kidney throughout the growth period[13,14] and also of the body as a whole. Since the dimensions of the body and its tissues are so different, the weight at fullterm birth has been taken as unity and all other values expressed in relation to this. Weights at birth that have been taken as unity are shown in Table 33–2.

The largest soft tissue in the body is skeletal muscle. It makes up 24% of the weight of the fetus at 20 to 24 weeks' gestation, 24% of the infant at term, and 40 to 50% of the adult.[15] Men have more muscle than women; muscle is approximately 50% of the weight of the "average" man and 40% of the weight of the "average" woman. The figures show that skeletal muscle increases more in weight after birth than the body as a whole or any of the other tissues considered here, and from the age of 10 the increase in weight of the muscle is greater in boys than in girls.

The rate in growth of heart muscle (Fig. 33–1) is much less than that of skeletal muscle. The hearts of boys increase more in weight than those of girls, but the difference is not apparent until age 14 years.

The increase in weight of the liver and brain is shown in Figure 33–2. The liver increases in weight by 10 or 11 times between birth and age 18 years, and sex differences are very small.

The growth of the brain is different. The rapid period of brain growth, or "growth spurt," occurs from midgestation to 18 months after birth, by which time the brain has reached a weight of about 1 kg, or more than 70% of its adult weight. At birth the brains of boys are slightly heavier than those of girls, and this difference persists throughout life. The increase in weight after birth is marginally greater in boys and in girls.

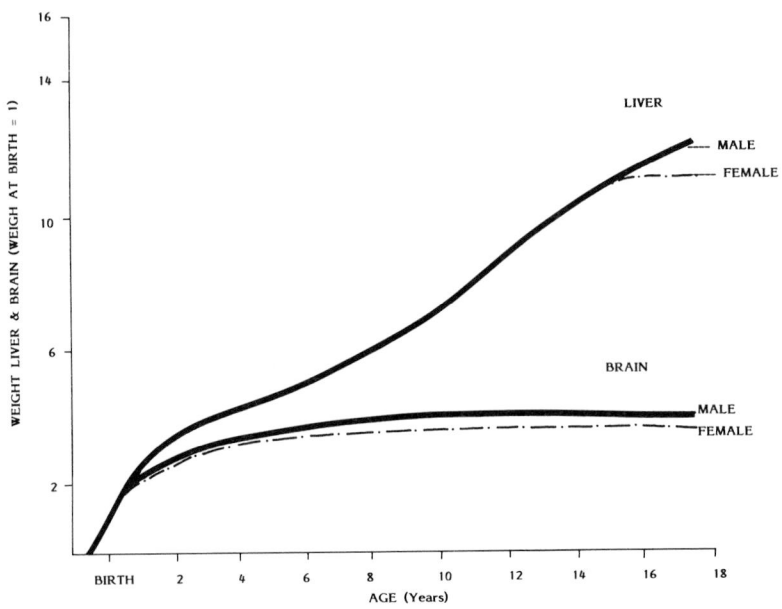

**Fig. 33–2.** Weight of liver and brain. Weight at birth = 1. Documenta Geigy Scientific Tables. 7th ed. (Diem, K., Lentner, C., Eds.) Basel, J.R. Geigy, S.A., 1970.

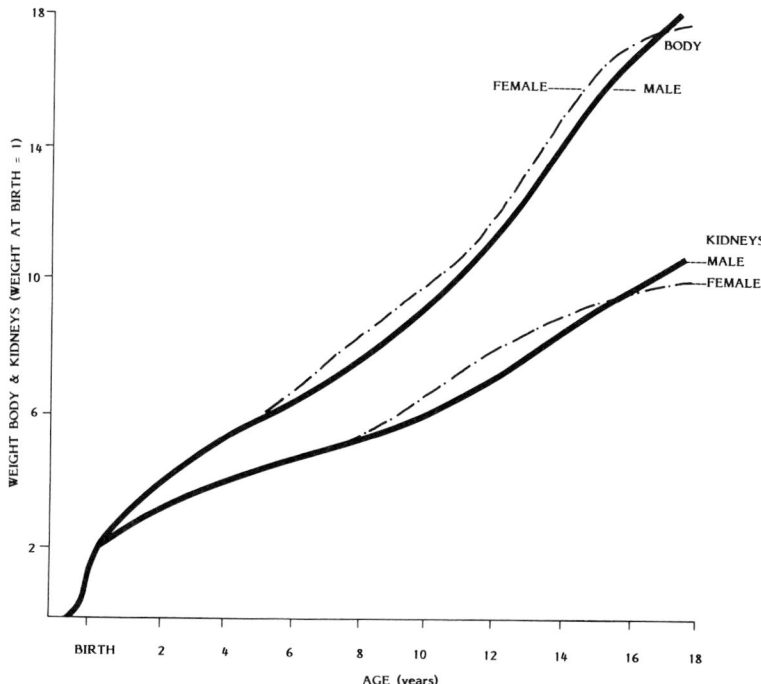

**Fig. 33–3.** Weight of whole body and kidneys. Weight at birth = 1. Documenta Geigy Scientific Tables. 7th ed. (Diem, K., Lentner, C., Eds.) Basel, J.R. Geigy, S.A., 1970.

The kidneys increase in weight in a similar fashion to the liver (Fig. 33–3). Both liver and kidneys increase in weight after birth less than the body so that they come to form a smaller percentage of the body weight.

## Cellular Development of Specific Organs and Tissues

**Skeletal Muscle.** Skeletal muscle changes considerably in chemical, anatomic, and cellular structure during development. Muscle fibers are believed to be formed from elongated precursor cells, called myoblasts, with single nuclei. During fetal development these fuse to form myotubes, which are long narrow cells with many nuclei. The nuclei are situated centrally in the myotubes and are large in proportion to the diameter of the cell. The spaces between the myotubes are filled

with the ground substance of the extracellular phase. The myotubes are converted to muscle fibers, the nuclei move to the periphery and lie immediately under the sarcolemma, and the muscle fibers become arranged in bundles. As in other tissues, there is an increase in number of cells or fibers up to the time of a full-term birth and probably into the first year. MacCallum[16] and Montgomery[17] considered that the adult number of fibers is reached early in postnatal development, but others believe that the number of fibers goes on increasing long after this.[18] Stickland's more recent study of fetal muscle suggests that the rate of increase in number of myofibers in the sartorius muscle starts to slow down at about 21 weeks' gestation and by term has become very slow indeed (Fig. 33–3).[19] The mean cross-sectional area of a myofiber, on the other hand, increases rapidly throughout gestation, reaching 90 $m\mu^2$ at term, and continues to increase all through the period of growth. At adolescence the mean area is about 2,000 $m\mu^2$.

There is evidence that the number of muscle fibers in an individual is genetically determined within species as well as between them.[21,22] Muscle fibers are much the same width in adult mammals of such different sizes as mice and cattle, 50 $\mu m$, which corresponds to an area of about 2,000 $m\mu^2$, the same as is found in man. The interspecies

**Table 33–2.  Weight of Body and Organs at Birth**

|  | Boys | Girls |
| --- | --- | --- |
| Skeletal muscle kg | 0.82 | 0.77 |
| Heart g | 20 | 20 |
| Liver g | 124 | 124 |
| Brain g | 353 | 347 |
| Kidneys g | 24 | 24 |
| Whole body kg | 3.4 | 3.2 |

*Compiled from references 13, 14, and 15. Weights are taken as unity in Figures 33–1, 33–2, and 33–3.

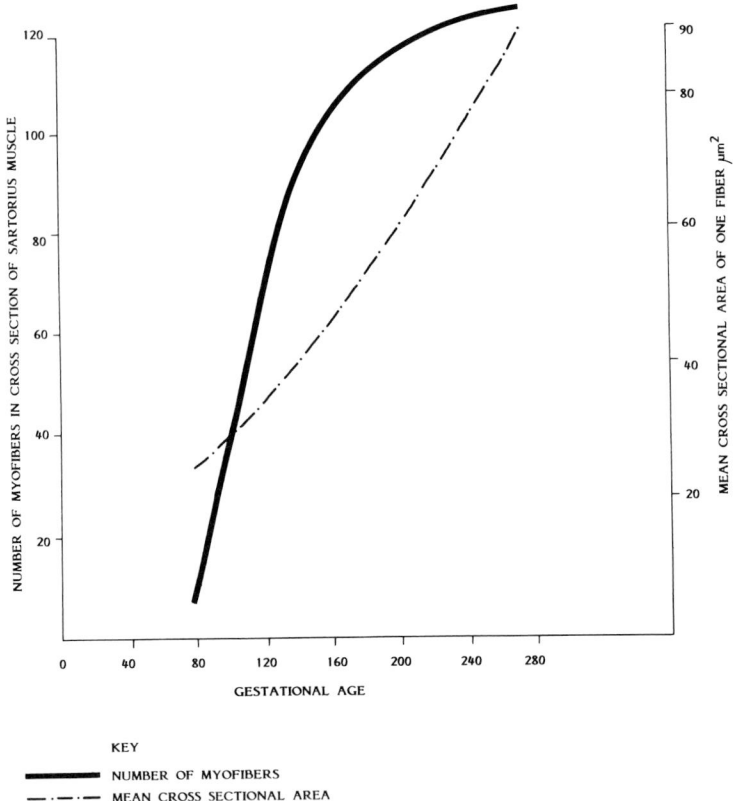

**Fig. 33–4.** Number and mean cross-sectional area of myofibers in sartorius muscle of the human fetus (age in days). Stickland, N.C.: J. Anat., *132*:557–579, 1981.

difference in size of muscles is due to a difference of several orders of magnitude in the number of fibers.[23] Growth of muscle after birth in man is caused primarily by an increase in the size of the fibers that already exist at birth, and this is influenced by nutrition and activity. As the muscle fibers grow in diameter and length, the extracellular material between them becomes less and less. This is seen in Table 33–3, which shows the chloride or extracellular space of human skeletal muscle at various ages and the intracellular fluid and protein per 100 g of muscle.[24] The number of

nuclei within the muscle fibers increases as the muscle grows, and this increase is brought about both by mitosis and by incorporation of satellite cells into the fiber. Figure 33–5 shows the total amount of DNA in two gastrocnemius muscles of the human fetus before and up to term. The amount of DNA and hence the number of nuclei in the gastrocnemius muscles increased by 10 between the 13th and 22nd weeks of gestation.[25] Between 22 and 40 weeks of gestation there was a further 4-fold increase, but the rate of increase was already slowing down. No values are avail-

**Table 33–3. Extracellular and Intracellular Compartments of Skeletal Muscle***

|  | Fetus | | Infant | | Adult |
| --- | --- | --- | --- | --- | --- |
|  | *13–14 weeks* | *20–22 weeks* | *Newborn at term* | *4–7 months* | *Adult* |
| Chloride or extracellular fluid space g/100g muscle | 67.2 | 57.7 | 35.0 | 29.3 | 18.3 |
| Intracellular fluid space g/100g muscle | 23.5 | 31.0 | 45.4 | 49.2 | 60.9 |
| Intracellular protein g/100g muscle | 6.6 | 7.5 | 9.1 | 13.6 | 16.9 |

*From Widdowson, E.M., Dickerson, J.W.T.: Chemical Composition of the body. *In* Mineral Metabolism Vol. 2A (Comar, C.L., Bronner, F., Eds.) New York, Academic Press, 1964, 1–247.

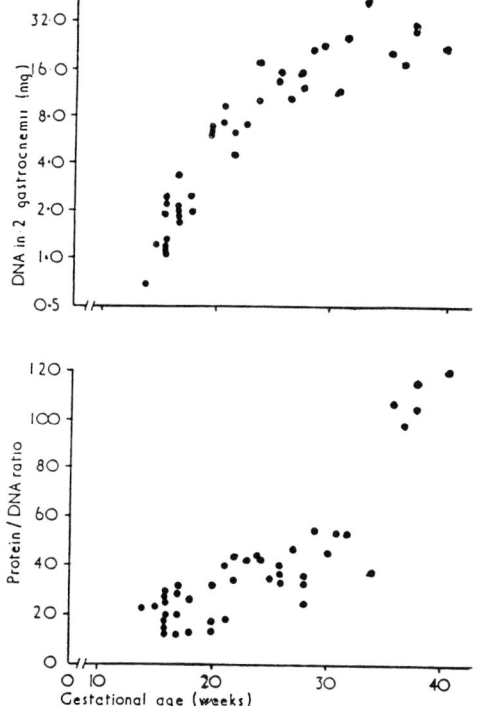

**Fig. 33–5.** DNA and protein/DNA ratio in gastrocnemius muscle of the human fetus. Widdowson, E.M., Crabb, D.E., Milner, R.D.G.: Arch. Dis. Child., *47*:652-655, 1972.

able for individual muscles after birth, but Cheek has calculated the amount of DNA and hence the number of nuclei in the total muscle mass of infants soon after birth and of older infants and children up to the age of 17.[13] The amount of DNA in a weighed biopsy sample of gluteal muscle was determined, and it was assumed that this was representative of all the muscle of the body, which may or may not be true.[26] The weight of muscle in the individual was estimated from the excretion of creatinine, taking each gram of urinary creatinine in 24 hours as being equivalent to 20 kg of muscle. Cheek's results suggest that the amount of DNA and the number of nuclei in muscle increase 6-fold between birth and 11 years of age in both sexes. There is a further 50% increase in girls between 11 and 17 years, but a 2½-fold increase in boys, which parallels the greater amount of skeletal muscle they lay down during adolescence.

The ratio of protein to DNA (mg/mg) in gastrocnemius muscle increased from 20 at 13 weeks' gestation to 120 at term[25] (Fig. 33–5). The ratio at adolescence was about 300.[13] Thus the amount of cytoplasm, as indicated by protein, that is associated with one nucleus, as indicated by DNA,

increased 6-fold in the last 26 weeks of gestation, but barely trebled between birth and maturity.

**Heart.** The heart is fully formed at 11 weeks of gestation, and heart sounds usually can be heard by 18 to 20 weeks. It develops early, too, in its chemical composition, the proportions of water and protein at birth being not very different from those of adult heart.

Figure 33–6 shows the amount of DNA found in the whole heart of human fetuses between 13 weeks of gestation and term.[25] There was a rapid increase between 13 and 30 weeks, the amount of DNA approximately doubling each three weeks. Then the rate of cell division fell off, and at the same time the ratio of protein to DNA rose from 10 at 13 weeks' gestation to 30 at 30 weeks' and 70 at term. There was a further increase of about 5-fold in DNA to 250 mg in adult heart, and more than a doubling of the protein/DNA ratio to 190 mg in the adult organ.

**Kidney.** The kidneys, like the heart, develop and begin to function early in fetal life, and by 9 weeks

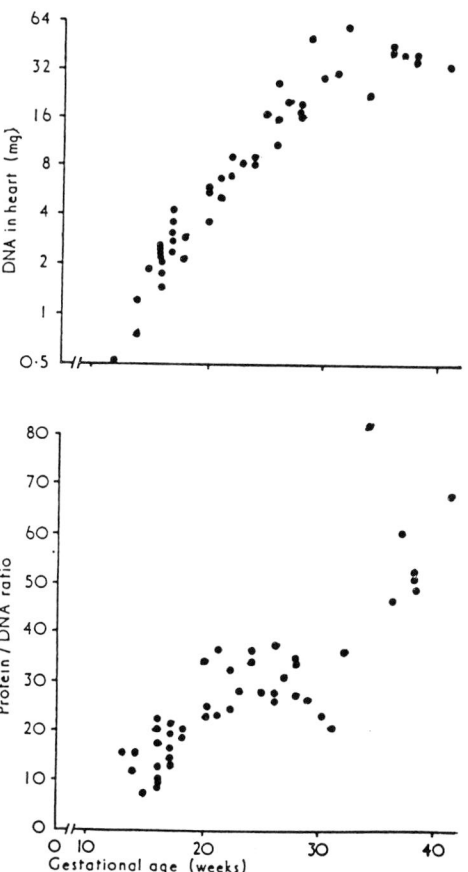

**Fig. 33–6.** DNA and protein/DNA ratio in heart of human fetus. Widdowson, E.M., Crabb, D.E., Milner, R.D.G.: Arch. Dis. Child., *47*:652-655, 1972.

of gestation they are already beginning to secrete urine. Kidney tissue always includes the fluid that was in the tubule at the time of death, and in the adult, who produces a hypertonic urine, the concentration of chloride is likely to be higher than the true value in the kidney tissue itself. In fetal life the urine is hypotonic with respect to sodium and chloride, and this may make fetal kidney tissue appear to contain less chloride and extracellular fluid than it really does. The concentration of protein increased from 9 g/100 g at 20 to 22 weeks of gestation to 12 g/100 g at term and further to 15 g/100 g in the adult.[27]

Figure 33–7 shows the total amount of DNA in the two kidneys before birth.[28] By 13 weeks' gestation the two kidneys already had about 1 mg of DNA in them, or the amount in the nuclei of 200 million cells. Five further divisions and redivisions were required to bring the amount of DNA to 40 mg at 26 weeks of gestation and perhaps one more division to arrive at the amount of 80 to 100 mg at term. Among the kidneys there was often one with twice as much DNA and therefore presumably twice as many cells as another of the same gestational age. Just the same was true of the

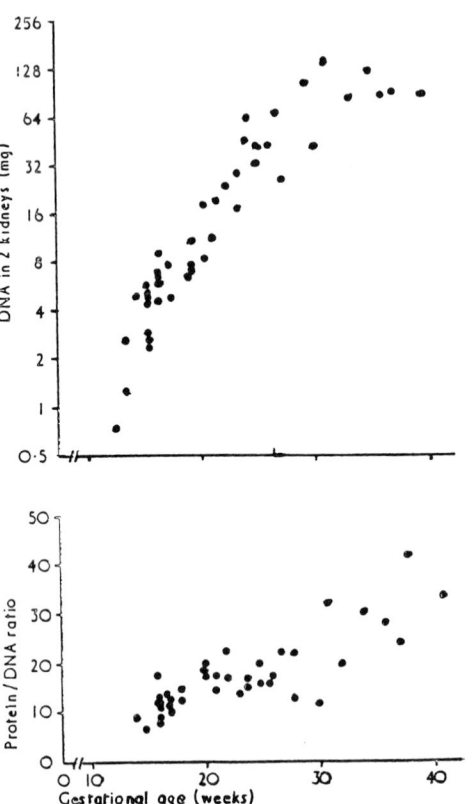

**Fig. 33–7.** DNA and protein/DNA ratio in kidneys of human fetus. Widdowson, E.M., Crabb, D.E., Milner, R.D.G.: Arch. Dis. Child., *47*:652–655, 1972.

heart, and indeed also of the gastrocnemius muscle. Those with the most DNA at any given age were in fact one cell division ahead of those with the least. In the adult, too, there was a wide variation in the amount of DNA in the organs from one individual to another. The mean value for DNA in adult kidneys was 736 mg, but the range was from 505 to 803 mg. In the adult, however, the bigger the body the bigger the organ, and on the whole, the bigger the organ the more cells in it, but this was not necessarily true in the active period of cell division before birth.

The ratio of protein to DNA in the kidneys rose fairly steadily from about 8 at 13 weeks' gestation to 35 at term and 45 in the adult. Thus, in the kidneys, as in the heart and muscle, there was a far greater increase in number of nuclei or cells between birth and adult life than there was in the size of the cells, which in the kidneys only increased by about 30%.

Morphologic studies of the development of the human kidney show that the number of functional units or nephrons is complete at the time of full-term birth.[28] The glomeruli are about half the adult size, and the tubules are short and not completely differentiated. They are all there, however, about 82,000 in each kidney, by the time the fetus reaches term; yet the cells have reached less than 20% of the adult number.

**Liver.** There are difficulties about using the total DNA and the protein/DNA ratio to measure the number and size of liver cells. The liver cells are not all diploid, and polyploidy occurs in hepatocytes at all ages. Further, some cells are binucleate, and both mononucleate and binucleate cells exhibit polyploidy. There is evidence, however, that the amount of cytoplasm in hepatocytes is proportioned to the ploidy of the cell,[29] so that the protein/DNA ratio may still be a valid index of changes in mean cell size. The fetal liver, however, is heterogeneous, containing both hepatic and hemopoietic tissue. Clearly, a chemical approach to measurement of cellular growth of the liver is limited in value, for this method can take no account of the differential growth of the different kinds of cells within the organ.

The liver increases in weight about 13-fold between birth and maturity; its protein increases rather more because the percentage of the organ that is occupied by cells increases. The amount of DNA in the livers of human fetuses increased from about 12 mg at 13 weeks' gestation to 320 mg at 30 weeks'[25] (Fig. 33–8), and then the rate of increase slowed down, while the ratio of protein to DNA had begun to rise. There was little change in the protein/DNA ratio in the liver up to 30 weeks' gestation, but then it rose from about

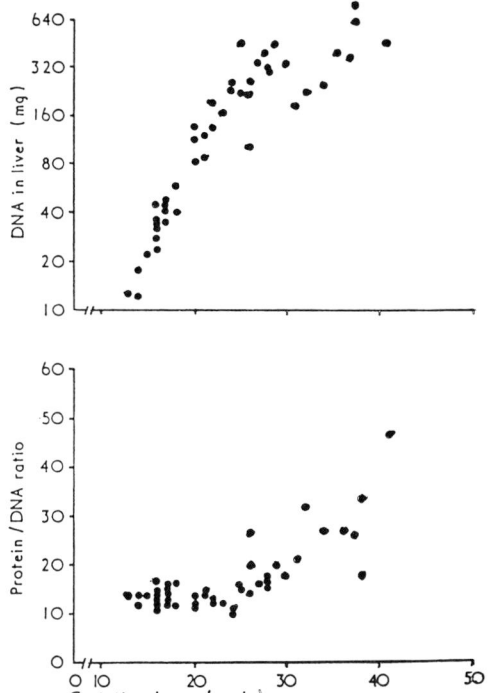

**Fig. 33–8.** DNA and protein/DNA ratio in liver of human fetus. Widdowson, E.M., Crabb, D.E., Milner, R.D.G.: Arch. Dis. Child., *47*:652-655, 1972.

15 to 30 at term. Thus, bearing in mind the complication arising from polyploidy and mononucleate and binucleate cells, it is perhaps unwise to make statements about the number of cells in the liver, but the amount of DNA in the liver, like that in the kidneys and heart, appeared to increase rapidly up to 25 or 30 weeks' gestation, and the rate of increase slowed down at about the same time as the ratio of protein to DNA began to increase. There was a 6-fold increase in DNA and a 2½-fold increase in protein/DNA ratio between the time of birth and adulthood, which suggests that more of the growth of the liver after birth is caused by an increase in the number of cells and less by an increase in their size.

We do not know when cell division normally ceases in the human liver, but we do know that, unlike skeletal muscle, the liver is capable of considerable cell division after birth, and in fact the cells retain the capacity to divide and arrange themselves into new functional units after growth has ceased. During pregnancy,[30] and to a much greater exent during lactation,[31] the liver of the rat enlarges in response to the increased food intake, and this is brought about by an increase in number and a small increase in size of cells. If part of the liver of a rat is surgically removed, the remainder grows by cell division to the original

size and functional efficiency, and this surgical operation has been repeated twelve times in the same animal in a year, each time followed by cellular division and liver growth.[32]

**Brain.** Much of our information about the cellular development of the human brain comes from the work of Dobbing and Sands.[33] They analyzed the brains of fetuses from 10 weeks' gestation to term, and from children of various ages up to maturity. There were 148 brains in all, and most of those of children after birth were from infants up to 1 year of age. The brains were from fetuses and children who were apparently growing normally when they died.

Much of Dobbing and Sands' interest was in cellular development in the three main regions of the brain, the forebrain or cerebrum, the cerebellum, and the brain stem. In the cerebrum the total number of cells, as measured by DNA, rises rapidly during fetal life and this rise continues after birth until the second year (Fig. 33–9). Then cell multiplication slows down, but it continues throughout the remainder of childhood, so that the total number of cells is approximately doubled between two years and maturity. The cells in the cerebellum begin their rapid multiplication later in fetal life than those in the forebrain, but the process is faster during the first year after birth, and the adult number of cells in the cerebellum is reached between one and two years (Fig. 33–10). The increase in number of cells in the brain stem follows a similar course to that of the cerebrum.

There are two main types of cells in the brain, those of the neurons and those of the glia. Dobbing and Sands were able to identify two phases of rapid cell multiplication in the forebrain (Fig.

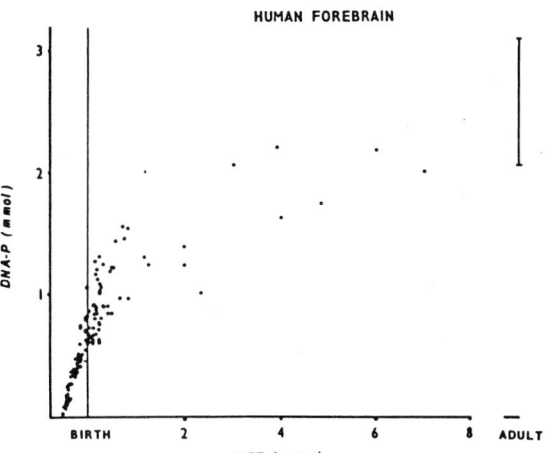

**Fig. 33–9.** DNA-P in human forebrain during growth. Dobbing, J., and Sands, J.: Arch. Dis. Child., *48*:757-767, 1973.

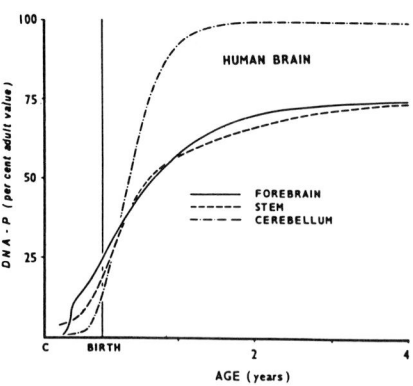

**Fig. 33–10.** DNA-P in human forebrain, cerebellum, and brain stem as a percentage of adult value. Dobbing, J., and Sands, J.: Arch. Dis. Child., *48*:757-767, 1973.

33–11). The first lasted from 10 to 18 weeks of gestation and corresponds to the multiplication of the neuroblasts; this process ceases at about 18 weeks of gestation when the neuroblasts are differentiated into neurons. About this time glial multiplication begins, and most further increase in number of cells is due to an increase in number of glia. As already stated, cell multiplication in all parts of the brain has slowed down by two years. Myelination follows glial multiplication, since the constituent lipids are synthesized by the glia. This process continues at a fairly rapid rate till about four years of age and then more gradually throughout childhood into adolescence.[34]

One striking point that arises from the results of Dobbing and Sands is the wide variation in number of cells in the forebrain from one individual to another of the same age. Thus one child of two years had twice as much DNA in its forebrain as another. It was the larger brains that had

the most DNA, but there is no evidence that there is any relationship between mental ability and the size of the brain or the number of cells in it.

**Adipose Tissue.** White fat, in the form of triglycerides, is contained in a specific type of connective tissue cells, which have a particular distribution in the body, in the subcutaneous tissue and around the internal organs. At about 6 months of gestation the rate of deposition of triglycerides begins to increase. Most of the fat cells are unilocular by this time and contain a single fat droplet. They are smaller than the cells at term, with a mean cell diameter of about 40 μm and a fat content of 0.03 μg.[12] As already stated, in the term infant the cells in the gluteal region averaged 68 μm in diameter and contained 0.17 μg lipid. In the anterior abdominal wall the corresponding figures were 50 μm and 0.06 μg. After birth the cells of adipose tissue from both regions continued to increase in size to about 120 μm diameter and 0.9 μg lipid between 6 and 12 months. Thus, in the gluteal region there was a 5-fold increase in the amount of lipid in the average cell, and in the adipose tissue from the abdominal wall a 14-fold increase. The total fat in the body increases about 4-fold during the first year after birth, which suggests that no increase in number of cells is required to accommodate it.

Between one year and maturity the amount of fat in the bodies of males increases by about five times and in females seven to eight times, whereas the mean fat content per cell rises by about 50%. There must therefore be a considerable increase in number of adipocytes during childhood and adolescence to accommodate all this fat. Brook reported a 5-fold increase in the number of cells containing fat in normal children between 1 and 15 years.[35]

## THE CESSATION OF GROWTH

At a predetermined age for each species growth slows down and ultimately stops. The skeleton is the tissue above all that determines the dimensions of the body, and in man the growth of the skeleton ceases when the epiphyses fuse at the end of the puberty growth spurt around 18 years. In some species, however, such as the rat, which reach puberty long before they reach their adult stature, the epiphyses never fuse; yet growth of the skeleton ultimately slows down and virtually ceases. In other species, such as the pig, which reaches puberty while still growing rapidly, the epiphyses do eventually fuse and growth of the skeleton ceases, but this occurs at 2 to 3 years, whereas puberty is reached at around 7 months when the pig is only half its adult weight.

The length of a muscle depends on the distance

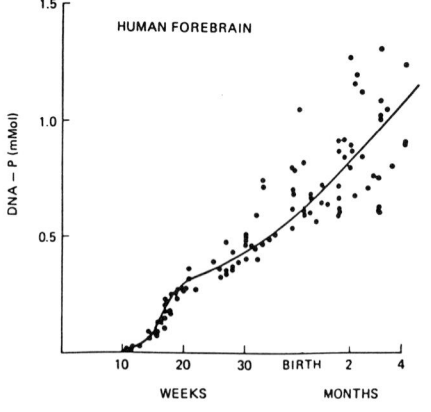

**Fig. 33–11.** DNA-P in human forebrain before and after birth. Dobbing, J., Sands, J., and Sands, J.: Arch. Dis. Child., *48*:757-767, 1973.

between its two points of attachment, most obvious in the limbs. Muscles attached to the long bones can grow only as long as the bones to which they are attached, and the size of the skeleton determines the lengths of the individual muscles. They too, therefore, cease growing in length when the skeleton reaches its final size. Excessive activity of particular parts of the body in all species leads to an increase in the width of the muscles, but not in their length.

Generally speaking, the internal organs of man and animals are appropriate to the size of the body. Thus, a genetically small man, a Yorkshire terrier, or a pony has smaller organs than a tall man, a Labrador dog, or a Shire horse. Some organs, the liver, the pancreas, adrenals, ovaries and testes, for example, can go on growing and multiplying the number of their cells long after growth of the skeleton has ceased. Yet they too stop growing when they have reached the appropriate size and functional capacity for the body they have to serve. How this is brought about still remains to be discovered.

## EFFECTS OF UNDER- AND OVERNUTRITION ON ORGAN AND CELL GROWTH

### Undernutrition

Undernutrition retards growth and this is true of all the different parts of the body. Some parts are affected more than others, adipose tissue losing its fat, and muscle and liver some of their protein. If the undernutrition is severe, the adipocytes become unrecognizable as cells and the spaces between the empty cells become filled with an extracellular "gel." The muscle fibers shrink, and again the spaces between them are occupied with extracellular material. There is less change in the composition of the kidneys and heart, and the brain is the least affected of all.

If undernutrition is imposed early in life, when growth is at its most rapid, then complete recovery in size may never be possible, even though the undernutrition is temporary and plentiful food is supplied thereafter. Winick and Noble explained this at a cellular level.[36] They postulated that if the animal is undernourished at the stage of development when the cells are dividing rapidly cell division is hindered, and the cell divisions lost during the period of undernutrition will never be regained. Thus, organs will have a smaller number of cells than they would have done had the animal been well nourished throughout, and they therefore cannot grow as large as those of their well-nourished counterparts, even after rehabilitation. Winick and Noble demonstrated that the smaller

organs of rats undernourished during the first 3 weeks after birth by being suckled in large numbers on one mother and then given plentiful food did indeed contain less DNA and hence fewer cells than those of larger animals originally suckled in groups of 3.[36] Rats undernourished for 3 weeks at a later stage of development do recover completely when rehabilitated. Winick and Noble's suggestion, which was based on their own observations[4] and those Enesco and Le Blond[2] that cellular growth takes place in 3 stages, hyperplasia, hyperplasia and hypertrophy, and then hypertrophy alone, seemed to be a breakthrough in our understanding of the observed effects of undernutrition and rehabilitation at different ages. But as time has gone on, it has been realized that matters are not quite as simple as they at one time seemed. From what has been said earlier, it is clear that there is a physiologic limit to the size an individual cell can grow, and the major contributor to growth of organs after birth, in man at any rate, is in the number of cells in them. Sands, Dobbing and Gratrix[5] repeated Winick and Noble's[4] original study on rats, and their results were somewhat different. In their animals the ratio of weight to DNA, which they took as a measure of cell size, had reached its mature value by 8 weeks after birth in the kidney, heart, and liver, but the total DNA was still increasing when the experiment terminated at 16 weeks. They concluded that cell multiplication continues until growth of the body comes to an end. Thus, they did not confirm Winick and Noble's[4] third stage of cellular growth consisting only of enlargement of already existing cells. However, an early phase of very rapid cell multiplication undoubtedly does occur, and this may well be the stage of development when the organism is particularly vulnerable to undernutrition.

Another problem that arises over the attempt to explain the failure of rats to recover completely after a period of undernutrition just after birth is that it is not the internal organs or even skeletal muscle that determines the dimensions of the body, but the skeleton. It is the failure of the skeleton to show "catch-up" growth after early undernutrition that results in the small body, and the small body has organs that are appropriate to its size. There is no reason to suppose that the livers of rats that are small because they were undernourished early in life could not regenerate themselves by hyperplasia after partial hepatectomy just as well as those of rats that were well nourished throughout their lives. The small kidneys of the small animals are perfectly capable of maintaining the constancy of the volume and composition of the body fluids even though, taken out of the body and analyzed, they might be condemned as having too few cells. We have to be careful about drawing conclusions about the efficiency of an organ from its size or the number of cells in it without considering its size, structure, and performance relative to the body from which it came. Organs of animals undernourished early in life and then rehabilitated may be small, but this is the consequence and not the cause of the failure of the body as a whole to show "catch-up" growth.

### Overnutrition

Just as it was believed in the early 1970s that a small number of cells in the internal organs somehow conferred a disadvantage on the individual, so it was thought that a large number of adipose cells did the same thing. Papers were published suggesting that obese children and adults have more fats cells than leaner ones.[37–39] The suggestion was made that fat cells are formed early in life and never lost later, so that fat infants tend to become fat adults, and adults whose obesity dated from infancy had an excess of fat cells which were inevitably with them for the rest of their lives. Brook et al. found that children who became obese during their first year had more cells with fat than those who had been of average weight, but this was not true of those who became obese later, although the amount of fat was similar in the two obese groups.[38] Those that became fat later had more fat in each cell. Salans et al. came to a similar conclusion,[40] and they and Brook et al.[38] agreed that once an excessively large number of adipose cells had been achieved, this was not reduced when weight was lost by dieting. Häger did not confirm these observations, and he could not find any relationship between the age of onset of obesity and the number of cells containing fat.[41] Knittle's later studies showed that it was not until two years that obese children had a significantly greater number of detectable adipose cells than those that were of normal size.[42] Moreover, fat is not necessarily lost from all cells equally when an individual becomes slim, and Ashwell and Garrow demonstrated in one obese patient who lost weight that the mean cell size actually increased because small cells lost what little fat they had and so disappeared from the reckoning.[43]

The errors involved in estimating the total number of fat cells in the body have already been discussed, and it is now generally held that weight and fatness and number of adipocytes during the first year after birth may not be an important determinant of shape, size, and obesity during later childhood.[44–46]

## THE HARMONY OF GROWTH

"The growth of a living organism is a highly complex affair, involving as it does a multitude of different processes working in harmony, each cutting in and cutting out at the appropriate time.... The general principles about growth apply to all species, but species vary very much among themselves, most obviously perhaps in the rate at which the body grows and the ultimate size that it becomes.... The rate of cell division is genetically determined, but its fulfilment depends upon the supply of food and to the ability of the animal to make use of it.... Within each species the growth and development of each part of the body is in perfect harmony with that of the rest, and it is exactly attuned at each age to the function it has to perform."[47]

### REFENENCES

1. Black, D.A.K.: Essentials of Fluid Balance. 2nd ed. Oxford, Blackwell Scientific Publications, 1960.
2. Enesco, M., Leblond, C.P.: J. Embryol. Exp. Morphol. *10*:530-564, 1962.
3. Osgood, E.E.: Pediatrics, *15*:733-751, 1965.
4. Winick, M., Noble, A.: Dev. Biol. *12*:451-466, 1965.
5. Sands, J. Dobbing, J., Gratrix, C.A.: Lancet *2*:503-505, 1979.
6. Schneider, W.C.: J. Biol. Chem. *161*:293-303, 1945.
7. Burton, K.: Biochem. J. *62*:315-323, 1956.
8. Boivin, A., Vendrely, R., Vendrely, C.: Compt. Rend. Acad. Sci. *226*:1061-1063, 1948.
9. Davidson, J.N., Leslie, I.: Nature *165*:49-53, 1950.
10. Brachet, J.: Biochemical Cytology. New York, Academic Press, 1957.
11. Durnin, J.V.G.A., Womersley, J.: Br. J. Nutr. *32*:77-79, 1974.
12. Dauncey, M.J., Gairdner, D.: Arch. Dis. Child. *50*:286-290, 1975.
13. Cheek, D.B.: Muscle cell growth in normal children. *In* Human Growth. (Cheek, D.B., Ed.) Philadelphia, Lea & Febiger, 1968, 337-351.
14. Documenta Geigy Scientific Tables. 7th ed. (Diem, K., Lentner, C., Eds.) Basel, J.R. Geigy S.A., 1970.
15. Wilmer, H.A.: Proc. Soc. Exp. Biol. Med. *43*:545-547, 1940.
16. MacCallum, J.B.: Bull. Johns Hopkins Hosp. *9*:208-215, 1898.
17. Montgomery, R.D.: Nature *195*:194-195, 1962.
18. Adams, R.D., DeRueck, J.: Basic Research in Myology. Proceedings of the II International Congress on Muscle Diseases, Part I, ICN Series No. 294. Amsterdam, Excerpta Medica, 1973.
19. Stickland, N.C.: J. Anat. *132*:557-579, 1981.
20. Hartman, W.H.: Histologic study of muscle cell size. *In* Human Growth. (Cheek, D.B., Ed.) Philadelphia, Lea & Febiger, 1968, 372-381.
21. Luff, A.R., Goldspink, G.: Life Sci. *6*:1821-1826, 1967.
22. Stickland, N.C., Widdowson, E.M., Goldspink, G.: Br. J. Nutr. *34*:421-428, 1975.
23. Burleigh, I.G.: Biol. Rev. *49*:267-320, 1974.
24. Widdowson, E.M., Dickerson, J.W.T.: Chemical composition of the body. *In* Mineral Metabolism Vol. 2A (Comar, C.L., Bronner, F., Eds.) New York, Academic Press, 1964, 1-247.

25. Widdowson, E.M., Crabb, D.E., Milner, R.D.G.: Arch. Dis. Child. *47*:652-655, 1972.

26. Enesco, M., Puddy, D., Am. J. Anat. *114*:235-244, 1964.

27. Widdowson, E.M., Dickerson, J.W.T.: Biochem. J. *77*:30-43, 1960.

28. Potter, E.L., Thierstein, S.T.: J. Pediatr. *22*:695-706, 1943.

29. Epstein, C.J.: Proc. Natl. Acad. Sci. *57*:327-334, 1967.

30. Campbell, R.M., Fell, B.F., Mackie, W.S.: J. Physiol. (Lond.) *241*:699-713, 1972.

31. Kennedy, G.C., Pearce, W.M., Parrott, D.M.: J. Endocrinol. *17*:158-160, 1958.

32. Ingle, D.J., Baker, B.L.: Proc. Soc. Exp. Biol. Med. *95*:813-815, 1957.

33. Dobbing, J., Sands, J.: Arch. Dis. Child. *48*:757-767, 1973.

34. Hoar, R.M., Monie, I.W.: Comparative development of specific organ systems. *In* Developmental Toxicology. (Kimmel, C.A., Buelke-Sam, J., Eds.) New York, Raven Press, 1981, 13-33.

35. Brook, C.D.G.: Lancet *2*:624-627, 1972.

36. Winick, M., Noble, A.: J. Nutr. *89*:300-406, 1966.

37. Hirsch, J., Knittle, J.L.: Fed. Proc. *29*:1516-1521, 1970.

38. Brook, C.G.D., Lloyd, J.K., Wolff, O.H.: Br. Med. J. *2*:25-27, 1972.

39. Brook, C.G.D.: Arch. Dis. Child. *46*:182-184, 1971.

40. Salans, L.B., Cushman, S.W., Weismann, R.E.: J. Clin. Invest. *52*:929-941, 1973.

41. Häger, A.: Postgrad. Med. J. *53*:101-107, 1977.

42. Knittle, J.L.: Adipose tissue development in man. *In* Human Growth Vol. 2, (Falkner, F., Tanner, J.M., Eds.) London, Baillière Tindall, 1977, 295-315.

43. Ashwell, M., Garrow, J.S.: Lancet *2*:1036-1037, 1973.

44. Melbin, T., Viulle, J.C.: Br. J. Prev. Soc. Med. *27*:225-235, 1973.

45. Fisch, R.O., Bilek, M.K., Ulstrom, R.: Pediatrics *56*:521-528, 1975.

46. Poskitt, E.M.E., Cole, T.J.: Br. Med. J. *1*:7-9, 1977.

47. Widdowson, E.M.: Lancet, *1*:901-905, 1970.

*Chapter* **34**

# DIET, NUTRITION AND DRUG REACTIONS

Daphne A. Roe

The gulf that formerly separated nutrition and pharmacology has closed, particularly since it has been realized that nutrients can behave as drugs, and drugs may have some of the properties of nutrients. An interscience of drug-nutrient interactions has been created. The concerns of this newer discipline must include nutrients as drugs. However, to the clinical pharmacologist, drug effects on food intake and dietary factors influencing the disposition of drugs are of primary importance. The toxicologist is concerned with nutritional factors in teratogenesis, as well as dietary and nutritional influences on the initiation and promotional phases of carcinogenesis. Pharmacologic problems related to change in body composition, drug-food and drug-nutrient incompatibilities, and alcohol-drug and alcohol-food interactions are of particular concern to the physician, whereas adverse or positive effects of drugs on nutrient absorption, transport, metabolism, cellular uptake and excretion, are of special importance to the nutritionist. The aims of this review are both to describe and classify drug-nutrient interactions and to discuss adverse outcomes.

## NUTRIENTS AS DRUGS

Vitamins and their analogues may have both pharmacologic and nutritional properties. The pharmacologic effect of vitamins has long been appreciated and has been utilized for therapeutic purposes. The inhibitory effects of massive doses of vitamin A on keratinization were utilized by Miescher in 1954.[1] In patients given daily doses of 200,000 to 400,000 IU of vitamin A, ichthyosis disappeared more or less completely within 2 to 3 months but recurred when treatment was discontinued. It was claimed that no side effects were encountered.

About the same time, however, the toxic effects of vitamin A overload were reported in children to include skeletal abnormalities and hemorrhages.[2] These side effects were observed to follow doses of vitamin A in the order of 500,000 IU daily. Sulzberger and Lazar reported signs of vitamin A intoxication in a woman of 44 years who took 600,000 IU daily for 18 months.[3]

Vitamin $D_3$ (calciferol) was advocated by Dowling and co-workers in England,[4] by Michelson in the United States[5] and by Charpy in France[6] for the treatment of tuberculosis of the skin (lupus vulgaris). Dosage ranges were between 100,000 and 600,000 IU vitamin $D_3$ daily. The clinical experience of these investigators was critically reviewed by Goldsmith and Hellier in 1954.[2] Toxic reactions, including fatalities, were frequently observed. Anning et al. reported that in a group of 200 cases of lupus vulgaris receiving vitamin $D_3$, 19% developed toxic symptoms including anorexia, vomiting, tiredness, malaise, nausea, headache, constipation, abdominal pain, and polyuria.[7] Laboratory tests revealed hypercalcemia and evidence of impaired renal function.

Three years after the isolation of niacin and its effective use at physiologic doses in the treatment of pellagra, studies were carried out by Bean and Spies to examine the vasodilator effect of niacin and several analogues.[8] Pyridine compounds, which produced vasodilatation, included nicotinic acid (niacin), sodium nicotinate, ammonium nicotinate, and ethyl nicotinate. It was early demonstrated that nicotinamide did not have vasodilator potency. Ruffin and Smith had observed that vasodilatation and headache occurred in normal subjects who took 250 mg niacin four times a day. Vasodilator effects of niacin were subsequently used therapeutically in the treatment of Raynaud's phenomenon.[9]

The vasodilatory effect of niacin has been considered as justification for administration to elderly patients with cerebrovascular disease. However, although there have been claims that the vitamin could cause dilatation of cerebral vessels and thereby improve memory and brain function, there is no scientific evidence to support such a claim.

Niacin has been and is still used in megadosages ($\geq 1$ g/day) for the treatment of familial hypercholesterolemia and other disorders of lipoprotein metabolism. The hypocholesterolemic effects of large doses of niacin were first reported by Altschul et al. in 1955.[10] Since that time, niacin has been in use as a hypocholesterolemic agent, and although its use for this function declined after the mid-1960s for several years, now again niacin is used as an adjunct drug with coadministration with a bile acid sequestrant. It has been demonstrated that niacin decreases total plasma triglycerides and very low density lipoprotein triglyceride. It also decreases plasma cholesterol and increases the hepatic secretion of biliary cholesterol.

Reported side effects occurring in patients receiving niacin therapy at dosages $\geq 300$ mg/day include flushing, dryness of the skin, nausea and diarrhea, and, rarely, the skin changes of acanthosis nigricans. Some patients have developed impaired hepatic function, hyperglycemia, and hyperuricemia. Hepatotoxicity with elevation of plasma transaminases and alkaline phosphatase is dose-dependent, occurring with greater frequency when the niacin dose exceeds 2.5 g/day. Glucose intolerance is usually moderate; hyperuricemia occurs in about one third of the patients receiving pharmacologic doses of niacin, but is

not usually associated with gout. Arrythmia has been described.[11–13]

The vasodilator effects of niacin, including the flushing and infrequently associated tachycardia, tinnitus, and pruritus, may be partially or completely inhibited by aspirin (0.3 g), but the hepatotoxic and other metabolic effects of niacin can be reversed only when the "drug" is discontinued.[14]

Limitation on the use of vitamins as drugs have been the toxic effects and the limited therapeutic effectiveness. The availability of vitamin analogues has reactivated interest in the use of vitamin-like substances as drugs. 13-*cis*-retinoic acid (isotretinoin) is currently being used in the treatment of acne vulgaris, particularly cystic and inflammatory forms of acne.[15] This "drug" is an oral synthetic vitamin A derivative, which is actually effective in controlling a wide variety of dermatoses characterized by defective keratinization. Long-term use (15 to 20 weeks) produces sustained remission of severe refractory cystic acne. However, higher doses and long-term administration of 13-*cis*-retinoic acid have been employed to control such keratinizing dermatoses as lamellar ichthyosis.[16]

Adverse side effects of 13-*cis*-retinoic acid at dosages of 1 to 2 mg/kg/day, as used in acne, include dry skin, fissuring of the lips, headache, dryness of the conjunctiva, and in some patients moderate elevation of plasma cholesterol and triglyceride. At daily dosages of 3 to 4 mg/kg/day taken over a prolonged period (1 to 2 years), this drug has caused hyperostoses with multiple bony outgrowths of the vertebral column.[17] Both 13-*cis*-retinoic acid and the related retinoid, etretinate, which has been shown to be of therapeutic benefit in psoriasis, have been shown to induce severe birth defects when women have taken these drugs in the first trimester of pregnancy.[17a]

## DRUGS AS CALORIC SOURCES AND NUTRIENTS

Whereas vitamins administered in high dosages can exert pharmacologic properties, drugs may have nutritional functions. Alcohol, now the most widely used social drug, was formerly a therapeutic drug used in the treatment of fevers and of diabetes mellitus.[18,19] By ancient tradition, beer and wine were given to acutely ill patients as sources of nourishment when solid food could not be tolerated. Atwater and co-workers, who carried out the first fundamental studies on the metabolism of alcohol, cited cases in which alcohol was used as the only means of nutritional support.[20] One of the cases cited was a girl in the Massachusetts General Hospital with pneumonia who received more than a gallon of brandy over a period of seven days and no other form of food. Atwater and Benedict's human studies, carried out in the years 1898 to 1900, were the first to provide information that alcohol is oxidized and serves as a fuel.[21] They found that alcohol spares protein, fat, and also possibly carbohydrates. The viewpoint held at the beginning of the twentieth century was that alcohol resembles food with respect to its oxidation but that it differs from foods in that it is not retained in the body for any considerable period.[22]

Today alcohol is seldom used as a therapeutic drug because better drugs are available and also because of its toxic properties. Becker et al. summarized the history and current position of alcohol as a therapeutic drug as follows:[23] "Alcohol has been used clinically as an appetite stimulant, as a sedative-hypnotic drug, and as a caloric source for intravenous alimentation. Such medicinal uses of alcohol have never been subjected to controlled evaluation. Health tonics contain substantial quantities of alcohol and may as a consequence be abused."

Alcohol is absorbed as a drug and is metabolized both as a macronutrient and as a drug. In high dosages it behaves as an antinutrient in that alcohol abuse can be associated with malabsorption and impaired utilization of a number of nutrients, particularly fat and water-soluble vitamins.[24] Today we use alternate synthetic food-energy sources that are free of the toxicity of alcohol, for example, glucose polymers, which are used as caloric sources in enteral formulas for acutely ill or chronically sick patients. In contrast to alcohol, these alternate energy sources can promote micronutrient absorption of riboflavin and the rate of folic acid absorption.[25]

## DIETARY FACTORS INFLUENCING THE DISPOSITION OF DRUGS

Absorption of most drugs occurs by diffusion through the mucosa of the gastrointestinal tract. Although absorption of drugs can occur through any portion of the tract, absorption of most orally administered drugs is maximal at the level of the proximal part of the small intestine. Absorption across the mucosa of this part of the intestine is enhanced by the large surface area provided by the folds of Kerckring, the villi, and the microvilli. However, before absorption can occur, solid formulations of drugs must first be disintegrated and dissolved in the stomach by the gastric juice. The drug solution then leaves the stomach at a rate that is dependent on the gastric emptying time.[25a]

Food components have been shown to affect drug absorption and bioavailability.[26] Three general mechanisms explain these effects: gastric emptying time, interactions with the gut lumen, and competitive inhibition.

**Gastric Emptying Time.** Absorption of drugs may be increased or decreased by physiologic changes in the gastrointestinal tract in the fed versus the fasted state. Gastric emptying time influences the rate of drug absorption. In the fasted state, or when there is little food in the stomach, drugs leave the stomach rapidly and will therefore soon reach the small intestine where they are optimally absorbed. Conversely, if a drug is formulated as a solid preparation—such that disintegration of drug particles as well as dissolution of the drug in stomach fluid must precede absorption—then rapid stomach emptying time will militate against efficient drug absorption. In this case, the drug may be better absorbed after food intake, particularly after intake of foods or forms of foods that delay stomach emptying. Slow stomach emptying time occurs after heavy meals, meals containing fat, and after hot meals.[26]

The volume of a beverage taken with a drug and the characteristics of such a beverage can also influence drug absorption. Drugs are more efficiently absorbed when they are in dilute solution and therefore when the drug is taken with a beverage.[27]

Postprandial conditions that delay gastric emptying may also enhance drug absorption because the drug is metered out more slowly and efficiently to its intestinal absorption site. This effect is believed to explain the enhanced absorption of the thiazide diuretic, chlorothiazide, after food intake, as well as the enhanced absorption of pharmacologic doses of riboflavin after food intake.[28,29] Dietary factors that enhance the absorption of pharmacologic doses of riboflavin include food as such, dietary fiber, cola beverages, and intake of a glucose polymer.[30]

**Interactions Within the Gut Lumen.** There may be a physical or chemical interaction of the food and drug within the gut lumen. For example, tetracycline is less well absorbed when taken with foods containing calcium, magnesium, iron, or zinc. The drug forms chelates with these minerals, which then are not absorbed.[31] Drugs can also interact with the components of enteral feeding formulas so that a gel or precipitate is formed, which can reduce drug or nutrient absorption and clog feeding tubes. In 1982 Bauer reported that when neurosurgical patients were given phenytoin during continuous nasogastric feeding, the plasma levels of the drug were reduced and there was escape from the desired anticonvulsant effects of the drug.[32] These effects were explained by direct interaction of formula constituents and this anticonvulsant within the gut lumen.

**Competitive Inhibition.** Food-induced increases in splanchnic blood flow may also increase the bioavailability of certain drugs after food. This effect is seen with some of the beta blocker drugs such as propranolol and metoprolol.[33] The absorption of drugs can also be influenced by individual nutrients. For example, absorption of L-dopa is reduced when this drug is taken with a high protein meal or with an amino acid mixture. Competitive inhibition of L-dopa absorption occurs when other amino acids absorbed from the same transport system are presented.[34] A similar protein or amino acid effect has been reported with methyldopa.[35]

A significant reduction of particular drug formulations by food has been reported in patients (Table 34–1). Slowing of drug absorption by food occurs with the drug formulations listed in Table 34–2. On the other hand, significant enhancement of the drugs listed in Table 34–3 occurs when the drug is taken with food. However, a recent report of different effects of food on different slow-release preparations of theophylline[35a] indicates a need to explore food effects on drug absorption further so that we may be better able to predict the direction of the food effect.

## DIETARY FACTORS INFLUENCING DRUG METABOLISM

Rates of drug metabolism in the intestine, as well as in the liver, are influenced by dietary composition. High protein diets enhance drug metabolism, and protein-deficient diets slow drug metabolism. Effects of protein restriction on the drug metabolizing activity of the liver have been reported in both in vitro and in vivo studies.[36,37]

Dietary factors that influence drug oxidation or conjugation reactions include protein quality, indolic compounds in vegetables of the *Brassica* family (cabbage and brussel sprouts), methylxanthine-containing beverages (coffee, tea, cocoa, chocolate), dietary fiber, and cooking method. Charcoal broiling of meats promotes drug metabolism in human subjects. Rapid effects of non-nutrient dietary components such as flavones on drug metabolism occur when a drug is taken concurrently or in close temporal proximity to food.[38]

Whereas in human subjects relatively few dietary factors have been examined for their effects on drug metabolism, in laboratory animals a wide range of macro- and micronutrients such as vitamins and trace elements, as well as other minerals, have been investigated with regard to this effect. In a 1981 review of the subject, McLean emphasized that there are major nutrient influences on the rate and direction of drug metabolism that are superimposed on the genetic determinants of drug metabolism.[39] McLean also pointed out that weaker nutritional influences may have significant effects on the response to foreign compounds in the natural environment.

Animal experiments have shown that not only the level but also the quality of dietary protein affect drug metabolism. When the level of dietary protein is reduced so that it is limiting for growth, the basal rate of the cytochrome P-450 linked drug metabolism, as well as the response to inducers of drug metabolism such as phenobarbital, is diminished. When animals are fed a low protein diet that is adequate in energy content, glucuronidation increases. Diets low in the sulfur-containing amino acids methionine and cystine cause a reduction in sulfate conjugation rates.[40,41]

Outcomes of protein restriction on drug or xenobiotic toxicity depend on whether the parent substance or the metabolite is more toxic. If the parent substance is more toxic, then protein restriction will increase toxicity, whereas if the metabolite is more toxic, then protein restriction may diminish toxicity. Reduction in toxicity by protein restriction has been dramatically demonstrated with respect to the pesticide heptachlor.[42] Previously it was considered that reduction in the metabolic activation of carcinogens (initiators of the carcinogenic process) by protein restriction explained the lessening of tumor development in animals on a low protein diet; it has now been shown that protein restriction has its major influence on the promotional phase of carcinogenesis.[43,44]

The level of dietary fat also influences drug metabolism, as does the quality of fats administered. When fat-free diets are fed to laboratory animals, there is a reduction in the cytochrome P-450 levels and in the activity of drug-metabolizing enzymes.[45,46]

In guinea pigs it has been shown that diets deficient in ascorbic acid cause a reduction in the level of hepatic cytochrome P-450 and also in the activity of drug metabolizing enzymes.[47]

Numerous animal studies have shown large effects of diet composition on drug metabolism and drug toxicity, but relatively few of these effects have as yet been demonstrated in human populations or in subjects enrolled in drug trials. Indeed, the need to carry out epidemiologic and metabolic studies of effects of diet composition on drug toxicity has been highlighted as a much needed area for research, particularly in aging populations and in elderly individuals in whom it is not clear whether the high prevalence of drug reactions can be explained by drug overuse or mis-

**Table 34–1.   Compounds Whose Absorption May be Reduced by Food or Food Supplements**

| Compound | Dosage Form |
|---|---|
| Amoxycillin | Capsules |
| Ampicillin | Capsules |
| Aspirin | Tablets |
| Aspirin, calcium | Tablets |
| Atenolol | Tablets |
| Captopril | Tablets |
| Cephalexin | Capsules, suspension |
| Demeclocycline (demethylchlortetracycline) | Capsules |
| Doxycycline | Capsules |
| Ethanol | Solution |
| Folic acid | Tablets* |
| Hydrochlorothiazide | Tablets |
| Iron | Solution, tablets |
| Isoniazid | Tablets |
| Ketoconazole | Tablets |
| Levodopa | Tablets |
| Lincomycin | Capsules |
| Methacycline | |
| Nafcillin | Tablets |
| Oxytetracycline | |
| Penicillamine | Tablets |
| Penicillin G | Tablets, suspension |
| Penicillin V (K) | Capsules, suspension, tablets |
| Penicillin V (Ca) | Tablets |
| Penicillin V (acid) | Tablets |
| Phenacetin | Suspension |
| Phenazone (antipyrine) | Syrup |
| Phenethicillin | Capsules, tablets |
| Phenylmercaptomethylpenicillin | Capsules |
| Phenytoin | Capsules† |
| Pivampicillin | Capsules |
| Propantheline | Tablets |
| Rifampicin | |
| Sotalol | Tablets |
| Tetracycline | Capsules |
| Theophylline | Capsules, controlled release‡ |

*Absorption reduced by calcium carbonate.
†Absorption reduced by folic acid and by enteral formula.
‡Absorption reduced by controlled release preparation of theophylline (Theo-Dur Sprinkle, Key Pharmaceuticals).
Adapted from Welling, P.: Nutrient effects on drug metabolism and action in the elderly. Drug-Nutrient Interac. 4(1/2):183, 1985.

use, by the effects of aging on drug disposition, or by diet-related factors.[47a]

## EFFECTS OF DIET ON DRUG EXCRETION

Low protein diets that decrease renal plasma flow and creatinine clearance can also reduce the renal clearance of certain drugs. For example, restriction of dietary protein decreases the clearance of the antigout drug allopurinol. Such diets also promote the renal tubular reabsorption of the chief metabolite of allopurinol, oxypurinol.[47b–47d] Practical implications of these findings are that elderly patients with gout should not be prescribed low-protein conventional or formula diets when they are receiving allopurinol, unless the drug dosage is reduced sufficiently to avoid the risk of toxicity, which is related to persistence of the parent drug and its metabolite in the body. This precaution is particularly important in elderly patients whose renal function is compromised. Indeed, it is well known that in such patients, the risk of allopurinol toxicity is increased. This toxicity is manifested by fever, a rash, peeling of the skin, hepatitis, and worsening of renal function.[47e]

A low protein diet can also lessen the rate of excretion of basic drugs such as the antibiotic, gentamicin, or the antiarrhythmic drug, procainamide. This is explained by the alkalinizing effect of the diet, which results in less of the ionized form of these drugs being presented in the renal tubule and therefore more of the drug being reabsorbed. A similar effect is produced by intake of antacids that are commonly taken by elderly patients. It is recommended that in patients receiving basic drugs, the urinary pH be monitored, and if the pH is increasing there is a need for the physician to reduce the drug dose or to consider an alternative drug.[47f]

**Table 34–2.  Compounds Whose Absorption May be Delayed by Food**

| Compound | Dosage Form |
|---|---|
| Alclofenac | Suspension |
| Amoxycillin | Tablets |
| Aspirin | EC tablets |
|  | Effervescent tablets |
| Cefaclor | Capsules, suspension |
| Cephalexin | Capsules |
| Cephradine | Capsules |
| Cimetidine | Tablets |
| Cinoxacin | Capsules |
| Diclofenac | EC tablet |
| Digoxin | Tablets |
| Furosemide | Tablets, solution |
| Glipizide | Tablets |
| Indoprofen | Capsules |
| Metronidazole | Tablets |
| Paracetamol (acetaminophen) | Tablets |
| Phenytoin | Capsule, powder or suspension* |
| Piroxicam | Capsules |
| Potassium ion | Tablets and solution |
| Quinidine |  |
| Sulfadiazine | Suspension |
| Sulfadiazine, sodium | Solution |
| Sulfadimethoxine | Tablets |
| Sulfafurazole (sufisoxazole) | Tablets |
| Sulfanilamide | Suspension |
| Sulfamethoxypyridazine | Tablets |
| Sulfasymasine | Tablets |
| Theophylline | Solution, sustained release tablet |
|  | Sustained release tablets |
|  | Sustained release tablets and capsules, enteric-coated tablets |
|  | Tablets |
| Valproic acid | Syrup, capsules |

*Absorption delayed by protein solution or enteral formula.
Adapted from Welling, P.: Nutrient effects on drug metabolism and action in the elderly. Drug-Nutrient Interact. 4(1/2):187, 1985.

Competition between drugs or between drugs and nutrients for a common renal secretory pathway can also change the rate of drug excretion. For example, the renal clearance of the antifolate drug, methotrexate, is markedly reduced by administration of aspirin.

## INFLUENCE OF FOOD AND NUTRIENTS ON PRESYSTEMIC CLEARANCE OF DRUGS

It has been pointed out by Melander and McLean that drugs can have a low degree of oral bioavailability in spite of the fact that gastrointestinal absorption is complete.[48] This is explained by the fact that some drugs undergo extensive presystemic metabolism during their first passage through the gut mucosa and the liver. The intake of specific nutrients has been found to influence the bioavailability of certain drugs that are known to undergo presystemic metabolic clearance. These drugs are lipophilic bases including propranolol, metoprolol, labetalol, and hydralazine, which are metabolized presystemically by hydroxylation, glucuronidation, and acetylation. Marley et al. reported that food-induced increases in the bioavailability of propranolol are related to the amount of protein in a meal.[49] This effect may be explained by the effect of the protein in the meal on splanchnic blood flow. It is not clear, however, from the published studies, whether this protein effect is of clinical significance when the drug is given in several doses per day and on a long-term basis.

Erratic responses to these drugs can be explained by administration in a haphazard way in relation to meal times, so that the food sometimes has an effect on their bioavailability and at other times does not. It is recommended therefore, that these drugs always be given with a meal and preferably always with a meal of similar composition.

## EFFECTS OF DIET ON MICROBIAL METABOLISM OF XENOBIOTICS

It has long been established that the gut microflora are capable of metabolizing foreign compounds as well as endogenous metabolites. Most

**Table 34–3. Compounds Whose Absorption May be Increased by Food or Formula**

| Compound | Dosage Form |
|---|---|
| Alafosfalin | Capsules |
| Canrenone | Tablets |
| Carbamazepine | Tablets |
| Chlorothiazide | Tablets |
| Dextropropoxyphene | Capsules |
| Diazepam | Tablets |
| Dicoumarol | Tablets |
| Diftalone | Capsules |
| Griseofulvin | Tablets or capsule |
| Hydralazine | Tablets |
| Hydrochlorothiazide | Tablets |
| Labetalol | Tablets |
| Lithium citrate | Tablets |
| Mebendazole | Tablets |
| Methoxsalen | Coated tablets |
| Metoprolol | Tablets |
| Nitrofurantoin | Capsules, tablets |
| Phenytoin | Capsules |
| Pivampicillin | Capsules |
| Propranolol | Capsules |
| Riboflavin* | Tablets, solution |
| Riboflavin-5′-phosphate* | Tablets, solution |
| Sulfamethoxydiazine | Tablets |
| Alpha-tocopherol nicotinate | Capsules |

*Absorption is slowed by increased by food by specific dietary fiber sources including bran and by a glucose polymer solution (Polycose.Ross).
Adapted from Welling, P.: Nutrient effects on drug metabolism and action in the elderly. Drug-Nutrient Interact. 4(1/2):193, 1985.

of the studies that have demonstrated metabolism of drugs by the gut microflora have been carried out in vitro. Prins has pointed out, however, that in vitro demonstration that the intestinal microflora metabolize a drug does not actually mean that this process takes place in vivo.[50] For in vivo metabolism of drugs to take place, the drug or its metabolites must actually be in contact with the bacteria within the lumen of the intestine. Criteria have been developed to indicate whether a drug is metabolized by the gut microflora in vivo. These criteria can be summarized as follows: (1) the reaction should occur more extensively after oral rather than parenteral administration of the drug; (2) the microbial drug metabolism should be decreased when antibiotics are given; and (3) the reaction should not occur in germ-free animals. Most metabolic activities of the gut microflora with respect to therapeutic drugs and other xenobiotics are degradative. In rodents, microbial metabolism of foreign compounds and endogenous metabolites is more extensive than in man both because the upper gastrointestinal tract is colonized with bacteria capable of these activities and also because the animals practice coprophagy so that drugs and their primary metabolites may be returned to the tract several times. In the human, as in other animals, most of the microbial metabolism of foreign compounds occurs after initial absorption of the parent drug and its con-

version by the microsomal drug metabolizing system to primary metabolites. These metabolites are absorbed into the enterohepatic circulation and are then excreted via the bile into the gut lumen. It is presumed that in human subjects the microbial metabolism of drugs is in the large intestine, because the major colonization of the gut by bacteria is in the large intestine, except under conditions of disease when the small intestine may be colonized.

## EFFECTS OF OBESITY ON DRUG PHARMACOKINETICS

Differences in body composition may influence drug disposition. The disposition of gentamicin and tobramycin have been studied in mildly obese subjects, and it has been found that the mean relative volume of distribution is similar to that in normal-weight subjects when normalized body mass is used in the calculation.[51] Following this study it was recommended by these and other investigators that dosing schedules for tobramycin and for other aminoglycosides should be based on ideal body weight.[52,53]

Tobramycin pharmacokinetics was studied by Blouin et al. in subjects who were 124.9 ± 36% S.D. overweight.[53] The volume of distribution of the drug ($v_{area}$) related to ideal body weight was approximately 1.7 times as high as in published reports on normal subjects. Specifically, Blouin et al. recommended that the loading dose of tobramycin in morbidly obese subjects should be based on a $v_{area}$ of 0.26 L/kg × (IBW + 58% adipose mass).[53] However, there is still a need to determine whether multiple doses or the duration of multiple doses would alter the volume of distribution of aminoglycosides at the steady state.

## DRUG EFFECTS ON FOOD INTAKE, BODY WEIGHT, NUTRIENT REQUIREMENTS, AND GROWTH

Drugs can reduce food intake because they cause a perversion or loss of appetite, because they induce sedation, or because they evoke an adverse response when food is taken. Drugs affecting appetite may do so by central or peripheral effect. Appetite-reducing drugs acting centrally include unsubstituted and substituted amphetamines, as well as related compounds. Although this class of drugs has not shown outstanding effectiveness in the treatment or control of obesity, it has been shown that, when children are given a similar drug, such as dextroamphetamine, for the control of hyperactivity, growth may be retarded while the drug therapy is maintained. Fortunately, rebound growth occurs when the drug is discontinued. Ethoxzolamide (Ethamide) has a similar effect to that of dextroamphetamine with respect to inhibition of growth.

Intentional or unintentional modulation of appetite by drugs has been a subject of much research in recent years and of several major reviews.[54,55] Whereas all reviews on appetitive control by drugs stress drugs that have been and are used in the treatment of obesity, our present concern is with other therapeutic drugs for which change in appetite and, hence, change in food intake are unwanted side effects. Any drug that induces nausea is likely to reduce food intake and hence contribute to weight loss. Digitalis, which is usually administered for long periods, if also prescribed at a high dosage level, can cause severe wasting (digitalis cachexia) because associated nausea diminishes the desire for food.[56]

Among all drug groups that reduce appetite, the cancer chemotherapeutic drugs are most important. At effective therapeutic dosages, these drugs commonly have an acute anorectic effect, which is an integral part of the systemic toxicity. However, there also may be reduced intake of food following administration of cancer chemotherapeutic drugs because of either oral or intestinal ulceration. A reduction in food intake is related to gastroenterologic toxicity. It is largely explained by the reluctance to eat, since food causes unpleasant symptoms, which may include pain and diarrhea.[57]

A wide range of environmental chemicals that have significant systemic toxicity induce a reduction in food intake. For example, experience has shown that in the Yusho disease that occurred in Fukuoka, Japan, as a result of exposure to polychlorinated biphenyls, poor appetite was a consistent symptom of intoxication.[58]

Risks from the effects of drug-induced anorexia depend on both the primary toxicity of the substance and the secondary effects of the anorexia or loss of desire to consume food. The latter includes not only weight loss, but also specific nutrient deficiencies that may ensue because of diminished intake of nutrients. A classification of anorectic drugs is given in Table 34–4.

Drugs that increase appetite include the phenothiazine and benzodiazepine tranquilizers and lithium carbonate, which is used as a psychotherapeutic agent in patients with manic depressive psychoses. Effects of these drugs, which increase appetite and food intake in psychotic patients, are due to both to direct pharmacologic effects and to the fact that administration of the drug reduces mental agitation. Cyproheptadine is another drug that can increase appetite. It is used as an antihistamine and serotonin antagonist. The hyperphagic effect of this drug has been utilized in the nutritional management of the debilitated individual whose appetite is precarious.[59]

## DRUG EFFECTS ON NUTRIENT REQUIREMENTS

In human subjects, as in laboratory animals, microbial nutrient synthesis occurs in the intestine. Contribution of this synthesis to the nutrition of the host has been considered to be modest in the human, whereas in rodents the nutrient synthesis in the small and large intestine is important in contributing to vitamin needs. However, there are

**Table 34–4.   Classification of Anorectic Drugs**

A. Primary → appetite suppression
  1. *Centrally acting*
    a) Catecholaminergic, e.g., dextroamphetamine
    b) Dopaminergic, e.g., levodopa
    c) Serotoninergic, e.g., fenfluramine
    d) Endorphin modulators, e.g., naloxone
  2. *Peripherally acting*
    a) Agents that inhibit gastric emptying, e.g., levodopa
    b) Bulking agents, e.g., methyl cellulose

B. Secondary → Adverse response to food → Loss of appetite
    a) Drugs causing nausea and vomiting, e.g., digoxin–toxic dose
    b) Drugs causing loss of taste, e.g., penicillamine
    c) Drugs causing stomatitis, e.g., fluorouracil
    d) Hepatotoxic agents, e.g., alcohol

Based on Pawan, G.L.S.[59]

circumstances in which microbial synthesis of specific nutrients becomes critical, particularly when intake of said nutrients is inadequate. For example, the synthesis of biotin in the intestine may supply needs for this vitamin in patients who are totally fed with a biotin-free enteral formula. A recent case report illustrates the development of biotin deficiency in an adult that was induced by lack of biotin intake as well as by suppression of the normal colonic bacterial flora by long-term antibiotic therapy. The patient who had inflammatory bowel disease of long standing may also have had gastrointestinal losses of biotin through fistulae. Food-energy and nutrient intake of this man was supplied by parenteral alimentation using a formula that did not contain biotin.[60]

Broad-spectrum antibiotics, such as tetracycline, can also depress vitamin K synthesis in the intestine. The impact of this nutrient effect of the antibiotic with respect to vitamin K status is not important unless concurrently the patient is vitamin K-deficient because of liver disease or a warfarin anticoagulant which is a vitamin K antagonist is also being administered.[61,62]

## DRUG-INDUCED MALDIGESTION AND MALABSORPTION

Drugs that may cause nutrient malabsorption include antacids, laxatives, antibacterial agents such as sulfasalazine, and also isoniazid (isonicotinic acid hydrazide, INH). Absorption induced by antacids is multifactorial. When the pH of the upper part of the jejunum is increased following ingestion of sodium bicarbonate, folate absorption is reduced. However, our own studies of peptic ulcer patients taking antacids suggest that folate deficiency is not very common and that when it does occur, it is more often associated with a very inadequate intake of the vitamin, rather than intake of sodium bicarbonate. A risk does exist, nevertheless, that if large doses of sodium bicarbonate are taken concurrently with food sources of folate, significant malabsorption could lead to folate depletion and deficiency.

A phosphate depletion syndrome is known to occur in elderly people taking heavy doses of antacids containing aluminum or magnesium hydroxide or mixtures of these substances. Dietary phosphate combines with aluminum and magnesium hydroxide to form insoluble aluminum and magnesium phosphates, which are excreted via the gastrointestinal tract. The risk of phosphate depletion is greatest when there is an interactive effect with a low phosphate diet. Some effects of phosphate depletion are muscle weakness, which may be limited to the proximal limb muscles, malaise, parasthesias in the limbs, an-

orexia, hemolytic anemia, and convulsions. Congestive heart failure may also occur. In a few patients with phosphate depletion, a low phosphate osteomalacia has developed.[63,64]

It has been proposed that folate malabsorption associated with intake of sulfasalazine is due to inhibition of folate enzymes in the gastrointestinal tract. Sulfasalazine is a competitive inhibitor of folate transport by the intestine.[65] Folate malabsorption in patients with inflammatory bowel disease who are receiving this drug depends not only on drug intake but also on whether they obtain a sufficiency or otherwise of dietary folate.[66]

Two drugs used in the treatment of tuberculosis, rifampicin and isoniazid, interfere with the normal metabolism of vitamin D and, hence, may impair calcium absorption. Isoniazid inhibits both the hepatic 25-hydroxylase and the renal 1-alpha-hydroxylase. Rifampicin is a microsomal enzyme inducer, which stimulates metabolism of 25-hydroxycholecalciferol with a resultant decrease in circulating levels of this vitamin D metabolite. Whether or not hypocalcemia and metabolic bone disease (osteomalacia) occur as a result of ingestion of these drugs depends on the age of the patient, physiologic stress (pregnancy or lactation), ultraviolet exposure, vitamin D or calcium intake, presence of alcoholic liver disease, administration of both isoniazid and rifampicin, and a previous partial gastrectomy.[67,68]

Malabsorption of protein-bound vitamin $B_{12}$ has been reported with intake of the $H_2$ receptor blocking drugs, cimetidine and ranitidine. Cimetidine, in a dosage of 1,000 mg/day (200 mg 3 times/day + 400 mg at night), has been shown to reduce the absorption of protein-bound cobalamin by peptic ulcer patients and also by normal subjects. When cimetidine was administered in a dosage of 400 mg/night, it had no significant effect on the absorption of the vitamin.[69] Ranitidine can also cause protein-bound vitamin $B_{12}$ malabsorption, but these effects are rapidly reversible when the drug is discontinued.[70]

The anticonvulsant drugs, phenytoin and phenobarbital, have been shown to cause hypocalcemia and rickets or osteomalacia in epileptic children and adults who receive these anticonvulsant drugs. The mechanisms responsible for the adverse effects of these drugs on calcium absorption are not entirely clear. The drugs may have a direct effect on bone growth, but also it has been found that both drugs inhibit the synthesis of calcium-binding protein and thereby will inhibit calcium absorption. It has been further proposed that these drugs stimulate the catabolism of 25-hydroxycholecalciferol to vitamin D metabolites, which are inactive in promoting calcium absorption.[71-73]

Mechanisms responsible for drug-induced maldigestion and malabsorption include interaction of the drug and nutrient in the gastrointestinal tract, change in gastrointestinal function, and drug-induced enteropathy with damage to the brush border of the intestinal villi, causing interference with active transport mechanisms for nutrients. Drug-induced maldigestion and malabsorption are classified in Table 34–5 together with mechanisms.

## VITAMIN ANTAGONISTS

Vitamin antagonists are those therapeutic drugs and environmental chemicals that have antinutrient function by virtue of the fact that they interfere with the metabolism and physiologic function of vitamins. The antivitamin effects of drugs may be utilized intentionally in the treatment of disease, or these effects may be an unwanted side effect of drug therapy.[74]

Drugs for which the therapeutic effect is related to vitamin antagonism include methotrexate, which is used in the treatment of choriocarcinoma, head and neck cancer, and acute lymphoblastic leukemia, and pyrimethamine, which is used in the prevention and treatment of malaria. Another class of therapeutic compounds that are vitamin antagonists are the coumarin anticoagulants. Methotrexate has several antifolate effects. In the tissues, this drug binds tightly to the dihydrofolate reductase enzyme. Folate from dietary sources is thereby displaced from the dihydrofolate reductase enzyme by the drug and is thereafter excreted in the urine. Methotrexate polyglutamates are formed, and synthesis of folate polyglutamates is diminished. Thymidylate synthetase is inhibited. The synthesis of DNA, RNA, and protein are thereby also inhibited. Methotrexate reduces the incorporation of deoxyuridine (dU) into DNA and favors incorporation of thymidine into DNA by the alternate pathway. The dU suppression test is abnormal in people who are receiving methotrexate.[75]

Methotrexate has a greater affinity for folate-binding protein at the pH optimum for the radiometric assay for plasma folate. It has therefore been proposed that this assay, which is by competitive protein binding in plasma and erythrocytes, should not be used to measure this vitamin in the plasma or erythrocytes of patients receiving the drug.[76]

Sulfasalazine is also a folate antagonist. Inhibitory actions of sulfasalazine include inhibition of three enzymes in vitro, including dihydrofolate reductase, methyltetrahydrofolate reductase, and serine transhydroxymethylase, which each catalyze a different reaction involving folate coenzymes. Sulfasalazine has been shown to act as a folate antagonist in intact lymphocytes.[77]

Nitrous oxide, long used as an anesthetic and more recently used in the management of patients after cardiac bypass surgery, has been shown to be a vitamin $B_{12}$ antagonist. Megaloblastic erythropoiesis and neurologic disorders have been reported both in man and in laboratory animals following exposures to high concentrations of this gas. Nitrous oxide causes multiple metabolic defects. It oxidizes vitamin $B_{12}$ and causes an inhibition of methionine synthetase. When inactivation of methionine synthetase is produced by nitrous oxide, there is displacement of cobalamin from the enzyme. Further, there is an increased formation of inactive cobalamin analogues.[78-81]

Vitamin antagonism is a significant side effect of a number of therapeutic drugs, including isoniazid and hydralazine. Both of these drugs are vitamin $B_6$ antagonists. Isoniazid can also induce a secondary niacin deficiency with development of pellagra. Such secondary niacin deficiency is rare, but it has been reported in tuberculous patients who have been on a marginal intake of niacin. It is thought that the deficiency in these patients

## Table 34–5. Drug-induced Maldigestion and Malabsorption

| Mechanism | Example of Inducing Drug(s) | Effect on Nutrient Absorption |
|---|---|---|
| Intraluminal interaction of drug and nutrient | Mineral oil | ↓ Absorption fat-soluble vitamins; ∴ solubilization and ↓ micelle formation |
| | Cholestyramine | ↓ Absorption of folic acid ∴ absorption onto drug |
| Change in milieu of GI tract or GI function | Sodium bicarbonate | ↓ Absorption of folic acid ∴ ↑ pH* |
| | Cimetidine | ↓ Absorption of vitamin $B_{12}$ ∴ ↓ gastric digestion |
| | Alcohol | ↓ Absorption of fat ∴ ↓ exocrine pancreatic function |
| Drug-induced enteropathy | Neomycin Colchicine | Disaccharide intolerance and fat malabsorption ∴ damage to brush border |

*∴ = "due to . . ."

results from an inhibition of the enzyme kynureninase in the pathway of nicotinamide nucleotide synthesis from tryptophan as a result of complex formation between isoniazid and pyridoxal phosphate (Schiff base formation).[82,83]

Vitamin K antagonists include coumarin drugs such as warfarin, dicoumarol, and phenprocoumon, as well as coumarins in plants, which sometimes are used in making herbal teas. These coumarin derivatives inhibit the hepatic reductase, which converts the storage form of vitamin K (vitamin K 2,3-epoxide) to the active form of the vitamin.[84] High doses of vitamin K decrease the anticoagulant effect of coumarin drugs and lessen their clinical effectiveness in the prevention of thromboses.[85]

Moxalactam, which is a beta-lactam cephalosporin antibiotic as well as a beta-lactam antibiotic, can decrease vitamin K-dependent clotting factors including prothrombin. Hemorrhagic events following use of these antibiotics are most frequent with moxalactam. This drug can interfere with blood clotting through three different mechanisms: production of hypoprothrombinemia, platelet dysfunction, and occasionally thrombocytopenia. Only hemorrhage that is associated with hypoprothrombinemia can be reversed or prevented by administration of vitamin K.[86,87]

The cancer chemotherapy drug doxorubicin (Adriamycin) produces a dose-dependent cardiomyopathy when the total cumulative dose is greater than 500 mg/meter$^2$. In laboratory animals, the histopathologic aspects of the cardiac lesion are similar to those of vitamin E deficiency. The lesions seen in vitamin E deficiency, and apparently in doxorubicin toxicity, are the result of free radical reactions that cause lipid peroxidation of membrane lipids. The incidence and severity of the doxorubicin-induced cardiac damage has been reduced by administration of vitamin E to laboratory animals, but this vitamin has not been effective in preventing doxorubicin cardiotoxicity in man.[88]

Adverse effects of alcohol excess on nutritional status include an impairment in the utilization of B vitamins.[89] For example, the Wernicke-Korsakoff syndrome is a thiamin dependency disease that occurs mainly in alcoholics. The acute phase of this disease (Wernicke's encephalopathy) responds to intravenous administration of high doses of thiamin.[90]

Wernicke's encephalopathy has also been reported in a diabetic patient following administration of the oral hypoglycemic agent tolazamide. Signs were reversed by administration of thiamin given as combined intramuscular and oral therapy. It was suggested that administration of this hypoglycemic agent to diabetic patients may increase the demand for thiamin because there is a sudden increase in utilization of glucose in an individual who previously is thiamin-depleted.[91] Drugs that have significant effects as vitamin antagonists are classified in Table 34–6.

## DRUG-INDUCED FETAL MALNUTRITION

All drugs given to a pregnant woman can be considered as being potentially harmful to the fetus because they cross the placental membrane. The highest risk for disruption in fetal development is during the period of embryogenesis.[92] The most important toxic effect of drug administration during the period of embryogenesis is the development of fetal malformations (teratogenic effect). The teratogenic potential of drugs is related to drug properties, including drug metabolism; to the time of administration during gestation; to dosage and maternofetal transfer; to the species, strain, and genetic susceptibility of the animal or individual; and to nutritional status. Drugs that are vitamin antagonists impose a high risk for teratogenic effects. Whereas fetal malformations result from an interruption in fetal growth and development during embryogenesis, specific associations between the change in nutritional status and the fetal malformations have been identified as follows: (1) A disturbance in DNA synthesis, such as that imposed by folacin deficiency, causes multiple malformations. Interference with DNA synthesis can be brought about by drugs such as methotrexate or pyrimethamine, which are folate antagonists. (2) Impaired glycosaminoglycan synthesis or sulfation can result in malformations related to the skeleton. Sulfation of the glycosaminoglycans in the fetal skeleton is dependent on substrate availability. When drugs that require sulfoconjugation, such as salicylamide, are administered during pregnancy, competitive utilization of sulfate for sulfoconjugation and sulfation of the skeletal elements occurs.[93] (3) Riboflavin deficiency induced by administration of the flavin antagonist, galactoflavin, can induce congenital anomalies in the fetus because of impairment of the electron transport system. Depressed function of the electron transport system during the critical period of development usually results in malformations.[94]

## DRUG EFFECTS ON MINERAL STATUS

Drug effects on mineral status include overload and depletion. Sodium overload with development of congestive heart failure can result from intake of antacids containing sodium bicarbonate.

**Table 34–6. Therapeutic Drugs That Are Vitamin Antagonists**

| Antagonists | Drug | Usage |
|---|---|---|
| Folacin | Methotrexate | Cancer chemotherapy |
| | Pyrimethamine | Antimalarial |
| | Triamterene | Diuretic |
| | Trimethoprim | Antibacterial |
| | Sulfasalazine | Anti-inflammatory |
| Vitamin B$_6$ | Isoniazid | Antituberculosis agent |
| | Hydralazine | Antihypertensive agent |
| Vitamin B$_{12}$ | Nitrous oxide | Anesthetic |
| Vitamin K | Warfarin | Anticoagulant |
| | Moxalactam | Antibiotic |

The risk is most severe in elderly people with pre-existing heart disease who are also consuming high-sodium diets. Intake of other high-sodium drugs can also cause sodium overload, particularly in cardiac patients. The antihypertensive agent, diazoxide, which increases the proximal tubular reabsorption of sodium, can also cause sodium overload.[74,95]

**Potassium Overload.** A number of drugs are known to produce hyperkalemia. Administration of succinylcholine can produce significant increases in serum potassium levels which may result in arrhythmia and cardiac arrest.[96] Hyperkalemia with development of metabolic acidosis can result from administration of a biguanide such as phenformin when this drug is given to a diabetic patient with impaired renal function.[97]

Hyperkalemia can follow use of potassium-sparing diuretics. Hyperkalemia resulting from administration of spironolactone, an aldosterone antagonist is caused by blocking of the distal tubular sodium-potassium exchange. Hyperkalemia due to spironolactone is more severe in patients with impaired renal function.[98] Triamterene, which is also a potassium-sparing diuretic, can cause hyperkalemia.[99] Increases in serum potassium have been reported with use of beta-blocking drugs.[100,101]

**Hypercalcemia.** Hypercalcemia may be drug-related, but usually this metabolic disorder is multifactorial. Hypercalcemia can occur with administration of thiazide diuretics; however, this is a relatively uncommon side effect of thiazide therapy and may only be temporary.[102]

It is known that the thiazide diuretics cause calcium retention, and the actual effect of these drugs on the mineral content of bone has been measured. Thiazide users have a greater bone mineral content than nonusers who have been matched. It has been suggested that thiazide drugs might have a therapeutic role in the management of osteoporosis.[103]

Pharmacologic doses of vitamin D and its metabolites cause hypercalcemia. In vitamin D intoxication, hypercalcemia is associated with polyuric renal failure and also soft tissue calcification. When high doses of vitamin D are taken, the hypercalcemic effect is potentiated by concurrent intake of calcium salts.[104,105]

The milk-alkali syndrome occurs as a complication of excessive ingestion of soluble alkali and milk. It is characterized by hypercalcemia with hypercalciuria. Renal insufficiency with azotemia can develop with alkalosis. Signs include band keratitis due to deposition of calcium in the cornea. The milk-alkali syndrome has been reported in people taking large amounts of sodium bicarbonate or calcium carbonate. Persons at particular risk are those with pre-existent renal insufficiency.[106]

When malignant tumors metastasize to bone, they may induce hypercalcemia, and it has been shown that when androgenic steroids are used in the treatment of metastases from breast tumors, hypercalcemia may thereby be increased.[107]

There has also been concern that chronically supplementing dietary calcium with calcium salts, as a means to delay age-related bone loss or to prevent hypertension, could also cause the milk alkali syndrome.[107a] Previous estimates of the amount of ingested calcium and alkali necessary to produce the syndrome were 4 to 5 g up to 60 g of calcium carbonate daily.[107b] The current extensive use of calcium carbonate tablets for osteoporosis and hypertension prevention may therefore lead to an increased prevalence of the syndrome such as was encountered in peptic ulcer patients when the Sippy diet and antacid treatment were in vogue.

**Magnesium Overload.** Magnesium intoxication has been reported in patients with chronic renal failure who have been taking magnesium-containing antacids. Signs include nausea, vomiting, flushing, impaired respiratory function, and partial or complete heart block. Lithium carbonate, used in the management of manic-depressive psychosis, may induce hypermagnesemia.[108,109]

**Drug-Induced Mineral Depletion.** Drug-induced mineral depletion is commonly multifactorial. For example, in the elderly it may be the outcome of concurrent use of several drugs that have this side effect, as well as intake of the mineral. Such common drugs causing potassium deficiency, for example, are diuretics, including both thiazide and loop-type diuretics, and in the elderly individuals who are taking one of these drugs, there may be concurrent use of laxatives, which also cause potassium depletion, and the same patient may have an inadequate potassium intake. Factors contributing to mineral depletion in such individuals include prolonged drug intake and renal disorder. Crooks and Stevenson drew attention to the relationship between an age-related decline in renal function and the potential for mineral depletion by nephrotoxic drugs.[110] Related diseases that potentiate drug-related mineral depletion include renal disease and catabolic diseases, including metastatic cancer. Drugs that cause potassium depletion may damage the renal tubule and thereby cause secondary depletion of magnesium and zinc.[74] Drug causes of mineral depletion as well as the sequelae of such depletion are classified in Table 34–7.

## DRUG-FOOD AND DRUG-ALCOHOL INCOMPATIBILITIES

Food and drug incompatibilities usually arise as outcomes of the drug-induced inhibition of enzymes acquired in the catabolism of potentially toxic endogenous metabolites. Many of the incompatibilities result in flush reactions. "Histamine poisoning" has been reported in individuals receiving isoniazid as an antituberculous drug during intake of certain kinds of fish, including tuna and skipjack. Signs include redness of the face, itching of the eyes, face, and palms, and severe headache. It is known that isoniazid is a potent histaminase inhibitor and it has therefore been suggested that eating fish that is not fresh and contains high levels of histamine, may produce these side effects.[111]

Chlorpropamide-alcohol flushing (CPAF) has been found in many patients with noninsulin-dependent diabetes. This type of flushing can be blocked by administration of prostaglandin inhibitor drugs such as aspirin and indomethacin. These findings have indicated an etiologic association between prostaglandins and the flush reaction.[112-114]

Tyramine reactions have occurred when fermented foods such as cheese have been consumed by people receiving monamine oxidase inhibitor drugs. These drugs include certain antidepressants such as phenelzine, the cancer chemotherapeutic drug procarbazine, and isoniazid. In these patients absorption of tyramine, because of inhibition of its metabolism in the intestine, triggers

**Table 34–7.   Drug Causes, Signs, and Sequelae of Mineral Depletion**

| Mineral Depletion | Drugs Causing | Signs and Sequelae |
|---|---|---|
| Sodium | Chlorpropamide | Hyponatremia, anorexia |
| | Tolbutamide | Nausea |
| | Vincristine | Vomiting |
| | Amitryptyline | Muscle weakness, seizures |
| | Mannitol | Loss of consciousness |
| | Thiazides | |
| | Spironolactone | |
| | Captopril | |
| Potassium | Thiazides | Hypokalemia, anorexia |
| | Furosemide | Muscle weakness |
| | Ethacrynic acid | Renal tubular damage |
| | Laxatives, e.g., phenolphthalein | Arrhythmias, hyperglycemia |
| | Nephrotoxic antibiotics, e.g., gentamicin | Magnesium and zinc depletion |
| Calcium | Aluminum hydroxide | Hypocalcemia, tetany, osteomalacia |
| | Phenytoin | |
| | Phenobarbital | |
| | Corticosteroids | Osteoporosis |
| Magnesium | Thiazides | Muscle weakness |
| | Furosemide | Tremors |
| | Ethacrynic acid | Seizures |
| | Gentamicin | Tetany |
| | Cisplatin | Psychotic behavior |
| | Neomycin | |
| | Colchicine | |
| Iron | Aspirin | Anemia |
| | Indomethacin | |
| Zinc | Penicillamine | Loss of taste |
| | | Dermatitis |
| | | Impaired wound healing |

release of catecholamines with resultant acute elevation in blood pressure. Attacks of hypertension of short duration are associated with headaches, palpitations, nausea, and vomiting. In some cases major cerebrovascular accidents have occurred. Severity of each attack is related both to the current drug dosage and also to the level of tryamine in the particular food ingested. Foods high in tyramine documented in these incompatibility reactions include not only aged cheese but also Chianti wine and chicken livers.[115–119] The amino acid dopa or its amine derivative, dopamine, present in broad beans may trigger the tyramine reaction in patients on monamine oxidase inhibitor drugs.[115]

The disulfiram reaction occurs when people receiving the drug disulfiram (Antabuse) either drink alcoholic beverages or consume foods containing alcohol, or apply alcohol-containing lotions or other solutions to the skin. The reaction is associated with flushing and headache followed by nausea, vomiting, and a variable degree of chest and/or abdominal pain. Since these symptoms are unpleasant, the drug has come to be used as an alchohol deterrent for alcoholics. Disulfiram-like reactions are caused by all drugs that are aldehyde dehydrogenase inhibitors. Disulfiram is such a drug. Other drugs in this category are: metronidazole, furazolidone, griseofulvin, quinacrine, tolazoline, and procarbazine. Inky-cap mushroom *(Coprinus atramentarius)* contains an aldehyde dehydrogenase inhibitor such that consumption of these mushrooms with or following an alcoholic beverage, including beer, causes a disulfiram reaction.[89,120–123]

Hypoglycemic reactions may occur when diabetic patients receiving hypoglycemic agents ingest alcohol. Symptoms are characterized by weakness, mental confusion, irrational behavior, and, if untreated, by loss of consciousness. Hypoglycemic attacks have occurred when sweet or semisweet drinks containing alcohol are ingested on an empty stomach.[124]

## SUMMARY

In this account of drug-nutrient interactions major emphasis has been on the impact on human health. Whereas drug-nutrient interactions can be defined as events and outcomes that ensue as a result of physical, chemical, physiologic, or pathophysiologic relationships between drugs and nutrients, the significance of drug-nutrient interactions is in their adverse or unwanted outcomes. Unwanted outcomes include reduction in the intended or expected response to a therapeutic drug because of diet-induced changes in drug bioavailability or metabolism, drug-induced-nu-

tritional deficiencies or overload, drug-induced fetal malnutrition, and drug-food and drug-nutrient incompatibility reactions. Risk of drug-nutrient interactions and their outcomes depends most on the characteristics of the exposed individual, including age, physiologic status, multiple drug exposure, hepatic and renal function, and diet. However, as emphasized in this account, whether or not a drug-nutrient interaction occurs depends largely on the concurrent use or exposure to drug and nutrients at the critical period. Avoidance of drug-nutrient interactions depends on a knowledge of the risk and also avoidance of temporal proximity of drug-nutrient, drug-alcohol, drug-food intake that imposes a high risk situation.

## REFERENCES

1. Miescher, G.: Dermatologica *108*:300-303, 1954,
2. Goldsmith, W.N., Hellier, F.F.: Recent Advances in Dermatology. 2nd. ed. New York, Blakiston Co. Inc., 1954.
3. Sulzberger, M.B., Lazar, M.P.: J.A.M.A. *146*:788-793, 1951.
4. Dowling, G.B., Gauvain, S., Macrae, D.E.: Br. Med. J. *1*:430-435, 1948.
5. Michelson, H.E.: Arch. Dermatol. Syphol. *58*:680-695, 1948.
6. Charpy, M.J.: Ann. Dermatol. Syphol. (Paris) *6*:310-346, 1946.
7. Anning, S.T., Dawson, J., Dolby, D.E., et al.: Qt. J. Med. *17*:203-228, 1948.
8. Bean, W.B., Spies, T.D.: Am. Heart J. *20*:62-75, 1940.
9. Ruffin, J.M., Smith, D.T.: South. Med. J. *32*:40-47, 1939.
10. Altschul, R., Hoffer, A., Stephen, D.: Arch. Biochem. Biophys. *54*:558-559, 1955.
11. Cook, P., James, I.: N. Engl. J. Med. *305*:1560-1564, 1981.
12. Grundie, S.M., Mok, H.Y.I., Zec, L., et al.: J. Lipid Res. *22*:24-36, 1981.
13. Illingworth, D.R., Phillipson, B.E., Rapp, J.H., et al.: Lancet *1*:296-298, 1981.
14. Havel, R.J., Kane, J.P.: Ann. Rev. Med. *33*:417-433, 1982.
15. Peck, G.L., Olsen, T.G., Yoder, F.W., et al.: N. Engl. J. Med. *300*:329-333, 1979.
16. Peck, G.L., Gross, E.G., Butkus, D.: *In* Retinoids: Advances in Basic Research and Therapy. (Orfanos, C.E., Ed.) New York, Springer-Verlag, 1981, pp. 279-286
17. Pittsley, R.A., Yoder, F.W.: N. Engl. J. Med. *308*:1012-1014, 1983.
17a. Morison, W.L.: Arch. Dermatol. *122*:133-134, 1986.
18. Anstie, F.E. On the Uses of Wines in Health and Disease. London, Macmillan Publishing Co., Inc., 1977.
19. Hutchison, R. Food and the Principles of Dietetics. New York, W. Wood. Co., 1905, pp. 335, 464-466.
20. Atwater, W.O., Woods, C.D., Benedict, F.G.: Bull. 44, Office of Experiment Stations, USDA, Washington, DC, 1903.
21. Atwater, W., Benedict, F.B.: Bull. 69, 109, USDA, Washington, DC, 1900.
22. Billings, J.S. (Ed.): The Nutritive Value of Alcohol.

*In* Psychological Aspects of the Alcohol Problem, vol. 2. Boston, Houghton-Mifflin and Co. (The Univ. Press, Cambridge), 1903, pp. 174-343.

23. Becker, C.E., Roe, R.L., Scott, R.A.: Alcohol as a Drug: A Curriculm on Pharmacology, Neurology and Toxicity. Baltimore, Williams & Wilkins Co., 1974.

24. Roe, D.A.: Alcohol and the Diet. Westport, CT., AVI Publishing Co., 1979.

25. Belko, A., Rotter, M., Roe, D.A.: J. Am. Coll. Nutr. *1*:413, 1982.

25a.Gibaldi, M. Biopharmaceutics and Clinical Pharmacokinetics, 2nd ed. Lea & Febiger, 1977, pp. 15-41.

26. Welling, P.G.: J. Pharmacokinet. Biopharmaceut. *5*:291-331, 1977.

27. Borowitz, J.L., Moore, P.F., Yim, G.K.W., et al.: Toxicol. Appl. Pharmacol. *19*:164-168, 1971.

28. Welling, P.G., Barbhaiya, R.H.: J. Pharm. Sci. *71*:32-35, 1982.

29. Jusko, W.J., Levy, G.: J. Pharmacol. Sci. *56*:56-58, 1967.

30. Roe, D.A.: *In* Nutrition and Drugs. (Winick, M., Ed.) New York, John Wiley & Sons, 1983, pp. 129-138.

31. Neovonen, P., Gothoni, G., Hackman, R.: Br. Med. J. *4*: 532-534, 1970.

32. Bauer, L.A.: Neurology *32*:570-572, 1982.

33. Melander, A., Danielson, K., Schersten, B., et al.: Clin. Pharmacol. Therap. *22*:108-122, 1977.

34. Goldin, B.R., Goldman, P. Fed. Proc. *32*:798, 1973. (Abs.)

35. Sved, A.F., Goldberg, I.M. and Fernstrom, J.D.: J. Pharm. Exp. Ther. *214*:147-151, 1980.

35a.Karim, A., Burns, T., Wearley, L., et al.: Clin. Pharmacol. Ther. *38*:77-83, 1985.

36. Anderson, K.E., Conney, A.H., Kappas, A.: Clin. Pharmacol. Ther. *26*:493-501, 1979.

37. Kato, R., Oshima, T., Tomizawa, S.: J. Pharmacol. *18*:356-366, 1968.

38. Conney, A.H., Pantuck, E.J., Pantuck, C.B., et al.: *In* Proceedings First World Conference Clinical Pharmacology and Therapeutics, London, U.K., Aug. 3-9, 1980. Macmillan Publishing Co., Inc. 1980.

39. McLean, A.E.M.: *In* Nutrition in Health and Disease and International Development. Symposium 12th International Congress Nutrition. New York, Alan R. Liss, Inc., 1981, pp. 729-737.

40. Woodcock, B.G., Wood, G.C.: Biochem. Pharmacol. *20*:2703, 1971.

41. Krijgsheld, K.R., Scholtens, E., Mulder, G.J.: Biochem. Pharmacol. *30*:1973-1981, 1981.

42. Campell, T.C., Hayes, J.R.: Pharm. Rev. *26*:181-197, 1974.

43. Weatherholtz, W.M., Campbell, T.C., Webb, R.E.: J. Nutr. *98*:90-94, 1969.

44. Campbell, T.C.: *In* Nutrition and Drug Interrelations. (Hathcock, J.N., Coon. J., Eds.) New York, Academic Press, 1978, pp. 409-422.

45. Marshall, W.J., McLean, A.E.M.: Biochem. J. *122*:569-573, 1971.

46. Nored, W.P., Wade, A.E.: Biochem. Pharmacol. *21*:2887-2897, 1972.

47. Sato, P.H., Zannoni, V.G.: J. Pharmacol. Exp. Ther. *198*:295-307, 1976.

47a.Conclusions and Perspectives of the International Conference on Nutrients, Medicine and Aging. Bellagio, Italy. Drug-Nutrient Interact. *4*:251-263, 1985.

47b.Berlinger, W.A., Park, G.D., Spector, R.: N. Engl. J. Med. *313*:771-776, 1985.

47c.Elion, G.B., Kovensky, A., Hitchings, G.H., et al.: Biochem. Pharmacol. *15*: 863-880, 1966.

47d.Hande, K.R., Noone, R.M., Stone, W.J.: Am. J. Med. *76*:47-56, 1984.

47e.Hande, K., Reed, E., Chabner, B.: Clin. Pharmacol. Ther. *23*:598-605, 1978.

47f.Reidenberg, M.M.: N. Engl. J. Med. *313*:816-818, 1985.

48. Melander, A., McLean, A.E.M.: Clin. Pharmacokinet. *8*:286-296, 1983.

49. Marley, T., Fagan, T.C., Wiley, K., et al.: Clin. Pharmacol. Ther. *30*:790-795, 1981.

50. Prins, R.A.: *In* Nutrition and Drug Interactions. (Hathcock, J.N., Coon, J., Eds.) New York, Academic Press, 1978.

51. Schwartz, S.N., Pazin, G.J., Lion, J.A., et al.: J. Infect. Dis. *138*:499-505, 1978.

52. Sarubbi, F.A., Jr., Hull, J.H.: Ann. Intern. Med. *89*:612-618, 1978.

53. Blouin, R.A., Mann, H.J., Griffen, W.O., et al.: Clin. Pharmacol. Ther. *26*:508-512, 1979.

54. Sullivan, A.C., Cheng, L.: *In* Nutrition and Drug Interrelations. (Hathcock, J.N., Coon, J., Eds.) New York, Academic Press, 1978. pp. 21-65.

55. Sullivan, A.C., Triscari, J., Cheng, L.: *In* Nutrition and Drugs. (Winick, M., Ed.) New York, John Wiley & Sons, 1983, pp. 139-167.

56. Pawan, G.L.S.: Proc. Nutr. Soc. *33*:239-244, 1974.

57. Pratt, W.B., Ruddon, R.W.: The Anticancer Drugs. New York, Oxford University Press, 1979.

58. Lindsey, D.G., Sherlock, J.C.: *In* Adverse Effects of Foods. (Jelliffe, F.P., Jelliffe, D.B., Eds.) New York, Plenum Press, 1982, p. 95.

59. Pawan, G.L.S.: Proc. Nutr. Soc. *33*:239-244, 1974.

60. McClain, C.J., Baker, H., Onstad, G.R.: J.A.M.A. *247*:3116-3117, 1982.

61. Gabuzda, G.J., Gocke, T.M., Jackson, G.G., et al.: Arch. Intern. Med. *101*:476-513, 1958.

62. Mezey, E. Gastroenterology *74*:770-783, 1978.

63. MacKenzie, J.F., Russell, R.I.: Clin. Sci. Mol. Med. *51*:363-368, 1976.

64. Russell, R.I., Dahr, G.J., Dutta, S.K., et al.: J. Lab. Clin. Med. *93*:428-436, 1979.

65. Selhub, J., Dahr, G.J., Rosenberg, I.H.: J. Clin. Invest. *61*:221-114, 1978.

66. Halstead, C.H.: Ann. Rev. Med. *31*:79-87, 1980.

67. Brodie, M.J., Boobis, A.R., Hillyard, C.J., et al.: Clin. Pharm. Ther. *30*:363-367, 1981.

68. Brodie, M.J., Boobis, A.R., Hillyard, C.J., et al.: Clin. Pharm. Ther. *32*:525-530, 1981.

69. Streeter, A.M., Goulston, K.J., Bathur, F.A., et al.: Dig. Dis. Sci. *27*:13-16, 1982.

70. Belaiche, J., Cattan, D., Zittoun, J., et al.: Dig. Dis. Sci. *28*:667-668, 1983.

71. Sotaniemi, E.A., Hakkarainen, H.K., Puranen, J.A., et al.: Ann. Intern. Med. *77*:389, 1972.

72. Dent, C.E., Richens, A., Rowe, D.J., et al.: Br. Med. J. *4*:69-72, 1970.

73. Hunter, J., Maxwell, J.D., Stewart, D.A., et al.: Br. Med. J. *4*:202, 1971.

74. Roe, D.A.: Clin. Lab Med. *1*:647-664, 1981.

75. Wickramasinghe, S.N., Saunders, J.E.: Acta Haematol. *58*:193-206, 1977.

76. Waxman, S.: *In* Folic Acid in Neurology, Psychology, and Internal Medicine. (Boter, M.I., Reynolds, E.H., Eds.) New York, Raven Press, 1979, p. 47.

77. Baum, C.L., Selhub, J., Rosenberg, I.H.: J. Lab. Clin. Med. *97*:778-784, 1981.
78. Amess, J.A.L., Burman, J.F., Reese, G.M., et al.: Lancet *2*:339-342, 1978.
79. Deacon, R., Lumb, M., Perry, J., et al.: Lancet *2*:1023-1024, 1978.
80. Agamolis, D., Chester, M., Victor, M., et al.: Neurology *26*:905-914, 1976.
81. Kondo, H., Osborn, M.L., Kolhouse, J.F., et al.: J. Clin. Invest. *67*:1270-1283, 1981.
82. Biehl, J.P., Vilter, R.W.: Proc. Soc. Exp. Biol. Med. *85*:389-395, 1954.
83. Bender, D.A., Russell-Jones, R.: Lancet *2*:1125-1126, 1979.
84. O'Reilly, R.A.: Pharmacology *7*:149, 1972.
85. Koch-Weser, J., Sellers, E.M.: N. Engl. J. Med. *285*:487-498, 1971.
86. Bang, U., Tessler, S.S., et al.: Rev. Infect. Dis., Suppl. 4. S546-S554, 1982.
87. Bruch, K.: Lancet *1*:535-536, 1983.
88. Legha, S.S., Wang, Y-M., MacKay, B., et al.: Ann. N.Y. Acad. Sci. *393*:411-418, 1982.
89. Roe, D.A. Alcohol and the Diet. Westport, CT., AVI Publishing Co., 1979, pp. 119-130.
90. Victor, M., Adams, R.D., Collins, G.H.: The Wernicke-Korsakoff Syndrome. A Clinical and Pathological Study of 245 Patients, 82 with Post Mortem Examination. Philadelphia, F.A. Davis Co., 1971.
91. Kwee, I.L., Nakada, T.: N. Engl. J. Med. *309*:599-600, 1983.
92. Krauer, B., Krauer, F.: Clin. Pharmacokinet. *2*:157-181, 1977.
93. Knight, E., Roe, D.A.: Teratology *18*:17-22, 1978.
94. Landauer, W.: J. Exp. Zool. *120*:469, 1952.
95. Bartorelli, C., Gargano, N., Leonnetti, G., et al.: Circulation *27*:895-903, 1963.
96. Gronert, G.A.: J.A.M.A. *211*:300, 1970 (letter).
97. Mestman, J.H., Pocock, D.S., Kirchner, A.: Calif. Med. *111*:181-185, 1969.
98. Herman, E., Rado, J.P.: Arch. Neurol. *15*:74-77, 1966.
99. Dorph, S., Olgaard, A.: Nord. Med. *79*:516-518, 1968.
100. Pederson, E.B., Kornerup, H.G.: Acta Med. Scand. *200*:263-267, 1976.
101. Pederson, O.L., Mikkelsen, E.: Clin. Pharmacol. Ther. *26*:339-343, 1979.
102. Duarte, C.G., Winnaker, J.L., Becker, K.L., et al.: N. Engl. J. Med. *284*:828-830, 1971.
103. Wasnich, R.D., Benfante, R.J., Yano, K., et al.: N. Engl. J. Med. *309*:344-347, 1983.
104. Milne, M.D.: *In* Clinical Effects of Interaction Between Drugs. (Cluff, L.E., Petrie, J.C., Eds.) New York, Elsevier Publishing Inc., 1974, p. 193.
105. Stewart, V.L., Herling, P., Dalinka, M.K.: J.A.M.A *250*:78-81, 1983.
106. Randall, R.E. Jr., Strauss, M.B., McNeeley, W.: Arch. Intern. Med. *107*:163-181, 1961.
107. Spencer, H., Lewin, I.: J. Chronic Dis. *16*:713-726, 1963.
107a. Editorial: Ann. Intern. Med. *103*:946-947, 1985.
107b. Orwoll, E.S.: Ann. Intern. Med. *97*:242-248, 1982.
108. Wacker, W.E.C., Parisi, F.: N. Engl. J. Med. *278*:658-663, 712-717, 771-776, 1968.
109. Nielson, J.: Acta Psychiatr. Scand. *40*:190-196, 1964.
110. Crooks, J. Stevenson, I.H.: Age Ageing *10*:73-80, 1981.
111. Uragoda, C.G.: Am. Rev. Resp. Dis. *121*:157-159, 1980.
112. Pike, D.A., Leslie, R.D.G.: Br. Med. J. *2*:1521-1522, 1978.
113. Strakosch, C.R., Jefferys, D.B., Keen, H.: Lancet *2*:394-396, 1980.
114. Barnett, A.H., Spiliopoulos, A.J., Pike, D.A.: Lancet *2*:164-166, 1980.
115. Blomley, B.J.: Lancet *2*:1181-1182, 1964.
116. Blackwell, B., Mabbit, L.A.: Lancet *1*:938-940, 1965.
117. Marley, E., Blackwell, B.: Adv. Pharmacol. Chemotherap. *8*:185-239, 1970.
118. Kent-Smith, C., Durack, D.T.: Ann. Intern. Med. *88*:520-521, 1978.
119. Spivack, S.D.: Ann. Intern. Med. *81*:795-800, 1974.
120. Seixas, F.A.: Ann. Intern. Med. *83*:86-92, 1975.
121. Penick, S.B., Carrier, R.N., Sheldon, J.B.: Am. J. Psychiat. *125*:1063-1066, 1969.
122. Bruck, R.W.: N. Engl. J. Med. *265*:681-686, 1961.
123. Reynolds, W.A., Lowe, S.H.: N. Eng. J. Med. *272*:630-631, 1965.
124. O'Keefe, S.J.D., Marx, V.: Lancet *1*:1286-1287, 1977.

# Part III
*Adequacy and Safety of the Food Supply*

*Chapter* **35**

# CRITERIA OF AN ADEQUATE DIET

George H. Beaton

Perhaps the earliest dietary standard was that prepared by Carl von Voit in 1881 although an earlier statement, expressed only in terms of carbon and nitrogen, had been prepared in England in 1862.[1] In the more than 100 years since those beginnings, much experimental and epidemiologic work has served to refine our knowledge of human nutrition requirements. Nevertheless, some would argue that we are only slightly further ahead in the art and science of interpreting requirement estimates and assessing the nutritional adequacy of observed intake. Certainly there is much confusion and controversy about what published requirement estimates really mean and how they should be used.

Much of this confusion stems from our failure to emphasize constructs for interpretation and application. In the last decade, major developments in this direction would suggest that we are in a much better position than we have thought.

This chapter will emphasize a set of concepts and constructs that underlies nutritional requirements and the application of these in approaches to assessing observed intake. The chapter first develops the constructs, providing illustrations in relation to individuals and to population intake distributions. It then addresses some of the limi-

tations that must be borne in mind in applying the constructs. The chapter draws heavily on three committee reports[2-4] that have explicitly addressed relevant aspects of the concepts and constructs. The reader is referred to those reports for further detail. Finally, brief comment is offered on a conceptual issue that has arisen recently: What do we mean by "recommended intake"?

Nutrient requirement information may be used in either a prescriptive (advising or counseling) mode or in a diagnostic (assessment) mode. Considerations relating to the former have dominated the adopted conventions for describing nutrient requirements. In the counseling mode it is appropriate to suggest, "To be safe his diet should provide . . ." That is, we would *recommend* a level of intake that we believe is sufficient for the individual, and for almost all similar individuals. If one examines the FAO/WHO/UNU report,[3] the Canadian report,[2] or United States RDA reports,[5,6] it is apparent that the published numbers represent attempts to define a level that is deemed adequate or safe for an individual of the specified type, and hence can be recommended for such an individual.

There are two critically important elements in this recognition. First is the realization that requirement estimates relate more closely to individuals than to populations.[3] This fact is in almost direct contradiction to the apparent meaning of statements found in the introductory passages of most previous nutrient requirement reports, including those from the United Nations[7] and Canada.[8] The basis of this change is simply the recognition that we derive requirement estimates by examining individuals; they must relate to individuals. Second is the realization that requirements vary among similar individuals, and hence that the application of requirement estimates to particular individuals must be made on a probability basis if it is to have meaning.[2-4] The "recommended intake" is one that has a low probability of being inadequate for a randomly selected individual. Of necessity, the "recommended intake" exceeds the actual requirements of almost all individuals in the specified class.[9] It follows that failure to ingest the "recommended intake" does not mean that the intake is inadequate to meet the individual's own requirement. Thus, assessment of observed intake must be based on an explicit recognition of the underlying variability of actual requirement among similar individuals. Probability theory can provide a reasonable approach to such assessment.

## VARIABILITY OF REQUIREMENT: EMERGENCE OF THE PROBABILITY APPROACH*

### Evolution of Concepts

All studies of human nutrient requirements that have ever been undertaken yield one common finding. Even after adjustment has been made for all of the customarily measurable variables (age, sex, physiologic state, activity profile, nature of the diet consumed), a variability of measured requirement among individuals remains. This finding should not be surprising. It is characteristic of the parameters of all biologic systems. To the experimental scientist it is a nuisance; he must increase group sizes to obtain a reliable mean for intergroup comparisons. The rule of thumb that has evolved on empiric evidence is that for many, if not most, biologic systems this variability has a coefficient of variation of about 15%. Early nutrition reports also tended to treat this variability

as a nuisance, a suggestion that we did not really know requirement and must add a "margin of safety."[10] Variability of requirement was recognized; however, the constructs of requirement and requirement description were inadequate to deal with it effectively. The search was for a single number that would describe "requirement." A 1948 Canadian report set forth the beginnings of a refinement of description of requirement.[11] Both an average need and a variability of need were recognized. However, the report went on to discuss requirements as a "nutritional floor," which led to further confusion. By the 1960s it was accepted that variability was a characteristic of nutrient requirements and that the appropriate approach to dealing with the individual was to recommend an intake that would be "sufficient . . . for the nutritional needs of practically all healthy persons in a population," even though it must be recognized that these intake levels "must of necessity be in excess of the (actual) requirements of most of them."[9]

During this period, many population nutrition studies involving dietary, biochemical, and clinical assessments were undertaken. An almost universal finding was that the dietary assessments were in major disagreement with the biochemical and clinical assessments. Failure to ingest nutrients at levels approximating the "recommended intake" did not associate with biochemical evidence of depletion or deficiency. This finding should not have been surprising but it was. Largely on this basis, published dietary requirement estimates fell into disrepute. In point of fact, the fault was not necessarily with the requirement estimates but with our failure to interpret them correctly. We had failed to deal in a meaningful way with the issue of variability of requirement. The door was open for recognition of a new approach, a probability approach to interpretation of nutrient requirements[12,13] and its application to individual and population assessment.[4]

Figure 35–1 illustrates the distribution of requirements for a nutrient among apparently similar individuals (i.e., persons of the same age, sex, body weight). Also portrayed is the most common convention for the selection of the "recommended intake."* Although it is customary to publish that

---

*Many of the calculations of risk assessment and nutrient energy ratios presented in this chapter have been made with an unpublished computer program prepared for the Apple IIe computer by the author. The program also illustrates and applies additional concepts relating to adjustment of variance of requirements and other aspects that are beyond the scope of this chapter. Readers interested in additional information on program and costs should contact the author.

---

*The terms "recommended intake,"[7] "recommended dietary allowance,"[6] "recommended daily nutrient intake,"[8] "recommended nutrient intake,"[2] and "safe level of intake"[3] have been used in various reports to describe that level of intake deemed adequate to meet the needs of all but a small proportion of individuals of the specified class. Where there have been estimates of the variability of requirement and it is assumed that the distribution is normal, almost all committees have set this level as the mean + 2 standard deviations. The terms are used interchangeably in this chapter.

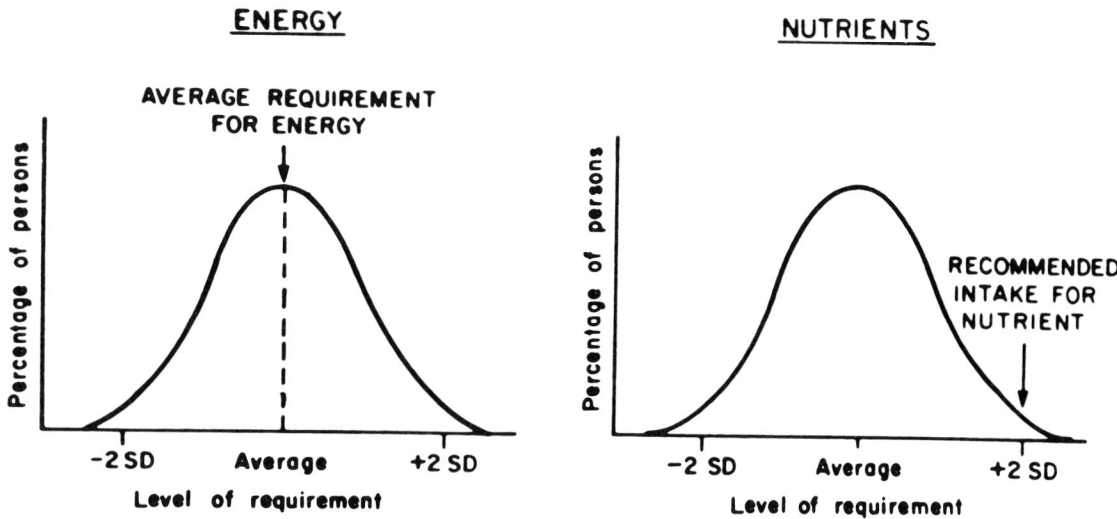

**Fig. 35–1.** The distribution of nutrient requirements among individuals of a homogeneous age and sex group. Portrayed are the conventions used in describing the distributions. For energy the *average* requirement is usually tabulated. For nutrients a *recommended* or *safe* level of intake, generally set at about the average + 2 standard deviations, is published. (From Recommended Nutrient Intakes for Canadians,[2] with permission of the Department of National Health and Welfare.)

single number in table form in dietary standards, in effect the recommended intake is a single point descriptor of an underlying distribution.[3] We tend to forget about the distribution and to focus on the single point.

For example, it has been generally assumed that protein requirement/kg body weight is normally distributed and has a coefficient of variation (CV) of about 15%.[2,5,6] The recent FAO/WHO/UNU committee critically examined the data from human balance studies and concluded (1) that there was no evidence to suggest that requirements are not distributed normally (the data set is not sufficiently large to *prove* that the distribution is gaussian) and (2) that after taking into account experimental error in the primary studies, the coefficient of variation in adult protein requirement/kg is about 12.5%, a little lower than the usual assumption.[3] (The argument of Sukhatme and Margen[14] that this included a major component of within person variation was not accepted.) Certainly, for protein, it is realistic to accept Figure 35–1 as portraying the distribution of requirements within a homogeneous group of individuals. Present evidence suggests that this distribution reflects traits of the individuals, persisting over time, no matter how these traits originally were conditioned.[3] Following existing convention, the recommended intake for protein has been set at the average need + 2 standard deviations (either 130% or 125% of the estimated average requirement). At this level of intake, the

needs of all but 2.3% of normal individuals would be met. It is a safe recommendation.

## Probability Approach Applied to Nutrients

If we now ask whether a particular level of observed intake is adequate for a randomly selected man, we can conclude that if the intake is equal to the recommended intake, only 2.3 men in 100 would have a higher requirement; there are 97.7 chances in 100 that it will be adequate for our randomly selected subject. We do not know his actual requirement, we only know the distribution in which his requirement fits (see Fig. 35–1). However, one *can* describe the probability that any particular level of intake would or would not meet his actual requirement. This can be done by simply looking at the areas of the requirement distribution to the left and right of the selected intake level (97.7% and 2.3% in the example). In this manner one can build a probability curve that describes the likelihood that an observed intake is not adequate to meet the *actual* requirement of a randomly selected individual. This curve depicts the "risk" of inadequacy for the individual (Fig. 35–2). With this curve we can assess any observed intake. A purely qualitative assessment is that the further the intake falls below the recommended intake, the greater is the chance that it is inadequate. However, if the requirement distribution is known or can be estimated with reasonable confidence, we can offer a quantitative probability statement.

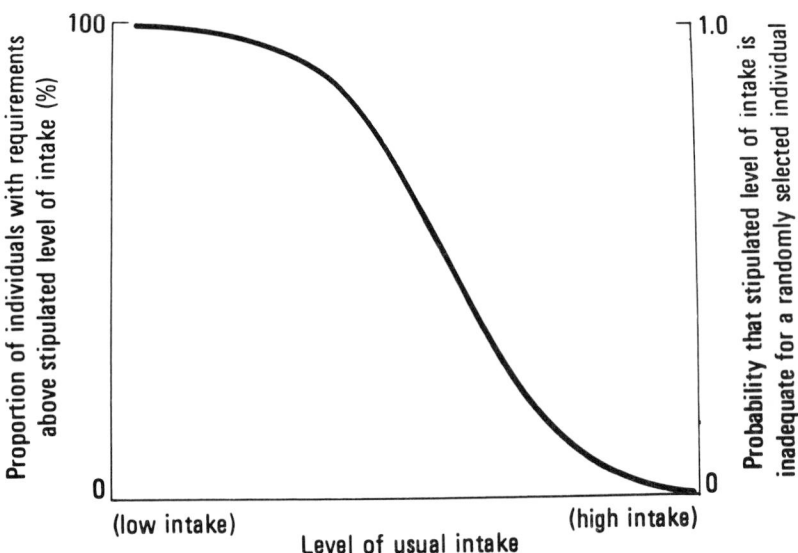

**Fig. 35–2.** The risk or probability that observed intake is inadequate for a randomly selected member of a specified age and sex group. The probability of inadequacy may be described as the risk that the intake is inadequate to meet the individual's actual requirement, or as the proportion of similar individuals who can be expected to have a requirement above the observed intake. (From FAO/WHO/UNU,[3] with permission.)

This statement is illustrated in Table 35–1. For each interval of intake, the associated probability of inadequacy has been computed using the type of relationship that is portrayed in Figure 35–2 and the Canadian protein requirement estimates.[2] Anderson et al.[15] applied this approach for one-week food intake records from a sample of Canadian children and adolescents using the requirement estimates of the 1975 Canadian Dietary Standard.[8] They made three assumptions: (1) that requirements, except for iron in menstruating women were normally distributed within classes of individuals, (2) that the coefficient of variation was 15% for all distributions, and (3) that the recommended intake had been set at the average + 2 standard deviations (130% of the average requirement for the specified class of individual). With these assumptions they constructed tables describing the probability of inadequacy associated with intervals of intake. It was then only a matter

of adding the probabilities, multiplied by the number of individuals with that interval of intake, to obtain an estimate of the expected *prevalence* of inadequate intakes in the population studied. Table 35–2 presents intake assessments conducted by probability analyses and contrasts these with a comparison of group mean intake to the recommended intake. A counting of individuals having intakes below the recommended intake is also included. These last two approaches (columns 1 and 2 of the table) are frequently presented in the literature. Given the foregoing discussion, it should be readily apparent which of the approaches is conceptually correct.

When an analogous approach was applied to intakes reported for young adult men in the USDA Nationwide Food Consumption Survey of 1977 to 1978, the results presented in Table 35–3 were obtained.[4] In actual practice, using computers, the probability of inadequacy can be computed for

**Table 35–1.** Computed Risk of Inadequacy Associated with Observed Protein Intakes*
(Adult Male, Age 25, Weight 70 kg, Intakes in g/d)

| *Observed Protein Intake* | *Associated Risk of Inadequacy (%)* | *Observed Protein Intake* | *Associated Risk of Inadequacy (%)* |
|---|---|---|---|
| 25 | 100 | 50 | 19 |
| 30 | 98 | 55 | 5 |
| 35 | 92 | 60 | 1 |
| 40 | 73 | 65 | 0 |
| 45 | 45 | | |

*Computations based on requirement description in Recommended Nutrient Intakes for Canadians.[2] The Recommended Nutrient Intake for this class of individual would be 57 g/day.

**Table 35–2.** **Comparison of Approaches to Dietary Assessment of Inadequacy***
(16–18 Years of Age, One-Week Dietary Records)

| Nutrient | Sex | Group Mean Intake as % of RDNI | Proportion of Individuals with Intakes Below RDNI (%) | Probability Prevalence Estimate† (%) |
|----------|-----|-------------------------------|------------------------------------------------------|--------------------------------------|
| Protein | M | 207 | 2 | 2 |
|         | F | 174 | 13 | 2 |
| Vitamin C | M | 597 | 2 | 0 |
|           | F | 437 | 5 | 3 |
| Thiamin | M | 137 | 31 | 14 |
|         | F | 118 | 44 | 24 |
| Riboflavin | M | 195 | 9 | 4 |
|            | F | 169 | 24 | 8 |
| Calcium | M | 150 | 24 | 11 |
|         | F | 147 | 34 | 21 |

n = 45 males, 38 females

*Requirement estimates used were those of the Dietary Standard for Canada, 1975.[8] RDNI = Recommended Daily Nutrient Intake. Based on Anderson, G.H., et al.[15]
†See text for description of this approach.

each intake rather than for an average probability across intervals of intake.[4]

Some nutrients do not exhibit normal distributions of requirements. Iron in menstruating women is a clear example. Hallberg and colleagues[16] and Cole et al.,[17,17a] working with total communities in Scandinavia and in Scotland, provided independent estimates of the distribution of blood losses of normal menstruating women. These distributions were similar. Beaton[18] combined the two data sets after blood losses had been converted to iron losses, using a normative value for hemoglobin concentration and thus disregard-

ing the anemia associated with high losses.[16,19] A lognormal distribution reasonably fitted the data set. The documentation is strong that while these losses show a high variation among women, there is high consistency from one menstrual period to the next within the same woman.[16,17,17a,19] The lognormal distribution then described the major source of variation in iron requirements of menstruating women. Provision was then made for the endogenous losses by the dermal, urinary, and fecal routes. If one uses the dietary iron absorption estimates of Recommended Nutrient Intakes for Canadians,[2] this lognormal distribution with

**Table 35–3.** **Apparent Prevalence of Inadequate Protein Intakes Among Young Adult Men in the United States***

| Intake Interval g/d | Proportion of Total Population with Observed Intake Falling in Interval* (%) | Probability of Inadequacy† | Estimated Proportion of Total Population with Inadequate Intake (%) |
|---------------------|------------------------------------------------------------------------------|----------------------------|---------------------------------------------------------------------|
| <24 | 0.4 | 1.0 | 0.4 |
| 24–28 | 0.1 | 0.995 | 0.1 |
| 28–32 | 0.2 | 0.97 | 0.19 |
| 32–36 | 0.2 | 0.90 | 0.18 |
| 36–40 | 0.5 | 0.74 | 0.37 |
| 40–44 | 0.9 | 0.50 | 0.45 |
| 44–48 | 1.1 | 0.26 | 0.29 |
| 48–52 | 1.3 | 0.10 | 0.13 |
| 52–56 | 1.8 | 0.03 | 0.05 |
| 56–60 | 3.5 | 0.005 | 0.02 |
| >60 | 91.0 | 0 | 0.0 |
| Estimated Prevalence of Inadequate Intakes (Sum) | | 2.2 | |

*Intakes from 1977–1978 Nationwide Food Consumption Survey. Intake distribution has been adjusted to remove effect of day-to-day variation.
†Based on United States Recommended Dietary Allowances.[6] Average protein requirement = 43 g/d; coefficient of variation = 15%. Probabilities are derived from a table of areas under the normal distribution (Table of Z values). The probability of inadequacy is the proportional area to the right of Z where Z = deviation from average/standard deviation.

Modified from Nutrient Adequacy: Assessment Using Food Consumption Surveys.[4]

added basal losses can be used to describe the risk curve for iron in menstruating women. The curve is portrayed in Figure 35–3.

The level part to the left marks the basal iron losses (dermal, fecal, and urinary) common to all women while the curve represents the variable iron loss associated with menstruation. Using slightly different requirement estimates[20] and a somewhat different estimate of the distribution of menstrual losses than portrayed in Figure 35–3, Beaton demonstrated that for a Canadian population of women, although about 75% had intakes below the recommended level, the apparent prevalence of inadequate intakes was only 12.5%.[12] Later he examined this finding in relation to hematologic data from the Ten State Nutrition Survey, using a probability approach to interpret the hematology, and showed general consistency in the two assessments of inadequacy[18] giving credibility to both the approach to interpreting requirement estimates and the approach to deriving the requirement estimates themselves. This is in direct contrast to the frequently heard allegation that estimates of iron requirements for women in the United States,[6] in Canada,[2] and international countries[20] are much too high. That impression derives from a notion that all individuals must ingest the recommended intake if they are to avoid deficiency–a clear misconception and misinterpretation.

When the curve portrayed in Figure 35–3 was applied to the observed iron intakes of young adult women reported in the 1977 to 1978 USDA Nationwide Food Consumption Survey (after the distribution was adjusted as described in section 5), the estimated prevalence of inadequate intakes was 23%.[4] This estimate can be compared to 95 + % of the intakes falling below the US RDA of 18 mg/d.[6] By the curve portrayed in Figure 35–3, the RDA would be associated with a probability of inadequacy of about 0.02. The apparent higher estimate of inadequate intakes in the USDA data than in the Canadian study reported previously[12] may have occurred because the USDA data did not include iron ingested as pharmaceutical supplements. It is also due to small differences in the requirement distributions assumed in the two analyses.

Conceptually, then, the "probability approach" is simply a statistical approach that takes into account the variability of nutrient requirement among seemingly similar individuals. Rather than developing fixed cut-off points to mark adequacy and inadequacy, researchers adopt a continuous variable function. In theory this approach can be applied to individuals or to collections of individuals in a population sample. In practice, as will be discussed later, there are important limitations in applying the approach to an individual. To a major degree, these limitations can be overcome in population studies.

An important advantage of the probability ap-

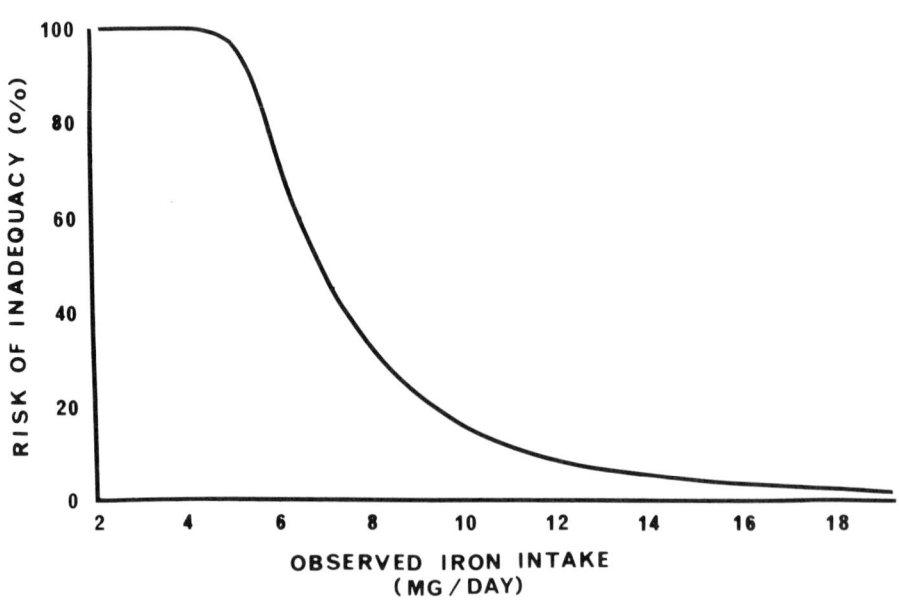

**Fig. 35–3.** Risk of inadequacy of iron intake in menstruating women. Requirements are based on Recommended Nutrient Intakes for Canadians.[2] The criterion of adequacy in setting iron requirement was the maintenance of iron stores; an upper limit of 19% for dietary iron absorption was accepted. (From Nutrient Adequacy: Assessment Using Food Consumption Surveys,[4] with permission of National Academy Press.)

proach is that it gives an estimate of prevalence of inadequate intakes that can be compared to estimates of the prevalence of depletion or deficiency assessed by biochemical or clinical means. If these different estimates of reality differ appreciably, then there is reason to challenge the requirement estimates (or the biochemical marker). The approach opens the door to the application of epidemiologic principles in the derivation or validation of requirement estimates. Do the estimates make sense epidemiologically?[2] A limitation inherent in the concepts underlying the probability approach is the realization that we cannot categorize particular individuals as having "adequate" or "inadequate" intake, an approach that has characterized too many of the dietary studies in the past. Similarly, it is difficult, if not impossible, to describe the proportion of subjects with multiple dietary inadequacies.[4] This approach to assessment has been attractive.[21]

## Energy: The Notable Exception

In Figure 35–1 the conventions used in selecting the single point descriptors of requirement distributions were portrayed. The difference between energy and the nutrients is clear. In the case of energy, the almost universal convention is to describe the *average* requirement with the implicit, if not explicit, recognition that individuals vary around this average. In the last revision of the United States Recommended Dietary Allowances, energy requirements were described in terms of both averages and ranges.[6] This format gave explicit recognition to the variability of requirement, although the ranges may not have portrayed the full extent of variability.

One cannot deal with energy requirements in the same way as has been described for the nutrients. Why is energy different?

A full and explicit discussion of the issues surrounding the definition and description of energy requirements may be found in the recently revised FAO/WHO/UNU report.[3] For the purpose of the present discussion, the key element in considering energy is the recognition that if external factors do not interfere, the human organism has the ability to adjust intake to match expenditure or to adjust expenditure to match intake over considerable ranges.[22] There may be functional consequences of these adjustments[23,24] that lead to a decision to incorporate normative judgments about desirable body weight or desirable profiles of physical activity into descriptions of energy requirements.[3] Nevertheless, the fact remains that among free-living subjects with unconstrained access to food and with unconstrained activity, one can expect that intake and expenditure will be

adjusted such that energy balance is approximated. This is done without conscious thought unless the individual is trying to change the status quo. Over moderate periods of time (but not day to day), there is a strong correlation between energy intake and energy expenditure (energy requirement) among individuals.

There is no evidence that, in the human, such regulatory adjustments are made for nutrients, i.e., that individuals select nutrient intakes to match their individual needs. Within age-sex groups, it is reasonable to assume that the correlation between intake and requirement is very low for the nutrients as long as common variables (such as body size, which can affect both intake and requirement) are eliminated.

The probability approach described herein depends on the assumption that the correlation between intake and requirement, within homogeneous groups of individuals, is very low or 0. Although it is possible to apply the approach to nutrients, it is not possible to apply it to energy unless a direct estimate of the correlation between intake and requirement is available.[3] In this circumstance, adequacy of energy intake must be judged not from assessment of dietary intake but rather from assessment of suitability of body size, body composition, growth rate in children, and both occupational and nonoccupational activities.[2,3,6,23,24]

It is unfortunate that the distinction between energy requirements and nutrient requirements, and its implication in interpretation and application, has not been widely understood. It is to be hoped that appreciation of the difference will gradually increase and that differentiated approaches to interpretation will progressively improve.

## PROBABILITY OF INADEQUACY VS. CONSIDERATION OF SEVERITY

The foregoing discussion has presented a statistical approach to the description of the likelihood that an observed intake is inadequate. The logical question that follows is "inadequate for what?" To address this question, one must consider the criteria of adequacy and nutritional health that underlaid the original requirement estimate. For example, one might consider the requirement for ascorbic acid that would prevent clinical symptoms of scurvy or the requirement for thiamin that would prevent manifestations of beriberi. One might also consider the requirement for ascorbic acid to maintain a predetermined metabolic pool size or turnover rate or the requirement for thiamin to maintain tissue levels or enzyme activities. Both sets of criteria are legitimate.

Both give rise to definable requirement distributions. With each of these distributions, probability statements and prevalence estimates could be generated. The statistical considerations are identical. However, the interpretation has changed. We are considering different "for what's" in describing the likelihood or prevalence of inadequacy.

The distinction is illustrated dramatically in Table 35–4, which is drawn from the National Academy of Sciences report on the assessment of nutritional adequacy.[4]

Earlier it was stated that one of the strong advantages of the probability approach applied to population groups is that it should yield a prevalence estimate that can be compared to prevalence of inadequacy estimated using biochemical or clinical indices. It facilitates an epidemiologic validation of requirement estimates. That is true, but only if the underlying criteria of dietary requirement, of biochemical adequacy, and of clinical health are identical. If the criteria differ, as they would in the portrayal presented in Table 35–4, then agreement between dietary, biochemical, and clinical assessments cannot be expected.

It follows also that when the adopted criteria change, the dietary requirement estimates must be expected to change. In Canada, for many years the recommended intake for ascorbic acid in the adult male was 30 mg/day.[8] This amount was based on white cell levels and other indices. In the last revision of the Canadian nutrient requirement estimates, the recommended intake for young adult males was set at 60 mg/day (average

requirement = 45 mg/day, CV = 15%). The committee changed the criterion of adequacy. This time requirement was based on metabolic turnover rates.[2] If one compares the Canadian and United States recommended intakes for the various nutrients, a number of differences are found. If one examines recommended intakes from around the world,[25] even more differences are found. Many of these differences are explicable in terms of different judgments about the appropriate criterion of adequacy as was the historical difference in ascorbic acid requirement estimates.

Two important points emerge. First, although the probability approach yields a mathematical estimate of "risk" for an individual or of prevalence of inadequate intake for a population group, the biological dimension, "risk of what" or "prevalence of what," must be addressed by examining the basis of the original requirement estimate. This may differ between reports. One should not be dismayed by the multiplicity of requirement estimates and hence multiplicity of prevalence estimates that can be generated. However, one must consider the multitude of possible conceptual definitions of nutritional adequacy, the dimension of "severity." The authors of requirement reports have an undeniable responsibility to be explicit in defining the criterion of adequate nutriture that was applied in deriving the requirement estimate.

The second point that emerges is that one should envisage a family of risk curves based on distributions of requirements for different criteria of adequacy. This might be exemplified most easily for iron. As body iron stores are depleted and as anemia develops, the efficiency of absorption of dietary iron increases. The risk curve portrayed in Figure 35–3 was based upon the maintenance of iron stores and assumed that iron can be absorbed by the person with need (intake close to actual requirement) at an efficiency of up to about 18 to 19%.[2,4] If instead we wished to describe the distribution of iron requirements among women who had no, or very small, iron stores and who exhibited mild anemia, we would have to accept that the efficiency of iron absorption from the same diet would increase. The distribution of iron losses would not be expected to change appreciably. The shape of the curve would be similar to that portrayed in Figure 35–3, but the curve would be shifted to the left. A hypothetical family of such curves is portrayed in Figure 35–4. These are all probability or risk curves for the same nutrient, but the "risk of what?" question takes on different answers. The family of curves represents the dimension of *severity* while any one curve portrays the dimension of *probability*. In judging observed intakes one finds that these two dimensions are

**Table 35–4. Estimated Prevalence of Inadequate Intake Employing Different Criteria of Nutritional Adequacy (Young Adult Males)***

| Criterion of Adequacy Adopted in Defining Nutrient Requirement | Estimated Prevalence of Inadequate Intakes | |
|---|---|---|
| | Ascorbic Acid (%) | Thiamin† (%) |
| Avoidance of clinically detectable signs of deficiency | 0.7 | 0 |
| Maintenance of normative tissue levels of metabolic pools | 39.6 | 3.4 |

*Intake data drawn from the 1977–1978 Nationwide Food Consumption Survey. Observed distribution adjusted as described in section on Practical Considerations.

†Thiamin intake and requirement both expressed as mg/1,000 kcal/d. No lower limit was placed on an adequate thiamin intake (such a limit is imposed in the Recommended Dietary Allowances).[6]

Modified from Nutrient Adequacy: Assessment Using Food Consumption Surveys.[4]

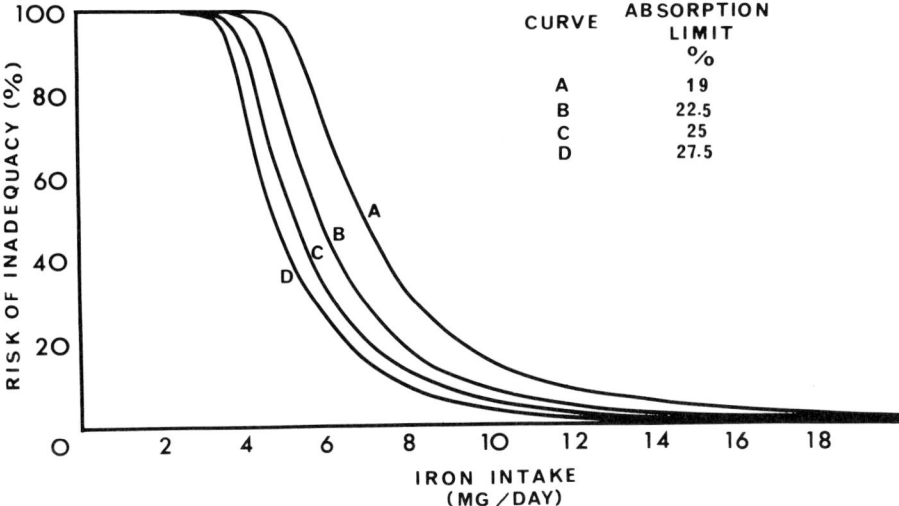

**Fig. 35–4.** Family of curves portraying the risk of inadequate iron intake in menstruating women. The curves assume different upper limits for iron absorption and thus conceptually reflect different physiologic criteria of adequacy in setting requirements. These criteria might range from maintenance of iron stores (curve A) to maintenance of a moderately anemic state (curve D). (From Beaton, G.H.,[24] with permission of John Libbey.)

not always differentiated, giving rise to apparent contradiction in interpretation. A particular observed intake may be associated with a *high* risk of failure to maintain iron stores and at the same time a comparatively *low* risk of being associated with anemia.

With recognition of these two dimensions in mind, it is to be hoped, and expected, that future reports on nutrient requirement will present multiple requirement estimates relating to different levels of nutriture, and that multitiered assessments will be made in the study of populations and population groups.[4] Such multilevel assessments, as portrayed in Table 35–4, offer a more meaningful portrayal of the situation of the population than does an assessment in relation to either criterion of adequate intake by itself.

## SOME RELATED CONCEPTS

A major theme of this chapter is the application of concepts of statistical probability to biological systems and biological variability. These considerations are relevant to two other issues in the field of nutrition. One issue is the recognition that parallel concepts *should* apply to the consideration of "toxicity," which must exhibit variability. The other issue is the recognition that in dealing with adequate (or excessive) concentrations of nutrients, we must address the variability of energy needs (a major source of variation in total food intake) as well as the variability of nutritional requirements. These two extensions are discussed below.

### Safe Range of Intake

Until recently, attention in the field of nutrient requirements has been focused on the amounts required to prevent depletion or deficiency. In the field of trace elements, there has been a long-standing awareness of the detrimental effects of high, as well as low, intakes, and attempts have been made to define ranges within which intake is neither too high nor too low.[6,26] Implicitly we have recognized the possible detrimental effects of high intakes of other nutrients, but this subject has not been systematized or incoporated into requirement reports. In their current revisions, both the Canadian[2] and FAO/WHO/UNU[3] requirement reports emphasize this concept and issue a plea for an evolution of thinking.

The risk curve relating to inadequate intakes of nutrients was portrayed in Figure 35–2. Conceptually, there is an analogous risk curve relating to excessive intakes and "toxic" effects. The duality of risk curves was operationalized in the consideration of suitable levels of water fluoridation.[27] Here one curve dealt with the relationship between "inadequate" concentrations and dental caries. The other curve was concerned with the relationship between "excessive" concentrations and dental mottling. The selected range (for temperate climates) of 0.5 to 1.5 ppm represented the "intake" range that was associated with low prevalence of both "deficiency" and "excess" in populations. It was a "safe range."

Figure 35–5 presents the same concept as it might be applied to nutrient intakes. The range

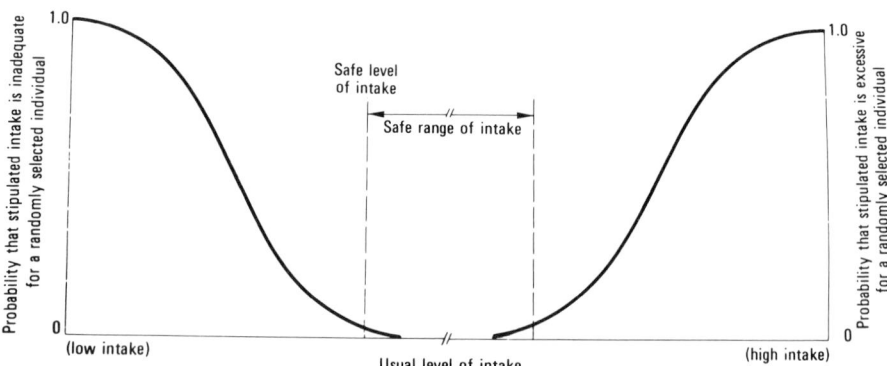

**Fig. 35–5.** The safe range of intakes. Through this range of intakes the homeostatic mechanisms of the body appear to utilize the nutrient effectively without recognized physiologic advantage associated with any particular level. At the ends of the range, the probability of inadequacy (low intakes) or of excess (high intakes) increases. Based on Recommended Nutrient for Canadians.[2]

through which the risk of inadequacy and the risk of excess are both low represents a "safe range of intake." In physiologic terms, it may be seen also as the range of effective operation of the homeostatic mechanisms of normal humans. Across this range there is neither physiologic advantage nor disadvantage to particular levels of intake; there is no "optimum intake."[2,3] (See later discussion of other effects of nutrients not encompassed within the usual conceptualization of nutritional requirements.) Nutrient requirements, as we think of them now, relate to the lower limit of this range of safe or appropriate intakes.

The portrayal and underlying concept emphasize a fundamental point: in spite of the name, we do not recommend that people consume the *recommended* intake! Specifically, for example, the United States Recommended Dietary Allowances do not advocate that protein intake be *lowered* to the recommended intake level. What we do mean is that people should consume levels *at or above* the "recommended" intake–intakes that would fall within the safe range of intakes in Figure 35–5. This is probably the correct interpretation of the early Canadian Dietary Standard,[11] which described the requirement estimates as being "nutritional floors beneath which maintenance of health in people cannot be assumed."

The portrayal has another significance. We are now moving into a situation in which legitimate concern about an "adequate diet" focuses upon the upper rather than lower limit. One example is the current situation in North America with reference to fat and fatty acids. There are concerns about inadequacies of intake and about essential fatty acid deficiencies. By and large, these concerns are restricted to clinical situations where fat and fatty acid intake may have been artificially

constrained (as in intravenous alimentation before suitable and approved fat emulsions became available), where essentially fat-free formulas were used for infant feeding, or where extreme restriction of dietary fat intake was advocated for clinical reasons. These issues warrant attention and action, but they are small issues in comparison to the questions that now surround the need to define upper limits to fat and fatty acid intake. In the case of dietary fat, serum lipid, and cardiovascular disease, one is concerned with the definition of the upper limit of the safe range of intakes. Here is a clear example of the importance of considering the concepts embodied in Figure 35–5. Ultimately the goal must be to describe the "safe range of intake" itself. Statements on this subject are found in current dietary standards in Canada,[2] in the United States,[6] and at the international level[28] but, with the possible exception of the last, the statements do not provide definite "requirement" estimates for both ends of the range.

It is hoped that research attention will be directed to the effects of high intakes of nutrients, not just fat and associated materials, and that it will be possible in the future to apply a probability approach to excess intakes, as now can be done for inadequate intakes, and to evaluate observed intakes in terms of "safe ranges of intake."

## Assessment of Dietary Quality: Nutrient-Energy Ratios

Recent years have seen a renewed interest in using "nutrient density" as a criterion of the nutritional quality of diets.[29–31] Use of nutrient density has been strongly advocated in the Nordic countries and was described in detail, for iron, by Wretlind.[32] Standards for nutrients per 1,000 kcal have been developed for several of the countries,[33] and a set of Nordic Nutrition Recommendations, including nutrient density standards for diets, has been accepted.[34]

The concept is not new. Platt and colleagues gave it prominence when they argued for the use of Net Dietary Protein as % Calories (NDPCals%) as a dietary criterion of adequacy.[35] The underlying concept has been that a diet that has an adequate *concentration* of nutrients will satisfy nutrient requirement when the individual stops eating because of satiation of energy requirement. That idea is eminently logical.

The issue that arises is how to define the criterion of an appropriate nutrient:energy ratio. For a few nutrients, such as thiamin, riboflavin, and niacin, it has been accepted that energy intake is a major variable of requirement, and the practice has been to define their requirements as units per 1,000 kcal. This then provides a direct reference criterion for the nutrient:energy ratio. For most other nutrients it must be assumed that, except for a common relationship to lean body mass, requirements for the nutrient and for energy are not related. There is no a priori base for a nutrient/ 1,000 kcal requirement reference. Thus, for example, Beaton and Swiss made a specific search of extant data sets as well as published papers and concluded that the correlation between protein requirement and energy requirement, both expressed per unit body weight, could not be higher than about 0.2.[36] The two requirement distributions were essentially independent of one another (unlike the situation for thiamin).

This independence of the requirement distributions leads to the issue of the approach to defining a reference criterion for the examination of dietary nutrient energy ratios. The most frequent practice has been to calculate the ratio of numbers appearing in reports such as the United States Recommended Dietary Allowances. However, this method has a tenuous basis. To derive a reference protein:energy ratio in this way, one would be dividing the average protein requirement + 2 standard deviations (the RDA) by the average energy requirement. This approach is not logical even though it is convenient. It does not convey the meaning of either the RDA for protein (sufficient for almost all individuals) or the average requirement for energy (sufficient for half the individuals). It would be possible to compute many other ratios as portrayed schematically in Figure 35–6. In this figure, the distributions of energy and protein requirements of young adult men (Canadian requirement estimates[2]) are portrayed along the axes. In the body of the figure are presented some ratios that could be computed by se-

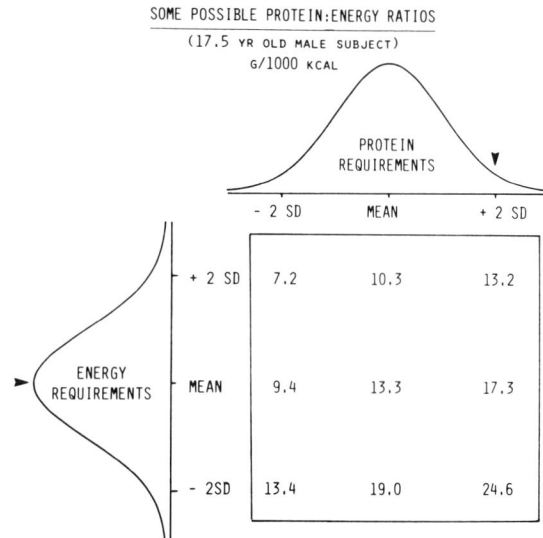

SOME POSSIBLE PROTEIN:ENERGY RATIOS

(17.5 YR OLD MALE SUBJECT)

G/1000 KCAL

PROTEIN REQUIREMENTS

|  |  | - 2 SD | MEAN | + 2 SD |
|---|---|---|---|---|
| | + 2 SD | 7.2 | 10.3 | 13.2 |
| ENERGY REQUIREMENTS | MEAN | 9.4 | 13.3 | 17.3 |
| | - 2SD | 13.4 | 19.0 | 24.6 |

BASED ON RECOMMENDED NUTRIENT INTAKES FOR CANADIANS, 1983.

**Fig. 35–6.** Calculation of protein:energy ratios. Distributions of both protein requirements and energy requirements are portrayed on the axes. The published average energy need and recommended protein intake are marked by arrows. Some examples of possible ratio calculations are shown, based on use of + 2 SD, the mean, and − 2 SD for each of the distributions. There is a distribution of possible ratios, each having a different probability of adequacy for the randomly selected individual of the specified age and sex class. This can be described as the bivariate distribution of energy and protein requirements. The values shown are based on Canadian requirement estimates.[2]

lecting various arbitrary points on the distributions. Consider, for example, an individual who had a low protein need and high energy need (in the upper left corner). His protein:energy need would be approximately 7.2 g/1,000 kcal (2.9% of energy as protein). With equal probability there could be another individual with high protein need and low energy (lower right corner). He would need to ingest a diet containing about 24.6 g/1,000 kcal (9.8% of energy as protein) to ensure that protein needs were met when energy needs were satiated. For the individual with average requirements for both energy and protein, the ratio would be 13.3 g/1,000 kcal (5.3% of energy as protein). The usual practice of dividing the recommended protein intake by the average energy requirement is portrayed as the middle value in the right-hand column: 17.3 g/1,000 kcal (6.9% of energy as protein).

Any of these values could be selected as a reference criterion. Which is the appropriate value? Certainly the likelihood that an individual lies at the extreme of both distributions (the situations portrayed in the four corners) is small. If mean requirements were used to compute the ratio, it would be inadequate for half the people and would be of doubtful merit as a criterion of adequacy.

Beaton and Swiss approached the issue by adopting a probability approach.[36] The presence of a bivariate distribution of possible protein:energy requirements was accepted. In a manner directly analogous to the probability approach discussed for univariate distributions of nutrient requirements, it is possible to assign to any selected ratio a risk or probability of inadequacy for the random individual. It is also possible to select the ratio that conveys a predetermined probability of inadequacy, i.e., a "safe" or "recommended" protein:energy ratio can be derived.[36] The mathematical approach was confirmed and reduced to a single, albeit complex, equation in the FAO/WHO/UNU report on energy and protein requirements.[3] The equation can be applied to other nutrients provided there is knowledge of, or reasonable assumption about, the primary requirement distributions. Table 35–5 presents illustrations of ratios derived by this approach, using the protein requirement estimates of Recommended Nutrient Intakes for Canadians[2] and the FAO/WHO/UNU[3] equation. Risk (probability) levels were set at values ranging from 0.025 to 0.9 (from the conventional level of a "recommended intake" to a level of almost certain inadequacy). The results, for 11 age groupings, are presented in Table 35–5. Within any age group, the "required" protein:energy ratio decreases as the risk level increases. The first column of the table approximates the risk level associated with the recommended intake of protein. Across age

groups, within any single risk category, the protein:energy ratio initially falls slightly and then climbs markedly. In contradiction to common notion, the table suggests that the elderly need a much higher protein concentration in their diet than the traditional "vulnerable group," the infant or young child.

There is, then, a probability theory basis for the derivation of criteria for the assessment of dietary quality by nutrient:energy ratios. The criteria can be derived for any level of "risk" that is desired, in theory.

Following the publication of protein:energy ratios by Beaton and Swiss,[36] Payne issued a strong and important criticism.[37] He pointed out that any of these approaches depended not only on the distribution of nutrient requirements but also, in the denominator, on the *position* of the distribution of energy requirements. As discussed previously, it is clear that individuals and populations can adjust energy intake and expenditure to maintain energy balance. A part of this adjustment is related to levels of physical activity. Inactive populations have lower energy needs, lower energy intakes, and consequently higher nutrient:energy ratio requirements. Thus, the nutrient:energy ratio "requirement" depends upon the activity level of the individuals in a population or group. This fact can be seen in part in Table 35–5 in which the nutrient:energy ratio for a given level of risk increases with age in adults even without a comparable rise in nutrient requirement per day; rather, the estimated energy requirement falls with increasing age. A similar phenomenon would be seen if one compared physically active

**Table 35–5.   Computed Protein:Energy Ratios for Different Levels of Risk of Inadequacy in Males***
**(Ratios are Expressed as g/1,000 kcal)**

| Age Group (yr) | Risk Level | | | | | |
|---|---|---|---|---|---|---|
| | *2.5%* | *10%* | *25%* | *50%* | *75%* | *90%* |
| 1 | 19 | 16 | 15 | 13 | 11 | 10 |
| 2–3 | 19 | 16 | 15 | 13 | 11 | 10 |
| 4–6 | 16 | 14 | 13 | 11 | 9.7 | 8.6 |
| 7–9 | 15 | 13 | 12 | 10 | 9.2 | 8.2 |
| 10–12 | 17 | 15 | 13 | 12 | 10 | 9.1 |
| 13–15 | 20 | 17 | 15 | 14 | 12 | 11 |
| 16–18 | 20 | 17 | 15 | 14 | 12 | 10 |
| 19–24 | 22 | 19 | 17 | 15 | 13 | 12 |
| 25–49 | 26 | 22 | 20 | 18 | 15 | 14 |
| 50–74 | 30 | 26 | 23 | 20 | 18 | 16 |
| 75 + | 32 | 28 | 25 | 22 | 19 | 17 |

*Requirement estimates based on Recommended Nutrient Intakes for Canadians, 1983.[2] Assumed correlation between protein and energy requirements is 0.2.[36] "Risk" is the probability that the protein requirement of a randomly selected individual will not have been met when sufficient food is eaten to satisfy his own energy requirement. Values have been computed from the bivariate distribution of protein and energy requirements using the equation published by FAO/WHO/UNU[3] and solving for the specified probabilities of inadequacy. Age groupings are those presented in the Canadian report.

and physically inactive subgroups in the population of, for example, young adult men.

The criticism by Payne[37] and the underlying issue that it displayed have serious implications for the use and interpretation of nutrient:energy ratios as criteria of adequate diets. To use them, one should ask for whom (what age/sex/weight group) they are adequate and for what activity level and plane of energy requirement. Conversely, if this aspect of the nutrient:energy ratio is understood, then consideration of the ratios may prove to be a useful adjunct in the epidemiology of nutritional problems, (e.g., to determine what sectors of the population are more likely to have inadequate intakes of nutrients if all consumed similar diets) or in operational terms (e.g., to determine for which segments of the population nutritional quality of the diet is likely to be particularly important).

## PRACTICAL CONSIDERATIONS: PRESENT CONSTRAINTS TO APPLICATION OF THE PROBABILITY APPROACH

The National Academy of Sciences report examined the application of the probability approach to population survey data.[4] In this report, the potential sources of error in the derived estimate of prevalence of inadequate intake were systematically examined both by statistical theory and by empirical sensitivity testing. Although the report focused upon population data, certain inferences can be drawn about application of the approach to individuals as well as to populations. These considerations can be divided into two broad groupings: those relating to the estimate of requirements and those relating to the estimate of intake. It will be apparent in the discussion that follows that although the approach can be applied with reasonable confidence to population data, there are serious limitations in applying it to particular individuals. In the latter instance, the concepts still hold and should underlie any approach to interpretation of observed intake, but the numeric derivations of risk may exhibit serious errors.

### Considerations Relating to Requirement Distribution

As was illustrated in Figures 35–2 and 35–3, the development of the probability approach depended on a knowledge of the distribution of requirements: the mean or median requirement and the characteristics of the distribution including its standard deviation. Without this knowledge, there is no way of assigning *precise* risk estimates to the observed intake of a particular individual; one could speak in relative terms but not with precision. Today we have such descriptions of requirement distributions for only a few nutrients and for only a few age-sex groups. In the examples presented in this chapter, major *assumptions* about the distributions have been made. The reader is left to judge whether or not these assumptions are reasonable. This, then, is a major limitation to application to the particular individual. Conversely, the National Academy of Sciences report demonstrated that use of intake distributions for populations resulted in prevalence estimates that were sensitive to the position of the mean requirement but relatively insensitive to either the variability of requirement or shape of the requirement distribution as long as the requirements were distributed relatively symmetrically about the mean.[4] The critical information needed, then, for most nutrients for population assessments is: (1) an estimate of average requirement, and (2) an assurance that requirements are equally distributed about the mean. Requirement reports[2,6] have not usually presented mean requirement estimates for nutrients; it has not been considered important in the past. Future reports may do so. The second important addition to future reports would be inclusion of requirement estimates associated with different defined states of nutriture. This change would then permit and encourage multitiered assessments of observed population intakes.[4] For population data, it is reasonable to suggest that the probability approach is feasible and that the requirement information needed is within our reach even if not now commonly presented.

One lesson that emerged from the National Academy of Sciences study was the importance of expressing requirements in terms of known variables. Specifically, thiamin requirement is commonly derived as mg/1,000 kcal because the energy flux is an important determinant of need. In dietary standards, it has been common practice to then convert this measurement to mg thiamin/day assuming some normative value for expected energy intake. The report[4] applied current United States requirement estimates[6] to the Nationwide Food Consumption Survey data. When both requirement and intake were expressed as mg/1,000 kcal, the apparent prevalence of inadequate intakes was 3.4% among young adult men. When both were expressed as mg/day, the prevalence estimate rose to 36.9%. The latter approach failed to take into account an important variable of requirement:energy intake. It also failed to recognize that this same variable would be expected to affect intake (the higher the energy need, the more food one ingests, and the higher is likely to be the thiamin intake). Thus a spurious correlation between intake of and requirement for thiamin was introduced and ignored in the analysis. The moral, of course, is to express both intake and requirement in relation to variables that are believed to influence both. (Another example would be body size where this is a known variable of requirement as for protein.)

## Considerations Relating to Estimation of Intakes

The obvious assumption of any assessment approach is that the intake has been correctly estimated. Any bias (under- or over-reporting) in the intake estimate will lead to a bias in the assessment. Chapter 47 addresses the methods for collecting food intake information. Methodology is not discussed here; rather, the present discussion focuses on more subtle issues.

In considering the approaches presented in this chapter, one must recognize that requirement estimates refer to intakes persisting over moderate periods of time. Although, by convention, they are expressed as *rates* of intake in units per day, none of the committees that establish the requirement estimates meant to infer that the intake on each day should be judged.[2,3] It follows, then, that the estimate of intake under examination must persist over moderate periods of time. Explicitly, when one-day intake data are used for this purpose, serious errors of interpretation can result. The intake on a single day is an inadequate descriptor of an individual's "usual" intake. Discussion of this point is beyond the scope of this chapter, but the reader will find an increasing volume of material on dietary methodology and on the impact day-to-day variation in intake on analyses of various types. One must select dietary methodology appropriate to the purpose at hand.[38]

To make a correct assessment of intake for an individual, one would have to sample his intake on a sufficient number of days to represent, with confidence, the persisting average intake across time. This is seldom feasible and, as a consequence, a built-in source of error is present in individual assessments.

Fortunately, the assessment of population data is less demanding of dietary methodology and has major implications for survey design.[39] Here it is possible to adjust the *distribution* of intakes to remove the effect of day-to-day variation. What is needed is a statistically appropriate sample of replicated intakes and an analysis of these replicates to estimate the variance attributable to the within-person day-to-day variation. With this knowledge, the general distribution of intakes (but not the individual intakes) can be adjusted.[4] Many of the

other potential sources of error that could pose serious concerns in assessment of an individual become less important in population assessments, as long as one can assume that the errors are randomly distributed across the individuals in the population. These potential errors include such sources as: variability of food composition (the food composition tables present average composition, not the composition of the specific item of food ingested), random under- and over-reporting, and even random variation in bioavailability.[4] The recommended approach to factoring out day-to-day variation will eliminate certain of these errors; others will resolve themselves in population data or will exert a relatively small effect on the prevalence estimate. Again we realize that application of the probability approach to population data is feasible and within our grasp even though we must express reservations about its precise application to individuals.

All discussions in this chapter refer to the judgment of adequacy of diets consumed by individuals or a group of individuals (data for each person available). They do *not* refer to population averages or per caput diets. To use a population average it would be necessary to recognize that not all individuals consume the average diet and a statistical adjustment for this variability in intake would be necessary.[3,36] To reemphasize a point made at the beginning of this chapter, one of the major changes that has taken place in the past decade has been the progressive realization that nutrient requirement estimates relate more to individuals than to populations—an apparent contradiction to the statements commonly found in dietary standards and general texts.

## NEWLY EMERGING CONCEPTS: "RECOMMENDED INTAKE"

The primary focus of this chapter has been the use of requirement estimates in the *assessment* of observed intake, a "diagnostic" approach. However, the point was made earlier that most national and international requirement reports have focused on deriving a "recommended nutrient intake," a level of intake that would be adequate to maintain nutriture among almost all normal subjects. This would be seen as a "prescriptive" recommendation for use in counseling. The distinction between these concepts is critically important. In recent years, a number of issues have arisen. There is every indication that they will continue to grow, and the ensuing confusion may be destructive to the progress that we have made.

## Conflict of Perspective Between Counselors and Assessors

Earlier we discussed the enormous difference between the proportion of women failing to ingest the "recommended intake" of iron and the proportion judged to have inadequate intakes by the probability approach. For the professional who is counseling individuals, conventional wisdom suggests that the objective is to counsel each individual toward a situation that conveys a low "risk" to that person. To that professional, the proportion of women with intakes below the "recommended intake" represents the magnitude of the problem he faces. In contrast, for the professional concerned with the health of the public as a whole, the problem he faces is better described by the estimated prevalence of inadequate intakes, a much smaller problem. It is understandable that a real and legitimate debate exists between persons with these two different perspectives of the same reality.[12]

There is no solution to this "conflict of perspective" and "conflict of mission." However, there is room for understanding and for open discussion of the programmatic and public health approaches that will be promoted. It is hoped that such discussion can take the form of intelligent dialogue rather than the confrontational and polarized form it sometimes adopts.

## Acceptable Level of "Risk"

If no clear resolution to the conflict presented previously is apparent, it is at least possible to discuss the acceptable level of risk that should be the objective of individual counseling. As noted earlier, when we have an informed judgment about the distribution of requirements, and think that is is gaussian in nature, the current convention is to set the "recommended intake" at the mean +2 standard deviations. This is a purely arbitrary decision, a convention based on a widespread statistical notion that a normal population is encompassed by the mean ±2 standard deviations and that abnormality lies outside these intervals. When we use a number set in this way we are counseling individuals to a "risk level" representing 97.7% assurance of no risk of inadequacy. Is this approach appropriate? Would an 84% assurance be adequate? If so, the recommended intake would be set at the mean +1 standard deviation (perhaps about 12% lower than at present). One could continue to lower and lower levels of assurance (or to higher and higher levels) with associated different "recommended intakes." An FAO/WHO committee[20] and a Canadian committee[2] declined to set recommended iron intakes to cover all but 2.3% of menstruating women; rather, they targeted the recommendation for 95% coverage, again by arbitrary decision. In the Canadian report, this lowered the "recommended intake" from about 18 mg/d to 14 mg/d. Why was it not lowered further? In counseling, what is an acceptable level of risk for the individual?

The second level of issue is embodied in the question of "requirement for what?" Over the years, we have progressively moved toward the definition of nutrient requirements for the maintenance of tissue levels judged appropriate. Clearly this is a normative approach. We have moved away from a functional criterion of need, i.e., the prevention of clinically detectable manifestations of deficiency. When we counsel (or assess) the client in terms of "risk," we have evolved the meaning of risk. The "risk of what" has changed. Again, although we can argue that maintenance of tissue levels offers assurance of satiation of nutrient fuctions and offers a "margin of safety" against unexpected shortfalls of intake or increases of need as during an illness, is it necessary or appropriate to have all people in a population—a basically healthy population—achieve these levels?

There are no clear answers to these questions. Nevertheless, they are issues that warrant some public policy debate to the extent that they drive public programs. It seems probable that in the next few years they are going to attract more public debate. To the present counselor, these issues warrant professional consideration. How hard should one push the client toward the "recommended intake" for what level of benefit?

## The "Abnormal" or Clinical Population

Dietary standards usually emphasize in the introductory paragraphs that the requirement estimates pertain to "the maintenance of health in already healthy individuals."[7] The concept of variability discussed previously is believed to incorporate the range of requirements that exists in the normal population; the arguments for a much wider range of variability are not generally accepted in the nutritional community. However, the accepted variability does not take into account the existence of the unusual genetic "inborn errors of metabolism" or "dependency syndromes" that have been documented in the literature. It also does not take into account the higher requirements of persons who are depleted and in need of rehabilitation (or children undergoing catch-up growth). Nor does it consider clinical patients showing evidence of malabsorption, of greatly increased requirement (e.g., the increase in energy requirement associated with febrile conditions), or of other disturbances of nutrient metabolism and requirement. Many of these situations are discussed in other chapters of this book.

The clinician or other practitioner, however, should not ignore published requirement estimates. Rather, he must exercise clinical judgment. The requirement estimates and the discussions in this chapter are relevant to most individuals living in North America. The clinician may use this as a baseline. The task then is to identify those situations, relatively small in number in the total population but potentially frequent in certain types of specialized practice, in which there is a need for adjustment of nutrient requirement estimates and hence in criteria of an adequate diet. It would be a disservice to the public and a promotion of a growing industry of specialized supplement manufacture and distribution to assume that the exceptions outnumber the general case.

## Recommended Intakes: A New Perspective

In 1985, all these issues and another major issue came to a head when the Food and Nutrition Board and the National Academy of Sciences announced that they would not publish the scheduled revision of the Recommended Dietary Allowances.* Buried in this decision were differences in judgment and opinion about the appropriate criteria of nutritional adequacy to be used in setting requirements (e.g., for ascorbic acid), the degree to which public policy considerations should affect the alteration of a "recommended intake," and the meaning of the numbers and their use.

These issues were not new. What was new was a serious issue about the meaning of a Recommended Dietary Allowance. Is this to be a figure based on nutrient requirements as we have understood them in relation to the physiologic and metabolic functions ascribed to *nutrients*? Or should a Recommended Dietary Allowance take into account the levels of a chemical that would be de-

sirable in the diet for another type of function that is not specifically related to its "nutrient" function as we have understood it?

A specific example is found in vitamin A. Studies in the past decade have given us a better basis for estimating the levels of dietary vitamin A required to maintain predetermined tissue levels and to relate these tissue levels to the periods of time that would be required for the development of functional abnormalities in the face of sudden deprivation. This new information might lead to a *reduction* in current requirement estimates. However, this comes at a time when an increase in the intake of vitamin A or β-carotene for the possible prevention of certain types of cancer is being advocated by other groups.[40]

We are suddenly faced with two completely different meanings: the traditional view that the purpose of the dietary standard reports is to describe "nutrient requirements" and the growing view that the reports should offer prescriptive advice about a desirable pattern of dietary intake. These meanings are based not only on conventional concerns about nutrient deficiencies (which are rare in the United States) but also on the relationship of diet-borne factors with chronic disease.[41] This debate will certainly grow in the next few years.

Perhaps the only workable solution for the future is to eliminate the term "recommended" from reports on nutrient requirements. We never did "recommend" that protein intakes be lowered to the "recommended" intake. If we followed such a path we might separate considerations of nutritional needs from considerations of desirable patterns of diet. It is hoped that a recommended diet would suffice to meet nutritional needs (and avoid nutritional excesses); conceivably it might also achieve other goals.

---

*In the fall of 1985 the National Research Council and the Food and Nutrition Board announced that the planned revision of the RDAs would not be published. Under the heading RDA Impasse, the American Institute of Nutrition published letters from F. Press, Chairman of the National Research Council, K. Isselbacher, Chairman of the Food and Nutrition Board, H. Kamin, Chairman of the Committee on Dietary Allowances, and J.A. Olson and R.E. Hodges, Members of the RDA Committee, all addressing the issues underlying the decision.[39a] That correspondence is complemented by articles in other publications.[39b,39c,39d,39e] Some members of this committee have published papers on an individual basis on various nutrients reflecting their opinions on *Recommended Dietary Intakes* (see Appendix Table A–1d).

## REFERENCES

1. Smith, E.: Fifth Report of the Medical Officer of the Privy Council, 1862, p. 320. *See also* J. (R.) Soc. Arts. *12*:212, 1894.
2. Department of National Health and Welfare: Recommended Nutrient Intakes for Canadians. Ottawa, Ontario, 1983.
3. FAO/WHO/UNU: Energy and Protein Requirement. Report of a Joint FAO/WHO/UNU Expert Consultation. Geneva, WHO Technical Report Series, No. 724, 1985.
4. Subcommittee on Criteria of Dietary Evaluation: Nutrient Adequacy: Assessment Using Food Consumption Surveys. Food and Nutrition Board, Commission on Life Sciences, National Research Council. Washington, D.C., National Academy Press, 1985.
5. Food and Nutrition Board: Recommended Dietary Allowances. Washington, D.C., National Academy of Sciences, National Research Council, 1974.
6. Food and Nutrition Board: Recommended Dietary Allowances. Washington, D.C., National Academy of Sciences, National Research Council, 1980.
7. FAO/WHO: Energy and Protein Requirements. Geneva, WHO Technical Report Series No. 522, 1973.

8. Department of National Health and Welfare: Canadian Dietary Standard. Ottawa, Ontario, 1975.

9. Department of Health and Social Services: Recommended Intakes of Nutrients for the United Kingdom. Reports on Public Health and Medical Subjects No. 120. London, Her Majesty's Printing Office, 1969.

10. Food and Nutrition Board: Recommended Dietary Allowances. Washington, D.C., National Academy of Sciences, National Research Council, 1943.

11. Canadian Council on Nutrition: A Dietary Standard for Canada. Department of National Health and Welfare, Ottawa, Ontario, 1948.

12. Beaton, G.H.: The use of nutritional requirements and allowances. *In* Proceedings: Western Hemisphere Nutrition Congress III. (White, P.L., Selvey, P.L., Eds.) Mount Kisko, N.Y., Futura Publishing Company, 1972.

13. FAO/WHO Joint Expert Committee on Nutrition: Eighth Report. Geneva, WHO Technical Report Series No. 477, 1971.

14. Sukhatme, P.V., Margen, S.: Am. J. Clin. Nutr. *31*:1237–1256, 1978.

15. Anderson, G.H., Peterson, R.D., Beaton, G.H.: Nutr. Res. *2*:409–415, 1982.

16. Hallberg, L., Hogdahl, A.-M., Nilsson, L., et al.: Acta Med. Scand. *180*:639–650; Acta Obstet. Gynecol. Scand. *45*:320–351, 1966.

17. Cole, S.K., Billewicz, W.Z., Thompson, A.M.: J. Obstet. Gynecol. Br. Commonwealth, *78*:933–939, 1971.

17a. Cole, S.K., Thompson, A.M., Billewicz, W.Z.: J. Obstet. Gynecol. Br. Commonwealth *79*:994–1001, 1972.

18. Beaton, G.H.: The epidemiology of iron deficiency. *In* Iron in Biochemistry and Medicine. (Jacobs, A., Worwood, M., Eds.) London, Academic Press, 1974.

19. Beaton, G.H., Myo Thein, Milne, H., et al.: Am. J. Clin. Nutr. *23*:275–283, 1970.

20. FAO/WHO: Requirements of Ascorbic Acid, Vitamin D, Vitamin B12, Folate and Iron. Geneva, WHO Technical Report Series No. 452, 1970.

21. Pao, E.M., Mickle, S.J.: Food Technology *35*:58–79, 1981.

22. James, W.P.T.: Appetite control and other mechanisms of weight homeostasis. *In* Nutrition Adaptation in Man. (Blaxter, Sir Kenneth, Waterlow, J.C., Eds.) London, John Libbey, 1985.

23. Beaton, G.H.: Nutr. Rev. *41*:325–340, 1983.

24. Beaton, G.H.: The significance of adaptation in the definition of nutrient requirements and for nutrition policy. *In* Nutrition Adaptation in Man. (Blaxter, Sir Kenneth, Waterlow, J.C., Eds.) London, John Libbey, 1985.

25. IUNS: Recommended Dietary Allowances Around the World. Report by Committee 1/5 of the International Union of Nutritional Sciences. Nutr. Abst. Rev. Clin. Nutr. *53*:939–1117, 1983.

26. WHO: Trace Elements in Human Nutrition. Geneva, WHO Technical Report Series No. 532, 1973.

27. Nikiforuk, G., Grainger, R.M.: Fluorine. *In* Nutrition: A Comprehensive Treatise, Vol. 1. (Beaton, G.H., McHenry, E.W., Eds.) New York, Academic Press, 1964.

28. FAO/WHO: Dietary Fats and Oils in Human Nutrition. Rome, FAO Food and Nutrition Paper No. 3, 1977.

29. Hansen, R.G., Wyse, B.W., Sorenson, A.W.: Nutritional Quality Index of Foods. Westport, Connecticut, AVI Publishing Co., 1979.

30. Hansen, R.G., Wyse, B.W.: J. Am. Diet. Assoc. *76*:223–227, 1980.

31. Windham, C.T., Wyse, B.W., Hansen, R.G.: J. Am. Diet. Assoc. *82*:34–43, 1983.

32. Wretlind, A.: Food iron supply. *In* Iron Deficiency: Pathogenesis, Clinical Aspects, Therapy. (Hallberg, L., Harwerth, H.-G., Vannotti, A. Eds.) London, Academic Press, 1970.

33. Wretlind, A.: Am. J. Clin. Nutr. *36*:366–375, 1982.

34. Bruce, A.: Nutrition Recommendations for the Nordic Countries. Personal communication. Uppsala, Sweden, The National Food Administration, 1981.

35. Platt, B.S., et al.: Protein values of human food. *In* Recent Advances in Clinical Nutrition. (Brock, J.F., Ed.) London, Churchill, 1961.

36. Beaton, G.H., Swiss, L.: Am. J. Clin. Nutr. *27*:485–504, 1974.

37. Payne, P.R.: Am. J. Clin. Nutr. *28*:281–286, 1975.

38. Beaton, G.H., Chery, A.: Can. J. Physiol. Pharmacol. *64*:772–780, 1986.

39. Food and Nutrition Board: Assessing Changing Food Consumption Patterns. Committee on Food Consumption Patterns, Washington, D.C., National Academy of Sciences. National Research Council, 1981.

39a. AIN: Nutrition Notes *21*:1–6, 1985.

39b. Guthrie, H.A.: J. Am. Diet. Assoc. *85*:1646–1648, 1985.

39c. Isselbacher, K.: J. Am. Diet. Assoc. *85*:1648–1649, 1985.

39d. Monsen, E.R., Owen, A.L.: J. Am. Diet. Assoc. *85*:1649, 1985.

39e. Marshall, E.: Science *230*:420–421, 1985.

40. National Research Council: Diet, Nutrition and Cancer. Report of the Committee on Diet, Nutrition and Cancer. Assembly of Life Sciences. Washington, D.C., National Academy Press, 1982.

41. Hegsted, D.M.: Statement concerning application of the recommended method. *In* Nutrient Adequacy: Assessment Using Food Consumption Surveys. Report of the Subcommittee on Dietary Evaluation, Food and Nutrition Board, Commission on Life Science, National Research Council. Washington, D.C., National Academy Press, 1985.

*Chapter* **36**

# FOOD FADS AND FADDISM

Philip L. White and Therese D. Mondeika

Mysticism and food faddism are probably as old as civilization itself. Constantly changing, man's belief in the curative, protective, and magical properties of foods has led to cultism that often becomes a blend of pseudoscience and a religion.[1-5] Unusual dietary patterns are adopted with the zeal of religious fanaticism by certain segments of our population as a means of creating a spiritual awakening or rebirth. Some of the philosophies no doubt provide satisfying emotional experiences for their followers. Man's belief in medical properties of foods is reinforced by modern emphasis on various components of foods as causative of or protective against the degenerative disorders. Nearly every nutrient or component of food has been implicated in one way or another. In some measure, frequent references to food components as risk factors for coronary heart disease and cancer undermines confidence in conventional foods and encourages fanaticism.

Urged on by the Surgeon General's report, *Healthy People*, individuals are encouraged to reduce their risks of disease.[6] Efforts to urge more healthful styles of life[7] have inadvertently spawned an array of unorthodox recommendations.

Many sensible, sincere people are also motivated to seek alternative food styles for ecologic reasons. They are worried about environmental pollution through the use of agricultural chemicals and have, thus, turned to "organic" and other types of "health" foods. The pressure of these ecologic concerns has increased both the number of people and the emotional intensity involved in this practice. This same concern about the natural environment and the food supply has existed through the generations. Although concern for environmental protection is commendable, a line must be drawn between healthy skepticism and paranoia.[8]

The health food movement produced persuasive leaders who charmed their followers with their own brand of proselytism. Examples may be found in the careers of Graham, Kellogg, and Post.[5] Frequently a lucrative business develops from fads and cults, as with the present-day health food enterprise. The power of advertising and communications helps to expand and to perpetuate the myths upon which the business was based. The enterprise builds upon the consumer's ignorance, desperation, or fear until mere interest evolves into zealotry.

## HEIGHTENED HEALTH AWARENESS

The current emphasis on health promotion and disease prevention, as attractive and desirable as that may be, has given opportunity to the health hustler for lucrative schemes. Personal efforts at risk reduction relate to abatement of tobacco use, alcohol and drug abuse, dietary immoderations, stress, and physical inactivity. Unfortunately, the emphasis on disease prevention, in addition to coining terms such as "preventive health" and "preventive nutrition," has produced a variety of dietary recommendations for avoiding degenerative disease.[7,9] The result has been specific diets for the management of the hyperlipidemias, hypertension, osteoporosis, obesity, and cancer. National nutrition policy is expressed in the form of U.S. Dietary Guidelines.[10] Antioxidants, such as ascorbic acid and selenium, plant fibers, and vitamin A and the retinoids are touted as inhibitors

**666**

of tumor development.[7] The polyunsaturated fatty acids, whether the omega-3 or omega-6 eicosapentaenoic acids from marine or vegetable sources, respectively, share the limelight as potential preventers of coronary heart disease and cancer. All of the aforementioned compounds are exploited by the health hustler.

The plethora of information about health promotion and disease avoidance has strained physicians' abilities to meet unrealistic patient expectations. This strain has bolstered the persuasiveness of the medical fringe. The new health awareness plays into the hands of the health hustler who promotes tailor-made products and systems to: (1) help one resist disease, (2) improve overall health, or (3) slow the aging process.[11] The heightened awareness has also spawned an exercise-equipment industry with an astounding variety of exercise machines and food supplements of dubious merit.

Heightened health awareness may have created expectations that at present exceed the ability of medical science to deliver. As a result, individuals turn to self-assessment and self-treatment, develop their own sets of health beliefs, lose confidence in the scientific method, and demonstrate willingness to accept anything new that sounds plausible.[11]

Public interest in health is influenced by a large number of stimuli ranging from personal or family experience to media-reinforced, often improperly reported, research discoveries. Often, patients are driven to try desperate treatment (such as Laetrile treatment for cancer or chelation therapy for atherosclerosis) by the failure of some physicians to communicate adequately when discussing anticipated outcomes of serious illnesses. Withholding hope or promising too much too soon can drive patients to try unorthodox treatments.

Unorthodox practitioners are persuasive, are not bound by codes of ethics, and generally hold simplistic views of disease. When their methods are challenged, the usual response is (1) an invitation to prove that their methods do not work, (2) a challenge to read their patients' testimonials and their literature (never published in peer-reviewed journals), or (3) a retreat to their simplistic views of disease that defy biologic explanation.[12]

White and Selvey captured the essence of "metabolic therapy" and the new wave of unorthodox therapies:

> *Metabolic therapy* is a generic term for an unconventional approach to healing that traces the degenerative diseases, as well as nutritional and psychological disorders, to some metabolic imbalance or another. "Optimum metabolic balance" is sought, e.g., by way of laetrile, severely restricted diets, mul-

tiple nutritional supplements of high dosage, enzymes, live cell injections, animal gland extracts, colonic irrigations, coffee enemas, and homeopathic supplements. Metabolic clinics are springing up all over the country.

"Nutritionally oriented" clinics and dentists now caught up in *nouveaux* metabolics use hair analysis, dietary review, and cursory blood analysis as "diagnostic" aids. The "diagnosis" usually yields a litany of trace mineral imbalances, subclinical vitamin deficiencies, and meaningless, albeit detailed, metabolic double-talk. The patient ends up with boxes and bottles full of nutritional supplements and sometimes animal gland extracts. If the hair analysis suggests "toxic" levels of heavy metals, chelation therapy will also accompany the supplements. Interestingly, whenever a vitamin or trace mineral deficiency is suspected, therapeutic trials would probably yield results before the analytic data are available from the hair analysis laboratory.

Superoxide dismutase (SOD) supplements have replaced "vitamin $B_{15}$" as the health aficionado's wonder supplement. What $B_{15}$ doesn't do for you, SOD will.

Superoxide dismutase is an enzyme that functions as a free radical superoxide scavenger, an important process for maintenance of cellular integrity. The univalent reduction of oxygen to water (not the usual biologic route of oxygen utilization) produces the intermediates: hydrogen peroxide, superoxide $(O_2^-)$, and the hydroxyl radical. The latter two are mutagenic, biologically destructive, free radicals and are thought to be created by ionizing radiation. Superoxide dismutase converts the superoxide radical to oxygen and hydrogen peroxide, the latter being eliminated by the action of catalase. Superoxide dismutase is ubiquitous in those life forms that are aerobes, human cells included.

Astounding claims are made for supplements of SOD, ranging from delayed aging to enhanced beauty. The dismutase enzymes, however, are proteins that, if taken by mouth, could not withstand the human digestive process and thus could not be absorbed biologically intact. They certainly could not reach our cells to do their wondrous things.[11]

Each generation is visited by what Herbert calls "the health hustlers."[13] Some are self-styled "experts" who know the protection inherent in the First Amendment to the Constitution and use it to further their own careers. Others are simply misguided laymen. Both mislead the public and undermine faith in medicine and nutrition as they promote their own brands of pseudonutrition. Those brands usually include the prescription of vitamins and/or minerals to prevent or cure whatever disease or condition is currently confounding the medical profession. So-called megavitamin therapy, or orthomolecular medicine, is a current panacea for everything from schizophrenia to cancer.[14,15] Because the health hustlers frequently are given the opportunity to promote their theories or products via mass communications, the public is often incapable of differentiating the "hustler" with inappropriate credentials from the qualified scientist.[16,17] As long as the health hustlers successfully avoid the infringement of laws and regulations concerned with protecting the public against pretended medical skills or unlawful medical practice, false and misleading food and drug claims on labels, or misuse of the United States mails, they are free to prey on the unsuspecting public.[13]

The Food and Drug Administration, the Federal Trade Commission, and the Post Office Department have the major regulatory responsibilities that could act to discourage illicit health practices. Each agency is handicapped by lack of adequate budget and manpower to control health fraud. Their efforts are further diminished by an amendment to the Food, Drug and Cosmetic Act (PL 94-278, Title V, 4/22/76) that significantly reduces FDA ability to regulate dietary supplements.[18] The composition of dietary supplements can be limited only by the manufacturer's imagination and FDA ability to show toxicity. The government must now evaluate the safety of dietary supplement components.

The amendment is the result of the entry of the health food industry into legislative affairs.[14] This marks a new era in the fight against health fraud that will warrant close scrutiny in the future.

The Secretary of Health and Human Services is authorized to regulate dietary supplements intended only for use by children under four years of age and by pregnant or lactating women. The amendment allowed the marketing of a wide variety of supplement products and high-concentration vitamin and mineral products. Provided no health claim appears on the product label, virtually anything edible can be marketed. Promotion of the product by advertising, booklets or pamphlets, lectures, and media stories brings it to public attention. In-store promotions, health magazine articles, and advice by store clerks seem to be effective and within the law if they are not done at the point of sale so that the claims made do not constitute product labeling. Thus, one can purchase an astounding array of worthless products highly touted for health benefit or disease avoidance. Unless the FDA can demonstrate toxicity and then regulate under food additive sections of the FDC act, or hold that the product is a drug and thus subject to regulations as a new drug, the FDA is powerless to regulate food supplements.

## SAFETY AND ADEQUACY OF FOOD SUPPLY

Real or imagined apprehension about the quality and safety of the food supply or specific concern about particular food manufacturing practices and food additives leads many people to seek alternative food practices and nonconventional approaches to personal nutrition. When one is dealing with alternative food practices that appear to be mere faddism, it is important to distinguish between debatable issues that have a basis in science and issues that represent personal philosophies. For example, people may be convinced that all chemicals used in foods are unsafe and unnecessary. That belief represents personal philosophy—they wish things as God made them, simple and pure. In reality, the issue is based in science relating to the particular chemical and the use it serves. The issue of risk and benefit relative to food chemicals cannot be debated solely on the basis of personal philosophy.

Cultism can emerge as a result of confusion between the significance of uncertain or implied environmental risk and that of unequivocal risk to health. The natural or organic food movement related to this as people became concerned about modern agricultural practices that rely on chemical sprays and other agricultural chemicals. Apprehension about the safety and quality of processed foods also contributes to faddism. Customers patronizing health food stores are led to believe that foods presumably grown without the use of pesticides or artificial fertilizers but with the application to the soil of natural fertilizers (manures) and other organic matter are more nourishing and less likely to be hazardous. "Natural foods" are those that have undergone little or no processing and do not contain additives.[19] In large measure, the movement is based upon distortion of fact and exploitation of the unwary. The movement has also produced an uncompromising situation related to the demand for absolute safety in our environment and our foods. Today, as the result of strong societal pressures, experts are asked to provide evidence of absolute safety, an unrealistic and unattainable goal, rather than evidence of hazard.[20]

The natural food concept is also based on the belief that naturalness or "organicness" lends particular health-giving properties to foods and nutrients. The unwary are led to believe that vitamins are not vitamins unless they are derived or extracted directly from plant or animal products. The consumer pays dearly for such products as vitamin C from rose hips or acerola berries. Perpetuation of the myth is necessary for the continued vitality of the health food movement.

It is unlikely that customers patronizing health food stores and paying for so-called organically grown or natural foods are unaware of the increased prices. Aside from the cost factor, there is more reason to be concerned about the health delusion that may have attracted the consumer initially.

Wolff pointed out that most people who patronize health food stores and restaurants know what they are doing and what they want.[21] They have their own beliefs about the cultural significance of food and about the quality and safety of more conventional foods. They do not believe and behave as they do because of the books they read; rather, what they read is determined by their beliefs.[21] Their motivation is generally a desire for a simpler diet not related to the highly processed, convenience foods produced by the American food industry.

> Foods most often bought in health food stores were (reported in descending order of frequency): whole grain products, whole wheat bread, fresh vegetables and fruits, raw nuts, wheat germ, brown rice, honey, yogurt, dried fruits, brewers' yeast, seeds. Foods most frequently avoided in the diet were (in descending order of frequency): refined sugar, processed and canned foods with chemical additives, white flour products and white bread, carbonated drinks, meat from animals raised in the United States, monosodium glutamate, processed meats such as hot dogs and luncheon meats, chocolate, processed cereals, white rice, coffee.[21]

What was once considered to be a fad (a regimen followed with great enthusiasm for a short period of time) may now be thought of as a subculture that is, in reality, only a departure from some conventionally defined norm.[21,22] According to Wolff, "what has been called the counterculture can perhaps best be understood as an expression of disaffection, alienation perhaps, or disappointment with an environment that is becoming increasingly man made and yet increasingly foreign, frustrating and incomprehensible."[21] Wolff states that health "foodists" (his coined word) believe and behave in opposition to the culture in which they were raised and are able to maintain their opposition because they receive strong reinforcements: "...a sense of community, a shared (counter) culture, and a feeling of well being."

The health counterculture is no longer a fringe force, but one that is moving rapidly toward center in our society.[23]

The willingness of segments of American industry to turn to its own advantage the words of the counterculture, "organic" and "natural," may have produced apparent confirmation of concern. Industry plays two sides by promoting such products as organic eye shadow and natural breakfast cereals. The immediacy of commerce and the ability to tailor-make products to capitalize on consumer interests or concerns may serve at times to confirm a given fear. Thus, the difference between the conventional food industry and the health food industry becomes confused. Perhaps in the confusion the words "organic" and "natural" will lose their significance.

The publication of books and articles pertaining to nutrition and health abounds in this country. Unfortunately, much of the information is erroneous or misleading. The public is being bombarded with nutrition misinformation at an alarming rate. What is more unfortunate is that no reliable mechanism exists to help the public evaluate this information and put it into proper perspective. In the absence of such a mechanism, the media and publishers should assume the responsibility for assuring that statements and recommendations made to the public are based on scientific fact rather than on personal opinion.

The chicanery practiced by the health food store "medicine man" who diagnoses ailments and dispenses roots, herbs, teas, or nutritional supplements to "cure" disease or relieve its symptoms differs only in degree from that involved in medical quackery.[24] Although the latter is more serious because the quack may deprive gravely ill patients of appropriate medical treatment, the rationale for turning to any charlatan is no doubt similar. Bernard succinctly appraised it:

> The need to believe in a therapeutic miracle, when medical science is or seems to be failing, can be so strong that it drives one's intelligence into twisting the facts to fit emotional necessity. Thus, faith in the quack, under such conditions, can be maintained without too much offense to reason by mobilizing such arguments as: the quack may have hit upon something of which medical science is still ignorant; the quack is a genius who is too far ahead of his time to be accorded recognition; the quack is a great healer who is the victim of organized medicine's vindictive jealousy or protection of a professional monopoly, and so on. Clearly, the psychological situation is very different for those who turn toward quackery in extremis when medicine is impotent than for the majority of those on whose gullibility and weakness quackery trades.[25]

The key words are "the need to believe in a therapeutic miracle" and "emotional necessity." It is on these needs that quackery thrives. The recipients are in reality paying for benefits that are not there. Their belief alone may be sufficient justification for action.

Unconventional or apparently bizarre dietary habits may reflect alternative styles of life or perhaps some long-standing cultural or religious practice that is simply different than the usual pattern. Many people have a rational argument for nutritional behavior that is based on a cultural or religious viewpoint rather than on misinformation of scientific knowledge of nutrition. Therefore, if attempts are made to change their behavior, it is imperative to understand their way of thinking and their point of view. When the resultant nutrient intake is appropriate, there is little reason to be concerned. At the same time, aberrant diets or exotic regimens derived from a given religious philosophy can be fraught with biologic hazard for the devotee. Health fraud can exist within a mask of culture or religion. By the same token, individuals perpetrating the fraud can hide behind religion to avoid persecution and prosecution. The only rational way to bring about behavior modification among followers of a sect or subculture that embraces a hazardous diet or dietary practice is to work within that system of beliefs. Within the value system, changes can be brought about that will improve the nutritional status.

## WEIGHT REDUCTION

Weight reduction regimens promoted to the public as the solution to obesity exemplify the fad diet. They are followed with great excitement for short periods. Their popularity is more directly related to the persuasiveness of the promotion and the personality of the "originator" than to the value of the diet. Essentially all reducing diets will help remove weight, especially if the dieter can be swept up in the lure of the regimen. Ultimately, the behavior pattern that precipitated the obesity in the first place takes over and failure begins. The dieter then becomes a candidate for the next highly publicized crash diet.

Most fad diets are based on imbalance, not necessarily calorie imbalance, which is the thermochemical logic of weight reduction, but rather on macronutrient imbalance. There have been diets that are excessive in fat, protein, or carbohydrate content at the expense of one or the other of these nutrients. The ketogenic diets contain minimal carbohydrate and excessive fat content. The body water loss, the reduced appetite associated with ketosis, and the inability to consume unlimited quantities of high-fat foods apparently explain the weight loss that occurs with such diets.

Starvation and semistarvation diets appear, disappear, and reappear regularly. Although short-term starvation as a means of losing weight has been incorporated into weight reduction programs by some physicians, the exploitation of extended fasting as a popular method of weight reduction is not in the public interest. Too many hazards are associated with unsupervised starvation to justify its popularization. Nevertheless, books and lecturers still extol the virtues of the extended fast for weight control. The protein-sparing modified fast based upon the provision of 1 to 2 g protein/kg ideal body weight, with or without a few hundred kcal from carbohydrate, is currently being used in the management of obesity.

Under medical guidance, such regimens have enjoyed success, but their ultimate development was not without pain and suffering brought on by inappropriate exploitation of the concept.[26]

## MEDICAL SCIENCE AND MIRACLES

Why in this enlightened age does the public fall prey to the counterculture of nutrition and medicine? Why is health fraud becoming more lucrative with little probability that public support will diminish? The answers seem to relate to a condition of human frailty: the expectation of miracles. Rational judgment is ruled out because even a total lack of scientific evidence does not eliminate the possibility that a treatment or practice may appear to benefit some users. Psychosomatic effects and unaided recovery, which occur frequently, reinforce faith in the results assumed from this uncritical trial-and-error approach. In addition, millions of people appear to be basing important health decisions on the idea that, because there are individual differences in people, there is a chance that almost any treatment may be beneficial. In other words, because it did not work for one does not mean that it might not work for another.

Bruch has discussed the possibility that quackery may be an expression of the relative failure of the scientific approach:

> The great progress of modern medicine during the nineteenth and twentieth centuries, based on the scientific method, has led in its extreme application to a model of medical practice in which the patient is dealt with as a passive object on whom the scientific physician practices his special knowledge. This model overlooks that the doctor-patient interaction rests on a number of shared assumptions and social roles. Talcott Parsons, the sociologist, feels there is need to consider the *function* of medical practice, what is ordinarily called therapy, not simply as the goal of the physical but as the *collectively*-constituted interaction by physician and patient taken together.[28] When a patient is treated 'purely' as an object, his contribution becomes zero, leaving him frustrated and dissatisfied....
>
> Many physicians may give in to the demands from patients for 'special' medications, and at least a few may convince themselves of that effectiveness in the absence of any real data. Thus, in its application, modern medicine may have a magical component called the placebo effect, which on closer and more specific definition should be called magical thinking....[27]

Rampant empiricism has as part of its basis the

well-known placebo effect mentioned by Bruch. It can be appreciated, if the increase in health fraud is related to the failure of the scientific approach, that nutrition to the health hustler is a philosophy, not a science. Unencumbered by science and the truth, hustlers know only those bounds defined by the law.

Following congressional hearings by the Senate Select Committee on Aging, Subcommittee on Health and Long-Term Care, May, 1984, the FDA, the United States Postal Service, and the Federal Trade Commission launched efforts to build coalitions to fight health fraud. By 1986, expenditures on fraudulent health care devices and supplements reached $25 billion annually. The aforementioned agencies sponsored 22 regional conferences on health fraud to enlist understanding and support from private, professional, and local agencies. The fruits of such labors should be easily measurable and deserve the support of the medical profession. Faddism, fraud, and cultism will always abound; the challenge is to control them in such a manner that followers suffer the least harm.

## REFERENCES

1. Smith, R.L.: The Health Hucksters. New York, Thomas Y. Crowell, 1960.
2. Young, J.H.: The Medical Messiahs. Princeton, Princeton University Press, 1967.
3. Trager, J.: The Bellybook. New York, Grossman Publishers, 1972.
4. Barrett, S., and Knight, G. (Eds.): The Health Robbers. Philadelphia, George F. Stickley Co., Publ., 1976.
5. Deutsch, R.: The New Nuts Among the Berries. Palo Alto, Bull Publishing Company, 1977.
6. U.S. Dept. of Health and Human Services: Healthy People: The Surgeon General's Report on Health Promotion and Disease Prevention. Publication 79-55071. Washington, D.C., U.S. Government Printing Office, 1979.
7. The Committee on Diet, Nutrition, and Cancer: Diet, Nutrition, and Cancer. Assembly of Life Sciences, National Academy of Sciences. Washington, D.C., National Academy Press, 1982.
8. Council on Foods and Nutrition, AMA: Conference on Food Faddism and Cultism. Unpublished data, 1971.
9. White, P.: JAMA *245*:2239, 1981.
10. U.S. Department of Agriculture and U.S. Department of Health and Human Services: Dietary Guidelines for Americans. 2nd ed. Washington, D.C., 1985.
11. White, P., and Selvey, N.: JAMA *247*:2914, 1982.
12. Soffer, A.: Arch. Intern. Med. *146*:457, 1986.
13. Herbert, V.: *In* The Health Robbers. (Barrett and Knight, Eds.). Philadelphia, George F. Stickley Co., Publ., 1976.
14. Jukes, T.: JAMA *233*:50, 1975.
15. Herbert, V.: Food Nutr. News *47*:March-April, 1976.
16. White, H.: Food Nutr. News *36*:October, 1973.
17. Gunther, M.: *In* The Health Robbers. (Barrett and Knight, Eds.). Philadelphia, George F. Stickley Co., Publ., 1976.
18. White, P.: Postgrad. Med. *6*:204, 1976.
19. White, P.: Food Tech. *26*:29, 1972.
20. White, P.: Food Drug Cosmet. Law J. *31*:497, 1976.
21. Wolff, R.V.: Am. J. Clin. Nutr. *26*:438, 1973.
22. Erhard, D.: Nutr. Today *8*:4, 1973; *9*:20, 1974.
23. Enloe, C.: Nutr. Today *16*:26, 1981.
24. Frankle, R.T., and Heussenstamm, F.K.: Am. J. Public Health *64*:11, 1974.
25. Bernard, V.W.: Am. J. Public Health *55*:1143, 1965.
26. Newmark, S., and Williamson, B.: Arch. Intern. Med. *143*:1423, 1983.
27. Bruch, H.: J. Am. Diet. Assoc. *57*:316, 1970.
28. Parsons, T.: Social Structure and Personality. Glencoe Free Press of Glencoe, 1964.

Chapter **37**

# EFFECTS OF PROCESSING AND PREPARATION ON THE NUTRITIVE VALUE OF FOODS

Benjamin Borenstein and Paul A. Lachance

Food processing serves to make perishable foods available year-round. Relatively "fresh" foods are also available from thousands of miles away because of refrigerated transportation. The technologies of controlled environments (e.g., hot houses) and hydroponic gardening on a large scale are an increasing source of off-season food. The consumer, therefore, has the choice of local "garden"-fresh foods in season, "market"-fresh foods grown and transported from elsewhere, as well as garden-fresh foods commercially preserved by heat processing and freezing, with an extended (months) shelf life, or commercially preserved by chilling with a shelf life of weeks. Fresh products continue to respire or spoil as do chilled products and, therefore, their nutritive value varies considerably and decreases as acceptability decreases. Garden-fresh products and commercially frozen foods retain higher nutritive values and flavor qualities. Important food ingredients such as flour, sugar, and vegetable oils are "refined" to standardize the products and to extend their shelf life; thus, these ingredients and the products derived from their incorporation into formulated foods such as bread or pudding have a relatively constant but diminished nutritive value in specific cases. Certain ingredients, especially wheat and corn flour, can serve as excellent carriers of highly stable fortification nutrients.

However, fortification is restricted or not allowed if the food product has a federal standard. This explains why, for example, ready-to-eat cereals and instant breakfast products have a number of added micronutrients, whereas "standard of identity" products such as pasta, bread, jam, jelly, and ketchup have few, if any, nutrients restored, i.e., added to a level one would have expected given the food composition of the starting foods.

Whether nutrients are naturally occurring in a food or added to a food, they are affected by the same physiochemical parameters that occur in the processing and/or the preparation of food. These parameters are temperature, oxygen, light, pH, and the extent (concentration and duration) of exposure to one or a combination of the parameters. In principle, exposure of food to a high temperature of 140°C for a short time (seconds) is less damaging to nutrient value than exposure to a moderate temperature of 90°C for a longer time (minutes). Similarly, commercial freezer storage at $-30$ to $-40°C$ is more favorable to extended shelf life than is freezer chest storage at $-15$ to $-20°C$.

Oxygen, even at very low levels (ppm), can be destructive to specific micronutrients such as vitamins A, E, C, and folacin. Some nutrients, e.g., riboflavin, and vitamin A, are extremely sensitive to sunlight or direct lighting for a few hours. Foods treated with sulfite to preserve (inactivate enzymes) and to enhance color suffer thiamin loss but retain ascorbic acid. Fermenting foods or using additives that shift the pH (usually to pH 4.5 or lower for microbial safety reasons) will aid retention of nutrients such as vitamin $B_6$ and thiamin that are stable at acid pH but not as stable at low acid or alkaline pH. The alkalinity of chocolate in chocolate cake is destructive to thiamin. Some nutrients (e.g., niacin and minerals) are stable to practically all types of treatments except for leaching from the product into the packing medium or into the cooking water. Substantial losses of all water-soluble nutrients occur in thawing exudates and dripping during cooking and leaching. The most significant losses of nutrients overall occur in the home and during food service preparation of foods.

The importance of institutional feeding is growing with the increase in fast food establishments, school feeding, day care centers, and health care facilities. Nutritional status is compromised not only by nutritive value losses with food service practices extending over hours, but also by the food combinations offered, elected, and/or eaten.

Canned foods (thermally processed) are sometimes overheated with respect to optimal texture, flavor, and micronutrient retention, and nutrients leached into the process medium of canned foods are frequently decanted and discarded. Fresh foods are frequently boiled rather than steamed, or excessive amounts of water in coverless pots are used to cook fresh or frozen foods. Fresh foods are often subdivided, thus increasing the surface area to expedite cooking or to meet some other cooking objective, but the practice accelerates leaching and destruction of nutrients. In food service, foods are heated or reheated and then held on steam tables at serving temperature (75°C) for time periods exceeding 20 minutes during slack cafeteria hours or when demand is low.

Superior nutrient retention occurs with frozen foods packaged in pouches that do not permit direct exposure of the food to water and oxygen when cooked, or with foods that are steamed in a steam basket, with cover, or with foods that are microwaved but not overcooked.

Insoluble protein, carbohydrates, lipids, minerals, vitamin K, biotin, and niacin are stable (85% retention) during the processing, preparing, and storing of foods. Vitamins A, D, E, $B_6$, $B_{12}$, riboflavin, pantothenic acid, and folacin are less stable. The vitamins thiamin and ascorbic acid are most likely to be seriously depleted during thermal processing, extended storage, and poor food handling practices during the preparation and service of foods. In addition, water solubles may be leached out of particulate foods during processing steps such as blanching.

The scientific literature is extensive but not comprehensive. The following is an example of data that demonstrate the principle just presented. Post-harvest handling of peas caused significant vitamin C losses from field to plant to process line (120 mg/100 g, to 110, to 93, respectively) before any further processing steps.[1] Simultaneously, the carotene, thiamin, riboflavin, and niacin values were essentially unchanged during hauling and handling. The blanching and canning steps caused further ascorbic acid losses of approximately 30%, but these losses were no greater than those that occur in home preparation of fresh peas. Thiamin, $B_6$, and niacin losses during blanching and canning were 30 to 40%. The newer processes of aseptic canning and thermal processing in retort pouches decrease heat stress on the thermolabile vitamins and improve stability.[2]

An extreme example of undesirable food preparation resulted in one of the earliest cases of diagnosed folacin deficiency in man. An individual subsisting on restaurant hamburgers, doughnuts, and coffee had megaloblastic anemia definitely traced to folacin deficiency. The hamburgers were thin and kept on a hot plate for several hours before consumption and had little residual folate.[3]

## VITAMINS

The vitamin content of raw foods can vary because crops vary with type, soil, climate, fertilizer, and other growing conditions. In addition, nutritive value varies with the maturity of the food commodity. Humans choose to consume mature bananas, fruits, berries, potatoes, beans, and peas, but prefer immature snap beans and spinach, semimature lima beans and kernel corn, and overmature broccoli and cauliflower. The area of highest nutritive value is often just under the peel of fruits and vegetables,[4] yet peelings are not always desirable because of the high concentration of naturally occurring toxicants and possible agricultural residues.

The requirements of nutrition labeling have accelerated the acquisition of nutritive value data by food manufacturers. The study of the kinetics of specific nutrient losses under controlled conditions is a relatively new area of research. The practice of calculating nutrient losses attributable to type of processing (raw vs. canned vs. frozen) from handbooks of nutritive values frequently exaggerates losses. Meaningful estimations cannot be made when the variety, processing conditions, and other parameters are unknown and not comparable. The most useful data are obtained by considering the properties of the individual vitamins as a guide to their stability in given foods under given conditions as reviewed by DeRitter[5] and Borenstein.[6]

**Vitamin C.** The term vitamin C is used to designate both ascorbic and dehydroascorbic acid. The former is easily oxidized to the latter, and the latter is heat-labile. Vitamin C is thus labile to oxygen and heat, as well as neutral and basic pH. The half-life of dehydroascorbic acid at pH 6.0 is less than 2 minutes at 70°C (158°F), irrespective of the presence of oxygen. The readily simple dye reduction titration for assaying reduced and total ascorbic acid was used extensively in early research and has resulted in this vitamin being used as an indicator of nutritive value and processing changes.

Fruit products, in particular, citrus juices, followed by potato products are the most significant sources of vitamin C in North America. Vitamin C in frozen orange juice concentrates or in juices packed in airtight cans and glass lose less than 10% in processing. However, juices in paperboard containers lined with wax or polyethylene lose up to 75% of their vitamin C in three weeks, even at refrigerator temperatures, because the packaging breathes and the oxygen in the head space continues to serve as an oxidant. Frozen juice concentrates after thawing and dilution into open containers fair no better, even if refrigerated. Carbonated products containing 10 to 20% juice have no vitamin C unless it is added.

Potatoes are the second most significant source of vitamin C in the United States diet. There are over 100,000 quick-service restaurants in the United States and an increasing number of outlets in most developed countries. Almost all of these limited-menu restaurants offer french fried potatoes. French fried products retain as much as 75% of their vitamin C but practically all of it is dehydroascorbic acid protected by the surface oil and dehydration effect (case hardening) of the potato during frying.[7]

Slicing fruits and vegetables accelerates ascorbic acid oxidation. Preparing cole slaw and holding for two hours causes 50% destruction, slicing cucumbers and holding for one hour leads to 30% loss, and slicing cantaloupes and refrigerating for 24 hours causes a 35% loss.[8]

In three meal systems, Hallberg et al. found a 50% vitamin C loss after warming peeled, boiled potatoes for one hour.[9] Equally significant, warming these meals for four hours decreased iron availability 34%. This effect was due entirely to vitamin C destruction because adding back the initial level of ascorbic acid to the meals increased the iron absorption to the same values as from freshly prepared meals. Preservice holding of whipped potatoes (holding period for 60 minutes at 82°C [180°F] in warmers before transport to a hospital tray assembly area) leads to a loss of 36% of vitamin C.[10] Instant potato products do not contain vitamin C unless it has been added.

## Water-Soluble Vitamins

**Thiamin.** Breads and cereal products made with enriched flour contribute approximately one third of the dietary thiamin in the United States. Meat, poultry, and fish contribute over one fourth of the dietary thiamin, with pork being one of the richest sources of this group. Fruits and vegetables contribute one fifth and dairy products one tenth of dietary thiamin.

Thiamin is the most unstable B vitamin, but it is more stable than thiamin pyrophosphate, the cocarboxylase bound form that accounts for over 50% of the native form in specific foods. Thiamin hydrochloride and mononitrate salts are used for fortification. Even at low temperatures, thiamin is readily degraded in neutral and alkaline environments. Retention in breads (pH 5.8) is 75 to 80%, whereas thiamin is completely degraded in chocolate cake (pH 8.0).

Retention of thiamin in cooked and processed meats ranges from 40% for irradiation products to about 85% for mild cured products. Cooking meat under home preparation conditions produces variable results; retention of 40 to 100% has been reported. The roasting temperature of beef and pork is a significant variable. High oven temperature decreases retention: 60% retention at low temperature vs. 50% at high temperature. This subject is well reviewed by Lachance and Erdman.[7] Sulfite splits thiamin into its pyrimidine and thiazole constituents. For this reason, the USDA does not permit the use of sulfite in meat products. Thiaminases in raw fish can degrade thiamin.

Thiamin and other water-soluble vitamins are distributed between the solids and liquid in canned vegetables. The liquid generally contains approximately 30% of the available thiamin, which the consumer usually decants. Canned vegetables and fruits stored for one year at 19°C (65°F) show minimal losses of thiamin, but at 29°C (85°F) losses are 15 to 25%. The sensitivity of thiamin to sulfite is shown by the comparative losses when cabbage is blanched with and without sulfite: 45% and 15%, respectively.[11] Similarly, the use of sulfite as a preservative in total parenteral feeding systems is destructive to vitamin $B_1$.

During bulk milk pasteurization, 10% of thiamin is destroyed; in heat processing evaporated milk, 30% or more is destroyed. High temperature short-time pasteurization decreases thiamin only 3 to 4%. Spray-dried milk powder suffers moderate losses of 5 to 15%.

Many of the degradation products of thiamin are volatile and have been associated with a green grass odor, but they also create the favorable flavor noted in coffee and cocoa.[12]

**Riboflavin.** Dairy products contribute over 40% of the United States dietary riboflavin. Meat, fish, poultry, and eggs contribute 30% of the dietary riboflavin. Cereals contribute 15%, and fruits and vegetables 10%. Broccoli and asparagus are rich sources that are often overlooked because of the emphasis on dairy products as the principal dietary source of riboflavin.

This vitamin is heat-stable in acid solution and in the presence of mild oxidizing agents, but it is sensitive to light, particularly at neutral and alkaline pH. In neutral solution, it is moderately heat-stable. Its retention (75% and 90%) during brine grading and blanching of lima beans is superior to and less variable than that of thiamin.[13] Retention in blanched cabbage is 80%, and losses during cabbage dehydration are negligible. Riboflavin is stable in the processing and cooking of meat (approximately 90% retention). Roasting beef and pork results in retention of 70 to 90% if the drippings are discarded. The drippings contain 15 to 20% of the original vitamin. Home cooking of legumes results in retention of 100% for fast-cooking lentils and 76 to 80% for longer-cooking products.[14] Although the vitamin is light-sensitive, it is stable in white bread wrapped in clear cellophane. It is also stable in home cooking procedures.

Pasteurization and sterilization of milk cause less than 10% degradation in milk products. Light exposure of fluid milk can cause losses of 20 to 80% in two hours, depending on temperature, surface area exposed, and light intensity. Fluorescent light is less harmful than sunlight.[15] The greatest destruction is caused by light in the wavelength range of 420 to 560 nm.

**Niacin.** In the United States, meat, fish, poultry, and eggs provide 45% of the dietary preformed niacin; cereals, raisins, and coffee provide another 37%; and fruits and vegetables provide 16%.[16] Whereas milk and eggs are low in preformed niacin, they contain high amounts of tryptophan and, as such, are a source of niacin. This biochemical conversion requires the presence of thiamin, riboflavin, and vitamin $B_6$. The vitamin is present as nicotinic acid in plant foods and as niacinamide in animal foods. Niacin has excellent heat and light stability in the entire pH range of foods. However, niacin leaches readily in blanching and washing operations and is thus reduced both in frozen and in canned vegetables. It can be enzymatically degraded in aging meats.

Niacin in cereal grains is substantially located in the husk, which is removed in the milling process. Restoration of niacin is now a feasible practice in developed countries, but not all countries permit the practice of fortifying flour. Niacin in wheat bran occurs as niacytin, a glycopeptide that is not bioavailable, and is excreted in the urine as a methylated derivative. Niacin in corn and rice occurs as niacinogen, a peptide. The alkali (lime water) pretreatment of corn in the preparation of tortillas increases the bioavailability of niacin and explains the rarity of pellagra in tortilla-eating cultures, in contrast to cultures consuming fermented corn (ogi) and other corn products (e.g., corn bread). Ogi, a common weaning food in Nigeria, also loses tryptophan during fermentation.[17] Niacin retentions vary among legumes, a finding that is probably also related to the chemical form and/or the structure of the legume. Although great northern beans and small white beans have the same cooking time, their niacin retentions are different: 73% and 60%, respectively.[14]

**Vitamin $B_6$.** In the United States, meat and eggs provide 49% of the dietary source of vitamin $B_6$, fruits and vegetables 28%, dairy products 10%, cereals 6%, and legume 5%.[16]

Vitamin $B_6$ occurs as six structurally related vitamins, the free bases, pyridoxine, pyridoxal, and pyridoxamine, and their corresponding phosphates. The stability of the overall $B_6$ content of food depends on the forms present and upon the extent of exposure to temperature, pH, and light. Interconversion occurs between the different forms. Gregory and Hiner observed formation of pyridoxal from pyridoxine.[18] Gregory and Kirk reported conversion of pyridoxamine to pyridoxal.[19]

Pyridoxamine, pyridoxal, pyridoxamine phosphate, and pyridoxal phosphate are less stable than pyridoxine. The different rates of degradation for each form of the vitamin and the effect of pH explain the different retentions of vitamin $B_6$ that have been reported in foods.[20] It can be predicted that foods with lower pHs will show greater retention of the free bases, and vegetables and other food groups containing high proportions of the vitamin as pyridoxine will retain greater levels than meats containing the more heat-labile forms: pyridoxal and pyridoxamine.

Everson et al. reported 100% retention of vitamin $B_6$ in tomato juice concentrate subjected to either conventional retorting or aseptic canning and nine-month storage.[21] Pyridoxine is the predominant vitamer and is extremely stable at pH 4.0 to 4.4. Fruits and vegetables contain pyridoxine and pyridoxal, whereas foods from animal sources are generally higher in pyridoxal and pyridoxamine.

Canning and subsequent storage of strained lima beans and strained beef lead to 22 to 26% losses of vitamin $B_6$.[21] There is a 20 to 30% destruction in cooking vegetables and similar losses in canning.

In milling wheat, 75 to 90% of the vitamin $B_6$ is lost.[22] Baking bread destroys 15% of the $B_6$, and an additional loss of 10% occurs after three days of storage.[23] Vitamin $B_6$ is stable during milk pasteurization and during manufacture and storage of milk powder. Canned evaporated milk retains only 50 to 65% of its initial content during heat processing. Sweetened condensed milk, which has a milder heat treatment, retains about 80%. Pyridoxal in milk is somewhat light-sensitive, with 21% loss after eight hours in sunlight. Ang measured the photodegradation rate of pyridoxine, pyridoxal, and pyridoxamine.[24] Pyridoxine was the most stable and pyridoxamine the least stable.

**Biotin.** Although the data on biotin stability in foods are scarce, all evidence indicates good stability to heat, dilute acids and alkalis, oxygen, and light. It is inactivated by lipid peroxides. Evaporated and powdered milk incur losses of 10 to 15% during processing. Biotin is stable during home cooking of frozen baby lima beans and does not leach in cooking water. In nature, biotin is usually bound. A protein complex, avidin, occurring in egg whites, reacts with and inactivates biotin. Avidin is denatured by heat so that cooked egg white is not a source of biotin antivitamin activity.

**Pantothenic Acid.** This vitamin is stable at pH 5 to 7, but is more heat-sensitive at pH 3 to 4. It occurs widely in foods primarily as coenzyme A, a conjugated nucleotide.

Although the available data suggest it is ubiquitous in foods, data also suggest it is only moderately stable in food processing and storage. More information is therefore required.

In home-cooked legumes, pantothenic acid retentions ranged from 46% for chick-peas to 81% for lentils.[14] Pantothenic acid is stable to home-cooking procedures in the preparation of frozen lima beans, with 90% retention with cooking in minimum water and 70% retention in excess water. Roasting meat causes degradation of only 7 to 10% pantothenic acid, but the meat drippings contain 20 to 25% of the original content. Cooking rice causes some leaching or destruction.

An interesting study on 75 commonly consumed United States foods was conducted by Walsh et al.[25] They used a radioimmunoassay preceded by an enzymatic procedure to release pantothenic acid from coenzyme molecules. The foods were assayed only after bringing each product to the ready-to-eat stage, and losses during processing and home preparation were not measured. The authors concluded that a relatively low amount of pantothenic acid occurs in many highly processed foods, including products made from refined grains, fruits, fat- and cereal-extended meats, and fish.

**Folacin.** In the United States, fruits and vegetables provide 43% of the dietary folacin. Meats, fish, poultry, and eggs provide 21%, legumes 19%, cereal products 13%, and dairy products 4% of dietary folacin.[16]

The folacins vary in their stability. The tetrahydro, dihydro, and 5-methyltetrahydro forms are heat-labile. The 5-formyl tetrahydro form is of intermediate stability, and the fully oxidized, unsubstituted form, pteroylglutamic acid, is most stable to heat.[26–28] The conjugate form of folacin also affects stability. The monoglutamate (unconjugated) form is moderately heat-stable in acid solution and at neutrality. The tri- and hepta-glutamate conjugates are heat-unstable. Therefore, the stability of folacin is affected by the folate composition present in foods. However, owing to the extreme difficulty in assaying the individual chemical forms of folacins in food products, this hypothesis has not been quantitatively tested. The added folacin in folacin-supplemented foods is stable because the pteroylglutamate form of the vitamin is used for fortification.

Natural inhibitors of folacin utilization may be present in specific foods. Folacin from cooked beef liver appears to be fully available as does raw cabbage folacin.[29] In contrast, 60% of the folacin in cooked cabbage is not biologically available; however, this loss may be associated with the concomitant loss of ascorbic acid. The thermal destruction of folacins is related to their oxidative state. The vitamin is stabilized by ascorbic acid, and its destruction is catalyzed by copper.

Folacin is only slightly water-soluble, but leaching of folacins into the cooking water with boiling and blending procedures occurs. Leichter et al. observed that the leaching of folates out of the vegetable into the cooking water varied with the type of vegetable, with a low of 22% for asparagus to a high of 84% for cauliflower.[30] In fact, in four of the six vegetables examined, the cooking water contained more folacin than the cooked vegetable retained.

Folacin is also lost during food holding at high temperatures. Thin hamburgers held warm for several hours have little residual folate.[6]

Unconjugated folic acid is stable during milk pasteurization. The folacin-binding protein of commercial pasteurized skim milk was partially denatured during pasteurization in one study.[31] This finding was presumed to explain the differences found between raw and pasteurized milk products in their ability to enhance folacin absorption.[32] Boiling milk five seconds decreases free folic acid activity 40 to 90%. Fermented dairy products have increased folacin levels.[33]

Native total folacin levels are approximately the same in baked bread as in the initial dough mix[34] because folacin increases during dough proofing by yeast synthesis, and approximately the same amout is then destroyed during baking. Added folic acid losses average about 10% during different bread-baking procedures.[34]

**Vitamin $B_{12}$.** In the United States, meat and eggs provide 78% of the dietary vitamin $B_{12}$. Dairy products provide 20% and cereal products only 2% of the dietary vitamin $B_{12}$.[16] All $B_{12}$ is of microbial origin. Microorganisms in the human intestine are also able to synthesize the vitamin, but since this process occurs in the colon and gastric intrinsic factor is not available, and the receptor is present at the ileal level, the vitamin is not absorbed. The strict vegetarian is at risk of $B_{12}$ deficiency, especially if soil microorganisms from "organic" fertilizers are thoroughly washed from roots and tuber plant foods.

The predominant forms of $B_{12}$ in animal products are methylcobalamin, adenosylcobalamin, and hydroxycobalamin. Vitamin $B_{12}$ has moderate to good heat stability at pH 4 to 5, but retorting at high pH causes rapid destruction, as does exposure to light. Pasteurizing milk has minimal effect on $B_{12}$ content, as do most methods of cooking. Evaporated milk has losses of 70 to 90%, and spray-dried milk has losses of 20 to 35%. Ferrous salts catalyze destruction. Fermented dairy products have slightly lower $B_{12}$ levels than their unfermented dairy components.

Controversy has developed concerning the possible effect of consuming 0.5- to 1.0-g quantities of ascorbic acid with meals on the stability of the $B_{12}$ contained in the food. In 1974 the Herbert group reported that megadoses of vitamin C may destroy substantial amounts of vitamin $B_{12}$ in food.[35] Other researchers believe this is an analytic problem caused by destruction of $B_{12}$ during sample extraction and analysis.[36] Amore recent report by Herbert et al. indicates that destruction of human serum $B_{12}$ can occur during serum analysis in the presence of high ascorbate levels and that this destruction is prevented by the addition of potassium cyanide (KCN).[37] A study of the effect of supplemental ascorbic acid (1 to 2 g daily) on the serum $B_{12}$ levels of myelomeningocele patients demonstrated no significant differences between the control and experimental groups except that the hemoglobin levels were slightly higher in the supplemental ascorbic acid group.[38] The authors concluded that it is highly improbable that megadoses of supplemental ascorbic acid would induce vitamin $B_{12}$ deficiency in man.

## Fat-Soluble Vitamins

**Vitamin A.** Vitamin A activity occurs in foods of animal origin, primarily as retinyl palmitate, and in plant foods as provitamin A carotenoids of which beta-carotene is the most important. Approximately 50% of the vitamin A activity of American diets comes from the vitamin A in foods such as beef, pork, chicken and calves liver, butter fat, and egg yolks. The remainder comes from carotenoid-rich plants such as carrots, sweet potatoes, broccoli, and spinach.[39] The conjugated double bond structure of both vitamin A and the provitamin carotenoids makes them susceptible to oxidation. Vitamin A oxidation not only lowers the nutritive value of milk but also has been implicated in the development of off-flavors in milk. Dehydrated foods are most likely to lose vitamin activity as a result of oxidation during storage. Freeze-dried carrots become white on exposure to air for one to two weeks.

Thermal processing and cooking of foods can result in a reduction of vitamin A activity owing to degradative changes occurring in the provitamin A carotenoids. Canning causes the conversion of the more potent all-trans carotenoids to the less biologically active cis-isomers, thus lowering the vitamin A activity. In one study, vitamin A potency was reduced 15 to 28% in canned green vegetables and 30 to 35% in canned yellow vegetables as a result of the thermal processing involved in canning.[40] Carotene absorption from high-fiber foods, such as carrots, may be increased by cooking. This phenomenon may offset the lowered vitamin A activity resulting from cis-trans isomerization, but the degree to which this occurs is not known.

The instability of vitamin A to light is marked. In one study, the vitamin A content of homogenized milk stored in glass under fluorescent light was reduced 20% after three hours of exposure.[41] Vitamin A-fortified low-fat and skim milks are more susceptible to light-induced vitamin A degradation than unfortified whole milk. Sixty percent of the vitamin A in low-fat milks fortified with retinyl palmitate was lost in samples stored for three hours in fluorescent light.[41] Total parenteral nutrition solutions are susceptible to vitamin A degradation by light. In another study, total parenteral nutrition solutions exposed to daylight lost 90% of their vitamin A in six hours.[42]

**Other Fat-Soluble Vitamins.** Vitamin D is sensitive to both oxygen and light. Analysis of D compounds is difficult at food occurrence levels, and conclusions about D stability require careful replication. Vitamin K compounds are light-sensitive. Vitamin $K_1$, which occurs in green plants, is the predominant form in foodstuffs. Alpha-tocopherol, the most important tocopherol with respect to vitamin E activity, is an effective fat-phase antioxidant and can oxidize readily. Oxidation is catalyzed by low levels of copper. Bunnell et al. reported the alpha-tocopherol and total tocopherol contents of a wide variety of foods showed that the ordinary processes used in preparing foods for the table do not involve large losses.[43] Alpha-tocopherol in dried milk or fortified dried milk was stable for two years at room temperature in one study.[44,45] However, Bunnel et al. found significant losses of tocopherol during the storage of foods that had been cooked in vegetable oil.[43] High losses occurred in a relatively short time, even during freezer storage at $-12°C$. The researchers also found almost complete loss of the tocopherols in various cooking oils heated to high temperature. Hirai et al. reported similar results.[46] Vegetable oils are the major dietary sources of vitamin E, and it is important that vegetable oil processors monitor and minimize vitamin E losses during refining steps. Kanematsu et al. reported total tocopherol in refined oil to be 60 to 70% of that in crude oil.[47] Sunflower and safflower oil contain less total tocopherol but a higher percentage of alpha-tocopherol than soybean or rapeseed oils.

Of major interest is research on the inhibition of nitrosamine formation in bacon by alpha-tocopherol.[48] The Food and Drug Administration and the Department of Agriculture have approved the addition of alpha-tocopherol during bacon processing to reduce the nitrosamine content of fried bacon. Tocopherols are currently under investigation to assess the inhibition of nitrosamine formation in the gut.

## MINERALS

The literature on the effects of processing and home preparation on minerals in food is sparse. The two major potential effects of processing are changes in bioavailability and leaching of water solubles, but little specific information is available.

Intestinal tract absorption of minerals depends on the oxidation state of the cation, on whether the cation is bound to organic compounds, on the type of binding, and on the type of anions present in the food and in the GI tract during digestion. Insoluble compounds such as iron oxalates are poorly absorbed. Zinc in human milk is bound to high-molecular-weight protein fractions and has greater bioavailability than that in cow's milk as measured by treatment of infants with acrodermatitis enteropathica, a genetic disease caused by zinc deficiency.[49]

The milling of cereal grains, especially wheat, to prepare flours leads not only to reductions (40 to 60%) in fiber content, but also to concomitant losses in vitamins and minerals.[50] The effects of processing on the sodium:potassium and calcium:phosphorus content of six canned products, four frozen products, peanuts, wheat, and french fried potatoes have been reported by Wyatt and Ronan.[51] One study of the effect of reheating canned, cooked frozen, microwaved, and boiled foods on mineral retention was conducted under defined laboratory conditions for apples, sweet potatoes, spinach, peas, yellow summer squash, lima beans, and carrots.[52] Retention could not be calculated for chromium, cobalt, molybdenum, and selenium because the quantity present was at or near the level of detection. Retention was calculated for calcium, copper, iron, magnesium, manganese, phosphorus, potassium, sodium, and zinc. The average retention was 80 to 100%, with highest retention for the cooked, previously frozen product and lowest retention for the cooked, previously canned product.

Bender points out that the uptake of minerals from processing and cooking water may actually be of dietary importance.[53] Special precautions must be taken in processing low-sodium foods because softened water may contain 50 mg Na/dl. Brining to prevent the discoloration of vegetables and for quality grading leaves sodium on the product even after rinsing. Meat preparation under Kosher regulations requiring the salting out of blood also augments sodium by several fold. With the advent of sodium labeling, more food companies are monitoring and, in many cases, slowly decreasing the amount of added sodium in canned and frozen foods.

In canned foods, sodium and other solutes tend to be distributed uniformly between the food and the liquid. Blanching peas before canning in one study had little effect on sodium, iron, calcium, magnesium, or phosphorus levels, but potassium was reduced 25%.[54] According to Meiners et al., the cooking water of legumes contains measurable amounts of all the minerals studied (nine) and surprisingly high amounts of magnesium, phosphorous, and potassium.[55] Their data are presented in such a manner that the percentage of leaching cannot be determined. Legume cooking may be an exceptional case with respect to leaching because of the lengthy cooking period required. In a study of beans, broad beans, cowpeas, chick-peas, and lentils, potassium retention after cooking was 70 to 77%, copper 57 to 85%, zinc 91 to 100%, and iron 90 to 100%.[14]

## Iron

Only a portion of dietary iron can be absorbed; therefore, it has been assumed that the bioavailability of dietary iron is a major determinant of body iron stores. According to Cook, although there is little direct evidence for this assumption, the high prevalence of iron deficiency in developing countries correlates better with the quality of the diet than with total iron intake.[56] We ingest both heme and non-heme iron, but their transport mechanisms from lumen to mucosal cell are different. The larger dietary iron source is non-heme iron, which must be reduced ($Fe^{++}$) and be soluble within the lumen to be absorbed. The absorption of iron is greatly influenced by the nature of the meal,[57] because foods differ in their content of factors that promote or inhibit reduction and solubility.

Heme iron is absorbed as the intact iron porphyrin complex and is catabolized in the mucosa. Heme iron in developed countries accounts for one third of the iron absorbed even though only 5 to 10% of dietary iron is from meat; therefore, the meat content of the diet correlates well with iron status in population studies.[58] Approximately one third of the meat products consumed in the United States are cured meats, i.e., products treated with nitrite to convert the heme pigments to the more stable nitroso derivatives. This group includes frankfurters, bologna, cured ham, bacon, and corned beef. Lee and Gregor assessed the effect of nitrite curing on iron bioavailability from bologna-type sausages in both rats and humans and concluded that the cured meat product studied had no significant difference in iron bioavailability compared to the uncured meat product.[59]

Non-heme iron absorption is enhanced two- to four-fold by the presence of animal protein in the meal.[60] The efficiency of fortifying the diet with iron depends on the nature of the diet to which iron is added.[55] The most effective enhancer of iron absorption is ascorbic acid. The absorption of iron in a meal can be increased three- to seven-fold by the presence of orange juice and/or fresh fruit or ascorbic acid per se.[61–63]

Inhibitors of iron absorption include tea, coffee, specific vegetable proteins, and bran. The formation of highly insoluble iron tannates makes tea the most potent inhibitor of iron absorption; coffee is less potent. The coffee inhibitors are probably polyphenolic compounds.[64] Various soy proteins inhibit non-heme iron absorption, and this inhibition can be significantly offset by ascorbic acid.[65] Bran, irrespective of phytate content, decreases iron absorption in a dose-dependent manner.[66] Pectin and cellulose do not inhibit absorption; therefore, the type of dietary fiber and not dietary fiber per se must be considered.[56] Camire and Clydesdale found that the addition of ascorbic acid to wheat bran completely inhibited the in vitro binding of added ferrous iron.[67]

Lee has reviewed the effects of processing on iron absorption,[68] and Clydesdale[69,70] as well as Smith[71] have studied and reviewed the physicochemical reactions in food on solubility and the free energy state of iron. For the most part, beneficial changes in chemical form and solubility have been demonstrated with processing and storage, as well as with processing that decreased pH, thus increasing solubility.

The industry is increasingly developing formulated and fabricated foods with added nutrients. The bioavailability of specific iron compounds was rated by the Select Committee on GRAS Substances.[72] Rated adequate were reduced (elemental) iron, ferrous sulfate, ferric carbonate, and organic ferrous salts (ascorbate, gluconate, lactate, citrate, and fumarate). Rated low were ferric phosphate, ferric pyrophosphate, ferric sodium pyrophosphate, oxides of iron, and ferrous carbonate. Iron in a mixed diet is considered 10% bioavailable, ranging from 2% of the iron in spinach, because of insoluble oxalates, to 40% of a reference dose of ferrous ascorbate in a borderline deficient individual.[73]

## PROTEIN AND AMINO ACIDS

The essential amino acid content of a protein is a relative indicator of its protein nutritive value provided the protein is digestible and/or the limiting essential amino acid is bioavailable. Processing can both increase and decrease the nutritive value of protein. Five types of changes attributable to processing can be identified: (1) Mild heat treatment, such as occurs in blanching (60°C), is sufficient to denature, that is, alter the tertiary structure of the protein, and this change has *no* effect on nutritive value; however, the specific enzymic or hormonal activity of protein molecules is lost, and considerable changes in the chemical properties of significance in food technology occur. Changes in solubility, elasticity, and viscosity, among others, alter the functional properties of the protein as a food. (2) Mild heat treatment in the presence of sufficient moisture and reducing substances (usually a monosaccharide) results in a linkage of the epsilon amino group of lysine with the reducing group, which cannot be hydrolyzed by the digestive enzymes. This is the Maillard or nonenzymatic browning reaction. This mechanism causes bread with a brown crust to have no protein nutritive value in contrast to the interior bread crumb that retains its protein value. (3) More severe heating (115°C) converts lysine and other amino acids, in particular cystine, to other compounds (e.g., methylmercaptan), decreasing the protein nutritive value and digestibility. (4) Excessive heat (180 to 300°C) over time leads to decomposition of the amino acids and formation of cross-linkages and compounds such as lysinoalanine and other polyamino acids. This process occurs to various degrees in roasting meat and baking biscuits and is the source of several flavor compounds. Nutritive value is decreased because essential amino acid decomposition has occurred. (5) Protein changes may also occur with alkali treatment and oxidation.

Mild heat treatment is an important method for inactivating naturally occurring toxicants such as hemagglutinins and trypsin inhibitors. Mild alkali treatment can be used to destroy toxins, to improve functional properties, and to solubilize protein in the preparation of protein isolates. Mild alkali treatment can either enhance or reduce protein nutritive value. Lachance and Molina developed a process based on the combined use of 0.075% sodium hydroxide for one hour and treatment with a proteolytic enzyme to extract coconut protein and then demonstrated its equivalency to casein as a protein source.[74] Sanderson et al. reported that the alkaline treatment of corn to prepare tortilla flour and hominy resulted in losses of arginine and cystine and led to the formation of lysinoalanine.[75] However, the alkaline treatment increases the bioavailability of the bound niacin, and there is no evidence of a decrease in protein nutritive value.[76] Proteins respond differently to alkali treatment depending on the number and positions of the reactive groups. Loss of amino acids, especially cystine and the formation of lysinoalanine, increases with severity of alkali treatment.

To assess effects on soy protein quality, DeGroot and Slump alkali-treated various soy protein products at pH 12 for eight hours at 60°C,[77] and Woodward and Short alkali-treated soy protein products at 40°C for four hours.[78] The protein nutritive value index fell from 63 to 41, whereas that of the isolate dropped to 24. Casein similarly treated dropped from 63 to 53. Lysinoalanine per se is nephrotoxic,[79] but it does not appear to be harmful when it is part of an intact protein.[80] Steinberg found lysinoalanine to be widely distributed in foods in amounts ranging from 50 ng/g to 50 mg/g.[81] Its occurrence in fried egg white is surprising.

Food storage may decrease protein quality by the nonenzymatic browning reaction of reducing sugars with protein, but it is difficult to evaluate the practical significance of this reaction in foods.

Potato protein contains satisfactory ratios of the nutritionally limiting amino acids in most human diets—lysine, threonine, tryptophan, and methionine. Theoretically, therefore, potato chips with a 5% protein content may be a good protein source, but there are no data on the effects of frying and browning reactions on the quality of potato chip protein.

When herring meal is stored in air, as opposed to in nitrogen, available lysine is decreased. Further evidence that lipid oxidation can affect protein quality is a study in which the use of oxidized oil to fry fish fillets decreased available lysine approximately 10% compared to a control product fried with fresh oil.[82]

## FAT

Three types of degradation changes can occur in fats and oils: (1) auto-oxidation (temperature up to 100°C), (2) thermal polymerization (200° to 300°), and (3) thermal oxidation ($\cong$200° with air). Many published nutrition studies on the effects of heated fats are based on findings with severely treated oils atypical of commercial and consumer practice. Such work is not of practical significance because the consumption of such severely damaged oil is not likely. The main symptoms observed in animal feeding experiments after ingestion of such overheated fats are decreased absorption of the fats and unsaturated fatty acids, growth depression that may be related to decreased food intake, decreased food efficiency, decreased motility of the GI tract, disturbances in chylomicron formation, enlarged livers and kidneys, and reduced fat stores of the body.[83]

Many decomposition products of severely heated fats have been isolated and identified. In one study, cottonseed oil was kept at 182°C for six 8-hour periods. After conversion to methyl esters, the distillable nonurea adductable fraction (DNUA) was separated into 136 components. Esters of alicyclic fatty acids made up 34% of the characterized material. These cyclic materials are probably responsible for the toxic effects seen when DNUA is isolated and fed to rats.[84] The actual content of cyclic fatty acid monomers in commercial frying oils used by fast food outlets in the United States and by street vendors in Egypt and Israel has been reported.[85] The United States samples ranged from 0.1 to 0.5% cyclic monomers and from 1 to 8% polar and noneluted thermal oxidation products. The Middle East samples showed significantly more heat abuse: cyclic monomers, 0.2 to 7% and polar products, 2 to 22%.

Heating corn oil, cottonseed oil, safflower oil, and shortening for 7.5 hours to fry potatoes caused linoleic acid losses of 4 to 11%.[86] Oxidative rancidity results in gradual loss of essential fatty acid activity in a fat and also an increase in the concentration of fatty acid peroxides that may be more or less toxic, accompanied by destruction of carotenoids, vitamin A, tocopherols, and vitamin E. Such oxidation may occur at any stage of storage, processing, or use of fats and oils. It also causes rancidity, so that the consumer is not likely to consume badly oxidized fat.

Thermal polymers, however, cannot be readily tested, and any process in which thermal polymerization is suspected should be thoroughly checked. A significant drop in the iodine value of fats and oils occurs with thermal polymerization. It is therefore easy for a processor to monitor potential polymerization by measuring the iodine value. This is not currently feasible for individual fast food restaurants, and additional work is necessary in this area of food supply.

Highly unsaturated oils have a shorter shelf life during home storage than do products such as olive oil and cottonseed oil. Tocopherols are the natural antioxidants of vegetable oils. Animal fats contain low tocopherol levels and may have a short oxidative shelf life even though they have low unsaturated fatty acid levels.

Vegetable oil refining (i.e., removing free fatty acids, bleaching, and deodorizing) almost completely removes the carotenes and reduces the tocopherols in oils. The tocopherol losses are minimal under proper processing conditions. These losses do not affect the quality of the triglycerides per se.

### *Trans* Fatty Acids

*Trans* fatty acids have been claimed to be implicated in hypercholesterolemia and atherosclerosis. The unsaturated fatty acids of naturally occurring fats and oils contain one or more double bonds in the *cis* position (i.e., the hydrogen atoms are on the same side of the double bond). During the hydrogenation process (usually partial) of various vegetable oils, such as in the manufacture of margarines, variable amounts of the *un*saturated fatty acids that are not hydrogenated are converted from the *cis* to the *trans* configuration (i.e., the hydrogen atoms are now on the opposite sides of the double bond). This process of isomerization from *cis* to *trans* also occurs naturally in the rumen of sheep and cattle; therefore, *trans* fatty acids are found in the milk and fat of these animals.

*Trans* fatty acids of various types *(trans* monoenoic acid; *trans, trans* dienoic acid; *cis, trans* or *trans, cis* dienoic acids) are present in hydrogenated oils, tub and stick margarines, as well as in products that incorporate these ingredients such as bakery products and puddings.[87] American human subjects have been reported to possess 2 to 6% total *trans* fatty acids in adipose tissue and 1 to 3% in liver tissue.[88] There is disagreement on the precise quantities present in food and their effect, if any, on human metabolism.[89–92]

The average daily intake per person has been estimated at 12.1 g/day or 8% of fat ingested.[93] The most comprehensive study of the *trans* fatty acid content of important foods was published by Enig et al.[94] The fat in 220 samples of 35 food types was analyzed. The *trans* content (by weight of fat) was: stick margarines, 16 to 31%; tub margarines, 7 to 18%; vegetable shortenings, 9 to 35%; diet margarines, 11 to 13%; bread mixes, 8 to 33%; cakes, candies, frostings, 2 to 33%; cream substitutes, 0.4 to 12%; cookies and crackers, 2 to 34%; and snack chips, 0.4 to 30%. Most mayonnaise samples, salad dressings, salad oils, and potato chips did not contain *trans* fatty acids, nor did peanut butter.

By far, the most prevalent *trans* fatty acid in food is *trans* 18:1. In Enig's study of 220 products, only six samples had a total of *trans* dienoic acids (c,t 18:2, t,c 18:2, and t,t 18:2) above 5% and 175 had levels below 3%. It is desirable to assess the metabolism of *trans* 18:1 separately from that of the three 18:2 *trans* compounds in light of the large differences in food content of these compounds.

*Trans* fatty acids are absorbed and digested as well as their *cis* counterparts, but *trans* fatty acids appear to behave in their metabolism as saturated rather than as unsaturated fatty acids. *Trans* fatty acids have been identified in human milk.[95]

There is no evidence to support the implication that accumulation of *trans* fatty acids in tissues may somehow be related to atherosclerosis. Human studies conducted in three countries revealed no differences in tissue levels of *trans* fatty acids between subjects who died from atherosclerosis and controls who died from other causes.[96] *Trans* fatty acids are metabolized completely by rats and there is no good experimental evidence of any harmful effects. In one major study, 46 generations of rats were maintained with no adverse effects on a diet in which the sole source of fat was a hydrogenated margarine fat containing 7% *cis*-9, *cis*-12-linoleic acid, 3% isomers of linoleic acid, and 35% *trans* isomers of oleic acid.[97] After removal of the *trans* fatty acids from the diet of rats for nine months, only negligible amounts remained in various tissues (except adipose tissue). The rats fed *trans* fatty acids as compared to corn oil or lard had lower serum free and total cholesterol levels.[98]

A major concern expressed about the biologic

effects of *trans* fatty acids is the influence on membrane-bound enzymes and on membrane permeability to cholesterol and, thus, a potential acceleration of atherosclerosis. Feeding 3.2% and 6.6% *trans* fatty acids to rabbits did not produce aortic atherosclerosis different from that produced by the control diet even though serum cholesterol and triglycerides were elevated in the rabbits fed 6% *trans* fatty acids.[99] Kritchevsky noted that currently available data suggest no special deleterious role of *trans* fatty acids and that they are not especially contributory to the development of atherosclerosis.[100]

The consumer needs to understand that there is no cholesterol in plant foods irrespective of the claims on the label that imply it might have been removed. In addition, saturated fatty acids, hydrogenated fatty acids, and *trans* unsaturated fatty acids are essentially metabolized as saturated fatty acids. If there is a clinical interest in increasing *cis* unsaturated fatty acid intake, the recommendation should be to encourage the use of oils other than coconut, palm, and palm kernel oils, such as in nondairy creamers, and also to avoid oils that are *partially* hydrogenated, which is stated on the ingredient label.

## Oral and Tube Nutrition Formulas

A major advance in clinical nutrition has been the development and manufacture of an array of parenteral[101] and enteral[102,103] nutrition products. Any patient can now be fed every day regardless of the function of the gastrointestinal tract by means of enteral nutrition.

The enteral defined-formula diets are product line extensions of infant formula preparations for which there is now considerable experience. These products are either in powder or in liquid forms. The parenteral products are invariably in liquid form or may be prepared by pharmacy from dry premixes. The nutrients most sensitive to deterioration are vitamins. Protein quality also can become a concern in liquid preparations because all the conditions except heat are present for the Maillard reaction between the epsilon amino group of lysine and a reducing sugar. If this reaction occurs, it can substantially reduce protein quality.

The stability of vitamins in well-packaged dry (low water activity) environments is good. Shelf life losses of sensitive nutrients such as ascorbic acid are anticipated by small overages at the time of formulation, and the label claim is guaranteed to the expiration date provided the conditions for storage are not abused. The same is true for hermetically sealed liquid products. Stability data that is part of the quality assurance data of the manufacturer is not widely disseminated in the open literature but is available by direct inquiry to the manufacturer. Analogous data have been published for dried or low-moisture products, namely six-month storage at 23°C of fortified flour for baked goods, including key nutrients such as vitamin A and folic acid.[104,105] Favorable clinical experience with protein and other nutrient bioavailabilities has been reported for some enteral formulas.[106,107]

The best guidance is to suspect any product whose history of storage cannot be ascertained or whose package integrity appears compromised (pin holes or poor seams in aluminum foil laminate pouches, or cans that are bulging or are dented).

## REFERENCES

1. Lee, C.Y., Massey, L.M., VanBuren, J.P.: J. Food Sci. *47*:961, 1982.
2. Rizvi, S.S.H., Acton, J.C.: Food Technol. *36*:105, 1982.
3. Zalusky, R., Herbert, V.: N. Engl. J. Med. *265*:1033, 1961.
4. Holman, W.I.M.: Nutr. Abstr. Rev. *26*:277, 1956.
5. DeRitter, E.: Food Technol. *30*:48, 1976.
6. Borenstein, B.: *In* Handbook of Food Additives. 2nd ed. (Furia, T., Ed.) Cleveland, CRC Press, 1972.
7. Lachance, P.A., Erdman, J.: *In* Nutritional Evaluation of Food Processing. (Harris, R., Karmas, E., Eds.) Westport, CT, AVI Publishing Co., 1975.
8. Harris, R.S.: *In* Nutritional Evaluation of Food Processing. (Harris, R.S. von Loesecke, H., Eds.) New York, John Wiley & Sons, 1960.
9. Hallberg, L., et al.: Am. J. Clin. Nutr. *36*:846, 1982.
10. Snyder, P.O., and Matthews, M.E.: J. Am. Diet. Assoc. *83*:454, 1983.
11. Mallette, M.F., et al.: Ind. Eng. Chem. *38*:437, 1946.
12. Dwivedi, B., Arnold, R.: J. Agric. Food Chem. *21*:54, 1973.
13. Cook, B.B., Gunning, B., Uchimoto, D.: J. Agric. Food Chem. *9*:316, 1961.
14. Haytowitz, D.B., Matthews, R.H.: Cereal Foods World *28*:362, 1983.
15. Sattar, H., deMan, J.M.: J. Can. Inst. Food Sci. Technol. *6*:170, 1973.
16. USDA: Economic Research Service National Food Review (NFR-1) D.C., 1978.
17. Makinde, M.A., Lachance, P.A.: Nutr. Rept. Intl. *14*:671, 1976.
18. Gregory, J.F., Hiner, M.E.: J. Food Sci. *48*:1323, 1983.
19. Gregory, J.F., Kirk, J.R.: J. Food Sci. *43*:1801, 1978.
20. Yonker, C.B., Lachance, P.A.: Food Quality. In Press, 1986. cf. Yonker, C.: Determination of B-6 vitamer degradation kinetics of HPLC. Ph.D. Thesis, Rutgers University, New Brunswick, N.J., 1983.
21. Everson, G.J., et al.: Food Technol. *18*:87, 1964.
22. Polansky, M.M., Toepfer, E.W.: Cereal Chem. *46*:664, 1969.
23. Perera, A.D., Leklem, J.E., Miller, L.T.: Cereal Chem. *56*:577, 1979.
24. Ang, C.Y.W.: J. Assoc. Off. Anal. Chem. *62*:1170, 1979.
25. Walsh, J.H., Wyse, B.W., Hansen, R.G.: J. Am. Diet. Assoc. *78*:140, 1981.

26. Paine-Wilson, B., Chen, T.S.: J. Food Sci. *44*:717, 1979.
27. Chen, T.S., Copper, R.G.: J. Food Sci. *44*:713, 1979.
28. Ervin, M.S., Lachance, P.A.: J. Food Quality. In press, 1986, cf. Ervin, M.: Determination of kinetic parameters of folacin analogs using an HPLC assay. Ph.D Thesis, Rutgers University, New Brunswick, N.J., 1983.
29. Ristow, K.A., Gregory, J.F., Damron, B.L.: J. Agric. Food Chem. *30*:801, 1982.
30. Leichter, J., Switzer, V.P., Landymore, A.F.: Nutr. Rep. Int. *18*:475, 1978.
31. Gregory, J.F.: J. Nutr. *112*:1329, 1982.
32. Colman, N., Hettiarachchy, N., Herbert, V.: Science *211*:1427, 1981.
33. Alm, L.: J. Dairy Sci. *65*:353, 1982.
34. Keagy, P.M., Stokstad, E.L.R., Fellers, D.A.: Cereal Chem. *52*:348, 1975.
35. Herbert, V., Jacob, E.: JAMA *230*:241, 1974.
36. Newmark, H., et al.: Am. J. Clin. Nutr. *29*:645, 1976.
37. Herbert, V., et al.: Am. J. Clin. Nutr. *31*:253, 1978.
38. Ekvall, S., Chen, I., Bozian, R.: Am. J. Clin. Nutr. *34*:1356, 1981.
39. FNB (Food and Nutrition Board, National Research Council): Recommended Dietary Allowances. 9th ed. Washington, D.C., National Academy of Sciences, 1980.
40. Sweeney, J.P., and Marsh, A.C.: J. Am. Diet. Assoc. *59*:238, 1971.
41. Thompson, J.N., Erdody, P.: J. Inst. Can. Sci. Technol. Aliment. *7*:157, 1974.
42. Allwood, M.C.: J. Parenter. Enter. Nutr. *7*:192, 1983.
43. Bunnell, R.H., et al.: Am. J. Clin. Nutr. *17*:1, 1965.
44. Metecka, M.: Zesk. Nauk.-Akad. Ekon, Paznamic (Poland) Ser. *1*:19, 1981.
45. Wollard, D.C., Edmiston, A.D.: N.Z. Dairy Sci. Technol. *18*:21, 1983.
46. Hirai, K., Ohtani, T., Miyagawa, K.: Osakashiritsu Daigaku Seikatsukagakubu *30*:1, 1982.
47. Kanematsu, H., et al.: Ykagaku *32*:122, 1983.
48. Fiddler, W., et al.: J. Agric. Food Chem. *26*:653, 1978.
49. Eckhert, C.D., et al.: Science *195*:789, 1977.
50. Lachance, P.A.: *In* Adding Nutrients to Food: Where Do We Go from Here? (Vetter, J., Ed.) Minneapolis, Am. Assoc. Cer. Chem., 1982, pp. 31–41.
51. Wyatt, C.J., Ronan, K.: J. Agric. Food Chem. *31*:415, 1983.
52. Dudek, J., et al.: Nutritional Quality of Processed Foods. Washington, D.C., National Food Processors Assoc. Research Foundation, 1982.
53. Bender, A.E.: Food Processing and Nutrition. New York, Academic Press, 1978, p. 82.
54. Lee, C.Y., Parsons, G.F., Downing, D.L.: J. Food Sci. *47*:1034, 1982.
55. Meiners, C.R., et al.: J. Agric. Food Chem. *24*:1126, 1976.
56. Cook, J.D.: Food Technol. *37*:124, 1983.
57. Layrisse, M., Martinez-Torres, C., Roche, M.: Am. J. Clin. Nutr. *21*:1175, 1968.
58. Bothwell, T.H., et al.: Iron Metabolism in Man. Oxford, Blackwell Scientific, 1979, p. 7.
59. Lee, K., Gregor, J.L.: Food Technol. *37*:139, 1983.
60. Cook, J.D., Monsen, E.R.: Am. J. Clin. Nutr. *29*:859, 1976.
61. Layrisse, M., Martinez-Torres, C., Gonzolez, M.: Am. J. Clin. Nutr. *27*:152, 1974.
62. Cook, J.D., Monsen, E.R.: Am. J. Clin. Nutr. *30*:235, 1977.
63. Hallberg, L., Rossander, L.: Am. J. Clin. Nutr. *39*:577, 1984.
64. Morck, T.A., Lynch, S.R., Cook, J.D.: Am. J. Clin. Nutr. *37*:416, 1983.
65. Morck, T.A., Lynch, S.R., Cook, J.D.: Am. J. Clin. Nutr. *36*:219, 1982.
66. Simpson, K.M., Morris, E.R., Cook, J.D.: Am. J. Clin. Nutr. *37*:1469, 1981.
67. Camire, A.L., Clydesdale, F.M.: J. Food. Sci. *47*:1296, 1982.
68. Lee, K.: *In* Nutritional Bioavailability of Iron (Kies, Ed.) Symp. Series No. 203, Washington, D.C., Am. Chem. Soc., 1982, p. 27.
69. Clydesdale, F.M.: *In* Nutritional Bioavailability of Iron. (Kies, Ed.) Symp. Series No. 203. Washington, D.C., Am. Chem. Soc., 1982, p. 55.
70. Clydesdale, F.M.: Food Technol. *37*:133, 1983.
71. Smith: Food Technol. *37*:115, 1983.
72. Life Sciences Research Office: Evaluation of the Health Aspects of Iron Salts as Food Ingredients. Bethesda, MD, Fed. of Am. Soc. for Expt. Biol., 1980.
73. Hallberg, L.: Annu. Rev. Nutr. *1*:123, 1981.
74. Lachance, P.A., Molina, M.: J. Food Sci. *39*:581, 1974.
75. Sanderson, J., et al.: Cereal Chem. *55*:204, 1978.
76. Bressani, R., et al.: J. Nutr. *97*:173, 1969.
77. DeGroot, A.P., Slump, P.: J. Nutr. *98*:45, 1969.
78. Woodward, J.C., Short, D.D.: J. Nutr. *103*:569, 1973.
79. Woodward, J.C., et al.: Food Cosmet. Toxicol. *15*:109, 1977.
80. VanBeek, L., Feron, V.J., DeGroot, A.P.: J. Nutr. *104*:1630, 1974.
81. Sternberg, M., Kim, C.V., Schwende, F.J.: Science *190*:992, 1975.
82. Tooley, W.H., Lawrie: J. Food Technol. *9*:247, 1974.
83. Perkins, E.G.: Rev. Fr. Corp. Gras. *23*:313, 1976.
84. Artman, N.R., Smith, D.E.: J. Am. Oil Chem. Soc. *49*:318, 1972.
85. Frankel, E.N., et al.: J. Am. Oil Chem. Soc. *61*:87,1984.
86. Kilgore, L., Bailey, M.: J. Am. Diet. Assoc. *56*:130, 1970.
87. Carpenter, D.L., Slover, H.T.: J. Am. Oil Chem. Soc. *50*:372, 1973.
88. Ohlrogge, J.B., Emken, E.A., Gully, R.M.: J. Lipid Res. *22*:955, 1981.
89. Kaunitz, H.: Z. Ernahrungswiss *15*:26, 1976.
90. Kummerow, F.A.: J. Food Sci. *40*:21, 1975.
91. Alfin-Slater, R., Aftergood, L.: *In* Geometric and Positional Fatty Acid Isomers. (Emken, Dutton, Eds.) Champaign, IL, Am. Oil Chem. Soc., 1979, p. 53.
92. Kinsella, I.E., et al.: Am. J. Clin. Nutr. *34*:2307, 1981.
93. Enig, M.G., Munn, R.J., Keeney, M.: Fed. Proc. *37*:2215, 1978.
94. Enig, M.G., et al.: J. Am. Oil Chem. Soc. *60*:1788, 1983.
95. Aitchison, J.M., Dunkeley, W.I., Canolty, N.L., et al.: Am. J. Clin. Nutr. *30*:2006, 1977.
96. Applewhite, T.H.: J. Am. Oil Chem. Soc. *58*:260–269, 1981.
97. Alfin-Slater, R., et al.: J. Nutr. *63*:241, 1957.
98. Moore, C.E., Alfin-Slater, R.B., Aftergood, L.: Am. J. Clin. Nutr. *33*:2318–2323, 1980.
99. Ruttenberg, H., et al.: J. Nutr. *113*:835, 1983.
100. Kritchevsky, D.: *In* Dietary Fats and Health. (Per-

kins, E.G., Visek, W.J. Eds.) Champaign, IL, Am. Oil Chem. Soc., 1983, pp. 403–413.

101. Wretlind, A.: History and overview of parenteral nutrition. *In* Human Nutrition—Clinical and Biochemical Aspects. (Garry, P.J., Ed.) Washington, D.C., Am. Assoc. Clin. Chem., 1981, pp. 323–351.

102. Bistrian, B.R., Wade, J.E.: Feeding the hospitalized patient. *In* Human Nutrition—Clinical and Biochemical Aspects. (Garry, P.J., Ed.) Washington, D.C., Am. Assoc. Clin. Chem., 1981, p. 352.

103. Shils, M.E. (Ed.): Defined Formula Diets for Medical Purposes. Chicago, American Medical Association, 1977.

104. Cort, W.M., Borenstein, B., Harley, J.H., et al.: Food Technol. *30*:52–62, 1976.

105. Emodi, A., Scialpi, L.: Cereal Chem. *57*:1, 1980.

106. Copelan, H., Lachance, P., Mohammed, K.: Nutr. Rep. Int. *8*:49–59, 1973.

107. Heymsfield, S.B., Bleier, J., Whitmire, L., et al.: Am. J. Clin. Nutr. *39*:243–250, 1984.

*Chapter* **38**

# NATURALLY OCCURRING FOOD-BORNE TOXICANTS

## Paul M. Newberne

Diet and nutrition are not synonymous; diet is the total of various substances consumed whereas nutrition includes only those substances that serve to nourish the individual. Toxic and non-nutritive substances are usually excluded from nutrition considerations even though they often interact with nutrients and exert enormous effects on the health of the individual.

Inadequate quality or quantity or an imbalance of nutrients as well as the presence of toxins in the diet may contribute to disease. Nutrition should, therefore, be concerned with the entire spectrum of health, including preventive and therapeutic medicine. This goal demands continued investigations about the metabolism and interactions of nutrients and other dietary components, including toxins.

Malnutrition occurs in the United States. It is particularly severe in other areas of the world where it appears at the end of a chain of conditions extending across national and political borders. Whatever actions may comprise appropriate solutions must include a worldwide increase in the production of food. This implies not only an increase in conventional sources but the introduc-

tion of new and novel foods and the continued use of pesticides that carry with them the potential, albeit small, for minor questions of safety.

There is a myth in the marketplace today about "all natural ingredients."[1] The identical food, containing safe food additives, stays on the shelf longer, tastes as good or better than the "all natural" foods, and is less expensive. Consumer gullibility is at an all-time high; "natural" means profits to packagers aware of the myth. Ninety-nine percent of food is natural. The remaining 1% is composed of intentional additives.

Public concern about food hazards centers on the dangers posed by such items as polychlorinated biphenyl compounds (PCBs) and mercury contamination, or red dye No. 2 and saccharin additives; however, it is naive to think that removing all additives, or purchasing only foods labeled "natural," eliminates poisons from food. On the contrary, numerous natural poisons occur in food.

For example, the potato contains 150 distinct chemicals including the alkaloid solanine, oxalic acid, arsenic, tannins, and nitrate, all of which are toxic. Carrots, nutmeg, and pepper contain myristicene, a narcotic and psychomimetic. Arsenic is found in shrimp. Some compounds in cabbage can cause goiters; others inhibit cancer. Bananas and cheese contain vasoactive amines, naturally occurring toxicants that can markedly increase blood pressure and cause other vascular effects.

What does natural mean? Natural is a vague term—a word that may be in need of legal definition. The Food and Drug Administration has not defined the word natural in relation to articles of food and drink. Its only policy prohibiting the term is with products containing artificial colors, artificial flavorings, and synthetic ingredients including chemical additives. This leaves a good deal of room for misrepresentation.

Nitrates and nitrites, famous as the additives used in cured meats, ham, and wieners, are possible carcinogens. What is less well known is that these famous putative hazards also occur naturally in many green leafy vegetables such as spinach. These ingested nitrates are also broken down into nitrite in saliva. Bacteria in the human intestine even synthesize this chemical. Thus, we could not avoid consuming nitrates, or prevent their synthesis in our bodies, no matter how we might try. The same could be said for most of the toxins that now occur in our foods. We have lived with most of them for centuries and will continue to live with them; they are not new to the human race.

There are thousands of chemical compounds in the diet of man, but only a few of them have important nutritional significance. The concept that toxicity may be produced by chemical entities that are normal ingredients of plant and animal foodstuffs continues to gain acceptance and documentation. The increasing complexity of our modern industrial society and the wide-ranging nature of the international food trade have increased the risk of contamination of foods by chemical and biologic agents. However, nature has exceeded man in the introduction of toxic substances into foods. In our broadening search for new sources of food and for additional uses for old sources of food, we must be alert to the potential for natural and man-made toxicity occasioned by harmful chemicals in foods eaten as they are grown, or by chemicals entering foods as accidental contaminants or as a result of food processing. We must not, however, ban the use of substances and procedures that enhance quality, quantity, and shelf life, nor should we entertain other unfounded fears of pollution.

Although food contamination may arise from man-made industrial pollution (mercury, lead, arsenic), agricultural technology (fertilizers, pesticides), or food processing (nitrosamines, poly-nuclear hydrocarbons), some of the more dangerous food contaminants occur naturally in plant and animal foodstuffs, such as plant toxins, pathogenic microorganisms, or fungal toxins, many of which we can do little or nothing about. Thus, the primary concern of this chapter is to address those components of the diet, natural or man-made, that have adverse effects on health. We do have control over some of these by one means or another; others we must accept.

Naturally occurring toxicants have been generally accorded a lower order of concern, in terms of human health, than have non-nutritive components, including contaminants. Increasing use of plant foodstuffs containing low levels of toxicants to which human populations may be exposed over long periods forces a reassessment of this area. Numerous surveys have identified large numbers of chemicals added to foods by man as well as those that are natural toxicants or contaminants. From this extensive assemblage, only a few have been chosen for examination in this chapter. A certain element of comfort is provided by the statement by a recent FDA commissioner that our food supply is "incredibly safe."[2]

## TOXINS FROM PLANT FOODS

Although large numbers of poisonous plants have compounds that have been chemically characterized, they have not been carefully examined, either chemically or biologically, as to their effects on health. They constitute only a small fraction of the total food supply and therefore are considered a low risk to human health.

When subjected to a variety of stress conditions, most commonly due to fungal invasion, many plants undergo metabolic changes that can result in the production and accumulation of abnormal, toxic metabolites. Most notable are those plant "stress" metabolites possessing antifungal activity (the phytoalexins).[3] Genetic manipulation to create new plant varieties may result in the introduction of the stress mechanism.

Specific examples of types of substances in food and feed plants considered important in human health are summarized here.

### Protease Inhibitors

Compounds that can inhibit the proteolytic activity of certain enzymes are found throughout the plant kingdom, mainly in legumes. One of the most studied inhibitors, trypsin inhibitor, is present in raw soybeans. This factor was first described by Read and Haas in 1938[4] and independently discovered by Ham and Sandstedt in 1944.[5] In 1917, Osborne and Mendel showed that rats grew better after the soybean had been heated.[6] Emphasis has shifted from the poor absorption of the sulfur amino acids in raw soybeans to a disturbance in the metabolism of cystine and methionine when raw soybeans are fed to rats.[7]

At present, there is no valid explanation for the growth-inhibiting action of raw soybeans. Most of the harmful biologic effects observed when raw soybeans are fed largely disappear when the meal is properly roasted. Trypsin inhibitors are well known for the effects observed with raw soybeans, but most of these effects are easily dealt with.

Protease inhibitors may have some unexpected beneficial effects; a number of investigations indicate that some of them may provide protection against induced carcinogenesis in animal models,[8,9] suggesting such a role in human populations.

## Hemagglutinins

Many botanical groups, including mono- and dicotyledons, molds, and lichens, contain substances that have the property of agglutinating red blood cells. These compounds have been collectively classified as phytohemagglutinins or lectins.[10]

The first of these compounds to be identified was extracted from castor beans by Stillmark.[11] It agglutinates the red cells from both human and animal blood. The nutritional significance of the phytohemagglutinins is detailed in a number of papers in the literature.[12] Much of the toxic fraction of hemagglutinins is destroyed or neutralized in the digestive tract, and only a relatively small amount appears to be absorbed.

In addition to the castor bean, other plant materials contain phytohemagglutinins; these include soybeans, peanuts, red kidney beans (phytohemagglutinin A), black beans (phaseolotoxin A), yellow wax beans (hemagglutinin), and jack beans (concanavalin A).[13] These compounds have profound effects on mitosis and constitute an important class of environmental toxins.

Some of the hemagglutinins, such as ricin from the castor bean, produce an intense inflammation with destruction of epithelial cells of the gastrointestinal tract; local hemorrhages may also be observed elsewhere. Liver, kidney, and heart damage have also been reported for several of them. The important effect on lymphocytes is the induction of mitosis. This effect has made some of these compounds (mitogens) useful in biomedical work, particularly in studies related to immunocompetence where exposure in vitro causes lymphocytes to increase DNA synthesis and to undergo changes equated with cell division. These proteins are associated in the plant with other protein material and thus are not easily detected by chemical analysis. Instead, they currently must be determined by their biologic activities.

## Lathyrism

Lathyrism is a neurologic disease seen in human subjects who have consumed large amounts of *Lathyrus sativus* (chickling vetch), *L. cicera* (flat-podded vetch), or *L. clymenum* (Spanish vetchling).[14] *L. sativus* is cultivated in India and grows wild in the Tian Shan mountains of western China. *L. cicera* is used to feed cattle in France, Italy, and Algeria and to make bread when wheat is in short supply. *L. clymenum* is grown in Spain, North Africa, and the Orient.

Human lathyrism is often referred to as neurolathyrism.[15] This condition usually develops in individuals between the ages of 15 and 30 years, more often in men.[16] The first symptom is a feeling of heaviness of the legs, with weakness setting in shortly thereafter. While the individual is standing, the leg muscles become tremulous, and when he starts to walk he may drag his feet. The leg muscles may become spastic and rigid. The gait becomes jerky; short steps are taken by walking on the balls of the feet. Tingling sensations are felt in various parts of the body. Complete loss of sensation to heat and pain may occur.[17] Most of these symptoms are associated with lesions of the lateral pyramidal tracts and funiculi of Goll of the spinal cord.[16] Attempts to associate lathyrism with dietary deficiencies of nutrients have not been fruitful, and evidence is overwhelming that the etiologic agent is in the seeds of various lathyrus plants.[18,19] The substance has not been identified.

The collagen of rats with odoratism (produced by feeding considerable amounts of *L. odoratus*) is abnormal both in form and distribution,[20] resulting in a reduction in its tensile strength. Studies with isotopic sulfur indicate that the primary change is a failure in the formation of chondroitin sulfates A and C and their complexes with proteins resulting in a defect in fibrogenesis.[21] The defect in odoratism involving primarily collagen formation is in sharp contrast to the human disease of lathyrism in which the essential lesion involves the nervous tissue.

## Favism

Sensitivity to fava or broad beans appears to be an example of an inherited metabolic disturbance. In sensitive individuals, inhalation of pollen from these plants or ingestion of the bean in either the cooked or raw state produces a hemolytic anemia. Such individuals have a deficiency of glucose-6-phosphate dehydrogenase and reduced glutathione levels in their blood.[22] The glutathione level in the red blood cells of sensitive individuals is still further reduced following the eating of fava beans; the mechanism of this action is unknown. The individuals recover once the hemolysis ceases.[23]

Most sensitive individuals are children of parents who originated from the Mediterranean area, Asia, or Taiwan.[24] Because the enzymatic deficiency in favism appears to be common to a number of other disturbances, it is assumed to be transmitted in the same way, i.e., sex-linked. The mother of the affected male carries the genetic defect.[24] The enzymatic defect is common in blacks in the United States, but favism is rarely seen in these individuals.

The toxic substance in fava beans may be vicine (2,4 diamino-6-hydroxypyrimidine-β-D-glycopyranose),[25] present in fava beans to the extent of about 0.5% of their dry weight, but this has not been firmly established.

### Hepatotoxins

At least 25 species of the *Senecio* genus of plants are poisonous to livestock and human beings. An important characteristic of toxins from these sources is the delayed liver damage in animals and man.[26] Senecio disease often occurs in human populations from breads contaminated with seeds from the poisonous plants.[27] The chemistry of several of these compounds has been established.[26]

In some areas of the United States, the seeds of Crotalaria are present in wheat and corn harvested from land where the plants grow interspersed among the grain plants. Mechanical harvesters collect both grain and the poisonous seeds of the Crotalaria.[28]

The alkaloids produced by the *Senecio* plants are potent liver toxins with a profound effect on mitosis. In low to moderate exposure they produce a delayed effect, including veno-occlusive disease and cirrhosis in man; in animals, liver cancer is also induced.[29,30]

Plants of the genus that produce the toxic alkaloids are used to make teas in the southeastern Unites States and in Curacao. Consumption of these teas has been associated with esophageal and other forms of cancer in man.[31] Only a few publications are available on mechanisms of actions of the toxins, and the data are not conclusive.[32] The hepatotoxicity appears to be due to the formation of pyrrolic metabolites.[33] Some of these toxins can be transferred via milk to a mother's offspring, constituting a potential hazard to children.[34]

### Mycotoxins

There are a large number of fungal toxins in foods but only a few of them appear to be of real or potential danger to the health of man. These include the aflatoxins, patulin, ochratoxin, penicillic acid, and trichothecene toxins. Only two of these families are of sufficient significance to be addressed here. They are the aflatoxins, now known to be hepatotoxic for man[35] and animals and carcinogenic for many animal species,[36] and Fusaria toxins.

**Aflatoxins.** Indications for man's susceptibility to aflatoxin poisoning derive from epidemiologic evidence, an outbreak in India, a childhood disease in Thailand (Reye's syndrome), and a limited number of experiments designed to define the pattern of aflatoxin metabolism by the liver in vitro. From this data it seems that, compared with some experimental animal species, man is relatively resistant to both the acute and chronic effects, although aflatoxin $B_1$ has been declared a human carcinogen by WHO.[37]

Interspecies differences and many other factors influence an individual's response.[38] Female animals and castrated males are more resistant to both the acute and chronic effects of aflatoxin; women are somewhat less susceptible than men to the carcinogenic effects of dietary aflatoxin.[37] Furthermore, in animals, nutrition plays an important role in both acute toxicity and chronic disease.[39–43] High-protein diets are generally protective from the acute toxic effects because they enable the detoxifying enzymes of the liver to function optimally. In some cases, however, they activate other procarcinogens to the active form. Protein deficiency or excess, certain vitamin deficiencies, and diets rich in saturated and unsaturated fats render the animal more susceptible to aflatoxin poisoning.

An assessment of man's likely exposure to aflatoxin can be based on the fact that cow's milk is a nearly universal major food and that animal feedstuffs are occasionally contaminated with aflatoxin.[37,48,49] When this happens it can be assumed that cow's milk will almost certainly contain the toxic metabolite aflatoxin M. With a typical analytic detection limit of 0.04 ppb, up to 0.02 ppb of this toxin could escape detection and yet be ingested by man in his daily half-liter of milk.[41,44]

Definite conclusions regarding the hazards of aflatoxin exposure to man cannot be drawn at this time. Earlier epidemiologic studies suggested a correlation between primary liver cancer and exposure to aflatoxin in parts of Africa, the Philippines, and Thailand.[24–48] However, more recent investigations strongly suggest that the development of primary liver cancer is correlated with hepatitis B virus infection.[49–51]

Sudden deaths from acute encephalopathy and

fatty degeneration of the viscera have been as-cribed to aflatoxicosis.

A serious outbreak of acute aflatoxin poisoning in man and dogs in India began in October, 1975 in several tribal villages of the western states of Gujarat and Rajasthan.[35] The presenting features were jaundice, rapidly developing ascites, portal hypertension, and a high mortality rate. In most cases death was caused by massive gastrointes-tinal tract bleeding. Examination of the various items of feed collected randomly from the affected households showed that the maize content of af-latoxin varied from 6 to 15 ppm, which means that the affected subjects must have consumed 2 to 6 mg of toxin daily for almost a month. Analyses of tissues from victims of the outbreak revealed aflatoxin and some of the metabolites, confirming the tentative diagnosis.

A promising area of research in the human tox-icoses is that in which the adducts of aflatoxins in urine and other body fluids are used to monitor individuals who may be exposed to aflatoxins.[52] These techniques permit identification of exceed-ingly small amounts of aflatoxin adducts and allow the tracking of individuals who are exposed to aflatoxins.[53]

The relation of aflatoxin to kwashiorkor has been raised[54] and discussed.[55] One explanation for the increased levels of the toxin in kwashiorkor is the inability of the malnourished liver to me-tabolize aflatoxin with consequent increase. The levels may possibly rise to an extent where they may cause the severe hepatic lesions occasionally seen in children with kwashiorkor and associated with a high fatality rate.[55]

**Fusaria Species.** A number of toxins isolated from *Fusaria* are important to human and animal health. Alimentary toxic aleukia (ATA) in the So-viet Union in 1944 was the cause of a large number of human fatalities. It was traced to consumption of overwintered cereals infected with species of *Fusarium*.[56] The clinical features of ATA are usu-ally divided into four stages, all of which have been described in detail.[56] Human intoxication with *Fusaria* continues to be a public health prob-lem in the Soviet Union.

**Trichothecene Toxins.** The trichothecene tox-ins are produced by at least 8 of the 9 species of *Fusarium* recognized in the Snyder and Hansen system of classification and, at least in the labo-ratory, by several other genera of fungi.[57] Before 1900 feed grains heavily invaded by some (20) of these species of *Fusarium* have been recognized as toxic to animals that consumed them. ATA, as described by Joffe,[56] is caused by one or more of the trichothecene toxins (T-2 toxin, neosolanol, T-2 tetraol) or perhaps anguidine (DAS).

In 1982, the United States government an-nounced that after eight years of investigating spo-radic reports of chemical warfare attacks in Laos, the evidence was such that the use of biologically active toxins on human populations could no longer be denied.[58] Thus began the saga of "yellow rain." The episodes were so named because the toxic materials were reported to be delivered from planes, helicopters, or artillery shells, often in the form of a yellow cloud that "came down from the sky." The story has been detailed by Watson et al.,[59] and the reader is referred to that source for further reading. A major toxic component of "yel-low rain" has been identified as trichothecenes, powerful radiomimetics that destroy bone marrow and the immunocompetence of individuals, and also severely injure the intestine.

Some in the scientific community do not be-lieve that mycotoxins are involved in "yellow rain" but rather that it is composed of bee feces.[59a,59b] This author accepts this view as a pos-sibility but believes that some of the data strongly support mycotoxins as etiologic factors.

The incidence and concentration of the tri-chothecene toxins in foods and crops have been described as more widespread and significant than those of the aflatoxins. Most of the data avail-able concern T-2 toxin. This is the mycotoxin most commonly recognized in foods, because the anal-ysis is relatively easy. More than half of the corn samples examined in the United States in 1973 were positive, making this family of toxins of con-siderable potential importance.[60]

**Zearalenone.** Zearalenone, or F-2 toxin, is pro-duced by *Fusarium graminearum (Gibberella zeae)*, *Fusarium tricinctum*, *Fusarium roseum*, *Fusarium gibbosum*, *Fusarium roseum equiseti*, and *Fusarium roseum graminearum*.[61] Stob[62] and Urry[63] elucidated its structure as 6-(10-hydroxy-6-oxo-trans-1-undecenyl)-B-resorcylic acid lac-tone. Zearalenone has strong uterotropic activity and has been implicated in estrogenism in pigs fed moldy corn. Feeding the toxin to pigs pro-duces true estrus. These changes are reversible when treatment is halted.

There are no reports implicating zearalenone in human illnesses following ingestion of food. Al-though zearalenone has not been known to cause any human health problems, however, it has been found in corn destined for human food in the United States, in amounts known to cause vul-vovaginitis in swine.[61]

### Goitrogens

Some natural products in plant foods consumed by man and animals are goitrogens. They cause hypothyroidism and a compensatory enlargement of the thyroid gland. The cause of goiter is iodine deficiency, or factors that induce it, and increased iodine consumption is used under most circumstances to prevent or cure the condition. There are factors, however, in some plant foods that can cause enlargement of the thyroid gland with symptoms of iodine deficiency. The *Brassica* genus includes a number of widely eaten plant foods: cabbage, turnips, rutabagas, mustard greens, horseradish, radishes, and white mustard. Most of these plants contain small quantities of thioglucosides, which serve as goitrogens. Other foods that are suspect are soybeans and peanuts.[64]

A number of investigators have observed that goitrogens are transmitted from the milk of cows to man.[64,65] The significance of this remains to be determined.

### Allergens

Allergic reactions to substances in food are spontaneous, peculiar to certain humans, and rarely demonstrable in lower animals; hence, there are no good animal models for evaluating such reactions. The most common affliction caused by a food allergy is of the skin and respiratory tract; the gastrointestinal tract is less frequently involved. Occasionally food allergy affects the central nervous system and produces a manifestation similar to migraine headaches or, in the most severe form it may predispose to convulsive seizures. Aberrant behavior in patients has been described as being associated with allergic disorders. Infants and children may complain of abdominal distress, and occasionally the genital and urinary tract as well as the cardiovascular system may be involved. The allergic response of individuals is evaluated by skin tests consisting of subcutaneous injection or patch testing of extracts of the suspected materials. If the individual is sensitive, a response is elicited after a specific period of time.

One of the better understood forms of food allergies is so-called celiac disease or gluten enteropathy, an adverse response by some individuals to certain fractions of wheat gluten. This disease has many of the symptoms seen in patients with idiopathic and tropical sprue.[66] A number of early investigators reported that the elimination of wheat from the diet produced an improvement in the condition of celiac patients. Even the so-called banana diet, as originally proposed by Haas,[67] was one that completely eliminated wheat.[68] The dramatic response observed by the Dutch investigators with one of their pediatric patients when wheat gluten was added to or removed from the diet was enough to establish this protein as the dietary factor associated with the characteristic symptoms.[69,70] When wheat gluten is removed from the diet, improvement occurs in all aspects of the disease, but as long as a year may pass before the individual is completely restored to normal functioning.[66]

### Saponins

The saponins have been identified in at least 400 different species belonging to more than 80 different plant families. These toxins, which occur as glycosides, have a bitter taste and characteristically hemolyze red blood cells. Although saponins have been studied from the point of view of hemolytic activity and, in some cases, for their therapeutic properties, those occurring in foods and feeds have been studied very little. The nutritional significance of soybeans and alfalfa, in which saponins occur, makes this area one of potential significance to human populations.[71,72]

### Oxalates

Increased interest in oxalates occurred in the 1930s when spinach was considered a valuable addition to the diet of children.[73] Analyses of foods showed that oxalic acid made up about 10% of the dry weight of such foods as spinach, New Zealand spinach, Swiss chard, beet tops, lamb's quarters, pokeweed, purslane, and rhubarb.[74] This was primarily in the form of insoluble calcium oxalate crystals, demonstrable in microscopic sections of the leaves.[75] Foodstuffs of animal origin contain only small amounts of oxalates.[76] Both animal studies and clinical trials with children[77] indicate that calcium in spinach is not available, especially when the calcium content of the diet is close to the minimum requirement. The presence of soluble oxalates in foods may decrease the absorption of calcium from other foods.

Individuals who develop mild symptoms of oxalic acid poisoning following the ingestion of rhubarb complain of gastroenteritis with abdominal pain. Diarrhea and vomiting, and occasionally hematuria, convulsions, collapse, noncoagulability of blood, and coma are seen in severe poisoning.[75] The *Dieffenbachia* plant commonly displayed in homes and offices may pose a danger to small children.

An interesting endemic episode of calcium oxalate stones in children has been described in Thailand.[79] This disease arises from the high content of oxalates in native food products. Highly effective preventive and therapeutic measures have been used to diminish the effects of oxalates in human populations of the affected areas, particularly the young.

## Thiaminase

The initial interest in this enzyme stemmed from the thiamine deficiency that appeared among foxes fed frozen carp as part of their ration. With the recognition that this enzyme was distributed in a wide variety of fish,[80–82] was the possibility that some individuals consuming large amounts of seafood might develop a thiamine deficiency. The closest approach to such a condition is Haff (or Yuksov) disease, reported from a number of areas in northern Europe among people consuming perch, bream, and lake trout.[83] Although some investigators have suggested a relation between Haff disease and thiaminase present in the fish consumed by these individuals, such a relationship may be more apparent than real because: (1) the symptoms appear within 24 hours after eating the fish, (2) the urine has a brownish-black color, and (3) recovery is usually complete 24 hours after eating the fish.[84] A deficiency of thiamine would not be associated with any of these characteristics.

Bracken fern *(Pteridium aquilinum),* which grows in upland pastures or in open woods, remains green even when most forage crops have succumbed to drought. If, at such times, monogastric animals consume considerable amounts over a few weeks, they exhibit symptoms of thiamine deficiency about four weeks after first eating the fern.[85] Most of the reported cases have involved horses and, even with animals of that size, only four weeks were required for a deficiency to become manifest. Complete recovery occurs if supplemental thiamine is given before the condition becomes terminal.

Bracken fern is known to be carcinogenic for cattle, guinea pigs, rats, and mice.[86] However, the young sprouts of some ferns (fiddlehead greens) are eaten as a delicacy by a number of populations. Studies in our laboratories demonstrated no effects when fed to rats for as long as two years at concentrations of 10% of the diet.[86] This finding is in contrast to reports of others who claim, without sufficient evidence, that the young sprouts are a health hazard.[87]

## Cycad

Cycads are palm-like trees consisting of nine species growing mainly in the tropics and subtropics. Peoples on various southwest Pacific islands use cycads because they are some of the few plants capable of surviving adverse climatic conditions. Prior to and during World War II, they provided a source of calories during droughts and following severe typhoons and served as a supplement when food supplies became low because of military action.[88]

The people of Guam use the seeds of the cycad both as an emergency source of food and, to a lesser extent, as a regular part of their diet. The starchy centers or the kernels of the seeds are used in thickening various dishes (soups, tortillas, fruit desserts), while the outer husk of the seed is used as a confection.

Widespread interest in cycad toxicity developed when amyotrophic lateral sclerosis was associated with consumption of flour prepared from cycad nuts. The incidence of amyotrophic lateral sclerosis is 100 times greater among the Chamoro Guamanians than among the inhabitants of the United States or Europe. Human patients suffering from amyotrophic lateral sclerosis become progressively paralyzed and die about five years after the onset of symptoms. At present there is no known cure for this disease.

The Guamanians have recognized for many years that the kernels of *Cycas circinalis* are toxic. They attempt to eliminate the toxin by soaking the kernel in vats of water for 7 to 10 days. The water may be changed several times during a soaking period. After soaking, the kernels are dried in the sun and then ground to a powder similar to that of wheat flour.[89]

The toxic substance in cycad stems and cycad seeds *(Cycas revoluta)* has been identified as methylazoxymethanol-β-glucoside. The aglycone of this glucoside, methylazoxymethanol, is common to the glycosides present in other species of cycad.[90,91] The latter glycosides have sugars other than glucose linked to the aglycone.

The beta-glycoside linkage in cycad explains why the glycoside is nontoxic when injected into conventional animals[92] or fed to germ-free animals.[93] Liberation of the active aglycone requires a beta-glucosidase present in bacterial but not in mammalian cells. When the bacterial action in the gastrointestinal tract is circumvented by parenteral injection or by feeding to germ-free animals, cycasin remains intact and, as such, is nontoxic. A possible exception to the absence of beta-glucosidases in mammalian tissues comes from the observation that cycasin injected into day-old rat pups was toxic.[94] These animals developed kidney tumors about five months after a single injection. The nature of the induction of cancer in rats under these conditions requires clarification.

## Herbs

The use of herbal products has increased greatly in recent years. These products include capsules, teas, and cigarettes and other smoking mixtures advertised as "natural and legal drugs" or "herbal highs."[95] Such products are available in health food stores and markets as well as by direct mail order from importers or suppliers. Many of the preparations contain significant amounts of psychoactive substances, the use of which has resulted in intoxications requiring clinical attention.

More than 200 distinct herbs are commercially available for smoking as cigarettes or as blended smoking mixtures. The most common of those containing psychoactive materials are spearmint, thyme, rosemary, yerba santa, mullein, and damiana. Many of these are advertised as nontobacco substitutes. Some are advertised as mimicking the effects of marihuana. A variety of clinical symptoms have been associated with smoking these mixtures, including pervasive "spaced-out" sensation, ataxia, slurred speech, blurred vision, dilated pupils, and dry mouth and throat. One such product, "mint bidis," imported from India, results in such responses. Analysis of the cigarettes revealed that a single cigarette contained 16 μg of atropine and 65 μg of scopolamine. Another cigarette made from *Datura stramonium* contained 250 μg of atropine and 220 μg of scopolamine. Some patients have consumed cigarettes in quantities to provide as much as 0.7 mg total alkaloids per day.

Teas are popular with a significant segment of the population of the United States, and currently 396 distinct herbs and spices are commercially available for use singly or as blended mixtures. Psychoactive agents are present in at least 43 of these, but generally in lower concentrations than in cigarettes. A leading product, kavabava tea, associated with confusion, ataxia, impaired breathing, dimmed vision, dulled hearing, and hallucinations, is made from crushed roots of the kava plant, *Piper methysticum,* indigenous to islands of the South Pacific. Nutmeg tea may also result in symptoms of nausea, dryness of mouth and throat, drowsiness, rapid pulse, flushed skin, disturbed vision, incoherent speech, vertigo, and hallucinations.[96,97]

Tea is also made from *Datura stramonium* or jimsonweed. It results in ataxia, restlessness, blurred vision, and severe hallucinations, much as the cigarette made from the same plant. The tea made from *Datura stramonium* contains large amounts of atropine and scopolamine, and the symptoms are typical of stramonium poisoning.

Another interesting tea that is widely advertised and consumed is made from the root bark of the sassafras tree *(Sassafras albidum).* The major constituent in sassafras tea is safrole (4-albyl, 1,2-methylenedioxybenzene), a hepatocarcinogen for laboratory animals. Aqueous and alcoholic extracts of sassafras root bark elicit a variety of pharmacologic responses in mice, including central nervous system depression, hypothermia, hypersensitivity, ptosis, and ataxia.[96]

In addition to the disturbing clinical symptoms and intoxications and real or potential health hazards, herb teas may change the bioavailability of foods and therapeutic drugs consumed concomitantly. The use of herbal cigarettes, teas, and capsules is to be discouraged.

## Mushrooms

Under ordinary circumstances, the consumption of the inky cap mushroom *Coprinus atramentarius* produces no unpleasant reactions. However, if an alcoholic beverage is drunk during or shortly after a meal that includes this mushroom, the face of the drinker and perhaps other parts of his body soon become purplish-red.[97] This mushroom apparently contains a compound with an action similar to that of disulfiram (Antabuse).[98]

Poisoning from the ingestion of other types of mushrooms has occurred for many centuries.[99,100] In the United States, fewer than 2% of the cases reported to the National Clearinghouse for Poison Control Centers involved mushrooms.[101] A partial explanation for the few cases of mushroom toxicity stems from the fact that only a few species are toxic. For instance, although over 800 species of these plants grow in New England, only 53 are considered poisonous.[102]

Domestically cultivated varieties of mushrooms *(Agaricus bisporus)* are free of any toxic substance. Moreover, the more poisonous species are not amenable to cultivation. Safety dictates that mushrooms should be purchased in the marketplace rather than harvested from the forest.

## TOXINS OF MARINE ORIGIN

### Paralytic Shellfish Poisoning (PSP)

Mussels, clams, and occasionally scallops and oysters from both the Atlantic and Pacific coastal areas and from such other areas as South Africa, New Zealand, Belgium, Germany, France, England, and Ireland have produced poisoning in man.[103] Poisoning is associated with the growth in the water of dinoflagellates. These unicellular organisms produce a poison that is retained in the dark gland or hepatopancreas of the mussel or other shellfish feeding on them. The shellfish show no disturbance as a result of the toxin; however, when the contaminated seafood is eaten by man, symptoms of toxicity usually develop in 1 to 3 hours.[104]

The symptoms associated with paralytic shellfish poisoning include a numbness of the lips and fingertips, an ascending paralysis and, finally, in severe poisoning, death from respiratory paralysis, which is reported to occur in about 8.5% of cases.[103] Death may occur in 3 to 20 hours after eating the shellfish. Should the person survive the first 24 hours, the prognosis for his complete recovery is good. In most areas, the poisoning is confined to local residents who dig for their own shellfish. In the Alaskan coastal area, the problem becomes of more importance to general public health, since the shellfish from this area are canned or frozen and widely distributed. Hazardous levels of PSP accumulate when the dinoflagellate undergoes rapid growth (i.e., "blooms") in the area where shellfish are feeding. The increase in organisms and the associated changes are referred to as the "red tide." As a protective measure along United States and Canadian coastal waters, a quarantine is posted whenever the toxicity of the shellfish becomes dangerous. The toxicity is determined by injecting an aqueous extract of the shellfish into mice.[103,104] Even this measure is not completely adequate, since sampling of shellfish from various areas in the same region may suggest low levels of toxicity while other areas nearby may have highly toxic shellfish.[103]

The compound isolated from both the Alaskan butter clams and axenic cultures of the dinoflagellates has been given the name saxitoxin. This word comes from the scientific name for the butter clams, *Saxidomus giganeus.* The toxin appears to block nerve transmission in the motor axon and not at the end-plate, presumably by blocking the increase of sodium conductance normally associated with excitation. On the basis of experiments with cats, it was estimated that the lethal dose of this toxin for an adult would be 0.4 mg given intravenously.[105] Orally, the toxic dose has been suggested as 8 mg.[106]

## Allergic Reactions

The problem of allergic reactions is subject to a great deal of conflicting testimony, partly because of the psychoneurotic factor in many reactions[107,108] and the confusion of classifying fish by the lay public. The commercial classification of fish frequently differs from that recognized by the ichthyologists. A related problem exists among the solutions used in testing for food sensitivity. Antigenically, the same preparation from a variety of sources exhibits a remarkable lack of uniformity in antigenic components.[109]

Fish and shellfish are known to serve as powerful allergens which, in some persons, may produce almost explosive reactions.[103] These reactions include urticaria, angioneurotic edema, gastrointestinal disturbances, and migraine. Asthma and coryza are seen less frequently. Attempts have been made to classify fish on the basis of those to which an allergic individual might be sensitive in order to avoid them. However, those allergic to cod might also react to trout, carp, herring, and sardines. Whether such a classification will survive is doubtful since there are reported cases of allergies to one specific type of seafood with no reactions to other closely related species.[103,108] Newer methods in immunologic detection should clarify these questions.

## Mercury in Fish

The United States Food and Drug Administration adopted, in May of 1969, a safe-level guideline of 0.5 ppm mercury in fish,[110] which applied to all fish in interstate commerce. The 0.5 ppm level was an interim guideline for internal use in deciding when to charge that a fish product was adulterated under the federal Food, Drug and Cosmetic Act, but it has remained in effect since its original application.

The action by the FDA was taken following reports of methylmercury poisoning in Japan and Sweden.[110–115] The level of 0.5 ppm for methylmercury in fish was based on a careful review of the limited information available to the FDA at that time. A major part of these data was observation of clinical symptoms and blood levels of mercury in victims of the Minamata Bay incident. Further data were developed from the calculations made by the Swedish Expert Committee[116] who accepted 30 μg Hg/day as the upper limit of acceptable daily intake.

The Japanese investigators traced the contaminating methylmercury in the Minamata Bay incident from shellfish and finfish back through the waters of the bay to the effluent pipes and the sludge expelled from the principal industry in the village. A year before the first people became ill, this industry had started producing acetaldehyde and vinyl chloride with the aid of mercury compounds as catalysts.[111,112] During the reactions, some of the mercury was converted to methylmercury and discharged with other wastes into Minamata Bay. Here the fish and shellfish, feeding on contaminated marine life and pumping water through their gills, absorbed and concentrated the methylmercury.

These longitudinal studies of Clarkson and others indicate that problems may arise in selected human populations from methylmercury poisoning when fish with normal background levels of methylmercury are consumed in large quantities over extended periods. However, it would appear that, except for such environmental accidents as that of Minamata Bay, mercury in fish constitute little if any problem for human populations.

## METALS, METALLOIDS, AND OTHER CHEMICALS

The largest part of the total body burden of most metals in biologic species is traceable to diet. Sources include constituents of rocks and minerals that weathered to produce the soil, water erosion of soil particles, metals as added ingredients or impurities in fertilizers, pesticides containing metals (arsenic, lead, copper, mercury, manganese, and zinc), metals in manure and sludge, and those present in airborne dust (industrial and mining wastes, fossil fuel combustion production, wind-eroded soil particles, radioactive fallout, pollen, sea spray, and meteoric and volcanic material).

The two naturally occurring toxic metals in foods believed to be of most practical importance are mercury and selenium, although mercury, lead, and cadmium are the most serious environmental pollutants.

### Selenium

Selenium is essential for domestic animals, but the margin of safety is relatively narrow. A low level of selenium is essential to prevent myopathies, liver injury, and congenital abnormalities in domestic and laboratory animals and poultry. There is little reason to believe that humans differ appreciably in this regard. The report from China regarding Keshan's disease confirms a human requirement for selenium.[117]

High dietary selenium is toxic to animals, and a defined set of signs and lesions has been established for acute and subacute exposure to toxic concentrations in several species. Chronic long-term studies have been limited primarily to feeding studies in the rat, and these have involved relatively high concentrations of the element.[118,119] More recent studies indicate that selenium is protective against some forms of experimental cancer.[120,121]

The toxicity of selenium can be altered extensively by interactions with sulfate, methionine, cystine, mercury, lead, zinc, cadium, copper, arsenic, and vitamin E, but little is known about these interactions. Human toxicity has resulted primarily from acute industrial exposure.[122] There is little evidence that human populations living in affected areas are as affected by selenium deficiency or toxicity as animals are. The difference between man's susceptibility and that of domestic animals to chronic selenium poisoning is unlikely to be associated with a higher tolerance in the human species, since species differences in tolerance to selenium appear to be small. Absence of obvious signs of chronic selenosis in man in seleniferous areas is probably attributable to the wide geographic source of many of the foods composing modern dietaries and the fact that most of these foods, unlike animal feeds, are subject to modification by processing and cooking.

Epidemiologic studies with children and experimental studies with animals have indicated that above-normal intakes of selenium during the development period of the teeth increase the incidence of cavities.[123] The results reported would be more convincing if the actual selenium intakes of the children in the different groups had been measured.

The important questions of selenium and cancer and of selenium and dental caries clearly need further study. The fact that the FDA now permits the addition of selenium salts to poultry and swine feeds, however, indicates that scientific judgment has concluded that this element is not carcinogenic.

### Arsenic

Arsenic is widely distributed in the waters of the United States, but generally in low concentrations (10 to 22 ppb). In a few instances, arsenic concentrations reach significant, even toxic, levels. From all sources, the general public of the United States consumes a calculated daily intake of 0.137 to 0.330 mg of arsenic. Epidemiologic studies have clearly shown that chronic excessive consumption of arsenic results in cutaneous lesions, including skin cancer and, in some cases, lung cancer.[124] However, the lack of uniformity of design and other defects in the studies indicate a need for international agreements on the best methods for collecting and disseminating data for more accurate evaluation from one location to another.

There is little information about arsenic in marine organisms or about methylation-demethylation processes in marine and terrestrial organisms. Likewise, the uptake of arsenic by plants is poorly understood, although it appears to be related to the amount of soluble arsenic in the soil, the nature of the soil, and the species of plant.

### Lead

Most human foods under standard environmental conditions contain less than 1 ppm lead (Pb). Cow's milk may contain 0.02 to 0.08 ppm Pb, and muscle meats approximately 0.1 ppm.[125,126] Lead has a marked affinity for bone, which sometimes contains between 5 and 20 ppm in the fresh state. Little is known of the natural levels of lead in foods of plant origin; these levels must be quite low, however, because average intakes from food by adult man have been variously estimated to range from 0.22 to 0.4 mg Pb per day, approximately 0.3 to 0.5 ppm of the dry diet. In addition, smaller amounts of lead are ingested with drinking water, and inhaled from the atmosphere and from cigarette smoke. As a result of such activities, the current average daily adult intake of lead from all food sources in the United States has been estimated to be about 300 μg.[127]

Because many epidemiologic studies and experimental animal investigations indicate a chronic neurologic problem with lead, the EPA announced in 1984 that lead in gasoline will be phased out over the next few years. This is the major source of exposure.

## Cadmium

Daily intakes of cadmium (Cd) by human adults have been estimated to be 0.2 to 0.5 g, with considerable variation, according to sources and types of food. These estimates now appear to be much too high. A mean total cadmium content of 0.013 mg was reported for school lunches served to sixth-grade children in 300 United States schools.[127]

The total dietary cadmium intakes of institutionalized children (ages 9 to 12 years) in 28 United States cities were found to average 0.092 mg per day, with a range of 0.032 to 0.158 mg per day.

Oysters are exceptionally rich in cadmium, with levels of 3 to 4 ppm compared with levels of one tenth or one hundredth as much in most other foods. Appreciable amounts of cadmium may also be obtained from the air and the water supply. Soft water remaining overnight in galvanized or black polyethylene pipes can take up 0.15 to 1.1 μg Cd/L, although total intakes from these sources are calculated to supply no more than 1 to 2 μg Cd/day. The cadmium level in the air of 28 United States cities was shown to range from undetectable to as high as 0.06 μg Cd/cu mm of air.[127]

Whether cadmium intakes from the food, air, and water supply present any long-term hazards to human health speculative at best. The relationship of cadmium to hypertension in man is unknown. Some hypertensive patients, however, exhibit a higher than normal urinary excretion of a range of metals, especially cadmium, and carry significantly higher renal cadmium concentrations and a higher Cd:Zn ratio in their tissues than do similar normotensive individuals.[128]

## TOXINS FROM ANIMAL FOODSTUFFS

Factors in animal foodstuffs that have a potential for inducing toxic responses in man and animals have generally been treated in a superficial manner in most comprehensive treatises devoted to the topic of naturally occurring toxicants. This reflects a lack of interest and research in this area of food safety. Naturally occurring toxicants in animal tissues are limited mainly to avian and fish eggs and to some shellfish and amphibia. There are many examples, however, of toxicity caused by the introduction of man-made chemicals into meat and dairy products.

## Milk and Dairy Products

Because some segments of the population of the United States are vegetarian and depend on dairy and vegetable sources for their food needs, more data are needed on the effects of milk products on selected hypersensitive individuals or those with enzyme deficits. Milk and dairy products are of concern, then, because of the intolerance of some individuals to constituents in milk and milk products (i.e., milk proteins, lactose). In addition, milk can contain estrogens, plant substances, nitrates and nitrites, antibiotics, pesticides, radionuclides, and mycotoxins as contaminants. Further, as noted in the following section, cheese can contain a number of amines that are pharmacoactive and cause serious problems in people who are sensitive to them. Those amines of importance are norepinephrine, epinephrine and 5-hydroxytryptamine (serotonin).[129]

## Cheese

The presence of various symptoms in patients receiving monoamine oxidase inhibitors is an illustration of a food toxicity seen in special groups of people. These individuals complain of hypertension, severe headache, and palpitation. Initially, these disturbances were considered to be side effects of the monoamine oxidase inhibitors. It was almost 10 years after the introduction of these drugs that the "side effects" became associated with the consumption of cheese.[130]

The monoamine oxidase inhibitors are used to treat patients in depressive states. These drugs inhibit the enzyme that "destroys" serotonin, norepinephrine, and related neurohormonal compounds. As a result of this and possibly other reactions, the drugs produce a euphoric state.

Tyramine in cheese is a potent vasopressor substance. Under normal circumstances, it is metabolized through the action of monoamine oxidases. When the activity of these enzymes is inhibited by drugs, the tyramine from the cheese acts to produce severe hypertension and its sequelae.

## SUMMARY

Although food is essential to life, it is the most complex chemical mixture to which man and animals are exposed, and it may contain substances that are harmful when ingested. Whether the substances are natural and native to a particular food or whether they are included as nonintentional additives does not alter the significance of their effects on biologic systems. A fascinating account of foods and their effects on people is recorded by Cosman[131] and is well worth the time needed to read it. Progress in nutrition, food science technology, and toxicology now permits us to consider interactions of nutrients and chemicals as an area of high priority. To identify real or potential problems and to understand interactions that may help unravel the enigma of some of our important chronic diseases will contribute significantly to public health.

## REFERENCES

1. Rhodes, M.E.: The Sciences May/June 1979, pp. 11–12.
2. US News & World Report: September, 1984.
3. Liener, I. (Ed.): Toxic Constituents of Plant Foodstuffs. New York, Academic Press, 1969.
4. Read, J., Haas, C.: Cereal Chem. *15*:59, 1938.
5. Ham, T., Sandstedt, J.: J. Biol. Chem. *154*:505, 1944.
6. Osborne, T.B., Mendel, L.B.: J. Biol. Chem. *32*:369, 1917.
7. Barnes, R., Kwong, L.: J. Nutr. *86*:245, 1965.
8. Kennedy, A.: Vitamins, Nutrition and Cancer. (Prasad, K.N., Ed.) Basel, S. Karger A.G., 1984, p. 166.
9. Troll, W., Klassen, C., Janoff, A.: Science *169*:1211, 1970.
10. Tobishka, J.: Die Phythamagglutinine. Berlin, Akademie Verlag, 1964.
11. Stillmark, J.: Arch. Pharmakol. Inst. Dorpat. *3*:59, 1889.
12. Liener, I.: Am. J. Clin. Nutr. *11*:281, 1962.
13. Jaffe, Y.: Hemagglutinins and Toxic Constituents of Plant Foodstuffs. (Liener, Ed.). New York, Academic Press, 1969, p. 69.
14. Strong, F.M.: Nutr. Rev. *14*:65, 1956.
15. Selye, H.: Rev. Can. Biol. *16*:1, 1957.
16. Gardner, Sakiewicz: Exp. Med. Surg. *21*:164, 1963.
17. Ressler, C., Redstone, R.A., Erenberg, R.H.: Science *134*:188, 1961.
18. Lewis, H.B., Fajans, R.S., Esterer, M.B., et al.: J. Nutr. *36*:537, 1948.
19. Geiger, B.J., Steenbock, H., Parsons, H.T.: J. Nutr. *6*:427, 1933.
20. Smalley, E.B.: J. Am. Vet. Med. Assoc. *163*:1278, 1973.
21. Weaver, A.L., Spittel, J.A.: Proc. Staff Meet. Mayo Clin. *39*:485, 1964.
22. Zinkham, W.H., et al.: Bull. J. Hopkins Hosp. *102*:169, 1958.
23. Beutler, E.: *In* The Metabolic Basis of Inherited Disease. (Stanbury, Wyngaarden, and Fredrickson, Eds.) New York, McGraw-Hill Book Co., 1966.
24. Beutler, E.: Br. Med. J. *2*:1140, 1965.
25. Lin, H., Ling, Y.: J. Formosan Med. Assoc. *61*:579, 1962.
26. Bull, L., Culvenor, I., Dick, A.T.: The Pyrrolizidine Alkaloids. New York, John Wiley & Sons, Inc., 1968.
27. Selzer, G., Parker, G.F.: Am. J. Pathol *27*:885, 1951.
28. Leiner, I. (Ed.): Toxic Constituents of Plant Foodstuffs. New York, Academic Press, 1969, p. 408.
29. Newberne, P., Rogers, A.: Plant Foods for Man *1*:23, 1973.
30. Svoboda, D., Reddy, J.: Cancer Res. *32*:908, 1972.
31. Schoental, R.: Isr. J. Med. Sci. *4*:1133, 1968.
32. Mattocks, A.R.: *In* Trace Substances in the Environment: A Handbook, Part II. (Newberne, P.M. Ed.) New York, Marcel Dekker, Inc., 1982.
33. IARC Monograph No. 10: Lyon, France, 1976, p. 333.
34. Candrian, U., Lüthy, J., Graf, U., et al.: Fd. Chem. Toxicol. *22*:223, 1984.
35. Krishnamachari, K.A.U.R., Nagarajan, V., Bhat, R.V., et al.: Lancet *1*:1061, 1975.
36. Newberne, P.M.: Environ. Health Perspect. *9*:23, 1974.
37. WHO Environmental Health Criteria for Mycotoxins: Vol. 1, Aflatoxins, January, 1977, p. 116.
38. Patterson, D.S.P.: Food Cosmet. Toxicol. *11*:287, 1973.
39. Newberne, P.M., Rogers, A.E.: J. Natl. Cancer Inst. *50*:439, 1973.
40. Newberne, P.M., Harrington, D.H., Wogan, G.N.: Lab Invest *15*:962, 1966.
41. Rogers, A.E., Newberne, P.M.: Cancer Res. *29*:1965, 1969.
42. Rogers, A.E., Newberne, P.M.: Nature *229*:62, 1971.
43. Newberne, P.M.: Cancer Detect. Prev. *1*:129, 1976.
44. Campbell, T.C., Caedo, J.P., Bulatao-Jayne, et al.: Nature *227*:403, 1970.
45. Alpert, E., Hutt, B., Wogan, G.N., et al.: J. Natl. Cancer Inst. *50*:549, 1973.
46. Peers, F.G., Linsell, C.A.: Br. J. Cancer *27*:473, 1973.
47. Shank, R.C., Bhamarapravati, N., Gordon, J.E., et al.: Food Cosmet. Toxicol. *10*:171, 1972.
48. Van Rensburg, S., Van der Watt, J., Purchase, I.F.H., et al.: S. Afr. Med. J. *48*:2508, 1974.
49. W.H.O., Scientific Group Meeting Report: Prevention of primary liver cancer. Lancet *1*:463–465, 1983.
50. Gerin, J.L.: Editorial. Gastroenterology *84*:869–870, 1983.
51. Arthur, M.J.P., Hall, A.J., Wright, R.: Lancet *1*:607–610, 1984.
52. Maugh, T.H. Science *226*:1184, 1984.
53. WHO-IARC Technical Report 84/003, Lyon, 1984.
54. Hendrickse, R.G.: Trans. R. Soc. Trop. Med. Hyg. *78*:427–435, 1984.
55. Editorial: Aflatoxins and kwashiorkor. Lancet *2*:1133–1134, 1984.
56. Joffe, H.: *In* Mycotoxins. (Purchase, Ed.) Amsterdam, Elsevier, 1974.
57. Smalley, E., Strong, F.: *In* Mycotoxins. (Purchase, Ed.) Amsterdam. Elsevier, 1974.
58. Haig, A.: Report to Congress from Secretary of State, March 22, 1982. U.S. Government Printing Office, Washington, DC.
59. Watson, S.A., Mirocha, C.J., Hayes, A.: Fund. Appl. Toxicol. *4*:700, 1984.
59a. Marshall, E.: Science *221*:526–529, 1983.
59b. Ashton, P.S.: Nature *315*:284, 1985.
60. Mirocha, C.J., Pathre, S.V., Schauerhamer, B., et al.: Appl. Environ. Microbiol. *32*:553, 1976.
61. Mirocha, C.J., Christensen, C.M.: Annu. Rev. Phytopathol. *12*:303, 1974.
62. Stob, M., Baldwin, R.S., Tuite, J., et al.: Nature *196*:1318, 1962.
63. Urry, W.H., Wehrmeister, H.L., Hodge, E.B., et al.: Tetrahedron Let. *27*:3109, 1966.
64. Van Etten, C.H.: *In* Toxicant Constituents of Plant

Foodstuffs. (Liener, Ed.) New York, Academic Press, 1969.

65. Clements, H., Wishart, J.: Metabolism *5*:623, 1956.
66. Frazer, A.C.: Adv. Clin. Chem. *5*:69, 1962.
67. Haas, W.: Am. J. Dis. Child. *28*:421, 1924.
68. Weijers, H.A. Van de Kamer, J.H.: Am. J. Clin. Nutr. *17*:51, 1965.
69. Dicke, J. Weijers, H.A. Van de Kamer, J.H.: Acta Paediatr. *42*:34, 1953.
70. Weijers, H.A., Van de Kamer, J.H., Dicke, J.: Adv. Pediatr. *9*:277, 1957.
71. Pederson, W., Aimmer, J.C., McAllister, C., et al.: Crop Sci. *7*:349, 1967.
72. Birk, Y.: *In* Toxicant Constituents of Plant Foodstuffs. (Liener, Ed.) New York, Academic Press, 1969.
73. Tisdall, M., Drake, E., Summerfeldt, J.F., et al.: J. Pediatr. *11*:374, 1937.
74. Kohman, E.F.: J. Nutr. *18*:233, 1939.
75. Jeghers, D.J., Murphy, R.: N. Engl. J. Med. *233*:208, 1945.
76. Zarembski, P.M., Hodgkinson, A.: Br. J. Nutr. *16*:627, 1962.
77. Editorial: J.A.M.A. *109*:1907, 1937.
78. Drach, G., Maloney, W.H.: J.A.M.A. *184*:1047, 1963.
79. Valyasevi, A., Dhanamitta, S.: Am. J. Clin. Nutr. *27*:877, 1974.
80. Deutsch, H.F., Hasler, A.D.: Proc. Soc. Exp. Biol. Med. *53*:63, 1943.
81. Melnick, D., Hochberg, M., Oser, B.L.: J. Nutr. *30*:81, 1945.
82. Jacobsohn, K.P., Azevedo, M.D.: Arch. Biochem. *14*:83, 1947.
83. Shewan. J.M.: *In* Fish as Food, Vol. 2. (Borgstrom, Ed.) New York, Academic Press, 1962.
84. Berlin, M.: Acta Med. Scand. *129*:560, 1948.
85. Kingsbury, J.M.: Poisonous Plants of the United States and Canada. Englewood Cliffs, Prentice-Hall, 1964.
86. Newberne, P.: J. Natl. Cancer Inst. *56*:551, 1976.
87. Pamukcu, A.M., Yalciner, J., Price, J.M., et al.: Cancer Res. *30*:2671, 1970.
88. Whiting, M.G.: Econ. Bot. *17*:271, 1963.
89. Campbell, M.E., et al.: J. Nutr. *88*:115, 1966.
90. Nishida, K., Kobayashi, A., Nagahama, T.: Bull. Agric. Chem. Soc. Japan, *19*:77, 1955.
91. Riggs, N.V.: Chem. Ind. *35*:926, 1956.
92. Nishida, K., Kobayashi, A., Nagahama, T., et al.: Seikagaku (Biochemistry), *28*:218, 1956 (in Japanese).
93. Laquer, G.: Fed. Proc. *23*:1386, 1964.
94. Magee, P.: Fourth Conference on the Toxicity of Cycads. (Whiting, Ed.) Bethesda, National Institutes of Health, 1965.
95. Siegel, R.K.: J.A.M.A. *236*:473, 1976.
96. Segelmen, A.B., Segelman, F.P., Karliner, J.K., et al.: J.A.M.A., 236, 477, 1976.
97. Kingsbury, J.M.: Poisonous Plants of the United States and Canada. Englewood Cliffs, Prentice-Hall, 1964, p. 96.
98. Weir, H., Tyler, J.: J. Am. Pharm. Assoc. *49*:426, 1960.
99. Van der Veer, J., Farley, M.: Arch. Intern. Med. *55*:773, 1935.

100. Grossman, C.M., Malbin, B.: Ann. Intern. Med. *40*:249, 1954.
101. Cann, J., Verhulst, H.: Am. J. Dis. Child. *101*:127, 1961.
102. Buck, R.W., N. Engl. J. Med. *265*:681, 1961.
103. Halstead, B.W.: Fish as Food, Vol. 2. (Borgstrom, Ed.) New York, Academic Press, 1962.
104. Schantz, E.J.: Ann. N.Y. Acad. Sci. *90*:834, 1960.
105. Kao, C.Y., Nishiyama, A.: J. Physiol. *180*:50, 1965.
106. Meyer, K.F.: N. Engl. J. Med. *249*:843, 1953.
107. Burden, S.S.: Ann. Intern. Med. *43*:1283, 1955.
108. Fenton, S.W.: *In* Practice of Allergy. (Vaughn, Black, Eds.) St. Louis, C.V. Mosby Co., 1948.
109. Cohen, S.: J. Allergy, *30*:267, 1959.
110. Kolbye, A.: Testimony Subcommittee on Energy, National Resources and the Environment of the Senate Committee on Commerce, May 8, 1970.
111. Irukayama, N.: Kumamoto Med. J. *15*:57, 1962.
112. Katsuna, S. (Ed.): Minamata Disease. Study Group of Minamata Disease, Kumamoto University, 1968.
112a.Clarkson, T.: Personal communication.
113. Kurland, J.K., Faro, A., Siedler, H.C.: World Neurol. *1*:370, 1960.
114. Lofroth, W.: Bull. No. 4, Ecological Research Committee, Swedish National Science Research Council, 1969.
115. Johnels, A.G., Westermark, T.: *In* Chemical Fallout. (Miller, Berg, Eds.) Springfield, Charles C Thomas, 1969, p. 221.
116. Berglund, D.E., Berlin, M., Mirke, J.K.: Nord. Hyg. Tidskr. Suppl. 4. Stockholm, National Institute of Health, 1971.
117. Chen, Y.N., Xang, C., Chan, P.K., et al.: Second International Symposium on Selenium. *In* Biol. Med. Westport, Connecticut, AVI Press, 1980.
118. Halverson, A.W., Monty, K.J.: J. Nutr. *70*:100, 1960.
119. Harr, J.R., Bone, J.F., Tinsley, I.J., et al.: Selenium in Biomedicine. (Muth, Ed.) Westport, Connecticut, AVI Press, 1967.
120. Griffin, A.C.: Mol. Interrelations of Nutrition and Cancer. (Arnott, Ed.) New York, Raven Press, 1982, p. 401.
121. Newberne, P.M., Suphakarn, V.: Vitamins, Nutrition and Cancer. (Prasad, K., Ed.) Basel, S. Karger, AG, 1984, p. 46.
122. Underwood, E.J.: Trace Elements in Human and Animal Nutrition, 4th ed. New York, Academic Press, 1977, pp. 545.
123. Hadjimarkos, D.M.: Caries Res. *3*:14, 1969.
124. Bennett, G.A., Heyman, C.: Principles of Internal Medicine. 5th ed. (Harrison, et al., Eds.) New York, McGraw-Hill Book Co., 1966, p. 1405.
125. Cantarrow, A., Trumper, M.: Lead Poisoning. Baltimore, Williams & Wilkins, 1944.
126. Murthy, G.K., Rhea, U., Peeler, J.T.: J. Dairy Sci. *50*:651, 1967.
127. NAS/NRC: Geochemistry of the Environment, Vol. I, 1974, p. 53.
128. Heyden , J.: J. Chronic Dis. *29*:149, 1976.
129. 144 Sapieka, N.: Toxic Constituents of Animal Foodstuffs. (Liener, Ed.) New York, Academic Press, 1974, p. 1.
130. Blackwell, B., Mabbitt, L.A.: Lancet *1*:938, 1965.
131. Cosman, M.P.: Feast for Aesculapius. Historical Diets for Asthma and Sexual Pleasure. Annual Reviews of Nutrition, 1983.

*Chapter* **39**

# FOOD ADDITIVES AND CONTAMINANTS

Frederic R. Senti

The urbanization of modern society and the introduction of advanced technology have led to the separation of food produced by the farmer and its consumer, not only by great distances, but also by the many steps involved in the handling, storage, transport, processing, packaging, and delivery of the food to the retail market. Foods may be exposed to chemicals at each of these steps, either intentionally or inadvertently. The farmer treats crops in the field with pesticides to protect them from insects, weeds, and other pests and also to produce the quality product that consumers expect to find in the marketplace. Similarly, stored cereal grains and other farm commodities may be treated with pesticides. The food manufacturer, to produce processed foods with the attributes that the consumer expects—pleasing texture and appearance, appetizing flavor, stability during storage, and economical price—uses a variety of synthetic and naturally occurring chemicals. These chemicals may be added directly to food or may enter food indirectly by migration from food contact surfaces or from packaging materials. In addition to the intentional use of chemicals for specific purposes, chemicals can inadvertently contaminate the food supply as a result of industrial accidents or environmental pollution, or from natural sources such as pathogenic and toxicogenic microorganisms.

Food laws and government regulations are designed to ensure that the amounts of substances added to food from the aforementioned sources are safe for human consumption. As technology,

toxicology, and food laws have evolved, different categories of added food constituents have been defined. This chapter discusses the different categories, gives examples of substances in each category and the functions they serve in their intended use, and reviews the scientific evidence and testing procedures applied to establish safety. Emphasis is given to substances intentionally added to processed food by the food industry because they constitute the greatest number and diversity of added food constituents. For more information concerning the use, properties, regulatory status, health aspects, and safety of added and natural food constituents, the reader is referred to the Selected Readings.

## FOOD ADDITIVES

Substances generally considered to be food additives are those that are added to foods by the food processor. They may be added directly to food or they may enter food by an indirect route. Direct additives are substances added intentionally to serve some functional purpose such as sweetness, flavor, leavening action, or color. A direct food additive may be a single chemical substance, e.g., sucrose or sodium chloride, or a mixture of chemicals, e.g., those found in vinegar, spices, or mustard. Indirect additives result from the contact of food with processing equipment, packaging materials, or other surfaces and the migration or extraction of components of these surfaces into the food. Indirect additives are generally present in the finished food in only trace amounts.

As used in this chapter, the term food additive has a broad connotation and includes all substances added by the food processor unless otherwise stated.

## Functions and Benefits

Food additives perform a variety of functions. The physical and technical functional effects for which substances are added to foods are illustrated by the types of agents permitted for direct addition.[1] These agents are listed in Table 39–1.

The principal benefits of the use of food additives are (1) improved food quality and attractiveness; (2) enhanced nutrient content or stabilization; (3) prevention of microbial contamination, spoilage, and waste; (4) user convenience in preparation of food for the table; (5) increased variety of foods available to consumers; and (6) cost reduction.

Examples of the use and benefits of food additives are numerous.[2] Development of modern mass production methods for bread and the resultant lowered production costs required emulsifiers and dough conditioners (oxidizing and reducing agents, proteases) to compensate for the variability in the properties of flour and to ensure satisfactory operation of the process and consist-

**Table 39–1. Types of Direct Food Additives According to Functional Effects**

Anticaking and free-flow agents
Antimicrobial agents
Antioxidants
Colors and coloring adjuncts
Curing and pickling agents
Dough strengtheners
Drying agents
Emulsifiers and emulsifier salts
Enzymes
Firming agents
Flavor enhancers
Flavoring agents and adjuvants
Flour treating agents
Formulation aids
Fumigants
Humectants
Leavening agents
Lubricants and release agents
Non-nutritive sweeteners
Nutrient supplements
Nutritive sweeteners
Oxidizing and reducing agents
pH control agents
Processing aids
Propellants, aerating agents, and gases
Sequestrants
Solvents and vehicles
Stabilizers and thickeners
Surface-active agents
Surface-finishing agents
Synergists
Texturizers

ent quality of the product. Propionates are used to protect bread against the growth of mold, extending its usable life after purchase. Acidulants are added to a variety of foods to prevent the germination of fungal spores and the growth of microorganisms, which lead to spoilage or cause food poisoning or disease. The success of cake mixes in ensuring the production of a good cake by the home baker is largely a result of the additives (emulsifiers and leavening agents) included in the formulation. Addition of small amounts of antioxidants protects margarine, shortening, and cooking and salad oils against rancidity resulting from air oxidation (and formation of possible toxic compounds), thereby providing the shelf life needed in today's production and distribution system. Enrichment of cereal products with niacin in the 1940s was a factor in the elimination of pellagra from the United States. In addition, the natural level of iron in the food supply is insufficient to provide the dietary intake of iron recommended by the Food and Nutrition Board for several population groups. Iron enrichment now provides about 25% of the iron in the United States diet.

## Specifications

To ensure the uniformity as well as the purity of food additives, the U.S. Food and Drug Administration (FDA) requires that they be of food-grade quality as defined by specifications for their chemical composition, identification and limits of impurities, methods of manufacture, and physical, chemical, and biologic properties. The Food Chemicals Codex, prepared by the Committee on Food Protection, National Academy of Sciences, contains specifications for both direct and indirect food additives.[3] The FDA requires that food additives meet the specifications defined in the Food Chemicals Codex or, for substances not included in this Codex, specifications defined by the FDA regulations. Uniformity of product resulting from the requirement that food additives conform to compositional and related specifications is important in food safety considerations because it ensures that the product used in food is the same, within the limits specified, as the product tested for safety.

The FDA has prescribed criteria of *good manufacturing practice* to ensure that processed foods are wholesome and safe for human consumption. Criteria for good practice apply to raw materials, plant facilities, methods, and controls used in the manufacturing, processing, packing, and holding of various types of foods. Good manufacturing practice also restricts the level of addition of a food additive to no more than that reasonably required to accomplish its intended physical, nutritive, or other technical effect.

## Legal Definition

The 1958 Amendment[4] to the Federal Food, Drug, and Cosmetic (FFD&C) Act[5] in its legal definition of the term food additive includes both direct and indirect additives and also formally defines any radiation treatment of food as a food additive. The amendment requires that food additives receive approval from the FDA before they may be added to foods. Approval must be based on scientific data provided by the petitioner (i.e., proposed user or manufacturer) that demonstrate the absence of hazard when the substance is used in the amount and manner proposed. Approval of a substance having carcinogenic activity is specifically precluded by the Delaney clause of the amendment, which states in part, "that no additive shall be deemed to be safe if it is found to induce cancer when ingested by man or animal, or is found, after tests which are appropriate for the evaluation of the safety of food additives, to induce cancer in man or animal."

Several categories of substances added to food by food processors are not included in the legal definition of a food additive. These categories were defined in the 1958 Amendment and were exempted from premarket safety approval or other requirements specified for a food additive. The major category excluded in this amendment includes substances generally recognized as safe (GRAS) under the conditions of their intended use in the judgment of scientists qualified by training and experience to evaluate food safety. The basis for such views may be either scientific evaluation procedures or, in the case of a substance used in food before January 1, 1958, experience based on common use in food. Also excluded are color additives and substances sanctioned or approved by the FDA or the U.S. Department of Agriculture (USDA) for use in meats or poultry before the enactment of the 1958 amendment. These excluded substances are not exempt from federal scrutiny for safety, but regulation is exercised under other sections of the FFD&C Act. Residues of pesticides and drugs that were added to food crops or animals by the producer are also regulated by the FFD&C Act.

**Examples of Food Additives as Legally Defined.** In general, food additives are substances that were approved as direct or indirect additives after the passage of the 1958 Amendment to the FFD&C Act. They were approved on the basis of scientific data submitted by petitioners to the FDA that (1) established the safety of the additives when used in the amount and manner proposed (e.g., the spe-

cific foods or food packaging materials in which the additives were proposed to be used and the levels of addition), (2) showed the additives to be effective for their intended uses, and (3) provided analytic methods to allow monitoring of their levels in foods.

The Code of Federal Regulations[1] provides the following classifications of additives permitted for direct addition to food:

1. *Food preservatives.* Examples are the antioxidants butylated hydroxyanisole (BHA), butylated hydroxytoluene (BHT), and ethoxyquin; the proxidant metal sequestering agent disodium ethylenediaminetetraacetate; and sodium nitrite and sodium nitrate as preservatives and color fixatives in smoked fish.

2. *Coatings, films, and related substances.* Substances in this category are used to provide protective coatings for fresh bananas, beets, citrus fruits, eggplant, melons, and similar fruits and vegetables. Included are fatty acids and their methyl esters, wood rosin, oxidized polyethylene, synthetic paraffin and its succinic derivatives, terpene resins, and petroleum naphtha as a vehicle for the application of coatings.

3. *Special dietary and nutritional additives.* The only vitamins regulated as food additives are folic acid (folacin), D-pantothenamide, the nicotinamide-ascorbic acid complex, the aluminum salt of nicotinic acid, and the calcium pantothenate-calcium chloride double salt. Most vitamins are classified as GRAS food ingredients, which indicates that they were commonly used before 1958.

Approved amino acids are glycine and the L-isomers of alanine, arginine, asparagine, aspartic acid, cysteine, cystine, glutamic acid, glutamine, histidine, isoleucine, leucine, lysine, methionine, phenylalanine, proline, serine, threonine, tryptophan, tyrosine, and valine, as well as DL-methionine (not for infant foods). If an amino acid is added to a food to improve its nutritional quality, several conditions must be met. The biologic quality of the protein of the food to which the amino acid or combination of amino acids is added must be significantly improved, and the addition must result in a protein efficiency ratio (PER) in the finished ready-to-eat food that is equivalent to the PER of casein. A reasonable daily adult intake of the finished food must furnish at least 6.5 g of naturally occurring, primarily intact protein. Limits also are placed on the amount of amino acids added for nutritive purposes plus the amounts naturally present expressed as a percentage by weight of total protein in the finished food.

Other substances approved as additives for nutritive purposes are bakers' yeast protein; the calcium, ferrous, magnesium, potassium, and sodium salts of fumaric acid as sources of minerals; kelp and potassium iodide as sources of iodine; and fish protein concentrates and isolates.

4. *Anticaking agents.* Four substances are approved in this category. Iron ammonium citrate and sodium ferrocyanide are permitted only in salt and at levels not in excess of 25 and 13 ppm, respectively. Calcium silicate and silicon dioxide are approved in only those foods in which the additive has been demonstrated to have an anticaking effect and in amounts not in excess of those reasonably required to produce the intended effect but not in excess of 2% of the weight of the food. However, up to 5% by weight of calcium silicate may be used in baking powder.

5. *Flavoring agents.* Two classes of flavoring agents are listed as approved food additives: natural (and natural substances used in conjunction with flavors) and synthetic. Both are to be used in the minimum quantity required to produce their intended effect and in accordance with the principles of good manufacturing practice. The natural flavorings consist of plant parts, extracts, oil, gums, resins, balsams, waxes, or distillates of some 130 plant species. The approximately 750 synthetic flavoring substances and adjuvants are specific chemical compounds, many of which are counterparts of substances present in natural flavors.

6. *Gums, chewing gum bases, and related substances.* Included in this category are the masticatory substances, natural (e.g., chicle, a plant gum) and synthetic (e.g., polyethylene, polyisobutylene) polymers, and plasticizers that are approved as chewing gum bases.

7. *Multipurpose additives.* This group of some 75 additives includes acetone peroxides (flour-maturing agents and dough conditioners), aspartame (sweetener and flavor enhancer), oxystearins (crystallization inhibitors in vegetable oils and release agents in vegetable shortenings), sodium lauryl sulfate (emulsifier, whipping agent, and surfactant), polysorbate 80 (solubilizing and dispersing agent, surfactant, emulsifier, wetting agent, or defoaming agent), propylene glycol alginate (emulsifier, stabilizer, or thickener), succinylated monoglycerides (emulsifiers in liquid shortenings, dough conditioners in bread baking), fatty acids (lubricants, binders, or defoaming agents), modified food starches (thickeners, stabilizers, or dispersing agents), and other specified compounds that may have two or more functional effects in foods.

8. *Secondary direct additives.* Members of this group are principally substances used as processing aids. In many cases, the additive is removed after treatment is completed. The group of about 120 substances is divided into four major categories: polymer substances for purification and clarification; enzyme preparations and microorganisms; solvents, lubricants, release agents, and related substances; and specific usage additives.

Included in polymer substances are ion-exchange resins employed in the purification of water and a variety of foods. Other resins are approved for use as flocculants to clarify liquids, e.g., polyacrylamides for cane and beet sugar juices and polyvinylpyrrolidone for beverages and vinegar.

Enzymes produced by specific microorganisms are approved as secondary direct food additives for use in producing glucose, distilled spirits, vinegar, citric acid, sucrose, and cheese and in processing clams and shrimp. Many other enzyme preparations are considered GRAS. Included are animal-derived enzymes such as pepsin and trypsin; plant-derived enzymes including papain and bromelain; and microbe-derived enzymes such as the glucose isomerases and carbohydrases.

The major permitted uses of approved solvents are for the extraction of flavors from spices and hops and for the decaffeination of coffee. Ethyl acetate, methylene chloride, and trichlorethylene are listed for the extraction of caffeine. However, the food processing industry discontinued use of trichloroethylene when it became a suspected animal carcinogen and the FDA proposed banning its use.[6] Permitted solvents for the extraction of flavors from hops in the manufacturing of beer and for the extraction of flavors from spices include acetone, isopropyl alcohol, and hexane. The safe use of these solvents is prescribed by specifying the maximum permitted residue in the product or the maximum amount that can be added in a food-processing operation.

Specific usage additives include substances that may be safely used as boiler-water additives in the preparation of steam that will contact food; chemical substances (e.g., detergents) for use in washing or in the lye peeling of fruits and vegetables; defoaming agents in food-processing operations (e.g., white mineral oil, silicon dioxide, or polyethylene glycol); and the combustion product gases from butane, propane, or natural gas for displacing or removing oxygen in the processing, storing, or packaging of foods other than meats.

9. *Indirect food additives.* Indirect food additives are substances approved as components of paper and paperboard, resinous and polymeric coating materials, and plastics and adhesives intended for use in or as articles that contact food. Such articles may provide an opportunity for the components to migrate into food. Included are

strippable food coatings; interior coatings of metal cans, paper, paperboard, and plastic packages; and other articles for packaging or holding food and heating prepared foods. Substances approved are synthetic and natural polymeric materials; numerous organic compounds used as plasticizers, bounding, and cross-linking agents; and preservatives. Test procedures are prescribed by the FDA for determining the amount of material extracted from resinous and polymeric coatings, paper and paperboard, and some of the rigid or semirigid plastics. Test extraction conditions stimulate the types of foods and beverages and the exposure conditions of the intended use of these materials. For approval as an indirect food additive, the amount of material that is extracted under the test conditions must not exceed a specified limit.

## GRAS SUBSTANCES

The GRAS concept provided a modified grandfather clause to accomplish the evaluation of several hundred food ingredients in common use before January 1, 1958, without requiring extensive testing. As noted previously, the 1958 Amendment to the FFD&C Act provided that substances in use at that time could be considered GRAS either through experience based on common use or through scientific evaluation procedures. In contrast to substances legally defined as food additives, which are required to have their safety demonstrated by industry before FDA approval, such evidence is not mandatory for GRAS substances that were in use before 1958. Food ingredients introduced after January 1, 1958 can be considered GRAS only on the basis of evidence developed through scientific procedures. In such instances, the FDA requires the same quantity and quality of scientific evidence for GRAS status as required to obtain approval of a food additive regulation for the ingredient. In addition, the FDA specifies that the recognition of safety shall ordinarily be based on published studies, which may be corroborated by unpublished studies and other data and information. An important distinction between food additives and GRAS food ingredients is that the Delaney clause applies to the former but not to the latter. However, other sections of the FFD&C Act give the FDA the authority to ban a GRAS food ingredient or to restrict its use to safe levels if evidence indicates that it may be injurious to health.

The exemption of biologic testing for GRAS food ingredients in use before 1958 was of concern to many. In 1969 the United States President, on recommendation of the White House Conference on Food, Nutrition, and Health, directed the FDA to critically evaluate the scientific literature on these substances. This study was initiated by the FDA in 1970, and to date the health aspects of some 500 GRAS substances have been evaluated.[7]

**The GRAS List.** The 1985 revision of The Code of Federal Regulations[1] lists about 600 substances currently considered to be in the GRAS category by the FDA. About 100 additional substances, not listed in the Code of Federal Regulations, were approved in letters issued by the FDA and are regarded by the FDA as unpublished GRAS substances. Not all substances that are generally regarded as safe for their intended use are listed in the Code of Federal Regulations. Other substances ordinarily regarded as GRAS are food ingredients of natural biologic origin that have been widely consumed for their nutrient properties in the United States before January 1, 1958, without known detrimental effects. They must be prepared by conventional processing as practiced before January 1, 1958.[1] Included in this category are common food commodities, e.g., cereal flours, meats, fruits, and vegetables, as conventionally processed.

The 1958 Amendment did not specify that the FDA be the sole judge of GRAS status of a substance; it required only that such recognition of safety be among experts "qualified by training and experience to judge its safety." One such group that has made additional GRAS classifications is a panel of experts formed by the Flavor and Extract Manufacturers' Association (FEMA) to evaluate the natural and synthetic substances used as flavoring agents in processed foods. The FEMA expert panel evaluated approximately 1,650 flavoring agents as GRAS.[8] Of this group, more than 700 were subsequently approved by the FDA as food additives and now appear in the Code of Federal Regulations.

The GRAS food ingredients perform functions similar to those of food additives. Most substances added to foods as sources of vitamins or minerals are GRAS nutrients, as shown in Table 39–2. With the exception of cuprous iodide, potassium iodide, and vitamins $D_2$ and $D_3$, maximum levels of the added GRAS nutrients are not specified, but levels are required to conform to good manufacturing practice, i.e., to not exceed that level needed to accomplish the intended nutritional effect. The maximum level of cuprous iodide or potassium iodide permitted in salt as a source of dietary iodine is 0.01%. After a comprehensive safety review of vitamins $D_2$ and $D_3$, the FDA affirmed their GRAS status but with specific limitations on the levels of addition and the foods in which their use is permitted.[9] Limitations on use were proposed in view of the relatively low margin of safety between the total intake of vitamin

**Table 39–2. Nutrients from the FDA GRAS List***

Ascorbic acid
Biotin
Calcium carbonate
Calcium citrate
Calcium glycerophosphate
Calcium pantothenate
Calcium phosphate
Calcium pyrophosphate
Carotene
Choline bitartrate
Choline chloride
Copper gluconate
Cuprous iodide
Ferric phosphate
Ferric pyrophosphate
Ferric sodium pyrophosphate
Ferrous gluconate
Ferrous lactate
Ferrous sulfate
Iron, reduced
Linoleic acid
Magnesium oxide
Magnesium phosphate
Magnesium sulfate
Manganese chloride
Manganese citrate
Manganese gluconate
Manganese glycerophosphate
Manganese hypophosphite
Manganese sulfate
Manganous oxide
Niacin
Niacinamide
D-Pantothenyl alcohol
Potassium chloride
Potassium glycerophosphate
Potassium iodide
Pyridoxine hydrochloride
Riboflavin
Riboflavin-5-phosphate
Sodium phosphate
Thiamin hydrochloride
Thiamin mononitrate
Tocopherols
α-Tocopherol acetate
Vitamin A
Vitamin A acetate
Vitamin A palmitate
Vitamin $B_{12}$
Vitamin $D_2$
Vitamin $D_3$
Zinc chloride
Zinc gluconate
Zinc oxide
Zinc stearate
Zinc sufate

*From Code of Federal Regulations. Title 21: Food and Drugs, Parts 170–199 rev. Washington, D.C., U.S. Government Printing Office, 1985.

D from all sources and the amounts that may produce toxic manifestations.

Another category of additional substances considered GRAS are the chemical preservatives (Table 39–3), which include substances having antimicrobial or antioxidant activity. BHA and BHT are listed both as food additives and as GRAS substances. In their GRAS use, maximum levels of total antioxidants (e.g., BHA and BHT combined) must not exceed 0.02% of the fat or oil content of the food. Approval as food additives extended their use to certain specified foods (e.g., potato flakes, dry breakfast foods) at higher levels, based on fat content, that are required to inhibit rancidification.

Because of the safety issues raised by the pharmacologic implications of the induction of hepatic microsomal enzymes in rats and monkeys fed BHT and the increased incidence of tumors in mice receiving BHT in their diet, the FDA issued a proposed interim food additive regulation on BHT in 1977.[10] This proposed regulation listed maximum usage levels of BHT in specified foods. It also directed interested persons to undertake appropriate feeding studies to resolve the issues. Subsequent studies of tumorigenesis have given conflicting results: two rat studies gave negative results;[11,11a] a third study showed an increased

**Table 39–3. Chemical Preservatives from the FDA GRAS List***

Ascorbic acid
Ascorbyl palmitate
Benzoic acid
Butylated hydroxyanisole
Butylated hydroxytoluene
Calcium ascorbate
Calcium sorbate
Dilauryl thiodipropionate
Erythorbic acid
Methylparaben
Potassium bisulfite
Potassium metabisulfite
Potassium sorbate
Propionic acid
Propyl gallate
Propylparaben
Sodium ascorbate
Sodium benzoate
Sodium bisulfite
Sodium metabisulfite
Sodium propionate
Sodium sorbate
Sodium sulfite
Sorbic acid
Stannous chloride
Sulfur dioxide
Tocopherols

*From Code of Federal Regulations. Title 21: Food and Drugs, Parts 170–199 rev. Washington, D.C., U.S. Government Printing Office, 1985.

incidence of hepatocellular carcinoma in male rats at the highest dose level, 250 mg/kg body weight, but not at 25 mg/kg body weight.[12] Estimated per capita daily human exposure is 0.037 mg/kg body weight. A more recent study with rats suggests that BHT is a weak promoter of liver carcinogenesis.[12,12a] Concern also has developed regarding BHA. It has caused tumors at high dietary levels in the stomach of rats[13] and Syrian golden hamsters,[14] both species having forestomachs, but not in the stomach of dogs[15] or monkeys,[15a] which, like humans, do not have forestomachs.

The Joint FAO/WHO Expert Committee on Food Additives in its June 1986 meeting set an Acceptable Daily Intake level of 0–0.5 mg/kg body weight for BHT and 0–0.3 mg/kg body weight for BHA.

Sulfiting agents have been used in foods for decades to inhibit oxidative discoloration and flavor changes without reports of adverse reactions. However, several reports indicate that individuals with asthmatic conditions are particularly sensitive to foods containing sulfites.[16–19] Sulfites as GRAS food ingredients are used in many processed foods, including fruit drinks, beer, wine, baked goods, some canned foods, and dried fruits.[19] In restaurant foods, sulfites have been used as preservatives for holding prepeeled potatoes and seafoods before cooking; for a few years sulfites were widely used on salad bars to keep vegetables and fruits looking fresh. Reports of severe reactions and deaths associated with the consumption of sulfite-treated foods, mainly raw fruits and vegetables eaten in restaurants, led the FDA to make consumers aware of products that contain sulfites, and to reduce consumer exposure.[20] A labeling regulation requires manufacturers to declare sulfites on the label of any food containing the substance at a level of 10 ppm or more.[21] If the sulfite is used specifically as a preservative or has a technical functional effect in the food, it must be declared on the label regardless of the amount in the finished product. A second regulation bans the use of sulfites on fruits and vegetables that are intended to be served or sold raw to consumers.[22]

## COLOR ADDITIVES

Rules concerning color additives were prescribed in the 1960 Color Additives Amendment to the FFD&C Act and have been incorporated into the Code of Federal Regulations.[23] This amendment provided requirements for FDA approval similar to those for food additives and made the food industry responsible for proving the safety of colors added. Approval of carcinogenic color additives was precluded. It required that safe conditions of use be established by regulation and that all color additives be batch-certified, i.e., a sample of each production lot must be tested and found to conform to FDA specifications unless exempted by the commissioner of the FDA. Color additives approved for use in food and exempt from certification are mostly plant materials such as dehydrated beets, β-carotene, grape color extract, fruit juices, carrot oil, paprika, saffron, and similar substances. Also included is the most widely used food color, caramel, produced by heat treatment of food-grade carbohydrates such as dextrose, sucrose, maltose, starch hydrolysates, and molasses with approved acids, alkalis, and salts. Caramel is also approved by the FDA as a GRAS flavoring substance.

All color additives requiring certification of identity and purity are synthetic organic compounds. They are often referred to as coal tar colors because the starting chemicals of most were originally derived from coal tar. Those on the market when the 1960 Color Additives Amendment was passed were provisionally listed; their use was permitted on an interim basis until their safety was established. Seven substances are now "permanently" approved for food use. Five of these, FD&C Blue No. 1, FD&C Green No. 3, FD&C Red No. 3, FD&C Red No. 40, and FD&C Yellow No. 5, are approved for general food use at levels consistent with good manufacturing practice. Uses and levels of addition of the other two substances are limited: Orange B is limited to casings or surfaces of frankfurters and sausages at levels no greater than 150 ppm based on the weight of the finished food, and Citrus Red No. 2 is limited to use in skins of oranges not intended for processing at levels no greater than 2 ppm based on the weight of the whole fruit. Two colors, FD&C Yellow No. 6 and FD&C Blue No. 2, are provisionally approved for use in foods. Three colors, FD&C Blue No. 2, FD&C Red No. 3, and FD&C Yellow No. 6, are provisionally listed for drug and cosmetic use. Information from animal feeding studies with these colors and other provisionally listed D&C colors is now being reviewed by the FDA.[24,25]

Because a number of studies have indicated an association between allergic reactions and ingestion of food colored with FD&C Yellow No. 5, labels on foods containing this substance must declare its presence by naming it as FD&C Yellow No. 5 in the list of ingredients. Other certified colors are not required to be listed by specific name, but may be listed as an artificial color, artificial coloring, or color added.

## CONSUMER EXPOSURE TO FOOD ADDITIVES

An important factor in determining the possible hazard of a food ingredient is the quantity ingested. Information on the dietary intake of GRAS food ingredients, color additives, and food additives has been provided by surveys of the food industry conducted by the National Research Council in 1970,[26] 1975,[27] and 1977.[28] Daily per capita usage was calculated from poundage data given in these reports for the food additives used in greatest amounts by industry.[2] For the 15 GRAS food ingredients used in greatest amounts, values ranged from 87 g of sucrose to 0.09 g of sodium aluminum phosphate (Table 39–4). Included in this group are substances also commonly used in the home: sucrose, corn syrup, salt, sodium bicarbonate, yeast, monosodium glutamate, and hydrolyzed vegetable proteins. Greatest per capita usage reported for a substance classified as a direct food additive was 0.180 g/day for the modified starch, starch diphosphate. This starch derivative is used as a viscosity stabilizer and thickening agent in canned foods. Few other additives were used in per capita amounts exceeding 6 mg/day.

Although flavoring agents comprise the majority of substances intentionally added to foods, they are added in relatively small amounts, generally at levels of a few parts per million. Those used in greatest quantity by the food industry and in the home are the natural flavoring substances (Table 39–5). Included are such common household condiments as mustard, pepper, nutmeg, oregano, caraway seed, cloves, and allspice. Daily

**Table 39–4. GRAS Food Ingredients Used by the Food Industry in Largest Quantities in 1975***

| Substance | Usage | |
|---|---|---|
| | *Million lb/yr* | *g/d per capita* |
| Sucrose | 14,900 | 87 |
| Corn syrup | 1,530 | 9.0 |
| Sodium chloride | 1,420 | 8.3 |
| Dextrose | 266 | 1.6 |
| Mono- and diglycerides | 86 | 0.50 |
| Hydrochloric acid | 82 | 0.46 |
| Caramel | 74 | 0.43 |
| Sodium bicarbonate | 60 | 0.35 |
| Yeasts | 57 | 0.33 |
| Citric acid | 57 | 0.33 |
| Calcium phosphate, mono-basic | 48 | 0.29 |
| Monosodium glutamate | 28 | 0.16 |
| Carbon dioxide | 27 | 0.16 |
| Hydrolyzed vegetable proteins | 23 | 0.14 |
| Sodium aluminum phosphate | 15 | 0.087 |

*Adapted from Senti, F.R.: I&EC Prod. Res. Dev. 20:237–246, 1981.

**Table 39–5. Natural Flavoring Substances Reported Used by the Food Industry in Largest Amounts in 1970 and 1976***

| Substance | Usage | |
|---|---|---|
| | *1,000 lb/yr* | *mg/d per capita* |
| Mustard, yellow | 31,000 | 176 |
| Pepper, black | 19,051 | 108 |
| Malt extract | 7,050 | 40 |
| Pepper, red | 2,334 | 14 |
| Caffeine | 2,000 | 11 |
| Lemon oil | 1,547 | 9 |
| Cassia | 1,147 | 7 |
| Oregano | 920 | 5 |
| Peppermint oil | 870 | 5 |
| Nutmeg | 770 | 4 |
| Caraway seed | 634 | 4 |
| Cocoa extract | 536 | 3 |
| Cloves | 519 | 3 |
| Allspice | 498 | 3 |

*Reprinted with permission from Senti, F.R.: I&EC Prod. Res. Dev. 20:237–246, 1981. Copyright 1981 American Chemical Society.

**Table 39–6. Synthetic Flavoring Substances: Adjuncts and Adjuvants Reported Used in the Largest Amounts in 1976***

| Substance | Usage | |
|---|---|---|
| | *1,000 lb/yr* | *mg/d per capita* |
| Monosodium glutamate | 18,000 | 104 |
| Isopropyl alcohol | 4,000 | 23 |
| Malic acid | 3,000 | 17 |
| Acetone | 570 | 3.3 |
| Ethyl acetate | 560 | 3.2 |
| Methyl salicylate | 280 | 1.6 |
| Ethyl acetoacetate | 63 | 0.36 |
| 4-(Methylthio)-2-butanone | 59 | 0.34 |
| Thiamin hydrochloride | 57 | 0.33 |
| Isobutyl acetate | 44 | 0.25 |
| Ethyl maltol | 38 | 0.22 |
| Isoamyl butyrate | 36 | 0.21 |
| Butyric acid | 27 | 0.15 |
| Triacetin | 20 | 0.13 |
| Acetaldehyde | 19 | 0.11 |

*Reprinted with permission from Senti, F.R.: I&EC Prod. Res. Dev. 20:237–246, 1981. Copyright 1981 American Chemical Society.

per capita use of the 14 agents used in greatest amounts ranged from 176 to 3 mg.

The 15 synthetic substances used in greatest amounts in flavorings by the processed food industry (Table 39–6) include substances that enhance or modify a flavor or that serve as solvents or carriers for flavors. Per capita exposure ranged from 104 to 0.11 mg/day. Of these 15 substances, only monosodium glutamate, the substance used in greatest amount, is commonly used in the home. Although prepared synthetically, many are natural constitutents of foods: for example, malic acid, ethyl acetate, thiamin, isobutyl acetate, iso-amyl butyrate, and butyric acid occur naturally in fruits, cheeses, and other foods.

Of all flavorings, natural and synthetic, 78% were reported used by the food industry in the 1970s in quantities less than 1,000 lb (0.006 mg/day/capita), 61% less than 100 lb, and 38% less than 10 lb.[2]

Some perspective on the level of consumption of synthetic chemicals added to foods for preserving, emulsifying, flavoring, or other functions may be gained by comparison with the level of consumption of naturally occurring substances that are toxic when consumed in excessive amounts. A safety factor of 100 has been traditionally applied to the highest "no-observed-adverse effect" level derived from studies in which a proposed food additive has been fed to animals at multiple dosage levels, at least one of which is associated with a toxic response. As an example of a naturally occurring toxic substance, potatoes normally contain 2 to 13 mg of the toxic alkaloid solanine per 100 g fresh weight.[29] In certain isolated cases, concentrations as high as 80 to 100 mg/100 g have been reported, as in the "greening" in smaller tubers exposed to light. Per capita daily consumption of potatoes is about 150 g, and normal per capita exposure to solanine is in the range of 3 to 20 mg/day. An oral dose of 200 mg solanine causes drowsiness, hyperesthesia, and dyspnea in humans; higher doses result in vomiting and diarrhea. Thus the safety factor for solanine is about 10.

Cyanogenetic glucosides that release hydrogen cyanide on enzymatic hydrolysis occur in lima beans, sweet potatoes, chickpeas, and other food plants.[30] One white-seeded American variety of lima beans produced 10 mg/100 g seed. The lethal dose for the adult human is reported to be in the range of 0.5 to 3.5 mg/kg body weight or 30 to 210 mg for a 60-kg individual. Chronic neurologic disease in certain tropical countries has been attributed to cyanide intoxication from dietary cassava.[30]

### Pesticides

Pesticides are widely used in modern agriculture for the control of insects, nematodes, fungi, weeds, and other pests. Pesticides may also be used in food-handling establishments where food products are stored, processed, prepared, or served. Maximum residual levels of pesticides on the raw commodity as harvested and in any processed food product are limited by tolerances set by the United States Environmental Protection Agency (EPA). Tolerances for some 90 pesticides

in foods and limitations on their use are given in the Code of Federal Regulations.[1]

Effectiveness of the regulations set for pesticide residues is monitored in the Total Diet Study Program for adults, toddlers, and infants conducted by the FDA. The adult total diet study involves determination of pesticide residues, polychlorinated biphenyls (PCBs), other industrial chemicals, and selected chemical elements in the diets of typical 16- to 19-year-old males. The study is based on food consumption patterns of this age group found in the USDA's 1965 food consumption surveys of the south, northeast, north central, and west geographic regions of the United States. In the FY 1981/1982 (October 1980 to March 1982) study of adults,[31] market baskets consisting of 120 food items (including drinking water) representing 14-day diets were collected through the year in 27 urban markets in the four geographic regions (5 to 8 market baskets per region). The individual food items were separated into 12 food groups (e.g., meat, poultry and fish, dairy products, grains and cereals, leafy vegetables). Each item was prepared in the manner usually consumed, foods in each group were combined into composites, and the composite was then analyzed.

Pesticides found in the FY 1981/1982 study of adults included organochlorine pesticides, e.g., DDT and dieldrin; organophosphorus pesticides including parathion and malathion; chlorophenoxy acid herbicide residues such as 2,4-D and 2,4,5-T; and carbaryl and orthophenylphenol residues. Sixty different pesticides and industrial chemicals (including degradation products) were detected in the adult study. The number of chemicals detected per food group ranged from 0 to 26, the most being found in garden fruit (26), fruit (22), and oils-fats (20), and the least being found in beverages (below detection limits). The maximum levels found were fractional parts per million, and the calculated total dietary intake of each of the pesticides, with the exception of dieldrin, was 2% or less of the acceptable daily intake (ADI) set by the United Nations' Food and Agriculture Organization and the World Health Organization (FAO/WHO).[32] The total dietary intake of dieldrin was 16% of the ADI.

The daily intakes of pesticides and industrial chemicals by adults for Fiscal Years 1978 to 1981/1982 were relatively constant.[31]

The FY 1981/1982 total diet studies for infants and toddlers[33] were similar to those for adults. Market baskets of 50 food items for 6-month-old infants and about 110 for 2-year-old toddlers, which represented the diet patterns in the four United States geographic regions, were collected in 13 cities. Individual food items of the market basket sample were separated into 11 groups and blended, and the composites were analyzed for selected pesticides, industrial chemicals, and elements. In the foods of infants, 36 organic chemicals were detected and in the food of toddlers, 48 were detected. In the infant diets, the greatest numbers of chemicals were detected in oils-fats (13), meat-fish-poultry (11), and potato (11) groups, and the least (below detection limits) in water and other beverages. In the toddler diet, the greatest numbers of residues were found in the oils-fats (24) and fruit-fruit juices (16) groups, and the least in the beverage group. The calculated total dietary intake of each of the pesticides did not exceed 4% of the ADI set by FAO/WHO, except for dieldrin, which was 20% of the ADI for infants and 23% for toddlers. Comparison with values obtained in the FY 1978 to FY 1980 surveys indicates that the daily intakes of pesticides and industrial chemicals were relatively constant over that period for both infants and toddlers.

## Contaminants

Contaminants in foods may arise from industrial and natural sources, and as a result of the reaction of food constituents. Industrial contaminants are principally chemicals that were inadvertently or accidently released into the environment as either end products or by-products of manufacturing processes.

**Industrial Chemicals.** Widely publicized examples of inadvertent or accidental release of industrial chemicals are the PCBs and the polybrominated biphenyls (PBBs). Both are stable compounds that resist biodegradation and produce adverse effects in animals when ingested at low levels. Before 1971, PCBs were used in a wide variety of applications primarily because of their excellent electrical and thermal properties.[34] Leakage of PCB fluids from heat exchangers in feed-processing plants contaminated poultry feeds, and in turn caused the contamination of meat and eggs intended for human consumption. Migration of PCBs into dairy cattle feed from paints used to coat the interior of silos also led to the contamination of milk with these compounds. Food packaging made from recycled paper that included carbonless copy paper containing PCBs in the paper mix resulted in the contamination of some food products with low levels of PCBs. Disposal of old transformers and other devices and materials containing PCBs resulted in their leakage into watersheds and lakes and the contamination of fish. Since 1971, levels of PCBs in foods have declined as a result of restrictions on their industrial use. Freshwater fish now appear to be the major residual source of PCBs in the United States diet. The maximum level permitted by the FDA in fish and shellfish (edible portion) is 2 ppm; in milk and processed dairy products, 1.5 ppm (fat basis); in poultry, 3 ppm (fat basis); and in eggs, 0.3 ppm. PCBs were not detected in infant and toddler diets in the FDA's FY 1981/1982 Total Diet Studies.[33] They were found only in the meat, poultry, fish group in the adult diet.[31] Estimated total daily intake per person decreased from 1.86 µg in FY 1978 to 0.21 µg in FY 1981/1982.

PBB contamination of foods, mainly animal products, resulted when a fire retardant product was unknowingly used in place of a feed supplement in the preparation of feeds in a manufacturing plant in Michigan in 1973.[34] Control measures included disposal of contaminated feed, livestock, and poultry. Production of the chemical was discontinued in 1974. The FDA set action levels for the seizure of PBB-contaminated products at 0.3 ppm for the fat of meat, milk, and dairy products and 0.05 ppm for eggs and animal feeds. Exposure to PBBs has been limited largely to the population of Michigan, as indicated by surveys conducted by the EPA.

**Natural and Industrial Chemicals.** Lead, cadmium, arsenic, mercury, and selenium are among the chemical elements known to present health risks at relatively low exposure levels. Signs of chronic poisoning may appear in animals given parts per million doses of these elements in their diets. The chemicals may enter food or the food chain from one or more sources including pesticide residues, food containers, natural background levels in plants and animals produced in environments largely unaffected by human activity, and industrial wastes that pollute soils and water, causing increased levels of contaminants in plants and animals. Pesticides containing lead, arsenic, and mercury formerly contributed to increased levels of these elements in food, but this contribution has been minimized since their replacement in most cases by organic chemicals.

The current use of lead for soldering the seams of tin cans for packaging foods is a significant dietary source of lead. In 1979, lead from the solder in canned foods was estimated to contribute about 14% of the lead in the average daily diet of persons over 1 year of age; an additional 7% came from the food itself.[35] With the encouragement of the FDA, industry has reduced lead levels in canned products. Because infants and children are at a substantially greater risk than adults of lead exposure, emphasis has been placed on infant foods, including canned evaporated milk. As a result of these efforts, the evaporated milk industry has replaced lead-soldered cans with welded cans. Improved soldering technology and increased use of nonsoldered containers have reduced lead levels in other canned foods. A 1983 retail market survey for lead content of 14 canned foods commonly fed to children showed an overall reduction of 39% since 1980 to a mean level of 0.19 ppm.[36] A similar survey in 1984 showed a further reduction to 0.12 ppm.[37]

Silver-plated hollowware and ceramic ware intended for holding liquid foods may also be sources of lead contamination. The FDA has placed limits on the amount of lead that may be leached from these articles under specified test conditions. Similar tests and limits for leachable cadmium apply to ceramic ware intended for holding liquid foods.

Levels of lead, cadmium, arsenic, and mercury in fish, lobsters, and shellfish reflect the concentration of contaminant in the waters from which they are taken, and this concentration is influenced by industrial wastes, erosion of geologic formations, and other factors.[38] Fish are a major dietary source of arsenic. Levels in fruits, vegetables, and cereal products rarely exceed 1 ppm, fresh basis, whereas levels of 2.7 to 56.4 ppm have been reported for marine fish.[39] In one study, flounder taken from a mineral area contained 18.3 ppm arsenic compared with 2.5 ppm in flounder from a nonmineral area, which illustrates the effect of geologic formation. Fish are also a major dietary source of mercury. Industrial activity over the past 100 years appears not to have substantially affected the mercury content of marine fish as indicated by comparing the mercury level in museum specimens of tuna with present levels.[40] However, examples of increased levels of mercury in fish associated with lakes contaminated with mercury from industrial wastes or geologic formations are available.[39]

Wolnik et al. reported background levels of lead, cadmium, selenium, and 11 other elements in six major food crops collected from fields in their respective principal producing areas in the United States.[41,42] The crops chosen—lettuce, peanuts, potatoes, soybeans, sweet corn, and wheat—provide the major portion of cadmium in the U.S. diet. Fields were selected to minimize contamination from human activities. Lead, cadmium, and selenium levels varied by crop and by location. The mean levels for lead and cadmium reported by Wolnik et al. are one sixth to one half of those found for the same foods collected from commercial assembly points in the FDA's 1977 study of metals in foods.[43] Wolnik et al. attribute the lower levels found in their study to collection from relatively uncontaminated fields, careful sampling and handling, and laboratory practices that reduce contamination during analysis.

The maximum levels (5.3 ppm) for selenium in wheat reported by Wolnik et al.[42] are equal to those reported to be toxic to livestock when present in forages grown on seleniferous soils. Wheat products, of course, constitute only a fraction of the human diet, whereas seleniferous forage may be the sole source of feed for livestock. Although toxic at relatively low levels in feed, selenium has been shown by studies with animals to be an essential nutrient. A level of 0.1 to 0.15 ppm based on dry matter in the diet of humans is recommended by the Food and Nutrition Board of the National Academy of Sciences.[44] The relatively small difference between the levels in wheat and the toxic forages indicates the small margin between safe and toxic levels. Concentrations of arsenic, cadmium, lead, mercury, and selenium in the various food groups were determined in the FY 1981/1982 Total Diet Studies.[31,33] In adult diets, the grain and cereal products and/or the meat, poultry, and fish food groups had the highest concentrations of arsenic, cadmium, mercury, and selenium. Potatoes and leafy vegetables also had relatively high concentrations of cadmium. Lead was present in highest concentration in the legume vegetables and garden fruits food groups. Of the food groups in the infant diets, fruits and fruit juices and grains and cereal products had the highest concentration of lead; vegetables and fruit and fruit juices were highest in the diets of toddlers.

The contribution of a food group to the total intake of an element depends on both the concentration of the element and the amount of the food group consumed. The importance of the latter factor is evident in the intake of cadmium and lead by infants and toddlers. Whole milk was the major source of cadmium in the diets of both and the second most important contributor (after fruits and fruit juices) in infant diets.

Estimated average intakes of arsenic, cadmium, lead, mercury, and selenium by 16- to 19-year-old males (3,900 kcal/day) in the FY 1981/1982 Total Diet Study were 46 (inorganic and organic arsenic), 28, 57, 3, and 139 $\mu$g/day, respectively. For toddlers, the respective daily intakes were 16, 16, 30, 1, and 54 $\mu$g, and for infants, 1, 11, 20, <1, and 22 $\mu$g. Values for arsenic (inorganic), cadmium, and mercury were substantially below the Provisional Tolerable Daily Intakes proposed by FAO/WHO for adults, toddlers, and infants.[45,46] Values for lead in the infant and toddler diets represented 13 and 20%, respectively, of the tolerable intake proposed by the FDA for lead from all sources.[47]

**Natural Contaminants.** Other sources of natural contaminants are bacteria, fungi, and other organisms that occur in foods. Of these, bacteria are responsible for most documented cases of food-borne illnesses.[48] Symptoms generally appear a few hours after ingestion of the contaminated food, and effects vary from temporary discomfort to the acutely toxic consequences of botulism. The principal species involved are *Salmonella* spp., *Staphylococcus aureus,* and *Clostridium perfringens.* Botulinal toxin produced by *Clostridium botulinum* is one of the most potent toxins known, and its ingestion is often fatal. Fortunately, its occurrence in food is infrequent.

It has been estimated that 1.4 to 3.4 million cases of food-borne (including water) diseases occur annually in the United States.[49] Most are the result of the mishandling of food in food service establishments and in the home. Mishandling includes improper holding temperature, inadequate cooking, and contaminated equipment.

Certain parasites can occur in foods. *Trichinella spiralis,* a nematode that sometimes occurs in pork, is the most common, and inadequate cooking of the meat results in a number of cases of infestation of humans by this parasite each year.[48] Other parasites may be found in oysters, crabs, and fish, although such findings are reported infrequently.

Mycotoxins are natural contaminants that generally result from mold growth on agricultural crops in the field or after harvest during storage. The best known of these is aflatoxin, a product of the widespread fungus *Aspergillus flavus.*[50] Aflatoxin is a potent carcinogen in rats. It is most frequently found in corn and peanuts, but has also been found in cottonseed, tree nuts, and a number of other commodities. Depending on the levels fed, aflatoxin and/or a metabolite, also carcinogenic, may be detected in the tissues of farm animals (particularly the liver) or in the milk of dairy animals. The FDA has set action levels of 20 parts per billion (ppb) in food products and 0.5 ppb in fluid milk. The Delaney clause does not apply to naturally occurring contaminants. The FDA acted under other provisions of the FFD&C Act recognizing that aflatoxin cannot be avoided by good manufacturing practices, but that technology changes may enable a further reduction of action levels.

Other mycotoxins found in food and feed crops are zearalenone, several trichothecenes, ochratoxin A, patulin, and penicillic acid.[50] Disease outbreaks in farm animals have been associated with the ingestion of feeds contaminated with these fungal metabolites. Many additional toxic metabolites have been isolated. Some are produced by molds that occur widely in foods and feeds and may be of potential health significance.

Both the USDA and the FDA conduct programs directed at controlling food-borne diseases associated with bacterial or parasitic contamination. The USDA monitors the slaughtering, handling, and processing of poultry and meat products. For other foods, the FDA regulations specify good manufacturing practice in processing, packing, and holding foods. Sanitation and food safety programs are also conducted cooperatively by the FDA and state health authorities in the areas of food service, milk, and shellfish safety.

**Reaction Products.** Another source of potentially toxic products in food is their formation through the reaction of food constituents during processing or home cooking. Benzo[*a*]pyrene and other carcinogenic hydrocarbons accumulate during the charcoal broiling of meats.[51] Carcinogenic nitrosamines can form in bacon during cooking when residual nitrite added as a curing agent reacts with secondary amines present in the meat. To minimize the extent of this reaction, the USDA limits the quantity of nitrite that can be added, requires the addition of ascorbic or erythorbic acid as an inhibitor of nitrosamine formation, and has set 10 ppb as the maximum permitted level of nitrosamines.[52] Mutagenic activity has been demonstrated in charred beef and fish,[53] boiled beef stock,[54] and grilled hamburger.[54] The significance of these findings to human health is not known.

## ESTABLISHING THE SAFETY OF FOOD ADDITIVES

The FFD&C Act requires that the safety of food additives be established before marketing by the evaluation of appropriate toxicologic information in light of probable consumer exposure to the substance. The FDA has described the toxicologic tests that are required for direct food and color additives, the guidelines for conducting these tests, and the necessary information about population exposure, molecular structure, purity, and specifications of the additive.[55] Minimum levels of testing are specified based on probable consumer exposure and estimates of toxicity of the proposed additive. These estimates are inferred from molecular structural similarities to compounds of known biologic activity, or from existing studies of the substance. Short-term genetic tests for carcinogenic potential are required for all substances.

The extent of testing required is determined by the effects observed in the basic tests. The tests to be conducted are ordered in a tiered system for deciding what further toxicologic information may be needed. Minimum tests for substances of highest concern are (1) carcinogenicity studies with two rodent species, (2) a chronic feeding study, of at least one year in duration with rodents, (3) a long-term (at least one year) feeding study with a nonrodent species, and (4) a multigeneration reproduction study (minimum of two generations) with a teratology phase in a rodent. These tests may also be required for any proposed additive, depending on the outcome of the tiered system of tests applied.

The aforementioned principles for assessing the safety of new food additives are being applied by the FDA in an ongoing review of currently approved additives in which the adequacy of existing toxicology data to meet current safety standards is being assessed.[56] Data on 1,332 synthetic flavors, 273 other direct additives, and 55 color additives and diluents used in foods, cosmetics, or drugs have been reviewed. The information on these substances also provides a data base for correcting chemical structure with toxicity parameters.[57,58]

Although many tests for safety were employed before passage of the Food Additives Amendment of 1958, extensive advances have since been made in toxicology, such as the development of short-term tests for genetic toxicity. Subtle chronic effects can be detected by employing today's protocols for testing, and current toxicologic criteria for food safety are more rigorous. Areas of continuing interest are hypersensitivity and the behavioral effects of food additives. Advances in cell biology and clinical immunology may aid in the development of simpler and more reliable procedures for the study of reactions to foods mediated through cytotoxic, antigen-antibody complex, and delayed hypersensitivity mechanisms.[59] Tests for behavioral effects are less developed. Much effort is needed for the development of reliable tests that provide quantifiable and reproducible information on behavioral effects of food ingredients. Future refinements of current tests and development of new tests will increase assurances of safety.

## REFERENCES

1. Code of Federal Regulations. Title 21: Food and Drugs, Parts 170–199 rev. Washington, D.C., U.S. Government Printing Office, 1986.
2. Senti, F.R.: I&EC Prod. Res. Dev. *20*:237–246, 1981.
3. National Research Council: Food Chemicals Codex. 3rd ed. Washington, D.C., National Academy Press, 1981.
4. Food Additives Amendment of 1958, P.L. 85–292, 72 Stat. 1984.
5. Federal Food, Drug, and Cosmetic Act, As Amended, and Related Laws. Washington, D.C., U.S. Government Printing Office, 1986.
6. Roberts, H.R.: Food additives. *In* Food Safety. (Roberts, H.R., Ed.) New York, John Wiley & Sons, Inc., 1981.
7. Select Committee on GRAS Substances: Appendix to Insights on Food Safety Evaluation. Springfield, Va., National Technical Information Service, PB83–154146, U.S. Department of Commerce, 1982.
8. Oser, B.L., Ford, R.A.: Food Technol. *33*:65–73, 1979.
9. Federal Register: *50*:30149–30152, 1985.
10. Federal Register: *42*:27603–27609, 1977.
11. National Cancer Institute. DHEW Publication No. (NIH) 79–1706, 1979.
11a. Hirose, M., Shibata, M., Hagiwara, A., et al.: Food Cosmet. Toxicol. *19*:147–151, 1981.
12. Olsen, P., Bille, N., Meyer, O.: Acta Pharmacol. Toxicol *53*:433–434, 1983.
12a. Olsen, P., Meyer, O., Bille, N., Würtzen, G.: Food Chem. Toxicol. *24*:1–12, 1986.
13. Ito, N., Fukushima, S., Hagiwara, A., et al.: J. Natl. Cancer Inst. *70*:343–352, 1983.
14. Grunow, W.: Food Chem. New *25*:33–34, 1983.
15. Grunow, W.: Food Chem. News *28*:7, 1986.
15a. Iverson, F., et al.: Cancer Lett. *26*:43–50, 1985.
16. Stevenson, D.D., Simon, R.A.: J. Allergy Clin. Immunol. *68*:26–32, 1981.
17. Baker, G.J., Collett, P., Allen, D.H.: Med. J. Aust. *2*:614–617, 1981.
18. Buckley, C.E., III, Saltzman, H.A., Sieker, H.O.: J. Allergy Clin. Immunol. *75*:144 (Abstract), 1985.
19. Ad hoc Review Group on the Reexamination of the GRAS Status of the Sulfiting Agents: Springfield, Va., National Technical Information Service, PB85–164044, U.S. Department of Commerce, 1985.
20. Lecos, C.: FDA Consumer. *19*:17–20, 1986.
21. Federal Register: *51*:25012–25020, 1986.
22. Federal Register: *51*:25021–25026, 1986.
23. Code of Federal Regulations. Title 21: Food and Drugs, Parts 1–99 rev. Washington, D.C., U.S. Government Printing Office, 1986.
24. Federal Register: *50*:26377–26383, 1985.
25. Federal Register: *50*:35783–35790, 1985.
26. National Research Council: Subcommittee on Review of the GRAS List—Phase II (1970). Washington, D.C., National Academy of Sciences, 1972.
27. National Research Council: Committee on GRAS List Survey—Phase III (1975). Washington, D.C., National Academy of Sciences, 1978.
28. National Research Council: Committee on GRAS List Survey—Phase III (1977). Washington, D.C., National Academy of Sciences, 1979.
29. Whittaker, J.R., Feeney, R.E.: Enzyme inhibitors in foods. *In* Toxicants Occurring Naturally in Foods. 2nd ed. Committee on Food Protection, National Research Council. Washington, D.C., National Academy of Sciences, 1973.
30. Montgomery, R.D.: Cyanogens. *In* Toxic Constituents of Plant Foodstuff. 2nd ed. (Liener, I.E., Ed.) New York, Academic Press, 1980.
31. Gartrell, M.J., Craun, J.C., Podrebarac, D.C., et al.: J. Assoc. Off. Anal. Chem. *69*:146–161, 1986.
32. Food and Agriculture Organization of the United Nations/World Health Organization: Guide to Codex Recommendations Concerning Pesticide Residues. Part 2. Maximum Limits for Pesticide Residues. 1984.
33. Gartrell, M.J., Craun, J.C., Podrebarac, D.S., et al.: J. Assoc. Off. Anal. Chem. *69*:123–145, 1986.
34. International Agency for Research on Cancer: Polychlorinated Biphenyls and Polybrominated Biphenyls. IARC Monographs. Vol. 18. Lyons, France, International Agency for Research on Cancer, 1978.
35. Federal Register: *44*:51233–51242, 1979.

36. National Food Processors Association: The NFPA-CMI 1983 Retail Market Survey for Lead in Canned Foods. Washington, D.C., National Food Processors Association, 1983.

37. National Food Processors Association: The NFPA-CMI 1984. Retail Market Survery for Lead in Canned Foods. Washington, D.C., National Food Processors Association, 1986.

38. Goldberg, E.D., Martin, J.H.: Metals in seawater as recorded by mussels. *In* Trace Metals in Sea Water. (Wong, C.S., Boyle, E., Bruland, K.W., et al., Eds.) New York, Plenum Publishing Corp., 1983.

39. Munro, I.C., Charbonneau, S.M.: Environmental contaminants. *In* Food Safety. (Roberts, H.E., Ed.) New York, John Wiley & Sons, Inc., 1981.

40. Miller, G.E., Grant, P.M., Kishore, R., et al.: Science *175*:1121–1122, 1972.

41. Wolnik, K.A., Fricke, F.L., Capar, S.G., et al.: J. Agric. Food Chem. *31*:1240–1244, 1983.

42. Wolnik, K.A., Fricke, F.L., Capar, S.G., et al.: J. Agric. Food Chem. *31*:1244–1249, 1983.

43. Food and Drug Administration: Compliance Program Report of Findings, FY-77 Pesticides and Metals Program. Springfield, Va., National Techical Information Service, PB82–260605, U.S. Department of Commerce, 1977.

44. Food and Nutrition Board: Recommended Dietary Allowances. Washington, D.C., National Academy of Sciences, 1980.

45. Joint FAO/WHO Expert Committee on Food Additives: 16th Report. World Health Organization, 1972.

46. Joint FAO/WHO Expert Committee on Food Additives: 27th Report. World Health Organization, 1983.

47. Mahaffey, D.R.: Pediatrics *59*:448–456, 1977.

48. Centers for Disease Control: Foodborne Disease Surveillance Annual Summary, 1981. Atlanta, Centers for Disease Control, 1983.

49. Hauschild, A.H.W., Bryan, F.L.: J. Food Protection *43*:435–440, 1980.

50. Rodricks, J.V., Hesseltine, C.W., Mehlman, M.A., (Eds.): Mycotoxins in Human and Animal Health. Park Forest South, Il., Pathotox Publishers, Inc., 1977.

51. Lijinsky, W., Shubik, P.: Ind. Med. Surg. *34*:152–154, 1965.

52. Federal Register: *43*:32136–32137, 1978.

53. Sugimura, T., Nagav, M.: CRC Crit. Rev. Toxicol. *6*:189–209, 1979.

54. Spingarn, N.E., Weisburger, J.H.: Cancer Lett. *7*:259–264, 1979.

55. Food and Drug Administration: Toxicological Principles for the Safety Assessment of Direct Food Additives and Color Additives Used in Food. Washington, D.C., Bureau of Foods, U.S. Food and Drug Administration, 1982.

56. Rulis, A.M., Hattan, D.G., Mergenroth, V.H. III: Reg. Toxicol. Pharmacol. *4*:37–56, 1984.

57. Rulis, A.M., Hattan, D.G.: Reg. Toxicol. Pharmacol. *5*:152–174, 1985.

58. Hattan, D.G., Rulis, A.M.: Reg. Toxicol. Pharmacol. *6*:181–191, 1986.

59. Buckley, R.H., Metcalf, D.: JAMA *248*:2627–2636, 1982.

## SELECTED READINGS

Furia, T.E. (Ed.): Handbook of Food Additives. 2nd Ed. Cleveland, CRC Press, 1972.

Liener, I.E. (Ed.): Toxic Constituents of Plant Foodstuffs. 2nd Ed. New York, Academic Press, 1980.

Roberts, H.R. (Ed.): Food Safety. New York, John Wiley & Sons, Inc., 1981.

Select Committee on GRAS Substances: Insights on Food Safety Evaluation. Springfield, Va., National Technical Information Service, PB83–154146, U.S. Department of Commerce, 1982.

Siu, R.H., Borzelleca, J.F., Carr, C.J., et al.: Fed. Proc. Fed. Am. Soc. Exp. Biol. *36*:2519–2562, 1977.

*Chapter* **40**

# NUTRIFICATION OF FOOD

### J. Christopher Bauernfeind

For some time, man has been nourished by consuming a variety of foods selected from available plant, animal, marine, and inorganic sources in the environment. Early man probably ate an average share of the digestible portion of whole living matter as influenced by variation in food availability with seasons of the year and other prevailing factors. Among the products he considered as his food supply were animal milks, products meant to nurture the young animal; honey, an energy food stored by and for the bee against unfavorable climatic conditions; and avian and turtle eggs destined to hatch into other creatures. Most foods consumed by early man were primarily intended for another purpose, and man, in common with omnivorous animals, competed for them. As man began to adapt and control plant and animal life to better suit his needs, food became involved in his economic, psychologic and social life. With time he further compounded the food selection process with folklore, religious taboos, and politics.

In man's historic struggle for food, he ate primarily whole foods or so-called natural foods that underwent little processing except prior to consumption.[1,2] Eventually food acquisition and distribution were delegated to certain individuals or groups: the farmer, butcher, baker, or fisherman. To preserve food for longer periods of time and to provide variety, food preservation and food processing programs were introduced. Throughout these changes the anthropocentric concept of

many individuals continued to exist: that the entire world's food supply was foreordained to serve man and one should not tamper too boldly with it.

## FOOD GUIDES

In the immediate past and somewhat at present, the consumer considered his nutritional needs in terms of meat, potatoes, milk, eggs, fruit, and so forth. Consumption of a variety of foods was emphasized. About 100 years ago menu planning was initiated, applying the early knowledge of nutrition.[3] Later guidelines by the USDA for the consumer were built around daily selections of seven types of foods that were reduced to four groups (milk and dairy products; meat, poultry, and fish; vegetables and fruit; bread and cereal products) for greater ease of understanding and use.[3] These groupings have served well as guides but have limitations.[4,5] With the accumulation of nutritional knowledge over the past century, we recognize that it is not just food per se but nutrients in the food that the human body requires. Proper balance of macronutrients (proteins, carbohydrates, fats, and water) and micronutrients (vitamins and minerals), components of foods in the strict sense, is required for the continued functioning of our bodies. Consequently, the more enlightened consumers have come to recognize that calcium and vitamin D are associated with milk, vitamin A with margarine and butter, the B vitamins with bread and cereals, vitamin C with fruit (particularly citrus), protein with meat, fish, chicken, eggs, and soybeans, and energy from cereal grains, sugars, and fats.

## NUTRITION AND FOOD SCIENCE

Food science and food technology predate the concept of modern nutrition.[6] While an awareness of the importance of nutrition was evolving, marked changes had been taking place in the food supply system. Food technology advances in the developed countries have imposed on the consumer the burden of selecting a balanced diet not only from the traditional, natural, processed, and refined food, but also from the new convenience, fabricated, and novel foods, some of which simulate known foods and others which have no traditional counterpart. The complexity of the type and number of these food items complicates the problem of segregating them into a guideline of a few food groups with recommended daily servings. Other advances in chemical and microbial engineering included the production of relatively pure inorganic and organic nutrients (the vitamins and amino acids) in an adequate volume and cheaply enough to permit their consideration as components of the human diet. It has been apparent for some time that part of the solution of the world's need for a nourishing food supply will depend on maximizing the combined benefits from food technologic and nutritional knowledge[6] and adapting these benefits toward human needs as influenced by social and political pressures within individual countries.

## NUTRITION RIGHTS

A primary motivating force of early mankind in forming a social structure was the greater assurance of an adequate food supply and with it the corollary of the greater well-being of its members.[7] Today's emphasis is on preventive measures, nutritional and otherwise, to maintain optimal health and resistance to disease.[8–15] Diet is being regarded as an important contributor to man's successes against disease and disability. Nutrition awareness among United States consumers, food processors, physicians, teachers, and government officials has increased during the last decade[16] with the greater recognition that food should be nutritious[17,18] in addition to being attractive and enjoyable. According to the 1976 Nutrition Bill of Rights framed by the American Dietetic Association,[19] every person has: the right to optimum nutritional health; the right to safe foods that will promote good nutrition and improve resistance to disease; and the right to make informed choices from available foods and to be protected against nutritional misinformation.

## FOOD PROCESSING AND FOOD HABITS

Nutrient content of food usually decreases when it is processed[20–26] because (1) some nutrients are sensitive to heat, oxygen, light, or a combination thereof, (2) some nutrients are extracted by liquids (solvents) or gases (water vapor), (3) some nutrients are altered by enzyme action, and (4) nutrients are lost by physically removing part of the food or fractionating it into two or more parts. Nutrient content may change through harvesting, storing, washing, trimming or peeling, blanching, extracting, straining, pasteurizing, boiling, sterilizing or canning, baking, dehydrating, irradiating, fermenting, brining, milling, bleaching, curing, frying, roasting, and steam table holding practices. The nutrient content of a food at the time of consumption, not that of the raw food product, is important. Living and eating habits influence dietary intake.[27–29] Skipped meals, high-fat snacks, high-sugar sweets and drinks, and high alcohol intake may lower micronutrient consumption. Unsound food faddism programs contribute to dietary insufficiencies.

## NUTRIENT NEEDS AND ALLOWANCES

Modern man is virtually unchanged biologically from his primeval origin. Consequently, his nutritional requirements are not believed to have changed much throughout the centuries. He has a monogastric intestinal tract; thus most of his nutritional essentials, in specific structural form, must be continually provided at short time intervals throughout his life cycle.

About 50 nutrients are now known to be needed for life, and nutrient daily allowances for man exist for approximately half of them.[30,31] The nutrients have been identified by chemical structure and by chemical reactions. Assay methods have been developed to determine the content of the nutrients in the food, thereby establishing the potential contribution that an individual serving of any food product makes in meeting the daily allowance or requirement for that nutrient. Publications are available on the composition of food,[32–35] but not for all known nutrients. No single food, even whole or natural foods, supplies all the nutrients required for human nutrition in the correct proportions to meet the daily nutrient needs. Hence, the earlier admonition to eat a variety of different foods, more recently expressed as eating a balanced diet, was and is a valid concept. If all the people in the world had a sufficient array and quantity of plant, animal, marine, and inorganic foods and chose to eat a correctly selected diet, there probably would be little or no insufficiency of required nutrient consumption. In reality, however, an insufficient volume of food and/or poor dietary practices bring about in the developing countries severe nutrient deficiencies of vitamin A,[36] iron,[37] and calories.[38] In addition, in developed countries there are marginal deficiencies of vitamins and minerals.[39–46]

## MEAL OR DIET PREPARATION

For the 50 or so known nutrients required for life, a food-labeling program can be set up, as is now in progress in the United States, in which a food label may show the content of one fourth to one half of the known nutrients on the container. Although food labeling is helpful in comparing food products within a given class of foods or against another class of foods, the consumer is puzzled[5] and rarely can be expected to prepare the daily menu from foods by tabulating each nutrient to determine whether the diet under consideration is adequate (balanced). Until nutritional knowledge becomes more complete from a quantitative nutrient aspect and interrelationships of nutrients are better understood, there is wisdom in concentrating on the limiting nutrients within population groups whether in developed or developing countries and providing nutrient delivery systems that require a minimum nutrition education effort. Under a future national food and nutrition policy, it is hoped that workable guidelines understood by the consumer will appear that will provide adequate diets for all consumers. Various countries are struggling with this problem.

## FOOD AND NUTRITION POLICY

Development and placement of a food and nutrition policy or guideline at the core of national planning[47] should and eventually will receive high governmental priority in most countries. The formulation of a food and nutrition policy integrated in national development plans aims at securing an adequate diet for each consumer irrespective of income level and with attention to approaching defined problems on a cost/benefit or a cost/efficiency basis. It involves forecasting, reconciliation, and coordination of economic, educational, legislative, and technical aspects. Its development and operation may be aided by use of systematic nutritional analysis (Fig. 40–1).[48,49] National nutrition planning policy and guideline development continue to undergo study in various parts of the world.[50–55] A political commitment to a national nutrition program is basic,[56–58] a most important determinant of the nature, magnitude, and success of programs addressed to malnutrition.

As a national nutrition objective it would seem appropriate to seek first (1) enough food to satisfy hunger for every child and adult, and closely following this objective with (2) a diet nutritionally adequate for each person. The second objective would eventually assure that each person receive the recommended daily allowance of each required nutrient, starting at the initiation of the program with the most significant nutrient deficiencies causing human misery.

## NUTRIFICATION

Among the nutritional interventions to be considered in a national nutrition program, nutrification,[59,60] defined as the addition of one or more nutrients to one or more commonly consumed foods or food mixtures, can, if properly introduced and controlled, improve the dietary intake of a given population. The terms "to nutrify" or the process of "nutrification" merely mean to make a food more nutritious. Nutrification is used here as a replacement term for fortification, enrichment, restoration, or supplementation, terms that originally were borrowed from disciplines or applications other than food use. The great potential offered by wise utilization of industrially produced nutrients, vitamins, minerals, amino acids, and protein isolates has rarely been utilized fully.[61]

## NUTRIFICATION PROGRAM CONSIDERATIONS

Whether a program is undertaken depends upon (1) local circumstances and (2) a consideration of alternate approaches. Once a nutrification policy is adopted it should remain dynamic, open to revision and to periodic updating of nutritional knowledge and standards. What foods to nutrify and what aspects to consider prior to initiating a nutrification program are suggested as follows:

**Food Vehicle(s) or Food Carrier(s) for Added Nutrient(s).** The carrier should be a food or food ingredient universally consumed by the targeted population, preferably with relatively little variation in pattern. More than one food carrier may be chosen.

**Sources of Added Nutrient(s).** They should possess acceptable chemical, physical, and organoleptic properties. More than one nutrient may be considered.

**Location(s) for Nutrification Process.** The addition of the nutrient(s) to the food carrier(s) in a uniform fashion, to produce an adequate volume of nutrified food(s), is necessary to serve the intended purpose. Equipment and required expertise need be provided.

**Production Controls for Nutrified Food(s).**

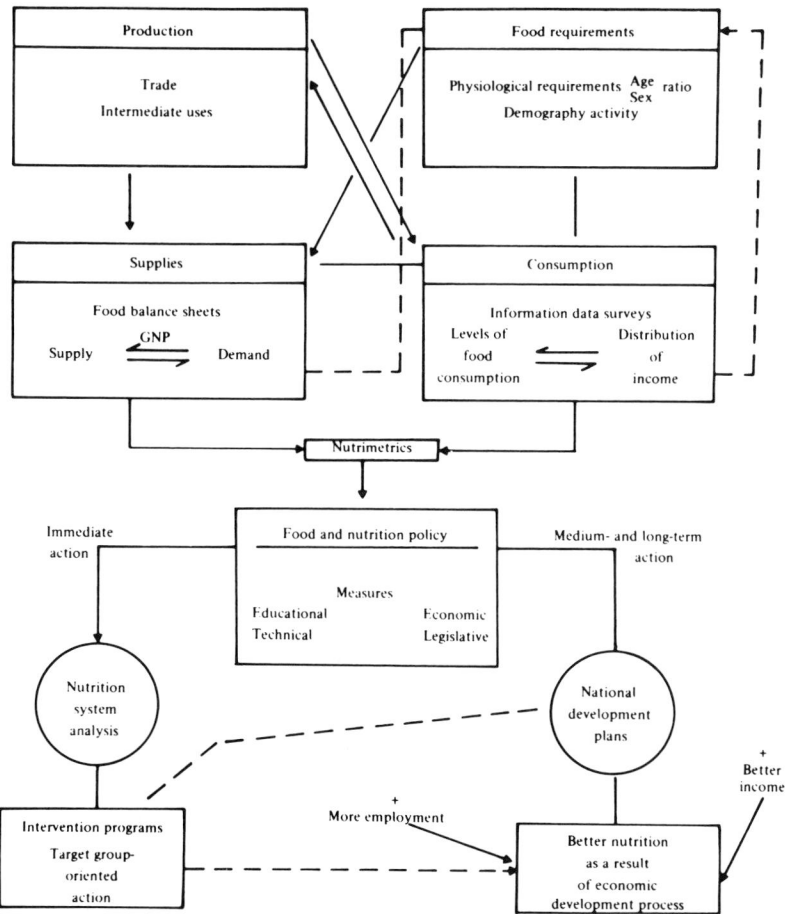

**Fig. 40–1.** Use of nutrition systematics in national planning. (Reprinted with permission from Ganzin, M., Perisse, J., Francois, P.: Need for food and nutrition policies. *In* Man, Food and Nutrition (Recheigl, M., Jr., Ed.) Boca Raton, CRC Press, 1973, pp. 275-286. Copyright CRC Press, Inc., Boca Raton, Fl.)

Qualitative control procedures at the site of the nutrification process and quantitative laboratory procedures, periodically applied, provide assurance of operations.

**Distribution of Nutrified Product.** Marketplace checkpoints are desirable to observe continued patterns of food use.

**Voluntary or Mandated Program.** Officials must determine whether the program is to be undertaken by government decree and whether there is support for such action. Acceptance of the program is of utmost importance.

**Overall Program Monitoring.** If the program is to remedy an existing health problem, suitable monitoring of the targeted population at time intervals will confirm whether the program is gradually correcting the problem.

**Cost of Program.** Prior decisions are necessary to determine whether the consumer or government pays for the program. If the food industry is

to absorb the cost initially, an understanding with government is desirable on prevailing policy under inflationary situations.

Nutrification of food could not be undertaken until the necessary active ingredients could be produced in sufficient quantities at commercially feasible prices. A technology has been developed over the years, and in most situations technical feasibility exists for the addition of nutrients to many foods or food ingredients.[62–65a] Adding micronutrients to a food for nutritional improvement is not a new concept.[66] Iodine was proposed as an additive to salt in the nineteenth century in South America.[67] The twentieth century saw nutrification of vegetable-fat spreads with vitamin A in Europe.[68] These and other nutrification programs were initiated in the United States and elsewhere. In 1939 the Council on Foods and Nutrition of the American Medical Association (AMA) published a policy on the addition of specific nutrients to foods, followed in 1941 by one from the Food and Nutrition Board of the National Research Council (NRC). In 1961, revised editions were issued by both the AMA and the NRC. The current NRC revision calls for evidence that the nutrified food would be nutritionally and economically beneficial for the population, that the food selected would be a proper carrier for effective distribution of the added nutrient, and that the added nutrient would be physiologically available, chemically stable, capable of being monitored, and nontoxic under usual conditions of dietary use.[69]

Nutrification is the most rapidly applied, most flexible, and most socially acceptable intervention method of changing the nutrient intake without a vast educational effort and without a change in the current food intake pattern of a given population. It usually has a favorable cost-benefit ratio compared to other methods. Once a nutrification program involving the addition of a single nutrient has been initiated, adding a second or subsequent ones is an easier task and costs are lower.[70,114] An educational effort along with any nutrification plan may be helpful to explain the goal of the program and to introduce, if warranted, other interventions such as improved agricultural and health practices.

## SITUATIONS FOR FOOD NUTRIFICATION

Nutrification of food can be considered as one possible intervention measure where a substantial segment of a population would benefit from the incorporation of a nutrient or nutrients in its diet, but preferably where the total quantity of food available is reasonably adequate. Nutrification with micronutrients adds to the nutritional quality of the diet, less so to the quantity of the diet. The detailed plans of the selected nutrification approach depend upon many factors, including governmental policies, time period to achieve the goal, economics, and safeguards to ensure that the efficacy and safety of the program are maintained. The following situations might call for nutrification with industrially produced nutrients.

**Changing Economic Conditions.** Industrially produced nutrients, appropriately utilized in combination with agricultural products, offer protective safeguards or alternate choice products in changing economic conditions.[61] Amino acids and more vegetable protein extenders are now utilized in foods in Japan and the United States, although the initial impetus for the increased use of vegetable protein concentrates in human foods came from the earlier concern of meeting a sus-

pected protein crisis in the developing countries by supplementing cereal grain products.

**Inadequate Supply or Intake of Protective Foods.** Some populations in the world do not have access to a sufficient quantity of protective foods or do not consume valuable or protective foods because of beliefs and taboos. Both practices can lead to dietary deficiencies. Although long-range approaches need to be introduced under these circumstances, in many instances a nutrification program can quickly introduce the missing nutrient or nutrients. An example is the insufficient consumption of vitamin A, iron, and foods containing iodine in some of the developing countries.

**Overconsumption of High-Calorie Foods.** With the passage of time, a greater percentage of the population has become involved in more sedentary occupations and hence has lowered caloric needs. On the other hand, advances in food technology have generated more kinds of high-energy food products, many of which have a refined or highly processed character or have been fabricated from refined food components. Although many of these foods provide calories, they do not contain an appropriate level of essential micronutrients. Examples of these high-energy items are high-calorie beverages and sweets made from sucrose, fructose, glucose, corn sugar syrups, and table syrups; high-calorie items made with fats, shortenings, and vegetable oils, some of which also have added sugar and/or starch; and alcoholic (ethanol) drinks. Substantial consumption of these high-calorie items can lead to underconsumption of important micronutrients.

One philosophy has been to add nutrients in amounts that will make the food self-sufficient metabolically.[71] If all foods contained the required micronutrients at levels comparable to their caloric contribution to the diet, there would be less difficulty with nutritional insufficiencies. Certain high-calorie foods fit less well into a meal pattern and fall more into a category of "snack, fun, or pleasure foods," that is, they are more frequently consumed between meals. Soft drinks can make up 30 to 35% of the caloric intake of 10 to 15-year-olds.[72] How then should they be considered in nutrification programs since foods consumed between meals may influence the consumption pattern of foods eaten at meal time?[72a] Because no recognized serving size exists, a nutrification program could best be guided by an adjusted caloric density approach.[62] The judicious nutrification of some high-caloric foods[61,62,71,73–75] along with a nutrition education program to control total caloric intake would seem helpful. Nutritious candy products have been prepared.[76–78]

**Food Class Standardization for Nutrient Content.** If a natural food for a given class of foods is serving as a substantial source of a micronutrient and another food containing little or none of that nutrient is promoted or recommended for the same purpose, some justification exists for adding the missing nutrient(s). One case in point is consumption of cranberry juice (naturally low in vitamin C) in place of citrus juice as a breakfast beverage. Since a good portion of daily vitamin C needs is consumed at breakfast, there is merit in having cranberry and other juices low in natural vitamin C, such as prune, apricot, and pineapple, contain standardized vitamin C levels. The consumer can then have variety of selection without forfeiting nutritional value. Another case is the vegetable protein food analogues adapted to serve as replacements for animal protein products wherein the vegetable product should be nutrified with nutrients to simulate the composition of the product imitated.[79] A third example is the meal replacers. When either a dietetic, instant, frozen, or dried meal packaged product is developed and promoted to replace a regular meal, a suitable approach to micronutrient nutrification would be to have the new product provide one fourth or one third of the daily allowance of micronutrients. When new food products are developed to replace an existing food, the new product should contain a reasonably complete and similar array of micronutrients found in the natural product to avoid product inferiority.

**Restoration of Nutrients.** Under the restoration concept, some micronutrients originally present in the whole natural food but lost in processing are returned to a processed food. For example, peanuts are roasted in the usual manufacture of peanut butter, a process that destroys the thiamin naturally present. It is technically feasible to add pure thiamin back to the butter during the grinding operation. Because of the volume consumed, freshly cooked white potatoes have made a substantial contribution of vitamin C and other nutrients to some populations. Currently, more potatoes are consumed in manufactured forms as convenience foods such as fries, powders, buds, flakes, chips, or crisps. In many instances, processing and storage on supermarket shelves degrade much of the natural vitamin C. Restoring vitamin C to these processed potato products is nutritionally justifiable.[80–83]

**Deficiencies in Geochemical Environments.** Soils in wide areas of the world are deficient in certain minerals. This situation can result in low concentrations of major or trace minerals in drinking water, plant crops, and even tissues of farm animals, thus contributing to marginal or deficient dietary intakes in humans.[73,73a] Minerals in this category are fluorine, iodine, molybdenum, and selenium; in some countries, the first two are added back to the diet in the form of fluoride-treated water and iodized salt. Trace mineral elements are gaining increased attention.[73,73a,84–86] Certain areas of the United States and New Zealand are known to be selenium-deficient,[73,73a] and estimated safe intakes of selenium have been determined. Nutrification with selenium in selected areas may be a consideration in the future. Copper, chromium, and zinc likewise may become future additives under certain conditions.

**Improvement in Bioavailability.** Concern is increasing about the biologic availability of mineral elements naturally present in the diet and mineral compounds added to food by the nutrification process.[84,87–90] When one is dealing with an insufficiency of a mineral element in the diet, two approaches are developing: (1) to increase the mineral content by the addition of a proper mineral source, and (2) to attempt to improve the bioavailability of the mineral already in the diet, for example, an approach gaining momentum is to improve the biologic availability of existing dietary iron supplies or added iron by incorporating in the diet some facilitating substance such as L-ascorbic acid or its sodium salt.[91–94] Cereal grain meals, soybean meal, sugar, MSG, coffee, tea, and milk are some suggested food carriers. Some investigators believe that in high-cereal diets ascorbic acid would be helpful. Enhancement by ascorbic acid is dose-dependent. An intake of as little as 25 mg at a meal may be significant,[93] but intakes of 100 mg or more daily may be the goal sought in severely iron-deficient populations.

Problems also influence the bioavailability of vitamins such as antagonists or antimetabolite, bound, or labile forms of the nutrient present in food or at times consumed with food.[94a,94b]

**Improvement of Cereal Grain Products.** Cereal grains and tuber foods provide the basic energy sustenance to most of mankind.[95] Cereal grains account for 52% of the global average per capita intake for calories and 47% of the average protein intake. About 26% of the daily caloric intake in the United States comes from products based on cereal grains.[96] This intake does not vary greatly relative to income and geographic region. In some developing countries cereal grain products provide up to 70% of the caloric intake. As a class of foods, cereal grains have considerable merit[95–97] because (1) they are universally consumed, (2) they are prime suppliers of calories and protein, (3) they provide diet variety by use of industrial and home processing for consumption, (4) they contain complex carbohydrates (indigestible fiber), which are believed to function as a health maintenance aid, and (5) they are a form of food easily stored if moisture content and insect infestation are controlled. Since they enjoy wide acceptability as a food and already contain some vitamins, minerals, and amino acids, they can be substantially improved by nutrification to make them into superior food products.[97a] In short, they are logical food products to serve as carriers of added nutrients to populations of both developed and developing countries. The number and amount of additives, vitamins, minerals, amino acids, and/or vegetable protein concentrates to be added to specific cereal grain meal or fractional grain products would depend upon geographic location and local problems.

A major contribution to an increased food supply can be made through developing nutritionally designed processed products based on cereal, tuber, and other primarily carbohydrate crops and utilizing nutrients that are produced by chemical and microbial processes.[61] In the United States, the Food and Nutrition Board of the National Research Council, on reviewing nutrition and dietary survey data, found evidence of potential risk of deficiencies of vitamin A, thiamin, riboflavin, niacin, vitamin $B_6$, folic acid, iron, calcium, magnesium, and zinc among some segments of the population. Believing cereal grain products to be suitable nutrient carriers, the Board has proposed that these nutrients be added to all products based on the major cereal grains (wheat, corn, and rice) where technically feasible[96] (Table 40–1).

From the early days of the addition of synthetic nutrients to processed foods, two schools of thought developed: (1) to restore nutrient levels only to the unprocessed food and (2) to add nutrients at levels to prevent disease and produce optimal health based on the use of the food product in the daily diet. In the past 40 years the trend has shifted from the former to the latter view as man's needs and goals have been more realistically recognized as evidence in the 1974 NCR proposals.

Between 1974 and 1985 studies have been conducted to determine the technical feasibility of the proposed 10-nutrient addition to wheat flour, farina, pasta, refrigerated and frozen dough, prepared mixes, corn flour, grits, corn meal, and white rice.[98–104] Although studies are not complete, the data generated so far indicate that with small modifications on specific carriers the proposed program may be quite feasible.[104–104d] Riboflavin, because of its yellow color and high calcium and magnesium additions, may have to remain in an optional classification for white rice until further feasible procedures are developed.

For the past two decades it has been the hope that the lower-quality proteins of the cereal grains would be supplemented with added amino acids, with isolated protein or with legume or oilseed meals to provide improved protein quality more comparable to human needs.[105–111] Supplementation of cereal grains with amino acids or dipeptides may be[111a] an attractive goal. At present, the more practical trend has been to prepare protein food mixtures that have the additional merit of providing calories when food is insufficient to meet protein-calorie needs.[112–118] The favorable effect of added protein, minerals, and vitamins on human nutrition has been observed in controlled clinical and field studies over the years.[118a–118f]

**Table 40–1. Comparison of Nutrification of Flour with Four Nutrients vs. Ten Nutrients**

| Nutrients[a] | Used at Present[b] | | Proposed[c] | |
|---|---|---|---|---|
| | In Flour | In Bread[d] | In Flour | In Bread |
| Thiamin | 2.9 | 1.8 | 2.9 | 1.8 |
| Riboflavin | 1.8 | 1.1 | 1.8 | 1.1 |
| Niacin | 24.0 | 15.0 | 24.0 | 15.0 |
| Iron | 13.0–16.5 | 8.0–12.5 | 40.0[e] | — |
| Calcium | — | — | 900 | 562 |
| Vitamin A[f] | None | None | 1.3 | 0.8 |
| | | | (4,300 IU)[g] | (2,700 IU) |
| Pyridoxine | None | None | 2.0 | 1.2 |
| Folic acid | None | None | 0.3 | 0.18 |
| Magnesium | None | None | 200.0 | 125.0 |
| Zinc | None | None | 10.0 | 6.2 |

[a]Expressed as milligrams per pound of flour.
[b]Minimums and maximums in Code of Federal Regulations. Title 21, Parts 136–137.
[c]NAS, NRC (1974).
[d]Bread is considered to contain 62.5% wheat flour based on the conversion of 100 lb of flour to 160 lb of bread.
[e]November 18, 1977, the FDA restored the provision for 13.0–16.5 mg lb.
[f]Retinol equivalent.
[g]The originally proposed level of 2.2 mg/lb (7,300 IU) was lowered to 1.3 mg/lb (4,300 IU)
From Emodi, A.S., Scialpi, L.,[102] with permission of Cereal Chem.

**Special Purpose Alimentation.** A number of unique dietary foods are designed to meet specific physiologic states or life cycle stages.[5,75,119,120] They may be sole sources of nutrient supplies for the time period. Others may be supplemental to the diet. Examples are diets for pregnancy and lactation, for diabetics, for allergy control, for control of hypertension, for weight control, for pre- or postoperative periods, and for infants. Those influencing most adult individuals are diets for weight control. Diets containing 900 to 1200 calories need close scrutiny regarding adequacy in essential amino acids, vitamins, and minerals. Nutrients in total parenteral nutrition are prepared either by synthetic means (e.g., many amino acids and vitamins) or by purification (e.g., minerals and trace elements).

**Addition for Non-nutritional Purposes.** Several nutrients have dual properties. In addition to serving as dietary essentials they contribute some technologic advantage to the food product to which they are added. L-ascorbic acid (vitamin C) may act as (1) an oxygen scavenging agent in bottled and canned food products, (2) an inhibitor of oxidative rancidity in frozen fish, (3) a stabilizer of color and flavor and an inhibitor of nitrosamine formation in cured meats, (4) a flour maturing agent and dough conditioner, (5) an oxygen acceptor in beer production, and (6) a reducing agent in wine.[121] α-Tocopherol (vitamin E) serves as a fat-soluble antioxidant in fats and oils and a retardant to nitrosamine formation.[121,122] β-Carotene and β-apo-8′-carotenal, carotenoid vitamin A precursors, also serve as food colors.[123,123a] Ferrous gluconate improves color in processed ripe olives.

## SUCCESSFUL NUTRIFICATION PROGRAMS

Over the past decade a number of articles have been published on the merits of nutrification of foods,[70,104a,114,124–128e] some of which are mentioned here. Iodine addition in the form of potassium iodide or iodate to salt (NaCl) as a goiter preventive is a practice still carried on in the United States and a number of other countries. Two instances of the effectiveness of iodine nutrification are the 1980 Thailand study, in which potassium iodate nutrification of salt reduced iodine deficiency in schoolchildren from 84% to practically zero within six years,[129] and the effect

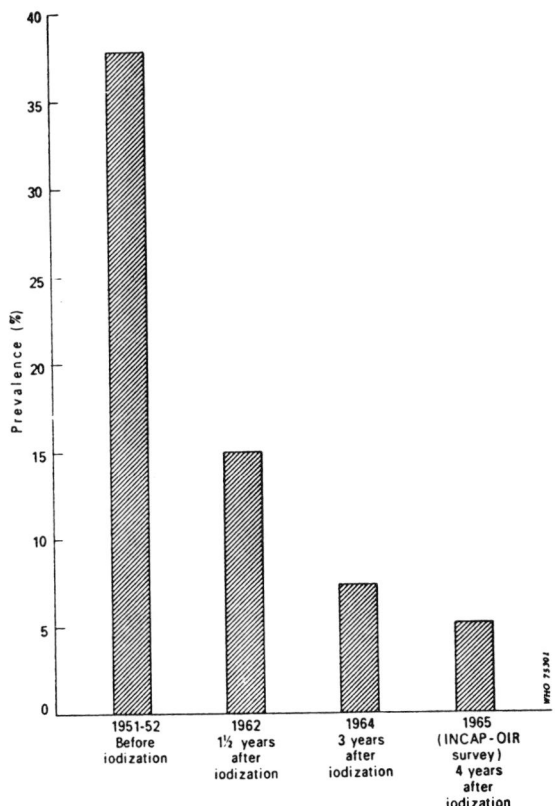

**Fig. 40–2.** Prevalence of endemic goiter found in Guatemala in surveys carried out before and after the compulsory iodization of salt. Data provided by the Institute of Nutrition of Central America and Panama (INCAP), Guatemala. (From Beaton, G.H.,[125] with permission of World Health Organization.

**Table 40–2. Vitamin Potency of Nutrified Margarine**

| *Vitamins A and D Commonly Added to Margarine* | | |
|---|---|---|
| *Country* | *Vitamin A (IU/kg)* | *Vitamin D IU/kg* |
| Australia | 30,000 | 4,000 |
| Austria | 20,000 | 1,000 |
| Belgium | 20,000 | 1,000 |
| Brazil | 15,000–50,000 | 500–2,000 |
| Canada | 33,000 | |
| Chile | 14,000–18,000 | 1,000 |
| Columbia | 20,000–30,000 | 2,000–4,000 |
| Denmark | 20,000 | 625 |
| Finland | 20,000 | 2,500–3,500 |
| Germany | 20,000–30,000 | 1,000 |
| Greece | 25,000 | 1,500 |
| Israel | 30,000 | 3,000 |
| Japan | 30,000–40,000 | |
| Mexico | 20,000 | 2,000 |
| Netherlands | 20,000 | 2,000 |
| Norway | 20,000 | 2,500 |
| Philippines* | 22,000 | 1,100 |
| Portugal | 20,000–35,000 | 875–1,000 |
| South Africa | 20,000 | 1,000 |
| Sweden | 30,000 | 1,500 |
| Switzerland | 30,000 | 3,000 |
| Turkey | 20,000 | 1,000 |
| United Kingdom | 30,000–33,000 | 2,900–3,500 |
| United States | 33,000 | 4,400 |

*100 mg vitamin $B_1$ also added.
From Morton, R.A.,[68] with permission of R. Soc. Health J.

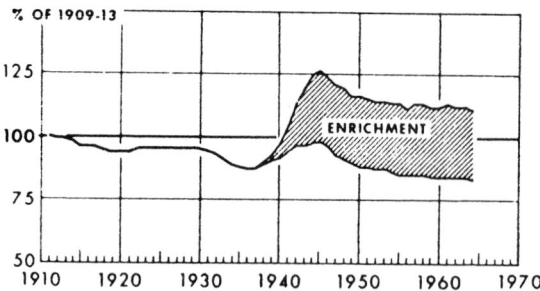

**Fig. 40–3.** Value of nutrification of cereal grain products in improving thiamin (vitamin $B_1$) intake. These figures are based on per capita civilian consumption. (Reprinted with permission from LeBovit, C.J.: Agric. Food Chem. *16*:153-157, 1968. Copyright 1968 American Chemical Society.)

of mandatory iodization based on health and nutrition survey observations in Central America[125] (Fig. 40–2). Another mineral, fluoride, has been added to drinking water to reduce dental caries. Although this practice has successfully lowered tooth decay for several decades,[30,130] it remains a debatable subject in some parts of the world.

Decades ago, when infants and young children developed rickets because of dietary deficiency of vitamin D, cod liver was fed to cows to increase the level of vitamin D in milk. Later, irradiated yeast and then irradiated ergosterol were fed; still later, cow's milk was irradiated with ultraviolet light. Now, vitamin D is added directly to fluid milk, a more economical and better controlled practice. The nutrification of cows' milk with vitamin D has been credited as the major factor in the disappearance of infantile rickets as a public health problem.[128] Nonfat milk (skim milk) in many instances has added vitamins A and D, whether in dry or fluid form. Today the major portion of the world's margarine production is nutrified with vitamin A[68] (Table 40–2). Vitamin A nutrification of margarine and wheat flour enrichment have been credited with significant health improvement in the people of Newfoundland.[131,132]

The addition of three vitamins and one mineral

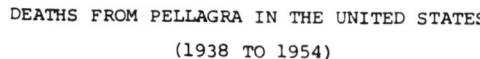

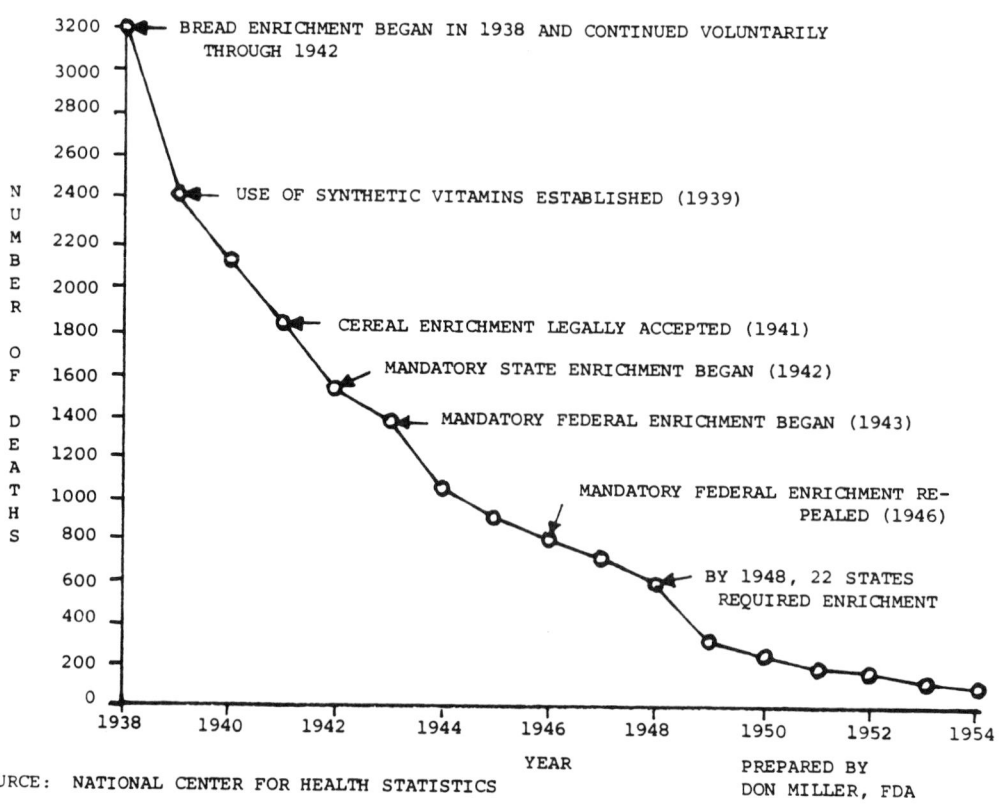

**Fig. 40–4.** Deaths from pellagra in the United States (1938 to 1954). (From Miller, D.F.[134] with permission of Am. Assoc. Cereal Chemists.)

## Table 40–3. Nutrification of Wheat Flour* (mg/kg)

| Country | Vitamin B₁ Min. | Vitamin B₁ Max. | Vitamin B₂ Min. | Vitamin B₂ Max. | Niacin Min. | Niacin Max. | Iron Min. | Iron Max. | Calcium Min. | Calcium Max. |
|---|---|---|---|---|---|---|---|---|---|---|
| Australia | 1.5 | — | 2.2 | — | 15 | — | 14 | — | 1,000 | |
| Canada† | 4.4 | 7.7 | 2.7 | 4.8 | 35 | 64 | 29 | 43 | 1,100 | 1,400 |
| Chile | 6.3 | — | 1.3 | — | 13 | — | 30 | — | — | — |
| Congo | 4 | 6 | 2.5 | 3.5 | 32 | 45 | 26 | 35 | 1,000 | 1,500 |
| Costa Rica‡ | 4.4 | 5.5 | 2.6 | 3.3 | 35 | 44 | 28 | 36 | 1,100 | 1,400 |
| Denmark | 5 | — | 5 | — | — | — | 30 | — | 2,000 | — |
| Dominican Republic | 4.4 | 5.5 | 2.6 | 3.3 | 35 | 44 | 29 | 38 | 1,100 | 1,400 |
| Guatemala‡ | 4.4 | — | 2.6 | — | 35 | — | 29 | — | 1,700 | — |
| Guyana | 4.4 | 5.5 | 2.7 | 3.3 | 35 | 44 | 29 | 36 | — | — |
| Israel | — | — | 2.5 | — | — | — | — | — | — | — |
| Japan | 5 | 8 | 3 | 5 | — | — | — | — | 1,500 | 3,000 |
| Kenya | 4.5 | 5.5 | 2.7 | 3.3 | 35 | 44 | 29 | 36 | — | — |
| Mexico | 4.4 | 8.8 | 2.6 | 5.2 | 35 | 70 | 29 | 57 | — | — |
| Nigeria | 5 | — | 3.5 | — | 50 | — | 35 | — | — | — |
| Panama‡ | 4.4 | — | 2.6 | — | 35 | — | 29 | — | 1,100 | — |
| Peru | 4 | — | 4 | — | 30 | — | 20 | — | 1,000 | — |
| Philippines | 4.4 | 5.5 | 2.6 | 3.3 | 35 | 44 | 29 | 36 | 1,100 | 1,400 |
| Portugal | 4.4 | 5.5 | 2.6 | 3.3 | 35 | 44 | 28 | 36 | — | — |
| Puerto Rico | 4.4 | 5.5 | 2.6 | 3.3 | 35 | 44 | 28 | 36 | — | — |
| Sweden | 4 | 8 | 1.5 | 3 | 40 | 80 | 65 | 90 | — | — |
| Switzerland | 4.4 | — | 2 | — | 50 | — | 29 | — | — | — |
| United Kingdom | 2.4 | — | — | — | 16 | — | 16.5 | — | 940 | 1,560 |
| USA§ | 6.4 | — | 4 | — | 55 | — | 44 | — | 2,120 | — |
| USSR | 2 | 4 | 4 | — | 10 | 30 | — | — | — | — |
| West Indies | 4.4 | 5.5 | 2.6 | 3.3 | 35 | 44 | 28 | 36 | 1,100 | 1,400 |

*Specifications exist in some countries for other cereal-grain products such as white rice, maize meal, corn grits, pasta products, and breakfast cereals.

†Other nutrients permitted are vitamin B₆, 2.5–3.1; folic acid, 0.04–0.05; d-pantothenic acid, 1–1.3; and magnesium 1,500–1,900 mg/kg.

‡Guatemala and Costa Rica started to add vitamin A palmitate (50 IU of 15 μg or retinol equivalent per gram) to refined sugar (sucrose) in 1975. Panama initiated the practice in 1976. El Salvador, Honduras, and Nicaragua are planning to introduce this nutrification practice.

§FDA regulations allow production of special-formula bread[136a,136b] containing added vitamin A, vitamin B₆, folic acid, magnesium, and zinc in addition to the above-listed nutrients. Nutrified food sent abroad from the USA under the USA-AID or Food for Peace (PL 480) have the following specifications: nonfat dried milk, 2,200 IU vitamin A and 440 IU vitamin D per 100 g; soy-fortified corn meal, 2–3 mg thiamin, 1.2–1.3 mg riboflavin, 16–24 mg niacin, 4,000–6,000 IU vitamin A, 13–26 mg iron, and 500–700 mg calcium per lb; soy-wheat flour blend, 2–2.5 mg thiamin, 1.2–1.5 mg riboflavin, 16–20 mg niacin, 4,000–6,000 IU vitamin A, and 500–1,107 mg (for 6% soy) or 750–1,364 mg (for 12% soy) calcium per lb; other foods have other specifications.

Note: This table of values taken from the literature serves as a guide. Up-to-date values need to be confirmed with the regulatory agency of the specific country.

to processed white flour and other processed cereal-grain products has been credited with substantial increases of these nutrients (Fig. 40–3) in the United States[133] and with the virtual disappearance of pellagra in the South[134,135] and beriberi and pellagra in urban centers (Fig. 40–4). In 1972 it was estimated that nutrification provided 40% of thiamin, 25% of iron, 20% of niacin, and 15% of riboflavin in the 1970 United States nutrient supplies.[136] A number of countries currently add these nutrients to cereal-grain products (Table 40–3). Flour enriched in Israel with riboflavin is credited with improved consumer status in that vitamin.[137] Enrichment of rice with thiamin was shown to solve the beriberi problem in Bataan.[138] Enrichment of maize meal with riboflavin and niacin during milling was shown to be highly effective in improving vitamin nutritional states in

Africa[139] and was recommended for national initiation. If the 10 nutrients[96,102] previously discussed (see Table 40–1) were added to the cereal-grain products in the United States, it is estimated that 15 to 50% of the RDA for the nutrients would be provided.[103]

Retention of nutrients added to cereal grains is quite good during storage.[98–104] The loaf volume, crumb color, grain, and proof time of nutrified bread compare favorably with those qualities of non-nutrified bread.[99,102] For years, micronutrients have been added to breakfast cereals in the United States. A developed technology allows micronutrients to be added in a stable and biologically available form without influencing flavor or color of the cereal product.[140,140a]

Successful nutrification projects are also underway in other parts of the world. The commer-

**Table 40–4. Food Mixtures, Schemes**

| Country | Exploratory State | Production Terminated | Production Irregular/Position not Known | In Regular Production |
|---|---|---|---|---|
| *Latin and Central America* | | | | |
| El Salvador | | Incaparina 1962* | | Incaparina 1961 |
| Guatemala | | | | Protea 1950s |
| Mexico | General Mills (?) 1969<br>General Foods 1969<br>Corn Products 1968 | | Soya Products (Conasupo) early 1960s | |
| Nicaragua | Quaker Oats 1968<br>Nutrition Development Corp. 1969 | Incaparina 1962 | | |
| Panama | | Incaparina 1966 | | |
| Cuba | United Nations agencies/Govt. 1971 | | | |
| St. Lucia | United Nations agencies/Govt. 1971 | | | |
| South Brazil | Coca-Cola 1968<br>General Foods 1968 | Saci 1968<br>Incaparina 1965/66<br>Multi-Purpose Food 1956 | Solein 1963<br>Fortifex 1963 | Cerealina 1965 |
| Chile | University of Chile 1968<br>US/AID | | | |
| Colombia | | Pochito 1967 | | Incaparina 1961/62<br>Colombinarina 1967<br>Duryea 1969<br>Puma 1969 |
| Guyana | | | | |
| Peru | Agrarian University 1968 | Peruvita 1965 | | |
| Venezuela | Nutrition Development Corp. 1969 | Incaparina 1965 | | |
| *Africa* | | | | |
| Algeria | | | | Superamine 1967 |
| Arab Republic of Egypt | United Nations agencies/Govt. 1969 | | | Supramine 1972 |
| Ethiopia | | | | Faffa 1967 |
| Kenya | | | | Simba 1959<br>Supro 1967 |
| Madagascar | United Nations agencies/Govt. 1970 | | | |

| Country | Product / Sponsor | Date |
|---|---|---|
| Mozambique | | |
| Nigeria | Amama | 1959 |
| | Arlac | 1963 |
| | Super Maeu | 1965 |
| Rhodesia | Nutresco | 1963 |
| Senegal | Ladylac | 1966 |
| South Africa | Pronutro | 1962 |
| | Protone | |
| | Kupangi Biscuits | 1961 |
| Tunisia | United Nations agencies/Govt. | 1968/69 |
| Uganda | Soya Products | 1968 |
| Zambia | Milk Biscuits | 1971 |
| *Near East* | | |
| Iran | Yoo Hoo | 1969 |
| | United Nations agencies/Govt. | 1969 |
| Turkey | Sekmanna | 1971 |
| | United Nations agencies/Govt. | 1968 |
| *Far East* | | |
| Hong Kong | Vitasoy | 1940 |
| India | Multi-Purpose Food (CFTRI) | 1965 |
| | Multi-Purpose Food (Chandra) | 1960 |
| | Multi-Purpose Food (Agrawal) | 1966 |
| | Protamin | 1966 |
| | Nutro Biscuits | 1950s |
| | Bal-Ahar | 1966 |
| | Mil-Tone | 1968 |
| | Milpro | 1969 |
| | Bal-Amul | 1969 |
| | Uni-Protein Biscuits | 1970 |
| Indonesia | Saridele | 1957 |
| Malaysia | Vitabean | 1952 |
| Pakistan | General Mills | 1968 |
| Singapore | Vitabean | 1962 |
| Taiwan, China | Wei Chuan | 1964 |
| | Soya Products | 1963 |
| Thailand | Poluk Milk | 1964 |
| | Vitamilk | 1960s |

*Dates refer to initiation of the scheme.
From Orr, E.,[154] with permission of Food Nutr.

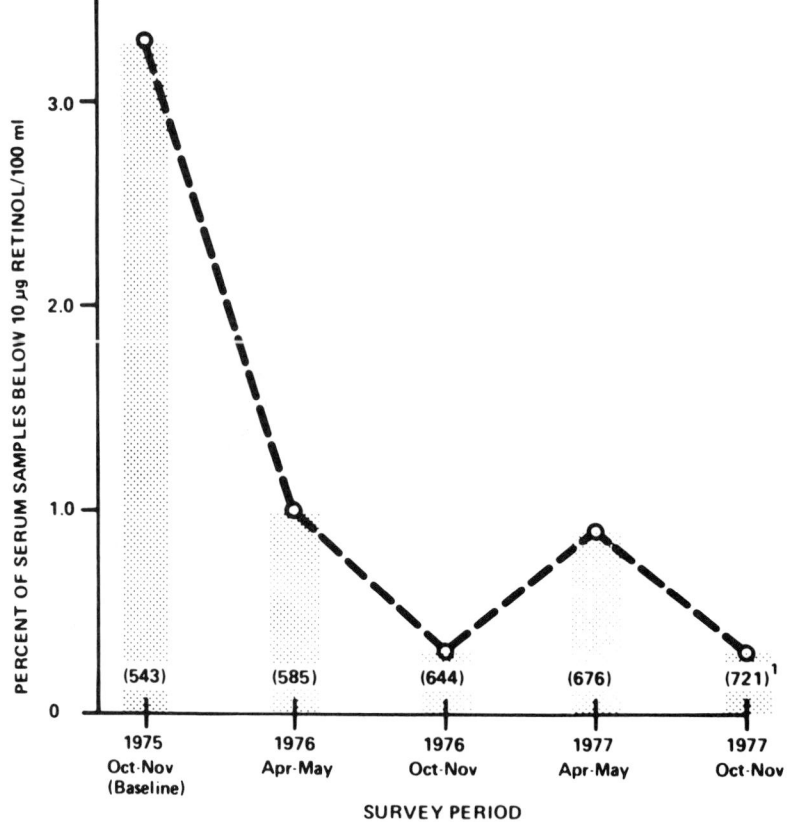

**Fig. 40–5.** Decrease in the percentage of children with "deficient" serum retinol levels as a result of nutrification of sugar with vitamin A initiated after the baseline period. (From Arroyave, G., Agular, J.R., Flores, M., et al.,[157] with permission of Pan American Health Organization.

cial production of amino acids, largely centered in Japan, has enabled nutrification of cereal-grain products with them.[108] During the past 10 years, oilseed protein mixtures have been prepared with wheat, corn, sorghum, oats, and bulgur.[141–145a] In these products, the oilseed or vegetable proteins supplement the proteins from cereal grains, which are inferior. Various baked goods have been developed with oilseed mixtures.[146,147] One of these is a leavened bread made from wheat flour and 12% soy flour, with the aid of the dough conditioner, stearoyl-2-lactylate.[147,148] Developed by Kansas State University, the bread has texture, color, and volume almost indistinguishable from those of regular bread. For some years a nutrified bun (Nutribun) made from soy-wheat flour and added micronutrients has been successfully used in the school nutrition program in the Philippines. In India and Ecuador, a soy-wheat flour has been used with success in production of bread. Other cereal-grain products improved through the addition of oilseed protein are CSM (corn-soy-milk blend), WSB (wheat-soy blend), SFSG (soy-fortified sorghum grits), SFCM (soy-fortified corn-

meal), and WSDM (whey-soy drink mix), designed to be used for infants, children, and pregnant and lactating women.[149–152b] Processing cereal grain-vegetable protein mixtures in low-cost extrusion cookers has introduced an appropriate technology in the production of nutritious food supplements.[153] High-protein pasta and high-protein cookies have elicited some interest. Blends of cereal products that have achieved some success in retail sales are Incaparina in Guatemala and Pronutro in South Africa.[154] A range of food mixtures and schemes exists worldwide (Table 40–4).

One form of blindness, xerophthalmia, occurs in infants and young children in areas of the world such as Asia, the Middle East, Africa, and Latin and South America where the intakes of vitamin A are inadequate.[154a] As many as 500,000 children around the world may go blind annually as a result of this nutritional deficiency. In addition to eye symptoms, other signs of vitamin A deficiency are growth depression, greater susceptibility to disease and, in many instances, eventual death. Through the cooperative efforts of the Agency for International Development, the World Health Organization, UNICEF, the International Vitamin A Consultative Group, the international blindness societies, and national groups, a concerted effort has been made to eradicate vitamin A deficiency. Programs of various types are underway or planned in India, Africa, Indonesia, Bangladesh, Pakistan, Sri Lanka, Haiti, Guatemala, Panama, Costa Rica, El Salvador, Brazil, and the Philippines. Part of these programs deals with distribution of foods nutrified with vitamin A. Among the foods[155] are dried milk, wheat flour, sugar (sucrose), tea dust and tea leaves, and seasonings such as monosodium glutamate and salt.[155a] The nutrification of sugar with vitamin A, developed by INCAP and practiced in Guatemala (Fig. 40–5), is an outstanding example of the nutrification concept converted to successful practice.[156,157]

Similar programs are underway for nutrifying foods with available forms of iron to combat another worldwide problem, iron deficiency anemia.[158,159] Some plans suggest putting both vitamin A and iron in the same food carrier. In other instances, addition of vitamin C, known to increase the bioavailability of iron, is being considered.

## NUTRIFICATION AND THE FUTURE

Knowledge of the requirements for and function of the essential nutrients is incomplete. The larger gaps in our knowledge of the major minerals are being filled in, and in the future more trace minerals may be included in nutrification programs. Zinc has already been proposed.[73] Greater use of the pure amino acids as additives as well as new sugars and fats may be involved in future nutrification programs. Appropriate mixtures of natural ingredients (cereal grains, oilseed products, and animal products) will continue for some time. New micronutrients can be incorporated only after detailed assessment of their past intake, the human requirement, the nutritional status of the population, and benefits to be derived. The possibility that more micronutrients will be incorporated into nutrification programs brings with it the following:

1. Continued pressures on the ingenuity of the chemist and food technologist to develop application forms that allow the nutrient to be uniformly incorporated and stable during the market distribution without altering flavor and biologic availability in the human body.

2. Continued biologic evaluation by the nutritionist of potential interactions among nutrients and among food components, which might alter performance in the body.

3. Continued search for food carriers to nutrify that minimize changes in food habits and hence reach an increasing percentage of the population.

4. Overcoming past barriers, real and created, to nutrification.

## SUMMARY

The ultimate goal of national and international nutrition food policies must be to make available to all people diets that meet all recognized nutrient allowances. The common objective in utilizing industrially produced nutrients is to supplement staple, agriculturally produced foods, or food ingredients to meet the required nutrient intake needs of a given population.

The economical production of micronutrients essential for life in pure or concentrated form by the chemical and fermentation industries has enabled nutritionists and food technologists to develop a nationwide nutrient delivery system that depends on the addition of missing or inadequate nutrients to existing food or food ingredients. This method for improving the nutritional and health status of a population is one of the great accomplishments in the nutrition of mankind and preventive medicine and hence ranks among the milestones in the history of public health. Nutrification, however, has its limitations and is certainly not a panacea for all malnutrition situations. Its continued success depends on: new scientific advances in the understanding of human requirements; continued dietary, biochemical, and clinical surveys; more extensive data on nutrient content of food, and a better understanding of nutrient interrelationships.

World needs demand the fullest application of technologies, knowledge, and resources both of agriculture and of industry for the efficient production and distribution of food.

## REFERENCES

1. Christensen, R.P.: USDA Yearbook of Agriculture. Doc. 349. Washington, D.C., U.S. Government Printing Office, 1966.
2. Buikstra, J.E.: West. Hemisphere Nutr. Congr. V, 297-305, 1978.
3. Hertzler, A.A., Anderson, H.L.: J. Am. Diet. Assoc. *64*:19-28, 1974.
4. King, J.C., Cohenour, S.H., Corruccini, C.G., et al.: J. Nutr. Educ. *10*:27-29, 1978.
5. Lachance, P.A.: Food Prod. Develop. *8*(5):63-70, 1974.
6. Chichester, C.O., Darby, W.J.: Food Technol. *29*:38-42, 1975.
7. Behar, M.: WHO Chronicle, *30*:140-143, 1976.
8. McGinnis, J.M.: J. Am. Diet. Assoc. *77*:129-132, 1980.
9. HEW: Healthy People. The Surgeon General's Report on Health Promotion and Disease Prevention. Publ. No. 79-55071. U.S. Dept. Health, Education

and Welfare. Washington, D.C., Public Health Service, 1979.

10. National Academy of Sciences: Toward Healthful Diets. Washington, D.C., 1980.

11. HEW: Nutrition and Your Health: Dietary Guidelines for Americans. Depts. Health, Education and Welfare and Agriculture. Washington, D.C., U.S. Government Printing Office, 1980.

12. Bourne, P.G.: Nutritional Policy as a Health Issue. Conference on Nutrition and the American Food System. Washington, D.C., June 1, 1978.

13. Symposium: Am. J. Clin. Nutr. *32*(Suppl.): 12, 1979.

14. U.S. Senate Select Committee on Nutrition and Human Needs: Dietary Goals for the United States. 2nd ed. Publ. No. 052-070-94376-8, Washington, D.C., U.S. Government Printing Office, 1977.

15. Taylor, T.G.: Importance of Vitamins to Human Health. Lancaster, England, MTP Press, 1979.

16. White House 1969 Conference on Food, Nutrition and Health: Final Report, Washington, D.C., U.S. Government Printing Office, 1970.

17. Society for Nutrition: Nutritional Claims for Foods. Berkeley, Calif., November, 1976.

18. Guthrie, H.A.: J. Am. Diet. Assoc. *71*:14-19, 1977.

19. J. Am. Diet. Assoc. *69*(5):Cover page, 1976.

20. Malini, R., Radhakrishnaiah, S.G., Saroja, S., et al.: Indian Food Packer *32*(6):26-61, 1978.

21. Fennema, O.: Food Technol. *31*(12):32-38, 1977.

22. Lachance, P.A., Erdman, J.W., Jr.: Effects of home food preparation practices on nutrified content of foods. *In* Nutritional Evaluation of Food Processing. (Harris, R.S., Karmas, E., Eds.) Westport, Conn., AVI Publishing Co., 1975, pp. 527-567.

23. Lund, D.B.: Effect of blanching, pasteurization and sterilization on nutrients. *In* Nutritional Evaluation of Food Processing. (Harris, R.S., Karmas, E., Eds.) Westport, Conn., AVI Publishing Co., 1975, pp. 205-240.

24. Lachance, P.A.: Effects of food preparation procedures in nutrient retention with emphasis upon food service practices. *In* Nutritional Evaluation of Food Processing. (Harris, R.S., Karmas, E., Eds.) Westport, Conn., AVI Publishing Co., 1975, pp. 463-528.

25. Schroeder, H.A.: Am. J. Clin. Nutr. *24*:562-573, 1971.

26. Harris, R.S., Von Loesecke, S.B.: Nutritional Evaluation of Food Processing. New York, John Wiley & Sons, Inc., 1960.

27. LeBovit, C.: Foods eaten away from home. National Food Situation, Washington, D.C., USDA Economic Research Service, 1970, pp. 25-31.

28. Lachance, P.A., Moskowitz, R.B., Winawer, H.H.: Food Technol. *26*(6):30-40, 1972.

29. Lowenberg, M.E.: Food Technol. *24*:751-756, 1970.

30. NRC: Recommended Dietary Allowances. 9th ed. Pub. 0-309-02941-1, Washington, D.C., National Academy of Sciences, 1980.

31. Report of the Committee on International Dietary Allowances of the International Union of Nutritional Sciences: Nutr. Abstr. Rev. *45*:89-111, 1975. Revised, Food Nutr. Bull. *4*:34, 1982.

32. Leung-Wu, W-T., Bussom, F., Jardin, C.: Food Composition Table for Use in Africa. Project U.S. Dept. HEW and FAO. Bethesda, Health, Education and Welfare, 1968.

33. Adams, C.F.: Nutritive Value of American Foods. Agriculture Handbook No. 456. U.S. Dept. Agric.

Washington, D.C., U.S. Government Printing Office, 1975.

34. Leung-Wu, W-T., Butrum, R.R., Chang, F.H., et al.: Food Composition Table for Use in East Asia. Project U.S. Dept. HEW and FAO. Rome. Food and Agriculture Organization, 1972.

35. Watt, B.K., Merill, A.L.: Composition of Foods—Raw, Processed, Prepared. Agriculture Handbook 8-12. Washington, D.C., U.S. Dept. Agric., 1963-1984.

36. WHO: Vitamin A Deficiency and Xerophthalmia. Report of Joint WHO/USAID Meeting. Tech. Rept. 590 and 672. Geneva, World Health Organization, 1976 and 1982.

37. WHO: Control of Nutritional Anaemia with Special Reference to Iron Deficiency. Report of Joint IAEA/USAID/WHO Meeting. Tech. Rept. 580. Geneva, World Health Organization, 1975.

38. Olson, R.E.: Protein-Calorie Malnutrition. Orlando, Academic Press, 1975.

39. Brubacher, G.: Bibl. Nutr. Dieta. *28*:176-183, 1979.

40. Pao, E.M., Mickle, S.J.: Food Technol. *35*(9):58-69, 78, 1981.

41. Brin, M.: Concept of Marginal Vitamin Deficiency in U.S. Population Presentation. 20th Annual Meeting American College Nutrition, St. Louis, June, 1979.

42. Davis, T.R.A., Gershoff, S.N., Gamble, D.F.: J. Nutr. Educ. *1*(Suppl.) : 41-57, 1969.

43. First Health and Nutrition Examination Survey (Hanes 1) 1971-1974: U.S. Dept. Health, Education and Welfare, Publ. No. 79-1657 (PHS), 1979.

44. Dietary Intake Source Data: United States 1976-1980. National Health Survey, Series 11, No. 231, DHHS Publ. No. 83-1683 (PBS), 1983.

45. Sabry, Z.I., Campbell, E., Campbell, J.A., et al.: Nutrition Canada–A National Nutrition Survey. Nutr. Rev. *32*:105-111, 1974; Can. Med. Assoc. J. *115*:775-777, 1976.

46. Truswell, A.S., and Apeagyi, F.: Incidence of Wernicke's Encephalopathy and Korsakoff's Psychosis in Sydney. Abstr. 3rd Asian Cong. of Nutr. (Jakarta) Oct. 1980, pp. 76-77.

47. Beaton, G.H.: Perspectives and priorities in food and nutritional planning. *In* Nutrition and Agricultural Development. (Scrimshaw, N.S., Behar, M., Eds.) New York, Plenum Publishing Corp., 1976, pp. 37-44.

48. Berg, A., Muscat, R.: Am. J. Clin. Nutr. *25*:939-954, 1972.

49. Ganzin, M., Perisse, J., Francois, P.: Need for food and nutrition policies. *In* Man, Food and Nutrition. (Recheigl, M., Jr., Ed.). Boca Raton, CRC Press, 1973, pp. 275-286.

50. Berg, A.D.: Am. J. Clin. Nutr. *23*:1396-1408, 1970.

51. Guidelines for a national nutrition policy. Nutr. Rev. *32*:153-157, 1974.

52. Hosoya, N.: Japan's National Nutrition Policy. Proc. Internat. Food Delivery Systems. Berkeley, Univ. Calif., 1975, pp. 91-103.

53. Santos, W.J.: National Food and Nutrition Plan–Planan. Proc. Internat. Food Delivery Systems. Berkeley, 1975, pp. 75-86.

54. Austin, J.E.: Wld. Rev. Nutr. Diet *25*:108-141, 1976.

55. Harper, A.E.: Food Nutr. News *52*(4):1-3, 1981.

56. Shaughnessy, D.E.: Ann. N.Y. Acad. Sci. *300*:92-95, 1977.

57. Field, J.O., Levinson, F.J.: Nutrition and development: The dynamics of commitment. *In* Nutrition

and Agricultural Development. (Scrimshaw, N.S., Behar, M., Eds.) New York, Plenum Publishing Corp., 1976, pp. 99-111.

58. Anderson, M.A., Grewal, T.: Nutrition planning in the developing world. Proc. Regional Workshop of CARE in India, Kenya and Columbia. Programas Editoriales, Carrera 28, No. 68-72, Bogota, Columbia, 1976.
59. Bauernfeind, J.C.: Vitamin fortification and nutrified foods. Proc. 3rd Internat. Congr. Food Sci. Technol., Washington, D.C., Aug. 9-14, 1970, pp. 217-232.
60. Lachance, P.A.: Food Technol. *24*(6):100, 1970.
61. Darby, W.J., Hambraeus, L.: Nutr. Rev. *36*:65-71, 1978.
62. Borenstein, B.: CRC Crit. Rev. Food Technol. *2*:171-186, 1971.
63. Klaeui, K.: Proc. IV Congr. Food Sci. Technol. *I*:740-762, 1974.
64. Bauernfeind, J.C., Cort, W.M.: Crit. Rev. Food Technol. *4*:337-375, 1974.
65. NRC: Technology of Fortification of Foods. Publ. ISBNO-309-02415-3. Washington, D.C., National Academy of Sciences, 1975.
65a. Yong, S.H.: Fortification technology. *In* Global Malnutrition and Cereal Fortification. (Austin, J.E., Ed.) Cambridge, Mass. Ballinger Publishing Co., 1979, pp. 43-80.
66. Cowgill, G.R.: Improving the quality of cheap staple foods. *In* Handbook of Nutrition. Chicago, American Medical Association, 1951, pp. 677-697.
67. Boussingault, M.: Ann. Chem. Phys. *54*:163-177, 1833.
68. Morton, R.A.: R. Soc. Health J. *90*(11):21-28, 1970.
69. General policies in regard to improvement of nutritive quality of foods. Nutr. Rev. *31*:324-326, 1973.
70. Teply, L.J.: Food fortification. *In* Man, Food and Nutrition. (Recheigl, M., Jr., Ed.) Boca Raton, CRC Press, 1973, pp. 243-250.
71. Navia, J.M.: J. Agric. Food Chem. *16*:172-176, 1968.
72. MacDonald, I.: Food Chem. *2*:193-197, 1977.
72a. Morgan, K.J.: Cereal Food World *28*:305-306, 1983.
73. Mertz, W.: Ann. N.Y. Acad. Sci. *300*:151-160, 1977.
73a. Mertz, W.: Food Prod. Develop. *12*(5):62, 67-72, 1977.
74. Kline, O.L.: What foods should be fortified. *In* Nutrients in Processed Foods: Vitamins and Minerals. Acton, Mass., American Medical Association Publishing Sciences Group Inc., 1974, pp. 129-136.
75. Kuebler, W.: Bibl. Nutr. Dieta, *18*:224-245, 1973.
76. Anonymous: Agric. Res. *22*(4):12, 1973.
77. Vandercook, C.E., Borden, C.M.: Food Prod. Develop. *7*(9): 58, 1974.
77a. Richardson, T.: Manufacturing Confectioner *60*(10):47-48, 50, 53-54, 1980.
78. Holsinger, V.H.: Cereal Science Today *19*:316-317, 1974.
79. Rosenfield, D.J.: Am. Diet. Assoc. *72*:475-477, 1978.
80. Klaeui, H.: Proc. IV Internat. Congr. Food Sci. Technol. *1*:740, 1974.
81. Cording, J., Eskew, R.K., Salinard, G.J. et al.: Food Technol. *15*:279-282, 1961.
82. Maga, J.A., Sizer, C.E.: Lebensm. Wiss. Technol. *11*:192-197, 1978.
83. Voirol, F.: Food Trade Rev. *44*(8):7, 1974.
84. Erdman, J.W., Jr.: Cereal Chem. *58*:21-26, 1981.
84a. Erdman, J.W., Jr., Forbes, R.M.: Food Prod. Develop. *11*(10):46, 48, 1977.

85. Mertz, W.: J. Am. Diet. Assoc. *77*:258-263, 1980.
86. Mertz, W.: Micronutrients needing better definition of requirements. *In* Nutrients in Processed Foods: Vitamins and Minerals. Acton, Mass., American Medical Association Publishing Sciences Group Inc., 1974, pp. 19-24.
87. Ranhotra, G.S., Lee, C., Gelroth, J.A.: Cereal Chem. *56*:552-554, 1979.
88. Cook, J.D.: Food Nutr. News *49*(3):1,4, 1978.
89. Lee, K., Clydesdale, F.M.: Crit. Rev. Food Sci. Nutr. *11*:117-153, 1979.
90. Rossander, L., Hallberg, L., Björn-Rasmussen, E.: Am. J. Clin. Nutr. *32*:2484-2489, 1979.
91. Lynch, S.R., Cook, J.D.: Contemp. Nutr. *5*(9):1-2, 1980.
91a. Lynch, S.R., Cook, J.D.: Ann. N.Y. Acad. Sci. *355*:32-44, 1981.
92. Olivares, M., Hertrampf, E., Cayazzo, M., et al. Brighton, Abstracts of XIII Internat. Congr. Nutrition, Aug. 1985, p. 130.
92a. Stekel, A., Olivares, M., Lopez, I., et al.: Pediatr. Res. *14*:74, 1980.
93. Björn-Rasmussen, E., Hallberg, L.: Nutr. Metab. *16*:94-100, 1974.
94. Cook, J.D., Monsen, E.R.: Am. J. Clin. Nutr. *30*:235-240, 1977.
94a. Bauernfeind, J.C., Miller, O.N.: Vitamin $B_6$: nutritional and pharmaceutical usage, stability, bioavailability, antagonists and safety. *In* Proceedings of a Workshop, Human Vitamin $B_6$ Requirements. Washington, D.C., National Academy Sciences, 1978, pp. 78-110.
94b. Machlin, L.J.: Handbook of Vitamins. New York, Marcel Dekker, Inc. 1984, pp. 269, 343, 406, 487, 505.
95. Austin, J.E.: Cereal Food World *23*:229-233, 265, 1978.
96. NRC: Proposed fortification policy for cereal-grain products. Publ. ISBN 0-309-02232-0. Washington, D.C., National Academy of Sciences, 1974.
97. Lachance, P.A.: Food Technol. *35*(3):49-60, 1981.
97a. Lorenz, K.: Lebensm. Wiss. Technol. *15*:121-125, 1982.
98. Cort, W.M., Borenstein, B., Harley, J.H., et al.: Food Technol. *30*(4):52-60, 1976.
99. Rubin, S.H., Emodi, A.E., Scialpi, L.: Cereal Chem. *54*:895-904, 1977.
100. Brooke, C.L.: J. Agric. Food Chem. *16*:163-167, 1968.
101. Hepburn, F.N.: Cereal Foods World, *21*:360, 1976.
102. Emodi, A.S., Scialpi, L.: Cereal Chem. *57*:1-3,1980.
102a. Ranum, P.M., Loewe, R.J., Gordon, H.T.: Cereal Chem. *58*:32-35, 1981.
103. Proc. Workshop on Technology of Fortification of Cereal-Grain Products. U.S. Dept. Comm. Nat. Tech. Information Ser. PB-281476, Springfield, VA, May, 1977.
104. Vetter, J.L.: Food Prod. Develop. *13*(4):37, 1979.
104a. Vetter, J.L., Adding Nutrients to Foods. St. Paul, American Association Cereal Chemists, 1982.
104b. Ranum, P.M.: Cereal Chem. *57*:70-72, 1980.
104c. Ranum, P., Kulp, K., Barrett, F.: Develop. Food Sci. *5B*:1055-1063, 1983.
104d. Ponte, J.G., Jr.: Develop. Food Sci. *5B*:1075-1079, 1983.
105. Anonymous: C&EN *48*(33):36-44, 1970.
106. Shukla, T.: Crit. Rev. Food Sci. Nutr. *6*:1-75, 1975.
107. Clark, H.E.: Wld. Rev. Nutr. Diet *32*:27-48, 1978.
108. Scrimshaw, N.S., Altschul, A.M.: Amino Acid For-

tification of Protein Food. Cambridge, MIT Press, 1971.

109. Howe, E.E., Jansen, G.R., Gilfillan, E.W.: J. Clin. Nutr. *16*:315-320, 1965.

109a. Howe, E.E., Jansen, G.R., Gilfillan, E.W.: Am. J. Clin. *20*:1134-1147, 1967.

110. Altschul, A.M.: New Protein Foods, Vol. 1. Orlando, Academic Press, 1974.

110a. Altschul, A.M.: New Protein Foods, Vol. 2. New York, Academic Press, 1976.

111. Milner, M.: Protein Enriched Cereal Foods for World Needs. St. Paul, Minn., Am. Assoc. Cereal Chemists, 1969.

111a. Sharifi, B.G.: Dissertation Abstracts International *B45*:1181, 1984.

112. Crowley, P.R. Supplementation of cereals with protein: State of the art in improving the nutrient quality of cereals. *In* Report of Second Workshop on Breeding and Fortification. (Wilcke, H.L., Ed.) Washington, D.C., Agency for International Development, 1976, pp. 220-224.

113. Barrett, F.: Fortification with protein supplements. *In* Report of Second Workshop on Breeding and Fortification.(Wilcke, H.L., Ed.) Washington, D.C., Agency for International Development, 1976, pp. 225-229.

114. WHO Tech. Report. Food fortification: Protein-calorie malnutrition. Report No. 477, World Health Organization. Geneva, FAO/WHO Joint Expert Committee on Nutrition, 1971.

115. Jansen, G.R., Harper, J.M., O'Deen, L.: Nutritional Evaluation of Blended Foods. Philadelphia, Meeting Institute Food Technologists, June, 1977.

116. Wilcke, H.L.: Improving the nutrient quality of cereals II. *In* Report of Second Workshop on Breeding and Fortification. Washington, D.C., Agency for International Development, 1976.

117. Milner, M.: Cereal Sci. Today *19*:509-512, 1974.

118. Parman, G.K.: J. Agric. Food Chem. *16*:168-171, 1968.

118a. Swaminathan, M., Daniel, V.A.: J. Nutr. Diet. *5*:316-336, 1968.

118b. Mejia, L.A., Arroyave, G.: Am. J. Clin. Nutr. *36*:87-93, 1982.

118c. Kamien, M., Woodhill, J.M., Nobile, S., et al.: Aust. N.Z. J. Med. *5*:123-133, 1975.

118d. Coleman, N.: Nutr. Rev. *40*:225-233, 1982.

118e. Rivera, R., Ruiz, R., Hegenauer, J., et al.: J. Clin. Nutr. *36*:1162-1169, 1982.

118f. James, C., Penfield, M.P., Andrews, F.E., et al.: Nutr. Repts. Internat. *27*:737-744, 1983.

119. Filer, L.J., Jr.: Agric. Food Chem. *16*:184-189, 1968.

120. Sarett, H.P.: Fortification of foods for general use vs. those for special dietary uses. *In* Nutrients in Processed Foods: Vitamins and Minerals. Acton, Mass. American Medical Association Publishing Sciences Group Inc., 1974, pp. 151-160.

121. Bauernfeind, J.C.: Ascorbic acid technology in agricultural, pharmaceutical, food and industrial applications. *In* Ascorbic Acid: Chemistry, Metabolism and Uses. (Seib, P.A., Tolbert, B., Eds.) Washington, D.C., American Chemical Society, 1982, pp. 395-498.

122. Bauernfeind, J.C.: Tocopherols in foods. *In* Vitamin E: A Comprehensive Treatise. (Machlin, L.J., Ed.) New York, Marcel Dekker, Inc., 1980, pp. 99-167.

123. Bauernfeind, J.C.: Carotenoids as Colorants and Vitamin A Precursors: Technology and Applications. Orlando, Academic Press, 1981.

123a. Gordon, H.T., Johnson, E.E., Borenstein, B.: Cereal Foods World *30*:274-276, 1985.

124. Arroyave, G.: Fortification of foods with nutrients. *In* Nutrition and Agricultural Development. (Scrimshaw, N.S., Behar, M., Eds.) New York, Plenum Publishing Corp., 1976, pp. 413-448.

124a. Quick, J.A., Murphy, E.W.: The fortification of foods: A review. USDA Agric. Handbook #598, Washington, D.C., USDA, 1982.

125. Beaton, G.H.: Food fortification. *In* Nutrition in Preventive Medicine. (Beaton, G.H., Bengoa, J.M., Eds.) Geneva, World Health Organization, 1976, pp. 370-388.

126. Rosenfield, D., Berntson, B.L.: Economics and Technology of Cereal Fortification. Los Angeles, American Chemical Society, March, 1971.

127. Sebrell, W.H., Jr.: Past experience in fortification of processed foods. *In* Nutrients in Processed Foods: Vitamins and Minerals. Acton, Mass., American Medical Association Publishing Sciences Group Inc., 1974, pp. 95-102.

128. Sebrell, W.H., Jr.: The concept of the fortification of foods with synthetic vitamins. *In* Amino Acid Fortification of Protein Foods. (Scrimshaw, N.S., Altschul, A.A., Eds.) Cambridge, MIT Press, 1971, pp. 63-76.

128a. Austin, J.E., Belding, T.K., Pyle, D., et al.: Nutrition Intervention in Developing Countries: Fortification and Formulated Foods. Cambridge, Mass., Oegleschlager, Gunn & Hain Publishers Inc., 1981.

128b. Levinson, F.J.: Food Nutr. Bull. *4*:24-33, 1982.

128c. Chauhan, B.M., Kapoor, A.C.: Sci. Cult. *50*(2):40-45, 1984.

128d. Leveille, G.A.: Food Technol. *38*:58-63, 1984.

128e. Brubacher, G.: Gordian *85*(½):14, 16-18, 1985.

129. Suwanik, R.: J. Natl. Res. Counc. (Thailand) *12*:1-45, 1980.

130. Present Knowledge in Nutrition. 5th ed. Washington, D.C., The Nutrition Foundation, Inc., 1984.

131. Miller, L.A.: What's New in Home Economics *16*(12):60-61, 144, 1952.

132. Wilder, R.M.: Recent Nutrition Surveys in Newfoundland: Significance of the Findings. Chicago, Wheat Flour Institute, 1952.

133. LeBovit, C.: J. Agric. Food. Chem. *16*:153-157, 1968.

134. Miller, D.F.: Cereal Enrichment/Pellagra–USA in Perspective 1977. San Francisco, American Association Cereal Chemists, Oct. 1977.

135. Miller, D.F.: Food Prod. Develop. *12*(4):30, 1978.

136. Friend, B.: Enrichment and Fortification of Foods, 1966-1970. Hyattsville, MD, National Food Situation USDA–ARS Form CFE (Adm.) 282, Jan., 1973.

136a. LaBell, F.M.: Food Proc. USA *45*(4):64-65, 1984.

136b. Gage, J.W.: Bakers Digest, March: 25, 1984.

137. Guggenheim, R., Brzezinski, A., Ilan, J., et al.: Am. J. Clin. Nutr. *7*:526-531, 1959.

138. Salcedo, J., Jr., Barnba, M.D., Carrosco, E.O., et al.: J. Nutr. *42*:501-523, 1950.

139. Duplessis, J.P., Wittmann, W., Groothof, G., et al.: S. Afr. Med. J. *48*:1641-1649, 1974.

140. Hayden, E.B.: Cereal Foods World *25*:141-143, 1980.

140a. Hayden, E.B.: Cereal Science Today *18*:120-123, 148, 1973.

141. Horan, F.E.: Cereal Science Today, *19*:112-117, 1974.

142. Weisberg, S.M.: Food Technol. *26*(9):60-68, 1972.

143. Elder, A.L., Weisberg, S.M.: High Nutrition-Low

Cost Foods: Their Impact in Developing Countries. Washington, D.C., 34th Internat. Congr. Food Sci. and Technol., Aug., 1970, pp. 91-104.

144. Altschul, A.M.: Low Cost Foods: Fortified Cereals and Protein Beverages. Washington, D.C., Amer. Soc. Cereal Chem. and Amer. Oil Chem. Soc., April, 1968.

145. Benevenga, N.J., Cieslak, D.G.: Some Thoughts on Amino Acid Supplementation of Proteins in Relation to Improvement of Protein Nutriture. Chicago, 174th Amer. Chem. Soc. Mtg., Sept., 1977.

145a. Cheigh, H.S., Ryu, C.H., Kwon, T.W.: J. Korean Soc. Food Nutr. *13*:377-380, 1984.

146. Weisberg, S.M.: Cereal Science Today, *18*:47-50, 1973.

147. Barrett, F.: Cereal Food World *20*:323-326, 1975.

148. Hoover, W.J.: A Case Study: Ecuador. Workshop on Breeding and Fortification. (Wilcke, H.L., Ed.) Washington, D.C., AID, 1976.

149. Hoover, S.R., Senti, F.R.: Enrichment and Fortification of U.S. Donated Foods. Prague, VIIIth Internat. Congr. Nutr. Aug., 1969.

150. Senti, F.R.: Formulated cereal foods in the U.S. food for peace program. *In* Protein-Enriched Cereal Foods for World Needs. St. Paul, Minn., American Association Cereal Chemists, 1969, pp. 246-254.

151. Senti, F.R.: Cereal Science Today *17*:157-161, 1972.

152. Shaughnessy, D.E.: Food for Peace Programs and the Marketplace. Portland, Oregon, The Oregon Wheat Growers League, Dec., 1976.

152a. Bookwalter, G.N.: Cereal Food World *28*:507-511, 1983.

152b. Bookwalter, G.N.: Develop. Food Sci. *5B*:1152-1159, 1983.

153. Jansen, G.R., Harper, J.M., O'Deen, L.: Nutritional Evaluation of Blended Foods Made with a Low-cost Extruder Cooker. Philadelphia, 37th Inst. Food Tech. Meeting, June, 1977.

154. Orr, E.: Food Nutr. *3*(2):2-10, 1977.

154a. Bauernfeind, J.C.: Vitamin A Deficiency and its Control. Orlando, Academic Press. (In press), 1986.

155. Bauernfeind, J.C.: Wld. Nutr. Diet. *41*:110-199, 1983.

155a. Husaini, M.A., Barizi, B., Djojosoebagio, S., et al.: Brighton, Abstract of XIII Internat. Congr. Nutr., Aug., 1985, p. 142.

156. Arroyave, G., Mejia, L.A., Aquilar, J.R.: Am. J. Clin. Nutr. *34*:41-49, 1981.

157. Arroyave, G., Agular, J.R., Flores, M., et al.: Evaluation of Sugar Fortification with Vitamin A at the National Level. Publ. No. 384. Washington, D.C., Pan. Am. Health Organ. Sci., 1979.

158. Cook, J.D., Reusser, M.E.: Am. J. Clin. Nutr. *38*:648-654, 1983.

159. Clydesdale, F.M., Weimer, K.L.: Iron Fortification of Foods. Orlando, Academic Press, 1985.

# Part IV
## *Malnutrition, Its Assessment and Therapy*

*Chapter* **41**

# CLINICAL MANIFESTATIONS OF NUTRITIONAL DISORDERS

Donald S. McLaren

Nutritional disorders result from an imbalance between the body's requirements for nutrients and energy and the supply of these substrates of metabolism. This imbalance may take the form of either deficiency or excess and may be attributable either to an inappropriate intake or to defective utilization.

Despite the extensive understanding of human nutritional requirements, malnutrition continues to be one of the main causes of morbidity and mortality in developing regions of the world, especially in young children. In technologically advances societies, malnutrition no longer constitutes a major hazard to health, but occurs in especially vulnerable groups in various ways. Some of these are related to the introduction and widespread use in recent years of techniques such as parenteral feeding and renal dialysis. Chronic alcoholism, drug abuse or even the medically supervised use of drugs, and food fadism may lead to deficiency disease states. The misuse of vitamins can cause toxicity.

This chapter is confined to nutritional disorders related to vitamins and essential elements. Disorders of protein and energy intake are considered elsewhere. A number of vitamin-dependency states have been identified in recent years. Their symptomatology relates to the metabolic abnormalities produced by the respective apoenzyme disorders, and not to vitamin deficiency, and they are considered under the appropriate vitamin.

The clinical manifestations of vitamin and element disorders will be discussed. These consist of the symptoms elicited from the patient and the signs observed on general physical examination, but not those requiring special investigations. Other aspects of these disorders are presented under the respective nutrients.

## VITAMINS

### Vitamin A (Retinol)

**Deficiency.** The symptoms and signs of vitamin A deficiency have been studied in greater detail than those of any other nutritional disorder.[1,2] The eye is primarily involved and predominantly in young children. Night blindness, an early feature, can be elicited by a careful history and some simple tests in a poorly illuminated room.[3] Color vision may also be affected. Dryness (xerosis) and unwettability of the bulbar conjunctiva follow. An advanced degree of this process is Bitot's spot, a heaping up of desquamated, keratinized epithelial cells (Plate I–*A*). This condition usually occurs on the temporal aspect of the interpalpebral fissure near the corneal limbus, but may less commonly also involve the nasal aspect and other parts of the bulbar conjunctiva. In older children and adults, Bitot's spots may be stigmata of earlier deficiency, or may be entirely unrelated to vitamin A deficiency. Corneal involvement, commencing as a superficial punctate keratopathy,[4] and proceeding to xerosis (Plate I–*B*) and varying degrees of "ulceration" and liquefaction (keratomalacia) (Plate I–*C*), frequently results in blindness. Punctate degenerative changes in the retina (xerophthalmic fundus) are a rare sign of chronic deficiency usually seen in older children.[5] Corneal scars have many causes, but one of these is previous vitamin A deficiency. They may be fine nebulae, denser leucomata, or may consist of total scarring of a shrunken globe (phthisis bulbi) or corneal ectasia amd anterior staphyloma.

Extraocular manifestations include perifollicular hyperkeratosis, a heaping up of hyperkeratinized skin epithelium around hair follicles. This condition is most commonly found on the outer aspects of the upper arms and thighs. It is also seen in starvation and has been attributed to B complex or essential fatty acid deficiency. Other changes, which include impaired taste, anorexia, vestibular disturbance, bone changes with pressure on cranial nerves, increased intracranial pressure, congenital malformations, and infertility, have been best demonstrated in animals.[6]

**Toxicity.** Acute toxicity causes a rise in intracranial pressure, leading to drowsiness, irritability, headache, vomiting, and peeling of the skin. In infants the anterior fontanelle bulges (see Fig. 50–21).

Chronic poisoning produces a bizarre clinical picture that may be misdiagnosed if excessive intake is not suspected. It is characterized by anorexia, headache, blurred vision and diplopia, dry skin and pruritus, painful extremities due to periosteal thickening of the long bones, (see Fig. 50–11) and hepatosplenomegaly.

Birth defects have been reported in the offspring of women receiving 13-*cis*-retinoic acid (isotretinoin) during pregnancy.[7]

**Hypercarotenosis.** This condition is caused by excessive intake of carotenoids. Yellow or orange discoloration of the skin (xanthosis cutis, carotenoderma) affects areas where sebum secretion is greatest (nasolabial folds, forehead, axillae, groins) and keratinized surfaces such as the palms

and soles. The sclerae and buccal mucous membranes are not affected.

## Vitamin D (Calciferol)

**Deficiency.** Vitamin D deficiency is manifested as rickets in children and osteomalacia in adults. Those forms not due to primary nutrient deficiency also exhibit signs and symptoms of the underlying disease and of hypocalcemia (to be discussed).

*Rickets.* The rachitic infant is restless and sleeps poorly. Consequently, the occipital hair is denuded. Craniotabes, softening of the bones of the skull and their ready depression on palpation, is often the earliest sign, but it must be present away from the suture lines to be diagnostic of rickets. Frontal bossing occurs and the fontanelles close late. Sitting, crawling, and walking are all delayed. If the disease is active when these activities occur, weight-bearing results in knock-knees or bowing of the arms or legs. Enlargement of the epiphyseal cartilages is most evident at the lower end of the radius and ulna and the upper ends of the tibia and fibula (see Fig. 50–5). The rachitic rosary, due to enlargement of the costochondral junctions of the ribs, is said to be smoother than that due to scurvy (see discussion of vitamin C). The chest may also show Harrison's sulcus or groove, a bilateral indentation of the lateral parts of the lower ribs. Other deformities of the chest, such as depression (funnel chest or pectus excavatum) and elevation (pigeon chest or pectus carinatum) of the sternum, are now considered to be congenital and not rachitic in origin.

*Osteomalacia.* The main features of this disease are bone pains and tenderness, skeletal deformity, and weakness of the proximal muscles. In severe cases all the bones are painful and tender, often sufficiently so to disturb sleep. Tenderness may be particularly marked over Looser's zones (see Chap. 13), usually occurring in the long bones, the pelvis, the ribs, and around the scapulae in a bilaterally symmetric pattern. Fractures of the softened bones are common. The proximal muscle weakness, the cause of which is uncertain, is more marked in some forms of osteomalacia than in others. Osteomalacia usually results in a waddling gait and difficulty in getting up and down stairs. In the elderly it may simulate paraplegia; in those younger, muscular dystrophy.

**Toxicity.** Some of the symptoms and signs are related to the hypercalcemia and are common to all causes of that condition. Anorexia, nausea, vomiting, and constipation are usually present. Weakness, hypotonia, stupor, and hypertension are less common. Polyuria and polydipsia are

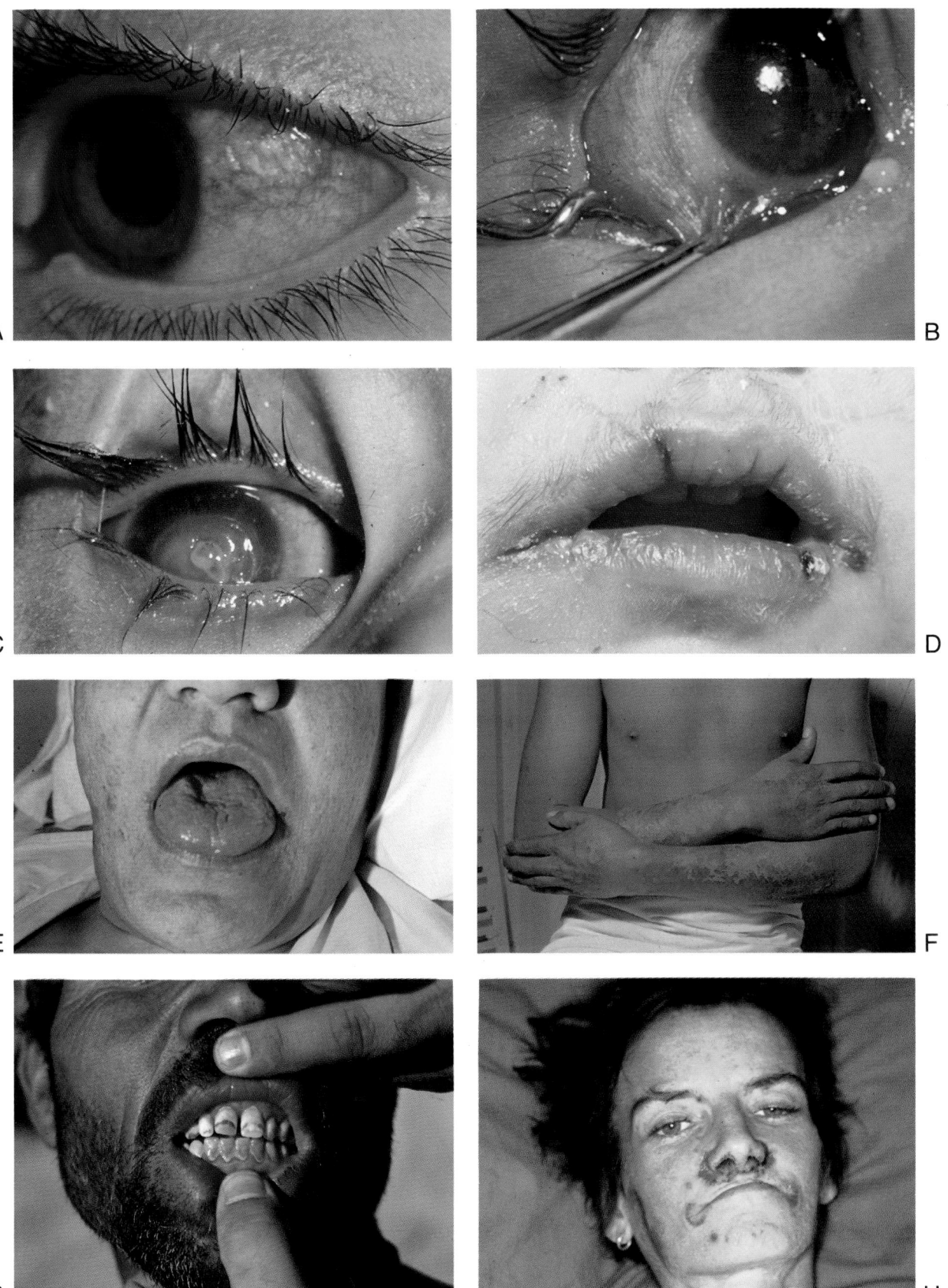

**Plate I**   *A,* Vitamin A deficiency. Bitot's spot in temporal interpalpebral fissure. *B,* Vitamin A deficiency. Conjunctival and corneal xerosis. *C,* Vitamin A deficiency. Keratomalacia. *D,* Riboflavin deficiency. Cheilosis and angular stomatitis. *E,* Riboflavin deficiency. Magenta tongue. *F,* Niacin deficiency. Symmetrical dermatosis of pellagra. *G,* Fluorosis. Early stage with brown mottling that is most marked on upper central incisors *H,* Zinc deficiency. Typical dermatosis associated with alcoholic cirrhosis in this patient. (From Ilchyshyn, A., Mendelsohn, Z.: Br. Med. J. *284*:1676, 1982.)

caused by hypercalciuria. Renal colic due to stone formation may result.

Vitamin D excess has been reported to take two forms: mild and severe. In the mild form, the patient is usually 3 to 6 months of age, and the symptoms and signs are those already described. In the severe form, in addition to the manifestations of hypercalcemia, there is mental retardation, stenosis of the aorta and the pulmonary arteries, and a characteristic facial appearance termed "elfin facies."[8]

## Vitamin E (Tocopherol)

Deficiency of this vitamin is usually confined to biochemical abnormalities. Substantial clinical changes are few. Low-birth-weight infants are particularly susceptible, especially if fed formulas high in polyunsaturated fatty acids after a hemolytic anemia made worse by iron supplements has occurred.[9,10] Lipofuscin deposition within muscle cells has been reported to account for the brown bowel syndrome.[11] The retinopathy of abetalipoproteinemia may be in part caused by vitamin E deficiency.[12] Spinocerebellar syndromes, similar to those seen in this disease, have shown a good response to vitamin E in children with cystic fibrosis and chronic cirrhosis. Ataxia and visual field defect were corrected with vitamin E supplementation in a 64-year-old man with chronic steatorrhea.[14] Retrolental fibroplasia, a cause of blindness in the low-birth-weight infant subjected to high postnatal incubation oxygen concentrations, is also influenced by the presence of vitamin E deficiency,[15] as are some cases of intraventricular hemorrhage and subependymal hemorrhage.[16]

**Toxicity.** Low-birth-weight infants receiving prolonged pharmacologic doses of vitamin E are prone to a high incidence of sepsis and necrotizing enterocolitis.[16a] Use of a new FDA-unapproved intravenous vitamin E product led to pulmonary deterioration, thrombocytopenia, liver and renal failure, and a high mortality.[16b]

## Vitamin K

**Deficiency (Hypoprothrombinemia).** Hemorrhagic disease of the newborn may result in bleeding anywhere in the body, but the most common sites are the gut, producing melena neonatorum, cephalhematomas, and the umbilical stump. Bleeding may also result from circumcision. Generalized ecchymoses, often without petechiae, intracranial bleeding, and intramuscular hemorrhages are less common.

In the adult, bleeding from this cause is most common in chronic liver disease, obstructive jaundice, and in patients receiving anticoagulants, prolonged antibiotic therapy, or certain cephalosporin antibiotics, e.g., moxalactam disodium (see Chap. 14).

Rare instances of deficiency have been attributed to dietary restriction[18] or total parenteral nutrition[19] when inadequate amounts were added to the solutions or injected. Cases have been reported in the United States in 4- to 6-week-old infants, often with intracranial hemorrhage, who were exclusively breast-fed and did not receive vitamin K in the newborn period, usually because of home delivery.[19a] Large doses of vitamin E may induce deficiency of vitamin K.[20]

**Toxicity.** Kernicterus (bilirubin encephalopathy) has occurred in low-birth-weight infants receiving large doses (75 mg) of menadione or its water-soluble derivatives; this has not occurred when vitamin K has been given. Lethargy, hypotonia, and loss of the sucking reflex are followed by opisthotonos, hypotonia, generalized spasticity, and frequently death from pulmonary complications. Survivors may develop the post-kernicterus syndrome: high-frequency nerve deafness, athetoid cerebral palsy, and dental enamel dysplasia.

## Thiamin (Vitamin B₁)

**Deficiency.** Beriberi in the adult occurs in two distinct forms, wet and dry beriberi, in which the cardiovascular and the nervous systems, respectively, are affected. For reasons that are not clear, the two forms rarely occur in the same patient. Infantile beriberi is described separately.

Cardiovascular beriberi takes two forms: the more common high-output state and the rare, but highly fatal, low-output state.

*High-Output State.* Signs and symptoms of biventricular heart failure are present. The right ventricle is more affected than the left, resulting in dyspnea, orthopnea, and pulmonary rales. There is sinus tachycardia, a wide pulse pressure and, before heart failure supervenes, a sweating and warm skin. In the presence of heart failure, peripheral vasoconstriction results in cold and cyanosed extremities in an attempt to maintain arterial pressure.[21]

*Low-Output State (Shoshin Disease).* This form is characterized by signs and symptoms of severe hypotension, lactic acidosis, and very low systemic vascular resistance. Peripheral edema is absent.[22]

### Beriberi of the Nervous System

*Cerebral Beriberi (Wernicke-Korsakoff Syndrome).* In its most severe form, mental confusion, accompanied by ophthalmoplegia due to paralysis of the sixth cranial nerve, leads to coma (Wernicke's encephalopathy). Korsakoff's psychosis is produced by lesser degrees of deficiency and consists of mental confusion, aphonia, and sixth nerve weakness, evidenced by nystagmus.[23]

*Peripheral Neuropathy.* The most characteristic features are symmetric footdrop, associated with marked tenderness of the calf muscles, and a mild disturbance of sensation over the outer aspects of the legs and thighs, and in patches over the abdomen, chest, and forearms. Ataxia with loss of position and vibration sense, burning paresthesias in the feet, and amblyopia are less common.

**Infantile Beriberi.** Early mainfestations are anorexia, vomiting, pallor, restlessness, and insomnia. The disease progresses typically to (1) an acute, cardiac form in infants 2 to 4 months of age; (2) a subacute, aphonic form in those 5 to 7 months old; and (3) a chronic, pseudomeningeal form between 8 and 10 months of age. The acute form presents with dyspnea, cyanosis, a rapid, thready pulse, and other signs of acute heart failure. In the subacute form, aphonia or a characteristic hoarse cry, dysphagia, vomiting, and convulsions predominate. The chronic form is characterized by neck retraction, opisthotonos, edema, oliguria, constipation, and meteorism.[24]

### Riboflavin

**Deficiency.** The skin and mucous membranes are affected in what is known as the orooculogenital syndrome. Areas of skin affected are those containing many sebaceous glands, mainly the nasolabial folds, alae nasi, external ears, eyelids, scrotum in the male, and labia majora in the female. They become reddened, scaly, greasy, painful, and pruritic. Plugs of inspissated sebum may accumulate in the hair follicles and give the appearance known as dyssebacea or shark skin (Fig. 41–1).

At the angles of the mouth there are painful fissures, known as angular stomatitis when active (Plate I–*D*). When chronic, they give rise to one form of rhagades. Vertical fissures of the vermilion surface of the lips constitute cheilosis. These and the angular lesions may become infected with *Candida albicans,* giving rise to the appearance known as perlèche. The tongue may be painful and may have a magenta color (Plate I–*E*). These changes are not specific for this deficiency.

Photophobia, lacrimation, and conjunctival injection are often present, but neovascularization of the cornea, common in experimental animals, is rare in man.

### Niacin

**Deficiency.** Pellagra affects primarily the skin, gastrointestinal tract, and nervous system.

The dermatosis is usually the earliest and most prominent manifestation. It is symmetric and appears on parts exposed to sunlight or trauma. Erythema progresses to keratosis and scaling with pigmentation (Plate I–*F*). The back of the hands, wrists, forearms, face, and neck (Casal's necklace) are typical situations. The skin and mucous membrane changes of riboflavin deficiency are also commonly present (see preceding section on riboflavin).

The tongue often has a "raw beef" appearance, is bright red, swollen, and painful. Symptoms of gastritis, bouts of diarrhea, and signs of malabsorption suggest similar changes in the gastrointestinal tract.

Nervous system involvement is suggested in the early stages by periods of depression, with insomnia, headaches, and dizziness. Later, tremulous movement or rigidity of the limbs occurs with loss of tendon reflexes, numbness, and paresis of the extremities, ultimately incapacitating the patient. In profound deficiency an encephalopathy has been described that resembles that of acute cerebral beriberi (see section on thiamin) but responds to some extent to niacin.

### Pyridoxine (Vitamin B<sub>6</sub>)

**Deficiency.** This deficiency is rarely severe enough to produce signs and symptoms. Volunteers receiving a deficient diet and a pyridoxine antagonist became irritable and depressed. Seborrheic dermatosis affected the nasolabial folds, cheeks, neck, and perineum. Several subjects also developed glossitis, cheilosis, angular stomatitis, blepharitis, and a peripheral neuropathy.

An uncommon form of sideroblastic anemia, often severe, has been reported to respond in some instances to pyridoxine, but most types appear to be due to dependency rather than to deficiency.[25] Convulsions occurred in infants fed a milk formula in which the pyridoxine had been destroyed during processing.[26]

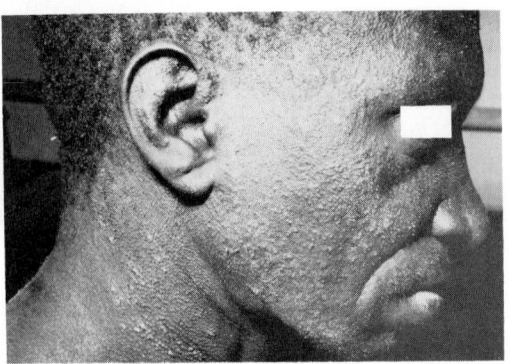

**Fig. 41–1.** Dyssebacea associated with riboflavin deficiency.

**Toxicity.** A sensory neuropathy has been attributed to the abuse of pyridoxine in megadoses.[27] Seven adults developed gradually progressive sensory ataxia and profound lower limb impairment of position and vibration sense. Touch, temperature, and pain were less affected. The motor and central nervous systems were unimpaired. One review noted that an impurity in the pharmaceutical product used might possibly have been responsible.[28]

## Biotin

**Deficiency.** This deficiency has occasionally been induced in patients who have consumed large amounts of egg white over a prolonged period.[29] Egg white contains avidin, which antagonizes the action of biotin. The skin of the face and hands becomes dry, shining, and scaling. The oral mucosa and tongue are swollen, magenta in color, and painful.

An infant with short-gut syndrome received total parenteral nutrition from 5 months of age. Five months later the infant lost all body hair and developed a waxy pallor, irritability, lethargy, mild hypotonia, and an erythematous rash. Biotin deficiency was confirmed biochemically, and all signs were reversed by supplementation.[30] Two adult patients receiving home parenteral nutrition after extensive gut resection developed severe hair loss that was reversed by 200 μg intravenous biotin daily.[31]

## Vitamin B$_{12}$ (Cobalamin)

**Deficiency.** This may be primary or secondary as in pernicious anemia.

*Pernicious Anemia.* This condition usually manifests after middle age. There is a slight female preponderance. It may be associated with signs of other autoimmune diseases. The most common complaints—those usually associated with anemia—ordinarily do not arise until the anemia is well advanced. Neurologic changes may long precede the hematologic changes. The tongue may be red, smooth, shining, and painful. Anorexia, weight loss, indigestion, and episodic diarrhea are also usually present.

The typical patient with pernicious anemia has prematurely grey hair, blue eyes, and wide cheek bones. Mild jaundice gives the so-called lemon yellow tint. A few patients have widespread brown pigmentation affecting nail beds and skin creases particularly, but sparing the mucous membranes.

In advanced cases there is usually pyrexia, enlargement of liver and spleen, and occasionally bruising due to thrombocytopenia. Older patients may present with congestive cardiac failure.

A distal sensory neuropathy with "glove and stocking" sensory loss, paresthesias, and areflexia may occur in isolation or more commonly together with a myelopathy known as subacute combined degeneration of the cord. In this condition the initial symptom is symmetric paresthesias of the feet or, occasionally, of the hands. There is increasing difficulty in walking, due to a combination of weakness and loss of postural sense. Psychiatric disturbances, especially mild dementia, may be the presenting or only feature. Visual loss from optic atrophy is not uncommon.

Congenital lack of intrinsic factor presents before the age of 2 with irritability, vomiting, diarrhea, weight loss, and anemia. An infant exclusively breast-fed by a mother with a latent pernicious anemia developed megaloblastic anemia and neurologic abnormalities.[31a]

**Primary Dietary Deficiency.** When this condition of malabsorption is the cause of deficiency, anemia is usually the most prominent feature, but glossitis, optic neuropathy, and subacute combined degeneration of the cord have also been described. Megaloblastic anemia developed in an infant exclusively breast-fed by a vegan mother.[31b]

## Folic Acid

**Deficiency.** The anemia has morphologic features similar to those of vitamin B$_{12}$ deficiency (see Chap. 21), but it develops more rapidly. Subacute combined degeneration of the cord does not occur, but about 20% of patients may have a peripheral neuropathy. The tongue may be red and painful in the acute stage. In chronic deficiency, the papillae atrophy, leaving a shiny, smooth surface. Hyperpigmentation of the skin, similar to that occurring in vitamin B$_{12}$ deficiency, is sometimes present.

Folic acid treatment before conception has prevented the recurrence of neural tube defects in the offspring,[32] and several large trials using multivitamin therapy, including folic acid, have given similar results in the United Kingdom.

Folate deficiency has been described in total parenteral nutrition with certain amino acid mixtures in the absence of supplementary folic acid.[33] An infant exclusively breast-fed by a mother taking estrogen-progestogen contraceptive pills developed megaloblastic anemia responsive to folic acid.[33a]

## Pantothenic Acid

**Deficiency.** In adult volunteers on a deficient diet, researchers claimed that the "burning feet syndrome" resulted and that this condition responded to the vitamin. In clinical practice this distressing complaint has rarely responded to this treatment.

### Carnitine

**Deficiency.** A 41-year-old male receiving long-term total parenteral nutrition developed jaundice, symptoms of hypoglycemia, and generalized skeletal muscle weakness associated with biochemical evidence of carnitine deficiency.[34] All the signs were reversed by carnitine therapy.

### Vitamin C (Ascorbic Acid)

**Deficiency.** Scurvy tends to affect either the very young or the elderly. The clinical picture differs in these two groups and requires separate consideration.

*Infantile Scurvy (Barlow's Disease).* The onset, usually in the second half of the first year of life, is presaged by a period of fretfulness, pallor, and loss of appetite. Localizing signs are tenderness and swelling, most marked at the knees or ankles. These symptoms result from characteristic bone changes demonstrable by roentgenogram (see Fig. 50–21). Enlargement of the costochondral junctions produces the scorbutic rosary, which has a sharper feel than that due to rickets (see section on vitamin D). The infant often adopts the "pithed frog" position of maximum comfort, with the legs flexed at the knees and the hips partially flexed and externally rotated. The arms are less commonly involved. Hemorrhage and spongy changes in the gums are confined to the sites of teeth that have recently erupted or are about to do so. Bleeding may occur anywhere in the skin (the orbit is a not infrequent site) or from mucous membranes, including the renal tract. Petechiae and ecchymoses, usually found in the region of the bone lesions, are less common than in the adult. A microcytic, hypochromic anemia is common. Older children may develop the characteristic perifollicular hemorrhages and hair changes seen in the adult.

*Adult Scurvy.* Early symptoms are weakness, easy fatigue, and listlessness, followed by shortness of breath and aching in bones, joints, and muscles, especially at night. These symptoms are followed by characteristic changes in the skin.[35] Acne, indistinguishable from that of adolescence, precedes defects in the hairs of the body. These defects consist of broken and coiled hairs and a "swan-neck" deformity resulting from their being flat instead of round in cross section. However, the true hallmark of scurvy in the adult is perifollicular hemorrhages and perifollicular hyperkeratosis, most common on the anterior aspect of the thorax, forearms, thighs, and legs and on the anterior abdominal wall (Fig. 41–2).

Frank bleeding is a late feature of scurvy. The classic gum changes are only associated with natural teeth or buried roots and are enhanced by poor dental hygiene and advanced caries. The interdental papillae become swollen and purple and bleed on trauma. In advanced scurvy the gums are spongy and friable, bleeding freely. Secondary infection leads to loosening of the teeth and gangrene (Fig. 41–3). Patients who are edentulous or whose teeth are in good repair have little or no evidence of scorbutic gingivitis. Hemorrhage commonly occurs deep in muscles and into joints. Multiple splinter hemorrhages may form a crescent near the distal ends of the nails. Old scars break down and new wounds fail to heal.

### Essential Fatty Acids

Although these are not considered as vitamins, it is convenient to consider the symptomatology of deficiency of these fatty acids here.

**Deficiency.** Growth retardation, sparse hair growth, a bran-like desquamation of the skin of the trunk, poor wound healing, and increased susceptibility to infection have been observed in infants receiving a formula deficient in essential fat or receiving long-term, lipid-free parenteral nutrition.

In adults reports have been associated with prolonged, usually lipid-free, total parenteral nutrition.[36] Sometimes there is only a dry, flaky skin, but more advanced deficiency results in a scaling, eczematoid dermatosis, usually starting on the nasolabial folds and eyebrows and spreading across the face and neck (Fig. 41–4). Anemia and enlarged fatty liver have also been reported.

*Linolenic Acid Deficiency.* A single report has claimed response to linolenic acid alone consisting of neurologic changes that included paresthesias, weakness, inability to walk, pain in the legs, and blurred vision.[37] The patient was a 6-year-old girl with extensive gut resection, receiving total parenteral nutrition rich in linoleic acid but low in linolenic acid. The claim has been challenged[38] and defended.[39]

### MINERALS

### Calcium

**Hypocalcemia.** Symptoms and signs of underlying disorders will be present. Hypocalcemia in clinical conditions is rarely caused by inadequate calcium ingestion but rather by disorders of calcium metabolism. The low blood calcium per se causes the nervous system to be affected. Depression and psychosis, progressing to dementia or encephalopathy, occur. The most characteristic syndrome is tetany, consisting of (1) paresthesias

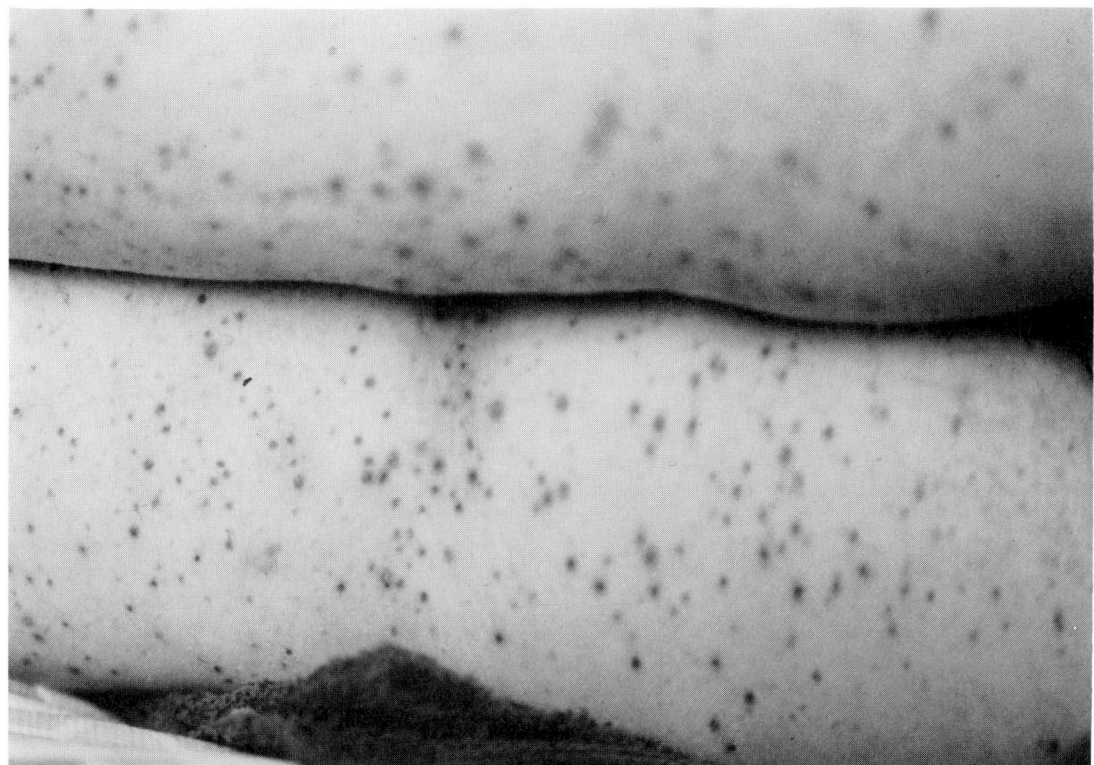

**Fig. 41–2.** Perifollicular hemorrhages of the legs in adult scurvy.

of the lips, tongue, fingers, and feet; (2) carpopedal spasm, resulting in the "obstetrician's hand," a deformity that may be painful and prolonged; (3) generalized muscle aching; and (4) spasm of facial musculature. At the earlier stage of latent tetany, the neuromuscular irritability may be elicited by provocative tests. Chvostek's sign is contraction of the facial muscles on light tapping of the facial

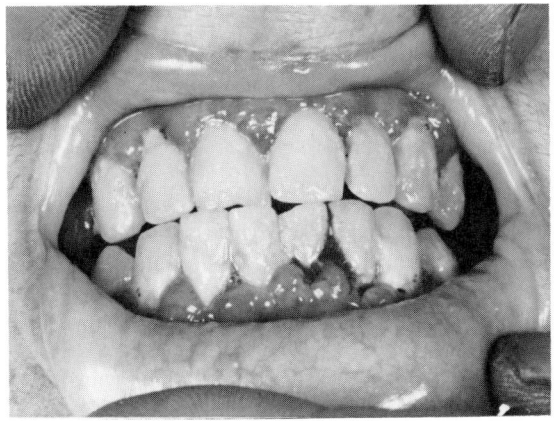

**Fig. 41–3.** Gum changes of scurvy in food fadism. (From Sherlock, P., Rothschild, E.O.: JAMA *199*:794–798, 1967.)

nerve. Trousseau's sign is carpopedal spasm induced by restriction of the blood supply to a limb by a tourniquet applied for about three minutes. Cataract may be the earliest feature.

In the neonate and older infant tetany may manifest as rhythmic, focal myoclonic jerks, sometimes followed by convulsions, cyanosis, and heart failure. Muscular spasms and laryngismus stridulus may occur in young children.

**Osteoporosis.** Calcium deficiency plays an ill-defined part in this condition of loss of bone mass. It is common in the elderly, especially in postmenopausal women. There is bone deformity, localized pain, and fracture. Osteomalacia may co-exist. The most common deformity is loss of height due to vertebral collapse, which accounts for most of the pain. Fractures of the neck of the femur and Colles' fracture above the wrist are most commonly due to trauma, which may be trivial, in the elderly with osteoporosis.

**Calcium-Deficiency Rickets.** Reports from South Africa have suggested that true rickets can be produced by dietary calcium deficiency in the presence of a normal vitamin D status.[40] The histologic changes of rickets were confirmed by biopsy and responded to calcium therapy alone.[41]

**Hypercalcemia.** This condition occurs from a

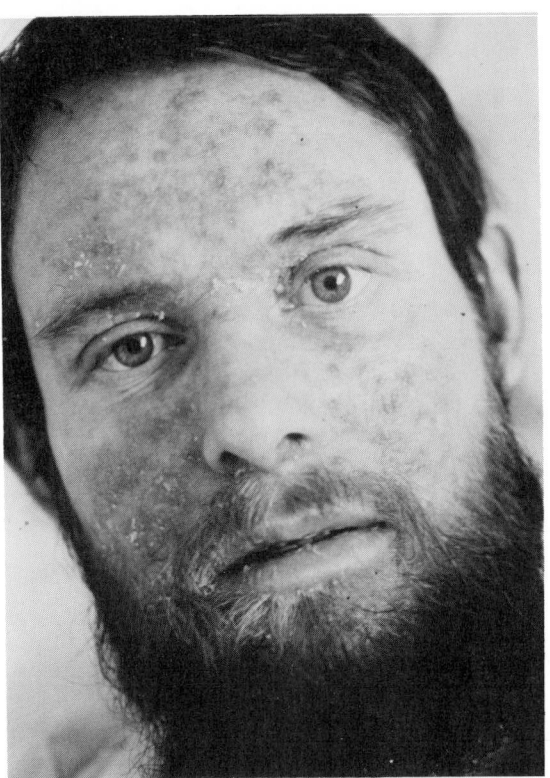

**Fig. 41–4.** Dermatosis of essential fatty acid deficiency associated with total parenteral nutrition. (Courtesy of Dr. R.E. Hodges.)

variety of causes and produces a symptom complex that is, to some extent, characteristic of this state. Gastrointestinal symptoms include anorexia, nausea, vomiting, constipation, abdominal pain, and ileus. Renal system involvement produces polyuria, nocturia, polydipsia, stone formation, and sometimes hypertension and signs and symptoms of uremia. Muscle weakness and myopathy occur. More advanced disease, which causes psychosis, delirium, stupor, and coma, may prove fatal.

**Osteopetrosis (Marble Bone Disease).** A severe, often fatal, form occurs in infancy and a milder form in later childhood.[42] Bones become more dense than normal and enlarge, encroaching on the marrow and foramina in the skull. Cranial nerve palsies, especially those leading to blindness and deafness, occur. There is anemia and splenomegaly.

## Magnesium

**Deficiency.** This condition is frequently accompanied by hypocalcemia, depletion of potassium, and other disturbances. The symptoms may vary. Magnesium depletion in volunteers has induced anorexia, nausea, vomiting, lethargy, weakness,

personality change, tetany, tremor, and muscle fasciculations. In young children, severe deficiency has been associated with generalized tonic-clonic seizures (see Chap. 6).

It has been suggested that increased vascular contractility in magnesium deficiency might be responsible for preeclampsia.[43]

**Toxicity.** Hypermagnesemia is common in renal failure patients receiving magnesium-containing drugs. Deep tendon reflexes disappear and ECG abnormalities appear. Hypertension, respiratory depression, narcosis, and ultimately cardiac arrest may occur with very high blood magnesium levels (see Chap. 6).

## Phosphorus

Patients on renal dialysis and with phosphate-restricted diets supplemented with phosphate-precipitating oral medications, parenteral nutrition with inadequate phosphate, diabetic keto-acidosis, and chronic alcoholism are at risk of phosphate depletion or symptomatic hypophosphatemia secondary to phosphate redistribution. Profound anorexia, nausea and vomiting, confusion, dysarthria, paresthesias, peripheral neuropathy, anemia, and signs of hypoxia have all been described.[44,45]

It has been claimed that rickets may be induced by phosphate deficiency, independent of calcium or vitamin D deficiency.[46] Hypophosphatemic rickets is a well-recognized entity.

## Iodide (Iodine)

**Deficiency.** Enlargement of the thyroid gland is the most common clinical sign. When due to iodine lack this condition is termed simple, endemic, colloid, or euthyroid goiter. It is more common in women and is often noted at the onset of puberty, during pregnancy, or at the menopause. Early on the enlargement is soft, symmetric, and smooth, but later multiple nodules and cysts may appear. Most patients are euthyroid or have hyperthyroidism, but goitrous hypothyroidism may occur.

When endemic goiter is severe, it is accompanied by endemic cretinism with delayed growth, fatigue, slow mental responses, hypotension, bradycardia, constipation, pretibial edema, and slow deep tendon reflexes. In its overt form this condition consists of three components: mental retardation, bilateral hearing defect, and neuromotor abnormalities. These are found to a varying extent in any one patient.[47] The neurologic abnormalities include sensory neuro-hearing defects, leading to deaf-mutism in advanced cases, proximal spasticity of the extremities, and certain release phenomena such as blepharospasm.[48]

**Toxicity.** Prolonged excessive intake of iodine leads eventually to iodide-goiter and myxedema, especially in patients with preexisting Hashimoto's thyroiditis.

## Iron

**Deficiency.** Deficiency of iron, in common with that of other hematopoietic agents, has its major impact on many systems through the reduction in tissue oxygenation consequent upon decreased hemoglobin concentration. The clinical picture depends upon the rapidity of the development of anemia.

After acute blood loss the symptomatology relates primarily to volume depletion. The typical syndrome of shock ensues, with collapse, dyspnea, tachycardia, thready pulse, hypotension, and marked vasoconstriction resulting in cold extremities with sweating.

Anemia of insidious onset manifests as increasing fatigue and slight pallor, best seen in the mucous membranes. Later, cardiorespiratory signs and symptoms include exertional dyspnea, tachycardia, palpitations, angina, claudication, night cramps, increased arterial and capillary pulsation, cardiac bruits, reversible cardiac enlargement and, if cardiac failure occurs, basal crepitations, peripheral edema, and ascites. Neuromuscular involvement is evidenced by headache, tinnitus, vertigo, cramps, faintness, increased cold sensitivity, and retinal hemorrhage. Gastrointestinal symptoms include anorexia, nausea, constipation, and diarrhea. Low-grade fever, menstrual irregularities, urinary frequency, and loss of libido may occur.

Iron deficiency per se has certain characteristics not usually associated with other forms of anemia. A nonspecific glossitis with almost complete loss of filiform papillae is common. Angular stomatitis is less frequent. Spoon-shaped nails, koilonychia, are characteristic of long-standing iron deficiency. The Paterson-Kelly (Plummer-Vinson) syndrome is the association of iron deficiency anemia, glossitis, dysphagia, and achlorhydria, usually seen in middle-aged women, but more rarely than formerly. In severe cases, postcricoid webs and malignant change in this region may occur. Signs of deficiency of other B group vitamins are often also present. Pica (geophagia) is an occasional feature of iron deficiency. Even mild degrees of iron deficiency are considered to be an important factor in decreased work efficiency.[49]

**Toxicity.** Acute vomiting, upper abdominal pain, pallor, cyanosis, diarrhea, drowsiness, and shock occur.

**Chronic Toxicity (Hemochromatosis).** Chronic iron overload affects many tissues. Diabetes, often the presenting manifestation, eventually develops in about 80% of patients. The skin has a characteristic slate-grey coloration. The liver becomes enlarged and then cirrhotic, and hepatoma may develop. Cardiomyopathy leads to heart failure in about 15% of patients and is a common cause of death in younger people. Arthropathy develops in about 50%. Pituitary failure may cause testicular atrophy and loss of libido. Focal hemosiderosis damages the lungs and kidneys.

## Copper

**Deficiency.** Although uncommon, copper deficiency may develop in young children who are malnourished or fed an exclusively milk diet. Anemia is the most common sign, but bone lesions have also been reported. A newborn maintained on total parenteral nutrition developed severe copper deficiency.[50] There was anemia, depigmentation of the skin and hair, and distended blood vessels due to changes in the elastin of the vessel walls. Hypotonia and psychomotor retardation were present. The long bones showed osteoporosis, cupping, flaring and fractures of the metaphyses, deposition of periosteal new bone, and calcifications of soft tissues (Fig. 41–5).

Menkes' kinky-hair syndrome (see Chap. 9) presents with a typical swollen appearance of the face and sparse and brittle grey hair. Growth is retarded, and developmental regression begins within a few months of birth. Muscle hypotonus and seizures are common. Arterial lesions and scurvy-like bone changes may be present.

**Toxicity.** In Wilson's disease (hepatolenticular degeneration) accumulation of copper in the liver leads to cirrhosis and signs of liver failure. Deposits in the brain result in tremors, choreathetoid movements, rigidity, dysarthria, and eventually dementia. Anemia and signs of renal failure are common. Characteristic changes in the eye are the Kayser-Fleischer ring, a brown or green ring near the limbus of the cornea, and a "sunflower" cataract.

Indian childhood cirrhosis is a common condition on the Indian subcontinent and has been reported in Indian children elsewhere.[51] It has been attributed to copper accumulation in the liver probably as the result of feeding animal milk contaminated by boiling and storing in brass and copper pots.[51a]

## Zinc

**Deficiency.** In Iran a syndrome of dwarfism, hypogonadism, anemia, hepatosplenomegaly, rough dry skin, and lethargy associated with geophagia has been reported.[52] A similar syndrome associated with parasitism occurs in Egypt.[53] Hy-

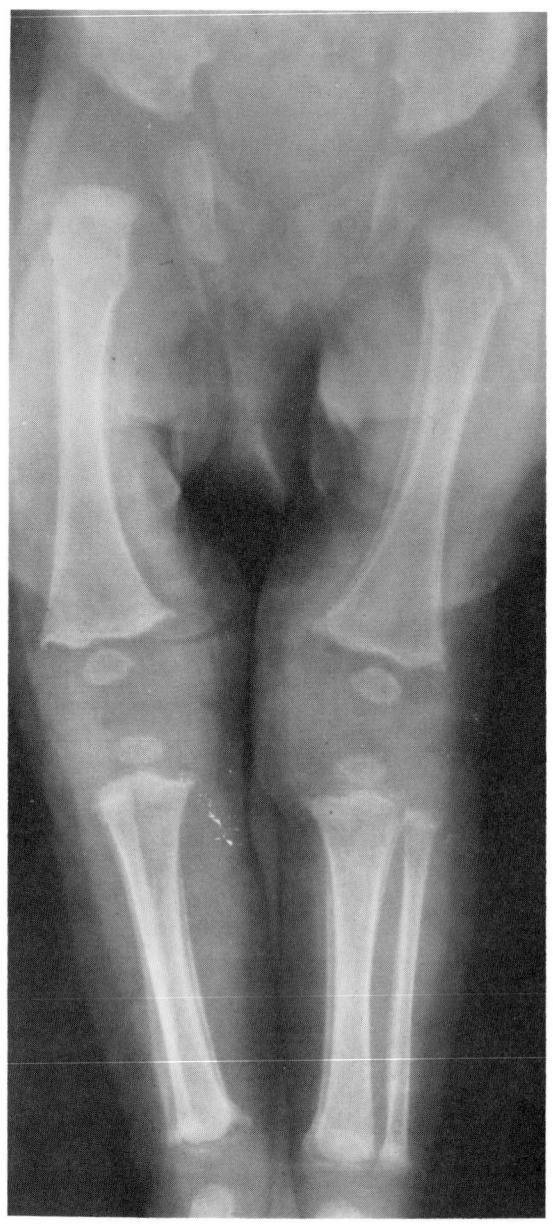

**Fig. 41–5.** Bone changes due to copper deficiency. (From Bennani-Smires, C., Medina J., Young, L.W.: Am. J. Dis. Child. *134*:1155, 1980.)

pogeusia (diminished taste) and growth retardation in children of immigrant families to parts of the United States have responded to zinc supplementation.[54] Some cases of night blindness and impaired dark adaptation, secondary to liver disease,[55] malabsorption,[56] and sickle cell anemia[57] have responded to zinc therapy. Taste abnormalities and gonadal dysfunction in uremic males receiving renal dialysis improved with zinc.[58] Wound healing is impaired. Hepatic encephalop-

athy has responded to zinc therapy.[58a] Total parenteral nutrition has on occasion been responsible for an acute deficiency syndrome, characterized by diarrhea, mental depression, alopecia, and dermatosis, usually around the orbits, nose, and mouth[59] (Plate I–G).

Acrodermatitis enteropathica, an inherited disorder manifest in artificially fed infants, caused by a defect in zinc absorption, is characterized by an extensive dermatitis, growth retardation, diarrhea, hair loss, and paronychia (see Chap. 9).

There is evidence that human maternal zinc deficiency may cause anencephaly in the offspring.[60]

**Toxicity.** Ingestion of the metal in large amounts, usually from an acid food or drink from a galvanized container, has caused vomiting and diarrhea. Metal fume fever is an industrial hazard caused by inhalation of zinc oxide fumes. A cause of neurologic damage, it is also called "brass-founders ague" or "zinc shakes."

### Fluorine (Fluoride)

**Deficiency.** Fluorine has not yet been proved to be an essential trace element for man, but areas with a low fluorine content of the water supply have high rates of dental caries. Fluoridation of the water has been associated with a significant fall in dental caries rates.

**Toxicity.** Fluorosis of the teeth is associated with high levels of fluoride in drinking water. It is most evident in permanent teeth that develop during high fluorine intake. Deciduous teeth are affected only at very high levels. The earliest changes, chalky white irregularly distributed patches on the surface of the enamel, become infiltrated by yellow or brown staining, giving rise to the characteristic "mottled" appearance (Plate I–H). Severe fluorosis weakens the enamel, resulting in surface pitting (Fig. 41–6).

Bone changes, consisting of deformity of the

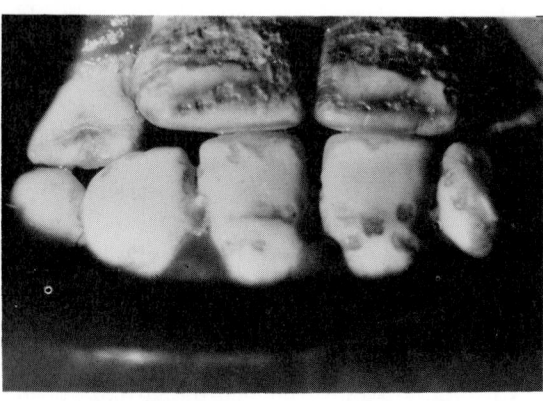

**Fig. 41–6.** Pitting of enamel in severe fluorosis.

spine and genu valgum, usually are seen only after prolonged high intake in adults.

## Selenium

**Deficiency.** Prominence has been given in recent years to a syndrome that is considered to be due primarily to selenium deficiency.[61] It has been named Keshan disease after the region in China where it is endemic. The symptomatology consists of a cardiomyopathy with a high mortality, affecting mainly children and women of childbearing age.

A number of studies have reported low selenium status in patients receiving long-term parenteral nutrition, but most of these individuals have been asymptomatic. Two fatal cases of cardiomyopathy developing under these circumstances have been reported in the United States.[62,63] One child had a cardiomyopathy that was regarded as responsive to selenium.[64] Another child also developed muscle pain and tenderness and white fingernail beds that responded to treatment with selenium.[65] Muscle tenderness and pain resolved in another case.[66]

**Toxicity.** Endemic selenosis, long recognized in animals, has been suspected in some human communities. The most convincing evidence has been reported from China.[67] The most frequently observed signs were loss of hair and nails. Skin lesions and polyneuritis were less certainly attributable to selenium toxicity. Alopecia and nail changes occurred in New York City from consumption of a "health store" supplement with excessive amounts of selenium.[67a]

## Chromium

**Deficiency.** A patient receiving total parenteral nutrition for more than 5 years unexpectedly developed 15% weight loss, a peripheral neuropathy, and glucose intolerance after 3½ years of nutritional support.[68] These conditions were all reversed with chromium therapy.

## Cobalt

There is little evidence for a role for cobalt in human nutrition other than as part of the vitamin $B_{12}$ molecule. One report claimed response of anemia to cobaltous chloride 1 g/day associated with geophagia in a 16-month-old girl living in an area of Wales, United Kingdom with cobalt-depleted soil.[69]

**Toxicity.** Cobalt has sometimes been recommended for the treatment of anemia of nephritis and infection in addition to the usual hemopoietic agents. In large doses it was reported to cause goiter, myxedema, and congestive heart failure in five patients.[70] A cardiomyopathy with a high mortality has been described after industrial exposure, during maintenance renal dialysis, and after drinking of beer contaminated during processing.[71]

## Molybdenum

**Deficiency.** A single case of nutritionally related depletion has been described. The tachycardia, tachypnea, headache, night blindness, nausea, vomiting, central scotomas, lethargy, disorientation and coma were reversed by molybdate therapy.[72] The abnormalities were similar to those described in a case of congenital deficiency of the molybdenum cofactor apoenzyme.[73]

## Manganese

One possible and unsubstantiated case of human deficiency has been reported to have occurred when manganese was inadvertently omitted from the vitamin K-deficient purified diet a patient was receiving as a volunteer. Clinical signs included weight loss, transient dermatitis, nausea and vomiting, changes in hair color, and slow growth of hair.[74]

**Toxicity.** This condition is usually limited to those who mine and refine ore. Prolonged exposure has caused neurologic changes resembling those of parkinsonism or Wilson's disease.

## Silicon

**Deficiency.** In rats and chickens, retarded growth and bone deformities have resulted, together with poorly characterized changes in cartilage and connective tissue. Deficiency in man has not yet been reported.

**Toxicity.** Therapy over many years with the antacid magnesium trisilicate has been reported to cause the formation of silicate urinary calculi.[75]

## REFERENCES

1. McLaren, D.S.: Nutritional Ophthalmology. New York, Academic Press, 1980.
2. Sommer, A.: Nutritional Blindness: Xerophthalmia and Keratomalacia. New York, Oxford University Press, 1982.
3. Sommer, A., Hussaini, G., Muhilal, et al.: Am. J. Clin. Nutr. *33*:887–891, 1980.
4. Sommer, A., Emran, N., Tamba, T.: Am. J. Ophthalmol. *87*:330–333, 1979.
5. Teng Khoen Hing: Ophthalmologica *137*:81–85, 1959.
6. International Vitamin A Consultative Group. The Symptoms and Signs of Vitamin A Deficiency and their Relationship to Applied Nutrition. Washington, D.C., IVACG, 1981.
7. Lammer, E.J., Chen, D.T., Hoar, R.M., et al.: N. Engl. J. Med. *313*:837–841, 1985.
8. Black, J.A., Bonham Carter, R.E.: Lancet *2*:745–749, 1963.
9. Melhorn, D.K., Gross, S.: J. Pediatr. *79*:569–580, 1971.

10. Melhorn, D.K., Gross, S.: J. Pediatr. *79*:581–588, 1971.
11. Foster, C.S.: Histopathology *3*:1–17, 1979.
12. Lloyd, J.K.: Disorders of lipid metabolism. *In* Textbook of Paediatric Nutrition. 2nd ed. (McLaren, D.S., Burman, D., Eds.) Edinburgh, Churchill Livingstone, 1982.
12a. Elias, E., Muller, D.P.R., Scott, J.: Lancet *2*:1319–1321, 1981.
13. Sokol, R.J., Heubi, J.E., Iannaconne, S.T., et al.: N. Engl. J. Med. *310*:1209–1212, 1984.
14. Howard, L., Oversen, L., Satya-Murti, S., et al.: Am. J. Clin. Nutr. *36*:1241–1249, 1982.
15. Hittner, H.M., Godic, L.B., Rudolph, A.J., et al.: N. Engl. J. Med. *305*:1365–1371, 1981.
16. Hittner, H.M., Speer, M.E., Rudolph, A.J., et al.: Pediatrics *73*:238–249, 1984.
16a. Johnson, L., Bowen, F.W., Jr., Abbasi, S., et al.: Pediatrics *75*:619–638, 1985.
16b. Lorch, V., Murphy, D., Hoersten, L.R., et al.: Pediatrics *75*:598–602, 1985.
17. Roberts, H.J.: J.A.M.A. *246*:129–131, 1981.
18. Kark, R., Lozner, E.L.: Lancet *2*:1162–1163, 1939.
19. Ryan, J.A., Jr.: *In* Total Parenteral Nutrition. (Fischer, E. Ed.) Boston, Little, Brown, and Co., 1976, pp 55–100.
19a. O'Connor, M.E., Livingstone, D.S., Hannah, J., et al.: Am. J. Dis. Child. *137*:601–602, 1983.
20. Corrigan, J.J., Marcus, F.I.: J.A.M.A. *230*:1300–1301, 1974.
21. McIntyre, N., Stanley, N.N.: Br. Med. J. *3*:567–569, 1971.
22. Jeffrey, F.E., Abelmann, W.H.: Am. J. Med. *50*:123–128, 1971.
23. Victor, M., Adams, R.D., Collins, G.H.: The Wernicke-Korsakoff Syndrome. Oxford, Blackwell, 1971.
24. Jelliffe, D.B.: Infant Nutrition in the Tropics and Subtropics. 2nd ed. Geneva, WHO, 1968.
25. Weintraub, L.R., Conrad, M.E., Crosby, W.H.: N. Engl. J. Med. *275*:169–176, 1966.
26. Coursin, D.B.: Vitam. Horm. *22*:756–786, 1964.
27. Schaumberg, H., Kaplan, J., Windebank, A., et al.: N. Engl. J. Med. *309*:445–448, 1983.
28. Rudman, D., Williams, P.J.: N. Engl. J. Med. *309*:488–489, 1983.
29. Bonjour, J.P.: Int. J. Vitam. Nutr. Res. *47*:107–118, 1977.
30. Mock, D.M., DeLorimer, A.A., Lieberman, W.M., et al.: N. Engl. J. Med. *304*:820–823, 1981.
31. Innis, S.M., Allardyce, D.B.: Am. J. Clin. Nutr. *37*:185–187, 1983.
31a. Johnson, P.R., Roloff, J.S.: J. Pediatr. *100*:917–919, 1982.
31b. Higginbottom, M.C., Sweetman, K., Nyhan, W.L.: N. Engl. J. Med. *299*:317–320, 1978.
32. Laurence, K.M., James, N., Miller, M.H., et al.: Br. Med. J. *282*:1509–1511, 1981.
33. Anonymous: Nutr. Rev. *41*:51–53, 1983.
33a. Mandel, H., Berant, M.: Arch. Dis. Child. *60*:971–972, 1985.
34. Worthley, L.I.G., Fishlock, R.C., Snoswell, A.M.: J. Parenter. Ent. Nutr. *7*:176–180, 1983.
35. Hodges, R.E., Hood, J., Canham, J.E., et al.: Am. J. Clin. Nutr. *24*:432–443, 1971.
36. Fleming, C.R., Smith, L.M., Hodges, R.E.: Am. J. Clin. Nutr. *29*:976–983, 1976.
37. Holman, R.T., Johnson, S.B., Hatch, T.F.: Am. J. Clin. Nutr. *35*:617–623, 1976.
38. Bozian, R.C., Moussavian, S.N.: Am. J. Clin. Nutr. *36*:1253–1254, 1982.
39. Holman, R.T., Johnson, S.B., Hatch, T.F.: Am. J. Clin. Nutr. *36*:1254–1255, 1982.
40. Pettifor, J.M., Ross, P., Wang, J., et al.: J. Pediatr. *92*:320–324, 1978.
41. Marie, P.J., Pettifor, J.M., Ross, F.P., et al.: N. Engl. J. Med. *307*:584–588, 1982.
42. Yu, J.S., Oates, R.K., Walsh, K.H., et al.: Arch. Dis. Child. *46*:257–263, 1971.
43. Altura, B.M., Altura, B.T., Carella, A.: Science *221*:376–378, 1983.
44. Coburn, J.W., Hartenbower, D.L., Kleeman, C.R.: Divalent ion metabolism. *In* The Year in Metabolism 1977. (Freinkel, N., Ed.) New York, Plenum Publishing Corp., 1978.
45. Knochel, J.P.: Arch. Intern. Med. *137*:203–220, 1977.
46. Bronner, P.: Am. J. Clin. Nutr. *29*:1307–1314, 1976.
47. Stanbury, J.B., Querido, A.: Policy and planning for endemic goiter control. *In* Nutrition in the Community. 2nd ed. (McLaren, D.S., Ed.) Chichester, Wiley, 1983.
48. Delange, F., Thilly, C., Pourbaix, P., et al.: Treatment of Idjwi island endemic goiter by iodized oil. *In* Edemic Goiter (Stanbury, J.B., Ed.) Washington, D.C., PAHO, 1969.
49. Andersen, H.T., Barkve, H.: Scand. J. Clin. Lab. Invest. *25*(Suppl):*114*:1–62, 1970.
50. Young, L.W.: Am. J. Dis. Child. *134*:1155–1156, 1980.
51. Portmann, B., Tanner, M.S., Mowat, A.P., et al.: Lancet *2*: 1338–1340, 1978.
51a. Tanner, M.S., Bhave, S.A., Kantarjian, A.H., et al.: Lancet *2*:992–995, 1983.
52. Prasad, A.S., Halsted, J.A., Nadimi, M.: Am. J. Med. *31*:532–546, 1961.
53. Prasad, A.S., Miale, A., Jr., Farid, Z., et al.: Arch. Intern. Med. *111*:407–428, 1963.
54. Hambidge, K.M., Hambidge, C., Jacobs, M., et al.: Pediatr. Res. *6*:868–874, 1972.
55. Morrison, S.A., Russell, R.N., Carney, E.A., et al.: Am. J. Clin. Nutr. *31*:276–281, 1978.
56. Morley, J.E., Russell, R.M., Reed, A., et al.: Am. J. Clin. Nutr. *34*:1489–1495, 1981.
57. Warth, J.A., Prasad, A.S., Zwas, F., et al.: J. Lab. Clin. Med. *98*:189–194, 1981.
58. Mahajan, S.K., Prasad, A.S., Briggs, W.A., et al.: Clin. Res. *28*(2):475A, 1980.
58a. Reding, P., Duchateau, J., Bataille, C.: Lancet *2*:493–495, 1984.
59. Younaszai, H.D.: J. Parenter. Ent. Nutr. *7*:72–74, 1983.
60. Cavdar, A.O., Arcasoy, A., Baycu, T.: Teratology *22*:141, 1980.
61. Chen, X., Yang, G., Chen, J., et al.: Biol. Tr. El. Res. *2*:91–107, 1980.
62. Johnson, R.A., Baker, S.S., Fallon, J.T., et al.: N. Engl. J. Med. *304*:1210–1212, 1981.
63. Fleming, C.R., Lie, J.T., McCall, J.T., et al.: Gastroenterology *83*:689–693, 1982.
64. Collipp, P.J., Chen, S.Y.: N. Engl. J. Med. *304*:1304–1305, 1981.
65. Kien, C.L., Ganther, H.E.: Am. J. Clin. Nutr. *37*:319–328, 1983.
66. van Rij, A.M., Thomson, C.D., McKenzie, J.M., et al.: Am. J. Clin. Nutr. *32*:2076–2085, 1979.
67. Yang, G., Wang, S., Zhou, R., et al.: Am. J. Clin. Nutr. *37*:872–881, 1983.

67a.Centers for Disease Control: Morb. Mort. Wkly. Rep. *33*:157–158, 1984.

68. Jeejeebhoy, K.N., Chu, R.C., Marliss, E.B., et al.: Am. J. Clin. Nutr. *30*:531–538, 1977.

69. Shuttleworth, V.S., Cameron, R.S., Alderman, G., et al.: Practitioner *186*:760–764, 1961.

70. Kriss, J.P., Carness, W.H., Gross, R.T.: JAMA *157*:117–121, 1955.

71. Sullivan, J.F., Egan, J.D., George, R.P., et al.: J. Lab. Clin. Med. *68*:1022–1023, 1966.

72. Abumrad, N.N., Schneider, A.J., Steel, D., et al.: Am. J. Clin. Nutr. *34*:2551–2559, 1981.

73. Johnson, J.L., Waud, W.R., Rajagopalan, K.U., et al.: Proc. Natl. Acad. Sci. *77*:3715–3719, 1980.

74. Doisy, E.A.: *In* Trace Substances in Environmental Health. VI. (Hemphill, D.D., Ed.) Minneapolis, University of Minnesota Press, 1972, pp. 193–199.

75. Levison, D.A., Banim, S., Crocker, P.R., et al.: Lancet *1*: 704–705, 1982.

## SELECTED READINGS

McLaren, D.S.: A Colour Atlas of Nutritional Disorders. London, Wolfe, 1981.

*Chapter* 42

# PROTEIN-ENERGY MALNUTRITION

## Benjamín Torún and Fernando E. Viteri

Protein-energy malnutrition (PEM) results when the body's needs for protein, energy fuels, or both cannot be satisfied by the diet. It includes a wide spectrum of clinical manifestations conditioned by the relative intensity of protein or energy deficit, the severity and duration of the deficiencies, the age of the host, the cause of the deficiency, and the association with other nutritional or infectious diseases. Its severity ranges from weight loss or growth retardation to distinct clinical syndromes, frequently associated with deficiencies of minerals and vitamins.

Dietary energy and protein deficiencies usually occur together, but sometimes one predominates and, if severe enough, may lead to the clinical syndrome of *kwashiorkor* (predominant protein deficiency) or *marasmus* (mainly energy deficiency). *Marasmic kwashiorkor* is a combination of chronic energy deficiency and chronic or acute protein deficit. It is difficult to recognize which deficit predominates in milder forms of the disease.

The origin of PEM can be primary, when it is the result of inadequate food intake, or secondary, when it is the result of other diseases that lead to low food ingestion, inadequate nutrient absorption or utilization, increased nutritional requirements, and/or increased nutrient losses. Its onset can be relatively fast, as in starvation due to abrupt withholding of food, or gradual. This chapter discusses primary PEM of a relatively chronic onset, where the metabolic alterations and clinical characteristics of protein and/or energy deficits predominate. PEM secondary to other diseases and the metabolic and clinical manifestations of starvation and of specific vitamin and mineral deficiencies are described in other chapters.

## HISTORICAL BACKGROUND

It has long been recognized that inadequate food intake produces weight loss and growth retardation and, when severe and prolonged, leads to body wasting and emaciation. It took much longer to understand the nature of the edematous forms of PEM, probably because they could be found among children who were not starving and in families in good socioeconomic position. Although the disease was possibly mentioned by Hippocrates[1], one of the earliest descriptions of edematous PEM, or of something resembling it, was written in Yucatan, Mexico by Patrón-Correa in 1908.[2] The disease was called "culebrilla" ("snake-like") because of the serpentine areas of skin hyper- and hypopigmentation. The dermatologic signs were further described with undue attention in later publications from Asia,[3,4] Africa,[5,6] and tropical America,[7,8] leading to the initial beliefs that the disease was caused by tropical parasites or a vitamin deficiency. The distinction of PEM from pellagra and other vitamin deficiencies and the absence of a causal relationship with parasites were suggested by various authors in the late 1920s and 1930s. The real nature of the disease received more attention, however, after Cicely Williams published in 1933 an extended note of a report she had written one year earlier in the Gold Coast.[9] In another publication, two years later, she referred to the disease by its local name, "kwashiorkor," used by the Ga tribe in the Gold Coast (now Ghana) for "the sickness the older child gets when the next baby is born."[10] This native term already suggested that the disease could be due to ignorance or inability to provide good foods to a child during the weaning period.

Several pediatricians who worked in tropical countries described various aspects of the disease in the 1930s and showed that it could be cured by feeding milk or other high-protein food, sometimes in combination with blood transfusions.[11,12] In the 1940s researchers showed that the concentration of serum proteins was low in most patients. Thus, the association of the disease with dietary protein intake became increasingly more evident. Hegsted and co-workers pointed out that the quality of dietary proteins could also affect serum protein concentration.[13] Nevertheless, it was not until the 1950s that the nature and importance of this disease gained worldwide recognition, partly owing to publications such as those of Brock and Autret,[14] Autret and Béhar,[11] and Trowell, Davies, and Dean.[12] By then, more than 40 names had been given to this clinical syndrome.[12] Some of them, such as "síndrome policarencial de la infancia" (infantile pluricarential syndrome), indicated that young children were mainly affected and that a deficit of various nutrients was involved. Others, such as "Mehlnahrschaden" ("damage by cereal flours"), "starch edema," and "sugar babies" indicated that it was caused by the intake of foods with high carbohydrate and low protein contents. Today, the more comprehensive term of "protein-energy (or protein-calorie) malnutrition"[15] is universally accepted, and its severe forms are most often called "marasmus," "kwashiorkor," and "marasmic kwashiorkor." The term "malnutrition" is usually used in lay language for PEM.

Studies done in the last 25 years have shown that marasmus and kwashiorkor have distinct metabolic features, that some manifestations, such as anemia and reduced physical activity, are due to adaptive mechanisms, that the immune response of severely malnourished patients is impaired, and that physical and emotional stimulation are important elements in treating malnourished children. These findings are the basis of current therapeutic measures.

## ETIOLOGY AND EPIDEMIOLOGY

Protein-energy malnutrition is the most important nutritional disease in the developing countries because of its high prevalence and its relationship with child mortality rates, impaired physical growth, and inadequate social and economic development. Associated deleterious effects on mental growth and maturation have been demonstrated in experimental animals and they seem to occur in humans, but it has not been possible to disassociate completely the nutritional factors from other environmental conditions, nor to ascertain the irreversibility of the nutritional mental damage. PEM occurs more frequently when infections impose additional demands or induce greater losses of nutrients and when living conditions demand greater energy expenditure, as in heavy physical work.

### Magnitude of the Problem

The global magnitude of PEM is difficult to estimate with precision because mild and moderate malnutrition usually is not recorded, and many patients with kwashiorkor or marasmus do not receive medical attention. Rough estimates made by the United Nations' Food and Agriculture Organization[16] and the World Bank,[17] based on the chronic consumption of food in amounts that provide less than the minimum energy to lead a sedentary life (i.e., 1.2 times basal energy expenditure), indicate that between 800 million and one billion persons have some degree of PEM. This may be a conservative estimate, as an energy intake of 1.2 times basal expenditure will still limit the functional performance and optimal development of most growing children and of adults with energy-intensive life-styles.[18–20]

As PEM mainly affects infants and preschool children, another estimate of its magnitude is based on considering it the main cause of growth retardation. The World Health Organization estimates that around 300 million children have growth retardation related to malnutrition.[21] If one uses weight deficit for a given age as indicator of present or past growth impairment, in many developing countries 20 to 75% of all children under 5 years of age have suffered from PEM.[22] An analysis of 25 different surveys in Asia, Africa, and Latin America indicated that about 3% (range: 0.5 to 20%) had severe PEM and about 20% (range: 4 to 46%) had a moderate form of the disease.[22] These figures increase markedly during severe food shortages, as in wars or droughts.

Most malnourished persons live in developing countries, about 30% each in Africa and the Far East, and 15% each in Latin America and the Near East.[16] The current differences between countries with different degrees of development will probably become wider, as projections for food demands in 1985, compared with 1970, show increases of 26% for developed countries and 75% for developing countries.[23] The situation is even more serious for the latter, since the distribution of food is usually unequal between more and less affluent groups in those societies.

## Causes of PEM

Primary PEM results from insufficient food intake or from the ingestion of foods with proteins of poor nutritional quality. These inadequate intakes are almost always linked to conditions such as poverty, ignorance, infectious diseases, and low food availability. Therefore, social, economic, biologic, and environmental factors must be considered as underlying causes of PEM.

**Social and Economic Factors.** Poverty almost always accompanies PEM. As its consequence there is low food availability for lack of means to produce or buy foods, overcrowded and unsanitary living conditions, and improper child care.

Ignorance, by itself or associated with poverty, is a frequent cause of PEM in some families or societies, leading to poor infant- and child-rearing practices, misconceptions about the use of certain foods, inadequate feeding conducts during illnesses, and improper food distribution within the family members.[24,25] A decline in the practice and duration of breastfeeding, combined with inadequate weaning practices when breast milk is withdrawn or when it can no longer provide sufficient dietary energy and protein to the infant, is associated with growing rates of infantile PEM.

Social problems such as child abuse, maternal deprivation, abandonment of the elderly, alcoholism, and drug addiction can result in PEM. Cultural and social practices that impose food taboos, some food and diet fads, particularly popular among adolescents and women,[26] and the migration from traditional rural settings to urban slums can also contribute to or precipitate the appearance of PEM.

**Biologic Factors.** Maternal malnutrition prior to and/or during pregnancy is more likely to produce an underweight newborn baby.[27] This intrauterine malnutrition can be compounded after birth by insufficient food to satisfy the infant's needs for catch-up growth, resulting in PEM.

Infectious diseases are major contributing and precipitating factors in PEM. Diarrheal disease, measles, and respiratory and other infections frequently result in negative protein and energy balance due to anorexia (reduced food intake), vomiting, decreased absorption (increased nutrient losses), and catabolic processes (increased requirements and metabolic losses).[28-32] Intestinal parasites apparently have little or no effect unless the infection is extensive or causes acute diarrhea.[33,34]

Diets with low concentrations of proteins and energy, as occur with overdiluted milk formulas or bulky vegetable foods that have low nutrient densities, can lead to PEM in young children whose gastric capacity does not allow the ingestion of large amounts of food. Foods with low protein quality (i.e., low contents of one or more essential amino acids) will be poorly utilized, and imbalanced diets can produce anorexia.[35] Moreover, foods poor in protein and rich in carbohydrates are particularly prone to produce kwashiorkor.

**Environmental Factors.** Overcrowded and/or unsanitary living conditions lead to frequent infections with deleterious nutritional consequences. This is an especially important cause of PEM among weanlings who develop severe or frequent episodes of diarrhea.[36]

Agricultural patterns, climatic conditions, and man-made catastrophes, such as wars and forced migrations, that lead to cyclic, sudden, or prolonged food scarcities can cause PEM among whole populations. Post-harvest losses of food due to bad storage conditions and inadequate food distribution systems contribute to PEM, even after periods of agricultural plenty.

## Age of the Host

PEM can affect all age groups but it is more frequent among infants, especially those born prematurely or weighing less than 2,500 g, and among preschool children. This is because dietary protein and energy requirements of young children are high per unit of body weight, they cannot obtain food by their own means and, when living under poor hygienic conditions, they frequently become ill with diarrhea and other infections.[37,38] Most infants from poor families in developing countries who are weaned prematurely from the breast or who are breast-fed for a prolonged time without adequate complementary feeding practices become malnourished for lack of adequate energy and protein intake. The chronic intake of insufficient food can result in marasmus, which is the most common form of severe PEM before one year of age. The edematous forms of the disease are more frequent after 18 months of age and typically occur in children who are fed diets consisting of starchy gruels, diluted cereal-based beverages, and vegetable foods that are rich in carbohydrates but almost devoid of proteins of good nutritional quality (i.e., lacking one or more essential amino acids). Children who consume large amounts of such diets can develop kwashiorkor. Most often, the severe protein deficit is associated with chronic dietary energy deficit and results in a combined form of marasmic kwashiorkor. The appearance of edema is frequently preceded or accompanied by acute diarrhea or other infectious disease.

Older children usually have milder forms of PEM because they can cope better with social and food availability constraints. Infections and other precipitating factors become less severe, and early survival may imply a natural selection of the more fit.

Pregnant and lactating women are also vulnerable to PEM because the increases in their nutritional requirements may not be accompanied by equivalent increments in food intake due to economic or cultural factors, nausea in early pregnancy, and gastric discomfort as pregnancy advances. Energy deficiency with or without proportional protein deficit predominates in this age group. However, the consequences of the dietary deficiencies usually have a greater impact on the growth, nutritional status, and survival rates of their fetuses, newborn babies, and infants.

The elderly who are unable to care properly for themselves due to physical or mental deterioration tend to suffer from PEM. Gastrointestinal alterations can be an important contributing factor. Their energy requirements fall as a consequence of reduced physical activity and reductions in maintenance energy metabolism, but their protein needs do not diminish at the same rate.[39] Consequently, protein deficiency may predominate in this age group.

Adolescents, men, and nonpregnant, nonlactating women usually have lowest prevalence and the mildest forms of the disease because of the greater opportunities to obtain food, and the cultural and social practices that protect the productive members of the family. Nevertheless, many weight-losing diets and food fads can predispose them to, or actually produce some degree of, PEM.

## PATHOPHYSIOLOGY AND ADAPTIVE RESPONSES

PEM develops gradually over many days or months. This process allows a series of metabolic and behavioral adjustments that result in decreased nutrient demands and a nutritional equilibrium compatible with a lower level of cellular nutrient availability. If the supply of nutrients becomes persistently lower than that to which the body can adapt, death supervenes. Metabolic equilibrium can also be disrupted during the progression of the disease or as a result of inadequate therapeutic measures. Therefore, the following characteristics of PEM must be considered:

1. PEM induces a metabolically dynamic, changing state to which the affected person adapts to survive in a compensated manner.
2. The cost of this adaptation includes functional limitations and decreased interactions with the physical and social environment.
3. Harmonic changes in the metabolism of proteins, energy, and other nutrients allow a better adaptation to current nutritional conditions.
4. Metabolic adjustments are more stable when PEM develops slowly, as in chronic mild-moderate cases or in marasmus, than more acutely, as in kwashiorkor of rapid onset.
5. Severe protein and energy deficiencies and sudden additional metabolic stress, such as dehydration, overloading with dietary proteins or energy, and acute infections, can cause decompensation with functional derangement and even death.

### Energy Mobilization and Expenditure

A decrease in energy intake is quickly followed by a decrease in energy expenditure, accounting for shorter periods of play and physical activity in children[40–42] and for longer rest periods and less physical work in adults.[43] When the decrease in energy expenditure cannot compensate for the insufficient intake, body fat is mobilized with a decrease in adiposity and weight loss.[44] Lean body mass diminishes at a slower rate, mainly as a consequence of muscle protein catabolism with increased efflux of amino acids, primarily alanine, that contribute to the energy sources. As the cumulative energy deficit becomes more severe, subcutaneous fat is markedly reduced, and protein catabolism leads to muscular wasting. Visceral protein is preserved longer, especially in the marasmic patients.

In marasmus, these alterations in body composition lead initially to increased basal oxygen consumption (i.e., basal metabolic rate) per unit body weight, and it decreases in more sereve stages.[45,46] In kwashiorkor, the severe dietary protein deficit leads to an earlier visceral depletion of amino acids that affects visceral cell function and reduces oxygen consumption; therefore, basal energy expenditure decreases per unit of lean or total body mass.

Blood glucose concentration remains normal, mainly at the expense of gluconeogenic amino acids and fats, and it falls in severe PEM or when complicated by serious infections or fasting.

### Protein Breakdown and Synthesis

The poor availability of dietary amino acids decreases protein synthesis in viscera and muscles. This is followed by increased muscle protein catabolism resulting in modified composition of the free amino acid pool and increased amino acid availability for viscera. A marked recycling of amino acids and a reduction in urea synthesis and excretion occur. In the steady state, the amount of free amino acids entering the body pool from dietary and tissue proteins is equal to the amount leaving it. The latter is represented by the amino acids synthesized into body protein and the amount of amino acid nitrogen that is excreted. On a normal protein intake, 25% of the amino acids leaving the total body pool are excreted as nitrogenous compounds and 75% are recycled or reutilized for protein synthesis. This latter fraction may rise to 90 to 95% when protein intake is reduced.[47,48] Therefore, the adaptive change is not so much a reduction of total nitrogen or amino acid turnover, but an increase in the proportion turned over that is used for synthesis and a corresponding reduction in the proportion of nitrogen that is excreted.

At the intracellular level there are changes in the activity of enzymes involved in the adaptive adjustments of energy and protein metabolism.[49-52] Table 42–1 shows some of the changes observed in leukocytes, muscle, and liver cells. These enzymatic changes result in energy mobilization from reserve depots (mainly fat), and in the provision of amino acids by muscle cells and their optimal utilization by viscera. Consequently, the synthesis, catabolism, and breakdown of proteins and specific amino acids differ in the various tissues and organs.

The half-life of some proteins increases. The rate of albumin synthesis decreases, but after a time lag of a few days the rate of breakdown also falls.[53] In addition to its increased half-life, a shift of albumin from the extravascular to the intravascular pool assists in maintaining adequate levels of circulating albumin in the face of reduced synthesis. Muscle breakdown also supplies amino acids to the liver for the synthesis of albumin, lipoproteins, and other serum proteins. When the adaptive mechanisms fail, the concentration of serum proteins, and especially albumin, decreases. The ensuing reduction in intravascular oncotic pressure and outflow of water into the extravascular space contribute to the development of the edema of kwashiorkor.

These adaptations lead to the sparing of body protein and the preservation of essential protein-dependent functions. The gradual and inevitable loss of body protein as a result of long-term dietary protein deficit is primarily from skeletal muscle. Some visceral protein is lost in the early development of PEM but then becomes stable until the nonessential tissue proteins are depleted; the loss of visceral protein then increases, and death may be imminent unless nutritional therapy is successfully instituted.

### Endocrine Changes

Endocrine changes may not be wholly explained by the circulating levels of hormones, because their secretion rates and half-lives and the cellular responses to hormonal stimulation may also be altered in PEM.[54] There are contradicting reports concerning many endocrine functions in malnutrition, probably because of differences in analytical techniques, type and severity of PEM, and conditions and timing of the studies.[54-56] Table 42–2 summarizes the most consistent changes reported in severe PEM. The functional capacities of the hypothalamic-pituitary axis and adrenal medulla are preserved, thus allowing en-

**Table 42–1. Selected Enzyme Activity Changes in Protein-Energy Malnutrition\*†**

| Cells | Enzymes | Change in Activity |
|---|---|---|
| Muscle and leukocytes | aldolase | decrease |
| | dehydrogenases | decrease |
| | pyruvic kinase | decrease |
| | aminotransferases | increase |
| Liver | phenylalanine hydroxylase | decrease |
| | urea cycle enzymes | decrease |
| | valine aminotransferase | decrease |
| | amino acid activating enzymes | increase |

\*Changes favor energy mobilization, muscle protein breakdown, and liver protein synthesis.
†Adapted from Viteri, F.E.[58]

**Table 42–2. Summary of Selected Hormonal Changes and Their Main Metabolic Effects Usually Seen in Severe PEM**

| Hormone | Influenced in PEM by | Hormonal Activity in | | Metabolic Effects of Changes in PEM |
|---|---|---|---|---|
| | | Energy Deficit | Protein Deficit | |
| Insulin | Low food intake (↓ glucose) (↓ amino acids) | Decreased | Decreased | ↓ muscle protein synthesis ↓ lipogenesis ↓ growth |
| Growth hormone | Low protein intake (↓ amino acids) Reduced somatomedin synthesis | Normal or moderately increased | Increased | ↑ visceral protein synthesis ↓ urea synthesis ↑ lipolysis |
| Somatomedins | Low protein intake? | Variable | Decreased | ↓ muscle and cartilage protein synthesis ↓ collagen synthesis ↓ lipolysis ↓ growth ↑ production of growth hormone |
| Epinephrine | Stress of food deficiency, infections (↓ glucose) | Normal but can increase | Normal but can increase | ↑ lipolysis ↑ glycogenolysis inhibits insulin secretion |
| Glucocorticoids | Stress of hunger Fever (↓ glucose) | Increased | Normal or moderately increased | ↑ muscle protein catabolism ↑ visceral protein turnover ↑ lipolysis ↑ gluconeogenesis |
| Aldosterone | ↓ blood volume ↑ extracellular K ? ↓ serum Na ? | Normal | Increased | ↑ sodium retention and ↑ water retention contribute to appearance of edema |
| Thyroid hormones | ? | T4 normal or decreased; T3 decreased | T4 usually decreased; T3 decreased | ↓ glucose oxidation ↓ basal energy expenditure ↑ reverse T3 |
| Gonadotropins | Low protein intake? Low energy intake? | Decreased | Decreased | delayed menarche |

↓ = low or reduced    ↑ = high or increased

docrine and metabolic responses to stress conditions.[57]

Hormones play important roles in the adaptive processes of energy and protein metabolism in severe PEM.[58] These can be summarized as follows: (1) The decreased food intake tends to reduce plasma concentrations of glucose and free amino acids which, in turn, reduce insulin secretion and increase epinephrine release; the latter further reduces insulin secretion. (2) The low plasma amino acid levels, seen mainly in kwashiorkor, also stimulate the secretion of human growth hormone; the low plasma somatomedin activity, also seen mainly in kwashiorkor, contributes to the high circulating levels of growth hormone, due to the absence of the feedback inhibition postulated for somatomedins.[59,60] (3)The increased levels of growth hormone and epinephrine influence the reduction of urea synthesis, thereby favoring amino acid recycling.[48,61] (4) The stress induced by the low food intake and further amplified by fever, water, and electrolyte losses,

and other manifestations of the infections that frequently accompany PEM, also stimulates epinephrine release and corticosteroid secretion, more so in marasmus than in kwashiorkor, probably because of the greater severity in energy deficit that characterizes marasmus.[62,63] (5) Resistance to the peripheral action of insulin increases,[64] probably due to the increase in plasma free fatty acid concentration resulting from the lipolytic activity of growth hormone, glucocorticoids, and epinephrine. (6) The plasma concentrations of $T_3$ and $T_4$ decrease, by mechanisms that are not clearly defined. The iodination of tyrosine and monodeiodination of $T_4$ are probably involved, as the reduction of $T_3$ (3,5,3'-triiodothyronine) is accompanied by an increase in the circulating levels of the metabolically inactive reverse-$T_3$ (3,5,5'-triiodothyronine).[65] (7) The secretion of hormones involved in nonvital, growth-related functions, such as gonadotropins, decreases.[66]

All these changes, illustrated in Figure 42–1,

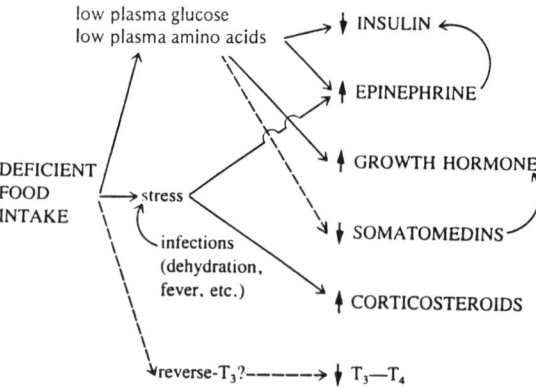

**Fig. 42–1.** Endocrine adaptive functions in severe PEM related to energy and protein metabolism. (From Torun, B., Viteri, F.E.,[149] with permission of McGraw Hill Book Co.)

contribute to the maintenance of energy homeostasis through increased glycolysis and lipolysis; increased amino acid mobilization; decreased storage of glycogen, fats and proteins; and decreased energy expenditure. Amino acids are spared for the synthesis of proteins that are essential for survival through preservation of visceral protein, growth retardation, and enhanced breakdown of muscle protein. The latter increases the availability and turnover of amino acids in viscera, particularly liver. In addition to being energy fuels and producing ketone bodies that can be used by the brain as energy sources, the increase in circulating fatty acids also reduces the peripheral actions of insulin.

## Hematology and Oxygen Transport

The reduction in hemoglobin concentration and red cell mass that almost always accompanies severe PEM is an adaptive phenomenon related to tissue oxygen needs.[46,67] Figure 42–2 illustrates the proposed responses. The reduction in lean body mass and the lower physical activity of malnourished patients lead to lower oxygen demands. The simultaneous decrease in dietary availability of amino acids results in reduced hematopoietic activity, which spares amino acids for synthesis of other more necessary body proteins. As long as the tissue's needs for oxygen are satisfied by the existing capacity for oxygen transport, this should be considered an adaptive response and not a "functional" anemia (i.e., with tissue hypoxia). When the tissue synthesis, lean body mass, and physical activity begin improving with dietary treatment, there is a rise in oxygen demands calling for accelerated hematopoiesis. If iron, folic acid, and vitamin $B_{12}$ are not available in sufficient

amounts, functional anemia with tissue hypoxia will develop.

Figure 42–3 shows that the administration of hematinics to a severely malnourished patient will not induce a hematopoietic response until dietary treatment produces an increase in lean body mass. Figure 42–4 shows that the reticulocyte response is related to the amount of protein intake when erythropoetic substances are not limiting.[58]

The severely malnourished patient may have relatively high body iron stores[68] and retains the ability to produce erythropoietin and reticulocytes in response to acute hypoxia. Nevertheless, these patients are prone to develop functional, severe anemia if there is a superimposed dietary iron or folic acid deficiency, or a chronic blood loss, as in hookworm infection.

## Other Physiologic and Metabolic Changes

Not all pathophysiologic changes lead to advantageous adjustments. Certain functions are affected and some nutrient reserves decrease, making the malnourished individual more susceptible to injuries that a well-nourished individual can withstand with little repercussion.

**Cardiovascular and Renal Functions.** Cardiac work decreases, as does functional reserve, and central circulation takes precedence over peripheral circulation.[69–71] Cardiovascular reflexes are altered, leading to postural hypotension and diminished venous return. In severe PEM, peripheral circulatory failure comparable to hypovolemic shock may occur. Hemodynamic compensation occurs primarily from tachycardia rather than from increased stroke volume. Renal plasma flow and glomerular filtration rates may be reduced as a consequence of the decreased cardiac output, but water clearance and the ability to concentrate and acidify urine appear unimpaired.[72–74]

**The Immune System.** The major defects seen in severe PEM seem to involve T-lymphocytes and the complement system.[75,76] A marked depletion of lymphocytes from the thymus and atrophy of the gland occur. In addition, cells from the T-lymphocyte regions of the spleen and lymph nodes are depleted, probably owing to decreases in thymic factors.[77,78] The production of several complement components, the functional activity of the complement system assessed by both the classic and alternative pathways, and the opsonic activity of serum are depressed in severe PEM.[76,79] These deficiencies may explain the high susceptibility of severely malnourished patients to gram-negative bacterial sepsis. Phagocytosis, chemo-

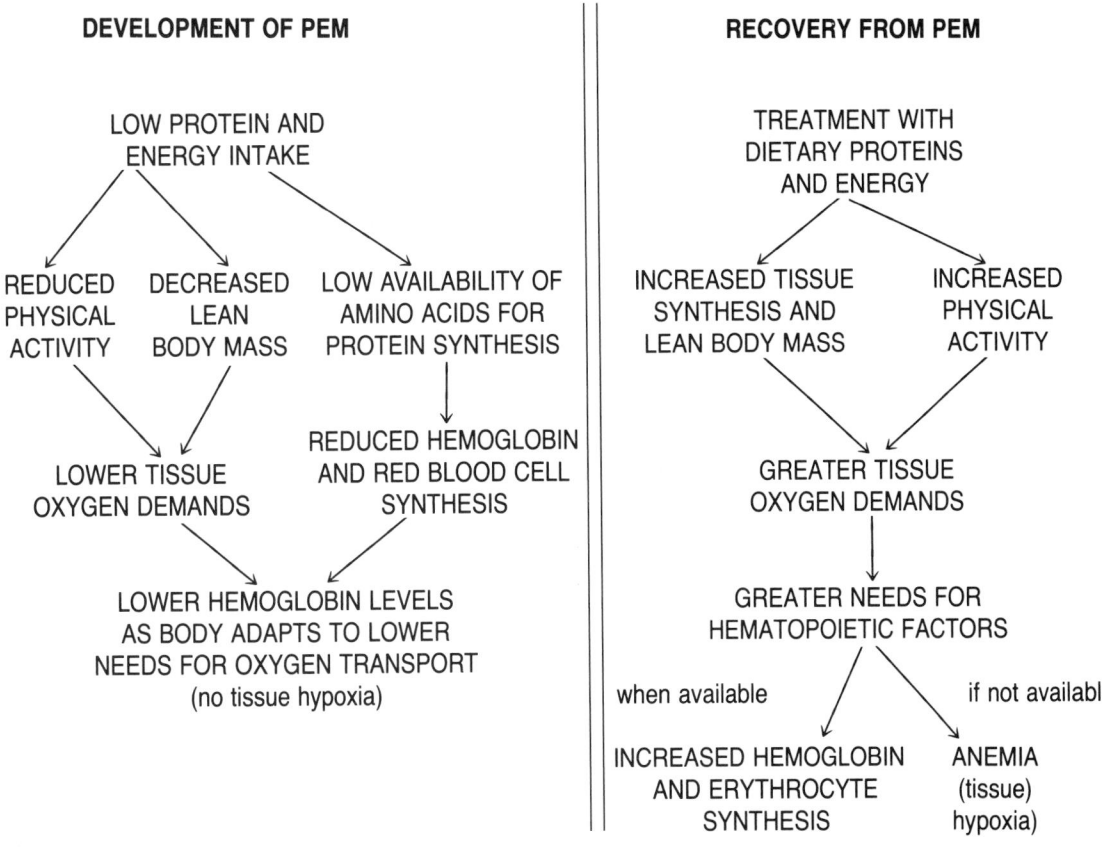

**Fig. 42–2.** Proposed hematologic responses in protein-energy malnutrition and during its treatment.

taxis, and intracellular killing are also impaired, partly due to the defects in opsonic and complement functional activities. The B-lymphocyte areas of spleen and lymph nodes and the circulating levels of B cells and immunoglobulins are relatively normal, but there may be defects in antibody production, such as secretory IgA.

The overall consequences of all these alterations in severe PEM are a greater predisposition to infections and to severe complications of otherwise less important infectious diseases. The defects in immune functions disappear with nutritional rehabilitation, except perhaps when they are due to intrauterine malnutrition.[80]

**Potassium and Sodium.** Total body potassium decreases in PEM because of the reduction in muscle proteins and loss of intracellular potassium. The low insulin action and diminished intracellular energy substrates reduce the availability of ATP and phosphocreatine.[81] This process probably alters the cellular exchange of sodium and potassium, leading to potassium loss and increased intracellular sodium.[82] Water accompanies the sodium influx, and although total body intracellular water is decreased because of losses

in lean body mass, there may be intracellular overhydration. These alterations in cell electrolytes and energy sources may explain, at least in part, the increased fatigability and reduced strength of skeletal muscle.[83]

**Gastrointestinal Functions.** Impaired intestinal absorption of lipids and disaccharides and a decreased rate of glucose absorption occur in severe protein deficiency. The greater the protein deficit, the greater the functional impairment. A decrease in gastric, pancreatic, and bile production is also observed, with normal to low enzyme and conjugated bile acid concentrations.[84–86] These alterations further impair the absorptive functions. Nevertheless, the ingestion of nutrients in high, therapeutic amounts usually allows for their uptake in sufficient quantity to permit nutritional recovery.[87] Malnourished persons, however, are prone to have diarrhea because of these alterations and possibly also because of irregular intestinal motility and gastrointestinal bacterial overgrowth. Diarrhea aggravates the malabsorption and can further impair nutritional status. Malabsorption disappears with nutritional recovery, unless there is an underlying food or nutrient intolerance unrelated to primary PEM.

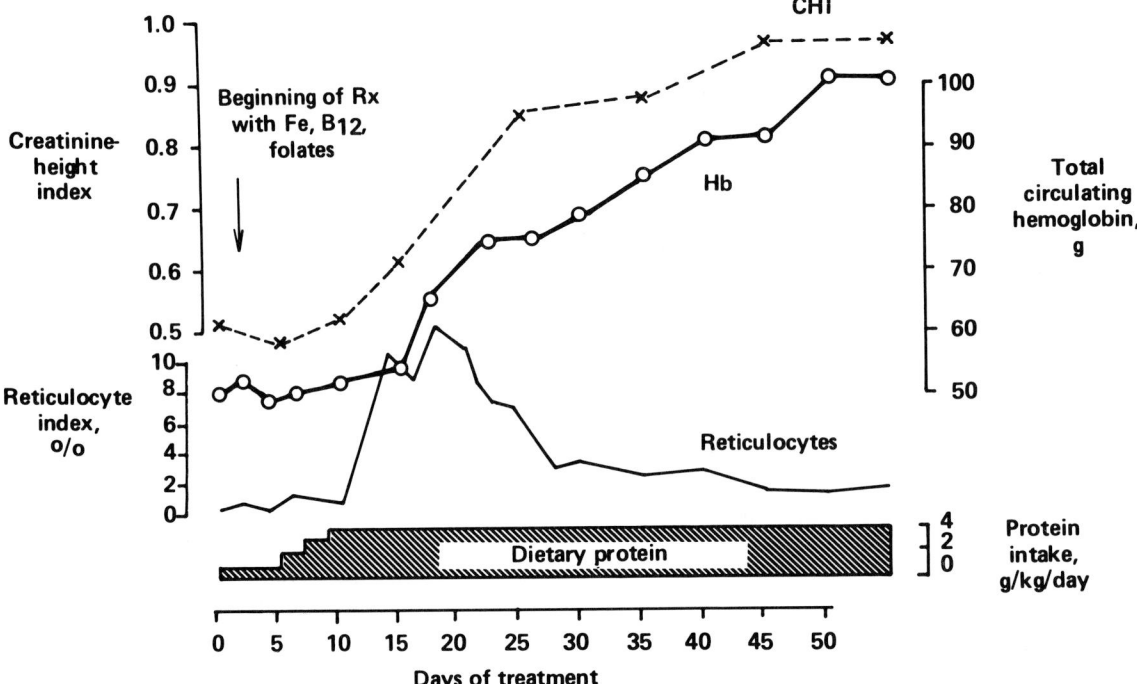

**Fig. 42–3.** Hematologic response of a child with severe protein-energy malnutrition. Treatment with iron, folic acid, and vitamin $B_{12}$ began on day 2; dietary energy and proteins were increased gradually to 150 kcal and 4 g protein/kg/day on day 9. There was no reticulocyte or hemoglobin response until lean body mass, assessed by the creatinine-height index, began increasing.

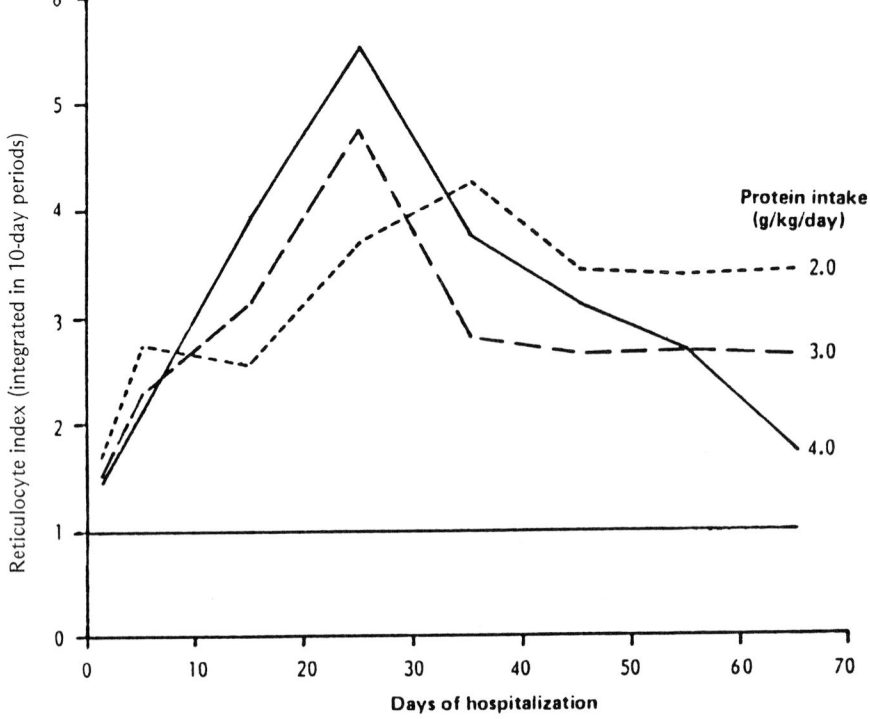

**Fig. 42–4.** Reticulocyte response of children treated for severe PEM with different amounts of dietary proteins, and adequate amounts of dietary energy and hematinics. (From Viteri, F.E.,[58] with permission of Raven Press.)

**Central and Peripheral Nervous System.** Individuals with severe PEM may have decreased brain growth, nerve myelination, neurotransmitter production, and velocity of nervous conduction, although the long-term functional implications of these alterations have not been clearly demonstrated. Neither have their causes and mechanisms been fully elucidated. The explanations proposed include reduced number of nervous cells when PEM occurs in utero or before six months of age, small cell size when it occurs at a later age, alterations in brain catecholamine production, defects in lipid metabolism, and decreased content of potassium in the brain.[88-93]

## METABOLIC FACTORS LEADING TO MARASMUS AND KWASHIORKOR

The concept that marasmus or kwashiorkor is the end result of either severe energy or protein deficiency[94,95] is too simplistic.[58,96] Other factors such as overloading a severely malnourished person with carbohydrates, or metabolic changes induced by infections, may cause or contribute to the appearance of kwashiorkor with its characteristic edema, hypoalbuminemia, and enlarged fatty liver. Some investigators have postulated that the evolution of PEM into either kwashiorkor or marasmus may be partly related to differences in adrenocortical response, whereby a greater response preserves visceral proteins more efficiently and leads to the better-adapted syndrome of marasmus.[97,98] Most probably, both endogenous and exogenous factors play a role in the development of marasmic or edematous PEM.[58,99,100] This might explain, at least in part, the fact that marasmus, kwashiorkor, and marasmic-kwashiorkor predominate in different parts of the world.

When there is a severe lack of food, endocrine adjustments mobilize fatty acids from adipose tissue and amino acids from muscle tissue, plasma protein concentration remains normal, and hepatic gluconeogenesis is enhanced.[101] An increase in carbohydrate intake when protein intake is very low can produce a breakdown of those adjustments, as follows: (1) Carbohydrate intake induces insulin release and a reduction in the production of epinephrine and cortisol.[102,103] (2) Lipolysis decreases and the action of insulin is enhanced due to the suppression of the inhibitory effects of free fatty acids on the peripheral action of insulin.[104] (3) Muscle protein breakdown is reduced and the body pool of free amino acids decreases. The decreased supply of muscle amino acids to the other organs results in less visceral protein synthesis.[105-107] (4) The decreased synthesis of plasma proteins in the liver, particularly albumin, reduces intravascular oncotic pressure. Plasma

water decreases and accumulates in extravascular tissues, tissue pressure rises, and cardiac output diminishes. As a consequence, perfusion pressure in the kidney is reduced with a fall in glomerular filtration, a rise in sodium retention, and juxtaglomerular ischemia. The latter results in more renin production, increased aldosterone, and further enhancement of sodium and water retention.[108-110] The ensuing dilution of plasma proteins further reduces oncotic pressure, more water goes into the extravascular space, and clinical edema appears or increases. (5) Increased hepatic fatty acid synthesis from the excess carbohydrate, impaired lipolysis, and reduced production of apo-beta-lipoproteins for lipid transport lead to fatty infiltration of the liver and hepatomegaly.

Infections in undernourished children also can precipitate the onset of kwashiorkor. The process by which this occurs has not been satisfactorily explained, but the following mechanisms may be involved: (1) Infections might divert the meager amino acid pool to the production of globulins and acute phase reactant proteins (AP), instead of albumin and transport proteins.[111-113] (2) The increase of APs that are proteinase inhibitors, such as alpha-1-antitrypsin and alpha-1-antichymotrypsin, may impair muscle protein breakdown.[114] (3) An impaired production and utilization of ketone bodies for energy during infections might lead to the use of more amino acids for gluconeogenesis.[115] (4) Protein catabolism and nitrogen losses are enhanced by many viral and febrile infections, probably through increased epinephrine and cortisol actions.[116,117] Regardless of the mechanisms involved, protein losses during severe infections can amount to as much as 2% of muscle protein per day.[118]

### Disruption of Adaptation

When the supply for tissue and cell energy can no longer be maintained by patients with severe energy deficiency, a serious decompensation occurs with hypoglycemia, hypothermia, impaired circulatory and renal functions, acidosis, coma, and death. These events can occur within a period of a few hours. Metabolic decompensation due to severe protein deficiency, in addition to the changes discussed in the onset of kwashiorkor, may include hemorrhagic diathesis and jaundice due to failure by the liver to synthesize several clotting factors and transport proteins; various degrees of renal failure with acidosis, and water and sodium retention; decreased cardiac work, pulmonary congestion, and increased susceptibility to pulmonary infections; coma, and death.

A high-carbohydrate, low-protein diet is not the only iatrogenic cause of serious metabolic disruption in patients who have or are prone to develop edematous PEM. The abrupt administration of too much protein to patients with edematous PEM can also have serious, life-threatening consequences. When such patients have been eating minute amounts of protein or none at all, and they are suddenly fed large amounts of proteins or given large transfusions of plasma or blood, they may experience a rapid increase in intravascular protein concentration and entry of extracellular fluid into the vascular compartment leading to cardiovascular insufficiency and pulmonary edema. In fact, a premature introduction of high-energy or high-protein diet to a severely malnourished patient may be fatal.[119,120]

## DIAGNOSIS

The clinical, biochemical, and physiologic characteristics of PEM vary according to the severity of the disease, the patient's age, the presence of other nutritional deficits and infections, and the predominance of energy or protein deficiency.

### Classification of PEM

The classifications shown in Table 42–3 are important for the diagnosis and treatment of PEM, and for the application and evaluation of public health measures. Intensity is determined mainly by anthropometry, since other clinical findings and biochemical indexes usually do not show changes unless the disease is well advanced. More accurate measurements, such as assessment of body composition, are not practical or feasible in most of the settings where PEM occurs, and the so-called functional indicators[121] are not as yet well standardized or may be too complex to measure routinely.

Classification of the disease as acute, chronic, or acute with a chronic background is also done by anthropometry to assess current nutritional status and degree of growth retardation in children. Dietary history is useful, especially in adults, as are dietary surveys in population groups. The relative contributions of dietary protein and energy deficits in the mild and moderate forms of PEM are assessed mainly by the individual's dietary

history or the population's dietary habits and food availability. Clinical characteristics and biochemical data confirm the diagnosis in severe PEM.

**Anthropometric Measurements.** The choice of anthropometric measurements depends on their simplicity, accuracy, and sensitivity; on the availability of measuring instruments; and on the existence of reference standards for comparison.

In order to allow international comparisons, it is sensible to use the same standard of reference for various populations. International or universal standards based on reliable anthropometric data can be used because: (1) Most children have similar growth potentials, regardless of ethnic background.[122,123] (2) The relationship of various anthropometric measurements, especially weight and height, is relatively constant in normal, healthy individuals of all age groups.[20] (3) The reference standards are merely for purposes of comparison and do not necessarily represent an ideal or a target. (4) The interpretation of the comparison (i.e., the values that separate "normal" from "deficient" and further divide the latter into "mild," "moderate," and "severe" forms) is a matter of judgment that comes into play when deciding whether the expected normal value for a given population should be 100%, 90%, or other proportion of the standard. Setting different cut-off points relative to a single standard is more practical than constructing local standards which, in a country with heterogeneous population groups, may pose the same problem as a "foreign" commonly used reference. At present, the World Health Organization recommends the data from the United States National Center for Health Statistics (NCHS)[124] as reference for weight and height.

The best anthropometric assessment of nutritional status and PEM is based on measurements of weight and height or length, and records of age, to calculate two indexes: *weight for height*, as an index of current nutritional status, and *height for age*, as an index of past nutritional history. Deficient height for age may represent a short period of growth failure at an early age or a longer period at a later age. Waterlow suggested the terms *wasting* for a deficit in weight for height, and *stunting* for a deficit in height for age.[125] Patients may then fall into four categories: (1) normal, (2) wasted but not stunted (suffering from acute PEM), (3) wasted and stunted (suffering from acute and chronic PEM), and (4) stunted but not wasted (past PEM with present adequate nutrition, or "nutritional dwarfs"). The intensity of wasting and stunting can be graded by calculating weight as percentage of the reference median weight for height, and

**Table 42–3. Classification of PEM According to Intensity of Disease, its Duration, and Predominant Nutrient Deficiency**

| Intensity | Duration | Main Deficit |
|-----------|----------|--------------|
| Mild | Acute | Energy |
| Moderate | Chronic | Protein |
| Severe | Both | Both |

height as percentage of the reference median height for age, as follows:

$$\frac{\text{\% wt for ht}}{\text{(or ht for age)}} = \frac{\text{observed weight (or height)}}{\text{reference wt for patient's ht}} \times 100$$
$$\text{(or reference ht for}$$
$$\text{patient's age)}$$

The grading shown in Table 42–4 is suggested for most countries, although some might find it convenient to use different cut-off points for specific groups. For example, the normal height for age in populations that are genetically short could be less than 95% of the reference. Some authors advocate the use of centiles or standard deviations from the mean, instead of percent deviations from the median. Although there may be a statistical advantage for the former, percent deviations are easier to understand by the general public, and to calculate by field workers. Color-coded charts and graphs have been devised to simplify the measurements and their interpretation.[126–128]

For adolescents and adults, weight for height alone is usually used to assess nutritional status, and the use of the *body mass index* (or Quetelet's index), weight/height$^2$, has been advocated as being independent of the person's height.[20]

The Gomez classification has probably been the most widely used index for children.[129] It classifies PEM into three grades based on *weight for age:* grade I = 90 to 75% of reference; grade II = 74 to 60%; grade III = less than 60% The use of this index does not differentiate between a truly underweight child (current PEM) and one who is short in stature but well proportioned in weight (past PEM); furthermore, the information about chronologic age is not always reliable. However, it is useful in public health and epidemiologic studies, as it indicates the proportion of children in a population group who at some time in their lives had malnutrition.

Other anthropometric indexes have been used, such as the developmental quotient for weight or height (weight-age or height-age divided by the chronologic age),[130] mid-arm circumference in absolute terms[131] or relative to height (QUAC-stick)[132] or weight, and ratio of arm circumference to head circumference.[133]

## Mild and Moderate PEM

The main clinical feature of mild and moderate PEM is weight loss. A decrease in subcutaneous adipose tissue may become apparent. When PEM is chronic, children show growth retardation in terms of weight (wasting) and height (stunting). Groups of populations in whom PEM is highly prevalent or "endemic" show slow weight gains, as illustrated in Figure 42–5.

Physical activity and energy expenditure of children decrease.[40–42] Other functional indicators of immunocompetence, gastrointestinal functions, and behavior may be altered, but their assessment is not yet practical for diagnostic purpose.[19,46,58,76,121] Nonspecific manifestations include more sedentary behavior, frequent episodes of diarrhea, and apathy, lack of liveliness, and short attention spans.

In adults, mild to moderate PEM results in leanness with reduction in subcutaneous tissue. The most common change in body composition is a reduction of adiposity below the average 12 and 20% expected in normal, well-nourished men and women, respectively. Capacity for prolonged physical work is reduced, but this change is usually apparent only in persons engaged in intense, energy-demanding, occupations.[18,43] Malnourished women have a higher probability of giving birth to infants with low birth weights.[134] As in children, there may be other functional alterations not yet well characterized.

Biochemical information is not consistent in mild and moderate PEM. Laboratory data related to low protein intakes may include low urinary excretion of creatinine, leading to a low creatinine-height index in children,[135] low urinary urea nitrogen and hydroxyproline excretions, altered plasma patterns of free amino acids with a decrease in branched-chain essential amino acids, slight decreases in serum transferrin and albumin, and reduced number of circulating lymphocytes.

**Table 42–4. Classification of Intensity of Current ("Wasting") and Past or Chronic ("Stunting") PEM Based on Weight for Height, and Height for Age***

| | *Normal* | *Mild* | *Moderate* | *Severe* |
|---|---|---|---|---|
| Weight for height (deficit = wasting) | 90–110† | 80–89 | 70–79 | <70, or with edema |
| Height for age (deficit = stunting) | 95–105 | 90–94 | 85–89 | <85 |

*Adapted from Waterlow, J.C.[125]
†Percentage relative to the median NCHS standards.[124]

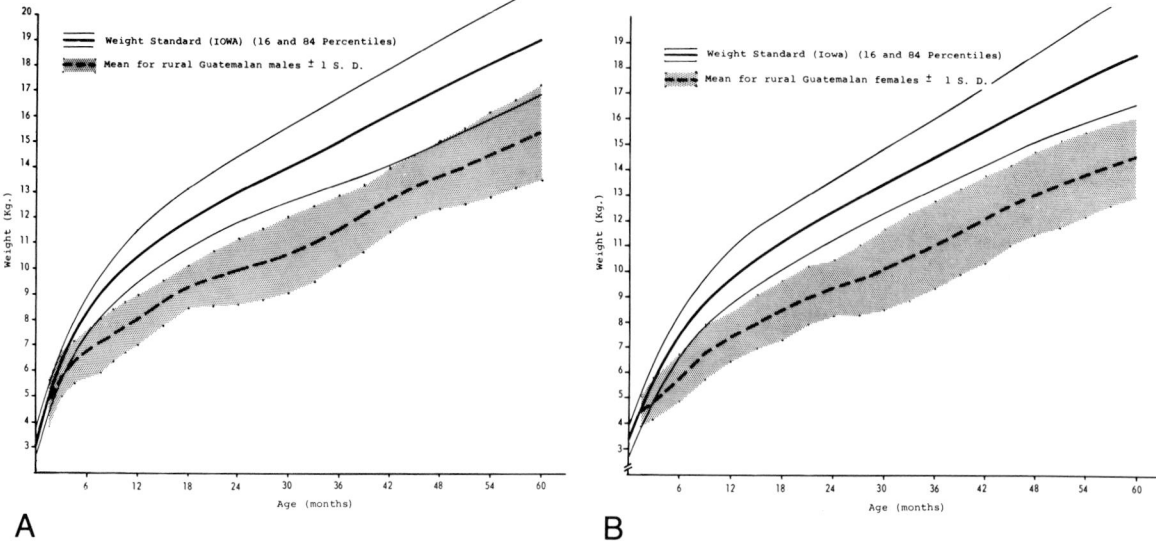

**Fig. 42–5.** Pattern of weight gain, from birth to 5 years, in 431 boys and 436 girls from low-income families in rural Guatemala. (From INCAP,[150] with permission.)

### Severe PEM

The diagnosis is principally based on dietary history and clinical features. Marasmus is usually associated with severe food shortage, prolonged semistarvation, or infrequent feeding of infants, and kwashiorkor with poor protein intakes. Chronic or recurrent diarrhea and infections are common features.

**Marasmus.** Generalized muscular wasting and absence of subcutaneous fat give the patient with severe, nonedematous PEM a "skin and bones" appearance (Figs. 42–6 and 42–7). Marasmic patients frequently have 60% or less of the weight expected for their height, and children have marked retardation in longitudinal growth. The hair is sparse, thin, and dry, without its normal sheen, and usually of a dull brown or reddish color; it is easily pulled out without causing pain. The skin is dry, thin, with little elasticity, and wrinkles easily. Patients are apathetic but usually aware and with a look of anxiety on their face. These features and the sunken cheeks caused by disappearance of the Bichat fat pads, which are among the last subcutaneous adipose depots to disappear, give the marasmic child's face the appearance of a monkey's or an old person's.

Some patients are anorexic while others are ravenously hungry, but they seldom tolerate large amounts of food and vomit easily. Constipation is frequent but diarrhea may be present. There is marked weakness and children frequently cannot stand without help. Heart rate, blood pressure, and body temperature may be low. Hypothermia of 35°C or less can occur, especially after fasting for 8 or more hours, and is often accompanied by hypoglycemia. The viscera are usually small. Abdominal distention may be present. The lymph nodes are easily palpable.

Differential diagnosis must be made from the secondary PEM of body-wasting diseases; dietary history plays an important role.

Common complicating features are acute gastroenteritis, dehydration, respiratory infections, and eye lesions due to hypovitaminosis A. Systemic infections can be present without an appropriate febrile response, tachycardia, or leukocytosis. These infections lead to septic shock or intravascular clotting with high mortality rates.

**Kwashiorkor.** The predominant feature is soft, pitting, painless edema, usually in the feet and legs, but extending to the perineum, upper extremities, and face in severe cases (Fig. 42–8). Most patients have skin lesions, often confused with pellagra, in the areas of edema, continuous pressure (e.g., buttocks and back), or frequent irritation (e.g., perineum and thighs). The skin may be erythematous, and it glistens in the edematous regions with zones of dryness, hyperkeratosis, and hyperpigmentation, which tend to become confluent. The epidermis peels off in large scales, exposing underlying tissues that are easily infected. Subcutaneous fat is preserved, and there may be some muscle wasting. Weight deficit, after accounting for the weight of edema, is usually not as severe as in marasmus. Height may be normal or retarded, depending on the chronicity of the current episode and on past nutritional history.

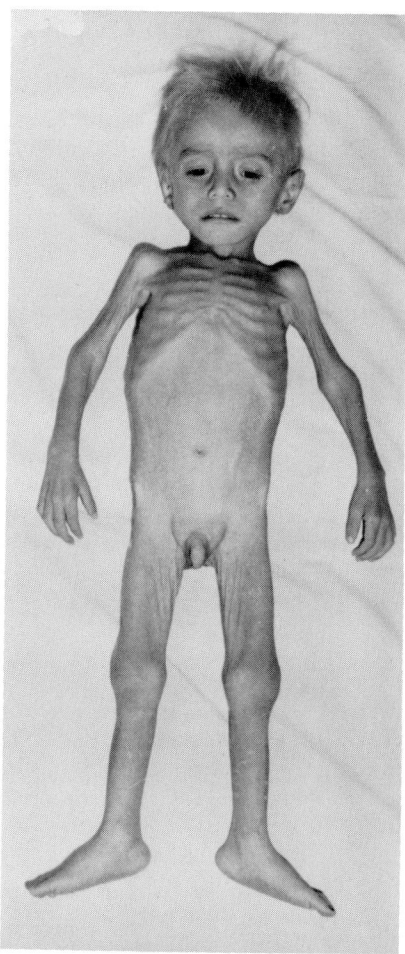

**Fig. 42–6.** Marasmus in a 21-month-old child. (From Viteri, F.E.,[58] with permission of Raven Press.)

The hair is dry, brittle, without its normal sheen, and can be pulled out easily without pain. Curly hair becomes straight, and the pigmentation usually changes to dull brown, red, or even yellowish-white. Alternating periods of poor and relatively good protein intake can produce alternating bands of depigmented and normal hair, which have been termed the "flag sign."

The patients may be pale, with cold and cyanotic extremities. They are apathetic and irritable, cry easily, and have an expression of misery and sadness. Anorexia, sometimes necessitating nasogastric tube feeding, postprandial vomiting, and diarrhea are common. These conditions improve without specific gastrointestinal treatment as nutritional recovery progresses. Hepatomegaly with a soft, round edge caused by severe fatty infiltration is usually present. The abdomen is frequently protruding because of distended stomach and intestinal loops. Peristalsis is irregular. Mus-

cle tone and strength are greatly reduced and tachycardia is common. Both hypothermia and hypoglycemia can occur after short periods of fasting.

Differential diagnosis must be made from other causes of edema and hypoproteinemia, and from secondary PEM due to impairment in protein absorption or metabolism.

The same complications occur as in marasmus, but diarrhea and respiratory and skin infections are more frequent and severe. Serious, fatal infections may occur, frequently without fever, tachycardia, respiratory distress, or appropriate leukocytosis. The most common causes of death are pulmonary edema with bronchopneumonia, septicemia, gastroenteritis, and water and electrolyte imbalances.

**Marasmic Kwashiorkor.** This form of edematous PEM combines clinical characteristics of kwashiorkor and marasmus. The main features are the edema of kwashiorkor, with or without its skin lesions, and the muscle wasting and decreased subcutaneous fat of marasmus (Fig. 42–9 and 42–10). When edema disappears during early treatment, the patient's appearance resembles that of marasmus. Biochemical features of both marasmus and kwashiorkor are seen, but the alterations of severe protein deficiency usually predominate.

### Biochemical and Histopathologic Features of Severe PEM

The most common biochemical findings are the following: serum concentrations of total proteins, and especially albumin, are markedly reduced in edematous PEM, and normal or moderately low in marasmus; hemoglobin and hematocrit are usually low, more so in kwashiorkor than in marasmus; the ratio of nonessential to essential amino acids in plasma is elevated in kwashiorkor and usually normal in marasmus; serum levels of free fatty acids are elevated, particularly in kwashiorkor; blood glucose level is normal or low, especially after fasting 8 to 12 hours; urinary excretions of creatinine, hydroxyproline, 3-methylhistidine, and urea nitrogen are low. Edematous children have markedly reduced urinary creatinine excretions in relation to their height, leading to a low creatinine-height index,[135] whereas marasmic children may have a normal or somewhat low index.

Plasma levels of other nutrients vary and tend to be moderately low. They do not necessarily reflect the body stores. For example, serum iron and retinol may be normal with almost depleted body stores, or in kwashiorkor they may be relatively low with adequate stores because of alterations in

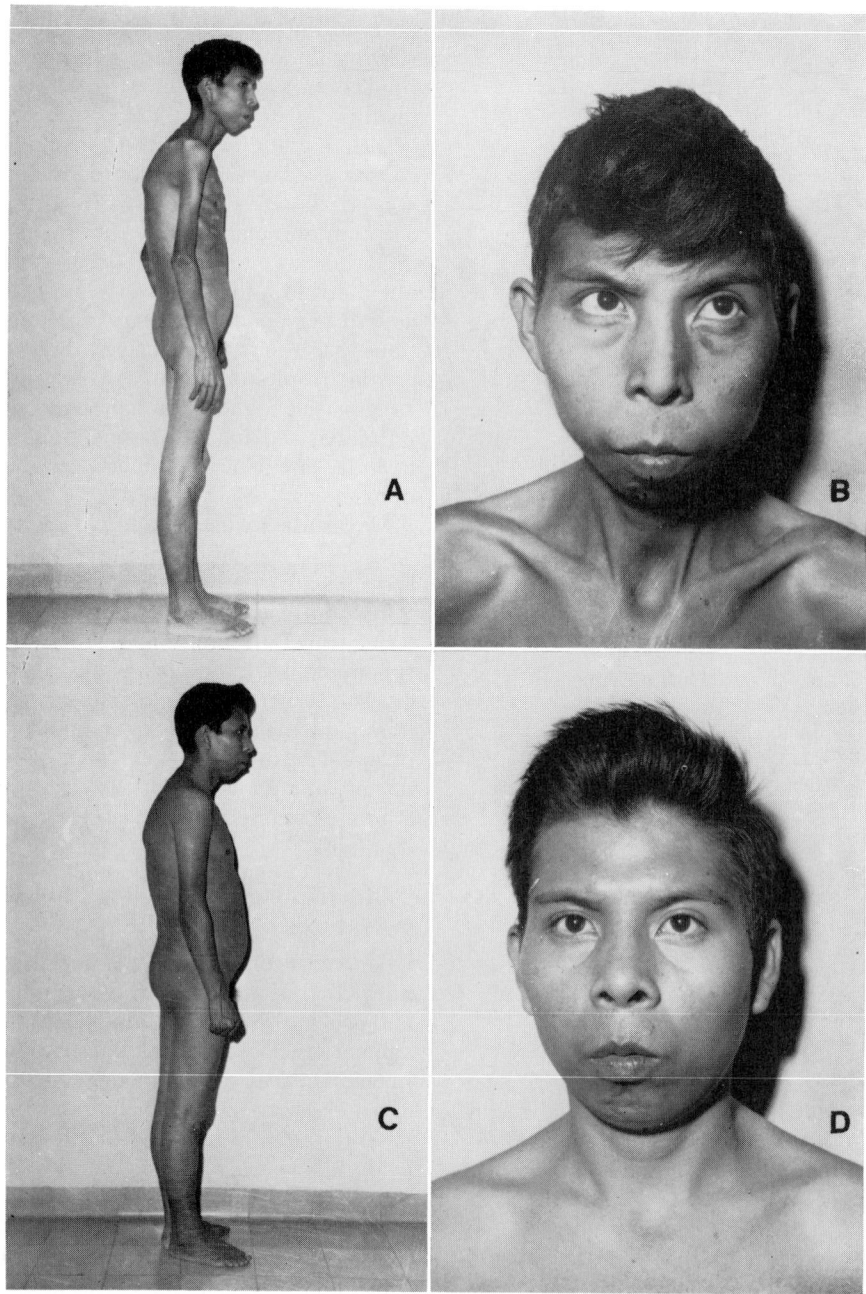

**Fig. 42–7.** *A,B,* Marasmic PEM in a 29-year-old man. *C,D,* Patient after three months of treatment.

the transport proteins, transferrin, and retinol-binding protein.

Many other biochemical changes have been described in severe PEM; some of them were discussed in the section on "Pathophysiology and Adaptive Responses." Others are listed in Table 42–5. Although they have little practical importance in diagnosing the disease, they allow a better understanding of the pathophysiologic modifications.

Body protein decreases at a slow rate, most of it from muscle, and the greater loss of adipose tissue results in a relative increase of total body water (i.e., per unit of body mass), mainly as intracellular water. In severe protein deficiency (kwashiorkor) extracellular water also increases. The intracellular concentrations of potassium and magnesium decrease and that of sodium increases, although the serum concentrations of electrolytes do not necessarily reflect these alterations.[81]

**Table 42–5.  Additional Selected Biochemical Changes Observed in Severe PEM§**

|  | Marasmus | Edematous PEM |
|---|---|---|
| Body composition |  |  |
| Total body water | High | High |
| Extracellular water | High | Higher |
| Total body potassium | Low | Lower |
| Total body protein | Low | Low |
| Serum or plasma |  |  |
| Transport proteins* | Normal or low | Low |
| Branched-chain amino acids | Normal or low | Low |
| Tyrosine/phenylalanine ratio | Normal or low | Low |
| Enzymes (in general)† | Normal | Low |
| Transaminases | Normal or high | High |
| Liver |  |  |
| Fatty infiltration | Absent | Severe |
| Glycogen | Normal or low | Normal or low |
| Urea cycle and other enzymes‡ | Low | Lower |
| Amino acid synthesizing enzymes | High | Not as high |

*For example, transferrin, ceruloplasmin, retinol-, cortisol-, and thyroxine-binding proteins, α- and β-lipoproteins.
†For example, amylase, pseudocholinesterase, alkaline phosphatase.
‡For example, xanthine oxidase, glycolic acid oxidase, cholinesterase.
§From Torun, B., Viteri, F.E.,[149] with permission of McGraw-Hill Book Co.

Histopathologic studies show nonspecific atrophy, mainly in tissues with greater cell turnover rates, such as intestinal mucosa, red bone marrow, and testicular epithelium; intestinal villi are flattened and enterocytes lose their columnar appearance.[136] In marasmus there is generalized atrophy of skeletal muscle. The skin changes consist of dermal atrophy, ecchymosis, ulcerations, and hyperkeratotic desquamation, seen primarily in areas subjected to irritation and not necessarily restricted to exposed areas, as in the case of pellagra. The liver in individuals with kwashiorkor is enlarged with fatty infiltration; periportal fat appears first and advances centripetally as severity increases. Other histologic analyses, special staining techniques, and electron microscopy reveal more alterations, not all of which result specifically from primary protein-energy malnutrition. All do reflect generalized atrophy, however. Lesions due to superimposed infections and other nutrient deficiencies often are evident macroscopically and upon histopathologic examination. These changes usually revert to normal with nutritional recovery, although some residual lesions may persist for some time.

## PROGNOSIS AND RISK OF MORTALITY

Treatment of mild and moderate PEM corrects the acute signs of the disease, but children's catch-up growth in height may take a long time or might never be achieved. It has been suggested that many children who have suffered from severe or moderate PEM are not normal even when they have recovered fully.[137] These children have been deprived not only of food but also of opportunities for development, and they have missed the critical periods for harmonic physical, mental, and social maturation. Weight for height can be restored easily, but the child may remain stunted, and a small body size may influence his maximal working capacity as an adult. Many severely malnourished children appear to have residual behavioral and mental problems in terms of creativity and social interaction. However, the causal roles of malnutrition and a poor living environment are difficult to disassociate, and there is no irrefutable evidence that the damage cannot be corrected in a good, stimulating environment.

Anthropometric characteristics are associated with mortality rates, as in the classification of severe PEM into first, second, or third degrees, based on weight for age.[129] A higher mortality rate is associated with the more intense anthropometric deficits but not with mild or moderate deficiencies.[138] Mortality rates in severe PEM can be as high as 40%; the immediate causes of death are usually infections. Table 42–6 lists the characteristics that generally indicate a poor prognosis. Mortality rate can decrease to 10% or less with the prevention and adequate treatment of infections and other complications, together with adequate dietary therapy.

### TREATMENT

#### Severe PEM

Patients with uncomplicated PEM should be treated outside the hospital whenever possible. Hospitalization increases the risk of cross-infec-

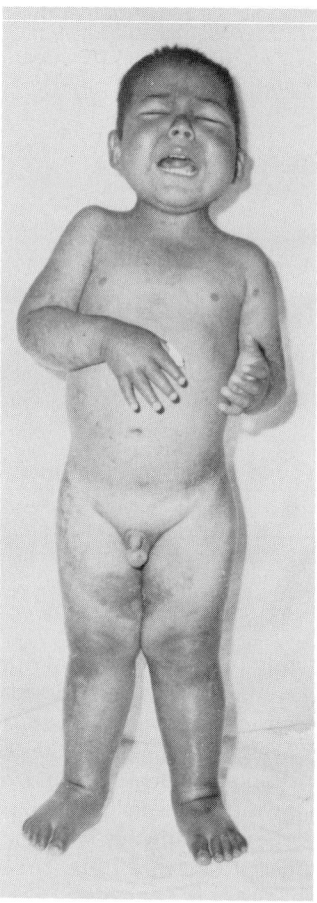

**Fig. 42–8.** Kwashiorkor in a 36-month-old child. Note that subcutaneous tissues were preserved in the trunk and face.

tions, and the unfamiliar setting may increase apathy and anorexia in children, making feeding more difficult. When hospitalization is necessary, treatment strategy can be divided into three stages: (1) resolving life-threatening conditions, (2) restoring nutritional status without disrupting homeostasis, and (3) ensuring nutritional rehabilitation.

**Resolving Life-Threatening Conditions.** Nutritional rehabilitation can be delayed until life-threatening conditions are solved. The most frequent are:

1. *Fluid and electrolyte disturbances.* The assessment of dehydration is not easy in severe PEM, as classic signs of dehydration, such as sunken eyeballs and decreased skin turgor, are frequently found in well-hydrated patients, while hypovolemia may coexist with subcutaneous edema. Useful signs are low urinary output, weak and rapid pulse, low blood pressure, and a declining state of consciousness. The therapeutic approach differs from that in well-nourished patients because of water and electrolyte peculiarities of severe PEM, namely: (1) hypo-osmolality with moderate hyponatremia, frequently with intracellular sodium excess; (2) intracellular potassium depletion, usually without hypokalemia; (3) mild-to-moderate metabolic acidosis, which decreases or disappears when the patient receives dietary or parenteral energy, and electrolyte balance is reestablished; (4) high tolerance to hypocalcemia, partly because the acidosis produces a relative increment in ionized calcium and partly because hypoproteinemia makes less protein available to bind calcium ions; and (5) decreased body magnesium, with or without hypomagnesemia.

Fluid repletion should allow a diuresis of at least 200 ml in 24 hrs in children and 500 ml in adults, or a micturition every 2 to 3 hrs. Whenever possible, oral or nasogastric rehydration should be used. Initially, 10 ml/kg/hr can be given every 1 to 2 hrs, and the volume should be modified according to patient response. Patients who are urinating should receive about 6 meq K, 2 to 3 meq Na, 2 to 3 meq Ca, and 20 to 30 kcal/day/kg of body weight. This can be accomplished by dissolving in 1 L of water, 3 g KCl, 1 g table salt (NaCl), 2 g $CaCl.6H_2O$ (or 4 g calcium gluconate), and 50 g glucose or sucrose (sugar). Potassium should be withheld when there is no diuresis. Additional fluids must be given to compensate for the losses of diarrhea and vomiting, providing about 35 meq Na and 30 meq K per Kg of excreta (i.e., 2 g table salt and 2 g KCl/L). Dietary formula with calcium should be started as early as possible, if necessary alternating with the electrolyte solution; this can usually be 4 to 6 hrs after beginning the oral rehydration therapy. Total K intake can be raised to 8 to 10 meq/kg/day.

Intravenous fluids must be used in severe dehydration with hypovolemia, impending shock, frequent vomiting, and persistent abdominal distention. Hypo-osmolar solutions (200 to 280 mOsm/L) must be used. K (when urinating) and Na should not exceed 6 and 3 meq/kg/day, respectively, and glucose must provide 15 to 30 kcal/kg/day. During the first hour, 10 to 30 ml/kg are infused, depending on the patient's condition. Subsequent volumes are calculated at 2- to 4-hr intervals. Additional losses through diarrhea and vomiting must be compensated with about 3 meq Na, 3 meq K, 6 meq Cl, and 15 kcal/100 g (i.e., 20 ml isotonic saline, 2 ml of 10% KCl, and 78 ml of 5% dextrose/100 g excreta). An increase in pulse and respiratory rate with weight gain after accounting for weight of excreta, pulmonary rales, and appearance or exacerbation of edema indi-

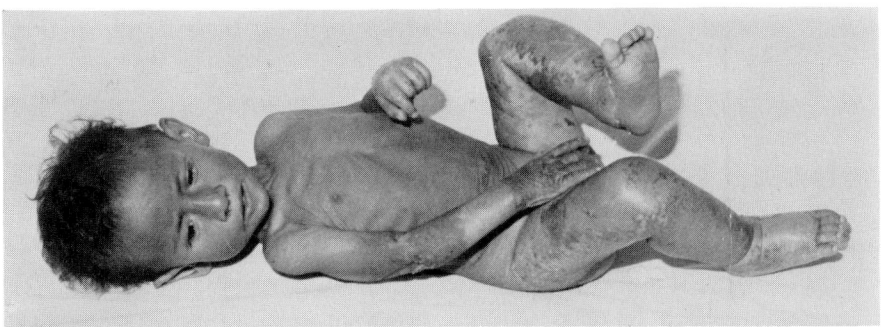

**Fig. 42–9.** Marasmic kwashiorkor in a 22-month-old child. Note the edema in the lower part of the body, the emaciated upper part, and the skin lesions. (From Torun, B., Viteri, F.E.,[149] with permission of McGraw-Hill Book Co.)

cates overhydration. An increase in pulse and respiratory rate with weight loss, low urine output, and continuing losses from diarrhea and vomiting suggests insufficient fluid therapy.

Some clinicians advocate the routine use of solutions containing lactate or bicarbonate. However, the mild metabolic acidosis of malnutrition usually disappears with energy intake. Therefore, treatment for acidosis should be withheld unless blood pH is below 7.25, urinary pH is below 5, or clinical signs of severe acidosis are present.

Small increases (0.5 to 1 g/dl) in plasma protein concentration help to prevent a rapid exit of water from the intravascular compartment in patients with severe hypoproteinemia (less than 3 g/dl), anuria, and signs of hypovolemia or impending circulatory collapse. This can be achieved by administering plasma intravenously, 10 ml/kg in 1 to 2 hrs, followed by 20 ml/kg/hr of a mixture of two parts of 5% dextrose and one part of isotonic saline, for 1 or 2 hrs. If diuresis does not improve, the dose of plasma can be repeated. Further treatment for circulatory collapse is similar to that of well-nourished patients.

Hypocalcemia may occur secondary to magnesium deficiency. When the patient has symptoms of hypocalcemia and serum magnesium determinations are not available, it is essential not only to give calcium infusion but also to give magnesium intravenously or intramuscularly. When the serum concentration of calcium rises to normal level or, in the absence of laboratory data, when the symptoms of hypocalcemia disappear, calcium infusion may be discontinued. Intramuscular or oral magnesium supplementation should follow the initial parenteral magnesium until the patient is repleted with this ion as indicated by maintenance of serum and urine magnesium concentrations. When there are no laboratory facilities to monitor Mg concentrations, a general therapeutic guideline is to give magnesium intramuscularly as a 50% solution of magnesium sulfate in doses of 0.5, 1, and 1.5 ml, respectively, for patients who weigh less than 7, between 7 and 10, and more than 10 kg. The dose can be repeated every 12 hours until there is no recurrence of the hypocalcemic symptoms and oral magnesium supplementation of 0.5 to 1 meq Mg/kg/day can be given, as described later. Certain antibiotics, such as amphotericin, can cause loss of magnesium and potassium into the urine, increasing the need for both ions.

2. *Infections.* Malnourished patients are particularly prone to infections. Although these are often severe and life-threatening, paradoxically, clinical manifestations may be mild and the classic signs of fever, tachycardia, and leukocytosis absent. Antigen-antibody reactions are often impaired and skin tests, such as tuberculin, often give falsely negative results.

Antibiotics should not be used prophylactically, but when an infection is suspected appropriate antibiotic therapy must be started immediately, even before obtaining the results of microbiologic cultures. The choice of drug will vary with the suspected etiologic agent, the severity of the disease, and the local pattern of drug resistance. When septicemia is suspected, a broad-spectrum antibiotic or a combination, such as ampicillin and gentamicin, is usually given intravenously. Other supportive treatment may also be necessary, as for respiratory distress, hypothermia, and hypoglycemia.

Repeated transfusions of fresh frozen human plasma, 10 ml/kg during the first 3 to 4 days of treatment, accelerate the recovery of impaired complement hemolytic activity in patients with edematous PEM.[79,139] Although this might reduce serious infections complications, clinical evidence is still lacking about the advantages of this treatment.

Clinicians should be aware that gastrointestinal,

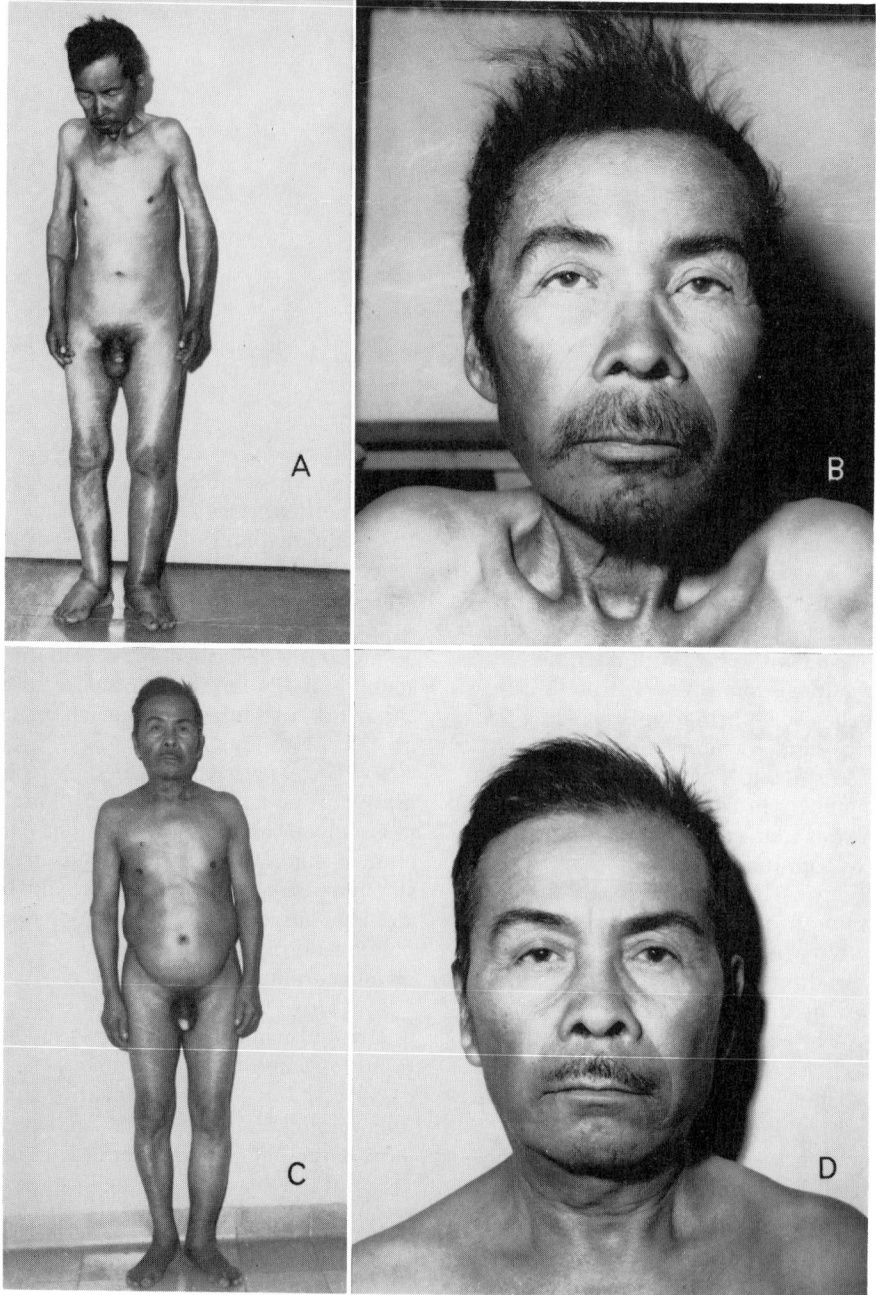

**Fig. 42–10.** *A,B,* Edematous PEM in a 46-year-old man. *C,D,* Patient after three months of treatment.

hepatic, and renal alterations that might accompany severe PEM could potentiate the toxic effects of a drug. Treatment for intestinal parasites is rarely urgent and can be deferred until nutritional rehabilitation is underway. This delay decreases the risks of potential toxicity, including the possibility of absorbing drugs normally not absorbed by a healthy intestine.

3. *Hemodynamic alterations.* Cardiac failure

may develop during or after administration of intravenous fluids, or shortly after the introduction of high-protein and high-energy feedings, leading to pulmonary edema and frequent secondary pulmonary infection. These alterations may be the result of impaired cardiac function, sudden expansion of the intravascular fluid volume, severe anemia, or impaired membrane function. Diuretics such as furosemide (10 mg intravenously or

**Table 42–6. Characteristics that Indicate Poor Prognosis in Patients with PEM**

—Age less than 6 months.
—Deficit in weight for height greater than 30%, or in weight for age greater than 40%.
—Stupor or coma.
—Infections, particularly bronchopneumonia or measles.
—Petechiae or hemorrhagic tendencies (purpura is usually associated with septicemia or a viral infection).
—Dehydration and electrolyte disturbances, particularly hyponatremia, hypokalemia, and severe acidosis.
—Severe tachycardia, signs of heart failure, or respiratory difficulty.
—Total serum proteins below 3 g/dl.
—Severe anemia with clinical signs of hypoxia.
—Clinical jaundice, increased serum bilirubin, and/or frankly elevated transaminases.
—Extensive exudative or exfoliative cutaneous lesions, or deep decubitus ulcerations.
—Hypoglycemia or hypothermia.

intramuscularly, repeated as necessary) should be given, as well as other supportive measures. Many clinicians advocate the use of digoxin (0.03 mg/kg intravenously, every 6 to 8 hrs). *The use of diuretics merely to accelerate the disappearance of edema in kwashiorkor is contraindicated.*

4. *Severe anemia.* Blood transfusions should be given *only in cases of severe anemia* with less than 4 g hemoglobin/dl, or with signs of hypoxia or impending cardiac failure. Whole blood (10 ml/kg) can be used in marasmic patients, but it is better to use packed red blood cells (6 ml/kg) in patients with edematous PEM. The transfusion should be given slowly, over 2 to 3 hrs, and repeated if necessary after 8 to 24 hrs. The routine use of blood transfusions endangers the patient. Hemoglobin levels will improve with proper dietary treatment supplemented with hematinics.

5. *Hypothermia and hypoglycemia.* Body temperature below 35.5°C and plasma glucose concentration below 60 mg/dl can be due to either impaired thermoregulatory mechanisms, reduced fuel substrate availability, or severe infection. Asymptomatic hypoglycemia can be prevented or treated by the frequent feeding of small volumes of glucose-containing diets and solutions. Severe symptomatic hypoglycemia must be treated intravenously with 10 to 20 ml of 50% glucose solution followed by oral administration of 25 to 50 ml of 5% glucose solution at 2-hr intervals for 24 to 48 hrs.

Body temperature usually rises in the hypothermic patient with frequent feedings of glucose-containing diets or solutions. Body temperature must be closely monitored when external heat sources are used to reduce the loss of body heat,

as these patients may rapidly become hyperthermic. It is best to keep the seminude patients in an ambient temperature of 30 to 33° C.

6. *Severe vitamin A deficiency.* Severe PEM is often associated with vitamin A deficiency. A large dose of vitamin A should be given on admission, since ocular lesions can develop as a result of increased demands for retinol when adequate protein and energy feeding begins. Water-miscible vitamin A should be given orally or intramuscularly on the first day, at a dose of 50,000 to 100,000 IU for infants and preschool children, or 100,000 to 200,000 IU for older children and adults, followed by 5,000 IU orally each day for the duration of treatment. The initial dose should be repeated two more days in symptomatic patients. Corneal ulcerations should be treated with ophthalmic drops of 1% atropine solution and antibiotic ointments or drops until the ulceration heals.

**Homeostatic Restoration of Nutritional Status.** The next objective of therapy is to replace nutrient tissue deficits as rapidly and safely as possible. Based on the premise that the patient is adapted to the malnourished state, nutritional treatment must be gradual to avoid disrupting his metabolic equilibrium. Various regimens provide a diet that meets daily maintenance requirements for a few days, followed by increases in nutrient delivery. Table 42–7 shows a therapeutic schedule for children, based on the experience of INCAP. The only difference between kwashiorkor and marasmus is that the latter often requires larger amounts of dietary energy, which can be provided by adding vegetable oil to increase the diet's energy density. Diets with as much as 60 to 75% of the energy from fats are usually well tolerated; there may be some steatorrhea without profuse diarrhea, and 85 to 92% of the fat is absorbed.[87] The intervals for the dietary increments in Table 42–7 can be lengthened to 3 to 5 days in severely malnourished children, especially those with plasma protein less than 3 g/dl or serious metabolic disturbances.

It is best to begin with a liquid formula fed orally or by nasogastric tube, divided equally into 5 to 12 feedings per day, depending on the patient's age and general condition. This frequent feeding of small volumes prevents vomiting and the development of hypoglycemia and hypothermia. For older children and adults with good appetite, the liquid formula can be partly substituted with solid foods that have a high density of good-quality, easily digestible nutrients.

Intravenous alimentation is rarely justified in primary PEM and can increase mortality rates.[140]

The diet must be supplemented to provide 8 to

**Table 42–7.  Dietary Therapeutic Regimen Based on Milk Formulas, for Infants and Preschool Children with Severe PEM***

| Days From Beginning of Treatment | Protein (g) | Energy (kcal) | Milk† oz. (g) | Sugar (g) | Oil‡ (g) | Water§ (ml) |
|---|---|---|---|---|---|---|
| 1 | 0.8–1 | 70–90 | 1 (3) | 15 | – – | 70 (100) |
| 3 | 1.5–2 | 105–115 | 2 (6) | 20 | – [1] | 40 (100) |
| 5 | 2.5–3 | 125–135 | 3 (9) | 20 | – [2] | 10 (100) |
| 7 | 3.5–4.5 | 145–160 | 4.5 (14) | 20 | – [3] | – (120) |
| Marasmus** | | | | | | |
| 12 | — | 175 | — | — | 2 [5] | — |
| 17 | — | 200 | — | — | 5 [8] | — |
| 22 | — | 220 | — | — | 7 [10] | — |
| etc. | 3.5–4.5 | ‖ | 4.5 (14) | 20 | ‖ | – (120) |

*Amounts are per kg body weight per day. The formulas must be supplemented with adequate amounts of vitamins, minerals, and electrolytes. Additional water must be given to provide at least 1 ml of total fluids per kcal in the diet.

†Amounts on the left are fluid ounces of whole fluid milk with 3% fat. Amounts in parentheses are g of dry, powdered milk.

‡IMPORTANT: When one is using powdered skim milk, vegetable oil must be added as indicated inside the brackets.

§Amounts on the left are added to fluid milk, amounts in parentheses to powdered milk.

**Marasmic patients may require more dietary energy. Two to three ml of vegetable oil per kg per day should be added at five-day intervals until the rate of weight gain becomes adequate.

10 meq K, 3 to 5 meq Na, 5 to 8 meq Ca, and 1 to 2 meq Mg/Kg of body weight per day. This can be accomplished by adding 0.3 g KCl and 0.1 g NaCl/dl to milk formulas, or by adding appropriate amounts of the mineral mixture shown in Table 42–8 to most other diets. Additional supplements should include daily doses of 60 to 120 mg elemental iron, 10 mg elemental zinc, 0.3 mg folic acid, 5,000 IU vitamin A, and other vitamins and trace elements in the doses provided by most commercial preparations.

The protein source must be of high biologic value and easily digested. Cow's milk is frequently available, but some clinicians worry about the possibility of lactose malabsorption in severe PEM. Cow's milk usually is well tolerated and assimilated by severely malnourished children and can be safely advocated.[141,142] Eggs, meat, fish, soy isolates, and some vegetable-protein mixtures are also sources of good protein. Most vegetable mixtures have protein digestibilities that are 10 to 20% lower than those of animal proteins, making it necessary to feed larger amounts, and their bulk might pose a problem in feeding small children.

The attitude of the person who feeds the patient and the appearance, color, and flavor of the foods are important to overcome the patient's lack of appetite.

The initial response to diet is either no change in weight or a decrease due to loss of edema, accompanied by large diuresis (Fig. 42–11). After 7 to 15 days, there is a period of rapid weight gain or "catch-up." The rate of catch-up usually is slower in marasmus than in kwashiorkor. In children, this initial rate of weight gain generally is 10 to 15 times that of a normal child of the same age, and it can be as high as 20 to 25 times greater. Some patients only show a four- or fivefold increase in catch-up. Most often this is associated with insufficient energy intakes (e.g., due to formula inadequately prepared, insufficient amounts of formula given at each feeding, too few feedings per day, anorexia, or lack of patience of the person who feeds the child) or with overt or asymptomatic infections, such as urinary infections and tuberculosis.

**Ensuring Nutritional Rehabilitation.** This last stage of treatment may begin in the hospital and continue on an outpatient basis, but the patient must continue to eat adequate amounts of protein, energy, and other nutrients, especially when traditional foods are introduced into the diet. Emotional and physical stimulation must be provided, and persistent diarrhea, intestinal parasites, and other minor complications must be treated. Children should be vaccinated during this period as well.

**Table 42–8.  Mineral Mixture to Complement Liquid Formulas***

| Salt | Amount (g) | 1 g mixture provides (meq) | |
|---|---|---|---|
| KCl | 44 | K+ | 8.5 |
| NaCl | 9 | Na+ | 3.5 |
| Na₂HPO₄ | 7 | Ca²⁺ | 1.4 |
| CaCO₃ | 5 | Mg²⁺ | 0.6 |
| MgSO₄·7H₂O | 5 | HPO₄²⁻ | 1.2 |

*From Torun, B., Viteri, F.E.,[119] with permission of Rev. Col. Med.

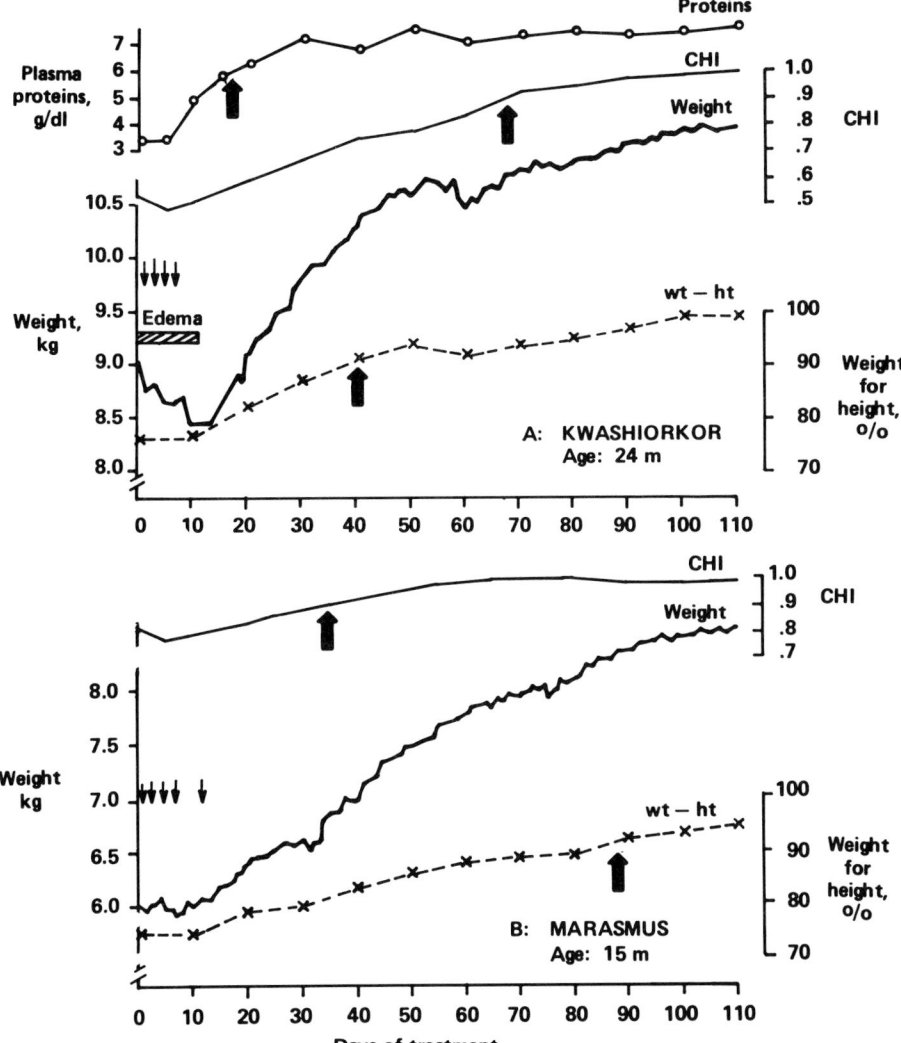

**Fig. 42–11.** Weight gain and improvement in weight-for-height, creatinine-height index (CHI), and plasma protein concentration of two children treated at INCAP for kwashiorkor *(A)* and marasmus *(B)*. The thin arrows ( ↓ ) indicate gradual increments in dietary proteins and energy, as described in Table 42–7. The thick arrows ( ↑ ) indicate the day when the lower limit of normal values was reached. The marasmic child had normal plasma protein concentration on admission. Weight-for-height was calculated for child A on admission after correcting for the weight of edema. Dietary energy was reduced on days 60 and 80 for child A, and on day 100 for child B.

1. *Introduction of traditional foods.* Other foods, especially those available at home, are gradually introduced into the diet in a combination with the high-energy, high-protein formula. This step should be taken when edema has disappeared, the skin lesions are notably improved, the patient becomes active and interacts with the environment, the appetite is restored, and adequate rates of catch-up growth have been achieved in children. A daily minimum intake of 3 to 4 g of protein and 120 to 150 kcal/kg of body weight (or more in marasmus) must be ensured. To achieve this, the energy density of solid foods must be

increased with oil or fat, and protein density and quality must be high, using animal proteins, soybean protein preparations, and good vegetable protein mixtures. Local traditional foods can be used in appropriate combinations[143–145] *in addition to the liquid formula,* as in the following examples: (1) One part of a dry pulse or its flour (e.g., black beans, soybeans, kidney beans, cowpeas) and three parts of a dry cereal or flour (e.g., corn, rice, wheat) may be used; fat or oil should be added to the mashed or strained pulse during or after cooking in amounts equal to the weight of the dry pulse or flour, and to the cereal preparations in amounts of 10 to 30 ml oil/100 g dry cereal product, depending on the type of preparation. (2) Four parts of dry rice and one part of fresh fish may be used; fat or oil should be added in amounts equal to 20 to 40% of the dry weights. The food can be served as separate dishes or it can be mashed or blended and fed as paps to infants and young children.

2. *Emotional and physical stimulation.* The malnourished child needs affection and tender care from the beginning of treatment. This requires patience and understanding by the hospital staff and the relatives. Involvement of parents or relatives is usually very helpful. Hospitals should be brightly colored, cheerful, with audible stimulation such as music. As soon as the child can move without assistance and is willing to interact with the staff and other children, he must be encouraged to explore, to play, and to participate in activities that involve body movements. Relatively small increments in physical activity and energy expenditure during the course of nutritional rehabilitation result in faster longitudinal growth and accretion of lean body tissues.[146] Parents should be encouraged to stimulate and teach their children by playing and talking. Toys and play materials can often be made from discarded local articles. Adult patients should exercise regularly with gradual increments in cardiorespiratory workload.

3. *Persistent diarrhea and other health problems.* Mild diarrhea does not interfere with nutritional rehabilitation as long as fluid and electrolyte intakes maintain satisfactory hydration. This condition often disappears without specific treatment as nutritional status improves.[147] However, persistent diarrhea can contribute to the development of a new episode of PEM and should be treated. Treatment is undertaken by determining the underlying cause of diarrhea, usually intestinal infections, excessive bacterial flora in the upper gut that ferment food substrates and deconjugate bile salts, intestinal parasites (particularly amebiasis, giardiasis, and trichuriasis), and intolerance to food components. Among the latter, lactose, milk protein, and gluten have often been held responsible. However, the apparent high prevalence of lactose malabsorption and intolerance in PEM is often founded on inadequate diagnostic procedures (e.g., intolerance to 2 g lactose/kg in aqueous solution, rather than to the 7 to 15 g lactose contained in a milk meal.)[85] When food intolerance is suspected, the diet should be modified, taking care to preserve its nutritional quality and density. Before a patient is deemed intolerant to a given food, it should be reintro-duced into the diet to confirm the diagnosis, and adequate diagnostic tests should be done.

4. *Criteria for recovery.* The most practical criterion is weight gain. A patient should be discharged from in-hospital or outpatient treatment when he has no edema and reaches a body weight equal to or near that expected for his height. As shown in Figure 42–11, however, weight-for-height does not necessarily indicate protein repletion, and it is best to use it in conjunction with body composition indices. If urine can be collected for 24 to 72 hours in children, the creatinine-height index (CHI) can be used as an indicator of body protein repletion. An increase in plasma protein or albumin concentration indicates a good response but not full recovery (see Fig. 42–11).

A premature termination of treatment increases the risk of a recurrence of malnutrition. As a general guideline, when body composition cannot be assessed, dietary therapy should continue for one month after the patient admitted with edematous PEM reaches an adequate weight-for-height without edema and his clinical and overall performances are adequate, or for 15 days after the marasmic patient reaches that weight. The minimum normal limits should be 92% of the weight expected for height and, especially in children, a creatinine-height index of 0.9. Some patients, however, do not reach those values because they are in the lower end of the normal distribution curve. If they continue growing at a normal rate and have no functional impairments, treatment can be terminated after one month of adequate dietary intake and weight-for-height and CHI stabilization. Specific treatment of other nutritional problems (e.g., iron deficiency) sometimes must be prolonged beyond discharge for PEM.

When discharged, patients or their parents must be taught about the causes of PEM, emphasizing rational and nutritious use of household foods, personal and environmental hygiene, appropriate immunizations, and early treatment of diarrhea and other diseases.

## Mild and Moderate PEM

The less severe forms of PEM should be treated in an ambulatory setting, supplementing the home diet with easily digested foods that contain proteins of high biologic value and a high energy density. In some instances, therapy can be achieved merely by instructing the adult patient about adequate eating habits and a better use of food resources, or by instructing mothers in improved child-feeding practices and in more nutritious culinary habits. It is almost always necessary, however, to provide both nutritious food supplements and instructions for their use.

The quantity of food supplements will vary depending upon the degree of malnutrition and the relative deficit of proteins and energy. As a general guideline, the goal should be to provide a total intake, including the home diet, of at least twice the protein and 1.5 times the energy requirements. For preschool children, this would signify a daily intake of about 2 to 2.5 g of high-quality protein and 120 to 150 kcal/kg of body weight, and for infants under 1 year, about 3.5 g protein and 150/kcal/kg/day.

The ingestion of the food supplement by the malnourished person must be ensured. This is more likely to occur if it is appetizing to both the child and the mother, if it is ready-made or easy to prepare, if additional amounts are provided to feed the siblings, and if it does not have an important commercial value outside the home that would make it easy and profitable for the family to sell the item for cash. A substitution effect on the home diet (i.e., a decrease in the usual food intake) is almost unavoidable, but it can be reduced by using low-bulk supplements with high-protein and -energy densities. Special attention should be given to avoid a decrease in breast-feeding. The supplements for breast-fed infants should be paps or solid foods that will not quench the infant's thirst and thus not change the infant's demand nor the mother's attitude toward lactation.

Adequate amounts of vitamins and minerals must be assured, although mild deficiencies can be overcome by the micronutrients in the food or by use of fortified vehicles such as iron-enriched bread or sugar fortified with retinol.

## PREVENTION AND CONTROL OF PEM

Poverty, ignorance, frequent infections, cultural customs, cyclic climatic conditions, and natural and man-made disasters are among the main causes of PEM. Therefore, its control and prevention require multisectorial approaches that include food production and distribution, preventive medicine, education, social development, and economic improvement. At a national or regional level, control and prevention can only be achieved through short- and long-term political commitments, and effective actions to enforce the measures to eradicate the underlying causes of malnutrition.

Nevertheless, the physician, nutritionist, public health worker, and educator *can* and *must* play an active role in the prevention of PEM, even though aimed at smaller population groups or individuals. Their efforts may have to be diverted toward those with higher risk to develop PEM. A profile of risk factors is then useful. The most likely victims are children under 2 years of age from low socioeconomic strata whose parents have misconceptions concerning the use of foods, who come from broken or unstable families, whose families have a high prevalence of alcoholism, who live under poor sanitary conditions in urban slums or in rural areas frequently subject to droughts or floods, and whose families have societal beliefs that prohibit the use of many nutritious foods.

Special attention must be given to the availability and rational use of foods that optimize nutrient utilization, the control or reduction of infections, and health and nutrition education programs for the individual, the family, and the community.

### Food Availability

Animal foods are the best protein sources but they tend to be expensive, unavailable, or prohibited by religious practices. Under such circumstances, the staple vegetable foods can be complemented with other vegetable foods combined in culturally acceptable ways to permit a good essential amino acid complementation and to improve the biologic value of dietary protein. For example, corn and black bean combinations that provide proteins in a proportion of about 60:40, equivalent to about three parts of dry corn and one part of dry beans, have an excellent amino acid composition and permit adequate growth and function.[148] The same is true of a series of other combinations of grains and pulses.[143–145] The relatively low nitrogen digestibility of these vegetable sources must be considered in recommending the amounts to be eaten. Energy density can be increased by adding fats or carbohydrates.

It is often necessary to convince parents about the safety of using foods which, in some cultures, are fed only to adults and older children. This is especially true of foods to complement mother's milk or to wean infants from the breast. Trials at INCAP have shown that it is feasible to feed paps based on black beans *(Phaseolus vulgaris)*, a cereal, and vegetable oil to babies as young as 3 months of age without intestinal discomfort and without decreasing breast milk intakes. Breast-fed infants from populations at risk of PEM should start receiving at 4 months of age paps prepared by mashing boiled rice, cooked corn products (e.g., tamale, tortilla), or bread soaked in about 50% water. At 6 months of age, one part of a cooked pulse (e.g., kidney beans, soybeans, chick peas) should be added for every three parts of rice, corn, or bread to provide a better protein mixture.

If the child is underweight, one teaspoon of vegetable oil or two teaspoons of sugar can be added to every 2 to 3 ounces of pap. Infants who are fully weaned or only occasionally breast-fed must receive energy- and protein-rich amounts of staples and, ideally, of animal foods to satisfy their nutritional needs and to allow adequate growth.

## Reduction of Morbidity Rates

This is a logical consequence of the interactions of nutrition with infection. Since young children are at a greater risk of malnutrition, high priority must be given to immunizations, sanitary measures to reduce fecal contamination, and early oral rehydration and feeding of children with diarrhea.

## Education

The presence of a malnourished child in a family suggests that other members of the household might also be at risk of malnutrition. Therefore, nutritional and health education must not be restricted to the rehabilitation of the index case, but to prevention of nutritional deterioration of other family members, especially siblings and pregnant and lactating women. Similarly, a high prevalence of children with malnutrition or growth retardation indicates that the entire community is at some risk of impaired nutrition. Consequently, education programs must be devised for community leaders, civic action groups, and the community as a whole. Such programs must emphasize promotion of breast-feeding, appropriate use of weaning foods, nutritional alternatives using traditional foods, personal and environmental hygiene, feeding practices during illness and convalescence, and early treatment of diarrhea and other diseases. Personal and communal involvement should be pursued through commitments to apply the recommendations. Toward this aim, it is important that all educational programs incorporate the people's own assessment of their nutritional problems and their feelings toward personal participation to contribute to the solution.

## REFERENCES

1. Adams, F.: Genuine works of Hippocrates. Cited by Trowell, H.C., Davies, J.N.P. Br. Med. J. *2*:796–798, 1952.
2. Patrón-Correa, J.P.: Rev. Med. Yucatán (México) *3*:89–96, 1908.
3. Normet, L.: Bull. Soc. Pathol. Exot. *19*:207–213, 1926.
4. Kerandel, J.: Bull. Soc. Pathol. Exot. *19*:302–311, 1926.
5. McConnell, R.E.: Uganda Ann. Med. San. Report, Appendix 2. Entebbe, Government Printer, 1918.
6. Procter, R.A.W.: Kenya Med. J. *3*:284, 1927.
7. Mann, W.L., Helm, J.B., Brown, C.J.: JAMA *75*:1416–1418, 1920.
8. Payne, G.C., Payne, F.K.: Am. J. Hyg. *7*:73–83, 1927.
9. Williams, C.D.: Arch. Dis. Child. *8*:423–433, 1933.
10. Williams, C.D.: Lancet *2*:1151–1152, 1935.
11. Autret, M., Béhar, M.: Síndrome Policarencial Infantil (Kwashiorkor) and its Prevention in Central America. FAO Nutr. Studies No. 13. Rome, FAO, 1954.
12. Trowell, H.C., Davies, J.N.P., Dean, R.F.A.: Kwashiorkor. London, Edward Arnold, Ltd., 1954.
13. Hegsted, D.M., Tsongas, A.G., Abbott, D.B., et al.: J. Lab. Clin. Med. *31*:261–284, 1946.
14. Brock, J.F., Autret, M.: Kwashiorkor in Africa. FAO Nutr. Studies No. 8. Rome. FAO, 1952.
15. Jelliffe, D.B.: J. Pediatr. *54*:227–256, 1959.
16. FAO: The Fourth World Food Survey. FAO Food Nutr Series No. 10. Rome, FAO, 1977.
17. Reutlinger, S., Alderman, H.: The Prevalence of Calorie-Deficient Diets in Developing Countries. World Bank Staff Working Paper No. 374. Washington, D.C., World Bank, 1980.
18. Viteri, F.E., Torun, B., Immink, M.D.C., et al.: Marginal malnutrition and working capacity. *In* Nutrition in Health and Disease and International Development. (Harper, A.E., Davis, G.K., Eds.) New York, Alan R. Liss, 1981.
19. Allen, L.H.: Clin. Nutr. *3*:169–175, 1984.
20. WHO: Energy and Protein Requirements. WHO Technical Report Series No. 724. Geneva, WHO. 1985.
21. WHO: Infant and Young Child Nutrition. Report by the Director General to the World Health Assembly. March, 1983 (Document WHA 36/1983/7).
22. DeMaeyer, E.M.: Protein-energy malnutrition. *In* Nutrition in Preventive Medicine. (Beaton, G.H., Bengoa, J.M., Eds.) Geneva, WHO, 1976.
23. United Nations: Assessment of the World Food Situation, Present and Future. Rome, U.N. World Conference, 1974.
24. Fonaroff, A.: Bull. Pan. Am. Health Organ. *9*:112–123, 1975.
25. Ojofeitimi, E.O., Adelekan, M.O.: Child Care Health Dev. *10*:61–66, 1984.
26. Rynearson, E.H.: Nutr. Rev. *32* (Suppl. 1):1–14, 1974.
27. Raman, L.: Am. J. Clin. Nutr. *34*:775–783, 1981.
28. Scrimshaw, N.S., Taylor, C.E., Gordon, J.E.: Interactions of Nutrition and Infection. WHO Monograph Series No. 57. Geneva, WHO, 1968.
29. Keusch, G.T., Katz, M. (Eds.): Proceedings of Symposium held in Haiti, 1977. Am. J. Clin. Nutr. *31*:2035–2126, 2202–2356, 1978.
30. Mata, L.J.: The Children of Santa Maria Cauque: A Prospective Field Study of Health and Growth. Cambridge, MIT Press, 1978.
31. United Nations University: Protein-Energy Requirements under Conditions Prevailing in Developing Countries: Current Knowledge and Research Needs. United Nations Univ. Food Nutr. Bull. (Suppl. 1), 1979.
32. Torun, B., Caballero, B., Flores-Huerta, S., et al.: United Nations Univ. Food Nutr. Bull. Suppl. *10*:216–231, 1984.
33. Brown, K.H., Gilman, R.H., Khatun, M., et al.: Am. J. Clin. Nutr. *33*:1975–1982, 1980.

34. Keusch, G.T. (Ed.): Rev. Infect. Dis. *4*:735–911, 1982.

35. Munro, H.N., Crim, M.C.: The proteins and amino acids. *In* Modern Nutrition in Health and Disease. 6th ed. (Goodhart, R.S., Shils, M.E., Eds.) Philadelphia, Lea & Febiger, 1980.

36. Gordon, J.E., Chitkara, I.D., Wyon, J.B.: Am. J. Med. Sci. *245*:345–377, 1963.

37. Rowland, M.G.M., Cole, T.J., Whitehead, R.G.: Br. J. Nutr. *37*:441–450, 1977.

38. Torun, B.: Environmental and educational interventions against diarrhea in Guatemala. *In* Diarrhea and Malnutrition. (Chen, L.C., Scrimshaw, N.S., Eds.) New York, Plenum Press, 1983.

39. Ordy, J.M.: Postmaturity differences in carbohydrate, lipid, and protein intake and metabolism. *In* Nutrition in Gerontology. (Ordy, J.M., Harman, D., Alfin-Slater, R.B., Eds.) New York, Raven Press, 1984.

40. Rutishauser, I.H.E., Whitehead, R.G.: Br. J. Nutr. *28*:145–152, 1972.

41. Viteri, F.E., Torun, B.: Nutrition, physical activity and growth. *In* The Biology of Normal Human Growth. (Ritzén, M., Aperia, A., Hall, K., et al., Eds.) New York, Raven Press, 1981.

42. Torun B: Physiological measurements of physical activity among children under free-living conditions. *In* Energy Intake and Activity. (Pollitt, E., Amante, P., Eds.) New York, Alan R. Liss, 1984.

43. Viteri, F.E., Torun, B.: Bol. Of Sanit. Panam. *78*:58–74, 1975.

44. Torun, B., Viteri, F.E.: United Nations Univ. Food Nutr. Bull. Suppl. *5*:229–241, 1981.

45. Kerpel-Fronius, E., Varga, F., Kun, K.: Ann. Paediatr. (Basel) *183*:1–28, 1954.

46. Viteri, F.E., Alvarado, J.: Rev. Col. Med. (Guatemala) *21*:175–230, 1970.

47. Waterlow, J.C.: Adaptation to low protein intakes. *In* Protein-Calorie Malnutrition. (Olson, R.E., Ed.) New York, Academic Press, 1975.

48. Waterlow, J.C., Garlick, P.J., Millward, D.J.: Protein Turnover in Mammalian Tissues and in the Whole Body. Oxford, North Holland, 1978.

49. Stephen, J.M.L.: Br. J. Nutr. *22*:153–163, 1968.

50. Pineda, O.: Metabolic adaptation to nutritional stress. *In* Calorie Deficiencies and Protein Deficiencies. (McCance, R.A., Widdowson, E.M., Eds.) Boston, Little, Brown and Co., 1968.

51. Waterlow, J.C., Alleyne, G.A.O.: Adv. Protein Chem. *25*:117–241, 1971.

52. Metcoff, J.: Cellular energy metabolism in protein-calorie malnutrition. *In* Protein-Calorie Malnutrition. (Olson, R.E., Ed.) New York, Academic Press, 1975.

53. James, W.P.T., Hay, A.M.: J. Clin. Invest. *47*:1958–1972, 1968.

54. Crim, M.C., Munro, H.N.: Protein-energy malnutrition and endocrine function. *In* Endocrinology. (DeGroot, L.J., Cahill, G.F., Odell, W.D., et al., Eds.) New York, Grune and Stratton, 1979.

55. Gardner, L.I., Amacher, P. (Eds.): Endocrine Aspects of Malnutrition. Santa Ynez, CA, Kroc Foundation, 1973.

56. Becker, D.J.: Hormones and malnutrition. *In* Infant Feedings-Deficiencies-Diseases. (Lifshitz, F., Ed.) New York, Marcel Dekker, Inc., 1982.

57. Prinsloo, J.G., Freier, E., Kruger, H., et al.: S. Afr. Med. J. *48*:2303–2305, 1974.

58. Viteri, F.E.: Primary protein-energy malnutrition: Clinical, biochemical, and metabolic changes. *In* Textbook of Pediatric Nutrition. (Suskind, R.M., Ed.) New York, Raven Press, 1981.

59. Parra, A., Klish, W., Cuellar, A., et al.: J. Pediatr. *87*:307–314, 1975.

60. Daughaday, W.H., Herington, A.C., Phillips, L.S.: Annu. Rev. Physiol. *37*:211–244, 1975.

61. Picou, D., Taylor-Roberts, T.: Clin. Sci. *36*:283–296, 1969.

62. Ferreyra de Spada, E., Rivarola, M.A., Beas, F.: Arch. Latinoam. Nutr. *27*:9–15, 1977.

63. Olusi, S.O., Orrell, D.H., Morris, P.M., et al.: Clin. Chim. Acta *74*:261–269, 1977.

64. Smith, S.R., Edgar, P.J., Pozefsky, T., et al.: Metabolism *24*:1073–1084, 1975.

65. Trimarchi, F., Melluso, R., Sobbrio, G., et al.: Ann. Endocrinol. (Paris) *41*:371–378, 1980.

66. Sreedhar, R., Ghosh, K.K., Chakravarty, I.: Hum. Nutr. Clin. Nutr. *37*:373–379, 1983.

67. Viteri, F.E., Alvarado, J., Luthringer, D.G., et al.: Vitam. Horm. *26*:573–615, 1968.

68. Caballero, B., Solomons, N.W., Batres, R., et al.: J. Pediatr. Gastroenterol. Nutr. *4*:97–102, 1985.

69. Viart, P.: Am. J. Clin. Nutr. *30*:334–348, 1977.

70. Viart, P.: Am. J. Clin. Nutr. *31*:911–926, 1978.

71. Heymsfield, S.B., Bethel, R.A., Ansley, J.D., et al.: Am. Heart J. *95*:584–594, 1978.

72. Alleyne, G.A.O.: Pediatrics *39*:400–411, 1967.

73. Paniagua, R., Santos, D., Munoz, R., et al.: Pediatr. Res. *14*:1260–1262, 1980.

74. Mahakur, A.C., Mishra, A.C., Panda, S.N., et al.: J. Assoc. Physicians India *31*:79–81, 1983.

75. Keusch, G.T., Wilson, C.S., Waksal, S.D.: Nutrition, host defenses and the lymphoid system. *In* Advances in Host Defense Mechanisms, Vol 2. (Gallin, J.I., Fauci, A.S., Eds.) New York, Raven Press, 1983.

76. Keusch, G.T.: Clin. Nutr. *3*:156–160, 1984.

77. Chandra, R.K.: Clin. Exp. Immunol. *51*:126–132, 1983.

78. Olusi, S.O., Thurman, G.B., Goldstein, A.L.: Clin. Immunol. Immunopathol. *15*:687–691, 1980.

79. Keusch, G.T., Torun, B., Johnson, R.B., et al.: J. Pediatr. *105*:434–436, 1984.

80. Chandra, R.K.: Pediatrics *67*:407–411, 1981.

81. Parra, A., Garza, C., Garza, Y., et al.: J. Pediatr. *82*:133–142, 1973.

82. Nichols, B.L., Alvarado, J., Hazlewood, C.F., et al.: J. Pediatr. *80*:319–330, 1972.

83. Lopes, J., Russell, D.M., Whitwell, J., et al.: Am. J. Clin. Nutr. *36*:602–610, 1982.

84. Viteri, F.E., Schneider, R.: Med. Clin. North Am. *58*:1487–1505, 1974.

85. Torun, B., Solomons, N.W., Viteri, F.E.: Arch. Latinoam. Nutr. *29*:445–494, 1979.

86. Lifshitz, F., Teichber, S., Wapnir, R.A.: Malnutrition and the intestine. *In* Nutrition and Child Health: A Perspective for the 1980's. (Tsang, R.C., Nichols, B.L., Eds.) New York, Alan R. Liss, 1981.

87. Torun, B.: Nutrient absorption in malnutrition. *In* Interactions of Parasite Diseases and Nutrition. Vatican, Pontificia Academia Scientiarum, 1986.

88. Winick, M.: Fed. Proc. *29*:1510–1515, 1970.

89. Winick, M.: Malnutrition and Brain Development. New York, Oxford University Press, 1976.

90. Wurtman, R.J., Wurtman, J.J., (Eds.): Nutrition and the Brain, Vol 2. New York, Raven Press, 1977.

91. Kumar, A., Ghai, O.P., Singh N: J. Pediatr. *90*:149–153, 1977.

92. Ghosh, S., Vaid, K., Mohan, M., et al.: J. Neurol. Neurosurg. Psychiatry *42*:760–763, 1979.
93. Anderson, G.H.: Br. Med. Bull. *37*:95–100, 1981.
94. McCance, R.A., Widdowson, E.M.: Lancet *2*:158–159, 1966.
95. Whitehead, R.G., Alleyne, G.A.O.: Br. Med. Bull. *28*:72–78, 1972.
96. Anonymous: Nutr. Rev. *37*:250–252, 1979.
97. Jaya-Rao, K.S.: Lancet *1*:709–711, 1974.
98. Reddy, V.: Protein-energy malnutrition: An overview. *In* Nutrition in Health and Disease and International Development. (Harper, A.E., Davis, G.K., Eds.) New York, Alan R. Liss. 1981.
99. Rosen, E., Buchanan, N., Hansen, J.D.L.: Lancet *2*:458, 1974.
100. Waterlow, J.C.: Lancet *2*:712, 1974.
101. Olson, R.E.: Am. J. Clin. Nutr. *28*:626–637, 1975.
102. Alleyne, G.A.O., Trust, P.M., Flores, H., et al.: Br. J. Nutr. *27*:585–592, 1972.
103. Munro, H.N.: General aspects of the regulation of protein metabolism by diet and by hormones. *In* Mammalian Protein Metabolism, Vol 1. (Munro, H.N., Allison, J.B., Eds.) New York, Academic Press, 1964.
104. Eisenstein, A.B., Singh, S.P.: Hormonal control of nutrient metabolism. *In* Modern Nutrition in Health and Disease. 6th ed. (Goodhart, R.S., Shils, M.E., Eds.) Philadelphia, Lea & Febiger, 1980.
105. Arroyave, G., Wilson, D., Funes, C., et al.: Am. Clin. Nutr. *11*:517–524, 1962.
106. Holt, L.E., Snyderman, S.E., Norton, P.M., et al.: Lancet *2*:1343–1348, 1963.
107. Vis, H.L.: Aspects de Mecanismes des Hyperaminoaciduries de L'Enfance. Paris, Editions Arsica, 1963.
108. Kirtzinger, E.E., Kanengoni, E., Jones, J.J.: Lancet *1*:412–413, 1972.
109. Beitins, I.Z., Graham, G.G., Kowarski, A., et al.: J. Pediatr. *84*:444–451, 1974.
110. Van der Westhuysen, J.M., Kanengoni, E., Jones, J.J., et al.: S. Afr. Med. J. *49*:1729–1731, 1975.
111. Cohen, S., Hansen, J.D.L.: Clin. Sci. *23*:351–359, 1962.
112. Beisel, W.R.: Annu. Rev. Med. *26*:9–20, 1975.
113. Koj, A.: Acute-phase reactants. Their synthesis, turnover and biological significance. *In* Structure and Function of Plasma Proteins, Vol 1. (Allison, A.C., Ed.) New York, Plenum Press, 1974.
114. Schelp, F.P., Migasena, P., Pongpaew, P., et al.: Am. J. Clin. Nutr. *31*:451–456, 1978.
115. Neufeld, H.A., Pace, J.A., White, F.E.: Metabolism *25*:877–884, 1976.
116. Beisel, W.R., Sawyer, W.D., Ryll, E.D., et al.: Ann. Intern. Med. *67*:744–779, 1967.
117. Beisel, W.R.: Am. J. Clin. Nutr. *30*:1236–1247, 1977.
118. Powanda, M.C.: Am. J. Clin. Nutr. *30*:1254–1268, 1977.
119. Torun, B., Viteri, F.E.: Rev. Col. Med. (Guatemala) *27*:43–62, 1976.
120. Patrick, J.: Br. Med. J. *1*:1051–1054, 1977.
121. Solomons, N.W.: Clin. Nutr. *3*:151–155, 1984.
122. Habicht, J.P., Martorell, R., Yarbrough, C., et al.: Lancet *1*:611–615, 1974.
123. Graitcer, P.L., Gentry, E.M.: Lancet *2*:297–299, 1981.
124. United States Dept. Health Education and Welfare: NCHS Growth Curves for Children from Birth to 18 Years. Hyattsville, DHEW Publ. PHS 78–1650, 1977.
125. Waterlow, J.C.: Classification and definition of protein-energy malnutrition. *In* Nutrition in Preventive Medicine. (Beaton, G.H., Bengoa, J.M., Eds.) Geneva, WHO, 1976.
126. Nabarro, D., McNab, S.: J. Trop. Med. Hyg. *83*:21–33, 1980.
127. Torun, B., Samayoa, C., Garcia, B.: Arch. Latinoam. Nutr. In press, 1987.
128. Torun, B., Samayoa, C.: Hum. Nutr. Appl. Nutr. Submitted, 1986.
129. Gomez, F., Ramos-Galvan, R., Frenk, S.: Adv. Pediatr. *7*:131–169, 1955.
130. Graham, G.G.: The later growth of malnourished infants: Effects of age, severity, and subsequent diet. *In* Calorie Deficiencies and Protein Deficiencies. (McCance, R.A., Widdowson, E.M., Eds.) London, Churchill, 1968.
131. Jelliffe, D.B., Jelliffe, E.F.P.: J. Trop. Pediatr. *15*:253–260, 1969.
132. Arnhold, R.: J. Trop. Pediatr. *15*:243–247, 1969.
133. Kanawati, A.A., McLaren, D.S.: Nature *28*:573–575, 1970.
134. Habicht, J.P., Lechtig, A., Yarbrough, C., et al.: Maternal nutrition, birth weight and infant mortality. *In* Size at Birth. (Elliott, K., Knight, J., Eds.) Ciba Foundation Symposium 27. Amsterdam, Associated Scientific Publishers, 1974.
135. Viteri, F.E., Alvarado, J.: Pediatrics *46*:696–706, 1970.
136. Miller, F.N.: Peery and Miller's Pathology. 3rd ed. Boston, Little, Brown and Co., 1978.
137. Bengoa, J.M.: Significance of malnutrition and priorities for its prevention. *In* Nutrition, National Development and Planning. (Berg, A., Scrimshaw, N.S., Calloway, D.A., Eds.) Cambridge, MIT Press, 1971.
138. Chen, L.C., Chowdry, A.K.M.A., Hoffman, S.L.: Am. J. Clin. Nutr. *33*:1838–1845, 1980.
139. Torun, B., Keusch, G.T., Cruz, J.R., et al.: INCAP Annual Report. Scientific Publication V-47. Guatemala, INCAP, 1984.
140. Janssen, F., Bouton, J.M., Vuye, A., et al.: JPEN *7*:26–36, 1983.
141. Solomons, N.W., Torun, B., Caballero, B., et al.: Am. J. Clin. Nutr. *40*:591–600, 1984.
142. Torun, B., Solomons, N.W., Caballero, B., et al.: Am. J. Clin. Nutr. *40*:601–610, 1984.
143. Cameron, C., Hofvander, Y.: Manual on Feeding Infants and Young Children. 2nd ed. New York, United Nations Protein-Calorie Advisory Group, 1976.
144. Torun, B., Young, V.R., Rand, W.M. (Eds.): Protein-Energy Requirements of Developing Countries: Evaluation of New Data. Tokyo, United Nations Univ. Food Nutr. Bull. (Suppl. 5) 1981.
145. Rand, W.M., Uauy, R., Scrimshaw, N.S. (Eds.): Protein-Energy Requirement Studies in Developing Countries: Results of International Research. Tokyo, United Nations Univ. Food Nutr. Bull. (Suppl. 10), 1984.
146. Torun, B., Schutz, Y., Bradfield, R.B., et al.: Effect of physical activity upon growth of children recovering from protein-calorie malnutrition (PCM). *In* Proceed. 10 Internat. Congr. Nutr. Kyoto, Victory-sha Press, 1976.
147. Torun, B.: Alimentación de niños con desnutrición proteínico-energética y diarrea, con énfasis en las

experiencias del INCAP. Pan Am Health Organization meeting on Feeding of Children Ill with Diarrhea. Washington, DC, PAHO, 1983.

148. Viteri, F.E., Torun, B., Arroyave, G., et al.: Food Nutr. Bull. Suppl. *5*:202–209, 1981.

149. Torun, B., Viteri, F.E.: Protein-energy malnutrition. *In* Tropical and Geographical Medicine. (Warren, K.S., Mahmoud, A.A.F., Eds.) New York, McGraw-Hill Book Co., 1984.

150. INCAP: Evaluación Nutricional de la Población de Centro América y Panamá: Guatemala. Guatemala, Inst. Nutr. Centro América y Panama, 1969.

*Chapter* **43**

# STARVATION

## L. John Hoffer

Graham Lusk in 1928 defined starvation as the deprivation of any element necessary for an organism's nutrition.[1] Nowadays, the term usually refers to a chronic, inadequate intake of dietary energy, protein, or both. In this chapter the modern definition is adopted, while recognizing that clinical starvation typically is accompanied by multiple nutrient deficiencies. Studies of normal weight or obese, but otherwise healthy subjects, provided most of the information discussed here, because they allow the clearest description of the metabolic response to starvation. Some of these studies, such as the one by Ancel Keys and his collaborators,[2] are acknowledged classics of physiologic research.

Although a biochemical understanding of the adaptation to starvation is the ultimate goal, at present this is still a remote ideal. Modern studies of starvation at the tissue level often require the removal of a part of the body from its normal nutritional and hormonal environment, so the results obtained may not be directly applicable to the physiologic situation. At our present stage of understanding, studies in the intact organism continue to be essential, and the best older writing of the earlier years of this century continues to be relevant for the contemporary student.

This chapter is divided into four sections. First, techniques for the study of human protein metabolism are described, since these were used to obtain much of the material described subsequently. Second, the concept of protein storage and labile protein is reviewed. Third, the general concepts of the adaptation to protein and energy malnutrition are outlined. Finally, human protein metabolism during total fasting and some related subjects are discussed.

## CLINICAL LABORATORY TECHNIQUES FOR THE STUDY OF STARVATION

### Fuel Utilization

The rates of consumption of protein, fat, and carbohydrate in the living organism may be calculated from the dietary intake, rate of energy expenditure, respiratory quotient, and body nitrogen (N) excretion. To illustrate: The N content of the mixed proteins of the body is 16%. Thus, 1 g of excreted N represents a loss from the body of 6.25 g of mixed proteins.[3] Intracellular protein exists in approximately a 20 to 25% aqueous solution in the lean tissue of the body (the fat-free, connective tissue-free and bone-free "wet" tissue). Assuming that 1 g protein is associated with 5 g of hydrated lean tissue, then 1 g of excreted nitrogen represents a loss of 6.25 × 5 = 31 g of lean tissue. A similar figure of 32 g of lean tissue/g nitrogen is a frequently used approximation to this value.[4] Extracellular (structural) protein makes up a large proportion of total body protein and is also lost in increased amounts during starvation.[5] However, losses of this metabolically inactive protein are small in comparison to those of lean tissue protein.[6]

Glycogen, the body's endogenous carbohydrate storage form, is found in muscle, liver, and to a lesser extent in other tissues. Stores of approximately 200 g in muscle and 100 g liver are typical for a resting average man following the overnight fast.[7] Glycogen is stored in a solution of 3 to 4 g water/g glycogen.[8] The rate of carbohydrate and fat oxidation can be determined by indirect calorimetry and their contribution to total weight loss thereby deduced. Other techniques more related to the study of body composition are covered in Chapter 30.

### Nitrogen Balance

In use for 150 years, nitrogen balance is one of the mainstays of starvation studies.[9,10] Recent work has defined its limitations and reconfirmed its value when meticulously carried out.[11,12] N balance detects small gains or losses of body protein in the whole organism.

### Organ Balance

With the organ balance technique the concentrations of nutrients in the blood vessels that supply and drain a particular tissue bed are sampled by means of indwelling catheters. Multiplication of the blood arteriovenous difference by the flow rate through the tissue yields the rate of organ uptake or output of the element of interest, provided that flow can be measured accurately and is not perturbed by the measurement technique itself.

Measurements of this kind demonstrate a dynamic transfer of nutrients among different tissues. However, the approach has a number of limitations. Extrapolation from arteriovenous differences across limb muscle beds to whole body muscle metabolism may be misleading because of different metabolic behavior of different

muscle types and groups and because of difficulty in estimating muscle mass precisely. Moreover, skin and adipose tissue also make a contribution to limb metabolism. In the intact organism one cannot separate the splanchnic circulation into its liver and intestinal components without resorting to portal vein catheterization, so arterial-hepatic venous differences reflect the combined influences of all the splanchnic organs. Furthermore, net uptake or release of substrates from a tissue bed does not reveal the metabolic handling within the tissue. This is of particular interest in the study of protein metabolism, for the rate of protein synthesis and protein breakdown (proteolysis) may be wholly or partly independent of the rate of amino acid uptake or release from the whole tissue. A tissue may go into negative amino acid balance even with an unchanged or decreased rate of proteolysis, as would occur if protein synthesis fell to a slower rate than breakdown. Indeed, this pattern is characteristic of chronic starvation. The distinction between "proteolysis" (which designates the absolute rate of protein breakdown) and "net proteolysis" (protein breakdown minus protein synthesis) must be borne in mind.[13]

### Methylhistidine Excretion

The methylhistidine excretion technique for measuring simple proteolysis in specific tissues is based on the observation that certain histidine residues of the contractile protein actomyosin are posttranslationally methylated at the 3 position. When the protein breaks down, the 3-methylhistidine is released into the tissues and thence into the circulation and subsequently is excreted almost quantitatively in the urine. Thus, the urinary 3-methylhistidine excretion rate indicates the rate of whole-body actomyosin proteolysis.[14,15] Because skeletal muscle tissue is the greatest reservoir of actomyosin, it has been assumed that 3-methylhistidine excretion is a measure of skeletal muscle proteolysis. However, studies in the rat indicate that protein turnover in the smooth muscle of the gastrointestinal tract may be so rapid that 3-methylhistidine from this source could contribute as much as 50% of the total urinary excretion.[16,17] In the human, skeletal muscle probably accounts for 75% of urinary excretion of 3-methylhistidine.[18–20] Clinical measurements require the short-term dietary exclusion of animal meat, a source of exogenous 3-methylhistidine.

### Tracer Studies

Turnover of substrates may be determined in the whole body and in selected tissues in vivo by techniques involving the administration of isotopic tracers. Figure 43–1 illustrates the features of a simple one-pool model for whole-body kinetics of leucine.[21,22] A leucine turnover study is conducted in the following manner. The tracer amino acid is administered at a constant, known

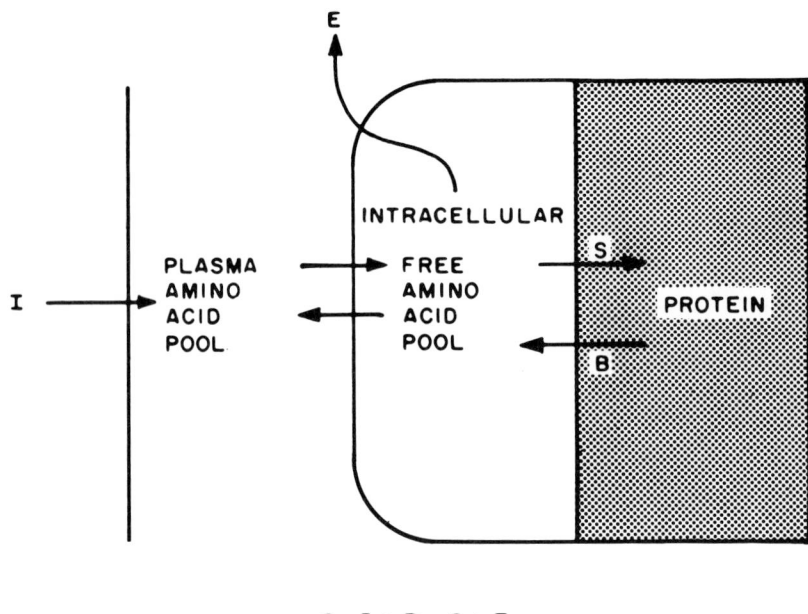

$$Q = I + B = S + E$$

**Fig. 43–1.** A model for body amino acid turnover. The plasma-free amino acid pool is assumed to be in rapid equilibrium with the intracellular pool. Amino acids enter this general free amino acid pool when dietary protein is consumed, or when tissue proteins are broken down to release their constituent amino acids. The sum of the dietary amino acid intake (I) and breakdown (B) is equal to the entry rate, or flux (Q), of amino acids into the pool. Amino acids leave the pool either to be taken up into newly synthesized proteins (S) or when they are oxidized or otherwise irreversibly biotransformed and their metabolic end products are excreted (E). In the steady state, the entry rate of amino acids equals the exit rate from the pool; thus, $Q = I + B = S + E$. As I and E can be measured, and Q determined using tracer methods, values relating to whole body protein synthesis (S) and breakdown (B) may be derived.

rate until its concentration in the sampled blood reaches a steady state as verified by serial measurements. Equilibrium is achieved within only 2 or 3 hours because, despite the large mass of body protein, the free amino acid pools are small. The concentration of the tracer in unlabeled free leucine is known as the "specific radioactivity" when the tracer is labeled with a radioactive isotope (such as [14]C) and the "isotopic enrichment" when the tracer is labeled with a stable isotope (such as [13]C). In the latter case, the tracer is distinguished from unlabeled leucine by the slightly greater mass of the labeled molecule, using the technique of mass spectrometry.[23,24] The specific activity (or isotopic enrichment) of leucine at steady state is determined by the (known) contribution of tracer and the (unknown) contribution of endogenous leucine, which, in the absence of food intake, is entirely derived from endogenous protein breakdown. Thus, for a radioisotope study,

$$\text{specific radioactivity (measured)} = \frac{\text{rate of administration of radioactivity (known)}}{\text{rate of appearance of endogenous leucine (unknown)}}$$

The equation is then solved for the unknown value, the rate of appearance of leucine in the plasma. In the steady state the rate of appearance of leucine (derived from protein breakdown) must equal its rate of removal from the circulation. Removed leucine has two possible fates: either to be taken up into newly synthesized protein or to be oxidized. The first irreversible step of leucine oxidation is decarboxylation. By labeling leucine at the carboxyl carbon and monitoring the rate of appearance of labeled carbon dioxide in expired air, one may derive a value for the rate of leucine oxidation.[21,22,24] If this value is subtracted from that for total removal from the circulation, the rate of leucine uptake into newly synthesized protein is obtained.

Another useful tracer methodology uses [15]N-glycine to determine N turnover. The labeled N distributes widely in the free amino acid pool and ultimately equilibrates in the pools of urea and ammonia, the excretion end products of amino acid oxidation. By measuring [15]N isotopic enrichment in the urea or ammonia pools, it is possible to calculate whole body N turnover and protein breakdown and synthesis using the same arguments as in the previous paragraph.[21,25] In this case, total amino acid oxidation is directly measured from urine N excretion rather than inferred from appearance of tracer in expired $CO_2$.

This simplified model for protein turnover has important practical and conceptual limitations.[22,26] The specific activity of plasma free amino acids is higher than that within the tissues, to an extent that varies for different amino acids and in different tissues. The result is the underestimation of leucine turnover.[26] The problem has been addressed in the case of leucine by measuring the specific activity of plasma 2-ketoisocaproate, leucine's transamination product generated intracellularly and subsequently released into the circulation (discussed later). Another limitation of the method is that extrapolation of plasma turnover figures for individual amino acids to whole protein turnover is risky because the turnover of individual amino acids may not always represent the fate of all proteins, and the molar contribution of a particular amino acid to the total in the proteins contributing to the turnover is at best an educated guess. Finally, the turnover value derived is an integrated value for all the proteins in the body and cannot by itself separate those turning over rapidly or slowly. However, these limitations are more than compensated for by the method's potential to give insight into the dynamic aspects of protein and amino acid metabolism in the intact organism. Several investigations are currently refining the model.[27,28] It has been found that the rate of plasma leucine oxidation (as determined by tracer infusion), correlates positively with the rate of total amino acid oxidation as determined from urinary N excretion.[29–31] This indicates that under certain circumstances, at least, the fate of administered tracer leucine truly reflects the rate of net protein degradation.

## LABILE PROTEIN

In metabolically stable adults on a maintenance diet adequate in protein and energy, total N output from the body approximates the intake, resulting in zero N balance, or "equilibrium." Following the transition from such a diet to one that is protein-free but still adequate in energy, urinary N decreases to reach, after a period of 6 to 10 days, a steady value of approximately 2 to 3 g/d, the so-called "obligatory" or "endogenous" rate of urinary N loss.[9,32,33] Obligatory N losses in the feces, secretions, and skin have likewise been determined to be approximately 1 g/d.[34,35] Historically, recommendations for protein intake have been based in part on the concept that replacement of the obligatory loss with an equivalent amount of

high-quality protein will meet the nutritional requirement.[34] This section deals with the significance of the protein rapidly mobilized during the period of adaptation from an adequate to a low protein diet.

Carl Voit first demonstrated in 1866 the existence, in the well-nourished animal, of a quantity of readily available protein determined by the protein content of the diet and excreted during the first several days of fasting or on changing from a higher to a lower protein intake.[32] This is now known to be a general phenomenon of body protein gain or loss over several days in response to variations in the protein intake level, energy level, or to a variety of hormonal and physiologic stimuli.[32] In the case of the human switched from a normal diet to a protein-free diet, when the original protein intake is resumed, N balance becomes positive and body protein is reaccumulated until the previous losses are made up (Fig. 43–2). This protein readily gained or lost from the body is termed *labile protein*.[32,33] It constitutes about 3% of the total body protein in well-nourished rats or humans.[32] In the human, labile protein is thus represented by about 50 to 60 g N (or 300 to 400

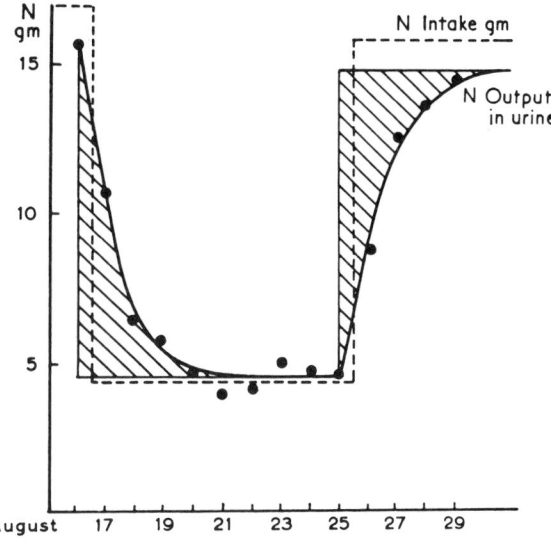

**Fig. 43–2.** Labile protein. The solid line indicates the N excretion of a human subject abruptly changed to a low-protein diet. The dashed line indicates the level of N intake. Initially, the N intake approximates its excretion, and the subject is close to N equilibrium. Upon switching to the lower N intake, N losses exceed the intake for several days until equilibrium is re-established. The N lost from the body during this period is shown in the first shaded area. On resuming the former intake, the subject stores N, as shown by the second shaded area. The two shaded areas are approximately equal. (Reproduced from Munro, H.N.,[32] with permission of the author and Academic Press.

g protein), an insignificant figure in terms of total body N economy but one which is important to recognize in assessing the adaptive response to starvation.

After a loss of labile protein in response to a dietary deprivation, protein loss will cease if the new level of intake is compatible with maintenance or continue at a lower, constant rate from less readily mobilized "endogenous" sources.[33] In the protein-deficient or fasted rat, the greatest acute loss of protein is from the liver, with the other visceral organs making large contributions as well. This is in accord with the more rapid turnover rates of proteins in these organs. With prolongation of the protein-deficient diet, subsequent losses occur as well from muscle, quantitatively the major nonstructural protein store.[32]

## Metabolic Significance

Although small, the amount of labile protein in the body is still larger than the free amino acid pool, which makes up only about 0.5 to 1.0% of total body amino acids.[36,37] The free amino acid pool, because of its disproportionately small size and rapid turnover, can be assumed to play an essential role in the regulation of synthesis and breakdown of protein tissue.[37] Labile protein undergoes the most rapid exchange with the free amino acid pool and must, therefore, be important in determining amino acid utilization, particularly of amino acids newly entering from the diet.[32]

In order to distinguish the effects of acute changes in labile protein from the chronic effects of the dietary change, studies on the effects of starvation must allow for a period of several days for the body to come into a new adapted state. During this time the content of enzymes in the liver and other tissues is altered to re-establish optimal metabolism of the amino acids and energy substrates in the new diet. The biochemical adaptation to a new diet may require only a few days, but even more rapid changes occur every day because food typically is consumed intermittently. In the course of meal consumption, the free amino acid and even protein content of the tissues undergoes cyclic oscillations within hours. Waterlow and Garlick draw an important distinction between "regulation," which they define as the usual short-term adjustments to internal and external changes (for example, to the intake of a *customary meal*), and "adaptation," which is the setting of a new, oscillating steady state (as in the response to a *new dietary pattern*). When observations are made at a given moment, it is necessary to distinguish the long-term effects of the diet from the short-term effects of the last meal or of the interval since the last meal.[38]

## Effect of Meals on Protein Metabolism

It is self-evident that the body can gain in protein (and energy) stores only when food is consumed. It is less obvious, but apparently true, that the fate of dietary amino acids—a choice between uptake into new protein synthesis or catabolism with formation of urea or ammonium—is largely determined during or shortly after their initial absorption into the body. Transient increases in plasma urea and urinary urea excretion follow meals.[39] Studies employing direct catheterization of the portal and hepatic veins demonstrate a large postprandial increase in urea output in association with the hepatic uptake of amino acids derived from dietary protein.[40]

Comparisons have been made between the fed (absorptive) and between-meal (postabsorptive) state in humans by means of labeled leucine infusions. The consumption of a protein-containing meal results in an increase both in whole-body leucine oxidation and its incorporation into protein, but different conclusions as to an effect on protein breakdown have been reached.[20,41–43]

Plasma concentrations of the essential amino acids are only modestly perturbed during protein meals, despite a large intake of amino acids in relation to the size of the free amino acid pool.[44] This relative stability of the free amino acid pool can be achieved by an increase in protein synthesis (thereby hastening removal of amino acids from their free pools), by a decrease in endogenous protein breakdown (decreasing entry into the pools), or by an increase in amino acid oxidation. In this setting, oxidation may be considered an overflow device that eliminates amino acids from the body when their free-pool size increases. Meal-related enhancement of protein synthesis and diminished protein breakdown, particularly in the liver, would divert amino acids from oxidation by limiting the increase in the size of the free amino acid pool. The result is a transient increase in the body's protein content—labile protein. The amount of labile protein present at any moment is determined by the activity of the amino acid metabolizing enzymes as programmed by the preceding habitual diet. In the interval between meals, a finer tuned regulation may occur, as some of the amino acids in the labile proteins accumulated acutely during the dietary influx are released and redistributed for the synthesis of more slowly turning over proteins.[32] Because amino acid oxidation does not cease during this period, the body still has an opportunity to retain or discharge some body protein.

Since leucine makes up about 8% by weight of the proteins turning over in the body,[45] total amino acid turnover in the postabsorptive state is estimated to be about 10 g/h.[46] This is a substantial rate when compared with an influx of 20 or 30 g of dietary amino acids over a few hours during a protein meal. The importance of the splanchnic tissues and labile protein become clear when it is considered that the splanchnic tissues are the primary recipients of this concentrated dose of amino acids, whereas postabsorptive turnover relates to the flux through all the tissues of the body.

It should not be assumed, however, that a meal-related enhancement in protein synthesis occurs only in the splanchnic organs. A recent study in humans demonstrates a rise in the fed-state synthesis rate of skeletal muscle protein as well.[20]

## RESPONSE TO PROTEIN- AND ENERGY-DEFICIENT DIETS

An energy-deficient diet is one that provides less utilizable food energy than the body expends. Adaptation to such a diet typically includes a decrease in physical activity and a decrease in the resting energy expenditure.[35] When these decreases do not re-equate the energy output to the limited intake, endogenous fuels must be used to balance the equation, and a net loss of body substance ensues. This states the long-recognized thermodynamic law of starvation.

### Body Fuel Stores

Fat is the major storage fuel of animals, and in fasting, the body fat supply appears to determine the length of survival. Fat makes up 20 to 25% of body weight in men and 25 to 30% in women. This would provide 60 to 70 days of fuel, assuming an energy expenditure of 2,000 kcal/day. In obesity, fat storage is far greater. One obese individual survived a fast of 310 days,[47] whereas the survival of nonobese fasting individuals coincides roughly with the predicted time of depletion of fat, approximately 60 days.[48]

In contrast, carbohydrate is a quantitatively insignificant storage fuel. The combined caloric value of liver glycogen (100 g), muscle glycogen (200 g) and circulating free glucose (20 g) amounts to 1,200 kcal, less than a single day's resting energy consumption.[7] Yet glucose has unique characteristics that make it an essential body fuel: (1) it is a rapidly mobilizable energy source; (2) it can be metabolized along the glycolytic pathway without oxygen (useful in oxygen-deprived tissues such as anaerobically exercising muscle); (3) it is the obligatory fuel for blood cells and, under most circumstances, for the brain. The brain's moment-to-moment dependence on carbohydrate has far-reaching consequences that account for much of the biochemical adaptation to total fasting (see below).

Body protein is present in amounts of about 12 kg, but only 6 to 7 kg of this are in actively metabolizing tissues, the rest being structural. The active protein tissue (30 to 40 kg of hydrated lean tissue) could theoretically supply about 2 weeks' worth of calories. But, unlike carbohydrate and fat, even a relatively modest depletion of the active protein store has profound adverse functional consequences. In the nonobese individual, weight loss in chronic starvation is roughly proportional to the lean tissue loss,[2] and weight or protein losses in the range of 50% or more are incompatible with survival.[49,50] The essentiality of body protein for survival has long been known from studies of prolonged starvation in animals. In the course of fatal starvation, fat loss is accompanied by a continuing drain of body protein, though the protein losses are increasingly curtailed as starvation progresses. After the fat is largely depleted, a reversal of protein economy and an outpouring of urinary N have been described by some (but not all) observers as a "premortal rise in N excretion" that signals the obligatory switch to protein as fuel, followed very shortly by death.[1,33] The importance of body protein for health and survival explains why efforts to understand protein metabolism and to ensure its maintenance are a major focus of research in starvation.

### Determinants of Protein Losses

If the intake of other nutrients is otherwise adequate, N balance after adaptation to a protein- and energy-deficient diet is determined by several factors: energy balance, protein intake, protein nutritional state, biologic individuality, and obesity.

**Energy Balance.** Under normal conditions, and over a range of fixed levels of protein intake, N balance at a constant protein intake is improved by an increase and worsened by a decrease in energy intake.[32,51] The energy effect is most potent in the modestly submaintenance range for both protein and energy.[52] Under most circumstances the source of the fuel (carbohydrate or fat) is immaterial.[10]

Kinney and Elwyn have refined this concept by emphasizing the importance of the *energy balance* (the difference between exogenous energy ingested and energy expended).[53] As this is the amount of dietary energy "left over" or in deficit after accounting for expenditure, the energy balance may be the specific physiologic variable that modifies the N balance. This would be particularly important to consider in hospitalized patients in whom energy expenditure rates may vary considerably.

**Protein Intake.** Over a wide range of energy intake, N balance is improved by an increased protein intake.[32] The protein effect is most marked for increases from very low to moderate levels of protein intake. As N intake increases into the maintenance range (and at maintenance energy), improvements in N balance continue but do not keep pace, implying less efficient retention of dietary protein in the high range of protein intakes.[34,35] The energy and protein effects are interactive. Thus, the beneficial effect of an increase in energy intake can be prevented by an inadequate protein intake. An improvement in N balance due to increased protein intake will be lessened if there is insufficient dietary energy.[32] In the United States the current recommended dietary allowance for protein assumes that the energy intake is at the maintenance level.[54]

**Protein Nutritional Status.** It has long been recognized that the efficiency of N retention at a given level of protein and energy is increased by prior protein depletion.[55] As already demonstrated, this phenomenon occurs with respect to depletion and repletion of labile protein (Fig. 43–2). It also applies to major (endogenous) protein loss as in prolonged starvation. One may speculate that the labile protein pool remains submaximal as long as the endogenous protein pools are depleted, providing a potential mechanism for the increased protein avidity that occurs under these conditions. Increased avidity for protein also occurs during active growth.

The effect on protein economy of diets that are submaintenance in both protein and energy is similar to that of low-protein, high-energy diets, except that fat loss occurs (because endogenous fuel must now make up the energy deficit) and N losses are greater because energy deprivation impairs the efficiency of protein retention. If the deficits are not ultimately lethal, prolonged negative N balance will persist until the continuing depletion of body protein enhances the body's avidity for protein sufficiently to re-establish N equilibrium. This new steady state is obtained at the expense of diminished body protein stores and a slowing of body protein turnover.[56,57] Therefore, the attainment of zero N balance on a particular diet does not, in itself, permit the conclusion that the diet is nutritionally adequate.[58]

The increased avidity of protein retention during prolonged protein depletion probably relates in part to a simple diminution of the mass of active body protein, without need to postulate other mechanisms to improve the efficiency of amino acid utilization.[35] The maintenance protein re-

quirement of a slight individual will be less than that of a large, muscular one. An appropriate minimum protein requirement is therefore most accurately defined in terms of body stature, and this is the recommendation for well-nourished individuals.[35,54]

**Biologic Individuality.** This is a convenient label for internal factors, presently unknown, which result in a large individual variation in the response to a given diet. When unexpected responses are observed, attention should always be directed to correctable factors in the environment such as the adequacy of micronutrient provision[59] and the possible presence of physiologic stress (e.g., to cold, infection, or trauma). Even when these factors are controlled, the variation in individual responses to starvation is wide.[60,61] This is consistent with the scope of biochemical individuality[62] and specifically with the wide variation in individual amino acid requirements of normal men.[63]

**Obesity.** Comparisons of N excretion by lean and obese individuals in different starvation studies have suggested to some observers that protein may be conserved more efficiently by obese individuals under these conditions.[2,64] In the rat, a short-term protein-sparing effect of obesity seems established.[65] Nevertheless, in human studies in which it is possible specifically to examine an effect of adiposity on protein loss in starvation, eliminating as much as possible the effects of sex, diet composition, and prior protein depletion, no important differences have been observed.[66–69]

Forbes has observed that the rate of weight loss at a given time during total fasting is directly proportional to body weight.[70] A similar relationship holds for the rate of N loss and lean body mass as estimated from urinary creatinine excretion.[71,72] In agreement, N losses of starving obese individuals on diets of fixed protein intake vary directly with the urinary creatinine excretion.[69,73,74] To the extent that the lean tissue mass is increased in very obese individuals, their absolute rate of N loss will therefore be greater than that of leaner individuals,[75] a finding compatible with the notion that protein requirements are proportional to the lean body mass.[54] Since similar rates of N loss occur in obese fasting individuals and in most normal-weight fasting individuals, both in early and adapted total fasting,[69] it is possible that relative to the total amount of lean tissue present, the *fractional* N loss could be somewhat slower in obesity. However, clearcut quantitation of this relationship is lacking.

## Adaptation of Protein Metabolism

In the rat, the feeding of a protein-deficient diet results in adaptive changes in the activities of amino acid-metabolizing enzymes in the liver and elsewhere, accompanied by changes in the rate of protein synthesis and breakdown. Protein deficiency decreases protein synthesis in muscle[76,77] and liver.[76,78,79] The decrease in liver protein synthesis in association with low-protein meals is consistent with in vitro findings of an activation of protein synthetic machinery in response to fluctuations in the amino acid supply comparable to those encountered normally during ingestion of protein meals.[80] The increased protein synthetic response to amino acids can also be evoked in the isolated perfused liver, showing that the hormonal responses evoked during meal absorption are not essential for liver protein synthesis.[80] Early in the feeding of a protein-deficient diet, liver protein breakdown rates are maintained.[79] This, together with slowed synthesis rates, accounts for the rapid loss of liver substance in early protein depletion.

When assessed on a whole-body basis by means of tracer leucine infusions, protein synthesis, oxidation, and breakdown all decrease during protein deficiency in both rats[77] and humans.[41] During the refeeding of previously starved patients, body protein turnover may increase to above-normal values at the same time that nitrogen balance becomes positive.[56] Even late in refeeding and when the characteristically depressed serum levels of most essential amino acids are near normal, the rate of release of many amino acids from peripheral tissues remains depressed, concurrent with continuing body protein accumulation.[81]

Protein turnover also increases in association with the marked negative N balance that accompanies severe physiologic stress.[82] For comparable stress, N loss is less in previously starved animals than in well-nourished ones.[83] One would predict that protein turnover, already depressed in starvation, would similarly show a blunted rise in response to physiologic stress. This has been confirmed in a recent human study.[84]

The determinants of the rate of protein turnover are not well understood. Kinney and Elwyn have noted a relationship between body N loss and energy expenditure,[85] and it is possible that the energy cost of whole body protein turnover plays a role in that relationship, for the energy requirements for protein synthesis and breakdown may make up a significant proportion of the resting energy expenditure.[86,87] The energy cost of protein synthesis must be even greater than accounted for by the sum of the ATP molecules hydrolyzed for amino acid transport, activation and incorporation into protein, because proteins are synthesized nonrandomly and regulated processes are energy consuming. Similarly, protein hydrolysis to its amino acids, although thermodynamically favored, consumes energy because it, too, is regulated.

Because protein turnover consumes energy, an important question is whether the known continuous recycling of body proteins in a seemingly "futile cycle" provides any biologic advantage. Newsholme has shown that substrate cycles of certain individual molecules at regulatory points of metabolic pathways permit a finely tuned control of metabolite flow.[88] Does the recycling of entire proteins similarly allow a rapid remodeling of body protein distribution and function in times of need? If this is so, then slowed rates of protein turnover characteristic of adapted starvation will confer a potential disadvantage on the organism. Sukhatme and Margen carried out a detailed analysis of the patterns of N balance of normal men on maintenance diets with different protein contents.[11] They demonstrated nonrandom cyclic fluctuations in N excretion with a periodicity of days, increasing in amplitude with increasing protein intake. The quantity of body protein clearly is regulated, and these recent observations may provide future insight into the "feedback" characteristics of the process. It is apparent that the greater the protein intake, the coarser (and perhaps, therefore, less efficient) the regulation. This could relate to the interaction between energy and protein in determining N balance during starvation. When the protein intake is high, protein turnover is maximal and dietary protein utilization as a consequence is inefficient. This state is associated with wide fluctuations in N excretion.[11] When the protein intake is low, protein turnover rates are slowed to maximize amino acid reutilization, a state manifested by low fluctuations in N excretion. Starvation is associated with a slower rate of body protein turnover because (1) slower rates of turnover are energy conserving and (2) rapid flux through the free amino acid pools is incompatible with the finest regulation (and efficiency) of amino acid oxidation. The effect of exogenous energy may be to increase the efficiency of amino acid utilization at any rate of turnover.[89]

## PROLONGED FASTING

The major emphasis of this section is on body protein metabolism in prolonged fasting. For details of other fasting responses, the reader is referred to review articles on endocrine,[7] metabolic,[90] fuel-metabolic,[91,92] fluid and electrolyte,[93] and the clinical[75] aspects.

### Comparison of the Fed and Postabsorptive States

A lucid description of fasting best proceeds from the last meal before the fast begins. Characteristic of the fed state are increased blood concentrations of glucose, fats (and their metabolic intermediates), and amino acids, as well as of urea (indicating acutely increased hepatic amino acid catabolism). Another characteristic is insulin secretion induced by the absorbed nutrients as well as by neural and gut hormone signals. Insulin regulates the disposition of the absorbed nutrients by stimulating glucose incorporation into glycogen in the liver, glucose transport and glycogen synthesis in muscle, triglyceride synthesis and amino acid transport and synthesis into proteins in the insulin-sensitive peripheral tissues (mainly muscle). Glucagon levels are unchanged or decreased during meals containing carbohydrate, but during the consumption of a protein meal low in carbohydrate, glucagon secretion is stimulated with the net effect that the liver continues glucose synthesis and glycogen breakdown, maintaining glucose levels in spite of the concurrent insulin stimulation driving glucose and amino acids into the peripheral tissues.

A protein-rich meal may contain quantities of amino acids comparable in size to the total free amino acid pool for some amino acids; yet meal-related fluctuations of most amino acid plasma levels are relatively small. As described earlier, the size of the free amino acid pool is maintained relatively constant by the rapid removal of absorbed amino acids into labile proteins and possibly by a decrease in the breakdown rate of endogenous proteins, particularly in the liver. The splanchnic tissues (gut and liver), being exposed to the greatest fluctuations of amino acid concentrations, play a vital role in regulating the fate of absorbed amino acids.

Three essential amino acids—leucine, isoleucine, and valine (the branched chain amino acids, so named because of their branched aliphatic side chains)—are handled differently from the others. Although there is a substantial uptake of most amino acids by the liver during the absorption of a protein meal, most ingested branched chain amino acids appear to pass relatively unimpeded into the peripheral circulation.[44] The enzyme that transaminates these amino acids is plentiful in muscle (but not in liver). It has therefore been assumed that these amino acids are largely catabolized in muscle. It has recently been recognized that the transamination products, the branched chain keto acids, are measurable in the peripheral circulation and derive from muscle tissues.[94] Their concentrations rise and fall in correspondence with those of the parent amino acids.[95–97] Branched chain ketoacid dehydrogenase, which catalyzes the next (and the first irreversible) step in catabolism, is more concentrated in liver than

in muscle[94] and a number of observations suggest that a portion of the branched chain amino acids absorbed into muscle tissues may recycle back to the liver as the ketoacids for final disposition.[94,98–101]

Some of the amino groups removed from the branched chain amino acids link with pyruvate, a product of glycolysis, to form the nonessential amino acid, alanine. Alanine is continuously released from peripheral tissues and taken up by the liver both in the fed and the fasted state.[100] Thus there is probably a cycle between liver and muscle by which N brought to muscle as a component of the branched chain amino acids is returned to the liver in alanine, and a proportion of the branched chain amino acids themselves return to the liver, but now minus their amino groups. The unique handling of the branched chain amino acids raises a suspicion that they have special regulatory functions. Indeed, all of them, or in some cases only leucine or its metabolites, affect rates of protein synthesis or breakdown in various isolated tissue preparations.[102,103]

The fed state ends when the last absorbed nutrient is disposed of and the transition to endogenous fuel consumption begins. The state, approximately 12 hours from the previous meal (corresponding to the condition following an overnight fast) has been found convenient for study and is termed the "postabsorptive state." The postabsorptive state is characterized by the release, interorgan transfer, and oxidation of endogenous fatty acids, glucose from liver glycogen, and muscle amino acids, all a result of (or facilitated by) low levels of circulating insulin. Even with high carbohydrate diets, the major postabsorptive fuel is fat, with $2/3$ of the resting energy expenditure being accounted for by fat oxidation.[1]

## Key Role of Glucose

In normal postabsorptive man, the plasma glucose appearance rate is about 8 g/h.[7] The free glucose pool of the body, about 16 g, is thus replaced every 2 hours. If the circulating glucose concentration falls rapidly below a critical value, altered mentation and coma result almost immediately, and prolonged hypoglycemia may destroy brain tissue. Consequently, there is no room for error in the regulation of rates of glucose delivery to the circulation by the liver. Indeed, blood glucose concentrations normally are tightly regulated within a narrow range by the action of at least three control systems. First, high insulin levels promote the uptake of glucose into muscle and fat, stimulate hepatic glycogen synthesis while inhibiting its breakdown, and inhibit the synthesis and discharge of newly synthesized glucose molecules from the liver. All these act to decrease circulating glucose levels. Second, glucagon stimulates hepatic glycogen breakdown and gluconeogenesis, thereby increasing blood glucose concentrations. Third, an autonomic nervous and hormonal counterregulatory system is activated in response to brain glucose deprivation, stimulating rapid glycogen breakdown and a rise in the blood glucose concentration.

In the postabsorptive state, the release of liver glucose equals the rate of utilization by the brain and other tissues, a total of about 250 g/d.[7] It has been estimated that about ¾ of the glucose released by the postabsorptive liver is derived from glycogen, the remainder being formed from noncarbohydrate sources.[7] One source of glucose precursors is the pool of 3-carbon intermediates: glycerol derived from triglyceride hydrolysis and lactate and pyruvate derived from the Embden-Myerhof glycolytic pathway. Because this source of lactate and pyruvate is pre-existing glucose, their biotransformation into glucose molecules in the liver constitutes a substrate cycle (known as the Cori cycle in the case of lactate) whose activity results in no net increase or decrease in the amount of glucose in the organism. The advantages of this cycle are twofold: (1) Tissues that derive energy only by means of the anaerobic Embden-Meyerhof pathway (such as blood cells) may operate without causing a loss to the body of precious glucose molecules. The lactate and pyruvate molecules produced as end products of glycolysis are returned to the liver for resynthesis into new glucose molecules, the energy cost of this process being borne by fatty acid oxidation in the liver. (2) Muscle tissue cannot release stored glucose, as it lacks glucose-6-phosphatase. Glucose-6-phosphate derived from muscle glycogen breakdown is glycolyzed to lactate and pyruvate, which may then leave that tissue to be used as a precursor for gluconeogenesis in the liver. The newly synthesized glucose is now available for use in the brain. Under usual dietary conditions, the brain oxidizes glucose completely to $CO_2$ and water and therefore irreversibly drains the body glucose pool. In the absence of dietary glucose or endogenous glycogen stores, the source of substrate to make up this requirement must come from elsewhere—from amino acids (except leucine, whose carbon atoms cannot be converted into glucose) and from glycerol derived from triglyceride hydrolysis. Although glycogen breakdown largely meets the needs of brain glucose oxidation postabsorptively, total body glycogen stores are inadequate to meet this requirement for more than 3 days. Liver biopsy studies confirm the depletion of liver glycogen that accompanies extended fasting.[104] Brain glucose needs must therefore increasingly be made up by amino acid conversion to glucose, and a typical observation in early total fasting is a marked increase in body N losses, approximately 12 g/d.[105]

### Protein Metabolism

As a fast is prolonged, liver glycogen becomes depleted, and so long as brain glucose oxidation continues unabated, gluconeogenesis from amino acids must increase to meet the glucose requirement. Changes in insulin and glucagon orchestrate a process by which increasing amounts of muscle amino acids become available, and their conversion to glucose in the liver is stimulated. In the first days of a total fast, insulin levels drop while glucagon levels remain constant or rise modestly and transiently. This combination primes enzymes in the liver to inhibit glycolysis and to convert gluconeogenic three-carbon intermediates into glucose, while blocking their oxidation through the Krebs cycle. The lowered ratio of insulin to glucagon also activates the liver for fatty acid oxidation, and the lowered circulating insulin level allows for a mobilization of free fatty acids from adipose tissue triglyceride. After such activation, the liver's rate of fatty acid oxidation is determined by the rate of presentation of the fatty acids.[106] Thus, along with diminished conversion of glucose and glucose precursors to acetyl coenzyme A (the entry substrate for the Krebs cycle), there is a marked increase in production of acetyl coenzyme A derived from fatty acid oxidation. Although some acetyl coenzyme A produced from fatty acid oxidation presumably is terminally oxidized through the intrahepatic Krebs cycle, most is converted to acetoacetate, which in turn gives rise reversibly to beta-hydroxybutyrate and to a lesser extent (irreversibly) to acetone. The appearance in the circulation of these three substrates, collectively known as "ketone bodies," is the hallmark of a low insulin-to-glucagon ratio and rapid hepatic fatty acid oxidation.

Recent evidence indicates that small amounts of acetoacetate are produced and utilized in the liver even in the fed state.[107] Circulating concentrations of ketone bodies are very low under these conditions (0.1 mM), and the export of ketone bodies from the liver is probably negligible. In the early days of fasting, the rate of acetoacetate synthesis increases greatly, and all, or almost all, synthesized acetoacetate and beta-hydroxybutyrate leaves the liver to be used as a fuel substrate in the other tissues, including muscle and brain. As ketone body concentrations rise, they largely replace glucose as a brain fuel, and the rate of brain glucose oxidation decreases substantially.

In a study carried out in 5-week fasting humans, glucose uptake by the brain was found to be equivalent to only 40 g/d, less than half the normal rate. Moreover, only 60% of the glucose taken up by the brain was oxidized to $CO_2$ and water; the remainder was returned to the circulation as reutilizable lactate and pyruvate.[108] This adaptation permits a 75% reduction in the irreversible loss of glucose through brain oxidation with a concurrent decrease in the need for gluconeogenesis from amino acids and glycerol.

Historically, the recognition that the brain glucose requirement can also be met by ketone bodies came by a different route. It was long known that the early stages of fasting are accompanied by glycogen depletion followed by a rise in body N loss and that provision of carbohydrate early in the fast inhibits the protein loss. Lusk demonstrated in living animals the efficient conversion of protein to glucose. There was no similar conversion of fat to glucose and, as predicted, if glucose was the energy source specifically required, equivalent amounts of fat had no protein-sparing effect.[1]

It was thus apparent that glucose is required in early fasting, and in the absence of glycogen the need is met by conversion of protein to glucose. When, subsequently, the obligate glucose requirement of the brain was understood, the maximum possible rate of gluconeogenesis, as calculated from body N and fat loss, fell far short of the presumed metabolic needs of the brain during fasting.[105] Finally, the human study described above by Owen and co-workers in 1967 demonstrated both utilization of ketone bodies and decreased oxidation of glucose in the human brain during prolonged fasting.[108] Biochemical studies in the rat confirmed that brain tissues readily metabolize ketone bodies, at a rate controlled by the prevailing concentration of the ketone bodies.[109]

The brain's need for glucose in the absence of ketone bodies and its ability to use them instead of glucose explain much of the adaptation to fasting. In prolonged fasting (2 weeks or more), rates of N loss diminish to 4 to 6 g/d, one-half to one-third those at the beginning. This adaptation is life-saving, for if N losses continued at the rate of early fasting, lethal protein depletion would result within a few weeks. As ketone body levels continue to rise over the first 2 weeks of a prolonged fast, it has been proposed that they increasingly displace glucose as brain fuel during this time, thereby diminishing the need for gluconeogenesis from amino acids and sparing body protein.

## Mechanism for Diminished Protein Losses

Unexplained in this scheme of protein metabolism in prolonged fasting is the mechanism early in fasting that makes body proteins available for conversion to glucose and the nature of the signal, later on, which "tells" the proteins they need no longer be broken down. Much research has been conducted to address this question, because of its relevance to clinical situations in which the sparing of body protein could be life-saving.

In the postabsorptive state, muscle is in negative amino acid balance.[110] The release of alanine and glutamine far exceeds that of the other amino acids, and, indeed, it can be estimated that only about one third of the alanine released from postabsorptive muscle is derived from the alanine of muscle protein itself.[100] The source of the alanine is pyruvate and an amine group, but uncertainty exists about both the source of the pyruvate carbon skeleton and the amine with which it links. According to one view, the pyruvate is derived almost entirely from glucose molecules. Alanine released by muscle, taken up by the liver, and converted into glucose would not then provide new glucose molecules to the body, because it derives from glucose in a cycle termed the *glucose-alanine cycle*.[111,112] *New* glucose molecules would be synthesized when amino acids other than alanine are delivered to the liver intact, or following their conversion within the muscle to glutamine. Another view maintains that most amino acids are converted within muscle tissue into pyruvate, then aminated to alanine, and released to the liver.[90,113] According to this view, alanine is largely an amino acid-derived gluconeogenic precursor and is not part of a substrate cycle. The amine group of alanine could either be derived from the branched chain amino acids,[114] a view consistent with the glucose-alanine cycle or, alternatively, alanine could be a carrier to the liver of N removed from any of the amino acids catabolized within the muscle to pyruvate.

In addition to alanine, postabsorptive muscle is in a negative balance of similar magnitude for glutamine, the nonessential amino acid that is the amide of glutamate.[115] About one third of the glutamine released from postabsorptive muscle can be accounted for by a concurrent uptake of glutamate, but, since each glutamine molecule contains two amine groups, glutamine is quantitatively a more important transporter of nitrogen from the muscle than alanine.[115] In the rat a large proportion of muscle-exported glutamine is taken up by the intestinal tissues and oxidized as a fuel substrate.[116] The kidney is also an important site of glutamine uptake, where it is used as a substrate for ammonia production.[100] In prolonged fasting, glutamine release by muscle diminishes by two thirds.[115]

Although the details are controversial, it is clear that during fasting the muscle mass decreases while amino acid carbons of muscle origin are directed within the liver (and kidney) into glucose synthesis and their N atoms are ultimately excreted as urea and ammonia.

Tracer studies indicate that large amounts of amino acids become available for catabolism early in fasting because the rate of body protein synthesis declines, but protein breakdown remains at postabsorptive rates or increases.[117] Confirming this, the rate of excretion of urinary 3-methylhistidine appears to remain at prefasting rates for a period of approximately one week, only later declining significantly.[118]

The decrease in muscle protein synthesis, which makes free amino acids available for catabolism, is probably due to the combined influence of falling insulin levels and an absence of exogenous amino acids. Both factors individually are known to inhibit muscle protein synthesis.[119] The fasting liver is already primed for gluconeogenesis by the altered glucagon-insulin ratio. In early fasting, plasma alanine levels actually fall, despite their augmented muscle release. Balance studies confirm that this decrease is due to exceptionally avid uptake of alanine by the liver and conversion to glucose.[7] In prolonged fasting, the liver's avidity for gluconeogenic precursors is unaltered. The protein-sparing mechanism of prolonged fasting appears to reside therefore in muscle, for as a fast is extended, the release of all the amino acids (and dramatically that of alanine and glutamine) declines due to a decrease in the net breakdown rate of muscle protein.[7] The question then remains: What "tells" net muscle protein breakdown to diminish in prolonged fasting, thereby diminishing the rate of loss of whole body protein?

Since brain metabolism adapted to oxidation of ketone bodies no longer requires as much glucose, and hence creates less need for amino acid catabolism, it is natural to ask whether the brain somehow "signals" the muscle to decrease its rate of proteolysis. In fact, it has not been demonstrated that the decrease in brain glucose oxidation is closely linked in time with the adaptive diminution of body protein losses, which becomes evident after about 10 to 14 days of total fasting (Fig. 43–3). Indeed, brain glucose oxidation probably declines as early as a few days after commencing a fast. The ketone-oxidizing enzymes in the brain are already active after an overnight fast,[7] and it is entirely possible that blood ketone body levels of 2mM, which may be achieved by 48 h of fasting, could permit efficient utilization of ketone bodies.[120]

Human studies with tracer glucose demonstrate a 50% decrease in plasma glucose turnover within a few days of fasting.[105] This is not due to a slowing of the Cori cycle, which is quantitatively unchanged in prolonged fasting.[121] It is therefore likely due to decreased oxidation of glucose to $CO_2$ and water. Confirming this, even large losses of body N of 12 g/d in the first week of fasting represent the loss to the body of only about 75 g of protein, which theoretically could give rise to a maximum 45 g of new glucose per day,[1] an inadequate amount to meet usual brain requirements once glycogen is used up. Therefore, consumption of brain fuel has probably switched substantially to oxidation of ketone bodies by, at the latest, one week of fasting and at a time when body protein catabolism is still nearly maximal.

If a diminution of brain glucose oxidation does not signal the muscle to diminish proteolysis, what may do so? A consistent observation in prolonged fasting is a continuing rise in blood ketone body levels for about 7 to 10 days, followed by a more gradual rise to a plateau of 6 to 8 mM after 2 to 3 weeks. Because production of liver ketone bodies is already maximal by day 3 or 4, the rise in levels must be due to decreased utilization or excretion. In fact, both occur. In the first 3 to 10 days of fasting, the efficiency of renal conservation of ketone bodies increases, thus limiting their losses in the urine. In later fasting, oxidation of muscle ketone bodies decreases, to be largely replaced by oxidation of fatty acids. In the face of continuing ketogenesis, this has the effect of raising the blood ketone body concentration.[7] It has been suggested that hyperketonemia itself may provide a protein-sparing signal to muscle.

Another possibility is that the process by which muscle metabolism switches from oxidation of ketone bodies to oxidation of fatty acid, as fasting progresses, is intimately involved in the decreased protein breakdown. Perhaps increased oxidation of muscle fatty acid spares the branched chain amino acids (which have structural similarity to fatty acids) and these spared branched chain amino acids (or their metabolites) bring about diminished proteolysis.[91] This is an attractive possibility since these molecules have been shown to have protein-sparing effects in tissue preparations.[103]

A third possibility is stimulation of insulin secretion by ketone bodies.[122,123] Even though circulating insulin levels remain low in prolonged fasting, it has been suggested that hyperketonemia may stimulate a rise in insulin levels too slight to be measured with present methods.[106,124] It is possible that a slight rise in insulin levels under these

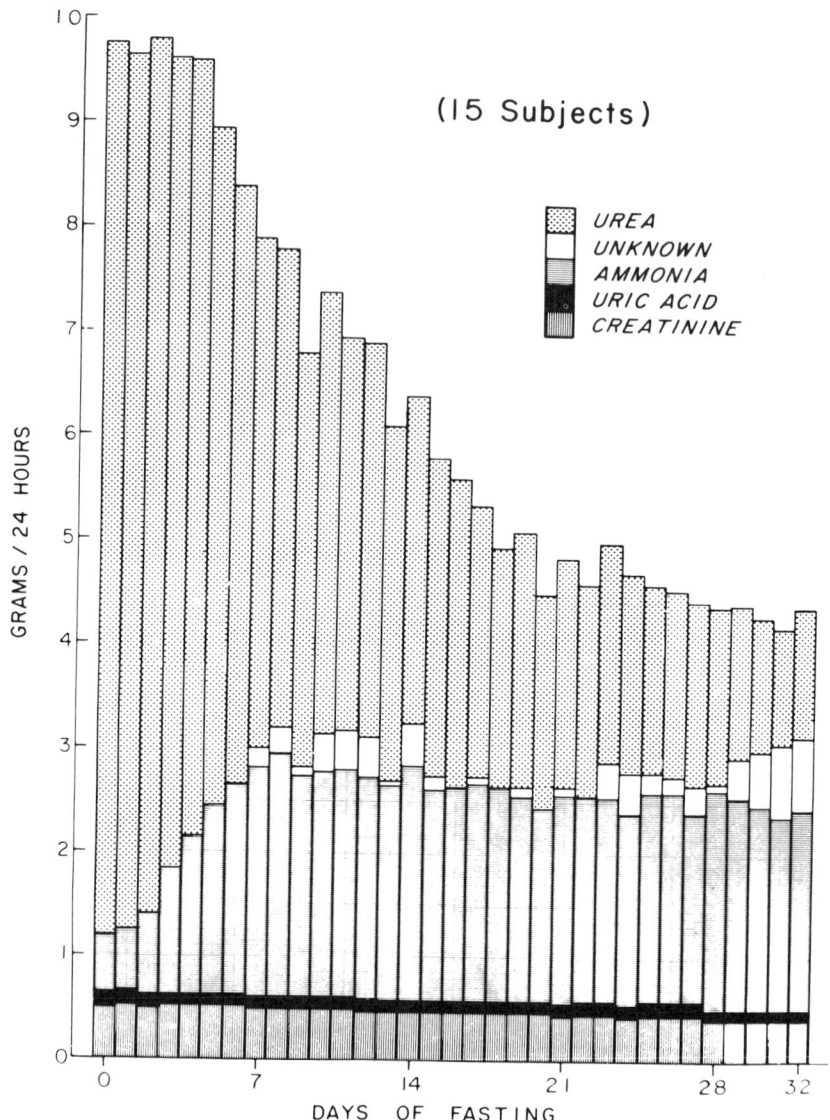

**Fig. 43–3.** Urinary N excretion during a total fast. After the first week of fasting N losses gradually fall to about 5 g/day in the third week. Initially, most N losses are in the form of urea, but ammonium excretion triples in the first week of fasting as urea excretion falls. In the third week, ammonium excretion accounts for approximately half of the total N loss. (Reproduced from Aoki, T.T.,[154] with permission of the author and Allen R. Liss, Inc.

conditions can have an important effect on the tissues to spare proteins.

Finally, the discharge of labile protein must be considered. In late fasting, urinary N excretion usually falls to 4 to 6 g/d.[1,125] and is associated with a major diminution in whole body protein and plasma leucine turnover.[126,127] This rate of excretion is not much greater than adapted total body N losses of 3 to 4 g/d on high-calorie, zero-protein diets. As described in the next section, some of the N losses of total fasting are due to

acidosis or potassium deficiency, and when these are corrected, fasting N losses may diminish to as low as 3 to 5 g/d. It is possible, therefore, that increased protein loss in early fasting and its later diminution occur by similar, but less efficient, mechanisms to those that mediate the adaptation to protein deficiency in the presence of ample carbohydrate and calorie provision and normal insulin levels. The general mechanisms for conserving body protein may function independently of hormone effects (beyond a small permissive insulin presence) and depend instead on the built-in protein-synthetic and degradative machinery of each individual tissue.[128,129]

## PROTEIN-SPARING TREATMENTS DURING FASTING

The identification of the following modifiers of protein metabolism during fasting has proven useful to the understanding of starvation and has provided important improvements in nutrition therapy.

### Carbohydrate

Protein is abruptly lost upon initiating a fast or upon withdrawing carbohydrate from an adequate diet (even if replaced isoenergetically by fat). In both cases the response is associated with lowered insulin levels (although, in the case of a carbohydrate-free but otherwise maintenance diet, zero N balance is re-established within a few days despite continuing low insulin levels).[10,130] On the other hand, administration of carbohydrate (which raises insulin levels) has long been known to spare proteins in early fasting, whereas pure fat given in the absence of any accompanying protein has only a slight[33,128] or undetectable[10] protein-sparing effect. Clinicians have long made use of carbohydrate's protein-sparing effect.[131] The most often cited demonstration was that by Gamble who showed that 100 g glucose/d diminished by half the anticipated N losses of normal volunteers undergoing a short-term total fast.[132] An additional 50 g of protein provided no additional protein-sparing effect. Dating from this time, it has been standard clinical practice to administer 5% glucose intravenously to patients temporarily unable to take food, with the goal of providing at least 100 g carbohydrate daily to spare body proteins by serving brain glucose needs.

As has long been appreciated,[91] glucose's protein-sparing effect late in fasting is far less than during the first few days,[91,133,134] because the metabolic adaptation to fasting brings about protein-sparing to an efficiency that cannot be substantially improved upon. Indeed, in the absence of dietary protein, body N losses could not be expected, by any maneuver, to diminish to less than the rate of the "protein minimum" of 2 to 3 g/day achieved on a protein-free diet that is adequate in all other respects.

There is evidence that the mechanisms of the protein-sparing effect of carbohydrate differ in early and late fasting. In early fasting, almost all the N lost from the body is in the form of urea. By two or three weeks of fasting, urea excretion has diminished dramatically while ammonium excretion has increased, so that 50% of N excreted

is in this form (Fig. 43–3). Increased generation of ammonia is an adaptation of the kidneys to the ketoacidosis of fasting. N derived from the degradation of amino acids is delivered to the kidneys mainly in the form of glutamine, where the amine groups are removed as ammonia and released into the renal tubular fluid. There the ammonia combines with hydrogen ions and is excreted in the urine as ammonium ions. The removal of the amine groups from glutamine is accompanied by the conversion of its carbon atoms into glucose. This metabolic activity of the kidney is so active that in late fasting, renal gluconeogenesis equals that of the liver.[125]

The typical effect of administration of carbohydrate in late fasting is to diminish ammonia excretion so as to diminish N losses by 1 g/d, an effect achieved with similar potency by 150 g of carbohydrate per day or by as little as 15 g.[134,135] The effect of the lower dose of carbohydrate is to diminish urinary excretion of ketone bodies dramatically without a systemic effect on circulating hormones, ketone bodies, or fatty acids. Glucose may therefore exert much of its action in late fasting by a direct effect on the kidney. This has important implications for the treatment of hospitalized patients. Until recent years, intravenous glucose solutions were commonly administered for prolonged periods to patients unable to eat, in the expectation that body proteins were being conserved. It is now recognized that, apart from a beneficial protein-sparing effect in the first 7 to 10 days of fasting, continued administration of glucose is barely more effective than that which the body could achieve through its own adaptation, and it also produces an undesirable side effect. With body protein stores being maximally conserved due to protein depletion, the continued administration of glucose stimulates insulin and results in a preferential shunting of amino acids into the insulin-sensitive peripheral tissues at the expense of the visceral tissues.[32] The consequence, after a few weeks of administration of glucose, is diminished circulating albumin levels and impaired immunologic reactivity. The disease produced by prolonged administration of glucose in this setting is reminiscent of kwashiorkor, the disease of protein-malnourished children with access to a carbohydrate supply. The modern approach to patients unable to obtain normal oral nutrition for prolonged periods is therefore to provide full parenteral nutrition.

### Potassium

Body potassium is almost entirely stored within the lean tissues, where it serves as the dominant intracellular cation. Muscle, which makes up most of the lean tissue (and certainly the bulk of the lean tissue lost in late fasting), contains about 3meq potassium/g N.[136] With N losses of about 5 g/d in late fasting, potassium losses of about 15 meq/d would therefore be anticipated and are typically observed.[75] In the early days of a total fast, potassium losses are substantially higher than this, due to the rapid rate of loss of visceral lean tissues (some of which are richer in N than muscle), losses of glycogen (1 meq potassium/3 g glycogen), and perhaps some potassium wasting associated with the sodium diuresis that accompanies early fasting.[93] Body potassium deficiency probably develops during early fasting and is stemmed, but not reversed, as the fast continues. Evidence for the existence of a deficiency is the potassium retention which occurs when the mineral is provided to prolonged fasting patients. Potassium deficiency causes urinary ammonium wasting, and treatment of obese patients on prolonged fasts with large doses of potassium chloride (0.5 meq/kg) diminishes urinary ammonium excretion by approximately one third, resulting in N sparing of about 0.6 g/d.[137]

### Bicarbonate

If the increased urinary ammonium loss of prolonged fasting is a response to ketoacidosis, then neutralizing the ketoacids may be protein-sparing. As predicted, when large daily doses of potassium bicarbonate are administered to obese patients on prolonged fasts (180 to 250 meq/d), urinary ammonium excretion falls to low levels, resulting in N sparing of 2.0 g/d.[137] A similar decrease in ammonium excretion occurs when only 150 meq of sodium bicarbonate is administered, together with 60 meq of potassium chloride.[138] In addition to its effect on ammonium excretion, the neutralizing treatment produces a modest, but definite, urea N sparing.[138] A decrease in excretion of urea N has also been observed in renal patients with chronic metabolic acidosis when sodium bicarbonate supplements of 72 to 120 meq/d were administered.[139] Although ammonium-N sparing with bicarbonate therapy is understandable during metabolic acidosis, there is no obvious explanation for the diminished urea synthesis that accompanies this therapy.

### Ketone Bodies

According to a theory cited above, rising circulating levels of ketone bodies exert a protein-sparing effect that would account for the diminution in N losses in prolonged fasting.[7] This theory has proven difficult to support or refute. In one study, the sodium salt of β-hydroxybutyric acid was infused into the circulation of prolonged fasting subjects, and urinary N excretion decreased.[140] However, the sodium salts of the ketoacids are actually alkalinizing agents, and it now appears that the N-sparing effect of the ketone body infusions could entirely be accounted for by the latter effect.[141]

In another study, ketone body infusions were carried out in normal postabsorptive individuals, and no change in leucine kinetics was observed.[142] However, this study, too, is inconclusive, because the postulated protein-sparing effect of ketosis would not be expected to occur until much later in fasting and with ketone body concentrations much greater than were achieved in the study. Moreover, leucine turnover studies are not a suitable substitute for measurements of urinary N when assessing small changes in stores of body proteins. Assuming that leucine makes up 8% of the body proteins being turned over, then a change in 2 g N lost/d, readily determined with the N balance technique, is equivalent to a change of less than 6 $\mu$mol/min in leucine oxidation—a change too small to be detected reliably with the leucine turnover method.

### Branched Chain Amino and Keto Acids

From 12 to 20 g leucine were infused intravenously over 12 h to obese patients after 3 days or 4 weeks of fasting. Even accounting for the 1.2 to 2.0 g N provided by this treatment, N balance improved by about 2 g/d in early fasting and about 1 g/d in late fasting.[127] Although it is possible that the leucine infusions in early fasting stimulated insulin secretion with a protein-sparing effect, this is an unlikely explanation for the result in prolonged fasting because the treatment actually increased circulating glucose levels. The effect was evident only during the 1 or 2 days of leucine administration. In contrast, when a mixture of essential amino acids plus the ketoacids of the branched chain amino acids, phenylalanine and methionine, was infused into prolonged fasting patients over 3h for each of 7 days (a dose of 0.4 g N/d), there was a gradual and steady decrease in urinary excretion of urea N (of about 1 g/d), which remained evident for at least a week after the final infusion.[143] It appears likely that branched chain amino acids or their keto acids exert a protein-sparing effect in late fasting, particularly in view of the biochemical evidence that they have an effect on protein synthesis or degradation at the tissue level. However, the present evidence does not permit any conclusion about the characteristics or importance of this effect in humans.

## Protein

As the previous discussion has shown, the rate of endogenous body N loss of about 3 g/d represents the best possible N-sparing effect achievable in the absence of dietary protein but with maintenance energy provision. Prolonged fasting N losses would not be expected to fall as low as this, even with maximum adaptation, because the efficiency of protein utilization is impaired by an energy deficit and because brain glucose oxidation, although drastically diminished, is still ongoing and therefore requires conversion of amino acids to glucose. Taking into account the effects of potassium and bicarbonate therapy in prolonged fasting, which may permit the sparing of as much as 2 g N/d, adapted N losses in the absence of any calories come surprisingly close to the "protein minimum." However, comparisons of this kind must be made cautiously, because N loss after several weeks of fasting may be increasingly curtailed by the continuing loss of endogenous lean tissue (thus increasing the efficiency of protein utilization), whereas typical measurements of endogenous N loss are carried out after only 10 days on a protein-free diet.

It is evident that only a diet providing protein can halt body protein loss or permit protein reaccumulation. Until recent years, it was widely assumed that even ample dietary protein would not permit zero N balance as long as there was an energy deficit. This conclusion was based on studies carried out for an insufficient time to permit adaptation to the test diet or at protein intake levels that, although adequate for N balance with maintenance dietary energy, now are known to be inadequate when the energy intake is restricted.[69] Indeed, Lusk, who based his conclusions on studies by Carl Voit,[1] long ago concluded that the organism could remain in zero N balance while remaining in negative "carbon" balance. Nitrogen equilibrium occurs commonly during weight reduction dieting, provided that the protein intake is sufficiently high.[144,145] It also may be achieved in nonstressed, malnourished hospitalized patients given low energy intravenous amino acid infusions, although the amount administered must be more than twice that which would be necessary if maintenance energy were also provided.[146]

## Very Low Calorie Weight Reduction Diets (See also Chapter 46)

Although anticipated by the early work of Evans and Strang,[147] the current interest in high protein, very low calorie weight reduction diets is a phenomenon of the last 20 years.[148] Without reviewing this clinical area in detail, certain general conclusions can be drawn from the large number of studies published in recent years. First, zero N balance can be achieved in some, but not all, obese patients subsisting on low energy, high protein diets. The initial pattern is an abrupt loss of body protein, followed over the ensuing 1 to 3 weeks by improved N balance. However, individual variability in the response is great, with some patients never attaining zero N balance over the period of observation. There is some suggestion that continuing N losses occur more frequently in men than in women, and in those with the greatest degree of overweight—those individuals with greater initial lean body mass. It should be recognized that some body N losses may be inevitable with weight reduction in the extremely obese, since loss of body fat decreases the need for extra muscles to move about and for extra supporting tissues to maintain the adipose tissue.

In addition to protein, the other nutrients needed for lean tissue synthesis must be supplied. This is well-known in the field of parenteral nutrition, where serious deficiencies of phosphorus, magnesium, and potassium occur unless they are provided along with amino acids and energy. These deficiencies may lead to serious physiologic disturbances, or (when the deficiency is only mild) to a failure to attain the positive N balance that would otherwise be anticipated.[59]

The likelihood of zero N balance is increased by administering large amounts of protein. A controlled comparison trial in which attention was paid to micronutrient supplementation indicated that on average, the N balance was zero with a protein level almost twice that of the U.S. recommended dietary allowance, but remained negative at a protein level equivalent to the recommended dietary allowance.[31] This result could be predicted from the concepts described earlier in this chapter.

The protein provided should be of high quality. Studies reviewed by Lusk in 1928 demonstrated that a protein of poor quality, such as collagen, did not permit N balance and instead was immediately converted to glucose.[1] Nevertheless, some 50 years later many thousands of Americans purchased and consumed low calorie "liquid protein" diets made from hydrolyzed collagen, sometimes for periods of several months. A small number died suddenly of cardiac disturbance, either while on their diet or shortly after ending it.[148] The epidemic of liquid protein deaths occurred in the late 1970s and has not recurred since the low quality protein products were abandoned. Nevertheless, contemporary physicians carefully monitor weight reduction diets providing less than 800 kcal/d, and give special attention to a high protein intake, with vitamin and mineral (particularly potassium) supplementation. It remains possible that supplementation of collagen products with certain essential amino acids (particularly tryptophan and the sulfur amino acids) may permit some protein sparing. This possibility, based on N balance data, was known to Lusk[1] and is supported by more modern studies.[150] Nevertheless, N balance provides insufficient information about the manner in which absorbed proteins are distributed within the body, and no expert at present recommends the use of low quality protein products.

Protein turnover as measured in the fed state is well-maintained with very low calorie diets, provided the protein intake is sufficiently high.[126,151] At a low protein intake or during the ingestion of a low quality protein, protein turnover is dramatically reduced.[25] At an intermediate protein intake, the evidence for a lowering of protein turnover is inconclusive.[25,31,152]

The pattern of weight loss with very low calorie, high protein diets is different from that during total fasting. If protein is introduced following a period of prolonged total fasting, a markedly positive N balance typically follows.[129] A cessation of weight loss or even some weight gain may occur under these circumstances, even if no carbohydrate is given along with the protein. Provision of carbohydrate causes renal retention of sodium and an increase of *extracellular* fluid. Protein, by stimulating lean tissue accretion, increases *intracellular* body water. Thus the obese patient may be faced with the dismaying paradox of a stable body weight despite an extremely low caloric intake while consumption of endogenous fat continues at a rapid rate. On the other hand, the rate of body weight loss with high protein, very low calorie diets is surprisingly similar to that during late total fasting, if one neglects about 0.15 kg/d of the total weight loss during fasting as undesirable lean tissue catabolism, which is avoided with the low-calorie diet when N equilibrium is achieved. Rates of fat loss in fasting and low-calorie dieting are similar because the metabolic rate decreases less drastically with low calorie diets (by about 10%) than during total fasting (about 25%).

## METABOLIC SIGNIFICANCE OF KETOSIS

The mention of ketosis and ketoacidosis most often brings diabetes mellitus to mind. In the most severe form of diabetes, destruction or absence of the beta cells of the pancreas produces a state of severe insulin deficiency. The result is increased mobilization of fatty acids and a priming of the liver for production of ketone bodies and gluco-

neogenesis.[106] Without insulin, little or no glucose is removed by muscle and adipose tissue, with the result that the concentration of blood glucose rises to high levels. In the normal fasting individual, a sufficiently high circulating level of ketone bodies probably stimulates insulin secretion.[106,122–124] The released insulin both inhibits production of free fatty acids and enhances peripheral utilization of ketone bodies, with the result that levels of ketone bodies do not rise above 6 to 8 mM. In severe diabetes, this presumed feedback mechanism is unavailable, and levels of ketone bodies may rise to 12 to 14 mM, imposing an acid load too great for the body's buffering system to handle. A life-threatening fall in pH occurs if insulin therapy is unavailable.

Prolonged fasting is characterized not by a high, but by a low blood glucose concentration, because peripheral glucose removal is unimpaired. The insulin level is low, not because of insulin deficiency as in diabetes, but because insulin secretion is not stimulated by any dietary carbohydrate (or other nutrients); the feedback mechanisms that permit euglycemia and control of the ketone body level are intact. Ketosis in fasting is physiologic and a manifestation of proper metabolic regulation. It does not lead to the severe condition typical of diabetic ketoacidosis.[7,106]

Glucose, because it stimulates secretion of insulin and acts directly on the liver,[106] prevents or abolishes ketosis and is said to be antiketogenic. Dietary protein is also antiketogenic, although it is less potent than glucose.[1] The blood concentration of ketone bodies on a high protein, carbohydrate-free diet is typically 2 to 3 mM, less than half that found in prolonged fasting.[31,129,130] The switch from a carbohydrate-rich to a carbohydrate-free diet results in a transient loss of body protein and the development of sustained, mild ketosis.[130] After the period of adaptation, a carbohydrate-free diet, so long as it is adequate in protein and total energy, is compatible with normal protein economy.[10,130] On the other hand, a diet providing only 100 to 200 g of glucose (400 to 800 kcal) per day is not typically ketogenic; yet it results in a sustained loss of body substance.[153] It is apparent, then, that ketosis is not a sensitive or specific marker for starvation or a necessary condition for fat mobilization. It is best considered simply as the manifestation of a low-insulin state, resulting (in the absence of a pathologic insulin deficiency) from a diet low in carbohydrate.

## CONCLUSION

The essential features of the metabolic response to starvation are altered rates and patterns of fuel utilization and protein metabolism, aimed at minimizing fuel needs and limiting lean tissue loss. The nature of the starvation diet determines the pattern of hormone levels and fuel consumption. A high carbohydrate, starvation diet is associated with normal glucose metabolism and insulin levels, even when the diet necessitates increased consumption of endogenous fat to make up any energy deficit. In total fasting (and in other states of carbohydrate deprivation) fat oxidation dominates in a metabolic setting of low insulin levels and ketosis. Fuel utilization by the brain, kidney, and muscle is markedly altered in total fasting. The brain switches from exclusively glucose to predominantly ketone body oxidation. The fuel of resting muscle switches from predominantly fatty acids to ketone bodies, finally returning, after weeks of total fasting, to fatty acid oxidation again. The metabolic acidosis of prolonged fasting induces a compensatory increase in renal production of ammonia in order to increase removal of hydrogen ions from the body. This change is associated with augmented renal gluconeogenesis and a somewhat greater loss of body N than would occur without the acidosis. Despite the important influence of dietary carbohydrate on hormones and on fuel consumption patterns, all types of starvation diets produce a similar alteration of overall protein metabolism. This is characterized by a rapid loss of labile body protein, followed by a prolonged period during which further protein losses are minimized in association with a slowed rate of synthesis and breakdown of body protein.

Unlike experimental starvation, the clinical diseases of protein-calorie malnutrition are greatly influenced by the composition of the starvation diet. Laboratory studies are never extended to the point of severe protein depletion, but this end-stage condition is common in the clinical setting. When extended long enough, a protein-deficient starvation diet will lead more rapidly to a state of functional protein deficiency, with its severe consequences, than one providing an equal number of calories but with more protein because the latter diet would be more effective in minimizing ongoing protein losses. Also, clinical starvation is commonly accompanied by many dietary deficiencies in addition to protein or energy, and it is wise to bear in mind Lusk's original definition of starvation, cited at the beginning of this chapter. Concurrent nutritional deficiencies, when flagrant, will produce characteristic clinical syndromes, but when mild, they may only impair the protein-sparing adaptation to a starvation diet or to a refeeding diet following starvation. Finally, the evolution of protein-calorie malnutrition is critically influenced by the effects of physiologic stress.

Labile protein makes up only a small amount of body lean tissue, but its gain or loss is in some way a marker for the adaptive response to a change in the protein or energy content of the diet. At the present time, the precise factors regulating protein economy in response to dietary change, under both short- and long-term conditions, remain poorly understood.

## ACKNOWLEDGEMENT

The suggestions of Professors E.B. Marliss and B.R. Bistrian are gratefully acknowledged.

## REFERENCES

1. Lusk, G.: The Elements of the Science of Nutrition. 4th ed. (1928). New York, Johnson Reprint Corporation, 1976.
2. Keys, A., Brozek, J., Henschel, A., et al.: The Biology of Human Starvation. Minneapolis, The University of Minnesota Press, 1950.
3. Merrill, A.L., Watt, B.K.: Energy Value of Foods. Agriculture Handbook No. 74. United States Department of Agriculture. Washington, D.C., U.S. Government Printing Office, 1973.
4. Reifenstein, E.C., Jr., Albright, F., Wells, S.L.: J. Clin. Endocrinol. *5*:367–395, 1947.
5. Ball, M.F., Canary, J.J., Houck, J.C.: J. Clin. Endocrinol. Metab. *35*:416–424, 1972.
6. James, H.M., Dabek, J.T., Chettle, D.R., et al.: Clin. Sci. *67*:73–82, 1984.
7. Felig, P.: Starvation. *In* Endocrinology. (DeGroot, L.J., et al., Eds.) New York, Grune & Stratton, 1979, pp. 1927–1940.
8. Van Itallie, T.B., Yang, M.-U.: N. Engl. J. Med. *297*:1158–1161, 1977.
9. Peters, J.P., Van Slyke, D.D.: Quantitative Clinical Chemistry Interpretations. Vol. 1. 2nd ed. Baltimore, Williams & Wilkins, 1946.
10. Munro, H.N.: Physiol. Rev. *31*:449–488, 1951.
11. Sukhatme, P.V., Margen, S.: Am. J. Clin. Nutr. *31*:1237–1256, 1978.
12. Oddoye, E.A., Margen, S.: J. Nutr. *109*:363–377, 1979.
13. Rennie, M.J., Harrison, R.: Lancet *1*:323–325, 1984.
14. Young, V.R., Munro, H.N.: Fed. Proc. *27*:2291–2300, 1978.
15. Lukaski, H.C., Mendez, J., Buskirk, E.R., et al.: Am. J. Physiol. *240*:E302–E307, 1981.
16. Wassner, S.J., Li, J.B.: J. Physiol. *243*:E293–E297, 1982.
17. Rennie, M.J., Millward, D.J.: Clin. Sci. *65*:217–225, 1983.
18. Afting, E.-G., Bernhardt, W., Janzen, R.W.C., et al.: Biochem. J. *200*:449–452, 1981.
19. Ballard, F.J., Tomas, P.M.: Clin. Sci. *65*:209–215, 1983.
20. Rennie, M.J., Edwards, R.H.T., Halliday, D., et al.: Clin. Sci. *63*:519–523, 1982.
21. Golden, M.H.N., Waterlow, J.C.: Clin. Sci. Mol. Med. *53*:277–288, 1977.
22. Waterlow, J.C., Garlick, P.J., Millward, D.J.: Protein Turnover in Mammalian Tissues and in the Whole Body. Amsterdam, North-Holland Publishing Co., 1978.
23. Matthews, D.E., Bier, D.M.: Ann. Rev. Nutr. *3*:309–339, 1983.

24. Wolfe, R.R.: Tracers in Metabolic Research. New York, Alan R. Liss, Inc., 1984.

25. Garlick, P.J., Clugston, G.A. Waterlow, J.C.: Am. J. Physiol. *238*:E235–E244, 1980.

26. Garlick, P.J., Clugston, G.A.: Measurement of whole body protein turnover by constant infusion of carboxyl-labelled leucine. *In* Nitrogen Metabolism in Man. (Waterlow, J.C., Stephen, J.M.L., Eds.) London, Applied Science Publishers, 1981, pp. 303–322.

27. Matthews, D.E., Bier, D.M., Rennie, M.J., et al.: Science *214*:1129–1131, 1981.

28. Tessari, P., Tsalikian, E., Schwenk, W.F., et al.: Am. J. Physiol. *249*:E121–E130, 1985.

29. Reeds, R.J., Harris, C.I.: Protein turnover in animals: man in his context. *In* Nitrogen Metabolism in Man. (Waterlow, J.C., Stephen, J.M.L., Eds.) London, Applied Science Publishers, 1981, pp 391–408.

30. de Benoist, B., Adbulrazzak, Y., Brooke, O.G., et al.: Clin. Sci. *66*:155–164, 1984.

31. Hoffer, L.J., Bistrian, B.R., Young, V.R., et al.: J. Clin. Invest. *73*:750–758, 1984.

32. Munro, H.N.: General aspects of the regulation of protein metabolism by diet and hormones. *In* Mammalian Protein Metabolism. Vol. 1. (Munro, H.N., Allison, J.B., Eds.) New York, Academic Press, 1964, pp 381–481.

33. Peret, J., Jacquot, R.: Nitrogen excretion on complete fasting and on a nitrogen-free diet - endogenous nitrogen. *In* Protein and Amino Acid Functions. (Bigwood, E.J., Ed.) Oxford, Pergamon Press, 1972, pp. 73–118.

34. Joint Food and Agriculture Organization/World Health Organization Expert Committee: Energy and Protein Requirements. WHO Technical Report Series No. 522, Geneva, World Health Organization, 1973.

35. Joint Food and Agriculture Organization/World Health Organization/United Nations University Consultation: Energy and Protein Requirements. WHO Technical Report Series No. 724, Geneva, World Health Organization, 1985.

36. Munro, H.N.: Free amino acid pools and their regulation. *In* Mammalian Protein Metabolism. Vol. 4. (Munro, H.N., Ed.) New York, Academic Press, 1970. pp. 299–386.

37. Waterlow, J.C.: Free amino acid pools and their regulation. *In* Nitrogen Metabolism in Man. (Waterlow, J.C., Stephen, J.M.L., Eds.) London, Applied Science Publishers, 1981, pp. 1–16.

38. Waterlow, J.C., Garlick, P.J.: Metabolic adaptions to protein deficiency. *In* Alcohol and Abnormal Protein Biosynthesis. (Rothschild, M.A., Oratz, M., Schreiker, S.S., Eds.) New York, Pergamon Press, 1975, pp. 67–94.

39. Raforth, R.J., Onstad, G.R.: J. Clin. Invest. *56*:1170–1174, 1975.

40. Elwyn, D.H.: The role of the liver in regulation of amino acid and protein metabolism. *In* Mammalian Protein Metabolism. Vol. 4. (Munro, H.N., Ed.) New York, Academic Press, 1970, pp. 523–558.

41. Motil, K.J., Matthews, D.E., Bier, B.N., et al.: Am. J. Physiol. *240*:E712–E721, 1981.

42. Clugston, G.A., Garlick, P.J.: Hum. Nutr. Clin. Nutr. *36C*:57–70, 1982.

43. Hoffer, L.J., Yang, R.D., Matthews, D.E., et al.: Br. J. Nutr. *53*:31–38, 1985.

44. Wahren, J., Felig, P., Hagenfeldt, L. J. Clin. Invest. *57*:987–999, 1976.

45. Block, R.J., Weiss, K.W. Amino Acid Handbook: Methods and Results of Protein Analysis. Springfield, IL, Charles C Thomas, 1956.

46. Matthews, D.E., Motil, K.J., Rohrbaugh, D.K., et al.: Am. J. Physiol. *238*:E473–E479, 1980.

47. Barnard, D.L., Ford, J., Garnett, E.S., et al.: Metabolism *18*:564–569, 1969.

48. Leiter, L.A., Marliss, E.B.: JAMA *248*:2306–2307, 1982.

49. Garrow, J.S., Fletcher, K., Halliday, D.: J. Clin. Invest. *44*:417–425, 1965.

50. Grant, J.P.: Clinical impact of protein malnutrition on organ mass and function. *In* Amino Acids: Metabolism and Medical Applications. (Blackburn, G.L., Grant, J.P., Young, V.R., Eds.) Boston, John Wright, 1983, pp. 347–358.

51. Elwyn, D.H., Gump, F.E., Munro, H.N., et al.: Am. J. Clin. Nutr. *32*:1597–1611, 1979.

52. Calloway, D.H.: Energy-protein relationships. *In* Protein Quality in Humans: Assessment and In Vitro Estimation. (Bodwell, C.E., Adkins, J.S., Hopkins, D.T., Eds.) Westport, CT, Avi Publishing Co., 1981, pp. 148–168.

53. Kinney, J.M.: Energy metabolism. *In* Surgical Nutrition. (Fischer, J.E., Ed.) Boston, Little, Brown and Co., 1983, pp. 97–126.

54. Committee on Dietary Allowances, Food and Nutrition Board: Recommended Dietary Allowances. 9th Rev. Ed. Washington, DC, National Academy of Sciences, 1980.

55. Lusk, G.: Physiol. Rev. *1*:523–552, 1921.

56. Golden, M.H.N., Waterlow, J.C., Picou, D.: Clin. Sci. Mol. Med. *53*:473–477, 1977.

57. Rennie, M.J., Edwards, R.H.T., Emery, P.W., et al.: Clin. Physiol. *3*:387–398, 1983.

58. Allison, J.B., Bird, J.W.C.: Elimination of nitrogen from the body. *In* Mammalian Protein Metabolism. Vol. 1. (Munro, H.N., Allison, J.B., Eds.) New York, Academic Press, 1964, pp. 483–512.

59. Rudman, D., Millikan, W.J., Richardson, T.J., et al.: J. Clin. Invest. *55*:94–104, 1975.

60. Howe, P.E., Mattil, H.A., Hawk, P.B.: J. Biol. Chem. *11*:103–127, 1912.

61. Passmore, R., Strong, R.A., Ritchie, F.J.: Br. J. Nutr. *12*:113–122, 1958.

62. Williams, R.J.: Biochemical Individuality. New York, John Wiley and Sons, 1956.

63. Hegsted, D.M.: Fed. Proc. *22*:1424–1430, 1963.

64. Van Itallie, T.B., Yang, M.-U.: Nitrogen balance during weight reduction: effect of body stores of protein and fat. *In* Recent Advances in Obesity Research: II. (Bray, G.A., Ed.) London, Newman Publishing Ltd., 1978, pp. 379–384.

65. Goodman, M.N., Lowell, B., Belur, E., et al.: Am. J. Physiol. *246*:E383–E390, 1984.

66. Young, C.M., Gehring, B.A., Merrill, S.H., et al. J. Am. Diet. Assoc. *36*:447–452, 1960.

67. Adibi, S.A., Livi, E.D., Prafulla, M.A.: J. Lab. Clin. Med. *77*:278–289, 1971.

68. Göshke, H., Stahl, M., Thölen, H.: Klin. Wschr. *53*:605–610, 1975.

69. Hoffer, L.J., Bistrian, B.R.: Journal of Obesity Weight Reg. *3*:35–47, 1984.

70. Forbes, G.B.: Am. J. Clin. Nutr. *23*:1212–1219, 1970.

71. Forbes, G.B., Bruining, G.J.: Am. J. Clin. Nutr. *29*:1359–1366, 1976.

72. Forbes, G.B., Drenick, E.J.: Am. J. Clin. Nutr. *32*:1570–1574, 1979.

73. Wilson, J.H.P. Lamberts, S.W.J.: Am. J. Clin. Nutr. *32*:1612–1616, 1979.

74. Contaldo, F., Presta, E., di Biase, G., et al.: Int. J. Obesity *6*:97–100, 1982.

75. Drenick, E.J.: Weight reduction by prolonged fasting. *In* Obesity in Perspective. Department of Health Education and Welfare Publication No. NIH 75–708. Bethesda, MD, John E. Fogarty International Center for Advanced Study in the Health Sciences, National Institutes of Health, 1973, pp. 341–360.

76. McNurlan, M.A., Pain, V.M., Garlick, P.J.: Biochem. Soc. Trans. *8*:283–285, 1980.

77. Laurent, B.C., Moldawer, L.L., Young, V.R., et al.: Am. J. Physiol. *246*:E444–E451, 1984.

78. Oratz, M., Rothschild, M.A.: The influence of alcohol and altered nutrition on albumin synthesis. *In* Alcohol and Abnormal Protein Synthesis. (Rothschild, M.A., Oratz, M., Schreiber, S.S., Eds.) New York, Pergamon Press, 1975, pp. 343–372.

79. Conde, R.D., Scornik, O.A.: Biochem. J. *158*:385–390, 1976.

80. Munro, H.N., Hubert, C., Baliga, B.S.: Regulation of protein synthesis in relation to amino acid supply—a review. *In* Alcohol and Abnormal Protein Biosynthesis (Rothschild, M.A., Oratz, M., Schreiber, S.S., Eds.) New York, Pergamon Press, 1975, pp. 33–66.

81. Smith, S.R., Pozefsky, T., Chhetri, M.K.: Metabolism *23*:603–618, 1974.

82. James, W.P.T.: Protein and energy metabolism after trauma: old concepts and new developments. Acta. Chir. Scand. (Suppl) *507*:1–16, 1982.

83. Munro, H.N., Chalmers, M.F.: Br. J. Exp. Pathol. *26*:396–404, 1945.

84. Tomkins, A.M., Garlick, P.J., Schofield, W.N., et al.: Clin. Sci. *65*:313–324, 1983.

85. Kinney, J.M., Elwyn, D.H.: Ann. Rev. Nutr. *3*:433–466, 1983.

86. Garrow, J.S.: Energy Balance and Obesity in Man. Amsterdam, North-Holland Publishing Co., 1974.

87. Flatt, J.P.: The biochemistry of energy expenditure. *In* Recent Advances in Obesity Research: II. (Bray, G., Ed.) Westport, CT, Food and Nutrition Press, 1978, pp. 211–228.

88. Newsholme, E.A., Start, C.: Regulation in Metabolism. New York, John Wiley and Sons, 1974.

89. Hoffer, L.J., Bistrian, B.R., Phinney, S.D., et al.: Whole body protein turnover, studied with ¹⁵N-glycine, during weight reduction by moderate energy reduction. *In* Amino Acids, Metabolism and Medical Applications. (Blackman, G.L., Grant, J.P., Young, V.R., Eds.) Boston, John Wright, 1983, pp. 48–54.

90. Levenson, S.L., Seifter, E.: Starvation: metabolic and physiologic responses. *In* Surgical Nutrition (Fischer, J.E., Ed.) Boston, Little, Brown and Co., 1983, pp. 423–478.

91. Cahill, G.F., Jr.: Clin. Endocrinol. Metab. *5*:397–415, 1976.

92. Aoki, T.T.: Hormone-fuel interrelationships in normal, fasting and diabetic man. *In* Joslin's Diabetes Mellitus. 12th ed. (Marble, A., Krall, L.P., Bradley, R.F., et al., Eds.) Philadelphia, Lea & Febiger, 1985, pp. 138–157.

93. Drenick, E.J. The effects of acute and prolonged fasting and refeeding on water, electrolyte, and acid-base metabolism. *In* Clinical Disorders of Fluid and Electrolyte Metabolism. 3rd ed. (Maxwell, M.H., Kleeman, C.P., Eds.) New York, McGraw-Hill, 1980, pp. 1481–1501.

94. Harper, A.E., Miller, R.H., Block, K.P.: Ann. Rev. Nutr. *4*:409–454, 1984.

95. Harper, A.E., Benjamin, E.: J. Nutr. *114*:431–440, 1984.

96. Schauder, P., Schröder, K., Langenbeck, U.: Ann. Nutr. Metab. *28*:350–356, 1984.

97. Schauder, P., Herbertz, L., Langenbeck, U.: Metabolism *34*:58–61, 1985.

98. Livesey, G., Lund, P.: Biochem. J. *188*:705–713, 1980.

99. Abumrad, N.N., Jefferson, L.S., Rannels, S.R., et al.: J. Clin. Invest. *70*:1031–1041, 1982.

100. Felig, P.: Inter-organ amino acid exchange. *In* Nitrogen Metabolism in Man. (Waterlow, J.C., Stephen, J.M.L., Eds.) London, Applied Science Publishers, 1981, pp. 45–62.

101. Anonymous: Nutr. Rev. *43*:59–60, 1985.

102. Adibi, S.A.: J. Lab. Clin. Med. *95*:475–484, 1980.

103. Walser, M., Williamson, J.R. (Eds.): Metabolism and Clinical Implications of Branched Chain Amino and Ketoacids. New York, Elsevier North Holland, 1981.

104. Nilsson, L.H., Hultman, E.: Scand. J. Lab. Clin. Invest. *32*:325–330, 1973.

105. Cahill, G.F., Jr. Herrera, M.G., Morgan, A.P., et al.: J. Clin. Invest. *45*:1751–1769, 1966.

106. Foster, D.W., McGarry, J.D.: N. Engl. J. Med. *309*:159–169, 1983.

107. Endemann, G., Goetz, P.G., Edmond, J., et al.: J. Biol. Chem. *257*:3434–3440, 1982.

108. Owen, O.E., Morgan, A.P., Kemp, H.G., et al.: J. Clin. Invest. *46*:1589–1595, 1967.

109. Williamson, D.H., Bates, M.W., Page, M.A., et al.: Biochem. J. *121*:41–47, 1971.

110. Felig, P.: Ann. Rev. Biochem. *44*:933–955, 1975.

111. Felig, P.: Metabolism *22*:179–207, 1973.

112. Chang, T.W., Goldberg, A.L.: J. Biol. Chem. *253*:3677–3684, 1978.

113. Snell, K., Duff, D.A.: Branched chain amino acids and muscle alanine synthesis. *In* Metabolism and Clinical Implications of Branched Chain Amino and Ketoacids. (Walser, M., Williamson, J.R., Eds.) New York, Elsevier North Holland, 1981, pp. 251–256.

114. Haymond, M.W., Miles, J.M.: Diabetes *31*:86–89, 1981.

115. Marliss, E.B., Aoki, T.T., Pozefsky, T., et al. J. Clin Invest. *50*:814–817, 1971.

116. Windmueller, N.G., Spaeth, A.E.: J. Biol. Chem. *253*:69–76, 1978.

117. Tsalikian, E., Howard, C., Gerich, J.E., et al.: Am. J. Physiol. *247*:E323–E327, 1984.

118. Young, V.R., Haverberg, L.N., Bilmazes, C.B., et al.: Metabolism *22*:1429–1435, 1973.

119. Jefferson, L.S.: Diabetes *29*:487–496, 1980.

120. Flatt, J.P., Blackburn, G.L., Randers, G., et al.: Metabolism *23*:151–157, 1974.

121. Streja, D.A., Steiner, G., Marliss, E.B., et al.: Metabolism *26*:1089–1098, 1977.

122. Robinson, A.M., Williamson, D.H.: Physiol. Rev. *60*:143–187, 1980.

123. Miles, J.M., Haymond, M.W., Gerich, J.E.: J. Clin. Endocrinol. Metab. *52*:34–37, 1981.

124. Williamson, D.H.: Proc. Nutr. Soc. *40*:93–98, 1981.

125. Owen, O.E., Felig, P., Morgan, A.P., et al.: J. Clin. Invest. *48*:574–583, 1969.

126. Winterer, J., Bistrian, B.R., Bilmazes, C., et al.: Metabolism *29*:575–581; 1980.

127. Sherwin, R.S.: J. Clin. Invest. *62*:1471–1481, 1978.

128. Marliss, E.B.: The physiology of fasting and semistarvation: roles of "caloristat" and "aminostat" mechanisms. *In* Recent Advances in Obesity Research: II. (Bray, G., Ed.) Westport, CT, Food and Nutrition Press, 1978, pp. 345–358.

129. Marliss, E.B., Murray, F.T., Nakhooda, A.F.: J. Clin. Invest. *62*:468–479, 1978.

130. Phinney, S.D., Bistrian, B.R., Wolfe, R.R., et al.: Metabolism *32*:757–768, 1983.

131. Strang, J.M., McCluggage, H.B., Evans, F.A.: Am. J. Med. Sci. *181*:336–349, 1931.

132. Gamble, J.L.: Harvey Lect. *40*:247–273, 1947.

133. O'Connell, R.C., Morgan, A.P., Aoki, T.T., et al.: J. Clin. Endocrinol. Metab. *39*:555–563, 1974.

134. Aoki, T.T., Muller, W.A., Brennan, M.F., et al.: Am. J. Clin. Nutr. *28*:507–511, 1975.

135. Sapir, D.G., Owen, O.E., Cheng, J.T., et al.: J. Clin. Invest. *51*:2093–2102, 1972.

136. International Commission on Radiological Protection: Report of the Task Group on Reference Man. Publication 23. Oxford, Pergamon Press, 1975.

137. Sapir, D.G., Chambers, N.E., Ryan, J.W.: Metabolism *25*:211–220, 1976.

138. Hannaford, M.C., Leiter, L.A., Josse, R.G., et al.: Am. J. Physiol. *243*:E251–E256, 1982.

139. Papadoyannikis, N.J., Stefanidis, C.J., McGeown, M.: Am. J. Clin. Nutr. *40*:623–627, 1984.

140. Sherwin, R., Hendler, R.G., Felig, P.: J. Clin. Invest. *55*:1382–1390, 1975.

141. Féry, F., Balasse, E.O.: J. Clin. Invest. *66*:323–331, 1980.

142. Miles, J., Nissen, S., Rizza, R., et al.: Diabetes *32*:197–205, 1983.

143. Sapir, D.G., Owen, O.E., Walser, M.: J. Clin. Invest. *54*:974–980, 1974.

144. Brown, E.G., Herman, C., Ohlson, M.A.: J. Am. Diet. Assoc. *22*:858–863, 1946.

145. Leverton, R.M., Rhodes, H.N.: J. Am. Diet. Assoc. *25*:1012–1016, 1949.

146. Greenberg, G.R., Jeejeebhoy, K.N.: J.P.E.N. *3*:427–432, 1979.

147. Evans, F.A., Strang, J.M.: J.A.M.A. *97*:1063–1069, 1931.

148. Wadden, T.A., Stunkard, A.J., Brownell, K.D.: Ann. Intern. Med. *99*:675–684, 1983.

149. Felig, P.: N. Engl. J. Med. *310*:589–591, 1984.

150. Fisler, J.S., Drenick, E.J., Blumfield, D.E., et al.: Am. J. Clin. Nutr. *35*:471–486, 1982.

151. Pencharz, P.B., Motil, K.J., Parsons, H.G., et al.: Clin. Sci. *59*:13–18, 1980.

152. Bistrian, B.R., Sherwin, M., Young, V.R.: J. Clin. Endocrinol. Metab. *53*:874–878, 1981.

153. Greenberg, G.R., Marliss, E.B., Anderson, G.H., et al.: N. Engl. J. Med. *294*:1411–1416, 1976.

154. Aoki, T.T.: Metabolic adaptations to starvation, semistarvation, and carbohydrate restriction. *In* Nutrition in the 1980's: Constraints on Our Knowledge. (Selvey, N., White P.L., Eds.) New York, Alan R. Liss, Inc., 1981, pp. 161–177.

*Chapter* **44**

# OBESITY

### F. Xavier Pi-Sunyer

## DEFINITION AND CLASSIFICATION

Obesity, characterized by an excess accumulation of fat, is a detriment to good health and well-being. It is easy for individuals to take on excess fat as soon as enough food and leisure are available in a society, causing an imbalance between energy intake and energy expenditure. Although there has been disagreement as to which side of this energy equation is more important in the epidemic of obesity, both sides are certainly involved.

### Criteria for Weight Normality

A population cannot be precisely divided into normal and obese, because with a gradually increasing fat accumulation, there is not a normal bell-shape curve of weights in Western industrialized societies. Rather, the curve is skewed to the right, with a trailing out of excess weights.

Even in a genetically homogenous population, weight is variable. In the modern world, with the great intermixing of ethnic and racial groups, wide genetic heterogeneity exists. The heterogeneity is manifested by differing heights, body circumference (chest, waist, hips), and heaviness of frame. It is undesirable to focus on a single number of kilograms for height in centimeters as the "normal" weight. This is particularly evident since it is not clear what the criterion for "normal" weight should be. Should it be low mortality, low morbidity, a combination of the two, or should it be the longest extended "optimal health" or "well-being" of the individual?

For lack of a better data-base, life insurance industry statistics have been used widely to develop tables of normality. These tables give weight ranges for height and frame size and are associated with the greatest longevity in individuals who were healthy at the time of initial examination when their height and weight were measured.

Although these are the best data available, they are inadequate in a number of ways. They predominantly reflect data from upper middle class Caucasian groups. They are sex- and height-specific but not age-specific. As such, they provide data on the basis of the predictive longevity of young persons weighed in their early twenties and followed to their death. The tables have been used on the assumption that whatever weight is desirable at age 21 years is also desirable at age 45 or 65. Yet, in Western society, weight changes with age in a normal population, with a gradual in-

**795**

crease in women from 20 to 60 and a more gradual increase for men from 20 to 50, with a fall after that.[1] In addition, body composition changes with age, with the gradual accretion of fat and loss of lean body mass. Therefore, it is unclear whether the "normal" weight should be the same as age advances or whether it should rise as percent body adipose tissue increases.

In an effort to clarify the confusion about how to classify overweight, Garrow has proposed a classification that is useful clinically.[2] It is based on two simple measurements: height without shoes and weight with minimal clothing. The weight/height$^2$ (W/H$^2$), called the Body Mass Index (BMI), is then calculated, with weight expressed in kilograms and height in meters. The population, whether male or female, can be divided for degree of obesity as follows:

$$\text{Grade III: W/H}^2 > 40$$
$$\text{II: W/H}^2 \text{ 30 to 40}$$
$$\text{I: W/H}^2 \text{ 25 to 29.9}$$
$$\text{O: W/H}^2 \text{ 20 to 24.9}$$

The major weakness of the use of W/H$^2$ (originally proposed by Quetelet in 1871) is that some very muscular individuals may be classified as obese when they are not. These numbers will be small, however. BMI is the relative weight index that shows the highest correlation with independent measures of body fat.[3] The BMI range of 20 to 24.9, classified as normal, coincides well with the normal mortality ratio derived from life insurance tables. The mortality ratio begins to increase at BMI levels above 25, and it is here that health professionals should be concerned.

Although the increase in mortality in Grade 1 obesity (W/H$^2$ = 25 to 29.9) is not great, it is of importance because it is transitional to Grades II and III, which truly create health risks for the individual.

Figure 44–1 presents a diagram of this classification by height and weight.[2]

## Other Relative Weight Measures

Another relative weight index, W/H, has been suggested, but it correlates less well with body fat.[3,4] In addition, neither the ponderal index, the cube root of the weight divided by height (W$^{0.33}$/H), nor the Rohrer index (W/H$^3$) has been helpful because neither is independent enough of height to accurately reflect overweight.

## Skinfolds

Over half the fat in the body is deposited under the skin, and the percentage increases with increasing weight. The thickness of this subcutaneous fat can be measured at various sites with the use of standardized skin calipers. The distribution and amount of subcutaneous fat change with age and are also quite different by sex. One difficulty with skinfold measurement is that there is no agreement on the number and sites that best reflect actual body fat content. Another is that it is easy to make large errors if the observer is inexperienced or careless.

Data on skinfolds for children are less reliable than for adults. They have been obtained on cross-sectional population studies. Arbitrary definitions of obesity (such as eighty-fifth percentile and above of weight) have been set. Sex differences in percentage total body fat occur early in life, so that by 5 years of age different standards are necessary for males and females. In adults, sex differences are marked. Subcutaneous fat is about 11% of body weight in men and 18% in women.[5] Tables are available for triceps and subscapular percentile distributions for boys and girls (Appendix Table A–11) and for adult men and women (Appendix Table A–12)[6] with provisional data for the elderly (Appendix Tables A–15 and A–16).

Because the amount of fat distributed from place to place in the body varies, some investigators have suggested that using the sum of skinfolds from different areas will better reflect total body fat. Durnin and Womersley derived tables, for instance, using the sum of four skinfolds (biceps, triceps, subscapular, and suprailiac) and related them to the fat content of the body[7] (Appendix Table A–17).

## Other Body Fat Measurements

Other measurements that can be used for measuring body fat and other body compartments are more difficult, expensive, and time-consuming and have generally been used for research purposes. These include indirect measurements of body fat done by measuring the fat-free compartment and subtracting this amount from total body weight to derive the weight of fat.

For instance, total body water can be measured by dilution of tritiated ($^3$H$_2$O) or deuterated (D$_2$O) water. Both deuterium and tritium oxides rapidly equilibrate in body water so that the test can be done in two to three hours. Deuterium is nonradioactive and therefore is preferentially used in children and women of childbearing age. Water is then assumed to be a fixed proportion of fat-free mass (FFM), that is, FFM = water mass/0.73. The calculated FFM is subtracted from total body weight to obtain total body fat.[8] Alternatively, the naturally occurring $^{40}$K in the body can be counted in a whole body counter. Total body $^{40}$K can be measured as an index of lean body mass because

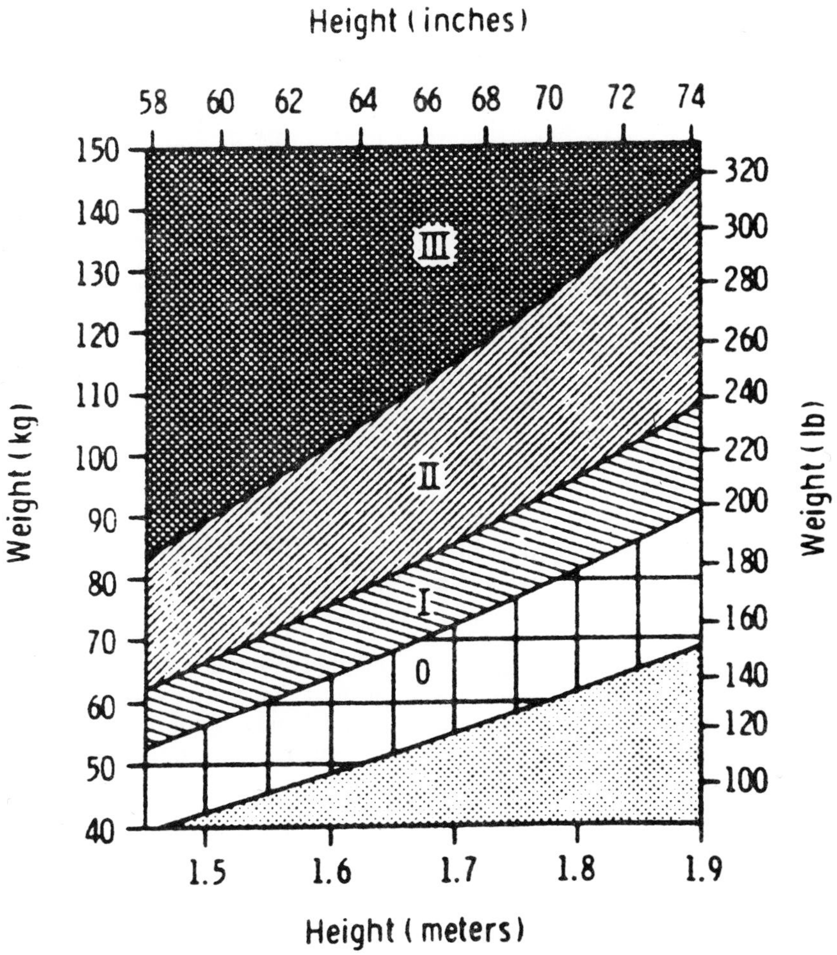

## Height (inches)

**Fig. 44–1.** Relation of weight to height defining the desirable range (O), and grades I, II, and III obesity, marked by the boundaries $W/H^2$ = 25 to 29.9, 30 to 40, and over 40 respectively. (From Garrow, J.S.,[2] with permission of Churchill Livingstone.)

potassium is present only in the fat-free compartments of the body. $^{40}K$ makes up 0.012% of the total potassium and since it is radioactive it can be detected by a sensitive counter. Using an estimated value for the meq of K in lean body, one can calculate the lean body mass and once again derive total body fat.[9]

### Body Density

The density of the whole body is derived from the density of the various body components (bone, water, fat, protein), which are all slightly different. It is easier to think of the body as divided into a fat and a fat-free mass, with fat having a density of 0.900 g/ml and the fat-free mass a density of 1.100 g/ml. Therefore, as the proportion of fat in the body increases, the density will decrease. The amount of fat in the body can be determined by measuring the density of the entire body. This re-

quires total submersion of an individual and accurate correction for lung and abdominal air.[10]

### Fat-Soluble Gases

The most tedious method for estimating fat is to use an inert gas, such as krypton or xenon, which is soluble in fat but poorly soluble in water. The gas must be breathed for a number of hours so equilibration with tissues can occur. The proportion of gas retained reflects the amount of fat in the body.[11]

### PREVALENCE

### Standards of Normality

Efforts to produce standards of obesity for the population against which individuals can be compared have generally concentrated on weight and have taken two forms. The first is the use of "desirable" weight, which is weight (stratified for sex and height and frame size) that is correlated to the greatest longevity. These weights come from life insurance data. The 1983 Tables of the Metropolitan Life Insurance Company[12] are presented in Appendix Table A–5. The second is the use of average weights of subsamples of a general population stratified by sex, age, and height. Obesity then is defined as some specific deviation from these averages. The data for these populations are often given in percentiles. Examples are the HANES tables produced by the National Center for Health Statistics in 1960 to 1962[1] and 1971 to 1974.[13] The 1971 to 1974 data are presented in Tables A–6 and A–7, in six age groupings from 18 to 74 years and by sex. In these tables, it becomes necessary to define what deviations from the average values will be considered abnormal.

Two points are evident from the Metropolitan Life tables and the HANES tables. The first is that, as a rule, the desirable weights of the insurance tables are lower than the average weights descriptive of the United States population, although this is less true using the 1983 Metropolitan Life Tables, which were set considerably higher than the 1959 tables. The second is that the HANES data show an increase of weight by age from 18 years to 54 years, with a plateau and then a fall after that. This shows that, in the United States population, weight is not static with age once maturity is reached, but is actually a function of age.

The insurance companies used the terms "ideal weight" or "desirable weight" to describe weights that actuarially were associated with the least mortality. In subsequent usage of these tables, the definition of overweight has been accepted as 10% above an ideal or desirable weight and of obesity as 20% or more above this point. Using such criteria, researchers found a high incidence of overweight in the HANES Survey of 1960 to 1962.[1] Data of the HANES Survey of 1971 to 1974 show that United States adults measured at that time were comparably obese.[13,14] These data are shown in Table 44–1.[15]

The tables make clear that an alarming percentage of Americans are overweight. This percentage increases with age, particularly among women.

## Obesity in Children

The prevalence of obesity in the Western world begins with infancy. Studies available, though imperfect, suggest that one third or more of infants in the Western industrialized world are too heavy.[16–18] Data for schoolchildren are less available and estimates have varied between 6 and 15%.[16,19,20] Adolescent obesity rates have been cal-

**Table 44–1. Prevalence of Overweight.\* United States Health Examination Survey 1960–1962 and Health and Nutrition Examination Survey 1971–1974**

| | Men (%) | | Women (%) | |
|---|---|---|---|---|
| Age | 1960–1962 | 1971–1974 | 1960–1962 | 1971–1974 |
| 20–74 | 14.5 | 14.0 | 25.1 | 23.8 |
| 20–24 | 9.6 | 7.4 | 9.1 | 9.6 |
| 25–34 | 13.3 | 13.6 | 14.8 | 17.1 |
| 35–44 | 14.9 | 17.0 | 23.2 | 24.3 |
| 45–54 | 16.7 | 15.8 | 28.9 | 27.8 |
| 55–64 | 15.8 | 15.1 | 38.6 | 34.7 |
| 65–74 | 14.6 | 13.4 | 38.8 | 31.5 |

\*Percentage of population deviating by 20% or more from desirable weight. Estimated from regression equation of weight on height for men and women ages 20–29 years, obtained from HANES I.
From Abraham, S., Johnson, C.L.: Overweight Adults 20–74 Years of Age: United States, 1971–74. Vital and Health Statistics. Advance Data No. 51. Hyattsville, Md., National Center for Health Statistics, Public Health Service, DHEW.

culated at the 20 to 30 % rate.[18,20–22] The studies suggest that young women are more likely to be obese than are young men. The prevalence of obesity seems to be relatively constant throughout childhood.

Whether obesity in childhood leads to obesity in the adult has been widely debated. Some retrospective studies have suggested that there is a direct progression from a fat child to a fat adult.[23] Rimm and Rimm report that 50% of adult women in every age group with weights greater than 18% of ideal body weight had been obese adolescents.[24] In addition, it has been stated that 30% of adults who are obese become obese during childhood. About 80% of obese adolescents become obese adults,[25] and they tend to be fatter than those who become obese as adults.[24] Although a recent workshop concluded that there is no evidence that the obese child becomes an obese adult, a still newer study showed that 26.5% of initially obese infants and children were still obese two decades later, compared with the 15% expected by chance.[26]

## Socioeconomic Influence

Epidemiologic studies have shown a strong association between socioeconomic status and the prevalence of obesity. This relationship is much stronger in women.

The effect of social environment on obesity was investigated in the "Midtown Manhattan Study," which studied a population with both high- and low-income groups. Socioeconomic status and the prevalence of obesity were found to be inversely related.[27] As many as 30% of women of lower socioeconomic class were obese, 16% of middle-status women, and 5% of upper status. Men showed similar but less exaggerated trends. Similar socioeconomic trends have been found in other countries.[28,29] Obesity was also related in the Manhattan study to ethnicity,[30] with Eastern Europeans being particularly heavy. Others have also found ethnicity to be an important variable.[31] In addition, religious affiliation was important, with the prevalence being higher among Jews, followed by Catholics, and lowest among Protestants.[32]

Although a relationship exists between prevalence of obesity and socioeconomic status, it is not all clear-cut. For example, an English study showed that the prevalence of overweight was low in males of lower socioeconomic status engaged in heavy manual labor.[33]

There is also an effect of race on obesity. In the United States, for instance, black women have a higher prevalence of obesity than white women whereas white men have a higher prevalence than black men.[34] The reasons for this finding are not at present evident.

## MORTALITY AND MORBIDITY

Overweight has been associated with excess mortality in many studies.[35–38] Table 44–2 summarizes mortality data for three such studies, the Build and Blood Pressure Study of 1959,[37] the American Cancer Society Study,[39] and the Build and the Blood Pressure Study of 1979.[38] All three studies show increasing mortality with increasing overweight, with higher mortality risks in men than in women.

The American Cancer Society Study, which was not an insurance study, counteracts the objection that insured lives are not typical of the general population because insured individuals tend to be richer and predominantly Caucasian, and also the objection that it is not valid to use weight at insurance to relate to death some 35 years afterward. Since the results of the American Cancer Society data are similar to the insured data, they validate the use of the actuarial data of insured lives.

Since insurance companies relate only to healthy persons, their data should exclude ill people. The American Cancer Society study in all likelihood overstated the mortality of underweight persons because it only lasted 12 years, and the general population it studied no doubt included some persons with illnesses and weight loss that could have caused early death.

The mortality rate increase is not linear with increasing weight. An accelerated mortality occurs as people get heavier, particularly for males.[40] In addition, in the insurance data, the relative mortality is higher in males who are overweight than in females, whereas this is not so in the general population, as reflected by the American Cancer Society Study. Many studies do not show increased risk of mortality at relative weights up to 20% above desirable level.[40–44]

Evidence now exists that the relationship between weight and mortality is different at different times of life. The Whitehall study of 18,000 English civil servants showed that the relationship between weight quintile and mortality changes with age so that for the youngest men coronary heart disease mortality shows a linear increase from lowest weight quintile to highest, whereas for the oldest men no relationship is evident.[45]

Three other studies have investigated this relationship of weight to mortality in the elderly. All seem to agree on a protective effect of increased weight in old age.[46–48]

The finding of a relationship between obesity and increased mortality at a young age and no such relationship at an older age implies that it is continuous obesity over many years that affects health and can lead to death.

The data on the relationship of obesity and mortality may be obscured by the fact that fatness may relate to the type of death as well as to overall

**Table 44–2.   Mortality According to Variations in Weight***

| Weight Group | Build and Blood Pressure Study 1959 | | American Cancer Society Study | | Build and Blood Pressure 1979 | |
|---|---|---|---|---|---|---|
| | *Male* | *Female* | *Male* | *Female* | *Male* | *Female* |
| 20% Underweight | 95 | 87 | 110 | 100 | 105 | 110 |
| 10% Underweight | 90 | 89 | 100 | 95 | 94 | 97 |
| 10% Overweight | 113 | 109 | 107 | 108 | 111 | 107 |
| 20% Overweight | 125 | 121 | 121 | 123 | 120 | 110 |
| 30% Overweight | 142 | 130 | 137 | 138 | 135 | 125 |
| 40% Overweight | 167 | | 162 | 163 | 153 | 136 |
| 50% Overweight | 200 | | 210 | | 177 | 149 |
| 60% Overweight | 250 | | | | 210 | 167 |

*Each study measured departures from its own set of average weights, where mortality would be 100.
From Van Itallie, T.B.,[213] with permission of Am. J. Clin. Nutr., American Society for Clinical Nutrition.

mortality. That is, the obese may be at a greater risk for some forms of death yet at lesser risk for others. In a study of 2,381 males between the ages of 45 and 75 from West Scotland, lean men were found to have a higher overall mortality rate than the obese,[49] with an excess of cardiovascular deaths. Thus it may not be possible to assign a single optimum weight or an optimum level of fatness. There may be "different optima for different causes of death at different time periods and ... no single value of weight or fatness is optimal for all."[49]

## Causes of Death and Morbidity

The causes of death in men 20% and 40% above average weight as derived from the data of the American Cancer Society Study[5] and the Build Study of 1979[4] are shown in Table 44–3.

**Cardiovascular Disease.** Prospective studies of cardiovascular morbidity and mortality have shown an association with obesity. The effect of obesity on cardiovascular disease has not always been an independent one, but has generally been through exacerbation of other risk factors such as hypertension, diabetes, and hyperlipidemia.[50] This finding is not surprising, since blood pressure, blood lipids, and glucose values increase when individuals gain substantial weight.[51] This predictable increase in cardiovascular risk factors by increasing weight has been well quantified in the Framingham study. For every 10% rise in relative weight, systolic blood pressure rises 6.5 mm, plasma cholesterol 12 mg/dl, and fasting blood glucose 2 mg/dl.[52] Although the association of these cardiovascular risk factors is not as strong in women as in men, the association of obesity to cardiovascular disease is as strong in women as in men.[53]

There is evidence that obesity, when it occurs at an earlier age (20 to 40 years) has a greater influence on cardiovascular disease than later-onset obesity.[54] The Manitoba Study, which compared the 26-year incidence of coronary heart dis-

ease (CHD) and had a young average entry age of 30.8 years, found that body mass index was significantly related to CHD.[55] Myocardial infarction, sudden death, and coronary insufficiency were all associated with a high body mass index. It is noteworthy that this association was not evident until the tenth year of follow-up. Thus, short-term studies, or studies concentrating on older individuals, may not show an independent effect of obesity because they are too short, or have not focused on the correct age group.

Similarly, studies by Chapman et al. using ponderal index as a measure of obesity found a higher rate of myocardial infarction in men under age 40 and not in those older.[56] In the Whitehall study, the ten-year coronary heart disease mortality showed an increase from the lowest- to the highest-weight quintiles for the younger men, but no effect of weight in the older men.[45] In addition, the effect of weight is small when blood pressure, cholesterol, and smoking are accounted for. For the older men, the highest mortality is in the lowest-weight quintile.

**Blood Lipids.** Although hypertriglyceridemia has been associated with obesity,[57] the association is not strong. Triglycerides are transported predominantly as very low density lipoproteins (VLDL).[58] Hypertriglyceridemia may be related to the insulin resistance and consequent hyperinsulinemia of obesity,[59] which increases plasma triglyceride secretion.[58,60] In addition, because FFA levels are raised in obesity, the increased hepatic uptake of FFA may increase the secretory rate of triglyceride.[61] Enhanced triglyceride production may also come from more glucose precursors extracted by the liver.[61] Despite this increased triglyceride production, the level of triglycerides in obese persons is often normal or only slightly elevated. Because lipoprotein lipase activity is elevated in obesity,[62] it is possible that this activity enhances VLDL clearance at the periphery. After weight reduction, plasma triglycerides that were high tend to fall.[58] This change is associated with a decreased VLDL-triglyceride production and a

**Table 44–3. Mortality Ratios (Factor of Increased Risk)***

| | Men 20% above Average Weight | | Men 40% above Average Weight | |
| | Build Study 1979 | American Cancer Society | Build Study 1979 | American Cancer Society |
|---|---|---|---|---|
| Cause of Death | | | | |
| Coronary heart disease | 118 | 128 | 169 | 175 |
| Cerebral "hemorrhage" (stroke) | 110 | 116 | 164 | 191 |
| Cancer | 100 | 105 | 105 | 124 |
| Diabetes | 250 | 210 | 500 | 300 |
| Digestive diseases | 125 | 168 | 220 | 340 |
| All causes | 120 | 121 | 150 | 162 |

*Each study measured departures from its own set of average weights, where mortality would be 100.
From Van Itallie, T.B.,[213] with permission of Am. J. Clin. Nutr., American Society for Clinical Nutrition.

decreased insulinemia.[58] It is interesting that, in families carrying the combined hyperlipidemia trait, obese relatives tend to manifest high levels of very low density lipoproteins (VLDL), whereas the nonobese individuals show elevated low density lipoproteins (LDL).[63]

There is much less evidence of cholesterol elevation in obesity. Only marginally significant correlations have been shown.[64,65] Total cholesterol levels may be raised, and the ratio of LDL to high density lipoproteins (HDL) is elevated. The elevation of this ratio enhances the risk of coronary heart disease.

**Diabetes Mellitus.** A strong association exists between obesity and diabetes mellitus. In fact, obesity can be considered the most important "environmental" determinant in the manifestation of diabetes. In epidemiologic studies including many geographic areas, races, and cultures, West et al. noted a marked correlation between prevalence of diabetes and overweight.[66] In some of these populations, diabetes has been found to be as much as threefold higher in females than in males. These sex differences can be corrected by matching for adiposity.[66]

Even moderate obesity can raise the risk of diabetes tenfold.[67] In the Framingham study, women in the upper quintile of weight were four times as likely to develop glucose intolerance as women in the lower quintile.[68]

Body fat distribution has been implicated as a predictor of glucose intolerance and hyperinsulinemia.[69–72] The size of fat cells in the abdominal area is related to metabolic disturbance; this is not so in the thigh area.[71,72] This increased risk with abdominal fat suggests that a "male" pattern of fat distribution poses a greater risk for diabetes than a "female" pattern. It is not yet clear whether the important factor is upper-body obesity or central obesity.

Obesity is associated with hyperinsulinemia[73] and, in general, the fatter an individual, the higher will be the basal or fasting insulin.[59] In addition, in nondiabetics, the height of the insulin response to glucose or other stimuli is related to basal insulin and therefore is closely correlated with the degree of obesity.[59] In obese subjects with an abnormal glucose tolerance, however, the percentage increase of insulin over basal values is actually decreased in comparison to lean subjects. Thus, the impairment of glucose disposal can often be explained by an accompanying impairment of insulin secretion. This impairment is first observed in the early phase of insulin response, but as carbohydrate tolerance deteriorates, the entire time course of the insulin response is affected.

*Insulin Resistance.* The phenomenon of excessive blood insulin levels in obesity, both basal and after stimuli, suggests that an insulin resistance or insensitivity is present. Studies of intra-arterial insulin infusion in the forearm have revealed insulin resistance in both adipose tissue and muscle.[74] Moreover, the insulin insensitivity of muscle in obesity extends to amino acid metabolism. Thus, the amino acids most sensitive to the action of insulin are elevated in the plasma of obese subjects, despite the hyperinsulinemia.[75] These elevated blood amino acids may constitute a possible feedback stimulus for hyperinsulinemia in obesity.[76]

The liver in obese subjects also manifests insulin resistance. When compared to lean normal subjects, obese individuals have a higher splanchnic uptake of glucose precursors and have a smaller inhibition in splanchnic glucose output with equivalent insulin elevations.[76]

*Insulin Receptor and Postreceptor Defects.* The first step in the action of insulin on the cell is the binding of the hormone to a specific receptor on the outer plasma membrane. This process then initiates a series of "postreceptor" biochemical events, such as glucose and amino acid transport, stimulation of protein DNA and RNA synthesis, and inhibition of protein degradation. Generally, where high levels of insulin prevail in the blood, low levels of insulin receptors are present. This self-regulation of the membrane insulin receptor, so that high insulin levels cause a lowering of insulin receptor number, is called down-regulation.[77] It now seems clear that cells from obese humans have a decreased number of insulin receptors.[78–79]

Although part of the insulin resistance in obesity can be attributed to changes in insulin receptor number and/or receptor affinity for insulin, the tissues of obese animal models show intracellular postreceptor defects in glucose metabolism that account for the major part of insulin resistance.

In obese humans, the degree of insulin resistance is much greater than can be predicted from the magnitude of the decrease of insulin receptors. Using the euglycemic glucose clamp technique, researchers can study in vivo insulin dose-response curves. The least hyperinsulinemic, least insulin-resistant patients show only a receptor defect, whereas the most hyperinsulinemic show the largest postreceptor defect.[80] The nature of the postreceptor defect is being actively investigated. It could be due to a decrease in the number of glucose transporters, a decrease in the affinity of the transporter for glucose, or a decrease in the accessibility of the transporter to the cell surface.

*Significance of Hyperinsulinemia.* The production of excessive quantities of insulin for a prolonged period may lead to pancreatic exhaustion in those who are genetically predisposed.[81] Eventually, insulin response can decrease, resulting in metabolic decompensation. Support for this position comes from data suggesting that the duration of obesity rather than the degree can be best correlated with carbohydrate intolerance in obese adults.

**Hypertension.** Blood pressure elevation is a common concomitant of obesity.[82–84] The causes of the association of obesity and hypertension are not clear. A relationship between weight gain and increase in blood pressure is well documented.[85,86] In hypertensive patients, weight reduction reduces blood pressure,[87–89] and weight regain raises pressure. The fall in blood pressure with weight reduction is associated with a decrease in blood volume, cardiac output, and sympathetic activity.[90]

The cardiac output and the peripheral vascular resistance are the most important determinants of the blood pressure. These in turn are affected by the total body sodium content and by neurohumoral factors. Data by Dahl et al. incriminated sodium loss rather than weight loss as the cause of the lowered blood pressure with caloric restriction.[91] Others, however, have reported that it is weight reduction that is important.

Insulin may play a role in the hypertension of obesity[92] since changes in the plasma insulin concentration can affect sodium transport in the human kidney.[93] Insulin reduces sodium excretion independent of changes in plasma glucose. This effect can be noted without concurrent changes in filtered load of glucose, glomerular filtration rate, renal blood flow, and plasma aldosterone levels.[94] Natriuresis occurs during fasting or hypocaloric diets, when insulin levels fall, and antinatriuresis occurs with refeeding, when insulin rises again.[95] The hyperinsulinemia of obesity may raise the blood pressure by increasing renal sodium absorption, which in turn expands the extracellular fluid volume, raising cardiac output, peripheral resistance, and blood pressure.[92]

Whether catecholamines play a role in the hypertension of obesity is unclear, although Landsberg has reported a decreased sympathetic nervous system activity during weight loss diets and an increase during refeeding.[96]

The distribution of fat in the body may have an important effect on blood pressure risk, as it does in diabetes, with central fat or upper body fat being more likely to raise blood pressure than the lower body fat of the gluteal and thigh region.[97] The reasons for this tendency are not clear.

**Respiratory Problems.** As an individual becomes more obese, the muscular work required for ventilation increases. If the limitation of movement of the chest wall is great enough, $CO_2$ retention occurs. This condition can lead to lethargy and somnolence. The $CO_2$ narcosis can also lead to periods of apnea that usually occur during sleep and exacerbate the problem of $CO_2$ retention. In addition, polycythemia may occur, which can enhance thrombosis. In severe cases of respiratory disease, pulmonary hypertension, cardiac enlargement, and congestive heart failure may develop.

**Gallbladder Disease.** The risk for gallbladder disease is higher as obesity increases and is greater for women than for men.[98] An increased body fat reservoir is associated with increased cholesterol production.[99] As a result, greater biliary excretion of cholesterol increases the cholesterol concentrations in bile, which can enhance cholesterol stone formation.[100]

**Arthritis.** The clinical impression is that the incidence of osteoarthritis of the weight-bearing joints is higher in obese than in lean persons and that this condition tends to become worse with higher weight.[101] However, no good prevalence studies are available.

**Gout.** The cause for the rise in uric acid levels with increasing weight is unclear. Usually this uric acid elevation is asymptomatic, but the occurrence of gouty attacks is higher in obese than in lean individuals, particularly when overweight reaches 30% above ideal.

**Cancer of the Breast and Endometrium.** Obesity has been suggested as a risk factor in the development of cancer of the endometrium.[102–104] It is possible that this association is related to endocrine abnormalities, and an increased conversion of estrone to androstenedione in adipose tissue has been implicated. In addition, obesity is correlated with increasing estrogenicity of cervical smears.[105] Although such increased estrogen activity could cause increased risk of breast cancer in postmenopausal women,[106–108] no proof of this effect is available.

## GENETICS AND ENVIRONMENT

Twin studies have been pursued to try to determine the relative importance of genetic inheritance vs. environmental influences in obesity. The weights of identical twins raised in separate homes have been reported to be similar,[109] thereby suggesting that heredity contributes significantly to weight. Although Newman et al. showed a greater difference in twins raised apart than in twins raised together, thereby implicating environment, they also found that fraternal twins raised apart showed a greater weight difference than did identical twins, suggesting a strong genetic component.[110]

The Ten-State Nutrition Study suggests that environmental factors may be most important in the obesity found in families. Skinfold thicknesses were compared in 429 adoptive parent-child pairs and in 198 genetically unrelated siblings. In addition, 6,372 pairs of biologic parent-child pairs and 3,713, biologic pairs of siblings were measured. No difference was found between the correlations for biologic sibling pairs as compared to genetically unrelated siblings.[111] In addition, the correlations in skinfolds between parents and children were high.[112] If parents were divided into lean, medium, or obese and placed in appropriate mother-father combinations (lean-lean, lean-obese, obese-lean, obese-obese), the children were fatter as the parents increased in fatness. This latter finding, however, does not prove a genetic risk; in households with fatter parents, food may be more plentiful and may lead to fatness in the children.

Studying adoptive parent-child pairs, Withers could find no evidence that the correlation of fatness between a parent and an adopted child was different from that between a parent and a biologic child.[113] However, Biron et al. studied 374 families with one or more adopted children.[114] There was no correlation in weight between adopted children and their adoptive parents and siblings.

Common environment seems to have less influence as children grow older. Rao et al., studying 1,068 families in Brazil, found that the influence of shared family environment on weight could account for only 18% of the variance.[115]

Thus, the relative importance of genetics and environment on weight is still unclear. To date, no specific genetic marker of obesity has been found.

## PATHOGENESIS

### Endocrinopathy in Obesity

Although popular thought ascribes obesity to glandular troubles, in actuality endocrinopathy is a rare cause of obesity. Overactivity of the adrenal gland, leading to Cushing's syndrome, causes central obesity. Why in this condition adipocytes located at the center of the body are stimulated to multiply and fill, whereas those at the extremities are not, is unclear. The central obesity is associated with hypertension and diabetes.

In severe hypothyroidism, some increased adipose mass may occur, but most of the increased weight is water. Few obese patients suffer from hypothyroidism.

Hypogonadism is sometimes associated with mild obesity, although the reason is not clear. Women with Stein-Leventhal syndrome (ovarian cysts) are generally overweight. The etiology of this syndrome is unclear. It is possible that the ovary may secrete steroids that simulate the action of adrenal steroids.

A hypothalamic lesion caused by tumor, infection or, rarely, trauma may lead to obesity. This is secondary to damage of nerve fibers in the ventromedial area important in food intake regulation.

In children, obesity may be seen with certain congenital syndromes. The cause of these obesities is unknown. They include Prader-Willi syndrome, Laurence-Moon-Biedl syndrome, adiposogenital dystrophy (Fröhlich's syndrome), Bongiovanni-Eisenmenger syndrome, and pseudohypoparathyroidism.

Whereas the cause of obesity is seldom due to a hormonal abnormality, obesity may lead to abnormalities of hormone levels.[116] Owing to the development of insulin resistance, insulin levels in the blood rise, as has already been discussed. Triiodothyronine ($T_3$) is elevated in conditions of high-caloric intake with adequate carbohydrate. Thyroxine levels are normal. The urinary excretion of free cortisol and of hydroxycorticoids, sometimes elevated in obesity, is probably related to an increase in cortisol turnover. These changes are related to the higher lean body mass in the obese. Blood cortisol levels are usually in the normal range in obesity, and diurnal patterns are generally normal. Growth hormone levels are in the low-normal range. Stimulatory tests with arginine, insulin hypoglycemia, or L-dopa demonstrate a poor growth hormone response. This growth hormone response reverts toward normal with weight loss.

### Thermogenesis

Obese individuals have been described as utilizing energy calories more "efficiently" than lean subjects. They have been characterized as requiring fewer calories per unit of lean body mass. If they eat a number of calories equal to those eaten by a lean subject, more of the calories will be available as extra energy to be deposited as fat. This subject, however, is controversial.

The expenditure of energy takes three forms: basal metabolic rate (BMR), activity, and the thermic effect of food.

**Basal Metabolic Rate.** The basal metabolic rate is that energy required for the basic maintenance of the cells of the body. Since the metabolic rate is defined by the cell mass of the body, it is reasonable to express it in terms of the lean body mass (LBM). The contribution of the LBM to the

BMR is three to five times greater per kg than that of body fat.[117] The correlation of BMR with LBM explains why men have higher metabolic rates than women and why metabolic rates decrease with age. The high metabolic rate of children can be ascribed to the energy cost of growth.[118,119]

There is, however, a difference in metabolic rate in individuals matched for age, sex, and LBM.[120] These differences can be as high as 30%. As a result, at a given fixed intake, one individual may gain weight while the other does not. Thus, different people will maintain weight on different caloric intakes.

The BMR of obese persons is higher than that of lean individuals.[121,122] Since obese people have a higher LBM than lean people, this finding is not surprising. The obese often have a BMR lower than that of lean individuals if it is expressed per kg of body weight. This phenomenon is reasonable since per unit of weight they have a relatively lower amount of metabolizing cell mass. If one expresses BMR as total energy expended per unit time, the obese expend more calories than lean people. In terms of basal or resting energetics, therefore, the obese are not more efficient.

**Thermic Effect of Foods.** The rise of metabolic rate above basal after eating has been called the thermic effect of food or dietary-induced thermogenesis (DIT). About 10% of the ingested diet that can be metabolized is lost as heat, which is used up in the intermediary metabolism of substrates, in the utilization of ATP, and in the formation of ATP from reduced coenzymes by oxidative phosphorylation.

Although some studies have suggested that obese people have a lower DIT than lean people,[123–125] others have reported no difference.[126–128]

Insulin may be required for a full diet-induced thermogenic effect.[129] Insulin deficiency and/or resistance could lead to defective glucose oxidation and impaired thermogenesis.[130] Thus, whether obese individuals show an impaired or delayed DIT may well depend on their insulin sensitivity or insulin response.

The evidence for diminished thermic effect of food in obese as compared to lean individuals is meager if one eliminates glucose-intolerant subjects. In addition, even in those studies showing a decreased DIT, if it is added to the elevated BMR all obese persons manifest, the total energy expenditure (BMR and DIT) is elevated over that of lean persons.

**Thermogenesis and Overfeeding.** Neumann suggested 84 years ago that if a lean individual overate, the excess calories eaten were dissipated as heat (luxus consumption) and normal weight was maintained.[130a] Garrow has summarized the results of 15 studies in which lean and obese subjects were overfed.[131] Most show fairly conclusive evidence that significant overfeeding (2,000 + extra calories per day) for at least 10 day leads to some energy wastage. In the four studies in which obese subjects were evaluated, however, no evidence of luxus consumption was found. Thus, it is possible that the lean people are more adept at burning off excess ingested energy than are the obese. However, even in lean people, instances of caloric wastage have only been documented with very large caloric overeating, much higher than is usual.

The case for deficient ability to increase thermogenesis with overingestion in obese humans has been attractive because it has been documented in genetically obese rodents.[132] This finding has been ascribed to brown fat activity, but there is doubt whether enough brown fat is available in adult man to produce such excess heat. The extrapolation of small animal data to man is not valid at this time.

**Exercise.** Does exercise potentiate DIT? Again, the data are contradictory. Some studies support this theory;[133,134] others do not.[135–137] Overfeeding has not been shown to potentiate the effect of exercise in two studies,[138–139] and even in studies suggesting a potentiating effect of exercise on food, the effect is small. If a difference is present between lean and obese individuals, it is smaller still.

In summary, almost no experimental evidence suggests a difference in lean and obese individuals in wasteful energy production to any stimulant. There are two exceptions. First, it is possible that with great overfeeding (2,000 kcal or more above the usual intake) for a long period of time (10 days or more) some wasteful energy production will occur and that this may be greater in the lean than the obese person. Second, it is possible that obese patients with insulin resistance or insulin deficiency may have a defective glucose oxidation and generate less heat after carbohydrate ingestion.

### Fat Cells

Fat cells or adipocytes are distributed throughout the body. They form a reservoir depot of energy that is elastic, being able to contract to accommodate the energy balance of the organism. The depot can expand in two ways: by increasing the size of the fat cells or by increasing their number. Although the size of the fat cell is generally between 0.3 and 0.9 µg, the number is more expandable, averaging from as low as $2 \times 10^{10}$ to as high as $16 \times 10^{10}$.[140] There is thus enormous flexibility for expansion of the adipose reservoir.

Fat cells develop from fat cell precursors called preadipocytes. It is unclear what stimulus activates the preadipocyte to differentiate into an adipocyte and begin to accumulate lipid. The size of adipocytes gradually increases if energy balance continues to be positive until a cell size of about 10 µg is reached. At this point, it does not seem possible for the adipocyte to enlarge further.

If positive energy balance then persists, a trigger for adipocyte proliferation occurs, and cell number begins to rise. Since the expansivity of numbers is virtually unlimited, the adipose reservoir can reach huge dimensions if caloric intake remains high.

Key time periods of adipose cell proliferation have been a controversial subject. Knittle and Hirsch reported that an increase in rat fat cell number occurred in the preweaning phase[141] and not in the postweaning phase.[142] However, others have since shown that rat fat cells can proliferate in the postweaning period.[143–145] Although the data in humans are more sparse, there is evidence for an increase in fat cell size in the initial year of life with a rise in fat cell number subsequently,[146] so that fat cell number increases fivefold between 1 and 22 years of age.

Whether fat cell number is fixed after reaching adulthood has been debated. Accumulating data favor the concept that fat cell number may continue to increase as long as nutritional excess occurs. Thus, excess storage energy is accommodated by enhancing fat cell number. However, once fat cells are formed, it seems to be difficult to dedifferentiate them. Number seems to remain fixed even if weight is lost.[147] The net effect of weight loss is then to bring fat cell size down toward normal and eventually to below normal.

If maximum fat cell size is attained by infants at one year of age and then additional fat reserves are created by increasing fat cell number, the chronically overfed child will develop an excess number of fat cells (hyperplasia). This condition has been well documented.

This hyperplastic child is not, however, destined inevitably to become a hyperplastic adult. Obesity at age 2 or 3 is not necessarily predictive of obesity at age 21. Even though a child who is hyperplastic has a greater number of fat cells than his lean contemporary, he has a lower total number than a lean adult. Thus he may "grow out" of his obesity by retaining his greater number of fat cells, which, if not increasing as he grows older, may gradually approach normality.

In summary, obesity can be classified as hypertrophic or as both hypertrophic and hyperplastic. Obese patients are not hyperplastic without being hypertrophic unless they have lost weight by dieting or illness. This classification may be important prognostically in treatment. Hypertrophic obese patients may be able to maintain weight loss better than hyperplastic ones.[148] This possibility requires further investigation.

## Lipoprotein Lipase

Adipose tissue lipoprotein lipase (LPL) is an enzyme that determines the rate of uptake by fat cells of circulating plasma triglyceride. It originates in adipocytes and muscle cells and then is secreted to the endothelium where it acts on circulating VLDL triglyceride. It enhances the breakdown of triglycerides to glycerol phosphate and free fatty acids. These smaller molecular weight substances can enter adipose cells, be re-esterified, and be stored as triglyceride.

Adipose tissue LPL activity is elevated in human obesity.[62,150] When adipose LPL is expressed per cell, it correlates significantly with fat cell size and with percent desirable weight.[62,150,151] This correlation is not true of postheparin LPL, muscle LPL, or hepatic lipase.[150] Racial differences also seem to exist in LPL. For instance, Pima Indians, a group renowned for their high prevalence of obesity, have lower levels than obese Caucasians.[151]

Whether the elevated adipose LPL is primary, that is, causative for obesity, or just a secondary consequence of the obese state is unclear. Obese individuals could have elevated LPL as a primary defect that enhances their ability to "pull" triglyceride into cells, or obesity could develop from some other etiology and the enhanced LPL activity could be secondary to the enlarged fat cells. Schwartz and Brunzell have suggested that the first hypothesis is correct, and that the LPL activity rises further with weight loss and returns to lower (though elevated) values with weight regain.[152,153] The further elevation of LPL with any weight drop tends to enhance lipid clearance, to raise stored triglyceride levels, and to restore the obese state.

Although this is an attractive hypothesis, recent data do not confirm it. Two studies have shown that after stabilized significant weight reduction, the elevated adipose tissue LPL activity drops,[150,154] whereas other tissues lipases are not affected.[150] In addition, with refeeding, the LPL activity rises rapidly to above previous baseline levels.[154] Thus, this change may enhance the capacity of storing triglycerides that are circulating owing to the enhanced food intake. It may therefore contribute to the efficient regain of weight in a refeeding obese patient who was previously on a hypocaloric regimen.

## Weight Regain

Of patients who lose significant amounts of weight, 80 to 100% regain it. The explanation for this dismal record is not readily evident, but a few hypotheses bear mentioning.

The first is that a reducing obese patient has decreased energy requirements. Patients on a reducing diet experience a significant drop of 15 to 30 percent in their metabolic rate.[155,156] As a result, it is more difficult for them to lose weight on the same hypocaloric diet in the second month than in the first, and in the third than the second.[155] This reduced metabolic rate also may make it easier to regain weight on returning to a more normal diet. After a fast or a hypocaloric diet, refeeding is associated with a supranormal tissue response to nutrients. This response is characterized by a "repletion reaction" that includes a generalized increased substrate utilization with an adaptive hyperlipogenesis in adipose tissue and liver. In adipose tissue, this hyperlipogenesis is characterized by a marked production of triglyceride and $CO_2$ from glucose.[157,158] The rapid transfer of glucose into the tissues, enhanced by increased insulin levels plus greater tissue insulin sensitivity, may cause enhanced lipogenesis and may also lead to lower blood glucose levels that may enhance hunger and stimulate greater food intake.[158]

The increased efficiency of rats after fasting has been documented. Animals fasted for 4 days and then refed could maintain their new lower weight (90% of baseline) if fed only 60% of the original daily calories.[159] In addition, fasted rats refed their original daily caloric intake could regain their lost weight without overeating. These reports suggest that during the refeeding period, animals are more efficient at utilizing the same number of calories.[160]

Suggestive evidence of a similar phenomenon is beginning to emerge from human studies. In morbidly obese patients who were significantly reduced (from an average 152 kg to 100 kg), seven-day energy intake requirements to maintain weight dropped from 1,432 kcal/m²/day to 1,021 kcal/m²/day.[161] The figure of 1,021 kcal/m²/day was significantly lower than the value of 1,341 kcal/m²/day found in normal lean individuals weighing a mean of 63 kg. Since this weight loss was a recent one, a second metabolic study was executed with reduced obese patients who had maintained their weight loss for 4 to 6 years. These four women also showed kilocalorie requirements averaging 1,031/m²/day to maintain their weight.

This finding suggests that at least some reduced-obese individuals have lowered caloric requirements that may persist for years and that if caloric intake is increased above the 1,000 kcal/m²/day range, weight regain will occur. This theory helps to explain the poor record in maintaining weight loss after dieting.

The regulation of adipose tissue mass may occur by an ability of the organism to sense the filling of adipose cells with triglyceride. That is, weight regain in a refeeding animal seems to continue until fat cells have once again returned to their original size. Some investigators have suggested that in this way adipose tissue exerts a regulatory function on energy intake and energy balance.[162] This process could explain why reduced obese patients have such difficulty staying on hypocaloric diets after they have dropped to a certain weight. At that point, their fat cells are at lower limits of normal size. To drop weight further, these cells would need to reduce to an abnormally low size. If hyperplastic obese persons do succeed in lowering their weight to an extent where fat cell size is below normal, they will be unable to remain at that weight, regain will occur, and fat cells will be filled to at least a "normal" size.[163]

The role of the fat cell in energy regulation is intriguing, and more investigative studies in this area are necessary.

## THERAPY FOR OBESITY

### Dietary Management

Many strategies for losing weight have been tried over the years because, as a rule, losing weight and keeping the weight off are extremely difficult. This is particularly true for those individuals who are 25% or more overweight.

**Reduced Efficiency of Utilization.** Protein was initially thought to be primarily responsible for diet-induced thermogenesis. A high-protein diet was therefore considered to be more "thermogenic" by causing more obligate heat production. As a result, fewer of these calories would be available for deposition as fat. However, this approach is incorrect, since it is now known that carbohydrate and fat contribute reasonably equivalently, calorie for calorie, to DIT.[164]

**Impaired Absorption.** Impairment of intestinal absorption of ingested calories has been a suggested strategy. Fiber has been particularly touted in this regard. There is, however, little evidence that fiber significantly affects total intestinal absorption.[165]

Nondigestible fat substitutes have been developed. An example is sucrose polyester, which can be used in the diet as a replacement for fat. Perfluoroactyl bromide, an inert synthetic product, can coat the gastrointestinal tract and prevent some caloric absorption. Also being developed are agents that slow the natural breakdown of macro-molecular nutrients into the smaller absorbable molecules. An example is the alphaglucosidase inhibitor acarbose, which inhibits hydrolysis of carbohydrate.[166] These "starch-blockers," however, have only been shown to delay absorption, not to inhibit it. As a result, no weight loss has been documented.

Because of the noxious side effects of fat and carbohydrate malabsorption, the acceptability and marketability of malabsorptive products have been low.

**Unbalanced Low-Calorie Diets.** These diets all have a marked imbalance of macronutrients that can also cause an imbalance of micronutrients. They emphasize particular food groups (carbohydrate, protein, or fat) and prohibit or deemphasize others. Because of their focused nature, they are easier for individuals to follow and this makes them popular.

They can be divided into different types. The most popular are high-protein, high-fat, low-carbohydrate diets. These are ketogenic diets. The carbohydrate generally makes up less than 20% of the diet. Proponents suggest that the ketosis causes appetite suppression. However, no adequate study of the effectiveness of ketones in inhibiting food intake is available.

Such diets tend to be low in vitamin C. Enhanced calcium loss can occur. The high uric acid produced may be dangerous for those predisposed to gout. These diets have a high cholesterol content, dangerous for people with hypercholesterolemia.[167] They often cause nausea, hypotension, and fatigue.[167]

The aforementioned diets have been modified to be high-protein (40 to 45%), low-fat (30 to 35%), and low-carbohydrate (20 to 25%). These diets tend to be lower in calories by the limiting of fat, a high-calorie item. They are still ketogenic, with the same side effects of nausea, hypotension, and fatigue. They tend to be high in saturated fats and cholesterol and low in vitamin A, C, thiamin, and iron. The amount of cholesterol may be triple that in a regular diet.[168]

A radically different type of diet is one that is high in carbohydrate, low in protein (35 g/day), and low in fat (as low as 10%).[169] The emphasis is on fruits, vegetables, breads, and cereals. No table fats, oil, or dairy products except skim milk are allowed. Often these diets prohibit sugar. If taken faithfully, such diets may be low in salt, iron, essential fatty acids, and fat-soluble vitamins.

**Total and Modified Fasts.** Some physicians have proposed total fasting as a way of losing weight.[170,171] Recent advocates have used it inter-mittently in treating obese type 2 diabetics. The problem with a total fast is that not only fat, but also much lean body mass, is lost.[172] Particularly in older individuals, lean body mass is difficult to regain. In addition, because of the diuresis induced, significant mineral losses occur.

Because of the deficiencies of total fasting, regimens called protein-supplemented modified fasts (PSMF) have become popular.[173] These are severely limited diets of 400 to 700 calories that generate a rapid weight loss. The protein is given in the form of either formula or natural foods such as lean meat, fowl, or fish. These diets have been given for extensive periods of time, although the consensus is that it is dangerous to allow them for longer than 16 weeks.[174]

Patients lose 1.5 to 2.3 kg/wk on these diets. The protein that the patients take needs to be of high biologic quality to help prevent the loss of body protein that occurs during a standard fast.[173]

It is well known that in a fasting subject the nitrogen excretion is initially high (11 to 23 g/d).[175] Nitrogen loss decreases steeply in the first few days to a nadir of obligate nitrogen excretion.[176] With total fasting, a cumulative nitrogen loss of 154 g of nitrogen or 963 g of protein occurs after 15 days.[177] Simply adding 100 g of carbohydrate per day decreases nitrogen loss by 40%.[178] Administering 55 g of high-quality protein per day causes negative nitrogen balance to occur initially for the first 10 days, but many patients achieve balance at about 20 days.[179] These low-calorie diets have been given large-scale trials by three groups.[180–182] One group gave 25 g of egg albumin and 40 g of oligosaccharides per day.[181] Another group gave 45 g of egg albumin and 30 g of sucrose per day.[182] The third gave 1.1 to 1.4 g of lean meat per kg ideal body weight, with the only carbohydrate being that in meat glycogen.[180] All required vitamin and mineral supplements daily as well as essential fatty acids.[181] They reported little morbidity. Vertes et al., with 1,200 outpatient years of experience, had 4 deaths, which they describe as less than expected for the population treated.[183]

It has been hypothesized that these diets spare protein by decreasing insulin level and enhancing ketonemia.[184] The ketonemia will in turn inhibit release of amino acids from muscle.[185] There is little experimental evidence that this hypothesis is correct, since insulin levels are not absolute determinants of protein sparing.[186,187]

With the popularization of these PSMF diets, numerous commercial preparations of liquid protein became available for over-the-counter purchase. Fifty-eight deaths have been associated with the use of these formulas.[188] Although the reason for these deaths in unclear, 17 of them have been investigated.[189,190] Patients seem to develop refractory ventricular arrhythmias. Whether this condition is secondary to myocardial protein atrophy, myocarditis, potassium deficiency, or other mineral losses is unclear.[189,191,192]

These deaths were most likely due to poor-quality protein in the commercial-formula diets. The proteins eaten in a regular diet, such as dairy products, meat, fish, and poultry, and grain and cereal products, provide about 87% of the calcium, 80% of the phosphorus, 60% of the magnesium, 74% of the iron, 80% of the zinc, 57% of the copper, 80% of the manganese, and 100% of the selenium in a usual diet. Many of the poor-quality hydrolyzed protein diets have not adequately replaced these minerals and others.

Besides the mortality, there is also morbidity with these diets. Orthostatic hypotension may be a problem with the sodium diuresis and volume depletion that occur.[193] This condition is probably secondary to the natriuretic effect of hyperketonemia[194] and the impaired norepinephrine secretion associated with it.[193] Other symptoms and signs include dehydration, cold intolerance, fatigue, dry skin, hair loss, and menstrual irregularities. Cholecystitis, pancreatitis, and peroneal nerve palsy occasionally have been reported.

Although it is true that nitrogen balance is better with PSMF than with starvation, there is little evidence that PSMF is better than a mixed diet. Comparisons of an 800-kcal mixed diet and an 800-kcal all-protein ketogenic diet and starvation in obese subjects have shown that while starvation gives the most negative nitrogen balance, nitrogen loss is less and not much different between the mixed and the all-protein diet.[195] Over a 10-day period, 2.8 kg of weight are lost with a mixed diet and 4.7 kg with the ketogenic diet, but all the extra weight lost with the ketogenic diet is water.[195] Longer 60-day studies show no difference in nitrogen balance between a mixed diet and a ketogenic diet.[196]

**Balanced Hypocaloric Diets.** In view of the aforementioned risks and problems of unbalanced diets, and the prolonged periods of time that restricted diets must be followed, a well-balanced mixed diet seems a sensible approach. Diets in the 1,100- to 1,200-kcal range can include appropriate macro and micro elements, vitamins, and protein.[197] They can be followed for months without specific supplements. The nutrients most likely to be deficient are iron, folacin, vitamin $B_6$, and zinc.[197] In such a diet, the percentage of protein is raised so that at least 240 calories or about 60 g per day are as protein. The protein should be of high quality and should make up about 25% of calories. At least 20% of the rest of the diet should be carbohydrate and at least 20% fat. In this way, fat-soluble vitamins and essential fatty acids will be available from fat and fiber and antiketogenic effect from carbohydrate.

In formulating a balanced diet for micronutrients and vitamins, one should use food items from the four food groups: (1) meat, fish, poultry, and meat substitutes; (2) milk and milk products; (3) cereals and cereal products; and (4) vegetables and fruits. The nutrients obtained are: (1) protein, fat, niacin, iron, and thiamin; (2) vitamins A and D, calcium, magnesium, and zinc; (3) carbohydrates, fat, phosphorus, magnesium, zinc, and copper; and (4) carbohydrate, vitamins A and C, iron, and magnesium.[197]

Since obese individuals need to be on a diet for a long time, it is crucial that the diet be acceptable. The diet must therefore fit the tastes and habits of the individual and be flexible enough to allow eating outside the home as well as in.

### Exercise

The therapeutic use of exercise to reverse obesity has been widely hailed. As has been previously mentioned, body weight is determined by a balance between energy intake and energy expenditure. If the energy expenditure can be increased by incremental physical activity and if energy intake is kept constant, weight will drop. A number of points must be emphasized. The first is that it requires a significant amount of physical effort to expend a significant number of calories. Calorie charts for expenditure are usually listed as the total caloric expenditure for a given period of time. It is clear, however, that an individual not doing the activity would not revert to an expenditure of zero calories but would expend at somewhat above basal levels (sitting, standing, or walking). For example, an obese woman exercising on a treadmill at 4 MPH would expend about 7.0 kcal/min or 210 calories if she were to continue this exercise for 30 minutes. Sitting in a chair, such a woman would expend about 1.3 kcal/min. or 39 kcal over 30 minutes. Thus, her exercise-induced expenditure would not be 210 kcal but 210 minus 39 or 171 kcal. Therefore, in looking at expenditure tables, one must always subtract between 1 and 1.5 kcal/min for the resting or sitting metabolic expenditure that would occur anyway.

The second point that must be clarified is the purported prolonged elevation of oxygen consumption for long periods after exercise. Such a sustained effect of exercise lasting for 7 to 48 hours has been described, but two reviews of the literature have concluded that no sustained increase could be demonstrated after exercise.[198,199] Studies have supported a lack of a sustained effect, using exercise levels that would be realistic for individuals on weight-control programs.[200–203] Since there is no appreciable caloric loss beyond that generated by the exercise period itself, claims for sustained effects of exercise on resting metabolic rate in weight-control programs are unwarranted.

The third point relates to the effect of exercise on food intake. Although it has been generally suggested that exercise inhibits food intake, this phenomenon has not been documented. In lean individuals, exercise generally leads to an increased energy intake and a maintenance of body weight.[204] This tendency is true with both mild (about 400 kcal/day) or moderate (about 775 kcal/day) exercise.[205] In obese individuals, it may be that in response to exercise, weight is defended to the same degree as in lean persons.

Most of the studies of the effect of exercise on obese subjects have only measured weight or body fat; they have not measured food intake. As mentioned previously, if expenditure is increased and food intake remains stable, weight loss will be commensurate with the increased expenditure. Such a result has been described.[206] Other studies, however, have documented amounts of weight loss that suggest that food intake was curtailed.[207,208] Some studies show no effect of exercise on weight at all.[209] Two metabolic ward studies over long periods of time, 19-day intervals[200] or 57-day intervals,[201] suggest that obese women tend to fix on an intake and remain at that intake even if the amount of activity is changed. The changes in intake seemed to relate more to the gustatory characteristics of the diet provided than to whether exercise was high or low.[209]

Despite these caveats, exercise is a valuable adjunct in a weight-reduction regimen. Although it is not invested with magical powers in sustaining an enhanced metabolic rate or in inhibiting food intake, every calorie expended can help in the net battle to utilize significantly more calories than are ingested. Exercise will help attain weight loss while allowing less stringent diets—a more acceptable regimen to many patients.

## Pharmacologic Treatment

Although the most widely used drugs for weight control are appetite suppressants, others have been tried that attack the food intake and metabolizing pathway at other sites, such as at digestion, absorption, lipid synthesis, or thermogenesis. The anorectic agents, which suppress appetite, will be discussed first.

The first, and a successfully marketed drug for many years, was amphetamine. Amphetamine is a β-phenethylamine and seems to induce anorexia via brain catecholamines, specifically norepinephrine and dopamine, although the relative importance of each in man is not yet clear. It causes not only anorexia, but also many other effects, among which are central stimulation, mood enhancement, cardiovascular excitation, and a selective effect on certain normal transmitter agents, especially catecholamines. Some of these effects can lead susceptible individuals to abuse and even to addiction.[210] In addition, in a small number of patients, discontinuing the drug seems to be associated with onset of depression.

Four anorexic drugs that seem to have fewer side effects and induce less dependence than amphetamine are most commonly used. There are diethylpropion, mazindol, fenfluramine, and phentermine.

Diethylpropion seems to have little effect on sleep and infrequent addiction has been reported. It is closest in structure to amphetamine, being modified by addition of a keto group on the β carbon and of ethyl groups on the N terminal. Mazindol is thought to act by prolonging the action of norepinephrine. It also causes central nervous system stimulation.[211] It is a tricyclic compound with a long plasma half life (33 to 55 hours). Fenfluramine has an ethyl group on the N terminal and a $CF_3$ on the phenyl ring. Its action is thought to be mediated by a central serotonergic system. It has no central stimulant effect.[212] Phentermine resin has had methyl groups substituted on the alpha carbon. The stimulant properties of this drug are less than those of amphetamine and yet it seems to be as effective. However, dry mouth, tachycardia, and increased blood pressure often occur.

Although we do not know enough yet to classify obesity in terms of etiology, there are probably differing causes. The drugs available are also different. It is not surprising, therefore, that the response is different from person to person.

These drugs may be a useful adjunct for treatment of obesity in some patients. The widespread beliefs in some medical circles that all appetite-suppressant drugs are useless and that tolerance quickly develops are not necessarily true. In addition, although side effects are common if excess dosage is taken, they do not necessarily occur at recommended dosage. An anorectic agent can be helpful in some people. One must remember, however, that the drug will be ineffective unless appropriate dosage is given and blood levels are adequate. It is also wise to individualize use to a patient's dietary habits. One would not administer a relatively short-acting drug in the morning if a patient eats no breakfast and is an evening and night eater.

Anorectic drugs will not work alone. Other therapy, such as diet and exercise, must also be stressed. Drugs may be helpful not only during weight loss but also in the difficult period of weight maintenance when many obese patients have their hardest time.

Although other pharmacologic agents have been tried, none has been shown to be successful enough to be marketed. These include inhibitors of dietary lipid absorption and inhibitors of lipid synthesis. An effort to develop thermogenic agents is underway, but no satisfactory drug is available to date.

Thyroid preparations, digitalis, or human chorionic gonadotrophin have no place in the treatment of obesity. Diuretics are rarely necessary, and certainly should never be used in combination with low-calorie diets.

Bulking agents, such as methylcellulose and other fibers, have been touted as aids in weight loss, but no evidence of this is available. They do not cause malabsorption and have not been shown to decrease food intake.[213]

In summary, though drugs may be helpful in some individuals at some periods in the weight loss and the weight maintenance periods, they do not hold first rank in any therapeutic program.

### Psychotherapy

The psychologic treatment of obesity has not enjoyed much success. Although there have been a few optimistic reports of the effect of psychoanalysis in producing weight loss,[214,215] particularly in adolescents,[214] therapeutic failure is the common result. Many obese patients may have emotional problems, but these vary. Some have anxiety, some are depressed, but some have no evident psychiatric problems at all, except for overeating and/or being underactive.[216] There is no particular personality type who is obese.

Although it has been suggested obesity may be protective for underlying neurotic behavior, this possibility has not been confirmed by patients undergoing obesity surgery. Some psychiatrists predicted that morbidly obese individuals would develop other addictive tendencies or overt neurotic or psychotic traits as weight loss occurred. This has not happened. Patients either have had no psychiatric change or have improved, but few have deteriorated.[217]

A distortion of body image does seem to exist in a minority of obese patients[216] with an overestimation of body size. In a study of morbidly obese subjects who were reduced enough to have significant changes in body size, the distortion of body image was persistent, particularly in those obese from childhood.[218]

Some psychiatrists have even reported evidence of low anxiety and depression in obese individuals,[219] and epidemiologic evidence suggests that they have a lower incidence of suicide than the general population.

Since there is no evidence that all or even most obese subjects are neurotic, it is incumbent on health professionals to individually evaluate each patient.

### Behavior Modification

Because of the poor record in the treatment of obesity by classical psychoanalysis and psychotherapy, behavior modification has grown in favor. Behavior modification programs grew out of the studies of Schachter, who suggested that the obese overeat because they are stimulus-bound. Schachter concluded that environmental food-relevant cues controlled eating rather than any psychogenic neurotic states.[220] This "externality theory" suggested that external environmental stimuli overrode whatever internal hunger or satiety cues generally caused lean individuals to initiate or stop eating.[221] This theory differentiating obese from lean has been questioned because others have not been able to duplicate the differences in the two groups.[222]

Nevertheless, the theory won wide recognition and stimulated interest in behavior modification programs to control food intake. Programs evolved whose intention was to greatly diminish the number of external cues that led to overeating.[223]

As a first step in a behavior modification program, the eating and activity patterns of an individual must be identified. As a result, careful diaries are kept. Patients record not only when and what was eaten, but where, with whom, how (sitting, standing, walking), their feelings, and hunger. In addition to the diary of food-related behavior, a diary of all activity-related behavior is kept, including when, with whom, where, and feelings at the time. Food management behavior must also be itemized, including buying, storing, preparing, serving, and cleaning up food. These diaries are analyzed to identify possible clues, whether environmental (such as television) or emotional (such as depression), that lead to overeating, so that these may be recognized and controlled. Once these cues have been identified, then techniques are invoked to try to control or evade them. Environmental stimuli to eating are controlled. Food shopping habits, visual cues, food preparation habits, and food storage habits are changed.

In addition, techniques to control the act of eating are also controlled. These include always eating in the dining room, sitting, concentrating on eating (no reading or watching television), eating more slowly, taking more and smaller bites, putting utensils down between bites, not skipping meals, not taking snacks, changing high-calorie foods for low-calorie ones, and eating at prescribed times only.

Besides these efforts to diminish environmental cues, new discriminative stimuli are introduced to develop new eating patterns. These include distinctive sites for eating, new and smaller plates, and eating with others as often as possible.

Finally, behavior modification programs try to change the consequences of eating. A reward system is introduced for changing behavior. The rewards are generally immediate and may be monetary or social feedback. Family, friends, group members, and group leaders can all contribute.

Mahoney has outlined the assumptions under which the behavior modification movement operates. They are

> (1) Obesity is a learning disorder, created by and amenable to principles of conditioning; (2) obesity is a simple disorder resulting from excess calorie intake; (3) the obese individual is an overeater; (4) obese persons are more sensitive to food stimuli than are nonobese individuals; (5) there are important differences in the "eating style" of obese and nonobese persons; (6) training an obese person to behave like a nonobese one will result in weight loss."[224]

Many if not all of these assumptions are now considered to be untrue, so that many of the strategies for weight loss in behavioral modification programs are founded on false assumptions. It can be argued, however, that though the theoretical background may be incorrect, the strategy developed is nevertheless effective. This argument is probably true. Stunkard reviewed 30 controlled trials and found that behavioral treatment was more successful in producing weight loss than a variety of other treatments.[225] Compared to group psychotherapy, nutrition education, and relaxation training, the behavior modification programs seemed to be more successful. It must be emphasized, however, that success is not universal, and some patients do well and others poorly. To date, it has not been possible to identify the characteristics that determine success.

Although some weight has been lost, it has not been impressive. Jeffrey et al. reviewed 21 studies and found a mean weight loss of 11.5 lb.[226] This amount; although a loss, is not enough to be clinically of much importance. In addition, the success in maintaining weight loss has been minimal.

Not many persons have lost weight after termination of the program,[227] and maintenance of weight loss for longer than a year has been poor.

In summary, it is difficult to be certain at this point whether behavioral treatment is better, and if so, how much better, than other forms of treatment. Well-controlled follow-up studies suggest that the same problem in recidivism that is true of other weight-control programs may be true of the behavior modification ones.

### Surgical Treatment

The refractoriness of many patients with morbid obesity to diet, psychotherapy, behavior modification, drugs, and exercise programs has led to a pessimistic outlook on the part of physicians concerning the likelihood of long-term therapeutic success. As a result, surgical treatment has been attempted. The surgical treatment is based on one of two principles: (1) a short bowel is created to produce malabsorption of ingested calories and (2) a small stomach is created so that the reduced reservoir for food will prevent much caloric intake at any one time.

**Short Bowel Procedure.** There are many variations of the jejunoileal bypass procedure.[228] These depend on how much jejunum and how much ileum is bypassed. The earliest procedure connected 12 to 15 inches of jejunum to 4 to 8 inches of ileum. Connections were end-to-end or end-to-side. The bypass loop was either left to drain where it was (end-to-side) or was reconnected to drain somewhere in the ascending or transverse colon (end-to-end). Various-sized segments have been left in continuity (14 in. to 4 in., 10 in. to 10 in., 14 in. to 8 in.). Weight loss does generally occur, although it is variable. A few patients lose only a small amount of weight. The bypass procedure creates malabsorption of both exogenous nutrients and endogenous gastrointestinal secretions. A number of complications have made this procedure suspect.[228] These include hypokalemia, hypocalcemia, vitamin $B_{12}$ deficiency, hepatic toxicity, renal calculi, and polyarthritis. In addition, there are the potential operative risks, including pulmonary embolus, pneumonia, wound infections, wound dehiscence, and phlebitis. Because of all these problems, this procedure has been largely discontinued.

**Gastric Bypass.** The gastric bypass operation was first described by Mason and Ito in 1967.[229] In this operation, the stomach was transected (or stapled) so that a small upper pouch (30 to 50 ml) was created. This pouch was anastomosed to a loop of jejunum. The opening between pouch and jejunum was 9 to 11 mm in diameter. This operation made a blind loop of much of the stomach, the duodenum, and the proximal jejunum.

More commonly now, a modification of this operation, the gastroplasty, is done. The stomach is stapled across, creating a small 50- to 60-ml reservoir on top and a small 1-cm outlet to the rest of the stomach on the lesser, middle, or greater curvatures.

Another recent procedure is the vertical banded gastroplasty.[230] In this procedure, a 20- to 30-ml stomach pouch is made by two longitudinal staple lines. In addition, wrapping of the pouch with Teflon mesh can be undertaken to prevent pouch distention and stoma widening.

These operations have been associated with considerably less morbidity than the intestinal operations. The problems are generally postoperative and include anastomotic leaks, transient gastrojejunostomy obstruction, and intra-abdominal abscess. Wound infection, dehiscence, pulmonary embolism, and atelectasis can also occur.

Subsequent to these early problems, late morbidity is greatly dependent on how much education the patient is given and how compliant he is. Vomiting is frequent if the speed or amount of eating is too great. Late complications consist primarily of revisions due to suture-line disruption or channel size problems. If chronic vomiting persists, esophagitis, hypokalemia, and malnutrition with dehydration can occur.

The success rate with gastroplasty has been variable, depending greatly on the surgeon. It is difficult to construct a stoma small enough to inhibit too rapid a transit from the small reservoir to the large, yet not so small that it will cause obstructive symptoms. Whereas Mason has reported a 36-kg average weight loss in 3 years, others have not done as well.[229]

In addition, patients can ensure failure by consuming high-caloric-density liquid or semisolid food that can easily pass through the small stoma.

**Truncal Vagotomy.** Truncal vagotomy has been attempted in an effort to reduce the stimulus to initiate or continue a meal. Although the physiologic rationale seemed sound, the results have been disappointing.[231]

**Jaw-Wiring.** The experience with the jaw-wiring technique has been scarce. It has been tried primarily in England, and success in significant weight loss has been reported.[232] The jaws must be unwired at some point (usually 6 to 9 months). At that point, weight regain can be rapid if no effort to change the underlying eating patterns and life-styles has been made.

**Lipectomy.** This treatment is not for obesity. It is surgical removal of adipose tissue for cosmetic purposes. Not enough fat can be removed to make a real impact on obesity, and it should not be performed for this reason. Lipectomy may be used to treat localized unsightly adiposity. A recent modification of this procedure is suction lipectomy, which is done nonsurgically. Long-term results of this procedure are unavailable.

## REFERENCES

1. National Center for Health Statistics, Roberts, J.: Weight by height and age of adults, United States, 1960–62. Vital and Health Statistics. Series 11, No. 14. PHS Pub. No. 1000. Public Health Service, Washington, U.S. Government Printing Office, May 1966.
2. Garrow, J.S.: Treat Obesity Seriously. Edinburgh, Churchill Livingstone, 1981, p. 3.
3. Womersley, J., Durnin, J.V.G.A.: Br. J. Nutr. *38*:271–284, 1977.
4. Keys, A., Fidanza, F., Karvonen, M.J., et al.: J. Chronic Dis. *25*:329–343, 1972.
5. Wilmer, H.A.: Proc. Soc. Exp. Biol. Med. *43*:386–388, 1940.
6. National Center for Health Statistics: Basic Data on Anthropometric Measurements and Angular Measurements of the Hip and Knee Joints for Selected Age Groups 1–74 years of Age, U.S. 1971–1975. Vital and Health Statistics. DHHS Publication No. (PH) 81–1669, Series 11, No. 219, Maryland, 1981. See also, Bishop, E.W., Bowen, P.E., Ritchey, S.J.: Am. J. Clin. Nutr. *34*:2530–2539, 1981.
7. Durnin, J.V.G.A., Womersley, J.: Br. J. Nutr. *32*:77–97, 1974.
8. Pace, N., Rathbun, E.: J. Biol. Chem. *158*:685–691, 1945.
9. Smith, T., Hesp, R., Mackenzie, J.: Phys. Med. Biol. *24*:171–175, 1979.
10. Behnke, A.R., Wilmore, J.H.: Evaluation of Body Build and Composition. Engelwood Cliffs, N.J., Prentice Hall, 1974.
11. Lesser, G.T., Deutsch, S., Markofsy, J.: Metabolism *20*:792–804, 1971.
12. 1983 Metropolitan Height and Weight Tables: Stat. Bull Metropolitan Life Insurance Co. *64*:2–9, 1984.
13. National Center for Health Statistics, Abraham, S., Johnson, C.L. and Najjar, M.F.: Weight by height and age for adults 18–74 years, United States, 1971–74. Vital and Health Statistics. Series 11, No. 208. DHEW Pub. No. (PHS) 79–1656. Public Health Service, Washington, U.S. Government Printing Office, Sept. 1979.
14. Bishop, C.W., Bowen, P.E., Ritchey, S.J.: Am. J. of Clin. Nutr. *34*:2530–2539, 1981.
15. National Center for Health Statistics, Abraham, S., Carroll, M.D., Najjar, M.F., Fulwood, R.: Obese and overweight adults in the United States. Vital and Health Statistics. Series 11, No. 230. DHHS Pub. No. (PHS) 83–1680. Public Health Service, Washington, U.S. Government Printing Office, Feb. 1983.
16. Taitz, L.S.: Br. Med. J. *1*:315–316, 1971.
17. Shukla, A., Forsyth, H.A., Anderson, C.M., et al.: Br. Med. J. *4*:507–515, 1972.
18. Jelliffe, D.B., Jelliffe, E.F.: Environ. Child Health Monogr. *41*:124–159, 1975.
19. Johnson, M.L., Burke, B.S., Mayer, J.: Am J. Clin. Nutr. *4*:231–238, 1956.
20. Hathaway, M.L., Sargent, D.W.: J. Am. Diet. Assoc. *40*:511–515, 1962.

21. Garn, S.M., Clark, D.C.: Pediatrics *57*:443–456, 1976.
22. Colley, J.R.T.: Br. J. Prev. Soc. Med. *28*:221–225, 1974.
23. Mossberg, H.: Acta Paediatr. Scand. (Suppl. II) *35*:1–122, 1948.
24. Rimm, I.J., Rimm, A.A.: Am. J. Public Health *66*:479–481, 1976.
25. Abraham, S., Nordsieck, M.: Public Health Rep. *75*:263–273, 1960.
26. Garn, S.M., LaVelle, M.: Am. J. Dis. Child. 139:181–185, 1985.
27. Goldblatt, P.B., Moore, M.E., Stunkard, A.J.: Social factors in obesity. JAMA *192*:1039–1044, 1965.
28. Baird, I.M., Silverstone, J.T., Grimshaw, J.J., et al.: Practitioner *212*:706–714, 1974.
29. Noppa, H., Bengston, C.: J. Epidemiol. Community Health *34*: 134–142, 1978.
30. Stunkard, A.J.: Fed. Proc. *27*:1367–1373, 1968.
31. Ross, C.E., Mirowsky, J.: J. Health Soc. Behav. *24*:288–296, 1983.
32. Moore, M.E., Stunkard, A.J., Srole, L.: JAMA *181*:962–966, 1962.
33. Silverstone, J.T., Gordon, R.P., Stunkard, A.J.: Practitioner *202*:682–688, 1969.
34. Height and weight of adults ages 18–74 years by socioeconomic status and geographic variables, United States. DHHS Publication No (PHS) 81–1674, National Center for Health Statistics, Hyattsville, Maryland, 1981.
35. Armstrong, D.B., Dublin, L.I., Wheatley, G.M., et al.: JAMA *147*:1007–1014, 1951.
36. Lew, E.A.: J. Am. Diet. Assoc. *38*:323–327, 1961.
37. Build and Blood Pressure Study, 1959, Vol 1. Chicago, Society of Actuaries, 1960.
38. Build Study 1979. Chicago, Society of Actuaries and Association of Life Insurance Medical Directors, 1980.
39. Lew, E.A., Garfinkel, L.: J. Chronic Dis. *32*:563–576, 1979.
40. Belloc, N.B.: Prev. Med. *2*:67–81, 1973.
41. Andres, R., Elahi, D., Tobin, J.D., et al.: Int. J. Obes. *4*:381–386, 1980.
42. Dyer, A.R., Stamler, J., Berkson, D.M., et al.: J. Chronic Dis. *28*:109–123, 1975.
43. Keys, A., Aravanis, C., Blackburn, G., et al.: Ann. Intern. Med. *77*:15–27, 1972.
*44. Keys, A.: Nutr. Rev. *38*:297–307, 1980.
45. Jarrett, R.J., Shipley, M.J., Rose, G.: Br. Med. J. *285*:535–537, 1982.
46. Libow, L.S.: Geriatrics *29*:75–88,1974.
47. Milne, J.S., Lauder, I.J.: Age and Ageing *7*:129–137, 1978.
48. Burr, M.I., Lennings, C.I., Milbank, J.E.: Age and Ageing *11*:249–255, 1982.
49. Garn, S.M., Hawthorne, V.M., Pilkington, J.J., et al.: Am. J. Clin. Nutr. *38*:313–319, 1983.
*50. Keys, A.: Overweight and the risk of heart attack and sudden death, Vol. 2. *In* Obesity in Perspective. (Bray, G.A., Ed.) Washington, D.C., Dept H.E.W., NIH. Publication No. 75–708, 1976. pp. 215–223.
51. Kannel, W.B., LeBauer, E.J., Dawber, T.R., et al.: Circulation *35*:734–744, 1967.
52. Kannel, W.B., Gordon, T.: Physiological and medical concomitants of obesity: the Framingham study. *In* Obesity in America. (Bray, G.A., Ed.), Washington, D.C., Dept. of H.E.W., NIH Publication No 79–359, 1979, pp. 125–163.
53. Shurtleff, D.: Some characterics related to the incidence of cardiovascular disease and death: the Framingham study, 18–year follow-up. *In* The Framingham Study, Section 30. (Kannel, W.B., Gordon, T., Eds.) Washington, D.C., Dept., H.E.W.N.I.H. Publication No. 76, 1974, p. 599.
54. Ostfeld, A.M., Gibson, D.C.: Epidemiology of Aging. Washington, D.C., Dept. H.E.W.N.I.H., Publication No. 75–711, 1975, pp. 217–219.
55. Rabkin, S.W., Mathewson, F.A.L., Hsu, P.H.: Am. J. Cardiol. *39*:452–458, 1977.
56. Chapman, J.M., Coulson, A.H., Clark, V.A., et al.: J. Chronic Dis. *23*:631–645, 1971.
57. Albrink, M.H., Meigs, J.W.: Am. J. Clin. Nutr. *15*:255–261, 1964.
58. Olefsky, J., Reaven, G.M., Farquhar, J.W.: J. Clin. Invest. *53*:64–76, 1974.
59. Bagdade, J.D., Bierman, E.L., Porte, D., Jr.: J. Clin. Invest. *46*:1549–1557, 1967.
60. Olefsky, J.M., Farquhar, J.W., Reaven, G.M.: Am. J. Med. *57*:551–560, 1974.
61. Havel, R.J., Kane, J.P., Balasse, E.O., et al.: J. Clin. Invest. *49*:2017–2035, 1970.
62. Pykalisto, O.J, Smith, P.H., Brunzell, J.D.: J. Clin. Invest. *56*:1108–1117, 1975.
63. Brunzell, J.D., Hazzard, W.R., Motulsky, A.G., et al.: Clin. Res. *22*:462a, 1974.
64. Rifkind, B.M., Begg, T.: Br. Med. J. *2*:208–210, 1966.
65. Montoye, H.J., Epstein, F.H., Kjelsberg, M.O.: Am. J. Clin. Nutr. *18*:397–406, 1966.
66. West, K.M., Kalbfkeisch, J.M.: Diabetes *20*:99–108, 1971.
67. Westlund, K., Nicholaysen, R.: Scand. J. Clin. Lab. Invest. *30* (Suppl. 127):3, 1972.
*68. Kannel, W.B.: Health and obesity: An overview. *In* Health and Obesity. (Conn, H.L., Jr., DeFelice, E.A., Kuo, P., Eds.) New York, Raven Press, 1983.
69. Feldman, R., Sender, A.J., Siegelaub, A.B.: Diabetes *18*:478–486, 1969.
70. Hartz, A.J., Rupley, D.C., Kalkhoff, R.D., et al.: Prev. Med. *2*:351–357, 1983.
71. Kissebah, A.H., Vydelingum, N., Murray, R.: J. Clin. Endocrinol. Metab. *54*:254–260, 1982.
72. Krotkiewski, M., Bjorntorp, P., Sjostrom, L., et al.: J. Clin. Ivest. *72*:1150–1162, 1983.
73. Karam, J.H., Grodsky, G.M., Forsham, P.H.: Diabetes *12*:197–204, 1963.
74. Rabinowitz, D., Zierler, K.L.: J. Clin. Invest. *41*:2173–2181, 1962.
75. Felig, P., Marliss, E., Cahill, G.F., Jr.: N. Engl. J. Med. *281*:811–816, 1969.
76. Felig, P., Wahren, J., Hendler, R., et al.: J. Clin. Invest. *53*:582–590, 1973.
77. Kahn, C.R., Neville, D.M., Jr., Roth, J.: J. Biol. Chem., *248*:244–250, 1973.
78. Archer, J.A., Gorden, P., Roth, J.: J. Clin. Invest. *55*:166–174, 1975.
79. Olefsky, J.M.: J. Clin. Invest. *57*:1165–1172, 1976.
*80. Roth, J., Kahn, C.R., Lesniak, M.A., et al.: Recent Prog. Horm. Res. *31*:95–126, 1976.
81. Pfeifer, M.A., Halter, J.B., Porte, D., Jr.: Am. J. Med. *70*:579–588, 1981.
82. Berchtold, P., Simms, E.A., Horton, E.S., et al.: Biomed. Pharmacother. *37*:251–258, 1983.
83. Stamler, J., Stamler, R., Romberg, A., et al.: J. Chronic Dis. *28*:499–525, 1975.
*84. Tobian, L.: N. Engl. J. Med. *298*:46–48, 1978.

85. Johnson, B.C., Karunas, T.M., Epstein, F.H.: Clin. Sci. Mol. Med. *45*(Suppl. 1):355–455, 1973.
86. Kannel, W.B., Brand, N., Skinner, J.J.: Ann. Intern. Med. *67*:48–59, 1967.
87. Oberman, A., Lane, N.E., Harlan, W.R., et al.: Circulation *36*:812–822; 1967.
88. Tyroler, H.A., Heyden, S., Harnes, C.G.: Weight and hypertension: Evans County studies of blacks and whites. *In* Epidemiology and Control of Hypertension. (Paul, O., Ed.) New York, Stratton Intercontinental Medical Book Corp., 1975, pp. 177–201.
89. Reisin, E., Abel, R., Modan, et al.: N. Engl. J. Med. *298*:1–6, 1978.
90. Reisen, E., Frolich, E.D., Messerli, F.H., et al.: Ann. Intern. Med. *98*:315–319, 1983.
91. Dahl, L.K., Silver, L., Christie, R.W.: N. Engl. J. Med. *258*:1186–1192, 1958.
92. DeFronzo, R.A.: Insulin and renal sodium handling: Clinical implications. *In* Recent Advances in Obesity Research, III. (Bjorntorp, P., Cairella, M., Howard, A.N., Eds.) London, John Libbey, 1980, pp. 32–41.
93. DeFronzo, R.A., Goldberg, M., Agus, Z.: J. Clin. Invest. *58*:83–89, 1976.
94. DeFronzo, R.A., Cooke, C.R., Andres, R., et al.: J. Clin. Invest. *55*:845–855, 1975.
95. Kolanowski, J., Bodson, A., Desmecht, P., et al.: Eur. J. Clin. Invest. *8*:277–282, 1978.
96. Landsberg, L., Young, J.B.: N. Engl. J. Med. *298*:1295–1301, 1978.
97. Weinsier, R.L., Norris, D.J., Birch, R., et al.: Hypertension *7*:578–585, 1985.
98. Rimm, A.A., White, P.L.: Obesity: Its risks and hazards. *In* Obesity in America. (Bray, G.A., Ed.), Washington, D.C., NIH Publication No. 79–359, 1979, pp. 103–124.
99. Miettinen, T.A.: Horm. Metab. Res. *14*:37–44, 1974.
100. Grundy, S.M., Metzger, A.L., Adler, R.D.: J. Clin. Invest. *51*:3026–3043, 1972.
101. Leach, R.E., Baumgard, S., Broom, J.: Clin. Orthop. *93*:271–273, 1973.
102. Blitzer, P.H., Blitzer, E.C., Rimm, A.A.: Prev. Med. *5*:20–31, 1976.
103. McMahon, B.: Gynecol. Oncol. *2*:122–129, 1974.
104. Dunn, L.J., Bradbury, J.T.: Am. J. Obstet. Gynecol. *97*:465–471, 1967.
105. DeWaard, F., Baanders-Van Halewijn, E.A.: Acta Cytol. *13*:675–678, 1969.
106. DeWaard, F.: Cancer Res. *35*:3351–3356, 1975.
107. Wynder, E.L., Bross, I.J., Hirayama, T.: Cancer *13*:559–601, 1960.
108. Beer, A.E., Billingham, R.E.: Lancet *1*:296, 1978.
109. Shields, J.: Monozygotic Twins Brought Up Apart and Brought Up Together. London. Oxford University Press, 1962.
110. Newman, H.H., Freeman, F.N., Holzinger, K.J.: Twins: A Study of Heredity and Environment. Chicago, University of Chicago Press, 1937.
111. Garn, S.M., Bailey, S.M.: Am. J. Clin. Nutr. *29*:1067–1068, 1976.
112. Garn, S.M., Clark, D.C.: Pediatrics *57*:443–455, 1976.
113. Withers, R.F.J.: Eugenic Rev. *56*:81–90, 1964.
114. Biron, P., Mongeau, J.G., Bertrand, D.: J. Pediatr. *91*:555–558, 1977.
115. Rao, D.C., MacLean, C.J., Morton, N.E., et al.: Am. J. Hum. Genet. *27*:509–520, 1975.

116. Sims, E.A.H., Danforth, E., Jr., Horton, E.J., et al.: Recent Prog. Horm. Res. *29*:457–476, 1973.
117. Bernstein, R.S., Thornton, J.C., Yang, M.U., et al.: Am. J. Clin. Nutr. *37*:595–602, 1983.
118. Millward, D.J., Garlick, P.J.; Proc. Nutr. Soc. *35*:339–349, 1976.
119. Spady, B.W., Payne, P.R., Picou D., et al.: Am. J. Clin. Nutr. *29*:1073–1088, 1976.
120. Boothby, W.M., Berkson, J., Dunn, H.L., et al.: Am. J. Physiol. *116*:468–484, 1936.
121. James, W.P.T., Trayhurn, P.: Br. Med. Bull. *37*:43–48, 1981.
122. Ravussin, E., Burnand, B., Schutz, Y., et al.: Am. J. Clin. Nutr. *35*:566–573, 1982.
123. Kaplan, M.L., Leveille, G.A.: Am. J. Clin. Nutr. *29*:1108–1113, 1976.
124. Shetty, P.S., Jung, R.T., James, W.P.T., et al.: Clin. Sci. *60*:519–525, 1981.
125. Pittet, P., Chappuis P., Acheson, K., et al.: Br. J. Nutr. *35*:281–288, 1976.
126. Strang, J.M., McClugage, H.B.: Am. J. Med. Sci. *182*:79–81, 1931.
127. Clough, D.P., Durnin, J.V.G.A.: J. Physiol. *207*:89P, 1970.
128. Felig, P., Cunningham, J., Levitt, M., et al.: Am. J. Physiol. *244*:E45–51, 1983.
129. Rothwell, N.J., Stock, M.J.: Metabolism *30*:673, 678, 1981.
130. Golay, A., Schutz, Y., Meyer, H.U., et al.: Diabetes *31*:1023–1028, 1982.
130a. Neumann, R.O.: Arch. Hyg. *45*:1–87, 1902.
131. Garrow, J.S.: The regulation of energy expenditure in men. *In* Recent Advances in Obesity Research, Vol 2. (Bray, G.A., Ed.) London, Newman, 1978, p. 200–210.
*132. James, W.P.T., Trayhurn, P.: Obesty in mice and men. *In* Nutritional Factors: Modulating Effects on Metabolic Processes. (Beers, R.F., Barrett, E.G., Eds.) New York, Raven Press, 1981, pp. 123–138.
133. Bradfield, R.B., Curtis, D.E., Margen, S.: Am. J. Clin. Nutr. *21*:1208–1210, 1968.
134. Segal, K.R., Gutin, B.: Metabolism *32*:581–589, 1983.
135. Swindells, Y.E.: Br. J. Nutr. *27*:65–73, 1972.
136. Hansen, J.J.: J. Appl. Physiol. *35*:587–591, 1973.
137. Warnold, I., Lenner, R.A.: Am. J. Clin. Nutr. *30*:304–315, 1977.
138. Strong, J.A., Shirling, D., Passmore, R.: Br. J. Nutr. *21*:909–919, 1967.
139. Sims, E.A.H., Goldman, R.F., Gluck, C.M., et al.: Trans. Assoc. Am. Physicians *81*:153–170, 1968.
*140. Sjostrom, L.: Fat cells and body weight. *In* Obesity. (Stunkard, A.J., Ed.) Philadelphia, W.B. Saunders Co., 1980.
141. Knittle, J.L., Hirsch, J.: J. Clin. Invest. *47*:2091–2098, 1968.
142. Hirsch, J., Han, P.W.: J. Lipid Res. *10*:77–82, 1969.
143. Braun, T., Kazdova, L., Fabry, P., et al.: Metab. Clin. Exp. *17*:825–832, 1968.
144. DiGirolamo, M., Mendlinger, S.: Am. J. Pysiol. *221*:859–864, 1971.
145. Lemmonier, D.: J. Clin. Invest. *51*:2907–2915, 1972.
146. Hager, A., Sjostrom, L., Arvidsson, B., et al.: Metabolism *26*:607–614, 1977.
147. Hager, A., Sjostrom, L., Arvidsson, B., et al.: Am. J. Clin. Nutr. *31*:68–75, 1978.
148. Krotkiewski, M., Sjostrom, L., Bjorntorp, P., et al.: Int. J. Obes. *1*:395–416, 1977.

149. Reference deleted.
150. Lithell, H., Boberg, J. Hellsing, K., et al.: Ups. J. Med. Sci. *83*:45–52, 1978.
151. Reitman, J.S., Kosmakos, F.C., Howard, B.V., et al.: J. Clin. Invest. *70*:791–797, 1982.
152. Schwartz, R., Brunzell, J.: Lancet *1*:1230–1231, 1978.
153. Schwartz, R., Brunzell, J.: J. Clin. Invest. *67*:1425–1430, 1981.
154. Rebuffe-Scrive, M., Basdevant, A., Guy-Grand, B.: Am. J. Clin. Nutr. *37*:974–980, 1983.
155. Apfelbaum, M., Bostsarron, J., Lacatis, D.: Am. J. Clin. Nutr. *24*:1405–1409, 1971.
156. Grande, F., Anderson, J.T., Keys, A.: J. Appl. Physiol. *12*:230–238, 1958.
157. Owens, J.L., Thompson, D., Shah, N.: J. Nutr. *109*:1584–1591, 1979.
158. Bjorntrop, P., Enzi, G., Karlsson, M., et al.: Int. J. Obes. *4*:11–19, 1980.
159. DiGirolamo, M., Smith, U., Bjorntorp, P.: Refeeding effects on adipocyte metabolism. *In* Recent Advances in Obesity Research. (Bjorntorp. P., Cairella, M., Howard, A.N., Eds.) London, John Libbey, 1980, pp. 99–105.
160. Bjorntorp, P., Yang, M.U.: Am. J. Clin. Nutr. *36*:444–449, 1982.
161. Leibel, R.L., Hirsch, J.: Metabolism *33*:164–170, 1984.
162. Faust, J.M., Johnson, P.R., Hirsch, J.: Science *197*:393–396, 1977.
163. Krotkiewski, M., Sjostrom, L., Bjorntorp, P.: Int. J. Obes. *1*:395–416, 1977.
164. Bradfield, R.B., Jourdan, M.H.: Lancet *2*:640–643, 1973.
*165. Van Itallie, T.B.: Am. J. Clin. Nutr. *31*:543–552, 1978.
166. Caspary, W.F.: Lancet *1*:1231–1233, 1977.
*167. Council on Foods and Nutrition: JAMA *224*:1415–1419, 1973.
168. Rickman, F., Mitchell, N., Dingman, J., et al.: JAMA *228*:54–58, 1974.
169. Pritikin, N.: Live Longer Now: The First One Hundred Years of Your Life. New York, Grosset and Dunlop, 1974.
170. Thompson, T.J., Runcie, J., Miller, V.: Lancet *2*:992–996, 1966.
171. Drenick, E.J., Swendseid, M.E., Blahd, W.H., et al.: JAMA *187*:100–105, 1964.
172. Felig, P., Owen, O.E., Wahren, J., et al.: J. Clin. Invest. *48*:584–594, 1969.
173. Lindner, P.G., Blackburn, G.L.: Obes. Bariatric Med. *5*:198–216, 1976.
*174. Wadden, T.A., Stunkard, A.J., Brownell, K.D.: Ann. Intern. Med. *99*:675–684, 1983.
175. Owen, O.E., Felig, P., Morgan, A.P., et al.: J. Clin. Invest. *48*:574–583, 1969.
176. Calloway, D.H., Odell, A.C.F., Margen, S.: J. Nutr. *101*:775–786, 1971.
177. Felig, P., Owen, O.E., Wahren, J., et al.: J. Clin. Invest. *48*:584–594, 1969.
178. Consolazio, C.F., Matoush, L.O., Johnson, H.L., et al.: Am. J. Clin. Nutr. *21*:803–812, 1968.
179. Apfelbaum, M., Bostsarron, J., Brigant, L., et al.: Gastroenterologia *108*:121–134, 1967.
180. Bistrian, B.R., Winterer, J., Blackburn, G., et al.: J. Lab. Clin. Med. *89*:1030–1035, 1977.
181. Baird, I.M., Parsons, R.L., Howard, A.N.: Metabolism *23*:645–657, 1974.

182. Genuth, S.M., Castro, J.H., Vertes, V.: JAMA *230*:987–991, 1974.
183. Vertes, V., Genuth, S.M., Hazelton, I.M.: JAMA *238*:2151–2153, 1977.
184. Flatt, J.P., Blackburn, G.L.: Am. J. Clin. Nutr. *27*:175–187, 1974.
185. Sherwin, R.S., Hendler, R.G., Felig, P.: J. Clin. Invest. *55*:1382–1390, 1975.
186. Marliss, E.B., Murray, F.T., Nakhooda, A.F.: J. Clin. Invest. *62*:468–479, 1978.
187. Landau, R.L., Rochman, H., Blix-Gruber, P., et al.: Am. J. Clin. Nutr. *34*:1300–1304, 1981.
188. Frattali, V.P.: FDA By-Lines 9:179, 1979.
189. Sours, H.E., Frattali, V.P., Brand, C.D., et al.: Am. J. Clin. Nutr. *34*:453–461, 1981.
190. Singh, B.N., Gaarder, T.D., Kanegae, T., et al.: JAMA *240*:115–119, 1978.
*191. Van Itallie, T.B.: JAMA *240*:144–145, 1978.
192. Jones, A.O.L., Jacobs, R.M., Fry, B.E., et al.: Am. J. Clin. Nutr. *33*:2545–2550, 1980.
193. DeHaven, J., Sherwin, R., Hendler, R., et al.: N. Engl. J. Med. *302*:477–482, 1980.
194. Sigler, M.H.: J. Clin. Invest. *55*:377–387, 1975.
195. Yang, M.U., Van Itallie, T.B.: J. Clin. Invest. *58*:722–730, 1976.
196. Yang, M., Barbosa-S, J.L., Pi-Sunyer, F.X., et al.: Int. J. Obes. *5*:231–236, 1981.
*197. Pi-Sunyer, F.X.: Obesity. *In* Conn's Current Therapy. (Rackel, R.E., Ed.) Philadelphia, W.B. Saunders Co., 1985.
198. Steinhaus, A.H.: Physiol. Rev. *13*:103–147, 1983.
199. Karpovitch, P.V.: Res. Q. *12*:423–431, 1941.
200. Woo, R., Garrow, J.S., Pi-Sunyer, F.X.: Am. J. Clin. Nutr. *36*:470–477, 1982.
201. Woo, R., Garrow, J.S., Pi-Sunyer, F.X.: Am. J. Clin. Nutr. *36*:478–484, 1982.
202. Freedman-Akabas, S., Colt, E., Kissileff, H.R., et al.: Am. J. Clin. Nutr. *4*:545–549, 1985.
203. Adams, R.P., Welch, H.G.: J. Appl. Physiol. *49*:863–868, 1980.
204. Passmore, R., Thomson, J.G., Warnock, G.M.: Br. J. Nutr. *6*:253–264, 1952.
205. Woo, R., Pi-Sunyer, F.X.: Metabolism *34*:836–841, 1985.
206. Dempsey, J.A.: Res. Q. *35*:275–287, 1964.
207. Williams, B.T.: J. Am. Geriatr. Soc. *16*:794–797, 1968.
208. Boileau, R.A., Buskirk, E.R., Horstman, D.H., et al.: Med. Sci. Sports *3*:183–189, 1971.
*209. Pi-Sunyer, F.X., Woo, R.: Am. J. Clin. Nutr. *42*:983–990, 1985.
210. Craddock, D.: Obesity and Its Management. 3rd Ed. Edinburgh, Churchill Livingstone, 1978, pp. 92–109.
211. Evans, E.R., Wallace, M.G.: Curr. Med. Res. Opin. *4*:132–137, 1975.
212. Sullivan, A.C., Cheng, L.: Appetite regulation and its modulation by drugs. *In* Nutrition and Drug Interrelations. (Hathcock, J.N., Coon, J., Eds.) New York, Academic Press, 1978.
*213. Van Itallie, T.B.: Am. J. Clin. Nutr. *32*:2723–2733, 1979.
214. Bruch, H.: Eating Disorders: Obesity, Anorexia Nervosa and the Person Within. New York, Basic Books, 1973.
215. Rand, C.S., Stunkard, A.J.: J. Am. Acad. Psychoanal. *5*:459–497, 1977.
216. Powers, P.S.: Obesity, the Regulation of Body Weight. Baltimore, Williams & Wilkins, 1980.

217. Halmi, K.A., Stunkard, J.A., Mason, E.E.: Am. J. Nutr. *33*:446–451, 1980.

218. Glucksman, M.L., Hirsch, J.: Psychosom. Med. *31*:1–7, 1969.

219. Crisp, A.H., McGuiness, B.: Br. Med. J. *1*:7–9, 1975.

220. Schachter, S.: Am. Psychol. *26*:129–144, 1971.

221. Schachter, S.: Emotion, Obesity and Crime. New York, Academic Press, 1971.

*222. Rodin, J.: The externality theory today. *In* Obesity. (Stunkard, A.J., Ed.) Philadelphia, W.B. Saunders Co., 1980.

223. Stuart, R.B.: Behav. Res. Ther. *5*:357–365, 1967.

224. Mahoney, M.J.: Phychiatr. Clin. North Am. *1*:651–660, 1978.

*225. Stunkard, A.J.: Int. J. Obes. *2*:237–249, 1978.

226. Jeffrey, R.W., Thompson, P.D., Wing, R.R.: Behav. Res. Ther. *16*:363–370, 1978.

227. Stalonas, P.M., Johnson, W.G., Christ, M.: J. Consult. Clin. Psychol. *46*:463–469, 1978.

228. Pi-Sunyer, F.X.: Am. J. Clin. Nutr. *29*:409–416, 1976.

229. Mason, E.E., Ito, C.: Surg. Clin. North. Am. *47*:1345–1351, 1967.

230. Tretbar, L.L., Sifers, E.C.: Int. J. Obes. *5*:538, 1981.

231. Kral, J.G.: Am. J. Clin. Nutr. *3*:416–419, 1980.

232. Garrow, J.S., Gardiner, G.T.: Br. Med. J. *282*:858–860, 1981.

*Review article.

*Chapter* **45**

# NUTRITIONAL ASSESSMENT BY CLINICAL AND BIOCHEMICAL METHODS

## Steven B. Heymsfield and Patricia J. Williams

The association of wasting and illness was made early in the history of medicine. Hippocrates provided a vivid description of the physical appearance of patients with severe heart failure in the fifth century: "The flesh is consumed and becomes water... the abdomen fills with water; the feet and legs swell; the shoulders, clavicles, chest, and thighs melt away."[1] The assessment of wasting illnesses moved form the descriptive phase with the classic experimental studies of Lavoisier and LaPlace in 1756.[2] Release of heat from organic fuels metabolized in vivo was shown to follow the same pattern of combustion observed in vitro. Loss of tissue mass during starvation was later shown to involve oxidation of endogenous fuel stores in order to generate energy required for life-sustaining metabolic activities.[3]

By mid-nineteenth century there was a general consensus that the diet must contain a source of energy in order to maintain health. A more comprehensive concept was developed in 1845 by J. Pereira, who suggested that an adequate diet must contain 13 elements that are essential components of the human body: C, H, O, N, S, P, Cl, Ca, Na, K, Mg, Fe, and Fl.[4] In 1912 Funk proposed the essentiality of "vitamines," and the list of essential nutrients has now grown to about 40 compounds.[5] An inadequate body content of one or more of the essential nutrients is associated with a specific deficiency syndrome. The most common deficiency syndrome observed in patients with underlying disease is protein-energy malnutrition, [6] and the assessment of this condition will be described in detail in this chapter. The other nutrient deficiencies will be referred to briefly, and detailed reviews are provided in other chapters throughout the book.

The state of health is characterized by a range of body compositions, tissue functions, and metabolic activities. The fundamental aim of nutritional assessment is to gather information on each of these three areas from the patient under study and then compare the results to the healthy reference population and to the individual followed over time. The basic principles of body composition and metabolism in health are reviewed in the first section of the chapter, with a special emphasis on the interrelations between the two. In the second portion of the chapter we review the derangements in body composition and metabolism observed in diseased patients. The third section provides currently available and practical indices of metabolism, body composition, and tissue function. The recommended clinical application of these tests is then provided in the final section of the chapter.

## BODY COMPOSITION AND METABOLISM IN HEALTH

### Tissue and Chemical Components of Body Weight

Tissue mass in humans can be chemically separated into fat and fat-free components. Fat is nearly all in the form of triacylglycerol, and this storage fuel is found mainly in adipose tissue. All that remains of body weight after ether extraction of fat is referred to as the fat-free body mass (FFM). The FFM in healthy humans is a mixture of water, protein, and bone mineral in the approximate proportions 0.725, 0.195, and 0.08.[7] A fourth and more variable component of FFM is glycogen, which represents a fraction of FFM that is between 0.01 and 0.02. Most protein and all of the glycogen mass are found within cells, referred to collectively as protoplasm or body cell mass.[8] The water component of FFM is distributed both in the intra- and extracellular spaces, and intracellular water is bound primarily by glycogen (4 to 5 ml $H_2O$/g) and protein ( 4.0 to 4.5 ml/g). The cells and bathing fluids within FFM form the organs and tissues, and representative weights are provided in Table 45–1.

The major determinants of body weight are water and organic fuels, the latter consisting of protein (5.65 kcal/g), carbohydrate (4.1 kcal/g), and fat (9.4 kcal/g).[10] The sum of these three classes of fuels is equal to the total body energy content. Although protein is 5.56 kcal/g, dilution of protein by water leaves FFM with an average

gross energy density of 1.16 kcal/g. Combustion of protein in vivo is imcomplete, and some of the gross energy in protein is lost in the form of urea. This lowers the usable fuel value of FFM to 1.0 kcal/g; the energy available from glycogen does not contribute significantly or reproducibly to the energy density of FFM. In summary, body weight is primarily equal to the sum of total body water and sources of fat + protein (Fig. 45–1). Weight loss occurs when water or energy balance, or a combination of the two, become negative.

### Energy Metabolism

The living cell is continuously releasing energy from organic fuels in order to maintain cellular function. The classic reaction taking place within the protoplasmic tissues is the following:

$$\text{Fuel} + O_2 \rightarrow \text{high energy intermediate}$$
$$+ CO_2 + H_2O + \text{heat} + \text{urea} \quad (1)$$

Oxidation of the three principal fuels generates a high-energy intermediate, with the additional release of $CO_2$, $H_2O$, heat, and urea in the case of protein metabolism. These metabolic reactions take place within the FFM, and all heat losses can be grouped into three metabolic states. The first is fasting, and this level of heat production is generally referred to as the basal or resting metabolic rate. In health, there is a close correlation between FFM and basal oxygen consumption, carbon dioxide production, and heat release (Fig. 45–2).

The second metabolic state occurs following the ingestion of a meal. Resting energy expenditure increases above the fasting level and then returns to baseline over several hours. Although the mechanism of the thermic effect of food is not fully understood, most workers agree that a major factor is the processing and storage of nutrients.[11] Another related effect on metabolic rate is an increase, when a patient is fed continuously by enteral or parenteral catheter, of the intraprandial resting metabolic rate in a steady-state fashion above the fasting level.[12] Termed the "thermic response to fuel" in order to distinguish it from the classic thermic effect of food, this increase in energy expenditure is a function of formula caloric infusion rate, diet composition,[12] and the patient's underlying illness.[13]

The third factor that increases fuel oxidation above the basal level is physical activity. The major determinants of the thermic response to activity are the size of the workload and the subject's body weight.[14]

The fat-free tissues thus convert endogenous fuel sources into metabolically useful forms of energy, which in turn allows survival of the orga-

**Table 45–1.　Reference Man: Summary of Anatomic Values***

| Organ/Tissue | Weight (g) | Organ/Tissue | Weight (g) |
|---|---|---|---|
| Adipose | 15,000 | Kidneys (2) | 310 |
| Subcutaneous | 7500 | Larynx | 28 |
| Separable | 5000 | Lenses (2) | 0.40 |
| Yellow marrow | 1500 | Liver | 1800 |
| Interstitial | 1000 | Lung tissue (plus arterial and ven- | |
| | | ous blood) | 1000 |
| Adrenal glands (2) | 14 | Lymphocytes | 1500 |
| Blood (total) | 5500 | Lymphatic tissue ("fixed") | 700 |
| Red blood cells | 2400 | Muscles (skeletal) | 28,000 |
| Plasma | 3100 | Palatine tonsils (2) | 4 |
| Bone marrow (total) | 3000 | Pancreas | 100 |
| Red bone marrow | 1500 | Parathyroid glands (4) | 0.12 |
| Yellow bone marrow | 1500 | Periarticular tissue (total) | 1500 |
| Brain | 1400 | Pineal gland | 0.18 |
| Breasts (2) | 26 | Pituitary gland | 0.60 |
| Bronchial tree | 30 | Prostate gland | 16 |
| Cartilage (skeletal) | 1100 | Pulmonary blood | 530 |
| Connective tissue | 5050 | Salivary glands (3 prs.) | 85 |
| Cartilage | 2500 | Parotid (2) | 50 |
| Tendons and fascia | 850 | Submaxillary (2) | 25 |
| Other | 1700 | Sublingual (2) | 10 |
| Esophagus | 40 | Skeleton | 10,000 |
| Eyes (2) | 15 | Bone | 5000 |
| Fat (total) | 13,500 | Marrow | 3000 |
| Nonessential | 12,000 | Other tissue | 2000 |
| Essential† | 1500 | Skin (total) | 2600 |
| Fingernails and toenails | 3 | Epidermis | 100 |
| Gallbladder | 10 | Dermis | 2500 |
| GI tract (without contents) | 1200 | Spinal cord | 30 |
| Esophagus | 40 | Spleen | 180 |
| Stomach | 150 | Stomach | 150 |
| Small intestine | 640 | Superficial fascia | 500 |
| Large intestine | 370 | Teeth | 46 |
| GI tract contents | 1005 | Tendons and deep fascia | 850 |
| Stomach | 250 | Testes (2) | 35 |
| Small intestine | 400 | Thymus | 20 |
| Upper large intestine | 220 | Thyroid | 20 |
| Lower large intestine | 135 | Tongue | 70 |
| Hair | 20 | Tonsils (2 palatine) | 4 |
| Heart (without blood) | 330 | Trachea | 10 |
| Heart (at end of diastole) | 570 | Ureters (2) | 16 |
| Heart (at end of systole) | 425 | Urethra | 10 |
| Hypodermis | 7500 | Urinary bladder | 45 |

*Weight 70 kg, body surface area 1.8 m², specific gravity 1.07 g/cc.
†Essential fat is the lipid component of cell membranes and lean tissue organelles.
Adapted from report of the Task Group on Reference Man. International Commission on Radiologic Protection. New York, Pergamon Press, 1984.

nism. Although heat is the major byproduct of these metabolic reactions, there are also other nonthermal losses of energy and protein. These can be grouped into digestive, urinary, and integumental losses.

Digestive losses occur even during fasting and include desquamated epithelial cells, bacteria, and unabsorbed intestinal secretions. With feeding, additional digestive juices are mixed with food and then reabsorbed. Some of this digestive mix and poorly absorbed dietary compounds passes into the feces, thus accounting for net intestinal energy and protein losses. Each dietary fuel differs in digestibility (%), which is calculated as:

$$\frac{(\text{Intake} - \text{Stool losses})}{\text{Intake}} \times 100 \qquad (2)$$

If 100 grams of fat are ingested per day, and if daily stool fat averages 5 grams, then the "apparent digestibility" of fat is 95%. On a mixed diet, the average digestibility of carbohydrate, protein, and fat is, respectively, 98, 93, and 95%.[15]

Urinary energy losses occur primarily in the form of urea (5.62 kcal/g), the end product of protein metabolism. Since the average nitrogen con-

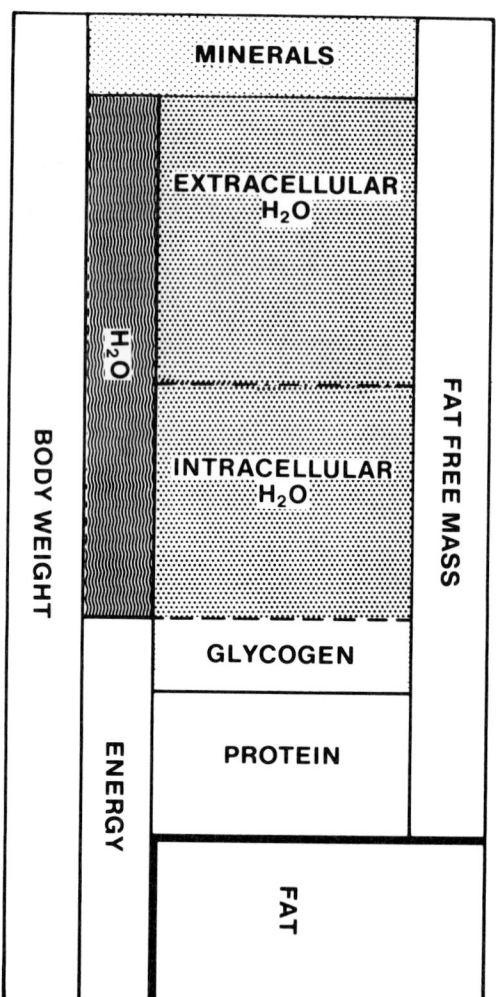

**Fig. 45–1.** The major components of body weight. Water, protein, and mineral within the fat-free body mass occur in the average proportions 0.725, 0.195, and 0.08; glycogen is variable at 0.01 to 0.02; and 50 to 55% of water is intracellular, with the remainder in the extracellular space.

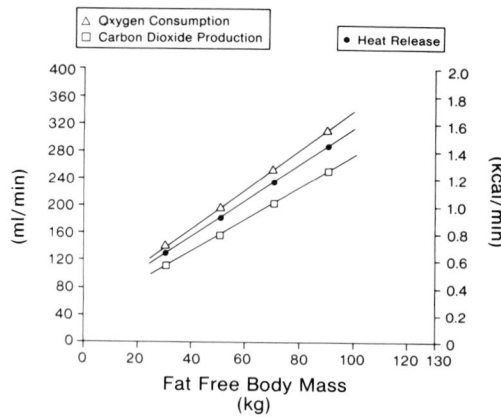

**Fig. 45–2.** Relationship between the fasting rate of oxygen consumption, carbon dioxide production, heat release (gradient-layer calorimeter), and fat-free body mass. The healthy subjects were between the ages of 20 and 70 years, and 90 to 115% ideal body weight. (From Heymsfield, S.B., et al.: Unpublished data.)

ergy and nitrogen loss. Climatic conditions,[17] physical activity,[18] and protein intake [19] are among the determinants of integumental losses.

To preserve body weight and total body energy content, the loss of endogenous fuels must be replaced by the diet. When energy intake is equal to losses, total body energy content remains constant. Similarly, when protein intake replaces protein and nitrogen losses, total body protein mass remains unchanged.

## PATHOPHYSIOLOGY OF WEIGHT LOSS

### Mechanisms

The major cause of weight loss in patients is an energy-protein intake that inadequately replaces losses. A low intake can be absolute or relative. If a patient decreases absolute food intake and there are no changes in energy or protein losses, the result will be negative energy and nitrogen balance. A relative reduction in food intake occurs when the absolute food intake remains unchanged, but energy and protein requirements are increasesd by fever, stress, and other pathologic states. The end result, negative balance, is the same. Clinically, food intake often falls simultaneously with an increase in nutrient requirements, creating a more severe degree of negative balance. In most chronic diseases associated with weight loss, a form of cyclic semistarvation is caused by periods of inadequate intake mixed with periods of normal or increased food ingestion. Integrated over time, balance is slightly negative, leading to gradual weight loss. Some rep-

tent of body protein is 16%, loss of one gram of urea nitrogen reflects oxidation of 1/0.16 or 6.25 grams of protein. Urea accounts for 80 to 85% of total urinary nitrogen, with the remainder accounted for by ammonia (7.4%), creatinine (6.4%), uric acid (2 to 3%), and other minor nitrogenous compounds (1 to 2%).[16] Since the primary source of nitrogen loss from the body is urea, and not protein, consideration of protein balance is usually simplified to nitrogen balance. This is acceptable because, under usual circumstances, nearly all of body nitrogen is incorporated into protein. Nitrogen balance is therefore considered synonymous with protein balance.

The skin, hair, sweat, nasal secretions, seminal discharge, and menstrual flow all account for enresentative intake patterns are depicted in Figure 45–3.

Energy losses in the form of heat are increased with fever, infection, severe injury, and endocrinopathies (pheochromocytoma, thyroid disease).[20] In addition to the loss of the thermal energy, there may also be abnormally large losses of energy and protein in chemical form. Energy and nitrogen losses in the stool are increased in patients with digestive and other debilitating diseases.[21] Representative examples of energy and protein digestibility are presented in Figure 45–4 for a variety of stable hospitalized patients. In some cases of malabsorption the losses are severe. For example, a protein digestibility of 50% in a patient with a jejunoileal bypass means that if 80 grams of protein were ingested, only a net of about 40 grams would remain after accounting for nitrogen losses in the stool. Marked steatorrhea also is associated with the loss of other essential nutrients, notably calcium, magnesium, and vitamins A, D, E, and K.

The urine, integument, and other fluid or tissue losses in disease contribute to negative balance and weight loss. Increased urinary losses occur in the presence of diabetes, proteinuria, aminoaciduria, and hematuria. The most striking increase in urinary energy losses occurs in diabetic ketoacidosis, when urinary energy content may increase to between 500 and 1000 kcal/d. Integumental losses are increased in patients with desquamating skin diseases, thermal injuries, or large open or draining wounds. Another loss of energy and nitrogen in pathologic states involves fluid or blood loss. Drainage of an effusion, ascitic fluid, or an abscess all contribute to overall energy and nitrogen losses.

## Pattern of Tissue Changes

The pattern of tissue change that occurs during the course of a wasting illness is determined by the magnitude of negative energy and nitrogen balance and by the underlying disease process. Only a general description and basic principles are presented in this section, and more specific details will be reviewed with the respective assessment indices.

**Chemical Composition.** Weight decreases in malnutrition are caused by a decline in fat and FFM. During the early phase of semi- or total starvation, the small supply of glycogen undergoes oxidation.[22] This depletion of fuel plus a release of glycogen-bound water accounts for a rapid fall in body weight over several days. Following this initial period, the two primary sources of fuel are triacylglycerol and amino acids. The rate of fat depletion is therefore closely related to energy and nitrogen balance, and these interrelations are described in Table 45–2.

Other than the initial loss of glycogen and water from lean tissues, the change in FFM as weight loss proceeds is determined largely by nitrogen balance. The obligatory water loss that accompanies protein catabolism proceeds at a slightly slower rate than the loss in nitrogen.[24] This rate differential causes a relative increase in the proportion of FFM as water and a decrease in the proportion as protein. An additional compositional change is that the profile of tissue proteins undergoes revision, with an increase in the pro-

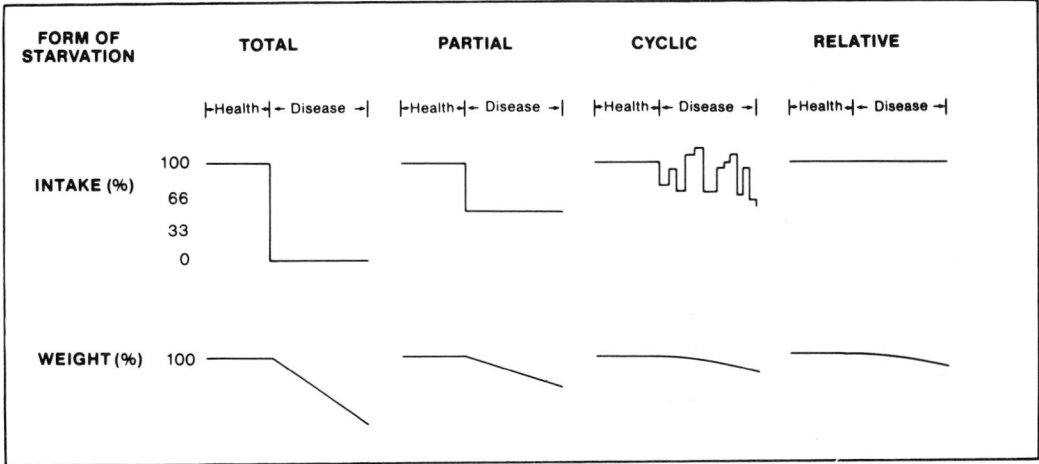

**Fig. 45–3.** Representative patterns of food intake. Total or partial starvation usually occurs in acute disease states or following injury. Cyclic starvation is characteristic of chronic disease, with negative balance resulting in gradual weight loss. In relative starvation, intake remains unchanged, but negative balance and weight loss are caused by an increase in energy and protein losses. (From Heymsfield, S.B., et al.: Unpublished data.)

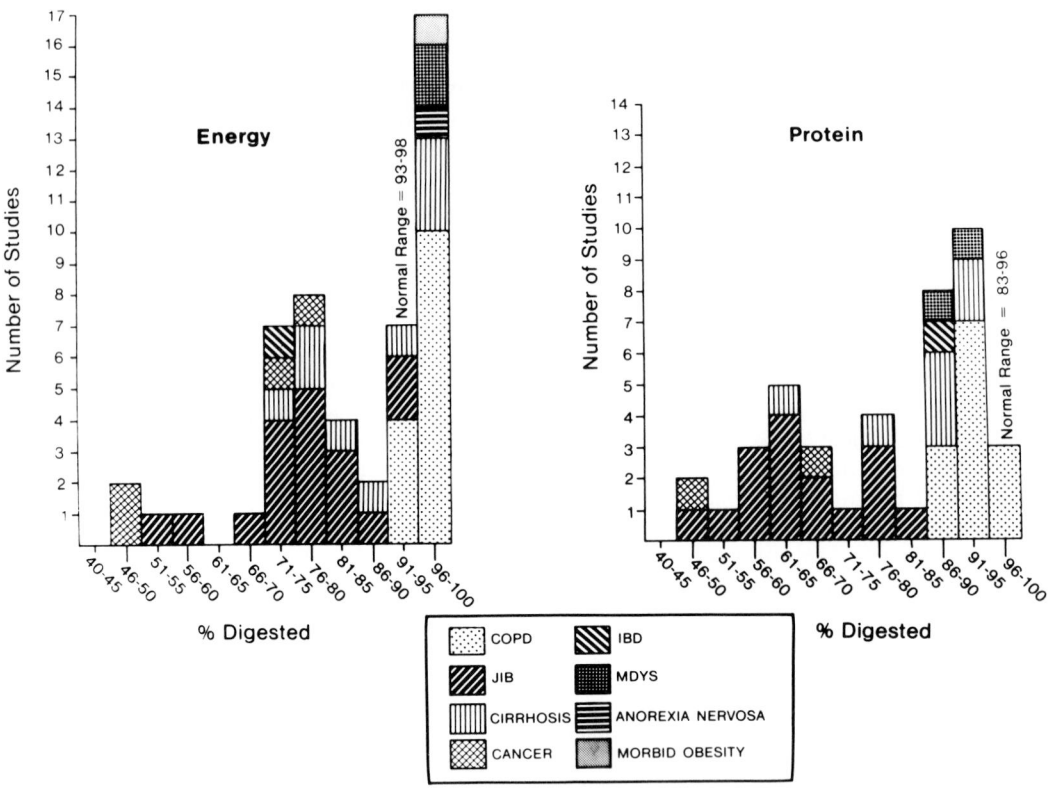

**Fig. 45–4.**   Apparent digestibility of energy and protein in a variety of hospitalized patients ingesting a general diet. COPD = chronic obstructive pulmonary disease; IBD = inflammatory bowel disease; JIB = jejunoileal bypass; and MDYS = muscular dystrophy. The normal ranges are from Southgate and Durnin.[15] (Modified from Heymsfield, S.B., Smith, J., Kasriel, S., et al.[21])

portion of connective tissue proteins and a relative reduction in cytoplasmic and extracellular soluble proteins.[25]

**Organ-Tissue Mass.**  At the organ and tissue level, rates and degree of atrophy differ during evolution of weight loss. The largest lean tissue component is skeletal muscle, which ranges between 30 and 50% of FFM in healthy subjects.[26] Skeletal muscle loses mass steadily throughout negative energy and nitrogen balance, and the relative rate of atrophy is more rapid than the loss in body weight.[27] In severe emaciation, up to two thirds of skeletal muscle tissue may be lost before the individual succumbs. Heart and kidney decrease in mass during periods of undernutrition at about the same relative rate as the loss in body weight.[28] Liver, spleen, and portions of the intestinal tract rapidly lose weight in the first few days of semistarvation, but changes thereafter are more gradual.[29] Overall, human liver and spleen decrease in mass by 60 to 65% during periods of severe weight loss.[29] Brain does not atrophy perceptibly, and skeletal mass remains unchanged, even in severe malnutrition.

**Influence of Disease Process.**  The combination of chemical changes in FFM and the differential rate and degree of organ atrophy in severe malnutrition imply that FFM departs substantially from the composition described earlier for healthy individuals. This simple scheme depicting otherwise uncomplicated malnutrition becomes vastly more complex in patients with underlying disease. The most important considerations are the following:

1. Edema or ascites may cause water balance to dissociate from nitrogen balance, and therefore total body weight and FFM in individuals afflicted with these disorders are poor indices of total body energy and nitrogen content, respectively.

2. Some organs and tissues within the FFM may not atrophy at the expected rate during semistarvation. There are two causes for this phenomenon. The first is that tissues may become infiltrated by abnormal constituents, such as tumors, connective tissue, fat, amyloid, and other pathologic material. The second cause is that the rate of organ atrophy is usually slowed by subjecting the tissue to an increased metabolic or mechanical

### Table 45–2.  Relationship between Metabolic Balance and Body Composition*

For a given change ($\Delta$) in energy-nitrogen balances (E, N), where

    (1) $\Delta E = E_{intake} - E_{losses}$,

and

    (2) $\Delta N = N_{intake} - N_{losses}$,

what are the changes in body fat, protein, and $H_2O$?

Basic information:

    (3) $\Delta$ protein (g) = $\Delta N$ (g) × 6.25 (g protein/gN)

    (4) $\Delta$ protein (kcal) = $\Delta$ protein (g) × 5.65† (kcal/g)

    (5) $\Delta$ fat (g) = $\Delta$ fat (kcal)/9.4† (kcal/g)

Method:

A. Estimate or measure energy-nitrogen balance in kcal/d and g/d, respectively.

B. Calculate $\Delta$ protein in g/d and kcal/d from $\Delta N$ (g/d), using equations 3 and 4.

C. Then:

    (6) $\Delta$ fat (kcal/d) = $\Delta E$ (kcal/d) − $\Delta$ protein (kcal/d).

D. Then: $\Delta$ fat (g/d) is calculated from equation 5.

E. The change in body weight ($\Delta BW$) is then used to calculate $\Delta H_2O$:

    (7) $\Delta H_2O$ (g/d) = $\Delta BW$ (g/d) − [$\Delta$ protein (g/d) + $\Delta$ fat (g/d)].

F. Summary:

    (8) $\Delta BW = \Delta$ protein + $\Delta$ fat + $\Delta H_2O$.

From Wright, R.A., Heymsfield, S.B.,[23] with permission of Blackwell Scientific Publications.

*The mass of bone mineral and glycogen are omitted from this simplified analysis.

†Caloric value of meat protein and animal fat.

workload, independent of overall nitrogen balance. For example, atrophy of a limb muscle in the undernourished rat can be prevented by subjecting the limb to vigorous exercise.[30] Infiltrative processes, or relative organomegaly, may cause body weight and FFM to lose their classic value in nutritional assessment.

3. Severe stress and hypercatabolic states change the rate and pattern of weight loss seen in uncomplicated semistarvation. The more severe degree of negative energy and nitrogen balance seen in stressed individuals increases the rate of fat and protein depletion, and, once again, the rate at which each component is lost depends directly on energy and nitrogen balance. In addition, the altered metabolic and hormonal profile in stress changes how the components of FFM respond during semistarvation. For example, renal mass may enlarge markedly in patients with severe burns;[31] and a marked increase may be observed in the biosynthetic rate of some of the serum proteins.[32] Renourishment during the early phase of the stress period may also differ from normal, with little or no repletion of protein mass, but excessive rates of glycogen and fat formation.[33] Identifying the presence of stress is important in properly

interpreting assessment indices at baseline and during nutritional therapy.

## COMPONENTS OF THE CLINICAL ASSESSMENT

In the clinical evaluation of nutritional status, the practitioner aims to define the patient's relationship to the scheme presented in Figure 45–5. Consider point A as the range of body composition and function compatible with health. Energy, nitrogen, and water balance are zero, and body weight is stable. A disease process now supervenes, and energy and nitrogen balance become negative. Weight now decreases until point $B_U$, when all available tissue fuels are depleted. The underweight patient then succumbs if negative balance persists beyond $B_U$. Not all individuals

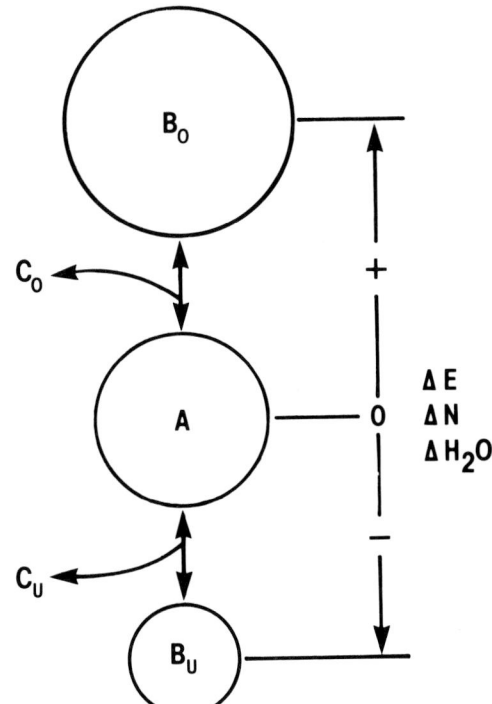

**Fig. 45–5.** Model depicting changes in metabolic balance and body composition in protein-energy malnutrition and obesity. Point A is the range of body composition and tissue function found in health. Weight is stable, and balance of energy, nitrogen, and water is zero. Disease causes negative metabolic balance, weight loss, and changes in body composition and tissue function. Point $B_U$ is the minimal range of body composition and tissue function that is compatible with survival. The course of a patient moving between points A and $B_U$ may be interrupted by a complication related to malnutrition, and this is indicated by point $C_U$. Positive balance leads to obesity, and a similar set of endpoints, $B_O$ and $C_O$, are designated. Nutritional assessment aims to define the patient's status between points A, B, and C.

survive malnutrition to its limits at point $B_U$; another possible outcome is for a complication of malnutrition to alter the natural history of the disease (point $C_U$). If the patient is fortunate, nutritional therapy will prevent weight loss or gradually correct protein-energy malnutrition already present. The aim of nutritional assessment is to determine the location, direction, and rate of change of the individual patient between points A, B, and C. Although not reviewed in this chapter, positive balance of energy, nitrogen, and water ultimately lead to obesity. Point $B_O$ defines the terminal upper limit of weight, and $C_O$ the associated morbid complications of obesity. The components of the clinical assessment are grouped into three main categories, energy and nitrogen balance, body composition, and tissue function.

### Energy and Nitrogen Balance

Disturbances in energy and nitrogen balance are related to reduced intake or increased losses as described earlier. The standard medical history and review of systems include information regarding appetite, food habits, and gastrointestinal symptoms. A more comprehensive assessment is performed by the dietitian, and three techniques are generally available: 24-hour recall with a food frequency cross-check, analysis of a food record or diary, and a calorie count.

In the 24-hour recall,[34] the patient is questioned regarding food intake and physical activity level during a one-day period. The activity history provides a rough estimate of the energy cost of physical exertion and also helps the patient recall food intake at different times of the day. Close relatives or friends should be asked to provide diet information, as the history often differs between the patient and family. Portion sizes are difficult to estimate accurately, and food models aid in this component of the analysis. Other than a representative intake, the questions regarding food habits and social conditions listed in Table 45–3 should be included in the evaluation.

The food frequency questionnaire is aimed at eliciting how often a food item is eaten during a specified time period, usually a week.[35] The food frequency and the 24-hour recall are used together, thus filling in gaps in the history and allowing for a cross-check of information. These two types of diet history are often compiled soon after admission to the hospital. Both the 24-hour recall and the food frequency techniques can also be used for outpatients.

Food records or diaries require that the patient keep a 3-to-5-day record of food intake, including all solids and liquids.[36] The patient estimates portion sizes or may actually weigh the foods prior

**Table 45–3.  Supplementary Components of the Food Intake History**

A.  The patient eats at home: Prepares own meals/Meals are prepared by ?
B.  Type of food preparation: Conventional/Convenience/Snack?
C.  The patient eats away from home: times per week? Restaurants/lCafeterias/Fast Foods?
D.  Is salt added: In cooking/At table?
E.  Weekend food intake differs from weekday: Yes/No; How?
F.  Takes: Vitamins/Minerals/Other supplements?
G.  Physical needs affecting nutrition: Visual/Auditory/Dexterity/Mobility/Smokes/Appetite Change/Pica/Dentures/Chewing or Swallowing Problems?
H.  Social needs affecting nutrition: Resides alone/Depression/Alcohol consumption/Budget limitations/Inadequate kitchen facilities?
I.  Previous diet counseling: Yes/No?
J.  Foods patient cannot eat: Allergies/Ethnic/Religious/Dislikes?
K.  Fad diets?

to consumption. Obtaining an accurate food record requires a cooperative patient, and generally one who can read and write.

The direct observation method is used in hospitalized patients and is generally referred to as a calorie count. Once the calorie count is requested, the assigned health care member is responsible for estimating the amounts of food a patient eats during the meal. This information is then recorded on the menu, and the results are calculated by the dietitian. In order to be accurate, all forms of nutrient supplied during the evaluation period must be tabulated. A high level of cooperation among medical care personnel is required to achieve an accurate calorie count. Among the valuable features of a calorie count are the following: chewing problems can be noted, food refusal can be documented, and direct observations can be correlated with the food intake history. Interpretation should be cautious, as patients under hospital surveillance may eat more or less than they do at home. The suggested minimal calorie count interval is three days.

Once collected, the diet information is processed either by use of food composition tables or by an exchange system.[37,38] The results are tabulated by hand or by available computer programs. The amount and adequacy of total energy, carbohydrate, fat, and protein are assessed by comparison to Recommended Daily Allowances. [39] Adjustments in energy and protein requirements based upon the patient's disease state may also be needed. Individual nutrients or groups of nutrients can be assessed for adequacy, and the patient identified as high risk for specific nutrient deficiencies.

Despite the limited accuracy of techniques aimed at assessing energy and nitrogen intake,[40] their value in nutritional assessment should not be overlooked. Even minor reductions in food intake lead to negative balance and weight loss when extended over long periods. The intake information often remains the only valid assessment index when other classic nutritional markers are confounded by factors related to the underlying disease process.

When determining caloric intake, the energy value of specific fuels or foods is measured by bomb calorimetry.[21] In the early twentieth century, average gross energy values (in kcal/g) were developed for the carbohydrate (4.1), protein (5.65), and fat (9.4) found in a general diet.[41] Since not all of this potential energy is available to balance losses of energy in the form of heat, early workers simplified fuel values in two additional steps.[41] First, the gross energy value of each fuel was adjusted for average net digestive losses. The digestible energy values thus became 4.0, 5.25, and 9.0 kcal/g of carbohydrate, protein, and fat. Second, the potential energy in protein lost as urea was accounted for by subtracting an additional 1.25 kcal/g of dietary protein. This resulted in the physiologic fuel values (in kcal/g) for carbohydrate (4.0), protein (4.0), and fat (9.0). For patients eating a regular diet who do not have abnormally large energy losses in stool or urine, use of these corrected fuel values simplifies calculation of energy balance; energy losses in stool and urine are eliminated from consideration. Similar corrected fuel values for specialized enteral or parenteral diets are not yet available, and the current practice is to use the physiologic fuel values developed for regular diets. Although this approach is technically incorrect, the errors involved in clinically estimating energy intake are relatively small.

The protein content of food is usually measured by assuming that protein has an average nitrogen content of 16% and then measuring protein nitrogen by the micro-Kjeldahl[42] or other newer techniques.[43] Food tables or product labels also provide protein values, which are then multiplied by 0.16 or divided by 6.25 in order to convert to nitrogen.

Abnormally large losses of energy and nitrogen are identified from the history and by laboratory studies. Nausea, vomiting, diarrhea, and a history of intestinal disease, renal abnormalities, diabetes, fever or serious injury are all clues to the presence of increased losses of energy and protein in chemical or thermal form.

The simplest method of assessing heat losses is to calculate approximate values for basal energy expenditure, thermic effect of food, physical ac-

tivity, and fever/injury as outlined in Table 45–4. No estimates are yet available for the thermic response to fuel, and it is likely that this form of heat loss is highly variable. When calorimetry equipment is available, the procedures outlined in Table 45–4 will provide measured values for daily heat losses.

Fecal energy and nitrogen losses are usually measured by bomb calorimetry[21] and the micro-Kjeldahl techniques,[42] respectively. Measurement is not required in patients who do not have a history of malabsorption. For energy, the physiologic fuel values are already adjusted for this loss. Prediction equations are available for calculating fecal N from protein intake,[54] but this approach is valid only for the diet upon which the mathematical expression was developed. A simple approach is to multiply orally ingested nitrogen by 1 minus an approximate value for apparent nitrogen digestibility (A2, Table 45–5).[55] The table presents the apparent digestibility of nitrogen in two groups of depleted hospitalized patients, one that had no prior history of malabsorption, and the other with moderate malabsorption. Balance studies lasted for one week, and the results include three types of tube feeding solutions and a general hospital diet. Daily fecal nitrogen losses during total parenteral nutrition in patients without malabsorption ranges between 0.3 and 0.8 g/d, or about 8 mg/kg.

For patients who are evaluated for malabsorption and weight loss, the simplest measureable index of absorption is daily stool weight. Normal values are less than 200 g/day, and values less than 100 g/day are more typical of low-residue tube feeding diets. A summary of additional absorption studies is presented in Table 45–6.

Urinary energy and nitrogen losses are measured by the same analytic methods described for diet and stool. For patients without an apparent cause for increased urinary energy losses, the adjusted fuel value of protein is already corrected for this loss. Proteinuria, glucosuria, and ketonuria all increase urinary energy losses, and rough estimates of the urine energy content in these subjects can be derived by qualitative laboratory studies. For example, a dipstick urine of 4+ means an approximate glucose of 20 g/dl. Multiplying by daily urine volume and the energy value of glucose (3.75 kcal/g) then provides an estimated value in kcal for glucosuria.

Several approaches are available for measuring nitrogenous losses in urine. The ideal method is to determine total urinary nitrogen on several 24-hour collections and then average the results. Often the hospital laboratory cannot measure total urinary nitrogen, and an alternative is to measure

**Table 45–4.   Clinical Estimation of Thermal Energy Losses**

| | *Calculate* | *Measure* |
|---|---|---|
| A. Basal energy expenditure* (BEE, kcal/d)† | 1. Tables of basal energy expenditure based on age, sex, height, weight, and FFM are available.[16]<br>2. Prediction equations* are available, and a few examples are as follows:<br>Males: BEE = 66.473 + 13.7516(W) + 5.0033(H) + 6.7550(A).[44]<br>Females: BEE = 655.0955 + 9.5634(W) + 84.96(H) + 4.6756(A).[44]<br>Males and females: BEE = 396 + 19.2(FFM)[45]<br>Males and females: BEE = 471 + 20.8(FFM).[46] | 1. Classic method: Following overnight 12-hour fast, the resting early morning oxygen consumption and carbon dioxide production are measured at thermoneutrality for 5–15 minutes. The caloric value of oxygen is determined from the respiratory exchange ratio, and energy production (kcal/min) is calculated from the equations of Zuntz and Schumberg.[47] A more complete approach includes collection of a 24-hr urine sample, and analysis for urea nitrogen. This allows a more precise calculation of the caloric value of oxygen.[48] Usually results are extrapolated to 24 hours. For the sleeping portion of the day, some workers recommend using the BEE × 0.9 × proportion of day asleep. |
| | A = age, years:<br>FFM = fat-free body mass, kg;<br>H = height, cm;<br>W = weight, kg. | 2. Alternative method: Rather than a single value, multiple fasting and resting measurements are made throughout the day. Results are then averaged, or the area beneath the energy expenditure curve is calculated. |
| B. Thermic effect of food (TEF, kcal/d)[49] | TEF = BEE × 0.1 | Measure BEE, and feed standard meal. Indirect calorimetry measurements continued for 3–6 hours following the meal allow calculation of TEF. The TEF varies with meal size, so a true estimate per day may require feeding several different sized meals. |
| C. Thermic response to fuel (TRF, kcal/d)[13,50] | TRF varies with formula type, infusion rate, and patient illness. | When indirect calorimetry is performed during continuous feeding, the resulting value includes the TRF. Either method 1 or 2 for BEE above is used to measure this combined basal and feeding thermal loss. |
| D. Physical activity (kcal/d)[14,20] | Sitting = duration × 0.08 BEE<br>Standing = duration × 0.17 BEE<br>Walking slowly = duration × 1.37 BEE<br>Duration is the time span of each activity (in minutes) as determined from a diary divided by 1440. | The energy cost of each activity can be measured by indirect calorimetry. A diary is then used to establish the duration of each activity. |
| E. Disease-related thermal losses (kcal/d)[20,51,52]<br>   Noncatabolic illness<br>   Elective surgery<br>   Skeletal trauma<br>   Blunt trauma<br>   Acute respiratory failure and sepsis<br>   Head injury<br>   Severe sepsis<br>   Burns[53]<br>      area involved = 0–20%<br>                >20≤40%<br>                >40≤100% | Multiply BEE by:<br><br>0.20<br>0.24<br>0.32<br>0.34<br><br>0.60<br>0.64<br>0.71<br><br>0.1–0.5<br>0.5–0.85<br>0.85–1.05 | Measure as described above for BEE. The result includes the thermal response to injury. |
| F. Fever (kcal/d)<br>[average temperature elevation (°C per day) − 37°] × [0.125 × BEE] | | |
| G. Summary:<br>Total thermal losses (kcal/d) = A + (B or C) + D + E + F.<br>Zero energy balance in eumetabolic ambulatory patient is usually achieved when intake is equal to 1.4–1.6 times the calculated or measured BEE. | | During continuous formula infusion in the resting injured patient, the measured energy expenditure includes A + C + E + F. The only remaining thermal loss is physical activity (D), which is often estimated at 0.2 BEE for inactive hospital patients. |

*Predicted values using different equations may vary by 10 to 20%.

†We have avoided using the term resting energy expenditure (REE), as there is no consensus on the definition of this measurement.

**Table 45–5. Nitrogen Balance Studies in Hospitalized Patients***

| Diet | N (g/d) Intake | N (g/d) Stool | N (g/d) Urine | N (g/d) Urine Urea | Urine Urea N Divided by Total Urine N | Total Urine N Minus Urea N (g/d) A1 | (mg/kg/d) A1 | Apparent Digestibility A2 | Stool N (mg/kg/d) A3 | Total N Losses† Minus Urea N (g/d) A4 | (mg/kg/d) A4 |
|---|---|---|---|---|---|---|---|---|---|---|---|
| *Enteral (Depleted patients)* | | | | | | | | | | | |
| General hospital diet, 40% fat (n=10) | 16.5 | 1.9 | 9.1 | 7.3 | 0.80 | 1.8 | (33) | 0.88 | 34 | 4.1 | (74) |
| Elemental—free amino acid, 2% fat (n=22) | 15.8 | 0.6 | 12.3 | 10.8 | 0.87 | 1.5 | (32) | 0.96 | 13 | 2.6 | (56) |
| Elemental—predigested protein, 2% fat (n=30) | 16.2 | 1.5 | 8.5 | 7.1 | 0.83 | 1.4 | (27) | 0.91 | 29 | 3.3 | (64) |
| Polymeric—intact protein, 40% fat (n=33) | 15.5 | 1.5 | 10.0 | 8.5 | 0.85 | 1.5 | (30) | 0.90 | 30 | 3.4 | (67) |
| Total formulas (n=85) | 15.3 | 1.2 | 10.2 | 8.7 | 0.85 | 1.5 | (30) | 0.92 | 24 | 3.1 | (62) |
| *Enteral (Depleted malabsorption patients)* | | | | | | | | | | | |
| General hospital diet 40% fat (n=4) | 14.8 | 3.7 | 12.4 | 10.2 | 0.83 | 2.2 | (31) | 0.77 | 52 | 6.4 | (90) |
| Elemental—free amino acid, 2% fat (n=6) | 14.4 | 1.6 | 12.8 | 11.4 | 0.87 | 1.4 | (23) | 0.88 | 26 | 3.4 | (56) |
| Elemental—predigested protein, 2% fat (n=6) | 14.9 | 2.5 | 9.5 | 7.5 | 0.78 | 2.0 | (33) | 0.82 | 41 | 4.9 | (80) |
| Polymeric—intact protein, 40% fat (n=4) | 13.7 | 1.6 | 9.4 | 7.1 | 0.75 | 2.3 | (35) | 0.88 | 25 | 4.3 | (66) |
| Total formulas (n=16) | 14.4 | 1.9 | 10.7 | 8.9 | 0.81 | 1.8 | (29) | 0.86 | 31 | 4.2 | (68) |
| *Parenteral* | | | | | | | | | | | |
| Healthy subjects D5W | | | | | 0.85 | 1.3 | | | 8‡ | | |
| Depleted patients D5W | | | | | 0.81 | 1.7 | | | | | |
| TPN§ | | | | | 0.92 | 2.1 | | | | | |
| Septic patients D5W | | | | | 0.74 | 3.3 | | | | | |
| TPN | | | | | 0.82 | 5.4 | | | | | |
| Trauma patients D5W | | | | | 0.78 | 3.7 | | | | | |
| Cystectomy D5W | | | | | 0.83 | 2.7 | | | | | |
| TPN | | | | | 0.88 | 3.3 | | | | | |

*Modified from Heymsfield, S.B., Tochilin, N., McManus, C.B., et al.[55] and Shaw, S., Askanazi, J., et al.[56]
†Stool N + Urine N + estimated integumental N.
‡Estimated value.
§Total parenteral nutrition.

**Table 45–6.  Nutrient Absorption Studies in General Use**

| | *Normal values* | *Comment* |
|---|---|---|
| *General* | | |
| Stool weight | Wet weight <200 g/d<br>Dry weight <66.4 g/d | Increased in maldigestion and malabsorption; may also be increased in secretory diarrhea due to water and electrolyte loss |
| *Carbohydrate* | | |
| Glucose (100 g orally) | Rise in blood glucose of >35 mg/dl | "Flat curve" in sucrose deficiency, diseases of the intestinal wall, and in monosaccharide malabsorption |
| Sucrose (100 g orally) | Rise in blood glucose of >20 mg/dl | Low to flat curve in diseases of the intestinal wall |
| Lactose (50–100 g orally) | Rise in blood glucose of >20 mg/dl | Low to flat curve in lactase deficiency and diseases of the intestinal wall |
| Xylose (25 g orally) | Urinary excretion ≥4.5 g/5 hrs | A good screening test of carbohydrate absorption; differentiates between maldigestion and malabsorption; diminished in mucosal diseases; does not predict how well an individual will be able to use carbohydrates or disaccharides |
| *Protein* | | |
| Stool nitrogen (general hospital diet × 3 days) | Apparent digestibility of ≥83% | Increased in malabsorption |
| *Energy* | | |
| Stool kcal (general hospital diet × 3 days) | Apparent digestibility of ≥90% | Increased in malabsorption |
| *Minerals* | | |
| Stool Mg, Ca, P, K, Fe, Zn, Na, Cl | Digestibilities vary | Methods include balance studies, isotopes, and flame photometry. Blood analysis of corresponding mineral supports the diagnosis of impaired retention |
| *Vitamins* | | |
| Vitamin B | Serum level 200–600 pg/ml | Diminished with gastric resection, intestinal stasis, ileal dysfunction, or resection; if low, consider Schilling test to elucidate mechanism |
| Folate | Serum level 6–15 ng/ml<br>RBC level 150–450 ng/ml | Diminished, especially in small bowel disease; RBC level better indicator of body stores of folate |
| K (prothrombin time) | Control value of prothrombin time | Prolonged |
| A (serum carotene) | Vitamin A, 20–100 µg/dl<br>Serum carotene 60–400 µg/dl | Diminished, especially in small bowel disease |
| *Fat* | | |
| Stool fat | | |
| Qualitative (Sudan stain) | Subjective interpretation of microscopic stool specimen | Presence of stool fat droplets suggest steatorrhea; if present, proceed to quantitative study |
| Quantitative (100 g fat diet × 3 days) | Fecal fat <6 g/d or apparent digestibility of ≥95% | Best test for diagnosing malassimilation; values are increased in maldigestion or malabsorption |

urinary urea nitrogen. Total urinary nitrogen can then be calculated by adding to the urea nitrogen an estimated value for non-urea losses (A1, Table 45–5). Note that A1 is influenced by diet, and the type and extent of injury. Other factors that influence A1 are body composition, acid base disturbances, and the presence of an aminoaciduria.[57]

Integumental losses must be estimated on the clinical ward, and in healthy individuals values range between 0.3 and 0.5 gN/day. Losses may increase markedly in diseases involving the skin, but little information is avaiable on this topic. The same applies to drainage fluid losses, which must undergo direct analysis to obtain accurate values for energy and nitrogen. Small or moderate amounts of typical drainage fluids contain less than 50 kcal and about 0.5 to 1.0 gN/day, and therefore omitting this measurement from the clinical estimate of energy and nitrogen balance does not cause major errors.

The last chemical consideration in clinically estimating nitrogen balance occurs in patients who have a change in blood urea nitrogen (BUN) level during the urine collection period. Urea distributes in the total body water space, and nitrogen balance must be corrected for this change in non-protein nitrogen.[58] The following equation is usually applied clinically:

$$\Delta \text{ Nonprotein nitrogen (g/d)} = [(BUN_f$$
$$- BUN_i) \times 0.6 \times BW_i + (BW_f - BW_i) \quad (3)$$
$$\times BUN_f]/(Day_f - Day_i)$$

where $i$ and $f$ are initial and final values at the beginning and end of the balance period, BW is body weight in kg, and BUN is in g/L. Note that the value for nonprotein nitrogen can be either positive or negative. The equation assumes that 60% of body weight is water and that changes in weight are due to changes in total body water. In lean patients or those with edema, the fraction of 0.6 is too low, and, conversely, obese individuals or the very young have a lower fraction of weight as water. No simple corrections are available for these groups.

In the clinical setting it is unusual to have all the facilities needed to perform metabolic balance studies. However, even qualitative information is useful when the observer recognizes the key components of energy and nitrogen balance, their derangements in disease, and the relationship of balances to observed changes in body composition. The composite metabolic profile is useful in selecting the type and amount of nutritional therapy and also aids in monitoring the effects of the selected treatment program.

Energy balance evaluated clinically relies on calculating the estimated or measured differences between intake and losses. When malabsorption and hypermetabolism are not present, the energy balance equation is simplified to:

$$\Delta \text{ Energy} = E_{intake} - [E_{basal} + E_{TEF} + E_{activity}] \quad (4)$$

where TEF is the thermic effect of food. Energy intake is calculated from the physiologic fuel values, and heat losses are calculated as described in Table 45–4. When malabsorption or increased urinary losses are present, then the calculated energy loss must include a measured or estimated value for energy in stool and urine. Energy intake must then be calculated from the gross energy values of the three respective fuels. When hypermetabolism or fever is present, the increase in energy losses can either be measured or estimated as described in Table 45–4.

For nitrogen balance, the basic question is:

$$\Delta N = N_{intake} - [N_{urine} + N_{stool} + N_{integument}] \quad (5)$$

If there are drainage fluid losses of nitrogen or if BUN rises during the evaluation period, then these two additional factors must be added to the equation. Intake of nitrogen is calculated from the diet history or observed calorie count, and under rigorous conditions diet nitrogen is chemically analyzed by available methods. Urinary nitrogen is either measured directly, or calculated by adding the nonurea nitrogen losses (A1, Table 45–5) to urea nitrogen.

Stool nitrogen is calculated either by multiplying enterally ingested nitrogen by one minus A2 (Table 45–5), or by multiplying body weight by an average value for stool N (A3, Table 45–5). A more accurate approach, especially for patients with malabsorption, is to measure stool nitrogen directly on a three-day (minimum) fecal collection. Integumental nitrogen is estimated at 7 and 8 mg/kg for men (A5) and women (A6), respectively.[59] A common practice is to measure only urinary urea nitrogen and then calculate nitrogen balance by adding approximate values for the remaining nonurea nitrogen losses:

$$\Delta N = N_{intake} - [N_{urea} + A1$$
$$+ A2 \text{ or } A3 + A5 \text{ or } A6] \quad (6)$$

A simplification is to add to urea nitrogen a composite value for the remaining nonurea nitrogen losses (A4, Table 45–5) and then calculate nitrogen balance as:

$$\Delta N = N_{intake} - [N_{E \text{ urea}} + A4] \quad (7)$$

Unfortunately, not all of the information needed for making these calculations in all patients was available during the preparation of this chapter. When published, this missing information can be used to fill in the gaps in Table 45–5.

Three important points in considering the results of balance estimates are that:

1. Clinical balance values are usually somewhat higher than actual balances because intake tends to be overestimated, whereas losses are often underestimated.[60]

2. Balance results observed shortly after a major change in intake may not reflect balances after a new steady state is achieved. Depending on the clinical circumstances, this may take as little as three days and as long as several weeks.[61]

3. The between-day variability in all balance terms is large, and therefore increasing the number of observations reduces this form of error.[62]

When balances are negative, the patient will lose fat and FFM as described in Table 45–2; positive balance indicates growth of new tissue. The magnitude of negative or positive balance will determine the rate of tissue loss or gain, respectively. These results will also aid in interpreting the clinical significance of measurements of body composition. For example, marked negative energy and nitrogen balance in a patient whose body composition is near point $B_u$ in Figure 45–5 would indicate a very significant problem. If this patient was then started on therapy, an estimate of the time needed to restore body composition to within the normal range (A, Fig. 45–5) could then be based on balance results. Even crude bedside balance calculations often help in gaining perspective on a patient's therapeutic course.

## Body Composition

**Anthropometric Methods.** Anthropometry, a technique developed in the late nineteenth century by anthropologists, employs simple measuring devices to quantify differences in human form. The potential of anthropometric methods in assessing nutritional status was first realized in the late nineteenth century by Richer, who used skinfold thickness as an index of fatness.[63] The modern era of nutritional anthropometry began with the studies of Matiegka during World War I.[64] Matiegka's interest in the physical efficiency of soldiers led him to develop methods of anthropometrically subdividing the human body into muscle, fat, and bone. The major anthropometric categories now in clinical use are body weight, fat, and FFM.

*Body Weight.* The weight of an individual is the sum of fat and FFM ($H_2O$ + protein + glycogen + mineral). The simplifying assumptions are that body weight is a measure of total body energy stores and that changes in weight parallel energy and nitrogen balance. In adults, weight usually varies less than $\pm$ 0.1 kg/day. A loss in weight of more than 0.5 kg/day either indicates negative energy or water balance, or a combination of the two. Clinically significant weight loss is considered a relative decrease in weight of greater than 10%.

The severity of weight loss in an individual is determined by two factors, the rate of weight change over time and the total reduction in weight. The rate of weight loss in total starvation is approximately 0.4 kg/d, and survival is sustained to about 70% of desirable (i.e., ideal) body weight.[65] Semistarvation, the more typical cause of negative energy balance in patients, results in a more gradual loss in weight compared to that in total starvation. In extreme cases of chronic disease, the weight change may occur over years or decades. The minimal survivable body weight in humans is between 48 and 55% of desirable body weight (i.e., point $B_u$ in Figure 45–5.[24] The body weight at this point consists of less than 5% fat; the remaining FFM has a relative increase in water and skeletal mass, with a corresponding decrease

in protein. Exhaustion of the remaining metabolically usable fat mass results in rapid depletion of lean tissues and death.

The absolute body weight and rate of change in weight have prognostic value, and two aspects are recognized. The first is that an absolute body weight of less than 55 to 60% of desirable places the subject at or near the survival limits of semistarvation. Further negative balance could not be tolerated for long. The second aspect is that a significant reduction from the pre-illness weight (>10 to 20%) places the patient at a high risk of an adverse outcome. This observation has been made in many medical conditions, ranging from cancer[66] and chronic lung disease[67] to elective surgery.[68] A later section in this chapter provides additional details regarding weight as a prognostic marker.

Body weight is measured longitudinally to establish the effectiveness of nutritional therapy. A change in weight reflects energy and water balance.

Measuring body weight in the hospital should be accomplished within $\pm$ 0.1 kg on a calibrated physician's scale. Special scales should be used in bedridden or wheelchair-bound patients. Edema, if present, should be recorded with the weight. The general procedure is to obtain a morning weight following evacuation of the bladder. The weight of the hospital gown can be subtracted from the total weight if the desired goal is nude weight. When comparing the patient to standard values, the attire is usually presented in a footnote on the table. Serial weights should be measured on the same or a carefully calibrated scale. Intake and output records may be useful in interpreting the significance of changes in daily weight.

Reference tables provide a standard weight for height, and in some cases there is an adjustment for frame size. Height is usually measured by a sliding bar attached to the physician's scale, although more accurate techniques are used for research purposes. The reference table will usually specify the technique used to establish frame size.

The patient's weight is evaluated using two reference sources. The first reference values are those of the patient, and these include a "usual weight" by history or previous measured weight. Equations for processing this information are provided in Addendum 1. The second reference source is the healthy population, and this is described along with other anthropometry reference values at the end of this section.

There are four conditions in which interpretation of body weight as an index of available energy supply must be used with caution:

1. Edema and ascites cause a relative increase in total body $H_2O$ and mask loss in fat and protein.

2. Massive tumor growth or organomegaly masks loss in fat and lean tissues, such as skeletal muscle.

3. Lean tissue atrophy is masked by residual fat in obese patients undergoing rapid or severe weight loss.

4. Large changes in energy intake cause corresponding changes in glycogen mass over a several day period. Each gram of glycogen binds 4 to 5 grams of water, and a weight change in this period may consist of an unusually large proportion of water.

For these reasons, and also to provide a more complete characterization of body composition, anthropometric methods are used to further compartmentalize the body.

*Fat.* Fat is nearly all in the form of triacylglycerol, which in humans has an energy density of 9.4 kcal/g. Most triacylglycerol is found in adipose tissue, which has an approximate composition of 80% fat, 18% water, and 2% protein.[69] Adipose tissue is distributed in two major locations, the subcutaneous space and the internal space. Age, sex, and individual differences exist in the proportion of adipose tissue at different subcutaneous sites,[70] and in the relation of subcutaneous to internal fat.[71]

The amount of fat in healthy subjects varies greatly, with relatively small amounts in some highly trained athletes and relatively large amounts during the later stages of pregancy. During protracted undernutrition, all but a small amount of total body fat can be utilized as metabolic fuel. Two factors determine the adequacy of fat: the amount of triacylglycerol present and energy balance. Very little fat is sufficient if the individual is healthy and in zero energy balance. Contrastingly, a small amount of fat in the presence of marked negative energy balance implies a limited survival time. The usual practice is to compare fat values from an individual patient to reference standards and also to follow trends over time. During nutritional therapy, the measurement of fat provides an indirect guide to energy balance, and the specific relations between the two are described in Table 45–2.

Three methods of assessing body fat are available: the one skinfold method, the limb fat area method, and the total body fat calculated from multiple skinfold measurements. The measurements common to all three techniques are now briefly reviewed, and the interested reader should consult additional references for added details.

Measuring body fat requires two instruments, a skinfold caliper and a tape measure. The caliper should be a rugged and light instrument, and jaw pressure should be maintained at 10 g/mm² throughout the skinfold range. The contact surface area of the jaws can vary between 30 and 100 mm², and the jaws on some calipers remain parallel as they are opened wider. A calibration block is usually supplied with the instrument. The tape measure should be durable, resist stretching, and have an accuracy of ± 0.1 cm. Plastic and fiberglass tapes meet these criteria, and calibration should be checked periodically against a meter stick.

Two types of measurement are usually made, skinfold thicknesses and limb circumferences. The location of six widely used skinfold sites and circumferences are described in Addenda 2 and 3. For arm measurements, the most important aspect is to make repeated measurements using the same arm. Some workers recommend evaluating the nondominant arm; when comparing to standard values, consult the arm selected in the reference table. The measuring techniques and methods of optimizing precision are presented in Addenda 4 and 5. Skinfold measurements are not accurate in the massively obese.

The absolute skinfold thickness can be used directly for comparison to reference tables and for longitudinal follow-up. The limitation of evaluating one skinfold thickness is that a single measurement is a relatively poor predictor of the absolute amount and rate of change in total body fat because (1) there are large interindividual differences in fat distribution,[70] (2) as total body fat changes, each skinfold site responds differently relative to changes in total body fat;[23] and (3) an exponential relationship exists between (A) subcutaneous skinfold thickness and total body fat, and (B) between subcutaneous fat and internal fat[71] (Fig. 45–6). Other factors that limit skinfold thickness as a measure of fat include: changes in the composition of adipose tissue with age and nutritional status; variation in skinfold distribution and compressibility with age; and the inclusion of nonfat tissues (e.g., skin) in the measurement. The final consideration is that the between-day variability in measuring the same skinfold is rather large,[72] even when the rigorous procedures outlined in Addenda 4 and 5 are followed. Measuring skinfold thickness should therefore be considered a qualitative measure of the amount and rate of change in total body fat. The advantages are ease and rapidity of measurement, especially in bedridden patients.

Combining a limb skinfold thickness with a corresponding circumference allows calculation of limb fat areas (Addendum 6). Most of the problems related to one skinfold measurement are also found with the limb fat area. The advantage gen-

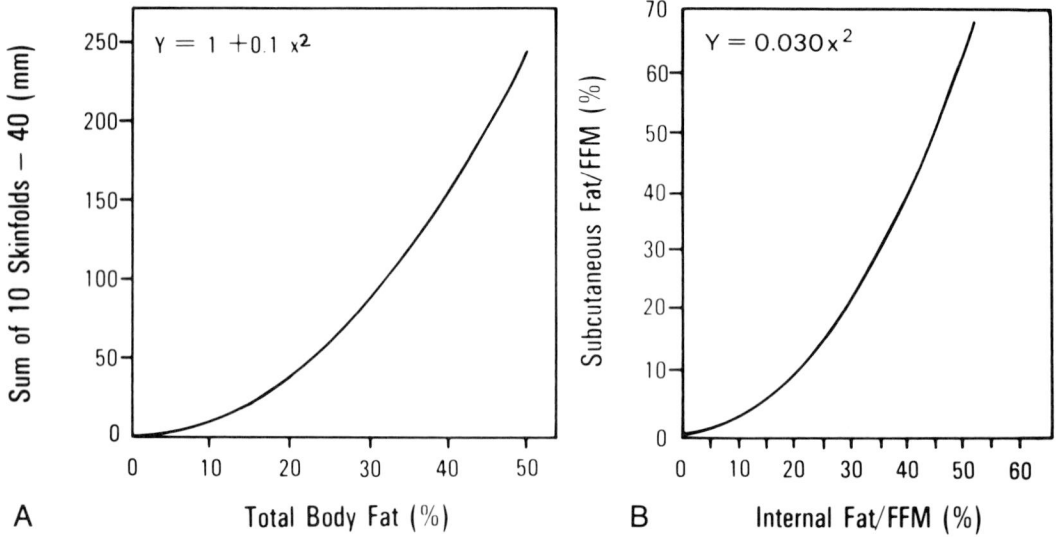

**Fig. 45–6.** *A,* The sum ($\Sigma$) of ten skinfolds versus percentage of total body fat. Forty millimeters were subtracted from $\Sigma$ to correct for skin thickness. Total body fat was measured by underwater weighing. The relationship is exponential. *B,* Subcutaneous fat versus internal fat, both expressed as a percentage of FFM. The relationship between the two major fat reservoirs is nonlinear. (Modified from Allen T.H., Peng, M.T., Chen, K.P., et al.[71])

erally ascribed to area calculations is that the result includes the contribution of limb circumference; two limbs with equal skinfolds but unequal circumferences will have different amounts of fat.

There are many prediction equations for calculating total body fat from measured skinfold thicknesses and body weight. The most widely applied equation in current use was developed by Durnin and Womersley[73] (Addendum 7); subtracting total body fat from body weight provides a value for FFM. The advantages of calculating total body fat are (1) more than one skinfold site is included in the calculation; and (2) the result (in kg) can be used directly to calculate energy reserves as fat. The latter values can then be integrated with estimated energy balance calculations, thus providing a more physiologic description of the patient's nutritional state. A cautionary note is that like all prediction equations, results are most accurate on populations upon which the equation was derived. The accuracy of the Durnin-Womersley equation is unknown in patients with severe weight loss, and the technique should not be applied when there is a gross distortion in body habitus or obvious fluid accumulation. As emphasized by Damon and Goldman,[74] skinfold measurements describe, but do not predict total body fat. More accurate methods of measuring fat are therefore usually applied in research studies of body composition.

*Fat-Free Body Mass.* The main constituents of FFM are water and protein, with lesser amounts of mineral and glycogen. The metabolically active component of FFM is referred to as the body cell mass, with extracellular fluid and structural elements accounting for the remainder.[8] Severe semistarvation results in up to a 50% loss in FFM, which reflects depletion of glycogen and negative balance of water, nitrogen, and minerals. The relative decrease in nonconnective tissue proteins during semistarvation is greater than the relative loss of FFM,[24,25] because the rate of decrease in this component of FFM exceeds the rate of depletion of water (notably extracellular fluid), structural proteins, and bone. Thus the active cell mass constitutes a smaller proportion of FFM in severe malnutrition than in health.

The two main soft tissue components of FFM are skeletal muscle and viscera, and the proportion of each depends upon sex and age; men have relatively more skeletal muscle than women, and the young have a larger muscle mass than the old.[75] As noted earlier, not all tissue components of FFM atrophy at the same rate or to the same degree during weight loss. Brain mass and skeletal weight are minimally affected by weight loss, while the rate of change of the remaining organs is about the same as (e.g., heart, kidney) or greater than (e.g., liver, skeletal muscle, spleen) the rate of change in body weight.[27–29]

In anthropometrically assessing the severity of malnutrition, a basic goal is to define the amount and rate of change in total body or skeletal muscle protein. The anthropometric indices used for this assessment are FFM and limb muscle areas. As lower limits compatible with survival are known for both types of measurement,[76] the severity of protein-energy malnutrition is usually judged as the patient's value relative to the normal range on the one hand and the minimal range on the other. In terms of prognostic value, these measurements will provide some index of potential survival time; given the patient's anthropometric FFM or muscle index and nitrogen balance, progression toward or away from potentially lethal starvation can be established. During nutritional therapy and follow-up, the anthropometric FFM indices are used as measures of nitrogen balance, and specific details regarding interpretation are presented below.

Measuring FFM is accomplished by the skinfold methods described earlier in the section on fat (Addendum 7). The same cautions in measurement technique and selection of patients noted in the earlier discussion for fat also apply to FFM. With regard to interpretation, in theory multiplying FFM (in g) by 0.195, 1.16, and 1.0 provides the amount of total body protein in grams, total kcal, and usable kcal, respectively.[23] Of the usable kcal in a healthy subject, about one half is available during prolonged periods of semistarvation. When combined with balance data and information on total body fat, these bedside calculations often provide an interesting insight into a patient's course. Unfortunately, the information needed for accurate prediction of total body protein cannot be derived from anthropometric FFM because of the changes in body hydration and the variability of skinfold measurements described earlier. A large tumor burden or organomegaly of any cause may also add mass (i.e., protein + $H_2O$ + mineral) to the FFM that is metabolically unavailable.[77] In patients with serious derangements in body composition, FFM can be used to calculate basal energy expenditure from the equations provided in Table 45–4. This calculation is useful because basal energy expenditure/kg FFM is independent of sex and age; therefore, only one equation is needed.

Calculating the amount of limb muscle tissue from anthropometric data requires only two measurements, the limb circumference and the corresponding skinfold thickness.[23] The midportion of the upper limb is usually studied, and little additional information is gathered by also measuring thigh and calf muscle areas. The latter would of course be useful in subjects whose upper extremities are burned, amputated, edematous, or immobilized by casts or traction devices. The upper arm muscles tend to atrophy slightly more rapidly than the muscles of the thigh or calf, but the differences are not large.[23] The equations for calcu-

lating the limb muscle indices are provided in Addendum 8.

The primary application of limb muscle measurements is to obtain a measure of the amount and rate of change in skeletal muscle protein. The following three factors should therefore be considered.

1. The mass of a skeletal muscle represents a three-dimensional measurement (i.e., volume), whereas limb muscle area and circumference are two- and one-dimensional indices, respectively.[76,78] As the muscle changes volume, the corresponding proportional changes in muscle area and circumference will be smaller than the change in volume. For example, a 50% decrease in muscle volume will correspond to a theoretical decrease in muscle area and circumference of 37 and 21%, respectively. As a rule, the relative change in muscle area will be larger than the change in muscle circumference. Therefore, although limb muscle area and circumference will be highly correlated with one another, the area measurement will provide a more realistic estimate of the relative change in muscle mass.

2. The equations for calculating limb muscle indices are based upon simple theoretical assumptions regarding arm geometry.[78] Actually, the calculated arm muscle area overestimates the amount of skeletal muscle by 15 to 25%.[76,78] One half of this overestimate is due to the inclusion of bone in the calculated area, and the remainder is due to errors in the assumptions and the inclusion of nonmuscle tissue (e.g., neurovascular bundle) in the result. Two methods of correcting this overestimate of muscle area are available. The first is to express results as a percentage of standard, as the standard value will also contain these "nonskeletal muscle" components. The second approach is to calculate a value for bone-free arm muscle area,[78] as described in Addendum 8 (equation 5). The advantages and limitations of the calculations are described in the addendum.

3. Atrophic skeletal muscle differs in chemical composition from normal tissue.[79,80] Per gram of muscle, the amounts of water, total lipid, and collagen are increased, while the noncollagen proteins are reduced (Fig. 45–7). Thus the concentration of functional proteins per unit arm muscle area or circumference is relatively lower in the atrophied muscle. Another chemical consideration is that muscle size can abruptly change by ± 5 to 10% in response to rapid changes in muscle glycogen[80] as a result of the water-binding properties of glycogen.

Thus both anthropometric FFM and muscle indices are truly indirect markers of the active protein component of body weight. The two lean tis-

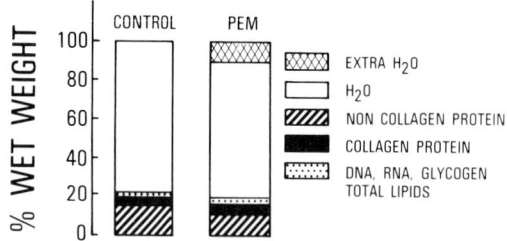

**Fig. 45–7.** Muscle composition per g of wet muscle weight in control and protein-energy malnourished (PEM) humans. Muscle specimens were collected at autopsy. There were relatively more water (including extra water), collagen proteins, and total lipids in undernourished patients compared to controls. The extra water was calculated by assuming that muscle dry weight is normally 21% of wet weight. (From Heymsfield, S.B., Stevens, B., Noel, R., et al.[80] with permission of the American Journal of Clinical Nutrition.)

sue indices should be considered approximate bedside guides to the amount of total body protein. Small changes in total body protein cannot be detected by anthropometry, and nitrogen balance and other techniques[81,82] must be used for this assessment.

*Aging and Anthropometric Indices.* Body composition changes throughout adulthood, and this must be considered when evaluating anthropometric indices. Height declines[83] and, assuming body weight remains unchanged, there is more fat and less FFM in an elderly subject compared to a younger individual of the same sex.[84] Most of the loss in FFM can be accounted for by a decrease in skeletal muscle mass.[75] Table 45–7 summarizes how body composition changes with age and how anthropometric measurements are affected.

A difficult problem in the elderly is estimation of height, especially in the wheelchair-bound, bedridden, or kyphotic subject. A useful approach

is to use the knee height (Addendum 9) to predict adult statutre. Knee height undergoes little change during adulthood, and this measurement provides a value for stature difficult to obtain by conventional methods. The predicted value for height can then be used in calculating other assessment indices and for comparison of these results to height adjusted reference values.

The basic relations between body composition and energy-nitrogen balance remain valid at any age. The best anthropometric methods of assessing the amount and rate of change in energy stores and protein mass in the aged patient remains an unanswered question and perhaps before long more specific guidelines will be available.

*Standard Values.* Three methods are used to process anthropometric data. The first method is to express the individual's values relative to a healthy reference population. This provides the anthropometric component used to assess if and to what extent the patient is malnourished. The reference tables can be divided into three types.

Type 1. Ideal or "desirable" reference tables are based upon mortality statistics and provide information only for body weight. Two desirable body weight tables are presented in Appendix Tables A–5a and A–5e, which represent studies performed in 1959[91] and 1979.[92] The description of desirable body weights presented in this chapter is based upon the 1959 study.

Type 2. Survey tables present the results of large surveys and usually describe the general population. Addenda 10, 12, 14 and 15 provide reference values for the United States population as a whole and Addenda 11, 13, and 16 for elderly persons.

Type 3. Local reference tables are useful when working with ethnic minorities or when publi-

**Table 45–7.  Effects of Aging on Body Composition and Anthropometric Measurements**

| Anthropometric Measurement | Comment |
| --- | --- |
| Weight | The average population value increases until the fifth decade, and then plateaus or declines.[85] |
| Height | Height decreases by 1–3 cm/20 years after maturity. The rate in height decline is race and sex dependent.[83,86] |
| Fat | Fat increases as a percentage of body weight; redistribution occurs from subcutaneous to internal fat, and between different subcutaneous sites.[70,87] |
| Skinfold | The compressibility of skinfolds changes with age.[88] There is a loss in the elastic recoil of skin and an increase in viscoelastic recovery time.[89] Skinfolds in the elderly are often pendulous and difficult to measure. |
| Fat-free body mass | Fat-free body mass decreases as a percentage of body weight mainly due to a loss in skeletal muscle mass.[75] The mass of visceral organs remains unchanged or decreases only sightly with age. The bone mineral and protein portion of FFM decreases, while $H_2O$ increases.[75] Skeletal muscle undergoes compositional changes, which include a relative increase in connective tissue and fat and relative loss in myofibrillar proteins.[90] |

From Wright, R.A., Heymsfield, S.B.,[23] with permission of Blackwell Scientific Publication.

cation of results is planned. The specific features of the reference group are then under the control of the practitioner, leaving no question as to the relevance of the data to the patients under study. An example set of reference tables is provided in Addendum 17.

Serious questions surround the concept of ideal body weight,[93] and the applicability of the currently available reference tables.[94,95] There are also notable gaps in reference values for selected groups, especially the elderly. We have provided provisional reference values for this latter group of subjects in Addenda 11, 13, and 16. Our suggestion is to select carefully and apply one set of reference values, preferably a data set upon which all results were generated from the same subject group.

The reference tables usually present data in three forms: as a mean ($\bar{x}$) value, as a $\bar{x}$ and standard deviation (SD), and as percentiles. Describing a population in term of a $\bar{x}$ and SD assumes the measurement under study is symmetrically distributed. Other equivalent terms for this type of distribution are Gaussian, bell-shaped, or normal. If data fit this model, then the $\bar{x} \pm 2\text{SD}$ includes 95% of the population. An abnormal value is more than 2 SD above or below the $\bar{x}$. Some tables provide only a $\bar{x}$, and the patient's value is then expressed as a percentage of the standard or reference value; weakness of this approach is that this type of table does not provide the observer with a method of determining if the result is within the normal range. The second type of table includes the SD, or 95% range of the healthy population, thus indicating if and to what degree the patient is abnormal. The third mode of expression is in terms of percentiles. The advantage of expressing results as a percentile rather than as a percentage of standard is that the reference population need not be symmetrically distributed. Often anthropometric surveys of populations produce "skewed" distributions (i.e., they are asymmetric), and therefore the easiest option is to present results in percentiles. In this approach, the values of the subject(s) exactly in the middle of the group is (are) at the 50th percentile. If the patient's value is between the 5th and 95th percentile, the result is considered normal; below or above these respective values is abnormal.

There is no simple method of judging the severity or potential morbidity of protein energy malnutrition from anthropometric data. Studies in adults have not yet clearly defined the "risk" of a subnormal anthropometric index, especially for results falling just below the normal range. Combining anthropometric data with the results of other components of the nutritional assessment provides some measure of potential morbidity, and this is described in the section on prognosis.

We emphasize again that body composition data should always be considered in relation to energy-nitrogen balance and other clinical factors. When semistarvation occurs gradually and without any other morbid complications, the individual reaches a minimum survivable body composition (point $B_u$, Fig. 45–5). No exact values are available for such a state, but approximations recently developed at our center are based upon a large pool of chronically undernourished patients (Addenda 17A and 17B).[23,76] This information may prove useful in determining the patient's position between the healthy range on the one hand and the clearly fatal range on the other.

The second method of expressing anthropometric data is in terms of the individual's total body energy content, fat, and FFM. When estimated energy and nitrogen balance are combined with these body composition data, a whole spectrum of potential calculations is possible. These, of course, are by necessity estimates, but their application in teaching and solving simple clinical questions often proves useful.

The third method of expressing anthropometric data is to follow trends over time. A previous value is needed and this is obtained from the history (e.g., body weight) or an earlier anthropometric examination.

*Clinical Applications.* The suggested applications of anthropometry are the following:

1. A weight and height should be recorded in the chart of every hospitalized patient. The weight indices described in Addendum 1 should be added to the data base for all patients who have a history of weight loss. The weight of all patients undergoing nutritional support should be measured daily.

2. The recommended uses of one skinfold measurement, limb fat area, and limb muscle area are:

a. When body weight is an invalid index of energy reserves due to edema or massive tumor burden. The upper limb is usually not affected by dependent edema.

b. When body weight is unmeasurable due to immobilizing devices, such as a cast or respirator.

c. When patients are seen for nutritional consultation or presented at rounds removed from the bedside, this provides a quantitative description of what is usually visible at the bedside. Although weight alone is useful in this regard, two patients of the same height and weight may differ markedly in body composition.

d. During short-term nutritional support of hospitalized patients. Although changes in fat and lean tissue will most likely not be detected over a 1- to 2-week period, the anthropometric data will become a permanent component of the nutritional data base. This information will then be available if a future re-evaluation is needed.

3. Total body fat and FFM are useful indices:

a. In patients who are undergoing long-term nutritional follow-up over months or years. Limb muscle area measurements should also be included in this group.

b. In groups of subjects forming the basis of nutritional studies, when a more critical assessment of body composition is often useful.

c. In calculating basal energy requirements based upon FFM (Table 45–4).

d. For teaching purposes, when the interrelation of metabolic balance, body composition, and nutritional therapy are the subject of discussion.

**Chemical Methods.** Several chemical methods of assessing body composition are available, but only one approach, the measurement of 24-hour urinary creatinine, has found widespread clinical acceptance.[96] Myers and Fine were the first to show that urinary creatinine output was proportional to the total body creatine content in humans.[97] Burger, assuming that nearly all body creatine was within muscle and that muscle possessed a constant creatine content, proposed that urinary creatinine was proportional to muscle mass.[98] Most workers now agree than 1 g of urinary creatinine is equal to between 17 and 20 kg of whole wet skeletal muscle.[99] A number of other investigators have shown a linear correlation between total FFM and 24-hour urinary creatinine. This correlation allows prediction of FFM from creatinine excretion, and a recent equation developed by Forbes and Bruining (100) is the following:

$$FFM \ (kg) \ = \ 29.08 \ creatinine \ (g/d) \ + \ 7.38 \quad (8)$$

As body size is a major determinant of the amount of muscle mass, the usual approach is to divide the 24-hour urinary creatinine by height, which is then referred to as the creatinine-height index.[101,102] Reference values for the latter are provided in Addendum 18.

The general approach is to measure between two and four consecutive daily urine samples for creatinine and then average the values. The results of obviously poor collections are discarded. The normal between-day variation on a metabolic ward is ±4 to 8%, and variability is larger on a clinical service.[99] An inadequate number of urine collections, especially in an unreliable patient, can lead to serious errors in the creatinine-height index.

The basic assumption of the creatinine method

is that the result is proportional to skeletal muscle mass or FFM; longitudinal changes should provide a measure of nitrogen balance. Although in general these are reasonable expectations, creatinine excretion is confounded by several factors, and therefore results are insufficiently accurate for use on a day-to-day basis. The large between-day variability on a clinical service has already been mentioned. A ±5 to 10% variability is also noted during emotional stress,[103] and results can be increased by 5 to 10% by strenuous exercise.[104] Another major factor is diet, as intake of creatine or creatinine in meat ultimately results in an increase in urinary creatinine that is independent from changes in FFM or skeletal muscle mass.[105,106] This factor is paricularly important to note in patients switching from a meat diet to a creatine-free feeding solution, or vice versa. The menstrual cycle also influences creatinine excretion, with a rise of between 10 and 15% during the second half of the cycle.[107] An increase in urinary creatinine excretion also occurs with severe infection, high fever, or trauma.[99] While the magnitude of this effect is variable, the range is between +20 and +100%. Finally, advanced renal disease (serum creatinine ≥6 mg/dL) is associated with an increase in nonrenal losses of creatinine, thereby disrupting any proportionality of the urinary losses of the compound to body composition.[108]

The following recommendations can therefore be made:

1. The urinary creatinine excretion in patients with advanced renal disease and severe catabolic states is not an accurate measure of skeletal muscle mass or FFM.

2. The creatine-creatinine content of the diet should not be changed during the evaluation period. When comparing to reference tables, check the table for the diet used in the control population.

3. Careful collection of several daily urine samples is important.

4. Anthropometric muscle indices are highly correlated with creatinine excretion;[99] as the former are easier, cheaper, and more practical, both are not usually required. Examples where creatinine can be substituted for anthropometry are the following: marked obesity, when skinfolds are inaccurate; inaccessibility of limbs for anthropometric measurement; and skin diseases, such as scleroderma, that invalidate skinfold measurements.

*Serum Proteins.* The serum proteins are readily sampled by venipuncture, and, for most species, measurement is simple and accurate. Selecting a protein for analysis and proper interpretation of results requires an understanding of two questions:

1. How does the concentration of the selected serum protein correlate with the total body amount and rate of change in the protein?

2. How does the serum protein relate to the amount and rate of change in total body protein?

These two questions will be examined using the classic marker of nutritional status, serum albumin.

Review of the first question requires an understanding of the determinants of serum protein concentration. The concentration of albumin in serum is normally determined by three independent factors: the rate of biosynthesis, the volume of distribution, and the rate of breakdown or catabolism. Two additional factors in diseased patients are the presence of abnormally large albumin losses and derangements in fluid status.

The hepatocytes within the human liver synthesize albumin at a daily rate of 120 to 200 mg/kg body weight.[109] The biosynthetic rate of albumin is determined by dietary protein intake, ambient temperature, and plasma oncotic pressure. The rate of albumin synthsis is low in the presence of hypothyroidism, excessive levels of serum cortisol, stress, and hepatic parenchymal disease.

Once the albumin molecule is synthesized, it enters the circulation and then distributes in the intravascular and extravascular spaces. The total body albumin pool is normally between 3 and 5 g/kg body weight, and 40% of this is in the intravascular space.[109,110] Extravascular albumin is found in all lean tissues, with about half of the total in skin. A shift of intravascular to extravascular albumin occurs in patients following surgery or a thermal injury.[111] The opposite occurs in semistarvation, with a movement of albumin from the extravascular to the intravascular space.[112]

The major catabolic sites of albumin are the intestinal tract and vascular endothelium, and 6 to 10% of the pool is catabolized per day.[109,110] The half-life of albumin ranges between 14 and 20 days, with an equal probability of destruction for new and old molecules. The rate of albumin catabolism is increased by stress and hypermetabolism and in Cushing's syndrome. Some malignant tumors also increase the catabolic rate of albumin. The rate of albumin catabolism is lowered by semistarvation[112] and hypometabolism.

Abnormally large losses of albumin occur in burns, nephrotic syndrome, and protein-losing enteropathy.[109–111] Finally, over- or underhydration causes corresponding changes in concentration of serum albumin. To summarize these determinants of serum albumin concentration, the measured value of the protein in serum is deter-mined by the rate of synthesis, the volume and nature of the distribution space, the rate of catabolism, the presence of abnormally large losses, and by the state of hydration.

How does the concentration of albumin in serum correspond to changes in total body albumin in the presence of uncomplicated protein-energy malnutrition? A general sequence of events can be recreated from animal and human studies.[112,113] The earliest change in albumin kinetics in response to dietary manipulation is an alteration in the rate of synthesis. With low protein-energy intake, the rate of synthesis falls rapidly; the result is negative albumin balance. If intake remains low, then the catabolic rate of albumin slows, thereby reducing the rate of loss of whole body albumin. This tends to preserve serum levels, along with a second major adaptation; there is a shift of albumin from the extravascular to the intravascular space. These two adaptations preserve the serum level of albumin, even though the synthesis rate of the protein is reduced. A reasonable conclusion is that the relative decrease in whole body albumin will be greater than the lowering of serum albumin.

Although the reduction in serum albumin is small in uncomplicated protein-energy malnutrition, severe hypoalbuminemia is observed in association with some forms of malnutrition, and the specific cause of this finding is not entirely clear.[114–116] Explanations include (1) the presence of other ongoing processes, such as infection; (2) depletion of extravascular albumin, indicating a severe stage of protein-energy malnutrition; (3) fatty infiltration of the liver, resulting in disturbed hepatocyte function; and (4) severe muscle atrophy, leading to depletion of amino acid precursors for albumin synthesis. Whatever the mechanisms, the finding of hypoalbuminemia in children or adults with protein-energy malnutrition usually signals other serious metabolic derangements and an adverse prognosis.[114–116] This is described in more detail in the section on prognosis.

Protein-energy malnutrition in hospitalized patients is often complicated by the presence of a traumatic injury or ongoing stress. During the acute catabolic phase of the injury there is a rise in serum levels of the acute phase reactants, such as fibrinogen, haptoglobin, and C-reactive protein. There is a decrease in the concentration of other serum proteins, and albumin is one of those affected. Serum albumin concentration remains low during the stress period, even when seemingly adequate levels of nutritional support are provided.[117] During this phase of an illness the serum level of albumin is a poor index to albumin balance or whole body albumin mass.

The second question is how does serum albumin relate to other proteins within the FFM? A number of studies show a strong degree of correlation between serum albumin and body cell mass (the metabolically active component of FFM), and limited information suggests that relative changes in serum albumin and total body protein are about equal.[113,118] There are, however, striking deviations from these generalizations. For example, the patient with anorexia nervosa may show severe muscle and liver atrophy, and yet the serum albumin level may be normal or near normal.

The nonspecificity and slow response of serum albumin level to nutritional factors has led to the investigation of other serum proteins. In general, relative to albumin, these proteins have lower absolute biosynthetic rates, smaller total body pools, shorter half-lives, and lower serum levels. The key aspects of each of these proteins are summarized in Table 45–8. Under ideal conditions, these proteins are more sensitive indices of dietary intake than serum albumin. Synthesis rates and plasma levels change rapidly in response to dietary protein intake. The serum concentration of these proteins also responds to many of the same nonnutritional factors described earlier for albumin. Interpretation must therefore be cautious.

The use of serum proteins in nutritional assessment can thus be summarized as follows:

1. Five potential factors determine the level of a protein in serum: the rate of synthesis and catabolism, the volume of and compartmental distribution, abnormal body losses, and the state of hydration.

2. The first aim of measuring serum protein concentration as an index of nutritional status is to determine the total amount and rate of change in the specific protein. In uncomplicated malnutrition the serum protein level will usually correlate with the whole body amount of the protein; note that the relative change in the concentration of the protein in serum may not be equal to the relative change in the total body amount of protein. Over time, changes in serum protein will reflect protein balance. More rapid changes will occur following nutritional intervention in the proteins with a short half-life.

3. The second aim is to provide a marker of total body or visceral protein nutriture. Although a correlation may exist between the serum protein and other indices of whole body protein, it is doubtful whether such inferences are meaningful. This is especially true of the short half-life proteins, which may rise and fall quickly in response to dietary change without a major change in total body protein.

4. All of the factors influencing serum protein concentration, other than nutritional status, that are listed in Table 45–8 may confound the results. Application and interpretation of the serum protein assay must therefore be very cautious.

5. The serum levels of some of the proteins listed in Table 45–8 correlate with disease outcome, and this information is reviewed in a later section.

**Tissue Function**

The health of an individual ultimately derives from collective tissue function. A major determinant of tissue function is nutritional status,[125] and therefore functional measurements are included in the assessment protocol. As each of the essential nutrients is associated with a number of bodily functions, the potential number of tests is large. Other chapters throughout the book review functional tests of vitamin and mineral nutriture, and details of these indices are provided in these reviews.

Several general principles regarding functional assessment indices are worth noting. First, each organ or system has multiple functions. For example, skeletal or cardiac muscle can be described in terms of electrical, mechanical, or metabolic functions. Not all of the functions of an organ or system are affected at the same rate or to the same degree during weight loss and subsequent recovery. An example is that with severe muscle atrophy the electrical potential of the myofiber undergoes little change,[126] but there is a marked loss in muscle strength.[127]

Most organs have a "global function," that is, an activity that characterizes that organ. The heart pumping blood, the lungs exchanging respiratory gases, and the kidneys excreting solute are a few examples of global organ activity. When undernutrition is uncomplicated by disease, the reduction in global function will usually be in proportion to the loss in organ mass and protein content. A classic example is the cardiac atrophy that occurs in severe protein-energy malnutrition that is accompanied by a proportional reduction in cardiac output.[128,129] This leads to a high degree of intercorrelation between functional tests and body composition indices, often making one of the measurements redundant and unnecessary. At times the functional measurement may be the preferred assessment technique due to a higher degree of accuracy or ease of measurement. Finally, many factors determine the function of an organ or system in addition to nutritional status, and therefore careful selection and interpretation of tests in this category is essential.

The first step in assessing bodily function is to

**Table 45–8.  Serum Proteins Used in Nutritional Assessment**

| Serum Protein | Approximate Molecular Weight (Dalton's) | Biosynthetic Site | Normal Value $\overline{X} \pm$ SD or (range)[†] | Half-life (days) | Function | Comment* |
|---|---|---|---|---|---|---|
| Albumin | 66,000 | Hepatocyte | 45 (35–50) | 14–20 | Maintain plasma oncotic pressure; carrier for small molecules | Serum levels are determined by the processes described in the text |
| Transferrin | 77,000 | Hepatocyte | 2.3 (2.0–3.2) | 8–9 | Binds $Fe^{++}$ in plasma and transports to bone | Iron nutriture strongly influences plasma level;[119] increases during pregnancy, during estrogen therapy, and acute hepatitis; reduced in protein-losing enteropathy and nephropathy, chronic infections, uremia, and acute catabolic states; often measured indirectly by total iron binding capacity[120] |
| Prealbumin | 61,000 | Hepatocyte | 0.30 (0.2–0.5) | 2–3 | Binds T3 and to a lesser extent T4. Carrier for retinol-binding protein | Increased in patients with chronic renal failure on dialysis.[121] Reduced in acute catabolic states, post surgery, hyperthyroidism; serum level determined by overall energy balance as well as nitrogen balance[122] |
| Retinol-binding protein | 21,000 | Hepatocyte | 0.0372 ± 0.0073[‡] | 0.5 | Transports vitamin A in plasma; binds noncovalently to prealbumin | Catabolized in renal proximal tubular cell; with renal disease RBP increases and T1/2 is prolonged; low in vitamin A deficiency, acute catabolic states, postsurgery, and hyperthyroidism |
| Somatomedin C | 7,400 | Hepatocyte | 0.83 IU/ml (0.55–1.4) | 0.1–0.3 | One of a family of insulin-like peptides that have anabolic actions on fat, muscle, cartilage, and cultured cells | Levels fall rapidly with fasting and quickly recover during refeeding.[123] Low values in hypothyroid patients and with estrogen administration |
| Fibronectin | 440,000 | Hepatocyte and other tissues | Plasma: 2.92 ± 0.2 Serum: 1.82 ± 0.16 | 0.5–1.0 | A glycoprotein found in many tissues; a soluble form appears in blood and behaves as an opsonic glycoprotein; may exert chemotactic activity and be involved in wound healing | Plasma fibronectin deficiency may contribute to host defense suppression with malnutrition;[124] may also be a sensitive marker during repletion. More clinical studies needed |

*All of the listed proteins are influenced by hydration and the presence of hepatocellular dysfunction.
†Units are g/L. Normal range varies between centers; check local values.
‡Normal values are age and sex dependent. Table value is for pooled subjects.

assemble information from the history and physical examination. Each system has specific historical features that are associated with impaired organ function; for example, frequent infections might be a clue to an immune system impaired by semistarvation. The physical examination offers many bedside opportunities to evaluate nutrition-related functions: the bradycardia of severe protein-energy malnutrition,[130] a slow or nonhealing surgical incision, and a weak hand grasp are all simple clues to systemic malfunction caused by the semistarvation process.[127] Available laboratory studies may support bedside impressions. The renal atrophy of malnutrition is associated with a low glomerular filtration rate and impaired concentrating mechanism, both easily measured indices in hospitalized patients.[131] Another example is that the atrophic myocardium of severe protein-energy malnutrition is easily documented by chest radiography and electrocardiography.[130] The latter changes include low electrical voltage of the QRS complex, a slow heart rate (<60 beats/min), and frequent arrhythmias.[132] Although an exhaustive listing of functional tests is beyond the scope of this section, the key point is that the routine examination often provides important clues to nutrition-related tissue function.

Another important aspect of functional testing occurs during monitoring of patients on nutritional support. A good example is the patient with severe chronic respiratory insufficiency and right-sided congestive heart failure who requires parenteral alimentation during an acute phase of the illness. The infusion of formula may precipitate cardiac[129] or respiratory failure,[133] and therefore close monitoring of symptoms, physical findings, and laboratory tests will provide early clues to worsening organ function during the feeding program. Specific functional tests during feeding may be considered, and these will be based upon the individual's underlying disease process.

Two categories of functional tests are worthy of a more extensive review; these are indices of muscle and immune function.

**Muscle Function.** A wide variety of tests are available for quantifying muscle function. Electrical activity can be measured by electromyography and electrocardiography. Other than the cardiac muscle atrophy and rhythm disturbances found in severe semistarvation, these tests have not found widespread clinical application. Muscle strength can be measured by handgrip dynamometry,[127] maximal respiratory pressure,[134] and echocardiography.[129] The handgrip technique is simple and its use is advocated by some workers.[127,135] A major problem with evaluating voluntary skeletal muscle strength is that a high level of cooperation is required from the patient. Another recent test that does not require patient effort is the pattern of muscle contraction and relaxation generated by the adductor pollicis muscle following electrical stimulation of the ulnar nerve.[136,137] This functional muscle index is advocated as an early and sensitive muscle assessment index. Unfortunately, a critical analysis of the technique cannot be provided at the present time, as the number of reports using the method is too limited.

**Immune Function.** Protein-energy malnutrition is an important and widespread cause of impaired immune function. This immunosuppression, recognized for centuries in the form of famine and plague, is an important cause of infection, morbidity, and mortality in hospitalized patients.[138] Early recognition and correction of specific nutrition-mediated defects in the immune system are desirable goals. While potential in this area is great, information from available tests is limited by the complexity of the interaction among nutrition, immunity, and infection. Six problems are significant in defining these relationships. (1) Undernutrition is associated with a depleted body content of protein, energy, minerals, and vitamins; nutrients other than protein and energy influence the immune response, and the degree of observed immunologic deficit depends upon the type and extent of other essential nutrient deficiencies.[139,140] (2) There are five major components of the immune system: skin and mucosal barriers, phagocytes, humoral immune response, cellular immune response, and complement; each of these is affected differently, depending upon the type and degree of nutritional deficiency.[139] (3) Although it is well known that malnutrition can lead to immunodeficiency and infection, it is also known that infection can cause malnutrition. Therefore, it is often difficult to determine if the relationship between malnutrition and infection is cause, effect, or merely an association. (4) Since much of the data relating nutrition to immunity is derived from animal models or studies of children in developing countries, extrapolation of results to hospitalized adults must be cautious. (5) Many abnormalities in immune function have been found in undernourished patients; however, identification of the clinically significant abnormalities is difficult. (6) The underlying disease process or therapy may cause derangements in the immune system independent of nutritional factors.

This multiplicity of confounding factors has made clinical evaluation of nutrition-mediated defects in the immune system extremely difficult to analyze. There is, however, almost universal agreement that the observation of lymphocytopenia or anergy is associated with a poor patient prognosis.[141–144]

The total lymphocyte count is derived from the complete blood count (% lymphocytes × white blood cell count), and the needed information is usually available on most hospitalized patients. Lymphocytopenia is defined as an absolute lymphocyte count of less than 1,000 cells/cubic mm. At least three common clinical disorders will reduce circulating lymphocytes:[139] trauma, infection or inflammation, and severe protein-energy malnutrition. Attempts to associate undernutrition with specific lymphocyte subpopulations has not improved the specificity of the test, although the constantly improving methodologies in this area may eventually produce clinically useful information.[145] A low lymphocyte count might provide supportive information when analyzed in the context of other clinical data.

Delayed cutaneous hypersensitivity is the most widely used index of immunodeficiency in malnourished hospitalized patients. This in vivo test of cell-mediated immunity can be used to document the presence or absence of anergy. The skin testing procedure is relatively simple, inexpensive, and widely available, but several authors have questioned its utility in nutritional assessment.[139,146] The problems concerning data on skin testing include poor study design, failure to control for nonnutritional influences, technical difficulties of skin testing, inadequately standardized recall antigens, varying definitions of anergy, and the inability to show consistent changes in delayed cutaneous hypersensitivity in mild to moderate malnutrition.

Many other immunologic tests have been studied in undernourished patients, and these include mitogen-induced lymphocyte proliferation, mixed lymphocyte cultures, immunoglobulin levels, antibody production, and complement function.[139] Results are generally inconclusive, and many of these studies suffer from the six limitations described earlier.

The multiplicity of problems in associating specific derangements in immune function and protein-energy malnutrition has led most workers to conclude that current tests add little to the routine nutritional assessment data base. Advances in this field are occurring at a rapid rate, and perhaps before long a useful clinical tool will emerge.

As noted earlier, lymphocytopenia and/or anergy in hospitalized patients is clearly associated with an increased risk of infectious and other morbid complications. The incorporation of this finding into prognostic indices is described in a later section.

## APPLICATION OF CLINICAL ASSESSMENT

The first two steps in the initial evaluation of a patient are (1) to determine if the individual has the potential of becoming or is already malnourished, and (2) to establish the patient's risk of developing a nutrition-related complication. Following the intial assessment, the next phase is to conduct a more in-depth evaluation of patients identified by the screening procedure.

### Screening Procedure

A collective effort among the physician, nursing staff, and clinical dietitian is required to identify patients in need of a more in-depth evaluation. A recommended approach is for the physician and nurse to enter the patient's diagnosis, present and past medical history, review of systems, drug and social histories, and physical examination into the hospital chart as usual. The dietitian then completes his/her respective portions of the intitial assessment data base, an example of which is provided in Table 45–9.[147] Patients who have the potential of developing malnutrition, those who show indicative signs of a deficiency state (Table 45–10), or individuals who are already clearly malnourished are then candidates for a more in-depth evaluation. The more complete assessment is undertaken only in those patients in whom nutritional therapy and/or follow-up will improve the clinical course of their disease. This often must be a subjective decision that is based upon a multiplicity of factors.

**Prognosis.** An important consideration in screening patients is to identify those whose disease outcome could be measurably improved by early nutritional management. In general, the outcome or prognosis of an illness is determined by the nature and severity of the underlying disease and by host factors such as age and sex. The basic considerations in this component of the medical evaluation are duration, morbid complications, and survival time of the disease process.

Historically, Studley was among the first to associate nutritional status and disease outcome.[68] In 1936 this pioneering investigator made the classic observation that marked weight loss prior to surgical procedures for peptic ulcer resulted in a higher postoperative mortality rate relative to that in weight-stable patients. Modern workers have identified weight loss as a major determinant of prognosis in many disease states, and some recent extensions of Studley's observations are: (1) weight loss is associated with reduced survival time in patients with carcinoma of the colon;[148] and (2) weight loss in patients with chronic ob-

**Table 45–9.  Memorial Sloan-Kettering Cancer Center Initial Nutrition Assessment Form**

1. a) What is your usual weight? _____lbs.
   b) What is your height? _____feet _____inches.
   c) In the last two months, have you gained weight?
      No _____Yes _____. If yes, how many pounds? _____.
      Lost weight? No _____Yes _____. If yes, how many pounds? _____.
2. Is your present appetite usual _____better _____or worse _____than normal?
3. a) Do you have a problem related to eating? No _____Yes _____. If yes, check the appropriate reason(s): Sore
      mouth _____Swallowing _____Chewing _____Choking _____Salivation _____Change in taste _____Food
      aversions _____Nausea _____Vomiting _____Diarrhea _____Constipation _____Other _____

   b) Do you need help in eating? No _____Yes _____.
4. Do you wear dentures? Upper _____Lower _____None _____.
5. a) Were you previously on a special diet? No _____Yes _____. If yes, specify: _____

   b) Do you take vitamins or minerals? No _____Yes _____. If yes, specify: _____

   c) Do you have any personal or religious dietary restrictions? Kosher _____Vegetarian _____Other ____
6. Do you have any allergies or intolerances for food? No _____Yes _____. If yes, please list: _____
7. Do you take any other special food regularly? No _____Yes _____. If yes, please list: _____
8. Do you have any major food dislikes? No _____Yes _____. If yes, please list: _____
9. What is the reason for this hospital admission? _____

---

### DO NOT WRITE BELOW THIS LINE—FOR DIETITIAN'S USE ONLY

Date of initial visit _____
1. Diagnosis: _____
2. Expected treatment plan: Surgery _____Radiation therapy _____Chemotherapy _____Other _____
3. Abnormal lab data (list): _____

4. Metabolic and other problems:

   | | |
   |---|---|
   | Diabetes _____ | Recurrent infections _____ |
   | Hypertension _____ | Hyperlipidemia _____ |
   | Heart disease _____ | Malabsorption |
   | Persistent fever _____ | Type _____ |
   | Severe trauma/burns _____ | GI obstruction |
   | Alcohol/Drug abuse _____ | Partial _____ |
   | Renal disease _____ | Complete _____ |
   | Liver disease _____ | GI fistula _____ |

5. Present medications: _____

6. Ht: _____cm  Adm wt: _____kg  Avg Std: _____kg
   Pre-illness wt: _____lbs _____ kg
   Percentage wt change (%): _____[(Pre-illness—Adm)/Pre-illness] × 100
7. Anticipated problems due to illness or treatment plan? No _____Yes _____

8. Edema/Ascites: (site) Degrees—0–4 +)
   Ascites: _____  Sacral edema _____
9. Nutritional care plan:
   a) No apparent problem _____
   b) Diet Rx _____
   c) Supplements Rx _____
   d) Date to re-evaluate _____
   e) Nutrition team consult _____
10. Discharge plan/Comments: _____

Signed: _____

---

(From Shils, M.E.,[147] with permission of Alan R. Liss, Inc.)

**Table 45–10. Signs of Clinical Deficiency States***

| Clinical Finding | Consider Deficiency | Comment |
|---|---|---|
| *Hair* | | |
| Easily pluckable, sparse | Protein, biotin | Loss of scalp and body hair may also occur |
| Straight, dull | Protein | Hair will be fine and silky |
| Flag sign | Protein | Reddening of normally black scalp; occurs in black-skinned children, possibly due to abnormal sebaceous gland activity |
| Coiled, corkscrew-like | Vitamin A, C | Due to follicular change; due to a keratinization disturbance and possibly abnormal sebaceous gland activity |
| *Skin* | | |
| Xerosis | Essential fatty acid | Dryness of skin |
| Petechiae | Vitamin A, vitamin C | Pin-headed sized hemorrhages |
| Pigmentation | Niacin | Sign of pellagra distributed symmetrically in sun-exposed areas; also seen in hemochromatosis, an iron storage disease |
| Desquamation | | |
| Follicular keratosis | Vitamin A, possibly essential fatty acid | Keratin plugs in follicles, sandpaper feel of skin |
| "Flaky-paint" dermatitis | Protein | |
| Subcutaneous fat loss, fine wrinkling | Protein-energy | Minimal fat reserves; low values for anthropometric indices |
| Poor tissue turgor | Water | |
| Edema | Protein, thiamin, vitamin E (in premature infants) | Seen in protein-energy malnutrition with hypoalbuminemia and in wet beriberi due to thiamine deficiency |
| Purpura (subcutaneous skin hemorrhage) | Vitamin C, vitamin K | |
| Perifollicular hemorrhage | Vitamin C | |
| Pallor | Folacin, iron, B12, copper, biotin | |
| Excessive hair growth | Protein-energy | Like fetal lanugo; noticeable in girls with anorexia nervosa; may be heat-retaining mechanism |
| Tendency toward excessive bruising (ecchymoses) | Vitamin C, vitamin K | Due to increased fragility of capillary walls |
| Pressure sores | Protein-energy | Common in pressure and bony points |
| Seborrheic dermatitis | Essential fatty acid, pyridoxine, zinc, biotin, riboflavin in infants | Also seen in acrodermatitis enteropathica due to a defect in zinc absorption |
| Poor wound healing | Protein-energy, zinc, and possibly essential fatty acids | Scrotal or vulvar in riboflavin deficiency; nasolabial in pyridoxine deficiency |
| Dermatitis | Biotin, possibly manganese | |
| Dry scaling | Nonspecific | |
| Thickening of skin | Essential fatty acid | |
| *Eyes* | | |
| Dull, dry (xerosis) conjunctiva | Vitamin A | Can lead to xerophthalmia in severe deficiency |
| Blepharitis | B-complex | Angular in riboflavin deficiency |
| Ophthalmoplegia | Thiamin | Wernicke's syndrome; prompt treatment necessary |
| Keratomalacia | Vitamin A | Softening of cornea |
| Bitot's spot | Vitamin A | Early evidence of deficiency |
| Corneal vascularization | Riboflavin | |
| Photophobia | Zinc | |
| *Lips and Oral Structures* | | |
| Angular fissures, scars, or stomatitis | B-complex, iron, protein, riboflavin | Also seen with ill-fitting dentures |
| Cheilosis | B-6, niacin, riboflavin, protein | Seen especially at corners of mouth |
| Ageusia, dysgeusia | Zinc | Also associated with altered sense of smell |
| Swollen, spongy, bleeding gums | Ascorbic acid | If not edentulous |

**Table 45–10.** *Continued*

| Clinical Finding | Consider Deficiency | Comment |
|---|---|---|
| *Tongue* | | |
| Magenta tongue | Riboflavin | Controversial; magenta color may also be due to poor general nutrition |
| Fissuring, raw | Niacin | |
| Glossitis | Pyridoxine, folacin, iron, B12 | Due to inadequate repair of epithelial tissues |
| Large size, swollen | Iodine, niacin | In niacin defiency the tongue can be deeply fissured and infected |
| Fiery red tongue | Folacin, B12 | Seen if anemia is not pronounced |
| Pale | Iron, B12 | Seen in severe cases |
| Atrophic lingual papillae | Riboflavin, niacin, iron | |
| *Teeth* | | |
| Higher frequency of tooth decay | Fluorine | May also be due to poor dental care |
| Loss of dental fillings, dental caries | Vitamin C | Scurvy |
| *Glands* | | |
| Parotid enlargement | Protein | Rare, seen in alcoholic patients |
| "Sicca" syndrome | Ascorbic acid | Includes changes in salivary and tear glands |
| Thyroid enlargement | Iodine | Seen in inland areas where deficiency has not been corrected by iodination of table salt. Rarely due to a goitrogenic agent such as cabbage or brussel sprouts |
| Hypogonadism, delayed puberty | Zinc | |
| *Nails* | | |
| Spoon-shaped nails (koilonychia) | Chromium, iron | Rare in the U.S. |
| Brittle, ridged, lined nails | Nonspecific | May be protein undernutrition |
| *Heart* | | |
| Tachycardia, cardiomegaly, congestive heart failure | Thiamin | "Wet" beriberi associated with high output congestive heart failure |
| Decreased cardiac function | Phosphorus | |
| Cardiac arrhythmias | Magnesium, potassium | |
| Cardiomyopathy | Selenium | Referred to as Keshan disease in the Orient. Occurrence in the U.S. with parenteral nutrition |
| Small heart, decreased output, bradycardia | Protein-energy | Prone to congestive heart failure during refeeding |
| Sudden failure, death | Ascorbic acid, thiamin | In ascorbic acid deficiency death may be due to small hemorrhages in the myocardium |
| *Abdomen* | | |
| Hepatomegaly (fatty liver) | Protein | Also commonly seen in alcoholics |
| Wasting | Energy | Found in marasmus |
| Enlarged spleen | Iron | Found in 15 to 25% subjects with a significant degree of iron-deficiency anemia |
| *Bones and Joints* | | |
| Epiphyseal thickening, deformities | Vitamin D | Rickets in children |
| Bone pain | Calcium, vitamin D, phosphorus, vitamin C | (Adult)—osteomalacia due to repeated pregnancies with poor $Ca^{++}$ intake, little sun, light steatorrhea<br>(Child)—superiosteal hemorrhage in scurvy |
| *Muscles, Extremities* | | |
| Wasting | Protein-energy | Evident in temporal area, dorsum of hand between thumb and index fingers, calf muscles |
| Pain in calves, weak thighs | Thiamin | |
| Edema | Protein, thiamin | |
| Muscular twitching | Pyridoxine | |
| Muscular pains | Biotin, selenium | |
| Muscular weakness | Sodium, potassium | |
| Muscle cramps | Sodium, chloride | |

**Table 45–10.** *Continued*

| Clinical Finding | Consider Deficiency | Comment |
|---|---|---|
| *Neurologic* | | |
| Ophthalmoplegia, foot-drop | Thiamin | Wernicke's encephalopathy |
| Disorientation | Thiamin, sodium, water | Korsakoff's psychosis; confabulation occurs in thiamin-deficient alcoholics |
| Decreased position, vibratory sense, ataxia, optic neuritis | B12 | Subacute combined cord degeneration |
| Weakness, paresthesia of legs | Thiamin, pyridoxine, pantothenic acid, B12 | Nutritional polyneuropathy, especially with alcoholism; "burning foot" syndrome with pantothenic acid deficiency |
| Hyporeflexia | Thiamin | |
| Mental disorders | Niacin, magnesium, B12 | In untreated B12 deficiency mental disorders may progress to severe psychosis |
| Convulsions | Pyridoxine, calcium, thiamin (infants), magnesium, phosphorus | |
| Depression, lethargy | Biotin, folacin, vitamin C | |
| Sleep disturbances, impaired coordination | Pantothenic acid | |
| Nonketonic hyperosmolar syndrome | Sodium | Due to large glucose infusions that result in an osmotic diuresis; occurs in TPN patients |
| Aphonia | Thiamin | Infants |
| Hyperesthesia | Biotin | |
| Peripheral neuropathy | Pyridoxine | |
| *Other* | | |
| Diarrhea | Niacin, folacin, B12 | |
| Delayed wound healing and tissue repair | Vitamin C, zinc, protein-energy. | |
| Anemia, pallor | Vitamin E, pyridoxine, $B_{12}$, iron, folacin, biotin, copper | |
| Anorexia | B12, chloride, sodium, thiamin, vitamin C | |
| Nausea | Biotin, pantothenic acid | |
| Fatigue, lassitude, apathy | Energy, biotin, pantothenic acid, magnesium, phosphorus, iron, potassium, vitamin C, (infants), sodium | |
| Growth retardation | Protein-energy, magnesium, zinc, vitamin D, calcium | |
| Constipation | Thiamin | GI atony |
| Headache | Pantothenic acid | |
| Glucose intolerance | Chromium | |
| Bleeding diathesis | Vitamin K | |

*This table was compiled from numerous sources.

structive lung disease is associated with early onset of right-sided congestive heart failure and shortened survival time.[149]

Often patient prognostic groups are identified by a "clustering" of more than one assessment index,[150] for example: A low caloric intake and a subnormal triceps skinfold thickness in patients with chronic obstructive lung disease are associated with an increased frequency of hospital admissions;[151] severe weight loss and a prolonged electrocardiographic QT interval are associated with serious arrhythmias and sudden death;[152,153] hypoalbuminemia and lymphocytopenia or anergy are associated with an increased morbidity and mortality in several different types of hospitalized patients;[141,142] subnormal weight, serum albumin, and midarm muscle circumference are associated with an increased mortality rate in patients with chronic renal failure undergoing hemodialysis;[154] and mortality rate is related to four patient clusters based upon a complex scheme of ten nutritional assessment indices developed by Nazari and his colleagues.[155]

Although these associations by themselves provide clinical prognostic information, a desirable goal is to have prediction equations that generate a numerical value for the risk of a subsequent complication or death. It should then be possible to show that improving nutritional status lowers risk and thus provides the patient with a more favorable outcome. This approach was used on patients admitted for major elective surgical procedures by investigators at the University of Pennsylvania Hospital.[156] Stepwise regression and discriminant analyses were used to develop an equation that identified patients whose course was complicated by postoperative organ failure, infection, wound dehiscence, or death. Four assessment indices were shown in this setting to have significant predictive value, serum albumin (ALB, g/dl), triceps skinfold thickness (TSF, mm), serum transferrin (TFN, mg/dl), and maximal skin test reactivity to any of three recall antigens (DH; 0 = nonreactive, 1- <5 mm reactivity, 2- ≥5 mm reactivity). The resulting prognostic nutritional index (PNI) was:

$$PNI\ (\%) = 158 - 16.6(ALB) - 0.78(TSF)$$
$$- 0.2(TFN) - 5.8(DH). \quad (9)$$

Patients classified as high risk according to this scheme have a PNI ≥50%; values for intermediate and low risk are, respectively, 40 to 49%, and <40%. In two follow-up studies on subjects undergoing major surgical procedures, Buzby and his co-workers confirmed the predictive value of the equation.[156] In a limited study of preoperative nutritional support, patients receiving >7 days of "adequate" total parenteral nutrition suffered less morbidity and mortality than either predicted or observed in a nontreated control group.

One of the major goals of modern clinical nutrition is to reduce the adverse consequences of protein-energy malnutrition in hospitalized patients. The studies described in this section should be considered the initial investigations aimed at fulfilling that goal. There are limitations present in all of the aforementioned studies, and these can be summarized as follows:

1. Assessment indices are often influenced by the nonnutritional factors described throughout the chapter; it therefore may not always be valid to infer cause-effect relations from the above associations.

2. The addition of many other nonnutritional items to the prediction data base may substantially improve the sensitivity and specificity of the risk analysis. In other words, overall prognosis or the risk of a specific complication may be determined by factors other than nutritional status.[157]

3. Follow-up studies at other centers often cannot confirm the associations described in the original report.

4. The reported associations are often not valid when applied to individuals who do not fit the selection criteria of the original study.

5. Some of the assessment procedures are not generally available, are time consuming, and expensive.

We recommend the following. First, the reader should closely monitor developments in this rapidly growing and important area of clinical nutrition. Secondly, the patient's diagnosis and overall prognosis should be established using the routine history, physical examination, and laboratory studies. In some cases, specialized tests related to the disease process may be needed to refine the prognostic estimate. The relationship of nutritional indices, as described above, to prognosis will weigh into this estimate.

### In-depth Evaluation

Three groups of patients require an in-depth evaluation of nutritional status. The first group consists of the patients indentified as at risk of becoming or who are already malnourished according to the initial screening survey. Also included in this group are patients considered "at risk" of nutrition-related complications. The second group of patients are those individuals who, during the course of a prolonged hospitalization, develop symptoms and signs of malnutrition. Rechecking patients at one- to two-week intervals is important in detecting this group. The third group are those patients on whom a nutritional consultation is requested during their hospital stay.

The aim of the in-depth assessment is to determine the patient's position in the scheme presented earlier in Figure 45–5. Questions asked are:

1. What are the causes of the observed or potential malnutrition? Answering this question requires a compilation of material from the history, physical examination, and laboratory studies that relate to the components of energy and nitrogen balance. Other essential nutrients should also be considered. The material evaluated may range from a simple qualitative description to complex and specialized measurements. The types of evaluation procedures used will depend, of course, on the setting, the patient's diagnosis, and the specific aim of the assessment.

2. How severely malnourished is the patient? Here the same sources of information are used to define body composition and tissue function. The examiner determines the distance, direction, and rate of change of each index relative to the patient's pre-illness status and the normal range. Assessing a rate requires data at two points in time, and this information is not available for all of the indices on the initial evaluation. The tests selected for evaluation will once again depend upon the ultimate use of the information. The data base can vary between hospitals, with different types

of patients, and according to the needs of the practitioner or investigator.

3. Is the patient at risk of developing a malnutrition-related complication? The potential of an individual succumbing from semistarvation is related to the rate and amount of fuel depletion. Data from all components of the assessment are used to evaluate this form of risk. The second group of complications occurs within specific patient groups, and the evaluation methods were described earlier in the initial assessment section.

4. Does the patient require nutritional therapy and, if so, what type? Much of the information needed to make this assessment is gathered during the in-depth evaluation, and specific recommendations are made in other chapters throughout the book.

5. Is the patient responding to nutritional therapy? This assessment is made by continuing to evaluate historical, physical examination, laboratory, and special test data during the course of treatment or follow-up. This information is synthesized into balance, body composition, and functional results that describe if and to what degree the patient's nutritional status is improving.

## CONCLUSION

Ongoing current research promises to produce major advances in the area of clinical nutritional assessment. Investigators are now exploring new techniques for evaluating body composition such as the use of stable isotopes,[158] impedance, total body electrical conductivity (TOBEC),[160] infrared interactance,[161] and magnetic resonance imaging.[162] Development of functional measures of nutritional status is a focus of several research groups. Workers are now recognizing the relation between health status and body fat distribution.[163] Major advances are occurring in the technology for measuring energy expenditure.[164] A recent conference addressed the need for specifically defining anthropometric measuring sites. The intense current interest in nutritional assessment can be readily appreciated from this diverse panorama of ongoing research.

In summary, nutritional assessment is a clinical science in an early phase of development. Our aim in this chapter is to provide a firm pathophysiologic basis for each component of the assessment. The value of a crude test can sometimes be improved when the examiner thoroughly understands the uses, strengths, and limitations of the method. More important, a newly developed test can be rationally inserted into a framework of understanding. The process of gradually replacing inaccurate and nonspecific indices will lead to an evolving science of nutritional assessment.

## REFERENCES

1. Pittman, J.G., Cohen, P: N. Engl. J. Med. *271*:403–409, 1964.
2. Leicester, H.M.: The Historical Background of Chemistry. New York, John Wiley and Sons, 1956.
3. Benedict, F.C., Miles, W.R., Roth, P., et al.: Human Vitality and Efficiency under Prolonged Restricted Diet. Carnegie Institute of Washington, Publication No. 280.
4. Pereira, J.: Treatise on Food and Nutrition. London, Longman, 1843.
5. Harrow, B.: Casimir Funk, Pioneer in Vitamins and Hormones. New York, Dodd, Mead & Co., 1955.
6. Bistrian, B.R., Blackburn, G.L., Hallowell, E.: JAMA *230*:858–860, 1974.
7. Garrow, J.S.: Energy Stores: Their composition, Measurement and Control. Energy Balance and Obesity in Man. Amsterdam, North Holland, 1974.
8. Moore, F.D., Olesen, K.O., McMurrey, J.D., et al.: The Body Cell Mass and Its Supporting Environment: Body Composition in Health and Disease. Philadelphia, W.B. Saunders, 1963.
9. International Commission on Radiologic Protection, Report of the Task Group on Reference Man. Adopted by the Commission in October, 1974, New York, Pergamon Press.
10. Allison, R.G., Senti, F.R.: A Perspective on the Application of the Atwater System of Food Energy Assessment. Bethesda, MD, Life Sciences Research Office, Federation of American Societies for Experimental Biology, 1983.
11. Brody, S.: Bioenergentics and Growth. New York, Reinhold Publishing Corp., 1945.
12. Hill, J.O., Heymsfield, S.B., DiGirolamo, M.: A New Approach for Studying the Thermic Response to Dietary Fuel. Am. J. Clin. Nutr. *42*:1290–1298, 1985.
13. Askanazi, J., Carpentier, Y.A., Elwyn, D.H., et al.: Ann. Surg. *191*:40–46, 1980.
14. Durnin, J.G.V.A., Passmore R.: Energy, Work, and Leisure. London, Heinemann Educational Books, 1967.
15. Southgate, D.A.T., Durnin, J.V.G.A.: Br. J. Nutr. *24*:517–535, 1970.
16. Lentner, C.: Geigy Scientific Tables. Vol. 1. 8th ed. Basel, Switzerland, Ciba-Geigy, Ltd., 1981.
17. Ashworth, A., Harrower, A.D.B.: Br. J. Nutr. *21*:833–843, 1967.
18. Calloway, D.H., O'Dell, A.C., Margen, S.: J. Nutr. *101*:775–786, 1971.
19. Cheng, A.H.R., Gomez, A., Bergan, J.G., et al.: Am. J. Clin. Nutr. *31*:12:22, 1978.
20. Long, C.L., Schaffel, N., Geiger, J.W., et al.: J. Parent. Ent. Nutr. *3*:452–456, 1979.
21. Heymsfield, S.B., Smith, J., Kasriel, S., et al.: Am. J. Clin. Nutr. *34*:1954–1960, 1981.
22. Cahill, G.F., Jr.: Clin. Endocrinol. Metab. *5*:397–415, 1976.
23. Wright, R.A., Heymsfield, S.B.: Nutritional Assessment of the Adult Hospitalized Patient. Boston, Blackwell Scientific Publications, 1984.
24. Keys, A.J., Brozek, J., Wenschel, O., et al.: *In* The Biology of Human Starvation. Minneapolis, MN, University of Minnesota Press, 1950.
25. Halliday, D.: Clin. Sci. *33*:365–370, 1967.

26. Cohn, S.H., Vaswani, A.N., Aloia, J., et al.: Metabolism 25:89–95, 1976.

27. Heymsfield, S.B., McManus, C., Smith, J., et al.: Am. J. Clin. Nutr. 35:1192–1199, 1982.

28. Stevens, V., Shoji, M., Heymsfield, S.: Clin. Res. 29:844A, 1981.

29. Addis, T., Poo, L.J., Lew, W.: J. Biol. Chem. 115:111–116, 1936.

30. Goldberg, A.L.: Biochemical events during hypertrophy of skeletal muscle. *In* Cardiac Hypertrophy. (Alpert, N.R., Ed.) New York, Academic Press, Inc., 1971.

31. Goodwin, C.W., Aulick, L.H., Becker, R.A., et al.: JAMA 244:1588–1590, 1980.

32. Belfrage, S.: Acta Med. Scand. 173 (Suppl):1–169, 1963.

33. Kinney, J.M., Long, C.L., Gump, F.E., et al.: Ann. Surg. 168:459–474, 1968.

34. Taylor, K.B., Anthony L.E.: Clinical Nutrition. New York, McGraw-Hill, 1983.

35. Cutrone, C.: The Dietary History Nutritional Assessment Series. Atlanta, Emory University School of Medicine, 1981.

36. Graham, A.M.: Proc. Nutr. Soc. 41:343–348, 1982.

37. Watt, B.K., Merrill, A.L.: *In* Composition of Foods, Raw, Processed, Prepared. U.S. Department of Agriculture Handbook No. 8 Washington, DC, U.S. Government Printing Office, 1963.

38. Posati, L.P., Orr, M.L.: *In* Composition of Foods–raw, processed, prepared–Dairy and Egg Products. U.S. Department of Agriculture Handbook No. 8–1. Washington, DC, U.S. Government Printing Office, 1976.

39. Recommended Dietary Allowances. 9th Edition.: Washington DC, Food and Nutrition Board, National Academy of Sciences, 1980.

40. Nutr. Rev. 34:310–311, 1976.

41. Atwater, W.O., Bryant, A.P.: Conn. (Storrs) Agr. Expt. Sta. 12th Ann. Rpt., 1899, pp. 73–110.

42. Steyermark, A., Alber, H.K., Aluise, V.A., et al. Anal. Chem. 23:523–528, 1951.

43. Ward, M.W.N., Owens, C.W.I., Rennie, M.J.: Clin. Chem. 26:1336–1339, 1980.

44. Mirtallo, J.M., Joch, L., Fabri, P.J.: Hosp. Formul. 18:57:64, 1983.

45. Heymsfield, S.B., Head, A., Grossman, G.: Manuscript in preparation.

46. Ravussin, E., Burnand, B., Schutz, Y., et al.: Am. J. Clin. Nutr. 35:566–573, 1982.

47. Lusk, G.: The Elements of the Science of Nutrition. 4th ed. Philadelphia, W.B., Saunders, 1928. p. 65.

48. Weir, J.B., de V.: J. Physiol. 109:1–9, 1949.

49. Hill, J.O., Heymsfield, S.B., McManus, C.B. III, et al.: Metabolism. 33:743–749, 1984.

50. Heymsfield, S.B., Grossman, G.D., Head, C.A., et al.: Am. J. Clin. Nutr. 40:116–130, 1984.

51. Wilmore, D.W.: The Metabolic Management of the Critically Ill. New York, Plenum Medical Book Company, 1977.

52. Duke, J.H., Jorgensen, S.B., Broell, J.R., et al.: Surgery 68:168–174, 1970.

53. Wilmore, D.W., Long, J.M., Mason, A.D., Jr.: Ann. Surg. 180:653–668, 1974.

54. Mueller, K.J., Crosby, L.O., Oberlander, J.L., et al.: J. Parent. Ent. Nutr. 7:266–269, 1983.

55. Heymsfield, S.B., Tochilin, N., McManus, C.B., et al.: Clin. Consult. 4:6–10, 1984.

56. Shaw, S., Gil, K., Askanazi, T., et al: Fed. Proc. 43:469, 1984.

57. Scriver, C., Rosenberg, L.: Amino Acid Metabolism and Its Disorders. Philadelphia, W.B. Saunders Co., 1973.

58. Harvey, K.B., Blumenkrantz, M.J., Levine, S.E., et al.: Am. J. Clin. Nutr. 33:1586–1597, 1980.

59. Calloway, D.H., Odell, A.C.F., Margen, S.: J. Nutr. 101:775–786, 1971.

60. Wallace, W.M.: Fed. Proc. 18:1125–1130, 1959.

61. Forbes, G.B.: Nutr. Rev. 31:297–300, 1973.

62. Rand, W.M., Scrimshaw, N.S., Young, V.R.: Conventional ("long-term") nitrogen balance studies for protein quality evaluation in adults: Rationale and limitations. *In* Protein Quality in Humans: Assessment and in vitro Estimation. (Bodwell, C.E., Adkins, J.S., Hopkins, D.T., Eds.) Westport, CT, AVI Publishing Co., 1981.

63. Richer, P.: Nouv. Inconogr. Salpetriere 3:20–26, 1890.

64. Matiegka, J.: Am. J. Phys. Anthropol. 3:223–230, 1921.

65. Leiter, L.A., Marliss, E.B.: JAMA 248:2306–2307, 1982.

66. Warren, S.: Am. J. Med. Sci. 184:610–615, 1932.

67. Boushy, S.F., Adhikari, P.K., Sakamoto, A., et al.: Dis. Chest 45:402–411, 1964.

68. Studley, H.O.: JAMA 106:458–460, 1936.

69. Keys, A., Brozek, J.: Physiol. Rev. 33:245–316, 1953.

70. Garn, S.M.: Hum. Biol. 27:75–79, 1955.

71. Allen, T.H., Peng, M.T., Chen, K.P., et al.: Metabolism 5:346–352, 1956.

72. Burkinshaw, L., Jones, P.R.M., Krupowicz, D.W.: Hum. Biol. 43:273–279, 1973.

73. Durnin, J.V.G.A., Womersley, J.: Br. J. Nutr. 32:77–79, 1974.

74. Damon, A., Goldman, R.F.: Hum. Biol. 36:32–44, 1964.

75. Cohn, S.H., Vartsky, D., Yasumura, S., et al.: Am. J. Physiol. 239:524–530, 1980.

76. Heymsfield, S.B., McManus, C.B., Smith, J., et al.: Am. J. Clin. Nutr. 35:680–690, 1982.

77. Theologides, A.: Cancer 29:484–488, 1972.

78. Heymsfield, S.B., Olafson, R., Kutner, M., Nixon, D.W.: Am. J. Clin. Nutr. 32:693–702, 1979.

79. Lopes, J.M., Russell, D.McR., Whitwell, J., et al.: Am. J. Clin. Nutr. 36:602–610, 1982.

80. Heymsfield, S.B., Stevens, V., Noel, R., et al.: Am. J. Clin. Nutr. 36:131–142, 1982.

81. Cohen, S.H., Ellis, K.J., Wallach, S.: Am. J. Med. 57:683–690, 1974.

82. Cohn, S.H., Sawitsky, A., Vartsky, D., et al.: Body composition as measured by in vivo activation analysis. *In* Nutritional Assessment–Present Status, Future Directions and Prospects, (Levenson, S.M.,) Columbus, OH, Ross Laboratories, 1981.

83. Trotter, M., Gleser, G.: Am. J. Phys. Anthropol. 9: 311–324, 1951.

84. Skerlj, B., Brozek, J., Hunt, Jr., E.: Am. J. Phys. Anthropol. 11:577–600, 1953.

85. Dequeker, J.V., Baeyens, J.P., Classens, J.: J. Am. Geriatr. Soc. 17:169–179, 1969.

86. Mitchelll, C.O., Lipschitz, D.A.: Am. J. Clin. Nutr. *35*:398–406, 1982.
87. Young, C.M., Blondin, J., Tensuan, R., et al.: J. Am. Diet. Assoc. *43*:344–348, 1963.
88. Brozek, J., Kinzey, W.: J. Gerontol. *15*:45–51, 1960.
89. Daly, C.H., Odland, G.F.: J. Invest. Dermatol. *73*:84–87, 1979.
90. Safiq, S.A., Lewis, S.G., Dimino, L.C., et al.: Electron microscopic study of skeletal muscle in elderly subjects. *In* Aging. 3rd ed. (Daldor, G., DiBattista, W.J., Eds.) New York, Raven Press, 1978.
91. Metropolitan Life Insurance Company: Statistical Bulletin, New Weights and Standards for Men and Women. Vol 40. November–December 1959.
92. 1979 Build Study: Society of Actuaries and Association of Life Insurance Medical Directors of America, 1980.
93. Simopoulos, A.P., Van Itallie, T.B.: Ann. Intern. Med. *100*:285–295, 1984.
94. Knapp, T.R.: JAMA *250*:506–510, 1983.
95. Bastow, M.D.: Proc. Nutr. Soc. *41*:381–388, 1982.
96. Bistrian, B.R., Blackburn, G.L., Sherman, M., et al.: Surg. Gynecol. Obstet. *141*:512–516, 1975.
97. Myers, V.C., Fine, M.J.: J. Biol. Chem. *14*:9–26, 1913.
98. Burger, M.Z.: Z. Ges. Exp. Med. *9*:361–399, 1919.
99. Heymsfield, S.B., Arteaga, C.L., McManus, C.B., Smith, J.: Am. J. Clin. Nutr. *37*:478–493, 1983.
100. Forbes, G.B., Bruining, G.J.: Am. J. Clin. Nutr. *29*:1359–1366, 1976.
101. Viteri, F.E., Alvarado, J.: Pediatrics *46*:696–706, 1970.
102. Blackburn, G.L., Bistrian, B.R., Maini, B.S., et al.: J. Parent. Ent. Nutr. *1*:11–22, 1977.
103. Scrimshaw, N.S., Habicht, J.P., Piche, M.L., et al.: Am. J. Clin. Nutr. *18*:321–324, 1966.
104. Srivastava, S.S., Mani, K.V., Soni, C.M., et al.: Ind. J. Med. Res. *55*:953–960, 1957.
105. Bleiler, R.E., Schedl, H.P.: J. Lab. Clin. Med. *59*:945–955, 1972.
106. Crim, M.C., Calloway, D.H., Margen, S.: J. Nutr. *106*:371–381, 1976.
107. Smith, O.W.: J. Clin. Endocrinol. *2*:1–12, 1942.
108. Goldman, R.: Proc. Soc. Exp. Biol. Med. *85*:446–448, 1954.
109. Kirsch, R., Frith, L., Black, E., et al.: Nature *217*:578–579, 1968.
110. Rothschild, M.A., Oratz, M., Schreiber, S.S.: N. Engl. J. Med. *286*:748–757, 1972.
111. Moore, F.D., Langohr, J.L., Ingebretson, M., et al.: Ann. Surg. *132*:1–19, 1950.
112. James, W.P., Hay, A.M.: J. Clin. Invest. *47*:1958–1972, 1968.
113. Rothschild, M.A., Waldmann, T.: Plasma Protein Metabolism. New York, Academic Press, 1970.
114. Hay, R.W., Whitehead, R.G., Spicer, C.C.: Lancet *24*:427–429, 1975.
115. Starker, P.M., Gump, F.E., Askanazi, J., et al.: Surgery *91*:194–199, 1982.
116. Reinhardt, G.F., Myscofski, J.W., Wilkens, D.B.: J. Parent. Ent. Nutr. *4*:357–359, 1980.
117. Skillman, J.J., Rosenoer, V.M., Smith, P.C.: N. Engl. J. Med. *295*:1037–1040, 1976.
118. Forse, R.A., Shizgal, H.M.: J. Parent. Ent. Nutr. *4*:450–454, 1980.
119. Ismadi, S.D., Suschella, T.P., Narasinga, Roe, B.S.: Nutr. Rev. *31*:135, 1973.
120. Miller, S.F., Morath, M.A., Finley, R.K.: J. Trauma *21*:548–550, 1981.
121. Young, G.A., Keogh, G.B., Parsons, F.M.: Clin. Chim. Acta *61*:205–213, 1975.
122. Golden, M.H.N.: Am. J. Clin. Nutr. *35*:1159–1165, 1982.
123. Clemmons, D.R., Klibanski, A., Underwood, L.E., et al.: J. Clin. Endocrinol. Metab. *53*:1247–1250, 1981.
124. Howard, L., Dillon, B., Saba, T.M., et al.: J. Parent. Ent. Nutr. *8*:237–244, 1984.
125. Solomons, N.W., Allen. L.H.: Nutr. Rev. *41*:33–50, 1983.
126. Bhatia, S., DeFelice, L., Heymsfield, S.: Clin. Res. *27*:725A, 1979.
127. Klidjian, A.M., Foster, K.J., Kammerling, R.M.: Br. Med. J. *281*:899–901, 1980.
128. Alleyne, G.A.O.: Clin. Sci. *30*:553–562, 1966.
129. Heymsfield, S.B., Bethel, R.A., Ansley, J.D., et al.: Am. Heart J. *95*:584–594, 1978.
130. Heymsfield, S.B., Nutter, D.O.: The heart in protein-calorie undernutrition. *In* Update I. The Heart. (JW Hurst, Ed.) New York, McGraw-Hill, 1979.
131. Alleyne, G.A.O.: Pediatrias *39*:400–411, 1966.
132. Gottdiener, J.S., Gross, H.A., Henry, W.L., et al.: Circulation *58*:425:433, 1978.
133. Covelli, H.D., Black, J.W., Oslen, M.S., et al.: Ann. Intern. Med. *95*:579–591, 1981.
134. Grant, J.P.: Clinical impact of protein malnutrition on organ mass and function. *In* Amino Acids. Metabolism and Medical Applications. (Blackburn, G.L., Grant, J.P., Young, V.R., Eds.) Boston, John Wright, PSG Inc., 1983.
135. Hunt, D., Rowlands, B.J., Wilkenfeld, K., et al.: Clin. Res. *32*:233A, 1984.
136. Russell, D.McR., Leiter, L.A., Whitwell, J., et al.: Am. J. Clin. Nutr. *37*:133–138, 1983.
137. Berkelhammer, C.H., Leiter, L.A., Jeejeebhoy, K.N., et al.: Am. J. Clin. Nutr. *42*:845–854, 1985.
138. Bistrian, B.R., Blackburn, G.L., Sherman, G.L., et al.: Arch. Intern. Med. *137*:1408–1411, 1977.
139. Miller, C.L.: J. Parent. Ent. Nutr. *2*:554–563, 1978.
140. Good, R.A., West, A., Fernandes, G.: Fed. Proc. *39*:3098–3104, 1980.
141. Harvey, K.B., Moldawer, L.L., Bistrian, B.R., et al.: Am. J. Clin. Nutr. *34*:2013–2022, 1981.
142. Meakins, J.L., Pietsch, J.B., Bubenik, O.: Ann. Surg. *186*:241–250, 1977.
143. Mullen, J.L., Gertner, M.J., Buzby, G.P., et al.: Arch. Surg. *114*:121–125, 1979.
144. Lewis, R.T., Klein, H.: J. Surg. Res. *26*:365–371, 1979.
145. Dionigi, R.: Proc. Nutr. Soc. *41*:355–371, 1982.
146. Twomey, P., Ziegler, D., Rombeau, J.: J. Parent. Ent. Nutr. *6*:50–58. 1982.
147. Shils, M.E.: Indices of the nutritional status of the individual. *In* Nutrition in the 1980's: Constraints on our knowledge. (Selvey, N., White, P.L., Eds.) New York, Alan R Liss, Inc., 1981.
148. Nixon, D.W., Heymsfield, S.B., Cohen, A.B., et al.: Am. J. Med. *68*:683–690, 1980.
149. Vandenbergh, E., Van de Woestijne, K.P., Gyselen, A.: Am. Rev. Respir. Dis. *195*:556–566, 1967.

150. Nazari, S., Dionigi, R., Dionigi, P., et al.: J. Parent. Ent. Nutr. *4*:499–500, 1980.
151. Braun, S.R., Dixon, R.M., Keim, N.L., et al.: Chest *85*:353–357, 1984.
152. Sours, H.E., Frattali, V.P., Brand, C.D., et al.: Am. J. Clin. Nutr. *34*:453–461, 1981.
153. Isner, J.M., Roberts, W.C., Heymsfield, S.B., et al.: Sudden death in anorexia nervosa associated with Q-T interval prolongation. Ann. Intern. Med. *102*:49–52, 1985.
154. Wolfson, M., Strong, C.J., Minturn, D., et al.: Am. J. Clin. Nutr. *39*:547–555, 1984.
155. Nazari, S., Comincioli, V., Dionigi, R., et al.: J. Parent. Ent. Nutr. *5*:307–316, 1981.
156. Buzby, G.P., Mullen, J.L.: Analysis of nutritional assessment indices–prognositic equations and clusters analyses. *In* Nutritional Assessment of the Adult Hospitalized Patient. (Wright, R.A., Heymsfield, S.B., Eds.) Boston, Blackwell Scientific Publications, 1984.
157. Nichols, R.M.: N. Engl. J. Med. *307*:1701–1702, 1982.

158. Schoeller, D.A., Kushner, R.F., Taylor, P., et al.: Measurement of total body water: isotope dilution techniques. *In* Body-Composition Assessments in Youth and Adults. (Roche, A.F., Ed.) Columbus, Ross Laboratories, 1985, pp 24–29.
159. Lukaski, H.C., Johnson, P.E., Bolonchuk, W.W., et al.: Am. J. Clin. Nutr. *41*:363, 1985.
160. Van Itallie, T.B., Segal, K.R., Yang, M-U., et al.: Clinical assessment of body fat content in adults: potential role of electrical impedance methods. *In* Body-Composition Assessments in Youth and Adults. (Roche, A.F., Ed.) Columbus, Ross Laboratories, pp 5–8, 1985.
161. Conway, J.M., Norris, K.H., Bodwell, C.E.: Am. J. Clin. Nutr. *40*:1123–1130, 1984.
162. Heymsfield, S.B., Rolandelli, R., Casper, K., et al.: Application of electromagnetic and sound waves in nutritional assessment. In press.
163. Krotkiewski, M., Bjorntorp, P., Sjostrom, L., et al.: J. Clin. Invest. *72*:1150–1162, 1983.
164. Lifson, N., Gordon, G.B., McClintock, R.: J. Appl. Physiol. *7*:704, 1955.

## Addendum 1.   Equations for Calculating Change in Body Weight (BW)

| Equation | Comment |
|---|---|
| (1) $\Delta BW\ (kg) = BW_p - BW_i$ | calculates weight loss from initial (i) to present (p) weight |
| (2) $\Delta BW\ (kg/d) = (BW_p - BW_i)/(day_p - day_i)$ | calculates rate of weight change |
| (3) $\Delta BW\ (kg) = BW_u - BW_p$ | calculates weight loss from usual (u) to present (p) body weight |
| (4) $\Delta BW\ (\%) = \dfrac{(BW_{u\ or\ i}) - (BW_p)}{BW_{u\ or\ i}} \times 100$ | calculates % weight loss from usual (u) or from initial (i) observation |

Reprinted from Wright, R.A., Heymsfield, S.B.,[23] with permission of Blackwell Scientific Publications, Inc.

## Addendum 2.   Skinfold Measurement Sites

1. **Biceps skinfold thickness.** Lift the skinfold on the anterior aspect of the upper arm, directly above the center of the cubital fossa, at the same level as the triceps skinfold and midarm circumference. The arm hangs relaxed at the patient's side, and the crest of the fold should run parallel to the long axis of the arm.
2. **Triceps skinfold thickness.** Grasp the skin and subcutaneous tissue 1 cm above the midpoint between the tip of the acromial process of the scapula and the olecranon process of the ulna. The fold runs parallel to the long axis of the arm. Care should be taken to assure that the measurement is made in the midline posteriorly, and that the arm hangs relaxed and vertical.
3. **Subscapular skinfold.** The skin is lifted 1 cm under the inferior angle of the scapula with the shoulder and arm relaxed. The fold should run parallel to the natural cleavage lines of the skin; this is usually a line about 45 degrees from the horizontal extending medially upwards.
4. **Suprailiac skinfold.** Pick up this skinfold 2 cm above the iliac crest in the midaxillary line. The crest of this fold should run horizontally.
5. **Thigh skinfold.** The skin is picked up on the posterior aspect at the same level as the thigh circumference. The crest of the skinfold should run parallel with the leg.
6. **Calf skinfold.** This skinfold is picked up on the posterior aspect of the calf at the same level as the calf circumference. The crest of the skinfold should run parallel to the leg.

## Addendum 3.   Circumferential Measurement Sites

1. Mid-upper arm. This circumference is taken at the midpoint between the acromial and olecranon processes of the scapula and the ulna, respectively. The arm should hang relaxed at the patient's side.
2. Midthigh. The subject stands with feet slightly apart, and with weight evenly distributed on both feet. The tape is placed around the thigh horizontally at the midpoint between the lower extent of the gluteal fold and the crease immediately posterior to the patella.
3. Midcalf. With the subject standing in the same position as for the thigh circumference, the measurement is made with the tape horizontal at the maximal circumference of the calf.

## Addendum 4.   Methods of Measuring Skinfolds and Circumferences

*Skinfolds*
1. Arrive at the anatomic site as defined in Addenda 2 and 3.
2. Lift the skin and fat layer from the underlying tissue by grasping the tissue with the thumb and forefinger.
3. Apply calipers about 1 cm distal from the thumb and forefinger, midway between the apex and base of the skinfold.
4. Continue to support the skinfold with the thumb and forefinger for the duration of the measurement.
5. After 2 to 3 seconds of caliper application, read skinfold to the nearest 0.5 mm.
6. Measurements are then made in triplicate until readings agree within ± 1.0 mm; results are then averaged.

*Circumferences*
1. The tape should be maintained in a horizontal position touching the skin and following the contours of the limb, but not compressing underlying tissue.
2. Measurements should be made to the nearest millimeter, in triplicate, as previously described for skinfolds.

**Addendum 5.   Methods for Optimizing Precision**

1. Train observers by skilled professionals.
2. Use one rather than multiple observers for the same subject over time.
3. Mark the anatomic site of the skinfold and circumferential measurement with indelible ink when repeatedly measuring the same patient over a short time span.
4. Learn the anatomic landmarks, how to grasp the skinfold, how long to compress the skinfold site, and how to properly read the caliper scale.
5. Periodically assess interobserver and between-day measurement differences of the staff.

**Addendum 6.   Equations for Calculating Limb Fat Areas**

| Extremity | Equation | Comment |
|---|---|---|
| (1) upper arm | arm fat area (cm²) $$= \left[ \frac{MAC \times TSF}{2} \right] - \left[ \frac{\pi \times (TSF)^2}{4} \right]$$ | This general equation assumes a circular limb and muscle compartment and a symmetrically distributed fat rim. The accuracy of this equation in predicitng mid upper arm fat area is unknown. TSF = triceps skinfold (cm); MAC = midarm circumference (cm) |
| (2) thigh | thigh fat area (cm²) $$= \left[ \frac{MTC \times THSF}{2} \right] - \left[ \frac{\pi \times (THSF)^2}{4} \right]$$ | THSF = thigh skinfold (cm); MTC = midthigh circumference (cm) |
| (3) calf | calf fat area (cm²) $$= \left[ \frac{MCC \times CSF}{2} \right] - \left[ \frac{\pi \times (CSF)^2}{4} \right]$$ | CSF = calf skinfold (cm); MCC = mid-calf circumference (cm) |

Reprinted from Wright, R.A., Heymsfield, S.B.,[23] with permission of Blackwell Scientific Publications, Inc.

**Addendum 7.   Calculation of Fat and Fat-Free Mass According to the Method of Durnin and Womersley[73]**

1. Determine the patient's age and weight (kg).
2. Measure the following skinfolds in mm: biceps, triceps, subscapular, and suprailiac (Addenda 2 and 4).
3. Compute $\Sigma$ by adding the four skinfolds.
4. Compute the logarithm of $\Sigma$.
5. Apply one of the following age and sex adjusted equations to compute body density (D, g/cc).

*Equations for men:*
Age range
17–19   $D = 1.1620 - 0.0630 \times (\log \Sigma)$
20–29   $D = 1.1631 - 0.0632 \times (\log \Sigma)$
30–39   $D = 1.1422 - 0.0544 \times (\log \Sigma)$
40–49   $D = 1.1620 - 0.0700 \times (\log \Sigma)$
50 +    $D = 1.1715 - 0.0779 \times (\log \Sigma)$

*Equations for women:*
Age range
17–19   $D = 1.1549 - 0.0678 \times (\log \Sigma)$
20–29   $D = 1.1599 - 0.0717 \times (\log \Sigma)$
30–39   $D = 1.1423 - 0.0632 \times (\log \Sigma)$
40–49   $D = 1.1333 - 0.0612 \times (\log \Sigma)$
50 +    $D = 1.1339 - 0.0645 \times (\log \Sigma)$

6. Fat mass is then calculated as: Fat mass (kg) = body weight (kg) $\times \dfrac{4.95}{D} - 4.5$.

7. Fat free mass is then calculated as: FFM (kg) = body weight (kg) − fat mass (kg).

Adapted from the data of Durnin, J.V.G.A., Womersley, J.,[73] and reprinted from Wright, R.A., Heymsfield, S.B.,[23] with permission of Blackwell Scientific Publications, Inc.

**Addendum 8.   Anthropometric Equations for Calculating Muscle Mass**

| Equation | Comment |
|---|---|
| (1)  Calf muscle area (cm²) = $$\frac{[MCC - \pi \times CSF]^2}{4\pi}$$ | Includes bone area; assumes a circular limb and muscle compartment and symmetrically distributed fat rim. |
| (2)  Thigh muscle area (cm²) = $$\frac{[MTC - \pi \times THSF]^2}{4\pi}$$ | Bone corrections are available.[24] |
| (3)  Arm muscle circumference (cm) = $$MAC - \pi \times TSF$$ | Same assumption as for equations 1 and 2; includes bone. Note that as muscle loses mass or volume in protein-energy malnutrition, circumferential measurements will change proportionately less than area measurements. The latter therefore more realistically depicts severity of muscle atrophy.[76] |
| (4)  Arm muscle area (cm²) = $$\frac{[MAC - \pi \times TSF]^2}{4\pi}$$ | Same assumption as equations 1 and 2; includes bone. Equation overestimates actual muscle area; by expressing absolute value as % of standard, the error is corrected.[78] |
| (5)  Arm muscle area (cm²) = <br> a.  Men $$\frac{[MAC - \pi \times TSF]^2}{4\pi} - 10$$ <br> b.  Women $$\frac{[MAC - \pi \times TSF]^2}{4\pi} - 6.5$$ | Same basic assumptions as equations 1 and 2; the overestimate in equation 4 is corrected, and the average value for bone area is also subtracted. Resulting value is therefore bone-free arm muscle area. As for all muscle derivatives on this chart, the resulting value remains an approximation ($\pm$ 8%) of actual muscle area.[24] |
| (6)  Available arm muscle area = <br> equation 5 (a or b) $- 9$ cm² | Subtracts approximate minimal value of arm muscle area compatible with survival.[27] Values at or less than zero are associated with life-threatening protein-energy malnutrition, and values above 5 cm but below normal range indicate muscle atrophy. |

From the data of Heymsfield, S.B., et al.[23] and Heymsfield, S.B. et al.[27] and reprinted from Wright, R.A. Heymsfield, S.B.,[23] with permission of Blackwell Scientific Publications, Inc.


**Addendum 9.   Prediction of Adult Stature from Knee Height**

This dimension is measured in centimeters using a broad-blade caliper, similar to the type of instrument used to measure infant length. The subject lies supine and bends the knee at a 90-degree angle. One blade of the caliper is placed over the anterior surface of the left thigh, above the condyles of the femur and just proximal to the patella. The caliper shaft is held parallel to the shaft of the tibia. Pressure is applied and two readings should agree within $\pm$ 0.5 cm. Height (in cm) is then calculated from the following two prediction equations:

Height (men) = 64.19 − (0.04 × age) + (2.02 × knee height)
Height (women) = 84.88 − (0.24 × age) + (1.83 × knee height).

From Chumlea, W.C., Roche, A.F., Mukherjee, D.: Nutritional Assessment of the Elderly through Anthropometry. Ross Laboratories, Columbus, Ohio, 1984.

**Addendum 10.   Age- and Sex-Specific Reference Values for Weight\***

| Age Group (yrs) | Percentile | | | | | | |
|---|---|---|---|---|---|---|---|
| | 5 | 10 | 25 | 50 | 75 | 90 | 95 |
| *American Men* | | | | | | | |
| 18–24 | 56.4 | 60.0 | 65.9 | 73.2 | 81.8 | 92.7 | 100.9 |
| 25–34 | 60.0 | 63.6 | 69.5 | 78.2 | 87.7 | 98.6 | 105.9 |
| 35–44 | 60.0 | 65.0 | 72.7 | 80.0 | 89.1 | 96.8 | 102.3 |
| 45–54 | 59.1 | 63.2 | 71.4 | 79.5 | 87.3 | 97.7 | 102.3 |
| 55–64 | 56.8 | 62.3 | 69.1 | 77.3 | 85.0 | 94.5 | 100.9 |
| 65–74 | 55.4 | 59.1 | 66.8 | 74.1 | 81.8 | 90.0 | 95.9 |
| *American Women* | | | | | | | |
| 18–24 | 45.4 | 48.2 | 51.8 | 58.2 | 64.5 | 74.1 | 83.2 |
| 25–34 | 46.8 | 49.5 | 54.1 | 60.0 | 69.1 | 82.3 | 91.8 |
| 35–44 | 49.5 | 51.8 | 56.4 | 63.2 | 74.1 | 88.6 | 97.7 |
| 45–54 | 49.5 | 51.8 | 57.7 | 65.9 | 74.5 | 86.8 | 96.8 |
| 55–64 | 47.3 | 50.4 | 58.2 | 65.4 | 75.1 | 86.8 | 92.3 |
| 65–74 | 47.7 | 50.9 | 57.3 | 64.5 | 74.1 | 83.2 | 86.6 |

Anthropometric reference values based on Health and Nutrition Examination Survey (Hanes II, 1971–1974). Reported by Bishop, C.W., Bowen, P.E., Ritchey, S.J.: (Am. J. Clin. Nutr. 34:2530–39, 1981). The samples of 28,043 persons represented the 194 million noninstitutionalized civilians living in the 48 contiguous states of the United States at the time of the survey. Anthropometric measurements were made on the right side of the body.
\*Values are in kg. Clothing worn.

**Addendum 11.   Provisional Age- and Sex-Specific Reference Values for Weight in Elderly Subjects in Kg (lbs)**

| Age Group (years) | 5% | 50% | 95% |
|---|---|---|---|
| *Men* | | | |
| 65 | 62.6 (138.0) | 79.5 (175.0) | 102.0 (224.9) |
| 70 | 59.7 (131.6) | 76.5 (168.7) | 99.1 (218.5) |
| 75 | 56.8 (125.2) | 73.6 (162.3) | 96.3 (212.3) |
| 80 | 53.9 (118.8) | 70.7 (155.9) | 93.4 (205.9) |
| 85 | 51.0 (112.4) | 67.8 (149.5) | 90.5 (199.5) |
| 90 | 48.1 (106.0) | 64.9 (143.1) | 87.6 (193.1) |
| *Women* | | | |
| 65 | 51.2 (112.9) | 66.8 (147.3) | 87.1 (192.0) |
| 70 | 49.0 (108.0) | 64.6 (142.4) | 84.9 (187.2) |
| 75 | 46.8 (103.2) | 62.4 (137.6) | 82.8 (182.5) |
| 80 | 44.7 (98.5) | 60.2 (132.7) | 80.6 (177.7) |
| 85 | 42.5 (93.7) | 58.0 (127.9) | 78.4 (172.8) |
| 90 | 40.3 (88.8) | 55.9 (123.2) | 76.2 (168.0) |

Data from 119 men and 150 women. The subjects were all ambulatory. (From Chumlea, W.C., Roche, A.F., and Mukherjee, D.: Nutritional Assessment of the Elderly through Anthropometry. Ross Laboratories, Columbus, Ohio, 1984.)

**Addendum 12. Triceps Skinfold Thickness**

| Age Group (yrs) | Sample Size | Estimated Population (millions) | Mean (mm) | Percentile | | | | | | |
|---|---|---|---|---|---|---|---|---|---|---|
| | | | | 5 | 10 | 25 | 50 | 75 | 90 | 95 |
| *Men* | | | | | | | | | | |
| 18–74 | 5261 | 61.18 | 12.0 | 4.5 | 6.0 | 8.0 | 11.0 | 15.0 | 20.0 | 23.0 |
| 18–24 | 773 | 11.78 | 11.2 | 4.0 | 5.0 | 7.0 | 9.5 | 14.0 | 20.0 | 23.0 |
| 25–34 | 804 | 13.00 | 12.6 | 4.5 | 5.5 | 8.0 | 12.0 | 16.0 | 21.5 | 24.0 |
| 35–44 | 664 | 10.68 | 12.4 | 5.0 | 6.0 | 8.5 | 12.0 | 15.5 | 20.0 | 23.0 |
| 45–54 | 765 | 11.15 | 12.4 | 5.0 | 6.0 | 8.0 | 11.0 | 15.0 | 20.0 | 25.0 |
| 55–64 | 598 | 9.07 | 11.6 | 5.0 | 6.0 | 8.0 | 11.0 | 14.0 | 18.0 | 21.5 |
| 65–74 | 1657 | 5.50 | 11.8 | 4.5 | 5.5 | 8.0 | 11.0 | 15.0 | 19.0 | 22.0 |
| *Women* | | | | | | | | | | |
| 18–74 | 8410 | 67.84 | 23.0 | 11.0 | 13.0 | 17.0 | 22.0 | 28.0 | 34.0 | 37.5 |
| 18–24 | 1523 | 12.89 | 19.4 | 9.4 | 11.0 | 14.0 | 18.0 | 24.0 | 30.0 | 34.0 |
| 25–34 | 1896 | 13.93 | 21.9 | 10.5 | 12.0 | 16.0 | 21.0 | 26.5 | 33.5 | 37.0 |
| 35–44 | 1664 | 11.59 | 24.0 | 12.0 | 14.0 | 18.0 | 23.0 | 29.5 | 35.5 | 39.0 |
| 45–54 | 836 | 12.16 | 25.4 | 13.0 | 15.0 | 20.0 | 25.0 | 30.0 | 36.0 | 40.0 |
| 55–65 | 669 | 9.98 | 24.9 | 11.0 | 14.0 | 19.0 | 25.0 | 30.5 | 35.0 | 39.0 |
| 65–74 | 1822 | 7.28 | 23.3 | 11.5 | 14.0 | 18.0 | 23.0 | 28.0 | 33.0 | 36.0 |

(From Bishop, C.W., Bowen, P.E., Ritchey, S.J.: Norms for nutritional assessment of American adults by upper arm anthropometry. Am. J. Clin. Nutr. 34:2530–39, 1981. Measurements were made in the right arm.)

**Addendum 13. Provisional Percentiles for Triceps Skinfold Thickness in the Elderly (in mm)**

| Age Group (years) | 5% | 50% | 95% |
|---|---|---|---|
| *Men* | | | |
| 65 | 8.6 | 13.8 | 27.0 |
| 70 | 7.7 | 12.9 | 26.1 |
| 75 | 6.8 | 12.0 | 25.2 |
| 80 | 6.0 | 11.2 | 24.3 |
| 85 | 5.1 | 10.3 | 23.4 |
| 90 | 4.2 | 9.4 | 22.6 |
| *Women* | | | |
| 65 | 13.5 | 21.6 | 33.0 |
| 70 | 12.5 | 20.6 | 32.0 |
| 75 | 11.5 | 19.6 | 31.0 |
| 80 | 10.5 | 18.6 | 30.0 |
| 85 | 9.5 | 17.6 | 29.0 |
| 90 | 8.5 | 16.6 | 28.0 |

Data are from 119 men and 150 women. All subjects were ambulatory, and measurements were made in the recumbent position on the left side. (From Chumlea, W.C., Roche, A.F., and Mukherjee, D.: Nutritional Assessment of the Elderly Through Anthropometry. Ross Laboratories, Columbus, Ohio, 1984.)

**Addendum 14.   Midarm Muscle Circumference**

| Age Group (yrs) | Sample Size | Estimated Population (millions) | Mean (cm) | Percentile | | | | | | |
|---|---|---|---|---|---|---|---|---|---|---|
| | | | | 5 | 10 | 25 | 50 | 75 | 90 | 95 |
| *Men* | | | | | | | | | | |
| 18–74 | 5261 | 61.18 | 28.0 | 23.8 | 24.8 | 26.3 | 27.9 | 29.6 | 31.4 | 32.5 |
| 18–24 | 773 | 11.78 | 27.4 | 23.5 | 24.4 | 25.8 | 27.2 | 28.9 | 30.8 | 32.3 |
| 25–34 | 804 | 13.00 | 28.3 | 24.2 | 25.3 | 26.5 | 28.0 | 30.0 | 31.7 | 32.9 |
| 35–44 | 664 | 10.68 | 28.8 | 25.0 | 25.6 | 27.1 | 28.7 | 30.3 | 32.1 | 33.0 |
| 45–54 | 765 | 11.15 | 28.2 | 24.0 | 24.9 | 26.5 | 28.1 | 29.8 | 31.5 | 32.6 |
| 55–64 | 598 | 9.07 | 27.8 | 22.8 | 24.4 | 26.2 | 27.9 | 29.6 | 31.0 | 31.8 |
| 65–74 | 1657 | 5.50 | 26.8 | 22.5 | 23.7 | 25.3 | 26.9 | 28.5 | 29.9 | 30.7 |
| *Women* | | | | | | | | | | |
| 18–74 | 8410 | 67.84 | 22.2 | 18.4 | 19.0 | 20.2 | 21.8 | 23.6 | 25.8 | 27.4 |
| 18–24 | 1523 | 12.89 | 20.9 | 17.7 | 18.5 | 19.4 | 20.6 | 22.1 | 23.6 | 24.9 |
| 25–34 | 1896 | 13.93 | 21.7 | 18.3 | 18.9 | 20.0 | 21.4 | 22.9 | 24.9 | 26.6 |
| 35–44 | 1664 | 11.59 | 22.5 | 18.5 | 19.2 | 20.6 | 22.0 | 24.0 | 26.1 | 27.4 |
| 45–54 | 836 | 12.16 | 22.7 | 18.8 | 19.5 | 20.7 | 22.2 | 24.3 | 26.6 | 27.8 |
| 55–64 | 669 | 9.98 | 22.8 | 18.6 | 19.5 | 20.8 | 22.6 | 24.4 | 26.3 | 28.1 |
| 65–74 | 1822 | 7.28 | 22.8 | 18.6 | 19.5 | 20.8 | 22.5 | 24.4 | 26.5 | 28.1 |

From Bishop, C.W., Bowen, P.E., Ritchey, S.J.: Norms for nutritional assessment of American adults by upper arm anthropometry. Am. J. Clin. Nutr. 34:2530–39, 1981. Measurements were made in the right arm.

**Addendum 15.   Midarm Muscle Area**

| Age Group (yrs) | Sample Size | Estimated Population (millions) | Mean (cm) | Percentile | | | | | | |
|---|---|---|---|---|---|---|---|---|---|---|
| | | | | 5 | 10 | 25 | 50 | 75 | 90 | 95 |
| *Men* | | | | | | | | | | |
| 18–74 | 5261 | 61.18 | 62.4 | 45.1 | 49.0 | 55.1 | 62.0 | 69.8 | 78.5 | 84.1 |
| 18–24 | 773 | 11.78 | 59.8 | 44.0 | 47.4 | 53.0 | 58.9 | 66.5 | 75.5 | 83.1 |
| 25–34 | 804 | 13.00 | 63.8 | 46.6 | 51.0 | 55.9 | 62.4 | 71.7 | 80.0 | 86.2 |
| 35–44 | 664 | 10.68 | 66.0 | 49.8 | 52.2 | 58.5 | 65.6 | 73.1 | 82.0 | 86.7 |
| 45–54 | 765 | 11.15 | 63.3 | 45.9 | 49.4 | 55.9 | 62.9 | 70.7 | 79.0 | 84.6 |
| 55–64 | 598 | 9.07 | 61.5 | 41.4 | 47.4 | 54.7 | 62.0 | 69.8 | 76.5 | 80.5 |
| 65–74 | 1657 | 5.50 | 57.2 | 40.3 | 44.7 | 51.0 | 57.6 | 64.7 | 71.2 | 75.0 |
| *Women* | | | | | | | | | | |
| 18–74 | 8410 | 67.84 | 39.2 | 27.0 | 28.7 | 32.5 | 37.8 | 44.3 | 53.0 | 59.8 |
| 18–24 | 1523 | 12.89 | 34.8 | 24.9 | 27.2 | 30.0 | 33.8 | 38.9 | 44.3 | 49.4 |
| 25–34 | 1896 | 13.93 | 37.5 | 26.7 | 28.4 | 31.8 | 36.5 | 41.8 | 49.4 | 56.3 |
| 35–44 | 1664 | 11.59 | 40.3 | 27.2 | 29.4 | 33.8 | 38.5 | 45.9 | 54.2 | 59.8 |
| 45–54 | 836 | 12.16 | 41.0 | 28.1 | 30.3 | 34.1 | 39.2 | 47.0 | 56.3 | 61.5 |
| 55–64 | 669 | 9.98 | 41.4 | 27.5 | 30.3 | 34.4 | 40.7 | 47.4 | 55.1 | 62.9 |
| 65–74 | 1822 | 7.28 | 41.4 | 27.5 | 30.3 | 34.4 | 40.3 | 47.4 | 55.9 | 62.9 |

Calculated from Bishop, C.W., Bowen, P.E., Ritchey, S.J.: Norms for nutritional assessment of American adults by upper arm anthropometry. Am. J. Clin. Nutr. 34:2530–39, 1981. Measurements were made in the right arm.

**Addendum 16.   Provisional Percentiles for Midarm Muscle Area (cm²) in the Elderly**

| Age Group (years) | 5% | 50% | 95% |
|---|---|---|---|
| *Men* | | | |
| 65 | 43.2 | 59.4 | 77.1 |
| 70 | 41.4 | 57.7 | 75.3 |
| 75 | 39.6 | 55.9 | 73.5 |
| 80 | 37.8 | 54.1 | 71.7 |
| 85 | 36.0 | 52.3 | 69.9 |
| 90 | 34.3 | 50.5 | 68.2 |
| *Women* | | | |
| 65 | 33.5 | 44.5 | 66.4 |
| 70 | 33.0 | 44.1 | 65.9 |
| 75 | 32.6 | 43.6 | 65.5 |
| 80 | 32.2 | 43.2 | 65.1 |
| 85 | 31.8 | 42.8 | 64.7 |
| 90 | 31.3 | 42.4 | 64.2 |

Data are from 119 men and 150 women. All subjects were ambulatory, and measurements were made in the recumbent position on the left side. (From Chumlea, W.C., Roche, A.F., and Mukherjee, D.: Nutritional Assessment of the Elderly through Anthropometry. Ross Laboratories, Columbus, Ohio, 1984.)

**Addendum 17.   Local Reference Values for Anthropometric Data**

Healthy subjects, who were between the ages of 20 and 70 years and within the desirable body weight range (1959 table) of ± 10%, were evaluated at the Emory University Clinical Research Facility. The data are presented for younger (age ≥20 to ≤45 years) and older (age ≥46 to ≤70 years) men (Addendum 17A) and women (Addendum 17B), respectively. The age cutoff was established arbitrarily and was intended for graphic presentation of results.

The data are plotted according to the method of Tukey (Tukey, J.W.: Exploratory Data Analysis. New York, Addison Wesley, 1977, p. 688). The 50th percentile is the small bar within the box. The upper and lower edges of the box are the 75th and 25th percentiles, respectively. The "whiskers" are the minimum and maximum values. Symmetric distributions are those where the 50th percentile bar is centered in the box and the lengths of whiskers are the same. Skewed distributions are detected by asymmetric placement of the 50th percentile mark.

A lower limit (shaded area) is provided for each index that represents an estimated minimal value for that dimension. Patients of similar height to the control group who suffered from severe emaciation were used to derive this information. The location, direction of movement, and the rate of change of the patient's value between the two ranges is used to establish severity and response to therapy of protein-energy malnutrition.

Adapted from the data of Heymsfield, S.B., et al.,[27] and reprinted from Wright, R.A., and Heymsfield, S.B.,[23] with permission of Blackwell Scientific Publications, Inc.

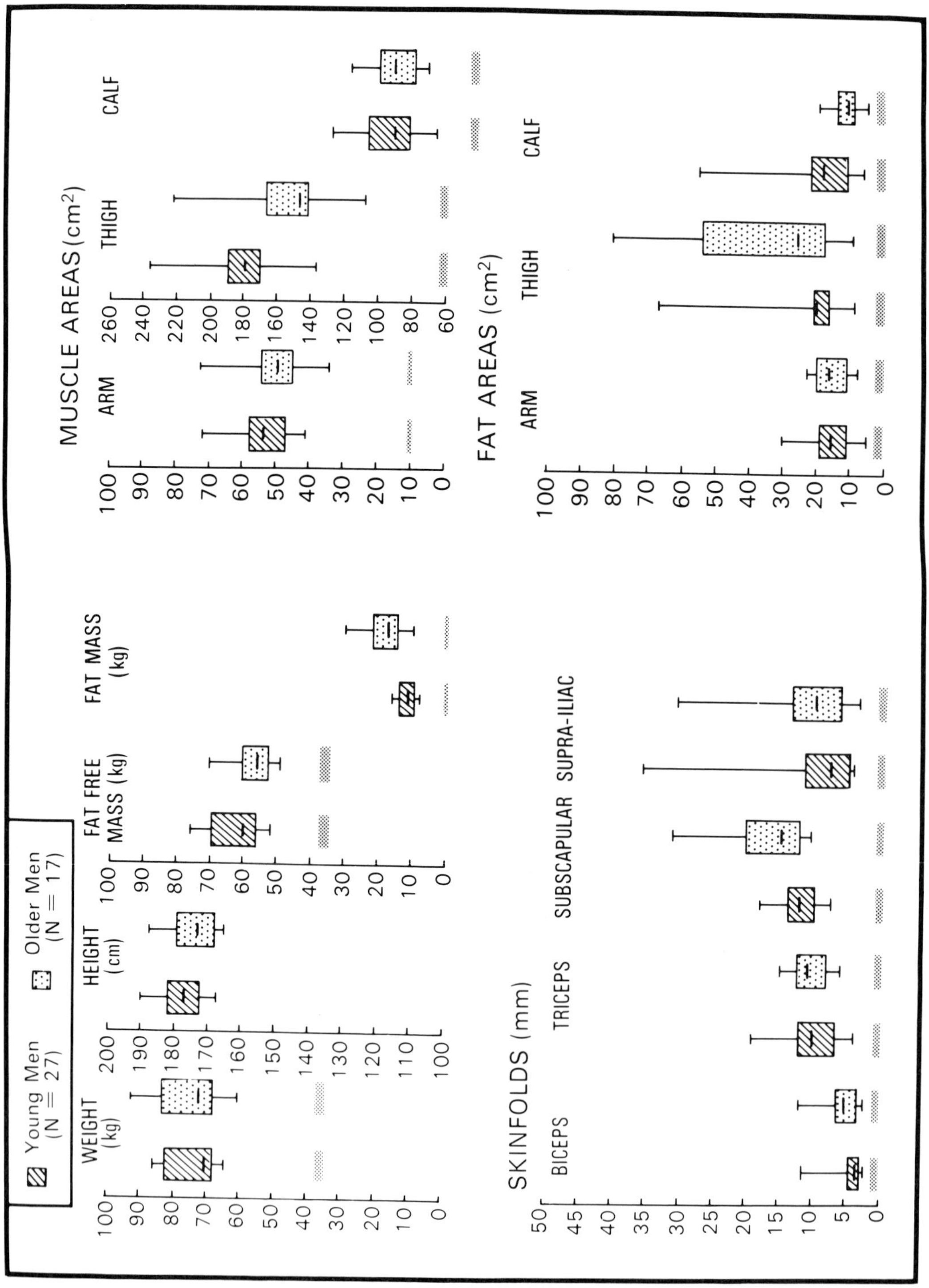

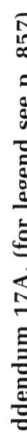

**Addendum 17A. (for legend see p. 857)**

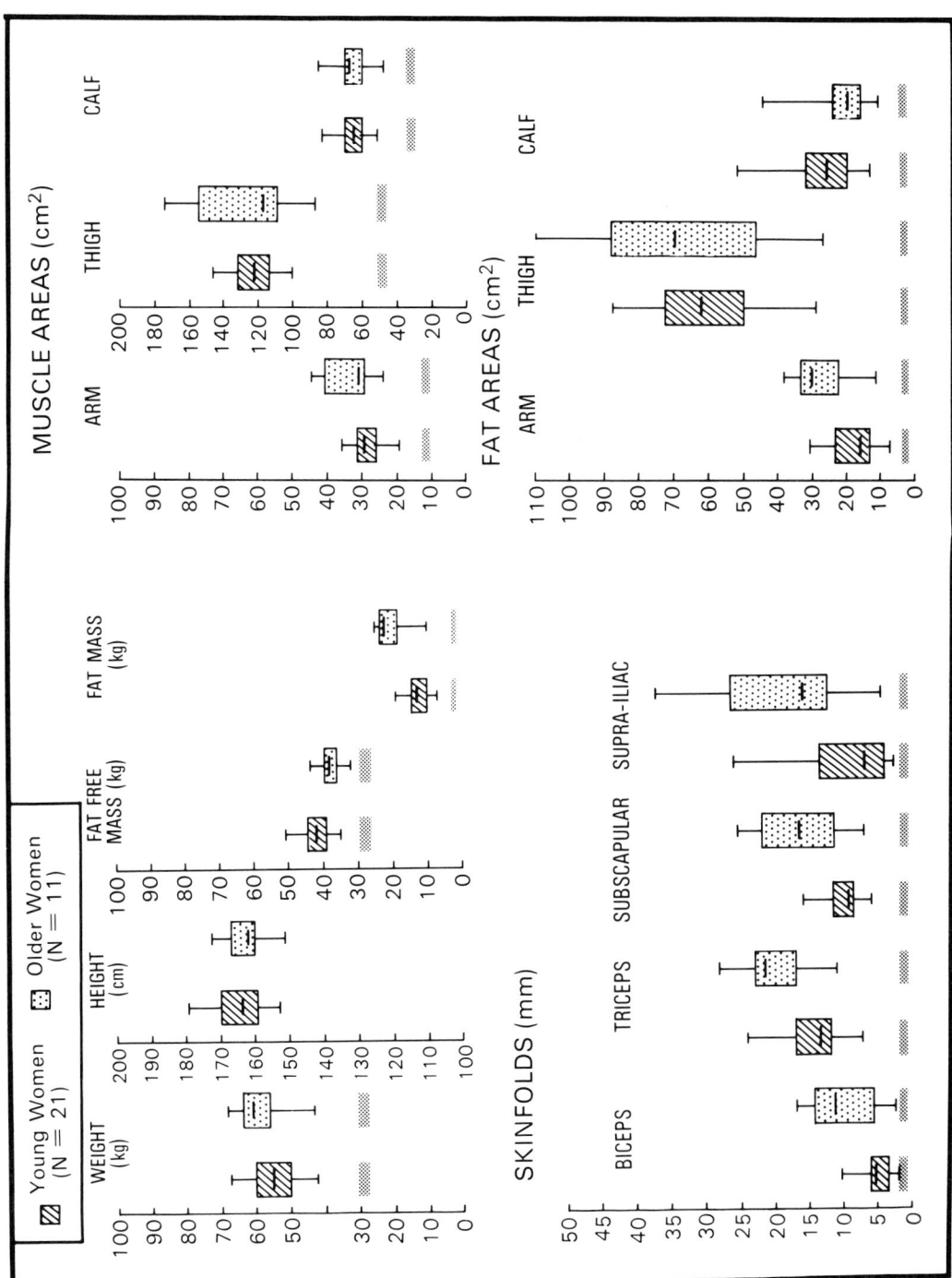

**Addendum 17B. (for legend see p. 857)**

**Addendum 18.  Urinary Creatinine Excretion of Normal Men and Women of Different Heights***

| | Men | | | | | Women | | | |
|---|---|---|---|---|---|---|---|---|---|
| Height in.   cm | Ideal Weight (kg) | Creatinine Coefficient (mg/kg) | 24-hr Urine Creatinine (gm) | | Height in.   cm | Ideal Weight (kg) | Creatinine Coefficient (mg/kg) | 24-hr Urine Creatinine (gm) |
| 62  157.5 | 56.0 | 23 | 1.29 | | 58  147.3 | 46.0 | 17 | 0.782 |
| 63  160.0 | 57.6 | | 1.32 | | 59  149.9 | 47.2 | | 0.802 |
| 64  162.5 | 59.0 | | 1.36 | | 60  152.4 | 48.6 | | 0.826 |
| 65  165.1 | 60.3 | | 1.39 | | 61  154.9 | 49.9 | | 0.848 |
| 66  167.6 | 62.0 | | 1.43 | | 62  157.5 | 51.3 | | 0.872 |
| 67  170.2 | 63.8 | | 1.47 | | 63  160.0 | 52.6 | | 0.894 |
| 68  172.7 | 65.8 | | 1.51 | | 64  162.6 | 54.3 | | 0.923 |
| 69  175.3 | 67.6 | | 1.55 | | 65  165.1 | 55.9 | | 0.950 |
| 70  177.8 | 69.4 | | 1.60 | | 66  167.6 | 57.8 | | 0.983 |
| 71  180.3 | 71.4 | | 1.64 | | 67  170.2 | 59.6 | | 1.01 |
| 72  182.9 | 73.5 | | 1.69 | | 68  172.7 | 61.5 | | 1.04 |
| 73  185.4 | 75.6 | | 1.74 | | 69  175.3 | 63.3 | | 1.08 |
| 74  188.0 | 77.6 | | 1.78 | | 70  177.8 | 65.1 | | 1.11 |
| 75  190.5 | 79.6 | | 1.83 | | 71  180.3 | 66.9 | | 1.14 |
| 76  193.0 | 82.2 | | 1.89 | | 72  182.9 | 68.7 | | 1.17 |

From Bistrian, B.R.: Nutritional Assessment and Therapy of Protein-Calorie Malnutrition in the Hospital, J. Am. Diet. Assoc., 71:393, 1977. Subjects were fed a creatinine and creatinine-free diet during the three days of urine collection.

*Creatinine:height index is defined as the 24-hour creatinine excretion of the patient divided by the expected 24-hour creatinine excretion of a normal adult of the same height. Table is for adults less than or equal to age 54. For older subjects, decrease value by 10% per decade (Rowe, J.W., et al.: The effect of age on creatinine clearance in men: A cross-sectional and longitudinal study. J. Gerontol. 31:155, 1976.)

*Chapter* **46**

# ASSESSMENT OF BONE STRUCTURE

## Michael D. Fallon

During the last two decades, several technical advances have permitted the more precise assessment of bone structure. Progress has stemmed from the development of biochemical methods for the measurement of circulating hormones and vitamins that influence bone. The noninvasive radiologic methods allowing quantitative determination of bone mass, such as single and dual photon absorptiometry, as well as computed tomography, now enhance the detection of changes in skeletal mass previously unrecognized by routine radiographs. These diagnostic tools, however, are indirect markers of skeletal structure. Consequently, the recently developed procedure for a simplified bone biopsy technique and the ability to prepare undecalcified histologic sections of bone have permitted the direct examination of skeletal tissue.

Examination of the microstructure of bone offers the advantage of determining not only the state of skeletal mineralization but also the level of bone remodeling activity.

## BONE AND NUTRITION

One of the major functions of the skeleton is related to nutrition. Bone is a dynamic organ that plays a role in calcium and mineral homeostasis.

To understand how skeletal abnormalities occur as a result of nutritional disorders, it is necessary to understand the relationships between normal mineral homeostasis, bone structure, and bone cell physiology.

## HISTOLOGIC FEATURES OF BONE

Bone is a specialized connective tissue of mineralized extracellular collagenous matrix. The skeleton functions not only to provide mechanical support and protection, but also to serve as a mineral reservoir for calcium homeostasis.

Cortical bone, also called compact bone, is located in the diaphyses of the long tubular bones and provides structural support (Fig. 46–1). Trabecular or cancellous bone consists of spicules of bone, known as trabeculae, that transverse the marrow spaces. Although trabecular bone constitutes only 20% of the skeleton, the three-dimensional arrangement of the cancellous network provides an enormous surface area (see Fig. 46–1).

There are three main types of bone cells (Fig. 46–2). Bone matrix is synthesized by *osteoblasts,* the cuboidal mononuclear cells found along bone surfaces. *Osteocytes* represent osteoblasts that have been incorporated into the previously syn-

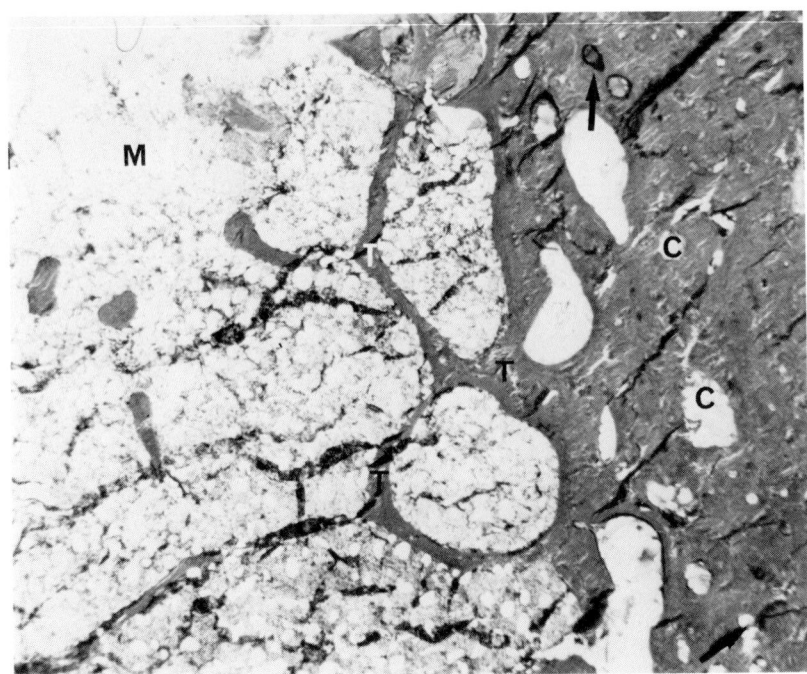

**Fig. 46–1.** Transcortical core biopsy of normal iliac bone. Cortical bone (C) is of normal thickness and contains haversian canals (arrow). Trabecular bone (T) forms interconnecting plates or ribbons of bone. M = marrow. (Undecalcified section, Masson trichrome stain; original magnification = 25 ×)

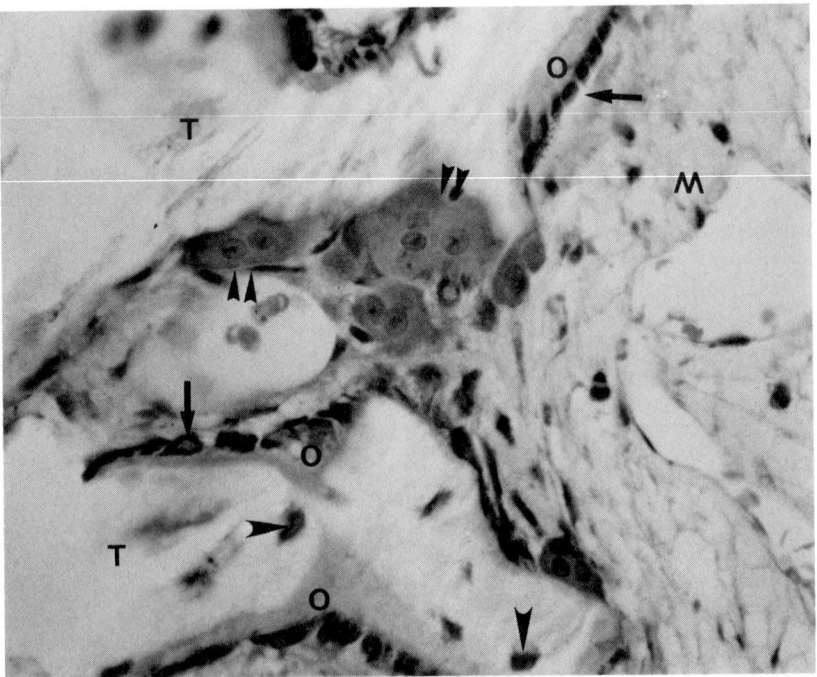

**Fig. 46–2.** Bone cells. Osteoblasts (arrow) line osteoid seams (O). Osteocytes (single arrowhead) are entrapped osteoblasts, now completely surrounded by matrix of the trabecular bone (T). Large multinucleated osteoclasts (double arrowhead) resorb bone. M = marrow. (Toluidine blue; original magnification = 340 ×)

thesized bone matrix. *Osteoclasts* are large multinucleated cells responsible for bone resorption.

Bone collagen is secreted in a highly organized manner, resulting in the formation of layers of bone matrix called lamellae. Bone matrix is composed of collagen and other noncollagenous proteins, which in the newly deposited unmineralized state are termed osteoid (Fig. 46–3). The osteoid layer found along trabecular bone surfaces is termed an osteoid seam. Mineralization of osteoid is an orderly process that begins with the deposition of amorphous calcium phosphate at the interface between the osteoid seam and mineralized bone (i.e., the mineralization front). These nascent mineral deposits subsequently "mature" into hydroxyapatite crystals, the mineral phase characteristic of adult bone.

The binding affinity of autofluorescent tetracycline antibiotics for immature mineral deposits, but not the mature crystal, enables the identification of calcification foci and subsequently permits the determination of the rate of bone mineralization.

### Tetracycline as an In Vivo Bone Marker

Tetracycline antibiotics are utilized as biologic markers of mineralization.[1] During the first labeling course, tetracycline (dimethylchlortetracycline, oxytetracycline, or demeclocycline (1 g/day in divided doses) is administered for three days. After a 14-day, drug-free hiatus, a second course of tetracycline is given over a three-day interval. The bone biopsy is obtained three to four days after the last dose of tetracycline.

Tetracycline fluorescence is evaluated on unstained nondecalcified tissue sections by ultraviolet light. The first course of tetracycline appears as a discrete fluorescent band within the mineralized bone (Fig. 46–4). The second, more recently administered, course of tetracycline is located at the current mineralization front. The distance between the two bands represents the amount of new bone synthesized and mineralized over the drug-free interval.

## GROWTH AND REMODELING

Growth refers to a net increase in skeletal mass occurring prior to epiphyseal plate closure. Modeling is the shaping process responsible for maintaining the characteristic morphology of the growing bone. Both growth and modeling require that bone formation (osteoblast activity) and resorption (osteoclast activity) occur at anatomically separate sites.

### Coupling

Despite the fact that the skeleton is composed predominantly of inorganic extracellular matrix,

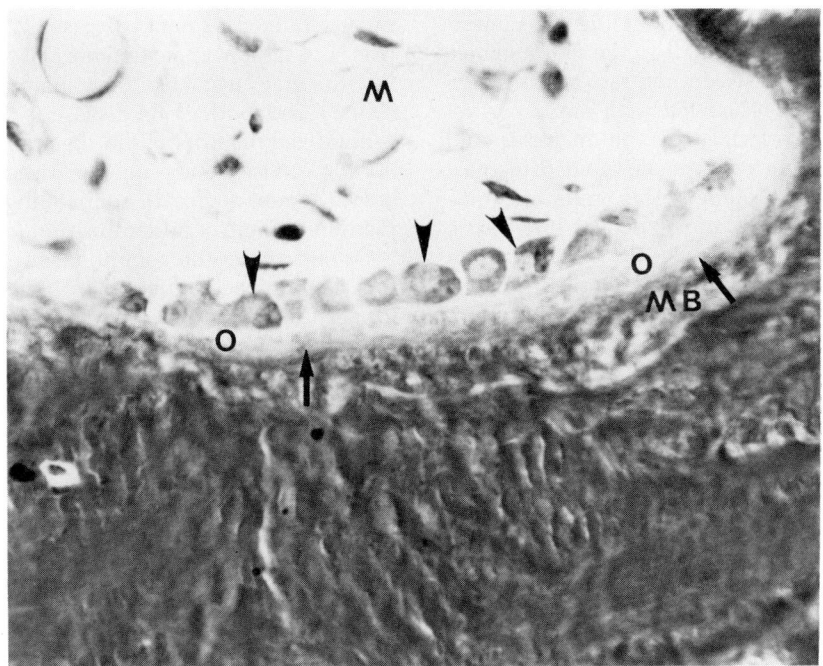

**Fig. 46–3.** Bone matrix synthesized by active, plump osteoblasts (arrowheads) forming an osteoid seam (O). Mineralization occurs at the junction between the mineralized bone (MB) and osteoid seam (arrows with O). M = marrow. (Masson trichrome stain; original magnification = 120 ×)

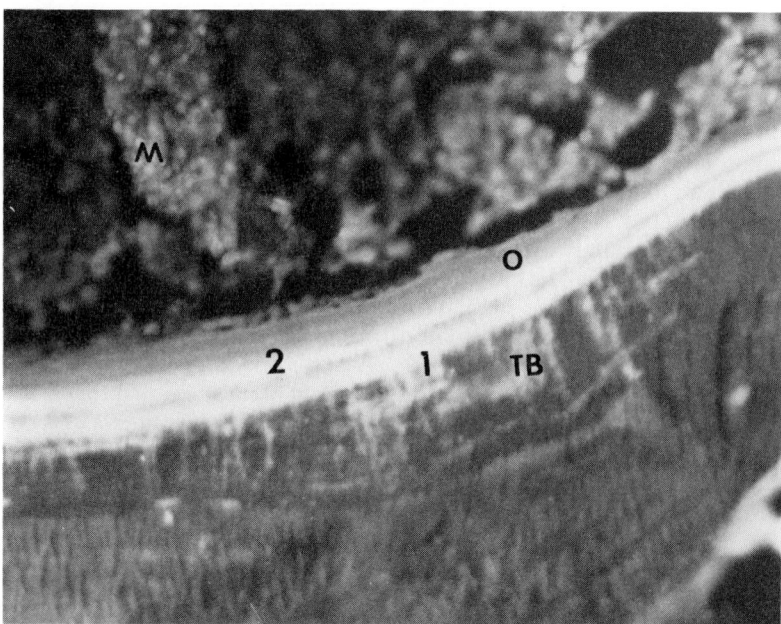

**Fig. 46–4.**   Similar field as in Figure 46–3, as viewed by fluorescent light to reveal the dual tetracycline labels. The first course of tetracycline (1) is buried in the mineralized trabecular bone (TB). The second course of tetracycline (2) marks the recent mineralization fronts at the osteoid seam interface (O). M = marrow.

bone is a dynamic organ, the microarchitecture of which is constantly being modified by two groups of hormonally responsive bone cells: osteoblasts and osteoclasts. The linked activation of osteoclasts and osteoblasts, termed coupling, is the basis of bone turnover or remodeling, the continuous skeletal activity related to the maintenance of mineral homeostasis. In contrast to the structural modification associated with modeling, remodeling is characterized by the anatomic and sequential coupling of osteoclast and osteoblast activity (Fig. 46–5). Remodeling units are initiated by the appearance of osteoclasts that resorb a packet of bone, creating a scalloped resorption bay or Howship's lacuna. Following osteoclastic activity, a reversal phase of varying duration ensues. A densely staining metachromatic line, the cement line, is formed at the limits of the resorption focus. The appearance of osteoblasts marks the end of the reversal phase as lamellar bone matrix is deposited in an appositional fashion, filling in the resorptive defect.

## METABOLIC BONE DISEASES: DEFINITIONS OF OSTEOPENIA, OSTEOPOROSIS, AND OSTEOMALACIA

The ability of the skeleton to provide structural support depends upon the skeletal mass, i.e., the amount of bone tissue, as well as the quality of that tissue, i.e., the degree of mineralization (Fig. 46–6). The amount of bone tissue is determined primarily by the location and extent of bone removal and formation during the remodeling cycle. Because the mineralization process and the level of bone remodeling are influenced by several systemic factors, disorders of these activities result in generalized skeletal disease. When the bone mass can no longer sustain normal forces, skeletal fracture may ensue, leading to pain and deformity. Thus, a metabolic bone disease is defined as any generalized disorder of the skeleton, regardless of etiology. Most metabolic bone diseases are due to either an imbalance in remodeling activity or a disorder of matrix mineralization (see Fig. 46–6).

Osteopenia is the generic term used to denote this generalized reduction in bone mass. By radiographic examination, the skeleton appears "washed out," or "demineralized." Osteoporosis and osteomalacia are the two major osteopenic syndromes. Osteoporosis is a group of diseases characterized by quantitatively low bone mass, but the composition of the remaining bone is chemically normal and, therefore, implies no assumption as to the pathogenesis. Osteomalacia, on the other hand, is a group of diseases characterized by bone that is qualitatively abnormal owing to an impaired state of mineralization. Defective mineralization of cartilage at the epiphyseal plate of growing bones is termed rickets.

### The Bone Biopsy

For any systemic skeletal disorder, a small sample of bone obtained from any skeletal site should

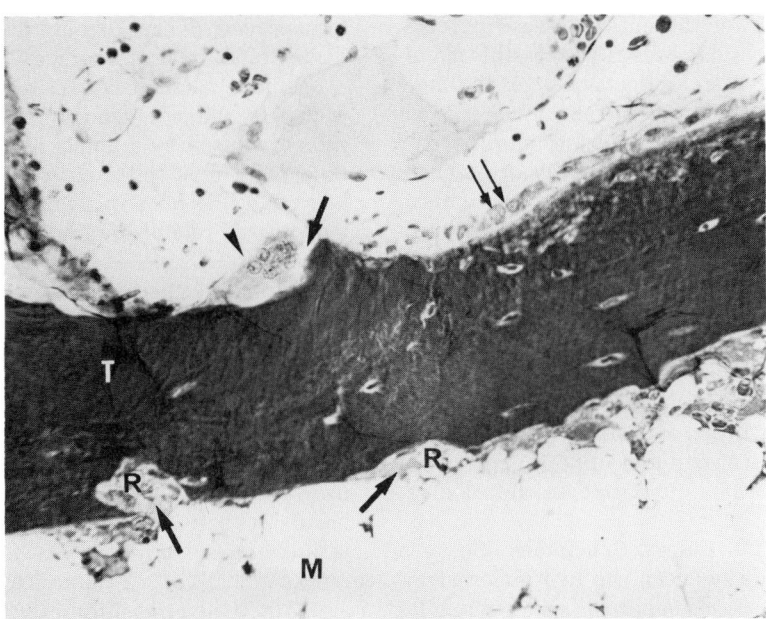

**Fig. 46–5.** The normal remodeling cycle. An osteoclast (arrowhead) resorbs a packet of bone, i.e., a Howship's lacuna (arrows). A reversal phase (R) denotes the transition phase between osteoclast activity and subsequent appearance of osteoblasts (double arrows). T = trabecular bone; M = marrow. (Masson trichrome stain; original magnification = 98 ×)

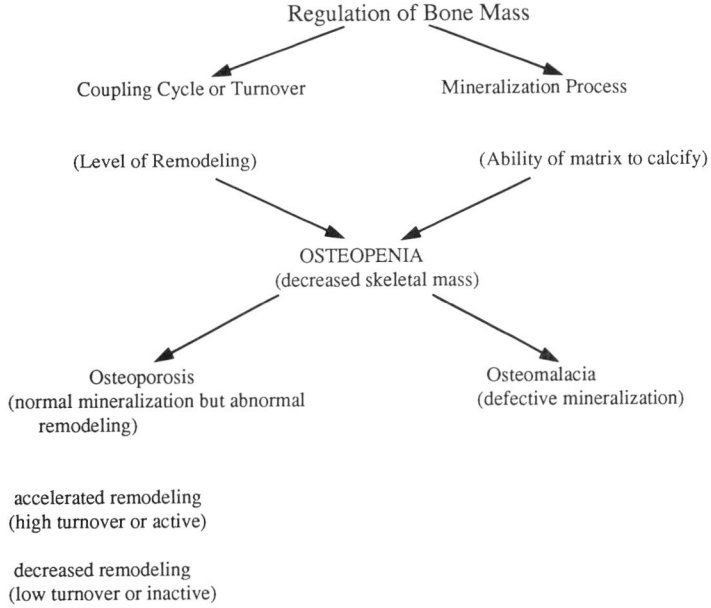

**Fig. 46–6.** Regulation of bone mass.

be representative of the entire disease process. The iliac crest region is a readily accessible standardized biopsy site and reflects changes that may be occurring at more clinically relevant sites, such as the spine or long bones. By examination of this representative bone tissue, the level of bone remodeling activity and the rate of bone mineralization may be determined. The bone biopsy procedure and the direct examination of bone tissue have become important tools in the differential diagnosis of metabolic bone diseases.

Trocars ranging from 5 to 8 mm in diameter are commercially available. A biopsy of the anterior iliac crest may be performed transcutaneously under local anesthesia, as shown in Figure 46–7, to produce a core or cylinder of bone. The actual biopsy procedure is described in detail elsewhere.[2]

**Processing Bone Biopsy Specimens.** Because the differentiation between the two major metabolic bone diseases, osteoporosis and osteomalacia, is based in part upon the quantity and quality of bone mineral, the ability to distinguish between calcified bone matrix and uncalcified bone matrix (osteoid) is critical. The traditional procedures for processing bone, acid decalcification and paraffin embedding, require the removal of inorganic matrix to facilitate histologic sectioning and, there-fore, prevent the subsequent determination of the degree of skeletal mineralization.

In nondecalcified bone sections, osteomalacia is usually characterized by the accumulation of osteoid caused by a defect in the mineralization process. It must be recognized, however, that excess quantities of osteoid may result not only from a decreased rate of mineralization, but also from an accelerated rate of bone matrix synthesis. In routine nondecalcified bone sections, these two forms of osteoid excess appear identical (Fig. 46–8). Differentiation between these states is based upon the determination of mineralization rates, using tetracycline as an in vivo bone marker.

The mean distance between the midpoints of the double tetracycline labels is measured with a linear reticle. This distance divided by the number of days between the two courses of tetracycline is the *mineral appositional rate* and normally ranges from 0.4 to 0.9 $\mu$m/day (mean 0.65 $\mu$m/day).

As the bone apposition rate increases, the distance between the labels grows wider (Fig. 46–9). In contrast, with a reduced mineralization rate, the parallel bands become narrow and may fuse to produce single labels.

Abnormal patterns of fluorescent label deposition are the hallmark of osteomalacia, and represent the morphologic expression of defective

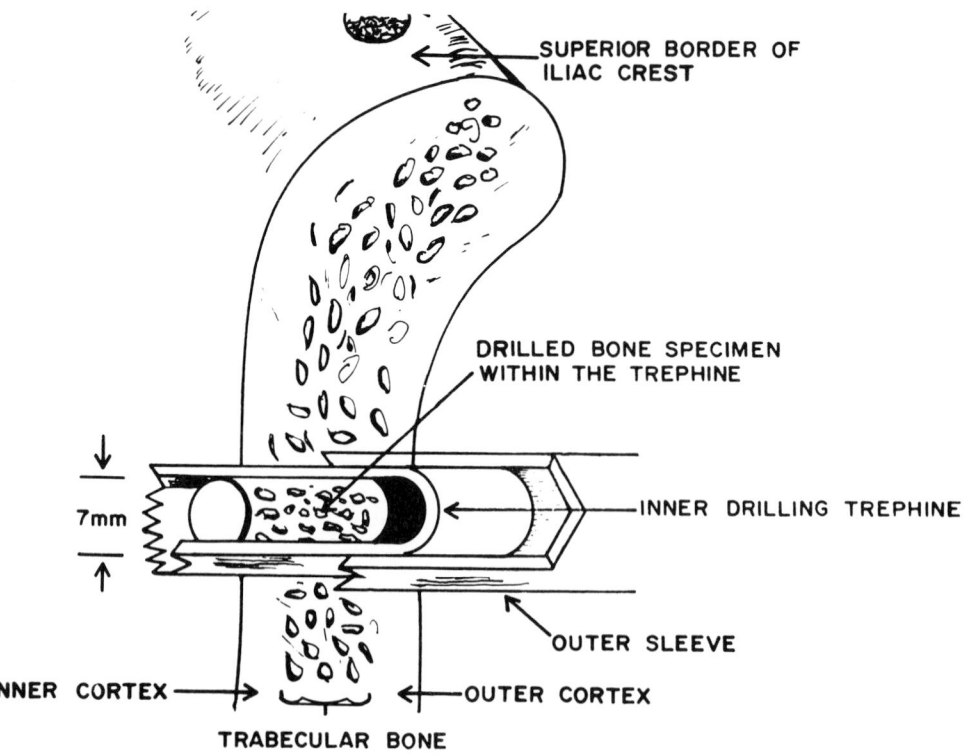

**Fig. 46–7.**   Diagram showing the standard biopsy procedure for obtaining a core of iliac bone.

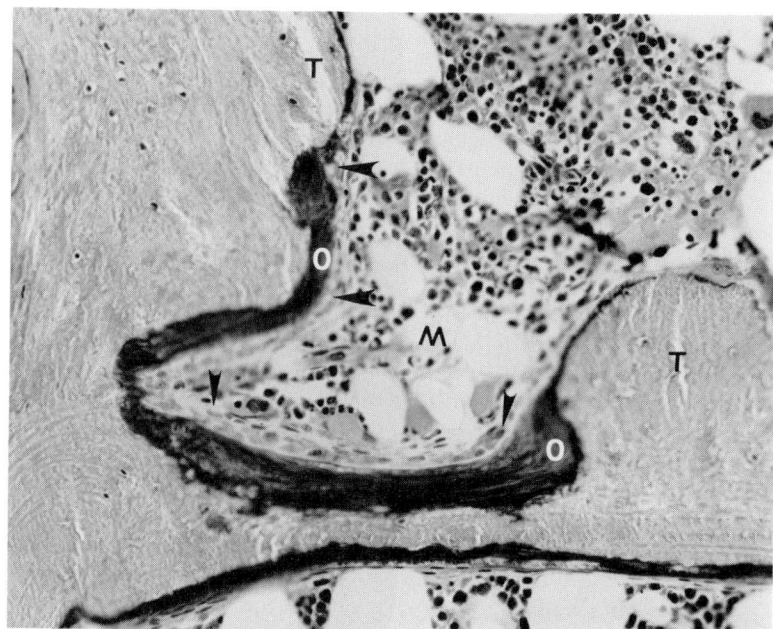

**Fig. 46–8.** Increased quantity of osteoid (O). Increased thickness of the osteoid seam may be due to accelerated matrix synthesis by osteoblasts (arrowheads) stemming from an abnormally high remodeling condition, or may result from defective mineralization secondary to an osteomalacic disorder. T = trabecular bone; M = marrow. (Goldner trichrome stain, original magnification = 250 ×)

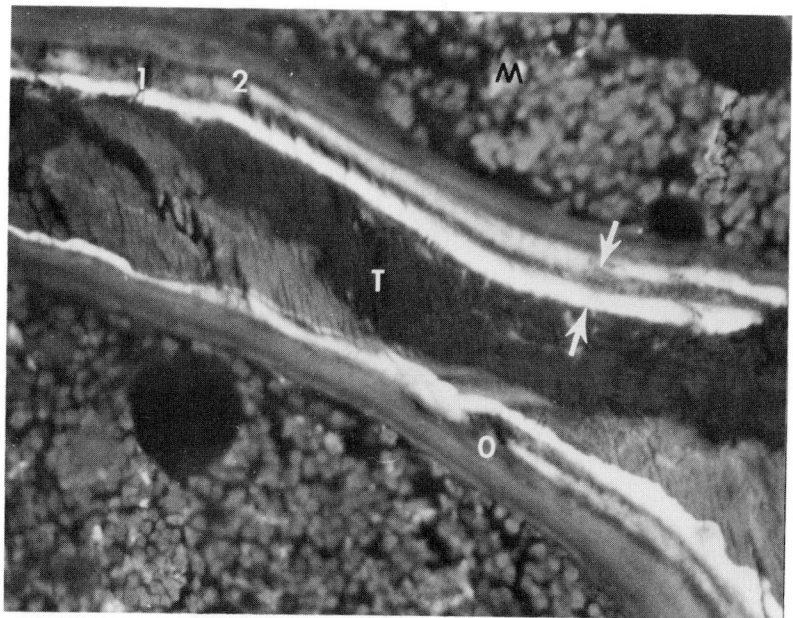

**Fig. 46–9.** The increased quantity of osteoid in Figure 46–8 was proven to reflect active bone remodeling, and not osteomalacia as revealed by the widely spaced dual tetracycline labels (arrows). Compare label distance to that of normal tissue in Figure 46–4. T = trabecular bone; M = marrow; O = osteoid; 1 = first course of tetracycline; 2 = second course of tetracycline.

mineralization.[3] The amount of tetracycline fluorescence is proportional to the amount of the immature amorphous calcium phosphate deposits in the mineralizing foci of the osteoid seam.

A common abnormal tetracycline pattern characteristic of osteomalacia is diffuse irregular fluorescence of an entire osteoid seam. Accumulation of immature bone mineral is thought to reflect a failure of maturation of amorphous calcium phosphate into hydroxyapatite crystals, thus permitting excessive tetracycline binding (Fig. 46–10). In some cases, osteoid seams are deficient in mineral and, therefore, osteoid is incapable of binding tetracycline, leading to an absence of fluorescence. As a result, the *mineralization front activity* (percentage of osteoid seams bearing normal tetracycline labels) is reduced (Fig. 46–11). It must be stressed that osteomalacia may occur with a normal quantity of osteoid (Fig. 46–12). Defective mineralization can only reliably be determined by kinetic tetracycline labeling.

The histologic techniques designed for the demonstration of bone mineral and tetracycline markers require the examination of nondecalcified tissue. Thus, specialized embedding and sectioning procedures have been developed.

To obtain nondecalcified tissue sections, bone is embedded without prior demineralization in methyl methacrylate (MM) plastic and sectioned on a heavy-duty, sledge microtome equipped with a carbide-tungsten-tipped steel blade.[4] This technique is laborious and requires rigorous tissue dehydration, careful attention to resin preparation, polymerization, and specialized equipment, thereby limiting ready application. Alternative simplified procedures utilize less expensive and more commonly available equipment.[5] The routine histologic evaluation of bone has been made possible by sectioning glycol methacrylate (GMA)-embedded tissue on glass knives.

**Bone Histomorphometry.** Bone histomorphometry is the quantitative analysis of undecalcified bone in which the skeletal remodeling parameters are expressed in terms of volumes, surfaces, and cell numbers[6] (Fig. 46–13)(Table 46–1).

To obtain this information from the two-dimensional format, principles of stereology are used to reconstruct the third dimension. This principle, described by the French mineralogist Delesse in 1848, simply states that if measurements are made at random on infinitely thin sections, the ratio of areas is equal to the ratio of volumes. Areas are measured by counting the number of cross-marks or "hits" formed by an array of points in the grid (see Fig. 46–13). The points are projected onto the field from a grid in the microscope eyepiece. The average number of cross-marks or hits that fall on the histologic feature of interest (as a fraction of the total number of possible hits) is equal to the volume of that component within the total unit volume. Measurements of bone surfaces or perimeter lengths are obtained by counting the number

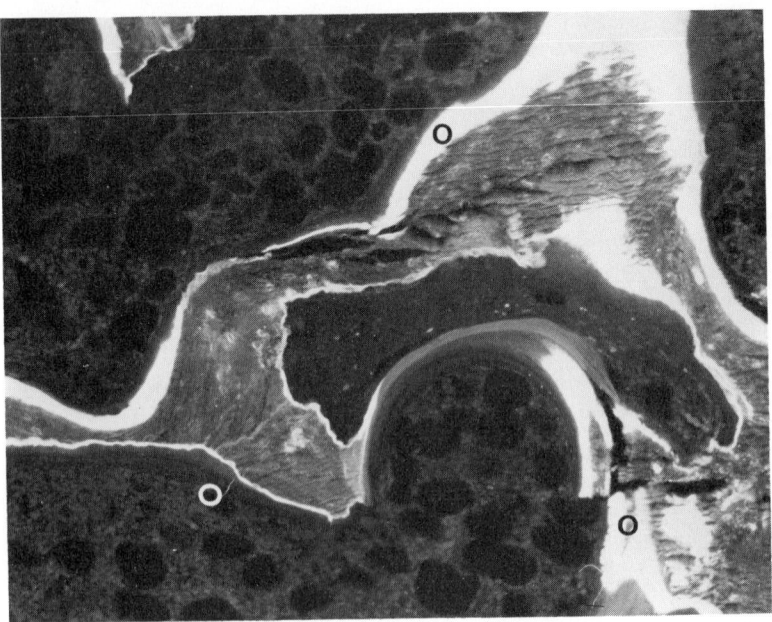

**Fig. 46–10.** Abnormal tetracycline fluorescent pattern diagnostic of osteomalacia. Defective mineralization in this instance is revealed by wide, diffuse uptake of tetracycline at the broad osteoid seams (O). (Unstained, fluorescent micrograph; original magnification = 60 ×)

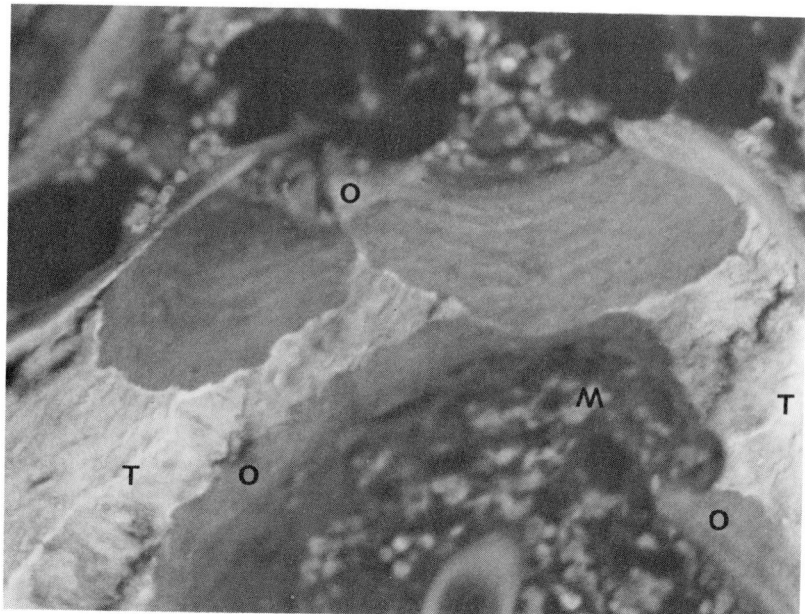

**Fig. 46–11.** A second common abnormal tetracycline in vivo reaction diagnostic of osteomalacia. Defective mineralization in this instance is characterized by an absence of tetracycline uptake, with failure of the osteoid seams (O) to fluoresce. T = trabecular bone; M = marrow; O = osteoid. (Unstained section; original magnification = 340 ×)

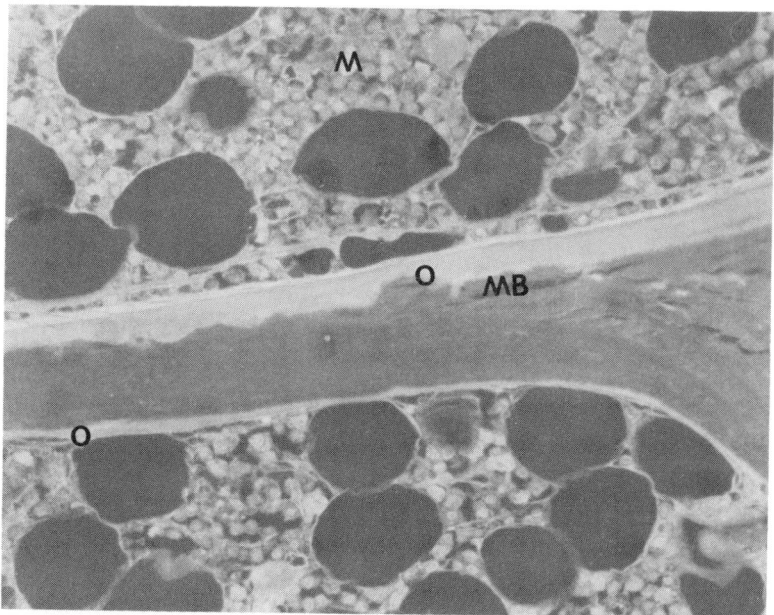

**Fig. 46–12.** This micrograph stresses the importance of performing in vivo tetracycline labeling prior to the biopsy. Despite a normal quantity of osteoid (O), the presence of a mineralization defect is demonstrated by the absence of tetracycline uptake at the mineralization fronts, i.e., the junction between the osteoid seams (O) and the mineralized bone interface (MB). Compare to Figures 46–8 and 46–9. M = marrow. (Unstained section; original magnification = 250 ×)

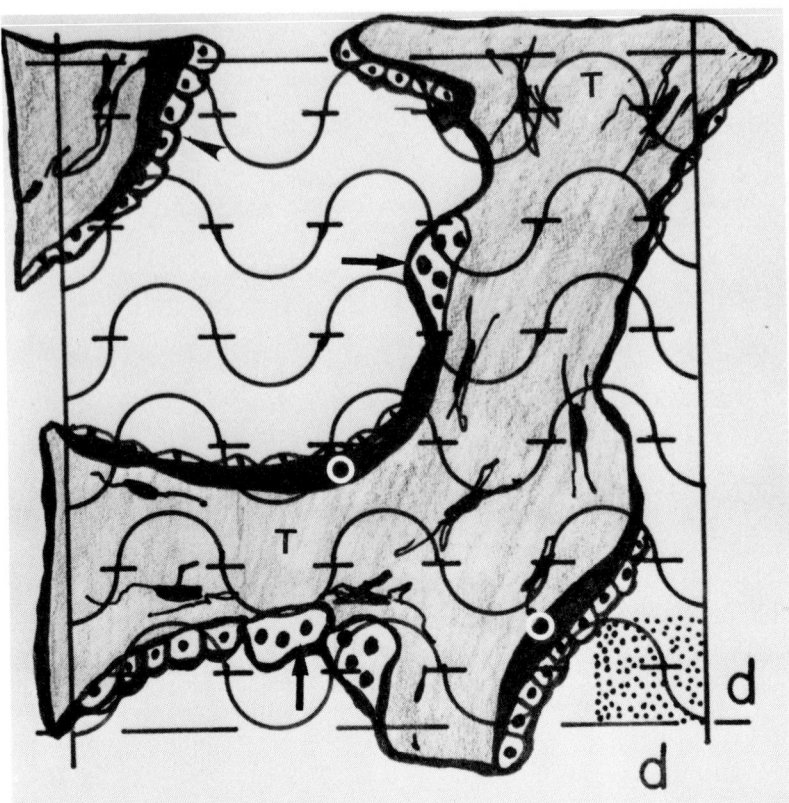

**Fig. 46–13.** Histomorphometry. A Merz-Schenk grid in the microscope eyepiece is shown projected onto a field of mineralized bone (light shading), osteoid (dark shading), and marrow (no shading). Of the cross-marks or hits in the grid, 13 are superimposed on mineralized bone, 3 on osteoid, 16 on marrow, 2 on osteoclasts, and 2 on osteoblasts. Therefore, 44.4% of the field is bone. Because 3 of the 16 hits on bone fall on osteoid, the relative osteoid volume is 18.8%. The absolute area occupied by the grid is 36 times the square of the distance (d) between the hits (area = $36d^2$). When viewed at 250 × magnification, "d" is measured by a calibrated ocular micrometer (the grid covers 0.155 $mm^2$). Approximately 200 fields (30 $mm^2$) should be measured for statistically valid results. The six semicircular parallel lines help compensate for nonrandomly oriented trabeculae, and the distance between the lines (d) is the same as that between hits. There are 18 intersections with the trabecular perimeter. Seven intersections are at osteoid surfaces, 5 are at resting mineralized surfaces, and 4 are at osteoclast-filled Howship's lacunae. Therefore, the osteoid surface is 38.9%, the resting surface 27.8%, and the active resorption surface 22.2% of the total number of intersections with the bone perimeter. O = osteoid; T = trabecular bone, arrow = osteoclast; arrowheads = osteoblasts lining osteoid seam.

of intersections between the bone perimeter and equidistant parallel grid lines. Distance between two items of interest, such as the distance between two tetracycline labels, is measured by a calibrated linear reticle.

**Bone Remodeling and Mineralization: Determinants of Bone Mass.** The level of bone remodeling activity is determined by a variety of calcium-regulating hormones (see Chapter 13). During states of calcium deficiency, parathyroid hormone is secreted, which stimulates osteoclastic bone resorption and liberates calcium and phosphate from apatite crystals. At the same time, renal tubular reabsorption of calcium is stimulated and urinary excretion of phosphate is enhanced. Elevated PTH is also a stimulus for increased 1,25 dihydroxyvitamin D production by

the kidney. Parent vitamin D, either produced in the skin by photoactivation or obtained by dietary sources, circulates in the blood and is converted to 25 hydroxyvitamin D by hepatic hydroxylase enzymes; 25 (OH) vitamin D serves as the renal substrate for further hydroxylation. This active dihydroxylated vitamin D stimulates intestinal absorption of calcium and, at supraphysiologic levels, stimulates osteoclastic activity.

Mineralization of osteoid matrix is promoted by optimum ambient calcium and phosphate levels maintained by the aforementioned hormones. Mineralization is facilitated by the enzyme alkaline phosphatase, which may remove endogenous crystallization inhibitors such as pyrophosphates. Other exogenous agents such as the diphosphonates, utilized in the treatment of Paget's disease

**Table 46–1.  Histomorphometric Parameters**

| Symbol | Determination | Range | Definition |
|---|---|---|---|
| TBV | trabecular bone volume | 15–25% | Percentage biopsy tissue occupied by mineralized and unmineralized bone tissue. |
| ROV | relative osteoid volume | 0.6–4.0% | Percentage trabecular bone volume composed of osteoid. |
| TOS | total osteoid surface | 4–20% | Percentage trabecular bone surface covered by osteoid seams. A function of the number of osteoblasts. |
| MOSW | mean osteoid seam width | 8–16 μm | Thickness of osteoid seams. A function of osteoblast cell activity. |
| OB | osteoblastic osteoid | 35–40% of osteoid or 2–8% of total trabecular surface | Percentage trabecular surface covered by osteoid lined by cuboidal osteoblasts. (Function of cell recruitment or number of osteoblasts.) |
| ARS | active resorptive surface | <0.5% | Percentage trabecular surface covered with osteoclasts. A function of the bone surface engaged in resorption. |
| OC | osteoclast number | 0.1–0.3/mm² | Number of osteoclasts per square millimeter of trabecular bone. |
| FIB | peritrabecular fibrosis | 0% | Percentage trabecular surface covered by fibrous tissue. |
| LEBF fract Lab | linear extent of bone formation or fractional labeled surface | 10–17% | Extent of tetracycline labeled surface, as a fraction of the total trabecular surface. A function of the number of active cells. |
| MF | mineralization front activity | 60–80% | Percentage mineralized bone-osteoid seam interfaces labeled with tetracycline. |
| AR,CR | appositional rate, calcification rate | .4–.9 μm/day | Average amount of new matrix deposited and mineralized over the tetracycline labeling period. A function of cell activity. |
| MLT | mineralization lag time | 11–23 days | Derived by dividing the mean osteoid seam width by the appositional rate. An index of the length of time that osteoid once synthesized becomes mineralized. |
| BFR | bone formation rate | 0.3–0.8 μm/day | Amount of bone made per day. Derived from the LEBF multiplied by the AR. A function, therefore, of cell activity and cell number. |

of bone, and sodium fluoride, an experimental agent utilized in osteoporosis therapy, may inhibit further crystal accumulation and may induce osteomalacia. It is unclear whether vitamin D metabolites play a direct role in osteoid maturation and mineralization, or whether they promote mineralization secondarily by maintaining serum calcium and phosphorus levels (see section on vitamin D deficiency states).

Bone cell activity is influenced by physical forces, endocrine-hormone levels, and nutritional-metabolic factors, all of which are summarized in Table 46–2. Normally bone resorption and formation are in balance (Figs. 46–14, 46–15). A net loss of bone tissue may occur from excessive bone resorption or deficient bone formation, or a combination of both, during the coupling cycle.

Bone remodeling activity may be categorized as either accelerated or reduced. Both of these high- and low-turnover states may result in a reduction of bone mass. Accelerated bone turnover is usually the result of an absolute increase in bone re-

**Table 46–2.  Determinants of Bone Turnover**

| | Resorption | Formation |
|---|---|---|
| Parathyroid hormone | ↑ | ↑ |
| Thyroxine | ↑ | ↑ |
| Calcitonin | ↓ | — |
| Estrogen | ↓ | — |
| Calcium | ↓ | — |
| Phosphate | ↓ | ↑ |
| 1,25 (OH)₂ vitamin D | ↑ | ↑ |
| Corticosteroids | ↓ or ↑ | ↓ |
| Growth hormone | ↑ | ↑ |

Determinants of Bone Mineralization

Promoters: Calcium, phosphate, vitamin D, alkaline phosphatase

Inhibitors: pyrophosphates, fluoride

sorption. At the cellular level, osteoclast activity is enhanced such that a greater volume of bone is removed at a given remodeling site. These unusually deep Howship's lacunae cannot be filled by normal osteoblast activity (see Fig. 46–14, B₁ and B₂). At the tissue level (see Fig. 46–15, B₁ and

# MECHANISMS OF REDUCED BONE MASS - CELL LEVEL
## (BONE REMODELING UNIT ACTIVITY)

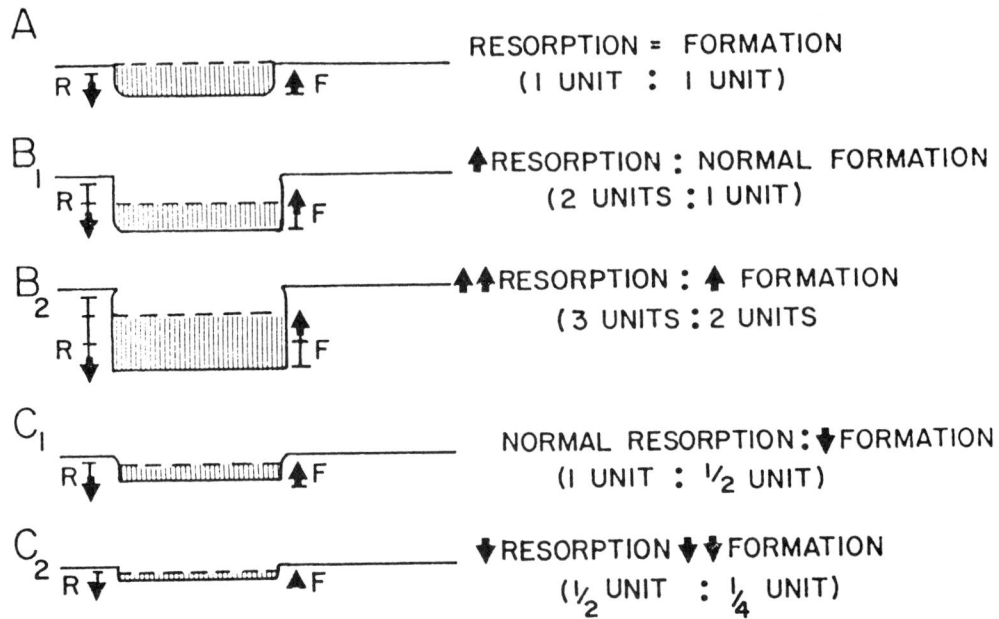

**Fig. 46–14.** Mechanisms of reduced bone mass at the cell level. A depicts skeletal balance (R = F); $B_1$ and $B_2$ depict negative balance (R>F) with high turnover; $C_1$ and $C_2$ depict negative balance (R>F) with low turnover (see text).

$B_2$) there may be a recruitment of new bone remodeling units such that the number of active resorbing sites increases. Given the normal coupling of bone formation to resorption, accelerated bone turnover is often accompanied by an increase in bone formation. Despite this compensatory increase in bone formation at the cell and tissue level, a net loss of bone ensues, owing to overriding bone resorptive activity (see Fig. 46–15, $B_2$).

Low bone remodeling states are often associated with a relative increase in bone resorption, such that the actual rate and extent of bone formation are reduced (see Figs. 46–14, 46–15, $C_1$ and $C_2$). Even if bone resorption is reduced, there is often a greater reduction in osteoblast function, resulting in a lower level of turnover, that nonetheless produces a steady loss of bone mass.

## Histopathologic Appearance of Metabolic Bone Diseases

Histologically, metabolic bone diseases appear as disorders of either increased remodeling activity, decreased remodeling activity, or defective mineralization (osteomalacia).

**Increased Bone Remodeling Activity (Accel-**

**erated Bone Turnover).** States of high turnover (see Fig. 46–15) are characterized by evidence of increased bone formation and increased resorption (Figs. 46–16, 46–17, 46–18). Histologic correlates of increased formation include: increased quantities of osteoid, increased osteoid surfaces, moderately increased osteoid seam thickness, and increased osteoblastic surfaces (Table 46–3). Tetracycline fluorescence may show an increase in the fraction of trabecular bone surfaces bearing double labels, indicating an increase in the linear extent of bone formation (Fig. 46–18B). The linear extent parameter is a function of the activation of additional osteoblasts. The mineralization rate (the distance between the double labels) may be increased, reflecting an augmentation of individual cell activity. Increased resorptive activity is manifested by an increase in the number of osteoclasts, and by the fraction of bone surfaces engaged in bone resorption resulting in Howship's lacunae complete with osteoclasts. Peritrabecular fibrous tissue deposition indicating osteitis fibrosa is a manifestation of general increased mesenchymal cell activity. This feature is not peculiar to hyperparathyroidism, but may be associated

# MECHANISMS OF REDUCED BONE MASS – TISSUE LEVEL
## (NUMBER OF BONE REMODELING UNITS)

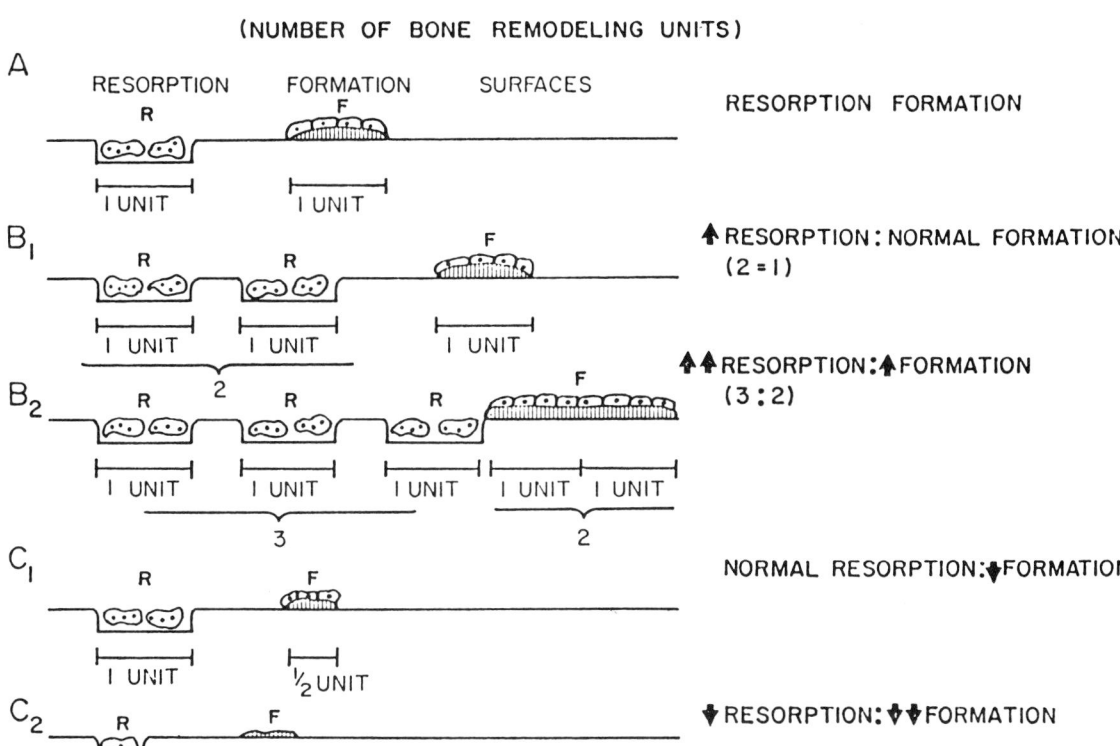

**Fig. 46–15.** Mechanisms of reduced bone mass at the tissue level. A depicts skeletal balance (R surface = F surface); $B_1$ and $B_2$ depict negative balance (R surface > F surface) with high turnover; $C_1$ and $C_2$ depict negative balance (R surface > F surface) with low turnover (see text).

with any condition resulting in accelerated tissue turnover (Fig. 46–19).

**Decreased Bone Remodeling Activity (Reduced Bone Turnover).** These states show little evidence of either bone formation or resorption (Table 46–4). Consequently, osteoid seams are thin and scanty, osteoblasts are flattened, and osteoclasts are reduced in number (Fig. 46–20A). Few tetracycline labels are apparent, consistent with the amount of osteoid seen by light microscopy. As a result, the *mineralization front activity* (fraction of tetracycline-labeled osteoid surface) is preserved, but is associated with a reduction in the linear extent of bone formation (fraction of labeled trabecular bone surfaces). Single fluorescent labels predominate (Fig. 46–20B), because the rate of bone matrix deposition is low enough to prevent spatial separation of the two courses of tetracycline.

**Osteomalacia.** Osteomalacia is usually characterized by excessive quantities of osteoid due to a failure of matrix calcification, despite continued matrix synthesis by osteoblasts (Table 46–5).

Marked increases in the thickness of osteoid seams are characteristic, but osteomalacia may be associated with normal or even reduced quantities of osteoid.[7] The static and dynamic parameters that characterize osteomalacia include an increase in the amount of osteoid, and a reciprocal decrease in the rate of mineralization, respectively. These two components allow one to distinguish osteomalacia from other disorders of bone remodeling activity manifesting abnormal quantities of osteoid. In low-turnover states, for example, the mineralization rate may be low, but the quantity of osteoid is appropriately reduced. If the mineralization rate is not low, the presence of a mineralization defect is unlikely, despite the presence of excess amounts of osteoid, as seen in high-turnover states when matrix synthesis is accelerated.

Although osteomalacia is usually associated with low bone remodeling activity, features of osteoblast activation, osteoclast proliferation, and peritrabecular fibrosis, all indicative of accelerated turnover, may be present. Osteomalacia is, therefore, often seen in the context of a mixed bone lesion, coexisting with osteitis fibrosa.

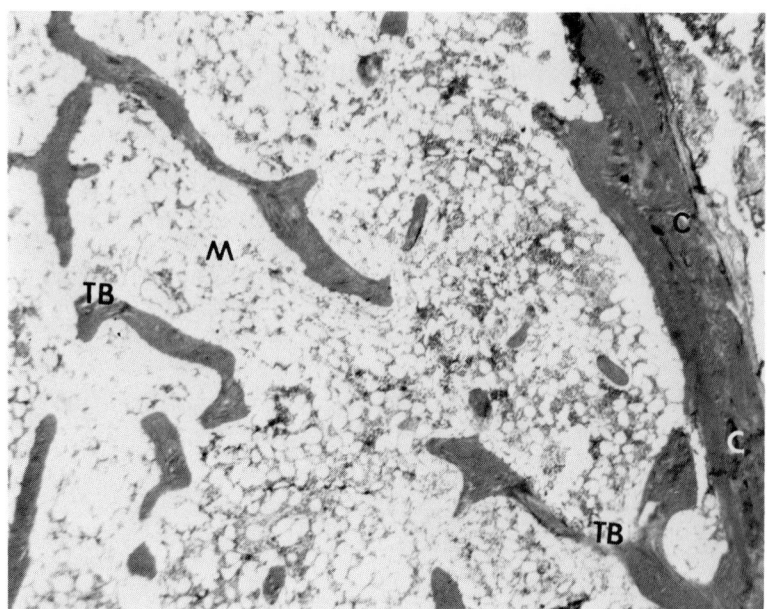

**Fig. 46–16.** Osteoporosis. Low-power photomicrograph shows a reduction in cortical width (C) and a loss of trabecular bone spicules (TB). Compare to Figure 46–1. M = marrow. (Masson trichrome stain; original magnification = 25 ×)

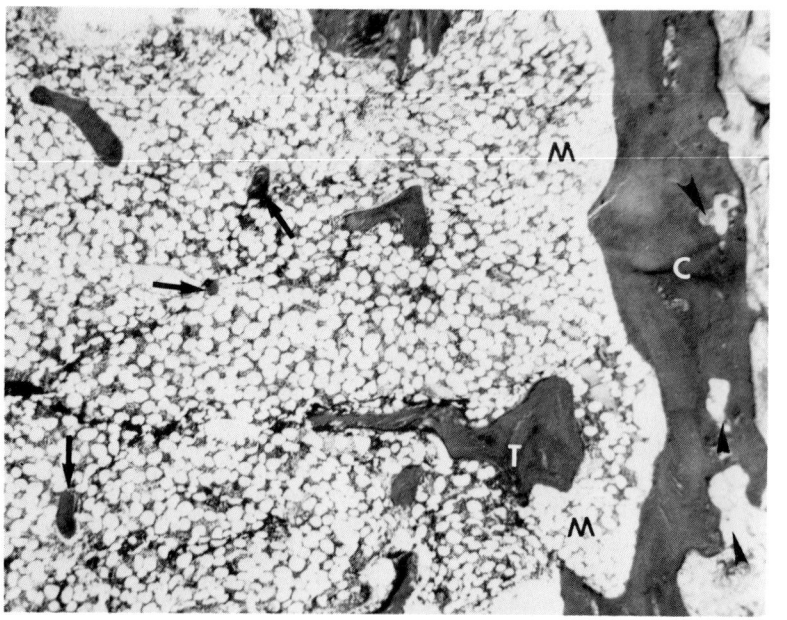

**Fig. 46–17.** Osteoporosis. Low-power photomicrograph illustrates a further progression of the osteopenic state. Trabecular bone is now reduced to islands and thin spicules (arrows) of bone, instead of intact struts or bars. Compare to Figure 46–1. Note the reduction in cortical thickness, and an increase in cortical porosity (arrowheads) due to resorption of bone by activated osteoclasts within haversian cutting cones. C = cortical bone; T = trabecular bone; M = marrow. (Masson trichrome stain; original magnification 25 ×)

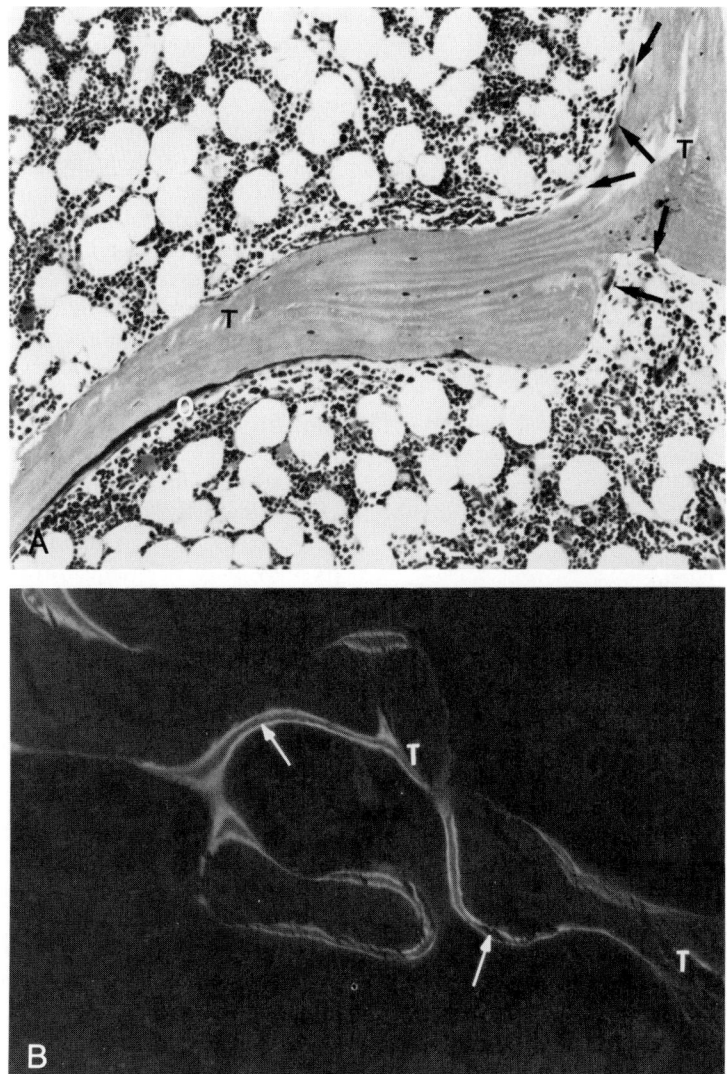

**Fig. 46–18.** *A,* Active remodeling osteoporosis. Notice the increased total osteoid surface (O), and the increased number of osteoclasts (arrows) along the trabecular bone (T). This biopsy was taken from a patient with postgastrectomy osteoporosis. (Masson trichrome stain; original magnification = 160 ×) *B,* Corresponding fluorescent photomicrograph showing an increase in the linear extent of bone formation as revealed by the extensive double tetracycline labeled surfaces (arrows). T = trabecular bone. (Unstained section; original magnification = 98 ×)

Examples of osteomalacia are shown in Figures 46–21*A* and *B.*

## SKELETAL MANIFESTATIONS OF NUTRITIONAL DISEASES

Bone plays a major role in calcium and mineral homeostasis and, as a result, the skeleton is sensitive to metabolic and hormonal imbalances. It is, therefore, not surprising that a wide variety of abnormalities of nutrition influence the skeleton (Table 46–6). Nutritional disorders either may result in defective mineralization producing osteomalacia or may manifest as osteoporosis. The os-

teoporotic conditions may result from either accelerated remodeling or reduced remodeling.

The skeleton is limited in the manner in which the tissue and cells respond to injury. The histologic differential diagnosis of metabolic diseases is, therefore, broad because various metabolic, endocrine, or nutritional disorders may produce similar morphologic changes in the skeleton.

The primary role of the bone biopsy procedure, therefore, is not to provide a diagnosis of a specific disease, but rather to establish the level of bone turnover and to confirm or to exclude the presence of a mineralization defect. In this manner, a list

**Table 46–3. Histologic Features of Increased Bone Remodeling Activity (Accelerated Turnover)**

Bone Formation Parameters
    Increased osteoid volume
    Increased osteoid surface
    Normal to increased osteoid seam width
    Increased osteoblastic surface

Tetracycline Kinetic Parameters
    Increased linear extent of bone formation
    Double fluorescent labels predominate
    Normal to increased appositional rate
    Mineralization front activity maximal
    Increased bone formation rate
    Normal or decreased mineralization lag time

Bone Resorption Parameters
    Increased osteoclast number
    Increased active resorbing surface
    Subperiosteal resorption

Other
    Increased cortical porosity
    Active cutting cones in cortex
    Decreased cortical width
    Osteitis fibrosa (peritrabecular fibrous tissue)
    Woven bone

of diagnostic possibilities is obtained, and the differential diagnosis is narrowed by a multidisciplinary approach involving clinical, laboratory, and radiologic findings.

## Idiopathic Osteoporosis

Idiopathic or primary osteoporosis is subdivided by the age at presentation and sex of the individual (e.g., postmenopausal or senile). The age-related or involutional bone loss for both sexes is well characterized, such that there is a progressive loss of cortical and trabecular bone (see Fig. 46–16, 46–17) with age in men and women, with a transient accelerated phase of loss that occurs in women after the menopause. Although involutional osteoporosis is heterogeneous and the etiology complex, bone loss is thought to be due to a variety of age-related factors including osteoblast senescence with reduced bone formation, decreased calcium absorption with decreased production of 1,25 $(OH)_2$ vitamin D and gastrointestinal resistance to its action, mild secondary hyperparathyroidism, calcitonin deficiency, and estrogen withdrawal. When calcium absorption from the diet is insufficient to offset fecal and urinary calcium losses, calcium must be withdrawn from the bone. The minimum daily requirement is currently set at 800 mg/day. The middle-aged and elderly may have actual daily intakes far less than this amount. Although normal adults adapt to decreased calcium intake by increasing the fraction of absorbed dietary calcium, this compensatory mechanism is blunted

by aging. Thus, the calcium requirement for postmenopausal women has been estimated to be as high as 1,500 mg/day to prevent negative calcium balance.

Although the importance of an adequate intake of calcium to promote growth is well known, the role of calcium intake in preventing osteoporosis is controversial.[8,9] Additional studies are required before final conclusions can be made.[10] In the meantime, prevention of osteoporosis should be directed at correcting low dietary calcium intakes (800 mg/day for adults and 1,500 mg/day for adolescents are minimum daily requirements). The National Institutes of Health Consensus Conference on Osteoporosis recommended a daily calcium intake of 1,000 to 1,500 mg for all postmenopausal women.[11]

Histologically, postmenopausal osteoporosis is a heterogeneous disorder. Bone remodeling activity may be accelerated, normal, or decreased.[12] Serum and urine biochemical tests fail to separate these groups. This heterogeneity of osteoporosis may be partly responsible for the current disappointing results of drug therapy trials. It has been postulated, based upon bone biopsy-derived tetracycline dynamics and the identification of active and inactive groups, that different therapies may be required. For example, calcium is known to inhibit osteoclast activity. Patients with inactive osteoporosis who are treated with vitamin D and calcium may undergo further depression of an already low bone remodeling status, such that the restoration of bone mass is unlikely.[13] The treatment of osteoporosis is described in detail elsewhere.[10]

## Calcium Deficiency, Chronic

The circulating calcium concentration is tightly regulated by a variety of hormones. The skeleton is the major reservoir for calcium, and during states of calcium deprivation, calcium homeostasis is maintained at the expense of the skeleton, even to the point of producing severe bone disease. The major response to hypocalcemia is the compensatory increase in parathyroid hormone secretion. Parathyroid hormone acts to increase bone resorption, and thereby to accelerate bone remodeling activity. Chronic hypocalcemia conditions such as chronic renal failure, vitamin D deficiency states, and mineral malabsorption secondary to gastrointestinal disease may exhibit evidence of increased bone turnover.

**Calcium Deficiency in Children.** Although calcium deficiency usually leads to secondary hyperparathyroidism with increased bone resorption, low dietary calcium intake in children may result in rickets and osteomalacia.[14] Defective

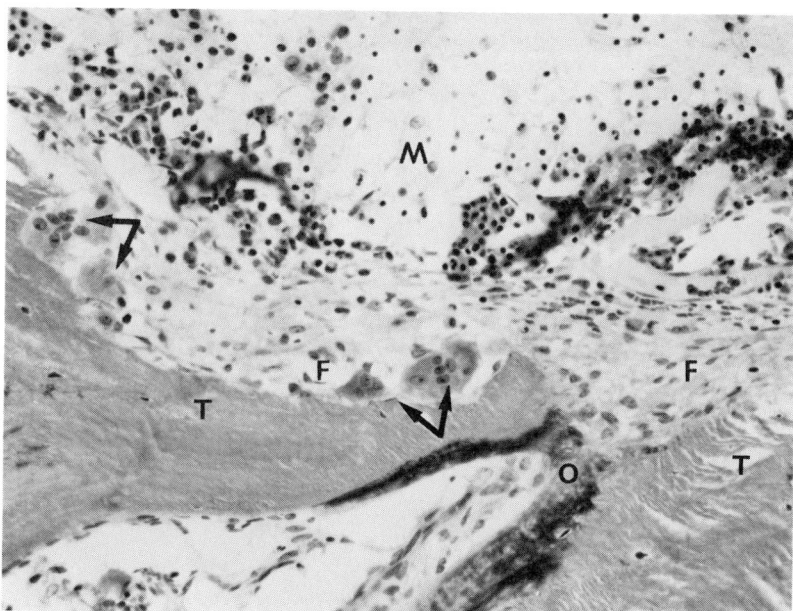

**Fig. 46–19.** Osteitis fibrosa, a manifestation of accelerated bone turnover, characterized by increased numbers of osteoclasts (arrows) and peritrabecular fibrosis (F). This biopsy was obtained from an osteoporotic patient with mineral malabsorption due to small intestinal disease with subsequent hypocalcemia and secondary hyperparathyroidism. T = trabecular bone; O = osteoid, M = marrow. (Goldner trichrome stain; original magnification = 250 ×)

mineralization is expressed more readily in this younger group than in adults because of the increased calcium demands required during skeletal growth.

## Hypophosphatemia

Mineralization of skeletal tissue requires phosphorus as well as calcium in the deposition of amorphous calcium phosphate and in the formation of hydroxyapatite crystals. Various clinical disorders are associated with hypophosphatemia. The skeletal disease consists of rickets in children and osteomalacia in adults. Histologi-

**Table 46–4. Histologic Features of Decreased Bone Remodeling Activity (Reduced Turnover)**

Bone Formation Parameters
    Normal to decreased osteoid volume
    Decreased osteoid surface
    Normal to decreased osteoid seam width
    Reduced osteoblastic surface

Tetracycline Kinetic Parameters
    Decreased linear extent of bone formation
    Single labels predominate
    Normal to reduced appositional rate
    Mineralization front activity low to normal
    Low bone formation rate
    Normal mineralization lag time

Bone Resorption Parameters
    Decreased osteoclast number
    Decreased active resorption surface

cally, osteomalacia exists in a pure form, i.e., low-turnover osteomalacia without evidence of osteitis fibrosa.

**X-Linked Hypophosphatemia (XLH).** XLH, also known as vitamin D-resistant rickets, familial hypophosphatemia, and phosphate diabetes, is the most common form of hereditary rickets and osteomalacia. XLH is characterized by a primary defect in renal transport of phosphorus resulting in hypophosphatemia. Histologically, osteoid excess is usually marked, with extremely widened osteoid seams covering virtually all bone surfaces, resulting in osteosclerosis. In addition, hypomineralized zones surround the osteocytes, producing a ring of osteoid (Fig. 46–22). This "halo" effect is thought to represent a mineralization defect around newly formed osteocytes, and a characteristic feature of this disorder.[15]

**Sporadic Hypophosphatemia.** Renal phosphorus wasting may also occur without a family history and may be present any time from infancy to adulthood.

### Oncogenic Osteomalacia

Oncogenic osteomalacia is caused by a secreted tumor product that inhibits renal tubular reabsorption of phosphorus and the 1-hydroxylation of 25-hydroxyvitamin D, resulting in hypophosphatemia and inappropriately low levels of 1,25 $(OH)_2$ vitamin D. This form of secondary hypo-

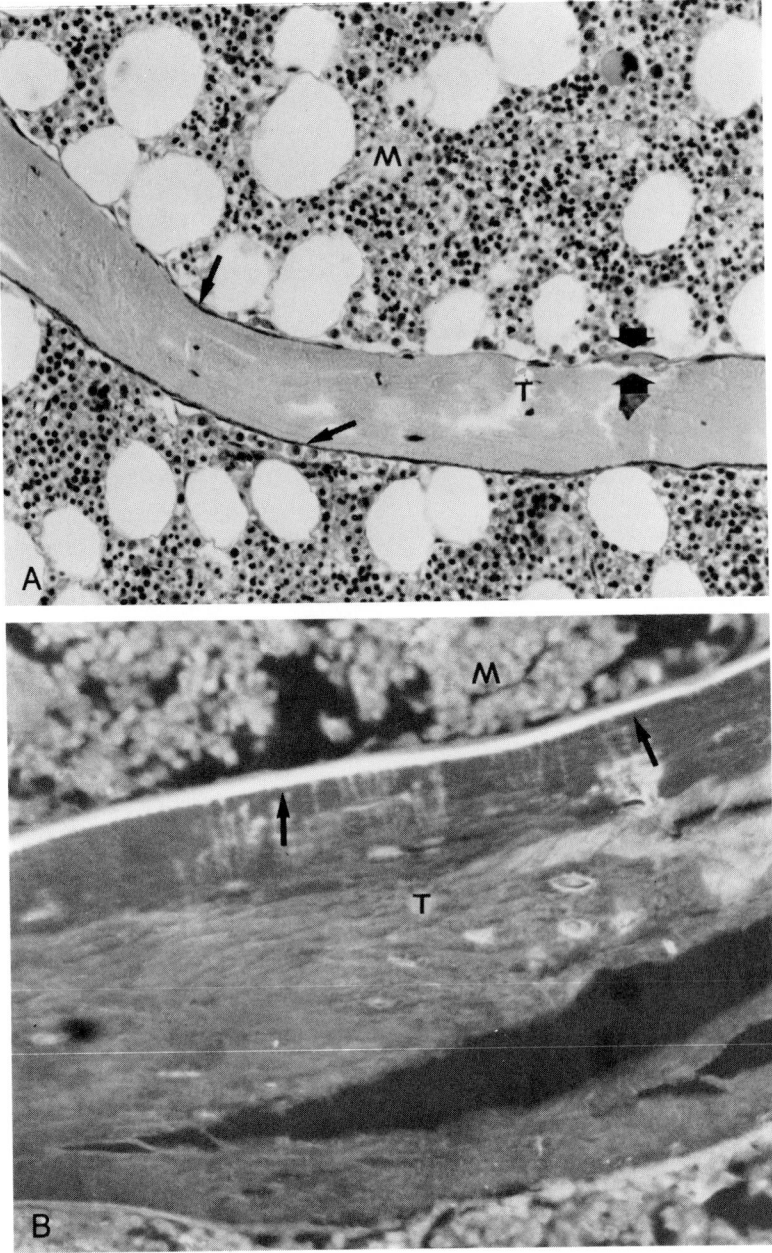

**Fig. 46–20.** *A,* Inactive osteoporosis. Note the thin almost nonexistent osteoid seams (arrows) and a single osteoclast (arrowheads). This biopsy is from a patient with anorexia nervosa and osteopenia. T = trabecular bone; M = marrow. (Goldner trichrome stain; original magnification = 160 ×) *B,* Corresponding fluorescent micrograph showing superimposed single linear tetracycline labels (arrows). Because the rate of bone turnover is so low, not enough matrix was synthesized over the two-week labeling period to allow spatial separation of the two fluorescent bands. T = trabecular bone; M = marrow.

phosphatemic osteomalacia has been described with a variety of bone and soft tissue mesenchymal tumors and prostatic adenocarcinoma.[16] The bone disease remits after complete resection of the coexisting neoplasm.

**Antacid-Induced Osteomalacia.** Chronic consumption of phosphate-binding antacids can cause hypophosphatemic osteomalacia.[17] Phos-phorus depletion is accompanied by hypophosphatemia with hypophosphaturia, hypercalciuria, and nephrolithiasis.

### Primary Vitamin D Deficiency

Adequate serum calcium and phosphorus levels are required for normal matrix mineralization. It remains unclear, however, whether vitamin D me-

**Table 46–5.   Histologic Features of Osteomalacia**

Bone Formation Parameters

Osteoid excess common:
    Increased osteoid volume
    Increased osteoid surface
    Markedly increased osteoid seam thickness
    Subperiosteal osteoid
    Cortical bone osteoid deposits

| | Bone Remodeling Activity Status | |
| --- | --- | --- |
| | Pure osteomalacia (low remodeling state) | Mixed osteomalacia osteitis fibrosa (high remodeling state) |
| Osteoblastic surface | Reduced | Normal to increased |
| Osteoblast number | Normal to decreased | Normal to increased |
| Active resorption surface | Normal to decreased | Normal to increased |
| Linear extent of bone formation | Reduced (may be 0) | May be reduced |
| Appositional rate | Reduced (often 0) | Reduced |
| Tetracycline labels | Predominantly abnormal Diffuse, unlabeled | Predominantly abnormal Diffuse, unlabeled |
| Mineralization front activity | Approaches 0 | Reduced |
| Bone formation rate | Reduced | Variable |
| Mineralization lag time | Increased | Increased |
| Peritrabecular fibrosis | Absent | Usually present |
| Subperiosteal resorption | Absent | May be present |

tabolites affect the mineralization process by a direct effect on the osteoblast, or by indirect mechanisms through augmentation of intestinal calcium and phosphorus absorption. Experimental studies utilizing vitamin D-deficient rats infused with calcium and phosphorus provided histomorphometric evidence that vitamin D was not essential for mineralization in growing rats.[18]

Because of the routine fortification of foodstuffs with vitamin D, dietary deficiency of this vitamin is now uncommon. Vitamin D deficiency, however, may still be encountered in certain clinical settings. Elderly individuals and institutionalized patients with poor diets and inadequate exposure to sunlight, food faddists, and alcoholics are prone to vitamin D deficiency. In addition to dietary restriction, vitamin D deficiency may occur following inadequate solar exposure.[19] Osteomalacia and rickets have been described in Asian immigrants who avoid exposure to sunlight.

Vitamin D functions to facilitate calcium absorption from the intestinal tract. Classic biochemical findings in Vitamin D deficiency include near-normal serum calcium and a low serum phosphorus, reflecting bone resorption and the renal phosphaturic effect of parathyroid hormone. In the face of a falling serum calcium concentration, homeostatic mechanisms attempt to preserve the normal extracellular calcium level, at the expense of the mineral-deficient skeleton. The histologic appearance of bone reflects this combination of osteomalacia and osteitis fibrosa.[20] The histologic changes may be variable, and may reflect the degree and duration of vitamin D de-

ficiency (see Fig. 46–21A, B). Milder forms of vitamin D deficiency may present as active bone remodeling disease resulting in osteoporosis, but not osteomalacia, because the mineralization may be ameliorated by compensatory secondary hyperparathyroidism.

**Hepatobiliary Disease**

Vitamin D deficiency, despite adequate intake, may result from impaired vitamin D metabolism. Hepatic disease may decrease production of 25-OH vitamin D, owing to inadequate microsomal hydroxylase activity.

**Alcohol-Associated Liver Disease.** Fractures in alcoholics are generally due to trauma. Chronic alcoholism may also alter calcium homeostasis and may predispose the skeleton to fracture. Several studies have shown a reduction in trabecular bone mass in alcoholics. Furthermore, drinking alcoholic beverages has been implicated as a risk factor for primary osteoporosis. Two histologic studies of bone from alcoholics found evidence of osteomalacia (increased osteoid volume), although the kinetics of bone remodeling using double tetracycline labeling were not reported.[20,21] A study of eight males with a 10-year history of alcohol abuse showed a reduction in vertebral trabecular bone mass, with preservation of appendicular cortical bone. Histologically, a reduction in active bone formation and resorption was seen without evidence of osteomalacia.[22] Several explanations could account for a reduction in bone mass in the alcoholic, including nutritional deficiencies of calcium and vitamin D, malabsorption of calcium and vitamin D secondary to pan-

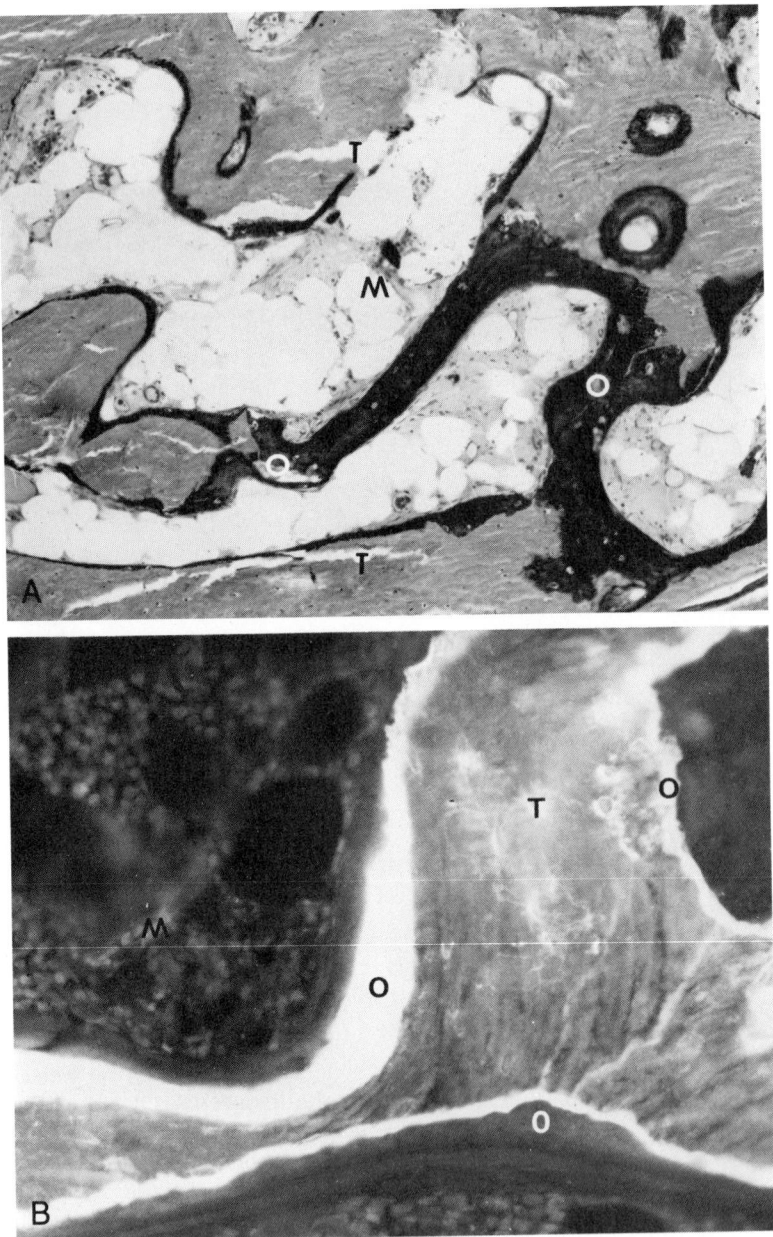

**Fig. 46–21.** *A*, Osteomalacia due to vitamin D deficiency. The mineralization defect is manifested by marked increases in the quantity of osteoid (O). The relative osteoid volume is increased as a result of an increase in the osteoid surface as well as an augmentation of the mean osteoid seam width. M = marrow; T = trabecular bone. (Goldner trichrome stain; original magnification = 120 ×) *B*, Corresponding fluorescent micrograph confirming the presence of a severe mineralization defect, as shown by the abnormal diffuse fluorescent tetracycline uptake at the osteoid seams (O). T = trabecular bone; M = marrow.

**Table 46–6.    Bone Histopathology Associated with Specific Nutritional Disorders**

| | |
|---|---|
| I. Accelerated Remodeling States (high-turnover or active osteoporosis) | Idiopathic Osteoporosis: involutional (postmenopausal; senile). |
| | Secondary Osteoporosis: calcium deficiency states; chronic (secondary hyperparathyroidism); small intestinal disease (early, compensated mineral malabsorption); postgastrectomy (mineral malabsorption). |
| II. Reduced Remodeling States (low-turnover or inactive osteoporosis) | Idiopathic osteoporosis: involutional (postmenopausal; senile). |
| | Secondary osteoporosis: hepatic disease (cholestatic liver disease, biliary cirrhosis; alcohol-associated); severe systemic disease, starvation, inanition, anorexia nervosa; total parenteral nutrition. |
| III. Osteomalacia—Pure | X-linked hypophosphatemia (vitamin D-resistant rickets); sporadic hypophosphatemia; antacid-induced osteomalacia; oncogenic osteomalacia; primary vitamin D deficiency; chronic pancreatitis; metabolic acidosis; renal osteodystrophy (aluminum-associated osteomalacia). |
| IV. Osteomalacia—Mixed (Osteomalacia/Osteitis Fibrosa) | primary vitamin D deficiency (nutritional, lack of solar exposure); small intestinal disease (vitamin D and calcium malabsorption); postgastrectomy (vitamin D and calcium malabsorption); renal osteodystrophy (mixed osteomalacia-osteitis fibrosa); calcium deficiency of children. |

creatic or liver disease, abnormal metabolism of vitamin D due to cirrhosis of the liver, abnormal parathyroid secretion, and a direct toxic effect of ethanol on calcium absorption.

**Cholestatic Liver Disease.** *The metabolic bone disease most commonly associated with cholestatic liver disease is osteoporosis.*[23] It is manifested by bone pain, fractures, and reduced bone volume. Even in the two series of patients that reported a high incidence of osteomalacia,[21,24] 50% or more of the patients with cholestasis who had radiographic evidence of osteopenia proved histologically to have a *reduction* in both mineralized bone and osteoid.

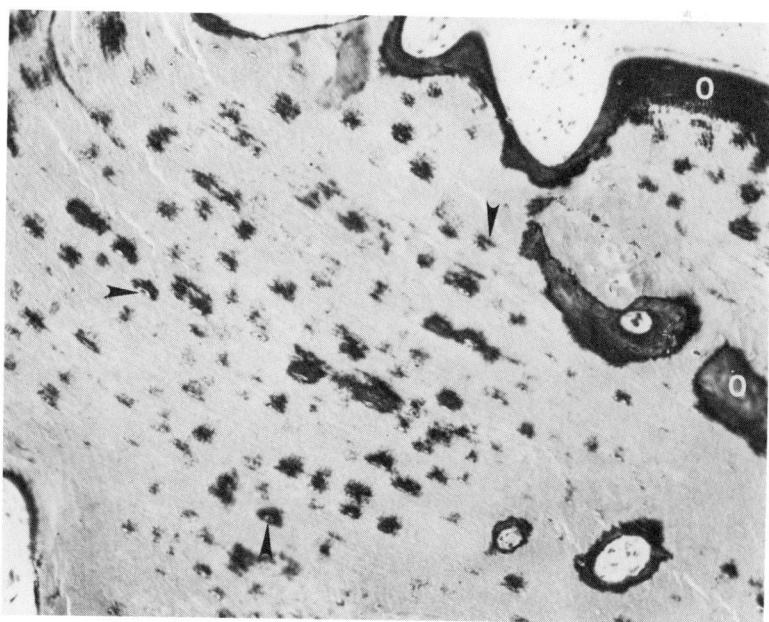

**Fig. 46–22.** Osteomalacia of x-linked hypophosphatemia (vitamin D-resistant rickets). Hypophosphatemia promoted osteomalacia as shown histologically by the increased volume of osteoid (O) and presence of osteoid around osteocytes creating a "halo sign" (arrowheads). This periosteocytic mineralization defect is typical of XLH. (Goldner trichrome stain; original magnification = 120 ×)

In one histologic study, accelerated remodeling features were seen in iliac crest biopsy specimens from patients with primary biliary cirrhosis.[25] Despite findings of low circulating levels of 25-hydroxyvitamin D, histomorphometric analysis of bone failed to reveal evidence of osteomalacia. Hyperosteoidosis was absent, as measured by fractional osteoid surface, osteoid volume, or fractional osteoid volume. In addition, mineral appositional rates and calculated bone formation rate were normal. These findings suggest that vitamin D deficiency (hyperosteoidosis) does not contribute significantly to hepatic osteodystrophy observed in patients with primary biliary cirrhosis.

### Partial Gastrectomy

Dietary deficiency, impaired absorption of calcium, and malabsorption of vitamin D with steatorrhea may be seen in gastrectomy patients. The skeletal lesion may, therefore, be variable, depending upon the relative contribution by malabsorption of minerals versus vitamin D. In contrast to those with small bowel resection, most patients following partial gastrectomy develop osteoporosis rather than osteomalacia (Fig. 46–18*A, B*). High-turnover features usually predominate in bone biopsy specimens.

### Small Bowel Disease

Currently, osteomalacia in adulthood is frequently associated with intestinal malabsorption.[26] Chronic inflammatory disease of the small intestine, such as gluten-sensitive enteropathy and regional enteritis, often result in malabsorption of vitamin D and minerals. Anatomic defects, such as small bowel resections and small bowel bypass operations, may also produce these functional disorders. Malabsorption of vitamin D and calcium may be selective and may not be reflected by the degree of steatorrhea or necessarily by the extent, severity, and duration of small bowel disease. Malabsorption states may present with a reduction in bone mass without marked increases in osteoid (i.e., osteoporosis). Because symptomatic osteomalacia in patients with gastrointestinal disease may occur with a paucity of clinical and laboratory clues, the bone biopsy procedure has become the most reliable method for establishing the type and severity of the skeletal disease.

### Total Parenteral Nutrition (TPN) (Hyperalimentation)

Patients receiving total parenteral nutrition have multiple derangements in mineral metabolism. Frequently, they have osteopenia, which may antedate their nutritional therapy. Rickets and osteomalacia have been associated with

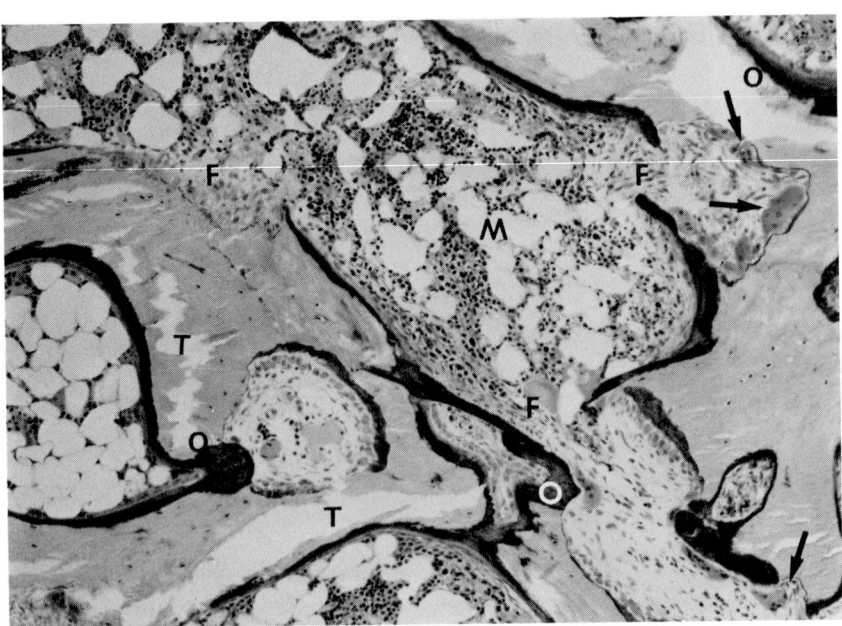

**Fig. 46–23.**   Renal osteodystrophy mixed with osteomalacia and osteitis fibrosa. Osteomalacia is suggested by the presence of a marked increased in the total osteoid surface (O), and was confirmed by abnormal tetracycline fluorescent patterns. Parathyroid hormone effect on the skeleton is evident by the presence of extensive peritrabecular fibrosis (F) and increased numbers of osteoclasts (arrows). T = trabecular bone; M = marrow. (Goldner trichrome stain; original magnification = 98 ×)

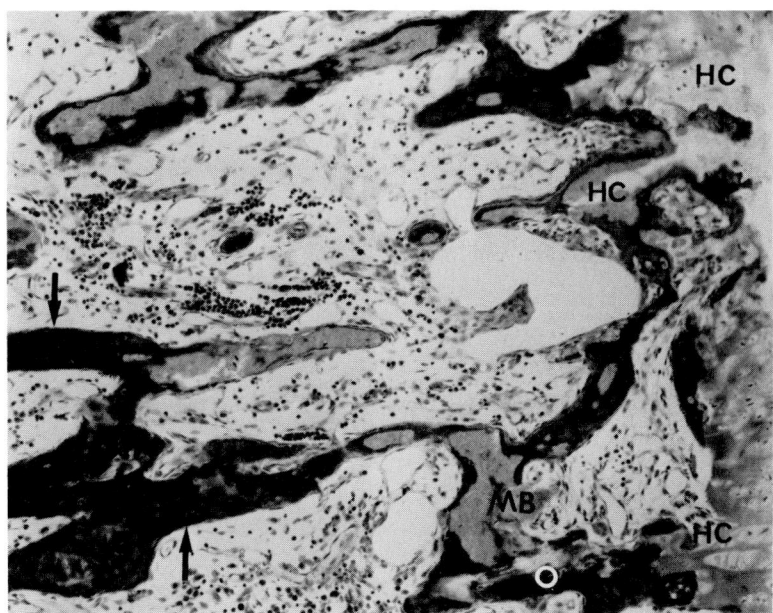

**Fig. 46–24.** Rickets and osteomalacia in a child with chronic renal insufficiency. The mineralization defect of the cartilage, characteristic of rickets, consists of irregular tongues of poorly calcified hypertrophic chondrocytes (HC). Defective mineralization of the metaphyseal bone represents osteomalacia, with marked increases in osteoid (O). In some instances entire trabeculae consist of unmineralized matrix (arrows). Rickets and osteomalacia, due to primary vitamin D deficiency, may also exhibit a similar histologic appearance, although of variable severity. MB = metaphyseal bone. (Goldner trichrome stain; original magnification = 250 ×)

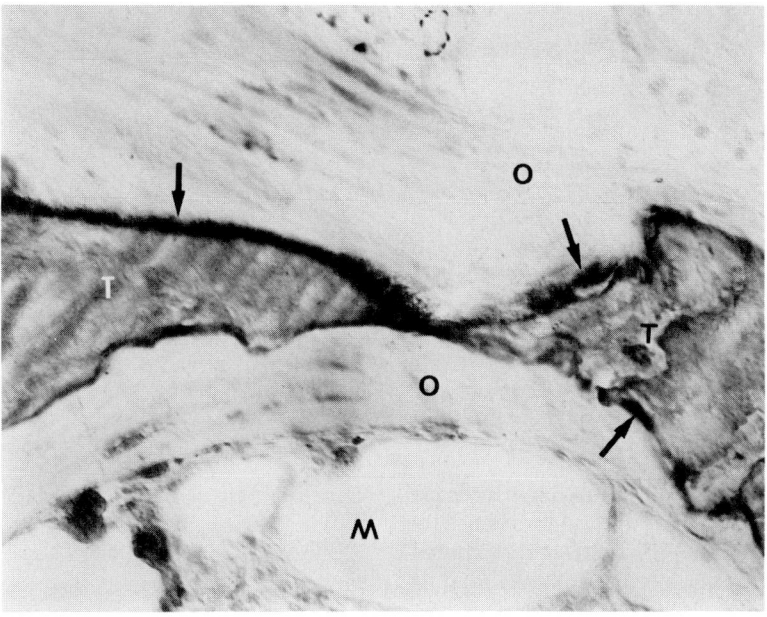

**Fig. 46–25.** Positive aluminum histochemical stain, in a biopsy from a patient with renal osteodystrophy exhibiting pure osteomalacia. Reaction product (arrows) lines the mineralization fronts. O = osteoid accumulation; T = trabecular bone; M = marrow. (Aluminum stain, no counterstain; original magnification = 250 ×)

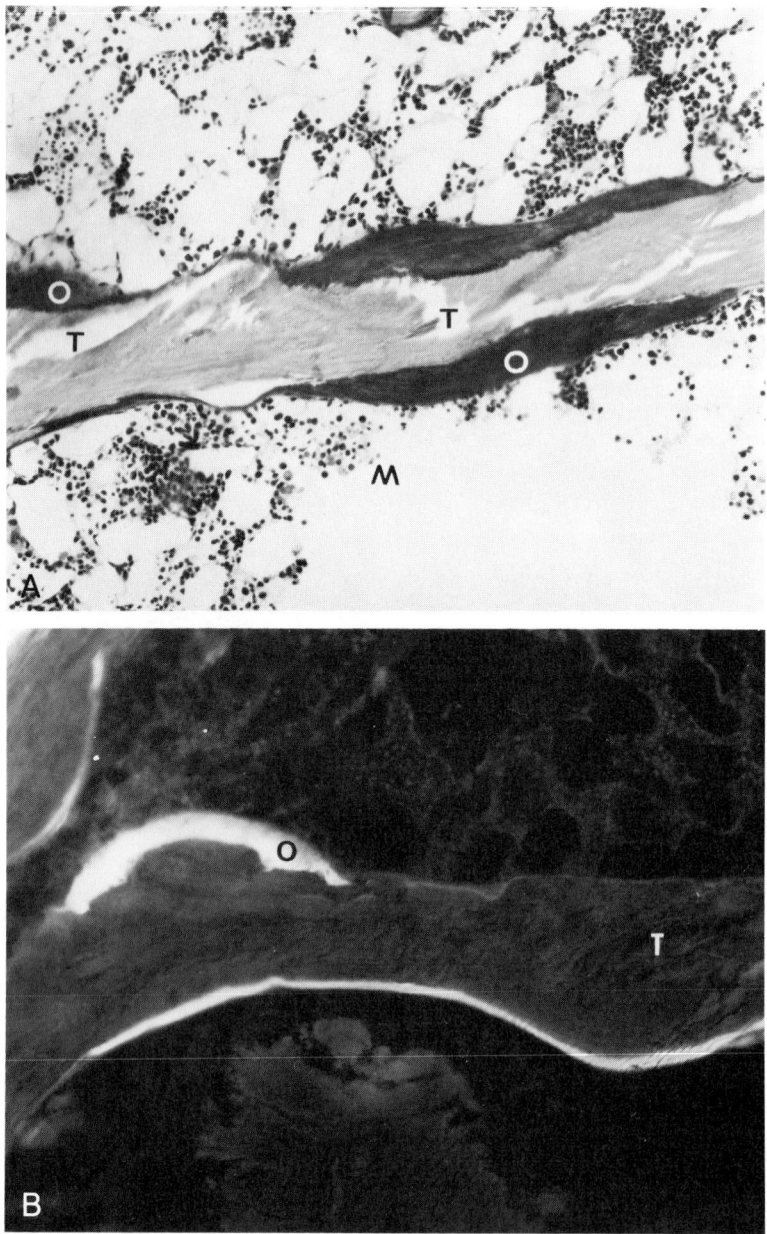

**Fig. 46–26.** *A,* Osteomalacia due to long-term high-dose sodium fluoride therapy for osteoporosis. Pattern of fusiform osteoid accumulation (O) around several of the trabecular spicules (T) is characteristic of sodium fluoride-induced mineralization defect. M = marrow. (Goldner trichrome sain; original magnification 250 ×) *B,* By fluorescent microscopy, the unusual osteoid deposits seen by light microscopy exhibit diffuse tetracycline uptake. O = osteoid; T = trabecular bone. (Unstained section; original magnification 120 ×)

TPN.[27] This syndrome is characterized by bone pain, fractures, hypercalciuria, intermittent hypercalcemia, normal 25-OH vitamin D, reduced $1,25(OH)_2$ vitamin D, and normal parathyroid hormone concentrations. The pathogenesis of the bone changes remains unknown. Factors postulated include recognized trace metal deficiency and excess or altered vitamin D metabolism.[28] Aluminum may play a pathogenetic role in the

development of the osteomalacia in patients receiving casein hydrolysates contaminated with aluminum.[29] Patients who are exposed to parenteral aluminum appear to develop a low-formation bone lesion that leads to symptoms and fractures. Total parenteral nutrition solutions should be carefully monitored to avoid aluminum contamination.

In one study of 13 home TPN patients, bone

histomorphometry showed reduced bone volume and reduced osteoid with normal resorption and calcification rates.[30] These abnormalities were associated with hypercalciuria, but the plasma levels of $1,25(OH)_2D$ were normal. Abnormalities in bone metabolism in these patients suggest a fundamental decrease in bone matrix formation rather than a mineralization defect as the underlying mechanism.

## Chronic Renal Failure

Renal osteodystrophy comprises the spectrum of skeletal and mineral alterations that attend chronic renal failure. The pattern of bone involvement may be categorized by histologic examination of tissue into three major groups: pure osteomalacia, mixed osteomalacia/osteitis fibrosis, and predominance of osteitis fibrosis. Mixed bone lesions and osteitis fibrosis-predominant lesions result from aberrations of vitamin D metabolism, calcium deficiency, phosphorus retention, and secondary hyperparathyroidism. In general, biochemical values and biologic changes are approximate indicators of the underlying bone changes. The type of skeletal lesions can only reliably be determined by direct examination of bone tissue.[31] Renal osteodystrophy is a complex disorder that is histologically heterogeneous. Osteomalacia may coexist with accelerated rate of mineralization in adjacent osteoid surfaces (Figs. 46–23, 46–24). Therefore, the proportion of abnormally mineralizing osteoid seams can only be determined by evaluation of kinetic tetracycline markers.

The pure-osteomalacia form of renal bone disease has been associated with the accumulation of aluminum in bone (Fig. 46–25). The retention of aluminum due to the inability to excrete this metal in chronic renal insufficiency is associated with the deposition of this ion in bone tissue.[32]

## Renal Tubular Acidosis

Rickets or osteomalacia may occur in patients with chronic hyperchloremic acidosis due to renal tubular diseases.[33] A renal tubular defect results in impaired hydrogen ion excretion, promoting systemic acidosis. Calcium is lost from bone as the skeleton attempts to buffer the responses to chronic acidosis. The mechanism of osteomalacia is unknown, but may involve alterations in vitamin D metabolism. Alkali treatment alone has resulted in healing of the mineralization defect.

## Starvation-Inanition

Bone formation may be affected not only at the level of mineralization but also during the earlier stage of organic matrix synthesis and secretion.

General inhibition of cellular protein synthetic capacity may be associated with inanition, starvation, or chronic systemic disease. Anorexia nervosa has been associated with inactive or low-turnover osteoporosis[34,35] (cf Fig. 46–20).

## Crystal Poisons, Drug Induced

Osteomalacia may be produced by drugs that inhibit hydroxyapatite crystal growth. Sodium fluoride (an experimental agent used in the treatment of osteoporosis) (Fig. 46–26*A, B*) as well as diphosphonates (agents used to treat the skeletal lesions of Paget's disease of bone) may produce a mineralization defect if given for prolonged periods and in high doses.

## Hypomagnesemia

Hypocalcemia is a frequent complication of hypomagnesemia. Three factors have been implicated: altered PTH secretion, impaired PTH responsiveness, and impaired calcium-magnesium exchange in bone. Hypomagnesemia appears to produce a form of PTH resistance, with hypocalcemia and blunted osteoclastic bone resorption to exogenous PTH administration.[36] Histologic evaluation of bone from magnesium-deficient dogs shows features of reduced bone turnover consistent with a skeletal resistance to the actions of PTH.[37]

## REFERENCES

1. Frost, H.M.: Calcif. Tissue Res. *3*:211–237, 1969.
2. Rao, S.D., Matkovic, V., Duncan, H.: Henry Ford Hosp. Med. J. *28*:112–115, 1980.
3. Fallon, M.D., Teitelbaum, S.L.: Hum. Pathol. *13*:416–417, 1982.
4. Baron, R., Vignery, A., Neff, L., et al.: Processing undecalcified bone specimens for bone histomorphometry. *In* Bone Histomorphometry: Techniques and Interpretation. (Recker, R.R., Ed.) Boca Raton, FL, CRC Press, 1983, p. 13–35.
5. Fallon, M.D., Teitelbaum, S.L.: Calcif. Tissue Int. *33*:281–283, 1981.
6. Merz, W.A., Shenk, R.K.: Acta Anat. *75*:54–66, 1970.
7. Teitelbaum, S.L.: Clin. Endocrinol. Metab. *9*:43–62, 1980.
8. Thompson, D.L., Frame, B.: Ann. Intern. Med. *85*:789, 1976.
9. Gallagher, J.C., Riggs, B.L.: N. Engl. J. Med. *298*:1935, 1978.
10. Riggs, B.L., Melton, L.J.: N. Engl. J. Med. *314*:1676–1686, 1986.
11. Consensus Conference: Osteoporosis. JAMA *252*:799–802, 1984.
12. Whyte, M.P., Bergfeld, M.A., Murphy, W.A., et al.: Am. J. Med. *72*:193–202, 1982.
13. Kleerekoper, M., Frame, B., Villanueva, A.R.: Treatment of osteoporosis with sodium fluoride alternating with calcium and vitamin D. *In* Osteoporosis: Recent Advances in Pathogenesis and Treatment. (DeLuca, H.F., Frost, H.M., Jee W.S.S., Eds.) Baltimore, University Park Press, 1981, pp. 441–448.

14. Marie, P.J., Pettifor, J.M., Ross, F.P., et al.: N. Engl. J. Med. *307*:584–588, 1982.
15. Choufoer, J.H., Steendijk, J.: Calcif. Tissue Int. *27*:101–104, 1979.
16. Taylor, H.C., Fallon, M.D., Valasco, M.E.: Ann. Intern. Med. *101*:786–788, 1984.
17. Carmichael, K.A., Fallon, M.D., Kaplan, F.S., et al.: Am. J. Med. *76*:1137–1139, 1984.
18. Weinstein, R.S., Underwood, J.L., Hutson, M.S., et al.: Am. J. Physiol. *246*:E499–505, 1984.
19. Kaplan, F.S., Soriano, S., Fallon, M.D., et al.: Clin. Orthop. Rel. Res. *205*:216–221, 1986.
20. Verbanck, M., Verbanck, J., Bravman, J., et al.: Calcif. Tissue Res. *22*(Suppl.):538, 1977.
21. Long, R.G., Meinhard, E., Skinner, R.K., et al.: Gut *19*:85, 1978.
22. Bikle, D.D., Genant, H.K., Cann, C., et al.: Ann. Intern. Med. *103*:42–48, 1985.
23. Paterson, C.R., Losowski, M.S.: Scand. J. Gastroenterol. *2*:293–300, 1967.
24. Reed, J.S., Meredith, S.C., Nemchausky, B.A.: Gastroenterology *78*:513–517, 1980.
25. Matloff, D.S., Kaplan, M.M., Neer, R.M., et al.: Gastroenterology *83*:97–102, 1982.
26. Parfitt, A.M., Miller, M.J., Frame, B., et al.: Ann. Intern. Med. *89*:193–213, 1978.
27. Shike, M., Harrison, J.E., Strutridge, W.C., et al.: Ann. Intern. Med. *92*:343–350, 1980.
28. Shike, M., Strutridge, W.C., Tam. C.S., et al.: Ann. Intern. Med. *95*:560–568, 1981.
29. Ott, S.M., Maloney, N.A., Klein, G.L., et al.: Ann. Intern. Med. *99*:910–914, 1983.
30. Shike, M., Shils, M.E., Heller, A., et al.: Am. J. Clin. Nutr. *44*:89–98, 1986.
31. Hruska, K.A., Teitelbaum, S.L., Kopelman, R., et al.: Metab. Bone Dis. Relat. Res. *1*:39–44, 1978.
32. Ott, S.M., Maldrey, W.A., Coburn, J.W., et al.: N. Engl. J. Med., *307*:709–713, 1982.
33. Brenner, R.J., Spring, D.B., Sebastian, A., et al.: N. Engl. J. Med. *307*:217–221, 1982.
34. Rigotti, N.A., Nussbaum, S.R., Herzog, D.B., et al.: N. Engl. J. Med. *311*:1601–1606, 1984.
35. Kaplan, F.S.K., Pertschuk, M., Fallon, M., et al.: Clin. Orthop. Rel. Res. *125*:64–68, 1986.
36. Breslau, N.A., Pak, C.Y.C.: Metabolism *28*:1261–1276, 1979.
37. Freitag, J.J., Martin, K.J., Conrades, M.B., et al.: J. Clin. Invest. *64*:1238–1244, 1979.

*Chapter* **47**

# ASSESSMENT OF DIETARY INTAKE

Johanna T. Dwyer

Dietary assessment has been a part of clinical medicine since ancient Chinese, Egyptians, and Greeks first recorded their theories of health and disease. However, not until the science of nutrition had identified the major nutrients was it possible to disaggregate data on food consumption into quantitative estimates of intakes of nutrients or other constituents found in food. By the mid-twentieth century, all the major dietary assessment methods had been developed. In the intervening years, theoretical and methodologic refinements, especially in food composition, in data processing, and in overall nutritional status assessment, have constituted the major advances in the area.

Four basic questions must be answered before choosing a dietary assessment method: Why is the dietary assessment being carried out? Who is to be assessed? What is being assessed? How must the factor of interest be measured? Table 47–1 summarizes some of the possibilities. The type of data that must be collected, the number of observations necessary, and the choice of methods vary accordingly.

## METHODOLOGIC ISSUES

### Selecting the Appropriate Dietary Survey Method

Five essential considerations in selecting between alternative methods are reliability, validity, respondent burden, costs, and other characteristics unique to the investigation. These considerations are especially important when large groups are being studied. The most appropriate choice of method ultimately depends on the objective of the study. Many excellent and detailed references on dietary assessment methods can be studied with profit by those who wish to learn more about specific applications.[1–27] The following discussion raises some of the major methodologic issues that are involved. They apply to dietary assessments of both individuals and groups.

Several sources of variation other than true differences must be considered: errors in measurements of current diet due to differences between usual diet and that measured in the study (representativeness), and errors of measurement attributable to characteristics of the respondent, the observer, or the instrument itself.[26] Table 47–2 summarizes these problems.

**Reliability (Representativeness).** In studies of individuals, it is important to assure that dietary intakes reflect typical patterns for the person because only these are likely to have nutritional significance. If generalizations are made, the individuals must be representative of the larger population. In studies of groups, representative samples of the population must be investigated so that findings can be generalized to the larger population. One common problem is that those who are being studied vary in their reliability and their willingness to cooperate. In most large-scale di-

**Table 47-1.   Questions to Be Considered in Choosing A Dietary Assessment Method**

| Issue | Possibilities |
|---|---|
| Why the dietary assessment is being carried out | Screening |
| | Assessment for clinical evaluation in conjunction with other indices |
| | Monitoring or surveillance |
| | Research: descriptive or experimental |
| Who is to be assessed | Single individual |
| | Group |
| What is to be assessed | Single food or food group |
| | Nutrient or constituent |
| | Many foods, food groups, nutrients, or constituents |
| | Entire diet |
| | Temporal patterns of consumption |
| | Associations of consumption with some other function |
| How precisely the factor of interest must be measured | Quantitative precision: may be high for some dietary constituents and low for others, high for all, or low for all |

etary assessment studies, the number of those who fail to volunteer or who prove to be noncooperative is considerable. Thus even when random sampling techniques are employed, unless additional steps are taken, the actual population studied may not be representative of the reference population, threatening reliability.

Another problem is characterizing the intakes of people who have variable food patterns. The variation from weekday to weekend and from season to season is usually recognized and attempts are made to measure it. Other types of variation may also need to be taken into account. For example, it it important to characterize the intakes of those who regularly embark on weight reduction diets. In order to develop a valid measure of typical intakes, these patterns must be identified and a suitable weighting system developed for sampling days involving each kind of behavior.

**Validity.** Methodologic, respondent and observer characteristics also contribute to errors in dietary assessment. Table 47-2 provides some examples. Retrospective assessments, such as dietary recalls and dietary histories, may involve errors related to forgetting. These errors threaten validity. The task of finding out what people eat on a regular basis in prospective studies is further complicated because the very act of assessing food intake often alters the phenomenon we are measuring. In prospective studies involving record keeping or collecting duplicate samples, people may unconsciously alter their habitual intakes to simplify the recording task during the observation period. If an observer is present, intakes may also change. Although in research settings such as metabolic units in hospitals, food intakes can be measured precisely, these intakes may also be atypical and may fail to reflect ad libitum intakes under everyday circumstances.

Some individuals are better respondents than others. These include nutritionists, graduate students, bank clerks, and others who are used to noticing detail, who have been trained to record and to remember, or who are especially interested in their food intakes. Those who commonly experience difficulties, particularly with certain types of assessments, are listed in Table 47-2. Even intelligent people may have difficulty remembering their food intakes in great detail without previous warning or practice. In addition, they may become bored or annoyed when the interviewer probes for better estimates of portion size, frequency of consumption, or number of helpings of food eaten. Poor respondents' reports make it more difficult to describe intakes validly and reliably. Some reports may be reliable but invalid, making them more difficult to recognize as inadequate.

The concurrent validity of dietary assessment measures is often low, that is, the correlation between a dietary measure and some other index such as a biochemical, clinical, or anthropometric measurement is poor. There are several reasons for this imperfect correspondence.

First, although dietary assessment data do not always represent deviations in nutritional status at the pathologic level, this deviation is likely to be most relevant to the clinician. Deviations in dietary intake represent an earlier stage in the onset of disease than do many biochemical, anthropometric, or clinical indices. A considerable length of time may elapse before disease actually becomes apparent at these other levels.

Second, measurement of diet is imprecise. It is highly dependent on the skill of the subject and the interviewer. It is extraordinarily difficult to obtain any dietary information at all from some individuals. In addition, clinicians probably vary

**Table 47–2. Causes of Variation Between Actual and Measured Diets in Dietary Assessments\***

| Causes of Variation | Examples |
| --- | --- |
| Differences between usual diet and that measured in the study | Study group is unrepresentative of the general population. |
| | Individual's diet is unrepresentative of usual diet because sampling method fails to capture the type of variability that is present (e.g., weekday vs. weekends, season to season, spells of illness, periodic episodes of weight reduction diets, binges among bulimics, eating at home vs. at business, travel, alternating day and night shifts). |
| | Inadequate numbers of observation employed. |
| Assessment method | Retrospective methods involve forgetting, which may be selective or nonuniform from food to food and by frequency of consumption (seldom eaten items remembered poorly),[19,28] "telescoping," or including two weekends in one week. |
| | Prospective methods may lead to unconscious alteration of usual diets during reporting periods, especially in the first few days. |
| | Errors in food composition tables or nutrient data base.[38] |
| Respondent | Underreporting common among: those who are nonadherent to therapeutic diets obese persons (especially early in reporting period for snacks, sweets, desserts)[29–31] heavy drinkers and alcoholics (for alcohol)[32–36] |
| | Overreporting common among: recipients of food or meal program benefits anorectics and parents of infants with nonorganic failure to thrive those embarrassed about meager intakes |
| | Alterations of a selective type: respondents report their preconceived notions of ideal or desirable intakes[37] respondents report what they think interviewers wish them to eat, especially respondents who have high needs for social approval[25] or who fear loss of benefits or chastisement from those in power |
| Observer | Characteristics making reporting difficult[38]: very old, very young persons (infants and children) ill, retarded, or confused persons (mentally ill, alcoholics, drug addicts) non-English-speaking persons or illiterates disinterest or lack of motivation desire to conceal true intake chaotic and/or unstructured food intakes |

\*The list of variations in this table is taken from Stallones, R.,[26] with permission of Am. J. Clin. Nutr., American Society for Clinical Nutrition. The examples presented are those of the author.

more in their skill in obtaining dietary information than they do in obtaining biochemical measurements, so that imprecision on the part of observers is an additional problem. Even when information is obtained, it may not reflect usual intakes, and even when food intakes are known precisely, the content of the constituent in the food supply may only be partially known.

Third, cutoff points differ for the point at which risk of dietary inadequacy is declared (e.g., inadequate intakes are defined as under 66%, under 80%, or as some other percentage of the Recommended Daily Allowance). Cutoff points for dif-

ferent nutrients may represent different points in the progress toward clinically apparent disease.

Fourth, the association between dietary intakes and individual nutritional status is influenced by factors other than intake itself, such as the bioavailability of the diet, and the presence of nutrient imbalances, diseases, or environmental stresses. Physical and biochemical indicators often better characterize individuals with respect to risk of malnutrition, but no single measurement usually provides definitive diagnosis in individual cases.[1,2] Among patients who are already ill, the disease itself or other factors, such as drugs, may affect the validity of other types of measurement of nutritional status, making it more important to augment the dietary assessment methods with the appropriate characteristics.

Thus it is usual for estimating individual nutritional status that a combination of dietary, biochemical, clinical, and anthropometric methods is needed. A greater number of measurements may be required to obtain acceptable estimates for an individual than for the population. Design considerations, particularly the number of dietary observations that are feasible, may make this difficult.[4] Interpretation is further complicated because, unlike metabolic experiments, many dietary variables change simultaneously.[12]

**Respondent Burden.** The difficulties in terms of time and psychologic burdens of different assessment procedures need to be considered. Time involved varies from a few minutes to several hours, depending on the method chosen. Psychologic burdens include the added work of remembering or recording food intake and the reporting of intakes that may be of a sensitive nature.

**Costs.** This consideration includes costs that are immediately apparent, such as the need for forms and food models, the time of respondent and interviewer, as well as hidden costs, such as the considerable amounts of time needed for developing protocols, interview training, checking, coding, calculating, and interpreting intakes. These time commitments are usually much greater than one imagines.[17]

**Other Characteristics.** Other characteristics that need to be taken into account in choice of method include the skill and training of the interviewers in dietary assessment techniques, limitations imposed by the setting in which the interviews are being done, and the time and facilities available for the considerable work involved in analyzing the data.

## Data Collection Period and Requirements

Table 47–3 summarizes factors that influence how long data must be collected to describe dietary intakes satisfactorily. The number of days needed to assess nutrient intakes with sufficient accuracy to describe usual intakes and to provide a definitive test that differences exist depends upon "intra-" and "interindividual" variation as well as the focus of the study (i.e., individuals or groups). Populations have different individual variations. Variations also occur by foods and nutrients.[4] If the "intra-" and "interindividual" variability in the intake of a particular dietary constituent is known, it is possible to calculate the measurement period necessary to correctly classify intakes into quantiles with satisfactory accuracy in a population.

"Intraindividual" variation, that is, day-to-day variation within a subject, is usually much larger than is the variation in means between individuals. Data provide some information on its size in studies of adults,[2,4,5,8,39–43] young infants,[31] and other special populations.[9,44–48]

A single day's intake usually gives erroneous estimates of ordinary intakes because diets and nutrient intakes vary greatly from day to day. Data on several days of intakes are usually necessary to characterize most diets. By utilizing the data in one review of several studies that involved different populations, one can estimate if a week's observations suffice for classifying various nutrients of interest reliably.[4] When the aim is to classify the nutrient intakes of individuals into tertiles, a week's worth of records is sufficient for many nutrients of interest. However, certain constituents, such as vitamin A, riboflavin, iron, and cholesterol, have large "intraindividual" variations, and a week of record-keeping would not suffice for them.[2,4] The practical significance of these observations is that so many days of observation may be needed for some constituents that respondent burden is excessive, and thus it may be impractical to attempt to estimate intakes with dietary techniques.[48] Although the estimates of how long data must be collected that are gleaned from the literature may be helpful, empirical evidence on the actual population to be measured is also necessary because "intraindividual" variation varies from one study to another.[49] Food frequency and dietary history questionnaires are sometimes employed to minimize "intraindividual" variation because they purport to report typical or usual intakes. However, they do not completely overcome the problems: intraindividual variation may be unknown, and threats to validity due to forgetting, unequal estimation errors, and different periods of time used as the interval for reporting all introduce errors.[50] Several reporting periods may also be necessary when they are used to overcome these difficulties.

"Interindividual" variation also affects estimates of how much data must be collected. Populations differ in their "interindividual" variability from one dietary constituent to another.

Finally, whether the focus of the study is to describe intakes of individuals or groups is important. The number of food records needed to describe an individual's typical intake satisfactorily is much larger than that required to characterize the mean intake of a group.[8,9] A single day's intake is inadequate to characterize an individual's usual intake correctly for placement

**Table 47–3. Factors that Influence How Long Data Must Be Collected**

| | |
|---|---|
| Size of "intraindividual" variation | The type, number, and spacing of diet observations may not be sufficient to reflect usual intakes.[3–7] |
| | Energy intakes have lowest "intraindividual" variation (25%), and variation for other nutrients is usually less than 50%.[2] Some constituents, such as cholesterol or vitamins, have large "intraindividual" variability. |
| | Single-day records give estimates—even of energy or protein—that are essentially meaningless (e.g., 50% deviation from individual sample means over a month).[3] |
| Size of "interindividual" variation | Groups differ in these respects: |
| | Examples of large "interindividual" variation: |
| |    alcohol intakes among teetotalers, social drinkers, and alcoholics |
| |    vitamin intakes among users and nonusers of nutrient supplements |
| | Examples of small "interindividual" variation: |
| |    groups in congregate dining facilities where everyone eats virtually the same food. |

into some range of nutrient distributions, such as quantiles. Several days of diet information are needed to make individual comparisons for exploring nutrient and disease or risk factor associations.[51]

## Special Problems in Assessing Diets of Individuals

The purpose of dietary assessment in clinical situations is usually to describe the "true" or habitual intake of a single individual. This poses particular problems. Table 47–4 summarizes these problems.

## Food Composition Tables

**Tables Available.** Many different food composition tables are in use in the United States today. They vary in the timeliness, completeness, and specificity of the information they provide with respect to foods, nutrients, and other food constituents. They also differ as to whether they are in the public domain (such as the information provided by updates of United States Department of Agriculture tables) or proprietary (such as many of the commercially available computerized nutrient data bases).

Most food composition tables rely heavily upon United States Department of Agriculture compilations at various times, the latest and most complete being the expanded recent version of USDA Handbook 8.[51] However, USDA data are frequently not identified as to source or brand name in the case of prepared foods, some proprietary food manufacturer data are not included, reports of additional research on food composition since publication of the tables may not be included, and not all constituents of possible interest are necessarily covered. For these reasons, other food tables that cover these issues are useful for some purposes.[52–54] Tables from other countries may also be helpful in special instances.[55,56]

**How Data are Collected.** The United States Department of Agriculture has the largest and most comprehensive program for collection of food composition data in the world. The Department utilizes methods that attempt to develop average values representative of the nutrient composition of foods available in this country, and they constantly upgrade the quality, quantity, completeness of information, and documentation provided.[57,58] Information on food composition is best when it is based on samples drawn for representativeness (as is done in the USDA program) rather than for convenience. The information in some other food composition tables and nutrient data bases can be criticized on the grounds that samples of convenience may have been employed, the documentation for values provided is not given, and the user has no way of knowing the quality of the data or how to estimate how much confidence can be placed in results obtained from the data.

New food products are being developed so rapidly that it is difficult to keep the ratio of the number of foods analyzed to the number of foods consumed constant or to increase it.[57] Similarly, the number of food components of potential interest is immense; few analyses are available for many components, and for others, good analytic methods are not yet developed.[59] Thus, complete information on each component of each food consumed in this country is unlikely to ever be available, and it is likely that missing values will always need to be calculated or imputed for many of them. This process involves errors, but if standardized procedures can be developed and

**Table 47–4. Problems in Assessing Dietary Intakes of Individuals**

| Issue | Implications and References |
|---|---|
| Individual requirements for nutrients are never known. | Adequacy of an individual's intake against a standard is a probabilistic statement because it is unknown whether the individual's requirement is high or low.[2] |
| Individual intakes are unrelated to individual requirements. | Those who have high requirements for a nutrient do not necessarily eat more of it than those with a low requirement.[2] |
| Characteristics of individuals may make it difficult or impossible to obtain valid data. | Some individuals may be unable or unwilling to report valid intakes (young children, the very sick, chronic alcoholics, drug addicts, mentally handicapped, or those with memory impairments or an inability to read and write). Others may fabricate information (patients with anorexia nervosa) or may alter actual intakes on reporting days (individuals on therapeutic diets). |
| Systematic errors in reporting may be present. | Systematic reporting errors in the same direction may exist. When individuals are the focus of the study, these errors are not balanced out. These can be discovered by reliance on direct observations of food intake or biochemical markers as well as on diet. |
| Usual intakes often vary within indices more than between indices. | The number of observations sufficient to reflect usual intakes is usually much greater for individuals than for groups.[3–9] |
| Estimates of usual intakes must be obtained. | Reporting days must reflect usual intakes; intakes should not change on reporting days. Spacing of reporting days must be sufficient to sample seasonal or other variations that must be reflected in intake estimates. |
| The precision necessary may vary from one nutrient to another. | Only one or a few nutrients may need to be assessed precisely. The precision necessary and the nutrients involved will affect frequency of diet record collection. |
| The length of time needed to obtain reliable estimates of usual intakes may exceed the individual's patience. | |
| Interpretation of dietary data is difficult. | Many factors other than intake influence nutritional status.[11,12] |
| Correct classification is essential. | Little information is available on specificity and sensitivity assessment methods by themselves. Usually additional measurements of nutritional status are needed to make a definitive diagnosis.[1] No single measurement provides a definitive diagnosis in individual cases. |
| Focus (individuals or groups). | More records are necessary to describe typical intakes of individuals than to describe groups.[3–8] Examples: With five nonsequential days, deviations of individuals exceed true energy and protein intakes by 20%, whereas deviations from group means are only 11%.[3] For energy, coefficients of variation for single days are 51% for usual intakes of individuals but only 36% for groups.[8] |

adopted, comparisons between studies will be facilitated and many methodologic errors will be avoided.[38,60]

**Variability of Data.** Technical errors relating to food composition include true random variability of composition of the individual food item, biased food composition data owing to sampling, and differences in bioavailability of individual nutrients, all of which can lead to variations in results.[60]

Samples of similar foods vary in their composition owing to genetics, and environmental, food processing, and preparation differences. The single numbers provided in most tables are only approximations and do not provide information on the statistical distribution of the constituent in foods. They should not be regarded as absolute or immutable quantities but rather as approximations. Comparisons between calculated and chemically analyzed values for diets are closer than comparisons of individual foods for most nutrients.

The variation of actual nutrient levels from published levels is much greater than many users of food composition tables realize. Among the causes of this variability are differences in the soil in which food plants are grown, the feed consumed by livestock, post-harvest or -slaughter time-related changes in nutrient composition, storage, food processing, cooking, and the effects of light, heat, humidity, and other environmental factors (see Chapter 37). The inherent variability and influences of these factors differ from one food constituent to another. Errors may also occur in deriving or compiling values from several sources to develop representative values for many nutrients.[61] In general, calculated and analyzed values for protein are closest. Values for total calories, carbohydrate, and fat are also fairly reliable, although the fat content of meat itself as well as cooking and eating practices vary greatly and may increase errors. In contrast, the vitamin and mineral content of foods, especially that of the trace elements, is subject to greater environmentally determined variation, and the differences between calculated and analyzed values are larger.

Differences also exist between values obtained from nutrient data bases among different industrialized countries. Some of these are real, and others are due to methodologic differences.[59,62] Therefore caution is indicated when information from various food tables is combined.

Although the completeness of information on food composition leaves much to be desired in the United States, the information available on food composition in developing countries is far more fragmentary and incomplete.[63]

**Precautions in Estimating Possible Ranges of Values.** In the light of the numerous aforementioned sources of error and the lack of information on the variability and representativeness of the data, prudence is recommended in drawing conclusions about intakes of nutrients calculated from tables of food composition and nutrient data bases, especially from proprietary sources.[64–67] They should be regarded as approximations to be confirmed by other measures, and not as immutable certitudes.

## Computerized Dietary Analysis Systems

In the past few years, computerized dietary assessment systems have become widely available.[68–70] The most sophisticated of these require large mainframe computers and permit the respondent or the interviewer to interact with the computer, posing and answering questions about foods consumed, food likes and dislikes, and constraints imposed by therapeutic considerations. Because the data are entered directly into the computer during the interview and the computation capacity of such mainframe systems is large, results expressed as intakes of various food groups or nutrients are available virtually instantaneously. Some programs also are capable of incorporating dietary prescriptions and anthropometric findings and producing menus or eating pattern plans that are tailored to therapeutic considerations as well as to the individual's dietary habits.

Other computerized systems consist solely of a nutrient data base based on food groups or individual food items and software for providing appropriate calculations when individual intakes are entered.

The most exciting development in the 1980s has been the rapid drop in the costs of microcomputer hardware with greatly expanded computer memories.[69] The simultaneous development of nutrition software programs that are suitable for these free-standing units holds great promise for revolutionizing the dietary assessment process, permitting clinical nutritionists who do not have access to mainframe computers to set up their own systems that will provide rapid feedback of results.[71,72] In the next decade, hardware and available microcomputer memory space will continue to expand. This expansion will permit the development of more sophisticated interactive computerized dietary assessment programs and the use of larger and more complete data bases. Better software programs are also now being developed utilizing the combined expertise of nutrition scientists, clinical nutritionists, and computer programmers.[73]

At present, however, these systems have their limitations. Those who are contemplating their purchase need to be sophisticated buyers. It is sometimes wrongly assumed that computerized dietary analysis systems "solve" all the problems associated with dietary assessment. They are actually computational aids, not panaceas.[69,71] Computerized systems cannot compensate for careless data collection, coding, or interpretation of results. Moreover, assumptions are made in some programs that may introduce errors and influence results, so it is important to study them closely before they are adopted. To illustrate, let us consider how various computerized systems differ in the nutrient data bases (the tables of food composition) they use. At present, computerized nutrient data bases differ in many ways, including the number of foods and nutrients they contain, the completeness of the information, and the frequency with which they are updated. Thus differences between systems can be expected even if the same records are analyzed.[74–77] These differences may in some cases be so large that they obscure the effects of treatments or changes in intakes.[74] These and other characteristics of computerized nutrient analysis systems need to be carefully assessed before a choice is made.

It is important to ensure that the data base used is relatively complete and that sufficient foods or groups of food are available so that all foods consumed can be coded correctly. The number of foods has increased at least five times in USDA tables of food composition over the past three decades, and the number of nutrients for which values are available has nearly doubled, so it is vital to ensure that the nutrient data base is up to date if the data will be used for research purposes.[58] The nutrient data bases used in microcomputer programs sometimes consist solely of average values for different groups of foods rather than individual food items, relying on the assumption that it is appropriate to use the "average" nutrient composition for a mixture of foods usually consumed within the food group by some reference population. However, if an individual's food choices within these food groups are atypical, his actual intakes may be quite different from results provided by the software program. Other nutrient data bases have missing data for the nutrient composition of many foods, but the program treats these unknowns as if they were zeros, and as a result nutrient intakes may appear to be lower than they really are. The shortcomings of nutrient composition data are well known to nutrition scientists. However, they may be unknown to the non-nutritionists who are often the individuals who develop or use computerized dietary analysis systems.[78] Often the result is that computerized analyses provide positive and definitive statements on nutrient intakes of sugars, biotin, vitamin K, or other nutrients for which data are still fragmentary and incomplete. The resulting analyses can be grossly misleading, and may be invalid.

### Errors in Calculating Nutrient Intakes

The first difficulty in computing intakes involves coding dietary records in a valid and reliable fashion. The errors that can be introduced by differences in coding are large, because foods are often described vaguely and many possible coding alternatives with different nutrient values for a given item are often available. Some method for handling unknowns is necessary other than simply omitting them from coding in order to obtain complete intakes. In research studies, it is often worth the effort to obtain additional infor-

mation from the cook, restaurant, or manufacturer, especially if the item is likely to be high in a nutrient of interest. In one study of fat intakes, for example, 15% of total fat intakes were of an unknown type and about half of this amount could be identified with further probing.[38] This finding is particularly important for nutrients such as fat that are commonly added to foods and differ in their composition.[79] Errors can be further reduced by checking records before and during coding to resolve additional ambiguities on portion size. Finally, development and use of coding protocols to assure uniformity of coding and training those who are coding records will further reduce errors.

For most methods, a second problem is that food composition tables only approximate the nutrient content of foods as actually consumed.[80,81] The difficulties associated with food tables for diet purposes also include missing values for certain nutrients.[78] Pennington has developed tables of food composition with imputed values that may be useful.[53] However, they may introduce additional errors due to interpolation.

The third difficulty in computing nutrient intakes is the great computational burden imposed by the calculations if several nutrients are of interest. The advent of computerized nutrient data bases has minimized the onerous task of making nutrient calculations from dietary records and has reduced computational errors.[82,83] At present the best reference for reviewing nutrient data base capabilities is that of Hoover and Perloff.[84] It is worthwhile to conduct such reviews before, rather than after, a choice is made on a dietary analysis system.

### Alternative Types of Analyses

A variety of means for describing dietary data are available other than simply calculating nutrient intakes or food frequencies. In some instances, these may provide additional information that is helpful not only for assessment but also for descriptive purposes. For example, indicators of dietary characteristics, such as dietary complexity, food diversity, and food quantity, are being developed for use in conjunction with nutrient intake assessments.[85,86] Alternative analytic methods, such as a dietary score based on food groups, diet complexity, and diversity, have shown good correlations in some studies and provide a single value that not only describes dietary habits but also correlates well with risks of deficiency in groups of elderly persons.[87] Other workers are developing short scoring methods for rapid dietary analysis[88,89] based on dietary patterns such as food groups. Despite their limited accuracy, the results are useful for screening purposes because they are extremely rapid.

## METHODS FOR ASSESSING NUTRIENT INTAKES

Dietary assessment methods are summarized in this section; they are reviewed elsewhere in great detail.[3,9–11,13,14,16–24,90–93] This section discusses some of the newer applications and retrospective methods (that are more commonly used clinically) in greater depth and prospective methods more briefly. Table 47–5 summarizes some systematic errors and biases present in these methods. Several studies contrast different methods used in estimating specific nutrients.[15,94–99]

### Retrospective Methods

These methods include the 24-hour recall, food frequency recalls, semiquantitative food frequency recalls, and dietary histories. All of them rely on the ability of the individual to recall diets

eaten in the near or more distant past and thus rely heavily upon memory.[131]

The assumption that people can remember what they ate over relatively long periods of time is important in case control studies of the associations between diet and chronic degenerative disease. Dietary data collection in these studies is predicated on the belief that the data are representative of long-term intake. Usual intakes obtained on individuals at the time when the disease became apparent are supplemented by whatever additional information can be remembered about changes in consumption over many years before the appearance of disease. If these assumptions are correct, then differences between cases and controls on timing, dose, frequency, or duration of exposure to the food components of interest may provide clues that will be helpful in sorting out the associations between diet and disease risks.

The accuracy of recall is related to interview setting, characteristics of the interviewer, effects

**Table 47–5. Systematic Errors and Biases in Dietary Methods**

| *Method and Problem* | *Comment* |
|---|---|
| RETROSPECTIVE METHODS | |
| Recall accuracy varies with method used. | Different methods are not directly comparable. |
| Selective forgetting of specific foods occurs. | Fruits, vegetables, breads, cereals, fats, oils, liquids, snacks, and alcohol are commonly forgotten.[19,28,39,42] |
| Failure to include diet alterations results from seasonal changes, reducing diets, sick days, or other variations. | Methods for obtaining representative samples of usual, *not* optimal or ideal intakes, must be employed.[118] |
| Confusion may be present about frequency of consumption (especially of items not eaten daily), number of helpings, and portion size. | |
| Current diet often biases recollections of past diet.[112,114–116] | |
| Recalls over more than one month are not quantitatively precise, and ability to classify individuals into groups may be doubtful after two years. | |
| PROSPECTIVE METHODS | |
| Alteration of intakes may occur on recording days. | Food intakes may actually be changed or actual food intakes may not be reported. |
| Failure to record intakes may occur on days requested. | Failure to record intakes may alter representativeness of records obtained. |
| Degree of stability of diet and thus number of observations may vary between subjects and groups. | |
| ALL METHODS | |
| Individuals differ in their reporting ability and motivation.[68] | |
| Socially acceptable rather than real intakes are reported owing to embarrassment, or attempts to please interviewers by following prescribed diets. | Underestimates of alcohol use are common, especially by heavy drinkers and alcoholics.[32–38] |
| | Obese persons often underreport desserts and snacks.[29–31] |
| | Patients may attempt to report intakes in line with prescribed diets or what they believe they should be eating.[68] |
| Usual intakes are difficult to obtain.[117] | |
| Sample sizes are often inadequate to detect true differences if they do exist.[119] | |

of instruction, respondent characteristics such as commitment, memory, sex, age, education, recent health status, and diet,[14] characteristics of the respondent's diet such as its stability over time, and a number of other factors.[10,100,101]

Given the proper incentives and training, most adults can recollect what they ate over the past day or week well enough for group recalls of intakes to correspond in rank by tertiles or sextiles to measured records of food intake collected at the same time.[4,102–104] Recalls of actual food consumption during the previous 24- to 48-hour period are the most reliable. The maximum period over which recalls of usual dietary intakes can be considered reliable is one month.[16,19,105–109] However, usual or customary habits going back much farther in time are probably also recalled.[103,104] The practical question is whether it is worthwhile to take the time to obtain such information from the distant past. Dietary methods, such as the Burke dietary history, have been used to obtain estimates of nutrient intakes 6 to 12 months before the interview.[106–109] Validity and reliability fall off rapidly over such an interval, so that precise estimates of individual intakes cannot be obtained. For example, when Morgan et al.[108] asked subjects to provide dietary histories for their current intakes and also for their intakes six months before, estimates for the latter period were lower for most nutrients than those for the former.[101] This finding may reflect true changes (e.g., reductions in food intake) in the past, but it also may reflect subjects' inability to recall precisely what they ate or drank at some earlier time. Retrospective estimates of usual intake of a year-long period were also poor in the studies of Houser and Bebb.[37] Subjects tended to overestimate their consumption, and intakes of some foods were remembered better than others.

For epidemiologic purposes it is often sufficient if stable, semiquantitative, relative rankings for groups of respondents can be obtained.[18] For such purposes, the accuracy of long-term recall data is better.[18,106,107,109] Results from several investigations that queried respondents about their intakes in periods from six months to five years before the follow-up assessment suggest that retrospectively collected dietary information does have some meaning; for most nutrients, differences in mean intakes were less than 10% from the various food groups studied. However, questions remain about whether the technique is valid enough for uses in some epidemiologic studies.[110–113] One problem is that the reliability of recall after two years is insufficient to classify individuals into tertiles or quantiles by their nutrient intakes.[106,107,109] In addition, current diet biases re-

calls of diet from the distant past, and such errors may affect cases differently than controls in epidemiologic studies.[112,114–116]

Table 47–6 discusses the strengths and weaknesses of some studies using each method.

**24-Hour Recalls.** This method is probably the most commonly used of all dietary assessment methods. The respondent is asked to recall all the foods and beverages consumed over the past day. The interviewer uses portion size models or measuring implements to assess estimates of portion sizes and probes in various ways to assure that all intake has been reported.[10]

The major difficulty with single 24-hour recalls is that they do not represent the usual food intakes of individuals.[2,117,124] They cannot identify with precision those individuals whose intakes are likely to be high or low in the population. Group mean intakes may be reliable, because those who report high intakes on a given day are balanced out by those who report low intakes, but it does not follow that individuals will maintain these rankings on a second occasion even though group means may be constant.[2,11,42]

Thus quantitative estimates of intakes from single 24-hour recall data are highly suspect for individuals. The use of several 24-hour recalls may be helpful, but the number of observations necessary may be large for obtaining valid estimates of some constituents.[50]

Single 24-hour recalls are often incorrectly used in surveys to report the number of individuals below some cutoff point for dietary adequacy.[60] In comparison to longer observation periods, distribution of nutrient intake obtained from them are more spread out, with more high and low values.[2] When 24-hour recalls are used to report the percentage of patients whose intakes were below or above some cutoff point, such as the Recommended Dietary Allowances, a larger proportion of the population will not meet the criterion than when other dietary assessment measures, such as diet histories of food frequencies that better reflect typical or usual intakes, are used.[2,11,124]

Such 24-hour recalls are also often used incorrectly in studies involving investigations of associations between intakes and biochemical or other health indices. When 24-hour recalls or other measures of diet on a single day are used to study associations with various biochemical parameters, the correlations are often extremely low or nonexistent.[8,48] It may be that a relatively strong association actually exists but that "intraindividual" variation is so great that it obscures these relationships. Expanding the size of the groups does not compensate by altering the distribution of intakes so that they are more similar to typical

**Table 47–6. Comparative Strengths and Limitations of Different Dietary Methods**

| Strengths | Limitations |
| --- | --- |
| **24-HOUR RECALL** | |
| Respondent burden is low. | Single 24-hour recall does not represent individual's usual intake.[3–7,120] |
| Well accepted by most respondents. | Interviewers must be trained. |
| No record keeping by respondent is required. | Some, such as the very young or old, cannot remember their intakes.[121,122] |
| Time for administration is short. | |
| Probability sampling within populations and individuals is possible. | Forgetting may introduce bias and may lead to incomplete records, especially for those who have poor memories.[23,24,105,121] |
| Bias introduced by record keeping is avoided. | |
| Costs are low, especially for computerized versions. | Desires to please interviewer may result in distorted intakes.[123] |
| Useful in clinical situations. | Recalls are likely to be incomplete for certain items and nutrients.[19] |
| More objective than dietary history. | |
| Does not alter usual diets. | Forgetting is especially high for liquids, snacks, alcohol, fats, and sweets, leading to errors in calories, fat, and alcohol. |
| Serial 24-hour recalls can provide estimates of usual intakes in individuals. | Group means of single 24-hour recalls are reliable, but individual rankings vary from one day to the next[42] and cannot identify individuals whose intakes are consistently high or low. Serial recalls are needed in this situation.[125] |
| | Often used incorrectly in surveys to identify individuals with inadequate intakes or to identify associations with other risk factors. |
| **FOOD FREQUENCY QUESTIONNAIRES** | |
| Provides description of how often foods are eaten. | Lists compiled for the general population are not useful for obtaining information on groups with different eating patterns (e.g., vegetarians or those on special ethnic or therapeutic diets). |
| Easy to standardize. | |
| Does not require highly trained interviewers, and some types may be self-administered. | Difficult to obtain information on total consumption because some foods are not included in lists. |
| Rapid | |
| Inexpensive | Respondent burden rises as number of items queried increases.[130] |
| Useful for describing food intake patterns[90] for diet and meal planning. | Many assumptions are necessary if food frequency estimates are to be used to estimate nutrient intakes, and special computer programs must be used. |
| Useful when purpose is to study associations of a specific food or small number of foods and disease, such as artificially sweetened beverages and bladder cancer,[127] coffee and birth defects[128] or pancreatic cancer,[129] or alcohol and birth defects.[32–36] | Reliability is lower for individual foods than for groups of foods.[130] |
| | Foods differ in extent to which they are over or underreported.[132–133] |
| Correlations with other methods or food is good when group is focus of analysis.[130] | Amount and frequency with which a food is consumed influence errors in estimation, staples and large quantities being better estimated than accessories or items eaten less frequently.[132] |
| Limited information about nutrient intakes may be obtained. | |
| Useful when purpose is to establish relative rankings with respect to intakes of certain food items or groups. | Intakes are underestimated because not all foods eaten are listed; forgetting occurs. |
| Does not alter usual diets. | Translation from intakes of food groups to nutrients requires that many assumptions be made. |
| Helpful for rapid estimates of single nutrients[136,137] or food groups. | Validity must be established for each questionnaire.[134,135] |
| | Longer lists may agree well with diet histories for single nutrients.[138] |
| **SEMIQUANTITATIVE QUESTIONNAIRES** | |
| Rapid to administer. | Utility in dietary assessment of individuals not yet ascertained. |
| Sometimes possible to self-administer. | |
| Do not alter usual diets. | Existing questionnaires differ as to their purpose and should only be used for their intended purposes. |
| Precoding and direct data entry to computer available to speed analysis on some versions. | Most instruments currently available are only for adults. |
| | Must be periodically updated. |
| Correlations between these questionnaires and other methods are satisfactory for food items and targeted nutrients when groups are the focus of analysis.[150] | Specific nutrient intakes, rather than all nutrient intakes or food constituents, are measured. |

**Table 47–6. Continued**

| Strengths | Limitations |
|---|---|
| Permit investigators in large epidemiologic investigations to obtain dietary information that would not be possible with longer methods.[150] <br><br> Costs of analysis are relatively low. | General population, not specific subgroups with different diets, is suitable target group. <br> As food consumption patterns change, questionnaires must be updated. <br> Not yet validated for those who eat modified or unusual diets. <br> Ability to monitor short-term changes in food intake (weeks or months) is unknown. <br> Correlations for individual nutrient intakes obtained with semiquantitative food frequency questionnaires[18,150,151] are poor when compared to diet histories and food records in household measures.[150,152] <br> Correlations between existing semiquantitative food frequency questionnaires and diet histories may be poor for ethnic groups eating unusual diets and for those on special diets. |

BURKE-TYPE DIETARY HISTORY

| | |
|---|---|
| Provides a more complete and detailed description of both qualitative and quantitative aspects of food intake than do food records, 24-hour recalls, or food frequency questionnaires.[18] <br> Correlations with other measures of nutritional status are good.[153] <br> Accounts for seasonal and other systematic variations in diet. <br> Useful in longitudinal studies.[153] <br> Does not alter usual diets.[154] <br> Provides some description of previous diet before beginning prospective studies. | Highly skilled research nutritionists are required to administer it.[131] <br> Highly dependent on subject's memory. <br> Time-consuming (1–2 hours). <br> Difficult to standardize. Differences among interviewers can be considerable.[155] <br> Costs of analysis are high because records must be checked, coded, and entered appropriately. <br> Time frame actually used by subject for reporting intake history is uncertain. <br> Subjects usually overestimate intakes owing to overestimating frequency and portion size and forgetting missed meals and sick days, so that dietary histories tend to be higher than food records collected over same period.[156] <br> Validity must be established in each study.[157,158] |

FOOD DIARY

| | |
|---|---|
| Record of what is eaten is recorded at time of consumption. <br> Subject can be instructed in advance so that recording errors are minimized. <br> Errors of recall are less than with retrospective methods. | Food intake may be altered during reporting periods. <br> Respondent burden is great. <br> Literacy required. <br> Respondent may not record intakes on assigned days, compromising representativeness. <br> Portion sizes are difficult to estimate.[159–161] Measuring helps. Models, pictures, or abstract shapes for sizing overcome some but not all inaccuracies.[162] <br> Underreporting is common.[163–169] <br> Number of days must be sufficient to provide usual intakes.[164–167] <br> Records must be checked and coded in a standardized manner.[168] <br> Measured food intakes are more valid than records above.[169] <br> Costs of coding and analysis are high. |

WEIGHED FOOD DIETARY

| | |
|---|---|
| Increased accuracy over food diaries with estimates of portions or household measures.[170–171] | Increased respondent burden. May alter consumption, especially away from home[91] and may increase number of dropouts. |

TELEPHONE INTERVIEWERS

| | |
|---|---|
| Face-to-face interviews are eliminated. <br> Respondent burden lowered. <br> Effects of forgetting minimized. <br> Validity good[175,176] <br> Respondent acceptance good. | Validation studies incomplete.[173,174] |

**Table 47–6.   Continued**

| Strengths | Limitations |
|---|---|
| **PHOTOGRAPHIC RECORDS** | |
| Validity good.[175,176] | Technical problems with estimating portion size and some foods from photographs. |
| | Necessary details may be lacking. |
| | Food waste may be ignored, leading to overestimates. |
| **ELECTRONIC RECORDS (SPECIALLY PROGRAMMED PORTABLE COMPUTER)** | |
| Decrease respondent burden.[179] | Require considerable instruction. |
| Preliminary validations good. | Special food groups must be constructed for population to be studied.[180] |
| | Portion size estimates may be imprecise. |
| **DUPLICATE PORTION COLLECTION AND ANALYSIS** | |
| Highly accurate in metabolic research studies. | May alter intakes.[184] |
| Duplicate portion can be analyzed chemically. | High respondent burden. |
| Helpful for validating other methods for constituents on which food composition data are incomplete.[185] | Expensive and time-consuming to analyze. |
| | Differences between duplicate portions and weighed records large (7% for energy, larger for other nutrients.[13,81] |

intakes, although it may help to alleviate other problems.[2]

Finally, it sometimes is not recognized that the errors of estimates of usual intake vary from one nutrient to the next when one-day intakes are used to assess nutrient intakes. The relative reliabilities of estimates of usual intake of different nutrients vary greatly with both single and multiple observations.

**Food Frequency Recalls.** The food frequency technique employs a list of various food items and inquires about usual intakes in terms of frequency with which they are (or were) consumed per day, per week, or per month. Thus, it is possible to collect and categorize data on the frequency of consumption of various food items by themselves or by various food groups that have been included on the inventory. The number of food items that are specified varies, depending upon the purpose of the study, but never includes all items that could possibly be eaten. Food frequency questionnaires available at present also vary as to whether they are self-administered or given in a personal interview, whether portion size is assumed or asked for, whether a day or some longer time unit is used as reference, and in many other ways.[126] Strengths and weaknesses of the method are summarized in Table 47–6.

Food frequency recalls have serious limitations for making statements about the nutrient intakes of individuals.[97] Time is saved by focusing on the frequency with which a limited number of specific foods or groups of food are eaten, but information on other foods consumed may be lost. Total dietary intakes of nutrients cannot be estimated unless the list of food items is extensive and information on portion size and number of servings per eating occasion is also obtained.[4,91] It is difficult to measure portion size. The use of "average" or usual portion sizes (which differ among men, women, and children) as reference standards may introduce further complications. Because total nutrient intakes are derived from both the frequency and amount of foods consumed, data will be biased unless portion size standards are relevant and estimation is appropriate.

When questionnaires focus only on intakes of food groups or food exchange lists, the assumptions involved in using estimates of "average" nutrient contributions from these groups further increase errors. Means for the nutrient contributions of food groups are based upon the usual mixture of foods eaten in a particular category by the population used to develop the food grouping system.[139,140] If the individual surveyed has different food choices from these, the nutrient contributions of the food groups to the individual's diet may be markedly different. This is often true when food frequency recalls based on healthy populations with "usual" eating habits are used to survey individuals who have unusual or markedly different diets.

To illustrate, let us assume that the averages derived for the exchange lists or some similar list for the "starch" group are based on averages for bread, rice, and other commonly eaten starch foods, each food given an equal weight in the average. Suppose, however, that one is dealing with a Mexican American population that eats mostly tortillas or a Chinese American population that eats mostly rice? These are obviously different and while their frequency estimates for starchy foods might be similar, the nutrient contributions of the starchy food would be different. If one simply applies average values to these frequency estimates, the nutrient values obtained are likely to be false. The correct procedure is to "weight" the various foods contributing nutrients and to develop averages for groups of foods for each population being studied. If there is any likelihood that the study population's "food choice mix" or portion size selected differs from that used for generating nutrient average values for the food groups, validity may be compromised in estimating nutrient intakes from such data.

If only a single nutrient is of interest, lists are now available of about 100 foods that, by virtue of their composition, portion size, and the frequency with which they are eaten, contribute the most to intakes of that nutrient in national surveys of representative samples of Americans.[141,142] These and other lists permit the clinical nutritionist to focus the interview on a relatively small number of foods that, because of their composition and the frequency of their consumption, are likely to account for most of the constituent's consumption.[143]

**Semiquantitative Food Frequency Questionnaires.** Until the late 1970s, food frequency questionnaires were used chiefly in epidemiologic studies of specific groups or in abbreviated versions based on food groups in clinical situations. Now more sophisticated methods have been developed using data on the foods that are the most common sources of nutrients in the general population. These methods permit semiquantitative estimates of nutrient intakes of groups. They differ from earlier food frequency recall questionnaires in that they have longer lists of foods, the lists are derived from national surveys of representative samples of the American adult population,[144] vitamin and mineral intakes from supplements are included, and some estimates of portion size are provided.

Table 47–6 represents the strengths and limitations of the existing method.

Two semiquantitative food frequency questionnaires in widespread use at present have been tested most extensively. They are the instrument developed by Willett et al. at Harvard University[145,146] and that developed by Block and co-workers at the National Cancer Institute.[147–149] They differ in their method of construction, the reference populations used to select foods, the extent to which they have been validated, the reference portion sizes used, the number of foods they contain, the nutrient intakes they are designed to assess, the extent to which they account for overall intakes of these nutrients and of other constituents, the questions they ask on vitamin, mineral, and other dietary constituents, the nutrient data bases that have been used for translating findings from them into nutrient intakes, and probably in other respects as well. The extent to which they yield similar results, how they compare to each other in their performance, how they behave with populations who consume modified diets and among ethnic subgroups in the population whose dieting patterns differ markedly from those of the general population, and their ability to monitor changes in food intake over relatively short periods (e.g., weeks or months) need to be assessed.

It is also important to evaluate the utility and performance of these questionnaires in the dietary assessment of individuals because they are now being widely used for this purpose.

The food supply and dietary habits are constantly changing, and such changes have large effects both on what foods are consumed and on the nutrient composition of foods that are eaten. Therefore, for such questionnaires to continue to include the major food contributors of nutrients or other constituents of interest, they must be periodically updated, as must the nutrient data bases used when nutrient intakes are calculated from them.

**Burke-Type Dietary History.** In the 1930s as part of the effort that went into describing factors known to affect the growth of children, Bertha Burke, who was the research nutritionist in the Harvard (Boston) longitudinal study of growth and development, created a method to describe usual intakes. Her name is often used in referring to this method. It attempted to establish the usual dietary intake of foods over several months or a year relying on the subject or his parent's recall. The respondent first was asked to report the foods and beverages consumed on a typical day. Then the interview progressed to questions about the frequency of consumption and the amount of these foods consumed and of other foods consumed in the diet. Usually respondents or their parents also provided some documentation of several days' intakes using food records that the nutritionist could use to ensure that recollected intakes agreed with reported intakes, and that all foods frequently consumed were included. Food models, cross checks on food consumption, careful nondirective probing, and other techniques were employed to do this. The usual dietary history takes one to two hours to obtain even when the interview is conducted by a highly skilled nutritionist.[102]

## Prospective Methods

A wide variety of methods for obtaining food records at the time the food is eaten are in use at present. They all possess the advantage of being less affected by the effects of memory than do retrospective methods. However, the very act of recording intake probably inadvertently stimulates a greater consciousness of what is being eaten on the respondent's part and may lead to altered intakes during recording periods. These methods are reviewed briefly in the following section. Additional information is available on them from other sources.[10,91,154,155] The strengths, limitations, and some examples of their use are presented in Table 47–6.

**Food Diaries.** The respondent is asked to record all food and drink consumed, estimating portion sizes in household measures after being instructed on how to fill out records. The records are usually collected for several days at a time. They are then checked out by the interviewer with the respondent so that ambiguous entries are clarified and analyzed.

**Weighed Intakes.** After careful instruction, the individual is provided with a small scale so that all food and drink consumed can be weighed and recorded. After records have been collected, they are checked and additional details are requested when necessary.[91] Weighed food intakes are frequently used in Great Britain for prospective assessment, but they have not been as popular in the United States, in part because foods are rarely weighed in households here.[45,172]

**Telephone Interviews.** Because personal interviews are so expensive and record keeping is so laborious, various alternatives for collecting immediate reports of food intake have been explored. These include telephone interviews for 24-hour recalls[173] and the contemporaneous reporting of three- or seven-day food records by telephone either to an interviewer or to a telephone answering service.[174]

**Photographic Records.** A photographic method of dietary assessment has been developed. The respondent photographs all meals at a standardized distance and records the meal number of the photograph and any meal preparation that would not appear in photograph (such as method of preparation) on a separate sheet.[175,176]

**Electronic Food Records.** This method involves the use of a specially programmed electronic recording device on which the subject can record his food intake.[177,178]

**Records for Monitoring Specific Foods.** In some instances all that is required is information on a few nutrients in the diet. Specific food inventory methods have been developed for monitoring the intakes of these nutrients by selecting foods or groups of foods that are known to be potent contributors of the nutrient in the population under study. Such methods permit easy and rapid quantification for monitoring purposes on therapeutic diets or for research.[181] The problem is that the sources of the food constituent must be well documented in the diets of the population under study. These techniques are most highly developed for fat-modified diets, but now self-monitoring food records are also being used for other applications such as modifications of sodium, potassium, and protein.

**Duplicate Portion Analysis.** The collection of duplicate portions of foods consumed by an individual and the subsequent chemical analysis of the foods to obtain direct measurements of a nutrient provide accurate measurements of intakes of nutrients or other constituents. When food composition tables do not provide information on the food constituent of interest, this may be the only way to obtain estimates of intakes.[182,183]

**Constant Observation by a Trained Observer.** In controlled or highly supervised environments and more rarely in field situations, intakes may be monitored directly by trained observers who use one of the aforementioned dietary assessment methods. This observation may be done in either an overt or covert fashion.[91,186] The strength of the method is that precise records can be obtained of foods eaten without a great respondent burden. The weaknesses are the altered food intakes that result from the very fact of being observed and the high costs of observation.

**Special Records.** Special records kept by respondents that involve elaborate reports of intakes as well as additional information, such as mood, time, and place of eating, are also employed for some clinical or research purposes. These are useful not only for documenting intakes but also for helping patients monitor their food intakes as they progress in dietary treatment. For example, they have been used extensively in behaviorally oriented treatment of obesity and bulimia, and for assisting patients to gain insight into the psychologic and social circumstances associated with consumption. The major strength is that they provide insight into the variables associated with consumption. Major limitations include the high respondent burden, high costs of analysis, and imprecision with respect to type and amount of food eaten unless special steps are taken to instruct subjects.

## Combination of Methods

Often it is helpful to combine several methods in a single study to obtain greater accuracy. For example, in one study of the elderly, weighed daily records were checked using 24-hour recalls, food frequency lists, and a general questionnaire to improve accuracy of the records and to provide some notion of how representative intakes were of usual dietary patterns.[81] Only slightly more time was needed with this combination than would have been necessary with a single method, and more accuracy was obtained. The USDA National Food Consumption Survey utilized a 24-hour recall combined with either two- or three-day written records, and the Department of Health and Human Service's Health and Nutrition Examination Survey used a 24-hour recall and food frequency information.[22] The monumental year-long diet study conducted by the USDA also used a variety of methods.[187,188] These combinations provide cross checks and better estimation of typical diets.

## SUMMARY

The voluminous literature that now documents the differences and comparisons between various methods for assessing food intakes may be helpful in planning dietary assessment studies. It is important to remember that all the methods are imperfect. In the end, the validity and reliability of all of them are heavily dependent upon the skill of the interviewer, careful instructions, and cooperative respondents. Comparisons can never reveal which method is "best." "Best" depends upon the purpose of the investigation. However, comparisons are helpful in showing the differences between the methods and the differences in apparent nutrient intakes that are likely to result.

All dietary assessment methods must fulfill the specific purpose of the study, assure that intakes are representative of typical diet over the time period being investigated, provide reliable, repeatable, and representative data that are capable of validation, and conform to the constraints imposed by respondents and interviewer characteristics and costs.[10] Considering these factors before beginning dietary studies will ultimately save a great deal of time.

In the next few years it is likely that dietary assessment methodologies and the indices derived from them will continue to expand to encompass more than simple associations between a single nutrient and health indices. Attempts will also be made to provide more complete descriptive data[189–191] as well as to develop better food guidance systems.[192–195]

## REFERENCES

1. Harrison, G.G.: Concepts of sensitivity and specificity; Their relevance to the nutritional assessment of the elderly. *In* Assessing the Nutritional Status of the Elderly—State of the Art. Columbus, Ross Laboratories, 1982.
2. Beaton, G.A.: What do we think we are estimating? *In* Proceedings of the Symposium on Dietary Data Collection, Analysis, and Significance. (Beal, V.A., Laus, M.J., Eds.) Amherst, Agricultural Experiment Station, 1982.
3. Todd, K.S., Hudes, M., Calloway, D.H.: Am. J. Clin. Nutr. *37*:139–146, 1983.
4. James, W.P.T., Bingham, S.A., Cole, T.J.: Nutr. Cancer *2*:203–212, 1980.
5. Balough, M., Medalie, J.H., Smith, H., et al.: Isr. J. Med. Sci. *4*:195–203, 1968.
6. Lechtig, A., Yarbrough, C., Martorell, R., et al.: Arch. Latinoamer. Nutr. *26*:243–271, 1976.
7. Linussen, E.E.I., Sanjur, D., Ericson, E.C. Arch. Latinoam. Nutr. *24*:277–294, 1974.
8. Beaton, G., Milner, J., Corey, P., et al.: Am. J. Clin. Nutr. *32*:2546–2559, 1979.
9. Rush, D., Kristal, A.: Am. J. Clin. Nutr. *35*:1259–1268, 1982.
10. Burk, M., Pao, E.: Methodology for Large Scale Surveys of Household and Individual Diets. Home Economics Research Report 40. Washington, D.C., U.S. Department of Agriculture, 1976.
11. Beaton, G.H.: Evaluation of dietary intake of the elderly. *In* Assessing the Dietary Intake of the Elderly: State of the Art. Columbus, Ross Laboratories, 1982.
12. Gordon, T., Fisher, M., Rifkind, B.M.: Am. J. Clin. Nutr. *39*:152–156, 1984.
13. Pekkarinen, M.: World Rev. Nutr. Diet. *12*:145–171, 1970.
14. Marr, J.W.: World Rev. Nutr. Diet. *13*:105–164, 1971.
15. Bingham, S., Wiggins, S., Helms, P., et al.: Nutr. Cancer. In press, 1986.
16. Bazarre, T.L., Meyers, M.D.: Nutr. Cancer *1*:22–45, 1978.
17. Black, A.E.: Pitfalls in dietary assessment. *In* Recent Advances in Clinical Nutrition. (Howard, A.N., Baird, I.M., Eds.) London, John Libbey 1981.
18. Block, G.: Am. J. Epidemiol. *115*:495–505, 1982.
19. Burr, M.L.: Hum. Nutr.: Appl. Nutr. *37A*:339–345, 1983.
20. Graham, A.M.: Proc. Nutr. Soc. *41*:343–348, 1982.
21. Miller, D.S.: Proc. Nutr. Soc. *29*:191–196, 1970.
22. Nesheim, R.G.: Am. J. Clin. Nutr. *35*:1292–1296, 1982.
23. Trulson, M.F.: J. Am. Diet. Assoc. *30*:991–995, 1954.
24. Trulson, M.F.: J. Am. Diet. Assoc. *31*:797–802, 1955.
25. Black, A.E.: Hum. Nutr.: Appl. Nutr. *36A*:85–94, 1982.
26. Stallones, R.: Am. J. Clin. Nutr. *35*:1290–1294, 1982.
27. Research Dietetic Practice Group, American Dietetic Association Validity and Relocapability in Dietary Methodology: An Annotated Bibliography Part Three. Chicago, American Dietetic Association, 1986.
28. Campbell, V.A., Dodds, M.L.: J. Am. Diet. Assoc. *51*:29–33, 1967.
29. Beudoin, R., Mayer, J.: J. Amer. Diet. Assoc. *29*:29–34, 1953.
30. Lansky, D., Brownell, K.: Am. J. Clin. Nutr. *35*:727–730, 1982.

31. Bray, G.A., Zachary, B., Dahms, W.T., et al.: J. Am. Diet. Assoc. *72*:24–27, 1978.

32. Ouelette, E.M., Rosett, H.L., Rosman, P.I., et al.: N. Engl. J. Med. *297*:528–533, 1977.

33. Watson, C., Tilleskjor, C., Hoodeshed-Schow, E., et al.: J. Stud. Alcohol *45*:344–348, 1984.

34. Pernanen, K.: Validity of survey taken on alcohol use. *In* Gibbons Red. Research Advances in Alcohol and Drug Problems, Vol 1. New York, John Wiley & Sons, Inc., 1977, pp. 355–374.

35. Poikolainen, K., Karkkainew, P.: J. Stud. Alcohol *46*:219–222, 1985.

36. Dams, G., Aitken, S., Malin, H.: J. Stud. Alcohol *46*:223–227, 1985.

37. Houser, H.B., Bebb, H.T.: Individual variation in intake of nutrients by day, month and season in relation to meal patterns and implications for dietary survey methodology. *In* Assessing Changing Food Consumption Patterns (Food and Nutrition Board, Committee on Food Consumption Patterns). Washington, D.C., National Academy Press, 1981.

38. Milner, J.P., McGuire, V.M., Little, J.A.: Am. J. Clin. Nutr. *38*:964–970, 1983.

39. Edholm, O.G., Fletcher, J.G., Widdowson, E.M., et al.: Br. J. Nutr. *9*:286–300, 1955.

40. Young, C.M., Franklin, R.E., Foster, W.D., et al.: J. Am. Diet. Assoc. *29*:459–464, 1953.

41. Hankin, J.H., Reynolds, W.E., Margen, S.: Am. J. Clin. Nutr. *20*:935–945, 1967.

42. Acheson, K.J., Campbell, I.T., Edholm, O.G., et al.: Am. J. Clin. Nutr. *33*:1147–1154, 1980.

43. Marr, J.W.: Individual variation in nutrient intake. *In* Preventive Nutrition and Society. (Turner, M., Ed.) New York, Academic Press, 1980.

44. Black, A.E., Cole, T.J., Wiles, S.S., et al.: New York, Hum. Nutr.: Appl. Nutr. *37A*:448–458, 1983.

45. Bingham, S.A., McNeil, I., Cummings, J.H.: Br. J. Nutr. *45*:23–35, 1981.

46. McGee, D., Rhoads, G., Hankin, J., et al.: Am. J. Clin. Nutr. *36*:657–663, 1982.

47. White, J.C., MacNamara, D.J., Ahrens, E.H.: Am. J. Clin. Nutr. *34*:199–203, 1981.

48. Liu, K., Stamler, J., Dyer, A., et al.: J. Chronic. Dis. *31*:399–418, 1978.

49. McGee, D., Rhoads, G., Honkin, J., et al.: Am. J. Clin. Nutr. *36*:657–660, 1982.

50. Liu, K.: Statistical issues related to design of dietary survey methodology for NHANES III. *In* NHANES III Dietary Survey Methodology Workshop. Washington, D.C., National Center for Health Statistics. In press, 1986.

51. Consumer and Food Economics Institute: Composition of Foods: Raw, Processed, Prepared. Agricultural Handbook Number 8-1 to 8-15. Washington, D.C., U.S. Department of Agriculture, 1976–1984.

52. Pennington, J.A.T., Church, H.N.: Bowes and Church's Food Values of Portions Commonly Used, 14th Ed. Philadelphia, J.B. Lippincott Co., 1985.

53. Pennington, J.A.T.: Dietary Nutrient Guide. Westport, CT, AVI Publishing Company, 1974.

54. Leveille, G.A., Zabik, M.E., Morgan, K.J.: Nutrients in Foods. Cambridge, MA, The Nutrition Guild, 1983.

55. Paul, A.A., Southgate, D.A.T.: McCance and Widdowson's The Composition of Foods, 4th Ed. New York, Elsevier/North Holland Biomedical Press, 1978.

56. Dories, N.T., Warrington, S.: Hum. Nutr.:Appl. Nutr. *40A*:49–59, 1984.

57. Stewart, K.K.: Food Nutr. Bull. *5*:54, 1983.

58. Hepburn, F.: Am. J. Clin. Nutr. *35*:1297–1299, 1982.

59. Rand, W.M.: J. Am. Diet. Assoc. *85*:1081–1082, 1985.

60. Subcommittee on Criteria for Dietary Evaluation: Errors in nutrient intake measurement. *In* Nutrient Adequacy: Assessment Using Food Consumption Surveys. Washington, D.C., National Academy Press, 1986, pp. 48–65.

61. Polacchi, W.: J. Am. Diet. Assoc. *85*:1134–1135, 1985.

62. Bagu, K., Rutishauser, I.H.E.: J. Food Nutr. *41*:17–20, 1984.

63. Southgate, D.A.T.: Food Nutr. Bull. *5*:30–33, 1983.

64. Stewart, K.K.: Nutrient analyses of food: A review and a strategy for the future. *In* Human Nutrition Research: Beltsville Agricultural Research Conference 4. (Beecher, G.R., Ed.) Allanhelf, Osmun, and Totowa, 1981, pp. 209–236.

65. Stewart, K.K.: Nutrient analysis of foods: A reexamination. *In* Trace Organic Analysis: A New Frontier in Analytical Chemistry. National Bureau of Standards Special Publication 519. (Herz, H.S., Chesler, S.N., Eds.) Washington, D.C., U.S. Department of Commerce, 1979, pp. 249–255.

66. Taylor, M.L., Kozlowski, B.W., Baer, M.T.: J. Am. Diet. Assoc. *85*:1136–1138, 1985.

67. Hoover, L.W.: Comparison of data banks. *In* Proceedings of the Symposium on Dietary Data Collection, Analysis, and Significance. (Beal, V.A., Laus, M.J., Eds.) Amherst, MA, Agricultural Experiment Station, College of Food and Natural Resources, 1982.

68. Witschi, J., Porter, D., Vagel, S., et al.: J. Am. Diet. Assoc. *69*:385–389, 1976.

69. Youngwirth, J.: J. Am. Diet. Assoc. *82*:62–67, 1983.

70. Dwyer, J.: Effective Use of Microcomputer Systems. *In* Proceedings of the Fourth Nutrient Data Base Conference. Amherst, University of Massachusetts College of Agriculture, 1984.

71. Dwyer, J.T., Suitor, C.W.: J. Am. Diet. Assoc. *84*:302–312, 1984.

72. McMurray, D., Hoover, L.W.: J. Nutr. Ed. *16*:39–45, 1984.

73. Bredbenner, C.B., Pelican, S.: J. Nutr. Ed. *16*:77–79, 1984.

74. Adelman, M.O., Dwyer, J.T., Woods, M., et al.: J. Am. Diet. Assoc. *83*:421–428, 1983.

75. Frank, G.C., Farris, R.P., Berenson, G.S.: J. Am. Diet. Assoc. *84*:818–821, 1984.

76. Jacobs, D.R., Elmer, P.J., Corder, D.D., et al.: Am. J. Epidemiol. *121*:580–592, 1985.

77. Shanklin, D., Endres, J.M., Sawicki, M.: J. Am. Diet. Assoc. *85*:308–311, 1985.

78. Stewart, K.K.: Nutrient Analysis of Foods: State of the Art for Routine Analyses. *In* Proceedings of the Symposium on State of the Art For Routine Analyses. Washington, D.C., American Association of Analytical Chemists, 1980.

79. Jain, M., Harrison, L., Howe, G.R., et al.: Am. J. Clin. Nutr. *36*:931–935, 1982.

80. Murphy, E.W., Watt, B.K., Rizek, R.L.: Food Technol. *27*:40–51, 1973.

81. Whiting, M.G., Leverton, R.M.: Am. J. Public Health *50*:815–823, 1960.

82. Hoover, L.W.: J. Am. Diet. Assoc. *82*:501–506, 1983.
83. Hoover, L.W., Perloff, B.P.: J. Am. Diet. Assoc. *82*:506–508, 1983.
84. Hoover. L.W., Perloff, B.P.: Model for Review of Nutrient Data Base System Capabilities. University of Missouri, Columbia, 1981.
85. Sanjur, D., Romero, E.: Nutrition *2*:214–222, 1975.
86. Caliendo, M.A., Sanjur, D., Wright, J., et al.: Ecol. Food Nutr. *5*:75–81, 1976.
87. Harrison, K.G., Bond, J.B.: J. Can. Diet. Assoc. *45*:26–29, 1984.
88. Guthrie, H.A., Scheer, J.C.: J. Am. Diet. Assoc. *78*:240–244, 1981.
89. Strohmeyer, S.L., Massey, L.K., Davidson, M.A.: J. Am. Diet. Assoc. *84*:428–432, 1984.
90. Krantzler, N.J., Mullen, B.J., Comstock, E.M., et al.: J. Nutr. Educ. *14*:108–119, 1982.
91. Fehily, A.M.: Hum. Nutr.: Appl. Nutr. *37A*:419–425, 1983.
92. Stuff, J.E., Garza, C., O'Brian-Smith, E., et al.: Am. J. Clin. Nutr. *37*:300–306, 1983.
93. Cannell, C.F., Marguis, K.H., Laurent, A.: A Summary of Studies of Interviewing Methodology. Vital and Health Statistics Series 2 No. 69. Washington, D.C., U.S. Department of Health Education and Welfare, 1977.
94. Gray, G.E., D.C., Paganini-Hill, A., Ross, R.K., et al.: Am. J. Epidemiol. *119*:581–590, 1984.
95. Russell Briefel, R., Caggiula, A., Kuller, L.H.: Am. J. Epidemiol. *122*:628–636, 1985.
96. Rider, A.A., Calkins, B.M., Arthur, R.S., et al.: Am. J. Clin. Nutr. *40*:906–911, 1984.
97. Chu, S.Y., Kolonel, L.N., Hankin, J.H., et al.: Am. J. Epidemiol. *119*:323–324, 1984.
98. Bull, N.L., Wheeler, E.F.: Hum. Nutr.: Appl. Nutr. *40A*:60–66, 1986.
99. Sorenson, A., Calkins, B., Connolly, M., et al.: J. Nutr. Educ. *17*:92–99, 1985.
100. Burke, B.S.: J. Amer. Diet. Assoc. *23*:1041–1044, 1947.
101. Epstein, L.M., Reshef, A., Abramson, J.H., et al.: Isr. J. Med. Sci. *6*:589–597, 1970.
102. Burke, B.S., Stuart, H.C.: Pediatrics *12*:493–497, 1938.
103. Paul, O., Lepper, M.H., Phelon, W.H., et al.: Circulation *28*:20–24, 1963.
104. Browe, J.H., Gofstein, R.M., Morley, D.M., et al.: J. Am. Diet. Assoc. *48*:95–99, 1966.
105. Meridith, A., Mathews, A., Zickefoose, M., et al.: J. Am. Diet Assoc. *27*:749–753, 1951.
106. Den Hartog, C., Van Schaik, T.F.S.M., Dalderup, L.M., et al.: Voeding *26*:184–187, 1965.
107. Hankin, J., Rhoads, G.G., Glober, G.A.: Am. J. Clin. Nutr. *28*:1055, 1975.
108. Morgan, R.W., Jain, M., Miller, A.B., et al.: Am. J. Epidemiol. *107*:488–498, 1978.
109. Dawber, T.R., Pearson, P., Anderson, G.V., et al.: Am. J. Clin. Nutr. *11*:226–234, 1962.
110. Jain, M., Howe, G.R., Johnson, K.C., et al.: Am. J. Epidemiol. *111*:212–219, 1980.
111. Cubeau, J., Pequignot, G.: Rev. Epidemiol. Sante Publique *24*:61–67, 1976.
112. Byers, T.E., Rosenthal, R.I., Marshall, J.R., et al.: Nutr. Cancer *5*:69–77, 1983.
113. Van Leeuwen, F.E., DeVet, H.C.W., Hayes, R.B., et al.: Am. J. Epidemiol. *118*:752–758, 1983.
114. Garland, B., Ibrahim, M., Grimson, R.: Assessment of Past Diet in Cancer Epidemiology. Unpublished

paper presented at Fifteenth Meeting of the Society for Epidemiologic Research. Morgantown University of West Virginia, 1982.
115. Van Leeuwen, F.E., DeVet, H.C.W., Hayes, R.B., et al.: Am. J. Epidemiol. *118*:752–755, 1983.
116. Byers, T.E., Rosenthal, R.I., Marshall, J.R., et al.: Nutr. Cancer *5*:69–77, 1983.
117. Subcommittee on Criteria for Dietary Evaluation: The use of short term dietary intake data to estimate usual dietary intake. *In* Nutrient Advisory: Assessment Using Food Consumption Surveys. Washington, D.C., National Academy Press, 1986, pp. 17–24.
118. Richear, L., Roberge, A.G.: Nutr. Res. *2*:661–668, 1982.
119. Hall, J.C.: Am. J. Clin. Nutr. *37*:473–477, 1983.
120. Garn, S.M., Cole, P.E.: Am. J. Clin. Nutr. *31*:1114–1115, 1978.
121. Bazarre, T.L., Yuhas, J.A., Wu, S.M.L.: J. Nutrition Elderly *2*:3–10, 1983.
122. Emmons, L., Hayes, M.: J. Am. Diet. Assoc. *62*:409–415, 1973.
123. Dwyer, J.T.: Analyzing dietary data. *In* Nutrition Assessment for Children and Youth Workshop Proceedings. Lansing, Michigan, Department of Health, 1977.
124. Beaton, G.H.: Am. J. Clin. Nutr. *35*:1280–1289, 1984.
125. Hegsted, D.M.: Am. J. Clin. Nutr. *35*:1302–1305, 1982.
126. Samet, J.M., Humble, C.G., Skipper, A.E.: Am. J. Epidemiol. *120*:572–581, 1984.
127. Morrison, A.S., Buring, J.: N. Engl. J. Med. *302*:537–541, 1980.
128. Linn, S., Schoenbaum, S.C., Monson, R.R., et al.: N. Engl. J. Med. *306*:141–146, 1982.
129. MacMahon, B., Yen, S., Trichopoulos, D., et al.: N. Engl. J. Med. *304*:630–633, 1981.
130. Marr, J.W., Heady, J.A., Morris, J.N.: Towards a method for large scale individual diet surveys. *In* Proceedings of the Third International Congress on Dietetics. London, Newman Books, 1961.
131. Young, C.M., Trulson, M.F.: Am. J. Public Health *50*:803–814, 1960.
132. Mullen, B.S., Krantzler, N.J., Grivetti, L.E., et al.: Am. J. Clin. Nutr. *39*:136–143, 1984.
133. Yarnell, J.W.G., Fehily, A.M., Milbank, J.E., et al.: Hum. Nutr.:Appl. Nutr. *37A*:103–112, 1983.
134. Axelson, J.M., Csernus, M.M.: J. Am. Diet. Assoc. *83*:152–154, 1983.
135. Greger, J.L., Ethyre, G.M.: Am. J. Public Health *68*:70–72, 1978.
136. Sandler, R.B., Slemenda, C.W., La Porte, R.E., et al.: Am. J. Clin. Nutr. *42*:270–274, 1985.
137. Colditz, G.A., Branch, L.G., Lipnick, R.J., et al.: Am. J. Clin. Nutr. *41*:32–36, 1985.
138. Byers, T., Marshall, J., Fieldler, R., et al.: Am. J. Epidemiol. *122*:41–50, 1984.
139. American Dietetic Association Handbook of Clinical Dietetics: New York, Yale University Press, 1981.
140. Stefanik, P.A., Trulson, M.: Am. J. Clin. Nutr. *34*:1121–1125, 1981.
141. Block, G., Dresser, C., Hartman, A., et al.: Am. J. Epidemiol. *122*:27–40, 1985.
142. Block, G., Dresser, C., Hartman, A., et al.: Amer. J. Epidemiol. *122*:12–26, 1985.
143. Pao, E.M., Fleming, K.H., Guenther, D.M., et al.: Foods Commonly Eaten By Individuals: Amount

Per Day and Per Eating Occasion. Human Nutrition Information Service, Home Economics Research Report 49. Washington, D.C., Department of Agriculture, 1982.

144. Dresser, C.M.V.: Food Consumption Profiles of White and Black Persons Aged 1–74 Years. United States 1971–74 DHEW Publication No(PHS)79–1658. Hurtsville, U.S. Department of Health Education and Welfare 1979.

145. Willett, W.C., Stampfer, M.J., Underwood, B.A., et al.: Am. J. Clin. Nutr. *38*:631–639, 1983.

146. Willett, W.C., Sampson, L., Stampfer, M.J., et al.: Am. J. Epidemiol. *122*:51–65, 1985.

147. National Cancer Institute Division of Cancer Prevention and Control: Health Habits and History Questionnaire, Bethesda, National Institutes of Health, 1985.

148. Dresser, C.M.V., Carroll, M.: Foods Most Often Reported in the Natural Health and Nutrition Examination Surveys Between 1971–74 and 1976–80. Unpublished manuscript. Hyattsville, Nutrition Statistics Branch, Division of Health Examination Statistics, National Center for Health Statistics, U.S. Department of Health and Human Services, 1984.

149. Dresser, C.M.V.: Use of a Food Frequency Questionnaire in Large Scale Studies. Unpublished manuscript. Hyattsville, Division of Health Examination Statistics, National Center for Health Statistics, U.S. Department of Health and Human Services, 1984.

150. Hankin, J.H., Stallones, R.A., Messinger, H.B.: Am. J. Epidemiol. *87*:285–292, 1968.

151. Balogh, M., Kahn, H.A., Medalie, J.H.: Am. J. Clin. Nutr. *24*:304–310, 1971.

152. Abramson, J.H., Slone, C., Kosovsky, C.: Am. J. Public Health *53*:1093–1101, 1963.

153. Reed, R.B., Burke, B.S.: Am. J. Public Health *44*:1015–1026, 1954.

154. Huenemann, R., Turner, D.: J. Am. Diet. Assoc. *18*:562–568, 1942.

155. National Dairy Council: Dairy Council Digest *53*:19–23, 1982.

156. Mhalko, J.R., Johnson, L.K., Gallagher, S.K., et al.: Am. J. Clin. Nutr. *42*:542–553, 1985.

157. Van Staveren, W.A., de Boer, J.O., Burema, J.O.: Am. J. Clin. Nutr. *42*:554–559, 1985.

158. Hankin, J., Kolonel, L., Hinds, M.W.: J. Natl. Cancer Inst. *73*:1417–1422, 1984.

159. Agricultural Research Service, U.S. Department of Agriculture: Portion Sizes and Day's Intakes of Selected Foods, Northeastern Region ARS-NE-67. Washington, D.C., Agricultural Research Service, 1975.

160. Guthore, H.A.: J. Am. Diet. Assoc. *84*:1440–1444, 1984.

161. Krebs-Smith, S.M., Smicilas-Wright, H.: J. Amer. Diet. Assoc. *85*:1139–1143, 1985.

162. Kircaldy-Hargreaves, G., Lynch, W., Santor, C.: J. Can. Diet. Assoc. *4*:102–105, 1980.

163. Sempos, C.T., Johnson, N.E., Smith, E.L., et al.: Am. J. Epidemiol. *121*:120–130, 1985.

164. Sempos, C.T., Johnson, N.E., Smith, E.L., et al.: J. Am. Diet. Assoc. *84*:1006–1110, 1984.

165. St. Jeor, S.T., Guthrie, H.A. Jones, M.B.: J. Am. Diet. Assoc. *83*:155–158, 1983.

166. White, J.C., Mac Namara, D.J., Ahrens, E.H.: Am. J. Clin. Nutr. *34*:199–203, 1981.

167. Guthrie, H.A., Crocetti, A.F.: J. Am. Diet. Assoc. *85*:325–329, 1985.

168. Frank, G.C., Hollatz, A.T., Webber, L.S., et al.: J. Am. Diet. Assoc. *84*:1432–1439, 1984.

169. Hallfrisch, J., Steele, P., Cohen, L.: Nutr. Res. *2*:263, 1982.

170. Nielson, M., Nettleton, P.A.: J. Human Nutr. *34*:325–329, 1980.

171. Nettleton, P.A., Day, K.C., Nelson, M.: J. Hum. Nutr. *34*:349–352, 1980.

172. Holdsworth, M.D., Davies, L., Wilson, A.: Hum. Nutr.: Appl. Nutr. *38A*:132–137, 1984.

173. Posner, B.M., Borman, C.L., Morgan, L., et al.: Am. J. Clin. Nutr. *36*:546–553, 1982.

174. Schucker, R.E.: Am. J. Clin. Nutr. *35*:1306–1309, 1982.

175. Bird, G., Elwood, P.C.: Hum. Nutr.:Appl. Nutr. *37A*:470–473, 1983.

176. Elwood, P.C., Bird, G.: Hum. Nutr.:Appl. Nutr. *37A*:474–479, 1983.

177. Stockley, L., Chapman, R.I., Holley, M., et al.: Hum. Nutr.:Appl. Nutr. *40A*:13–18, 1986.

178. Stockley, L., Hurren, C.A., Chapman, R.I., et al.: Hum. Nutr.:Appl. Nutr. *40A*:19–23, 1986.

179. Stockley, L.: Direct measurements of intake. In Dietary Assessment of Populations. London, Medical Research Council Special Report 4, 1984, pp. 1–4.

180. Stockley, L., Faulks, R.M., Broadhurst, A.J., et al.: Hum. Nutr.:Appl. Nutr. *39A*:339–348, 1985.

181. Frank, G.C., Nicolich, J., Voors, A.W., et al.: Am. J. Clin. Nutr. *38*:474–480, 1983.

182. Akesson, B., Johansson, B.M., Svensson, M., et al.: Am. J. Clin. Nutr. *34*:2517–2520, 1981.

183. Bransly, E.R., Daubney, D.G., King, J.: Br. J. Nutr. *2*:89–110, 1948.

184. Kim, W.W., Mertz, W., Judd, J.T., et al.: Am. J. Clin. Nutr. *40*:1333–1338, 1984.

185. Rider, A.A., Arthur, R.S., Calkins, B.M.: Am. J. Clin. Nutr. *40*:914–917, 1984.

186. Tulinius, H.: Nutr. Cancer *2*:200–204, 1981.

187. Miles, C.W., Brooks, B., Barnes, R., et al.: Am. J. Clin. Nutr. *40*:1361–1367, 1984.

188. Kim, W.W., Kelsay, J.L., Judd, J.T., et al.: Am. J. Clin. Nutr. *40*:1327–1331, 1984.

189. Schutz, H.G.: Am. J. Clin. Nutr. *35*:1310–1328, 1982.

190. Schwerin, H.S., Stanton, J.L., Smith, J.L., et al.: Am. J. Clin. Nutr. *35*:1319–1326, 1982.

191. Campbell, C., Roe, D.A., Eickwort, K.: J. Am. Diet. Assoc. *81*:687–694, 1981.

192. Dodds, J.M.: J. Nutr. Educ. *13*:50–52, 1981.

193. Pennington, J.A.T.: J. Nutr. Educ. *13*:53, 1981.

194. Guthrie, H.A., Scheer, J.C.: J. Nutr. Educ. *13*:46–49, 1981.

195. King, J.C., Cohenaur, S.H., Corruccini, C.G., et al.: J. Nutr. Educ. *10*:27–31, 1978.

*Chapter* **48**

# RADIOLOGIC FINDINGS IN NUTRITIONAL DISTURBANCES

## Robin C. Watson, Herman Grossman, and Morton A. Meyers

The roentgenographic findings in nutritional disorders are somewhat varied. They may be distinctive, as in scurvy or rickets, but they are often nonspecific, as in osteoporosis and osteomalacia, and the diagnosis may depend upon secondary manifestations.[1-3] In addition, any radiographic abnormality occurs only in the face of prolonged deficiency or excessive intake. In all probability, the most striking changes are seen today as the result of malabsorption rather than deficient intake. However, particularly in underdeveloped areas, the latter is still a dominant factor. Generally, the earliest and most specific findings are seen in the child and adolescent, rather than in the adult, although with gastrointestinal abnormalities this tendency probably is reversed.

### OSTEOPOROSIS

Over the years the meaning of "osteoporosis" has blurred and it has become a vague, all-embracing word.[4,5]

In the normal subject there is a balance between osteoporosis and osteolysis and an adequate degree of bone mineralization. Osteoporosis represents a breakdown in this mechanism; osteogenesis is defective while osteolysis proceeds at the normal rate and the process of bone mineralization is unimpaired. The result is an overall loss of bone mass with respect to the volume of bone present. The bone elements, therefore, become sparse and brittle.

Radiographically the cortical bone thins, with an overall loss of bone density. The distance between the normally mineralized longitudinal, but thin, trabeculae increases (hence the term *porotic*), while there is a concomitant loss of transverse trabeculae.[6] These changes are usually first apparent in the spine; however, in advanced cases, the process may be seen to involve all bones. Fractures resulting from brittle quality of the bone are common and deformities may result. Most often seen are crush fractures of the spine with collapse of the vertebral end-plates and anterior wedging of the bodies, resulting in increased lordotic curves. Pseudofractures are not seen in this condition.

Osteoporosis may be seen in relation to:
1. senile and postmenopausal patients
2. malnutrition
3. hypovitaminosis C
4. endocrine disorders, such as Cushing's disease, acromegaly, hypothyroidism, and hyperthyroidism
5. the congenital defect of osteoporosis imperfecta
6. idiopathic conditions.

Interpretation is difficult because loss of the mass of bone must be extensive before this condition becomes radiographically apparent. Furthermore, the findings are nonspecific and there is no way of differentiating postmenopausal osteoporosis, for example, from that found in multiple myeloma.

Osteoporosis is, perhaps, most often seen in elderly patients, often in reduced circumstances, who have an associated dietary insufficiency, including that of vitamin C. Although there are perhaps fewer of these individuals than in the past, they exist in both rural and urban areas.

## SCURVY

Abnormalities in the skeleton in infantile scurvy have been studied by Park.[7] A disturbance of endochondral bone growth occurs, with subperiosteal hemorrhagic manifestations occurring without associated trauma. The bone changes occur symmetrically throughout the skeleton and are more widely distributed than are gross subperiosteal or intramedullary hemorrhages. As are the changes in rickets, those of scurvy are most marked where growth in length is normally most rapid: at the sternal end of the middle ribs, the lower end of the femur, the upper end of the humerus, both ends of the tibia and fibula, and the lower end of the radius and ulna, in approximately the order given.

The columns of cartilage cells in the proliferative cartilage in infantile scurvy tend to be irregular rather than linear. Whether this change represents a purely scorbutic process or whether it depends in part on an associated or antecedent rickets is not entirely certain. Scurvy interferes with the mechanism for removal of calcified cartilage matrix. It suppresses the formation of new trabeculae and, wherever there is bone already formed, resorption proceeds. These changes, morphologically important in themselves, affect the structure of bone also from a functional point of view by diminishing its capacity to withstand mechanical stress.

Roentgenographic changes are often diagnostic or suggestive. The costochondral junctions of the ribs are wide (Fig. 48–1*A* and *B*). The abrupt bony swelling culminates in a ridge where bone and cartilage meet. The sternochondral plate may be displaced posteriorly by atmospheric pressure where the cartilage has been pushed backward at the line of its separation from the bony shaft.

In the early stages, the changes in the bone are nonspecific, presenting poorly discernible trabeculae and thin cortices. As the disease progresses, a thick white line at the metaphysis develops (Figs. 48–2, 48–3). Spurs develop at the cartilage shaft junction, and subepiphyseal atrophy casts a transverse line or band of diminished density[8] (Fig. 48–2). This zone of rarefaction is a linear break in the bone proximal and parallel to the white line. Peripheral metaphyseal clefts, the so-called corner sign, are characteristic of scurvy[7] (Fig. 48–3). Ossification centers have central rarefaction with heavy ring shadows (Fig. 48–2) on

the margins. Epiphyseal separation may occur along the line of destruction, with linear displacement or compression of the epiphysis against the shaft.

Subperiosteal hemorrhages often appear on the larger long bones[8,9] (Fig. 48–4*A* and *B*). During healing the elevated periosteum becomes calcified (Fig. 48–4*B*), creating a heavy shell of subperiosteal bone. This shell of bone gradually shrinks and forms a new cortex. Subperichondrial hemorrhages over the epiphysis are said not to occur in scurvy.

## OSTEOMALACIA

In most countries osteomalacia is now considered to be the adult form of rickets. It represents an abnormality of the mineralizing process, whereas both osteogenesis and osteolysis proceed at a normal rate.[10] The result of the mineral deficiency is that the bone becomes soft and pliable. Whereas in osteoporosis the thin and brittle bones fracture easily, in osteomalacia there is more likely to be bending of the bony structures. The bone mass is still of normal volume, but a loss of bone density occurs.[11]

Most often osteomalacia is related to malabsorption as a result of a variety of conditions: sprue, steatorrhea, pancreatic insufficiency, Crohn's disease, gastric or small bowel resections, fistulas, or chronic ulcerative colitis. Radiographically the bone density is decreased; however, this may be hard to recognize. The trabeculae are poorly defined and coarse, with widening of the intertrabecular spaces. The most striking feature is that, in areas of stress, pseudofractures appear as thin radiolucent lines extending across the cortex at right angles to the long axis of the bone.[12] These fractures are most often symmetrical and bilateral. With treatment, the margins become sclerotic, but angulation often occurs at the site. One theory is that the fractures are related to pulsating periosteal blood vessels; however, this relationship seems unlikely. In partially treated or untreated cases, these zones of lucency remain for considerable periods. The bones most commonly affected are the first or lower ribs, the pubic rami, the transverse processes of the lumbar vertebrae, the lateral scapular borders, the tibiae and fibulae and the shafts of the femoral necks. In chronic and untreated cases, gross skeletal deformities may result.

## RICKETS

Rickets, a disease of infancy and childhood, is a metabolic disorder of bone characterized by formation of normal collagen, matrix, and osteoid with a disturbance in calcium and phosphorus

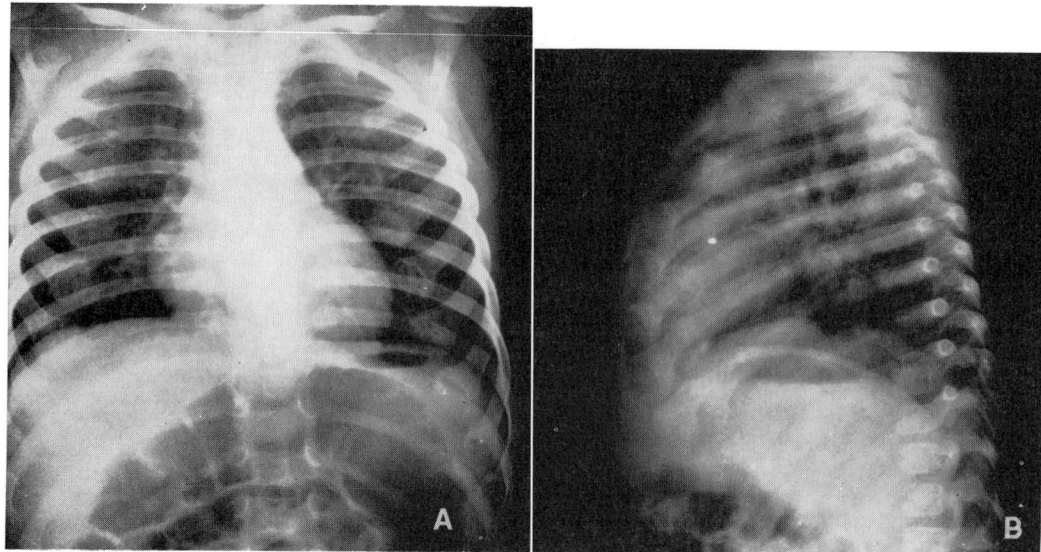

**Fig. 48–1.** A 27-month-old male with scurvy. Frontal *(A)* and lateral *(B)* chest roentgenograms demonstrate bony swelling at the costochondral junctions of the ribs.

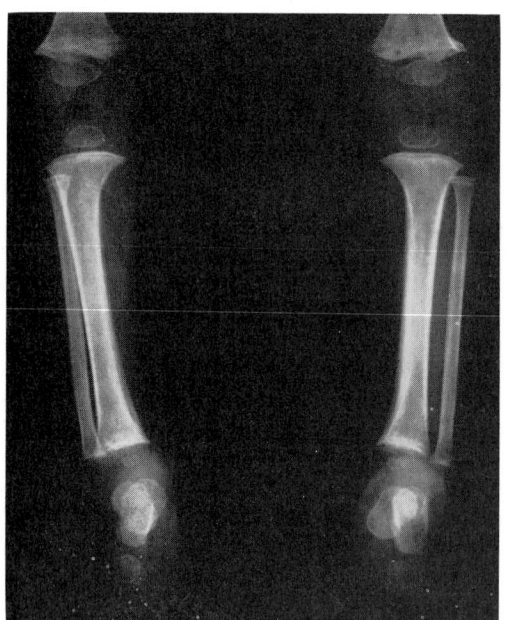

**Fig. 48–2.** A 10-month-old male with scurvy. A thick white line occurs at the metaphyses of the long bones of the knees. Linear breaks are present in the bones proximal and parallel to the white lines of the distal femur. Spurs are present and best seen at the ends of the femurs and medial aspect of the right tibia. The ossification centers have central rarefaction with heavy ring shadows on the margins. Periosteal new bone is along the medial aspects of the tibias

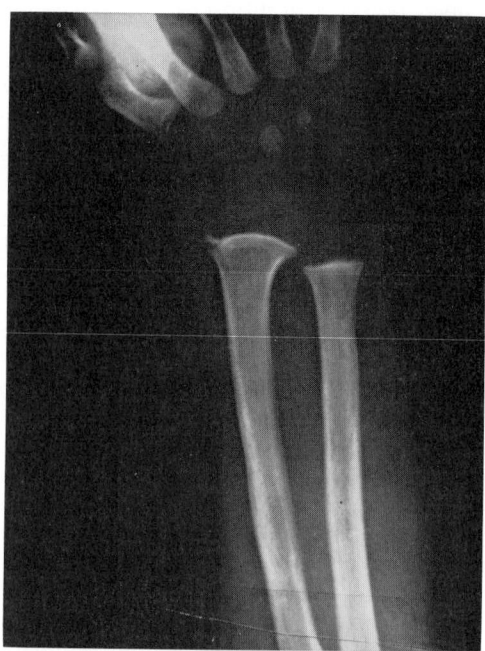

**Fig. 48–3.** An 8-month-old female with scurvy. Dense white lines and rarefaction are present at the distal ends of the radius and ulna. The "corner sign" of scurvy, noted at the distal lateral aspect of the radius, is the result of a defect at the angle between the provisional zone of calcification and the cortex.

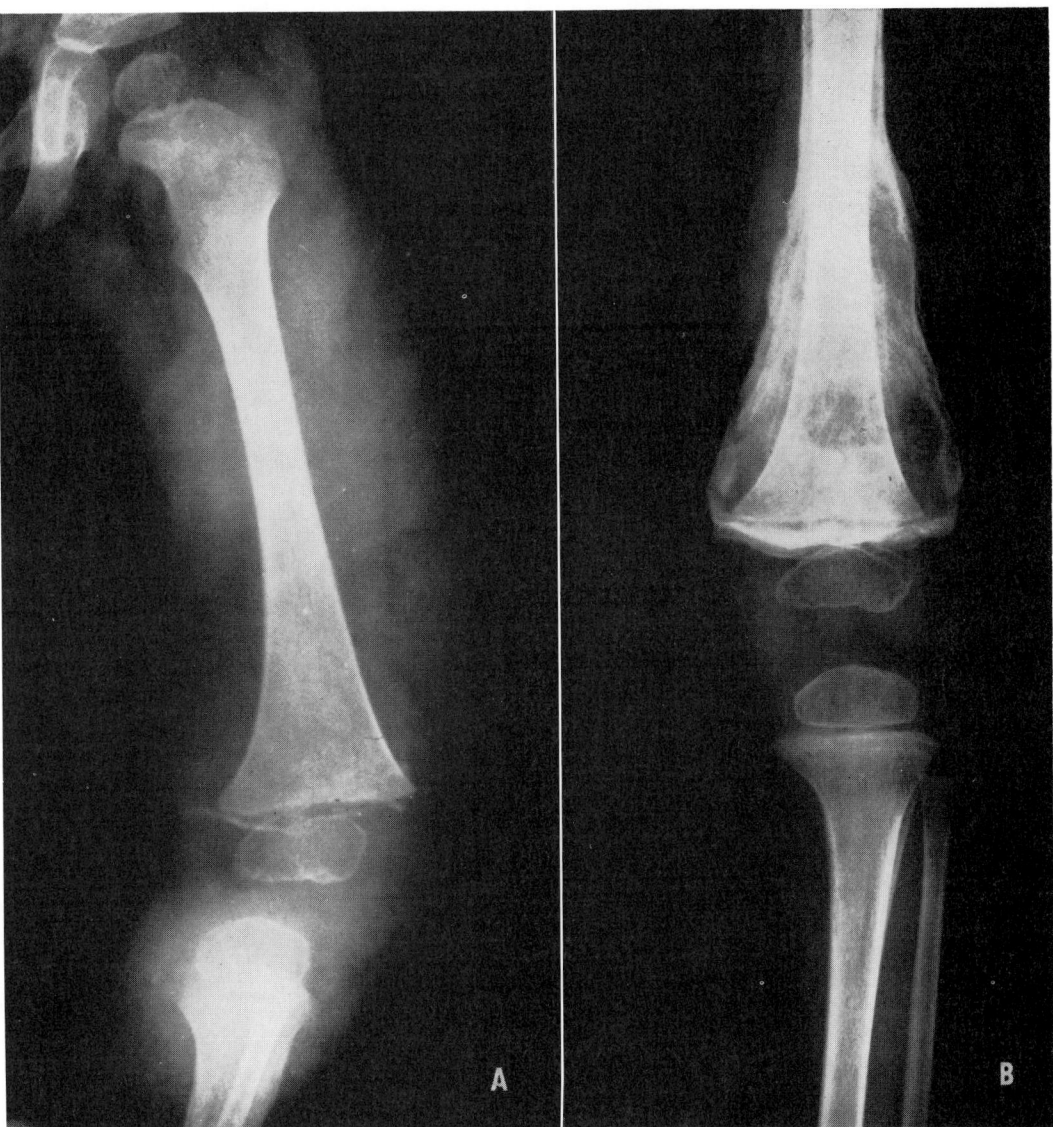

**Fig. 48–4.** A 12-month-old male with healing scurvy. *A*, Fracture of the provisional zone of calcification of the distal femur with early calcification is apparent. Displacement of the soft tissues is due to hematoma, which has not begun to calcify. *B*, Extensive calcification of elevated periosteum occurs after two weeks of vitamin C therapy.

metabolism that prevents the normal deposition of calcium salts in the growing parts of the skeleton. The skeleton becomes weak, is unable to withstand the stress and strain to which it is ordinarily subjected, and yields and deforms. For the development of ordinary rickets, a deficiency must exist both in the short ultraviolet radiations of the sun and in the vitamin D present in certain foods. Osteomalacia is merely deficiency rickets occurring after endochondral growth has ended.

The roentgenograms give the most accurate information regarding rickets. The costochondral junctions, the most actively growing bones, are not accessible for clear radiographic study early in the course of rickets. The lower end of the femur is too thick and the junction of the epiphysis with the diaphysis is too uneven for slight changes to show distinctly. The lower ends of the radius and ulna are most useful for the study of rickets by x-ray pictures because of their small size and convenient location. Significant changes are often visible in the ulna when the radius appears to be normal.

The changes at the cartilage shaft junction are characterized by total or partial lack of calcification of the terminal segment of the shaft. This "invisible" provisional zone of calcification is seen only in rickets (Fig. 48–5*A*). Cupping,

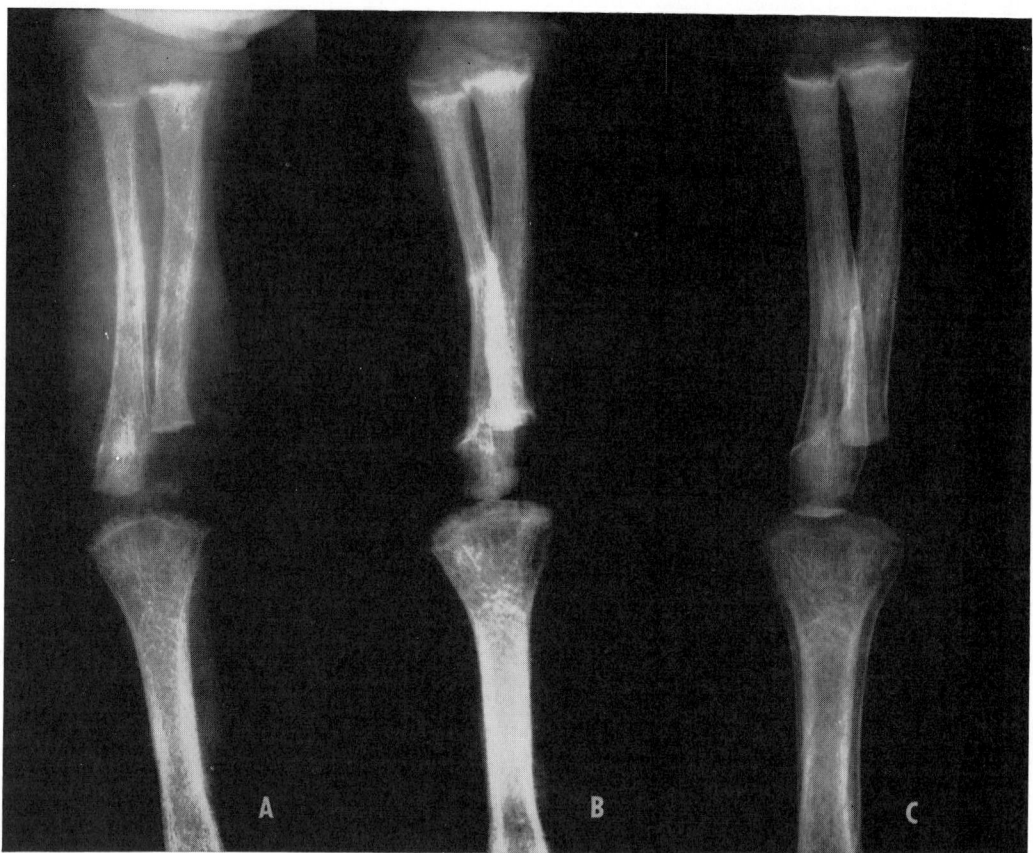

**Fig. 48–5.** A 10-month-old male during various stages of rickets. *A*, Noncalcified provisional zone, and fraying of the distal humerus are evident. Strands of calcified osteoid project from the sides of the bone. *B*, Cupping, spread metaphysis, fraying, and cortical spurs occur. Transverse linear recalcified density develops in rachitic metaphysis. A fracture is present in the midshaft of the radius. Greenstick fractures are common in the long bones. *C*, Metaphyseal spongiosum recalcifies and fuses with that of the provisional zone of calcification. Diffuse layer of recalcified cortex is present.

spreading, cortical spurs, and fraying at the ends of bones are also seen in rickets, but not one of these changes itself is characteristic of this disease. Each may be seen in other conditions such as congenital syphilis or scurvy.

Cupping may not be evident until treatment is begun because of the lack of lime salts in the organic tissue that forms the cup (Fig. 48–5*B* and *C*). Cupping may be seen in scurvy, to a slight degree, in the ulnae of young, especially premature, infants whose bones are growing rapidly.

Cortical spurs are linear shadows that extend as prolongations of the shadows of the cortex along the sides of the proliferative cartilage[13] (Fig. 48–5*B*). They are not always in the direct line of the cortex but are external to it, since they lie in the perichondrial-periosteal layer that envelops the cortex. Such shadows may be found on one or both sides; they may be straight and in line of the cortex or they may arch outward. The shape

and direction of the spurs are determined by the configuration of the proliferative cartilage. X-ray films often show the spurs lying external to the cortex, overlapping, and seeming to splint the cartilage shaft junction. This represents a new cortical layer forming outside the old. Spur formation also occurs in congenital syphilis.

Fraying consists of thread-like calcified shadows extending from the end of the shaft into the transparent cartilage[14] (Fig. 48–5*B*). These frayed densities are neither straight nor parallel but extend in various directions, exactly as would be expected from the disorder in the underlying pathologic condition.

In severe rickets, the shaft of the bone shows a diffuse rarefaction caused by the loss of lime. The cortex may be thin and, in places, invisible. Strands of osteoid may extend from the poorly defined cortex to the almost invisible periosteum, which contains enough lime salts to cast hair-like shadows sticking out from the sides of the bones (Fig. 48–5*A*). Other changes in the shaft that may be visible are complete or partial fracture, callus formation, curvature of the shaft, with great thickening on the concave side, or displacement of the epiphysis on the diaphysis.

Healing rickets is first observed in the provisional zone of calcification. A transverse linear recalcified density develops in the rachitic metaphysis beyond the visible end of the shaft and at a level the epiphyseal plate would have reached in the absence of rickets (Fig. 48–5*B*). As healing continues, the new provisional zone of calcification thickens. The metaphyseal spongiosum also recalcifies and fuses with that of the provisional zone of calcification. The cortex heals more slowly and is less conspicuous roentgenographically. However, when layers of osteoid have been deposited under the periosteum, recalcification of this osteoid discloses a diffuse layer or cortex, which may be of uniform density or lamellated (Fig. 48–5*C*).

Complete healing can be achieved in deficiency rickets. Distortion and sclerosis in the bone remain visible in the same level of the shaft for years, and cortical thickening on the concave surfaces of curvature deformities may also remain. Most bowing and angulation deformities result from displacement of the epiphyseal cartilage. Angulation deformities may also be secondary to pathologic fractures.

Rickets may be distinguished from scurvy by the tenderness and pain present with scurvy, which exceeds anything found in rickets. The various hemorrhagic phenomena seen with scurvy do not occur in rickets. Difficulty may be encountered in distinguishing the enlargement of the costochondral junctions found in scurvy from that found in rickets. Differentiation may be impossible.

Vitamin D and C deficiencies occur commonly together, since both vitamins must be given as accessories to the diet. If one is not given, it often happens that the other is omitted also. The association is thus due to chance, not to any chemical interrelationship between the two vitamins. However, a deficiency in one vitamin may prevent deficiency in the other from expressing itself by characteristic symptoms and signs. If vitamin D deficiency is sufficiently severe and prolonged, the lattice of calcified matrix framework, which is a characteristic feature of scurvy, cannot form at all or forms imperfectly. In scurvy the collapse of the brittle lattice framework is responsible for the fractures and the development of subperiosteal hemorrhage—and probably the pain and tenderness. Thus, as a result of suppressing the de-

velopment of the lattice, vitamin D deficiency may prevent or modify important symptoms of scurvy, typical roentgenographic signs, and characteristic histology.

## IRON DEFICIENCY ANEMIA

Roentgenographic changes in the skeleton in association with congenital hemolytic anemia result from increased proliferation of hematopoietic tissue in the bone marrow.

In 1936 Sheldon first described a child with changes in the skull in association with iron deficiency anemia.[15] In the 1960s many other reports described such changes.[16–20] Lanzkowsky[21] reported several children with iron deficiency anemia who had changes in the metacarpals as well as in the skull.

The degree of change in the roentgenograms of the skull and metacarpals is variable. Children with marked changes are similar to those seen with severe congenital hemolytic anemias. The diploic space of the skull is widened in a nonuniform manner. The squama occipitalis is usually not wide, a result of normally deficient marrow in this portion of the skull. The trabeculae may be perpendicular to the inner table, presenting a radial pattern that may have a "hair-on-end" appearance (Fig. 48–6*A* and *B*).

## HYPERVITAMINOSIS A

Early roentgenographic findings of chronic vitamin A poisoning may be limited to widened sutures in the skull and a bulging anterior fontanelle (Fig. 48–8*A* and *B*). The long bones (Fig. 48–9*A* and 48–10) may be normal at this stage of the disease. The 2-year-old patient represented in Figures 48–8 to 48–10 was seen for anorexia and vomiting. Because her fontanelle was full, a skull x-ray film was taken and demonstrated sutural diastasis. The dense line at the metaphyses of all long bones suggested lead poisoning. The history of a "poor eater" raised the possibility of pica, but careful questioning revealed that "extra" cod liver oil had been given, 100,000 units of vitamin A and 15,000 units of vitamin D, one to three times a day, intermittently during the previous six months. Serum vitamin A level was elevated. The dense line was considered to be caused by excess vitamin D. Two weeks after the diagnosis and the cessation of vitamin A, cortical hyperostosis was present on the ulnae (Fig. 48–9*B*) and the fibulae. The bone changes are usually symmetrical. Three weeks after admission of the child to the hospital, the serum vitamin A became normal but the hyperostosis continued.

When soft tissue swellings are noted in association with clinical symptoms of vitamin A tox-

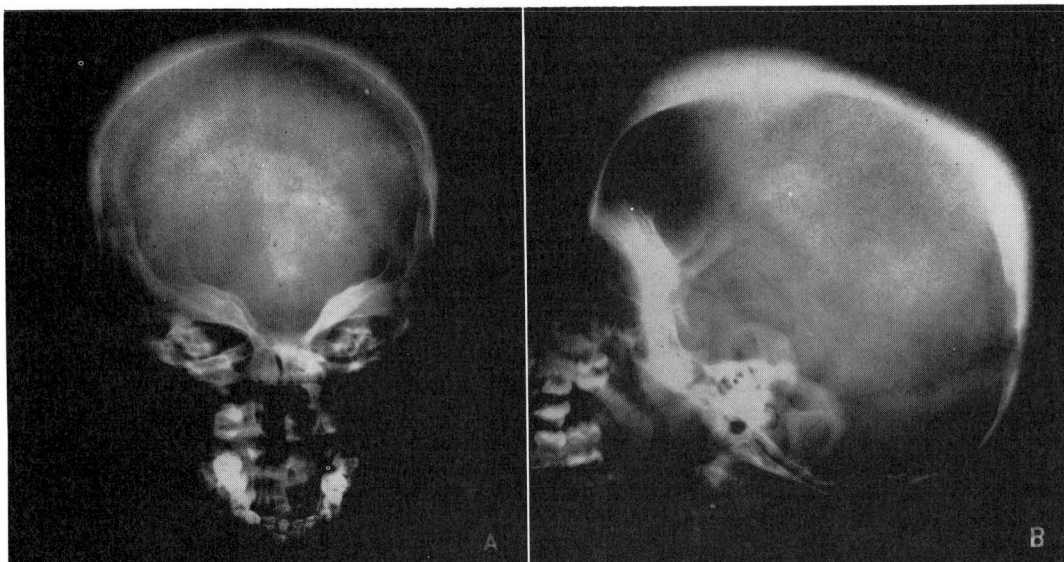

**Fig. 48–6.** Frontal *(A)* and lateral *(B)* views of the skull in a young child with iron deficiency anemia demonstrating nonuniform widening of the diploic space with a "hair-on-end" appearance. (Courtesy of Dr. Philip Lanzkowsky.)

icity (e.g., anorexia, pruritus, alopecia, desquamation of the skin), cortical thickening of long bones is present (Fig. 48–11*A*). Although vitamin A then is eliminated from the diet, the changes in the bones continue. The subperiosteal new bone continues to thicken (Fig. 48–11*B*). These cortical thickenings usually stop short of the ends of the shafts. In some patients metaphyseal cupping, splaying of the affected end of the shaft, hypertrophy of the contiguous epiphyseal ossification center, and premature fusion of this center with the shaft are found (Fig. 48–11*B* and C). Premature fusion of the center with its shafts is most often seen at the distal ends of the femurs and results in arrested growth, with permanent shortening of the affected bones. Although these changes at the metaphyses and epiphyses were demonstrated in experimental animals,[23,24] it was not until Pease[25] reported seven patients in 1962 that this complication of vitamin poisoning was universally accepted. Cortical hyperostosis of ribs also occurs with vitamin A poisoning (Fig. 48–12).

Caffey reviewed the many diseases that cause cupping of the metaphyses.[26] He believes that the basic defect is a reduced growth in the arterial segment of the epiphyseal plate. The "walls" of the cup are dependent on the periosteal and metaphyseal arteries, not on the epiphyseal arteries. Therefore, the peripheral zones of the bones continue to grow. Caffey suggests that in vitamin A poisoning, spontaneous immobilization is caused by exquisite pain and hyperesthesia. Immobilization causes slowing and stagnation of the blood,

which lead to thrombosis of the arteries of the epiphyseal plate.

## HYPERVITAMINOSIS D

In the presence of an excess of vitamin D, an increased mobilization of mineral occurs with secondary hypercalcemia and phosphatemia.[27] Calcific deposits occur in the renal tubules with secondary renal failure, and sometimes death results. In the growing child, the zone of provisional calcification becomes relatively dense in comparison to the adjacent metaphyseal region. In addition, extensive periarticular and vessel calcification may be present with, in some cases, premature vascular calcification.[28,29] When the calcium intake is correspondingly high, thickening of the bony cortex may result so that, instead of decreased density, the bones may in fact be more dense. Distinguishing between this entity, hypercalcemia, and hypovitaminosis D can be difficult radiographically.

## SUTURAL DIASTASIS FOLLOWING RAPID WEIGHT GAIN

Sutural diastasis has been considered a sign of acute raised intracranial pressure in children, especially those under the age of 10 years. Capitanio and Kirkpatrick described three children with nutritional deprivation who developed increased head circumference and cranial sutures following the correction of malnutrition.[30] In 1970, two other reports added nine more children with these changes related to nutrition.[31,32] The increased

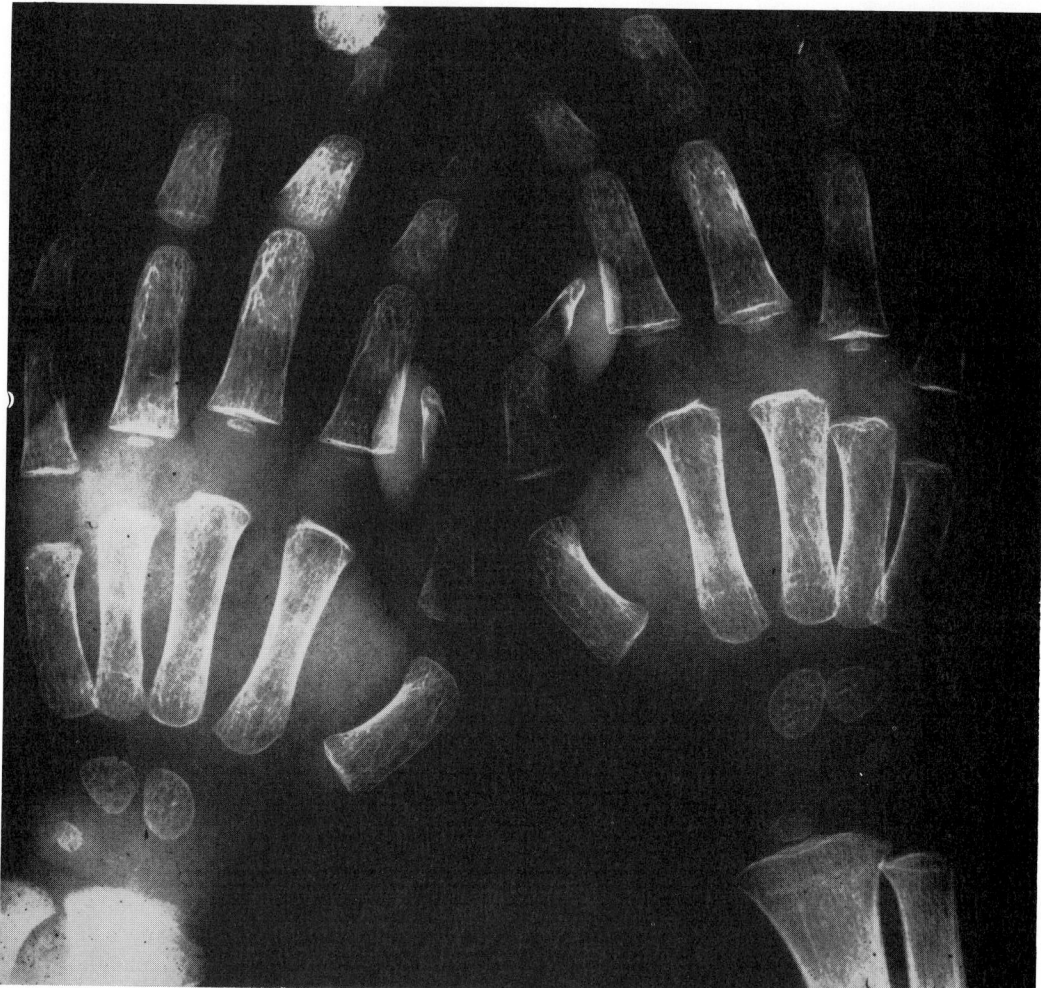

**Fig. 48–7.** The hands of a child with iron deficiency anemia. Widening of the metacarpals, prominent trabeculae of the bones of the hands, and thin cortices are evident. (Courtesy of Dr. Philip Lanzkowsky.)

head circumference and separation of the cranial sutures (Fig. 48–13*A* and *B*) are caused by cellular growth of the brain when nutrition is improved in previously malnourished young children.[33] Although the sutural diastasis simulates increased intracranial pressure, there are no abnormal neurologic signs or symptoms. No increased intracranial pressure has been noted and, in the one patient who had a pneumoencephalogram, the lateral ventricles were normal.

Distention of the stomach may be apparent on abdominal roentgenogram in nutritional deprivation. One patient had a small bowel study done as part of the workup for "failure to thrive." Thickened valvulae conniventes and separation of loops, noted on an early examination (Fig. 48–14*A*), were normal on an examination one month later (Fig. 48–14*B*). The pathogenesis of the gastrointestinal changes is not known, but it

was thought that these findings were the result of edema, although the serum albumin was normal.

## MILK-ALKALI SYNDROME

With excessive ingestion of milk and alkali, usually related to peptic ulcer disease, insoluble calcium and phosphate precipitates may occur,[34] resulting in a renal tubular deposition of calcium with visible demonstration of nephrocalcinosis. To a certain extent, the condition can be relieved by limiting the intake of calcium. Soft tissue calcification, usually periarticular in nature, is also a feature of this syndrome; however, the most common finding is that of calculi within the upper urinary tracts.[35]

## FLUOROSIS

When fluorine is used to excess, probably above levels of 4 million ppm in water, or in the treat-

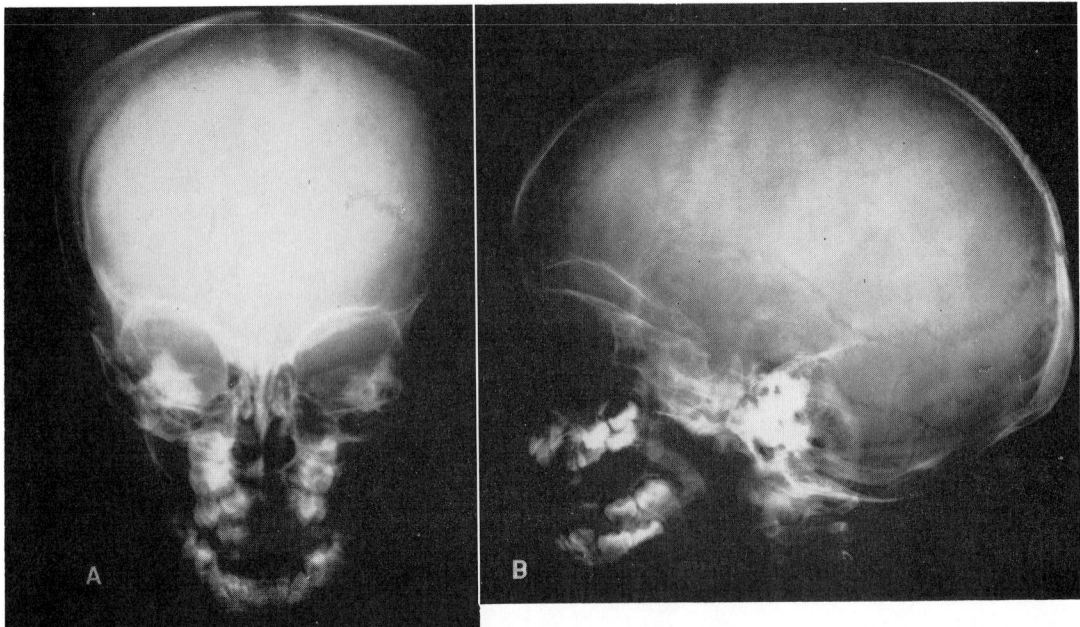

**Fig. 48–8.**   *A* and *B*. Skull of a 2-year-old female, in frontal and lateral projections, with hypervitaminosis A showing wide sagittal and coronal sutures.

ment of osteoporosis, multiple myeloma, or Paget's disease, certain side effects may be demonstrated.[36] Arguments persist as to the exact mechanism by which fluorine exerts its effects, but in all probability it acts by decreasing the solubility of bone salts, thus impairing the process of osteolysis. Radiographically, thickening and coarsening of the trabeculae and similar changes in the cortex are seen. The overall result is one of increased density of the bony structure, although the underlying abnormality is sometimes difficult to visualize. Similar changes, of course, are seen in cases of myelosclerosis and myelofibrosis.

## LEAD AND BISMUTH POISONING

Both these heavy metals have an affinity for bone and act by replacing calcium. In these days the effects of bismuth are rarely seen, as it is seldom used for the treatment of syphilis in the growing child except when the mother has been treated during pregnancy. However, cases of lead poisoning still occur where eating lead paint has been the causative factor. In the growing child, deposition of heavy metals is principally seen in the region of the metaphyses of long bones, particularly where there is accelerated growth, i.e., the knee, ankle, and wrist. Intoxication makes itself evident by zones of increased density in this region. Confirmation may be obtained by the visualization of heavy metal content in the GI tract,

together with widening of the skull sutures, indicating increased intracranial pressure.

## GASTROINTESTINAL DISTURBANCES

Although the clinical presentation of gastrointestinal abnormalities that may lead to nutritional disturbances is often nonspecific, gastrointestinal contrast studies may be crucial in making the correct initial diagnosis, in outlining the site and extent of disease, or in indicating the likely underlying entities requiring furthur investigation. In many of these conditions, x-ray interpretation relies upon subtle but characteristic findings. It must be emphasized that x-ray abnormalities may reflect pathologic anatomic changes or physiologic disturbances.

### Malabsorption Syndromes

**Sprue.** This group of diseases includes celiac diseases of children, nontropical sprue (gluten-induced enteropathy, idiopathic steatorrhea), and tropical sprue. Characteristic radiologic changes in the small intestine are present in almost all patients during the active phase of the disease.[37,38] The essential elements of this deficiency state include: (1) dilatation of small bowel loop, either diffusely or more markedly in the middle and distal jejunum, and (2) hypersecretion, shown by dilution of the barium suspension, often with striking flocculation and segmentation (Fig. 48–15*A* and *B*).

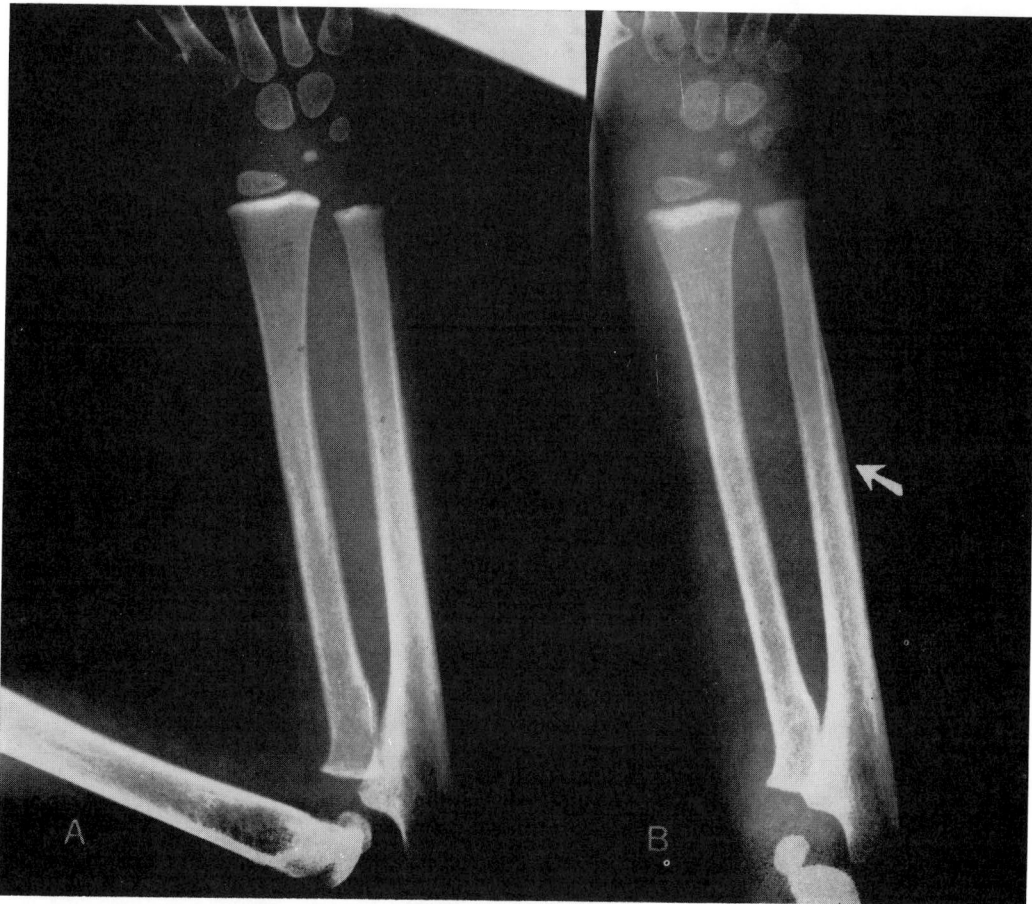

**Fig. 48–9.** Same patient as in Figure 48–8. *A,* Dense line occurs at the distal end of radius and ulna. No subperiosteal new bone is present. *B,* Three weeks later periosteal new bone is seen on the lateral aspect of the ulna.

Frazier et al. have shown that the classic "deficiency pattern" of segmentation within the small bowel is not necessarily associated with disordered motor function of the intestinal wall but is dependent upon the quality of the contents of the intestinal lumen.[39] The loops are flaccid and contract poorly, so that the transit time through the small bowel may be delayed. Little intrinsic change occurs in the mucosal folds. Their appearance is dependent upon the amount of secretions and peristaltic disorder. Short nonobstructive intussusceptions may transiently occur.[40]

The peculiar relationship of sprue and lymphosarcoma of the bowel[41] must be kept in mind. Not only may lymphoma demonstrate sprue-like malabsorption,[42] but the incidence of lymphoma complicating well-documented chronic cases of adult celiac disease is about 7%.[43] Roentgenographic study may be helpful in the distinction.[38]

Malabsorption and a sprue-like radiologic pattern may result from vascular insufficiency of the small bowel.[44,45] This condition must be sus-

pected clinically if malabsorption appears in middle or later life, particularly if accompanied by abdominal angina or manifestations of atherosclerotic occlusive disease elsewhere. Abdominal aortography and selective arteriography may be crucial in establishing the diagnosis. Revascularization procedures have been shown to reverse the steatorrhea.[45]

**Whipple's Disease (Intestinal Lipodystrophy).** Although the multisystem involvement of this disease is shown by the major clinical manifestations of diarrhea, steatorrhea, arthralgias, increased skin pigmentation, lymphadenopathy, and serous effusions, the intestinal symptoms are usually predominant by the time the diagnosis is established.

Small intestinal series demonstrate definite thickening of the mucosal folds in the jejunum and duodenum and only occasionally in the ileum (Fig. 48–16). The coarsened folds are frequently wild and redundant in outline and may present slightly nodular contours. No significant hyperse-

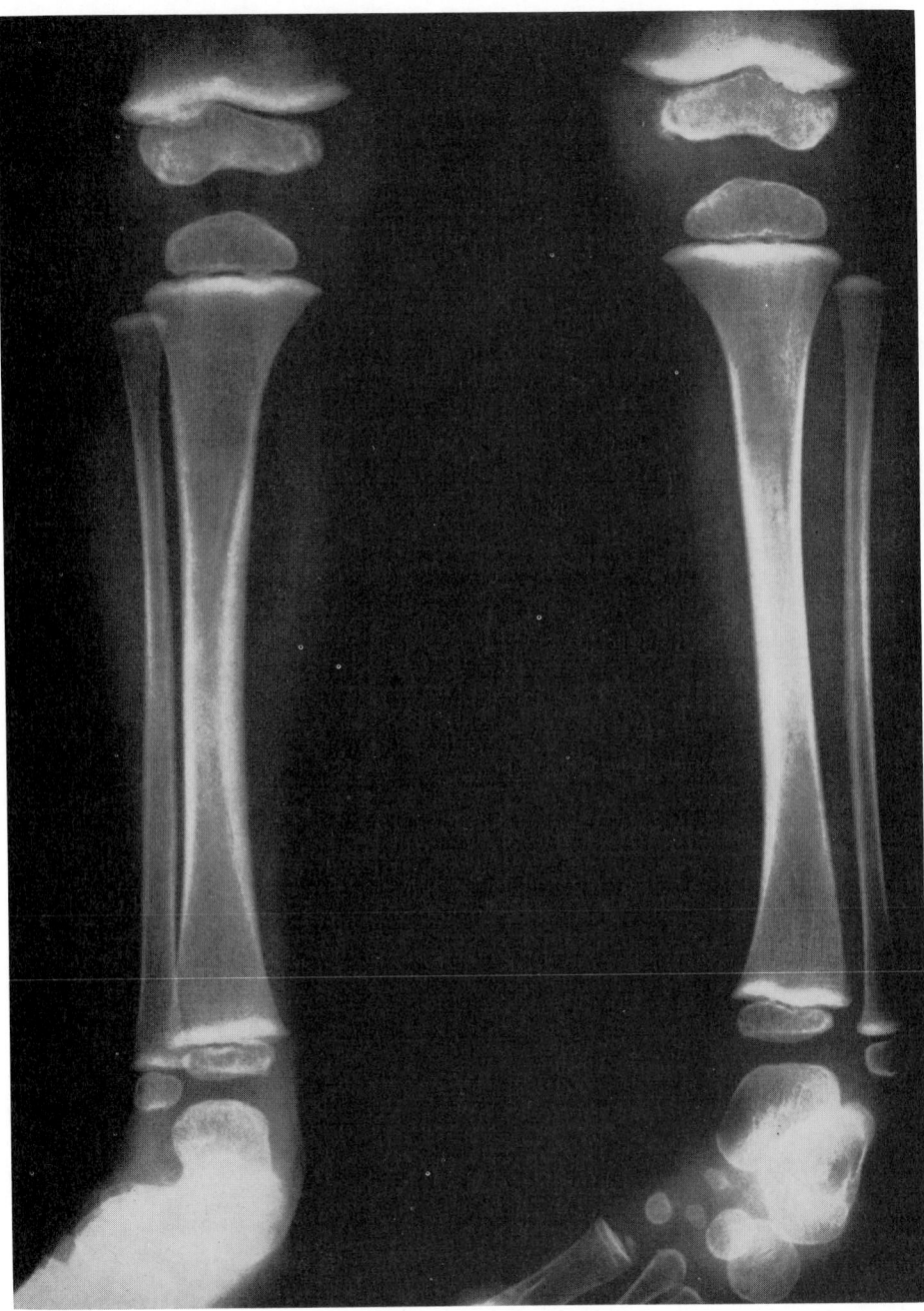

**Fig. 48–10.**   Same patient as in Figure 48–8. Initial roentgenograms of the metaphyses at the knees and ankles demonstrate dense lines. No periosteal new bone is present.

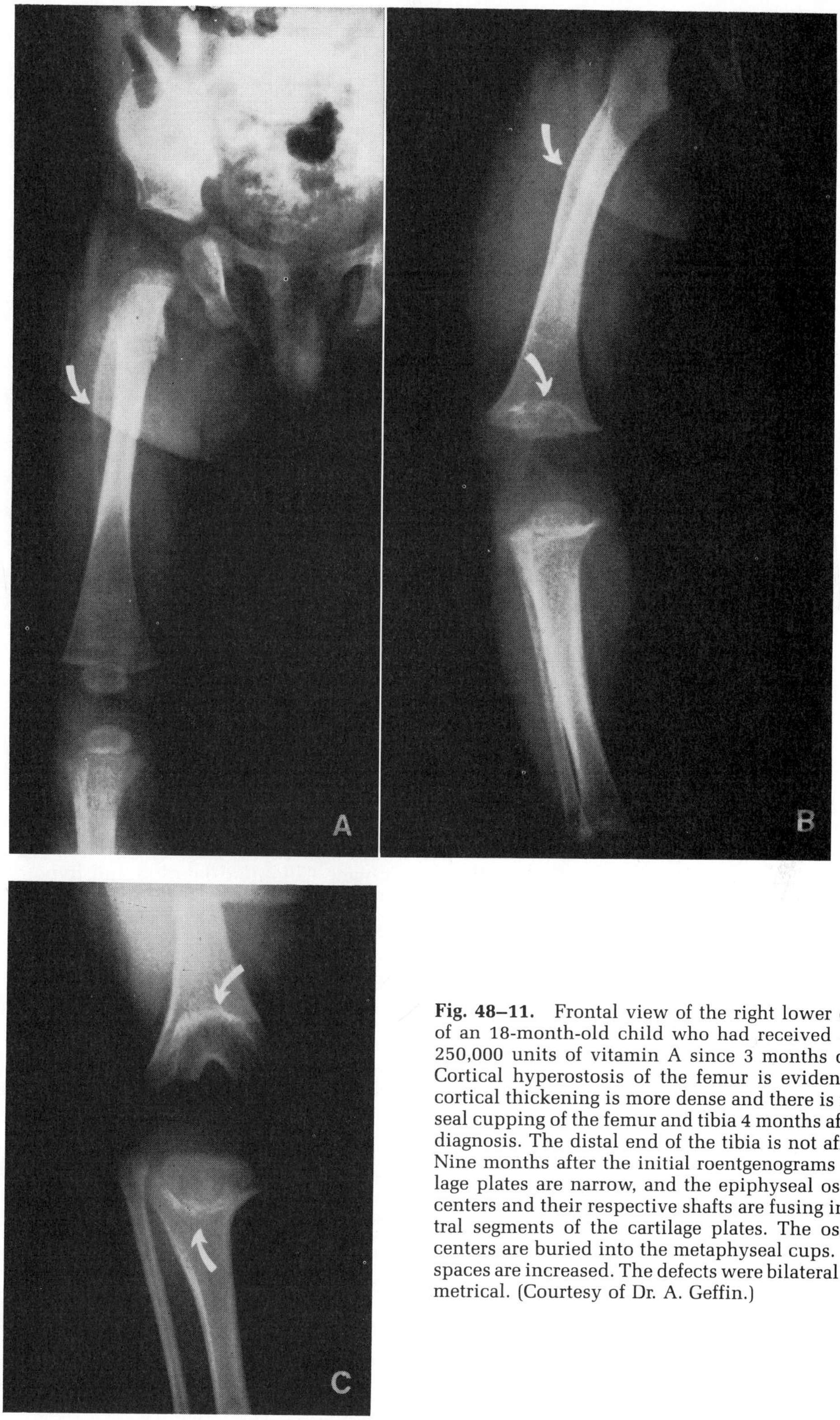

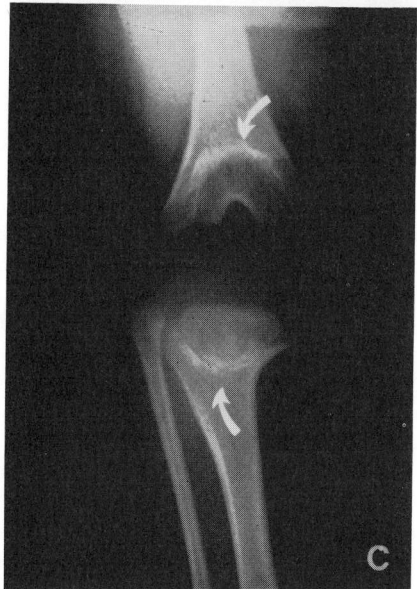

**Fig. 48–11.** Frontal view of the right lower extremity of an 18-month-old child who had received 50,000 to 250,000 units of vitamin A since 3 months of age. *A*, Cortical hyperostosis of the femur is evident. *B*, The cortical thickening is more dense and there is metaphyseal cupping of the femur and tibia 4 months after initial diagnosis. The distal end of the tibia is not affected. *C*, Nine months after the initial roentgenograms the cartilage plates are narrow, and the epiphyseal ossification centers and their respective shafts are fusing in the central segments of the cartilage plates. The ossification centers are buried into the metaphyseal cups. The joint spaces are increased. The defects were bilateral and symmetrical. (Courtesy of Dr. A. Geffin.)

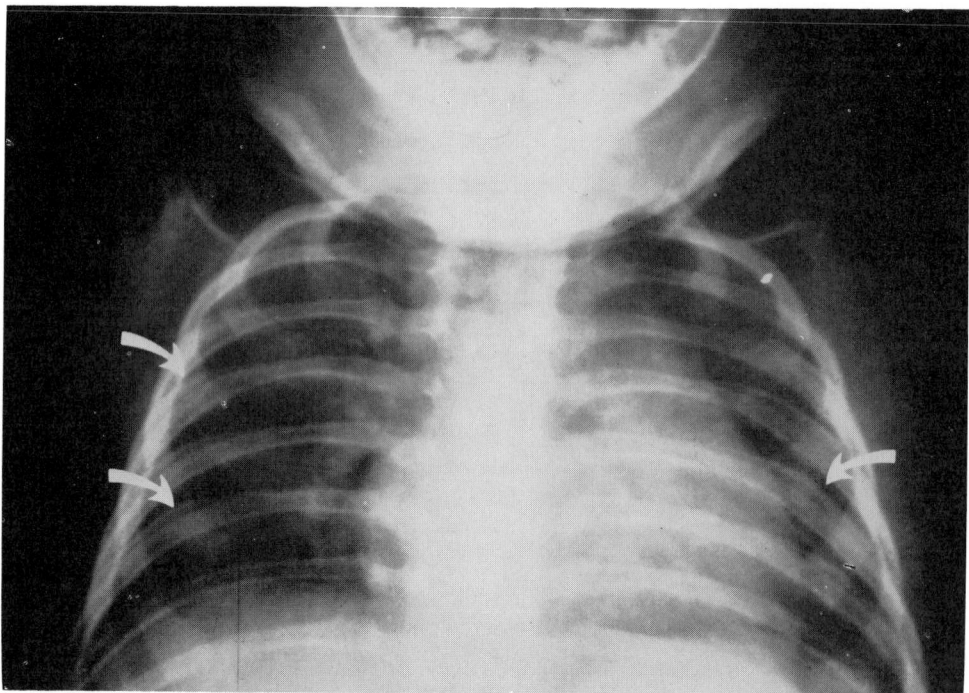

**Fig. 48–12.** Same patient as in Figure 48–11. Chest roentgenogram shows cortical hyperostosis of many ribs caused by vitamin A poisoning.

cretion or dilatation is shown; any flocculation or segmentation is minimal. There is normal peristaltic activity, and transit time from stomach to cecum is within normal limits.[46,47]

The diagnosis can be established by intestinal mucosal or lymph node biopsy. The small bowel villi are swollen and the lamina propria is infiltrated with macrophages containing PAS-positive bodies. These have been shown to be bacteria.[48] Improvement in the radiologic picture may parallel the clinical remission on long-term antibiotic therapy.[47]

**Scleroderma (Diffuse Systemic Sclerosis).** The hallmarks of sclerodermatous involvement of the alimentary tract are dilatation and a marked diminution in peristaltic activity. These symptoms reflect the underlying pathologic changes of collagen replacement of the muscular layers. Bacterial overgrowth in the intestinal lumen is now recognized as a major cause for steatorrhea in patients with scleroderma.

The esophagus is most commonly involved and presents hypomotility and some dilatation. Poor drainage results. Characteristic roentgenographic findings include failure of the esophagus to empty on prone films and stasis even in the erect position, with air-fluid levels (Fig. 48–17A).

In the intestines, large flaccid loops are seen without hypersecretion. The dilatation may appear most striking in the descending duodenum (Fig. 48–17B). Transit time is often markedly prolonged. Colonic dilatation and hypotonicity may also be present, with characteristic secondary pseudosacculations projecting from the antimesenteric border of the transverse colon (Fig. 48–17C).

**Amyloidosis.** The presence of malabsorption in some patients with amyloidosis has been well established.[49] In a report from the Mayo Clinic, Herskovic et al. reviewed 103 patients with amyloidosis and found 6 with documented steatorrhea.[50] With known gastrointestinal involvement, the incidence of malabsorption may approach 50%.[51] Radiologically, markedly diminished motility, conspicuous valvulae conniventes and, rarely, tumor-like deposits scattered throughout the intestinal tract may be present.[51]

**Disaccharidase Deficiency.** This condition is probably the most common abnormality of the small bowel in man, the only known mammal in whom lactase activity in the small intestine is maintained after weaning. Diarrhea, cramps, and flatulence after milk ingestion clinically indicate the disorder, which can be easily confirmed roent-

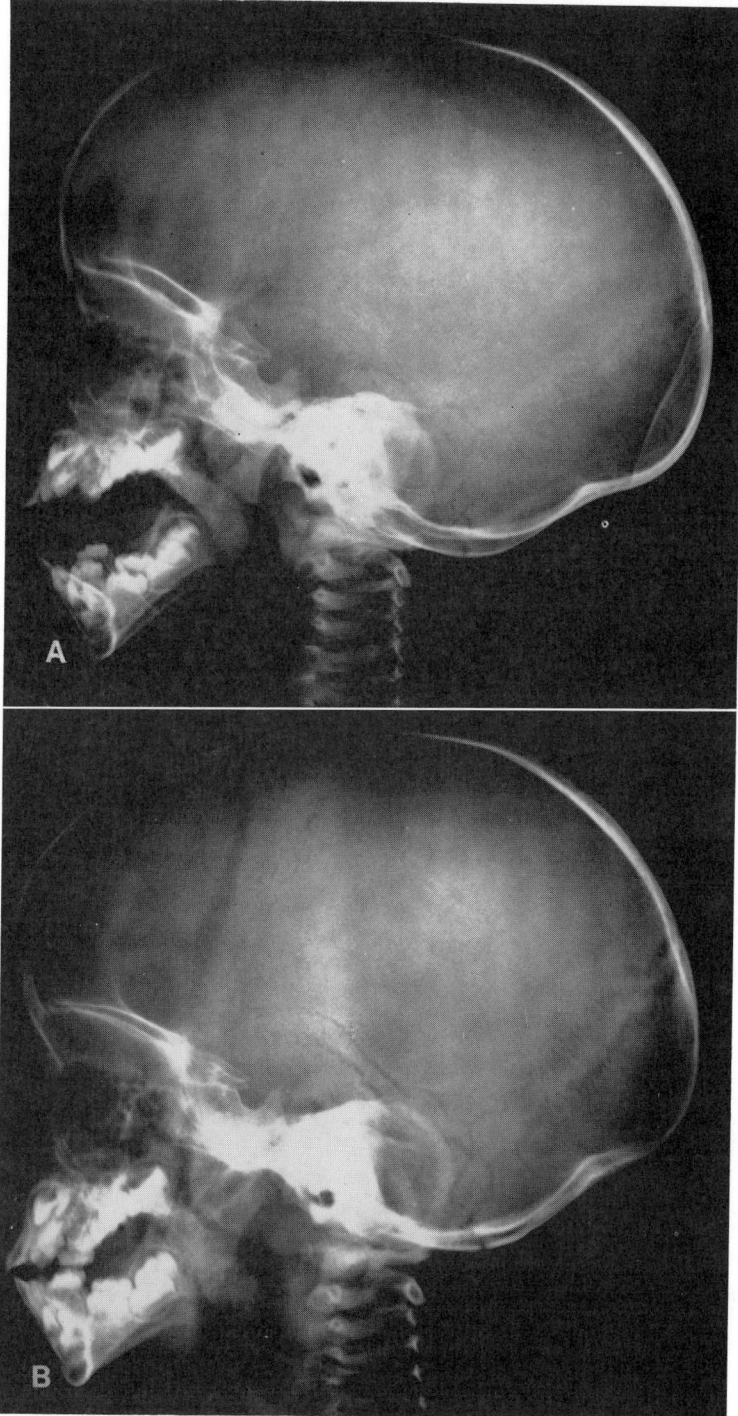

**Fig. 48–13.** A 30-month-old male hospitalized for failure to thrive. *A,* Lateral skull roentgenogram at time of admission is normal. *B,* Two months later, when the child had gained weight and was well, the lateral skull roentgenogram demonstrates wide coronal and lambdoid sutures.

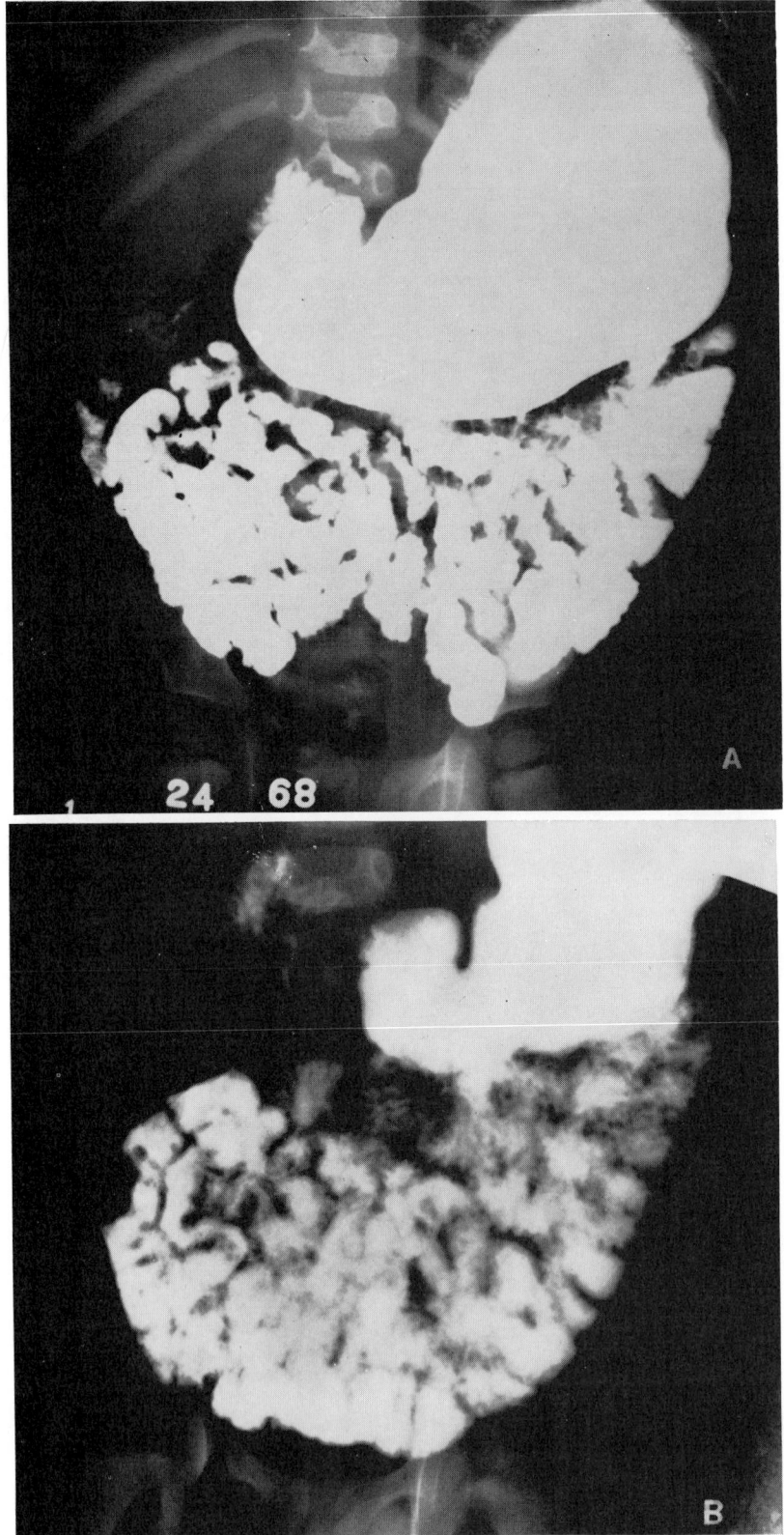

**Fig. 48–14.**    *A,* Gastrointestinal series two weeks after admission demonstrates a large stomach and separated loops of small intestine with thickened valvulae conniventes. *B,* Four weeks after the original study, when the patient was well, repeated intestinal studies show the small intestine to be normal.

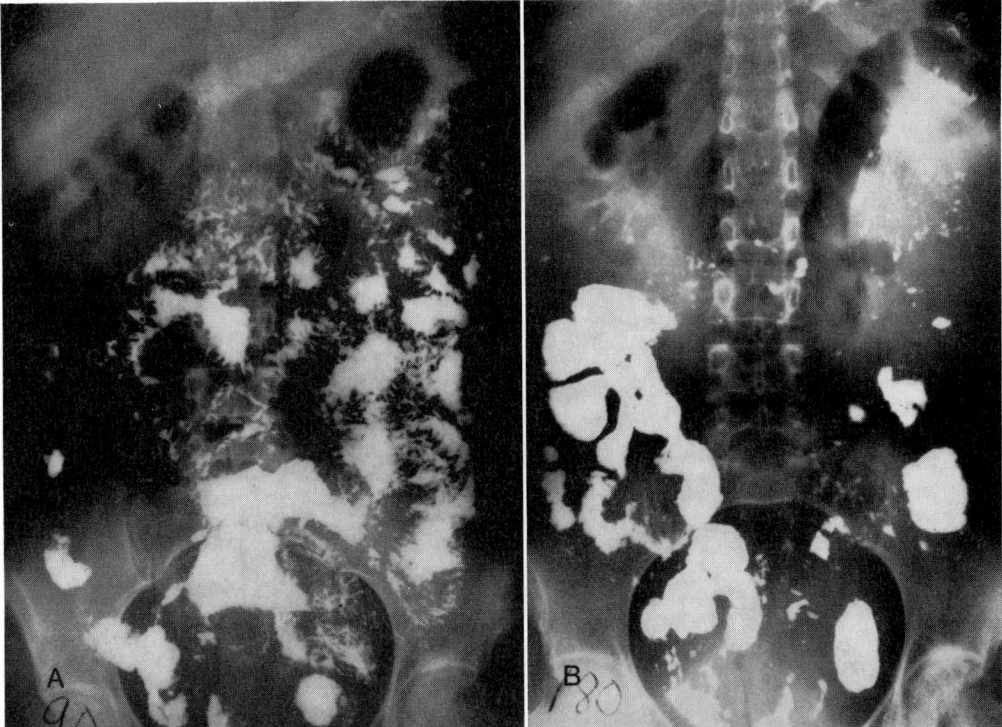

**Fig. 48–15.** Nontropical sprue. *A,* At 90 minutes, conspicuous fragmentation and flocculation of the barium suspension are seen. Disordered motor activity is apparent. *B,* At 180 minutes, segmentation of the contrast within ileal loops, further reflecting hypersecretion.

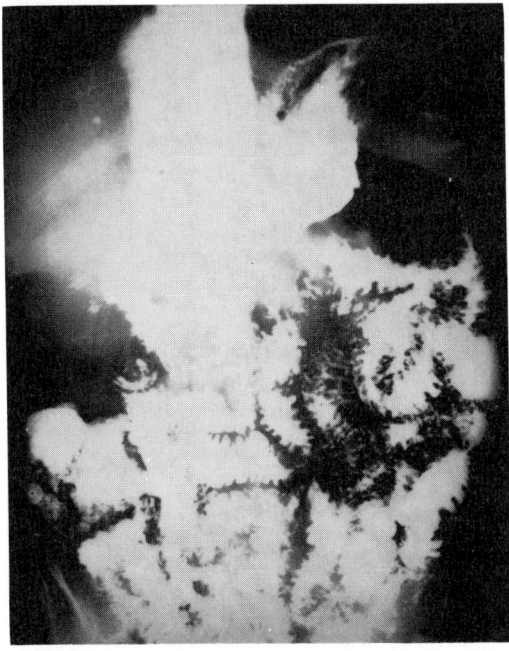

**Fig. 48–16.** Whipple's disease. Markedly prominent valvulae conniventes without hypersecretion or dilatation are present.

genologically.[52,53] When 50 g of lactose are added to the usual barium mixture, characteristic changes occur in the small bowel series. These changes include dilution of the barium, particularly noticeable in the ileum and colon, and dilatation of the small bowel (Fig. 48–18). These effects are secondary to the ingress of water into the bowel lumen in response to the osmotic forces of the disaccharide. Rapid intestinal motility accompanies the dilatation.

Intestinal lactase deficiency occurs on a genetic basis and is also common in a variety of intestinal disorders. This radiologic technique is the most valuable screening aid for it. The addition of lactose to the barium sulfate mixture does not interfere with the examination of the small bowel in patients without disaccharidase deficiency. When a lactase deficiency is discovered, a conventional small bowel examination with barium alone is indicated to identify any morphologic abnormality.[53]

**Small Bowel Resection.** The severity of malabsorption after small bowel resection generally depends on the extent and site of resection, presence of the ileocecal valve, and the condition of the remaining small bowel and other digestive organs.[54] These parameters of the "short-gut syn-

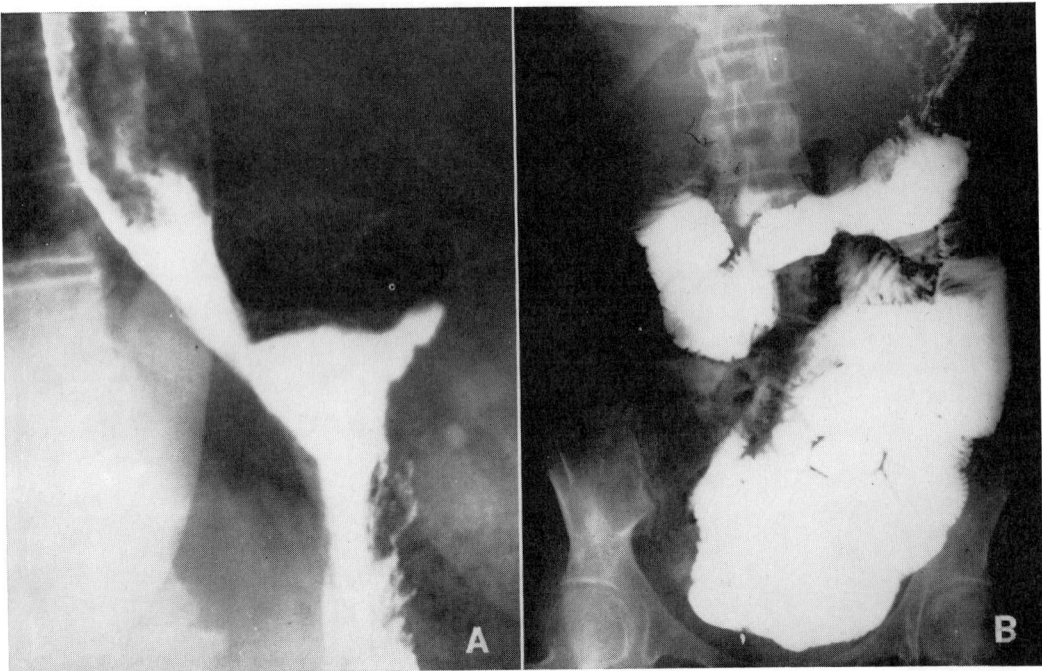

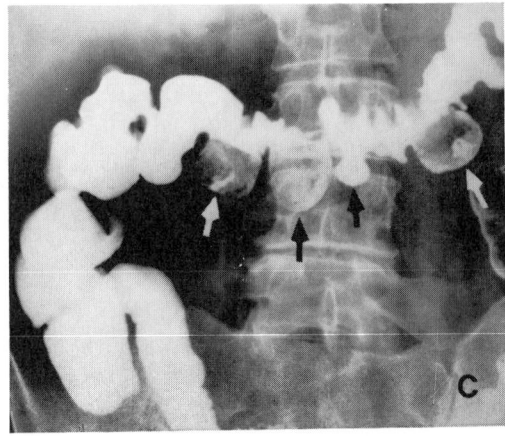

**Fig. 48–17.** Scleroderma. *A,* Despite a nonobstructed lumen, differential fluid levels persist in the esophagus and stomach in the upright position. *B,* Diffuse involvement of the small bowel results in gross dilatation, most evident in the descending duodenum and jejunum. *C,* Asymmetrical involvement of the colon is shown by large wide-mounted pseudosacculation *(arrows).*

drome" can be evaluated by roentgenographic study (Fig. 48–19). On occasion, the exact extent of resection performed in the past is not known when malabsorption becomes a serious problem of management. Since the normal length of small intestine is variable, more important than knowledge of the length of bowel *removed* is an accurate appraisal of the length in the *remaining* functioning loops. Measurements derived from x-ray study after the passage of an opaque tube obviate the inaccuracy inherent in measuring the continuity of superimposed barium-filled loops.

Enteric fistulas and inadvertent gastro-ileostomy[55] result in a similar condition by bypassing the absorptive mechanisms of the small bowel (Fig. 48–20*A* and *B*).

**Diverticula, Blind Loops, and Strictures.** Common to all these conditions, which may result in malabsorption, is stasis of intestinal contents and bacterial overgrowth. Normally, the small bowel flora consists of predominantly gram-positive and anaerobic organisms. The ileocecal valve serves to separate two distinct groups of organisms: above, mainly streptococci, lactobacilli and fungi; below, coliforms, bacteroides, and anaerobic lactobacilli.[56] In a variety of disease states, an overgrowth of bacteria—especially the anaerobic bacteroides, lactobacilli, and clostridia—may occur and cause steatorrhea by deconjugating and/or dehydroxylating primary bile salts in the intestinal lumen.[57]

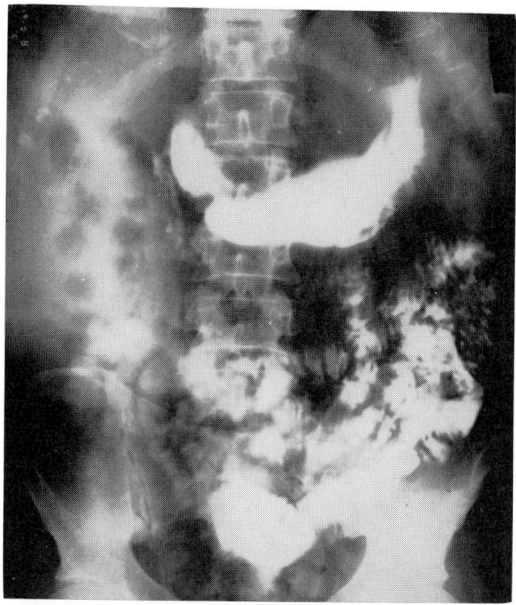

**Fig. 48–18.** Lactase deficiency. A barium-lactose mixture results in progressive dilution and hypermotility.

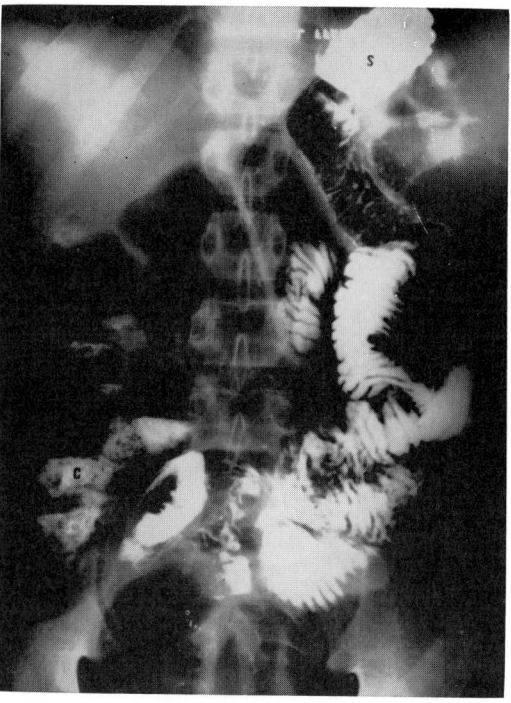

**Fig. 48–19.** Massive small bowel resection for volvulus following gastrojejunostomy. Few small bowel loops, primarily jejunal as shown by their mucosal pattern, remain between the stomach pouch (S) and the cecum (C).

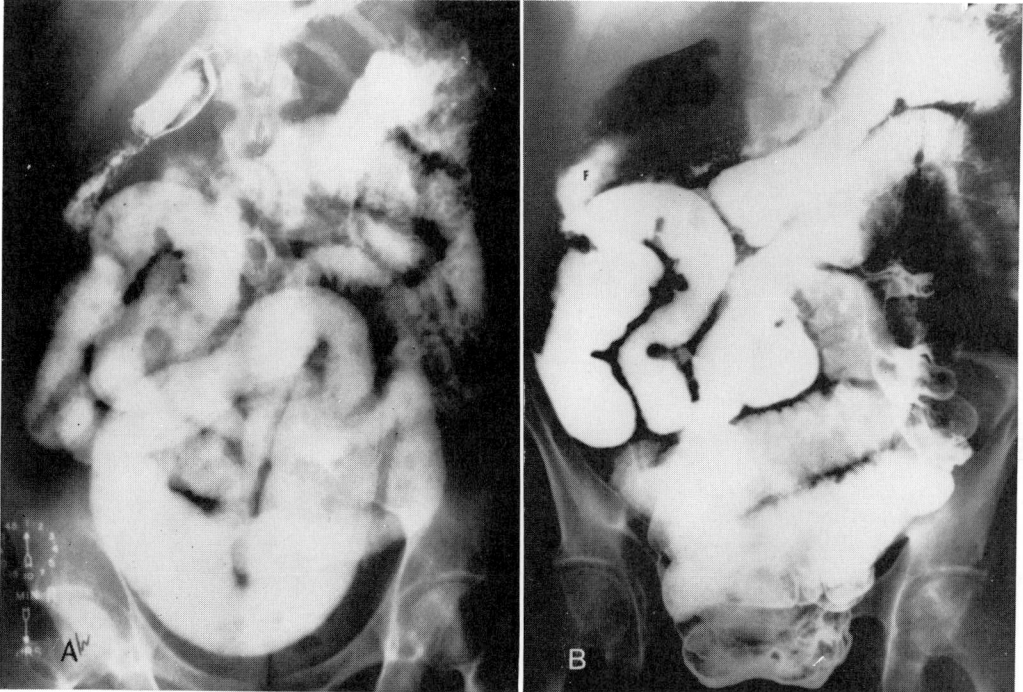

**Fig. 48–20.** Enteric fistula producing malabsorption following ileotransversostomy. *A,* Dilatation and hypersecretion of small bowel loops. Although there is no flocculation or segmentation, these changes constitute a sprue-like pattern. *B,* During another examination, the fistula (F) between the distal ileum and descending duodenum is demonstrated.

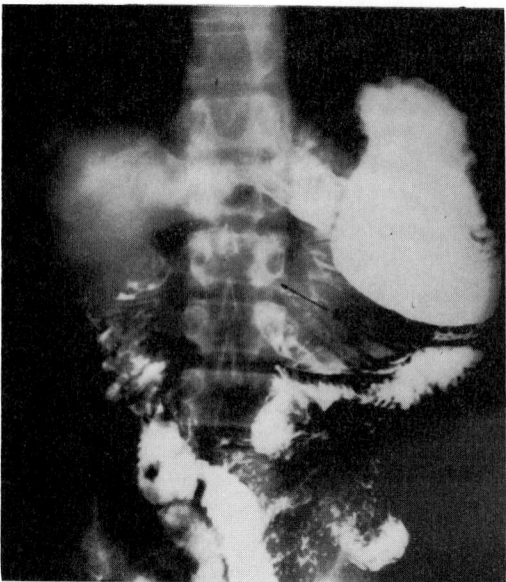

**Fig. 48–21.** Afferent loop syndrome. The massively distended, obstructed afferent loop following a Billroth II gastrojejunostomy constitutes a blind loop leading to malabsorption.

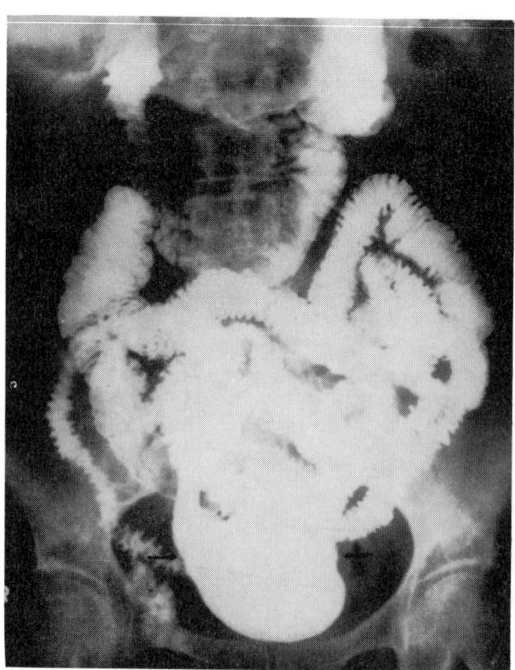

**Fig. 48–22.** Blind loop secondary to radiation effects. Stasis within a fixed, distended loop occurs as a consequence of multiple strictures.

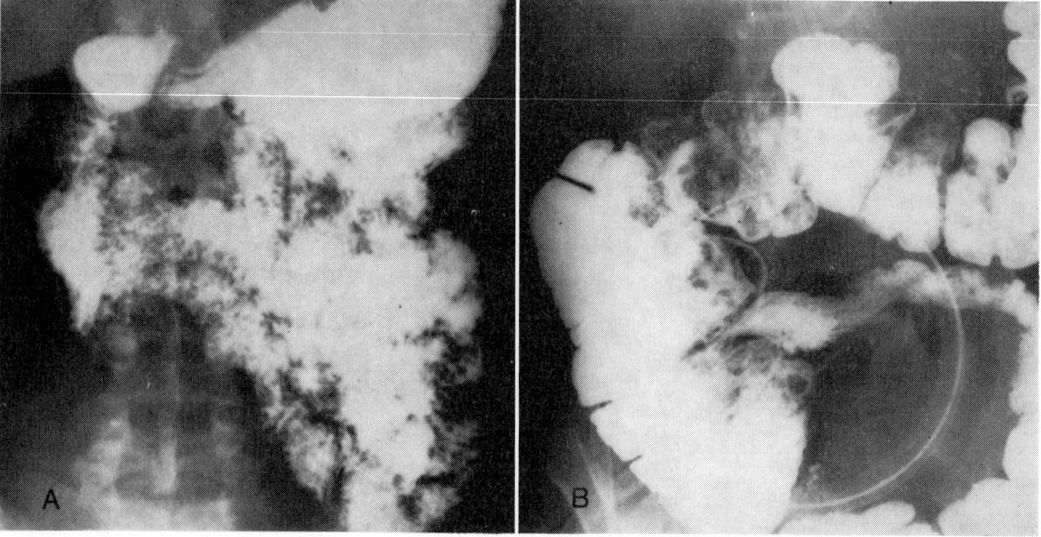

**Fig. 48–23.** Nodular lymphoid hyperplasia of the small intestine associated with hypogammaglobulinemia. Two different cases illustrate multiple punctate to nodular submucosal filling defects in the jejunum *(A)* and terminal ileum *(B)*.

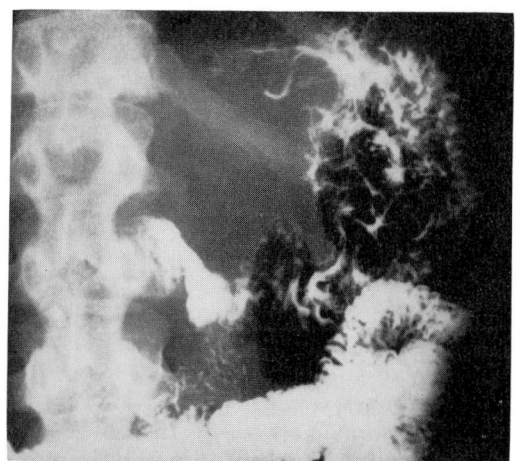

**Fig. 48–24.** Menetrier's disease. Markedly enlarged gastric folds are particularly prominent in the upper two thirds of the stomach.

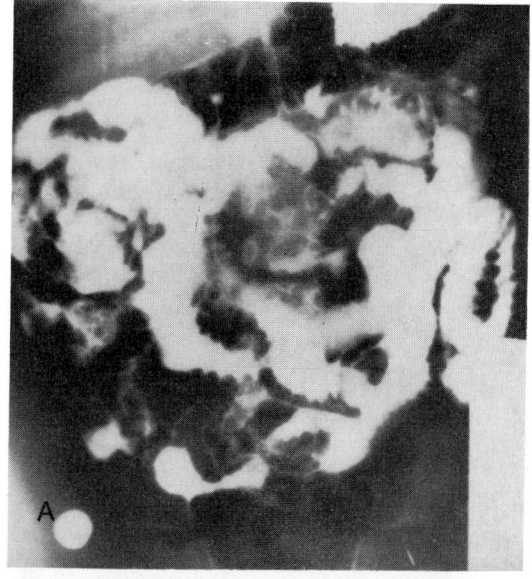

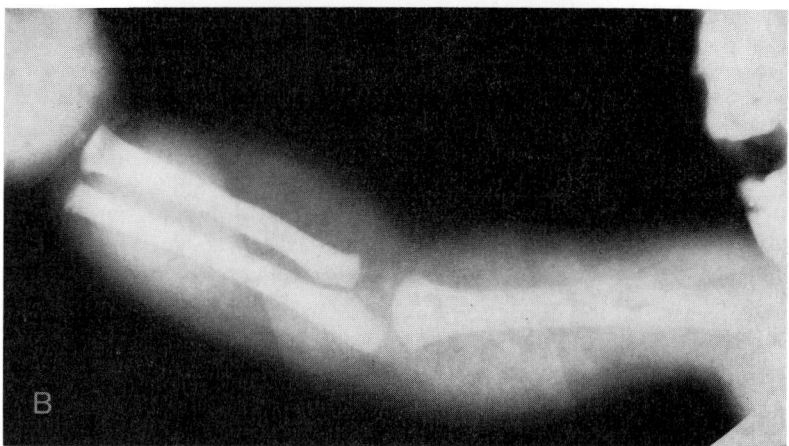

**Fig. 48–25.** Intestinal lymphangiectasia in a 3-year-old child with severe protein-losing enteropathy. *A,* Prominent mucosal folds occur within mildly dilated small bowel loops containing increased secretions. *B,* Edematous involvement of the right upper extremity is apparent.

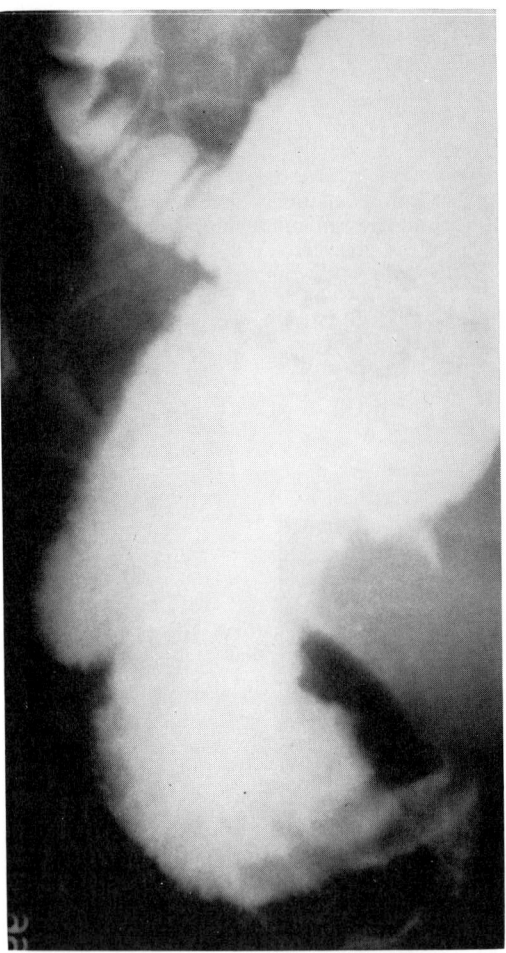

**Fig. 48–26.** Villous adenoma of the rectum. Large circumferential mucosal mass with diffusely irregular contours is present.

Diverticulosis of the small bowel is readily recognized as multiple outpouchings without gross intrinsic contractility from the mesenteric borders of the loops. Blind loops may be a result of (side-to-side) intestinal anastomoses, an obstructed postoperative loop, as in the afferent-loop syndrome following a Billroth II gastrojejunostomy (Fig. 48–21), multiple strictures of the intestine, as in the stenotic phase of regional enteritis,[38] or postradiation changes (Fig. 48–22). In radiation enteritis, lymphatic dilatation, bowel thickening, and avascularity may also contribute to the malabsorption.[58]

**Parasitic Diseases.** The enteritis caused by infestation with *Giardia lamblia*[59] or *Strongyloides stercoralis*[60] is reflected by roentgenographic alterations, which may first draw the attention of the clinician to the diagnosis.

**Dysgammaglobulinemia.** Hypogammaglobuli-

nemia may underlie a clinical pattern of repeated infections and chronic or intermittent diarrhea and mild steatorrhea. In 1966, Hermans and his co-workers noted the association of nodular lymphoid hyperplasia of the small intestine, with or without giardiasis, in cases of dysgammaglobulinemia with a disproportionate deficiency of the IgA and IgM components.[61] These nodular hyperplastic lymphoid follicles in the lamina propria can be recognized as tiny, 1- to 3-mm filling defects, primarily in the duodenum and jejunum[62] (Fig. 48–23*A* and *B*). Their recognition may be an important clue in directing the clinician to evaluation of the gamma globulins and to intestinal biopsy for information necessary in management.

**Uncommon Constitutional Disorders.** In recent years, a number of uncommon systemic diseases in which malabsorption may be a significant complication have been recognized. Radiologic abnormalities in the gastrointestinal tract have been noted or are a conspicuous feature in the Canada-Cronkhite syndrome,[63] mastocytosis,[64] Degos' disease,[65] abetalipoproteinemia (Bassen-Kornzweig syndrome),[66] and Waldenström's macroglobulinemia.[67]

## PROTEIN-LOSING ENTEROPATHY

There is now widespread recognition that excessive gastrointestinal protein loss is a major cause of hypoproteinemia seen in association with a wide variety of disorders. Loss of protein secondary to exudation through an inflamed or ulcerated mucosa (as in regional enteritis or ulcerative colitis) or secondary to obstructed outflow of the gastrointestinal lymphatics (as in lymphoma or Whipple's disease) is well known. In an excellent review, Waldmann has compiled over 40 such gastrointestinal disorders and emphasizes that, in many of these patients with clearly defined gastrointestinal tract diseases, hypoproteinemia and edema may be the only clinical manifestations.[68]

**Giant Hypertrophy of the Gastric Mucosa (Menetrier's disease).** Massively enlarged gastric rugae may be the site of loss of plasma proteins, particularly albumin, into the lumen.[69] They characteristically are more prominent along the greater curvature and usually do not extend to involve the gastric antrum. The hypertrophied folds maintain pliability and are not nodular or ulcerated (Fig. 48–24).

**Intestinal Lymphangiectasia.** This syndrome reflects a generalized disorder of the development of lymphatic channels. First defined by Waldmann in 1961, it is characterized by excessive loss of serum protein into the intestine with massive edema (often asymmetrical), chylous effusions, hypoalbuminemia, and hypogammaglobuline-mia. The dilated lymphatic vessels invariably present in the intestinal wall may leak protein through an intact epithelium or may rupture and discharge their contents into the lumen of the gut. Isotopic studies are helpful in documenting the serum protein loss into the intestine.

The condition is being recognized with increased frequency, and x-ray study plays an important role in its diagnosis. The characteristic appearance in the small bowel series consists of enlargement of the valvulae conniventes of both jejunum and ileum, increased secretions, and minimal or absent dilatation of the bowel (Fig. 48–25*A* and *B*). The fold enlargement may assume a "cobblestone" pattern. Punctate filling defects occasionally seen may represent the enormously enlarged villi secondary to dilated submucosal lymphatics.[70]

Hypoalbuminemia itself, below a level of 2.5g/dl resulting from other causes (e.g., nephrosis or hepatic cirrhosis), may result in edema of the bowel with diffusely thickened intestinal folds,[71] but usually does not exhibit increased intraluminal secretions.

Lymphangiographic findings support the concept that this disease is a systemic lymphatic dysplasia.[70,72] In the lower extremities, either hypoplasia of lymph vessels or dilated varicose lymphatics are present. In the abdomen, hypoplasia of lymph nodes or moderate contrast reflux into mesenteric lymphatics, associated with possible obstruction of the cisterna chyli and enlarged nodes, has been demonstrated.

**Villous Adenoma of the Colon.** Among the neoplasms of the gastrointestinal tract that may produce excess secretion of mucus to result in severe protein loss, villous adenoma of the colon is one of the most prominent. It is most common in the rectum where, because of its usual soft consistency, it may be easily missed on digital palpation. On barium enema examination, it is revealed by its characteristically irregular polypoid or flame-shaped contours as the contrast agent fills in the interstices between its frond-like projections (Fig. 48–26).

## REFERENCES

1. Gould, D.M.: Am. J. Med. Sci. *223*:569, 1952.
2. Barnett, E., Nordin, B.E.C.: Br. J. Radiol. *34*:683, 1961.
3. Shapiro, R.: Clin. Radiol. *13*:238, 1962.
4. Harrison, M., Fraser, R., Mullan, B.: Lancet *1*:1015, 1961.
5. Park, E.A.: Pediatrics *33 (Suppl.)*:815, 1964.
6. Steinbach, H.L.: Radiol. Clin. North Am. *2*:191, 1964.
7. Park, E.A., Guild, H.G., Jackson, D., et al.: Arch. Dis. Child. *10*:265, 1935.
8. McLean, S., McIntosh, R.: Am. J. Dis. Child. *36*:875, 1928.
9. Kato, K.: Radiology *18*:1096, 1932.
10. Albright, F., Burnett, C.H., Parson, W., et al.: Medicine *25*:399, 1946.
11. Lasser, E.C.: Dynamic Factors in Roentgen Diagnosis, Baltimore, Williams & Wilkins, 1967.
12. Milkman, L.A.: A.J.R. *32*:622, 1934.
13. Park, E.A.: Harvey Lect. *34*:157, 1938–1939.
14. Park, E.A., Jackson, D.A.: J. Pediatr. *13*:748, 1938.
15. Sheldon, W.: Proc. R. Soc. Med. *29*:743, 1936.
16. Shahidi, N.T., Diamond, L.K.: N. Engl. J. Med. *262*:137, 1960.
17. Britton, H.A., Canby, J.P., Kohler, C.M.: Pediatrics *25*:621, 1960.
18. Moseley, J.E.: J. Mt. Sinai Hosp. *29*:109, 1962.
19. Burko, J., Mellins, H.Z., Watson, J.: A.J.R. *86*:447, 1961.
20. Ryan, B.: Med. J. Aust. *1*:844, 1962.
21. Lanzkowsky, P.: Am. J. Dis. Child. *116*:16, 1968.
22. Holt, J.F., Hodges, F.J.: Year Book of Radiol. 1958–1959 Series. Chicago, Year Book Medical Publishers, 1958, p. 51.
23. Wolbach, S.B.: J. Bone Joint Surg. *45*:171, 1947.
24. Maddock, C.L., Wolbach, S.B., Maddock, S.: J. Nutr. *39*:117, 1949.
25. Pease, C.N.: J.A.M.A. *182*:980, 1962.
26. Caffey, J.: A.J.R. *108*:451, 1970.
27. Christiansen, W.R., Liebman, C., Sosman, M.: A.J.R. *65*:27, 1951.
28. Bauer, J.M., Freyberg, R.H.: J.A.M.A. *130*:1208, 1946.
29. Danowski, T.S., Winkler, A.W., Peters, J.P.: Ann. Intern. Med. *23*:22, 1945.
30. Capitanio, M.A., Kirkpatrick, J.A.: Radiology *92*:53, 1969.
31. Sondheimer, F.K., Grossman, H., Winchester, P.: Arch. Neurol. *23*:314, 1970.
32. DeLevie, M., Nogrady, M.B.: J. Pediatr. *76*:523, 1970.
33. Wincik, M., Rosso, P.: J. Pediatr. *14*:774, 1969.
34. Wenger, J., Kersner, J.B., Palmer, W.L.: Am. J. Med. *24*:161, 1958.
35. Burnett, C.H., Commons, R.R., Albright, F., et al.: N. Engl. J. Med. *240*:787, 1949.
36. Leone, N.C., Stevenson, C.A., Hilbish, T.F., et al.: A.J.R. *74*:874, 1955.
37. Laws, J.W., Booth, C.C., Shawdon, H., et al.: Br. Med. J. *1*:1311, 1963.
38. Marshak, R.H., Lindner, A.E.: Semin. Roentgenol *1*:138, 1966.
39. Frazier, A.C., French, J.M., Thompson, M.D.: Br. J. Radiol. *22*:123, 1949.
40. Ruoff, M., Lindner, A.E., Marshak, R.H.: A.J.R. *104*:525, 1968.
41. Sherlock, P., Winawer, S.J., Goldstein, M.J., et al.: Progress in gastroenterology. Vol. II. New York, Grune & Stratton, 1970, pp. 367–391.
42. Sleisenger, M.H., Almy, T.P., Barr, D.P.: Am. J. Med. *15*:66, 1953.
43. Harris, O.E., Cooke, W.T., Thompson, H., et al.: Am. J. Med *42*:899, 1967.
44. Shaw, R.S., Mayard, E.P.: N. Engl. J. Med. *258*:874, 1958.
45. Watt, J.K., Watson, W.C., Haase, S.: Br. Med. J. *3*:199, 1967.
46. Clemett, A.R., Marshak, R.H.: Radiol. Clin. North Am. *7*:105, 1969.
47. Rice, R.P., Roufail, W.N., Reeves, R.J.: Radiology *88*:295, 1967.

48. Trier, J.S., Phelps, P.C., Edelman, S., et al.: Gastro-enterology *48*:684, 1965.
49. Gilat, T., Spiro, H.M.: Am. J. Dig. Dis. *13*:619, 1968.
50. Herskovic, T., Bartholomew, L.G., Green, P.A.: Arch. Intern. Med. *114*:629, 1964.
51. Legge, D.A., Carlson, H.C., Wollaeger, E.E.: A.J.R. *110*:406, 1970.
52. Laws, J.W., Neale, G.: Lancet *2*:139, 1966.
53. Preger, L., Amberg, J.R.: A.J.R.: *101*:287, 1967.
54. Winawer, S.J., Broitman, S.A., Wolochow, D.A., et al.: N. Engl. J. Med. *274*:72, 1966.
55. Katz, I, Karp, F.L.: A.J.R. *99*:162, 1967.
56. Gorbach, S.L., Plaut, A.G., Nahas, L., et al.: Gastro-enterology *53*:856, 1967.
57. Rosenberg, I.H., Hardison, W.G., Bull, D.M.: N. Engl. J. Med. *276*:1391, 1967.
58. Tankel, H.I., Clark, D.H., Lee, F.D.: Gut *6*:560, 1965.
59. Marshak, R.H., Ruoff, M., Lindner, A.E.: A.J.R. *104*:557, 1968.
60. Louisy, C.L., Barton, C.L.: Radiology *98*:535, 1971.
61. Hermans, P.E., Huizenga, K.A., Hoffman, H.N., et al.: Am. J. Med. *40*:78, 1966.
62. Hodgson, J.R., Hoffman, H.N., Huizenga, K.A.: Radiology *88*:883, 1967.
63. Orimo, H., Fujita, T., Yoshikawa, M., et al.: Am. J. Med. *47*:445, 1969.
64. Clemett, A.R., Fishbone, G., Levine, R.J., et al.: A.J.R. *103*:405, 1968.
65. Strole, W.E., Clark, W.H., Isselbacher, K.G.: N. Engl. J. Med. *276*:195, 1967.
66. Stacy, G.S., Loop, J.W.: A.J.R. *92*:1072, 1964.
67. Khilnani, M.T., Keller, R.J., Cuttner, J.: Radiol. Clin. North Am. *7*:43, 1969.
68. Waldmann, T.A.: Gastroenterology *50*:422, 1966.
69. Reese, D.F., Hodgson, J.R., Dockerty, M.B.: A.J.R. *88*:619, 1962.
70. Shimkin, P.M., Waldmann, T.A., Krugman, R.L.: A.J.R. *110*:827, 1970.
71. Marshak, R., Khilnani, M.T., Eliasoph, J., et al.: A.J.R. *101*:379, 1967.
72. Bookstein, J.J., French, A.B., Pollard, H.M.: Am. J. Dig. Dis. *10*:573, 1965.

**Part V**
*Nutrition in Growth, Aging, and Physiologic Stress*

*Chapter* **49**

# PREGNANCY AND LACTATION

R.G. Whitehead

Nutritional requirements of women during pregnancy and lactation, as defined by various national and international committees, have largely been derived on an incremental basis. To the nonpregnant, nonlactating allowances are added the dietary amounts that, on theoretical grounds, would be needed to cover completely the metabolic cost to the mother of these physiologic processes. It has been tacitly assumed that the metabolic ability of the mother to handle nutrients during these periods remains unaltered. These basic concepts will be reviewed together with recent research, which seems to indicate a need to modify some of our current approaches.

## DIETARY ENERGY

Satisfying dietary energy requirements is the cornerstone of practical nutrition: unless this is achieved, determining protein and other nutrient needs has little or no meaning. It is not surprising, therefore, that a major scientific effort has been directed toward providing an adequate estimate of how much extra energy is required during pregnancy and lactation.

**Pregnancy.** Table 49–1 summarizes the typical type of approach that has been adopted for pregnancy. The total energy cost of pregnancy is usually assumed to be of the order of 80,000 kcal. How this energy cost is believed to accumulate during successive trimesters is illustrated in Figure 49–1. It will be noted that one major component arises from the accumulation of some 3.5 kg of fat most of which has been laid down by the 30th week.[2] This is at a time when the actual fetus

and maternal reproductive organs are increasing in weight only slowly and it is generally accepted that its physiologic role is to protect the fetus against the particularly high energy costs encountered in the last trimester of pregnancy and during the first six months of lactation. The other major energy component in Figure 49–1 is concerned with theoretical increases in the amount of energy required for maintenance metabolism. Functions consuming this energy include a raised cardiac output and respiratory rate plus the demands imposed by an increased cellular mass in the uterus, placenta, fetus, and breasts. Kidney function is also greatly increased.[2] The theoretical net energy needs for this increased maintenance amount to some 36,000 kcal over pregnancy as a whole, virtually the same as that for fat synthesis. However, the developmental pattern of these two processes

**Table 49–1. Incremental Method for Calculating the Energy Requirements of Women During Pregnancy***

| Energy Cost of Pregnancy | kcal |
|---|---|
| Fat stores | 36,000 |
| Maintenance metabolism and tissue synthesis | 36,000 |
| Allowance for efficiency of conversion (90%) | 8,000 |
| | 80,000 |
| 1st trimester allowance (150 kcal/d) | 14,000 |
| 2nd and 3rd trimester allowance 350 kcal/d) | 65,300 |
| | 79,300 |

*From FAO/WHO[1]

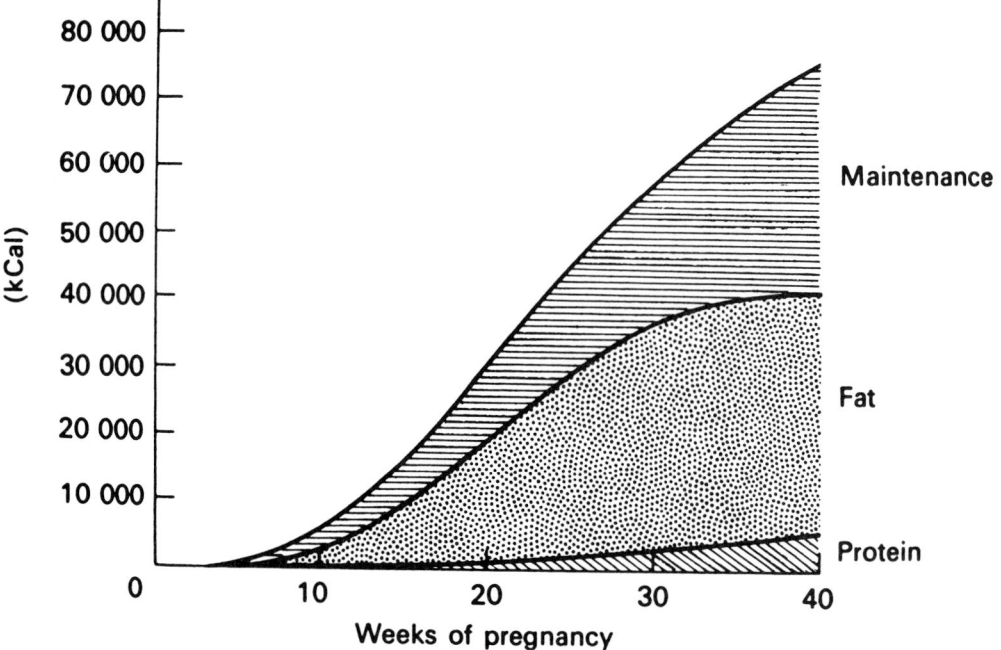

**Fig. 49–1.** The cumulative energy cost of pregnancy and its components. (From Hytten, F., Chamberlain, G.,[2] with permission of Blackwell Scientific Publications.)

is different with fat synthesis dominating the early part of pregnancy and a raised maintenance metabolism the second. It has been reasoned that throughout the second and third trimesters increased energy requirements are essentially constant and usually an extra 350 kcal/d is recommended. For the first trimester a rather arbitrary 150 kcal/d is a common allowance (see Table 49–1).

In the latest recommendations on this topic from FAO/WHO/UNU,[1a] it is stated that if women cannot reduce their previous level of activity, every effort should be made to provide the full energy allowance during pregnancy. The report suggests, however, that there is little evidence that the extra energy requirement varies between the three trimesters and advise an average addition of 258 kcal daily throughout pregnancy. If the mothers are healthy and are lucky enough to be able to reduce their activity by a reasonable amount, it was considered that an average additional allowance of 200 kcal/d might be more appropriate.

**Lactation.** The extra energy requirements needed to support lactation are theoretically greater than for pregnancy, but to some extent subcutaneous fat reutilization is believed to balance part of the energy deficit. A typical incremental calculation is shown in Table 49–2. If a mother delivers 850 ml of milk each day for 6 months, the total amount of energy required is of the order of 135,000 kcal, assuming that dietary energy is

converted into milk energy with an efficiency of 90%. If, as described for pregnancy, the mother has laid down 36,000 kcal as body fat during pregnancy and this is totally utilized during the first 6 months of lactation, the mother needs to provide from her diet only an extra 100,000 kcal or, on average, about 550 kcal/d. Since the energy requirements of an average moderately active woman are 2,300 kcal/d, the total recommendation becomes 2,750 kcal/d.

Although explained in the text to tables of recommended dietary allowances, it is not always

**Table 49–2. Typical Incremental Calculation for Energy Needs during Lactation***

| | |
|---|---|
| Volume of milk per day | 850 ml |
| Six months' lactation | 155 L |
| Energy content plus cost of synthesis | 135,000 kcal |
| Energy derived from maternal fat stores | 36,000 kcal |
| Net dietary requirements (approx.) | 100,000 kcal |
| OR | 550 kcal/d |
| Energy needs of moderately active women | 2,200 kcal/d |
| Total allowance for first 6 months of lactation | 2,750 kcal/d |
| Total after 6 months | 2,950 kcal/d |
| If doing heavy manual work (approx.) | 3,300 kcal/d |

*From FAO/WHO[1]

realized that the above assumptions apply only up to six months; where breast-feeding extends beyond this time, the total increment of 750 kcal/d is theoretically required. This is by no means an exceptional situation; the majority of rural African women would breast-feed up to two years as a matter of course.

Table 49–2 was the approach adopted in the FAO/WHO recommended allowances.[1] The one recently used by FAO/WHO/UNU is essentially similar,[1a] except more notice was taken of variations in milk excretion during the course of infancy. The calculations were based on the average milk intakes of Swedish children on the assumption that milk contains 70 kcal/100 ml. As in the previous report,[1] it was also assumed that the utilization of body fat would provide 200 kcal/day and that the efficiency of conversion of dietary energy into maternal milk energy proceeded with an efficiency of 80%. Up to six months the average recommended energy increment was thus about 700 kcal/day less 200 kcal from body fat or a net 500 kcal. If breast-feeding continued after this time, 500 kcal/day continued to be the recommendation because, although milk ouput has on average dropped by then, there is in theory, progressively less stored maternal fat to augment the diet. When there was more than one child to be fed, the requirement would need to be increased accordingly.

**Effect of Pattern of Activity.** Apart from considerations relating to duration of lactation, the aforementioned calculations make a number of additional assumptions. It has been assumed that mothers remain as active throughout pregnancy and lactation as their nonpregnant, nonlactating counterparts and that a gradually increasing weight, distributed in a rather cumbersome fashion, makes no additional energy demands. In traditional societies in the developing world the first assumption is perhaps not an unreasonable one because many women have to work regardless of their condition. Indeed it is debatable whether for such active women a baseline energy requirement of 2200 kcal/d is correct: a value of 2500 kcal/d has been considered more appropriate (see Table 49–2). How much an extra 12 kg in body weight affects a mother's energy needs for different types of activity, however, has not been adequately investigated.

In western environments it should be recognized that conditions are rather different. Culturally it is accepted that mothers may need to rest more during pregnancy and lactation, and often they become relatively listless. A general relaxation of voluntary muscle tone and a reduction in free thyroid hormone possibly allow maternal tissue to function at a slightly reduced tempo.[2] After considering these complexities, the most recent United States NRC recommended dietary allowances point out there must, in practice, be a range of dietary needs depending on the pattern of activity of the mother.[3] They quote, for example, a range of 2,100 to 2,900 kcal/d for women over 23 years of age during lactation. The lowest values are, in fact, no higher than baseline values for nonpregnant, nonlactating mothers.

## PROTEIN

During the course of pregnancy about 950 g of protein have to be synthesized by the mother to support the development of her fetus and maternal reproductive tissues. The net accumulation of this protein is not regularly distributed throughout pregnancy, and Hytten and Leitch have estimated from an analysis of fetuses, stillborn children, and placental tissues that the rates of protein accretion during the successive ten-week quarters of pregnancy are 0.6, 1.8, 4.8 and 6.1 g/d, respectively.[4] Some authorities have largely ignored these differences. The Department of Health in the United Kingdom (DHSS), for example, has reasoned that an increase of 5 g protein/d during only the second and third trimesters provides an adequate extra allowance.[5] Adopting a contrary approach, FAO/WHO in 1973 recommended only an extra 1 g protein/d for the first quarter of pregnancy, but 4, 8, and 9 g/d during the final three quarters.[1]

In the FAO/WHO/UNU Report published in 1985,[1a] however, it is suggested that making separate allowances for the different trimesters may be arbitrary, and it is estimated that protein requirements should be increased by an average of 6 g/day *throughout* pregnancy. This amount is expressed in terms of milk or egg protein and would further need to be corrected for digestibility.

In the United States the National Research Council (NRC) has taken a radically different stance and actually recommends an additional 30 g/protein/day for the whole of pregnancy[3] (Table 49–3). This step was taken on the basis of nitrogen balance studies carried out by Calloway and colleagues.[6] Exactly what the significance is of the high nitrogen retentions they reported still has to be determined: they certainly represented more than twice that which can be accounted for on theoretical grounds. The response of the NRC is a good example of the course of action that has had to be adopted by many expert committees—when in doubt, err on the side of caution. Scientifically speaking, however, it is clearly undesirable to leave in doubt such an enigma affecting this vitally important sector of the community.

**Table 49–3.  Extra Daily Nutrient Allowances For Pregnancy***

| Nutrient | Nonpregnant | Pregnant | Increase |
|---|---|---|---|
| Energy (kcal) | 2100 | 2400 | 300 |
| Protein (g) | 44 | 74 | 30 |
| Retinol ($\mu$g) | 800 | 1000 | 200 |
| Vitamin D ($\mu$g) | 7.5 | 12.5 | 5 |
| Vitamin E (mg) | 8 | 10 | 2 |
| Vitamin C (mg) | 60 | 80 | 20 |
| Riboflavin (mg) | 1.3 | 1.6 | 0.3 |
| Nicotinic acid (mg) | 14 | 16 | 2 |
| Vitamin $B_6$ (mg) | 2.0 | 2.6 | 0.6 |
| Folate ($\mu$g) | 400 | 800 | 400 |
| Thiamin (mg) | 1.1 | 1.5 | 0.4 |
| Calcium (mg) | 800 | 1200 | 400 |
| Iron (mg) | 18 | S† | S† |
| Zinc (mg) | 15 | 20 | 5 |

*From NRC,[3] with permission of the National Academy of Sciences.
†The increased requirement cannot be obtained from the diet and thus supplemental iron was recommended.

More detailed studies are urgently needed to clarify the situation.

Fortunately, calculating maternal protein allowances for lactation is not nearly so complicated nor are the conclusions of different expert committees as diverse. Most authorities base their recommendations on an average daily milk output of 850 ml. If the protein content of human breast milk is 1.2 g/100 ml and the efficiency of dietary nitrogen utilization remains unaffected, it can be calculated that an extra 24 g/d of dietary protein is needed to compensate for nitrogen secreted in milk if the diet has a chemical protein score of 70, the latter being the value adopted by FAO/WHO.[1] In the United States, where usually the average protein score is higher than this, an increment of 20 g/d was adopted by the NRC.[3] (Table 49–4).

In the latest FAO/WHO/UNU recommendations account is taken of the fact that the volume of milk secreted does change with the age of the infant.[1a]

Initially it was assumed to rise from an average of 719 ml/day at 0 to 1 months up to 848 ml at 2 to 3 months. After this time a fall occurs as mixed feeding is introduced and for calculation purposes a value of 600 ml/day was adopted for 6 to 12 months and 550 ml for 12 to 24 months. Expressed in the form of milk or egg protein the mean extra protein requirement, plus two standard deviations to cover individual variability, became about 16 g/day during the first six months of lactation, 12 g/day during the second six months and 11 g/day thereafter. As with the pregnancy requirements these are to be added to the normal estimate of the woman's protein requirement and corrected for the digestibility of the dietary protein.

It will be noted that for both pregnancy and lactation the percentage increase in the recommended dietary intake is greater for protein than for energy. FAO/WHO in 1973, for example, recommended only an additional 26% energy during lactation but 60% more protein.[1] These dietary

**Table 49–4.  Extra Daily Nutrient Allowances for Lactation***

| Nutrient | Nonpregnant, nonlactating | Lactating | Increase |
|---|---|---|---|
| Energy (kcal) | 2100 | 2600 | 500 |
| Protein (g) | 44 | 64 | 20 |
| Retinol ($\mu$g) | 800 | 1200 | 400 |
| Vitamin D ($\mu$g) | 7.5 | 12.5 | 5 |
| Vitamin E (mg) | 8 | 11 | 3 |
| Vitamin C (mg) | 60 | 100 | 40 |
| Riboflavin (mg) | 1.3 | 1.8 | 0.5 |
| Nicotinic acid (mg) | 14 | 19 | 5 |
| Vitamin $B_6$ (mg) | 2.0 | 2.5 | 0.5 |
| Folate ($\mu$g) | 400 | 500 | 100 |
| Thiamin (mg) | 1.1 | 1.6 | 0.5 |
| Calcium (mg) | 800 | 1200 | 400 |
| Iron (mg) | 18 | S† | S† |
| Zinc (mg) | 15 | 25 | 10 |

*From NRC[3], with permission of National Academy of Sciences.
†The increased requirement cannot be obtained from the diet and thus supplemental iron was recommended.

guidelines would imply that for women living on diets marginal in protein content, the quality of their food should markedly improve during lactation. The same is true of pregnancy. In the developing world there is very little sign of this occurring in practice; indeed, it is rare anywhere for the diet of mothers during the reproductive phase of their lives to be any different from that of the family fare in general.

## VITAMINS

All expert committees on dietary allowances have advised that there needs to be a substantial increase in the intake of most vitamins and minerals during pregnancy and lactation. The group that has provided the most comprehensive recommendations is the NRC,[3] and its views on pregnancy are summarized in Table 49–3 and for lactation in Table 49–4. The increased allowances made for lactation in particular make the total the highest for any sector of the community. Once again, the percentage increase with many vitamins and minerals is greater than for energy, 67% in the case of vitamin C, 40% for riboflavin, and 50% for calcium. Thus the comments about dietary quality and protein are valid considerations in terms of vitamins and minerals as well.

Extra allowances have again been derived largely on an incremental basis after taking into account the physiologic costs of pregnancy and lactation. Usually, conclusions of expert committees are easier to justify in the latter condition than in the former. Another generalization is that, when in doubt, the United States NRC has tended to be more generous than other expert groups.

**Retinol.** Retinol intake is a good example of this attitude of the NRC. The DHSS in the United Kingdom decided not to make an addition during pregnancy,[5] in contrast to the NRC, which recommended a further 200 μg of retinol/d.[3] With lactation there is more agreement. Breast milk contains about 50 μg of retinol/100 ml, and on the assumption that a mother will secrete 850 ml milk/day, an extra allowance of 400 μg of retinol and its equivalents has been recommended by most authorities. One of the difficulties in defining retinol needs is that the body contains substantial stores that may not become dangerously depleted for months or even years.

**Vitamin D.** The other major fat-soluble vitamin, D, is also associated with a fundamental physiologic complication that makes a completely confident recommendation difficult. Most authorities differ in their views about the relative proportions of vitamin D that one can expect to be synthesized via sunlight and the amount that needs to come from the diet of healthy nonpregnant, nonlactating

women. They agree, however, that an increased exogenous source is needed for pregnancy and lactation, and the 5 μg/d recommended by the NRC is typical.[3]

**Vitamins E and K.** NRC also recommends an extra 2 mg of vitamin E for pregnancy, and this is increased to 3 mg/d during lactation.[3] No special allowances are made in the case of vitamin K. It was assumed the 70 to 140 μg/d recommended for adults plus that coming from vitamin K synthesized by gut bacteria should assure adequate amounts. The newborn baby is protected against any risk of vitamin K deficiency by NRC recommendations that 0.5 to 1 mg of vitamin K should administered intramuscularly immediately after birth to assist adequate blood clotting function.[3]

**Vitamin C.** Vitamin C requirements during pregnancy are difficult to define, as indeed they are in the nonpregnant state. Allowances vary widely from country to country, and each edition of different national recommendations seems to show more alteration with this nutrient than any other. The general allowance for young females in the United States is now 60 mg/d, an increase of 15 mg/d over what it was in the previous NRC guidelines.[7] For pregnancy the recommendation is raised by a further 20 mg/d and thus becomes a total of 80 mg/d. In the United Kingdom,[5] which has the lowest vitamin C recommended allowances of all countries, the pregnancy increment is 30 mg/d, making the total 60 mg/d.

Breast milk contains on average 40 to 55 mg of ascorbic acid per liter, and the NRC allowance is raised by 40 mg/d to 100 mg/d during lactation.[3] The British maintain the same value as for pregnancy, in other words 60 mg/d.[5]

**Thiamin.** Recommended allowances for thiamin also vary widely for young adults, with American values again higher than most. The British adhere to the 1967 WHO/FAO recommended norm of 0.3 mg thiamin/1000 kcal of energy consumed.[8] Thus, for normal young women, after the addition of a safety margin, the requirement is placed at 0.9 mg/d. In contrast, in the United States the NRC set its corresponding baseline level at 1.1 mg/d for women up to 23 years of age.[3] Additionally, the British allow only an extra 0.1 mg/d to cover pregnancy and 0.2 mg for lactation,[5] whereas the NRC reasoned that as much as an extra 0.4 mg/d was necessary for pregnancy and 0.5 mg/d for lactation, thus bringing the totals to 1.5 and 1.6 mg/d,[3] respectively, in contrast to the British values of only 1.0 and 1.1 mg/d. Breast milk contains no more than 0.2 mg of thiamin in a typical day's secretion, and it is not wholly apparent why such large increments were deemed desirable by the American experts.

**Riboflavin.** With riboflavin the differences in recommendation are not nearly so great. Both in the United States[3] and in Britain[5] the baseline recommendation is 1.3 mg/d and both national authorities recommend an extra 0.3 mg during pregnancy and 0.5 mg for lactation. About 0.3 to 0.5 mg of riboflavin are secreted in breast milk each day.

Recent work in The Gambia, West Africa, and in Cambridge, United Kingdom, however, has suggested this amount may not be sufficient.[9] Using a community-based approach, Bates et al. determined under prevailing circumstances the intake of riboflavin needed to achieve conventional biochemical normality—an erythrocyte glutathione reductase coefficient of not more than 1.3. During both pregnancy and lactation it was concluded that 2.5 mg/d was necessary before even 70% of women achieved this desired level of function. Parallel investigations in the United Kingdom indicated that much the same level of intake was necessary there too.

**Folate.** Folic acid is the only vitamin for which the recommended increment is greater for pregnancy than for lactation because of the major role this vitamin plays in one carbon unit metabolism, a key process in the synthesis of the purine and pyrimidine bases of the nucleic acids. Once again, however, there is a considerable difference between British and American scientists in terms of exactly how much extra is required. The NRC adds an extra 400 μg of folic acid onto the baseline value of 400 μg for pregnancy, making a total of 800 μ/d,[3] whereas the corresponding British increment is only 200 μg/d, making a total of 500 μg/d.[5]

For lactation the British recommend only an increment of 100 μg/d, and for once there is general agreement between the two sets of authorities. The increment in the United States used to be an extra 200 μg/d,[7] the reason being that breast milk contains 50 μg of folate per liter and it was assumed that the efficiency of conversion of dietary folate to milk folate was only 25%. The NRC now holds that a 100 μg/d increment is more compatible with the folate content of breast milk. The calculation exhibits a major problem with recommendations for folate: namely, the complex nature of the folate derivatives found in food.[10] The efficiency of digestion and absorption of these derivatives is known to be variable, and the processes involved are far from completely understood. Be that as it may, it is clear that neither an intake of 500 μg or the 800 μg recommended for pregnancy is likely to be achieved from dietary sources alone, and oral folate supplements, often coupled with iron, are now the usual routine.

**Nicotinic Acid.** Nicotinic acid is another vitamin which occurs in foods in a bound form and the availability of these derivatives too is not known with certainty, but it is thought this could be limited. The vitamin is also synthesizable from the amino acid tryptophan and it is usually assumed that for every 60 mg of the amino acid consumed 1 mg of the vitamin becomes available.[11] During the course of pregnancy and lactation, however, the conversion of tryptophan to nicotinic acid may occur with greater efficiency, but this is by no means certain. This crucial gap in our knowledge clearly merits further investigation. Because of the complex dietary sources of nicotinic acid, allowances are usually quoted in niacin equivalents—the equivalent of 1 mg of free nicotinic acid. The British recommendations[5] are more than the American,[3] being 18 and 16 mg/d during pregnancy and 21 and 19 mg/d for lactation, respectively. There is no fundamentally important reason for this difference, however, just different ways of linking vitamin and energy intakes together.

**Vitamin B$_6$.** Vitamin B$_6$ also presents a number of unsolved problems, and any recommendations must be regarded with some caution. The recommendations for pregnancy and lactation are even more arbitrary than with most nutrients. NRC suggests an extra 0.6 mg/d for pregnancy and 0.5 mg/d for lactation.[3]

**Vitamin B$_{12}$.** With vitamin B$_{12}$, also, the extra 1 μg/d allowed by the NRC for pregnancy is largely arbitrary,[3] but the same increment for lactation has rather more factual justification because it is related to the amount found in a natural day's secretion of milk.

## MINERALS

**Calcium.** Breast milk contains an appreciable amount of calcium, about 300 mg in a typical day's supply.[12] Calcium also represents a major requirement during pregnancy, particularly during the last trimester when bone growth becomes rapid. The difficulty in determining requirements is complicated, however, by apparent differences in efficiency of digestion and utilization of calcium depending on customary levels of intake.[12] For the nonpregnant, nonlactating women for example, 300 mg/d seems perfectly adequate in many developing world countries, whereas 800 to 900 mg/d is necessary for zero balance in industrialized countries like the United Kingdom.[13] In studies carried out in Sweden adaptation to low intakes has been shown to occur,[14] but this can be slow and more research needs to be carried out before it can be said with any certainty whether it is safe to assume that similar adaptations apply during pregnancy and lactation. So far no national or international group of experts has dared make this assumption.

The NRC recommends an extra 400 mg/day during both pregnancy and lactation, which makes a total of 1,200 mg/d.[3] DHSS in the United Kingdom recommends the same total but gets there by a different process of calculation;[5] the baseline is only 500 mg/d, in agreement with FAO recommendations,[12] but for no very good reason their increment is 700 mg/d. Such an intake is improbable for women receiving only a small amount or no cow's milk in their diet. FAO acknowledges this but has stated that their high recommendation of 1,200 mg/d is compatible with the best system of diet that can be given to mothers even though, unfortunately, such advice cannot always be put into practice.[12] It has to be borne in mind that the loss of calcium from the bones that afflicts women after the menopause and that can ultimately lead to disabilities such as fractured femurs might well be exacerbated by a poor diet during the reproductive phase.[15] It is one of the world's nutritional enigmas, however, that women in the developing countries, who go through as many as 10 to 12 pregnancies and breast-feed their children up to two years on an intake of calcium only a quarter of the recommended amount, seem not to have an excessive incidence of osteoporosis and consequent high fracture rates.

**Iron.** Another mineral of major consideration for pregnancy and lactation is iron. Here too availability from different food sources is a key issue.[16] During pregnancy a number of physiologic processes, but in particular those involved in blood manufacture, clearly demand iron, but to some extent this need is countered by a cessation of iron losses through menstruation. Furthermore, it is known that the gut is the major regulatory organ in terms of iron homeostasis and that when subjects run into a state of iron deficiency then a greater proportion of dietary iron tends to be absorbed. It has not been convincingly demonstrated, however, that this latter process plays a major role in correcting iron balance during pregnancy. It might be reasoned that for the majority of women the net extra iron requirements might be low, and indeed this was the view of the British committee reviewing dietary requirements who merely raised the recommended amount by a nominal 1 mg/d, from 12 mg to 13 mg/d.[5] In the United States recommended iron allowances for nonpregnant, nonlactating women are already considerably higher than those in the United Kingdom,[3] 18 mg/d, the aim having been to cover the needs of all women, even those who have regularly high menstrual losses.[17] The British had

reasoned it was impracticable to take this broad approach and that such women really needed to be treated by daily administration of medicinal iron. The NRC believed that even 18 mg/d would not cover the needs of most women during pregnancy, but recognizing that raising *dietary* recommendations above this value would be virtually impossible to achieve with the habitual American diet, thus recommended the use of 30 to 60 mg/d supplemental iron.

Considerations during lactation are similar to those for pregnancy, especially during the period of amenhorrea. The loss of iron in the breast milk during lactation is rather less than that during menstruation, however, and DHSS reasoned that any losses could well be made good on a standard diet containing 1.3 mg iron per MJ (5 μg/kcal) taking into account the extra energy intake recommended for lactation.[5] The NRC also reasoned that iron needs during lactation were not substantially different from those of nonpregnant women but recommended that the iron supplementation initiated during pregnancy should be continued for 2 to 3 months after parturition in order to replenish any iron stores that have been depleted by pregnancy.[3]

**Zinc.** As well as iron and calcium, a whole range of other minerals theoretically need to be consumed at increased levels during pregnancy and lactation. Zinc has been of increased interest to nutritionists in recent years. The most detailed recommendations for this and other trace elements are contained in the NRC dietary allowances.[3] Increased allowances are made for pregnancy (5 mg/d) and lactation (10 mg/d) bringing the total estimated requirement up to as high as 25 mg/d. It is difficult to interpret these recommendations, however, because many women from both the industrialized and the developing countries have far lower measured intakes and seemingly suffer no major harm. As with calcium it seems likely that physiologic demand and efficiency of utilization might be interlinked, but this connection needs to be subjected to critical scientific evaluation.

**Other Trace Elements.** As far as other cations are concerned, such as copper, manganese, chromium, selenium, and molybdenum, the NRC attempted only to provide ranges of intake levels within which they would like to see community values fall. Because of the poverty of information available, no attempts were made to provide special recommendations for pregnancy and lactation.

## UNDERNUTRITION AND PREGNANCY

It is becoming increasingly obvious that women's diets do not respond as they theoretically should during pregnancy and lactation, and this is true both in the relatively affluent industrialized countries and in the developing world.[18]

Table 49–5 provides representative energy intake values for the third world, and in Table 49–6 corresponding levels are reported for various more affluent countries. It is readily apparent that in the former no values come anywhere near the recommended level, and even in the latter group of countries only data collected 10 to 20 years ago conform to the recommendations. It would seem that in many communities women go through pregnancy exhibiting either no or only minimal increases in food intake and that even during lactation any increments are only a fraction of that recommended. In spite of this, birth weights are remarkably little affected unless intakes fall to disastrously low levels, and even then the effect directly attributable to diet rarely exceeds 300 g, a fall of only 10%.[49]

The effect on the mother of undernutrition during pregnancy is less clear. Total weight gain during pregnancy does not appear to have been dramatically affected by the switch to mean intakes of about 2,000 to 2,200 kcal/d in the western world. In Cambridge, United Kingdom, for example, we have demonstrated that the mothers still gain an average of 12.6 kg and the theoretical

**Table 49–5.   Reported Energy Intakes of Poorly Nourished Childbearing Women**

| Country | Energy Intake (kcal/day) | Source |
|---------|--------------------------|--------|
| *Pregnancy* | | |
| The Gambia* | 1,350–1,450 | (19) |
| New Guinea | 1,360 | (20) |
| India | 1,400 | (21) |
| India | 1,410 | (22) |
| Guatemala | 1,500 | (23) |
| Ethiopia | 1,540 | (24) |
| India | 1,570 | (25) |
| Colombia | 1,620 | (26) |
| The Gambia† | 1,600–1,700 | (19) |
| Guatemala | 1,720 | (27) |
| Tanzania | 1,850 | (28) |
| Iraq | 1,880 | (29) |
| India | 1,920 | (30) |
| Thailand | 1,980 | (31) |
| Guatemala | 2,060 | (32) |
| *Lactation* | | |
| The Gambia* | 1,200–1,300 | (19) |
| India | 1,300 | (33) |
| India | 1,400 | (34) |
| India | 1,440 | (35) |
| Guatemala | 1,600 | (27) |
| India | 1,620 | (25) |
| The Gambia† | 1,600–1,750 | (19) |
| Mexico | 1,950 | (36) |

*Wet season.
†Dry season.

**Table 49–6.   Energy Intakes of Pregnant and Lactating Women from Industrialized Countries**

| Country | Energy Intake (kcal/day) | Source |
|---------|--------------------------|--------|
| *Pregnancy* | | |
| Scotland | 2,503 | (37) |
| Australia | 2,090 | (38) |
| Sweden | 2,154 | (39) |
| United Kingdom— Leeds | 1,957 | (40) |
| United Kingdom | 2,152 | (41) |
| United Kingdom— Cambridge | 1,980 | (42) |
| *Lactation* | | |
| Australia | 2,460 | (39) |
| Scotland | 2,716 | (43) |
| United Kingdom— London | 2,930 | (44) |
| United Kingdom— London | 2,728 | (45) |
| Sweden | 2,280 | (46) |
| United States | 2,124 | (47) |
| United Kingdom— Cambridge | 2,295 | (42) |
| Australia | 2,306 | (48) |

total energy store is of the order of 39,000 kcal, i.e., the same levels that were recorded when food intakes were apparently much higher.[42] On the much lower energy intakes reported from the developing world, smaller weight gains are encountered, and it is apparent that the fetus is being protected at the expense of the mother.[50] Since we do not have satisfactory data covering changes in body composition, it is not possible to state precisely the true functional significance of this failure to gain weight at conventially approved rates.

## UNDERNUTRITION AND LACTATION

The effect of undernutrition on breast-milk output and upon its composition is also uncertain. Table 49–7 shows a typical selection of values from prospective studies on output, which have been carried out in different parts of the developing world. These are substantially lower volumes than those quoted in Table 49–8, which shows a contrasting selection from the industrialized world. The interpretation of this data is not completely straightforward, since, if one adjusts the values for body weight of the child, some of the differences become less marked. It is open to question as to whether the reduced demands of a smaller baby control the amount of milk or whether a low output of milk results in a reduced rate of growth.[55] The simplest way of testing the latter hypothesis is to improve the maternal diet. In a recent review of this subject it was concluded that maternal dietary supplementation during lac-

**Table 49–7. Milk Output (ml/24h) of Women from the Developing World**

| Country (Ref.) | Month of Lactation | | | | | | | |
|---|---|---|---|---|---|---|---|---|
| | 1 | 2 | 3 | 4 | 5 | 6 | 7–9 | 9–12 |
| Zaire (51) | 436 | 405 | 380 | 417 | 415 | — | 323 | — |
| Zaire (52) | 517 (250–780) | — | 605 (390–920) | — | — | 525 (180–1,080) | 580 (210–950) | 582 (270–850) |
| Kenya (53,54) | — | 675 (271–1,079) | — | — | 555 (189–921)* | — | 487 (153–821)* | — |
| Mexico (36) | — | 577 (433–842) | — | 537 (455–663) | — | 561 (432–850) | — | 462 (377–670) |
| Gambia (19) | — | 677 (525–1,055) | — | — | 617 (355–885) | — | 595 (435–744) | 542 (210–730) |

*Ranges calculated from mean ± 2 SD.

**Table 49–8. Milk Output (ml/24h) of Well-nourished Mothers from Industrialized Societies**

| Country (Ref.) | Month of Lactation | | | | | |
|---|---|---|---|---|---|---|
| | 1 | 2 | 3 | 4 | 5 | 6 |
| Sweden (56)* | 610 (416–839) | 727 (508–964) | 766 (497–1,029) | 784 (577–1,065) | – | 778 (510–1,123) |
| Sweden (57) | 724 (490–958)§ | 752 (575–929)§ | – | – | 756 (476–1.036)§ | – |
| Sweden (58)† | 660 (380–860) | 755 (575–985) | 780 (600–930) | 795 (560–1,045) | 566 (170–950) | 450 (50–1,145) |
| UK (59)† | 740 (480–1,059) | 785 (380–1,235) | 784 (280–1,114) | 717 (210–1,091) | 588 (183–1,020) | 493 (135–906) |
| Canada (60)* | – | – | 793 (651–935)§ | 856 (658–1,054)§ | 925 (701–1,149)§ | 873 (602–1,124)§ |
| Australia (48)†·‡ | 1,187 (799–1,611) | 1,238 (862–1,543) | – | – | – | 1,128 (608–1,610) |
| USA (61)† | 569 (398–989) | – | 523 (242–1,000) | – | – | 436 (147–786) |
| USA (62)* | 606 (336–876)§ | 601 (355–847)§ | 626 (392–860)§ | – | – | – |

*Exclusively breast-fed.
†Includes mixed feeding.
‡Data obtained by weighing the mother, not the child.
§Ranges calculated from mean ± 2 SD.

tation had led to disappointing results in terms of improving milk yield.[63] Although a number of groups of investigators have satisfactorily demonstrated that giving extra food to undernourished pregnant women will reverse the birth-weight deficit, a similar positive effect has not been convincingly demonstrated in lactation.[49] This is such an important topic, however, it would be unwise to regard any study so far carried out as being absolutely definitive in terms of the world as a whole.

As far as milk composition is concerned, it would appear that except in extreme maternal undernutrition the concentrations of total energy and protein in breast milk are maintained at remarkably normal levels in the developing world. In The Gambia, for example, where in the good times of the year measured energy intakes are only 1,700 kcal/d,[19] the average energy content is maintained at almost the same level as in the well-to-do British mother.[64] Even when mean energy intakes fall to 1,100 kcal/d, the energy content of the mother's breast milk fell only by about 10%.[19]

## REPRODUCTION AND ENERGY HOMEOSTASIS

Exactly how mothers manage to maintain energy homeostasis when they do not exhibit all the theoretically required increments during pregnancy and lactation is currently the subject of intensive study. A number of different hypotheses are being tested. Some investigators believe that the low intakes are merely artifacts arising from measurement error. It has to be admitted that it is difficult to quantitate food intake to the level of

accuracy needed without running the risk of distorting the normal feeding pattern of the subject. It would not be surprising if when the energy input-output equations are finally balanced that error in the measurement of food intake does prove to be one factor. Be this as it may, it is equally improbable that it will account for all the energy gap. Other scientists reason that reductions in the pattern of activity of the mother during pregnancy or changes in the economy of effort she puts into customary tasks will prove to be the major component balancing the low energy intake. Data have been published establishing that in the western world women do indeed gradually spend more time lying down and sitting, especially in the last trimester of pregnancy.[65] In traditional rural communities in the developing world the situation is more complex. Some societies do protect pregnant women, but most do not and even during the last trimester women may well be faced with a heavy farming load. So far there is little information on adaptations in the economy of effort required for these tasks, and hypotheses associated with this idea clearly need to be tested by rigorous scientific investigation.

Patterns of work activity during the course of lactation have been even less objectively studied than in pregnancy. The issue is particularly relevant in agricultural communities in the developing world where mothers traditionally breast-feed for up to 2 years. In a study carried out in The Gambia, West Africa, by Roberts and colleagues,[66] it was demonstrated that the proportions of time spent working did drop somewhat in the seventh, eight, and ninth months of pregnancy and in the first month of lactation but from then on levels of work activity returned to non-pregnancy values (Fig. 49–2.)

The third set of hypotheses concerning energy balance during pregnancy and lactation proposes that physiologic and metabolic changes improve the actual efficiency of energy utilization. Controlled scientific studies to test this hypothesis are only at a preliminary stage. The most revealing are perhaps those recently carried out by Durnin and colleagues in Glasgow, Scotland,[65] in which they demonstrated that the rate of increase in maintenance energy consumption (resting metabolic rate, RMR) during pregnancy was not anything like that postulated in Figure 49–1. Indeed, it was not until the eighth and ninth months of pregnancy that any significant response in RMR was detectable. To what extent this can be explained on grounds of increased physiologic efficiency still needs to be decided. When changes in RMR during pregnancy found by Durnin[65] were confirmed among a group of rural mothers studied in The Gambia, the difference from the theoretical pattern shown in Figure 49–1 was even more marked.[65a] Of particular significance was the fact that the RMR response was sensitive to dietary status: maternal dietary supplementation during pregnancy resulted in RMR rising by a greater amount and more in line with that predicted on theoretical grounds.

## VITAMIN AND MINERAL DEFICIENCIES

In contrast to the proximal constituents, the vitamin content of milk, particularly that of the water-soluble vitamins, is sensitive to dietary intake. It has been demonstrated that a maternal diet low in thiamin can result in infantile beriberi.[67] Riboflavin content is also affected by maternal diet and, despite the existence of mechanisms that favor the fetus at the expense of maternal stores, a baby who is born deficient in riboflavin will remain so throughout infancy if the mother's diet is not appropriately fortified.[68] It has also been shown that the vitamin C content of milk parallels closely the seasonal variations in vitamin intake.[69] Folic acid is likewise affected.[19] The situation with the fat-soluble vitamins is less dramatic but nevertheless clear-cut. A comparative study of breast milk samples from well-nourished Swedish mothers and underprivileged Ethiopian ones has shown a significantly higher vitamin A level in the former and a greater concentration of β-carotene in the latter.[70]

The mineral content of human milk in relation to diet has been insufficiently studied. The calcium content of breast milk is variable, and there have been suggestions that malnourished mothers do produce milk with a lower average calcium content. The iron in breast milk, although relatively low in concentration, is also of crucial im-

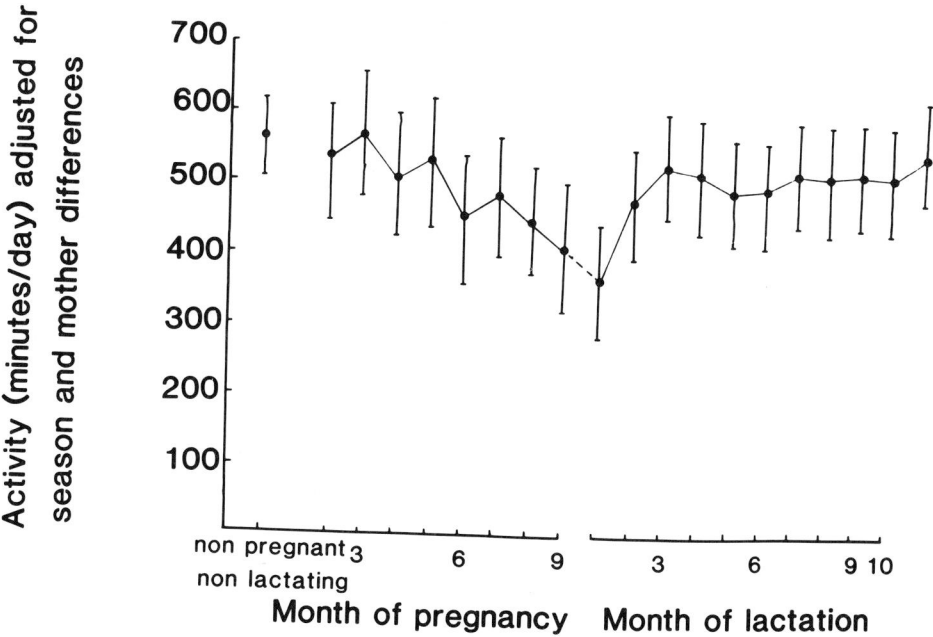

**Fig. 49–2.** Time spent working (mean and SE) by month of pregnancy and lactation in a rural Gambian village. (From Roberts, S.B., et al.,[66] with permission of the Royal Society of Tropical Medicine and Hygiene.)

portance to the young baby because of the high degree of efficiency with which it is absorbed.[71] This is partly, although not completely, so because of the association of milk iron within a lactoferrin-protein complex. It has been demonstrated in Ethiopia that mothers on a high iron intake have high concentrations of lactoferrin and vice versa.[72]

Deficiencies in both vitamins and minerals in breast milk can be readily reversed by supplementing the mother's diet. This is an important consideration when designing a maternal dietary supplement. Perhaps nutritionists, particularly those in the developing world, have tended to think too narrowly and only consider energy and protein intake. The balance of the diet as a whole is of critical importance.

## CONCLUSIONS

There can be few areas of nutrition more important than that concerned with the health and well-being of the mother and the survival of the very young baby. In the developing world, in particular, the only truly safe way of feeding a baby, at least up to the age of four months, is from the breast. We need to know more about the nutritional and physiologic complexities involved during both pregnancy and lactation to ensure that the child has an adequate start in life and at the same time the mother's health is not affected. It is to be hoped that the shortcomings in our knowledge highlighted in this chapter will be given the research priority they deserve.

## REFERENCES

1. FAO/WHO.: Energy and Protein Requirements. WHO Technical Report Series, No. 522. Geneva, WHO, 1973.
1a. FAO/WHO/UNU: Energy and Protein Requirements. WHO Technical Report Series No. 724. Geneva, WHO, 1985.
2. Hytten, F., Chamberlain, G.: Clinical Physiology in Obstetrics. Oxford, Blackwell Scientific Publications, 1980.
3. NRC.: Recommended Dietary Allowances, 9th ed. Washington, D.C., National Acacemy of Sciences, National Research Council, 1980.
4. Hytten, F.E., Leitch, I.: The Physiology of Human Pregnancy, 2nd ed. Oxford, Blackwell Scientific Publications, 1971.
5. DHSS: Recommended Daily Amounts of Food Energy and Nutrients for Groups of People in the UK. Reports on Health and Social Subjects, No. 15. London, Her Majesty's Stationery Office, 1979.
6. Calloway, D.H.: Nitrogen balance during pregnancy. *In* Nutrition and Fetal Development. (Winick, M., Ed.) New York, John Wiley & Sons, 1974.
7. Food and Nutrition Board, National Research Council: Recommended Dietary Allowances. 8th ed. Washington, D.C., National Academy of Sciences, 1974.
8. Joint FAO/WHO Expert Group on Requirements of

Vitamin A.: Thiamin, Riboflavine, and Niacin. FAO Nutrition Meetings Report Series, No. 41. United Nations, New York. WHO Technical Reports Series, No. 362, Geneva 1967.
9. Bates, C.J., Prentice, A.M., Paul, A.A., et al.: Am. J. Clin. Nutr. *34*:928–935, 1981.
10. Philips, D.R., Wright, A.J.A.: Br. J. Nutr. *49*:181–186, 1983.
11. Goldsmith, G.A., Miller, O.N., Unglaub, W.G.: J. Nutr. *73*:172–176, 1961.
12. FAO/WHO: Calcium Requirements. WHO Technical Reports Series, No. 230. Rome, WHO, 1962.
13. Marshall, D.H., Nordin, B.E.C., Speed, R.: Proc. Nutr. Soc. *35*:163–173, 1976.
14. Malm, O.J.: Calcium Requirement and Adaptation in Adult Man. Oslo, Oslo University Press, 1958.
15. Newton-John, H.W., Morgan, D.B.: Lancet *1*:232–233, 1968.
16. Layrisse, M., Martinez-Torres, C., Roche, M.: Am. J. Clin. Nutr. *21*:1175–1183, 1968.
17. Monsen, E.R., Kuhn, I.N., Finch, C.A.: Am. J. Clin. Nutr. *20*:842–849, 1967.
18. Whitehead, R.G., Paul, A.A.: Diet and the pregnant and lactating women. *In* Nutrition and Health, a Perspective. (Turner, M.R. Ed.) London, M.T.P. Press Ltd., 159–162, 1982.
19. Prentice, A.M.: Variations in maternal dietary intake, birth weight and breast milk output in The Gambia. *In* Maternal Nutrition during Pregnancy and Lactation. (Aebi, H., Whitehead, R.G., Eds.) Berne, Hans Huber, 1980, pp. 167–183.
20. Oomen, H.A.P.C., Malcolm, S.: Nutrition of the Papuan child. *In* South Pacific Commission Technical Paper, No. 118. Noumea, New Caledonia, South Pacifc Commission, 1958.
21. Gopalan, C.: Bull. WHO *26*:203–211, 1962.
22. Venkatachalan, P.S.: Bull WHO *26*:193–201, 1962.
23. Lechtig, A., Habicht, J.P., Yarbrough, C., et al.: Proc. 9th Int. Congr. Nutr., Mexico, *2*:44–52, 1972.
24. Gebre-Medhin, M., Gobezie, A.: Am. J. Clin. Nutr., *28*:1322–1329, 1975.
25. Rajalakshmi, R.: Trop. Geogr. Med. *23*:117–125, 1971.
26. Mora, J.O., de Navarro, L., Clement, J., et al.: Nutr. Rep. Int. *17*:217–228, 1978.
27. Arroyave, G.: Am. J. Dis. Child. *129*:427–430, 1975.
28. Maletnlema, T.N., Bavu, J.L.: East Afr. Med. J. *51*:515–528, 1974.
29. Demarchi, M., Isa, A., Al-Saide, S., et al.: J. Fac. Med. Baghdad *8*:20–30, 1966.
30. Bagchi, K., Bose, A.K.: Am. J. Clin. Nutr. *11*:586–592, 1962.
31. Thanangkul, O., Amatyakul, K.: Am. J. Dis. Child. *129*:426–427, 1975.
32. Mata, L.J., Urrutia, J.J., Garcia, B.: Proc. 9th Int. Congr. Nutr., Mexico *2*:175–192, 1972.
33. Karmarkar, M.G., Rajalakshmi, R., Ramakrishnan, C.V.: Acta Paediatr. Scand. *52*:473–480, 1963.
34. Devadas, R.P., Murthy, N.K.: World Rev. Nutr. Diet. *27*:1–33, 1977.
35. Karmarker, M.G., Kapur, J., Deodhar, A.D., et al.: Indian J. Med. Res. *47*:344–351, 1959.
36. Martinez, C., Chavez, A.: Nutr. Rep. Int. *4*:139–149, 1971.
37. Thompson, A.M.: Br. J. Nutr. *12*:446–453, 1958.
38. English, R.M., Hitchcock, N.E.: Br. J. Nutr. *22*:615–624, 1968.
39. Lunell, N.O., Persson, B., Sterky, G.: Acta Obstet. Gynecol Scand. *48*:187–195, 1969.

40. Smithells, R.W., Ankers, C., Carver, M.E., et al.: Br. J. Nutr. *38*:497–506, 1977.
41. Darke, S.J., Disselduff, M.M., Try, G.P.: Br. J. Nutr. *44*:243–252, 1980.
42. Whitehead, R.G., Paul, A.A., Black, A.E., et al.: UNU/Food and Nutr. Bull. Suppl. *5*:259–264, 1981.
43. Thomson, A.M., Hytten, F.E., Billewicz, W.Z.: Br. J. Nutr. *24*:565–572, 1970.
44. Naismith, D.J., Ritchie, C.D.: Proc. Nutr. Soc. *34*:116A–117A, 1975.
45. Whichelow, M.J.: Proc. Nutr. Soc. *35*:62A–65A, 1976.
46. Abrahamsson, L., Hofvander, Y.: Naringsforskning *21*:93–94, 1977.
47. Sims, L.S.: J. Am. Diet. Assoc. *73*:139–146, 1978.
48. Rattigan, S., Ghisalberti, A.V., Hartmann, P.E.: Br. J. Nutr. *45*:243–249, 1981.
49. Prentice, A.M., Whitehead, R.G., Watkinson, M., et al.: Lancet *1*:489–492, 1983.
50. Prentice, A.M., Whitehead, R.G., Roberts, S.B., et al.: Am. J. Clin. Nutr. *34*:2790–2799, 1981.
51. Holemans, K., Lambrechts, A., Martin, H.: Rev. Med. Liege *9*:714–723, 1954.
52. Hennart, Ph., Vis, H.L.: J. Trop. Paediat. *26*:177–183, 1980.
53. Van Steenbergen, W.L., Kusin, J.A., Voorhoeve, A., et al.: Trop. Geogr. Med. *30*:505–522, 1978.
54. Van Steenbergen, W.L., Kusin, J.A., Vans Rens, M.M. J. Trop. Paediatr. *27*:155–161, 1981.
55. Whitehead, R.G., Paul, A.A., Cole, T.J.: Acta Paediatr. Suppl. *291*:43–50, 1982.
56. Wallgren, A.: Acta Paediatr *32*:778–790, 1945.
57. Lonnerdal, B., Forsum, E., Gebre-Medhin, M., et al.: Am. J. Clin. Nutr. *29*:1134–1141, 1976.
58. Hofvander, Y., Hagman, U., Sjolin, S.: Var Foda, *31* (Suppl. 3):182, 1979.
59. Whitehead, R.G., Paul, A.A.: Lancet *2*:161–163, 1981.
60. Chandra, R.K.: Nutr. Res. *1*:25–31, 1981.
61. Pao, E.M., Himes, J.M., Roche, A.F.: J. Am. Diet. Assoc. *77*:540–545, 1980.
62. Picciano, M.F., Calkins, E.J., Garrick, J.R., et al. Acta Paediatr. Scand. *70*:189–194, 1981.
63. Whitehead, R.G.: UNU Food and Nutrition Bulletin, Suppl. *6*:1–107, 1983.
64. Whitehead, R.G., Paul, A.A., Rowland, M.G.M.: Topics in Paediatrics 2, Nutrition. Tunbridge Wells, UK, Pitman Medical, 22–33, 1980.
65. Durnin, J.V.G.A.: Nestle Foundation Annual Report, pp 13–22 and 47–62, 1982.
65a.Lawrence, M., Lawrence, F., Lamb, W.H., et al.: Lancet *1*:363–365, 1984.
66. Roberts, S.B., Paul, A.A., Cole, T.J., et al.: Trans R. Soc. Trop. Med. Hyg. *76*:668–678, 1982.
67. Jelliffe, D.B.: *In* Infant Nutrition in the Subtropics Tropics. WHO Monogr. Ser., No. 29. Geneva, WHO, 1968.
68. Bates, C.J., Prentice, A.M., Paul, A.A., et al.: Trans. R. Soc. Trop. Med. Hyg. *76*:253–258, 1982.
69. Bates, C.J., Prentice, A.M., Prentice, A., et al.: Trans. R. Soc. Trop. Med. Hyg. *76*:341–347, 1982.
70. Gebre-Medhin, M., Valquist, A., Hofvander, Y., et al. Am. J. Clin. Nutr. *29*:441–451, 1976.
71. McMillan, J.A., Landaw, S., Oski, F.A.: Pediatrics *58*:686–690, 1976.
72. Lonnerdal, B., Forsum, E., Gebre-Medhin, N., et al.: Am. J. Clin. Nutr. *29*:1134–1141, 1976.

## SELECTED READINGS

Aebi, H., Whitehead, R.G. (Eds.): Maternal Nutrition during Pregnancy and Lactation. Bern, Hans Huber, 1980.

Hambreus, L., Sjölin, S. (Eds.): The Mother/Child Dyad—Nutritional Aspects. Stockholm, Almqvist & Wiksell, 1979.

Hytten, F., Chamberlain, G. (Eds.): Clinical Physiology in Obstetrics. Oxford, Blackwell, Scientific Publications, 1980.

Jelliffe, D.B., Jelliffe, E.F.P.: Human Milk in the Modern World. Oxford, University Press, 1978.

*Chapter* **50**

# NUTRITION IN INFANTS AND CHILDREN

## William C. Heird and Arthur Cooper

Those concerned with the feeding of infants and children must keep in mind this population's unique nutritional needs for supporting both the inevitable increase in size (growth) and the changes in organ function and body composition (development). Further, because the metabolic rate of infants and children is greater and the turnover of nutrients more rapid than in the adult, the nutritional needs for growth and development are superimposed upon maintenance requirements that are higher than those of the adult. Moreover, provision of these greater needs, particularly to the smaller members of this population, is hindered by the lack of teeth as well as the limited digestive and metabolic processes.

This chapter discusses the nutritional needs of the normal infant as well as those of some subsets of the total pediatric population (i.e., low-birth-weight infants and infants and/or children with a number of disease states thought to alter nutritional needs). Because the nutritional management of low-birth-weight (LBW) infants presents some of the most pressing problems encountered by those involved in the feeding of infants and children, the nutritional needs of this subpopulation are discussed initially. This discussion is followed by less detailed discussions of the nutritional needs of the normal infant as well as those of infants and children with specific diseases. General approaches to providing the nutritional needs both of LBW infants and of compromised infants and children also are discussed. The final section is a detailed discussion of parenteral nutrition in pediatric patients.

## NUTRITIONAL REQUIREMENTS OF THE LOW-BIRTH-WEIGHT INFANT

Approximately 8 to 10% of infants born in the United States each year weigh less than 2,500 g at birth. Although the number of such births has not increased over the past few decades, survival has improved steadily. Today, for example, the survival rate of even the smallest such infants (i.e., those weighing <1,000 g at birth) approaches 75%, whereas as recently as a decade ago, few of these infants survived; survival of larger LBW infants today approaches 100%. The increasing number of such infants that must be fed, in turn, has heightened awareness of the problems encountered in meeting their nutritional needs.

The importance of adequate early nutritional management of the LBW infant is best illustrated by a consideration of the energy metabolism of the fasted infant. As in the adult, energy to meet ongoing needs during fasting is derived from endogenous stores of various nutrients. Initially, hepatic glycogen stores are utilized. However, these stores are limited in amount and are depleted rapidly; thus, fat stores become the major source of endogenous energy. Protein stores also are called upon to provide amino acids from which glucose can be synthesized (i.e., gluconeogenesis) for use by those tissues that have an absolute requirement for glucose. Therefore, assuming that hydration is adequate, the available endogenous stores of fat and protein are the ultimate determinants of the length of time a fasting infant can survive.

As illustrated in Table 50–1, the body content

**Table 50–1.** **Intrauterine Accretion Rates of Various Nutrients During Last Trimester of Pregnancy***

| Component | Accumulation During Various Stages of Gestation† | | |
| --- | --- | --- | --- |
| | *26–31 wk* | *31–34 wk* | *34–38 wk* |
| Weight (g) | 600 | 750 | 950 |
| Protein (g) | 68 | 97 | 126 |
| Fat (g) | 60 | 95 | 145 |
| Water (g) | 459 | 539 | 627 |
| Calcium (g) | 3.4 | 5.12 | 8.7 |
| Phosphorus (g) | 2.2 | 3.3 | 5.4 |
| Magnesium (mg) | 93 | 131 | 193 |
| Nitrogen (meq) | 46 | 53 | 64 |
| Potassium (meq) | 25 | 31 | 39 |
| Chloride (meq) | 35 | 37 | 37 |

*Adapted from Ziegler, E.E., et al.[1]
†Body weight increases from 880 g at 26 weeks to 3,160 g at 38 weeks.

of both protein and fat, particularly fat, increases throughout gestation. Thus, an infant weighing 2,000 g at birth has more extensive endogenous nutrient reserves than one weighing 1,000 g, and an infant weighing 3,500 g has more extensive reserves than one weighing 2,000 g. In other words, the smaller the infant, the more marked is his inability to withstand starvation. The extent of this inability is illustrated in Figure 50–1. Under conditions of total starvation, the 1,000-g infant has sufficient endogenous reserves to survive for only 4 to 5 days, the 2,000-g infant has sufficient reserves to survive for approximately 12

days, and the term infant has sufficient reserves to survive for approximately a month.[2] Daily provision of glucose intravenously (e.g., 7.5 g/kg/day, the amount provided by 150 ml/kg/day of a 5% glucose solution or 75 ml/kg/day of a 10% glucose solution) theoretically will prolong survival of the 1,000-g, 2,000-g, and 3,500-g infant, respectively, by 7, 18, and 50 days.

These theoretical calculations depict in a semi-quantitative manner the general clinical observations concerning the LBW infant's susceptibility to starvation and, hence, the necessity of careful attention to early nutritional management. In addition to this practical role of early adequate nutrition for the LBW infant, there is concern that inadequate nutrition at any time during the period of cellular proliferation of various organ systems, particularly the central nervous system, may result in nonrecoupable cellular deficits. This concern is based on evidence obtained primarily in rodents,[3] but probably is applicable to all species.[4] It is particularly applicable to the prematurely born infant whose brain undergoes considerable growth during the period corresponding to the last trimester of intrauterine life. Although the period of cellular proliferation of the entire human brain encompasses at least the first 18 months of life,[5] and although transient cellular deficits apparently can be reversed if adequate nutrition is provided before the end of this period, little is known concerning the duration of cellular proliferation within specific regions of the brain. This uncertainty coupled with the persistently high incidence of neurodevelopmental deficits in surviving LBW infants[6] suggests that better nutritional management, in addition to decreasing mortality, may also decrease morbidity.

The aforementioned factors are now recognized by neonatologists, and the importance of early adequate nutritional management of the LBW infant is generally accepted. As a result, the general sub-

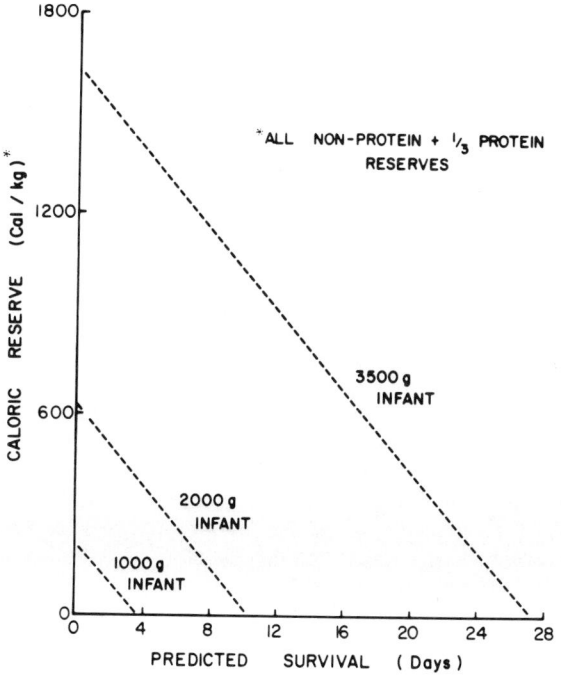

**Fig. 50–1.** Caloric reserves of 1,000-g, 2,000-g, and 3,500-g infants and predicted survival without exogenous nutrients. Adapted from Heird, W.C.[2]

ject of the LBW infant's nutritional requirements is an area of active investigation. Such investigation, however, is just beginning and much remains to be learned. The discussion that follows is an attempt to summarize the present state of knowledge.

**Goals of Nutritional Management.** The most generally accepted goal for nutritional management of the LBW infant is to provide sufficient amounts of all nutrients to support continuation of the intrauterine growth rate. Thus, the LBW infant's requirements for various nutrients are assumed to be the amounts necessary to allow their accumulation at intrauterine rates (see Table 50–1). This concept figures prominently in the recommended nutrient intakes for LBW infants proposed by the Committee on Nutrition of the American Academy of Pediatrics (Table 50–2). It also was taken into account in the design of a number of formulas introduced over the past few years for feeding the hospitalized LBW infant (Table 50–3).

Opposing views concerning the goals for nutri-

tional management of LBW infants include, on the one hand, the fear that the intake of protein required to assure its accumulation at the intrauterine rate may overwhelm the LBW infant's ability to utilize protein and, on the other, the desire to produce the most rapid growth rate possible, preferably even more rapid than the intrauterine rate, thereby reducing the duration and the cost of hospitalization. Proponents of the former view advocate feeding human milk because of its lower protein content and its theoretical non-nutritional benefits, e.g., enhanced infant bonding and protection against infection. Proponents of the latter view advocate providing sufficient nutrients to permit the most rapid growth rate possible.

**Energy Requirements.** It is usually assumed that LBW infants require approximately 120 kcal/kg/day—75 kcal/kg/day for resting expenditure and the remainder for specific dynamic action (10 kcal/kg/day), replacement of inevitable stool losses (10 kcal/kg/day), and growth (25 kcal/kg/day).

The 75 kcal/kg/day usually allotted for meeting

**Table 50–2.  Recommended Nutrient Intakes for Low-Birth-Weight Infants\*†**

| Nutrient | Recommended Intake (Amount/100 kcal) |
|---|---|
| Protein (g) | 2.7–3.1 |
| Fat (g) | 4.3–5.4 |
|  | (300 mg essential fatty acids) |
| Carbohydrate | — |
| Electrolytes and Minerals |  |
| Sodium (meq) | 2.3–2.7 |
| Potassium (meq) | 1.8–1.9 |
| Calcium (mg) | 140–160 |
| Magnesium (mg) | 6.5–7.5 |
| Phosphorus (mg) | 95–108 |
| Chloride (meq) | 2–2.4 |
| Trace Minerals |  |
| Iron | ‡ |
| Zinc (mg) | 0.5 |
| Copper (μg) | 90 |
| Manganese (μg) | 5 |
| Iodine (μg) | 5 |
| Vitamins | *Amount/day* |
| A (IU) | 1400 |
| D (IU) | 500 |
| E (IU) | 5–25 |
|  | (1.0 IU/g linoleic acid) |
| C (mg) | 35 |
| Thiamin (μg) | 300 |
| Riboflavin (μg) | 400 |
| Niacin (mg) | 6 |
| $B_6$ (μg) | 300    (15 μg/g protein) |
| Folic acid (μg) | 50 |
| $B_{12}$ (μg) | 0.3 |
| Pantothenic acid (mg) | 2 |
| Biotin (μg) | 35 |

\*From Committee on Nutrition, American Academy of Pediatrics,[7] with permission of Pediatrics.
†Lower values are the recommended intakes for larger infants; higher values are the recommended intakes for smaller infants (BW <1,250 g).
‡See text.

**Table 50–3. Composition (Amount/100 kcal) of Standard Formulas for Low-Birth-Weight Infants**

| Component | Similac Special Care* | Enfamil Premature† | SMA Premie‡ |
|---|---|---|---|
| Protein (g) | 2.71 (bovine milk, whey) | 3 (bovine milk, whey) | 2.4 (bovine milk, whey) |
| Fat (g) | 5.43 (MCT, soy and coconut oils) | 5.1 (MCT, soy and coconut oils) | 5.4 (coconut, oleic and soy oils, oleo, MCT) |
| Carbohydrate (g) | 10.6 (lactose, glucose polymers) | 11 (lactose, corn syrup solids) | 10.1 (lactose, glucose polymers) |
| Calcium (mg) | 180 | 117 | 90 |
| Phosphorus (mg) | 90 | 59 | 50 |
| Magnesium (mg) | 12 | 4.9 | 8.6 |
| Iron (mg) | 0.37 | 0.25 | 0.38 |
| Zinc (mg) | 1.5 | 1.5 | 1.0 |
| Manganese (mg) | 12 | 13 | 25 |
| Copper (mcg) | 250 | 160 | 86 |
| Iodine (mcg) | 20 | 7.9 | 10 |
| Sodium (mg) | 50 | 39 | 40 |
| Potassium (mg) | 140 | 111 | 90 |
| Chloride (mg) | 90 | 85 | 66 |
| Vitamin A (IU) | 680 | 1200 | 300 |
| Vitamin D (IU) | 150 | 330 | 60 |
| Vitamin E (IU) | 4.0 | 4.6 | 1.9 |
| Vitamin K (mcg) | 12 | 13 | 8.6 |
| Thiamin (mcg) | 250 | 250 | 100 |
| Riboflavin (mcg) | 620 | 350 | 160 |
| Vitamin $B_6$ (mcg) | 250 | 250 | 60 |
| Vitamin $B_{12}$ (mcg) | 0.55 | 0.3 | 1.3 |
| Niacin (mcg) | 5000 | 4000 | 750 |
| Folic acid (mcg) | 37 | 35 | 12.5 |
| Pantothenic acid (mcg) | 1900 | 1200 | 450 |
| Vitamin C (mg) | 37 | 35 | 8.6 |

*Ross Laboratories.
†Mead Johnson Nutritional Division.
‡Wyeth Laboratories.

resting needs includes the basal requirement (about 50 kcal/kg/day) as well as additional requirements imposed by activity and response to cold stress. However, LBW infants are relatively inactive and, with careful control of the environmental temperature, energy expenditure in response to cold stress is minimal. In fact, studies in relatively inactive infants maintained in a strictly thermoneutral environment suggest that the resting requirement rarely exceeds 60 kcal/kg/day.[8–10]

The energy required for specific dynamic action, or the thermic effect of food (i.e., the difference between resting energy expenditure of the fed infant and that of the fasted infant), may be a function of the composition of the diet. At one time it was thought that protein content of the diet was the primary determinant of this thermic effect, but more recent studies suggest that the energy content of the diet is equally important.[10,11]

Fecal losses of nutrients, especially fat, appear to be inevitable in the fed LBW infant. The extent of these losses is a function of the nature of the fat intake (see section on fat requirements). In infants fed either human milk or modern formulas, stool fat losses rarely exceed 15 to 20% of the fat intake, or 7.5 to 10% of the total energy intake.

The precise energy requirement for growth is unknown. This requirement includes two components: the energy cost of synthesizing new tissue, which is probably measured as a part of either resting expenditure or the thermic effect of food, and the energy value of stored nutrients. Values of 3 to 6 kcal/g weight gain have been reported for the latter component.[10–12] Because this value obviously depends upon the composition of the newly synthesized tissue (e.g., deposition of calorically dense fat tissue requires more calories than deposition of lean body mass), such a range is to be expected. The calculated energy value of tissue deposited by the fetus between the thirtieth and thirty-eighth weeks of gestation is 2.0 to 2.5 kcal/g (see Table 50–1), whereas the calculated energy value of tissue deposited by the normally growing term infant between birth and 4 months of age[13] is approximately 4.5 kcal/g.

The range of energy requirements for each category is summarized in Table 50–4. Depending upon the conditions, the energy requirement may range from 95 to 160 kcal/kg/day. Aside from growth, the factors of greatest quantitative impor-

**Table 50–4. Range of Energy Requirements of Low-Birth-Weight Infants**

| Category | Range of Requirement (kcal/kg/day) |
|---|---|
| Resting expenditure | 50–75 |
| Thermic effect of diet | 5–10 |
| Fecal losses | 10–15 |
| Growth | 30–60 |
| TOTAL | 95–160 |

**Table 50–5. Essential Amino Acid Requirements of Low-Birth-Weight Infants\***

| Amino Acid | Minimal Requirement (mg/kg/day) |
|---|---|
| Histidine | 48 |
| Isoleucine | 128 |
| Leucine | 216 |
| Lysine | 155 |
| Methionine | 52 |
| Phenylalanine | 104 |
| Threonine | 92 |
| Tryptophan | 30 |
| Valine | 138 |
| Cysteine | 85 |
| Tyrosine | 50 |

\*From Snyderman, S.E., et al.[18] with permission of Pediatrics.

tance are the infant's activity state and the environmental conditions under which it is nursed. For most LBW infants, an energy intake of 120 kcal/kg/day is adequate.

**Protein Requirements.** The common practice of feeding low-birth-weight infants with human milk was largely abandoned approximately 40 years years ago following the demonstration that protein intakes higher than those provided by human milk resulted in a greater rate of weight gain.[14] However, formulas used in this study also contained more electrolytes and minerals (ash) than human milk; thus, it was suggested that the greater weight gain was due to increased water retention secondary to the greater ash intake rather than to the greater protein intake. Indeed, subsequent studies demonstrated that both total body water and extracellular fluid of infants fed high-protein, high-solute intakes were greater than those observed in infants fed low-solute formulas.[15] Nonetheless, it is clear that there is also a direct relationship between protein intake and weight gain.[16,17]

In general, a protein intake of approximately 3 g/kg/day, or somewhat less, appears to be adequate for the LBW infant. On the other hand, higher intakes appear to be well tolerated metabolically and also support a greater rate of weight gain.[17] The protein, of course, must be of such quality as to provide sufficient amounts of all essential amino acids (Table 50–5) including those that are essential only for the premature infant (i.e., histidine,[18] tyrosine,[19] and cysteine).[20] In this regard, current LBW infant formulas contain "humanized" bovine milk protein (60% whey proteins and 40% caseins). However, despite a higher cyst(e)ine content, there is little evidence that this protein is more efficacious than unmodified bovine milk protein (18% whey protein and 82% caseins), particularly with respect to growth.[21] Of theoretical interest is the fact that plasma threonine concentrations of infants fed "humanized" bovine milk formulas are approximately double those observed in infants fed unmodified bovine milk protein, whereas plasma tyrosine concentrations are higher in infants fed unmodified bovine milk formulas.[21–23]

**Fat Requirements.** Although fat accounts for 40

to 50% of the total energy content of most diets, including those designed for LBW infants, the only known requirement for fat in human nutrition is to provide essential fatty acids. In general, this requirement can be met by provision of 2 to 4% of the total energy intake as linoleic acid. The possibility that linolenic acid also may be required has received considerable attention.[24] If so, this nutrient may be particularly important for the LBW infant. Because the developing brain contains relatively large amounts of linolenic acid metabolites, failure to provide the precursor of these potentially important fatty acids may contribute to suboptimal central nervous system development.

The role of fat in infant feeding has received considerable attention for two additional reasons. First, neither the LBW infant nor the newborn term infant absorbs fat well. Second, there is considerable concern regarding the effect of fat intake on serum lipid concentrations and the effect of serum lipid concentrations on subsequent development of arteriosclerosis.

Compared to adults and even term infants, the LBW infant has a limited bile salt pool and a low intraduodenal bile salt concentration.[25] This limitation, in fact, appears to be the major factor in the LBW infant's poorer fat absorption. Although pancreatic lipase is also limited,[26] the presence of salivary and/or gastric lipases provides adequate lipase activity for hydrolysis.[27] Infants fed unprocessed human milk, of course, have the additional benefit of human milk lipase. Mucosal uptake of the products of hydrolysis seems to proceed normally in suckling animals[28] but has not been studied in infants. The status of the process of chylomicron formation and secretion in the LBW infant is not known, but there is no suggestion that it is inadequate.

Fat absorption is also a function of the chemical nature of the fat. Triglycerides containing poly-unsaturated fatty acids (e.g., human milk fat, vegetable oils) are better absorbed than those containing saturated fatty acids.[29] The position of the fatty acid on the triglyceride molecule also seems to play a role in fat absorption.[30] Because mono-glycerides are better absorbed than fatty acids and because lipase preferentially cleaves fatty acids from the 1- and 3-positions, triglycerides containing poorly absorbed fatty acids in these positions are more likely to be associated with poor overall fat absorption. Triglycerides of short-and medium-chain fatty acids are absorbed directly into the portal circulation, regardless of the intraluminal bile salt and lipase activities.[31] Thus, substitution of a major portion of the fat content of infant formulas with medium-chain triglycerides results in enhanced absorption.[32–34] Interestingly, this substitution does not necessarily result in improved weight gain.[34]

The fat content of infant diets, particularly the cholesterol content, has received considerable attention because of its possible relationship to later development of arteriosclerosis. Cholesterol is not an essential nutrient for either the preterm or term infant; thus, there is no absolute requirement for cholesterol, and currently available infant formulas do not contain cholesterol. Natural milks, however, contain abundant amounts of cholesterol, and infants fed these milks have higher serum cholesterol concentrations than infants fed artificial formulas.[35] This observation has given rise to two arguments. One concerns the possible deleterious effect of high serum cholesterol concentration during infancy with respect to subsequent development of arteriosclerosis. The other is based on the concept that the higher serum cholesterol concentration of infants fed natural milks may be desirable because it results in induction of enzymes necessary for cholesterol catabolism. Studies in swine show that animals fed low-cholesterol diets in early life have higher serum cholesterol concentrations when fully grown.[36] However, such studies in humans do not demonstrate a conclusive effect of cholesterol intake during infancy on serum cholesterol concentration in later life.[37] Thus, there is no conclusive evidence, at present, that the cholesterol content of the infant's diet is either harmful or beneficial.

**Carbohydrate Requirements.** The central nervous system and the hematopoietic tissue are largely dependent upon glucose as a metabolic fuel. However, glucose can be produced from either exogenously administered protein or endogenous protein stores (e.g., gluconeogenesis). Thus, in contrast to requirements for specific amino acids and fatty acids, there appears to be no absolute requirement for carbohydrate. On the other hand, the various gluconeogenic mechanisms of LBW infants are not well developed.[38] Exogenous glucose is therefore necessary to prevent hypoglycemia, particularly during the immediate neonatal period.

Carbohydrates comprise approximately 40–50% of the total energy content of most dietary regimens designed for LBW infants. Although the predominant carbohydrate of most natural milks is lactose, most current LBW infant formulas contain a mixture of lactose and glucose polymer (see Table 50–3). Despite the fact that development of intestinal lactase activity lags behind development of other disaccharidases,[39] most viable infants tolerate lactose well. In fact, satisfactory clinical progress has been observed with formulas that contain only lactose, only sucrose, only glucose, only glucose polymers, and mixtures of these sugars.

**Fluid Requirements.** Several bases of reference have been suggested for estimating maintenance fluid requirements, e.g., body weight, body surface area, and energy expenditure. Of these, energy expenditure, which focuses attention on the physiologic and nonphysiologic factors most likely to modify fluid requirements (e.g., body temperature, ambient temperature, ambient humidity, activity, and respiratory rate), seems the most relevant. In the nongrowing older infant, the maintenance fluid requirement is approximately 1 ml/kcal expended.[40] This allotment replaces insensible water losses through the lungs and skin as well as obligatory renal and gastrointestinal losses.

Insensible water loss varies considerably in all infants, particularly LBW infants. Moreover, both pulmonary and cutaneous components of insensible water loss are related inversely to ambient humidity. Under usual nursery conditions, the insensible water loss of term infants is approximately 30 ml/100 kcal. In the very small infant, cutaneous losses may be considerably greater than those of the term infant, possibly because of altered skin permeability to water,[41] whereas the common practice of nursing LBW infants in relatively high humidity probably tends to decrease insensible pulmonary losses. Phototherapy, a commonly used modality in LBW infants with hyperbilirubinemia, also increases insensible water losses.[42] Thus, the insensible water loss of most LBW infants probably exceeds that of the term infant.

Obligatory renal losses of the LBW infant also are variable. Although even immature infants can regulate the volume of urine excreted according to the solute load and the available water, both renal concentrating and diluting mechanisms are limited.[43] In general, allowance for a urinary volume of 50 to 60 ml/100 kcal permits excretion of the usual range of solute loads at urine concentrations of 150 to 450 mosm/L, which are easily achieved even by an immature kidney.

In unfed infants, fluid losses via the gastrointestinal tract are minimal. If the infant is fed, however, approximately 10% of the fluid intake is lost in stool. These losses are even greater in infants receiving phototherapy.[42]

The LBW infant's fluid requirement for growth, of course, is a function of both the rate of growth and the water content of the newly synthesized tissue. The water content of tissue synthesized during the last trimester of gestation is approximately 70% (see Table 50–1), whereas the water content of the tissue synthesized by the reference infant between birth and 4 months of age is 40 to 45%.[13] An estimate of 50 to 60% for the growing LBW infant seems reasonable.

The water requirements for insensible (30 ml/100 kcal) and obligatory (50 to 60 ml/100 kcal) losses as well as for growth (10 to 20 ml/100 kcal) are reduced by the endogenously produced water of oxidation, i.e., approximately 12 ml/100 kcal. Thus, the LBW infant, like the term infant, seems to have a minimum water requirement of 1 ml/kcal utilized. The fasting infant, therefore, requires at least 65 to 75 ml/kg/day while the growing infant requires at least 120 ml/kg/day. However, the very immature infant and the infant undergoing phototherapy may require much more water. In general, a fluid intake of 140 ml/kg/day is well tolerated by most infants; intakes above this amount are associated with an increased likelihood of developing patent ductus arteriosus.[44]

**Electrolyte Requirements.** The daily obligatory electrolyte losses of the term infant have been estimated to be approximately 0.5 meq/kg of both sodium and chloride and approximately 0.75 meq/kg of potassium. Because renal reabsorption mechanisms are not fully developed in the LBW infant, the renal losses are likely to be greater. Losses probably are greater also in infants with increased fluid losses secondary to phototherapy.

The electrolytes required for tissue synthesis depend upon the rate of growth. Assuming continuation of the intrauterine growth rate (see Table 50–1), the daily requirement of these nutrients for tissue synthesis will be approximately the amounts that accumulate during the last trimester of gestation, i.e., 1.0 to 1.5 meq/kg of sodium and 0.5 to 1.0 meq/kg of both potassium and chloride. If the rate of weight gain is more or less than the intrauterine rate, or if the composition of weight

gain is different, the requirements obviously change proportionally.

The minimal daily sodium, potassium, and chloride requirements of the LBW infant receiving adequate protein and energy intakes and growing at the intrauterine rate are, respectively, 1.5 to 2.0 meq/kg, 1.25 to 1.75 meq/kg, and 1.0 to 1.5 meq/kg. The quantities of potassium and chloride present in the volumes of both human milk and commonly used formulas usually ingested are sufficient to provide these requirements. However, the sodium content of human milk (approximately 1.2 meq/100 kcal), even if completely absorbed, is insufficient. On the other hand, the growth rate of LBW infants fed human milk is somewhat less than the intrauterine rate; therefore, their sodium requirement for growth probably is less than 1.5 meq/kg/day. The intakes recommended by the Committee on Nutrition of the American Academy of Pediatrics are considerably greater than these minimal intakes (see Table 50–2).

**Mineral Requirements.** Until recently, studies of calcium and phosphorus needs were directed toward defining the intakes necessary to prevent hypocalcemia. Because this condition develops more commonly in infants fed formulas with a high content of phosphorus relative to calcium (i.e., a low calcium/phosphorus ratio), emphasis has been placed on the ratio of calcium to phosphorus intake rather than on absolute amounts of either mineral. Experience has shown that a ratio of roughly 1.5 to 2.0 is satisfactory (Table 50–6).

The amount of calcium retained during the latter part of normal intrauterine growth is approximately 14 meq/day, whereas the calcium content of human milk is only ~20 meq/L. Thus, if the LBW infant's requirement for calcium is assumed to be the amount necessary to allow continuation of the rate of accumulation that occurs in utero, human milk obviously contains inadequate calcium. Moreover, LBW infants fed human milk have less dense skeletons radiographically than those fed formulas containing large amounts of calcium; many, in fact, develop rickets and/or fractures.[45] Thus, LBW infants fed human milk, including those fed their own mother's milk require supplemental calcium for optimal skeletal mineralization. LBW infants growing more rapidly than the fetus probably also require more phosphorus than provided by usual intakes of human milk.

Iron requirements depend upon the existing body stores and the rate of growth. The LBW infant obviously has more limited stores of iron than the term infant and, therefore, is more susceptible to the development of iron deficiency, especially during periods of rapid growth. It has been estimated that the LBW infant's endogenous iron stores, in the absence of exogenous intake, will be depleted sometime during the second to third month of life rather than during the fifth month of life as appears to be the case in the term infant. For this reason, it is generally suggested that the LBW infant receive iron supplements or iron-fortified formulas as early as possible. Such supplements, however, increase the infant's susceptibility to vitamin E deficiency[46] especially when formulas high in polyunsaturated fatty acids are fed. In addition, the bactericidal properties of the iron-binding proteins of human milk (i.e., lactoferrin and lactoglobulin) are abolished if saturated with iron.[47]

In light of these considerations, it seems unnecessary and perhaps undesirable to fortify the formulas of LBW infants with iron during the first two months of life. Alternatively, formulas that contain moderate amounts of polyunsaturated fats and ample vitamin E may be supplemented with 1 mg of iron/100 kcal.[48]

Little information is available concerning the LBW infant's requirements for other trace minerals. In general, the recommendations for intake of these various minerals are based on either the amounts provided by human milk or the amounts recommended for term infants.

The Food and Nutrition Board of the National Academy of Sciences-National Research Council recommends a daily zinc intake of 3 mg[49] (Appendix Table A1a). The American Academy of Pediatrics Committee on Nutrition recommends that formulas for term infants contain 0.5 mg of zinc/100 kcal[50] (see Table 50–6). This level of zinc intake, assuming 50% absorption from the gastrointestinal tract, should allow accumulation of zinc at the intrauterine rate. The concentration of zinc in human milk is approximately 3 to 5 mg/L; thus, it provides minimally adequate zinc to allow accumulation at the intrauterine rate. On the other hand, the zinc content of human milk is absorbed more efficiently than that of bovine milk.[51]

The daily iodine intake recommended by the Food and Nutrition Board of the National Academy of Science-National Research Council is 35 μg.[49] The minimal requirement recommended by the American Academy of Pediatrics Committee on Nutrition for normal infants is 5 μg/100 kcal,[50] also the iodine content of human milk. Because the uptake of radioiodine by the thyroid of LBW infants is in the same range as that of term infants, older children, and adults,[52] this recommended intake is probably adequate.

The recommended copper content of infant formulas is 60 μg/100 kcal.[50] Although this intake might not allow accumulation of copper at the intrauterine rate, it is approximately the amount present in human milk. Although some have recommended a copper intake of 90 μg/100 kcal for LBW infants,[53] such intakes are probably not necessary owing to the large hepatic stores of copper. In one study, in fact, a copper intake of only 14 μg/kg/day for 60 days did not provoke manifestations of deficiency.[54]

**Vitamin Requirements.** Specific recommendations concerning either requirements or advisable allowances of vitamins for LBW infants are not available; thus, it is usually suggested that the RDAs for term infants be given (Appendix Table A1a). Infants fed sufficient amounts of either human milk or artificial formulas to produce adequate growth usually receive sufficient amounts of all vitamins, although human milk (and unfortified bovine milk) may be deficient in vitamin D. Nonetheless, because the consumption of sufficient volumes of formula to satisfy vitamin requirements may not be attained for several weeks, a supplement containing vitamins A, C, and D is recommended. In addition, the LBW infant may have special needs for vitamin E and folic acid.

Vitamin E functions as an antioxidant to prevent peroxidation of polyunsaturated fatty acids in various cell membranes. Thus, it is not surprising that inadequate vitamin E intake results in erythrocyte hemolysis.[55] Because the polyunsaturated fatty acid content of all membranes is related to intake of these fatty acids, infant formulas containing vegetable oils of high polyunsaturated fatty acid content impose a greater vitamin E requirement. Such formulas, therefore, should have a higher vitamin E content. In general, the aim should be to provide a total of 1 I.U. of vitamin E per gram of polyunsaturated fatty acids, i.e., an E/PUFA ratio of 1.

LBW infants fed formulas containing polyunsaturated fats and given therapeutic doses of iron also have a greater incidence of erythrocyte hemolysis and lower serum vitamin E levels than infants fed formulas containing less iron and polyunsaturated fats.[56] Thus, the relationship between the vitamin E and iron contents of the formula as well as the relationship between the vitamin E and polyunsaturated fat contents of the formula are important. For this reason, careful attention must be given to vitamin E intake if iron supplements are given.

Large doses of vitamin E have been recommended to prevent both retrolental fibroplasia[57] and bronchopulmonary dysplasia.[58] However, it is not clear whether these recommendations are warranted, particularly considering the potential toxicity of the large doses.

Folic acid functions as a coenzyme in many

metabolic reactions including the synthesis of purines and pyrimidines; thus, it is essential for production of new cells. Studies of folate metabolism in preterm infants show that serum values fall from approximately normal adult levels at birth to levels below this range by a few weeks of age. These values remain low until around 3 months of age at which time levels rise again to those observed in normal adults. Although this decrease in serum folate values can be prevented by oral supplements of 50 μg/day, neither growth nor hemoglobin concentration of supplemented infants differs from that of unsupplemented infants.[59] Unsupplemented infants, however, have more hypersegmented neutrophils and lower erythrocyte folate levels. Thus, the recommendation that LBW infants be supplemented with 50 μg/day of folic acid[60] is endorsed.

**Delivery of Nutrient Requirements to LBW Infants.** For most LBW infants, the foregoing discussion of nutrient requirements is largely academic. Underlying illnesses as well as a number of neurophysiologic deficiencies (e.g., poor or unsustained suck, uncoordinated swallowing mechanism, delayed gastric emptying, and poor intestinal motility) make delivery of any enteral nutritional regimen virtually impossible, particularly during the first week of life. During the immediate neonatal period, a nutritional regimen that prevents catabolism and allows some increment in lean body mass probably is satisfactory. This more realistic goal for the first several days of life can be achieved in sick LBW infants with a parenteral regimen that provides as few as 60 kcal/kg/day, an amino acid intake of 2.5 g/kg/day, and necessary electrolytes, minerals, and vitamins.[61] A similar regimen delivered enterally should be equally efficacious provided intestinal absorption is not severely compromised.

Various methods of delivering nutrients by the intravenous route (total parentral nutrition) as well as by the gastrointestinal tract (e.g., continuous nasogastric or transpyloric infusions) have been proposed as alternatives to more conventional feeding techniques. Although no one method is likely to be ideal for all situations, use of a combination of these methods of nutrient delivery, allowing the particular clinical problems of an individual infant to be the basis for selecting the method of delivery, should improve nutritional management. In many infants, a combination of conventional and these less conventional methods of feeding permits delivery of sufficient nutrients to support "normal" growth.

Within reason, every infant should be given a trial at conventional feeding, i.e., tolerated nipple or gavage feedings of either human milk or a standard formula plus intravenous supplmentation with 5 to 10% glucose solutions. If adequate nutrients cannot be delivered in this way, a trial of continuous nasogastric or transpyloric feedings is warranted. Tolerated enteral feedings delivered conventionally or by continuous infusion also can be supplemented by intravenous infusions of appropriate mixtures of glucose, amino acids, and/or lipid. In the event that enteral feedings are not tolerated, parenteral administration of a balanced nutritional mixture deserves serious consideration. A regimen that provides 75 kcal/kg/day plus amino acids, electrolytes, minerals, and vitamins can be delivered by peripheral vein infusion without imposing an unreasonable fluid load. Such a regimen usually maintains existing body composition; thus, it is particularly applicable for infants who are likely to tolerate enteral intake within a brief priod. Use of a central vein catheter allows delivery of a more concentrated nutrient mixture and is particularly useful in situations associated with prolonged intolerance of enteral feedings.

**Role of Human Milk in Feeding the LBW Infant.** Currently, there is a widespread interest in providing human milk for feeding the LBW infant, and even in establishing human milk banks to ensure an adequate supply of this product. However, evidence that human milk is nutritionally superior for this population is lacking. On the contrary, as discussed previously, growth rates of LBW infants fed human milk are considerably lower than those of infants fed formulas. This observation has been ascribed in part to the relatively low protein concentration of human milk, i.e., about 1 g/100 ml (an intake of approximately 2 g/kg/day at the volumes tolerated by most LBW infants). Milk of mothers who deliver prematurely has an approximately 20% higher protein concentration[62] and appears to support greater growth rates.[63] Nonetheless, this milk contains insufficient amounts of other nutrients, namely sodium, calcium, and phosphorus.[64]

In contrast to the nutritional disadvantages of human milk in feeding the LBW infants, its immunologic properties may be a distinct advantage. These properties (i.e., cellular as well as humoral components) theoretically could confer passive immunity and/or enhance immunologic maturation thereby providing some protection against infections and, perhaps, necrotizing enterocolitis. Although no concrete clinical evidence exists that feeding human milk either prevents necrotizing enterocolitis or is associated with a lower incidence of infection, there are potentially beneficial differences in stool pH and fecal flora between infants fed human milk and those fed formulas.

It must be remembered, however, that the immunologic properties of human milk are altered by storage and processing methods. Cellular elements do not survive either freezing or pasteurization, and many of the humoral factors, although not altered by freezing, are heat-labile.

Despite the possible immunologic advantages of fresh human milk, the additional steps involved in collection, storage, and dispensing of expressed human milk make inadvertent contamination likely. Thus, stringent hygienic techniques and bacterial screening are mandatory to assure bacteriologic safety. Viral contamination is also a major concern. For example, cytomegalovirus (CMV) excretion in the milk of seropositive women is relatively common,[65] and CMV infection has been reported in infants fed CMV-positive milk.[66] Moreover, one case of HTLV III infection transmitted by human milk has been reported.[67] Herpes and rubella viruses and hepatitis B surface antigen also have been detected in human milk, but transmission of these viruses via milk has not been demonstrated.

More research is necessary to elucidate the role of human milk, provided either by the infant's mother or by a donor (or donors), in feeding the LBW infant. This research should be well underway before enormous expense and effort are spent in establishing milk banks to supply safe human milk for routine feeding of LBW infants. On the other hand, if an individual mother wishes to provide milk for her infant, the potential psychologic benefits of her involvement in the infant's care as well as the benefits with respect to eventual success in nursing are strong reasons for encouraging milk expression until the infant can be breast-fed. Even in these situations, however, the infant must be carefully monitored for development of specific nutrient deficiencies of protein, calcium, phosphorus, sodium, and vitamin D.

## NUTRITIONAL REQUIREMENTS OF THE NORMAL INFANT

In contrast to the situation of the LBW infant, the nutritional requirements of the normal infant have been addressed by a number of investigators over several years, and recommended dietary allowances for most nutrients have been established. These recommendations are summarized in Table 50–6. The requirements of some nutrients are discussed briefly here.

Energy requirements of the normal infant, per unit of body weight, are three to four times greater than those of the adult, i.e., 90 to 120 kcal/kg/day vs. 30 to 40 kcal/kg/day. These greater needs, like the greater needs of the LBW infant, are a result of both the infant's relatively high resting metabolic rate and the special needs for growth and development. However, even in the normal infant, relatively inefficient intestinal absorption mechanisms contribute. Individual variations in energy requirements can be considerable.

So far as the source of energy is concerned, there is no evidence to suggest that either carbohydrate or fat is superior, provided total energy intake is adequate. Sufficient carbohydrate to avoid development of ketosis and/or hypoglycemia is required ($<5$ g/kg/day) as is enough fat to avoid development of essential fatty acid deficiency ($\sim$0.5 g/kg/day of linoleic acid plus, perhaps, a smaller amount of linolenic acid).

In concert with the recommendation that the dietary fat intake of the general population be reduced, particularly that of cholesterol and saturated fat, some agencies have suggested that this guideline be applied to infants. Because fat is important both as a major source of energy and as a source of essential fatty acids, however, groups responsible for making recommendations for infants have not endorsed this recommendation. After 1 to 2 years of age, however, attention to this general guideline is warranted.

The protein requirement of the normal infant per unit of body weight also is greater than that of the adult, but is not as great as the requirement of the LBW infant. The normal infant, like the LBW infant, also requires a higher proportion of essential to nonessential amino acids than the adult (Table 50–7). The minimal intakes of essential amino acids consistent with normal growth were determined under conditions of maximal nitrogen sparing. Thus, if the required intakes of the essential amino acids are met, the total intake of nitrogen is more important than the particular mixture of amino acids provided. Indeed, the overall protein requirement is probably two to three times the aggregate requirement for essential amino acids. Obviously, the required intake of a specific protein is a function of its quality. In general, the more closely the amino acid pattern of a specific protein resembles that of human milk, the more closely the requirement for that protein approaches the absolute minimum requirement for human milk. It also follows that the overall quality of a specific protein can be improved by supplementing it with the essential amino acid that is lacking. An example is soy protein which, in the native state, has insufficient methionine but, when fortified with methionine, approaches or equals the overall quality of bovine milk protein.[69]

Although the amino acid composition of human milk is ideal, its overall protein content, approximately 1.0 g/dl, is such that ingestion of 180 to 200 ml/kg/day is required to ensure a protein in-

**Table 50–6.**    **Recommended Nutrient Intakes for Normal Infants\*†**

| Nutrient | Recommended Intake (Amount/100 kcal) |
|---|:---:|
| Protein (g) | 1.8–4.5 |
| Fat (g) | 3.3–6.0 |
| | (3% of calories as linoleic acid) |
| Carbohydrate | — |
| Electrolytes and Minerals | |
|    Calcium (mg)‡ | 50 |
|    Phosphorus (mg)‡ | 25 |
|    Magnesium (mg) | 6 |
|    Sodium (meq) | 0.9–2.6 |
|    Potassium (meq) | 2.1–5.1 |
|    Chloride (meq) | 1.5–4.2 |
| Trace Minerals | |
|    Iron (mg) | 0.15 |
|    Iodine (μg) | 5 |
|    Zinc (mg) | 0.5 |
|    Copper (μg) | 60 |
|    Manganese (μg) | 5 |
| Vitamins | |
|    A (IU) | 250–700 |
|    D (IU) | 40–100 |
|    K (μg) | 4.0 |
|    E (IU) | 3.0 |
|    C (mg) | 8.0 |
|    Thiamin (μg) | 40.0 |
|    Riboflavin (μg) | 35.0 |
|    Pyridoxine (μg)§ | 35.0 |
|    $B_{12}$ (μg) | 0.15 |
|    Niacin (mg) | 250 |
|    Folic acid (μg) | 4.0 |
|    Pantothenic acid | 300 |
|    Biotin (μg) | 1.5 |
|    Choline (mg) | 7.0 |
|    Inositol (mg) | 4.0 |

\*From Committee on Nutrition, American Academy of Pediatrics,[50] with permission of Pediatrics.
†Lower values are minimal recommended intakes; higher values are maximum recommended intakes.
‡Calcium to phosphorus ratio should be between 1.1 and 2.0.
§0.7 IU vitamin E/g linoleic acid; 15 μg pyridoxine/g protein.

**Table 50–7.**    **Essential Amino Acid Requirements of the Term Infant\***

| Amino Acid | Requirement (mg/kg/day) |
|---|:---:|
| Leucine | 76–229 |
| Isoleucine | 103–119 |
| Lysine | 88–102 |
| Methionine | 33–45 |
| Phenylalanine | 47–90 |
| Threonine | 45–87 |
| Tryptophan | 15–22 |
| Valine | 85–105 |
| Histidine | 16–34 |

\*From Holt, L.E., Jr., Snyderman, S.E.,[68] with permission of J.A.M.A.

take equal to the recommended intake of 2.0 to 2.2 g/kg/day. This fact has led some to question the adequacy of the protein content of human milk and others to question the validity of the recommended intake. On balance, the high quality and easy digestibility of human milk protein appear to compensate for any quantitative deficiency. On the other hand, bovine milk protein, the protein source of most infant formulas, also is a high-quality protein and, if properly processed, is utilized nearly as well as human milk protein. Thus, the actual requirement for protein when bovine milk is the source may be only slightly higher, if at all, than when human milk is the source.[70]

The electrolyte, mineral, and vitamin requirements of the normal infant are better defined than those of the LBW infant but not as well defined as those for energy and protein. Nonetheless, recommended intakes for most have been established (see Table 50–6), and infants who receive these intakes experience few problems. In recent years, the concept that limitation of sodium intake may decrease the incidence of hypertension later in life has increased in popularity. However, there are few hard data on which to base a definitive conclusion.

Iron deficiency is the most common nutrient deficiency syndrome in infancy. This finding is somewhat surprising because the normal infant has sufficient stores of iron at birth to meet requirements for 4 to 6 months. However, these stores as well as the absorption of iron are variable. Although human milk contains less iron than most formulas, iron deficiency is less common in breast-fed infants. To prevent development of iron deficiency, routine iron supplementation of most formula-fed infants over 2 months of age is recommended. Some also recommend supplementation of infants who are less than 2 months of age. As discussed more fully in the earlier section addressing iron requirements of the LBW infant, the amount required may be related to the vitamin E and polyunsaturated fat contents of the diet.

If protein intake is adequate, deficiencies of most vitamins are rare; if it is inadequate, deficiencies of nicotinic acid and choline, which are synthesized, respectively, from tryptophan and methionine, may develop. In contrast, hypovitaminosis D would be endemic among formula-fed infants if bovine milk and bovine milk formulas were not supplemented with vitamin D. The breast-fed infant may be relatively better protected from development of vitamin D deficiency,[71] but vitamin D supplementation of breast-fed infants also is recommended. Routine perinatal administration of vitamin K is recommended as prophylaxis against hemorrhagic disease of the newborn.

The normal infant's absolute requirement for water is probably 75 to 100 ml/kg/day. However, because of higher obligate renal, pulmonary, and dermal water losses as well as a higher overall metabolic rate, the infant is more susceptible to dehydration, particularly with vomiting and/or diarrhea. Thus, provision of 150 ml/kg/day is recommended. The typical breast-fed infant as well as the typical formula-fed infant usually consumes at least this volume.

**Human Milk vs. Artificial Formula.** Because of its ready availability, its relative safety, and the theoretical possibility that it may enhance both resistance to infection and bonding between the mother and infant, human milk usually is considered the perfect food for the normal infant.[72] For most infants, there is no evidence that this is not true. On the other hand, certain theoretical and practical hazards of breast-feeding must be considered.

The major theoretical hazard is that human milk may contain too little calcium and phosphorus for optimal skeletal development of the growing infant. In this regard, there is little doubt that the breast-fed infant has a less mineralized skeleton than the infant fed formulas of higher calcium content.[73] On the other hand, unlike the situation in LBW infants, these lower calcium and phosphorus intakes and the less mineralized skeleton secondary to these intakes apparently are not detrimental to the normal infant.

Another theoretical hazard of human milk concerns its association in some infants with hyperbilirubinemia. The resulting hyperbilirubinemia, however, usually is a transient phenomenon; thus, unless hyperbilirubinemia persists or unless plasma bilirubin concentration exceeds 12 mg/dl, most feel that proscription of breast-feeding is not necessary.

The possibility that certain noxious or infectious agents may be present in breast milk (e.g., chemicals, drugs, foreign proteins) also must be borne in mind. The risk of infection secondary to the mode of feeding is far greater in formula-fed than in breast-fed infants, particularly if the artificial formula is prepared under less than optimal hygienic conditions.

The most important potential disadvantage of breast-feeding concerns the lack of constancy and adequacy of maternal milk supply. With proper counseling, this usually is not a problem. Nonetheless, breast-fed infants must be followed closely, particularly over the first few weeks of life, to ensure that growth and development are proceeding as expected. This requirement is crucial for first-born infants.

In large part, the historical problems associated with feeding the infant who cannot be breast-fed have been solved. In fact, considering the safety and easy digestibility of modern infant formulas, it is difficult to understand the current emphasis that governmental and nongovernmental agencies are placing on the promotion of breast-feeding. Although the economic advantages and microbiologic safety of breast-feeding for less developed and less affluent locales are obvious, these factors are of lesser importance in affluent, developed countries in which most of the current generation were fed artificial formulas during infancy. Thus, a reasonable and conservative approach is to allow the mother to make an educated choice of how she wishes to feed her infant and support her in that decision. On the other hand, evidence that the breast-fed infant has fewer common and serious infections during early life than the formula-fed infant is increasing.[74] If this difference is established to be due to breast feeding, per se, rather than to a myriad of other factors (e.g., socioeconomic status), breast-feeding, clearly, should be encouraged more avidly.

A number of formulas are available for feeding the normal infant. The composition of the most commonly used ones is shown in Table 50–8. Most are available in both a "ready to use" and a concentrated liquid form. Powdered products also are available; these are used infrequently in the United States but in many parts of the world are the only products available.

The most commonly used formulas contain either unmodified or modified bovine milk protein in a concentration of 1.5 g/dl. Thus, the infant who receives 180 ml/kg/day receives a protein intake of 2.7 g/kg/day, somewhat more than the breast-fed infant. Unmodified bovine milk protein has a whey:casein ratio of 18:82, whereas modified bovine milk protein has a whey:casein ratio of 60:40, which is similar to that of human milk. The latter products are prepared from either a mixture of bovine milk protein and bovine whey proteins or a mixture of bovine milk whey proteins and caseins. For the normal term infant, there is no convincing evidence that either the modified or unmodified bovine milk protein is more efficacious than the other. Formulas containing soy protein also are available for feeding the rare infant who is intolerant to bovine milk protein.

The major carbohydrate of the most commonly used bovine milk formulas is lactose. The soy protein formulas, however, contain either sucrose or a glucose polymer; thus, they are useful for the infant with either transient or congenital lactase deficiency. The fat content of both bovine milk and soy protein formulas is a blend of vegetable oils. In general, these oils are easily absorbed; most studies suggest that intestinal absorption approaches 90%.

The electrolyte, mineral, and vitamin contents of most formulas are similar. When fed in adequate amounts (150 to 180 ml/kg/day), all provide the recommended daily allowances for all these nutrients. Both iron-supplemented and nonsupplemented formulas are available. The former contain ~12 mg/L, whereas the latter contain only ~1 mg/L. As mentioned previously, it is usually recommended that infants receive iron-supplemented formulas, particularly after 2 to 3 months of age. Vitamin supplementation, although frequently recommended, is not required if intake of these formulas is adequate.

The goal of both breast-feeding and formula feeding, of course, is delivery of enough milk to support adequate weight gain. As a rule of thumb, the normal term infant's weight should double over the first 3 to 5 months of life and triple over the first 12 months. For the breast-fed infant, adequacy of intake can be assessed by periodic weighing immediately before and after feeding (1 g of weight gain = 1 ml of milk ingested). For the formula-fed infant, adequacy of intake can be determined by recording the quantity of formula ingested.

Demand feeding may be preferable during the early weeks of life, but most infants adjust easily to a 4-hour schedule; after 2 months of age, the night feedings usually can be omitted. Introduction of solid foods and administration of multivitamin supplements are unnecessary before 4 to 6 months of age; thereafter, most physicians recommend addition of a multivitamin supplement as well as strained or blenderized foods. The latter should be added stepwise, beginning with cereals, vegetables, and fruits. By approximately 1 year of age, most infants should have graduated successfully to table food and should be eating 3 to 4 meals daily. Once teeth have erupted and solid food is tolerated without difficulty, weaning should have been completed.

## NUTRITIONAL MANAGEMENT OF SPECIFIC DISEASES AND/OR CONDITIONS

The generalized deficiency of all nutrients, i.e., protein-energy malnutrition, is by far the most common nutritional deficiency in the world today. Although this condition is rare in developed countries, it occurs in a number of infants and/or children with underlying medical problems, some of which are discussed in this section. Thus, it is helpful to consider the special nutrient needs and nutritional management of these children within the framework of protein-energy malnutrition as encountered in many underdeveloped parts of the world (see also Chap. 42).

Protein-energy malnutrition results from a lack, in varying proportions, of protein and energy. It is seen most frequently in infants and young children and may occur in epidemic (famine-related) or endemic (disease-related) forms. Whether the cause is primary (i.e., insufficient food supply) or secondary (i.e., poor absorption, increased excretion, increased requirements), the physicochemical pattern of the tissues, defensive capacity to environmental aggressors, and the efficiency and ability for work are affected adversely. Moreover, the condition is associated with a high mortality rate.

Protein-energy malnutrition includes two distinct syndromes, marasmus and kwashiorkor, as well as a mixed syndrome, often termed marasmic kwashiorkor. Marasmus refers to the state of chronic total undernutrition (i.e., a deficiency of

**Table 50–8. Composition (Amount/100 kcal) of Standard Formulas for Normal Infants**

| Component | Similac* | Enfamil† | SMA‡ |
|---|---|---|---|
| Protein (g) | 2.22 (bovine milk) | 2.2 (bovine milk, whey) | 2.2 (bovine milk, whey) |
| Fat (g) | 5.37 (soy and coconut oils) | 5.6 (coconut and soy oils) | 5.3 (oleo, coconut, oleic and soy oils) |
| Carbohydrate (g) | 10.7 (lactose) | 10.3 (lactose) | 10.6 (lactose) |
| Calcium (mg) | 75 | 69 | 63 |
| Phosphorus (mg) | 58 | 47 | 42 |
| Magnesium (mg) | 6 | 7.8 | 7 |
| Iron (mg) | 1.8 | 1.88 | 1.8 |
| Zinc (mg) | 0.75 | 0.78 | 0.8 |
| Manganese ($\mu$g) | 5 | 15.6 | 22 |
| Copper ($\mu$g) | 90 | 94 | 70 |
| Iodine ($\mu$g) | 15 | 10.2 | 9 |
| Sodium (mg) | 32 | 27 | 22 |
| Potassium (mg) | 120 | 108 | 83 |
| Chloride | 75 | 62 | 55.5 |
| Vitamin A (IU) | 300 | 310 | 300 |
| Vitamin D (IU) | 60 | 62 | 60 |
| Vitamin E (IU) | 3.0 | 3.1 | 1.4 |
| Vitamin K ($\mu$g) | 8 | 8.6 | 8 |
| Thiamin $B_1$ ($\mu$g) | 100 | 78 | 100 |
| Riboflavin $B_2$ ($\mu$g) | 150 | 156 | 150 |
| Vitamin $B_6$ ($\mu$g) | 60 | 62.5 | 62.5 |
| Vitamin $B_{12}$ ($\mu$g) | 0.25 | 0.23 | 0.2 |
| Niacin ($\mu$g) | 1050 | 1250 | 750 |
| Folic acid ($\mu$g) | 15 | 15.6 | 7.5 |
| Pantothenic acid ($\mu$g) | 450 | 470 | 315 |
| Vitamin C (mg) | 9 | 8.1 | 8.5 |

| Component | Isomil*§ | Prosobee† | Nursoy‡ |
|---|---|---|---|
| Protein (g) | 2.66 (soy protein isolate) | 3 (soy protein isolate) | 3.1 (soy protein isolate) |
| Fat (g) | 5.46 (soy and coconut oils) | 5.3 (coconut and soy oils) | 5.3 (oleo, coconut, oleic and soy oils) |
| Carbohydrate (g) | 10.1 (corn syrup, sucrose)§ | 10 (corn syrup solids) | 10.2 (sucrose) |
| Calcium (mg) | 105 | 94 | 90 |
| Phosphorus (mg) | 75 | 74 | 63 |
| Magnesium (mg) | 7.5 | 10.9 | 10 |
| Iron (mg) | 1.8 | 1.88 | 1.7 |
| Zinc (mg) | 0.75 | 0.78 | 0.8 |
| Manganese ($\mu$g) | 30 | 31 | 30 |
| Copper ($\mu$g) | 75 | 94 | 70 |
| Iodine ($\mu$g) | 15 | 10.2 | 9 |
| Sodium (mg) | 47 | 43 | 30 |
| Potassium (mg) | 140 | 116 | 105 |
| Chloride | 65 | 81 | 56 |
| Vitamin A (IU) | 300 | 310 | 300 |
| Vitamin D (IU) | 60 | 62 | 60 |
| Vitamin E (IU) | 3.0 | 3.1 | 1.4 |
| Vitamin K ($\mu$g) | 15 | 15.6 | 15 |
| Thiamin $B_1$ ($\mu$g) | 60 | 78 | 100 |
| Riboflavin $B_2$ ($\mu$g) | 90 | 94 | 150 |
| Vitamin $B_6$ ($\mu$g) | 60 | 62 | 62.5 |
| Vitamin $B_{12}$ ($\mu$g) | 0.45 | 0.31 | 0.3 |
| Niacin ($\mu$g) | 1350 | 1250 | 750 |
| Folic acid ($\mu$g) | 15 | 15.6 | 7.5 |
| Pantothenic acid ($\mu$g) | 750 | 470 | 450 |
| Vitamin C (mg) | 9 | 8.1 | 8.5 |

*Ross Laboratories.
†Mead Johnson Nutritional Division.
‡Wyeth Laboratories.
§Isomil-SF (sucrose-free) has a similar composition except that glucose polymers are substituted for corn syrup and sucrose.

both protein and energy). It results in growth failure, gradual emaciation, and inanition. Kwashiorkor, derived from the Ga language of Ghana, was used initially to refer to the protein deficiency of weanling infants, i.e., "the disease that the first child gets when the second is on the way."[75] It is characterized by edema, ascites, and growth failure.

Both conditions occur in varying degrees in the groups of pediatric patients discussed later in this section. Mild and moderate forms of both distinct syndromes are subclinical and are characterized only by growth failure and possibly some retardation of mental development. Whether these consequences are permanent is a matter of debate; on balance, it appears that most can be ameliorated with appropriate treatment.

**Cystic Fibrosis and Other Chronic Pulmonary Diseases.** Cystic fibrosis is characterized by progressive deterioration of pulmonary and pancreatic function. The former may increase nutrient requirements somewhat, but probably affects nutrition more by adversely affecting intake; this is particularly true during acute exacerbations and in older children with severe pulmonary disease. Pancreatic insufficiency severely limits the absorption of fat, the chief energy source of most diets. Thus, the cause of malnutrition in infants and children with this disease is both primary (i.e., inadequate nutrient intake) and secondary (i.e., fecal losses of protein, and particularly, fat).

Traditionally, nutritional management of patients with cystic fibrosis has stressed a high-protein low-fat diet. However, with appropriate pancreatic enzyme replacement, most patients can maintain a reasonable nutritional status with a reasonably "normal" diet. Younger patients usually have a good appetite, but older patients with advanced pulmonary disease may have a poor appetite. In many of these individuals, intakes of both protein and energy are far less than recommended amounts.

There is some concern that malnutrition may hasten deterioration of pulmonary function, but there is no definitive proof that this is the case. Nonetheless, it is clear that acute improvement of nutritional status improves pulmonary muscle strength.[76] Thus, attempts either to improve nutritional status or to prevent even minimal deterioration of nutritional status are warranted.

**Congenital Heart Disease.** Chronic protein-energy malnutrition, manifested chiefly by growth failure, also is a common finding in patients with congenital heart disease, particularly with conditions associated with congestive heart failure. Although not studied extensively, the nutrient needs of patients with heart disease do not appear

to be much greater, if at all, than those of similar patients without heart disease. Rather, in most patients, the cause of the accompanying malnutrition can be traced to inadequate intake. In some individuals, this is a result simply of poor appetite; in others, it appears to be due to excessive tiring during feeding. In addition, fluid and sodium intakes frequently are restricted as a part of treatment, and use of diuretics is common. Either, of course, may limit growth even if intake of protein and energy is adequate.

The most common form of nutritional therapy for infants with congenital heart disease is use of a high-nutrient-density formula thereby reducing the volume that must be ingested. Tube feedings via either a nasogastric tube or gastrostomy are frequently necessary, particularly in infants whose disease is sufficiently severe to cause excessive tiring during feeding. In general, if sufficient nutrients are delivered, most such patients will grow at a reasonably "normal" rate.

**Gastrointestinal Disorders.** Malnutrition is endemic among infants and children with a variety of gastrointestinal disorders. The cause is usually loss of nutrients secondary to a specific derangement in gastrointestinal function, either diarrhea or vomiting. However, both diarrhea and vomiting are frequently "treated" by withholding all nutrients except water. This practice contributes to the development of malnutrition. Brief discussions of the nutritional management of these common gastrointestinal disorders follow.

*Diarrhea.* Diarrhea caused by most common organisms is usually self-limiting, rarely persisting for more than 4 to 5 days. During this phase, the major goal of nutritional therapy is to maintain a normal state of hydration. This can be accomplished with use of oral rehydration solutions and/or special formulas (Table 50–9). Hospitalization and intravenous fluid therapy may be necessary, particularly if fever or vomiting accompanies the diarrhea.

What to feed as well as whether to feed the child with acute diarrhea have been subjects of considerable controversy for many years, and both have remained unresolved. In general, stool output is greater in the patient who is fed, but this does not necessarily mean that feeding should be proscribed. In most patients, at least some nutrient intake is possible; however, the nature of this intake must be selected carefully taking into account the probable etiology of the diarrhea. The approach followed by the authors is outlined here; other approaches, of course, may be equally successful.

In general, the etiology of most acute diarrhea is either bacterial or viral. Thus, a stool culture to

**Table 50–9. Composition (Amount/100 kcal) of Special Formulas for Infants with Deranged Intestinal Function**

| Component | RCF* | Pregestamil† | Nutramigen† |
|---|---|---|---|
| Protein (g) | 4.95 (soy protein isolate) | 2.8 (casein hydrolysate) | 3.3 (casein hydrolysate and tryptophan) |
| Fat (g) | 8.91 (soy and coconut oils) | 4 (corn oil, MCT) | 3.3 (corn oil) |
| Carbohydrate (g) | 0 | 13 (corn syrup solids, modified tapioca starch) | 13.5 (sucrose, modified tapioca starch) |
| Calcium (mg) | 173 | 94 | 94 |
| Phosphorus (mg) | 124 | 62 | 70 |
| Magnesium (mg) | 12.4 | 10.9 | 10.9 |
| Iron (mg) | 0.37 | 1.88 | 1.88 |
| Zinc (mg) | 1.2 | 0.62 | 0.62 |
| Manganese (mcg) | 50 | 30 | 31 |
| Copper (mcg) | 124 | 90 | 90 |
| Iodine (mcg) | 25 | 7 | 7 |
| Sodium (mg) | 80 | 47 | 47 |
| Potassium (mg) | 190 | 109 | 102 |
| Chloride (mg) | 145 | 86 | 70 |
| Vitamin A (IU) | 500 | 310 | 250 |
| Vitamin D (IU) | 100 | 62 | 62 |
| Vitamin E (IU) | 5 | 2.3 | 1.6 |
| Vitamin K (mcg) | 25 | 15.6 | 15.6 |
| Thiamin $B_1$ (mg) | 100 | 80 | 80 |
| Riboflavin $B_2$ (mcg) | 150 | 90 | 90 |
| Vitamin $B_6$ (mcg) | 100 | 60 | 60 |
| Vitamin $B_{12}$ (mcg) | 0.75 | 0.31 | 0.31 |
| Niacin (mcg) | 2230 | 1250 | 1250 |
| Folic acid (mcg) | 25 | 15.6 | 15.6 |
| Pantothenic acid (mcg) | 1240 | 470 | 470 |
| Vitamin C (mg) | 13.6 | 8.1 | 8.1 |

*Ross Laboratories
†Mead Johnson Nutritional Division.

detect the presence of bacterial pathogens is indicated. However, in most parts of this country, diarrhea secondary to the presence of common enteropathogenic bacteria (*Salmonella, Shigella,* and enteropathogenic *E. coli*) is rare. The organism responsible for most acute bacterial diarrhea is more likely to be one of the many toxicogenic strains of most gram-negative organisms. Thus, a routine stool culture, unless it suggests a predominant organism, is not usually helpful. On the other hand, since the pathogenesis of toxicogenic bacterial diarrhea (i.e., a secretory diarrhea resulting from stimulation of the adenylate cyclase system, as occurs in cholera)[77] is different from that of viral diarrhea (i.e., an osmotic diarrhea secondary to inhibition of glucose transport as described for rotavirus),[78] testing the stool for pH and the presence of reducing substances can be helpful. In general, a low pH (<6.0) and the presence of reducing substances suggest a viral etiology. The stool must be tested following a period of adequate intake of a reducing sugar (e.g., a 5% glucose solution or a rehydration solution).

If the etiology of the diarrhea appears to be viral, a carbohydrate-free formula (see Table 50–9) is usually tolerated. However, such formulas result in ketosis and sometimes hypoglycemia; thus, some carbohydrate intake is necessary. In the hospitalized child, this can be provided intravenously. Most infants who do not require hospitalization usually tolerate at least some enteral sugar intake. In general, 0.5 g of glucose or sucrose per ounce of formula, provided intake is adequate but not excessive, is well tolerated and is sufficient to prevent ketosis and/or hypoglycemia. If this preparation is tolerated, the amount of carbohydrate can be increased daily or every other day as tolerance for carbohydrate increases. Once full carbohydrate content (i.e., approximately 2 g/ounce) is tolerated, the patient can be switched to a formula containing carbohydrate.

If the diarrhea appears to be of toxicogenic bacterial etiology, feeding usually does not affect the volume of stool output. In many cases, in fact, a glucose-electrolyte solution appears to decrease the volume of stool output. In such patients, therefore, decisions concerning feeding must be based on clinical experience.

The general tendency to avoid feedings containing lactose in all infants with diarrhea, regardless of etiology, is probably unnecessary. If stool pH is normal and reducing substances are not present, lactase deficiency is an unlikely contributor to the diarrhea.

In a small number of patients, the acute episode of diarrhea does not resolve in the usual 4 to 5 days. Nutritional management then becomes a more important consideration. Although most infants can tolerate a 4- to 5-day period with little or no nutritional intake, few can tolerate a period of more than 2 weeks without becoming somewhat malnourished and developing secondary intestinal changes due to both persistent diarrhea and malnutrition. Such infants are more likely to develop secondary deficiencies of mucosal hydrolases (e.g., lactase deficiency and, less commonly, sucrase deficiency). In these infants, management without hospitalization is more difficult. Formula must be chosen on the basis of the suspected etiology of the diarrhea; in addition, the greater likelihood of secondary mucosal hydrolase deficiencies must be taken into account. If small volumes of a particular formula appear to be reasonably well tolerated, it frequently is possible to deliver sufficient amounts to meet nutritional needs by use of a continuous infusion technique. In small infants, this regimen usually requires hospitalization.

*Vomiting.* Most acute episodes of vomiting are of short duration and present few nutritional problems. However, chronic vomiting accompanies a number of conditions. The most common of these conditions intrinsic to the gastrointestinal tract is gastroesophageal reflux, or achalasia of infancy. To some extent, this condition is physiologic in infancy; it assumes pathologic significance only when it results in failure to thrive and/or recurrent pulmonary aspiration.

In the early stages, nutritional management of this condition includes maintaining the patient in an upright position during and immediately following feeding and reassuring the parents that the persistent vomiting is causing no harm so long as the infant is gaining weight normally and is not having respiratory symptoms. If either growth failure or a decrease in weight for height develops despite optimal medical management, remedial nutritional therapy, e.g., feedings delivered continuously into the jejunum to minimize the risk of further reflux, is indicated. In some patients, corrective surgery may be necessary.

*Short Bowel Syndrome.* Functionally, short bowel syndrome can be considered in the same way as chronic diarrhea. In this condition, the alterations of gastrointestinal motility, secretion, digestion, and absorption are secondary to massive small intestinal loss rather than to bacterial and or viral invasion and the secondary effects of both these organisms and malnutrition. In general, the severity of the short bowel syndrome is related inversely to the length of the remaining intestinal segment; however, loss of the ileocecal valve, which acts as a physiologic sphincter to slow transit time and to prevent backwash ileitis, also increases severity.[79] Specific symptoms also result from removal of specific segments of intestine. Because disaccharidase activity is greater in jejunal cells and because cholecystokinin is secreted by jejunal sites, removal of the jejunum results in more severe carbohydrate malabsorption and probably decreased biliary and pancreatic secretion. Ileal loss, on the other hand, is associated with selective impairment of both bile salt uptake and absorption of vitamin $B_{12}$. In general, jejunal loss is better tolerated than ileal loss. The latter has a slower transit time as well as transport sites for bile salts and vitamin $B_{12}$; in addition, the potential of the ileum for adaptation appears to be superior to that of the jejunum.

Nutritional management of the short bowel syndrome includes three phases. During the early phase, which usually is associated with massive fluid and electrolyte losses, effective enteral alimentation is rarely possible. Although some enteral intake usually is tolerated during the intermediate phase, most of the nutrient requirements must be provided parenterally. As the small bowel gradually adapts, enteral intake usually can be advanced, but this stage must proceed slowly. In general, continuous feedings via either an indwelling tube or gastrostomy are better tolerated during this phase than bolus feedings. In addition, elemental formulas generally are better tolerated than nonelemental formulas.

Eventually, maximum adaptation is achieved and more complex proteins and carbohydrates can be introduced. Even during this final phase, however, frequent small feedings may be necessary. During all phases, pharmacologic manipulations may provide symptomatic as well as physiologic improvement, e.g., cholestyramine to chelate bile acids; loperamide and/or paregoric to slow transit time; antibiotics to eradicate significant bacterial overgrowth.

## GENERAL APPROACH TO NUTRITIONAL THERAPY

**Assessment.** Accurate determination of nutritional status obviously is the first step in all types of nutritional therapy. However, assessment of the nutritional status of infants is difficult, primarily because of the lack of a precise definition of malnutrition. To some extent, the magnitude of this problem depends upon the purpose for which nutritional assessment is being used. If the purpose is simple nutritional screening, the definition used may be somewhat arbitrary; on the other hand, if its purpose is to provide a definitive nutritional diagnosis on which a decision regarding nutritional therapy is to be made, the definition must be more precise. In addition, the fact that the earliest changes of malnutrition are subtle adaptations that tend to ameliorate effects of malnutrition makes even moderately advanced protein-energy malnutrition difficult to recognize.

Despite these caveats, some objective evaluation of nutritional status should be applied to every child who is a potential candidate for nutritional therapy. If for no other reason, this evaluation provides a baseline for monitoring the results of therapy. Many anthropometric and biochemical assessment techniques are available; their specific advantages and disadvantages as well as their limitations have been discussed extensively.[80]

Because each stage in the development of overt malnutrition gives rise to distinct abnormalities, certain techniques may be more useful for detecting malnutrition at some times than others. In general, however, there is no ideal single test or combination of tests. Indeed, clinical judgment, based upon knowledge of the disease process and the status of the body's nutritional reserves, appears to be as reliable as any of the commonly used "objective" tests.[81] In the authors' experience, assessment of weight in relation to height (length) is one of the most useful indices of nutritional status. A child who falls below the tenth percentile on this standard curve, regardless of either weight for age or height (length) for age, can be assumed to be malnourished and in need of nutritional intervention.

The situation of the child whose weight is appropriate for height (length) but whose weight and height are low for age (i.e., the stunted child) is more problematical. There is no convincing evidence that such a child is malnourished and in need of aggressive nutritional intervention. On the other hand, attempts to permit the child to achieve his growth potential are warranted. This usually requires both a nutritional history and a more extensive medical evaluation, including evaluation of endocrinologic status.

**Nutritional Management.** In general, the approach advocated for nutritional management of the LBW infant is equally applicable for any malnourished infant or child—indeed, for any infant or child with an underlying condition predisposing to development of malnutrition. Initially, particularly in less severely affected individuals, attempts should be made to increase nutrient intake

by conventional means. If this approach is unsuccessful and/or if conventional foods are not tolerated, use of special formulas delivered by tube, either as a bolus or continuously, is the next step. The choice of both formula and method of delivery must be dictated by the patient's underlying condition. Tube feedings can be given throughout the day or only during part of the day (e.g., at night), with or without regular meals, depending upon the patient's condition and nutritional status. If gastrointestinal tolerance of even elemental formulas is severely limited and/or if the patient's condition (e.g., pulmonary disease) makes use of an indwelling tube inadvisable, parenteral nutrients can be used, either as the sole source of nutrition or as a supplement to tolerated enteral nutrients.

## PARENTERAL NUTRITION

The now widespread use of parenteral nutrition usually is considered to be the major contributing factor to the reduction over the past several years in the mortality of infants born with surgically correctable lesions of the gastrointestinal tract (e.g., omphalocele, gastroschisis, intestinal perforation) and infants with intractable diarrhea. Although the role of parenteral nutrient delivery in decreasing the mortality and morbidity of other groups of pediatric patients (e.g., LBW infants) is less clear, the technique is used in a wide variety of such patients. Moreover, despite the many hazards of the technique, most agree that the obvious anabolism achieved is preferable to continued catabolism of infants in whom delivery of adequate nutrients by other routes is impossible. This is particularly true if careful attention is paid to every aspect of the technique thereby minimizing the hazards and maximizing its benefits.

**Route of Administration.** Parenteral nutrients can be delivered by either central vein or peripheral vein infusion. An energy intake of 100 to 120 kcal/kg/day can be delivered by the central venous route, whereas only 70 to 80 kcal/kg/day can be provided consistently and safely by the peripheral venous route. Acceptable intake of amino acids and other nutrients is possible by either route.

Although there is much discussion concerning the advantages and disadvantages of these two routes of delivery, both are efficacious when used in the appropriate circumstances. In general, the length of time that parenteral nutrients are likely to be required and the nutrient needs of the patient should be the determining factors for choosing one route of administration over the other. If it is likely that parenteral nutrients will be required for more than approximately 10 days, central venous delivery usually is preferable because peripheral infusions rarely can be maintained for much longer than this period. In such patients, therefore, it seems reasonable to provide the greater amounts of nutrients the central route permits from the outset rather than resort to the use of a central catheter, primarily for venous access, late in the course of treatment. This is particularly true for nutritionally depleted patients. On the other hand, if nutritional status is not compromised and it is likely that adequate enteral intake can be achieved relatively quickly, peripheral vein delivery is preferable.

In LBW infants, the infusate frequently is delivered by umbilical vessel catheters. This route of delivery, however, cannot be recommended. The flow characteristics of the umbilical artery do not permit sufficient dilution of the nutrient infusate to circumvent vessel damage. In addition, the incidence of thrombosis with umbilical arterial catheters is high. Further, malposition of either arterial or venous umbilical catheters can result in severe consequences. The incidence of sepsis appears to be greater when nutrients are delivered by umbilical vessels than when they are delivered by either central or peripheral veins.

**The Nutrient Infusate.** The nutrient infusate should include a nitrogen source as well as sufficient energy (glucose and lipid), electrolytes, minerals, and vitamins. Suitable infusates for both central vein and peripheral vein delivery are shown in Table 50–10. Although these are acceptable for most infants and children, modification may be required to reflect the specific needs of individual patients.

Currently, crystalline amino acid mixtures are usually used as the nitrogen source for parenteral nutrition. Several such mixtures are available (Table 50–11), all of which contain most essential amino acids (exceptions are cystine and tyrosine both of which are insoluble in aqueous solution) and varying amounts of nonessential amino acids. An amino acid intake of 2.5 to 3.5 g/kg/day is recommended. Higher intakes, although tolerated by most infants, are more likely to result in elevated plasma amino acid concentrations and azotemia. Some advocate amino acid intakes of less than 2.5 g/kg/day for the LBW infant, particularly during the initial few days of therapy when nonprotein energy intake is low (due to glucose and lipid intolerance). There is no reason to advocate this practice unless concomitant energy intake is less than 25 to 30 kcal/kg/day.

Although glucose is the preferred parenteral energy source, the ability of some infants to metabolize it is limited. Many infants, particularly during the early period of parenteral nutrition, develop hyperglycemia and osmotic diuresis with concomitant loss of electrolytes when the amount of glucose infused exceeds tolerance. Because hyperglycemia has been implicated in the pathogenesis of intraventricular hemorrhage, this complication should be avoided.

Most LBW infants tolerate 5 to 7% solutions of dextrose (3.5 to 5.0 mg/kg/min or 17 to 24 kcal/kg/day), even during the first few days of life; thus, in very small and/or unstable infants, it is wise to begin parenteral nutrition with these lower glucose intakes and to increase the intake as the infant's glucose tolerance improves. In older more stable infants, initial glucose intakes of 13 to 15

**Table 50–10.   Composition of Suitable Parenteral Nutrition Infusate(s)**

| Component | Daily Amount (per kg) |
|---|---|
| Amino acids | 2.5–3.5 g |
| Energy | 60–120 kcal |
| Glucose* | 15–30 g |
| Lipid† | 0.5–3.0 g |
| Electrolytes and Minerals | |
| Sodium (as chloride) | 2–4 meq |
| Potassium (as phosphate and chloride)‡ | 2–4 meq |
| Calcium (as gluconate) | 1–4 meq |
| Magnesium (as sulfate) | 0.25 meq |
| Phosphorus (as potassium phosphate)‡ | 1.36 mmoles |
| Zinc (as sulfate) | 100–300 μg |
| Copper (as sulfate) | 20 μg |
| Vitamins§ | 1–3 ml/day |
| Volume | 120–150 ml |

*For peripheral vein infusion, glucose concentration should not exceed 10 to 12.5%.
†Lipid must be infused separately (see text).
‡Potassium, as phosphate, should be limited to 2 meq/kg/day unless chemical monitoring suggests need for more; additional potassium, if required, should be provided as the chloride salt.
§Use of Pediatric MVI (Armour Pharmaceutical, Kankakee IL) is suggested. The volumes suggested provide the following vitamin intakes: vitamin A, 460–1380 IU; vitamin D, 40–120 IU; thiamin, 0.24–0.72 mg; niacin, 3.4–10.2 mg; riboflavin, 0.28–0.84 mg; vitamin $B_6$, 0.2–0.6 mg; vitamin $B_{12}$, 0.2–0.6 μg; pantothenic acid, 1–3 mg; biotin, 4–12 μg.

**Table 50–11.** Amino Acid Content (mg/2.5 g) of Commercially Available Amino Acid Mixtures

| Amino Acid | Aminosyn* | Aminosyn-PF* | Travasol (B)† | Travasol (C)†§ | FreeAmine III‡ | Trophamine‡ |
|---|---|---|---|---|---|---|
| | (10%) | (7%) | (8.5%) | (10%) | (10%) | (6%) |
| Isoleucine | 180 | 191 | 120 | 150 | 175 | 204 |
| Leucine | 235 | 297 | 155 | 182 | 228 | 350 |
| Lysine | 180 | 170 | 145 | 145 | 182 | 204 |
| Methionine | 100 | 45 | 145 | 100 | 132 | 83 |
| Phenylalanine | 110 | 107 | 155 | 140 | 140 | 121 |
| Threonine | 130 | 129 | 105 | 105 | 100 | 104 |
| Tryptophan | 40 | 45 | 45 | 45 | 38 | 50 |
| Valine | 200 | 161 | 115 | 145 | 165 | 196 |
| Histidine | 75 | 79 | 109 | 120 | 71 | 121 |
| Cystine | 0 | 0 | 0 | 0 | <6 | <8 |
| Tyrosine | 11 | 16 | 10 | 10 | 0 | 58 |
| Taurine | 0 | 18 | 0 | 0 | 0 | 6 |
| Alanine | 320 | 175 | 518 | 518 | 178 | 133 |
| Aspartic acid | 0 | 132 | 0 | 0 | 0 | 79 |
| Glutamic acid | 0 | 206 | 0 | 0 | 0 | 125 |
| Glycine | 320 | 96 | 518 | 258 | 350 | 92 |
| Proline | 215 | 204 | 104 | 170 | 280 | 171 |
| Serine | 105 | 124 | 0 | 125 | 148 | 96 |
| Arginine | 245 | 308 | 258 | 286 | 238 | 304 |

*Abbott Laboratories.
†Travenol Laboratories.
‡Kendall-McGaw Laboratories.
§Available in Canada and some other non-USA countries.

g/kg/day (44 to 51 kcal/kg/day) usually are well tolerated. These intakes can be delivered easily by the peripheral route without exceeding a glucose concentration of 10%. With central venous delivery, much greater intakes (25 to 30 g/kg/day or 85 to 102 kcal/kg/day) are eventually tolerated. Even in the most stable patients, however, these higher intakes should be achieved gradually with daily increments of no more than 3 to 5 g/kg/day. In all patients, close monitoring of glucose tolerance is necessary as glucose intake is being increased. Once achieved, the higher intakes usually are well tolerated unless the infant's condition changes abruptly.

Electrolyte requirements vary from patient to patient; thus, the amounts suggested in Table 50–10 should not be interpreted as absolute requirements. Adjustments, which usually are necessary, should be made on the basis of close monitoring.

The amounts of calcium and phosphorus required for optimal skeletal mineralization, i.e., 120 to 150 mg/kg/day and 60 to 75 mg/kg/day, respectively, in the "normally growing" LBW infant, cannot be incorporated into the parenteral nutrition infusate because of the chemical incompatibility of calcium and phosphate. In general, the amounts suggested in Table 50–10 are compatible and cause no problems over the short term. However, if parenteral nutrition is required for weeks to months, skeletal mineralization is likely to be inadequate; this is particularly true for the LBW infant.

Addition of trace minerals to the infusate is recommended if exclusive parenteral nutrition is likely to exceed 7 to 10 days. Suggested intakes of zinc and copper are given in Table 50–10. It is likely that other trace minerals (e.g., manganese, chromium, selenium) will be needed if parenteral nutrients are required for a prolonged period or if the patient is depleted at the onset of TPN. However, the amounts of these nutrients that should be given are not well established.

Parenteral vitamin requirements also are not known with certainty. The usual RDAs have been used as general guides but these may not apply when administration is by the parenteral route. A multivitamin preparation designed for use in pediatric patients is now available. This preparation permits provision of the RDAs of all vitamins.

**Use of Parenteral Lipid Emulsions.** Infants who receive fat-free parenteral nutrition, particularly LBW infants and nutritionally depleted infants, develop essential fatty acid (EFA) deficiency quickly (within days) when growth or regrowth is initiated.[82] Thus, use of lipid emulsions to prevent this deficiency, which becomes apparent biochemically, i.e., an elevated ratio (>0.2) of eicosatrienoic to arachidonic acid, before clinical signs appear, is desirable. Parenteral lipid emulsions also are a useful source of energy. Emulsions of either soybean oil (Intralipid, Travamulsion, IV Fat Emulsion) or a mixture of safflower and soybean oils (Liposyn II) are available in both 10% and 20% concentrations (see Chap. 54). A dose of only 0.5 g/kg/day of soybean oil is sufficient to prevent EFA deficiency; because the linoleic acid content of the safflower oil emulsion is even greater, a smaller dose may be sufficient. However, the linolenic acid content of the safflower emulsion is somewhat lower.

All infants, including LBW infants, probably can tolerate the small dose of parenteral lipid emulsion necessary to prevent EFA deficiency. However, the ability of an individual infant to tolerate larger doses is variable. In general, the ability to metabolize intravenous fat emulsions is related directly to maturity,[83] but the stressed and/or malnourished patient (i.e., the small for gestational age LBW infant and the nutritionally depleted older child) also has difficulty metabolizing these preparations.[84]

Administration of doses of fat emulsion in excess of the infant's ability to metabolize it results in accumulation of triglyceride in the blood. This, in turn, decreases pulmonary diffusion capacity secondary, presumably, to accumulation of small lipid droplets within the pulmonary capillaries.[85] It also results in the recruitment of the reticuloendothelial system for lipid clearance. Lipid accumulation in these cells, which also has been demonstrated at post-mortem,[86] may explain the impaired host defense mechanisms reported in patients receiving lipid emulsions.[87] Metabolism of the infused lipid results in increased serum concentrations of free fatty acids that compete with bilirubin and other substances for binding to albumin.[88] Thus, administration of large doses of lipid emulsion may be hazardous for infants with pulmonary disease, infection, and/or hyperbilirubinemia.

Considering the difficulties of monitoring serum concentrations of both triglyceride and free fatty acids, it probably is wise to limit the dose of lipid emulsion given to patients who are likely to be intolerant to 0.5 g/kg/day. In most other patients, a dose of 3 g/kg/day or more usually is well tolerated; however, even in these patients, it probably is wise to use a smaller dose initially (1 to 1.5 g/kg/day). In LBW infants, administration of lipid emulsions should be initiated with a relatively low dose and increased gradually to a maximum dose of 2 g/kg/day. In all patients, the emulsion should be infused as slowly as possible, preferably at a considerably slower rate than the recommended rate of 0.15 g/kg/hr. Because even the higher rate usually is exceeded when 20% emulsions are used, these more concentrated emulsions offer minimal, if any, advantages. This is particularly true for the LBW infant.

Filters should not be used for the infusion of fat emulsions. Nor should the emulsions be mixed directly with other components of the infusate.

The size of the lipid particles of the emulsions (0.4 to 0.5 $\mu$) exceeds the pore size (0.22 $\mu$) of an effective filter, whereas mixing the emulsions with the other infusate components may either destroy the emulsion or inhibit detection of chemical incompatibilities within the complicated infusate (e.g., precipitation of calcium phosphate).

**Complications of TPN.** Despite its obvious nutritional efficacy, total parenteral nutrition is associated with a number of complications, both catheter- or infusion-related and metabolic.

At the time of central vein catheter insertion, pneumothorax, hemothorax, injury to an artery, and/or hematoma may occur. Thrombosis, dislodgement, perforation, infusion leaks (pericardial, pleural, mediastinal), and infections have been reported during use of central vein catheters. The most common infusion-related problem is infection. Phlebitis and soft tissue sloughs are the most frequent complications of peripheral vein infusions.

Although all the aforementioned complications can be controlled, it is difficult to prevent them completely. Careful attention to care of the central catheter, including frequent dressing changes, is particularly important for controlling infection. Frequent observation of the infusion site is necessary to prevent infiltration of infusates delivered by peripheral vein as well as to insure proper long-term function of central vein catheters.

Metabolic complications result either from the limited metabolic capacity of the patient for the various components of the nutrient infusate or from the infusate itself. The metabolic complications most commonly observed and their probable cause are listed in Table 50–12. One of the most troublesome of these is the occurrence of abnormal plasma amino acid patterns with use of many of the currently available amino acid mixtures.[89] Cyst(e)ine and tyrosine, both of which are essential amino acids for the newborn and probably essential for all patients receiving parenteral nutrients,[90] are only sparingly soluble; hence, none of the mixtures marketed at present contains appreciable amounts of these amino acids and all result in low plasma cyst(e)ine and tyrosine concentrations. Moreover, many available mixtures have large amounts of only a few nonessential amino acids (e.g., glycine) rather than a mixture of all nonessential amino acids. Thus, extremely high plasma concentrations of the amino acid(s) present in excess are commonly seen. Whether these abnormal plasma amino acid patterns are hazardous is not known. However, considering the well-known relationship between abnormally high plasma amino acid concentrations and mental retardation in infants with errors of metabolism

**Table 50–12.  Metabolic Complications of Total Parenteral Nutrition and Their Probable Etiology**

| Complication | Probable Etiology |
|---|---|
| Disorders related to metabolic capacity of patient: | |
| Hyperglycemia | Excessive intake (either excessive concentration or infusion rate); change in metabolic state (e.g., infection, surgical stress) |
| Hypoglycemia | Sudden cessation of infusion |
| Azotemia | Excessive nitrogen intake |
| Electrolyte disorders | Excessive or inadequate intake |
| Mineral (major and trace) disorders | Excessive or inadequate intake |
| Vitamin disorders | Excessive or inadequate intake |
| Essential fatty acid deficiency | Failure to provide essential fatty acids |
| Hyperlipidemia | Excessive intake, change in metabolic state (e.g., stress, sepsis) |
| Disorders related to infusate components: | |
| Acid-base disorders (hyperchloremic metabolic acidosis) | Use of hydrochloride salts of cationic amino acids |
| Hyperammonemia | Inadequate arginine intake |
| Abnormal plasma aminograms | Amino acid pattern of nitrogen source |
| Hepatic disorders | Unknown; suggested etiologies include prematurity, malnutrition, sepsis, decreased stimulation of bile flow, toxic effects of amino acids, specific amino acid deficiency, excessive amino acid and/or carbohydrate intake, nonspecific response to refeeding |

(e.g., phenylketonuria), normalization of plasma amino acid patterns seems warranted. Some of the newer amino acid mixtures (e.g., TrophAmine) accomplish this to a large extent.[91]

Although some of the metabolic complications are unavoidable, many can be controlled by careful chemical monitoring and appropriate adjustment of the infusate. A suggested monitoring schedule is given in Table 50–13. The monitoring required to ensure safe and efficacious use of lipid emulsions is the most problematical. The most common practice (e.g., inspection of the plasma for turbidity either visually or by nephelometry) does not permit detection of elevated plasma triglyceride and free fatty acid concentrations.[92] For this purpose, actual chemical determinations are required. Because this usually is not practical, a reasonable compromise is to observe the plasma frequently (at least three times a day), either visually or by nephelometry, for evidence of lipid accumulation (primarily triglyceride). This observation is particularly important while the lipid dose is being increased, while the infant is unstable, and when the infant's condition changes. If turbidity is observed, the rate of infusion should be decreased or the infusion stopped completely until the turbidity clears. Usually, infusion can then be resumed at a lower rate. Once the desired dose of intravenous fat is achieved, serum turbid-

ity should be checked once a day (unless the patient becomes unstable). If feasible and practical, actual determinations of serum triglyceride and free fatty acid concentrations are preferable.

**Weaning Infants From Parenteral Nutrition.** In most infants, administration of parenteral nutrients need not interfere with introduction of enteral feedings as soon as they are tolerated. Once enteral feedings are started, the volume can be advanced as tolerated by the infant and the volume of parenteral nutrients decreased. During the period of combined enteral and parenteral nutrition, care should be taken to assure both that nutrient requirements are met as nearly as possible and that tolerance for both fluids and nutrients is not exceeded. This requires careful attention to the total (parenteral *plus* enteral) intake and frequent adjustment downward of the parenteral intake as enteral intake increases.

**Home Parenteral Nutrition.** With increasing frequency, patients who require parenteral nutrients for a long time are being allowed to leave the hospital and receive this therapy at home. Considering the many difficulties of in-hospital parenteral nutrition discussed previously, the potential problems of home total parenteral nutrition seem formidable. Nonetheless, patients who can tolerate some enteral intake and patients who can tolerate only parenteral nutrients have been

**Table 50–13.  Suggested Monitoring Schedule During Total Parenteral Nutrition**

| Variables to be Monitored | Suggested Frequency (per week)* | |
| --- | --- | --- |
| | Initial Period | Later Period |
| Growth Variables | | |
|   Weight | 7 | 7 |
|   Length | 1 | 1 |
|   Head circumference | 1 | 1 |
| Metabolic Variables | | |
|   Plasma sodium, potassium, chloride | 3–4 | 2 |
|   Plasma calcium, magnesium, phosphorus | 2 | 1 |
|   Blood acid-base status | 3–4 | 1 |
|   Blood urea nitrogen | 2 | 1 |
|   Plasma albumin | 1 | 1 |
|   Liver function studies | 1 | 1 |
|   Serum lipids† | | |
|   Hemoglobin | 2 | 2 |
|   Urinary glucose | 2–6/day | 2/day |
| Variables for Detection of Infection: | | |
|   Clinical observations (activity, temperature) | daily | daily |
|   WBC count | as indicated | as indicated |
|   Cultures | as indicated | as indicated |

*Initial period is the time during which the desired energy intake is being achieved or the time(s) of metabolic instability.
†See text.

treated successfully at home for several months to years.[93] In many cases, sufficient nutrients can be administered during only a portion of the day, allowing the older patient to pursue reasonably normal daytime activities and the younger patient (as well as his parents) to sleep with little danger of accidental disconnection of the infusion system. Small portable infusion pumps are available such that the necessary apparatus can be enclosed in vests or backpacks allowing even the patient who requires constant infusion of parenteral nutrients to pursue a reasonably normal life. Obviously, home parenteral nutrition is more likely to be successful for the older child, adolescent, or adult. However, with careful patient selection, infants as young as 1 year of age, perhaps even younger, can be managed successfully at home.

In general, the catheter used for home total parenteral nutrition is the Broviac catheter, which can be used for several months and frequently for years. Standard nutrient infusates are obtained from the hospital pharmacy or from a number of commercial concerns and stored in a small home refrigerator. Catheter care is managed by the patient or by a family member after careful training before discharge.

All the usual metabolic and catheter-related complications of parenteral nutrition can occur at home as well as in the hospital. However, patients who can be managed successfully with home parenteral nutrition usually have reached the point at which requirements are reasonably stable. Thus, less frequent monitoring to detect metabolic problems is required. Nonetheless, successful

home parenteral nutrition, particularly for the young pediatric patient, requires frequent outpatient visits and frequent telephone contact. Some commercial home parenteral nutrition services include frequent home visits by a visiting nurse.

On balance, administration of parenteral nutrients at home has been more successful than initially envisioned. Certainly, this practice improves the quality of life for patients who require long-term parenteral nutrition.

## REFERENCES

1. Ziegler, E.E., O'Donnell, A.M., Nelson, S.E., et al.: Growth *40*:329–340, 1976.
2. Heird, W.C.: Nutritional support of the pediatric patient including the low birth weight infant. *In* Nutritional Support of the Seriously Ill Patient. (Winters, R.W., Greene, H.C., Eds.) New York, Academic Press, 1983, pp. 157–179.
3. Fish, I., Winick, M.: Exp. Neurol. *25*:534–570, 1969.
4. Winick, M., Rosso, P.: Pediatr. Res. *3*:181–184, 1969.
5. Winick, M., Rosso, P., Waterlow, J.: Exp. Neurol. *26*:293–300, 1970.
6. Ross, G., Lipper, E.G., Auld, P.A.M.: Pediatrics *76*:885–891, 1985.
7. American Academy of Pediatrics Committee on Nutrition: Pediatrics *75*:976–986, 1985.
8. Whyte, R.K., Haslam, R., Vlainic, L., et al.: Pediatr. Res. *17*:891–898, 1983.
9. Reichman, B.L., Chessex, P., Putet, G., et al.: Pediatrics *69*:446–451, 1982.
10. Schulze, K.F., Stefanski, M., Masterson, J., et al.: J. Pediatr. In press, 1986.
11. Van Aerde, J., Sauer, P., Heim, T., et al.: Pediatr. Res. *19*:368A, 1985.
12. Brooke, O.G., Alvear, J., Arnold, M.: Pediatr. Res. *13*:215–220, 1969.
13. Fomon, S.J.: Pediatrics *40*:863–870, 1967.

14. Gordon, H.H., Levine, S.Z., McNamara, H.: Am. J. Dis. Child. *73*:442–452, 1947.
15. Kagan, B.M., Stanincova, V., Felix, N.S., et al.: Am. J. Clin. Nutr. *25*:1153–1167, 1972.
16. Davidson, M., Levine, S.Z., Bauer, C.H., et al.: J. Pediatr. *70*:695–713, 1967.
17. Kashyap, S., Forsyth, M., Zucker, C., et al.: J. Pediatr. *108*:955–963, 1986.
18. Snyderman, S.E., Boyer, A., Rothman, E., et al.: Pediatrics *31*:786–801, 1963.
19. Snyderman, S.E.: The protein and amino acid requirements of the premature infant. *In* Metabolic Processes in the Fetus and Newborn Infant. (Jonxis, J.H.P., Visser, H.K.A., Troelstra, J.A., Eds.) Leiden, Steinfert Kruesse, 1971, pp. 128–141.
20. Sturman, J.A., Gaull, G.E., Raiha, N.C.R.: Science *169*:74–76, 1970.
21. Kashyap, S., Okamoto, E., Kanaya, S., et al.: Pediatrics. In press, 1986.
22. Rassin, D.K., Gaull, G.E., Heinonen, K., et al.: Pediatrics *59*:407–422, 1977.
23. Rassin, D.K., Gaull, G.E., Raiha, N.C.R., et al.: J. Pediatr. *90*:356–360, 1977.
24. Holman, R.T., Johnson, S.B., Hateh, T.F.: Am. J. Clin. Nutr. *35*:617–623, 1982.
25. Watkins, J.B., Szczepanik, P., Gaull, G.E., et al.: Gastroenterology *69*:706–713, 1975.
26. Zoppi, G., Andreotti, G., Pajno-Ferrara, F., et al.: Pediatr. Res. *6*:880–886, 1972.
27. Hamosh, M.: *In* Textbook of Gastroenterology and Nutrition in Infancy. (Lebenthal, E., Ed.) New York, Raven Press, 1981, pp. 445–463.
28. Simmonds, W.J.: Lipid Absorption: Biochemical and Clinical Aspects. (Rommel, K., Goebell, H., Bohmer, R., Eds.) Lancaster, MTP Press, 1976, pp. 51–61.
29. Tidwell, H.L., Holt, L.E., Jr., Fararow, H.L., et al.: J. Pediatr. *6*:481–489, 1935.
30. Filer, L.J., Jr., Mattson, F.H., Fomon, S.J.: J. Nutr. *99*:293–298, 1969.
31. Greenberger, N.J., Skillman, T.G.: N. Engl. J. Med. *280*:1045–1058, 1968.
32. Tantibhendyangkul, P., Hashim, S.A.: Pediatrics *55*:359–370, 1975.
33. Roy, C.C., Ste-Marie, M., Chartrand, L., et al.: J. Pediatr. *86*:446–450, 1975.
34. Okamoto, E., Muttart, C.R., Zucker, C.L., et al.: Am. J. Dis. Child. *136*:428–431, 1982.
35. Berenson, G.S., Scrinivasan, S.R., Frank, G.C., et al.: Prog. Clin. Biol. Res. *61*:73–94, 1981.
36. Reiser, R.: Circulation *II*:3, 1971.
37. Jensen, R.G., Hagerty, M.M., McMahon, K.E.: Am. J. Clin. Nutr. *31*:990–1016, 1978.
38. Williams, P.R., Fiser, R.H., Sperling, M.A., et al.: N. Engl. J. Med. *292*:612–614, 1975.
39. Boellner, S.W., Beard, A.G., Panos, T.C.: Pediatrics *36*:542–550, 1965.
40. Wallace, W.M.: Am. J. Clin. Pathol. *23*:1133–1141, 1953.
41. Hammerlund, K., Nilsson, G.E., Oberg, P.A., et al.: Acta Paediatr. Scand. *72*:721–728, 1973.
42. Oh, W., Kareoki, H.: Am. J. Dis. Child. *124*:230–232, 1972.
43. Aperia, A., Broberger, O., Herin, P., et al.: Acta Paediatr. Scand. (Suppl.) *305*:61–65, 1983.
44. Stevenson, J.G.: J. Pediatr. *90*:257–261, 1977.
45. Steichen, J.J., Gratton, T.L., Tsang, R.C.: J. Pediatr. *96*:528–534, 1980.
46. Melborn, D.K., Gross, S.: J. Pediatr. *79*:569–580, 1971.
47. Bullen, J.J., Rogers, H.J., Leigh, L.: Br. Med. J. *1*:69–75, 1972.
48. Lundstrom, U., Siimes, M.D., Dallman, P.R.: J. Pediatr. *91*:878–883, 1977.
49. National Academy of Sciences-National Research Council Food and Nutritional Board Committee on Dietary Allowances: Recommended Dietary Allowances. Washington, D.C., National Academy of Sciences, 1980.
50. American Academy of Pediatrics Committee on Nutrition: Pediatrics *57*:278–289, 1976.
51. Sandstrom, B., Cedeblad, A., Lonnerdal, B.: Am. J. Dis. Child. *137*:726–729, 1983.
52. Martmer, E.E., Corrigan, K.E., Charbeneau, H.P., et al.: Pediatrics *17*:503–509, 1956.
53. Cordano, A.: Pediatrics *54*:524, 1974.
54. Wilson, J.F., Lakey, M.E.: Pediatrics *25*:40–49, 1960.
55. Oski, F.A., Barness, L.A.: J. Pediatr. *70*:211–220, 1967.
56. Williams, M.L., Shoot, R.J., O'Neal, P.L., et al.: N. Engl. J. Med. *292*:887–890, 1975.
57. Mintz-Hittner, H., Godio, L.B., Rudolph, A.J., et al.: N. Engl. J. Med. *305*:1366–1371, 1981.
58. Ehrenkranz, R.A., Ablow, R.C., Warshaw, J.B.: N. Engl. J. Med. 564–569, 1982.
59. Burland, W.L., Simpson, K., Lord, J.: Arch. Dis. Child. *46*:189–194, 1971.
60. Dallman, P.R.: J. Pediatr. 742–752, 1974.
61. Anderson, T.L., Muttart, C.R., Bieber, M.A., et al.: J. Pediatr. *94*:947–951, 1979.
62. Atkinson, S.A., Anderson, G.H., Bryan, M.H.: Am. J. Clin. Nutr. *33*:811–815, 1980.
63. Gross, S.J.: N. Engl. J. Med. *308*:237–241, 1983.
64. Forbes, G.: Nutritional adequacy of human breast milk for premature infants. *In* Textbook of Gastroenterology and Nutrition. (Lebenthal, E., Ed.) New York, Raven Press, pp. 328–329, 1981.
65. Stagno, S., Reynolds, D.W., Pass, R.F., et al.: N. Engl. J. Med. *302*:1073–1076, 1980.
66. Ballard, R.A., Drew, W.L., Hufnagle, K.G., et al.: Am. J. Dis. Child. *133*:482–485, 1979.
67. Ziegler, J.R., Cooper, D.A., Johnson, R.O., et al.: Lancet *1*:896–897, 1985.
68. Holt, L.E., Jr., Snyderman, S.E.: JAMA *175*:100–103, 1961.
69. Fomon, S.J., Thomas, L.N., Filer, L.J., et al.: Acta Paediatr. Scand. *62*:33–45, 1973.
70. Raiha, N.C.R.: Pediatrics *75*:136–141, 1985.
71. Lakdewala, D.R., Widdowson, E.M.: Lancet *1*:167–168, 1977.
72. American Academy of Pediatrics Committee on Nutrition: Pediatrics *65*:657–658, 1980.
73. Minton, S.D., Steichen, J.J., Tsang, R.C.: J. Pediatr. *95*:1037–1042, 1979.
74. Cunningham, A.J.: J. Pediatr. *90*:726–729, 1977.
75. Wiliams, C.D.: Arch. Dis. Child. *8*:423–433, 1933.
76. Mansell, A.L., Andersen, J.C., Muttart, C.R., et al.: J. Pediatr. *109*:700–705, 1984.
77. Sack, R.B.: Bacterial and parasitic agents of acute diarrhea. *In* Acute Diarrhea: Its Nutritional Consequences in Infancy. (Bellanti, J.A., Ed.) New York, Raven Press, 1983, pp. 53–65.
78. Hamilton, J.R.: Viral enteritis: A cause of disordered small intestinal epithelial renewal. *In* Chronic Diarrhea in Children. (Lebenthal, E., Ed.) New York, Raven Press, pp. 269–276, 1984.
79. Wilmore, D.W.: J. Pediatr. *80*:88–95, 1972.

80. Cooper, A., Heird, W.C.: Am. J. Clin. Nutr. *35*:1132–1141, 1982.

81. Baker, J.P., et al.: N. Engl. J. Med. *306*:969–972, 1982.

82. Paulsmud, J.R., Pensler, L., Whitten, C.F., et al.: Am. J. Clin. Nutr. *25*:897–904, 1972.

83. Shennan, A.T., Bryan, M.D., Angel, A.: J. Pediatr. *91*:134–137, 1977.

84. Ricour, C., Hatemi, N., Etienne, J., et al.: Acta Chir. Scand *466*:114–115, 1976.

85. Greene, H.L., Hazlett, D., Demaree, R.: Am. J. Clin. Nutr. *29*:127–135, 1976.

86. Friedman, Z., Marks, M.H., Maisels, J., et al.: Pediatrics *61*:694–698, 1978.

87. Loo, L.S., Tang, J.P., Kohl, S.: J. Infect. Dis. *146*:64–70, 1982.

88. Odell, G.B., Cukier, J.O., Ostrea, E.M., Jr., et al.: J. Lab. Clin. Med. *89*:29–307, 1977.

89. Winters, R.W. Heird, W.C., Dell, R.B., et al.: Plasma amino acids in infants receiving parenteral nutrition. *In* Clinical Nutrition Update: Amino Acids. (Greene, H.L., Holliday, M.A., Munro, H.N., Eds.) Chicago, American Medical Association, 1977, pp. 147–154.

90. Stegink, L.D.: Am. J. Dis. Child. *137*:1008–1016, 1983.

91. Heird, W.C., Dell, R.B., Helms, R.A., et al.: Pediatrics In Press, 1986.

92. Schreiner, R.L., Glick, M.R., Nordschow, C.W., et al.: J. Pediatr. *94*:197–200, 1979.

93. Stroebel, C.T., Byrne, W.J., Fonkalsrud, E.W., et al.: Ann. Surg. *188*:394–403, 1978.

*Chapter* **51**

# DIET, NUTRITION, AND ADOLESCENCE

Elizabeth J. Gong and Felix P. Heald

The nutritional requirements of adolescents are influenced primarily by the normal events of puberty and the simultaneous spurt of growth. Puberty is an intensely anabolic period, with increases in height and weight, alterations in body composition resulting from increased lean body mass and changes in the quantity and distribution of fat, and enlargement of many organ systems. Adolescence is a unique period of development of physiologic, psychosocial, and cognitive levels, all of which impact on the nutritional needs of the adolescent. The teenager is a rapidly changing biologic organism, with very individual growth patterns, biologic makeup, and psychosocial development.

The nutritional management of adolescents must consider the rapid growth, maturation, and psychosocial changes of each individual. Three aspects of growth must be emphasized: the intensity and extent of the pubertal growth spurt; the sexual differences in the timing of growth, as well as the nature of change of body composition; and individual variation in the timing of the pubertal growth spurt.

The velocity of growth exerts a major influence on the nutrient requirements during adolescence. Adolescence is the only time in extrauterine life when growth velocity increases. The average American female experiences her most rapid spurt in linear growth between ages 10 and 13 years;

the average American male's growth spurt occurs about 2 years later, between 12 and 15 years. This is frequently termed the year of maximum growth, which for both height and weight is greatest in girls in the year prior to menarche. The linear spurt during adolescence contributes about 15% to final adult height; its contribution to the adult weight is approximately 50%. Therefore, it is obvious that nutrition plays a significant role in the doubling of body mass during pubescence. Since nutritional requirements are closely related to the rapid increase in body mass, it is of little surprise that peak nutritional requirements appear to occur during the year of maximum growth.

Although both adolescent males and females gain significant weight, there are marked sex differences with respect to the rate, quantity, composition, and distribution of tissues. During adolescence, boys tend to gain more weight at a faster rate, and their skeletal growth continues for a longer period of time than girls'. Girls deposit relatively more total body fat, whereas boys deposit more muscle mass. Patterns of body composition and distribution diverge during adolescence. Boys become leaner and paradoxically increase the number of actual adipose tissue cells while decreasing the percentage contribution of fat to total body mass, whereas girls have a steep rate of increase in actual fat deposition, as well as an increase in the percentage of fat to total body mass

This work is supported in part by Maternal and Child Health Grant MCJ 000980.

**969**

and an increase in lean body mass. As a result of pubertal changes, males have a larger lean body mass, a larger skeleton, and less adipose tissue as total body mass than females. As lean body mass has more active metabolic function than adipose tissue, sex differences in body composition produce sex differences in the nutritional requirements of adolescents.[1,2]

The large individual variance in the time at which the growth spurt begins, as well as the intensity of growth, makes chronologic age a poor index of nutritional requirements. Physiologic growth, or maturational age, is a better indicator for establishing requirements or evaluating intakes. Figure 51–1 illustrates three normal males and three normal females in prepubertal, midpubertal, and postpubertal stages of development.[3] Although each group is at the same chronologic age, each individual is at different

physiologic age; each adolescent has a different rate of growth and different body composition, both important determinants of nutrient needs. Standards for assessing physiologic age have been developed. Tanner's Sexual Maturity Ratings are widely used clinically and are helpful in describing the stage of development of individual adolescents.[4]

## NUTRITIONAL REQUIREMENTS

There are few actual data from adolescents on which to base the recommendations for their nutrient needs. Most recommendations are based on estimates of intakes associated with good health and growth, extrapolations from animal research, or interpolation from studies on children and adults. The most recent recommended dietary allowances (RDA) of the Food and Nutrition Board of the National Research Council for adolescents

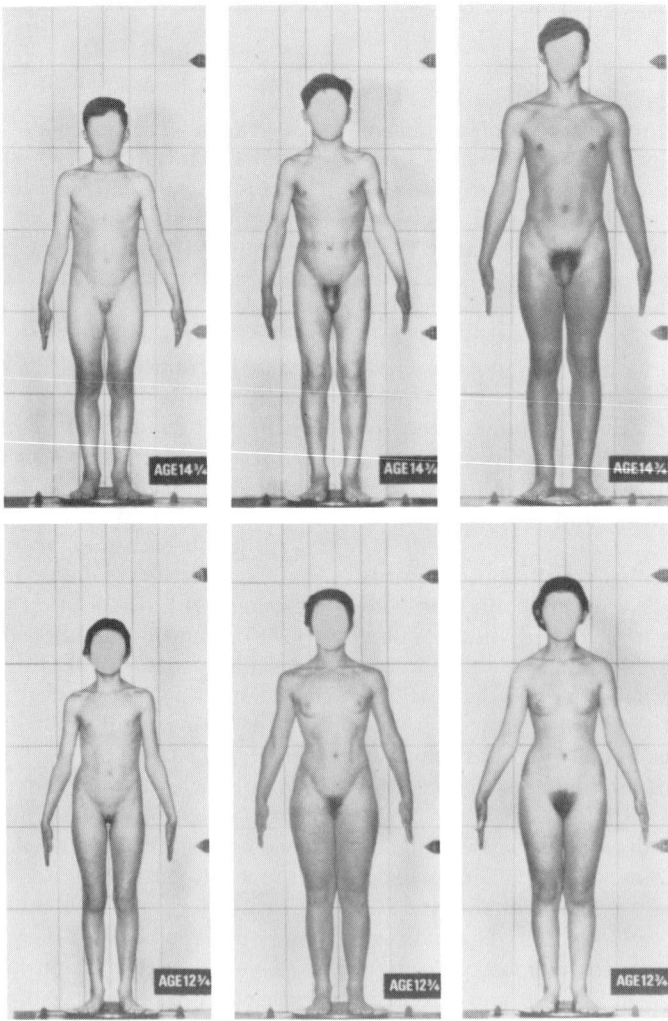

**Fig. 51–1.** Differing degrees of adolescence at the same chronologic age. *Top,* 3 boys all aged 14.75 years. *Bottom,* 3 girls all aged 12.75 years. (From Tanner, J.M.,[3] with permission of W.B. Saunders.)

are given in terms of age (4-year intervals), weight, and sex.[5]

## Energy

The caloric requirements for the growing adolescent have not been studied enough to give an accurate expression of the energy needs of individual teenagers. Some of the best data come from a study done by Wait, Blair, and Roberts.[6] Energy intake data from bomb calorimetry determinations support the thesis that the relationship of total calories to height or calories per unit of height per age were the preferred indices for determining caloric needs. From these observations, as well as supporting findings of Widdowson,[7] it appears that increments in height during adolescence may best represent the anabolic effect of this growth period.

The practical application of determining the individual requirements using the kcal/cm has been described. The RDAs calculated on kcal/cm of height for males and females are shown in Table 51–1.

In a group of normally growing teenagers followed longitudinally, Beal noted that when actual intake was compared to the RDAs, there were some teens whose energy intake fell outside the range of the RDAs.[8] Thus even when using the parameter for calculating calories best supported by data, kcal/cm height, there is considerable margin of error. Nevertheless, kcal/cm height may represent the best way of calculating individual energy requirements of adolescents at the present time.

A review of studies of energy intake of children and adolescents in the United States shows that girls appear to consume their peak caloric intake, about 2,550 kcal, at the time of menarche (around 12 years). This peak demand is followed by a slow decline. In boys, the caloric intake appears to parallel the adolescent growth spurt, increasing until age 16 years to approximately 3,400 kcal and then decreasing by 500 kcal by age 19 years.[9]

The most accepted way of assessing adequacy of energy intake is to evaluate growth and body composition. As previously discussed, the normal variability of pubertal growth patterns makes ideal weight during puberty an untenable concept. A common practice is to plot height and weight on the National Center for Health Statistics (NCHS) growth chart with the percentiles for each age group.[10] This plot tells us the relative position of that teenager to the NCHS sample.[11] The growth data gathered in the NCHS survey published in 1973 form the basis for the growth charts currently used in the United States.[11] (cf Appendix Table A–9e and d.) If multiple measurements over time are available, any significant changes in rates of linear growth or body mass can be detected by percentile shifts. However, the teenager in the 90th percentile for height may or may not be appropriately in the 90th percentile for weight. For example, a male at the 90th percentile weight for height with a triceps skinfold in the lower percentiles would be muscular. Another teenager in the 90th percentile weight for height with a triceps skinfold in the 75th percentile would be classified as obese (cf survey data summarized in Appendix Tables A–6, A–7, and A–11 to A–14).

The National Center for Health survey data have been analyzed in such a sophisticated way that accurate assessment of growth and simple measures of body composition are available to measure the impact of energy excess or scarcity on the growing teenager. We must be aware, however, that the effects of marginal energy deficits have a subtle effect on growth. One of the few studies available to us in the United States describing the long-term effect of chronic mild malnutrition on growth is that of Dreizen, et al.[12] The net effect over time was to diminish the rate of growth during late childhood and adolescence and delay puberty by 2 years, but ultimately this group of malnourished youth in southeastern United States reached similar heights and weights as those of a comparison group.

Acute energy deprivation is more easily recognized by rapid weight loss and diminished synthesis of carrier proteins, such as albumin, transferrin, retinol-binding protein, and prealbumin.

Keeping in mind the great variation in timing and intensity of growth seen in adolescents, one

**Table 51–1. Recommended Energy Intakes for Adolescents**

| Age (years) | Daily Total (kcal/cm height) | |
|---|---|---|
| | Median* | Range† |
| **Males** | | |
| 11–14 | 17.2 | 14.8[a,b]–20.7 |
| 15–18 | 15.9 | 13.2[b] –21.0 |
| 19–22 | 16.4 | 14.9[c] –17.7 |
| **Females** | | |
| 11–14 | 14.0 | 11.1[a,b]–17.6 |
| 15–18 | 12.9 | 7.9[b] –17.5 |
| 19–22 | 12.9 | 11.0[c] –14.6 |

*median: median energy intake and height (RDA)
†range: 10th and 90th percentiles of energy intake (RDA) and height
[a]Hamill, P.V.V., et al.: Am. J. Clin. Nutr. 32:607–629, 1979.
[b]Height and weight of youths 12–17 years, United States, 1973.
[c]Division of Health Examination on Statistics. Unpublished data from Second National Health and Nutrition Survey, 1976–1980.

must emphasize the large variation in caloric intake in this group. Physical activity also contributes significantly to an individual's total energy requirement, as does previous growth and nutritional status. Therefore, in considering the energy requirements of adolescents, the importance of individual variation from one adolescent to another in making nutritional recommendations must be recognized. Table 51–2 presents energy expenditure, expressed in three different body weights, for different activities.[13] The different activities have highly variable energy costs and can be used to guide dietary advice or weight management. (Appendix Table A–3d compares calculated average energy expenditure and observed intakes in comparison with the WHO Committee for adolescents.)

## Protein

As in energy recommendations, protein needs for an adolescent can be more useful when physiologic age is considered, rather than chronologic age. Using the RDA for protein as it is related to height is probably the most useful method for determining protein needs for adolescents.[5] For adolescent males, the daily protein recommendation is 0.29 and 0.32 g/cm height for 11 to 14 and 15 to 22 years, respectively. For adolescent females, the daily recommendation is 0.29, 0.28, and 0.27 g/cm height for 11 to 14, 15 to 18, and 19 to 22 years, respectively. Besides the physiologic state of the individual, other factors influencing protein metabolism in the body include: dietary intake, amino acid composition of the dietary protein, the adequacy of caloric intake, the nutritional status of the adolescent, and any disease state.

The requirement for proteins is determined by the amount needed for maintenance plus that needed for growth of new tissue, which during adolescence may represent a substantial portion of the total nitrogen needs. Unfortunately, data on either of these determinants of requirements are lacking in adolescents and have been interpolated from results of studies on infants and adults.[5,14]

The RDA for daily protein intake for adolescents ranges from 44 to 56 g.[5] Peak intakes of protein coincide with the peak in energy intake. The proportion of total energy intake represented by protein remains fairly constant, between 12 to 14%, throughout childhood and adolescence.[9]

Studies show that average intakes of protein in adolescents are above the recommended levels.[9,15,16] Although it appears most adolescents in the United States have sufficient intake of protein, some teenagers who restrict food intake because of a desire to lose weight, eating disorders such as anorexia nervosa and bulimia, or because of socioeconomic problems may be at risk of poor protein intake. Without adequate caloric intake, protein will be utilized in gluconeogenesis and be unavailable for tissue synthesis. Heald and Hunt demonstrated that, in the rapidly growing adolescent, protein metabolism is particularly sensitive to caloric restriction.[17]

Anthropometric measurements are generally simple to perform in order to assess protein status. Height, weight, and midarm circumference measurements (used to assess lean body mass) can be used as indicators of growth. Midarm circumference measurements and arm muscle area between the 25th and 75th percentile probably represent good nutritional status.[18]

Biochemical assessments of protein nutriture include creatine/height index and serum concentrations of certain proteins. Creatinine excretion reflects the total lean body mass of an individual.[19] With chronic malnutrition, skeletal muscle mass and creatinine excretion decrease simultaneously.[20] Low serum levels of these proteins—albumin, transferrin, prealbumin, and retinol-bind-

**Table 51–2. Energy Expenditure of Selected Activities\* (Calories Expended/Minute Activity)**

| Activity | | kcal/min/kg | 45 kg | 55 kg | 65 kg |
|---|---|---|---|---|---|
| Basketball | | 0.138 | 6.2 | 7.6 | 9.0 |
| Cycling 5.5 mph | | 0.064 | 2.9 | 3.5 | 4.2 |
| 9.4 mph | | 0.100 | 4.5 | 5.5 | 6.5 |
| Dancing (twist) | | 0.168 | 7.6 | 9.2 | 10.9 |
| Football | | 0.132 | 5.9 | 7.3 | 8.6 |
| Running 11.5 min./mile | | 0.135 | 6.1 | 7.4 | 8.8 |
| 8 min./mile | | 0.208 | 9.4 | 11.4 | 13.6 |
| Sitting quietly | | 0.021 | 0.9 | 1.2 | 1.4 |
| Walking, normal pace | | 0.080 | 3.6 | 4.4 | 5.2 |
| Writing, sitting | | 0.029 | 1.3 | 1.6 | 1.9 |
| Vacuuming | Females | 0.045 | 2.0 | 2.5 | 2.9 |
| | Males | 0.048 | 2.2 | 2.6 | 3.1 |
| Ironing | Females | 0.033 | 1.5 | 1.8 | 2.1 |
| | Males | 0.064 | 2.9 | 3.5 | 4.2 |

\*Adapted from McArdle, W.D. et al.[13]

ing protein—indicate depletion of body protein or decreased availability of amino acids for protein synthesis. Albumin and transferrin (with half-lives of 21 days and 8 days, respectively) are readily accessible measurements.[21,22] Clinically, however, their relative lack of sensitivity and specificity limit their use as the only biochemical measurement in assessment of nutritional status. Determinations of prealbumin and retinol-binding protein are much more sensitive indicators of subclinical malnutritional changes in diet.[22,23,24] Because of their relatively short half-lives (2 to 3 days for prealbumin[25] and 12 hours for retinol-binding protein[23]), these proteins may be the most valuable tools in the early diagnosis of subclinical malnutrition. A detailed evaluation of assessment procedures is given in Chapter 45.

## Minerals

Because of the adolescent growth spurt, the need for three minerals is of particular importance. There is increased need for calcium to sustain increased skeletal mass, iron to aid expansion of red cell and muscle mass, and zinc to generate new skeletal and muscle tissues. In addition to significant increases in need, intake of these nutrients has been shown to be below the recommended levels for adolescents.[15,16,26–28]

For example, the calcium intake of boys is higher than that for girls and is closer to achieving the recommended intakes.[29] Daily iron intakes as reported by the Ten State Nutrition Survey were found to be relatively lower. The majority (80%) of the girls 10 to 16 years of age were below the recommended 18 mg iron/day.[15] There is some evidence of an association between low concentrations of zinc in hair and poor growth. An analysis of food intake suggests poor eating habits.[30] The full extent of zinc deficiency and its adverse effect on puberty needs considerable more inquiry.

**Calcium.** With approximately 99% of the total body calcium in the skeleton,[31] the adolescent growth spurt associated with increased skeletal length and mass obviously has a significant impact on dietary requirements for calcium. Skeletal growth during adolescence accounts for approximately 45% of the adult skeletal mass. Since the absolute amount of calcium in the skeleton of a boy in the 95th percentile for height compared to that for another boy in the 5th percentile for height will differ by 36%, the calcium needs of these two boys will sharply differ because of the difference in skeletal size. The problem is further compounded by the normal differences in pubertal development, making age and sex alone poor predictors of individual calcium needs. Lastly, growth of the skeletal mass and gains in height

and muscle mass continue after adolescence until the third decade of life.[32,33]

Table 51–3 shows the average increments of body calcium for adolescence, as compared to the amount of daily increments of body calcium at the peak of the growth spurt.[34] At the peak of growth, the daily deposition of calcium is approximately double that for the average increment during the adolescent period. The daily peak increment of calcium during the growth spurt is greater, occurs later, and lasts longer in boys than in girls.[31]

The amount of calcium absorbed from different dietary sources varies. During peak periods of growth in adolescence, the average calcium retention is approximately 300 mg/day. The amount of calcium absorbed from different dietary sources varies; since the lower range of absorption is approximately 30%, a minimum of 900 mg calcium/day would be necessary during active skeletal growth.[35]

There is a wide difference in the daily allowances of calcium recommended by the two expert committees. The World Health Organization recommends intakes of 600 to 700 mg/day for 11- to 15-year-old adolescents and 500 to 600 mg/day for 16- to 19-year-old adolescents.[36] In contrast, the National Research Council recommends 1200 mg/day for these age groups.[5] It is apparent from these differences in recommended intakes that the amount of dietary calcium needed to sustain growth, as well as to provide maintenance, requires much more study.

It is difficult to establish requirements for the teenage group because of (1) the ability of many individuals to achieve equilibrium on a wide range of dietary intakes and (2) the large error likely to occur in calculating calcium balance because of errors in measuring intakes and excretions. In addition, because of differences among

**Table 51–3.  Increments in Body Content Due to Growth***

|  |  | Average for Period 10–20 yr (mg) | At Peak of Growth Spurt (mg) |
|---|---|---|---|
| Calcium | M | 210 | 400 |
|  | F | 110 | 240 |
| Iron | M | 0.57 | 1.1 |
|  | F | 0.23 | 0.9 |
| Nitrogen | M | 320 | 610 (3.8 g protein) |
|  | F | 160 | 360 (2.2 g protein) |
| Zinc | M | 0.27 | 0.50 |
|  | F | 0.18 | 0.31 |
| Magnesium | M | 4.4 | 8.4 |
|  | F | 2.3 | 5.0 |

*From Forbes, G.B.,[34] with permission of Raven Press.

individuals in rate of biologic maturation, it is difficult to establish guidelines. Other nutrients, such as protein and phosphorus,[37] affect calcium balance, making it even more difficult to study calcium metabolism.

Surveys in the United States reveal that adolescent girls are less likely to meet the recommended levels of calcium than are teenage boys.[15,16,29]

**Iron.** Iron deficiency is found in all races, both sexes, and in all socioeconomic groups. Teenagers require additional amounts of iron to synthesize substantial amounts of new myoglobin and hemoglobin. As puberty is initiated, boys accumulate more lean body mass than girls. In fact, at the end of puberty boys have twice the lean body mass of girls. Thus Hepner has calculated that for each additional kg of added tissue, males require 42 mg iron/kg body weight compared to 31 mg iron/kg body weight for girls.[38] In addition to the described sex differences, the normal biologic differences in body size make a tremendous difference in iron requirements. For example, a boy in the 97th percentile for body weight would require twice as much iron as a boy in the 3rd percentile.

The dietary intake of iron must be sufficient to account for the losses in feces, urine, skin, and menstruation, as well as provide for expansion of red cell volume and for tissue growth in adolescence. With menarche, the adolescent girl has additional iron loss from menstruation, so that the NRC recommended daily intake for both adolescent boys and girls is 18 mg.[5]

Unfortunately, iron requirements of adolescents have been studied very little. In a comprehensive review of iron requirements, Bowering et al. could find only one report on a controlled study with adolescents.[39] In the iron balance study of 6 adolescent girls, Schlaphoff and Johnson found that 0.62 to 1.82 mg/day (mean 1.0 mg/day) was retained, which included iron required to replace menstrual losses.[40] Assuming a rate of 10% absorption, they recommended a daily intake of 12 to 13 mg iron. Similar balance data are not available for boys. Finally, the amount of iron available in the American diet is estimated at 6 mg/1,000 calories. Therefore, teenage girls whose caloric intake varies between 2,000 and 2,400 calories find it difficult to ingest 18 mg of iron from dietary sources alone.

In the Ten State Nutrition Survey between 5% and 10% of the teenagers had hemoglobin or hematocrit levels below normal.[15] The results of other studies vary,[41,42] generally reporting more iron deficiency than iron deficiency anemia of the adolescents.

Results of several large surveys—the Ten State Nutrition Survey,[43] the Health and Nutrition Examination Survey I (HANES I),[42] and the Health and Nutrition Examination Survey II (HANES II)[44]—have shown a racial difference in hemoglobin level in adolescents. Blacks have approximately 1 g less hemoglobin than whites that is apparently unrelated to socioeconomic level, education, diet,[43] or obesity.[45] These differences have led many to recommend race-specific standards in screening for anemia.[45–48] Although use of different standards for hemoglobin concentration has been proposed, the biochemical basis for the racial difference of hemoglobin is unknown. The factors affecting hemoglobin differences, including genetic, socioeconomic, and dietary, are complex. At the present time, no data indicate that iron needs of black and white adolescents are different.

It is clear that the standards for normal values used in any study will determine the amount of iron deficiency in any population. As a matter of fact, hematocrit or hemoglobin alone are relatively insensitive indicators of iron deficiency and iron deficiency anemia. A detectable hemoglobin response to a therapeutic trial with iron is a reliable diagnostic test for iron deficiency.[49] If the hemoglobin does not rise after a three-week trial with iron, then iron deficiency is not present. The diagnosis of iron deficiency can be made if serum ferritin is below 12 $\mu$g/L and the serum transferrin is below 16% saturation. Iron deficiency anemia is strongly suspected when microcytosis (MCV in Coulter Model S $<70$ $\mu m^3$) and hypochromia (MCHC $<30\%$) are present.[50] Until more sophisticated studies are available, the true incidence of iron deficiency anemia in adolescents awaits clarification.

**Zinc.** Zinc affects protein synthesis and is essential for the growth process. Zinc is particularly important in adolescence because of the rapid rate of growth and sexual maturation. From Table 51–3, it is apparent that with the adolescent growth spurt there is greatly increased retention of zinc in both males and females, as compared to the average for the adolescent period. This striking increase in zinc retention during adolescence is related to the increase of lean body mass observed during this period.[51]

Zinc deficiency has been associated with growth retardation and hypogonadism in adolescents.[52,53] Zinc supplementation resulted in accelerated growth and sexual maturation.[52,54] Poor dietary zinc sources and inhibition of zinc absorption from phytates in high cereal diets contributed to the evolution of zinc deficiency and were major factors responsible for growth retardation and delayed sexual maturation.[53]

Evidence that adolescents undergoing rapid growth may be highly susceptible to inadequate dietary zinc is provided by Butrimovitz and Purdy.[55] These investigators found low plasma zinc concentrations during infancy and puberty, both periods of rapid growth. For adolescent girls and boys, plasma zinc levels were lowest at the ages when puberty was expected to occur.

Mild zinc deficiency has been reported in the United States. Hambidge, et al. studied zinc status in apparently healthy children in Denver and found an association of low growth percentiles, diminished taste acuity, and low hair zinc levels.[56] Apparently, marginal zinc status may be a health problem in American children.

Adolescents undergoing rapid growth are at high risk of inadequate zinc. Pregnant teenagers may be particularly susceptible to zinc deficiency, since there is rapid cell division and growth of the developing fetus, as well as continued growth of the biologically immature teenager.

## Vitamins

Data on vitamin requirements for adolescents are even more limited than those for mineral requirements. The vitamin requirements for youth are interpolated from data on infant and adult allowances. Very little data are derived directly from studies on adolescents.

**Vitamin A.** In a comprehensive review of vitamin A requirements, Rodriquez and Irwin found no reports of controlled experiments on the retinol requirements of adolescents.[57] Vitamin A intake is frequently cited in nutritional surveys as being considerably below the requirements for adolescents.[15,16,58,59] Low plasma levels of vitamin A have been found in 10 to 40% of the teenagers studied in the Ten State Nutrition Survey.[15] The clinical implications of these findings in adolescence are unknown.

**Vitamin D.** Vitamin D is involved in maintaining homeostasis of calcium and phosphorus in the mineralization of bone. There are no data on the vitamin D needs of adolescents. The exact requirement for this vitamin has not yet been established. Because of rapid rate of skeletal growth, the recommended daily allowance for vitamin D remains at 10 $\mu$g until adulthood when skeletal growth ceases and daily allowances are decreased to 7.5 and 5.0 $\mu$g for the age range of 19 to 22 and 23 to 50 years, respectively.[5]

**Vitamin C.** With the present knowledge of ascorbic acid metabolism, it is difficult to define precisely an adolescent's requirement for the vitamin. However, surveys have shown that fruits, vegetables, and salads are frequently on teenagers' lists of low preference foods.[60,61] With reports that vitamin C intakes in adolescents are often below the recommended levels, the unknown demands of growth, and changes in ascorbic acid metabolism due to smoking[62] and oral contraceptive use,[63] some teengers may have problems in vitamin C adequacy.

**Folacin.** Because of its role in DNA synthesis, this vitamin is important during periods of increased cell replication and growth. Folacin status may be at risk in some adolescents, particularly low income populations[64] and pregnant teenagers.[65] Low plasma concentrations of folacin, as well as low folacin intakes, have been found in these populations.

**Vitamin B$_{12}$.** Vitamin B$_{12}$ is required for the rapid growth of cells. Adolescents would appear to have increased need for vitamin B$_{12}$, particularly during the growth spurt. This vitamin is also involved in fat, carbohydrate, and protein metabolism. Because of the paucity of data for adolescents, the recommended intakes of vitamin B$_{12}$ for this group are similar to those of adults.

**Vitamin B$_6$.** This vitamin is involved in a large number of enzyme systems associated with nitrogen metabolism. The recommendations for adolescents are interpolated from data gathered from infants and adults. Vitamin B$_6$ intake has been found to be low,[59,66] with as many as 50% of the female adolescents selecting diets with less than two thirds of the RDA for vitamin B$_6$. In addition, approximately 30% of the adolescents had improvement of the vitamin-dependent enzyme erythrocyte alanine aminotranferase activity upon addition of vitamin B$_6$ to the diet.[66]

**Niacin, Riboflavin, and Thiamin.** These three vitamins are involved in energy metabolism; therefore, recommendations of intake of these B vitamins have been based on caloric intake. Data on these vitamins are extremely limited, and there is still considerable debate about the amount required for normal adolescent growth. Riboflavin status of adolescents has been studied by Lopez et al.[67] and Sauberlich et al.,[68] using erythrocyte glutathione reductase activity. Because this enzyme's activity is altered by dietary riboflavin, inadequate intake of riboflavin was found in 11%[67] and 27%[68] of the adolescents studied. Girls appear to be at higher risk of inadequate riboflavin intake than boys.[68] Black girls are particularly at high risk, with almost 40% of the black girls in Sauberlich's study having biochemical evidence of inadequate intake of riboflavin.[68] Unfortunately, the low biochemical values reported for some vitamins during adolescence do not have clinical correlates at this time. Only further research will reveal the importance of marginal vitamin deficiencies as currently defined.

## SPECIAL NUTRITIONAL PROBLEMS

### Obesity

Regulation of the amount of body fat in children and teenagers has been the matter of much discussion and misunderstanding. It is only in the last decade that a clearer picture of regulation of fat storage in the juvenile period has emerged. In the past, obesity was thought to be a pure eating disorder and tinkering with the diet was a cure-all. As any health care worker knows, obesity is particularly difficult to treat successfully over a long period.

A better understanding of the anatomy now clearly reveals the complexities of regulating adipose tissue organs. There are an estimated 5 billion adipocytes at birth. Primarily as a result of hyperplasia, but also influenced by some hypertrophy, the adipose tissue enlarges during growth until there are an estimated 30 billion adipocytes in young adult life. The crucial issue in excessive adipose tissue development in teenagers is the nature versus nurture issue. Is excessive eating for whatever reason the cause of adiposity? Or is the response of the child or teenager to food genetically modified to result in adiposity? Our best information comes from studies of monozygotic and dizygotic twins. The Swedish study of skinfold thickness in mono- and dizygotic twins estimated heritability of 0.88.[69] There was little evidence of prenatal growth or environment playing a significant role in the development of skinfold thickness. Parental influence can be dramatic, as reported by Garn and Clark.[70] At age 17 years children of obese parents are three times fatter than the teenagers of lean parents.

That nutrition can affect adipocyte development has been demonstrated. When overfed rats increase their lipid storage to a critical size, new adipocytes are recruited to be filled with triglyceride.[71] There is evidence of a humoral factor being released from mature cells that may aid in recruiting preadipocytes to be filled with lipid.[72] Until the anatomic, physiologic, and genetic aspects of adiposity are better understood, the treatment of juvenile obesity will be difficult.

The long-term results of treatment of juvenile obesity utilizing dietary counseling, anorectic drugs, and semistarvation have been dismal. The recent work of Brownell and his co-workers gives some promise for the future.[73] Utilizing the schools and involving the mothers, a well-structured behavioral modification program led to significant and long-term weight loss. The implications for this program are important and suggest, if their work can be replicated, a method for incorporating a practical public health program for adiposity control in the community.

### Atherosclerosis

Much evidence suggests that atherosclerosis begins during the juvenile period. This was first described in 1911, but only recently has much interest been focused on the disease process in children and adolescents. Serum cholesterol and serum lipoproteins have received the most attention, and a number of field studies have made available population studies on serum cholesterol. The most representative is the National Health Survey published in 1976. During adolescence, serum cholesterol in the male falls from 180.2 mg/100 ml to 166.7 mg/100 ml for 16-year-old white males. For females there is little change during adolescence, being 177.7 mg/100 ml for 16-year-old white females. Black males had 7.8 mg/100 ml more cholesterol than their white counterparts, and black females had 2.7 mg/100 ml more serum cholesterol than white females.[74]

More important, and less understood, is the nature of arterial disease during adolescence. There appears to be considerable support for the hypothesis that arterial disease we call atherosclerosis represents a reaction to injury.

The major risk factors associated with atherosclerotic disease appear to be elevated cholesterol, cigarette smoking, and hypertension. The exact mechanism of arterial injury is not known, but clearly there is a significant association with elevated cholesterol levels. Of recent interest are the oxidation products of cholesterol, which may be found in cholesterol-containing compounds exposed to heat or light. Some of the oxidation products, such as 25 hydroxycholesterol, are highly cytotoxic to the endothelium of arteries.[75] Their role in human disease has yet to be determined.

Few studies have been reported on dietary cholesterol restriction and the effect on blood cholesterol levels in adolescents. McGandy et al. studied a free-living population of adolescent boys in a Boston boarding school.[76] Lowering dietary cholesterol and saturated fat for two 3-month periods significantly lowered blood cholesterols in both periods. However, controlled studies are needed to understand better the quantitative aspects of dietary cholesterol and other lipids on blood levels in the adolescent population.

The recent NIH Consensus Development Conference (1984) Statement, "Lowering Blood Cholesterol to Prevent Heart Disease,"[77] recommends a moderate fat and moderate cholesterol diet (approximately 30% of the caloric intake from fats, total saturated fat intake of 10% or less of total calories, and no more than 250 to 300 mg cholesterol/day) for healthy adolescents. In growing adolescents, intakes should provide adequate nutrients, qualitatively and quantitatively, to ensure growth and development. This amount will be particularly important for adolescents going through their growth spurt. Adolescents with a family history of hypercholesterolemia or premature coronary heart disease should be considered high risk and should have their blood cholesterol levels evaluated. Presently, mass screening of cholesterol levels is not recommended because of unavailability of laboratories, costs, and management problems of large numbers of patients.[77]

In summary, there is a gathering consensus that every effort should be made to reduce saturated fat and high concentrations of cholesterol in our diet. Whether this is the correct course remains to be seen.

## Hypertension

Identifying, evaluating, and treating adolescents with high blood pressure is important. Not only is the prevalence of hypertension due to secondary causes higher in adolescents than adults,[78] hypertension is a major risk factor in the development of cardiovascular disease.[79] Ellison and his colleagues reported that there is increasing evidence that childhood and adolescence may be appropriate times to consider measures for the prevention of hypertension later in life.[80]

The Task Force on Blood Pressure Control in Children recommends that a history of three elevated blood pressures (above the 95th percentile for age and sex, obtained on separate occasions) should be considered abnormal.[81] For practical use, a blood pressure of 140 mm Hg systolic and 90 mm Hg diastolic during adolescence is often used as the cut-off point for hypertension.[78,82] Loggie and Rauh have summarized data from seven reports of studies of adolescent hypertension.[82] The prevalence of hypertension in this group ranges from 0.4 to 8.9% (systolic) and 1.4 to 12.2% (diastolic). These data should be interpreted with caution, taking into consideration differences in definition of hypertension, as well as geographic and methodologic differences used by the investigators.

The Joint National Committee on Detection, Evaluation, and Treatment of High Blood Pressure recently recommended that nonpharmacologic therapy "should be pursued aggressively" in the treatment of mild hypertension and should be an adjunct in the pharmacologic therapy of more severe hypertensive patients.[79] The nonpharmacologic approaches related to nutrition include weight reduction in overweight persons, moderate dietary restriction of sodium, and reduction of dietary saturated fat.

Nutritional counseling should be an integral part of the treatment plan of the adolescent hypertensive. Dietary intervention at this time can help establish good eating habits early. Weight reduction in overweight individuals with hypertension often results in substantial decrease in blood pressure,[79] even if desirable body weight is not achieved. Moderate sodium restriction (to approximately 2 g sodium or 5 g salt) is also recommended. Although restriction of dietary sodium will not help reduce blood pressure in all hypertensive persons, there is no health hazard from moderate sodium restriction. Recent studies report that reduction in saturated fat intake is associated with lower blood pressures. Although this association needs to be studied further, any reductions in the blood levels of triglycerides and cholesterol may help reduce the risk of cardiovascular disease.

Calcium has been studied in its role in the development and management of hypertension.[83] Data suggest that some hypertensive individuals may have differences in calcium metabolism compared to normotensive individuals.[84,85] In addition, low intake of calcium has been associated with increased blood pressure.[86,87] Calcium supplementation has decreased blood pressure in a group of healthy young individuals.[88] These data suggest calcium may be a factor in the development and management of hypertension in the adolescent. Additional research is needed, however, to explore the relationship of calcium and hypertension.

Changes in diet can be effective with many patients; however, not everyone will respond. Adolescents with severe hypertension should use dietary methods as an adjunct to pharmacologic therapy. Patients with moderate or mild hypertension may benefit in controlling blood pressure by an aggressive diet program. Because many foods popular with teenagers are high in sodium content and saturated fat,[89–91] educating the patient to select more foods with low to moderate salt content should be a part of the counseling. Present eating habits, considerations of adolescent development, and the role food can play in issues of independence and peer acceptance should be a part of setting realistic goals for the hypertensive adolescent.

## Pregnancy

The nutritional care of the pregnant adolescent must consider the health of both mother and infant. Knowledge of the role of nutrients is vital, as well as consideration of the principles of adolescent growth and development. Physiologically, the adolescent is at risk if she has not completed her growth.[92,118] Individual variability is great, but the majority of growth occurs prior to menarche in most females. Linear growth in the adolescent female typically is not completed until four years after the onset of menarche. Although the rate of growth after menarche has decelerated considerably, growth allowances should still be considered.

Gynecologic age (the difference between chronologic age and age at menarche) can give some indication as to the importance of the mother's growth in estimating nutrient needs. Because of the increased nutritional needs of her own growth, as well as fetal growth, nutrient requirements of the pregnant teenager are higher than those of adult women. The younger the adolescent and the lower her gynecologic age, the higher her nutrient requirements.[6]

The few studies that have focused on the energy needs of pregnant teenagers generally report that the teenagers frequently do not achieve the National Research Council's recommendation for caloric intake.[5] Naeye has raised the hypothesis that optimal weight gains for fetal survival may be higher in young teenagers, since both mother and infant compete for nutrients.[93] Recent reports of Frisancho et al.[94] and Meserole et al.[95] also suggest that optimal pregnancy weight gains for adolescents, particularly biologically immature ones, are greater than the adult recommendations of 25 to 30 pounds. Inadequate weight gain during pregnancy has been associated with low birth weight infants.[96]

Preliminary data from our research using anthropometric measurements as predictors of low birth weight outcome in pregnant teenagers, show that mothers of low birth weight infants tended to demonstrate a prenatal depletion of fat reserves (estimated from tricep skinfold measurements and calculating arm fat area) as compared to the mothers of normal birth weight infants, who accumulated fat.[97] In addition, prenatal protein stores of mothers of low birth weight infants changed little, whereas mothers delivering normal birth weight infants gained protein stores (estimated from midarm circumference measurements and arm muscle area calculations). Estimates of energy requirements indicate that sedentary adolescents needed at least 2,400 to 2,600 kcal/day. Physically active or rapidly growing adolescents needed additional energy, perhaps 50 kcal/kg of pregnant body weight per day.[98]

The issue of protein requirement for the pregnant adolescent is a complex one. King et al., using careful nitrogen balance studies on pregnant teenagers, presented the best experimental data on which to base protein recommendations.[99] Their data suggested that nitrogen retention was much greater than previously reported. In addition, maternal lean tissue of these adolescents increased during pregnancy, particularly during the last half of pregnancy.

Therefore, on the basis of more recent data it appears that pregnant teenagers, particularly those who are still in their own growth phase, do have increased needs for nutrients during pregnancy. The pregnant adolescent needs an additional 300 calories and 30 more grams of protein each day.[5] These additional calories and protein can be supplied with the addition of foods, such as those shown in Table 51–4.[100]

## Vegetarian Diets

During a time of increased independence and decision-making, as well as greater influences exerted by peers and role models, adolescents may use food as part of the process of individuation. Vegetarianism may be adopted for individuation, as well as for religious, moral, ecologic, economic, and health reasons. Because adolescence is a period of rapid physical growth and development, the nutritional needs are high. Vegetarian teenagers may be at risk of nutritional deficiencies, particularly at the time of the growth spurt.

Growing adolescents who are vegetarians may have problems in meeting their energy requirements because of the high-bulk content of vegetarian food patterns. In addition, many vegetarian diets are low in fat content.[101,102] Without sufficient energy intake, protein is used as an energy source and thus is unavailable for tissue synthesis and growth. It is necessary to assess the protein

**Table 51–4.  Foods to Increase Calories and Protein for the Pregnant Adolescent***

| Food | Calories |
|---|---|
| Peanut butter (2 tbsp) sandwich | 320 |
| Cereal (1 c), 8 oz lowfat milk, banana | 325 |
| 2 slices of 12″ cheese pizza | 290 |
| 8 oz flavored yogurt and 4 crackers | 320 |
| Hamburger (plain) | 305 |

| Food | Protein (gm) |
|---|---|
| Peanut butter (2 tbsp.) sandwich, 12 oz milk | 29 |
| 3 oz serving meat or poultry, 8 oz milk | 31 |
| Cheeseburger | 33 |
| 1 c spaghetti (meat sauce), 2 tbsp Parmesan cheese, 8 oz milk. | 32 |

*Nutritive Value of Foods, USDA.[100]

quality, protein quantity, and the energy intake of the individual. Other nutrients of concern in the teenage vegetarian include calcium, iron, zinc, vitamins D and $B_{12}$.[101-103]

Lacto-ovovegetarians (those consuming plant foods, dairy products, and eggs and excluding meat, poultry, and fish) who carefully plan and select their foods may have nutritionally adequate diets. However, strict vegetarians or vegans (those excluding all foods of animal origin) are unlikely to meet their nutritional needs. Energy requirements are not likely to be met during the growth spurt; vitamins $B_{12}$, $B_6$, and intake of riboflavin may be low, as well as calcium, iron, and zinc. The nutritional status of calcium, iron, and zinc may also be affected by high fiber intake, which can decrease absorption of these minerals.[103,104,106] Conscious effort and careful planning is necessary to insure adequacy of these nutrients. Supplements may be necessary to meet the recommended allowances. This is particularly true for vitamin $B_{12}$, which is found only in animal products. The vegetarian should carefully plan a diet from a variety of foods. Protein complementation (the combining of different plant foods so that low essential amino acids of one protein source are complemented by the essential amino acids of another protein source, resulting in a complete protein) can ensure that the qualitative aspects of protein adequacy are met. An evaluation of the quantitative aspects of protein adequacy of the vegetarian is also necessary. The RDA for total protein intake during adolescence ranges from 44 to 56 g/day,[5] providing energy requirements are met.

A food guide for the lacto-ovovegetarian and vegan adolescent can be found in Marino and King[107] and Smith.[108] The University of California offers practical guidelines, including food guides, menu plans, and recipes for older adolescents wanting more information on vegetarian diets.[109]

## Oral Contraceptive Use

With the widespread use of synthetic hormones as oral contraceptive agents, attention to the potential effects of these compounds on the adolescent's nutritional status is an important consideration in the health of the individual. The use of oral contraceptive agents has been shown to affect a number of metabolic processes, including alterations in lipid, carbohydrate, protein, vitamin, and mineral metabolism.[110-115] Ingestion of oral contraceptive agents may increase plasma levels of triglycerides and cholesterol, blood glucose and insulin, and plasma levels of vitamin A, iron, and copper. Oral contraceptive usage has been shown to decrease plasma albumin levels, as well as the circulating levels or function of riboflavin, pyri-

doxine, folacin, vitamin $B_{12}$, ascorbic acid, and zinc.[110-115] The metabolic changes appear to reverse when these agents are discontinued.

Some women using combination oral contraceptive agents have been shown to have higher total serum triglycerides and cholesterol levels. Elevations of blood glucose and plasma insulin have been reported, as well as a tendency toward impaired glucose tolerance. The major problems appear to be associated with high-dose formulations.[115] Low-dose formulations of oral contraceptives may minimize the adverse effects of these alterations. Women with a family history of hypercholesterolemia and diabetes will have increased risk of these elevations in lipid and carbohydrate metabolism.[115]

The effects of oral contraceptives on vitamin nutrition include decreased plasma or serum levels of riboflavin, pyridoxine ($B_6$), folacin, vitamin $B_{12}$, and ascorbic acid. However, clinical signs of vitamin deficiencies have rarely been detected. A very small group of women may experience biochemical signs of vitamin $B_6$[116] or folacin[117] deficiency. These women may respond to vitamin $B_6$ or folacin supplementation; however, widespread supplementation does not appear necessary. Hormonal contraceptive therapy appears to affect the metabolism of many nutrients, but the clinical significance of these changes remains inconclusive and controversial. Presently, there is not enough evidence to suggest all oral contraceptive users need supplementation to prevent nutritional deficiencies. Consumption of an adequate diet appears to be sufficient to meet the dietary needs of oral contraceptive users. Nutritional counseling to encourage good dietary habits is recommended to all oral contraceptive users. Nutritional supplements are certainly indicated for those with deficiency symptoms not correctable through dietary adjustments.

## REFERENCES

1. Marshall, W.A., Tanner, J.M.: Arch. Dis. Child. *44*:291–304, 1969.
2. Marshall, W.A., Tanner, J.M.: Arch. Dis. Child. *45*:13–24, 1970.
3. Tanner, J.M.: Growth and endocrinology of the adolescent. *In* Endocrine and Genetic Diseases of Children and Adolescents. 2nd ed. (Gardner, L.I., Ed.) Philadelphia, W.B. Saunders, 1975.
4. Tanner, J.M.: Growth of Adolescence. 2nd ed. Oxford, Blackwell Scientific Publications, 1962.
5. Food and Nutrition Board, National Research Council, Recommended Dietary Allowances, 9th rev. ed. Washington, DC, National Academy of Sciences, 1980.
6. Wait, B., Blair, R., Roberts, L.: Am. J. Clin. Nutr. *22*:1383–1396, 1969.
7. Widdowson, E.M.: Medical Research Council Spe-

cial Report Series No. 257. London, His Majesty Stationery Office, 1947.

8. Beal, V.A.: Nutritional intake. *In* Human Growth and Development. (McCammon, R.W., Ed.) Springfield, IL, Charles C Thomas, 1970.

9. Heald, F.P., Remmell, P.S., Mayer, J.: Caloric, protein and fat intake in children and adolescents. *In* Adolescent Nutrition and Growth. (Heald, F.P., Ed.) New York, Appleton-Century-Crofts, 1969.

10. National Center for Health Statistics: NCHS Growth Charts, 1976. Monthly Vital Statistics Report *25*(3) Suppl. (HRA) 76–1120, Rockville, MD, 1976.

11. National Center for Health Statistics: Height and weight of youths, United States. *In* Vital and Health Statistics Series 11, No. 132, Health Services and Mental Health Administration. Washington, D.C., Government Printing Office, 1973.

12. Dreizen, S., Spirakis, C.N., Stove, R.E.: J. Pediatr. *70*:256–263, 1967.

13. McArdle, W.D., Katch, F.I., Katch, V.L.: Exercise Physiology. Energy, Nutrition, and Human Performance. Philadelphia, Lea & Febiger, 1981.

14. Johnson, J.A.: Ann. N.Y. Acad. Sci. *69*:881–901, 1958.

15. Center for Disease Control: Ten State Nutrition Survey in the United States, 1968–1970. Atlanta, Health Services and Mental Health Administration, 1972.

16. National Center for Health Statistics: Caloric and Selected Nutrient Values for Persons 1–74 Years of Age. First Health and Examination Survey, 1971–1974. DHEW Publication (PHS) 79–1657, Hyattsville, MD, 1979.

17. Heald, F.P., Hunt, S.M.: J. Pediatr. *66*:1035–1041, 1965.

18. Frisancho, A.R.: Am. J. Clin. Nutr. *27*:1052–1058, 1974.

19. Forbes, G.B., Bruining, G.J.: Am. J. Clin. Nutr. *29*:1359–1366, 1976.

20. Jensen, T.G., Englert, D., Dudrick, S.J.: Nutritional Assessment. A Manual for Practitioners. Norwalk, CT, Appleton-Century-Crofts, 1983.

*21. Rothschild, M.A., Oratz, M., Schreiber, S.: N. Engl. J. Med. *286*:748–757, 816–621, 1972.

22. Ingenbleck, Y., Van Den Schrieck, H., DeNayer, P.H., et al.: Clin. Chim. Acta *63*:61–67, 1975.

23. Igenbleck, Y., Devisscher, M., DeNayer, P.H., et al.: Lancet *2*:106–108, 1972.

24. Shetty, P.S., Watrasiewicz, K.E., Jung, R.T., et al.: Lancet *2*:230–232, 1979.

25. Oppenheimer, J.H., Surks, M.I., Bernstein, G., et al.: Science *149*:748–750, 1965.

26. Hodges, R.E., Krehl, W.A.: Am. J. Clin. Nutr. *17*:200–210, 1965.

27. Hampton, M.C., Huenemann, R.L., Shapiro, L.R., et al.: J. Am. Diet. Assoc. *50*:385–396, 1967.

28. Wharton, M.A.: J. Am. Diet. Assoc. *42*:306–310, 1963.

*29. Irwin, M.I., Kienholz, E.W.: J. Nutr. *103*:1019–1095, 1973.

30. Henkin, R.I.: Trace Elements in Nutrition. New York, Marcel Dekker, 1971.

31. Committee on Nutrition: American Academy of Pediatrics. Pediatrics *62*:826–834, 1978.

32. Garn, S.M., Wagner, B.: The adolescent growth of the skeletal mass and its implications to mineral requirements. *In* Adolescent Nutrition and

Growth. (Heald, F.P., Ed.) New York, Appleton-Century-Crofts, 1969.

33. Roche, A.F., Roberts, J., Hamill, P.V.: Vital Health Stat. *11*(167):1–98, 1978.

34. Forbes, G.B.: Nutritional requirements in adolescence. *In* Textbook of Pediatric Nutrition. (Suskind, R.M., Ed.) New York, Raven Press, 1981.

*35. Greenwood, C.T., Richardson, D.P.: World Rev. Nutr. Diet. *33*:1–41, 1979.

36. World Health Organization: Handbook on Human Nutritional Requirements. Monograph Series No. 61. Geneva, WHO, 1974.

37. Linkswiler, H.M.: Calcium. *In* Present Knowledge of Nutrition. (Hegsted, D.M., Ed.) New York, Nutrition Foundation, 1976.

38. Hepner, R.E.: Nutrient Requirements in Adolescence, Cambridge, MIT Press, 1976.

*39. Bowering, J., Sanchez, A.M., Irwin, M.I.: J. Nutr. *106*:985–1074, 1976.

40. Schlaphoff, D., Johnson, F.A.: J. Nutr. *39*:67–82, 1949.

41. National Academy of Sciences: Food and Nutrition Board: Iron Nutriture in Adolescence. U.S. Department of Health, Education, and Welfare, DHEW Publication No. (HSA) 77–5100, 1976.

42. Johnson, C.L., Abraham, S.: Hemoglobin and Selected Iron-Related Findings of Persons 1–74 Years of Age: United States, 1971–74. U.S. Department of Health, Education, and Welfare, No. 46, January, 1979.

43. Garn, S.M., Smith, N.J., Clark, D.C.: J. Natl. Med. Assoc. *67*:91–96, 1975.

44. Yip, R., Johnson, C., Dallman, P.R.: Am. J. Clin. Nutr. *39*:427–436, 1984.

45. Dallman, P.R., Barr, G.D., Allen, C.M., et al.: Am. J. Clin. Nutr. *31*:377–380, 1978.

46. Garn, S.M., Smith, N.J., Clark, D.C.: Am. J. Clin. Nutr. *28*:563–568, 1975.

47. Owen, G.M., Yanochik-Owen, A.: Am. J. Public Health *67*:865–866, 1977.

48. Daniel, W.A., Jr.: Nutritional requirements of adolescent. *In* Adolescent Nutrition. (Winick, M., Ed.) New York, John Wiley & Sons, 1982.

49. Vartiainen, E., Widholm, O., Tenhunen, T.: Acta Obstet. Gynecol. Scand. (Suppl.) *46*:49–54, 1967.

50. Lanzkowsky, P.: Iron deficiency in adolescents. *In* Adolescent Nutrition. (Winick, M., Ed.) New York, John Wiley & Sons, 1982.

*51. Sandstead, H.H.: Am. J. Clin. Nutr. *26*:1251–1260, 1973.

52. Prasad, A.S., Schulert, A.R., Miale, A., Jr., et al.: J. Lab. Clin. Med. *61*:537–549, 1963.

53. Sanstead, H.H., Prasad, A.S., Schulert, A.R., et al.: Am. J. Clin. Nutr. *20*:422–442, 1967.

54. Prasad, A.S., Halsted, J.A., Nadimi, M.: Am. J. Med. *31*:532–545, 1961.

55. Butrimovitz, G.P., Purdy, C.: Am. J. Clin. Nutr. *31*:1409–1412, 1978.

56. Hambidge, K.M., Hambidge, C., Jacobs, M., et al.: Pediatr. Res. *6*:868–876, 1972.

*57. Rodriquez, M.S., Irwin, M.I.: J. Nutr. *102*:909–968, 1972.

58. Canada National Survey: Nutrition. A National Priority, Ottawa Dept. of National Health and Welfare, 1973.

59. Schor, B.C., Sanjur, D., Erikson, E.C.: J. Am. Diet. Assoc. *61*:415–420, 1972.

60. Huenemann, R.L., Shapiro, L., Hampton, M.C., et al.: J. Am. Diet. Assoc. *53*:17–24, 1968.

61. Nelson, M.: Dietary practices of adolescents. *In* Adolescent Nutrition. (Winick, M., Ed.) New York, John Wiley & Sons, 1982.

62. Pelletier, O.: Am. J. Clin. Nutr. *23*:520–524, 1970.

63. Rivers, J.M.: Am. J. Clin. Nutr. *28*:550–554, 1975.

64. Daniel, W.A., Gaines, E.G., Bennett, D.L.: Am. J. Clin. Nutr. *28*:363–370, 1975.

65. Vande Mark, M.S., Wright, A.C.: J. Am. Diet. Assoc. *61*:511–516, 1972.

66. Kirksey, A., Keaton, K., Abernathy, R.P., et al.: Am. J. Clin. Nut. *31*:946–954, 1978.

67. Lopez, R., Schwartz, J.V., Cooperman, J.M.: Am. J. Clin. Nutr. *33*:1283–1286, 1980.

68. Sauberlich, H.E., Judd, J.H., Jr., Nichoalds, G.E., et al.: Am. J. Clin. Nutr. *25*:756–762, 1972.

69. Borjeson, M.: Acta Paediatr. Scand. *65*:279–287, 1976.

70. Garn, S.M., Clark, D.C.: Pediatrics *57*:443–455, 1976.

71. Faust, I.M., Johnson, P.R., Stern, J.S., et al.: Am. J. Physiol. *235*:279–286, 1978.

72. Novakofski, J.E., Hausman, G., Martin, R.J.: Adiposity and Obesity Symposium (Abstract 9), Toronto, 1982.

73. Brownell, K.D., Kelman, J.H., Stunkard, A.J.: Pediatrics *71*:515–523, 1983.

74. U.S. Dept. of Health, Education and Welfare: Total Serum Cholesterol Values of Youths 12–17 Years. National Health Survey. DHEW Pub. No. (HRA) 76–1638, Series 11, No. 156, 1976.

*75. Taylor, C.B., Peng, S.K., Werthessen, N.T., et al.: Am. J. Clin. Nutr. *32*:40–57, 1979.

76. McGandy, R.B. Hall, B., Ford, C., et al.: Am. J. Clin. Nutr. *25*:61–66, 1972.

77. National Institutes of Health Concensus Development Conference Statement: Lowering Blood Cholesterol to Prevent Heart Disease. Vol. 5, No. 7. (December 10–12, 1984 Conference).

78. Neinstein, L.S.: Adolescent Health Care. A Practical Guide. Baltimore, Urban & Schwarzenberg, 1984.

79. The 1984 Report of the Joint National Committee on Detection, Evaluation and Treatment of High Blood Pressure. Arch. Intern. Med. *144*: 1045–1057, 1984.

80. Ellison, R.C., Newburger, J.W., Gross, D.M.: J. Am. Diet. Assoc. *80*:21–25, 1982.

81. Recommendatios of the Task force on Blood Pressure Control in Children. Pediatrics (Suppl.) *5*:797–820, 1977.

*82. Loggie, J.M.H., Rauh, L.W.: Med. Clin. North Am. *59*:1371–1383, 1975.

*83. Parrott-Garcia, M., McCarron, D.A.: Nutr. Rev. *42*:205–213, 1984.

84. Strazzullo, P., Nunziata, V., Cirillo, M., et al.: Clin. Sci. *65*:137–141, 1983.

85. McCarron, D.A.: N. Engl. J. Med. *307*:226–228, 1982.

86. Ackley, S., Barrett-Connor, E., Suarez, L.: Am. J. Clin. Nutr. *38*:457–461, 1983.

87. McCarron, D.A., Morris, C.D., Henry, H.J., et al.: Science *224*:1392–1398, 1984.

88. Belizan, J.M., Villar, J., Pineda, O., et al.: JAMA *249*:1161–1165, 1983.

89. Morgan, K.J., Bundy, K.T.: Cereal Foods World *26*:69–72, 1981.

90. Consumer Reports, pp. 508–513, September 1979.

91. Jacobson, M., Liebman, B.F., Moyer, G.: Salt. The Brand Name Guide to Sodium Content. New York, Workman Publishing, 1983.

92. Jacobson, M.S., Heald, F.P.: Nutritional risks of adolescent pregnancy and their management. *In* Premature Adolescent Pregnancy and Parenthood. (McAnarney, E.R., Ed.) New York, Grune and Stratton, 1983.

93. Naeye, R.L.: Pediatrics *67*:146–150, 1981.

94. Frisancho, A.R., Matos, J., Flegel, P.: Am. J. Clin. Nutr. *38*:739–746, 1983.

95. Meserole, L.P., Worthington-Roberts, B.S., Rees, J.M., et al.: J. Adolesc. Health Care *5*:21–27, 1984.

96. Eastman, N.J., Jackson, E.: Obstet. Gynecol. *23*:1003–1025, 1968.

97. Maso, M.J., Jacobson, M.S., Heald, F.P.: J. Adolesc. Health Care *3*:139, 1982.

98. Blackburn, M.L., Calloway, D.H.: J. Am. Diet. Assoc. *65*:24–30, 1974.

99. King, J.C., Calloway, D.H., Margen, S.: J. Nutr. *103*:772–775, 1973.

100. Nutritive Value of Foods, USDA Home and Garden Bulletin, No. 72, Washington, DC, 1981.

101. Raper, N.R., Hill, M.M.: Nutr. Rev. *32* (suppl.)29–33, 1974.

*102. MacLean, W.C., Graham, G.G.: Am. J. Dis. Child. *134*:513–519, 1980.

103. Carruth, B.R.: J. Current Adolesc. Med. *2*:44–47, 1980.

*104. Allen, L.H.: Am. J. Clin. Nutr. *35*:783–808, 1982.

105. Monsen, E.R., Hallberg, L., Layrisse, M., et al.: Am. J. Clin. Nutr. *31*:134–141, 1978.

*106. Solomons, N.W.: J. Am. Diet. Assoc. *80*:115–121, 1982.

*107. Marino, D.D., King, J.C.: Pediatr. Clin. North Am. *27*:125–139, 1980.

108. Smith, E.B.: J. Nutr. Educ. *7*:109–111, 1975.

109. University of California: The Creative Eater's Handbook. Better Nutrition Through Vegetarian Eating. Berkeley, University Student Health Service, 1982.

*110. King, J.C.: J. Am. Pharm. Assoc. *17*:181–182, 1977.

111. Massey, L.K., Davison, M.A.: Am. Fam. Physician *19*:119–123, 1979.

*112. Worthington, B.S.: Nurs. Clin. North Am. *14*:269–283, 1979.

113. Webb, J.L.: J. Reprod. Med. *25*:150–156, 1980.

114. Tyrer, L.B.: J. Reprod. Med. *29* (suppl.):547–550, 1984.

115. Brooks, P.G.: J. Reprod. Med. *29* (suppl.):539–546, 1984.

116. Adams, P.W., Rose, D.P., Folkard, J., et al.: Lancet *1*:897–904, 1973.

117. Lindenbaum, J., Whitehead, N., Reyner, F.: Am. J. Clin. Nutr. *28*:346–353, 1975.

118. Rees, J.M., Worthington-Roberts, B.: Adolescence, nutrition, and pregnancy interrelationships. *In* Nutrition in Adolescence. (Mahan, L.K., and Rees, J.M., Eds.) St. Louis, Times Mirror/Mosby College Publishing, 1984.

*Review article.

*Chapter* **52**

# NUTRITION AND AGING

## Ronni Chernoff and David A. Lipschitz

Since the mid-1970s, there has been a growing interest in the problems and needs of the population of the United States over the age of 65. Although human life span, approximately 100 years, has not changed, human life expectancy has increased from approximately 47 years in 1900 to 73 years in 1980.[1] At present, 25 million Americans are 65 years of age or older. It is projected that by the year 2030, approximately 57 million Americans will be over the age of 65 and approximately 25 million will be over the age of 75[2] (Fig. 52–1). Elderly persons are the greatest consumers of health care resources, at present accounting for 40% of acute care hospital days, 25% of all prescription drugs, and more than half of the federal health budget.[3] As the population base shifts its mean age upward, it becomes increasingly important for health care practitioners, managers, and planners to understand the normal process of aging, the impact of disease on aging, the role that nutrition has in aging, and the impact of age on nutrition requirements and nutritional status.[4]

Elderly individuals are more different from each other than any other group of people. The rate and manner in which people age are related to myriad factors that are difficult to distinguish, or possibly identify. The effects of environmental, genetic, social, economic, and health factors combine to impact on the process of aging so that we see frail, debilitated 60-year-olds, and 80-year-olds who are running marathons. The role that nutrition plays in growth and development, health maintenance, disease prevention, and normal aging cannot be underestimated, but it is also difficult to quantify.

Aging is an inevitable process that begins with the cessation of growth and development.[5] Changes that occur in body composition, organ function, physical performance, and cognition that are age-related will occur in all humans. However, there is great variability from person to person, and even within individuals in whom various organs may age at different rates (Fig. 52–2). Theories on aging usually focus on the role of deoxyribonucleic acid (DNA), the genetic material of all cells. Many theories of aging suggest a central genetic mechanism. Random errors occurring during DNA replication may cause the gradual accumulation of abnormalities that lead to the eventual death of cells.[6] Another theory suggests that DNA transcription errors produce imperfect RNA molecules that then code for aberrant proteins; these proteins eventually accumulate and compromise organ function.[7] Loss of functional cells eventually leads to organ or organism death.

Yet another theory suggests that changes in structural protein, primarily collagen, may impair organ function.[8] Studies in mice have suggested the free radical theory of aging, in which appropriate dietary antioxidants increase life span and decrease the incidence of spontaneous carcinoma.[9] These studies have not yet been confirmed in other species.

All these theories focus on the concept of cell loss and a concomitant reduction in cellular metabolism with increasing age. An overall reduction in total body protein is demonstrated by fewer actively functioning tissue structures, i.e., renal

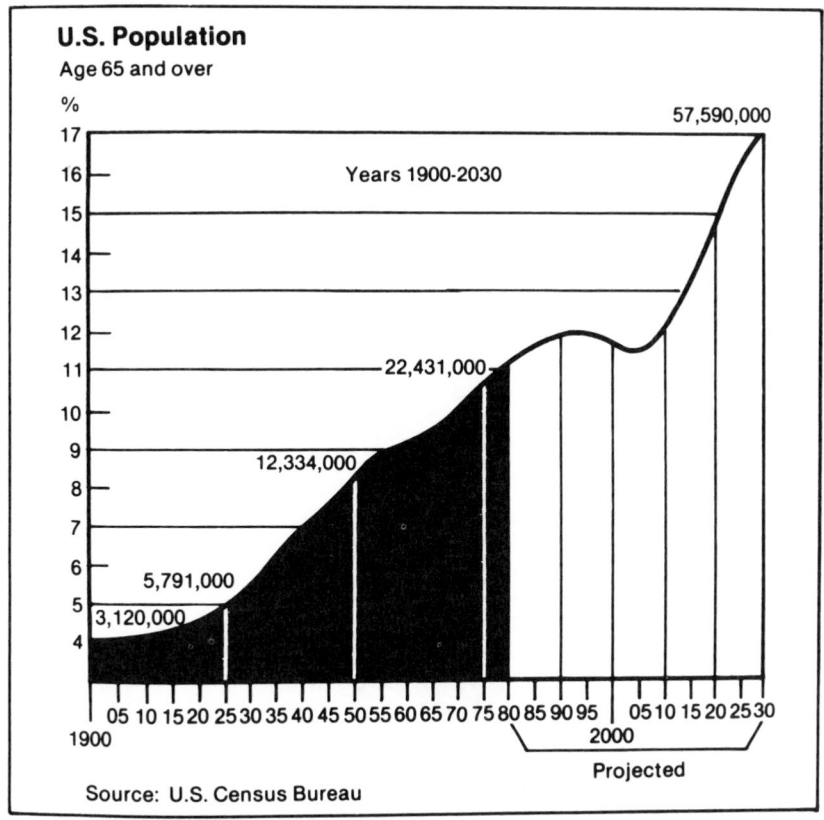

**U.S. Population**

Age 65 and over

Years 1900-2030

57,590,000

22,431,000

12,334,000

5,791,000

3,120,000

05 10 15 20 25 30 35 40 45 50 55 60 65 70 75 80 85 90 95  05 10 15 20 25 30

1900                                                        2000

Projected

Source: U.S. Census Bureau

**Fig. 52–1.** Percentage of U.S. population aged 65 and over from 1900 to 2030. (From Haynes, S.G., Feinleib, M. (eds.): Second Conference on the Epidemiology of Aging. Washington, D.C., USDHHS, NIH Publication No. 80–969, 1980.)

function is decreased owing to a loss of functioning nephrons.[10] These changes contribute to the decrease in adaptability to sudden changes in the environment and to longer response time to return to basal levels after a stressful event. The aforementioned theories all address the process of normal uncomplicated aging. Most of the studies conducted on aging populations are cross-sectional. This methodology does not contribute to a comprehensive understanding of the process of aging, but rather provides a compilation of the possible outcomes of aging at one point in time.

Longitudinal studies, where multiple measurements can be taken on each subject over time, contribute more significantly to identifying the progressive effects of chronic disease and other life events. They are, however, difficult studies to conduct. The Baltimore Longitudinal Study of Aging,[11] begun in 1958, has attempted to record the effects of aging on humans. The interim report, published in 1984, indicates that aging is a highly individual process. The effects of age are highly specific not only between individuals but for different organ systems within the same subject.

Those physiologic functions that require complex interactions among organ systems appear to be more affected by age than are more simple functions.[11] Because of the variability in aging demonstrated in this longitudinal study, it has become apparent that chronologic age is not a reliable predictor of functional age.

The impact of physiologic aging on metabolic and nutrition-related functions is also variable. Some of the changes associated with aging affect nutritional requirements, yet some functions remain stable throughout life unless affected by disease processes.

## ENERGY REQUIREMENTS

For decades, it has been recognized that total energy production falls progressively with age.[12,13] This reduction in energy metabolism is related to the production of protein tissue, which in turn appears to be related to a reduction in muscle mass rather than to a decrease in the metabolic activity of specific tissues.[14] Because basal energy requirements represent the needs of the metabolic processes involved in maintaining cell

## AGE DECREMENTS IN PHYSIOLOGIC PERFORMANCE

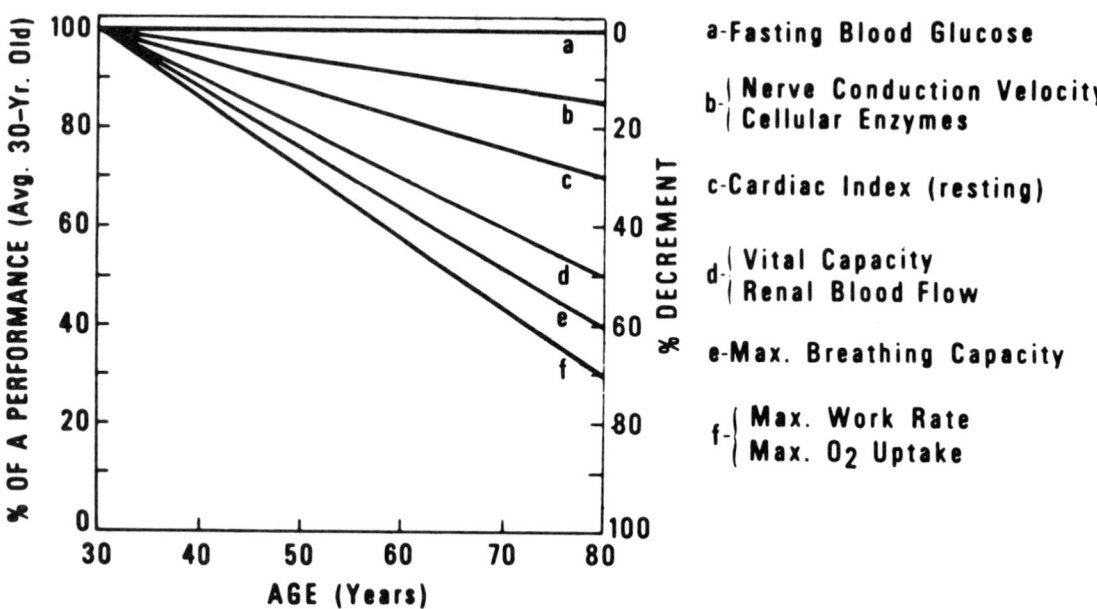

**Fig. 52–2.** Age decrements in physiologic performances. Average values for 30-year-old subjects taken as 100%. Decrements shown are schematic. a, Fasting blood glucose; b, nerve conduction velocity and some cellular enzyme activities; c, resting cardiac index; d, vital capacity and renal blood flow; e, maximum breathing capacity; f, maximum work rate and maximum $O_2$ uptake. (From Shock, N.W., et al.[11])

function, a decreased metabolically active cell mass will result in decreased energy needs. In studies performed to measure a "slowing" of the metabolic rate by examining potential age-related changes in the thyroid gland, the primary regulator of metabolic rate, the results showed no age-related decline in the plasma protein-bound iodine.[15]

Along with the reductions in energy requirements due to a decreased muscle mass, energy needs may be altered as a result of changes in activity level or energy expenditure. In a study conducted as part of the Baltimore Longitudinal Study of Aging, McGandy and others demonstrated an age-related reduction in physical activity in men.[16] These data were confirmed in studies performed on women.[17] Changes in level of activity may be related to decreases in strength associated with the decrement in muscle mass; the onset of joint and bone disease; loss of postural stability resulting in falls;[18] the progression of chronic disease such as angina pectoris, emphysema, coronary artery disease, or chronic obstructive pulmonary disease; intermittent claudication related to smoking or diabetes; neurologic disorders such as parkinsonism; or precipitous occur-

rences such as stroke, myocardial infarction, or fracture. Interestingly, the reduction in energy requirements is affected more by a decrease in activity-related energy expenditure than by the fall in basal metabolic rate.[16] (Fig. 52–3).

Caloric intake, measured in both cross-sectional[19] and longitudinal[20] studies, shows an inverse relationship with age; caloric intake decreases as age increases (see Fig. 52–3). Fewer calories ingested offset lower requirements for maintenance and prevent the onset of obesity. Until recently it has been generally accepted that obesity contributes to early mortality and, therefore, leanness contributes to longer life expectancy. These conclusions were drawn from life insurance actuarial data and were supported by animal studies. In rats, caloric restriction after weaning increased life span[21–26] whether caloric restriction was effected on day 21 of life or instituted at a later time after a period of ad libitum feeding. Similar studies in humans would be difficult to perform. Epidemiologic research underscores the difficulty that would ensue separating real effects of caloric restriction from effects of environmental, social, psychological, and genetic factors.

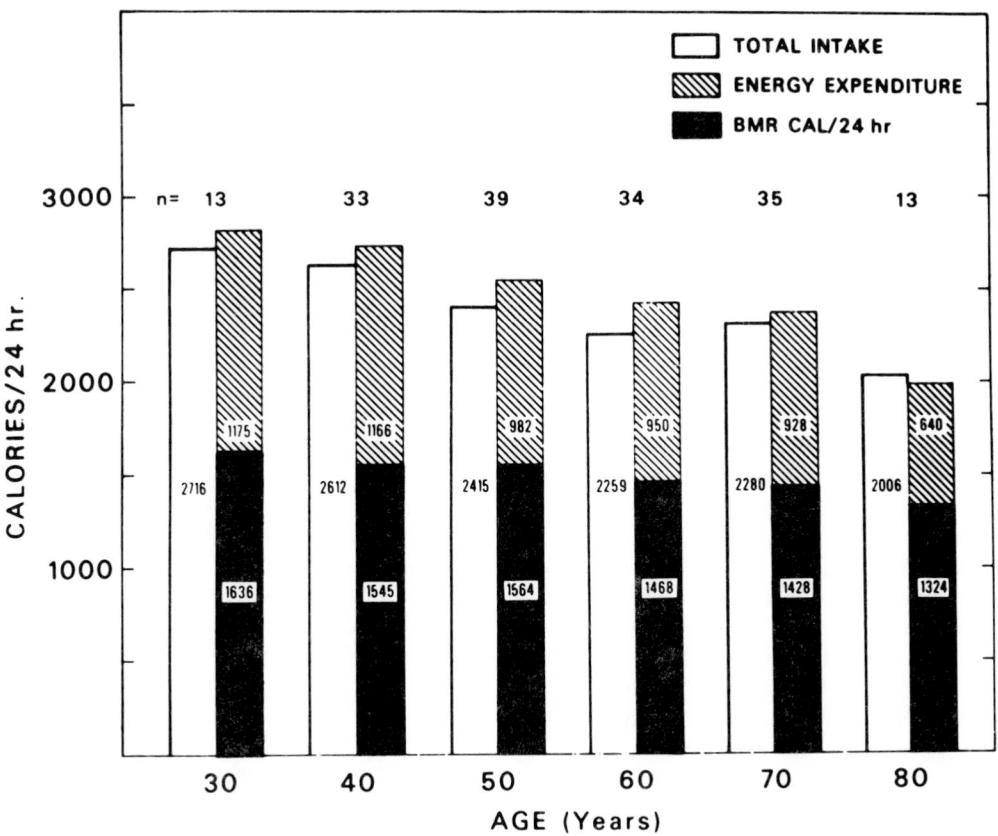

**Fig. 52–3.** Average daily energy balance in normal males aged 30 to 80 years. ☐, total dietary intake cals/24 hrs; ■, basal metabolism cals/24 hrs; ▨, caloric expenditure per 24 hrs calculated from activity history. (From McGandy, R., et al.,[16] with permission of J. Gerontol.)

In one interview, Stunkard explored the complex relationships that exist among nutrition, aging, and obesity.[27] Several challenges to the long-held belief that "thinner is better" have been raised. Andres has suggested from his studies that moderately overweight subjects have lower mortality rates.[28] Keys et al. concluded that obesity was not a risk factor for serious coronary heart disease when they presented the results of a 10-year epidemiologic study on middle-aged men.[29] Stunkard observed that the problems with these and other studies[30–33] are both methodologic and theoretical. The example given of a methodologic problem is the role of cigarette smoking. A higher proportion of smokers exists in the thinner group in the Framingham Study, leading to the higher mortality rate in this group. Stunkard has suggested that the theoretical problems with the reviewed studies are related to the complications of obesity, hypertension, diabetes, and hyperlipidemia, and their role in mortality. To dismiss obesity or relative body weight as a factor in mortality is a theoretical flaw. Because many of these

diseases can be controlled by a reduction in body weight, obesity must be considered a factor in mortality related to these diseases.

Energy balance should be a goal in elderly individuals. Maintenance of weight, unless weight reduction is desirable for control of hypertension, diabetes, hyperlipidemia, or chronic pulmonary disease, should be a priority in setting caloric needs. It is important to recognize that there are increased needs to be compensated for when illness, sepsis, stress, surgery, or trauma occurs. Adequate calories should be provided to hospitalized individuals to accommodate increased requirements during episodes of stress.[34]

## PROTEIN REQUIREMENTS

The subject of protein requirements for elderly individuals is controversial. It would seem a priori that protein requirements would decrease in association with a shrinking pool of total body protein as muscle mass decreases with age. Some studies seem to support this theory;[35–37] however, other more recent work indicates that the elderly may require more protein than do their younger counterparts.[38] Investigators found negative nitrogen balances in 15 elderly men and women studied for 30 days on metabolic diets. The subjects received 0.8 g egg protein/kg body weight/day—the amount required to meet the National Academy of Science/National Research Council Recommended Dietary Allowances. These investigators suggest that lower energy intake results in reduced retention of dietary nitrogen.[38]

Evidence suggests that protein metabolism changes with age. Muscle protein turnover appears to decrease as expressed as a percentage of total body protein, measured using urinary 3-methylhistidine excretion.[39] The decrease in muscle protein turnover may be related to a protein component shift to visceral protein metabolism. However, whether total body protein turnover changes with advancing age is not known with certainty. Experiments using $N^{15}$ glycine infusions[40] seem to indicate that it decreases.

Another issue associated with protein requirements for elderly individuals is the relationship between dietary protein and the progression of renal disease. Renal function in healthy individuals declines progressively after age 30, with renal blood flow and glomerular filtration rates being one half to one third those of younger adults by age 80. If renal disease develops, loss of functioning renal tissue occurs more rapidly.[41] It has been suggested that dietary protein restriction early in the course of renal disease will slow the loss of glomerular filtration associated with the disease processes.[41,41a] However, other investigators have challenged the hypothesis that dietary protein contributes to changes in glomerular filtration associated with aging.[41b] In subjects being followed longitudinally, these researchers found no relation between dietary protein intakes and changes in glomerular filtration measured as creatinine clearance. These subjects were aging individuals with no evidence of progressive renal disease. In individuals who do not have a disease-associated decline in renal function, protein intake will neither contribute to nor induce rapid deterioration of renal function. In individuals who do have renal disease, therapeutic regimens should be followed to manage their conditions.

Protein requirements are affected by the presence of acute or chronic disease.[34] Increased needs are related to surgery, sepsis, and trauma, whereas decreased needs may be associated with renal or hepatic disease. The long-term effects of diabetes, cardiovascular disease, pulmonary disease, and other chronic illnesses have not been explored. Protein needs must be evaluated on an individual basis with the primary focus on maintaining nitrogen equilibrium.

## FAT REQUIREMENTS

With the age-related decline in protein tisssue, there is a corresponding increase in total body fat. An overabundance of fat tissue leads to obesity, which is associated with the development of many chronic diseases such as diabetes, hypertension, cardiovascular disease of many types, renal disease, and biliary tract and hepatic diseases.

Fat, being the most calorically dense of the nutrients, is important for its contribution to the caloric adequacy of the diet and also for its role in the development of certain diseases. Diets that are high in saturated fats have been linked to the development of atherosclerosis[42] and certain cancers.[43–47] Although it seems apparent that fat in the diet of elderly Americans should be reduced to lower overall caloric intake while making the least decrease in overall nutrient content, altering dietary fat to reduce the risk of these serious diseases is controversial.[48,49]

Coronary artery disease has been associated with elevated serum total cholesterol levels; however, little is known about lipoprotein-cholesterol fractions in elderly persons.[49a] Serum total cholesterol values tend to stabilize in men after the age of 60 and in women after the age of 70.[49b] Low-density lipoprotein, the atherogenic component, tends to rise in the serum of individuals in their 60s and then declines with advancing age. Therefore, the impact of serum total cholesterol as a risk factor in coronary heart disease lessens as age advances. In a study comparing 10 healthy old women, mean age 93 years, with 10 healthy young women, mean age 36 years, the elderly women demonstrated a minimal plasma triglyceride elevation, an increase in high-density lipoprotein cholesterol concentration, and reduced platelet aggregation following ingestion of a saturated fat-rich meal.[49c] The investigators concluded that the elderly subjects had an advantage in reducing atherosclerotic risk.

High intakes of dietary fat and sodium are known to be risk factors for cardiovascular disease. It is doubtful, however, that the fibrocalcific lesions found in older adults are reversible. Dietary fat modification may benefit elderly individuals, but with many risk factors contributing to the incidence of coronary heart disease, it is difficult to attribute reduced coronary heart disease mortality to only one.[49d]

Beyond the age of 50 or 60, the presence of hypertension is the most important predictive factor of coronary heart disease.[49e] Because obesity is associated with hypertension, as well as increased levels of low-density lipoprotein-cholesterol, triglycerides, and blood glucose, reduction of weight or avoidance of obesity should be primary components of any therapeutic or disease prevention regimen for coronary heart disease.

For individuals who require weight reduction, decreasing the fat content of the diet is one of the most efficient ways to reduce overall calories.

## CARBOHYDRATE REQUIREMENTS

Carbohydrate is usually the major source of calories in the American diet, contributing 45 to 70% of total calories. It has been known for many years that the ability to metabolize carbohydrate decreases with advancing age.[50,51] This phenomenon is evident when subjects are tested both orally and intravenously.[52] Carbohydrate tolerance may be influenced by the size and route of the glucose load given, the time of the last meal, medications, activity level, chronic illnesses, and age of the subject.[52] If standard ranges of normal are used for older subjects, approximately half of them would be categorized as diabetic.[52,53] This possibility seems unlikely. Andres and colleagues have suggested that subjects be measured against their age cohorts using percentile ranks by means of a nomogram (Fig. 52–4) and a reporting form (Table 52–1).[52] Others suggest that fasting blood glucose levels greater than 140 mg/dl indicate diabetes.[53] Using the nomogram for a 65-year-old individual, one observes that 140 mg/dl is at the fiftieth percentile.

Many acute illnesses and many medications may be associated with impaired glucose tolerance. Hypoglycemia may remain undetected in elderly individuals owing to a lack of symptoms such as sweating, tachycardia, or pallor, but may present as progressive confusion. Uncontrolled hyperglycemia in the elderly may result in hyperosmolar nonketotic coma with extracellular fluid volume depletion and neurologic symptoms.[53]

Dietary carbohydrate intake in the elderly should be shifted away from refined products toward more complex starches. This practice would avoid large doses of simple sugars that raise postprandial circulating glucose, contribute to reduction of serum triglycerides and cholesterol,[54] and aid in bowel motility to resolve constipation.[55]

## FLUID REQUIREMENTS

In aged persons, fluid balance becomes an important factor in homeostasis and deserves serious consideration as part of nutritional monitoring. Usual requirements are estimated at 1 ml/kcal ingested or 30 ml/kg of body weight. In elderly individuals, inadequate fluid intake to compensate for normal observable output (sweat, feces, urine) and insensible losses (lungs, skin) may lead to problems associated with dehydration. Many elderly patients have symptoms of dehydration that are unrecognized or are attributed to other causes (Table 52–2).

Inadequate fluid intake may be related to excessive needs due to fever, diarrhea, vomiting, fistulous losses, or hemorrhage. Patients who are comatose, paralyzed, severely arthritic, confused or demented, immobile, or who have central nervous system dysfunction may not have ready access to fluid. Diuretic therapy, laxative abuse, and hypertonic intravenous infusions may also contribute to dehydration. Individuals with bladder control difficulties, i.e., incontinence, tend to limit their fluid intake in an attempt to compensate for their loss of control. Physiologic causes of dehydration may be related to the impaired capacity of elderly individuals to conserve water or of the aging kidney's inability to concentrate urine efficiently.[56]

Excess fluid in elderly persons is usually attributable to problems such as renal inability to excrete fluid, congestive heart failure, fluid retention due to hypoalbuminemia, or inappropriate antidiuretic hormone (ADH) secretion.[57] The syndrome of inappropriate ADH (SIADH) is common in elderly persons and may be associated with pulmonary and central nervous system problems such as pneumonia, tuberculosis, meningitis, and stroke.[58] Excess ADH secretion and subsequent water retention lead to hyponatremia which, if severe (below 110 meq/L), may cause seizures.[57]

Fluid balance should be regularly monitored in institutionalized older patients to avoid the aforementioned problems. Intake and output records should be kept if possible. These measures are often subjective estimates and are generally inaccurate, but they may alert caregivers to gross intake and output inequities. Weighing patients at regular, frequent intervals aids in monitoring fluid balance by noting rapid shifts in weight usually due to loss or gain of fluid. Physical examination of patients for signs of edema or dehydration should also be part of routine care for elderly institutionalized individuals. In free-living elderly, adequate fluid intake may also be a problem. Owing to thirst and osmoregulatory mechanism disturbances, excessive diuretic therapy, immobility, or infection will lead to intercompartmental fluid shifts resulting in rapid dehydration.[59] During periods of excessive climatic heat, elderly people should be checked regularly for signs and symptoms of dehydration to avoid heat-related deaths.

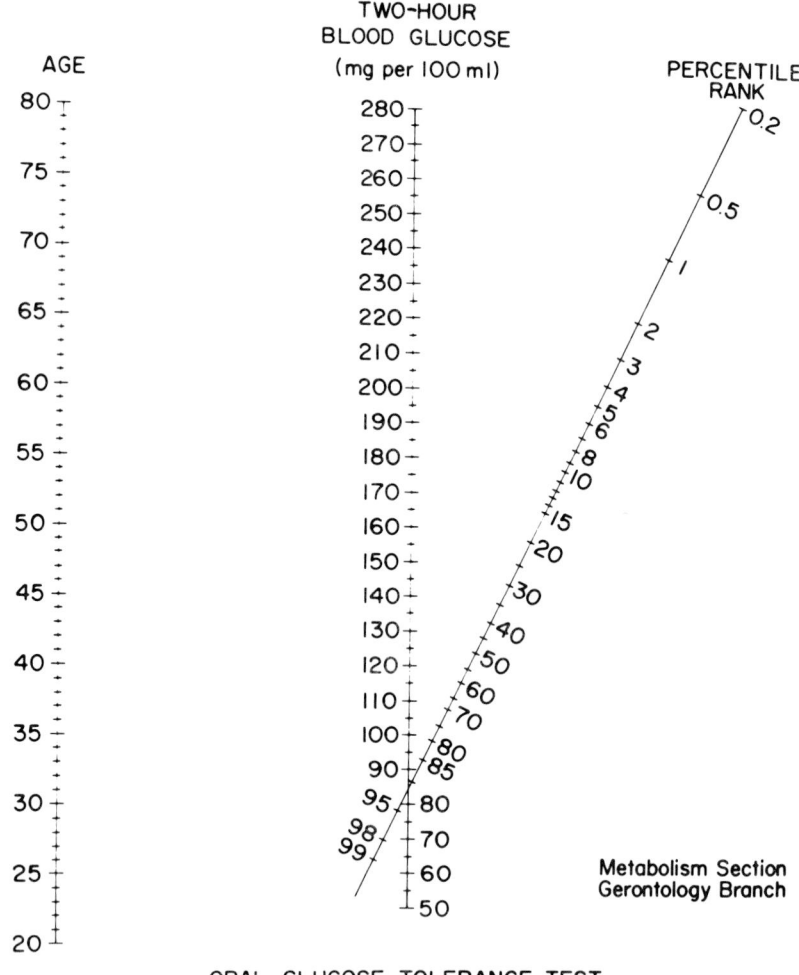

AGE

TWO-HOUR
BLOOD GLUCOSE
(mg per 100 ml)

PERCENTILE
RANK

**Fig. 52–4.** Oral glucose tolerance nomogram compares an individual's two-hour blood glucose concentration to those of his age cohorts. A line extending from the subject's age to two-hour blood glucose will intersect the percentile rank. Interpretation can be made by using the form on Table 52–1.

## MINERAL AND VITAMIN REQUIREMENTS

The recommended dietary allowances (RDAs) are published and updated periodically by the National Academy of Sciences' Food and Nutrition Board. The tenth edition, originally due in 1985, was delayed in part because of additional review needed to examine the relationship between nutrition and aging.[60] The RDAs published in 1980 offer recommendations for infants, children, and adults[61] (Appendix A–1). Older Americans are grouped together in the category "51 or older." If one knows the physiologic changes that occur with aging, the inappropriateness of this grouping becomes readily apparent. In establishing guidelines for nutrient requirements in older persons, consideration must be given to the interrelationships among lifelong nutritional intake, age-

dependent changes in body composition and physiologic functioning, and age-related diseases. Adequate intake recommendation should exceed levels required for the maintenance of health but, for elderly individuals, should accommodate nutrient needs for prevention of disease such as certain cancers, osteoporosis, obesity, atherogenesis, hypertension, and diabetes. In order to do this, longitudinal studies that follow nutrient intake, physiologic changes, and disease development must be conducted so that the relationships among these factors can be observed. By definition, these studies demand committed resources over extended periods. Present knowledge is primarily based on data collected from cross-sectional studies and will be subject to change over time.

**Calcium.** The requirements for calcium in aging

**Table 52–1.   Report Form For Oral Glucose Tolerance Test\***

U.S. PUBLIC HEALTH SERVICE

National Institutes of Health

National Institute of Child Health and Human Development

Gerontology Research Center

ORAL GLUCOSE TOLERANCE TEST

Name: _____

Date: _____Glucose Dose: 1.75 grams per kg body weight

| Time (min) | Blood Glucose Conc. (mg per 100 ml) | COMMENTS |
|---|---|---|
| 0 | _____ | |
| 20 | _____ | |
| 40 | _____ | |
| 60 | _____ | |
| 80 | _____ | |
| 100 | _____ | |
| 120 | _____ | |

INTERPRETATION: Abnormal _____Borderline _____Normal _____

PERCENTILE RANK: _____

The percentile rank compares the subject's performance to that of his own age cohorts. Thus, a rank of 50% is an exactly average performance and a rank of 2% is poor since it indicates that 98% of subjects of the same age will perform better than the subject tested. This type of ranking is necessary because of the marked decrease in tolerance which accompanies aging and because of uncertainty as to standards for the diagnosis of diabetes. The table below is a simple a rule of thumb for current use; it may need to be adjusted in the future.

| | | *Percentile Rank* | |
|---|---|---|---|
| *Age Group* | *Abnormal* | *Borderline* | *Normal* |
| 20–29 | 0–2 | 3–4 | 5 and over |
| 30–39 | 0–3 | 4–6 | 7 and over |
| 40–49 | 0–4 | 5–8 | 9 and over |
| 50–59 | 0–5 | 6–10 | 11 and over |
| 60–69 | 0–6 | 7–12 | 13 and over |
| 70–plus | 0–7 | 8–14 | 15 and over |

\*Percentile rank is explained on the form. From Andres, R.,[52] with permission of Med. Clin. N. Am.

**Table 52–2.   Signs of Dehydration in Aged Persons**

Dryness of lips or mucosa
Turbidity of the tongue
Sunken eyeballs
Elevated temperature
Hypotension
Decreased urine output
Constipation
Nausea and vomiting
Confusion

people has been receiving attention in recent years, especially because of the role of calcium in the development and prevention of osteoporosis.

Many studies indicate that calcium intake in the elderly is insufficient, based on the 1980 RDAs.[62–65] However, adequacy of calcium intake is more complex than quantitating dietary content. Other factors that determine availability and utilization of dietary calcium are the efficiency of gastrointestinal absorption, renal function, skeletal metabolism, nutrient-nutrient interactions, drug-nutrient interactions, and hormone produc-

tion.[65,66] It has been reported that the efficiency of intestinal absorption of calcium decreases after middle age.[67,68] Both passive and active transport systems are involved in calcium absorption. Active transport occurs in the upper part of the small intestine and is mediated by 1,25-$(OH)_2$ vitamin D (calcitriol).[65] Impaired calcium absorption in elderly persons may be related to inadequate production of calcitriol. This phenomenon may be due to age-related decreases in renal function or an imbalance between bone resorption and bone formation where excess circulating calcium (calcium released from bone is greater than calcium taken up by bone) suppresses parathormone secretion with a consequent reduction of calcitriol synthesis.[65,66]

In postmenopausal females, estrogen reduction may be related to a defect in the formation of calcitriol or to an estrogen deficiency-related skeleton sensitivity to parathormone leading to an increase in bone resorption, an elevation of serum ionized calcium, suppression of parathormone secretion, decreased calcitriol production, and decreased intestinal calcium resorption.[66] Reduction of osteoporotic fractures in postmenopausal females is often dependent on estrogen-replacement therapy, which provides greater protection against bone loss and the occurrence of new vertebrae deformities than does calcium supplementation therapy.[68a] The effects of calcium supplementation in the prevention of osteoporotic fractures are controversial. Some investigators have demonstrated that supplementary calcium improves calcium balance and reduces the rate of bone loss.[68b–d] However, the effects of calcium supplementation without estrogen replacement in the prevention of osteoporotic fractures are not clear.[68a] Prevention and treatment of senile osteoporosis, particularly in elderly males, have not been thoroughly investigated and, because of the inadequate dietary intake and physiologic changes associated with aging, should be areas of future investigation. These interrelationships of calcium intake, calcium metabolism, and aging are complex and still require elucidation through controlled metabolic studies.

Other dietary factors have an effect on calcium metabolism. Some studies indicate that high levels of dietary protein are associated with increased levels of urinary calcium.[69–71a] This increase occurs as a result of an increase in glomerular filtration rate and a decrease in renal calcium reabsorption.[65] However, studies performed by Spencer and colleagues seem to indicate that high levels of dietary protein do not have such an effect and that, in subjects who had hypercalciuria, the effect was transitory.[71b–74d] These observations are intriguing and would be strengthened if repeated with the use of an appropriate female cohort.

Dietary phosphorus is another nutrient shown to have an effect on calcium metabolism. Most studies indicate that skeletal integrity is supported by a Ca:P ratio of 1:1.[66] A slight inverse ratio of dietary phosphorus to urinary calcium does not seem to result in appreciable calcium binding.[65] Fluctuations in phosphorus intake impact on both calcium handling and bone remodeling, but the effects cancel each other.

In recent years, the level of fiber in the diet of many Americans has increased, particularly because of its role in the control of serum lipids or in glucose absorption in diabetics. Some studies have demonstrated that unrefined cereal products may be associated with a more negative calcium balance.[72,73] Reasonable amounts of fiber in the diet appear to affect calcium balance, perhaps increasing calcium requirements.[65] In elderly individuals, this finding may be noteworthy as they are often encouraged to increase their dietary fiber intake to enhance bowel motility and, as previously mentioned, their calcium intake is probably inadequate.

Other substances reported to interact with calcium metabolism include drugs, such as diuretics, alcohol, and antacids. Aluminum hydroxide antacids, in particular, may have serious adverse side effects such as hypercalciuria, bone resorption, and phosphorus depletion, which may all contribute to bone disease in the elderly.[65]

Of particular importance in elderly people is the effect of reduced physical activity on bone mass. In studies performed on immobilized human subjects, bone loss occurs with increased urinary loss and decreased dietary calcium absorption.[74,75] Increased intake does not reverse the loss, but with increased phosphorus intake, the loss slows.[65] Exercise has positive effects on calcium balance by reducing the rate of loss in immobilized persons and by increasing bone mass in elderly individuals taking part in exercise programs.[76]

There has been some controversy over appropriate allowances for dietary calcium.[65] The 1980 RDAs are 800 mg/day for nonpregnant, nonlactating adults. It has been suggested that allowances for calcium be raised to 1,200 to 1,500 mg/day,[65,66] especially for postmenopausal women.

One issue of potential concern is the possible toxic effects of higher levels of calcium intake. Potential side effects include hypercalciuria, urinary calculi, soft tissue calcification, and suppression of bone remodeling.[65,77] Dietary calcium intakes of 2,500 mg/day do not result in deleterious side effects in elderly persons.[65] Hypercalcemia most commonly occurs from hyperparathyroidism,[78] cancers,[79] or drug therapy.

**Sodium.** Sodium is a nutrient that is important to elderly individuals because it is often restricted in their diets. It has become fairly routine medical practice to restrict dietary sodium for patients who have hypertension, congestive heart failure, chronic renal disease, or cirrhosis. Many of the conditions for which dietary sodium is restricted are treated with drugs that diminish the need for more than mild sodium intake reduction. In fact, more severe restrictions may lead to hyponatremia. There is an age-related, impaired kidney response to dietary sodium reduction. Most aged individuals are able to conserve sodium and maintain salt balance, but it takes them a greater time to do so.[79,80] This is a particularly important factor because older patients lose their sense of thirst, and may become confused and disoriented when ill, which may contribute to anorexia or decreased dietary intake.[81]

The syndrome of inappropriate antidiuretic

hormone (SIADH) previously described, and therapies of certain drugs,[82] may also lead to water retention, contributing to hyponatremia.

Hypernatremia occurs most frequently in elderly patients who are nonambulatory, have thirst sensation impairment due to central nervous system dysfunction, or have diabetes insipidus, vomiting, or diarrhea.[79] A severe consequence of hypernatremia can be cerebral edema if hypernatremia is corrected by rapid large infusion of fluids.[83]

**Potassium.** Potassium requirements in elderly persons do not seem to be mediated by age per se, but rather are more related to changes due to diseases and treatments. Hypokalemia occurs in elderly persons in association with diuretic therapy compounded by an inadequate intake of dietary potassium.[79] Although this is the most common cause of hypokalemia in elderly persons, vomiting, diarrhea, excessive use of purgatives, renal tubular acidosis, and other causes may contribute to an abnormal decrease in serum potassium levels.

Consequences of hypokalemia include polyuria and polydipsia due to tubulointerstitial nephritis, electrocardiographic abnormalities with arrhythmia, depression, anorexia, fatigue, disorientation, confusion, abdominal distention, paralytic ileus, and glucose intolerance.[79]

Hyperkalemia in elderly people is related to impaired renal function. Decreases in renin and aldosterone production and in glomerular filtration rate tend to diminish urinary potassium excretion; therefore, increased serum potassium levels may result.[81] Administration of potassium supplements or unusual losses such as hemorrhage will compound the problem. Hyperkalemia may result in severe cardiac arrhythmia leading to sudden death. For a more detailed discussion, see Chapter 4.

**Iron.** Iron status measurements in healthy elderly individuals suggest that iron requirements are lowest in old age. Even under conditions where dietary intake is low, bone marrow iron stores and serum ferritin concentration increase with advancing age.[84] Hemoglobin (Hb) concentration remains within normal limits in healthy persons until the age of 70, after which Hb seems to decrease in men.[84] Nutritional adequacy of the diet may be affected by the source of the dietary iron. Studies have indicated that the bioavailability of dietary iron must be evaluated when one is determining adequacy of dietary intake.[85,86] Heme iron, found in meats, is readily absorbed, but nonheme iron, which requires an acid medium to be absorbed (needs reduction), may be less well absorbed unless ascorbic or other acid

is present. In the elderly, gastric achlorhydria may decrease absorption of nonheme iron considerably.[79,83]

Iron deficiency is manifested as iron deficiency anemia, which contributes to easy fatigability and lethargy. However, significant anemia in elderly persons should be carefully investigated to rule out bleeding.[83]

**Other Minerals.** Zinc deficiency has been associated with loss of taste acuity, impaired wound healing, and depressed immune function in humans.[87] Although several studies have indicated that elderly people may have inadequate dietary zinc intakes[88] or impaired absorption of zinc,[89] there does not seem to be any reason to increase the recommended allowance of 15 mg/day.[90] However, low plasma zinc concentrations may be found in elderly patients who have alcoholic cirrhosis, malabsorption, bacterial or parasitic infections, renal failure, or hemolytic anemias or in those who are being treated with parenteral hyperalimentation, chelating drugs, or antimetabolites.[79]

Copper deficiency rarely occurs in humans[90] unless an individual is on a copper-deficient diet for a long time e.g., on total parenteral nutrition without added trace elements. Serum copper and ceruloplasmin concentrations may be increased in patients who have liver disease, rheumatoid arthritis, atherosclerosis, hypertension, infections, or cancers, all of which may be found in the elderly.[79]

Chromium is another trace mineral that may be of interest for future investigations in elderly subjects. Chromium may be related to impaired glucose tolerance and ischemic heart disease;[91] however, these relationships have not been demonstrated conclusively. Tissue chromium levels may decline with age, but the mechanism for this process has not been identified.

As a group, the elderly may be at risk for mineral deficiencies due to inadequate intake, drug-nutrient interactions, impaired absorption, or the effects of chronic disease processes. At this time, there has been no indication of any increased requirements for minerals in the elderly, with the possible exception of calcium.

**Fat-Soluble Vitamins.** The Recommended Dietary Allowances for vitamin A intake are often not met by elderly individuals;[92] however, there is little evidence suggesting that vitamin A deficiency exists in this population.[83] Risk of hypervitaminosis A is more likely in elderly people who use high-potency vitamin supplements than risk of a deficiency disease.

Vitamin E, requirements and supplementation, continues to be a nutrient surrounded by controversy in the scientific community.[93] Claims for the benefits of supplemental vitamin E (which are mostly unproven) include protection against the development of heart and vascular diseases.[94-98] There is some evidence that vitamin E supplementation may play a role in the management of intermittent claudication;[99] however, this effect requires more investigation. Vitamin E has been attributed to have properties that slow biologic aging,[100] but this theory has not yet been demonstrated. Because there is virtually no reported incidence of vitamin E deficiency in man nor is there any compelling data to indicate any benefit from vitamin E supplementation, following the present RDAs for vitamin E for individuals 51 years of age and older seems appropriate.

Studies indicate that elderly people tend to be deficient in dietary vitamin D.[101,102] Compensation for the lack of dietary vitamin D, which is due to a decreased intake of milk and milk products because of gastrointestinal intolerance, is usually balanced by sunlight-dependent endogenous vitamin D synthesis.[101] Elderly persons may not receive adequate sunlight exposure, especially during months when severe weather (either heat or cold) may be expected.[103] In addition, elderly individuals may have impaired intestinal absorption of vitamin D, suppressed hepatic synthesis of 25-OHD, impaired renal conversion to 1,25-OHD, and increased metabolic requirements.[101,104] Prolonged and severe vitamin D deficiency causes osteomalacia. An individual with osteomalacia not only has bone pain, but may also experience muscle weakness and hypocalcemic tetany.[104] In addition, vitamin D deficiency may also contribute to the development of osteoporosis.

Individuals who use vitamin D supplementation in excess are at risk of developing hypercalcemia, soft tissue calcification with possible kidney damage, and increased plasma cholesterol levels.[104]

Vitamin K deficiency does not occur because of inadequate dietary intake, but may develop as a result of iatrogenic causes. Sulfa drugs or antibiotics, which may reduce the vitamin K-producing microflora in the intestine, and vitamin K antagonists, used to prevent intravascular clotting, may lead to a vitamin K deficiency.[83] Because these substances are commonly used in elderly people, they may be at risk for vitamin K deficiency.

Another etiologic factor that may contribute to a potential fat-soluble vitamin deficiency in elderly individuals is the use of cathartics and laxatives. These substances tend to increase bowel transit time or to interfere with absorption as occurs with the habitual use of mineral oil.

**Water-Soluble Vitamins.** In healthy, free-living elderly, thiamin deficiency is not a widespread problem.[105] Alcoholics, however, may experience interference with absorption, and an inadequate intake may occur in people who frequently consume alcoholic beverages.[105,106] Thiamin deficiency leads to anorexia, irritability, and weight loss. These symptoms in elderly people may remain unnoticed or may be attributed to many other causes. Untreated thiamin deficiency leads to the classic symptoms of beriberi, including peripheral neuritis, paresthesias, muscle cramping, mental changes and, ultimately, cardiac failure.[107] Chronically ill institutionalized elderly may be at greater risk of developing thiamin deficiency than are free-living, healthy elderly.[108] Dietary thiamin adequacy is related to overall caloric intake, which tends to diminish with age and illness.[105] In addition, drugs, such as anticonvulsants or antacids,[109] may interfere with vitamin absorption and utilization.

Healthy elderly persons do not appear to experience any significant problems with niacin or riboflavin deficiencies.[110] Deficiencies may appear in chronically ill, severely stressed, or malnourished elderly patients.

Although not extensively studied, folate deficiency does not seem to be a problem in free-living elderly people.[111] Megaloblastic anemia due to folate deficiency seems to be related more to alcoholism than to purely dietary inadequacy, and there is little evidence to indicate that gastrointestinal absorption is impaired in aging.[111] Folate deficiency, however, has been reported in patients with dementia.[112] It is unclear whether their neuropsychiatric illness contributes to a poor nutritional intake leading to a folate deficiency or whether the folate deficiency contributes to a worsened mental status.[113] The same relationship seems to exist in elderly individuals who are prone to depressive episodes.[112] Where folate deficiency is suspected, it is wise to examine vitamin $B_{12}$ status because hematologic manifestations of folic acid and vitamin $B_{12}$ manifestations are difficult to distinguish morphologically.[112] The incidence of vitamin $B_{12}$ deficiency in a healthy elderly population is not significant,[114] but this does not preclude deficiencies appearing in chronically or critically ill, malnourished, older patients.

Vitamin $B_{12}$ deficiency may occur as a consequence of ascorbic acid supplementation.[115] Although this possibility may seem somewhat obscure, many people take megadoses of vitamin C because it has been touted as a prevention against diagnoses as diverse as the common cold and cancer.[83] In one study,[116] fewer than 2% of the study population had plasma ascorbic acid concentrations below 0.2 mg/dl. Despite apparently adequate intake of vitamin C, more than half of the people studied were taking ascorbic acid supplements. Other than in severely malnourished individuals, the nutritional problems encountered in elderly people seem to be more related to megadose supplementation. Possible consequences of large doses of ascorbic acid include interference with vitamin $B_{12}$ absorption,[115] formation of uric and oxalic acid lithiasis,[117] erythrocyte hemolysis,[118] and false negative fecal occult blood tests.[119]

Most of the studies cited have examined samples of healthy elderly people, usually living in a home environment. The impact of chronic illness and living and economic circumstances cannot be easily dismissed or underestimated. The effects of life events, however difficult to quantitate, are considerable. When these factors are added to the age-related physiologic changes that have been described, identifying nutritional deficits in elderly people, especially those who have chronic illnesses or are institutionalized in acute or long-term care facilities, becomes difficult.

## NUTRITION ASSESSMENT

Identifying nutritional needs of individuals and groups has challenged clinicians and investigators for years. Because of its great individual diversity, the aging segment of the population presents unique problems in the assessment of nutritional status and requirements. So many factors have to be integrated to provide a comprehensive picture of the nutritional status of aged individuals that the process becomes complex and multidimensional.

Most nutritional assessments rely on standard measurements of anthropometric, biochemical, hematologic, and immunologic indices. Combinations of some of these measures have been selected by most clinicians to assess nutritional status in their patients. Most of the measures commonly used do not have normal ranges for older age groups or age-adjusted standards.

**Anthropometric Measures.** Of all the parameters used at present to assess nutritional status, anthropometric measures are the ones most apparently affected by the aging process. Changes in height or stature are the most noticeable.

Height is important in nutrition assessment as it is one of the measures that is expected to be a constant and therefore a reference point against which other measures are compared. However, height decreases with age.[120–122] Estimates of height loss range from 1.2 cm/20 yrs[123] to 4.2 cm/20 yrs.[124] Loss of height is due to thinning of the vertebrae, kyphosis, and osteoporosis.[120] Obtain-

ing accurate height measures may be difficult in some elderly people who cannot stand erect or who require help standing because of paralysis or other neuromuscular disorders. Some attempt should be made to measure height or recumbent length to have an anthropometric reference. Reliance should not be placed on the patient's report of his height as these values are notoriously inaccurate.

Changes in weight, either gains or losses, over short time spans are signals that the clinical status of an individual is changing. Regularly monitoring weight may alert a clinician to shifts in fluid balance and alterations in disease processes. Weight is also affected by normal aging. Weight tends to increase until the early 40s in males and the early 50s in females, stabilizes for the ensuing 15 to 20 years, and then decreases progressively.[120]

In addition to height and weight, other anthropometric measurements are also used to assess nutritional status by estimating body compartment sizes. Aging is associated with changes in body composition; lean body mass decreases, total fat increases, and intracellular water decreases. Interpretation of the routinely used anthropometric measures is impaired not only by shifts in body composition but also by shifts in body compartments. Fat is deposited around internal organs and tends to become more truncal.[125] As a predictor of body fat, subscapular and suprailiac skinfold measurements may be more reliable in males; triceps skinfold measurements correlate with fat stores in females.[126] Other factors that may make skinfold measurements less reliable are alterations in skin thickness, elasticity, and compressibility.[121] Only a few reference tables are available that were developed on samples of older subjects.[127,128]

**Biochemical Measures.** Biochemical parameters are known to be affected by age.[120] When reviewing these measures, one must remember that factors such as age-related decline in renal function efficiency, over- or underhydration, drug-drug or drug-nutrient interactions, and coexisting diseases will affect various biochemical indices.

Serum albumin is only minimally altered by aging; the range of values broadens, but the distribution remains normal.[129] Serum albumin is, therefore, a fairly reliable measure to use in nutritional assessment of the elderly as long as hydration status, drug profile, and primary diagnosis are considered. Even recognizing that prolonged bed rest may decrease levels, serum albumin is a good indicator of protein nutriture.[130]

Serum transferrin is often evaluated as part of a nutritional screening. In elderly subjects, the factors that may affect serum transferrin occur more frequently.[120] For example, tissue iron stores increase with age and, as a result, serum transferrin levels are reduced. This change should not be mistaken as a sign of malnutrition in elderly subjects.

Twenty-four-hour urinary creatinine excretion is often used to assess lean body mass. Owing to the loss of lean body mass associated with normal aging, creatinine excretion decreases.[120] In addition, renal function may decline; if this is the case, urinary creatinine excretion will not be a reliable measure to use for assessing lean body mass. To compensate for these changes, a creatinine/height index as a function of age was developed.[131] Creatinine excretion must be related to height to appropriately assess musculature; therefore, the value of this index is questionable when changes in height that occur as part of normal aging are considered. Total arm length has been suggested as an alternative for height as a constant in the creatinine/height calculations.[132]

Unless there is an underlying ongoing disease process or drug interaction, most biochemical measures will usually remain within reference normal ranges in elderly persons.

**Hematologic and Immunologic Measures.** Hematologic measures, such as hemoglobin, hematocrit, mean serum iron, total iron-binding capacity, and others, are often used as part of a comprehensive nutritional assessment. A higher percentage of below-normal hemoglobin and hematocrit values occurs with the increasing age of the subjects.[120,133,134] Usual causes for anemia seem to be rare in elderly persons. Because of the cross-sectional decline noted in hemoglobin for elderly males, a lower limit of normal for hemoglobin of 12 g/dl for both males and females is suggested.

Lymphocytopenia and anergy to intradermal antigens are often used as measures of immune function because malnutrition results in compromised host-defense mechanisms.[120] However, it has been reported that the incidence of anergy and lymphocytopenia increases with age.[135-137] In addition, cancer, trauma, general anesthesia, surgery, and other acute illness will alter cell-mediated immunity. Therefore, the efficacy of using immunologic testing as a measure of nutritional status is questionable in elderly individuals[120] (Fig. 52–5).

**Other Measures.** Although not measures in the sense of objective evaluation, assessments of socioeconomic and environmental circumstances should be included when one is attempting to determine nutritional status of elderly individuals.[130] Such factors as mobility, food preparation facilities, dentition, finances, isolation, loss of spouse, climate, proximity to family, friends, and church, and drug/medication and alcohol use contribute to overall nutritional status. These factors determine food selection, food preparation, exercise, appetite, and psychologic state, all of which contribute to nutritional intake.

## PROTEIN-ENERGY MALNUTRITION

Assessing nutritional status in elderly individuals is a difficult task because of all the age-related changes that impact on the commonly used nutritional assessment parameters described previously. The incidence of protein-energy malnutrition (PEM) in hospitalized patients ranges from 35 to 65%,[138-140] and most hospitalized patients are over the age of 65.[141] The scope of the problem of PEM in elderly hospitalized patients, therefore, demands attention.

PEM is usually secondary or subclinical until a primary disease develops or existing chronic problems are exacerbated. For example, PEM may develop secondary to chronic heart, lung, renal, or hepatic disease. The presence of these chronic conditions confounds the diagnosis of PEM.[141] An acute episode of illness severely stresses an elderly individual; for a patient with PEM, age-impaired responses to stress are even more delayed. Elderly patients respond appropriately to systemic insults, although a return to basal levels takes longer. Undiagnosed PEM impacts on wound healing, infection defense, and metabolic response to stress.

The most common presenting symptom of PEM in elderly patients is confusion or an altered mental state.[141] Changes in mental status may be associated with cardiac failure, cerebrovascular accidents, sepsis, or various metabolic dysfunctions. However, dehydration is probably the single most common cause of acute confusional states in elderly hospitalized patients.[141] Patients who have PEM usually have inadequate fluid intakes. Hydration status can be easily followed by monitoring changes in weight. Infection is a frequent complication of PEM and often is the precipitating factor necessitating hospitalization.

The physical signs of malnutrition, such as hair loss, flaky paint dermatitis, glossitis, dry skin, and sunken eyeballs, should be evaluated regularly in elderly patients. The presence of any of the risk factors (Table 52–3) should alert the clinician to the possibility of PEM.

## NUTRITION SUPPORT

Many elderly patients are managed using nutritional support methods that include oral supplementation, enteral feeding, and parenteral nutrition. Most clinicians are not trained in geriatrics

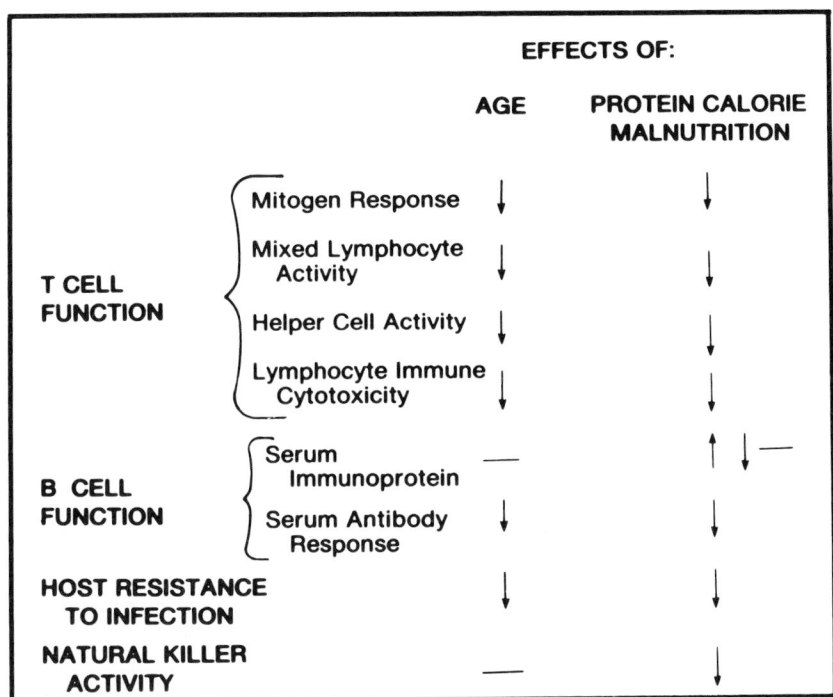

**Fig. 52–5.** A comparison of the effects of age or protein-calorie malnutrition on lymphocyte function. (From Adler, W.H.,[137] with permission of Ross Laboratories.)

and may not recognize the special needs of aged individuals. Elderly patients do have unique requirements that must be addressed when they are provided with nutrition support.

**Oral Supplementation.** When necessary, supplementation of inadequate dietary intake may be accomplished by providing food through federal or local government or charitable agencies. The federal government supports programs that are designed to help needy people obtain a quality diet. These include the food stamp program, surplus food distribution program, and the Administration on Aging, established as part of the Older

**Table 52–3.** **Risk Factors for Protein-Energy Malnutrition in Elderly Individuals**

Chronic or intercurrent illness
Edentulous
Vision impairment
Loss of mobility, independence
Alcohol abuse
Polypharmacy
Social isolation
Loss of spouse, bereavement
Depression
Poverty
Mental impairment, confusion
Surgery
Acute illness episode

Americans Act. Title VII of the Older Americans Act resulted in the development of congregate meal programs that provide one hot meal a day in a community setting. In addition, the Administration on Aging established state Agencies on Aging that function through regional or county Area Agencies on Aging. Many of these regional or county agencies provide home-delivered meal service for the disabled or frail elderly who are unable to participate in community congregate meal programs. Studies have shown that these programs do improve the nutritional intake of recipients.[142–144]

Oral liquid diet supplements, used in patients who are unable to ingest adequate nutrients as food, are another option for elderly patients (see Appendix Tables A–40, A–41). These products have been shown to improve nutritional status and to be tolerated well by this group.[59,145–147]

**Enteral Feeding.** One survey demonstrated that at least 50% of hospitalized patients who receive enteral or tube feeding are over the age of 65.[148] Surprisingly few research studies have been conducted on elderly patients receiving enteral nutrition support. Those that have been undertaken have indicated efficacy and tolerance of this procedure.[149–152] Elderly patients require careful monitoring to assure adequate intake and to avoid any complications associated with tube feeding (see Chap. 54). Perhaps the most commonly encountered complication seen in the enterally fed elderly patient is fluid and electrolyte imbalance.[141] Fluid shifts may occur rapidly in these patients, potentially resulting in peripheral edema or, at the most severe, cardiac failure.

An issue that has become the focus of some controversy in recent years is the withholding of nutrition and hydration therapy.[153–157] Many elderly, frail, terminally ill patients are maintained nutritionally using nutrition support modalities, usually by enteral feeding. Questions that have been raised focus on the provision of food and water as a basic human right. Some health care practitioners question whether administering nutrition support is prolonging life in a patient with a hopeless prognosis. The cessation of enteral feeding becomes an emotionally difficult situation for patients' caregivers, including professional staff and families. The problem has been stated as a definition of *ordinary* versus *extraordinary* care.[158] Enteral feeding is generally not viewed as being the same as other technologically advanced life support procedures and, therefore, presents a dilemma in making the distinction between ordinary and extraordinary care.[159] Perhaps the most important considerations are the wishes of the patient and family and the patient's comfort.[160,161] It is evident that the legal, ethical, and moral issues regarding enteral feeding of elderly individuals will remain a topic of discussion.

**Parenteral Feeding.** For severely malnourished, critically ill elderly patients, parenteral feeding may be required. Extensive research has not been conducted on nutrient requirements or the metabolic demands associated with aging. Basal caloric requirements are lower in elderly persons; however, adjustments for increased protein needs for healing wounds, fighting infections, and responding to the metabolic demands of stress must be balanced against a reduced rate of protein synthesis and turnover and possibly impaired renal or hepatic function.[162] In addition, high-protein diets may be associated with bone resorption in patients with osteoporosis.

The primary source of calories in most parenteral solutions is hypertonic glucose. Decreased glucose tolerance is common in elderly persons and should be monitored closely in patients receiving parenteral nutrition. If lipid is substituted for glucose as a calorie source, especially in fluid-restricted patients, serum lipid clearance should be followed regularly because some older patients have an impaired ability to clear lipids from their blood.[162]

Vitamin requirements for elderly patients supported on parenteral nutrition are not known to differ from dosages used for younger adults.[163] In severely vitamin-depleted patients, caution should be taken when one is administering therapeutic doses of vitamins parenterally; some vitamins, such as vitamin C and niacin, may cause cardiac arrhythmias or other deleterious side effects when given in moderately large doses.[164]

Mineral content of parenteral solutions can be adjusted to meet the specific needs or restrictions of individual patients. In elderly individuals, serum mineral or electrolyte levels should be evaluated in the context of hydration status and adjustments made accordingly.

Age is not a contraindication for the use of total parenteral nutrition if adequate consideration is given to the physiologic changes that occur as part of normal aging, of chronic disease, and of critical illnesses.

## DRUG-NUTRIENT INTERACTIONS

An important factor in the nutritional status and requirements of elderly people is related to medications, both prescription and over-the-counter, that they may be using. The older segment of the population is prescribed more drugs than any other population group.[165] Polypharmacy, or use of multiple drugs concurrently, is potentially dangerous in elderly patients because there is greater variability, and less predictability, in their responses to drugs.[166] Even if a clinician is aware of these potential adverse effects, control of the problem may be difficult because many elderly patients see different physicians for various ailments and may not give complete drug histories to all the physicians visited.

In elderly patients, the risk of adverse side effects due to overdosing or to decreased clearance capabilities[167] is compounded by the problem of potential drug-drug and drug-nutrient interactions (see Chap. 34). Not only do nutritional factors alter absorption, metabolism, and excretion of drugs, but drugs affect nutritional status (Table 52–4). The most significant drug-induced nutritional deficiencies occur in patients least likely to adapt: those having marginal dietary intake and those with chronic diseases.[168] Mineral depletion is probably the most common example of drug-induced nutritional deficiencies in elderly patients.[168]

Approximately half the drugs used by elderly persons are over-the-counter drugs.[168] Antacids, laxatives, analgesics, and even vitamin and mineral supplements may lead to untoward side effects in elderly patients. These may remain undetected for long periods because their effects may be subclinical until the patient is stressed or until

**Table 52–4. Drug Interferences with Nutritional Status***

| Drugs | Mechanism | Effect |
|---|---|---|
| Antihistamines | Appetite stimulation | Weight gain |
| Antihypertensives (ganglionic blockers) | GI motility effects | Generalized malabsorption |
| Anti-infectives | | |
| aminoglycosides | Enzyme inactivation | Reduced carbohydrate metabolism |
| chloramphenicol | Impaired nutrient metabolism and utilization | Protein-binding inhibition |
| isoniazid | Altered nutrient excretion | Pyridoxine deficiency |
| neomycin | Bile acid activity Interference | Iron, sugar, triglyceride absorption |
| Antineoplastics | | |
| aminopterin | Damage to intestinal mucosa | Reduced vitamin $B_{12}$, carotene, cholesterol, lactose, D-xylose absorption, megaloblastic anemia, steatorrhea |
| methotrexate | Damage to intestinal mucosa; impaired nutrient absorption | Same as above; decreased folic acid synthesis |
| Antirheumatoids (colchicine) | Damage to intestinal mucosa | Same as above |
| Central-nervous-system drugs | | |
| amphetamines | Appetite suppression | Weight loss |
| benzodiazepines | Appetite stimulation | Weight gain |
| levodopa | Competition for uptake at blood-brain barrier | Reduced phenylalanine and tyrosine absorption |
| Phenobarbital | Impaired nutrient metabolism and utilization | Vitamin D deficiency |
| Phenothiazines | Appetite stimulation | Weight gain |
| Phenytoin | Impaired nutrient metabolism and utilization | Osteomalacia |
| Tricyclic antidepressants | Appetite stimulation | Weight gain |
| Gastrointestinal drugs | | |
| aluminum hydroxide gel | Complex formation with nutrients | Reduced phosphate absorption |
| antacids | Altered GI pH | Thiamin deficiency |
| anticholinergics | GI motility effects | Generalized malabsorption |
| cathartics | GI motility effects | Calcium and phosphorus loss |
| cholestyramine | Bile acid activity interference | Vitamin A, D, E, and K deficiencies |
| clofibrate | Enzyme inactivation | Reduced carbohydrate absorption |
| | Appetite suppression | Weight loss |
| | Bile acid activity | Reduced vitamin $B_{12}$, carotene, iron, sugar, triglyceride absorption |
| Immunosuppressives | | |
| cytotoxic agents | Appetite suppression | Weight loss |
| steroids | Altered nutrient excretion | Sodium depletion in adrenally suppressed patients |

*From Chernoff, R.,[130] with permission of Ger. Med. Today.

an alert clinician takes a comprehensive history of drug and supplementation use.

## SUMMARY

A great deal is unknown about nutrition in aging. Research is needed in assessing nutritional status, in determining normal nutrient requirements, in quantifying the effects of chronic disease on nutritional status and requirements, in defining the optimum use of nutrition support modalities, and in identifying drug-drug and drug-nutrient interactions. Elderly individuals, being more different from each other than any other group of people, present constant challenges for their caregivers. Because the elderly are the most rapidly growing segment of the American population and are the users of the greatest portion of the health care resources, it is imperative that information regarding aging and nutrition be gathered through scientific endeavor and be disseminated to all health care practitioners.

## REFERENCES

1. Kovar, M.G.: Elderly people: The population 65 years and over. DHEW Publication No. HRA 77-1232, 1977.
2. Butler, R.N., McQuire, E.A.H.: Am. J. Clin. Nutr. *36*:977–978, 1982.
3. Besdine, R.W.: The data base of geriatric medicine.

*In* Health and Disease in Old Age. (Rowe, J.W., Besdine, R.W., Eds.) Boston, Little, Brown and Co., 1982.

4. McGandy, R.B.: Clin. Ther. *6*:728–729, 1984.

5. Gilchrest, B.A., Rowe, J.W.: The biology of aging. *In* Health and Disease in Old Age. (Rowe, J.W., Besdine, R.W., Eds.) Boston, Little, Brown and Co., 1982.

6. Hart, R.W., Settow, R.B.: Proc. Natl. Acad. Sci. USA *71*:2169, 1974.

7. Orgel, L.E.: Proc. Natl. Acad. Sci. USA *49*:517, 1963.

8. Bjorksten, J.: Finska Kenists Medd. *80*:23, 1971.

9. Harman, D.: J. Gerontol., *16*:247, 1961.

10. Davies, D.E., Shock, N.W.: J. Clin. Invest. *29*:496, 1950.

11. Shock, N.W., Greulich, R.C., Andres, R., et al.: Normal human aging: The Baltimore Longitudinal Study of Aging. U.S. Department of Health and Human Services, NIH Publication No. 84-2450, Nov., 1984.

12. Boothby, N.M., Berkson, J., Dunn, H.L.: Am. J. Physiol. *116*:468, 1936.

13. Shock, N.W.: Energy metabolism, caloric intake and physical activity of the aging. *In* Nutrition in Old Age. (Carlson, L.A., Ed.) X Symposium Swedish Nutrition Foundation. Uppsala, Almquist and Wiksell, 1972.

14. Tzankoff, S.P., Norris, A.H.: J. Appl. Physiol. *43*:1001–1006, 1977.

15. Gaffney, G.W., Gregerman, R.I., Yiengst, M.J., et al.: J. Gerontol. *15*:234, 1960.

16. McGandy, R., Barrows, C.H., Spanias, A., et al.: J. Gerontol. *21*:581, 1966.

17. LaPorte, R.E., Black-Sandler, R., Cauley, J.A., et al.: J. Gerontol. *38*:394–397, 1983.

18. Wyke, B.: Age Ageing *8*:251, 1979.

19. McGandy, R., Barrows, C.H., Spanias, A., et al.: J. Gerontol. *21*:581–587, 1966.

20. Elahi, V.K., Elahi, D., Andres, R., et al.: J. Gerontol. *38*:162–180, 1983.

21. Ross, M.H.: Nutrition *75*:197–210, 1961.

22. Ross, M.H.: Am. J. Clin. Nutr. *25*:834–837, 1972.

23. Stuchlikova, E., Juricava-Horakova, M., Deyl, F.: Exp. Gerontol. *10*:141–144, 1975.

24. Nolen, G.: J. Nutr. *102*:1477–1493, 1972.

25. Beauchene, R.E., Bales, C., Smith, C., et al.: Physiologist *22*:8a, 1979.

26. Masoro, E.J.: J. Am. Geriatr. Soc. *32*:296–300, 1984.

27. Stunkard, A.J.: Int. J. Obes. *7*:201–220, 1983.

28. Andres, R.: Int. J. Obes. *4*:381–386, 1980.

29. Keys, A., Aravanis, C., Blackburn, H., et al.: Seven Countries: A Multivariate Analysis of Death and Coronary Heart Disease. Cambridge, Harvard University Press, 1980.

30. Borhani, N., Hechter, H., Breslow, L.: J. Chronic Dis. *16*:1251–1266, 1963.

31. Dyer, A., Stamler, J., Berkson, D.M.: J. Chronic Dis. *28*:109–123, 1975.

32. Keys, A.: Nutr. Rev. *38*:297–307, 1980.

33. Belloc, N.: Prev. Med. *2*:67–81, 1973.

34. Scrimshaw, N.S., Young, V.R.: Sci. Am. *235*:50–64, 1976.

35. Vauy, R., Scrimshaw, N.S., Young, V.R.: Am. J. Clin. Nutr. *31*:771, 1978.

36. Watkin, D.M., Froeb, H.E., Hatch, F.T., et al.: Am. J. Med. *9*:441, 1950.

37. Tontisirin, K., Young, V.R., Miller, M, et al.: J. Nutr. *104*:495–505, 1974.

38. Gersovitz, M., Motil, K., Munro, H., et al.: Am. J. Clin. Nutr. *35*:6–14, 1982.

39. Vauy, R., Winterer, J.C., Bilmazes, C., et al.: J. Gerontol. *33*:663–671, 1978.

40. Winterer, J.C., Steffee, W.P., Davy, W., et al.: Exp. Gerontol. *11*:79–87, 1976.

41. Brenner, B.M., Meyer, T.W., Hostetter, T.H.: N. Engl. J. Med. *301*:652–659, 1982.

41a. Blachley, J.D.: Am. J. Med. Sci. *288*:228–234, 1984.

41b. Tobin, J., Spector, D.: Gerontologist *26*:59A, 1986.

42. Albrink, M.J.: Am. J. Med. *31*:4, 1961.

43. Carroll, K.K., Khor, H.T.: Dietary fat in relation to tumorigenesis. *In* Progress in Biochemical Pharmacology: Lipids and Tumors. (Carroll, K.K., Ed.) Karger, New York, 1975.

44. Wynder, E.L.: Diet and Killer Diseases with Press Reaction and Additional Information. Washington, D.C., U.S. Government Printing Office, 164–191, 1977.

45. Hill, P., Chan, P., Cohen, L., et al.: Cancer *39*:1820–1826, 1977.

46. Chan, P., Cohen, L.: Cancer Res. *35*:3384–3386, 1975.

47. Wynder, E.L.: Fed. Proc. *35*:1309–1315, 1976.

48. Bilheimer, D.W.: N. Engl. J. Med. *296*:508, 1977.

49. Mann, G.V.: N. Engl. J. Med. *297*:644, 1977.

49a. Kannel, W.B.: J. Am. Geriatr. Soc. *34*:27–36, 1986.

49b. Kritchevcky, D.: Postgrad. Med. *63*:133–137, 1978.

49c. Winterstein, G., Brook, J.G., Pillar, T., et al.: J. Am. Geriatr. Soc. *34*:569–572, 1986.

49d. McGandy, R.B.: *In* Health Promotion and Disease Prevention in the Elderly. (Chernoff, R., Lipschitz, D.A., Eds.) In press, 1987.

49e. Kannel, W.B., Gordon, T.: The Framingham Study. An Epidemiologic Investigation of Cardiovascular Disease, Section 27. Pub No 1740–0320. USDHEW, PHS, NIH, Washington, D.C., U.S. Government Printing Office, 1971.

50. Smith, L.E., Shock, N.W.: J. Gerontol. *4*:27, 1949.

51. Swerdloff, R.S., Pozefsky, T., Tobin, J.D., et al.: Diabetes *16*:161, 1967.

52. Andres, R.: Med. Clin. N. Am. *55*:835–846, 1971.

53. Rowe, J.W., Besdine, R.: Endocrine and metabolic systems. *In* Health and Disease in Old Age. (Rowe, J.W., Besdine, R.W., Eds.), Boston, Little, Brown and Co., 1982.

54. Hodges, R.E., Krehl, W.A.: Am. J. Clin. Nutr. *17*:334, 1965.

55. Minaker, K., Rowe, J.W.: Gastrointestinal system. *In* Health and Disease in Old Age. (Rowe, J.W., Besdine, R.W., Eds.) Boston, Little, Brown and Co., 1982).

56. Rowe, J.W., Shock, N.W., DeFronzo, R.: Nephron *17*:279, 1976.

57. Rowe, J.W.: Renal system. *In* Health and Disease in Old Age. (Rowe, J.W., Besdine, R.W., Eds.) Boston, Little, Brown and Co., 1982.

58. Schwartz, W.B.: Disorders of fluid electrolyte and acid base balance. *In* Textbook of Medicine, 15th Ed. (Beeson, P.B., McDermott, W., Wyngaarden, J., Eds.) Philadelphia, W.B. Saunders, 1979.

59. Beaumont, D.M., James, O.F.W.: Clin. Gastroenterol. *14*:811–827, 1985.

60. Schneider, E.L., Vining, E.M., Hadley, E.C.: N. Engl. J. Med. *314*:157, 1986.

61. Food and Nutrition Board: Recommended Dietary Allowances. 9th Ed. Washington, D.C., National Academy of Sciences, 1980.

62. Garry, P.J., Goodwin, J.S., Hunt, W.C., et al.: Am. J. Clin. Nutr. *36*:319–331, 1982.

63. Albanese, A.A.: Postgrad. Med. *63*:167–172, 1978.

64. Jowsey, J.: Geriatrics *32*:41–50, 1977.

65. Heaney, R.P., Gallagher, J.C., Johnston, C.C., et al.: Am. J. Clin. Nutr. *36*:986–1013, 1982.

66. Marcus, R.: Metabolism *31*: 93–102, 1982.

67. Gallagher, J.C., Riggs, B.L., Eisman, J., et al.: J. Clin. Invest. *64*:729–736, 1979.

68. Ireland, P., Fordtran J.S.: J. Clin. Invest. *52*:2672–2681, 1973.

68a. Cummings, S.R., Kelsey, J.L., Nevitt, M.C., et al.: Epidemiol. Rev. *7*:178–208, 1985.

68b. Recker, R.R., Saville, P.D., Heaney, R.P.: Ann. Intern. Med. *87*:649–655, 1978.

68c. Heaney, R.P., Recker, R.R., Saville, P.D.: J. Lab. Clin. Med. *92*:953–963, 1978.

68d. Nordin, B.E.C., Horsman, A., Crilly, R.G., et al.: Br. Med. J. *280*:4451–4454, 1980.

69. Allen, L.H., Oddoye, E.A., Margen, S.: Am. J. Clin. Nutr. *32*:741–749, 1979.

70. Margen, S., Chu, J.-Y., Kaufman, N.A., et al.: Am. J. Clin. Nutr. *27*:584–589, 1974.

71. Chu, J.-Y., Margen, S., Costa, F.M.: Am. J. Clin. Nutr. *28*:1028–1035, 1975.

71a. Seeman, E., Riggs, B.L.: Geriatrics *36*:71–76, 1981.

71b. Spencer, H., Kramer, L., Osis, D., et al.: J. Nutr. *108*:447–457, 1978.

71c. Spencer, H., Kramer, L., Osis, D., Norris, C.: Am. J. Clin. Nutr. *31*:2167–2180, 1978.

71d. Spencer, H., Kramer, L., DeBartolo, M., et al.: Am. J. Clin. Nutr. *37*:924–929, 1983.

72. Reinhold, J.G., Faradji, B., Abadi, P., et al.: J. Nutr. *106*:493–503, 1976.

73. Kelsay, J.L., Behall, K.M., Prather, E.S.: Am. J. Clin. Nutr. *32*:1876–1880, 1979.

74. Dietrick, J.E., Whedon, G.D., Shorr, E.: Am. J. Med. *4*:3–36, 1948.

75. Donaldson, C.L., Hulley, S.B., Vogel, J.M., et al.: *19*:1071–1084, 1970.

76. Aloia, J.F.: J. Am. Geriatr. Soc. *29*:104–107, 1981.

77. Zawada, E.T., Lee, D.B.N., Kleeman, C.R.: Postgrad. Med. *66*:91–100, 1979.

78. Heath, H., Hodgson, S.F., Kennedy, M.A.: N. Engl. J. Med. *302*:189–193, 1980.

79. Lindeman, R.D.: J. Am. Coll. Nutr. *1*:49–73, 1982.

80. Epstein, M., Hollenberg, N.K.: J. Lab. Clin. Med., *87*:411, 1976.

81. Rowe, J.W.: In Health and Disease in Old Age. (Rowe, J.W., Besdine, R.W., Eds.) Boston, Little, Brown and Co., 1982.

82. Lindeman, R.D.: *In* Nutrition, Aging, and Health. (Young, E.A., Ed.) New York, Alan R. Liss, Inc., 1987.

83. Watkin, D.M.: Handbook of Nutrition, Health, and Aging. Park Ridge, New Jersey, Noyes Publications, 1983.

84. Lynch, S.R., Finch, C.A., Monsen, E.R., et al.: Am. J. Clin. Nutr. *36*:1032–1045, 1982.

85. Monsen, E.R., Hallberg, L., Layrisse, M., et al.: Am. J. Clin. Nutr. *31*:134–141, 1978.

86. Hallberg, L.: Am. J. Clin. Nutr. *34*:2242–2247, 1981.

87. Sandstead, H.H., Henriksen, L.K., Greger, J.L., et al.: Am. J. Clin. Nutr. *36*:1046–1059, 1982.

88. Gregory, J.L., Sciscoe, B.S.: J. Am. Diabetes Assoc. *70*:37–41, 1977.

89. Spencer, H., Osis, D., Kramer, L., et al.: *In* Trace Elements in Human Health and Disease. Vol. 1.

90. (Prasad, A.S., Ed.) New York, Academic Press, 1976.

90. Turnlund, J., Costa, F., Margen, S.: Am. J. Clin. Nutr. *34*:2641–2647, 1981.

91. Bunker, V.W., Lawson, M.S., Delves, H.T., et al.: Am. J. Clin. Nutr. *39*:797–802, 1984.

92. Brin, M., Bauernfeind, J.C.: Postgrad. Med. *63*:155–163, 1978.

93. Horwitt, M.K.: Am. J. Clin. Nutr. *29*:569–578, 1976.

94. Vogelsang, A., Shute, E.V.: Nature *157*:772, 1946.

95. Toone, W.M.: N. Engl. J. Med. *289*:979–980, 1973.

96. Vracchio, J.F., Calenda, D.G.: N. Engl. J. Med. *249*:689–698, 1953.

97. Tappel, A.L.: Nutr. Today *8*:4–12, 1973.

98. Benson, H., McCallie, D.P.: N. Engl. J. Med. *300*:1424–1429, 1979.

99. Haeger, K.: Am. J. Clin. Nutr. *27*:1179–1181, 1974.

100. Tappel, A.L.: Am. J. Clin. Nutr. *23*:1137–1139, 1970.

101. Omdahl, J.L., Garry, P.J., Hunsaker, L.A., et al.: Am. J. Clin. Nutr. *36*:1225–1233, 1982.

102. Lee, C.J., Lawler, G.S., Johnson, G.H.: Am. J. Clin. Nutr. *34*:819–823, 1981.

103. Nutr. Rev. *43*: 78–80, 1985.

104. Parfitt, A.M., Gallagher, J.C., Heaney, R.P., et al.: Am. J. Clin. Nutr. *36*:1014–1031, 1982.

105. Iber, F.L., Blass, J.P., Brin, M., et al.: Am. J. Clin. Nutr. *36*:1067–1082, 1982.

106. Thomson, A.D., Baker, H., Leevy, C.M.: Am. J. Clin. Nutr. *21*:537–538, 1968.

107. Williams, R.D., Mason, H.L., Power, M.H., et al.: Arch. Intern. Med. *71*:38–53, 1943.

108. Baker, H., Frank, O., Jaslow, S.P.: J. Am. Geriatr. Soc. *28*:42–45, 1980.

109. Older, M.W.J., Dickerson, J.W.T.: Age Ageing *11*:101–107, 1982.

110. Garry, P.J., Goodwin, J.S. Hunt, W.C.: Am. J. Clin. Nutr. *36*:902–909, 1982.

111. Rosenberg, I.H., Bowman, B.B., Cooper, B.A., et al.: Am. J. Clin. Nutr. *36*:1060–1066, 1982.

112. Marcus, D.L., Freedman, M.L.: J. Am. Geriat. Soc. *33*:552–558, 1985.

113. Hurdle, A.D.F., Picton-Williams, T.C.: Br. Med. J. *2*:202, 1966.

114. Garry, P.J., Goodwin, J.S., Hunt, W.C.: J. Am. Geriatr. Soc. *32*:719–726, 1984.

115. Herbert, V., Jacob, E., Wong, K.T.J., et al.: Am. J. Clin. Nutr. *31*:253–258, 1978.

116. Garry, P.J., Goodwin, J.S., Hunt, W.C., et al.: Am. J. Clin. Nutr. *36*:332–339, 1982.

117. Smith, L.H.: N. Engl. J. Med. *298*:856, 1978.

118. Mengel, C.A., Greene, H.Z.: Ann. Intern. Med. *84*:490, 1976.

119. Jaffe, R.M. Kasten, B., Young, P.S., et al.: Ann. Intern. Med. *83*:824–826, 1975.

120. Mitchell, C.O., Lipschitz, D.A.: Am. J. Clin. Nutr. *35*:398–406, 1982.

121. Bowman, B.B., Rosenberg, I.H.: Am. J. Clin. Nutr. *35*:1142–1151, 1982.

122. Mitchell, C.O., Lipschitz, D.A.: Am. J. Clin. Nutr. *36*:340–349, 1982.

123. Trotter, M., Gleser, G.: Am. J. Phys. Anthropol. *9*:311–324, 1951.

124. McPherson, J.R., Lancaster, D.R., Carroll, J.C.: J. Gerontol. *33*:20–25, 1978.

125. Borkan, G.A., Norris, A.H.: Hum. Biol. *49*:495–514, 1977.

126. Vir, S.C., Love, A.H.G.: Gerontology *26*:1–8, 1980.

127. Master, A.M., Lasser, R.P., Beckman, G.: JAMA *172*:658–662, 1980.

128. Frisancho, A.R.: Am. J. Clin. Nutr. *40*:808–819, 1984.

129. Greenblatt, D.J.: J. Am. Geriatr. Soc. *27*:20, 1979.

130. Chernoff, R., Mitchell, C.O., Lipschitz, D.A.: Ger. Med. Today *3*:129–141, 1984.

131. Driver, A.G., McAlevy, M.T.: Am. J. Clin. Nutr. *33*:2057, 1980.

132. Mitchell, C.O., Lipschitz, D.A.: J. Parenter. Enter. Nutr. *6*:226–229, 1982.

133. Myers, M.A., Saunders, C.R.G., Chalmers, D.G.: Lancet *2*:261–263, 1968.

134. Lipschitz, D.A., Mitchell, C.O., Thompson, C.: Am. J. Hematol. *11*:47–54, 1981.

135. Roberts-Thomason, I.C., Whittinham, S., Youngchaiyred, U., et al.: Lancet *2*:368–370, 1974.

136. Weksler, M.E., Hutteroth, T.M.: J. Clin. Invest. *53*:99–104, 1974.

137. Adler, W.H.: *In* Assessing the Nutritional Status of the Aging—State of the Art, Report of the Third Ross Roundtable on Medical Issues. Columbus, Ohio, Ross Laboratories, 1982.

138. Bistrian, B.R., Blackburn, G.L., Hallowell, E., et al.: JAMA *230*:858–860, 1974.

139. Bistrian, B.R., Blackburn, G.L., Vitale, J., et al.: JAMA *235*:1567–1570, 1976.

140. Weinsier, R.L., Hunker, F.M., Krumdieck, C.L., et al.: Am. J. Clin. Nutr. *432*:418–426, 1979.

141. Lipschitz, D.A.: Primary Care *9*:531–543, 1982.

142. Kohrs, M.B., O'Hanlon, P., Eklund, D.: J. Am. Diet. Assoc. *72*:487–492, 1978.

143. Kohrs, M.B., Nordstrom, J., Plowman, E.L., et al.: Am. J. Clin. Nutr. *33*:2643–2656, 1980.

144. Lipschitz, D.A., Mitchell, C.O., Steele, R.W., et al.: J. Parenter. Enter. Nutr. *9*:343–347, 1985.

145. Banerjee, A.K., Brocklehurst, J.C., Wainwright, H., et al.: Age Ageing *7*:237–243, 1978.

146. Lipschitz, D.A., Mitchell, C.O.: J. Am. Coll. Nutr., *1*:17–26, 1982.

147. Katakity, M., Webb, J.F., Dickerson, J.W.T.: Hum. Nutr. Appl. Nutr. *37A*:85–93, 1983.

148. Lipschitz, D.A., Chernoff, R.: Unpublished data, 1985.

149. Ching, N., Grossi, C., Zurawinsky, H., et al.: J. Am. Geriatr. Soc. *27*:491–494, 1979.

150. Kaminski, M.V., Nasr, N.J., Freed, B.A., et al.: J. Am. Coll. Nutr. *1*:35–40, 1982.

151. Steffee, W.P.: Bull. NY Acad. Med. *56*:564–574, 1980.

152. O'Hara, J.G., Kennedy, S., Lizewski, W.: Can. Med. Assoc. J. *108*:977–980, 1973.

153. Dresser, R.S., Boisaubin, E.V.: Arch. Intern. Med. *145*:122–124, 1985.

154. Meyers, D.W.: Arch. Intern. Med. *145*:125–128, 1985.

155. Paris, J.J., Reardon, F.E.: JAMA *253*:2243–2245, 1985.

156. Siegler, M., Weisbard, A.J.: Arch. Intern. Med. *145*:129–131, 1985.

157. Mishkin, B.: Nutr. Clin. Pract. *1*:209, 1986.

158. Watts, D.T., Cassel, C.K.: J. Am. Geriatr. Soc. *32*:237, 1984.

159. Wood, J.S.: Clin. Geriatr. Med. *2*:601–615, 1986.

160. Wanzer, S.H., Adelstein, S.J., Cranford, R.E., et al.: N. Engl. J. Med. *310*:955–959, 1984.

161. Lo, B., Dornbrand, L.: N. Engl. J. Med. *311*:402, 1985.

162. Chernoff, R., Lipschitz, D.A.: *In* Clinical Nutrition, Vol. 2. Parenteral Nutrition. (Rombeau, J.L., Caldwell, M.D., Eds.) Philadelphia, W.B. Saunders Co., 1986.

163. American Medical Association: J. Parenter. Enter. Nutr. *3*:258–262, 1979.

164. Roe, D.A.: Geriatric Nutrition. Englewood Cliffs, New Jersey, Prentice-Hall, 1983.

165. Lamy, P.P.: Clin. Nutr. *2*:9–14, 1983.

166. Lamy, P.P.: Bull. NY Acad. Med. *57*:718, 1981.

167. Schmucker, D.L.: Pharmacol. Rev. *37*:133–148, 1985.

168. Roe, D.A.: Pharmacol. Rev. *36*:1095–1225, 1984.

*Chapter* **53**

# WORK AND EXERCISE

Eric Hultman, James A. Thomson, and Roger C. Harris

Interest in the relation between diet and activity, whether athletic, combatative, or occupational, is not new, although the current explosion of literature in the field would seem to suggest this. An adequate intake of foodstuffs is fundamental to the maintenance of health and to the survival of the individual. Reportedly both the Greeks and Romans were interested in the best foodstuffs for maximal performance, but it would be surprising if even earlier man did not have a similar interest in such matters. Understanding of the significance of different foodstuffs and rationalization of this to the energy requirements of different levels of activity, however, only really began in the last century with the work of the German physiologist Von Liebig.[1] Von Liebig considered that muscle proteins were the main provider of energy in working skeletal muscle, though by the end of the nineteenth century it was clear that this was incorrect and the main sources were in fact carbohydrate and possibly also fat.[2,3]

The first positive evidence of the importance of fat as a substrate for energy production during contraction of muscle was presented by Himwich and Rose.[4] This was in the form of respiratory quotient (RQ) measurements of muscle in dogs, which in the well fed state was found to be 0.92 at rest and 0.94 during exercise. Following 5 to 15 days of starvation these values decreased to 0.80 both at rest and during exercise. If one re-

members that oxidation of carbohydrate results in an RQ of 1.00 and fat 0.70, the results clearly indicated an increased utilization of fat by the muscle following starvation. A decade later, Christensen and Hansen in their now classic study of the influence of diet on work performance in man similarly observed a lower RQ both at rest and during exercise following a high fat diet, and a 30% reduction in endurance time compared to that when a mixed diet was given.[5] In contrast, a high carbohydrate diet resulted in an increase in exercise RQ, and although this did fall during the course of exercise (showing an increase in fat utilization), it never went below the resting value measured after the mixed diet. Endurance time after the carbohydrate diet was about twice that after the mixed diet.

Today it is accepted that some of the energy expenditure during exercise can also be derived from protein utilization especially when the work time is prolonged. The amount of energy covered, however, is only a few percent of the total, and in the isocaloric state carbohydrate and fatty acids constitute the major energy sources. Final proof of this was eventually provided by direct measurement of the different substrates in the working muscles using the needle biopsy technique introduced by Bergström and Hultman in the middle of the 1960s. Initially for the purpose of studying water and electrolytes in kidney patients,[6] the biopsy technique was subsequently used in the study of muscle glycogen in diabetic patients[7] and in studies of the local energy stores in normal muscle at rest and during exercise.[8-21] The introduction of the needle biopsy technique had a major, almost catalytic effect upon the growth of exercise biochemistry and physiology as scientific disciplines. In 1970 the closely similar liver biopsy technique was used to measure the second major carbohydrate store in the body.[22-26] In combination with muscle, blood, and respiratory measurements it became possible to obtain an almost complete picture of substrate utilization in exercising man.

An understanding of substrate utilization by the body during exercise and work is, of course, basic to a rational assessment of the nutritive needs of an individual. Today, with the rapid growth of recreational exercise, there is perhaps a greater awareness than ever before of the effects of adequate nutrition upon work performances. However, even among the most fastidious of us—the elite athletes and their trainers—there still exists a plethora of nutritive practices that would seem to owe more to the early work of Von Liebig than to any other subsequent studies.

## ENERGY SUBSTRATES AVAILABLE FOR WORK

When a muscle such as the quadriceps femoris is stimulated from rest to near maximal activity, the increase in rate of energy expenditure is approximately 300-fold. The energy used by the body to perform work is chemical, and the immediate energy source for the muscle contraction is adenosine triphosphate (ATP). ATP, however, is stored only in small amounts in the muscle cells (circa 5.5 mmol·kg$^{-1}$) and must be continually resynthesized from ADP and inorganic phosphate ($P_i$). The energy for rephosphorylation can be derived from several reactions that can be divided into those requiring oxygen, i.e., aerobic metabolism, and those that can proceed in the absence of oxygen, i.e., anaerobic metabolism.

Aerobic resynthesis of ATP occurs only within the mitochondria of the cells, the rate of synthesis being governed largely by the size and number of mitochondria per muscle cell and rate of oxygen uptake. Basic fuels that can supply substrates for oxidation are glucose transported from the liver via the blood, locally stored glycogen, and free fatty acids (FFA) taken up from the blood or to a limited extent derived from triglyceride depots within the muscle. Each of these fuels may be metabolized within the cytoplasm to smaller subunits, which then enter the tricarboxylic cycle within the mitochondria.

When oxidative energy production is insufficient to cover the expenditure as in the early stages of exercise before full readjustment of the blood supply or during very high intensity exercise, resynthesis of ATP is essentially anaerobic, and for this there are two metabolic pathways. The first is from phosphocreatine (PCr) which in the presence of creatine kinase can directly rephosphorylate ADP to ATP. The second route is from glycogen or glucose with formation of lactate. This is energetically far less efficient than when either substrate is metabolized completely to $CO_2$ and $H_2O$; anaerobic utilization generates only 3 ATP compared to 38 to 39 ATP per glucose unit when oxidized.

The contribution of the different fuel supplies to the total energy output by the muscle will vary both with the intensity and duration of the exercise and will be further influenced by the fitness of the individual, the nutritional status both before and during exercise, the level of anxiety, and even by the environment (altitude, temperature, and humidity). Morphologic differences between individuals in their muscle fiber makeup may also affect their use of the different fuels available during a standard exercise.

The maximum theoretical rate of utilization of a particular fuel for muscle contraction is determined by the activity of those enzymes concerned with its metabolism. Estimates of the maximum power available from phosphagen, carbohydrate, and fat utilization by muscle are presented here both as the maximum rate of energy phosphate ($\sim$P) that may be generated per kg of fresh muscle per second, and as the maximum rate calculated for the whole muscle mass. This is assumed to be 28 kg in a 70 kg man. Values in this latter case are given as mol $\sim$P per minute.

$$ATP, PCr \rightarrow ADP, Cr \qquad (1)$$

a. Max. rate of degradation: 2.6 mmol $\sim$P (kg muscle)$^{-1}$·s$^{-1}$ corresponding totally to 4.4 mol $\sim$P·min$^{-1}$

b. Amount available (quadriceps muscle): 24 mmol $\sim$P (kg muscle)$^{-1}$ totally 0.67 mol in 28 kg of muscle

The estimate of 2.6 mmol $\sim$P (kg muscle)$^{-1}$·s$^{-1}$ has been calculated from direct measurements in needle biopsy samples obtained from human quadriceps muscle during near maximum voluntary isometric contraction[27,28] or during tetanic electrical stimulation.[29] Other workers have suggested a figure nearer to 6 mmol $\sim$P (kg muscle)$^{-1}$·s$^{-1}$ based on less direct measurements.[30-32]

This is a figure close to the maximum velocity of creatine kinase measured in human muscle.[33]

$$\text{Glycogen} \rightarrow \text{lactate} \qquad (2a)$$

a. Max. rate of $\sim$P generation: 1.4 mmol $\sim$P (kg muscle)$^{-1} \cdot$s$^{-1}$corresponding totally to 2.35 mol $\sim$P$\cdot$min$^{-1}$

b. Amount available (quadriceps muscle): 240 mmol $\sim$P$\cdot$kg$^{-1}$ or totally 6.7 mol in 28 kg of muscle

The estimate of 1.4 mmol $\sim$P (kg muscle)$^{-1} \cdot$s$^{-1}$ was calculated from direct measurements of the metabolite changes during near maximum isometric contraction of the quadriceps muscle.[27,28] The total amount of $\sim$P available from glycogen was calculated, assuming that 90% of the normal store (i.e., 80 mmol glucose units$\cdot$kg$^{-1}$) is utilized[13] and that 3 mmol$\cdot\sim$P is formed per mol glucose in glycolysis. Total utilization of the muscle glycogen stores, however, never occurs, because of the increased acidosis in the muscle. According to Margaria et al., the accumulation of 1 mol of lactate is the maximum the body is able to tolerate.[34] This would limit the total amount of $\sim$P from anaerobic utilization of glycogen to 1.5 mol during heavy continuous work.

$$\text{Glycogen} \rightarrow CO_2 + H_2O \qquad (2b)$$

a. Max. rate of $\sim$P generation: 0.51 to 0.68 mmol $\sim$P (kg muscle)$^{-1} \cdot$s$^{-1}$ corresponding totally to 0.85 to 1.14 mol $\sim$P$\cdot$min$^{-1}$

b. Amount available (quadriceps femoris); 3,000 mmol $\sim$P$\cdot$kg$^{-1}$ or totally 84 mol in 28 kg of muscle

The limiting factor for the rate of glycogen oxidation is most probably mitochondrial electron transport determined by the availability of oxygen and/or the maximum velocity of the electron transfer mechanism. The rates of 0.51 to 0.68 were calculated assuming maximum rates of oxygen utilization available for glycogen oxidation of 3 l$\cdot$min$^{-1}$ in an untrained individual and 4 l$\cdot$min$^{-1}$ in a marathon runner. Aerobic glycogen degradation gives 38 mmol $\sim$P per mol glucose.

$$\text{Glucose} \rightarrow CO_2 + H_2O \qquad (2c)$$

a. Max. rate of $\sim$P generation: 0.22 mmol $\sim$P (kg muscle)$^{-1} \cdot$s$^{-1}$ corresponding totally to 0.16 mol $\sim$P$\cdot$min$^{-1}$

b. Total amount available: 18 mol $\sim$P

The maximum rate of utilization is very approximate and assumes a maximum output from the liver of 5 mmol glucose per minute of which 4 mmol$\cdot$min$^{-1}$ are available to the working muscles (calculated in this study as 11 kg).[20,35] During a short period of exercise most of this glucose will be derived from the utilization of liver glycogen, which corresponds to 500 mmol glucose totally in the resting state after a mixed diet.[36] This will amount to 18 mol $\sim$P.

$$\text{Fatty acids} \rightarrow CO_2 + H_2O \qquad (3)$$

a. Max. rate of $\sim$P generation: 0.24 mmol $\sim$P (kg muscle)$^{-1} \cdot$s$^{-1}$ corresponding totally to 0.4 mol $\sim$P$\cdot$min$^{-1}$

b. Amount available: in adipose tissues about 4,000 mol$\sim$P.

The maximum rate of $\sim$P generation, which was calculated by McGilvery,[37] is based upon experimental results published by Pernow and Saltin.[38] As pointed out by McGilvery, the low rate of $\sim$P generation from FFA oxidation must be due to a limiting step located before formation of acetyl CoA, since the later steps are also used when carbohydrates are oxidized.

## SUBSTRATE UTILIZATION IN RELATION TO WORK LOAD

The mechanisms by which the muscle cells regulate the use of the different fuels are complex. In essence FFAs constitute the main energy substrate at rest and are utilized in preference to carbohydrate, principally muscle glycogen, and at supramaximal work loads phosphagens are the major fuels. At no one work load, however, does the muscle utilize just one single fuel.

Some examples of energy demands during different types of exercise are given in Table 53–1. The rate of energy expenditure and the amount of energy needed for the activity will determine the choice of substrate. The table is modified from Fox,[39] who calculated that the maximum rate during a 100 m sprint was 2.6 mol $\sim$P$\cdot$min$^{-1}$. This is below the maximum rate obtainable from PCr breakdown but above that from anaerobic glycolysis. On energetic grounds, therefore, ATP and PCr will be obligatory fuels for this level of activity, though supply will be augmented by some anaerobic glycolysis. It used to be thought that during intense exercise there was an alactic acid period of up to 10 sec but we have recently shown that lactic acid accumulation may in fact begin within as little as 1.3 sec.[29] Other athletic activities dependent upon mainly PCr breakdown are shot put, tossing the caber, and hammer throw.

During a 400 m sprint PCr breakdown will again be necessary to meet the rate of $\sim$P expenditure (2.3 mol$\cdot$min$^{-1}$) but in itself is insufficient to cover the total energy requirement of 1.72 mol $\sim$P. To meet this demand some anaerobic glycolysis must

**Table 53–1.   Energy Demands and Fuels Used During Track Events**

| Activity | ~P used (mol) | Rate of ~P (mol·min⁻¹) | Fuel Combination |
|---|---|---|---|
| Rest (5 min) | 0.36 | 0.07 | Mostly fat |
| 100 m sprint | 0.43 | 2.6 | ATP & PCr |
| 400 m sprint | 1.72 | 2.3 | PCr & anaerobic glycolysis |
| 800 m run | 3.43 | 2.0 | PCr & anaerobic & aerobic glycolysis |
| 1,500 m run | 6.00 | 1.7 | PCr & anaerobic & aerobic glycolysis |
| 42,200 m marathon | 150.00 | 1.0 | Carbohydrate & fat |

Energy demand is modified from Fox, E.L.[39]

occur. The same is true both for 800 and 1500 m runs, but in these races total expenditure will exceed even the combined total possible from PCr breakdown and tolerable from the accumulation of lactate. At these distances energy demand will require also oxidative utilization of muscle glycogen. At ultra long distances such as the marathon the ATP turnover rate in an elite athlete lies just below the rate sustainable by aerobic utilization of carbohydrate; however, the total demand would require considerable utilization of fat as well.

The above calculations are of course drawn from athletic performances, but undoubtably the same spectrum of fuel utilization also exists in occupational work ranging from light office work to hard intermittent manual labor.

Because of delays in the mobilization of the different fuel sources and adjustments of the circulation, some utilization of PCr will occur whenever the rate of energy demand is suddenly increased. When the rate of energy demand, however, is less than the maximum rate from anaerobic glycolysis, resynthesis of PCr, even during continuation of the work, is possible. The increase in lactate and resultant decrease in pH will also affect the PCr level. This is because the increase in hydrogen ions will displace the equilibrium of the creatine kinase reaction towards creatine. Net utilization of PCr will therefore always occur when lactate is accumulating.

Accumulation of lactate is, however, self limiting, since the decrease in muscle pH will in turn inhibit further glycolysis and/or muscle contraction at the end of work with maximum power output. Under these conditions total utilization of the glycogen store will never occur. At work rates close to the subject's maximum oxygen uptake ($\dot{V}O_2$max) total glycogen utilization in the working muscles can occur (Fig. 53–1), and the amount of glycogen initially present will be a determinant of work capacity. If work is continued beyond this point, the work rate will decline as the muscles become progressively more dependent upon FFA and blood-borne glucose for their supply of energy. As previously discussed, the maximum rate

of ~P production from these two sources is appreciably lower than that from local muscle glycogen degradation.

During any form of prolonged exercise in excess of one hour, the utilization of fat will progressively increase with time due to increased availability of FFA. For instance, in a study of Ahlborg et al. a 4-hour exercise at a work load corresponding to 30% of $\dot{V}O_2$max resulted in an energy contribution by FFA of 37% during the first 40 min, and this increased to 62% during the final hour (Fig. 53–2).[40]

It should be noted that the estimates of maximal fuel utilization given earlier were calculated for a normal individual. In endurance trained subjects maximum fuel utilization from FFA can be higher due to an increased capacity to oxidize FFA.[41–44] Thus the maximum power output that can be sus-

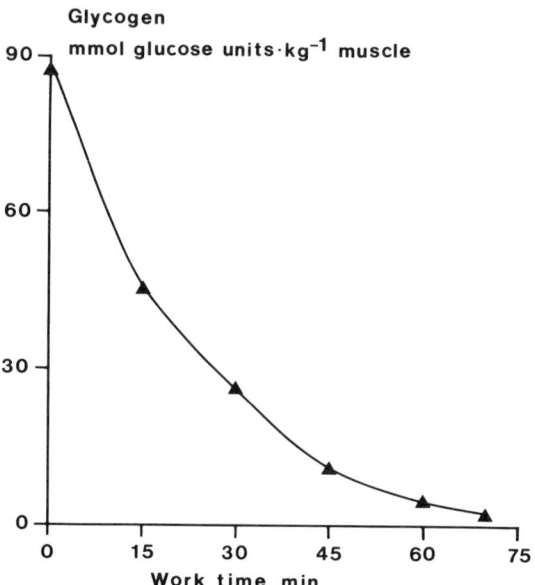

**Fig. 53–1.**   The glycogen content in the quadriceps femoris muscle during continuous bicycle exercise maintained at a load corresponding to 80% $\dot{V}O_2$max.[17] Each point is the mean value determined on 10 subjects. In each case the exercise was continued until exhaustion at which time depletion of the muscle glycogen stores was virtually complete.

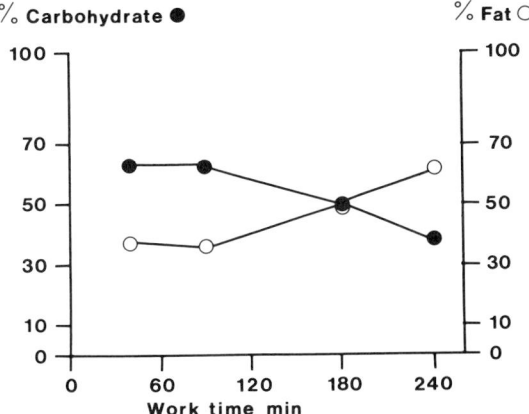

**Fig. 53–2.** The utilization of carbohydrate (predominantly muscle glycogen) and fat during prolonged exercise, i.e., bicycle exercise at a work load of 40% $\dot{V}O_2$max.[40]

tained by FFA utilization will be higher, increasing from 55 to 65% of the subject's $\dot{V}O_2$max. Above this level, however, work performance will still be limited by availability of muscle glycogen. The relation between glycogen degradation rate and work intensity is shown in Figure 53–3. The almost exponential rise in rate of glycogen degradation with increase in work load is consistent with: (1) high utilization of other energy sources

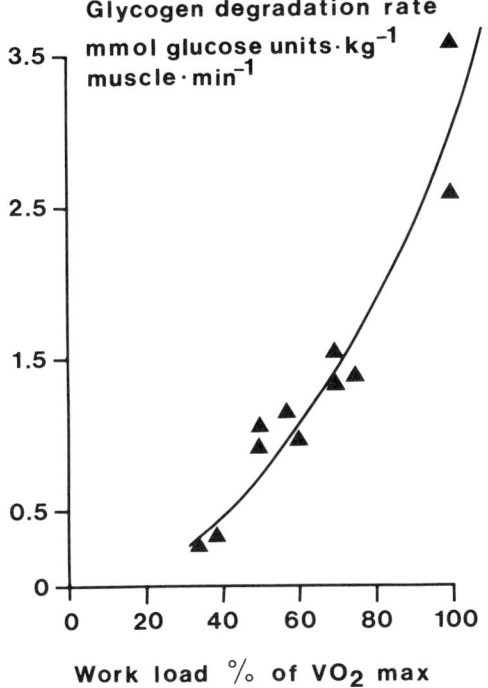

**Fig. 53–3.** The rate of muscle glycogen degradation during bicycle exercise sustained at different work loads.[45]

(predominantly fat) at low work loads; (2) principally oxidative utilization of glycogen at middle loads; and (3) rapid but energetically inefficient anaerobic utilization of glycogen at the highest work loads.

## UTILIZATION OF PROTEIN

The quantitative role of protein as an energy substrate in the isocaloric state is small, contributing at most about 5 to 10% of the total energy turnover. Nonetheless, during periods of prolonged exercise or training the degradation of protein can be of importance with respect to whole body homeostasis and as such merits further discussion here.

Recent studies have shown that there is an increase in the extracellular level of urea nitrogen during prolonged exercise[46–49] and an increased urinary output of urea during the rest period immediately after exercise.[48–51] In addition, measurements of the uptake and release of amino acids over the working muscles and over the splanchnic area and of the metabolism of isotopically labeled amino acids also indicate a significant contribution by protein to total energy turnover during exercise. Transport of amino acids from the working muscles in the form of alanine was first shown by Felig and co-workers.[52–54] The carbon skeleton of alanine was apparently derived from pyruvate and the amino group from deamination of amino acids in the muscle. It was also shown that branched chain amino acids were released from the liver and taken up by working muscle.[40]

It has been further shown that the carbon skeleton of the branched chain amino acid leucine is utilized for production of $CO_2$ during exercise[55–57] and that the rate at which this occurs is related to the work output.[58,59] Utilization of leucine, however, is modified by the amount of glycogen available in the muscles; a high glycogen content depresses the rate of leucine utilization.[47] Glucose infusion during exercise will also decrease the use of leucine,[58] whereas increased availability of FFA has been shown to have the opposite effect.[60] Apparently increased oxidation of fat as a result of increased availability of FFA or decreased utilization of carbohydrate during prolonged exercise will increase the oxidation of the carbon skeleton of branched chain amino acids, possibly by direct stimulation of the oxidative decarboxylation of the ketoacids formed.[60]

Possible sources of amino acids for energy production are the free amino acid pool in muscle or plasma or those released from protein catabolism. A decrease of the amino acids in plasma has been observed during prolonged exercise.[50,61,62] Similarly, Rennie et al. found a decrease in the content

of free amino acids in muscle at the end of prolonged exercise and calculated that the decrease
in the amino acid pool in plasma and muscle corresponded to 20% of the total nitrogen loss.[49] Thus
80% of the nitrogen in this study must have been
derived from the degradation of body protein. The
origin of this protein, however, is not known.
Studies of 3-methylhistidine excretion, as a
marker of muscle protein turnover, have given
conflicting results,[50,58,63] but generally indicate
that the contractile proteins are not broken down
in exercise bouts if there is no apparent damage
to the muscle cells. Studies of Millward et al. have
indicated that the liver may be an important
source of protein for utilization by the working
muscles.[58] Most probably the utilization of protein
as a fuel represents a general effect in which the
normal protein synthesis rate (about 300 g pro-
tein/day$^{-1}$)[64] is decreased and part of the amino
acids released through normal protein degradation is directed to the supply of energy in working
muscle cells. During recovery after prolonged exercise an increase in the rate of protein synthesis
has been observed.[49]

## ENERGY STORES
## AND EXERCISE CAPACITY

**Phosphagen.** At supra maximum loads with endurance times of just a few seconds energy supply
is mainly from utilization of phosphagen supplemented by anaerobic glycolysis. The phosphagen
stores, however, are seemingly impervious to dietary manipulation, and consequently there is no
easy way of increasing maximum power output
by this means.

**Carbohydrate.** At work intensities close to or
above the subject's $\dot{V}O_2$max lactate accumulation
with attendant decrease in muscle pH will inhibit
energy production and work output before depletion of the local glycogen stores. However, at work
intensities corresponding to 65 to 85% $\dot{V}O_2$max
the whole muscle store of glycogen may be utilized, if the exercise is sufficiently prolonged,
after which the power output from the muscle will
decline. In this range any increase in the muscle
glycogen store will help to improve performance.
Increased glycogen storage can, as will be discussed later, be achieved by one or more regimens
of exercise and diet.

**Fat.** Because of the almost limitless stores of
FFA in the well-fed individual, there are no
grounds for supposing that increase in the lipid
stores will increase endurance even during excessively prolonged exercise periods. The limitation to work at low work loads appears to be
due to factors other than the lack of substrate.
Onset of hypoglycemia can limit prolonged per-

formance, however, if the liver glycogen store at
the start of exercise is low and no carbohydrate is
taken during the work.

**Protein.** In contrast to fat and carbohydrates
there is no evidence today of any specific body
protein store available for exercise that can be increased by diet. A dietary effect of sorts, however,
is the protein sparing effect of carbohydrates as
shown by a lower utilization of protein at high
blood glucose levels and the presence of ample
glycogen in the muscle cells themselves[47,58]
Lemon and Mullin have shown that the protein
share of the energy substrates used during a 60
min exercise was 4% if the glycogen store in the
muscle was increased, but 10% if it was depleted
before the start of exercise.[47]

## NUTRITION FOR INCREASED
## WORK PERFORMANCE

**The Muscle Glycogen Store and Diet.** Initial
studies on the influence of diet upon the muscle
glycogen stores showed that the feeding of a
carbohydrate-rich diet or a carbohydrate-poor diet
or even total starvation over a period of days had
little effect upon the stores at rest (Fig. 53–4).[16]
There was, however, a remarkable difference between diets in the rate of glycogen synthesis when
feeding was preceded by depletion of the stores
by exercise. Total starvation or a carbohydrate-free
diet resulted in low rates of resynthesis, and normal values were not achieved for several days,
whereas a carbohydrate-rich diet resulted in a

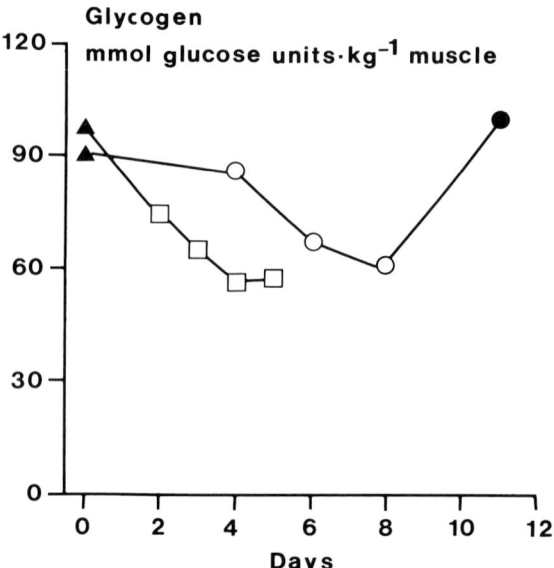

**Fig. 53–4.** Glycogen content in the quadriceps femoris
muscle after mixed diet: ▲ = during 5 days of total
starvation; □ and during 8 days of carbohydrate-free
diet; ○ = followed by a carbohydrate-rich diet. (●).[16]

rapid resynthesis to values above the normal range (Fig. 53–5). From studies in which one leg only was exercised it was shown that rapid resynthesis of glycogen to supernormal values was a local phenomenon restricted to the exercised muscles only (Figs. 53–6 and 53–7).[9]

The mechanism by which "supercompensation" in glycogen is brought about is not known. Enzyme studies have shown that the enzyme, glycogen synthetase, responsible for glycogen formation is transformed from inactive D form to active I form when the glycogen store is depleted. After one day of carbohydrate refeeding the I form is decreased to normal.[65] Other forms of the enzyme, intermediate between active and inactive, however, have been discovered[66] and these could account for the continuation of glycogen synthesis to supernormal values.[67]

The dramatic effect of increased muscle glycogen content upon work capacity is illustrated in Figure 53–8. In this study exhaustive exercise was repeated three times with three days' interval between bouts. The diet given before the first ex-

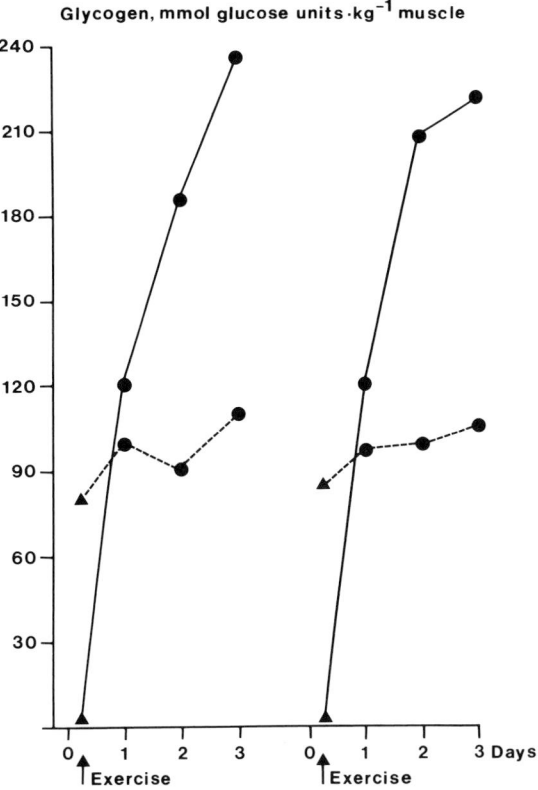

Glycogen, mmol glucose units·kg$^{-1}$ muscle

**Fig. 53–6.** One-leg exercise study showing the glycogen content of the exercised (——) and the rested (---) leg in two subjects. Biopsies were obtained immediately after the exercise and during 3 days during which subjects were fed a carbohydrate-rich diet.

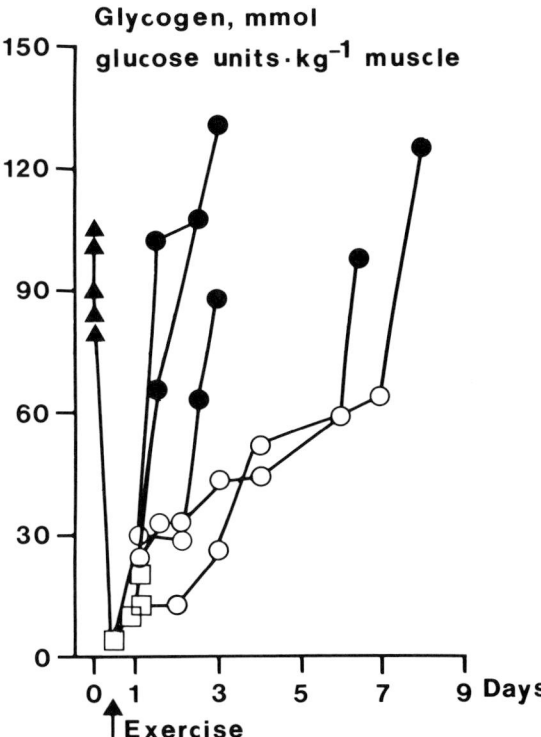

**Glycogen, mmol glucose units·kg$^{-1}$ muscle**

**Fig. 53–5.** Muscle glycogen content before and after exercise. Before exercise the diet was normal mixed (▲) and on the following days either total starvation (□) or a carbohydrate-free diet (○) was used followed by one or two days of a carbohydrate-rich diet (●).[16] Note the slow rate of glycogen resynthesis when the diet is carbohydrate-free compared to the rate when the diet is rich in carbohydrate. (See also Fig. 53–7.)

ercise was a normal mixed diet, and this was followed by a carbohydrate-free diet and finally (before the last exercise) by a carbohydrate-rich one.[18] The effect of the different diets was an increase in work time from 1 hour after the carbohydrate-free diet to 3 hours or more after the carbohydrate-rich diet. The study was originally done to demonstrate the relation between work capacity and the size of the muscle glycogen stores, but the method used to increase the muscle glycogen content has since been adopted as a procedure by athletes to increase these stores. A drawback to this regimen is that it leaves athletes with extremely low muscle glycogen stores for a period of 2 to 3 days, and this state could interfere with training. Sherman et al. have proposed a modified regimen of diet and exercise that avoids any period of carbohydrate-free diet, yet still results in equally high glycogen levels.[68] For subjects in regular training it is probably sufficient if they perform a depleting exercise twice during a period of mixed diet and thereafter change to a carbohydrate-rich diet during the final three days before

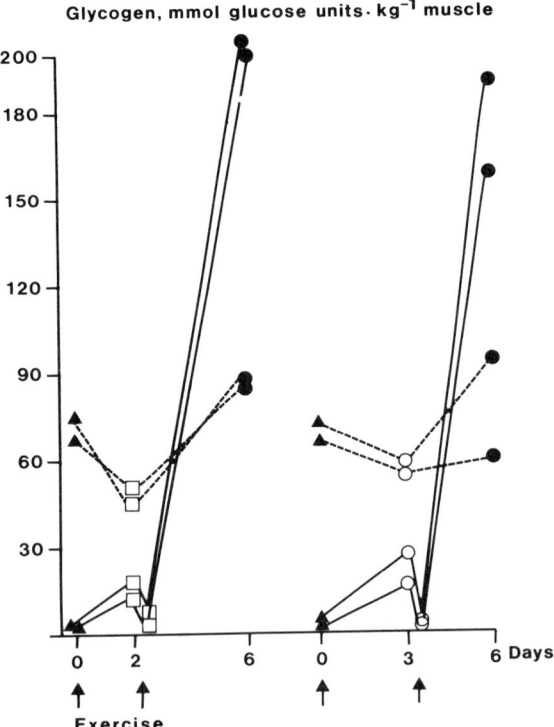

**Fig. 53–7.** The same "one-leg exercise" procedure as in Figure 53–6 showing the glycogen content in the exercised (——) and the rested leg (---). The diet was either total starvation (□) or carbohydrate-free diet (○) during 2 and 3 days, respectively. This was followed by a second one-leg exercise, and thereafter a carbohydrate-rich diet (●) was given.

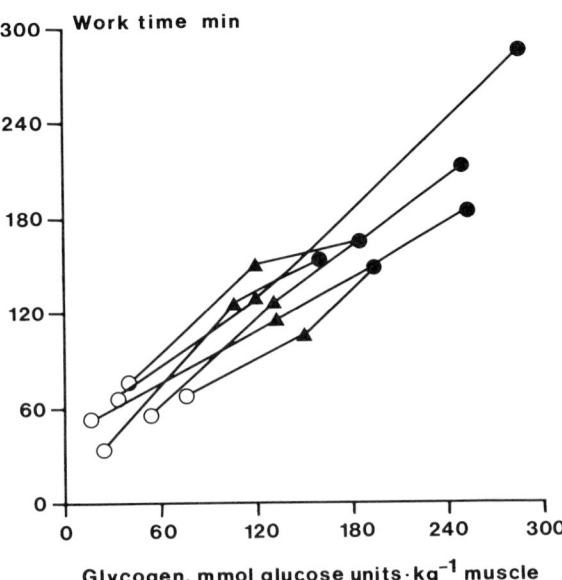

**Fig. 53–8.** The relation between the initial glycogen content in quadriceps femoris muscle and work time. Bicycle work was performed to exhaustion at a work load corresponding to 75% of $\dot{V}O_2$max. Each subject worked three times, and the experiments were preceded by 3 days of dietary regime: initially mixed normal diet (▲), followed by carbohydrate-free diet (○), and thereafter a carbohydrate-rich diet (●). The energy content of the diets was the same.[18]

competition. During the first two of these days light exercise can be done, leaving only the last day for total rest.

It should be noted that glycogen is stored in muscle together with water and potassium ions; 1 g (6 mmol) being associated with 2.7 g of water and 0.45 mmol of potassium.[21,69,70] As a result, supercompensation in glycogen will result in considerable increases in muscle water conent, which will increase body weight and may induce feelings of heaviness and stiffness in the muscle. Supercompensation cannot therefore be recommended to athletes needing only limited supplies of glycogen, e.g., sprinters.

**The Liver Glycogen Store—the Effect of Diet.** Unlike muscle, the liver glycogen store is extremely labile even in the resting state; the content in normal subjects following 12 to 16 hours of overnight fast varies from 90 to 500 mmol glucose units·kg⁻¹ liver tissue (circa 14 to 80 g glycogen).[36] This corresponds to a total liver glycogen store of 160 to 900 mmol glucose units in a 1.8 kg liver, which is the normal liver weight. Measurements of glycogen in repeated liver biopsy samples taken

in the postprandial state showed a continuous decrease amounting to 0.3 mmol glucose units·kg⁻¹·min⁻¹, from which it can be calculated that just one day of starvation would empty the liver glycogen store.[23] This was indeed found to be the case in two subjects from whom biopsies were taken after one day without food intake. The liver glycogen stores decreased from 155 to 24 and 345 to 48 mmol glucose units·kg⁻¹ In one of the two subjects the period of starvation was continued for a further two days with biopsies being taken each morning. Liver glycogen contents in these were found to be 15 and 21 mmol glucose units·kg⁻¹ (Fig. 53–9).[23]

It is known, however, that during even short periods of starvation there is an increase in both fat and protein degradation, which will result in an increase in gluconeogenic substrate brought to the liver. Evidently, this is not sufficient for de novo synthesis of glycogen to occur in the liver. To increase the supply of gluconeogenic substrates we gave a diet consisting of protein and fat with a caloric content of 8,400 kJ (2,000 kcal) per day. There was, however, still no increase in liver glycogen content during a 10-day period (Fig. 53–9).[23] When the diet was changed to one rich in carbohydrates with the same caloric content,

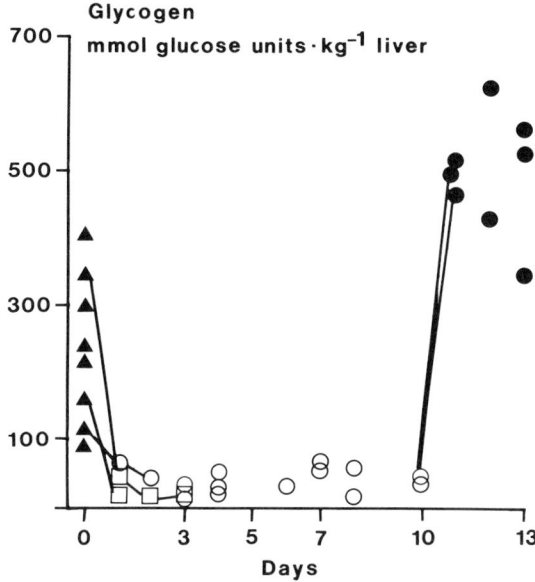

**Fig. 53–9.** The glycogen content in the liver determined in needle biopsy specimens from normal subjects after different diets: normal mixed diet (▲) followed by 1 or 3 days of starvation (□) or 1 to 10 days of carbohydrate-free diet (○). The period was ended by 1 or 3 days of carbohydrate-rich diet (●).

there was an immediate increase in liver glycogen content up to 500 to 600 mmol glucose units·kg.$^{-1}$ Carbohydrate intake through the diet is obviously necessary for preservation of the liver glycogen store. In these studies the fat and protein diet consisted of bacon, eggs, meat, vegetable oils, butter, and small amounts of tomatoes and lettuce, and the carbohydrate-rich diet contained 90% carbohydrate in the form of bread, spaghetti, potatoes, sugar, fruit, and juice. Spices and meat extract were added for taste.

The blood glucose concentration during fasting or during the period of carbohydrate-free diet decreased only marginally, from 5.2 to 4.3 mmol·l$^{-1}$ (94 to 77 mg/dl) after 10 days with the lowest value on day 5 to 3.8 mmol/l (68 mg/dl). Only light office work was done during the experimental period. The glucose output by the liver decreased, however, by 60%, which is the share normally derived from glycogen degradation.[24] The fact that the blood glucose concentration shows only a small change is the result of various adaptations in body metabolism, including an increased output of ketone bodies from the liver[24] and a shift from glucose utilization to ketone body oxidation by the brain.[71,72] Apparently this adaptation by the brain is a rapid process.

**The Liver Glycogen Store—Glucose Release and the Effect of Exercise.** During exercise glucose output from the liver increases. In one study of

heavy bicycle exercise a continuous increase in output was seen from 1 mmol·min$^{-1}$ before exercise up to 5 mmol·min$^{-1}$ during the last min of the work.[20] The average output over the whole of the exercise period was 2.4 mmol·min.$^{-1}$ In a further study in which liver biopsies were taken, one hour of hard bicycle exercise resulted in a mean glycogen degradation rate of 2.1 mmol glucose units ·kg$^{-1}$min$^{-1}$.[25] This means that up to half the normal liver glycogen store is lost during one hour of heavy exercise and that most of the glucose output is derived from glycogen and only a small fraction from the uptake and utilization of lactate, amino acids, and glycerol.

If exercise is performed after a carbohydrate-free diet, glucose output from utilization of liver glycogen is decreased and this decrease is only partially compensated for by increased glyconeogenesis. The effect, therefore, is a decrease in blood glucose content during exercise. This is illustrated by reference to the earlier mentioned study of Bergström et al. in which a pronounced decrease in blood glucose concentration was seen shortly after the start of the exercise performed after the period of carbohydrate-free diet.[18] The mean glucose content decreased during the first hour of exercise from 5.0 to 2.8 mmol·l$^{-1}$ (90 to 50 mg/dl) blood, and several of the subjects suffered from headache and dizziness during the later part of the exercise. In one of the subjects the work had to be stopped because of the effects of the low blood sugar blood content on the central nervous system. His blood glucose value was then 1.7 mmol·l$^{-1}$ (31 mg/dl), and he could not continue the exercise due to severe dizziness and headache. The corresponding blood glucose level after the carbohydrate-rich diet was 4.4 mmol·l$^{-1}$ (79 mg/dl) after 1 hour of exercise and 3.5 mmol·l$^{-1}$ (63 mg/dl) at the end of work (after 3 h).

Glucose production from gluconeogenesis is normally not increased during short-term exercise, but can increase during prolonged work to values nearly twice those of the resting level.[40] An increased rate of gluconeogenesis, however, does occur during short hard exercise if this is preceded by a period of carbohydrate-free diet,[35,73] although total glucose output, as previously mentioned, is still lower than after a normal mixed diet. After a carbohydrate-free diet approximately 50% of the glucose release from the liver can be accounted for by utilization of gluconeogenic substrates, whereas after a carbohydrate-rich diet the corresponding figure is only 5 to 10%. Following the carbohydrate-free diet an increase in oxygen uptake by the liver was observed,[73] which is consistent with the increased rate of glyconeogenesis, this being an ATP-consuming process.

In summary it would appear that dietary increase of the liver glycogen stores would be beneficial in most types of continuous or prolonged intermittent exercise/work. During work of several hours' duration a high level of liver glycogen will act as a buffer against development of hypoglycemia, which may lead to loss of central nervous function and exhaustion. One day of carbohydrate-rich diet before a competition is sufficient to produce high levels of glycogen in the liver.

## ENERGY REQUIREMENTS

**During Occupational Work.** The caloric need *at rest* has been calculated by Passmore and Durnin to be 105 kJ (25 kcal)·kg$^{-1}$ b.w.·day$^{-1}$ for men and 100 kJ (24 kcal)·kg$^{-1}$ b.w.·day$^{-1}$ for women.[74] The FAO/WHO defines of the energy needs for occupational work as indicated in Table 53–2.

These estimates are for subjects with body weights of 65 and 55 kg, respectively, and aged 20 to 39 years. Energy requirement decreases with increasing age; subjects aged 40 to 49 years require 95% of the above estimates, 50 to 59 years 90%, 60 to 69 years 80%, and above 70 years old 70%. These figures are similar to those presented by others such as Norgan and Ferro-Luzzi for Italian shipyard workers engaged in occupational work requiring light activity.[76] The same authors also studied horticulturalists in Papua-New Guinea and found a similar requirement in dietary energy of 160 to 190 kJ (38 to 45 kcal)·kg$^{-1}$ b.w.·day$^{-1}$. Total energy requirements are obtained by multiplying the above estimates by body weight. Thus, for occupational work with light activity, total daily requirements for a 65 kg man and 55 kg woman would be 10.9 MJ (10,900 kJ or 2,600 kcal) and 8.4 MJ (2,000 kcal), respectively.[75]

**During Exercise.** The energy requirement during athletic performance or training is of course determined by the type of activity and its duration. Several studies of the relative caloric costs of different sports have been published,[74,77] but no details of these will be given here; suffice to say that requirements vary from 12.5 MJ to 25 MJ (3,000 to 6,000 kcal), the higher values being for athletes engaged in high intensity endurance sports such as cross-country running or skiing and marathon running. High energy intakes of the same order are also required in the course of sports requiring intense repeated effort such as team sports (football, ice hockey, basketball), tennis, and fencing. In sports requiring sustained intense effort but over much shorter periods, such as swimming events over 100 yd, wrestling, downhill skiing, and running for 1 to 2 miles, the average daily expenditure is of the order of 12.5 to 21 MJ (3,000 to 5,000 kcal). The lowest energy requirement, up to 16.7 MJ (3,980 kcal) per day, is observed in low intensity sports of long duration such as baseball or golf, and when strenuous or maximal efforts are produced during very short periods, i.e., hurdles, long jump, 50-to-100 yd swimming events, discus, hammer throw, high jump, and javelin.

The total caloric need is influenced also by the body weight, the frequency of repetition of the event, and the length of practice during training. Training itself increases the daily caloric need by 5 to 40% depending upon the nature of the exercise and and length of practice (for further details see references[77]). The above estimates of energy expenditure have been adapted from Buskirk and are calculated to cover the caloric needs of 75% of all male subjects.[77] Women athletes require 10% fewer calories to cover the energy need for each type of sport, or during training.

## RECOMMENDED USE OF MACRONUTRIENTS DURING OCCUPATIONAL WORK

Estimates of energy expenditure during normal occupational work were given in the previous section. This energy can be derived from a variety of combinations of carbohydrate, fat, and protein.

**Carbohydrate.** Only carbohydrate may be totally omitted, since it can be synthesized from protein or glycerol contained in the food or from stores in the body itself. However, as discussed

**Table 53–2.   Energy Needs for Occupational Work***

| Activity | Men | Women |
|---|---|---|
| Light | 167 kJ · kg$^{-1}$ · day$^{-1}$ (39.8 kcal · kg$^{-1}$) | 157 kJ · kg$^{-1}$ · day (37.4 kcal · kg$^{-1}$ |
| Moderate | 192 kJ · kg$^{-1}$ · day$^{-1}$ (45.7 kcal · kg$^{-1}$ · day$^{-1}$) | 167 kJ · kg$^{-1}$ · day$^{-1}$ (39.8 kcal · kg$^{-1}$ · day$^{-1}$) |
| High | 225 kJ · kg$^{-1}$ · day$^{-1}$ (53.6 kcal · kg$^{-1}$ · day$^{-1}$) | 194 kJ · kg$^{-1}$ · day$^{-1}$ (46.2 kcal · kg$^{-1}$ · day$^{-1}$) |
| Exceptionally high | 257 kJ · kg$^{-1}$ · day$^{-1}$ (61.2 kcal · kg$^{-1}$ · day$^{-1}$) | 225 kJ · kg$^{-1}$ · day$^{-1}$ (53.6 kcal · kg$^{-1}$ · day$^{-1}$ 0 |

*From Ref 75.

previously, dietary carbohydrate is essential both for the maintenance of the liver glycogen store and for the rapid resynthesis of muscle glycogen. A loss of liver glycogen will result in decrease in the blood glucose content, and a lack of muscle glycogen will decrease the exercise capacity. Omitting carbohydrate from the diet for more than one day will result in increased ketone-body production, degradation of body protein, and loss of cations and water. These effects are counteracted by a minimum intake of about 100 g of carbohydrate (600 mmol glucose units) per day.

Generally, however, it is recommended that 55 to 60% of the energy content of the diet be included as carbohydrate. In a 70 kg man given a normal mixed diet, 70 to 150 g carbohydrate are stored as glycogen in the liver and 300 to 500 g in the muscles. The energy equivalents of these stores are 1.25 to 2.5 MJ and 5.0 to 8.3 MJ, respectively. As discussed previously, these stores may be greatly increased using a combination of diet and exercise. If the carbohydrate intake is higher than the capacity for storage and its immediate requirement as an energy source, transformation to fat and subsequent storage as such will occur.

To obtain optimal usage of carbohydrates these should be included in the diet as complex saccharides such as starch in bread, pasta, potatoes, rice, and cereals, and not as simple sugars such as glucose and sucrose. The reason is that starch and similar carbhoydrates are digested slowly in the intestine and absorbed over a longer time, with the result that a larger fraction is deposited in the glycogen stores and less as fat.

**Fat.** Fat in the form of FFA can be directly utilized as an energy substrate by most of the tissues in the body. Exceptions are the cells in the central nervous system (CNS) and the red blood cells. CNS cells are able to use both carbohydrate and ketone bodies if available, but the red blood cells and some other small cell compartments are totally reliant upon carbohydrate. FFA constitutes the largest energy reserve in the body and is stored in the form of triglycerides in adipose tissue. The store in an average 70 kg man amounts to about 9 kg, which corresponds to approximately 338 MJ (80,000 kcal). It is generally recommended that the diet should contain 8 to 10% of the total energy in the form of polyunsaturated FFA, and the total fat intake should not exceed 30% of the dietary energy.

**Protein.** Dietary proteins provide amino acids for the de novo synthesis of proteins and other tissue constituents in the body. Replacement of protein is a continuously ongoing process in the body. This results in a daily loss of nitrogen in the form of urea and amino acids, which must be covered by the intake of nitrogen-containing nutrients.

Amino acids taken up in the diet are used primarily for synthesis, but in excess they are rapidly degraded because there is no protein or amino acid store in the body. An intake in excess of the body's needs for synthesis of proteins will result in increased formation of urea, which is excreted via urine and sweat. The carbon skeleton of the amino acids, however, is retained and used as an energy substrate.

Energy production by the body is fundamental to life, and amino acids will be used preferentially as an energy source if the total intake of energy is lower than the amount needed. Calculation of the minimum requirement of protein in the diet thus requires that the caloric need is adequately met by other sources in the food. The mean daily utilization of body protein in a normal individual fed a protein-free diet is of the order of 0.45 g·kg$^{-1}$ b.w.[78] When a high-quality protein is given, such as egg protein, the efficiency of utilization is about 70%, which increases the estimate of protein required to 0.59 g·kg$^{-1}$ b.w. For the North American diet the average efficiency of utilization for the mixture of proteins ingested is still lower, with the result that the recommended protein intake is increased to 0.8 g·kg$^{-1}$ b.w.[78] A 70 kg man would thus require 56 g protein a day, and a 55 kg woman 44 g.

**Dietary Protein Intake in Different Diets.** The actual protein intake in the average Swedish diet with a energy content of 11.7 MJ (2,786 kcal) is 84 g of protein, corresponding to 1.2 g·kg$^{-1}$ b.w. for a 70 kg man. This is 50% higher than the recommendations by the Committee on Dietary Allowances and Food and Nutrition Board (RDA).[78] The energy value of the protein intake corresponds to 12% of the total content in the Swedish diet. The corresponding value for protein intake for Italian shipyard workers is 12.5 to 12.8%,[79] the mean Japanese diet is reported to contain 14.4% of the energy in the form of protein,[80] and the West German diet 11.1%.[81]

## PROTEIN REQUIREMENTS FOR ATHLETES DURING TRAINING

As discussed earlier, there is only a marginal increase in the utilization of protein during exercise. According to RDA no increase in protein intake is needed when energy output is increased during training or competition, or even during heavy exercise.[78] The increased loss of protein during prolonged heavy exercise/work was estimated by Lemon and Mullin to amount to only 4% of the total energy expenditure when performed with adequate levels of glycogen in both muscle and liver, but about 10% when these were depleted.[47] Similar figures were presented by Rennie et al., who calculated the contribution of amino acid oxidation as 4 to 8% of the total energy expenditure during prolonged exercise (3 ¾ h).[49] Thus if protein is to be increased during heavy endurance training, then it would seem reasonable to limit the increase maximally to 10% of the extra requirement of energy intake. Since the protein content of a normal diet comprises 11 to 14% of the total energy, then it will be sufficient to simply increase the amounts consumed to comply with the increase in energy requirement. No adjustment to the actual makeup of the diet will be required.

In calculating the increase in protein required, however, it was assumed that there is no preferential loss of essential amino acids (possible exception, leucine) and thus for dietary protein. If a preferential loss occurs, this would result in a negative nitrogen balance during longer periods of training, since the normal protein synthesis rate would decrease due to a lack of essential amino acids. Although there are a few studies in support of this,[46,51] most indicate that nitrogen balance is maintained during training,[83–87] and may even be positive during heavy weight training,[88] when subjects are given a moderate protein intake of 0.8 to 1.4 g·kg⁻¹·day⁻¹. In the study of Marable and his colleagues an increase in lean body mass of 2 kg was observed after 28 days of heavyweight training with a protein intake of 0.8 g·kg⁻¹·day⁻¹.[88] A protein intake of 2.4 g·kg⁻¹ resulted in a large increase in urinary nitrogen loss but the same rate of body protein synthesis. Similarly Torún et al. found that total body potassium, as an indicator of muscle mass, was unchanged or increased after 4 to 6 weeks of isometric exercise training when the subjects were given an egg protein intake of 1 g·kg⁻¹·day⁻¹.[83]

Much higher intakes of protein, however, are often seen in athletes. A dietary survey of Italian athletes showed an intake of protein corresponding to 17 to 18% of the energy content of the food or 2.2 to 2.8 g·kg⁻¹ b.w.[79] Laritcheva et al. reported a protein intake of 2.12 to 2.76 g·kg⁻¹ in weight lifters during training, though this decreased to 1.36 to 1.80 g·kg⁻¹ between training sessions.[89] Russian athletes studied by Rogozkin were recommended an intake of 13% of the dietary nutrients as protein for a total intake of 18.8 to 21 MJ, 12% for 23 to 27 MJ, and 11% at about 33 MJ.

The excess of protein in an athlete's food is often of the order of 100 g a day. If that protein were quantitatively used for muscle protein synthesis, muscle mass wold increase by 500 g a day. This is of course not the case. The extra protein taken will only increase the production and release of urea and thus increase the metabolic and excretory work by the liver and kidney. The calculation shows that extra intake of protein concentrates and protein pills, which is usual today among athletes and muscle builders, is of no meaning when the normal diet already contains protein in excess of that needed both for energy production and for muscle protein synthesis.

**Diet Composition.** Depending upon work rate, the recommended daily energy intake for men is 160 to 250 kJ (38 to 60 kcal) per kg b.w., and 130 to 220 kJ (31 to 52 kcal) per kg b.w. for women. Between 55 and 60% of the energy intake should be in the form of complex carbohydrates, 30% as fat (about half of which should be supplied as vegetable fat), and the remaining 12 to 15% in the form of high quality protein. Athletes in training can use essentially the same diet but with an increase in energy intake to meet the increase in energy expenditure. Exceptions to this are long-distance runners and cross-country skiers, who during prolonged bouts of training will need especially to increase their carbohydrate intake. In such cases 70 to 75% of the extra energy should be in the form of carbohydrate and a maximum of 10% as protein.

## DIET IN PREPARATION FOR COMPETITION

When an athlete is preparing for a competition involving prolonged heavy exercise of more than 60 minutes' duration, the muscle glycogen stores may be increased to maximum if the following program of diet and exercise is adopted. On the first day, i.e., 6 days before competition, an exhausting exercise should be performed, followed by 2 days of a carbohydrate-low diet with further bouts of exhausting exercise. Thereafter, a carbohydrate-rich diet (75 to 80% carbohydrate) should be given for 3 days during which no hard exercise should be performed. To avoid excessive depletion of the muscle glycogen stores, Sherman et al. recommended that the diet for the first 3 days should be a normal mixed diet (50% carbohydrate) after which the carbohydrate-rich diet is given. At the same time, shorter periods of exercise should be performed also on days 4 and 5, and rest taken only on the day preceding the competition. This procedure is probably sufficient for regularly training athletes.

For competitions lasting less than 1 hour a normal mixed diet will be adequate during the final day of preparation. The protein intake recommended in the normal diet is sufficient for resistance sports even during intensive training periods provided the total caloric intake is adequate to meet the energy needs.

On the day of competition a carbohydrate-rich meal should be given, but preferably at least 2 hours before the start of the event. Intake of rapidly absorbed sugars, notably glucose, prior to and during competition may result in increased release of insulin leading to a decrease in blood glucose levels, inhibition of FFA release,[91] and in the long run may evoke greater use of the muscle glycogen stores. In longer events of 2 or more hours' duration, where replacement of water and electrolytes will require increased intake, it has been shown that repeated intake of a glucose polymer solution can delay the onset of fatigue.[92] The carbohydrate-electrolyte solution should be taken in small amounts at frequent intervals.

## WATER AND ELECTROLYTE BALANCE IN PHYSICAL ACTIVITY

Water is of great importance to those performing physical activity. Indeed, it is the only nutrient whose lack presents an immediate and serious health risk, or even the possibility of death to the participant.[93–95] There is no question that dehydration can bring about a decrease in performance.[96] Water balance, therefore, should be of concern to all involved with physical activity.

**Role of Water.** The central role of water in the performance of exercise is a direct consequence of its involvement in the cardiovascular, metabolic, and thermoregulatory systems of the human body. During exercise, oxygen and fuel substrates must be delivered to the working cell, and metabolites removed. Consequently, a redistribution of cardiac output to the working muscles must occur. A consequence of the elevated metabolic rate of work is additional heat production, which must be dissipated if a tolerable increase in body temperature is to be realized. Therefore, the cardiac output is redistributed to the periphery for heat transport.[97]

In intense activity both the cardiovascular and thermal responses to exercise can become compromised. Inevitably, as exercise continues, the evaporation of sweat results in water loss to the body as a whole, and associated fluid shifts between the body's water compartments. Mounting water losses threaten the functional integrity of the systems and can bring about a decrease in performance, fatigue, or heat injury.[98,99,99a] The extent to which this occurs is governed by many factors, including the type and the mode of exercise, the intensity and duration of the work, the environmental conditions under which the work is performed, and the physical characteristics of the athlete (age, sex, weight, height, state of nutrition, hydration, and training).

Water metabolism during activity cannot be separated from the body's mineral balance. Water shifts between intracellular and extracellular spaces are accompanied by shifts also in sodium, potassium, magnesium, and chloride ions ($Na^+$, $K^+$, $Mg^{2+}$, $Cl^-$, respectively), and sweat losses provide a means for electrolyte loss as well.[100–102] Disturbance of water and electrolyte balance occurs not only during single exercise bouts, but also over prolonged periods of training.

**Types of Stress.** Two different situations stress water balance. In "make weight" sports such as wrestling, the competitor deliberately restricts his intake of food and fluid and strives to lose water by exercise, heat exposure, laxatives, and diuretics. The aim is to lower body weight rapidly and acutely, obstensibly to meet a smaller and weaker opponent.[103] This practice has been rejected for health reasons by professional associations.[96] Even so, the abuse continues and is prevalent in intense activities of brief duration that emphasize strength and coordination.

In contrast to such activities are endurance events such as road racing. These may last for several hours, and the exertional and environmental heat load imposed on the body may produce rectal temperatures in excess of 40.6°C.[94] Under such conditions athletes may lose fluid at rates of 2.0 to 2.8 $l \cdot h^{-1}$, resulting in a water deficit of 6 to 8% of body weight.[104,105,105a]

**Effects of Dehydration.** Numerous studies have been performed to assess the effects of dehydration on performance; the data reported include physiologic and biochemical variables and measures of muscular strength and endurance, anaerobic capacity, and aerobic power. Dehydration states have been produced thermally or in combination with exercise. The results depend upon the extent of the dehydration, which is expressed as the % body weight loss (%BWL).

As little as 2% BWL imposes an increased strain on the cardiovascular[106] and thermoregulatory systems[102]; a 2.5% decrease in plasma volume and a 1% decline in muscle water typically occurs for each 1% BWL. Plasma water accounts for 10 to 11% of the total water deficit.[100] Rectal temperature increased 0.4 to 0.5°C for each 1% BWL.[107] A 4% BWL has been shown to result in an approximate 30% decline in isometric and isotonic strength[108] through peak isokinetic torque declined only 13% when an 8% BWL was induced by food and fluid restriction.[103] However, 5% BWL, was without effect in an anaerobic cycling test,[109] and no impairment was noted at 8% BWL in an anaerobic running test.[103] A 4 to 5% BWL produced no change in $\dot{V}O_2$max, although a decrease in the maximal work time was seen.[106] Similarly, during activities of long duration, dehydration has invariably been reported to result in a decreased ability to work.[96,99,105,106,110] In other studies a decreased capacity is strongly suggested.[101,107] No positive benefits of weight reduction by hypohydration have been shown.

Electrolyte shifts have been reported with a 5.8% BWL, but calculations do not suggest any alteration in cell membrane potential.[100] Electrolyte losses occur together with water loss, but since sweat is hypotonic, the loss in water exceeds the loss of $Na^+$, $K^+$, $Mg^{2+}$, or $Cl^-$. The net result is that the plasma becomes hypertonic. The principal ions lost in sweat are $Na^+$ and $Cl^-$. A sweat loss causing a 5.8% BWL was found to produce a deficit of 5.7% in body $Na^+$ and $Cl^-$, but a 1% loss of $K^+$ and $Mg^{2+}$.[99] This small reduction in body stores is unlikely to lead to any impairment in neuromuscular function.

**Replacement Strategies.** Rehydration strategies to prevent, compensate for, or replace water loss are important in avoiding hypohydration. The aim of rehydration is either to quickly replace and reestablish water and electrolyte balance, as in the case of a dehydrated performer about to enter an event, or to prevent or retard water loss that occurs during an endurance event. Studies reveal that several factors are involved in fluid replacement, such as fluid composition, drinking frequency, volume intake, and fluid temperature.[111] The rate of gastric emptying provides a measure of rehydration efficiency, since almost all absorption of sugar, electrolytes, and water proceeds from the intestine.[105]

*Effect of Fluid Composition.* Sugar concentrations (glucose, sucrose, fructose) above 25 g·l$^{-1}$ significantly retard gastric emptying, thus preventing rapid rehydration. If water replacement is not a priority, more concentrated sugar solutions can be useful in providing a slow release of energy to the body over a prolonged period.[99] Because the fluid's osmolarity should be kept low (200 mOsmol·l$^{-1}$), salt concentrations at or below 20 g·1$^{-1}$ (10 to 30 mmol·1$^{-1}$) are recommended.[94,105,110] At these low concentrations electrolyte composition appears neither to help nor to hinder gastric emptying.[111]

*Fluid Volume.* Although large volumes of ingested fluid (up to 600 ml) increase the emptying rate, gastric discomfort may result. Drinking 150 to 250 ml every 10 to 15 min would therefore seem to be appropriate.[111]

*Fluid Temperature.* Chilled fluids (6 to 12°C) empty from the stomach more quickly than warm ones and can reduce body temperatures.[107,111]

*Drinking Schedule.* It is recommended that 400 to 500 ml of fluid be taken 10 to 15 min prior to competition,[94] although this does not replace the need for drinking during the event.[107] Rapid rehydration after dehydration can precipitate diuresis,[112] hyperhydration 40 to 80 min before an event produces a similar result.

*Electrolyte Replacement.* Hypertonic solutions of any kind, including the use of salt tablets, are not recommended, since they cause a fluid shift into the gastrointestinal tract.[110] Similarly, potassium supplements are considered dangerous.[113]

**Efficacy of Rehydration.** Rehydration before or during an event has been shown to be of significant benefit. Consuming 150 ml of fluid every 10 min during a 2 h cycling task in the heat dramatically limits the reduction in plasma volume, elevation of heart rate, and increase in body temperature.[99] Rectal temperature was about 0.7°C lower at the end of 2 h exercise when 200 ml of fluid was drunk every 20 min.[107]

The problems of dehydration may be partially alleviated during activity by the availability of water produced by metabolism and liberated during the breakdown of glycogen. Similarly, $K^+$ is released as glycogen is used.[11,21,69] These effects should help in maintaining fluid and electrolyte balance during exercise. Carbohydrate oxidation provides more metabolic water than does fat metabolism, and as the fuel source shifts in favor of muscle glycogen at higher work loads, plasma volume and thermoregulatory control are maintained. In practice, however, production of metabolic water has been shown to play only a minor role.[114]

Unfortunately, rehydration is often only partially complete during exercise; during moderate to heavy work, a water deficit occurs that canot be matched by increased fluid intake.[105a,111,115] Inevitably, there is a delay in drinking sufficient fluid because of increased exercise/thermal stress. This is termed *involuntary dehydration*.[116] Rules of a given event may also impede drinking.[92] Between 800 to 1500 ml·h$^{-1}$ of fluid can be replaced,[110,111] but fluid deficits of 400 to 800 ml during even light exercise (with free drinking) have been reported.[116] Forced drinking before the onset of thirst may be undertaken to minimize dehydration.[99]

It has been reported that after thermal dehydration even a 4 h rehydration period is insufficient to restore fluid and electrolyte balances.[112] During repeated, heavy exercise normal fluid balance was regained within 12 h, but sodium conservation by the kidneys continued for 24 h.

Recovery of performance following acute dehydration is still not complete after 3 to 4 h of rehydration. At such time isometric and isotonic endurance are still impaired by 13% and 21%, respectively.[108]

**Training Adaptation and Its Implications.** In response to endurance training and heat exposure athletes adapt and improve their work-heat tolerance.[117] Hypervolemia develops over several days of prolonged training or with three or more bouts of very intense, intermittent work. This expansion of plasma volume may contribute to the cardiovascular and thermoregulatory adaptations resulting from training.[118–120] These adaptations reduce the extent of body fluid shifts during exercise in the trained person.[98] Sweat rates increase as an adaptive response.[116,117,120] but water and electrolyte balances appear to be maintained. Together with an increase in voluntary fluid ingestion, the effect is a reduction in fluid deficit during work.[116] Hormonal control mechanisms operate to cause renal conservation and minimize the disturbance of water and electrolyte balance.[115,119] Indeed, given free access to food and fluid, trained runners have been shown to be able to maintain body weight and normal fluid balance during 20 days of severe prolonged exercise in warm temperatures.[115]

Concern about mineral depletion, in particular that of $K^+$, during exercise has been expressed. During short-term heavy exercise an increase in plasma $K^+$ is frequently seen together with a loss of intracellular $K^+$. The loss in intracellular $K^+$ follows, however, the degradation of glycogen; 0.4 mmol $K^+$ is lost per g of glycogen.[11] Studies have shown that subjects lost less than 2% of their total body potassium during four days of heavy exercise and sweating, even though they were consuming a diet low in $K^+$.[121] The very small loss in $K^+$ was accounted for by a reduction in $K^+$ excretion. Plasma $K^+$ concentration during chronic exercise may decline somewhat as a result of expanding plasma volume,[121] or show little change.[115] It would seem that $K^+$ depletion is not a concern within the normal range of diet and exercise levels.

Fluid ingestion before and particularly during intense, prolonged endurance activity will reduce the debilitating effects of dehydration and offer protection against exertional heat injury. Dehydration at the level of 4 to 8% of body weight decreases performance, and this loss cannot be completely restored in a 4 h period. Effective replacement fluids should contain only low concentrations of sugar and salt; if these are present at all, fluids should be served chilled and drunk in small amounts at frequent intervals. It may take from 12 to 24 h to reestablish normal water and electrolyte balance after cessation of intense exercise and/or thermal stress. Given normal food and fluid intake, however, this balance can be restored and maintained even during chronic exercise exposure by the neurohormonal regulation processes of the body.

## IRON BALANCE IN PHYSICAL ACTIVITY

Iron balance and metabolism in humans has been recently reviewed;[122,123] the subject is complex and is not fully understood yet. Its importance to persons engaged in physical activity derives from the central role of iron in cell metabolism. Iron is essential in the transport and delivery of $O_2$ to the mitochondria of the working cell via the proteins hemoglobin and myoglobin. It is also a component of many other protein systems, including the cytochromes and $\alpha$-glycerophosphate oxidase.[124] Iron deficiency, with or without anemia, is widespread in the population and is generally associated with decreased work performance[125] and other discomforting symptoms.[122] The ambiguous term "sports anemia" is used in connection with iron deficiency and exercise to imply both suboptimal performance and an exercise-induced causation.[125,126]

**Incidence of Iron Deficiency in Athletes.** Surveys of athletic groups have shown that both males and females, particularly those involved in intense endurance sports, have hemoglobin concentrations in the low to mid range of the population norms.[125,127–132] The number of athletes with clinical anemia, however, is low though significant; to cite two studies, 11% of the females in a small group[130] and 10% of the males and no women in a larger sample[128] had anemia.

A few studies have followed hematologic parameters in subjects during repeated bouts of exercise training. As the intensity or the total amount of physical activity sustained was increased, a temporary dilutional- or pseudoanemia was observed, based on hemoglobin levels.[133–135] This may be an initial response only, since a return toward normal values has been seen after eight to nine weeks of training.[136] No alterations were reported over ten weeks of cycle training.[137] The type of training, however, appears to influence the change in iron status; runners training at high intensity and over long distances appear more prone to developing low concentrations of hemoglobin in blood.[135,138]

Serum ferritin, transferrin saturation, and bone marrow iron are sensitive indicators of prelatent and latent iron deficiency and are used in assessing the state of the tissue iron stores.[122] From the measurement of these it has been found that many endurance runners, both male and female, are at risk to depletion of the iron stores. Studies using a range of sample sizes have reported 8 to 58% of male athletes and 40 to 80% of female athletes to be iron deficient.[125,128,130,135,138,138a,139,139a,139b] Since running elevates serum ferritin levels, the actual incidence could be even higher.[135] The extent of iron deficiency in athletes is clearly far higher than in the general population.[130,135]

**Factors Influencing Iron Balance in Exercise.** Several mechanisms have been proposed to account for the diminished iron status seen in athletes. The dilutional pseudoanemia seen in the early stages of training most likely reflects exercise-induced hypervolemia and as such is of no real concern.[118,120,131,133,135] Destruction of erythrocytes at this stage has also been suggested.[126]

Clearly, inadequate ingestion of iron to meet body needs could be a potential cause, particularly in rapidly growing adolescents, most notably in females and those engaged in activities that by their nature encourage dieting and low body weights.[128,130] Exercise has been shown to interfere with the normal increase in iron absorption, which occurs when the iron stores are depleted.[132] Increased elimination of iron in athletes has also been shown,[132] and a high sweat loss of iron is thought to be important.[132,139,140] Accelerated hemolysis, hemoglobinuria, hematuria, and fecal loss have been suggested and do occur,[126,128,129,134,138] but the importance of these has been questioned.[133]

Magnusson, Hallberg, and co-workers have carried out the most comprehensive studies to date on iron metabolism and sports anemia in male endurance athletes. They dismiss three commonly held views of the iron-exercise interaction:[126a] i.e., that sports anemia is an adaptation to reduce peripheral vascular resistance, is caused by increased mechanical destruction of red blood cells, and is due to enhanced iron loss. Instead, they view sports anemia as an altered iron metabolism, emphasizing liver hepatocytes as an adaptation strategy to large training volumes by elite runners.[140a] These workers show that no true sports anemia exists and that their athletes are not iron deficient when all markers of iron status are considered.[138a]

**Effects on Performance.** The ability to perform aerobic work has been studied over a wide range of hemoglobin levels from severe anemia to induced erythrocythemia, or blood doping.[141,141a,142] It it clear that $\dot{V}O_2$max and the capacity for intense endurance work are correlated with hemoglobin concentration in anemia. It is less certain, however, how work capacity and $\dot{V}O_2$max are affected when hemoglobin levels are above those for clinical anemia.[125] Compensatory mechanisms (total blood volume, total blood hemoglobin, circulatory adjustments, 2,3-bisphosphoglycerate concentration) come into play, so that variations in hemoglobin concentration within the normal range may have little real effect on performance.[131,141,141a,142] Recent results from blood doping studies suggest that hemoglobin levels below the mean of the population are suboptimal for maximum athletic performance.[125,142] Reinfusion of blood into trained athletes was first shown by Ekblom et al. to significantly increase both $\dot{V}O_2$max and work performance,[143] but the results were not so clear in a later study.[142]

Impairment of work performances due to iron deficiency, but without anemia, has been shown in rats,[124] but not so far in man. In the rat studies this was attributed to low activity of α-glycerophosphate oxidase and marked lactate accumulation due to enhanced anaerobic energy production in the iron-deficient state.

**Treatment of Iron Deficiency.** When iron deficiency anemia has been diagnosed in athletes, oral iron therapy has corrected the condition, and athletic performance has improved.[129,130] Oral iron treatment for iron deficiency without anemia has shown more inconsistent results. Hematologic variables of elite long-distance runners failed to show uniform improvement with iron therapy over a two-year period during which a rich dietary source and supplemental iron were given. Iron stores remained depleted, although iron balance was maintained.[132] Iron supplementation restored measures of mild iron deficiency to normal and lowered blood lactate levels during maximal exercise after iron therapy, but it had no effect on performance.[143a] When iron deficiency has not been diagnosed, iron supplementation has had little or no effect on hematologic measures or performance.[125,131,138,144]

Endurance athletes of both sexes, particularly runners who undergo prolonged, intense training, are suspectible to iron deficiency, with or without anemia. Impairment of performance may result. Iron status should be monitored regularly by serum ferritin and hemoglobin analysis. If latent or manifest iron deficiency is seen, supplemental oral iron treatments appear justified. When several measures of iron status reveal no true iron deficiency, routine iron supplementation is not indicated.[140a] A diet rich in iron, ascorbic acid, meats and protein, cobalamin and folacin should be consumed, to maintain iron balance and to prevent the occurrence of sports anemia and suboptimal hemoglobin levels.

## SELECTED VITAMINS AND OTHER MINERALS AND PHYSICAL ACTIVITY

The use of selected vitamins and other minerals remains controversial. The conservative recommendations of most recognized scientific authorities contrast sharply with the practice of athletes and coaches who experiment with a wide range of diets and supplements in the hope of maximizing performance. There is no doubt that physical work capacity is reduced by deficient nutrition and that an adequate diet is an important base for optimal work performance. Yet in over four decades of investigation, conflicting opinions still exist as to whether physical activity itself increases nutrient need above population norms, or whether levels of certain vitamins taken in excess of need can positively affect performance. In part, the confusion arises from the fact that experimental studies in this area are difficult to design.

Critical reviews of the literature relating to nutrition and exercise show a consensus with respect to recommendations on vitamins.[145,145a,146] Since one review is complete,[146] only recent work will be cited in the brief comments concerning selected vitamins and minerals.

**The Vitamin B Complex.** Thiamin, riboflavin, and niacin are three of the "energy releasing" vitamins functioning as cofactors in energy metabolism. In both the United States and Canada, daily recommended nutient intakes are related to energy intake.[147] If the demands of training increase the athlete's energy intake, the intake of these vitamins should also be increased, but in the same proportion as in the general population. The typically high protein intake of athletes suggests that sufficient niacin will in most cases be ingested.

Studies have suggested that a biochemical deficiency in thiamin and riboflavin and in pyridoxine can occur in groups of athletes.[148–151] This may be caused by the activity itself resulting in an increased elimination.[149] The riboflavin requirements of an active group were found to be higher than current standards needed for maintenance of normal activity of erythrocyte glutathione reductase.[150] Exercise increases the circulating levels of pyridoxine and pyridoxal phosphate, but it is uncertain if this increase has any effect on pyridoxine requirements.[151] It is still not clear whether a deficient state in any of these B vitamins has a negative effect on high intensity exercise[148] or if increases above physiologic need augment performance.

Cobalamin (vitamin $B_{12}$) supplementaion by athletes has been reported, though vitamin $B_{12}$ supplementation appears to have no effect upon performance.[152,153]

**Ascorbic Acid.** Because of its association with stress, such as exercise, and it's general notoriety, ascorbic acid supplementation has been recommended for athletes. This advice follows mainly from older work of European origin and perhaps reflects low dietary levels within the population studied as well as experimental design problems. One study used 1 g doses administered daily for two weeks following two weeks of placebo administration. No effect on work output was seen, but the administration of ascorbic acid resulted in a lower heart rate with exercise and lower blood glucose concentrations; an increase in plasma FFA. Training effects, however, would also have explained these findings.[154] Other studies, most of which are recent work employing more rigorous designs, suggest that little benefit to performance is gained with ascorbic acid supplementation.[155–157]

**Vitamin E.** The influence of this controversial vitamin on physical activity has been the subject of many investigations. Recent studies have uniformly failed to show any effect upon performance by vitamin E supplementation.[158–161]

**Excess Ingestion.** The toxic effects of overdoses of vitamins A and D are well known.[162] Disorders have been attributed to the ingestion of vitamin E in doses above 800 mg daily.[163] Ascorbic acid has been shown to destroy cobalamin (in vitro); it was suggested that daily doses of ascorbic acid should not exceed 500 mg.[164] Intake of large amounts of niacin are known to block the release of FFA from adipose tissue. This has been shown to increase the use of muscle glycogen during prolonged exercise and is experienced as earlier development of fatigue.[165]

**Minerals.** Several minerals serve as cofactors in enzyme systems that are involved in energy metabolism (e.g., zinc in lactate dehydrogenase, copper in cytochrome $aa_3$) or function in other important roles related to work (e.g., copper involvement in hemoglobin synthesis). Since sweat is one mechanism for loss, mineral balance for athletes in heavy training and/or a warm climate is of some interest. The diets of athletes, although rich in carbohydrate, may be poor in certain minerals such as zinc.[166] At present, few studies have been published, though there have been some recent reports of mineral deficiency in athletes involving zinc[166] and magnesium.[167] There is no agreement as to which biochemical indices related to performance or how and to what degree body levels of minerals affect exercise performance.

Plasma and erythrocyte concentrations of magnesium, copper, and zinc have been investigated to determine if a relationship to $\dot{V}O_2max$ exists.[168] Plasma magnesium, but not copper or zinc, was found to be weakly associated with $\dot{V}O_2max$ in athletes. A relatively high loss of copper by sweating has been shown, but sweat loss represents only a small percentage of the daily intake for zinc and iron[169] and magnesium.[99] A homeostatic conservation mechanism for zinc, which regulates whole body sweat loss in relation to varied zinc intake, has recently been indicated.[170] The results to date do not support the view that physical training interferes significantly with the status in the body of this second group of minerals.

In some athletes it is currently in vogue to supplement the diet with "pangamic acid" ("B[15]"; calcium gluconate and N, N-di-methylglycine). This may be considered also as calcium supplementation. However, no significant changes in short-term maximal treadmill performance were seen with "pangamic acid" supplementation in a recent, well-controlled study.[171]

**Conclusions.** At present, it appears that physical training does not increase vitamin or mineral requirement beyond levels that can be met by a balanced and adequate diet. Current research has failed to show any enhancement of performance when vitamin and mineral supplements are given in megadoses.[171a] Since excessive levels of nutrients can be toxic and nutrients in very high dosages may produce adverse side effects, megadose supplementation of vitamins or minerals cannot be recommended.

## SUMMARY AND COMMENTS

The recent interest concerning nutrition and diet in work and exercise stems not so much from our interests in occupational work but from those of high caliber training and competition in sports. It seems that we have come full circle from the times of the Greeks and Romans. Today's elite athlete experiments with a wide range of so-called ergogenic aids, including nutrients and foodstuffs, in what is often an irrational attempt to succeed.[172] It is at this level of exercise, which in the modern world places the greatest degree of physical stress on the human body, that the connection between nutrition and performance is best seen.

Scientific investigation have provided a sound understanding of the physiologic and biochemical events that occur in a variety of exercise situations; these studies form the basis for the recommendations on energy and fluid intake for optimization of performance and avoidance of exertional injury. Research has shown that dietary supplementation with vitamins and minerals above physiologic need is both ineffective and an unnecessary ergogenic aid and, with abuse, may actually impair performance and health.

Studies have shown, however, that physical activity can make one susceptible to micronutrient deficiency states that ultimately may impair performance. Accompanying any increase in energy requirement there is an increased need for thia-min, riboflavin, and niacin. Thus, the athlete's diet must maintain proper nutrient density as well as energy content. Exercise, by affecting absorption and/or elimination of nutrients, can upset the nutrient balance. This is suggested for riboflavin and for minerals such as iron. At present the risk of iron deficiency is best documented in young athletes. Continued research in this area is needed to define better the proper analytical measures as they relate to exercise performance, the effects of exercise on nutrient balance, and the means of preventing the occurrence of suboptimal nutritional state.

A factor complicating general recommendations on nutrition and diet for athletes is the variety of activities comprising what is known as sport. This variety is highlighted in a recent detailed four-year study of the dietary intake of university athletes.[173] At one extreme are strength sports (American football) in which one 118 kg player consumed 61.2 MJ (14,600 kcal) on one day. At the other end of the continuum are light weight-class wrestlers, gymnasts, and dancers with small bodies and dietary patterns that fluctuate widely in energy content but average 8.5 MJ (2,000 kcal) daily. This extensive analysis of athletic diets across the range of sports revealed two points: that proper diet can provide the nutrition required for performance across the sports spectrum and that many of the athletes were at risk because of poor intake of one or more nutrients. Trends in these athletic diets reflect certain modern concerns, such as a high intake of saturated fat, cholesterol, and sodium and appreciable vitamin and mineral supplementation.[173a] Studies reveal the need for more education programs about nutrition for athletes, trainers, and coaches and show that these groups are eager for factual information.[173,174]

Obviously, nutritional advice must be tailored to the demands of the specific work and exercise.[173] The statement by the American Dietetic Association provides a good model.[175] In it, recommendations for the general public and for athletes involved in training or competition are separated, yet span the categories of athletic, combatative, or occupational activity. The recommendations and overall viewpoint within the present review are in basic agreement with the succinct recommendations contained in the statement. The significance of diet, nutrition, work, and exercise is best summarized:

1. An adequate, balanced diet is necessary for an effective performance but does not guarantee it, since nutrition is but one aspect of performance.
2. A poor diet, on the other hand, will guarantee substandard performance.

3. Being a fit, trained athlete does not alter dietary requirements for most nutrients. Energy (carbohydrates), water, iron, and certain B vitamins are possible exceptions whose increased needs may be met by a proper diet.

4. Ingestion of one or more nutrients in amounts much greater than body needs will not enhance performance and may actually impair it.

## REFERENCES

1. von Liebig, J.: Animal Chemistry or Organic Chemistry in its Application to Physiology and Pathology. London, Taylor and Walton. 1842.
2. Zuntz, N.: Arch. Anat. Physiol. (Physiol 6th) 538–542, 1986.
3. Zuntz, N.: Arch. Gesamte Physiol. Menschen Tiere *83*:557–571, 1901.
4. Himwich, H.E., Rose, M.I.: Am. J. Physiol. *81*:485–486, 1927.
5. Chistensen, E.H., Hansen, O.: Skand. Arch. Physiol. *81*:160–175, 1939.
6. Bergström, J.: Scand. J. Clin. Lab. Invest. *14* (suppl. 68):1–110, 1962.
7. Bergström, J., Hultman, E., Roch-Norlund, A.E.: Nature (Lond.) *198*:97–98, 1963.
8. Bergström, J. Hultman, E.: Scand. J. Clin. Lab. Invest. *18*:16–20, 1966.
9. Bergström, Hultman, E.: Nature, *210*:309–310, 1966.
10. Hultman, E., Bergström, J., McLennan Anderson, N.: Scand. J. Clin. Lab. Invest. *19*:56–66, 1967.
11. Ahlborg, B., Bergström, J., Ekelund, L.-G., Hultman, E.: Acta Physiol. Scand. *70*:129–142, 1967.
12. Hultman, E.: Circ. Res. 20 & 21(suppl. 1):1–99, 1967.
13. Hultman, E.: Scand. J. Clin. Lab. Invest. *19*:209–217, 1967.
14. Bergström, J., Hultman, E.: Scand. J. Clin. Lab. Invest. *19*:218–228, 1967.
15. Bergström, J., Hultman, E.: Acta Med. Scand. *182*:93–107, 1967.
16. Hultman, E., Bergström, J.: Acta Med. Scand. *182*:109–117, 1967.
17. Hermansen, L., Hultman, E., Saltin, B.: Acta Physiol. Scand. *71*:129–139, 1967.
18. Bergström, J., Hermansen, L., Hultman, E., Saltin, B.: Acta Physiol. Scand 71:140–150, 1967.
19. Ahlborg, B., Bergström, J., Brohult, J., et al.: Förvarsmedicin *3*:85–100, 1967.
20. Hultman, E.: Scand. J. Clin. Lab. Invest. *19* (suppl. 94):1–63, 1967.
21. Bergström, J., Beroniade, V., Hultman, E., Roch-Norlund, A.E.: Symp. Über Transport and Funktion Intracellulärer Elekrolyte am ¾ Juni in Schüren/Saar. 108–117, 1967.
22. Nilsson, L., H:son: Studies on Liver Glycogen Metabolism in Man with Special Reference to Diet and Sugar Infusion. Thesis 1974.
23. Nilsson, L.H:son., Hultman, E.: Scand. J. Clin. Lab. Invest. *32*:325–330, 1973.
24. Nilsson, L., H:son, Fürst, P., Hultman, E.: Scand. J. Clin. Lab. Invest. *32*:331–337, 1973.
25. Hultman, E., Nilsson, L.H:son.: Adv. Exp. Med. Biol. *11*:143–151, 1971.
26. Nilsson, L.H:son., Hultman, E.: Scand. J. Clin. Lab. Invest. *33*:5–10, 1974.
27. Bergström, J., Harris, R.C., Hultman, E., Nordesjö, L.-O.: Adv. Exp. Med. Biol. *11*:341–355, 1971.
28. Harris, R.C.: Muscle Energy Metabolism in Man in Response to Isometric Contraction. A Biopsy Study. Thesis. University of Wales 1981.
29. Hultman, E., Sjöholm, H.: Substrate availability. *In* International Series on Sports Sciences Vol. 13. (Knuttgen, H.G., Vogel, J.A., Poortmans, J., Eds.) 1983.
30. Fletcher, J.G.L., Lewis, H.K.: Ergonomics *2*:114–115, 1959.
31. Wilkie, D.R.: Ergonomics *3*:1–8, 1960.
32. Davies, C.T.M.: Ergonomics *14*:245–256, 1971.
33. Kleine, T.O.: Z. Klin. Chem. *5*:244–247, 1967.
34. Margaria, R., Cerretelli, P., Mangili, F.: J. Appl. Physiol. *19*:623–628, 1964.
35. Hultman, E.: Regulation of carbohydrate metabolism in the liver during rest and exercise with special reference to diet. 3rd Int. Symp. on Biochemistry of Exercise. (Landry, F., Orban, W.A.R. Eds.) *3*:99–126, 1979.
36. Nilsson, L.H:son.: Scand. J. Clin. Lab. Invest. *32*:317–323, 1973.
37. McGilvery, R.W.: The use of fuels for muscular work. *In* Metabolic Adaption to Prolonged Physical Exercise. (Chowald, H., Portmans, J.R., Eds.) 1973.
38. Pernow, B., Saltin, B.: J. Appl. Physiol. *31*:416–422, 1971.
39. Fox, E.L.: Sports Physiology. 2nd Ed. CBS College Publishing. Philadelphia, W.B. Saunders Company, 1984.
40. Ahlborg, G., Felig, P., Hagenfeldt, L., et al.: J. Clin. Invest. *53*:1080–1090, 1974.
41. Holloszy, J.O.: Biochemical adaptations to exercise: aerobic metabolism. *In* Exercise and Sport Science Review. (Wilmore, J.H., Ed.) 1973.
42. Holloszy, J.O., Booth, F.W.: Ann. Rev. Physiol. *38*:273–291, 1976.
43. Holloszy, J.O., Winder, W.W., Fitts, R.H., et al.: Energy production during exercise. *In* Regulatory Mechanisms in Metabolism During Exercise. (Landry, F., Orban, W.A.R., Eds.) 1978.
44. Holloszy, J.O.: Arch. Phys. Med. Rehabil. *63*:231–234, 1982.
45. Hultman, E.: Muscle glycogen store and prolonged exercise. *In* Frontiers of Fitness. (Shephard, E.J., Ed.) Springfield, Il, Charles C Thomas Publisher, 1971.
46. Yoshimura, H., Inoue, T., Yamada, T., Shivaki, K.: World Rev. Nutr. Diet. *35*:1–86, 1980.
47. Lemon, P.W.R., Mullin, J.P.: J. Appl. Physiol. *48*:624–629, 1980.
48. Refsum, H.E., Strömme, S.B.: Scand. J. Clin. Lab. Invest. *33*:247–254, 1974.
49. Rennie, M.J., Edwards, R.H.T., Krywawych, S., et al.: Clin. Sci. *61*:627–639, 1981.
50. Décombaz, J., Reinhardt, P., Anantharaman, K., et al.: Eur. J. Appl. Pysiol. *41*:61–72, 1979.
51. Gontzea, I., Sutsesco, R., Dimitrache, S.: Nutr. Rep. Int. *11*:231–236, 1975.
52. Felig, P.E., Wahren, J.: J. Clin. Invest. *50*:2703–2714, 1971.
53. Felig, P.: Metabolism *22*:179–207, 1973.
54. Felig, P.: Annu. Rev. Biochem. *44*:933–955, 1975.
55. Young, V.R., Bier, D.M.: Stable isotopes ($^{31}$C and $^{15}$N) in the study of human protein and amino acid metabolism and requirements. *In* Nutritional Fac-

tors: Modulating Effects on Metabolic Processes. (Beers, R.F., Bassett, E.G., Eds.) Raven Press, New York, 1981.

56. Hägg, S.A., Morse, E.L., Adibi, S.A.: Am. J. Physiol. *242*:407–410, 1982.

57. Wolfe, R.R., Goodenough, R.D., Wolfe, M.H., et al.: J. Appl. Physiol. *52*:458–466, 1982.

58. Millward, D.J., Davies, C.T.M., Halliday, D., et al.: Fed. Proc. *41*:2686–2691, 1982.

59. White, T.P., Brooks, G.A.: Am. J. Physiol. *240*:155–165, 1981.

60. Buse, M.G., Biggers, J.F., Friedrici, K.H., Buse, J.F.: J. Biol. Chem. *247*:8085–8096, 1972.

61. Haralambie, G., Berg, A.: Eur. J. Appl. Physiol. Occup. Physiol. *36*:231–236, 1976.

62. Refsum, H.E., Gjessing, L.R., Strømme, S.B.: Scand. J. Clin. Lab. Invest. *39*:407–413, 1979.

63. Dohm, G.L., Williams, R.T., Kasperek, G.J., van Rij, A.M.: J. Appl. Physiol. *52*:26–33, 1982.

64. Munro, H.N.: Control of plasma amino acid concentrations. *In* Aromatic Amino Acids in the Brain. (Ciba Found, Symp. 22). New York, Elsevier, 1974.

65. Hultman, E., Bergström, J., Roch-Norlund, A.E.: Adv. Exp. Med. Biol. *11*:273–288, 1971.

66. Brown, J.H., Thompson, B., Mayer, S.E.: Biochemistry *16*:5501–5508, 1977.

67. Kochan, R.G., Lamb, D.R., Lutz, S.A., et al.: Am. J. Physiol. *236*:660–666, 1979.

68. Sherman, W.M., Costill, D.L., Fink, W.J., Miller, J.M.: Int. J. Sports Med. *2*:114–118, 1981.

69. Bergström, J., Guarnieri, G., Hultman, E.: J. Appl. Physiol. *30*:122–125, 1971.

70. Bergström, J., Guarnieri, G., Hultman, E.: Changes in muscle water and electrolytes during exercise. *In* Limiting Factors of Physical Performance. (Keul, J., Ed.) Stuttgart, Georg Thieme Publishers, 1973.

71. Owen, O.E., Morgan, A.P., Kemp, H.G., et al.: J. Clin. Invest. *46*:1589–1595, 1967.

72. Owen, O.E., Felig, P., Morgan, A.P., et al.: J. Clin. Invest. *48*:574–583, 1969.

73. Hultman, E., Nilsson, L.: Liver glycogen as a glucose-supplying source during exercise. *In* Limiting Factors of Physical Performance. (Keul, J., Ed.) Stuttgard, Georg Thieme Publishers, 1973.

74. Passmore, J.V.G.A., Durnin, J.V.: Energy, Work and Leisure. London, Heineman, 1967.

75. FAO/WHO Expert Committee Report: Energy and Protein Requirements. WHO Technical Report Series. WHO Geneva, 522, 1973.

76. Norgan, N.G., Ferro-Luzzi, A.: Int. Ser. Sport Sciences *7*:167–193, 1978.

77. Buskirk, E.R.: Nutrition for the athlete. *In* Sports Medicine. (Ryan, A.J., Allman Jr., F.L., Eds.) pp. 141–159, New York, Academic Press, 1974.

78. Recommended Dietary Allowances, 9th ed. Washington, DC, National Academy of Sciences, 1980.

79. Ferro-Luzzi, A., Venerando, A.: Int. Ser. Sport Sciences *7*:145–154, 1978.

80. Suzuki, S., Oshima, S., Tsuji, E., et al.: Int. Ser. Sport Sciences *7*:194–214, 1978.

81. Wirths, W.: Int. Ser. Sport Sciences *7*:227–235, 1978.

82. Young, V.R., Torún, B.: Prog. Clin. Biol. Res. *77*:57–85, 1981.

83. Torún, B., Scrimshaw, N.S., Young, V.R.: Am. J. Clin. Nutr. *30*:1983–1993, 1977.

84. Consolazio, C.R., Johnson, H.L., Nelson, R.A., et al.: Am. J. Clin. Nutr. *28*:29–35, 1975.

85. Darling, R.C., Johnson, R.E., Pitts, G.C., et al.: J. Nutr. *28*:273–281, 1944.

86. Pitts, G.C., Johnson, R.E., Consolazio, F.C., et al.: Am. J. Physiol. *142*:253–259, 1944.

87. Rasch, P.J., Pierson, W.R.: Am. J. Clin. Nutr. *11*:530–532, 1962.

88. Marable, N.L., Hickson Jr., J.F., Korslund, M.K., et al.: Nutr. Rep. Int. *19*:795–805, 1979.

89. Laritcheva, K.A., Yalovaya, N.I., Shubin, V.I., Smirnov, P.V.: Int. Ser. Sport Sciences *7*:155–163, 1978.

90. Rogozkin, V.A.: Int. Ser. Sport Sciences *7*:119–123, 1978.

91. Koivisto, V.A., Karonen, S.-L., Nikkilä, E.A.: J. Appl. Physiol. *51*:783–787, 1981.

92. Coyle, E.F., Hagberg, J.M., Hurley, B.F., et al.: J. Appl. Physiol. *55*:230–235, 1983.

93. Hughson, R.L., Green, H.J., Houston, M.E., et al.: Can. Med. Assoc. J. *122*:1141–1144, 1980.

94. American College of Sports Medicine: Med. Sci. Sports *7*(1):VII–IX, 1975.

95. Canadian Association of Sports Sciences: Can. J. Appl. Sport Sci. *6*:99–100, 1981.

96. American College of Sports Medicine: Med. Sci. Sports *8*(2):XI–XIII, 1976.

97. Milvy, P. (Ed.): The Marathon: Physiological, medical, epidemiological and psychological studies. Ann. N. Y. Acad. Sci. *301*: Parts I, II and III, 1977.

98. Senay, L.C., Jr.: Med. Sci. Sports *11*:42–48, 1979.

99. Costill, D.L., Miller, J.M.: Int. J. Sports Med. *1*:2–14, 1980.

99a.Sawka, M.N., Young, A.J., Francesconi, R.P., et al.: J. Appl. Physiol. *59*(5):1394–1401, 1985.

100. Costill, D.L.: Muscle water and electrolytes during acute and repeated bouts of dehydration. *In* Nutrition, Physical Fitness and Health. (Parizkova, J., Rogozkin, V.A., Eds.) Baltimore, University Park Press, 1978.

101. Sjøgard, G.: Am. J. Physiol. *245*:R25–R31, 1983.

102. Senay, L.C., Jr.: J. Appl. Physiol. *47*:1–7, 1979.

103. Houston, M.E., Marrin, D.A., Green, H.J., et al.: Phys. Sportsmed. *9*:73–78, 1981.

104. Costill, D.L.: Ann. N.Y. Acad. Sci. *301*:175–189, 1977.

105. Saltin, B.: Fluid, electrolyte and energy losses and their replenishment in prolonged exercise. *In* Nutrition, Physical Fitness and Health. (Parizkova, J., Rogozkin, V.A., Eds.) Baltimore, University Park Press, 1978.

105a.Myhre, L.G., Hartung, G.H., Nunneley, S.A., et al.: J. Appl. Physiol. *59*(2):559–563, 1985.

106. Saltin, B.: J. Appl. Physiol. *19*:1125–1132, 1964.

107. Gisolfi, C.V., Copping, J.R.: Med. Sci. Sports *6*:108–113, 1974.

108. Torranin, C., Smith, D.P., Byrd, R.S.: J. Sports Med. Phys. Fitness *19*:1–9, 1979.

109. Jacobs, I.: Int. J. Sports Med. *1*:21–24, 1980.

110. Bergström, J., Hultman, E.: JAMA *221*:999–1006, 1972.

111. Costill, D.L., Saltin, B.: J. Appl. Physiol. *37*:679–683, 1974.

112. Costill, D.L., Sparks, K.E.: J. Appl. Physiol. *34*:299–308, 1973.

113. Knochel, J.P.: Ann. N.Y. Acad. Sci. *301*:175–189, 1977.

114. Pivarnik, J.M., Leeds, E.M., Wilkerson, J.E.: J. Appl. Physiol. *56*:613–618, 1984.

115. Wade, C.E., Dressendorfer, R.H., O'Brien, J.C., et al.: J. Appl. Physiol. *50*:709–712, 1981.

116. Greenleaf, J.E., Brock, P.J., Kiel, L.C., et al.: J. Appl. Physiol. *54*:414–419, 1983.

117. Gisolfi, C.V., Wilson, N.C., Claxton, B.: Ann. N.Y. Acad. Sci. *301*:129–150, 1977.

118. Green, H.J., Thomson, J.A., Ball, M.E., et al.: J. Appl. Physiol. *56*:145–149, 1984.

119. Convertino, V.A., Brock, P.T., Keil, L.C., et al.: J. Appl. Physiol. *48*:665–669, 1980.

120. Convertino, V.A.: Med. Sci. Sports Exerc. *15*:77–82, 1983.

121. Costill, D.L., Cote, R., Fink, W.J.: Am. J. Clin. Nutr. *36*:266–275, 1982.

122. Conrad, M.E., Barton, J.C.: Am. J. Hematol. *10*:199–225, 1981.

123. Finch, C.A., Huebers, H.: N. Engl. J. Med. *306*:1520–1528, 1982.

124. Finch, C.A., Gollnick, P.D., Hlastala, M.P., et al.: J. Clin. Invest. *64*:129–137, 1979.

125. Pate, R.R.: Phys. Sportsmed. *11*:115–131, 1983.

126. Yoshimura, H.: Nutr. Rev. *10*:251–253, 1970.

126a.Hallberg, L., Magnusson, B.: Acta Med. Scand. *216*:145–148, 1984.

127. Clement, D.B., Asmundson, R.C., Medhurst, C.W.: Can. Med. Assoc. J. *17*:614–616, 1977.

128. Clement, D.B., Asmundson, R.C.: Phys. Sportsmed. *10*:37–43, 1982.

129. Hunding, A., Jordal, R., Paulev, P.E.: Acta Med. Scand. *209*:315–318, 1981.

130. Nickerson, H.J., Tripp, A.D.: Phys. Sportsmed. *11*:60–66, 1983.

131. Brotherhood, J., Brozovic, B., Pugh, L.G.C.: Clin. Sci. *48*:139–145, 1975.

132. Ehn, L., Carlmark, B., Högland, S.: Med. Sci. Sports. Exerc. *12*:61–64, 1980.

133. Dressendorfer, R.H., Wade, C.E., Amsterdam, E.A.: JAMA *246*:1215–1218, 1981.

134. Radamoski, M.W., Sabiston, B.H., Isoard, P.: Aviat. Space Environ. Med. *51*:41–45, 1980.

135. Dickson, D.N., Wilkison, R.L., Noakes, T.D.: Int. J. Sports Med. *3*:111–117, 1982.

136. Puhl, J.L., Runyan, W.S.: Res. Quart. *51*:533–541, 1980.

137. Wirth, J.C., Lohmann, T.G., Avallone, J.P. Jr., et al.: Med. Sci. Sports *10*:223–226, 1978.

138. Dufaux, B., Hoederath, A., Strietberger, I., et al.: Int. J. Sports Med. *2*:43–46, 1981.

138a.Magnusson, B., Hallberg, L., Rossander, L., et al.: Acta Med. Scand. *216*:149–155, 1984.

139. Paulev, P.E., Jordal, R., Pedersen, N.S.: Clin. Chim. Acta *127*:19–27, 1983.

139a.Par, R.B., Bachman, L.A., Moss, R.A.: Phys. Sportsmed. *12*(4):81–86, 1984.

139b.Wishnitzer, R., Vorst, E., Berrebi, A.: Int. J. Sports Med. *4*:27–30, 1984.

140. Vellar, O.D.: Scand. J. Clin. Lab. Invest. *21*:157–167, 1968.

140a.Magnusson, B., Hallberg, L., Rossander, L., et al.: Acta Med. Scand. *216*:157–164, 1984.

141. Gardner, G.W., Edgerton, V.R., Senewiratne, B., et al.: Am. J. Clin. Nutr. *30*:910–917, 1977.

141a.Perkkiö, M.V., Jansson, L.T., Brooks, G.A., et al.: J. Appl. Physiol. *58*(5):1477–1480, 1985.

142. Gledhill, N.: Med. Sci. Sports Exerc. *14*:183–189, 1982.

143. Ekblom, B., Goldbarg, A.N., Gullbring, B.: J. Appl. Physiol. *33*:175–180, 1972,

143a.Schoene, R.B. Escourrou, P., Robertson, H.T., et al.: J. Lab. Clin. Med. *102*:306–312, 1983.

144. Cooter, G.R., Mowbray, K.W.: Res. Quart. *49*:114–118, 1978.

144a.Hegenauer, J., Strause, L., Saltman, P., et al.: Eur. J. Appl. Physiol. *52*:57–61, 1983.

145. Vitousek, S.H.: Nutr. Today *14*:10–17, 1979.

145a.Van der Beck, E.J.: Sports Med. *2*:175–197, 1985.

146. Williams, M.H.: Vitamins, Iron and calcium supplementation: Effect on human physical performance. *In* Nutrition and Athletic Performance (Haskell, W., Scala, J., and Whittan, J., Eds.) Palo Alto, Bull Publishing Co., 1982.

147. Canada, Dept. of National Health and Welfare, Health Protection Branch, Food Directorate, Bureau of Nutritional Sciences: Recommended Nutrient Intakes for Canadians, Ottawa, 1983.

148. Haralambie, G.: Nutr. Metabol. *20*:1–8, 1976.

149. Van Dam, B.: Br. J. Sports Med. *12*:74–79, 1978.

150. Belko, A.Z., Obarzanek, E., Kalkwarf, H.J., et al.: Am. J. Clin. Nutr. *37*:509–517, 1983.

151. Leklem, J.E., Schultz, T.D.: Am. J. Clin. Nutr. *38*:541–548, 1983.

152. Montoye, H., Spata, P.J., Pinckney, V., et al.: J. Appl. Physiol. *7*:589–592, 1955.

153. Tin-May-Than, Ma-Win-May, Khin-Sann-Aung, et al.: Br. J. Nutr. *40*:269–273, 1978.

154. Howald, H., Segesser, B., Korner, W.F.: Ann. N.Y. Acad. Sci. *258*:458–463, 1975.

155. Gey, G.O., Cooper, K.H., Bottenberg, R.A.: JAMA *211*:105, 1970.

156. Keren, G., Epstein, Y.: J. Sports Med. Phys. Fitness *20*:145–148, 1980.

157. Keith, R.E., Driskell, J.A.: Am. J. Clin. Nutr. *36*:840–845, 1982.

158. Lawrence, J.D., Smith, J.L., Bower, R.C., et al.: J. Am. Coll. Health Assoc. *23*:219–222, 1974.

159. Lawrence, J.D., Bower, R.C., Riehl, W.P., et al.: Am. J. Clin. Nutr. *28*:205–208, 1975.

160. Sharman, I.N., Down, M.T., Sen, R.N.: Br. J. Nutr. *26*:265–276, 1971.

161. Shepard, R.J., Campbell, R., Pimm, P., et al.: Eur. J. Appl. Physiol. *33*:119–126, 1974.

162. DiPalma, J.R., Ritchie, D.M.: Ann. Rev. Pharmacol. Toxicol. *17*:133–148, 1977.

163. Roberts, H.J.: JAMA *246*:129–131, 1981.

164. Herbert, V., Jacob, E.: JAMA *230*:241–242, 1974.

165. Bergström, J., Hultman, E., Jorfeldt, L., et al.: J. Appl. Physiol. *26*:170–176, 1969.

166. Dressendorfer, R.H., Sockolov, R.: Phys. Sportsmed. *8*:97–100, 1980.

167. Liu, L., Borowski, G., Rose, L.I.: Phys. Sportsmed. *11*:79–80, 1983.

168. Lukaski, H.C., Bolonchuk, W.W., Klevay, L.M., et al.: Am. J. Clin. Nutr. *37*:407–415, 1983.

169. Jacob, R.A., Sandstead, H.A., Munoz, J.M., et al.: Am. J. Clin. Nutr. *34*:1379–1383, 1981.

170. Milne, D.B., Canfield, W.K., Mahalko, J.R., et al.: Am. J. Clin. Nutr. *38*:181–186, 1983.

171. Gray, M.E., Titlow, L.W.: Med. Sci. Sports Exerc. *14*:424–427, 1982.

171a.Barnett, D.W., Conlee, R.K.: Am. J. Clin. Nutr. *40*:586–590, 1984.

172. Percy, E.C.: Med. Sci. Sports *10*:298–303, 1978.

173. Short, S.H., Short, W.R.: J. Am. Dietet. Assoc. *82*:632–645, 1983.

173a.Ellsworth, N.M., Hewitt, B.F., Haskell, W.L.: Phys. Sportsmed. *13*:78–92, 1985.

174. Bedgood, B.L., Tuck, M.B.: J. Am. Dietet. Assoc. *83*:672–677, 1983.

175. American Dietetic Association: J. Am. Dietet. Assoc. *76*:437–443, 1980.

## SELECTED READINGS

Apple, D.F., Cantwell, J.D.: Medicine for Sport. Chicago, Year Book Medical Publishers, 1979.

Astrand, P.O.: Nutrition and physical peformance. World Rev. Nutr. Diet. *16*:59–79, 1973.

Bergström, J., Hultman, E.: Nutrition for maximal sports performance. JAMA *221*:999–1006, 1972.

Brotherhood, J.R.: Nutrition and Sports Performance. Sports Med. *1*:350–389, 1984.

Buskirk, E.R.: Some nutritional considerations in the conditioning of athletes. Ann. Rev. Nutr. *1*:319–350, 1981.

Clement, D.B., Sawchuk, L.L.: Iron status and sports performance. Sports Med. *1*:65–74, 1984.

Durnin, J.V.G.A., Passmore, R.: Energy, Work and Leisure. London, Heineman Educational Books. 1967.

Encyclopedia of Physical Education, Fitness and Sports: Training, Environment, Nutrition and Fitness. (Stull, G.A., Cureton, T.K., Jr., Eds.). Salt Lake City, Brighton, 1980.

Ergogenic Aids in Sport (Williams, M.H., Ed.). Champaign, IL, Human Kinetics, 1983.

Fox, E.L.: Sports Physiology. 2nd ed. Philadelphia, CBS College Publishing, Saunders College Publishing, 1984.

Hanley, D.F., Jr.: Athletic training, and how diet affects it. Nutr. Today *14*:5–9, 1979.

Haskell, W., Scala, J., Whittam, J.: Nutrition and Athletic Performance. Palo Alto, Bull, Publishing Co., 1982.

Lincoln, A.: Food for Athletes. Chicago, IL, Contemporary Books, 1979.

National Dairy Council. Nutrition and Human Performance. Dairy Counc. Dig. *51*:13–17, 1980.

National Research Council. Committee on Dietary Allowances: Recommended Dietary Allowances (RDA). 9th ed. Washington, DC: National Academy of Sciences, 1980.

Newsholme, E., Leech, R.: The Runner. Energy and Endurance. Roosevelt, New Jersey, Fitness Books. Walter L. Meagher. 1984.

Nutrition, Physical Fitness and Health. (Parizkova, J., Rogozkin, V.A., Eds.). Baltimore, University Park Press, 1978.

Smith, N.J.: Food for Sports. Palo Alto, Bull, Publishing Co. 1976.

Vitousek, S.H.: Is more Better? Nutr. Today *14*:10–17, 1979.

Vranic, M., Berger, M.: Exercise and diabetes mellitus. Diabetes *28*:147–163, 1979.

Young, D.R., Physical Performance, Fitness and Diet. Springfield, IL, Charles C Thomas, 1977.

*Chapter* **54**

# ENTERAL (TUBE) AND PARENTERAL NUTRITION SUPPORT

## Maurice E. Shils

The problem of assuring adequate nutrition is forced onto the physician who is confronted by the patient who will not eat, who cannot eat (i.e., because of obstruction), who cannot retain food (i.e., because of severe vomiting or obstruction) or who, for various reasons, cannot digest or absorb sufficient amounts of ingested nutrients. The solution to each of these problems is the use of one of the two methods of forced, involuntary, or artificial feeding, as the methods are often termed. The terms forced or involuntary are not necessarily correct because the patient often voluntarily accepts one of these two methods—tube feeding or parenteral feeding.

Regardless of the nutritional therapeutic method, the objective is to provide energy and nutrients in amounts that meet the needs of the individual patient. The needs may be high, as in the very hypercatabolic patient, or relatively low, as in the obese patient on a weight reduction diet. The term hyperalimentation entered into the nutrition lexicon in various ways to indicate the need for very large amounts of calories and certain other nutrients. Turner[1] stated that the term was first used by Co Tui in 1945 in describing "intravenous hyperalimentation" with moderately large amounts of casein hydrolysate and glucose or fructose to patients with peptic ulcer or pyloric obstruction.[2] In 1965, "hyperalimentation" was used to describe supplementary IV lipid feeding to cancer patients.[3] It was reintroduced by the University of Pennsylvania group as a general term for total parenteral nutrition[4] and became used widely in that sense, often being shortened to "hyperal." Because it was applied also to tube feeding, the terms "IV hyperalimentation" and "enteral hyperalimentation" appeared in the literature.

From both the historical and etymologic aspects, the term came to mean, to at least some physicians, the need for and provision of relatively large amounts of energy and protein. As information and experience have increased it has become apparent that the term hyperalimentation carries an inaccurate and potentially misleading connotation in terms of optimum nutrition support. In my view, the term should be either abandoned or relegated to mean the uncommon and undesirable provision of energy and other nutrients in amounts appreciably in excess of individual needs. More accurate and preferable are the general terms enteral (tube) feeding (or nutrition), parenteral nutrition, or parenteral alimentation.

## ENTERAL (TUBE) NUTRITION

### History

In a recent historical review of tube feedng, Randall noted that the place of tube feeding in nutrition support has been recognized for well over 100 years.[5] Initially, either a nasopharyngeal or a rectal feeding tube was used widely; after Einhorn pointed out the inadequacies of rectal feeding in 1910,[6] the nose became the primary entry site, with the tube tip placed in the esophagus, stomach, or upper small bowel. Tube feeding enterostomies developed later; the history of these procedures has been documented.[5,7] Tubes have been surgically placed into the pharynx, esophagus, duodenum, stomach, and jejunum. More recently they have been placed by percutaneous endoscopic gastrostomy (PEG)[8a,b] or, less commonly, by percutaneous endoscopic jejunostomy (PEJ).

Initially, tube feedings consisted of natural liquid foods or solid foods reduced to a relatively fine consistency by grinding or blending and dispersed in liquid. By the late 1930s a casein hydrolysate became available prepared initially by acid hydrolysis and later by enzymatic hydrolysis, and reports appeared of its clinical use by the intravenous route[9,10] and by the enteral route.[11–14]

As early as 1918, Andresen initiated jejunal feedings after gastroenterostomy while the patient was on the operating table.[15] Co Tui et al. also instituted feedings within a few hours after surgery.[14] This practice has a sound physiologic basis; while the stomach or colon tends to be hypoperistaltic immediately following surgery, the small bowel retains good peristalsis.[16–21] These observations were associated with renewal of interest in postoperative jejunal feedings in the 1970s by placement of jejunostomies intra- or postoperatively including the use of a needle catheter.[19,20] Andersson et al. compared the absorption of many nutrients from two types of complete, defined formula diets (soy proteins hydrolysate of osmolality 364 and intact protein of osmolality 250) infused for a 3- to 5-day period into the duodenum in the immediate postoperative period following colorectal surgery. Both formulas were well tolerated and had equally good absorption of amino acids, fat, carbohydrate, electrolytes, iron, and zinc.[21]

A number of the older studies yielded important basic information concerning caloric and nitrogen needs and indicated clearly the nutritional and metabolic value to the patient of enteral feeding.[5,11,13,14] The report of Smith and Lee in 1956 is one of the clinical landmarks in this field in light of their successful use of tube feeding in 11 consecutive patients with lateral duodenal fistulas; with the tip of the tube introduced into the efferent limb of the gastrojejunostomy, the fistulas closed spontaneously within 1 month in all patients.[22]

The first commercial defined-formula diet developed for clinical use was Nutramigen (Mead Johnson), introduced in 1942 and designed to treat children with allergies and intestinal disturbances. A major clinical advance in this field was Lofenalac (Mead Johnson), which, designed for phenylketonuric patients, included a phenylalanine-low protein hydrolysate. It was the prototype for what has become a group of special formulations for the nutrition support of children with inherited metabolic diseases (Chap. 63).*

An early report on the development and use of polymeric (i.e., containing intact protein) formulations for human metabolic and nutrition studies was that of Olson, et al. in 1953.[23] At about the same time, Ahrens initiated long-term studies of specific formulations primarily for oral use in metabolic studies.[24] A highly purified, laboratory-made, tube-fed formulation of intact purified casein with certain additional amino acids, vitamins, minerals, and trace elements was used beginning in 1961 for inducing human experimental magnesium deficiency.[25]

Investigators studying the nutritional requirements of laboratory animals had, since before the first World War, increasingly been purifying food sources as components of experimental diets, thereby bringing to light the existence of an increasing number of essential nutrients. In a brief history of the development and limitation of "elemental diets," Shapiro noted the work of Greenstein, et al. which extended the work of W.C. Rose and colleagues by developing experimental diets containing only the L-isomers of essential amino acids and by preparing the complete diets in liquid form.[26] The first long-term human feeding studies with such diets were conducted by Winitz, et al. in the mid 1960s in a project sponsored by the National Aeronautics and Space Administration (NASA).[27]

Beginning in 1969, Randall and associates began to publish a series of clinical investigations in patients with nutritional problems utilizing a commercially available formula (Vivonex) that was based on the work of Winitz et al.[5] These and other studies indicated that such tube-fed formulas could be useful for patients with a variety of nutritional problems and that tube feeding was a simpler, less expensive, and potentially less hazardous procedure than total parenteral nutrition (TPN). This conclusion lead to an explosion of commercial liquid formulations and the devel-

---

*The casein hydrolysate-based defined-formula diets that were used in early studies[9–14] and have been used clinically were based on the work of Warren M. Cox, Jr. and his staff at Mead Johnson and Company; they developed first, the casein acid-hydrolysate and then the enzymatic hydrolysate.

opment of improved and more acceptable feeding tubes and ancillary equipment such as bags and pumps. The state of the art in 1975 was summarized in the proceedings of a symposium on Defined-Formula Diets for Medical Purposes.[28]

The terminology of certain complete enteral formulations appearing on the market presents a problem. Although such terms as elemental, chemically defined, and synthetic are used, none of these diets are "elemental" in the chemical sense; few are "chemically defined" implying that all components have a precise chemical analysis and purity; and none are totally "synthetic." Because of these objections, the more general term *defined-formula diets* was recommended[29]; "defined" was used in the sense that the ingredients (including nutrients processed from foods and/or relatively purified compounds, simple or complex) are prepared commercially by designated procedures so that their composition is established fairly well although not necessarily with chemical precision. "Defined-formula" diets is useful as a general designation for a variety of nutritionally complete formulations with differing compositions, complexity, degrees of purification, and, perhaps, digestion and absorption characteristics. Under this general term, a given formulation may be characterized more specifically—e.g., as "chemically defined" (or "monomeric") "protein-hydrolysate," "with intact protein," or "with protein isolate" (or "polymeric").

## Indications

Some form of tube feeding is indicated primarily in those situations in which voluntary oral intake either is likely to be unsuccessful or is contraindicated. These situations include (1) persistent anorexia; (2) comatose or uncooperative status; (3) persistent nausea and/or vomiting; (4) severe persistent odynophagia (mucositis, pharyngitis, esophagitis) of any cause; (5) mechanical or functional impairment of swallowing mechanisms with serious risk of aspiration; (6) stable partial obstruction (functional or mechanical) of the esophagus, stomach, or intestinal tract; (7) fistulas of the alimentary tract with major fistula losses; (8) severe malabsorption of any cause in which diarrhea is exacerbated seriously by oral intake; and (9) increased or altered metabolic needs that cannot be met fully by voluntary oral intake (e.g., severe hypercatabolic states). All of these situations except persistent nausea and vomiting and severe persistent odynophagia are indications for a trial of tube feeding with certain qualifications. The adage "when the gut works, use it" is a useful but not infallible guide. Tube feeding is certainly merited and is a desirable procedure with persistent anorexia; the hypercatabolic patient whose total needs cannot be met by oral feeding alone; persistent upper small-bowel fistulas that can be successfully bypassed by a tube; or malabsorption syndromes of moderate severity in which adequate digestion and absorption can be achieved by slow-drip tube feeding of a proper formula.

Tube feeding is contraindicated in a patient who has total intestinal obstruction; a fistula with major drainage, especially a fistula of the upper alimentary tract, that cannot be bypassed by a tube or that has unacceptable exacerbation of fluid losses despite slow-drip tube feeding; severe diarrhea secondary to malabsorption; or persistent vomiting. The patient with one of these problems is instead a candidate for parenteral feeding. In addition, a patient who is comatose or has unpredictable serious vomiting (or hiccuping), has significant pulmonary disease, and lacks a gag refexis, in my view, a candidate for parenteral feeding to minimize the danger of aspiration pneumonia. On the other hand, the comatose patient with a gag reflex and without pulmonary disability is a candidate for tube feeding with the danger of aspiration minimized by placing the tip of the tube in the jejunum and using slow-drip tube feeding.

Tube feeding may be useful for the patient with odynophagia on swallowing liquid or solid food, such as in a patient with radiation or Candida esophagitis. When the discomfort is secondary to mucositis or pharyngitis associated with drug toxicity or leukemia with accompanying leukopenia and thrombocytopenia, the situation is different. In my experience, many physicians believe that insertion of a nasal tube for feeding is highly undesirable for those patients with severe bone marrow depression because of an increased risk of bleeding. de Vries, et al. investigated the impact of nasogastric tube feeding in adults being treated with intensive chemotherapy for acute leukemia; they concluded that the risk of digestive tract bleeding is not enhanced by tube feeding as compared to a control group on oral intake.[30] However, more evidence in children and adults is needed. Another contraindication to tube insertion is the discomfort of the tube in the patient with pharyngitis; a more important concern is the danger of aspiration with periodic emesis of the toxic patient.

Even if a patient is deemed suitable for tube feeding, he not uncommonly dreads tube insertion because of prior experience with a stiff, large nasogastric tube following surgery. The patient's level of anxiety may be such that the parenteral route is deemed preferable for relatively short periods and a surgically or endoscopically placed feeding gastrostomy is indicated for longer periods. I have found, however, that often a patient initially opposed to tube feeding agrees to allow insertion of a very small caliber flexible tube with the understanding that the tube will be removed if significant distress is present after 2 or 3 hours. Quite often the patient allows the tube to remain in place. For the individual who is an outpatient or is about to become an outpatient, a tube is often accepted if it is demonstrated that he or a member of the family can learn to insert and remove the tube easily so that the tube need not stick out of the nose at other times. The proviso is that the patient or family member must be reliable enough to carry out the usual testing to ensure that the tube tip is properly placed before feeding is instituted. When the outpatient continuously opposes the nasopharyngeal tube, insertion of the tube elsewhere by surgical or endoscopic means is indicated.

Sites of tube insertion are indicated in Fig. 54–1. The procedures and complications of surgical[7,31] or endoscopic[8] placement have been discussed. Esophagostomy is an alternative to jejunostomy for unobstructed patients needing long-term tube feeding who have had esophagectomy or a high subtotal gastrectomy with a stomach remnant in the chest or who have had a total gastrectomy. Placing a gastrostomy tube surgically or endoscopically is a desirable procedure for patients who are likely to need tube feedings for a long time. When intestinal surgery with intestinal resection is likely to result in significant persistent malabsorption, a feeding gastrostomy should be constructed at that time. The usual gastrostomy closes spontaneously and fairly quickly when no longer needed. Insertion of a jejunostomy tube by surgical or endoscopic means is indicated when there is obstruction at a higher level or when a gastrostomy is inadvisable.

## Composition of Formulas

Nutritionally complete defined formula diets may be classified into the following catagories: (1) mixtures of natural foods or mixtures of natural food and more purified nutrients sources (e.g., protein isolates) (Appendix Table A–40a), (2) formulas with protein in the form of isolates (e.g., soybean, egg white, lactalbumin, or casein) and with moderately to highly purified sources of carbohydrates, fats, vitamins, and minerals, (polymeric formulas) (Appendix Table A–40b); (3) formulas made with hydrolyzed proteins with moderate to highly purified sources of carbohydrates, fats, vitamins, and minerals (Appendix Table A–40c); (4) formulas made from crystalline amino acids and purified sources of carbohydrates, fats, vitamins, and minerals (chemically defined or monomeric diets) (Appendix Table A–40c); and (5) formulations for special metabolic needs (Appendix Tables A–42, A–43, and A–45).

The protein or protein equivalent (as hydrolysate or free amino acids) in commercial formulas varies from between 12 and 18% of total calories. Formulas with natural food mixtures including fat have the protein caloric contribution mostly in the range of 16 to 24%. Arguments have been advanced for the therapeutic value of formulas with 20% or more of protein calories in conditions of old age, catabolic states, and protein depletion.[32] In my view, most patients in these categories who are able to be fed by tube are not likely to be so catabolic that their needs cannot be met by formulas with protein in the 16 to 18% category, provided that they are given sufficient nonprotein calories; such formulas have a nitrogen to energy ratio of 1:156 or 1:139, which are relatively high nitrogen to energy ratios. Metabolic studies were conducted in malnourished patients with anorexia nervosa who were fed isocaloric diets with either 10% or 20% of energy as protein; weight gain and nitrogen retention were similar in both groups.[33]

## Nutritional and Physiologic Studies

A number of nutritional, biochemical, and physiologic studies using various commercial formulations have been performed since the studies in the 1950s of Winitz's group with their water-soluble chemically defined diets. Caution is needed in interpreting results because of the var-

### TUBE FEEDING SITES

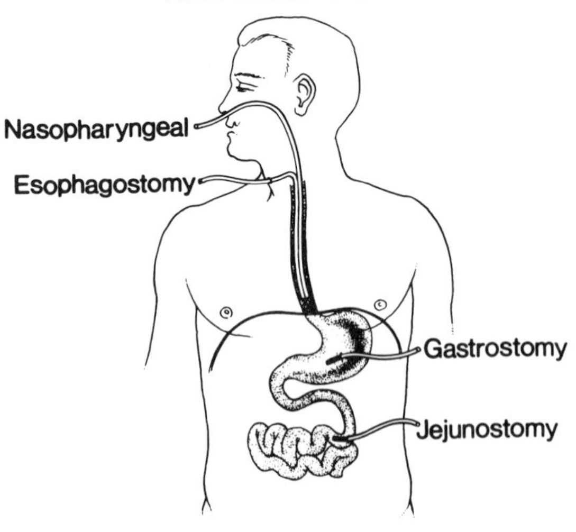

**Fig. 54–1.** Diagram of feeding tube insertion sites (From Shils, M.E., unpublished.)

iabilities in caloric density and concentrations of protein and other nutrients. However, some generalizations can be made.

**Nutritional Comparison.** When liquid defined-formula diets were given isocalorically either orally or intragastrically over a 2-week period, rats fed orally gained more weight than those fed intragastrically.[34] However, differences were significant for only three of the five diets—control, Vivonex (amino acids), and Flexical (hydrolysate); the differences for rats on Vital (hydrolysate) or Vivonex HN were not significant. Some investigators have found lower body-weight gain in rats maintained on commercial defined-formula diets when compared to their isocalorically chow-fed controls[35–38]; others have found no difference.[39] In comparative studies in which the formula and chow diets were allowed to be eaten ad libitum, growth was found to be similar[40] or greater[38] in the formula-fed rats.

Comparison has been made of nutritional parameters when a (TPN-type) formula high in carbohydrate was given to rats either IV or intragastrically in similar amounts. In some studies, weight and nitrogen balance were better maintained by the enteral route.[41–43] In another report, weight gain was equal with the IV and intragastric routes.[44] The causes for the difference in efficiency are not clear. One possible reason, bypass of the portal vein in systemic TPN, has been ruled out by other experiments in which the solution was infused into a branch of the portal vein with no advantage being observed.[41] While fat deposition in the liver was greater with the IV infusion,[41] it is known that increased fat does occur with the excessive feeding of high-carbohydrate formula diets.[34]

**Physiologic Functions.** A number of studies have been done in experimental animals as well as in human subjects on the influence of various formulations on gastrointestinal functions. Reviews of the literature have noted the complexity and variability of the data and the problems of interpretation.[45–46]

It is difficult to compare the effect of formula diets on gastric secretion or emptying because of the influences of differences in calorie content, osmolality, the amounts of glucose or fat, and the amino acid amounts and form (intact or hydrolyzed protein or free amino acids). For example, free amino acid formulas bind more gastric acid than does intact protein. The emptying of fluid meals is also controlled by hydrolytic products acting on receptors in the small intestine.[45] Induction of more gastric secretion can increase the rate of gastric emptying on a volume basis. Hence, predicting the effect of a given liquid formula is

problematic. It is likely that any differences that may occur would not have any practical physiologic significance in the individual with a normally functioning upper alimentary tract. For example, meals containing corn oil, sucrose, and one of three proteins emptied from the stomach of rats at about the same rates as a similar meal in which an isonitrogenous mixture of amino acids was substituted for the intact protein.[47]

It is well known that amino acids infused into the intestine individually or as mixtures stimulate pancreatic enzyme or protein secretion in humans and dogs. In comparison with regular food fed orally to dogs, a defined-formula diet containing protein hydrolysate fed orally resulted in an appreciably lower volume of secretion without any difference in enzyme concentration as measured by pancreatic fistulas.[48] Similarly, duodenal administration of Vivonex also decreased the water and bicarbonate secretion below that observed with oral administration of the formula[49]; the authors concluded that the difference in response between the oral and the duodenal routes arose mainly from the addition of secreted acid to the intragastric contents. In comparison to intraduodenal Vivonex, intravenous TPN produced only minor increases in pancreatic secretions. The data suggest that it is the route of the infusion of the formula, and not necessarily the composition, that influences the response of the pancreas. In any case, it would appear that intravenous rather than tube feeding is desirable if the objective is to minimize pancreatic secretion to the greatest extent.

Rats on diets with free amino acids (Vivonex) or protein hydrolysate (Flexical) fed isocalorically or ad libitum had decreased bile acid excretion compared with the control rats fed a standard diet and had increased bile salt half-life so that the bile acid pool remained unchanged.[38]

**Small Intestine Functions.** When fiber-free defined-formula diets were infused in rats intragastrically, the total mucosal weight, total protein, and mucosal DNA were appreciably decreased as compared to those of rats given chow diets isocalorically but by mouth.[36] When rats were given a continuous intragastric infusion of amino acid formula (Vivonex), an intravenous nutrient formula, or an oral rat chow (caloric intake being similar), the mucosal DNA and protein of the small intestine was least in the intravenously fed animals, greatest in the chow-fed animals, and midway for the intragastrically fed animals.[37] When a defined-formula diet and a chow diet were adjusted to contain a similar protein content, no significant differences were noted in the villus heights.[46] When a diet containing free amino acids was compared with the same formula with bulk added as alpha-cellulose[36] or as pectin,[50] the bulk-expanded diet induced greater dimensions of the bowel mucosa parameters.

Atrophy of the small bowel has been reported frequently in starvation and with parenteral feeding, presumably as the result of a prolonged interdigestive state. Entry of food into the alimentary tract increased weight, DNA, protein, and glycolytic and disaccharidase enzyme concentrations in the small bowel both in the intact animal and in the residual bowel following intestinal resection, when compared to animals fed solely intravenously.[46] Carbohydrate, long-chain fat (to a greater extent than medium-chain fat),[51] fatty acids (oleic, linoleic),[52] short-chain fatty acids,[53] and bulk formers[36,50] can each induce intestinal mucosal proliferation.

Cholecystokinin and secretin given intravenously to dogs prevented hypoplasia of the small-bowel mucosa,[54] and enteroglucagon is reported to stimulate such growth,[55] although there is some conflicting evidence.[52] Regardless of the issue of cause and effect of peptide hormones, it has been demonstrated that certain defined-formula diets given orally to rats did not maintain gastrointestinal structure and growth as effectively as did orally fed chow diets; however, gastrointestinal structure and growth were better maintained than they were with intravenous feeding.[35,39,40,56,57] Glutamine with a TPN formula given intravenously to rats improved villous heights as compared to the TPN solution alone.[58] Despite a decrease in gastrin, animals on a variety of defined-formula diets fed oral formula maintained a positive nitrogen balance with a good weight gain.[56] With defined-formula diet intake, hormone levels approach 70% of the plasma level observed postprandially.[57]

Pancreaticobiliary secretions have been demonstrated by various experimental procedures to play a role in the maintenance of both intestinal mucosal architecture and function in experimental animals and man.[45,59,60]

Thus, in addition to luminal nutrition and neurovascular stimuli,[61] certain hormones have been implicated as important factors in the maintenance of normal intestinal structure and function.

## The Form of Amino Acids in Diets

Despite isolated evidence to the contrary, the concept that amino acids in intact protein had to be hydrolyzed to free amino acids prior to the amino acids' absorption persisted until the late 1960s and into the early 1970s.[62] This belief was held at the time that Winitz, et al. developed the L-amino acid–containing formulas; thus, a formula with free amino acids was deemed preferable to one with hydrolysates or intact protein.

**Efficiency of Absorption.** It is known now that mechanisms of transport of free amino acids differ from those of dipeptides and, in some degree, from tripeptides; the absorption of the tripeptides appears to be mediated partially or totally by dipeptide carriers. The small peptides that enter the epithelial cells are hydrolyzed by proteases and then are either used in the cell or transferred into the systemic circulation. The majority of animal studies have indicated that tetrapeptides (or higher peptides) are not absorbed intact but require hydrolysis by brush-border hydrolases to di- or tripeptides prior to absorption.[63] When nitrogen and amino acid absorption was measured using jejunal perfusion techniques in human volunteers, absorption from the protein hydrolysates containing increased tri-, tetra-, and pentapeptides were absorbed more slowly than those from hydrolysates consisting mainly of di- and tripeptides.[64,65] These data suggest that direct absorption of tetrapeptides and higher residues in perfusion experiments is limited and tend to confirm earlier studies in experimental animals that brush-border hydrolysis of tetrapeptides to di- and tripeptides is necessary prior to absorption.[62,63,66]

With the knowledge that small peptides were absorbed form the lumen without hydrolysis, the issue of absorptive advantage was again raised. Ordinarily, individuals with normal transit time and normal digestive and absorptive capacity have no problem absorbing adequate amounts of amino acids from intact protein. However, several earlier studies had indicated an absorptive advantage for several dipeptides over their free amino acids by some patients with malabsorption.[67,68] The concept developed that small oligopeptides would have certain advantages over free amino acids or whole protein for oral feeding of individuals with intestinal dysfunction,[69] because, first, the dipeptides and tripeptides are only one half or one third as active osmotically as the same amount of amino acids in free form; even though osmolarity is ordinarily not a problem, under abnormal conditions decreased osmolarity may be helpful. Second, absorption of amino acids and protein in a meal may take several hours or more for completion; thus, where malabsorption with rapid transit occurs, such time delay could decrease the absorption of amino acids whereas dipeptides and tripeptides would tend to be more rapidly absorbed. Third, pancreatic proteolytic enzymes are not required for hydrolysis of small oligopeptides because this hydrolysis occurs by mucosal peptide hydrolases; hence, the small peptides would be absorbed in pancreatic insufficiency, whereas intact protein hydrolysis would be less efficient.

When the absorption of hydrolysates of casein, fish protein, and lactalbumin was compared to their respective simulated mixtures of free amino acids, significant differences were noted in the degree and variability of absorption of the various amino acids; some amino acids were absorbed better in peptide form, whereas other amino acids, provided in the free form, were absorbed as well as or even better than those in peptide form under the experimental conditions.[68–72] These comparative human intestinal perfusion studies indicated also that greater proportions of the infused alpha amino nitrogen were absorbed during perfusion of certain hydrolysate preparations of casein and lactalbumin than during the perfusion of their respective free amino acids mixtures. The studies also indicated that hydrolysates were often not equal; for example, fish protein hydrolysates were not superior to their amino acid mixtures in their ability to absorb alpha amino nitrogen; furthermore, absorption of all of the individual amino acids was less from the fish hydrolysates than from the casein hydrolysates. Casein and lactalbumin hydrolysates had a stimulatory effect on jejunal absorption of water and electrolytes, whereas the fish protein hydrolysate seemed to cause a net secretion of fluids and electrolytes.[69,71]

Such in vivo intestinal perfusion methods have several disadvantages: a steady state of absorption has to be reached before intestinal contents can be sampled, and the osmotic loads used were high and in excess (perhaps three times as much) of that which would be presented during constant infusion into the intestinal tract over a 24-hour period.[66]

The issue of the influence of concentration on the percentage and absolute absorption of amino acids in lactalbumin, its hydrolysate, and its simulated amino acid mixtures was studied in healthy volunteers using the intestinal perfusion technique with three different nutrient concentrations in solutions of 290 to 300 mosm/kg; the concentrations were 40 mmol/L (0.53 g/dl), 70 mmol/L (0.92 g/dl), and 100 mmol/L (1.32 g/dl).[73] The hydrolysate had 20% of its amino acids in free form and 30 to 35% as di-, tri-, and tetrapeptides; the remainder were polypeptides.

At the 100 mmol/L-concentration, the observations of Silk, et al.[68–72] were confirmed in that there was a significantly greater percentage absorption from the hydrolysate of those amino acids that were absorbed less well from amino acid mixtures (i.e., phenylalanine, tyrosine, serine, histidine, threonine, and glutamine) (Table 54–1). However, at the lower concentrations (40 mmol), this pattern was altered; those amino acids that at the 100-mmol concentration were absorbed to an equal extent from amino acid mixtures and hydrolysate were, at the 40-mmol concentration, absorbed more rapidly in free amino acid form than in peptide form (e.g., isoleucine), and there was no significant difference in absorption at 40 mmol of the six amino acids listed above.

Calculation of the *absolute* amounts absorbed (rather than the percentages of amino acids absorbed in the hydrolysate form) at 100 mmol suggested that absorption is related more to the concentration of substrate than to the presence of specialized transport systems. Earlier work supports this concept; glycine and methionine were absorbed more rapidly from glycylmethionine than from their free amino acid mixture only at high peptide concentrations; the same pattern was observed for lysyl-lysine and its amino acid mixture. Others have found that at lower concentrations (30 mmol/L), the absorption of amino acids from hydrolysate containing 80% of its amino acids as di- and tripeptides was not better than absorption from its simulated free amino acid mixture, whereas at 100 mmol/L the hydrolysate amino acids were better absorbed.[65] Hegarty, et al. concluded that the nutritional advantage of peptides transport compared with that of free amino acids is doubtful.[73]

**Metabolic Studies.** The claim that mixtures of free amino acids or di- and tripeptides are more easily absorbed than formulas with hydrolysates or even those with intact protein remains unsettled, but evidence against this general proposition is increasing. A number of metabolic studies have been reported in recent years comparing the nitrogen availability from formulas containing intact protein, protein hydrolysates of differing manufacture, and free amino acid formulations. Some of these are reviewed here briefly.

When fed by a tube positioned in the proximal jejunum, nitrogen was as well absorbed from a formula with intact protein (Isocal) as it was from isocaloric isonitrogenous amounts of a hydrolysate-containing formula (Criticare HN) in undernourished but nonmalabsorbing subjects.[74] Better nitrogen *retention* was observed in subjects given Criticare than those given the free amino acid formula (Vivonex HN)[75,76] Jones, et al. showed that only small differences existed between a free amino acid formula (Vivonex HN) and the intact protein diet (Clinifeed 400) when infused by tube over 24 hours in randomized fashion in 70 malnourished patients needing nutrition support after a period of inadequate intake;[77] with similar nitrogen and caloric intakes, nutritional parameters

**Table 54–1. Amino Acid Absorption (% of perfused load) During Jejunal Perfusion of Equimolar Concentrations (40, 70, 100 mmol ∝NH₂N/l) of Lactalbumin Hydrolysate and Equivalent Amino Acid Mixture[73]***

| Amino acid | 40 mmol ∝NH₂N/l (0·53 g/100 ml) | | | 70 mmol ∝NH₂N/l (0·92 g/100 ml) | | | 100 mmol ∝NH₂N/l (1·32 g/100 ml) | | |
|---|---|---|---|---|---|---|---|---|---|
| | Amino acid mixture | P | Lactalbumin hydrolysate | Amino acid mixture | P | Lactalbumin hydrolysate | Amino acid mixture | P | Lactalbumin hydrolysate |
| ILEU | 90·0± 4·2 | <·05 | 75·6±3·1 | 76·8±4·1 | <·05 | 50·4±2·6 | 66·2± 6·3 | NS | 68·3± 6·1 |
| LEU | 89·2± 6·1 | <·05 | 76·9±3·2 | 79·6±3·2 | NS | 66·0±2·8 | 66·1± 6·3 | NS | 62·4± 7·1 |
| MET | 85·2± 2·9 | <·05 | 70·3±6·8 | 77·2±3·1 | <·05 | 69·6±3·1 | 73·1± 4·2 | NS | 65·1±10·4 |
| ARG | 71·1± 5·1 | <·05 | 45·1±6·4 | 67·1±4·3 | NS | 67·2±3·8 | 58·1± 8·4 | NS | 47·6± 7·9 |
| PRO | 68·2± 6·2 | <·05 | 52·3±3·8 | 63·4±3·0 | <·05 | 38·8±2·7 | 59·9± 8·0 | NS | 43·2±10·6 |
| VAL | 70·5±10·8 | NS | 55·1±4·0 | 70·0±3·4 | <·05 | 53·6±2·9 | 50·2±·9·6 | NS | 58·6± 6·7 |
| ALA | 71·0± 5·9 | NS | 60·1±6·0 | 60·3±3·3 | NS | 53·3±2·9 | 44·3±10·4 | NS | 54·3± 9·3 |
| LYS | 61·2± 8·2 | NS | 56·2±3·6 | 47·5±2·7 | NS | 46·8±1·8 | 39·7± 5·9 | NS | 43·9± 8·6 |
| GLY | 48·5± 6·8 | NS | 49·7±6·1 | 39·0±3·7 | NS | 34·7±3·1 | 30·6± 6·2 | NS | 37·2± 7·3 |
| TYR | 64·1±10·1 | NS | 68·0±5·6 | 60·7±3·2 | NS | 57·2±6·8 | 39·8± 4·8 | <·05 | 55·1± 9·5 |
| SER | 62·8± 5·6 | NS | 59·3±3·3 | 45·1±4·1 | NS | 35·4±5·3 | 28·8± 8·2 | <·05 | 43·8± 7·9 |
| PHE | 60·1± 7·6 | NS | 66·0±4·8 | 62·6±3·8 | NS | 62·7±3·2 | 44·6± 5·8 | <·05 | 65·1± 5·9 |
| THR | 57·9± 7·3 | NS | 53·6±2·9 | 39·8±2·9 | NS | 37·1±2·6 | 23·3± 4·8 | <·05 | 40·1± 7·8 |
| HIS | 56·4± 7·6 | NS | 61·8±5·2 | 40·1±3·8 | NS | 34·9±2·7 | 24·6± 6·8 | <·05 | 51·5±10·8 |
| GLU | 43·6± 7·1 | NS | 51·4±5·6 | 24·2±4·1 | <·05 | 31·9±1·6 | 14·2± 5·1 | <·05 | 31·5± 6·1 |
| ASP | 21·8± 3·8 | <·05 | 49·6±3·2 | 12·1±3·1 | <·05 | 34·8±1·1 | 12·5± 5·0 | <·05 | 30·6± 4·8 |

*Results are mean of six studies ± SEM

were about the same, but the intact protein formula allowed somewhat better nitrogen balance. These authors point out that increased nitrogen excretion (as urea) noted in their study and elsewhere[75] may be accounted for as a secondary effect of the large amounts of glutamine in Vivonex HN.

Using the same intact lactalbumin, its hydrolysate, and its free amino acid mixture that were employed in perfusion experiments by Hegarty, et al.,[73] two healthy subjects were maintained for 38-day periods on each of these three preparations in a complete formula at 36 kcal/kg/day. A relatively low nitrogen content, i.e., 47 mg/kg/day equivalent to 0.3 g protein per kg (20 g for a 70-kg individual) was used to stimulate nitrogen conservation.[78] There were no significant differences among the three amino acid sources, with slight negative nitrogen balances occurring with each.

A comparative metabolic study was performed in seven patients with a short-bowel syndrome (less than 150 cm of residual jejunum ending in a stoma).[79] Absorption was evaluated with each patient being tested on each diet, namely a defined-formula diet with protein isolate, a protein hydrolysate (15 to 20% free amino acids; 80 to 85% 2 to 6 amino acid peptides), and three solid diets. The diets varied in fat, fiber, and carbohydrate. Two patients were fed the liquid formulas by tube; the other sipped the formula. All ate the solid diets, While there were marked variations in absorption among patients, almost all had similar percentages of caloric and nitrogen absorption when on the two defined-formula diets, and four

of six had about the same percentage fat absorption; caloric and nitrogen absorption were generally better with the defined-formula diets than with the solid diets. Stoma effluent volumes were similar in six of the seven subjects. The investigators concluded that a liquid diet consisting of peptides, oligosaccharides, and medium-chain triglycerides is not more beneficial than a polymeric diet in patients with a high jejunostomy. This similarity of response does not mean that the diets were adequate for all of these malabsorbing patients, because additional electrolytes were often necessary and some subjects needed continuing parenteral nutrition.

In a comparative study using gastrostomy-fed malnourished chair-adapted primates given a hydrolysate formula (Criticare HN) or Vivonex HN (made isonitrogenous), the hydrolysate diet resulted in greater weight gain, less decrease in serum albumin, larger increase in iron binding capacity, and a more positive nitrogen balance.[80]

A comparative study of whey protein and its simulated amino acid mixture was peformed in hypercatabolic burned guinea pigs (30% of total body surface area burned).[81] While immediate enteral feeding of both formulations reduced postburn hypermetabolic response significantly, the intact protein maintained body weight better and resulted in more nitrogen retention, significantly better carcass, liver, and gastrocnemius muscle weights, and higher serum albumin, transferrin, and complement C3 levels than did the free amino acid formula.

The various defined-formula diets differ not

only in their sources and amounts of amino acids, but also in their sources of energy and their content of carbohydrates, fats, and other nutrients (Appendix Tables A–40b, A–40c, A–42). This point should be remembered in the evaluation of results of comparative experiments because these variables are essentially uncontrolled. Furthermore, in most of the comparison experiments that have been reported, the amino acid composition of free amino acid formulation was different from that of the protein hydrolysate or protein in the respective formulations.[78,81] Randall has reviewed the plasma amino level patterns occurring with various enteral and parenteral formulas.[82]

A defined-formula diet for general use (Vivonex-TEN) has extra branched-chain amino acids (BCAA), accounting for 33% of the total amino acids (Appendix Table A–40c). Hepatamine, the formula used for special metabolic situations, also has a larger than usual amount of BCAA, as well as other amino acid modifications (Appendix Table A–42). The effectiveness of formulations with additional BCAA and reduced aromatic amino acids in improving hepatic encephalopathy is controversial (see Chaps. 56E, 65, and 67). The critically important issue of diagnosis and treatment of children with intolerance for various amino acids is considered in Chapter 63, with appropriate formulations given in Appendix Table A–43.

## Carbohydrates

A variety of carbohydrates have been included in commercial formulations, all of which are eventually hydrolyzed to glucose in the small intestine. Starches vary in glucose units from 400 to many thousands. Hydrolysis forms polymers with decreasing numbers of glucose units. In general, the term polysaccharides includes carbohydrates with more than 10 units; the term oligosaccharides includes those with 4 to 10 units. Glucose syrup is defined by FDA standards (paragraph 168.120) as the purified concentrated aqueous solution of nutritive saccharides obtained from edible starch with the solids content not less than 70%; the reducing sugar content (dextrose equivalent), expressed as D-glucose, is not less than 20% calculated in a dry basis.[83] When the starch is derived from corn grain, its syrup is designated corn syrup. It also includes maltose, isomaltose, and triose. In commercial practice, the dextrose equivalent of corn syrup solids generally is 24% but can be as high as 65%.[84] Sucrose may be added to the formula. Maltodextrins are defined by the FDA (paragraph 184.1444) as a nonsweet saccharide polymer that consists of D-glucose units linked primarily by α-1-4 bonds and that has a dextrose equivalent (DE) of less than 20.[83] In commercial practice they have a DE between 10 and 20.

The osmolality of a formula is influenced to a major extent by the sources and amounts of glucose, sucrose, and the shorter chain glucose units and to a lesser extent by free amino acid and electrolyte concentrations. Osmolality of current defined-formula diets varies from a low of about 150 mosm/kg (in a low-salt dilute formula) up to about 800 mosm/kg (Appendix Tables A–40, A–42).

The defined-formula diets (i.e., those that do not include natural foods and, specifically, milk) do not contain lactose, thus eliminating the problem of intolerance to this disaccharide or to galactose for those with primary or secondary lactose deficiency or galactosemia. Primary sucrose-isomaltase deficiency is usually detected when oral feedings are instituted in early infancy. Secondary deficiency can occur in individuals with severe disorders of the small intestine in association with rapid transit (e.g., gastrectomy, short-bowel syndrome, Crohn's disease, gluten enteropathy, and villus atrophy of any cause); this deficiency should be considered when intestinal symptoms occur and persist even with slow-drip feedings.

In the individual with normal gastrointestinal function, hydrolysis of starch and long-chain glucose polymers is rapid. With marked pancreatic insufficiency with possible amylase insufficiency, oligosaccharides are useful because they are hydrolyzed to glucose by the brush-border enzymes, alpha dextrinase (isomaltase), and maltases (see Chap. 2A).

Insulin responses to glucose given enterally or intravenously differ. The acute insulin response to glucose given enterally was appreciably higher than the response when it was given intravenously.[85] However, insulin was found to be higher when high-glucose TPN infusions were given intravenously and persistently than when the same formula was given enterally by tube.[86] Others have found hepatic extraction of glucose was several fold higher when glucose was given enterally than when it was given intravenously. This difference is noted even if the plasma levels of insulin are made comparable, suggesting that unknown factors related to intraluminal enteral feedings play an important role in glucose disposal after such administration. The enterocyte converts some glucose to triglycerides, so that, following enteral feeding with carbohydrate without fat, serum triglycerides are greater than when an equal amount is given intravenously over the same period using the same diet.

The initial rapid infusion into the stomach or jejunum of large volumes of high osmolality is to be avoided in those patients with vagotomy (which also occurs with esophagectomy), gastrectomy, and intestinal dysfunction, because this infusion can induce rapid transit, glucose malabsorption, intestinal discomfort, and diarrhea. Hyperosmolar nonketotic coma can occur with high carbohydrate feedings just as with parenteral feeding; coma is most likely to develop in the diabetic patient who has become infected and dehydrated. Excess carbohydrate calories in enteral feeding—as in parenteral nutrition—can result in hypercarbia in patients with respiratory difficulties and in a rise in metabolic rate.

### Lipids

The concentration of fat in defined-formula diets varies from less than 2% of the total calories to up to 45% (Appendix Tables A–40, A–42). The lipids, usually corn oil or soy oil, have a large proportion of polyunsaturated fatty acids; some have lecithin added (presumably as an emulsifier). Others have medium-chain-length triglycerides (MCT) (see Chap. 3) that may vary as the major or minor fat. Some manufacturers add some mono- and diglycerides. The relatively large amounts of polyunsaturated fat (usually corn oil or soy oil) in most formulas provides more than an adequate amount of essential fatty acids; the need for the latter is estimated at about 3 to 4.5% of the total calories, with somewhat more needed for pregnant and lactating females (see Chap. 3).

As with other nutrients, the efficiency of absorption of lipids will depend on the rate of infusion, the concentration of the nutrient, and the digestive and absorptive capacities of the alimentary tract. (Lipid characteristics and other factors affecting digestion, absorption, and metabolism are reviewed in detail in Chapter 3. Aspects of abnormal fat absorption and the use of defined-formula diets in gastrointestinal disease are considered in Chapter 56, particularly in sections B and C.) Patients with exocrine pancreatic insufficiency may absorb more than 50% of dietary fat despite the absence of measurable pancreatic lipase activity. This absorption appears to be related to roles of lingual and gastric lipases.[87] Nevertheless, administration of pancreatic extracts is useful in patients with such insufficiency.

A report compared the effectiveness of five different levels of fat (from 10 to 50% of nonprotein calories) in tube-fed formulas given to guinea pigs with 30% total body surface full-thickness burns;[88] it was concluded that lipid levels between 5 and 15% nonprotein calories were optimal for nutritional support. (The utilization of fat and its effectiveness in nitrogen utilization in seriously hypercatabolic patients is discussed further in the section on parenteral nutrition in this chapter.)

### Vitamins

All complete defined-formula diets contain the full range of vitamins with the exception of vitamin K. The levels stated on the container label are given in Appendix Tables A–40, A–41, and A–42 for many formulations. The volumes of intake needed to provide the RDA for adults are also given.

Several issues must be considered. The first has to do with limits of vitamin stability in commercial liquid formulas during shelf life as stated by the manufacturer. There is essentially no data in the published literature on this specific and important subject. However, FDA standards and the quality-control programs of reputable manufacturers stipulate that at the expiration date, the content of each vitamin shall be at the level (within defined limits) indicated on the label.[89] Because some deterioration of some of the vitamins occurs, the initial amounts are higher than indicated on the label, the variation depending on the stability characteristics of the specific vitamins under the conditions prevailing. Various factors affecting solubility and stability of vitamins have been reviewed.[89]

Periodic sampling of the vitamin A content of two formulas (Osmolite and Vivonex) placed in polyvinylchloride (PVC) plastic bags and allowed to stand over 6 hours indicated that the vitamin was stable.[90] Storage in plastic bags of a formula with hydrolyzed protein that was frozen for 3 months, then thawed in warm water and allowed to stand at room temperature did not significantly change the content of riboflavin or of vitamins A and E.[91]

Another issue concerns absorbability of the various vitamins. Again, published data are absent; however, older data on absorption of nutrients from solutions would support the concept that the nutrients are absorbable from liquid formulas by the normal intestinal tract.[89] One aspect of this possible absorption is related to the impact of malabsorption on absorbability of vitamins. Data on the efficiency of absorption of formula vitamin content are lacking especially absorption of fat-soluble vitamins when fat absorption is seriously compromised. For such patients, slow drip of the formula would undoubtedly improve absorption. One wonders, however, about the efficiency of absorption of fat-soluble vitamins present in formulas with only 1% or 2% of their calories as fat in patients with major resection or bile salt depletion as the result of ileal bypass, resection, or damage.

When vitamin K is absent and administration is not contraindicated, and when the formula is the primary source of nutrition, especially in patients on long-term antibiotics or when bile salt depletion is present, the vitamin should be given; with bile salt depletion, vitamin K is best given in the water-soluble form as menadiol sodium diphosphate. In such patients not receiving this vitamin, periodic prothrombin levels should be obtained.

### Electrolytes, Acid-Base Balance, and Trace Elements

As with all nutritional support, provision of suitable amounts of sodium, potassium, chloride, calcium, phosphate, and magnesium is essential. Such requirements vary greatly depending on the nutritional needs and the clinical problems that may be present, such as malabsorption, diarrhea, and cardiac, hepatic, renal, and endocrine abnormalities.

**Electrolytes.** Review of the levels of electrolytes in the various commercial formulations (Appendix Tables A–40, A–42) reveals that most have adequate amounts while some have quite high levels per 1000 kcal of formula. The variations are large. Choice of formulas should take these differences into account in accordance with clinical need. Adequate care requires periodic measurements of serum electrolyte levels, particularly in unstable patients.

**Acid-Base Balance.** The composition of the formula in the context of the metabolic processes can affect the acid-base status of the patient. This consideration is particularly important in infants and in adults with difficulties in maintaining normal acid-base balance.[92,94a,b] The metabolic aspects of diets that contribute to the net acid base are the load of potential bicarbonate delivered; the amount of sulfuric acid derived from catabolized sulfur-containing amino acids; the load of metabolically produced organic acids in the child or malnourished adult being nutritionally repleted; and the release of hydrogen ion. Two additional but relatively insignificant contributions to net acid load are deposition of body water and new cell solids. In health, the total net acid load contributed by all of these processes is matched by the urinary net acid renal excretion, which is defined as urinary ammonium ion plus titratable acidity minus bicarbonate. An excessive net acid load, particularly in infants or in those with compromised renal function, should be avoided. Examples of acid-base data from various formulas are given by Heird.[92]

**Trace Elements.** The increasing knowledge of trace elements has focused interest on their quantities in defined-formula diets. The use of relatively purified ingredients in those formulas not containing natural foods restricts the presence of trace elements and necessitates their addition if desirable and safe levels are to be present. In Appendix A–40 and A–42, the contents of all formulations are listed per 1000 kcal for iron, iodine, copper, and zinc; the amounts are such that the RDA (or estimated safe and adequate daily intake) for adults will be achieved or exceeded when ingested in the volumes stated at the bottom of the column for each formulation. At this time, figures for the content of chromium, selenium, molybdenum, and manganese are not available for a significant percentage of formulations. Several reports have pointed out the low levels of selenium present in a number of defined-formula diets.[95,96] This and other newer trace elements listed above may be added by additional manufacturers in 1988.

When the formula is the primary source of nutrition and when the degree of malnutrition or malabsorption has been significant, review of the label will provide information on trace element content. A change of formula or supplementation of the low level of certain elements is indicated when requirements exceed those of the formulation. As with parenteral nutrition, with patients subsisting for prolonged periods primarily on formulations, analyses should be performed for serum levels of those trace elements most likely to be needed, i.e., zinc, copper, iron, and selenium. Nursing home, hospital, or home-made formulas based primarily on low-fat milk are likely to be deficient in essential fatty acids (notably linolenic acid,[96a] iron, and copper.

### Fiber

Some of the newer formulas have added fiber to provide bulk (Appendix Table A–40). A soy polysaccharide that is used is 75% carbohydrate and 12% crude protein, with some moisture, ash and 2% fat. The carbohydrate fraction contains 60% total dietary fiber or 30% neutral detergent fiber (NDF) and is composed of various complex polysaccharides.[97] When 25 g/day of fiber was ingested by healthy volunteers with an adequate low-fiber diet, average total fecal weight increased by about 25% over that of the control period; this increase was accounted for almost entirely by increased fecal water. Transit time was not modified. Approximately 80% of this fiber disappeared in the digestive tract.

A similar soy polysaccharide (27% NDF) was added to the intact protein formula Ensure at either 30 g or 60 g per 1500 kcal and compared with Enrich (containing 30 g fiber) (Appendix Table A–40) and ingested randomly by healthy young adult males.[98] Fecal net weight was greater with the fiber intake than with Ensure alone; the largest weight noted was with the formula Enrich. Transit time was reduced with the fiber. Variations were very large within all groups in both studies and the findings differed. No studies were done on patients with malabsorption or other bowel dysfunction.

### Considerations in Clinical Management

Table 54–2 lists clinical situations for which such diets have been advocated. For some situations the evidence for diet efficacy is strong; for others, proof of value is lacking or is questionable; for others the evidence is negative.

Winitz, et al. claimed that the formula with free amino acids markedly reduced the concentrations and types of microorganisms in the large bowel.[99] If correct, this report has important clinical implications because such a formula could, by eliminating or markedly depressing pathogenic organisms, decrease their entry into the bloodstream through intestinal mucosa damaged by toxic agents or radiation or facilitated by suppressed immune function. Subsequent investigations have been unable to duplicate these results, however.[100–102] While fecal weight was decreased over

that with normal diets and the total number of organisms from the large bowel decreased with the formula, the number of organisms was still enormous; furthermore, the change in types of organisms was not consistent among individuals. The value of such diets in protecting the intestinal mucosa against toxic agents such as cancer chemotherapeutic drugs and radiation is controversial (see Chap. 64).

Physicians, dietitians, and nutritionists must evaluate the nutritional and clinical status of the patient in order to use defined-formula diets effectively; these considerations have been considered in various chapters on clinical care. Route of administration and flow rate must also be considered so that the nutritional and physiologic needs of the patient are met appropriately. For example, the composition of a specific formulation in terms of osmolality and the type and amount of carbohydrates, amino acids, and fats may be critical factors when the formula is fed rapidly to certain patients such as those with high subtotal gastrectomy or those on jejunostomy feedings. These same factors may pose little or no problem in the same patient when a formulation is fed by slow drip over many hours. Hence, the technique of

**Table 54–2.   Clinical Situations for which Defined-Formula Diets have been Recommended**

| Situations | Reference Chapters |
|---|---|
| Anorexia | 50, 56, 64, 66 |
| Alimentary tract disorders | |
|     Chewing and swallowing disorders | 64 |
|     Malabsorption syndromes | 54, 56 |
|     Chronic partial bowel obstruction | 64 |
|     Inflammatory bowel disease | 56 |
|     Short-bowel syndrome | 56 |
|     Radiation enteritis | 64 |
|     Fistulas | 56, 64 |
|     Pancreatic insufficiency, pancreatitis | 54, 56 |
|     Hepatic failure | 56, 65 |
| Pediatric problems | |
|     Infantile diarrhea | 50 |
|     Prematurity; failure to thrive | 50 |
|     Malabsorption | 50 |
|     Inflammatory bowel disease | 56 |
|     Anorexia | 50, 54, 65 |
|     Cystic fibrosis | 56 |
|     Inborn errors of metabolism | 63 |
| Hypercatabolic states | |
|     Severe trauma, burns, sepsis | 54, 62 |
| Renal failure | 54, 58 |
| Miscellaneous uses | |
|     Nonallergic food source | 61 |
|     Preoperative bowel preparation[83] | 54 |
|     Postoperative feeding | 54 |
|     Protection of intestinal mucosa against toxic agents (controversial) | 64 |
|     Coma, paralysis, or handicapped states | 54 |
|     Toilet management | 54 |
|     Reduction of intestinal flow | 54, 56 |
|     Food supplementation | 54, 56 |
|     Decrease type and concentration | 54 |

feeding will play a role in the choice of certain preparations.

Because a formula may be needed in fairly large amounts and over an extended period of time, the physician and dietitian should consider cost when planning nutritional support. Costs may be reduced for the patient treated at home by developing a diet that can be prepared by the patient or family, thus avoiding charges for packaging, labor, and delivery, particularly when the materials can be purchased in bulk. However, ordinary blending of foods is not sufficient to reduce particles to a size at which they will pass through fine-caliber tubes.

Defined-formula diets are both a boon and a potential problem to the patient, physician, and dietitian. Advantages include the ready availability of nutritionally complete formulas in stable form with little or no preparation. They flow readily through very small caliber tubes and when purchased in bulk are relatively inexpensive. A significant problem arises from their fixed composition. Patients having certain metabolic problems may be unable to tolerate the amounts of one or more nutrients when the formula is given in the volume needed to meet overall fluid and other nutritional requirements; hence, the formula may be potentially or actually deleterious. Diabetics given large amounts of carbohydrate may suffer hyperosmolar nonketotic coma. For the renally impaired patient, the levels of protein and certain electrolytes, as well as the acid load, may be excessive with usual formulas.

Excessive amounts of nutrients can be diluted by addition of water (although this approach dilutes all nutrients) or by addition of nutrients other than the potentially deleterious ones. Alternatively, a formula can be prepared from "modular" components, which are now commercially available.[103a–c] Calculation of such formulas requires special expertise provided by a nutrition team dietitian and physician, and a specialized unit in the nutrition or food service.

Although comparative studies of different types of formulas in some clinical situations are reported occasionally,[104a–c] rarely have well-controlled comparative studies been done in a number of the problem areas for which defined-formula diets have been recommended. The reasons for this lack are apparent; the required metabolic studies are very expensive, and the requisite number of individuals with the desired clinical characteristics frequently are either clinically unstable or unwilling to stay in a metabolic unit for any significant period. Furthermore, to test a component (e.g., protein source), only that component's characteristics should vary in the test and control diets.

Reports of complications in patients on tube feedings are available.[105a,105b,106] They include equipment failure, too-rapid feeding by staff, diarrhea for many reasons, contamination, infection, aspiration, over- and underhydration, abnormalities (high or low) of various substrates, electrolytes, and other nutrients, and the development of liver abnormalities. Adequate knowledge of the patient and of the formula with sufficiently close follow-up of the patient by the physician, nurse, and dietitian will minimize complications.

## PARENTERAL NUTRITION

Knowledge of human requirements, the availability of various essential nutrients, and the means for their parenteral delivery over protracted periods is such that nutritional status can be improved and adequately maintained solely or primarily using intravenous feeding for long periods. For a given patient, proper intravenous feeding requires expertise in formulation to assure adequate provision of the necessary nutrients and the sterility, compatibility, and stability of all components. These efforts must go hand in hand with close monitoring of the patient to detect quickly any significant changes in the biochemical and clinical status that may require modification of formula. Adequate training of the nursing staff and patient will minimize infection and catheter complications.

The nutritional needs of the patient can if necessary be met completely by the intravenous route. Venous access may be gained through a central catheter or by peripheral vein. For the individual whose nutritional needs can be partially met by mouth or tube, supplementary parenteral nutrition is a useful adjunct.

### History

World War II stimulated much research into the metabolic changes induced by trauma and infection and the importance of nutrition in critically ill patients. Advances in biochemistry, physiology, and endocrinology led to better understanding of the important relationships among caloric intake, nitrogen intake, and nitrogen utilization. These requirements were increasingly recognized by clinical investigators in the 15 years after the end of the WW II.[107–109] Peripheral (or occasionally central) 5% or 10% glucose, protein hydrolysates, intravenous fat (IV Lipomul), electrolytes, and multivitamins were used in the decade 1955–65 by some clinicians for limited periods, although IV Lipomal was withdrawn from the market because it could produce serious side effects with prolonged daily use. The lack of a safe fat emulsion for provision of adequate calories by peripheral vein for periods of weeks or longer created a serious problem because the substitute very hypertonic glucose solutions could not be given by this route. While central catheters threaded into veins had been used as early at 1944, these were not commonly used. (See Selected Reading 12.)

Widespread interest in and appreciation of parenteral nutrition developed following the reports of Dudrick, et al., who used percutaneous central catheters and demonstrated in growing dogs and in malnourished infants and adults that parenteral nutrition alone resulted in good growth, development of positive nitrogen balance, and dramatic clinical rehabilitation.[4]

Dependence on glucose as the sole source of non-nitrogen calories in the United States ended in 1977 with approval by the FDA of a 10% IV soybean emulsion (Intralipid) (see below). Intralipid had been used extensively and satisfactorily in many other countries before its approval for use in the United States.[110]

The consistent use of concentrated glucose solutions (i.e., 10%) in parenteral nutrition requires their infusion via an indwelling catheter with its tip in a vessel with rapid and copious blood flow (e.g., the superior vena cava). Alternatively, when fat calories (as a 10% or 20% emulsion) are given with glucose at 5% or 10% concentration, amino acids, and other nutrients, infusion of the nutrient solutions through a peripheral vein is feasible because the fat emulsons are isotonic and a major energy source. Hence, peripheral total parenteral nutrition is possible by using large amounts of fat emulsion.

### Indications

The primary purpose of parenteral nutrition is maintenance of an adequate nutritional state or its improvement in a previously undernourished individual when oral or tube feeding is contraindicated or is grossly inadequate, and when routine hypocaloric parenteral support is no longer deemed sufficient. With these indications and with the guidelines indicated below, this form of nutrition may be lifesaving in a variety of clinical situations. These are (1) mechanical obstruction of the alimentary tract when immediate surgical or other intervention is delayed, contraindicated, or ineffective; (2) disordered peristalsis leading to persistent functional obstruction, e.g., pseudointestinal syndromes or ileus; (3) severe malabsorption of any cause not amenable to tube feeding; (4) hypercatabolic states when oral or enteral feedings are inadequate or precluded, e.g., major burns or severe trauma with infection; (5) persistent nausea and vomiting secondary to central nervous system lesions or drug effects or when aspiration is likely, especially in a patient with serious pulmonary disease; (6) severe mucositis or esophagitis associated with severe thrombocytopenia secondary to cancer chemotherapy or immune deficiency diseases; (7) heavy sedation or coma in critically ill patients on respirators and unable to be fed by tube; and (8) one or more of these indications in a pediatric disorder or in congenital intestinal anomalies, intractable diarrhea, prematurity, or failure to thrive. In short, parenteral nutrition is used for patients who cannot eat or be tube fed, should not eat or be tube fed, or cannot be fed enough orally or by tube, and who are likely to remain in such a state for some time.

The availability of parenteral therapy should not be an excuse for delaying initiation of more-definitive therapy when it could be begun without significantly increasing the risk to the adequately nourished or mildly malnourished patient. Deficits of hemoglobin, water, electrolytes, vitamins, and minerals can usually be reversed in a matter of hours or days, after which surgery, radiation therapy, or chemotherapeutic agents can proceed. The situation is very different for the seriously malnourished patient, because lean body mass takes much longer to replace and such patients are less likely to tolerate therapeutic intervention at this stage.

The development of a pre- or postoperative or other complication precluding oral or tube feeding cannot be predicted. When such complications do occur, there is a tendency to hope for the best, often causing an undesirable delay in the initiation of adequate parenteral feeding, which may lead to serious weight loss or actual debilitation.

Serious malnutrition, manifested by major loss of lean body mass, both muscle and visceral—usually in association with depletion of body fat, decreased levels of albumin and other plasma proteins, depressed phagocytosis and cell-mediated immunity,[111,112] electrolyte and fluid problems, and secondary nutrient depletions[109]—is associated with marked increases in infection, respiratory difficulties, skin breakdown with ulceration, weakness, edema, psychologic problems (especially apathy and/or irritability), and eventually poor wound healing. There is increased morbidity and mortality in patients with serious gastrointestinal disorders, prolonged postoperative complications, serious trauma, and sepsis in adults (Chaps. 56, 62) and children (Chap. 50).

As short a period as 10 days with 5% glucose as the sole caloric intake can depress the response to hypoxia in previously well-nourished adults.[113]

Impaired nutrition may lead to increased infection of the lower airway and to a role in the pathophysiology of respiratory failure.[114,115] There is ample evidence that the occurrence of serious trauma, burns, and sepsis markedly accelerates the metabolic rate and depletion of lean body tissues.[109,116] (see Chap. 62) Failure to act to meet the increased demands in such patients will result in progressive deterioration as the hypercatabolic stress continues.

The decision to undertake TPN requires the weighing of a number of factors and due consideration for the patient's diagnosis and prognosis. When the clinical situation is such that improvement in nutritional status will assist in full recovery of the patient or will permit significant palliation of underlying disease, the TPN program has obvious merit and should be pursued vigorously. It is not a defensible substitute for oral or tube feeding when either is feasible and it has no place in prolonging life in the hopelessly ill patient or in short-term postoperative care of the reasonably well-nourished patient who can be managed by hypocaloric fluids with adequate electrolytes.

**Peripheral Versus Parenteral Nutrition.** Experience with peripheral parenteral nutritional infusions in which fat emulsion provides the major proportion of calories is considerable.[117,118] Peripheral infusion has the advantage of not requiring the insertion and maintenance of a central catheter and may be useful for the patient who needs parenteral nutrition and has a goodly supply of patent peripheral vessels. However, because many patients requiring parenteral nutrition have had numerous peripheral infusions and venesections previously, their peripheral veins are often in a poor state. As a result, this route often becomes unreliable before the need for parenteral nutrition is ended. Furthermore, the seriously ill or unstable patient must have a reliable venous access at all times; hence, a central catheter in such a patient is a necessity.

**Guidelines for Parenteral Nutrition.** The initiation and route of parenteral nutrition must be determined for each patient. There are no absolute guidelines for deciding when to initiate the program for all patients. However, assuming that the criteria mentioned in the preceding paragraphs have been met, certain recommendations can be made:

1. Prevent nutritional debilitation by initiating TPN in patients who are obviously going to be unable to ingest food orally or by tube for some time, regardless of why. In particular, the presence of hypermetabolic factors such as serious infection and trauma dictate early

and vigorous nutritional therapy. Lean body mass should be retained or regained insofar as appropriate nutritional and other support and therapeutic measures will allow.

2. Nontraumatized, noninfected, previously well-nourished individuals may be maintained on routine IV fluids for periods of 5 to 7 days without significant debility. Beyond this period, more aggressive nutritional therapy is indicated by peripheral or central routes.

3. Young children should not be permitted to lose weight and preferably should be fed intravenously early in situations in which serious interruption of food intake is likely (Chap. 50).

4. Older children and adult patients having a loss of more than 10% of their usual weight and in whom continued impaired oral or tube feeding is likely should be given adequate IV nutritional therapy.

Adherence to guidelines such as these will prevent the most common cause of malnutrition in patients unable to be fed orally or by tube—namely, physician procrastination in the hope that the patient's condition will improve and permit regular food intake "within the next few days."

### Infusion Routes

For the infusion of very hypertonic glucose solutions, the catheter tip should be in a vessel with high blood flow where rapid dilution occurs; this placement minimizes the occurrence of phlebitis and thrombosis. A number of approaches to vascular access have been used (Table 54–3). Popularized by Dudrick et al., the percutaneous subclavian approach in adults and the duodenal or external jugular approach in infants were adopted widely.[119] Percutaneous peripheral vein placement of a long catheter threaded into the superior vena cava has been used. Arteriovenous (AV) fistulas of the internal type, usually with a bovine graft or external fistulas, have been used; some of the early patients discharged on TPN had one or another of these fistulas. The other vascular approaches have been adopted in situations in which the usual vessels have not been patent or otherwise available. In an effort to reduce infection, tunneled central catheters were introduced in 1973; these are usually placed surgically within the subclavian or jugular vein with the tip in the superior vena cava and the entrance brought out some distance away from the vessel often anchored with a Dacron cuff to eliminate the need for persisting sutures in the skin.[120,121] More recently, subcutaneously placed chambers (ports)

**Table 54–3.  Vascular Access Routes for Parenteral Nutrition**

| Route | Reference |
|---|---|
| Peripheral vein—percutaneous approach | 118 |
| Jugular vein (internal or external)—percutaneous approach | 119 |
| Jugular vein (internal or external)—surgical approach* | 120 |
| Subclavian vein or tributary—percutaneous approach | 119 |
| Subclavian vein or tributatry—surgical approach† | 121 |
| Portal vein | 122a–c |
| Arteriovenous (AV) fistulas | |
|     Internal | 123–125 |
|     External | 125, 126 |
| Femoral or iliac vein | |
| Azygos vein (via right thoracotomy) | 127 |
| Common facial vein | 120, 128 |
| Inferior epigastric vein | 129 |
| Saphenous vein | 130 |
| Right atrium | 131 |

*Used in placement of tunneled catheter
†Used in placement of subcutaneous port

with silicone rubber or other elastomer dia-phragms have been developed with the chamber connected by tubing, usually directed via the sub-clavian vein with its tip in the superior vena cava.[132,133] The infusion flows into the chamber through special needles penetrating the skin. Such chambers are a development from an earlier con-cept using a hydrocephalus shunt in this man-ner.[134]

The insertion and use of an indwelling central venous catheter imposes significant risks to the patient including risk of pneumothorax, hemo-thorax, microbial contamination and colonization of the catheter, phlebitis, or thrombosis of the vein.[135] Thromobogenicity varies with the cathe-ter material; polyvinyl[136] and polyethylene[137] catheters are associated with more thrombus for-mation than silicone elastomer types, while poly-urethane catheters induced appreciably less plate-let adherence and thrombophlebitis than silicone catheters.[137]

These complications tend to occur less fre-quently when experienced personnel, preferably members of a clinical nutrition team, exercise pre-cautions, which include aseptic techniques in catheter insertion and maintenance, assurance of proper placement (checked by x-ray study prior to use), the delivery of sterile solutions, and over-seeing of formulation prescriptions and of the bio-chemical and clinical status of the patient.[138–140a–c] Insertion of the catheter or port should be treated as a serious surgical procedure. Recommenda-tions for infection control in association with par-enteral nutrition have been published.[141]

In general, bacteremia or fungemia with the pos-sibility of catheter colonization should be seri-ously considered when the patient experiences sudden spiking fever and shaking chills. A sus-tained elevated fever is more likely to be related

to an abscess somewhere without catheter colo-nization. With the onset of fever, other sources of infection should be sought. Appropriate cultures should be taken both from the peripheral vein and through the catheter and appropriate antibiotic treatment instituted as indicated.

When colonization is suspected in a percuta-neously placed catheter, the use of a modified Seldinger technique is extremely valuable;[142,143] this technique involves rapid replacement of a central catheter over a flexible wire using appro-priate sterile technique but without another ven-ipuncture. If the original catheter is in proper po-sition, this procedure, if properly performed, assures that the new catheter also will be correctly positioned. X-ray study is indicated, nevertheless, before resuming infusion of the hypertonic glu-cose solutions. This technique greatly reduces the need for further venipunctures and the possibility of complications and is particularly valuable for the patient who is expected to require long-term TPN and in whom continued vascular access is critical. Because of some evidence (not well documented[139]) that the use of tunneled catheters is associated with less infection and fewer tech-nical problems (e.g., dislodgement) and because double- and even triple-lumen catheters of this type have become available, their use has been increased markedly, particularly in hospitalized patients at increased risk of infection because of depressed immunity secondary to drugs and ra-diation and for patients at home undergoing can-cer chemotherapy or TPN.

Use of subcutaneously placed ports is increas-ing, presumably based on the assumption that the risk of infection is reduced by the chamber's po-sition and with the only external entry site being a needle that is in place for only 8 to 16 hours during the infusion. No controlled comparative data are available to allow an objective appraisal of this technique as against other types of catheters. Such devices are very expensive and prone to cause infection and technical problems. Our experience and that of many others indicates that, with good placement technique, good solution preparation, and proper maintenance, indwelling catheters of the percutaneous or tunneled type can remain in place safely for months and years without infection or disruption. The situation is less sanguine in patients with chronic infection, debility, or diseases affecting immune mechanisms.

Particularly at risk of infection are those cancer patients treated with aggressive chemotherapy or those with cancer or aplastic anemia in a bone marrow transplant program. Summaries of mechanical and infection complications associated with the use of tunneled central catheters (Hickman type) have been reported;[144,145] 84% (300 of 357) initial catheters were in place for a median of 93 days (range 16-209) without complications and were removed electively, while 9.6% of all catheters were removed for infections unresponsive to antibiotics and 5.9% for mechanical complications (half of these because of accidental dislodgement).[195]

Internal fistulas or external arteriovenous (AV) shunts may be considered for long-term infusion of hypertonic solutions under special conditions when other prolonged venous access is limited (Table 54-3). Thrombosis with occlusion has been the major factor causing removal or requiring thrombectomy. Engels, et al. have reviewed their experience with eight AV fistulas in seven patients and the literature on 30 AV fistulas in 25 patients.[125] In their patients were six thromboses, three caused by intimal proliferation in the vein. The literature review indicated that 13 of 30 fistulas thrombosed. However, many fistulas were useful for many months or years. Coumarin anticoagulation did not appear to be very effective, but perhaps use of aspirin and low-dose heparin may decrease clotting.

## Delivery Systems

The nutrient solutions for peripheral parenteral nutrition (PPN) are delivered from bottles or plastic bags by gravity with or without drop counters. TPN solutions are generally delivered using propulsion pumps of various types. Pumps assure an even flow rate, overcome the increased resistance of filters of small porosity (especially with continued use), and minimize the likelihood of clotting at the catheter tip. Because pumping of fluids—especially from bottles—presents the danger of air embolism, it requires either constant supervision or, preferably, a controlling photo-

electric monitor attached to the drip chamber or a weight-sensing device. Pumps have become increasingly sophisticated and expensive, with an additional expense in many instances related to required special tubing.

Although their value is not agreed upon, in-line membrane filters have been used in an effort to provide greater assurance of sterile delivery of parenteral fluids and to prevent introduction of particulate matter; currently, 0.22-μm filters are used when "triple-mix" infusions with lipid are not used.

The use of pliable plastic bags of various sizes eliminates the danger of breakage, simplifies transportation, and greatly reduces storage space requirements prior to and after filling, compared to glass or formed-plastic bottles. Unlike other nutrients that are dissolved in water solutions, albumin, lipids, and blood can extract plasticizers or stabilizers used in the manufacture of most pliable plastic bags and tubes.[146] Plasticizer-free tubing and bags are available for fat emulsions but are currently more expensive.

### Parenteral Components: Nutritional and Metabolic Considerations

#### General Requirements

Approximately 30 kcal (7.17 kilojoules [kj]/kg of body weight/day should be sufficient to maintain weight for the relatively unstressed middle-aged adult patient in an acceptable weight range with restricted activity and without fever or other hypermetabolic condition. A nitrogen-kilocalorie ratio of approximately 1:250 to 1:300 (1:60 to 1:72 N/kj) is appropriate based on the RDA. (Appendix Table A-1). It has been demonstrated that malnourished nonhypercatabolic adults can be placed into positive nitrogen balance on a caloric intake approximately equal to resting energy expenditure (REE) (29 kcal/kg = 1.3 × REE) while on parenteral solutions supplying 5 g of amino acids/kg (180 mg N/kg) per day or twice that amount; nitrogen retention was better at the higher nitrogen intake. Hence, such patients appear to behave like growing children in this respect.[147] For weight gain to occur, more calories would be required, depending on the weight desired. Shaw, et al. present a graphic presentation of the effects of nitrogen and energy intake on nitrogen and fat balance in depleted patients. To minimize or help regain loss of lean body mass in those patients acutely stressed by trauma, burns, or infection inducing severe catabolic problems, the nitrogen/calorie ratio may have to be modified to 1:150 to begin to approach nitrogen equilibrium and, later, positive balance (Chap. 62). Caloric provision per kg of such patients may have to be at or above 45 kcal. (The goals for infants and children and adolescents have been reviewed in Chapters 50 and 51, respectively.)

All of the essential and sufficient nonessential amino acids should be provided in amounts needed for adequate protein synthesis. Essential fatty acids should be supplied regularly, particularly to malnourished and hypercatabolic adults and to all children. Macromineral, trace elements, and vitamin intakes should meet individual requirements without excessive wastage or toxicity. A key point to remember in all nutrition support is that a deficiency of any essential nutrient—no matter how adequate the formula is in other respects—can lead to negative balance of nitrogen and various nutrients. For example, Rudman, et al. found that a single deficiency, e.g., phosphate, potassium, sodium, or nitrogen, impaired or abolished retention of other elements,[148] while Wolman, et al. found that depletion of zinc induced negative nitrogen balance.[149] Water should be administered in volumes consistent with the renal and cardiovascular requirements of the patient and adequate to cover abnormal fluid losses.

### Water

The fluid component must be sufficient to meet individual needs, avoiding the dangers of over- and underhydration in patients who may have difficulty in excreting or retaining needed water. The close interrelationships of water, electrolytes, and other factors have been considered in Chapter 4.

The water derived from the metabolism of energy substrates is as significant in enteral and parenteral nutrition as it is with oral diets. It is sodium-free water and the volumes involved are usually a significant addition to the total volume infused (Table 54–4).

Expansion of extracellular fluid (ECF) is common in hospitalized patients with malnutrition.[150] Starker, et al. described two consistent patterns of body weight and serum albumin in the first week of TPN.[151] One response, occurring in patients who had previously been on an intake of only 5% dextrose solution and who had previous weight loss of 16%, was marked by a loss of weight and an increase in serum albumin; this change was interpreted as the consequence of sodium loss with diuresis. The other response occurred in a group of patients who with TPN had a gain in weight and no change in their albumin levels; these patients had various inflammatory processes. A third group of patients studied subsequently had severe malnutrition with a weight loss of more than 30% but no inflammatory proc-

esses.[152] After a week of TPN with caloric provision of 1.25 to 1.75 times the resting energy expenditure, they were in positive nitrogen balance and had a 2-kg weight gain that was associated with a cumulative gain of 390 meq of sodium. The estimated increase in ECF in addition to the increase in body cell mass accounted for essentially all of the weight gain; there was only a small decrease in serum albumin. Thus, severe malabsorption as well as inflammatory processes are associated with sodium and fluid retention in the early period of nutritional rehabilitation. Such clinical factors must be considered in evaluating the significance of changes in weight and serum albumin concentration.

### *Energy Sources and Requirements*

**Carbohydrate.** Glucose is the most commonly used carbohydrate for caloric replacement and is usually the major source of energy. Parenteral glucose is in the form of the monohydrate, with 1 g providing about 3.4 kcal. It is readily available in various concentrations in liquid form, is relatively inexpensive, and is rapidly metabolized by the great majority of patients. To achieve a glucose energy contribution of 2000 kcal in a tolerable fluid volume requires a very hypertonic solution (Table 54–5); hence the need for its infusion into a major vein with a rapid flow.

Other carbohydrates given intravenously are metabolized in whole or part. Because fructose is converted to glucose in the liver, it requires insulin for utilization. When fructose as an energy source is given in the necessary large quantities, it raises serum lactate, urate, and bilirubin and depresses hepatic ATP.[153a] It has a low renal threshold and, like glucose, it depresses serum phosphate. Sorbitol, a hexose hydroxyalcohol used in some countries other than the United States, is converted to fructose. Xylitol[153b] is a pentose hydroxyalcohol that bypasses insulin-dependent glucose pathways;[153b] like sorbitol, it is not available in the United States. Some intravenous maltose is metabolized but a significant proportion is excreted unchanged.[154] When infused over 12 hours at 2.5 mg/kg/min, 39.3% of the administered labeled dose was excreted as total sugars; at 5 mg/kg/min, 70.8% was excreted in these forms. A glucose oligosaccharide mixture with only α-D-1-4 linkage (80% as 2-8 glucose chain length) was infused IV in labeled form over 12 hours; at rates of 1.75, 2.5, and 5.0 mg/kg/min, 21%, 43%, and 62% of the infused oligosaccharides were excreted in the urine, respectively.[155] About 14% of postsurgical patients had good utilization.[155a] Neither IV maltose nor IV oligosac-

**Table 54–4.  Water Formed in the Metabolism of Tissue and Caloric Sources**

| Source | Amount |
|---|---|
| Muscle | 1 g yields 0.85 ml |
| | (0.1 ml from protein + 0.75 ml cellular |
| | water) |
| Mixed tissue | 100 kcal yields 10 ml |
| Fat | 1 g yields 1.0 ml |
| Protein | 1 g yields 0.4 ml |
| Glucose | 1 g yields 0.64 ml |
| Glucose H₂O | 1 g yields 0.60 ml |
| Mixed diet | 100 kcal yields 20 ml |

| Example: High-Glucose TPN Solution | |
|---|---|
| 750 ml 10% amino acids | = 300 kcal yields 30 ml H₂O |
| 1175 ml 50% glucose/water | = 2000 kcal yields 353 ml H₂O |
| 143 ml 10% lipid | = 157 kcal yields 14 ml H₂O |
| Total: 2063 ml | = 2457 kcal yields 397 ml H₂O |

| Example: Glucose–Lipid TPN Solution | |
|---|---|
| 750 ml 10% amino acids | = 300 kcal yields 30 ml H₂O |
| 750 ml 50% glucose/water | = 1275 kcal yields 225 ml H₂O |
| 500 ml 20% lipid | = 1000 kcal yields 100 ml H₂O |
| Total: 2000 ml | ¿ 2575 kcal yields 355 ml H₂O |

**Table 54–5.  Osmolalities and Energy Values of Intravenous Glucose and Lipid Preparations**

| Solution % | | mosm/kg H₂O* | kcal/L |
|---|---|---|---|
| Glucose† | 5 | 278 | 170 |
| Glucose | 10 | 523 | 340 |
| Glucose | 20 | 1250 | 780 |
| Glucose | 50 | 3800 | 1700 |
| Glucose | 70 | 5320 | 2380 |
| Lipid | 10 | 280 | 1100 |
| Lipid | 20 | 330 | 2000 |

*Plasma = 290; 0.9% NaCl = 308 mosm/kg H₂O
†Monohydrate form

charides are currently utilized in TPN because of their urinary losses.

*Glucose Metabolism.* The influences of glucose in individuals with normal and abnormal hormone status have been reviewed in Chapter 31. Byrne, et al. studied the adaptation in patients who were being prepared for or were already on home TPN to increasing loads of parenteral glucose and other nutrients as the duration of infusion was shortened; the patients were presumably in a fairly stable clinical state without a history of obesity, diabetes, liver disease, or glucocorticoids.[156] After the patients adapted to successive periods of 24-, 17-, and 12-hour infusions of the same TPN formulas, glucose as well as various hormones was studied in the course of each infusion and during the periods when the glucose infusion rate tapered to zero (Fig. 54–2). With the 24- and 17-hour infusions, all subjects responded well, with the major response to abrupt initiation of the infusion being a brisk insulin secretion. Tapering resulted in a fall of glucose to fasting levels with a rapid decline in insulin. No signif-

icant changes in glucagon, cortisol, or growth hormone were noted. With the 12-hour infusion, one of the five patients developed marked hyperglycemia, hyperglucagonemia, and increased growth hormone and cortisol levels; the elevated hormone levels persisted beyond the tapering period. Because glucose-intolerant patients are not uncommon, tolerance to glucose should be checked before infusing large amounts in cyclic fashion.

An individual has a limited ability to oxidize glucose. The limits are markedly different for individuals with little or no trauma as compared to seriously traumatized patients and particularly those with injury and sepsis. (This subject has been discussed in Chapter 62 and elsewhere.[157–160]) Infusion rates of glucose below approximately 4 mg/kg/min in normal subjects maximally suppressed gluconeogenesis.[157] In postoperative patients, glucose production was suppressed to 17% of the basal level at an infusion rate of 4 mg/kg/min.[159] The reasonably stable patient can oxidize glucose to CO₂ efficiently up to approximately 14 mg/kg/min, whereas the criti-

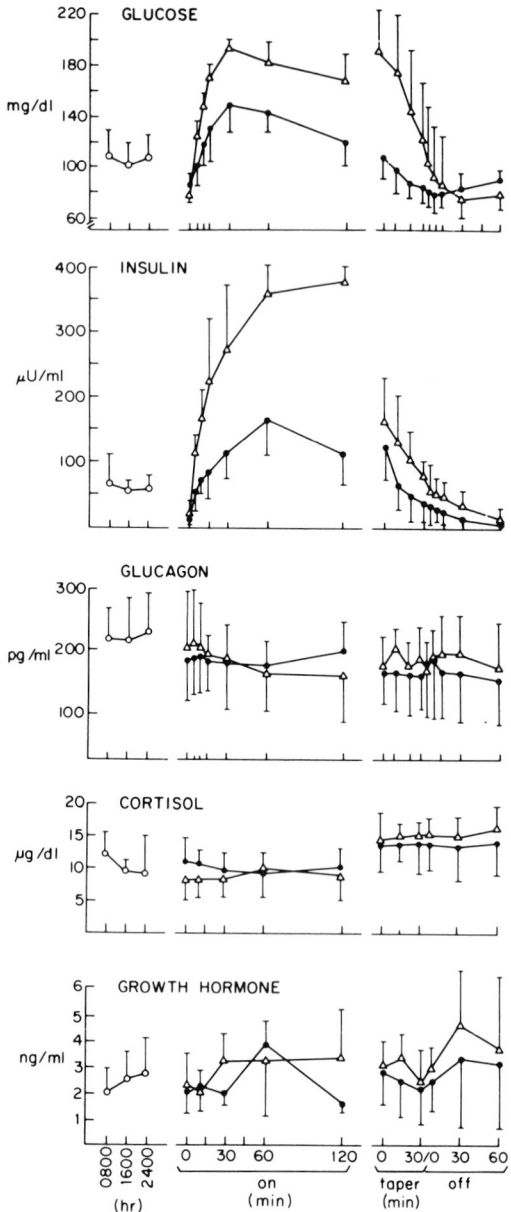

**Fig. 54–2.** The responses of glucose, insulin, glucagon, cortisol, and growth hormone to infusions of TPN solution in the same five adapted patients over 24 hours (○—○), 17 hours (●—●) and 12 hours (△—△), and over a 30-min period during which the infusions were tapered and stopped and over the first 60 min following cessation of infusion. Mean ± SEM is depicted for all 5 patients at 24 and 17 hours and for 4 patients at 12 hours. (Reprinted with permission from Byrne, W.J., et al., Gastroentrology, Vol. 80, pp. 947–956. Copyright 1981 by The American Gastroenterological Association.)

cally ill patient has a capacity of at most half of that amount, i.e., 5 mg/kg/min in burn patients[157] and 6- to 7-mg/kg/min in postoperative patients.[158] Infusion above the limiting rate will result in conversion of the glucose to fat with an increase in energy expenditure and an increase above 1 of the respiratory quotient (RQ). When glucose is given in excessive amounts, its conversion to fat is energy dependent and, with oxidation of the resultant fat, results in an ATP source that is 30% of that theoretically obtained by direct oxidation of the glucose involved.[161]

In addition to these limits on the body's ability to derive more energy from glucose and to exert further nitrogen-sparing effect, there are potentially detrimental effects of glucose excess. Wolfe, et al. have calculated that at an infusion rate of 9 mg/kg/min, 206 g/day of triglyceride were synthesized in the liver; only a small fraction of newly synthesized fat would have to remain in the liver to account for the development of fatty liver.[159] Fatty liver has been reported fairly commonly during TPN with large glucose infusions.[162]

Other undesirable effects of excess glucose relate to hyperglycemia and glycosuria with resultant water and sodium losses and, particularly in the dehydrated and infected diabetic, the danger of hyperosmolar nonketotic coma. Glucose intolerance in the TPN patient can be managed by either substituting a significant proportion of non-nitrogen calories as IV lipid or adding intravenous insulin to the parenteral solution in the proper ratio. While approximately half of added insulin is rapidly made unavailable by absorption, the remainder is stable for at least 24 hours. Intravenous insulin has a biologic half-life of about 40 minutes. The simultaneous infusion of insulin with glucose, together with the shorter half-life of the IV insulin, allows good control when a reasonable ratio has been established for a given patient.

As noted above, the infusion of excessive quantities of glucose (i.e., above that which is oxidized, or approximately that of REE plus activities) results in lipogenesis; this is associated with increased carbon dioxide production with a rise in the nonprotein RQ as $O_2$ oxygen consumption increases by a smaller amount[163a] (Fig. 54–3). Elwyn, et al. demonstrated that in malnourished individuals no increase in REE occurred with increasing glucose intake when intake was below that needed for energy equilibrium; however, when that amount of glucose was exceeded, REE increased by 1 kcal for each 5 kcal of intake; i.e., fat deposition resulted and was associated with a rise in RQ above 1.[163b] This fat deposition can be desirable for a relatively short period in the se-

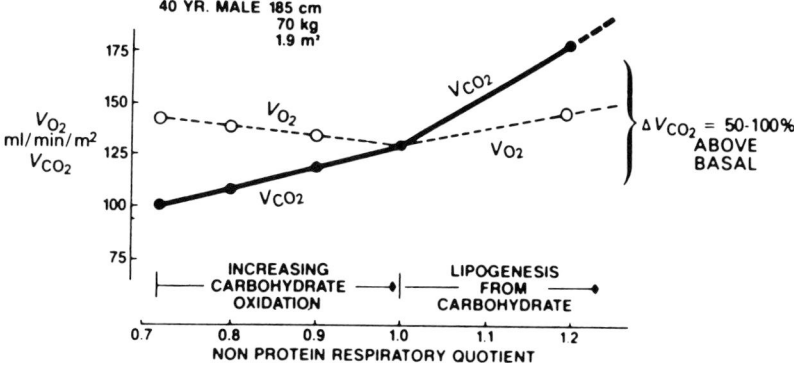

**Fig. 54–3.** Average values of $O_2$ consumption and $CO_2$ production for a normal middle-aged male as the nonprotein respiratory quotient (RQ) was raised by increasing carbohydrate administration. Conversion of carbohydrate to fat is associated with a large RQ; hence, a large increase occurs in $CO_2$ production as glucose is given above that needed for energy equilibrium. In this individual, $CO_2$ production was raised by 50 to 100% above normal basal levels with the high glucose infusion, producing a nonprotein RQ between 1.1 and 1.2. Because there was a small energy expenditure associated with lipogenesis, $O_2$ consumption increased by a much smaller amount with the larger glucose infusion. (From Kinney, ref 163a, with permission.)

riously malnourished but otherwise healthy stable individual.

The injured or septic patient given large amounts of glucose with lipid-free TPN reacted differently, exhibiting major increases not only in resting $CO_2$ production, but also in resting $O_2$ consumption; hence, the nonprotein RQ remained below 1.[164] This finding is compatible with other evidence indicating that some fat oxidation persists despite a glucose intake that normally abolishes fat oxidation and produces net lipogenesis.[159,165] In a study of surgical patients on TPN, a group on high-glucose formula was compared to a group on an isocaloric glucose-fat formula with 60% of non-nitrogen calories as fat. When the high-glucose formula was given at an infusion rate of 4 mg/kg/min, the energy increase was 11% of the mean daily energy intake and 21% of the mean resting expenditure; those patients on the glucose fat formula had an increase of 3% and 7%, respectively.[166]

*Ventilatory Response to Glucose.* With glucose infusion above REE in the malnourished individual with resultant lipogenesis (RQ rising above 1), minute ventilation at rest was found to increase by about 32%. In individuals with a low or normal metabolic rate prior to TPN, minute volume increased by 121%. Hypermetabolic patients who had an elevated resting ventilation before TPN, had a further increase of about 71% during administration of high-glucose TPN (Fig. 54–4).[167] Most of the increase in minute ventilation in these three groups resulted from an increase in tidal volume with little or no change in frequency. In patients with a decreased sensitivity to $CO_2$ or in patients with compromised lung function or who were already hyperventilating, the added ventilatory stimulus of the high-glucose TPN may aggravate the pre-existing pulmonary situation. It may occasionally precipitate respiratory failure and may make weaning the patient from the mechanical venilator more difficult.[168]

It is apparent that in the traumatic septic patient a glucose-fat formula has advantages when the glucose is restricted to amounts and rates that permit efficient utilization. Glucose in an amount contributing approximately 60% of non-nitrogen calories (or approximately 35 kcal/kg/hr) seems reasonable.

TPN solutions with glucose as the non-nitrogen energy source are associated with low serum cholesterol and triglyceride levels. Such a TPN solution was associated with a 26% increase in the fractional catabolic rate of low-density lipoprotein (LDL) with an associated reduction of plasma cholesterol levels through changes in both LDL and high-density lipoprotein. The enhanced LDL catabolism may result from the TPN-induced hyperinsulinemia.[169]

**Intravenous Lipid Emulsions.** These emulsions consist of very tiny droplets of triglyceride with a very small amount of cholesterol derived from egg yolk phosphatides serving as the core, surrounded by a solubilizing and stabilizing surface layer of the emulsifying phospholipids. Intravenous fat emusions have been used extensively since Intralipid 10% was introduced in 1961 in Sweden and approved by the FDA in the United States in 1977.[170] Both 10% and 20% concentrations of several preparations are available and serve as a source of calories and of essential fatty acids (EFA) (Table 54–6). Other preparations are available in the United States and Europe. They contain purified phosphatides from egg yolk or

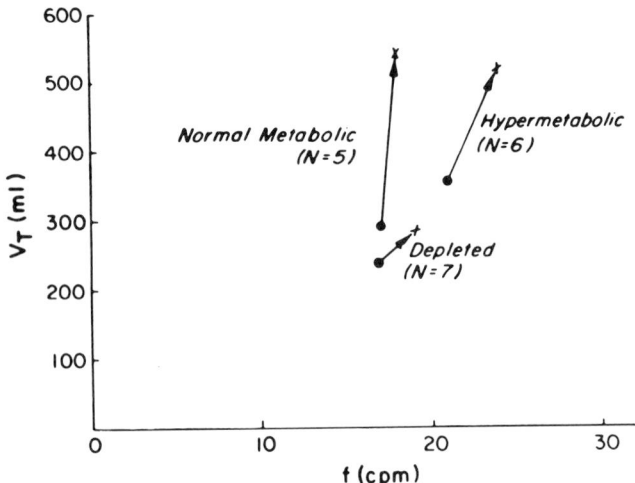

**Fig. 54–4.** Changes in tidal volume and frequency of ventilation are indicated for each of three groups of patients studied before and during TPN with glucose calories appreciably greater than the energy expenditure. The depleted and hypometabolic individuals (bottom arrow) showed a 32% increase in minute ventilation; patients with a normal metabolic rate prior to TPN had a 121% increase, and hypermetabolic patients had an elevated resting ventilation prior to TPN, which was further increased by 71% during TPN. Most of the increase in minute ventilation of these latter groups was due to an increase in tidal volume with little change in frequency. (From Askanazi, et al., ref 167, with permission.)

from soy as the emulsifier, and glycerol, which makes the emulsions isotonic and also serves as a carbohydrate source. The isotonicity and tolerance of the endothelium of small vessels to the IV lipid preparation permits the peripheral infusion of a large amount of calories; the equivalent amount of the 2000 kcal in 1 L of 20% lipid emulsion would require 1 L of 59% glucose solution, a degree of hypertonicity requiring a central venous catheter for its infusion.

As noted in Table 54–6, Intralipid contains appreciably more linolenic acid (Cl8:3, n–3) than Liposyn II, while Liposyn II has more linoleic acid (C18:2, n–6). The precursor of Liposyn II (Liposyn) had safflower oil as its only fat source and contained only a very small percentage of linolenic acid. Although the human requirement for linolenic acid is unknown and may be quite low, the low content of linolenic acid in Liposyn and the possibility of Liposyn's prolonged use, espe-

**Table 54–6.  Parenteral Lipid Emulsions: Approximate Compositions**

| Fat Source | Soybean Oil* | | Soybean Oil† plus Safflower Oil | |
|---|---|---|---|---|
| Concentration % | 10 | 20 | each 5 | each 10 |
| kcal/ml | 1.1 | 2.0 | 1.1 | 2.0 |
| Vitamin E activity (mg/L) | 18# | 36# | 20§–44‖ | 40§–88‖ |
| Egg phosphatides % | 1.2 | | 1.2 | |
| Glycerol | 2.25 | | 2.5 | |
| Linoleic acid %‡ | 50–60 | | 65.8 | |
| Oleic acid %‡ | 20–26 | | 17.7 | |
| Palmitic acid %‡ | 9–13 | | 8.8 | |
| Linolenic acid %‡ | 6–9 | | 4.2 | |
| Cholesterol (mg/L) | 200–300 | | 13–22 | |
| Phosphorus (mg/L) | 150–200 | | 150–200 | |
| mosm/L | 260–350 | | 300–340 | |
| pH | 8.0 | | 8.0 | |

*Commercial Products: Intralipid (Kabi-Vitrum); Travamulsion (Travenol): IV Fat Emulsion (McGaw): Soyacal (Alpha Therapeutic)
†Commercial Product: Liposyn II (Abbott)
#Tocopherol isomers in Intralipid in mg/L (and E activity): α7.7 (7.7); δ383(0.38); β + α = 51.1 (10.2); total = 97.1 (18.3) From Gutscher, G.R., Lax, A.M., Farrell, P.M.: J. Parenter. Enteral Nutr. *8*:269–273, 1984.
‡As % of total fatty acids
§Data from Bell, E.F., Filer, L.J. Jr.: Am. J. Clin. Nutr. *34*:412–422, 1981.
‖Calculated from data in Table 15–2

cially in infants, as the only lipid source was a cause of concern and presumably was the reason for the change of formula to that of Liposyn II. (The role of EFA in nutrition, their metabolism, and requirements are discussed in Chap. 3.) An oral intake for nonpregnant adults of 3 to 4.5% of total calories as EFA is recommended. EFA deficiency is prevented by average daily provision of about 3.2% of total calories as intravenous fat.[171] Administration of both formulas may result in an increase in serum cholesterol, as noted below. Soy oil has appreciably lesser amounts of α-tocopherol and larger amounts of the γ isomer than does safflower oil. As noted in the footnote to Table 54–6, the activity of vitamin E of the γ isomer is 0.1 or 0.3 that of the α form, depending on method and reference (see Chap. 15).

*Total Nutrient Admixture (TNA).* Intravenous lipids have generally been given by piggybacking the emulsion's tubing into the tubing from a water-based TPN or PPN solution. Mixing in one container amino acids, dextrose, minerals, and vitamins with a fat emulsion (TNA or "triple mix") has long been practiced by some European physicians; it has only relatively recently been gaining acceptance in the United States. The admixture is potentially unstable and requires adherence to certain principles of formulation (see below). In addition, certain aspects of TNA cause concern in terms of clinical safety. Table 54–7 lists advantages and disadvantages.

Davis and Brown, et al. reviewed in detail relevant aspects of the properties of the phosphatide emulsifiers and various factors influencing the stability of the fat emulsions in the presence of various additives in the admixture.[172a,b] Dextrose solutions reduce the pH of the mixture and in certain volumes may reduce the surface (zeta) potential of the charged fat particles to the point of instability. Divalent and especially trivalent ions, to a much greater degree than monovalent ions, can do the same. The major stages of progressive emulsion instability are aggregation, creaming, and breaking (oiling).[122a,122b] The cumulative effect of different electrolytes can be predicted using the formula $X < a + 64b + 729c$ where a, b, and c are the concentrations of mono-, di- and trivalent cations in mmol/L and where X is the critical aggregation number, i.e., the concentration of NaCl in mmol/L required to aggregate the emulsion system; this number is 130.[172a,172b] Hence, to help assure stability, the critical aggregation number should be less than 130. Davis cited an example of an unstable admixture that had the following electrolytes in mmol/L: $Na^+ = 50$; $K^+ = 40$; $Ca^{2+} = 7.5$; $Mg^{2+} = 3$; $Fe^{3+}$ 0.05. Using the above formula, the total was 798 mmol in 2520 ml, or 317

mmol/L, which is far above the critical figure of 130 mmol.

Davis pointed out that "as soon as an emulsion is administered to the blood, plasma components are absorbed to the surface extremely rapidly; the nature of the absorbed material changing with the surface properties of the particle," and that "there is the possibility that administered fat droplets from a mixed system may be coated in a different way to the same droplets given directly using an unmixed system and are thus handled differently by the body."[172a] Of interest in this connection is a brief note reporting catheter blockage in some patients receiving long term (70 to 402 days) an admixture of European TPN constituents. The occlusions could not be overcome with Urokinase; dissection revealed creamy lipid-like material that stained as fat.[173a]

Experimental and clinical experiences with TNA in the United States and abroad have been reviewed.[172a,172b,173a–c] While significant advantages accrue to the patient, nursing staff, and pharmacist, there are also disadvantages, including the potentially serious situation in which an increased bacterial growth in the admixture is complicated by an inability to utilize a 0.22-μm filter. The other uncertainties of this procedure require close nurse and physician surveillance, especially in patients at home, until more data are accumulated on potential problems.

*Metabolism of IV Lipids.* Unlike intestinally derived chylomicrons, an IV fat emulsion, as administered, does not contain surface apoproteins. Once in the circulation, the droplets acquire certain apoproteins, including apoprotein C (Apo C), from other circulating apoproteins. As with circulating chylomicrons, lipoprotein lipase (LPL) on the surface of capillary endothelial cells is activated by Apo C on the lipid droplet and hydrolyzes the triglyceride in the core, releasing FFA and glycerol. This is the rate-limiting step in clearance. The released FFA enter tissues; in adipose tissues they are re-esterified to triglycerides and stored, whereas in muscle they are oxidized; they also bind to albumin and circulate as metabolic fuel to the heart, the liver, and skeletal muscle. In the liver they are converted to very low density lipoprotein and are secreted into plasma.[174] Unlike chylomicrons, which undergo further metabolism (see Chap. 3), the remnant of the IV lipid particle is composed of a portion of the phospholipid in the emulsion (mesophase phospholipid).

Infusion even at rates low enough to avoid hypertriglyceridemia causes changes in plasma lipoprotein and cholesterol in infants, adults, and experimental animals.[175] Elevated plasma free

**Table 54–7.  Advantages and Disadvantages of the TNA System\***

| *Advantages* | *Disadvantages* |
|---|---|
| 1) Decrease in nursing personnel time and subsequent cost savings resulting from simplification of administration. | 1) TNA systems appear to support the growth of a variety of microorganisms significantly better than the conventional dextrose/amino acid solutions. |
| 2) Increased patient compliance for home patients resulting from ease of administration. | 2) Undesired effects (i.e., oiling-out) could result when base solutions ratios and/or additives exceed the amounts tested by the manufacturer. |
| 3) Decrease in training time for home patients requiring daily lipid emulsion. | 3) Changes in TNA formulations would necessitate remaking the remaining days' supply, which would increase waste and cost. |
| 4) Potential decrease in rate of extrinsic contamination because of a reduced number of manipulations of IV delivery system by nursing personnel. | 4) TNA systems cannot be filtered with a 0.22-μm bacterial retention filter. |
| 5) Less likelihood of lipid toxicity caused by increased dilution and duration of lipid infusion. | 5) Total membrane sampling cannot be used on TNA systems for a pharmacy quality assurance sterility testing program. |
| | 6) The consequences of long-term administration of larger particle size (greater than 0.4 μm) that exists in TNA systems are not definitely known. |
| | 7) TNA systems are difficult to inspect for particulate matter. |
| | 8) Peristaltic pumps may not be suitable for delivery of TNA systems to patients. In one report, a peristaltic pump delivered a TNA 50–75 ml/hour slower than the rate set. |
| | 9) Requires plasticizer-free bags with increased expense. |
| | 10) Shorter shelf-life in current home care practice with more frequent delivery and cost. |

\*Items 1–8 from Brown, R., Quercia, R.A., and Sigman, R.: J. Parent. Enter. Nutr. *10*:650–658, 1986, ©by Amer. Soc. of Parenteral and Enteral Nutrition.

cholesterol and phospholipids occurred in association with the LDL fraction. The LDL was altered and a particle appeared closely resembling the lipoprotein-characteristic of biliary obstruction and of inherited deficiency of the esterifying enzyme lecithin/cholesterol acyltransferase (LCAT). The Lp-X in infants infused with lipid in TPN contained 64% phospholipid, 26% free cholesterol, 3% albumin, and 3% apoprotein.[176] While the excess phospholipid was accounted for by the phospholipid in the TPN solution, the excess free cholesterol could have come only from endogenous sources.[176] Similar changes in LDL composition and the appearance of Lp-X have been demonstrated in rats given Intralipid.[175] In adults on TPN given either 9 or 12 g of phospholipids as Intralipid (10% or 20%), Lp-X could be detected in plasma within 2 days, and its increase was correlated with that of phospholipid and cholesterol in plasma and the amount of lipid given.[177] Lp-X was not correlated with LCAT activity.

Innis and Boyd found that in rats infused with either lipid-containing TPN or glucose TPN, tissue activities of key enzymes involved in the synthesis of cholesterol or in its conversion to bile salts differed.[175] Their findings suggested that the liver

in the lipid-infused rats, rather than being the source of excess plasma free cholesterol, was involved in its clearance, because the increasing influx into the liver resulted in a feedback inhibition of 3-hydroxyl-3-methylglutaryl coenzyme A reductase. They and also Rigaud, et al. tend to confirm the hypothesis of Griffin, et al. that Lp-X arises by an intravascular physicochemical union of phospholipid with leached membrane cholesterol either before or after combining with plasma albumin.[176,177] Lp-X particles are eventually cleared after cessation of the lipid infusions; the clearance mechanism or mechanisms are unknown but may involve phagocytosis. The half-life of Lp-X appears to be 2 to 4 days, with small amounts still present 7 days after termination of IV lipid.[177]

*Tolerance.* When the concentration of lipid increases to the level at which binding sites on LPL are saturated, a maximum elimination capacity has been reached. In normal adults, this maximum rate is about 3.8 g of fat/kg/24 hours corresponding to about 35 kcal/kg/24 hours.[174] The rate increases in starvation (by approximately 50%) and even more with trauma (up to 250%).[174] However, as discussed below, the clearance rate from plasma is not equivalent to the oxidative rate. As noted in Chapter 50 and elsewhere,[174] the sick infant or one who is small for gestational age has been found to clear fat very slowly; for these patients, IV fat must be given in small amounts and carefully.

Daily infusion of the fat emulsion over a period of a week or more is associated with increased tolerance as indicated by decreased preinfusion serum triglycerides. Serum FFA are cleared more rapidly when carbohydrate is administered simultaneously. Daily infusion of Intralipid in adults to provide 40–60% of calories with TPN resulted in a relative decrease in serum triglycerides with an absolute rise in cholesterol, as compared to infusion of high-glucose TPN without lipid.[177] Intralipid given to patients to provide 83% of calories caused a major rise in cholesterol.[178] A 3-month study of dogs comparing 10% and 20% emulsions in isocaloric amounts clearly demonstrated markedly lower serum cholesterol, triglyceride, and phospholipid with the latter over the entire course of the study.[179] As noted in Table 54–6, the total amount of phospholipids in 20% emulsion is half the amount in the 10% emulsion on an equal volume basis.

Cases of bleeding dyscrasia primarily in young children have occurred in association with high plasma levels of lipid and lipid-engorged platelets.[180] Decreases in pulmonary diffusion capacity have been reported during acute hyperlipidemia.[181] Other investigators have found no changes in lung dynamics but noted a decrease in arterial oxygenation,[182] while others have found no oxygenation impairment in neonates despite high triglyceride levels.[174] Increased amounts of circulating FFA have been reported to compete with albumin in the binding of bilirubin with possible increased risk of kernicterus in infants.[183] Though more recent studies have tended to minimize this risk,[184] any jaundiced neonate receiving IV lipid must be adequately monitored.

Various fat emulsions given intravenously are known to result in the presence of lipid particles and deposition of a ceroid pigment in reticuloendothelial cells of the bone marrow, lymph nodes, and spleen and in the Kupffer cells and hepatocytes of the liver of adults, children, and laboratory animals.[185a–c,186a,b] Giant cells, microgranulomas, and fibrosis may develop. To date, no effect of these histologic changes on hepatic function has been discovered. However, the changes have caused concern about possible depression of immune functions[186] and have led to many studies with variable findings. Inhibition of neutrophil chemotaxis has been reported in in vitro studies and in vivo studies.[187a] Other studies have found inhibition in infants only with very high lipid infusion rates,[188] while still others have found no effect in human studies.[189a,b] Comparison of the effects of glucose TPN with those of glucose-lipid TPN revealed no differences in the phagocytic activity of cultured Kupffer cells from infused septic rats.[189c] Detailed studies of various immune functions in malnourished cancer patients on either high-glucose TPN or glucose-lipid TPN noted depressed cell-mediated immunity prior to TPN but no alteration in immune parameters with either TPN solution.[189d] There is evidence that lipids can influence the adherence to antigen-antibody complement complexes of a variety of immune effector cells. Red cells and neutrophils were affected;[190] red cell immune adherence was augmented in 5 of 10 patients given Intralipid and was inhibited in 4; cytotoxic red cell transformations occurred in 5 patients with 4 of these having depression of immune adherence.

*Influence of Burns, Trauma, and Sepsis on Metabolism of Parenteral Lipids.* A significant amount of literature now indicates that hypercatabolic states affect the degree of lipid metabolism. As noted above, trauma is associated with increased clearance of exogenous lipid;[174,191] hence, parenteral fat has been used commonly in hypercatabolic patients, particularly as a result of the finding that glucose oxidation is limited in such patients.[157–166] However, Long, et al. claim that lipid infusion into burn patients did not exert the nitrogen-sparing effect of glucose;[192] this controversial finding is discussed below.

Goodenough and Wolfe studied fat metabolism in eight patients with major burns and significant open wounds 13 to 56 days postburn.[193] FFA turnover and oxidation were compared using $^{13}C$-palmitate with the patient in the fasting state and then at 1 hour and 72 hours of TPN administration while supplying calories at twice the predicted basal metabolic rate (BMR); glucose was given at the rate of 5 mg/kg/min and amino acids at 2.5 g/kg/day, with Liposyn 10% as the lipid source. Endogenous FFA turnover and oxidation were rapidly and markedly suppressed at the *onset* of TPN—presumably as the result of increased insulin release induced by the glucose. At 72 hours, a modest increase occurred in fat oxidation but not in turnover. Fat oxidation accounted for about 25% of $CO_2$ production (rather close to the percentage of fat calories given to the patients, which was in the range 23 to 46% with an average of 32%). Most of the fat oxidized was from endogenous fat stores and not primarily from the cleared exogenous lipid. The authors point out that, from the standpoint of metabolism in these patients, "it makes little difference. . . . whether the balance of energy requirements—above that supplied by 5 mg/kg/min of glucose—is supplied by the infusion of lipid emulsion or extra glucose. The primary difference of the two approaches is therefore the means by which the fat stores are maintained. With glucose infusion alone, oxidized fat is replaced via hepatic synthesis from glucose. In the other case, oxidized fat is replaced with intact triglycerides."

Studies in young dogs with [14]C-palmitate as a lipid label indicated a decreased ability to metabolize parenteral fat during septic shock as compared to a control period.[194] Kinney's group had demonstrated earlier that, unlike nutritionally depleted subjects, the acutely ill hypermetabolic patient responded to high-glucose TPN with a minimal reduction in net lipolysis and continuing fat oxidation.[163a,195]

*Non-Nitrogen Calories and Nitrogen Retention.* Solid evidence exists for the nitrogen-sparing effect of carbohydrate (including glycerol) in both the absence and presence of amino acids.[196,197] In the absence of amino acids, fat does not appear to spare nitrogen beyond its glycerol release and metabolism as a carbohydrate precursor.[196,198] There is disagreement on the nitrogen-sparing effect of fat in the presence of amino acids in hypercatabolic subjects. Certainly on a mixed American type of diet, positive nitrogen balance occurs with a considerable proportion of calories coming from fat; however, usually an equal or greater proportion of calories is derived from carbohydrate. In subjects with an inadequate calorie intake, the effect of added carbohydrate on nitrogen sparing was more pronounced than the effect of an isocaloric amount of fat.[197] Older studies with orally fed patients with typhoid fever or with burns indicated that carbohydrate, rather than fat, exerted a dominant effect on nitrogen retention.[197]

In studies of parenteral nutrition using stressed, burned, or traumatized patients, Long, et al. were unable to achieve nitrogen equilibrium or positive balance when fat was supplied as the non-nitrogen calorie source.[192] Calories from carbohydrate were required in an amount equal to the resting metabolic rate in order to achieve maximum nitrogen retention. Contradictory evidence is available. Jeejeebhoy, et al. alternated the same patients with gastrointestinal disease from high-glucose (91% of calories) to high-fat infusions (75% of calories as triglyceride); they noted that there was an adjustment period of 3 to 5 days after the patients were placed on the high-fat diets during which nitrogen excretion increased and then decreased to levels comparable to the level observed with the high-carbohydrate diet.[199] Rhesus monkeys with pneumococcal sepsis were shown to use IV

fat at 55 kcal/kg/day when it was *added* to dextrose at 32 kcal/kg in a TPN solution; weight gain and nitrogen sparing occurred with extra calories as fat.[200] The presence of substantial amounts of glucose may have played a role in the effectiveness of the added fat.

*Newer Fat Sources.* Medium chain-length triglycerides have an established role in oral and enteral nutrition (see Chap. 3) but have only recently become an object of research interest in parenteral nutrition.[201] A battery of reasons are advanced in favor of MCT's replacing long-chain triglycerides (LCT) in parenteral nutrition. These include the rapid oxidation of MCT in the liver with formation of ketones, MCT's utilization by extra hepatic tissues, and the claim that the fatty acids from MCT do not need carnitine to cross the mitochondrial membrane of extra hepatic tissues.[202]

Observations began in the early 1970s on the tolerance and metabolism of IV fat emulsions containing both MCT and LCT.[201,204,205] In general, ketonemia and production of labeled $CO_2$ indicated that rapid metabolism occurred.

Short-term studies were conducted in normal subjects given a 10% fat emulsion mixture containing 75% MCT (primarily octanoic and capric acids), 25% soybean oil with soy phosphatide, and 25% sorbitol over 6 hours at a rate of 0.12 g/kg/hour.[205] Comparison was made with 10% soybean emulsion (LCT). The triglyceride peak was appreciably less with the MCT mixture. The estimated half-life after completing the infusion was 17 min for MCT and 33 min for LCT. Serum β hydroxybutyrate was somewhat higher with MCT than with LCT during the infusion but not thereafter. The fat mixture appeared to be well tolerated in short-term observations in patients.[204,205]

A series of studies used rats to compare the relative effectiveness of TPN with LCT, with MCT, with mixtures of LCT and MCT, with structured triglycerides (TG) containing 60% medium-chain and 40% safflower oil fatty acids. Rats with burns given LCT or the structured TG had weight gain; those on MCT or a 1:1 mixture of MCT:LCT experienced weight loss; all groups were in positive nitrogen balance, but those given structured TG had significantly higher balances. The rats given MCT alone had markedly increased energy expenditure (30%). Estimated protein energy expenditure was significantly less with the structured TG.[206] In contrast to this study, rats with nonsterile femur fractures on TPN with these various lipids had weight loss somewhat greater with MCT and structured TG than with LCT, and the positive nitrogen balance was less.[207] Rats with nonsterile fractures differed in the presence of bacteremia; those given a mixed lipid emulsion with TPN (75% MCT/25% LCT) were not bacteremic; those with glucose or LCT with TPN were bacteremic. Following intravenous $^{59}$Fe-labeled E. coli, the MCT/LCT group had significantly less label in the lung and more in the liver than did either glucose TPN or labeled TPN. There was no difference in spleen uptake or in nitrogen balance on these three infusions.[208]

The issue of carnitine independence of MCT is raised by a report in which rats were infused with TPN, half on MCT and half on LCT; half of each group was given in addition 100 mg of L-carnitine. Those rats given MCT had appreciably higher excretions of the dicarboxylic acids (C6, C8, and C10) than did the LCT rats; carnitine markedly reduced their excretion from both lipid sources;[209] hence, MCT transport may depend on carnitine.

Patients having abdominal surgery of mild to moderate severity were observed with regard to nitrogen sparing and tolerance over 3 postoperative days during infusion of 10% soybean lipids (LCT), 5% MCT/5% LCT (29.5 kcal/kg/day), or 5% glucose (as the sole caloric intake).[210] The MCT/LCT emulsion, unlike the LCT, had to be infused into a central vein because peripheral vein infusion caused thrombophlebitis at this rate. Triglycerides and essential fatty acids were appreciably higher with LCT than with MCT/LCT. Total blood ketones were similar during all three infusions.

These studies testing various new lipid sources are intriguing and their role in parenteral nutrition deserves further definition.

**Ethanol.** Ethanol had been used occasionally as a source of calories. Its acute and chronic metabolic and toxic effects, however, together with the easy availability of superior energy sources, has made its use undesirable.

**Amino Acids.** Intravenous amino acid solutions have evolved from the original hydrolysates of casein or blood fibrin to solutions of formulations of crystalline L-amino acids of somewhat different compositions and varying concentrations, based in part on the amino acid composition of hydrolysates or modifications of high-quality dietary proteins. Variations of formulations continue to appear. More recently, formulations of crystalline L-amino acids for specific clinical use have been developed that claim superiority over general formulas in conditions of renal and hepatic failure, in trauma, and for growth in infants. Their development has been summarized (see Selected Reading 14). (The composition of a number of commercially available solutions are given in Table 50–11 and in Appendix Table A-39.) The eight

essential amino acids are present in all, as are histidine and arginine. Glycine and alanine are present in large concentrations in the general adult formulations as sources of non-essential amino nitrogen. The ratio by weight of essential to total amino acids in the pediatric and general adult solutions varies between 0.41 and 0.48. Taurine has been included in several formulations on the basis of certain observations in infants (see below).

Achievement of nitrogen equilibrium or positive nitrogen balance requires sufficient essential amino acids, some nonessential amino nitrogen, and some semiessential amino acids (e.g., histidine and arginine), depending on the patient's age and clinical status, in order to permit optimum new tissue synthesis. Caloric requirements for nitrogen utilization have been discussed above. The issue of optimum amino acid requirement has been and continues to be of great interest to researchers[213,214] (see Chaps. 1, 50, and 62 and Selected Reading 14).

Plasma or whole-blood free amino acid patterns (aminograms) have been used to assess the nutritional value of parenteral amino acid solutions in efforts to maximize protein anabolism in infants, children, and malnourished or catabolic adults, and to minimize the effects of diseases in which organ failure is related to amino acid needs. Plasma free amino acid levels are a very small proportion (<3%) of the total body free amino acids, and plasma free essential amino acids are only about one fourth of this small fraction.[211] As noted in Chapter 1, the total free amino acids in the body are only about 0.5% of the total body amino acid pool; their physiologic and nutritional significance are reviewed in that chapter and elsewhere.[211]

Plasma free amino acid concentrations may not reflect tissue needs at a given time. However, investigations regarding the concentrations under varying conditions continue, with various formulations indicating requirements. The levels of postprandial plasma amino acids have been used to develop formulations for infants (see Selected Reading 14).

Monitoring of serum free amino acids was performed in stable adult patients on continuous or cyclical TPN on a glucose–amino acid formula. Studying the amino acid formulation Synthamin (Travenol), Philcox, et al. concluded that, according to aminograms of healthy subjects, the supply of branched-chain amino acids (BCAA), lysine, and histidine was suboptimal; they concluded also that taurine was synthesized adequately from the relatively large amounts of methionine present.[212] After 12 hours of cyclic TPN, cysteine fell from fasting levels by an average of 13% and tyrosine by 24% (neither of these is present in the formulation); however, with both amino acids, there was one major outlyer among the eight patients so that the changes for most were not large. On these bases they designed an amino acid additive mixture containing additional BCAA, histidine, and lysine for long-term home TPN patients.

The serum and urinary concentrations of amino acids were determined in patients who had abdominal surgery and who for 14 hours/day were given TPN solutions containing different amino acid formulations. These formulations providing 9.3 g of amino acids, corresponded to the formulation in either egg protein or human milk protein.[213] The authors note that the patterns of some of the amino acids resembled those reported in malnourished patients and in postoperative patients on glucose-rich nitrogen-free TPN; they suggested that these common changes were related more to endocrine status than to postoperative nutrition. Despite some plasma amino acid differences, cumulative nitrogen losses were similar.

Comparison of two TPN solutions with differing proportions of BCAA in critically ill patients indicated that the higher BCAA concentration (44.6%) was associated with higher arterial levels of these three BCAA compared to the control solution, which had 19% BCAA; their femoral AV differences were more positive with the 19% solution. There were no sigificant differences in nitrogen balance.[214] A similar lack of difference in nitrogen balance between two different levels of BCAA (25% versus 45%) has been recorded in postoperative patients; it was noted that the ratio of individual BCAA to the amount of leucine was more critical to nitrogen-sparing efficiency than was the percentage of total BCAA infused.[215]

*Requirements.* Assuming an adequate composition of the amino acid solution, the daily requirement for growth, maintenance, or rehabilitation depends on age, nutritional status, metabolic needs, and the caloric contribution of non-nitrogen sources.

Infants and older children require an appreciably greater proportion of their total amino acid requirement as essential amino acids than do adults. Based on oral intakes, the fraction of essential to total amino acids as essential amino acids for each of these age groups is 0.43 for infants, 0.36 for older children, and 0.19 to 0.20 for adults (see Fig. 1–27). The ratios for parenteral feeding are not known with precision. However, as noted above, the fractions in pediatric and general adult formulations are between 0.41 and 0.48. An optimum ratio for repletion of lean body mass

in seriously debilitated adults is probably similar to that for the growing child. As has been stressed above, amino acid needs must be related to the level of provision of non-nitrogen calories and to the current nutritional status of the individual. For example, malnourished patients on TPN given a fixed amount of amino acids (averaging 173 mg N/kg) had, at *zero* energy balance, only slight positive nitrogen balance (this amount is about double that of nitrogen required to maintain zero nitrogen balance in normal adults). Nitrogen retention increased 1.7 mg for each additional kcal of increased non-amino acid energy.[216]

For infants, the range of amino acid requirements is 2.5 to 3.5 g/kg/day. The lower figure is preferable, since it permits positive nitrogen balance and weight gain equivalent to those gained with higher intakes but with less risk of azotemia (see Chap. 50). This figure (2.5 g/kg/day) is only slightly higher than the RDA of 2.2 g/kg/day suggested for infants less than 6 months of age (Appendix Table A–1). For nonhypermetabolic older children of normal height and weight and for adults requiring TPN, the RDA figures of 1.2 to 1.5 g/kg and 0.8 g/kg, respectively, appear adequate. Because most patients on TPN suffer from various degrees of stressful conditions, the provision of amino acids should be appropriate to need. Examples of needs for the spectrum of adult patients are given in Chapter 62.

Lundholm, et al. pointed out that in seriously ill traumatized or postoperative patients in an intensive care unit, the large amount of blood products (blood, plasma, albumin) given was sufficient to overcome negative nitrogen balance caused by administration of incomplete and unbalanced amino acid solutions (essential amino acids or BCAA) compared to administration of complete and balanced amino acid solutions;[217] they noted that infusion of blood products is often not considered when nitrogen balance studies in such patients are reported.

*Dipeptide Utilization.* Vazquez, et al. studied the direct utilization of peptides by the intravenous route. They compared adolescent baboons' responses to a 4-week infusion of TPN solutions with 16 amino acids either in free forms or as dipeptides, primarily as the glycyl peptides.[218] There were no significant differences with respect to weight gain, nitrogen balance, plasma and muscle amino acid concentration, plasma concentrations of various proteins, or leucine incorporation into muscle. Only trace amounts of the dipeptides were lost in the urine. Liver, kidney, and immune functions were well maintained. They concluded that, in this species, dipeptide mixtures were used safely and effectively.

**Carnitine.** The roles of carnitine in metabolism were reviewed in Chapter 24B. Patients on enteral and parenteral formulas lacking carnitine tend to have plasma and tissue carnitine levels below normal, although the pathophysiologic significance, if any, of such reductions is not clear, and more data are needed to allow judgment on this issue. Low carnitine levels were noted in cirrhotic patients. Septic patients may have reduced plasma free carnitine and short-chain acylcarnitine.[219] In several case reports of patients with serious liver dysfunction on long-term TPN, liver function improved with added carnitine.[220,221] In one of these patients, symptoms of muscle weakness and reactive hypoglycemia improved.[221] This patient had received additional lysine over a long period; hence, the response to carnitine suggests an inability to synthesize the latter compound. A patient on long-term TPN with muscle weakness, lethargy, and scleroderma but with normal liver function also improved with carnitine.[222]

**Taurine.** Neonates on TPN may be depleted of this amine sulfonic acid (see Chap. 24D) because parenteral solutions lack cysteine and neonates have low activity of the cystathionase needed to convert TPN methionine to cysteine. The report of abnormal electroretinograms in children on long-term parenteral nutrition led to the addition of taurine to several amino acid formulas[223] (Appendix Table A–39). Adults on long-term parenteral nutrition with significant malabsorption had their taurine concentrations reduced to 35 to 49% of normal values in plasma, platelets, lymphocytes, and erythrocytes but not in granulocytes.[224] The pathophysiologic significance of chronically low taurine levels in adults is not apparent at this time.

### Ionic Components

The macrominerals—sodium, potassium, calcium, magnesium, phosphate, and chloride—are essential nutrients. Because a significant proportion of patients on or needing parenteral nutrition have malabsorption and large fluid losses, mineral anions and cations, together with bicarbonate, tend to be chronically lost in significant quantities. Hence, a major and continuing concern in the care of such patients is the adequacy of fluid and electrolyte balance. These important issues have been considered in some detail in Chapters 4, 42, 50, 56, and 58 and earlier in this chapter. Table 54–8 suggests macromineral levels with the caution that age and clinical and metabolic status are critical factors requiring adequate monitoring of acid-base status and estimating losses of body fluids.

**Trace Elements.** Direct evidence exists for the essentiality for humans of iron, iodide, zinc, copper, chromium ($Cr^{3+}$), and selenium (see Selected Reading 13 and appropriate chapters in this volume). Manganese ($Mn^{2+}$) has been found to be essential for all experimental species studied, though clear evidence of manganese deficiency in man has not occurred. There is a single well-documented report of a case of molybdenum deficiency occurring in a long-term TPN patient with bizarre symptoms.[226]

Trace elements are not added deliberately by the manufacturer to intravenous nutrient solutions but are present in various quantities as contaminants. The degree of contamination varies greatly with manufacturer, component, and batch. In estimating patient intake, one must consider the trace elements present in infused drugs, blood products, and ancillary fluids as well as those absorbed from food and drink. Analytic data have been published in various papers with varying detail for zinc, copper, and manganese.[227–231] The minimum and maximum manganese contents of complete TPN solution were 8.1 μg and 21.8 μg, respectively.[231] Selenium is not detectable in TPN solutions by fluorometric analysis (<10 ng/ml).[232–233] A pediatric TPN solution contained 4.0 μg of chromium as a contaminant;[234] analysis in our laboratory of the mineral and vitamin content of complete TPN solutions indicated a minimum of 7 μg/day of chromium.

The issue of toxicity of parenteral lead, cadmium, and mercury merits serious consideration because of the administration of large amounts of fluids bypassing the normal barriers of the gastrointestinal tract and lungs.[235] The 20 components of a TPN solution used by me were analyzed individually for mercury; all values were below the quantitative detection limit. The complete solution had less than 0.001 μg/ml of mercury (the lower detection limit); the cadmium content was 0.08 ng/ml, and that of lead was 2.0 ng/ml. Potassium chloride and phosphate solutions contained 135 and 77 ng/ml of lead, respectively.

Aluminum is of special concern because of its adverse effects on neurologic, bone, and hematopoietic functions as originally described in renal patients being treated with antacids or hemodialysis (see Chap. 58). Reports of serious metabolic bone disease in a group of patients in California on home TPN for 6 to 72 months were followed by the discovery that the casein hydrolysate being used contained relatively large amounts of this element.[236,237] There were 2313 ± 149 μg/L of aluminum in the 10% hydrolysate (providing 3471 μg in 3 L of TPN) as compared to 26 ± 20 μg in a 10% free amino acid solution (providing 33 μg in 3 L of TPN). The aluminum concentrations in

**Table 54–8.  Suggested Approximate Daily Intravenous Requirements\* for Macrominerals**

| Ion | Units | Infants and Young Children per kg/day | Adults (per day) |
|---|---|---|---|
| Sodium* | meq | 3–5 | 60 and up |
| Potassium* | meq | 3–5 | 60 and up |
| Magnesium* | meq | 0.3–0.5 | 12–20 or higher |
| Calcium | meq | 1–2 | 10–25† |
| Phosphorus‡ | mg | 15–30 | 450 and up |
| Sulfur | § | § | § |

\*For patients with normal cardiovascular, renal, and intestinal function. The higher ranges are suggested for children with rapid growth rate and for adults with large gastrointestinal losses and adequate renal functions. In such patients, periodic evaluation of serum, stool, and urine levels are indicated.
†The higher calcium intakes are indicated for children with rapid growth and adults with conditions predisposing to prior bone demineralization and chronic acidosis.
‡As inorganic phosphate. Increased amounts are indicated when initiating TPN with large amounts of glucose to counteract resulting hypophosphatemia with serial serum monitoring. Phosphorus as phosphatide is present in I.V. fat (Table 54–6). Increased amounts of phosphate have been recommended to decrease calciuria.[225]
§Supplied as methionine.

plasma, urine, and bone were markedly elevated in all patients studied, and the bone morphology showed mild to severe osteomalacia.

Even though free amino acid solutions have small amounts of aluminum, other TPN ingredients may have significant amounts and contribute to the total burden.[238,239a] Premature infants on TPN with free amino acids for more than 3 weeks had increased urine, plasma, and bone aluminum as a result of their parenteral exposure and poor renal clearance.[238] Wu, et al. analyzed a large number of parenteral nutrients and found widely varying concentrations of aluminum in the same nutrient from different manufacturers or in different salts of the same mineral; hence, careful selection of products can reduce the aluminum dosage from 288 μg/L of TPN solution with high-level components to 10.9 μg/L with low-level components.[239a] Long-term TPN patients (14 to 53 months) ages 14 to 73 years given 2 to 3 L of solutions with free amino acids containing 16 to 24 μg of aluminum per liter had normal plasma, urine, and bone aluminum.[239b] Factors other than aluminum appear to play roles in bone metabolism of long-term TPN patients, as noted below.

*Trace Element Needs.* Following the recommendation of an expert committee of the Nutrition Advisory Group of the AMA to the FDA,[227] commercial intravenous solutions of zinc, copper, manganese, and chronium became available, ending an unfortunate period in which such solutions were available only to those physicians or pharmacists who personally prepared them. The committee's suggested intakes are given in Table 54–9. I recommend alterations based on newly available information. For infants above 3 kg, zinc may be provided in the range of 100 to 300 μg/kg. Man-

ganese suggested in the table levels can be reduced for both infants and adults; for infants, 5 μg/kg, and for adults, 0.06 to 0.12 mg/day would seem satisfactory. The latter figures are based on the finding of approximately 8 to 22 μg in a daily TPN solution[231] and achieving long-term serum levels within the normal range with these adult daily dosages.[240]

Serum iodides with no added iodide remain normal in infants[241] and adults;[242] adults on home TPN have been followed at least 5 years. This effect is explained by contamination of TPN salts with iodide and the efficient absorption of iodides present in ingested foods in addition to use of an iodine-containing topical antimicrobial agent. For the occasional previously depleted patient with malabsorption who may have an initially low serum iodide, 1 μg/kg appears adequate during the repletion period.

*Selenium.* As noted in Chapter 10A, major advances have been made since 1973 in our understanding of the metabolic and nutritional importance of selenium. Though Keshan disease in China is related to selenium depletion, there is reason to believe that selenium depletion is not the only factor. Similarly, although in the United States approximately four deaths have been reported in TPN patients with low blood and tissue selenium levels, a number of patients have remained on TPN for years with serum selenium levels in the extremely low range without any symptoms or signs suggestive of this deficiency. However, one cannot and should not ignore the deaths associated with cardiomyopathy[243] and the reports of muscle tenderness and weakness responding to selenium.[232,243,244]

The clinical consequences, assessment of selen-

**Table 54–9.  Suggested Daily Intravenous Intake of Essential Trace Elements***

|  | Pediatric Patients, μg/kg[†] | Stable Adult | Adult in Acute Catabolic State[§] | Stable Adult With Intestinal Losses[§] |
|---|---|---|---|---|
| Zinc | 300[‡]<br>100[¶] | 2.5–4.0 mg | Additional 2.0 mg | Add 12.2 mg/L of small-bowel fluid losses and 17.1 mg/kg of stool or ileostomy output |
| Copper | 20 | 0.5–1.5 mg | — | — |
| Chromium | 0.14–0.2 | 10–15 μg | — | 20 μg |
| Manganese | 2–10 | 0.15–0.8 mg | — | — |

*From ref 227, with permission. See original paper for further comments. See suggested modifications by author and data on other trace elments in text of this chapter.
†Limited data available for infants weighing less than 1500 g.
‡For premature infants (L 1500 g) up to 3 kg body weight; thereafter, recommendations for full-term infants apply.
§Frequent monitoring of blood levels in these patients is essential to guide proper dosage.
¶For full-term infants and children up to 5 years old. Thereafter the recommendations for adults apply up to a maximum of 4 mg/day.

ium status, and types of selenium compounds that could be used parenterally were considered in a 1986 A.S.P.E.N. workshop.[245] Selenous acid (selenite) for intravenous use is now available. It is stable with the AMA-FDA vitamin formula.[245a,245b] In my experience, 100 μg/day of selenium as selenite in TPN returns very low serum selenium levels to normal within 7 to 10 days; 40 μg/day will maintain normal levels in those eating or absorbing poorly. For infants and children, 2 to 3 μg/kg/day appear adequate to maintain normal levels. Not all patients on TPN require added selenium; in general, blood selenium correlates inversely with the requirement for TPN calories.[246] I found that an estimate of selenium need relates inversely to the efficiency of xylose absorption.

*Iron.* When iron must be administered IV, it can be given as a dilute Imferon (iron dextran) solution in varying amounts after a test dose has ensured that the patient is not hypersensitive. Because many patients on parenteral nutrition have had previous surgery and blood transfusions, their body stores must be determined before instituting iron therapy. This testing can be done by measuring serum iron or ferritin or by staining for iron in a bone marrow biopsy. Assuming that iron is needed (see Chap. 7), it can be replenished by addition in appropriate amounts to the TPN solution prior to infusion. Iron in blood lost from persistent venipuncture for various tests may be replaced on the basis of 10 mg of iron for every 25 to 30 ml of whole blood in a patient with normal hematocrit. The stable adult male on home TPN requires about 1 mg/day, the menstruating female about 2.5 mg, and infants and young children 1 to 2 mg/day.

*Molybdenum.* The metabolic and nutritional roles of molybdenum (Mo) were reviewed in Chapter 11. The single reported case of nutritional deficiency in a long-term TPN patient was successfully treated with 300 μg of molybdenum as ammonium molybdate.[226] No other dosages were tested, however, and it appears likely to me that much lower doses could prevent depletion. Data on the molybdenum content of TPN solutions are not currently available and should be developed because molybdenum is probably present as a contaminant. Molybdate is reasonably well absorbed (see Chap. 11).

*Ultratrace Elements.* These elements are reviewed in Chapter 11. Currently there is no evidence favoring the addition to TPN of arsenic, boron, nickel, silicon, vanadium, and others of this class, although the essentiality for man of one or more (e.g., arsenic or boron) is likely.

### Vitamins

The inadequacies of intravenous multivitamin solutions[247] (see Selected Reading 13), combined with pressure on the FDA for change through a court order,[248] resulted in major changes in parenteral vitamins. Recommendations to the FDA in December, 1975 by the Nutrition Advisory Group of the AMA for intravenous vitamin formulations[247,249] were approved by the FDA in 1979 for the adult formulation;[250] the adult formulation is designated here as the AMA-FDA adult formula. In 1984, the recommended pediatric formula was approved. Both formulas are now in general use (Table 54–10). The pediatric formula provides all known essential vitamins, while the adult formula omits vitamin K; this must be added separately at a recommended dosage of 5 mg once weekly in the TPN solution. The manufacturers add excess nutrients at production time (within limits set by the FDA) in order to meet label requirements at the time of the expiration date.

Vitamins must be in solution for parenteral use. Their association and interactions with numerous other nutrients, solubilizers, and stabilizers, their

**Table 54–10.    Composition of Parenteral Vitamin Formulation\***

|  |  | MVI Concentrate (5 ml) | AMA-FDA Formulas | |
|  |  |  | Adult† | Pediatric‡ |
|---|---|---|---|---|
| Vitamin A | (mg) (IU)§ | 3.5 (10,000) | 0.99 (3300) | 0.7 (2300) |
| Vitamin $D_2$ | (μg) (IU) | 25.0 (1,000) | 5.0 (200) | 10.0 (400) |
| Vitamin E | (mg) (IU)‖ | 5.0 (5) | 10.0 (10) | 7.0 (7) |
| Vitamin $K_1$ | (mg) | 0 | 0 | 0.2 |
| Thiamin# | (mg) | 50.0 | 3.0 | 1.2 |
| Riboflavin¶ | (mg) | 10.0 | 3.6 | 1.4 |
| Niacin | (mg) | 100.0 | 40.0 | 17.0 |
| Pyridoxine# | (mg) | 15.0 | 4.0 | 1.0 |
| Pantotheneate\*\* | (mg) | 25.0 | 15.0 | 5.0 |
| Biotin | (μg) | 0 | 60.0 | 20.0 |
| Folic Acid | (μg) | 0 | 400.0 | 140.0 |
| Cyanocobalamin ($B_{12}$) | (μg) | 0 | 5.0 | 1.0 |
| Ascorbic acid | (mg) | 500.0 | 100.0 | 80.0 |

\*See Table 54–11 for list of excipients
†10-ml volume (in divided form) from most producers; Roche Berroca PN has 2-ml volume
‡Lyophilized
§Vitamin A as retinol by most producers; as retinol palmitate in Roche Berocca PN
‖Vitamin E as dl-alpha tocopherol acetate by most producers; as dl-alpha tocopherol in Roche Berroca PN
#As the hydrochloride
¶As phosphate
\*\*As dexpanthenol

contact with glass or plastic containers, tubes, and filters, and their exposure to light and heat might allow absorption or destruction to varying degrees. DeRitter has reviewed in detail factors affecting the solubility and stability of vitamins in various pharmaceutical preparations.[251] Several studies have been reported on the degree of stability of a number of vitamins in parenteral solutions of varying compositions and test conditions. The majority of studies in the United States have used the old MVI solution or its concentrate (Table 54–10). Appreciable amounts of vitamin A appear to be lost from solution,[252–254] particularly when flow through tubing is slow[253,254] or when the vitamin solution is present in the TPN solution for many days, even under refrigeration.[255] Losses with sorption of this vitamin and perhaps other fat solubles is a matter of particular concern. Retinyl palmitate (present in the Roche PN version of the AMA-FDA formula) is more stable than retinol (present in the other formulations) or retinyl acetate;[253] however, others have found with this palmitate ester significant losses that are partially reduced by protection against light.[256] Vitamins D and E can also be lost from MVI;[252] the latter is present as dl-α-tocopherol acetate. dl-α-tocopherol in Berocca Parenteral Nutrition was not absorbed by infusion sets.[253]

Thiamin is split and so loses biologic activity in the presence of sodium bisulfite, which is a component of United States amino acid solutions; appreciable amounts can be lost with prolonged contact.[257] Ascorbic acid is unstable in adult AMA-FDA adult formula, particularly in the presence of cupric ion and oxygen.[258] Folate is very stable when the TPN solution has a pH above 5.0, which is usually the case;[259] it is stable also to room and fluorescent light, as thiamin, riboflavin, and $B_6$ were in the old MVI preparation.[260] Riboflavin and $B_6$ are unstable over a matter of hours in direct sunlight at room temperature.[260]

Although more data on stability are needed for the current vitamin preparations, it is obvious that the multivitamin solution should be added to the TPN solution just prior to infusion to ensure that the patient receives as much of the dose as possible of the less stable nutrients. Direct sunlight should be avoided.

Parenteral multivitamins contain a variety of excipients serving as emulsifiers, stabilizers, antioxidants, buffers, and preservatives. Their presence and concentrations in various commercial preparations of the AMA-FDA formulas are given in Table 54–11. The American Academy of Pediatrics recently reviewed the issue of excipients as "inactive ingredients" in pharmaceutical products with particular reference to infants and children because some are not inert ingredients.

The issue of vitamin needs for sick and injured patients has long been of concern. A National

**Table 54–11.  Intravenous Multivitamins—Excipient Component Comparison***

| | | | Amounts per Total Daily Dose | | | |
|---|---|---|---|---|---|---|
| | | | Adult | | | Pediatric† |
| Ingredient | | Function | MVI-12 (Armour) (10 ml) | MVC 9+3 (LyphoMed) (10 ml) | Berocca (Roche) (2 ml) | MVI (Armour) (10 ml) |
| Polysorbate 80 | (mg) | Surfactant, emulsifier | 80 | — | — | 50 |
| Polysorbate 20 | (mg) | Surfactant, emulsifier | 1.4 | 240 | — | 0.8 |
| Polyoxyethylated vegetable oil‡ | (mg) | Surfactant, emulsifier | — | — | 100 | — |
| Gentisic acid ethanolamide | (mg) | Stabilizer, preservative, solubilizer | 100 | 100 | 40 | — |
| Propylene glycol | (mg) | Stabilizer | 3000 | 3000 | 500 | — |
| Ethanol | (ml) | Stabilizer | — | — | 0.1 | — |
| Benzyl alcohol | (mg) | Preservative | — | — | 20 | — |
| BHT§ | (mg) | Lipid antioxidant | 0.1 | 0.09 | — | 0.058 |
| BHA‖ | (mg) | Lipid antioxidant | 0.025 | 0.02 | — | 0.014 |
| Citric acid | (mg) | Buffer | present | present | 17 | — |
| Sodium citrate | (mg) | Buffer | present | present | — | — |
| EDTA (disodium) (edetate) | (mg) | Metal chelator, stabilizer, antioxidant | — | — | 0.2 | — |
| Mannitol | (mg) | Lyophilization aid | — | — | — | 375 |

*Modified (with pediatric formulation data added) from tabular material of H. Newmark, with permission
†Upon reconstitution of lyophilized product
‡Emulphor EL-620
§BHT = Butylated hydroxytoluene
‖BHA = Butylated hydroxyanisole

Academy of Sciences publication of 1952 (which began the trend to higher dosage of therapeutic vitamins) stated, "The vitamin requirements under stress situations have never been completely determined."[262] Although exact quantitation for various disease states for all vitamins still is not at hand, the existing data for adult patients permit a relatively narrow range of values for a number of these nutrients to emerge.[258,263] Although much of the information obtained in seriously ill patients is based on short-term data of a few weeks to a few months, for the great majority this is the critical time range. Nevertheless, uniform agreement among physicians is lacking, and, for some, vitamin dosages reflect the "art" rather than the "science" with very large doses being given of certain of the water-soluble vitamins.[263]

Varying amounts of vitamins have been administered to postoperative and other patients on parenteral nutrition with differing intervals between the times of vitamin infusion and those of blood sampling; in most patients, blood levels were the usual criteria for adequacy, although some investigators used enzymatic methods. Very few investigators have performed a complete survey of the 13 vitamins. A review of data on vitamin levels in TPN patients suggests that adequate blood levels or related enzyme activities may be attained in hypercatabolic patients with daily infusion dosages for a number of vitamins that are appreciably less than those dosages of the old MVI formula and, in some cases, are below, at, or not far above the AMA-FDA adult dosages.[264–268]

Vitamin needs of long-term stable home TPN patients have been examined by several groups of investigators. Two reports were based on supplemented earlier MVI-based formulas.[269a,269b] More recently, 16 adult patients on home TPN for 1 to 9 years were studied serially over many months on the AMA-FDA formulation (MVI-12).[258] In this study, blood sampling was performed at least 36 hours after the preceding infusion of vitamins was terminated. Mean values for plasma vitamin A were near or above the upper limit of reference values, in part because five of the subjects had renal insufficiency; the high values were associated with elevated retinol-binding protein levels. Thiamin, pyridoxine, nicotinate, biotin, riboflavin, vitamin $B_{12}$ and folate levels were within the reference ranges for all subjects; pantothenate levels tended to be within or above the reference ranges; thiamin tended to be toward the lower half of the reference range, as did vitamin E levels. The vitamin E levels in the lower range (0.5 to 0.95 mg/dl, with the normal range being 0.5 to 1.6 mg/dl) occurred in association with low plasma lipids, which tend to decrease circulating E levels. A few subjects tended to have their ascorbic acid values persistently below 0.3 mg/dl, perhaps because half of the bags with this vitamin stood for 30 hours. Levels of 25-OH vitamin D and 1,25(OH)$_2$ vitamin D in eight individuals after 430 to 588 days on MVI-12 were within the reference range, as were PTH levels. Prothrombin times were normal with 5 mg of vitamin K$_1$ oxide added once every week.

The adequacy of the pediatric AMA-FDA formulation (Table 54–10) was studied by Greene, et al. in premature and full-term infants and in children up to 11 years of age.[270a,270b] The latter two groups received one vial per day; premature infants received 65% of this dose. Vitamin A levels in term infants and children on home TPN were increased from baseline levels with good correlation with retinol-binding protein levels. Levels in premature infants did not change, perhaps because of retinol loss in the delivery system (tubing, etc.) exacerbated by special lighting used in the intensive care unit.[270a] Dissolving the multivitamins in Intralipid reduced the retinol loss to 10% from 80%.[270c] 25-OH vitamin D levels were maintained within or above the reference range.[270b]

Vitamin E levels were maintained above 1.1 mg/dl;[270b] however, those infants weighing less than 1000 g given 65% of a vial had high levels.[270b] It has been noted that small infants on this product had blood tocopheral levels that were elevated higher than may be desirable.[270b,271a,271b] For this reason, the FDA and the manufacturer successively recommended reductions to 65% and later to 30% of a vial for infants less than 1000 g.[271a,272] The amount of vitamin E in 30% may be insufficient, however; with the 30% volume, 56% of such infants had serum levels less than 1 mg/dl, while only 6% of those given 65% of a vial had levels less than 1 mg/dl.[273a] Blood levels between 1 and 2 mg/dl have been recommended.[273b]

Thiamin, riboflavin, and B$_6$ (all evaluated by their appropriate enzymatic activities) and niacin and red cell folate were maintained in all patients.[271] Pantothenate, biotin, and ascorbate were maintained within reference levels for term infants and children for 2 to 4 weeks or longer. Ascorbate increased significantly to high levels in premature infants as did pantothenate and biotin, while B$_{12}$ was maintained above the reference range in all groups.

The AMA-FDA Pediatric formula that is now available contains no propylene glycol (PG) but does contain mannitol, polysorbate 80, and polysorbate 20 (Table 54–11). This formulation avoids the serum hyperosmolarity noted in low-birth-weight infants caused by the PG contained in the adult MVI and MVI-12, which were used prior to the advent of the pediatric formula.[272] Mannitol did not cause significant diuresis when the new formula was given at 65% of a vial per day.

The adequacy of parenteral vitamin D dosage has been considered. When 25 IU/dl of solution (maximum dose, 31 IU/kg) were infused on a daily basis in infants requiring TPN for surgery as the only source of nutrition, the serum 25-OH vitamin D rose and remained normal up to 6 months, together with normal growth and calcium and phosphorus homeostasis.[274]

The new vitamin regimens mark an advance in completeness and ability to maintain vitamin nutrition well above deficient ranges for the great majority of patients. Their use should bring to an end reports of iatrogenic vitamin deficiency in TPN patients. On the other hand, more controlled investigations of quantitative requirements are needed, particularly in premature infants and in severely catabolic individuals, together with improved methods of preventing losses, especially of vitamins A and C.

## Complications in Hospital and at Home

Relevant categories include (1) fluid and electrolyte abnormalities; (2) other nutrient deficiencies or excesses; (3) metabolic problems including abnormal plasma amino acids, organ failure (e.g., liver dysfunction or bone abnormalities), and gallstones; (4) hyper- or hypoglycemia; (5) infection; (6) problems associated with insertion and functioning of catheters or ports; (7) financial burden and employment difficulties imposed by this procedure; and (8) psychologic problems (associated frequently with financial difficulties). The first five problems are best managed by prevention and early detection. This requires experienced physicians, nurses, and pharmacists working as a team and exercising close supervision of both inpatients and outpatients. A patient being trained for TPN administration at home must be in a reasonably stable clinical condition prior to discharge, and the home situation must be duplicated prior to discharge in terms of the duration of TPN, amounts and types of foods likely to be eaten, measurement and replacement of fluid and electrolyte contents of gastrointestinal losses, and insulin needs, if any. The home orders must include frequent and adequate laboratory follow-up, particularly in the first weeks at home, in association with visits by a nurse and appointments with the physician. *A physician's allocation to a home care company of responsibility for providing nutrition solutions and supplies and monitoring the patient does not relieve that physician of responsibility for the patient's nutritional welfare.*

**Infection.** The issue of prevention and treatment

of infection requires careful supervision of the patient with respect to insertion techniques, care of the insertion site, connection and disconnection of infusions, and formula preparation. Strict aseptic technique in the pharmacy associated with inspections and random testing for contamination are essential. Endogenous or exogenous infections do occur, however, especially in patients with various types of immune suppression. Experience with patients on TPN who are on cancer chemotherapy and/or total body irradiation has demonstrated that close supervision, good technique, and aggressive and rational antibiotic coverage allow excellent results.

Optimum functioning of catheters requires selection of proven equipment, placement by an experienced physician, strict adherence to rules for sterility and assurance of proper placement, avoidance of contamination and clotting, and close attention to patients' complaints about malfunction.

**Psychologic Problems.** These are prevented or ameliorated by strong supportive efforts with the patient and family by the staff, especially a trained nurse who knows the patient well and is accepted by the patient, and by the patient's ability to communicate easily and at all times with team members. Concern and supportive efforts about financial problems are needed, and psychotherapy with family members or friends may be needed. Especially necessary are minimization of time on TPN, encouragement and assistance for the patient to return to maximum activities and responsibilities commensurate with the state of the underlying disease, and his ability to resume gainful employment without incurring additional financial penalities. To achieve the latter, Medicare restrictions must be revised.

**Abnormal Amino Acid Levels.** These are of particular importance to the newborn to avoid both deficiencies and excessively high levels (see Chap. 50). Amino acid mixtures are being modified. Supplementation of missing amino acids for certain types of pediatric and adult patients (e.g., cysteine, taurine, carnitine) should be instituted when indicated. The changes in organ function associated with TPN—particularly over the long period—are of special concern because etiologic factors are not well understood.

**Hepatic Dysfunction.** Biochemical and morphologic evidence of hepatic dysfunction have been observed in both children and adults on TPN. Infants and young children show biochemical and histologic evidence of cholestasis; progressive jaundice with hepatic fibrosis have been noted primarily in low-birth-weight or premature infants.[275] Cholestasis has been reported in various series to occur in anywhere from 7.4 to 42.1% of infants, with wide variations among differing populations, criteria, hospital practice, and clinical conditions.[276] In one series of 46 children with cholestasis, two distinct processes were involved; one had to do with an apparent influence of TPN in children with hypoxia (i.e., intracranial hemorrhage or patent ductus arteriosus); the other involved gastrointestinal surgery, sepsis, or both.

In adults on TPN, hepatic dysfunction is often associated with mild to moderate rises in alkaline phosphatase and amino transferases; bilirubin abnormalities are variable, and progressive liver disease can occur (see below).

Factors influencing fat deposition have been studied in rats on TPN. Keim has reviewed this literature and studied the relative importance of the adequacy of amino acids, the amount of nonprotein energy, and various glucose-lipid-calorie ratios.[277] The most marked effect of nitrogen inadequacy was a threefold increase in liver lipid with excessive calorie-high fat infusates. Wih adequate amino acids and adequate calories (250 kcal/kg/day), a high fat intake (90% of non-nitrogen kcal) resulted in liver fat only slightly higher than that with an isocaloric low fat (10%) intake. With excessive calories (350 kcal/kg/day) and adequate amino acids, high glucose infusion (90% of non-nitrogen kcal) resulted in approximately 60% more lipid in the liver than the isocaloric high fat diet did. Steatosis was minimized in diets providing adequate calories, nitrogen, and low fat (only 4% more than in rats fed stock diet). The greatest amounts of liver lipid have been found in rats with fat contributing 50% or 100% of the non-nitrogen calories.[278]

Surgical patients, who had normal liver function tests on initiation of TPN, developed elevated γ-glutamyl trans-peptidase in all 26 cases by week 4.[279] Most abnormalities were transient, but alkaline phosphatase was prolonged beyond week 9. Abnormal liver function tests occurred in almost twice as many septic patients as in nonseptic patients. Malnourished patients at the beginning of TPN were more likely to develop abnormalities in aminotransferases, alkaline phosphatase, and glutamyltranspeptidase. Stein, et al. noted that preoperative patients with gastrointestinal tract malignancies given TPN could be divided into those with low and those with high levels of liver fat after 7 to 10 days; the high-fat group had lower pre-TPN total plasma proteins, albumin, and iron-binding capacity than the low-fat group and a failure to improve plasma albumin levels on TPN.[280]

In patients with other biochemical evidence of liver dysfunction, reports of abnormal bilirubin vary greatly. Some investigators have found little or no rise in bilirubin;[279,281] however, large blood transfusions have been associated with hyperbilirubinemia.[279] Others have found hyperbilirubinemia, but this is confounded by the definition of normality and pre-existing liver disease.[279]

Data are accumulating on the long-term effects of TPN on hepatic function. Of 60 patients with gastrointestinal problems requiring home parenteral nutrition (average duration 29 months, range 4 to 122 months), 51 patients had either no abnormalities or a mild and transient elevation of liver chemistries,[275] nine patients (15%) had liver test abnormalities that persisted for 8 to 95 months and led to liver biopsies, and three patients had prolonged jaundice (two died with significant liver disease, while the survivor had chronic liver disease). Although only a small number of patients were involved, the findings suggest that steatohepatitis in these patients may progress to chronic liver disease.

In a study of 18 patients with varying degrees of resection of the intestine who were followed while on parenteral nutrition for 1 year, four of six who had massive loss of the intestine (from the ligament of Treitz to the midtransverse colon) developed progressive and marked increases in liver biochemistries with hepatic cholestasis and fibrosis.[282] This type of complication obviously deserves further investigation and preventive intervention. Metronidazole has been reported by several investigators to prevent hepatic-derived serum enzyme abnormalities during TPN.[283] Careful prospective studies are indicated because this drug has been found to induce peripheral neuropathy and chromosomal aberrations.[284]

**Metabolic Bone Disease.** Osteomalacia and osteoporosis can be associated with chronic gastrointestinal and liver diseases.[285] The osteomalacia is accounted for by malabsorption resulting in vitamin D deficiency and impaired calcium absorption; the osteoporosis occurs when corticosteroids are given chronically.

Metabolic bone diseases occur also in patients on parenteral nutrition. Rickets has been described in infants on parenteral nutrition.[286,287] The primary problem appears to be the need for more calcium and phosphate in the small fluid volume required by the neonate, rather than the need for more vitamin D.

Bone abnormalities can occur in adults on prolonged parenteral nutrition. Reports document abnormalities in series of patients from three different institutions with somewhat different parenteral nutrition formulas and differing findings. Reference has been made above to the issue of aluminum contamination. Of 15 adults (9 of the 13 women were postmenopausal), 12 had symptomatic bone disease that was not present pre-TPN.[288,289] In another group, severe symptoms of intense periarticular and lower extremity pain developed in 5 months in 5 of initial 11 patients, despite improvement in their overall nutritional state.[288] These patients had received their amino acids in the form of casein hydrolysate together with 1000 IU of vitamin $D_2$ per day. Patchy osteomalacia with impaired mineralization and decreased bone turnover were noted in bone histomorphometric studies. In another study, osteoid was present in increased amounts in 2 of 7 patients. Serum calcium, phosphorus and 25-OH vitamin D were generally normal; calcitriol was markedly diminished;[289] hypercalcemia was common, and PTH was normal to low. Discontinuation of TPN for 1 to 2 months in some of these patients (an unlikely procedure for individuals with very severe malabsorption) was associated with improvement in symptoms. Five children 0.9 to 3.7 years of age on TPN for 9 to 26 months did not develop symptomatic bone disease (the source of amino acids in these children is not clearly indicated).

Later publications by these investigators noted that 14 of 16 patients had been on casein hydrolysate-containing TPN solutions contaminated with aluminum; 3 L providing approximately 3.5 mg of aluminum had been given for 1 to 7 years.[290] Stainable aluminum was detected in the bone biopsy of those given casein hydrolysate but was not present in bone from those receiving crystalline amino acids. The rate of bone formation was negatively correlated with the amount of stainable aluminum. When a patient given casein hydrolysate for 2 years was switched to amino acids, the aluminum stain became negative, and histology and symptoms improved.[291] The authors concluded that their data "suggest that aluminum may be involved in the pathogenesis of this low-turnover bone disease."[291]

A second series of home TPN patients were observed prospectively in Toronto. In these studies, crystalline amino acids were used. Vitamin $D_2$ (500 IU) was given every other day as MVI-1000; all other vitamins were included daily except biotin.

In the first report, 16 patients (6 males, 10 females) were observed while on parenteral nutrition (because of serious gastrointestinal diseases) for 7 to 89 months (including the duration of the metabolic study).[292] Twelve had some degree of osteomalacia in their bone biopsies; 7 had hypercalcemia, while 10 were hypercalciuric and in negative calcium balance. Serum phosphorus was normal and plasma PTH levels were normal or low. Six of the 16 had somewhat elevated 25-OH vitamin D levels. Three had bone pain (not further described), and 2 of those had compression of lumbar vertebrae. Initially, the bone biopsies* showed predominantly a hyperkinetic pattern, compatible with hyperparathyroidism that may have been present on a secondary basis with their malabsorption and initial malnutrition. For most, the bone histology changed to that of osteomalacia at 6 to 73 months on HTPN.

More detailed bone histomorphometric data were published on 11 patients before and after withdrawal of vitamin D and by other vitamin modifications that included removal of MVI-1000 and replacement of its water soluble vitamins, with Solu-Zyme; this replacement eliminated from the formula vitamin A for 6 months (although serum vitamin A levels were maintained) as well as vitamin $D_2$ for approximately 6 to 16 months at which time the patients were studied again. Withdrawal of vitamin $D_2$ (and A) was associated with a significant reduction in the elevated osteoid index in 6 of 10 individuals, and with a significant increase in tetracycline uptake. However, after 6 months there was continuing evidence of a high turnover rate. In the three symptomatic patients, bone pain subsided, fractures healed, and urinary losses of calcium and phosphate decreased with the vitamin modification.[292,293] It was recommended that "vitamin D solutions not be added to total parenteral nutrition of home patients,"[293] although the possible adverse role of this vitamin was not specifically delineated. Aluminum was not detectable in the amino acid or MVI-1000 solutions used in this investigation.

A third series of 12 patients studied in New York, NY who had been on home TPN for 9 to 123 months consisted of 5 males ages 25 to 67 and 7 females ages 39 to 77.[294] (A thirteenth patient had been maintained on a different nutritional formulation for 120 months in another institution and is not included in this discussion.) Crystalline amino acids had been used throughout the study for all but several of the subjects on TPN for the longest time who had previously received casein hydrolysate but were switched to crystalline amino acids 6 years earlier. Of the 12 patients, 6 had minor bone complaints, mainly vertebral and usually associated with known osteoarthritis. One of the 12 had suffered trauma after 4 years on TPN (2 years prior to the study) with resultant multiple fractures, which healed. The vitamin that had been administered to many patients was MVI concentrate (5 ml) given twice weekly in addition to folate, $B_{12}$, biotin, and vitamin K, with an average daily infusion of vitamin $D_2$ of 284 IU and of vitamin A of 2800 IU. Three to ten months prior to initiating the study, MVI-12 replaced the MVI concentrate for all subjects and provided 200 IU of vitamin $D_2$ and 3300 IU of vitamin A. Bone histomorphometry revealed a different histologic picture than that of the two studies reviewed above; namely, osteopenia with reduced bone and cortical volume, subnormal osteoid volume, normal trabecular osteoid seam width, and tetracycline labeling. Calcification rate was normal. Two patients had some aluminum staining; both had been exposed to casein hydrolysate 6 years before and both had renal dysfunction; the bone aluminum of these two patients was slightly elevated in relation to bone calcium. The others had low bone and serum aluminum. The TPN solutions with amino acids had very low aluminum content. Serum plasma calcium, phosphorus, vitamin D metabolites, and PTH were normal; urinary calcium and phosphate were increased.

The reasons for the marked difference in bone histology between the Toronto and New York studies are not apparent. Appreciably less fat calories and proportionatey more glucose calories, different vitamins including biotin, and more normal serum calcium, PTH, and calcitriol values were obtained in the New York study. Which, if any, of these variables played a causative role remains to be determined.

A significant proportion of patients were in negative calcium and/or phosphate balance. This situation may reflect persistent bone abnormalities, at least in some patients, including the effect of estrogen deficiency in postmenopausal women. It is known that amino acid infusion per se is associated with hypercalciuria;[295] whether the observed short-term effect persists with prolonged parenteral nutrition is unknown. Increased phosphate in the infusion has been noted to decrease urinary calcium losses.[296]

**Gallbladder Abnormalities.** A number of risk factors for gallbladder disease have been examined in patients on long-term parenteral nutrition. Of 109 patients on TPN for a mean of 13.5 months, 23% developed gallbladder disease.[297] TPN patients with ileal disorders had a higher than expected incidence (40%) of cholecystitis and cholelithiasis. Prolonged fasting, use of narcotics and cholinergics, and ileal dysfunction were risk factors; however, IV lipids, antibiotics, $H_2$ inhibitors, steroids, and abnormal liver function tests were not significant risk factors.

In 23 adults on TPN with severe intestinal disorders, the percentage of gallbladder sludge-

---

*See Chapter 46 for discussion of techniques and standards in bone histomorphometry and illustration of findings in various conditions.

positive patients increased from 6% during the first 3 weeks to 50% between the fourth and sixth weeks of TPN.[298] Gallstone formation was demonstrated in 6 of 14 sludge formers but not in those who were sludge negative. Bowel rest and bile stasis with parenteral nutrition appeared to be risk factors.

**Pancreatitis.** Manufacturers of parenteral lipids suggest caution in their use in patients with dyslipoproteinemias and acute pancreatitis. In contrast to oral or enteral feeding, parenteral nutrition given to dogs either induces no increase in pancreatic secretions or induces less increase than oral or enteral feeding. In patients with pure pancreatic fistulas, glucose-TPN resulted in a decreased secretion in one study;[299] two of three other studies with lipid-TPN indicated no change, while the third showed increased secretion. The value of parenteral nutrition in management of pancreatitis has been reviewed in Chapter 56, section B2).[299] TPN is a useful adjunct to a supportive regimen in acute pancreatitis and has a therapeutic role in chronic complications of the disease. There are reports that hyperlipidemic patients may be more prone than normal individuals to pancreatitis with an oral fat load. The data on the effect of IV fat in hyperlipidemic patients is scanty, but caution is advised in such patients. The data suggesting a deleterious effect of fat in patients who have normal lipids is unconvincing. Data from both experimental animals and man suggest that use of lipids did not exacerbate existing pancreatitis; however, individual case histories report occurrence of pancreatitis with lipid. Hypercalcemia occurring with TPN may be a primary factor.[300]

**Pulmonary Complications.** Attention was given earlier to exacerbation of pre-existing serious pulmonary problems by high-glucose infusions in excess of caloric needs and of the effect of amino acids in increasing respiratory drive. Caution must be exercised in providing amounts of these nutrients to meet the special needs in patients with such pulmonary disabilities. On the other hand, failure to provide adequate nutrition to patients with respiratory problems can depress respiratory function, increase infection, and increase morbidity and mortality.[113,301,302]

## Home Parenteral Nutrition

Since the first patient was discharged from the hospital in 1969 on home TPN,[126] this means of outpatient nutritional support mushroomed and is now accepted by physicians and insures as an effective procedure. Some of the data collected and distributed by the Home TPN Registry at the New York Academy of Medicine under my direc-

tion has been published.[303] There is now a very significant literature on this subject.[303–305]

Precautions and complications of prolonged parenteral nutrition were discussed earlier in this chapter, and its use in various clinical situations has been discussed in numerous chapters in this book concerned with specific clinical issues. As has been emphasized, optimum care, before discharge and at home, requires care by physicians knowledgeable in home TPN and clinical nutrition, generally working with other trained health professionals in a team setting.

## REFERENCES

1. Turner, F.P.: JAMA *223*:441, 1973 (letter).
2. Co Tui, Wright, A.M., Mulholland, J.H., et al.: Gastroenterology *5*:5–17, 1945.
3. Watkin, D.M., Steinfeld, J.L.: Am. J. Clin. Nutr. *16*:182–212, 1965.
4. Dudrick, S.J., Wilmore, D.W., Vars, H.M., et al.: Ann. Surg. *169*:974–984, 1969.
5. Randall, H.T.: J. Parenter. Enteral Nutr. *8*:113–136, 1984.
6. Einhorn, M.: Med. Rec. *78*:92–95, 1910.
7. Torosian, M.H., Rombeau, J.L.: Surg. Gynecol. Obstet. *150*:918–927, 1980.
8a. Ponsky, J.L., Gauderer, M.W.L.: Gastrointest. Endosc. *27*:9–11, 1981.
8b. Kirby, D.F., Craig, R.M., Tsang, T-K, et al.: J. Parenter. Enteral. Nutr. *10*:155–159, 1986.
9. Elman, R., Weiner, D.O.: JAMA *112*:796–802, 1939.
10. Elman, R.: Parenteral Alimentation in Surgery. New York, P.B. Hoeber, 1947, Chap. 9.
11. Shohl, A.T., Butler, A.M., Blackfan, K.D., et al.: J. Pediatr. *15*:469–475, 1939.
12. Elman, R.: Am. J. Digest. Dis. *10*:48–50, 1943.
13. Abbott, W.O.: Ann. Surg. *112*:584–593, 1940.
14. Co Tui, Wright, A.M., Mulholland, J.H., et al.: Ann. Surg. *120*:99–122, 1944.
15. Andresen, A.F.R.: Ann. Surg. *67*:565–566, 1918.
16. Wells, G., Tinkler, L.F., Rawlinsen, K., et al.: Lancet *1*:4–10, 1964.
17. Glucksman, D.L. Kalser, M.H., Warren, W.D.: Surgery *60*:1020–1025, 1966.
18. Editorial: Postoperative ileus. Lancet *2*:1186–1187, 1978.
19. Delany, H.M., Carnevale, N., Garvey, J.W.: Surgery *73*:786–790, 1973.
20. Page, C.P., Ryan, J.A. Jr, Haff, R.C.: Surg. Gynecol. Obstet. *142*:184–188, 1976.
21. Andersson, H., Hulten, L. Magnusson, O., et al.: J. Parenter Enteral Nutr. *8*:497–500, 1984.
22. Smith, D.W., Lee, R.M.: Surg. Gynecol. Obstet. *103*:662–672, 1956.
23. Olson, F., Michaels, G., Partridge, J.W., et al.: Am. J. Clin. Nutr. *1*:134–139, 1953.
24. Ahrens, E.H. Jr.: Adv. Metab. Disorders. *4*:297–332, 1970.
25. Shils, M.E.: Am. J. Clin. Nutr. *15*:133–143, 1964.
26. Shapiro, R.: Historical development and limitations of "elemental" diets. *In* Defined Formula Diets for Medical Purposes (Shils, M.E., ed.). AMA, Chicago, 1977, pp. 1–5.
27. Winitz, M., Seedman, D.A., Graff, J.: Am. J. Clin. Nutr. *23*:525–545, 1970.
28. Shils, M.E. (ed.): Proceedings of Conference: De-

fined-Formula Diets for Medical Purposes, Chicago, AMA, 1977.

29. Shils, M.E. (ed): Introduction: Proceedings of Conference: Defined-Formula Diets for Medical Purposes, Chicago, AMA, 1977.

30. de Vries, E.G.E., Mulder, N.H., Houwen, B., et al.: Am. J. Clin. Nutr. *35*:1490–1496, 1981.

31. Rombeau, J.L., Barot, L.R., Low, D.W., et al.: Feeding by tube enterostomy. *In* Enteral and Tube Feedings (Edited by J.L. Rombeau, M.D. Caldwell). Philadelpia, W.B. Saunders, 1984.

32. Heimburger, D.C., Young, V.R., Bistrian, B.R., et al.: J. Parenter. Enteral Nutr. *10*:425–430, 1986.

33. Forbes, G.B., Kreipe, R.E., Lipinski, B.A., et al.: Am. J. Clin. Nutr. *40*:1137–1145, 1984.

34. Young, E.A., Cioletti, L.P., Traylor, J.B., et al.: Am. J. Clin. Nutr. *35*:715–726, 1982.

35. Johnson, L.R., Copeland, E.M. Dudrick, S.J., et al.: Gastroenterology *68*:1177–1183, 1975.

36. Ecknauer, R., Sircar, B., Johnson, L.R.: Gastroenterology *81*:781–786, 1981.

37. Morin, C.L., Ling, V., Bourassa, D.: Dig. Dis. Sci. *25*:123–128, 1980.

38. Nelson, L.M., Russell, R.L.: J. Parenter. Enteral Nutr. *10*:399–404, 1986.

39. Ryan, G.P., Dudrick, S.J., Copeland, E.M., et al.: Gastroenterology *77*:658–663, 1979.

40. Janne, P., Carpentier, Y., Willems, G.: Am. J. Digest. Dis. *22*:808–812, 1977.

41. King, W. W-K., Boelhouer, R.V., Kingsnorth, A.N., et al.: J Parenter. Enteral Nutr. *7*:443–446, 1983.

42. Bury, K.D., Grayston, M., Kanarens, J.: Surg. Forum *25*:75–77, 1976.

43. Lanza-Jacobey, S., Sitren, H.S., Stevenson, N.R., et al.: J. Parenter. Enteral Nutr. *6*:496–502, 1982.

44. Levine, G.M., Deren, J.J., Steiger, E., et al.: Gastroenterology *67*:975–982, 1974.

45. Koretz, R.L., Meyer, J.H.: Gastroenterology *78*:393–410, 1980.

46. Young, E.A., Weser, E.: Animal models for enteral feeding of defined formula diets. *In* Enteral and Tube Feeding (Edited by J.E. Rombeau, M.D. Caldwell). Philadelphia, W.B. Saunders, 1984.

47. Gupta, J.D., Dakroury, A.M., Harper, A.E.: J. Nutr. *64*:447–456, 1958.

48. McArdle, A.H., Echave, W., Brown, R.A., et al.: Am. J. Surg. *128*:690–692, 1974.

49. Kelly, G.A., Nahrwald, D.L.: Surg. Gynecol. Obstet. *43*:87–91, 1976.

50. Koruda, M.J., Rolandelli, R.H., Settle, R.G., et al.: J. Parenter. Enteral Nutr. *10*:343–350, 1986.

51. Vanderhoof, J.A., Grandjean, C.J., Kaufman, S.S., et al.: J. Parenter. Enteral Nutr. *8*:685–689, 1984.

52. Gray, V.L., Garafolo, C., Greenberg, G.R., et al.: Am. J. Clin. Nutr. *40*:1235–1242, 1984.

53. Miazzi, B.M., Al-Mukktar, M.Y.T., Salmeron, M., et al.: Gut *26*:518–524, 1985.

54. Hughes, C.A., Bates, T., Dowling, R.H.: Gastroenterology *75*:34–41, 1978.

55. Dowling, R.H., Hosomi, M., Stace, N.H., et al.: Scand. J. Gastroenterology *20*(Suppl 112):84–95, 1985.

56. Sircar, B., Johnson, L.R., Lichtenberger, L.M.: Am. J. Physiol. *238*:G376–G383, 1980.

57. Greenberg, G.R., Wolman, S.L., Christofides, M.D., et al.: Gastroentrology *80*:988–993, 1980.

58. Hwang, T.L., O'Dwyer, S.T., Smith, R.J., et al.: Surg. Forum *37*:56–58, 1986.

59. Weser, E., Drummond A., Tawil, T.: J. Parenter. Enteral Nutr. *6*:39–42, 1982.

60. Damge-Stocke, C., Aprahamian, M., Raul, F., et al.: Scand. J. Med. *21*:1115–1123, 1986.

61. Dworkin, L.D., Levine, G.M., Farby, N.J., et al.: Gastroenterology *71*:626–630, 1976.

62. Matthews, D.M., Adibi, S.A.: Gastroenterology *71*:151–161, 1976.

63. Burston, D., Taylor, E., Matthews, D.M.: Biochim. Biophys. Acta *553*:175–178, 1979.

64. Grimble, G.K., Rees, R.G., Keohane, P.P., et al.: Gastroenterology *92*:136–142, 1987.

65. Grimble, G.K., Keohane, P.P., Higgins, B.C., et al.: Clin. Sci. *71*:65–69, 1986.

66. Smithson, K.W., Gray, G.M.: J. Clin. Invest. *60*:665–674, 1977.

67. Adibi, S.A., Fogel, M.P., Agrawal, R.M.: Gastroenterology *67*:586–591, 1974.

68. Silk, D.B.A., Kumar, P.J., Perrett, D., et al.: Gut *15*:1–8, 1974.

69. Keohane, P.P., Silk, D.B.A.: Peptides and Free Amino Acids In Enteral and Tube Feeding (Edited by J.L. Rombeau and M.D. Caldwell). Philadelphia, W.B. Saunders, 1984.

70. Silk, D.B.A., Fairclough, P.D., Clark, M.L., et al.: J. Parenter. Enteral Nutr. *4*:548–553, 1980.

71. Fairclough, P.D., Hegarty, J.E., Silk, D.B.A., et al.: Gut *21*:829–831, 1980.

72. Keohane, P.P., Grimble, G.K., Brown, B., et al.: Gut *26*:907–913, 1985.

73. Hegarty, J.E., Fairclough, P.D., Moriarty, K.J., et al.: Gut *23*:304–309, 1982.

74. Heymsfield, S.B., Bleir, J., Whitmir, L., et al.: Am. J. Clin. Nutr. *39*:243–250, 1984.

75. Smith, J.L., Arteaga, C., Heymsfield, S.B.: N. Engl. J. Med. *306*:1013–1018, 1982.

76. Beer, W.H., Halsted, C.H.: Am. J. Clin. Nutr. *39*:689, 1984 (Abstr.).

77. Jones, B.J.M., Lees, R., Andrews, J., et al.: Gut *24*:78–84, 1983.

78. Moriarty, K.J., Hegarty, J.E., Fairclough, P.D., et al.: Gut *26*:694–696, 1985.

79. McIntyre, P.B., Fitchew, M., Lennard-Jones J.E.: Gastroenterology *91*:25–33, 1986.

80. Albina, J.E., Jacobs, D.O., Melnik, G., et al.: J. Parenter. Enteral Nutr. *9*:189–195, 1985.

81. Trocki, O., Mochizuki, H., Dominioni, L.: J. Parenter. Enteral Nutr. *10*:139–145, 1986.

82. Randall, H.T.: J. Parenter. Enteral Nutr. *8*:113–136, 1984.

83. Food and Drug Admin. Dept. of Health, Human Services: 21 CFR Ch. 1 (4/1/86 Ed) Washington, D.C.

84. Guy, D.G.: Mead Johnson Nutritional Group, Personal Communication.

85. McIntyre N., Holdsworth C.D., Turner, D.S.: J. Clin. Endocrinol. Metab. *25*:1317–1324, 1968.

86. McArdle, A.H., Palmason, C., Morency, I., et al.: Surgery *90*:616–623, 1981.

87. Abrams, C.K., Hamosh, M., Dutta, S.K., et al.: Gastroenterology *92*:125–129, 1987.

88. Mochizuki, H., Trocki, O., Dominioni, L., et al.: J. Parenter. Enteral Nutr. *8*:638–646, 1984.

89. DeRitter, E.: J. Pharm. Sci. *71*:1073–1096, 1982.

90. Bryant, C.A., Neufeld, N.J.: J. Parenter. Enteral Nutr. *6*:403–405, 1982.

91. Davis, A.T., Fagerman, K.E., Douner, F.D., et al.: J. Parenter. Enteral Nutr. *10*:245–246, 1986.

92. Heird, W.C.: Acid-base effects of defined-formula

diets. *In* Defined Formula Diets for Medical Purposes. (Edited by M.E. Shils). Chicago, AMA, 1977, pp. 43–47.

93. Lemann, J., Jr., Lennon, E.J.: Kidney Int. *1*:275–279, 1972.

94a. Kildeberg, P., Winters, R.: Pediatrics *49*:801–802, 1972.

94b. Healy, C.E.: Pediatrics *49*:910–911, 1972.

95. Zabel, N.C., Harland, J., Gormican, A.T., et al.: Am. J. Clin. Nutr. *31*:850–858, 1978.

96. Martin, R.F., Young V.R., Janghorbani, M.: J. Parenter. Enteral Nutr. *10*:213–215, 1986.

96a. Bjerve, K.S., Mostad, I.L., Thoresen, L.: Am. J. Clin. Nutr. *45*:66–77, 1987.

97. Tsai, A.C., Mott, E.L., Owen, G.M., et al.: Am. J. Clin. Nutr. *38*:504–511, 1983.

98. Slavin, J.L., Nelson, N.L., McNamara, B.S., et al.: J. Parenter. Enteral Nutr. *9*:317–321, 1985.

99. Winitz, M., Adams, R.F., Seedman, D.A., et al.: Am. J. Clin. Nutr. *23*:546–559, 1970.

100. Attebery, H.R., Sutter, V.L., Finegold, S.M.: Am. J. Clin. Nutr. *25*:1391–1396, 1972.

101. Crowther, J.S., Draser, B.S., Goddard, P., et al.: Gut *14*:790–793, 1973.

102. Bornside, G.H., Cohn, I., Jr.: Ann. Surg. *181*:58–60, 1975.

103a. Shils, M.E. (ed.): Proceedings of Conference: Defined-Formula Diets for Medical Purposes. Epilogue. Chicago, AMA, 1977, p. 153.

103b. Smith J.L., Heymsfield, S.B.: J. Parenter. Enteral Nutr. *7*:280–288, 1983.

103c. Macburney, M.M., Jacobs, D.O., Apelgren, K.N., et al.: Modular feeding. *In* Enteral and Tube Feeding (Edited by J.L. Rombeau and M.D. Caldwell). Philadelphia, W.B. Saunders, 1984.

104a. Mock, D.M.: (Editorial). Gastroenterology *91*:1019–1023, 1986.

104b. Moore, M.C., Greene, H.L., Donald, W.D., et al.: Am. J. Clin. Nutr. *44*:33–41, 1986.

104c. Glotzer, D.J., Boyle, P.L., Silen, W.: Surgery *74*:703–707, 1973.

105a. Vanlandingham, S., Simpson, S., Daniel, P., et al.: J. Parenter. Enteral Nutr. *5*:322–324, 1981.

105b. Cataldi-Betcher, E.L., Seltzer, M.H., Slocum, B., et al.: J. Parenter. Enteral Nutr. *7*:546–552, 1983.

106. Barnard, M., Forlaw, L.: Complications and their prevention. *In* Enteral and Tube Feeding (Edited by J.L. Rombeau, M.D. Caldwell). Philadephia, W.B. Saunders, 1984.

107. Ellison, E.H., McCleery, R.S., Zollinger, R.M., et al.: Surgery *26*:374–383, 1949.

108. Rice, C.O., Orr, B., Treloar, A.E., et al.: Arch. Surg. *61*:977–991, 1950.

109. Moore, F.D.: Metabolic Care of the Surgical Patient. Philadelphia, W.B. Saunders, 1959, pp. 1011.

110. Wretlind, A.: Current status of intralipid and other fat emulsions. *In* Fat Emulsions in Parenteral Nutrition (Edited by H.C. Meng, D.W. Wilmore.) Chicago, American Medical Association, 1976, pp. 109–122.

111. Law, D.K., Dudrick, S.J., Abderi, N.I.: Ann. Intern. Med. *79*:545–550, 1973.

112. Pietsch, J.B. Meakins, J.L., MacLean, L.D.: Surgery *82*:349–355, 1977.

113. Doekel, R.C., Zwillich, C.W., Scoggins, C.H., et al.: N. Engl. J. Med. *295*:358–361, 1976.

114. Niederman, M.S., Merrill, W.W., Ferranti, R.D., et al.: Ann. Intern. Med. *100*:795–800, 1984.

115. Askanazi, J., Weissman, C., Rosenbaum, S.H., et al.: Crit. Care Med. *10*:163–172, 1982.

116. Wilmore, D.W.: The Metabolic Management of the Critically Ill. New York, Plenum Med. Book Co., 1977.

117. Freeman, J.B., Fairful-Smith, R.J.: Physiologic approach to peripheral parenteral nutrition. *In* Surgical Nutrition (Edited by J.E. Fischer). Boston, Little, Brown & Co., 1983, pp. 703–717.

118. Hoshal, V.: Arch. Surg. *110*:644–646, 1975.

119. Dudrick, S.J., Wilmore, D.W, Vars, H.M., Rhoads, J.E.: Ann. Surg. *169*:974–984, 1969.

120. Jeejeebhoy, K.N., Zohrab, W.J., Langer, B., et al.: Gastroenterology *65*:811–820, 1973.

121. Broviac, J.W., Cole, J.J., Scribner, B.H.: Surg. Gynecol. Obstet. *136*:602–606, 1973.

122a. Solassol, C., Joyeux, H.: Ann. Anesth. Franc. Special *2*:75, 1974.

122b. Joyeux, H., Astruc, B., Martin, G., et al.: J. Chir. (Paris) *107*:335–366, 1974.

122c. Fairman, R.M., Crosby, L.O., Stein, T.P., et al.: J. Parenter. Enteral Nutr. *7*:237–243, 1983.

123. Zincke, H., Hirsche, B.L., Amamoo, D.G., et al.: Surg. Gynecol. Obstet. *139*:350–352, 1974.

124. Heizer, W.D., Orringer, E.P.: Gastroenterology *72*:527–532, 1977.

125. Engels, L.G.J., Skotnicki, S.H., Buskens, F.G.M., et al.: J. Parenter. Enteral Nutr. *7*:412–414, 1983.

126. Shils, M.E., Wright, W.L., Turnbull, A., et al.: N. Engl. J. Med. *283*:341–344, 1970.

127. Malt, R.A., Kempter, M.: J. Parenter. Enteral Nutr. *7*:580–581, 1983.

128. Kosloske, A.M., Klein, M.D.: Surg. Gynecol. Obstet. *154*:395–399, 1982.

129. Danahoe, P.K., Kim, S.H.: J. Pediatr. Surg. *15*:737–738, 1980.

130. Fonkalsrud, E.W., Berquist, W., Burke, M. et al.: Am. J. Surg. *143*:209–211, 1982.

131. Oram-Smith, J.C., Muller, J.L., Harken, A.H., et al.: Surgery *83*:274–276, 1979.

132. Lokich, J.J., Bothe, A., Jr., Benotti, P.: J. Clin. Oncol. *3*:710–717, 1985.

133. Beck, S.L., Rose, N.R., Zagoren, A.J.: Nutr. Clin. Practice *2*:26–29, 1987.

134. Belin, R.P., Koster, J.K., Bryant, L.J., et al.: Surg. Gynecol. Obstet *134*:491–493, 1972.

135. Bozetti, F., Scarpa, D., Terno, G., et al.: J. Parenter. Enteral Nutr. *7*:560–562, 1983.

136. Curelaru, I., Gustavsson, B., Hansson, A., et al.: Acta Anesthesiol. Scand. *27*:158–169, 1983.

137. Linder, L-E., Curelaru, I., Gustavsson, E, et al.: J. Parenter. Enteral Nutr. *8*:399–406, 1984.

138. Nehme, A.E.: JAMA *243*:1906–1908, 1980.

139. Keohane, P.P., Jones, B.J.M., Attrill, H., et al.: Lancet *2*:1388–1390, 1983.

140a. Tomford, J.W., Hershey, C.O., McLaren, C.E., et al.: Arch. Intern. Med. *144*:1191–1194.

140b. Dalton, M.J., Schepers, G., Gee, J.P., et al.: J. Parenter. Enteral Nutr. *8*:146–152, 1984.

140c. Traeger, S.M., Williams, G.B., Milliren, R., et al.: J. Parenter. Enteral Nutr. *10*:408–412, 1986.

141. Williams, W.W.: J. Parenter. Enteral Nutr. *9*:735–746, 1985.

142. Shils, M.E.: Am. J. Clin. Nutr. *28*:1429–1435, 1975.

143. Newsome, H.H., Jr., Armstrong, C.W., Mayhall, G.C., et al.: J. Parenter. Enteral Nutr. *8*:560–562, 1984.

144. Press, O.W., Ramsey, P.G., Larson, E.B., et al.: Medicine *63*:189–200, 1984.

145. Petersen, F.B., Clift, R.A., Hickman, R.O., et al.: J. Parenter. Enteral Nutr. *10*:58–62, 1986.
146. Jaeger, R.J., Rubin, R.J.: Environ. Health Perspect. *1*:95–102, 1973.
147. Shaw, S.N., Elwyn, D.H., Askanazi, J., et al.: Am. J. Clin. Nutr. *37*:930–940, 1983.
148. Rudman, E., Millikan, W.J., Richardson, T.J., et al.: J. Clin. Invest. *55*:94–104, 1975.
149. Wolman, S.L., Anderson G.H., Marliss, E.B., et al.: Gastroenterology *76*:458–467, 1979.
150. Elwyn, D.H., Bryan-Brown, C.W., Shoemaker, W.C.: Ann. Surg. *182*:76–85, 1975.
151. Starker, P.M., LaSala, P.A., Askanazi, J., et al.: Ann. Surg. *198*:720–724, 1983.
152. Starker, P.M., LaSala, P.A., Forse, A., et al.: J. Parenter. Enteral Nutr. *9*:300–302, 1985.
153a.Woods, H.F., Alberti, K.G.M.M.: Lancet *2*:1354–1357, 1972.
153b.Georgioff, M., Moldawer, L.L., Bistrian, B.R., et al.: J. Parenter. Enteral Nutr. *9*:199–209, 1985.
154. Young, E.A., Drummond, A., Cool, D.A., et al.: J. Clin. Endocrinol. Metab. *50*:764–772, 1980.
155. Young, E.A., Fletcher, J.T., Cioletti, L.A., et al.: J. Parenter. Enteral Nutr. *5*:369–377, 1981.
155a.Stegink, L.D., Zike, W.L., Andersen, D.W., et al.: Metabolism *35*:519–523, 1986.
156. Byrne, W.J., Lippe, B.M., Strobel, C.T., et al.: Gastroenterology *80*:947–956, 1981.
157. Wolfe, R.R., Allsop, J.R., Burke, J.F.: Metabolism *28*:210–220, 1979.
158. Burke, J.F., Wolfe, R.R., Mullany, C.J., et al.: Ann Surg. *190*:274–283, 1979.
159. Wolfe, R.R., O'Donnell, T.F., Jr., Stone, M.D., et al.: Metabolism *29*:892–900, 1980.
160. Wolfe, R.R.: J. Burn Care and Rehabilitation *6*:408–418, 1985.
161. Flatt, J.P.: The biochemistry of energy expenditure. *In* Recent Advances in Obesity Research II. (Edited by G. Bray). Lancaster, Pa., Technomic Publ. Co., 1978, pp. 211–228.
162. Lowry, S.F., Brennan, M.F.: J. Surg. Res. *26*:300–307, 1979.
163a.Kinney, J.M.: The carbohydrate content of parenteral nutrition. *In* Advances in Clinical Nutrition (Edited by I.D.B. Johnson). Boston, MTP Press Ltd., 1983.
163b.Elwyn, D.H., Grump, F.E., Munro, H.N., et al.: Am. J. Clin. Nutr. *32*:1597–1611, 1979.
164. Askanazi, J., Carpentier, Y.A., Elwyn, D.H., et al.: Ann. Surg. *191*:40–46, 1980.
165. Nordenstrom, J., Carpentier, Y.A., Askanazi, J., et al.: Ann. Surg. *198*:725–735, 1983.
166. MacFie, J., Halmfield, J.H.M., King, R.F.G., et al.: J. Parenter. Enteral Nutr. *7*:1–5, 1983.
167. Askanazi, J., Rosenbaum, S.H., Hyman, A.I., et al.: JAMA *243*:1444–1447, 1980.
168. Askanazi, J., Nordenstrom, J., Rosenbaum, S.H., et al.: Anesthesiology *54*:373–377, 1981.
169. Chait, A., Foster, D., Miller, D.G., et al.: Proc. Soc. Exp. Biol. Med. *168*:97–104, 1981.
170. Wretlind, A.: J. Parenter. Enteral Nutr. *5*:230–235, 1981.
171. Barr, L.H., Dunn, G.D., Brennan, M.F.: Surgery *193*:304–311, 1981.
172a.Davis, S.S.: The stability of fat emulsions for intravenous administration. *In* Advances in Clinical Nutrition (Edited by I.D.A. Johnson). Boston, MTP Press Ltd., 1983, pp. 213–239.
172b.Brown, R., Quercia, R.A., Sigman, R.: J. Parenter. Enteral Nutr. *10*:650–658, 1986.
173a.Main, J., Pennington, C.R.: J. Parenter. Enteral Nutr. *10*:247, 1986 (letter).
173b.Harrie, K.R., Jacob, M., McCormick, D., et al.: J. Parenter. Enteral Nutr. *10*:381–387, 1986.
173c.Ang, S.D., Canham, J.E., Daly, J.M.: J. Parenter. Enteral Nutr. *11*:23–27, 1987.
174. Adamkin, D.H., Gelke, K.N., Andrews, B.F.: J. Parenter. Enteral Nutr. *8*:563–567, 1984.
175. Innis, S.M., Boyd, M.C.: Am. J. Clin. Nutr. *38*:95–100, 1983.
176. Griffin, E., Breckenridge, W.C., Kuksis, A., et al.: J. Clin. Invest. *64*:1703–1712, 1979.
177. Rigaud, D., Serog, P., Legrand, A., et al.: J. Parenter. Enteral Nutr. *8*:529–534, 1984.
178. Sanderson, I., Kuksis, A., Jeejeebhoy, K.N.: Gastroenterology *64*:A796, 1973 (abst.).
179. Izzo, R.S., Larcker, S., Remis, W., et al.: J. Parenter. Enteral Nutr. *8*:160–168, 1984.
180. Campbell, A.N., Freedman, M.H., Pencharz, P.B., et al.: J. Parenter. Enteral Nutr. *8*:447–449, 1984.
181. Greene, H.C., Hazlett, D., Demaree, R.: Am. J. Clin. Nutr. *29*:127–135, 1975.
182. Pereira, G.R., Fox, W.W., Stanley, C.A., et al.: Pediatrics *66*:26–30, 1980.
183. Andrew, G., Chan, G., Schiff, D.: J. Pediatr. *88*:279–284, 1976.
184. Burckart, G.J., Whitington, P.F., Helms, R.A.: Am. J. Clin. Nutr. *36*:521–526, 1982.
185a.Hessov, I., Flemming, M., Haug, A.: Arch. Surg. *114*:66–68, 1979.
185b.Thompson, S.W.: Pathology of Parenteral Nutrition with Lipids. Springfield, IL, CC Thomas, 1974.
185c.Paswell, J.H.,David, R., Katznelson, D., et al.: Arch. Dis. Child. *51*:366–368, 1976.
186a.Fischer, G.W., Hunter, K.W., Wilson, S.R., et al.: Lancet *1*:819–820, 1980.
186b.Cleary, T.G., Pickering, L.K.: J. Clin. Lab. Immunol. *11*:21–26, 1983.
187a.Hawley, H.P., Gordon, G.B.: Lab. Invest. *34*:216–222, 1976.
187b.Nordenstrom, J., Jarstrand, C., Wiernik, A. Am. J. Clin. Nutr. *32*:2416–2422, 1979.
187c.Wiernik, A., Jarstrand, C., Julander, I.: Am. J. Clin. Nutr. *37*:256–261, 1983.
187d.Fraser I., Neoptolemos, J., Darby, H., et al.: J. Parenter. Enteral Nutr. *8*:381–384, 1984.
188. English, D., Roloff, J.S., Lukens, J.N., et al.: J. Pediatr. *99*:913–916, 1981.
189a.Palmblad, J., Brostrom, O., Lahnborg, G., et al.: Am. J. Clin. Nutr. *35*:1430–1439, 1982.
189b.Escudier, E.F., Escudier, B.J., Henry-Amar, M.C., et al.: J. Parenter. Enteral Nutr. *10*:596–598, 1986.
189c.Nishiwaki, H., Iriyama, K., Asami, H., et al.: J. Parenter. Enteral Nutr. *10*:614–616, 1986.
189d.Ota, D.M., Jessup, J.M., Babcock, G.F., et al.: J. Parenter. Enteral Nutr. *9*:23–27, 1985.
190. Siegel, I., Liv, T.L., Zaret, P., et al.: JAMA *251*:1574–1579, 1984.
191. Wilmore, D.W., Moylan, J.A., Hlemkamp, G.M., et al.: Ann. Surg. *178*:503–509, 1973.
192. Long, J.M., Wilmore, D.W., Mason, A.D., et al.: Ann. Surg. *185*:417–422, 1977.
193. Goodenough, R.D., Wolfe, R.R.: J. Parenter. Enteral Nutr. *8*:357–360, 1984.
194. Coran, A.G., Drongouski, R.A., Lee, G.S., et al.: J. Parenter. Enteral Nutr. *8*:652–656, 1984.

195. Carpentier, Y.A., Askanazi, J., Elwyn, D., et al.: J. Trauma *19*:649–653, 1979.
196. Brennan, M.F., Moore, F.D.: J. Surg. Res. *14*:501–504, 1973.
197. Wilmore, D.W.: Energy requirement for maximum nitrogen retention. *In* Clinical Nutrition Update— Amino Acids (Edited by H.L. Greene, M.A. Holliday, H.N. Munro.) Chicago, AMA, 1977, pp. 51–53.
198. Brennan, M.F., Fitzpatrick, G.F., Cohen, K.H., et al.: Ann. Surg. *182*:386–393, 1975.
199. Jeejeebhoy, K.N., Anderson, G.H., Nakhooda, A.F., et al.: J. Clin. Invest. *57*:125–136, 1976.
200. Wannemacker, R.W. Jr., Kaminski, M.V., Dinterman, R.E., et al.: J. Parenter. Enteral Nutr. *6*:100–105, 1982.
201. Bach, A.C., Babayan, V.K.: Am. J. Clin. Nutr. *36*:950–962, 1982.
202. Brenner, J.: Trends Biochem. Sci. *2*:207–209, 1980.
203. Reference deleted.
204. Eckart, J., Adolph, M., Van der Mühlen, V., et al.: J. Parenter. Enteral Nutr. *4*:360–366, 1980.
205. Sailer, D., Muller, M.: J. Parenter. Enteral Nutr. *5*:115–119, 1981.
206. Mok, K.T., Maiz, A., Yamazaki, K., et al.: Metabolism *33*:910–915, 1984.
207. Yamazaki, K., Maiz, A., Solvado, J., et al.: J. Parenter. Enteral Nutr. *8*:361–366, 1984.
208. Hamawy, K.J., Moldawer, L.L., Georgieff, M., et al.: J. Parenter. Enteral Nutr. *9*:559–565, 1985.
209. Böhles, H., Akcetin, Z., Lehnert, W.: J. Parenter. Enteral Nutr. *11*:46–48, 1987.
210. Crowe, P.J., Dennison, A.R., Royle, G.T.: J. Parenter. Enteral Nutr. *9*:720–724, 1985.
211. Abumrad, N.N., Miller, B.: J. Parenter. Enteral Nutr. *7*:163–170, 1983.
212. Philcox, J.C., Hartley, T.F., Worthley, L.I.G., et al.: J. Parenter. Enteral Nutr. *8*:535–541, 1984.
213. Jacobson, S.: J. Parenter. Enteral Nutr. *6*204–213, 1982.
214. Woude, P.V., Morgan, R.E., Kosta, J.M., et al.: Crit. Care Med. *14*:685–688, 1986.
215. Bonau, R.A., Ang, S.D., Jeevanandam, M., et al.: J. Parenter. Enteral Nutr. *8*:622—627, 1984.
216. Elwyn, D.H., Gump, F.E., Munro, H.N., et al.: Am. J. Clin. Nutr. *32*:1597–1611, 1979.
217. Lundholm, K., Bennegård, K., Wickström, I., et al.: J. Parenter. Enteral Nutr. *10*:29–33, 1986.
218. Vazquez, J.A., Paleos, G.A., Steinhardt, H.J., et al.: Am. J. Clin. Nutr. *44*:24–32, 1986.
219. Nanni, G., Pittiruti, M., Giovannini, I., et al.: J. Parenter. Enteral Nutr. *9*:483–490, 1985.
220. Palombo, J.D., Schnure, F., Bistrian, B.R., et al.: J. Parenter. Enteral Nutr. *11*:88–91, 1987.
221. Worthley, L.I.G., Fishlock, R.C., Snoswell, A.M.: J. Parenter. Enteral Nutr. *7*:176–180, 1983.
222. Worthley, L.I.G., Fishlock, R.C., Snoswell, A.M.: J. Parenter. Enteral Nutr. *8*:717–719, 1984.
223. Geggel, H.S., Ament, M.E., Heckenlively, J.R., et al.: N Engl. J. Med. *312*:142–146, 1985.
224. Vinton, N.E., Laidlow, S.A., Ament, M.E., et al.: Am. J. Clin. Nutr. *44*:398:404, 1986.
225. Wood, R.J., Sitrin, M.D., Cusson, G.J., et al.: J. Parenter. Enteral Nutr. *10*:188–190, 1986.
226. Abumrad, N.N., Schneider, A.J., Steel, D., et al.: Am. J. Clin. Nutr. *34*:2551–2559, 1981.
227. Shils, M.E., Burke, A.W., Greene, H.L., et al.: Guidelines for essential trace element preparations for parenteral use. A statement by an expert panel. JAMA *241*:2051–2054, 1979.
228. Jetton, M.M., Sullivan, J.F., Burch, R.E.: Arch. Intern. Med. *136*:782–784, 1976.
229. Phillips, G.D., Garnys, V.P.: J. Parenter. Enteral Nutr. *5*:11–14, 1981.
230a. Shils, M.E. (ed.): Working Conference on Parenteral Trace Elements II, Sept. 14–15, 1982. Bull. N.Y. Acad. Med. *60*:117–212, 1984.
230b. Shike, M.: Working Conference on Parenteral Trace Elements II, Sept. 14–15, 1982. (Edited by M.E. Shils.) Bull. N.Y. Acad. Med. *60*:132–143, 1984.
231. Kurkus, J., Alcock, N.W., Shils, M.E.: J. Parenter. Enteral Nutr. *8*:254–257, 1984.
232. Van Rij, A.M., Thomson, C.D., McKenzie, J.M., et al.: Am. J. Clin. Nutr. *32*:2076–2085, 1979.
233. Lane, H.W., Barroso, A.O., Englert, D., et al.: J. Parenter. Enteral Nutr. *6*:426–431, 1982.
234. Kien, C.L., Veillon, C., Patterson, K.Y., et al.: J. Parenter. Enteral. Nutr. *10*:662–664, 1986.
235. Makaffey, K.R.: Working Conference on Parenteral Trace Elements II, Sept. 14–15, 1982. (Edited by M.E. Shils.) Bull. N.Y. Acad. Med. *60*:196–209, 1984.
236. Klein, G.L., Targoff, C.M., Ament, M.E., et al.: Lancet *2*:1041–1044, 1980.
237. Klein, G.L., Alfrey, A.C., Miller, N.L., et al.: Am. J. Clin. Nutr. *35*:1425–1429, 1982.
238. Sedman, A.B., Klein, G.L., Merritt, R.J., et al.: N. Engl. J. Med. *312*:1337–1343, 1985.
239. Wu, W.W.K., Kaplan, L.A., Horn, J., et al.: J. Parenter. Enteral Nutr. *10*:591–595, 1986.
239. Heyman, M.B., Klein, G.L., Wong, A., et al.: J. Parenter. Enteral Nutr. *10*:86–87, 1986.
240. Shils, M.E., Shike, M.: Unpublished data.
241. Greene, H.C.: Personal communication.
242. Shils, M.E., Jacobs, D.H.: Am. J. Clin. Nutr. *37*:731, 1983 (abst.).
243. Fleming, C., Lie, J., McCall, J., et al.: Gastroenterology *83*:689–693, 1982.
244. Brown, M.R., Cohen, H.J., Lyons, J.M., et al.: Am. J. Clin. Nutr. *43*:549–554, 1986.
245. Levander, O.A., Burk, R.F.: J. Parenter. Enteral Nutr. *10*:545–549, 1986.
245a. Shils, M.E., Levander, O.A.: Am. J. Clin. Nutr. *35*:829, 1982 (abst.).
245b. McGee, C.D., Mascarenhas, M.G., Ostro, M.J., et al.: J. Parenter. Enteral Nutr. *9*:568–570, 1985.
246. Lipkin, E., Schumann, L., Young, J.H., et al.: J. Parenter. Enteral Nutr. *10*:40–44, 1986.
247. Vanamee, P., Shils, M.E., Burke, A.W., et al.: J. Parenter. Enteral Nutr. *3*:258–262, 1979 (Adaptation of the Original AMA "Guidelines for Multivitamin Preparations for Parenteral Use," 1977).
248. Federal Register: *37* No. 241, 15027 (July 1972) and 26623 (Dec. 14, 1972).
249. Shils, M.E.: Bull. Parent. Drug Assoc. *30*:226–233, 1976.
250. Federal Register: *44*:40933–40936, 1979.
251. DeRitter, E. J. Pharm. Sci. *71*:1073–1096, 1982.
252. Gillis, J., Jones, G., Pencharz, P.: J. Parenter. Enteral Nutr. *7*:11–14, 1983.
253. Gutcher, G.R., Lax, A.A., Farrell, P.M.: Am. J. Clin. Nutr. *40*:8–13, 1984.
254. Riggle, M.A., Brandt, R.B.: J. Parenter. Enteral Nutr. *10*:388–392, 1986.
255. Howard, L., Chu, R., Feman, S., et al.: Ann. Intern. Med. *93*:576–577, 1980.

256. Kishi, H., Yamaji, A., Kataoka, K., et al.: J. Parenter. Enteral Nutr. *5*:420–423, 1981.
257. Scheiner, J.M., Aranjo, M.M., DeRitter, E.: Am. J. Hosp. Pharm. *38*:1911–1913, 1982.
258. Shils, M.E., Baker, H., Frank, O.: J. Parenter. Enteral Nutr. *9*:179–188, 1985.
259. Barker A., Hebron, B.S., Beck, P.R., et al.: J. Parenter. Enteral Nutr. *8*:3–7, 1984.
260. Chen, M.F., Boyce, H.W. Jr., Triplett, L.: J. Parenter. Enteral Nutr. *7*:462–464, 1983.
261. Am. Acad. Pediatrics Comm. on Drugs: Pediatrics *76*:635–643, 1985.
262. Pollack, H., Halpern, S.L.: Therapeutic Nutrition Publ. 234. Washington, D.C., Natl. Acad. Sci.–Natl. Res. Council, 1952.
263. Jeppson, B., Gimmon, Z.: Vitamins. *In* Surgical Nutrition (Edited by J.E. Fischer). Boston, Little, Brown & Co., 1983.
264. Shils, M.E., Randall, H.T.: Diet and Nutrition in the Care of the Surgical Patient. *In* Modern Nutrition in Health and Disease. 6th Ed. (Edited by R.S. Goodhart, M.E. Shils). Philadelphia, Lea & Febiger, 1980, pp. 1111–1113.
265a.Nichoalds, G.E., Meng, H.C., Caldwell, M.D.: Arch. Surg. *112*:1061–1064, 1977.
265b.Bradley, J.A., King, R.F.J.G., Schorah, C.J., et al.: Br. J. Surg. *65*:492–494, 1978.
266. Stromberg, P., Shenkin, A., Campbell, R.A., et al.: J. Parenter. Enteral Nutr. *5*:295–299, 1981.
267. Kirkemo, A.K., Burt, M.E., Brennan, M.: Am. J. Clin. Nutr. *35*:1003–1009, 1982.
268. Kishi, H., Nishii, S., Ono, T., et al.: Am. J. Clin. Nutr. *32*:332–338, 1979.
269a.Jeejeebhoy, K.N., Langer, B., Tsallas, G., et al.: Gastroenterology *71*:943–953, 1976.
269b.Howard, L., Bigaouette, J., Chu, R., et al.: Am. J. Clin. Nutr. *37*:421–428, 1983.
270a.Moore, M.C., Greene, H.L., Phillips, B.L., et al.: Pediatrics *77*:530–538, 1986.
270b.Greene, H.L., Courtney-Moore, M.E., Phillips, B.L., et al.: Pediatrics *77*:539–546, 1986.
270c.Greene, H.L., Phillips, B.L., Franck, L., et al.: Pediatrics *79*:894–900, 1987.
271a.MacDonald, M.G., Fletcher, A.B., Johnson, E.L., et al.: J. Parenter. Enteral Nutr. *11*:169–171, 1986.
271b.DeVito, V., Reynolds, J.W., Benda, G.I., et al.: J. Parenter. Enteral Nutr. *10*:63–65, 1986.
272. Greene, H.L., Phillips, B.L. (Letter): Pediatrics *79*:655, 1987.
273a.Phillips, B.L., Franck, L.S., Greene, H.L., et al: Pediatrics 80: Oct. 1987 (in press).
273b.Poland, R.L. (Letter): Pediatrics *77*:787–788, 1986.
274. Koo, W.W.K., Tsang, R.C., Steichen, S.J., et al.: J. Parenter. Enteral Nutr. *11*:172–176, 1987.
275. Bowyer, B.A., Fleming, C.R., Ludwig, J., et al.: J. Parenter. Enteral Nutr. *9*:11–17, 1985.
276. Bell, R.L., Ferry, G.D., Smith, E.O, et al.: J. Parenter. Enteral Nutr. *10*:356–359, 1986.
277. Keim, N.L.: J. Parenter. Enteral Nutr. *11*:18–22, 1987.
278. Jacobs, D.O., Settle, R.G., Trerotola, S.O., et al.: J. Parenter. Enteral Nutr. *10*:177–183, 1986.
279. Robertson, J.F.R., Garden, O.J., Shenkin, A.: J. Parenter. Enteral Nutr. *10*:172–176, 1986.
280. Stein, T.P., Buzby, G.P., Gertner, M.H., et al.: Am. J. Physiol. *239*:G280–G287, 1980.
281. Host, W.R., Serlin, O., Rush, B.F.: Am. J. Surg. *123*:57–62, 1972.
282. Stanko, R.T., Nathan, G., Mendelow, H., et al.: Gastroenterology *92*:197–202, 1987.
283. Lambert, J.R., Thomas, S.M.: J. Parenter. Enteral Nutr. *9*:501–503, 1985.
284. Goldman, P.: N. Engl. J. Med. *303*:1212–1218, 1980.
285. Kaplan, M.M.: Viewpoints Dig. Dis. *15*:9–12, 1983.
286. Knight, P.J., Buchanan, S., Clarworthy, H.W.J.: JAMA *243*:1244–1246, 1980.
287. Kien, C.L., Brouring, C., Jona, J., et al.: J. Parenter. Enteral Nutr. *6*:152–156, 1982.
288. Klein, G.L., Targoff, C.M., Ament, M.E., et al.: Lancet *2*:1041–1044, 1980.
289. Klein, G.L., Horst, R.L., Norman, A.W., et al.: Ann. Intern. Med. *94*:638–643, 1981.
290. Klein, G.L., Alfrey, A.C., Miller, N.L.: Am. J. Clin. Nutr. *35*:1425–1429, 1982.
291. Ott, S.M., Maloney, N.A., Klein, G.L., et al.: Ann. Intern. Med. *98*:910–914, 1983.
292. Shike, M., Harrison, J.E., Sturtridge, W.C., et al.: Ann. Intern. Med. *92*:343–350, 1980.
293. Shike, M., Sturtridge, W.C., Tam. C.S., et al.: Ann. Intern. Med. *95*:560–568, 1981.
294. Shike, M., Shils, M.E., Heller, A., et al.: Am. J. Clin. Nutr. *44*:89–98, 1986.
295. Bengoa, J.M., Sitrin, M.D., Wood, R.J., et al.: Am. J. Clin. Nutr. *38*:264–269, 1983.
296. Wood, R.J., Sitrin, M.D., Cusson, G.J., et al.: J. Parenter. Enteral Nutr. *10*:188–190, 1986.
297. Roslyn, J.J., Pitt, H.A., Many, L.L., et al.: Gastroenterology *84*:148–154, 1983.
298. Messing, B., Bories, C., Kunstlinger, F., et al.: Gastroenterology *84*:1012–1019, 1983.
299. Kirby, D.F., Craig, R.M.: J. Parenter. Enteral Nutr. *9*:353–357, 1985.
300. Izsak, M., Shike, M., Roulet, M., et al.: Gastroenterology *79*:555–558, 1980.
301. Driver, A.G., LeBrun, M.: JAMA *244*:2195–2196, 1980.
302. Nederman, M.S., Merrill, W.W., Ferranti, R.D., et al.: Ann. Intern. Med. *100*:795–800, 1984.
303. Howard, L., Michalek, A.V.: Ann. Rev. Nutr. *4*:69–99, 1984.
304. Steiger, E. (ed): Home Parenteral Nutrition Proc. Symposium, Feb. 17–18, 1980. Silver Springs, Md, Am. Soc. Parent. Enter. Nutr., 1981, pp. 49.
305. Jejeebhoy, K.N. (ed.): Total Parenteral Nutrition in the Hospital and at Home. Boca Raton, Fl, CRC Press, 1983, pp. 255.

## SELECTED READINGS

1. Pareira, M.D.: Therapeutic Nutrition with Tube Feeding. Springfield, Il, CC Thomas, 1959.
2. Shils, M.E. (Ed.): Defined Formula Diets for Medical Purposes. Proc. Symp. 1975. Chicago, AMA, 1977, p. 154.
3. Torosian, M.H., Rombeau, J.L.: Feeding by tube enterostomy. Surg. Gynecol. Obstet. *150*:918–927, 1980.
4. Koretz, R.L., Meyer, J.H.: Elemental Diets—facts and fantasies. Gastroenterology *78*:393–410, 1980.
5. Randall, H.T.: Tube feeding in acute and chronic illness. J. Parenter. Enteral Nutr. *8*:113–136, 1984.
6. Elman, R.: Parenteral Alimentation in Surgery. New York, P.B. Hoeber, 1947, pp. 284.
7. Geyer, R.P.: Parenteral nutrition. Physiol. Rev. *40*:150–186, 1960.
8. Meng, H.C., Law, D.H. (Eds.): Parenteral Nutrition. Proc. Internat. Symp., 1968. CC Thomas. Springfield, Il, 1970, pp. 594.
9. White, P.L., Nagy, M.E. (Eds.): Total Parenteral Nutrition. Proc. Internat. Symp., 1972. Publ. Sci. Gp., Acton, Ma., 1974, pp. 477.

10. Rhoads, J.E., Vars, H.M., Dudrick, S.J.: The development of intravenous hyperalimentaiton. Surg. Clin. North Am. *61*:429–435, 1981.

11. Day, H.G. (Ed.): Total Parenteral Nutrition Symposium Fed Proc. *43*:1390–1411, 1984.

12. Levenson, S.M., et al.: Early History of Parenteral Nutrition, pp. 1391–1406.

13. Shils, M.E.: Historical aspects of minerals and Vitamins in Parenteral Nutrition, pp. 1412–1416.

14. Winters, R.W., et al.: History of Parenteral Nutrition in Pediatrics with Emphasis on Amino Acids, pp. 1407–1411.

15. Howard, L., Michalek, A.V.: Home Parenteral Nutrition (HPN) Ann. Rev. Nutr. *4*:69–99, 1984.

**Part VII**
*Diet and Nutrition in the Prevention and Treatment of Disease*

*Chapter* **55**

# NUTRITION IN RELATION TO DENTAL MEDICINE

Edward A. Sweeney and James H. Shaw

Dental medicine is that specialty concerned with the welfare of the teeth and soft tissues of the oral cavity and with the diagnosis of systemic diseases that have oral manifestations.

By reason of the location and functions of the oral cavity, its tissues are subjected to a wider variety and more stringent series of trauma and stresses than tissues in other moist internal cavities of the body. Consider, for example, the wide variety in:

• physical texture of the food that has to be chewed into a form suitable for swallowing and the physical pressure on the teeth and supporting structures that is needed to subdivide the food in the masticatory process;

• temperature of common foods as ingested; and

• chemical stimuli to which the tissues of the oral cavity are exposed periodically.

In addition, the temperature and humidity of the oral cavity, coupled with food passing through it frequently, provide ideal circumstances for the growth and multiplication of the many microorganisms that normally reside there. The subdivision of food by the teeth and the buffering and diluting capacity of the saliva greatly reduce the intensity of these stresses before the food-saliva mixtures are passed on to the lower areas of the gastrointestinal tract.

The soft tissues of the mouth are unusually susceptible to current metabolic abnormalities of nutritional origin, in large part because of the rapidity of cellular turnover that results at least partially from the previously listed trauma. During the early years of nutritional science in which characteristic signs of nutrient deficiencies were being recognized, the soft tissues of the oral cavity were particularly important by reason of their susceptibility to nutritional disturbances and their easy accessibility for examination. The classic signs of nutritional deficiencies in the oral tissues are described in the chapters concerned with B complex deficiencies and scurvy.

The mineralized (hard) tissues of the oral cavity, enamel, dentin, and cementum are subjected to different types of influences during two phases of their life history: *development,* when the tooth is forming within the jaw, and *posteruptively,* when the external surfaces are bathed continually with mixtures of saliva, microorganisms, and food and are colonized by microorganisms. During development, the enamel and dentin are influenced by systemic abnormalities that may alter the elaboration of the organic matrices or mineralization of these matrices. Visual or chemical evidence of such abnormalities is imprinted in the enamel and dentin permanently and disappears only with the destruction of these tissues. Posteruptively, after the crowns erupt into the oral cavity, the enamel and dentin may be destroyed progressively by microbial action in the characteristic pattern of tooth decay. The tooth also may be lost due to destruction of the periodontal structures with or without any previous breakdown of the enamel or dentin. When the cementum is exposed by periodontal breakdown and recession, it is colonized by microorganisms, and root caries may occur.

In any discussion of the relationship of nutrition to the integrity of the mineralized structures, the dietary influences upon both the oral environment and the nutritional status as mediated through one or more systemic pathways must be considered and integrated. Attention needs to be directed in an increasing degree to those nutritional abnormalities that occur during development or over prolonged periods of adult life, but that may not be detected until long after the actual nutrient imbalance may have begun.

Some diseases of the oral cavity are especially good examples of diseases with delayed etiologic components. Dental caries in particular has been shown to be related to specific nutritional abnormalities that occur during tooth development and maturation (e.g., inadequate fluoride during mineralization and in the early posteruptive periods results in high caries experience). In industrialized countries, dental caries prevalence decreased significantly between 1960 and 1980.[1] However, the reverse appears to have been occurring in numerous developing countries.[2] The diseases of the periodontal tissues may likewise have nutritional components that are at present unknown or ill-defined. In all probability, the prevalence of periodontal disease will increase as the average age of the population increases and as the number of teeth surviving into old age increases. The latter results from decreased caries prevalence and increased availability and utilization of preventive and restorative techniques. This possibility of increased prevalence of periodontal diseases should spur more diligent investigation of the possible ways in which systemic influences are mediated.

Before a discussion of the oral diseases that are related to nutritional abnormalities, let us consider the structure of the teeth and their surrounding tissues and the uniqueness of the mineralized tissues.

## STRUCTURE OF TEETH

The teeth are composed of three highly mineralized tissues: enamel, dentin, and cementum

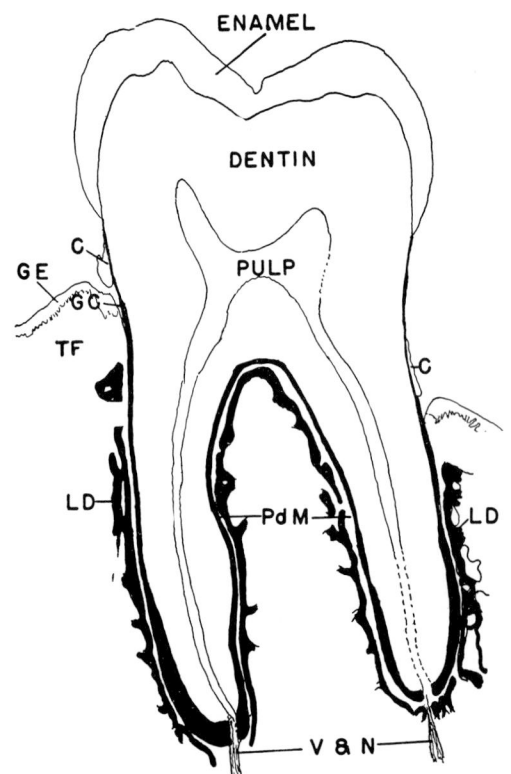

**Fig. 55–1.** Mesiodistal section of a lower molar tooth. Normally the gingival epithelium (GE) is in close apposition to the cervix of the tooth and acts as a barrier to decrease bacterial invasion of the underlying dermis. Transverse fibers (TF) form another barrier against bacterial penetration. In this case, a small amount of salivary calculus (C) was deposited and caused the formation of an abnormally deep gingival crevice (GC). This is the beginning of periodontitis. At a later stage, periodontitis causes destruction of the lamina dura (LD), a compact bony plate lining the alveolus as well as the periodontal membrane (PdM), which attaches the entire tooth root to the surrounding bone. V and N = vessels and nerves supplying the dental pulp.

(Fig. 55–1). Enclosed within these rigid tissues is a highly vascular connective tissue, the dental pulp, which is frequently called the "nerve" by laymen because of its sensitivity to heat, cold, pressure, and other stimuli.

The teeth are retained in their bony sockets (alveoli) by means of the highly fibrous structure termed the periodontal membrane or ligament. Influences that affect the integrity of this structure and bone surrounding the socket result in periodontal disease that may progress sufficiently to cause loosening and loss of the teeth.

Enamel is the hardest, most highly mineralized structure in the body, containing 97 to 98% hydroxyapatite, less than 1% organic matter, and about 2% water. The organic matter secreted by the ameloblasts (enamel-forming cells) is finely divided into sheaths around the mineral crystals.[3] Enamel is amazingly well designed to withstand food mastication for the several decades of life, but by reason of its composition is subject to demineralization when exposed excessively to microbially produced acids or to vomitus.

Dentin is more similar to bone than enamel, containing about 70% hydroxyapatite, 20% organic matter, most of which is collagen, and 10% water. The dentin is traversed by tubules that radiate from the pulp to the dentoenamel junction. Organic processes from the odontoblasts (dentin-forming cells) and nerve fibers penetrate the entire width of the dentin.

The life history of a tooth may be divided into three main eras: (1) the period during which its crown is forming and mineralizing in the jaw, (2) the period of maturation when the tooth is erupting into oral cavity and its root or roots are forming, and (3) the maintenance period while it is functioning in the oral cavity. The extended period during which a human tooth is developing and maturing prior to its functional responsibilities is often forgotten. For example, the first permanent molar, the 6-year molar, is one of our more important teeth by reason of its large masticating surface: its histologic primordia begin to be elaborated about the eighteenth week in utero. From then until 2½ to 3 years of age, the organic matrices of enamel and dentin in the crown are being deposited and mineralized. By 3½ to 4 years of age, the crown has attained its adult size. Eruption into the oral cavity begins between 6 and 7 years, and its roots are completed around 9 to 11 years of age. Thus about 10 years elapse between initiation of this tooth and attainment of its final form. Comparable data for the primary and permanent teeth are presented in Table 55–1.

## Dental Structures vs. Other Tissues

At least three striking differences exist between the mineralized tissues of the teeth and other tissues of the body. First, enamel contains no capillary or lymphatic vessels to act as transport systems. However, the intimate relationships between the organic and the inorganic components of enamel suggest that pathways in the enamel exist for diffusion of ions and small molecules from saliva, and possibly from blood. Although the dentin likewise contains no formed vascular elements, it is more readily permeable to the passage of extracellular fluids from the blood, by reason of the dentinal tubules that traverse the dentin. Studies with radiotracers indicate that enamel and dentin are permeable to various inorganic ions.[4] The inorganic elements of each area of mature teeth participate in slow exchange with comparable elements carried to the area by body fluids. The interchange between elements in the enamel takes place through the bathing of its external surface with saliva. In contrast, the interchange in the dentin occurs by reason of the ions in the blood supply to the pulp or periodontal membrane.

Second, owing to the absence of cells, mineralized dental tissues do not have a microscopically or chemically detectable ability to repair improperly formed or mineralized areas, and the tooth does not have the ability to repair itself after a portion has been destroyed by tooth decay or mechanical injury. An exception to the latter statement is the ability for remineralization of slightly demineralized, superficial areas of the enamel where the organic matrix and surface integrity are still intact, commonly referred to as "white spots." In addition, secondary dentin is formed by the odontoblasts, which persist throughout life on the pulpal surface of the dentin, in response to chemical stimuli from an advancing carious lesion in an effort to wall off the noxious influence. Lack of ability to repair dental tissues is in direct contrast to bone with its continual remodeling by the haversian systems.

Third, unlike other tissues, the mineralized tissues of teeth have a partial change of environment midway in their life. When the tooth begins to emerge into the oral cavity, the vascular supply to the enamel organ is severed, and the enamel surface comes in contact with a complex mixture of saliva, microorganisms, food debris, and epithelial remnants. Thus, instead of a systemic environment only, the erupted tooth has, in addition, an oral or external environment. As a consequence, the enamel surfaces on which carious lesions are initiated by microbial action are largely outside the influences of humoral immune systems so that immune relationships to the caries process are limited to those in saliva.

## CURRENT CONCEPTS OF NUTRITIONAL RELATIONSHIPS TO DENTAL CARIES

Three major parameters, systemic and local environmental influences and microbial agents need to interact simultaneously for sufficiently long periods of time for carious lesions to be discernible (Fig. 55–2). Carious lesions are initiated on the enamel surface as a result of interaction between metabolic products of the microorganisms and the enamel. The primary reaction is between the microbially produced acids and hydroxyapatite, which dissolves at pH values of approximately 5.5 or less. The lesion progresses through the enamel and dentin toward the pulp,

**Table 55–1.   Chronology of Development of the Human Dentition***

| | *Primary Dentition* | | |
|---|---|---|---|
| *Tooth* | *Mineralization Begins (wk. in utero)* | *Crown Completed (mo.)* | *Eruption (mo.)* |
| Central incisors | 14–14½ | 1½–2½ | 7½–9⅓ |
| Lateral incisors | 16–16½ | 2½–3 | 11–13¼ |
| Cuspid | 17–17½ | 9 | 19½–19⅔ |
| 1st molar | 15–15½ | 5½–6 | 15⅔–16 |
| 2nd molar | 18–19 | 10–11 | 26½–28 |
| | *Permanent Dentition* | | |
| *Tooth* | *Mineralization Begins* | *Crown Completed (yr.)* | *Eruption (yr.)* |
| Cental incisors | 3–4 mo | 3½–4½ | 6–7½ |
| Lateral incisors | 4–12 mo | 4–5½ | 7¼–8½ |
| Cuspid | 4–5 mo | 5½–6½ | 9¾–11⅔ |
| 1st premolar | 1½–2 yr | 6½–7½ | 10–10¾ |
| 2nd premolar | 2–2½ yr | 7–8½ | 10¾–11½ |
| 1st molar | 32 wk in utero | 3½–4½ | 6–6¼ |
| 2nd molar | 2½–3 yr | 7–8 | 11¾–12¼ |
| 3rd molar | 7–10 yr | 12–16 | 20–20½ |

*Adapted from Moyers, Hartsook, Kopel: *In* Growth and Development of Children. 6th ed. (Lowrey, Ed.) Chicago, Year Book Medical Publishers, 1973.

ultimately causing pulpal infection unless the forward progress of the lesion is arrested by restorative treatment or by a striking dietary change. Carious lesions probably do not progress continuously, but progression is in an interrupted fashion related to the availability of food to support microbial metabolism. The rate of progression in early lesions is the end result of the balance between demineralization when microbial metabolism is rapid and remineralization in intervening quiescent periods.

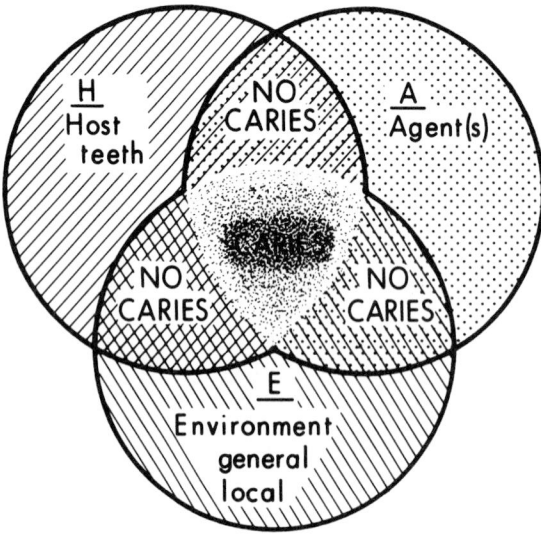

**Fig. 55–2.** Interaction of three major parameters to cause development of caries.

## Microbial Agents

Microorganisms are required to cause the destruction of tooth substance in the characteristic fashion termed "tooth decay." Caries-susceptible rats maintained on a caries-producing diet under germ-free conditions did not develop carious lesions.[5] Monoinoculation by several species of microorganisms caused characteristic carious lesions.[6] Under certain conditions in hamsters and rats, dental caries can be considered an infectious and transmissible disease.[7] For example, carious lesions can be induced in caries-inactive hamsters by oral inoculation with single or pooled cultures from hamsters with active lesions or by caging caries-active and caries-inactive hamsters together.[8] Some strains of streptococci isolated from human carious lesions were immunologically similar to those isolated from the oral cavities of rats and hamsters and were capable of causing carious lesions when inoculated into these animals.[9,10]

*Streptococcus mutans* has received special attention in recent years by reason of the recognition that this microorganism was important in the causation of dental caries in hamsters. This species is not detectable in the mouth before teeth are present but colonizes to the surfaces in infants soon after the tooth erupts.[11] It is present in many carious lesions in children.[12] The mother appears to be a primary source of the microorganisms found in her infant's mouth.[13] In addition, rigorous procedures to reduce the *S. mutans* count in the mother's mouth before the infant's birth and during the first years of life greatly reduced the likelihood that the infant would be heavily infected[14] and the young child highly susceptible to caries.[15]

*S. mutans* has the interesting ability to synthesize a polyglucose, dextran, from dietary sucrose. This ability enables this organism to colonize tooth surfaces and form plaque, which also can be colonized by other microorganisms.[10] A thoroughly cleaned tooth is immediately coated with saliva and colonized by microorganisms. Under this conglomerate, the interaction between the metabolites of the microorganisms and tooth substance can occur to cause dental caries. Demineralization probably occurs whenever the pH falls to 5.5. Because *S. mutans* may not be sufficiently aciduric to metabolize readily at substantially lower pH values in deep lesions, this microorganism may be particularly harmful in superficial lesions, whereas more aciduric microorganisms, such as *Lactobacilli acidophilus,* may be more harmful in deeper carious lesions.

Metabolism of oral microorganisms is dependent upon the food passing through the oral cavity, some of which is retained in plaque, on tooth surfaces, and on soft tissues. Both the composition of food and the frequency of use are related to caries and will be discussed later.

## Nutritional Influences During Tooth Development

With this background about tooth structure and development, and the etiology of dental caries, let us examine relationships between nutrition and dental caries in the three eras in the tooth's life history. Unquestionably the most striking influences occur as a result of nutritional deficiencies during tooth development. Three classic nutritional deficiencies influence tooth development in histologically discernible ways: (1) avitaminosis-A, (2) scurvy, and (3) rickets attributable to deficiencies of vitamin D, calcium, or phosphorus or to a gross imbalance of the calcium/phosphorus ratio. In addition, inadequate levels of fluoride and disturbed calcium/phosphorus ratios result in abnormalities of the chemical composition, at a submicroscopic level, which are related to caries susceptibility.

**Vitamin A.** Just as vitamin A deficiency influences the integrity of epithelial tissue throughout the body, this deficiency also influences ameloblasts of epithelial origin.[16,17] The first histologically visible change was observed in the odontoblasts. However, it is believed that the first abnormality during the early stages of vitamin A deficiency was the loss of the physiologic ability of the ameloblasts to stimulate the differentiation of odontoblasts from the adjacent connective tissue. The odontoblasts did not arrange themselves

in normal linear fashion parallel to the ameloblasts. Later, profound degeneration and atrophy of the ameloblasts were observed. In late stages, these cells resembled squamous metaplasia with virtually no recognizable ameloblasts and a great reduction in the rate of organic matrix formation. Enamel hypoplasia is a prominent manifestation of severe and prolonged vitamin A deficiency in experimental animals.

Repair patterns in the teeth of rodents recovering from vitamin A deficiency were straightforward and rapid. The odontogenic epithelium regained its function and morphologic appearance; the formation of normal odontoblasts and the deposition and mineralization of normal dentin followed.

In vitamin A deficiency in infants, Dinnerman reported abnormalities in the enamel and the enamel-forming organs consistent with those lesions in experimental animals.[18] In addition, the dentin was poorly mineralized and contained scattered globules of unusual size; the predentin was extraordinarily wide. Harris and Navia produced vitamin A deficiency in rat pups during critical periods of tooth development.[18a] They observed increased caries susceptibility without any evidence of changes in the structure or physiology of the salivary glands or of alterations in the solubility of surface enamel. In organ cultures of third molars of rats, a vitamin A deficiency produced major aberrations in enamel and dentin formation.[18b]

No conclusive body of information indicates that enamel hypoplasia in human beings is directly attributable to vitamin A deficiency during tooth development. However, linear enamel hypoplasia of deciduous incisors has been reported in as many as 50% of children from some developing countries that commonly have endemic vitamin A and protein-calorie deficiencies.[19,20] The etiology of this perinatally timed enamel hypoplasia may have its basis in malnutrition-infection interrelationships. With a cariogenic diet, these affected teeth demonstrated a high susceptibility to a type of decay that has been called odontoclasia.

**Vitamin C.** Scurvy has been described in other chapters. In frank vitamin C deficiency, the gingival lesions are particularly striking.[21]

Vitamin C deficiency primarily affects the ability of cells of connective tissue origin to elaborate and assemble their collagenous products. The odontoblasts that form the dentin are of mesodermal origin and are readily affected by this deficiency.[22] When guinea pigs were maintained on a scorbutic diet, the odontoblasts soon became atrophic and resembled the nearby pulp cells with a decrease in their orderly polar arrangement, a decrease in height, and eventually complete disorganization. The decreased height of the odontoblasts and the rate of dentin formation were sufficiently closely related to the amount of vitamin C consumed that they were used as bioassay criteria before the advent of chemical analyses.[23] The dentin was laid down irregularly with the dentinal tubules lacking their normal parallel arrangement. In severe deficiencies, dentin deposition stopped entirely, and predentin was hypercalcified. At late deficiency stages, the ameloblasts atrophied and hemorrhages occurred.

The pathologic condition in the pulp and in the odontoblastic layer in scorbutic human beings was nearly identical with the pathologic changes in the scorbutic guinea pig, according to Westin.[24] In scorbutic adults, the dentin began to resorb and was porotic. The small amount of replacement dentin formed was of the osteodentin type. The pulp was atrophic and hyperemic.

Although the relationship of vitamin C deficiency to gingival changes and to bone pathology has been demonstrated repeatedly, no clear demonstration of a relationship between scurvy and dental caries has been described in numerous trials.

**Vitamin D, Calcium, and Phosphorus.** Lady May Mellanby in 1918 observed that deficiency of a fat-soluble vitamin, later designated vitamin D, in young puppies had a profound effect on the developing enamel and dentin of secondary teeth, on the eruption rate, and also on tooth position in the jaw.[25,26]

The changes that occurred in teeth during the rachitic process were appreciably less complex than those in bones. The first and most prominent change in rickets in rats was a calciotraumatic line, a line of disturbed mineralization of the dentin, accompanied by retardation in the formation of dentin and pronounced disturbance in mineralization of dentin and cementum.[27]

Grossly visible enamel hypoplasia did not occur except in the more severe cases of rickets in the dog, whereas inadequate mineralization of both the enamel and dentin could be demonstrated in relatively mild rickets. Gross hypoplasia has not been described in the rat as a result of rickets.

The bony structures supporting the teeth (alveolar bone) developed changes in rickets characteristic of those in bone elsewhere in the body. Wide osteoid borders were found on the trabeculae of the alveolar bone, and the number and size of the trabeculae were greatly decreased.

In human beings, more than one cause of enamel hypoplasia is probable (Figs. 55–3, 55–4). In a thorough survey of the case histories of indi-

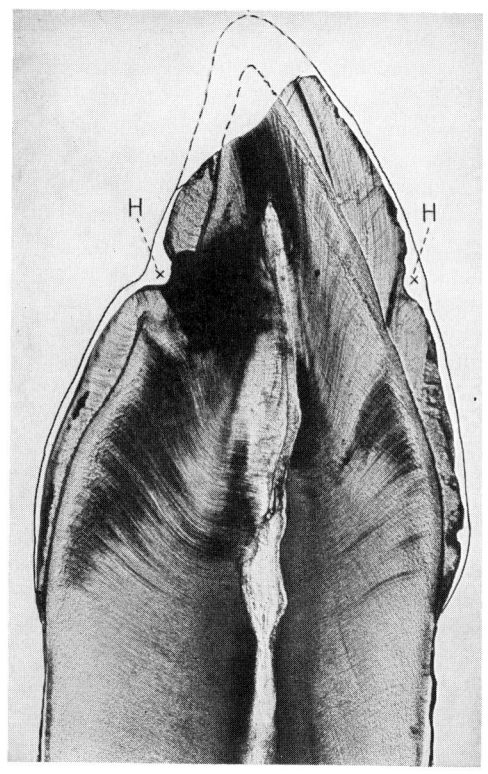

**Fig. 55–3.**  Section of an upper canine tooth. A severe systemic disturbance, which occurred when the patient was about 3 years old, caused the hypoplasia of the enamel (H). As shown by poor calcification and rills in the subsequently formed enamel (near the cervix of the tooth), the condition improved but did not become normal. Solid line = extent of normal enamel; dotted lines = loss of tooth structure from attrition.

viduals with enamel hypoplasia, Sarnat and Schour reported that only a small number had any evidence of a rachitic process during development.[28]

Nikiforuk and Fraser proposed a "unifying concept" of enamel hypoplasia in humans.[29] On the basis of a series of patients with abnormalities of calcium and phosphorus metabolism, they reported that enamel hypoplasia occurred only in those patients with grossly depressed serum calcium levels. Elevations of serum phosphate were not associated with hypoplasia, even though Ca/P ratios were perturbed. A perplexing part of their hypothesis, however, concerns the severe hypocalcemia (6.0 mg/dl) necessary to produce enamel hypoplasia.

Mellanby conducted studies in an era when rickets was prevalent to evaluate the possibility of a correlation between the structure of human teeth as studied microscopically and the susceptibility to decay. As standards for comparison, various stages of increasing severity of microscope

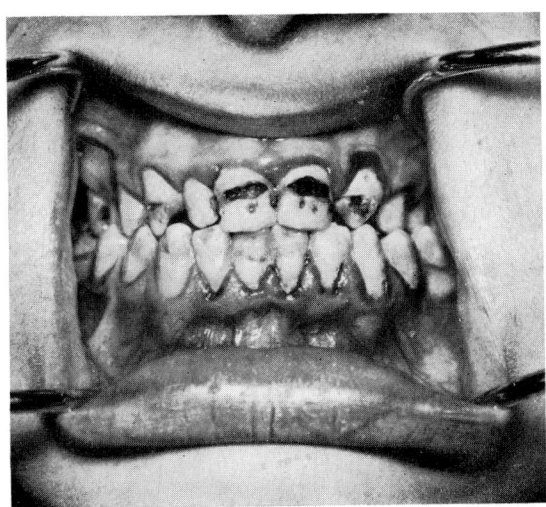

**Fig. 55–4.** Excessive enamel hypoplasia of the anterior teeth of a 16-year-old girl may have been caused by severe malnutrition in early childhood. The marked gingivitis on lower anterior gingiva cleared up quickly as a result of vitamin C therapy. (From Cahn: Pathology of the Oral Cavity. Baltimore, Williams & Wilkins, 1941.)

defects were described and correlated with the degrees of caries incidence in the same teeth. The minor defects that Mellanby described—referred to as Mellanby hypoplasia—were visible only microscopically and could be clinically discerned only by a careful exploration of the tooth surface with a sharp explorer.[30] Thus this class of defects could be readily differentiated from grossly visible hypoplasia. Mellanby reported that 78% of primary teeth with well-mineralized enamel and dentin were free from caries, whereas only 6% of teeth with appreciable degrees of microscopic abnormalities were free of tooth decay. This correlation should not be interpreted to mean that grossly hypoplastic teeth will decay for that reason, nor is the corollary true that teeth appearing to be microscopically perfectly mineralized will never decay.

The effect of vitamin D supplementation upon the initiation and progress of carious lesions has been studied a great deal more intensively than the effect of any other essential nutrient. The studies conducted by Mellanby and co-workers in England, which lasted from 1932 through 1936, suggested that vitamin D supplements might cause some reduction in dental caries incidence.[31] Both positive and negative findings have been reported by other investigators.[32–36a]

Evidence from epidemiologic studies suggests that vitamin D may be important for the maintenance of teeth in children. Efforts have been made to determine if there is any correlation between the incidence of dental caries and the hours of sunshine in a given community, the latitude of the locality, and its winter temperature.[37] For example, in a statistical evaluation based on dental caries data collected by many individuals with varying degrees of training under supervision of the United States Public Health Service, Mills reported a definite increase in dental caries among 12- to 14-year-old boys as the latitude increased.[37] This increase amounted to approximately 15 carious lesions per 100 children for each degree of latitude. Increases were reported from 289 decayed, missing, or filled (DMF) teeth per 100 children in the cities between 25° and 36° latitude in the southern states to 491 DMF teeth per 100 children in the cities between 43° and 46° latitude just south of the Canadian border.

On the basis of the same dental caries data, East observed a correlation between the annual mean hours of sunshine and the average dental caries experience.[38] Other studies suggested a correlation between dental caries and mean winter temperature, with more tooth decay where the winter temperature was lower. The most likely explanation of these effects would be increased exposure of the children to sunlight to provide more vitamin D. Other more subtle factors than the simple irradiation of the skin, such as the geographic distribution of naturally available fluoride in the water, may contribute to this end result.

Studies with rodents have shown that the calcium/phosphorus ratio of the diet during tooth development is an important factor in determining the composition of the inorganic fraction of the enamel and dentin. A diet with a high calcium/phosphorus ratio resulted in the formation of teeth in the white rat and the cotton rat with a high carbonate/phosphate ratio.[39–41] In contrast, teeth of animals fed a diet with a low calcium/phosphorus ratio during tooth development had a much lower carbonate/phosphate ratio. The calcium/phosphate ratios of these diets were appreciably more drastic than would ordinarily be encountered in human dietaries. The relation of these studies to human beings is unknown.

**Fluoride in Foods.** Fluoride is the nutrient that has been demonstrated most clearly to reduce the caries susceptibility of teeth when consumed in optimal amounts during tooth development and the early posteruptive periods. No current chapter on the relation of nutrition to oral health would be complete without a discussion of the role of fluoride in the etiology of dental caries. Fluoride is ubiquitous, occurring in minute amounts in all foodstuffs and water supplies. Surveys of the fluoride content of more than 130 foods are available.[42–44] Most foods, such as vegetables, meats, cereals, and fruits, contain between 0.2 and 1.5 ppm of fluorides. Outstanding exceptions to this lower range are the products containing mechanically deboned meat and fowl; seafood, the edible portion of which may contain 5 to 15 ppm of fluoride; and tea leaves, which contain 75 to 100 ppm. A cup of tea supplies approximately 0.1 mg of fluoride. Analyses of the fluoride contribution by food in common human dietaries in Toronto, Minneapolis, and Washington, D.C. indicate that an average diet supplies between 0.1 and 0.6 mg of fluoride daily, without the use of unusual amounts of either seafoods or tea.

Because of the widespread fluoride distribution, production of an experimental diet extremely low in fluoride is laborious. Schwarz used an ultraclean isolator system and a highly purified diet in which all ingredients, including the amino acids, had been purified to an extent not normally needed in dietary studies.[45] Under these circumstances, young rats fed the basal diet grew slowly and the orange pigment of incisor enamel was not produced. The addition of 2.5 μg fluoride per g of diet caused a significant increase in growth rate and normal formation of the incisor pigment.

**Fluoride in Water Supplies.** In data from many epidemiologic surveys in human populations and from rodent studies, a close correlation has been demonstrated between the amount of fluoride ingested during tooth development and the amount of tooth decay occurring in the teeth after eruption. Possibly the first evidence of this relationship was provided in 1929 by Bunting and co-workers, who conducted a survey in Minonk, Illinois.[46] The amount of tooth decay among children born and raised in this community was much lower than that of children who moved into Minonk after tooth development was complete. The investigators recognized that this striking difference must be related to the water supply, but the active agent was undefined. Later it was found that the drinking water in Minonk contained 2.5 ppm fluoride.

In 1939, more extensive information was provided by Dean and his co-workers from a survey of 1,581 children in 4 communities in Illinois where the water supplies contained varying amounts of fluoride.[47] Later a more comprehensive survey was reported for 4,425 children from 13 cities and 4 states by the same investigators. The data from the latter study are presented in Figure 55–5 in terms of the number of DMF permanent teeth observed in the 12- to 14-year-old children.[48] Where the water contained 1 ppm of fluoride or more during tooth development, the children had less tooth decay than children in

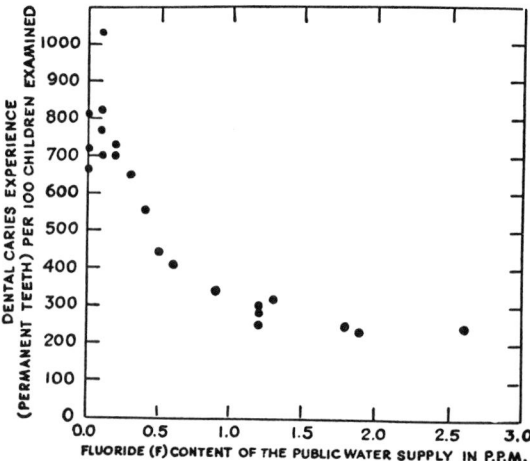

**Fig. 55–5.** Relationship between fluoride content of water supply and the number of decayed, missing, or filled teeth in children.

nearby communities where the water contained appreciably less fluoride. These findings have been corroborated in numerous areas of the United States, as well as in Canada, England, and other countries.

Although these studies were concerned with the permanent teeth of the children, the primary teeth, likewise, have been shown to benefit from the ingestion of fluoride-bearing water during tooth development.[49] In addition, the beneficial effect from the consumption of fluoride-bearing water continued into adult life.[50] Worldwide surveys have demonstrated that exposure to naturally borne fluoride during tooth development continued to manifest itself by a lower incidence of tooth decay in adult life. The ingestion of optimal fluoride during tooth development appears to be as effective in an area of relatively low caries incidence such as Hungary as in areas of high caries incidence such as England and the United States.

The fluoride content of teeth developed in areas where different amounts of fluoride were present in the water supply closely parallels the amount of fluoride in the water.[51] Where drinking water contained 0 to 0.3 ppm fluoride, as in Washington, D.C. before water fluoridation, the teeth of the native continuous residents had approximately 0.01% fluoride in enamel and 0.024% in dentin. Where the water supply contained 1.0 to 1.2 ppm of naturally occurring fluoride, as in Aurora, Illinois, the teeth of residents contained 0.014% fluoride in enamel and 0.036% in dentin. Comparable increases in bone fluoride occurred as the fluoride concentrations in the water supply increased.

Presumably the caries resistance of the teeth is related, at least partially, to their fluoride content.

The exact nature of this relationship is not known. In an x-ray diffraction study of bone samples with various levels of fluoride, Zipkin, Posner, and Eanes observed that increasing fluoride concentrations were associated with increased "crystallinity" of the hydroxyapatite as evidenced by larger crystal size and more nearly perfect crystals.[52] These changes in "crystallinity" reduce the effective surface area of the crystals, reduce the reactivity of the crystals, and provide less area for deposition and surface orientation of carbon dioxide and citrate, in particular. The inverse relationship between fluoride concentration and the carbonate and citrate concentrations in bone has been demonstrated.[53] Zipkin and Posner postulated that, if this inverse relationship existed in enamel as well as in bone, a new concept could be introduced to explain the relationship between fluoride concentration in enamel and susceptibility in dental caries.[54]

In addition, Jenkins and Speirs noted that a very thin surface layer of enamel consistently had a much higher fluoride level than deeper layers.[55] This difference in fluoride distribution in enamel was detectable in unerupted as well as in erupted teeth, which indicates that the fluoride gradient was established during development and before the teeth had erupted into the oral cavity and were contacted with saliva. These observations have been corroborated by Brudevold and co-workers, who demonstrated an additional posteruptive acquisition of fluoride by the surface layers of enamel in proportion to the fluoride concentration in the drinking water.[56,57] Cooper and Ludwig observed decreases in the mesiodistal and buccolingual diameters and in cuspal height of molars in children who grew up in an area with fluoridated water.[58] This observation is consistent with earlier studies in rats and with the smaller crystal lattice in bones with elevated fluoride levels. Optimal fluoride during tooth development has also been reported to result in more perfectly formed fissures between molar cusps.[59]

**Supplemental Fluoride.** The first survey to determine whether the introduction of comparable amounts of fluoride into low-fluoride waters would be equally efficacious was begun at Grand Rapids, Michigan in January, 1945. The fluoride content of the water supply was increased to 1.2 ppm at first and later to 1.0 ppm. Muskegon, Michigan served as the control low-fluoride city. Soon after this, similar surveys were begun in other cities. Some of the impressive data that are now available from the older surveys are presented in Table 55–2.[60]

The dental caries experience in teeth formed during the survey period averaged 60% lower than the caries experience in otherwise comparable teeth formed prior to the increased fluoride content of the water supply, or in those teeth formed in children in neighboring cities where the fluoride content of the water supply was not adjusted. The greatest benefits were in the youngest age groups and in the teeth of older children formed after fluoride adjustment. These facts are clearly shown in Figure 55–6 for the children of Newburgh and Kingston 10 years after fluoridation began in Newburgh.[61]

These data in cities where water fluoridation was initiated are strikingly similar to those in communities where fluoride is naturally present. It is also noteworthy that comparable decreases in dental caries experience did not occur during that time interval in children of nearby communities where the fluoride content of the communal waters was not increased.

In rural areas or urban communities where the drinking water contains less than the optimal level of fluoride, supplemental drops or tablets may be provided daily at home or school throughout the period of tooth development. This procedure is as effective as water fluoridation provided it is followed faithfully from birth through the middle teens when the crowns of the teeth are fully formed.[62] The recommended levels for daily supplementation are shown in Table 55–3. Unfortunately, compliance in the provision of the fluoride supplement is difficult to obtain over such a long period.

Fluoridation of the water supplies in schools is another effective way to provide an appropriate amount of fluoride systemically. Since children are only present in school about 7 hours per day and 180 days per year, the level of fluoride incorporated must be appreciably higher (e.g., 5.0 ppm).[63]

**Pathologic Effects of Excess Fluoride.** The most sensitive cells in the body to excessive fluoride ingestion appear to be the ameloblasts. When the drinking water contains 2.0 ppm or more of fluoride, the prevalence of visibly discernible mottled enamel (chronic endemic dental fluorosis) increases.[64] This problem occurs only when high fluoride ingestion takes place during tooth development, and cannot occur after tooth development has been completed. The degree of mottling varies from slight, aesthetically insignificant amounts to an extensive chalkiness of the surface with large opaque areas, which may erode rapidly and which in severe cases become heavily stained. However, even severely mottled teeth are highly resistant to dental caries. In Figure 55–7, the freedom from fluorosis at optimal fluoride levels in the water is clearly demonstrated.[65]

**Table 55–2. Reduction in Tooth Decay Observed in Various Fluoridation Study Projects***

| Community | Fluoridation Date Started | Report Period (yr) | Age Group (yr) | Reduction in Decay† (%) |
|---|---|---|---|---|
| Grand Rapids, Mich. | Jan. 1945 | 8 | 6 | 70.8 |
| | | | 7 | 52.5 |
| | | | 8 | 49.2 |
| | | | 9 | 48.1 |
| | | | 13 | 39.7 |
| Brantford, Ont. | June 1945 | 7 | 6 | 59.4 |
| | | | 7 | 69.5 |
| | | | 8 | 51.5 |
| | | | 9 | 46.2 |
| | | | 13 | 32.9 |
| Newburgh, N.Y. | May 1945 | 7 | 6 | 69.4 |
| | | | 7 | 67.8 |
| | | | 8 | 40.4 |
| | | | 9 | 51.4 |
| Evanston, Ill. | Feb. 1947 | 4 | 6 | 73.6 |
| | | | 7 | 56.4 |
| | | | 8 | 35.4 |
| Sheboygan, Wis. | Feb. 1946 | 6 | 9–10 (4th grade) | 35.3 |
| | | | 12–14 (8th grade) | 29.7 |

*Adapted from Ast, Smith, Wachs, et al.[61]
†Decayed, missing, and filled teeth.

As the fluoride content of the water increases, the severity and the extent of mottled enamel increase until at levels of 8 to 10 ppm in the communal water almost all individuals who grow up in an area have aesthetically disfiguring mottled enamel. At fluoride levels from 2.0 ppm or more, the water supply is in need of treatment, either by the development of a new source, by dilution with low-fluoride waters, or by removal of the fluoride.

On the basis of numerous epidemiologic surveys, 1.0 ppm fluoride in the water supply has been shown to be no detriment to the health of the public in north temperate regions. In hotter

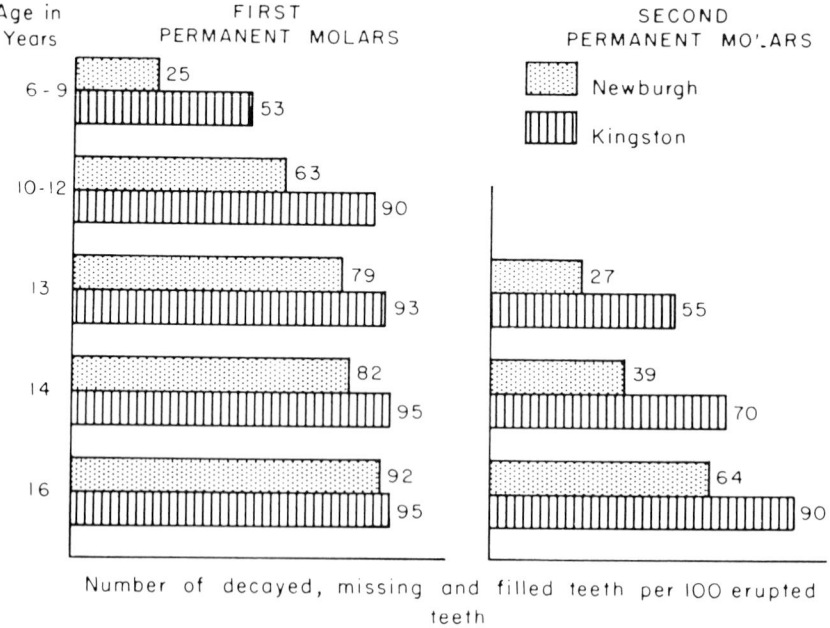

**Fig. 55–6.** The relation of added fluoride in the water supply for 10 years to the incidence of dental caries in first and second permanent molar teeth of children from 6 to 16 years of age. (From Ast, Smith, Wachs, et al.[61] Courtesy of J. Am. Dent. Assoc.)

**Table 55–3.   Recommended Fluoride (F) Supplementation‡**

| Water Supply F Concentration (ppm) | Desirable Fluoride Supplementation (mg/day) by Age | | | | |
|---|---|---|---|---|---|
| | *(0–6 mo)* | *(6–18 mo)* | *(18–36 mo)* | *(3–6 yr)* | *(>6 yr)* |
| <0.2 | 0* | 0.25 | 0.5 | 0.75 | 1.0 |
| 0.2–0.4 | 0* | 0* | 0.25 | 0.5 | 0.75 |
| 0.4–0.6 | 0* | 0* | 0 | 0.25 | 0.5 |
| 0.6–0.8 | 0* | 0* | 0 | 0 | 0.25 |
| >0.8 | 0* | 0* | 0 | 0 | 0† |

*0.25 for fully breast-fed infants.
†In this age group, the hazard of fluorosis is low and some additional protection will probably be afforded by fluoride supplementation. However, fluoride supplementation is not desirable when drinking water provides more than 1.1 ppm.
‡From Wei, S., Fomon, S.J., Anderson, T.A.: Nutrition in dental health. *In* The Food that Stays: An Update on Nutrition, Diet, Sugar and Caries. (Sweeney, E.A., ed.) New York, Medcom Inc., 1977.

climates, where water consumption is appreciably higher, the optimal level of fluoride ingestion may need to be as low as 0.6 to 0.7 ppm.[66]

Controlled fluoridation at the recommended levels has not resulted in aesthetically disfiguring mottling among children of any community. Where fluoride is being added to a water supply, continual monitoring is needed to ensure that excessive amounts are not incorporated, but more importantly, that adequate amounts to obtain dental benefits are being introduced.

Abnormalities other than mottled enamel have been sought in various surveys in the United States and elsewhere throughout the world. Probably the most important and extensive surveys evaluating general systemic influence of fluoride ingestion were made in Bartlett and Cameron, Texas.[66] The former community had a water supply that contained approximately 8 ppm fluoride, whereas the latter community, situated some 30 miles distant, had a water supply with about 0.1 ppm fluoride. In 1943 a series of inhabitants who had resided at least 15 years in each community was selected at random and carefully examined by skilled physicians: 116 in Bartlett and 121 in Cameron. These individuals ranged from 15 to 68 years of age in 1943: 57.8% of the Bartlett participants and 47.2% of those from Cameron were over 55 years of age. X-ray films of various portions of the skeletal system and full case histories were taken. As many of these individuals as possible were studied again in 1953.

The data in these surveys indicated no significant difference in any phase of health between individuals of the two communities, with two exceptions. Many individuals who had resided in

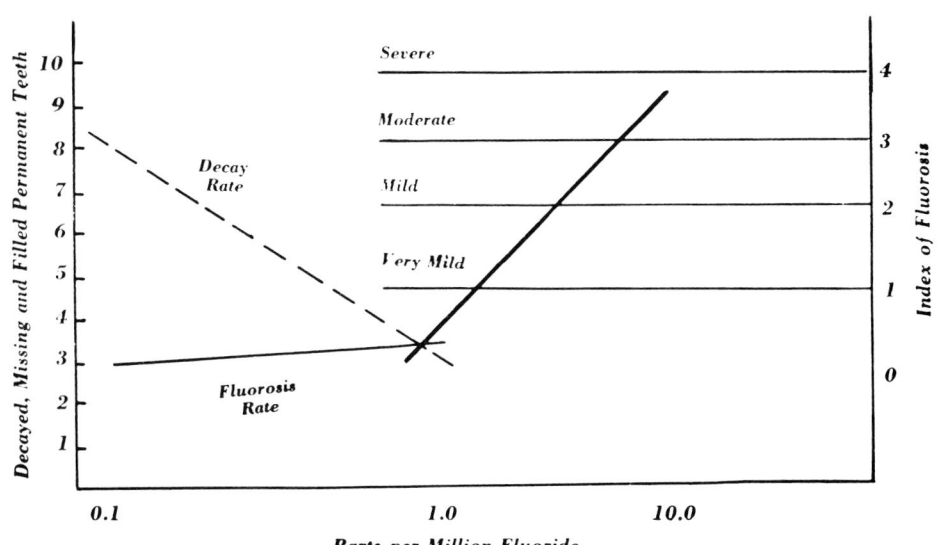

**Fig. 55–7.**   Relation between DMF teeth (dotted line), severity of dental fluorosis (solid line), and fluoride concentration of the water expressed on a logarithmic scale. (Adapted from Hodge and Smith: *In* (Fluoridation as a Public Health Measure. (Shaw, Ed.) Washington, American Association for the Advancement of Science, 1954.)

Bartlett during childhood had severely mottled teeth. In addition, a slightly higher incidence of cardiovascular disease was observed in Cameron, the low-fluoride community. In all other regards, no detectable abnormalities could be attributed to the different fluoride contents of these two water supplies.

Though this survey is undoubtedly the most intensive of all that have been conducted, many other surveys on different phases of the fluoride problem as related to systemic disease have been conducted. In all cases, levels of 1.0 ppm or more, up to 8.0 ppm, in the United States have been shown to be negative with respect to any correlation of a systemic abnormality to the fluoride content of the water.

Claims have been advanced that increased incidence of cancer occurred in communities where water fluoride was increased to the recommended level. These claims and the data on which they were based have been studied intensively by biostatisticians of the National Institutes of Health[67] and the Royal Society of Statistics (England).[68] They concluded that the analyses of the data presented by opponents of fluoridation were invalid. Instead, appropriate analyses indicated that water fluoridation had had no adverse influence on the incidence of cancer.

The case for both the dental benefits and the systemic safety of controlled fluoridation of public water supplies at recommended levels has been unequivocally established. Possibly the ingestion of inadequate levels of fluoride over prolonged periods may be disadvantageous for bone. Leone identified 279 cases of osteoporosis among 546 persons in a radiographic study in Framingham, Massachusetts where the water contained 0.1 ppm fluoride.[69] In addition, a higher frequency of other bone abnormalities was noted than had been observed in either Bartlett or Cameron, Texas. Leone concluded that the data support "the hypothesis that disadvantageous effects on the bone structure of the adult population may be associated with the prolonged use of drinking water that contains an insufficient concentration of fluoride."

Bernstein et al. conducted a survey in two towns in North Dakota where the water supplies contained 4.0 to 5.8 ppm fluoride and in three towns where the water contained 0.15 to 0.30 ppm fluoride.[70] Reduced bone density was more prevalent in the low-fluoride than in the high-fluoride communities. In addition, the males in the low-fluoride towns had a much higher frequency of mineralization in the abdominal aorta.

In a recent study, Simonen and Laitinen reported a significantly decreased bone fragility as measured by the incidence of femoral-neck fracture in inhabitants over 50 years in a Finnish community fluoridated at 1 ppm since 1959 as compared to a control town with only 0.1 ppm F. The differences noted were striking for men over age 50 and for both sexes after age 70.[70A]

Rich and Ensinck have reported improvements in calcium balance in six patients with osteoporosis and one with Paget's disease when fluoride was given orally in several divided doses daily.[71,72] The average improvement in calcium balance was 802 mg per week during the tenth to fourteenth weeks of therapy. Jowsey and coworkers[73] and Hanson and Roos[74] have also shown significant increases in bone mineral mass in patients with osteoporosis, using as much as 100 mg of sodium fluoride per day in combination with vitamin D and calcium supplementation. Calcium supplementation probably avoids the problem of osteomalacia associated with secondary hyperparathyroidism. Kyle et al. have also shown similar beneficial results in patients with multiple myeloma by using the same therapeutic regimen.[75] More study is needed in this area of fluoride metabolism, but these preliminary findings may indicate the existence of more widespread benefits to the skeleton from fluoride ingestion than had been previously expected.

Over 3 million individuals in the United States have consumed natural fluoride-bearing waters in excess of 1.0 ppm for decades, and an additional 5 million individuals have consumed amounts between 0.5 and 1.0 ppm.[76] The fluoridation of community water supplies has been widely instituted throughout the United States and elsewhere in the world. In 1983, fluoride was being added to the water supplies in 8,000 cities and towns in the United States with a total population of 120,000,000 or 52% of the population. Major cities with central water supplies that are not optimally fluoridated are San Diego, Los Angeles, Phoenix, Tucson, and San Antonio.[77]

In a carefully controlled extensive evaluation of preventive dental procedures in five fluoridated and five nonfluoridated communities over a four-year period, the overwhelming importance of water fluoridation was reaffirmed as an extremely effective and inexpensive (less than $1 per person per year) preventive procedure.[77] The treatments evaluated were: pit and fissure sealants; a professional cleaning with a fluoride gel followed by a fluoride gel application twice yearly; a weekly fluoride mouth rinse coupled with daily fluoride tablets if the community did not have water fluoridation; education in plaque control, diet regulation, and dental health; and combinations of these treatments. When a comprehensive treatment regimen was followed, the cost was as high as $54.92 per child per year. One of the interesting incidental observations in this study was that 60% of the decay observed was present in only 20% of the children.

**Other Systemic Relationships to Dental Caries.** In humans in whom salivary glands are congenitally missing or are destroyed by disease or radiation of the head and neck region, xerostomia occurs with an invariably increased susceptibility to dental caries.[78] Similarly, in experimental animals, the surgical removal of the major salivary glands results in spectacular increases in tooth decay.[79] In human studies, the quantity and consistency of the saliva have not yet been shown conclusively to have a definite relation to caries incidence except in cases of xerostomia. The total amounts of certain salivary constituents secreted may be more important than the total volume in which they are secreted.

Genetic relationships to caries suceptibility have not been demonstrated to be strong in man. The relationship between the genetic and environmental factors in experimental dental caries has been described by Larson.[80] Probably the most striking experimental evidence of a genetic factor was provided by a double-mating of female rats from a white caries-susceptible strain with males of the same strain and males of a black, less caries-susceptible strain.[81] The white strain had a tendency to eat more frequently than the black strain. Despite identical intrauterine environmental conditions, the heterozygotic offspring had fewer dental caries than the homozygotic littermates. Human twin studies also suggest moderate genetically determined influences on caries susceptibility.[82] Identical twins tended to have more similar caries experiences than dizygotic twins.

## Tooth Maturation and Maintenance in the Oral Environment

**Tooth Maturation.** The maturation period of a tooth is the era about which the least is known. There are several demonstrations that the caries susceptibility of the molar teeth of rodents decreases as the tooth age increases.[83-85] In children, if a tooth is protected from decay during its early months in the oral cavity, it becomes less liable to be attacked by the carious process later. These findings suggest a change in tooth structure or in permeability of the tooth after emergence into the oral cavity.

Radioisotope studies show that the recently erupted tooth has a high ability to incorporate inorganic ions into its structure.[86] The rate at which this occurs is 10 to 20 times faster than the exchange in teeth that have been in the oral cavity

for longer periods. In addition, the rate of exchange in recently erupted teeth is only about one half the rate in developing crowns of teeth within the jaw. This relatively small difference between unerupted and recently erupted teeth is in striking contrast to the concept that the enamel of erupted teeth is an inert region.

Another influence upon tooth maturation has been demonstrated in histologic studies. The enamel of rats exposed to a cariogenic diet during the early posteruptive period was more permeable to histologic stains than the enamel of littermates fed their entire ration by stomach tube.[87] The changes that take place during tooth maturation may be influenced by the salivary secretions, with the saliva providing the ions needed for tooth maturation.

Briner et al. made an interesting observation concerning the presence of hypomineralized (and presumably developmentally immature) areas of sulcal enamel in rat molars at the time of eruption.[88,89] When a nutritionally adequate noncariogenic diet was fed, these hypomineralized areas slowly mineralized to sound enamel. However, when a cariogenic diet was fed, these hypomineralized areas increased dramatically and progressed to form gross carious lesions.

**Tooth Maintenance.** The truism that "a clean tooth never decays" and the difficulty in obtaining such a condition have been demonstrated by experiments in both normal and sialoadenectomized rats where the caries-producing diet was introduced directly into the stomach by tube-feeding.[86] Oral flora was observed in those animals, but carious lesions did not develop. When the same caries-producing diet was eaten in the usual fashion by littermates, a high incidence of tooth decay was observed.

Of all the dietary components, carbohydrates, particularly the sugars, are essential in the oral cavity for the production of experimental tooth decay. When a carbohydrate-free diet was fed for prolonged periods, either to intact or to sialoadenectomized rats, carious lesions did not develop.[90] Mono- and disaccharides as the sole carbohydrates in purified diets usually caused more dental caries in experimental animals than the same quantities of starches or dextrins.[91] Mixtures of sucrose with starch in similar diets caused high rates of caries formation; as little as 1% sucrose in the presence of 65% starch was adequate to cause caries.[92] Under experimental conditions where *Streptococcus mutans* predominated, dietary sucrose permitted a more rapid progression of carious lesions than glucose and greater recoveries of cariogenic streptococci.[93] The latter microbiota produced large quantities of insoluble dextrans exclusively from sucrose, which enabled the microorganism to adhere to and metabolize on tooth surfaces.[94,95]

Such studies led to the hypothesis that sucrose was uniquely cariogenic and that its replacement by other disaccharides or by monosaccharides in the human diet might be beneficial. Some laboratory data have not supported that position. For example, in the rat, other carbohydrates such as glucose and maltose were as cariogenic as sucrose, and the mixed flora in these rats was able to form insoluble dextrans from glucose and maltose.[96] The likelihood is high in experimental animals that sucrose was of greater cariogenicity than other mono- and disaccharides only when *S. mutans* was the predominant cariogenic organism, as in the hamster and in rats inoculated heavily with the microorganisms.

The frequency of eating and the length of time that a caries-producing diet was made available to rats each day were directly related to the amount of dental caries.[97] Total sugar consumption and percentage of sugars in foods were not as closely related to caries incidence. These laboratory observations closely paralleled epidemiologic studies in children where correlations have been observed between frequency of eating cariogenic snacks and caries activity.

An analysis of the NHANES I survey data found a significant association between the frequency of at-meal and between-meal consumption of soft drinks and high dental decay experience. The associations remained after accounting for concurrent sugar consumption in other foods and other confounding variables.[97a]

Animal studies have advantages by reason of the ability to maintain highly controlled experimental situations and to conduct experiments that are unethical in human populations. However, findings from animal studies must not be transferred directly to a human population, but must be checked in as suitable circumstances as possible. The available human studies can be divided into two general categories: epidemiologic surveys and clinical trials. Numerous surveys have been conducted to determine the incidence of dental caries among primitive populations and to determine the extent to which their dental caries experience has been modified as they came in contact with civilization. One of the most definitive of these surveys concerned the prevalence of tooth decay in primitive and civilized groups of Eskimos in Greenland.[98] The overall prevalence of caries increased dramatically from 1914 to 1945. The prevalence was routinely at least twice as high in each of the four surveys for Eskimos living in contact with main trade stations in com-

parison to those living in more remote areas (Fig. 58–8).

Extensive dental caries statistics were collected on children from European countries during World Wars I and II (Fig. 58–9).[99] Studies representing a total of about 750,000 children from 11 countries have been summarized and evaluated in detail by Sognnaes. Possibly the most detailed data are available from the children in Norway, where almost complete reduction in carbohydrate intake from sugar and highly refined flours occurred in 1939. Progressive increases in caries-free permanent teeth among 7-year-old children occurred until 1945. The teeth that erupted 6 to 8 years after hostilities enforced drastic changes in food habits had much less incidence of caries than the teeth that erupted during prewar and the earlier war years.

In World War I the maximum reduction in caries incidence was not observed until 1922 and 1923, that is, after the cessation of hostilities and the partial return of refined foods and sugar to the European diet. In other words, the teeth that were benefited most were those that were just beginning to form when the wartime dietary change was imposed.

These reductions in dental caries incidence were comparable for the two wars and in the several countries from which data were available, which suggests that the data have a high degree of validity. The active factors in this effect on dental caries incidence are unknown. Since children of the same ages were being compared, the expectation would be that the teeth had been exposed to the oral environment for the same length of time. However, in the later years of World War II, the permanent teeth erupted much later and the primary teeth were retained in the mouth longer than in the prewar period.[100,100a] Therefore, those

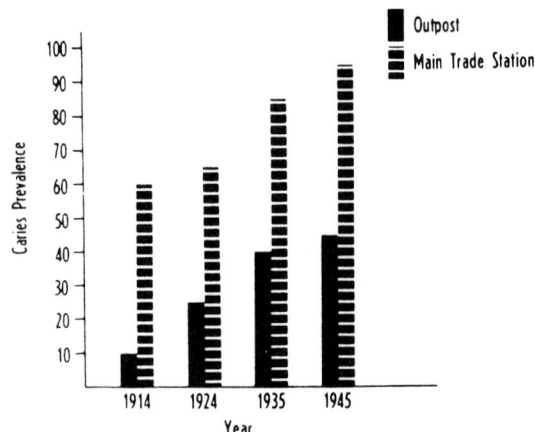

**Fig. 55–8.** Prevalance of tooth decay in primitive and civilized groups of Eskimos in Greenland.

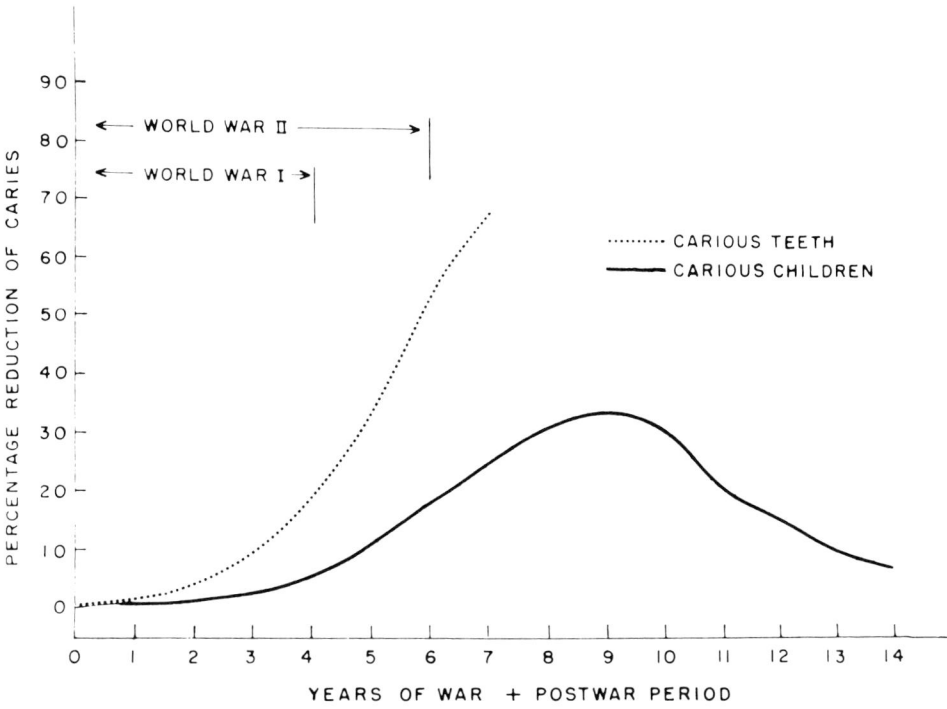

**Fig. 55–9.** The percentage reductions in decayed, missing, and filled teeth and in the number of children with carious lesions are plotted for the periods during World Wars I and II. The data on carious teeth represent averaged observations from Norway, Denmark, Finland, Sweden, and Britain. The curve for reductions in children with caries presents the averaged findings from Norway, Denmark, Britain, France, and Germany. (From Sognnaes.[99])

teeth examined in the later years of the war in any age group had had a shorter exposure to the oral environment than those of children of the same age in prewar and early war years.

In extensive clinical trials in a Swedish mental institution, sucrose was fed in several forms at high levels to residents for relatively prolonged periods of time.[101] When high amounts of sucrose were fed in solution at meals, the increase in dental caries incidence was barely perceptible. However, when sucrose was fed in the form of sticky candy, such as caramels or toffees, between meals, large increases in caries occurred. Comparable amounts of sugar in chocolates between meals or in bread at meals caused intermediate increases in dental caries incidence. As soon as the between-meal supplements were stopped, the frequency of new carious lesions decreased to the preexperimental level. These studies uniformly point toward the rate of oral clearance of carbohydrates and the frequency of their consumption as strong determinants of the extent of tooth decay.

Whereas the Vipeholm Sweden study focused attention on the importance of the timing in the relationship between consumption of sugar and dental caries, a number of studies since then have attempted to study the relationships between the

consumption of high sugar-containing foodstuffs such as candies, cakes, and icing. Samuelson et al. found a high correlation between consumption of sweets, buns, and cakes and the caries index in 4-, 8-, and 12-year-olds.[102–105] These are inclusive ages of high caries activity, and the caries rates reported are probably reflective of current caries activity and are not merely a record of what may have been true 10 or 20 years in the past. Bagramian and Russell examined the between-meal snacking habits of 14- to 17-year olds and did not find an association between caries and snacking frequency.[106]

The previous finding stands in contrast to two reported by Garn[107,108] and another by Weiss and Trithart.[109] Garn et al. examined the sugar-containing food-eating patterns of the children in the upper and lower 15% of dental caries experience in the Ten State Nutritional Survey and found a highly significant association between sugar consumption and incidence of caries.[107] The same result was found when they examined over 700 children who were in the upper and lower 15% of body weight as estimated by skin fold thickness.[108] Weiss and Trithart also reported a direct relationship between the frequency of snacking and caries prevalence.[109]

Another study of dietary variables in institutionalized individuals was reported from Australia in 1953.[110] Hopewood House was the residence of children who lived there continually for slightly longer than the first decade of their life. The diet of the institution was essentially ovo-lacto-vegetarian with carbohydrate provided in the form of whole grains, soy beans, rice, and potatoes without any added sugar. Only minimal amounts of honey or molasses were consumed. Dental caries prevalence throughout this period averaged 1.1 DMF tooth per child, which was approximately only 10% of the prevalence of other schoolchildren in the area.

After the children left the home at age 12 or 13 and began to consume the usual Australian diet, their decay rates increased and assumed the same graphic shape as those in the general population. This fact is the reverse of that demonstrated in the Vipeholm study where decay rates returned to normal after the cessation of the large sucrose supplements. This study also demonstrated that the lowered decay rate observed during the residence period at Hopewood House was not due to significant tooth developmental or nutritional influences but merely to local environmental influences on dental plaque and acid formation.

Additional persuasive data on the importance of fermentable carbohydrate and the frequency of its use in the initiation and progression of carious lesions have been obtained from an "experiment of nature." Hereditary fructose intolerance is a rare genetic abnormality that results in inability to metabolize fructose.[111] After consumption of any food containing fructose, subjects with this disorder can exhibit severe physical symptoms of nausea, vomiting, headache, tremor, and even coma or seizures. The affected individuals rapidly learn, by aversive conditioning, to avoid fructose-containing substances such as sucrose and fruits. Diet analyses of such affected individuals reveal that the carbohydrates consumed are mainly the starches found in cereal products, rice, and potatoes with relatively small amounts of glucose and lactose. Newbrun et al. summarized the dental caries status of the subjects reported by him and others and indicated that 15 of 27 individuals from age 6 to 54 were caries-free and that most of the rest had extremely low caries rates of 1 to 2 DMF teeth, in marked contrast to the population at large.[111]

The data from these surveys and numerous others point to the fact that the increasing use of refined foods resulted in increased dental caries incidences among the populations consuming these diets.

Whether sucrose in man is uniquely cariogenic in any sense other than being the predominant simple sugar in human diets remains to be evaluated in clinical trials. Replacement of sucrose by glucose, fructose, or maltose in the human diet does not seem likely to result in major caries reductions. In two human studies in Finland, the use of the five-carbon polyol, xylitol, was evaluated in the diet[112,112a] or in chewing gum.[113] In the first trial as much of the sucrose in the diet as possible was replaced by either xylitol or fructose. Major reductions in caries occurred in the xylitol group and minor reductions in the fructose group. In the second study, xylitol was used in chewing gum in place of sucrose without any attempt to change the sucrose content of the diet. Again, a major reduction in caries was observed, which is in keeping with Loesche's recent data indicating a reduction in cariogenic streptococci with xylitol gum chewing.[114]

Since approximately three quarters of all sugars entering commerce are introduced into foods during processing, the homemaker is greatly restricted in the ability to control the amount of sugar available for consumption by the family members. It is axiomatic that carious lesions cannot occur without fermentable carbohydrates and the appropriate microbial flora. As the availability and frequency of carbohydrate consumption increase, the potential for the development and progression of caries increases.

In a discussion of ethical considerations of human experimentation on dental caries, Horowitz stated that many previous studies with children have increased our knowledge about the effects on dental caries of ingesting various types of refined carbohydrates.[115] However, now that the relationship of the frequency and amount of candy and other sugar-rich, orally retained items to dental caries incidence has been established with sufficient clarity, regimens with such requirements are now considered to be ethically unacceptable.

**Dietary Calcium and Phosphorus Supplements.** Stralfors reported that the supplementation of cariogenic diets with phosphates caused major reductions in caries in the hamster.[116] Many additional studies on dietary phosphates and experimental dental caries in rodents have been conducted and are reviewed by Nizel and Harris.[117] Salts of trimetaphosphate have been the most effective of the many phosphates tested.[118]

Although the influence of phosphates in reducing dental caries in laboratory animals has been consistent, human trials on dietary supplementation have been inconsistent: one indicated a good reduction[119] whereas two had negative results.[120,121] In the comparison of a population normally consuming tortillas made from lime-soaked corn that contained large amounts of calcium and phosphate with a similar population consuming bread, fewer carious lesions were found in areas of the mouth that are not self-cleansing and in areas where the susceptible enamel pits had become plugged with calcified material.[122]

## LESIONS OF ORAL MUCOUS MEMBRANES AND SUPPORTING STRUCTURES OF TEETH

In the diagnosis and treatment of the various diseases of the oral mucous membranes, and of the supporting tissues of the teeth, all local conditions that might subject the oral tissues to excessive physical or chemical trauma should be evaluated. The presence of any systemic abnormality, whether nutritional, infectious, endocrine, constitutional, or psychologic, which might alter the resistance of the oral tissues, should be ascertained. A thorough visual examination of the oral tissues, eyes, hair, and skin should determine if any classic signs of nutritional deficiency are present. When none of these signs is found to exist as an indication of frank deficiency, evidence of subclinical dietary deficiency should be sought through discussions with the patient about his diet and also by laboratory tests and whatever clinical methods of evaluation are applicable for each individual case. Frequently such subclinical deficiencies may predispose to a sufficiently low tissue tone and resistance to traumatic or infectious processes that ordinarily tolerable oral conditions become overwhelming.

### Periodontitis

The major cause of tooth loss in the adult is periodontitis, a condition in which progressive destruction of the collagenous periodontal ligament that anchors the teeth to bone is accompanied by resorption of the surrounding alveolar bone. The process ultimately results in loosening of the teeth and pockets of bacterial infection between the remaining gingiva and root. The process is chronic, but the initial stages always involve inflammation of the gingiva.

The gingiva, that portion of the oral mucosa that surrounds the necks of the teeth, is fixed to the underlying bone by collagenous and elastic fibers. The gingiva surrounds each tooth to create a moat (gingival sulcus). The oral surface of the gingiva is keratinized and gradually blends into the oral mucosa. On the inside of the moat in contact with the tooth, the gingiva is not keratinized and gradually thins out as it approaches the crown of the tooth to a very thin layer of cells. This thin layer

essentially sits on a basement membrane that is attached very loosely to the tooth itself by hemidesmosomes. Most investigators believe that this area of junctional epithelium may be the susceptible site that allows the penetration of products of microbial metabolism such as enzymes, endotoxins, and other substances into the subjacent connective tissue, causing a chronic inflammatory response, gingivitis.

Gingivitis can routinely be produced in man and experimental animals by the omission of oral hygiene measures for as little as three to four days.[123] In the area of the junctional epithelium, the small blood vessels initially become dilated and large numbers of polymorphonuclear leukocytes migrate into the area and pass into the gingival sulcus. Selective histologic stains show that up to 15% of the collagen that was present is resorbed and the space created is filled with edema. Fluid resembling edema can be found traversing the junctional epithelium and flowing into the gingival sulcus and out into the oral cavity. If the condition is not reversed by reinstitution of adequate oral hygiene, the histologic apearance begins to shift such that after one week the copious cellular infiltrate is predominantly composed of cells for the lymphoid line. Further loss of collagen occurs and the cellular morphology of fibroblasts is altered. The cell types involved at this stage and the pathologic changes observed are consistent with the hypothesis that cellular hypersensitivity is present at the early stage of gingivitis. After about a month of inflammation, plasma cells and antigen-antibody complexes can be demonstrated in the deeper connective tissue. If the condition remains uncorrected, the gingiva may become fibrotic with gross alteration of its architecture.[124]

Gingivitis may be present for months or years without evidence of further involvement or destruction of the periodontal ligament and resorption of the alveolar bone. In many individuals, some of these areas may progress to complete periodontitis with gradual migration of the junctional epithelium and epithelial attachment toward the root tip and with the loss of collagenous attachment and the surrounding alveolar bone. The pathologic picture closely resembles that of chronic inflammatory disease of connective tissue, such as rheumatoid arthritis.

The processes that trigger the transition from gingivitis to periodontitis are not well known but certainly involve local factors, such as the presence of calculus or faulty dental restorations and the composition of the microbial subgingival plaque, and systemic factors, such as endocrine status, psychologic stress, and nutritional problems.

The multifactorial etiology of periodontitis and the likelihood that its progress is intermittent make it very difficult to sort out and study the components of the disease. However, it is clear that if the bacterial plaque, even in moderately advanced cases, can be eliminated by local or chemotherapeutic measures singly or in combination, the progress of bone loss and epithelial migration can be arrested.

The epidemiologic findings of the distribution of periodontitis in industrialized nations and the emerging nations are somewhat equivocal, but clearly indicate the large number of adults affected in the latter countries. It is not easily determined in a disease as chronic and complex as periodontitis whether this high prevalence is due to the usually concomitant poor nutrition of inhabitants of these countries or to the lack of oral hygiene or of dental care, and presence of large amounts of dental plaque and local disease-promoting factors such as dental calculus.

The host factors that operate to reduce or prevent periodontitis, such as immunoresponsiveness and cellular turnover and repair, have both been shown to be influenced by nutritional status. Although the subtleties of interaction among nutrients and these processes may be elusive in a marginally deficient population, some of the more acute forms of periodontal disease, such as acute necrotizing ulcerative gingivitis (ANUG) and noma, can be seen to have clearer associations between malnutrition, stress, and infection.

ANUG is an acute form of gingivitis characterized by erythema and edema of the gingiva followed rapidly by necrosis and sloughing of the interdental gingival papillae. Microscopically, spirochetes invade the deeper tissues, and large collections of fusobacteria occur in the coronalsulcular areas. The disease, often associated with psychologic stress, affects younger individuals (late teen to early adult). It is not known whether emotionally stressful situations create eating patterns leading to acute deficiencies, thus lowering the host's response to the spirochetes and fusobacteria normally found in most mouths.

### Noma

Noma is also a rapid, highly destructive condition manifested by gangrenous lesions of the orofacial structure, including bone and the soft tissues of the oral cavity and cheek. This disease appears to be initiated in the same manner and with the same microorganisms as those involved in ANUG.[125] While occasionally observed in severely debilitated or immunocompromised individuals in the developed countries, it is more commonly seen in children in less developed countries who are malnourished and who have recently experienced a metabolically stressful event such as an exanthematous or viral disease. Like ANUG, the process is highly responsive to penicillin, but the tissue destruction may be extensive if therapy is not instituted rapidly.

Given the presence of similar etiologic conditions of agent and stress, the clinical courses of ANUG and noma seem to be dependent on the nutritional immunocompetency of the host, as has been observed in other conditions and as discussed in the major review of the interrelationships of nutrition and infection by Scrimshaw, Taylor, and Gordon.[126]

In the usual chronic forms of periodontitis, the role of nutritional factors is neither clear nor persuasive. What is known can be considered under local effects of diets and generalized nutritional effects.

### Local Effects

As indicated earlier, the removal of supragingival plaque by mechanical means will prevent or reverse simple gingival inflammation. A common misconception has implied that chewing firm, fibrous foods will remove food debris and plaque from teeth, resulting in enhanced gingival cleanliness and keratinization. The contour of the normal human tooth is such that the cleansing action of such foods does not include the gingival moat, where the process of gingivitis appears to be initiated (sulcular epithelium is not keratinized). Hence, enhancement of keratinization of the gingiva on the outside of the "moat" (attached epithelium) by frictional stimulation could not be expected to reduce whatever inflammatory process is occurring on the inner aspect of the gingival moat.

The supragingival plaque composition in terms of the numbers and distribution of bacterial species can be affected by diet in essentially the same ways as was indicated for dental caries. However, the subgingival plaque, with or without bone loss and pocket formation, appears to be both quantitatively and qualitatively a function of the nutrients available in the gingival exudate fluid and the systemic distribution of such nutrients via vascular means. Whether aqueous extracts of foods can penetrate the sulcular junctional epithelia and elicit immune responses is controversial, but has been reported.

### Systemic Effects

The systemic effects of nutritional deficiency may affect local barrier responses of the gingiva to infection and the penetration of products of infection, such as bacterial enzymes, or the action of cellular lysosomal enzymes elaborated in the process of inflammation. Alfano has discussed the importance of "barrier function" in the prevention of the penetration of noxious substances into and through the gingival epithelial barrier.[127] He emphasized that any nutritional deficiency that can affect cell turnover rates may have an influence on periodontal disease because of the rapid turnover of cells of the sulcular epithelium occurring every four to six days.[127]

In studies on the effects of folate supplementation, Vogel et al. noted decreases in gingival fluid flow (an indication of inflammation) when 2.0 mg of folic acid was given as a daily supplement to a group of subjects with normal serum folate levels.[128] They postulated an end organ defect perhaps related to an increased local requirement due to rapidity of cellular turnover or an increased nutrient need due to such substances as oral contraceptives. They also suggested that an end organ deficiency of any nutrient that can affect cellular division and maturation or tissue repair may manifest itself in the development or progression of the periodontal lesion. Deficiencies of nutrients such as iron, ascorbate, and amino acids may exacerbate the inflammatory process in periodontitis because of the critical nature of the fibroblast and collagen in the maintenance and repair of the periodontal structures. Despite the experimental evidence that such nutritional inadequacies may influence the progression of the disease to some ill-defined degree, Alfano clearly states that... "none of the common-place periodontal diseases results exclusively from primary nutrient deficiencies..."[129]

Indeed, one analysis of ascorbic acid intakes and periodontal disease status of over 8,000 participants in the NHANES I survey between 1971 and 1974 indicated only a weak positive association between periodontal disease and low ascorbic acid intakes. The ingestion of ascorbic acid supplements provided no benefit to periodontal disease status.[130]

## Oral Cancer

Some recent findings indicate in the hamster cheek pouch and tongue cancer models induced by 9, 10 dimethyl -1,2 benzanthracene that certain nutrients may play a role in tumor development. When 10 mg of 13-cis-retinoic acid was provided orally twice weekly, tongue tumor development was significantly delayed.[131] At the end of the experimental period, both the size and invasive extent of the tumors were diminished in the retinoic acid-supplemented groups. Similar results were obtained in a parallel experiment using the cheek pouch model.[132] In similarly designed experiments, vitamin E (DL-L tocopherol) supplementation resulted in fewer and smaller tumors with less invasion of underlying tissues and less surface necrosis than in unsupplemented controls.[133]

## Calcium and Phosphorus

Some data suggest that interferences in calcium and phosphorus metabolism may play a role in the loss of bone associated with periodontal disease. Krook's group suggested that low calcium intakes or low calcium to phosphorus ratios in the diet might lead to nutritional secondary hyperparathyroidism and an increase in mobilization of the bone reserves of calcium.[134-136] It seems improbable that bone resorption due to abnormal Ca/P ratios can fully account for initiation of the type of alveolar resorption found in periodontitis, but the concept is interesting and may in some individuals have a bearing on the rapidity or progression of the disease.

## RELATIONSHIP OF CHEWING ABILITY AND NUTRITIONAL STATUS

Examples of interrelationships between the availability and quality of dentures and malnutrition have been reported. Mann and co-workers studied 160 edentulous patients with a longstanding multiple deficiency disease who had been under their observation for at least 3 years.[137] All had previous histories or present evidence of chronic pellagra, beriberi, scurvy, or riboflavin deficiency as identified by the presence of characteristic mucosal membrane lesions of pellagra; the peripheral neuritis of beriberi; the gingival lesions of scurvy; and the angular cheilosis and ocular lesions of riboflavin deficiency.

The vertical dimension of the face had decreased in 140 of the 160 individuals. Of the 74 patients who had only one denture or none, 57 had monilial cheilitis. Of the 66 patients who were wearing dentures with decreased vertical dimension, 52 gave evidence of monilial cheilitis. In contrast, only 7 of 20 patients with a normal vertical dimension had angular cheilosis. Ninety-eight patients with a reduced vertical dimension complained of symptoms arising from the alimentary tract: "burning of the mouth and tongue, epigastric burning and pain, nausea and vomiting, intermittent diarrhea, cramping and anorexia." Only 8 of 20 patients with normal vertical dimension mentioned these subjective symptoms. In most cases, dentures had been constructed poorly or of inferior materials, which resulted in much irritation that was ultimately augmented by the unsanitary condition of these appliances. Under these circumstances, in many patients, the consumption of adequate amounts of a variety of foodstuffs was either difficult or impossible. When patients with a reduced vertical dimension were given riboflavin, cheilotic lesions decreased, but at no time did these lesions disappear if a reduced vertical dimension was still present. Niacin and pyridoxine did not have any effect on angular cheilosis, although they aided in the reduction of other symptoms characteristic of these particular deficiencies.

These data indicate the necessity to provide adequate dental function by well-fitted dentures that restore and maintain the normal vertical dimension. Even dentures that are perfect when originally fitted must be examined periodically to determine whether the alveolar ridges have been resorbed sufficiently to alter the original normal relationships. If such a reduction in dental function is allowed to persist, monilial cheilitis may result from the decreased vertical dimension of the face, and a complex nutritional deficiency disease may arise from the inability to masticate an adequate amount or an adequate variety of food.

In a continuation of these studies, Greene and co-workers surveyed the prevalence of impaired mastication ability in 446 consecutive patients at the Nutrition Clinic of the Hillman Hospital in Birmingham, Alabama.[138] "Masticatory insufficiency" was the term used to describe a variable clinical condition that resulted for some reason in the inadequate ability to chew food. Thirty of the 446 patients had various degrees of masticatory insufficiency, and only 145 had natural or artificial well-functioning dentitions according to the definitions used by the investigators. The incidence of masticatory insufficiency was observed to increase with age.

A further problem with patients who have been edentulous for prolonged periods is the difficulty in designing and making dentures that are comfortable and efficient for chewing. After prolonged periods of edentulousness, the resorption of the alveolar and basal bones may be so extensive as to make impossible the proper fitting and wearing of dentures. The mucous membranes of the mouth atrophy sufficiently to make wearing dentures difficult.

### Xerostomia (Dry Mouth)

Although xerostomia is rare in young people, older individuals have gradually decreased salivary flows as a function of aging and the replacement of acinar tissue with oncocyte cell types. In the elderly, this gradual decrease in flow usually does not seem to provoke any serious conse-

quences. However, in one form, Sjögren's syndrome, in addition to the usually profound xerostomia, a decrease in lacrimation usually occurs that may lead to keratoconjunctivitis sicca. Frequently associated with this syndrome is evidence of autoimmune disease, usually rheumatoid arthritis. Sjögren's syndrome is generally believed to be an autoimmune disorder.

Xerostomia has also been reported in the following conditions: aplasia of one or more of the salivary glands, systemic diseases with an accompanying high fever or inducing a state of dehydration, menopause, psychic stimulation (fear, anxiety), certain drugs (atropine, antihistamines, rauwolfia alkaloids, sympathomimetic drugs), and postradiation fibrosis of salivary glands.

### Pain

Oral pain may vary from the annoyance of a "burning" sensation in the tongue to the excruciating manifestations of tic douloureux. Burning tongue is one of the most difficult problems with which the dentist and physician must cope. Each case is a diagnostic problem in itself. The condition, usually localized in the lateral margins and the tip of the tongue, is described as a peppery or burning sensation. Burning tongue is commonly an early sign of pernicious anemia, and also occurs early in pellagra, sometimes in diabetes, early pregnancy, and alcoholism. In all these situations a deficiency of one or more members of the vitamin B complex may be involved. If the underlying factor can be diagnosed, the burning tongue is easily corrected. If faulty absorption of nutrients is suspected, the parenteral route is advisable. In all cases, treatment is likely to be prolonged.

Various claims have been made for specific effects of thiamin and pyridoxine. However, no data corroborate these statements with any degree of accuracy, although isolated patients may have responded to therapy in this line. From available data, it cannot be deduced that supplementation with these vitamins is specific for the treatment of such sensations as are described under the terms burning tongue or tic douloureux. In these conditions, it is important to treat local problems that may contribute to the breakdown of the adjacent tissues but, in addition, systemic conditions of a general nature must be considered and evaluated. It is relatively rare that individual nutrients are responsible for any of these manifestations.

### Recommended Dietary Treatment

By far the preferred means of treating dietary abnormalities that may accompany or predispose toward these local lesions of the oral mucous membranes or of the supporting structures of the teeth is the prescription of a well-balanced diet composed of the four basic food groups with a distribution of the foods generously among the several groups. When clear-cut evidence of prolonged deficiency of one or more nutrients exists, they should obviously be supplied in purified form in high enough amounts to replete the body supplies. However, by and large, supplementation is neither necessary nor desirable. Where cases of faulty absorption or accompanying disease requirements are demonstrated, supplementation at appropriate levels is in order. It is noteworthy, too, in connection with postoperative healing, especially when there are extensive needs in the oral cavity, that a diet adequate with respect to all the nutrients should be prescribed.

## SUMMARY

Our knowledge about the relationships of nutrition to the diseases of the oral cavity has been rapidly expanding during the past decades. This is best exemplified by the increased factual information about the relationship of nutrition to the development, the maturation, and the maintenance of the teeth and to their caries susceptibility. Insofar as the influence of nutrition upon the lesions of the oral mucous membranes and of the supporting structures of the teeth is concerned, a much smaller collection of established facts is available than is needed. We can assume by reason of the rapidly expanding horizons in nutritional research that the next decades may provide as many substantial answers to the latter category of oral problems as have been added to our pool of knowledge about tooth decay in the past quarter century. It is noteworthy, although not surprising in view of the chronic nature of most oral problems, that many nutritional problems of the mouth involve metabolic abnormalities that create predispositions to disease entities manifested years or decades later.

The best advice for any age group about the dietary regimen that will provide the best opportunity for normal oral tissues is simple and straightforward. Each of the basic four food groups should be represented liberally in each day's diet, and as many as possible in each of the day's three meals. The best selection of foods for dental health is one where as many foods as possible are purchased in their natural state without excessive refining and where the cooking procedures conserve the maximum of the original nutritive value. The diet should also include a frequent and varied series of foods that require vigorous mastication as a means to stimulate and exercise the various tissues and organs involved in the comminution

of food. In addition, a liberal source of vitamin D should be provided daily throughout the entire period of an individual's growth and development. A minimum of sticky, adherent, high-carbohydrate foods with a low rate of clearance from the oral cavity should be consumed. In addition to the amount of such foods, the frequency of their ingestion each day should be kept to a minimum. After one eats foods with a slow oral clearance, the teeth should be cleaned thoroughly by the procedure recommended by the individual's dentist. As between-meal snacks, fresh fruits, vegetables, fruit juice, milk, and other dairy products are to be preferred to sticky high-carbohydrate foods. In the overall nutritional planning for improved dental health, one of the most important facets to be urged is the fluoridation of public water supplies.

## REFERENCES

1. Glass, R.L.: J. Dent. Res. *61*:1304, 1982.
2. Barmes, D.E.: J. Clin. Periodontol. *4*:80, 1977.
3. Scott, D.B., Ussing, M.J., Sognnaes, R.F., Wyckoff, R.W.G.: J. Dent. Res. *31*:74, 1952.
4. Sognnaes, R.F., Shaw, J.H.: J. Am. Dent. Assoc. *44*:489, 1952.
5. Orland, F.J., Blayney, J.R., Harrison, R.W., et al.: J. Dent. Res. *33*:147, 1954.
6. Orland, F.J., Blayney, J.R., Harrison, R.W., et al.: J. Am. Dent. Assoc. *50*:259, 1955.
7. Keyes, P.H.: Arch. Oral. Biol. *1*:304, 1960.
8. Fitzgerald, R.J., Keyes, P.H.: J. Am. Dent. Assoc. *61*:9, 1960.
9. Fitzgerald, R.J., Jordan, H.V., Stanley, H.R.: J. Dent. Res. *39*:923, 1960.
10. Gibbons, R.J., Berman, K.S., Knoettner, P., et al.: Arch. Oral Biol. *11*:549, 1966.
11. Berkowitz, R.J., Jordan, H.V., White, G.: Arch. Oral Biol. *20*:171, 1975.
12. Gibbons, R.J., dePaola, P.F., Spinell, D.M., et al.: Infect. Immun. *9*:481, 1974.
13. Berkowitz, R.J., Jordan, H.V.: Arch. Oral Biol. *20*:725, 1975.
14. Köhler, B., Brathall, D., Krasse, B.: Arch. Oral Biol. *28*:225, 1983.
15. Köhler, B., Andreen, I., Jonsson, B.: Arch. Oral Biol. *29*:879, 1984.
16. Wolbach, S.B., Howe, P.R.: J. Exp. Med. *42*:753, 1925.
17. Wolbach, S.B., Howe, P.R : Am. J. Pathol. *9*:275, 1933.
18. Dinnerman, M.: Oral Surg. *4*:1024, 1951.
18a. Harris, S.S., Navia, J.M.: Arch. Oral Biol. *25*:415, 1980.
18b. Navia, J.M., Snider, C., Punyasingh, J., et al.: Arch. Oral Biol. *29*:911, 1984.
19. Sweeney, E.A., Cabrerra, J., Urrutia, J, et al.: J. Dent. Res. *48*:1275, 1969.
20. Sweeney, E.A., Saffir, A.J., deLeon, R.: Am. J. Clin. Nutr. *24*:29, 1971.
21. Dalldorf, G.: *In* The Vitamins. Chicago, American Medical Association, 1939. p. 339.
22. Wolbach, S.B., Howe, P.R.: Proc. Soc. Exp. Biol. Med. *22*:400, 1925.
23. Crampton, E.W.: J. Nutr. *33*:491, 1947.
24. Westin, G.: Dent. Cosmos *67*:868, 1925.

25. Mellanby, M.: Lancet *2*:767, 1918.
26. Mellanby, M.: Br. Dent. J. *44*:1031, 1923.
27. Weinman, J.P., Schour, I.: Am. J. Pathol. *21*:821, 1945.
28. Sarnat, B.G., Schour, I.: J. Am. Dent. Assoc. *28*:1989, 1941; *29*:67, 1942.
29. Nikiforuk, G., Fraser, D.: J. Pediatr. *98*:888, 1981.
30. Mellanby, M.: Special Report Series, Medical Research Council, Report No. 191. London, His Majesty's Stationery Office, 1934.
31. Committee for the Investigation of Dental Disease: Special Report Series, Medical Report Series, Medical Research Council, Report No. 211. London, His Majesty's Stationery Office, 1936.
32. Agnew, M.C., Agnew, R.G., Tisdall, F.F.: J. Am. Dent. Assoc. *20*:193, 1933.
32a. Agnew, M.C., Agnew, R.G., Tisdall, F.F.: J. Pediatr. *2*:190, 1933.
33. McBeath, E.C.: Am. J. Public Health *24*:1028, 1933.
34. McBeath, E.C. Verlin, W.A.: J. Am. Dent. Assoc. *29*:1393, 1942.
35. Anderson, P.G., Williams, C.H.M., Halderson, H., et al.: J. Am. Dent. Assoc. *21*:1349, 1934.
36. Day, C.D.M., Sedwick, H.J.: J. Dent. Res. *14*:213, 1934.
36a. Day, C.D.M., Sedwick, H.J.: J. Nutr. *8*:309, 1934.
37. Mills, C.A.: J. Dent. Res. *16*:417, 1937.
38. East, B.R.: Am. J. Public Health *29*:777, 1939.
39. Sobel, A.E., Hanok, A.: J. Biol. Chem. *176*:1103, 1948.
40. Sobel, A.E., Hanok, A.: J. Dent. Res. *37*:631, 1958.
41. Sobel, A.E., Hanok, A., Shaw, J.H.: Abstracts, 124th Meeting American Chemical Society, Abstract No. 173, 1953, p. 72.
42. Armstrong, W.D., Knowlton, M.: J. Dent. Res. *21*:326, 1942.
43. Singer, L., Ophaug, R.J.: Fluoride intake in humans. *In* Fluoride Effects on Vegetation, Animals, and Humans. (Shuper, J.L., Peterson, J.B., and Leone, N.C., Eds.) Salt Lake City, Paragon Press, 1983.
44. McClure, F.J.: Public Health Rep. *64*:1061, 1949.
45. Schwarz, K.: Fed. Proc. *33*:1748, 1974.
46. Bunting, R.W., Crowley, M., Hard, D.G., et al.: Dent. Cosmos *70*:1002, 1928.
47. Dean, H.T., Jay, P., Arnold, F.A., Jr., et al.: Public Health Rep. *54*:862, 1939.
48. Dean, H.T., Arnold, F.A., Jr., Elvove, E., Public Health Rep. *57*:1155, 1942.
49. Dean, H.T.: Public Health Rep. *53*:1443, 1938.
50. Russell, A.L., Elvove, E.: Public Health Rep. *66*:1389, 1951.
51. McClure, F.J., Likins, R.C.: J. Dent. Res. *30*:172, 1951.
52. Zipkin, I., Pozner, A.S., Eanes, R.D.: Biochim. Biophys. Acta *59*:255, 1962.
53. Zipkin, I., McClure, F.J., Lee, W.A.: Arch. Oral Biol. *2*:190, 1960.
54. Zipkin, I., Posner, A.S.: International Association for Dental Research, 40th General Meeting. Preprinted Abstracts, 28, 103, 1962.
55. Jenkins, G.N., Speirs, R.L.: J. Physiol. *121*:21, 1953.
56. Brudevold, F., Gardner, O.E., Smith, F.A.: J. Dent. Res. *35*:420, 1956.
57. Isaac, S., Brudevold, F., Smith, F.A., et al.: J. Dent. Res. *37*:318, 1958.
58. Cooper, V.K., Ludwig, T.G.: N. Z. Dent. J. *61*:33, 1965.
59. Simpson, W.J., Castaldi, C.R.: Odontol. Rev. *20*:1, 1969.
60. Sognnaes, R.F., Arnold, F.A., Jr., Hodge, H.C., et al.: Washington, National Research Council, Publications No. 294, 1953.
61. Ast, D.B., Smith, D.J., Wachs, B., et al.: J. Am. Dent. Assoc. *52*:314, 1956.
62. Horowitz, H.S.: Pediatr. Dent. *4*:286, 1982.
63. Newbrun, E.: Cost-effectiveness and practicality features in the systemic use of fluorides. *In* The Relative Efficiency of Methods of Caries Prevention in Dental Public Health. (Burt, B.A. Ed.) U. Michigan, Ann Arbor. 1978.
64. Moulton, F.R. (Ed.): Fluorine and Dental Health. Washington, American Association for the Advancement of Science, 1942.
65. Galagan, D.J., Vermillion, J.R.: Public Health Rep. *72*:491, 1957.
66. Shaw, J.H. (Ed.): Fluoridation as a Public Health Measure. Washington, American Association for the Advancement of Science, 1954.
67. Hoover, R.N., McKay, F.W., Fraumeni, J.F., Jr.: J. Natl. Cancer Inst. *57*:757, 1976.
68. Oldham, P.D., Newell, D.J.: Appl. Stat. *26*:125, 1977.
69. Leone, N.C.: Arch. Ind. Health *21*:324, 326, 1960.
70. Bernstein, D.S., Sadowsky, N., Hegsted, D.M., et al.: J.A.M.A. *198*:499, 1966.
70a. Simonen, O., Laitinen, O.: Lancet *2*:432, 1985.
71. Rich, C., Ensinck, J.: Nature *191*:184, 1961.
72. Rich, C., Ensinck, J.: Clin. Res. *10*:118, 1962.
73. Jowsey, J., Riggs, B.L., Kelly, P.J., et al.: Am. J. Med. *53*:43, 1972.
74. Hansson, T., Roos, B.: Am. J. Roentgenology *126*:1294, 1976.
75. Kyle, R.A., Jowsey, J., Kelly, P.J., et al.: N. Engl. J. Med. *293*:1334, 1975.
76. Hill, I.N., Jelinek, O.E., Blayney, J.R.: J. Dent. Res. *28*:398, 1949.
77. Preventing Tooth Decay: Results from a four-year national study. Special Report #2, Robert Wood Johnson Foundation, 1983.
78. Dreizen, S., Brown, L.R., Daly, T.E., et al.: J. Dent. Res. *56*:99, 1977.
79. Schwartz, A., Weisberger, D.: Salivary factors in experimental animal caries. *In* Advances in Caries Research. (Sognnaes, R.F., Ed.) Washington, American Association for the Advancement of Science, 1955.
80. Larson, R.H.: Genetic and environmental factors in experimental dental caries. *In* Environmental Variables in Oral Disease. Washington, American Association for the Advancement of Science, Publication No. 181, 1966.
81. Larson, R.H., Simms, M.E.: Science *149*:982, 1965.
82. Kent, R.L., Jr., Moorrees, C.F.A.: Proceedings International Association for Dental Research, Abstract #526, 1979.
83. Hodge, H.C.: J. Dent. Res. *22*:275, 1943.
84. Braunschneider, G.E., Hunt, H.R., Hoppert, C.H.: J. Dent. Res. *27*:154, 1948.
85. Constant, M.A., Sievert, H.W., Phillips, P.H., et al.: J. Nutr. *53*:29, 1954.
86. Sognnaes, R.F., Shaw, J.H., Bogoroch, R.: Am. J. Physiol. *180*:408, 1955.
87. Kite, O.W., Shaw, J.H., Sognnaes, R.F.: J. Nutr. *42*:89, 1950.
88. Francis, M.D., Briner, W.W.: Arch. Oral Biol. *11*:349, 1966.

89. Briner, W.W., Rosen, S.: Arch. Oral Biol. *12*:1077, 1967.
90. Shaw, J.H.: J. Nutr. *53*:151, 1954.
91. Schweigert, B.S., Shaw, J.H., Phillips, P.H., et al.: J. Nutr. *29*:405, 1945.
92. Michalek, S.M., McKee, J.R., Shiota, T., et al.: Infect. Immun. *16*:712, 1977.
93. Krasse, B.: Arch. Oral Biol. *10*:215, 1965.
94. Wood, J.M., Crichley, P.: Arch. Oral Biol. *11*:1039, 1966.
95. Gibbons, R.J., Banghart, S.B.: Arch. Oral Biol. *12*:11, 1967.
96. Shaw, J.H., Krumins, I., Gibbons, R.J.: Arch. Oral Biol. *12*:755, 1967.
97. Konig, K.G., Schmid, P., Schmid, R.: Arch. Oral Biol. *13*:13, 1968.
97a. Ismail, A.I., Burt, B.A., Eklund, S.A.: J. Am. Dent. Assoc. *109*:241, 1984.
98. Baarregaard, A.: Oral Surg. *2*:995, 1949.
99. Sognnaes, R.F.: Am. J. Dis. Child. *75*:792, 1948.
100. Toverud, G.: Milbank Mem. Fund Q. *34*:354, 1956.
100a. Toverud, G.: Milbank Mem. Fund Q. *35*:127, 373, 1957.
101. Gustafsson, B.E., Quensel, C.E., Lanke, L.S., et al.: Acta Odontol. Scand. *11*:232, 1954.
102. Samuelson, G.: Acta Paediatr. Scand. (Suppl.) *2*:14, 1971.
103. Samuelson, G.: Nutr. Metab. *12*:321, 1970.
104. Samuelson, G.: Acta Paediatr. *60*:653, 1971.
105. Samuelson, G., Grahnen, H., Lindstrom, G.: Odontol. Rev. *22*:189, 1971.
106. Bagramian, R.A., Russell, A.L.: J. Dent. Res. *52*:42, 1973.
107. Garn S.M., Cole, P.E., Schaefer, A.E.: Ecol. Food Nutr. *9*:135, 1980.
108. Garn, S.M., Solomon, M.A.: Am. J. Clin. Nutr. *33*:1890, 1980.
109. Weiss, R.L., Trithart, A.H.: Am. J. Pub. Health *50*:1097, 1960.
110. Lilienthal, B., Goldsworthy, N.E., Sullivan, H.R., et al.: Med. J. Aust. *21*:878, 1953.
111. Newbrun, E., Hoover, C., Mettraux, G., et al.: J. Am. Dent. Assoc. *101*:619, 1980.
112. Scheinin, A., Mäkinen, K.K., Ylitalo, K.: Acta Odontol. Scand. *32*:381, 1974.
112a. Scheinin, A., Mäkinen, K.K., Ylitalo, K.: Acta Odontol. Scand. (Suppl.) *33*:67, 1975.
113. Scheinin, A., Mäkinen, K.K., Tammisalo, E., et al.: Acta Odontol. Scand. *33*:269, 1975.
114. Loesche, W.W., Grossman, N.S., Earnest, R., et al.: J. Am. Dent. Assoc. *108*:587, 1984.
115. Horowitz, H.S.: J. Dent. Res. *56*:154, 1977.
116. Strålfors, A.: Tandlak, Tidskr. *49*:108, 1956.
117. Nizel, A.E., Harris, R.S.: J. Dent. Res. *43*:1123, 1964.
118. Shaw, J.H.: J. Dent. Res. *59*: 644, 1980.
119. Strålfors, A.: J. Dent. Res. *43*:1137, 1964.
120. Ship, I.I., Mickelsen, O.: J. Dent. Res. *43*:1144, 1964.
121. Averill, H.M., Bibby, B.G.: J. Dent. Res. *43*:1150, 1964.
122. Sutfin, L.V., Sweeney, E.A., Ascoli, W.: J. Dent. Res. *49*:772, 1970.
123. Löe, H., Theilade, E., Jensen, S.B.: J. Periodontol. *36*:177, 1965.
124. Payne, W.A., Page, R.C., Oglivie, A.L., et al.: J. Periodont. Res. *10*:51, 1975.
125. Tempest, M.N.: Br. J. Surg. *53*:949, 1966.
126. Scrimshaw, N.S., Taylor, C.E., Gordon, J.E.: Effect of malnutrition on resistance to infection. *In* Interactions of Nutrition and Infection. Geneva, World Health Organization, 1968.
127. Alfano, M.C.: J. Prev. Dent. *5*:26, 1978.
128. Vogel, R.I., Fink, R.A., Schneider, L.C., et al.: J. Periodontol. *47*:667, 1976.
129. Alfano, M.C.: Nutrition in periodontal diseases. *In* New Horizons in Nutrition for the Health Professions. (Slavkin, J.C., Ed.) Los Angeles, U.S.C. Press, 1981.
130. Ismail, A.I., Burt, B.A., Eklund, S.A.: J. Am. Dent. Assoc. *107*:927, 1983.
131. Shklar, G., Marefat, P., Kornhauser, A., et al.: Oral Surg. *49*:325, 1980.
132. Shklar, G., Schwartz, J., Graw, D., et al.: Oral Surg. *50*:45, 1980.
133. Shklar, G.: J. Natl. Cancer Inst. *68*:791, 1982.
134. Krook, L., Lutwak, L., Whalen, L.P., et al.: Cornell Vet *6*:32, 1972.
135. Krook, K., Whalen, L.P., Lesser, G.V., et al.: Cornell Vet. *62*:371, 1972.
136. Lesser, G.V., Krook, L.: Ann. Dent. *33*:7, 1974.
137. Mann, A.W., Mann, J.M., Spies, T.D.: J. Am. Dent. Assoc. *32*:1357, 1945.
138. Greene, H.I., Dreizen, S., Spies, T.D.: J. Am. Dent. Assoc. *39*:561, 1949.

Chapter **56**

# NUTRITION AND DIET IN MANAGEMENT OF DISEASES OF THE GASTROINTESTINAL TRACT

*(A) ESOPHAGUS, STOMACH, AND DUODENUM*
  *(1) Nutrition and Esophageal Disease*

## Mukesh B. Desai and Khursheed N. Jeejeebhoy

The eosophagus transmits swallowed food to the stomach and prevents the reflux of gastric contents. Thus, diseases of the esophagus may result in malnutrition because of a profound effect on one's ability to ingest a normal oral diet. On the other hand, the diet can influence esophageal function. For example, the composition of food and the use of cigarettes[1] and alcohol[2] all affect the tone of the lower esophageal sphincter (LES), which is important in preventing reflux.

## EFFECT OF ESOPHAGEAL DISEASE ON NUTRITIONAL STATE

Organic obstruction of the esophagus is commonly associated with a history of weight loss, which is usually proportional to the degree of reduced food intake. However, despite esophageal obstruction in some instances, weight loss may not occur because the patient has learned to augment his caloric intake with liquid supplements such as milk or ice cream. In patients with carcinoma of the esophagus, weight loss is profound as a result of wasting of adipose tissue and muscles. In one study, 93% of patients had dysphagia for 4.1 months and 46% had weight loss.[3] In another study, 20 patients with upper esophageal carcinoma who weighed on average only 46.8 kg had lost a mean of 11 kg. Nutritional support, without reducing the tumor load, resulted in weight gain. The mean weight increased to 50.7

kg, and was associated with a positive nitrogen balance.[4]

Other conditions associated with marked weight loss due to esophageal obstruction are peptic stricture of the esophagus, stricture resulting from caustic chemical burns of the esophagus, reflux esophagitis, rings and webs, achalasia, and candidal esophagitis. In addition to starvation, conditions causing patients with esophageal obstruction to lose weight include sepsis resulting from an aspiration pneumonia or from the spread of carcinoma of the esophagus.

Iron deficiency anemia is seen in esophageal disease (e.g., reflux esophagitis, achalasia, and chemical injury). The Plummer-Vinson (Paterson-Kelly) syndrome is associated with iron deficiency, but also consists of dysphagia and a web in the upper 2 to 4 cm of the esophagus. The pathogenesis is unexplained.[5]

## TREATMENT OF THE OBSTRUCTED PATIENT

The ideal treatment is to relieve the obstruction. However, if this option is not possible, then the following routine should be adopted. With a minor degree of obstruction, the patient should eat small pieces of food, chewed well. When obstruction is more serious, defined-formula diets, fortified milk shakes, and pureed foods can be used to provide the patient with nutrients.

When obstruction is almost complete, there are

two possibilities. Either the patient is given a percutaneous feeding gastrostomy or jejunostomy or, alternatively, home parenteral nutrition may be used. Because these patients have an intact intestinal tract, the indications for home parenteral nutrition are rare, and the former approach is preferred.

Patients with severe esophageal obstruction are often wasted, and the question arises whether a short period of preoperative nutritional support might be beneficial in improving postoperative outcome. Haffejee et al. have shown an improvement in immune function by giving preoperative total parenteral nutrition (TPN) to these patients.[4] Muller[6] showed that a short period of preoperative TPN in patients with cancer of the gastrointestinal tract significantly reduced postoperative morbidity and mortality.[6] Although similar data exclusively for esophageal carcinoma are not available, it appears that severely malnourished patients may benefit from a short course of TPN.[7,8]

## NUTRITION AND ESOPHAGEAL REFLUX

Esophageal reflux occurs with moderate frequency in otherwise healthy persons. However, when it is frequent and prolonged, it becomes symptomatic. In addition, the nature of the refluxed fluid determines the degree of epithelial injury. A combination of acid and bile is more injurious than one or the other alone.[9] The injured epithelium becomes sensitive to the pH and osmolarity of the food and fluid ingested, and the patient finds that swallowing a variety of foods may cause pain, thus limiting intake. In particular, patients experience discomfort from drinking citrus fruit juices, tomato juice, and alcohol. The avoidance of citrus fruits and vegetables may result in vitamin C deficiency.[10]

The cause of reflux is multifactorial. However, reduced tone of the lower esophageal sphincter (LES) is a major cause of the reflux of gastric contents into the esophagus, although it may occur even with normal LES pressures. In such patients, inability to clear the lower esophagus of acid, reduced gastric emptying, and pyloric obstruction may contribute to reflux.

Although a variety of pharmacologic and neurohormonal factors affect LES, certain dietary factors do play a role in enhancing reflux and/or symptoms in patients with reflux.

**Factors Affecting LES Pressure.** Fat has been shown to reduce LES pressures[11] and accounts for the frequently experienced phenomenon of reflux after large fatty meals. Smoking, a potent inhibitor of LES pressure, enhances reflux.[1] Chocolate,[12] coffee,[13] and mint may reduce LES pressure. Coffee seems to have this effect independent of caffeine.[13]

**Factors Affecting Gastric Emptying.** Because gastric retention aids reflux, dietary fat (especially together with protein), the ingestion of hypertonic solutions, and fiber may be associated with reduced gastric emptying, and thus enhance reflux.

**Factors Irritating Sensitized Esophageal Mucosa.** The ingestion of orange and lemon juices, tomato juice, and alcohol may cause discomfort in patients with reflux and a sensitized epithelium. The discomfort is not simply due to the presence of organic acid, as it occurs even when these drinks are neutralized with alkali.

**Body Weight.** Obesity enhances reflux, and weight reduction is an important measure for the control of reflux.

## DIETETIC TREATMENT OF ESOPHAGEAL REFLUX

Treatment of patients with esophageal diseases is based on the principles of enhancing LES pressure, promoting gastric emptying, and avoiding foods likely to irritate the sensitized esophagus. Low fat intake is advised to avoid reducing LES pressure and to promote gastric emptying. Smoking, coffee, chocolate, mint, alcohol, and citrus and tomato juices should be avoided. Patients with gastric obstruction and those recovering from gastric surgery are likely to form bezoars. In such patients, fiber intake should be reduced.

Finally, in patients who are obese or above their ideal body weight, reduction of weight is important in improving symptoms of reflux.

## REFERENCES

1. Dennish, G.W., Castell, D.O.: N. Engl. J. Med. *284*:1136–1137, 1971.
2. Hogan, W.J., Viegas de Andrade, S.R., Winship, D.H.: J. Appl. Physiol. *32*:755–760, 1972.
3. Ojala, K., Sorri, M, Jokisien, K., et al.: Postgrad. Med. J. *58*:264–267, 1982.
4. Haffejee, A.A., Angorn, I.B.: Ann. Surg. *189*:475–479, 1979.
5. Chisholm, M.: Postgrad. Med. J. *50*:218, 1974.
6. Muller, J.M., Brenner, U., Dienst, C., et al.: Lancet *1*:68–71, 1982.
7. Lim, S.T.K., Choa, R.G., Lam, K.H., et al.: Br. J. Surg. *68*:69–72, 1981.
8. Heatley, R.V., Williams, R.H.P., Lewis, M.H.: Postgrad. Med. J. *55*:541–545, 1979.
9. Henderson, R.D., Mugashe, F., Jeejeebhoy, K.N., et al.: Can. J. Surg. *17*:112–116, 1974.
10. Hiebert, C.A.: Ann. Thorac. Surg. *24*:108–112, 1977.
11. Nebel, O.T., Castell, D.O.: Gut *14*:270–274, 1973.
12. Joel, E., Richter, M.D., Castell, D.O.: Med. Clin. North Am. *65*:1223–1234, 1981.
13. Cohen, S., Booth, G.H.: N. Engl. J. Med. *293*:897–899, 1975.

*Chapter* # 56

# NUTRITION AND DIET IN MANAGEMENT OF DISEASES OF THE GASTROINTESTINAL TRACT

## (A) ESOPHAGUS, STOMACH, AND DUODENUM
### (2) Nutritional Effects of Disease of the Stomach and Duodenum

Stephen L. Wolman

Diseases of the stomach affect nutritional status in a number of ways, one or more of which may be operative in any particular disease state. The stomach serves as a reservoir for food. Its inability to perform this function causes symptoms that decrease food consumption and result in weight loss. This condition is often seen as early satiety, nausea, and vomiting. It may occur as a result of delayed gastric emptying with no apparent gastric lesion as in viral gastroenteritis,[1] anorexia nervosa,[2] or diabetes mellitus.[3] These symptoms can be seen in postgastric surgery patients who have small gastric remnants or vagotomies and subsequently decrease their oral intake. Mechanical obstruction may result from inflammation, ulceration, or tumor and may cause the same symptoms or symptom complex. Patients with peptic disease with obstruction have a higher incidence of weight loss, although fully one third of obstructed patients have no weight loss.[4] Pain, which is often associated with inflammation and ulceration, may increase with food intake and will contribute to decreased consumption and weight loss. When these diagnoses, as well as diabetes, scleroderma, chronic renal failure, and Chagas' disease, have been excluded, the delayed gastric emptying may be idiopathic or a result of antral tachygastria.[5,6]

If the reservoir function of the stomach is compromised, rapid gastric emptying may occur. This condition most often occurs in 15 to 49% of patients after gastric surgery.[7,8] The symptoms of dumping syndrome, including anxiety, weakness, tachycardia, sweating, cramps, and diarrhea soon after meals, result in the avoidance of food or alteration in eating habits and subsequently weight loss.

The gastric function of grinding and pumping results in the entrance of food particles of approximately 1.0 mm diameter into the duodenum.[9] Liquids empty more rapidly than solids. Gastric emptying slows with increased osmolality, fat content, and acidity.[10] This process results in the delivery of food matter to the small bowel in a more efficient manner so that normal fat, carbohydrate, and protein absorption occurs. Surgery of the stomach can disturb this process by (1) allowing larger particles to empty; (2) causing inadequate mixing with pancreatic juice and bile; and (3) presenting large high-osmotic loads.

These alterations and their significance will be discussed in the section on specific diseases.

The acid production of the stomach does not appear to perform a major nutritional role. Patients with spontaneous achlorhydria or long-term acid reduction therapy only rarely show any nutritional abnormalities. The decrease in gastric acid after gastric surgery for ulcer disease may facilitate bacterial overgrowth in a patient who has predisposing stasis in the distal gut. Inadequate solubilization may also contribute to the malabsorption of calcium and iron.[11,12]

The intrinsic factor production of the stomach can be decreased as a result of autoimmume pernicious anemia and less often as a result of antral gastritis and antral resection. This change results in a megaloblastic anemia when $B_{12}$ stores are depleted.

## SPECIFIC DISEASE STATES

For the most part, specific diseases have not been studied with the criteria of malnutrition used in more recent clinical nutrition. These parameters are many and include weight loss, triceps skinfold thickness, midarm muscle circumference, creatinine height index, serum albumin level, serum transferrin, total lymphocyte count, serum complement level, serum immunoelectrophoresis, lymphocyte rosettes, neutrophil migration, delayed cutaneous hypersensitivity (DCH), hemoglobin, vitamin C, $B_2$, or $B_6$ levels, total body potassium, hand grip dynamometry,[13,14] total body nitrogen,[15] muscle strength, force-frequency ratio, relaxation rate, and fatigability.[16] The following will highlight specific entities where the published data are truly informative in the comparison of malnutrition in these situations.

## GASTRIC SURGERY

Peptic ulcer disease and gastric cancer are often treated by surgical means. Treatment may consist of proximal vagotomy, vagotomy and pyloroplasty, vagotomy and antrectomy, the subtotal gastrectomies Billroth I and II, and total gastrectomy. All of these procedures result in some degree of malnutrition that tends to vary with the extent of the operative procedure. As mentioned previously, these treatments produce weight loss as a result of decreased caloric intake and malabsorption, and iron, folate, $B_{12}$, calcium, and vitamin D deficiencies.

Reports show that three years after vagotomy and drainage procedures, weight loss occurs in 5 to 39% of patients. After vagotomy with antrectomy, weight loss occurs in 10 to 42%, and after Billroth II anastomosis, the results increase to 25 to 44%.[17] Billroth II anastomosis apparently has more severe effects and produces greater weight loss than Billroth I.[18,19] Others report that approximately 60% of subtotal gastrectomy patients fail to regain their optimum weight.[20] Total gastrectomy seems to cause the most severe loss with 90% losing weight,[21] the average amount being 24% of preoperative weight.[22] The quantity of weight loss with total gastrectomy does not appear to be influenced by the type of reconstruction. A Roux-en-Y and a Longmire-Mouchet are equivalent after approximately 2 years, although the loss is more rapid with the Roux-en-Y.[22a]

The most important cause of this weight loss is decreased consumption. After total gastrectomy, dietary history has revealed daily intake to be 1,800 kcal, whereas the recommended intake for these male patients was estimated to be 2,400 to 2,800 kcal per day.[23] It has been observed that patients in hospital may voluntarily ingest an adequate diet as compared with the recommended dietary allowances (RDA); in the home environment, however, these patients may change to a diet that is well below the RDA.[24] Subsequent balance studies on an enforced 80-g protein/100-g diet revealed that 8 of 10 patients could consume enough to achieve a positive nitrogen balance. This finding demonstrates that these patients usually have the necessary absorptive capacity. Other studies have confirmed this observation. It is interesting that diarrhea and weight loss are more prevalent in less affluent patients, such as those at a Veterans Administration hospital in the United States, than in private patients.[25]

Absorption studies found that in vagotomy or any anastomotic procedure of the upper gastrointestinal tract steatorrhea was limited to 10 to 12% (i.e., 10 to 12 g daily).[26] Even in total gastrectomy, fat malabsorption was present in 69% of patients and averaged 16.5%, ranging from 10 to 25%. Nitrogen wasting was observed in 42%, averaging 2.3 g/day. Breath hydrogen studies reveal excessive malabsorption of carbohydrates as well as fat and protein. This malabsorption has not been quantitated. However, patients with ongoing weight loss show increased transit rate compared to those without a continuing problem.[26a] Gut hormone release from the distal small bowel is also increased, but this may reflect the rapid transit. The total calculated caloric loss was less than 60 kcal/day.[27] This caloric deficit is so minimal that, in the absence of factors that inhibit intake, it would not be expected to cause weight loss.

The malabsorption results from the factors previously mentioned. The accelerated gastric emptying impairs gastric dispersion of food,[8,28] creates inadequate mixing, and continues as rapid small intestinal transit.[29] In addition, truncal vagotomy results in a 50% decrease in pancreatic response.[27,28,30]

Malabsorption may be considerably more severe in a lesser number of patients owing to secondary complications of surgery. Blind loop syndrome may occur whenever gastric acidity is decreased. Stasis of intestinal contents most often occurs in Billroth I anastomosis where a blind loop is formed. Subsequently, deconjugation of bile salts leads to steatorrhea; binding of vitamin $B_{12}$ leads to megaloblastic anemia, and deamination of amino acids and toxic bacterial metabolites contribute to hypoaluminemia.[31] The rapid delivery of nutrients to the small bowel may uncover previously subclinical gluten-sensitive enteropathy with its mucosal damage and panmalabsorption. Uncontrolled delivery of lactose may cause excessive fluid secretion in the upper small bowel that may result in increased malabsorption owing to intestinal hurry and excessive fluid. The exaggerated fluid shifts, flatulence, and diarrhea may also inhibit oral intake. Pancreatic insufficiency causing protein malnutrition after partial gastrectomy has been reported,[32] but is apparently rare. Other more obvious complications that may inhibit oral intake are recurrent ulcer, recurrent tumor, bezoar, stricture, and stasis.

Anemia is commonly seen after gastric surgery. It may be due to iron, folate, or $B_{12}$ deficiency or may be mixed in pathogenesis.

The cause of iron deficiency anemia is not clear-cut. Although total food intake is reduced, patients appear to ingest sufficient quantities of iron.[33] These patients also absorb pure iron salts normally,[34,35] whereas they do not absorb iron salts incorporated into food.[35-37] Hemoglobin iron is absorbed normally.[38] These studies as a whole do not support a single malabsorptive etiology. Certainly most anemia in these patients is due to bleeding.[39,40] Contributory factors include rapid transit across the major iron absorptive area in the duodenum, larger particle size, and decreased solubilization by acid. Considering these factors, it is reasonable that Billroth II partial gastrectomy would be the most common cause of anemia because the anatomy allows for bile reflux gastritis as well as a bypassed segment of duodenum. Fully 50% of patients with subtotal gastrectomies suffer from anemia.[41] Vagotomy and pyloroplasty do not cause anemia as frequently.[42,43]

Vitamin $B_{12}$ deficiency is less common and results from either decreased intrinsic factor production or bacterial overgrowth. Intrinsic factor is produced in large excess, and thus the development of deficiency occurs with larger resections. Bacteria bind $B_{12}$ thereby inhibiting absorption by the body.

Folate deficiency occurs at least partially by decreased intake, but also perhaps by inadequate hydrolysis in the upper small intestine. Bone disease of a major degree was found to be extremely common after partial gastrectomy.[43a] Many patients having undergone Billroth II procedures have severe bone pain.[43b] One study reported the incidence of fractures in men 20 years after a gastrectomy to be almost double that found in controls.[43c] The abnormalities found in men may resemble osteoporosis or osteomalacia or may have features of both. Certainly malabsorption of calcium and vitamin D plays a role in the pathogenesis, most likely because of steatorrhea in which vitamin D is malabsorbed and calcium is bound intraluminally. Bone mineral content of patients with Billroth I gastrectomy is approximately 89% of normal and correlates with 1,25 dihydroxy vitamin D levels, which are relatively high while PTH levels are normal. This may represent a compensatory mechanism.[43d]

Gastric stapling procedures are done with the intention of producing weight loss. Other nutrient deficiencies may be produced as a side effect. Neuromuscular weakness of unknown origin has been reported in two cases.[43e,43f]

## GASTRIC ULCER

Malnutrition has been reported as a consequence of gastric ulcer, but reports primarily document weight loss. Peptic ulcer that includes duodenal ulcerations has been evaluated more critically, primarily in comparison with gastric cancer. Specific information can be found in Table 56A2–1.

## GASTRIC CANCER

Quantitative measurements of nutritional status have been made in patients with gastric cancer. To give the reader some perspective, comparison with a group with peptic ulcer is made. Dionigi et al. evaluated the major criteria used in clinical nutritional assessment.[44] (See Table 56A2–1). They observed that hemoglobin, total proteins, albumin, iron percentage, usual body weight, and delayed cutaneous hypersensitivity (DCH) were significantly more abnormal in patients with gastric cancer. The study was carried out in Italy, and the author noted that it was unlikely that the normal North American anthropometric standards would apply. Delayed cutaneous hypersensitivity was more often abnormal in cancer patients with subsequent sepsis. In addition, depressed DCH was consonant with greater spread of tumor. The abnormalities found in this study may represent specific tumor effects or a greater severity of disease and decrease in nutrient intake.

Symreng et al. found that 60% of their gastric cancer patients were malnourished by limiting criteria[45] (Table 56A2–2). These patients were subsequently grouped into normal, near normal, and malnourished. Within the population with gastric carcinoma, only 15% had an abnormal weight index, and 19% had severe weight loss; 72% had subnormal albumin and 82% had decreased prealbumin. These findings may reflect

**Table 56A2–1.　Percentage of Abnormal NA Parameters in Patients with Gastric Cancer and Peptic Ulcer**

| Parameters | Abnormality | Peptic Ulcer (n = 24) | Gastric Ulcer (n = 32) | Significance (x² test) |
|---|---|---|---|---|
| Hemoglobin | F <12 g%–M <14 g% | 46 | 75 | p <0.01 |
| Total serum proteins | <6.5 g% | 29 | 59 | p <0.05 |
| Albumin | <3.5 g% | 13 | 66 | p <0.001 |
| Ceruloplasmin | >40 mg% | 54 | 53 | NS |
| Retinol binding protein (RBP) | <3.7 mg% | 17 | 41 | NS |
| Transferrin | <200 mg% | 13 | 9 | NS |
| Fe | F <60 μg%–M <80 μg% | 50 | 87.5 | p <0.01 |
| Urine creatinine | F <18 mg/kg–M <23 mg/kg | 50 | 59 | NS |
| Creatinine/height index | <90% | 56 | 57 | NS |
| % Arm muscle circumference | <90% | 17 | 28 | NS |
| % Ideal body weight | <90% | 17 | 22 | NS |
| % Usual body weight | <90% | 50 | 94 | p <0.001 |
| % Standard arm circumference | <90% | 25 | 38 | NS |
| % Standard triceps skinfold | <90% | 67 | 63 | NS |
| Lymphocytes | <1,500/mm³ | 4 | 9 | NS |
| WBC | <4,000/mm³ | 0 | 6 | NS |
| C3 complement | >120 mg% | 33 | 44 | NS |
| Skin tests | % hypoanergic | 18 | 55 | p <0.01 |

From Dionigi, P., et al.[44] with permission of JPEN *6*:128–133, 1982

**Table 56A2–2.　Limits Between Normal and Severe Malnutrition for Anthropometric and Biochemical Variables* in Patients with Gastric Carcinoma**

| Variables | Normal | | Malnutrition | | | |
|---|---|---|---|---|---|---|
| | | | Moderate | | Severe | |
| Weight-index (%) | ≥80 | (22)* | 60–79 | (4)* | ≥59 | (0)* |
| WL (% month) | — | (21) | — | — | >5 | (5) |
| Triceps skin fold (percentiles) | >10th | (15) | ≤10th >5th | (1) | ≤5th | (5) |
| Arm muscle circumference (percentiles) | >10th | (20) | ≤10th >5th | (0) | ≤5th | (1) |
| Albumin (g/L) | ≥37 | (7) | 29–36 | (11) | ≤28 | (7) |
| Transferrin (g/L) | ≥2.2 | (20) | 1.5–2.1 | (5) | ≤1.4 | (0) |
| Prealbumin (g/L) | ≥0.25 | (3) | 0.20–0.24 | (9) | ≤0.19 | (13) |
| Cholinesterase (μkat/L) | ≥37 | (19) | 20–36 | (5) | ≤19 | (1) |
| Fibronectin (%) | ≥60 | (24) | 20–59 | (0) | ≤19 | (0) |

*Figures in parentheses indicate the number of patients (total = 26) regarded as being normal, moderately malnourished, or severely malnourished for each variable.
From Symreng, T., et al.,[45] with permission of Ann. Surg.

alterations in visceral protein status that are more severe than alterations in muscle bulk or gastric mucosa leaking plasma protein. Despite the preservation of muscle bulk in the malnourished group, significant reduction of muscle adenine nucleotides, phosphorylcreatine, creatine, and glycogen was found. This finding was interpreted as indicating that malnutrition results in abnormal muscle energy metabolism.

## GASTRITIS

Malnutrition due to gastritis is comparable to that observed with gastric ulcer. No formal studies of this entity have been performed. When alcohol is a factor in the etiology, the nutritional consequences may be exaggerated. Acetylsalicylic acid and nonsteroidal anti-inflammatory medication do not appear to produce a different outcome in those patients with no exacerbating factors. Corrosives and radiation gastritis may produce severe gastritis. The result may be permanent damage to the stomach with resulting long-term effect on the ingestion of nutrients, and the production of acid and intrinsic factor.

## OTHER CONDITIONS

Other diseases of the stomach and duodenum affect nutritional status. The pathogenesis is most likely similar to that for the conditions discussed. There is little collected data for these conditions, which include gastric lymphoma, polyps, benign tumors, abnormal motility, Zollinger-Ellison syndrome, and benign hypertrophic gastropathy.

### REFERENCES

1. Meeroff, J.C., Schreiber, D.S., Trier, J.S., et al.: Ann. Intern. Med. *92*:370–373, 1980.

2. Dubois, A., Gross, H.A., Ebert, M.H., et al.: Gastroenterology *77*:319–323, 1979.

3. Campbell, I.W., Heading, R.C., Tothill, P., et al.: Gut *18*:462–467, 1977.

4. Kozoll, B.D., Meyer, K.A.: Arch. Surg. *91*:983–994, 1965.

5. Telander, R.L., Morgan, K.G., Keulen, D.L., et al.: Gastroenterology *75*:497–501, 1978.

6. You, C.H., Lee, K.Y., Chey, W.Y., et al.: Gastroenterology *79*:311–314, 1980.

7. Cox, A.G., Spencer, J., Tinker, J.: Review of clinical results. *In* After Vagotomy. (Alexander-Williams, J., Cox, A.G., Eds.) London, Butterworths, 1969, pp. 119–130.

8. Nelson, P.G.: Aust. N.Z. J. Surg. *37*:283–285, 1968.

9. Meyer, J.H., Okaski, H., John, D., et al.: Gastroenterology *80*:1489–1496, 1981.

10. Hunt, J.N., Knox, M.T.: Regulation of gastric emptying. *In* Handbook of Physiology, Vol. IV. (Code C.F., Ed.) Washington, American Physiological Society, 1968, pp. 1917–1983.

11. Harvald, B., Krogsgard, A.R., Louis P.: Acta Med. Scand. *172*:497–503, 1962.

12. Meyer, J.H.: Chronic morbidity after ulcer surgery. *In* Gastrointestinal Disease, Vol. 1 (Fordtran, J.S., and Schleisenger, M.H., Eds.) Philadelphia, W.B. Saunders Co., 1983, pp. 757–779.

13. Klidjian, A.M., Foster, K.J., Kammerling, R.M., et al.: Br. Med. J. *281*:899–907, 1980.

14. Mullen, J.L., Gerner, M.H., Buzby, G.P., et al.: Arch. Surg. *114*:121–125, 1972.

15. McNeill, K.G., Mernagh, J.R., Jeejeebhoy, K.N., et al.: Am. J. Clin. Nutr. *32*:1955–1961, 1979.

16. Lopes, J., Russell, D.M., Whitwell, J., et al.: Am. J. Clin. Nutr. *3*:602–610, 1982.

17. Meyer, J.H.: Chronic morbidity after ulcer surgery. *In* Gastrointestinal Disease, Vol. 1. (Fordtran, J.S., and Schleisenger, M.H., Eds.) Philadelphia, W.B. Saunders Co., 1983, p. 770.

18. Butler, T.J.: Ann. R. Coll. Surg. Engl. *29*:300–327, 1961.

19. Wall, A.J., Ungar B., Baird, C.W., et al.: Am. J. Dig. Dis. *12*:1077–1086, 1967.

20. French, J.M., Crane, C.W.: Undernutrition, malnutrition and malabsorption after gastrectomy. *In* Post Gastrectomy Complications and Metabolic Consequences. (Stammes, F.A.R., Alexander-Williams, J., Eds.) London, Butterworths, 1963.

21. Adams, J.F.: Scand. J. Gastroenterol. *2*:137–149, 1967.

22. Kelly, W.P., Maclean, L., Perry, J.F., et al.: Surgery *35*:964–981, 1954.

22a.Basso, N., Materia, A., Gizzonio, D., et al.: Ital. J. Surg. Sci. *15*(4):335–40, 1985.

23. Roberts, K.E., Randall, H.T., Bane, H.N., et al.: N.Y. State J. Med. *55*:2897–2902, 1955.

24. Bradley, E.L., Isaacs, J.T., Hersh, T., et al.: Ann. Surg. *182*:415–429, 1975.

25. Meyer, J.H., Schwabe, A., Isenberg, J.I., et al.: West. J. Med. *126*:273–287, 1977.

26. Haubrich, W.S.: Sequelae of gastric surgery for peptic ulcer. *In* Gastroenterology. (Bockus, H.L., Ed.) Philadelphia, W.B. Saunders Co., 1974, pp. 906–937.

26a.Kotler, D.P., Sherman, D., Bloom, S.R., et al.: Dig. Dis. Sci. *30*(3):193–9, 1985.

27. Bradley, E.L., III: Total gastrectomy. *In* Clinics in Gastroenterology, Vol. 8. (Blum, A.L., Siewert, J.R., Eds.) Philadelphia, W. B. Saunders Co., 1979, pp. 354–371.

28. Mayer, E.A., Thomson, J.B., Jehn, D., et al.: Gastroenterology *83*:184–192, 1982.

29. Lundh, G.: Acta Chir. Scand. (Suppl.) *231*:1–83, 1958.

30. MacGregor, I., Parent, J.A., Meyer, J.H.: Gastroenterology *72*:195–205, 1977.

31. Isaacs, P.E.T., Kim, Y.S.: Blind loop syndrome and small bowel bacterial contamination. *In* Clinics in Gastroenterology, Vol 12. (Schleisenger, M.H., Ed.) Philadelphia, W.B. Saunders Co., 1983, pp. 395–414.

32. Neale, G., Antcliff, A.C., Welbourn, R.B., et al.: Q. J. Med. *36*:469–494, 1967.

33. Baird, I.M., Blackburn, E.K., Wilson, G.M.: Q. J. Med. *28*:21, 1959.

34. Turberg, L.A.: Q. J. Med. *35*:107–118, 1966.

35. Magnusson, B.E.: Scand. J. Haematol. (Suppl.) *26*:1–111, 1976.

36. Choudhury, M.R., Williams, J.: Clin. Sci. *18*:527–532, 1959.

37. Hallberg, L., Solvell, L., Zederfeldt, B.: Acta Med. Scand. (Suppl.) *445*:26A, 1966.

38. Hallberg, L, Solvell, L.: Acta Med. Scand. *181*:335–354, 1967.

39. Baird, I.M., Sutton, D.R.: Gut *13*:634–637, 1972.

40. Kimber, C., Patterson, J.F., Weintraub, L.R.: J.A.M.A. *202*:935–938, 1967.

41. Hines, J.D., Hoffbrand, A.V., Mollin, D.L.: Am. J. Med. *43*:555–569, 1967.

42. Wastell, C.: Ann. R. Coll. Surg. Engl. *45*:193–211, 1969.

43. Wheldon, E.J., Venables, C.W., Johnston, I.D.S.: Lancet *1*:437–440, 1970.

43a.Clark, C.G.: Partial gastrectomy. *In* Vagotomy on Trial. Cox, A.G., and Alexander-Williams, J. (Eds.), pp. 53–65, 1973.

43b.Alexander-Williams, J.: J. Abdominal Operations. pp. 491–516, 1971.

43c.Nelson, B.E., and Vastlin, L.E. Acta Chirurgica. Scand. *137*:533, 1971.

43d.Nilas, L., and Christiansen, C.: Calcif. Tissue Int. *37*:461–6, 1975.

43e.Paulson, G.W., Martin, E.W., Mojzisik, C., et al.: Arch. Neurol. *42*(7):675–7, 1985.

43f.Somer, H., Bergstrom, L., Mustajoki, P., et al.: Acta. Med. Scand. *275*(5):575–6, 1985.

44. Dionigi, P., Nazari, S., Bonoldi, A.P., et al.: J. Parenter. Enteral Nutr. *6*:128–133, 1982.

45. Symreng, T., Larsson, J., Schildt, B., et al.: Ann. Surg. *198*:146–150, 1983.

*Chapter* **56**

# NUTRITION AND DIET IN MANAGEMENT OF DISEASES OF THE GASTROINTESTINAL TRACT

## (A) ESOPHAGUS, STOMACH, AND DUODENUM
### (3) Diet and Peptic Ulcer Disease

Mukesh B. Desai and Khursheed N. Jeejeebhoy

Peptic ulcer refers to a break in the mucosa that occurs in juxtaposition to an acid-secreting area of the stomach. Peptic ulcers usually occur in non-acid-secreting mucosa adjacent to acid-secreting mucosa. Thus, they are found in gastric mucosa that is nonacid-secreting, in the duodenum, in the esophagus, and in the small intestine when anastomosed to stomach. The formation of an ulcer depends on two opposing factors operating at the site of ulceration: acid peptic secretion injuring the mucosa and factors such as mucus secretion and surface glycoproteins protecting it. Ulceration is caused by an imbalance between those two factors, the exact nature of which is as yet unresolved. In general, patients with duodenal ulcer tend to have a higher acid output than normal,[1] increased secretory drive during the nonstimulated state,[2] rapid gastric emptying uninhibited by acid,[3] and decreased duodenal pH. In these patiets, the dominant element is mucosal injury due to acid secretion. In contrast, patients with gastric ulcer have normal or low acid output,[4] although factors altering mucosal defense are probably more important. These conditions are duodeno-gastric reflux of bile, causing bile salt-induced mucosal injury,[5] aspirin ingestion,[6] and altered mucosal blood flow.[7]

It is now recognized that irrespective of the cause, suppression of acid secretion by the use of the new $H_2$-blockers heals the ulcer in most patients.

## DIET AND EATING HABITS IN ULCEROGENESIS

There is little scientifically sound information to support the folklore that diet contributes to peptic ulcer disease. Nevertheless, a few interesting observations require comment. Duodenal ulcer is more common in South India, where rice is the staple diet; in contrast, it is uncommon in the wheat-eating northern region.[8] This difference has been ascribed to the diet because, in a randomized trial, duodenal ulcer patients fed a wheat diet had a significantly lower recurrence rate than those fed the usual rice.[9] The lower rate was attributed to the need to secrete more saliva to chew the wheat. The same author had believed previously that a more liquid diet might predispose to ulcer formation.[10] This theory has also been supported by Gregory[11] for other reasons, namely, that saliva has an epidermal growth factor, urogastrone,[12] that inhibits acid secretion and enhances healing of experimental ulcer.[13] More recently, it has been claimed that high-fiber diets may protect against gastric ulcer.[14]

Coffee is a strong stimulant of acid secretion, which is not due to its caffeine content.[15] In addition, coffee may aggravate or induce nonspecific symptoms of abdominal discomfort.[16] Increased coffee consumption has been associated with a higher incidence of peptic ulcer.[17] The intake of other caffeine-containing beverages (colas and diet soft drinks) also increases acid secretion,[18] but evidence for their inducing peptic ulcer is not available.

Alcohol ingestion has not been shown to increase the incidence of peptic ulceration,[19] but in one study, patients in whom the ulcer had healed on a placebo were less likely to have taken alcohol.[20] Cigarette smoking is one of the most common factors associated with increased risk of duodenal and gastric ulceration, reduced ulcer healing, and increased relapse after treatment.[21,22]

## DIET IN THERAPY OF PEPTIC ULCER DISEASE

Folklore ascribes a major role to strict diet in the treatment of peptic ulcer disease. Despite evidence to the contrary, Isenberg found that, out of 326 hospitals surveyed in the United States, 250 (77%) still prescribed "peptic ulcer diets."[22] This folklore is based upon a long tradition. Celsus in the first century ordered smooth diets, and later practitioners wrote about the special healing properties of milk.[23] It is thus not surprising that in 1915 Sippy advocated a rigidly outlined program of milk, cream, and soft foods.[24] Modifications of milk-based "soft" bland diets continue to be advocated today.[25]

What is the evidence for the efficacy of dietetic treatment in ulcer healing, and what diet should be recommended? To understand the advantages and disadvantages, it is necessary to consider the effect of a mixed meal on acid secretion and gastric pH. The advent of $H_2$-blockers (cimetidine and ranitidine) has clearly shown that, if the pH of the stomach is maintained at a higher level, the ulcer heals. Lennard-Jones and Barbouris showed that the buffer effect of each meal raises the pH for approximately an hour,[26] and indeed, patients with ulcer disease experience relief of pain immediately after intake of food. However, the effect of a meal alone in raising the pH above 3.0 in patients with duodenal ulcer is either absent or short-lived.[27] During the night, when the patient is fasting, the pH falls to 1.5 to 1.7. By contrast, effective doses of an $H_2$-blocker such as cimetidine, which promotes peptic ulcer healing, increase the pH to 3.5 or better and, in particular, maintain a high pH at night. Similarly, intragastric pH is raised more when antacids are given one to three hours after meals than when they are given hourly on an empty stomach.[28] Thus, food by itself does not raise the pH in patients with duodenal ulcer disease to sufficiently high levels, and the effects are short-lived.

What is the role of milk, the substance supposed to have special healing properties in patients with ulcer? After a transient buffering effect lasting for 20 minutes,[29] milk, because of its calcium content, increases the secretion of acid to a greater extent than it can buffer (Table 56A3–1).[30] Thus, it is not surprising that clinical trials of so-called peptic ulcer diets have shown no effect on the healing of peptic ulcers, either gastric or duodenal.[31–33]

What is the role of diet in peptic ulcer disease? In the uncomplicated disease, it has no role. Patients with uncomplicated disease treated with an $H_2$-blocker are rapidly able to eat and tolerate all foods without discomfort. However, avoidance of cigarettes, coffee, or caffeinated soft drinks that induce increased acid secretion may prevent heartburn and discomfort due to reflux. Milk is neither necessary nor desirable for this purpose, especially if the patient is lactose-intolerant.

## DIET AND NUTRITION IN PATIENTS WITH COMPLICATIONS

Complications associated with peptic ulceration include hemorrhage, perforation, penetration, and obstruction. Two of these complications (hemorrhage and perforation) are medicosurgical emergencies, and the other two affect the ability to eat. Thus they are associated with changes in our ability to nourish the patient.

**Hemorrhage.** During acute continuing hemorrhage, it is impossible to feed by mouth because of the need to monitor bleeding through nasogastric suction. In many instances, a patient is admitted with a history of mild bleeding that has ceased. Such patients need not be practically starved by keeping them NPO (nil per os) and infusing hypocaloric electrolytes and dextrose (DSW). As early as 1935 Meulengracht showed that early feeding was beneficial to patients with hemorrhage.[34]

Once the need for nasogastric suction has passed (i.e., bleeding has been well controlled for over 12 hours), the patient should be refed as quickly as possible to help replace the protein and iron that have been lost. Later, if there is evidence of anemia, iron supplementation should be given.

In cases where the patient requires surgery, the question of postoperative parenteral nutrition arises. It is not known whether such support is necessary and/or effective in promoting recovery. The following guidelines are recommended in the absence of data. Clearly if there is previous malnutrition, significant weight loss (over 15%), and hypoproteinemia, then parenteral nutrition should be started as soon as possible in the postoperative period. However, if weight loss has been less than 10% and there is no hypoalbuminemia, then parenteral nutrition need not be given routinely. If complications occur that prevent oral alimentation for periods exceeding a week, then total parenteral nutrition (TPN) should be given. In this

**Table 56A3–1.** **Mean (± SEM) Basal and 2-hour Gastric Acid Output after Various Forms of Milk, 0.15 Mol NaCl, and Peptone**

|  | *Whole (meq/hour)* | *Low-fat (meq/hour)* | *Nonfat (meq/hour)* | *Low-calcium (meq/hour)* | *0.15 Mol NaCl (meq/hour)* | *Peptone (meq/hour)* |
|---|---|---|---|---|---|---|
| Patients with duodenal ulcer |  |  |  |  |  |  |
| Basal hour | 9.9 ± 3.7 | 7.0 ± 1.6 | 8.8 ± 2.5 | 7.9 ± 1.7 | 8.8 ± 2.2 | 10.1 ± 2.4 |
| First hour | 16.0 ± 5.0 | 11.9 ± 3.9 | 13.4 ± 3.6 | 13.4 ± 3.3 | 8.9 ± 2.8 | 14.8 ± 4.1 |
| Second hour | 13.8 ± 4.5 | 12.8 ± 2.2 | 14.7 ± 4.3 | 13.1 ± 3.8 | 11.5 ± 3.7 | 14.0 ± 3.1 |
| Normal subjects |  |  |  |  |  |  |
| Basal hour | 3.6 ± 1.3 | 2.3 ± 0.5 | 4.1 ± 1.4 | 6.4 ± 2.7 | 2.8 ± 1.0 | 2.3 ± 0.5 |
| First hour | 8.9 ± 2.1 | 7.0 ± 1.9 | 8.2 ± 3.0 | 4.7 ± 2.1 | 1.2 ± 0.5 | 7.8 ± 0.9 |
| Second hour | 7.7 ± 1.9 | 7.2 ± 2.5 | 6.0 ± 2.8 | 6.5 ± 2.8 | 3.1 ± 0.8 | 3.0 ± 0.3 |

From Ippoliti, A.F., Maxwell, V., Isenberg, J.I.,[30] with permission of the Ann. Intern. Med.

situation, it is preferable to give nutritional support early because of the evidence that functional changes occur within two weeks of nutrient deprivation and precede significant weight loss.[35]

**Perforation.** Perforation is a surgical emergency, and the question of nutritional support only arises in the postoperative period. The aforementioned guidelines are appropriate. The onset of peritonitis may result in prolonged ileus, necessitating TPN in the postoperative period.

**Gastric Outlet Obstruction.** Gastric obstruction results in early satiety and later vomiting. Both these factors reduce the intake of food and prevent it from entering the small bowel. Marked weight loss occurs unless the patient learns to adapt to a liquid diet. Clearly the only way to treat this problem is to correct the obstruction surgically. However, the physician is often faced with the patient who is malnourished and is not suitable for an operation. The question of nutritional support as a preoperative measure has to be considered. Although there are no controlled trials to prove or disprove the benefits of preoperative preparation, the following are practical guidelines.

Patients who have lost less than 10% body weight and who are not hypoproteinemic should be prepared for surgery simply by correcting dehydration, chloride and potassium deficits due to vomiting, and any anemia.

In patients who have more than 10% weight loss, preoperative nutritional support is advisable. Initially it is necessary to clean out retained gastric contents using an Ewald tube and lavage of the stomach. Emptying the stomach, leaving a clear passage for liquid feeds, is of great importance in allowing the patient to tolerate liquid formula feeds without vomiting. Following clearing of the stomach, liquid diets should be fed orally, or by continuous intragastric infusion. Continuous infusion often permits greater intake of calories because the uniform rate of infusion into the stomach may equal outflow and may avoid distending the stomach.

In persons with complete pyloric obstruction or in those with severe vomiting, a period of TPN is used to improve the nutritional status of the patient while allowing edema in the obstructed stomach to subside. The TPN may be given as a peripheral infusion for 7 to 10 days using an amino acid, glucose, and fat mixture. Following this period, nasogastric feeding could again be attempted if the patient is still markedly malnourished. If prolonged nutrition must be given via the parenteral route, then TPN infused through a central venous catheter should be used.

## REFERENCES

1. Kirkpatrick, J.R., Lowrie, J.H., Forrest, A.P.M., et al.: Gut *10*:760–762, 1969.
2. Hunt, J.M., Kay, A.W.: Br. Med. J. *2*:1444–1446, 1954.
3. Lam, S.K., Isenberg, J.I., Grossman, M.I., et al.: Dig. Dis. Sci. *27*:598–604, 1982.
4. Grossman, M.I., Kirsner, J.B., Gillespie, I.E.: Gastroenterology *45*:14–26, 1963.
5. Rhodes, J., Barvardo, D.E., Phillips, S.F., et al.: Gastroenterology *57*:241–252, 1969.
6. MacDonald, W.C.: Gastroenterology *65*:381–389, 1973.
7. Ritchie, W.P., Jr.: Surgery *76*:363–366, 1974.
8. Pulvertaft, C.N.: Br. J. Prev. Soc. Med. *13*:131–138, 1959.
9. Malhotra, S.L.: Postgrad. Med. J. *54*:6–9, 1978.
10. Malhotra, S.L.: Gut *5*:412–416, 1964.
11. Gregory, H.: Nature *257*:325–327, 1975.
12. Elder, J.R., Ganguli, P.C., Gillespie, I.E., et al.: Gut *16*:887–893, 1975.
13. Hoffman, C.G., Berry, J., Elder, J.B.: Br. J. Surg. *64*:830–836, 1977.
14. Cleave, T.L.: Peptic Ulcer. Bristol, John Wright, 1962.
15. Cohen, S., Barth, G.H.: N. Engl. J. Med. *293*:897–899, 1975.
16. Cohen, S.: N. Engl. J. Med. *303*:122–124, 1980.
17. Pfeffenburger, R.S., Jr., Wing, A.L., Hyde, R.T.: Am. J. Epidemiol. *100*:307–315, 1974.
18. McArthur, K., Hogan, D., Isenberg, J.I.: Gastroenterology *83*:199–203, 1982.
19. Friedman, G.D., Siegelaub, A.B., Seltzor, C.C.: N. Engl. J. Med. *290*:469–473, 1974.
20. Koo, J., Lam, S-K.: Gastroenterology *35*:413–419, 1983.

21. Sonnenberg, A., Muller-Lissner, S.A., Vogel, E., et al.: Gastroenterology *81*:1061–1067, 1981.

22. Isenberg, J.I.: Peptic ulcer: Epidemiology, nutritional aspects, drugs, smoking, alcohol and diet. *In* Nutrition and Gastroenterology. (Winick, M., Ed.) New York, John Wiley & Sons, Inc., 1980, pp. 141–151.

23. Williams, S.R.: Nutrition and Diet Therapy. St. Louis, The C.V. Mosby Co., 1981.

24. Sippy, B.W.: JAMA *64*:1625–1630, 1915.

25. Spiro, H.M.: J. Clin. Gastroenterol. *3*:219–220, 1981.

26. Lennard-Jones, J.E., Barbouris, M.: Gut *6*:113–117, 1965.

27. Peterson, W.L., Barnett, C., Feldman, M., et al.: Gastroenterology *77*:1015–1020, 1979.

28. Fein, H.D.: Nutrition in disease of the stomach, including related areas of the esophagus and duodenum. *In* Modern Nutrition in Health and Disease. 6th ed. (Goodhart, R.S., Shils, M.E., Eds.) Philadelphia, Lea & Febiger, 1980, pp. 892–911.

29. Bingle, J.P., Lennard-Jones, J.E.: Gut *1*:337–344, 1960.

30. Ippoliti, A.F., Maxwell, V., Isenberg, J.J.: Ann. Intern. Med. *84*:286–289, 1976.

31. Baron, J.H., Wastell, C.: Medical treatment. *In* Chronic Duodenal Ulcer. (Wastell, C., Ed.) London, Butterworth, 1972, pp. 117–133.

32. Evans, P.R.C.: Br. Med. J. *1*:612–616, 1954.

33. Doll, R., Pygott, F.: Lancet *1*:171–175, 1952.

34. Meulengracht, E.: Lancet *2*:1220–1222, 1935.

35. Russell, D.McR., Leiter, L.A., Whitwell, J., et al.: Am. J. Clin. Nutr. *37*:133–138, 1983.

*Chapter* **56**

# NUTRITION AND DIET IN MANAGEMENT OF DISEASES OF THE GASTROINTESTINAL TRACT

## *(A) ESOPHAGUS, STOMACH, AND DUODENUM*
### *(4) Nutrition and Surgery for Peptic Ulcer*

### Mukesh B. Desai and Khursheed N. Jeejeebhoy

The stomach subserves specific functions that are altered by gastric surgery. These alterations result in the development of various postgastrectomy symptoms, which in turn affect the ability to eat.

The functions of the normal stomach are summarized in this section.

**Reservoir.** The stomach can hold up to one liter of contents and, under normal circumstances, it relaxes receptively to receive the meal.[1] Thus, it is possible to eat large meals at infrequent intervals when the individual has an intact stomach.

**Trituration of Food.** The antrum grinds the food into small particles that are released into the duodenum only when the particle size falls to 2 mm or less.[2] For example, digestion proceeds more rapidly when particles of ingested liver have been reduced to a size below 1 mm than it does with larger pieces.[2,3]

**Controlled Release of Ingested Food.** In the stomach, the food is diluted to an isotonic state before it enters the duodenum. Gastric emptying is controlled by complex interactions between pressure and resistance, both within and beyond the stomach.[4] Osmoreceptors in the duodenum also control gastric emptying.[5] They prevent hypertonic fluids from entering the small intestine. One study showed that the rate of gastric emptying is controlled by the rate at which calories enter the duodenum. A variety of liquid meals all emptied at a rate of 2.3 kcal/min.[6]

**Digestion of Protein.** Acid and pepsin break proteins down into peptides. The gastric mucosal barrier prevents autodigestion of the gastric lining.

**Intrinsic Factor and R Protein.** Intrinsic factor, secreted by parietal cells in the fundus, combines with exogenous vitamin $B_{12}$ to facilitate its absorption in the terminal ileum. Another substance, called R protein, also binds cobalamin (vitamin $B_{12}$). At an acid pH, R proteins have more affinity for vitamin $B_{12}$ than intrinsic factor. Thus, in the stomach vitamin $B_{12}$ binds to R protein. In the proximal small intestine, pancreatic protease releases vitamin $B_{12}$ from its complex with R protein. The released vitamin $B_{12}$ at the higher pH of the intestine binds to intrinsic factor. The ileal mucosa then absorbs vitamin $B_{12}$ from its complex with intrinsic factor. Thus, apart from resection of terminal ileum, malabsorption of vitamin $B_{12}$ can also be caused by pancreatic insufficiency because the $B_{12}$ is then not released from its complex with R protein.

## PATHOPHYSIOLOGIC EFFECTS OF VAGOTOMY AND GASTRECTOMY

Truncal vagotomy alters the resting tone of the stomach and makes it noncompliant.[7,8] After gastric resection, liquid emptying is accelerated irrespective of the nutrient fed.[9] However, solids of a large particle size leave the stomach early only after antral resection.[10,11] The procedure of gastric drainage and vagotomy has a variable effect on solid gastric emptying,[10] but emptying of liquids is rapid,[12] and hypertonic fluids leave the stomach without dilution.

Disruption of the pylorus and the effect of gravity[13] accelerate the flow of hypertonic fluids into the duodenum after pyloroplasty. As far as solid emptying is concerned, in contrast to rapid emptying in some patients, others may have gastric retention[14] due to vagotomy. Parietal cell vagotomy or highly selective vagotomy only mildly accelerates liquid emptying and does not alter the emptying of solids. Finally, all gastric resections reduce the size of the stomach and thus reduce the amount that can be eaten at any one time.

## CLINICAL EFFECTS OF GASTRIC SURGERY

**Dumping.** The most common effect of all gastric surgical procedures that injure or bypass the pyloric mechanism (e.g., Billroth II and esophagojejunostomy) is termed dumping. Within 20 to 90 minutes of eating, the patients develops upper abdominal pain, distention, and early satiety, and may become nauseated and vomit. These symptoms are related to distention of the proximal jejunum.[15] Following these symptoms are vasomotor (sympathetic) effects such as flushing, palpitations, sweating, dizziness, and hypotension. Finally the patient may feel an urge to have a bowel movement or may have copious diarrhea, followed by relief of symptoms. It is believed that some aspects of the vasomotor phenomenon are due to extravascular fluid depletion resulting from the rapid influx into the jejunum of hypertonic gastric contents requiring dilution. Nevertheless, the symptoms are not entirely abolished by simultaneous expansion of the vascular and extracellular fluid volume by intravenous infusions.[16,17] Release of intestinal hormones is believed to contribute to the production of the symptoms.[18] Among these agents are serotonin, bradykinin,[19] and substance P.[20] The levels of enteroglucagon,[21] gastric inhibitory peptide,[22] and neurotensin[23] are raised during dumping.

Thus the patient recognizes the association between food intake and discomfort. He finds that the larger the meal, the greater the problem and that lying down helps relieve the symptoms.

**Diarrhea.** Diarrhea is the next most important symptom. The primary cause of diarrhea is the rapid entry of hypertonic fluids into the jejunum.[24] Hypertonicity is associated with a marked inflow of fluid and electrolytes because the "tight junctions" between the enterocytes in this area of the bowel are relatively permeable. The process is an exaggeration of the phenomenon seen in normal subjects who have ingested a hypertonic meal of soluble carbohydrates composed of milk and doughnuts.[25] It tends to be worse after ingestion of liquids. Taking hypertonic liquids such as soup, soft drinks, and syrups is likely to cause more marked symptoms. Because of rapid intestinal transit, these patients may be unable to hydrolyze lactose in milk[26] and thus they develop diarrhea after taking milk and milk products such as ice cream, milkshakes, and milk-containing desserts. In addition, these patients may have a high output of bile acid.[27] Although one study showed no significant difference between fecal outputs of bile acid in postvagotomy patients with and without diarrhea, fecal chenodeoxycholic acid output was higher in the former group.[27] Thus excessive bile acid output into the colon also may be a factor in the pathogenesis of postvagotomy diarrhea. Diarrhea occurs because bile acids stimulate peristalsis, preventing the colon from absorbing water and salt. Diarrhea after gastric surgery may also be due to other factors. One such cause is the unmasking of subclinical celiac sprue.[28] Finally, diarrhea can be a result of inadvertent gastroileostomy, short-circuiting the bowel.

**Malabsorption.** In contradistinction to postprandial diarrhea, some patients may develop malabsorption after gastric surgery. The malabsorption may be of macronutrients such as proteins, fats, and carbohydrates or may be selective for micronutrients such as iron, calcium, vitamin D, and vitamin $B_{12}$.

*Macronutrient.* Although reduced gastric acid and pepsin could in theory cause reduced digestion, this is not the cause in practice, since acid reduction has to be marked in order to influence digestion. In addition, pancreatic secretions can complete hydrolysis of food even when gastric digestion is impaired.

The reduced acid plus stasis in the afferent loop can cause bacterial growth and a stagnant loop syndrome.[29] Bacterial contamination of the upper bowel can also occur as a result of gastrocolic fistula developing from a recurrent ulcer. In some instances there may be an asynchrony between the release of food from the stomach and the secretion of pancreatic juice, resulting in a functional pancreatic insufficiency.[13] Gastric surgery, when superimposed on patients with existing short bowel, causes rapid transit and can result in an insurmountable degree of malabsorption and diarrhea.

Despite the aforementioned possibilities, in most patients who have had gastric surgery, steatorrhea usually does not exceed 20 g/day on a moderately high fat diet[30,31] unless there is a preexisting celiac sprue, short bowel, or inadvertent gastroileostomy. In addition, fecal nitrogen output rarely exceeds 20% of nitrogen intake.[30]

*Micronutrient.* Iron deficiency is common after gastric surgery,[32] especially in women who are menstruating.[33] Iron deficiency is casued by a lack of gastric acid, which reduces the release of iron bound to protein.[34] Another cause of iron deficiency in patients with a vagotomy or gastric resection is the inadequate release of ferrous iron from coated tablets taken after meals. In addition, the tablets are rapidly emptied from the gastric remnant.[33] In contrast, absorption of heme iron from meat is normal.[35]

Imbalance of calcium metabolism is also common after gastric surgery, and 30% of patients have metabolic bone disease.[36] However, this bone disease is often subclinical.[37] Occult fractures are uncommon, although there is a greater tendency to fracture bones with only moderate trauma in patients who have a long-standing postgastrectomy state.[38] Osteomalacia also has been observed in these patients, but the cause is not clear since significant steatorrhea is absent and vitamin D absorption is normal.[39] Although serum vitamin $B_{12}$ levels are low, pernicious anemia is rare[40] unless the patient has had a "high" subtotal or total gastrectomy.

## NUTRITIONAL CONSEQUENCES AND THERAPY OF THE POSTGASTRECTOMY STATE

**Weight Loss.** Significant weight loss is common, especially after gastric resection.[41] It is less so after vagotomy and drainage, but does occur if dumping is severe. The weight loss may be extreme— 25 to 30% after a total gastrectomy. The cause of this weight loss is unlikely to be malabsorption alone, since the loss of 15 g of fat plus 10 g of protein in a person eating a 100-g fat and 80-g protein diet would result in a loss of only 199 kcals. This loss can easily be overcome if the patient increases his food intake. If the intake is not increased, however, then even such a small difference can add up to a substantial amount lost over a year. For example, if the patient has a deficit of 100 kcal/day, he will lose a kilogram a month until a new equilibrium is established between the metabolic rate of the now lighter patient and the reduced availability of energy.

However, in patients with gastrectomy and associated celiac disease[28] or preexisting short bowel, the weight loss may be severe owing to a combination of early satiety, anorexia, and marked malabsorption.

**Nutritional Therapy.** The dietetic treatment of early satiety and dumping is based on the fact that they are largely caused by the entry of hypertonic fluids into the upper jejunum. Thus, feeding a dry solid meal, low in simple sugars but high in complex carbohydrates and pectin,[42] slows the output of liquid gastric contents. Use of fiber, such as pectin, may especially aid this process. Avoidance of simple sugars reduces the tonicity of contents leaving the stomach because most of it will be composed of large molecular-weight starch, peptides, dextrins, and triglycerides. Significant amounts of milk and milk products should be avoided because of a functional lactose deficiency unless lactose has been hydrolyzed by the enzyme lactase or by bacteria (e.g., yogurt).

The patient is given an hour or two to allow the "dry" food to leave the stomach and then is permitted to take a hypotonic fluid drink such as water or tea without sugar. An increase in the intake of red meat should be encouraged to provide more heme iron (which is readily absorbed.)

This proposed diet is also advisable for other reasons. Even in normal persons, a steak-and-salad meal results in less jejunal volume than a milk-and doughnut meal.[25] In this study, the eating of both meals was followed by an increased volume in the duodenum. However, the former meal (steak) was associated with a reduced jejunal volume. In contrast, the doughnut-milk meal continued to be diluted along the small intestine, and the volume reaching the colon was enhanced.

Although small frequent meals low in simple sugars are popularly recommended to patients who dump (cf. Appendix Table A-31), it should be recognized that in the absence of major gastric resection, the main problem is jejunal distention with hypertonic fluid. Thus, separation of solids and liquids should take priority over eating frequent meals and snacks. Otherwise it becomes difficult to obtain sufficient time for one meal to leave the stomach before the next meal is taken. In addition, the intake of a diet containing complex carbohydrates and fiber should be emphasized. Because bile salt loss into the colon causes choleraic diarrhea, and patients with gastric surgery have an increased output of bile salts, use of a bile salt binding agent, such as cholestyramine resin, is useful in patients with diarrhea after gastric surgery.[27]

Patients who do not respond to these simple measures should be investigated to rule out associated (1) celiac disease, (2) pancreatic insufficiency, and (3) abnormal small bowel anatomy, such as gastroileostomy, blind loops, a long afferent loop, or a fistula.

Oral supplements of iron and folic acid and vitamin $B_{12}$ by injection, when indicated, should be given to prevent anemia.

The degree of malabsorption, and particularly whether steatorrhea is in excess of 15%, should be noted. In the presence of significant malabsorption, treatment should be directed to correcting celiac disease with a gluten-free diet, to correcting bacterial overgrowth with antibiotics, and to correcting anatomic abnormalities by reoperation.

The most difficult patients are those with a small gastric remnant, severe dumping, and malabsorption, and those with a total gastrectomy. In the last, the usual reason for the gastrectomy is a malignant lesion. However, improved chemotherapy and early operation are resulting in an increasing number of long-term survivors who become chronically malnourished. Such patients, especially if they have marked weight loss (>25%) and inability to gain weight, need nutritional support by artificial means. There are two ways of giving such support: home enteral and home parenteral feeding.

*Home Enteral Nutrition.* Because these patients have difficulty handling liquid osmotic loads, nasogastric feeding of a defined formula diet may not be tolerated in bolus feeding. However, the use of a continuous regulated infusion (with a pump) of a defined formula diet through a nasogastric tube is usually tolerated well without diarrhea. The regulation of the infusion avoids entry of peak loads of hypertonic fluids into the jejunum and contributes to successful feeding (see Chapter 54).

*Home Parenteral Nutrition.* Patients with gastric resection associated with small bowel resection may need home parenteral nutrition because the combined disability causes intractable diarrhea and/or severe malabsorption (see Chapter 54).

**Specific Nutritional Supplementation and Precautions.** Iron deficiency is the most common problem and needs attention. It can be avoided by eating more red meat and using iron supplements, especially in menstruating women and those with a previous history of anemia. Chelated iron is better tolerated when it is given at night after lying down.[33] Regular determination of hemoglobin levels should be undertaken as required. An increased calcium intake should be encouraged, especially since the patient often has difficulty in taking dairy products. Use of calcium supplements may be necessary if the patient cannot consume low-lactose dairy products such as hard cheese or lactose-treated milk or yogurt. Medium-chain triglycerides may be valuable as a dietary replacement for long-chain triglycerides since they have been shown to improve the absorption of calcium after gastrectomy.[43] Vitamin $B_{12}$ should

be given by injection to all patients who have had a total gastrectomy.

Weight loss is a common symptom owing to the reduced intake of food caused by early satiety and the aversion to eating caused by postcibal symptoms of dumping and diarrhea. The treatment is control of the dumping and diarrhea.

Patients who complain of early satiety, constant upper abdominal pain, and pain immediately postprandially may have a bezoar, a mass of retained food and vegetable matter in the stomach. Treatment consists of washing out the bezoar through a large-bore tube and later putting the patient on a diet restricted in vegetables and fruits. When the problem is recurrent, the patient is well advised to blend all fruits and vegetables before consumption. In the occasional patient, even blended vegetables and fruits are retained, and in that case they should all be avoided and supplementary multivitamins, including folic acid, should be given to avoid deficiencies of these nutrients. In patients receiving folic acid, it is necessary to ensure that vitamin $B_{12}$ deficiency does not occur concurrently. This is especially important, for the hematologic features of the deficiency are masked by the intake of folate. Vitamin $B_{12}$ absorption should be measured, and if abnormal, injections of the vitamin given.

## REFERENCES

1. Guyton, A.C.: *In* Textbook of Medical Physiology. 6th ed. Philadelphia, W.B. Saunders Co., 1981, p. 792.
2. Meyer, J.H., Thomson, J.B., Cohen, M.B., et al.: Gastroenterology *76*:804–813, 1979.
3. Meyer, J.H., Ohashi, H., Helin, D., et al.: Gastroenterology *80*:1489–1496, 1981.
4. Miller, J., Kauffman, G., Elashoff, J., et al.: Am. J. Physiol. *241*:G403–G415, 1981.
5. Hunt, J.N.: J. Physiol. (Lond.) *132*:267–288, 1956.
6. Brener, W, Hendrix, T.R., McHugh, P.R.: Gastroenterology *85*:76–82, 1983.
7. Carter, D.C., Whitfield, H.N., MacLeod, I.B.: Gut *23*:874–879, 1971.
8. Jahnberg, T.: Scand. J. Gastroenterol. (Suppl. 46) *12*:1–32, 1977.
9. MacGregor, I.L., Parent, J.A., Meyer, J.H.: Gastroenterology *72*:195–205, 1977.
10. MacGregor, I.L., Parent, J.A. Meyer, J.H.: Gastroenterology *72*:206–211, 1977.
11. Buckler, K.G.: Gut *8*:137–147, 1967.
12. Clarke, R.J., Alexander-Williams, J.: Gut *14*:300–307, 1973.
13. McKelvey, S.T.D.: Br. J. Surg. *57*:741–748, 1970.
14. Dragstedt, L.R., Schafer, P.W.: Surgery *17*:742–749, 1945.
15. Machella, T.E.: Gastroenterology *14*:237–252, 1950.
16. Butz, R: Ann. Surg. *154*:225–234, 1961.
17. LeQuesne, L.P., Hobsley, M., Hand, B.M.: Br. Med. J. *1*:141–147, 1960.
18. Editorial: Lancet *2*:1173–1174, 1980.
19. Zeitlin, I.J., Smith, A.N.: Lancet *2*:986–991, 1966.

20. Pernow, B., Wallenstein, S.: Acta Chir. Scand. *128*:530–540, 1964.
21. Bloom S.R., Royston, C.M.S., Thompson, J.P.S.: Lancet *2*:789–791, 1972.
22. McLaughlin, J.C., Buchanan, K.D., Alan, M.J.: Lancet *2*:603–605, 1979.
23. Blackburn, A.M., Christoficles, N.D., Ghatei, A., et al.: Clin. Sci. *59*:237–243, 1980.
24. Ladas, S.D., Isaacs, P.E., Quereshi, Y., et al.: Gastroenterology *85*:1088–1093, 1983.
25. Fordtran, J.S., Locklear, T.W.: Am. J. Dig. Dis. *11*:503–521, 1966.
26. Condon, J.R., Westerholm, P., Tanner, N.C.: Gut *10*:311–314, 1969.
27. Allan, J.G., Gerskowitch, V.P., Russel, R.I.: Br. J. Surg. *61*:516–518, 1974.
28. Hedberg, C.A., Melnyk, C.S., Johnson, C.F.: Gastroenterology *50*:796–804, 1966.
29. Booth, C.C., Brain, M.C., Jeejeebhoy, K.N.: Proc. R. Soc. Med. *57*:582–585, 1964.
30. Lawrence, W., Jr., Vanamee, P., Peterson, A.S., et al.: Surg. Gynecol. Obstet. *110*:601–616, 1960.
31. Edwards, J.P., Lyndon, P.H., Smith, R.B., et al.: Gut *15*:521–525, 1974.
32. Clark, C.G.: Compr. Ther. *7*:26–32, 1981.
33. Hobbs, J.R.: Gut *2*:141–149, 1961.
34. Wheldon, E.J., Venables, C.W., Johnston, I.D.A.: Br. J. Surg. *62*:356–359, 1975.
35. Hallberg, L., Solvell, L., Zederfeldt, B.: Acta Med. Scand. *179*(Suppl. 445):269–275, 1966.
36. Eddy, R.L.: Am. J. Med. *50*:442–449, 1971.
37. Bordier, P., Matrajt, H., Hioco, D., et al.: Lancet *1*:437–440, 1968.
38. Nilsson, B.E., Westlin, N.E.: Acta Chir. Scand. *137*:533–534, 1971.
39. Schwartz, M.K., Bodansky, O., Randall, H.E.: Am. J. Clin. Nutr. *4*:51–60, 1956.
40. Deller, D.J., Witts, L.J.: Q. J. Med. *31*:71–88, 1962.
41. Goligher, J.C., Domball, F.T.D., Pulvertaft, C.M., et al.: Br. Med. J. *2*:781–787, 1968.
42. Leeds, A.R., Ralphs, D.N.L., Ebied, E., et al.: Lancet *1*:1075–1078, 1981.
43. Agnew, J.E., Holdsworth, L.D.: Gut *12*:973–977, 1971.

*Chapter* **56**

# NUTRITION AND DIET IN MANAGEMENT OF DISEASES OF THE GASTROINTESTINAL TRACT

## (B) PANCREAS

### (1) The Exocrine Pancreas: Nutrient Interactions with Function and Structure

### Gordon R. Greenberg

The exocrine pancreas plays a key role in the assimilation of food. By secreting an alkaline juice comprised predominantly of digestive enzymes, the pancreas allows nutrients to be hydrolyzed within the intestinal lumen and subsequently absorbed. The first part of this section is concerned with the components of pancreatic juice and the maner in which they act on nutrients reaching the small intestine. The second part deals with the complex interplay between neural and hormonal regulatory mechanisms that control pancreatic exocrine secretion. Finally, the manner by which nutrients may affect pancreatic structure is considered.

## COMPONENTS OF PANCREATIC JUICE

**Pancreatic Enzymes.** Over a dozen enzymes and isoenzymes are secreted from the acinar cells that comprise about 90% of the functional mass of the pancreas. The proteolytic enzymes, including trypsin and chymotrypsin, constitute the largest component and are responsible for the hydrolysis of protein peptide bonds to oligopeptides and amino acids. These proteases are secreted as inactive precursors and are activated in the small intestinal lumen. Enterokinase, a peptidase found in the small intestinal mucosa, converts trypsinogen to trypsin, which in turn activates other proenzymes by a cascade process. Lipolysis is achieved by lipase, an enzyme secreted in the active form, which hydrolyzes triglycerides to monoglycerides and free fatty acids. Emulsification of fat by bile salts is necessary for optimal lipase activity. However, the pH of bile salts also inhibits the action of lipase. This reaction is circumvented by colipase, a small-molecular-weight cofactor secreted in pancreatic juice, which combines with lipase to reduce the optimal pH activity to 6.5 and thus below the pH of bile.[1] From a clinical standpoint, lipase is perhaps the most essential enzyme because its absence is manifested by steatorrhea with potentially deleterious nutritional consequences. It is also the enzyme most susceptible to inactivation by gastric juice. This finding has led to the use of $H_2$-receptor antagonists in the management of pancreatic insufficiency to reduce postprandial gastric acid secretion, thereby improving the therapeutic efficacy of pancreatic enzyme replacement therapy.[2] Amylase hydrolyzes starch to form disaccharides, trisaccharides (maltose and maltotriose), and dextrins.[3] These products are then broken down into glucose by enzymes in intestinal mucosa.

**Pancreatic Electrolytes.** The exocrine pancreas also secretes an isotonic juice, composed of water and electrolytes, which is thought to arise from centroacinar cells of the ductal system. The major cations are $Na^+$ and $K^+$; $HCO_3^-$ and $Cl^-$ are the principal anions. At maximal secretory rates, as would be observed after a meal, $HCO_3^-$ concentration greatly exceeds $Cl^-$ concentration. This difference helps to neutralize acidic gastric chyme and to achieve an optimal duodenal pH for the action of pancreatic enzymes. Pancreatic juice also contains small quantities of calcium, magnesium, and zinc, although their role is unknown.

## REGULATION OF PANCREATIC SECRETION

Pancreatic exocrine secretion is regulated by a complex interplay of neural and hormonal mechanisms triggered by the exposure and subsequent ingestion of nutrients.

### Response to Nutrients

The pancreatic response, as determined by enzyme output, peaks within the first hour after ingestion and then declines progressively as nutrients leave the duodenum. Thus, seeing or smelling food, as well as tasting or chewing, initiates the "cephalic phase" of pancreatic secretion through vagal pathways, and may account for up to one third of maximal secretion.[4,5] Subsequently, when food reaches the stomach, the "gastric phase," mediated in part by gastric distention (through a gastropancreatic neural reflex) and perhaps in part through gastrin release, also stimulates pancreatic secretion.[6] However, the most important stimulants to pancreatic secretion are the products of protein and fat digestion in the intestinal lumen, which participate in the "intestinal phase" of pancreatic secretion. In man, maximal enzyme secretion has been observed with either solid or homogenized meals, provided they contain these two principal dietary nutrients.[7] Dextrose has no effect on pancreatic secretion.

Fat is the single most potent stimulus to pancreatic secretion. Although intact triglycerides and glycerol are without effect, fatty acids are among the strongest stimulants.[8,9] The degree of stimulation is determined by the chain length, as long-chain fatty acids (C18) are more effective than those of medium-chain length (C8). Moreover, there is a direct correlation between the length of small bowel exposed to fatty acids and the degree of pancreatic enzyme output, suggesting that the load is more important than the concentration. Consequently, factors that modify the rate of fatty acid absorption, such as bile salt concentration, may also influence the degree of pancreatic stimulation.

Products of protein digestion are also potent stimuli for pancreatic secretion. As with fat, undigested protein is ineffective, but polypeptides, oligopeptides, and essential amino acids (in man, particularly phenylalanine, valine, tryptophan, and methionine) elicit an enzyme response that is about 60% of maximal pancreatic enzyme output.[10] This response is somewhat less than has been observed with fatty acids, a difference that might be explained either because amino acids are weaker stimulants of enzyme secretion or, alternatively, because protein concomitantly releases humoral inhibitors. The pancreas responds to amino acids only by secreting enzymes; there is no stimulation of bicarbonate. This contrasts with the response to fatty acids where the ratio of bicarbonate to enzyme secretion increases with the concentration and saturation of fatty acids exposed to the intestinal lumen.[8] Although the perfusion of the small intestine with hydrolytic products of fat and protein digestion stimulates pancreatic secretion, experimental studies in man with chyme diversion techniques indicate that stimulation of the stomach and duodenum is sufficient to elicit a normal pancreatic enzyme response to a meal.[11] This finding accords with observations that pancreatic enzyme replacement has no effect on the malabsorption of patients with short bowel syndrome.[12]

In addition to nutrients, the load of hydrogen ions reaching the duodenum after a meal is also a major determinant of pancreatic volume and bicarbonate secretion. Although hydrogen is initially buffered in the stomach, when it reaches the duodenum it gradually becomes dissociated from protein. This accounts for the somewhat delayed output of bicarbonate when compared with the pancreatic enzyme in response to a meal.[13] In man, cimetidine has no effect on the pancreatic enzyme secretion to a nutrient load, suggesting that in the physiologic setting of a meal, duodenal acid load may not be an important determinant of pancreatic enzyme secretion.[14]

**Postabsorptive Phase.** Reports on the effects of absorbed products of digestion on pancreatic secretion are conflicting. Infusion of intravenous glucose sufficient to achieve hyperglycemia appears to inhibit the trypsin output in response to a liquid meal.[15] In dogs, intravenous amino acids stimulate,[16] inhibit,[17] or have no effect[18,19] on protein output. In man, intravenous amino acid infusion stimulates gastric acid by a gastrin-independent mechanism,[20] but effects on pancreatic exocrine function have not been reported. In the dog, intravenous fat stimulates pancreatic enzyme secretion,[16] but in man, intravenous lipid (Intralipid) in amounts used for total parenteral nutrition has no effect on either pancreatic enzyme or bicarbonate secretion.[21] Although species variation may account for these differences, the observations in man support the efficacy of intravenous fat emulsions in patients with pancreatic disease.

**Fasting Secretion.** Basal pancreatic exocrine secretion is an active process that is coordinated with several other gastrointestinal events. Cyclic elevations in pancreatic enzyme, bicarbonate, and volume secretion have been recorded during late phase II of the interdigestive motor complex and are associated with plasma increments of certain of the gut hormones, notably gastrin and pancreatic polypeptide (PP).[22] Peak pancreatic enzyme outputs approaching one third maximal rates of secretion have been reported.[22] Subsequently it has been determined that phase II activity of the interdigestive motor complex, along with PP and gastrin release, is mediated by a vagal excitatory pathway.[23] Similarly, pancreatic enzyme but not bicarbonate secretion is controlled by tonic vagal stimulation.[23a]

### Neurohumoral Mechanisms

Recent advances support the concept that both neural and hormonal mechanisms interact in a complex fashion to modulate postprandial pancreatic exocrine secretion.

**Hormonal Control.** Several of the recently isolated hormones from the gut and pancreas influence pancreatic exocrine secretory responses. Many are stimulatory, whereas others selectively or jointly inhibit protein and bicarbonate outputs (Fig. 56B1–1). One of the major limitations in ascribing a physiologic role to these hormones in the modulation of pancreatic function has been the failure to detect a rise in circulating plasma concentrations after a meal. Methodologic modifications in radioimmunoassay techniques to measure hormones in plasma have, in part, resolved some of the controversy. For example, fasting and postprandial plasma levels of secretin are characterized by rapid and short-lived increments that coincide with intermittent falls in duodenal pH.[24] These plasma increments are very small indeed, ranging from 2.5 to 7 pmol/L. However, when such levels are reproduced by intravenous infusion of bolus injection of secretin, significant elevations in pancreatic bicarbonate can be achieved.[25,26] The intimate relationship between secretin and acid delivery to the duodenum suggests that secretin may function most effectively during fasting and in the late postprandial period because these are times when gastric acid is least likely to be buffered.

The humoral regulation of pancreatic enzyme secretion is most widely ascribed to cholecystokinin (CCK). Only amino acids produce a pancreatic enzyme response qualitatively similar to exogenous infusions of CCK. The response to fatty acids can best be accounted for by invoking the release of large amounts of CCK against a small background of secretin, whereas the reverse relationship is true for hydrochloric acid.[27] This potentiating response between secretin and CCK is one of the more important gut hormone interactions and has been well documented in man.[28] Although CCK circulates in several molecular forms, significant plasma increments after food

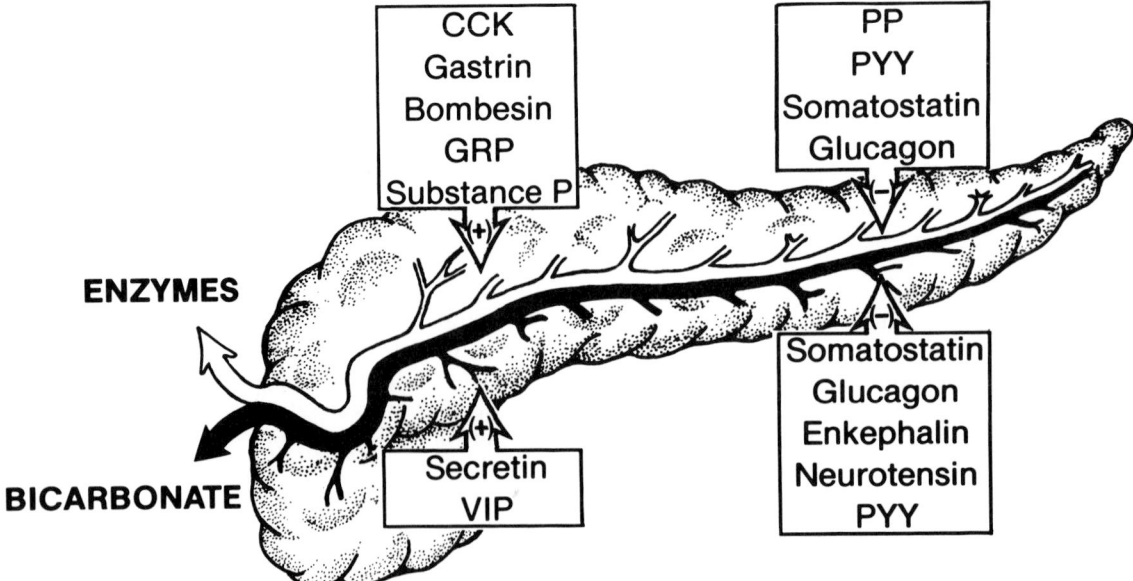

**Fig. 56B1–1.** Hormones from the gut and pancreas that influence pancreatic exocrine secretory responses. CCK = cholecystokinin; PP = pancreatic polypeptide; VIP = vasoactive intestinal peptide.

are found only with CCK$_8$[29,30] and CCK$_{33}$.[31] Infusion of CCK$_8$ to reproduce postprandial levels has been reported to achieve 50% maximal pancreatic enzyme output.

As noted previously, the pancreatic enzyme response to intestinal perfusion of amino acids is about 60% of that observed after maximal stimulation with CCK. The release into the circulation of a peptide that is inhibitory to pancreatic enzyme secretion could provide an explanation for this observation. A recently identified pancreatic hormone, pancreatic polypeptide (PP), seems one likely candidate. This hormone rises rapidly in plasma after a meal; protein is one of the major stimulants for its release. When infused in man, PP is a potent inhibitor of both basal and stimulated pancreatic enzyme outputs.[32] A second candidate hormone, peptide YY (PYY), found in highest concentrations in the mucosa of the ileum and colon, is structurally very similar to PP. PYY also potently inhibits both secretin and CCK-stimulated pancreatic exocrine secretion.[32a] Since this action occurs at plasma concentrations equivalent to those observed after a meal, PP and PYY are strong contenders for participation in the humorally mediated inhibitory modulation of pancreatic exocrine secretion.

The preceding hormones are thought to act via the circulation in a traditional endocrine mode of control. However one hormone, somatostatin, is found in pancreatic endocrine cells (D cells) characterized by long cytoplasmic processes that are adjacent to neighboring effector cell types. It is postulated, therefore, that somatostatin may act via a local or paracrine mechanism of release. Somatostatin is a potent inhibitor of pancreatic exocrine secretion both directly and as a consequence of the inhibition of endogenous secretin release.[33] Hormones also participate in the regulation of pancreatic exocrine secretion via a neurocrine mechanism of control as discussed later.

**Neural Control.** A complex network of nerves arising from the sympathetic, parasympathetic, and peptidergic components of the autonomic nervous system innervates the pancreas. Cholinergic neural reflexes that participate in the regulation of pancreatic secretion are mediated via the vagus nerves and through direct neural connections between the small intestine and pancreas. Several lines of investigation have shown that the vagus influences pancreatic secretion. In man, truncal vagotomy reduces the pancreatic enzyme and bicarbonate response to all intestinal stimulants.[34] These observations were originally explained by the suggestion that vagotomy blunts the release of those hormones involved in pancreatic stimulation. More recently, it was shown

that in the autotransplanted extrinsically denervated canine pancreas, enzyme secretion was as sensitive to CCK as was observed with vagally intact animals.[35] This finding supports the concept that the interruption of an enteropancreatic reflex best explains the effects of vagotomy.

Moreover, electrical stimulation of the vagus nerves in animal preparations is a potent stimulus of enzyme and bicarbonate secretion from the pancreas. Although atropine abolishes the enzyme secretion, indicating control via a vagal cholinergic excitatory pathway, bicarbonate output is only moderately reduced. It has been proposed that this atropine-resistant component of bicarbonate output in response to vagal stimulation is mediated by vasoactive intestinal peptide (VIP). Present in nerves throughout the gastrointestinal tract, this hormone is one of the candidate neurotransmitters of the newly described peptidergic component of the autonomic nervous system. VIP is released during vagal stimulation and produces a profuse bicarbonate output in the presence of atropine.[36]

The predominant effects of the sympathetic innervation to the pancreas are inhibitory, and appear to be a consequence of vasomotor actions on the circulatory supply.[37]

## FACTORS AFFECTING PANCREATIC STRUCTURE

Either nutrient deprivation of alterations in nutrient composition may affect the structural characteristics, and thus the functional capacity, of the exocrine pancreas.

**Nutrient Deprivation.** Prolonged starvation produces a marked reduction in pancreatic weight[38] and a decrease in protein and amylase content.[39] Proteolytic and lipolytic enzymes seem to be spared. The selective reduction in amylase has been postulated to be a consequence of a decrease in circulating levels of glucose and insulin, since a critical ratio of both substances is required to reverse this effect in rats.[40] Longstanding protein-calorie malnutrition in man similarly produces significant exocrine dysfunction,[41] which is rapidly restored on feeding.[42] Moreover, both in dogs[43] and in man,[44] the maximal enzyme and bicarbonate response to secretin-CCK stimulation is reduced after a period of total parenteral nutrition. The mechanisms for these changes are not entirely clear. However, the observations with total parenteral nutrition (TPN) suggest that, in addition to possible direct alterations in pancreatic structure during nutrient deprivation, changes in small intestinal function (secondary to the absence of intraluminal nutrient supply) may be a contributing factor. During TPN, several of the gastrointestinal hormones are maintained at plasma levels equivalent to those observed in the fasted state.[45] It is well established that certain of these gut hormones, notably CCK, are trophic to the pancreas.[46] Thus, a prolonged absence of release, as would otherwise normally occur in the postprandial state, may contribute to the morphologic and functional changes observed with the exocrine pancreas in settings where the gastrointestinal tract is deprived of nutrients.

**Nutrient Composition.** Studies in rats have suggested that feeding increases pancreatic enzyme synthesis, but confirmatory evidence in other species has not been reported. The postulated mechanisms may in part be related to the release of gastrointestinal hormones after a meal, and possibly the stimulation of neural reflexes. Thus both CCK and the cholinergic analogue, carbachol, enhance pancreatic protein synthesis by a mechanism that is dependent upon elevation of cytoplasmic calcium.[47] The particular composition of the diet also influences the composition of various digestive enzymes within the acinar cell. For example, protease activity increases markedly on a casein diet, whereas a high-sucrose or -fat diet increases, respectively, pancreatic amylase and lipase content.[48-50] Selective stimulation of one or more gastrointestinal hormones also appears to participate in the modulation of these enzymes. Thus, changes in amylase on a high-carbohydrate diet have been postulated to reflect higher circulating levels of insulin, whereas the effects of protein and fat are believed to be a CCK-mediated action. Prolonged administration of defined formula (elemental) diets also reduces pancreatic amylase activity in rats.[51] The long-term effect of these diets on pancreatic function in man has not been studied, although they have been used successfully in the management of patients with acute pancreatitis.[52]

## REFERENCES

1. Borgstrom, B., Erlansom, C.: Eur. J. Biochem. *37*:60–65, 1973.
2. Durie, P.R., Bell, L., Linton, W., et al.: Gut *21*:778–786, 1980.
3. Beck, I.T.: Am. J. Clin. Nutr. *26*:311–325, 1973.
4. Sarles, H., Dani, R., Prezelin, G., et al.: Gut *9*:214–221, 1968.
5. Novis, B.H., Bank, S., Marks, I.N.: Scand. J. Gastroenterol. *6*:417–422, 1971.
6. Vagne, M., Grossman, N.I.: Gastroenterology *57*:300–310, 1969.
7. Malagelada, J.R., Go, V.L.W., Summerskill, W.H.J.: Dig. Dis. Sci. *24*:101–110, 1979.
8. Meyer, J.H., Jones, R.S.: Am. J. Physiol. *226*:1178–1187, 1974.
9. Malagelada, J.R., DiMagno, E.P., Summerskill, W.H.J., et al.: J. Clin. Invest. *58*:493–499, 1976.
10. Malagelada, J.R., Go, V.L.W., DiMagno, E.P.: J. Clin. Invest. *52*:2160–2165, 1973.
11. Miller, L.J., Clain, J.E., Malagelada, J.R., et al.: Dig. Dis. Sci. *24*:150–154, 1979.
12. Go, V.L.W., Miller, L.J.: Scand. J. Gastroenterol. *18*:135–142, 1983.
13. Itoh, Z., Honda, R., Hiwatashi, K.: Am. J. Physiol. *238*:G332–G337, 1980.
14. Longstreth, G.F., Go, V.L.W., Malagelada, J.R.: Gastroenterology *72*:9–13, 1977.
15. McGregor, I.L., Deveney, C., Way, L.W., et al.: Gastroenterology *70*:197–202, 1976.
16. Konturek, S.J., Taster, J., Cieszkowski, M., et al.: Am. J. Physiol. *236*:E678–E684, 1979.
17. DiMagno, E.P., Go, V.L.W., Summerskill, W.H.J.: J. Lab. Clin. Med. *82*:241–248, 1973.
18. Stabile, B.E., Debas, N.T.: Surg. Forum *32*:224–226, 1981.
19. Fried, G.M., Ogden, D.W., Rhea, A., et al.: Surgery, *92*:902–905, 1982.
20. Isenberg, J.I., Maxwell, V.: N. Engl. J. Med. *298*:27–29, 1978.
21. Edelman, K., Valenzuela, J.E.: Gastroenterology *85*:1063–1066, 1983.
22. Keane, F.B., DiMagno, E.P., Dozois, R.R., et al.: Gastroenterology *78*:310–316, 1980.
23. Hall, K.E., Greenberg, G.R., El-Sharkaway, T.Y., et al.: Can. J. Physiol. Pharmacol. *61*:1289–1298, 1983.
23a. Anagnostides, A., Chadwick, V.S., Selden, A.C., et al.: Gastroenterology *87*:109–114, 1984.
24. Greenberg, G.R., McCloy, R.F., Baron, J.H., et al.: Eur. J. Clin. Invest. *12*:361–372, 1982.
25. Pelletier, M.J., Chayvialle, J.A.P., Minaire, Y.: Gastroenterology *75*:1124–1132, 1978.
26. Schaffalitzky de Muckadell, O.B., Fahrenkrug, J., Matzen, P.: Scand. J. Gastroenterol. *14*:55–90, 1979.
27. Meyer, J.H.: Control of pancreatic exocrine secretion. *In* Physiology of the Gastrointestinal Tract. (Johnson, L.R., ed.) New York, Raven Press, 1981, pp. 821–829.
28. Greenberg, G.R., Domschke, S., Domschke, W., et al.: Acta Hepato. Gastroenterol. *26*:478–481, 1979.
29. Walsh, J.H., Lamers, C.B., Valenzuela, J.E.: Gastroenterology *82*:438–444, 1982.
30. Calam, J., Ellis, A., Dockray, G.J.: J. Clin. Invest. *69*:218–225, 1982.
31. Greenberg, G.R., McCloy, R.F., Adrian, T.E., et al.: Lancet *2*:1280–1282, 1978.
32. Chang, T.-M., Chey, W.Y.: Dig. Dis. Sci. *28*:456–468, 1983.
32a. Pappas, T.N., Debas, H.T., and Taylor, I.L.: Gastroenterology *89*:1387–1392, 1985.
33. Hanssen, L.E., Hanssen, K.F., Myren, J., et al.: Scand. J. Gastroenterol *12*:391–394, 1977.
34. Malagelada, J.R., Go, V.L.W., Summerskill, W.H.J.: Gastroenterology *66*:22–27, 1974.
35. Solomon, T.E., Grossman, M.I.: Am. J. Physiol. *236*:E186–E190, 1979.
36. Holst, J.J., Knuhsten, S., Jensen, S.L., et al.: Scand. J. Gastroenterol. *18*:85–99, 1982.
37. Vayasse, N., Batie, M.J., Pascal, J.P., et al.: Gastroenterology *72*:711–718, 1977.
38. Mainz, D.L., Parks, N.M., Webster, P.D.: Proc. Soc. Exp. Biol. Med. *156*:340–344, 1977.
39. Viera-Matos, A.N., Tenenhouse, A.: Can. J. Physiol. Pharmacol. *55*:90–97, 1977.
40. Solomon, T.E.: Regulation of exocrine pancreatic cell proliferation and enzyme synthesis. *In* Physi-

ology of the Gastrointestinal Tract. (Johnson, L.R., ed.) New York, Raven Press, 1981, pp. 873–892.

41. Tandon, B.N., Banks, P.A., George, P.K., et al.: Gastroenterology *58*:358–362, 1970.

42. Kumar, R., Banks, P.A., George, P.K., et al.: Gastroenterology *68*: 1593–1595, 1975.

43. Johnson, L.R., Schanbacher, L.M., Dudrick, S.J., et al.: Am. J. Physiol. *233*: E524–E529, 1977.

44. Koflen, D.P., Levine, G.M.: N. Engl. J. Med. *300*:241–242, 1979.

45. Greenberg, G.R., Wolman, S.L., Christofides, N.D., et al.: Gastroenterology *80*:988–993, 1981.

46. Mainz, D.L., Black, O., Webster, P.D.: J. Clin. Invest. *52*:2300–2304, 1973.

47. Kvoc, M.: Am. J. Physiol. *243*:G69–G75, 1982.

48. Robberecht, P., Deschodt-Lanckman, M., Camus, J., et al.: Am. J. Physiol. *221*:376–381, 1971.

49. Snook, J.T.: Am. J. Physiol. *221*:1383–1387, 1971.

50. Bourdel, G.: Am. J. Physiol. *244*:G125–G130, 1983.

51. Young, E.A., Croletti, L.A., Winborn, W.B., et al.: Am. J. Clin. Nutr. *33*:2106–2118, 1980.

52. Voitk, M.D., Brown, R.A., Echave, V., et al.: Am. J. Surg. *125*:223–227, 1973.

*Chapter* **56**

# NUTRITION AND DIET IN MANAGEMENT OF DISEASES OF THE GASTROINTESTINAL TRACT

## (B) PANCREAS
### (2) Nutritional Support of Patients with Pancreatic Diseases

### Robin I. Russell

Pancreatic insufficiency, or dysfunction of the pancreas, can occur in any disease process affecting the pancreas. Nutritional deficiency may be associated with all types of pancreatic disorders; these include acute pancreatitis, chronic pancreatitis and cystic fibrosis, tumors of the pancreas, pancreatic abscesses, pseudocysts, and fistulas. This chapter will consider each of these conditions, by examining the type and severity of nutritional insufficiency that may occur, and will assess the most appropriate form of nutritional therapy or support in each.

Nutritional therapy ranges from alterations in diet and the use of dietary or nutrient supplements to full enteral or intravenous nutrition regimens.

Enteral feeding can be given by the normal oral route, by nasogastric tube or, if required, by gastrostomy or jejunostomy tubes. The most effective and standard method of providing enteral nutrition is by nasogastric tube, and when enteral feeding is considered in this section, nasogastric tube feeding, set up and monitored in an organized manner, is recommended. Enteral nutrition preparations include nutritional supplements, the defined formula diets comprising polymeric diets, and "elemental" diets (rapidly absorbed in the upper small intestine with minimal digestion). There have been major advances in recent years in the types of preparations and regimens available for both enteral and intravenous feeding, their logical and scientific application, and the techniques available for their safe and effective use. These subjects have all been reviewed.[1-4] (see also Chapter 54).

## ACUTE PANCREATITIS

Patients with severe or complicated pancreatitis may rapidly develop nutritional insufficiency. This condition is compounded by sepsis, metabolic abnormalities, cardiovascular problems and, in some patients, surgical procedures. Although surgery is not commonly performed in patients with acute pancreatitis, a laparotomy may be necessary to confirm the diagnosis. Occasionally, surgically correctable lesions are associated with acute pancreatitis, requiring urgent operation. These patients commonly develop severe or protracted acute pancreatitis that in itself leads to marked nutritional insufficiency. Thus patients requiring surgery are generally those who are most severely malnourished.

**Table 56B2–1.   Value of Various Methods of Nutritional Support in Acute Pancreatitis**

| | |
|---|---|
| Dietary alterations | No value |
| Nutrient supplements | No value |
| Enteral nutrition* | Polymeric diets require full digestion and do not rest the pancreas<br>"Elemental" diets require minimal digestion and may improve nutritional insufficiency, but do not fully rest the pancreas |
| Intravenous nutrition | Provides nutritional support and pancreatic rest |

*Usually by tube feedings.

## Nutritional Changes

Nutritional depletion produced by severe acute pancreatitis has been reported by several groups.[5-7] The nutritional changes in patients with acute pancreatitis have been compared with those in other severe gastrointestinal disorders; the pancreatitis patients differed only slightly from those with generalized gastrointestinal disease with nutritional deficiency.[7] The nutritional deficiency in such patients may be worsened by the fact that specific amino acid deprivation and malnutrition can itself exacerbate pancreatic inflammatory processes.[8] Patients with acute pancreatitis associated with alcoholism may have more severe nutritional insufficiency owing to a preexisting poor nutritional status.

## Nutritional Support

The value of various methods of nutritional support in acute pancreatitis is set forth in Table 56B2–1.

**Dietary Alterations and Nutrient Supplements.**
The nature and severity of acute pancreatitis preclude any value of dietary alterations or oral nutrient supplements in the acute stages of the disease.

More specific nutritional support may be required in acute pancreatitis for two possible reasons. First, this support can improve nutritional insufficiency in the presence of severe illness, especially if surgery may be required or if the patient is at risk of developing other catabolic complications such as abscess, fistula, or pancreatic pseudocyst. A second possible use may be as primary therapy; in this respect, nutritional support may represent active intervention in the pathologic processes that exacerbate the acute disease, improving malnutrition, preventing complications, and decreasing pancreatic exocrine secretion.

The two principal ways of providing such nutritional support are enteral nutrition and intravenous nutrition.

**Enteral Nutrition.** Because acute pancreatitis is generally accompanied by duodenal ileus and gastrointestinal dysfunction that may be prolonged, there would appear to be little place for enteral feeding in the management of nutritional insufficiency associated with acute pancreatitis. Ordinary food and complete oral (whole protein) liquid diets require digestion and are likely to stimulate the pancreas, thus potentially worsening the acute pancreatitis; pancreatic rest is not provided by these preparations. In addition, the associated gastrointestinal dysfunction is likely to prevent the effective use of adequate enteral nutritional support. "Elemental" diets do provide adequate nutrition without the requirements of full digestive processes. However, a number of studies, especially in normal human volunteers, suggest that elemental diets such as Vivonex* and Flexical* do stimulate pancreatic function, although it is possible that stimulation may be less than with normal food. These preparations thus do not wholly rest the pancreas.

The effectiveness of an elemental diet in the pretreatment prophylaxis of experimental canine pancreatitis induced by injection of a bile-saline solution mixture in a retrograde manner into the pancreatic duct has been studied.[9] After the preoperative procedure, half of the dogs from each group were fed Vivonex 100 and the other half ordinary animal laboratory chow. Both nutritional preparations were given preoperatively and postoperatively, thus creating four groups. The successful induction of pancreatitis was assessed by the difference between preoperative and postoperative amylase values. No ultrastructural evidence was found for the modification of zymogen granules with pretreatment by the elemental diet, nor was there evidence histologically or electron-

---

*In the United States, Vivonex has been mainly replaced by Vivonex TEN and Flexical has been completely replaced by Criticare by their respective companies (see Appendix Table A-40 for composition). The composition of Vivonex and Flexical are given in Table A31 of the 6th Edition of this book.

microscopically of any difference in the severity of pancreatitis between the pretreated and non-pretreated groups. Mortality figures demonstrated no efficacy of the Vivonex preparation for pretreatment prophylaxis of acute pancreatitis in this study.

However, a beneficial effect of an "elemental" diet in reducing pancreatic exocrine secretion while providing nutritional support has been reported in patients with severe pancreatitis.[6] Of 11 patients with severe acute pancreatitis who had undergone surgery, 9 completely recovered after receiving jejunostomy feeding exclusively with elemental diets.[10] Blackburn and his colleagues used the polymeric low-fat diet Precision LR (see Appendix Table A40 for composition) in severe acute pancreatitis in patients unable to tolerate a normal diet.[7] These patients were maintained on the diet until the disease allowed consumption of regular food. This stage took 35 ± 23 days, and allowed good nutritional support with minimal requirement for intravenous feeding. In this study, the efficacy of the defined formula diet was repeatedly demonstrated by the failure of many of the patients studied to tolerate regular food and by the prompt recovery from brief attacks of the pancreatitis when the elemental diet was restarted. This study reemphasizes the long time that may be necessary for complete restoration of lean body mass with this form of therapy.

With intravenous nutrition, the principal effect is the improvement of lean body mass and caloric reserves in peripheral tissue.[11] The greater insulin response to intravenous feeding rather than oral feeding and the insulin storage effect on adipose and muscle tissue are largely responsible for the peripheral sequestration of administered proteins. With enteral feeding using defined formula diets, restoration of the distal compartment occurs slowly; in severe stress and sepsis with insulin resistance, further loss of visceral protein is reflected in decreased serum albumin levels. Thus, nutritional repletion could preferentially precede artificially produced hypercatabolic states in the nutritionally depleted patient.

This situation together with the prolonged hospitalization and time required for nutritional improvement using defined formula diets in such patients, makes the use of intravenous feeding the nutritional therapy of choice in severe acute pancreatitis, especially in the more acute phase of the disease. Enteral feeding may be successfully used in the recovery stages of the disease. Furthermore, the associated paralytic ileus may effectively preclude adequate enteral feeding, and most normal foods and complete tube feeds are likely to have undesirable pancreatic stimulatory effects, even if the feeds are tolerated.

**Intravenous Nutrition.** Correction of nutritional insufficiency must be achieved without stimulation of the pancreas, which in turn would lead to further exacerbation of the acute pancreatitis. Intravenous feeding does not significantly stimulate exocrine pancreatic function.[12–17]

Intravenous nutrition can prevent loss of body nitrogen even in the early catabolic phase of injury, but its effectiveness in correcting depleted body protein stores is reduced in this period. The duration and timing of nutritional support are important factors, with short-term support being only able to cover the acute phase of pancreatitis. Longer therapy would be required before any major operative procedure, such as resective surgery, could be undertaken.

Several studies have now been published reporting the effect of intravenous nutrition in the treatment of acute pancreatitis. A reduction was reported of overall mortality from 22 to 14%, which was attributed to improvement of nutritional insufficiency with intravenous feeding.[6] Of 77 patients with severe protracted acute pancreatitis, 13 required surgical therapy such as distal pancreatectomy or total pancreatectomy.[7] These were mostly patients with alcoholism. After preoperative identification of the specific lesion and adequate correction of nutritional insufficiency with intravenous feeding, 11 of the 13 patients without severe disease were operated on with no deaths or significant complications.

Of 15 critically ill patients with acute pancreatitis and with nonfunctioning gastrointestinal tracts, 12 were treated with intravenous nutrition for periods ranging from 1 to 3 months with an overall survival rate of 80%.[18] Intravenous feeding in the early phase of acute pancreatitis was associated with a higher incidence of catheter-related sepsis than is normally seen.[18] Otherwise, there were few technical or metabolic complications. This report suggested that the benefit of intravenous nutrition in these patients lies entirely in the nutritional support and that it has no effect as primary therapy on the acute pancreatitis itself. The treatment had no effect on complications of pancreatitis such as renal failure or respiratory failure. Intravenous nutrition cannot therefore be regarded as primary therapy in acute pancreatitis, but purely as supportive therapy in maintaining or improving the general nutritional state of the patients.

Intravenous nutrition has also been successfully used in a patient with acute relapsing pancreatitis and hypertriglyceridemia during the last two weeks of pregnancy. The therapy reversed maternal weight loss, rapidly settled the pancreatitis, and did not induce further hypertriglyceridemia.[19]

The intravenous feeding regimen used in acute pancreatitis need not differ from those used for ordinary intravenous nutritional support. Silberman and his colleagues studied the safety of a lipid-based intravenous nutrition regimen in patients with acute pancreatitis, and studied lipid profiles in some patients.[20] No exacerbations of the pancreatitis were attributable to intravenous feeding, and the condition resolved or improved in 8 of the 11 patients studied. A positive nitrogen balance was achieved, and nutritional parameters improved. Significant hyperlipidemia was not observed before or during lipid infusions.

## CHRONIC PANCREATIC INSUFFICIENCY

Nutritional insufficiency is commonly present in severe chronic exocrine pancreatic insufficiency.[21]

### Nutritional Changes

Longstanding maldigestion and malabsorption may occur, often with chronic debilitating disease. Even when patients are on maximal pancreatic enzyme supplementation, fecal fat excretion may remain significantly elevated.[22] Deficiency of fat-soluble vitamins is common even in those persons considered adequately treated with pancreatic supplements.[23]

Trace element deficiency may also occur, and one study has demonstrated the importance of pancreatic function in maintaining normal zinc metabolism in man.[24] These authors demonstrated impaired handling of orally administered zinc sulfate, but not zinc dipicolinate, in patients with pancreatic insufficiency. A decrease of zinc output in duodenal aspirate after secretin stimulation of the pancreas in patients with pancreatic insufficiency has also been reported.[25] There is thus abundant evidence of both severe nutritional insufficiency and latent nutritional deficit in patients with chronic pancreatic insufficiency.

### Nutritional Support

The value of various methods of nutritional support in chronic pancreatic insufficiency is set forth in Table 56B2–2.

**Dietary Alterations and Nutrient Supplements.** When maldigestion and malabsorption are present, a diet with a high calorie intake (2,000 to 5,000 kcal/day) is required. This diet should consist principally of carbohydrate and protein. A high-carbohydrate content (400 g/day or more) and a high-protein diet (100 to 150 g/day) is usually desirable. Because steatorrhea may be a problem in such patients, a low-fat diet has attractions, and a diet containing 40 to 50 g of fat per day may be given. To maintain a high calorie content, however, fat is required in the diet and may be best provided by using medium-chain triglycerides. These are more easily absorbed than ordinary dietary fat because hydrolysis using pancreatic lipase is unnecessary for their absorption.

When diabetes mellitus is present, carbohydrate restriction in relation to other diabetic treatment may be necessary.

Supplements of fat-soluble vitamins such as vitamins A, D, and K may also be required. In addition, vitamin $B_{12}$ supplements may be necessary.

**Enteral Nutrition.** In mild cases of pancreatic insufficiency, nutritional supplements and adequate amounts of pancreatic enzyme preparations are all that are necessary to replace any deficiencies that may be present as a result of the pancreatic disease.

In more severe deficiency states, full enteral

**Table 56B2–2.　Value of Various Methods of Nutritional Support in Chronic Pancreatic Insufficiency**

| | |
|---|---|
| Dietary alterations | High-calorie intake<br>　high-protein, high-carbohydrate<br>　medium-chain triglycerides |
| Nutrient supplements | Fat-soluble vitamins (A,D,K)<br>　vitamin $B_{12}$ may also be necessary<br>Pancreatic enzyme supplements |
| Enteral nutrition* | Polymeric diets require digestive capability<br>　from pancreas but may improve nutritional<br>　status if given with pancreatic enzyme<br>　supplements<br>"Elemental" diets, improve nutritional status<br>　without requiring exocrine pancreatic<br>　function |
| Intravenous nutrition | Rarely necessary, but effective if required |

*Usually by tube feedings.

**Table 56B2–3.    Effect of "Elemental" Diets on Pancreatic Enzyme Secretion in Dogs**

| Preparation | Route of Administration | Effect | Reference |
|---|---|---|---|
| Flexical | Oral | Inhibits enzyme secretion | 26 |
| | Oral | Inhibits pancreatic trypsinogen | 27 |
| Flexical | Oral | Inhibits pancreatic trypsinogen and reduces secretion | 28 |
| Vivonex | Intrajejunal | Inhibits secretion | 29 |
| | Intragastric | Stimulates secretion | |
| Vivonex | Intraduodenal | Stimulates volume and protein output | 30 |
| Vivonex | Intrajejunal | Reduces enzyme concentration | 31 |
| Vivonex | Oral | Stimulates pancreas | 32 |
| Vivonex | Oral and intraduodenal | Stimulates protein response and reduces water and bicarbonate production | 33 |
| Vivonex | Oral | Stimulates pancreas | 9 |
| Vivonex | Oral | Inhibits enzyme response | 34 |
| Flexical Vivonex | Oral | Both stimulate enzyme response; less stimulation occurs with Vivonex | 35 |
| Vivonex HN | Oral Gastrostomy Jejunostomy | Reduces synthesis and release of enzymes | 36 |

**Table 56B2–4.    Effect of "Elemental" Diets on Exocrine Pancreatic Secretion in Normal Human Subjects**

| Preparation | Route of Administration | Effect | Reference |
|---|---|---|---|
| Flexical | Oral | Stimulates enzyme secretion to same level as control diet | 37 |
| Vivonex | Intraduodenal | Stimulates enzyme secretion | 38 |
| Vivonex | Oral | Stimulates enzyme secretion | 39 |
| Vivonex | Intraduodenal | Reduces trypsin concentration | 40 |

nutrition regimens given by nasogastric tube may be indicated. Complete oral (whole protein) liquid diets require reasonable exocrine pancreatic function to allow adequate digestion and therefore adequate absorption of nutrients. Thus, in many patients with chronic pancreatic insufficiency, these preparations may not be adequate to correct nutritional insufficiency, although the use of concomitant pancreatic enzyme supplements may be helpful. (These preparations may be destroyed by acid in the stomach; antacids or H2-receptor antagonists should thus be given with them for long-term use.) Elemental diets, however, present nutrients to the alimentary tract in a predigested form, thus requiring minimal digestion before adequate absorption. A number of studies have examined the effect of these preparations on pancreatic exocrine secretion in animals and man.[3] These results are summarized in Tables 56B2–3 and 56B2–4, respectively.

Many of the early animal studies suggested a reduction or even absence of pancreatic exocrine stimulation by these preparations. Some later animal work, however, has shown that some pan-

creatic stimulation does occur. There have been few good studies in man, but they have generally shown exocrine pancreatic stimulation with both Vivonex and Flexical. This stimulation may be somewhat less than with normal food.

Amino acids are stimulators of pancreatic secretion when infused into the upper small intestine, but intragastric administration of amino acids causes less marked pancreatic stimulation. Intrajejunal glucose inhibits pancreatic secretion. However, there is no clear indication that less pancreatic stimulation occurs when elemental diets are administered directly into the duodenum compared with the oral route. Any reduction of pancreatic enzyme activity may be related to the lower nitrogen content of the elemental diet, although further work is required on this aspect.

Differing results would be expected in such a widely varying series of studies. Different formulations and concentrations of preparations have been used. Rates of infusion were different, and the results may vary depending upon the method of giving the preparations—orally, intragastrically, or by direct intraduodenal or intrajejunal infusion. Different ways of measuring exocrine pancreatic secretion have also been employed in these studies.

The principal value of elemental-type diets in chronic pancreatic insufficiency may thus lie in allowing effective absorption of nutrients in the absence of normal pancreatic enzyme secretory function.

Vivonex has been reported to be successful in the management of patients with chronic pancreatic insufficiency.[41] These patients presented with marked steatorrhea, weight loss, and weakness and had not improved with pancreatic supplements. The use of this diet, either as the sole source of nutrition or as a supplement of normal food, improved the nutritional status of seven of the eight patients. However, some evidence suggests that the apparent biologic value of the amino acid content of this preparation may be less in terms of nitrogen balance efficacy than that of other amino acid sources in liquid formulas (e.g., casein hydrolysate).[41a]

Because patients with chronic pancreatic insufficiency may also have diabetes mellitus, the additional glucose load supplied by Vivonex may complicate diabetic control and may necessitate an adjustment of insulin dosage.

A formula such as Flexical has also been successfully used as the sole source of nutrition in patients with chronic pancreatic insufficiency, some of whom have complications.[5]

**Intravenous Nutrition.** In a few instances, intravenous feeding is indicated in patients with chronic pancreatic insufficiency. The use of intravenous nutrition infers either a major degree of urgency of correction of nutritional insufficiency and/or major dysfunction of the gastrointestinal tract. Although maldigestion with subsequent malabsorption occurs in these patients, this condition is rarely severe enough to preclude the use of the alimentary tract for adequate nutritional support, even in the presence of nutritional insufficiency.

If intravenous feeding is required in a patient with chronic pancreatic insufficiency, the issue of the safety of IV fat arises. Some reports (mainly case reports) associate high-concentration IV lipid with onset or exacerbation of pancreatitis.[41b] Furthermore, IV fat has been used in treating acute pancreatitis without untoward effects[6,7,18–20] and, despite its wide general use, reports of induction of pancreatitis are uncommon. IV lipid given to rats with experimental pancreatitis did not exacerbate pancreatic changes or increase mortality as compared to controls.[41c]

The use of fat to provide significant calories decreases the need for insulin in the patient who has diabetes mellitus. In addition, intravenous insulin in the IV container allows good diabetes control after a brief adjustment period to establish the patient's need for regular insulin in relation to the glucose load. Glucose replacements (e.g., fructose or sorbitol used in some countries outside the United States) may be used to minimize insulin needs.

There are no reported series of patients with chronic pancreatic insufficiency treated with intravenous nutrition. Occasionally, and as a last resort in the management of pain associated with chronic pancreatitis, total pancreatectomy may be performed. During and following this procedure, a full program of intravenous nutritional support is required.

## CYSTIC FIBROSIS

Children with cystic fibrosis have long been known to suffer from chronic nutritional deficiency.

### Nutritional Changes

Children with cystic fibrosis frequently have poor growth,[42] may develop deficiency of fat-soluble vitamins (A, D, E, and K), and have low serum concentrations of albumin and urea nitrogen.[43] Trace element deficiency may also occur. Negative retention of zinc in metabolic studies of children with cystic fibrosis has been reported.[44] Growth failure in cystic fibrosis is more closely related to chronic pulmonary disease than to malabsorption,[45] which can generally be well controlled with efficient use of pancreatic supplements. However, deficient energy intake is also a reason for growth failure in cystic fibrosis. Many children consume only 80% of their requirements of energy and protein. This finding becomes more important in the presence of chronic infection, when energy intake requires an increase of 30% to satisfy increased metabolic needs.

### Nutritional Support

The value of various methods of nutritional support in cystic fibrosis is set forth in Table 56B2–5.

**Dietary Alterations and Nutrient Supplements.** Many patients with cystic fibrosis have chronic exocrine pancreatic insufficiency and associated maldigestion and malabsorption. A high caloric intake with a high-protein, high-carbohydrate, and low-fat diet may be of value in these patients.[46] Medium-chain triglycerides may be of particular value in view of their more effective absorption in the presence of exocrine pancreatic insufficiency. If secondary disaccharidase deficiency is present, a lactose-free diet is indicated. Fat-soluble vitamin supplements (A, D, K) may

**Table 56B2–5.    Value of Various Methods of Nutritional Support in Cystic Fibrosis**

| | |
|---|---|
| Dietary alterations | High-caloric intake<br>high-protein, high-carbohydrate<br>medium-chain triglycerides |
| Nutrient supplements | Fat-soluble vitamins (A,D,K)<br>Pancreatic enzyme supplements<br>Sodium chloride |
| Enteral nutrition* | Polymeric diets require pancreatic digestive capability but may be of value with pancreatic enzyme supplements<br>"Elemental" diets effective in improving nutritional status; palatability problem is overcome by tube feeding |
| Intravenous nutrition | Effective if required |

*Usually by tube feeding.

also be required. Owing to the excess loss of sodium in patients with cystic fibrosis, sodium chloride supplements, 2 to 3 g/day, may be necessary.

**Enteral Nutrition.** The effective use of various full enteral nutritional preparations given by nasogastric tube—polymeric diets and elemental diets—is similar to that in chronic pancreatic insufficiency. Polymeric preparations require digestion and, in theory, they may not be effective in improving nutritional status unless adequate pancreatic enzyme supplementation is also given. Elemental diets, however, that require minimal digestion may be of value in these patients. The importance of nutritional support has been well recognized in children with cystic fibrosis. Growth has been satisfactorily stimulated and nutrition improved by the use of enteral nutrition regimens using nasogastric feeding in several studies.[46–49] In most patients, long-term nutritional support is required, often using the technique of home enteral feeding.[50] There is no evidence of improvement of pulmonary problems by nutritional support.[51] The use of elemental diets would seem likely to be more effective than polymeric diets in cystic fibrosis, and improvement has been reported using these preparations.[47,52] However, palatability difficulties may preclude their fully effective use. Polymeric diets can also be helpful in cystic fibrosis. In one study, 10 patients with malnutrition resistant to oral supplementation and moderate to severe lung disease were fed a polymeric diet via a jejunostomy tube.[53] The nutritional state improved but little change in lung function occurred; few technical problems were found.

**Intravenous Nutrition.** In some patients with cystic fibrosis in whom severe nutritional deficiency is unresponsive to dietary alterations, nutrient supplements, or various specific forms of enteral nutrition, intravenous feeding may be

required. Nutritional improvement can be achieved with such feedings in these children,[46] and may be used to initially improve nutritional status before the introduction of long-term enteral nutrition.

## TUMORS OF PANCREAS

Many nutritional and metabolic changes occur with pancreatic tumors, as with other cancers.

### Nutritional Changes

Most patients with advanced pancreatic tumors have demonstrable abnormalities of carbohydrate, fat, and protein metabolism, together with vitamin and mineral deficiencies. The combination of these metabolic abnormalities is a factor in causing cancer cachexia; this finding accounts for a number of deaths from malignant disease and is characterized by a hypercatabolic state associated with anorexia and resulting in malnutrition, weight loss, and wasting of lean body mass.[54,55] Cancer cachexia is frequently worsened by the therapeutic modalities employed in the treatment of the cancer: surgery, radiotherapy, and cytotoxic chemotherapy. Reduced oral food intake associated with severe anorexia or aversion to food in patients with malignant tumors also contribute to protein-calorie malnutrition.

In patients with carcinoma of the pancreas, weight loss is almost invariable, frequently dramatic and progressive, and may precede other symptoms. Aversion to food is common early in the course of the disease. Pain, diabetes mellitus, maldigestion, and malabsorption all contribute to the nutritional deficiency. Pancreatic cancer may itself be associated with chronic pancreatic insufficiency, and indeed may follow from preexisting chronic pancreatic insufficiency. A background of nutritional deficiency may exist in these patients before the development of the tumor. Maldigestion and malabsorption may dominate the clinical picture for 9 to 12 months before the onset of the other features of the tumor. Severe nutritional deficiency contributes to weakness and debility, delayed wound healing, predisposition to bed sores, impaired immunity, and increased morbidity and mortality.

## Nutritional Support

Because untreated tumors of pancreas are almost invariably progressive, nutritional support in these patients has concentrated on its application as an adjunct to cancer therapy. The rationale for nutritional support in such patients is to reduce the complications of nutritional insufficiency, possibly to improve the therapeutic response of the malnourished patient, and to reduce the morbidity from treatment.[54] When surgery is performed, further catabolic influences worsen the nutritional state of the patient. Regional pancreatectomy may be performed for tumors of the pancreas in these patients, the operation being commonly followed by severe diarrhea and malabsorption, the development of severe nutritional deficiency with magnesium and zinc deficiency, and impairment of protein and fat absorption.[55,56] Prolonged diarrhea and malabsorption may occur, but may improve after some months of nutritional support.

**Dietary Alterations and Nutrient Supplements.** Good general oral nutritional support together with the correction of any deficiencies of vitamins, minerals, and trace elements is important. A major problem, however, is the persistent aversion to food that may be present. Some improvement may be possible with good dietary advice and encouragement, but in many instances alternative means of providing nutritional support will be required.

**Enteral Nutrition.** Enteral nutrition may have less part to play in the management of patients with pancreatic tumors than in the management of those with other malignant tumors. Associated chronic pancreatic insufficiency may cause sufficient maldigestion and consequent malabsorption to preclude the effective use of whole-protein liquid diets in many patients, and there is no reported series of patients with pancreatic tumors treated in this way.

Elemental diets have been used to improve the nutritional status of patients with pancreatic tumors with accompanying exocrine pancreatic insufficiency,[57,58] their value being increased in such patients because of their minimal digestion requirements. These preparations have also been used to improve nutritional status in patients with other tumors, although palatability problems reduce their practical effectiveness. Polymeric preparations are likely to be more palatable than elemental diets, and may be at least as effective in nutritional improvement.

Because nutritional support generally needs to be rapidly effective in such patients to improve nutritional status before surgery, radiotherapy, or chemotherapy, enteral nutrition is unlikely to have a major role to play in patients with pancreatic tumors.

**Intravenous Nutrition.** In patients with pancreatic tumors in whom rapid nutritional improvement is required, intravenous feeding may be necessary. The alimentary tract may be functioning satisfactorily in such patients, although some pancreatic insufficiency may be present and may affect the prospects of effective enteral nutritional support. In many instances, however, the necessary medical workup interferes with tube feeding; furthermore, rapid improvement is required before surgery, radiotherapy, or chemotherapy. In these patients, intravenous feeding is the most effective and certain way of improving nutritional support within a short period. When surgery such as regional pancreatectomy is performed, intravenous nutrition is generally required, not only to cover the operation itself, but also to maintain the nutritional state worsened by prolonged severe diarrhea and malabsorption (perhaps over several months, after which time improvement may occur).[59] Occasionally complete pancreatectomy is performed for tumor, with full intravenous nutritional support required to cover the period of surgery and often for the time following the operation.

As with other tumors, there is no evidence to suggest that the provision of nutritional support, either intravenous or enteral, has any primary effect on the tumor itself.

## ABSCESSES, PSEUDOCYSTS, AND FISTULAS OF THE PANCREAS

Abscesses of the pancreas are an infrequent but serious complication of acute pancreatitis and are associated with significant morbidity and mortality.[54] These patients often develop severe nutritional insufficiency, due initially to the acute pancreatitis and thereafter to the continuing catabolic effect of chronic infection associated with the abscess. The mortality rate is high.

Management of the nutritional insufficiency is complicated by markedly delayed gastric emptying that may persist even after drainage of the abscess.[60,61] The use of intravenous nutrition with a central venous line may be more hazardous than usual in patients with sepsis. In one report, three patients with pancreatic abscess were given satisfactory nutritional support with an elemental diet using Vivonex. This diet was administered via a feeding jejunostomy introduced at the time of drainage of the abscess, together with a gastrostomy for gastric decompression.[62] This treatment allowed progressive nutritional improvement over four weeks.

Pancreatic pseudocysts are commonly associated with prolonged ill health, weight loss, and deterioration of nutritional status. In such patients, the diagnosis may be delayed, thus leading to a further deterioration of the patient's nutritional state. When the diagnosis has been made, surgical drainage is required. Before surgery and postoperatively, the nutritional status may need to be improved. This change is best achieved by intravenous feeding, which provides effective nutritional support and rapid nutritional improvement. In one study, Flexical was successfully used in the management of pancreatic pseudocysts associated with pancreatic fistulas.[5]

Pancreatic fistulas can follow acute pancreatitis and can be particularly resistant to treatment, leading to progressive nutritional insufficiency and ill health. These fistulas are notoriously difficult to treat. The use of nutritional support together with bowel rest has been of value in promoting healing of a wide range of gastrointestinal fistulas. Pancreatic fistulas have been reported to heal with intravenous feeding and bowel rest.[63,64] Most reports, however, have been of small numbers of patients. No detrimental effect of fat emulsions has been reported in the intravenous regimens of patients with pancreatic fistulas.[16]

It would seem unlikely that enteral nutrition with ordinary food or polymeric diets would be of value in providing bowel and pancreatic rest with improvement of nutritional insufficiency in patients with pancreatic fistulas. However, the use of an elemental diet may be of value, and encouraging nutritional improvement has occurred with the use of Flexical in individual patients.[65] Flexical has also been used effectively in the management of individual patients with pancreatic fistulas associated with pancreatic pseudocysts.[5] A positive nitrogen balance, weight gain, resolution of sepsis, and closure of the pancreatic fistulas were achieved in five of the six patients. Improvement of nutritional status, the low-residue nature of the preparations, and pancreatic rest provided by the elemental diet may have been beneficial. However, controlled studies comparing the use of elemental diets and intravenous feeding, with respect to nutritional support and bowel and pancreatic rest in the healing of pancreatic fistulas, have not yet been performed.

## REFERENCES

1. Tweedle, D.E.F.: Metabolic Care. London, Churchill Livingstone, 1982.
2. Russell, R.I.: Intravenous nutrition and elemental diets. *In* Scientific Foundations of Gastroenterology. London, Heineman, 1980, pp. 130–140.
3. Russell, R.I.: Elemental Diets. Boca Raton, Florida, CRC Press, 1981.
4. Russell, R.I.: Enteral feeding. *In* Clinical Nutrition and Gastroenterology. (Heatley, V., Kelleher, J., Losowsky, M.S., Eds.) London, Churchill Livingstone, 1987, pp. 97–115.
5. Voitk, A., Brown, R.A., Echave, V., et al.: Am. J. Surg. *125*:223–227, 1973.
6. Feller, J.H., Brown, R.A., Toussaint, G.P., et al.: Am. J. Surg. *127*:196–201, 1974.
7. Blackburn, G.L., Williams, L.F., Bistrian, B.R., et al.: Am. J. Surg. *131*:114–124, 1976.
8. Farber, E., Popper, H.: Proc. Soc. Exp. Biol. Med. *74*:838–840, 1950.
9. Kerstein, M.D., Tonkens, R.M.: Surg. Gynecol. Obstet. *143*:253–256, 1976.
10. Baulieux, J., Boulez, J., Peix, J.L., et al.: Chirurgie *107*:59–63, 1981.
11. Blackburn, G.L., Bistrian, B.R., Flatt, J.P., et al.: Clin. Res. *23*:315A, 1975.
12. Lawson, L.J.: Br. J. Surg. *52*:795–800, 1965.
13. DenBesten, L., Reyna, R., Connor, W., et al.: J. Clin. Invest. *75*:1384–1393, 1973.
14. Adler, N., Pieroni, P.L., Takeshima, T., et al.: Surg. Forum *26*:445–446, 1975.
15. Johnson, L.R., Schandbacher, L.M., Dudrick, S.J., et al.: Am. J. Physiol. *233*:E.524–529, 1977.
16. Grundfest, S., Steiger, E., Selinkoff, P., et al.: J. Parenter. Enter. Nutr. *4*:27–31, 1980.
17. Hughes, C.A., Prince, A., Dowling, R.H.: Clin. Sci. *59*:329–336, 1980.
18. Goodgame, J.T., Fischer, J.E.: Ann. Surg. *186*:651–658, 1977.
19. Weinberg, R.B., Itrin, M.D., Adkins, G.M., et al.: Gastroenterology *83*:1300–1305, 1982.
20. Silberman, H., Dixon, N.P., Eisenberg, D.: Am. J. Gastroenterol. *77*:494–497, 1982.
21. Brooks, F.P.: Chronic and relapsing pancreatitis. *In* Diseases of the Exocrine Pancreas. Philadelphia, W.B. Saunders Co., 1980, pp 4–83.
22. DiMagno, E.P., Malagelada, J.R., Go, V.L.W., et al.: N. Engl. J. Med. *296*:1318–1322, 1977.
23. Dutta, S.K., Bustin, M.P., Russell, R.M., et al.: Ann. Intern Med. *97*:549–552, 1982.
24. Boosalis, M.G., Evans, G.W., McClain, C.J.: Am. J. Clin. Nutr. *37*:268–271, 1983.
25. Adler, P.J., Robbrecht, P., Mestdagh, M., et al.: Clin. Biol. *4*:441–449, 1980.
26. Bounous, G., Sutherland, N.G., McArdle, A.H., et al.: Surg. *166*:312–343, 1967.
27. Brown, R.A., Thompson, H.E., McArdle, A.H., et al.: Surg. Forum *21*:391–393, 1970.
28. McArdle, A.H., Echave, W., Brown, R, et al.: Am. J. Surg. *128*:690–692, 1974.
29. Ragins, H., Levenson, S.M., Signer, R., et al.: Am. J. Surg. *126*:606–614, 1973.
30. Wolfe, B.M., Keltner, R.M., Kaminsky, D.L.: Surg. Gynecol. Obstet. *140*:241–245, 1975.
31. Cassim, M.M., Allardyce, D.P.: Ann. Surg. *180*:228–231, 1974.
32. Kerstein, M.D., Neviackas, J.A.: Am. J. Gastroenterol. *66*:460–463, 1976.

33. Kelly, G.A., Nahrwold, D.L.: Surg. Gynecol. Obstet. *143*:87–91, 1976.
34. Neviackas, J.A., Kerstein, M.D.: Surg. Gynecol. Obstet. *142*:71–74, 1976.
35. Lewis, J.W., Freeman, J.B.: Can. J. Surg. *20*:345–350, 1977.
36. Traverso, L.W., Abou-Zamzam, A.M., Maxwell, D.S., et al.: J. Parenter. Enter. Nutr. *5*:496–500, 1981.
37. Perrault, J., Devroede, G., Bounous, G.: Gastroenterology *64*:569–576, 1973.
38. Vidon, N., Hecketsweiler, P., Butel, J., et al.: Gut *19*:194–198, 1978.
39. Atherton, S.T., Nelson, L.M., Russell, R.I.: Scott. Med. J. *23*:115, 1978.
40. Panayiotides, T., Christofides, N., Bjornsson, O.G., et al.: Gut *20*:A450, 1979.
41. Pincus, I.J., Citron, P.P., Haverback, B.J.: *In* Balanced Nutrition and Therapy. Stuttgart, George Thieme Verlag, 1971, pp. 77–80.
41a. Smith, H., Arteaga, C., Heymsfield, S.B.: N. Engl. J. Med. *306*:1013–1018, 1982.
41b. Lashner, B.A., Kirsner, J.B., Hanauer, S.B.: Gastroenterology *90*:1039–1041, 1986.
41c. Raasch, R.H., Hak, L.J., Benaim, V., et al.: J. Parenter. Enter. Nutr. *7*:254–256, 1983.
42. Sproul, A., Huang, N.: J. Pediatr. *65*:664–676, 1964.
43. Berry, H.K., Kellogg, F.W., Hunt, M., et al.: Am. J. Dis. Child. *129*:165–171, 1975.
44. Aggett, P.J., Thorn, J.M., Delves, H.T., et al.: Monogr. Pediatr. *19*:8–11, 1979.
45. Kraemer, R., Rudeberg, A., Hadorn, B., et al.: Acta Paediatr. Scand. *67*:33–37, 1978.
46. Shepherd, R, Cooksley, W.G.E., Domville-Cooke, W.D.: J. Pediatr. *97*:351–357, 1980.
47. Bertrand, J.M., Morin, C.L., Lasalle, R., et al.: J. Pediatr. *104*:41–46, 1984.
48. Shepherd, R.W., Thomas, B.J., Bennett, D., et al.: J. Pediatr. Gastroenterol. Nutr. *2*:439–446, 1983.
49. Levy, L.D., Durie, P., Pencharz, P.B., et al.: J. Pediatr. *107*:225–230, 1985.
50. Main, A.N.H., Morgan, R.J., Hall, M.J., et al.: Scot. Med. J. *25*:312–314, 1980.
51. Editorial: Lancet *1*:249–251, 1986.
52. Yassa, J.G., Prosser, R., Dodge, J.A.: Arch. Dis. Child. *53*:777–783, 1978.
53. Boland, M.P., Stoski, D.S., MacDonald, N.E., et al.: Lancet *1*:232–234, 1986.
54. Copeland, E.M., MacFadyen, B.V., Dudrick, S.J.: J. Surg. Res. *16*:241–247, 1974.
55. Fortner, J.G.: Cancer *47*:1712–1718, 1981.
56. Fortner, J.G., Kim, D.K., Cubilla, A., et al.: Ann. Surg. *186*:42–50, 1977.
57. Calman, K.C.: Proc. Nutr. Soc. *37*:87–93, 1978.
58. Trotter, J.M., Calman, K.C.: *In* Elemental Diets. (Russell, R.I., Ed.) Boca Raton, Florida, 1981, pp. 175–186.
59. Holden, J.L., Berne, T.V., Rosoff, L.: Arch. Surg. *11*:858–861, 1976.
60. Evans, F.C.: Am. J. Surg. *117*:537–540, 1969.
61. Miller, T.A., Lindenauer, S.M., Frey, C.F., et al.: Arch. Surg. *108*:545–551, 1974.
62. Paloyan, D., Simonowitz, D., Bates, R.J.: Am. J. Gastroenterol. *69*:97–100, 1978.
63. Dudrick, S.J., Wilmore, D.W., Steiger, E., et al.: J. Trauma *10*:542–553, 1970.
64. Owings, J.M., Bomar, W.E., Ramage, R.C.: Ann. Surg. 1975: 712–718, 1972.
65. Bury, K.D., Stephens, R.V., Randall, H.T.: Am. J. Surg. *121*:174–183, 1971.

*Chapter* **56**

# NUTRITION AND DIET IN MANAGEMENT OF DISEASES OF THE GASTROINTESTINAL TRACT

## (C) SMALL INTESTINE
### (1) Effects of Intestinal Disease on Digestion and Absorption

### Mukesh B. Desai and Khursheed N. Jeejeebhoy

## LUMINAL ABNORMALITIES OF DIGESTION

**Blind Loop Syndrome.** The normal human small bowel is sterile or has few bacteria. With the exception of the terminal ileum, there are few anaerobic organisms in the small bowel. Conditions that reduce the motility of the bowel and promote stasis, such as scleroderma, intestinal pseudo-obstruction, or small bowel diverticulosis promote the growth of anaerobic bacteria in the upper small intestine. This condition also occurs with strictures of the small intestine and fistulous communications between the small and large bowel.

The presence of a heavy bacterial growth, especially of anaerobes, results in deconjugation (removal of amino acid groups) and 7-dehydroxylation of bile salts. These deconjugated and dehydroxylated bile salts are either insoluble and precipitate or, because they have lost a polar group (amino acid), become lipid-soluble and diffuse back through the intestinal mucosal surface. Because of back diffusion, deconjugation reduces the intestinal concentration of bile salts to below the critical micellar concentration, thus decreasing fat absorption.[1]

Bacteria utilize dietary vitamin $B_{12}$, causing a deficiency of this vitamin and thus a megaloblas-tic anemia.[2] Bacterial deamination of amino acids also affects the availability of protein and may cause hypoproteinemia.[3] In addition, there is bacterially mediated injury to the enterocyte.[4]

## ABNORMALITIES OF INTESTINAL SURFACE ENZYMES

The most common deficiency of intestinal surface enzymes is lactase deficiency. The lack of lactase results in the malabsorption of dietary lactose, which then enters the colon and is metabolized by colonic bacteria into short-chain fatty acids. The malabsorbed lactose and its bacterial decomposition products cause diarrhea when persons who are lactase-deficient drink sufficient amounts of milk or milk products. The diagnostic clinical features of lactase deficiency are the development of bloating, cramps, and diarrhea after the ingestion of milk or milk-containing foods. Newer fabricated foods may have sources of lactose. In addition, drugs may contain lactose as "binders." The patient may not recognize that his diarrhea is due to lactose intolerance when this disaccharide is present in less obvious forms. Appendix Table A-34 provides a list of the concentrations of lactose in various foods.

Sucrase deficiency is a rare condition where ingestion of sucrose (a disaccharide of fructose and glucose) causes diarrhea. Occasionally, sucrase deficiency may be masked in early life and present later when patients may become addicted to drinking tea or coffee with much sugar. Honey, which has invert sugar (i.e., hydrolyzed sucrose) does not require sucrase.

## DIFFUSE MUCOSAL DISEASE

Various diseases can cause diffuse damage to the small intestine by a variety of processes. These may result in (1) mucosal atrophy, as in celiac and tropical sprue, (2) infiltration, as in Whipple's disease, amyloidosis, or lymphoma, (3) diffuse ulceration, as with microulcerative jejunitis, or (4) extensive parasitic colonization, as with *Giardia lamblia* infestation in a person with a common varied immunoglobulin deficiency. All these processes cause malabsorption of various substances. Mucosal disease is also associated with a reduction in the levels of disaccharidases with resultant inhibition of the hydrolysis of disaccharides. Diffuse mucosal disease inhibits the transport of proteins, carbohydrates, fats, vitamins, and minerals in a nonselective way. Such patients have diarrhea, severe weight loss, and signs of vitamin deficiency with glossitis, stomatitis, edema, and neuropathy. They may have tetany due to magnesium deficiency and resulting hypocalcemia. Metabolic bone disease may occur, as well as osteomalacia. In addition, vitamin K deficiency may cause hypoprothrombinemia and edema.

**Celiac Sprue (Gluten Enteropathy).** This is the most common and most important member of the group of conditions that cause diffuse mucosal lesions. It has an incidence of 1:3,000 (1:300 in Ireland),[5] is most common in HLA B1 and B8 tissue types, and may present at all ages from infancy to senescence. The disease is characterized by villous atrophy, predominantly affecting the proximal small bowel, and is caused by exposure to a specific wheat peptide called gliadin. Gliadin is a constituent of gluten, which is present in wheat, rye, barley, and oats.[6] The mechanism of villous damage is still uncertain but may be mediated by immune injury in response to the ingestion of gluten.[7,8] A genetic predisposition may exist.[9] By definition, exclusion of gluten from the diet causes a return to normal of the intestinal epithelium. Although steatorrhea is usually present, selective deficiency of other nutrients such as iron also may occur. In the full-blown disease, there is malabsorption of fat, protein, calcium, magnesium, vitamins A, D, and K, and folates. Even vitamin $B_{12}$ can be malabsorbed in severe cases in which the villous atrophy involves the whole small bowel. In addition to these deficiencies, several other complications may arise. These include an increased incidence of esophageal cancer, reticulum cell sarcoma of the intestine,[10] ulcerative jejunoileitis,[11] intestinal pseudo-obstruction,[12] and pulmonary fibrosis.

Celiac disease is diagnosed by (1) demonstrating malabsorption of fat and D-xylose, (2) showing dilation of the small intestine with flocculation and segmentation of barium in a small bowel meal, (3) demonstrating villous atrophy on small bowel biopsy, and (4) its returning to normal on a gluten-free diet.

Partial villous atrophy also occurs in other conditions, which include severe malnutrition, dermatitis herpetiformis (DH),[13] tropical sprue,[14] intestinal lymphoma,[15] and hypogammaglobulinemia.[16] The villous atrophy of DH appears to be identical to that of celiac disease and responds to gluten exclusion.[17]

**Tropical Sprue.** This condition affects inhabitants of, and visitors to, tropical countries,[18] but curiously is rare in Africa. It is believed to be caused by infection of the intestinal mucosa by an unidentified organism and is characterized pathologically by villous atrophy similar to, but less severe than, that of celiac disease. Usually it presents with diarrhea, weight loss, steatorrhea, and folate deficiency. Although symptoms generally commence in the tropics, they are delayed occasionally until return to more temperate climes. Diagnosis is based on travel history, an abnormal intestinal biopsy, and a good response to treatment with folic acid and a broad-spectrum antibiotic.

**Infiltrative Lesions.** These lesions include those of lymphoma, Whipple's disease, amyloidosis, and tuberculosis.

*Lymphoma of Small Intestine.* This condition may be confined to the gut, may be part of a generalized reticulosis, or may occur as a complication of long-standing celiac disease.[19] It presents with weight loss, diarrhea, abdominal pain, or perforation and, in the case of celiac disease, an increase in IgA level may occur. Any part of the gut may be involved, especially the distal ileum where the richest aggregation of lymphatic tissue exists. Diagnosis is often difficult, but ulceration, mucosal infiltration, and irregular dilatation may be demonstrated by a small bowel barium meal. In many cases, laparotomy is required for confirmation.

*Whipple's Disease.* This is a rare condition caused by infection with a bacilliform organism that is present not only in the lamina propria but also in the heart, lymph nodes, and central nervous system.[20] The usual clinical presentation is with weight loss, arthritis, pigmentation, splenomegaly, diarrhea, and sometimes dementia and myoclonus. Small bowel biopsy reveals large numbers of PAS-positive macrophages in the lamina propria together with intracellular bacteria. Treatment with penicillin and streptomycin usually elicits a good response.

*Amyloid Infiltration of Small Bowel.* This condition may occur in both primary and secondary types of amyloidosis. Such involvement is rarely of clinical significance, but occasionally gives rise to mild malabsorption. Small bowel barium studies show thickened folds that produce a "picket fence" appearance. However, this appearance is also found in patients with Whipple's disease, intestinal edema, ischemia, lymphoma, and macroglobulinemia. The presumptive diagnosis is confirmed by small bowel biopsy that shows perivascular depositions of amyloid.

## INTESTINAL INFECTIONS AND INFESTATIONS

Malabsorption may be caused by infestation, most commonly with *Giardia lamblia.* In patients with AIDS syndrome, intractable diarrhea and malabsorption may occur as a result of cryptosporidial and other infections, resulting in intestinal villous atrophy, steatorrhea, and diarrhea.[21]

## ABNORMALITIES OF INTESTINAL LYMPHATIC FUNCTION

Failure of normal intestinal lymphatic drainage results in steatorrhea, iron deficiency, and enteric loss of protein. Lymphatic dysfunction occurs in many diseases including intestinal lymphangiectasia,[22] tuberculosis,[23] Crohn's disease,[24] severe heart failure,[25] lymphoma, and retroperitoneal fibrosis. Apart from intestinal lymphangiectasia, the features of lymphatic obstruction are usually overshadowed by those of the underlying disease. In primary lymphangiectasia, there is a congenital defect in the lymphatic system affecting not only the gut but also other parts of the body such as the legs and arms. A mild degree of steatorrhea is present, edema occurs secondarily to hypoproteinemia, hematologic examination reveals iron deficiency anemia and lymphopenia, and tests of enteric protein loss are abnormal. Small bowel biopsies show cystic dilatation of the villous lymphatics.

Immune surveillance is defective as a result of intestinal loss of lymphocytes and gammaglobulin, and patients with lymphangiectasia have an increased incidence of reticulosis. A similar degree of protein loss can complicate many other gastrointestinal diseases. The more important of these are Menetrier's disease, Crohn's disease, celiac disease, lymphomas, and ulcerative colitis.

Protein-losing gastroenteropathy can be confirmed by measuring fecal radioactivity after the intravenous administration of $^{51}CrCl_3$.

## RADIATION INJURY

The gastrointestinal tract is the second most sensitive organ to the effects of radiation, the first being bone marrow.

### Morphologic Changes Following Radiation[26,27]

**Acute Changes.** The effect of radiation is evident within 24 to 48 hours. The villi gradually shorten in length, and the total thickness of the mucosa is reduced. The lamina propria gradually becomes infiltrated with inflammatory cells and plasma cells. The inflammatory response is sometimes severe enough to result in crypt abscesses. Mitoses in the crypts decrease, and this change slows renewal of villous cells, leading to mucosal ulcerations. Megalocytosis of the epithelial cells occurs, and the absorptive surface is reduced. The mucosal morphologic changes are limited to the bowel directly exposed. They usually heal within two weeks of cessation of radiation.

**Subacute Lesions.** These changes, which usually appear during the first year after radiation, involve swelling and degeneration of arteriolar endothelium. Fibrin plugs and thrombosis follow. The reduction in blood supply is associated with thickening and fibrosis of the submucosa.

**Chronic Changes.** These changes can progress over several years and consist of ischemic stenosis and bowel obstruction, chronic bowel ulceration, and fistula formation.

### Functional Disturbance

The function of the gastrointestinal tract may be affected severely by irradiation. In severe radiation enteritis, water and electrolyte transport across the mucosa can be markedly inhibited, resulting in loss of fluid and electrolytes and leading to dehydration, electrolyte depletion, and death if uncorrected. There is malabsorption of fats, sugars, calcium, magnesium, iron, and vitamins. The malabsorption may begin early with marked enteritis, is still present in the middle of irradiation treatment, and may disappear following its termination. On the other hand, if chronic changes occur, malabsorption for water, minerals, fat, and other nutrients may persist and even intensify. The malabsorption may occur because of morphologic changes of the mucosa that decrease its absorptive power, reduction of enzymatic digestion in both lumen and cell, emergence of a pathologic flora or an increase in the virulence of existing flora, and an increase in gastrointestinal motility. Malabsorption may appear only months or years after treatment when it may be due to chronic enteritis, intestinal stricture, or fistula.[26]

## DIET IN TREATMENT OF MALABSORPTION

The nutritional treatments of patients with malabsorption due to gastric, pancreatic, and liver disease, and those with a short bowel, are given elsewhere in this chapter. Specific dietary therapy is primarily of therapeutic benefit in three conditions: celiac disease, intestinal lymphangiectasia, and disaccharidase deficiency.

**Celiac Disease.** The withdrawal of dietary gluten (from wheat, barley, rye and, preferably, oats) is therapeutic in most patients with true caliac sprue. The diet should be gluten-free and not just gluten-reduced, because the most common cause of dietary failure is the inadvertent intake of wheat in sources such as sauces, salad dressing, ice cream, and canned foods. Appendix Table A-32 provides detailed information about gluten-free diets. It is a life-long commitment that is not justified without a biopsy-proved diagnosis demonstrating an abnormal jejunum. The patient should show clinical improvement within a few weeks of starting the diet. If improvement does not occur, and careful assessment fails to indicate that there is inadvertent intake of gluten, then another agent may be a possible cause of a similar lesion.[28] With prolonged treatment, the bowel recovers and, in 50% of patients, the jejunal mucosa returns to normal.

*Supplemental Dietary Therapy.* In patients who already have severe deficiencies when examined, it may be necessary to supplement the individual's food intake while waiting for the gluten-free diet to take effect. Anemic patients should receive parenteral vitamin $B_{12}$, folate, and iron. The last may have to be given in intramuscular doses of the iron-sorbitol complex if oral iron tends to exacerbate diarrhea or is otherwise not tolerated.

Those with dehydration and tetany and/or hypokalemia need intravenous infusions of half normal saline plus potassium and magnesium. It is a common mistake to treat tetany with calcium alone. The problem is not a deficiency of calcium, but an inability to maintain plasma levels of ionized calcium. This difficulty is caused by a lack of response to parathormone, due in turn to magnesium deficiency.[29] Intramuscular magnesium sulfate in doses of 25 meq/day for 1 to 3 days rapidly corrects the problem.

Patients with bone disease should receive supplemental calcium (1 g/day) together with oral vitamin D in doses of 4,000 to 12,000 units orally until the condition has improved clinically. It is advisable to monitor the serum calcium to avoid toxicity. If hypercalcemia occurs, then vitamin D should be withdrawn.

In severely ill patients who are malnourished and intolerant of adequate oral or tube-fed diets because of their debilitated state, intravenous feeding may be required for a few weeks until the condition of the individual has reached a point where he can benefit from an oral diet.

**Intestinal Lymphangiectasia.** Patients with this condition have a loss of protein into the bowel owing to rupture of mucosal lymphatics. The increase in lymph flow that occurs during fat absorption enhances protein loss. The use of very-low-fat diets of less than 10 g/day markedly reduces the protein loss, and enhances serum protein levels.[30] Such low-fat diets are unpalatable and can be made more appealing by substituting some medium-chain triglycerides (MCT) for long-chain triglycerides. MCT have special value by virtue of having fatty acids with chain lengths of 8 to 12 carbons; these are absorbed almost exclusively through the portal circulation rather than the lymphatics.

**Disaccharidase Deficiency.** The most common disaccharidase deficiency is lactase deficiency. In patients with this condition, there is a wide range of tolerance to lactose-containing products. The degree of restriction of milk or milk products should not be based solely on the demonstration of lactase deficiency, but on the degree of tolerance to lactose-containing products. In patients with mild intolerance, up to 15 g of lactose can be taken within a short time without symptoms. This amount is equivalent to 1-½ cups of milk or a cup of chocolate milk, ice cream, or yogurt. Amounts in excess of this may cause symptoms in such patients. The lactose content of cheeses and yogurts is low. Patients with lactose intolerance should be encouraged to eat these and related dairy products so that they can receive the nutrients in milk without gastrointestinal discomfort. A lactase enzyme is available. One such product is called LactAid. Milk treated with this enzyme is almost indistinguishable from untreated milk. The lactose content is reduced to about 3 g/cup after one day of treatment, and to only 1 g/cup after two to three days of treatment (the milk is refrigerated until used). Such milk can be taken by most lactose-intolerant persons without causing symptoms. In some areas, LactAid-treated milk is commercially available.

## NUTRITIONAL SUPPORT OF PATIENTS WITH MALNUTRITION

Because of the deranged ability of the patient with malabsorption to digest and absorb food, the diet needs special consideration. The goal is to make the best possible use of the remaining digestive and absorptive functions, by giving the types of foods that are most readily absorbed (and avoiding those poorly absorbed)—as small frequent feedings given either orally or by drip feeding by tube if necessary—and by providing supplements, e.g., vitamins and minerals or, in more extreme cases, by providing parenterally those nutrients not absorbed from the gut. One may need to resort to one or more of these approaches in a given patient (see Chapter 54).

Fat absorption usually suffers the greatest derangement, so that changes in fat intake are frequently the most important. Because a substantial decrease in the amount of fat ingested may seriously affect adequate caloric intake, the nature of the fat ingested is altered, rather than drastically decreasing total intake. Long-chain fatty acids may be replaced in part with medium-chain triglycerides. These are hydrolyzed more rapidly than those of normal fat,[31] and the fatty acids are absorbed directly into the portal system. Moreover, in the event that pancreatic lipase is absent, the triglycerides are absorbed directly without hydrolysis, thus permitting their use in patients with pancreatic insufficiency. Similarly, bile salts are not essential for their absorption. However, the ability of the patient to tolerate MCT should be ascertained by progressively increasing the fat, since some individuals do not tolerate sudden ingestion of a large amount. The overall fat content should be reduced depending on the severity of the steatorrhea. Because a high fiber content in a diet will exacerbate any existing diarrhea, the diet should be low in fiber.

Because steatorrhea and diarrhea reduce the absorption of fat-soluble vitamins and ions such as calcium, magnesium, and iron, increased amounts of these substances need to be added orally. Iron may be given intramuscularly if the diarrhea is severe and the iron deficiency is acute. Where distal ileal damage is serious, oxalate intake must be restricted when the colon is present, since such a patient is at increased risk of renal oxalate stones (see Appendix Table A-35).

In some patients in whom a significant part of the gut is involved, such minor modifications in diet are not sufficiently helpful. In these patients, special defined-formula diets containing hydrolyzed protein, oligosaccharides, vitamins, minerals, and some source of essential fatty acids may be needed (see Chapter 54). These nutrients are more rapidly absorbed from the upper part of the gastrointestinal tract leaving only a minor residue in the lower part. They probably do not stimulate much intestinal secretion, thus reducing diarrhea.

In still more seriously ill patients who have lost significant weight, who show signs of nutritional deficiency, and cannot rely upon the gut for significant absorption, parenteral nutrition may be considered.

## REFERENCES

1. Kim, Y.S., Spritz, N., Blum, M., et al.: J. Clin. Invest. *45*:956–962, 1966.
2. Welkos, S.A., Toskes, P.P., Baer, H.E., et al.: Gastroenterology *80*:313–320, 1981.
3. Varcoe, R., Halliday, D., Tavill, A.S.: Gut *15*:898–902, 1974.
4. Toskes, P.P., Giannella, R.A., Jervis, H.R., et al.: Gastroenterology *68*:1193–1203, 1975.
5. McCarthy, C.F., Mylotte, M., Stevens, F., et al.: Family studies on coeliac disease in Ireland. *In* Coeliac Disease. (Hekkens, W.T.J.M., Pena, A.S., Eds.) Leiden, Stenfert Kroese, Proceedings of the Second International Coeliac Symposium, 1974, pp. 311–319.
6. Kowlessar, O.D., Sleisenger, M.H.: Gastroenterology *44*:357–362, 1963.
7. Falchuk, Z.M., Gebhard, R.L., Sessoms, C., et al.: J. Clin. Invest. *53*:487–500, 1974.
8. Ferguson, A., MacDonald, T.T., McClure, J.P., et al.: Lancet *1*: 895–897, 1975.
9. Pena, A.S., Mann, D.L., Hague, N.E., et al.: Gastroenterology *75*:230–235, 1978.
10. Selby, W.S., Gallagher, N.D.: Dig. Dis. Sci. *24*:684–688, 1979.
11. Bayless, T.M., Kaplewitz, R.F., Shelly, W.M., et al.: N. Engl. J. Med. *276*:996–1002, 1967.
12. Faulk, D.L., Anuras, S., Christensen, J.: Gastroenterology *74*:922–931, 1978.
13. Brow, J.R., Parker, F., Weinstein, W.M., et al.: Gastroenterology *60*:355–361, 1971.
14. Brusner, O., Eidelman, S., Klipstein, F.A.: Gastroenterology *58*:655–668, 1970.
15. Eidelman, S., Parkins, R.A., Rubin, C.E.: Medicine *45*:111–137, 1966.
16. Ament, M.E., Ochs, H.C., Davis, S.D.: Medicine *52*:227–248, 1973.
17. Weinstein, W.M., Brown, J.R., Parker, F., et al.: Gastroenterology *60*:362–369, 1971.
18. Gardner, F.H.: N. Engl. J. Med. *258*:791–796, 1958.
19. Weingrad, D.N., DeCosse, J.J., Sherlock, P., et al.: Cancer *49*:1258–1265, 1982.
20. Maizel, H., Ruffin, J.M., Dobbins, W.O.: Medicine *49*:175–205, 1970.
21. Sloper, K.S., Dourmaskin, R.R., Bird, R.B., et al.: Gut *23*:80–82, 1982.
22. Mistilis, S.P., Skyring, A.P., Stephen, D.D.: Lancet *1*:77–79, 1965.
23. Popovic, O.S., Brkic, S., Bojic, P., et al.: Gastroenterology *78*:119–125, 1980.
24. Steinfeld, J.L., Davidson, J.D., Gordon, R.S., Jr., et al.: Am. J. Med. *29*:405–415, 1960.
25. Davidson, J.D., Waldmann, T.A., Goodman, D.S., et al.: Lancet *1*:899–902, 1961.
26. Dalla Palma, L.: Intestinal malabsorption in patients undergoing abdominal radiation therapy. *In* Gastrointestinal Radiation Injury. Report of a symposium, Richland, Washington, Sept. 25-28, 1966, (Sullivan, M.E., Ed.) Amsterdam, Excerpta Medica Foundation, 1968, pp. 261–275.
27. Berthrong, M., Fajardo, L.F.: Am. J. Surg. Pathol. *5*:153–178, 1981.

28. Baker, A.L., Rosenberg, I.H.: Ann. Intern. Med. *89*: 505–508, 1978.

29. Anast, C.S., Winnaeker, J.L., Forte, L.R.: J. Clin. Endocrinol. Metab. *42*:707–717, 1978.

30. Jeffries, J.H., Chapman, A., Sleisenger, M.H.: N. Engl. J. Med. *270*:761–766, 1964.

31. Greenberger, N.J., Rodgers, J.B., Isselbacher, K.J.: J. Clin. Invest. *45*:217–227, 1966.

*Chapter* **56**

# NUTRITION AND DIET IN MANAGEMENT OF DISEASES OF THE GASTROINTESTINAL TRACT

## (C) SMALL INTESTINE
### (2) Fluid and Electrolyte Exchange in the Intestinal Tract

### Mukesh B. Desai and Khursheed N. Jeejeebhoy

In this section, the total handling and mechanisms of absorption of water and electrolytes by the gut and the role of individual parts of the gut are discussed (see also Chap. 26).

Apart from digesting and absorbing the nutrients in food, the gastrointestinal tract serves another important function: dealing with the water and electrolytes ingested. An average man consumes about 1.5 liters of fluid in 24 hours. However, the bulk of water and electrolytes in the gastrointestinal tract comes from the gastric, biliary, and pancreatic secretions, which measure about 7 liters/day.

Table 56C2–1 summarizes water and electrolyte entry into and losses from the gut. An adult gut can absorb a maximum of 15 to 20 liters of water and 1,500 to 3,000 meq of sodium, in the form of isotonic saline, when given over 24 hours.

The major part of the digested diet is absorbed in the proximal 100 to 150 cm of jejunum.[1] The ileum and colon absorb water and electrolytes and concentrate the intestinal contents. The normal colon receives about 1,500 ml of fluid and absorbs all but 100 to 200 ml.[2] In patients with established ileostomies, the ileum may adapt to increase its absorption[3] (Table 56C2–2). By comparing the contents of ileostomy fluid and feces, one can estimate that the colon absorbs 1,300 to 1,400 ml of water and 132 to 206 meq of sodium, and that it secretes potassium.

**Table 56C2–1.** **Mean Quantity of Water, Sodium, Chloride, and Potassium Entering the Gut in 24 Hours***

| | Water $H_2O$ (ml) | Sodium $Na^+$ (meq) | Chloride $Cl^-$ (meq) | Potassium $K^+$ (meq) |
|---|---|---|---|---|
| Input | | | | |
|   Diet | 1,500 | 150 | 150 | 80 |
|   Gut secretions | 7,500 | 1,000 | 750 | 40 |
|   Total | 9,000 | 1,150 | 900 | 120 |
| Output | | | | |
|   Ileostomy | 450 | 60 | 45 | 4 |
|   Feces | 150 | 5 | 3 | 12 |

*Adapted from Kramer, P., et al.: Gastroenterology *42*:535, 1962; and Wrong, O.M., et al.: Clin. Sci. *28*:357, 1965.

**Table 56C2–2.** **Comparison of Approximate Daily Water and Electrolytes Delivered to and from Normal Colon***

| | Fluid Delivered to Colon† | | Fluid Delivered to Stool | |
| | Amount | Concentration meq/L | Amount | Concentration meq/L |
| --- | --- | --- | --- | --- |
| Water | 600 ml | | 100 ml | |
| Sodium | 75 meq | 125 | 4 meq | 40 |
| Potassium | 5 meq | 9 | 9 meq | 90 |
| Chloride | 36 meq | 60 | 2 meq | 15 |
| Bicarbonate | 44 meq | 74 | 3 meq | 30 |

*From Fordtran, J.S.: Fed. Proc. 26:1408, 1967 with permission.
†Based on patients with ileostomy. The quantities listed vary from those noted in the text because of substantial adaptation of the small bowel following ileostomy. This change results in underestimation of the contents delivered to the colon normally, and therefore of the work done by this organ. Despite this matter of degree, the direction and relative changes seen here correctly illustrate the role of the colon in absorption and excretion.

## MECHANISMS OF ABSORPTION

**Electrogenic Sodium Absorption.** The $Na^+ - K^+ ATPase$ at the basolateral membrane pumps sodium out of the cytosol into the intercellular space[4] (Fig. 56C2–1). This process keeps the cytosolic sodium concentration low (15 mmol) and thus maintains a gradient across the brush border and the inside of the enterocyte. Thus there is a constant inward movement of sodium into the cell along the electrochemical gradient, which in theory should occur until the luminal sodium concentration falls below the low cytosolic concentration. However, the luminal concentration in vivo at which sodium movement stops is 133 mmol in the jejunum, 75 mmol in the ileum, and 30 mmol in the colon. This difference is due to differences in back diffusion across the intercellular tight junctions (Fig. 56C2–2, 56C2–3).

**Passive Diffusion.** Passive back diffusion is greatest in the jejunum, which has permeable tight junctions, and least in the colon, which has the "tightest" tight junctions.[5] The magnitude of the leak determines the final potential difference (PD)

# NORMAL FLUID AND SOLUTE ABSORPTION

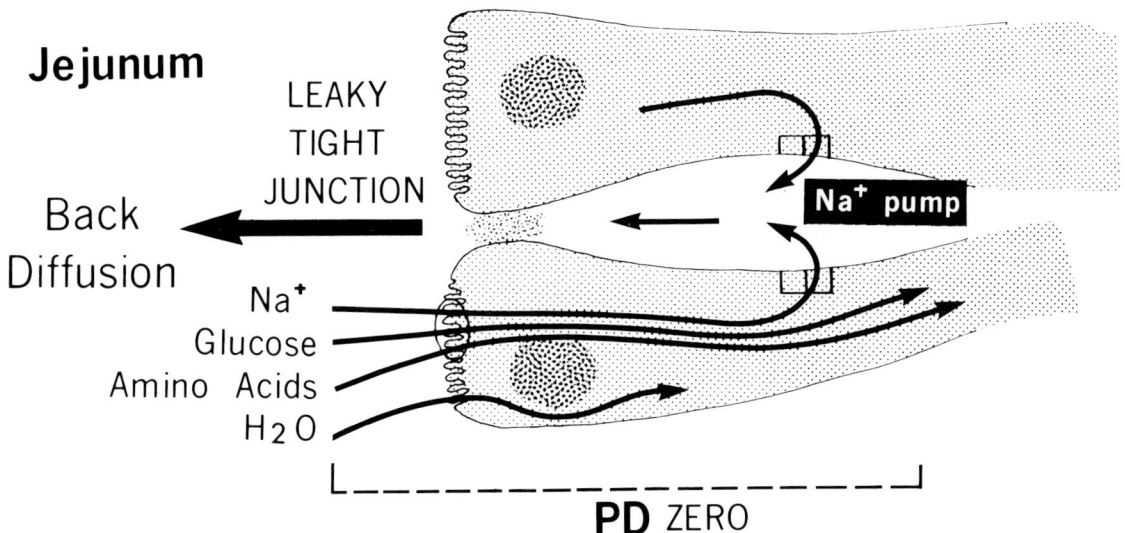

**Fig. 56C2–1.** Absorption in the jejunum. Note that "leaky" tight junctions between enterocytes result in so much back diffusion of water and electrolytes that the resulting potential difference between lumen and basal membrane is only ⁻3V, and luminal contents remain essentially isotonic. Note also the assistance given to absorption of glucose and amino acids by the inward transport of sodium.

# Ileum

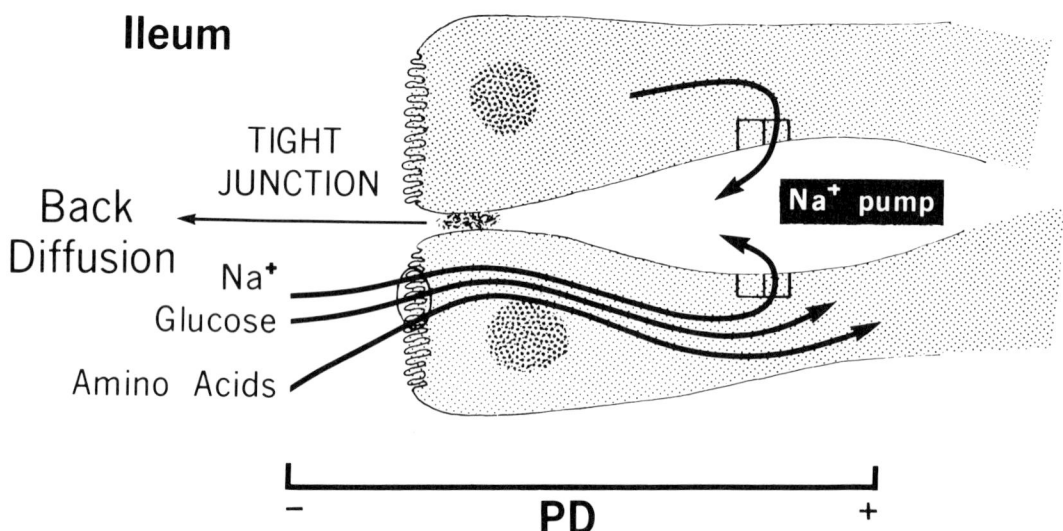

**Fig. 56C2–2.** Absorption in the ileum. Here "tighter" tight junctions allow less back diffusion and therefore a greater potential difference and some concentration of luminal contents.

between the lumen and the basal membrane. The PD is only −3V (lumen negative) in the jejunum, and −20V in the colon. The magnitude of the PD determines how low the luminal sodium can fall before transport ceases. Thus in the case of the jejunum, the luminal sodium cannot be reduced below isotonic levels. In the ileum it can be half that of the plasma, and the colon can resorb most of the sodium and concentrate its contents.

**Glucose-amino Acid Stimulated Transport.** Because the sodium transporter at the brush bor-der membrane is coupled to glucose and/or to amino acid transport,[6] absorption of glucose and amino acids enhances sodium flux (see Fig. 56C2–1).

**Coupled Exchange Transport: Na+ − H+ Exchange.** In both jejunum and ileum, Na+ is exchanged for H+. Thus sodium transport is enhanced if bicarbonate is added to the luminal side to keep luminal H+ concentration low by neu-tralization.[7]

**Short-chain Fatty Acid (SCFA) Absorption.** In

# Colon

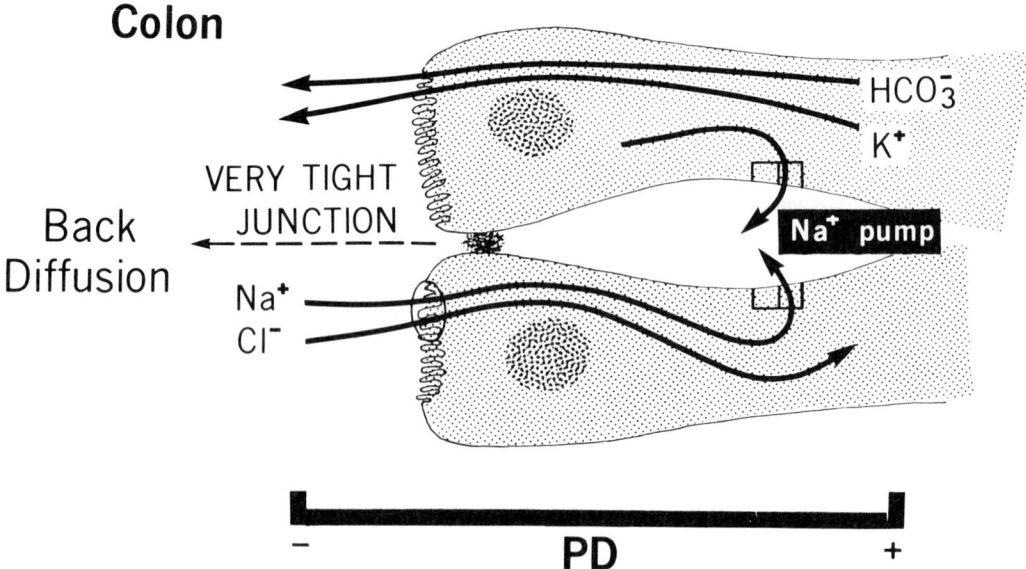

**Fig. 56C2–3.** Absorption in the colon. Here the tight junctions are "tightest," resulting in a potential difference of about -20V and substantial concentration of luminal contents.

the colon, SCFAs formed from the bacterial degradation of nonabsorbed carbohydrates increase water and $Na^+$ absorption in this section of the gut.[8]

$Na^+ - H^+$ **and** $Cl^- - HCO_3^-$ **Exchange.** In the human ileum, there is a dual exchange, and the overall result is comparable to neutral NaCl absorption.

**Convection.** The movement of $Na^+$ into the intercellular spaces draws water through the permeable mucosa. This process is most important in the jejunum where the intercellular tight junctions are permeable as indicated earlier.

## ROLE OF STOMACH AND DUODENUM

Although individually serving different functions, both stomach and duodenum achieve a common goal, i.e., making the intraluminal contents isotonic with plasma. The stomach does this by a gradual and coordinated release (probably through duodenal osmoreceptors)[9] of gastric contents into the duodenum. Little fluid is absorbed from the stomach although exchange of fluid takes place in both directions in the gastric mucosa.[10] The movement of diffusible ions (mainly $Na^+$ and $Cl^-$) and bulk movement of water bring the hypertonic gastric contents into iso-osmotic equilibrium before emptying into the duodenum.[11] Because the total contribution of nonelectrolytes to the tonicity of postprandial jejunal contents is less than 50 mosm/L (irrespective of the meal)[12] compared with the approximately 300 mosm/L of plasma, the jejunal contents are in approximate ionic equilibrium with plasma.

Although net absorption of fluid and electrolytes in the gastroduodenal region is minimal, the upper gastrointestinal secretions are mixed thoroughly with the luminal contents and both are brought to isotonicity with plasma.

## JEJUNAL FUNCTION

The jejunum serves the following main functions: (1) Absorption of products of carbohydrate, protein, and fat digestion. (2) Neutralization of pancreatic bicarbonate ($HCO_3^-$) via sodium ion-hydrogen ion ($Na^+ - H^+$) exchange. This process keeps the $H^+$ concentration in the jejunum low and promotes $Na^+$ absorption. (3) Rapid absorption of sodium chloride (NaCl) by coupling its movement to the active transport of dietary sugars and amino acids via solvent drag, thus conserving energy.

Although little absorption occurs from a perfusion of pure isotonic saline,[12] the presence of intraluminal products of digestion, such as glucose,[13] galactose,[14] and some amino acids such as leucine,[15] promotes absorption of $H_2O$, $Na^+$, and $Cl^-$ from the lumen due to coupled sodium transport. Bicarbonate neutralization in the lumen also promotes absorption of $Na^+$, even in the absence of other products of digestion.

Most of the $HCO_3^-$ disappears from the lumen by its reaction with gastric $H^+$ to form water and $CO_2$. Thus, the "absorption" of pancreatic $HCO_3^-$ is probably as carbon dioxide ($CO_2$) (as suggested by Turnberg).[16] Although little is known regarding the absorption of $K^+$ in the jejunum, it is probably passive, owing to solvent drag.

Thus in the upper jejunum, products of digestion and related amounts of $Na^+$, $Cl^-$, and $H_2O$ are absorbed. $HCO_3^-$ is absorbed as $CO_2$ and $K^+$ is absorbed because of solvent drag. The fluid subsequently presented to the ileum still contains significant quantities of water and electrolytes.

## ROLE OF ILEUM AND COLON

Although the mucosa of both ileum and colon is relatively impermeable to bulk movement of water as compared with jejunal mucosa, significant water absorption still occurs in the lower bowel.

$Na^+$ is absorbed by active transport. Part of $Cl^-$ is absorbed with $Na^+$ with the rest being absorbed in exchange for $HCO_3^-$. Although the relative $K^+$ concentration in the lower bowel is high (because of the relative impermeability of colonic mucosa and/or active secretion), the luminal fluid is still hypotonic. This condition promotes passive water absorption, following $Na^+$ and $Cl^-$. Table 56C2–2 provides data about colonic function.

## WATER AND ELECTROLYTE ABSORPTION IN DISEASE

More than one of the aforementioned mechanisms may be deranged, but it is easier to understand the pathologic lesion if dysfunction is considered regionally.

**Gastroduodenal Dysfunction.** When the regulatory mechanism for gastric emptying is deranged, for example, in gastroduodenal surgery or in thyrotoxicosis, the result is usually the rapid gastric emptying of hypertonic contents into the duodenum, giving the latter insufficient time to make the luminal contents isotonic. This process results in a rapid influx of fluid into the lumen of the upper jejunum, which exceeds the jejunal absorptive capacity. This is a factor in the dumping syndrome and also causes diarrhea.

Excessive gastric, biliary, or pancreatic secretion can theoretically cause fluid diarrhea if the intestines are loaded with more fluid than they can absorb. Diarrhea in the Zollinger-Ellison syndrome may be caused by fluid load or by increased acidity that reduces intestinal water and Na$^+$ absorption.[17] Apart from this, various hormones have been incriminated in causing diarrhea in animals.[18]

**Jejunal Dysfunction.** Because the jejunum normally absorbs digestion products and, coupled with them, water and sodium, it is clear that in any disorder of malabsorption where these digestion products are not absorbed, water and Na$^+$ will remain in the lumen, thus presenting the ileum with more fluid than is normal. If ileal absorptive capacity is exceeded, diarrhea results. This occurs transiently in infantile gastroenteritis with temporary failure of absorption of sugars, and in kwashiorkor. The mechanism of diarrhea is similar in regional enteritis.

In adult celiac disease and cholera, there is secretion of fluid rather than failure of absorption. Especially in the latter disease, a massive outpouring of fluid occurs, easily exceeding lower bowel absorptive capacity and so causing severe diarrhea.

**Ileal and Colonic Dysfunction.** Following ileal resection or bypass, there is failure of the normal absorption of bile acids by the terminal ileum. In turn these bile acids decrease water and Na$^+$ absorption in the colon, thus causing diarrhea. This diarrhea can be treated by giving cholestyramine resin to bind the bile acids if ileal function is not too seriously deranged.

In ulcerative colitis and regional colitis, diarrhea is caused by decreased water and Na$^+$ absorption by the diseased colonic mucosa.

## SECRETORY DIARRHEA

There is a constant passive inflow of NaCl into the cell at the basal membrane because of Na$^+$ − K$^+$ATPase activity maintaining a high concentration of Na$^+$ in the intercellular spaces. The Cl$^-$ ion flowing in with the sodium does not diffuse back into the lumen because the brush border membrane is impermeable to Cl$^-$. However, activation of cellular cyclic AMP (cAMP), toxins (cholera and *Escherichia coli*), an increase in vasoactive intestinal polypeptide (VIP) levels (as with a tumor secreting VIP), and a rise in cytosolic Ca$^{++}$ levels will increase permeability to Cl$^-$, allowing the inflowing chloride to be secreted into the intestinal lumen causing diarrhea.[19]

## HORMONAL CONTROL OF ELECTROLYTE AND WATER ABSORPTION

Aldosterone enhances sodium absorption and potassium secretion in the colon[20] but not in the small bowel. Glucocorticoids enhance sodium absorption in the small intestine. Opiates[21] and somatostatin[22] enhance sodium chloride absorption in the ileum and the colon.

## REFERENCES

1. Borgstrom, B., Dahlqvist, A., Lundh, G., et al.: J. Clin. Invest. *36*:1521–1536, 1957.
2. Phillips, S.E., Giller, J.: J. Lab. Clin. Med. *81*:733–746, 1973.
3. Wright, H.K., Cleveland, J.C., Tilson, M.D.: Am. J. Surg. *117*:242–244, 1969.
4. Schultz, S.G., Zalusky, R.: J. Gen. Physiol. *47*:567–584, 1964.
5. Fordtran, J.S., Rector, F.C., Jr., Ewton, M.F., et al.: J. Clin. Invest. *44*:1935–1944, 1965.
6. Goldner, A.M., Schultz, S.G., Curran, P.F.: J. Gen. Physiol. *53*:362–384, 1969.
7. Turnberg, L.A., Fordtran, J.B., Caster, N.W., et al.: J. Clin. Invest. *49*:548–556, 1970.
8. Bond, J.H., Levitt, M.D.: J. Clin. Invest. *57*:1158–1164, 1976.
9. Hunt, J.N.: J. Physiol. (Lond.) *132*:267–288, 1956.
10. Scholar, J.F., Code, C.F.: Gastroenterology *27*:565–577, 1954.
11. Fordtran, J.S., Locklear, J.W.: Am. J. Dig. Dis. *11*:503–521, 1966.
12. Whalen, G.E., Harris, J.A., Geenen, J.E., et al.: Gastroenterology *51*:975–984, 1966.
13. Sladen, G.E., Dawson, A.M.: Clin. Sci. *36*:119–132, 1969.
14. Fordtran, J.S., Rector, F.C., Jr., Carter, N.W.: J. Clin. Invest. *47*:884–900, 1968.
15. Adibi, S.A.: J. Appl. Physiol. *28*:753–757, 1970.
16. Turnberg, L.A., Biederdorf, E.A., Morawski, S.G.: J. Clin. Invest. *49*:557–567, 1970.
17. McHardy, G.J.R., Parsons, D.S.: Q. J. Exp. Physiol. *42*:33–48, 1957.
18. Gardner, J.D., Peskin, G.W., Cerda, J.J., et al.: Am. J. Surg. *113*:57–64, 1967.
19. Frizzell, R.A., Heintze, K., Stewart, C.P.: Mechanism of intestinal chloride secretion. *In* Secretory Diarrhea. (Field, M., Fordtran, J.S., Schultze, S.G., Eds.) Bethesda, MD, American Physiological Society, 1980, pp. 11–19.
20. Levitan, R., Ingelfinger, F.J.: J. Clin. Invest. *44*:801–808, 1965.
21. Racusen, L.C., Binder, H.J., Dobbins, J.W.: Gastroenterology *74*:1081, 1978 (Abstract).
22. Dharmasthaphorn, K., Binder, H.J., Dobbins, J.W.: Gastroenterology *78*:1559–1565, 1980.

*Chapter* **56**

# NUTRITION AND DIET IN MANAGEMENT OF DISEASES OF THE GASTROINTESTINAL TRACT

## *(C) SMALL INTESTINE*
### *(3) Nutrient Interactions with Structure*

Gordon R. Greenberg

The intestine is the vehicle by which nutrients are assimilated and absorbed. Although the reserve capacity of this structure is significant, functional alterations caused either by mucosal disease or by surgical resection may dramatically compromise the nutritional status of the host. In such settings, optimal restitution of protein and energy requirements becomes a major therapeutic challenge. Fundamental to the achievement of this goal is a basic understanding of the mechanisms by which nutrients promote structural adaptation of the intestine.

Morphologic and functional adaptation is well recognized after massive small bowel resection. This process, characterized by an increase in both crypt depth and villous height, is due to true hyperplasia of the remaining intestinal remnant rather than hypertrophy, as evidenced by increased incorporation of [3]H thymidine into mucosal DNA.[1] The net result is a substantial increase in absorptive surface area, which occurs for all nutrient substrates. The site of resection does, however, determine the degree of adaptation. Thus, the response to jejunectomy is substantially greater, since trophic indices in the ileum increase up to 100%. This response is in contrast to findings in the jejunal remnant after ileal resection, where changes approximating 25% are observed.[2] In rats such adaptive responses occur within a few days; however, in man clinical observations, such as fecal fat excretion and stool weight, suggest that the process is more prolonged and may not be complete for up to one year. Three major mechanisms are postulated to account for the intestinal adaptation of resection: luminal nutrition, pancreaticobiliary secretion, and hormonal factors.

## LUMINAL NUTRITION

The exposure of the small intestinal mucosa to nutrients is one of the prerequisites for normal mucosal growth and for the adaptive response that is observed following small bowel resection. Complete starvation reduces the intestinal mass by over half in rats and is associated with decreased numbers of proliferating enterocytes, a prolongation of the cell cycle, and a delay in cell migration.[3–5] Alternatively, intestinal villous hyperplasia has been reported in several experimental models of hyperphagia, as for example with chronic exposure to low temperatures.[6]

Similarly, oral nutrients play a major role in the adaptive changes after intestinal resection. In dogs, hyperplasia of the ileum after jejunal resection is well recognized provided nutrients are given orally, but fails to occur with intravenous nutritional support.[7] Moreover in man, following jejunoileal bypass for morbid obesity, the excluded segment becomes hypoplastic while that portion of the intestine in continuity shows mucosal hyperplasia.[8] Laboratory animals receiving nutritional support totally by parenteral nutrition develop hypoplastic mucosa,[9] but similar morphologic studies in man have not been reported to date. It is known, however, that in man, after a relatively short period of TPN, functional parameters seem to be preserved as is evidenced by a normal postprandial gut hormone profile after three weeks of TPN.[10]

The type of oral nutrient may also influence the adaptive hyperplasia that follows resection. In jejunectomized rats, intragastric infusion of carbohydrate or protein does not entirely prevent the intestinal mucosal hypoplasia associated with TPN.[11] The most potent stimulus for intestinal growth in this experimental setting is fat. Long-chain triglycerides, in contrast to protein or glycogen, are capable of maintaining normal structure and function in parenterally fed rats when only 20% of total daily energy requirements are provided as corn oil. Subsequently these same investigators have demonstrated that an even smaller amount (10%) of a mixture of free fatty acids is as effective as a standard diet in achieving adaptation and is more stimulatory than an equivalent amount of long-chain triglycerides.[12] The mechanisms by which oral nutrients promote this response are not completely resolved. It is known that the effect of carbohydrate does not require active absorption but rather seems to be dependent only on mucosal contact.[13] As discussed later, the stimulation of pancreaticobiliary secretion and the release of one or more hormones that are trophic to the intestine have both been implicated.

## PANCREATICOBILIARY SECRETION

The presence of nutrients within the intestinal lumen provides a potent stimulus for pancreatic and biliary secretion. The mechanisms regulating pancreatic secretion are complex. At least in part, they involve the release of many of the gut hormones including secretin and cholecystokinin (CCK). Studies by Altmann were the first to demonstrate that transplantation of the duodenal papilla into an isolated loop of ileum could promote ileal mucosal hyperplasia, thus pointing to pancreaticobiliary secretion alone as a trophic factor.[14] Of interest, however, is the subsequent observation that transplanting the bile duct into the ileum additionally results in significant growth of the mucosa in the proximal jejunum remote from the transplant.[15] Thus, pancreaticobiliary diversion appears to cause adaptive hyperplasia not only in the ileum, but also in the jejunum deprived of those secretions. The factors in pancreaticobiliary secretions that might be responsible for these observations have not been identified, although bile and pancreatic juice are independently trophic to the ileum.[16] A specific heat-labile trophic factor in pancreatic juice has been excluded.[17]

## HORMONAL FACTORS

To assess one of the mechanisms by which pancreaticobiliary secretion might be trophic, Hughes and colleagues studied CCK-secretin infusions in dogs that had developed intestinal hypoplasia on TPN.[9] These hormonal infusions totally prevented the villous hypoplasia observed with TPN. Such experiments could implicate CCK and/or secretin as direct trophic agents to the small intestine, similar to the marked effects of CCK on pancreatic growth. Alternatively, since both these hormones potently stimulate pancreatic and biliary secretion, the effect of these hormones may be indirect.

Other studies support this latter concept. In parenterally fed rats, CCK and secretin have no trophic effect on a bypassed jejunal segment that is excluded from endogenous pancreatic secretions.[18] Other gut hormones have also been advanced as candidates for a trophic role to small intestinal mucosa. Foremost of these is enteroglucagon, a hormone found predominantly in the ileum and colon. After a meal, plasma enteroglucagon rises rapidly, with its release stimulated mainly by carbohydrates and long-chain triglycerides. Striking elevations of plasma enteroglucagon have been observed in patients with untreated celiac disease[19] and in those who have undergone massive small resection.[20] In experimental models of resection, higher crypt cell production rates have been associated with substantial elevations of enteroglucagon.[21,22] Moreover, a single patient with an enteroglucagon-producing tumor had marked mucosal hyperplasia.[23] Although preliminary experiments with a partially purified enteroglucagon preparation have shown the stimulation of DNA synthesis in cultured jejunal mucosa,[24] confirmation of its trophic actions awaits sufficient quantities of the pure peptide for study. A trophic role for gastrin had been previously postulated, but several studies now support the concept that this hormone has no trophic action beyond the ligament of Treitz.[25]

## REFERENCES

1. Williamson, R.C.N., Bauer, F.L.R., Ross, J.S., et al.: Gastroenterology *74*:16–23, 1978.
2. Williamson, R.C.N., Bauer, F.L.R.: Br. J. Surg. *65*:736–739, 1978.
3. Steiner, M., Bourges, H.R., Freedman, L.S., et al.: Am. J. Physiol. *215*:75–77, 1968.
4. Hopper, A.F., Rose, P.M., Wannemacher, R.W.: J. Cell Biol. *53*:225–230, 1972.
5. Hagemann, R.F., Stragand, J.J.: Cell Tissue Kinet. *10*:3–14, 1977.
6. Heroux, O., Gridgeman, N.T.: Can. J. Biochem. Physiol. *36*:209–216, 1958.

7. Feldman, E.J., Dowling, R.H., McNaughton, J., et al.: Gastroenterology *70*:712–719, 1976.

8. Gleeson, M.H., Cullen, J., Dowling, R.H.: Clin. Sci. *43*:731–742, 1972.

9. Hughes, C.A, Bates, T., Dowling, R.H.: Gastroenterology *75*:34–41, 1978.

10. Greenberg, G.R., Wolman, S.L, Christofides, N., et al.: Gastroenterology *80*:938–993, 1981.

11. Morin, C.L., Grey, V.L., Garofalo, C.: Influence of lipids on intestinal adaptation after resection. *In* Mechanisms of Intestinal Adaptation. (Robinson, J.W.L., Dowling, R.H., Riecken, E.D., Eds.) Lancaster, U.K., MTP Press Ltd., 1982, pp. 175–184.

12. Morin, C.L., Grey, V.L., Garofalo, C., et al.: Gastroenterology *84*:1253, 1983.

13. Weser, E., Vandeventer, A., Tawil, T.: Scand. J. Gastroenterol. (Suppl.) *17*:105–113, 1982.

14. Altmann, G.G.: Am. J. Anat. *132*:167–178, 1971.

15. Weser, E., Heller, R., Tawil, T.: Gastroenterology *73*:524–529, 1977.

16. Williamson, R.C.N., Bauer, F.L.R., Ross, J.S., et al.: Surgery *83*:570–576, 1978.

17. Hughes, C.A, Ducker, D.A., Warren, I.F.: Gut *20*:A924–A925, 1979.

18. Fine, H., Levine, G.M., Shiau, Y.F.: Am. J. Physiol. *245*:G358–G363, 1983.

19. Besterman, H.S., Bloom, S.R., Sarson, D.L., et al.: Lancet *1*:785–788, 1978.

20. Bloom, S.R., Besterman, H.S., Adrian, T.E., et al.: Gastroenterology *76*:1101, 1979.

21. Al-Mukhtar, M.Y.T., Sagor, G.R., Ghatei, M.A.: Br. J. Surg. *70*:398–400, 1983.

22. Sagor, G.R., Al-Mukhtar, M.Y.T., Ghatei, M.A., et al.: Br. J. Surg. *69*:14–18, 1982.

23. Gleeson, M.H., Bloom, S.R., Polak, J.M., et al.: Gut *12*:773–782, 1971.

24. Uttenthal, L.O., Batt, R.M., Carter, M.W., et al.: Regul. Pept. *3*:84, 1982.

25. Morin, C.L., Ling, V.: Gastroenterology *75*:224–229, 1978.

*Chapter* **56**

# NUTRITION AND DIET IN MANAGEMENT OF DISEASES OF THE GASTROINTESTINAL TRACT

*(C) SMALL INTESTINE*
   *(4) Nutritional Support in Inflammatory Bowel Disease*

   Irwin H. Rosenberg

Inflammatory bowel disease refers to idiopathic chronic inflammatory conditions of the intestine, principally ulcerative colitis and Crohn's disease. Ulcerative colitis is an inflammatory ulcerating process of the colon. Crohn's disease is a transmural granulomatous enteritis that may involve any part of the intestine, but primarily involves the distal small intestine and the colon.

The chronic inflammatory bowel diseases (IBD), ulcerative colitis, and Crohn's disease, by their direct involvement of the gastrointestinal tract and by their effects on food intake, are commonly associated with nutritional depletion. Proper management of these diseases requires persistent attention to nutritional maintenance and/or repletion, often concurrent with dietary restrictions designed to "rest" the inflamed bowel and allow healing to proceed.

## NUTRITIONAL DEFICIENCIES IN IBD

From Table 56C4–1, one can appreciate the challenge to patients with IBD in maintaining an adequate nutritional state. Spontaneous oral intake is reduced in the presence of postprandial exacerbation of symptoms. Crohn's disease, by affecting the small bowel, may lead to malabsorption. Both Crohn's disease and ulcerative colitis may cause increased nutrient utilization in the face of heightened cell turnover and excessive en-

teric losses of protein, iron (bleeding), and zinc (diarrhea). Drugs may interfere with nutrient absorption or utilization.

A wide range of nutritional problems may develop in patients with IBD (Table 56C4–2).[1] Most patients, especially those with Crohn's disease, suffer from some degree of calorie/protein depletion. Weight loss is reported in most individuals with Crohn's disease and in many with ulcerative colitis. Micronutrient depletion is less prevalent, but as diagnostic techniques improve, the risk of deficiency of fat-soluble vitamins and folate and of minerals and trace minerals, iron and zinc in particular, becomes apparent.

## PRINCIPLES OF NUTRITION MANAGEMENT

The principle is to set dietary goals that are adequate for the nutritional needs of the patient and, at the same time, to minimize stress on the inflamed and often narrowed segments of bowel. Evidence of lactose intolerance should be documented when possible and dietary restriction imposed as needed. In many patients with cramping and diarrhea, decreasing the intake of dietary fiber or residue is beneficial. In those with steatorrhea, a decreased fat intake may substantially improve diarrhea. Once these restrictions are imposed, it is important to replenish the diet with

**Table 56C4–1.   Causes of Malnutrition in Inflammatory Bowel Disease**

| Etiology | Examples |
|---|---|
| Decreased oral intake | Disease-induced (abdominal pain, diarrhea, nausea, anorexia)<br>Iatrogenic (restrictive diets without supplementation) |
| Malabsorption | Decreased absorptive surface due to disease or resection<br>Bile salt deficiency after ileal resection<br>Bacterial overgrowth<br>Drugs (see below) |
| Increased secretion and nutrient loss | Protein-losing enteropathy<br>Electrolyte, mineral, and trace metal loss in diarrhea<br>GI blood loss |
| Increased utilization and increased requirements | Inflammation, fever, infection<br>Increased intestinal cell turnover<br>Hemolysis (see sulfasalazine) |
| Drug interference | Corticosteroids and calcium absorption/protein metabolism<br>Sulfasalazine and folate absorption/hemolysis<br>Cholestyramine and fat-soluble vitamin absorption |

**Table 56C4–2.   Reported Nutritional Deficiencies in Hospitalized Patients with Inflammatory Bowel Disease[†]**

Calorie-protein deficiency
Iron deficiency anemia
Low serum vitamin $B_{12}$
Low serum folate
Low serum magnesium
Low serum potassium
Low serum vitamin A
Low serum vitamin C
Low serum 25-OH-vitamin D
Low serum zinc
Low serum copper
Metabolic bone disease
Pellagra
Hypoprothrombinemia (vitamin K deficiency)

[†]Modified from Driscoll, R.H., Rosenberg, I.H.[1]

other foods that will provide sufficient calories, protein, vitamins, and minerals to restore and maintain desirable body weight and nutritional status. In some patients this goal can be attained only by the use of vitamin, mineral, and caloric supplements.

In general, the diet should be liberal in protein with calories sufficient to maintain or restore weight, or to support growth in children and adolescents. The diet should usually be supplemented by a multivitamin preparation containing one to five times the normal Recommended Dietary Allowances.[2] The higher (therapeutic) dose is indicated if there is clinical or laboratory evidence of deficiency of any of the several nutrients

that may be poorly absorbed or whose requirements may be increased.

The techniques for identification of nutritional deficiencies and for monitoring efficacy of therapy are not unique to patients with IBD. Appropriate nutritional assessment and monitoring techniques are discussed elsewhere in this book (see Chap. 45).

## RATIONALE FOR MODIFYING FOOD INTAKE

Nutritional maintenance by diet may be difficult at times of symptomatic activity of IBD. Most patients report postprandial worsening of symptoms. Diarrhea, which may lead to depletion of electrolytes and other micronutrients, is worsened by eating. Eating increases the likelihood of certain complications of IBD. The impaction of bulky food in a narrowed or inflamed loop of bowel in Crohn's disease may precipitate obstruction. Likewise, fistulas will not heal in the presence of active flow of bowel contents.

In order to decrease these eating-associated symptoms and decrease bowel activity during healing, patients hospitalized for IBD are sometimes placed on a "bowel rest" program. It is reasoned that the elimination of oral intake can decrease the absorptive work of the bowel, minimize the mechanical trauma caused by food passage, and decrease diet-associated secretions and the inflammation that can be attributed in part to growth of bacterial organisms. In addition, because the pathogenesis of ongoing inflammation may involve continued antigenic stimulation in the gut, cessation of oral intake may be effective not only by decreasing luminal flora, but also by avoiding exposure to antigenically complex food-stuffs.

On the other hand, a diet that is highly restrictive in dietary residue owing to withdrawal of fruits, vegetables, and milk products is often inadequate in some B vitamins, folate, vitamin C, and calcium unless these are reintroduced by specific intention. Proper management of Crohn's disease or ulcerative colitis *must* accomplish both goals of lessening symptoms and maintaining nutritional adequacy.

## SPECIAL DIETARY CHANGES IN IBD

**Lactose Restriction.** In a group of children and adolescents with Crohn's disease, Kirschner et al. found that 34% failed to absorb physiologic doses (32 or 25 g) of lactose.[3] Nearly half of black and Jewish children had positive tests. Furthermore, the diffuse functional and structural small bowel abnormalities of Crohn's disease are reflected in significantly reduced specific activities of lactose and other mucosal enzymes.[4] In most such patients, elimination of dietary lactose decreases abdominal cramps and diarrhea.

Most patients with lactose malabsorption require only diminution of milk or ice cream to one cup per day. For the especially fastidious patient, guidelines for greater restriction of lactose are available elsewhere in this text (Appendix Table A34). Because the major dietary source of lactose (milk and milk products) is also the major source of calcium, however, prolonged adherence to a milk-free diet may contribute to negative calcium balance.[5] In some, especially in growing children or adolescents, use of bacterial lactase (LactAid) to hydrolyze the lactose in milk may be indicated. LactAid-treated milk is now available in many food stores.

**Low-residue (Fiber) Diets.** In patients with inflammatory narrowing of the lumen or chronic stenosis, the rationale for restricting dietary fiber is apparent: by avoiding substances that are not digested in the gastrointestinal tract, the probability of worsening symptoms of intestinal obstruction is reduced. In addition, physical irritation of the inflamed bowel should be lessened. The other physiologic effects of a low-residue diet include reduced stool weight and frequency and slower rate of intestinal transit.

Because available data on fiber content of food are incomplete, this diet is usually described in qualitative terms (see Chap. 2B and Appendix Table A26). Fiber intake can be reduced by avoiding coarse whole-grain breads and cereals, nuts, and most fruits and vegetables. As a result, this diet may be marginal in folic acid, ascorbic acid, other vitamins, and some minerals.

The benefits of a fiber-restricted diet are controversial. A retrospective study of 32 patients with Crohn's disease treated with an unrefined carbohydrate, fiber-rich diet failed to support the impression that dietary fiber worsens symptoms. Hospital admissions were significantly fewer and shorter in the fiber-enriched patients, and only one experimental subject (versus five controls) required surgery during the study period.[6] No patient on the test diet developed obstruction. If a change in dietary fiber intake is recommended to patients, the change should be made carefully and gradually, and the individual response of the patient must guide continuing use of this aspect of diet management. Increased fiber intake would not usually be appropriate for patients with evidence of intestinal narrowing.

**Fat Restriction.** Patients with Crohn's disease involving the small bowel, particularly with resections, have fat malabsorption of varying severity. Steatorrhea is a major factor in the diarrhea of these patients, with fatty acids and their hydroxylated derivatives exerting a cathartic effect upon the colonic mucosa.[7] In addition, there is a direct correlation between loss of fat in stools and the loss of calcium, magnesium, and possibly zinc. Also related to the formation of fatty acid-calcium complexes in the stool is the excessive absorption of uncomplexed oxalate and the hyperoxaluria and increased risk of calcium oxalate stone formation. Diarrhea with persistent serious fluid loss, if not adequately replaced, may lead to acidic concentrated urine and to systemic acidosis that predisposes also to urate stone formation.

Patients with steatorrhea experience symptomatic benefit from decreasing intake of dietary fat. Often modifications of intake from the usual 100 to 120 g or more of fat in the Western diet to 70 to 80 g will suffice to lessen diarrhea and improve calcium and magnesium balances without serious impairment of palatability. In patients with more severe malabsorption, especially those with short bowel syndrome, further reduction may be needed with consequent depressed palatability and total calorie intake. It is critical that the calories lost by removal of calorie-dense fat from the diet be replaced by more easily absorbed calorie sources if the diet is to remain adequate in energy. The most ready sources of calories for substitution are the carbohydrates—sugars and starches. Some patients will benefit also from the use of medium-chain triglycerides (MCT) in substitution for some fat in the diet (salad dressing, some baked and cooked foods) as MCT are more efficiently absorbed. Similarly, calorie intake can be increased with commercially available carbohydrates derived from corn solids by partial hydrolysis (e.g., Polycose). The broader use of formula supplements to augment dietary intake or to provide a complete source of enteral nutrition in selected patients is discussed later.

## TREATMENT OF SPECIFIC DEFICIENCIES

In some patients, specific nutritional supplementation is necessary in addition to dietary change and multivitamins. Sometimes this supplementation requires special enteral or intravenous formulas, which are discussed later, particularly when there are special problems in meeting calorie and protein requirements. When deficiencies in micronutrients are the concern, targeted regimens of supplementation may be indicated. For example, folate deficiency, which has been observed in patients with IBD, especially in those taking sulfasalazine, an inhibitor of folate absorption,[8] can be readily reversed or prevented by the use of 1 mg of folic acid daily either as a separate supplement or as part of a multivitamin preparation containing folate. Patients with extensive disease and/or resection of terminal ileum for Crohn's disease usually have a deficit in vitamin $B_{12}$ absorption. Such patients require supplementation with intramuscular vitamin $B_{12}$ at a dose of 500 to 1,000 µg at least every three months and, in some, every month. Patients with persisting watery diarrhea may have difficulty maintaining adequate zinc status by dietary means.[9] In such patients, supplementation with zinc at a usual dose of 60 mg/day of zinc as sulfate may be indicated.

Iron deficiency is a challenge in the presence of intermittent or chronic blood loss and altered absorption. Iron supplements in full therapeutic dose may exacerbate symptoms. Slower supplementation using 30 to 60 mg of iron daily may be a useful strategy.

The causes of metabolic bone disease in patients with Crohn's disease, in particular, are multiple. Chronic corticosteroid therapy results in chronic negative calcium balance; malabsorption of vitamin D and calcium may result from small bowel disease. In such patients, measuring 25-hydroxyvitamin D levels may be the best way to screen for patients at risk of deficiency. In most patients with low values, doses of oral vitamin D between 2,000 and 10,000 I.U. daily will restore normal 25-hydroxyvitamin D levels and correct osteomalacia, as documented by bone biopsy.[10]

In some patients, protein deficits, which reflect enteric protein loss as much as dietary deficiency or malabsorption, can be reversed by selective increase in sources of high-quality protein (protein supplements).

## INTENSIVE NUTRITIONAL SUPPORT

Thus far, this discussion has focused primarily upon ambulatory patients who represent the large majority of individuals with moderate to mild symptoms. For patients with more severe symptoms unresponsive to medical therapy, the challenge of medical management and consideration of surgery both increase. In that setting, more intensive nutritional support may be mandatory.

**Liquid Formulas.** Liquid formulas have been reported to be effective in managing some patients with ulcerative colitis or Crohn's disease, even with fistulas, growth retardation, or short bowel. Some enthusiastic proponents believe that the "partial bowel rest" provided by these nutritionally complete, minimal-residue, liquid diets, which involve considerably fewer risks and less expense than parenteral nutrition, may be the preferred management.

Either parenteral nutrition or liquid formula diets can be used to restore nutritional status and achieve weight gain, and each has particular advantages in some situations. Experience with such diets and total parenteral nutrition is reviewed in the sections that follow.

Lactose-free, fiber-free nutritional liquid formulas can be administered by mouth as a complete diet or as a dietary supplement, or such formulas can be administered by feeding tube to meet calorie and nutritional goals. Administration of a total liquid formula diet by tube is well tolerated and can be performed at home for extended periods. Nutritional deficits can be reversed by such a regimen while symptoms are ordinarily kept in control with the additional use of drug therapy. A controlled trial of the use of liquid formula supplements in patients with Crohn's disease demonstrated a clear benefit over unsupplemented controls in measures of nutritional status including weight, arm circumferences, and albumin.[11] However, the symptomatic response was similar in both supplemented and control groups.

Enteral formulas have been used successfully in the management of patients with fistulas in Crohn's disease with a clear decrease in fistula drainage and healing in some individuals. Enteral formula supplements have been used effectively to meet calorie requirements and to restore growth in children with growth retardation complicating Crohn's disease.[12]

**Parenteral Nutrition.** In the management of many hospitalized patients with severely active ulcerative colitis or Crohn's disease, physicians tend to place the patient on a nothing-by-mouth regimen, together with medications including corticosteroids, in an effort to control symptoms of diarrhea, abdominal pain, and sometimes fever. Such patients may be managed with the use of central line and total parenteral nutrition for nutritional repletion and maintenance. In ulcerative colitis, the combined reported experience in uncontrolled studies demonstrates clinical remission in approximately one third of severely symptomatic patients managed with total parenteral nutrition, while the remainder usually requires surgery eventually.[13] In one controlled study of patients with colitis comparing total parenteral nutrition with hospitalization and drug therapy alone, no greater incidence of remission was observed in those on parenteral nutrition.[14]

In Crohn's disease, the experience with the use of total parenteral nutrition is more extensive and more positive. About 70% of patients in reported series will undergo clinical remission in hospital, and reversal of nutritional deficits is regular.[13] However, the duration of symptomatic remission is highly variable. Controlled studies comparing total parenteral nutrition to enteral nutrition to other forms of hospital management are required.

Total parenteral nutrition is often used to manage patients with enterocutaneous fistulas in Crohn's disease. In the reported series, approximately one third of fistulas healed in hospital on such a regimen.[13]

## NUTRITIONAL MANAGEMENT OF GROWTH RETARDATION

When inflammatory bowel disease begins in childhood, persistently active disease may affect growth and sexual maturation in as many as one third of such children. Although retarded growth may reflect the chronic use of high doses of daily corticosteroids in some, the major cause of growth retardation is the calorie deficit, particularly in view of the increased caloric requirement for growth in children who modify their eating patterns to lessen postprandial symptoms. Consistently, growth-retarded children ingest less than two thirds of the projected requirements in calories.[12] Increased demand for protein because of high losses into the inflamed intestine must also be met. Vitamin deficiencies are not common in this population, and iron and zinc deficiencies are no more prevalent than in patients with normal growth.

To reestablish growth and sexual maturation in the growth-retarded adolescent, nutritional needs, particularly those for adequate calories, must be met. In many patients, these goals can be met by aggressive attention to dietary caloric intake once symptoms are controlled by medication to the

extent possible.[12] In some, liquid dietary supplements are required in addition to foods. A small percentage of patients requires intensive nutritional support by nasoenteral tube feeding of defined formula diets or total parenteral nutrition. When surgery is indicated, particularly for severe narrowing or obstruction in Crohn's disease, symptomatic improvement is associated with an improved dietary intake to meet the needs for growth. The principle is that growth retardation or arrest can be reversed if nutritional requirements are met. Sometimes, because of the delay in bone age that accompanies growth retardation, the adolescent growth spurt is delayed by as much as two or three years, and growth may continue well beyond the usual adolescent span.

## HOME PARENTERAL NUTRITION

There is a growing experience with the use of home total parenteral nutrition in the management of patients with severe and intractable Crohn's disease. Home total parenteral nutrition was first used in such patients who had had recurrent and extensive small bowel resections and could not meet their nutritional requirements by diet alone.[15] As the technique of home total parenteral nutrition has become more widely available, this approach is sometimes used as a substitution for a bowel rest and total parenteral nutrition regimen in hospital for patients with uncontrolled disease or unhealing fistulas or for those requiring extensive nutritional repletion in preparation for surgery. There are few published series of such an approach. Experience with adolescents with Crohn's disease in Los Angeles demonstrated that home parenteral nutrition was capable of producing symptomatic remissions in most patients, but symptomatic recurrences required reinstitution of home therapy in many of these patients within less than a year.[16] This approach still appears to have advantages in some patients as an alternative to repeated hospitalizations.

## REFERENCES

1. Driscoll, R.H., Rosenberg, I.H.: Med. Clin. North Am. *62*:185–201, 1978.
2. Food and Nutrition Board: National Research Council, Recommended Dietary Allowances. 9th ed. Washington, D.C., U.S. National Academy of Sciences, 1980.
3. Kirschner, B.S., de Favara, M.V., Jensen, W.: Gastroenterology *81*:829–832, 1981.
4. Arvanitakis, C.: Digestion *19*:259–266, 1979.
5. Meredith, S.C., Rosenberg, I.H.: Clin. Endocrinol. Metab. *9*:131–150, 1980.
6. Heaton, K.W., Thornton, J.R., Emmett, P.M.: Br. Med. J. *2*:764–766, 1979.
7. Ammon, H., Phillips, S.F.: Gastroenterology *65*:744–749, 1973.

8. Franklin, J.L., Rosenberg, I.H.: Gastroenterology *64*:517, 1973.
9. Wolman, S.L., Anderson, G.H., Marliss, E.B., et al.: Gastroenterology *76*:458–468, 1979.
10. Driscoll, R.H., Jr., Meredith, S.C., Sitrin, M., et al.: Gastroenterology *83*:1252–1258, 1982.
11. Harries, A.D., Danis, V., Heatley, R.V., et al.: Lancet *1*:887–890, 1983.
12. Kirschner, B.S., Klich, J.R., Kalman, S.S., et al.: Gastroenterology *80*:10–15, 1981.
13. Bengoa, J.M., Rosenberg, I.H.: Parenteral nutrition therapy in gastrointestinal disease. *In* Year Book of Medicine, 1983, pp. 363–385.
14. Dickinson, R.J., Ashton, M.G., Axon, A.T.R., et al.: Gastroenterology *79*:1199–1204, 1980.
15. Jeejeebhoy, K.N., Langer, B., Tsallas, G., et al.: Gastroenterology *71*:943, 1976.
16. Strobel, C.T., Byrne, W.J., Ament, M.E.: Gastroenterology *77*:272, 1979.

*Chapter* **56**

# NUTRITION AND DIET IN MANAGEMENT OF DISEASES OF THE GASTROINTESTINAL TRACT

## (C) SMALL INTESTINE
### (5) Nutritional Support of Patients with Short Bowel Syndrome and Malabsorption

### Mukesh B. Desai and Khursheed N. Jeejeebhoy

Resection of small intestine is required in situations associated with tumors, vascular insufficiency, inflammation, trauma, and congenital abnormalities. Frequent causes of bowel resection are Crohn's disease in young people and intestinal infarction in older individuals.

Resection of only short lengths of small bowel causes little disturbance of function, particularly when the ileocecal junction remains intact. This is chiefly because of the considerable intestinal reserve in normal man. Furthermore, even with resection that compromises absorption, the adaptation of the remaining bowel increases its function and substantially restores its ability to absorb normally. Impairment of absorption tends to be prolonged or permanent, however, when more than half of the small bowel has been removed. Because the malnutrition resulting from excision is the result of several factors, knowledge of the length of bowel removed is not sufficient in itself to forecast the degree and specific type of functional disability.

For a given individual following bowel resection, the nutritional support regimen will depend upon the site and length of resection, the degree of adaptation, and existing disease. Consequently, this regimen may change as adaptation of the remaining bowel progresses.

## NORMAL ABSORPTION AND MOTILITY OF SMALL INTESTINE

To understand better the subsequent clinical effects of resection, one needs to review pertinent features of small bowel function.

**Motility.** Following a meal, transit through the gastrointestinal tract depends upon a complex interrelationship modulating gastric, small bowel, and colonic motility.

**Gastric Emptying.** The nature of the chyme entering the small intestine alters gastric emptying. In general, the ingestion of nutrients, especially fat, but also protein and, to a lesser extent, carbohydrate, inhibits gastric emptying. This inhibition depends upon stimulation not only of duodenal receptors but also of receptors that are further down the intestine. Experimental reinfusion of chyme collected from the duodenum into the jejunoileum inhibits gastric motility. It seems too that the inhibition is prolonged with a larger meal.[1]

**Small Intestinal Motility.** Small bowel transit has been studied in rats using nonabsorbable isotopes.[2] Such studies have shown the importance of the ileum in slowing transit. The marker traverses the first 50% of the bowel in a third of the time it takes to pass through the next 30%. Similarly in man, Connell demonstrated that passage of chyme through the jejunum was clearly more rapid than passage through the succeeding ileum.[3]

**Ileocecal Valve.** The nature of this valve and its control over intestinal motility is controversial; nevertheless, when the ileum is resected, excision of the valve speeds up small bowel transit, and reconstruction of the valve reduces the diarrhea and fluid loss found in this situation.[4,5]

**Colonic Motility.** Motility of the gastrointestinal tract is slowest at the level of the colon. The mean transit time through the colon varies widely (between 24 and 150 hours), depending on the fat and fiber content of the diet eaten. Thus the colon is important in slowing intestinal transit.

**Interdigestive Motility and Secretion.** Periodically, during the NPO (nil per os) state, the stomach and small bowel become active, being swept by waves of electrical activity called the interdigestive migratory myoelectric complexes (MMC). At these times, secretion of bile and pancreatic juice is significant[6]—as much as 30% of the maximum.

**Secretion and Absorption of Fluid and Electrolytes.** Each day a total of 5 to 6 liters of endogenous secretions enters the small bowel: 1 liter or so each of saliva and bile, and 1.5 to 3 liters of gastric and pancreatic juices. All of this, except for a liter, is absorbed in the small intestine. The absorption site varies with the nature of what is eaten. Following a meat and salad meal, most of the fluid is absorbed high in the jejunum, whereas following a meal of milk and doughnuts, when more water is secreted into the bowel, more of the fluid is absorbed distally.[7] In each of the three major areas of the intestine, namely jejunum, ileum, and colon, the absorption of fluid and electrolytes is significantly different depending partly on the nature of the electrolyte transport processes, and partly on the permeability of the intercellular spaces. Successful management of someone with resection of proximal and/or distal bowel depends on a good understanding of the difference between the effects of these resections, with due recognition also of the role of the colon following intestinal resection.

In general, water absorption is a passive process resulting from the active transport of nutrients and electrolytes. Sodium transport is the main electrolyte process that helps create an electrochemical gradient across the mucosa and thereby aids the uptake of amino acids and sugars.[8] Two main processes result in the absorption of sodium and chloride. One is coupled to the absorption of carbohydrates and amino acids, and the other to the absorption of isotonic sodium chloride. In the jejunum,[9] the first process is dominant whereas in the ileum[10] and colon the second one is the more active.

These mechanisms not only aid transport of electrolytes across the intestinal epithelium, but they also help in the absorption of nutrients through the aforementioned coupling of sodium transport with that of amino acids and sugars. The net effect on intraluminal contents depends upon this absorption, as well as upon back diffusion through the intercellular junctions. In the jejunum, where these junctions are "leaky," back diffusion readily occurs, resulting in the maintenance of isotonicity of jejunal contents. In contrast, the "tightness" of ileal and colonic junctions increases progressively distally so that back diffusion occurs less and less readily as one moves along the gastrointestinal tract. This change results in the intraluminal contents becoming concentrated with respect to plasma, thus conserving body fluid.

**Nutrient Digestion and Absorption.** Products of digestion not absorbed by the jejunum are taken up by the ileum. In man, absorption of nutrients is commonly completed within the first 150 cm of the bowel,[11] so that usually little nutrient reaches the ileum.

**Unique Functions of the Ileum.** Notwithstanding the foregoing, the ileum is involved with the absorption of certain specific items: vitamin $B_{12}$ and bile salts. Being unique to this section of small intestine, these functions have special implications for patients with ileal resection. Most of the bile salts secreted during a meal are reclaimed by their ileal reabsorption, and are then recycled to the jejunum by way of the portal blood, liver, and gallbladder (the enterohepatic circulation). With increasing length of ileal resection or bypass, such recycling is progressively less efficient. If the loss of ileum is greater than 100 cm, synthesis of bile salts in the liver never catches up to the demands of a whole day. This inadequacy causes altered digestion and absorption of fat in the jejunum.

When the distal ileum has been extirpated, bile salt synthesis increases the bile salt pool during the night when the bowel is quiescent; hence, for the first meal of the day there may be sufficient bile for its fat absorption. However, because ileal reabsorption is minimal, the bile salt pool quickly becomes depleted, and progressive malabsorption of the fat occurs in subsequent meals. When any portion of the distal ileum is resected or bypassed, decreased absorption of bile salts causes an increased amount to enter the colon, resulting in a reduced absorption of water and sodium, giving rise to cholera-like diarrhea. Deoxy-bile acids also cause fluid secretion from the colon, so that the fluid and electrolyte losses are increased.

## EFFECTS OF INTESTINAL RESECTION

### Motility

**Gastric Motility.** Earlier it was noted that the presence of nutrients in the small intestine inhibits gastric motility; conversely, the rate of gastric emptying is increased with small bowel resection.

**Small Bowel Motility.** Because motility is rapid in the jejunum but slow in the distal ileum, resection of proximal bowel alone does not result in an increased rate of intestinal transit.[12] By contrast, following ileal resection, the remaining bowel has a short transit time.[12,13] Fed as a marker, [51]Cr is almost completely excreted within a few hours.[14]

**Colonic Motility.** The region of the intestinal tract with the slowest motility is colon, Hence, an intact colon is most important for maintaining transit rates that are close to normal. Distal resections that include some or all of the colon tend to shorten intestinal transit time.

### Absorption of Fluid and Electrolytes

Both the extent of intestinal resection and its location govern consequent changes in fluid and electrolyte absorption. Losses of fluid and electrolytes will not be excessive unless (1) the fluid load delivered to the colon following small bowel resection exceeds its reserve absorptive capacity, or (2) the contents of the small intestinal dejecta reaching the colon inhibit colonic absorption. The reserve capacity of the normal colon is about 5 liters per day,[15] but bile salts[16] and free fatty acids[17] reduce its ability to absorb both water and sodium. Colonic bacteria can degrade certain forms of vegetable residue and carbohydrate into titratable acids that increase the osmotic load and thereby the water output.[18,19]

Proximal resection causes little diarrhea because the ileum is able to reabsorb the increased fluid and electrolyte load, and any excess still remaining is taken up by the colon. Because bile salts have been taken up by a still intact ileum, the colon does not receive any substances preventing water and electrolyte absorption. Following distal resection (i.e., of the ileum), diarrhea occurs because the colon receives a larger fluid load that is not only unconcentrated but also isotonic, and because additional substances (bile salts, fatty acids, unabsorbed carbohydrate) reach the colon and so reduce the reabsorption of water and electrolytes.

Should the colon be partially or completely resected, that section of bowel that is capable of taking over at least some of the fluid and electrolyte absorption of the extirpated small bowel is lost. The importance of the colon in modifying the severity of the diarrhea after resection has been emphasized.[20,21] Should both ileum and colon be resected, the loss of isotonic water and salt becomes a major problem, with resultant dehydration, hypokalemia and hypomagnesemia.

### Nutrient Absorption

Because absorption of nutrients occurs throughout the small bowel following jejunectomy, the ileum can assume, with hyperplasia, the proximal absorptive function and there is little malabsorption.[22] Resections of ileum, however, need exceed only 100 cm to cause steatorrhea.[23]

Malabsorption, and its effect on the nutritional status of the patient, increases with increasing length of resection[24] while an assortment of nutrients is malabsorbed.[14,25] A literature review indicates that despite considerable variability, resections up to 33% cause no malnutrition, and up to 50% are tolerable without special aids. However, when resection exceeds 75% of the bowel, nutritional status can only be maintained with special help.[26–30] When resection leaves but a few inches of jejunum, survival is limited, and survivors usually are severely depleted nutritionally[31,36] unless total parenteral nutrition is instituted.

## ADAPTATION OF SMALL INTESTINE

Flint in 1912 first demonstrated a significant postresection increase in villus height in man, and calculated that the absorptive surface area increased four-fold.[37] Since then, this phenomenon has been shown to occur in studies in man[38] and in animals.[39,40]

In parallel with anatomic changes, absorption in animals[41] and in humans is improved.[42] Morphologic effects after resection include increases in cell proliferation[43,44] and cell migration to the villus tip. The former appears to result from an increase in size of the crypt zone where cell replication occurs.[44,45] Morphologic changes then could be responsible for the functional compensation. Additionally, individual cells may show alterations, as in increased Na-K ATPase activity.[46]

The cause of these functional and morphologic changes may be grouped into four major categories: (1) the increased work load for the remaining bowel, (2) local nutrition, (3) the effect of endogenous secretions (e.g., bile and pancreatic juice), and (4) hormonal effects.

Hyperplasia occurs, presumably as a result of the aforementioned factors, when the ileum (normally not exposed to a large nutrient load) is transposed to the area of the jejunum.[47] Instillation of non-nutritive agents, such as NaCl, $\alpha$-methylglucoside, and lactose, which are transported by the mucosa, is most effective in promoting cell proliferation.[48] Thus, increased functional demand rather than local nutrition may be more important for adaptation. Further, crypt cells, where stimulation would be expected to occur,[49] do not take up enterally fed amino acids. Therefore, it seems unlikely that orally fed amino acids stimulate mucosal protein synthesis at these sites of cell proliferation. Parenterally administered amino acids, however, are taken up by crypt cells.

Endogenous secretions have been implicated in promoting villus hypertrophy through experiments where transplantation of the duodenal papilla into the ileum (with resultant local influx of pancreatic and biliary secretions) resulted in ileal hyperplasia.[50] Lastly, the role of humoral factors has been recognized following observations in parabiotic animals, where intestinal resection in one of the pair resulted in hyperplasia of the intestine in the other.[51] Enteroglucagon is an interesting candidate hormone for this phenomenon as suggested by observations in man.[52]

## NUTRITIONAL THERAPY OF INTESTINAL RESECTION

On the basis of the foregoing discussion, the approach to a patient with intestinal resection depends on the amount and site of resected bowel, the presence of continuing intestinal disease (which reduces the functional length of the intestine), and the time required for adaptation. With time, the progress of the patient may lead to modifications of treatment. Nevertheless, several therapeutic avenues are applicable to all patients.

General approaches will be considered first, and then specific applications.

### Initial Treatment after Resection

**Control of Diarrhea.** Diarrhea is caused by a combination of increased secretions, increased motility, and osmotic stimulation of water secretion due to malabsorption of luminal contents. The first step in achieving control of severe diarrhea is to decrease or stop oral intake to reduce any osmotic component, and to treat presenting dehydration effectively. Even when the patient is NPO, fluid loss may be substantial owing to gastric hypersecretion and malabsorbed endogenous secretions stimulated by interdigestive migratory myoelectric complexes (MMC). Reduction of secretion, particularly gastric secretion, can be

achieved by infusing $H_2$ blockers. Our preference is to give the $H_2$ blocker initially as a continuous IV infusion (cimetidine 300 mg over 6 hours), rather than as a bolus, because of its short half-life. Use of opiates as well aids in slowing intestinal propulsion and in increasing ion transport.[53] Locally acting loperamide should be tried in increasing doses. If this agent is ineffective, codeine or diphenoxylate may be used.

**Oral Feeding.** The next step is to determine the nature and amount of oral diets that might be instituted. The degree of concern and the rigor of these measures depend upon the amount of bowel resected. Even for those patients with massive resection, some oral intake (or tube feeding) should be instituted in order to stimulate hyperplasia of the remaining bowel. For patients who have more than 60 to 80 cm of their bowel remaining (>15 to 20% of normal length),[54,55] refeeding should be progressive so that eventually they will eat a normal or modified oral diet. In sharp contrast, for patients whose only remaining small bowel is duodenum, the initial target must be small liquid feeds in addition to parenteral nutrition.

For those having intermediate lengths of bowel, procedures for feeding vary. One program for progressive feeding starts with a carbohydrate-electrolyte mixture that is flavored and isotonic, and contains an oligosaccharide (e.g., Caloreen 3.4% or Polycose, $Na^+$ 85 meq/L, $K^+$ 12 meq/L, $HCO_3^-$ 9 meq/L, and $Cl^-$ 109 meq/L). Such a mixture is well absorbed by patients with massive resection who previously were dependent on intravenous fluids.[56]

The next stage of oral feeding involves a choice between a normal diet and a defined-formula diet. Again, as a rule of thumb, when resection leaves the patient with more than 60 to 80 cm of small intestine, a normal oral diet should be tried. When testing such a diet, the patient should be given fairly dry solids, with isotonic fluids being allowed not less than one hour after the solids. The separation of solids from liquids is critical in view of the marked increase in speed of gastric emptying noted with resection. With this plan, the nature of the diet fed does not change the diarrhea or total malabsorption in patients with massive resection.[14] On the other hand, in patients who fail to tolerate a normal diet using this plan, and in those with very little bowel, one should test a constant infusion of a defined-formula diet. The pertinent aspect is the use of controlled, well-modulated rates of infusion, commencing with 25 ml/hour, and gradually increasing to 100 to 125 ml/hour. This procedure can ensure that the rate at which the osmotic load is received by the intestine is constant. With this approach, many patients who would otherwise need intravenous feeding can in fact be managed entirely by the enteral route (see Chap. 54).

**Parenteral Electrolytes and Nutrients.** Following a major resection, all patients need intravenous fluid and electrolyte replacement, especially sodium chloride, potassium, and magnesium. These are infused to meet needs as judged by a urine flow that exceeds 1 liter per day, and by the ability to maintain normal serum electrolyte levels, central venous pressure, and blood pressure. There should be no postural hypotension if hydration is adequate.

A gradual decrease in the intravenous infusion is balanced by an equivalent increase in the oral intake in an effort to achieve the goal of meeting all needs orally. This regimen requires patience and may need several weeks or more of adaptation and modification.

**Parenteral Nutrition.** For patients whose remaining small bowel is less than 60 to 80 cm, parenteral nutrition should be started immediately in order to avoid malnutrition during the period of oral refeeding. Here too parenteral nutrient intake may be reduced gradually if oral intake increases. Although most nutrient requirements are met orally eventually, in some situations it may continue to be necessary to give electrolytes parenterally. An area often neglected in parenteral nutrition is trace elements. With small bowel resection and severe diarrhea, the need for zinc increases to 12 to 15 mg/day because of endogenous losses.[57] These amounts are computed by measuring the volume of intestinal fluid lost per day in the NPO state and adding 12 to 17 mg of zinc for every liter of such loss.

## Long-Term Nutritional Support

Long-term nutritional support is a dynamic process (i.e., the patient is likely to adapt with time, even measured in years) and thus should be reevaluated periodically. There are four possible outcomes: (1) a normal oral diet, or one modified by separating solids from liquids; (2) defined-formula diets; (3) an oral diet with parenterally administered electrolytes and fluids; or (4) parenteral nutrition that is total, or partial with variable oral intake.

Because the objective is to try to stabilize the patient on an oral diet with or without supplements, it is necessary to continually reevaluate the patient on parenteral nutrition in order to determine whether bowel adaptation has occurred. In difficult cases the following approach is taken by the authors. The patient's resting metabolic rate is determined, and a target calorie intake (TCI) of

130% of that rate is chosen to allow extra calories for activity. Then a fecal fat excretion is measured on a standard fat intake. Because two earlier studies have shown that the percentage of fat absorbed approximates the percentage of carbohydrates and protein absorbed,[14,58] we can determine how many calories of a balanced diet need to be eaten to meet the TCI. For example, if the TCI is 1,800 kcal/day, and absorption is 50%, then the patient must eat 3,600 kcal/day. If this intake can be achieved without discomfort, then macronutrient requirements are judged to be met by an oral diet. The next problem is micronutrient, water, and electrolyte needs. These needs are judged by gradually reducing IV intake and observing the levels of serum electrolytes, trace elements, prothrombin time, and especially fat-soluble vitamins. In many instances, the patient can meet macronutrient requirements orally, but needs electrolyte, trace element, and vitamin supplementation by the parenteral route.

Enthusiasm for the goal of progressing toward the first outcome listed should be tempered by appreciating the following. Although the system must allow the patient to maintain normal nutritional status, it should also be free of serious diarrhea or bowel frequency so that he may work and achieve social rehabilitation. For example, it is indeed possible for a patient to eat 10 to 12 meals a day, have a similar number of bowel movements, including nocturnal ones, and remain free of parenteral support. However, life for such a person is an oral-anal existence, leaving little time for anything else. The option chosen must avoid such an outcome and permit social and work rehabilitation. The successes with home enteral[59] and parenteral nutrition[60–62] have revolutionized the prognosis of patients with major intestinal resection (see Chap. 54).

## Special Considerations

Special considerations may be needed depending on the length and site of resection.

**Jejunal Resection with Intact Ileum and Colon.** Patients in this category can be fed orally immediately and rarely have any problems. However, initial feedings should be advanced and tolerance tested as ileal hyperplasia develops.

**Ileal Resection of Less than 100 cm with Colon Largely Intact.** Patients in this situation have so-called choleraic diarrhea, and are best helped by an initial administration of 4 g of cholestyramine three times daily to bind the bile salts left unabsorbed by the resected ileum. Vitamin $B_{12}$ absorption should be measured and, if low, parenteral vitamin $B_{12}$ should be injected intramuscularly in a dose of 100 to 200 μg per month. These patients also may have hyperoxaluria because of enhanced colonic absorption of oxalate.[63] Thus they need both a low-oxalate diet and cholestyramine. Because bile salts enhance colonic oxalate absorption,[64] the binding of the salts by the cholestyramine reduces the oxalate absorption.

**Ileal Resection of More than 100 to 200 cm with Colon Largely Intact.** This group of patients has little difficulty in maintaining nutrition with an oral diet, but has steatorrhea with fatty acid diarrhea. For such a patient, fat restriction is mandatory. With the larger resection, so much in the way of bile salts is lost in the postoperative period that liver compensation cannot occur, and luminal bile salts are low;[16] hence, cholestyramine may be of little or no value. This group benefits from dietary advice concerning the separate eating of solids and liquids to reduce diarrhea. Hyperoxaluria, with danger of oxalate stones, and vitamin $B_{12}$ malabsorption must be considered and managed appropriately.

**Resection in Excess of 200 cm of Small Bowel and Lesser Resection with Associated Colectomy.** Patients of this class require the graduated adaptation program indicated previously under the section on general considerations. Regimens will differ depending upon the amount of bowel left and on what adaptation occurs.

**Resection Leaving Less than 60 cm Small Bowel or only a Duodenum; Massive Bowel Resection with Short Bowel Syndrome.** Patients in this most severely affected category need parenteral nutrition at home on an indefinite basis. Infusion rate and caloric intake are gradually reduced if the patient is able to maintain his weight with an oral diet. When to reduce intravenous feeding is decided on the basis of weight gain beyond desired limits and the fact that reduced infusion does not cause electrolyte and fluid imbalances.

## REMAINING PROBLEMS

For patients with major intestinal resection, micronutrient and vitamin requirements constitute an area needing further study, for those receiving total parenteral nutrition and also for those taking their nutrition orally. Although macronutrient requirements can be largely estimated from body composition, the need for many micronutrients and for oral supplementation is not well defined.

## REFERENCES

1. Malagelada, J-R.: Gastric, pancreatic and biliary responses to a meal. *In* Physiology of the Gastrointestinal Tract. (Johnson, L.R., Ed.) New York, Raven Press, 1981, pp. 893–924.
2. Summers, R.W., Kent, T.H., Osborne, J.W.: Gastroenterology *59*:731–739, 1970.
3. Connell, A.M.: Rend. Gastro-Enterol. *2*:38–46, 1970.
4. Singelton, A.O., Redmond, D.C., McMurray, J.E.: Ann. Surg. *159*:690–694, 1964.
5. Ricotta, J., Zuidema, G.D., Gadacz, T.R., et al.: Surg. Gynecol. Obstet *152*:310–314, 1981.
6. Vantrappen, G.R., Peeters, T.L., Janssens, J.: Scand. J. Gastroenterol. *14*:663–667, 1979.
7. Fordtran, J.S., Locklear, T.W.: Am. J. Dig. Dis. *11*:503–521, 1966.
8. Goldner, A.M., Schultz, S.G., Curran, P.F.: J. Gen. Physiol. *53*:362–384, 1969.
9. Fordtran, J.S., Dietschy, J.M.: Gastroenterology *50*:263–285, 1966.
10. Turnberg, L.A., Bieberdorf, F.A., Morawski, S.G., et al.: J. Clin. Invest. *49*:557–567, 1970.
11. Borgstrom, B., Dahlquist, A., Lundh, G., et al.: J. Clin. Invest. *36*:1521–1536, 1957.
12. Nylander, G.: Acta Chir. Scand. *133*:131–138, 1967.
13. Reynell, P.C., Spray, G.H.: Gastroenterology *31*:361–368, 1956.
14. Woolf, G.M., Miller, C., Kurian, R., et al.: Gastroenterology *84*:823–828, 1983.
15. Debongnie, J.C., Phillips, S.F.: Gastroenterology *74*:698–703, 1978.
16. Hofmann, A.F., Poley, J.R.: N. Engl. J. Med. *281*:397–402, 1960.
17. Binder, H.J.: Gastroenterology *65*:847–850, 1973.
18. Williams, R.D., Olmsted, W.H.: J. Nutr. *11*:433–449, 1936.
19. Bond, J.H., Levitt, M.D.: J. Clin. Invest. *57*:1158–1164, 1973.
20. Cummings, J.H., James, W.P.T., Wiggings, H.S.: Lancet *1*:344–347, 1973.
21. Mitchell, J., Zukerman, L., Breuer, R.I.: Gastroenterology *72*:1103, 1977.
22. Booth, C.C., Alldis, D., Read, A.E.: Gut *2*:168–174, 1961.
23. Hofmann, A.E., Poley, J.R.: Gastroenterology *62*:918–934, 1972.
24. Nylander, E., Ladefoged, K., Jarnum, S.: Scand. J. Gastroenterol. *15*:853–858, 1980.
25. Ladefoged, K.: Am. J. Clin. Nutr. *36*:59–67, 1982.
26. Haymond, H.E.: Surg. Gynecol. Obstet. *61*:693–705, 1935.
27. McClenahan, J.E., Fisher, B.: Am. J. Surg. *79*:684–688, 1950.
28. Trafford, H.S.: Br. J. Surg. *44*:10–13, 1956.
29. West, E.S., Montague, J.R., Judy, F.R.: Am. J. Dig. Dis. *5*:690–692, 1938.
30. Pilling, G.P., Cresson, S.L.: Pediatrics *19*:940–948, 1957.
31. Maring, J.R., Pattee, C.J., Gardner, C., et al.: Can. Med. Assoc. J. *69*:429–433, 1953.
32. Kinney, J.M., Goldwyn, R.M., Barr, J.S., et al.: J.A.M.A. *179*:529–532, 1962.
33. Walker-Smith, J.: Med. J. Aust. *1*:857–860, 1967.
34. Clayton, B.E., Cotton, D.A.: Gut *2*:18–22, 1961.
35. Anderson, C.M.: Br. Med. J. *1*:419–422, 1965.
36. Meyer, H.W.: Surgery *51*:755–759, 1962.
37. Flint, J.M.: Johns Hopkins Hosp. Bull. *23*:127–144, 1912.
38. Porus, R.L.: Gastroenterology *48*:753–757, 1965.
39. Booth, C.C., Evans, K.T., Menzies, T., et al.: Br. J. Surg. *46*:403–410, 1959.
40. Nygaard, K.: Acta Chir. Scand. *133*:233–248, 1967.
41. Stassoff, B.: Beitr. Klin. Chir. *89*:527–586, 1914.

42. Althausen, T.L., Doig, R.K., Uyeyama, K., et al.: Gastroenterology *16*:126–139, 1950.
43. Loran, M.R., Althausen, T.L.: J. Biophys. Biochem. Cytol. *7*:667–672, 1960.
44. Obertop, H., Nundy, S., Malamud, D., et al.: Gastroenterology *72*:267–270, 1977.
45. Cairnie, A.B., Lamerton, L.F., Steel, G.G.: Exp. Cell Res. *39*:528–538, 1965.
46. Tilson, M.D., Wright, H.K.: Surg. Forum *21*:326–327, 1970.
47. Altmann, G.G., Leblond, C.P.: Am. J. Anat. *127*:15–36, 1970.
48. Clarke, R.M.: Digestion *15*:411–424, 1977.
49. Alpers, D.H.: J. Clin. Invest. *51*:167–173, 1972.
50. Weser, E., Heller, R., Tawil, T.: Gastroenterology *73*:524–529, 1977.
51. Williamson, R.C.N., Buckholtz, T.W., Malt, R.A.: Gastroenterology *75*:249–254, 1978.
52. Gleeson, M.H., Bloom, S.R., Polak, J.M., et al.: Gut *12*:773–782, 1971.
53. McKay, J.S., Linaker, B.D., Turnberg, L.A.: Gastroenterology *80*:279–284, 1981.
54. Cook, G.C., Carruthers, R.H.: Gut *15*:545–548, 1974.
55. Backman, L., Hallberg, D.: Acta. Chir. Scand. *140*:57–63, 1974.
56. Griffin, G.E., Fagan, E.F., Hodgson, A.J., et al.: Dig. Dis. Sci. *27*:902–908, 1982.
57. Wolman, S.L., Anderson, G.H., Marliss, E.B., et al.: Gastroenterology *76*:458–467, 1979.
58. Woolf, G.M., Jeejeebhoy, K.N.: Dig. Dis. Sci. In Press, 1986.
59. Bastian, C.H., Driscoll, R.S.: Enteral tube feedings at home. *In* Enteral and Tube Feeding. (Rombeau, J.L., Caldwell, M.D., Eds.) Philadelphia, W.B. Saunders Co., 1984, pp. 494–512.
60. Jeejeebhoy, K.N., Zohrab, W.J., Langer, B., et al.: Gastroenterology *65*:811–820, 1973.
61. Broviac, J.W., Scribner, B.H.: Surg. Gynecol. Obstet. *139*:24–28, 1974.
62. Shils, M.E.: Am. J. Clin. Nutr. *28*:1429–1435, 1975.
63. Andersson, H., Jagenburg, R.: Gut *15*:360–366, 1974.
64. Chadwick, V.S., Gaginella, T.S., Carlson, G.L., et al.: J. Lab. Clin. Med. *94*:661–674, 1979.

*Chapter* **56**

# NUTRITION AND DIET IN MANAGEMENT OF DISEASES OF THE GASTROINTESTINAL TRACT

*(C) SMALL INTESTINE*
  *(6) Factors Influencing Absorption of Natural Diets*

David J.A. Jenkins

In the treatment of gastrointestinal disease, emphasis has been placed on improving absorption of nutrients in conditions such as Crohn's disease, celiac disease, short bowel and stagnant loop syndromes, radiation enteropathy, postgastrectomy, and Whipple's disease. However, there are also situations in which therapies have attempted to reduce the rate or amount of nutrients absorbed. These include the treatment of diabetes, hyperlipidemia, or obesity using, for example, high-fiber diets, enzyme inhibitors, ileal bypass, or jejunoileal bypass.

Manipulations that increase or decrease the rate of absorption are likely to have a number of physiologic consequences as illustrated in Figures 56C6–1 and 56C6–2. Where the absorption rate is reduced, a larger length of small intestine is likely to be exposed to the nutrient, with an increased proportion absorbed more distally (see Fig. 1a). On the other hand, rapidly absorbed foods are likely to be taken up more proximally in the small intestine and over a shorter segment (see Fig. 1b). After oral intake the consequences of the slower flux of nutrient into the system will result in lower

circulating nutrient levels, and consequently lower endocrine responses, (see Fig. 56C6–2a) as opposed to the sharper rises and falls seen with the more rapid fluxes (see Fig. 56C6–2b). In addition, differences can be expected in nutrient absorption characteristics (e.g., chylomicra synthesis) depending on the region of the bowel in which this takes place. Regional specialization also occurs in terms of the gut endocrine responses to nutrients absorbed in different parts of the bowel. For example, more gastric inhibitory polypeptide (GIP) will be secreted when carbohydrates are absorbed proximally and more enteroglucagon when they are absorbed distally.

The food factors that influence the absorption of nutrients relate not only to the nature of the nutrients themselves but also to their interaction with each other and with the nonabsorbable components of the food, the dietary fiber, and associated antinutrients. All these factors combined produce the form or physical state of the food which itself exerts a major influence on the handling of a food by the gastrointestinal tract. Some of these effects are acute, but food constituents

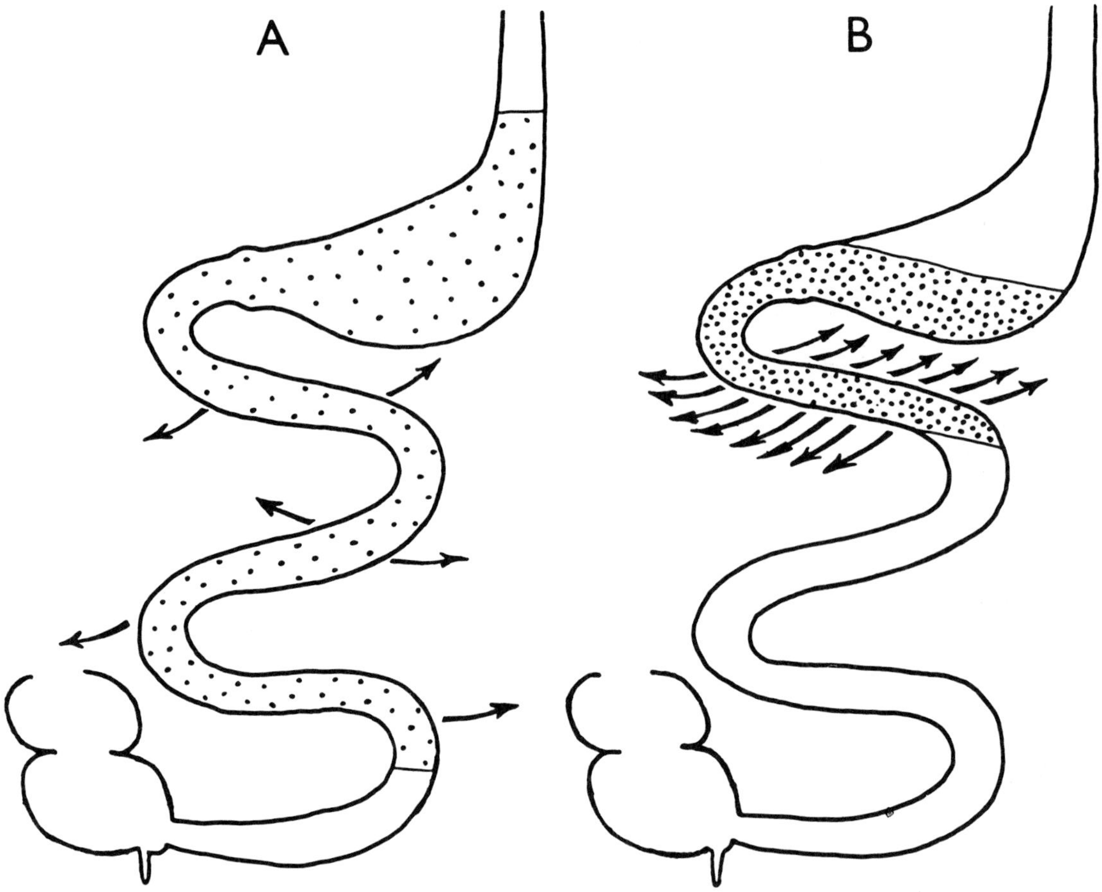

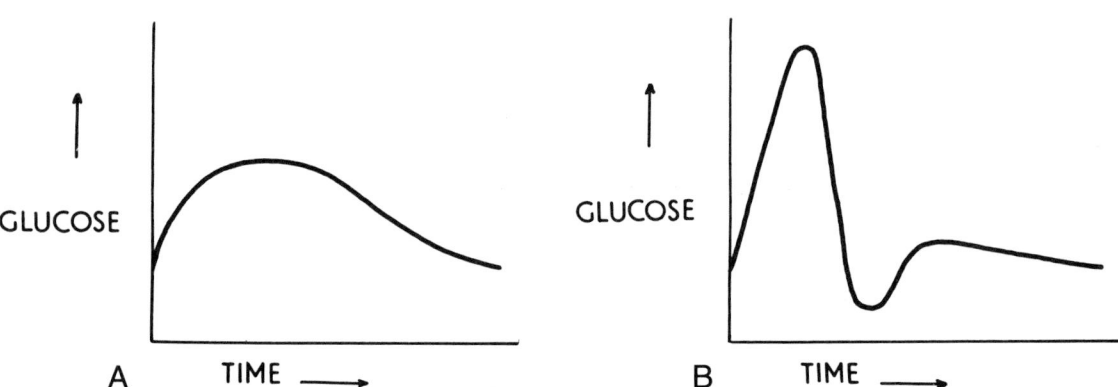

**Fig. 56C6–1.**   Schematic representation of stomach and small intestine showing *(A)* slow digestion and absorption of energy-dilute food in a "fiber-rich" diet and *(B)* rapid digestion and absorption of energy-dense food from a low-fiber diet.

**Fig. 56C6–2.**   Schematic representation of the postprandial glycemia following *(A)* slow absorption of starchy fiber-rich meals and *(B)* rapid absorption with undershoot due to excessive insulin release following refined, fiber-depleted carbohydrate foods.

also have chronic effects. They may influence the absorptive capacity of the gut either by enzyme induction or by effects that may be stimulatory, inhibitory, or toxic to mucosal cell growth turnover and villus structure.

## EFFECT OF MACRONUTRIENTS AND FIBER

Before we discuss the effects of food form and the so-called antinutrients in influencing the absorbability of natural diets, it is useful to consider both the similarities and differences that exist within the three macronutrient groupings and their relationships to each other and to fiber.

### Carbohydrate

Traditionally it has been held that "complex" carbohydrates (starches) are absorbed more slowly than "simple" carbohydrates.[1] Meals, therefore, that contain a higher proportion of their carbohydrates as sugars were considered to result in more rapid absorption and higher blood glucose rises.[2] This view has been challenged by a number of studies. Using solutions of starch (a glucose polymer), caloreen (predominantly 5 glucose units), and glucose itself, Wahlquist and colleagues demonstrated similar glucose and insulin rises following consumption of 50-g carbohydrate loads of each of these glucose sources by healthy volunteers.[3]

**Starch.** Such results should have been predictable since earlier work of Dahlquist and Borgstrom[4] and Fogel and Gray[5] had indicated that luminal hydrolysis of starch is not rate-limiting for starch digestion. Fogel and Gray had stated that even patients with chronic pancreatitis and significant exocrine pancreatic insufficiency (10% amylase secretion rate compared with normal) nevertheless hydrolyzed starch in vivo at a similar rate to normals.[5] Their studies involved feeding 50-g starch loads and aspirating the residual hydrolytic contents at the ligament of Treitz (duodeno-jejunal junction). Nevertheless, this finding does not indicate that luminal events are unimportant in the digestion of foods of complex composition. Rather it indicates that differences in absorption are unlikely to be seen between meals containing sugars or highly processed, low amylose or soluble starches (25 to 30% amylose and 70 to 75% amylopectin).[6] Such a statement does not cover the important effects of differences in food form or indigestible food components that may have a profound effect on the rate of luminal digestion.

If, however, the proportion of amylose (1-4 linked straight chain starch) to amylopectin (1-6 linked branched starch) varies in a food, then alterations in digestibility may be seen. Traditionally it was considered that such branching was nutritionally significant because α-amylase has poor specificity for 1-6 branch points and produces α-limit dextrins.[7] Digestion was considered to proceed more slowly for this reason. However, it now appears the brush border α-glucosidases are so efficient that it makes no difference in terms of rates of uptake whether the substrate for absorption is glucose, maltose, or α-limit dextrins.[8] There is even some evidence that absorption is more rapid as chain length increases up to G-10.[8] Part of the explanation may be related to the reduced osmotic effect.

Nevertheless differences do exist between amylose and amylopectin but in the opposite direction to that first expected. This phenomenon may relate to the more compact structure and hydrogen bonding of the glucose chains in amylose which render it physically less accessible to amylolytic attack than the more open and branched amylopectin.[9] In this respect, raw legume starch (higher in amylose) has been shown in rats to be less digestible than corn starch (higher in amylopectin), and the rate of hydrolysis of legume starch in vitro is less than that of corn starch.[10,11] Possible differences in the nature of starches from different foods have been emphasized by Crapo and co-workers.[12–15] In vivo studies of whole legumes (30 to 40% amylose) have indicated that they produce lower glycemic responses than cereals (25 to 30% amylose).[16,17] They are also digested less rapidly in vitro[18,19] than other starchy foods. As expected from their higher amylose content, they produce more glucose and less maltotriose on digestion.

Furthermore, the degree of hydration of the starch is a major determinant of digestibility,[20] and this is a function of both cooking and other forms of processing. Cooked starch produced higher blood glucose responses than raw starch (Fig. 56C6–3).[21] In addition, processing (milling) prior to cooking legumes was more effective in increasing digestibility than grinding after cooking,[22] and damp heat had more effect than dry heat in making both the carbohydrate[22–24] and protein[25,26] more readily absorbed. Comparisons of legumes and cereal foods illustrate many of the facets of foods that influence absorbability. Studies have clearly demonstrated the slower digestibility of legumes by comparison with cereal products[26,27] and the relationship of digestibility to the glycemic response in both normal and diabetic volunteers.[19,28] Nevertheless, such studies also highlight the other factors of possible importance including food form, fiber, and non-nutritive food factors (including the so-called antinu-

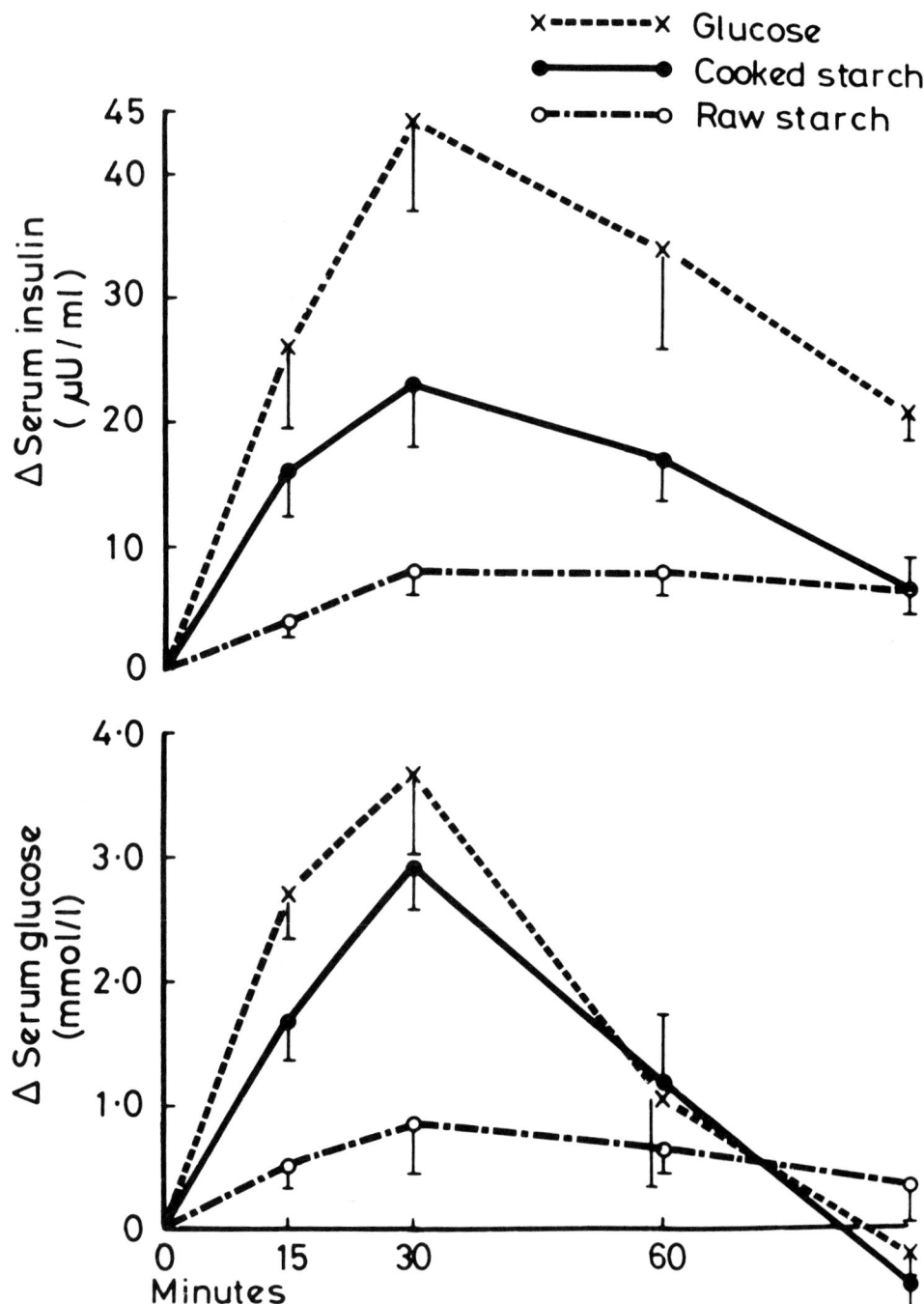

**Fig. 56C6–3.**   Mean serum insulin and glucose concentrations after ingestion of glucose monohydrate (1.1 g/kg body weight) and cooked and raw corn starch (0.91 g/kg body weight) in healthy volunteers. Conversion (SI to traditional units): Glucose: 1 mmol/L ≃ 18 mg/dl. (From Collings, P., Williams, C., MacDonald, I.,[21] with permission of Br. Med. J.)

trients) in determining absorbability or carbohydrate from foods.

**Sugars.** Efficient transport systems exist for maltose, maltotriose, $\alpha$-limit dextrins, sucrose, lactose, glucose, and galactose. Fructose absorption is less efficient and the transport maxima may be exceeded with large amounts of the sugar. The pentose, D-xylose, is only approximately 50% absorbed, and considerable malabsorption is found with the sugar alcohols or polyols, sorbitol and xylitol.[29] There are, therefore, great differences between sugars in the rate and proportions likely to be absorbed.

Recently there has been much interest in the comparative effects of sugars and starches on the blood glucose response. Contrary to many previous assumptions, numerous studies have shown that the response to sucrose in both normal and diabetic volunteers is lower than that after an equivalent amount of starch.[30,31] Nevertheless, large differences are apparent between the degree to which different sugars raise the blood glucose: fructose causes a comparatively small rise, lactose and sucrose are intermediate, and glucose and maltose cause the highest rises.[30,32–35] This effect appears to relate to the proportion of the sugar molecule that is glucose, with nonglucose components raising the blood glucose minimally.

Thus, although both the type of starch and the nature of the sugar source are likely to affect their absorption, other attributes of sugars in addition to their rates of absorption will determine their physiologic effects (e.g., glycemic and endocrine responses).

### Fats

Although much work has been done on the absorption of fatty acids, most fat in the human diet is in the form of triglycerides. Studies by Calloway and Kurtz indicated comparable digestibility of a wide range of edible fats including butter, lard, and soybean, coconut, corn, and cotton seed oils.[36] Early work had already demonstrated that butter, lard, shortening, and cod liver and corn oils were all absorbed to the same extent with maximum absorption occurring within 6 to 8 hours[37] at a time when the chylomicra rise would also have peaked.[30–40] It was estimated that 24 to 41% of the fat was absorbed by 2 hours, 53 to 71% by 4 hours, 68 to 86% by 6 hours, and 97 to 99% after 12 hours.[37] In comparisons of lymphatic absorption of long-chain fatty acids, including palmitic, oleic, linoleic, and stearic acids in man, there was a slight discrimination against triglyceride synthesis from stearic acid and in favor of cholesterol ester synthesis from oleic acid.[41] In addition, other studies suggest that triglycerides

composed of the saturated dietary fatty acids (palmitic and stearic) are less well absorbed in the presence of high calcium, whereas triglycerides containing the unsaturated fats of lower melting point (oleic and linoleic) are unaffected.[42,43] It has been suggested that, in general, either palmitic or stearic acid in the 1,3 positions of the triglyceride molecule reduce the absorption of that fat.[44,45]

Through the use of medium-chain triglycerides (MCT) in drinks, baked foods, and enteral feeds, however, attempts have been made to increase the absorption of dietary fat. Their advantage lies in their direct absorption without micelle formation with uptake as the fatty acid into the portal vein and clearance by the liver. They can, therefore, be absorbed even in the absence of bile salts or when lipoprotein synthesis necessary for chylomicra production is impaired or absent. Animal studies suggest that their efficiency of absorption is four times that of long-chain triglycerides.[46]

The use of MCT has been advocated in various situations, including small intestinal disease or damage, short bowel syndrome, pancreatic and biliary insufficiency (biliary atresia), and $\alpha$-beta-lipoproteinemia (Tangier disease). Their disadvantages are several. They do not stimulate chylomicra formation, and fat-soluble vitamins are therefore not transported out of the enterocyte. In addition, in experiments on rats, dietary substitution of MCT for corn oil resulted in 20% less weight gain largely through lack of deposition of carcass fat.[47] In man weight gain has been variable,[41] and the early clinical use of MCT was in the control of obesity.[48,49] Saunders even questioned the increased absorptive efficiency of the gut for MCT, pointing out that the widely used solvent system for stool lipid extraction in the Van de Kamer method[50] only extracts up to 68% of the medium- to short-chain fatty acids.[51] Senior responded that in the titrimetric determination, where the assumed mean fatty acids molecular weight is 284, the conversion factor is twice that which should be applied to the MCT (mean molecular weight, 144) to derive the grams of fat malabsorbed. The two errors should therefore balance out.[52] However, cramping abdominal pain and increased diarrhea together with increased steatorrhea have been reported in the short bowel syndrome following MCT.[53] In addition, MCT should not be used in decompensated cirrhosis because poor clearance of short- and medium-chain fatty acids may exacerbate encephalopathy.[54,55] Further cautioning against possible associations with liver disease is a report of two instances in which cirrhosis evolved in young patients with $\alpha$-beta-lipoproteinemia who were fed diets that were chronically high in MCT[56] (see Chap. 56E2).

Thus in terms of dietary fats, foods and dishes containing oleic or linoleic acid appear to be well absorbed. MCT may have an advantage in specific states but should be monitored with caution. At the same time as the dietary fat load is increased, there are proportionate increases in fecal fat losses.[57]

### Protein

Comparatively little is known of the intrinsic digestibility of proteins from different food sources independent of other factors in the food such as enzyme inhibitors. Data are scarce to indicate whether individual differences exist between such common protein foods as, for example, eggs, meats, poultry, fish, or cheeses that might favor their specific incorporation into the therapeutic diets of patients with limited absorptive capacity. Surprisingly, in studies of patients with cirrhosis, nitrogen balance studies have indicated no advantage of conventional animal protein foods over protein from cereal and legumes[58–60] (see Chap. 56E1).

There are, however, ways in which foods may be processed that may influence the digestibility of their constituent proteins. Nevertheless, studies have focused on the total amount absorbed or retained rather than on how the rate of absorption may be modified.

It has been noted that when protein foods are heated, cross linking may occur between amino acids or between amino acid side chains and sugars. In this last reaction, the free $NH_2$ groups on the lysine chains combine with the reducing groups of sugars, especially in the presence of heat, such as in baking of breads or cereal products and the manufacture of breakfast cereals. This synthesis (Maillard reaction) reduces the effectiveness of tryptic digestion and in experimental animals reduces the biologic value of the protein. The effect on blood amino acid responses in man remains to be assessed.

In addition, much work is being carried out on modifying proteins such as those of soy,[61] fish,[62] casein, and whey[63] to improve such functional properties as solubility, emulsifying capacity, and heat stability so that they may be used in human foods. However, their nutritional and digestibility properties will be reduced because common methods involve succinylation or acetylation of the ξ-amino group of lysine, the hydroxyl group of serine and threonine, the sulfhydryl group of cysteine, the phenol group of tyrosine, or the imidazole group of histidine.[64] It has been shown in vitro that succinylated proteins have low digestibility owing to resistance of the succinyl-lysyl bonds to pancreatic digestion.[64,65]

In terms of processing, the predominant effect is therefore to reduce the digestibility of the proteins. Nevertheless, these same processes (e.g., heat) may be essential to remove the antinutrients from other food sources (e.g., legumes, cereals, and tubers) and to enhance digestibility. Thus, use of heat in the achievement of this latter objective is likely to have a net positive rather than negative nutritional impact.

### Dietary Fiber

Many of the differences in the digestibility of foods that cannot be explained by intrinsic differences in their macronutrient components are attributable to differences in their dietary fiber or antinutrient constituents.

Large differences exist in the physical form and the physiologic effect of various classes of dietary fiber (see Chap. 2B). In general, purified viscous fibers such as the gums, gels, and mucilages reduce the rate of nutrient absorption, whereas the particulate fibers (e.g., cereal brans) have little effect on nutrient absorption in the small intestine but have a major impact on colonic function (see end of this section).

Dietary fiber of the viscous type, such as the gums and pectic substances, delays gastric emptying[66–69] and slows small intestinal uptake of sugars, amino acids,[70,71] and drugs such as acetaminophen and digoxin.[66,72] Fiber is also associated with increased fecal losses of bile acids.[73,74] The small intestinal effect of fiber is thought to be due to its ability to increase the thickness of the unstirred water layer, which acts as a barrier to diffusion of nutrients to the enterocyte brush border. Nevertheless, although slow absorption has been observed, malabsorption has not resulted as judged by urinary recoveries of xylose,[71] acetaminophen,[66] and the lack of breath $H_2$ evolution.[75] In addition, only minimally raised fat and protein losses have been reported, as judged by the marginally increased outputs of protein and fat from the termimal ileum[76] after bran supplementation (see Chap 56D1). In fact, it is of interest that viscous fiber preparations, possibly due to their lipid emulsion stabilizing property, are associated with enhanced chylomicronemia and higher postprandial fat-soluble vitamin levels.[77,78]

Viscous fiber preparations have been used in the management of diabetes[79–82] and to reduce serum cholesterol levels in hyperlipidemia.[83–85] They also improve symptomatology in the dumping syndrome following gastric surgery.[68,86,87] Detailed studies have demonstrated that addition of viscous fiber to test meals resulted in a blunting of the glucose, insulin, and GIP responses when taken with a glucose load,[87] less of an undershoot in blood glucose,[86] and less hemoconcentration assessed by hematocrit[68] as an index of the reduction in hypovolemia. In this situation, the hypovolemia is associated with the dumping of an osmotically active load into the duodenum.

The results are less clear in terms of the effect of fiber in reducing the rate of absorption and altering associated metabolic events. No significant differences were found between white bread, pasta, and rice and their wholemeal or bran equivalents in terms of glycemic response[88,89] (Fig. 56C6–4) or digestibility.[19] In addition, when over 50 foods of equivalent carbohydrate content were compared, the flattening in postprandial glycemia was significantly negatively related to their fat and protein contents but not to fiber[30] (Fig. 56C6–5). This may have been due to the large number of high-cereal fiber foods examined. Because cereal fiber appears to have little effect on small intestinal absorption, the effect of other types of fiber may have been obscured.

Studies with purified fiber, therefore, indicate that certain types of fiber may markedly affect the absorbability of foods. However, fiber in unprocessed foods is also likely to influence the absorption of the macronutrient components in a Western diet through its effect on food form (to be discussed later). (For a general account of fiber see Chap. 2B.)

### Nutrient-Nutrient Interactions in Foods

The nutrient-nutrient interactions have a significant effect on the digestibility of foods. Studies using breath hydrogen measurement to assess carbohydrate malabsorption have indicated significant (10% to 20%) malabsorption from white bread and other farinaceous products.[90] When gluten-free flour was used, no malabsorption was seen, nor was malabsorption produced by adding back purified gluten to the same level as that found originally in the white bread (Fig. 56C6–6). It was concluded that the natural physical interaction of the starch and protein in wheat limited its rate of digestion, resulting in a proportion being malabsorbed.[90] The implication of this study is that patients without definite evidence of celiac disease who are placed on a gluten-free diet and appear to improve may do so because of the enhanced availability of dietary starch rather than the elimination of the gliadin component of wheat protein. Such a measure may therefore have general therapeutic applicability where malabsorption of carbohydrate (starch) is a problem.

Conversely the presence of protein in the small intestine aids in the stabilization of fat emulsions and enhances micelle formation and fatty acid uptake.[91,92] This finding has been demonstrated with casein given with olive oil to dogs,[91,92] in mixtures of proteins (bovine albumin and bovine hemaglobin/ovalbumin mixture), and in various digests of these administered to rats.[91] In addition, the effect of fiber in reducing the glycemic response to carbohydrate has been reported to be diminished as the level of dietary protein is increased.[93]

Fat, on the other hand, has long been recognized as being able to delay gastric emptying[94] and thus will slow the digestion and absorption of other nutrients. However, the degree to which this is achieved may depend on the stability of the fat-food mixture because separation of fat into an upper lipid phase may result in fat having little effect on the gastric emptying of the carbohydrate and protein lying below.

Lipid-lipid interactions are also important. For example, lecithin may enhance triglyceride absorption through facilitating micelle formation.[92,95] Similarly, owing to their effect in stimulating chylomicra formation, long-chain fatty acids increase cholesterol absorption[96] and, most importantly, the absorption of fat-soluble vitamins.[97]

### Micronutrient Interactions

The discussion has so far focused on the factors affecting the absorption of the so-called macronutrients from foods rather than the minerals, trace elements, and vitamins. At this level there are another series of interrelationships. A variety of types of fiber have been shown to reduce the absorbability of $Ca^{++}$, $Fe^{++}$, and $Mg^{++}$.[98–101] Phytate, a fiber-associated antinutrient, may also be an important factor, although the relationship of this substance to deficiency states is not clear (see Chap. 2B). Consumption of long-chain fatty acids facilitates fat-soluble vitamin uptake. High levels of fat in the diet may increase $Ca^{++}$ losses in the feces.[102] Raising the dietary protein intake may diminish the absorption of $Zn^{++}$, $Cu^{++}$, and $Ca^{++}$ in the presence of modest amounts of fiber.[93] In the colon, the reduction of pH by carbohydrate fermentation favors the absorption of $Mg^{++}$[103] and vitamin K.[104] Many other such interrelationships are discussed in their respective sections.

### INFLUENCE OF FOOD FORM AND NON-NUTRIENT FOOD COMPONENTS

Many of the studies showing differences in the absorbability of natural diets have been carried out in relation to those factors concerned with the absorption of carbohydrate from foods. Much of the present discussion will therefore concentrate on carbohydrate digestibility as illustrating the general principles. The factors involved include

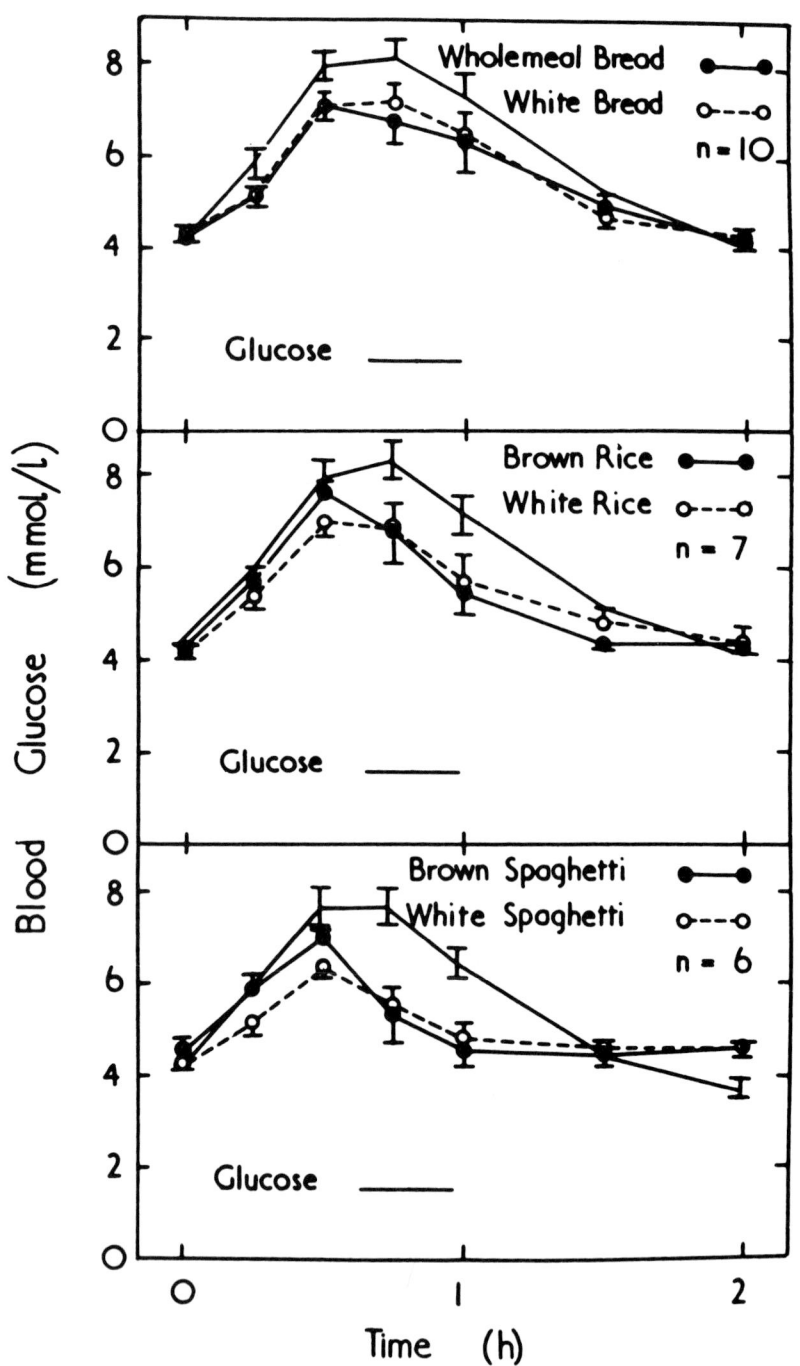

**Fig. 56C6–4.**   Effect of fiber depletion on the mean blood glucose curves after eating 50-g carbohydrate portions of bread, rice, and spaghetti compared with 50-g glucose tolerance tests. (From Jenkins, D.J.A., Wolever, T.M.S., Taylor, R.H., et al.,[88] with permission of Diabetes Care.)

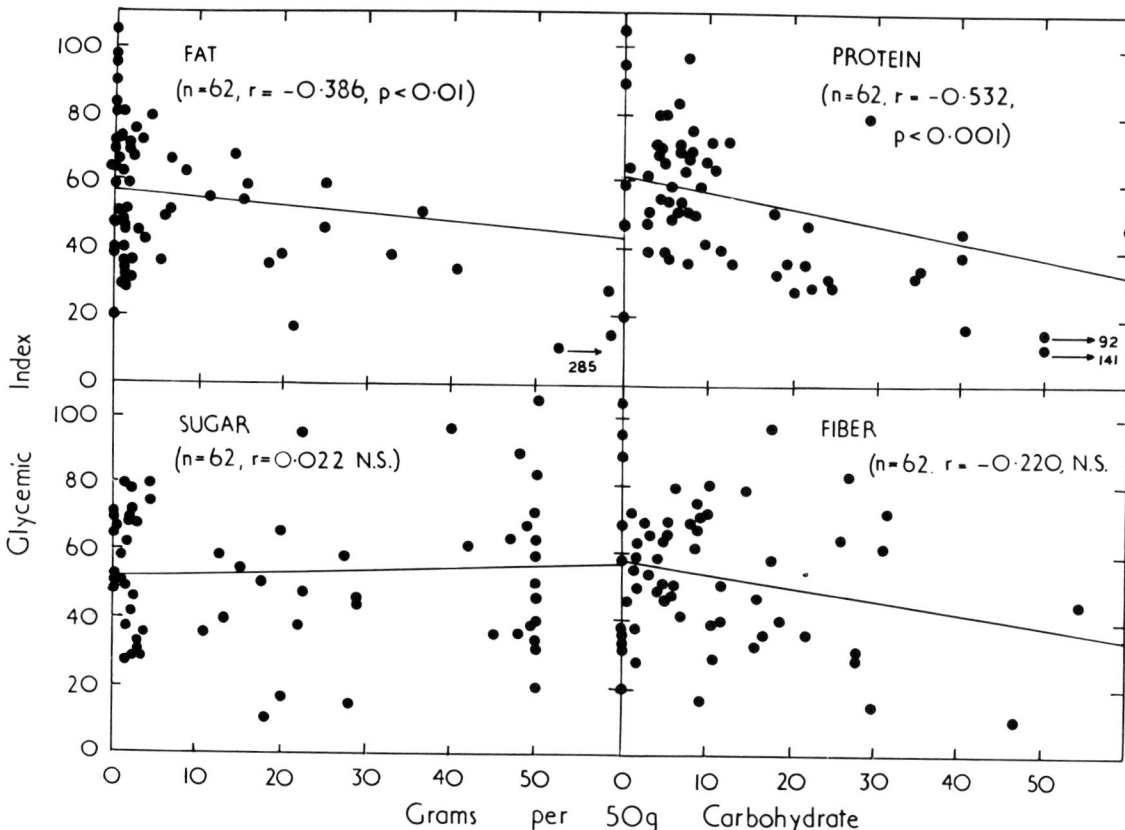

**Fig. 56C6–5.** Relationship of fat, protein, and fiber content of 62 foods and sugars to the glycemic index of 50-g carbohydrate portions. (From Jenkins, D.J.A., Wolever, T.M.S., Taylor, R.H.,[30] with permission of Am. J. Clin. Nutr.)

food form, fiber content, and the presence of lectins, tannins, saponins, and phytates. The possible role of fiber has already been mentioned.

### Food Form

The form in which a food is eaten has been shown to be a major determinant of its rate of digestion and absorption. Apples eaten whole as opposed to blended produced flatter blood glucose and insulin responses as an indication of the slower rate of absorption.[105] Crapo and co-workers demonstrated differences in glucose and insulin responses to a range of starchy foods including baked potato, boiled rice, bread, and corn that in part might be attributed to food form.[12,13] Maize and rice produced the least responses, representing whole seeds, whereas baked potato, a less "compact" food, approximated the blood glucose rise seen when the equivalent amount of carbohydrate was given as glucose.[12–14] The importance of this finding was further brought out by studies demonstrating that rice that was ground and then cooked gave rises in blood glucose and insulin approximating those for glucose[106] together with a more rapid rate of in vitro digestion compared

with whole rice. Though this may be important for some foods, the application of this principle may not be universal. Studies with lentils indicated that blending to a smooth paste after cooking made no difference to the in vitro rate of digestion or the glycemic response,[107] nor did boiling for an additional 40 minutes. Heat treatment for 12 hours was required to increase the digestibility of the lentils.[107]

### Enzyme Inhibitors

Enzyme inhibitors in foods, although common in storage organs such as seeds, cereal grains, and beans, are usually effectively destroyed by the heat treatment of conventional cooking practices.[108] Their relevance to human nutrition is therefore likely to be limited. In terms of animal nutrition, however, the antitryptic activity of uncooked bean meal has attracted attention as limiting the protein quality of animal feeds. In rats it was associated with impaired growth and pancreatic hypertrophy.[94]

On the positive side, purified enzyme inhibitors are beginning to find a use in modifying small intestinal absorption. Inhibitors of carbohydrate

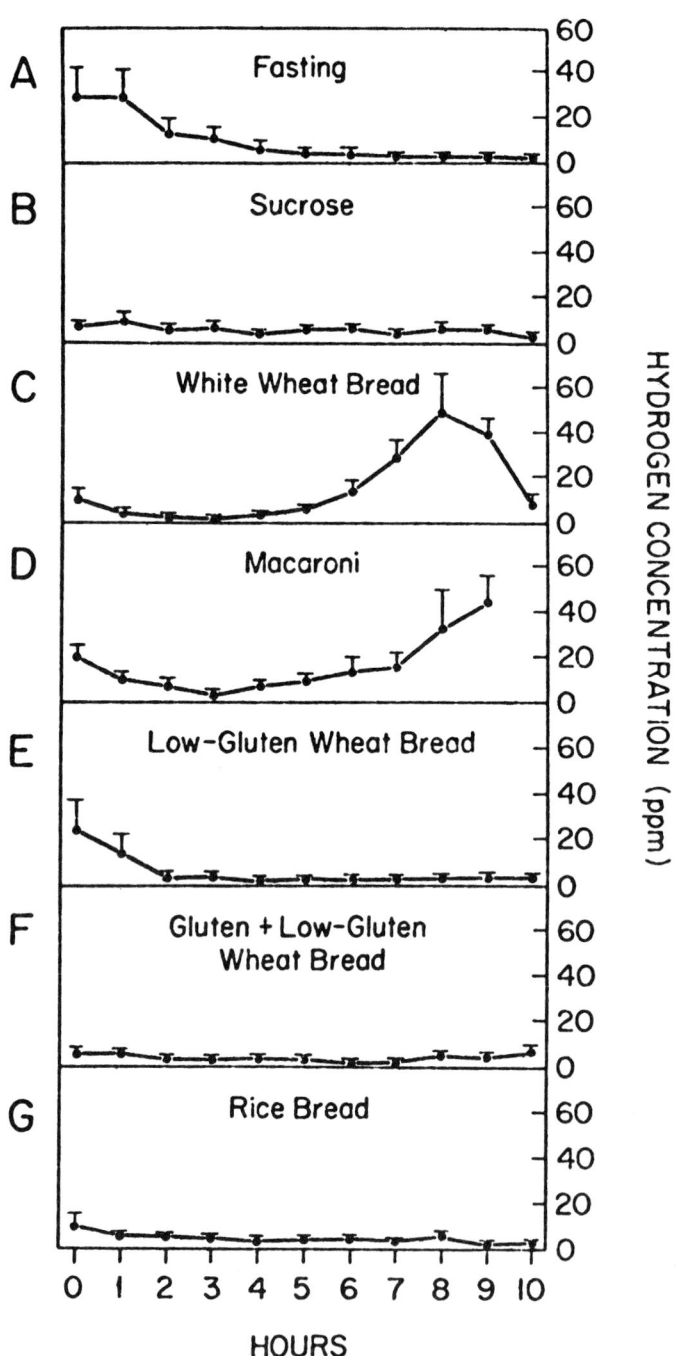

**Fig. 56C6–6.** Breath hydrogen concentration as a measure of carbohydrate malabsorption in healthy volunteers during 10-hr fast (A) and after ingestion of 100 g carbohydrate (B through G). (Ref. 90 with permission N. Engl. J. Med.)

absorption have been developed specifically to control the rate of carbohydrate absorption. An anti-α-amylase isolated from wheat was shown to reduce the rate of starch digestion and the glycemic response to a starch meal in rats, dogs, and man.[109] Subsequently, commercial development of an α-glycoside hydrolase inhibitor with anti-sucrase, -maltase and -amylase activity was shown to have application in the treatment of diabetes[110] and in the dumping syndrome.[111] In the latter instance, relief was obtained despite enhanced carbohydrate losses.[111] Presumably the reduction in glycemic excursions due to dampening the carbohydrate flux offered a large measure of relief to the patients concerned and outweighed the discomfort of carbohydrate malabsorption to which they were already accustomed. Thus, although enzyme inhibitors may be of little relevance in the context of commonly eaten foods and dietetic manipulators, the pharmacologic development of these agents may in the future provide a further means of modifying small intestinal absorption in the same way as addition of enzymes is currently used to enhance absorption of foods in pancreatic insufficiency.

## Saponins

These steroidal or triterpenoid amphiphilic glycosides with surface active and emulsion stabilizing properties are relatively heat-resistant and thus their levels are maintained in fat-containing plant foods and oils. Under normal circumstances they are not absorbed. They have attracted attention as possibly precipitating cholesterol and interfering with micelle formation in the small intestine by enhancing the binding of bile acids to fiber.[112] There is no suggestion that they would induce major changes in fat absorption, but it is possible in view of their effects on cholesterol absorption that they may interfere with fat-soluble vitamin uptake. The exact effect of these surface active agents on the enterocyte or digestive enzymes remains to be documented.

## Tannins

These are large condensed polyphenols. They are powerful reducing agents widely distributed in plant foods. Because they are heat stable, however, they survive cooking procedures and have been shown to complex with dietary proteins reducing their digestibility.[113] They are also known to reduce the activity of the digestive enzymes trypsin and amylase.[114,115] They may therefore reduce the rate or total absorption of both dietary starch and protein from foods. Although tannins occur in quite high concentrations in certain natural diets, their effects have

never been studied directly in man. However their concentration in foods has been shown to relate negatively with the digestibility and glycemic response of a wide range of foods tested.[116]

## Phytates

The most important of these substances is *myo*-inositol 1,2,3,4,5,6 hexakis dihydrogen phosphate. It is found in relatively high concentrations in many high-fiber foods (cereals, legumes, and vegetables). Its levels are reduced by the action of yeast in the leavening of bread. Nevertheless, phytates have the ability to bind metal ions[117,118] and to bind to protein[117,118] and possibly to starch, thereby reducing macro- and micro-nutrient digestibility. As a consequence, phytates have been implicated in causing calcium and zinc deficiency in man.[119] Their exact role, however, seems to be of lesser importance than that of fiber.[120] Nevertheless, phytates have been shown to reduce carbohydrate digestibility when added to white bread at the same concentration as found in legumes (Fig. 56C6–7).[121] This effect is likely to be due to the binding of $Ca^{++}$, which catalyzes the action of amylase[122] since addition of excess $Ca^{++}$ minimizes the effect.[121] Although phytate may also bind to proteins and so reduce protein digestibility,[117,118] the significance of this to commonly eaten foods is not clear. It is possible that phytates may play a major role in determining starch digestibility in foods since they have been shown to have a highly significant negative relationship with digestibility and glycemic response to a wide range of foods tested in man.[121] Their levels are especially high in legumes, which show some of the slowest rates of in vitro digestion.[19]

## Lectins

These substances are a diverse family of proteins and glycoproteins found ubiquitously in plant foods.[123] Lectins bind to carbohydrate receptors on cell surfaces and, in very high concentrations, have been shown to cause small intestinal mucosal damage in rats.[124] Apart from retrospective studies by Bender concerning raw kidney bean consumption,[125] no toxic effects have been reported in man at levels commonly found in the diet. However, preliminary studies indicate that, as with many of the antinutrients, the lectin content of a food and its digestibility both in vitro and in vivo are related.[126] The exact significance of this finding awaits further elaboration.

## DIFFERENCES IN DIGESTIBILITY OF FOODS AND PHYSIOLOGIC IMPLICATIONS

Owing to the wide range of factors that may alter the digestion and absorption of foods, the present

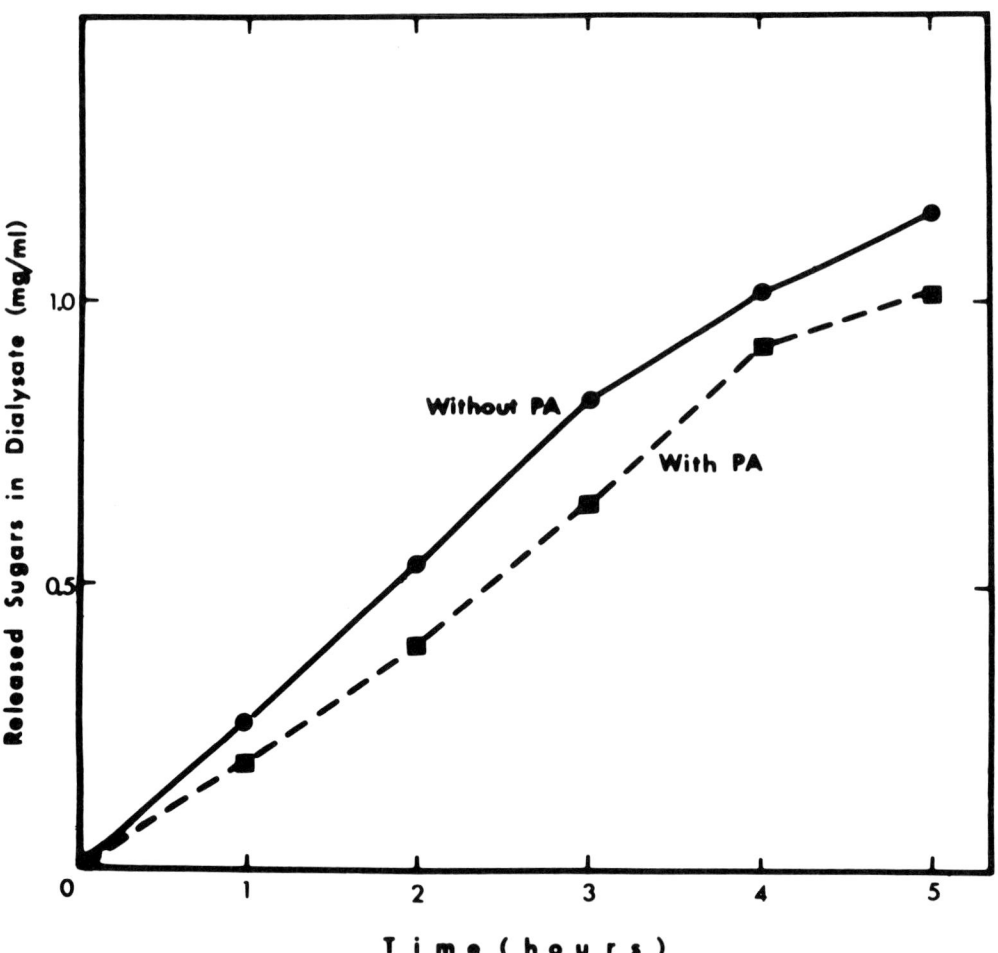

**Fig. 56C6–7.** Rate of digestion of starch in unleavened breads with and without addition of sodium phytate. (From Yoon, J.H., Thompson, L.U., Jenkins, D.J.A.,[121] with permission of Am. J. Clin. Nutr.)

state of knowledge is not sufficiently comprehensive to predict the rate at which a food will be digested simply by knowing its constituents. Nevertheless, as illustrated by starch-containing foods, large differences in the rates of in vitro amylolytic digestion are seen between different foods (Table 56C6–1).[27] Predictably the legumes that are relatively high in soluble fiber and antinutrients are digested more slowly than the cereal foods and potato.[27] In addition, they release a greater proportion of glucose and maltose and a smaller proportion of maltotriose. As mentioned earlier in this section, this in turn may reflect their higher content of the less readily digested amylose form of starch. On the other hand, the comparison of cereal fiber in white and wholemeal bread demonstrates clearly the lack of effect of this form of fiber in reducing the rate of digestion of bread. Again, by contrast, foods of similar composition (e.g., white bread and white spaghetti) differ markedly, presumably due to differences in food form.

Since rate of digestion relates well to the glycemic response to foods,[19] the physiologic implications of these differences are large. Flatter glycemic responses are seen (expressed as a glycemic index) in response to feeding foods that are digested less rapidly (Fig. 56C6–8).[19] As data accumulate, it should be possible to select diets on the basis of rates of digestion to achieve the desired physiologic and metabolic effects.

## Colonic Absorption

Food residues not completely absorbed in the small intestine may be absorbed in the colon. In terms of overall protein metabolism, $NH_3$ and the bacterial metabolites of amino acids may have little impact apart from their deleterious effects in the genesis of encephalopathy in liver disease. In the case of malabsorbed carbohydrate, however, the situation is different. A small proportion of the starch in many commonly consumed foods escapes absorption in the small intestine and

**Table 56C6–1.    Differences in Digestion Rates and Sugars Released from Common Foods\***

| Food | Sugar Concentration (mg/L) at 3 hr Total | % of Total as Glucose | Maltose | Maltotriose |
|---|---|---|---|---|
| White bread standard | 866 | 6.9 | 76.6 | 16.5 |
| Whole wheat bread | 811 | 6.2 | 76.6 | 17.2 |
| Rice | 652 | 3.9 | 71.7 | 24.4 |
| Cornflakes | 954 | 4.9 | 73.5 | 21.7 |
| Porridge oats | 424 | 6.3 | 76.5 | 17.3 |
| Spaghetti | 583 | 5.6 | 73.4 | 21.0 |
| Potato | 638 | 8.8 | 74.2 | 17.1 |
| Mean SEM | 707 | 6.0 | 74.6 | 19.4 |
| Kidney beans | 263 | 6.9 | 79.8 | 13.3 |
| Chick peas | 263 | 8.7 | 79.1 | 12.3 |
| Lentils | 258 | 10.6 | 84.0 | 5.4 |
| Mean SEM | 261 | 8.7 | 81.0 | 10.3 |
| Significance of difference between beans and other foods | 0.005 | 0.05 | 0.005 | 0.005 |

\*Mean concentration and percentage of sugars released into 800 ml dialysate after 3 hr salivary digestion of 2-g carbohydrate portions of 10 foods.

enters the colon. This is especially true for foods that are slowly absorbed. Breath $H_2$[96,107] and ileostomy studies[127,128] indicate that 7 to 20% of the starch in bread enters the colon. With other foods, such as legumes, the percentage lost may be higher. Although these losses related to the in vitro

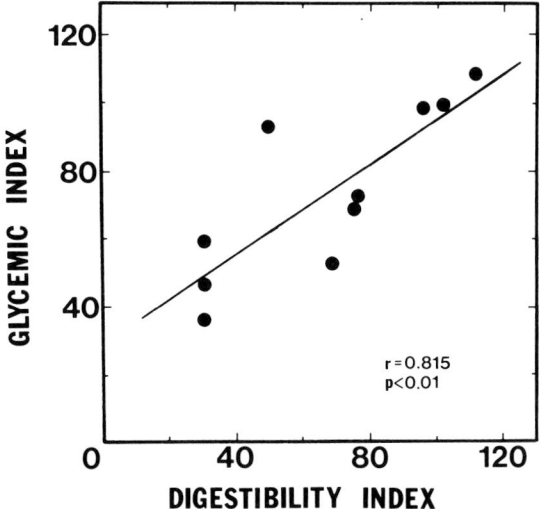

**Fig. 56C6–8.** Relationship between the mean glycemic index and mean digestibility index for each of the 10 foods studied. The glycemic and digestibility indices were calculated by ascribing to white bread a value of 100 both for the glycemic response areas observed over 3 hr after consumption of the test foods and for the total sugars liberated at 3 hr during in vitro digestion (descending order of digestibility: cornflakes, white and wholemeal breads, rice, potato, spaghetti, porridge, kidney beans, chick peas, and lentils). (From Jenkins, D.J.A., Ghafari, H., Wolever, T.M.S.,[19] with permission of Diabetologia.)

rate of digestion, the differences in the percentage of carbohydrate malabsorbed between foods are of a much smaller magnitude than the percentage difference in their glycemic responses.[16,17] Carbohydrate losses, therefore, do not appear to account for the flatter glycemic responses of starchy foods of low glycemic index.

In terms of energy losses from carbohydrate foods (starch, sugars, and fiber), much may be salvaged by colonic absorption of the resulting volatile fatty acids.[129,130] It has been estimated that these may contribute 10% or more of dietary calories[130] (see Chap. 56D1). Factors, therefore, that alter the rate of carbohydrate digestion may not be reflected in malabsorption so much as an altered balance of different parts of the gut including the colon.

### Long-Term Effects

Not only is it possible to produce specific acute effects in terms of gastrointestinal function and absorption by using specific foods or food processes, but important long-term effects may be associated with specific diets and dietary components. For example, feeding diets high in carbohydrate induces sucrase-isomaltase and enhances the absorption of sucrose, whereas removal of carbohydrate from the diet rapidly reverses this trend.[131] Diets high in specific dietary fibers have been shown to reduce sucrase levels in rats.[132] Pectin reduced sucrase and lactase, tannin and galactomannan reduced lactase, and cellulose was without effect.[132] Other studies have demonstrated that increasing the protein or the carbohydrate in the diets of diabetic rats either decreased or increased the absorption of cholesterol respectively.[133] Changes in small intestinal morphology may also be produced by diet. In view of the broad leaf-like jejunal villi seen in inhabitants of high-fiber areas not associated with tropical sprue, researchers wondered what effect unprocessed vegetable material had on villus structure. Studies with rats demonstrated that standard chow and pectin feeding resulted in a flattening of villous structure that was not seen when cellulose or cholestyramine was the only unabsorbable component of the diet.[134] An unexplored but possibly analogous situation might be seen in those habitually consuming diets high in the glycoproteins (lectins). Certainly this is evident in extreme form in susceptible individuals (celiacs) following exposure to the glycoprotein, gliadin, of wheat.

Dietary components apparently may be used to induce changes not only in morphology, enzyme levels, and absorptive function of the upper gastrointestinal tract but also in motor activity. Studies have indicated that after four weeks of pectin supplementation gastric emptying of a pectin-free meal in healthy volunteers was decreased by two-fold by comparison with the original control. This, too, may have important nutritional and metabolic consequences. Cellulose supplementation was without effect.[135]

## SUMMARY

The nature of dietary carbohydrates, fats, and proteins is acutely important in influencing the absorption of natural diets. Perhaps less well recognized is the role of food form and food preparation procedures, especially those that alter either the absolute amount of fiber and antinutrients within a food or their relationship with the macronutrients. In addition, the long-term adaptation of small intestinal and indeed colonic function to the maneuvers described is only now beginning to be explored.

It is likely that active modification of small intestinal absorption has the potential for becoming an important therapeutic modality in the future.[136]

## REFERENCES

1. Allen, F.M.: J. Exp. Med. Balt. *31*:381–402, 1920.
2. Christakis, G., Miridjanian, A.: *In* Diabetes Mellitus. Theory and Practice. Edited by M. Ellenberg and H. Ritkin. New York, McGraw-Hill Book Co., 1970, pp. 594–623.
3. Wahlquist, M.L., Wilmshurst, E.G., Richardson, E.N.: Am. J. Clin. Nutr. *31*:1998–2001, 1978.
4. Dahlquist, A., Borgstrom, B.: Biochem. J. *81*:411–418, 1961.
5. Fogel, M.R., Gray, G.M.: J. Appl. Physiol. *35*:263–267, 1973.
6. Wolfrom, M.L., Khoden, H.E.: *In* Chemistry and Technology. New York, Academic Press, 1965, p. 254.
7. Gray, G.M., Fogel, M.R.: *In* Modern Nutrition in Health and Disease. 6th Ed. (Goodhart, R.S., Shils, M.E., Eds.) Philadelphia, Lea & Febiger, 1980, pp. 99–112.
8. Silk, D.B.A., Sawson, A.M.: International Reviews of Physiology: Gastrointestinal Physiology III. Vol. 19. (Crane, R.H., Ed.) Baltimore, University Park Press, 1979, pp. 151–204.
9. Leach, H.W.: *In* Starch Chemistry and Technology. New York, Academic Press, 1965, p. 292.
10. Geervani, P., Theophilus, F.: J. Food Sci. *46*:817–828, 1981.
11. Shurpalekar, K.S., Sunderavalu, D.E., Rao, M.N.: Nutr. Rep. Rev. *19*:111–117, 1979.
12. Crapo, P.A., Reaven, G., Olefsky, J.: Diabetes *25*:741–747, 1976.
13. Crapo, P.A., Reaven, G., Olefsky, J.: Diabetes *26*:1178–1183, 1977.
14. Crapo, P.A., Kolterman, O.G., Waldeck, N., et al.: Am. J. Clin. Nutr. *33*:1723–1728, 1980.
15. Crapo, P.A., Insel, J., Sperling, M., et al.: Am. J. Clin. Nutr. *34*:184–190, 181.
16. Jenkins, D.J.A., Wolever, T.M.S., Taylor, R.H., et al.: Am. J. Clin. Nutr. *34*:362–366, 1981.
17. Jenkins, D.J.A., Wolever, T.M.S., Jenkins, A.L., et al.: Diabetologia *24*:257–264, 1983.
18. Jenkins, D.J.A., Wolever, T.M.S., Taylor, R.H., et al.: Br. Med. J. *281*:14–17, 1980.
19. Jenkins, D.J.A., Ghafari, H., Wolever, T.M.S., et al.: Diabetologia *22*:450–455, 1982.
20. Bocher, C.E., Behan, I., McNeans, E.: J. Nutr. *45*:75, 1951.
21. Collings, P., Williams, C., MacDonald, I.: Br. Med. J. *282*:1032, 1981.
22. Kon, S., Wagner, J.R., Booth, A.N., et al.: J. Food Sci. *36*:635–639, 1971.
23. Geervani, P., Theophilus, F.: J. Sci. Food Agric. *32*:71–78, 1981.
24. Devados, R.P., Leela, R., Chanchasilearan, K.N.: J. Nutr. Dietet. *1*:84–86, 1964.
25. Geervani, P., Theophilius, F.: J. Food Sci. *46*:817–828, 1981.
26. Alli, I., Baker, R.E.: J. Sci. Food Agric. *31*:1316–1322, 1980.
27. Pak, C.W., Belea, C.S., Bartter, F.C.: N. Engl. J. Med. *290*:175–178, 1974.
28. Jenkins, D.J.A., Wolever, T.M.S., Thorne, M.J., et al.: Am. J. Clin. Nutr. *40*:1125–1191, 1984.
29. Felber, J-P.: Beta Release *7*:6–9, 1983.
30. Jenkins, D.J.A., Wolever, T.M.S., Taylor, R.H.: Am. J. Clin. Nutr. *34*:362–366, 1981.
31. Bantle, J.P., Laine, D.C., Castle, G.W.: N. Engl. J. Med. *309*:7–12, 1983.
32. Schauberger, G., Brinck, U.C., Guldner, G., et al.: Diabetes *26*:415, 1977.
33. Crapo, P.A., Scarlett, J.A., Kolterman, O.G., et al.: Diabetes Care *5*:512–517, 1982.
34. Swan, D.C., Davidson, P., Albrink, M.J.: Lancet *1*:60–63, 1966.
35. Bohannon, N.V., Karana, J.H., Forsham, P.H.: Diabetes *27*(Suppl. 2):438, 1978.
36. Calloway, D.H., Kurtz, G.W., McMullen, J.J., et al.: Food Res. *21*:621, 1956.
37. Steenbock, H., Irwin, M.H., Weber, J.: J. Nutr. *12*:103–111, 1936.
38. Turner, D.A.: Am. J. Digest. Dis. *3*:594–708, 1958.

39. Jenkins, D.J.A., Gassull, M.A., Leeds, A.R., et al.: Int. J. Vitam. Nutr. Res. *46*:226–230, 1976.
40. Gassull, M.A., Blendis, L.M., Jenkins, D.J.A., et al.: Int. J. Vitam. Nutr. Res. *46*:211–214, 1976.
41. Bloomstrand, R., Gurtler, J., Werner, B.: J. Clin. Invest. *44*:1766–1777, 1965.
42. Werner, M., Lutwak, L.: Fed. Proc. *22*:553–563, 1963.
43. Cheng, A.L.S., Morehouse, M.G., Davel, H.J.: J. Nutr. *37*:237–250, 1949.
44. Tomarelli, R.M., Meyer, B.J., Waeber, J.R., et al.: J. Nutr. *95*:583–590, 1968.
45. Filer, L.J., Mattson, F.H., Formon, S.J.: J. Nutr. *99*:293–298, 1969.
46. Bennett, S.: Q.J. Exp. Physiol. *49*:210–218, 1964.
47. Geliebter, A., Torbay, N., Braeco, E.F., et al.: Am. J. Clin. Nutr. *37*:1–4, 1983.
48. Winawer, S.J., Broitman, S.A., Wolochow, D.A.: N. Engl. J. Med. *274*:72–78, 1966.
49. Kaunitz, H., Slanetz, C.A., Johnson, R.E., et al.: J. Nutr. *64*:513, 1958.
50. Van de Kamer, J.H., ten Bokkel Huinink, H., Weyers, H.A.: J. Biol. Chem. *177*:347–355, 1949.
51. Saunders, D.R.: Gastroenterology *52*:135–136, 1967.
52. Senior, B.: *In* Medium Chain Triglycerides. (Senior, B., Van Italie, T.B., Greenberger, N., Ed.) Philadelphia, University of Pennsylvania Press, 1968, p. 38.
53. Greenberger, N.J., Ruppert, R.D., Tzagousis, M.: Ann. Intern. Med. *66*:727–734, 1967.
54. Muto, Y., Takahaski, Y.: Postgrad. Med. *37*:A158, 1965.
55. Zieve, L.: Arch. Intern. Med. *118*:211–223, 1966.
56. Partin, J.S., Partin, J.C., Schubert, W.K., et al.: Gastroenterology *67*:107–118, 1974.
57. Cummings, J.H., Wiggins, H.S., Jenkins, D.J.A., et al.: J. Clin. Invest. 953–962, 1978.
58. Uribe, M., Marquez, M.A., Ramos, G.G., et al.: Dig. Dis. Sci. *27*:1109–1116, 1982.
59. de Bruijn, K.M., Blendis, L.M., Zilm, D.H., et al.: Gut *24*:53–60, 1983.
60. Shaw, S., Wroner, T.M., Lieber, C.S.: Am. J. Clin. Nutr. *38*:59–62, 1983.
61. Franzen, K., Kinsella, J.E.: J. Agric. Food Chem. *24*:788–795, 1976.
62. Mehychyn, P., Stapley, R.B.: US Patent 3764711, 1973.
63. Creamer, L.K., Roeper, J., Lahrey, E.N.: N.Z.J. Dairy Sci. Technol. *6*:107, 1971.
64. Siu, M., Thompson, L.U.: J. Agric. Food. Chem. *30*:743–747, 1982.
65. Matoba, T., Doi, E.: J. Food Sci. *44*:537, 1979.
66. Holt, S., Heading, R.C., Carter, D.C., et al.: Lancet *1*:636–639, 1979.
67. Leeds, A.R., Ralphs, D.N.L., Bonlos, D., et al.: Proc. Nutr. Soc. *37*:33, 1978.
68. Leeds, A.R., Ralphs, D.N.L., Ebied, F., Metz, G., Dilawari, J.B.: Lancet *1*:1075–1078, 1981.
69. Taylor, R.H.: Lancet *1*:872, 1979.
70. Elsenhans, B., Sufke, V., Blume, R., et al.: Clin. Sci. *59*:373–380, 1980.
71. Jenkins, D.J.A., Wolever, T.M.S., Leeds, A.R., et al.: Br. Med. J. *1*:1392–1394, 1978.
72. Kasper, H., Zilly, W., Fassl, H., et al.: Am. J. Clin. Nutr. *32*:2436, 1979.
73. Eastwood, M.A., Hamilton, D.: Biochem. Biophys. Acta *152*:165–173, 1968.
74. Kay, R.M., Truswell, A.S.: Am. J. Clin. Nutr. *30*:171–175, 1977.
75. Jenkins, D.J.A., Leeds, A.R., Gassull, M.A., et al.: Ann. Intern. Med. *86*:20–23, 1972.
76. Sandberg, A-S., Andersson, H., Hallgren, B., et al.: Br. J. Nutr. *45*:283–294, 1981.
77. Jenkins, D.J.A.: *In* International Conference on Atherosclerosis. (Carlson, L.A., Paoletti, R., Sirtori, C.R., et al., Eds.) New York, Raven Press, 1978, pp. 173–182.
78. Kasper, H., Rabast, U., Fassl, H., et al.: Am. J. Clin. Nutr. *38*:1847–1849, 1979.
79. Jenkins, D.J.A., Wolever, T.M.S., Hockaday, T.D.R., et al.: Lancet *2*:779–780, 1977.
80. Jenkins, D.J.A., Wolever, T.M.S., Nineham, R., et al.: Br. Med. J. *2*:1744–1746, 1978.
81. Aro, A., Uusitupa,M., Voutilainen, E., et al.: Diabetologia *21*:29–33, 1981.
82. Doi, K., Matsuura, M., Kawara, A., et al.: Lancet *1*:987–988, 1979.
83. Fahrenbach, M.J., Riccardi, B.A., Saunders, J.L., et al.: Circulation *31/32* (Suppl. 2):1141, 1965.
84. Miettinen, T.A., Tarpila, S.: Clin. Chim. Acta *79*:471–477, 1977.
85. Jenkins, D.J.A., Reynolds, D., Slavin, B.: Am. J. Clin. Nutr. *33*:575–581, 1980.
86. Jenkins, D.J.A., Gassull, M.A., Leeds, A.R., et al.: Gastroenterology *73*:215–217, 1977.
87. Jenkins, D.J.A., Bloom, S.R., Albuquerque, R.H., et al.: Gut *21*:574–579, 1980.
88. Jenkins, D.J.A., Wolever, T.M.S., Taylor, R.H., et al.: Diabetes Care *4*:509–513, 1981.
89. Jenkins, D.J.A., Wolever, T.M.S., Jenkins, A.L., et al.: Diabetes Care *6*:155–159, 1981.
90. Anderson, I.H., Levine, A.S., Levitt, M.D.: N. Engl. J. Med. *304*:891–892, 1981.
91. Meyer, J.H., Stevenson, E.A., Watts, H.D.: Gastroenterology *70*:232–239, 1976.
92. Turner, D.A.: Am. J. Dig. Dis. *3*:594–708, 1958.
93. Monoz, J.M.: *In* Dietary Fiber in Health and Disease. (Vahouny, G.V., Kritchevsky, D., Eds.) New York, Plenum Publishing Corp., 1982, pp. 85–89.
94. Thomas, E.J.: Physiol. Rev. *37*:453–474, 1957.
95. Augur, V., Rollman, H.S., Deuel, H.J.: J. Nutr. *33*:177–186, 1947.
96. Sylven, C., Borgstrom, B.: J. Lipid Res. *10*:351–355, 1969.
97. Roels, D.A., Trout, H., Dujacquier, R.: J. Nutr. *65*:115–127, 1958.
98. Reinhold, J.G., Faradji, B., Abadi, P., et al.: J. Nutr. *106*:493–503, 1976.
99. Cummings, J.H., Hill, M.J., Jivraj, T., et al.: Am. J. Clin. Nutr. *32*:2086–2093, 1979.
100. Jenkins, D.J.A., Hill, M.J., Cummings, J.H.: Am. J. Clin. Nutr. *28*:1408–1411, 1975.
101. Kelsay, J.: *In* Dietary Fiber in Health and Disease. (Vahouny, G.V., Kritchevsky, D., Eds.) New York, Plenum Publishing Corp, 1982, pp. 91–103.
102. Nicolaysen, R., Eeg-Larsen, N., Malm, O.J.: Physiol. Rev. *33*:424–444, 1953.
103. Rayssiguier, Y., Remesy, C.: Ann. Rech. Vet. *8*:105–110, 1977.
104. Hollander, D., Rim, E., Ruble, P.E.: Gastroenterology *72*:A48/1071, 1977.
105. Haber, E.B., Heaton, K.W., Murphy, D., et al.: Lancet *2*:679–682, 1977.
106. O'Dea, K., Nestel, P.J., Antionoff, L.: Am. J. Clin. Nutr. *33*:760–765, 1980.

107. Jenkins, D.J.A., Thorne, M.J., Camelon, K., et al.: Am. J. Clin. Nutr. *36*:1093–1101, 1982.

108. Leiner, I.E.: Proc. Nutr. Soc. *38*:109–113, 1979.

109. Puls, W., Keup, V.: Diabetologia *9*:97–101, 1973.

110. Walton, R.J., Sherif, I.T., Noy, G.A., et al.: Br. Med. J. *1*:220–221, 1979.

111. Jenkins, D.J.A., Barker, H.M., Taylor, R.H., et al.: Lancet *1*:109, 1982.

112. Oakenfull, D.G., Fenwick, D.E.: Br. J. Nutr. *40*:299–309, 1978.

113. Bressani, R., Elias, L.G.: *In* Polyphenols in Cereals and Legumes. (Hulse, J.H., Ed.) Canada, I.D.R.C., 1980.

114. Singh, D., Jambunathan, R.: J. Food Sci. *46*:1364–1367, 1981.

115. Griffiths, D.W., Moseley, G.: J. Sci. Food Agric. *31*:255–259, 1980.

116. Thompson, L.U., Yoon, J.H., Jenkins, D.J.A., et al.: Am. J. Clin. Nutr. *39*:745–751, 1984.

117. Erdman, J.W.: J. Am. Oil Chem. Soc. *56*:736–740, 1979.

118. Cheryan, M.: C.R.C. Crit. Rev. Food Sci. Nutr. *13*:297–335, 1980.

119. Reinhold, J.G., Lahimgarzodeh, A., Nasr, K., et al.: Lancet *1*:28–33, 1973.

120. James, W.P.T.: *In* Medical Aspects of Dietary Fiber. (Spiller, G.A., Kay, R.M., Eds.) New York, Plenum Publishing Corp., 1980, pp. 239–259.

121. Yoon, J.H., Thompson, L.U., Jenkins, D.J.A.: Am. J. Clin. Nutr. *38*:835–842, 1983.

122. Alfonsky, D.: *In* Saliva and its Relation to Oral Health. Birmingham, University of Alabama Press, 1966.

123. Nachbar, M.S., Oppenheim, J.D.: Am. J. Clin. Nutr. *33*:2338–2345, 1980.

124. Puzstai, A., Clarke, E.M.W., King, T.P.: Proc. Nutr. Soc. *38*:115–120, 1979.

125. Noah, N.D., Bender, A.L., Reaidi, G.B., et al.: Br. Med. J. *281*:236–237, 1980.

126. Rea, R., Thompson, L.U., Jenkins, D.J.A.: Nutr. Res. *5*:919–929, 1985.

127. Wolever, T.M.S., Thorne, M.J., Thompson, L.U., et al.: Proc. Nutr. Soc. *5*:919–929, 1985.

128. Stephen, A.M., Haddad, A.C., Phillips, S.F.: Gastroenterology *85*:589–595, 1983.

129. Bond, J.A., Currier, B.E., Buchwald, H., et al.: Gastroenterology *78*:444–447, 1980.

130. Cummings, J.H.: Gut *22*:763–779, 1981.

131. Rosensweig, N.S., Herman, R.: J. Clin. Invest. *47*:2253, 1968.

132. Thomsen, L.L., Tasman-Jones, C.: Digestion *23*:253, 1982.

133. Thomson, A.B.R., Rajotte, R.: Am. J. Clin. Nutr. *37*:244–252, 1983.

134. Tasman-Jones, C., Owne, R.L., Jones, A.L.: Dig. Dis. Sci. *27*:519, 1982.

135. Schwartz, S.E., Levine, R.A., Singh, A., et al.: Gastroenterology *83*:812–817, 1982.

136. Creutzfeldt, W.: *In* Delaying Absorption as a Therapeutic Principle in Metabolic Diseases. (Creutzfeldt, W., Folsch, U.R., Eds.) New York, Thieme-Stratton, Inc., 1983, p. 1.

*Chapter* **56**

# NUTRITION AND DIET IN MANAGEMENT OF DISEASES OF THE GASTROINTESTINAL TRACT

## (D) COLON
### (1) Diet and Colonic Function

### David J.A. Jenkins

The functions of the human colon are many. They include: storage of intestinal contents prior to their elimination; fermentation of the residues of digestive processes with production of short-chain fatty acids (SCFA), ammonia, amines, and other fermentation products, together with the liberation of physically trapped or chemically bound materials (e.g., water and minerals); and absorption of water, the production of bacterial metabolism, minerals, and bile acids.

In many ways there are parallels between the storage function of the colon and that of the stomach. Both are storage organs at either end of the gastrointestinal tract. The latter takes in nutrient over short segments of the day, in part as dictated by social behavior, and releases it slowly at a rate appropriate to the small intestinal absorptive capacity. The colon, on the other hand, receives the residue of the digestion process over the course of the day and discharges it over brief periods, again, in part, as dictated by social behavior. They differ in that the stomach secretes whereas the colon absorbs fluid. In addition, the cells lining both contain carbonic anhydrase. In the stomach this substance is associated with secretion of $H^+$ ion with release of $HCO_3$ into the blood. In the colon it is the $HCO_3$ that is secreted. Finally, the function of both is profoundly influenced by the diet.

## BALANCE OF DIETARY COMPONENTS ACROSS THE COLON

By definition, the food residues that are likely to influence colonic function by their presence in the lumen of the colon are those that are not absorbed in the small intestine. Much may therefore be learned by attempting to draw together balance data or input and output data, to define the gross functions of the colon in relation to dietary constituents (Tables 56D1–1 and 56D1–2).[1–3]

### Macronutrients and Fiber

In this respect dietary fiber has attracted much attention as a major component of the solids discharged from the terminal ileum. It now appears, especially on certain diets, that substantial amounts of "available" carbohydrate (starches and sugars) may also enter the colon together with a significant loss of protein (Table 56D1–1).[1–3] In general, fat losses appear to be of small magnitude.[1–3]

**Fiber.** By definition all the fiber in the diet should enter the colon. On a Western diet this

**1167**

**Table 56D1–1.   24-Hour Ileostomy Outputs from Studies in the Literature**

|  | Study 1[1] (g) | Study 2[2] (g) | Study 3[3] a (g) | b* (g) |
|---|---|---|---|---|
| Wet weight | 507 | 760 | 363 | 457 |
| Dry weight | 39 | 62 | 32 | 41 |
| Fat | 2.2 | 5.5 | 1.0 | 1.5 |
| Protein | 5.6 | — | 11.9 | 12.5 |
| Carbohydrate | (25) | 7.5† | 11.8 | 17.9 |
| Ash | (6) | — | 5.3 | 6.6 |

Figures in parentheses are estimates. Studies 1 and 3 include patients with colectomy for ulcerative colitis only. Study 2 includes patients with colectomy for Crohn's disease.
*Study 3b is similar to study 3a, but 10 g wheat bran have been added to the diet.
†Measured as starch and sugars.

**Table 56D1–2.   Representative Values for Colon Absorption and Secretion of $H_2O$ and Electrolytes (per day)**

|  | $H_2O$ (ml) | $NA^+$ (meq) | $K^+$ (meq) | $CL^-$ (meq) | $HCO_3^-$ (meq) |
|---|---|---|---|---|---|
| Stool | 125 | 5 | 11 | 2 | 3* |
| Terminal ileum | 1,650 | 200 | 5 | 137 | 63 |
| Balance | −1,525 | −195 | +6 | −135 | −60 |

*$HCO_3^-$ secreted but in the colon most $HCO_3^-$ is converted to $CO_2$
Adapted from Smith, E.W., Sleisenger, M.H.[24]

amount is approximately 20 g daily. Ileostomy studies suggested that 27 to 100% of the pectin[4] and noncellulosic fiber[3,5] and 75 to 100% of the cellulosic components were recovered in the ileostomy effluent.[3,5] Failure to recover 10 to 20% of the ingested bran fiber in some ileostomates is perhaps due to its digestion by gastric juice, or to bacterial fermentation in the ileum, or both.[3] This otherwise high recovery of cereal fiber in ileal effluent has been confirmed by other studies.[6] In feeding studies it has been estimated that the fecal recovery for fiber may be as high as 93% for certain types of cellulose[7] and as low as zero for noncellulosic fiber.[8] The losses of noncellulosic polysaccharides were greatest, and these studies also indicated that the smaller the particle size the greater the losses.[9] Studies with pectin, a purified noncellulosic polysaccharide component of fruit and vegetables, indicated that as much as 15 to 46% of ingested pectin disappears from the small intestinal contents. After passage through the colon only 4 to 5% of the ingested dose was recovered in the feces.[4] On the other hand, hemicellulosic materials from certain fruits and vegetables do not appear to reach the terminal ileum.[5] The type and form of the fiber will then determine the amount entering the colon and whether it contributes as a substrate for colonic bacterial metabolism or as a source of bulk for the colon with implications in water holding and colonic motility.

**Starch and Sugars (Available Carbohydrate).** The arrival of fiber in the colon was predicted by definition. Studies of its effects on colonic metabolism, motor activity, morphology, and histology have already contributed enormously to our understanding of colonic function. However, it has only recently been appreciated that quantitatively "available" carbohydrates (largely starches) may make an even more important contribution as a bacterial substrate than fiber. Early studies by Kramer indicated daily dry weight losses in ileostomates of 39 g/day (see Table 56D1–1).[1] Fat and protein losses were estimated at 22 and 5.6 g respectively. Assuming 5 g ash and 20 g dietary fiber, then the remaining 6 g were probably starch. More recently, in studies where the dry weight losses of ileostomates were 32 g/day, only .5 g starch was reported to be present.[2] Breath $H_2$ studies in normal volunteers first drew attention to the substantial "available" carbohydrate losses that may occur in man.[10] Hydrogen is evolved when colonic bacteria break down carbohydrate. Since mammalian cells do not produce $H_2$ and since gut $H_2$ diffuses into the blood and is exhaled in the breath, its measurement can indicate the carbohydrate load arriving in the colon.[11] Such studies using white bread indicated that perhaps between 10 and 20% of the starch in bread was not absorbed, possibly due to a protein-starch interaction.[10] Subsequent studies have confirmed these findings. Stephen and associates, using normal subjects intubated to the cecum with a triple lumen tube, demonstrated that between 2 and 20% of the meal carbohydrate (approximately three fourths as starch) entered the cecum.[12] At the same time studies in ileostomates indicated 7% available carbohydrate losses after wholemeal bread and as much as 18% losses after cooked split red lentils.[13] These results agreed with indirect assessments made in normal volunteers using breath $H_2$ measurement.[13] Since the fiber content of red lentils is only 11%, the starch losses may have constituted a large proportion of the total carbohydrate entering the colon.

The emerging picture, therefore, is one where potentially large amounts of fermentable carbohydrate substrates may be presented to the colon. Whereas the amount of fiber from many foods can be predicted using the appropriate food tables, however, this is not possible for available carbohydrate losses because the factors responsible have not as yet been determined. In addition, unless the carbohydrate load is the result of large quantities of osmotically active sugars delivered rapidly to the colon, carbohydrate in the form of starch and sugars is completely fermented in the colon. Carbohydrate foods may therefore be major determinants of colonic metabolism and colonic retrieval of calories not absorbed in the small intestine.

**Protein.** Ileostomy studies have indicated that assuming mean protein intakes of 75 g[1] and 110 g per day[3] the ileal losses were 7.5%[1] and 10.8%[3] respectively (see table 56D1–1). In the ileostomy study of Kramer, the protein losses ranged from 4 to 7.4 g per day on a wide range of different foods.[1] However, the presence of other materials in the diet, such as 16 g of wheat bran daily, appears to have only a small effect on the ileal protein losses, which were 11.9 g/day on the control diet and 12.5 g/day on the control plus bran diet.[3] These ileostomy protein losses are comparable to the 8 g fecal protein losses, reported as nitrogen, in metabolic studies of student volunteers on Western diets who consumed approximately 90 g protein daily.[14,15] Addition of fiber as pectin or as wheat bran raised the fecal excretion to 9.9 g[14] and 12.5 g daily,[15] respectively, while increasing dietary protein from 63 to 136 g/day raised fecal $NH_3$ levels from 15 to 30 mmol/kg.[16] The dietary protein probably contributes to colonic bacterial metabolism but many factors may influence fecal nitrogen loss. Such losses may rather indicate bacterial cell multiplication and bacterial protein synthesis secondary to substrate availability in the form of fiber and other sources of nutrients entering the colon. In addition, blood urea has been shown to diffuse into the colon, and in the rat it is an important source of nitrogen in the cecum.[17] The blood urea level may thus be another diet-related variable influencing colonic metabolism.

**Fat.** Studies in which fat has been measured in ileostomy effluents have indicated relatively small fat losses of 1 to 2 g (see table 56D1–1) on intakes ranging from 70 to 130 g daily.[1,3] Fecal losses on metabolic diets containing 62 and 152 g daily gave mean values of 1.1 and 3.1 g daily in healthy volunteers.[18] As with the ileostomy losses, the fecal losses are small but reflect the levels of intake. It therefore appears that under normal circumstances quantitative changes in fat across the colon are likely to be small because bacteria do not use long-chain fatty acids as an energy source.[19] There is evidence, however, that qualitative changes may take place in the nature of the fatty acids because unsaturated bonds tend to become saturated.

## Bile Acids, Water, and Electrolytes

The role of the colon in water and electrolyte balance has long been recognized, and there is now much interest in the effect of diet on colonic bile acid metabolism and fecal losses.

**Bile Acids.** The entry of bile acids into the colon also appears to be affected by nutrient intake. Increased intakes of fat or of certain types of fiber have been shown during metabolic balance studies to greatly increase the losses of bile acids in the feces. These increased colonic bile acid losses, associated with fat[18] and certain types of fiber,[20–22] are likely to be due to increased small intestinal losses. In the latter instance this phenomenon is probably the result of bile salt binding by fiber.[23] Diet may therefore alter the load of bile acids arriving in the colon. Since it is estimated that the human colon also absorbs 300 to 350 mg of bile acids daily,[24] the degree to which the luminal contents render bile acids unavailable[23] for colonic uptake will also determine the bile salt loss. In addition, free bile acids deconjugated by colonic bacteria have a function in enhancing colonic losses of water and electrolytes.[25,26] Thus the degree to which dietary factors enhance ileal losses of bile acids and the degree to which bile acids remain bound to the colon may have important effects on colonic function. Little data exist, however, on the relationship between individual foods and the balance of bile salts across the human colon.

**Water and Electrolytes.** The importance of the colon in water and salt retrieval cannot be overstressed. This fact is particularly significant in ileostomates who may be more easily depleted of salt and water. Normally the colon absorbs over a liter of water daily but, with time if the need arises, its capacity to absorb may increase considerably.

The 24-hour outputs of dry matter, Na[+], and K[+] in ileostomates range from 36 to 45 g, 35 to 90 mmol, and 3.4 to 3.6 mmol per day respectively.[1,2] These amounts compare with the larger outputs estimated as entering the normal colon and shown in Table 56D1–2.[24] As shown in this table, the balance of water and electrolytes across the colon is such that this organ plays a major role in absorption and secretion. It is suggested that daily the colon absorbs 1,350 to 1,700 ml water, 175 to 215 meq Na[+], and 115 to 155 meq Cl and secretes 4 to 8 meq K[+] and 60 meq HCO$_3$. Dietary constituents, such as fiber acting directly or through bile acid metabolism, may influence these functions of the colon.

In addition to the absorption of electrolytes, the potential effect of the colon on mineral balance has been illustrated in another monogastric animal, the pig. Using reentrant cannulae in the terminal ileum to distinguish between absorption from the small intestine and colon, Partridge ascribed the proportion of the absorption attributable to each part of the gut.[27] The potential importance of the colon in this animal is evident by its major role in magnesium and zinc absorption (Table 56D1–3).[28]

Kramer et al. have examined the effects of different foods on the small intestinal losses of water and electrolytes and thus have indicated how diet might modify this aspect of colonic function.[1] Values obtained from ileostomates indicated qualitative differences between various foods[1] and also gave lower small intestinal losses of water Na[+] and K[+] than those accepted as representing the losses in normal man.[24] Studies demonstrated that of the limited number of foods tested only prune juice, cooked cabbage,[1] and wheat bran[1,2] altered ileal output by increasing the losses of water, Na[+], and K.[+] Orange juice, milk, black pepper, fried foods, corn, pork, carbonated beverages, and rye bread were without effect.[1] Baked beans, however, tended to increase the dry weight.[1] These studies suggested a role for fiber but did not allow firm conclusions to be reached.

## DIET AND COLONIC BACTERIA

The recognition of the essential role of colonic bacteria in healthy colonic function and their relationship to diet is an area where much new information has been gathered over the past decade.

### Diet and Bacterial Numbers

One way in which foods may alter colonic function is by altering bacterial cell mass. This may change both metabolic activity and physical events in the colon through increasing the fecal bulk. Alterations in fat[18] and protein[16] content of the diet are not associated with alterations in fecal output. However, the effects of fiber may be marked. Different fibers appear to increase bacterial yields to different extents, depending on the degree to which they themselves are degraded.[29]

### Diet and Alterations in Type of Colonic Flora

The possibility has also been explored that food residues entering the colon may alter bacterial type or metabolism. These changes may in turn modify synthesis, degradation, and absorption of the products of fermentation of fat, protein, and carbohydrate. Much of the work carried out in this area has been aimed at determining how dietary components may influence carcinogen synthesis within the colon with special reference to the genesis of colonic carcinoma. In general, short-term changes in diet have failed to alter fecal microflora assessed by classic bacteriologic techniques of counting, culturing, and identifying species.[29–37] Studies in which the level of intake of dietary cereal fiber,[29,32–34] fat,[18] or protein[36] was changed also failed to alter colonic microflora as did pro-

**Table 56D1–3.    Dietary Fiber and Mineral Absorption**

| Mineral | Intake (g) | Low-Cellulose Diet* | | |
|---|---|---|---|---|
| | | Small Intestine Absorption (%) | Colonic Absorption (%) | Total Absorbed (%) |
| Sodium | 5 | 46 | 53 | 99 |
| Potassium | 5 | 90 | 7 | 97 |
| Calcium | 14 | 43 | 31 | 74 |
| Phosphate | 10 | 64 | 17 | 81 |
| Magnesium | 1 | −1 | 74 | 73 |
| Zinc | 0.1 | 10 | 50 | 60 |

*The Fraction of Dietary Minerals and Phosphate Absorbed in the Small and Large Intestine of Pigs Fed Low Fiber Diets[27]
Table adapted by James, W.P.T.[28]

longed fasting.[37] In addition, feeding different sources of soluble fiber and changing the nature of the fat were also without effect.[31]

## Diet and Colonic Bacterial Metabolism

It is possible that classic bacteriologic methods are inappropriate to detect the effects of dietary change and that assessment of the metabolic capabilities of colonic bacteria is a more relevant measurement. Questions arise as to whether habituation increases colonic ability to degrade fiber with consequent effects on mineral and $NH_3$ metabolism. Similarly enhanced bacterial capacity to metabolize bile acids and other steroidal molecules would increase their absorption.

In this respect a clear picture has not emerged, and few studies have reported differences in metabolic activity as a consequence of diet. One study, however, did show a fall in $\alpha$-glucosidase activity on changing from a high meat to a meatless diet.[38] More recently, alterations in carbohydrate enzymes have been reported after bran was added to the diet.[39]

In addition studies have indicated that fermentation of unabsorbable carbohydrate (in the form of lactulose) could inhibit certain aspects of bacterial metabolism by reducing intraluminal pH. Evidence for this finding derives from the observation of Perman et al. that as the fecal pH falls, less $H_2$ is produced from the fermentation of a given amount of lactulose.[40] Diet may therefore influence this aspect of colonic function acutely by the provision of fermentable substrate rather than longer-term effects on the type or metabolic capabilities of colonic bacteria.

## BACTERIAL FERMENTATION IN THE COLON

Through this process nutrients are made available within the colon for absorption. It is a process that both produces toxic substances and degrades them. It influences mucosal cell metabolism and ultimately fecal bulk and colonic motor function.

### Fermentable Substrates

As already discussed, the major variables in terms of dietary residue arriving in the colon (and leaving it) are the carbohydrate components, fiber, starch, and sugars. The amounts of protein and fat entering the colon are relatively small over a wide range of dietary intakes. These substances form the major substrates for colonic bacterial fermentation.

In general, the more a potential substrate increases fecal bulk, the less it is degraded. Thus the noncellulosic components of fiber, starches, and sugars, which have little influence on fecal

output, are largely metabolized by colonic microflora. An exception is when the quantities delivered to the colon per unit are in excess of the colonic capacity to ferment them completely. This situation may occur, for example, with large doses of lactulose or lactose and sucrose in hypolactasia and hyposucrasia respectively.

Specifically, starch from wheat and other cereal products and legumes, together with their unabsorbable sugars (raffinose, stachyose, verbascose, and melibiose), and the major part of the fiber from fruit, vegetables, legumes, and, to a much lesser extent, cereals form the common carbohydrate sources for colonic bacterial fermentation. The degree to which different fibers are fermented was investigated early on by Williams and Olmsted in 1936[41] and similar results have been obtained more recently (Table 56D1–4).[42] The lower fermentability of cereal fiber is well illustrated in a study by Calloway and Kretsch where six healthy American men digested 77% of the fiber in a Guatemalan diet of beans, tortillas, rice, fruit, and vegetables, but only 52 to 55% of the fiber in oat bran.[43] The Guatemalan diet, besides being high in fermentable fiber, is likely to contain nonabsorbable sugars. In addition, the percentage of starch malabsorption is likely to be significant but remains undocumented. The exact fermentable load from given foods or diets is difficult to assess. It may be as little as 20 g/day (15 g fiber and 5 g starch) or as much as 60 g (15 g fiber and 45 g starch) on a Western diet depending on the method of calculation.[44] The load will be far greater in those on high-fiber diets, or in those who have jejunoileal bypass or short bowel syndrome.

### Fermentation Products

With respect to contribution to the products of bacterial fermentation in the colon, the greatest

**Table 56D1–4.  Fate of Fiber in the Gut**

| Source of Fiber | Disappearance (%)* |
|---|---|
| Carrot | 74 |
| Cabbage | 66 |
| Sugar-beet pulp | 65 |
| Agar | 60 |
| Corn germ meal | 60 |
| Peas | 53 |
| Wheat bran | 30 |
| Cottonseed hulls | 18 |
| Celluflour | 10 |
| Alfalfa leaf meal | 9 |

*Disappearance of water-insoluble "cellulose" and "hemicellulose" from the digestive tract of three subjects. Results are given as mean percentage digested.[41] From Cummings, J.H.,[42] with permission of MTP Press, Ltd.

contribution is made by dietary carbohydrate sources, although in liver disease the relatively small contribution made by dietary proteins and amino acids may be physiologically significant.

The overall equation for carbohydrate fermentation may be given as[45]

$$34.5\ C_6H_{12}O_6 \rightarrow 64\ SCFA + 23.75\ CH_4 \\ + 24.23\ CO_2 + 10.5\ H_2O$$

assuming that short-chain fatty acids (SCFA) are the sole nongaseous end products and that all individuals are methane producers (when in fact only 30 to 60% of American and British populations are).[46–48] The SCFA produced include propionate, butyrate, and acetate. Lactate also accumulates when carbohydrate loads are large because the utilization by gut bacteria of lactate produced during fermentation is inhibited by a fall in pH.[49,50] Thus, levels of lactate of up to 50 mmol/L have been reported in the feces of infants with lactose deficiency or in those fed milk who are suffering with acute infectious diarrhea.[51–53] In addition, ethanol, methanol, and formate are intermediates in the breakdown of carbohydrate in the colon. Formate is rapidly broken down to $CO_2$ and water,[54] and the alcohols are absorbed as such.

The gases produced include $CO_2$, $H_2$ (used clinically as a measure of carbohydrate malabsorption), and $CH_4$ (produced by 30 to 60% of American and British individuals and 75 to 80% of Nigerians).[44] In terms of gas production the finding of Perman et al. is of interest.[40] As already discussed, they demonstrated that reduction in the pH of colonic contents, as would follow carbohydrate fermentation, reduced $H_2$ production. Such changes may be part of the adaptation to high-fiber diets.

Dietary protein losses are small, as already described, yet they may play a significant part in colonic metabolism. Thus, serum albumin given by mouth to cirrhotic patients is as coma-inducing as other proteins. This effect can be prevented by antibiotic therapy and is not seen with intravenously administered albumin unless amounts large enough to elevate serum levels are given.[55] In the colon, bacterial metabolism of amino acids contributes to ammonia production together with the volatile derivatives of amino acids. These derivatives have been implicated in hepatic encephalopathy. Normally after absorption from the gut the major proportions of these volatiles are extracted by the liver, but in hepatic dysfunction they bypass the liver and accumulate in the blood to be excreted in the urine and exhaled in the breath.[55] Examples of these are the metabolites of

methionine: methylmercaptan, methane, ethane thiol, methionine sulfoxide, and dimethyl sulfide. In addition, 3-methyl butanal may be produced from leucine, and 3-methyl butanal has been found significantly elevated in encephalopathic cirrhotics.[56] Gut bacterial degradation is apparently the source of the volatiles. Recognition of this finding has resulted in the successful use of antibiotics in the treatment of hepatic encephalopathy.

As with protein, fat losses to the colon are relatively small. However, elevated levels of the short-chain fatty acids, valeric and octanoic acid, are also associated with hepatic coma.[57,58] Rather than being derived from fat, these too may be the result of bacterial action on amino acids in the gut and their subsequent absorption. Although it has been suggested that the longer-chain SCFA (valeric and octanoic) may be derived from incomplete oxidation of long-chain fatty acids,[59] researchers have also proposed that long-chain fatty acids are relatively inert in terms of bacterial degradation.[19]

## ABSORPTION OF NUTRIENTS

Studies by Bond and Levitt in man have demonstrated that intubation to the cecum and infusion of [14]C-labeled glucose resulted in as rapid a rise in [14]C in the breath as when the [14]C-labeled glucose was taken by mouth.[60] This finding emphasized the speed with which the products of glucose metabolism had been absorbed from the cecum of man. Using conventional and germ-free rats and a similar experimental design, researchers demonstrated that bacteria were necessary for this effect. The results indicated that whereas [14]C lactate and acetate could be taken up from the colon of germ-free animals in a fashion similar to that of conventional animals, glucose could not.[60] It appeared that bacterial fermentation of glucose was first required to produce the SCFA (e.g., acetate, propionate) that could then be readily absorbed. The exact mechanism by which the colon absorbs SCFA is not certain,[43] but it seems to involve $HCO_3$. Colonic epithelium (like the rumen of herbivores) contains high concentrations of carbonic anhydrase.[61,62] The $HCO_3$ found in the gut during absorption of SCFA may come either from the plasma, from hydration of $CO_2$ by carbonic anhydrase, or from luminal hydration of $CO_2$. It is possible that fatty acids are absorbed in the ionized form by exchange with $HCO_3$ or, due to the greater permeability of the un-ionized acid, as the protonated acid resulting from luminal hydration of $CO_2$.[44]

## Short-Chain Fatty Acids and Diarrhea

The accumulation of SCFA is now not generally considered to lead to diarrhea either by a direct action on the colonic mucosa or by an osmotic effect. Although fiber may contribute to an increased stool output, the breakdown of unabsorbed carbohydrate leads only to a relatively small increase in osmotic pressure since the fatty acids produced are among the most rapidly absorbed ions in the colon.[63] In fact, it is perhaps more appropriate to consider the action of the colonic bacteria as reducing the diarrheal effect of malabsorbed sugars.[60]

## Colonic Fermentation

**Contribution to Energy Metabolism.** As mentioned, depending on how the potential substrate available for colonic fermentation is calculated, the figure for this substrate is either 20 g (15 g fiber and 5 g starch) or 60 g (15 g fiber and 45 g starches and sugars).[44] This amount would yield SCFA with energy equivalents of 224 KJ (56 kcals) or 600 to 700 KJ respectively. In the latter instance approximately 7% of normal energy intake would be derived from the colon. On high-starch diets with high-fiber intakes, a three-fold increase in colonic production of SCFA may occur, and the colon would therefore play a valuable role in energy balance.

**Ammonia Absorption.** Another important aspect of colonic fermentation of carbohydrate is its effect in reducing $NH_3$ uptake. Not only is this effect important in the physiology of the enterohepatic circulation of nitrogen, but it is also relevant to the goal of reducing blood ammonia levels in liver disease (see 56E1). In patients with cirrhosis, urea production fell and fecal N excretion rose when they were given lactulose as a fermentable carbohydrate source.[64] This finding suggests that $NH_3$ was channeled away from absorption into the portal blood and diverted into bacterial protein synthesis in the gut. Two separate mechanisms may be operating. First, SCFA production reduces luminal pH, and renders $NH_3$ in a more ionized and therefore less absorbable form. The $NH_4^+$ is thus trapped within the lumen of the bowel.[65,66] Second, the presence of SCFA stimulates bacterial cell multiplication, and the luminal $NH_4^+$ level falls as $NH_3$ is used for bacterial protein synthesis. Visek has pointed out that this may be the way in which fiber offers protection from colonic cancer since $NH_3$ can induce changes in colonic epithelium that it is hypothesized favor the development of cancer.[66,67]

## Mucosal Cell Growth

It is also possible that SCFA are important in promoting normal mucosal cell growth. In man

the colonic mucosa is known to be dependent on butyrate as an energy source,[68] particularly in the distal colon.

The defect in butyrate uptake by mucosal cells of individuals with ulcerative colitis has even suggested impaired butyrate uptake as a factor in the etiology of this colitis.[69]

## DIET AND MOTOR FUNCTION OF THE COLON

Primary motor functions of the colon are concerned with the accommodation and the onward passage of materials delivered from the small intestine. The colonic contraction patterns measured by tubes with various sizes of balloons, open-ended perfused tubes, radio telemetering capsules, and time-tape cinefluorography have been classified into wave types I to IV. However, division into propulsive (peristaltic) and segmentation (nonpropulsive phasic contractions) may be more useful.[70] Propulsive movements are infrequent and may be triggered by food (the "gastrocolic reflex"). Although the exact mechanism is not known, they usually start in the transverse colon and in a few seconds may result in fecal material entering the pelvic colon. The segmentation or phasic activity consists of periodic, relatively stationary uncoordinated contractions with pressures of 10 to 60 mmHg and frequencies of 2 to 3 contractions per minute.[71] They too appear to be stimulated by eating and are diminished in constipation and diarrhea.

As discussed, to a large extent the volume of colonic contents is determined by the nature and amount of unabsorbed carbohydrate from the diet. This also acts as a stimulus to propulsive motor activity. Its contribution to fecal bulk relates to the degree to which the material is fermented (see Chap. 2B). Bran that is slightly fermented has the ability to increase fecal bulk and significantly reduces transit time. On the other hand, a carbohydrate source such as pectin, which is completely fermented, has little effect on motor activity (see Chap. 56D2). In general, fecal bulk in turn relates negatively to the transit time for stool weights below 140 g.[72] Above this no such relationship is seen.[72] Much of the work on dietary modification of colonic motor function has involved the use of wheat bran, which appears to be one of the best fecal bulking agents. Its consumption has been associated with a shortened gastrointestinal transit time plus a reduction in segmentation wave height and frequency.[73] Although the relevance of transit time to disease is not clear, the effect of fecal bulk in reducing intracolonic pressures has been of considerable interest in relation to diverticular disease where pressure may be high[73] (see Chap. 56D2).

## SUMMARY

Much of the renewed interest in diet and colonic function has resulted from studies of the physiologic effects of dietary fiber. In recent years information has been acquired not only on the motor functions of the colon but on the absorptive functions as well. In this capacity, in addition to water and electrolyte salvage, it is also acknowledged to have a significant role in maintaining $Ca^{++}$, $Mg^{++}$, and $Zn^{++}$ balance. The SCFA formed as a result of bacterial fermentation of carbohydrates are now seen as potentially valuable energy sources that are rapidly taken up by colonic mucosa. The important symbiotic role of the colonic bacteria themselves is becoming increasingly recognized, but it is in this area, especially in relation to the effects of dietary changes, that further research is required.

## REFERENCES

1. Kramer, P., Kearney, M.M., Ingelfinger, F.J.: Gastroenterology *42*:535–546, 1962.
2. McNeil, N.I., Bingham, S.A., Grant, A.M., et al.: Gut *18*:A958, 1977.
3. Sandberg, A-S., Andersson, H., Hallgren, B., et al.: Br. J. Nutr. *45*:283–294, 1981.
4. Holloway, W.D., Tasman-Jones, C., Maher, K.: Am. J. Clin. Nutr. *37*:253–255, 1983.
5. Holloway, W.D., Tasman-Jones, C., Lee, S.P.: Am. J. Clin. Nutr. *31*:927–930, 1978.
6. Cohen, Z., Wolever, T.M.S., Thompson, L.U., et al.: Gastroenterology *84*:1127, 1983.
7. Williams, T.D., Olmsted, W.H.: J. Nutr. *2*:433–449, 1936.
8. Cummings, J.H.: Br. Med. Bull. *37*:65–70, 1981.
9. Heller, S.N., Hackler, L.R., Rivers, J.M., et al.: Am. J. Clin. Nutr. *33*:1734–1744, 1980.
10. Anderson, I.H., Levine, A.S., Levitt, M.D.: N. Engl. J. Med. *304*:891–892, 1981.
11. Bond, J.A., Levitt, M.D.: J. Clin. Invest. *51*:1219–1225, 1972.
12. Stephen, A.M., Haddad, A.C., Phillips, S.F.: Gastroenterology *85*:589–595, 1981.
13. Wolever, T.M.S., Cohen, Z., Thompson, L.U., et al.: Am. J. Gastro. *81*:115–122, 1986.
14. Cummings, J.H., Southgate, D.A.T., Branch, W.J., et al.: Br. J. Nutr. *41*:477–485, 1979.
15. Cummings, J.H., Hill, M.J., Jenkins, D.J.A., et al.: Am. J. Clin. Nutr. *29*:1468–1473, 1976.
16. Cummings, J.H., Branch, W.J., Houston, H., et al.: Gut *18*:A411–A412, 1977.
17. Demigne, C., Remesy, C.: Ann. Biol. Anim. Biochem. Biophys. *19*:929–935, 1979.
18. Cummings, J.H., Wiggins, H.S., Jenkins, D.J.A., et al.: J. Clin. Invest. *61*:953–963, 1978.
19. Prius, R.A.: *In* Microbial Ecology of the Gut. (Clarke, R.T.J., Nauchop, E., Eds.) New York, Academic Press, 1977, p. 185.
20. Kay, R.M., Truswell, A.S.: Br. J. Nutr. *37*:227–235, 1977.
21. Walters, R.L., Baird, I.M., Davies, P.S., et al.: Br. Med. J. *2*:536–538, 1975.
22. Eastwood, M.A., Hamilton, D.: Biochem. Biophys. Acta *152*:165–173, 1968.
23. Story, J.A., Kritchevsky, D.: J. Nutr. *106*:1292–1294, 1976.
24. Smith, F.W., Sleisenger, M.H.: *In* Gastrointestinal Disease. (Sleisenger, M.H., Fordtran, J.S., Eds.) Philadelphia, W.B. Saunders Co., 1978, pp. 1523–1548.
25. Mekhjian, H.S., Phillips, S.F.: Gastroenterology *59*:120–129, 1970.
26. Mekhjian, H.S., Phillips, S.F., Hofmann, A.F.: J. Clin. Invest. *50*:1569–1577, 1971.
27. Partridge, I.G.: Br. J. Nutr. *39*:539–545, 1978.
28. James, W.P.T.: *In* Medical Aspects of Dietary Fiber. (Spiller, G.A., Kay, R.M., Eds.) New York, Plenum Publishing Corp., 1980, pp. 239–259.
29. Cummings, J.H.: *In* IV. Factors Influencing the Composition and the Activity of the Intestinal Flora. XV Symp. Swed. Nutr. Found. 1981, pp. 77–86.
30. Draser, B.S., Hill, M.J.: Human Intestinal Flora. New York, Academic Press, 1974.
31. Draser, B.S., Jenkins, D.J.A.: Am. J. Clin. Nutr. *29*:1410–1416, 1976.
32. Draser, B.S., Jenkins, D.J.A., Cummings, J.H.: J. Med. Microbiol. *9*:423–431, 1976.
33. Floch, M.H., Fuchs, H.M.: Am. J. Clin. Nutr. *30*:833, 1977.
34. Fuchs, H.M., Dorfmann, S., Floch, M.H.: Am. J. Clin. Nutr. *29*:1443–1447, 1976.
35. Attebery, H.R., Sutter, V.L., Finegold, S.M.: Am. J. Clin. Nutr. *25*:1391–1398, 1972.
36. Hentges, D.J., Mader, B.R., Burton, G.C., et al.: Cancer Res. *37*:568–571, 1977.
37. Finegold, S.M., Sutter, V.L.: Am. J. Clin. Nutr. *31*(5):S116–S122, 1978.
38. Reddy, B.S., Weisburger, J.H., Wynder, E.L.: Science, *1983*:416–417, 1974.
39. Bourke, G., Neale, G.: Ir. J. Med. Sci. *149*:38, 1980.
40. Perman, J.A., Molder, S., Olson, A.C.: J. Clin. Invest. *57*:643–650, 1981.
41. Williams, T.R.D., Olmsted, W.H.: J. Nutr. *11*:433–449, 1936.
42. Cummings, J.H.: *In* Colon and Nutrition. (Kasper, H., Goebell, H., Eds.) MTP Press Ltd., 1982, pp. 91–103.
43. Calloway, D.H., Kretsch, M.J.: Am. J. Clin. Nutr. *31*:1118–1126, 1978.
44. Cummings, J.H.: Gut *22*:763–799, 1981.
45. Miler, T.L., Wolin, M.J.: Am. J. Clin. Nutr. *32*:164–172, 1979.
46. Bond, J.H., Engel, R.R., Levitt, M.D.: J. Exp. Med. *133*:572–588, 1971.
47. Pitt, P., Bruijn, K.M., De Beeching, M.F., et al.: Gut *21*:951–959, 1980.
48. Haines, A., Metz, G., Diliawari, J., et al.: Lancet *2*:481–483, 1977.
49. Hungate, R.E.: *In* Handbook of Physiology (Code, C.F., Ed.) Section 6, Vol. V. Baltimore, Williams & Wilkins, 1968, p. 2725.
50. Dunlop, R.H.: *In* Advances in Veterinary Science and Comparative Medicine. (Brandley, C.A., and Cornelius, C.C., Eds.) New York, Academic Press, 1972, p. 259.
51. Torres-Pinedo, R., Lavastida, M., Rivera, C.L., et al.: J. Clin. Invest. *45*:469–480, 1966.
52. Weijers, H.A., Van De Kamer, J.H.: Acta Paediatr. *52*:329–337, 1963.
53. Weijers, H.A.: Acta Paediatr. *50*:55–71, 1961.
54. Hungate, R.E.: The Lumen and its Microbes. New York, Academic Press, 1966.
55. Conn, H.O., Lieberlhal, M.M.: The Hepatic Coma

Syndromes and Lactulose. Baltimore, Williams & Wilkins, 1979, p. 410.

56. Goldberg, E.M., Sandler, S., Blendis, L.M.: Model simulators, *10*:167–173, 1979.
57. Walker, C.O., Schenker, S.: Am. J. Clin. Nutr. *23*:619–632, 1970.
58. Chen, S., Zieve, L., Mahadevan, V.: J. Lab. Clin. Med. *75*:628–635, 1970.
59. Derr, R.F., Zieve, L.: J. Neurochem. *21*:1555–1557, 1973.
60. Bond, J.H., Levitt, M.D.: J. Clin. Invest. *57*:1158–1164, 1976.
61. Carter, M.J., Parsons, D.S.: Nature (Lond.) *219*:176–177, 1968.
62. Carter, M.J., Parsons, D.S.: J. Physiol. *220*:465–478, 1972.
63. Argensio, R.A.: J. Am. Vet. Med. Assoc. *1973*:662–672, 1978.
64. Weber, F.L.: Gastroenterology, *78*:518–523, 1979.
65. Down, P.F., Agostini, L., Murison, J., et al.: Clin. Sci. *43*:101–114, 1972.
66. Visek, W.J.: Fed. Proc. *31*:1178–1193, 1972.
67. Visek, W.J.: Am. J. Clin. Nutr. *31*:S216–S220, 1978.
68. Roedinger, W.E.W.: Gut *21*:793–798, 1980.
69. Roedinger, W.E.W.: Lancet *2*:712–715, 1980.
70. Hagihara, P.F., Griffen, W.O.: Surg. Clin. North Am. *52*:797–805, 1972.
71. Misiewicz, J.J.: Gut *16*:311–314, 1975.
72. Cummings, J.H., Branch, W.J., Bjerrum, L., et al.: Nutr. Cancer *1*:61–66, 1982.
73. Brodribb, A.J.M., Humphreys, D.M.: Br. Med. J. *1*:424–425, 1976.

*Chapter* **56**

# NUTRITION AND DIET IN MANAGEMENT OF DISEASES OF THE GASTROINTESTINAL TRACT

*(D) COLON*
### (2) Fiber and Colonic Disease

## David J.A. Jenkins

Because of its effect on colonic function, fiber is possibly the most relevant dietary component in relation to human colonic disease. The newness of the topic and its impact on current clinical practice therefore warrant further detailed discussion. Interest in this aspect of dietary fiber owes much to Denis Burkitt, Hugh Trowell, and Neil Painter. The dietary fiber hypothesis they proposed to explain differences in disease patterns between industrialized and nonindustrialized nations is discussed in Chapter 2B. So also are the general implications of the hypothesis. The present discussion will therefore focus specifically on practical aspects of possible therapeutic and prophylactic roles of fiber in colonic disorders.

## CONSTIPATION

It has long been recognized that certain types of fiber have a marked laxative effect of increasing stool weight, enhancing the output of fecal water and electrolytes, and reducing transit time (see Chap. 2B). In general, much simple constipation can be helped by increasing the fiber content of the diet, especially by the use of wholemeal or whole wheat products (bread, biscuits, breakfast cereals) that are high in cereal fiber.

In most instances, then, current treatment of constipation includes advice to increase fiber consumption, possibly with the additional use of bulk laxatives.

Devroede has recommended a dietary trial where a crude fiber intake of 14.4 g daily is the goal.[1] This amount would be considerably higher in terms of dietary fiber content but, as pointed out, with the exception of McCance and Widdowson's tables,[2] dietary fiber values (which include the noncellulosic polysaccharides) are not generally available. Bockus advises that individualization is required in a dietary prescription the principles of which are "ample fluid, sufficient fiber and enough laxative foods."[3]

Concern has been expressed that the most obstinate types of nonspastic constipation may be associated with colonic irritability induced by laxative abuse and enemas.[3] In this situation a bland diet with a hydrophilic colloid such as psyllium husk (Metamucil) has been advised[3] (Table 56D2–1).

The emphasis, nevertheless, has been on the use of fiber either in the diet (food fiber) or as supplements (vegetable mucilloids) in the management of simple constipation, (see Table 56D2–1). A wide range of vegetable mucilloids or vegetable gums has been used including agar, gum arabic, acacia, tragacanth, and sterculia gum. In addition, modified dietary fibers or cellulose products have been developed for the treatment of constipation (and induction of satiety) including methylcellulose, carboxymethyl cellulose, and ethylhydroxyethyl cellulose.

**Table 56D2–1.　Bulking (Swelling) Agents***

| Source | Name of Product Manufacturer | Form Available | Daily Dose |
|---|---|---|---|
| Psyllium plantago ovata | Konsyl (Burton Parsons) | Power | 1–3 tsp |
| Psyllium plantago ovata | Metamucil (Searle) | Powder | 1–3 tsp |
| Psyllium plantago ovata | Instant Mix Metamucil (Searle) | Powder (effervescent) | 1–2 packets |
| Plantago with B | Siblin (Parke-Davis) | Powder | 1–3 tsp |
| Psyllium plantago loeflingii | Mucilose (Winthrop-Breon) | Powder | 1–3 tsp |

*Partial list. Those containing bowel irritants and drug laxatives are omitted.
From Bockus, H.L.,[3] with permission of W.B. Saunders Co.

Of the "natural" products, coarse wheat bran either alone or in wholemeal products appears to have the greatest laxative effect on a weight-for-weight basis compared with other food sources.[4,5] A change from white to wholemeal wheat products may prove useful, and additional bran may be taken in high-fiber breakfast cereals. If further bran is required, this may be sprinkled over breakfast cereals or mixed with yogurt or mashed banana. The dose should be increased gradually one dessert spoon at a time since abdominal distention and flatulence may make the treatment unacceptable. A large intake of bran may also give rise to pruritus ani. This condition is likely to result from the abrasive nature of the coarse bran particles. The problem may be relieved by dilution of the bran through consumption of additional fiber sources such as cabbage, where the increase in fecal bulk is largely bacterial in origin,[5,6] or by the addition of legumes to the diet as a nonparticulate high-fiber source. In patients with celiac disease, rice bran is an acceptable source of fiber, although its fecal bulking effect is less pronounced.

## IRRITABLE BOWEL

In the irritable bowel, especially when dominated by constipation, use of fiber in the form of hydrophilic mucilloids has been recommended.[1,2] As with pain in diverticular disease, the increased bulk induced by fiber may reduce intraluminal pressures within the colon.[7] Although not all studies have yielded convincing results, a controlled study of 26 patients supplemented with 20 g wheat bran daily (as bran or as 170 g wholemeal bread, i.e., 4 slices, or a combination to make 20 g bran) demonstrated some improvement in symptoms and reduced colonic motor activity.[7]

On the other hand, when diarrhea proves a problem, bran, as well as accelerating slow transit, may also decelerate rapid transit.[8,9] In addition,

kaolin and pectin have been recommended in mild cases and diphenoxylate (Lomotil) in the more severe.[10] The use of the purified fiber pectin here is of interest in emphasizing the difference between different fiber sources. With pectin, a source of fiber metabolized in the colon, fecal bulk is not increased and its addition to the diet may be constipating (see Chap. 2).

## DIVERTICULAR DISEASE

In 1971 Painter and Burkitt published their hypothesis linking reduced fiber consumption in the West with the increased incidence of diverticular disease.[11] They suggested that fiber, by maintaining intraluminal bulk, reduced the development of high intracolonic pressures. Hence it prevented the production of diverticula produced by mucosal evagination along the track of blood vessels piercing the muscular coat of the bowel (Fig. 56D2–1).[12] As Almy noted,[13] the law of La Place may apply to the bowel such that tension (t) in the wall must be greater to exert a given pressure (p) when the radius (r) of the bowel is large: $p = \dfrac{t}{r}$.

However, the association of dietary fiber deficiency in the etiology of diverticular disease has been criticized. Epidemiologic studies in Africa suggesting a protective role for dietary fiber were followed by studies in Greece that appeared to refute the relationship between fiber intake and the incidence of diverticular disease.[14] Only cellulosic intake was assessed, however, and this is unlikely to give a meaningful picture of fiber consumption.[15] The population with a low incidence (rural) had higher fecal weight and faster transit times than the population with the higher incidence (urban, Western diet) suggesting true dietary fiber intakes may well have been different.[15] Subsequently, Brodribb and Humphreys demonstrated that the fiber intake of 40 British patients

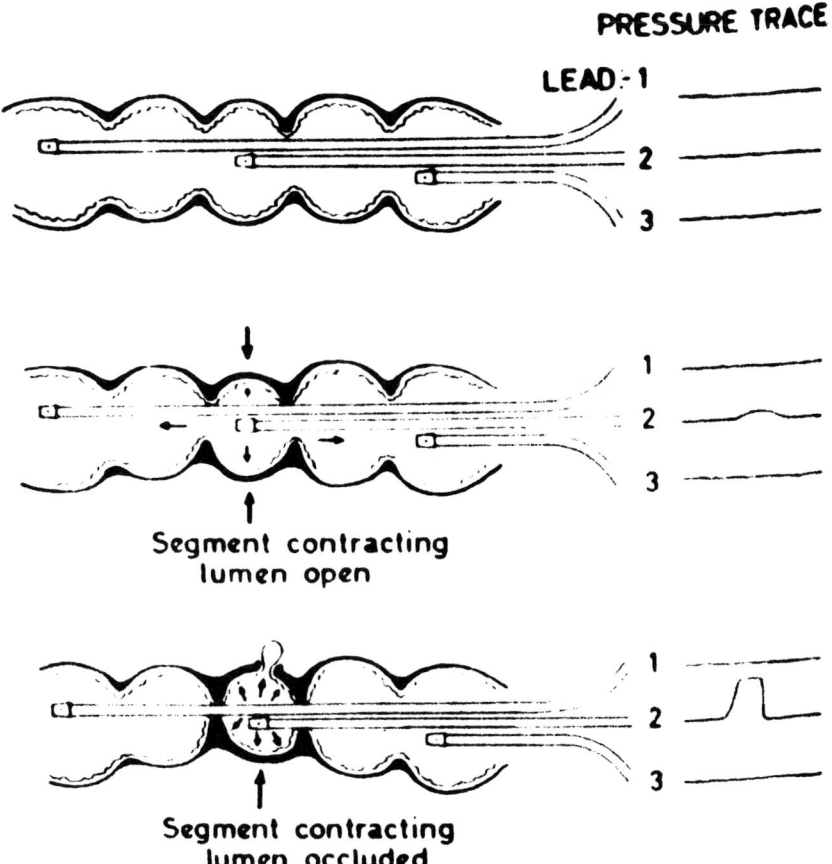

PRESSURE TRACE

**Fig. 56D2–1.**   Illustration showing how raised segmenting pressures may result in the formation of a diverticulum. Pressure tracings recorded from a triple lumen are also evident. The three panels indicate a sequence showing a progressive increase in intraluminal pressure. Finally, when the lumen is occluded, a sphere is isolated where pressures are sufficiently high to result in the formation of a diverticulum by mucosal evagination along the track of vessels that enter the bowel from without. (From Painter, N.S.,[12] with permission of The Royal College of Surgeons.)

with symptomatic disease was half that of matched controls,[16] and similar results have been obtained using vegetarian groups.[17] More recently, further reports from Japan suggest that a reduction in fiber intake in the population relates well to the increasing incidence of diverticular disease.[18] These changes may possibly also be explained by other changes such as the increase in fat and protein in the diet.[19] There is also concern that no appropriate animal model has been studied.[20]

Nevertheless, the last decade has seen a general change from the low-fiber diets once advocated in the management of diverticular disease[21] to therapeutic trials of high fiber. This change has been the result of the importance placed on colonic volume in the hypothesized mechanisms for the generation of diverticula, the implication of fiber in the epidemiology and, to a lesser extent, clinical trials.

One of the first trials was that of Painter and colleagues in which patients on a high-fiber, low-sugar diet with enough bran to ensure defecation at least once daily showed 88% improvement of symptoms over a follow-up period of 22 months.[22] Others have shown similar results.[23–29]

The first double-blind controlled trial also indicated a reduction in pain score, although other dyspeptic symptoms (nausea, vomiting, heartburn, eructation, and abdominal distention) or bowel function scores (excessive flatulence and defecation-related problems) were not significantly different.[30]

More recently the use of fiber has been questioned by a trial involving bran, ispaghula, and placebo where just over 4.5 or 6.5 g of dietary fiber were added to the diets of patients with symptomatically mild diverticular disease. No significant improvement in symptoms was observed over a 4-month period despite a 15 to 30% increase in fecal weight.[31]

In both these controlled studies the increase in fecal weight was relatively small. For consistency, larger fiber intakes may be required. In addition, it is possible that the relatively milder symptoms in the second study and absence of pain as a dominant feature may be reasons why a significant change was not seen. Flatulence and abdominal distention from the fiber itself may also have produced some of the milder symptoms in the treatment group. However, such studies caution that future advice may focus on other types of fiber, in addition to wheat bran, and possibly other dietary modifications (e.g., in terms of fat or protein).

Smith and his colleagues in a prospective trial demonstrated that five years after sigmoid myotomy only patients who had been placed on bran maintained their reduced mean motility indices.[32] Many other studies have also indicated reduction in segmenting pressures on fiber supplementation.[26-29] In view of our understanding of pain and the proposed etiology of the diverticula in diverticular disease, there appears good reason why high-fiber diets should continue to be used in the management of diverticulosis.

## CROHN'S DISEASE

Little attention has been paid to the possible use of fiber in the prophylaxis or treatment of inflammatory bowel disease. In exacerbations of both ulcerative colitis and Crohn's disease, bland low-residue diets are advised. In ulcerative colitis, where depressed lactose levels may exist, physicians often attempt to reduce further the fermentable carbohydrate substrates entering the colon by eliminating milk or using low-lactose diets. In Crohn's disease, the presence of strictures would appear to be a logical contraindication to the use of high-fiber diets for fear of causing obstruction. In the acute phase, complete bowel rest has been advocated. Nevertheless, it has been reported that, as with diverticular disease, patients with Crohn's disease also consumed less fiber and more sugar prior to diagnosis than did controls.[33,34] Such retrospective evidence prompted a prospective trial of dietary modification including a reduction in sugar intake and an increase in fiber consumption in Crohn's disease patients. No fiber supplements were advocated, but fiber intake was increased by the use of whole-grain foods and increased fruit and vegetable consumption. White flour products were eliminated and sugar intake was reduced. Over a five-year period, the test group required one fifth the time in hospital of the control group and was subjected to fewer operations.[35] The trial was undertaken irrespective of the presence of strictures although, as stated earlier, these would seem to be an obvious contraindication. The apparent success of this trial

suggests that the role of fiber in the outpatient management of Crohn's disease warrants further attention.

## COLONIC CANCER

Many associations link colonic cancer with diet and many theories have been advanced to explain these. High-fat, high-protein, and low-fiber intakes are found in those populations in whom the incidence of colonic cancer is highest.[36,37] Dietary fat, it has been suggested, acts either directly by the toxic effect of unabsorbed fatty acids on colonic mucosa[38] or indirectly by enhancing colonic bile acid losses. Fecal bile acid concentrations, highest in populations with the greatest risk of colonic cancer,[39] may act directly on the colonic mucosa or after bacterial degradation to promote neoplastic change.

The reason for the association with protein may also be secondary to the bacterial metabolism of protein within the lumen of the colon with the production of volatile derivatives of amino acids, nitrosamines, or $NH_3$. $NH_3$ has been proposed as a promoter of tumor growth.[40] With increased protein intake, it has been suggested that colonic bacterial production of volatile phenols and ammonia will increase to fulfill this role.[41,42]

Despite the fact that the epidemiologic associations are not as strong for fiber as for fat and protein, additional hypotheses have been proposed to suggest a rationale for a protective role of fiber in relation to colonic cancer. In fact, most of the properties of fiber have been ascribed a function in this respect. These include the ability of fiber to increase fecal bulk, to reduce gastrointestinal transit time, to trap or bind materials within the bowel lumen, to lower colonic pH, and to provide substrates for colonic mucosa and for bacterial cell growth (see Chaps. 2B and 56D1).

The ability of fiber to increase fecal bulk resulted in the suggestion that fiber may dilute potential carcinogens in the colon. Where careful measurements have been made between increased fecal bulk and freedom from colonic cancer,[43] this relationship holds true. Comparisons made in four Scandinavian populations with a three- to fourfold difference in risk of colonic cancer showed a significant negative relationship between fecal weight and incidence of colonic cancer.[43] The dietary data on fiber intake supported the physiologic measurements.[43] In this same study, it was of interest that no relationship was seen with gastrointestinal transit time despite the hypothesis that the more rapid the transit time the less time was available for the bacterial production of potential carcinogens. A similar lack of difference was seen between the Japanese in Hawaii, who are more prone to colon carcinoma, and the inhabitants of Japan, who are less prone to carcinoma.[44] Part of the reason for this finding may lie in the fact that at fecal outputs of more than 140 g/day the significant relationship between fecal weight and transit time no longer exists.[43]

Fiber and other nonabsorbed carbohydrate sources on being metabolized by bacteria to short-chain fatty acids (SCFA) reduce colonic pH.[45,46] This in turn may limit uptake of $NH_3$ by epithelial cells.[47,48] Low pH may also reduce $\alpha$-dehydroxylation of bile acids as potential carcinogens.[49]

In addition, the provision of energy in the form of SCFA may promote bacterial growth and so result in the lowering of possible toxic compounds in the colon either through their metabolism for nontoxic forms (e.g., formic acid to $CO_2$ and water) or through their uptake for bacterial synthetic purposes (e.g., $NH_3$ incorporation into bacterial protein).

In addition, SCFA have been shown to protect colonic epithelial cells in vitro from neoplastic change, and it was suggested that SCFA per se are antineoplastic. Conflicting evidence, however, is now being uncovered about the role of SCFA in the genesis of chemically induced colon cancer in rats;[50-52] tumor yield is enhanced when feeding fiber forms that are readily degraded by colonic bacteria to SCFA with accompanying falls in pH.[53] The model is difficult to interpret, however, because of the very large amounts of fiber fed relative to the animal's body (10 to 20% of the diet), and because the carcinogen administered causes tumors in the small intestine and ascending colon, a situation very different from the colorectal cancer seen in man.

These results further conflict with what is known of the human disease from epidemiologic studies. In these studies, diets rich in legumes were found to relate negatively to colonic cancer rates in different countries;[54] some diets (rich in dried beans), however, are among the richest sources of soluble fiber and therefore are substrates for colonic SCFA production.

Although all these possibilities remain as speculation in relation to human colonic carcinogenesis, they have acted as a great stimulus to the investigation of many underexplored aspects of colonic metabolism in health and disease.

## SUMMARY

The aim of this chapter has been to discuss the five possible areas (constipation, the irritable bowel, diverticular disease, Crohn's disease, and colonic cancer) where fiber may be relevant. For constipation and diverticular disease, dietary fiber is generally accepted as having a useful role in treatment. The involvement of fiber in the treatment of the irritable bowel is less clear, although a trial of increased fiber consumption in some cases may prove worthwhile and merits attention in the absence of more successful therapies. A role of fiber in Crohn's disease remains to be confirmed. Fiber in the prophylaxis of colonic cancer continues to be of great speculative interest. For a more mechanistic discussion of the action of fiber, see Chapter 2B.

## REFERENCES

1. Devroede, G.: *In* Gastrointestinal Disease. (Sleisenger, M.H., Fordtran, J.S., Eds.) Philadelphia, W.B. Saunders Co., 1978, pp. 368–386.
2. Paul, A.A., Southgate, D.A.T.: *In* The Composition of Foods. (McCance, R.A., Widdowson, E.M., Eds.) London, HMSO, 1978.
3. Bockus, H.L.: *In* Gastroenterology. (Bockus, H.L., Ed.) Philadelphia, W.B. Saunders Co., 1976, pp. 936–953.
4. Williams, R.D., Olmsted, W.H.: J. Nutr. *2*:433–449, 1936.
5. Cummings, J.H., Branch, W., Jenkins, D.J.A., et al.: Lancet *1*:5–9, 1978.
6. Stephen, A.M., Cummings, J.H.: Nature (London) *2*:283–284, 1980.
7. Manning, A.P., Heaton, K.W., Harvey, R.F., et al.: Lancet *2*:417–418, 1977.
8. Harvey, R.F., Pomare, E.W., Heaton, K.W.: Lancet *1*:1278–1280, 1973.
9. Payler, D.K., Pomare, G.W., Heaton, K.W., et al.: Gut *16*:209–213, 1975.
10. Haubrich, W.S.: *In* Gastroenterology. (Bockus, H.L., Ed.) Philadelphia, W.B. Saunders Co., 1976, pp. 895–917.
11. Painter, N.S., Burkitt, D.P.: Br. Med. J. *2*:450–455, 1971.
12. Painter, N.S.: Ann. R. Coll. Surg. Engl. *34*:98–119, 1964.
13. Almy, T.P.: Gastroenterology *49*:109–112, 1965.
14. Manousos, O.N., Vrachliotis, G., Delosakis, E., et al.: Am. J. Dig. Dis. *18*:174–176, 1973.
15. Brodribb, A.J.M.: *In* Medical Aspects of Dietary Fiber. (Spiller, G.A., Kay, R.M., Eds.) New York, Plenum Publishing Corp., 1980, pp. 43–66.
16. Brodribb, A.M.J., Humphreys, D.M.: Br. Med. J. *1*:424–425, 1976.
17. Gear, J.S.S., Ware, A., Fursdon, P., et al.: Lancet *1*:551–554, 1979.
18. Ohi, G., Minowa, K., Oyama, T., et al.: Am. J. Clin. Nutr. *38*:115–121, 1983.
19. Mendeloff, A.J.: Am. J. Dig. Dis. *21*:109–112, 1976.
20. Loeb, P.M.: *In* Gastrointestinal Disease. (Sleisenger, M.H., Fordtran, J.S., Eds.) Philadelphia, W.B. Saunders Co., 1978, pp. 1745–1771.
21. De La Vega, J.M.: *In* Gastroenterology. (Bockus, H.L., Ed.) Philadelphia, W.B. Saunders Co., 1976, pp. 973–1000.
22. Painter, N.S., Almeida, A.Z., Colebourne, K.W.: Br. Med. J. *2*:137–140, 1972.
23. Plumley, P.C., Francis, B.: J. Am. Diet. Assoc. *62*:527, 1973.
24. Hodgson, J.: Br. Med. J. *3*:729–731, 1972.
25. Parks, T.G.: Proc. R. Soc. Med. *67*:1037–1040, 1974.
26. Srivastava, G.S., Smith, A.N., Painter, N.S.: Br. Med. J. *1*:315–318, 1976.
27. Taylor I, Duthie, H.L.: Br. Med. J. *2*:988–990, 1976.

28. Tarpila, S., Miettinen, T.A.: Scand. J. Gastroenterol. *10*:27, 1975.
29. Brodribb, A.J.M., Humphreys, D.M.: Br. Med. J. *1*:424–425, 1976.
30. Brodribb, A.J.M.: Lancet *1*:664–666, 1977.
31. Ornstein, M.H., Littlewood, E.R., McLean Baird, I., et al.: Br. Med. J. *1*:1353–1356, 1981.
32. Smith, A.N., Kirwan, W.O., Sheriff, S.: Proc. R. Soc. Med. *67*:1041–1043, 1974.
33. Kasper, H., Somner, H.: Am. J. Clin. Nutr. *32*:1898–1901, 1979.
34. Thornton, J.R., Emmett, P.M., Heaton, K.W.: Br. Med. J. *2*:762–764, 1979.
35. Heaton, K.W., Thornton, J.R., Emmett, P.M.: Br. Med. J. *2*:764–766, 1979.
36. Armstrong, B., Doll, R.: Int. J. Cancer *15*:617–631, 1975.
37. Doll, R., Peto, R.: J. Natl. Cancer Inst. *66*:1191–1308, 1981.
38. Newmark, H.L., Wargovich, M.J., Bruce, W.R.: *In* A Decade of Achievements and Challenges in Large Bowel Cancer Research. (Mastromarino, A.J., Bratlain, M.G., Eds.) Westport, CT, Praeger Scientific, 1983, pp. 2–15.
39. Hill, M.J., Crowther, J.S., Draser, B.S., et al.: Lancet *1*:95–100, 1971.
40. Visek, W.J., Clinton, S.K., Truex, C.R.: Cornell Vet. *68*:3–39, 1978.
41. Bone, E., Tamin, A., Hill, M.J.: Am. J. Clin. Nutr. *29*:1448–1454, 1976.
42. Cummings, J.A., Hill, M.J., Bone, E.S., et al.: Am. J. Clin. Nutr. *32*:2094–2101, 1979.
43. Cummings, J.A., Branch, W.J., Bjerrum, L., et al.: Nutr. Cancer *4*:61–66, 1982.
44. Glober, G., Klein, K.L., Moore, J.O., et al.: Lancet *2*:80–81, 1974.
45. Walker, A.R.P., Walker, B.F., Segal, I.: S. Afr. Med. J. *5*:495–498, 1979.
46. Brown, R.L., Gibson, J.A., Sladen, E.E., et al.: Gut *15*:999–1004, 1974.
47. Down, P.F., Agostini, L., Murison, J., et al.: Clin. Sci. *43*:101–114, 1972.
48. Brown, R.L., Gibson, J.A., Fenton, J.C.B., et al.: Clin. Sci. Mol. Med. *48*:279–287, 1975.
49. Narasawa, T., Magadia, N.E., Weisburger, J.H., et al.: J. Natl. Cancer Inst. *53*:1093–1097, 1974.
50. Denter, D.L., Les, K., McKendall, G.R., Mitchell, P., et al.: Histochem. J. *16*:137–149, 1984.
51. Kruh, J.: Mol. Cell Biochem *42*:65–82, 1982.
52. Ryan, G.P., Dudrick, S.J., Copeland, G.M., et al.: Gastroenterology *77*:658–663, 1979.
53. Jacobs, L.R., Lupton, J.R.: Cancer Res. *46*:In Press, 1986.
54. McKeown-Eysse, G.: Prev. Med. In Press, 1986.

*Chapter* **56**

# NUTRITION AND DIET IN MANAGEMENT OF DISEASES OF THE GASTROINTESTINAL TRACT

## (E) LIVER
### (1) Nutritional Support in Liver Disease

### Laurence M. Blendis and David J.A. Jenkins

The prevalence of serious liver disease and annual death rate from it are increasing dramatically throughout the world, especially in Europe and North America, where the principal causes of liver disease are chronic alcoholism and viral hepatitis. The causes of death in individuals with these diseases are mainly the consequences of portal hypertension, such as bleeding from esophageal varices, or hepatic failure. The degree to which nutritional factors contribute to the progress of the hepatic lesion is not clear at present. Nevertheless, an understanding of the possible nutritional implications of liver disease is crucial to most therapeutic maneuvers undertaken in this condition. A common clinical picture of the cirrhotic patient who requires nutritional attention is one with a large distended abdomen and thin extremities. The patient looks clearly malnourished, and the malnutrition is due to several factors including anorexia with reduced caloric and nutrient intake, maldigestion, and malabsorption. These conditions in turn may be associated with multiple dys-

functions including abnormal amino acid and carbohydrate metabolism, alcoholic gastritis, a decrease in bile acid output,[1] and pancreatic insufficiency secondary to chronic pancreatitis.

The picture is therefore often one of protein-calorie malnutrition with deficiencies of trace elements and vitamins, both fat- and water-soluble.

The spectrum of these deficiencies and hence the therapeutic options vary with the etiology and stage of the liver disease. Alcoholic hepatitis and cirrhosis are associated with the most common clinical nutritional problems.

## PROTEINS AND AMINO ACIDS

The major nutritional dilemma in liver disease is how much protein should be given to the malnourished patient with hepatic insufficiency. The goal is to avoid overloading the liver and hepatic encephalopathy, and at the same time, to give sufficient exogenous protein to maintain body protein stores and to allow tissue repair.

## Etiology of Liver Injury

The early theory that liver injury in chronic alcoholics was due not to alcohol but to malnutrition was rejected following the demonstration that alcohol per se induced steatosis in nonalcoholic volunteers on isocaloric diets.[2] However, the concept that liver injury in chronic alcoholism may also be due to nutritional deficiency, in particular to protein-calorie malnutrition, resurfaced after the observation that patients undergoing jejunoileal bypass[3] developed a lesion identical to that of alcoholic hepatitis. The role of nutrition in liver injury was supported by an epidemiologic study that found that the only difference between alcoholic patients with cirrhosis and those without cirrhosis was a significant decrease in calorie and protein consumption in the former.[4] However, the role of nutrition in liver injury is not entirely proven because population studies in France[5] and West Germany[6] have shown that the incidence of cirrhosis is related directly to the average daily alcohol intake and the number of years of drinking. Furthermore, more recent studies have not confirmed a correlation between the severity of liver disease, diet, and nutritional status.[6a]

## Alcoholic Hepatitis

Patients with acute alcoholic hepatitis are often anorexic and wasted. In one study, 100% of 284 patients had some evidence of marasmus or kwashiorkor.[6b] All patients may have nausea and vomiting if there is associated alcoholic gastritis, so that feeding them can be a problem. In addition, the more severely ill patients are often encephalopathic, necessitating protein restriction. Although enteral or parenteral feeding is frequently indicated, there are theoretical contraindications to both, principally that of encephalopathy.

**Increased Caloric Intake or Steroids.** The efficacy of treatment of acute severe alcoholic hepatitis with steroids remains controversial.[7,8] An early study had shown significant benefit with prednisone,[9] which was later thought to be due to the improved appetites of steroid-treated patients. A subsequent study was then performed comparing the effects of prednisone with those of caloric supplementation without prednisone in patients with severe alcoholic hepatitis and encephalopathy.[10] Fourteen patients were randomized to take prednisone and to eat "ad libitum," or to receive at least 1,600 nonprotein calories daily administered orally as high-calorie lemonade and hard candy, together with an intravenous infusion of 25% glucose solution if necessary. The result was that all seven patients with this high-calorie intake alone died compared with two out of seven receiving prednisone. This study indicated that the beneficial effect of prednisone was unlikely to be due to increased caloric intake.

**Enteral Feeding.** The problem of anorexia in the patient with alcoholic cirrhosis was overcome in one study by tube feeding.[11] However, the commercially available formulas used in this study either in maintenance doses (2 L, 2,000 kcal, with 80 g protein) or repletional doses (3 L, 3,000 kcal, with 120 g protein) resulted in increased ascites and precipitation of, or deterioration in, encephalopathy.

In another preliminary study, four patients were given 1 to 1.5 L of a formula with 1,580 kcal/L (15% of calories from protein, 50% from carbohydrate, and 35% from fat). None of the patients developed encephalopathy, and three out of four improved their appetite.[12] Urinary creatinine excretion increased, and mean serum albumin levels rose from 2.4 g to 3.4 g/dl over an unspecified period. Liver enzymes and prothrombin times fell.

In another study on a small group of malnourished patients, enteral feeding achieved protein intakes of greater than 80 g per day and positive nitrogen balance without exacerbation of encephalopathy.[12a]

In a more recent study, 64 patients with acute alcoholic hepatitis with or without underlying cirrhosis were randomized regardless of encephalopathy to receive a controlled diet alone or with supplementation. The diet was administered orally, nasogastrically, or intravenously as necessary with 2,000 kcal and 10 g nitrogen daily with further randomization into a conventional protein source or branched-chain amino acids (BCAA). The median periods of observation were 14 to 18 days. Twenty-four-hour nitrogen balances were significantly correlated with nitrogen intake, and daily intakes of 10 g or more of protein were invariably associated with a positive balance. The nutritional therapy did not affect mortality in the series as a whole or in the subgroups and did not have any consistent effect on encephalopathy.[12b]

These preliminary studies suggested that enteral feeding can be well tolerated in anorexic patients with acute alcoholic hepatitis, that it does not precipitate encephalopathy, and that is is associated with an improvement in well-being and nutritional status.

**Parenteral Nutrition.** The deterrent to the earlier use of parenteral nutrition, especially with amino acids, was generated by concern over precipitating encephalopathy. This occurred particularly after the introduction of the "false neurotransmitter" hypothesis[13] involving high levels of circulating aromatic amino acids, especially phenylalanine, tryptophan,[14] and methionine, with production of toxic metabolites such as mercaptans.[15] The infusion of standard amino acid mixtures in patients with portocaval anastomoses caused mental deterioration.[16]

In patients who can ingest at least 700 calories, 900 mosm/L solutions infused in a peripheral vein can have the same nutritional effect on nitrogen metabolism as the 1,800 mosm/L central nutritional therapy in the same patients.[17] Based on this observation, Galambos showed first that this regimen was safe, i.e., did not induce encephalopathy, in patients with alcoholic hepatitis.[12] The infusion rate was gradually increased to 2 L/day to provide between 50 and 77 g protein daily. Encephalopathy was not present, anorexia subsided, urinary urea excretion increased, serum albumin concentration rose, and at the same time liver enzyme levels improved.

These findings prompted a randomized controlled trial of IV amino acid therapy of 35 consecutive patients with alcoholic hepatitis.[18] All patients were offered a 300-kcal, 100-g protein diet and were studied for 28 days. The "treatment" group received IV amino acids (70 to 85 g of 7% Aminosyn or 8.5% Travasol). Both groups appeared to have similar biochemical features. The treated patients did not develop encephalopathy or ascites more frequently, serum bilirubin levels fell, serum albumin levels rose significantly, and none of the treated patients died compared with four of the controls ($P<0.02$). Unfortunately, the only evidence that the 4-week course of IV amino acids actually changed the nutritional status of the patient was the change in serum albumin concentration, which was more likely to be due to improved liver function. This first trial of its type so far reported is nevertheless suggestive that IV amino acid therapy may be therapeutic in acute alcoholic hepatitis. A subsequent controlled randomized study was performed for one month in 15 patients with biopsy-proven alcoholic hepatitis. Five patients received a parenteral amino-acid-glucose solution while 10 received the glucose solution alone. The former group experienced a greater improvement in nitrogen balance. However, amino acid therapy had no effect on nutritional assessment criteria in a composite clinical index or on histologic improvement, apart from fatty infiltration.[18a]

## Cirrhosis

In patients with cirrhosis but without alcoholic hepatitis, the problem of the ideal intake for maintenance and repair remains. In an early metabolic study, Gabuzda and Shear showed that with an intake of at least 1,500 to 3,500 calories per day,

nitrogen balance is maintained by taking only 35 to 50 g protein daily or 0.6 to 0.7 g/kg body weight/ day.[19] In a more recent study in cirrhotic patients, the average minimum protein requirement was 48 g/day or 0.74 g/kg/day whether natural or BCAA-enriched protein was used. At 60 g protein/day, the patients were in positive nitrogen balance with an average of + 1.2 g/day.[20]

**Enteral Nutrition.** Eight malnourished alcoholics and two postnecrotic cirrhotics with ascites were treated with a low-sodium (1 g/2,000 kcal), high-caloric-density formula (2 kcal/ml), supplying at the start 40 g of protein/day.[21] Nine patients tolerated this regimen well with significant improvement in serum albumin levels from 2.7 to 3.4 g/dl, in serum transferrin levels from 140 to 183 mg/dl, and in creatinine/height ratio from 5.3 to 6.1 mg/cm. The midarm muscle and fat areas also increased. Six of seven patients even tolerated increases in protein intake to 80 g and then to 143 g without adverse effect.

**Parenteral Nutrition: Amino Acid Requirements.** Because of the chronicity of the cirrhotic state, parenteral nutritional support has not been undertaken as part of long-term therapy, nor indeed has the routine use of enteral feeding, although this may warrant attention. On the other hand, considerable information has been gained on the derangements of amino acid metabolism in cirrhosis and the nutritional implications. Such information may help in defining not only the amount but also the nature of the protein best suited to the maintenance of cirrhotic patients.

*Hypotyrosinemia.* The effect of total parenteral nutrition (TPN) on the nutritional status of cirrhotics is unknown. The effect of TPN, using FreAmine II as the source of amino acids, on patients with malabsorption and on those with alcoholic cirrhosis was compared for 4 weeks.[22] After a baseline period of oral feeding, the patients began a 4- or 5-week course of TPN. Each liter contained 20% glucose, vitamins, and minerals as well as amino acids. All 6 patients with malabsorption and 8 of the 12 cirrhotic patients developed positive nitrogen balance (average + 6.2 g/ 70 kg ideal body weight [IBW]/day) associated with nutritional repletion and an improvement in liver blood tests. By contrast, in four cirrhotic patients, nitrogen balance remained close to zero, nutritional repletion did not occur, liver blood tests detriorated, and plasma cystine and tyrosine levels fell. When oral supplements of cystine and tyrosine were given during the fifth week of TPN, plasma levels became normal and nitrogen balance became positive at + 5.8 g/70 kg IBW per day, with improvement in anthropomorphic measurements, urinary creatinine/height ratios, and liver blood tests.

Eight essential amino acids are needed by normal adults. Thus, cystine and tyrosine are normally nonessential in the diet because they can be synthesized endogenously in the liver from adequate amounts of methionine and phenylalanine. However, a subgroup of cirrhotics who received FreAmine II (which contains little of these two amino acids) remained in negative nitrogen balance. Probably they were unable to synthesize these amino acids. Thus, when cystine and tyrosine were added to their oral diet, the plasma levels became normal and the patients developed positive nitrogen balance.

*Hypertyrosinemia.* In contrast, many cirrhotics have hypertyrosinemia.[23,24] In addition to a deficiency of phenylalanine hydroxylase, cirrhotic patients have a further block in tyrosine metabolism that may[24] or may not[25] be associated with decreased tyrosine transaminase activity as manifested by delayed tyrosine clearance after oral loading.

*Branched-Chain Amino Acid (BCAA) Supplements.* The abnormal plasma amino acid profile, high in aromatic amino acids (AAA), phenylalanine, tyrosine, and free tryptophan and low in BCAA first described in encephalopathy is also found commonly in nonencephalopathic cirrhotics.[26,27] Protein calorie intake can influence the ratio of AAA to BCAA in normal subjects.[28] The reason for this pattern is not clear, but one dietary study demonstrated that the ratio of tryptophan to neutral amino acids, for example, can be increased by protein restriction both in normal subjects and in cirrhotics.[29]

Initially, it was suggested that this pattern of plasma amino acids in liver disease was due to changes in muscle amino acid metabolism induced by the hyperinsulinemia present in these patients,[30] the cause of which may be peripheral insulin resistance.[31] However, this concept is not supported by more recent studies.[32,33] Thus in chronic liver failure when glucose oxidation becomes impaired, BCAA can be used as an alternative source of energy, with the resulting increased BCAA oxidation in muscle and adipose tissue leading to decreased plasma levels. Furthermore, the catabolic state stimulates protein breakdown with release of amino acids into the circulation, and the reduction in the capacity of the liver to metabolize amino acids leads to elevated amino acid levels.[34] However, increased postprandial BCAA levels are seen after a protein meal. This finding related significantly to the postprandial hyperglycemia seen after an oral glucose load,[33] indicating that this latter effect is associated with insulin resistance. Infusion of an amino acid mixture rich in BCAA (F080) has caused encephalopathic patients to achieve nitrogen balance.[35] In one study, enriched BCAA solutions were infused in nonencephalopathic cirrhotics who were within 10% of ideal body weight.[36] The solution was similar to the F080 solution, which also has less phenylalanine and tryptophan than usual amino acid solutions and contains no tyrosine. The patients received 500 ml over 5 hours for 3 days, after a 3-day basal period, while continuing on their oral diet that provided 25 to 30 kcal and 1 g protein/kg body weight/day. In a consecutive 3-day period, the patients received the same amino acid solution daily with 1,000 ml 25% dextrose solution over 10 hours. During both treatment periods, BCAA did not significantly change and phenylalanine, tyrosine, and free tryptophan fell, whereas the decreased plasma alanine levels rose.

The only assessment of nutritional change was the measurement of urinary 3 methylhistidine (3MH), which was slightly increased in the basal period and fell significantly to normal from 288 $\mu$mol/day to 210 and 182 $\mu$mol/day together with a decrease in 3MH/creatinine ratio. Measurement of urinary 3MH assesses myofibrillar protein catabolism,[37,38] but is also affected by muscle protein intake,[39] which in metabolic studies should therefore be excluded from the diet if possible. The patients in this study ate 80 g of meat at lunch daily. Thus, conclusions from this study must be guarded. The authors claim that BCAA-enriched solutions, especially leucine, may reduce excessive muscle catabolism. Alternatively, BCAA may stimulate protein synthesis. However, when 1-14C leucine was used in protein turnover studies in stable, noncatabolic cirrhotic patients, no difference was found between BCAA solution containing 60 mmol leucine and a standard amino acid solution containing 25 mmol leucine.[40]

Therefore, the role of intravenous (BCAA-enriched) amino acid solutions or TPN in cirrhosis is unclear. Over a relatively short period, i.e., four weeks, TPN can improve nutritional status and nitrogen balance in these patients, providing certain nonessential amino acids are supplemented. These data are not yet confirmed, and the place of such therapy over the course of years of a cirrhotic's life has yet to be evaluated.

## Complications of Cirrhosis

**Hepatic Encephalopathy (HE).** The classic treatment of cirrhotic patients with chronic encephalopathy (HE) is in direct conflict with the patient's nutritional requirements.

*Etiology.* A widely held theory is that a major

factor influencing the development of HE is ammonia. Ammonia is derived from intestinal nitrogen, which in turn is influenced by protein intake.[41] Although the negative influence of dietary protein is clear, the variability of blood ammonia levels in patients with HE makes it unlikely that it is the sole factor in the pathogenesis of this condition.[42] Ammonia is not the only nitrogenous substance implicated. Methionine ingestion causes mental deterioration in patients with a history of HE associated with the characteristic hepatic fetor.[43] This phenomenon was later identified as being due to metabolites of methionine in particular, mercaptans[44] or methanethiol (produced by bacterial metabolism of methionine), which is the most comatogenic.

*Branched-Chain Amino Acids (BCAA).* As already mentioned, amino acid metabolism is abnormal in cirrhosis. There is elevation of plasma levels of the aromatic amino acids phenylalanine and tyrosine, as well as of tryptophan and methionine, together with a depression of the BCAA.[45] These abnormalities are associated with the circulatory disturbances found in patients with decompensated cirrhosis and HE and prompted the false neurotransmitter hypothesis.[13] In brief, this hypothesis states that an abnormal plasma amino acid pattern causes a deficiency of catecholamines in the brain, associated with the production of sympathomimetic amines such as tyramine and octopamine from phenylalanine by alternative metabolic pathways in the brain. These sequences of events result from increased entry of the aromatic amino acids into the brain consequent to reduced levels of the BCAA. These amines might then interfere with normal neurotransmission by blocking neuronal receptor sites. The implication for therapy was to "normalize" the plasma aminogram by infusion of amino acid solutions rich in BCAA, and this attempt appeared to work in both experimental animals and in patients with HE.[35]

The role of BCAA in the pathogenesis and treatment of HE has been evaluated in seven randomized controlled trials using IV solutions[46–52] and in seven studies using oral BCAA supplementation.[53–59] In the case of IV BCAA in acute HE, the studies differed in various aspects. The entry criteria for the patients included the severity of liver disease and associated or precipitating factors such as alcohol or variceal bleeding. The mode of presentation, the study designs, and the treatment protocols all varied. Nevertheless, the presence of the control groups may at least make within-study comparison acceptable. BCAA were associated with a significant outcome in three studies,[42,43,47]

nonsignificant improvement in two,[44,46] and no significant benefit in two[45,48,48a] (Table 56E1–1).

As far as oral BCAA supplementation is concerned, in two studies BCAA supplementation improved HE, whereas in five studies there was no effect of BCAA treatment of HE (Table 56E1–2).

*Dietary Management.* Regardless of pathogenetic theories, dietary protein intake has been uniformly implicated in the etiology of HE, and thus restriction of protein intake has become standard practice. Shakespeare was perhaps one of the first to observe through Sir Andrew Aguecheek in Twelfth Night that meat protein was harmful: "...but I am a great eater of beef and I believe that does harm to my wit." It was Pavlov and his coworkers, however, who first pointed out that meat protein induced mental changes in dogs with Eck fistulas, whereas milk protein did not.[60] The reasons for this phenomenon were not clear except that red meat contains a certain amount of blood, and blood is more ammoniogenic than either fish or milk protein.[61] This finding prompted the use of a milk and cheese diet in the treatment of HE, with apparently some success. Another rationale for this diet was the possible change in colonic bacterial flora, from urease-containing bacteria (which form ammonia from urea) to predominantly lactobacilli.

With the advent of highly successful oral therapy for HE, such as lactulose and neomycin, the need for special diets has diminished. However, the fact remains that these patients need protein but are being treated by protein restriction. Intakes of 40 g of protein daily or less may be below requirements.

*Nature of the Protein.* Greenberger and his colleagues found that vegetable protein was less encephalogenic than animal protein.[62] However, they only studied three patients, the protocol varied, and two of the patients were on antiencephalopathic therapy, including lactulose. In a subsequent study, Uribe et al. reported that cirrhotic patients with encephalopathy on a daily intake of 80 g protein showed great improvement when vegetable was substituted for animal protein in their diet.[63] In this instance, no patients were treated with lactulose.

Following this investigation, deBruijn and his colleagues performed a crossover study in eight patients in a metabolic unit, four alcoholic and four postnecrotic shunted cirrhotics, using a standard five-week protocol.[64] After an initial period of one week, the patients ate a mixed diet for one week and then randomly alternated between one-week periods on equicaloric, isomacronutrient diets containing animal or vegetable protein, and one-week periods on a mixed

**Table 56E1–1. The Effects of IV BCAA on the Management of Porto Systemic Encephalopathy (PSE)***

| Study | Number of Patients | BCAA Additional Treatment | Control "Treatment" | Mortality (%) | | Improved Mental State (%) | |
|---|---|---|---|---|---|---|---|
| | | | | BCAA | Controls | BCAA | Controls |
| 1. Rossi-Fanelli et al.[50] | 34 | Glucose | Glucose Lactulose | 24 | 41 | 70 | 47 |
| 2. Wahren et al.[52] | 50 | 30 kcal/kg/day 50% glucose + 20% intra-lipid | Glucose | 40 | 20 | 56 | 48 |
| 3. Cerra et al.[46] | 75 | Glucose †Oral nutrition as tolerated <1,500 kcal/d | Glucose Neomycin | 17 | 55 | 77 | 45 |
| 4. Fiaccadori et al.[47] | 48 | Glucose †With or without lactulose | Glucose Lactulose | 0 | 0 | 94 | 62 |
| 5. Michel et al.[49] | 70 | †Lipids (100 g) | Conventional AA solution Lipids | 20 | 20.9 | 33 | 29 |
| 6. Strauss et al.[51] | 30 | †Oral protein to tolerance | Neomycin Enemas | 12 | 12 | 87 | 87 |
| 7. Gluud et al.[48] | 20 | | Glucose | 20 | 10 | 70 | 60 |

* Adapted from Ferenci, P., et al.[48a]
† All groups received a modified AA solution enriched with BCAA + glucose IV.

**Table 56E1–2.   The Effects of Oral BCAA on the Management of PSE***

| Study | Number of Patients | Treatment | | Duration of Treatment (days) | Type of Study | Outcome |
|---|---|---|---|---|---|---|
| | | BCAA | Controls | | | |
| 1. McGhee et al.[53] | 4 | "Hepataid" Casein 21 g | Casein 50 g | 11 | Sequential | No change None developed HE |
| 2. Horst et al.[54] | 37 | "Hepataid" | Oral Diet + glucose solution | 21 | Controlled Randomized | BCAA better HE became more severe in controls with increasing protein intake |
| | | 20 g protein diet | | | | |
| 3. Erikson et al.[55] | 7 | BCAA + sucrose | Maltodextrin diet | 14 | Crossover | BCAA better Improved psychometrics only |
| | | 40–100 g protein lactulose | | | | |
| 4. Egberts et al.[56] | 22 | BCAA | Casein | 7 | Crossover | No change |
| | | 1 g protein/kg/day | | | | |
| 5. Riggio et al.[57] | 28 | BCAA | Lactulose | 60 | Controlled Randomized | No difference |
| | | 0.5 g protein/kg/day | | | | |
| 6. Simko et al.[58] | 10 | "Hepataid" | Placebo | 90 | Controlled Randomized | No change |
| | | Standard unrestricted diet | | | | |
| 7. Sieg et al.[59] | 14 | BCAA Carbohydrates | Placebo isocaloric Carbohydrate intake | 90 | Crossover | No change |
| | | 40 g protein diet lactulose | | | | |

* Adapted from Ferenci, P., et al.[48a]

diet. All patients had subclinical HE as assessed by a standard neurologic examination, routine and computer-assessed EEG (CAEEG), psychometric tests (trailmaking part A or B), and raised fasting arterial ammonia levels.[65] During the crossover study, the only significant change occurred with CAEEG, which improved significantly with vegetable protein, with the peak frequency increasing from a mean of 6.6 Hz to 7.1 Hz. As previously reported, the ratio of BCAA to aromatics was decreased in these patients and did not change with the diets.

Shaw et al. demonstrated in five encephalopathic patients that substitution of vegetable for animal protein (largely as kidney and lima beans) for one-week periods, in diets containing approximately 50 g protein daily, did not alter nitrogen balance, fasting plasma amino acid levels, or the results of psychometric tests.[66] No assessments of EEG status were reported, but four of the five patients were maintained on lactulose (30 ml four times a day) throughout the study period.

The body of evidence therefore indicates that providing the vegetable protein substitution can be achieved in an acceptable form when the use of vegetable protein produces no deleterious effects and has some possible benefits. This therefore represents a reversal of conventional advice where, because of its superior biologic value, animal protein sources are usually recommended for the treatment of patients with hepatic encephalopathy.

What are the possible mechanisms by which the benefits of vegetable protein might occur? In terms of the false neurotransmitter theory, there is no significant difference in the BCAA or aromatics with any of the diets. However, the vegetable diets are higher in arginine. The basic amino acids arginine and ornithine may be beneficial in the treatment of HE based on the fact that increasing these amino acids in the Krebs urea cycle may lead to increased uptake of ammonia and decreased blood ammonia levels in normal subjects[67] and cirrhotics.[68] However, one controlled trial of oral arginine ingestion failed to show a beneficial effect.[69]

Other factors also may lead to differences between the effects of animal and vegetable protein diets. Animal protein diets contain significantly more methionine, which could have been detrimental owing to the formation of mercaptans. Vegetable protein diets may reduce the absorption of nitrogen because of the increased fiber content. Nitrogen balance studies have shown an increase in fecal nitrogen excretion on vegetable diets.[70] In addition, urinary urea[70] and total nitrogen excretion[64] were significantly reduced owing to a reduction in urea production. Thus, the mecha-

nism of the possible beneficial effect of vegetable protein remains complex.

**Amino Acid Analogues.** With the conflicting result of BCAA, an alternative approach is the administration of amino acids as the alphaketoanalogues. The administration of five essential amino acids (valine, leucine, isoleucine, methionine, and phenylalanine) as the calcium salts in gelatin capsules has resulted in a significant improvement in essential to nonessential amino acid ratio and in clinical improvement in mental status and psychologic testing.[71]

Finally, when the oral administration of ornithine salts of branched-chain ketoacids (34 mmol/day) was compared with that of branched-chain amino acids (68 mmol/day) in a double-blind crossover study, the ornithine salts produced significant improvement.[72] In contrast, patients receiving calcium salts of branched-chain ketoacids (34 mmol/day) or ornithine alphaketoglutarate showed either no change or deterioration, respectively.

**Salt and Water Retention.** Another common complication of portal hypertension is salt and water retention, leading to the development of massive ascites with or without peripheral edema. Routine management of this problem requires appropriate restriction of salt and fluid intake together with diuretic therapy. Patients with only a moderate amount of ascites require restriction of sodium intake to 2 g or 100 meq daily, particularly if they respond to potassium-sparing diuretics. However, as the patients become more resistant to these drugs and require additional "loop" diuretics such as furosemide, sodium intake must be restricted further to 50 meq/day. The more refractory patients then require hospitalization with bed rest and restriction of sodium intake to the lowest palatable level, which is generally 20 meq/day, together with one liter of fluid. These patients usually excrete less than 10 meq sodium/day in the urine and often less than 3 meq/day. The diets can be made more palatable with salt substitutes such as potassium chloride.

In a small group of patients who become virtually refractory to all diuretic regimens, a peritoneovenous shunt may result in an impressive diuretic response.[73] Over one to five years, ascites either disappears or is easily controlled with a no-added-salt diet with or without small doses of diuretics.[74]

In addition, the patients appear to regain body tissue, thus improving their emaciated appearance. In one study of body composition in seven patients, the initial diuresis was associated with a mean loss of 9 kg in weight. The natriuresis and kaliuresis were associated with a decrease in total body potassium (TBK) but not in total body nitrogen (TBN), resulting in a significant decrease in TBK/TBN ratio from 2.12 to 1.66 (p<0.01). By a mean of 14 months there were significant increases in mean TBN and the nitrogen index (ratio of actual amount to that predicted on the basis of body size).[75] These increases were associated with a significant increase in nonalcohol calories but not in protein consumption.[76] Thus, these studies indicate that TBK may be less satisfactory than TBN as a measure of lean body mass. It is also possible that ascites may affect nitrogen metabolism as well as diminish food intake.

## CARBOHYDRATES

Because the liver is so intimately involved in carbohydrate metabolism, it is not surprising that such metabolism is so frequently disturbed in patients with liver disease.

### Impaired Carbohydrate Metabolism and Diabetes

An association between cirrhosis and an increased incidence of diabetes has long been recognized. As many as 70% or more of cirrhotic patients have impaired carbohydrate tolerance[77–79] with up to 32% being frankly diabetic.[80,81] Diabetes in cirrhotic patients is usually controlled by diet and oral hypoglycemic agents. Only a few require insulin. Conversely, an increased incidence of cirrhosis has been found in diabetics at autopsy.[82] In addition, pericentral hepatic fibrosis and intracellular hyaline have been reported in nonalcoholic diabetics.[83]

In general, patients with cirrhosis have high fasting and postprandial serum insulin levels. The increased insulin levels are secondary to a number of factors including portosystemic shunting, increased peripheral insulin resistance, raised levels of glucagon, free fatty acids, growth hormone, and a low total body potassium.[79–86] Studies have indicated that individuals with "hepatogenous diabetes" illustrate many of the features of noninsulin-dependent diabetics. These include down-regulation of insulin receptors, increased fasting levels of insulin, and hyperinsulinism in response to oral glucose.[31] In addition, there may be a prolonged half-life of insulin-administered IV.[87]

A similar picture of deranged carbohydrate metabolism is also seen in chronic active hepatitis independently of cirrhosis. The derangement improves with steroid therapy and consequent improvement of liver function.[88]

In general, the diabetes associated with cirrhosis does not result in the complications seen with primary diabetes. It may, nevertheless, prove difficult to control. The raised serum insulin levels enhance the abnormal pattern of plasma amino acids already present in cirrhotics, namely raised levels of aromatic amino acids and methionine and depressed levels of branched-chain amino acids.

### Therapeutic Implications

Principles of dietary management currently being applied to noncirrhotic diabetics should apply equally well to cirrhotic patients with diabetes, although such complicating factors as ascites need additional salt restriction. The recommended increase in carbohydrate intake to 50% of dietary calories in the form of high-fiber foods[89–91] may have definite advantages for the diabetic cirrhotic. By virtue of their unabsorbable carbohydrate components, such foods may complement the use of antiencephalopathic therapy, such as lactulose, through enhancing the laxative effect and altering colonic metabolism by reducing the pH of intraluminal contents. These measures in themselves limit ammonia and amine production and their colonic absorption. This possibility was not mentioned by Shaw and colleagues[66] in explaining the claimed improvement by other investigators in hepatic encephalopathy upon substitution of vegetable for animal protein using legumes (dried beans).[63]

The provision of such foods to noncirrhotic diabetics has resulted in improved carbohydrate tolerance in acute studies and, in the longer term, has improved all aspects of diabetic control.[92–97] Preliminary studies in patients with cirrhosis have also indicated reduced postprandial glucose, insulin, and gastric inhibitory peptide (GIP) responses after legume-based to bread-based meals.[98] This finding may be due to a slower absorption of these foods, a concept that is supported by higher enteroglucagon and neurotension levels associated with the intake of legumes.[98] In addition, flatter amino acid responses were also seen after the legume-based meals.[98a]

Incidental evidence that these dietary maneuvers may have general application comes from the studies of Uribe and associates. They showed that the provision of 40 g of vegetable protein, in the form of legumes, in the diets of diabetic cirrhotic patients receiving insulin, resulted in reduction in insulin requirement. The fall in insulin requirements was sufficient to cause episodes of hypoglycemia.[63] These investigators followed up these observations with a crossover study in patients with chronic encephalopathy and diabetes using equicaloric diets of vegetable protein and of animal protein supplemented with 35 g of fiber daily.

They found significant reductions in fasting blood glucose levels on vegetable protein diets.[99]

Studies in this area are still in their infancy. Nevertheless, at present it seems reasonable to treat cirrhotic patients with impaired glucose tolerance or diabetes with higher-carbohydrate, high-fiber diets with or without vegetable protein in a fashion similar to the treatment of noncirrhotic individuals. Not only may there be advantages in terms of carbohydrate tolerance, but a reduction in insulin levels may help normalize amino acid abnormalities. In addition, increased consumption of high-fiber or more slowly digested vegetable foods may reduce ammonia absorption through effects in the colon.

## FAT

Unlike the other macronutrients, disturbances in fat metabolism may be deranged not only by hepatic parenchymal dysfunction, but also by cholestasis resulting in malabsorption of both fat and fat-soluble vitamins.

### Fat Malabsorption

Impaired fat absorption has been noted in patients with alcoholic cirrhosis as evidenced by modest increases in fecal fat output.[100] The previous observation of increased postprandial hypertriglyceridemia[101] has not been confirmed in one study. Indeed, in cirrhotic patients with low lecithin cholesterol acyl transferase (LCAT) activity, the triglyceride response was reduced.[102] No gross changes have been seen in small intestinal morphology on light microscopy or in absorptive capacity as judged by D-xylose tests. Pancreatitis and neomycin administration have been considered to be major causes of malabsorption,[100] although changes suggestive of small intestinal damage have been seen by electron microscopy. Additional reasons for the impaired fat absorption include the reduced bile salt pool size noted in cirrhosis[103] despite the absence of obvious intra- or extrahepatic obstruction. Nevertheless, in terms of the magnitude of fat malabsorption, this factor is small, as would be predicted from studies of biliary diversion where bile salts have been excluded from the small intestine.[104] Of possibly greater nutritional significance, however, is that the reduced luminal concentration of bile salts may impair the absorption of fat-soluble vitamins.[104,105] These factors lead to their deficiencies in primary biliary cirrhosis (PBC). In PBC, deficiency of fat-soluble vitamins may be exacerbated by cholestyramine given to treat the pruritis. This matter is discussed further in the context of the individual fat-soluble vitamins.

### Fatty Liver

Fatty liver is associated with a wide range of clinical states, including excessive alcohol ingestion, diabetes, obesity, jejunoileal bypass, weight reduction, toxemia of pregnancy, and TPN, some of which may be associated with progression to more serious forms of liver dysfunction. However, the relationship of fatty liver to the development of cirrhosis is not clear, and a fatty change may be a marker of liver injury rather than a causative factor in itself. Thus, for example, although excessive alcohol intake is associated with fatty liver, the deleterious effects of ethanol in producing cirrhosis[106] may result from a combination of various factors associated with excessive alcohol consumption. These include induction of the microsomal ethanol oxidizing system with the synthesis of toxic compounds and free radicals, and the production of an alcoholic hepatitis and altered collagen metabolism.[107,108]

In acute situations in which fatty liver results from overingestion of alcohol or exposure to toxins, such as chloroform and acetone, the lipid source is likely to be predominantly endogenous in origin. Fatty acid mobilized from adipose tissue after ethanol ingestion appears to be related to increased sympathetic activity and catecholamine release because it is blocked by adrenalectomy or adrenergic blockers.[109] The accumulation of lipid is further accentuated by the enhanced redox potential of the liver (raised $NADH/NAD^+$),[110] which favors lipogenesis rather than fatty acid oxidation. This phenomenon is related to the hepatic conversion of alcohol to acetaldehyde and is further illustrated by the accumulation of lactate in situations in which alcohol is being metabolized.[111] The level of alcohol intake that has been demonstrated to cause fatty infiltration in healthy volunteers ranges from 68 to 130 g daily (7 to 13 oz 86° whiskey) for one to two weeks or 270 g (27 oz 86° whiskey) for two days.[112]

In the long term, much of the fat that accumulates in alcoholic hepatic steatosis appears to be of dietary origin. Increases in hepatic triglyceride content have been found when fat in the diet constituted 36% of calories as opposed to 5% (a low-fat diet).[113] Furthermore, the fatty acid pattern reflected that of the diet, with increases in myristate and laureate from coconut oil and linoleate from dietary linseed oil, as compared with the endogenously synthesized oleate and palmitate seen with the low-fat diet. These researchers simply continued to feed rats alcohol in the presence of 10% fat.[113] Furthermore, substituting medium-chain triglycerides (MCT) for long-chain fatty acids in the diet[114] can also reduce steatosis because of the tendency for MCT to be oxidized to ketone bodies rather than being incorporated into tissue glyceride.

**Fat Absorption.** Part of the mechanism for fat absorption may also relate to the reduced bile salt pool seen in cirrhosis.[103] As mentioned already, under normal conditions, long-chain fatty acids are absorbed from bile salt micelles. In the absence of bile salts, micelles are not formed, chylomicra are not synthesized, and thus fatty acids are not absorbed by the lymphatic route. Instead, long-chain fatty acids are absorbed directly into the portal blood from the more distal small intestine. These albumin-bound fatty acids are extracted by the liver where they may either accumulate or act as substrates for metabolism.[115–119] Despite the fact that feeding medium-chain triglycerides appears to reduce hepatic steatosis, their use in states of decreased hepatic protein synthetic ability is questionable. In abetalipoproteinemia, treatment with MCT is associated with the development of cirrhosis.[118] It therefore appears prudent to advise fat restriction to patients with hepatic steatosis as has been advised for the general population (less than 35% of dietary calories). Studies by Forsgren in 1969 in man indicated that as much as 70% of ingested fatty acid was absorbed by the portal route in the absence of bile acids in the lumen of the small intestine.[105] Studies in bile fistula may have also shown that despite the absence of chylomicrons, steatorrhea is only modest, accounting for approximately 30% of ingested fat. Feeding fat is unlikely to cause cirrhosis.

## FAT-SOLUBLE VITAMINS

### Vitamin A

Vitamin A is essential for the maintenance of human life. Because it cannot be synthesized, it must be ingested either as vitamin A alcohol (retinol), its ester, or as beta-carotene. Carotene is a provitamin that is converted endogeneously to vitamin A. It is found in fruits and vegetables such as peaches, apricots, sweet potatoes, carrots, green vegetables, and dairy products containing butter fat. Cirrhotic patients may become deficient owing to poor dietary intake. In addition, in patients with fat malabsorption due to bile acid deficiency, vitamin A, along with other fat-soluble vitamins is malabsorbed. This phenomenon may be due to defective bile acid synthesis, as in alcoholic cirrhosis, or chronic cholestasis, as in primary biliary cirrhosis (PBC). In both conditions, reduced circulating vitamin A levels have been reported.[119,120] More recently, hepatic vitamin A levels were found to be decreased in patients with all histologic stages of alcoholic liver disease.[121]

Hepatic vitamin A was low even in those in whom the serum vitamin A and retinol-binding protein concentrations were normal.

Vitamin A deficiency may have at least three effects in patients with liver disease. First, it may be partially responsible for defective spermatogenesis.[122] Second, it can cause a deficiency of retinal, an aldehyde that, as the 11-cis isomer, is necessary for rhodopsin formation, which in turn is necessary for dark adaptation.[123] Thus, in one study, 9 of 11 patients with PBC and low vitamin A levels had an abnormally elevated dark adaptation threshold. None had overt night blindness, although four had xerophthalmia. To restore serum vitamin A levels, 25,000 to 50,000 units daily were required. Xerophthalmia was reversed, but dark adaptation remained abnormal in three individuals. Xerophthalmia in the remaining patients was restored with oral zinc therapy after zinc deficiency was identified in them.[120] The mechanism of the action of zinc was presumed to be on the restoration of zinc-related alcohol dehydrogenase with increased conversion of vitamin A to its active form, retinaldehyde.

Third, hepatic vitamin A deficiency in humans and rats is associated with increased numbers of microvesicular lysosomes in the liver,[124] although the long-term effects of these findings are unknown.

Thus it is recommended that both alcoholic and PBC patients routinely have their night vision tested, and that PBC patients supplement their diet with 5,000 to 15,000 units of vitamin A daily. This amount is well below the toxic dose of at least 100,000 units daily reported to have resulted in collagenization of the space of Disse with proliferation of Ito cells, resulting in portal hypertension.[125] (See Chapter 65 concerning caution in the selection of dosage of vitamin A in the alcoholic.)

### Vitamin D and Osteopenia

**Alcoholic Cirrhosis.** Osteopenia has been described both in alcoholic cirrhotics[124,125] and in patients with chronic cholestasis, i.e., PBC.[126–128] In alcoholic cirrhosis, the most frequent abnormality descibed is osteoporosis[129] with or without fractures,[130] whereas in PBC both osteomalacia and osteoporosis occur.[131] It is postulated that either malabsorption of vitamin D in cholestasis or deficient 25-hydroxylation of D in cirrhosis due to a reduced liver cell mass will lead to a reduction in serum 25-hydroxy vitamin D (25-OHD) levels.[132] Of 32 patients with severe advanced alcoholic cirrhosis, low serum 25-OHD levels were found in 14 (44%),[133] but the levels did not correlate with the reduction in bone density. There was no significant difference in dietary history, malabsorption, or sunlight exposure in those with normal versus low levels, but one or all of these factors may well contribute to the reduction. Thirteen patients with low serum 25-OHD levels were treated with oral vitamin $D_2$ (50,000 alternate days or weekly), which raised the mean levels from 7 to 116 ng/ml within one month, and the normal or supranormal levels persisted for the six-month treatment period. However, despite significant rises in serum calcium levels, bone density indices did not improve. Thus, defective hepatic 25-hydroxylation did not appear to be the limiting factor in these patients.

**Osteopenia.** Osteopenia is now regarded as one of the most important and disabling complications of chronic cholestasis, such as primary biliary cirrhosis (PBC), giving rise to bone pain and fractures (Table 56E1–3).[129] Classically it was thought to be due to osteomalacia secondary to vitamin $D_2$ malabsorption[134] as a consequence of intestinal bile acid deficiency.[135] Against this concept are the poor correlations among calcium absorption, 25-hydroxyvitamin D levels (+0.45), and fecal fat (+0.3).[136] Although it was claimed that patients with PBC could not 25-hydroxylate vitamin D[137] and that osteomalacia could be reversed with oral 25-OHD$_2$,[134] subsequent studies have shown that monthly injections of 100,000 IU of vitamin $D_2$ cause a significant rise in 25-OHD.[138,139]

Serum 25-OHD is the main form of circulating vitamin D. This measurement is a total of the 25-OHD$_3$ formed from the action of ultraviolet light on skin 7-dehydrocholesterol, plus preformed vitamin $D_2$ ingested in the diet. Measurements in PBC patients who were symptomatic with either icterus or pruritus tend to be low or in the low-normal range,[132,134,140] whereas asymptomatic patients have levels that are not significantly different from those of controls.[141]

Liver disease per se in the absence of cholestasis may affect vitamin D metabolism. For example, patients with either alcoholic hepatitis and/or cirrhosis or chronic active hepatitis may have low-normal serum 25-OHD levels.[132,138] Low levels are due in part to low serum albumin levels, possibly to defective hepatic 25-hydroxylation of vitamin D,[133,138] and also to defective bile acid formation. Cholic acid deficiency may lead to steatorrhea,[101] but more importantly to impaired vitamin D absorption.[103]

Other mechanisms for disturbances in vitamin D metabolism include interruption of the enterohepatic circulation of 25-OHD[142] (which may be of less importance than previously thought) increased urinary excretion of D metabolites,[143,144] and the administration for pruritus of cholestyramine, which binds vitamin D among other substances.[145]

The problem is further compounded by the finding that bone histology shows osteoporosis to be far more common in PBC patients than is osteomalacia,[131,136] and that it is of the "high-turnover" type. The reason for this type of bone histology is unclear. The observed increased bone erosion cannot be explained, since neither serum parathyroid hormone concentrations nor urinary cyclic AMP or hydroxyproline excretion is increased. The incidence and severity of osteoporosis in PBC, which is essentially a disease occurring in middle-aged females, raise the possibility of an exacerbation of postmenopausal estrogen-deficiency osteoporosis in these patients. Yet patients with

**Table 56E1–3. The Etiology of Hepatic Osteopenia***

| Etiologic Factor | Comment |
|---|---|
| Calcium malabsorption | |
| Phosphatase malabsorption | Correlated to decreased serum 25-OHD |
| | Absorption improved with 25-OHD |
| Vitamin D malabsorption | Insignificant in absence of steatorrhea |
| Reduced 25-hydroxylation of D? | Controversial; some studies showed 25-OHD to be normal |
| Other hydroxylation abnormalities? | For example, deficient 24:25-dehydroxylation |
| Disturbances of enterohepatic circulation? | D in bile mainly inactivation products; only 4% 25-OHD |
| Increased urinary excretion of D? | May be mostly inactivation products |
| Renal tubular acidosis | PBC contributory to osteomalacia; bicarbonate therapy beneficial here |
| Medical therapy | Cholestyramine, steroids |
| Osteoblast dysfunction? | Reduced life span |
| Abnormal parathyroid hormone metabolism (PTH)? | Kupffer cell dysfunction, reduced cleavage of inactive PTH |
| Environment and nutrition | Dietary lack of D and calcium |
| | Deficient sunlight, inactivity postmenopause |

*From Heaf, J.G.,[115a]

chronic liver disease have hyperestrogenemia.[146] In two studies, the incidences of bone pain and fractures were higher in younger patients.[131,147]

*Prevention of Osteopenia.* What is the optimal way of preventing and then treating metabolic bone disease in PBC? It is appropriate to encourage asymptomatic patients to ingest a high-calcium diet and appropriate sources of vitamin D to ensure normal calcium absorption. Where possible, the patient should take advantage of the sunlight available. Nevertheless, it is disappointing that in the latest two studies osteoporosis continued to progress in symptomatic patients who were given 100 μg of 25-OH D$_3$ orally[131] or 20 μg daily with adjustment of the dose to maintain supranormal serum levels of 25-OH D$_3$ at 1.5 to 2 times normal, resulting in final doses of 40 μg to 120 μg/day. The value of large doses of vitamin D supplements is therefore questionable. The role of such agents as sodium fluoride is unknown but one cannot be optimistic because these are effective mainly in states of "low-turnover" osteoporosis.

### Vitamin E

The average North American diet cotains 8 to 11 mg of α-tocopherol equivalents (12 to 16 IU).[148] Like other fat-soluble vitamins, its absorption is dependent on lymphatic fat absorption and thus adequate bile acids for micelle formation. After lymphatic transport in chylomicrons, tocopherols rapidly equilibrate with other plasma lipoproteins, the bulk being in low-density lipoproteins.[149] Tocopherol depletion occurs with fat malabsorption secondary to longstanding cholestasis, such as congenital biliary atresia. The mechanism is due to impaired intestinal absorption associated with low intraluminal bile acid concentrations. At the same time, plasma transport and tissue uptake of vitamin E remain intact[150] despite associated low levels of the major transport protein, β-lipoprotein.[151] The manifestations of E deficiency were once thought to be largely subclinical with shortened red cell survival without anemia.[152] However, neuropathologic and myopathic abnormalities have been described.[153] A pathognomonic syndrome has now been identified with areflexia, gait disturbance, diminished proprioception and vibration senses, and ophthalmoplegia.[154,155] The pathologic lesion is thought to be axonal dystrophy in the gracile nucleus, and the incidence of this lesion has diminished with routine vitamin E supplementation in infants with congenital biliary atresia.[156]

Thus infants and children with biliary atresia and cystic fibrosis should have their diet supplemented with vitamin E, up to 100 IU IM daily until the serum tocopherol levels are twice normal.

Side effects from overdosage vary from transient gastrointestinal disturbance to interference with vitamin K absorption and prolonged prothrombin time,[157] but the latter has occurred only with massive supplementation (11,200 IU daily).

### Vitamin K

Vitamin K deficiency is most likely to occur secondary to cholestasis and fat malabsorption due to failure of bile acid micelle formation. Nevertheless, even in complete bile duct obstruction, a percentage of fat-soluble vitamins is absorbed, presumably via the portal vein. Vitamin K deficiency can also be due to failure of normal hepatic prothrombin synthesis. The consequence of vitamin K deficiency is a prolongation of the prothrombin time due to deficiencies in factors VII, IX, and X, eventually resulting in overt pathologic bruising and bleeding. The differentiation of vitamin K deficiency as being due to cholestasis or deficient hepatic synthesis of prothrombin is simply determined by assessing the response of prothrombin time to vitamin K injections. In the absence of cholestasis, defective production of prothrombin is a more common cause of deficiency than dietary deficiency.

Vitamin K appears to be involved in the modification of the amino-terminal portion of a hepatic prothrombin precursor necessary for calcium binding with the formation of gamma-carboxyglutamic acid (G/a).[158] Furthermore, Factors IX, X, and VII also contain G/a with its calcium-binding properties.[159] G/a appears to form metal-dependent reversible, noncovalent bonds that stabilize the polypeptide backbone of prothrombin. Using crossed immunoelectrophoresis, researchers observed abnormal prothrombin not containing G/a in six patients with prolonged biliary obstruction.[160] The authors were unable to detect any abnormal plasma prothrombin in patients with hepatitis. By contrast, using sensitive radioimmunoassays for native and abnormal prothrombins, Blanchard et al. detected low levels of abnormal prothrombin in patients with both acute hepatitis and cirrhosis,[161] and vitamin K therapy failed to decrease the abnormal prothrombin levels. In addition, decreased native prothrombin without concomitant elevations of abnormal prothrombin suggests that both decreased synthesis of prothrombin and defective vitamin K decarboxylation occur in these patients.[162]

### WATER-SOLUBLE VITAMINS

Deficiencies of members of the vitamin B complex are common in liver disease.

# Thiamin

**Deficient Dietary Intake.** Thiamin deficiency has been recognized in alcoholic patients for many years[163] associated with the Wernicke-Korsakoff syndrome, peripheral neuropathy, and high-output cardiac failure. The recommended daily consumption is 0.5 mg/1,000 kcal, but alcoholic patients may consume less than 0.3 mg/1,000 kcal.[164]

**Decreased Intestinal Transport.** Thiamin absorption is impaired in severe alcoholics.[165] Thiamin is thought to be absorbed by an active, energy-requiring process against a concentration and electrochemical gradient, involving a carrier at the mucosal cell membrane and Na-K ATPase at the basolateral membrane.[166] Thiamin accumulates in the enterocyte as phosphorylated compounds. Feeding alcohol chronically to experimental animals resulted in decreased exit of thiamin from the serosal side of inverted intestinal sacs in association with a reduction in NA-K ATPase activity. This process was only observed when serum alcohol levels rose to over 200 mg/dl.[167] This effect of alcohol may be related to changes of membrane fluidity.

**Decreased Thiamin Pyrophosphate Formation.** Conversion of thiamin to thiamin pyrophosphate is impaired in alcoholic liver injury associated with decreased pyruvate decarboxylase and transketolase activity, so that red cell transketolase activity is decreased in malnourished alcoholic cirrhotics[168] and contstitutes a test for the deficiency of the vitamin.

**Decreased Hepatic Storage.** Hepatic thiamin content may be reduced by 75% in alcoholic cirrhosis[163] from a normal range of 2 to 8 mg/g wet weight.

Thiamin absorption may be diminished by other nutritional deficiencies, such as folate deficiency, commonly found in alcoholic cirrhosis.[169]

**Management.** In overt or suspected deficiency states including acute confusional states, thiamin may be given as part of an IV preparation of B vitamins or as 100 mg IV prior to administration of glucose and then daily until a normal diet is restored. For treatment of neurologic disorders including Wernicke-Korsakoff syndrome see Chapters 65 and 67.

# Pyridoxine (B$_6$) Deficiency

Low levels of serum pyridoxine were found in 25% of patients with alcoholic cirrhosis.[167] However, diets deficient in pyridoxine are uncommon in such patients. The biologically active form of vitamin B$_6$ is pyridoxal-5-phosphate (PLP). It has a key role in transamination and heme synthesis, and its deficiency has been implicated in both peripheral neuropathy[170] and sideroblastic anemia.[171] In addition, chronic B$_6$ deficiency is associated with the development of fatty liver and cirrhosis in the monkey. Decreased PLP levels and hepatic B$_6$ content have been found in alcoholic cirrhotics.

**Mechanisms.** Although low serum PLP levels were found in alcoholic cirrhotics, a high incidence of PLP deficiency was also found in alcoholic patients without liver impairment.[172] Acetaldehyde and not alcohol is perhaps responsible for the impaired formation of PLP from pyridoxine in erythrocytes[173] and hepatocytes.[174] Low PLP levels may also be due to decreased protective protein binding[175] and increased PLP clearance.[176]

**Supplementation.** The level of supplementation required by the alcoholic is not known but it is likely that the blanket B vitamin supplementation recommended to redress thiamin deficiency would also be reasonable, the aim being to overcome the aldehyde inhibition of PLP formation. Alternatively, 50 mg daily may be given until a normal diet is restored.

# Folic Acid

Low levels of serum and red cell folate have been described in patients with mainly alcoholic liver disease.[177]

**Mechanisms.** Probably the most important reason for this phenomenon is a reduced intake of folate-containing food in chronic alcoholic patients[178] (Table 56E1–4). Less important causes include malabsorption of folate, possibly from local damage by alcohol[179] and also from the effect of folate deficiency itself[180] on small intestinal mucosa. Severe hepatic insufficiency may lead to a reduction in dihydrofolate reductase activity with reduced conversion of dihydrofolate to tetrahydrofolate, the active form, and to "trapping" in the hepatic pool.[181] Furthermore, possibly owing to decreased affinity for binding sites, de-

**Table 56E1–4. Causes of Folate Deficiency in Liver Disease**

Decreased intake of offal, raw green leafy vegetables, pulses, bread, oranges, nuts, bananas.

Decreased absorption of pteroyl polyglutamates, deconjugated, reduced, and methylated.

Decreased hepatic uptake and storage as 5-methyl tetrahydrofolate (5 methyl THFA) or increased hepatic "trapping."

Decreased utilization of folate in hematogenesis leading to increased excretion of formiminoglutamic acid (FIGLU).

Decreased affinity for folate-binding protein leading to increased urinary folate excretion.

creased saturation of folate-binding protein[182] may lead to increased urinary folate excretion.[183]

**Pathology.** Macrocytosis is a common finding in chronic alcoholics, but even in those with liver disease only about one third is due to folate deficiency.[184] Because megaloblastosis may occur in the presence of normal folate and vitamin $B_{12}$ levels, it is postulated to be due to inability of red cells to utilize folate in the presence of alcohol with resultant increase in urinary folate excretion.

**Treatment.** Folate deficiency in liver disease should be managed with a diet high in folate (see Table 56E1–4). If this treatment proves difficult, then 5 mg folate once a week should be adequate to maintain folate requirements. In the presence of severe liver deficiency and decreased dihydrofolate reductase activity, folinic acid (5-formyl tetrahydrofolic acid) should be substituted.

## TRACE MINERALS

### Copper

In liver diseases, copper excess rather than copper deficiency is the problem, whether it is in the form of the recessively inherited disease, hepatolenticular degeneration (Wilson's disease), or in the form of chronic cholestasis such as primary biliary cirrhosis.

Only in the former are dietary considerations required. Patients with Wilson's disease have a life-long problem with copper. The drug of choice, D-penicillamine, which chelates copper and excretes it in the urine, must be taken throughout life. If treatment is started early enough, however, patients can be rendered asymptomatic. The medication should be supported by a low-copper diet, e.g., reduced ingestion of chocolate, shellfish, liver, pork, dark chicken, nuts, peas, and beans. Penicillamine chelates zinc, in addition to copper. Providing zinc intake is adequate, however, these patients will increase absorption. They rarely become sufficiently clinically zinc-deficient to require zinc supplementation with zinc sulfate.

On the other hand, increased oral zinc intake will result in a reduction in copper absorption and increased fecal copper excretion.[184a] Therefore, in the rare cases of penicillamine toxicity or difficulty in administration, zinc sulfate 100 to 200 mg t.i.d. (three times daily) can be given orally, resulting in a more satisfactory control of body copper stores by reducing copper absorption.[184a]

### Zinc

It has been suggested that zinc deficiency occurs in alcoholic liver disease with repeated demonstration of low serum zinc levels.[185,186] However,

because there may be a poor correlation between plasma zinc and body zinc status,[187] this claim is doubtful. More recent studies, however, have shown that leukocyte zinc content correlates well with muscle zinc[188] and that leukocyte zinc is reduced in liver disease.[189] In addition, hepatic zinc is reduced, even taking into account hepatic collagen content.[190]

**Mechanism of Deficiency.** Factors thought to be involved in the mechanism of zinc deficiency include increased urinary zinc excretion associated with excessive alcohol intake, rather than hepatic disease,[191] and alterations in zinc protein binding, with a decrease in albumin binding and increases in alpha$_2$-macroglobulin binding.[192] Perhaps of greater importance is that the low-protein diet taken by many alcoholics results in a low zinc intake because of the close correlation between oral zinc and protein intake.[193]

**Consequences of Deficiency.** What are the consequences of zinc deficiency? It has been postulated that it would result in decreased activity of hepatic zinc metalloenzymes, alcohol dehydrogenase, and glutamate dehydrogenase, thus possibly rendering the liver more susceptible to damage from continued alcohol ingestion. In zinc deficiency in rats, low plasma zinc concentrations are accompanied by low levels of vitamin A,[194] which are thought to be due to defective hepatic production of retinol-binding protein by alcohol dehydrogenase.[195] Zinc supplementation can result in elevations of vitamin A both in animals[196] and children.[197]

Defective dark adaptation occurring in cirrhotic patients and associated with decreased leukocyte zinc content[198] may be refractive to vitamin A therapy.[199] The reason for this phenomenon may be the presence of zinc deficiency.[200]

**Supplementation.** In addition, zinc deficiency is associated with impaired taste perception and immune response. Zinc supplementation seems to have improved liver function, with a reduction in sulfobromophthalein retention.[201] However, two controlled trials with zinc sulfate have showed either no improvement in hepatic function[202] or significant improvement in other measurements (plasma prothrombin, serum bilirubin levels, and taste function), but no change in dark adaptation.[203] Nevertheless, with prior supplementation with vitamin A, administration of 220 mg zinc sulfate for two weeks has improved dark adaptation.[204]

These confusing findings with zinc supplementation may be explained by one study that used the isotope tracer $^{65}$Zn in stable well-compensated cirrhotics. Although hepatic zinc content was reduced in association with a lower level of hepatic alcohol dehydrogenase, and zinc elimination in the urine increased, zinc absorption also increased. In addition, whole body zinc content increased.[205] This finding may indicate redistribution of body zinc with increased accumulation in the skeleton.[206]

The need for zinc supplementation in different degrees of hepatic disease is unclear, especially since assessment of zinc status remains difficult and uncertain in these patients. The use of a reasonably adequate protein diet with its naturally occurring zinc should remain the backbone of therapy. In patients with suggestive evidence of zinc deficiency such as abnormalities of dark adaptation or taste acuity, a trial of zinc supplementation is indicated although care must be taken not to inadvertently induce reciprocally low serum copper levels.[207]

In conclusion, the patient with liver disease presents many nutrition-related problems, some clinically obvious, others subclinical and subtle. Nevertheless, these problems may contribute to his feeling of ill health, and may require considerable effort and care on the part of the health team if successful diagnosis and treatment are to be attained.

# REFERENCES

1. Vlahcevic, Z.R., Bell, C.C., Buhac, I., et al.: Gut *11*:420–422, 1970.
2. Rubin, E., Lieber, C.S.: N. Engl. J. Med. *278*:869–876, 1968.
3. Galambos, J.T., Wills, C.E.: Gastroenterology *74*:1191–1195, 1978.
4. Patek, A.J., Toth, I.G., Saunders, M.G.: Arch. Intern. Med. *135*:1053–1057, 1975.
5. Pequignot, G., Chabert, C., Eydoux, H., et al.: Rev. Alcohol *20*:191–202, 1974.
6. Lelbach, W.K.: Epidemiology of alcoholic liver disease. *In* Progress in Liver Disease. (Popper, W., Schaffner, F., Eds.) New York, Grune and Stratton, 1976, pp. 476–493.
6a. Mills, P.R., Shenkin, A., Anthony, R.S. et al.: Am. J. Clin. Nutr. *38*:849–859, 1983.
6b. Mendenhall, C.L., Anderson, S., Weesner, M., et al.: Am. J. Med. *76*:211–222, 1984.
7. Maddrey, W.C., Boitnott, J.K., Bedine, M.S., et al.: Gastroenterology *75*:193–199, 1979.
8. Depew, W., Boyer, T., Omata, M., et al.: Gastroenterology *78*:524–529, 1980.
9. Helman, R.A., Tamko, M.H., Nye, S.W., et al.: Ann. Intern. Med. *74*:311–321, 1971.
10. Lesesne, H.R., Bozymski, E.M., Fallon, H.J.: Gastroenterology *74*:169–173, 1978.
11. Bethel, R.A., Jansen, R.D., Heymsfield, S.B.: Am. J. Clin. Nutr. *32*:1112–1120, 1979.
12. Galambos, J.T., Hersh, T., Fulenwider, J.T., et al.: Am. J. Gastroenterol. *72*:535–541, 1979.
12a. Smith, J., Horowitz, J., Henderson, J.M., et al.: Am. J. Clin. Nutr. *35*:56–72, 1982.
12b. Calvey, H., Davis, M., Williams, R.J.: Hepatology *1*:141–151, 1985.
13. Fischer, J.E., Baldessarini, R.J.: Lancet *2*:75–79, 1971.
14. Fischer, J.E., Funovics, J.M., Aguirre, A., et al.: Surgery *78*:276–290, 1975.
15. McClain, C.J., Zieve, L., Doizaki, W.M.: Gut *21*:318–323, 1980.
16. Fischer, J.E., Yoshinura, N., Aquirre, A., et al.: Am. J. Surg. *127*:40–47, 1974.
17. Isaacs, J., Millikan, W., Stackhouse, J.: Am. J. Clin. Nutr. *30*:552–559, 1977.
18. Nasrallah, S.M., Galambos, J.T.: Lancet *2*:1276–1277, 1980.
18a. Diehl, A.M., Boitnott, J.K., Herlong, F.: Hepatology *5*:57–63, 1985.
19. Gabuzda, G.J., Shear, L.: Am. J. Clin. Nutr. *23*:479–484, 1970.
20. Swart, G.A., Frenkel, M., Van den Berg, J.W.O.: *In* Metabolism and Clinical Implications of Branched Chain Amino and Ketoacids. (Walser, M., Williamson, J.R., Eds.) New York, Elsevier Science Publishing Co., 1981, pp. 427–432.
21. Smith, J., Horowitz, J., Henderson, J.M., et al.: Am. J. Clin. Nutr. *35*:56–72, 1982.
22. Rudman, D., Kutner, M., Ansley, J., et al.: Gastroenterology *81*:1025–1036, 1981.
23. Levine, R.J., Conn, H.O.: J. Clin. Invest. *46*:2012–2020, 1967.
24. Nordlinger, B.M., Fulenwider, J.T., Ivey, G.L., et al.: J. Lab. Clin. Med. *94*:832–840, 1979.
25. Hendersen, J.M., Faraj, B.A., Ali, F.M., et al.: Dig. Dis. Sci. *26*:124–128, 1981.
26. Morgan, N.Y., Milsom, J.P., Sherlock, S.: Gut *19*:1068–1073, 1978.
27. Shaw, S., Lieber, S.C.: Gastroenterology *74*:677–682, 1978.
28. Swendseid, M.E., Yamada, C., Vinyard, E., et al.: Am. J. Clin. Nutr. *21*:1381–1383, 1968.
29. Anderson, G.H., Blendis, L.M.: Am. J. Clin. Nutr. *34*:377–385, 1981.
30. Johnston, D.G., Alberti, K.G.M., Faber, O.K.: Lancet *1*:10–13, 1977.
31. Blei, A.J., Robbins, D.C., Drobney, E., et al.: Gastroenterology *83*:1191–1199, 1982.
32. Ferenci, P., Bratusch-Marrain, P., Waldhausl, W.K., et al.: Eur. J. Clin. Invest. *14*:255–261, 1984.
33. Marchesini, G., Bianchi, G., Zoli, M., et al.: Gastroenterology *85*:283–290, 1983.
34. Owen, O.E., Reichle, F.A., Mozzoli, M.A., et al.: J. Clin. Invest. *68*:240–252, 1981.
35. Fischer, J.E., Rosen, H.M., Ebeid, A.M., et al.: Surgery *80*:77–91, 1976.
36. Marchesini, G., Zoli, M., Dondi, C., et al.: Hepatology *2*:420–425, 1982.
37. Long, C.L., Haverberg, L.N., Young, V.R.: Metabolism *24*:929–935, 1975.
38. Bilmazes, C., Uauy, R., Haverberg, L.N.: Metabolism *27*:525–530, 1978.
39. Marliss, E.B., Wei, C.N., Dietrich, L.L.: Am. J. Clin. Nutr. *32*:1617–1621, 1979.
40. Weber, F.L., Bogby, B.S., Licate, L., et al.: Gastroenterology (Abstract) *90*:1780, 1986.
41. Conn, H.O., Lieberthal, M.M.: *In* The Hepatic Coma Syndromes and Lactulose. Baltimore, Williams & Wilkens, 1979, pp. 46–84.
42. Alexander, R.W., Berman, E., Balfour, D.C.: Gastroenterology *289*:1107–1111, 1973.
43. Phear, E.A., Ruebner, B., Sherlock, S., et al.: Clin. Sci. *15*:93–117, 1956.
44. Chen, S., Zieve, L., Mahadevan, V.: J. Lab. Clin. Med. *75*:628–635, 1970.

45. Rosen, H.M., Yoshimura, N., Hodaman, J.M., et al.: Gastroenterology *72*:483–487, 1977.
46. Cerra, F.B., Cheung, N.K., Fischer, J.E.: J. Parenter. Enter. Nutr. *9*:288, 1985.
47. Fiaccadori, F., Ghinelli, F., Pedretti, G., et al.: Branched chain amino acid enriched solutions in the treatment of hepatic encephalopathy in a controlled trial. *In* Hepatic Encephalopathy in Chronic Liver Failure. (Capocaccial, L., Fischer, J.E., Rossi-Fanelli, F., Eds.) New York, Plenum Publishing Corp., 1984, pp. 323–333.
48. Gluud, C., Dejgaard, A., Hardt, F., et al.: Scand. J. Gastroenterol. *18*(Suppl 86):19, 1983.
48a.Ferenci, P., et al.: *In* Recent Advances in Hepatology II. (Thomas, H.C., Jones, E.A., Eds.) London, Churchill-Livingstone, 1985.
49. Michel, H., Pommier-Layrargues, G., Aubin, J.P., et al.: Liver *5*:282–289, 1985.
50. Rossi-Fanelli, F., Riggio, O., Cangiano, C., et al.: Dig. Dis. Sci. *27*:929–935, 1982.
51. Strauss, E., Santos, W.R., Cantapalti, E., et al.: Hepatology *3*:862, 1983 (abstract).
52. Wahren, J., Denis, J., Desurmont, P., et al.: Hepatology *3*:475–480, 1983.
53. McGhee, A., Henderson, J.M., Millikan, W.J., et al.: Ann. Surg. *197*:288–293, 1983.
54. Horst, D., Grace, N.D., Conn, H.O., et al.: Hepatology *4*:279–287, 1984.
55. Eriksen, L.S., Persson, A., Wahren, J.: Gut *23*:801–806, 1982.
56. Egberts, E.H., Schomerus, H., Hamster, W., et al.: Gastroenterology *88*:887–895, 1985.
57. Riggio, O., Canciano, C., Cascino, A., et al.: Long term dietary supplement with branched chain amino acids; a new approach in the prevention of hepatic encephalopathy, results of a controlled study in cirrhotics with portocaval anastomosis. *In* Hepatic Encephalopathy in Chronic Liver Failure (Capocaccia L., Fischer, J.E., Rossi Fanelli, F., Eds.) New York, Plenum Publishing Corp., 1984, pp. 183–192.
58. Simko, V.: Nut. Rep. Int. *27*:765–773, 1983.
59. Sieg, A., Walker, S., Czygan, P., et al.: Z. Gastroenterol. *21*:644–650, 1983.
60. Nencki, M., Pavlov, J.P., Zaleski, J.: Arch Exp. Pathol. Pharmacol. *37*:26–51, 1896.
61. Bessman, A.N., Mirick, C.S.: J. Clin. Invest. *37*:990–998, 1958.
62. Greenberger, N.J., Carley, J., Schenker, S., et al.: Am. J. Dig. Dis. *22*:845–855, 1977.
63. Uribe, M., Marquez, M.A., Ramos, G.G., et al.: Dig. Dis. Sci. *27*:1109–1116, 1982.
64. deBruijn, K.M., Blendis, L.M., Zilm, D.H., et al.: Gut *24*:53–60, 1983.
65. Rikkers, L., Jenko, P., Rudman, D., et al.: Gastroenterology *75*:462–469, 1978.
66. Shaw, S., Worner, T.M., Lieber, C.S.: Am. J. Clin. Nutr. *38*:59–62, 1983.
67. Bessman, S.P., Shear, S., Fitzgerald, D.J.: N. Engl. J. Med. *256*:941–943, 1956.
68. Najarian, J.S., Harper, H.A.: Am. J. Med. *21*:832–842, 1956.
69. Reynolds, T.B., Redeker, A.G., Davis, P.: Am. J. Med. *25*:359–367, 1958.
70. Weber, F.L., Minco, D., Fresard, K.M., et al.: Gastroenterology *89*:538–544, 1985.
71. Maddrey, W.C., Weber, F.L., Coulter, A.W., et al.: Gastroenterology *71*:190–195, 1976.

72. Herlong, H.F., Maddrey, W.C., Walser, M.: Ann. Intern. Med. *93*:545–550, 1980.
73. Blendis, L.M., Greig, P.D., Langer, B., et al.: Gastroenterology *77*:250–256, 1979.
74. Greig, P.D., Blendis, L.M., Langer, B., et al.: Gastroenterology *80*:119–125, 1981.
75. Harrison, J.E., McNeil, K.G., Strauss, A.L.: Nutr. Res. *4*:209–224, 1984.
76. Blendis, L.M., Harrison, J.E., Russell, D. McR.: Gastroenterology *90*:127–134, 1986.
77. DeMoura, M.C., Cruz, A.G.: Am. J. Dig. Dis. *13*:893–897, 1968.
78. Rehfeld, J.R., Juhl, E., Hilden, M.: Gastroenterology *64*:445–451, 1973.
79. Berkowitz, D.: Am. J. Dig. Dis. *14*:691–699, 1969.
80. Megyesi, L., Samols, E., Marks, V.: Lancet *2*:7525–7528, 1967.
81. Conn, H.O., Schreiber, W., Elkington, S.G., et al.: Am. J. Dig. Dis. *14*:837–852, 1969.
82. Jacques, W.E.: N. Engl. J. Med. *16*:68–78, 1953.
83. Falchuk, K.R., Fiske, S.C., Haggitt, R.C., et al.: Gastroenterology *78*:535–541, 1980.
84. Podolsky, S., Zimmerman, J.H., Burrow, B.A., et al.: N. Engl. J. Med. *3*:644–648, 1973.
85. Collins, J.R., Lacy, W.W., Stiel, J.N., et al.: Arch. Intern. Med. *126*:608–614, 1970.
86. Marco, J., Diego, J., Villaneuve, M.L., et al.: N. Engl. J. Med. *289*:1107–1111, 1973.
87. Shankar, T.P., Solomon, S.S., Duckworth, W.C., et al.: J. Lab. Clin. Med. *102*:459–469, 1983.
88. Alberti, K.G.M.M., Record, C.O., Williamson, D.H., et al.: Clin. Sci. *42*:591–605, 1972.
89. Nuttall, F.Q.: Am. J. Clin. Nutr. *33*:1311–1312, 1979.
90. Special Report Committee of the Canadian Diabetes Association 1980: J. Can. Dietet. Assoc. *42*:110–118, 1981.
91. The Nutrition Sub-Committee of the British Diabetic Association's Medical Advisory Committee: Hum. Nutr.: Appl. Nutr. *36A*:378–394, 1982.
92. Anderson, J.W., Ward, K.: Diabetes Care *1*:77–82, 1979.
93. Anderson, J.W., Midgley, W.R., Wedman, B.: Diabetes Care *2*:329–389, 1979.
94. Jenkins, D.J.A., Wolever, T.M.S., Bacon, S., et al.: Am. J. Clin. Nutr. *33*:1729–1733, 1980.
95. Simpson, H.C.R., Carter, R.D., Lousley, S., et al.: Diabetologia *23*:235–239, 1982.
96. Rivellese, A., Giacco, A., Genovese, S., et al.: Lancet *1*:447–449, 1980.
97. Simpson, H.C.R., Lousley, S., Geekie, M., et al.: Lancet *1*:1–5, 1981.
98. Jenkins, D.J.A., Thorne, M.J., Taylor, R.H., et al.: Clin. Sci. *66*:649–657, 1984.
98a.Blendis, L.M., Jenkins, D.J.A.: Personal observations.
99. Uribe, M., Dibilodox, M., Malpica, S., et al.: Gastroenterology *88*:901–907, 1985.
100. Main Geobd, A., Clark, M.L., Senior, J.R.: Gastroenterology *56*:727–735, 1969.
101. Borowsky, S.A., Perlow, W., Baraona, E., et al.: Dig. Dis. Sci. *25*:22–27, 1980.
102. Avgerinos, A., Chu, P., Greenfield, C., et al.: Hepatology *3*:349–355, 1983.
103. Vhlachevic, Z.R., Buhac, I., Farrar, J.J., et al.: Gastroenterology *60*:491–498, 1971.
104. Jenkins, D.J.A., Gassull, M.A., Leeds, A.R., et al.: Int. J. Vitam. Nutr. Res. *46*:226–230, 1976.

105. Forsgren, L.: Acta. Chir. Scand. (Suppl.) *339*:3–29, 1969.
106. Leiber, C.S.: Clin. Gastroenterol. *10*:315–342, 1981.
107. Mezey, E.: Am. J. Clin. Nutr. *33*:2709–2718, 1980.
108. Horning, M.G., Williams, E.A., Maling, M.H., et al.: Biochem. Biophys. Res. Commun. *3*:635–640, 1960.
109. Brodie, B.B., Maickel, R.P.: Ann. N.Y. Acad. Sci. *104*:1049–1058, 1963.
110. Lieber, C.S., Schmid, R.: J. Clin. Invest. *40*:394–399, 1961.
111. Krebs, H.A., Cunningham, D.J.L., Stubbs, M., et al.: Isr. J. Med. Sci. *5*:959–962, 1969.
112. Lieber, C.S., Jones, D.P., Mendelson, J., et al.: Trans. Assoc. Am. Physicians *76*:289, 1963.
113. Lieber, C.S., Spritz, N.: J. Clin. Invest. *45*:1400–1411, 1966.
114. Malagelada, J.R., Linscheer, W.G., Houtsmuller, V.M.T., et al.: Am.J. Clin. Nutr. *26*:738–743, 1973.
115. Bloomstrand, R., Karlberger, G., Forsgren, L.: Acta Clin. Scand. *135*:329–339, 1969.
115a.Heaf, J.G.: Scand. J. Gastroenterol. *20*:1035–1040, 1985.
116. Saunders, D.R., Dawson, A.M.: Gut *4*:254–260, 1963.
117. Porter, H.P., Saunders, D.R., Brunser, O., et al.: Gastroenterology *58*:984, 1970 (Abstract).
118. Partin, J.S., Partin, J.C., Schubert, W.K., et al.: Gastroenterology *67*:107–118, 1974.
119. Smith, J.C., Jr., Brown, E.D., White, S.C., et al.: Lancet *1*:1251–1252, 1975.
120. Herlong, H.F., Russell, R.M., Maddrey, W.C.: Hepatology *1*:348–351, 1981.
121. Leo, M.A., Lieber, C.S.: N. Engl. J. Med. *307*:597–601, 1982.
122. VanThiel, D.H., Lester, R.: Gastroenterology *71*:318–327, 1976.
123. Wald, G.: Science *162*:230–239, 1968.
124. Leo, M.A., Sato, M., Lieber, C.S.: Gastroenterology *84*:562–572, 1983.
125. Russell, R.M., Boyer, J.L., Bagheri, S.A., et al.: N. Engl. J. Med. *291*:435–440, 1974.
126. Nilssau, B.E., Westlin, N.E.: Clin. Orthop. *90*:229–232, 1973.
127. Dalen, N., Feldreich, A.L.: Clin. Orthop. *99*:201–202, 1974.
128. Atkinson, M., Nordin, B.E.C., Sherlock, S.: Q. J. Med. *25*:299–213, 1956.
129. Paterson, C.R., Losowski, M.S.: Scand. J. Gastroenterol. *2*:292–300, 1967.
130. Summerskill, W.H.J., Kelly, P.J.: Proc. Mayo Clin. *38*:162–174, 1963.
131. Long, R.G., Meinhard, E., Skinner, R.K., et al.: Gut *19*:85–90, 1978.
132. Long, R.G., Wills, M.R., Skinner, R.K.: Lancet *2*:650–652, 1976.
133. Posner, D.B., Russell, R.M., Absood, S., et al.: Gastroenterology *74*:866–870, 1978.
134. Reed, J.S., Meredith, S.C., Nemchausky, B.A.: Gastroenterology *78*:513–517, 1980.
135. Badley, B.W.D., Murphy, G.M., Bouchier, I.A.D., et al.: Gastroenterology *58*:781–789, 1970.
136. Herlong, H.F., Becker, R.R., Maddrey, W.C.: Gastroenterology *83*:103–108, 1982.
137. Wagonfield, J.B., Nemchausky, B.A., Bolt, M.: Lancet *2*:391–394, 1976.
138. Hepner, G.W., Roginsky, M., Moo, H.F.: Am. J. Dig. Dis. *21*:527–532, 1976.

139. Skinner, R.K., Long, R.G., Sherlock, S.: Lancet *1*:720–721, 1977.
140. Kaplan, M.M., Goldberg, M.J., Matloff, D.S.: Gastroenterology *81*:681–685, 1981.
141. Long, R.G., Scheuer, P.J., Sherlock, S.: Gastroenterology *72*:1204–1207, 1977.
142. Compston, J.E., Thompson, R.P.H.: Lancet *1*:721–724, 1977.
143. Krawitz, E.L., Grundman, M.J., Mawer, E.B.: Lancet *2*:1246–1249, 1977.
144. Jung, R.T., Davie, M., Siklos, P.: Gut *20*:840–847, 1979.
145. Thompson, W.G., Thompson, G.K.: Gut *10*:717–722, 1969.
146. Pentikainen, P.J., Pentikainen, L.A., Azarnoff, D.L.: Gastroenterology *69*:20–27, 1975.
147. Matloff, D.S., Kaplan, M.M., Neer, R.M., et al.: Gastroenterology *83*:97–102, 1932.
148. Bieri, J.G., Evarts, R.P.: J. Am. Diet. Assoc. *62*:147–151, 1973.
149. McCormick, E.C., Cornwell, D.G., Brown, J.B.: J. Lipid Res. *1*:221–228, 1960.
150. Sokol, R.J., Heubi, J.E., Iannaccone, S., et al.: Gastroenterology *85*:1172–1182, 1983.
151. Gordansson, G., Norden, A., Akesson, B.: Scand. J. Gastroenterol. *8*:21–25, 1973.
152. Leonard, P.J., Losowky, M.S.: Am. J. Clin. Nutr. *24*:388–393, 1971.
153. Guggenheim, M.A., Ringel, S.P., Silverman, A., et al.: Ann. N.Y. Acad. Sci. *393*:84–93,1982.
154. Rosenblum, J.L., Keating, J.P., Prensky, A.L., et al.: N. Engl. J. Med. *304*:503–508, 1981.
155. Elias, E., Muller, D.P.R., Scott, J.: Lancet *2*:1319–1321, 1981.
156. Sung, J.H., Park, S.H., Mastri, A.R., et al.: J. Neuropathol. Exp. Neurol. *29*:584–597, 1980.
157. Corrigan, J.J., Marcus, F.I.: JAMA *230*:1300–1301, 1974.
158. Stenflo, I., Fernlund, P., Egan, W., et al.: Proc. Natl. Acad. Sci. USA *71*:2730–2733, 1974.
159. Bucher, D., Nebelin, E., Thosen, J., et al.: FEBS Lett. *68*:293–296, 1976.
160. Ganrot, P.O., Nilehn, J.E.: Scand. J. Clin. Lab. Invest. *28*:245–249, 1971.
161. Blanchard, R.A., Furie, B.C., Jorgensen, M., et al.: N. Engl. J. Med. *305*:242–248, 1981.
162. Liebman, H.A., Furie, B.C., Furie, B.: Hepatology *2*:488–494, 1982.
163. Leevy, C.M., Baker, H., Tenhove, W., et al.: Am. J. Clin. Nutr. *16*:339–346, 1965.
164. Neville, J.N., Eagles, J.A., Samson, G., et al.: Am. J. Clin. Nutr.*21*:1329–1339, 1968.
165. Tomasulo, P.A., Kater, R.M.H., Iber, F.L.: Am. J. Clin. Nutr. *21*:1340–1344, 1968.
166. Hoyumpa, A.M.: Am. J. Clin. Nutr. *33*:2750–2761, 1980.
167. Hoyumpa, A.M., Nichols, S., Henderson, G.I., et al.: Am. J. Clin. Nutr. *31*:938–945, 1978.
168. Fennelly, J., Frank, O., Baker, H., et al.: Am. J. Clin. Nutr. *20*:946–949, 1967.
169. Howard, L., Wagner, C., Schenker, S.: J. Nutr. *104*:1024–1032, 1974.
170. Walshe, F.M.R.: Q. J. Med. *12*:320–335, 1918.
171. Hines, J.D., Cowan, D.H.: N. Engl. J. Med. *283*:441–446, 1970.
172. Lumeng, L., Li., T.K.: J. Clin. Invest. *53*:693–704, 1974.
173. Veitch, R.L., Lumeng, L., Li, T.K.: J. Clin. Invest. *55*:1026–1032, 1975.

174. Kakuma, S., Leevy, C.M., Frank, O., et al.: Proc. Soc. Exp. Biol. Med. *168*:325–329, 1981.

175. Lumeng, L.: J. Clin. Invest. *62*:286–293, 1978.

176. Mitchell, D., Wagner, C., Stone, W.J., et al.: Gastroenterology *71*:1043–1049, 1976.

177. Klipstein, F.A., Linderbaum, J.: Blood *25*:443–456, 1965.

178. Herbert, V.I., Zalusky, R., Davidson, C.S.: Ann. Intern. Med. *58*:977–988, 1963.

179. Halstead, C.H., Griggs, R.C., Harris, J.W.: J. Lab. Clin. Med. *69*:116–131, 1967.

180. Hermos, J.A., Adams, W.H., Lin, Y., et al.: Ann. Intern. Med. *76*:957–965, 1972.

181. Halstead, C.H.: Am. J. Clin. Nutr. *33*:2736–2740, 1980.

182. Colman, N., Herbert, V.: Annu. Rev. Med. *31*:433–439, 1980.

183. Retief, F.P., Huskisson, Y.J.: Br. Med. J. *2*:150–152, 1969.

184. Wu, A., Chanarin, I., Slavin, G., et al.: Br. J. Haematol. *29*:469–478, 1975.

184a.Hoogenraad, T.V., Koerot, R., DeRvyter Korver, E.G.W.M. Eur. Neurol. *18*:205–211, 1979.

185. Vallee, B.L., Walker, W.E.C., Bartholomay, A.F., et al.: N. Engl. J. Med. *255*:403–408, 1956.

186. Sullivan, J.F., Heaney, R.P.: Am. J. Clin. Nutr. *23*:170–177, 1970.

187. Halsted, J.A., Smith, J.C.: Lancet *1*:322–324, 1970.

188. Jones, R.B., Keeling, P.W.N., Hilton, P.J., et al.: Clin. Sci. *60*:237–239, 1981.

189. Keeling, P.W.N., Jones R.B., Hilton, P.J., et al.: Gut *21*:561–564, 1980.

190. Boyett, J.D., Sullivan, J.F.: Am. J. Dig. Dis. *15*:797–802, 1970.

191. Sullivan, J.F., Lankford, H.G.: Am. J. Clin. Sci. *10*:153–157, 1962.

192. Schechter, P.J., Giroux, E.L., Schlienger, J.L., et al.: Eur. J. Clin. Invest. *6*:147–150, 1976.

193. Blendis, L.M., Wesson, D., Doody, M., et al.: Gastroenterology *75*:956, 1978 (Abstract).

194. Smith, J.C., McDaniel, E.G., Fan, F.F., et al.: Science *181*:954–955, 1973.

195. Smith, J.E., Brown, E.D., Smith, J.C.: J. Lab. Clin. Med. *84*:692–697, 1974.

196. Brown, E.D., Chan, W., Smith, J.C.: J. Nutr. *106*:563–568, 1976.

197. Shingwear, A.G., Mohanram, M., Reddy, V.: Clin. Chim. Acta. *93*:97–100, 1979.

198. Keeling, P.W.N., O'Day, J., Ruse, W., et al.: Clin. Sci. *62*:109–111, 1982.

199. McClain, C.J., VanThiel, D.H, Parker, S., et al.: Alc. Clin. Exp. Res. *3*:135–141, 1979.

200. Henkin, R.I., Bradley, D.F.: Life Sci. *9*:701–709, 1970.

201. Vallee, B.L., Wacker, W.E.C., Bartholomay, A.F., et al.: N. Engl. J. Med. *257*:1055–1065, 1957.

202. Hammond, J.B., Black, H.R., Collison, J.L.: Am. J. Dig. Dis. *5*:923–930, 1960.

203. Weisman, K., Christensen, E., Dreyer, V.: Acta. Med. Scand. *205*:361–366, 1979.

204. Russell, R.M.: Am. J. Clin. Nutr. *33*:1741–1749, 1980.

205. Mills, P.R., Fell, G.S., Bessent, R.G., et al.: Clin. Sci. *64*:527–535, 1983.

206. Gvozdanovic, S., Gvozdanovic, D., Crofton, R.W., et al.: Nuc. Med. Comm. *3*:127, 1982.

207. Prasad, A.S., Brewer, G.J., Schoomaker, E.G., et al.: JAMA *240*:2166–2168, 1978.

*Chapter* **57**

# NUTRITION MANAGEMENT OF DIABETES MELLITUS

James W. Anderson

Diabetes mellitus poses a major health threat in developed countries. In the United States alone, 5.5 million persons are known to have diabetes and an estimated 5 million have undetected disease.[1] Diabetes affects 0.2% of children, 1% of young adults, 6% of middle-aged adults, and 8 to 10% of the elderly.[2] Diabetes is not a benign disease. It causes 50% of all amputations of the lower extremities in adults, 25% of all kidney failure, and is the leading cause of blindness in adults in the United States.[3] Diabetes ranks sixth as a primary cause of death in the United States; when its complications are considered, it ranks third. The estimated economic impact of diabetes exceeds 16 billion dollars annually in the United States.[1] Proper care of diabetes is essential because no known cure exists and good management reduces the frequency of complications.[4] Diabetes management requires education and communication; patient knowledge is vital because diabetes health care is primarily self-care.

The nutrition plan serves as the cornerstone of any successful diabetes management plan. This chronic disease requires a strategy with short-term and long-term goals. The diabetic individual and the health care team jointly create a plan that fosters an optimal lifestyle while maintaining desirable blood glucose concentrations.

## HISTORICAL OVERVIEW[5]

Ancient civilization in Egypt, Greece, Rome, and India recognized diabetes and recommended diet modifications. Early medical writers reported the weight loss, excessive urination, and sweet taste of urine. Aretaeus (70 A.D.), a Roman citizen, noted the polydipsia and polyuria and named the condition *diabetes*, which means "to flow through." Thomas Willis (1675), a London physician, described the sweet taste of urine and introduced the term *mellitus*, meaning "honeylike." Most early physicians recommended carbohydrate replacement for the management of diabetes.

During previous centuries, recommendations regarding the dietary carbohydrate for diabetic individuals were based on theoretical considerations or beliefs rather than on scientific data. Consequently, supporters of the carbohydrate replacement thesis have debated supporters of the carbohydrate-restriction thesis. Believers in low-carbohydrate, high-fat diets logically argued that since diabetic individuals have too much sugar in their blood and urine they should eat less sugar and carbohydrate. Believers in carbohydrate replacement and high-carbohydrate diets argued that dietary carbohydrate should replace the sugar lost in the urine. One important feature still relevant to the management of most diabetic individuals today was endorsed by both sides: diabetes is best treated by energy-restricted diets.

**The Preinsulin Era.** John Rollo (1797), a British Army Surgeon-General, launched the modern era of nutrition therapy for diabetes by recommending a low-carbohydrate, high-fat diet.[6] He advised the complete avoidance of dietary carbohydrate and abstinence from every kind of vegetable. Therapy was directed at minimizing glycosuria. He noted that small quantities of bread allowed "saccharine matter" to return to the urine. When his patients improved, he allowed them to resume a cautious intake of vegetables. Charles Henry Pike (1860) of Philadelphia reiterated the "strict use of animal foods alone."[5]

The French clinician Appolinaire Bouchardat (1865) subsequently developed a more palatable low-carbohydrate, high-fat diet by eliminating milk and allowing some boiled vegetables. He observed that the limited food supplies during wartime were accompanied by less glycosuria for his diabetic patients. Consequently, in addition to limiting carbohydrate intake, he introduced a major nutrition principle: the restriction of energy intake. He also initiated the practice of intermittent fasting to control glycosuria.[5] His reports galvanized the widely accepted practice of using a low-carbohydrate, energy-restricted diet for diabetic individuals in the preinsulin era.

The German physician and investigator Bernhard Naunyn (1906) introduced carefully measured diets. He noted that dietary protein increased glycosuria and recommended restriction of protein as well as carbohydrate. He also reported that intermittent 24-hour fasts reduced glycosuria for less severe cases.[5] Subsequently, Frederick M. Allen (1912) of New York developed the famous "Allen Starvation Treatment" of diabetes. Using 1,000-kcal diets containing 10 g carbohydrate, he was able to sustain the lives of a few young men until insulin became available.[7] Thus, just prior to the discovery of insulin, diabetes was treated with low-carbohydrate, semistarvation regimens.

High-carbohydrate, energy-restricted diets were advanced by Thomas Willis in 1675.[5] He developed the milk diet that became standard treatment until the time of Bouchardat. Plorry (1875) of Paris, like Willis, argued that the sugar lost in the urine should be replaced with dietary carbohydrate. Donkin (1869) recommended skim milk, and others developed "cures" using other carbohydrate sources.[5] Van During (1875) used rice,

while Dujardin-Beaumetz (1889) and Mosse (1898) used potatoes.[5] Carl Hanko van Noorden (1902) developed an "oatmeal cure" for diabetes.[5] His report sustained the minority view that high-carbohydrate, energy-restricted diets were the treatment of choice for diabetes.

**Insulin Era.** Even after the discovery of insulin in 1921 most Western diabetologists used low-carbohydrate, high-fat diets to treat lean diabetic individuals. The few clinicians to report that high-carbohydrate, low-fat diets benefited diabetic individuals included Geyelin (1923),[8] Sansum (1928),[9] Rabinowitch (1935),[10] and Kempner (1968).[11] Table 57–1 outlines the changes in nutrition recommendations over the past 50 years. As discussed later, considerable clinical and experimental data have emerged recently to support recommendations of national diabetes associations for a generous carbohydrate, fat-restricted diet.

## CLASSIFICATION

Diabetes mellitus is a chronic metabolic condition characterized by derangements in the metabolism of glucose as well as abnormalities in the metabolism of fat, protein, and other substances. Hyperglycemia is its hallmark. Pathologic changes of the small blood vessels of the eyes, kidneys, and other tissues as well as degeneration of peripheral nerves develop with time. This condition, usually inherited, results from an absolute or relative deficiency of insulin, the hormone secreted by beta cells of the pancreas. Diabetes can be primary or secondary (Table 57–2.)

Insulin-dependent diabetes mellitus (IDDM or type 1) accounts for 10% of all cases and usually develops during childhood, although it can develop for the age of 20 years. About 1 of every 700 schoolchildren in North America develops type I diabetes. Characterized by a proneness to ketoacidosis, these individuals have virtually no capacity to secrete insulin after their diabetes is entrenched. Diabetes often develops acutely owing to the sudden cessation of insulin secretion, which is usually related to an autoimmune insult to the pancreatic beta cells in a genetically susceptible individual. This insult is usually triggered by a viral injection.[12] Viral destruction of the beta cells is a rare cause of type 1 diabetes; usually the virus evokes an autoimmune response that destroys the pancreatic beta cells. A small percentage of individuals with this type of diabetes have strong family histories of autoimmune conditions such as autoimmune thyroid disease (e.g., Grave's disease) or adrenal disease (Addison's disease). They apparently develop diabetes

**Table 57–1. Changes in Nutrition Recommendations for Persons with Diabetes**

|  | *1930* | *1955* | *1970* | *1985* |
|---|---|---|---|---|
| Carbohydrate, total (g/d) | 70 | 176 | 225 | 275 |
| % of energy | (14) | (35) | (45) | (55) |
| simple (g/d) | 40 | 71 | 112 | 125 |
| complex (g/d) | 30 | 105 | 113 | 150 |
| Fat, total (g/d) | 153 | 99 | 82 | 60 |
| % of energy | (69) | (45) | (37) | (27) |
| saturated (g/d) | 87 | 46 | 35 | 15 |
| monounsaturated (g) | 50 | 37 | 31 | 15 |
| polyunsaturated (g) | 9 | 11 | 13 | 25 |
| Cholesterol (mg/d) | 1,060 | 690 | 550 | 150 |
| Protein (g/d) | 85 | 101 | 90 | 90 |
| Dietary fiber (g/d) | 8 | 15 | 20 | 40 |

**Table 57–2. Classification of Diabetes Mellitus**

*Spontaneous diabetes mellitus (DM)*
   Insulin-dependent (IDDM or type I)
   Noninsulin-dependent (NIDDM or type II)
      Nonobese NIDDM
      Obese NIDDM
*Secondary diabetes*
   Pancreatic disease (pancreatitis, pancreatic insufficiency, or surgical pancreatectomy)
   Hormonal: Excess counter-regulatory hormones (growth hormone as with acromegaly, glucocorticoids as with Cushing's syndrome, catecholamines as with pheochromocytoma, or thyroid hormones as with thyrotoxicosis)
   Drug or chemical-induced (as with potassium-wasting diuretics, beta blocking agents, or diphenylhydantoin)
   Insulin receptor abnormalities
   Structurally abnormal insulin
   Certain genetic disorders (e.g., myotonic dystrophy)
*Impaired glucose tolerance*
*Gestational diabetes: glucose intolerance discovered during pregnancy*

from beta cell destruction by their own autoantibodies without a triggering virus infection.[12]

Noninsulin-dependent diabetes mellitus (NIDDM or type II) usually develops insidiously owing to a gradual reduction in insulin secretion. This genetic disorder is often associated with resistance of certain tissues, especially skeletal muscle, to the action of insulin. Obesity is a major cause of insulin resistance, although some lean individuals are insulin-resistant. Even in insulin-resistant individuals, impaired insulin secretory capacity is responsible for the diabetic state.[13–15] In type II diabetes, the pancreatic beta cells act like an aging factory whose production steadily declines. The only way for the body to manage with limited output is to reduce requirements. Individuals susceptible to type II diabetes can enhance their insulin sensitivity by weight loss, diet, and exercise, thereby decreasing their insulin requirements.

In North America about 90% of individuals with

primary diabetes have the type II variety; approximately 80% of them are obese. This form usually develops after the age of 40 years. Diabetes afflicts an estimated 3% of North American adults and almost 15% of nursing home residents. The prevalence of diabetes is about 10% higher in women than in men. In the United States, rates of diabetes are twofold higher in black than in white individuals, middle-aged black women being especially vulnerable. Individuals with lower income or education attainments have twice the rate of diabetes as those with higher income or education attainments. Thus, obesity, race, income, and education all correlate with rates of diabetes.[3]

Secondary factors account for the development of diabetes in 10% of cases in Western countries and up to 25% of case in Eastern countries such as India.[16] Total pancreatectomy obviously leads to insulin-dependent diabetes, whereas other secondary causes may produce conditions that resemble either the insulin-dependent or noninsulin-dependent forms. Hormonal disorders or drug therapy may trigger diabetes in the genetically susceptible individual. As in the management of the primary form, persons with secondary diabetes are managed with insulin or oral hypoglycemia agents, if required, and an appropriate diet.

## DIAGNOSIS

Classic symptoms such as polydipsia, polyuria, and rapid weight loss associated with gross and unequivocal elevation of blood glucose make the diagnosis of diabetes mellitus. Fasting plasma glucose concentrations exceeding 140 mg/dl on two or more occasions also are diagnostic. An oral glucose tolerance test is unnecessary and is actually contraindicated because of the risk of severe hyperglycemia.[17]

The oral glucose tolerance test (OGTT) identifies individuals with diabetes, impaired glucose tolerance, and gestational diabetes. For proper interpretation the individual must be ambulatory, otherwise healthy, and on no medications that impair the glucose tolerance (see National Diabetes Data Group).[17] For at least three days prior to the test, the individual should use a weight-maintaining diet that provides at least 150 g of carbohydrate daily. After an overnight fast of 10 to 16 hours, an oral glucose load of 50 to 100 g (or 40 g/M²) is given. The subject remains seated during the test. Water is permitted but smoking is not. Blood is taken before glucose administration and one half, one, one and one half, and two hours later for plasma glucose measurements.

Nondiabetic adults have fasting plasma glucose values <140 mg/dl and values during the OGTT <140 mg/dl at two hours and <200 mg/dl at one half, one, and two hours. Diabetes mellitus is present in nonpregnant adults when two or more OGTT are abnormal with plasma glucose values exceeding 200 mg/dl at two hours and one other time (one half, one, or one and one half hours).[17]

Impaired glucose tolerance is present in non-pregnant adults meeting all three of these criteria: fasting plasma glucose <140 mg/dl; the two-hour value at 140 to 200 mg/dl; and one other value (at one half, one, or one and one half hours) exceeding 200 mg/dl. The National Diabetes Data Group provides criteria for the diagnosis of diabetes in children and during pregnancy.[17]

## BODY FUEL REGULATION

**Role of Hormones.** Insulin, the major hormonal regulator of fuel storage and release, is synthesized in the pancreatic beta cells and secreted in response to specific stimuli. After its synthesis, proinsulin splits, producing the connecting peptide (C-peptide) and insulin (51 amino acids). Ordinarily insulin and C-peptide are released in equimolar quantities.[18]

Healthy lean adults secrete approximately 31 units of insulin daily. Because of peripheral resistance to the action of insulin, obese nondiabetic adults secrete an average of 114 units daily, three-fold more insulin than lean nondiabetic persons. Individuals with type I diabetes release only 4 units of insulin daily, on average, whereas lean type II diabetic individuals produce approximately 14 units daily, less than half the insulin produced by obese nondiabetic individuals. These estimates of insulin secretory capacity[19] support other evidence[13–15] that diabetes usually results from an absolute or relative deficiency of insulin.

Insulin serves as the main signal to the body regarding the "fed" or "fasting" state. After a large meal, the high blood levels of insulin in the fed state stimulate fuel and energy storage in certain tissues. After an overnight fast, the low blood insulin levels of the fasted state permit the mobilization of fuel and energy from storage depots. Glucagon, the pancreatic alpha cell hormone, plays a supporting role and facilitates fuel and energy release when blood insulin levels are low (Fig. 57–1). Under stressful circumstances such as hypoglycemia or trauma, glucagon and other "counter-regulatory" hormones (so named because they oppose the action of insulin) are released. These hormones, including glucagon, catecholamines, glucocorticoids, and growth hormone, act in specific ways to decrease glucose use, to promote glucose production, and to mobilize fatty acids from storage depots. In the fasting state and under stressful conditions, fatty acids emerge as the major source of energy.[20,21]

**Energy Stores.** A healthy 70-kg man stores approximately 70 g of liver glycogen, 200 g of muscle glycogen, and 30 g of glucose in the body fluids for a total of 300 g of glucose or 1,200 kcal of potential energy.[22] Thus, available glucose stores can meet energy requirements for only 12 to 18 hours of fasting. However, adipose tissue stores of triglycerides typically represent energy depots of over 120,000 kcal, roughly 100-fold greater than glucose energy reserves. Thus, with starvation or stress, fatty acids are released for

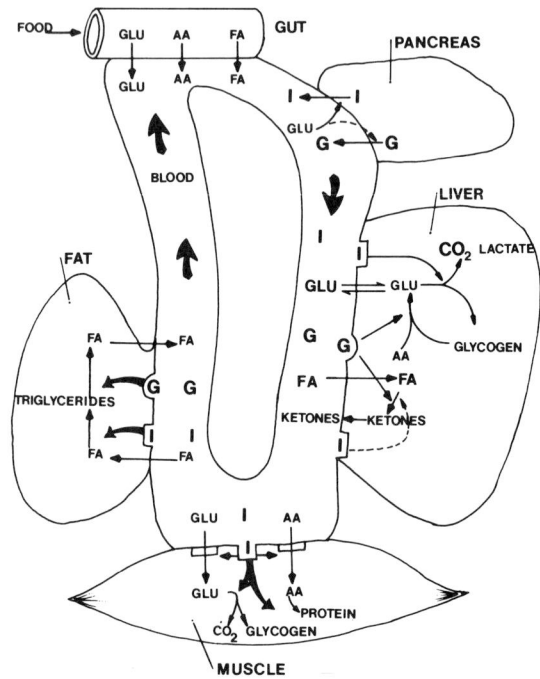

**Fig. 57–1.** Action of insulin and glucagon shown schematically. GLU = glucose; AA = amino acids; FA = fatty acids; I = insulin; G = glucagon. Solid arrows indicate stimulation and broken arrows indicate inhibition.

energy. Body proteins, skeletal and visceral structures, as well as enzymes and other vital components are unavailable for energy except under dire conditions of prolonged starvation or severe stress.

**The Fed State.** After meals gastrointestinal enzymes hydrolyze carbohydrates and proteins to their component monosaccharides and amino acids. After absorption these nutrients pass into the portal vein and stimulate insulin secretion. Thus sugars and amino acids enter liver cells that have high ambient insulin concentrations. In liver cells insulin stimulates glycogen synthesis, aerobic and anaerobic glycolysis, protein synthesis, and fatty acid synthesis. Insulin also inhibits glycogenolytic, gluconeogenic, proteolytic, and lipolytic processes. After activation by phosphorylation, glucose enters glycogen depots, generates energy in glycolytic and Kreb's cycle pathways, and yields precursors for fatty acid and protein synthesis. Other simple sugars enter the glycogen pool, generate energy, or serve as precursors for various synthetic processes. Amino acids enter the precursor pool designated for protein synthesis.

Muscle, fat cells, and other tissues receive a large percentage of the glucose and amino acids released after a large meal. High serum levels of insulin specifically stimulate the transport of glucose and amino acids into muscle cells and glucose into adipose sites. In muscle cells, under the influence of insulin, glucose enters glycogen depots and generates energy while amino acids serve as precursors for protein synthesis. Insulin also facilitates the conversion of glucose products to fatty acids for storage as triglycerides in fat cells. Most other tissues are freely permeable to glucose as well as amino acids and use the nutrients for glycogen formation, energy, and protein synthesis.

Ingested fat is handled quite differently by the gut, liver, and other tissues than are glucose and amino acids. The gut hydrolyzes fats to fatty acids, glycerol, cholesterol, phospholipids, and other constituents. Short- and medium-chain fatty acids are absorbed and enter the portal vein for use in the liver. Long-chain fatty acids, cholesterol, and phospholipids are repackaged in the gut mucosal cells and enter the lymphatic circulation as components of chylomicrons or very low-density lipoprotein (VLDL) particles. These fat transport particles travel via lymphatics and enter the superior vena cava via the thoracic duct. In the systemic circulation, chylomicrons and VLDL particles release fatty acids for use by liver, muscle, fat, and other cells.[23]

High circulating insulin levels affect lipid me-

tabolism in several ways. Insulin stimulates the synthesis of lipoprotein lipases that are secreted onto capillary membranes.[24] These lipases extract fatty acids from the triglyceride-rich circulating lipoproteins and facilitate the entry of these fatty acids into various tissue cells. In the fed state, a large proportion of these fatty acids are extracted by adipose tissue where they are incorporated into triglyceride storage depots. Liver cells exposed to generous amounts of insulin extract fatty acids from chylomicrons and repackage them as VLDL particles that are secreted into the systemic circulation. The VLDL also deliver fatty acids to adipose tissue for deposition as triglycerides.

**The Fasting State.** The transition from the fed to the fasted state is accompanied by a gradual fall in serum insulin levels and a rise in serum glucagon levels. The falling ratio of insulin to glucagon concentrations slowly switches the liver enzyme machinery from glucose utilization to glucose production. After an overnight fast of 12 hours or longer, about half of liver glycogen stores are depleted. With starvation for longer periods, hepatic glycolytic rates and activities of key glycolytic enzymes decline over 48 to 96 hours and then stabilize, whereas hepatic gluconeogenesis rates and activities of key gluconeogenic enzymes generally rise in a mirror-image fashion. After 72 hours of fasting, the liver has low glycolytic rates and has completely retooled for maximal rates of gluconeogenesis.[25]

The brain, other nervous tissues, red blood cells, and the renal medulla have ongoing requirements for glucose as an energy source while other tissues begin using fatty acids and ketones for energy. The low serum insulin levels stimulate lipolysis in adipose tissue. Fatty acids are released from these depots at rates required for energy by various tissues. Lipolysis is further stimulated by high serum levels of glucagon and catecholamines. The liver burns fatty acids to meet its energy needs and to fuel gluconeogenesis. Ketones are hepatic by-products of this active fatty acid oxidation process. Glucogenic amino acids released by muscles and other tissues provide the major substrates for this active gluconeogenic process. When the glycogen reserves of liver and muscle are exhausted, most tissues are totally dependent on fatty acids and ketones to meet their energy needs.

High levels of free fatty acids decrease the number of insulin receptors on various tissues and act in other ways to block insulin action. Because of low serum insulin and high serum free fatty acid levels, glucose and other amino acids are not transported into muscle cells. Protein synthesis ceases, and proteolysis is activated with amino acid release into circulation. Glucocorticoids also foster the mobilization of the amino acids required to support gluconeogenesis in the liver.

Thus, during a short-term fast, serum insulin and glucagon concentrations orchestrate changes in fuel homeostasis resulting in a steady supply of glucose to brain and other glucose-dependent tissues while mobilizing free fatty acids to meet energy needs of other tissues. After 7 to 10 days of fasting, the brain develops the capacity to use ketones for fuel and the need for conversion of amino acids to glucose abates, allowing the body to adjust to long-term fasting with sparing of skeletal and visceral proteins.

## METABOLIC DERANGEMENTS

The diabetic state resembles the fasting state, especially in the responses of the liver, muscle cells, and adipose tissues. Because of the low ratio of insulin to glucagon and the high levels of fatty acids, the liver produces glucose while other tissues use fatty acids and ketones instead of glucose. Muscle cells and adipose tissues respond to the diabetic state by using ketones and fatty acids. Even though these resemblances between the fasting state and the diabetic state are striking, pathologically low insulin levels disrupt the efficient responses seen in the fasting state.

Without the sustaining influence of insulin, activities fall for key glycolytic enzymes, such as glucokinase (in liver), hexokinase (in muscle and fat), phosphofructokinase, and pyruvate kinase (Fig. 57–2). Glucose utilization falls to levels far below those in the fasting state. At the same time, hepatic gluconeogenic enzymes such as phosphoenolpyruvate carboxykinase increase fivefold and gluconeogenic rates rise to extremely high levels. Bombarded with these free fatty acids, the liver sustains high rates of gluconeogenesis, secreting large amounts of VLDL while accumulating fatty acids in droplet forms. This simple metabolic derangement leads to a deposition of 25% more lipid than normal in the liver, a chronic toxic effect of diabetes. In the diabetic state the liver oxidizes these fatty acids and produces acetone, acetoacetate, and beta hydroxybutyrate.[25]

The muscle cells and adipose tissue experience a similar exaggerated reaction to the diabetic state. Muscle glycogen almost disappears and muscle protein is broken down to support gluconeogenesis. Cardiac and skeletal muscles meet their energy needs from ketones and fatty acids. Fat cells actively release fatty acids and deplete their storage depots under the combined lipolytic stimuli of glucagon and catecholamines accompanied by insulin deficiency.

Other tissues that are not insulin-dependent re-

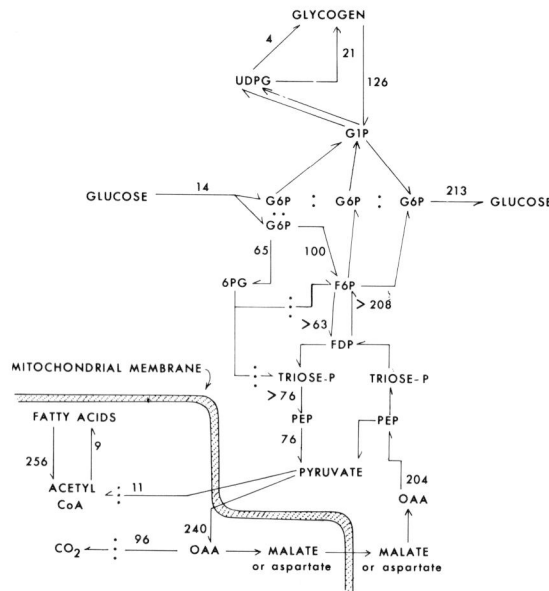

**Fig. 57–2.** Biochemical derangements in diabetes. The selective effects of insulin-deficient diabetes on hepatic glucose metabolism in rat are indicated. Numbers indicate enzyme activity as percentage of values for healthy controls. Note the range for key glycolytic enzymes from 14% activity for glucokinase converting glucose to G6P to 76% activity for pyruvate kinase activity converting PEP to pyruvate. Key gluconeogenic enzymes are stimulated (see glucose phosphatase activity at 213%). Glycogen synthesis from glucose is inhibited (4%) as is fatty acid synthesis (9%). Glycogenolysis (at 124%) and lipolysis (at 256%) are stimulated. See Anderson, J.W.[25] for further information.

spond to the diabetic state in a different way. Hexokinase, the key stimuli of glucose use, is increased in jejunal mucosa, renal cortex, and peripheral nerves of diabetic animals. These tissues respond to hyperglycemia with increased glucose utilization and accumulation and thus are influenced more by the diabetic hyperglycemic state than by the hypoinsulinemic state.[26]

Metabolic derangements in nondependent tissues are produced by the excess glucose accumulation. The carcass of a diabetic rat has almost 30% more glycogen than that of a nondiabetic rat.[26] Glycogen accumulates in renal tubules of diabetic rats in concentration nearly 50 times greater than in nondiabetic rats.[26] This accumulation of glucose contributes to tubular dysfunction and may increase the susceptibility to tubular damage resulting from toxins such as x-ray contrast dyes. The unimpeded entry of glucose into many tissues results in excess intracellular glucose. This condition produces linkage of glucose to tissue proteins (glycosylation). The diabetic state wreaks destruction on these noninsulin-dependent tissues, including glomerular capillaries, retinal vessels, nerves, and circulating cells in the blood.

## DIABETIC COMPLICATIONS

**Acute Problems.** Diabetes is usually recognized when an individual either exhibits symptomatic hyperglycemia or appears with a medical emergency due to severe hyperglycemia or ketoacidosis.[27,28] Most of the symptoms of diabetes are related to the hyperglycemia or the accumulation of glucose or glucose products in various tissues. As hyperglycemia develops, individuals develop increased polyuria, thirst, lack of energy, irritability, blurred vision, and weight loss. Adults usually develop these symptoms over weeks to months whereas children develop them in hours or days. If hyperglycemia remains undetected or if stress or illness intervenes, the individual develops stupor or coma (Table 57–3).

Adults with type II diabetes are likely to develop the hyperglycemic nonketotic state characterized by plasma glucose values exceeding 750 mg/dl without significant ketonemia.[29] Presumably, these individuals are protected from ketoacidosis because of low but measurable levels of insulin in the circulation. The hyperglycemic nonketotic condition may be precipitated by excessive sugar intake, moderate to severe dehydration, heat exposure, illness, or drug therapy with agents such as glucocorticoids, potassium-wasting diuretics, or diphenylhydantoin.[29]

Individuals with type I diabetes are vulnerable to diabetic ketoacidosis characterized by moderate to severe hyperglycemia and substantial ketonemia with heavy ketonuria. This condition occurs with either insulin deficiency (low circulating levels or an omission of an insulin injection) or stress, with high levels of counter-regulatory hormones such as catecholamines, glucagon, glucocorticoids or growth hormone.[30] Either the hyperglycemic nonketotic state or ketoacidosis can be fatal. Vigorous therapy with insulin, fluids, and electrolytes is the emergency treatment.

**Short-Term Complications.** Sustained hyperglycemia alters glucose metabolism in virtually all tissues. Cells that are not insulin-dependent are particularly vulnerable. In these cells, sugar alcohols (polyols) accumulate and proteins become heavily glycosylated. Most tissues gradually convert glucose to polyols that are used slowly (Fig. 57–3). Hyperglycemia causes high levels of intracellular glucose leading to more rapid formation of polyols. Despite rapid accumulation, however, they are still degraded slowly. As sorbitol and fructose (the major polyols) accumulate, they draw water into the cells and cause cell distention.[31,32] This condition combined with some toxic properties of polyols leads to cell dysfunc-

**Table 57–3. Diabetic Complications and Pathophysiologic Considerations**

| Complication | Pathophysiologic Considerations |
|---|---|
| *Acute* | |
| Moderate hyperglycemia | Polydipsia, polyuria, weight loss, fatigue, blurred vision |
| Severe hyperglycemia | Hyperglycemic nonketotic state |
| Ketogenesis | Diabetic ketoacidosis |
| *Short-term* | |
| Protein glycosylation | Premature aging of collagen, lens, and other tissue proteins; functional abnormalities of hormones, lipoproteins, and membrane proteins |
| Polyol accumulation | Nerve and lens dysfunction |
| Mucopolysaccharide abnormalities | Alterations in arterial walls |
| Glycogen accumulation | Renal tubular lesions |
| Hypercholesterolemia/hypertriglyceridemia | Accelerated atherosclerosis |
| Vascular permeability abnormalities | Protein leakage from capillaries |
| Microcirculation defects | Abnormal renal and muscle blood flow |
| White blood cell abnormalities | Altered response to infection and immune challenges |
| Platelet abnormalities | Contributing factor to micro and macrovascular abnormalities |
| Erythrocyte abnormalities | Stiffness and altered 2, 3-diphosphoglycerate |
| Nerve dysfunction | Decreased nerve conduction velocity |
| *Chronic* | |
| Renal glomeruli | Nodular or diffuse thickening |
| Retinal vessels | Hemorrhage, ischemia, new vessel proliferation |
| Neurologic abnormalities | Peripheral and autonomic neuropathies |
| Capillaries | Basement membrane thickening and microcirculation abnormalities |
| Arterial abnormalities | Generalized and accelerated atherosclerosis |

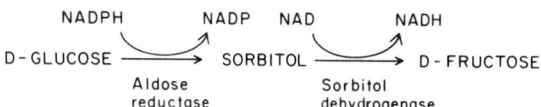

**Fig. 57–3.** Polyol pathway.

tion and even cell damage. Blurred vision, for example, is caused by distention of the lens, which reduces the ability to accommodate from near to distant vision. Polyol accumulation can alter the function of peripheral nerves. Blocking the accumulation of sorbitol in nerves using an enzyme inhibitor may diminish neuropathy.[33]

Excess glucose also affects the production of glycoproteins, which are proteins that contain sugar side chains (Fig. 57–4). The condensation reaction between glucose and an amino acid component of protein follows two stages: (1) The aldehyde group of glucose links to the amino group of an amino acid forming an aldimine (Schiff base). (2) The unstable aldimine releases glucose or undergoes an Amadori rearrangement to form the stable ketoamine linkage. This process occurs spontaneously without requiring enzyme action and is termed nonenzymatic glycosylation. Hemoglobin, serum albumin, and many other tissue proteins are glycosylated. In the diabetic state the rate of nonenzymatic glycosylation is related to the magnitude and duration of hyperglycemia.[34,35]

The sugar content of hemoglobin, the best characterized glycoprotein, is normally less than 8%. With sustained hyperglycemia, the percentage of glycosylated hemoglobin can exceed 25% of total hemoglobin.[35] When normal erythrocytes are incubated in glucose solutions, the glycohemoglobin content doubles within hours. Most of the glucose is attached by the unstable aldimine linkage, which can be dissociated if the erythrocytes are incubated in solutions with low glucose content. Chronic exposure to high levels of glucose causes formation of the irreversible ketoamine linkage that persists until the cell is degraded. Thus, glycohemoglobin measurements reflect glycemic control over the previous six to eight weeks. With excellent glycemic control, glycohemoglobin concentrations are normal. Poor diabetic control yields glycohemoglobin values exceeding 13% of total hemoglobin.

The degree of glycosylation of circulating proteins, hormones, lipoproteins, plasma membranes

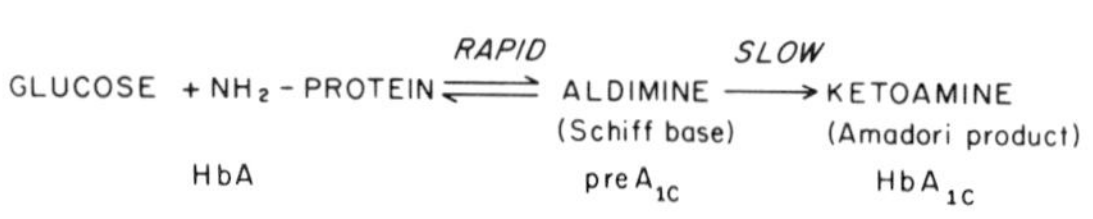

of cells, basement membranes, and other proteins in diabetes has not been determined. Moderate or severe hyperglycemia causes widespread nonenzymatic glycosylation in blood and tissues. It may contribute to basement membrane thickening, vascular permeability, microcirculation defects, and functional abnormalities of erythrocytes, leukocytes, and platelets.

Hyperglycemia induces a host of other metabolic derangements. Glycogen accumulates in a variety of noninsulin-dependent tissues. The increased flux of glucose through insulin-insensitive pathways such as mucopolysaccharide synthesis leads to qualitative and quantitative abnormalities of mucopolysaccharides, contributing to atherosclerosis and other derangements of tissues.[26] Hyperglycemia alters the orderly formation of glycoproteins in the kidney and other tissues, producing a disproportionate amount of glucose in these glycoproteins. This abnormality contributes to basement membrane thickening in glomerular capillaries and diabetic glomerulosclerosis.[36] Evidence suggests that many short-term problems of hyperglycemia can be avoided entirely by maintaining satisfactory plasma glucose concentrations.[37] In some cases, derangements can be reversed by good glycemic control.[38]

**Chronic Complications.** The pathogenesis of the chronic manifestations of diabetes (see Table 57–2) remains controversial. Metabolic, genetic, and other factors affect major diabetic complications such as retinopathy, nephropathy, and neuropathy. Based on comprehensive studies of diabetic animals and less rigorous observations of humans, most authorities maintain that chronic hyperglycemia accelerates the development of these complications.[37] Pirart carefully documented the prevalence of diabetic complications among 4,400 diabetic patients followed for an extensive period[39] (Fig. 57–5). After 25 years, most patients had complications of some type; however, the prevalence of complications was much lower in those patients who had achieved fairly good average glycemic control than in those who had sustained poor diabetic control. The individual genetic diathesis toward these complications also influences their frequency. Some diabetic individuals develop complications at an accelerated rate despite reasonable glycemic control; others show little tendency toward these complications. The prudent course is to achieve the best glycemic control possible without undue hypoglycemic episodes or severe limitation of lifestyle.

## ATHEROSCLEROSIS

Macrovascular disease is the most common complication of diabetes. Deaths due to athero-

GLUCOSE + NH₂ – PROTEIN ⇌ ALDIMINE → KETOAMINE

**Fig. 57–4.** Pathway for nonenzymatic glycosylation.

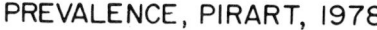

PREVALENCE, PIRART, 1978

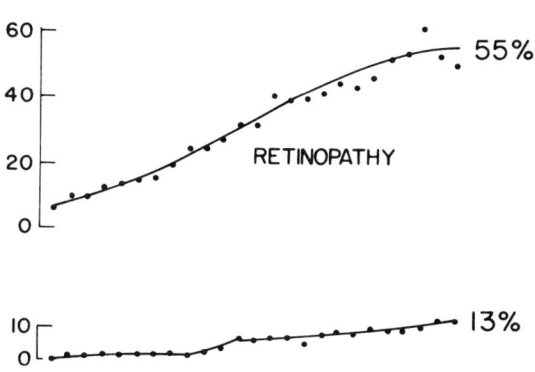

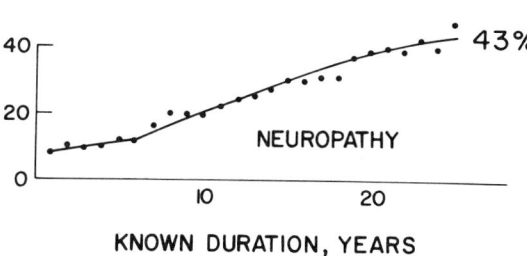

**KNOWN DURATION, YEARS**

**Fig. 57–5.** Prevalence of diabetic complications. (From Pirart, J.[39])

DIABETES AND ATHEROSCLEROSIS

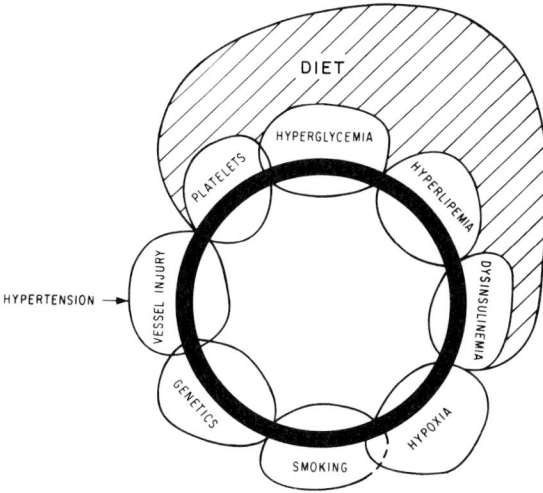

**Fig. 57–6.** Relationship of diabetes and atherosclerosis.

sclerosis are two- to threefold more common in diabetic than in nondiabetic individuals.[40] The mechanisms responsible for the pathogenesis of accelerated vascular disease are poorly understood. Figure 57–6 shows the major factors contributing to atherosclerosis in diabetes. Reducing the frequency of vascular disease requires improved glycemic control, avoidance of cigarette smoking, normal blood pressure, and desirable levels for blood lipids.

Hypertension is the major risk factor for ischemic heart disease for type I diabetic individuals and may be the most important contributor to vascular disease for all persons with diabetes.[41] Diabetic individuals, particularly women, develop hypertension more frequently than the general population.[41] Hypertension-induced physical stress on the vascular tree may act synergistically with abnormalities of the arterial wall, lipoproteins, and platelets in diabetes to accelerate atherosclerosis.

Hypercholesterolemia is the major lipid risk factor for atherosclerosis. Serum cholesterol values above 180 mg/dl confer a progressive increasing risk for coronary artery disease. In addition to

a variety of abnormalities in lipoproteins, diabetic individuals have higher serum cholesterol values than matched nondiabetic controls.[42]

Low-density lipoproteins (LDL) are the most atherogenic type of lipoproteins. Although specific defects in the production or removal of LDL have not been identified in diabetes, this lipoprotein may become glycosylated in diabetic individuals with poor glycemic control, decreasing binding to its receptor and causing intracellular accumulation of cholesterol esters.[43] Thus, glycosylation of LDL in diabetes may foster atherosclerosis.

Certain high-density lipoproteins (HDL) protect against atherosclerosis by extracting cholesterol from the artery wall. Serum HDL-cholesterol values may be low, normal, or high in diabetic patients.[44] HDL-cholesterol values are inversely related to serum triglyceride value since triglycerides displace cholesterol from this lipoprotein. Because hypertriglyceridemia is fairly common among diabetic individuals, it may contribute to reductions in serum HDL-cholesterol.

The platelet abnormalities of diabetes also contribute to the atherosclerotic process.[45] In experimental models of atherosclerosis, thrombocytopenia greatly inhibits or prevents atherosclerotic lesion development. Following aggregation, platelets release a growth factor, called a mitogen, that promotes smooth muscle cell proliferation. Thus, proliferation followed by lipid accumulation is a prominent feature of most current theories of the pathogenesis of atherosclerosis. The lipid-laden smooth muscle cells may become the foam cells in the atheroma.

Thromboxanes and prostacyclins modulate platelet effects at the arterial wall.[46] Thromboxanes are potent platelet aggregators and vasoconstrictors released by platelets. Prostacyclins are potent antiaggregators and vasodilators synthesized and released by endothelial cells. Sticky platelets that aggregate spontaneously or with minimal stimulation are features of poorly controlled diabetes. Not only does diabetes enhance platelet aggregation, it also increases platelet release of thromboxane and decreases endothelial synthesis of prostacyclin.

The endothelial cell of the arterial wall is the target of the atherosclerotic attack. HDL vs. LDL and prostacyclins vs. thromboxanes are only two of the sets of opposing forces. Endothelial injury by physical, chemical, or immunologic events followed by smooth muscle cell proliferation eventuating in foam cell accumulation are early stages of atherogenesis.[47] In diabetes a host of abnormalities potentiates this process. Platelet aggregation and fibrin deposition occur more readily in diabetes because of the hypercoagulable state and hyperaggregatable platelets. Vascular endothelial function may be impaired by hypoxia or polyol accumulation. Decreased platelet survival in diabetes may be due, in part, to more extensive aggregation in blood vessels. The resultant increased release of platelet growth factors would act in concert with greater amounts of serum growth factors to stimulate smooth muscle proliferation. Abnormal lipoproteins such as glycosylated LDL or VLDL remnants associated with diabetes contribute to lipid accumulation in smooth muscle cells. Abnormal structural components of the arterial wall, such as mucopolysaccharides, glycoproteins, or collagen, may enhance trapping or lipoproteins in this region with the diabetic state. Other perturbations, such as immune reactions, stiffening of the vascular tree, and decreased prostacyclin production, may aggravate the atherogenic tendency in diabetes.[48,49]

Epidemiologic evidence in humans and experimental studies in animals suggest hyperinsulinemia may exaggerate the risk for atherosclerosis in diabetes.[50] Most type II diabetic individuals have hyperinsulinemia due to insulin resistance or excessive insulin use. Many type 1 diabetic individuals have abnormally high serum-free insulin concentrations due to the timing or route of insulin administration. Insulin may stimulate smooth muscle proliferation, promote glucose incorporation into lipids of the arterial wall, or foster subtle derangements of serum lipoproteins.

Hyperinsulinism also may contribute to hypertension by inducing renal sodium retention[51] or other mechanisms. Circulating insulin antibodies in insulin-treated individuals may contribute to immunologic injury of vascular endothelial cells. Although further work is required to support this hypothesis, the proposed link between hyperinsulinism and atherosclerosis is an attractive concept.

## GOALS FOR NUTRITION THERAPY

A healthy individual with a full lifestyle and normal longevity is the ultimate goal for nutrition intervention. The diabetes nutrition plan attempts to diminish the effects of the disease by maintaining a normal metabolic state. Table 57–4 lists the specific and general goals for nutrition therapy. Diabetes management includes short, intermediate, and long-range goals. While maintaining desirable blood glucose values over the short range, one must also consider the intermediate effects of any program on the psychologic adjustment and general well-being of the individual. Although the long-term effects of specific diets on the outcome for individuals with diabetes are not known, one should use diets that, in the light of current medical knowledge, have the greatest potential for sustaining life with minimal complications.

Specifically, the primary goal of nutrition therapy is to achieve normal or physiologic blood glucose levels by optimizing glucose use, normalizing glucose production, and enhancing insulin sensitivity. Usually these efforts will maintain normal blood levels of other fuels such as fatty acids, ketones, and amino acids. Undue hyperglycemia as well as consequential hypoglycemia that is stressful and hazardous should be minimized by diet. Second in priority is achieving and maintaining desirable levels for plasma lipids.

**Table 57–4.   Goals for Nutrition Therapy of Diabetes**

| | |
|---|---|
| Specific | Achieve physiologic blood glucose levels |
| | Maintain desirable plasma lipids |
| | Reduce likelihood of specific diabetic complications |
| | Retard development of atherosclerosis |
| General | Provide optimal selection of nutrients |
| | Attain and maintain desirable body weight |
| | Meet energy needs in a timely manner |
| | Individualize to preferences and food available |
| | Address special requirements (such as pregnancy) |
| | Tailor for therapeutic needs (such as renal failure) |

Although recommended serum cholesterol values are still controversial, many authorities believe that desirable serum cholesterol levels range from 130 to 190 mg/dl.[52,53] I use a desirable serum cholesterol value of 150 mg/dl plus the age in years and a desirable fasting serum triglyceride value of less than 200 mg/dl. Third, a long-term goal of nutrition therapy is to reduce the frequency of specific diabetic complications such as retinopathy, nephropathy, and neuropathy. Although the pathogenesis of these disorders is not fully understood, success with the first goal should reduce the development of these complications. The last vital goal addresses the causes of atherosclerosis. Appropriate nutrition measures reduce the risk for hypertension, hypercholesterolemia, hypertriglyceridemia, and hyperinsulinemia. Theoretically, measures that normalize platelet aggregation, restore desirable serum levels for LDL- and HDL-cholesterol, and avoid hyperinsulinemia will retard the atherosclerotic processes.

In general terms, first the diet provides appropriate amounts and varieties of nutrients to ensure optimal nutrition. Recommended daily dietary allowances (RDAs) are presented in the Appendix. Second it provides appropriate energy and nutrient intakes to achieve desirable body weights. The lean adult wants to maintain a healthy weight while the obese individual should lose to a more desirable weight. Third, the diet provides three reasonable meals and snacks, as required, to meet energy needs between meals. Fourth, it is as consistent as possible with the established eating patterns of the individual, although the nutrition counselor should not be hesitant to recommend moderate to drastic changes in eating patterns for good cause. Breakfast, for example, is essential; other habits such as excessive intake of fat, sugar, or alcohol may need to be changed. Diet modifications can be achieved when the diabetic individual and his family work with the health care team. Through education and communication the patient learns the purpose of recommended changes and adapts these goals as his own. Fifth, special requirements for growth, pregnancy, or lactation are incorporated into the nutrition plan. Finally, it incorporates modifications for problems such as hypertension, congestive heart failure, osteopenia, or renal disease. Thus, the diabetes nutrition plan focuses not only on the diabetic state but also on overall health and well-being.

## THE NUTRITION PLAN

### Carbohydrate

**Amount.** Recommendations concerning the optimum carbohydrate content of the diet for dia-

betes are controversial. Currently, national diabetes associations in several countries recommend a nutrition plan that provides generous amounts of complex carbohydrate and fiber and restricts fat.[54] The advantages and disadvantages of these consensual recommendations merit discussion.

The advantages of higher carbohydrate intake appear to outweigh the disadvantages (Table 57–5). Individuals are more sensitive to endogenous or exogenous insulin when using high-carbohydrate as opposed to high-fat diets.[55] Increased numbers of insulin receptors on circulating monocytes and in adipose tissue accompany this increased sensitivity.[56] Rats fed high-carbohydrate diets have more insulin receptors per liver cells than rats fed high-fat diets.[57] Of greater importance is the enhanced intracellular metabolism of glucose associated with high-carbohydrate diets. Most of these findings are documented in experimental animals, but selected measurements in humans are confirmatory. Rates of glycogen synthesis and glycogen accumulation in liver, skeletal muscle, and jejunal mucosa are greater with high- rather than low-carbohydrate diets. Rates of glycolysis and activities of key glycolytic enzymes are higher in several tissues with high-carbohydrate diets. These diets also are associated with lower rates of gluconeogenesis in liver and lower activities of rate-limiting gluconeogenic enzymes. Thus, many metabolic changes accompany high-carbohydrate, low-fat diets that facilitate glucose use.[55,59]

The long-term use of high-carbohydrate diets for diabetic individuals is well documented.[10,11,59,60] Earlier studies documented that increasing carbohydrate intake did not worsen glycemic control and decreased serum cholesterol concentrations.[61,62] More recent studies document the beneficial effects of diets high in carbohydrates and fiber for diabetic individuals.[63–68] These diets also

**Table 57–5. Generous Carbohydrate Intakes: Advantages and Disadvantages**

| | |
|---|---|
| Advantages | Stimulate glucose use (glycolysis and glycogenesis) in many tissues |
| | Attenuate hepatic glucose production |
| | Increase tissue insulin sensitivity |
| | Increase insulin receptor number |
| | Lower postprandial and average serum triglycerides |
| Disadvantages | May increase postprandial plasma glucoses |
| | Temporarily may worsen glycemic control |
| | Tend to increase fasting serum triglycerides |

Modified from Anderson, J.W.[58]

lower serum cholesterol concentrations. Most of the improvement in glycemic control associated with higher carbohydrate, higher fiber diets appears related to the increased intake of carbohydrate and decreased intake of fat. Increasing fiber intake appears to play only a small role in these benefits.[69]

The disadvantages of high-carbohydrate diets low in dietary fiber include higher postprandial blood glucose values, temporarily worsening of glycemic control, and increases in fasting serum triglycerides. None of these disadvantages appears when high-carbohydrate, high-fiber diets are used. Postprandial plasma glucose values are lower for diabetic individuals on high-carbohydrate (70% of energy), high-fiber (70 g), low-fat (12%) diets than values on control (43% carbohydrate, 20 g fiber, and 38% fat) diets.[69a] Worsening of glycemic control can occur when diabetic individuals change from low-carbohydrate, high-fat diets to higher carbohydrate, low-fat diets. Although this condition is not well documented scientifically, experienced clinicians indicate it is of short duration (less than one week). Under metabolic ward conditions we have never seen worsening of diabetic control or increased insulin requirements when lean adult diabetic subjects were switched from control diets (43% carbohydrate) to high-carbohydrate (70% carbohydrate), high-fiber (70 g/day) diets. Thus, for diabetic individuals there is no scientific evidence that the long-term use of high-carbohydrate diets adversely affects glycemic control.

Hypertriglyceridemia is the major concern of experienced diabetologists who caution against the use of high-carbohydrate diets for diabetic individuals.[70] High-carbohydrate, low-fiber diets induce significant increases in fasting serum triglyceride values of nondiabetic and diabetic subjects.[71–73] However, these diets lower postprandial serum triglyceride values resulting in a decrease in ambient or average triglyceride values throughout the 24-hour day.[74,75] In sharp contrast, high-carbohydrate, high-fiber diets lower fasting and postprandial triglycerides of diabetic or hypertriglyceridemic patients over the short term (two weeks) and long term (three years).[75] Figure 57–7 illustrates our experience using high-carbohydrate (70%), high-fiber (70 g/day) diets for the short term and generous carbohydrate (55 to 58%), high-fiber (50 g/day) maintenance diets for longer term for diabetic patients. This experience suggests that higher-carbohydrate diets generous in plant fiber do not jeopardize the triglyceride metabolism of most individuals with diabetes.

**Type.** Simple carbohydrates from commonly used foods tend to raise blood glucose more than

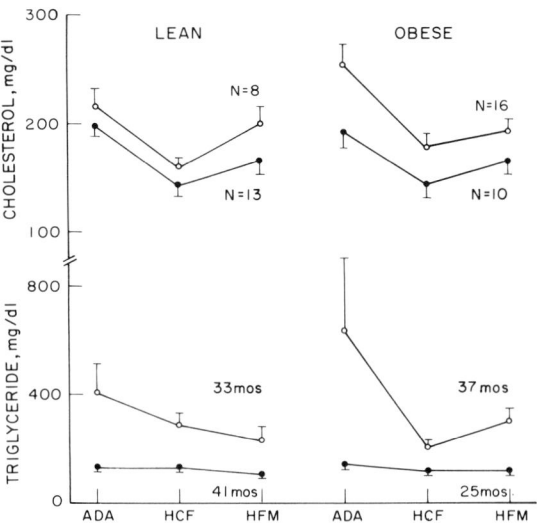

**Fig. 57–7.** Response of serum cholesterol triglyceride concentration to high-carbohydrate, high-fiber (HCF), and high-fiber maintenance (HFM) diets of lean and obese diabetic individuals. Open circles represent individuals with elevated serum triglyceride concentration on American Diabetes Association diet. Duration of follow-up is indicated in months.

do complex carbohydrates from starchy foods. Clearly, the glycemic response to 50 g of glucose is much greater than the response to a variety of foods providing 50 g of starch. This effect provides the foundation for most nutrition plans and exchange lists for use by diabetic individuals.[76] Although glucose, maltose, and sucrose produce large increases in the blood glucose, fructose does not (Fig. 57–8A). Fructose, metabolized without requiring insulin, evokes little increase in serum insulin concentrations in nondiabetic subjects. It produces only minimal increases in blood glucose for nondiabetic as well as diabetic subjects with reasonable glycemic control. Therefore, fructose may play a role as a sweetener for selected individuals with diabetes.[77–79]

Complex carbohydrates in different forms also evoke different glycemic responses. Bread or potatoes raise blood glucose more than beans (Fig. 57–8B.) Many individuals have compared the glycemic responses to foods rich in complex carbohydrate.[80–83] Jenkins and colleagues introduced the term "glycemic index" to describe these responses.[82] Table 57–6 compares the glycemic response to some selected foods.

Many factors influence the glycemic response to foods (Table 57–7). Sipping 50 g glucose slowly over several hours produces a smaller increase in blood glucose than does rapid intake of the same amount.[83] Eating three apples takes 15 minutes while their juice can be consumed in 1.5 min-

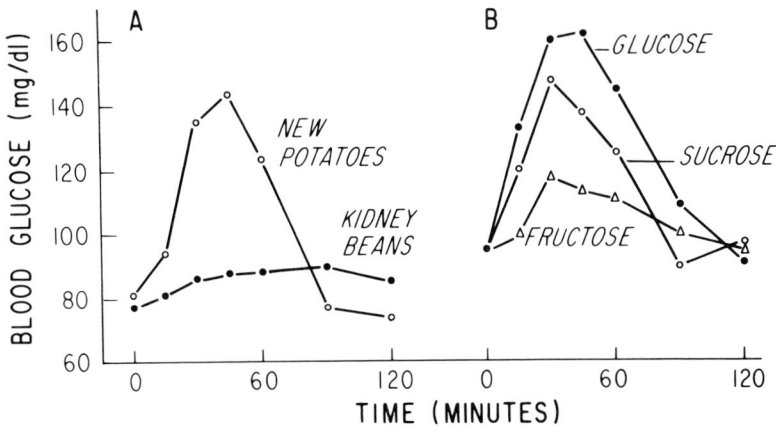

**Fig. 57–8.** *A,* Glycemic response of healthy individuals to 50 g carbohydrate from new potatoes or kidney beans. *B,* Glycemic response of healthy individuals to 50 g glucose, sucrose, or fructose.

**Table 57–6.   Glycemic Response to 50 g Carbohydrate Provided by Different Foods**

| Exchange | Food | No. of Servings* | KCAL | Glycemic Index† |
|---|---|---|---|---|
| Sugars | Glucose | 12 tsp | 200 | 100 |
| | Maltose | 12 tsp | 200 | 105 |
| | Sucrose | 12 tsp | 200 | 59 |
| | Fructose | 12 tsp | 200 | 20 |
| Milk | Skim milk | 4 | 336 | 32 |
| | Whole milk | 4 | 596 | 34 |
| | Yogurt (skim, plain) | 4.5 | 350 | 36 |
| Vegetable | Beets | 7 | 233 | 64 |
| | Carrots, cooked | 16 | 245 | 36‡ |
| | raw | 16 | 238 | 31‡ |
| Fruit | Apples | 5 | 208 | 39 |
| | Bananas | 4.5 | 216 | 62 |
| | Oranges | 6 | 209 | 40 |
| | Orange juice | 6 | 214 | 46 |
| | Raisins | 5 | 193 | 64 |
| Bread | Bread (white) | 4 | 255 | 69 |
| | (wholemeal) | 4 | 223 | 72 |
| | Bran (100%) cereal | 4 | 280 | 51 |
| | Cornflakes | 3 | 210 | 80 |
| | Oatmeal | 4.5 | 319 | 49 |
| | Wheat (shredded) | 3.5 | 245 | 67 |
| | Wheat flour | 3 | 258 | 59 |
| | Kidney beans | 4 | 376 | 29 |
| | Baked beans | 3 | 210 | 40 |
| | Lentils | 3.5 | 338 | 29 |
| | Peas, frozen | 5 | 315 | 51 |
| | Corn | 4 | 258 | 59 |
| | Lima beans | 4 | 250 | 36 |
| | Parsnips | 6 | 237 | 97 |
| | Potato, instant | 3 | 241 | 80 |
| | Potato, new | 3 | 240 | 70 |
| | Potato chips | 3 | 480 | 51 |
| Fat | Peanuts | 63 | 3,300 | 13 |
| High-fat foods | Ice cream | 4 | 640 | 36 |
| | Sausages | 68 | 7,276 | 28 |

*Number of servings (rounded to nearest half) to provide 50 g carbohydrate.
†Glycemic response compared to glucose. From Jenkins, et al.: Diabetologia *23*:477, 1982.
‡From Vaaler, et al.: Diabetes Care *7*:221, 1984.

**Table 57–7. Factors Affecting the Glycemic Response to Food**

Rate of ingestion
Prestomach hydrolysis
Stomach hydrolysis
Gastric emptying rate
Intestinal hydrolysis and absorption
  Food form
  Starch characteristics
  Fiber content
  Food ingredients
  Intestinal response
Hormone response
  Pancreatic hormones
  Gut hormones
Colon effects

utes.[84] Differences in both fiber content and the ingestion time influence the resultant glycemic response. Fat, water-soluble fiber, and other factors influence gastric emptying time. The food form may make a major impact on digestion time. For example, bread can be digested more rapidly than pasta. Foods with higher ratios of the amylopectin to the amylose form of starch are digested more rapidly than those with low ratios.[76]

Although plant fiber has attracted much attention in the last decade, it is only one of the many components of food that influence the glycemic response. Beans, one of the richest sources of soluble fiber, have lower glycemic indices than any other group of carbohydrate-rich foods.[82] The low glycemic response to beans is probably related to the high soluble fiber content, the food form (usually eaten as cooked beans rather than in bakery products), and their naturally occurring starch blockers (inhibitors of digestive enzymes responsible for hydrolysis of starch). Finally, fiber fermentation products, such as short-chain fatty acids, are absorbed from the colon into the portal vein; in the liver they may directly affect glucose metabolism.[85] The interactions of the many factors that influence the glycemic response to foods require more investigation.

### Fat

Traditionally, carbohydrate restriction led to high-fat diets (see Table 57–1). Although these diets provide distinct short-term advantages, the long-term consequences are still being tabulated. Substituting fat for carbohydrate in a meal lowers the postprandial glycemic response. Over a one-day period, replacing most of the dietary carbohydrate with fat decreases apparent insulin requirements.[86] When insulin-dependent subjects changed from generous-carbohydrate, low-fat diets to high-fat, low-carbohydrate diets, no changes in insulin requirements were observed

over two[87] or three weeks.[88] Thus, high-fat diets offer short-term benefits for glycemic control and have no discernible adverse effects on insulin requirements over two- or three-week periods.

Dr. Elliott P. Joslin expressed concern about the long-term consequences of high-fat diets in 1928,[89] suggesting they might increase the risk of heart attacks for individuals with diabetes. We have compared the effects of high-fat (50% of energy), low-carbohydrate (20%) diets with high-carbohydrate (70%), high-fiber (70 g/day), low-fat (12%) diets or serum lipid values of six insulin-dependent diabetic subjects.[87] As illustrated in Table 57–8, fasting serum cholesterol and free fatty acid values were significantly higher on high-fat than on high-carbohydrate diets. Many share the concerns of Joslin, but only limited epidemiologic evidence indicates high-fat diets contribute to the atherosclerosis so common in persons with diabetes.[90,91]

The metabolic disadvantages of high-fat diets are clear (Table 57–9.) They cause insulin resistance and impair intracellular glucose metabolism by a variety of mechanisms. Animal studies show dietary fat not only antagonizes the use of glucose but also stimulates inappropriate glucose production. High-fat diets decrease the number of insulin receptors in several tissues, decreasing glucose transport into muscle and adipose tissue and decreasing activities of insulin-stimulated processes. Rates of glycolysis and activities of key glycolytic enzymes are lower in a variety of tissues with high-fat versus high-carbohydrate diets. Glycogen synthesis rates, glycogen accumulation, and glucose oxidation are also lower with high-fat diets. A major problem for many diabetic individuals is unrestrained gluconeogenesis, which is the unrelenting production of glucose by the liver even though the blood glucose level is abnormally elevated. High-fat diets stimulate rates of gluconeogenesis and increase activities of rate-limiting gluconeogenic enzymes.[58]

High serum levels of free fatty acids (FFA) may mediate some of the adverse effects of high-fat diets on glucose metabolism.[92] High FFA levels may act directly to reduce the number of insulin receptors for certain tissues. The intracellular metabolism of FFA inhibits the essential glycolytic enzyme phosphofructokinase and still further acts to stimulate gluconeogenesis.[85] Thus, the two- to threefold rise in serum FFA associated with high-fat diets (see Table 57–8) antagonizes the state.

### Fiber

In the last quarter century fiber has emerged as an important dietary component with respect to

**Table 57–8. Serum Lipids with Control (ADA), High-Carbohydrate, High-Fiber (HCF), and High-Protein Diets***

| Serum Measurement | ADA Diet | HCF Diet | High-Protein Diet |
|---|---|---|---|
| Cholesterol (mg/dl) | 183 + 16† | 139 + 12 | 191 + 14† |
| Triglyceride (mg/dl) | 120 + 13 | 123 + 13 | 119 + 12 |
| Free fatty acids (μEq/L) | 530 + 94† | 218 + 51 | 439 + 86† |

*Six lean insulin-dependent diabetic men were fed each diet for two weeks.
†Differs from HCF values, p<0.05.
From Anderson, J.W.,[87] with permission of J. Am. Coll. Nutr.

**Table 57–9. Metabolic Disadvantages of High-Fat Diets***

| Measure | Change |
|---|---|
| Insulin sensitivity | Decreased |
| Insulin receptor number | Decreased in liver, skeletal muscle, adipose tissue |
| Glucose uptake | Decreased in skeletal muscle, adipose tissue |
| Glycolysis | Decreased in liver, skeletal muscle, adipose tissue |
| Glucokinase activity | Decreased in liver |
| Hexokinase activity | Decreased in skeletal muscle, adipose tissue |
| Phosphofructokinase activity | Decreased in liver |
| Pyruvate kinase activity | Decreased in liver |
| Glucose-6-phosphate dehydrogenase activity | Decreased in liver |
| Glycogen synthesis | Decreased in liver, skeletal muscle |
| Glucose oxidation | Decreased in skeletal muscle, adipose tissue |
| Gluconeogenesis | Increased in liver |
| Phosphoenolpyruvate carboxykinases activity | Increased in liver |

*Observations in humans and experimental animals summarized previously.[55]

diabetes. It not only may reduce the prevalence of diabetes but also may have therapeutic value. In 1960 Trowell reported diabetes was rare among African hospital patients.[93] The next year Walker postulated that high levels of cereal fiber intake might prevent the development of diabetes.[94] Subsequently, Walker and colleagues documented that healthy Bantu schoolchildren in South Africa had lower fasting blood glucose concentrations and lower glycemic responses to oral glucose than urban children.[95] Additional studies suggested that these differences were related to dietary fiber intake.[96] Based on these and other observations, Trowell speculated that the prolonged intake of fiber-depleted starch promoted the development of diabetes in the genetically susceptible individual.[97] He then formulated the dietary fiber hypothesis of the etiology of diabetes. Epidemiologic data support the concept that a low-fiber intake correlates with a higher prevalence of diabetes.[98]

The therapeutic value of fiber for diabetic individuals became evident over the last decade. In 1976 the Oxford group reported that fiber supplements reduced postprandial glycemic responses[99] while the Kentucky group reported that high-fiber diets decreased insulin requirements of lean diabetic individuals.[100] Both groups have extended their studies,[82,83,101,102] and many other groups have confirmed and extended the observations that either fiber-supplemented diets or high-fiber

diets benefit individuals with diabetes (Table 57–10).

Table 57–11 summarizes the pros and cons for recommending an increased fiber intake for diabetic individuals. For many individuals the advantages outweigh the disadvantages. Increased fiber intake usually improves glycemic control and reduces insulin requirements. Obviously, individuals with insulin resistance or type II diabetes obtain greater benefits from high-fiber diets than do insulinopenic individuals with type I diabetes. Our group reports major benefits for adults with type I or II diabetes.[115] We observe reductions in insulin requirements of 25 to 100% for these individuals. Children may receive small benefits (reductions in insulin requirements of up to 25%, better glycemic control, and lower blood lipids), but the disadvantages (those listed in Table 57–11 plus those associated with any strict regimentation of food selection) must be weighed with the advantages.

The benefits of increased fiber intake are seen most clearly when higher-carbohydrate, lower-fat diets composed of commonly available food are used. Soluble fiber supplements in palatable forms also offer benefits.[116,117] Most authorities recommend that increases in fiber intake should focus on fiber-rich foods rather than on fiber supplements for individuals with diabetes.

Concerns about increased fiber intake relate to

**Table 57–10.** **Response of Diabetic Subjects to High-Carbohydrate High-Fiber (HCF) or High-Fiber (HF) Diets Fed for 10 Days or Longer**

| Author | No. of Subjects | Type of Diet | Duration (Days)* | Glucose† | Response of Blood Cholesterol | Triglyceride | Body Weight |
|---|---|---|---|---|---|---|---|
| Anderson[63] | 10 | HCF | 639 | ↓ | ↓ | ↓ | ↓ |
| Anderson[101] | 20 | HCF | 16 | ↓ | ↓ | ↓ | → |
| Anderson[102] | 21 | HCF | 27 | ↓ | ↓ | ↓ | ↓ |
| Anderson[75] | 11 | HCF | 22 | ↓ | ↓ | ↓ | → |
| Anderson[64] | 14 | HCF | 1,940 | ↓ | ↓ | ↓ | → |
| Barnard[103] | 60 | HCF | 26 | ↓ | ↓ | ↓ | ↓ |
| Barnard[104] | 69 | HCF | 913 | ↓ | ↓ | → | → |
| Hjollund[56] | 9 | HCF | 21 | ↓ | ↓ | → | → |
| Karlstrom[68] | 14 | HF | 21 | ↓ | → | → | → |
| Kay[105] | 5 | HF | 14 | ↓ | | | → |
| Kinmonth[67] | 10 | HF | 42 | ↓ | | | |
| Kiehm[100] | 13 | HCF | 21 | ↓ | ↓ | ↓ | ↓ |
| Lindsay[106] | 12 | HCF | 14 | → | | | ↑ |
| Ney[65] | 20 | HCF | 119 | ↓ | | | |
| Pedersen[107] | 40 | HCF | 28 | ↓ | ↓ | → | ↑ |
| Riccardi[108] | 14 | HCF | 10 | ↓ | ↓ | ↓ | |
| Rivellese[109] | 8 | HCF | 10 | ↓ | ↓ | ↓ | |
| Rosman[110] | 10 | HF | 91 | ↓ | | | |
| Simpson[111] | 14 | HCF | 42 | ↓ | ↓ | → | → |
| Simpson[112] | 11 | HCF | 42 | ↓ | ↓ | | |
| Simpson[66] | 27 | HCF | 42 | ↓ | | | |
| Simpson[113] | 10 | HCF | 42 | ↑ | → | → | |
| Taskinen[114] | 21 | HCF | 42 | ↓ | ↓ | → | |

*Average number of follow-up days.
†Mean plasma glucose values or insulin requirements.

**Table 57–11.** **High-Fiber Intake: Advantages and Disadvantages**

| | |
|---|---|
| Advantages | Slows nutrient digestion and absorption |
| | Decreases postprandial plasma glucose |
| | Increases tissue insulin sensitivity |
| | Increases insulin receptor number |
| | Stimulates glucose use |
| | Attenuates hepatic glucose output |
| | Decreases counter-regulatory hormone release (such as glucagon) |
| | Lowers serum cholesterol |
| | Lowers fasting and postprandial serum triglycerides |
| | May attenuate hepatic cholesterol synthesis |
| Disadvantages | Increases intestinal gas |
| | Temporarily may cause abdominal discomfort of GI distress |
| | May alter availability of minerals |

gastrointestinal side effects and possible mineral depletion.[118] Increasing fiber intake increases intestinal gas production, with more eructations and more flatulence—social liabilities in Western society. Our group has approximately 6,000 patient years of experience with high-fiber diets in both inpatients (250 patients studied on a metabolic ward) and outpatients (over 1,000 outpatients followed for up to 10 years). All of our hospitalized patients tolerated individualized high-fiber diets providing 65 to 70 g fiber daily for periods of two to six weeks of study. All patients have more gas, most notice increased stool bulk, some have more frequent bowel movements, and occasionally they complain of diarrhea. For the first one to four days some have mild abdominal distention and occasionally complain of abdominal discomfort. These symptoms subside, and they continue the diet.

Outpatients note more symptoms related to increased fiber intake than do inpatients. Although the diets used for outpatients are lower in fiber (50 g or 20 to 25 g/1,000 kcal daily), these individuals have less experience with using high-fiber foods and may overbalance their diet in the use, for example, of wheat bran. Several women, perhaps with underlying irritable bowel disease, have been unable to tolerate increased fiber intake because of gastrointestinal symptoms. The majority of our patients accept and tolerate the two- to threefold increase in fiber intake quite well. When they complain of excessive gas, we advise them to avoid wheat bran and moderate legume use. These simple instructions usually permit them to continue the diet without undue symptoms.

Mineral or vitamin depletion has not been observed in our patients.[119] Others report high-fiber diets using commonly available foods are not associated with alterations in vitamin or mineral status.[120] Nevertheless, as a precaution, we prescribe a therapeutic vitamin and mineral supplement (e.g., Theragram M).

## A Prudent Nutrition Plan

After generations of controversy, many diabetologists appear to have reached a consensus regarding the diet prescription. In the last decade national diabetes associations from several countries recommended a nutrition plan that includes generous amounts of complex carbohydrate and fiber with restrictions of fat and cholesterol.[121–123] Table 57–12 summarized these recommendations. To reduce the risk for atherosclerotic heart disease, the American Heart Association recommends that the general public increase complex carbohydrate intake and restrict fat and cholesterol intake.[53] To reduce the risks for certain forms of cancer (especially colon, breast, and prostate), the American Cancer Society and National Cancer Institute recommend a general increase in complex carbohydrate and fiber intake and a reduction in fat intake.[124,125] Thus, current nutrition recommendations for persons with diabetes include all the nutriton principles of a prudent or health-promoting diet.

Carbohydrates should usually provide 50 to 60% of energy for diabetic persons, but up to 70% is well tolerated. This level of carbohydrate intake facilitates diabetes management in children as well as adults, in type I as well as type II diabetes. Complex carbohydrate should account for approximately two thirds of total carbohydrate. Unrefined carbohydrates in their natural fiber packages have advantages over highly refined carbohydrates. In the education process, many unfounded concerns about carbohydrate intake need to be addressed. Current recommendations do not consider the different glycemic responses to different foods.[82] Individuals should be alerted to these differences (see Table 57–6) to monitor their own response to specific items in their diet.

Protein should provide 12 to 20% of energy intake. When diets include substantial quantities of vegetables, cereals, breads, and legumes, 25 to 50% of the protein comes from vegetable sources. Some are concerned that generous intakes of protein may be associated with intrarenal hypertension and may contribute to development of azotemia and renal failure.[126] This hypothesis, based on studies in experimental animals, has not been substantiated in humans. To accommodate the usual eating patterns that include regular intake of red meat and poultry and to meet the need for vegetables, grains, and beans, we usually prescribe diets providing 18 to 20% of energy as protein.[127]

Fat intake should not exceed 35% of energy; intakes ranging from 20 to 30% are desirable. Saturated fat intake should not exceed 10% of energy intake, and cholesterol intake should not exceed 300 mg/day.[121] Polyunsaturated fats, (e.g., vegetable oil) are preferred to saturated fats (e.g., butter), but both should be restricted. Intake of polyunsaturated fats also should not exceed 10% of energy intake. These recommendations are consistent with those of the American Heart Association and several other groups.[53,124,125,128] One of the most important elements of a prudent diet is a reasonable restriction of fat intake.

Generous intakes of dietary fiber improve glycemic control and lower serum lipid values of diabetic individuals.[115,118] However, no specific recommendations for fiber intake have been developed. We have used diets providing approximately 50 g of fiber daily (about 25 g/1,000 kcal) for 10 years (approximately 6,000 patient years of experience).[127] Based on our experience, these diets are effective and have no consequential side effects or discernible effects on vitamin or mineral status.[119] Intake of total dietary fiber in several Western countries averages about 20 g/day (8 to 12 g/1,000 kcal).[129] A dietary fiber intake of 30 to 50 g/day should be safe and well tolerated. The measurable benefits appear to outweigh the potential side effects. High-fiber intakes are not recommended for individuals with inflammatory bowel disease.

Most recommend that an increase in fiber intake

**Table 57–12.  Comparison of Nutrition Recommendations for Persons with Diabetes**

| Component | Diabetes Associations Recommendations | High-Fiber Maintenance Diet |
|---|---|---|
| Carbohydrate (CHO) | 45–60% | 55–60% |
|  | Complex CHO emphasized | 60–70% complex CHO |
|  | Simple CHO restricted | 30–40% simple CHO |
| Protein | 12–25% | 15–20% |
| Fat | 30–38% | 20–30% |
| Cholesterol | <400 mg/d to not limited | <300 mg/d |
| Fiber | Encouraged from food sources | 35–60 g/d |
|  |  | ~20–25 g/1,000 kcal |

come from high-fiber foods rather than from purified fiber supplements. Guar supplements have well-documented benefits but are not available in palatable form at present. The benefits of other fiber supplements, ranging from wheat bran to formulated fiber supplements for diabetic individuals, are not established.

### Sweeteners

Most people consume sweetened beverages, baked goods, desserts, or other "sweets." Diabetic individuals should avoid foods that worsen their glycemic control or foster weight gain, but they should not be denied foods they enjoy that are safe and compatible with their nutrition plan. Although diabetic individuals cannot entirely avoid foods containing glucose, sucrose, or fructose, they should use discretion in the amount used. Foods containing high amounts of these sugars may produce hyperglycemia and weight gain. These foods often have high fat and energy contents as well. The use of modest amounts of sorbitol, mannitol, or xylitol probably poses no risk to diabetic or nondiabetic individuals.[130]

Fructose offers advantages over sucrose for diabetic individuals because it tastes sweeter, is metabolized without insulin, and produces less hyperglycemia. Although fructose may increase the blood glucose in poorly controlled diabetic individuals, it is well metabolized by well-controlled diabetic and nondiabetic persons. It produces only 20% of the glycemic response of glucose and 33% of the response of sucrose in well- or fairly well-controlled persons with type I or type II diabetes.[82] Thus, substituting fructose for glucose and sucrose in the diet lowers average blood glucose values in diabetic individuals. When fructose displaces fat from the diet, improved sensitivity to insulin results. However, the long-term safety of fructose for persons with diabetes is not established. We incorporated 50 g of fructose daily into a prudent diet for 12 diabetic men with IDDM or NIDDM.[131] Over a 24-week period we observed no adverse effects other than a significant weight gain. These and other studies indicate that diabetic individuals can include modest to moderate amounts of fructose with reasonable safety provided they do not gain weight.

Noncaloric or non-nutritive sweeteners enjoy wide use in beverages and other products. Saccharin, in use for over 80 years, may be associated with increased risk for bladder cancer.[132] At present, we recommend that pregnant women avoid saccharin, that children do not exceed two cans of saccharin-sweetened soft drinks daily, and that adults exercise moderation in its use. Although not available in the United States, cyclamates appear somewhat safer than saccharin and are preferred by many users. Aspartame, a dipeptide containing aspartic acid and phenylalanine, appears reasonably safe for individuals without phenylketonuria.[133] This sweetener with negligible caloric value appears to offer major advantages for diabetic individuals provided they avoid excessive energy intake. Practical guidelines for patients outline the availability of United States sweeteners.[134]

### Alcohol

Alcohol in moderation poses no greater health risk for diabetic than for nondiabetic individuals provided they follow sensible guidelines.[135,136] In addition to the general concerns about the habituating and toxic effects of alcohol, the person with diabetes has these specific concerns: moderate or severe hypoglycemia due to alcohol inhibition of hepatic glucose output; excessive energy intake; disruption of usual eating patterns; flushing, dizziness, and nausea when alcohol and oral sulfonylurea agents are used by some individuals; and aggravation or production of hypertriglyceridemia. However, most diabetic adults can safely have an occasional drink with meals.

Alcohol drinks are rich in energy and poor in nutrients. The average mixed drink provides 110 kcal from alcohol, or energy equivalent to 2.5 fat exchanges. A glass of dry wine contains 70 to 90 kcal, equivalent to 1.5 to 2 fat exchanges, and a 12-ounce glass of "light" beer has 90 to 110 kcal, equivalent to 2 fat exchanges. Because the energy contribution of alcohol should not exceed 6% of daily intake,[135] most individuals should not consume more than two glasses of dry wine or one mixed drink or two beers daily.

Individuals who wish to use alcohol should be given the following practical guidelines: 1. Discuss the use of alcohol with your physician and nutrition counselor. 2. Do not drink with an empty stomach. 3. Drink slowly. 4. Avoid sugary, sweetened drinks. 5. Estimate the caloric value of alcohol drinks and make appropriate changes in food intake. 6. Do not drive after drinking. 7. Use moderation and never drink to the extent that judgment is impaired.

### Other Considerations

**Obesity.** Obesity is the major contributor to diabetes in adults. Weight loss using diet and exercise is the treatment of choice; insulin use to control hyperglycemia is controversial. Oral hypoglycemic agents are useful for selected individuals as an adjunct to diet and exercise. Neither insulin nor drugs, however, should substitute for a strong emphasis on weight reduction.

The obese individual must be self-motivated to lose weight. We offer intensive weight-reduction programs to diabetic individuals but do not enroll them until they express enthusiasm and demonstrate commitment. Diaries of food intake, exercise, and blood or urine glucose values are important parts of the weight-loss regimen. Group sessions at weekly intervals and behavior modification techniques assist in maintaining motivation.[137] In addition to weight loss, favorable changes in glycemic control, insulin or drug requirements, blood pressure, or blood lipids provide positive reinforcement. Elimination of insulin need enables some individuals to lose weight more rapidly because they feel less hungry (from a physiologic or psychologic basis) and can exercise without fear of hypoglycemia. Enhancing and sustaining motivation require perception and ingenuity for the therapist.

Many safe diet choices are available. The safest program is one that modestly restricts energy and provides adequate amounts of protein, carbohydrate, minerals, and vitamins. For outpatients with reasonable glycemic control we use a generous carbohydrate and fiber diet. With modest caloric restriction (about 9 kcal/lb) and exercise, weight losses of 1 to 2 pounds weekly can be achieved. This regimen slowly improves glycemic control and sometimes decreases the need for exogenous insulin.

With poor glycemic control, despite large insulin doses, more vigorous intervention is indicated. We usually hospitalize persons for severe energy-restricted diets (about 3 kcal/lb). These diets (600 to 1,000 kcal/day) supply 55% of energy as carbohydrate, 45 to 60 g protein per day, and the remainder of energy from fat. We also provide vitamin and mineral supplements. With this program, individuals lose about 5 pounds per week and have improved blood glucose and lipid values with lower insulin needs. Insulin can be discontinued in 80 to 90% of type II diabetic individuals treated in this manner (Fig. 57–9). After 7 to 14 days of intensive therapy in the hospital, individuals are discharged on diets providing about 5 kcal/lb of current body weight. Other centers use very low-calorie diets,[138] supplemented fasts,[139] or protein-sparing modified fasts[140] with similar results for poorly controlled individuals.

Regular exercise plays a key part of the weight-loss regimen of most individuals. Exercise recommendations are individualized. Walking is the best exercise for most obese persons. They can usually begin walking 10 to 30 minutes once or twice daily and increase this amount gradually over a few weeks to 30 minutes twice daily. A treadmill is a good alternative to walking. Swimming or use of an exercise bicycle or rowing machine are satisfactory alternatives if arthritis or other problems do not favor walking. Exercise after meals enhances diet-induced thermogenesis, thus promoting a greater energy deficit. In addition to weight loss, cardiovascular fitness as well as blood glucose and lipids improve with exercise.

**Hyperlipidemia.** Diabetic individuals show more tendency toward undesirably high serum cholesterol or triglyceride values than nondiabetic individuals.[40] Good glycemic control, attaining and maintaining a desirable body weight, regular exercise, moderation in alcohol use, and a prudent diet—practices recommended for all diabetic individuals—reduce hyperlipidemia. Ideally, fasting serum cholesterol and triglyceride values should be less than 200 mg/dl. When values exceed these targets, the diabetic individual receives specific nutrition counseling directed at lowering serum cholesterol or triglyceride values. When serum cholesterol values exceed 260 mg/dl or triglycerides exceed 400 mg/dl, intensive nutrition management is instituted.

Hypercholesterolemia responds to nutrition management. Those with serum cholesterol concentrations below 350 mg/dl can usually achieve desirable serum cholesterol values with dietary measures, whereas individuals with higher values require dietary and pharmacologic intervention. The effective nutrition management of hypercholesterolemia includes: a generous intake of complex carbohydrate and fiber with carbohydrate contributing more than 55% of energy; limiting of cholesterol intake to less than 300 mg/day; restriction of fat intake to less than 30% of energy; and the inclusion of adequate quantities of water-soluble fiber from oat products and beans. Soluble fibers have specific hypocholesterolemic effects.[141] Our studies indicate the generous intake of oat bran or beans lowers serum cholesterol concentrations by 20% initially and maintains these reductions for up to two years.[142,143] Weight reduction to a lean body weight, regular exercise, and other measures are also useful.

Hypertriglyceridemia responds well to nutrition intervention, although good glycemic control takes first priority. Persons with hypertriglyceridemia should avoid alcohol, reduce fat intake, restrict energy intake, and include generous amounts of complex carbohydrate and fiber. Using a prudent diet (55% of energy from carbohydrate) that provides plant fiber from a variety of sources (about 50 g/day or 25 g/1,000 kcal) effectively lowers serum triglycerides for most individuals.[115] Weight loss to a lean weight, exercise, and avoiding excessive intake of simple carbohydrates are also helpful measures. Hypertriglyceridemia can

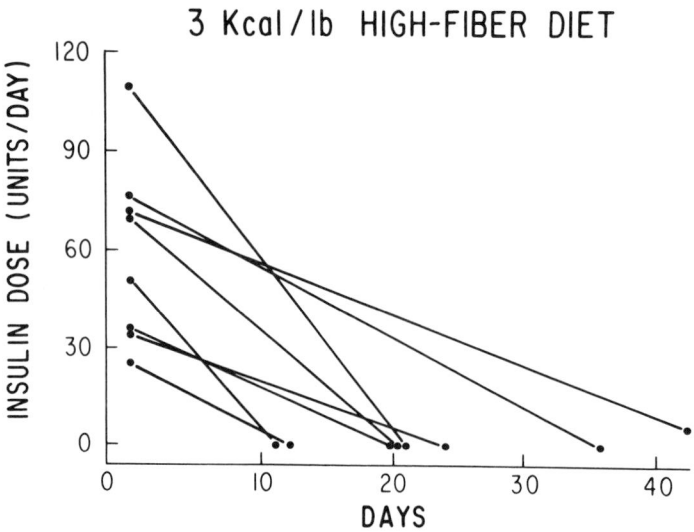

**Fig. 57–9.** Reduction of insulin dose for obese diabetic men fed high-fiber weight-reduction diets (3 kcal/lb).

usually be controlled by intensive nutrition intervention alone.[144]

**Pregnancy.** Pregnancy changes eating habits, exercise patterns, emotional states, insulin sensitivity, and hormone secretions.[145–147] These changes alter blood glucose control and insulin requirements. As placental and ovarian hormones decrease insulin sensitivity, the nondiabetic woman secretes more insulin to maintain satisfactory blood glucose levels. Between 1 and 3% of women lack the pancreatic reserve to meet this challenge and develop gestational diabetes. This condition usually abates after delivery, but these women are more likely to develop diabetes during subsequent pregnancies or later life. In pregnancy, thus, the most common diabetes problems are gestational diabetes and pregestational insulin-requiring diabetes. For all diabetic women the reduction of maternal, fetal, and perinatal risks requires excellent blood glucose control.

Insulin requirements change dramatically during pregnancy. To sustain a healthy fetus, the diabetic individual must adjust her nutrient intake and insulin dose to maintain excellent blood glucose levels and avoid ketosis. Maternal ketonemia causes more harm to the fetus than does hypoglycemia. During the first half of pregnancy, insulin requirements drop by 20 to 30% owing to decreased food intake and increased glucose uptake by the fetus and placenta. During the second half of pregnancy, insulin requirements rise by 60 to 100% above prepregnancy levels because of placental hormone production and insulin resistance related to other factors. After delivery

and removal of the placenta, insulin requirements drop precipitously. Much smaller doses are required the week after delivery, but requirements gradually increase to prepregnancy levels by six weeks after delivery. Proper adjustment of insulin therapy during the pregnancy and postpartum period requires careful blood glucose monitoring.

The nutrition goals during pregnancy include meeting nutrition needs and maintaining excellent blood glucose control. In time sequence these goals are: to achieve excellent blood glucose control before gestation and during the early weeks of pregnancy to reduce the risks of congenital malformations; to provide energy intake for a weight gain of approximately 25 pounds; to meet the increased protein needs; to provide carbohydrate to minimize ketosis and to meet the needs of the fetus and placenta; to optimize tissue sensitivity to insulin; and, during the critical three to four weeks prior to delivery, to maintain excellent blood glucose control.

Requirements for most nutrients increase with pregnancy and are similar for diabetic and nondiabetic women. During the first trimester most women should gain two to four pounds; this gain can be achieved by increasing energy intake by 100 kcal/day. During the second and third trimesters they should gain about one pound per week, which is achieved by increasing energy intake by 15% or 300 kcal/day. To meet increased needs, the intake of high-quality protein is increased by 30 g/day to at least 1.3 g protein/kg of body weight. Carbohydrate should provide at least 50% of the energy intake. Some individuals benefit from higher intakes of complex carbohydrate and fiber.[65] Fat should provide the remaining percentage of energy intake (25 to 30%). Most women require supplemental iron and folic acid; a multiple vitamin and mineral supplement including these is usually provided. A sound nutrition plan increases the likelihood of a successful pregnancy.

## GESTATIONAL DIABETES

Gestational diabetes presents a special challenge. These individuals usually remain unaware they have diabetes until it is discovered during pregnancy. They need intensive education. Furthermore, they are often obese and require a diet permitting a steady weight gain of 20 to 25 pounds but limiting excessive gains. Pregnancy is not the time for weight reduction. These individuals must also maintain good blood glucose control and, if necessary, use insulin to reduce risks of fetal macrosomatia, neonatal hypoglycemia, and perinatal mortality. Glucose tolerance tests and periodic blood glucose measurements are important for high-risk individuals because early control of hyperglycemia decreases the risks for the fetus and neonate.

## PREGNANCY AND INSULIN-DEPENDENT DIABETES

With type I diabetes, a successful pregnancy requires planning, investment of time and money, and commitment. Because poorly controlled diabetes threatens the health of the mother and the safety of the fetus and newborn, most women make these commitments. To reduce the risks of congenital malformations, excellent glycemic control prior to conception and during early pregnancy is necessary. Maintaining excellent glycemic control throughout pregnancy demands careful attention to diet, exercise, and insulin dose adjustments. Health professionals take responsibility for educating women about the special needs during pregnancy, with the patient, physician, dietitian, and nurse educator working as a team to accomplish goals.

Nutrition management plans for pregnant and nonpregnant women with insulin-dependent diabetes are similar, but pregnancy necessitates greater attention to the day-to day nutrition plan. Guidance during early pregnancy includes special consideration for food cravings or nausea. An individualized nutrition plan that evolves throughout pregnancy is essential to meet changing nutrition needs and insulin requirements. Three meals and three snacks usually supply energy requirements in a timely fashion to avoid hypoglycemia.

The pregnant diabetic woman requires intensive management to achieve a successful outcome. Frequent office visits and vigorous nutrition therapy are necessary. Using frequent home blood glucose measurements, the individual maintains fasting blood glucose values below 100 mg/dl and random values less than 150 mg/dl while avoiding frequent or severe hypoglycemic reactions. The health care team monitors the fetus and assesses fetal maturity to select the optimal time and mode for delivery. Hospitalization may be necessary to reestablish blood glucose control; early hospitalization for glycemic control prior to delivery is advisable. Finally, intensive neonatal management is essential. Employing these principles reduces maternal risk to that of the nondiabetic woman and reduces fetal and neonatal risk to near that of their offspring.

## DIABETES IN CHILDREN

Diabetes affects 1 in 700 school-age children in the United States. Children with diabetes cannot be treated as small adults; they have special needs and should not be immersed in an adult-oriented therapeutic program. Health care team members need special skills and interests to communicate effectively with the child and his parents. A nutrition plan must be practical and tailored to the needs of the individual child. Management strategies incorporate short, intermediate, and long-term goals.[148,149]

Immediate treatment should alleviate symptoms and restore a sense of "feeling good." Short-term objectives include eliminating polydipsia, polyuria, and polyphagia; preventing ketonuria, ketonemia, and ketoacidosis; avoiding hypoglycemia; and minimizing energy losses associated with heavy glycosuria. After elimination of symptoms, therapy helps the children resume their usual activities.

Intermediate objectives include: satisfactory glycemic control, normal serum cholesterol and triglyceride values, and normal physical growth and development without obesity. Other aims are the development of a prudent nutrition plan incorporated into the child's life-style and a high level of physical fitness. Both the child and parents are educated about diabetes so they can participate intelligently in its management. Gradually children assume increased responsibilities for their own daily care and management. The child should develop increasing self-reliance, and parents should avoid overprotectiveness. The child with diabetes should function as a normal family member and should not be singled out for special attention at school.

The ultimate goal in the management of the diabetic child is the development of a well-adjusted, healthy adult without physical or psychosocial limitations. Long-term objectives include: maturing to adulthood with appropriate intellectual, emotional, and physical capabilities; preventing diabetic complications; and minimizing the likelihood of atherosclerotic vascular disease.

To achieve these goals, one must make the nutrition plan individualized and flexible. It must evolve to meet changing requirements with growth and be continually reassessed. The nutrition plan must promote acceptable glycemic control and normal blood lipids. A generous carbohydrate and fiber intake coupled with a restricted fat intake offers the same advantages for children as for adults with diabetes. During periods of rapid growth or high energy requirements, more refined carbohydrates (starches and, to a limited extent, sugars) and fat can be included to meet energy needs. Carbohydrates need not be distributed evenly throughout the day. As a general rule, each main meal provides at least 20% of daily energy requirements. Using this guideline, one develops meal plans according to the preferences of the child. After the meal plan is established, insulin doses are adjusted to achieve suitable glycemic control; we do not manipulate meal patterns to attain glycemic control. The child receives guidelines to increase or decrease energy intake with snacks in anticipation of variable physical activity. Insulin doses also are adjusted for unusually active or sedentary (rainy) days. Adjusting food intake and insulin doses according to energy needs requires ingenuity and meticulous attention to blood glucose levels.

## INSULIN THERAPY[150]

Human insulin, available since 1980, represents a major breakthrough for the treatment of diabetes. Human insulin is manufactured either by biosynthesis in bacterial cells using recombinant DNA technology or by chemical conversion of pork insulin into human insulin. Both products are virtually free of impurities. Currently, highly purified pork, beef, or beef-pork mixtures also are available. These highly purified human or pork insulins have major clinical advantages over the less purified preparations used before 1980.

Many different insulin preparations are now marketed. Table 57–13 compares preparations widely used in the United States. The clinical effects of NPH insulin, an intermediate-acting insulin, differ from those of Lente insulin, another intermediate-acting insulin. Furthermore, the clinical effects of human NPH insulin differ from those of pork NPH insulin. Because of these differences, health professionals must be careful in changing treatment programs; they must be alert

to what preparation the person is using and ensure that he follows the recommendations accurately.

Physicians commonly prescribe the following regimens (their use and limitations are listed):

*Single dose.* From 5 to 30 units of intermediate-acting (e.g., NPH) insulin daily is often an adequate program for the type II diabetic individual with limited endogenous insulin secretion who needs supplemental insulin. Rarely is this approach suitable for the type I individual. When taken before breakfast, NPH insulin can cause hypoglycemia before the evening meal, before bedtime, or during the night; large doses (over 30 units) of NPH insulin before breakfast commonly cause nocturnal reactions. Individuals taking NPH insulin before breakfast may require a mid-afternoon or bedtime snack.

*Single injection, two insulins.* Using a mixture of intermediate-acting (e.g., NPH) and rapid-acting (e.g., regular) insulin in the same syringe before breakfast is a suitable program for some type II individuals, but rarely is adequate for the type I individual. With this regimen, persons often need mid-morning, mid-afternoon, and bedtime snacks.

*Two Injections.* Most persons with type I diabetes require at least two insulin injections and measurements of their own blood glucose daily for acceptable glycemic control. They commonly use a mixture of intermediate-acting (e.g., NPH) and rapid-acting (e.g., regular) insulins before breakfast and a second injectin (e.g., NPH plus regular insulin) before the evening meal. With this insulin regimen, they eat three meals at regularly scheduled times and have mid-morning, mid-afternoon, and bedtime snacks. Each meal provides 20 to 35% of daily energy intake, and each snack provides 5 to 15% of energy intake. Carbohydrate intake dose not need to be distributed because a generous carbohydrate intake (50 to 60% of energy) and a sensible meal plan ensure a reasonable distribution throughout the day.

*Three or more injections.* Certain type I individuals require three or more insulin injections and two or more blood glucose measurements daily to maintain satisfactory glycemic control. Some use insulin infusion pumps and frequent blood glucose measurements. These programs require injections or bolus infusions of rapid-acting (e.g., regular) insulin before each meal. One or two injections of intermediate (e.g., NPH) or long-acting (e.g., Ultralente) insulin may be used daily. These persons need three meals and usually three snacks daily. The timing of meals is more flexible, and the pre-meal dose of rapid-acting insulin can be adjusted for the energy and carbohydrate content of the meal.[151]

**Table 57–13.   Insulin Preparations**

| Action | Preparation | Peak Activity (hrs.) | Duration (hrs.) |
|--------|-------------|---------------------|-----------------|
| Fast | Regular | 1–3 | 5–7 |
|  | Semilente | 3–6 | 12–16 |
| Intermediate | NPH | 6–14 | 18–28 |
|  | Lente | 6–14 | 18–28 |
| Long | Ultralente | 18–24 | 30–40 |
|  | Protamine zinc (PZI) | 14–24 | 30–40 |

Home blood glucose monitoring is essential for achieving satisfactory glycemic control for most persons with diabetes.[151] This development is one of the most important advances since the discovery of insulin. With appropriate finger-pricking devices, a large drop of blood can be obtained with minimal discomfort. This is applied to a blood glucose test strip, and the blood glucose value is read visually or with a blood glucose meter in 1 to 2 minutes. When carefully done, these glucose measurements are as accurate as those taken in the clinical laboratory. This tool enables many diabetic individuals to maintain good to excellent glycemic control and still have a flexible schedule.

## ORAL HYPOGLYCEMIC AGENTS[152]

Sulfonylurea agents are widely used for adults with diabetes. They lower blood glucose values by increasing insulin secretion and enhancing peripheral sensitivity to insulin. Individuals who develop diabetes after 40 years of age, who have had diabetes for less than five years, and who either have not received insulin therapy or are well controlled with 20 units or less daily are likely to respond well to oral agent therapy. Normal-weight and obese persons are better candidates for drug therapy than underweight individuals.

Six agents are widely available (Table 57–14). All sulfonylureas appear to have the same mechanisms of action, but they differ in potency, duration of action, and metabolic fate. The second-generation drugs are more potent than the first-generation agents and have other advantages. Individuals who do not have good glycemic control on first-generation agents may be tried on the second-generation ones before starting insulin therapy.

For noninsulin-dependent (type II) persons with diabetes, diet and exercise remain the cornerstones of management. Sulfonylurea drugs are adjunctive. Unfortunately, diabetic individuals frequently gain weight after starting these drugs. Weight gain further worsens insulin resistance and increases the risk for atherosclerotic vascular disease. Thus, oral agents do not replace the need for a prudent diet but rather are combined with diet to avoid insulin need for some individuals. The critical importance of diet needs to be reinforced when oral agents are initiated.

## INDIVIDUALIZATION

To be effective over the long term, the health care team must tailor the nutrition plan to the needs of the individual. Preprinted diet sheets, readily available, provide clues to changes in eating habits but allow no flexibility and are doomed to eventual failure. Although the effects of diet components (carbohydrate and fat, especially) have been extensively studied, implementing the

**Table 57–14.   Selected Characteristics of Sulfonylureas**

| Compound | Daily Dose (mg/day) | Metabolism | Duration of Hypoglycemic Action/Hours | Doses/ Day |
|----------|---------------------|------------|---------------------------------------|------------|
| FIRST-GENERATION |  |  |  |  |
| Tolbutamide | 250–3,000 | Hepatic | 6–12 | 2–3 |
| Tolazamide | 100–1,000 | Hepatic | 12–14 | 1–2 |
| Acetohexamide | 250–1,500 | Hepatic | 12–18 | 1–2 |
| Chlorpropamide | 50–500 | Not metabolized | 60 | 1 |
| SECOND-GENERATION |  |  |  |  |
| Glyburide | 2.5–20 | Hepatic | 24 | 1–2 |
| Glipizide | 2.5–40 | Hepatic | 12–24 | 1–2 |

Adapted from Lebovitz, H.E.: Clinical Diabetes, July/August, 1984.

diet has received less attention. Good nutrition plans don't work if people don't follow them.

Initially, the physician or health care team member must realistically assess the motivation and capabilities of the diabetic individual and his family or support group. An optimistic approach is imperative; previous failures do not necessarily breed failure with a nutrition plan at this point. The individual may be unable to learn an exchange system and may need to be taught a "no-added-sugar" plan. Shortly after the diagnosis of diabetes, some individuals are best taught a "survival" diet, with more detailed nutrition education provided when they are better able to cope with their condition.

After this general evaluation, the dietitian or nutritionist assesses exercise habits, work schedule, socioeconomic level, living situation, and past eating habits. Diet recalls, food records, or surveys of the frequency of food use provide useful information on eating habits. A history or recall of food eaten in the past 24 hours is a practical way to estimate energy intake and percentge contribution of carbohydrate, protein, and fat. A seven-day survey of the frequency of food use offers a better overview of food intake. To obtain accurate information, the interviewer uses non-judgmental questions. "What do you usually have for breakfast?" is preferable to "Do you always have eggs for breakfast?" A diet diary kept for one or more days before the nutrition interview also provides a window for viewing the energy and nutrient intake. Finally, the food preferences, likes and dislikes, are elicited. All of this information about prior food use forms the foundation for building a solid nutrition plan.

Desirable body weight estimations also are made during the initial nutrition assessment. After obtaining a weight history (lightest and heaviest adult weights, recent weight changes, prior use of weight-reducing regimens), we often ask the individual how much he would like to weigh or what a "good" weight for him is. Ideally the individual identifies a good weight goal and we avoid having to designate a weight that he considers unrealistic. Desirable body weight estimations from tables or formulas provide guidance in setting weight goals. The diabetic individual and dietitian must work together to develop mutual targets for short- and long-term weight. The simple process of establishing an estimate of desirable body weight signals to the diabetic individual that the management of his condition is a partnership venture.

Developing the specific nutrition plan is the next step. Based on the available information, the dietitian and physician decide which nutrition

strategy best suits the individual. For some, a plan avoiding sucrose and foods rich in sucrose and other sugars (a "no-added-sugar" diet) works best. For others a plan using food exchanges is more appropriate. The next section outlines steps used to develop such a plan. Some individuals are good candidates for high-fiber diets. Once the team establishes a basic plan, they need to modify it for other conditions such as congestive heart failure. They also determine the energy level of the diet.

Tailoring the diet to the specific individual is probably the most difficult task in the management of diabetes. In doing so, the dietitian must consider treatment regimen (frequency and type of insulin injections or use of oral hypoglycemic agents), activity level, work schedule, meal schedule, food preferences, and other factors. The individualized nutrition plan should be as compatible as possible with the food habits and lifestyle of the patient. However, an effective nutrition plan usually requires ·change. The dietitian should develop the most therapeutically effective plan and train the diabetic individual and support persons to use this plan.

## FOOD EXCHANGES

Flexibility, a critical element, emerged slowly as an integral part of the diabetes nutrition plan. Joining forces, the American Diabetes Association and the American Dietetic Association released the Exchange Lists for Meal Planning in 1950. These "ADA Exchanges" were revised in 1976 (see Appendix). Other exchanges have been developed using the same principles. Exchange nutrition plans provide flexibility and choice while maintaining consistency from day to day.

Exchanges include foods of similar nutrient composition; all serving sizes or portions in one exchange provide similar amounts of energy, carbohydrate, protein, and fat. Using an ADA Exchange Diet, an individual chooses a certain number of items from each of six food groups daily. Since each exchange group includes many different foods, the individual's diet can be quite varied.

Although several methods of diet instruction are available, Exchange Nutrition Plans are widely used by health professionals. When individuals change health care providers, use of a universally understood nutrition plan facilitates communication and continuity of care.

**A Step-by-Step Guide to Exchange Diet Calculations.** First, estimate the energy needs of the patient for weight maintenance, tables (see Appendix) or diet histories provide guidance. As a rough approximation, allow 13 kcal/lb (present or current weight) for sedentary adults, 15 to 16 kcal/lb for moderately active adults, and 20 kcal/lb for very active adults. This estimation may need to be modified at a subsequent visit. For weight reduction, eliminate approximately 500 kcals daily for a weight loss of roughly one pound per week. Weight loss can be enhanced by exercise after meals.

Second, distribute energy intake between carbohydrate, protein, and fat. Carbohydrate usually contributes 50 to 60% of energy intake, protein contributes 12 to 20%, and fat provides the balance (20 to 30%). For example, a 2,000-kcal diet to provide 55% carbohydrate, 18% protein, and 27% fat would have: 55% carbohydrate = 1,100 kcal or 275 g (1,100 ÷ 4); 18% protein = 360 kcal or 90 g (360 ÷ 4); 27% fat = 540 kcal or 60 g (540 ÷ 9).

Third, set the number of servings from the exchange list to provide the desired grams of carbohydrate, protein, and fat. With experience, you can quickly estimate the number of exchanges required to approximate the target amounts. Food preferences also are incorporated at this stage. Table 57–15 illustrates a work sheet used to develop exchange lists for the sample 2,000-kcal diet. On the bottom line, list the target grams of carbohydrate, protein, and fat. Then estimate the number of exchanges needed to meet the target amounts by assigning servings of milk, then vegetables, fruits, and grain products to meet the carbohydrate target; meat required to meet the protein target; and finally fat. Many alternative exchange lists can be developed, including ones without milk (for the lactose-intolerant individual) and ones without meat (for the vegetarian).

Fourth, assign these exchanges to meals and snacks. Our group routinely develops meal plans to include three meals and an evening snack. For most persons taking insulin, we develop plans with mid-morning and mid-afternoon snacks as well. Distribute energy intake according to these guidelines: the three main meals should provide at least 65% of energy intake and snacks should provide up to 35%. Breakfast has 20 to 30%, the noon meal has 20 to 35%, and the evening meal has 25 to 40% of energy intake. Snacks provide 0 to 15% at mid-morning, 0 to 15% at mid-afternoon, and 0 to 15% in the evening. Insulin-treated individuals should be advised how to increase their food intake in response to exercise.

As an optional fifth step, compute the fiber content of the diet. Based on the fiber values (see Appendix), one can calculate that the diet example provides 12 g of fiber from vegetables, at least 22 g from breads and starches, and 12 g from fruits for a total of at least 46 g. This is a generous fiber diet; higher fiber intakes can be attained using the HCF Exchanges.[153]

## EDUCATION AND COUNSELING

Nutrition instruction and counseling are central to the control of diabetes. Unfortunately, many diabetic individuals do not follow a diet plan either because they have not received adequate education or because they lack the required skills. The low success rate with nutrition therapy in diabetes management has led to a degree of therapeutic nihilism. Some physicians believe nutrition counseling is a waste of time, and many dietitians are frustrated because of the poor dietary adherence of patients. These attitudes and frustrations often undermine the effectiveness of the nutrition program. In our experience, when the entire health care team is enthusiastic and supportive about a nutrition plan, diabetic individuals can change their eating patterns and closely adhere to a diet plan. Approximately 75% of a small selected group of patients adhered closely to a high-fiber maintenance diet for four years, while only 25% adhered poorly to the diet.[64]

The team approach to diabetes management enhances effectiveness. Successful diabetes control requres a partnership between the diabetic and the health care team. The physician, dietitian, and nurse act as coaches who train and assist the individual in the diabetes arena. Effective communication and education require multiple sessions with different team members. The physician and nurse must reinforce the message of the dietitian, just as each team member must be poised

**Table 57–15. Work Sheet for Developing Exchange Lists**

| Exchange | Servings | Carbohydrate | Protein | Fat |
|---|---|---|---|---|
| Milk | 2 | 24 | 16 | 0 |
| Vegetable | 6 | 30 | 12 | 0 |
| Bread | 11 | 165 | 22 | 0 |
| Meat | 6 | 0 | 42 | 18 |
| Fruit | 6 | 60 | 0 | 0 |
| Fat | 8 | 0 | 0 | 40 |
| TOTAL | — | 279 | 92 | 58 |
| TARGET | — | 275 | 90 | 60 |

to reinforce any aspect of the diabetes care program when the opportunity occurs. Education and management of diabetes have become more prevention-oriented and less crisis-oriented. Realizing that teaching is not synonymous with education, more professionals are interacting with patients to transmit knowledge that leads to behavior changes. Diabetes education, though time-consuming, is cost-effective in achieving the long-term goals of diabetes management.

The individualized nutrition plan is a key element of the diabetes education program. Usually the physician introduces the plan by discussing the role of diet in diabetes management and by outlining its critical features. The dietitian then collects information to tailor the diet to the patient. Although group sessions strengthen learning, the dietitian must provide individual instruction for the diabetic individual and others involved in meal preparation. A minimum of two sessions is necessary to initiate diet instruction, and follow-up visits are critical. Ideally, the newly diagnosed diabetic person should receive 6 to 12 hours of nutrition education. Instruction sessions should be short but frequent, allowing the person to assimilate new information, ask questions, and test this information. All team members should be familiar with the main features of the individual's diet plan and provide encouragement and reinforcement at every opportunity. The nurse, for example, will incorporate elements of the individual's diet when discussing prevention and treatment of insulin reactions. Nutrition counselors should also reinforce other features of the treatment plan.

Many hospitals and practice groups channel the expertise of health care team members from different disciplines into diabetes classes. Table 57–16 lists some important topics for consideration in developing diabetes education programs. High-priority items for discussion for a diabetes class include: (1) a description of diabetes, its inheritance, pathogenesis, and aggravating factors (e.g., obesity); (2) medicines for diabetes, such as insulin and oral hypoglycemic agents, and hypoglycemia; (3) meal planning; (4) control of diabetes, with blood and urine testing, and complications; (5) living with diabetes, including exercise, flexibility, and an upbeat discussion on how taking care of diabetes improves health. The diabetes health care team includes a physician, dietitian or nutritionist, and nurse educator; a pharmacist, social worker, psychologist, physical therapist, podiatrist, and exercise physiologist may complement the core team. Effective diabetes education involves communication between

**Table 57–16. Diabetes Education Topics**

Cause and inheritance
Nature of diabetes
Nutrition therapy
Meal planning: exchanges
Desirable body weight maintenance
Insulin and oral hypoglycemic agents
Insulin reactions: recognition, prevention, and treatment
Diabetic ketosis and hyperglycemia
Home glucose testing of blood or urine
Laboratory assessment: glycohemoglobin
Desirable serum lipid levels
Hazards of cigarette smoking
Exercise
Food intake during illness
Eating in restaurants
Adjusting insulin doses
Long-term complications
Foot care
Living with diabetes
Self-motivation
Good health measures
Community resources

experienced and empathetic health professionals and the individual with diabetes.

## CONCLUSION

An individualized nutrition plan is vital to the successful management of diabetes. The diabetic individual and the health care team integrate the nutrition plan into the daily schedule of activities to match the available insulin. Diet, physical activities, and available insulin (endogenous or exogenous) change constantly. The diabetic individual and health care team need the maximal amount of information, experience, and education to respond to these changes. Both short-term and long-term considerations influence the nutrition plan. Feeling good and avoiding trouble, while desirable attributes, should not persuade the diabetic individual or his health care team that the diet plan is optimal. Good glycemic control, desirable serum lipids, and reduction of risk for metabolic, microvascular, and macrovascular complications are the key goals for a diabetes nutrition plan.

## REFERENCES

1. American Diabetes Association: Diabetes Care *7*:505–506, 1984.
2. West, K.M.: Epidemiology of Diabetes and its Vascular Lesions. New York, Elsevier North-Holland, 1978.
3. National Diabetes Advisory Board: Sixth Annual Report. U.S. Department of Health and Human Services. NIH Publication No. 84-1587, May, 1984.
4. Raskin, P., Pietri, A.O., Unger, R., et al.: N. Engl. J. Med. *309*:1546–1550, 1983.
5. Wood, F.C., Jr., Bierman, E.L.: Nutr. Today *7*:4–12, 1972.

6. Rollo, J.: A General View of the History, Nature and Appropriate Treatment of Diabetes Mellitus. T. Gillet for C. Dilly, printer, London, 1798.

7. Allen, F.M.: JAMA *63*:639–643, 1914.

8. Geyelin, H.R.: JAMA *104*:1203–1208, 1935.

9. Sansum, W.D.: Blatherwick, N.R., Bowden, R.: JAMA *86*:178–181, 1926.

10. Rabinowitch, I.M.: Can. Med. Assoc. J. *33*:136–140, 1935.

11. Kempner, W., Peschel, R.L., Schlayer, C.: Postgrad. Med. J. *24*:359–371, 1958.

12. Cahill, G.F., Jr., McDevitt, H.O.: N. Engl. J. Med. *304*:1454–1464, 1981.

13. De Fronzo, R.A., Ferrannini, E., Koivisto, V.: Am. J. Med. *74*(Suppl. 1):52–81, 1983.

14. Ward, W.K., Beard, J.C., Halter, J.B., et al.: Diabetes Care *7*:491–502, 1984.

15. Reaven, G.M. (Ed.): Am. J. Med. 74 (Suppl.): 1–112, 1983.

16. Podolsky, S., Viswanathan, M.: Secondary Diabetes: The Spectrum of the Diabetic Syndrome. New York, Raven Press, 1980.

17. National Diabetes Data Group: Diabetes *28*:1039–1057, 1979.

18. Robbins, D.C., Tager, H.S., Rubenstein, A.H.: N. Engl. J. Med. *310*:1165–1175, 1984.

19. Genuth, S.M.: Quoted by Cahill, G.F., Jr. *In* Harrison's Principles of Internal Medicine, 9th ed. 1980, pp. 1053–1072.

20. Hales, C.N., Randle, P.J.: Lancet *1*:790–794, 1963.

21. Schellenberg, B., Oster, P., Vogel, G., et al.: Nutr. Metab. *23*:316–326, 1979.

22. Felig, P.: Am. J. Med. *60*:117, 1976.

23. Goldstein, J.L., Kita, T., Brown, M.S.: N. Engl. J. Med. *309*:288–296, 1983.

24. Nikkila, E.A., Huttinen, J.K., Ehnholm, C.: Diabetes *26*:11–20, 1977.

25. Anderson, J.W.: Am. J. Clin. Nutr. *27*:746–755, 1974.

26. Anderson, J.W.: Am. J. Clin. Nutr. *28*:273–280, 1975.

27. Schade, D.S., Eaton, R.P.: Diabetes Care *2*:296–306, 1979.

28. Kreisberg, R.A.: Ann. Intern. Med. *84*:681–695, 1978.

29. Khardori, R., Soler, N.G.: Am. J. Med. *77*:889–904, 1984.

30. Gerich, J.E., Cryer, P., Rizza, R.A.: Metabolism *29*:1165–1175, 1980.

31. Clements, R.S., Jr.: Diabetes *28*:604–611, 1979.

32. Brownlee, M., Cerami, M.: Annu. Rev. Biochem. *50*:385–432, 1984.

33. Greene, D.A.: Metabolism *32*(Suppl. 1):118–123, 1983.

34. Brownlee, M., Klassora, H., Cerami, A.: Ann. Intern. Med. *101*:527–537, 1984.

35. Bunn, H.F.: Diabetes *30*:613–617, 1981.

36. Spiro, R.G.: N. Engl. J. Med. *288*:1337–1347, 1973.

37. Siperstein, M.D.: N. Engl. J. Med. *309*:1577–1579, 1983.

38. Camerini-Davalos, R.A., Velasco, C., Glasser, M., et al.: N. Engl. J. Med. *309*:1551–1556, 1983.

39. Pirart, J.; Diabete Metab. 3:97–107, 1977.

40. Anderson, J.W.: Hyperlipidemia and diabetes: Nutrition considerations. *In* Nutrition and Diabetes. (Jovanovic, L., Ed.) New York, Alan R. Liss, 1985.

41. Christlieb, A.R., Warram, J.H., Krolewski, A.S., et al.: Diabetes *30*(Suppl. 2):90–96, 1981.

42. Saudek, C.D., Young, N.L.: Diabetes *30*(Suppl. 2):76–81, 1981.

43. Lewis, B.: Diabetes *30*(Suppl. 2) 88–89, 1981.

44. Nikkila, E.A.: Diabetes *30*(Suppl. 2):82–87, 1981.

45. Colwell, J.A.: Winocour, P.D., Lopez-Virella, M., et al.: Am. J. Med. *75*(Suppl. 5B):67–80, 1983.

46. Weksler, B.B.: Am. J. Med. *71*:331–332, 1981.

47. Wall, R.T., Rubenstein, M.D., Cooper, S.L.: Diabetes *30*(Suppl. 2):39–43, 1981.

48. Moore, S.: Diabetes *30*(Suppl. 2):8–13, 1981.

49. Steiner, G.: Diabetes *30*(Suppl. 2):1–7, 1981.

50. Stout, R.W.: Diabetologia *16*:141, 1979.

51. DeFronzo, R.A.: Diabetologia *21*:165–171, 1981.

52. Connor, W.E., Connor, S.L.: Dietary treatment of hyperlipidemia. *In* Hyperlipidemia: Diagnosis and Therapy. (Rifkind, B.M., Levy, R.I., Eds.) New York, Grune and Stratton, 1977.

53. Grundy, S.M., Bilheimer, D., Blackburn, H., et al.: Circulation *65*:839A–854A, 1982.

54. Arky, R.A., Wylie-Rosett, J., El-Beheri, B.: Diabetes Care *5*:59, 1982.

55. Anderson, J.W., Sieling, B.: Nutrition and diabetes. *In* Nutrition Update. (Weinenger, J., Briggs, G., Eds.) New York, John Wiley & Sons, 1985.

56. Hjollund, E., Petersen, O., Richelsen, B.: Metabolism *32*:1067, 1983.

57. Sun, J.V., Tepperman, H.M., Tepperman, J.A.: J. Lipid Res. *18*:533–539, 1977.

58. Anderson, J.W.: High-carbohydrate diet effects on glucose and triglyceride metabolism of normal and diabetic men. *In* Metabolic Effects of Utilizable Carbohydrates. (Reiser, S., Ed.) New York, Marcel Dekker, Inc., 1982.

59. Viswanathan, M.: J. Indian Med. Assoc. *70*:275–279, 1978.

60. Singh, I.: Lancet *1*:422–424, 1975.

61. Stone, D.B., Connor, W.E.: Diabetes *12*:127–135, 1963.

62. Weinsier, R.L., Seeman, A., Herrera, G.: Ann. Intern. Med. *80*:332, 1974.

63. Anderson, J.W., Ward, K.: Diabetes Care *2*:77–82, 1978.

64. Story, L., Anderson, J.W., Chen, W.L.: J. Am. Diet. Assoc. *85*:1105–1110, 1985.

65. Ney, D., Hollingsworth, D.R., Cousins, L.: Diabetes Care *5*:529, 1981.

66. Simpson, H.C.R., Lousley, S., Geekie, M., et al.: Lancet *1*:1, 1981.

67. Kinmonth, A-L., Angus, R.M., Jenkins, P.A., et al.: Arch. Dis. Child. *57*:187–194, 1982.

68. Karlstrom, B., Vessby, B., Asp, N.G., et al.: Diabetologia *26*:272, 1984.

69. Anderson, J.W.: High carbohydrate, high fiber diets for patients with diabetes. *In* Treatment of Early Diabetes. (Camerini-Davalos, R.A., Hanover, B., Eds.) New York, Plenum Publishing Corp., 1979.

69a. Anderson, J.W.: Unpublished observations.

70. Reaven, G.M.: Diabetologia *19*:409–413, 1980.

71. Bierman, E.L., Hamlin, J.T.: Diabetes *12*:432, 1961.

72. Herman, R.H., Zakim, D., Stifel, F.B.: Fed. Proc. *29*:1302, 1970.

73. Anderson, J.W.: Am. J. Clin. Nutr. *30*:402–408, 1977.

74. Schlierf, G., Reenheimer, W., Strossberg, V.: Nutr. Metab. *13*:80–91, 1971.

75. Anderson, J.W., Chen, W-J.L., Sieling, B.: Metabolism *29*:551–558, 1980.

76. Anderson, J.W.: Clin. Nutr. *3*:59–64, 1984.

77. Crapo, P.A., Kolterman, O.G., Olefsky, J.M.: Diabetes Care *3*:575, 1980.
78. Akgun, S., Ertel, N.H.: Diabetes Care *3*:583, 1980.
79. Bohannon, N.V., Karam, J.H., Forsham, P.H.: J. Am. Diet. Assoc. *76*:555, 1980.
80. Crapo, P.A., Reaven, Olefsky, J.: Diabetes *25*:741, 1976.
81. Crapo, P.A., Reaven, G., Olefsky, J.: Diabetes *26*:1178, 1979.
82. Jenkins, D.J.A., Wolever, T.M.S., Taylor, R.H., et al.: Am. J. Clin. Nutr. *34*:362, 1981.
83. Jenkins, D.J.A., Wolever, T.M.S., Jenkins, A.L., et al.: Diabetologia *24*:257, 1983.
84. Haber, G.B., Heaton, K.W., Murphy, D., et al.: Lancet *2*:679, 1977.
85. Anderson, J.W., Bridges, S.R.: Proc. Soc. Exp. Biol. Med. *177*:372–376, 1984.
86. Nuttall, F.Q.: Diabetes Care *6*:197–207, 1983.
87. Anderson, J.W.: J. Am. Coll. Nutr. *2*:307, 1983.
88. Ernest, I., Hallgren, B., Svanborg, A.: Metabolism *11*:912–919, 1962.
89. Joslin, E.P.: The Treatment of Diabetes Mellitus. 4th ed. Philadelphia, Lea & Febiger, 1928.
90. Paisey, R.B., Arredondo, L.N., Villalobos, A., et al.: Diabetes Care *7*:421–427, 1984.
91. West, K.M., et al.: Diabetes Care *6*:361–369, 1983.
92. Randle, P.J., Garland, P.B., Hales, C.N., et al.: Lancet *1*:785, 1963.
93. Trowell, H.C.: Non-infective Disease of Africa. London, Edward Arnold, 1960.
94. Walker, A.R.P., S. Afr. Med. J. *35*:114, 1961.
95. Walker, A.R.P., Walker, B.F., Richardson, B.D.: Lancet *2*:51, 1970.
96. Wapnick, S., Wicks, A.C.B., Kanengoni, E., et al.: Lancet *2*:300, 1972.
97. Trowell, H.C.: Diabetes *24*:762–764, 1975.
98. Trowell, H.: Am. J. Clin. Nutr. *31*:S53, 1978.
99. Jenkins, D.J.A., Leeds, A.R., Gassull, M.A., et al.: Lancet *2*:172–174, 1976.
100. Kiehm, T.G., Anderson, J.W., Ward, K.: Am. J. Clin. Nutr. *29*:895–899, 1976.
101. Anderson, J.W., Chen, W-J.L., Sieling, B.: Metabolism *29*:551–558, 1980.
102. Anderson, J.W., Sieling, B.: Obesity/Bariatric Med. *9*:109–113, 1980.
103. Barnard, R.J., Lattimore, L., Holly, R.A., et al.: Diabetes Care *5*:370–374, 1982.
104. Barnard, R.J., Massey, M.R., Cherny, S., et al.: Diabetes Care *6*:268–273, 1980.
105. Kay, R.M., Grobin, W., Track, N.S.: Diabetologia *20*:18, 1981.
106. Lindsay, A.N., Hardy, S., Jarrett, L., et al.: Diabetes Care *7*:63–67, 1984.
107. Pedersen, O., Hjollund, E., Lindkov, H.O., et al.: Diabetes Care *5*:284–291, 1982.
108. Riccardi, G., Rivellese, A., Pacioni, D., et al.: Diabetologia *26*:116–121, 1984.
109. Rivellese, A., Riccardi, G., Giacco, A., et al.: Lancet *2*:447–450, 1980.
110. Rosman, M.S., Smith, C.J., Jackson, W.P.U.: S. Afr. Med. J. *63*:310, 1983.
111. Simpson, R.W., Mann, J.I., Eaton, J., et al.: Br. Med. J. *1*:1753, 1979.
112. Simpson, R.W., Mann, J.I., Eaton, J., et al.: Br. Med. J. *2*:53, 1979.
113. Simpson, H.C., Mann, J.I., Chakrabarti, R., et al.: Br. Med. J. *284*:1608, 1982.
114. Taskinen, M., Nikkila, E.A., Allus, A.: Diabetes Care *6*:224, 1983.
115. Anderson, J.W.: Can. Med. Assoc. J. *123*:975–979, 1980.
116. Jenkins, D.J.A., Wolever, T.M.S., Nineham, R., et al.: Br. Med. J. *2*:1744–1746, 1978.
117. Jenkins, D.J.A., Wolever, T.M.S., Taylor, R.H., et al.: Br. Med. J. *1*:1353–1354, 1980.
118. Anderson, J.W., Midgley, W.R., Wedman, B.: Diabetes Care *2*:369–379, 1979.
119. Anderson, J.W., Ferguson, S.K., Karounos, D., et al.: Diabetes Care *3*:38–40, 1980.
120. Rattan, J., Levin, N., Graff, E., et al.: J. Clin. Gastroenterol. *3*:389–393, 1981.
121. American Diabetes Association: Diabetes Care *2*:520–523, 1979.
122. British Diabetes Association: Hum. Nutr. Appl. Nutr. *36A*:378–394, 1982.
123. Canadian Diabetes Association: J. Can. Diet. Assoc. *42*:110–118, 1981.
124. Nutrition and Cancer: Cause and Prevention: American Cancer Society, January, 1984.
125. Committee on Diet, Nutrition and Cancer: Cancer Res. *43*:3018–3023, 1983.
126. Brenner, B.M., Meyer, T.W., Hostetter, T.H.: N. Engl. J. Med. *307*:652–659, 1982.
127. Anderson, J.W.: Nutrition Management of Metabolic Conditions. Lexington, Kentucky, HCF Diabetes Research Foundation, 1985.
128. U.S. Department of Agriculture and U.S. Department of Health and Human Services: Nutrition and Your Health: Dietary Guidelines for Americans. U.S. Department of Agriculture Home and Garden Bulletin, No. 232, Washington, D.C., U.S. Department of Agriculture, 1980.
129. Bright-See, E., McKeown-Eyssen, G.E.: Am. J. Clin. Nutr. *39*:821–829, 1984.
130. Talbot, J.M., Fisher, K.D.: Diabetes Care *1*:231–240, 1978.
131. Anderson, J.W., Story, L., Zettwoch, N.: Diabetes *33*(Suppl. 1):5A, 1984.
132. Nightingale, E.O.: Am. J. Med. *71*:9–12, 1981.
133. ADA: Aspartame, A Summary and Annotated Bibliography. Chicago, American Dietetic Association, 1982.
134. Crapo, P.A., Powers, M.A.: Diabetes Forecast, 1981.
135. Lieber, C.S.: N. Engl. J. Med. *310*:846–848, 1984.
136. McDonald, J.: Diabetes Care *3*:629–637, 1980.
137. Wadden, T.A., Strunkard, A.J., Brownell, K.D.: Ann. Intern. Med. *99*:675–684, 1983.
138. Howard, A.N.: Int. J. Obes. *5*:195–208, 1981.
139. Genuth, S.M.: Am. J. Clin. Nutr. *32*:2579–2586, 1979.
140. Bistrian, B.R., Blackburn, G.L., Flatt, J.-P., et al.: Diabetes *25*:494–504, 1976.
141. Chen, W.-J.L., Anderson, J.W.: Hypocholesterolemic effects of soluble fibers. *In* Basic and Clinical Aspects of Dietary Fiber. (Vahouny, G., Kritchevsky, D., Eds.) New York, Plenum Publishing Corp., 1986.
142. Anderson, J.W., Story, L., Sieling, B.: Am. J. Clin. Nutr. *40*:1146–1155, 1984.
143. Anderson, J.W., Story, L., Sieling, B.: J. Can. Diet. Assoc. *45*:140–149, 1984.
144. Anderson, J.W.: Spec. Topics Endocrinol. Metab. *2*:1–42, 1981.
145. Ney, D., Hollingsworth, D.R.: Diabetes Care *4*:647–655, 1981.
146. Carpenter, M.W., Coustan, D.R.: Am. J. Obstet. Gynecol. *144*:768–773, 1982.

147. Whalley, P.J., Leveno, K.J.: Clin. Diabetes *2*:49–55, 1984.
148. Ehrlich, R.M.: Clin. Endocrinol. Metab. *11*:195–210, 1982.
149. Hadden, D.R.: Clin. Endocrinol. Metab. *11*:503–525, 1982.
150. Campbell, R.K.: Practical Cardiology *8*:66–74, 1984.
151. Schade, D.S., Santiago, J.V., Skyler J., et al.: Intensive Insulin Therapy. Amsterdam, Excerpta Medica, 1983.
152. Skillman, T.G., Feldman, J.M.: Am. J. Med. *70*:361–372, 1981.
153. Anderson, J.W.: User's Guide to HCF Diets, Lexington, Kentucky, HCF Diabetes Foundation, 1984.

*Chapter* **58**

# NUTRITION, DIET, AND THE KIDNEY

## Joel D. Kopple

## KIDNEY FUNCTION

The kidney has three primary functions: excretory, endocrine, and metabolic. Because all three functions may be impaired in renal disease and may impact on the patient's nutritional status and management, these three activities will be briefly reviewed.

### Excretory Function

The kidney is the primary organ for the excretion of metabolic waste products, except for the role of the lung in the removal of carbon dioxide. The kidney excretes a wide array of compounds. In addition, the kidney precisely regulates body water and the concentrations of many electrolytes including sodium, potassium, calcium, phosphorus, chloride, bicarbonate, and many biologically valuable organic compounds such as glucose and amino acids. It helps to regulate body pH by excreting acid or base. Normally, about 70 to 100 meq/day of acid are produced from ingested foods, metabolism, and fecal alkali losses; thus for the maintenance of homeostasis, excretion of acid is usually more important than excretion of base. The kidney excretes most of the hydrogen ion as inorganic acids, particularly phosphate, sulfate, and ammonium; organic acids and free hydrogen ion are quantitatively less important sources of urinary acid excretion.

Removal of metabolic waste and regulation of the body's content of minerals and organic compounds are carried out by a combination of ultrafiltration through the glomerulus and selective reabsorption or secretion by the tubular cells of the nephrons. Normally, compounds that are not protein-bound and that have a molecular weight of 5,000 or less are completely filtered by the glomerulus; there is a small degree of filtration of some compounds weighing greater than 100,000 daltons.[1] There are two recognized barriers to the filtration of molecules by the glomerulus: the pore size and the electrical charge on the glomerular basement membrane.

The mechanisms by which the normal kidney controls the excretion of electrolytes, water, and acid are remarkably sensitive and precisely regulated phenomena that are controlled by complex processes occurring within and without the kidney.[1–3] An example of this degree of precision for a normal adult who has a typical dietary intake of sodium, potassium, chloride, and water and who is in neutral balance for these substances is shown in Table 58–1. The quantity of sodium, potassium, chloride, bicarbonate, and water filtered by the kidney each day is often several times greater than the total amount in the body but only a small fraction is excreted.[3] With the exception of potassium, over 99% of the quantity of these electrolytes and water filtered by the glomerulus normally is reabsorbed by the tubules, and less than 1.0% is excreted in the urine. Potassium is extensively reabsorbed in the proximal tubule and ascending limb of the loop of Henle, but is secreted in the distal tubule. Reabsorption of filtered calcium, magnesium, and phosphorus is less complete. Tubular secretion is a major mechanism for the excretion of hydrogen ion, uric acid, and many other organic compounds. The kidney responds to changing intakes or body burdens of water or minerals by altering reabsorption or secretion in order to maintain homeostasis. If the dietary intake of water or any one of a number of minerals increases, a smaller proportion of the quantity filtered by the glomerulus is reabsorbed, and a greater fraction of the amount filtered is excreted in the urine. If either the potassium intake rises or acidemia (lowering of blood pH) occurs, renal tubular secretion of potassium or hydrogen ion increases.

The renal clearance of a compound is an indicator of the kidney's ability to transfer it from plasma to urine. The clearance of a compound refers to the volume (ml) of plasma that is completely cleared of the compound in a given time.

Renal clearance can be determined from the following equation:

$$C_x = \frac{U_x V}{P_x T}$$

$C_x$ is the clearance of compound x usually given in ml/minute, $U_x$ is the concentration of compound x in urine expressed per ml, V is the ml of urine volume (it is often collected for 24 hours), $P_x$ is the concentration of compound x in one ml of plasma, and T is the time of the urine collection, usually expressed in minutes.

Some plasma compounds are completely filtered by the glomerulus and are neither reabsorbed nor secreted by the renal tubules. The clearance of these compounds is equal to the rate of filtration of plasma through the glomerulus and can be used to measure the glomerular filtration rate (GFR). Such substances include inulin and iodothalamate. The normal GFR for young men and women is 125 ± (SD) 15 ml/min/1.73 m² of body surface area and 110 ± (SD) 15 ml/min/1.73

**Table 58–1.** **Approximate Quantities of Electrolytes and Water Filtered, Reabsorbed and Excreted by Normal Man***

| | Plasma Concentration (meq/L) | Glomerular Filtration Rate (L/24 hrs) | Gibbs-Donnan Factor | Quantity Filtered‡ | Quantity Excreted (meq/24 hrs) | Quantity Reabsorbed | Percent Reabsorbed |
|---|---|---|---|---|---|---|---|
| Sodium | 140 | 180 | 0.95 | 23,940 | 103 | 23,837 | 99.6 |
| Potassium | 4 | 180 | 0.95 | 684 | 51 | 633§ | 92.5§ |
| Chloride | 105 | 180 | 1.05 | 19,845 | 103 | 19,742 | 99.5 |
| Bicarbonate | 27 | 180 | 1.05 | 5,103 | 2 | 5,101 | 99.9 |
| | L/L | L/24 hrs | | | L/12 hrs | | % |
| Water | 0.94† | 180 | — | 169.2 | 1.5 | 167.7 | 99.1 |

*These values assume normal renal function (glomerular filtration rate of 125 ml/min), an approximate daily intake of 6 g/day of sodium chloride, 2 g/day of potassium, and 2.0 L/day of water, and neutral balance of the subject. Data from Pitts, R.F.[3]

†Plasma is composed of approximately 94% water and 6% protein.

‡The product of the plasma concentration, the glomerular filtration rate, and the Gibbs-Donnan factor gives the quantity of electrolyte or water filtered each day.

§The absolute quantity reabsorbed is actually greater because potassium is secreted in the distal convoluted tubule.

m², respectively.[3] The GFR is the most commonly used direct measurement of renal function.

Measurement of GFR with inulin or iodothalamate is time-consuming because these compounds are not normally present in serum and must be infused intravenously or, at the least, injected. Creatinine is the most commonly used measurement of GFR because it occurs naturally in plasma and urine and is easy to measure. Creatinine is completely filtered by the glomerulus, but in man it is also secreted by the renal tubules. The common method for measurement of creatinine with picric acid does not distinguish between creatinine and the Jaffe chromagens in plasma. The presence of the chromagens in normal serum may falsely elevate the creatinine measurement. These noncreatinine chromagens are poorly filterable, and very little is found in urine. For estimation of GFR, the falsely elevated serum creatinine measurement tends to cancel out the contribution of tubular secretion to creatinine excretion. Thus, under normal conditions, the creatinine clearance is a fair indicator of GFR and usually overestimates it only slightly. In renal failure, the creatinine clearance can overestimate the GFR by a greater and less predictable degree, and it is therefore less reliable. Urea clearance also has been used to estimate the GFR. Urea is completely filtered by the glomerulus. However, it is reabsorbed to a variable degree in the renal tubules and therefore consistently underestimates the GFR in an unpredictable fashion. More urea is reabsorbed by the tubules and less is cleared at lower urine flows. Hence, urea clearance, by itself, is not commonly used to ascertain the GFR.

Serum creatinine and serum urea nitrogen (SUN) have been employed to estimate the GFR.[4] Their relationship to GFR can be described as a rectangular hyperbola (Fig. 58–1). Although serum creatinine reflects the GFR less precisely than does the creatinine clearance, it usually reflects the GFR accurately enough to be used for clinical purposes. Because the SUN is also affected by the rate of protein degradation and urine flow as well as by the GFR, it is a poor indicator of the GFR.

When injury and necrosis of the renal parenchyma cause a loss of renal function, the quantity of the substances that are filtered by the kidney falls. However, many aspects of renal function undergo changes that act to preserve homeostasis and to minimize the derangements in plasma and tissue concentrations of substances that normally are excreted by the kidney. First, the remaining functional nephrons undergo an increase in function and size so that the magnitude of the reduction in GFR is proportionately less than the re-

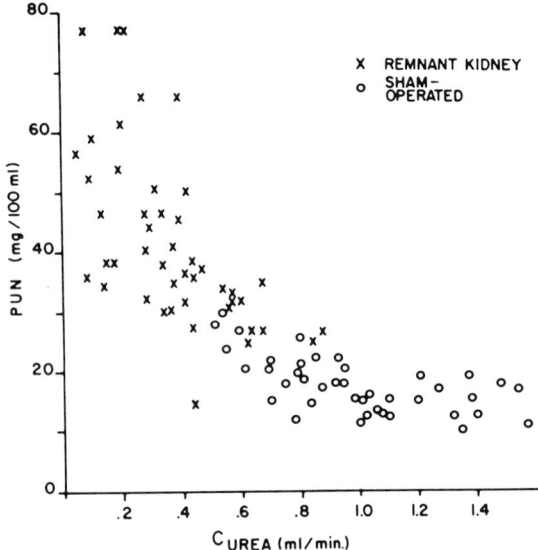

**Fig. 58–1.**   Relation between the plasma urea nitrogen (PUN) and glomerular filtration rate, as indicated by the urea clearance, in Sprague-Dawley rats with chronic renal insufficiency and sham-operated controls. Chronic renal failure was produced by ligation of two thirds to three fourths of the arterial supply to the left kidney and contralateral nephrectomy. (From Kopple, J.D.,[5] with permission of Plenum Publishing Corp.)

duction in functional parenchymal mass. A second mechanism is concerned with compounds that are primarily excreted by glomerular filtration with little or no reabsorption or secretion by the renal tubules. As indicated by the clearance equation previously discussed, at a given GFR, the greater the plasma levels of these compounds, the more that is filtered and excreted. This mechanism prevents the body's content of these compounds from increasing infinitely, as long as some glomerular filtration remains. Another adaptive mechanism in renal failure is a reduction in the renal tubular reabsorption of compounds or electrolytes that normally are filtered by the glomerulus and reabsorbed by the tubules. In addition, for substances that are normally secreted by the kidney tubules, the secretion rate (expressed per ml/min of GFR) may increase. These adaptive changes by the remaining functional nephrons serve to reduce the accumulation of compounds in renal failure; the adaptations are mediated by the dietary protein intake, hormonal factors, and physicochemical changes within the kidney.

A large number of organic compounds accumulate in renal failure.[6] Most of these compounds are products of amino acid and protein metabolism. Quantitatively, the most prominent of these compounds are urea, creatinine, other guanidino compounds, and uric acid. It is generally believed that a number of these compounds are toxic in high concentrations. Eventually renal failure may become so severe that the aforementioned adaptive mechanisms are no longer adequate to maintain homeostasis, even with special dietary therapy that restricts the intake of fluid, electrolytes, and protein. The accumulation of these toxic substances, the endocrine and metabolic disturbances, and the clinical signs and symptoms that result from renal failure are referred to as uremia. If this condition is not treated by hemodialysis, peritoneal dialysis, or renal transplantation, death will eventually supervene.

Excretion and regulation of body water, minerals, and organic compounds are clearly the most important functions of the kidney. Without renal excretory function, patients rarely live longer than 4 to 5 weeks and often less than 10 days, particularly if they are hypercatabolic. In contrast, anephric patients can be kept alive for years with intermittent hemodialysis or peritoneal dialysis, even though endocrine and metabolic functions of the kidney are not replaced.

## Endocrine Function

The kidney elaborates a number of hormones that have diverse metabolic effects. These effects have been the subject of many excellent and comprehensive reviews.[6a–9] The following is a brief summary of these hormonal actions. Renin, an enzyme with a molecular weight of approximately 42,000, is secreted by the juxtaglomerular apparatus of the kidney. Renin cleaves a circulating alpha$_2$-globulin, angiotensinogen, to form angiotensin I, a decapeptide.[7] Angiotensin I is cleaved by a converting enzyme present in blood and tissues to form angiotensin II. Angiotensin causes vasoconstriction and raises blood pressure. It also stimulates aldosterone secretion and plays a major role in the regulation of an intrarenal blood flow and glomerular filtration rate.

The kidney plays an essential role in vitamin D metabolism.[8] Vitamin D$_3$ (cholecalciferol) is hydroxylated in the liver to form 25-hydroxycholecalciferol. This compound is then converted in the kidney to 1,25-dihydroxycholecalciferol (1,25-dihydroxyvitamin D). The actions of 1,25-dihydroxyvitamin D are discussed in Chapter 13. In renal failure, the impaired synthesis of 1,25-dihydroxyvitamin D contributes to a vitamin D-deficient state associated with impaired intestinal calcium absorption, hyperparathyroidism, and the development of renal osteodystrophy.

The kidney synthesizes a number of eicosenoids including prostaglandins. These compounds have pervasive effects on renal function. Prostaglandins inhibit sodium and water reabsorption by the kidney, modify intrarenal blood flows and pressures, lower blood pressure, and have other intrarenal physiologic effects.[6a,7] The prostglandins synthesized in the kidney do not seem to have direct physiologic effects outside the kidney.

Erythropoietin, a glycoprotein with a molecular weight of 39,000 that stimulates erythropoiesis in bone marrow, is also produced by the kidney.[9,10] There is a well-known inverse relationship between the degree of kidney failure and erythropoiesis. The anemia of chronic renal failure is primarily caused by impaired erythropoiesis. Decreased red cell formation is mainly due to reduced erythropoietin production in the diseased kidneys, although other compounds that accumulate in renal failure also may suppress erythropoiesis. A mild hemolysis often contributes to the anemia. Certain kidney disease (e.g., kidney cysts or tumors) are occasionally associated with increased hemoglobin and hematocrit due to increased synthesis of erythropoietin.

The kidney, as well as other organs, produces kallikreins, a group of enzymes that cleave alpha$_2$-globulin (kininogen) to form kinins.[7] Kinins are peptides that are potent vasodilators and vasoconstrictors of different blood vessels and that can stimulate the inflammatory response. They also may act to regulate renal blood flow and sodium excretion.

## Metabolic Function

The kidney directly affects amino acid and protein metabolism because of its capability to synthesize or catabolize certain hormones and amino acids, to degrade peptides and small proteins, and to produce or utilize certain amino acids.[11,12] Peptides and low-molecular-weight proteins (e.g., up to 50,000 daltons) readily traverse the glomerulus and are reabsorbed and degraded by renal tubular cells. The kidney degrades many peptide hormones including insulin,[13] glucagon,[14] parathyroid hormone,[15] thyrotropin,[16] and gastrin.[17] After the liver, the kidney is the most important organ for degrading peptide hormones. The failing kidney has a reduced capacity to degrade peptides and small proteins, and this condition may lead to elevated plasma concentrations of many peptides and small proteins. Urinary excretion of some proteins may be increased in the diseased kidney.[18] Some of these proteins are secreted by the damaged renal tubules, but others may be excreted because of diminished ability of the renal tubular cells to catabolize the increased quantity of proteins that are often filtered by the diseased glomerulus.

About 2.5 moles of amino acids are delivered to the kidney each day by renal blood flow; this amount represents about 70 times the amino acid content of extracellular fluid. Approximately 0.5 moles of these amino acids are filtered by the kidney and are almost entirely reabsorbed in the proximal tubule. Only a few hundred milligrams of amino acids are excreted in the urine each day.

There is a net uptake or release into the circulation by the kidney of a number of amino acids. This process may help to regulate the pools of certain amino acids, particularly for serine, alanine, glycine, and glutamine.[11,12] The kidney converts glycine to serine and is a major source for serine in humans and animals. The abnormally low plasma serine level and ratio of plasma serine/glycine in renal failure may reflect impaired synthesis of serine from glycine by the diseased kidney.[11,12] The quantity of amino acids in renal arterial blood influences the renal uptake or release of many amino acids by the kidney. When an individual passes from the postabsorptive to the postprandial state, the pattern of production and utilization of amino acids changes, and many more amino acids are metabolized by the kidney. For example, after a meal or an amino acid load, the kidney removes alanine from the circulation, but during the postabsorptive period, alanine is released from the kidney.[11]

Glutamine is the major source of renal ammonia production, although glycine, alanine, glutamic acid, and other amino acids may be transaminated or deaminated and may generate ammonia. Chronic acidosis markedly increases renal glutamine uptake and urinary ammonia production. In chronic alkalosis, glutamine utilization and ammonia production decrease. An intriguing interrelationship between urea production in the liver and ammonia production in the kidney has been demonstrated in rats.[19] When rats ingesting a constant nitrogen intake are given an acid load, the ensuing increase in urinary ammonia excretion is associated with decreased production of urea. Despite the urinary excretion of ammonia, the kidney releases more ammonia into the general circulation than it takes up from the renal artery. Hence, in renal failure blood ammonia levels usually do not rise.

The kidney both degrades and synthesizes glucose. Normally, these processes are virtually equal, and there is little release of glucose by the kidney. However, with prolonged starvation, the kidney becomes an important net producer of glucose.[20] The kidney also catabolizes choline.[21]

## INTERRELATIONSHIPS BETWEEN NUTRIENTS AND KIDNEY FUNCTION

Kidney function both regulates and is influenced by the body's pools and concentrations of water, minerals, and many other nutrients and their metabolites. This section provides a brief overview of some of the more important of these interactions.

### Water and Electrolytes

The field of water and electrolyte metabolism is vast, and many books have been devoted to this subject. This section provides a brief overview of some of the interactions between water and electrolyte metabolism and renal function. No attempt has been made to be comprehensive or to present in-depth information. The reader is referred to several textbooks for more complete reading.[2,22–24]

**Water.** Dehydration can be caused by decreased fluid intake, vomiting, diarrhea, enhanced sweating, fistula drainage, or increased urine losses induced by diuretics or deficiency in or resistance to antidiuretic hormone (diabetes insipidus). Diuretic agents may be osmotic, such as glucose (e.g., in uncontrolled diabetes mellitus), mannitol, or urea, or may act chemically by inhibiting the renal tubular absorption of certain ions, particularly sodium and chloride. Dehydration can lead to decreased intravascular volume, hypotension, and a fall in renal blood flow and GFR. Sodium, chloride, and albumin provide the major colloidal osmotic forces in extracellular or intravascular fluid. If losses of these substances occur with dehydration, the decrease in intravascular fluid volume will be greater, and the effects of dehydration will be more profound. If disproportionately more water than sodium is lost from the body, serum sodium may increase to abnormally high levels. This change can lead not only to low blood pressure but also to central nervous system dysfunction. Replacement with water and sodium chloride reverses the volume depletion. However, sufficiently severe or prolonged reduction in renal blood flow may cause acute tubular necrosis and acute renal failure.

Retention of water in excess of sodium can lower serum sodium concentrations and cause water intoxication. Normally, the kidney can markedly dilute urine, to 50 to 60 mosm/L. The osmolality of normal plasma is 285 ± 10, and intake of large amounts of water can be handled safely by excretion of large quantities of dilute urine. However, many clinical conditions show impairment in the ability of the kidney to excrete free water (i.e., water in excess of the amount necessary to make urine isosmotic with plasma). These conditions include acute or chronic kidney, heart, or liver failure, certain diuretic drugs, and increased circulating levels of antidiuretic hormone. Plasma antidiuretic hormone can rise with surgery or trauma, many medicines, ethanol, heart or liver failure, and physiologic or psychologic stress. When a large fluid intake is superimposed on any of the foregoing conditions, dilution of serum sodium is more likely to occur and to progress to frank water intoxication.

**Sodium.** The kidney can conserve sodium efficiently, and under some conditions urinary sodium excretion can fall to less than 1 meq/day. Patients who have impaired kidney function or who receive diuretics often cannot conserve sodium normally, and low-salt diets can lead to sodium depletion. Addison's disease (adrenocortical insufficiency), vomiting, diarrhea, and renal diuretic agents can also cause sodium wasting and can lead to decreased extracellular and plasma volume and impaired renal function. The normal kidney can also excrete massive quantities of sodium by reducing the percentage of sodium reabsorbed in the renal tubules (see Table 58–1). This process can occur with potent diuretics, with massive sodium loading (if the individual does not develop salt and water retention), and in rare kidney disorders. Liver, heart, or kidney failure can impair sodium excretion and can lead to salt and water retention, particularly if sodium intake is large.

**Potassium.** If serum potassium rises or falls by as little as 2 to 4 meq/L, serious but potentially reversible disorders in cardiac and skeletal muscle function may occur. Although the kidney plays a central role in the regulation of extracellular potassium concentrations, the most immediate mechanisms for controlling extracellular levels are transcellular shifts in potassium. After an oral or intravenous potassium load, enhanced intracellular movement of potassium prevents or blunts the development of increased plasma potassium levels. Insulin and epinephrine play a major role in mediating this intracellular potassium shift. Alkalosis also promotes the intracellular movement of potassium, whereas acidosis promotes a shift of potassium to the extracellular space. Renal tubular secretion of potassium also rises following a potassium load. Factors that enhance renal potassium secretion include greater quantities of filtered sodium delivered to the distal tubule (e.g., from increased dietary intake or decreased sodium reabsorption in the proximal tubule due to diuretics), alkalosis, increased potassium concentrations in the distal tubular cells and the adrenocortical hormones, aldosterone, deoxycorticosterone (DOCA), and 18-hydroxy-deoxycorticosterone.

Urinary potassium excretion falls when there is reduced potassium intake, increased extrarenal potassium losses, potassium deficiency, acidosis, decreased circulating levels of adrenocortical hormones, renal tubular resistance to these hormones, medicines that inhibit the actions of these hormones, reduced sodium delivery to the distal tubule, and a large decrease in GFR.

Potassium deficiency is usually caused by diuretics, loss of gastrointestinal fluids by vomiting or diarrhea, or markedly impaired intake. Thiazide diuretics or loop diuretics such as furosemide are probably the most common causes of potassium depletion. These diuretics increase urinary potassium losses by their effects on sodium and chloride excretion. The sodium chloride losses stimulate aldosterone secretion. The combination of elevated aldosterone levels and increased delivery of sodium to the distal tubule, due to diuretic-induced decreased sodium reabsorption in the proximal nephron, leads to enhanced potassium excretion. Licorice ingestors or tobacco chewers occasionally develop potassium deficiency because glycyrrhizic acid in licorice or chewing tobacco has an aldosterone-like effect, and in large doses it can cause hypertension, salt and water retention, and enhanced urinary potassium excretion.

Potassium depletion is associated with impaired urinary concentrating ability and an inappropriately acid urine. The tubular cells may become vacuolated, particularly in the proximal tubule. Interstitial fibrosis, tubular dilation, and atrophy may occur; it is not clear to what extent these latter changes are due to pyelonephritis that may occur in association with potassium depletion.

**Calcium.** Increased serum calcium can be caused by hyperparathyroidism, neoplastic diseases, vitamin D intoxication, sarcoidosis, hyperthyroidism, hypothyroidism, adrenocortical insufficiency, the milk-alkali syndrome, and other disorders. Elevated serum calcium may cause nausea, vomiting, impaired renal concentrating ability, and polyuria. The nausea, vomiting, and polyuria can lead to a vicious cycle with dehydration, contraction of extracellular fluid volume, a fall in GFR and, with decreased renal excretion of calcium, further elevation of serum calcium. Hypercalcemia may also cause hypertension, obtundation and other central and peripheral nervous system abnormalities, decreased hydrogen ion secretion, and enhanced urinary magnesium excretion.

Elevated serum calcium can cause kidney damage by calcium deposition and possibly by the vasoconstrictive actions of calcium on arteriolar smooth muscle. Calcium tends to be deposited in the medulla where the concentration of calcium is greatest, particularly in the collecting ducts and ascending limb of the loop of Henle. Calcium deposition causes destruction of renal tubular cells, obstruction of the tubular lumen, intrarenal hydronephrosis, and interstitial scarring and fibrosis. Renal infection and hypertension may occur. If the hypercalcemia is not corrected, renal failure may ensue. Hypercalcemia may also cause calcium stones in the urinary tract. Hypocalcemia does not appear to have specific effects on kidney function.

**Phosphorus.** The clinical syndromes of hypophosphatemia and/or phosphorus depletion are well described.[25,26] These conditions occur not uncommonly in a variety of disorders including total parenteral nutrition with little or no phosphate intake, alkalosis (particularly respiratory), alcoholism, excessive intake of phosphate-binding antacids, diabetic ketoacidosis, and severe burns. Phosphate depletion may cause hypophosphatemia. However, serum phosphorus can be low without phosphate depletion if there is an intracellular shift of serum phosphorus. In general, hypophosphatemia is associated with hypocalciuria, decreased intestinal calcium absorption, and increased secretion of parathyroid hormone. Urinary phosphate excretion may be low or high, depending on the cause of the hypophosphatemia.

Kidney function is affected in phosphate depletion; hypophosphaturia, hypercalciuria, hypermagnesiuria, decreased renal gluconeogenesis, a fall in the GFR, and disorders in renal tubular function may occur.[26] Intestinal absorption of calcium increases, and serum parathyroid hormone may fall. The increased calcium in urine appears to be derived from enhanced calcium absorption from the intestine and bone. An unidentified circulating humoral factor may cause the hypercalciuria. The role of phosphorus intake in the progression of renal failure is discussed later.

**Magnesium.** Magnesium depletion can be caused by inadequate dietary intake, intestinal malabsorption, losses of gastrointestinal fluid, diuretic-stimulated urinary losses, primary hyperaldosteronism, hyperthyroidism, hyperparathyroidism, other hypercalcemic states, and rare genetic disorders in renal conservation of magnesium. Magnesium depletion occurs commonly in alcoholism, probably from inadequate magnesium intake and enhancement of urinary magnesium excretion by alcohol. Certain antibiotics and other drugs may increase urinary losses by inducing renal tubular dysfunction. Magnesium may also shift out of extracellular fluid into other body compartments. Magnesium depletion causes excessive urinary potassium excretion, potassium depletion, and decreased secretion and increased resistance to the actions of parathyroid hormone.

Thus, magnesium depletion is associated with hypomagnesemia, hypokalemia, and hypocalcemia. The hypokalemia and hypocalcemia are resistant to increased potassium and calcium intake until magnesium depletion is corrected.

Clinically important hypermagnesemia occurs almost exclusively in renal insufficiency and usually only when there is an abnormally high intake from magnesium-containing antacids or laxatives. Hypermagnesemia suppresses neuromuscular transmission and can cause hypotension, loss of deep tendon reflexes, weakness, paralysis, conduction disturbances in the heart, and possibly drowiness and coma. Cardiac arrest may occur.[27]

**Trace Elements.** The excessive intake of certain trace elements, primarily heavy metals, may alter kidney metabolism and may produce renal injury or failure. Trace elements primarily affect the renal tubular cells and interstitium, although gold, mercury, bismuth, and silicon toxicity can cause glomerular disease.[28–30]

Lead, cadmium, uranium, and copper can cause an interstitial nephritis and a Fanconi-like syndrome with impaired tubular reabsorption of glucose, amino acids, and phosphorus and decreased secretion of para-aminohippurate.[31–35] Lead, cadmium, and lithium may cause chronic interstitial nephritis, and beryllium may cause a granulomatous interstitial nephritis. Mercury, bismuth, uranium, cadmium, arsenic, gold, platinum, copper, thallium, antimony, and large doses of iron can produce acute tubular necrosis and acute renal failure. In animals, potassium dichromate can cause renal failure. The toxic effects of trace elements appear to be due to their propensity to bind to protein, often to the sulfhydryl groups; this may impair such cellular enzyme functions as respiration and oxidative phosphorylation.

### Effects of Malnutrition on the Kidney

Malnutrition can have important but usually reversible effects on renal function. In humans, malnutrition decreases GFR[36,37] and the capacity to concentrate and to acidify urine.[37–39] If nutritional intake improves, these functions become more normal. GFR falls reversibly in obese subjects placed on weight reduction diets containing no protein or calories but providing water, vitamins, and small quantities of minerals. This phenomenon is at least partly due to a reduction in extracellular body water, circulating blood volume, and renal blood flow. Increased salt and water intake rapidly reverses this condition. It is possible that the low or absent protein intake may contribute to the lower renal blood flow and GFR.[36,37]

Ichikawa and co-workers investigated the

mechanisms responsible for reduction in GFR with protein malnutrition.[40] These investigators found that in rats pair-fed a low (6%) protein diet as compared to an isocaloric high (40%) protein diet, there was almost a 35% reduction in GFR. Increased resistance was evident in the arterioles leading into (afferent) and out of (efferent) the glomerulus. There was also about a 25% reduction in the glomerular capillary plasma flow rate and almost a 50% decrease in the glomerular capillary ultrafiltration coefficient. Glomerular transcapillary hydraulic pressure differences were similar in the two groups.

Malnourished individuals often have the lower specific gravity of random urine specimens and increased daily urine volumes. Impaired concentrating ability probably contributes to the nocturia that occurs in malnutrition. The inability of the malnourished patient to concentrate urine normally appears to be due to the low protein intake and consequent low rate of urea synthesis.[38] Urea is critical for normal urinary concentration. Some urea filtered by the glomerulus is reabsorbed in the renal tubule and accumulates in the interstitium of the renal medulla. The high concentration of urea and also sodium chloride in the medullary interstitium makes it hypertonic. When plasma antiduiretic hormone rises, the distal tubule and collecting duct become more permeable to water that diffuses into the hypertonic renal medulla. The loss of water from the collecting duct lumen increases the concentration of urine. When protein intake is low, urea synthesis falls and SUN decreases; less urea is filtered by the glomerulus and reabsorbed into the renal medulla. Thus, medullary hypertonicity falls, and there is less tendency for water to move from the distal tubule and collecting duct to the medulla; hence, maximum renal concentrating ability is reduced. Ingestion of urea or protein by subjects who are malnourished or eating low-protein diets improves renal concentrating ability.[38] The capacity to dilute urine is normal in malnutrition.

Malnourished subjects are more likely to develop acidosis after an acid load.[39] Urinary phosphate and ammonia are primary carriers of acid in the urine. Hydrogen ion secretion into the lumen of the distal nephron lowers the pH of tubular fluid and converts $HPO_4^=$ to $H_2PO_4^-$ and ammonia to $NH_4^+$. In individuals who have a low phosphorus intake, the phosphate filtered in the kidney is largely reabsorbed to conserve body phosphate pools, and less is excreted in the urine. Thus, the capacity to excrete acid is reduced. Infusion of phosphate markedly improves urinary excretion of titratable acid in malnourished patients.[39] In malnutrition, renal production and excretion of ammonia are also reduced, both under basal conditions and after an acid load.[39] It is not clear why this capacity of the kidney to synthesize and to excrete ammonia is reduced.

During prolonged starvation, the kidney may account for up to 45% of endogenous glucose production (although part of the rise in the renal contribution to glucose synthesis is due to a fall in total body glucose production).[20] With extended starvation, there is also net renal extraction of lactate, pyruvate, amino acids, and glycerol.[20] The carbon skeleton in these compounds is virtually completely converted into glucose. During prolonged starvation, free fatty acids and beta-hydroxybutyrate are also extracted by the kidney, and acetoacetate is released.[20]

Acute starvation and others conditions associated with increased catabolism of nucleic acids, purines, and amino acids (e.g., chemotherapy of leukemias and certain other tumors) can cause a marked increase in uric acid production. Hyperuricemia and deposition of uric acid sludge in the kidney and lower urinary tract may occur and may cause acute renal failure. Treatment consists of allopurinol, which inhibits the synthesis of uric acid, maintenance of good hydration and a large urine flow, and alkalinization of the urine because urate is far more soluble in alkaline solutions.[41]

### Effect of Protein and Amino Acid Intake on Renal Function

Protein intake appears to engender both an immediate and a more long-term increase in renal blood flow (RBF) and GFR in humans. A transient increase in RBF and GFR occurs following a protein meal.[42,43] The rise occurs about two hours after the meal and generally lasts about one hour. RBF and GFR also increase transiently following an intravenous infusion of a mixture of essential and nonessential amino acids,[44] or a 30-minute infusion of arginine hydrochloride.[45] The elevation with arginine HCl is maximal by the end of the infusion. This more rapid rise in RBF and GFR may reflect the fact that the amino acids enter the blood immediately during an amino acid infusion as compared to a protein meal. The mechanisms underlying this increase in RBF and GFR are not well defined. Infusion of somatostatin blocks the rise induced by an amino acid infusion, indicating that peptide hormones may mediate the amino acid and protein enhancement of RBF and GFR.[44] Infusion of glucagon increases renal function and, since many amino acids stimulate glucagon secretion, this hormone may play a role in the amino acid or protein-induced increase in RBF and GFR. Acromegalic patients have an abnormally high GFR,[46] and infusion of growth hormone into normal humans for several days is reported to increase GFR.[47] However, when arginine hydrochloride was infused into growth hormone-deficient patients, the rise in renal plasma flow and GFR was similar to that of normal controls.[45] These observations suggest that growth hormone does not mediate the acute rise in GFR induced by protein and amino acids. Growth hormone causes a slower rise in RBF and GFR[47a]; this effect is probably mediated through IGF I.

Protein intake also has more prolonged effects on RBF and GFR. Pullman and co-workers fed three different levels of protein intake for two weeks each to young men and women.[36] The diets provided 0.1 to 0.4, 1.0 to 1.4, and 2.3 to 3.0 g protein/kg body weight/day. The three diets were isocaloric for each subject and were fed in random order. Effective renal plasma flow and GFR, measured after an overnight fast at the end of each two-week protein diet, varied directly with protein intake and were 640 ± 83 SD and 117 ± 19 ml/min/1.73 m², respectively, with the highest protein diet and 538 ± 94 and 95 ± 14 ml/min/1.73 m² with the lowest protein intake. The mechanism responsible for this longer-term effect of protein intake on renal function is unknown. It is probably not related to change in renal size. Studies in rats suggest that it is not due to urea excretion, although this concept has been challenged.[48]

### Effect of Nutritional Intake on the Rate of Progression of Renal Failure

It has been known for many years that patients with chronic renal disease who have sustained a substantial loss of GFR often continue to lose renal function inexorably until they develop terminal renal failure.[49–51] Although the rate of progression of renal failure varies greatly among different patients, in many individuals the decline in kidney function is linear.[49–51] It is not known what percentage of patients with renal insufficiency will progress to renal failure, but the suspicion is that, at the least, most patients who sustain a loss of 50% in GFR will show continued progression of their renal failure. Renal failure may progress because of continued activity of the underlying renal disease or because of superimposed disorders such as hypertension, kidney infection, obstruction, adverse effects of nephrotoxic medicines (e.g., antibiotics, radiocontrast material), hypercalcemia, or hyperuricemia. However, in innumerable instances the progression continues even after the initial cause of the renal disease seems to have disappeared.[52–55] For example, this phenomenon may occur in patients who have relief of urinary tract obstruction, control of hypertension, discontinuation of nephrotoxic medications,

or partial recovery from acute renal failure. Moreover, the continued progression of renal failure may occur when no associated causes of impaired renal function are identified. Several theories have been advanced to explain this phenomenon. These include the hypothesis that scarring and fibrosis of the diseased kidney cause obstruction of the renal tubules or small vessels, which in turn leads to intrarenal obstruction of tubular fluid and blood flow. It has also been suggested that the injured renal tissue elicits a secondary autoimmune response that causes further renal injury.[56] None of these theories has been confirmed.

Traditionally, dietary protein restriction has been used to minimize uremic toxicity.[57] In the first half of the twentieth century, a number of research studies in rats indicated that protein restriction could retard progression of renal failure.[58–60] The experimental design of these studies was often faulty, and the data were not considered to be applicable to humans. Studies in humans with renal disease were also not well controlled, and the results were inconsistent.

In the 1970s and 1980s, studies in both humans and rats indicated that dietary control can retard the state of progression of renal failure in a variety of renal diseases. In rats, several models of renal insufficiency were studied. These included surgical removal of the upper and lower poles of one kidney or ligation of about two thirds to three quarters of the arteries to one kidney; in some cases, experimental glomerulonephritis was created.[61–65] In these animals, diets low in protein and/or phosphorus retard or prevent progression of renal failure.[61–65] In addition, a diet low or high in certain fats may retard progressive renal damage.[66–69] Moreover, administration of prostaglandins may affect the progression of chronic renal disease in animals.[70–72]

Considerable effort has been directed toward elucidating the mechanisms by which dietary manipulations may alter the rate of progression of renal failure in rats. Before describing these studies, we shall briefly review the normal response to loss of renal function. Studies in animals with renal injury indicate that when the loss of functioning nephrons becomes sufficient to cause renal insufficiency, the remaining individual functioning nephrons undergo an increase in the glomerular plasma flow and GFR and an enlargement in size of both the glomeruli and the tubules.[73,74] As a result of these changes, the reduction in function of the kidney is proportionately less than the percentage loss of nephrons. In the injured or diseased kidney, an increase in the capillary blood flow of the remaining glomeruli and in the blood pressure gradient across the capillary wall has been reported.[74,75] In addition, the chemical and electrical (as well as pore size) barriers to the movement of plasma proteins across the glomerulus into the renal tubule are impaired.[76,77]

The mechanism responsible for these functional and anatomic changes in the diseased kidney are not well elucidated. It is known that a high-protein diet stimulates the increase in glomerular filtration rate, capillary blood flow, blood pressure gradients across the glomerular capillary wall, and enlargement of individual nephrons, whereas a low-protein diet blunts or prevents this response.[74] Moreover, rats with renal injury who are fed a high-protein diet develop renal failure, and when such animals are fed a low-protein diet, the progression of renal failure is retarded or arrested. A current theory postulates that a high-protein intake, by increasing both glomerular capillary blood flow and transcapillary glomerular hydraulic pressure, causes progressive renal injury to the basement membrane (filtering wall) of the glomerulus and allows protein and other chemicals to filter through the glomerulus.[74,78,79] This process in turn leads to disposition of protein-like chemicals in the glomerulus, an inflammatory response in some cases, and scarring. A low-protein diet retards or stops progressive renal damage by preventing these high flow rates and pressures.

Brenner, Meyer, and Hostetter proposed a "final common pathway" as the mechanism causing progressive renal failure.[78] They suggested that the loss of functioning nephron mass caused by many renal diseases leads to increased glomerular capillary plasma flow rate, increased glomerular transcapillary hydraulic pressure, and increased GFR in the remaining functional nephrons. These alterations, in turn, cause increased capillary permeability, enhanced movement of large molecules across the glomerular basement membrane, deposition of these compounds in the mesangium, mesangial expansion, induction of an inflammatory response in the glomerulus, scarring, and glomerulosclerosis. A normal or high dietary protein intake causes these hemodynamic and morphologic alterations, and a reduced protein intake may prevent or retard these changes. Diabetic rats with moderate hyperglycemia develop similar changes,[80] and similar abnormalities appear to occur in the intact kidney of humans with diabetes mellitus. Early during the course of diabetes mellitus, patients develop increased RBF, increased GFR, and large kidneys.[81] Ultimately, in a large proportion of these individuals, glomerulosclerosis occurs and renal failure supervenes.[82,83] Preliminary studies in rats and humans with diabetes mellitus indicate that either tight control of the serum glucose levels or a protein-restricted diet

in rats may retard the development or progression of the renal disease of diabetic mellitus.[83,84]

One may view the hyperfiltration response to renal insufficiency as both beneficial and harmful. It is advantageous because it maintains a more normal GFR in the face of renal injury. However, the intraglomerular hyperfiltration and hypertension that accompany the increased function of the remaining healthy nephrons may cause continued injury, scarring, and acceleration of the loss of renal function.

Other research has raised questions as to whether the hyperfiltration is solely responsible for progressive renal failure in the absence of apparent underlying causes. As previously indicated, low phosphorus intake independent of protein intake seems to retard progression of renal failure. The mechanism of action of the low phosphorus intake is unclear. One theory is that a low phosphorus intake decreases the deposition of calcium phosphate in kidney tissue, which may cause further renal damage.[85,86] However, the renal calcification may occur at the sites of necrotic cells and may be the result of cell death rather than its cause. This renal sparing effect of phosphorus restriction may be due to prevention or amelioration of hyperparathyroidism, but further evidence has not confirmed this theory.[87]

The role of fat metabolism in progressive renal injury is complicated and is still being elucidated by scientific investigation. A study in guinea pigs fed a diet containing 1% cholesterol demonstrated a high incidence of glomerular sclerosis, other renal lesions, and anemia in comparison to animals fed a control diet.[66] The essential fatty acid, arachidonic acid, can be metabolized in the kidney to several families of eicosenoids including prostaglandins. Prostaglandins have far-reaching effects on the blood flow and blood pressure inside the glomerulus, the propensity for platelets to clot in the glomerulus, and the inflammatory process. Certain eicosenoids have antagonistic effects; some increase glomerular blood flow and pressure and may impair platelet clotting, whereas others do the opposite. In renal insufficiency, elaboration of certain eicosenoids is increased in the kidney,[69,88] and they appear to play an important role in the complex adaptive processes that the nephron undergoes as kidney function deteriorates.[6a,89]

Rats and mice with pre-existing impaired renal function or renal disease demonstrated decreased progression of renal injury and a more normal GFR with the following treatments: supplemental dietary linoleic acid,[69] injections of prostaglandins $E_1$ or $E_2$[70,71] (drugs that inhibit synthesis of thromboxane, a prostaglandin that causes intrarenal vasoconstriction and platelet aggregation[89]), or anticoagulants that inhibit platelet clotting.[90] These experimental studies suggest that eicosenoids may play an important role in the progression of renal failure.

Experimental studies in NZB/NZW mice also suggest that dietary manipulation may ameliorate a renal disease resembling lupus erythematosus that occurs in these animals. A diet fed to these animals that is restricted in essential fatty acids decreases the severity of glomerulonephritis, lowers serum antinuclear antibody and anti-DNA antibody levels, and markedly prolongs life.[67,68,91] Diets deficient in essential fatty acids reduce synthesis of eicosenoid compounds, including PGE.[67] Subcutaneous injections of prostaglandins $E_1$ or $E_2$ in NZB/NZW mice also reduce the severity of renal disease, decrease the incidence of proteinuria, and prolong survival even though they do not alter serum immunoglobulin levels or antinuclear or anti-DNA antibodies.[70,71] Moreover, supplementing the diet with eicosopentanoic acid reduces proteinuria and prolongs survival in these NZB/NZW $F_1$ mice.[92] The mechanism of action of eicosopentanoic acid may be related to its propensity to impair platelet aggregation, which may, in turn, be due to the ability of this lipid to inhibit the synthesis of prostaglandins and thromboxanes from arachidonic acid.

McLeish and co-workers reported that injections of $PGE_1$ ameliorated the inflammatory and cellular response to immune-complex glomerulonephritis and may reduce deposition in the glomerulus of IgG and $C_3$, but not IgM.[72] The glomerular synthesis of leukotriene $B_4$, a lipoxygenase product of arachidonic acid released during inflammation, is increased in rats with immune-complex glomerulonephritis.[93] Preliminary evidence suggests that this compound may cause glomerular constriction and may participate in the reduced glomerular function that accompanies glomerular inflammatory injury.[94] In rats with Heymann nephritis, dietary protein restriction itself reduces eicosenoid synthesis.[95] Hence, it is possible that the beneficial effects of dietary protein restriction may be partly related to its effects on eicosenoid production.

Purkerson and co-workers postulate that chronic renal injury not only leads to glomerular hyperfusion and intraglomerular hypertension, but also promotes platelet aggregation.[89] According to their theory, platelet aggregation is facilitated by the endothelial damage that is caused by the hyperfiltration and increased glomerular capillary pressure. The platelet aggregation, in turn, may cause intraglomerular coagulation, further injury to the glomerulus, and increased glomerular

capillary permeability to proteins. The hyperfiltration, in association with increased capillary permeability, increases the flow of macromolecules into the glomerular mesangium where they may be deposited causing mesangial expansion and glomerular sclerosis. The platelet aggregation and deposition of macromolecules induce platelets and probably macrophages and monocytes to release growth factors and enzymes modifying collagen, elastic tissue, and other components of the mesangium and basement membranes. This process causes further damage to the mesangium. It is also possible that the stimulation of platelets, monocytes, and/or resident macrophages may induce proliferation of mesangial cells. The foregoing factors, in turn, promote mesangial expansion, sclerosis, and proliferative changes in the glomerulus. A schema for this hypothesis is shown in Figure 58–2.

Glomerular perfusion and pressure, platelet aggregation, and the inflammatory response each may be mediated by eicosenoid compounds. Hence, administration of diets or drugs that alter synthesis of various eicosenoids and anticoagulants may retard progressive renal disease. This schema for progressive renal disease is still largely unproven and represents the results of study in animal models of renal disease. There are major differences between most types of renal disease in humans and these animal models of renal disease, and it is not yet known to what extent the animal models represent progressive renal disease in humans.

Although the foregoing studies in animals indicate an important role for dietary control of protein, phosphorus, and certain fats to control progressive renal failure, there is evidence that certain medicines may be capable of substituting for the restriction of nutrients. Enalapril, a drug that decreases blood pressure by inhibiting the conversion of angiotensin I to angiotensin II, also lowers glomerular capillary blood flow and blood pressure gradients across the glomerular capillary wall in rats with renal insufficiency.[96] This agent also appears to retard progressive renal failure in these animals.[96,97] These findings are further evidence that intraglomerular hypertension does play a role in progressive renal failure. Captopril, an antihypertensive medicine that has a mechanism of action similar to that of enalapril, lowers but does not abolish marked urinary protein excretion in patients with diabetic kidney disease.[98] As described earlier, certain prostaglandins as well as drugs that prevent blood clotting or inhibit the synthesis of other eicosenoids also seem to reduce scarring and loss of renal function in rats.[89,90] Moreover, medicines that bind phospho-

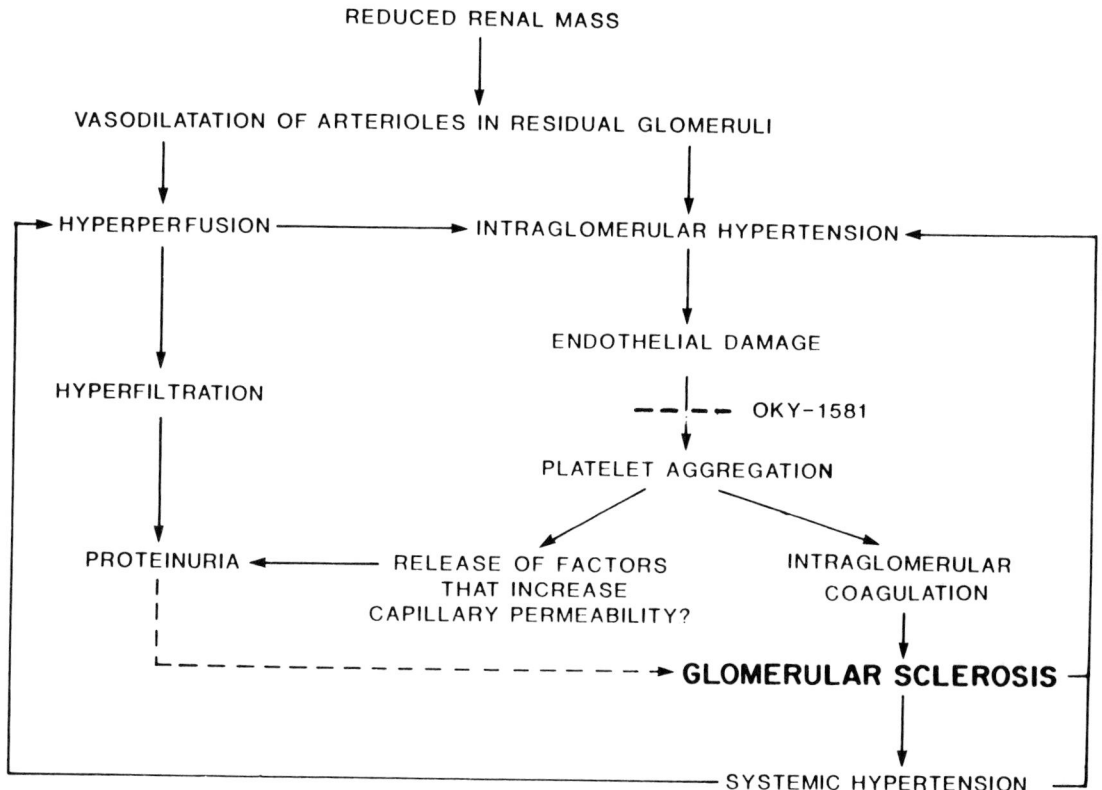

REDUCED RENAL MASS

VASODILATATION OF ARTERIOLES IN RESIDUAL GLOMERULI

HYPERPERFUSION → INTRAGLOMERULAR HYPERTENSION

ENDOTHELIAL DAMAGE

OKY-1581

PLATELET AGGREGATION

HYPERFILTRATION

PROTEINURIA ← RELEASE OF FACTORS THAT INCREASE CAPILLARY PERMEABILITY?

INTRAGLOMERULAR COAGULATION

**GLOMERULAR SCLEROSIS**

SYSTEMIC HYPERTENSION

**Fig. 58–2.** Proposed schema for mechanisms causing progressive glomerulosclerosis in rats with partial ablation of the kidneys. (From Purkerson, M.L., et al.,[89] with permission of Proc. Natl. Acad. Sci.)

rus in the intestinal tract can enhance the effectiveness of dietary phosphorus restriction.[61,99] These latter drugs are of particular value as a supplement to dietary phosphorus restriction because it is difficult to lower the dietary phosphorus intake to the necessary levels without making the diets highly restrictive, unpalatable, and difficult for adherence.

To what extent are the animal data applicable to patients? Virtually all recent dietary studies in humans with renal insufficiency indicate that a low dietary protein and phosphorus intake is effective in retarding the progression of renal failure.[100–106] There is some evidence that a low protein and phosphorus intake may each act separately to slow progressive renal failure.[200a]

Every study, however, suffers from one or more defects in experimental design. Particularly noteworthy among these defects are the retrospective nature of many studies, inadequate or complete lack of control groups, poor documentation of the patient's actual intake, and paucity or absence of data concerning whether these restrictive diets induce malnutrition. The need for adequate controls is particularly important because not all patients with renal insufficiency progress to advanced

renal failure, and the rate of progression can vary markedly from individual to individual. Nonetheless, it is striking that virtually all recent studies in humans show that low-protein, low-phosphorus diets retard progression.

Some investigators have used a modification of a low-protein diet in which the patient is prescribed a very low protein diet (e.g., about 16 to 25 g protein/day). This diet is supplemented with 10 to 20 g/day of the nine essential amino acids or of mixtures of some essential amino acids and ketoacid or hydroxyacid analogues of other essential amino acids.[100,102–105] The ketoacid or hydroxyacid analogue is structurally identical to its corresponding essential amino acid except that the amino ($NH_2$) group attached to the second (alpha) carbon of the amino acid is replaced with a keto group or hydroxy group, respectively (Fig. 58–3).

The ketoacid and hydroxyacid analogues can be transaminated in the body to the respective amino acids, although a proportion of the analogues are oxidized rather than transaminated. Because the ketoacids and hydroxyacids lack the nitrogen-containing amino group on the alpha carbon, these compounds provide a lesser nitro-

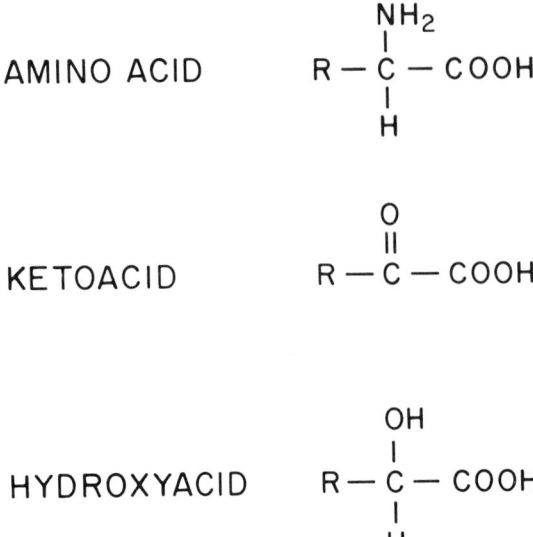

AMINO ACID

KETOACID

HYDROXYACID

**Fig. 58–3.** The prototype structure of an amino acid and of a ketoacid and hydroxyacid analogue of the amino acid. R refers to the side chain, which is different for each individual compound.

gen load to the patient. As they are broken down in the body, they should engender fewer waste products that will accumulate in renal failure. Certain ketoacids may be particularly likely to promote protein anabolism, possibly by decreasing protein degradation.[107,108] Hence, it is possible but not yet demonstrated that these ketoacids may play a beneficial role in maintaining protein mass in renal failure patients.

Walser et al. developed a mixture of ketoacids, hydroxyacids, and amino acids that was fed to patients with chronic renal failure in association with a diet that provided about 0.28 g protein/kg/day.[105] This combined low-protein, ketoacid, and amino acid diet had a marked effect in retarding or stopping progression of renal failure for up to three years. No concurrent control diet was evaluated in this study. However, the results were so dramatic as to suggest that this diet may be more effective at arresting progressive renal failure than any other diet that has been evaluated. It is noteworthy that the nitrogen content of this ketoacid-supplemented diet is not substantially lower than a 40-g protein diet. This finding suggests, but does not prove, that the ketoacid diet may exert a specific protective effect on progression of renal failure that may be independent of its nitrogen content. The ketoacid formulation contains no tryptophan or phenylalanine, which are both essential amino acids, although substantial amounts of tyrosine will replace most of the need for phenylalanine. Further studies are there-

fore necessary to carefully document that this diet will not engender malnutrition.

In humans, the role of dietary fat intake, prostaglandins, or drugs that alter eicosenoid metabolism in preventing progressive renal failure is virtually unstudied. Urinary prostaglandins are increased in patients with chronic renal disease.[88] Administration of inhibitors of prostaglandin synthesis to such patients (e.g., nonsteroidal anti-inflammatory drugs) may result in an acute reduction in RBF and GFR, particularly if they are volume-depleted.[109,110] These findings suggest that prostaglandins play an important role in maintaining renal function in patients with renal disease. Whether dietary lipid intake affects renal function acutely or chronically in humans is not known.

An interesting sidelight to these studies of the effect of diet on progression of renal failure is the question whether diet may promote or retard the development of renal failure in individuals with no underlying renal disease. Rats without renal disease or with only one kidney that are allowed to eat ad libitum or that are fed high-protein diets throughout life have a higher incidence of renal disease in old age.[111–114] In normal humans, after about the fourth decade of life, renal function falls progressively with age,[115] and it is possible that high-protein diets may play a role. In healthy young men and women, a high-protein intake increases RBF and GFR.[36] Moreover, there are similarities between the type of scarring that occurs in normal aging human kidneys and the kidneys of rats fed high-protein diets. In adults who have had a congenital absence, failure of development, or surgical removal of one kidney during childhood, there is an abnormally high incidence of spontaneous glomerular scarring in the remaining kidney.[116] The cause of this phenomenon is not known. However, it is possible that the typical protein intake of Americans, which is considerably higher than the Recommended Dietary Allowances for dietary protein,[117] may increase glomerular capillary blood flow and pressure and cause progressive renal injury.

### Nephrotic Syndrome

The nephrotic syndrome is a kidney disorder characterized by losses of large quantities of protein in the urine (at least 3.0 g/day), low serum albumin concentrations, high blood levels of certain fats, and accumulation of body water to form frank edema.[118] This condition is caused by diseases that affect the glomerulus and increase glomerular permeability to protein. Patients with the nephrotic syndrome are often wasted and debilitated. Because of their large protein losses and the frequent presence of poor appetite, such patients often develop protein malnutrition. Because certain vitamins and most trace elements are protein-bound in plasma, these individuals are also at risk for developing deficiencies of these nutrients. Vitamin D deficiency has been reported in patients with the nephrotic syndrome.[118,119] Wasting and malnutrition may occur in nephrotic patients even when they do not have advanced kidney failure. Studies suggest that both protein-restricted diets and angiotensin-converting enzyme inhibitors reduce proteinuria in nephrotic patients without causing a reduction in serum albumin levels or albumin pools.[98,120,121]

## NUTRITIONAL AND METABOLIC CONSEQUENCES OF CHRONIC RENAL FAILURE

Chronic renal failure causes pervasive nutritional and metabolic disorders that may affect virtually every organ system. These abnormalities will be reviewed briefly.

### Clinical, Nutritional, and Metabolic Disorders

Patients with chronic renal failure develop azotemia and uremia. Azotemia refers to the accumulation of nitrogenous metabolites in the blood. Uremia is the combination of azotemia with the clinical signs and symptoms of advanced renal failure. Chronic advanced renal failure is a complex disorder caused by a marked reduction in the excretory, endocrine, and metabolic functions of the kidney.

The many symptoms of uremia include weakness, a feeling of ill health, insomnia, fatigue, loss of appetite, nausea, vomiting, diarrhea, itching, muscle cramps, hiccups, twitching or jerking of the extremities, fasciculations, tremors, emotional irritability, and decreased mental concentration and comprehension. A characteristic fetid breath is often present. The fluid and electrolyte disturbances associated with renal failure can lead to congestive heart failure and hypertension or, if excessive sodium depletion occurs, reduction in extracellular fluid volume and a fall in blood pressure.

Altered serum electrolyte concentrations and acidosis can also occur, and these complications can have profound and life-threatening effects on the physiology and metabolism of the body. Disorders in water and electrolyte balance and acidosis are caused by impaired ability of the failing kidney to regulate the content of water, salts, and acids in the body. Most of these symptoms can be controlled or prevented with dietary therapy or dialysis. When untreated, uremia can lead to lethargy, loss of consciousness, coma, convulsions, and death.

Chronic advanced renal failure causes pervasive disorders in the absorption, excretion, or metabolism of many nutrients. These disorders include the accumulation of chemical products of protein metabolism;[6,122] a decreased ability of the kidney either to excrete a large salt load or to conserve salt rigorously when dietary sodium is restricted;[123] impaired renal ability to excrete water, potassium, calcium, magnesium, phosphorus, trace elements, acids, and other compounds;[124] a tendency to retain phosphorus;[125] decreased intestinal absorption of calcium[125,126] and possibly iron;[127] and a high risk for developing certain vitamin deficiencies, particularly for vitamin $B_6$, vitamin C, folic acid, and the most potent known form of vitamin D, 1,25-dihydroxycholecalciferol.[125,128] The chronic renal failure patient is also likely to accumulate certain potentially toxic chemicals, such as aluminum, that normally are ingested in small amounts and excreted in the urine.[129]

Uremia is also a polyendocrinopathy, and many of the metabolic and clinical manifestations of uremia are caused by the endocrine disorders. A large number of hormones are elevated in renal failure, particularly the peptide hormones, because of the impaired ability of the kidney to degrade peptides. These include parathyroid hormone, glucagon, insulin, growth hormone, prolactin, luteinizing hormone, often follicle-stimulating hormone (FSH), and gastrin.[13–17,125,130–133] Chronically uremic patients have altered thyroid hormone levels, although they probably are not hypothyroid.[134] Of the hormones elaborated by the kidney, plasma erythropoietin and 1,25-dihydroxycholecalciferol are reduced,[8–10,125] and plasma renin activity may be either increased, normal, or decreased. Serum somatomedin levels, measured by radioreceptor or radioimmunoassay, are usually reported to be normal in renal failure, but the biologic activity of somatomedins may be inhibited by uremic sera.[135,136] There is increased sensitivity to the actions of glucagon, which is reversed by hemodialysis, although hyperglucagonemia persists.[14] Resistance to the peripheral action of insulin occurs.[137] These effects on insulin and glucagon contribute to the mild glucose intolerance that is usually present in chronic renal failure.[137]

The ability of the failing kidney to synthesize or to metabolize many compounds, including amino acids, is impaired. Thus, there is reduced catabolism of glutamine, impaired synthesis of alanine, and decreased conversion of glycine to serine.[11,12,122]

Many products of metabolism accumulate in renal failure; the majority of these are derived from amino acids and proteins.[138] Most of these compounds accumulate as the result of decreased excretion, although in some instances enhanced synthesis or impaired degradation by the diseased kidney or other organs plays a role.[122] Abnormal metabolism in the gastrointestinal tract and probably the liver also contributes to increased levels of certain metabolites in renal failure.[122,139]

Quantitatively, the most important end product of nitrogen metabolism is urea.[138] In a clinically stable patient with chronic renal failure who is eating at least 40 g/day of protein, the net quantity of urea produced each day contains an amount of nitrogen equal to about 80 to 90% of the daily nitrogen intake. Guanidines are the next most abundant end product of nitrogen metabolism. These compounds include creatinine, creatine, and guanidinosuccinic acid. The "middle molecules" are a class of compounds that are midway in size between the small, readily dialyzable substances that accumulate in renal failure and small proteins. Most middle molecules are considered to have molecular weights of approximately 300 to 2,500 and contain amino acids. Some middle molecule compounds are increased in uremic sera.[138] Despite decades of study, the compounds that cause the uremic syndrome have not been well defined. Probably many compounds contribute to uremic toxicity. Prime suspects for uremic toxins include urea, guanidino compounds, phenolic acids, middle molecules, and some of the hormones that elevated in uremic plasma, especially parathyroid hormone and glucagon.[138]

Altered gastrointestinal function may affect nitrogen metabolism in uremic patients. The gastrointestinal tract metabolizes urea, uric acid, creatinine, and choline and synthesizes or releases from larger molecules dimethylamine, trimethylamine, ammonia, sarcosine, methylamine, and methylguanidine.[122] The quantity of intestinal bacterial flora is increased in uremia.[139]

Some of the metabolic alterations in uremia are adaptive homeostatic responses that offer both benefits and disadvantages to the patient. Hyperparathyroidism is an example. As the kidneys fail, impaired excretion of phosphorus leads to phosphorus retention. Concomitantly, the diseased and scarred renal parenchyma is less able to convert 25-hydroxycholecalciferol to the most potent metabolite of vitamin D, 1,25-dihydroxycholecalciferol.[125,126] Deficiency of 1,25-dihydroxycholecalciferol causes resistance to the actions of parathyroid hormone in bone. These alterations, in turn, promote hypocalcemia and lead to the development of hyperparathyroidism. The elevated serum parathyroid hormone reduces renal tubular reabsorption of phosphorus (enhancing urine phosphorus excretion), lowers serum phosphorus, promotes renal synthesis of 1,25-dihydroxycholecalciferol, mobilizes calcium from bone, and increases intestinal calcium absorption (although intestinal calcium absorption usually remains low or, in mild renal insufficiency, normal). The benefits derived from these homeostatic actions are that more normal concentrations of plasma phosphorus and calcium are maintained. The "tradeoff" is the development of hyperparathyroidism.[140] Parathyroid hormone has been implicated as a pervasive uremic toxin that affects many organs and tissues and contributes to the uremic syndrome.[141]

With the institution of appropriate dietary therapy or treatment with hemodialysis or peritoneal dialysis, blood levels of many metabolic products that accumulate in uremic plasma decrease, and the patient may experience clinical improvement. With maintenance hemodialysis or peritoneal dialysis, patients may live for many years with essentially no renal function. However, despite such improvement, many clinical and metabolic disorders may persist or even progress. These include: (1) a type IV hyperlipidemia,[142] (2) a high incidence of cardiovascular disease,[143] (3) osteodystrophy with disordered bone architecture, osteoporosis, or osteomalacia (aluminum toxicity often contributes to the osteomalacia),[125,126,129] (4) anemia,[9,10,127] (5) mildly impaired peripheral and central nervous system function, (6) muscle weakness and atrophy, (7) frequent occurrence of viral hepatitis,[144] (8) sexual impotency and infertility, (9) generalized wasting and malnutrition,[122,145–157] (10) a general feeling of ill health or depression, and (11) poor rehabilitation.[158] Most of these complications can be aggravated by poor nutritional intake or improved with good nutrition. When kidney failure is a complication of an underlying systemic disease, such as diabetes mellitus, hypertension, or lupus erythematosus, other manifestations of these underlying diseases may also adversely affect the patient. These manifestations may be progressive. It is important to recognize that all of the foregoing problems do not seriously affect every patient, and many chronically uremic and dialysis patients lead full and productive lives.

The foregoing considerations indicate that the intestinal absorption, excretion, and/or metabolism of virtually every nutrient may be altered in renal failure. In addition, the decreased intake of food and excessive intake of certain minerals (such as aluminum from the ingestion of aluminum phosphate binders) may alter nutritional status. Moreover, medicine therapy may adversely affect nutrient metabolism in renal failure. For example, anticonvulsant medicines may cause deficiencies of vitamin D and folic acid; hydralazine, isoniazid, and other medicines may cause vitamin $B_6$ deficiency.[128] Part of the challenge of dietary therapy for patients with renal failure is to provide for the altered nutritional requirements of many nutrients that occur in this condition.

## The Wasting Syndrome

The patient with chronic renal failure frequently shows evidence for wasting or protein-calorie malnutrition (Table 58–2).[122,145–157] The evidence includes decreased relative body weight (i.e., the patient's body weight divided by the weight of normal people of the same age, height, and sex), skinfold thickness (an estimate of total body fat), arm muscle mass, total body nitrogen, low growth rates in children, decreased serum concentrations of many proteins including albumin, transferrin, and certain complement proteins, and low muscle aklali soluble protein. The plasma amino acid pattern, which is pathognomonic for renal failure, also has similarities to that found in malnutrition. Total body potassium is reported to be low in patients with chronic renal failure and normal in those undergoing long-term maintenance hemodialysis. These findings are sometimes observed in nondialyzed patients with chronic renal failure, but are more prevalent in patients undergoing maintenance hemodialysis, intermittent peritoneal dialysis, and continuous ambulatory peritoneal dialysis. Not every dialysis patient has evidence for these disorders; however, virtually every survey of maintenance dialysis patients indicate that, as a group, they show evidence of malnutrition. In most patients who have wasting and malnutrition, it is only of mild to moderate severity. About 10 to 15% of dialysis patients have evidence of severe wasting.

There are many causes for wasting in chronic renal failure.[122,157] First, dietary intake is often inadequate, particularly for energy requirements.[122,146,155,156] The low dietary intake is caused by anorexia due to uremic toxicity, the debilitating effects of chronic illnesses, emotional depression, and the effects of acute superimposed illnesses on the patient's ability to eat or to accept tube feeding. In addition, the dietary prescription in renal failure, which is low in protein and other nutrients and which may be difficult to prepare or not palatable, can lead to low nutrient intakes. Second, in renal failure, there is a high incidence of superimposed catabolic illnesses.[158–160] Third, the dialysis procedure itself may induce wasting.

**Table 58–2.    Evidence for Wasting or Protein-Calorie Malnutrition in Patients with Advanced Chronic Renal Failure**

| Anthropometry, Body Composition, and Isotope Dilution Studies* | Biochemistry* |
|---|---|
| Decreased | Decreased |
|   Body weight |   Serum |
|   Height (children) |     Total protein |
|   Growth (children) |     Albumin |
|   Body fat (skinfold thickness) |     Transferrin |
|   Fat-free solids |     Prealbumin |
|   Intracellular water |     C3 |
|   Muscle mass (midarm muscle circumference) |     C3 Activator |
|   Total body potassium (nondialyzed patients) |     Cholinesterase |
|   Total body nitrogen (CAPD patients) |     Pseudocholinesterase |
|   Total albumin mass, synthesis, and catabolism |   Plasma |
|   Valine pools (nondialyzed patients) |     Leucine |
| |     Isoleucine |
| |     Total tryptophan |
| |     Valine |
| |     Tyrosine |
| |     Valine/glycine ratio |
| |     Essential/nonessential ratio |
| |   Muscle |
| |     Alkali-soluble protein |
| |     RNA:DNA ratio |
| |     Valine |
| |     Tyrosine |
| | Increased |
| |   Plasma |
| |     Glycine |

*Patients with chronic renal failure may have normal values for these parameters, but statistical comparisons indicate that the levels are often abnormal in these individuals.

During hemodialysis and peritoneal dialysis, there are losses of free amino acids, peptides or bound amino acids,[161–163] water-soluble vitamins,[128] proteins (with peritoneal dialysis),[164] glucose (during hemodialysis with glucose-free dialysate),[162] and probably other bioactive compounds. Hemodialysis also seems to increase net protein breakdown.[165] Fourth, renal failure patients sustain blood losses. Because blood is a rich source of protein, these losses might contribute to protein depletion. The blood losses occur from frequent blood drawing for laboratory testing, occult gastrointestinal bleeding, which is common in renal failure, and sequestration of blood in the hemodialyzer and blood tubing.[166]

Other possible but no established causes of wasting include (1) altered endocrine activity, particularly insulin resistance, hyperglucagonemia,[14] inhibition of somatomedin activity,[136] hyperparathyroidism, and deficiency of 1,25-dihydroxycholecalciferol[125]; (2) endogenous uremic toxins; (3) exogenous uremic toxins (e.g., aluminum); and (4) loss of metabolic functions of the kidney. Because the kidney is a metabolic organ that synthesizes or degrades many biologically valuable compounds, including amino acids, peptides, carbohydrates, and fatty acids,[122] it is possible that the loss of these activities in kidney failure could disrupt the body's metabolism and promote wasting.

There has been surprisingly little research concerning the adverse effects of wasting and malnutrition in renal failure. Several investigators have shown an inverse relationship between dietary protein consumption, as determined by the patient's urea nitrogen appearance or average SUN level, and morbidity and mortality in maintenance hemodialysis patients.[167,168] The lower the protein intake, the higher the incidence of morbidity and mortality. These were not prospective studies with randomized controls, and it is likely that the patients' underlying illnesses contributed to both their high mortality and the low protein intake. Nonetheless, the data are consistent with the thesis that poor nutrient intake and malnutrition adversely affect the prognosis in chronic hemodialysis patients.

## DIETARY MANAGEMENT OF CHRONIC RENAL DISEASE AND FAILURE

A recommended nutrient intake is given in Table 58–3 for patients with chronic renal failure who are not undergoing dialysis therapy as well as for patients undergoing maintenance hemodialysis or continuous ambulatory peritoneal dialysis. The following text explains our approach to the dietary management of these patients.

### General Principles of Dietary Therapy

The widespread metabolic and nutritional disorders, frequent occurrence of protein calorie wasting, and evidence that diet may retard the progression of renal failure indicate that nutritional management is a critical aspect of the treatment of chronic renal failure. There are three goals for dietary therapy: (1) to retard or to stop the rate of progression of renal failure, (2) to maintain good nutritional status, and (3) to prevent or to minimize uremic toxicity and the metabolic derangements of renal failure.

Adherence to specialized diets is a difficult and stressful endeavor for most patients and their families. Generally, it requires patients to undergo a major change in their behavior patterns and to forsake many of their traditional sources of daily pleasure. The patient must procure special foods, prepare special recipes, usually forego or severely limit his intake of many favorite foods, and is often compelled to eat foods that he may not desire. Demands are made on the time, effort, and emotional support system of his family or close associates. Therefore, it is incumbent on the physician not to prescribe radical changes in dietary intake unless there is a clear indication that they may be beneficial to the patient. In order to ensure successful dietary therapy, patients with renal failure must undergo extensive training concerning the principles of nutritional therapy and the design and preparation of diets, and they need continuous encouragement regarding dietary adherence. They must receive repeated retraining regarding their nutritional therapy. When nutritional intake is not carefully monitored, patients tend to adhere poorly to dietary prescription. They may eat too little rather than too much.

A team approach to dietary management may improve adherence. The team should include the physician, dietitian, close family members, the nursing staff and, where available, psychiatrists or social workers. The diet plans should be designed specifically for the individual tastes of the patient. At each visit, the physician should monitor dietary intake and should discuss the results with the patient.

The physician must strongly support the dietitian's efforts to train and to counsel the patient and to obtain dietary compliance. Generally, the spouse or other close relatives or friends should work closely with the patient to provide moral support and to assist with acquisition and preparation of foods. To promote dietary adherence, the entire medical team should assume an ener-

**Table 58–3. Recommended Nutrient Intake for Nondialyzed Patients with Chronic Renal Failure and for Patients Undergoing Maintenance Hemodialysis or Continuous Ambulatory Peritoneal Dialysis**

| | *Chronic Renal Failure*[a,b] | *Hemodialysis (HD) or Continuous Ambulatory Peritoneal Dialysis (CAPD)* |
|---|---|---|
| Protein source | Low-protein diet: 0.55–0.60 g/kg/day ≥0.35 g/kg/day of high-biologic-value protein<br>Very low-protein diet: About 0.28 g/kg/day of protein of any biologic value supplemented with either a ketoacid and amino acid mixture or essential amino acid mixture[d] | Hemodialysis[c] 1.0–1.2 g/kg/day ≥50% high-biologic-value protein<br>CAPD[c] 1.2–1.5 g/kg/day ≥50% high-biologic-value protein |
| Energy[e] | ≥35 kcal/kg/day unless the patient's relative body weight is greater than 120% or the patient gains unwanted weight | |
| Fat (% of total energy intake)[f,g] | 40–55 | 40–55 |
| Polyunsaturated: saturated fatty acid ratio[g] | 1.0:1.0 | 1.0:1.0 |
| Carbohydrate[h] | Rest of nonprotein calories | |
| Total fiber intake[g] | 20–25 g | 20–25 g |
| **Minerals** | *Range of Intake* | |
| sodium | 1,000 to 3,000 mg/day[i] | 750 to 1,000 mg/day[i] |
| potassium | 40 to 70 meq/day | 40 to 70 meq/day |
| phosphorus | 4 to 10 mg/kg/day[j,k] | 8 to 17 mg/kg/day[k] |
| calcium | 1,400 to 1,600 mg/day[l] | 1,400 to 1,600 mg/day[l] |
| magnesium | 200 to 300 mg/day | 200 to 300 mg/day |
| iron | ≥10 to 18mg/day[m] | ≥10 to 18 mg/day[m] |
| zinc | 15 mg/day | 15 mg/day |
| Water | up to 3,000 ml/day as tolerated[i] | usually 750 to 1,500 ml/day[i] |
| **Vitamins** | *Diets to be Supplemented with These Quantities* | |
| thiamin | 1.5 mg/day | 1.5 mg/day |
| riboflavin | 1.8 mg/day | 1.8 mg/day |
| pantothenic acid | 5 mg/day | 5 mg/day |
| niacin | 20 mg/day | 20 mg/day |
| pyridoxine HCl | 5 mg/day | 10 mg/day |
| vitamin $B_{12}$ | 3 μg/day | 3 μg/day |
| vitamin C | 60 mg/day | 60 mg/day |
| folic acid | 1 mg/day | 1 mg/day |
| vitamin A | no addition | no addition |
| vitamin D | see text | see text |
| vitamin E | 15 IU/day | 15 IU/day |
| vitamin K | None[n] | None[n] |

[a]GFR above 4–5 ml/min/1.73m² and less than 15–25 ml/min/1.73m².

[b]See text for discussion of dietary intake for patients with less severe renal insufficiency.

[c]Protein intake for hemodialysis patients generally should be closer to 1.2 g/kg/day; for CAPD patients who are not malnourished, it should be about 1.2–1.3 g/kg/day.

[d]There is no unanimity concerning the optimal quantity and formulation of the ketoacid and amino acid supplements. The values listed here are representative of the amounts used by nephrologists working in this field.

[e]This includes energy intake from dialysate in the CAPD patients.

[f]Refers to percentage of total energy intake (diet plus dialysate); if triglyceride levels are elevated, the percentage of fat in the diet may be increased to about 50% of total calories; otherwise, close to 40% of total calories is preferable.

[g]These dietary recommendations are considered less crucial than the others.

[h]Should be primarily complex carbohydrates, if tolerated by the patient.

[i]Can be higher in CAPD patients or in those nondialyzed patients with chronic renal failure and hemodialysis patients who have greater urinary losses.

[j]Phosphorus intake should be 4–9 mg/kg/day for patients ingesting a very-low-protein diet supplemented with ketoacids or amino acids; with the 0.55–0.60 g protein/kg/day diet, a phosphorus intake of 5–10 mg/kg/day is more tolerable.

[k]Phosphate binders (aluminum carbonate, aluminum hydroxide, calcium carbonate, or citrate) are often needed as well.

[l]Dietary intake usually must be supplemented to provide these levels.

[m]≥10 mg/day for males and nonmenstruating females; ≥18 mg/day for menstruating females.

[n]Vitamin K supplements may be needed for patients who are not eating and who are receiving antibiotics.

getic, positive, and sympathetic approach. If dietary therapy is prescribed to a patient, it requires a major commitment and effort by the patient and the medical staff to attain good results.

Because the prescribed diets are often marginally low in some nutrients (e.g., protein) and high in others (e.g., calcium) and malnutrition is not infrequent, it is important to periodically evaluate the adequacy of the diet and the patient's nutritional status. Nutritional evaluation should include assessment of dietary intake by interviews, dietary diaries, and measurement of urea nitrogen appearances (UNA) and evaluation of nutritional status by anthropometry, biochemical measurements, bone radiography, and other parameters[149] (see Table 58–2). The dietitian is often the person best qualified to perform anthropometric measurements of nutritional status because of training, interest in nutritional therapy, and access to the patient. In general, to maintain good dietary compliance and to monitor fluid and electrolyte disorders and clinical and nutritional status, patients with advanced renal failure should be seen monthly by the physician and the dietitian. Patients with slowly progressive mild or moderate renal insufficiency under some circumstances may see the physician less frequently, but they should still see the dietitian approximately monthly in order to promote better dietary adherence.

Recent evidence suggests that chronically uremic patients are at greatest risk for wasting and malnutrition during the period when the GFR falls below 5 ml/min and when the patient is commencing maintenance dialysis therapy.[157] Moreover, the nutritional status of patients at the onset of chronic dialysis treatments appears to be a good predictor of nutritional status two to three years later.[157,169] Hence, particular effort should be given to preventing malnutrition as the patient approaches the time when dialysis should be instituted and during the first few weeks of chronic dialysis therapy. Such effort should be directed toward maintaining a good nutritional intake during this period, rapidly instituting therapy for supervening illnesses, and maintaining good nutritional intake during such illnesses.

## Urea Nitrogen Appearance and Serum Urea Nitrogen/Serum Creatinine Ratio

The control of protein intake is pivotal for the nutritional management of patients with acute or chronic renal failure. Hence, it is of enormous importance to accurately monitor nitrogen intake. Fortunately, this is possible for most patients. Patients who are in nitrogen balance should have a total nitrogen output that is equal to nitrogen intake minus about 0.5 g nitrogen/day for unmeasured losses from growth of skin, hair, and nails, sweat, respiration, flatus, and blood drawing.[170] Thus, nitrogen output should accurately reflect nitrogen intake in patients who are more or less in nitrogen balance. For clinical purposes, slightly positive or negative balance does not substantially alter the use of the nitrogen output to estimate intake. If patients are in very positive or negative nitrogen balance (e.g., from pregnancy or severe infection), nitrogen output may not reflect intake. However, it is usually readily apparent to the clinician whether the patient is in very positive or negative balance and whether the nitrogen output will reflect intake.

The measurement of total nitrogen output is too laborious and expensive to be widely applied for clinical uses. However, because urea is the major nitrogenous product of protein and amino acid degradation, the UNA can be used to estimate total nitrogen output and, hence, nitrogen intake.[160,171,172] UNA refers to the amount of urea that appears or accumulates in body fluids and all outputs (e.g., urine, dialysis, fistula drainage). The term UNA is employed rather than urea production or generation because some urea is degraded in the gastrointestinal tract; the ammonia released from urea is largely transported to the liver and converted back to urea.[173,174] Thus, the enterohepatic urea cycle has little effect on urea or total nitrogen economy, and this cycle can be ignored without compromising the ability of the UNA to accurately estimate total nitrogen output or intake. Moreover, the recycling of urea cannot be measured without costly and time-consuming isotope studies.

UNA is calculated as follows:

Equation 1:

$$UNA \ (g/day) = urinary \ urea \ nitrogen \ (g/day)$$
$$+ \ dialysate \ urea \ nitrogen \ (g/day)$$
$$+ \ change \ in \ body \ urea \ nitrogen \ (g/day)$$

Equation 2:

$$Change \ in \ body \ urea \ nitrogen \ (g/day) = (SUN_f$$
$$- \ SUN_i, \ g/L/day) \times BW_i \ (kg) \times (0.60 \ L/kg)$$
$$+ \ (BW_f - BW_i, \ kg/day) \times SUN_f \ (g/L)$$
$$\times \ (1.0 \ L/kg)$$

where i and f are the initial and final values for the period of measurement, SUN is serum urea nitrogen (grams per liter), BW is body weight (kilograms), 0.60 is an estimate of the fraction of body weight that is water, and 1.0 is the volume of distribution of urea in the weight that is gained or lost.

The estimated proportion of body weight that is water may be increased in patients who are edematous or lean and decreased in individuals who are obese or very young. Changes in body weight during the one- to three-day period of measurement of UNA are assumed to be due entirely to changes in body water. In patients undergoing hemodialysis or intermittent peritoneal dialysis, the urea concentration in dialysate is low and difficult to measure accurately, and UNA is usually calculated during the interdialytic interval and then normalized to 24 hours. Because many dialysis patients have little or no urinary excretion, the equation for calculating their UNA during the interdialytic interval often can be simplified to Equation 2.

In our metabolic studies, the relationship between UNA and total nitrogen output in chronically uremic patients not undergoing dialysis is as follows:

Equation 3:

Total nitrogen output (g/day)

$$= 0.97 \text{ UNA (g/day)} + 1.93$$

If the individual is more or less in neutral nitrogen balance, the UNA also will correlate closely with nitrogen intake. Equation 4 describes our observed relationships between UNA and dietary nitrogen intake in clinically stable nondialyzed chronically uremic patients.

Equation 4:

Dietary nitrogen intake (g/day)

$$= 0.69 \text{ UNA (g/day)} + 3.3$$

When both nitrogen intake and UNA are known, nitrogen balance can be estimated from the difference between nitrogen intake and nitrogen output estimated from the UNA. If the patient is pregnant, Equation 4 will underestimate nitrogen intake. For patients who have large protein losses (e.g., from nephrotic syndrome or peritoneal dialysis) or who are acidemic and have sufficient kidney function to excrete large quantities of ammonia, Equations 3 and 4 will underestimate both nitrogen output and nitrogen intake. In most circumstances, however, these conditions are not present, and the UNA provides a powerful tool for monitoring nitrogen output and intake or estimating balance. Maroni et al. and Sargent and Gotch have described similar techniques for monitoring these parameters.[172,175]

The ratio of the SUN to serum creatinine also correlates closely with dietary protein or amino acid intake in chronically uremic patients who are not undergoing dialysis treatment.[4] This relationship can be used to estimate the recent daily intake of such patients. Although it is not as precise as the UNA and is influenced by a number of clinical factors, it is easy and inexpensive to measure. This ratio can also be used to select an appropriate protein intake for a given level of renal function.[4]

## Protein, Amino Acid, and Ketoacid Intake

**GFR Greater Than 70 ml/min/1.73m².** There are virtually no data concerning the optimal dietary protein and phosphorus intakes for patients with chronic renal disease and mild impairment in renal function. As information becomes available, dietary guidelines doubtless will change. At present, we do not routinely restrict protein for patients with a GFR greater than 70 ml/min/1.73m² unless renal function is continuing to decline. In the latter case, the patient is treated as indicated in the next paragraph. (Note: When the recommended nutrient is given in terms of body weight, the latter refers to desirable body weight as determined from the 1983 Metropolitan Life Insurance Tables.[176]

**GFR 25 to 70 ml/min/1.73m².** The studies indicating that low-protein, low-phosphorus diets may retard the rate of progression of renal failure are sufficiently convincing to warrant offering patients the opportunity for dietary therapy. Currently, our policy is to discuss with the patient the evidence that such diets retard progression and to indicate that the data justify undergoing dietary protein restriction. If the patient agrees to dietary therapy, he is offered a diet providing about 0.60 to 0.70 g protein/kg/day of which at least 35 g/kg/day is high-biologic-value protein to ensure a sufficient intake of the essential amino acids. This quantity of protein should maintain neutral or positive nitrogen balance and, for many patients, it should not be excessively burdensome.

**Chronic Renal Failure (GFR less than 25 ml/min/1.73m²) Without Dialysis: Role of Low-Protein Diets Supplemented with Amino Acids and Ketoacids.** The amino acid- and ketoacid-supplemented diets, as currently employed, generally provide about 16 to 20 g protein/day (about 0.28 protein g/kg/day) supplemented with amino acids or mixtures of amino acids, ketoacids, and sometimes hydroxyacids.[100,102–105,177–180] The quantity of essential amino acids or their ketoacid or hydroxyacid analogues in the supplements is sufficiently great so that it is not necessary to ingest food proteins of high biologic value. This allows patients a greater freedom of food selection. The essential amino acid supplements are usually composed of the nine essential L-amino acids (including histidine) and usually are given in doses of 14 to 21 g/day.[102,177–180] Traditionally, the essential amino acids have been proportioned according to the Rose daily amino acid requirements for healthy young adults.[177,178,180] Amino acid formulations have been modified to normalize the concentrations of several plasma and muscle intracellular amino acids.[179]

Furst reported, on the basis of [15]N studies, that patients with chronic renal failure may not be able to synthesize histidine, whereas normal adults can.[180a] However, we have evidence that neither normal nor chronically uremic adults are able to synthesize sufficient histidine for their needs.[180b] Moreover, we have not observed any difference in the metabolism of histidine in chronically uremic patients as compared to normal individuals, although the renal histidine clearance is less in the uremic patients.[180b–180d]

The ketoacid formulations have generally included mixtures of four essential L-amino acids (histidine, lysine, threonine, and tryptophan) and alpha-ketoacid or alpha-hydroxyacid analogues of the five other essential amino acids.[100,102–105] The ketoacids and hydroxyacids have the same structure as the respective essential amino acids except that the alpha-amino nitrogen is removed and a keto or a hydroxy group is substituted (see Fig. 58–3). The ketoacids and hydroxyacids generally are formulated as calcium salts or are bound to certain nonessential amino acids, especially ornithine.[100,103–105]

There are several potential advantages to using amino acid or ketoacid formulations in patients with renal insufficiency.[181] The relative quantities of these compounds can be modified to normalize plasma or tissue amino acid concentrations[179] or to increase the content of one or more essential amino acids or amino acid precursors that may improve nitrogen balance.[107,182–184] Several studies have indicated that an increased daily intake of leucine or all three branched-chain amino acids or ketoacid analogues may promote protein anabolism.[107,182,184–186] Because the ketoacids and hydroxyacids lack the alpha-amino group, for the same intake of amino acid equivalents less nitrogen is provided, and less generation of potentially toxic nitrogenous compounds results. Another advantage of the amino acid and ketoacid diets is that reducing the quantity of protein in the diet lowers the phosphorus intake.

There is no definitive evidence whether one type of low-nitrogen intake is more likely to retard the progression of renal failure. Clinical trials indicate that the worsening of kidney failure can be slowed in patients prescribed diets providing about 0.40 to 0.60 g protein/kg/day,[101,106] about 16 to 20 g protein/day supplemented with essential amino acids,[102] or 16 to 20 g protein/day supplemented with ketoacids.[103–105] There are few controlled comparisons between low-nitrogen diets. Jungers and colleagues found in a small number of patients that a ketoacid-supplemented diet may retard progression more effectively than a dietary prescription of about 0.60 g protein/kg/day.[187] In addition, the studies of Mitch and co-workers using a low-protein diet and the ketoacid-amino acid formulation, referred to as EE, showed a dramatic slowing of progression of renal failure.[105] Although the authors did not have a concurrent control group, their results with this ketoacid-amino acid formulation were more striking than the published reports with other types of low-nitrogen diets. Thus, it is likely, but not proven, that diets providing about 0.28 g protein/kg/day supplemented with certain ketoacid mixtures may be more effective at lowering the rate of progression of renal failure. Prospective clinical trials are currently underway to test this hypothesis.

Based on the foregoing considerations, it seems reasonable that when the GFR decreases to about 25 ml/min/1.73m[2], patients should be prescribed a diet providing 0.28 g protein/kg/day supplemented with a mixture of about 10 to 20 g of ketoacids and amino acids (Table 58–3). In the United States, ketoacid supplements have not yet been approved for clinical use. Where ketoacids are not available, essential amino acid supplements may be substituted for the ketoacid mixture, or patients may be prescribed 0.55 to 0.60 g protein kg/day with at least 0.35 g/kg/day of high-biologic-value protein (see Table 58–3). All three of these diets generally maintain neutral or positive nitrogen balance and generate a low UNA.[100,177,180,182,188] It is easier to obtain low phosphorus intakes with the essential amino acid diet, but many patients prefer the 0.55 to 0.60-g protein/kg/day diet. The latter diet is also less expensive than the essential amino acid diet. Each of the diets prescribed to patients with mild to severe renal failure should be increased by 1.0 g/day of high-biologic-value protein for each gram of protein excreted in the urine each day.

When the GFR falls below 5 ml/min/1.73m[2], there is no conclusive evidence that patients fare as well with low-nitrogen diets as with regular dialysis therapy and higher protein intakes. Because these latter patients may be at high risk for wasting or malnutrition,[157] it is recommended that maintenance dialysis treatment or renal transplantation be inaugurated at this time.

## Nephrotic Syndrome

Formerly it was recommended that patients with the nephrotic syndrome be prescribed high-protein diets to prevent protein malnutrition.[189] The current evidence that a high-protein intake may accelerate the progression of renal failure has caused a rethinking of the dietary protein prescription for nephrotic patients. Moreover, there is now evidence that low-protein diets (e.g., 0.80 g protein/kg/day plus 1.0 g for each gram of urine protein loss each day) may decrease urine protein excretion and may maintain or actually increase slightly the serum albumin levels.[120,121] Until more information is available, it is recommended that patients with the nephrotic syndrome be prescribed a diet containing 0.60 g protein/kg/day and 1.0 g/day of high-biologic-value protein for each gram of urinary protein lost each day. If the patient's GFR is less than 25 ml/min/1.73m², then ketoacid-supplemented diets, where available, may be employed. Patients with the nephrotic syndrome must be monitored closely for depletion of protein, vitamin D analogues, and other nutritional deficiencies.

## Maintenance Dialysis Therapy

Although there are few studies of dietary protein requirements for patients undergoing maintenance hemodialysis,[190] it seems clear that they have greater protein needs because of the removal of amino acids and peptides by the dialysis procedure[161,162] and possibly because of other metabolic factors that occur with end-stage renal disease, such as the catabolic stimulus of hemodialysis.[165] Based upon the available evidence from nitrogen balance studies and clinical monitoring of outpatients, it is recommended that patients undergoing maintenance hemodialysis receive 1.0 to 1.2 g protein/kg/day (Table 58–3). Because many maintenance dialysis patients have evidence for protein wasting, a protein intake of 1.2 g/kg/day is preferable for most individuals.

Patients undergoing continuous ambulatory peritoneal dialysis (CAPD) lose about 9 g protein/day into dialysate as well as a small amount of peptides and about 2.5 to 4.0 g/day of amino acids.[163,164] Nitrogen balance studies suggest that CAPD patients should, in general, be prescribed 1.2 to 1.3 g protein/kg/day.[190a] Patients undergoing CAPD who are protein-depleted may be prescribed up to 1.5 protein/kg/day. At least 50% of the daily protein intake of all maintenance dialysis patients probably should be of high biologic value.

## Energy

Studies in nondialyzed chronically uremic patients and those undergoing maintenance hemodialysis indicate that energy expenditure is normal during resting and sitting, following ingestion of a standard meal, and with defined exercise.[191,192] Nitrogen balance studies in nondialyzed chronically uremic patients ingesting 0.55 to 0.60 g protein/kg/day indicate that the amount of energy intake necessary to assure neutral or positive nitrogen balance is approximately 35 kcal/kg/day.[191] However, virtually every survey of energy intake in nondialyzed chronically uremic and hemodialysis patients indicates that, on average, the amount is lower than this level and usually 30 kcal/kg/day or less.[122,146,149,156] In nondialyzed patients with advanced chronic renal failure or patients undergoing maintenance hemodialysis, the finding that decreased body fat is one of the more prominent alterations in nutritional status supports the contention that these patients require more energy than they usually ingest.[149,152,156]

Current recommendations are that nondialyzed chronically uremic patients and patients undergoing maintenance hemodialysis or CAPD should ingest at least 35 kcal/kg/day. Patients who are obese with an edema-free body weight greater than 120% of desirable body weight may be treated with lower calorie intakes. Some patients, particularly those with mild renal insufficiency and young or middle-aged women, may become obese on this energy intake or may refuse to ingest the recommended calories out of fear of obesity. These individuals may require a lower energy prescription to avoid alienation from the staff.

Many commercially available high-calorie foodstuffs are low in protein, sodium, and potassium. A nephrology dietitian can recommend these foodstuffs as well as other low-protein, high-calorie foods that can be prepared easily at home.

### Lipids

Nondialyzed chronically uremic patients and maintenance dialysis patients have a high incidence of type IV hyperlipoproteinemia with elevated serum triglyceride levels, a low serum high-density lipoprotein (HDL) cholesterol, and elevated serum low-density lipoproteins (LDL) and very low-density lipoproteins (VLDL).[142,193] Because these alterations may contribute to the high incidence of atherosclerosis and cardiovascular disease in uremic patients, attention has been directed toward reducing serum triglycerides and increasing HDL cholesterol. Elevated serum triglyceride levels in uremia appear to be caused primarily by impaired clearance from blood. In addition, because diets in renal failure are usually restricted in protein, sodium, potassium, and water, it is often difficult to provide sufficient energy without resorting to a large intake of purified sugars that may increase triglyceride production. Serum triglycerides may be lowered by feeding a diet in which the carbohydrate content is reduced to about 35% of total calories, the fat content is increased to about 55% of total calories, and the polyunsaturated/saturated fatty acid ratio is raised to about 1.5:1.0 (Table 58–3).[194,195]

Some investigators report that serum triglycerides may be decreased if dialysis patients take L-carnitine, a compound that is often low in their plasma and possibly muscle.[196,197] Ingestion of activated charcoal may lower serum cholesterol and triglycerides in chronically uremic rats.[198] Clofibrate also lowers serum triglycerides in uremic patients, but owing to the altered pharmacokinetics of this drug in renal failure, there is a high risk of developing myopathy or other toxicities.[199]

Studies have not been performed to evaluate whether lowering serum triglycerides will improve morbidity and mortality in uremic patients, and high fat intakes might increase the risk of atherosclerotic vascular disease in these patients. It is our current policy to treat hypertriglyceridemia by dietary modification when serum triglycerides are more than slightly elevated (for example, at least 50 mg/dl above the upper given limit of normal). The carbohydrate content should be reduced to supply 35% of calories, the fat content raised to provide about 50% of calories, and the polyunsaturated:saturated fatty acid ratio should be 1.0:1.0. The patient's energy intake should be monitored with this diet to ensure that it does not fall. If serum triglycerides are not increased, it may be preferable to maintain fat intake at closer to 40% of total calories. If serum triglycerides are elevated, serum carnitine should be measured. If serum carnitine is low, patients may receive a trial of L-carnitine, 0.5 to 1.0 g/day orally for nondialyzed chronic failure and maintenance dialysis patients. Alternatively, hemodialysis patients may be given L-carnitine, 1.5 g at the end of each dialysis. There is no established treatment for the low serum concentrations of high-density lipoproteins in uremic patients, although a small amount of alcohol (one glass of wine per day) and exercise may increase levels.[195a]

## Carbohydrates

The patient should be encouraged to eat complex rather than purified carbohydrates to reduce triglyceride synthesis and, where pertinent, to improve glucose tolerance.

## Phosphorus

In renal failure patients, a high dietary phosphorus intake can lead to a high plasma calcium-phosphorus product with increased risk of calcium phosphate deposition in soft tissues.[200] As previously discussed, both animal and human studies indicate that a low phosphorus intake may reduce the rate of decline in renal function in chronic renal disease.[85–87,200a]

The degree to which dietary phosphorus should be reduced is not well established. For the nondialyzed patient, one approach would be to attempt to maintain normal renal tubular reabsorption of phosphorus, to prevent elevated serum parathyroid hormone levels. This approach would require a very low phosphorus intake, lower than can usually be obtained with the combination of a low-phosphorus diet and phosphate binders, unless ketoacid- or essential amino-acid-supplemented very-low-protein diets are used and the GFR is above 15 ml/min (Table 58–3). At the very least, in both nondialyzed and dialyzed patients, the morning fasting serum phosphorus concentrations should always be maintained within the normal range. Because there is a rough correlation between the protein and phosphorus content of the diet, it is easier to restrict phosphorus if protein intake is reduced.

For nondialyzed patients with a GFR below 25 ml/min/1.73m² who are prescribed a 0.55- to 0.60-g/kg/day protein diet, the phosphorus intake generally can be decreased to 5 to 10 mg/kg/day without substantially increasing the burdensomeness of the diet. This level of dietary phosphorus restriction usually does not maintain serum phosphorus levels within normal limits in patients with a GFR under about 15 ml/min, even with a reduction in the renal tubular reabsorption of phosphorus. Hence, phosphate binders are also employed. Traditionally, the two most commonly used phosphate binders have been aluminum carbonate and aluminum hydroxide. Usually, two to four 500-mg capsules taken three to four times per day are needed. Greater doses may be used if necessary. Evidence that aluminum-induced osteomalacia may be causally related to the intake of aluminum phosphate binders has made many nephrologists uneasy about using such binders.[201,202] However, the hazards of severe uncontrolled hyperparathyroidism would seem to outweigh the potential dangers of aluminum-induced osteomalacia. Thus, if serum phosphorus levels cannot be maintained within normal limits by diet alone, phosphate binders are used. Several nonaluminum phosphate binders are under investigation.[203] At present, the most commonly used is calcium carbonate. Calcium carbonate is taken in divided doses with meals and should not be given unless the serum phosphorus level is normal to avoid precipitation of calcium phosphate in soft tissues. Thus, hyperphosphatemic patients may be treated with an aluminum binder of phosphate until serum phosphorus falls to within normal limits, and at that time, they may be changed to calcium carbonate. Normally, patients should not receive more than about 5.0 g/day of calcium carbonate to prevent excessive accumulation of calcium in soft tissues.

As previously indicated, one advantage to the diets providing amino acids or ketoacids with about 0.28 g protein/kg/day is the greater ease with which the phosphorus intake can be lowered, often to as low as 4 to 6 mg/kg/day. If future studies confirm that these lower phosphorus intakes are both safe and beneficial for patients with mild or moderate renal insufficiency, this would provide additional justification for the use of these semi-synthetic diets at earlier stages of renal failure.

For patients with a GFR between 25 and 70 ml/min/1.73m$^2$ or with a higher GFR and a progressive loss of renal function, 7 to 12 mg phosphorus/kg/day may be prescribed with the 0.60- to 0.70-g protein/kg/day diet. Even this level of reduction in phosphorus intake will be difficult for some patients to accept, and lower phosphorus intakes will make the diet too restrictive for virtually all patients. These individual generally are not given phosphate binders unless the serum phosphorus levels rise above normal. The recommended phosphorus intake for the maintenance hemodialysis or CAPD patient is about 17 mg/kg/day or less. This higher upper limit was chosen because dialysis patients, with their greater protein intakes, cannot readily ingest less phosphorus without making the diet too restrictive. Maintenance dialysis patients usually require phosphate binders to prevent hyperphosphatemia.

At present, there is no defined lower safe limit for the serum phosphorus level in renal failure. Experience suggests that if the fasting serum phosphorus is maintained above the lower limit of normal, patients will not develop evidence for phosphate depletion. More work is necessary to examine whether this perception is valid.

## Calcium

Patients with chronic renal failure, including those undergoing maintenance dialysis therapy, usually have an increased dietary calcium requirement because they have both vitamin D deficiency and resistance to the actions of vitamin D. These disorders, which lead to impaired intestinal calcium absorption, are compounded by the low calcium content of diets for uremic patients. A 40-g protein diet, for example, generally provides only about 300 to 400 mg/day of calcium. Dietary calcium intake is low because many foods that are high in calcium are high in phosphorus (e.g., dairy products) and are therefore restricted for uremic patients.

Nondialyzed chronically uremic patients usually require 1,200 to 1,600 mg/day of calcium for neutral or positive calcium balance.[204] The current recommendation is to provide a total daily calcium intake (diet plus supplement) of 1,400 to 1,600 mg/day. Thus, the low-protein diets need to be supplemented with 1,000 to 1,400 mg/day of elemental calcium. Supplemental calcium should not be initiated unless the serum phosphorus concentration is normal (i.e., 2.5 to 4.5 mg/dl) in order to prevent calcium phosphate deposition in soft tissues. In addition, frequent monitoring of serum calcium is important because hypercalcemia may develop, particularly if serum phosphorus should fall to low-normal or low levels. Patients undergoing maintenance hemodialysis or peritoneal dialysis may require 1.0 g/day of supplemental calcium even though there is net calcium uptake from dialysate. The supplemental calcium should be taken in two or three divided doses each day.

Calcium comprises 40% of calcium carbonate, 18% of calcium lactate, and 9% of calcium gluconate. Calcium chloride should be avoided in uremic patients because of its acidifying properties. Calcium carbonate is inexpensive. It has a chalky taste but the flavor is easily masked, and it is usually well tolerated. Many calcium carbonate preparations available over the counter can be purchased without prescription. Caution should be exercised because some calcium carbonate preparations contain small amounts of amino acids. Treatment with vitamin D analogues may decrease the daily calcium requirement by enhancing intestinal calcium absorption.

## Magnesium

In chronic renal failure, there is net absorption of approximately 50% of ingested magnesium from the intestinal tract (net absorption is the difference between dietary intake and fecal excretion).[204] The absorbed magnesium is excreted primarily by the kidney. Hence, in renal failure, hypermagnesemia may occur.[27] Because the restricted diets of uremic patients are low in magnesium (usually about 100 to 300 mg/day for a 40-g protein diet), their serum magnesium levels are usually normal or only slightly elevated unless the patient takes substances that are high in magnesium content, such as magnesium-containing antacids and laxatives.[27,204] Nondialyzed chronically uremic patients require about 200 mg/day of magnesium to maintain neutral magnesium balance.[204] The optimal dietary magnesium allowance for the dialysis patient has not been well defined.

### Sodium and Water

Sodium is freely filterable by the glomerulus. In the normal kidney, the renal tubules reabsorb well over 99% of the filtered sodium (see Table 58–1). As renal insufficiency progresses, both the glomerular filtration and fractional reabsorption of sodium fall progressively. Thus, many patients with renal failure are able to maintain sodium balance with a normal salt intake. Normally, only about 1 to 3 meq/day of sodium are excreted in the feces, and in the nonsweating individual, only a few meq/day of sodium are lost through the skin. Despite an adaptive reduction in the renal tubular reabsorption of sodium when end-stage renal disease supervenes, patients may be unable to excrete the quantity of sodium ingested, and they may develop edema, hypertension, or congestive heart failure. This syndrome is particularly likely to occur when the GFR is below 4 to 10 ml/minute. When renal insufficiency is complicated by congestive heart failure, the nephrotic syndrome, or advanced liver disease, the propensity for sodium retention is increased. With decreased ability to excrete sodium, restriction of sodium and water intake and the use of diuretic medications may be necessary. In renal failure, hypertension often is more easily controlled with sodium restriction and may be accentuated with increased sodium intakes, possibly because of expansion of the extracellular fluid volume.[205]

In addition, nondialyzed patients with chronic renal failure often have an inability to conserve sodium normally.[123] A low sodium intake may not be sufficient to replace urinary and extrarenal sodium losses, and the patient may develop sodium depletion, a decrease in extracellular fluid volume, blood volume, and renal blood flow, and a further reduction in GFR. Volume depletion may be difficult to recognize. An unexplained weight loss or decrease in blood pressure may be signs of this condition. Nondialyzed patients with chronic renal failure who do not have evidence for fluid overload, hypertension, or heart failure may be cautiously given a greater sodium intake to determine whether their GFR can be improved slightly by extracellular volume expansion.

In general, when sodium balance is well controlled, thirst will regulate water balance adequately. However, when the GFR falls below 2 to 5 ml/minute, there is a particular risk of overhydration, and water intake should be controlled independently of sodium to prevent overhydration. In diabetics, hyperglycemia may also increase thirst and enhance positive water balance. For patients with far-advanced renal failure whose total body water is at the desired level (as indicated by normal or near-normal blood pressure, absence of edema, and normal serum sodium), urine volume may be a good guide to water intake. The daily water intake should equal the urine output plus approximately 500 ml to replace insensible losses.

In most nondialyzed patients with advanced renal failure, a daily intake of 1,000 to 3,000 mg (40 to 130 meq) of sodium and 1,500 to 3,000 ml of fluid will maintain sodium and water balance. The requirement for sodium and water varies markedly, and each patient must be managed individually. Patients undergoing maintenance hemodialysis or peritoneal dialysis usually are oliguric or anuric. For hemodialysis patients, sodium and total fluid intake generally should be restricted to 1,000 to 1,500 mg/day and 700 to 1,500 ml/day, respectively. Patients undergoing CAPD usually tolerate a greater sodium and water intake because salt and water can be easily removed by using hypertonic dialysate, which increases the flow of salt and water from the body into the peritoneal cavity, from which they are drained. Maintaining a large dietary sodium and water intake allows the quantity of fluid removed from the CAPD patient and, hence, the daily dialysate volume to be increased. This increase may be advantageous because the daily clearance of small molecules with CAPD is directly related to the volume of dialysate outflow. In nondialyzed chronically uremic patients or in those undergoing maintenance dialysis who are not anuric and who gain excessive sodium or water despite attempts at dietary restriction, a potent diuretic, such as furosemide, may be tried to increase urinary sodium and water excretion.

### Potassium

Normally, the kidney provides the major route for potassium excretion. In renal failure, potassium retention may occur and may lead quickly to fatal hyperkalemia. Two factors may prevent this occurrence in renal failure. First, as long as urine output remains at approximately 1,000 ml/day or greater, tubular secretion of potassium in the remaining functioning nephrons tends to be increased, and therefore the renal potassium clearance does not fall as markedly as the GFR. Second, fecal excretion of potassium is increased owing to enhanced intestinal secretion.[188] Thus, patients with chronic renal failure usually do not become hyperkalemic unless there is (1) excessive intake of potassium; (2) acidosis, oliguria, hypoaldosteronism (e.g., secondary to decreased renin secretion by the diseased kidney or renal tubular resistance to the actions of aldosterone); or (3) catabolic stress. Patients with chronic renal failure and those undergoing maintenance hemodialysis, in general, should receive no more than 70 meq of potassium per day.

## Trace Elements

Excesses and deficiencies of certain trace elements may be prevalent in renal failure. Dietary requirements for trace elements have not been well defined in uremic patients. Iron deficiency is common because intestinal iron absorption is sometimes impaired, there are often substantial blood losses, and iron may bind to the dialyzer membrane.[166,206] Both chronically uremic and dialysis patients may be given oral iron supplements. Ferrous sulfate, 300 mg three times a day, one half hour after meals, may be used. In some patients, other oral iron salts are better tolerated. Patients who are intolerant to oral iron supplements or who have iron deficiency may be best treated with intramuscular or intravenous iron.

Although the zinc content of most tissues is normal in renal failure,[207] serum and hair zinc may be low and red cell zinc is increased. Some reports indicate that dysgeusia, poor food intake, and impaired sexual function, which are common problems of uremic patients, may be improved by giving them zinc supplements.[208,209] Additional studies in this area are clearly indicated.

As previously indicated, increased body burden of aluminum has been implicated in nondialyzed chronically uremic and maintenance dialysis patients as a cause of a progressive dementia syndrome (particularly in hemodialysis patients), osteomalacia, weakness of the muscles of the proximal limbs, and anemia.[129,210,210a] Although contamination of dialysate with aluminum previously was the major source of aluminum toxicity in many dialysis centers, current methods of water treatment have removed virtually all aluminum from dialysate. At present, ingestion of aluminum binders of phosphate is probably the major cause of the excess body burden of aluminum. Consequently, many nephrologists now use aluminum binders more sparingly and rely more upon low-phosphorus diets and nonaluminum phosphate binders—particularly calcium carbonate—to control serum phosphorus levels.[203] The amount of phosphate that is bound by calcium salts is small, particularly if the total daily calcium intake is restricted to no more than two or three grams in order to avoid excessive calcium absorption. More efficient and nontoxic phosphate

binders are needed. Aluminum toxicity may be treated by reduction of aluminum intake and by intravenous infusions of desferrioxamine, a chelator of aluminum.[129] This chelator can be removed from the body by hemodialysis or peritoneal dialysis.

Many trace elements are bound avidly to serum proteins and, when present even in small quantities in dialysate, they may be taken up into blood and cause toxicity. It is therefore recommended that, as a routine practice, dialysate should be purified of trace elements prior to use. In certain circumstances, therapeutic doses of trace elements might be administered through dialysis, as has been done for zinc.[209]

## Vitamins

Chronically uremic patients are prone to develop deficiencies of water-soluble vitamins unless supplements are given. There are specific reasons for this tendency. First, vitamin intake is often low because of anorexia and poor food intake and also because many foods that are high in water-soluble vitamins are often restricted owing to the elevated potassium content. The typical diet for nondialyzed chronic renal failure and maintenance dialysis patients is frequently below the Recommended Daily Allowances for certain water-soluble vitamins.[128] Second, the metabolism of certain water-soluble vitamins tends to be altered in chronic renal failure.[211,212] Third, many medicines interfere with the intestinal absorption, metabolism, or actions of vitamins.[128] Vitamin $B_6$, vitamin C, and folic acid are the water-soluble vitamins most likely to be deficient in nondialyzed patients with chronic renal failure and in maintenance dialysis patients. Vitamin $B_{12}$ deficiency is uncommon in uremia because the daily requirement is small (3 $\mu g$/day for nonpregnant, nonlactating adults),[117] the body can store large quantities of this vitamin, and vitamin $B_{12}$ is protein-bound in plasma and hence is poorly dialyzed.

Many of the studies that indicated a need for routine vitamin supplementation in nondialyzed chronic renal failure or maintenance dialysis patients were carried out in the 1960s and early 1970s, at a time when the incidence of poor nutritional intake of these patients may have been greater than it is today.[128] Indeed, some more recent studies have suggested that many maintenance hemodialysis patients may subsist for months with no vitamin supplementation and without developing deficiencies of water-soluble vitamins.[213] However, these latter studies have not demonstrated that a small but sizable proportion of patients will not develop water-soluble vitamin deficiencies, particularly after one or more years of dialysis treatment. Because several different factors promote water-soluble vitamin deficiencies in these patients and because the water-soluble vitamin supplements are safe, it would seem prudent to continue to routinely use them until these issues are more completely resolved.

The daily supplements for most vitamins are not well defined in renal failure. There is evidence that, in addition to vitamin intake from foods, the following daily supplements of vitamins will prevent or correct vitamin deficiency (see Table 58–3): pyridoxine hydrochloride, 5 mg in nondialyzed patients and 10 mg in maintenance hemodialysis or peritoneal dialysis patients; folic acid, 1 mg; and the Recommended Daily Allowance for normal individuals for the other water-soluble vitamins.[117] It is probable that renal failure patients may need less than 1.0 mg/day of folic acid. However, since this vitamin is safe and some evidence suggests that there may be competitive interference with its actions in uremia,[128,211] it may be advisable to prescribe this dose of folic acid until more definitive studies of the requirements are carried out. A supplement of only 60 mg/day of vitamin C (the Recommended Daily Allowance[117]) is advised because ascorbic acid can be metabolized to oxalate. Large doses of ascorbic acid have been associated with increased plasma oxalate levels in renal failure patients.[214,215] Oxalate is highly insoluble, and there is substantial concern that high plasma oxalate concentrations can lead to precipitation in soft tissues, including the kidney, and can cause further impairment in renal function in the nondialyzed patient with renal insufficiency.

Because serum retinol-binding protein and vitamin A are elevated in uremia,[216] the routine use of supplemental vitamin A is not recommended, particularly because even relatively small doses of vitamin A (i.e., 7,500 to 15,000 IU/day) may cause bone toxicity.[217] Additional vitamin E and K are probably not necessary. However, patients who receive antibiotics for extended periods and who do not ingest foods containing vitamin K may need vitamin K supplements.[218]

Although in renal failure, many of the beneficial effects of $1,25\text{-}(OH)_2D_3$ can be reproduced by administration of other vitamin D analogues, such as dihydrotachysterol, cholecalciferol, or 25-hydroxycholecalciferol, $1,25\text{-}(OH)_2D_3$ has the advantage that it is the most potent agent. Because it is given in smaller doses and has a shorter half-life, there is little storage of this compound. Hence, it may be a safer agent to use. The high potency of $1,25\text{-}(OH)_2D_3$, however, increases the risk of hypercalcemia and hyperphosphatemia.[125,126]

Treatment with oral $1,25\text{-}(OH)_2D_3$ increases intestinal calcium and phosphorus absorption, raises serum calcium, lowers serum parathyroid hormone, decreases serum alkaline phosphatase activity, reduces bone reabsorption, decreases endosteal fibrosis, and often improves osteomalacia.[125,126] Therapy with $1,25\text{-}(OH)_2D_3$ is indicated for hyperparathyroidism, osteitis fibrosa, mixed osteomalacia and osteitis fibrosa, and severe hypocalcemia.[125] Some chronically uremic patients with vitamin D deficiency develop a myopathy, primarily of the proximal limb muscles, and may present with severe weakness. Strength may improve with vitamin D therapy.

Treatment with $1,25\text{-}(OH)_2D_3$ usually is started at 0.25 to 0.50 µg/day. The serum calcium must be monitored carefully, and if it is low and does not rise by at least 0.5 mg/dl with any particular dosage, the dose may be increased by 0.25 to 0.50 µg/day every four to six weeks. Hypercalcemia is treated by temporary withdrawal of $1,25\text{-}(OH)_2D_3$. Ultimately, the best criterion for effective treatment with $1,25\text{-}(OH)_2D_3$ is improvement in bone anatomy as determined by bone histology, radiographs, and densitometry. Improvement in muscle function or abolition of severe hypocalcemia also may indicate appropriate dosage of $1,25\text{-}(OH)_2D_3$. With time, the requirements for $1,25\text{-}(OH)_2D_3$ and the tolerance for this vitamin may decrease, and the maintenance dosage may have to be reduced. This change may occur after there has been sufficient bone healing so that the skeleton no longer serves as a sink for calcium and phosphorus. It is important that $1,25\text{-}(OH)_2D_3$ not be started unless serum calcium and phosphorus are not elevated and the calcium-phosphorus product is below 45. Serum calcium and phosphorus should be monitored during therapy to ensure that the concentrations are normal.

Slatopolsky and co-workers have reported that in maintenance hemodialysis patients, intravenous $1,25\text{-}(OH)_2D_3$ lowers serum parathyroid hormone levels more effectively than does the oral preparation, by an average of 70%.[219] The greater effect of intravenous $1,25\text{-}(OH)_2D_3$ may occur because a lower fraction of the dose may be taken up by the small intestine where it promotes calcium absorption and hypercalcemia. Because a lower fraction of infused $1,25\text{-}(OH)_2D_3$ is bound by and acts upon the intestine, greater amounts can be administered safely. Hence, with intravenous treatment, higher blood $1,25\text{-}(OH)_2D_3$ concentrations can be obtained, and the parathyroid glands may be suppressed more readily.

Vitamin D analogues currently are administered routinely only to patients with chronic renal failure who have clinical signs or symptoms of vitamin D deficiency and to uremic children to promote growth. It is likely that eventually all uremic patients who have low vitamin D levels will be given these agents.

## Acidosis

Metabolic acidosis occurs frequently in nondialyzed patients with chronic renal failure because the ability of the kidney to excrete acidic metabolites is impaired. In the earlier stages of chronic renal failure, metabolic acidosis can also be caused by excessive renal losses of bicarbonate. The rate of acid production is probably normal or below normal in stable chronically uremic patients. Acidosis can cause bone reabsorption and such symptoms as lethargy and weakness. Ingestion of low-nitrogen diets may prevent or reduce the severity of the acidosis by decreasing the endogenous generation of acidic products of protein metabolism. Alkali supplements are usually effective for preventing or treating the acidosis of chronic renal failure. Calcium carbonate, 5 g/day, may correct mild acidosis, provide needed calcium, and reduce intestinal phosphate absorption. For more severe acidosis, sodium bicarbonate or citrate may be administered orally or intravenously. If the nondialyzed chronically uremic patient is not oliguric and is not likely to develop edema, sodium is usually readily excreted when administered as sodium bicarbonate or citrate. Alkali therapy should probably be initiated if the arterial pH is below 7.35 or the serum bicarbonate is less than 20 meq/L. Before alkali therapy is implemented, it must be ascertained that the low serum bicarbonate is not a compensatory response to chronic respiratory alkalosis. If acidosis is severe and not controlled by the foregoing measures, hemodialysis or peritoneal dialysis may be employed.

## Fiber

Studies in the normal population suggest that a high dietary fiber intake may cause a lower incidence of constipation, irritable bowel syndrome, diverticulitis, and neoplasia of the colon, and possibly a greater glucose tolerance.[220] A high dietary fiber intake also may reduce the SUN by decreasing colonic bacterial ammonia generation and enhancing fecal nitrogen excretion.[221] Because the patient with renal failure may benefit from fiber intake, we currently prescribe 20 to 25 g/day of total dietary fiber; this amount may not be tolerated because of its potassium content.

## Prioritizing Dietary Goals

The number and magnitude of dietary modifications for chronically uremic patients are so great that if they are all presented to the patient at one time, demoralization and noncompliance may result. Hence, we often list goals for dietary treatment according to priority. Control of protein, phosphorus, sodium, energy, potassium, calcium, and magnesium intake generally is emphasized. On the other hand, unless the patient has a lipid disorder that carries a high risk of atherosclerotic disease, the types of carbohydrates and fats ingested and the ratio of the carbohydrate to fat intake are usually given lower priorities. A high dietary fiber intake also is not emphasized as strongly.

## NUTRITIONAL THERAPY IN ACUTE RENAL FAILURE

Acute renal failure is characterized by a sudden reduction or cessation in GFR. The most common causes of acute renal failure include shock, severe infection, trauma, medicines, obstruction, and certain types of glomerulonephritis. In most instances, if the patient survives the underlying diseases he will recover from the acute renal failure. When patients sustain acute renal failure, they are likely to develop fluid and electrolyte disorders, uremic toxicity, and wasting. These disorders are particularly prone to develop when the patient is both oliguric and hypercatabolic, which are common complications of acute renal failure.

Patients with acute renal failure, and particularly those with underlying catabolic illnesses, frequently undergo metabolic changes that promote degradation of protein and amino acids and consumption of fuel substrates. Energy expenditure is often increased.[222] In vitro studies with rat muscle tissue indicate that protein degradation is enhanced and protein synthesis is reduced.[223,224] In addition, hepatic gluconeogenesis is increased. If the liver from these animals is perfused or incubated with amino acids, the elevated hepatic glucose and urea production is further enhanced.[225] These findings have important implications for the nutritional management of patients with acute renal failure. As a result of the metabolic derangements, these patients are often unable to utilize protein, amino acids, and energy substrates efficiently. Hence, it may be difficult to maintain and to improve the nutritional status of these patients by enteral or parenteral nutrition.[226,227]

## General Principles

Because the available data concerning optimal nutritional therapy for acute renal failure are both limited and conflicting, it is not possible to strongly justify any treatment plan for such patients. The following therapeutic approach, summarized in Table 58–4, is based upon our analysis of the literature and personal experience.

Fluid and mineral balance should be carefully monitored in acute renal failure to prevent over-hydration or electrolyte disorders. Water intake, in general, should equal output from urine and all other measured sources (e.g., nasogastric aspirate, fistula drainage) plus 400 ml/day. This regimen takes into account the contributions of endogenous water production from metabolism and the insensible water losses (from respiration, skin losses) to water balance. In general, if the patient is catabolic, weight should be allowed to decrease by 0.2 to 0.5 kg/day to avoid excessive accumulation of fluid. Sodium, potassium, phosphorus, and magnesium intake should be restricted to prevent accumulation of these minerals. Energy and, if feasible, protein intake should satisfy the patient's nutritional requirements, which may exceed normal. By controlling the water and electrolyte intake and lowering the UNA, one may be able to reduce the need for dialysis treatments.

The patient's desirable nutrient intake will depend on the nutritional status, catabolic rate, residual GFR, and the indications for initiating dialysis therapy. For example, in a patient who is wasted, one might be more inclined to give a surfeit of nutrients and to provide dialysis as needed. A patient with acute renal failure who has a high residual GFR also may receive larger quantities of nutrients, because there is less risk of developing fluid and electrolyte disorders or accumulating potentially toxic metabolites. On the other hand, for a patient who has little or no urine flow and is not very catabolic or uremic, the intake of small quantities of water, minerals, and amino acids may reduce the need for dialysis. This latter approach may be particularly beneficial if it is anticipated that the patient will not tolerate dialysis well. Similarly, a patient who is starting to recover from acute renal failure may be given this latter regimen in order to avoid the need for a dialysis for a few days until renal function becomes adequate; in this patient, a high-calorie diet providing small amounts of essential amino acids or ketoacids with little or no protein may be used for short periods.

Whenever feasible, patients with acute renal failure should receive oral nutrition. If the patient will not eat adequately, the use of liquid formula diets, elemental diets, and tube or enterostomy feeding should be considered. Often parenteral nutrition is the only technique that will provide adequate nutrient intake.

### Specific Nutrient Intakes

**Protein and Amino Acid Intake.** The quantity of nitrogen and the composition of the amino acid

formulations that are administered enterally or parenterally to patients with acute renal failure are the subject of controversy. Abel and associates carried out a series of studies that suggested benefits of parenteral nutrition for patients with acute renal failure.[228–230] The patients were infused with solutions containing D-glucose and 12 to 30 g/day of essential amino acids but no nonessential amino acids. The authors reported that the SUN and serum potassium, phosphorus, and magnesium often stabilized or decreased and dialysis therapy sometimes could be postponed or avoided. In a prospective, randomized double-blind study, these investigators compared infusion of glucose and essential amino acids to treatment with an isocaloric infusion of hypertonic glucose that contained no amino acids.[230] The patients receiving glucose and essential amino acids had significantly greater survival until renal function recovered; hospital survival was slightly but not significantly increased. Retrospective studies with nonconcurrent controls reported by other investigators suggest that parenteral nutrition providing essential and nonessential amino acids improved morbidity and mortality, particularly in the patients with the more complicated clinical courses.[231–232]

Leonard et al. reported that parenteral nutrition with glucose and about 21 g/day of essential amino acids compared to isocaloric infusions with glucose alone had no advantages with regard to SUN levels, nitrogen balance, or survival in patients with acute renal failure.[233] Feinstein and co-workers carried out a randomized prospective double-blind study of individuals with acute renal failure who were unable to eat adequately.[226] Thirty patients were treated with one of three isocaloric parenteral nutrition formulations: hypertonic glucose with no amino acids, hypertonic glucose with 21 g/day of essential amino acids, or hypertonic glucose with 21 g/day of essential and 21 g/day of nonessential amino acids. The mean duration of study was 9.2 days per patient. The metabolic balance data indicated that many of these patients were severely catabolic with net rates of protein degradation, determined from the difference between nitrogen intake and the UNA, that were as high as 240 g/day. The UNA, nitrogen balance, and mortality rate were not different with any of the three infusion regimens.

It has been argued that more than 40 g/day of a mixture of essential and nonessential amino acids may be more effective at improving nitrogen balance. Feinstein and co-workers tested this hypothesis in a randomized prospective trial.[227] Patients received TPN providing 21 g/day of essential amino acids or TPN with essential and

**Table 58–4. Typical Composition of Solutions for Total Parenteral Nutrition in Patients with Acute Renal Failure***

| | | *Daily Quantity or Concentration to be Infused* |
|---|---|---|
| Volume | (L) | 1.0 |
| Essential and nonessential free crystalline amino acids (4.25–5.0%) or | g/L | 42.5–50 |
| Essential amino acids (5%)† | g/L | 12.5–25 |
| Dextrose (D-glucose)‡ | g/L | 350 |
| Energy (approx.)‡ | kcal/L | 1,140 |
| Electrolytes§ | | |
|   Sodium‖ | mmol/L | 40–50 |
|   Chloride‖ | mmol/L | 25–35 |
|   Potassium | mmol/day | ≤35 |
|   Acetate | mmol/day | 35–40 |
|   Calcium | mmol/day | 5 |
|   Phosphorus | mmol/day | 8 |
|   Magnesium | mmol/day | 4 |
|   Iron | mg/day | 2 |
|   Trace Elements | | (see text) |
| Vitamins | | |
|   Vitamin A** | | see text |
|   Vitamin D | | see text |
|   Vitamin K†† | mg/week | 7.5 |
|   Vitamin E‡‡ | IU/day | 10 |
|   Niacin | mg/day | 20 |
|   Thiamin HCl (B$_1$) | mg/day | 2 |
|   Riboflavin (B$_2$) | mg/day | 2 |
|   Pantothenic acid (B$_3$) | mg/day | 10 |
|   Pyridoxine HCl (B$_6$) | mg/day | 10 |
|   Ascorbic acid (C) | mg/day | 60–100 |
|   Biotin | mg/day | 200 |
|   Folic acid†† | mg/day | 2 |
|   Vitamin B$_{12}$†† | μg/day | 3 |

*These nutrients are present in each bottle containing 500 ml of 8.5 to 10% crystalline amino acids or 250 to 500 ml of 5% essential amino acids and 500 ml of 70% dextrose. The vitamins and trace elements are an exception because they are added to only one bottle per day. The patient's fluid status and serum electrolytes and glucose must be monitored closely. The composition and volume of the infusate may need to be changed if the patient is very uremic, acidotic, or volume-overloaded, if the serum electrolyte concentrations are not normal or if they are changing, or if dialysis therapy is not readily available or is particularly hazardous to the patient (see text).

†For patients who are more catabolic (e.g., UNA ≥5 g/day), are undergoing regular dialysis treatments (particularly for two or more weeks), or who are wasted, essential and nonessential amino acids may be infused: about 1.0–1.2 g/kg/day for hemodialysis patients and 1.2–1.3 g/kg/day for intermittent or CAPD patients (see text). For patients who are less wasted, are less catabolic, are not undergoing regular dialysis therapy, and will not be receiving TPN for more than two or three weeks, 21 to 40 g/day of the nine essential amino acids may be infused. See text for discussion of the formulations of amino acids. Only solutions of crystalline amino acids should be used.

‡To obtain an energy intake of 35 to 50 kcal/kg/day, 70% dextrose is added as necessary (see text). Lower energy intakes may be used in very obese patients. For the higher levels of energy intake (i.e., 45–50 kcal/kg/day), additional 70% dextrose may be added to the solutions. To balance the sources of calories and to prevent essential fatty acid deficiency, 50 to 100 g of lipids are infused each day or at least on two days each week. Usually a 20% lipid emulsion (250–500 ml) is used to reduce the water load. The approximate calorie values are dextrose monohydrate, 3.4 kcal/g; amino acids, 3.5 kcal/g.

§When one is adding electrolytes, the amounts intrinsically present in the amino acid solution should be taken into account.

‖Refers to the final concentrations of electrolytes after any additional 70% dextrose or other solutions have been added.

**Vitamin A is best avoided unless TPN is continued for more than two or three weeks (see text).

††Should be given orally or parenterally and not in the total parenteral nutrition solution because of antagonisms.

‡‡May need to be increased with use of lipid emulsions.

nonessential amino acids provided in a 1.0 to 1.0 ratio. With the latter treatment, attempts were made to infuse a quantity of nitrogen equal to the UNA. Thirteen patients with acute renal failure were randomly assigned to one of the two treatments. The results indicated that although the nitrogen intake was five times greater with the latter regimen, the nitrogen balance, determined from the difference between intake and urea nitrogen appearance, was not different. The UNA fell significantly only in the patients receiving the essential amino acids, whereas it tended to rise in the other group.

These data suggest that high-calorie solutions providing about 21 g/day of essential amino acids may be used more efficiently than isocaloric preparations containing larger quantities of essential and nonessential amino acids (e.g., 40 to 70 g/day) provided in an essential to nonessential ratio of 1.0:1.0. The essential amino acid solutions seem to reduce the UNA and total nitrogen output more than the essential and nonessential amino acids. Consequently, nitrogen balance seems to be no more negative with the former preparations, but the accumulation of nitrogenous metabolites is less. It would be of interest to examine the response to a TPN regimen that provides larger quantities of essential and nonessential amino acids but that contains a greater proportion of essential amino acids.

The data from rat studies are also inconclusive. Toback and associates caused acute renal failure in rats by injection of mercuric chloride.[234,235] The rats infused with glucose and a mixture of essential and nonessential amino acids had greater regeneration of renal cortical cells, as determined by [14]C-choline incorporation into phospholipids, than rats who were infused with glucose alone. Amino acids promoted intracellular protein synthesis as determined by [14]C-leucine uptake.[236] The maximum serum creatinine concentration also was lower in the rats infused with glucose and amino acids, suggesting that these nutrients enhanced the recovery of renal function. However, Oken and co-workers were unable to show a consistent beneficial effect of glucose and essential amino acids or glucose and essential and nonessential amino acids as compared to glucose alone on the rate or incidence of recovery of renal function or survival in rats with acute renal failure.[237]

These conflicting observations are probably the result of the following factors: (1) The clinical course of patients with acute renal failure is so complex and variable that it would be necessary to study large numbers of patients to show statistically significant benefits of nutritional therapy, if they exist. (2) Many of these studies were ret-

rospective or not randomly controlled. This fact may have led to unintentional biases in the results. (3) The optimal composition of nutrients in the TPN solutions has not been defined, and the use of suboptimal formulations of nutrients may reduce the clinical benefits of nutritional therapy. (4) It is probable that catabolic patients or rats with acute renal failure may need both good nutrition and metabolic intervention to suppress catabolic processes and to promote anabolism. Providing nutrients without metabolic intervention may not have a beneficial effect on nutritional status or clinical outcome, particularly in the first days after the onset of acute renal failure.

It is pertinent that the prospective studies of parenteral nutrition in patients with acute renal failure compared different regimens of nutritional therapy (i.e., infusion of high-calorie solutions containing amino acids versus isocaloric infusions without amino acids; administration of isocaloric solutions with essential amino acids as compared to essential and nonessential amino acids). No study has compared the clinical course of patients receiving nutritional therapy to those receiving no special nutritional support. The foregoing studies in patients with acute renal failure did not examine whether parenteral nutrition is beneficial. They only compared the response to different formulations of parenteral nutrition for these patients.

Our current policy for amino acid or protein intake in patients with acute renal failure is as follows: patients may be prescribed a low enteral or intravenous nitrogen intake if there is a low UNA (i.e., equal to or less than 4 to 5 g N/day), no evidence for severe protein malnutrition, and the anticipation that the patient will recover renal function within the next one or two weeks. A severely reduced glomerular filtration rate or the desire to avoid dialysis therapy are other factors that would suggest the use of a low nitrogen intake. Under these conditions, we may use 0.3 to 0.5 g/kg/day of primarily high-quality protein or essential amino acids, with or without arginine. We do not give more than 40 g/day of essential amino acids because there is evidence that larger quantities of the nine essential amino acids may cause serious amino acid imbalances.[238] Diets providing 0.10 to 0.30 g/kg/day of miscellaneous protein and 10 to 20 g/day of essential amino acids or ketoacids may also be used in patients who can eat. These regimens should minimize the rate of accumulation of nitrogenous metabolites and, unless the patient is severely catabolic, will usually maintain neutral or only mildly negative nitrogen balance. Hence, the need for dialysis therapy may be minimized or avoided. If the patient has substantial residual renal function (e.g., GFR of 5 to 10 ml/min) and is not very catabolic, he may be treated as a nondialyzed patient with chronic renal failure. The individual would receive 0.55 to 0.60 g/kg desirable body weight/day of protein or amino acids.

For patients who are more catabolic and have a higher UNA (greater than 5 g N/day), are severely wasted, or are undergoing regular dialysis therapy and either have or are anticipated to have acute renal failure for more than two weeks, we are inclined to prescribe a higher protein or amino acid intake, up to 1.0 to 1.2 g/kg desirable body weight/day. In comparison to small quantities of essential amino acids, these larger nitrogen intakes may improve nitrogen balance, particularly after the first one or two weeks of dialysis treatments. However, the UNA almost invariably rises, and the increased azotemia and, in those patients receiving TPN, the larger volumes of fluid necessary to provide this amount of amino acids may increase the need for dialysis.

If acute renal failure persists for more than two to three weeks, patients undergoing regular dialysis treatment are treated as maintenance dialysis patients, with about 1.0 to 1.2 g/kg/day of protein or amino acids for hemodialysis or 1.2 to 1.5 g/kg/day for maintenance intermittent or continuous ambulatory peritoneal dialysis.

Because the metabolic status of patients with acute renal failure often is organized to facilitate the catabolism of protein, amino acids, and other energy substrates,[222–225,239] there may be advantages to administering agents that promote anabolic processes or reduce catabolic pathways. Anabolic steroidal compounds, many of which are androgenic and resemble testosterone, have been used in patients with acute renal failure.[240,241] These agents can reduce UNA and increase nitrogen balance; they also have been reported to decrease the need for dialysis treatments. In vitro studies of skeletal muscle from rats with acute renal failure indicate that insulin may increase synthesis and reduce degradation of protein.[224] Studies in catabolic patients who do not have renal failure indicate that insulin may decrease the UNA.[242,243] As mentioned previously, the nitrogen intake appears to be utilized more efficiently if a greater proportion of the administered amino acids are essential.[226,227] This hypothesis has not yet been tested clinically. In addition, studies in catabolic patients without renal failure suggest that intravenous infusions in which a large proportion of the amino acids are branched chain (i.e., isoleucine, leucine, and valine) may have a specific anabolic effect.[244,245] Not all studies confirm these findings. Ketoacid analogues of the branched-chain amino acids in in vitro preparations and in nonuremic individuals who are not hypercatabolic also promote anabolism.[107,108] The intravenous infusion of the salt complex of alpha-ketoglutarate and ornithine in postoperative patients receiving total parenteral nutrition is reported to reduce UNA and to increase nitrogen balance.[246] The mechanism of action of this drug is not well understood. More research is clearly necessary to investigate the anabolic effects and clinical value of these agents for patients with acute renal failure.

**Energy.** Several lines of evidence suggest that patients with acute renal failure may benefit from a high energy intake. Because patients with acute renal failure are frequently in negative energy and nitrogen balance,[222,226,227,233] it has been argued that a greater energy intake may reduce the protein wasting. Moreover, unlike the nonuremic acutely ill patient who may receive large quantities of amino acids, patients with acute renal failure are usually given relatively small amounts of amino acids because of their excretory impairment. It is possible, although not proven, that higher energy intakes may improve the utilization of low nitrogen intakes. In one nonrandomized study, the patients with acute renal failure who died were found to have a higher energy expenditure and more negative energy balance than those who survived.[222]

As a result of these findings, we usually administer about 35 to 50 kcal/kg desirable body weight/day (see Table 58–4), except in patients who are extremely obese (e.g., greater than 125% desirable body weight). The higher energy intakes (i.e., 50 kcal/kg/day) are used for patients who have a higher UNA, who are severely ill, and who are less obese. For example, if nitrogen balance, estimated from the difference between the patient's nitrogen intake and the nitrogen output calculated from the UNA is negative, we try to provide an energy intake close to 50 kcal/kg/day.

Larger intakes are not used because there appears to be little nutritional advantage to administering more than 3,500 to 5,000 kcal/day to catabolic patients. Indeed, because high energy intakes generate more carbon dioxide from the infused carbohydrate and fat, they can promote hypercapnia if pulmonary function is impaired.[247] Carbon dioxide retention is particularly likely to occur with very high carbohydrate loads. In addition, high energy intakes may cause obesity and fatty liver and may increase the water load to the patient.[248]

Because most patients with acute renal failure do not tolerate large water intakes, glucose is usually administered in a 70% solution. The glucose and amino acid solutions are mixed so that the amino acids and energy are provided simultaneously (see Table 58–4). Patients receiving TPN for more than five to seven days should receive lipid emulsions. Preferably, 25 to 50 g of lipids should be infused daily, but no less than twice weekly to prevent essential fatty acid deficiency and to provide a more normal fuel mix. More recent evidence suggests that in nonuremic stressed patients, energy may be used more effectively if a higher proportion of the energy (25 to 50%) is provided each day as fat (see Chapter 54). In some pharmacies, the lipid emulsions are mixed with the glucose and amino acid solutions, whereas in others the lipids are administered separately (see Chapter 54).

**Minerals.** The mineral prescription for parenteral nutrition in acute renal failure is shown in Table 58–4. Any recommended intake of minerals is tentative and must be adjusted according to the clinical status of the patient. If the serum concentration of an electrolyte is increased, it may be advisable to reduce the quantity infused or to not administer it at the onset of parenteral nutrition. The patient must be monitored closely, because the hormonal and metabolic changes that often occur with initiation of parenteral nutrition may cause the serum electrolytes to fall rapidly. This occurrence is particularly likely for serum potassium and phosphorus. On the other hand, a low concentration of a mineral may indicate a need for greater than usual intake of that element. Again, metabolic changes and the impaired GFR can lead to a rapid rise in the serum concentrations during repletion.

Trace elements are probably not necessary in parenteral nutrition solutions unless this is the sole source of nutrition support for at least two to three weeks. The nutritional requirements for trace elements have not been established for uremic patients receiving total parenteral nutrition.

**Vitamins.** The vitamin requirements have not been well defined for patients with acute renal failure; more research on this subject is needed. Tentative recommendations for vitamin intake for patients receiving parenteral nutrition are shown in Table 58–4. Much of the recommended intake is based on information obtained from studies in chronically uremic patients, normal individuals, or nonuremic acutely ill patients. Vitamin A is probably best avoided because in chronic renal failure, serum vitamin A levels are elevated and small doses of vitamin A have been reported to cause toxicity to chronically uremic patients.[216,217] In addition, since most patients with acute renal failure receive parenteral nutrition for only a few

days to weeks, it is unlikely that a deficiency will occur for this fat-soluble vitamin.

The nutritional requirement for vitamin D in patients with acute renal failure has not been defined. Although vitamin D is fat-soluble and vitamin stores should not become depleted during the few days to weeks that most patients with acute renal failure receive parenteral nutrition, the turnover of its most active analogue, 1,25-dihydroxycholecalciferol, is much faster. Hence, this analogue may be needed in patients with acute renal failure. An intravenous preparation of 1,25-dihydroxycholeciferol should be available in the future.[219] Although vitamin K is fat-soluble, vitamin K deficiency has been reported in nonuremic patients who are not eating and are receiving antibiotics.[218] Vitamin K supplements therefore should be given routinely to patients receiving parenteral nutritional (see Table 58–4). Ten mg/day of pyridoxine hydrochloride (8.2 mg/day of pyridoxine) is recommended because studies in clinically stable or sick patients undergoing maintenance hemodialysis indicate that this quantity may be necessary to prevent or to correct vitamin $B_6$ deficiency.[249] Patients should probably not receive more than 60 to 100 mg/day of ascorbic acid because of the risk of increased oxalate production.[214,215]

The nutrient intake of patients with acute renal failure must be carefully reevaluated each day and sometimes more frequently. This reevaluation is particularly important because these patients may undergo rapid changes in their clinical and metabolic condition.

## Peripheral Parenteral Nutrition

Parenteral nutrition through a peripheral vein avoids the risks of inserting a catheter into the superior vena cava. Because the osmolality of the infusate must be restricted to no more than about 600 mosm to reduce the risk of thrombophlebitis, it is necessary to use a larger volume of fluid and/or a lower intake of nutrients. Both approaches may have undesirable consequences for patients with acute renal failure. The financial cost of total parenteral nutrition administered through a peripheral vein is about the same or greater than the cost of administration through a central vein because of the large quantities of expensive isotonic lipid emulsions used to provide the energy needs when peripheral veins are used.

Peripheral partial parenteral nutrition may be advantageous for these patients with acute renal failure who are able to ingest or be tube-fed only part of their daily nutritional requirements. The peripheral infusions may enable these patients to receive adequate nutrition without resorting to total parenteral nutrition through a large flow vein. In these latter patients, it is often most practical to infuse an 8.5 to 10% amino acid solution or a 20% lipid emulsion into a peripheral vein and to administer as much as possible of the other essential nutrients, including carbohydrates, through the enteral tract.

The peripheral vascular access used for hemodialysis can also be used for parenteral nutrition. Because there is a high blood flow through the vascular access used for hemodialysis, hypertonic solutions can be used, and the water load to the patient can be reduced. However, this technique probably increases the risk of infection in the vascular access, and it should not be used in patients who will need a hemodialysis access for extended periods.

### Supplemental Parenteral Nutrition

Infusion of amino acids and glucose may be given as a nutritional supplement to patients with acute or chronic renal failure who eat poorly. Supplemental amino acids and glucose can be infused conveniently during the hemodialysis procedure. Some physicians have recommended infusion of 20 to 30 g of the nine essential amino acids near the end of the dialysis therapy.[250] Because most patients in need of nutritional supplements have decreased intake both of essential and nonessential amino acids and of energy, however, we infuse 40 to 42 g of essential and nonessential amino acids and 200 g of D-glucose (150 g of D-glucose if the hemodialysate contains glucose). This preparation is infused throughout the hemodialysis procedure at a constant rate into the blood leaving the dialyzer. Such a technique minimizes the normal fall in amino acid and glucose pools that occurs as a result of dialysis of these nutrients. Most of the infused glucose and amino acids are retained; the amino acid losses into dialysate increase by only about 4 to 5 g.[162] The fact that the nutrients are not infused as a bolus may also enhance efficient utilization.

Patients who have low serum phosphorus or potassium concentrations at the onset of dialysis treatment may require supplements of these electrolytes during the amino acid and glucose supplementation. To prevent reactive hypoglycemia, the infusion should not be stopped until the end of hemodialysis, and the patient should eat a carbohydrate source 20 to 30 minutes before the end of the infusion. Although routine supplementation with intravenous or oral amino acids and an energy source has been recommended for hemodialysis patients, it is probably only of value for patients who have a suboptimal intake of these nutrients.[251,252]

### Continuous Arteriovenous Hemofiltration

Because many patients with acute renal failure are overhydrated, receive large quantities of intravenous solutions, and have impaired ability to excrete water and salt, a new technique called continuous arteriovenous hemofiltration (CAVH) has been used to control salt and water balance.[253] With CAVH, catheters are placed into a large artery and vein, such as the femoral artery and vein.[253] The blood flows through a small filtering apparatus where some of the plasma water is filtered; the remaining concentrated blood is returned to the vein. Some physicians combine parenteral nutrition therapy with CAVH in order to provide intravenous nutrition and, at the same time, to control the water and salt balance and to remove a small amount of the metabolic products that accumulate in renal failure. When CAVH is not used, patients with acute renal failure who receive parenteral nutrition may require treatment with a hemodialyzer as often as every day rather than three times weekly, which is the usual treatment for clinically stable maintenance hemodialysis patients. The more frequent use of a hemodialyzer is particularly likely if the patients receive the larger quantities of glucose and amino acids.

### Nutritional Dialysis

Some investigators have proposed adding amino acids and additional glucose to the dialysate of patients undergoing CAPD or maintenance hemodialysis.[254,255] The nutrients would then diffuse into the body during dialysis. At present, it appears that these techniques may provide supplemental nutrition but cannot be used routinely for total nutritional support. Further work should clarify the role for these treatments in patients who do not ingest adequate quantities of nutrients.

### Amino Acids That May Predispose to Acute Renal Failure

Several studies in rats suggest that amino acid or protein intake may increase the susceptibility to acute renal failure caused by ischemia or aminoglycoside nephrotoxicity.[256–259] The nutrients seem to increase both the incidence and the severity of acute renal failure induced by these agents. Although some studies have demonstrated this effect with large doses of intravenous amino acids or dietary protein,[256,259] the quantities of amino acids and proteins that might be prescribed for patients can also predispose to renal failure.[257,259] D-serine, DL-ethionine, and L-lysine appear to be particularly nephrotoxic.[257,258] It is not known whether amino acid or protein intake will predispose to renal failure in humans. If either one does, then patients who receive nephrotoxic medicines or who are at high risk for renal ischemia might benefit from low amino acid or protein intakes. Clearly more research is needed in this area.

## REFERENCES

1. Brenner, B.M., Dworkin, L.D., Ichikawa, I.: Glomerular ultrafiltration. *In* The Kidney. 3rd Ed. (Brenner, B.M., Rector, F.C., Jr., Eds.) Philadelphia, W.B. Saunders Co., 1986, pp. 124–144.
2. Brenner, B.M., Rector, F.C., Jr.: The Kidney. 3rd Ed. Philadelphia, W.B. Saunders Co., 1986.
3. Pitts, R.F.: Physiology of the Kidney and Body Fluids. Chicago, Year Book Medical Publishers, 1974.
4. Kopple, J.D., Coburn, J.W.: JAMA *227*:41–44, 1974.
5. Kopple, J.D.: Nutrition and the kidney. *In* Human Nutrition—A Comprehensive Treatise, Vol. 4. (Alfin-Slater, R.B., Kritchevsky, D., Eds.) New York, Plenum Publishing Corp., 1979, pp. 409–457.
6. Kopple J.D.: Nitrogen metabolism. *In* Clinical Aspects of Uremia and Dialysis. (Massry, S.G., Sellers, A.L., Eds). Springfield, Charles C Thomas 1976, pp. 241–283.
6a. Dunn, M.J.: Hormones and autacoids produced in the kidney. *In* Renal Endocrinology. (Dunn, M.J., Ed.) Baltimore, Williams & Wilkins, 1983.
7. Ballermann, B.J., Levenson, D.J., Brenner, B.M.: Renin, angiotensin, kinins, prostaglandins, and leukotrienes. *In* The Kidney. 3rd Ed. (Brenner, B.M., Rector, F.C., Jr., Eds). Philadelphia, W.B. Saunders Co., 1986.
8. Audran, M., Kumar, R.: Mayo. Clin. Proc. *60*:851–866, 1985.
9. Fisher, J.W.: Kidney Hormones, Vol. II. New York, Academic Press, 1977.
10. Caro, J., Brown, S., Miller, O., et al.: J. Lab. Clin. Med. *93*:449–458, 1979.
11. Kopple, J.D., Fukuda, S.: Am J. Clin. Nutr. *33*:1363–1372, 1980.
12. Tizianello, A., De Ferrari, G., Garibotto, et al.: J. Clin. Invest. *65*:1162–1173, 1980.
13. Rabkin, R., Simon, N.M., Steiner, S., et al.: N. Engl. J. Med. *282*:182–187, 1970.
14. Sherwin, R.S., Bastl, C., Finkelstein, F.O., et al.: J. Clin. Invest. *57*:722–731, 1976.
15. Vajda, F.J.E., Martin, T.J., Melick, R.A.: Endocrinology *84*:162–164, 1969.
16. Cuttelod, S., Lemarchand-Beraud, T., Magnenat, P., et al.: Metabolism *23*:101–113, 1974.
17. Davidson, W.D., Moore, T.C., Shippey, W., et al.: Gastroenterology *66*:522–525, 1974.
18. Strober, W., Waldmann, T.A.: Nephron *13*:35–66, 1974.
19. Oliver, J., Bourke, E.: Clin. Sci. Mol. Med. *48*:515–520, 1975.
20. Owen, O.E., Felig, P., Morgan, A.P.: J. Clin. Invest. *48*:574–583, 1969.
21. Rennick, B., Acara, M., Hysert, P., et al.: Kidney Int. *10*:329–335, 1976.
22. Schrier, R.W.: Renal and Electrolyte Disorders. 2nd Ed. Boston, Little, Brown and Co., 1980.
23. Arieff, A.I., DeFronzo, R.A.: Fluid, Electrolyte, and Acid-Base Disorders. New York, Churchill Livingstone, 1985.
24. Maxwell, M.H., Kleeman, C.R., Narius, R.G.: Clinical Disorders of Fluid and Electrolyte Metabolism. 4th Ed. New York, McGraw-Hill Book Co., 1987.
25. Lee, D.B.N., Kleeman, C.R.: Phosphorus Depletion in Man. (Banks, G., Ed.) Irvine, McGaw Laboratories, 1976.
26. Massry, S.G.: Effect of phosphate depletion on renal function and metabolism. *In* Proceedings of the VIIth International Congress of Nephrology. (Barcelo, R., Bergeron, M., Carriere, S., et al., Eds.) Basel, S. Karger, 1978, pp. 625–633.
27. Randall, R.E., Jr., Cohen, M.D., Spray, C.C., Jr., et al.: Ann. Intern. Med. *61*:73–78, 1964.
28. Munck, O., Nissen, N.I.: Acta Med. Scand. *153*:307–975, 1964.
28a. Czerwinski, A.W., Ginn, H.E.: Am. J. Med. *37*:969–975, 1964.
29. Silverberg, D.S., Kidd, E.G., Shnitka, T.K., et al.: Arthritis Rheum. *13*:812–825, 1970.
30. Saldanha, L.F., Rosen, V.J., Gonick, H.C.: Am. J. Med. *59*:95–103, 1975.
31. Charlas, R., Benabadji, A.: Maroc Med. *41*:1180–1182, 1962.
32. Schreiner, G.E., Maher, J.F.: Am. J. Med. *38*:409–449, 1965.
33. Beton, D.C., Andrews, G.S., Davies, H.J., et al.: Br. J. Ind. Med. *23*:292–301, 1966.
34. Stuve, J., Galle, P.: J. Cell Biol. *44*:667–676, 1970.
35. Giberson, A., Vaziri, N.D., Mirahamadi, K., et al.: Arch. Intern. Med. *136*:1303–1304, 1976.
36. Pullman, T.N., Alving, A.S., Dern, R.J., et al.: J. Lab. Clin. Med. *44*:320–332, 1954.
37. Klahr, S., Tripathy, K.: Arch. Intern. Med. *118*:322–325, 1966.
38. Klahr, S., Tripathy, K., Garcia, F.T., et al.: Am. J. Med. *43*:84–96, 1967.
39. Klahr, S., Tripathy, K., Lotero, H.: Am. J. Med. *48*:325–331, 1970.
40. Ichikawa, I., Purkerson, M.L., Klahr, S., et al.: J. Clin. Invest. *65*:982–988, 1980.
41. Gutman, A.B., Yu, T.-F.: Am. J. Med. *45*:756–779, 1968.
42. Bosch, J.P., Saccaggi, A., Lauer, A., et al.: Am. J. Med. *75*:943–950, 1983.
43. Bosch, J.P., Lauer, A., Glabman, S.: Am. J. Med. *77*:873–879, 1984.
44. Castellino, P., Hunt, W., DeFronzo, R.A.: Regulation of renal hemodynamics by plasma amino acid and hormone concentrations. Proceedings of the Fourth International Congress on Nutrition and Metabolism in Renal Disease. Kidney Int. (In press), 1987.
45. Hirschberg, R., Kopple, J.D.: Kidney Int. (In press), 1987.
46. Ikkos, D., Ljunggren, H., Luft, R.: Acta Endocrinol. *21*:226–236, 1956.
47. Christiansen, J.S., Gammelgaard, J., Orskov, H.: Eur. J. Clin. Invest. *11*:487–490, 1981.
47a. Rabb, H., Hirschberg, R., Bergamo, R, and Kopple, J.D.: Abstracts, Xth Intl Congress of Nephrology (in press).
48. Bouby, N., Trinh-Trang-Tan, M.-M., Kriz, W., et al.: Possible role of the thick ascending limb and of the urine concentrating mechanism in the protein-induced increase in GFR and kidney mass. Proceedings of the Fourth International Congress on Nutrition and Metabolism in Renal Disease. Kidney Int. (In press), 1987.

49. Mitch, W.E., Walser, M., Buffington, G.A., et al.: Lancet *2*:1326–1328, 1976.
50. Rutherford, W.E., Blondin, J., Miller, J.P., et al.: Kidney Int. *11*:62–70, 1977.
51. Barsotti, G., Guiducci, A., Ciardella, F., et al.: Nephron *27*:113–117, 1981.
52. McCormack, L.J., Beland, J.E., Schnekloth, R.E., et al.: Am. J. Pathol. *34*:1011–1022, 1958.
53. Kleinknecht, C., Grunfeld, J-P., Gomez, P.C., et al.: Kidney Int. *4*:390–400, 1973.
54. Rodriguez-Iturbe, B., Garcia, R., Rubio, L., et al.: Clin. Nephrol. *5*:198–206, 1976.
55. Torres, V.E., Velosa, J.A., Holley, K.E., et al.: Ann. Intern. Med. *92*:776–784, 1980.
56. Fishberg, A.M.: Hypertension and Nephritis. Philadelphia, Lea & Febiger, 1954.
57. Kopple, J.D., Shinaberger, J.H., Coburn, J.W., et al.: Am. J. Clin. Nutr. *21*:508–515, 1968.
58. Blatherwick, N.R., Medlar, E.M.: Arch. Intern. Med. *59*:572–596, 1937.
59. Farr, L.E., Smadel, J.E.: J. Exp. Med. *70*:615–627, 1939.
60. Addis, T.: Glomerular nephritis. *In* Diagnosis and Treatment. New York, Macmillan Publishing Co., Inc., 1948.
61. Ibels, L.S., Alfrey, A.C., Haut, L., et al.: N. Engl. J. Med. *298*:122–126, 1978.
62. Karlinsky, M.L., Haut, L.L., Buddington, B., et al.: Kidney Int. *17*:293–302, 1980.
63. Haut, L.L., Alfrey, A.C., Guggenheim, S., et al.: Kidney Int. *17*:722–731, 1980.
64. Laouari, D., Kleinknecht, C., Gubler, M-C., et al.: Kidney Int. *24*(Suppl. 16):S248–S253, 1983.
65. Kenner, C.H., Evan, A.P., Blomgren, P., et al.: Kidney Int. *27*:739–750, 1985.
66. French, S.W., Yamanaka, W., Ostwald, R.: Arch. Pathol. *83*:204–210, 1967.
67. Hurd, E.R., Johnston, J.M., Okita, J.R., et al.: J. Clin. Invest. *67*:476–485, 1981.
68. Howie, J.B., Helyer, B.J., Casey, T.P., et al.: Renal disease in autoimmune strains of mice. *In* Proceedings of the Third International Congress of Nephrology, Vol. 2. Basel, S. Karger, 1967, pp. 150–163.
69. Barcelli, U.O., Weiss, M., Pollack, V.E.: J. Lab. Clin. Med. *100*:786–797, 1982.
70. Zurier, R.B., Damjanov, O., Sayadoff, D.M., et al.: Arthritis Rheum. *20*:1449–1456, 1977.
71. Kelley, V.E., Winkelstein, A., Izui, S.: Lab. Invest. *41*:531–537, 1979.
72. McLeish, K.R., Gohara, A.F., Cunning, W.T., III: J. Lab. Clin. Med. *96*:470–479, 1980.
73. Deen, W.M., Maddox, D.A., Robertson, C.R., et al.: Am. J. Physiol. *227*:556–562, 1974.
74. Hostetter, T.H., Olson, J.L., Rennke, H.G., et al.: Am. J. Physiol. *241*:F85–F93, 1981.
75. Hostetter, T.H., Troy, J.L., Brenner, B.M.: Kidney Int. *19*:410–415, 1981.
76. Olson, J.L., Hostetter, T.H., Rennke, H.G., et al: Altered charge and size selective properties of the glomerular wall: A response to reduced renal mass. *In* Proceedings of the American Society of Nephrology. Thorofare, N.J., Charles B. Slack, Inc., 1979, p. 87A.
77. Olson, J.L., Hostetter, T.H., Rennke, H.G., et al.: Kidney Int. *22*:112–126, 1982.
78. Brenner, B.M., Meyer, T.W., Hostetter, T.H.: N. Engl. J. Med. *307*:652–659, 1982.
79. Meyer, T.W., Lawrence, W.E., Brenner, B.M.: Kidney Int. *24*(Suppl. 16):S243–S247, 1983.
80. Hostetter, T.H., Meyer, T.W., Rennke, H.G., et al.: Influence of strict control of diabetes on intrarenal hemodynamics. *In* Proceedings of the American Society of Nephrology. Thorofare, N.J., Charles B. Slack, Inc., 1982, p 122A.
81. Mogensen, C.E.: Diabetes *25*:872–879, 1976.
82. Mogensen, C.E., Steffes, M.W., Deckert, T., et al.: Diabetologia *21*:89–93, 1981.
83. Mogensen, C.E., Christensen, C.K., Vittinghus, E.: Diabetes *32*(Suppl. 2):64–78, 1983.
84. Pennell, J.P., Meinking, T.L.: Kidney Int. *21*:709–713, 1982.
85. Ibels, L.S., Alfrey, A.C., Huffer, W.E., et al.: Am. J. Med. *71*:33–37, 1981.
86. Alfrey, A.C., Tomford, R.C.: Phosphate and prevention of renal failure. *In* Prevention of Kidney Disease and Long-Term Survival. (Avram, M.M., Ed.) New York, Plenum Publishing Corp., 1982.
87. Tomford, R.C., Karlinsky, M.L., Buddington, B., et al.: J. Clin. Invest. *68*:655–664, 1981.
88. Suzuki, S., Shapiro, R., Mulrow, P.J., et al.: Prostaglandins Med. *4*:377–382, 1980.
89. Purkerson, M.L., Joist, J.H., Yates, J., et al. Proc. Natl. Acad. Sci. *82*:193–197, 1985.
90. Purkerson, M.L., Joist, J.H., Greenberg, J.M., et al.: Thromb. Res. *26*:227–240, 1982.
91. Dubois, E.L., Horowitz, R.E., Demopoulos, H.B., et al.: JAMA *195*:285–289, 1966.
92. Prickett, J.D., Robinson, D.R., Steinberg, A.D.: J. Clin. Invest. *68*:556–559, 1981.
93. Rahman, M.A., Nakazawa, M., Emancipator, S.N., et al.: Kidney Int. *29*:343, 1986.
94. Badr, K.F., Brenner, B.M., Wasserman, M., et al.: Kidney Int. *29*:328, 1986.
95. Schambelan, M., Hutchinson, F.N., Kaysen, G.A., et al.: Kidney Int. *29*:344, 1986.
96. Anderson, S., Meyer, T.W., Rennke, H.G., et al.: J. Clin. Invest. *76*:612–619, 1985.
97. Beukers, J.J.B., Hoedemaeker, P.J., Weening, J.J.: Kidney Int. *29*:265, 1986.
98. Taguma, Y., Kitamoto, Y., Futaki, G., et al.: N. Engl. J. Med. *313*:1617–1620, 1985.
99. Gimenez, L., Walker, W.G., Tew, W.P., et al.: Kidney Int. *22*:36–41, 1982.
100. Walser, M.: Clin. Nephrol. *3*:180–186, 1975.
101. Maschio, G., Oldrizzi, L., Tessitore, N., et al.: Kidney Int. *22*:371–376, 1982.
102. Alvestrand, A., Ahlberg, M., Bergstrom, J.: Kidney Int. *24*(Suppl. 16):S268–S272, 1983.
103. Barsotti, G., Morelli, E., Giannoni, A., et al.: Kidney Int. *24*(Suppl. 16):S278–S284, 1983.
104. Gretz, N., Korb, E., Strauch, M.: Kidney Int. *24*(Suppl. 16):S263–S267, 1983.
105. Mitch, W.E., Walser, M., Steinman, T.I., et al.: N. Engl. J. Med. *311*:623–629, 1984.
106. Rosman, J.B., Meijer, S., Sluiter, W.J., et al. Lancet *2*:1291–1295, 1984.
107. Mitch, W.E., Walser, M., Sapir, D.G.: J. Clin. Invest. *67*:553–562, 1981.
108. Tischler, M.E., Desautels, M., Goldberg, A.L.: J. Biol. Chem. *257*:1613–1621, 1982.
109. Donker, A.J.M., Arisz, L., Brentjens, J.R.H., et al.: Nephron *17*:288–296, 1976.
110. Arisz, L., Donker, A.J.M., Brentjens, J.R.H., et al.: Acta Med. Scand. *199*:121–125, 1976.
111. Striker, G.E., Nagle, R.B., Kohnen, P.W., et al.: Arch. Pathol. *87*:439–442, 1969.

112. Lalich, J.J., Faith, G.C., Harding, G.E.: Arch. Pathol. *89*:548–559, 1970.

113. Everitt, A.V., Porter, B.D., Wyndham, J.R.: Gerontology *28*:168–175, 1982.

114. Zucchelli, P., Cagnoli, L., Casanova, S., et al.: Kidney Int. *24*:649–655, 1983.

115. Rowe, J.W., Anres, R., Tobin, J.D., et al.: Ann. Intern. Med. *84*:567–569, 1976.

116. Kiprov, D.D., Colvin, R.B., McCluskey, R.T.: Lab. Invest. *46*:275–281, 1982.

117. Committee on Dietary Allowances, Food and Nutrition Board, National Academy of Sciences: Recommended Dietary Allowances, Ninth Revised Edition, Washington, D.C., 1980.

118. Glassock, R.J., Adler, S.G., Ward, H.J., et al.: Primary glomerular diseases. *In* The Kidney. 3rd ed., Vol. 1. (Brenner, B.M., Rector, F.C., Jr., Eds.) Philadelphia, W.B. Saunders Co., 1986, pp. 929–1013.

119. Massry, S.G., Feinstein, E.I., Goldstein, D.A., et al.: Metabolic and endocrine complications of the nephrotic syndrome. *In* Textbook of Nephrology, Vol. 1. (Massry, S.G., Glassock, R.J., Eds.) Baltimore, Williams & Wilkins, 1983, pp. 6.7–6.11.

120. Kaysen, G.A., Gambertoglio, J., Jimenez, I., et al.: Kidney Int. *29*:572–577, 1986.

121. Zeller, K.R., Raskin, P., Rosenstock, J., et al.: Kidney Int. *29*:209, 1986.

122. Kopple, J.D.: Kidney Int. *14*:340–348, 1978.

123. Gonick, H.C., Maxwell, M.H., Rubini, M.E., et al.: Nephron *3*:137–152, 1966.

124. David, D.S., Hochgelerent, E., Rubin, A.L. Lancet *2*:34–37, 1972.

125. Coburn, J.W., Slatopolsky, E.: Vitamin D, parathyroid hormone, and renal osteodystrophy. *In* The Kidney, Vol. II, 3rd Ed. (Brenner, B.M., Rector, F.C., Jr., Eds.) Philadelphia, W.B. Saunders Co., 1986, pp. 1657–1729.

126. Coburn, J.W., Hartenbower, D.L., Brickman, A.S., et al.: Intestinal absorption of calcium, magnesium and phosphorus in chronic renal insufficiency. *In* Calcium Metabolism in Renal Failure and Nephrolithiasis. (David, D.S., Ed.) New York, John Wiley & Sons, Inc., 1977, pp. 77–109.

127. Lawson, D.H., Boddy, K., King, P.C., et al.: Clin. Sci. *41*:345, 1971.

128. Kopple, J.D., Swendseid, M.E.: Kidney Int. Suppl. *2*:S79–S84, 1975.

129. Ott, S.M., Maloney, N.A., Coburn, J.W., et al.: N. Engl. J. Med. *307*:709–713, 1982.

130. Samaan, N., Freeman, R.M.: Metabolism *19*:102–113, 1970.

131. Nagel, T.C., Frenkel, N., Bell, R.H., et al.: J. Clin. Endocrinol. Metab. *36*:428–432, 1973.

132. Lim, V.S., Fang, V.S.: Am. J. Med. *58*:655–662, 1975.

133. Tourkantonis, A., Spiliopoulos, A., Pharmakioltis, A., et al.: Nephrons *27*:271–272, 1981.

134. Hershman, J.M., Krugman, L.G., Kopple, J.D., et al.: Metabolism *27*:755–759, 1979.

135. Schiffrin, A., Guyda, H., Robitaille, P., et al.: J. Clin. Endocrinol. Metab. *46*:511–514, 1977.

136. Phillips, L.S., Kopple, J.: Metabolism *30*:1091–1095, 1981.

137. Feldman, H.A., Singer, I.: Medicine *54*:345–376, 1975.

138. Kopple, J.D.: Nitrogen metabolism. *In* Clinical Aspects of Uremia and Dialysis. (Massry, S.G., Sellers, A.L., Eds.) Springfield, Charles C Thomas, 1976, pp. 241–273.

139. Simenhoff, M.L., Burke, J.F., Saukkonen, J.J., et al.: Lancet *2*:818–821, 1976.

140. Bricker, N.S.: N. Engl. J. Med. *286*:1093–1099, 1972.

141. Massry, S.G.: Semin. Nephrol. *3*: 306–328, 1983.

142. Golper, T.A.: Nephron *38*:217–225, 1984.

143. Rutsky, E.A., Rostand, S.G.: Kidney *16*:1–8, 1983.

144. Briggs, W.A., Lazarus, J.M., Birtch, A.G., et al.: Arch. Intern. Med. *132*:21–28, 1973.

145. Bianchi, R., Mariani, G., Toni, M.G., et al.: Am. J. Clin. Nutr. *31*:1615–1626, 1978.

146. Kluthe, R., Luttgen, F.M., Capetianu, T., et al.: Am. J. Clin. Nutr. *31*:1812–1820, 1978.

147. Young, G.A., Oli, H.I., Davidson, A.M., et al.: Am. J. Clin. Nutr. *31*:1802–1807, 1978.

148. Attman, P.O., Isaksson E.J.: Am. J. Clin. Nutr. *33*:801–810, 1980.

149. Blumenkrantz, M.J., Kopple, J.D., Gutman, R.A., et al.: Am. J. Clin. Nutr. *33*:1567–1585, 1980.

150. Guarnieri, G., Faccini, L., Lipartiti, T., et al.: Am. J. Clin. Nutr. *33*:1598–1607, 1980.

151. Bansal, V.K., Popli, S., Pickering, J., et al.: Am. J. Clin. Nutr. *33*:1608–1611, 1980.

152. Thunberg, B.J., Swamy, A.P., Cestero, R.V.: Am. J. Clin. Nutr. *34*:2005–2012, 1981.

153. Heide, B., Pierratos, A., Jhanna, R., et al.: Peritoneal Dialysis Bull. *3*:138–141, 1983.

154. Young, G.A., Swanepoel, C.R., Croft, M.R., et al.: Kidney Int. *21*:492–499, 1982.

155. Salusky, I.B., Fine, R.N., Nelson, P., et al.: Am. J. Clin. Nutr. *38*:599–611, 1983.

156. Wolfson, M., Strong, C.J., Minturn, D., et al.: Am. J. Clin. Nutr. *37*:547–555, 1984.

157. Kopple, J.D.: Causes of catabolism and wasting in acute or chronic renal failure. *In* Nephrology, Vol. II. Proceedings of the IXth International Congress of Nephrology. (Robinson, R.R., Ed.) New York, Springer-Verlag, 1984, pp. 1498–1515.

158. Carlson, D.M., Duncan, D.A., Naessens, J.M., et al.: Mayo Clin. Proc. *59*:769–775, 1984.

159. Evans, R.W., Manninen, D.L., Garrison, L.P., Jr., et al.: N. Engl. J. Med. *312*:553–559, 1985.

160. Grodstein, G.P., Blumenkrantz, M.J., Kopple, J.D.: Am. J. Clin. Nutr. *33*:1411–1416, 1980.

161. Kopple, J.D., Swendseid, M.E., Shinaberger, J.H., et al.: Trans. Am. Soc. Artif. Intern. Organs *19*:309–313, 1973.

162. Wolfson, M., Jones, M.R., Kopple, J.D.: Kidney Int. *21*:500–506, 1982.

163. Kopple, J.D., Blumenkrantz, M.J., Jones, M.R., et al.: Am. J. Clin. Nutr. *36*:395–402, 1982.

164. Blumenkrantz, M.J., Gahl, G.M., Kopple. J.D., et al.: Kidney Int. *19*:593–602, 1981.

165. Borah, M.F., Schoenfeld, P.Y., Gotch, F.A., et al.: Kidney Int. *14*:491–500, 1978.

166. Linton, A.L., Clark, W.F., Driedger, A.A., et al.: Nephron *19*:95–98, 1977.

167. Shapiro, J.I., Argy, W.P., Rakowski, T.A., et al.: Trans. Am. Soc. Artif. Intern. Organs *29*:129–132, 1983.

168. Acchiardo, S.R., Moore, L.W., Latour, P.A.: Kidney Int. *24*(Suppl. 16):S199–S203, 1983.

169. Salusky, I.B., Fine, R.N., Nelson, P., et al.: American Society of Nephrology 15th Annual Meeting, December 1982, p. 66A (abstract).

170. Calloway, D.H., Odell, A.C.F., Margen, S.: J. Nutr. *101*:775–786, 1971.

171. Kopple, J.D., Grodstein, G.: Clin. Res. *28*:597A, 1980.

172. Maroni, B.J., Steinman, T.I., Mitch, W.E.: Kidney Int. *27*:58–65, 1985.
173. Varcoe, R., Halliday, D., Carson, E.R., et al.: Clin. Sci. Mol. Med. *43*:379–390, 1975.
174. Walser, M.: J. Clin. Invest. *53*:1385–1392, 1974.
175. Sargent, J.A., Gotch, F.A.: J. Am. Diet. Assoc. *75*:547–551, 1979.
176. Weigley, E.S.: J. Am. Diet. Assoc. *84*:417–423, 1984.
177. Bergstrom, J., Furst, P., Noree, L.-O.: Clin. Nephrol. *3*:187–194, 1975.
178. Noree, L.-O., Bergstrom, J.: Clin. Nephrol. *3*:195–203, 1975.
179. Furst, P., Alvestrand, A., Bergstrom, J.: Am. J. Clin. Nutr. *33*:1387–1395, 1980.
180. Kopple, J.D.: *In* Proceedings VIIIth International Congress of Nephrology. (Barcelo, R., Bergeron, M., Carriere, S., et al., Eds.) Basel, S. Karger, 1978, pp. 497–507.
180a.Furst, P.: Scan J. Clin. Lab. Invest. *30*:307–312, 1972.
180b.Kopple, J.D., Swendseid, M.E.: J. Clin. Invest. *55*:881–891, 1975.
180c.Kopple, J.D., Swendseid, M.E.: J. Nutr. *111*:931–942, 1981.
180d.Jones, M.R., Kopple, J.D., Swendseid, M.E.: Am. J. Clin. Nutr. *35*:15–23, 1982.
181. Kopple, J.D., Swendseid, M.E.: Nephron *18*:1–12, 1977.
182. Walser, M., Coulter, A.W., Dighe, S., et al.: J. Clin. Invest. *52*:678–690, 1973.
183. Kopple, J.D., Swendseid, M.E.: Am. J. Clin. Nutr. *27*:806–812, 1974.
184. Sapir, D.G., Owen, O.E., Pozefsky, T., et al.: J. Clin. Invest. *54*:974–980, 1974.
185. Freund, H., Hoover, H.C., Atamuriam, S., et al.: Ann. Surg. *190*:18–23, 1979.
186. Sherwin, R.S.: J. Clin. Invest. *61*:1471–1481, 1978.
187. Jungers, P., Chauveau, B., Lebkiri, C., et al.: Prospective randomized comparison of ketoacids (KA) and low protein diet (LPD) on progression of advanced chronic renal failure (CRF). Proceedings of the Fourth International Congress on Nutrition and Metabolism in Renal Disease. Kidney Int. In press, 1987.
188. Kopple, J.D., Coburn, J.W.: Medicine *52*:583–595, 1973.
189. Blainey, J.D.: Clin. Sci. *13*:567–581, 1954.
190. Kopple, J.D., Shinaberger, J.H., Coburn, J.W., et al.: Trans. Am. Soc. Artif. Intern. Organs *15*:302–308, 1969.
190a.Blumenkrantz, M.J., Kopple, J.D., Moran, J.K., et al.: Kidney Int. *21*:849–861, 1982.
191. Kopple, J.D., Monteon, F.J., Shaib, J.K.: Kidney Int. *29*:734–742, 1986.
192. Monteon, F.J., Laidlaw, S.A., Shaib, J.K., Kopple, J.D.: Energy expenditure in patients with chronic renal failure. Kidney Int. *30*:741–747, 1986.
193. Cramp, D.G., Moorhead, J.F., Wills, M.R.: Lancet *1*:672–673, 1975.
194. Sanfelippo, M.L., Swenson, R.S., Reaven, G.M.: Kidney Int. *14*:54–61, 1977.
195. Sanfelippo, M.L., Swenson, R.S., Reaven, G.M.: Kidney Int. *14*:180–186, 1978.
195a.Goldberg, A.P., Geltman, E.M., Hagberg, J.M., et al.: Kidney Int. *24*(Suppl. 16):S303–S309, 1983.
196. Ciman, M., Rizzoli, V., Moracchiello, M., et al.: Am. J. Clin. Nutr. *33*:1489–1492, 1980.

197. Bellinghieri, G., Savica, V., Mallamace, A., et al.: Am. J. Clin. Nutr. *38*:523–531, 1983.
198. Manis, T., Deutsch, J., Feinstein, E.I., et al.: Am. J. Clin. Nutr. *33*:1485–1488, 1980.
199. Pierides, A.M., Alvarez-Ude, F., Kerr, D.N.S., et al.: Lancet *2*:1279–1282, 1979.
200. Massry, S.G., Coburn, J.W.: Divalent ion metabolism and renal osteodystrophy. *In* Clinical Aspects of Uremia and Dialysis. (Massry, S.G., Sellers, A.L., Eds.) Springfield, Charles C Thomas, 1976, pp. 304–387.
200a.Barsotti, G., Giannoni, A., Morelli, E., et al.: Clin. Nephrol. *21*:54–59, 1984.
201. Cannata, J.B., Briggs, J.D., Junor, B.J.R.: Br. Med. J. *286*:1937–1938, 1983.
202. Sedman, A.B., Miller, N.L., Warady, B.A., et al.: Kidney Int. *26*:201–204, 1984.
203. Hercz, G., Coburn, J.W.: Prevention of phosphate retention and hyperphosphatemia in uremia: A consideration of "newer" phosphate-binding agents. Proceedings of the Fourth International Congress on Nutrition and Metabolism in Renal Disease. Kidney Int. In Press, 1987.
204. Kopple, J.D., Coburn, J.W.: Medicine *52*:597–607, 1973.
205. Koomans, H.A., Roos, J.C., Boer, P., et al.: Hypertension *4*:190–197, 1982.
206. Lawson, D.H., Boddy, K., King, P.C., et al.: Clin. Sci. *41*:345–351, 1971.
207. Rudolph, H., Alfrey, A.C., Smythe, W.R.: Trans. Am. Soc. Artif. Intern. Organs *19*:456–465, 1973.
208. Atkin-Thor, E., Goddard, B.W., O'Nion, J., et al.: Am. J. Clin. Nutr. *31*:1948–1951, 1978.
209. Antoniou, L.D., Shalhoub, R.J., Sudhakar, T., et al.: Lancet *2*:895–898, 1977.
210. Alfrey, A.C.: Kidney Int. *29*(Suppl. 18):S53–S–57, 1986.
210a.Touam, M., Martinez, F., Lacour, B., et al.: Clin. Nephrol. *19*:295–298, 1983.
211. Jennette, J.C., Goldman, I.D.: J. Lab. Clin. Med. *86*:834–843, 1975.
212. Spannuth, C.L., Jr., Warnock, L.G., Wagner, C., et al.: J. Lab. Clin. Med. *90*:632–637, 1977.
213. Sharman, V.L., Cunningham, J., Goodwin, F.J., et al.: Br. Med. J. *285*:96–97, 1982.
214. Balcke, P., Schmidt, P., Zazgornik, J., et al.: Ann. Intern. Med. *101*:344–345, 1984.
215. Pru, C., Eaton, J., Kjellstrand, C.: Nephron *39*:112–116, 1985.
216. Smith, F.R., Goodman, D.S.: J. Clin. Invest. *50*:2426–2436, 1971.
217. Yatzidis, H., Digenis, P., et al.: Br. Med. J. *ii*:352–353, 1975.
218. Roe, D.A.: Drug-Induced Nutritional Deficiencies. Westport, Ct., AVI Publishing Company, 1976.
219. Slatopolsky, E., Weerts, C., Thielan, J., et al.: J. Clin. Invest *74*:2136–2143, 1984.
220. Symposium on Role Dietary Fiber in Health. Am. J. Clin. Nutr. *31*:S1–S291, 1978.
221. Rampton, D.S., Cohen, S.L., Crammond, V.De.B., et al.: Clin. Nephrol. *21*:159–163, 1984.
222. Mault, J.R., Bartlett, R.H., Dechert, R.E., et al.: Trans. Am. Soc. Artif. Intern. Organs *29*:390–394, 1983.
223. Flugel-Link, R.M., Salusky, I.B., Jones, M.R., et al.: Am. J. Physiol. Soc. *244*:E615–E623, 1983.
224. Clark, A.S., Mitch, W.E.: J. Clin. Invest. *72*:836–845, 1983.

225. Frohlich, J., Scholmerich, J., Hoppe-Seyler, G., et al.: Eur. J. Clin. Invest. *4*:453–458, 1974.

226. Feinstein, E.I., Blumenkrantz, M.J., Healy, H., et al.: Medicine *60*(2):124–137, 1981.

227. Feinstein, E.I., Kopple, J.D., Silberman, H.: Kidney Int. *26*(Suppl. 16):S319–S323, 1983.

228. Abel, R.M., Abbott, W.M., Beck, C.H., Jr., et al.: Am. J. Surg. *128*:317–323, 1974.

229. Abel, R.M., Shih, V.E., Abbott, W.M., et al.: Ann. Surg. *180*:350–355, 1974.

230. Abel, R.M., Beck, C.H., Jr., Abbott, W.M., et al.: N. Engl. J. Med. *288*:695–699, 1973.

231. Baek, S.M., Makabali, G.G., Bryan-Brown, C.W., et al.: Surg. Gynecol. Obstet. *141*:405–408, 1975.

232. McMurray, S.D., Luft, F.C., Maxwell, D.R., et al.: Arch. Intern. Med. *138*:950–955, 1978.

233. Leonard, C.D., Luke, R.G., Siegel, R.R.: Urology *6*:154–157, 1975.

234. Toback, F.G.: Kidney Int. *12*:193–198, 1977.

235. Toback, F.G., Teegarden, D.E., Havener, L.J.: Kidney Int. *15*:542–547, 1979.

236. Toback, F.G., Dodd, R.C., Maier, E.R., et al.: Clin. Res. *27*:432A, 1979.

237. Oken, D.E., Sprinkel, F.M., Kirschbaum, B.B., et al.: Kidney Int. *17*:14–23, 1980.

238. Motil, K.J., Harmon, W.E., Grupe, W.E.: J. Parenter. Enter. Nutr. *4*(1):32–35, 1980.

239. Kopple, J.D., Feinstein, E.I.: Proceedings EDTA *19*:129–140, 1983.

240. McCracken, B.H., Parsons, F.M.: Lancet *2*:885–886, 1958.

241. Gjorup, S., Thaysen, J.H.: Acta Med. Scand. *167*:227–238, 1960.

242. Hinton, P., Allison, S.P., Littlejohn, S., et al.: Lancet *1*:767–769, 1971.

243. Woolfson, A.M.J., Healtley, R.V., Allison, S.P.: N. Engl. J. Med. *300*:14–17, 1979.

244. Daly, M., Mihranian, M.H., Kehoe, J.I., et al.: Surgery *94*:151–159, 1983.

245. Cerra, F.B., Upson, D., Angelico, R., et al.: Surgery *92*:192–200, 1982.

246. Leander, U., Furst, P., Vesterberg, K., et al.: Clin. Nutr. *4*:43–51, 1985.

247. Askanazi, J., Elwyn, D.H., Silverberg, B.S., et al.: Surgery *87*(5):596–598, 1980.

248. Jeejeebhoy, K.N., Langer, B., Tsallas, G., et al.: Gastroenterology *71*:943–953, 1976.

249. Kopple, J.D., Mercurio, K., Blumenkrantz, M.J., et al.: Kidney Int. *19*:694–704, 1981.

250. Heidland, A., Kult, J.: Clin. Nephrol. *3*:234–239, 1975.

251. Hecking, E., Port, F.K., Brehm, H., et al.: Kidney Int. *12*:482, 1977.

252. Ulm, A., Neuhauser, M., Leber, H.-W.: Am. J. Clin. Nutr. *31*:1827–1830, 1978.

253. Golper, T.A.: Am. J. Kidney Dis. *6*:373–386, 1985.

254. Williams, F.P., Marliss, E.B., Anderson, G.H., et al.: Peritoneal Dialysis Bull. *2*:124–130, 1982.

255. Feinstein, E.I., Collins, J.F., Blumenkrantz, M.J., et al.: Prog. Artif. Organs *1*:421–426, 1984.

256. Zager, R.A., Johannes, G., Tuttle, S.E., et al.: J. Lab. Clin. Med. *101*:130–140, 1983.

257. Zager, R.A., Venkatachalam, M.A.: Kidney Int. *24*:620–625, 1983.

258. Malis, C.D., Racusen, C., Solez, K., et al.: J. Lab. Clin. Med. *103*:660–676, 1984.

259. Andrews, P.M., Bates, S.B.: Dietary protein prior to renal ischemia dramatically affects postischemic kidney function. Proceedings of the Fourth International Congress on Nutrition and Metabolism in Renal Disease. Kidney Int. In press, 1987.

*Chapter* **59**

# NUTRITION AND DIET IN HYPERTENSION

## Daniel Einhorn and Lewis Landsberg

Elevated arterial blood pressure, or hypertension, is a major public health problem in developed countries throughout the world. In recent years, scientific, political, and public interest in dietary treatment of hypertension has increased. As a consequence of the enormous public-health and financial impact of hypertension, the literature examining the relationship between dietary intake and blood pressure has expanded substantially, and a number of new concepts have emerged since the last edition of this text. For no single nutrient has a conclusive and unique relation to blood pressure been demonstrated for all population groups, however. Except for the well-established association of obesity and hypertension and of sodium chloride and hypertension in certain individuals, much of the literature summarized in this chapter must be considered suggestive, rather than conclusive, of a relationship between nutrient ingestion and blood pressure.

The difficulty in drawing conclusions about diet and hypertension stems from methodologic problems inherent in this area of research. Hypertension is not a single disease, but rather a heterogeneous group of diseases. Therefore, one subgroup of hypertensives might be sensitive to a dietary modification that has no impact on another subgroup, and study across a large population might obscure the impact of dietary modification on the sensitive subgroup. Furthermore, it is difficult to isolate a single nutrient and its unique impact on blood pressure because changing one nutrient generally produces changes in the overall composition of the diet. Criteria for establishing whether a nutrient affects blood pressure have been summarized,[1] but this burden of proof is not likely to be met for many nutrients of interest. These caveats should be kept in mind as this chapter examines the evidence linking diet and hypertension.

### HYPERTENSION: AN OVERVIEW

Actuarial data show that morbidity and mortality from cardiovascular, cerebrovascular, and renovascular disease increase with higher systolic and diastolic blood pressure. Even within the normal range, higher blood pressure is associated with higher morbidity and mortality, and it has been argued that everyone should strive to lower their blood pressure, even if it requires formal "treatment." The medical treatment of hypertension has potential risks, however. Definitions of hypertension have therefore been established to identify people whose benefit from medical therapy outweighs the potential risks. The generally accepted criteria for hypertension are: a systolic blood pressure greater than 130 mm Hg in people less than age 45; and systolic blood pressure greater than 150 mm Hg in people above age 45.

Numerous drug-treatment trials have shown that even with blood pressure changes of less than 5%, a significant decrease in morbidity and mortality from cardiovascular, cerebrovascular, and renovascular disease can be demonstrated among those who have hypertension by the foregoing criteria. It has been suggested, but not definitively shown, that a linear correlation exists between the degree of blood pressure reduction and the degree of reduction of morbidity and mortality. Most clinicians assume this correlation and treat all hypertensives as aggressively as needed to achieve normal blood pressure by the foregoing criteria. It has been argued, however, that the risk of drug therapy may not outweigh the benefits for people with diastolic blood pressures less than 100 mm Hg,[2] and that only a "risk-free therapy," such as dietary modification, might prove beneficial in the milder forms of hypertension. Treatment of isolated systolic hypertension, especially in the elderly, is more controversial and problematic. Systolic hypertension may be resistant to management with medications and is often associated with the higher incidence of side effects, such as orthostatic hypotension and dehydration.

### Causes

By the criteria listed previously, at least 10 to 20% of Americans may be considered hypertensive. Over 90% of people with hypertension have no identifiable cause of elevated blood pressure and are said to have "primary" or "essential" hypertension. It is likely that a number of different pathophysiologic processes contribute to elevated blood pressure in this group and that factors unrelated to diet are involved. These factors include advancing age, lower education and income levels, psychosocial stresses, and heredity.

Approximately 4 to 8% of people with hypertension do have an identifiable cause(s) for elevated blood pressure and are said to have "secondary hypertension." Renal diseases account for approximately 40% of cases of secondary hypertension and include parenchymal diseases such

as glomerulonephritis, chronic pyelonephritis, polycystic kidney disease, and obstructive uropathy, as well as renal vascular diseases. Another large percentage of secondary cases may be accounted for by use of oral contraceptives in women.[3,4] Endocrine diseases account for approximately 10 to 15% of cases of secondary hypertension, including such diseases as hyperaldosteronism, acromegaly, Cushing's syndrome, hypothyroidism, and pheochromocytoma. Patients with hyperaldosteronism are sensitive to variations in dietary sodium and potassium intake. Pheochromocytoma is especially interesting from a nutritional standpoint in that dietary tyramine, acting as an indirect sympathomimetic amine, may precipitate severe paroxysms of hypertension. Tyramine is found in many foodstuffs, including Chianti wine and fermented cheeses.

### Management

The evaluation of a person for causes and consequences of hypertension is beyond the scope of this chapter and has been well reviewed elsewhere.[5] Treatment of secondary hypertension usually requires correcting the underlying cause. Treatment of primary hypertension generally involves caloric restriction in the obese, salt restriction in salt-sensitive hypertensives, moderate exercise, and lifelong therapy with antihypertensive medications when other measures fail. Side effects of these antihypertensive medications are of great concern to physicians and public health officials and have been recently reviewed.[6] These side effects include carbohydrate intolerance; increased uric acid; increased triglycerides; increased calcium; increased VLDL cholesterol; increased LDL cholesterol; decreased potassium; decreased HDL cholesterol; decreased sodium; dehydration; metabolic alkalosis; and, possibly, increased atherogenesis. The known and potential risks of drug therapy, coupled with the importance of treating hypertension, contribute to the impetus to finding dietary methods of blood pressure control that may be cheaper and safer than antihypertensive drugs.

Both primary and secondary hypertension may be detected in their earliest forms during childhood.[7–9] Because drug therapy may have additional and currently unknown risks in young children, and because the risks of lifelong drug therapy beginning in childhood are unknown, the possibility of dietary modification to treat blood pressure in this group is especially important. The earlier hypertension is treated, the more likely it is that complications can be prevented.

## Mechanisms of Hypertension in Relation to Dietary Intake

A variety of physiologic mechanisms, some of which may be influenced by diet, can contribute to the development and maintenance of hypertension. The most striking example is the sympathetic nervous system. Increased caloric intake, especially in the form of carbohydrates and fat, has been shown to increase sympathetic nervous system activity to a significant degree.[10] Increased sympathetic nervous system activity can elevate blood pressure by means of direct vasoconstriction, increased cardiac contractility and heart rate,[11,12] expanded blood volume,[13,14] diminished venous capacitance,[15] enhanced sodium reabsorption by the kidney,[16-19] and increased levels of renin and angiotensin II.[20] This responsiveness of the sympathetic nervous system to high caloric intake suggests one important mechanism whereby blood pressure may be elevated in obese subjects.

Another important mechanism that may contribute to hypertension and may be amenable to dietary change involves the kidney and has been labeled the "natriuretic handicap."[21-24] In some people with hypertension, the kidneys may be unable to excrete normal amounts of sodium at normal blood pressures. As a consequence, body sodium and intravascular volume increase, and blood pressure rises, until a threshold pressure is reached at which sodium excretion by the kidney equals ingestion. This hypothesis has been demonstrated experimentally in an animal model of salt-sensitive hypertension, the Dahl-S rat.[25,26] The reason for this natriuretic handicap is not known, and circulating "natriuretic factors" have been sought for decades, thus far without success. Recent studies offer exciting promise that this natriuretic factor(s) may soon be identified.[27] One potential natriuretic factor may be plasma insulin, which has been associated with increased sodium reabsorption in the distal tubule of the kidney and may have special relevance to dietary manipulations.[28]

## OBESITY AND BLOOD PRESSURE

Throughout the industrialized world, obesity is a major cause of hypertension.[29-34] Because control of obesity could be both safe and cost effective (if difficult to achieve), great interest has been shown in understanding the mechanisms of obesity-related hypertension and in finding methods to control this problem.

The association between obesity and hypertension begins early in life; children and adolescents in the highest centile for body weight usually have the highest blood pressures.[35,36] Even in those who are normotensive during their youth, significant weight gain after young adulthood is associated with hypertension later in life,[37-39] and it may contribute to a higher rate of cardiovascular morbidity and mortality.[40] In societies where weight does not rise with age, blood pressure usually remains stable.[41] In the Framingham study, an increase of 10% in "relative weight" was a predictor of a 7-mm Hg rise in blood pressure,[42] an effect confirmed in a similar, unrelated study.[43] This finding suggested that weight gain itself, as distinct from absolute body weight, contributes to hypertension.

Weight reduction consistently lowers blood pressure in obese people with primary hypertension.[44-50] In the normotensive obese, weight reduction causes only a modest lowering of blood pressure.[49,53] The method used for weight reduction appears to be less important than simply losing the weight. The fall of blood pressure with weight reduction appears to be independent of sodium intake and occurs even if sodium intake is kept constant or is increased.[47,54-56]

The degree of blood pressure reduction is correlated with the height of the initial blood pressure,[51,52] as well as with the amount of weight lost.[43] Reductions of greater than 40 mm Hg systolic and 20 mm Hg diastolic blood pressure are common, and such reductions may be underestimated because subjects are often withdrawn from their antihypertensive medications during weight loss. Because a reduction in mean blood pressure of only a few mm Hg across the general population can produce a large decrease in the risk of cardiovascular complications of hypertension, the epidemiologic significance of weight loss in the general population is of great importance. For a given individual, weight loss is often accompanied by improvement in the plasma lipid profile and glucose tolerance, which also have a significant impact on cardiovascular risk.

## Mechanisms of Obesity-Related Hypertension

A number of mechanisms may contribute to the fall in blood pressure with weight loss. During weight loss in obese hypertensives, blood pressure falls before normal weight is achieved.[56,57] This finding suggests that the metabolic adaptations to hypocaloric feeding, rather than the absolute reduction in body mass, are primarily responsible for reducing blood pressure. One such adaptation involves the sympathetic nervous system. Hypocaloric feeding reduces sympathetic nervous system activity.[58-61] Because sympathetic nervous system activity can change rapidly with caloric restriction, and because the activity of this system plays a major role in blood pressure regulation, suppression of the sympathetic nervous system during hypocaloric feeding may contribute to blood pressure reduction.

Another important mechanism may be a change in the "natriuretic handicap," as outlined previously. In the obese hypertensive, this change may be influenced by higher plasma insulin levels; because insulin is responsive to caloric intake, it is possible that hypocaloric feeding lowers blood pressure partly by diminishing the effect of insulin on the kidney.

Other postulated mechanisms include decreased cardiac output, increased endogenous opiate activity, and reduction in plasma renin activity, but none of these have been firmly established. Regardless of the mechanism, however, caloric restrictions must be considered a major therapeutic tool in the treatment of hypertension in obese patients.

## SODIUM CHLORIDE AND BLOOD PRESSURE

Sodium chloride, or "salt," has been an important commodity throughout human history because of its properties as a preservative and taste enhancer. Salt was integral to trade routes and religious customs and was considered a favorite of the gods by Homer and Plato. To "sit above the salt" was a position of honor in which one could use as much salt as desired. To make a "covenant of salt" was to seal a bond among individuals. Salt was a major currency; our word "salary" derives from the Roman word "salarium," an amount of salt paid to Roman soldiers. Salt has continued to be valued in the modern era, but recent concern over the excessive use of salt in developed countries and its possible link to hypertension has generated much scientific and public controversy.

Sodium has often been considered, especially in the lay press, synonymous with sodium chloride; however, most of the "sodium controversy" actually concerns sodium chloride. Because research in this area has been done primarily on sodium chloride, rather than other sodium salts, and because chloride may have important effects on blood pressure,[62] this section focuses on sodium chloride and the evidence linking it to human hypertension.

The proper amount of dietary sodium has not been fully defined; the requirement depends on genetic factors and climate, among other factors. The total daily need in man is remarkably low, however. The kidney has the capacity to excrete a urine that is almost sodium-free. Other normal losses of sodium chloride, such as from perspiration, are usually small. In children, the daily requirement of sodium has been estimated to be as low as 9 meq/day,[63] and for adults it has been variously estimated to be between 30 and 90 meq/day.[64-67] In the United States, an average sodium intake is between 170 and 225 mg/day;[68] this "excess" intake may relate to hypertension. In populations where the sodium intake is less than 60 meq/day, hypertension virtually does not exist. At the higher sodium intakes, the incidence of hypertension is between 9 and 20%.

### Evidence Linking Sodium Chloride to Blood Pressure

Sodium chloride has dominated the literature relating diet to hypertension since the mid nineteenth century, when observations suggested that sodium chloride was linked to body fluid volume.[69] In 1904, Ambard and Beaujard showed that sodium chloride deprivation produced a fall in blood pressure in hypertensives.[12] Interest accelerated during the 1940s with further reports that dietary restriction of sodium chloride could lower blood pressure,[70-73] as well as with epidemiologic studies in isolated societies where low blood pressure and low sodium chloride intake appeared to be related. The association of renal disease with hypertension and the efficacy of diuretics added support to the hypothesis of a central role for sodium chloride in hypertension.[69]

Beginning in the 1920s, epidemiologic studies of isolated populations suggested an association between dietary sodium chloride intake and blood pressure.[66,69,74-89] Over 20 populations with low blood pressures were described.[74] These include culturally homogeneous people, relatively isolated people, lean people, people who gain little weight with age, physically active people, people consuming a high-potassium diet, and people consuming a low-sodium diet. Although these epidemiologic studies had enormous impact, they were plagued by methodologic problems and have been challenged accordingly. Furthermore, a number of these studies, especially in Western societies, failed to show an association between sodium chloride intake and hypertension. Intrasocietal studies did not show differences in sodium chloride consumption between normotensive and hypertensive subjects, and for both the general and the hypertensive population, sodium chloride intake was not shown to be linearly related to blood pressure. Thus, the evidence for a broad impact of sodium chloride on the blood pressure of the general population is still not firmly established.

One reason for the difficulty in demonstrating a definite relationship between sodium chloride and blood pressure in Western societies may be the heterogeneity of these societies. The current hypothesis is that some population subgroups are genetically susceptible to hypertension (perhaps 10% of the population of the United States), and only in these subgroups does a strong correlation between sodium chloride intake and blood pressure exist.[90-93] This genetic susceptibility has been suggested even in the normotensive offspring of hypertensive parents.[94] For example, blacks, as a group, appear to have an increased susceptibility to the hypertensive effects of sodium chloride.

The elderly are also more susceptible to the hypertensive effect of sodium chloride,[95,96] most likely because of diminished renal function, rather than genetic predisposition. Blood pressure and sodium chloride intake are strongly correlated in the elderly.[97,98]

In experimental trials, sodium chloride restriction has reduced blood pressure and has potentiated the hypotensive effect of diuretics and beta blockers. Not only has drastic sodium chloride restriction lowered blood pressure,[99-102] but also milder restriction has produced more modest blood pressure reductions.[97,103,104] For example, modifying the sodium chloride content in a water supply appeared to influence blood pressure in children in one study,[105] but this result has not been widely replicated. The blood pressure lowering effect of sodium chloride restriction has been demonstrated even when weight loss is taken into account.

Conversely, a high sodium intake may raise blood pressure, at least on a short-term basis, in normotensive individuals,[106] as well as in borderline hypertensives,[107] and it may blunt the hypotensive effect of thiazides.

The quantitative effects of sodium restriction on blood pressure are less dramatic and reproducible than the effect seen with weight reduction in the obese. Except in extreme situations in which diets are modified to either less than 1 g sodium/day or greater than 10 to 15 g sodium/day, the reductions in blood pressure are usually under 10 to 15 mm Hg systolic and 5 to 10 mm Hg diastolic pressure. Because those dietary extremes are often associated with weight changes and numerous effects on other nutrients, the isolated effect of sodium is difficult to ascertain. From an epidemiologic standpoint, however, it requires a reduction of only a few mm Hg in mean blood pressure to demonstrate a decrease in risk from complications of hypertension, and therefore, the potential contribution to public health of widespread reduction of dietary sodium may prove of value.

## Possible Mechanisms of Sodium Chloride's Effect on Blood Pressure

The best physiologic evidence linking sodium chloride to blood pressure involves renal sodium handling and intravascular volume, the "natriuretic handicap" discussed previously. High sodium intake has also been thought to increase arteriolar smooth muscle reactivity and sodium content. Sodium intake has been related to prostaglandin metabolism; high sodium intake has been suggested to lower levels of prostaglandin $E_2$ ($PGE_2$) and thus to increase blood pressure. Red blood cell membrane sodium and sodium potassium adenosine triphosphatase (ATPase) activity may be different in hypertensives, but whether this activity is affected by sodium exposure is not well defined.

The Dahl salt-sensitive (Dahl-S) rat is the major animal model of salt-sensitive hypertension, although a number of other animal models have been made hypertensive by high-salt feeding.[108-110] The Dahl-S rat develops mild hypertension on a regular diet and severe hypertension on a 4% sodium chloride diet; the Dahl salt-resistant rat does not develop hypertension even with an 8% sodium chloride diet.[111] As noted previously, the natriuretic handicap appears to occur in the Dahl-S rat. In addition, a diet high in sodium chloride may affect the sympathetic nervous system of this animal, to increase blood pressure.[92,112-115]

## Public Policy Issues

In the lay press and in public policy, sodium chloride has been the most conspicuous "villain" relating diet to hypertension. Numerous recommendations for lowering the sodium chloride content of processed foods, drinking supplies, medicines, and infant formulas have been proposed. Most current government programs focus on improved packaging labeling, consumer education to diminish salt intake, and monitoring food-consumption patterns; mandatory controls have been proposed if voluntary ones prove unsuccessful.

A few have questioned the wisdom of this approach,[116] although most would agree to the need to identify those at highest risk of salt-sensitive and other forms of hypertension.[117,118] Risk factors for hypertension include borderline hypertension, age greater than 65, black race, positive family history, impaired kidney function, increased weight gain with age, and being in a high percentile for blood pressure as a youth.

Attempts to modify salt taste are interesting in this regard and have been recently reviewed.[119] It appears that a newborn infant has a developed taste for sour, bitter, and sweet, but is neutral to salt by both neurophysiologic and behavioral data. By age two, however, sodium preference is established. It is not clear whether this sodium preference is based on dietary exposure or on maturation of the nervous system. Encouraging studies suggest that salt intake can be modified and that a gradual reduction in salt intake leads to a diminished salt preference over time.

## POTASSIUM AND BLOOD PRESSURE

In 1679, Thomas Willis described the diuretic effect of "salt of niter" (potassium nitrate) for treatment of dropsy.[120] In 1928, Addison suggested that potassium salt supplementation lowered blood pressure in hypertensive humans, including himself, and he attributed the high prevalence of hypertension in North America to the low "potash" content of the diet.[121] A few years later, Priddle demonstrated a similar effect of potassium supplementation in combination with a low sodium diet,[122] and McQuarrie and co-workers showed that potassium supplementation could attenuate the blood pressure elevation during high-salt feeding in diabetic children.[123,124] Many other writers have since advanced the hypothesis that increased dietary potassium may ameliorate hypertension,[125,129] especially hypertension that is sensitive to sodium chloride intake.[130]

### Evidence Linking Dietary Potassium to Blood Pressure

Dietary potassium salt supplementation has reduced blood pressure in several animal models of experimental hypertension.[126,127,131,132] Increased dietary potassium has also lowered blood pressure in normotensive animals,[125,133,134] but this result has not been found consistently.[135–138]

Epidemiologic evidence suggests a negative correlation between dietary potassium intake and blood pressure in both normotensive and hypertensive men.[139] In normotensive men, dietary supplementation with a 64 to 100 mmol/day of potassium chloride produced slight reduction of systolic and diastolic blood pressure, as well as natriuresis, when it was added to an unaltered diet,[140] to a sodium-chloride-restricted diet,[141] and to a 1,500-mmol/day-sodium-chloride diet.[142] Other work in normotensive humans, however, has shown no relationship between dietary potassium and blood pressure,[135,138,143] or no reduction of blood pressure with dietary potassium supplementation.[144–146]

Dietary potassium supplementation has lowered blood pressure in hypertensive humans,[147–151] as well as in their normotensive offspring.[152] In short-term studies, potassium supplementation lowered blood pressure in hypertensives consuming high levels of sodium and in those consuming low to normal sodium levels.[128] In a double-blind randomized trial of mildly hypertensive men, 4 weeks of 60 mmol/day potassium chloride supplementation reduced blood pressure and increased urinary sodium excretion.[148] This result, however, has not been consistently reported among hypertensive adults. It may be the higher ratio of dietary potassium to sodium chloride, rather the amount of potassium itself, that is responsible for the fall in blood pressure;[126,153–156] discrepancies among studies of potassium supplementation may relate to differences in this ratio. The high potassium intakes in the foregoing studies have generally been associated with increases in plasma potassium levels of approximately 0.6 meq/L.

### Potassium Depletion

Although the foregoing literature suggests efficacy of potassium supplementation for blood pressure control, several papers have suggested that potassium depletion may lower blood pressure in hypertensive[128,157,158] as well as normotensive,[135,159–161] animals, even when nutritional variables were tightly controlled.[159,162–164] Adverse long-term consequences of potassium depletion, however, such as on heart rhythm or muscle strength, generally preclude considering it as a form of dietary therapy.

### Possible Mechanisms of Potassium's Effect on Blood Pressure

Dietary potassium can influence blood pressure in a number of ways. First is sodium balance. The natriuretic action of potassium supplementation has been recognized for many years,[165–170] and it may be a direct effect of potassium on the nephron.[171–173] Although the hypotensive action of potassium has been closely linked to this natriuretic effect,[128] several studies have shown a fall in blood pressure with potassium, despite a lack of change in plasma volume, exchangeable sodium, or body weight.[131,148,152,174] A second mechanism is sympathoadrenal activity. Potassium supplementation may attenuate sympathoadrenal activity by blunting the blood pressure response to circulating norepinephrine.[126] This effect may be different in hypertensive than in normotensive men.[152] A third possible mechanism of potassium is a direct effect. Potassium may modify the excitability of vascular tissue and may relax arteriolar smooth muscle directly,[175,176] perhaps through an effect on smooth muscle membrane sodium-potassium ATPase.[177] Alterations in sodium-potassium ATPase in a variety of tissues have been considered in the etiology of primary hypertension. A fourth possible mechanism involves renin. Potassium supplementation generally decreases renin secretion,[178,179] despite natriuresis. Potassium depletion elevates renin levels.[160,180] Although it has been thought that this potassium effect on renin is a direct effect on the kidney rather than on sodium balance,[181,182] renin will rise in the face of high potassium intake if the natriuresis is severe enough.[183] The high chloride intake associated with potassium chloride supplementation may be integral to this observed effect on renin.[184]

In conclusion, evidence is mounting that dietary potassium supplementation lowers blood pressure. Before potassium supplementation is widely prescribed, however, one must realize that it may cause clinically dangerous hyperkalemia in hypertensive patients with renal insufficiency or diabetes, or those who are taking potassium-sparing diuretics or beta-adrenergic blocking drugs.

## DIVALENT CATIONS AND BLOOD PRESSURE

### Calcium

High dietary calcium intake has been associated with lower blood pressure in man,[185,186] and dietary calcium supplementation has lowered blood pressure in normotensive humans,[187] as well as in animals.[188,189] The positive calcium balance induced by thiazide diuretics and sodium restriction has been postulated to contribute to the antihypertensive effect of these drugs.[190] Calcium is involved in the regulation of numerous physiologic processes that influence blood pressure, but whether dietary calcium intake can influence these mechanisms remains to be determined. In vitro experiments have shown an interaction of calcium with sodium,[191] with vascular smooth muscle,[192,193] with volume regulation,[194] with neurotransmitter synthesis,[195] and with sympathoadrenal activity.[196,197] Ongoing studies from other investigators may soon provide more-conclusive evidence that dietary calcium supplementation lowers blood pressure.

### Magnesium

In 1925, Blackfan and Hamilton reported that high doses of magnesium salts lowered blood pressure.[198] Since then, a number of studies have suggested that low dietary magnesium levels may be associated with higher blood pressures.[199,200] Large doses of magnesium salts are still occasionally used to treat the hypertension of eclampsia in pregnancy.[201] In animal studies, magnesium-deficient diets raised blood pressure in normotensive rats and were associated with accelerated cardiovascular disease.[202] Magnesium may influence blood pressure by several mechanisms, but,

as with calcium, it is not known whether dietary modifications of magnesium within the physiologic range can affect these mechanisms. Magnesium homeostasis can affect multiple aspects of cellular and membrane physiology. Magnesium may influence vascular smooth muscle reactivity,[203,204] neurotransmitter synthesis and release,[205] intravascular volume, and the renin-angiotensin system.[206]

### Phosphorus

Whether dietary phosphorus affects blood pressure is not known. In normotensive individuals, an inverse relationship may exist between serum phosphorus and blood pressure.[207] Serum phosphorus levels, in turn, are sensitive to dietary phosphorus intake in individuals with normal renal and parathyroid function.

### Trace Elements

Although no firm evidence in humans suggests that alteration of dietary intake of trace elements within the physiologic range can affect blood pressure,[208] the growing evidence that membrane cation transport may be altered in certain subsets of hypertensives has led to interest in the impact of dietary trace elements on blood pressure.[209] Certain heavy-metal-binding agents do appear to exert antihypertensive effects in animals. Furthermore, some trace elements are part of metaloenzymes that may affect blood pressure through their involvement in the biosynthesis and degradation of peptides (such as zinc in angiotensin-converting enzyme), catecholamines (such as copper in dopamine beta-hydroxylase) and steroids (iron in mixed function oxidases for aldosterone synthesis). It is not known, however, whether dietary changes affect these enzyme systems, and research in this area is complicated by the interdependence of trace elements.[210]

**Cadmium.** Increased environmental exposure to cadmium has been associated with increased blood pressure.[211–214] Interpretation of these studies, however, is confounded by the question of what constitutes a proper control group. Other studies have shown no effect of cadmium exposure on blood pressure.[215,216] An interaction of cadmium exposure with salt-sensitive hypertension has been suggested.[217]

**Lead.** Chronic lead exposure can produce renal damage and elevated blood pressure in animals and in man.[218,219] Lead toxicity, even in the absence of overt renal insufficiency, may produce renal tubular dysfunction that may contribute to hypertension.[220,221] No correlation, however, exists between blood lead level and blood pressure in children,[222] or between lead levels in drinking water and blood pressure in adult communities.[223]

**Zinc.** One study of hypertensive patients showed an elevated zinc content of red blood cells, but not elevated plasma zinc levels.[224] Zinc deficiency may alter salt taste, but no evidence suggests that this change leads to increased sodium chloride consumption.[225] Toxemia in pregnancy has been associated with lower-than-normal zinc levels.[226] Thiazide diuretics used to treat hypertension can increase urinary zinc excretion and so may produce relative zinc deficiency.[227]

**Other Trace Elements.** Even less is known about other trace elements. Vanadium, added to the chow of rats with one kidney, raised blood pressure in proportion to plasma vanadium levels,[228] and intravenous vanadate raised blood pressure in cats.[229] Arsenic fed to male rats for a year caused no effect on blood pressure, but it did affect cardiovascular reflexes.[230] Trace amounts of nickel chloride induced coronary vasoconstriction in isolated dog heart,[231] but the effect of nickel chloride ingestion on blood pressure is not known. Iron deficiency has been associated with increased cardiac output,[232] as well as with increased sympathetic nervous system activity, but no clear evidence indicates that this deficiency affects blood pressure, and no correlation has been found between levels of iron in drinking water and blood pressure. Acute and chronic mercury poisoning may be associated with elevated blood pressure.

## NUTRIENTS AND BLOOD PRESSURE

### Dietary Fat

The ratio of polyunsaturated to saturated fat in the diet (the P/S ratio) may affect blood pressure. In normotensive and mildly hypertensive patients, an increase in the P/S ratio to 1 or more in a diet consisting of approximately 25% fat has been associated with lower blood pressure.[233,234] A higher total dietary fat content,[235] or a lower P/S ratio,[236] may not produce this blood pressure lowering effect. The effect on blood pressure of the increased P/S ratio appears to be independent of sodium balance or body weight.[237,238] Similar observations have been made in experimental animal studies.[239]

The mechanism(s) of this blood pressure lowering effect is thought to involve prostaglandin metabolism. Dietary linoleic acid, the usual source of polyunsaturated fat in experimental diets, is a precursor of arachidonic acid, which, in turn, is a precursor of prostaglandin biosynthesis.[240] Prostaglandins appear to have important effects on blood pressure regulation,[241] and linoleic acid is thought to influence blood pressure through changes in prostaglandin metabolism.[242,243] Most studies thus far have been short term and have used a small number of subjects, however.

### Carbohydrate

Glucose and sucrose raise blood pressure on a short-term basis under experimental conditions in both animals and man.[244–246] The rise in blood pressure may be due to increased sodium retention,[247] which may be produced by increased insulin secretion,[248] decreased glucagon levels,[249] or sympathetic nervous system stimulation[250–252] and related mechanisms.[28,253] The effect of other forms of carbohydrate on blood pressure and the long-term effects of glucose and sucrose in human beings are not known.[254]

### Protein

Evidence for the effect of protein intake on blood pressure in human beings is conflicting. In a controlled trial with vegetarians, the isocaloric addition of 250 g beef/day for 4 weeks resulted in elevation of systolic blood pressure by 3% over control values.[255] In some studies, low-protein feeding has been accompanied by lowering of blood pressure.[256,257] On the other hand, vegetarians in Western society appear to have blood pressures equal to those of meat eaters when they are matched by weight.[258] Furthermore, in recent work with a hypertensive animal model, low-protein feeding actually increased blood pressure and sympathetic nervous system activity.[259,260] Specific amino acids, such as tyrosine, have been shown to lower blood pressure under experimental conditions.[261–263]

### Vitamins

No clear evidence links vitamin intake with blood pressure in humans. For vitamin E, the data are conflicting. A diet low in vitamin E retarded the onset of hypertension in one group of spontaneously hypertensive rats,[264] but tocopheryl esters reduced blood pressures in another study involving both spontaneously hypertensive rats and those in whom hypertension was induced with desoxycorticosterone acetate (DOCA).[265] Spontaneously hypertensive rats have been reported to have low tissue vitamin E levels.[266] Vitamin D excess, even with hypercalcemia, is not universally associated with hypertension and 25-dihydroxy vitamin D levels in plasma are not different in hypertensive than in normotensive men when medication is taken into account.[267] No evidence links vitamin A or K or any of the water-soluble vitamins to blood pressure in man.

## OTHER DIETARY COMPONENTS AND BLOOD PRESSURE

### Fiber

Several studies have suggested blood pressure may be lowered by increased dietary fiber intake.[268,269] Vegetarians usually consume a high-fiber diet and as a whole have lower blood pressures, but numerous differences in vegetarians' diets and body weight may account for such variations.[270] In rabbits, the addition of dietary cellulose attenuated the hypertensive effect of a high-fat diet.[271] Several mechanisms through which dietary fiber may influence blood pressure are known. High-fiber diets are associated with lower postprandial insulin levels,[272] with greater fecal water and electrolyte excretion and probably with altered absorption rates of nutrients, especially of fats. For the most part, experiments with alteration in dietary fiber have been performed in the setting of other dietary modifications often associated with weight loss, so it remains to be determined whether dietary fiber can influence blood pressure in an independent manner.

### Alcohol

A strong association appears to exist between moderate-to-heavy alcohol consumption (greater than 3 oz. whiskey or equivalent/day) and hypertension;[273–276] it has been suggested that 5% of hypertension in the general population is attributable to the consumption of alcohol. The effect of alcohol on blood pressure appears to be more pronounced in the elderly than in the young.[277] The consumption of 2 to 3 oz. or less/day of 40% alcohol or its equivalent has been associated with lower blood pressure,[278–281] as well as with reduced cardiovascular risk,[282–285] as compared with nondrinkers. These observations suggest that alcohol begins to exert a hypertensive effect only when this threshold amount has been reached. Several other studies, however, suggest that blood pressure increases with the smallest degree of alcohol intake.[286–288]

This association of alcohol with hypertension may be due to an indirect, rather than to a direct, effect of alcohol. One possibility is that the increased prevalence of hypertension detected in alcoholic populations reflects alcohol withdrawal at the time of blood pressure measurement.[278,289,290] Second, alcohol consumption may be a marker of increased psychologic stress. Third, alcohol consumption may be correlated with high caloric intake and obesity. Alcohol may also directly affect terminal arterioles and venules,[291] or it may increase their sensitivity to circulating vasopressor agents by affecting calcium accumulation in vascular smooth muscle.[275] In one study of the neuroendocrine effects of alcohol, no change was seen in levels of catecholamines, renin, angiotensin II, aldosterone, or cortisol.[292] That the consumption of alcohol does bear some direct relation to blood pressure is suggested by the observation that formerly heavy drinkers who remain abstinent have blood pressures similar to those of nondrinkers.[287,290]

### Caffeine

Although not considered a nutrient, caffeine forms a common part of the American diet and may have effects on blood pressure. In doses as low as that found in a single cup of regular coffee, caffeine can produce a short-term, significant increase in both systolic and diastolic blood pressure.[293–295] Evidence for a long-term effect of caffeine on blood pressure is less clear, however. Although two studies have suggested that long-term caffeine intake is associated with higher blood pressures,[296,297] others have shown that tolerance develops to the pressor effect of caffeine during long-term administration.[298–300] Caffeine may exert its effects partly, but not entirely, through increased sympathoadrenal activity.[265]

## CONCLUSIONS

There is a growing consensus in American society that proper nutrition can help with both prevention and treatment of illness. Hypertension, and attendant cardiovascular disease, have drawn particular attention because of their prevalence, impact on public health, and potential responsiveness to nutritional therapies. The rapid advances in scientific knowledge over the past decade have still not kept pace with the pressures to formulate public policy and to provide guidance to health-care consumers, who expect clear recommendations from health professionals. As the evidence in this chapter summarizes, many current dietary recommendations are not of proved efficacy and may even have long-term negative nutritional consequences yet to be ascertained. Accordingly, it is not possible to write a dietary prescription that provides a scientifically proved public policy position. Given such uncertainty, however, a number of guidelines can be formulated as part of a working hypothesis based on evidence presented in this chapter. These include calorie restriction in obese individuals; moderate sodium chloride restriction in those with, or at risk for, salt-sensitive hypertension; an increased potassium to sodium ratio; increased fiber intake; a polyunsaturated to saturated fat ratio > 1; limited alcohol intake; and, possibly, increased calcium intake.

Research may benefit from a focus on overall composition of a therapeutic diet, rather than on manipulation of individual nutrients in the prevention and management of hypertension. With the rapid growth of knowledge and interest in this area, some of the questions raised in this chapter may soon be resolved.

## SUGGESTIONS FOR FURTHER READING

McCarron, D.A., Kotchen, T.A. (eds.): Nutrition and blood pressure control: current status of dietary factors and hypertension. Symposium Intern. Med., *98*:5(2), 697–890, 1983.

Kaplan, N.M.: Systemic hypertension: therapy. *In* Heart Disease: A Textbook of Cardiovascular Medicine. Edited by E. Braunwald. Philadelphia, W.B. Saunders, 1980.

## REFERENCES

1. McCarron, D.A., Henry, H.J., Morris, C.D.: Hypertension *4*:III2–III3, 1982.
2. Kaplan, N.M.: Arch. Intern. Med. *143*:255–259, 1983.
3. Pfeffer, R.I.: J. Chronic. Dis. *31*:389, 1978.
4. Weir, R.J., Briggs, E., Mack, A.: Br. Med. J. *1*:533, 1974.
5. Kaplan, N.M.: Systemic hypertension: therapy. *In*: Heart Disease: A Textbook of Cardiovascular Medicine. Edited by E. Braunwald. Philadelphia, W.B. Saunders, 1980.
6. Flamenbaum, W.: Ann. Intern. Med. *98*:875–880, 1983.
7. Voors, A.W., Webber, L.S., Berenson, G.S.: Hypertension *2(Suppl. 1)*:I102–I108, 1980.
8. Harlan, W.R., Oberman, A., Mitchell, R.E., et al.: A 30-year-old study of blood pressure in a white male cohort. *In* Hypertension: Mechanisms Management. Edited by Onesti, G., Kim, K.E., Moyer, J.H. New York, Grune & Stratton, 1973.
9. Heyden, S., Bartel, A.G., Hames, C.G., et al.: JAMA *209*:1,683–1,689, 1969.
10. Schwartz, J.H., Young, J.B., Landsberg, L.: J. Clin. Invest. *72*:361–370, 1983.
11. Frohlich, E.D.: Mayo Clin. Proc. *32*:361–368, 1977.
12. Korner, P.I, Fletcher, P.J.: Cardiovasc. Med. *2*:139–155, 1977.
13. Safar, M.E., Weiss, Y.A., Levenson, J.A., et al.: Am. J. Cardiol. *31*:315–319, 1973.
14. Safar, M.E., Weiss, Y.A., London, G.M., et al.: Clin. Sci. Molec. Med. *47*:513–514, 1974.
15. Simon, G.: Circ. Res. *38*:412–418, 1976.
16. Hollenberg, N.K., Epstein, M., Guttman, R.D., et al.: J. Appl. Physiol. *28*:312–317, 1970.
17. Bello-Reuss, E., Trevino, D.L., Gottschalk, C.W.: J. Clin. Invest. *57*:1104–1107, 1976.
18. Besarab, A., Silva, P., Landsberg, L., et al.: Am. J. Physiol. *233*:F39–F45, 1977.
19. Prosnitz, E.H., DiBona, G.F.: Am. J. Physiol. *235*:F557–F563, 1978.
20. Thames, M.D.: Fed. Proc. *37*:1,209–1,213, 1978.
21. Guyton, A.C., Coleman, T.G.: Circ. Res. *24*:1–26, 1969.
22. Dahl, L.K., Knudsen, K.D., Iwai, J.: Circ. Res. *25(Suppl.)*:I21–I33, 1969.
23. Haddy, F.J., Overbeck, J.W.: Life Sci. *19*:935–948, 1976.
24. De Wardner, H.E., MacGregor, G.A.: Kidney Int. *18*:1–5, 1980.
25. Tobian, L., Lange, J., Azar, S., et al.: Circ. Res. *43(Suppl.)*:I92–I97, 1978.
26. Iwai, J., Ohanian, E., Dahl, L.K.: Circ. Res. *40*:I131–I134, 1977.
27. Blaustein, M.P., Hamlyn, J.M.: Ann. Intern. Med. *98*:785–792, 1983.
28. Defronzo, R.A., Cooke, C.R., Andres, R., et al.: J. Clin. Invest. *55*:845–855, 1975.
29. Chiang, R.N., Perlman, L.V., Epstein, F.H.: Circulation *39*:403–421, 1969.
30. Kannel, W.B., Gordon, T.: Physiological and medical concomitants of obesity: the Framingham study. *In* Obesity in America. Edited by G.A. Bray. New York, National Institutes of Health Publication, 1979.
31. Stamler, J., Rhomberg, P., Schoenberger, J.A., et al.: J. Chronic Dis. *28*:527–548, 1975.
32. Stamler, R., Stamler, J., Riedlinger, W.F., et al.: JAMA *240*:1,607–1,610, 1978.
33. Havlik, R.J., Feinleib, M.: Hypertension *4*:III121–III127, 1982.
34. Berglund, G., Ljungman, S., Hartford, M., et al.: Hypertension *4*:692–696, 1982.
35. Havlik, R.J., Hubert, H.B., Fabsitz, R.R., et al.: Ann. Intern. Med. *98*:855–859, 1983.
36. Siervogel, R.M., Frey, M.A., Kezdi, P., et al.: Hypertension *2*:83–92, 1980.
37. Kannel, W.B., Brand, N., Skinner, J.J., et al.: Ann. Intern. Med. *67*:48–59, 1967.
38. Higgins, M.W., Keller, J.B., Metzner, H.L., et al.: Hypertension *2*:I117–I123, 1980.
39. Paffenbarger, R.S., Jr., Wing, A.L., Hyde, R.T.: Am. J. Epidemiol. *117*:245–257, 1983.
40. Hubert, H.B., Feinleib, M., McNamara, P.M., et al.: Circulation *67*:968–977, 1983.
41. Dustan, H.P.: Salt and hypertension. *In* Cardiology Update 1983. Edited by E. Rapaport, New York, Elsevier Biomedical, 1983.
42. Ashley, R.W., Jr., Kannel, W.B.: J. Chronic Dis. *27*:103–114, 1974.
43. Reed, D., McGee, D., Yano, K.: Hypertension *4*:406–414, 1982.
44. Stamler, J., Farinaro, E., Mohonnier, L.M., et al.: JAMA *242*:1,819–1,823, 1980.
45. Raison, J., Achimastos, A., Bouthier, J., et al.: Am. J. Cardiol. *51*:165–170, 1983.
46. Reisin, E., Frohlich, E.D., Messerli, F.H., et al.: Ann. Intern. Med. *98*:315–319, 1983.
47. Jung, R.T., Shetty, P.S., Barrand, M., et al.: Br. Med. J. *1*:12–15, 1979.
48. Sims, E.A., Phinney, S.D., Vaswani, A.: Int. J. Obes. *2*:215–223, 1978.
49. DeHaven, J., Sherwin, R., Hendler, R., et al.: N. Engl. J. Med. *302*:477–482, 1980.
50. Tuck, M.L., Sowers, J., Dornfeld, L., et al.: N. Engl. J. Med. *304*:930–933, 1981.
51. Stokholm, K.H., Nielsen, P.E., Quaade, F.: Int. J. Obes. *6*:307–312, 1982.
52. Young, J.B., Landsberg, L.: J. Chronic Dis. *35*:879–886, 1982.
53. Fagerberg, B., Andersson, O.K., Isaksson, B., et al.: Br. Med. J. *288*:11–14, 1984.

54. Young, J.B., Mullen, D., Landsberg, L.: Metabolism *27*:1,711–1,714, 1978.
55. Reisin, E., Frohlich, E.D.: J. Chronic Dis. *35*:887–891, 1982.
56. Berchtold, P., Jorgens, V., Kemmer, F.W., et al.: Hypertension *4*:III50–III55, 1982.
57. Eliahou, H.E., Iaina, A., Gaon, T., et al.: Int. J. Obes. *5(Suppl. 1)*:157–163, 1981.
58. Sowers, J.R., Nyby, M., Stern, N., et al.: Hypertension *4*:686–691, 1982.
59. Kopopeschaar, H.P., Meinders, A.E., Schwartz, F.: Int. J. Obes. *7*:569–574, 1983.
60. Jung, R.T., Shetty, P.S., James, W.P., et al.: Int. J. Obes. *6*:131–141, 1982.
61. Sowers, J.R., Whitfield, L.A., Catania, R.A., et al.: J. Clin. Endocrinol. Metab. *54*:1,181–1,186, 1982.
62. Kotchen, T.A., Luke, R.G., Ott, C.E., et al.: Ann. Intern. Med. *98*:817–822, 1983.
63. Amercian Academy of Pediatrics Committee on Nutrition: Pediatrics *53*:115–121, 1974.
64. Page, L.B., Danion, A., Moellering, R.C., Jr.: Circulation *49*:1,132–1,146, 1974.
65. Dahl, L.K.: N. Engl. J. Med. *258*:1,152–1,157, 1958.
66. Page, L.B., Danion, A., Moellering, R.C., Jr.: Circulation *49*:1,132–1,146, 1974.
67. Conn, J.W.: Adv. Intern. Med. *3*:373–393, 1949.
68. Fregly, M.S., Fregly, M.J.: The estimates of sodium intake by man. *In* The Role of Salt in Cardiovascular Hypertension. Edited by M.J. Fregly and M.R. Kare. New York, Academic Press, 1982.
69. Porter, G.A.: Ann. Intern. Med. *98*:720–723, 1983.
70. Maddocks, I.: Med. J. Aust. *1*:1,123, 1967.
71. Miall, W.E., Oldham, P.D.: Clin. Sci. Molec. Med. *17*:407–444, 1958.
72. Michell, A.R.: Perspect. Biol. Med. *21*:335–347, 1978.
73. Meneely, G.R., Batterbee, H.D.: Sodium and potassium. *In* Present Knowledge in Nutrition. Edited by D.M. Hegsted, et al. Washington, D.C., Nutrition Foundation, 1976.
74. Page, L.B.: Hypertension and atherosclerosis in primitive and acculturating societies. *In* Hypertension Update: Mechanisms Epidemiology Evaluation and Management. Edited by J.C. Hunt, et al. Bloomfield, NJ, H.L.S. Press, 1980.
75. Fodor, J.G., Abbott, E.C., Rusted, I.E.: Can. Med. Assoc. J. *108*:1,365–1,368, 1973.
76. Takahashi, E., Sasaki, N., Takeda, J., et al.: Hum. Biol. *29*:139, 1957.
77. Sinett, P.F., Whyte, H.M.: J. Chronic Dis. *26*:265–290, 1973.
78. Oliver, W.J., Cohen, E.L., Neel, J.V.: Circulation *52*:146–151, 1975.
79. Fukuda, T.: Chiba Igakkai Zasshi *29*:490–502, 1954.
80. Takamatsu, M.: Rodo Kagaku *31*:349–370, 1955.
81. Thomas, W.A.: JAMA *88*:1,559–1,560, 1927.
82. Hicks, C.S., Matters, R.F.: Aust. J. Exp. Biol. Med. Sci. *11*:177–183, 1933.
83. Kean, B.H.: Am. J. Trop. Med. *24*:341–343, 1944.
84. Kaminer, B., Lutz, W.P.W.: Circulation *22*:289–295, 1960.
85. Maddocks, I.: Med. J. Aust. *1*:1,123–1,126, 1967.
86. Morse, W.R., Beh, Y.T.: Lancet *1*:966–967, 1937.
87. Miall, W.E.: Br. Med. J. *2*:1,205–1,210, 1959.
88. Lowenstein, F.W.: Lancet *1*:389–392, 1961.
89. Prior, I.A.M., Evans, J.G., Harvey, H.P.B., et al.: N. Engl. J. Med. *279*:515–520, 1968.
90. Mark, A.L., Lawton, W.J., Abboud, F.M., et al.: Circ. Res. *36(Suppl. 1)*:I194–I198, 1975.
91. Langford, H.G., Watson, R.L.: Circulation *66(Suppl. II)*:II–105, 1982.
92. Gleibermann, L.: Ecol. Food Nutr. *2*:143–156, 1973.
93. Kawasaki, T., Delea, C.S., Bartter, F.C., et al.: Am. J. Med. *64*:193–198, 1978.
94. Falkner, B., Onesti, G., and Hayes, P.: The role of sodium in essential hypertension in genetically hypertensive adolescents. *In* Hypertension in the Young and the Old. Edited by G. Onesti and K.E. Kim. New York, Grune & Stratton, 1981.
95. Parijs, J., Joosens, J.V., Van der Linden, L., et al.: Am. Heart J. *85*:22–34, 1973.
96. Beretta-Piccoli, C., Davies, D.L., Boddy, K., et al.: Clin. Sci. *63*:257–270, 1982.
97. Morgan, T., Adam, W., Gillies, A., et al.: Lancet *1*:227–230, 1978.
98. Morgan, T.O., Myers, J.B.: Med. J. Aust. *2*:396–397, 1978.
99. Chapman, C.B., Gibbons, T.B.: Medicine *29*:29–69, 1950.
100. Watkins, D.M., Froeb, H.F., Hatch, F.T., et al.: Am. J. Med. *9*:441–493, 1950.
101. Grollman, A., Harrison, T.R., Mason, M.F., et al.: JAMA *129*:533–536, 1945.
102. Murphy, R.J.F.: J. Clin. Invest. *29*:912–917, 1950.
103. Magnani, B., Ambrosioni, E., Agosta, R., et al.: Clin. Sci. Molec. Med. *51*:625s–626s, 1976.
104. MacGregor, G.A., Markandu, N.D., Best, F.E., et al.: Lancet *1*:351–355, 1982.
105. Calabrese, E.J., Tuthill, R.W.: The influence of elevated levels of sodium in drinking water on elementary and high school students in Masssachusetts. *In* The Role of Salt in Cardiovascular Hypertension. Edited by M.J. Fregly and M.R. Kare. New York, Academic Press, 1982.
106. Luft, F.C., Rankin, L.I., Bloch, R., et al.: Circulation *60*:697–706, 1979.
107. Mark, A.L., Lawton, W.J., Abboud, F.M., et al.: Circ. Res. *36-37(Suppl. I)*:I194–I198, 1975.
108. Lenel, R., Katz, L.N., Rodbard, S.: Am. J. Physiol. *152*:557–562, 1948.
109. Meneely, G.R., Ball, C.O.T.: Am. J. Med. *25*:713–725, 1958.
110. Sapirstein, L.A., Brandt, W.L., Drury, D.R.: Proc. Soc. Exp. Biol. Med. *73*:82–85, 1950.
111. Ganguli, M., Tobian, L., Iwai, J., Johnson, M.A.: Clin. Sci. *61(Suppl.)*:73S–75S, 1981.
112. Ikeda, T., Tobian, L, Iwai, J., Goossens, P.: Clin. Sci. Molec. Med. *55*:225s–227s, 1978.
113. Goto, A., Ganguli, M., Tobian, L., et al.: *243*:H614–618, 1982.
114. Takeshita, A., Mark, A.L.: Circ. Res. *43(Suppl. I)*:I86–I91, 1978.
115. Takeshita, A., Mark, A.L., Brody, M.J.: Am. J. Physiol. *236*:H48–HJ52, 1979.
116. Swales, J.D.: Lancet *1*:1,177–1,179, 1980.
117. Altschul, A.M., Grommet, J.K.: Nutr. Rev. *38*:393–401, 1980.
118. Luft, F.C., Weinberger, M.H., Grim, C.E.: Am. J. Med. *72*:726–736, 1982.
119. Beauchamp, G.K., Bertino, M., Engleman, K.: Ann. Intern. Med. *98*:763–769, 1983.
120. Willis, T.: Pharmaceutica Rationalis. London, 1679.
121. Addison, W.L.T.: Can. Med. Assoc. J. *18*:281–285, 1928.
122. Priddle, W.W.: Can. Med. Assoc. J. *25*:5–8, 1931.

123. McQuarrie, I., Thompson, W.H., Anderson, J.A.: J. Nutr. *11*:77–101, 1936.
124. Thompson, W.H., McQuarrie, I.: Proc. Soc. Exp. Biol. Med. *31*:907, 1933.
125. Meneely, G.R., Lemley-Stone, J., Darby, W.J.: Am. J. Cardiol. *8*:527–532, 1961.
126. Dahl, L.K., Leitl, G., Heine, M.: J. Exp. Med. *136*:318–330, 1972.
127. Suzuki, H., Kondo, K., Saruta, T.: Hypertension *3*:566, 1981.
128. Parfrey, P.S., Wright, P., Goodwin, F.J., et al.: Lancet *1*:59, 1981.
129. Skrabal, F., Aubock, J., Hortnagi, H.: Lancet *2*:895, 1981.
130. Treasure, J., Ploth, D.: Hypertension *5*:864–872, 1983.
131. Dietz, R., Schomig, A., Rascher, W., et al.: Clin. Sci. *61*:69s–71s, 1981.
132. Suzuki, H., Kondo, K., Saruta, T.: Acta Endocrinol. *97*:525–532, 1981.
133. Battarbee, H.D., Funch, D.P., Dailey, J.W.: Proc. Soc. Exp. Biol. Med. *161*:32, 1979.
134. Tannen, R.L.: Ann. Intern. Med. *98*:773, 1983.
135. Reid, W.D., Laragh, J.H.: Proc. Soc. Exp. Biol. Med. *120*:26–29, 1965.
136. Meneely, G.R., Ball, C.O.T., Youmans, J.B.: Ann. Intern. Med. *47*:263–273, 1957.
137. Goto, A., Tobian, L., Iwai, J.: Hypertension *3*:128–134, 1981.
138. Young, J.B., McCaa, R.E., Pan, Y.J., et al.: Circ. Res. *38*(6 Suppl 2):84–89, 1976.
139. Langford, H.G.: Ann. Intern. Med. *98*:770–772, 1983.
140. Khaw, K.T., Thom, S.: Lancet *2(B)*:1,127–1,129, 1982.
141. Skrabel, F., Aubock, J., Hortnagl, H., et al.: Clin. Sci. *59*:157s, 1980.
142. Luft, F.C., Rankin, L.I., Bloch, R., et al.: Circulation *60*:697, 1979.
143. Campbell, W.B., Schmitz, J.M.: Endocrinology *103*:2,098–2,104, 1978.
144. Hollenberg, N.K., Williams, G., Burger, B., et al.: Clin. Sci. Molec. Med. *49*:527–534, 1975.
145. Burstyn, P., Hornall, D., Watchorn, C.: Br. Med. J. *281*:537, 1980.
146. Mickelson, O., Makdani, D., Gill, J.L., et al.: Am. J. Clin. Nutr. *30*:2,033, 1977.
147. Iimura, O., Kijima, T., Kikuchi, K., et al.: Clin. Sci. *61*:77s–80s, 1981.
148. MacGregor, G.A., Smith, S.J., Markandon, N.D.: Lancet *2*:567–570, 1982.
149. McQuarrie, I., Thompson, W.H., Anderson, J.A.: J. Nutr. *11*:77–101, 1936.
150. Tobian, L.: Am. J. Clin. Nutr. *32*:2,739, 1979.
151. Meneely, G.R., Battarbee, H.D.: Am. J. Cardiol. *38*:768–785, 1976.
152. Holly, J.M., Goodwin, F.J., Evans, S.J.W., et al.: Lancet *2*:1,384–1,387, 1981.
153. Altschul, A.M., Grommet, J.K.: Nutr. Rev. *38*:393, 1980.
154. Priddle, W.W.: Can. Med. Assoc. J. *86*:1–9, 1962.
155. Meneely, G.R., Ball, C.O.T.: Am. J. Med. *25*:713–725, 1958.
156. Skrabal, F., Aubock, J., Hortnagl, H., et al.: Clin. Sci. Molec. Med. *59*:157s–160s, 1957.
157. Fisher, E.R., Funckes, A.J.: Lab. Invest. *16*:539, 1967.
158. Rosenman, R.H., Freed, S.C., Friedman, M.: Proc. Soc. Exp. Biol. Med. *78*:77–79, 1951.
159. Freed, S.C., Friedman, M.: Science *112*:788–789, 1950.
160. Linas, S.L., Dickmann, D.: Kidney Int. *21*:757–764, 1982.
161. Freed, S.C., Friedman, M.: Proc. Soc. Exp. Biol. Med. *78*:74–77, 1951.
162. St. George, S.M., Freed, S.C., Rosenman, R.H.: Circulation *6*:371–372, 1952.
163. Abbrecht, P.H.: Am. J. Physiol. *223*:555–560, 1972.
164. Bahler, R.C., Ralcita, L.: Am. Heart J. *81*:650–657, 1971.
165. Keith, N.M., Binger, M.W.: JAMA *105*:1,584, 1935.
166. Brunner, H.R., Baer, L., Sealey, J.E.: J. Clin. Invest. *49*:2,128, 1970.
167. Baner, J.H., Gaunter, W.: Kidney Int. *15*:286, 1979.
168. Basset, S., Elden, C.A., McCann, W.S.: J. Nutr. *5*:1–27, 1932.
169. Wilks, S., Taylor, A.S.: Guy's Hosp. Rep. *9*:173–179, 1963.
170. Tannen, R.L., Wedell, E., Moore, R.: J. Clin. Invest. *52*:2,089–2,101, 1973.
171. Schneider, E.G., Lynch, R.E., Willis, L.R.: Kidney Int. *2*:197–202, 1972.
172. Stokes, J.B.: J. Clin. Invest. *70*:219–229, 1982.
173. Cardinal, J., Duchesneau, D.: Am. J. Physiol. *234*:F381–F385, 1978.
174. Lonis, W.J., Tabei, R., Spector, S.: Lancet *2*:1,283–1,286, 1971.
175. Haddy, F.J.: Life Sci. *16*:1,489–1,498, 1975.
176. Webb, R.C., Bohr, D.F.: Blood Vessels *16*:71–79, 1979.
177. Brace, R.A.: Proc. Soc. Exp. Biol. Med. *145*:1,389, 1974.
178. Stephens, G.A., Davis, J.O., Freeman, R.H., et al.: Am. J. Physiol. *234*:F10–F15, 1978.
179. Dluhy, R.G., Greenfield, M., Williams, G.H.: J. Clin. Endocrinol. Metab. *45*:141–146, 1977.
180. Douglas, J., Hansen, J., Catt, K.J.: Endocrinology *103*:60–65, 1978.
181. Flamenbaum, W., Kleinman, J.G., McNeil, J.S., et al.: Am. J. Physiol. *229*:370, 1975.
182. Kirchner, K.A., Mueller, R.: Am. J. Physiol. *242*:F463–469, 1982.
183. Treasure, J., Work, J., Palmer C., et al.: Hypertension *5*:521, 1983.
184. Kotchen, T.A., Galla, G.G., Luke, R.G.: Am. J. Clin. Nutr. *231*:1,050, 1976.
185. Ackley, S., Barrett-Connor, E., Suarez, L.: Am. J. Clin. Nutr. *38*:457–461, 1983.
186. McCarron, D.A., Cole, C., Morris, C.: Clin. Res. *29*:267a, 1981.
187. Belizan, J.M., Villar, J., Pineda, O., et al.: JAMA *249*:1,161–1,165, 1983.
188. Ayachi, S.: Metabolism *28*:1,234–1,238, 1979.
189. McCarron, D.A., Yung, N.N., Ugoretz, B.A., et al.: Hypertension *3*:I162–I167, 1981.
190. Popvitzer, M.M., Subryan, V.L., Alfrey, A.C., et al.: J. Clin. Invest. *55*:1,295, 1975.
191. Lee, C.O., Vassalle, M.: Am. J. Physiol. *244*:C110–C116, 1983.
192. Hurwitz, L., McGuffer, L.J., Smith, P.M., et al.: J. Pharmacol. Exp. Ther. *220*:382–388, 1982.
193. Rasmussen, H.: Ann. Intern. Med. *98*:809–816, 1983.
194. Rasmussen, H.: Science *170*:404, 1970.
195. Marone, C., Beretta-Piccoli, C., Weidmann, P.: Kidney Int. *20*:92, 1981.
196. Rasmussen, H.: Ann. N.Y. Acad. Sci. *356*:346, 1980.

197. Sowers, J.R., Barrett, J.D.: Am. J. Physiol. *242*:E–3230, 1982.

198. Blackfan, K.D., Hamilton, B.: Boston Med. Surg. J. *193*:617, 1925.

199. Petersen, B., Schrell, M., Christiansen, C., et al.: Acta Med. Scand. *201*:31, 1977.

200. Whang, R., Chrysant, S., Dillard, B., et al.: J. Am. Coll. Nutr. *1*:317, 1982.

201. Dyckner, T., Wester, P.O.: Br. Med. J. *286*:1,847, 1983.

202. Burch, G.E., Giles, T.D.: Am. Heart J. *94*:649, 1977.

203. Haddy, F.J., and Seelig, M.S.: *In* Magnesium in Health and Disease. Edited by M. Cantin, and M.S. Seelig. New York, Spectrum, 1980.

204. Ohhashi, T., Azuma, T.: Am. J. Physiol. *242*:C–25, 1982.

205. Altura, B.M., Altura, B.T.: Fed. Proc. *40*:2,672, 1981.

206. Resnick, L.M., Laragh, J.H., Sealey, J.E., et al.: N. Engl. J. Med. *15*:888–891, 1983.

207. Ljunghall, S., Hedstrand, H.: Br. Med. J. *1*:533, 1977.

208. Saltman, P.: Ann. Intern. Med. *98*:823–827, 1983.

209. Woods, K.L., Beevers, D.G., West, M.: Br. Med. J. *282*:1,186–1,188, 1981.

210. Saltman, P.: Ann. Intern. Med. *98*:823, 1983.

211. Kopp, S.J., Glonek, T., Perry, H.M., Jr., et al.: Science *217*:837–839, 1982.

212. Perry, H.M., Jr., Erlanger, M., Perry, E.F.: Am. J. Physiol. *232*:H114–H121, 1977.

213. Fehily, A.M., Milbank, J.E., Yarnell, J.W., et al.: Am. J. Clin. Nutr. *36*:890–896, 1982.

214. Kopp, S.J., Perry, H.M., Jr., Perry, E.F., et al.: Toxicol. Appl. Pharmacol. *69*:149–160, 1983.

215. Moreau, T., Orssaud, G., Lellouch, J., et al.: Arch. Environ. Health. *38*:163–167, 1983.

216. Perry, H.M., Jr., Kopp, S.J.: Sci. Total Environ. *26*:223–232, 1983.

217. Ohanian, E.V., Iwai, J.: Environ. Health Perspect. *28*:261–266, 1979.

218. Aviv, A., John, E., Bernstein, J., et al.: Kidney Int. *17*:430–437, 1980.

219. Lilis, R., Gavrilescu, N., Nestorescu, B., et al.: Br. J. Ind. Med. *25*:196–202, 1968.

220. Underwood, E.J.: Trace Elements in Human and Animal Nutrition, 4th Ed. New York, Academic Press, 1977.

221. Aviv, A., John, E., Bernstein, J., et al.: Kidney Int. *17*:430–437, 1980.

222. Friedlander, M.A., Brooks, C.T., Sheehe, P.R.: Arch. Environ. Health. *36*:310–315, 1981.

223. Sparrow, D., Sharrett, A.R., Garvey, A.J., et al.: J. Chronic. Dis. *37*:59–65, 1984.

224. Frithz, G., Ronquist, G.: Acta Med. Scand. *205*:647–649, 1979.

225. Beauchamp, G.K., Bertino, M., Engelman, K.: Ann. Intern. Med. *98*:763, 1983.

226. Cherry, F.F., Bennett, E.A., Bazzano, G.S.: Am. J. Clin. Nutr. *34*:2,367–2,375, 1981.

227. Reyes, A.J., Olhaberry, J.V., Leary, W.P., et al.: S. Afr. Med. J. *64*:936–941, 1983.

228. Steffen, R.P., Pamnani, M.B., Clough, D.L., et al.: Hypertension *3*:I173–I178, 1981.

229. Bochard, U., Greeff, K., Hafner, D., et al.: J. Cardiovasc. Pharmacol. *3*:510–521, 1981.

230. Carmignani, M., Boscolo, P., Iannaccone, A.: Br. J. Ind. Med. *40*:280–284, 1983.

231. Koller, A., Rubanyi, G., Ligeti, L., et al.: Acta Physiol. Acad. Sci. Hung. *59*:287–290, 1982.

232. DeHaven, J., Sherwin, R., Hendler, R., et al.: N. Engl. J. Med. *302*:477–482, 1980.

233. Iacono, J.M., Puska, P., Dougherty, R.M.: Am. J. Clin. Nutr. *38*:860–869, 1983.

234. Iacono, J.M., Dougherty, R.M., Puska, P.: Hypertension *4*:III34–III42, 1982.

235. Iacono, J.M., Marshall, M.W., Dougherty, R.M., et al.: Prev. Med. *4*:426, 1975.

236. Judd, J.T., Marshall, M.W., Canary, J.J.: Changes in blood pressure and blood lipids of adult men consuming modified fat diets. *In* Proceedings of the Beltsville Symposia in Agricultural Research. Vol. IV. Edited by G.R. Beecher, Montclair, New Jersey, Osmun and Company, 1981.

237. Iacono, J.M., Dougherty, R.M.: Prev. Med. *12*:60–69, 1983.

238. Puska, P., Iacono, J.M., Nissinen, A., et al.: Lancet 1–5, 1983.

239. Hoffman, P., Taube, C., Ponicke, K., et al.: Acta Biol. Med. Ger. *37*:5–6, 1978.

240. Sprecher, H.: Biosynthesis of polyunsaturated fatty acids and its regulation. *In* Polyunsaturated Fatty Acids. Edited by W.H. Kunau and R.T. Holman. Champaign, Illinois, American Oil Chemists' Society, 1977.

241. McGiff, J.C.: Prostaglandins as regulators of blood pressure. *In* Hypertension: Mechanism, Diagnosis and Management. Edited by J.O. Laragh, J.H. Davis, and A. Selwyn. New York, HP Publishing Co., 1977.

242. Camberg, H.-U., Heyden, S., Hames, C.E., et al.: Prostaglandins *15*:193–197, 1978.

243. Scherhag, R., Kramer, H.J., Dusing, R.: Prostaglandins *23*:369–382, 1982.

244. Rebello, T., Hodges, R.E., Smith, J.L.: Am. J. Clin. Nutr. *38*:84–94, 1983.

245. Young, J.B., Landsberg, L.: Metabolism *30*:421–424, 1981.

246. Jung, R.T., Shetty, P.S., Barrand, M, et al.: Br. Med. J. *1*:12–13, 1979.

247. Bloom, W.L., Azar, G.J.: Arch. Intern. Med. *112*:333–337, 1963.

248. Defronzo, R.A.: Diabetologia *21*:165–171, 1981.

249. Pullman, T.N., Lavender, A.R., Aho, I.: Metabolism *16*:358–373, 1967.

250. Besarab, A., Silva, P., Landsberg, L., et al.: Am. J. Physiol. *233*:F39—F45, 1977.

251. Young, J.B., Landsberg, L.: Nature *269*:615–617, 1977.

252. Welle, S., Lilavivathana, U., Campbell, R.G.: J. Clin. Endocr. Metab. *29*:806–809, 1980.

253. Landsberg, L., Young, J.B.: N. Engl. J. Med. *298*:1,295, 1978.

254. Prenss, H.G., Fournier, R.D.: Life Sci. *30*:879–886, 1982.

255. Sacks, F.M., Donner, A., Castelli, W.P., et al.: JAMA *246*:640–644, 1981.

256. Elias, J.W., Villescas, R., Palet, J.L., et al.: Exp. Aging Res. *4*:535–541, 1978.

257. Moreland, R.S., Webb, R.C., Bohr, D.F.: Hypertension *4*:III99–III107, 1982.

258. Armstrong, B., Clarke, H., Martin, C., et al.: Am. J. Clin. Nutr. *32*:2,472–2,476, 1979.

259. O'Hare, J.A., Young, J.B., Landsberg, L.: Clin. Res. *32*:1984.

260. Young, J.B., Kaufman, L.N., Saville, M.E., et al.: Increased sympathetic nervous system activity in rats fed a low-protein diet. Am. J. Physiol. *248*:R627–R637, 1985.

261. Sved, A.F., Goldberg, I.M., Fernstrom, J.D.: J. Pharmacol. Exp. Ther. *214*:147–151, 1980.
262. Sved, A.F., Fernstrom, J.D., Wurtman, R.J.: Proc. Natl. Acad. Sci. U.S.A. *76*:3,511–3,514, 1979.
263. Bresnahan, M.R., Hatzinikolaou, P., Brunner, H.R., et al.: Am. J. Physiol. *239*:H206–H211, 1980.
264. Pace-Asciak, C.R., Carrara, M.D.: Experientia *35*:1,561–1,562, 1979.
265. Igarshi, T., Nakajima, Y., Kobayashi, M., et al.: *25*:159–173, 1979.
266. Bendich, A., Gabriel, E., Machlin, L.J.: Proc. Soc. Exp. Biol. Med. *172*:297–300, 1983.
267. Kokot, F., Pietrek, J., Srokowska, S., et al.: Clin. Nephrol. *16*:188–192, 1981.
268. Anderson, J.W.: Ann. Intern. Med. *98*:842–846, 1983.
269. Kelsay, J.L., Behall, K.M., Prather, E.S.: Am. J. Clin. Nutr. *31*:1,149–1,153, 1978.
270. Armstrong, B., Van Merwyk, A.J., Coates, H.: Am. J. Epidemiol. *105*:444–449, 1977.
271. Burstyn, P.G., Husbands, D.R.: Cardiovasc. Res. *14*:185–191, 1980.
272. Anderson, J.W.: Dietary fiber and diabetes. *In* Medical Aspects of Dietary Fiber. Edited by G.A. Spiller and R.M. Kay. New York, Plenum Press, 1980.
273. Klatsky, A.L., Friedman, G.D., Siegelaub, M.S., et al.: N. Engl. J. Med. *296*:1,194–2,000, 1977.
274. Cairns, V., Keil, U., Kleinbaum, D., et al.: Hypertension *6*:124–131, 1984.
275. Knochel, J.P.: Ann. Intern. Med. *98*:849–854, 1983.
276. Friedman, G.D., Klatsky, A.L., Siegelaub, A.B.: Hypertension *4*:III143–III150, 1982.
277. Barboriak, P.N., Anderson, A.J., Hoffmann, R.G., et al.: Alcoholism *6*:234–238, 1982.
278. Wallace, R.B., Lynch, C.F., Pomrehn, P.R., et al.: Circulation *64*:III41–III47, 1981.
279. Ashley, M.J., Rankin, J.G.: Aust. N.Z. J. Med. *9*:201–206, 1979.
280. Ramsay, L.E.: Scott. Med. J. *27*:207–211, 1982.
281. Wallace, R.B., Barrett-Connor, E., Criqui, M., et al.: J. Chronic Dis. *35*:251–257, 1982.
282. Kagan, A., Yano, K., Rhoads, G.G., et al.: Circulation *64*:III27, 1981.
283. Klatsky, A.L., Friedman, G.D., Siegelaub, A.B.: Ann. Intern. Med. *81*:294, 1974.
284. Barboriak, J.J., Rimm, A.A., Anderson, A.J., et al.: Br. Heart J. *39*:239, 1977.
285. Klatsky, A.L., Friedman, G.D., Siegelaub, A.B.: Alcoholism *3*:33–39, 1979.
286. Saunders, J.B., Beevers, D.G., Paton, A.: Clin. Exp. Pharmacol. Physiol. *8*:451–454, 1981
287. Arkwright, P.D., Beilin, L.J., Rouse, I., et al.: Circulation *66*:60–66, 1982.
288. Criqui, M.H., Wallace, R.B., Mishkel, M., et al.: Hypertension *3*:557–565, 1981.
289. Turlapaty, P.V., Altura, B.M.: Science *208*:198–200, 1980.
290. Saunders, J.B., Beevers, D.G., Paton, A.: Clin. Sci. *57(Suppl.)*:295s–298s, 1979.
291. Altura, B.M., Ogunkoya, A., Gebrewold, A., et al.: J. Cardiovasc. Pharmacol. *1*:97–113, 1979.
292. Arkwright, P.D., Beilin, L.J., Vandongen, R., et al.: Circulation *66*:515–519, 1982.
293. Freestone, S., Ramsay, L.E.: Am. J. Med. *73*:348–353, 1982.
294. Smits, P., Hoffmann, H., Thien, T., et al.: Clin. Pharmacol. Ther. *34*:153–158, 1983.
295. Robertson, D., Frolich, J.C., Carr, R.K., et al.: N. Engl. J. Med. *298*:181–186, 1978.
296. Lang, T., Degoulet, P., Aime, F., et al.: Am. J. Cardiol. *52*:1,238–1,242, 1938.
297. Lang, T., Bureau, J.F., Degoulet, P., et al.: Eur. Heart J. *4*:602–607, 1983.
298. Izzo, J.L., Jr., Ghosal, A., Kwong, T., et al.: Am. J. Cardiol. *52*:769–773, 1983.
299. Robertson, D., Wade, D., Workman, R., et al.: J. Clin. Invest. *67*:1,111–1,117, 1981.
300. Ammon, H.P., Bieck, P.R., Mandalaz, D., et al.: Br. J. Clin. Pharmacol. *15*:701–706, 1983.

*Chapter* **60**

# NUTRITION AND DIET IN RELATION TO HYPERLIPIDEMIA AND ATHEROSCLEROSIS

Edwin L. Bierman and Alan Chait

## ATHEROSCLEROSIS

Atherosclerosis, a disorder of the larger arteries that underlies most coronary artery disease, aortic aneurysm, arterial disease of the lower extremities, and cerebrovascular disease, is responsible for the majority of deaths in the United States and most industrialized societies. It is characterized by accumulation of lipids (primarily cholesterol esters) in cells (smooth muscle cells and macrophages) and extracellular tissues of the inner lining of the walls of medium and large arteries.

Atherosclerosis is by far the leading cause of death in the United States in all persons above age 45 and in males after age 35. About 5 million Americans have clinically manifest coronary artery disease (CAD). Subclinical coronary artery atherosclerosis is likely to be more prevalent and may affect the majority of adult Americans, because a high prevalence in males in their second and third decades has been documented from autopsies of war casualties in Korea and Vietnam. Premature deaths from CAD, arbitrarily defined as appearing before age 65, occur predominantly in men, and a third of all deaths from CAD in males occur before age 65. In fact, nearly all the excess premature mortality in American males is due to CAD. Between the ages of 35 and 55, the death rate is five times higher in white men than in white women in the United States. The exceptions are women with hypertension, diabetes, hyperlipidemia, or premature menopause who are at increased risk and often share the risk of the male. Both sexes have more than a fivefold increase in the average annual incidence of myocardial infarction between ages 40 and 60.[1]

### International Comparisons

There are marked differences in premature death rates from CAD among most industrialized countries. The eight having the highest rates in males between 35 and 74 years of age are Finland, the United States, Scotland, Northern Ireland, Ireland, Australia, New Zealand, and England (Fig. 60–1).[2] Much lower age-adjusted death rates from CAD are found in some European countries, especially in Eastern Europe, and in Japan. The rates in Japan are about one fifth of those in the United

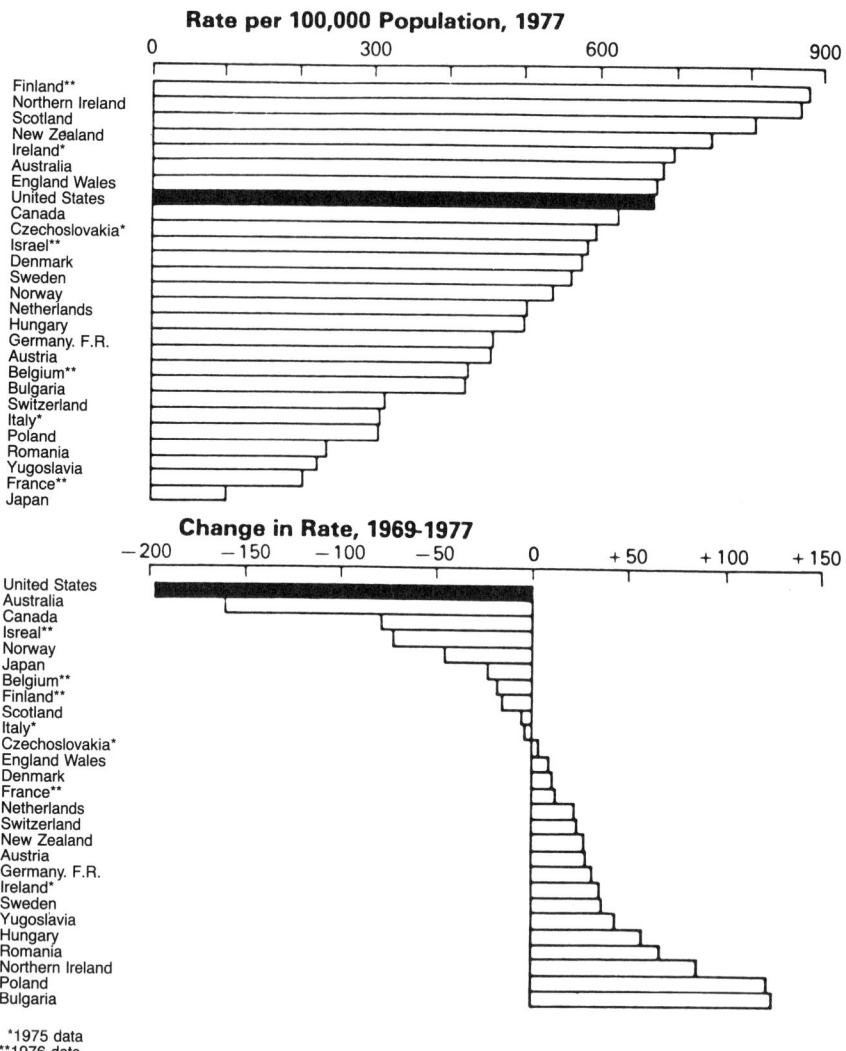

**Fig. 60–1.** Death rates from coronary heart disease by country in 35- to 74-year-old males. (From Levy, R.I.: Arteriosclerosis *1*:312, 1981.)

States. Subsamples obtained in many countries convey the strong impression that upper socio-economic classes that have adopted the culture and diet of Western industrialized countries have far more CAD than lower socioeconomic classes. Among the most obvious differences between these classes are total calories, fat content of the diet, and amount of physical work. Extensive epidemiologic studies have not revealed the reasons for differences between cultures that are superficially similar, suggesting that genetic factors play a role. However, migrants to the United States tend to have a higher risk of death from premature CAD than age-matched relatives who remain at home. A classic example is the Japanese migrants to the United States who have rapidly assumed the atherosclerosis risk of the American popula-

tion. Japanese migrants to Hawaii have a risk intermediate between those in Japan and those on the United States mainland. Although there are many instances in which different ethnic groups in the same locality have widely differing prevalences of CAD, the available evidence suggests that cultural and environmental factors including diet may be at least as important as genetic determination of CAD. Nevertheless, genetic heterogeneity probably underlies many of the striking differences in susceptibility seen among individuals sharing the same ethnic and cultural setting.

### Risk Factors

A number of conditions and habits are present more frequently in individuals who develop atherosclerosis than in the general population; these

**Table 60–1. Risk Factors for Atherosclerosis**

A. Not reversible
   Aging
   Male sex
   Genetic traits: positive family history of premature atherosclerosis

B. Potentially reversible
   Cigarette smoking
   *Hypertension
   *Obesity
   *Hyperlipidemia: hypercholesterolemia and/or hypertriglyceridemia
   *Hyperglycemia and diabetes mellitus
   *Low levels of high-density lipoprotein (HDL)

C. Other possible factors
   Physical inactivity
   Body build
   Emotional stress
   Personality type

*Risk factors that can be influenced by diet.

factors have been termed *risk factors*. Most people below age 65 afflicted with atherosclerosis have one or more identifiable risk factors other than aging per se (Table 60–1). The risk factor concept implies that a person with at least one risk factor is more likely to develop a clinical atherosclerotic event and to do so earlier than a person with no risk factors. The presence of multiple risk factors further accelerates the development of atherosclerosis. Risk factors vary in terms of importance in the population of the United States. There is general agreement from an epidemiologic perspective that hypercholesterolemia, hypertension, and cigarette smoking may be the most potent factors involved in causation of atherosclerosis. Risk factors also vary in terms of their potential reversibility with current techniques of preventive management.

**Reversibility.** Thus age, sex, and genetics are currently considered to be irreversible risk factors. Continually emerging evidence suggests that elimination of cigarette smoking and treatment of hypertension reverse the high risk for atherosclerosis attributable to those factors. Life insurance policyholder data suggest that reduction of marked obesity reduces total mortality, presumably by diminishing the sequelae of atherosclerosis. Although other risk factors including hyperglycemia and the various forms of hyperlipidemia are potentially reversible, the impact of treatment of diabetes or hyperlipidemia is not known. However, the data from the Lipid Research Clinics' coronary primary prevention trial indicate that hypercholesterolemia should be added to the list of reversible risk factors.[3] Other possible risk factors include physical inactivity, body build, emotional stress, and body type. Little is known regarding their potential reversibility.

**Interrelations Among Risk Factors.** These risk factors (see Table 60–1) clearly interact. For example, obesity appears to be causally associated with hypertension, hyperglycemia, hypercholesterolemia, and hypertriglyceridemia. Genetic factors may play a role by exerting direct effects on arterial wall cell structure and metabolism, or they may act indirectly via hypertension, hyperlipidemia, diabetes, and obesity. Furthermore, evidence suggests that the inheritance of several risk factors (e.g., diabetes and obesity) may be genetically linked.[4] Aging appears to be one of the more complex mechanisms associated with the development of atherosclerosis, because many of the risk factors in themselves are related to age (e.g., elevated blood pressure, hyperglycemia, and hyperlipidemia). Thus, in addition to the possible involvement of intrinsic aging in atherogenesis (perhaps through effects on arterial wall metabolism), a variety of associated metabolic factors are also age-dependent.[5]

### Role of Diet

Nutritional influences also underlie many of these risk factors. For example, hypertension, obesity, diabetes mellitus, hypercholesterolemia, hypertriglyceridemia, and decreased high-density lipoprotein (HDL) levels all may be strongly influenced by diet.

Hypertension appears to result from an interaction between genetic and environmental influences. Dietary sodium and perhaps potassium and calcium appear to modulate the expression of hypertension in genetically susceptible individuals. Obesity and weight gain can adversely affect blood pressure and hyperlipidemia, and are important in the clinical expression of disease in subjects with a genetic predisposition to noninsulin-dependent diabetes. Dietary cholesterol content and the nature of dietary fat can profoundly influence plasma lipid levels in hyperlipidemic individuals, as discussed subsequently.

Many of these risk factors respond favorably to dietary interventions. Dietary sodium restriction results in normalization of blood pressure in some salt-sensitive hypertensive individuals. Weight loss and maintenance of lowered body weight are associated with reversal of several risk factors, such as blood pressure reduction, lowering of elevated plasma glucose, cholesterol, and triglyceride levels, and elevation of HDL cholesterol. The direct impact of reversal of risk factors on mortality and CAD is, in some instances, now clear. As emphasized in this chapter, elevated plasma lipid levels also respond to therapeutic diets and, in many instances, normal levels can be achieved by dietary intervention alone.

## HYPERLIPIDEMIA

Hyperlipidemia consists of increased plasma levels of cholesterol and/or triglycerides, the major lipid components of lipoprotein particles in the circulation. Elevated plasma lipid levels result from one or more abnormalities of lipid metabolism or transport. Both *hypercholesterolemia* and *hypertriglyceridemia* appear to be important risk factors for the development of atherosclerosis.

### Definition and Normal Values

Although there is no absolute quantitative definition of hyperlipidemia, statistical definitions, based on the upper 5% of the distribution of plasma lipid levels within a population, are widely used. Such definitions are likely to detect affected individuals from families with one of the familial hyperlipidemias or hyperlipidemia secondary to other diseases or drugs. They also are useful for detection of individuals susceptible to premature atherosclerosis in whom preventive measures should be instituted. However, these statistical upper limits of "normality" are far above those plasma lipid levels associated with increasing risk of CAD in whole populations because an exponential gradient of risk is associated with increasing cholesterol levels (Fig. 60–2).

From a biologic standpoint, normal values could be regarded as those above which the risk of developing atherosclerosis is increased. Correlations between the cholesterol concentrations in young men in the United States and the incidence of premature CAD indicate that an increasing risk can be detected when the cholesterol level is higher than 200 mg/dl, a value close to the mean for men from 40 to 49 years of age in this population, and rises sharply above 260 mg/dl.[6] Thus normolipidemia, as defined statistically, does not imply freedom from an increased risk of atherosclerosis consequent to high lipid levels. Because populations vary, the selection of arbitrary limits of normality that can be usefully applied to all populations is meaningless. Plasma lipid levels vary with age and sex (Table 60–2), making the definition of disease somewhat arbitrary. From a practical standpoint, age- and sex-stratified statistical definitions of normality can be used such that values above the ninety-fifth percentile of that stratum are defined as hyperlipidemia. Genetic forms of hyperlipidemia associated with a markedly increased atherosclerosis risk (Table 60–3) often raise lipid levels above the ninety-ninth percentile for age and sex.

Adiposity may play a key role in the age-associated rise in triglyceride and cholesterol levels because the increases in triglyceride, cholesterol, and body weight with age in whole populations occur concurrently.[7] In primitive people who remain thin throughout adulthood, plasma lipids do not increase with age.[8] Metabolic mechanisms have been postulated whereby obesity, which is associated with insulin resistance of peripheral tissues and compensatory hyperinsulinemia, promotes enhanced production of triglyceride- and cholesterol-rich lipoproteins by the liver.[9] Current concepts of plasma lipoprotein transport suggest that accumulation of cholesterol in the circulation may in part be secondary to excessive production of triglyceride-rich lipoproteins.

### Lipoproteins

The increases in cholesterol are associated mainly with a rise in low-density lipoprotein (LDL) concentration, and the increases in triglyceride with a rise in very low-density lipoprotein (VLDL). Five main lipoprotein classes can be separated by ultracentrifugation or electrophoresis. Nomenclature is based on these two procedures. The predominantly triglyceride-rich lipoproteins are chylomicrons, which transport dietary (exogenous) triglyceride, and VLDL, which transports endogenous triglycerides. Both transport triglycerides to the tissues for energy utilization or storage. Remnant lipoproteins are formed during the catabolism of the triglyceride-rich lipoproteins; the intermediate-density lipoprotein (IDL) class consists largely of these remnant particles. The two predominantly cholesterol-containing lipoproteins are LDL and HDL. LDL transports cholesterol to tissues for use for membrane synthesis or steroid hormone formation. HDL appears to transport cholesterol from peripheral tissues back to liver, either directly or through intermediary lower-density lipoproteins; this process has been termed reverse cholesterol transport. Because a low HDL cholesterol level is an independent risk

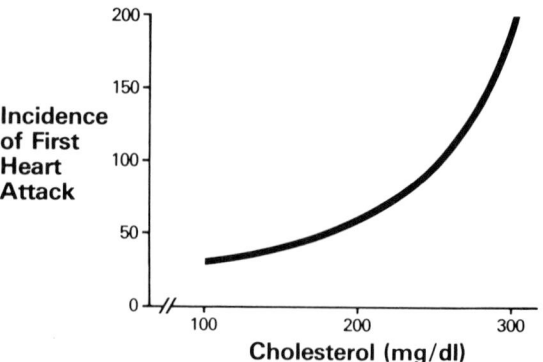

**Fig. 60–2.** Risk of coronary heart disease as a function of serum cholesterol. (Data from Dawber, T.R.[6])

**Table 60–2.** **Mean and Upper Ninety-Fifth Percentile Values for Fasting Plasma Cholesterol and Triglyceride Levels***

| Age (yrs.) | Cholesterol | | Triglyceride | |
|---|---|---|---|---|
| | (mg/dl) | | | |
| | Mean | 95th Percentile | Mean | 95th Percentile |
| Males | | | | |
| 0–9 | 160 | 200 | 55 | 100 |
| 10–19 | 155 | 200 | 70 | 140 |
| 20–29 | 175 | 230 | 110 | 225 |
| 30–39 | 195 | 260 | 135 | 290 |
| 40–49 | 210 | 270 | 150 | 320 |
| 50–59 | 215 | 275 | 145 | 305 |
| 60–69 | 215 | 275 | 140 | 280 |
| 70+ | 205 | 270 | 130 | 260 |
| Females | | | | |
| 0–9 | 160 | 200 | 60 | 110 |
| 10–19 | 160 | 200 | 75 | 130 |
| 20–29 | 165 | 220 | 75 | 140 |
| 30–39 | 180 | 235 | 85 | 160 |
| 40–49 | 200 | 260 | 100 | 200 |
| 50–59 | 225 | 295 | 120 | 250 |
| 60–69 | 230 | 300 | 130 | 240 |
| 70+ | 230 | 290 | 130 | 235 |

*From data derived from cross-sectional plasma lipid distributions among 48,431 white participants in Visit 1 of the Lipid Research Clinics Prevalence Study of 11 North American populations (The Lipid Research Clinics Program Data Book: Selected Variables in 11 North American Populations. Vol. I. Physiologic and Sociodemographic Characteristics, 1979). Ninety-fifth percentile values approximate + 2 standard deviations above the mean for cholesterol. Because triglyceride levels are not normally distributed, mean values will be higher than median values. Data for females are restricted to those not taking estrogen-containing drugs because females taking sex hormones have altered plasma lipid levels.

factor for CAD (see Table 60–1), its measurement may guide a physician to be more or less aggressive in the management of hypercholesterolemia. The ratio of LDL to HDL cholesterol has been used by some as an index of CAD risk; however, caution is necessary since many laboratories cannot measure HDL cholesterol accurately, and levels are always low in hypertriglycemia regardless of risk.

## Hyperlipidemia and Coronary Artery Disease

**Hypercholesterolemia.** Hypercholesterolemia is associated unequivocally with increased incidence of premature CAD; however, its importance varies in relation to age. In the Framingham study, cholesterol levels in males below age 40 were closely related to the future development of CAD; this relation was much less pronounced in older individuals.[6] For both sexes combined, the relative incidence of myocardial infarction in individuals between the ages of 30 and 49 with cholesterol levels greater than 260 mg/dl was three to five times that for individuals with cholesterol levels less than 220. These data are supported by comparisons of the prevalence of CAD and cholesterol (or LDL) in many other populations.[1]

**Hypertriglyceridemia.** There is a significant relationship of triglycerides and VLDL to CAD; however, this association is confounded by a rise in

cholesterol as VLDL increases. Nevertheless, in several but not all population studies, increased triglycerides (or VLDL) are independently correlated with premature CAD.[10] Hypertriglyceridemia may be associated with premature atherosclerosis in some specific disorders; this association may be masked in studies of whole populations. Patients with high VLDL who come from families with familial combined hyperlipidemia (see Table 60–3) appear to be at the same increased risk as those affected members of these families with elevated LDL levels.[11] In contrast, patients with comparably elevated VLDL levels who come from families with pure monogenic familial hypertriglyceridemia do not appear to have an increased risk. In addition, high VLDL levels may increase the risk for premature atherosclerosis in patients with other risk factors for coronary artery disease, such as diabetes, and in patients on chronic hemodialysis who smoke and are hypertensive. Individuals in whom remnant lipoproteins accumulate, with resulting elevations in both cholesterol and triglycerides, also seem to be at risk for early development of atherosclerosis.[12]

## Genetic Forms of Hyperlipidemia

Some of these relationships were clarified in a comprehensive study in Seattle of the role of the

**Table 60–3.   Genetic Hyperlipoproteinemias**

| Disorder | Plasma Lipoprotein Pattern | Genetic Mechanism | Estimated Frequency | Expression in Children | Premature Atherosclerosis |
|---|---|---|---|---|---|
| Familial hypercholesterolemia (monogenic) | II-A, II-B | Autosomal dominant | Common (1/500) | Yes | Yes |
| Familial hypercholesterolemia (polygenic) | II-A, II-B | Polygenic | — | — | Probable |
| Familial hypertriglyceridemia | IV, V | Autosomal dominant | Very common | Rare | Possible |
| Familial combined hyperlipidemia | II-A, II-B, IV, V | Autosomal dominant | Very common | Rare | Yes |
| "Broad-beta" disease | III | Mixed | Rare | Rare | Yes |
| Lipoprotein lipase deficiency | I, V | Autosomal recessive | Very rare | Yes | No |

genetics of hyperlipidemia in clinical atherosclerosis in which 500 consecutive survivors of myocardial infarction were tested.[13] Hyperlipidemia was present in about one third of the group. Approximately one half of the males and two thirds of the females below the age of 50 had either hypertriglyceridemia, hypercholesterolemia, or both. On the other hand, in individuals over the age of 70 the prevalence of atherosclerotic coronary disease was high, yet virtually no males (and only about one fourth of the females) had hyperlipidemia. Thus, in both sexes there appeared to be a progressive decline with age in the association of hyperlipidemia with myocardial infarction. More than half of the hyperlipidemic atherosclerotic survivors appeared to have simple monogenic familial disorders inherited as an autosomal dominant trait (familial combined hyperlipidemia, familial hypertriglyceridemia, and familial hypercholesterolemia, in descending order of frequency)[14] (see Table 60–3). These simply inherited hyperlipidemias (particularly hypercholesterolemia) were more frequent in myocardial infarction survivors below the age of 60 than in those who were older. In contrast, nonmonogenic forms of hyperlipidemia occurred with equal frequency in patients above and below age 60.

Thus, it appears that genes associated with the simply inherited hyperlipidemias accelerate changes seen with age, leading to manifestations of atherosclerotic complications at an earlier age than usual. All studies indicate that hyperlipidemia is a more meaningful risk factor in patients below the age of 50 and that it operates independently of, and in addition to, hypertension, diabetes, obesity, and other factors. For men and women over the age of 65, there is no evidence of a correlation between hyperlipidemia and atherosclerosis or its complications.

## Classification

The primary forms of hyperlipidemia, i.e., those forms in which known factors (other diseases or drugs) do not have a causative role, are usually divided into two categories: "familial," in which clear evidence of a genetic predisposition is based on the presence of the disorder in closely related family members, and "sporadic," in which neither known genetic nor known secondary factors play a role. Differentiation between primary and secondary hyperlipidemia is important because the secondary hyperlipidemias (Table 60–4) may be corrected simply by withdrawal of the inciting drug or, when possible, by treatment of the causative disease. Secondary hyperlipidemias, therefore, do not require specific dietary therapy.

Hyperlipidemia has been classified into six types (I, IIA, IIB, III, IV, and V) based on the specific electrophoretic patterns of the various lipoproteins in plasma.[15] In the past, approaches to dietary management of hyperlipidemia have been based on this physicochemical classification. However, these types or patterns are not specific because they do not reflect specific pathophysiologic mechanisms or genetic abnormalities responsible for the disorders. Furthermore, the plasma lipoprotein pattern can change over time in any individual, in part owing to effects of dietary changes and other metabolic influences on lipoprotein transport. Thus, a single lipoprotein pattern can reflect different diseases. Conversely, a single disease mechanism can lead to a variety of patterns (e.g., types IIA, IIB, IV, and V patterns can all occur in familial combined hyperlipidemia). Hyperlipidemia can be classified according to pathophysiologic characteristics[16] (see Table 60–4) as well as by genetic characteristics[17] (see Table 60–3). Diagnostic and therapeutic approaches can be profitably focused further as pathophysiologic mechanisms and molecular defects responsible for hyperlipidemia continue to be defined.

## TREATMENT OF HYPERLIPIDEMIA

A diet remains the first approach to therapy in most patients with hyperlipidemia. These patients still at high risk are then candidates for drugs.

### Goals

Goals of therapy include prevention of episodes of acute pancreatitis, which are associated with marked hypertriglyceridemia and the accumulation of chylomicrons in plasma ("chylomicronemia syndrome"), a condition that can be life-threatening. The major goal of treatment for most individuals is reduction of the risk for atherosclerosis, particularly when the increased risk is associated with plasma lipid abnormalities. Lipid lowering therapy may also help reduce atherosclerosis risk primarily due to other disorders such as diabetes mellitus or hypertension by reducing the compounding effects of multiple risk factors.

### Reversal of Atherosclerosis

Direct proof is still lacking that reduction of hyperlipidemia by diet results in a decrease in progression of atherosclerosis in humans. It has been demonstrated directly in nonhuman primates, however. In addition, several controlled trials of different diets that have been accompanied by a fall in mean cholesterol levels in small

**Table 60–4.  Pathophysiologic Defects Resulting in Hyperlipidemia**

| Defect | Primary | Secondary | Plasma Lipid Increased |
|---|---|---|---|
| VLDL overproduction | Familial hypertriglyceridemia<br>Familial combined hyperlipidemia<br>Sporadic (?) | Alcohol<br>Hyperinsulinemic states:<br>  obesity<br>  estrogens<br>  glucocorticoids<br>  mild noninsulin-dependent diabetes<br>  acromegaly | Triglyceride |
| Reduced lipoprotein lipase (LPL) activity | Primary LPL deficiency<br>Absence of LPL activator | Untreated diabetes mellitus<br>Hypothyroidism<br>Uremia | Triglyceride |
| Defective remnant removal | Remnant removal disease ("broad beta" disease) | Hypothyroidism<br>Liver disease | Cholesterol and triglyercide* |
| LDL overproduction | Familial combined hyperlipidemia | | Cholesterol |
| Impaired LDL catabolism | Familial hypercholesterolemia | Hypothyroidism | Cholesterol |

*The combined increase in plasma cholesterol and triglyceride results from accumulation of remnants. More commonly, combined elevations of cholesterol and triglyceride are due to the simultaneous increase in LDL and VLDL.

**Table 60–5. Studies of Dietary Manipulation in Adult Males for Lowering CAD Risk**

| Population | Diet | n | Diet % Fat Calories | Diet mg Cholesterol | Diet P/S | % Change Plasma Cholesterol | % Change CAD from Control |
|---|---|---|---|---|---|---|---|
| Los Angeles, VA Hospital* | Exptl. | 424 | 39 | 365 | 1.7 | −20 | −24 |
| | Control | 422 | 40 | 653 | 0.3 | −7 | — |
| Helsinki, Mental Hospital† | Exptl. | 313 | 32 | 271 | 1.5 | −8 | −56 |
| | Control | 241 | 36 | 498 | 0.3 | +6 | — |
| Oslo, MI subjects‡ | Exptl. | 206 | 39 | 264 | 2.4 | −18 | −33 |
| | Control | 206 | — | — | — | −4 | — |

*Dayton, S., Pearce, N.L., Hashimoto, S., et al: N. Engl. J. Med. 266:1017, 1962.
†Miettinen, M., Turpeinen, O., Karvonen, M.J., et al.: Lancet 2:7782, 1972.
‡Hjermann, I., Velve, B., Holme, I., et al.: Lancet 2:1303, 1981.

test populations have shown a favorable effect on the incidence of the overall complications of CAD[18] (Table 60–5). Drug studies have been more revealing. Results of the large WHO clofibrate trial in a normal population have provided evidence favoring the lipid hypothesis, because cholesterol lowering (and presumably triglyceride lowering) using this drug was associated with a reduced incidence of nonfatal myocardial infarctions.[19] The increase in total mortality in that study remains unsettling, however, and its relevance to the management of specific hyperlipidemic states is unknown. Nicotinic acid given to patients without regard to the presence of hyperlipidemia reduced the incidence of repeat myocardial infarctions in the Coronary Drug Trial, but did not reduce total mortality.[20] On the basis of these studies, the decision as to whom should be treated and when has been vigorously debated. Several reports suggest that lipid lowering therapy effecting a decrease in LDL and an increase in HDL inhibits progression of preexisting coronary or femoral atherosclerosis studies angiographically.[21,22]

The most convincing evidence to date favoring lipid-lowering therapy in high-risk patients for primary prevention of morbidity and mortality from atherosclerotic disease has emerged from the multicenter Lipid Research Clinics coronary primary prevention trial. Using both diet and drug therapy (cholestyramine) to reduce plasma cholesterol levels for at least five years in hypercholesterolemic middle-aged men, investigators demonstrated conclusively that sustained reduction of LDL decreased morbidity and mortality from atherosclerosis, with the decrease being directly proportional to the degree of LDL reduction.[3]

Thus, the weight of evidence at present strongly favors the use of safe measures to control hyperlipidemia in patients through middle age. Further definition of candidates for lipid-lowering drugs must await the results of additional studies needed to define the long-term efficacy and safety

of lipid-lowering agents and procedures for identification of subsets of individuals (e.g., women, younger men, those with specific familial disorders) who should be treated by lipid-lowering management for the prevention of atherosclerosis and its sequelae.

## Candidates for Treatment

In deciding whom to treat, how vigorously, and by what modalities, many factors should be taken into consideration. Because not all patients with hyperlipidemia are likely to benefit from treatment, factors including age, other diseases, clinically manifest atherosclerosis, the presence of other cardiovascular risk factors, and the nature of the underlying condition need to be considered (Table 60–6). The family history often is critical in making the decision whether to treat. For instance, a young person with hyperlipidemia who has a strongly positive family history of premature atherosclerosis, is fit, and is free of clinical manifestations of cardiovascular disease is likely to derive more benefit from lipid-lowering therapy than a patient who already has had a myocardial infarction or an elderly patient who has hyperlipidemia but no evidence of vascular disease.

Treatment is usually life-long because short-term therapy is unlikely to have lasting benefit. A decision to intervene with drugs after diet has been tried must be considered carefully and reserved for those at exceptionally high risk for development of accelerated atherosclerosis, particularly because compliance with dietary regimens over long periods frequently is unsatisfactory, and because some of the medications used for hyperlipidemia (especially the bile acid-binding resins) are rather unpleasant. On the other hand, an ominous family history could presumably be a powerful motivating force in promoting compliance with the therapeutic program. Aside from chylomicronemia syndrome, which must be treated vigorously, individuals who are younger,

**Table 60–6.  Factors to Consider in Treating Patients with Hyperlipidemia**

1.  Age
2.  Diseases that cause hyperlipidemia
    untreated insulin-dependent (type I) diabetes mellitus
    hypothyroidism
    uremia
    nephrotic syndrome (hypoproteinemia)
    obstructive liver disease
    dysproteinemia (multiple myeloma, lupus erythematosus)
    glycogen storage disease
    anorexia nervosa
    endocrine disorders (Cushing's disease, acromegaly)
    acute intermittent porphyria
3.  Drugs that produce hyperlipidemia
    estrogens
    oral contraceptives
    glucocorticoids
    antihypertensive agents (thiazides, beta adrenergic blocking agents)
4.  Dietary factors
    caloric intake (recent weight gain)
    dietary content of cholesterol and saturated fats
5.  Suspicion of genetic disorders
    family history of hyperlipidemia or xanthomas
    history of pancreatitis or recurrent abdominal pain
    family history of early atherosclerosis
6.  Presence of other cardiovascular risk factors

have a positive family history, or have associated risk factors for atherosclerosis, such as diabetes or hypertension, generally are candidates for consideration of treatment of hyperlipidemia.

## Hypertriglyceridemia

With hypertriglyceridemia, regardless of cause, fasting plasma triglyceride levels above 1,000 mg/dl are associated with a high risk for the development of pancreatitis and other clinical manifestations of the chylomicronemia syndrome. Because pancreatitis is potentially fatal and repeated triglyceride measurements vary widely when levels above 500 mg/dl are reached, such levels usually indicate that lipid-lowering management is indicated (see section on diet and forms of hyperlipidemia).

Individuals with fasting plasma triglyceride levels between 250 and 500 mg/dl present a different problem because in the aggregate such levels are associated with a twofold excessive risk of cardiovascular disease.[23] About 5% of United States males above the age of 30 have levels exceeding 250 mg/dl (see Table 60–2). In an individual patient these levels may be normal, may reflect lifestyle influences (e.g., obesity) or may be a marker for an underlying genetic form of hyper-

lipidemia that might be associated with an increased risk of accelerated atherosclerosis and might require some form of therapy.[23] Therefore, if such a patient has a positive family history for hyperlipidemia or premature cardiovascular disease (e.g., myocardial infarction in a first-degree male relative before the age of 50 or female relative before the age of 60) or coexistent hypercholesterolemia, further investigation is indicated to define the nature of the disorder before institution of appropriate therapy. Other than the promotion of lifestyle changes including dietary modification, most patients with triglyceride levels within this range do not require a specific form of therapy.

## Hypercholesterolemia

Plasma cholesterol levels above about 240 mg/dl also are associated with excess risk of cardiovascular disease, particularly when coupled with other risk factors. Most of these individuals have polygenic hypercholesterolemia, and dietary modification is generally sufficient to lower cholesterol levels.[24] More intensive therapy beginning with a dietary approach is usually advised for patients found to have hypercholesterolemia on the basis of one of the familial disorders (see Table 60–3).

## DIET

Dietary intervention alone can be effective in lowering blood lipids in many individuals with hyperlipidemia and should be the first approach to therapy.[24] Some genetic disorders, such as familial hypercholesterolemia, respond minimally; optimally diet alone rarely achieves more than a 20% reduction in cholesterol levels. Nevertheless, in all primary familial or sporadic disorders, dietary therapy should always be attempted initially. Only when the hyperlipidemia proves refractory, and the patient is at high risk for the development of atherosclerosis, should drugs be considered.

### Diet and Forms of Hyperlipidemia

Marked hypertriglyceridemia with chylomicronemia in fasting plasma, rarely due to primary lipoprotein lipase (LPL) deficiency, is more frequently due to the concomitant presence of genetic and secondary forms of hypertriglyceridemia. Treatment of the aggravating disorder usually lowers triglycerides to safer levels. Primary LPL deficiency (see Table 60–4), in which hypertriglyceridemia is aggravated by dietary fat, is best handled by stringent restriction of fat intake to reduce chylomicron input. The optional substitution of medium-chain triglycerides also may be helpful. The rationale for this substitution depends on the fact that medium-chain triglycerides, in contrast to long-chain triglycerides, are absorbed directly via the portal vein, bypassing chylomicron formation and transport through intestinal lymphatics. Dietary adherence is critical because none of the available drugs is effective in this disorder, although clofibrate or nicotinic acid, by lowering VLDL levels, can help prevent frequent episodes of life-threatening severe chylomicronemia and acute pancreatitis.[25]

Because fasting chylomicronemia most frequently results from a combination of a genetic form and a secondary form of hyperlipidemia, elucidation and treatment of the secondary cause,[25] including dietary measures where appropriate, are the mainstay of therapy. If this plan is not feasible and plasma triglyceride levels remain persistently above 1000 mg/dl, clofibrate or gemfibrozil should be prescribed. Abstinence from alcohol often helps to maintain lower plasma triglyceride levels. A reduced fat intake occasionally may be required in addition. When severe insulin deficiency is causing LPL deficiency (a frequent secondary cause of marked hypertriglyceridemia), the patient should be vigorously treated with insulin. In hypertriglyceridemia associated with modestly impaired LPL activity in conjunction with hyperglycemia, insulin or oral hypoglycemic agents may be effective in correcting the disorder.[26]

Most other types of hyperlipidemia respond to a basic diet that is low in cholesterol and saturated fat.[24] Such a diet most likely will contain a high proportion of carbohydrate (more than 50% of total calories). Because obesity aggravates many hyperlipidemias by promoting production of VLDL, this diet should be hypocaloric until the patient achieves ideal body weight, although maintenance of lowered body weight is notoriously difficult.

### Carbohydrate

In most instances, the higher percentage of total calories consumed as carbohydrate is of little concern, even in patients with hypertriglyceridemia. Although basal triglyceride levels are reportedly highest on high-carbohydrate diets, this phenomenon occurs only transiently during periods of a few weeks of adaptation. Studies of 24-hour patterns of triglyceride levels in patients with hypertriglyceridemia after a period of adaptation have shown them to be actually lower on higher-carbohydrate diets compared with diets higher in fat.[27] If control of hypertriglyceridemia is meant to imply lowering of all-day levels, as in diabetic therapy, evidence suggests that a calorie-restricted, relatively low-fat, high-carbohydrate diet would be desirable for the control of the

hypertriglyceridemias. Studies have shown that even for overnight fasting triglyceride levels, a low-fat diet may be more effective than a low-carbohydrate diet for long-term management.[28] Thus a disproportionate restriction of carbohydrates in the diet of these patients is not usually justified.

### Alcohol and Drugs

Alcohol, which may increase triglyceride production by altering the caloric balance and directly stimulating hepatic syntheses, should be discouraged in patients with any disorder in the transport of VLDL. Dietary management will be ineffective unless drugs such as estrogen, glucocorticoids, thiazide diuretics, or beta adrenergic blockers, which aggravate many forms of hypertriglyceridemia, can be withdrawn or the dosage lowered.

### Cholesterol and Saturated Fat

In patients with hypercholesterolemia, particular emphasis must be placed on lowering the intake of cholesterol-containing foods (Table 60–7, see also Appendix table A–20). Decreasing the dietary intake from the average American consumption of 400 to 700 mg/day to less than 300 mg/day is an essential step in therapy because dietary cholesterol will accumulate beyond the body's ability to compensate by reducing the amount synthesized and increasing the amount secreted, thus leading to an increase in plasma cholesterol.[29] Furthermore, cholesterol feeding increases LDL synthesis and reduces receptor-mediated LDL catabolism.[30] Saturated fat intake should also be curtailed to less than 10% of total calories because these fatty acids also appear to raise serum cholesterol levels, primarily by decreasing LDL clearance.[31] Cholesterol and saturated fat usually occur in many of the same foods, however, so that the dietary regimen would probably be similar. Because they have such a high risk of developing premature atherosclerosis, children of patients with familial hypercholesterolemia should be screened in infancy and childhood and appropriate dietary management instituted as early in life as possible, although improvement in outcome has not yet been proved. Dietary management reduces cholesterol levels during the first year of life in infants with familial hypercholesterolemia.[32]

### Polyunsaturated Fat

The value of substituting polyunsaturated for saturated fat in diets for patients with hypercholesterolemia is debatable. A diet high in polyunsaturated fats appears to be less efficient in low-

**Table 60–7.  Cholesterol and Saturated Fat Content in Some Common Foods***

| Food | Cholesterol mg/100 g food | Saturated Fat g/100 g food |
|---|---|---|
| Eggs | >500 | 3 |
| Organ meats (liver, kidney) | 300 | 2 |
| Butter | 230 | 50 |
| Shrimp, crab, lobster | 110 | 1 |
| Cheese | 110 | 21 |
| Meat (beef, pork, lamb) | 90–100 | 5–13 |
| Poultry (no skin) | 90 | 1 |
| Fish | 70 | 1 |
| Ice cream (10% fat) | 40 | 7 |
| Sherbet, frozen yogurt | 4 | <1 |
| Milk, whole (3.5% fat) | 14 | <2 |
| Milk, skim | 2 | 0 |
| Cottage cheese | 6 | 1 |
| Margarines, soft | 0 | 16 |
| Vegetable oil | 0 | 13 |
| Coconut oil, cocoa butter | 0 | 75 |

*Adapted from Connor, W.E., Connor, S.L.[38]

ering cholesterol levels than a diet restricted in cholesterol and saturated fats without the substitution. Furthermore, the long-term effects of highly unsaturated fat diets remain unknown.[33] A particular type of highly polyunsaturated fat containing long-chain fatty acids of the omega-3 series, such as eicosapentenoic acid (found in large amounts in certain fish oils such as salmon or mackerel) (see Appendix Table A–20b), in contrast to the fatty acids of the omega-6 series, such as linoleic acid (found in vegetable oil), will markedly lower VLDL and LDL levels in normal subjects and has been associated with the very low lipid levels and virtually absent atherosclerosis in populations that subsist on high-fish diets.[34] The role of these highly polyunsaturated marine fats in the management of various hyperlipidemic states is currently being evaluated. High dietary levels of omega-3 fatty acids prolong bleeding time in conjunction with altered prostaglandin synthesis.[34]

## Summary of Dietary Recommendations

Current recommendations of the American Heart Association (1984) for the population at large limit intake of polyunsaturated fats to no more than 10% of total calories.[18] Increase of the polyunsaturated/saturated fat (P/S) ratio to about 1.0 from the usual value of about 0.3 is achieved mainly by reduction of saturated fat intake. Thus, foods rich in animal fat should be avoided, and the use of margarine, nonfat milk, and vegetable oils encouraged. Reduction of the proportion of fat calories to 30 to 35% of the total would therefore require a reciprocal increase in the proportion of carbohydrate calories to 50% or more. This diet is also the recommended first phase in the dietary management of all hyperlipidemic states[24] (phase I, Table 60–8) (see also Appendix Table A–24). Additional steps (phases II and III, Table 60–8) employ a progressive reduction in total fat, saturated fat, and cholesterol and, when obesity is

**Table 60–8.  Dietary Approach to Prevention of Atherosclerosis and Treatment of Hyperlipidemia**

| Fat Phase* | Fat (% Calories) | Saturated Fat (% Calories) | Cholesterol (mg/day) | Practical Measures |
|---|---|---|---|---|
| I | 30 | 10 | 300 | Avoid foods rich in animal fats and cholesterol<br>Use margarine, nonfat milk, and vegetable oils |
| II | 25 | 8 | 200–250 | Eat <6–8 oz. meat per day<br>Use less fat and cheese<br>Use more grains, fruit, and vegetables |
| III | 20 | 7 | 100–150 | Eat mainly cereals, legumes, fruit, and vegetables<br>Eat meat as a condiment<br>Use low-cholesterol cheeses |

*Phase I is appropriate for the use of the population at large. Greater restriction of dietary fat and cholesterol (phase II) is required in subjects with genetic forms of hyperlipidemia, especially familial hypercholesterolemia and familial combined hyperlipidemia. Even greater fat and cholesterol restriction (phase III) may be required in the presence of other risk factors or when there is a strong family history of premature atherosclerotic complications.

present, caloric restriction. Phase II diets should be used in patients with genetic forms of hyperlipidemia, especially familial hypercholesterolemia and familial combined hyperlipidemia, or in subjects with multiple risk factors. Phase III diets should be reserved for use in those conditions with a strong family history of premature atherosclerosis.

### One-Diet Concept

According to this concept there is a *single basic diet* for all the common forms of hyperlipidemia. This low-calorie, low-saturated-fat, low-cholesterol diet that is appropriate for patients with hyperlipidemia is a prudent diet for the population at large. In practice, it translates into limitation of animal fats and emphasis on vegetable oils, fish, and carbohydrates. It carries little known risk in adults and is effective in lowering both cholesterol and triglyceride-rich lipoproteins. It should be individualized to fit the particular lipid disorder in the patient: for example, special attention should be paid to dietary cholesterol restriction for patients with familial hypercholesterolemia (to as little as 20 to 25% fat calories and 100 to 150 mg cholesterol) (Phase III, Table 60–8) and to alcohol and caloric restriction for those with hypertriglyceridemia and elevated VLDL. The role of various dietary fibers in the dietary management of hyperlipidemic patients is currently being evaluated. It does appear that increasing habitual physical activity is a useful adjunct to the dietary management of many hyperlipidemic states.

### DRUGS

When dietary management is not completely effective, drugs may be added to the therapeutic regimen (Table 60–9). Drugs often need to be added for the management of patients with monogenic forms of hyperlipoproteinemia, particularly those with familial hypercholesterolemia, familial combined hyperlipidemia, and/or a positive family history of early atherosclerosis, or prior episodes of acute pancreatitis. There is no evidence to support the use of lipid-lowering drugs for the prevention of atherosclerosis in the general population.[35]

### Hypertriglyceridemia

Drugs that act by reducing hepatic VLDL triglyceride production (e.g., clofibrate, gemfibrozil, nicotinic acid) are effective in treating several forms of hypertriglyceridemia. *Clofibrate* is an effective drug for prevention of recurrent bouts of abdominal pain in many patients with chylomicronemia syndrome. It is also particularly useful in the therapy of dysbetalipoproteinemia, in which it markedly reduces triglyceride and cholesterol levels and the β-VLDL that accumulates as a result of a defect in remnant removal. Such therapy induces regression of xanthomas, improves peripheral blood flow, and reduces symptoms (intermittent claudication and angina pectoris). *Gemfibrozil*, another fibric acid derivative, has similar effects on lipid transport. These drugs raise HDL cholesterol levels. *Nicotinic acid* probably acts primarily by inhibition of VLDL production, secondarily lowering LDL. As a result of decreased HDL catabolism, nicotinic acid also raises HDL cholesterol levels.

### Hypercholesterolemia

By directly diverting cholesterol and bile acids from the intestine to the feces, bile acid-binding resins, such as *cholestyramine* and *colestipol*, enhance cholesterol excretion, reduce body cholesterol pools, reduce enterohepatic recycling, and increase hepatic LDL receptor activity and thus receptor-mediated catabolism. Consequently, these agents are useful in lowering

**Table 60–9. Drug Treatment of the Hyperlipidemias**

| Class of Drug | Drugs Available | Major Lipoprotein Decreased | Mechanism |
|---|---|---|---|
| Fibric acid derivatives | Clofibrate Gemfibrozil | VLDL (LDL) | Decreases VLDL synthesis; enhances LPL action |
| Nicotinic acid | Nicotinic acid | VLDL (LDL) | Decreases VLDL synthesis |
| Bile acid-binding resins | Cholestyramine Colestipol | LDL | Promotes sterol excretion; increases LDL receptor-mediated removal |
| Nonabsorbable sterol binders | Neomycin Sitosterol | LDL | Promotes sterol excretion |
| Probucol | Probucol | LDL | Unknown |
| Steroids | Norethindrone Oxandrolone | Chylomicrons (VLDL) | Enhances LPL action |
| HMG-coA reductase inhibitors | Lovostatin | LDL | Blocks cholesterol synthesis; increases LDL receptor-mediated removal |

**Table 60–10.** **Secular Trends in Mean Dietary Fat and Cholesterol Intake and Plasma Cholesterol Levels in U.S. Adults**

| Decade | % Calories from Fat | Dietary Cholesterol (mg/day) | P/S Ratio | Plasma Total Cholesterol (mg/dl) |
|---|---|---|---|---|
| Men | | | | |
| 1950s* | 40 | 530 | 0.35 | 230 |
| 1970s† | 40 | 540 | 0.50 | 200 |
| Women | | | | |
| 1950s | 40 | 500 | 0.35 | 230 |
| 1970s | 40 | 325 | 0.50 | 194 |

*Gordon, T., Kagan, A., Garcia-Palmieri, N.R., et al.: Circulation 63:400, 1981.
†Gordon, T., Fisher, N., Ernst, N., et al.: Arteriosclerosis 2:505, 1982.

plasma cholesterol levels in patients with hypercholesterolemia due to increased LDL levels. *Probucol*, which also lowers LDL levels, is being used in the treatment of hypercholesterolemia; however, in contrast to bile acid binders, it also lowers HDL cholesterol levels.

Thus a bile acid-binding resin (colestipol or cholestyramine) is the treatment of choice for patients with familial hypercholesterolemia, and a fibric acid derivative (clofibrte or gemfibrozil) or nicotinic acid for patients with hypertriglyceridemia at high risk (see Table 60–9). *Combined therapy* with a resin and nicotinic acid has achieved dramatic normalization of LDL cholesterol levels in patients with heterozygous familial hypercholesterolemia, even when plasma cholesterol levels have exceeded 400 mg/dl.[36] The effect of this combined drug approach on regression (or interruption of progression) of atherosclerotic lesions and its use in the treatment of familial combined hyperlipidemia are currently being evaluated.

## PREVENTION

Prevention of atherosclerosis is the main goal of treatment of hyperlipidemia. Although an effective program has not been established with certainty, enough is known to guide in both identification of those with a higher risk and in development of conservative measures that probably will reduce that risk. Thus prevention currently is equated with risk factor reduction. Dietary management of hyperlipidemia and dietary adjustments in the population at large are fundamental features of any prevention program.

Several trials of dietary intervention aimed at long-term reduction of serum cholesterol have shown in the aggregate a favorable trend toward lowering of CAD morbidity and mortality rates (see Table 60–5), although each of the study designs can be criticized. Of particular interest, the results of the Lipid Research Clinics Coronary Primary Prevention Trial suggest that the hypercholesterolemic men treated with only diet and placebo sustained a reduction in CAD risk proportional to the degree of LDL cholesterol lowering.[3,37] Unfortunately, a dietary trial extended to a free-living normal population would require prohibitive numbers of subjects and exorbitant costs.

The decline of American death rates from premature CAD today[2] (Fig. 60–1) coincides with two trends in health practices. One is the increasing acceptance of the importance of detecting and attempting to correct some of the risk factors correlated with atherosclerosis. The other is a greater awareness of the dietary sources of cholesterol and saturated fats and a tendency of the public to restrict their intake. Over the past several decades, American adults appear to have decreased their dietary cholesterol and saturated fat intake and have lowered their average plasma total cholesterol levels (Table 60–10). Whether these trends are causally related to the decline in death rate is not known. Although a rigorous approach to changes in life-style for the general population may be debated, it is desirable to continue finding and helping those most susceptible to early atherosclerosis. The health professional's role in risk factor reduction involves treating hypertension and dispensing advice regarding diet, body weight, smoking, and exercise. Drug treatment of hyperlipidemia should be limited to those individuals at risk who do not respond adequately to dietary management. There is no treatment of atherosclerosis, only of its complications. Technical advances in the treatment of end-stage complications have reduced morbidity and mortality, but prevention remains the long-term goal of both research and health care practice.

## REFERENCES

1. Arteriosclerosis, 1981: U.S. Department of HHS, PHS, NIH Publication No. 81-2034, June 1981.
2. Levy, R.I.: Arteriosclerosis *1*:312–325, 1981.
3. Lipid Research Clinics Program: JAMA *251*:351–374, 1984.

4. Mandrup-Poulsen, T., Mortensen, S.A., Meinertz, H., et al.: Lancet *1*:250–252, 1984.
5. Bierman, E.L.: Fed. Proc. *37*:2832, 1978.
6. Dawber, T.R.: Risk factors for atherosclerotic disease. *In* Current Concepts. Kalamazoo, MI, Upjohn, 1975.
7. Bierman, E.L., Ross, R.: Aging and atherosclerosis. *In* Atherosclerosis Reviews. (Paoletti, R., Gotto, A.M., Jr., Eds.) New York, Raven Press, 1977.
8. Goldrick, R.B., Sinnett, P.F., Whyte, H.M.: An assessment of coronary heart disease and coronary risk factors in a New Guinea Highland population. *In* Atherosclerosis, Proceedings of the 2nd International Symposium. (Jones, R.J., Ed.) New York, Springer-Verlag, 1970.
9. Olefsky, J.M., Farquhar, J.W., Reaven, G.M.: Am. J. Med. *57*:551–560, 1974.
10. Hulley, S.B., Rosenman, R.H., Bawd, R.D., et al.: N. Engl. J. Med. *302*:1383–1389, 1980.
11. Brunzell, J.D., Schrott, H.C., Motulsky, A.G., et al.: Metabolism *25*:313–320, 1976.
12. Morganroth, J., Levy, R.I., Fredrickson, D.S.: Ann. Intern. Med. *82*:158–174, 1975.
13. Goldstein, J.L., Hazzard, W.R., Schrott, H.G., et al.: J. Clin. Invest. *52*:1533–1543, 1973.
14. Goldstein, J.L., Hazzard, W.R., Schrott, H.G., et al.: J. Clin. Invest. *52*:1544–1578, 1973.
15. Beaumont, J.L., Carlson, L.A., Cooper, G.R., et al.: Bull. WHO *43*:891–915, 1970.
16. Brunzell, J.D., Chait, A., Bierman, E.L.: Metabolism *27*:1109–1127, 1978.
17. Motulsky, A.G.: N. Engl. J. Med. *294*:823–827, 1976.
18. AHA Nutrition Committee: Arteriosclerosis *2*:177–191, 1982.
19. World Health Organization (WHO): Lancet *2*:379–384, 1980.
20. The Coronary Drug Project Research Group: JAMA *231*:360–381, 1975.
21. Levy, R.I.: Arteriosclerosis *3*:481a, 1983.
22. Duffield, R.G.M., Miller, N.E., Brunt, J.N.H., et al.: Lancet *2*:639–641, 1983.
23. NIH Consensus Development Conference Summary: Arteriosclerosis *4*:296–301, 1984.
24. Recommendations for the Treatment of Hyperlipidemia in Adults. Arteriosclerosis *4*:443A–468A, 1984.
25. Brunzell, J.D., Bierman, E.L.: Med. Clin. N. Am. *66*:455–468, 1982.
26. Brunzell, J.D., Porte, D., Jr., Bierman, E.L.: Metabolism *24*:1123–1127, 1975.
27. Schlierf, G., Reinhemer, W., Stosberg, V.: Nutr. Metab. *13*:80–91, 1971.
28. Sommariva, D., Scotti, L., Fasoli, A.: Atherosclerosis *29*:43–51, 1978.
29. Bierman, E.L., Glomset, J.A.: Disorders of lipid metabolism. *In* Williams' Textbook of Endocrinology, 7th ed. (Wilson, J.D., Foster, D.W., Eds.) Philadelphia, W.B. Saunders Co., 1985.
30. Packard, C.J., McKinney, L., Carr, K., et al.: J. Clin. Invest. *72*:45–51, 1983.
31. Shepherd, J., Packard, C.J., Grundy, S.M., et al.: J. Lipid Res. *21*:91–99, 1980.
32. Glueck, C.J., Tsang, R.C.: Am. J. Clin. Nutr. *25*:224–230, 1972.
33. Ahrens, E.H., Jr.: Lancet *2*:1345–1348, 1979.
34. Goodnight, S.H., Jr., Harris, W.S., Connor, W.C., et al.: Arteriosclerosis *2*:87–113, 1982.
35. Oliver, M.F.: N. Engl. J. Med. *306*:297–298, 1983.
36. Kane, J.P., Malloy, M.J., Tun, P., et al.: N. Engl. J. Med. *304*:251–258, 1981.
37. Glueck, C.J.: Arteriosclerosis *4*:543a, 1984.
38. Connor, W.E., Connor, S.L.: Med. Clin. North Am. *66*:485–518, 1982.

*Chapter* **61**

# FOOD ALLERGY

### Ranjit Kumar Chandra

## DEFINITIONS

The topic of food allergy is shrouded in myth, mystique, empiricism, and charlatanry. Adverse reactions to foods are common enough to be considered in the differential diagnosis of a wide variety of symptoms and signs, particularly in young children. At the same time, food allergy is both underdiagnosed and overdiagnosed. This apparent paradox stems from the inclusion of all types of intolerance reactions to food constituents in the all-inclusive popular term of food allergy. This tendency may lead to incorrect diagnosis, the indiscriminate use of elimination diets, and the potential danger of nutritional deficiencies. On the other hand, the rigorous application of scientifically sound diagnostic criteria is beginning to provide incontrovertible evidence that true allergy to dietary components may underlie a variety of symptom-complexes involving the gastrointestinal tract, upper and lower respiratory systems, central nervous system, skin, behavior, urinary tract, and musculoskeletal system.

The following definition of terms is generally accepted by most health professionals:

**Food Intolerance.** This general term describes an abnormal physiologic response to an ingested food component, constituent, or additive. Such a reaction can include immunologic, idiosyncratic, metabolic, pharmacologic, or toxic response.

**Food Allergy.** An adverse reaction to foods involving an immune mechanism, food allergy is a pathogenetic process that can include one or more of the following types: type I IgE-mediated immediate hypersensitivity, type II complement-mediated cell injury, type III antigen-antibody complexes, and type IV T cell-dependent delayed hypersensitivity.

**Food Toxicity.** Food toxicity is an adverse reaction caused by the direct action of a food or food additive and may involve nonimmune release of chemical mediators. The toxic component may be present in the food or may be released by microorganisms contaminating food products.

**Food Idiosyncrasy.** This quantitatively disproportionate response to a food substance or additive occurs only in some patients after a small amount of the substance is ingested. Food idiosyncrasy is unrelated to any physiologic, pharmacologic, or immune effects.

The lack of uniform definitions has handicapped the objective evaluation of the scientific and general literature on adverse reactions to foods and of claims for remedies used in the management of such reactions.

No single figure can give an accurate incidence of food allergy. The confounding variables include genetic predisposition, age, gestation and weight at birth, prevalent mode of infant feeding and age of introduction of solids, presence of primary immunodeficiency, adjuvant effect of gut microflora, and cultural factors impinging upon food habits.

## PATHOPHYSIOLOGY

The three major variables determining the occurrence of food allergy are antigen, host, and environment. The terminology, basic concepts, and procedures in clinical immunology are reviewed in Chapter 32.

### Antigen

Little information is available on the chemical nature of the antigen(s) involved in the adverse immunologic reaction to a given food. What makes a food protein more allergenic than others is largely unknown. Anaphylaxis to peanuts is more common than similar reaction to other legumes. Cross-reactions may occur between food substances within the same botanical family. For example, plum belongs to the same group as almond, peach, apricot, cherries, prunes, and nectarines. Similarly, eggs, chicken, duck, turkey, goose, pheasant, and grouse are grouped together. There is partial cross-reactivity across species. For instance, some children who are allergic to cow's milk protein are able to tolerate goat's milk, although this response is variable. Allergy to crustaceans does not imply that the patient will react to other seafoods such as bony fish.

The immunochemical characteristics of allergens are not well defined. Food allergen are generally glycoproteins with variable molecular weight and stability. Physicochemical properties of a few common food allergens are listed in Table 61–1. It is possible that heat denaturation and enzymic digestion may reduce or even eliminate antigenicity. Alternatively, digestion may give rise to other allergens.

Complete purification of food allergens has been seldom attempted. This has handicapped research as well as diagnosis. The availability of purified allergenic extract will aid in correct diagnosis and a better understanding of the pathophysiologic processes underlying clinical manifestations of food allergy.

### Host and Environment

The risk of developing allergic disease or atopy is largely inherited. In about 70% of patients with documented allergic symptoms, history of allergy in one or more first- and second-degree relatives can be elicited. The nature of the inherited susceptibility is not clear and could lie in differences in immune responses, presence of immunodeficiency, gastrointestinal uptake of macromolecules, and other variables.

The amount of antigen absorbed in the gastrointestinal tract is an important determinant of food hypersensitivity. Gastric acid, secretory IgA, pancreatic secretions, liver filtration, lysosomal function, mucus, ciliary activity, glycocalyx, and gut microflora contribute to the mucosal barrier. In the newborn, significant amounts of macromolecules derived from foods can enter the blood. Some physiologic and pathologic states associated with increased antigen uptake are listed in Table 61–2. For example, preterm low-birth-weight infants absorb twice the amount of bovine serum albumin compared with full-term neonates. A bout of viral gastroenteritis damages the gut barrier and can permit increased uptake of food proteins for several weeks.

### Types of Hypersensitivity

Four types of hypersensitivity reactions may underlie food allergic reactions. It is important to recognize that in one individual and in a particular disease, more than one process may be at work. The food macromolecules absorbed intact incite both systemic and mucosal immune response. Antibodies against food antigens are present in the serum of a large percentage of the normal population and are not diagnostic of food allergy. The mucosal immune response consists primarily of secretory IgA against that particular antigen and retards the further absorption of that antigen. It is hypothesized that T-suppressor cells cause systemic tolerance to that antigen and also

**Table 61–1. Immunochemical Characteristics of Allergens***

| Characteristic | Codfish | Tomato | Egg White | Cow's Milk | Antigen E |
|---|---|---|---|---|---|
| Active component | Glycoproteins | Glycoproteins | Glycoproteins | Glycoproteins | Glycoproteins |
|   Amount of component (mg) isolated from 100 g | 200 | 2.5 | 225 | 100 | 40 |
|   Quantity ($\mu$g) giving positive skin test | 0.0001 | 0.15 | 0.0025 | 0.10 | 0.001 |
| Molecular weight | 18,000 | 20,000 | 31,500 | 36,000 | 38,000 |
| Stability to: | | | | | |
|   heat (100°C) | + | + | + | + | − |
|   acid (pH 2) | + | + | + | + | − |
|   enzymes (proteolytic) | − | + | + | + | ± |

*Adapted from Bleumink, E.: World Rev. Nutr. Diet 12:505, 1970.

**Table 61–2.  Clinical States Associated with Increased Intestinal Uptake of Unaltered Food Proteins**

Physiologic
　Newborns
　Low-birth-weight infants
　　preterm
　　small-for-gestation

Pathologic
　Gastroenteritis
　IgA deficiency
　Inflammation of GI tract due to parasites
　Malnutrition
　Portal hypertension of hepatic origin

suppress deleterious cell-mediated immune response in the gut.

*Type I hypersensitivity* is mediated by IgE and is generally immediate in onset (Fig. 61–1). The cytophilic antibody binds to mast cell. Subsequent exposure of a sensitized individual to the appropriate antigen leads to sequential activation of intracellular metabolic events, mast cell degranulation, and release of the chemical mediators of inflammation. This process causes edema of the epithelium, vasodilation, smooth muscle contraction, and increased permeability of the mucosa. The histopathologic picture may be normal. The manifestation depends on the target organ and can vary in severity from fatal anaphylaxis to mild skin rash. Gastroscopic examination of food-allergic patients after ingestion of the offending antigen have demonstrated hyperemia, nodularity, edema and thickening of rugal folds, diminished peristalsis, and excessive production of mu-

TYPE I. IMMEDIATE HYPERSENSITIVITY

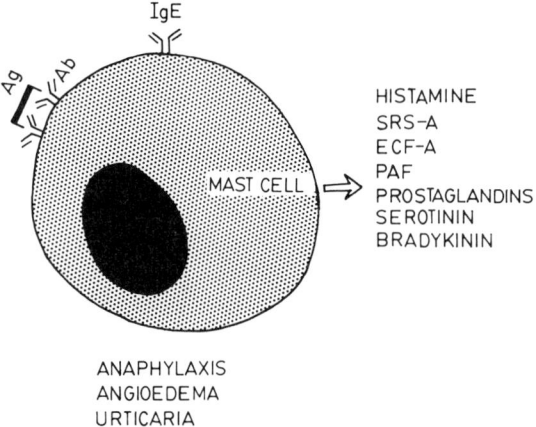

**Fig. 61–1.**  Type I hypersensitivity. Immediate hypersensitivity reaction. SRS-A = slow-reacting substance of anaphylaxis, also known as leukotriene D; ECF-A = eosinophil chemotactic factor of anaphylaxis; PAF = platelet-aggregating factor.

TYPE II.  COMPLEMENT-MEDIATED CYTOLYSIS

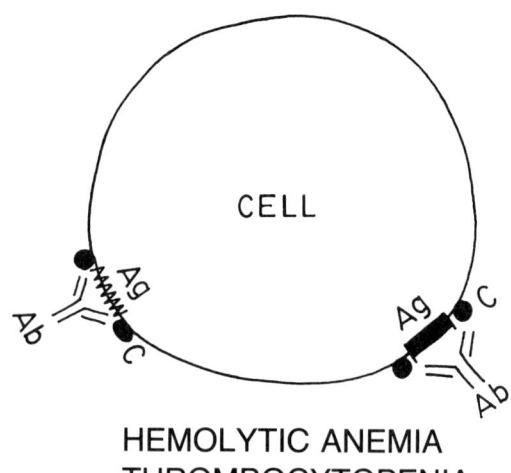

HEMOLYTIC ANEMIA
THROMBOCYTOPENIA
LEUKOPENIA

**Fig. 61–2.**  Type II hypersensitivity. Complement-mediated cytolysis.

cus. The food-specific IgE can often be detected in the serum by radioimmunoassay or enzyme-linked immunoassay and by skin tests.

*Type II hypersensitivity* is the result of complement-fixing antibodies combining with antigens fixed to the surface of cells (Fig. 61–2). Examples of this type of reaction are leukopenia and thrombocytopenia. *Type III hypersensitivity* consists of interaction between food antigen, antibody, and complement components, resulting in the formation of immune complexes (Fig. 61–3). In healthy subjects, these complexes consist predominantly of IgA; in food-allergic patients, IgG and IgE complexes may also be found. The IgA complexes are rapidly cleared, but other complexes may be deposited in the bowel wall and other parts of the body where they activate com-

TYPE III. ANTIGEN-ANTIBODY COMPLEXES

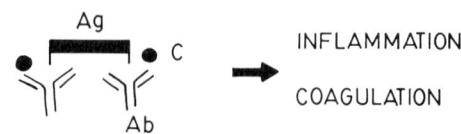

SERUM SICKNESS  (Ag Excess)
ARTHUS REACTION  (Ab Excess)

**Fig. 61–3.**  Type III hypersensitivity. Antigen-antibody complexes.

plement. Immune complex deposition in the gut leads to the accumulation of polymorphonuclear leukocytes, generation of anaphylatoxins, and enhancement of bowel wall permeability. Activation of complement by IgG against food antigen, shown in patients with egg-white and fish allergy, results in acute or chronic diarrhea, asthma, and urticaria. *Type IV hypersensitivity* is mediated by T-lymphocytes and release of a conglomerate of chemicals collectively called lymphokines (Fig. Fig. 61–4). Manifestations include skin rash, stomatitis, and proctitis.

## CLINICAL MANIFESTATIONS

Food allergy can produce symptoms and signs referred to one or more organs. The most frequently involved are the gastrointestinal and respiratory tracts and the skin. Evidence for the involvement of other organs, such as the central nervous system, musculoskeletal system, and others, is less firm and requires further proof. It is also essential to exclude nonimmunologic factors—toxic, biochemical, microbiologic, and psychologic processes—that may underlie certain adverse reactions. A list of illustrative examples is given in Table 61–3. Both quantitative and qualitative aspects should be considered. Enzyme deficiencies can result in profound intolerance to certain carbohydrates and amino acids. Some persons with such enzymopathies might still be able to tolerate small quantities of the offending food with few symptoms. Shellfish contain toxins that can produce swelling and numbness of lips, mouth, face, and limbs, as well as nausea, vomiting, incoordination, speech difficulty, dizziness, headache, and weakness. Fatal outcome can occur. The incubation time is about one hour. A heat-stable neurotoxin, saxitoxin, having curarelike activity is responsible for the symptoms. Aflatoxin in peanuts, cyanide in fruit pits, pressor amines in bananas, as well as pesticides, ergot, penicillin, dyes, and nitrites can be the source of food-associated nonimmunologic reactions. Histamine-containing and histamine-releasing foods (Table

61–4) produce "allergic" symptoms and signs, even though no immunologic process in involved. The same applies to foods containing tyramine, which can precipitate migraine in a sensitive individual (see Chaps. 38 and 39 for other data on food-borne toxicants).

Symptoms and signs due to food allergy can be broadly divided into reaginic and nonreaginic reactions. *Reaginic* responses are generally mediated by IgE and occur within a short time after ingestion of the offending food. Examples include anaphylaxis, abdominal pain, nausea, vomiting, diarrhea, urticaria, dermatitis, angioedema, rhinitis, and wheezing. *Nonreaginic* responses occur 6 to 24 hours after exposure to the allergenic food. Manifestations caused by this type of mechanism include GI bleeding resulting in iron deficiency anemia, malabsorption, allergic gastroenteropathy, urticaria, eczema, pneumonitis, pulmonary hemosiderosis, and wheezing.

A listing of the common manifestations of food allergy is given in Table 61–5. The frequency of common manifestations in a group of patients with proven food allergy is given in Figure 61–5.

## DIAGNOSIS

The accurate identification of the offending food is extremely difficult. One should begin with the history. It should include a description of the symptoms, time lapsed since ingestion of food, and the nature and amount of food required to provoke symptoms. When severe allergic symptoms follow soon after food intake, patients themselves make the association and avoid that specific food. In other cases, there might not be a clear association, such as when the offending food is eaten frequently and is, therefore, disregarded as a causative agent. Symptoms usually depend on the quantity of food ingested and may occur intermittently, even though the food is ingested daily. Symptoms generally occur within 48 hours of the ingestion of food, but may rarely be delayed. Other foods consumed in this time period make identification of the offending food difficult. In some patients, raw food may provoke symptoms but cooked food can be eaten with impunity. Symptoms can be due to food additives or contaminants.

### Diet Diary

In patients with occasional symptoms or in those with delayed onset of manifestations, an accurate record of all foods, beverages, and drugs ingested within 96 hours of each episode may provide a clue to the offending substance. Diet diary can also measure compliance when patients are advised to follow a hypoallergenic diet.

TYPE IV. DELAYED HYPERSENSITIVITY

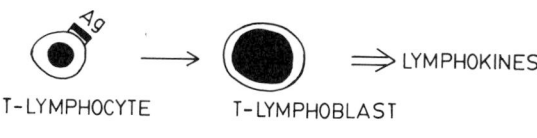

CONTACT DERMATITIS

**Fig. 61–4.** Type IV hypersensitivity. Delayed hypersensitivity.

**Table 61–3. Examples of Nonimmunologic Adverse Reactions to Foods**

| Clinical Features | Predisposing Factor | Offending Substance |
|---|---|---|
| Diarrhea, abdominal cramps | Lactase deficiency | Lactose in milk |
| Vomiting, neurologic problems | — | Saxitoxin in shellfish |
| Vomiting, diarrhea, neurologic symptoms | — | Botulinal toxin derived from *Clostridium botulinum* |
| Diarrhea, pain, fever, dizziness, weakness | — | *Salmonella* or *Staphylococcus* poisoning |
| Vomiting, pain, salivation, diarrhea, sweating, blurred vision | — | Mushroom poisoning |
| Headache, fever, gastrointestinal upset, depression, weakness | — | Solanine alkaloid in potato skins |
| Hemolytic anemia | Glucose-6-phosphate dehydrogenase deficiency | Fava beans, drugs |
| Paroxysmal atrial tachycardia | — | Caffeine |
| Bronchospasm | — | Meta-bisulfite in wine and salads |
| Urticaria | — | Benzoates and food dyes |
| Headache | — | Wine, cocoa, cheese, monosodium glutamate (MSG) |
| Migraine | — | Tyramine in cheese, pickled herring, marmite |
| Urticaria | — | Histamine in wine and beer, sauerkraut; or histamine released by chocolate, strawberries |
| Skin rash | — | Octopamine in citrus fruits; dihydrophenylalanine in broad beans |

**Table 61–4. Foods Containing Histamine and Tyramine**

*Histamine-containing foods*
  Beer and wine
  Cheese
  Other fermented foods
  Sauerkraut
  Canned foods
  Spinach
  Tomatoes
  Sardines

*Histamine-releasing foods*
  Strawberries
  Chocolate
  Eggs
  Fish
  Tomatoes

*Tyramine-containing foods*
  Cheese
  Pickled herring
  Marmite
  Avocados
  Raspberries

## Skin Tests

Prick or scratch tests using 10% w/v solution are done on the forearm so that a tourniquet can be applied in case of a systemic reaction. Intradermal tests produce a high incidence of false positives and should not be done. The reliability of skin tests depends on the quality of extracts and testing procedures. Food reagents should not cause nonspecific irritant reactions, and they should react with specific antibody. Reliability also depends on the food in question. The foods correlating most reliably with skin tests include peanuts, eggs, milk, soy, fish, and shellfish. Skin tests are usually positive with immediate hypersensitivity reactions, but may be negative with reactions of delayed onset. Confirmation of the positive skin test response with a positive double-blind food challenge would also validate the quality and specificity of food extracts being used.

## Intestinal Biopsy

In patients with gastrointestinal manifestations, jejunal mucosal biopsy may reveal abnormalities of villus shape and height, and infiltration with

**Table 61–5. Clinical Manifestations of Food Allergy**

| *Gastrointestinal System* | *Respiratory System* |
|---|---|
| Vomiting | Rhinorrhea |
| Abdominal pain | Postnasal discharge |
| Abdominal distention | Sneezing |
| Diarrhea | Cough |
| Malabsorption | Recurrent croup |
| Occult bleeding | Bronchospasm |
| Protein-losing enteropathy | Chronic pneumonitis |
|  | Serous otitis media |
| *Skin* | *Hematologic System* |
| Dermatitis | Anemia |
| Eczema | Eosinophilia |
| Urticaria | Thrombocytopenia |
| Angioedema |  |
| *Neurologic System and Behavior* | *Other Manifestations* |
| Irritability | Sudden infant death syndrome |
| Restlessness | Enuresis |
| Hyperactivity | Arthritis |
| Fatigue | Anaphylaxis |
| Migraine | Nephrotic syndrome |
| Depression |  |

inflammatory cells including eosinophils. In addition, immunofluorescence examination may show deposition of immunoglobulins and complement and presence of IgE-producing plasma cells. Ideally, one should repeat the biopsy after symptoms subside and again on relapse following challenge with the suspected food allergen.

### In Vitro Tests

The *radioallergosorbent test (RAST)* is the most commonly used in vitro test to measure levels of antibodies of IgE or other immunoglobulin classes to specific antigens in the serum or secretions. The technique uses antigen bound to a solid phase, usually paper disk. The test serum is added to permit binding of antibody to antigen, followed by incubation with radiolabeled anti-IgE. The amount of bound radioactivity gives an estimate of antigen-specific IgE in the patient's serum. The advantages of RAST include ability to test several samples in one sitting, to evaluate patients with dermatographism or severe skin disease, to standardize allergenic extracts, to detect antibodies or immunoglobulin isotypes other than IgE, to evaluate patients with anaphylactic reactions, and to test poisonous materials. The concurrent use of antihistaminics does not interfere with RAST results. The disadvantages are that RAST is expensive, requires the use and measurement of a radiolabelled agent, measures free rather than cell-bound IgE, and is variable in background binding; in addition, test results are not immediately available and are affected by the level of total IgE as well as blocking IgG and IgA antibody. Finally, RAST is unable to evaluate the extent of antigen-induced mediator release.

Two other tests show promise: elevated *plasma histamine* following challenge with the offending food and *lymphocyte mediator release* in the presence of the suspected food protein.

*Eosinophil* count >400/mm³ suggests the presence of allergy. Some patients with food allergy may show eosinophils in stools. *Complement activation* can be demonstrated in fewer than 5% of all patients. The presence of serum precipitins or hemagglutinins and coproantibodies is of little diagnostic help. *Leukocyte histamine release* in the presence of suspected allergen lacks specificity.

### Elimination Diet

Occasionally, the common diagnostic approaches outlined previously fail to identify the

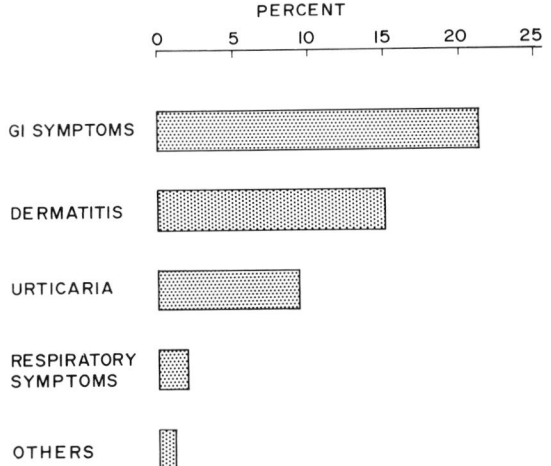

**Fig. 61–5.** Proportion of symptoms referable to different organs in patients with proven food allergy.

foods producing symptoms. This situation may warrant the use of an elimination diet excluding all suspected food allergens for at least two weeks followed by reintroduction of the omitted foods one by one until symptoms reappear.

A sample of such a diet is given in Table 61–6. The food elimination diet is a simple and inexpensive method of pinpointing the causative foods producing adverse reactions. It has the advantage of screening multiple foods and food combinations using menus applicable to a particular patient. The drawbacks include the fact that the procedure is not a double-blind method and involves subjective description of symptoms by patient or guardian. It is not a safe procedure if previous history suggests serious adverse reactions.

### Food Challenge

Food challenge should be undertaken in a double-blind objective manner so that unbiased observations can confirm or refute the diagnosis of food allergy. Both the doctor and the patient are unaware of the nature of the food being tested, and a neutral observer is present to record the findings. In older children and adults, dehydrated foods can be placed in opaque, nonallergenic capsules. In younger children, the suspected foods can be hidden in nonoffending foods. The challenge food is administered in increasing amounts, beginning with 10 to 100 mg depending upon the severity of symptoms. The symptoms are observed and recorded carefully. Medications, particularly antihistaminics and corticosteroids, should be withheld for about one week before the food challenge. Patients with a history of anaphylaxis to food should not be challenged. Hospitalization might be required when the suspected reaction is delayed by several hours. If a dose of 8 g is tolerated blindly, the food is then offered openly in

generous amounts prepared by conventional means so that the effects of cooking and preparation are also evaluated.

## MANAGEMENT AND PREVENTION

### Management

Avoidance of foods proven to cause clinical problems and symptomatic relief are the mainstays of effective management. The ease with which an elimination diet can be advised and executed depends upon the number of foods involved. In severe allergy to a wide variety of foods, it may be difficult to devise a nutritionally adequate diet, and the advice of a trained dietitian should be sought. In young children, growth failure secondary to a severely restricted diet is not rare and should be considered. Infants with cow's milk allergy must be switched to a hydrolysate

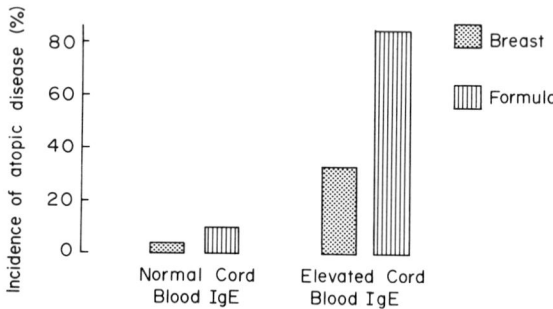

**Fig. 61–6.** Incidence of atopic eczema in infants by cord blood IgE and mode of feeding.

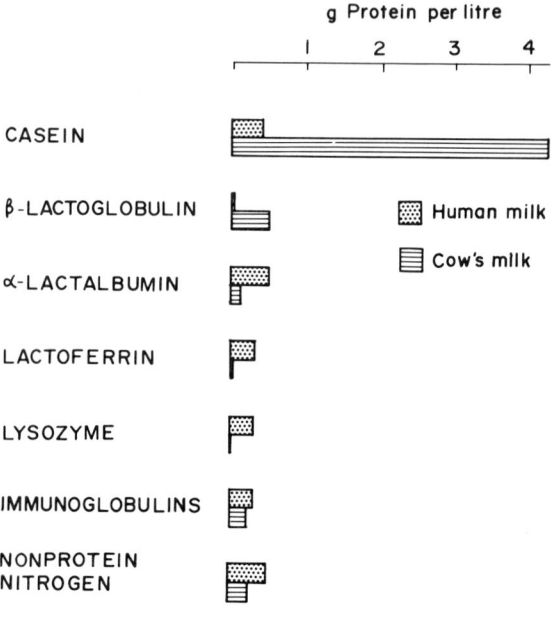

**Fig. 61–7.** Protein composition of human milk and cow's milk.

**Table 61–6.  Elimination Diet***

| Food Group | Item |
| --- | --- |
| Meat | Lamb, mutton, or pork |
| Vegetable | Cabbage, brussel sprouts, or cauliflower |
| Fruit | Apple, banana, or pear |
| Cereal | Rice |
| Fat | Sunflower oil or milk-free margarine |
| Carbohydrates | Sugar, sago, or tapioca |
| Others | Tea, coffee, or water |
| Supplement | Complete vitamin mineral supplement containing approximate minimum daily requirement of each nutrient |

*One new food should be introduced each week and a daily diary of symptoms and signs kept.

**Table 61–7. Substitute Formula for Patients with Cow's Milk Allergy**

| Product | Manufacturer | Protein Source | Carbohydrate Source | Fat Source |
|---|---|---|---|---|
| Nutramigen | Mead Johnson | Enzymatic hydrolysate of casein | Sucrose, tapioca | Corn |
| Pregestimil | Mead Johnson | Enzymatically hydrolyzed milk protein | Glucose, tapioca | Coconut, corn |
| Isomil | Ross | Soy-protein isolate | Corn sugar, sucrose, corn starch | Corn, coconut, soy |
| Mull-Soy | Syntex | Soy flour | Sucrose, invert sucrose | Soy oil |
| Neo-Mull-Soy | Syntex | Soy-protein isolate | Sucrose | Soy oil |
| Nursoy | Wyeth | Soy-protein isolate | Corn syrup, sucrose | Oleo, coconut, safflower, soy |
| ProSobee | Mead Johnson | Soy-protein isolate | Corn sugar, sucrose | Soy |

formula or a soy preparation (see Table 61–6). Almost 45% of infants allergic to cow's milk eventually become sensitized to soy as well. Hyposensitization or immunotherapy is of unproven value. Orally administered disodium cromoglycate prevents mast cell release of histamine and other chemicals and may provide symptomatic relief in some patients.

### Prophylaxis

Prevention of food allergy in infants has reawakened interest in breast-feeding. Most prospective studies on this subject have shown that prolonged (more than 4 to 6 months) exclusive breast-feeding is associated with a significant reduction in the incidence of eczema among high-risk infants (Fig. 61–6). In infants with no family history of atopy, the mode of feeding has little impact. This finding is not surprising because the food protein most frequently causing allergy in young infants is β-lactoglobulin, which is virtually absent in human milk (Fig. 61–7). If the mother elects not to breast-feed, it would be useful to consider a hydrolysate formula, or less satisfactorily, a soy-based formula (Table 61–7). There are no controlled trials evaluating the relative beneficial effects of the "hypoallergenic" substitutes.

### SELECTED READINGS

American Academy of Allergy and Immunology, and National Institute of Allergy and Infectious Disease: Adverse Reactions to Foods. NIH Document 84–2442, 1984.

Bleumink, E.: Food allergy; the chemical nature of the substance eliciting symptoms. World Rev. Nutr. Diet. *12*:505–570, 1970.

Brostoff, J., Challacombe, S.J (Eds.): Food allergy. Clin. Immunol. Allergy *2*:1–260, 1982.

Chandra, R.K. (Ed.): Food Allergy. St. John's, Newfoundland, Nutrition Research Education Foundation, 1986.

Chandra, R.K. (Ed.): Food Intolerance. New York, Elsevier, 1984.

Heiner, D.C. (Ed.): Food allergy. Clin. Rev. Allergy *2*:1–93, 1984.

May, C.D., Block, S.A.: A modern clinical approach to food hypersensitivity. Allergy *33*:166–188, 1978.

*Chapter* **62**

# DIET AND NUTRITION IN THE CARE OF THE PATIENT WITH SURGERY, TRAUMA, AND SEPSIS

Wiley W. Souba and Douglas W. Wilmore

No discipline in medicine has benefited more from the current advances in nutritional support of hospitalized patients than has surgery. As recently as 15 years ago, some surgical patients would have died from malnutrition, sepsis, and multiple-system organ failure because enteral feedings were not possible or were inadequate. Such patients now routinely survive major surgical procedures, multiple trauma, severe, debilitating gastrointestinal disease, and complications such as sepsis and enterocutaneous fistulae. Virtually all hospitalized patients may now be fed safely, with varying degrees of effectiveness, because of three recent developments: (1) the technique of central venous cannulation and infusion of hypertonic nutrient solutions into the superior vena cava;[1] (2) the development of specific enteral formula diets, usually delivered by a feeding tube;[2] and (3) the availability of fat emulsions for safe intravenous administration.[3]

Other major advances in the nutritional management of patients have also reduced mortality rates. These advances include the development of new antibiotics, the ability to screen, preserve, and administer blood and blood products, and the improvements in anesthesia and ventilatory support. Nonetheless, the ability to feed the patient who cannot or will not eat is a major advance in surgical care.[4]

Initially, it was suggested that 20 to 50% of patients in major hospitals had a moderate-to-severe degree of malnutrition. It was proposed that much of this undernutrition was iatrogenic, resulting from the provision of sophisticated medical care without concern for satisfying nutritional requirements.[5] Indeed, many patients lose weight during hospitalization, as the result of witholding of meals for diagnostic tests or other periods of inadequate nutrient intake associated with acute illness, major operation, or medical therapy. These patients can now be fed; however, controlled trials in patients with normal body composition who undergo elective operations or chemotherapy show that such nutritional support produces little improvement in outcome. Therefore, limited weight loss in selected hospitalized patients is acceptable because short-term undernutrition does not prolong a life-limiting illness, nor does it complicate convalescence following major operation or other therapy.

Not all hospitalized patients are malnourished because of diagnostic and therapeutic measures however; the disease process is often the major culprit. Critically ill patients are frequently anorexic secondary to illness and confinement. Patients who have multiple injuries, with or without complications such as sepsis, rarely take adequate calories spontaneously from a food tray.[6] Others often initially have some degree of gastrointestinal ileus and hence cannot or should not eat. Patients with inflammatory bowel disease or those who are critically ill frequently cannot tolerate adequate feedings; enteral feeding results in pain, fever, bloating, or diarrhea. Cancer patients have a diminished appetite secondary to the tumor burden or concomitant treatment regimens, and weight loss is a sign of disease progression.

This chapter reviews the metabolic alterations that occur in patients undergoing elective operations, in patients with accidental injury, and in patients with sepsis. Methods of nutritional assessment of individuals in each of these general groups are provided, along with current knowledge of the nutritional requirements of patients with these illnesses. The basis for selecting the safest and most effective route of nutrient administration is discussed.

## ELECTIVE OPERATIVE PROCEDURES

### Physiologic Responses to Surgery

**Endocrine Changes and Their Metabolic Consequences.** Improvements in anesthesia, surgical technique, and perioperative care have reduced the mortality rates for elective surgical procedures. A recent evaluation of the outcome of major operations reported low mortality rates (<1%), even in patients traditionally regarded as poor surgical candidates.[7]

Most patients undergoing elective operations are adequately nourished. Following an operation of the magnitude of cholecystectomy with common duct exploration, aneurysmectomy, or colectomy, oral feedings are generally not tolerated for 2 to 6 days. In a patient without postoperative complications, the duration of postoperative ileus depends on the extent of manipulation of the abdominal viscera and the length of the operation. Nasogastric decompression is frequently required, and the patient is routinely supported by 2 to 4 L intravenous fluids, usually containing 5% dextrose and appropriate electrolytes. Unless the patient has suffered significant preoperative mal-

nutrition, characterized by a weight loss >10%, or has had a major intraoperative or postoperative complication, solutions containing 5% dextrose may be administered for 5 to 7 days before the initiation of enteral nutrition, with no detrimental effect on outcome. With no dietary nitrogen and with insufficient calories, negative nitrogen balance occurs, in which urinary nitrogen excretion averages 10 to 15 g/day for 2 to 3 days, and then gradually diminishes. This nitrogen excretion is associated with a loss of potassium and phosphorus and indicates a loss of lean body mass.[8]

One of the earliest consequences of a surgical procedure is the rise in levels of circulating cortisol that occurs in response to a sudden outpouring of adrenocorticotropic hormone (ACTH) from the anterior pituitary gland. Activation of the pituitary gland occurs when afferent nervous signals from the operative site reach the hypothalamus to initiate the stress response. The rise in ACTH stimulates the adrenal cortex to elaborate cortisol. This hormone remains at 2 to 5 times normal levels for approximately 24 hours after a major operation.[9] Cortisol has generalized effects on tissue catabolism and mobilizes amino acids from skeletal muscle that provide substrates for wound healing and serve as precursors for the hepatic synthesis of acute-phase proteins or new glucose. Associated with the activation of the adrenal cortex is stimulation of the adrenal medulla through the sympathetic nervous system, with elaboration of epinephrine. This circulating neurotransmitter plays an important role in circulatory adjustment, but it may also elicit metabolic responses if the augmented secretion rate continues over a prolonged period of time.

In addition to increased circulating levels of epinephrine, norepinephrine levels rise during and following elective operative procedures.[10] The excitement, pain, fear, and hypovolemia that may accompany the surgical procedure are potent stimulators of the sympathetic nervous system. Urinary catecholamines may be elevated for 24 to 48 hours after operation and may then return to normal. The major catabolic role of this regulatory system may be the stimulation of hepatic glycogenolysis and gluconeogenesis in concert with glucagon and glucocorticoids.

The neuroendocrine responses to operation also modify the various mechanisms in salt and water excretion. Alterations in serum osmolarity amd tonicity of body fluids secondary to anesthesia and the operative stress stimulate the secretion of aldosterone and antidiuretic hormone (ADS).[10,11] Aldosterone is a potent stimulator of renal sodium retention, whereas ADH stimulates renal tubular water reabsorption. Although the neural and humoral mediators that result from tissue trauma may stimulate aldosterone release, afferent signals from volume receptors appear to be the major stimuli for these hormonal adjustments.

The ability to excrete a water load after elective surgical procedures is restricted.[12] The usual postoperative patient concentrates urine to 1 to 2 ml water/mosm solute excreted, corresponding to a urine osmolarity of 500 to 1,000 mosm/L, even in the presence of adequate hydration. Hence, weight gain secondary to salt and water retention is usual following operation. Edema occurs to a varying extent in all surgical wounds, and this accumulation is proportional to the extent of tissue dissection and local trauma. Administration of sodium-containing solutions during operation replaces this functional volume loss as extracellular fluid redistributes in the body. This "third-spaced" fluid eventually returns to the circulation as the wound edema subsides and diuresis commences 2 to 4 days following the operation.

Alterations occur in the response of the endocrine pancreas following elective operation. In general, insulin elaboration is diminished, and glucagon concentrations rise.[10,13] This response may be related to increased sympathetic activity or to the rise in levels of circulating epinephrine, which is known to suppress insulin release.[14] The increased elaboration of glucagon may be related to increased sympathetic nervous system stimulation or to alterations in circulating mediators. The rise in glucagon and the corresponding fall in insulin are a potent signal to accelerate hepatic glucose production, and, with other hormones (epinephrine and glucocorticoids), gluconeogenesis is maintained.

The postoperative hormonal responses are thought to orchestrate physiologic and biochemical changes that benefit the host. Salt and water conservation support the circulating blood volume. Augmented hepatic glucose production provides adequate essential fuel for the nervous system, red and white blood cells, and the healing wound. Skeletal muscle proteolysis provides amino acid precursors for gluconeogenesis and hepatic protein synthesis. Postoperative lipolysis provides abundant quantities of free fatty acid, as an additional energy source. Current techniques of postoperative care minimize, but do not reverse, these responses.

**Stage of Surgical Convalescence.** The period of catabolism initiated by operation, a combination of inadequate nutrition and alteration of the hormonal environment, has been termed the "adrenergic-corticoid phase."[8] This period is followed by the onset of anabolism, which occurs at a variable time in the patient's convalescence. In general, in the absence of postoperative complications, this phase starts 3 to 6 days after an abdominal operation of the magnitude of a colectomy or gastrectomy, often concomitant with the commencement of oral feedings. This "turning point" from catabolism to anabolism is referred to as the "corticoid-withdrawal phase" because it is characterized by a spontaneous sodium and free-water diuresis, a positive potassium balance, and a reduction in nitrogen excretion. This transitional phase usually lasts only 1 to 2 days.

The patient then enters a prolonged period of early anabolism characterized by positive nitrogen balance and weight gain. Protein synthesis is increased as a result of sustained enteral feedings, and this change is related to the return of lean body mass and muscular strength. The positive nitrogen balance is usually in the range of 2 to 4 g of nitrogen/day in the average adult, a range representing a daily gain of 60 to 120 g lean tissue. The total amount of nitrogen ultimately gained equals the amount lost, but the rate of gain is much slower than the rate of initial loss.

The fourth and final phase of surgical convalescence is late anabolism, the hallmark of which is much slower weight gain. During this period, the patient is in nitrogen equilibrium but in positive carbon balance, which results from the deposition of body fat.

**Usual Course: Case Example.** A 56-year-old, nonobese man is admitted to the hospital for a left colectomy for multiple polyps diagnosed following an episode of rectal bleeding. The patient has not lost weight and feels well. He has no significant history of other past illnesses, and all laboratory studies are within the normal range. His weight is 170 lb (77 kg), and his height is 5'9" [body surface area (BSA), 1.9 m$^2$]. He tolerates anesthesia and the operative procedure without complications.

Following the operation, the patient is hydrated with 5% dextrose, with appropriate electrolytes, at the rate of 125 ml/hour (3 L/day). His urine output on the first postoperative day is 1,200 ml, his nasogastric losses are 400 ml, and he gains 2 lb from fluid retention (Fig. 62–1). On the third postoperative day, the patient starts to diurese spontaneously and has a urine output of 2,800 ml. On the fifth postoperative day, the patient's nasogastric tube is removed, and he starts taking clear liquids. He is discharged from the hospital on the seventh day following the operation.

Nitrogen balance studies done from postoperative day 1 through postoperative day 5 show a cumulative 4-day negative nitrogen balance of 54 g. During this 5-day period, the patient had 0 nitrogen intake and approximately 600 kcal glu-

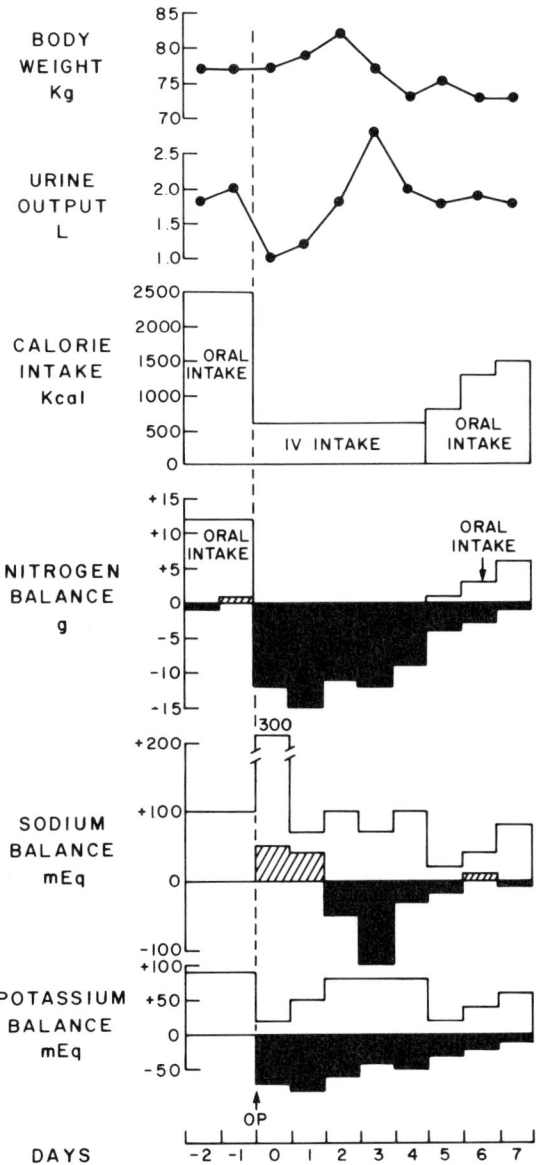

**Fig. 62–1.** The metabolic response of a previously healthy subject to an elective operative procedure. Intake is plotted upward from zero, output downward from the top of the intake line. Negative balance is represented by the solid black, with positive balance shaded.

cose/day. On the fifth postoperative day, he had lost approximately 5 lb, half of which was lean body tissue (50 g nitrogen* ≃ 300 protein ≃ 1,200 g lean body mass ≃ 2.5 lb) and half was body fat. On a follow-up 4 weeks later, he had returned to his usual weight.

---

*1 g nitrogen = 6.25 g protein; 1 g protein = 4 g lean body mass because tissue proteins exist in an aqueous state.

## Effects of Nutritional Support on Postoperative Metabolism

Early investigators who studied the catabolic responses to operation concluded that the negative nitrogen balance was "obligatory" and an irreversible consequence of the metabolic response to injury. This view was challenged by data from 2 studies in postoperative patients. Riegel and associates fed patients who had undergone gastrectomy and neurosurgical procedures with tube-feeding techniques and showed that nitrogen equilibrium could be achieved when 0.30 g nitrogen and 30 cal/kg were provided daily.[15] Subsequently, Holden and colleagues nutritionally supported gastrectomy patients in the early postoperative period with intravenous nutrients and noted that body weight was maintained and near nitrogen balance was achieved when adequate calories and nitrogen were administered. These investigators concluded that the catabolic response to operation is due in large part to inadequate food intake and is not an obligatory consequence of operative stress.[16]

The patient in the previous case example undergoes the same operation and has an identical postoperative course, except nutritional support is now provided in the postoperative period. He receives 3 L of a parenteral solution that delivers maintenance calories (2,200 kcal/day) and 12 g nitrogen/day as a balanced amino acid mixture.

Nitrogen balance studies show cumulative losses of 67 g from postoperative day 1 through postoperative day 5, so the patient's net balance for the 5 days equals −7 g. The patient has not lost weight during his hospital course (Fig. 62–2).

In general, if the patient is well nourished preoperatively and is expected to eat by the fifth to seventh postoperative day, 5% dextrose solutions will provide adequate calories to prevent detrimental losses of endogenous body protein. Although a balanced nutrient intake administered in the postoperative period reduces the brief negative nitrogen balance associated with elective surgery and may maintain body weight, such an approach appears to be unwarranted in most patients undergoing elective operation.[17,18] Such feedings have not improved recovery rates or diminished postoperative complications in this particular group; therefore, the increased cost of feedings and the potential complications associated with intravenous nutrition cannot be justified.

## Other Methods of Modifying Postoperative Responses

Attempts to modulate the physiologic and biochemical responses to an elective operative pro-

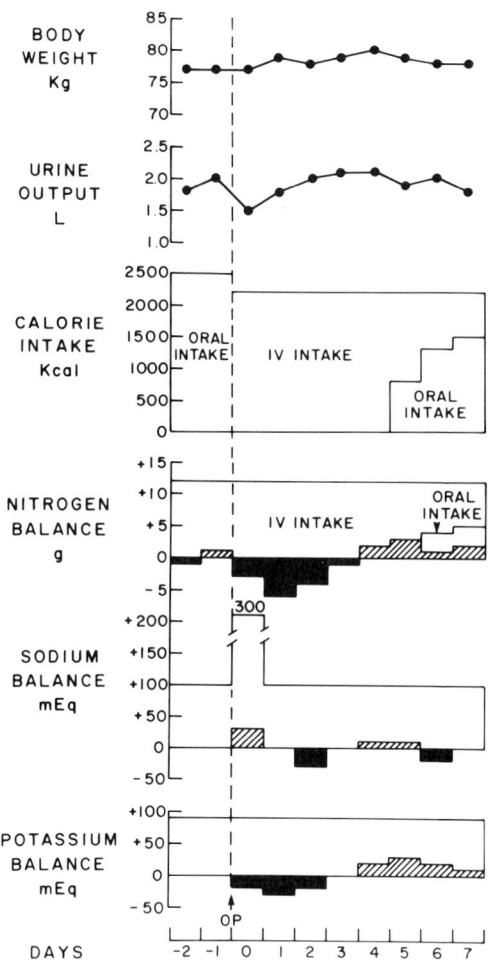

**Fig. 62–2.** The metabolic response to an elective operative procedure with constant intravenous nutrition.

cedure have been studied in an effort to reduce the magnitude of the stress of operations and to provide insight into mechanisms in these responses. To date, such modulation has altered efferent signals from the operative site, affected central (hypothalamic) integration of these signals, or used competitive blocking drugs to diminish the effects of adrenergic outflow.

**Afferent Blockade.** In a series of classic studies, Hume and Egdahl measured adrenal versus 17-hydroxycorticosteroids in experimental animals and demonstrated that adrenocorticoid secretion was not elicited after trauma to a denervated hindlimb.[19] The adrenocortical response to injury was not observed after transection of the peripheral nerve to the area of trauma, transection of the spinal cord above the injury, or section through the medulla oblongata. Other studies showed that the post-traumatic rise in ACTH could be abolished in animals subjected to standard operative

trauma with previously placed electrical lesions in the anterior medial eminence or following hypophysectomy.

A variety of human studies have shown that many postoperative responses can be ablated following denervation of the wound. Kehlet and colleagues used epidural or spinal anesthesia in women undergoing elective abdominal hysterectomy.[20] With epidural anesthesia extending from S5 to T4, plasma concentrations of cortisol, aldosterone, glucose, and free fatty acids remained normal, in contrast to increased concentrations in patients receiving general anesthesia alone. Other workers have extended these observations and have reported that low spinal anesthesia blocks the elevation of catecholamines, hyperglycemia, and inhibition of insulin release observed in patients undergoing surgical procedures on the lower half of the body.[21] These effects are not solely the consequence of reduced postoperative pain because these stress responses occur in pain-free patients without neuromuscular blockade.[20] These observations suggest that regional anesthetic techniques block afferent signals from the wound and interrupt sympathetic nervous efferent signals to the adrenal gland and possibly the liver. The effect of sympathetic blockade is a reduction in the apparent magnitude of the stress response.

These techniques have also been used during the postoperative period. Bromage and colleagues suppressed hyperglycemia and hypercortisolism with maintenance of an epidural anesthetic for the first 24 hours after operation.[22] Brandt and associates reported improved 5-day cumulative nitrogen balance in patients undergoing elective abdominal hysterectomy with epidural anesthesia, as compared to a similar group receiving general anesthesia.[23]

**Sympathetic Blockade.** Several investigators have studied stress responses in sympathectomized animals by blocking the efferent limb of the neuroendocrine reflex response. Although improved survival rates have been reported in sympathectomized dogs following hemorrhagic hypotension,[24] other investigators have reported a 100% mortality rate in cold-exposed animals given beta blockers.[25] These disparate results complicate the rationale for this approach in humans.

The effects of beta-adrenergic blockade on the metabolic response to surgery have also been studied in patients undergoing elective operative procedures. Cooper and associates studied the effects of intravenous propranolol (0.15 mg/kg body weight) and noted only a lower insulin concentration.[26] On the other hand, Tsuji and associates administered a higher dose of propranolol (0.30

mg/kg body weight) and noted inhibition of the usual elevations of glucose, lactate, and nonesterified fatty acids.[27]

**Central Blockade.** Brandt and colleagues reported that large doses of morphine (4 mg/kg) given prior to skin incision diminished the normal rise in plasma ACTH, cortisol, growth hormone, and glucose in patients undergoing aortic valve replacement.[28] These reports indicate that central nervous system blockade interrupts afferent signals stimulated by operative procedures.

## Malnourished Patient: Role of Preoperative Feeding

Nutritional support is a primary therapy for patients who develop malnutrition secondary to intestinal disease such as enterocutaneous fistulas, short bowel syndrome, inflammatory bowel disease with systemic sepsis, or slow-growing malignant tumors associated with oropharyngeal or esophageal obstruction. Patients with these disease processes, with greater than 10% weight loss, and requiring an operative procedure should be considered candidates for preoperative nutritional support. These patients are usually normometabolic and gain weight when provided with adequate calories and nitrogen. With weight gain and anabolism, they become better surgical candidates. Both past and recent investigations serve as the basis for this conclusion. In 1936, Studley reported that postoperative mortality rates increased in patients with duodenal ulcer disease when weight loss exceeded 20%.[29] Recent prospective studies have shown that adequate preoperative nutrition reduces postoperative morbidity and mortality rates in selected patients. Daly and colleagues reviewed operative therapy in 244 patients with esophageal cancer, some of whom received preoperative parenteral nutrition.[30] Those patients who received at least 5 days of preoperative parenteral nutrition lost less weight during treatment (3 versus 11 lb) and had fewer overall major postoperative complications (24 versus 41%). Significant reductions in major wound infections and other postoperative complications were noted in these patients, as compared with those who received only postoperative nutrition or no perioperative nutritional support.

Müller and associates studied 160 patients with cancer of the gastrointestinal tract who were matched for nutritional status and tumor site and who were then randomized to receive either free oral diet or the oral diet plus 10 days of preoperative parenteral nutrition.[31] Patients who received intravenous preoperative feedings had a reduced incidence of major postoperative complications (17 versus 32%). Furthermore, the mortality rate in the unfed group was more than 3 times that observed in the fed group (18 versus 5%).

Rombeau and colleagues suggested, from a retrospective analysis, that preoperative parenteral nutrition was beneficial in patients requiring operation for inflammatory bowel disease.[32] Patients who received preoperative parenteral nutrition for at least 5 days had fewer postoperative complications than patients who were fed for fewer than 5 days. All patients with postoperative complications had either a preoperative serum albumin concentration of less than 3.5 g/dl or a serum transferrin concentration less than 150 mg/dl. Other investigators have suggested that these laboratory indices reflect preoperative nutritional status.[33]

The specific mechanisms by which preoperative feedings produce clinical benefit are unknown. Nutritional deficits are not entirely replenished with 5 to 10 days of preoperative feeding. Such therapy may replete hepatic glycogen stores and the "labile" amino acid pool, however, and may thus aid liver function.[34] Enzyme induction may occur, and hormonal responses may be stimulated. Host defense mechanisms may also be restored, but none of these factors have clearly been linked to improved outcome of the nutritionally depleted patient undergoing operation.

## Indications for Postoperative Feedings

**Complications Following Operation in the Well-Nourished Patient.** In a small percentage of healthy patients undergoing elective operative procedures, complications preclude the use of the gastrointestinal tract.

One common complication is prolonged postoperative ileus. Despite enemas and ambulation, the absence of peristalsis persists, and nasogastric tube losses occur. If the ileus continues for more than 5 to 7 days, intravenous feedings, usually by a peripheral vein, should be initiated.

More frequently, ileus is the hallmark of an intra-abdominal inflammatory process, be it secondary to infection, pancreatitis, or active inflammatory bowel disease. Unlike the unstressed postoperative patient with simple ileus, these individuals are often febrile and hypermetabolic. In conjunction with appropriate treatment of the intra-abdominal process, nutritional support should be instituted; the nutritional goal is maintenance of body weight and protein stores and provision of adequate quantities of vitamins and micronutrients. The insertion of a central venous catheter for the delivery of hypertonic nutrient solutions provides 2,200 to 2,500 kcal and 14 to

17 g nitrogen/day with a calorie-to-nutrition ratio of approximately 150:1.

When an intra-abdominal abscess develops, drainage is required. When an abscess is associated with a gastrointestinal anastomosis, the formation of an enterocutaneous fistula may occur. Adequate nutritional care, coupled with prompt surgical care (drainage) and appropriate antibiotics, has reduced the mortality rate from this complication from 40 to 60% to as low as 6%.[35]

**High-Risk Surgical Patients.** Only an occasional previously healthy patient undergoing elective operation develops complications and subsequently requires nutritional support. The majority of surgical patients requiring nutritional support are individuals at increased operative risk. Many of these patients are malnourished; preoperative nutritional support should be a major objective. Other high-risk patients are those with diabetes, cirrhosis, heart disease, renal failure, marked obesity, or those known to abuse drugs or alcohol. In addition, immunocompromised patients should be carefully evaluated, and their nutritional deficits should be restored before operation.

A major complication of the high-risk patient is wound dehiscence.[36] This separation of the wound is most spectacular when it occurs following laparotomy. When abdominal evisceration occurs, the patient should be taken to the operating room, and the wound should be debrided and approximated. Because wound disruption is frequently associated with infection and results in a massive inflammatory reaction, calorie and nitrogen demands increase and should be provided by intravenous feedings.

When acute renal failure follows a major operation, the kidneys are unable to excrete waste solute (nitrogen) or solvent, although occasionally, polyuric renal failure occurs. Provision of the usual amounts of amino acids in the diet exacerbates the already elevated level of blood urea nitrogen. In these patients, adequate calories should be provided to minimize protein breakdown, and nitrogen intake should be restricted if the patient does not require hemodialysis.[37] Levels of potassium, magnesium, and zinc are monitored frequently, and these elements are administered with caution.

A special solution of essential amino acids (Nephramine) may improve protein synthesis and may reduce urea generation.[37] These amino acids are mixed with a 50 to 70% dextrose solution, to minimize fluid intake. This mixture is administered through central venous catheters. This renal failure formula has been evaluated in patients with postoperative acute renal failure. Abel and

associates reported that such parenteral nutrition improved survival rates and diminished renal dysfunction in patients with acute renal failure following aortic aneurysmectomy.[38] In this prospective, randomized, double-blind trial, patients given glucose and essential amino acids had a better chance of surviving acute renal failure than those receiving only glucose (75 versus 44%; p = 0.02). Because patients were carefully selected for entry into this study, these results may only be applicable to a select group of individuals with postoperative acute renal failure. Other studies generally support the conclusions of Abel and colleagues, however[37] (see also Chap. 58).

Hepatic failure occurs most commonly in the alcoholic cirrhotic patient who has a major gastrointestinal hemorrhage that requires operative intervention. Although the origin of hepatic encephalopathy is unknown, central nervous system function may be influenced by circulating levels of amino acids.[39] The branched-chain amino acids (leucine, isoleucine, and valine) circulate at unusually low levels in patients with liver failure, whereas levels of the aromatic amino acids (phenylalanine, tyrosine, and tryptophan) are elevated. The hypothesis states that branched-chain amino acids compete with neutral amino acids for uptake across the blood-brain barrier. Because of the low blood levels of the branched-chain amino acids, uptake of several of the amino acids that serve as precursors for the synthesis of false neurotransmitters may be increased. Correction of the abnormalities in plasma amino acid levels should improve outcome, and some investigators have reported improvement of hepatic coma following treatment with solutions high in branched-chain and low in aromatic amino acids.[40] This therapeutic effect has not consistently been observed,[41] and appropriate nutritional therapy for encephalopathic patients is currently under investigation (see also Chaps. 56E, 65, 67).

## Nutritional Support of Elective Surgical Patients

**Nutritional Assessment.** The two major objectives of nutritional assessment are: (1) to determine the patient's nutritional status; and (2) to determine energy, protein, and macro- and micronutrient requirements.

The nutritional status of a patient is determined by a careful history and physical examination, followed by additional tests to confirm the clinical impression. The medical history should include inquiries about associated disease processes, medication, and history of weight loss and dietary habits. The physical examination may establish the diagnosis of cachexia, protein-energy malnutrition, or specific nutrient deficiencies. Weight loss greater than 10% of the patient's weight before illness may compromise the patient's ability to combat infection or to heal wounds.

Anthropometric measurements include measurement of body weight and height. The features are compared with population norms.[42] Measurements of skinfold thickness are helpful to determine fat mass,[43] and a 24-hour urine collection with measurement of creatine allows determination of the creatinine-height index (CHI), a factor proportional to the size of muscle mass.[43] More sophisticated techniques to determine body composition include isotopic dilution methods, underwater weighing, total-body computerized axial tomography, and gamma-neutron activation; these methods are not generally practical in the routine screening of most elective surgical patients. A detailed evaluation of assessment procedures is given in Chapter 45.

Immunologic status had recently been used to evaluate nutritional status; total peripheral lymphocyte count, delayed hypersensitivity using a skin-test response to common antigens, and lymphocyte transformation have all been used as indicators of immunocompetence in the critically ill patient.[44] The depressed immune function often returns to normal with nutritional repletion, but altered immunologic responses are not specific for nutritional deficiencies and are observed in patients with advanced malignant disease or in those who have had a severe injury. Moreover, delayed hypersensitivity may return on resolution of the disease process, despite inadequate nutrient intake.

Laboratory tests are useful to confirm the clinical suspicion of malnutrition. Serum albumin and transferrin are the most common serum proteins measured, and they correlate well with body protein deficiency in isolated cases of malnutrition. Most nutritional deficits in surgical patients are secondary to a disease process, however, and the presence of an inflammatory or neoplastic process may alter these indicators. Other laboratory studies that may be useful in nutritional assessment include red blood cell indices to determine iron and micronutrient deficiencies, plasma glucose to assess insulin resistance, blood urea nitrogen to determine renal status, and liver function tests to evaluate hepatic function.

**Determining Nutritional Requirements.** Nutritional therapy should be directed to a specific goal; depending on the patient's nutritional status, this goal should be: (1) to diminish the rate of weight loss and body protein breakdown; (2) to maintain body weight and protein stores; and (3) to achieve weight gain and anabolism. In general,

patients with a normal body composition (no major nutritional deficiencies) and who are not hypercatabolic do not develop significant nutritional deficits during 5 to 7 days of undernutrition. For example, the uncomplicated postoperative patient may receive intravenous infusions of 5% dextrose in water or inadequate oral intake for this period of time without any detrimental effect on recovery or ultimate health. The malnourished patient who has lost greater than 10% of normal preillness weight requires vigorous nutritional support, however. The immediate goal in such an individual is nutritional maintenance, whereas the ultimate goal is restoration of body mass, which generally occurs in the later phases of surgical convalescence.

Total energy requirements are based on several factors: (1) the basal metabolic rate; (2) the degree of stress imposed by the disease process; and (3) the amount of energy expended with activity. Available nomograms relate normal metabolic requirements to a person's age, sex, height, and weight.[42] Once basal metabolic requirements of the nonstressed individual have been determined, additional factors such as the stress of the disease and hospital activity should be considered. These relationships are expressed in Table 62–1.

The principal influences on nitrogen balance in surgical patients are total energy intake, nitrogen intake, and the metabolic state of the patient. Energy and nitrogen relationships are altered in nutritionally depleted and hypermetabolic patients. Persons with nutritional deficits have intact protein-conserving mechanisms that allow nitrogen equilibrium when 7 to 8% of the total caloric needs are provided as protein. This translates into a calorie-to-nitrogen ratio of approximately 350:1. Hypermetabolic, catabolic patients, on the other hand, have a diminished protein economy and require much more protein. For example, Duke and associates showed that, in injured patients, protein contributes 15 to 20% of the total energy expenditure, such that the optimal calorie-to-nitrogen ratio is approximately 150:1.[45]

The provision of more protein to yield a calorie-to-nitrogen ratio of 100 to 150:1 may improve nitrogen balance, but such enthusiastic protein loading may result in an elevated blood urea nitrogen level. Electrolytes, vitamins, and other essential nutrients should be added to the patient's diet as required.

**Routes of Feeding.** Enteral or intravenous feedings are prescribed, depending on the patient's conditions.

*Enteral Feedings.* For patients who can eat and who have a functional gastrointestinal tract, adequate nutrition can best be provided by the regular

**Table 62–1.   Formulas for Determinations of Total Energy Requirements**

Daily Energy Requirement for Weight Maintenance =
Normal BMR[a] × Stress Factor[b] × 1.25[c]

Daily Energy Requirement for Weight Gain =
Maintenance Energy + 1,000 kcal[d]

[a]Normal BMR (basal metabolic rate, usually 1,500 to 1,800 kcal/day) can be determined using standard nomograms or formulas.[42] The approximate values of the basal metabolic rate for adults of average size are given below:

| Body Weight (kg) | 50 | 55 | 60 | 65 | 70 | 75 | 80 |
|---|---|---|---|---|---|---|---|
| Normal BMR (kcal/day) | 1,316 | 1,411 | 1,509 | 1,602 | 1,694 | 1,784 | 1,872 |

[b]Stress factor is the term used to correct the normal BMR for the effects of a disease process:

| Condition | Stress Factor |
|---|---|
| Mild starvation | 0.85–1.00 |
| Postoperative recovery (no complications) | 1.00–1.05 |
| Cancer* | 1.10–1.45 |
| Long-bone fracture | 1.25–1.30 |
| Peritonitis | 1.05–1.25 |
| Severe infection of multiple trauma* | 1.30–1.55 |
| Burns >40% body surface area | 2.0 |

*Proportional to the extent of the disease.

[c]The basal caloric requirements of the stressed patient are adjusted upward an additional 20 to 25% for hospital activity and the stress associated with treatment. This adjustment is unnecessary for patients receiving artificial ventilation who are paralzyed or are heavily sedated.

[d]If anabolism and weight gain are the goals, an additional 1,000 kcal/day may be added to maintenance requirements to provide for a weight gain of approximately 1 kg (2 lb)/week. Weight maintenance, not weight gain, should be the primary objective in most critically ill patients.

hospital diet. This diet may be supplemented with between-meal snacks if necessary. Daily calorie counts and body weight determinations are necessary to monitor intake and the response to therapy.

Some patients with a functional intestinal tract will not or cannot eat. Such patients include neurosurgical patients, those with oropharyngeal or esophageal obstruction, the elderly, and small children. In these patients, nasogastric or nasojejunal feedings may be indicated. Gastric feedings can be delivered 5 to 6 times daily by bolus feedings. Jejunal feedings require continuous administration. When permanent feedings are anticipated, a gastrostomy or feeding jejunostomy should be considered.[46] A variety of nutrient formulas are now available for enteral feedings. In general, intact or partially hydrolyzed nutrients are most appropriate. These diets should be nutritionally complete and free of lactose (see Chap. 54).

*Intravenous Feedings.* Frequently, surgical patients require nutritional support, but have a diseased or nonfunctional gastrointestinal tract. These persons are candidates for parenteral nutrition, which can be infused through a peripheral or central vein. Peripheral venous feedings provide dilute nutrients in a large fluid volume and rely on fat emulsions as a principal calorie source.

Central venous feedings consist of hypertonic glucose and amino acid solutions infused through a catheter placed in the superior vena cava. Ade-

quate calories can be administered in a small fluid volume, but this method of feeding requires placement and care of a central venous catheter (see Chap. 54).

**Formulating a Nutrition Support Plan.** Most patients undergoing elective operative procedures recover quickly, resume oral feedings early in the postoperative period, and require no specialized nutritional support. Other surgical patients do not fit this description and require formal nutritional care. This group includes patients with preoperative malnutrition, those with dysfunctional gastrointestinal tracts (prolonged ileus, inflammatory bowel disease), or those with specific diseases associated with a catabolic course (severe infection, major injury). These patients generally fall into one of three categories. In normally nourished patients, the nutritional goal is to maintain body weight and protein stores. In malnourished, nonstressed patients, weight gain and repletion of lean body tissue are indicated and are usually accomplished by providing an extra 1,000 cal/day. Anabolism is difficult to achieve in stressed catabolic patients, but body mass is generally restored simultaneously on resolution of the disease process. Hence, the nutritional goal in these patients is weight maintenance and treatment of the underlying disease process.

## TRAUMA

Accidental injury is a major cause of death and disability and is the leading cause of death in persons between 5 and 35 years of age in the United States.[47] Although trauma may affect persons of all ages, young, healthy, and potentially productive individuals are most commonly injured. Optimal care of the injured patient is often intensive and prolonged; survival may be followed by years of rehabilitation. Metabolic and nutritional support of the injured patient is a major component of overall care and is the focus of this section.

## Usual Response to Moderate Injury

**General Overview and Time Course.** Accidental injury is followed by a well-described pattern of physiologic responses. The events are generally related to the severity of injury; that is, the greater the insult, the more pronounced the specific response (Fig. 62–3). Although alterations following injury were first described in the 1860s, not until the 1930s were changes in injured humans carefully studied and an integrated response pattern described. David Patton Cuthbertson studied patients with long-bone fractures. He noticed that these patients lost large quantities of nitrogen, potassium, and phosphorus in their urine following injury, and this accelerated excretion rate could not be reversed by vigorous oral feedings.[48] Cuthbertson noted that the injured patient's oxygen consumption gradually rose, with simultaneous elevation in body temperature. Because no apparent site of infection was identified, this febrile response was referred to as "post-traumatic fever." Cuthbertson described the time course for many of the post-traumatic responses, and two distinct periods were identified, an early "ebb phase" and a subsequent "flow phase."[49] The ebb or shock phase was usually brief in duration (12 to 24 hours) and occurred immediately following injury. Blood pressure, cardiac output, body temperature, and oxygen consumption were reduced. These events were often associated with hemorrhage and resulted in hypoperfusion and lactic acidosis. With restoration of blood volume, ebb-phase alterations gave way to more accelerated responses. The flow phase was then characterized by hypermetabolism, increased cardiac output, increased urinary nitrogen losses, altered glucose metabolism, and accelerated tissue catabolism (Table 62–2).

The flow-phase responses to accidental injury are similar to those seen following elective operation. The response to injury is usually much more intensive and extends over a long period of time, however. For example, following soft tissue injury, patients often have an impaired ability to excrete a water load because of the heightened elaboration of aldosterone and ADH. The retention of large quantities of sodium and water that may occur during fluid resuscitation results in a dramatic increase in body weight, which may rise 10 to 20% over the patient's weight before injury.[8]

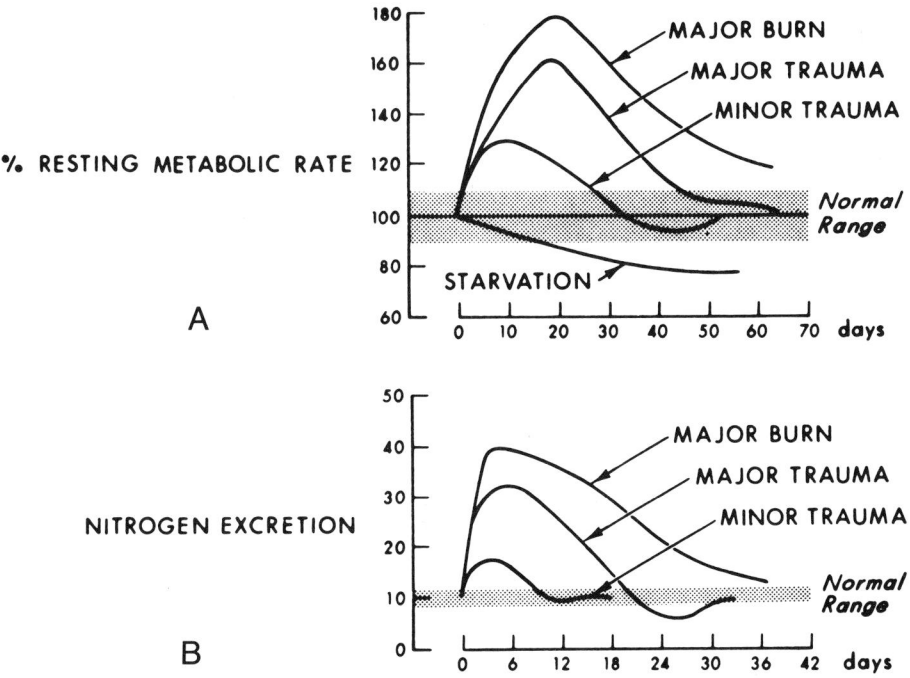

**Fig. 62–3.** Metabolic rate (*A*) and nitrogen excretion (*B*) are related to the extent of injury. The 2 responses generally parallel each other. Patients received 12 g nitrogen/day. (From Wilmore, D.W.[42])

**Table 62–2.  Metabolic Alterations Following Injury**

| Ebb Phase | Flow Phase |
|---|---|
| Blood glucose elevated | Glucose normal or slightly elevated |
| Normal glucose production | Increased glucose production |
| Free fatty acids elevated | Free fatty acids normal or slightly elevated; flux increased |
| Insulin concentration low | Insulin concentration normal or elevated |
| Catecholamines and glucagon elevated | Catecholamines high normal or elevated; glucagon elevated |
| Blood lactate elevated | Blood lactate normal |
| Oxygen consumption depressed | Oxygen consumption elevated |
| Cardiac output below normal | Cardiac output increased |
| Core temperature below normal | Core temperature elevated |

During recovery, the edema fluid reenters the vascular compartment, and the salt and water load is gradually excreted by the kidneys. Although sodium and water retention may occur following elective operation, the magnitude is much less great, and subsequent events (fluid mobilization followed by volume expansion and diuresis) are much less dramatic than in injured patients.

**Characteristics of the Flow Phase of the Injury Response.** This phase is characterized by hypermetabolism and by alterations in the metabolism of glucose, protein, and fat.

*Hypermetabolism.* Hypermetabolism is defined as an increase in basal metabolic rate (BMR) above that predicted on the basis of age, sex, and body size. Metabolic rate is usually determined by measuring the exchange of respiratory gases and by calculating heat production from oxygen consumption and carbon dioxide production (see Chap. 28). The degree of hypermetabolism (increased oxygen production) is generally related to the severity of the injury. Patients with long-bone fractures have a 15 to 25% increase in metabolic rate, whereas the metabolic needs of patients with multiple injuries increase by 50%. Patients with severe burn injury (greater than 50% of BSA) have resting metabolic rates that may reach twice basal levels.[42] These rates of heat production in trauma patients are contrasted with those in postoperative patients, who rarely increase their BMR by more than 10 to 15% following operation.

Concomitant with the development of hypermetabolism, the trauma patient usually develops a 1 to 2° C elevation in body temperature. This post-traumatic fever is a well-recognized component of the injury response and represents an upward shift in the thermoregulatory set point of the brain.[50] In general, if this febrile response is not marked (38.5° C) and if the patient is asymptomatic, the fever will rarely be treated.

*Altered Glucose Metabolism.* Hyperglycemia commonly occurs following injury, and the elevation of fasting blood sugar levels generally parellels the severity of stress in the ebb phase. At that time, insulin levels are low, and glucose production is only slightly elevated.[51] Later, during the flow phase, insulin concentrations are normal or elevated; yet, hyperglycemia persists. This phenomenon suggests an alteration in the relationship between insulin sensitivity and glucose disposal. Hepatic glucose production is increased,[52] and the accelerated gluconeogenesis is generally related to the extent of the injury. Studies in injured patients show that much of the new glucose generated by the liver arises from 3-carbon precursors (lactate, pyruvate, amino acids, and glycerol) released from peripheral tissues[52] (Fig. 62–4).

To determine which peripheral tissues use the large quantity of glucose produced by the liver, investigators measured substrate exchange across injured and uninjured extremities of severely burned patients matched for age, weight, and extent of total-body-surface burn.[53] That net glucose flux across uninjured extremities was low suggests that fat, not glucose, is the primary fuel for resting skeletal muscle in the postabsorptive state. Similar observations have been made in a study of normal volunteers; however, glucose uptake was increased across the burned extremity. In addition, the injured extremity released large quantities of lactate, which accounted for as much as 80% of the glucose consumed. This finding is consistent with our knowledge of the biochemistry of the specialized cells of the wound and inflammatory tissue (fibroblasts, macrophages, leukocytes), which undergo anaerobic metabolism and have a large capacity for lactate production. Additional measurements of blood flow and substrate concentration differences across the kidney and brain further characterize the glucose disposal in stable trauma patients.[53,54] The glucose

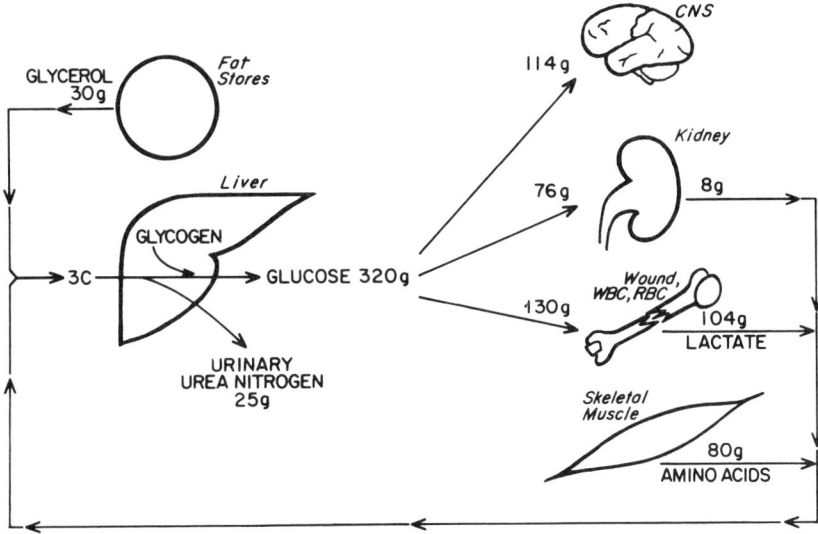

**Fig. 62–4.** The 24-hour flux of glucose and glucose (3-carbon) precursors following severe injury. (From Wilmore, D.W., Black, P.R., Muhlbacher, F.: Nutritional Support of the Seriously Ill Patient. New York, Academic Press, p. 44, 1983.)

consumed by the central nervous system in the injured patient is approximately normal (120 g/day) whereas that consumed by the kidney is approximately twice normal (75 g/day). Only a small fraction of the glucose is taken up by the resting skeletal muscle, and the remainder is consumed by the wound (Fig. 62–4). The wound converts most of the glucose to lactate, which is recycled to the liver in the Cori cycle.

These alterations in glucose metabolism have a profound impact on the handling of exogenously administered glucose contained in enteral or parenteral feedings. To characterize glucose disposal during the flow phase of injury, 6 traumatized patients who did not have sepsis were studied by means of the hyperglycemic glucose "clamp" technique for 5 to 10 days after the injury. The results were compared with 11 age-matched control subjects.[55] After an overnight fast, a 20% glucose solution was infused intravenously to elevate plasma glucose concentrations suddenly 125 mg/dl above basal levels. This elevation was maintained for 2 hours with bedside glucose monitoring and negative feedback servocontrol. The results showed a progressive increase in glucose disposal with time in normal control subjects, whereas the injured patients maintained a constant glucose disposal throughout the study (Fig. 62–5). Moreover, the quantity of insulin elaborated by the patients was greater than in control subjects; nonetheless, these rising insulin concentrations failed to increase glucose clearance in these patients.

Other studies have demonstrated a failure to suppress hepatic glucose production in trauma patients during glucose loading or insulin infusion.[55,56] Either of these perturbations usually inhibits hepatic glucose production in normal subjects. Wolfe and colleagues, using tracer methods, found that endogenous suppression comprised only 73% of the infused glucose load in burn patients (2.6 mg/kg/min).[57] This rate of glucose infusion completely suppresses glucose production in normal subjects. When investigators used the hyperglycemic glucose "clamp" technique combined with tracer methods, endogenous glucose production was only partially reduced in trauma patients, in spite of high concentrations of both glucose and insulin.[55]

To quantitate the extent of insulin resistance in peripheral tissues, Brooks and associates measured glucose uptake across the uninjured forearm in conjunction with hyperinsulinemic-euglycemic clamp studies in 11 normal subjects and 5 patients with multiple trauma.[58] Glucose uptake by uninjured forearm skeletal muscle of trauma patients was much less than that observed in control subjects (Fig. 62–6).

Thus, profound insulin insensitivity occurs in injured patients. Direct measurements show that liver and skeletal muscle are resistant tissues, and studies by Carpentier and associates suggest that lipolysis is not attenuated in trauma patients after glucose administration.[59] The cause of this marked insensitivity to insulin is unknown; however, similar effects are observed following alterations in the hormonal environment. For example, insulin-mediated forearm glucose uptake is

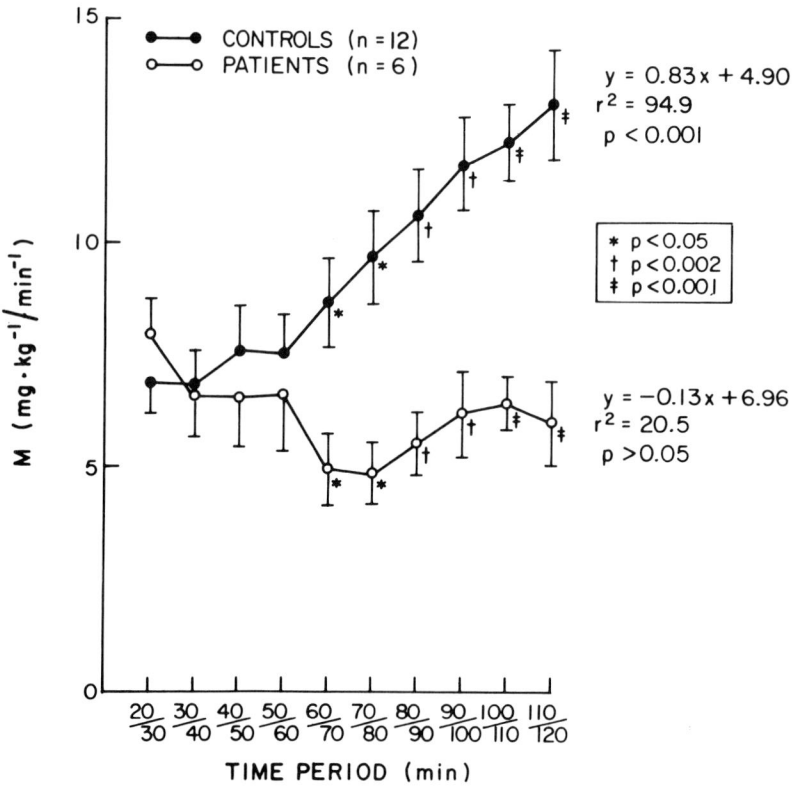

**Fig. 62–5.** With time, the rate of glucose disposal (M) progressively increases in the control subjects during the hyperglycemic glucose clamp. In contrast, glucose removal was constant in the patients over the 2 hours of study and averaged approximately 7 mg/kg/min. (From Black, P.R., Brooks, D.C., Bessey, P.Q., et al.[55])

diminished in normal subjects following 2 hours of epinephrine infusion.[60] Similarly, 3 days of glucocorticoid administration will decrease glucose consumption.[61]

*Alterations in Protein Metabolism.* Extensive urinary nitrogen loss occurs following major injury. Because of the magnitude of these losses and the progressive wasting of skeletal muscle mass and associated muscle weakness, it was originally hypothesized that the nitrogen loss represented a generalized and accelerated breakdown of muscle protein. Like other responses, the loss of nitrogen following injury is related to the extent of the trauma, but it also depends on the previous nutritional status, as well as the age and sex, of the patient, because these factors determine, in part, the size of muscle mass.

Although nitrogen balance studies demonstrate marked negative nitrogen balance following injury, these studies reflect only net nitrogen catabolism, not the absolute rate of nitrogen breakdown. In normal subjects, nitrogen equilibrium is maintained by a careful balance between rates of protein synthesis and rates of degradation. Negative nitrogen balance will occur if the breakdown

rate increases and protein synthesis remains the same, or if the breakdown rate remains the same and the rate of synthesis decreases. The use of isotopically labeled, nonradioactive amino acids allows quantification of the alterations in synthesis and breakdown rates associated with many disease processes.

Herrmann and associates administered [15]N glycine to achieve a steady state and measured [15]N urea nitrogen enrichment using the two-pool model of Picou and Taylor-Roberts.[62,63] Turnover rates of protein were measured, and rates of synthesis and catabolism were calculated in fed and fasted states in normal subjects. During feeding, synthesis and catabolism were equal, and the subjects maintained nitrogen equilibrium. Restriction of food intake caused a marked reduction in synthesis, with minimal impact on rates of protein catabolism.

Birkhahn and associates described protein kinetics in 4 patients following multisystemic injury, including long-bone fractures.[64] In contrast to patients undergoing elective orthopedic operations, these patients had a marked increase in catabolic rate and a slight increase in synthesis;

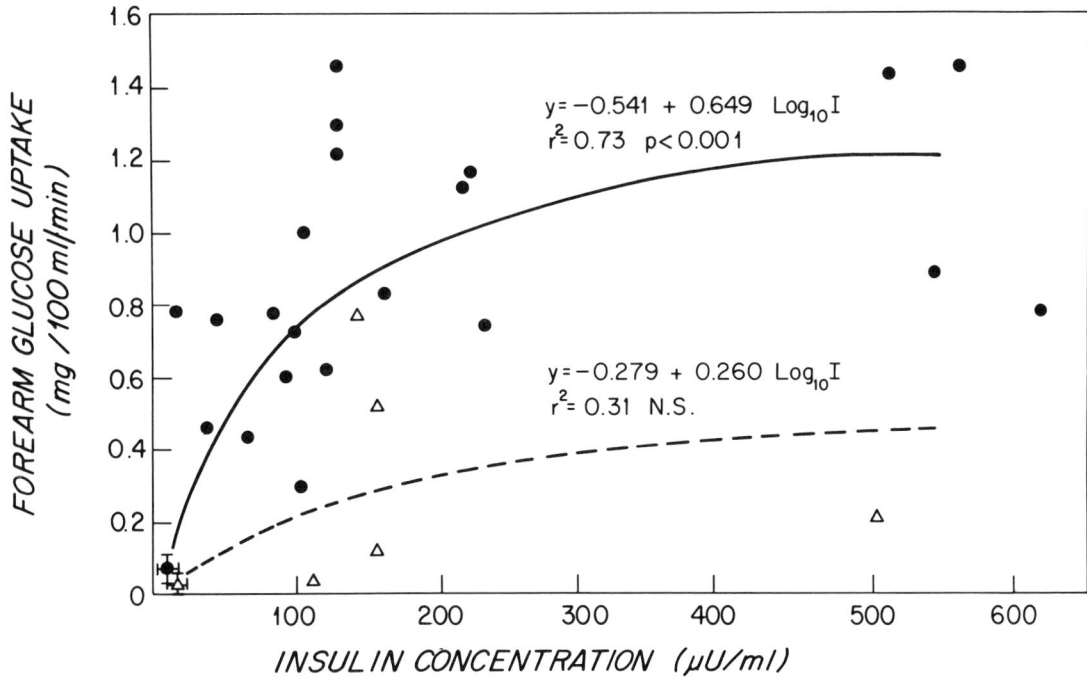

**Fig. 62–6.** Dose-response curves of forearm glucose uptake of various plasma insulin concentrations achieved during insulin infusion and euglycemia. The dose-response curves differ by co-variant analysis. Circles indicate control subjects,·and triangles represent patients. (From Brooks, D.C., Bessey, P.Q., Black, P.R., et al.[58])

because catabolism exceeded synthesis, the patients were in marked negative nitrogen balance while receiving standard infusions of 5% dextrose and water.

Thus, trauma accelerates nitrogen turnover. In unfed patients, breakdown rates exceed synthesis, and negative balance results. Providing exogenous calories and nitrogen increases synthesis, and, when adequate nutrients are provided, the two rates are matched, and nitrogen balance is maintained (Table 62–3).

That muscle is the origin of the nitrogen that is

lost in the urine following extensive injury was initially suggested by Cuthbertson.[48] In his patients with long-bone fractures, he suggested that this reaction was a uniform response of the entire muscle mass, and nitrogen was not lost solely from damaged muscle at the site of injury. This concept has been supported by a variety of studies that measured important markers of muscle catabolism, such as creatinine, creatine, zinc, and 3-methylhistidine.[65] Further evidence of net skeletal muscle breakdown has been demonstrated by quantification of the loss of amino acids from extremities of severely injured patients. Aulick and Wilmore used plethysmographic techniques to measure leg blood flow and simultaneously to determine arterial and femoral venous amino acid concentrations in traumatized patients.[66] They found a three- to fourfold increase in amino acid flux from the extremities of injured patients over that of normal subjects. Alanine efflux was the most highly elevated of the amino acids measured; glutamine was not measured. The increase in alanine release from the legs of the severely traumatized patients was generally related to the extent of injury and the oxygen consumption of the patient, but it was not related to the size of the limb injury or to blood flow in the leg. The accelerated rate of alpha-amino nitrogen release from the limbs of these patients appeared

**Table 62–3.   Alterations in Rates of Protein Synthesis and Catabolism that May Affect Hospitalized Patients**

|  | Synthesis* | Catabolism* |
|---|---|---|
| Normal: patient starved | ↓ | ○ |
| Normal: patient fed, during bedrest | ↓ | ○ |
| Elective surgical procedure | ↓ | ○ |
| Injury/sepsis: patient receiving intravenous Dextrose | ↑ ↑ | ↑ ↑ ↑ |
| Injury/sepsis: patient fed | ↑ ↑ ↑ | ↑ ↑ ↑ |

* ↓ = decrease; ○ = no change; ↑ = increase.

to be a generalized catabolic effect of injury, rather than a response to local inflammatory or metabolic events in the injured extremities. This response may be the result of chronic hypercortisolism, which occurs in injury.

Using dogs catheterized on a long-term basis to study hindquarter amino acid metabolism, Muhlbacher and colleagues observed that the long-term administration of dexamethasone (a potent glucocorticoid) resulted in a fourfold increase in glutamine and alanine release from skeletal muscle.[67] Although glutamine stores in muscle were reduced by 50% within 10 to 14 days, the accelerated glutamine release was exceeded by an accelerated consumption of this amino acid, and plasma glutamine levels fell by 30%.

Although it is now recognized that amino acids are released by muscle in increased quantities following injury, it has only recently been appreciated that the composition of amino acid efflux does not reflect the composition of muscle protein. Alanine and glutamine comprise 50 to 60% of amino acids released, whereas each makes up only about 6% of muscle protein. The branched-chain amino acids (valine, leucine, and isoleucine), on the other hand, make up approximately 6% of the released amino acids, but constitute nearly 15% of muscle protein. To explain these observations, Goldberg and Chang proposed that the branched-chain amino acids serve as amino donors for alpha-ketoglutarate, yielding the corresponding branched-chain ketoacids and glutamate.[68] The ketoacids can be converted to tricarboxylic-cycle intermediates in skeletal muscle, or they can be exported through the circulation. Glutamate may be a precursor for glutamine synthesis or an amino donor for alanine synthesis. These coupled reactions could explain the synthesis and increased release of alanine and glutamine as well as the diminished release of branched-chain amino acids (Fig. 62–7). Oxidation of branched-chain amino acids by skeletal muscle is accelerated following injury,[69] and skeletal muscle release of glutamine and alanine is increased.

Glutamine is also extracted by the kidney, where it contributes ammonium groups for ammonia generation, a process that excretes acid loads.[70] This effect can be augmented in the dog by the administration of glucocorticoids. Glutamine is taken up by the gastrointestinal tract and serves as an oxidative fuel.[71] The gut enterocytes convert glutamine primarily to ammonia and alanine, and these two substances are released into the portal venous blood. This ammonia is then removed by the liver and is converted to urea; the alanine may also be removed by the liver and may serve as a gluconeogenic precursor. Follow-

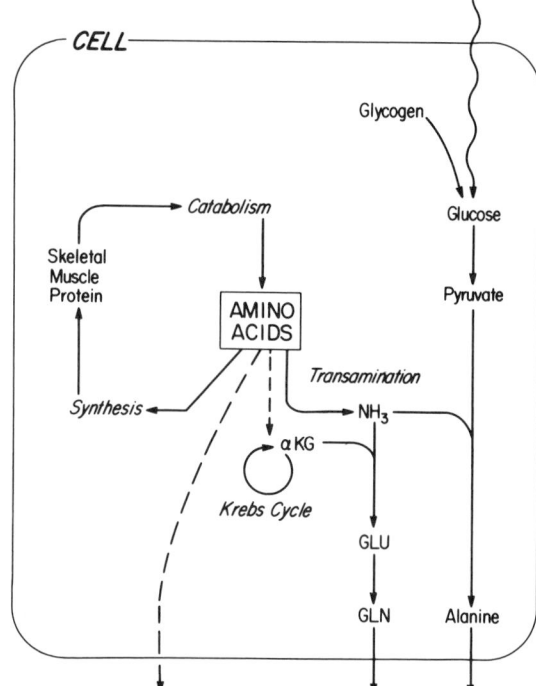

**Fig. 62–7.** Major biochemical reactions that lead to the synthesis of glutamine (GLN) and alanine in skeletal muscle.

ing experimental injury, glutamine consumption by the bowel and the kidney is accelerated,[72] a reaction that appears to be regulated by the increased elaboration of the glucocorticoids.[73] Although skeletal muscle releases alanine at an accelerated rate, the gastrointestinal tract and kidney also speed the production of alanine. This amino acid is extracted by the liver and is used in the synthesis of glucose and acute-phase proteins. Hence glutamine and alanine are important participants in the transfer of nitrogen from skeletal muscle to visceral organs; however, their metabolic pathways favor the production of urea and ammonia, both of which are lost from the body (Fig. 62–8).

*Alterations in Fat Metabolism.* To support hypermetabolism, increased gluconeogenesis and interorgan substrate flux, stored triglyceride is mobilized and is oxidized at an accelerated rate. Lipolysis is poorly attenuated following glucose administration;[59] this phenomenon may be the result of continuous stimulation of the sympathetic nervous system. Although mobilization and use of free fatty acids are accelerated in injured subjects, ketosis during brief starvation is blunted, and the accelerated protein catabolism remains unchecked.[74] If unfed, severely injured patients rapidly deplete their fat and protein stores. Such

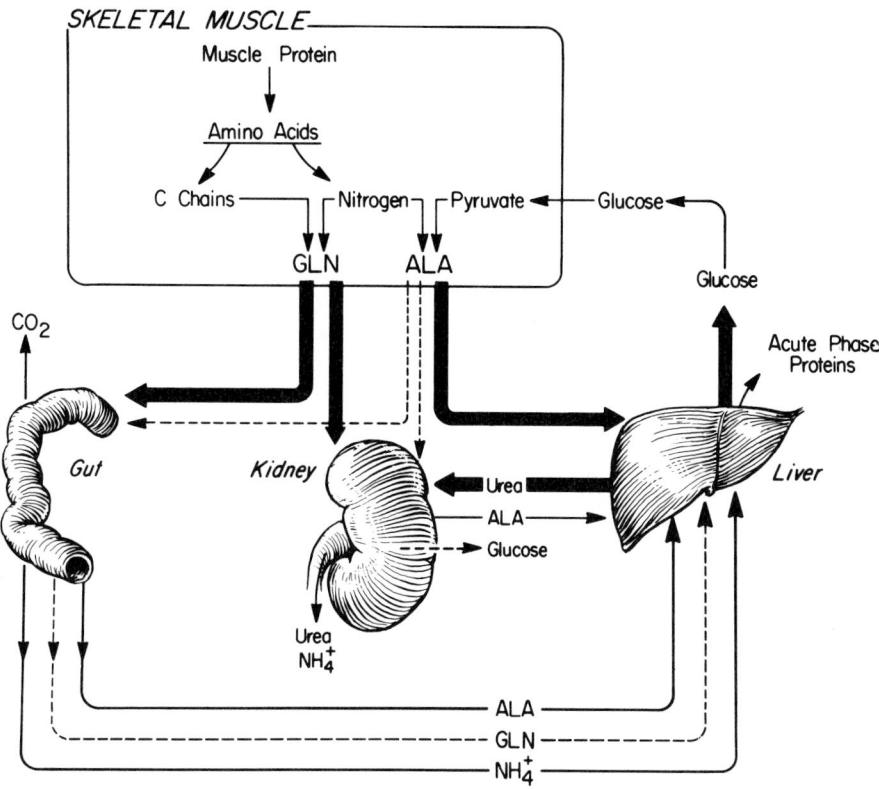

**Fig. 62–8.** Major pathways of "obligatory" loss of nitrogen from the body. ALA = Alanine; GLN = glutamine.

malnutrition increases their susceptibility to added stresses of hemorrhage, operations, and infection and may contribute to organ system failure, sepsis, and death.

**Hormonal Environment Associated with the Injury Response.** A variety of hormonal alterations occur in patients following injury; yet, the cause-and-effect relationships have only recently been established. In all phases of injury, one sees a marked rise in the counterregulatory hormones glucagon, glucocorticoids, and catecholamines.[75] During the ebb phase of injury, the sympathoadrenal axis primarily maintains the pressure-flow relationships necessary for an intact cardiovascular system. With the onset of hypermetabolism, characteristic of the flow phase, these and other hormones exert a variety of metabolic effects. Glucagon has potent glycogenolytic and gluconeogenic effects on the liver, and these effects signal the liver to make new glucose from hepatic glycogen stores and gluconeogenic precursors. Cortisol mobilizes amino acid from skeletal muscle, increases hepatic gluconeogenesis, and maintains body fat stores. The catecholamines stimulate hepatic gluconeogenesis and glycolysis and increase lactate production from peripheral tissues (skeletal muscle). Catecholamines also

increase metabolic rate and stimulate lipolysis. The level of growth hormone is elevated, even in the presence of hyperglycemia, and thyroid levels are reduced to low-normal concentrations.

Other blood-borne products may mediate the metabolic response to injury. Serum from uninfected burn patients contains a fever-producing substance that has been identified as endogenous pyrogen (interleukin-1).[75,76] This endogenous substance may produce fever by altering the hypothalamic temperature set point and may act directly on the liver to increase uptake of plasma amino acids and zinc used for synthesizing acute-phase proteins. Direct in vitro effects on skeletal muscle catabolism have also been reported. The role of this substance in catabolic responses is discussed in more detail in the section of this chapter on infection.

**Usual Course: Case Example.** A 28-year-old, nonobese male (6' tall; 170 lb; BSA, 2.0 m²) is admitted to the hospital with a pelvic fracture and soft tissue injury following a motor vehicle accident. He has always been in good health prior to this accident. He is resuscitated without incident with intravenous fluids and blood products. The patient is admitted to the trauma intensive care unit of the hospital, and a nasogastric tube is placed. Over the next 24 hours, his blood volume is restored, and he is given maintenance solutions with 5% dextrose and appropriate electrolytes at the rate of 125 ml/hour (3 L/day). His urine output on his first hospital day is 1,500 ml, and he gains 5 kg following fluid resuscitation. Because of a prolonged ileus, the patient is not fed, and he continues to receive intravenous fluids. On the seventh day of the injury, the ileus resolves and a spontaneous diuresis of 3,000 ml ensues. On the eighth day following the accident, the patient starts taking clear liquids and is gradually advanced to a regular diet over the next 4 days. He is discharged from the hospital 4 weeks later, when his fractures have stabilized.

Nitrogen balance studies from hospital day 1 through day 7 reveal a cumulative 7-day nitrogen loss of 108 g. During this 7-day period, the patient had 0 nitrogen intake and 600 cal glucose/day. On the eighth day of hospitalization, the patient lost 5 kg. Approximately half the weight represented loss of lean body mass,* and the remainder the loss of fat. On discharge from the hospital a month later, the patient had regained his initial body weight (Fig. 62–9).

## Response to Fixed Enteral or Parenteral Nutrition

Whereas the elective surgical patient can tolerate the mild catabolic responses following operation and with inadequate food intake, the trauma patient cannot because of accelerated tissue catabolism. This "obligatory" nitrogen loss can, in part, be reversed by nutritional means, but the accelerated excretion of nitrogen only returns to normal when the wound is closed or the fracture is stabilized and is healing. Nutritional support does not affect the hypermetabolic response associated with severe trauma, but provision of adequate calories and amino acids does reduce the magnitude of net lipogenesis, skeletal muscle proteolysis, and negative nitrogen balance.

Suppose the patient previously described sustains the same injury, but his postinjury period is modified by administration of all essential nutrients. The patient receives 3 L parenteral solution that delivers, 2,800 cal plus 15 g nitrogen/day as a balanced amino acid mixture (Fig. 62–10). This caloric intake is judged to be adequate to maintain body weight. Nitrogen balance studies

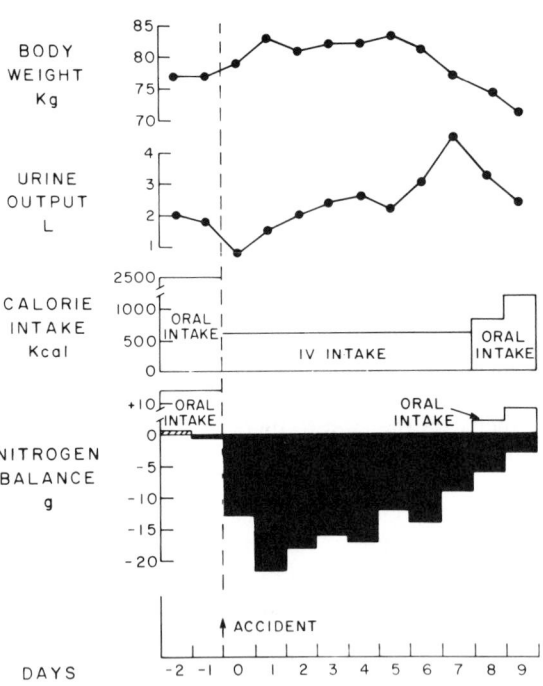

**Fig. 62–9.** The metabolic response of a previously healthy individual to an injury of moderate severity.

*108 g nitrogen = 675 g protein; 675 protein = 2.5 kg lean body mass.

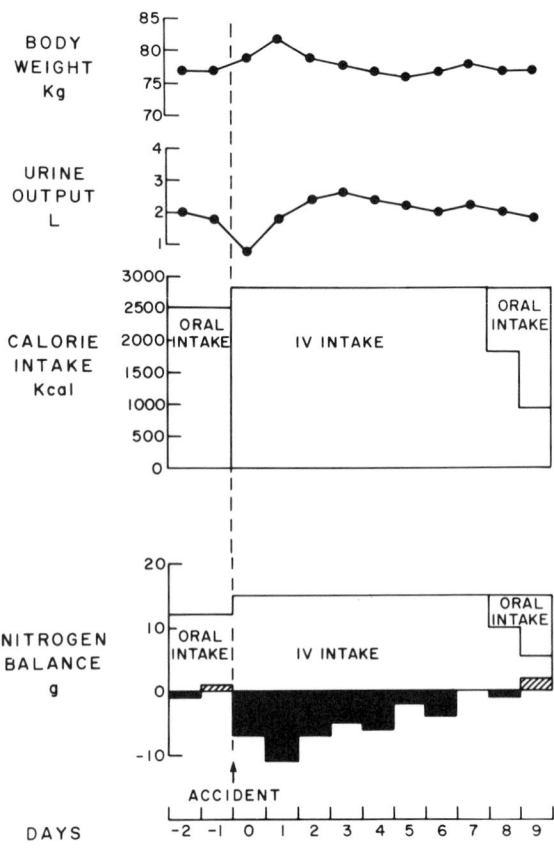

**Fig. 62–10.** The injury response with nutrition provided by central vein infusions.

show cumulative losses of 140 g from hospital day 1 through hospital day 7, so the patient's net loss for the 7 days equals 35 g. The patient lost 1 kg during this time, primarily lean body tissue.

In this patient, the administration of nutrients is designed to combat the negative nitrogen balance and weight loss associated with injury. The benefits of such feedings in patients with extensive injury have been translated into reduced morbidity and mortality rates when nutritional support is combined with other improvements in intensive care.

## Nutritional Support of the Injured Patient

**Consequences of Malnutrition.** The metabolic response to injury results in an increased energy expenditure. If energy intake is less than expenditure, oxidation of body fat stores and erosion of lean body mass will occur, with resultant loss of weight. Most injured patients can tolerate a loss of 10% of their weight prior to injury without a significant increase in the risks of injury. When weight loss exceeds 10% body weight, the complications of undernutrition interact with the disease process, with increased morbidity and mortality rates. Undernutrition to this extent following injury may impair the body's ability to respond appropriately to the injury and to inhibit responses to added stress such as infection.

The major impact of nutritional support in the trauma patient is to aid host defense. These patients are exposed to a variety of infectious agents in the hospital, and their injuries and requirements of care increase the risk of infection. The normal barrier defense mechanisms are disrupted by multiple indwelling catheters, nasotracheal and nasogastric tubes, and breakdown of skin and mucous membrane. Undernutrition may compromise the available host defense mechanism and may thus increase the likelihood of invasive sepsis, multiple organ system failure, and death. Additional consequences of malnutrition include poor wound healing, decreased mobility and activity, the occurrence of pressure sores and decubitus ulcers, altered gastrointestinal function, and the occurrence of edema secondary to reduced colloid osmotic pressure. Whereas these complications are most frequently observed in patients with severe malnutrition (> 15% body weight loss), adequate nutritional support helps to prevent them.

**Priorities of Care.** Nutrition should be integrated into the overall care of the critically ill patient to maximize the benefits of nutrition support, yet minimize complications in a complex intensive care setting. Priorities in care should be established at various points following injury. Resuscitation, oxygenation, and arrest of hemorrhage are immediate priorities for survival. Wounds should then be repaired or stabilized as expeditiously as possible. During wound repair, a patient's intensive metabolic demands abate, and nutrients become more effective in achieving anabolism. Early excision and grafting of burns and internal fixation of fractures are examples of early definitive wound care; yet even these procedures may be followed by several weeks of post-traumatic hypermetabolism. While the wound is treated, care should be taken to minimize other potential stresses that heighten metabolic demands in addition to those imposed by the injury alone. Such factors include pain, fear, mild cold exposure, acidosis, and hypovolemia. The greatest acceleration of catabolism occurs with infection, however, and every effort should be made to prevent sepsis.

Nutritional support is an essential part of the metabolic care of the critically ill trauma patient. Adequate nutrition allows normal responses that optimize wound healing and recovery. Nutritional support should be instituted before significant weight loss occurs. The development of techniques for intravenous administration of hypertonic nutrient solutions, the use of peripheral venous feedings with fat emulsions, and the availability of specific enteral diets have made it possible for virtually all injured patients to receive safe and effective nutritional support.

**Goals of Nutritional Support.** The majority of injured persons are not malnourished at the time of injury. The increased metabolic demands following injury will quickly lead to a malnourished state if the patient is not nutritionally supported (Fig. 62–11). Thus, nutritional support should be considered in all injured patients. The provision of full nutritional support early after injury may be fraught with metabolic complications, however. Hyperglycemia, hyperosmolality, and electrolyte disorders are frequently observed. Therefore, intravenous feedings are not usually begun immediately following the admission of the patient to the hospital. On stabilization of the patient's condition and development of a care plan, nutritional support can be gradually initiated. The goal of nutritional support is the maintenance of body cell mass and the limitation of weight loss to less than 10% of preinjury weight.

**Feeding the Patient.** Considerations include nutritional evaluation, requirements, monitoring, routes of administration, and specific formulas.

*Nutritional Assessment and Requirements.* Nutritional assessment of the trauma patient helps to determine energy and protein requirements. A

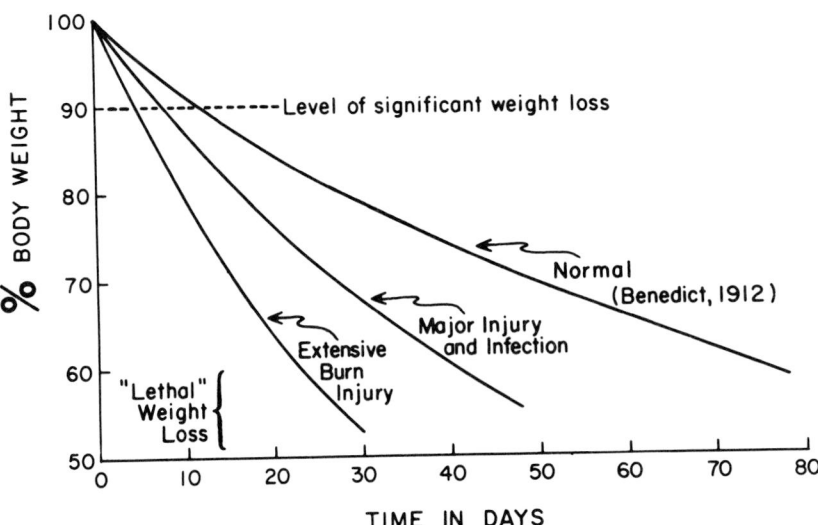

**Fig. 62–11.** Weight loss with starvation is accelerated following major injury and infection.

careful medical history and physical examination are essential, but the usual indicators of malnutrition are frequently misleading in the trauma patient. For example, body weight is increased in these patients because of edema, and serum albumin and transferrin decrease in concentration because of an enlarged distribution space. Hence nutritional support should be considered for all injured patients, with the goal to maintain usual (preinjury) body weight and body tissue mass.

Basal energy requirements are determined from standard tables based on age, sex, and BSA.[42] These requirements are adjusted for the increase in metabolic rate due to the injury or disease process by multiplication of a stress factor based on the severity of injury (see Table 62–1). An additional 25% is added to account for the energy expenditure associated with treatment and activity, but this addition is not required in inactive patients, such as those sedated or paralyzed while receiving artificial ventilation. The product of the factors (BMR times stress factors times 1.25, if needed) is an estimate of the patient's energy requirements.

The next step is to calculate nitrogen requirements. In normal subjects, the ratio of nitrogen to nonprotein calorie intake is usually 1:300 to 350; that is, for every 300 to 350 kcal, 1 g nitrogen is provided. Because of the heightened protein catabolism associated with the post-traumatic response, more dietary protein is required to achieve nitrogen balance. For critically ill patients, the optimal nitrogen-to-calorie ratio is thought to range between 1:100 and 1:200. This ratio indicates that approximately twice the quantity of protein is required to achieve "balance" in

the injured patient than in healthy persons. Approximately 15 to 20% of calorie intake should be protein.

Once energy and nitrogen requirements have been determined, the proportions of fat and carbohydrate need to be estimated, to maximize nitrogen retention. Long and associates studied the nitrogen-sparing effects of different isocaloric mixtures of glucose and fat in patients receiving 11.7 g nitrogen/m²/day.[77] They found no additional nitrogen-sparing effects when glucose calories exceeded the measured metabolic rate. Nitrogen equilibrium was aproached when glucose comprised 60 to 70% of the caloric needs, approximately 7 mg/kg/min. In addition, Wolfe and colleagues studied oxidation rates of postoperative patients receiving glucose.[78] No increase in oxidation of administered glucose was observed when patients received glucose infusions above 7 mg/kg/min. Black and colleagues, using the glucose clamp technique, demonstrated that injured patients had an upper limit to glucose disposal of approximately 6 to 7 mg/kg/min, a value that represented 60 to 70% of the estimated caloric needs.[55] In contrast, normal subjects could dispose of increasing quantities of glucose and approached an upper limit of 15 to 17 mg/kg/min. The results of these 3 independent studies using different techniques point to the same conclusion: no clear-cut gain is made in providing glucose calories in excess of 60 to 70% of daily metabolic requirements to injured patients. The administration of larger glucose loads, however, has been associated with an increasing incidence of complications such as hyperglycemia, hyperosmotic states, hepatic dysfunction, and respiratory insufficiency.[79] For patients who are intolerant of large caloric loads, the provision of 60% of caloric needs as glucose and the rest as fat should minimize complications and should maximize protein synthesis.

Multivitamins are administered daily, along with supplemental vitamin C, which is believed by some to be required in increased amounts following injury[80] (see Chap. 54). Electrolytes are present in standard diets or tube feedings; trace elements are variably present (cf Appendix Table A–40c); they must be added to parenteral infusions. Potassium, magnesium, and phosphate supplements in addition to those in tube formulas, may be required to maintain normal serum concentrations of these electrolytes. They must be added to parenteral fluids to meet needs except when present in amino acid–electrolyte combinations. Although the need for zinc has been demonstrated experimentally, clinical reports of zinc-replacement therapy in burn patients provide no definitive answers on the benefit of this supplement following injury.[81] Zinc supplements should be administered to severely malnourished individuals or to those with a history of poor nutrient intake (alcoholic patients) who have a major injury or major intestinal fluid losses. (See Chap. 54 concerning other trace elements.)

In summary, the nutritional requirements of the trauma patient can be determined as follows:

1. Determine BMR for age, sex, and BSA from the tables of Fleisch or the Harris-Benedict equation (BMR in kcal/day).[42]
2. Determine the percentage of increase in metabolic rate due to the injury (see Table 62–1), multiply by BMR, and add to 1 (% × BMR + BMR).
3. Add 25% × BMR for hospital activity (walking, physical therapy, sitting, treatment).
4. The sum of steps 1 to 3 is an estimated daily caloric requirement for maintenance of body weight.
5. Divide step 4 by 150 to determine nitrogen requirements (protein = 6.25 × nitrogen).
6. Give approximately 60% of caloric requirement (determined in step 4) as glucose.
7. Give remaining caloric requirement as fat (glucose can be used if tolerated by the patient). Glucose is much less expensive, and a central venous catheter will be necessary to administer the glucose solution. If glucose is used as the remaining caloric source, insulin may need to be given to avoid hyperglycemia. Fat emulsion should then be given 2 to 3 times/week to provide essential fatty acid requirements.

8. Reassess energy and nitrogen needs at least twice weekly. Weigh the patient daily.
9. If nutritional support seems unsatisfactory because of progressive weight loss, consider direct measurement of oxygen consumption or measurement of nitrogen loss and calculation of nitrogen balance.

*Nutritional Monitoring.* Once the trauma patient is nutritionally assessed, feedings can be gradually commenced. Protein and calorie intake should be measured and recorded daily. If nutritional requirements are not met by current therapy, then other feeding techniques should be used. Combined nutritional support techniques may be necessary during the convalescence of a severely injured patient (Fig. 62–12).

If the patient continues to lose more weight than can be attributed to a postresuscitation diuresis, then additional nutritional assessment techniques, such as indirect calorimetry or nitrogen balance testing, should be performed. Plasma glucose levels should be determined regularly, especially when one is beginning or increasing nutritional support. Insulin should be administered to maintain a plasma glucose level of 100 to 150 mg/dl. Urine sugar content should be evaluated by the hospital nursing staff every 6 to 8 hours. Levels of serum electrolytes, blood urea nitrogen (BUN), and creatinine and liver function should be determined regularly, as consistent with proper care. Serum potassium concentrations may need to be followed more closely because of increased potassium losses after injury and a tendency toward metabolic alkalosis.

*Additional Nutritional Assessment Techniques.* Energy requirements may be estimated with reasonable accuracy in 85% of hospital patients. If estimated requirements are delivered by current nutritional support, but therapy seems inadequate because of persistent weight loss in excess of estimated net fluid losses or an unsatisfactory clinical course, energy requirements may be measured by indirect calorimetry. Oxygen consumption ($\dot{V}_{O_2}$) and carbon dioxide production ($\dot{V}_{CO_2}$) are determined under resting, unstressed, basal conditions. These respiratory parameters are interrelated to energy expenditure by the following relationships:

Metabolic rate (kcal/hour)
$$= 3.9 \times \dot{V}_{O_2} \text{ (L/hour)} + 1.1 \times \dot{V}_{CO_2} \text{ (L/hour)}$$

This value is the resting energy expenditure of the patient and should be increased 20 to 30% to account for minimal daily activity when used to determine energy requirements.

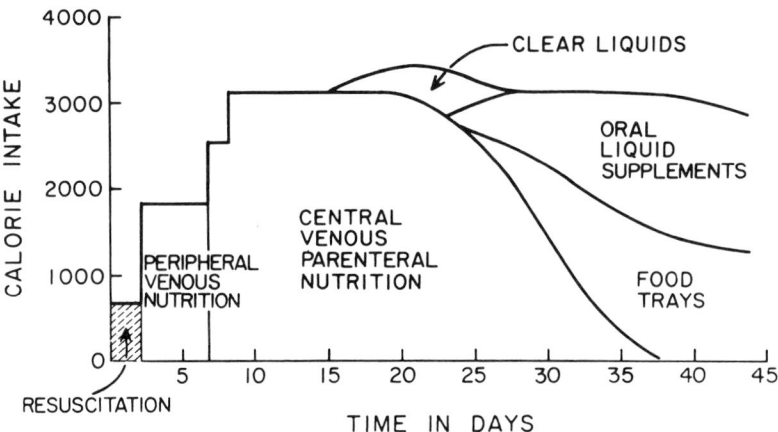

**Fig. 62–12.** In subjects with moderate-to-severe injury, a variety of techniques are necessary to provide safe and efficient nutrition.

Nitrogen balance studies help to define the effectiveness of nutritional support. These should be performed in patients whose clinical course is unsatisfactory or in whom nutritional efficacy cannot be estimated on clinical grounds alone. Nitrogen balance is the quantity of nitrogen taken in or administered to the patient minus the quantity of nitrogen lost:

$$N_{bal} \text{ (g/day)} = N_{in} - N_{out}$$

Most nitrogen is lost in the urine, mainly as urea. The urine is collected for 24-hour periods and is stored in acidified containers. Urinary urea nitrogen (UUN) is measured. This represents approximately 80% of urinary nitrogen. Additionally, about 2 g/day are lost in the feces and from the skin. If the BUN changes during the 24-hour period, the whole body change in urea nitrogen (ΔBUN) should be estimated as follows:

$$\Delta BUN \text{ g/day} = [(BUN \text{ day } 2 \text{ mg/dl} \\ - BUN \text{ day } 1 \text{ mg/dl}^a) \times 0.6 \times \text{body weight kg}^b \\ \div 1,000$$

where $^a$ = Change in concentration and
$^b$ = Estimated quantity of total body water

$$N_{out} \text{ (g/day)} = \frac{UUN}{0.8}$$

g/day + 2 g/day$^c$ + ΔBUN g/day$^d$
where $^c$ = Estimate for stool and skin and
$^d$ = Other loss from wounds or drains, as measured or estimated

Nitrogen is conventionally taken to be 16% of the total protein intake; that is, $N_{in}$/day = protein intake g/day × 0.16.

*Routes of Nutritional Support and Nutrient Formulas.* The routes of nutritional support are the same as those described elsewhere: oral, enteral, and parenteral. In general, oral and enteral routes are preferred over intravenous administration. Injured patients rarely take the required quantity of calories spontaneously from their hospital food tray. Hence oral liquid supplements should be administered. Nutrient intake is monitored daily by the dietitian, and each nursing shift is assigned a quantity of supplement to be provided. Free water or low-calorie drinks are not offered. All liquid is a calorie-dense nutrient supplement.

The patient's injuries may, however, preclude the use of oral feedings; for example, patients with facial trauma may have their jaws wired together. Children, older adults, patients with head injuries, and those receiving artificial ventilation are all potential candidates for tube feedings. Retro- or intraperitoneal hematomas, intra-abdominal sepsis, severe gastrointestinal injury and extensive repair, or other factors may lead to reduction in intestinal motility (ileus) or intolerance to enteral feedings. Jejunal or duodenal tube feedings are often successful even if the stomach must be continuously decompressed. Thus, for all patients who have undergone abdominal operations, feeding jejunostomy placement should be considered.[46] Alternatively, the jejunum or duodenum can be intubated perorally with special tubes, with or without the aid of fluoroscopy. The development of diarrhea in a patient receiving enteral feedings may limit the caloric load given by these routes. When the nutritional needs of the patient cannot be met by oral and enteral feedings, intravenous techniques can be used.

Enteral formulas are usually balanced mixtures of fat, carbohydrate, and protein. Several recently developed formulas are particularly rich in calories and protein, yet have low osmolality. In light of the injured patient's nutritional requirements, these formulas would seem to be particularly advantageous; however, a variety of formulas are available and may be preferred in selected cases.

Intravenous feedings may be necessary to supplement enteral feedings, or they may be required to provide adequate nutritional intake if enteral feedings cannot be tolerated or are inadequate. Peripheral nutrient solution can be given to supplement enteral feedings. These dilute solutions of glucose and amino acids should be minimized, and fat infusion should be maximized, while high-carbohydrate tube feeding is provided. Such an approach ensures adequate carbohydrate loads in a minimal fluid volume. Trauma patients, and particularly burn patients, are usually young adults without cardiovascular disease and with large daily fluid requirements. Thus, these patients are ideal candidates for peripheral-vein nutrient infusion. Unfortunately, however, adequate carbohydrate calories can rarely be provided solely by this route, and when parenteral nutrition is required, central venous feedings are usually indicated. The hypertonic solution provides glucose, amino acids, and other essential nutrients. Fat emulsion and supplemental fluids are easily administered through a second intravenous access site, usually a peripheral vein.

## SEPSIS

In spite of numerous advances in the treatment of infection and a better understanding of its mediators and pathophysiology, the mortality and morbidity rates for septicemia remain high. Unlike in elective operations and uncomplicated trauma, the response patterns following major infection are often unpredictable. The variability in the metabolic and physiologic responses is related in part to the patient's age, previous state of health, pre-existing disease, previous stresses, site of infection, and specific pathogens. Moreover, organ-system failure, such as septic shock or pulmonary insufficiency, may mask the more subtle manifestations of systemic infection.

In general, two physiologic response patterns have been described, based on cardiac output.[82] The first is characterized by an increased cardiac output and heightened systemic perfusion. This state varies, depending on the patient's physiologic compensation and administered fluid volume. The second response pattern is characterized by cardiac decomposition, inadequate tissue perfusion, and profound acidosis. This pattern is described as "low-flow sepsis." Both these responses reflect the body's reaction to systemic infection. These patterns are also modified by the underlying disease process and the physiologic reserve of the particular patient. In this section, we review the metabolic responses to sepsis and the priorities for safe nutritional support. Sepsis is defined as the presence of infection, resulting in systemic signs and symptoms, and diagnosed by bacteremia. Low-flow sepsis is difficult to reverse and usually results in death. Most of this discussion focuses on the metabolic responses that occur during the hyperdynamic high-flow state.

## Usual Physiologic Response to Systemic Infection

**General Overview and Time Course.** The invasion of the body by microorganisms initiates many host responses. Local penetration of tissues stimulates mobilization of phagocytes, initiates an inflammatory response at the local site, and may activate additional host immunologic mechanisms. If the infection progresses, fever, tachycardia, and other systemic responses occur; these more generalized reactions may reflect direct or indirect effects of the inflammatory response. Systemic events during the hyperdynamic phase of sepsis can be categorized into two general types of responses: (1) those related to the host's immunologic defenses; and (2) those related to the body's general metabolic and circulatory adjustments to the infection. The predominant alterations in host defense mechanisms include fever, leukocytosis, changes in acute-phase protein synthesis, and activation of a variety of immunologic reactions. The changes in metabolism relate to alterations in glucose, nitrogen, and fat metabolism, as well as those related to the redistribution of trace metals. These events are initiated by invasion of the microorganism and evolve as the infectious disease progresses through its period of incubation, initiation of metabolic responses and fever, and into early convalescence and recovery.

Several general characteristics describe the systemic events that occur after infection, as follows:

1. These responses appear stereotyped and can be produced after administering many microorganisms or their toxins. The systemic responses to infection are similar in many respects to events that follow injury, but these processes are not the same.

2. The magnitude of the responses varies with the extent and duration of the infection.

3. The complex sequence of systemic events that follows infection appears to change with time, and hence sequential studies must be performed to locate the responses precisely within that time.

4. Although the systemic responses to infection are stereotyped, these processes are modulated by the physiologic reserves of the individual. The magnitude of the responses to infection depends on the patient's age and sex, previous nutritional state, function of vital organs, immunologic memory, and associated disease processes. The classic response to infection has been observed in young, previously healthy, well-nourished, active adults with no other medical problems. These patients are rarely admitted to surgical services, however. Surgeons usually see patients at extremes of life or those who are hospitalized because of disease processes and who have additional stress, usually an operation or injury, that limits physiologic, biochemical, or immunologic responses to infection. Thus, infection complicating the recuperative course of a surgical patient may not evoke standard systemic responses. Limitations in the patient's capacity to respond to infection may affect recovery or survival.

5. As infection progresses, additional functional limitations may be imposed on one or more specific organs and may further impair the host systemic response. These limitations can be observed in patients with severe pneumonia and marked pulmonary dysfunction causing hypoxemia, associated with circulatory failure and hypotension related to severe gram-negative sepsis.

In spite of the complexities of unraveling and understanding the systemic responses to infection in critically ill surgical patients, a large body of investigative and clinical data is available to aid our understanding of these host defense mechanisms.

Beisel has described the time course of metabolic and immunologic responses during the course of a typical febrile illness.[83] Phagocytic activity is an early response that occurs shortly after the moment of exposure to the pathogen. The febrile period is the hallmark of systemic effects. With the onset of fever, negative nitrogen balance, accelerated losses of potassium, phosphate, and magnesium, and retention of salt and water all occur. On resolution of the sepsis, one sees spontaneous diuresis and a return to positive nitrogen balance. Associated with the losses of elements from the body is an internal redistribution of substances, particularly iron and zinc, which are sequestered in the body, presumably to make them unavailable to the invading organisms (Fig. 62–13).

**Systemic Metabolic Responses.** Many of the metabolic responses to infection are similar to those observed following injury. Hence investigators have speculated that a final common pathway may apply to all catabolic states. Severe infection is characterized by prolonged fever, hypermetabolism, diminished protein economy, altered glucose dynamics, and accelerated lipolysis. Anorexia is commonly associated with systemic infection and contributes to the loss of body tissue. These effects are compounded in the patient with sepsis by multiorgan system failure, which includes the gastrointestinal tract, liver, heart, and lungs.

*Hypermetabolism.* Oxygen consumption is usually elevated in the infected patient. The extent of this increase is related to the severity of infection, with peak elevations reaching 50 to 60% above normal.[42] Such responses often occur in the postoperative and postinjury periods secondary to severe pneumonia, intra-abdominal infection, or wound invasion. If the patient's metabolic rate is already elevated to a maximal extent because of severe injury, no further increase will be observed.[52] In patients with only slightly accelerated rates of oxygen consumption, the presence of infection causes a rise in metabolic rate that appears additive to the pre-existing state. A portion of the increase in metabolism may be ascribed to the increase in reaction rate associated with fever (Q10 effect). Calculations suggest that the metabolic rate increases 10 to 13% for each elevation of 1° C in central temperature. On resolution of the infection, the metabolic rate returns to normal.

*Altered Glucose Dynamics.* Blood glucose levels are generally elevated in the infected patient, but the descriptive term "diabetes of infection" is inappropriate because plasma insulin concentrations are generally normal or elevated in previously healthy individuals who develop infection.[84] That glucose production is increased in infected patients appears to be additive to the augmented gluconeogenesis that occurs following injury.[52] For example, uninfected burn patients have an accelerated glucose production rate approximately 50% above normal; with the onset of bacteremia in similar individuals, hepatic glucose production increases to twice basal levels. Glucose dynamics following infection are complex, and profound hypoglycemia and diminished hepatic glucose production have also been described in both animals and human patients.[85,86] The best clinical example of the imbalance in hepatic glucose production and tissue glucose consumption is found in neonatal hypoglycemia associated with gram-negative sep-

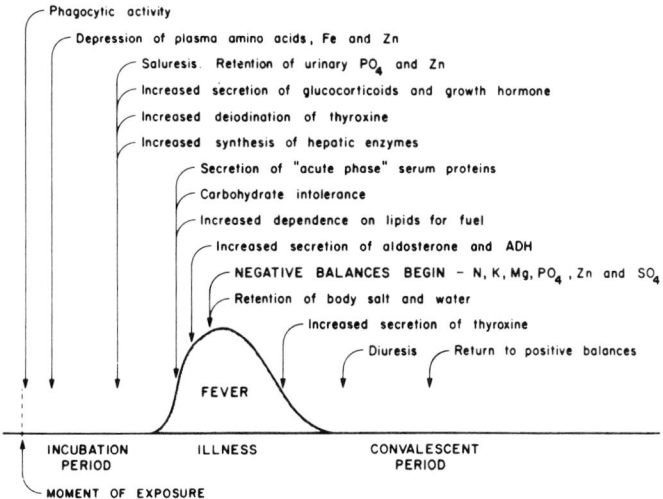

**Fig. 62–13.** Nutritional responses that evolve following a generalized febrile, infectious illness. (From Beisel, W.R.: Am. J. Clin. Nutr. *30*:1,236, 1977.)

ticemia.[87] Studies in animals and in human patients show that deterioration in glucogenesis is associated with more progressive stages of infection and may be related to alterations in splanchnic blood flow.[52] Hepatic dysfunction this profound is usually associated with other complications of sepsis, such as respiratory insufficiency and renal failure, and usually heralds impending cardiovascular instability and death.

*Alterations in Protein Metabolism.* Accelerated proteolysis, increased nitrogen excretion, and prolonged negative nitrogen balance occur following infection, and the response pattern is similar to that described for injury. Long and associates noted that the protein catabolic rate in infected patients was accelerated,[88] and Herrmann and colleagues showed that protein synthesis could be augmented in the infected patient by vigorous feeding.[62] Amino acid flux from skeletal muscle is accelerated in patients with sepsis,[89] and this flux is matched by accelerated visceral amino acid uptake. In infected burn patients, splanchnic uptake of amino acids is increased 50% above rates in uninfected burn patients with injuries of comparable size.[52] These amino acids serve as glucose precursors and are used for the synthesis of acute-phase proteins. In addition, acidosis frequently occurs in the patient with sepsis, and this stimulus serves as a signal for accelerated glutamine uptake by the kidney. Glutamine liberates an ammonia ion that combines with a hydrogen ion and is excreted in the urine, thus participating in acid base homeostasis.[70] Because the glutamine arises from skeletal muscle proteolysis, this complication of sepsis is yet another stimulus of heightened skeletal muscle breakdown.

*Alterations in Fat Metabolism.* Fat is a major fuel oxidized in infected patients, and the increased metabolism of lipids from peripheral fat stores is especially prominent during a period of inadequate nutritional support. Lipolysis is most probably mediated by the heightened sympathetic activity that is a potent stimulus for fat mobilization and accelerated oxidation. Serum triglyceride levels reflect the balance between rates of triglyceride production by the liver and use and storage by peripheral tissues. Marked hypertriglyceridemia has been associated with gram-negative infection,[90] but plasma triglyceride concentrations are usually normal or low. The use of free fatty acids is coupled with increased hepatic fat clearance. During starvation, hepatic uptake of free fatty acids is associated with ketosis, and the concentrations of beta-hydroxybutyrate and acetoacetate rise. This change does not occur in infected patients, and it has been hypothesized that the accelerated proteolysis seen during infection is a consequence of this hypoketonemic state. This hypothesis was tested by the infusion of beta-hydroxybutyrate into infected animals, however.[91] Following this infusion, the accelerated gluconeogenesis and proteolysis were not diminished; this finding suggests that these factors are governed by regulators other than the simple regulation of the oxidation of fat and carbohydrate. Other investigators have suggested that the hypoketonemic state of infection may be a consequence of the hyperinsulinemia associated with catabolic states.[92] Studies in rats and in human patients lend credence to this argument.[92,93]

*Changes in Trace Mineral Metabolism.* Changes

in the balance of magnesium, inorganic phosphate, zinc, and potassium generally follow alterations in nitrogen balance. Although the iron-binding capacity of transferrin is usually unchanged in early infection, iron disappears from the plasma, especially during severe pyrogenic infections; similar alterations are observed with serum zinc levels. These decreases cannot be totally accounted for by losses of the minerals from the body. Rather, both iron and zinc accumulate within the liver, and this accumulation appears to be another host defense mechanism. The administration of iron to the infected host, especially early in the disease, is contraindicated because increased serum iron concentrations may impair resistance. Zinc may be required during a prolonged, infective illness because zinc is both sequestered in body tissues and excreted in the urine. Zinc deficiency, however, is not reflected in serum concentrations, which are usually diminished as an initial host response. Unlike iron and zinc, copper levels generally rise, and the increased plasma concentrations can be ascribed almost entirely to the increase in ceruloplasm produced by the liver.

### Mediators of the Catabolic Response

**Hormones.** The hormonal responses during the hypermetabolic phase of infection are similar to those described following injury. Serum cortisol levels are elevated and lose their usual circadian rhythm.[83,94] Glucagon levels are increased, and insulin levels are normal or even elevated.[95] The insulin-to-glucagon ratio, a hormonal relationship considered to indicate hepatic stimulation of gluconeogenesis, remains below normal, however. Levels of catecholamines,[96] growth hormone, ADH, and aldosterone are all elevated.[97] The growth hormone level persists into convalescence, presumably to promote anabolism. These hormonal responses to infection are the subjects of recent reviews.[83,97]

**Circulating Toxins and Pyrogens.** It is well known that injection of pus or exudate from infected tissue into a test animal stimulates systemic responses. A constant feature of many early bacterial studies was that microorganisms secreted a substance into the culture medium that was regularly pyrogenic in animals and would often evoke a leukocytic response. At the turn of the century, it was realized that bacteria produced pyrogenic factors in addition to exotoxins. This new toxin was described as being tightly anchored to, if not part of, the cell wall. This substance was called endotoxin and was later biochemically characterized as a lipopolysaccharide. Endotoxins have many effects.[98] They cause fever, increase erythropoiesis, cause leukopenia and thrombocytopenia, and alter complement. They also cause the release of vasoactive substances and may play a central role in vascular collapse related to overwhelming infection. Endotoxins increase ACTH and growth hormone release, but have no effect on thyroid-stimulating hormone or luteinizing hormone. They stimulate a variety of the responses of the immune system, cause hyperglycemia and hyperlipidemia, and stimulate liver protein synthesis and redistribution of trace elements such as iron. Thus, this substance was thought for a long time to be the major mediator of the response to infection.

In spite of this belief, however, a recurring theme of many studies was that other mediators, which were products of the host's own cells, served as signals to stimulate fever and other responses to infection. In 1953, Bennett and Beeson developed techniques to exclude endotoxin from their test system and reported that a fever-induced substance could be extracted from rabbit granulocytes.[99] Further studies showed that this leukocytic substance was regularly pyrogenic, whereas similar extracts from many tissues had no fever-inducing effect. In addition, the host pyrogen, referred to as "endogenous pyrogen," differed in many respects from the pyrogens of microbial origin.

A variety of metabolic properties have been attributed to endogenously produced pyrogens, now referred to as interleukin-1. Interleukin-1 produces fever and has direct effects on the liver; it promotes hepatic uptake to plasma zinc and iron, increases plasma copper levels, and stimulates hepatic uptake of plasma amino acids.[100] It also stimulates the synthesis of acute-phase proteins. More recently, what appears to be a breakdown product of interleukin-1 has been shown in vitro to cause marked proteolysis.[76] Inflammatory cells in phagocytosis appear to regulate, either by direct or indirect effects, body redistribution of trace elements and nitrogen and stimulate acute-phase globulin synthesis to participate in the host defense mechanisms.

### Complications: Multisystem Organ Failure

The most severe complication of sepsis is the failure of essential organs, which may result in death. The current treatment of systemic infection consists of: (1) bacteriologic control by removal and drainage or containment of the source; (2) use of appropriate antibiotics; (3) support of cardiovascular and respiratory function; (4) supportive therapy of specific organ failure, whether cardiac, pulmonary, hepatic, renal, or gastrointestinal; and

(5) vigorous support of the host through nutritional means.

Septic shock may be associated with a fall or an increase in peripheral resistance. A hyperdynamic cardiac output is associated with a more favorable outcome. When mild hypotension occurs, vigorous fluid loading ensures a full blood volume and supports a hyperdynamic circulatory state.

The next most common problem associated with systemic infection is oxygenation and elimination of carbon dioxide. A variety of endotoxins and vasoactive factors mediated by the infectious process can alter pulmonary vascular permeability and may lead to pulmonary insufficiency. Patients often require intubation and vigorous ventilatory support with volume cycle ventilation and positive expiratory pressure. Ongoing problems include the development of infected pulmonary infiltrate, with resulting pneumonia and another source of infection.

The origin of renal failure associated with sepsis is unclear. Circulating factors are associated with increasing blood flow to the kidney. However, if cardiac output is inadequate, such a response will not be possible, and this failure, coupled with redistribution of blood flow, may cause progressive deficiency of the cortical portion of the kidney. In addition, the use of aminoglycoside antibiotics, which are nephrotoxic, may also cause progressive impairment and malfunction. When renal failure becomes progressive, the early use of hemodialysis, with or without filtration, minimizes the effects of uremia superimposed on the metabolism of sepsis. Adequate caloric support limits ureagenesis and normalizes alterations in serum electrolyte levels. Because uremia itself is a potent catabolic signal,[101] this condition further impairs the hypercatabolic infected host.

Sepsis causes marked changes in gastrointestinal function. The most common abnormality is ileus, which can result from intra-abdominal disease or from the effects of bacteria elsewhere. Stress ulcers lead to upper gastrointestinal bleeding, which may require operative treatment.

Hepatic dysfunction is a common manifestation of septicemia. The degree of dysfunction is variable and may appear early as a slight elevation of liver enzymes, or it may cause severe jaundice and hyperbilirubinemia. Specific bacteria, however, overwhelm the reticuloendothelial system of the liver and result in fulminant hepatic failure. Localized infections, such as hepatic abscesses, pylephlebitis, and hepatitis, may cause profound liver dysfunction because of the direct effect of infection on this organ. Occasionally, hypoglycemia accompanies ascending cholecystitis because of the direct effect of hepatic inflammation.

## Usual Course: Case Example

It is difficult to outline the usual response pattern following infection because of the many possible variations. The following case example illustrates the value of nutritional support in the overall integrated care of a patient with prolonged sepsis.

A 65-year-old man (6' tall; 175 lb; BSA, 2.0 m²) appeared in the hospital emergency ward with right-upper-quadrant pain, a temperature of 103° F, and mild jaundice. A recent ultrasonic study had shown the presence of gallstones, but the patient was otherwise well nourished and in good health. Initial laboratory studies showed a white blood cell count of 17,000, with a left shift, total bilirubin level of 5 mg/dl, and an alkaline phosphatase level of 550 Bodansky units. Shortly after hospital admission, the patient became confused, and his blood pressure fell to 70 mm Hg systolic. His skin was warm and pink, and a diagnosis of ascending cholangitis and septic shock was made. Intravenous fluid was administered, and the patient's blood pressure returned to normal. Antibiotics were started, and shortly thereafter the patient was taken into the operating suite, where he was found to have an impacted gallstone in the common bile duct. A cholecystectomy and common duct exploration were performed, and the impacted stone was removed. Pus was present in the gallbladder and the biliary tract.

Postoperatively, the patient required ventilatory support. On postoperative day 1, he was no longer dependent on cardiotonic agents to maintain normal blood pressure. He had a marked ileus and remained febrile. He received 5% dextrose solutions containing appropriate electrolytes. He gradually became alert, but remained dependent on the ventilator. On postoperative day 5, the patient's fever increased to 103.6° F, and he had marked leukocytosis. Diagnostic studies showed an intra-abdominal abscess, and the patient returned to the operating room for surgical drainage. Postoperatively, the patient received large doses of antibiotics, and 3 days after the second operation, he was weaned from the ventilator. Results of liver function tests gradually returned to normal, and the patient's ileus resolved. On postoperative day 15, the patient started a clear-liquid diet, and he was discharged from the hospital on postoperative day 22. Nitrogen balance studies from postoperative day 1 to day 16 showed a cumulative 15-day negative nitrogen balance of 225 g (Fig. 62–14). The patient had lost 11 lb by postoperative day 15, half of which was lean tissue and the remainder fat. By day 15, the patient had started oral intake, and by discharge day (day 22), he was clearly afebrile and anabolic, taking adequate quantities of nutrients.

### Response to Fixed Nutrient Intake

To evaluate the effects of fixed nutrient intake in sepsis, a patient with ascending cholangitis was supported vigorously throughout his course with parenteral nutrition. A combination of sepsis, anesthesia, and tissue trauma in this patient increased the metabolic rate by 50%, so the energy needs were approximately 2,900 cal/day. The patient received 3 L central venous nutrition, which provided 21 g nitrogen and 3,000 cal/day. Nitrogen balance studies from postoperative day 1 to day 16 showed a cumulative nitrogen loss of 375 g, and cumulative nitrogen balance for this 15-day period was −60 g. On postoperative day 16, the patient had lost only 4 lb, half of which was body fat, and the remainder lean body mass (Fig. 62–15).

Prompt initiation of nutritional support in patients with sepsis who cannot eat enough or should not eat is mandatory. On the other hand, provision of nutrients requires integration into the patients' management and support plan. The patient in the case example was started gradually on nutritional feedings, to avoid untoward complications of hyperglycemia, and the infusion was diminished during the second septic interval. Fat

should compose a moderate proportion of the infused energy, to avoid the complications of hyperglycemia and to diminish the possibilities of increased carbon dioxide production complicating hypercaloric glucose infusions. Because of the severe erosion of lean body mass possible in such a patient, nutrition support helps to diminish such erosion of body mass. This provision of calories and nitrogen cannot attenuate the hypermetabolism characteristic of sepsis, but it does reduce accelerated catabolism.

### Specific Feeding Problems

**Renal Failure.** Metabolic studies in patients with acute and chronic renal failure have limited the intake of nonessential amino acids, in an attempt to lower urea production. Proteins of high biologic value, but in much smaller quantities (<0.5 g/kg/day) than usually given, are administered along with adequate calories, usually in the form of glucose. When enteral feedings are not feasible, a central venous infusion of an essential amino acid solution and hypertonic dextrose provides calories and a small quantity of nitrogen, to reduce protein catabolism while simultaneously controlling the rise in BUN. Whether such nutritional therapy reduces mortality rates for renal failure associated with sepsis remains controversial. During dialysis, protein intake is liberalized, but the BUN is maintained below 100 mg/dl.

**Hepatic Failure.** Fulminant hepatic failure in

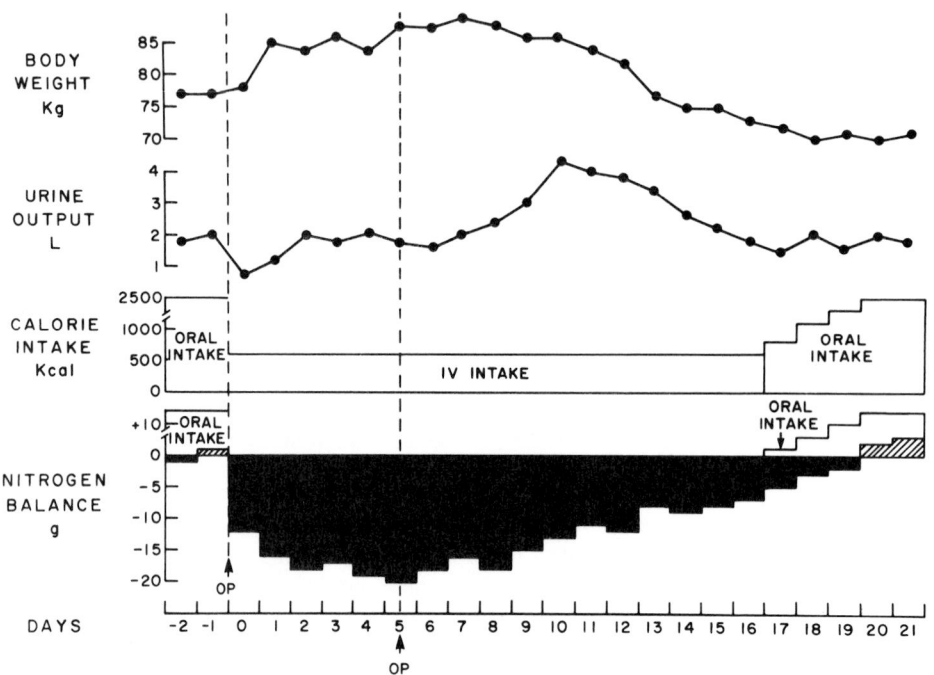

**Fig. 62–14.** The metabolic responses to sepsis.

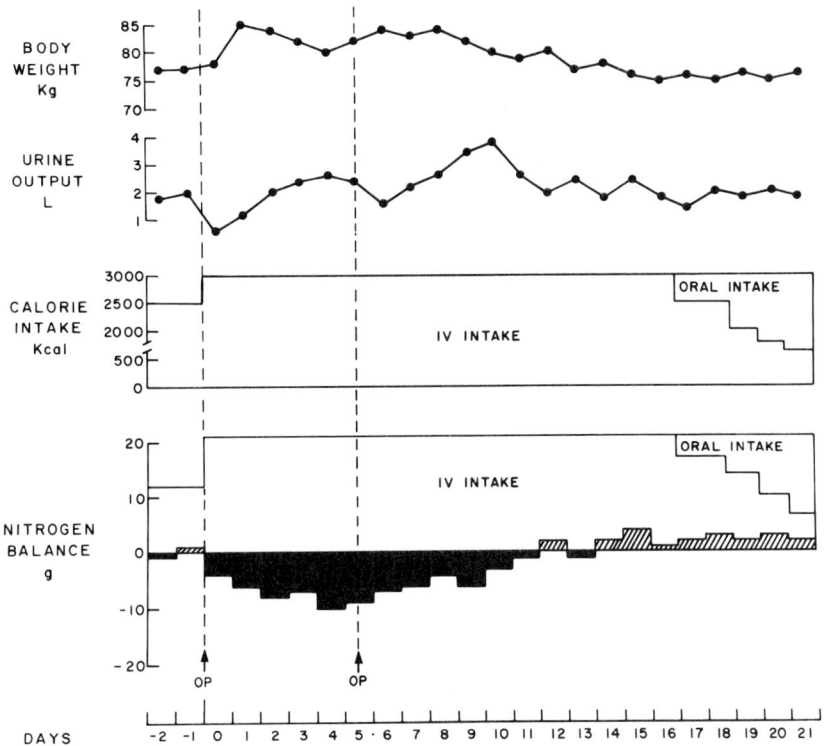

**Fig. 62–15.** The metabolic responses to sepsis with constant intravenous nutrition.

the patient with sepsis has a high mortality rate, especially when hepatic encephalopathy occurs. As discussed in the section on trauma, the effects of normalization of amino acid concentration and reversal of hepatic coma remain controversial. More common, however, are alterations in liver function studies, such as elevations in levels of alkaline phosphatase, hepatic enzymes, and serum bilirubin, which appear secondary to the septic event, but may worsen with intravenous feedings.[102] Hepatic dysfunction generally resolves on resolution of the sepsis, but if the inflammatory process persists, adjustments in the feeding formulation will be necessary. The carbohydrate load is usually reduced to consist of no more than 50% of metabolic requirements, and the additional calories should be provided as fat emulsion. If the patient's serum bilirubin level becomes elevated (generally above 12 mg/dl), the patient should be observed for the presence of encephalopathy, if this complication occurs, then the protein load should also be reduced.

**Cardiac Failure.** The myocardial dysfunction that occurs in sepsis is usually secondary to the elaboration of myocardial depressant factor or to heart failure secondary to pulmonary insufficiency. Malnourished patients with sepsis may be sensitive to volume overload, and use of a con-

centrated solution of hypertonic dextrose (D-70%) mixed with amino acids may be indicated to maximize calories and to minimize volume. In addition, 20% fat emulsion can be administered to provide additional energy.

**Respiratory Insufficiency.** Infected patients may develop pulmonary insufficiency secondary to increased capillary permeability. Most of the enteral and parenteral formulas used to provide nutritional support for critically ill patients contain large amounts of carbohydrate, which generate large quantities of carbon dioxide following oxidation. Such a large carbon dioxide load may worsen pulmonary function or may delay weaning from the ventilator.[79] If this factor becomes a problem, the carbohydrate load should be reduced to 50 to 60% of metabolic requirements. Fat emulsion is administered to provide additional calories.

### Associated Therapy

The integrated care of the patient with sepsis often requires the cooperation of many members of the health-care team. The nutritional and metabolic management of patients with serious infections is just one aspect of care and should be integrated into the overall care and treatment, which may include operative intervention, antibiotic therapy, dialysis, hormone administration, cardiopulmonary support, and physical therapy.

## Nutritional Assessment and Requirements

As with accidental injury, the onset of sepsis is generally sudden and unplanned. On the other hand, although most victims of trauma are well nourished and healthy prior to their injury, infected patients are often nutritionally depleted when bacteremia develops because of an underlying chronic disease, such as inflammatory bowel disease or chronic renal failure, or a complex and complicated postoperative course. Malnutrition is inseparable from the occurrence and effects of infectious diseases, and their interaction is synergistic.

As with all patients, the primary objectives of nutritional assessment are to evaluate the patient's present nutritional status and to determine energy, protein,and macro- and micronutrient requirements. Assessment of patients with sepsis should start with a medical history and physical examination, which are frequently difficult to obtain and perform because of the severity of the patient's illness. Use of anthropometric measurements is helpful, but weight may be an inaccurate reflection of nutritional status because of fluid retention. Serum protein concentrations (albumin and transferrin) are low because of redistribution secondary to the infection; hence these values are not useful indicators of malnutrition.

The immediate goal of nutritional therapy is weight maintenance. Weight gain and anabolism are generally difficult to achieve during the septic process, but they do occur once the disease process has abated. Total energy requirements can be calculated using the stress equation; mild-to-moderate infections increase energy requirements 20 to 30%, and severe infection increases caloric needs ≈50% above basal levels. The optimal calorie-to-nitrogen ratio is approximately 150:1, although providing more nitrogen has been proposed.

### Routes of Feeding

The routes of nutrient administration are similar to those for the elective surgical patient and the trauma victim. The enteral route should always be used when possible, but patients with sepsis usually have an ileus and therefore require parenteral nutrition. In general, this condition requires central venous nutrition because peripheral nutritional support cannot provide adequate calories in a moderately restrictive fluid volume. The risks of catheter sepsis are minimized by dedicating the central line solely to the infusion of

the hypertonic nutrient solutions and maintenance of strict asepsis at the catheter entrance site. In addition, the catheter may be changed over a guidewire using strict aseptic technique, and the catheter tip may be cultured.[103] This culturing is done at intervals of approximately 5 days and ensures that the catheter has not become the focus of the septic process.

## REFERENCES

1. Dudrick, S.J., Wilmore, D.W., Vars, H.M., et al.: Surgery *64*:134–142, 1968.
2. Stephens, R.V., Randall, H.T.: Ann. Surg. *170*:642–667, 1969.
3. Wretlind, A.: Nutr. Metab. *14(Suppl.)*:1–57, 1972.
4. Shires, G.T.: Ann. Surg. *192*:269–281, 1980.
5. Butterworth, C.E., Blackburn, G.L.: Nutr. Today *10*:8–18, 1975.
6. Wilmore, D.W., McDougal, W.S., Peterson, J.P.: Am. J. Clin. Nutr. *30*:1,498–1,505, 1977.
7. Bessey, P.Q., Wilmore, D.W.: Am. Soc. Reg. Anaesth. *7(Suppl.)*:5,178–5,187, 1982.
8. Moore, F.D.: Metabolic Care of the Surgical Patient. Philadelphia, W.B. Saunders, 1959.
9. Burke, G., Francsson, C., Plaintin, C.O.: Acta Endocrinol. *18*:201–209, 1955.
10. Traynor, C., Hall, G.M.: Br. J. Anaesth. *53*:153–160, 1981.
11. Deutsch, S.: Surg. Clin. North Am. *55*:775–786, 1975.
12. Philbin, D.M., Coggins, C.H.: Anesthesiology *49*:95–98, 1978.
13. Russell, R.C., Walker, C.J., Bloom, S.R.: Br. Med. J. *1*:10–12, 1975.
14. Porte, D., Jr., Graber, A.L., Kuzuwa, T., et al.: J. Clin. Invest. *45*:228–236, 1966.
15. Riegel, C., Koop, C.E., Drew, J., et al.: J. Clin. Invest. *26*:18–23, 1947.
16. Holden, W.D., Krieger, H., Levey, S., et al.: Ann. Surg. *146*:563–579, 1957.
17. Holter, A.R., Fischer, J.E.: J. Surg. Res. *23*:31–34, 1977.
18. Heatley, R.V., Williams, R.H.P., Lewis, M.H.: Postgrad Med. J. *55*:541–545, 1979.
19. Hume, D.M., Egdahl, R.H.: Ann. Surg. *150*:697–712, 1959.
20. Kehlet, H., Brandt, R.M., Rem, J.: J. Parenter. Enter. Nutr. *4*:152–155, 1980.
21. Engquist, A., Brandt, M.R., Fernandes, A., et al.: Acta Anaesthesiol. Scand. *21*:330–335, 1977.
22. Bromage, P.R., Shibata, H.R., Willoughby, H.W.: Surg. Gynecol. Obstet. *132*:1,051–1,056, 1971.
23. Brandt, M.R., Fernandes, A., Mordhorst, R., et al.: Br. Med. J. *1*:1,106–1,108, 1978.
24. Bloch, J.H., Pierce, C.H., Lillehei, R.C.: Annu. Rev. Med. *17*:483–504, 1966.
25. Estler, C.-J., Ammon, H.P.T.: Can. J. Physiol. Pharmacol. *47*:427–434, 1969.
26. Cooper, G.M., Paterson, J.L., Mashiter, K., et al.: Br. J. Anaesth. *52*:1,231–1,236, 1980.
27. Tsuji, H., Asoh, T., Shirasaka, C., et al.: Br. J. Surg. *67*:503–505, 1980.
28. Brandt, M.R., Korshin, J., Prange Hansen, A., et al.: Acta Anaesthesiol. Scand. *22*:400–412, 1978.
29. Studley, H.O.: JAMA *106*:458–460, 1936.
30. Daly, J.M., Massar, E., Giacco, G., et al.: Ann. Surg. *196*:203–208, 1982.

31. Müller, J.M., Dienst, C., Brenner, U., et al.: Lancet *1*:68–71, 1982.
32. Rombeau, J.L., Barot, L.R., Williamson, C.E., et al.: Am. J. Surg. *143*:139–143, 1982.
33. Buzby, G.P., Mullen, J.L., Matthews, D.C., et al.: Am. J. Surg. *139*:160–167, 1980.
34. Goldschmidt, S., Vars, H.M., Ravdin, I.S.: J. Clin. Invest. *18*:227–289, 1939.
35. McFadyen, B.V., Jr., Dudrick, S.J., Ruberg, R.L.: Surgery *74*:100–105, 1973.
36. Hunt, T.K.: Wound healing. *In* Current Surgical Diagnoses and Treatment. Edited by L.W. Way. Los Altos, CA, Lange Medical Publications, 1983.
37. Wesson, D.E., Mitch, W.E., Wilmore, D.W.: Nutritional considerations in the treatment of acute renal failure. *In* Acute Renal Failure. Edited by B. Brenner, and J.M. Lazarus. Philadelphia, W.B. Saunders, 1983.
38. Abel, R.M., Beck, C.H., Jr., Abbott, W.M., et al.: N. Engl. J. Med. *288*:695–699, 1973.
39. Fischer, J.E., Rosen, H.M., Ebeid, A.M., et al.: Surgery *80*:77–91, 1976.
40. Cerra, F.B., McMillen, M., Angelico, R., et al.: Surgery *94*:612–619, 1983.
41. Wahren, J., Denis, J., Desurmont, P., et al.: Intravenous administration of branched-chain amino acids in the treatment of hepatic encephalopathy. *In* Amino Acids: Metabolism and Medical Applications. Edited by G.L. Blackburn, et al. Boston, John Wright, 1983.
42. Wilmore, D.W.: The Metabolic Management of the Critically Ill. New York, Plenum Medical Book, 1977.
43. Grant, A.: Nutritional Assessment: Guidelines for Dietitians, 2nd Ed. Seattle, 1979.
44. Meakins, J.H., McLean, A.P.H., Kelly, R., et al.: J. Trauma *18*:240–247, 1978.
45. Duke, J.H. Jr., Jorgensen, S.B., Broell, J.R., et al.: Surgery *68*:168–174, 1970.
46. Page, C.P., Ryan, J.A. Jr., Haff, R.C.: Surg. Gynecol. Obstet. *142*:184–188, 1976.
47. Cowley, R.A.: J. Trauma *19*:354–357, 1979.
48. Cuthbertson, D.P.: Q. J. Med. *1*:233–246, 1932.
49. Cuthbertson, D.: Tilstone, W.J.: Adv. Clin. Chem. *12*:1–55, 1969.
50. Wilmore, D.W., Orcutt, T.W., Mason, A.D., Jr., et al.: J. Trauma *15*:697–703, 1975.
51. Wilmore, D.W.: Carbohydrate metabolism following injury. *In* Clinics in Endocrinology and Metabolism. Edited by K.G.M.M. Alberti. Philadelphia, W.B. Saunders, 1976.
52. Wilmore, D.W., Goodwin, C.W., Aulick, L.H., et al.: Ann. Surg. *192*:491–504, 1980.
53. Wilmore, D.W., Aulick, L.H., Mason, A.D., Jr., et al.: Ann. Surg. *186*:444–458, 1977.
54. Goodwin, C.W., Aulick, L.H., Powanda, M.C., et al.: Eur. J. Surg. Res. *12(Suppl. 126)*:126–127, 1980.
55. Black, P.R., Brooks, D.C., Bessey, P.Q., et al.: Ann. Surg. *196*:420–433, 1982.
56. Wilmore, D.W., Aulick, L.H., Goodwin, C.W., et al.: Acta Chir. Scand. *498 (Suppl.)*:43–47, 1980.
57. Wolfe, R.R., Durkot, M.J., Allsop, J.R., et al.: Glucose metabolism in severely burned patients. Metabolism *28*:1,031–1,039, 1979.
58. Brooks, D.C., Bessey, P.Q., Black, P.R., et al.: J. Surg. Res. *34*:100–107, 1984.
59. Carpentier, Y.A., Askanazi, J., Elwyn, D.H., et al.: J. Trauma *19*:649–654, 1979.
60. Bessey, P.Q., Brooks, D.C., Black, P.R., et al.: Surgery *94*:172–179, 1983.
61. Bessey, P.Q., Watters, J.M., Aoki, T.T., et al.: Ann. Surg. *200*(3):264–281, 1984.
62. Herrmann, V.M., Clark, D., Wilmore, D.W., et al.: Surg. Forum. *31*:92–94, 1980.
63. Picou, D., Taylor-Roberts, T.: Clin. Sci. *36*:283–296, 1969.
64. Birkhahn, R.H., Long, C.L., Fitkin, D., et al.: Am. J. Physiol. *241*:E64–E71, 1981.
65. Threlfall, C.J., Stoner, H.B., Galasko, C.S.B.: J. Trauma *21*:140–147, 1981.
66. Aulick, L.H., Wilmore, D.W.: Surgery *85*:560–565, 1979.
67. Muhlbacher, F., Kapadia, C.R., Colpoys, M.F., et al.: Am. J. Physiol. *247*:E75–E83, 1974.
68. Goldberg, A.L., Chang, T.W.: Fed. Proc. *37*:2,301–2,307, 1978.
69. Moldawer, L.L., Echenique, M.M., Bistrian, B.R., et al.: The importance of study design to the demonstration of efficacy with branched-chain amino acid enriched solutions. *In* Advances in Clinical Nutrition. Edited by I.D.A. Johnson. Boston, MTP Press, 1983.
70. Pitts, R.F.: Am. J. Med. *36*:720–742, 1964.
71. Windmueller, H.G., Spaeth, A.E.: J. Biol. Chem. *249*:5,070–5,079, 1974.
72. Souba, W.W., Wilmore, D.W.: Surgery *94*:342–350, 1983.
73. Souba, W.W., Kapadia, C.R., Smith, R.J., et al.: Surg. Forum. *34*:74–78, 1983.
74. Birkhahn, R.H., Long, C.L., Fitkin, D.L., et al.: J. Trauma *21*:513–519, 1981.
75. Wilmore, D.W., Aulick, L.H., Becker, R.A.: Hormones and the control of metabolism. *In* Surgical Nutrition. Edited by J.E. Fischer. Boston, Little, Brown, 1983.
76. Clowes, G.H.A., Jr., George, B.C., Villee, C.A., Jr., et al.: N. Engl. J. Med. *308*:545–552, 1983.
77. Long, J.M., III, Wilmore, D.W., Mason, A.D., Jr., et al.: Ann. Surg. *185*:417–422, 1977.
78. Wolfe, R.R., Allsop, J.R., Burke, J.F.: Metabolism *28*:210–220, 1979.
79. Askanazi, J., Rosenbaum, S.H., Hyman, A.I., et al.: JAMA *243*:1,444–1,447, 1980.
80. Levenson, S.W., Green, R.W., Taylor, F.H.L., et al.: Ann. Surg. *124*:840–856, 1946.
81. Brodribb, A.J.M., Ricketts, C.R.: Injury *3*:25–29, 1971.
82. Clowes, G.H.A., Jr., Vucinic, M., Weidner, M.G.: Ann. Surg. *163*:866–885, 1966.
83. Beisel, W.R.: Annu. Rev. Med. *26*:9–20, 1975.
84. Gump, F.E., Long, C., Killian, P., et al.: J. Trauma *14*:378–388, 1974.
85. LaNoue, K.F., Mason, A.D., Jr., Daniels, J.P.: Metabolism *17*:606–611, 1968.
86. McFadzean, A.J.S., Yeung, R.T.T.: Trans. R. Soc. Trop. Med. Hyg. *59*:179–185, 1965.
87. Yeung, C.Y.: J. Pediatr. *77*:812–817, 1970.
88. Long, C.L., Jeevanandam, M., Kim, B.M., et al.: Am. J. Clin. Nutr. *30*:1,340–1,344, 1977.
89. Duff, J.H., Viidik, T., Marchuk, J.B., et al.: Surgery *85*:344–348, 1979.
90. Gallin, J.I., Kaye, D., O'Leary, W.M.: N. Engl. J. Med. *281*:1,081–1,086, 1969.
91. Radcliffe, A.G., Wolfe, R.R., Colpoys, M.F., et al.: Am. J. Physiol. *244*:R667–R675, 1983.
92. Neufeld, H.A., Kaminski, M.V., Jr., Wannemacher, R.W., Jr.: Am. J. Clin. Nutr. *30*:1,357–1,358, 1977.

93. Watters, J.M., Wilmore, D.W.: Br. J. Surg. *73*:108–110, 1986.

94. Egdahl, R.H.: J. Clin. Invest. *38*:1,120–1,125, 1959.

95. Rocha, D.M., Santeusanio, F., Falonna, G.R., et al.: N. Engl. J. Med. *288*:700–703, 1973.

96. Groves, A.C., Griffiths, J., Leung, F., et al.: Ann. Surg. *178*:102–107, 1973.

97. Wilmore, D.W., Aulick, L.H.: Thermoregulatory responses and metabolism in surgical infectious diseases. *In* Surgical Infectious Disease. Edited by R.L. Simmons and R.J. Howard. New York, Appleton-Century-Crofts, 1982.

98. Berry, L.J.: Bacterial toxins. *In* Critical Reviews in Toxicology. Edited by L. Goldberg. Cleveland, Chemical Rubber Press, 1977.

99. Bennett, I.L., Jr., Beeson, P.B.: J. Exp. Med. *98*:477–492, 1953.

100. Dinarello, C.A.: Rev. Infec. Dis. *6*:51–95, 1984.

101. Garber, A.J.: J. Clin. Invest. *62*:623–632, 1978.

102. Kaminski, D.L., Adams, A., Jellinek, M.: Surgery *88*:93–100, 1980.

103. Graeve, A.H., Carpenter, C.M., Schiller, W.R.: Am. J. Surg. *142*:752–755, 1981.

*Chapter* **63**

# NUTRITION SUPPORT OF INHERITED METABOLIC DISEASES

## Louis J. Elsas, II and Phyllis B. Acosta

## GENETIC PERSPECTIVE

Geneticists approach the general subject of nutrition and the specific requirement for nutrients with the view that no minimum or recommended daily dietary allowances for an essential nutrient is optimum for all individuals. Rather, there is a continuum of individuals in a population with genetically determined variations in their nutrient requirements that extend over a wide range. This concept arose historically from two older scientific disciplines: human biochemical genetics and nutrition science. The former discipline originated with Sir Archibald Garrod's Croonian lectures of 1908. Garrod defined four "inborn errors of metabolism" as blocks in the normal flow of metabolic processes. Biochemical and clinical expression of these metabolic blocks demonstrated patterns of inheritance consistent with Mendel's prediction for transmission of single genes with large effect on the phenotype. Thus arose the concept that genes controlled metabolism and that disease states were created by blocks in this metabolic flow yielding accumulated precursors and deficient products.

Today, we recognize that "inborn errors" are discontinuous traits resulting from variation in the structure and function of enzymes or protein molecules. These enzymes are controlled by genes whose DNA structure, transcription, translation, post-translational events, and degradative rates all control enzymatic expression. Over 3,000 monogenic human disorders were cataloged in 1983 and, of these, about 250 have a defined biochemical basis.[1] The extent of normal variation in genes controlling enzyme activity suggests that about 30% of our population is heterozygous for common alleles.[2] Within this continuous diversity, mutations produce discontinuous, relatively rare traits that are expressed as disease under normal environmental conditions. Mutant gene frequencies vary in populations; for example, mitochondrial branched-chain alpha-ketoacid dehydrogenase deficiency (maple syrup urine disease) occurs in one of approximately every 250,000 newborns worldwide, but occurs in 1 of 176 in an inbred Mennonite population.[3,4] The mutation produces extreme toxicity due to accumulated branched-chain alpha-ketoacids if affected newborns are fed the RDA for branched-chain amino acids. However, normal growth and development are expected if dietary leucine, isoleucine, and valine are restricted to 20 to 40% of the RDA early in life depending on the degree of enzyme impairment.[5,6]

Considerable human variation occurs in the

structure and activity of enzymes involved in the catabolism of essential amino acids, but only a few are so impaired that ingestion of the RDA will create severe disease. Population-based newborn screening and dietary intervention are now applied through public health programs to at least five rare inborn errors where newborn screening predicts genetic susceptibility to a normal diet.[7,8] By contrast to these relatively rare inborn errors, all humans lack the enzyme that converts L-gluconogammalactone to ascorbic acid, but scurvy does not occur provided sufficient vitamin C is ingested and absorbed.[9] Thus, the frequency of genetic susceptibility to a "normal" diet ranges from rare to common and extends to the metabolism of aminoacids, carbohydrates, lipids, pyrimidines, minerals, and vitamins.

## GENETIC DISORDERS BENEFITED BY NUTRITION SUPPORT

Over 200 genetic disorders have been reported in which harmful manifestations relate to toxicity, deficiency, or overproduction of normally occurring substrates and products of metabolic flow. In many of them, modifications of the dietary supply alleviate the manifestations. In a large number, however, irreversible damage has already occurred by the time symptoms appear. Optimum management of these disorders depends on identifying affected subjects while they are presymptomatic or before irreversible disease has occurred. Because the disorders are genetic in origin, markers are theoretically present from the moment of conception, and thus the genetic power of prediction and prevention is applicable. In practice, a number of disorders can be detected in the fetus in the sixteenth to eighteenth weeks of gestation by studies on amniotic fluid cells. Prenatal diagnosis has been pushed forward to the eighth to twelfth weeks of gestation through the use of chorionic villus biopsy.[10] Some intrauterine sequelae of the inborn error, such as congenital cataracts in galactosemia, can be prevented by removing lactose from the mother's diet. Other inherited metabolic alterations are detected postnatally in the presymptomatic infant by analysis of blood, urine, erythrocytes, leukocytes, or cultured skin fibroblasts.

A search for presymptomatic genetic disease is most often undertaken only when there is a previous family history. Selective screening for inherited disease is also initiated for relatively common symptoms such as failure to thrive in childhood. Early treatment has proved effective

**Table 63–1. Criteria for Nonselective Newborn Screening**

| |
|---|
| The disorder should produce a high burden to the affected individual yet be preventable. |
| Methods for screening, retrieval, diagnosis, and management must be practical and available to the population as a whole. |
| Inheritance and pathogenesis of the disease should be understood. |
| Benefit-to-cost ratio of the program should be greater than one. |
| Patients' rights should be protected. |
| False-negative laboratory screening results should not occur. |
| False-positive laboratory results should be minimized. |

for many diseases such as phenylketonuria, galactosemia, isovaleric acidemia, homocystinuria, maple syrup urine disease (MSUD), argininosuccinic aciduria, and citrullinemia. Irreversible brain damage occurs if treatment is not initiated before the third week of life. To prevent this, population-wide screening of newborns has been instituted for phenylketonuria, MSUD, galactosemia, homocystinuria, and tyrosinemia. In MSUD, galactosemia, isovaleric acidemia, and disorders of the urea cycle, irreversible damage to the brain may occur within the first 7 to 10 days of life. Thus speed in diagnosis and treatment is of the utmost importance.

In the future, population-based presymptomatic detection will be extended to other disorders. However, before screening is initiated as a public health program, several principles should be fulfilled (Table 63–1). Note that knowledge of the pathogenesis and availability of therapy must precede the initiation of routine screening programs. Table 63–2 lists genetic disorders in which modification of nutrient intake has been employed. Effectiveness in preventing clinical sequelae is experimental in some of the therapies listed.

Although many inherited disorders benefit from nutrition support, each would require a chapter for adequate discussion. Thus, this chapter emphasizes disorders for which population-based screening, retrieval, diagnosis, and nutrition support are available to prevent their irreversible, severe pathologic problems.

## GENERAL PRINCIPLES OF GENETIC DISEASE MANAGEMENT

Specific proteins produced under the direction of individual genes form enzymes that catalyze specific reactions as noted in the following genetic and metabolic sequences:

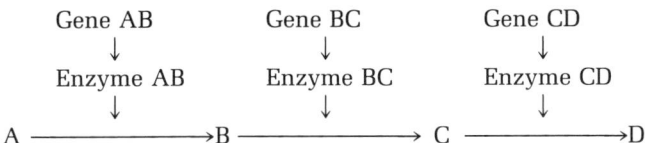

At least five pathologic effects could result from impaired enzyme CD in the above reaction sequence:

1. Lack of formation of D or some compound derived only from D. For example, in phenylketonuria (PKU) when phenylalanine is not hydroxylated to form tyrosine, not only is accumulated phenylalanine toxic, but tyrosine becomes an essential nutrient. Tyrosine must be supplemented to maintain proper infant growth in the dietary management of PKU. If product D normally functions in feedback control, overproduction of another product may occur because D is not present in amounts necessary to regulate production of intermediates "B" and "C." Exemplary of this phenomenon is excessive ACTH and androgen production in inborn errors of hydrocortisone production, such as steroid 21-hydroxylase deficiency. The consequence is overproduction of androgens and virilization of the female fetus or child.

2. Accumulation of C, the immediate precursor of the blocked reaction. In maple syrup urine disease, toxic branched-chain alpha-ketoacids accumulate because they cannot be decarboxylated and transacylated to their coenzyme A-simple acyl acid derivatives. The consequence in the neonate is severe central nervous system depression with apnea, stupor, coma, and death. If the neonate survives, severe mental retardation ensues if the child is not treated by diet restriction within two weeks of life.

3. Accumulation of A or B, remote precursors of the blocked reaction sequence CD. If the preceding reactions are freely reversible, a precursor, in addition to that proximal to the block, will accumulate. This process is illustrated in maple syrup urine disease by increased leucine, isoleucine, and valine, which are formed by reamination of the branched-chain alpha-ketoacids: alpha-ketoisocaproic, alpha-keto-beta-methylvaleric, and alpha-keto isovaleric acids, respectively.

4. Increased production of alternative normal products through little-used metabolic pathways. As illustrated in Figure 63–1, when phenylalanine is not hydroxylated to form tyrosine, phenylpyruvic, phenylacetic, and phenyllactic acids are produced in greater than normal amounts through existing pathways that normally do not function at physiologic concentrations of cellular phenylalanine.

5. Depressed production of needed nutrients through inhibition by accumulated substrate (i.e., C in CD enzyme impairment) of different metabolic pathways. For example, neurotransmitter synthesis may be depressed in PKU owing to increased blood phenylalanine that inhibits tyrosine hydroxylase (EC 1.14.16.2) and tryptophan hydroxylase (EC 1.14.16.4) in the central nervous system. Another example is type I tyrosinemia. The accumulation of succinylacetone inhibits delta aminolevulinic acid dehydratase (EC 4.2.1.24) (Fig. 63–2) and results in attacks of acute porphyria with peripheral neuropathy, hypertension, and bizarre behavior.

Eleven approaches to therapy of inherited metabolic disease are discussed here. The appropriate approach is dependent on the pathophysiology of disease expression. Several therapeutic approaches may be used simultaneously:

1. Correction of the primary imbalance in metabolic relationships. This correction involves a reduction through dietary restriction of accumulated substrate(s) that are toxic. Examples are PKU, MSUD, and galactosemia where phenylalanine; leucine, isoleucine, and valine; or lactose are limited, respectively.

2. Enhance excretion of accumulated substances that are overproduced. Treatment of gout with uricosuric agents leads to lower blood uric acid levels by blocking renal reabsorption. The tissue deposits of uric acid salts are then mobilized.

3. Provision of alternate metabolic pathways to decrease accumulated toxic precursors in blocked reaction sequences. For example, the accumulated ammonia in enzyme defects of the urea cycle is reduced by removing nitrogen through administration of therapeutic amounts of benzoic acid to form hippuric acid from glycine. Another example is isovaleric acidemia. Innocuous isovalerylglycine is formed from accumulating isovaleric acid if supplemental glycine is provided to drive glycine-N-transacylase (EC 2.3.1.13). Isovalerylglycine is excreted in the urine.

4. Use of metabolic inhibitors to lower overproduced products. Allopurinol inhibits xanthine oxidase (EC 1.2.3.2) and decreases overproduction of uric acid in gout. Lovastatin and compactin suppress hydroxymethylglutaryl CoA reductase (EC 1.1.1.34) and reduce excess cholesterol biosynthesis in familial hypercholesterolemia.

**Table 63–2.   Genetic Disorders for Which Nutrient Intake Should be Modified**

| Disorder | Therapy |
|---|---|
| Abetalipoproteinemia | Medium-chain triglycerides and vitamins A, E supplements |
| Acrodermatitis enteropathica | Zinc sulfate supplement |
| Alkaptonuria (ochronosis) | Ascorbic acid supplement; phenylalanine, tyrosine restriction |
| Anemia: hypochromic, sideroblastic | Pyridoxine supplement |
| Argininemia | Protein restriction; essential amino acids supplement; ornithine supplement |
| Argininosuccinic aciduria | Arginine, benzoic acid supplements; protein restriction |
| Beta-methylcrotonylglycinuria | Leucine restriction |
| β-sitosterolemia | Plant sterol restriction |
| Biotinidase deficiency | Biotin supplement |
| Branched-chain α-ketoaciduria | Branched-chain amino acid restriction; thiamin supplement |
| Carbamylphosphate synthetase deficiency | Arginine, benzoic acid supplements; protein restriction; essential amino acids |
| Chédiak-Higashi syndrome | Ascorbic acid supplement |
| Chloride diarrhea | Sodium chloride supplement |
| Citrullinemia | Protein restriction; essential amino acids; arginine and benzoic acid supplements |
| Combined hyperlipidemia | Calorie, carbohydrate, saturated fatty acid restriction; nicotinic acid and lovastatin and compactin therapy; cholestyramine |
| Cystathioninuria | Pyridoxine supplements |
| Cystic fibrosis | Enteric enzyme supplements (trypsin, lipase, chymotrypsin) |
| Cystinosis | Alkali; cysteamine; phosphate; vitamin D supplements |
| Diabetes insipidus | Water; low-solute diets; vasopressin |
| Diabetes mellitus | Insulin; controlled diet |
| Diabasic aminoaciduria | Arginine supplement; protein restriction |
| Ehlers-Danlos syndrome; lysyl hydroxylase defect | Ascorbic acid supplement |
| Folic acid reductase deficiency | $N^5$-formyltetrahydrofolic acid supplement |
| Folic acid transport defect | Parenteral folate supplement |
| Fructose intolerance | Fructose-free diet |
| Fructose-1, 6-diphosphatase deficiency | Frequent glucose; folate supplement; reduced fructose intake |
| Galactokinase deficiency | Galactose-restricted diet |
| Galactosemia | Galactose-restricted diet |
| Glucose-galactose malabsorption | Glucose, galactose restrictions; fructose supplement |
| Glucose-6-phosphate dehydrogenase deficiency | Avoidance of fava bean and drugs that cause erythrocyte hemolysis |
| Glutamate-aspartate transport defect | Glutamine supplement |
| Glutaric acidemia | Protein restriction |
| Glycogen storage | |
|    type I (glucose-6-phosphatase deficiency) | Frequent feeding; complex starch supplement |
|    type III (amylo-1,6 glucosidase deficiency) | Frequent feeding; high-protein diet |
|    type VI (phosphorylase deficiency) | Frequent feeding |
|    type VIII (phosphorylase kinase deficiency) | Avoid fasting, high-protein diet |
| Gout | Purine restriction; allopurinol |
| Hartnup disease | Nicotinamide supplement |
| Homocystinuria | |
|    cystathionine β-synthase deficiency | Methionine restriction; cysteine supplement; pyridoxine and betaine supplements |
|    $N^5,N^{10}$-methylenetetrahydrofolate reductase deficiency | Folic acid supplement |
|    $CH_3$-cobalamin deficiency | Parenteral $B_{12}$ |
| Hydroxykynureninuria | Nicotinic acid supplement |
| Hyperbeta-alaninemia | Pyridoxine supplement |
| Hypercholesterolemia | Restriction of saturated fatty acids and cholesterol; lovastatin and compactin, nicotinamide, cholestyramine supplementation |

**Table 63-2. Genetic Disorders for Which Nutrient Intake Should be Modified** *Continued*

| Disorder | Therapy |
| --- | --- |
| Hyperlipoproteinemia I | Fat-free diet; medium-chain triglyceride and essential fatty acid supplements |
| Hyperphenylalaninemia | Phenylalanine restriction; carbidopa; 5-hydroxytryptophan; |
|   dihydropteridine reductase deficiency |   $BH_4$ |
|   biopterin biosynthetic blocks | Tetrahydrobiopterin, carbidopa; 5-OH-tryptophan |
| Hypertriglyceridemia | Weight reduction; carbohydrate restriction |
| Hypophosphatemia | Vitamin D, phosphorus supplements |
| Isovaleric acidemia | Leucine restriction; glycine supplements |
| Ketoacidosis of infancy | Alkali, glucose supplements |
| Lactic acidosis, intermittent | |
|   (pyruvate decarboxylase deficiency) | High-fat, low-carbohydrate diet; thiamin supplement; alkali |
|   (pyruvate carboxylase deficiency) | Frequent feeds; alkali, thiamin and biotin supplements |
| Lactose intolerance | Lactose restriction |
| Lysine intolerance (hyperlysinemia) | Protein restriction |
| Methionine malabsorption | Methionine restriction; cysteine supplement |
| Methylmalonic aciduria | |
|   defective reduction or transport of cobalamin | $B_{12}$ supplement, megadoses parenterally |
|   impaired synthesis of 5′-deoxyadenosylcobalamin | Parenteral $B_{12}$, megadoses |
|   methylmalonyl-CoA mutase deficiency | Isoleucine, methionine, threonine, valine restriction |
| | $B_{12}$ |
|   methylmalonyl-CoA racemase deficiency | Biotin supplement |
| Multiple carboxylase deficiency | Biotin supplement |
| Nonketotic hyperglycinemia | Protein restriction, calorie supplements; strychnine |
| Ornithine transcarbamylase deficiency | Arginine, benzoic acid supplements; protein restriction; essential amino acids |
| Orotic aciduria | Uridine supplements |
| Oxalosis | Pyridoxine, magnesium, orthophosphate, water supplements |
| Periodic paralysis | |
|   hypokalemic | Carbohydrate restriction, potassium salts, sodium chloride |
|   hyperkalemic | Increased carbohydrates |
|   normokalemic | Sodium chloride |
| Phenylketonuria | Phenylalanine restriction, tyrosine supplement |
| Porphyria, acute intermittent | High glucose, hematin infusions |
| Propionicacidemia | Isoleucine. methionine, threonine, valine restriction; biotin supplement |
| Pyridoxine dependency with seizures | Pyridoxine, parenterally |
| Pyroglutamic aciduria | Alkali, protein restriction |
| Pyruvate dehydrogenase deficiency, partial | Thiamin supplement, carbohydrate restriction; energy supplement (lipids) |
| Refsum's disease | Phytanic acid restriction (diet low in dairy and ruminant fats) |
| Renal tubular acidosis | Alkali supplements |
| Sucrose-isomaltose malabsorption | Sucrose restriction |
| Tryptophanuria with dwarfism | Nicotinic acid |
| Tyrosinemia, type I | Phenylalanine-tyrosine restriction, high calorie; hematin infusions if porphyric symptoms persist |
| Tyrosinemia with keratosis and corneal dystrophy | Phenylalanine and tyrosine restriction |
| Valinemia | Valine restriction |
| Vitamin A defect (beta-carotene 15, 15′-dioxygenase) | Vitamin A |
| Vitamin $B_{12}$ defect (conversion of $B_{12}$ to precursor of 5′-deoxyadenosyl-$B_{12}$ and methyl-$B_{12}$ | Vitamin $B_{12}$ |
| Vitamin D-dependent rickets | 1,25 dehydroxy D |
| Vitamin K-dependent coagulation defect | Vitamin K |
| Xanthinuria | Purine restriction; allopurinol, fluids, alkali supplements |
| Xanthurenic aciduria | Pyridoxine |

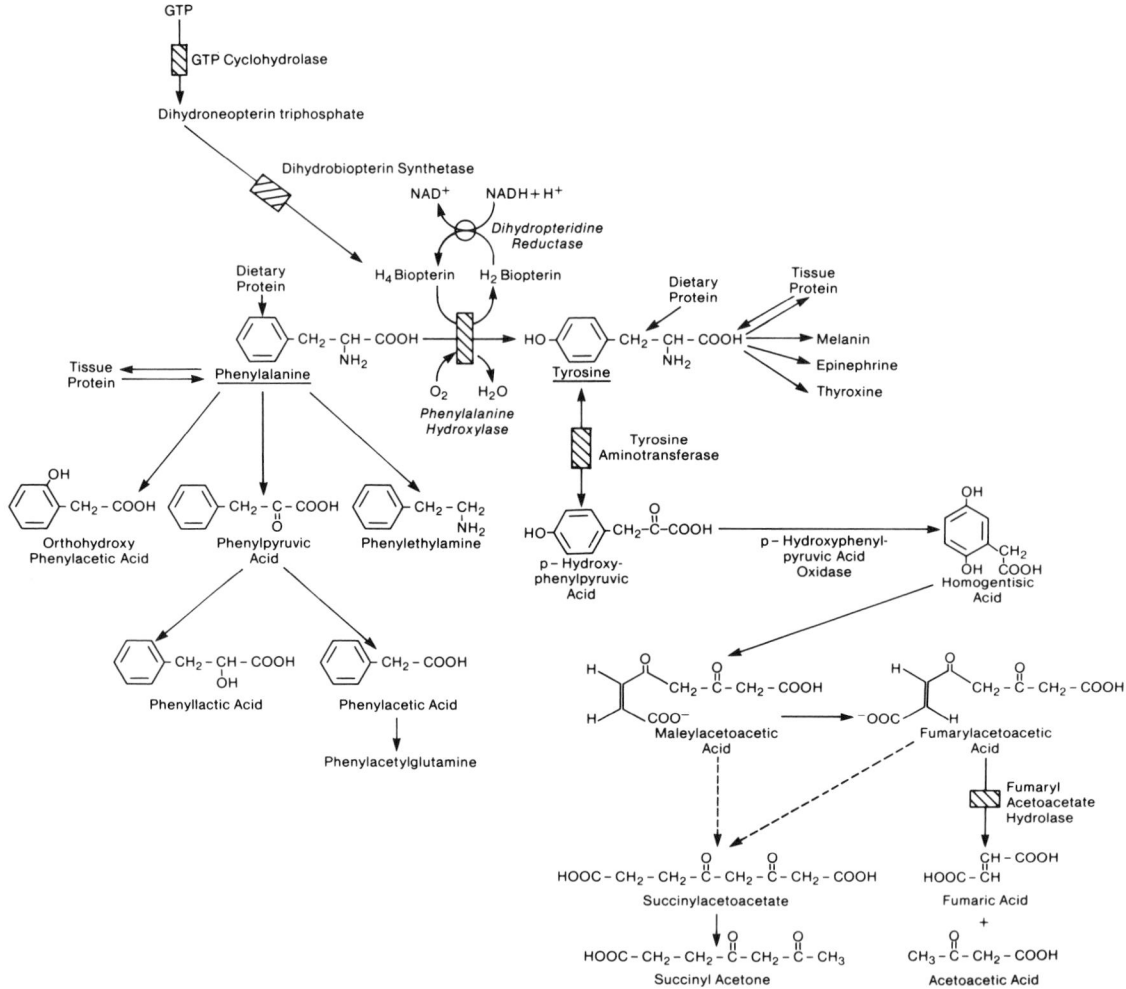

**Fig. 63–1.** Metabolism of aromatic amino acids. The metabolic flow and nutrient interaction in disorders of phenylalanine and tyrosine are schematized. Crosshatched bars represent impaired enzymes involved in biopterin biosynthesis, phenylketonuria, and tyrosinemia. See text for discussion.

5. Supplying products of blocked secondary pathways. In cystic fibrosis, the exocrine pancreas does not function in a normal manner to produce and secrete digestive enzymes. Administration of these pancreatic enzymes partially corrects the digestive defect in cystic fibrosis. Similarly, supplying hematin alleviates some neurologic deficits in tyrosinemia, type I where succinylacetone has inhibited delta-aminolevulinic acid dehydratase (EC 4.2.1.2.4) and consequently heme biosynthesis (see Fig. 63–2).

6. Stabilization of altered enzyme proteins. The rate of biologic synthesis and degradation of holo-enzymes is dependent on their structural conformation. In some holoenzymes, saturation by coenzyme increases their biologic half-life and, thus, overall enzyme activity at the new equilibrium. This therapeutic mechanism is exemplified in homocystinuria and maple syrup urine disease. Pharmacologic intake of vitamin $B_6$ in homocystinuria and vitamin $B_1$ in maple syrup urine disease increases intracellular pyridoxal phosphate and thiamin pyrophosphate and increases the specific activity of cystathionine beta-synthase (EC 4.2.1.22) and branched-chain alpha-ketoacid dehydrogenase complex, respectively.[11,12]

7. Replacement of deficient cofactors. A variety of vitamin-dependent disorders are due to blocks in coenzyme production and are "cured" by pharmacologic intake of a specific vitamin precursor. This mechanism presumably involves overcoming a partially impaired enzyme reaction by mass action. Variously impaired reactions required to produce either methylcobalamin and/or adenosylcobalamin result in homocystinuria and/or methylmalonic aciduria. Daily intakes of milli-

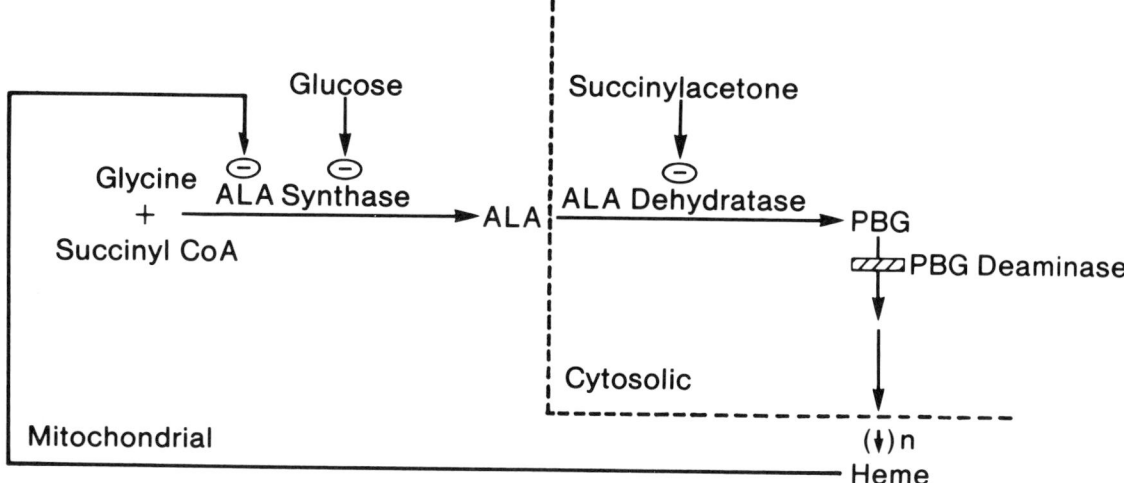

ALA = δ – Aminolevulinic Acid
PBG = Porphobilinogen
⊖ = Negative feedback or inhibition

**Fig. 63–2.** Inhibition site in heme biosynthesis of relevance to diagnosis and treatment of tyrosinemia, type I. Hatched bar represents, schematically, the partial block in acute intermittent porphyria with resultant overproduction of ALA (δ-aminolevulinic acid) and PBG (porphobilinogen) with decreased heme biosynthesis. In type I tyrosinemia, succinylacetone is produced and inhibits ALA dehydratase with accumulation of ALA alone, which is neurotoxic. ALA accumulation can be reduced by addition of excess dietary glucose (calories) and by hematin infusions that negatively control ALA synthase (EC 2.3.1.37) at levels of both enzyme and gene expression.

gram quantities of vitamin B$_{12}$ may cure the disease.[13] Reviews on "vitamin dependency syndromes" have been published.[14,15,145a,150]

8. Artificial induction of enzyme production. If the structural gene or enzyme is intact, but suppressor, enhancer, or promoter elements are not functional, abnormal amounts of enzyme may be produced. It should be possible to "turn on" or "turn off" the structural gene and enable normal enzymatic production to occur. In the acute porphyria of type I tyrosinemia, excessive delta-aminolevulinic acid production may be reduced by suppressing transcription of the delta-ALA synthase gene with excess glucose and hematin (see Fig. 63–2).

9. Enzyme replacement therapy. Many attempts to replace deficient enzymes by organ transplant, plasma infusions, and microencapsulation have been tried with limited success. Organ transplantation, such as kidney transplant in Fabry's disease and liver transplant in type I glycogen storage disease, may benefit systemic metabolism with the return of organ function through replacing deficient enzyme activity.

10. Correction of the underlying defect in DNA so that the body can manufacture its own functionally normal enzymes. This experimental approach has great possibility for the future. The DNA for several enzymes, such as phenylalanine

hydroxylase (EC 1.14.16.1), adenosine deaminase (EC 3.5.4.17), hypoxanthine-guanine phosphoribosyl transferase (EC 2.4.2.22), and argininosuccinic acid lyase (EC 4.3.2.1), has been cloned and retroviral constructs made by which gene transfer into dividing somatic cells has been accomplished. Human gene therapy is currently contemplated for these inborn errors, although several barriers to application in man must be solved first.[15a]

11. Limiting the frequency of inherited diseases through genetic counseling. This approach might decrease the number of affected individuals resulting from high-risk matings by developing tests for the heterozygous or carrier states, providing risks and alternatives to potential parents and providing prenatal detection where two heterozygous mates are contemplating having children.

Some practical considerations for nutritional control of inherited metabolic disorders should be considered. Dietary restrictions required to correct imbalances in metabolic relationships often require the use of chemically defined or elemental foods.[16] These chemically defined products are normally accompanied by small amounts of whole natural protein that supply the restricted amino acid(s). Natural foods seldom supply more than 25% and often much less of the protein requirements of patients. Other nitrogen-free natural foods that provide energy are limited in their range of nutrients. Consequently, care must be taken to provide food constituents often considered to be contaminants because their essentiality has been demonstrated through long-term use of total parenteral nutrition.[17] Thus, in addition to nutrients for which an RDA is established, other nutrients must be supplied in adequate amounts. These include the trace metals chromium, manganese, molybdenum, and selenium, the vitamins biotin and pantothenic acid and also choline and inositol. Other possible conditionally essential nutrients for patients with phenylketonuria have been described.[18]

Chemically defined diets consist of small molecules that often provide an osmolality greater than the physiologic tolerance of the patient. Abdominal cramping, diarrhea, distention, nausea, and vomiting have resulted from use of hyperosmolar feeds.[19] Aside from gastrointestinal distress, more serious consequences can occur such as hypertonic dehydration,[20] hypovolemia,[21] hypernatremia,[22] and death.[23] Osmolalities of selected chemically defined products intended for inherited diseases of amino acid metabolism have been published.[24,25]

## AROMATIC AMINO ACIDS

Inborn errors of the aromatic amino acids were historically the first to respond to nutritional support. Phenylketonuria was discovered 50 years ago, and the prevention of its resultant mental retardation by dietary intervention is classic. By contrast, the rare disorders of tyrosine metabolism remain problematic.

### Biochemistry

The essential amino acid phenylalanine is utilized for two major purposes: tissue protein synthesis and hydroxylation to form tyrosine. The hydroxylation reaction requires phenylalanine hydroxylase (EC 1.14.16.1), $O_2$, tetrahydrobiopterin, dihydropteridine reductase (EC 1.6.99.7), and NADH + H$^+$ (see Fig. 66–1). In the normal adult, only 10% of the RDA for phenylalanine is required for new protein synthesis, whereas approximately 90% is hydroxylated to form tyrosine. In the growing child, 60% of the phenylalanine required is used for new protein synthesis and 40% is hydroxylated to form tyrosine. Mass spectrometry and stable isotope studies of patients with phenylketonuria provide information on other pathways available for phenylalanine metabolism. These alternate pathways, outlined in Figure 63–1, are minor in the metabolism of phenylalanine at 50 µmol concentration in the plasma

of normal individuals. However, by-products become apparent when phenylalanine cannot be hydroxylated to tyrosine and accumulates to over 1,000 µmol.[26]

Tyrosine is the normal immediate product of phenylalanine and is essential to five pathways (see Fig. 63–1). These include synthesis of protein, catecholamines, melanin pigment, and thyroid hormones. Tyrosine also provides energy when catabolized through para-hydroxyphenyl pyruvate to fumarate and acetoacetate. Enzymes required in this latter degradative pathway include tyrosine aminotransferase (EC 2.6.1.5), *p*-hydroxyphenyl-pyruvic acid oxidase (EC 1.14.2.2), homogentisic acid oxidase (EC 1.13.11.5), and fumarylacetoacetic acid hydrolase (EC 3.7.1.2) (see Fig. 63–1).

### Phenylketonuria

**Definition.** Phenylketonuria (PKU) is a group of inherited disorders of phenylalanine metabolism caused by impaired phenylalanine hydroxylase activity. The disease is expressed at three to six months of age and is characterized by developmental delay, microcephaly, abnormal electroencephalogram, eczema, musty odor, and hyperactivity. If not treated before three weeks of age, the metabolic imbalance produces irreversible mental retardation. The defect in metabolism in classic PKU is associated with less than 2% activity of normal phenylalanine hydroxylase.[27] The enzyme is expressed primarily in liver, but not in peripheral blood cells, bone marrow, or cultured cells. Considerable heterogeneity exists for mutations affecting this apoenzyme. Heterozygous parents for "classic" PKU have 50% enzyme activity but are clinically normal even though mild in vivo differences from normal are observed in semifasting phenylalanine to tyrosine plasma concentration ratios.[28] Additionally, variant forms with less severe enzymatic loss require less stringent diet therapy. An attempt is being made to associate phenotype with variation in phenylalanine hydroxylase through the use of DNA analysis. If restriction fragment-length polymorphisms of DNA can define these variations, it will be easier to predict the need for nutrition support and genetic recurrence risks in families.[29] The gene for phenylalanine hydroxylase is located on chromosome 12q.

Other forms of PKU may result from defects in other enzymes involved in the overall reaction. Dihydropteridine reductase (EC 1.6.99.7) is an enzyme normally present in many tissues. It reduces the quininoid form of dihydrobiopterin to tetrahydrobiopterin (see Fig. 63–1). Several other types of PKU result from defects in the synthesis of tetrahydrobiopterin (See Fig. 63–1).[30] In addition to functioning as coenzyme for phenylalanine hydroxylase, tetrahydrobiopterin is also required by tyrosine hydroxylase and tryptophan hydroxylase[31,31a] (See Fig. 63–1). Because these enzymes produce essential neurotransmitters, defects in biopterin synthesis are associated with progressive neurologic disease unless tetrahydrobiopterin, L-DOPA, and serotonin are replaced.[31]

Although the precise pathogenesis of mental retardation in classic PKU is not known, the accumulation of phenylalanine or its catabolic byproducts, a deficiency of tyrosine or its products, or all four circumstances may produce central nervous system damage. The pathologic consequence varies with the time in brain development at which the chemical insult occurs. Deficient myelination and abnormalities in brain proteolipids and/or proteins occur in late gestation and during the first six to nine months of life.[32] During this period, oligodendroglia migration may also be impaired, resulting in irreversible brain damage later in childhood. Protein synthesis in the brain is also depressed, probably owing to competitive inhibition by high phenylalanine on blood-brain barrier transport with consequent imbalance in intraneuronal amino acid concentrations.[33] In the mature brain, behavioral difficulties and prolonged performance times may result from depressed neurotransmitter synthesis.[26] Impairment of these neuropsychologic functions in mature brain is reversible when phenylalanine returns toward normal concentrations in cells and blood.[26]

**Screening.** The disorders of phenylalanine metabolism require identification, diagnosis, and appropriate therapy before clinical expression of the disease is apparent. Nutrition and/or other therapy should be instituted before the third week of life. Thus a tetrapartite public health program involving screening, retrieval, diagnosis, and treatment must be coordinated and efficient to accomplish the objective of preventing mental retardation. A screening test utilizing the bacterial inhibition assay[34] detects potential cases in the newborn population. One laboratory can effectively screen 20,000 to 200,000 samples per year using these methods. Although other methods such as fluorometry are more quantitative, the Guthrie test is used worldwide because of its ease of application. Newborns with blood phenylalanine concentrations greater than 4 mg/dl on the screening test are restudied. The actions taken in "retrieval" depend on the concentration of blood phenylalanine, days of age, and protein intake at the time of screening. Repeat screening at 14 days of age is suggested.[35]

Newborn screening in most of the 50 states, in conjunction with aggressive approaches to retrieval and diagnosis, has led to early institution of diet therapy. To be successful, state-mandated screening programs must allow for easy collection and rapid evaluation of specimens while providing an organized, efficient retrieval system of babies having positive screening tests.[36] With the present early discharge from hospital and nursery of both mother and baby after delivery, lower phenylalanine concentrations of 2 to 4 mg/dl are considered to be positive and follow-up is initiated.

Approximately 1 in 10,000 white newborns is affected with PKU while 1 in 132,000 in the black population is affected. Data in Table 63–3 detail the number of cases of PKU diagnosed since the inception of an exemplary state-wide screening program in Georgia. The mean frequency of PKU is based on a population of newborn screenees that is 63% white. Retrieval time and age at initiation of treatment for PKU cases diagnosed in 1985 are given in Table 63–4. Outcome and accountability for preventing mental retardation are dependent on the speed with which nutritional management is implemented. Very little public health data of the type presented in Table 63–4 are available to evaluate dietary results in various programs.

**Diagnosis.** Patients with initial blood phenylalanine concentrations of 4 to 8 mg/dl should have the test repeated immediately. If the initial or follow-up screening test is greater than 8 mg/dl, plasma amino acids should be quantitated by ion exchange chromatography with the infant on a known phenylalanine intake from natural protein sources. A precise diagnosis is necessary to establish the mode of therapy.

Differential diagnosis requires several laboratory methods. These include ion exchange chromatography for quantitation of plasma phenylalanine, tyrosine, and other amino acid concentrations, determination of genotype of parents and proband,[28] and assays of biopterin and dihydropteridine reductase.[30] Assessment of phenylalanine hydroxylase activity in liver biopsy material[37] has been attempted in the past but is invasive and not ethical for routine diagnosis. DNA analysis using restriction fragment-length polymorphisms (RFLP) and cDNA probes for the phenylalanine hydroxylase gene will be helpful in the future.[29] For families with an affected child, prenatal diagnosis is now available using RFLP for the cDNA of phenylalanine hydroxylase.[38] Because phenylalanine hydroxylase is not expressed in cultured amniotic fluid cells, and because phenylalanine concentrations do not rise in am-

**Table 63–3.  Cases Diagnosed in 1985 and Since Inception of Comprehensive Newborn Screening Program, State of Georgia***

| Disease | 1985 Cases Diagnosed | 7-Year Total Cases Diagnosed | Incidence | Rate/100,000 |
|---------|:---:|:---:|:---:|:---:|
| PKU (Total) | 7 | 34 | 1/19,490 | 5.1 |
|     classic | 4 | 20 | 1/33,133 | 3.0 |
|     hyperphenylalaninemia | 3 | 14 | 1/47,333 | 2.1 |
| Homocystinuria | | | | |
|     classic | 0 | 3 | 1/220,887 | 0.5 |
|     other methionine abnormalities | 2 | 12 | 1/55,222 | 1.8 |
| MSUD | 1 | 8 | 1/82,833 | 1.2 |
| Tyrosinemia | | | | |
|     hereditary, type I | 0 | 4 | 1/165,665 | 0.6 |
|     transient | 60 | 384 | 1/1,726 | 57.9 |
| Galactosemia (Total) | 3 | 36 | 1/17,414 | 5.7 |
|     classic | 0 | 11 | 1/56,992 | 1.8 |
|     variant | 3 | 25 | 1/25,076 | 4.0 |

*Total screenees were 663,000 of which 37% were black.

niotic fluid until the last trimester, prenatal monitoring was impractical in the past.

**Treatment.** Patients with plasma phenylalanine concentrations of greater than 150 μmol and plasma tyrosine concentrations below 50 μmol require prompt treatment with a phenylalanine-restricted, tyrosine-supplemented diet. The objective of nutrition support in the child with classic PKU is to maintain blood phenylalanine concentrations that will allow optimum growth and brain development by supplying adequate energy, protein, and other nutrients while restricting phenylalanine and supplementing tyrosine intake.

Although the effects of moderately elevated plasma phenylalanine are not yet known, optimum blood levels should be as close to normal (50 μmol) as possible. This objective is met through use of a combination of proprietary, chemically defined, medical and natural foods. Some investigators have supplemented the phenylalanine-restricted diet with isoleucine, leucine, and valine[39] and have found improvement in behavior and decreased plasma phenylalanine. This may be related to inhibition of phenylalanine transport by competition at either the intestinal

or blood brain barrier uptake steps.[33] Gene replacement therapy using recombinant viruses containing the phenylalanine hydroxylase gene may be useful in the future as one approach to management of individuals with PKU. Recombinant retroviruses may be used to introduce a functioning phenylalanine hydroxylase gene into liver or bone marrow cells and thus may enable an individual with PKU to metabolize excess phenylalanine to tyrosine.[40] However, these latter approaches are still under study, and difficulty will be encountered in coordinating dihydropteridine reductase and biopterin synthesis to accomplish the overall reaction. Thus, this approach is not yet applicable in practice.

Therapy of the child with biopterin-deficient forms of hyperphenylalaninemia requires administration of tetrahydrobiopterin and use of the phenylalanine-restricted, tyrosine-supplemented diet in combination with L-DOPA and carbidopa.[31] Serotonin that is derived from tryptophan may also improve behavior if tryptophan hydroxylase is secondarily impaired by the absence of tetrahydrobiopterin.[31,31a,41]

*Initiation of Nutrition Support.* Rapid decline

**Table 63–4.  Retrieval Time (Days) for Cases Diagnosed in 1985 in Georgia**

| Disease | N | Age at First Test | Age at Second Test | Retrieval Time | Age at Start of Treatment |
|---------|:---:|:---:|:---:|:---:|:---:|
| PKU (classic) | 4 | 3.5 (2–7)* | 9.8 (7–16) | 6.3 (5–9) | 11.3 (8–17) |
| Hyperphenylalaninemia | 3 | 2.7 (2–4) | 12.7 (9–16) | 10.0 (7–12) | 23.0 (23) |
| Galactosemia (variant) | 3 | 7.0 (3–16) | 18.0 (11–27) | 10.3 (8–14) | 27.3 (15–33) |
| MSUD (variant) | 1 | 3 | 10 | 7 | 10 |

*Numbers in parentheses indicate range of age in days.

of blood phenylalanine concentration at the time of diagnosis may be obtained by feeding the infant a 20 kcal/oz (67 kcal/dl) low-phenylalanine or phenylalanine-free formula.[42] Within a mean of four days (SD ±3), blood phenylalanine concentration should drop to treatment range. Treatment should be initiated in hospitalized infants to enable adequate parental information transfer and to monitor blood amino acids daily. Laboratory results should be available promptly to prevent precipitation of phenylalanine deficiency and to enable rapid replacement of phenylalanine and tyrosine to optimum blood concentrations.

In the event that the infant or child is not hospitalized for initiation of nutrition support or if only weekly blood phenylalanine concentrations are obtained, a maintenance formula containing adequate phenylalanine from an appropriate source (Appendix Table A-43a) should be prescribed. Blood phenylalanine concentration will fall to treatment range within a mean of 10 days (SD 5) with this approach.[42] Choice of initial nutrition support should be predicated on producing controlled blood phenylalanine concentrations no later than the third week of life.

*Chronic Care.* Long-term care of the patient with classic PKU dictates that proprietary chemically defined products (medical foods) and natural foods provide all nutrients in required amounts.

*Nutrient Requirements.* Data in Table 63–5 outline the suggested amounts of phenylalanine, tyrosine, protein, energy, and fluid to offer. A formal prescription must be written that is individualized to the specific degree of impaired enzyme activity, growth rate, and consequent needs of each patient. Weekly adjustments in the diet prescription may be necessary, particularly during the first six months of life, based on hunger, growth, development, and laboratory analyses of plasma phenylalanine and tyrosine concentrations. The phenylalanine provided should maintain the three- to four-hour postprandial blood phenylalanine concentration as close to 50 μmol (50 to 150 μmol) as possible. Phenylalanine is an essential amino acid[43] and cannot be deleted from the diet without producing death.[44] Excess restriction produces growth failure, skin rashes, bone changes, and mental retardation.[44]

Phenylalanine required for growth by the infant with classic PKU is 20 to 70 mg/kg of body weight, with the younger infant requiring the larger amount.[45] Phenylalanine requirement declines rapidly between three and six months of age as growth rates plateau. Requirements for phenylalanine in the 6- to 12-month-old patient with classic PKU may fall to 15 mg/kg/day, but they vary considerably (see Table 63–5). Careful monitoring of blood phenylalanine concentration and intake is required to prevent excess intake when growth rate decelerates and inadequate intake when growth rate is at its peak.

Tyrosine is an essential amino acid for children with PKU. For this reason, plasma tyrosine values must be monitored and L-tyrosine supplements given. The supplement required is between 20 and 35 mg/kg/day in addition to that already present in chemically defined formula and food to reach a total of 120 to 150 mg/kg/day. Tyrosine supplements alone will not prevent mental retardation in classic phenylketonuria.[46]

**Table 63–5.** **Approximate Daily Requirements for Selected Nutrients\* for Infants and Children with Inherited Disorders of Amino Acid Metabolism**

| | | Age | | | | | | |
|---|---|---|---|---|---|---|---|---|
| Nutrient | Unit | 0<6 mo. | 6<12 mo. | 1<4 yr. | 4<7 yr. | 7<11 yr. | 11<15 yr. | 15<19 yr. |
| Fluid | ml/kg | 120–115 | 100 | 95 | 90 | 75 | 50 | 50 |
| Energy | kcal/kg | 145–95 | 135–80 | — | — | — | — | — |
| | kcal/day | — | — | 1,300 | 1,700 | 2,400 | 2,200–2,700 | 2,100–1,800 |
| | (range) | | | (900–1,800) | (1,300–2,300) | (1,650–3,300) | (1,500–3,700) | (1,200–3,900) |
| Protein | g/kg | 2.5 | 2.2 | — | — | — | — | — |
| | g/day | — | — | 25 | 30 | 35 | 45–50 | 45–55 |
| Carbohydrate | g/day | kcal × 0.35 – 0.30 ÷ 4 ←————————————— kcal × 0.50 – 0.60 ÷ 4 —————————→ | | | | | | |
| Fat | g/day | kcal × 0.50 ÷ 9 | | 4 ←————————————— kcal × 0.35 ÷ 9 ——————————→ | | | | |
| Isoleucine | mg/kg | 90–30 | 90–30 | 85–20 | 80–20 | 30–20 | 30–20 | 30–10 |
| Leucine | mg/kg | 100–60 | 75–40 | 70–40 | 65–35 | 60–30 | 50–30 | 40–15 |
| Methionine | mg/kg | 50–20 | 40–15 | 30–10 | 20–10 | 20–10 | 20–10 | 10–5 |
| Phenylalanine | mg/kg | 70–20 | 50–15 | 40–15 | 35–15 | 30–15 | 30–15 | 30–10 |
| Tyrosine | mg/kg | 80–60 | 60–40 | 60–30 | 50–25 | 40–20 | 30–15 | 30–10 |
| Valine | mg/kg | 95–40 | 60–30 | 85–30 | 50–30 | 30–25 | 30–20 | 30–15 |

\*All known essential amino acids, essential fatty acids, minerals, and vitamins must be provided in adequate amounts.

The protein content of the diet for infants with PKU has traditionally been greater than normal. Protein requirements are increased when either an L-amino acid mix or a casein hydrolysate is the primary protein source rather than natural protein.[47] Thus, recommendations for protein for nutrition support during infancy are greater than the RDA.[48] During childhood, because a greater amount of protein from natural foods is offered, the RDA for protein for age is adequate.[49] Recommendations for energy and fluid intake (see Table 63–5) are the same as those for normal infants and children.[48,50]

*Low-Phenylalanine and Phenylalanine-Free Chemically Defined Medical Foods.* Adequate protein cannot be obtained from natural foods without ingesting excess phenylalanine (natural proteins contain 2.4 to 9% by weight of phenylalanine.[51–56] Thus, special proprietary chemically defined medical foods are used to provide protein.[57–61] Sources and formulations of these products are given in Appendix Tables A-43b and A-43c; their composition is given in Appendix Table A-43d-1. Analog XP, designed for the infant, consists of L-amino acids, a blend of fat and carbohydrate that produces a fatty acid profile similar to breast milk, minerals, trace elements (including chromium, molybdenum, and selenium), and vitamins. Carnitine and taurine have also been added. Analog XP is free of phenylalanine (Appendix Table A-43c). Lofenalac, formulated from a specially treated enzymatic hydrolysate of casein, is low in phenylalanine and contains fat and carbohydrates. Minerals, vitamins, and four L-amino acids are also added. The phenylalanine content of Lofenalac is between 0.06 and 0.1% and is approximately 75 mg/100 g. Lofenalac has no added chromium, molybdenum, or selenium. Maxamaid XP, designed for the two- to eight-year-old child, is an orange-flavored powder free of phenylalanine that contains L-amino acids, carbohydrate, minerals, trace elements, and vitamins. It does not contain fat, chromium, selenium, or vitamin K. Maxamum XP is formulated for children eight years of age and older and for pregnant women. It is fat-free but has added carnitine, taurine, chromium, molybdenum, selenium, and vitamin K. Phenyl-Free is an L-amino acid mix containing carbohydrate, fat, minerals, trace elements (except chromium and molybdenum), and vitamins. It is designed for children and adolescents. PKU-1, PKU-2, and PKU-3 are L-amino acid mixes that are free of fat, chromium, and selenium. PKU-1 is designed for the infant, PKU-2 for the child, and PKU-3 for the adolescent and the pregnant woman.

*Natural Foods.* Serving lists are available to simplify the phenylalanine-restricted diet for families and professional persons guiding them (Appendix Table A-43e). The lists are similar to diabetic exchange lists in that foods of similar phenylalanine content are grouped together and can be exchanged one for another within a list to give variety to the diet.[62]

*Management Problems.* Management problems described for children with PKU occur in other children with inherited disorders of metabolism. Principles described here apply to children with other disorders as well but will not be reiterated in other sections.

Maintenance of an adequate intake of protein and energy is important for the child with PKU even though phenylalanine must be restricted. Protein is obtained from chemically defined medical foods; therefore, the amount of chemically defined formula offered must be varied to provide protein needed. Nonprotein sources of energy such as Duocal, corn syrup, Moducal, sugar, Protein Free Diet Powder (Appendix Table A-43d-5), and pure fats can be added to maintain energy intake and to satisfy the child's hunger without affecting blood phenylalanine concentrations. Natural foods should be prescribed in numbers of servings and introduced at the appropriate ages and in the usual textures as they would be for any child. Children should be given a variety of foods at the appropriate age so that these foods may be included in the diet later in life. In this way, increasing total phenylalanine requirements may be met, jaw muscles needed for speech can develop, and exercise for gums and teeth is provided.

A variety of factors may influence blood phenylalanine levels. Those that may produce an elevated blood phenylalanine concentration include acute infections with concomitant tissue catabolism, excessive or inadequate phenylalanine intake, and inadequate protein or energy intake. Infection affects plasma amino acids in normal adults.[63] Similar increases in blood phenylalanine occur in febrile, treated PKU patients. Because of this fact, any infection should be promptly diagnosed and appropriately treated. The best approach to nutrition support during short-term infections is to increase the intake of fluids and carbohydrates through use of fruit juices, high-carbohydrate protein-free beverages, and soft drinks that do not contain caffeine.

Excess phenylalanine intake is the most common cause of elevated blood phenylalanine concentration in the older child with PKU. This condition may be due to overprescription, misunderstanding of the diet by the caretaker, or "snitching" of food by the child. Frequent evaluations of blood phenylalanine with accompanying accurate diet records for calculation of intake are used to determine the dietary phenylalanine prescription. Diet records are also useful in determining parenteral understanding. Misunderstanding of diet requires additional education of parents. One of the most common "misunderstandings" in older children is the total amount of an exchange group allowed. In extended families living in close proximity, the child may receive three to four times the allowed amount of food from different well-intentioned but uninformed relatives. "Snitching" of food by the child is the most difficult problem to handle. The child should be given sound reasons for avoiding foods not allowed on his diet, and this responsibility should be shifted to the child by four to six years of age. Appropriate disciplinary action by the parents should also be supported if the patient is unwilling to accept this responsibility. Lifetime nutrition support should be emphasized to the parents at the onset of the therapy and at recurring intervals to both parents and child.

Phenylalanine deficiency associated with inadequate phenylalanine intake has three specific stages of development.[64] The first stage is characterized biochemically by decreased blood and urine phenylalanine. Clinically, the child may appear lethargic or anorectic. Failure to gain linear length or weight may occur. In the older child, increases in blood alanine and mild lactic and beta-hydroxybutyric acidemia occur as a consequence of muscle alanine production and beta-lipolysis. In the second stage, blood phenylalanine is increased as a result of muscle protein degradation. Increased branched-chain amino acid concentrations with decreases in other plasma amino acids occur. Aminoaciduria appears as a consequence of renal tubular malabsorption.[65] In this stage, body protein stores are catabolized, energy sources are depleted, and "active" membrane functions impaired.[65] Eczema is common. In the third stage of phenylalanine deficiency, blood phenylalanine is decreased below normal as are other amino acids. Accompanying clinical manifestations include failure to gain weight, failure to gain height, osteopenia, anemia, sparse hair, and finally death if the deficiency is not corrected by supplements of dietary phenylalanine.

Insufficient protein intake results in an inadequate supply of essential amino acids and/or nitrogen for growth. When protein synthesis is decreased, phenylalanine is no longer used for growth and accumulates in the blood. If catabolism occurs due to prolonged lack of nitrogen and/or amino acid intake, blood phenylalanine concentration increases because tissue protein contains approximately 5.5% phenylalanine. In case of protein insufficiency, chemically defined medical food intake should be increased to supply the required nitrogen and/or essential amino acids.

Energy, the first requirement of the body, is necessary for growth. When energy is provided as carbohydrate and fat, and if adequate nitrogen is available, nonessential amino acids may be synthesized from the keto-acid metabolites. Further, carbohydrate ingestion leads to insulin secretion, and insulin promotes amino acid transport into the cell and protein synthesis.[66,67] This amino acid transport and regulation by insulin are dependent on development of muscle. When energy intake is inadequate, tissue catabolism occurs to meet energy needs. Such catabolism releases phenylalanine, leading to elevated blood phenylalanine concentrations. Provision of sufficient energy through generous use of nonprotein and low-protein foods is important in order to assure a normal growth rate.

Low blood phenylalanine concentrations ($<25$ $\mu$mol) may lead to depressed appetite,[68] decreased growth[69] and, if prolonged, to mental retardation.[44] Low blood phenylalanine concentrations are often due to inadequate prescription of phenylalanine for the affected child. In such cases, the prescription for phenylalanine can be increased by addition of measured amounts of milk and/or solid foods. In some situations, chemically defined medical food may be diluted to a volume that is too great for the child to consume in the allotted time. The volume will need to be decreased to the amount the child is able to ingest. Concentrated chemically defined medical foods are frequently used without any untoward side effects. They may be mixed as a paste and spoon-fed, even to the young infant. The practice could begin at three to four months of age when tongue thrust is no longer evident. Extra fluid must then be offered between feedings to maintain appropriate water balance.

*Assessment of Nutrition Support.* Along with biweekly assessment of growth through measurement of height, weight, and head circumference and evaluation of development by appropriate developmental scales, the adequacy of phenylalanine and tyrosine intake is determined by twice-weekly quantitation of the blood phenylalanine and tyrosine concentrations. The first year is the period of most rapid growth and of greatest vulnerability to nutrition insult. Therefore, blood tests are suggested two times weekly during the first three months and weekly thereafter until the child is one year of age. After one year of age, twice-monthly blood tests are sufficient for monitoring diet. If, however, blood phenylalanine concentrations are greater than 250 μmol (4 mg/dl), more frequent determinations should be obtained. Where indicated, the prescription for phenylalanine is decreased and frequent blood tests are obtained until blood phenylalanine concentrations are between 50 and 150 μmol. In order for blood tests to be of use in adjusting the prescription, laboratory methods must be both accurate and prompt. Quantitative methods of phenylalanine determination using automated ion exchange chromatography and liquid blood are preferable. This method allows evaluation of all amino acids. The microbiologic (Guthrie) method is acceptable for screening, but is nonquantitative and invalid if antibiotics are used. Fluorimetric methods are quantitative and preferred to the Guthrie test to monitor blood phenylalanine.[70] If properly instructed, parents may be given responsibility for obtaining the specimens on filter paper or in microcapillary tubes and mailing them to a central laboratory.

A record of food ingested before and during blood sampling for blood phenylalanine measurement is essential and should be kept by the child's caregiver. The correlation between the child's intake of phenylalanine, tyrosine, protein, and energy, his clinical status, and the blood phenylalanine and tyrosine concentrations is considered when the diet is altered.

The success of early diet management rests with the parents and depends upon their understanding of the disease and their ability to cope with the diet. Later the child's understanding of the diet and ability to assume responsibility for it are critical. These factors in turn are related to the support the parents and patient receive from various professional members of the genetic team. Roles and functions of some team members have been described.[71]

*Results of Therapy.* Early diagnosis and treatment of infants with PKU with a nutritionally adequate, phenylalanine-restricted, tyrosine-supplemented diet have promoted normal growth and have prevented severe mental retardation. Mean height, weight, and head circumference of 111 children treated from before 120 days of age were the same as those of normal children at four years of age.[72] Assessment of mental development in these same children at four years of age yielded a mean I.Q. score of 93 on the Stanford Binet Intelligence Scale.[73] Delay in treatment and suboptimal control of blood phenylalanine concentration produced lower IQ than projected from parental IQ. More recent programs have improved overall outlook for normal IQ.

The semisynthetic nature of the phenylalanine-

restricted diet has led to questions concerning its adequacy. Calculation of intake of major nutrients indicates that these amounts are adequate[74] when compared to the RDAs. Balance studies of calcium, phosphorus, magnesium, and iron in eight girls, six to eight years of age, on Lofenalac suggested that magnesium may be inadequate to provide for optimal nutrition.[75] Studies by the authors of plasma zinc, copper, and hair zinc in 15 treated patients one month to seven years of age on Lofenalac imply that one fourth to one half the children may have subclinical zinc deficiency.[76,77] Studies of blood and/or plasma of children with PKU ingesting Phenyl-Free revealed low concentrations of chromium, selenium, and zinc.[78] Inadequate intake, poor absorption, or inefficient utilization may all be responsible. When Lofenalac is the protein source, the intake of vitamin E is sufficient to provide for normal plasma concentrations despite the high intake of polyunsaturated fatty acids.[79] Adequacy of niacin status in children on Lofenalac is questionable because of limited intakes of tryptophan and disturbances in tryptophan metabolism.[80]

*Diet Discontinuation.* A number of clinicians have suggested that diet might be discontinued at four, six, or 12 years of age with no adverse effects.[81–83] Investigators have questioned this possibility because studies have shown significant differences in performance and intelligence in children who discontinued diet at or above six years of age and those who remained on diet.[26,84,85]

In studies using the same patient as his own control, elevated plasma phenylalanine concentrations prolonged the performance time on neuropsychologic tests of higher integrative function, reduced the mean power frequency of the electroencephalogram, and decreased urinary dopamine excretion and plasma L-dopa in older treated patients with PKU.[26,86] A correlation was found between high plasma phenylalanine concentration, prolonged performance time on the neuropsychologic tests, and decreased urinary dopamine in 10 patients.[26] In a study of eight additional patients,[86] statistically significant decreases were found in the mean power frequency of the electroencephalogram and in plasma L-dopa when plasma phenylalanine increased. These effects were reversible and correlated in the reverse direction when plasma phenylalanine was reduced. Elevated plasma phenylalanine may be concentrated by the blood brain barrier in neural cells and may inhibit L-dopa and serotonin synthesis by competing for tyrosine hydroxylase and tryptophan hydroxylase.

For the female with PKU, diet discontinuation poses special problems. Few PKU women, untreated before and during pregnancy, who have carried the fetus to term have delivered normal infants. Congenital malformations, microcephaly, and retarded physical and mental growth are associated with in utero elevations of phenylalanine.[87] Active transport of amino acids by the placenta to the fetus leads to a fetal blood phenylalanine concentration two to three times that found in the maternal blood.[88] Such elevated fetal plasma phenylalanine concentrations may again be concentrated by the fetal blood brain barrier. Intraneuronal phenylalanine at 600 μmol interferes with brain development by one or more of the several previously described mechanisms including abnormal oligodendroglial migration and/or myelin and other protein synthesis.[89] Thus it is extremely important to maintain normal plasma phenylalanine concentrations in the reproductive female before and after conception.

### Tyrosinemias

**Definition.** Several known disorders of tyrosine metabolism (Table 63–6) may be amenable to nutrition support (see Fig. 63–1, Table 63–2). Precise biochemical diagnosis is important because other disorders such as liver disease, scurvy, prematurity, and general malabsorption may produce increases in blood tyrosine.

Two well-recognized forms of hereditary tyrosinemia have been reported. Type I was thought to be due to a deficiency of p-hydroxyphenylpyruvic acid oxidase (EC 1.13.11.27). More recently, secondary impairment in this enzyme has been attributed to a primary defect of hepatic fumarylacetoacetate hydrolase (EC 3.7.1.2) with the production of an abnormal metabolite, succinylacetone.[90] Succinylacetoacetate and succinylacetone are formed from the accumulated substrate fumarylacetoacetate (see Fig. 66–1). Succinylacetone is extremely toxic and is associated with impaired active transport function, disordered hepatic enzymes, including p-OH-phenylpyruvic acid oxidase and delta-aminolevulinic acid de-

hydratase (EC 4.2.1.24).[91] Decreased activity of both hepatic and erythrocyte delta-aminolevulinic acid dehydratase has been reported in these patients and is postulated as the mechanism by which acute porphyric-like episodes develop (see Fig. 63–2).[92–94]

Type I tyrosinemia is characterized by failure to thrive, hypophosphatemic rickets, renal tubular dysfunction, progressive liver failure, hypertension, episodic behavioral and peripheral nerve deficiencies, and elevated concentrations of blood phenylalanine and tyrosine.[95] This disease demonstrates an autosomal recessive mode of inheritance.

Tyrosinemia type II is characterized by greatly elevated concentrations of blood and urine tyrosine, and increases in urinary phenolic acids, N-acetyltyrosine, and tyramine. A deficiency of hepatic cytosolic tyrosine aminotransferase (EC 2.6.1.5) has been demonstrated.[95] An unusual set of symptoms is characterized by corneal erosions and plaques and bullous lesions. Persistent keratitis and hyperkeratosis occur on the fingers and palms of the hands and soles of the feet. These skin abnormalities respond to restriction of dietary phenylalanine and tyrosine. Intracellular crystallization of tyrosine is thought to cause these inflammatory responses. Mental retardation may occur. This disease is inherited via an autosomal recessive mode.

Neonatal tyrosinemia, associated with increased plasma and urinary concentrations of tyrosine and its metabolites, occurs in 0.2 to 10% of neonates.[95] Short-term protein restriction to 1.5 to 2.0 g/kg body weight/day has lowered plasma tyrosine concentrations in most patients within four weeks of life. Whether added ascorbate will stabilize and increase the activity of P-hydroxyphenylpyruvate oxidase in this disorder is not clear. Persistence of hypertyrosinemia in this disorder may lead to impaired mental function; short-term diet and ascorbate therapy are indicated.[96]

**Table 63–6. Inherited Disorders Producing Increased Plasma Tyrosine**

| Designation | Enzyme Defect | Clinical Features |
|---|---|---|
| Neonatal tyrosinemia | p-OHPPA oxidase* | prematurity ?benign? |
| Tyrosinemia (type I) | Fumarylacetoacetate hydrolase | cirrhosis, Fanconi syndrome, acute porphyria, (succinylacetone) |
| Tyrosinemia (type II) | Hepatic, cytosol tyrosine amino transferase | mental retardation eye, skin disorders |
| Tyrosinosis (Medes) | Probably type I | myasthenia (possibly acute porphyric attack) |

*p-OHPPA oxidase is p-OH-phenylpyruvic acid oxidase. Variation in neonatal development alters the control of expression of this enzyme. Monogenic impairment over a long term has not been confirmed.

**Diagnosis.** Differential diagnosis is imperative for institution of appropriate therapy. Quantitation of plasma amino acids by ion exchange chromatography and urinary organic acids by gas chromatography and mass spectrometry (GC/MS) are necessary approaches to diagnosis. The more severe type I tyrosinemia may not be detected by newborn screening using the bacterial inhibition assay because newborn blood tyrosine may not be above 8 mg/dl. Many newborn screening programs consider 8 mg/dl within normal limits and do not retrieve these babies for further diagnosis. We routinely retest newborns with blood tyrosine above 4 mg/dl if no other cause is clinically evident. If blood tyrosine is above 8 mg/dl at 14 days of age, we evaluate renal tubular and hepatic function as well as urine by organic acid analysis for the presence of parahydroxyphenyl acids and succinylacetone (Fig. 63–3). Prenatal diagnosis of type I hereditary tyrosinemia has been made by measurement of succinylacetone in amniotic fluid[97] and by measurement of fumarylacetoacetase activity in cultured amniotic fluid cells.[98]

**Treatment.** The objective of nutrition support for the hereditary tyrosinemias is to provide a biochemical environment that allows normal growth and development of intellectual potential and that prevents pathophysiologic changes. Plasma phenylalanine concentrations should be maintained between 40 and 80 μmol, and plasma tyrosine concentrations between 50 and 150 μmol. Plasma methionine should not be regulated by dietary means. Rather than restricting methionine below RDA, we follow plasma methionine as an index of S-adenosyl methionine transferase deficiency produced by liver damage.

Nutrition therapy of the hereditary tyrosinemias requires a firm diagnosis because the approaches to therapy for types I and II are different. The phenylalanine and tyrosine restriction is less severe and prognosis is excellent for type II. In type I, however, progressive liver and renal failure may occur as well as acute episodes of porphyria. Treatment of kidney impairment is also needed in type I tyrosinemia. Thus, generalized renal tubular failure may result in metabolic acidosis, hypophosphatemia, rickets, and hypokalemia unless replacement of bicarbonate, phosphate, 1,25-dihydroxycholecalciferol, and potassium is instituted. Rapid treatment of infections is required to prevent a "catastrophic" catabolic state with overproduction of succinylacetone.

Many of the "porphyric" symptoms may be due to overproduction of delta-aminolevulinic acid (ALA) secondary to the inhibitory effect of succinylacetone on ALA dehydratase and/or decreased heme biosynthesis (see Fig. 63–2). Specifically, hypertensive crises, behavior changes, and peripheral neuropathies that are acute abate with dietary control through high-carbohydrate feeds. Parenteral nutrition with 20 to 25% dextrose solutions may control these acute porphyric attacks.[98a] Continued or progressive loss of energy-requiring functions that involve loosely bound heme to heme-proteins (plasma membrane transporters, cytochrome $P_{450}$) may be due to rapid turnover and insufficient heme biosynthesis (see Fig. 63–2). Infusions of Hematin have produced transient decreases in delta-ALA and have improved acute attacks of intermittent porphyria.[99,99a] No published studies are available for this therapy in type I tyrosinemia, but we have successfully aborted attacks and have prolonged intervals between attacks in two patients with this treatment.

*Nutrition Requirements.* When one is planning nutrition support for the infant or child with tyrosinemia, a formal prescription that recommends amounts of phenylalanine, tyrosine, protein, energy, and fluid for the day should be written. The prescription for phenylalanine and tyrosine is based on blood analyses correlated with intake that indicate the child's requirement and/or tolerance for each amino acid. Data in Table 63–5 describe amounts of amino acids, protein, energy, and fluid to offer as beginning therapy.

Because a large portion of phenylalanine is normally hydroxylated to form tyrosine,[100] phenylalanine must be restricted in the diet of patients with tyrosinemia. Phenylalanine requirements appear to be greater for children with tyrosinemia than for children with PKU. In general, the more distal the block is in the catabolic pathway, the more normal is the amino acid requirement. Tyrosine needs of children with tyrosinemia have been inadequately described[101] and will vary with the metabolic state of the child and the accumulation of succinylacetone.

Some investigators suggest that patients with type I tyrosinemia have decreased ability to metabolize methionine, whereas others believe that the elevated plasma methionine concentrations are secondary to liver damage.[95] Whatever the cause for hypermethioninemia, some have recommended methionine restriction when blood methionine concentrations are above 40 μmol in the absence of hepatocellular damage. Although the extent of methionine restriction to maintain normal blood methionine concentration is unknown, one recommendation is 50 mg/kg of body weight for a 15-month-old child.[102] L-cysteine supplementation is also recommended for children with tyrosinemia type I, particularly if methionine restriction is implemented.[103]

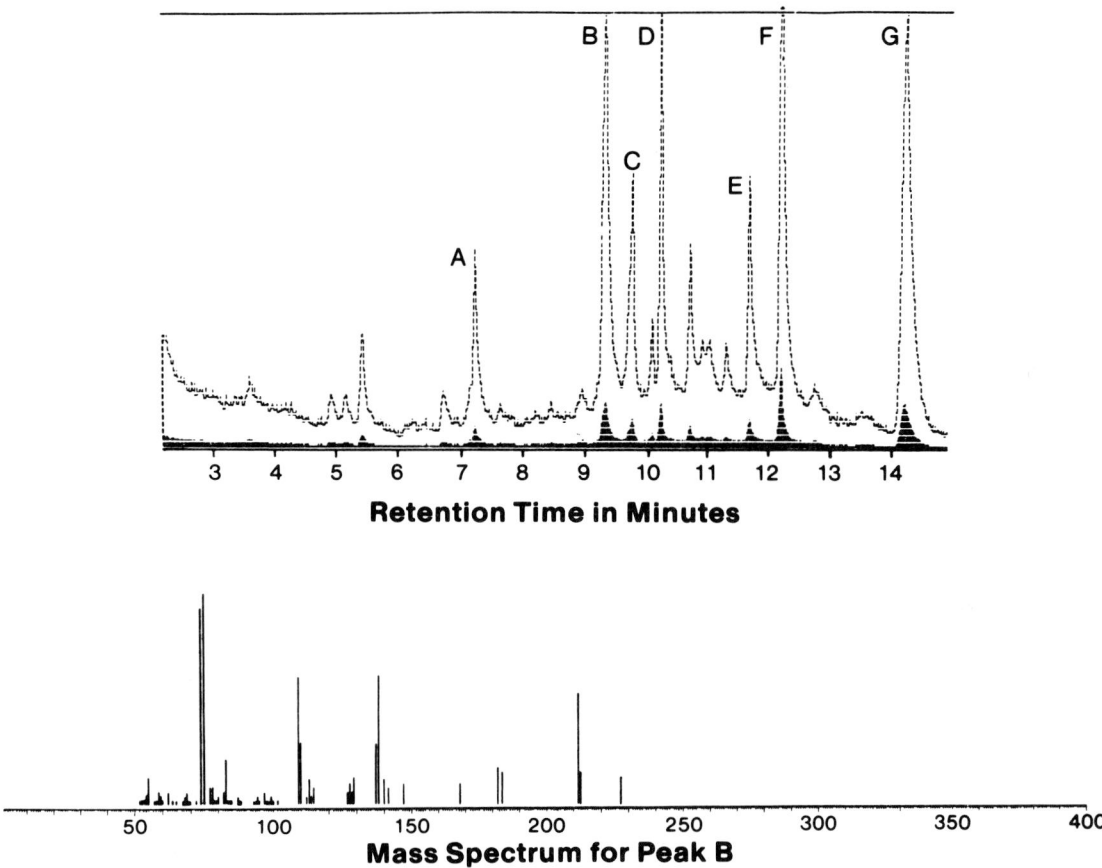

**Fig. 63–3.** Chromatogram and mass spectrum of succinylacetone from urine of a patient with tyrosinemia, type I. A volume of urine equivalent to 210 μg of creatinine was oximated with NaOH and hydroxyl amine hydrochloride. After acidification, organic acids were extracted, dried, and derivatized to their volatile silyl derivatives. Gas chromatography then separated organic acids by their mass (upper panel). Labeled peaks were identified from the mass spectrum of their oximated o-methyl ester derivatives and were: A, succinic acid; B, succinylacetone; C, α-ketoglutaric acid; D, p-OH-phenylacetic acid; E, p-OH-phenyllactic acid; F, p-OH-phenylpyruvic acid; G, tetracosane external standard. In the lower panel is the mass spectral analysis of peak B using a computer-integrated gas chromatography/ mass spectroscopy system. This spectrum is identical to chemical standards for succinylacetone treated like the urine specimen with characteristic fragments of mass 227, 212, 138, 109, and 82. (Courtesy of R. Salvo, Division of Medical Genetics, Emory University.)

Recommended protein intakes for infants and children with tyrosinemia are given in Table 63–5. Because the primary protein source used for the infant is either an L-amino acid mix or a casein hydrolysate, recommended intake is greater than for the normal infant.[47]

For tyrosinemia type I, high-carbohydrate feeds supplying 65 to 75% of kilocalories are recommended to suppress activity of delta-aminolevulinic acid synthase (EC 2.3.1.37).[104–106] For the infant up to two years of age, 150 kcal/kg/day is a minimum need. We try to maintain greater than 100 kcal/kg/day throughout childhood.

*Medical Foods Low in or Free of Phenylalanine and Tyrosine.* Adequate protein cannot be obtained from natural foods without ingesting excess phenylalanine and tyrosine (protein contains by mass 1.4 to 5.8% tyrosine). Thus, special medical foods are used in which there is little or no phenylalanine or tyrosine. Several medical foods are available to provide protein.[57–61] Sources and formulation of Analog XT Low P, Low Phe/Tyr Diet Powder, Maxamaid XT, Tyr 1, and Tyr 2 are given in Appendix Tables A-43b and A-43c. Their composition is given in Appendix Table A-43d-2. Formulation and composition of Analog XT Low P and Maxamaid XT are the same as for Analog XP and Maxamaid XP except for amino acids removed.

Low Phe/Tyr Diet Powder is an enzymatic hydrolysate of casein processed to remove most of the phenylalanine and tyrosine. Phenylalanine content is 75 mg/100 g powder, and tyrosine content is less than 38 mg/100 g powder. Taurine (36 mg/100 g) has been added. Fat and carbohydrate as well as minerals and vitamins are included in appropriate amounts to meet most nutrient needs of infants. Chromium, molybdenum, and selenium are not added to Low Phe/Tyr Diet Powder.

Phenylalanine- and tyrosine-free Tyr 1 and Tyr 2 are formulated from L-amino acids, sucrose, minerals, and vitamins. These two products contain no fat, chromium, or selenium and only a small amount of sucrose.

The methionine content of Analog XT Low P, Low Phe/Tyr Diet Powder, Maxamaid XT, Tyr 1, and Tyr 2 (Appendix Table A-43d-4) is too great for use alone if dietary methionine must be restricted. In such a situation, Analog XPXTXM and Maxamaid XPXTXM (Appendix Table A-43d-2), which contain no phenylalanine, tyrosine, or methionine, could be used.

*Serving Lists.* Serving lists are available for the phenylalanine-tyrosine-restricted diet (Appendix Table A-43e).[107] Methionine content is given for each list in the event that methionine restriction is required for type I.

*Initiation of Nutrition Support.* The most rapid decline of blood tyrosine concentration at the time of diagnosis may be obtained by feeding a 20 kcal/ounce (67 kcal/dl) low-phenylalanine or phenylalanine- and tyrosine-free formula with no added source of phenylalanine and tyrosine. Laboratory results of blood phenylalanine and tyrosine should be rapidly available, or a deficiency of phenylalanine and tyrosine[108] could be precipitated. This condition is particularly undesirable in treating type I tyrosinemia because a catabolic phase with overproduction of succinylacetone will worsen the clinical state. Protein sources containing 20 to 70 mg phenylalanine and 60 to 80 mg tyrosine/kg body weight/day are usually required after three to four days of total restriction in the newborn period.

*Assessment of Nutrition Support.* Frequency of assessment is dictated by the type of tyrosinemia and clinical course of the patient. In type I tyrosinemia, vital signs, height, weight, head circumference, neurologic examination and development are documented weekly for the first three months, biweekly for the second three months, and monthly between six months and one year of life. Plasma amino acids are quantitated by ion exchange chromatography; succinylacetone and the parahydroxyphenyl organic acids by GC/MS. Additional laboratory studies include urinary delta-aminolevulinic acid, renal and liver function tests, blood and urine phosphate, potassium, and bicarbonate. Clinical status, dietary intake, and laboratory data should be monitored and cor-

related in managing type I tyrosinemia at intervals indicated previously.

*Outcomes of Nutrition Support.* Outcomes, to date, have been variable with tyrosinemia, type I. Some of this "variation" is caused by lack of clear diagnostic criteria in the past to delineate the various types of tyrosinemia. Early detection and diagnosis using GC/MS (see Fig. 63–3), low-phenylalanine and -tyrosine high-carbohydrate diets, hematin infusions, and the early replacement of renal tubular losses have brought some success in treating type I tyrosinemia. The low-phenylalanine low-tyrosine diet has been successfully used in several patients with type II tyrosinemia with rapid resolution of clinical signs and symptoms.[95] Neonatal tyrosinemia requires early but transient protein restriction. Controlled outcome data are not yet available.

## BRANCHED-CHAIN AMINO ACIDS

Disorders of branched-chain amino acid metabolism provide an interesting interface between clinical and fundamental science. Using the nutritional model of preventing mental retardation through screening and management of newborns, many rare experiments of nature have become available and advanced our knowledge concerning nutritional needs and metabolic utilization of leucine, isoleucine, and valine.

### Biochemistry

The branched-chain amino acids isoleucine, leucine, and valine are essential nutrients. In the newborn 75% of the amounts ingested are used for protein synthesis. Those present in the body in excess of need for synthetic purposes are degraded through many steps to provide energy (Fig. 63–4). The initial step in catabolism is reversible transamination, requiring a specific transaminase and the coenzyme pyridoxal phosphate. The second step is irreversible oxidative decarboxylation, which utilizes the branched-chain alpha-ketoacid dehydrogenase complex. This four-protein, three-enzyme complex is located on the inner mitochondrial membrane and requires the coenzymes thiamin pyrophosphate, lipoic acid, coenzyme A, and NAD$^+$.[109–113] Figure 63–4 schematizes this overall reaction, which is impaired in maple syrup urine disease. Two cDNA clones, one for the transacylase protein (E2) and one for E–1 alpha of the decarboxylase of the branched-chain alpha-ketoacid dehydrogenase complex, have been isolated from a human fetal liver cDNA expression library.[110]

Elsas and Danner proposed a model for the role of thiamin in stabilizing the biologic turnover of the branched-chain alpha-ketoacid dehydrogen-

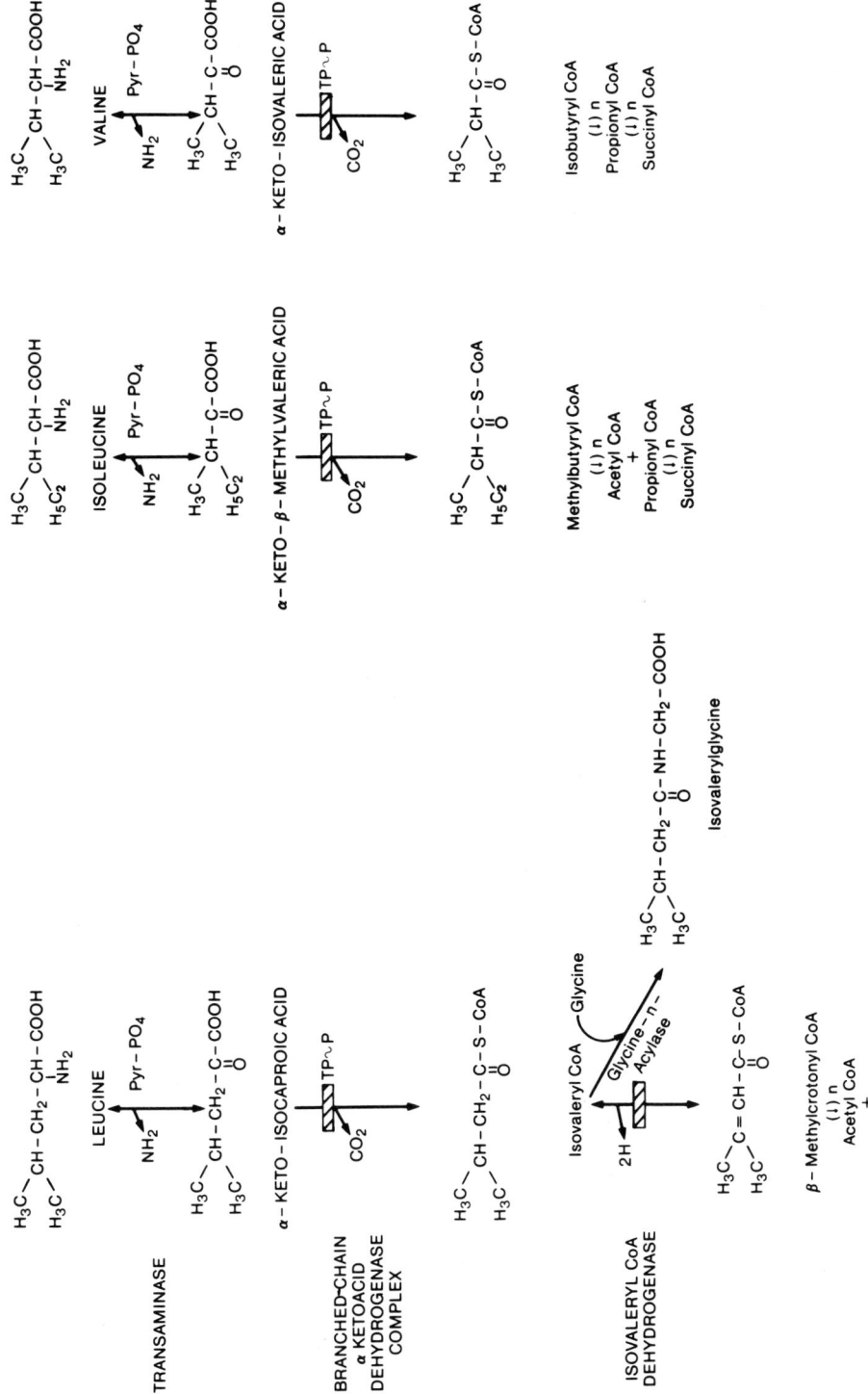

**Fig. 63–4.** Catabolism of branched-chain amino acids. Crosshatch bars represent blocks in maple syrup urine disease (branched-chain α-ketoacid dehydrogenase complex) and in isovaleric acidemia (isovaleryl CoA dehydrogenase). TP~P = the cofactor thiamin pyrophosphate; (n) = several catalyzed intermediate steps.

ase complex.[111] By increasing thiamin ingestion, intracellular thiamin pyrophosphate (TPP) is increased and the TPP binding sites on the decarboxylase (E–1–alpha) moiety of the branched-chain alpha-ketoacid dehydrogenase complex become saturated. When these TPP binding sites are occupied, the multienzyme complex undergoes a conformational change making it more resistant to degradation. The biologic half-life of the enzyme and overall activity are increased when a new equilibrium of enzyme synthesis and degradation is reached. This model has been tested and is confirmed at both functional and structural levels in vitro and in vivo (Fig. 63–5).[112–114]

### Branched-Chain Ketoaciduria

**Definition.** Maple syrup urine disease (MSUD) is a group of inherited disorders of isoleucine, leucine, and valine metabolism.[115] These disorders result from several different mutations that impair branched-chain alpha-ketoacid dehydrogenase (see Figs. 63–4 and 63–5). Although most mutant enzymes are immunologically present, one reported patient had absent branched-chain acyl transferase (E2) as a cause of thiamin-resist-

ant MSUD.[109,116] An autosomal recessive mode of inheritance is defined for most of the reported cases suggesting nuclear rather than mitochondrial genomic mutations. The cellular mechanism by which the products of these nuclear genes assemble as a multienzyme complex in mitochondria is a subject of considerable importance and current research effort.

Infants with MSUD appear normal at birth and are clinically well until after a protein-containing feed. The most severely impaired enzymes may produce seizures, apnea, and death within 10 days of life. The disorder is characterized by elevated blood, urine, and cerebrospinal fluid concentrations of the branched-chain alpha-ketoacids and their amino acid precursors. Progressive neurologic dysfunction and the production of fragrant urine with the odor of burnt sugar (caramel) or maple syrup follow. The sweet smell may only be evident in earwax, easily sensed after otoscopic examination. Neurologic impairment in the newborn is manifested by poor sucking, irregular respiration, rigidity alternating with periods of flaccidity, opisthotonos, progressive loss of Moro reflex, and seizures.

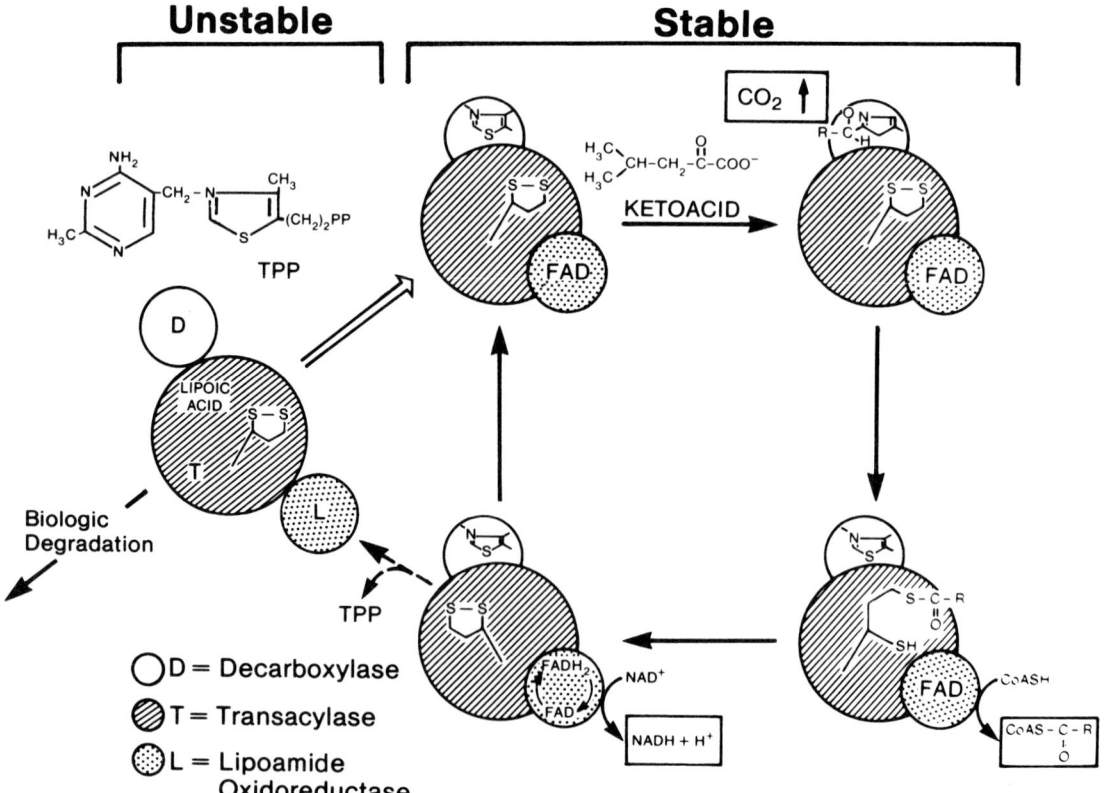

**Fig. 63–5.** A model for the stabilization of the branched-chain α-ketoacid dehydrogenase by thiamin pyrophosphate. The multienzyme complex branched-chain α-ketoacid dehydrogenase has a configuration that is more stable to degradation when thiamin pyrophosphate (TPP) binding sites on its decarboxylase moiety are occupied.

Several variants with a spectrum of impaired mitochondrial branched-chain alpha-ketoacid dehydrogenase have been reported. Clinical manifestations are expressed intermittently upon protein loading or with febrile illness in patients with partial enzyme activity between 5 and 15% of normal.[115]

Untreated patients with classic MSUD who survive beyond early infancy have retarded physical and mental development.[5,6] Early diagnosis and therapy lead to normal growth and development. If death occurs in the first few days of life, few unique abnormalities are seen in the brain. With prolonged survival, deficient myelination is thought to be due to enzymes involved in myelin formation, inhibition of amino acid transport, and inhibition by branched-chain alpha-ketoacids of oxidative phosphorylation.[5,115]

**Screening.** Because apnea and death may be the first clinical manifestations of the classic disorder, newborn screening, retrieval, diagnosis, and initiation of therapy are urgent, and all four processes must be completed within the first week of life. Nonselected screening of the newborn population is currently in progress (in some states) using bacterial inhibition assays for blood leucine concentrations.[36] Bedside screening in selected children uses the urinary dinitrophenylhydrazine (DNPH) reaction for branched-chain alpha-ketoaciduria. This reaction can also be used to monitor dietary progress. The incidence figure for MSUD based on international newborn screening appears to be about 1 in 216,000.[117] Incidence in Georgia, based on five years of newborn screening where 37% of newborns are black, is approximately 1 in 83,000 live births (see Table 63–3). Little information comparing frequency among ethnic groups is available, although some inbred communities have a high frequency.

**Diagnosis.** Any infant with a blood leucine concentration greater than 4 mg/dl on the newborn screening test should immediately be further evaluated. Most infants with the classic disease have greater than 8 mg/dl leucine at 72 hours of age. Diagnosis is confirmed using ion exchange chromatography to quantitate plasma isoleucine, leucine, valine, and alloisoleucine, and gas chromatography/mass spectrometry (GC/MS) to identify urinary branched-chain alpha-ketoacids (Fig. 63–6). The extent of enzyme impairment should be determined by rapid quantitative enzyme assay of peripheral lymphocytes and therapy accordingly altered. Prenatal monitoring is available if the cellular phenotype is confirmed in fibroblasts cultured from the patient's skin.[118] In some families with severely impaired enzyme function, heterozygotes are also identifiable from enzymatic assays of cultured dermal fibroblasts.[116]

**Treatment.** Although peritoneal dialysis with nitrogen-free dialysate[119,120] or exchange transfusion[121] may be required when diagnosis is delayed, if screening, retrieval, and diagnosis are completed within 8 to 10 days of life, this action is seldom necessary. Because peritoneal dialysis superimposes iatrogenic risk, it is not recommended. Branched-chain amino acid-free orogastric feeding of protein and energy should begin as soon as the diagnosis is made. The objective is to produce anabolism in the infant and thereby prevent accumulation of neurotoxic branched-chain alpha-ketoacids. If orogastric feeding is not acceptable, gastrostomy or a central line for hyperalimentation with dextrose and lipid should be initiated for initial care of classic MSUD during the neonatal period. Except during illness, reducing protein intake to 1.5 g/kg/day may be adequate therapy for those patients with 15% or more of enzyme activity.

Chronic therapy for MSUD is by means of diet. The objective of chronic nutrition support in the child with MSUD is to maintain plasma concentrations of branched-chain amino acids that will allow maximal development of intellect while supplying adequate energy, protein, and other nutrients for optimal growth. Plasma concentrations of branched-chain amino acids (three to four hours postprandial) should be maintained between the following ranges: isoleucine, 40 to 90 μmol, leucine 80 to 200 μmol; valine 200 to 425 μmol.

The objectives of nutrition support are met through use of a combination of medical foods (Appendix A-43d-3) and natural foods (Appendix A-43b). Most patients with MSUD who have the multienzyme complex present immunologically will respond to thiamin administration of 100 to 1,000 mg daily.[114,122] In classic MSUD, thiamin is only an adjunct therapy, and a diet restricted in isoleucine, leucine, and valine must also be given. Supraphysiologic amounts of thiamin should be added for at least a three-month trial period because its mechanism is to stabilize the enzyme complex. Increased residual specific activity of mitochondrial membrane-bound enzymes may require this prolonged period owing to the duration of the biologic half-life of this subcellular organelle. During this period, decreased sensitivity to dietary branched-chain amino acids is usually observed and more can be added to the diet.

*Nutrient Requirements.* Data in Table 63–5 outline the suggested amounts of branched-chain amino acids (BCAAs), protein, energy, and fluid to offer the infant or child with MSUD. Because the BCAAs are essential, they cannot be deleted from the diet without producing growth failure and death. In planning nutrition support of the infant or child with MSUD, a formal prescription should be written that includes recommended amounts of BCAAs, protein, energy, and fluid for the day. Frequent adjustments in the diet prescription are necessary. Adjustments are needed daily during the first few weeks and biweekly during the first six months of life, based on appetite, growth, development, and laboratory analyses of plasma BCAAs and alpha-ketoacids. Because leucine residues are more prominent than isoleucine and valine in most proteins, supplemental L-isoleucine and L-valine as free amino acids may be necessary in the newborn period to prevent deficiency of these two essential amino acids. However, competition between the free BCAAs at the intestinal cell can cause imbalances in plasma amino acids.[123]

Requirements for isoleucine, leucine, and valine vary considerably depending on age, growth rate, and extent of the enzyme deficit.[45] Younger infants normally have greater requirements per unit of body weight than older infants. A rapid decline occurs in requirements for BCAAs between birth and three to six months of age. Careful monitoring of plasma concentrations and intake of BCAAs is required to prevent excess intake when growth rate declines.

The recommended protein intake for infants with MSUD (see Table 63–5), after the initial acute period during which it is greater,[124] is slightly larger than that for normal infants because the primary protein source consists of L-amino acids. After infancy, when the diet contains a variety of food proteins, the RDA for protein may be adequate.

Recommended energy intakes, after the initial acute period, are the same as for normal infants and children but may vary considerably (see Table 63–5).[48] During the neonatal acute period, up to 170 kcal/kg/day may be required.[124]

*Branched-Chain Amino Acid-Free Medical Foods.* Adequate protein cannot be obtained from ordinary foods without ingesting more branched-chain amino acids than are required in classic maple syrup urine diseases. The BCAA content of foods as a percentage of protein ranges from approximately 3.5 to 8.5%.[51–56] Because of the BCAA content of most proteins, special medical foods are used that are formulated from L-amino acids free of BCAAs. In the United States, several products are available to provide protein.[57–61] Sources and formulations of these products are given in Appendix Table A-43b and A-43c. Composition is given in Appendix Table A-43d-3.

Analog X Isoleuc, Leu, and Val; Maxamaid X Isoleuc, Leu, and Val, MSUD Diet Powder; MSUD 1; and MSUD 2 are all formulated from L-amino acids. For a complete description of the Analog and Maxamaid range of products see the earlier section on low-phenylalanine and phenylalanine-free chemically defined medical foods. MSUD Diet Powder contains fat, carbohydrate, minerals, and vitamins and is intended to be a complete formula except for the BCAAs. However, the nitrogen-to-calorie ratio of MSUD Diet Powder is very low. This leads to inadequate nitrogen intake, especially when energy intake is low. L-Carnitine (8 mg/100 g) and taurine (36 mg/100 g) have been added to MSUD Diet Powder, but chromium, molybdenum, and selenium are not included. MSUD 1 and MSUD 2 contain, in addition to L-amino acids, a small amount of carbohydrate along with minerals and vitamins. Fat, chromium, and selenium are not added.

*Equivalent Lists.* Equivalent lists of foods are available to provide variety and needed natural protein in the diet.[107] The lists are similar to diabetic exchange lists in that foods of similar content of leucine are grouped together and may be exchanged for one another within the same list. Average isoleucine, leucine, valine, protein, and energy contents of these lists are given in Appendix Table A-43f.

*Initiation of Nutrition Support.* A rapid decline of plasma isoleucine and valine can be achieved at the time of diagnosis by feeding formula free of branched-chain amino acids. However, plasma leucine will continue to increase over the first four days of life even if dietary BCAA restriction is implemented at birth.[125] Most patients are not anticipated at birth, and positive screenees are treated at 7 to 14 days of life. In our experience, branched-chain ketoacidosis can be averted by high caloric intake with no added BCAAs over a 72-hour period if instituted between 8 and 11 days of age. There is an association among degree of α-ketoisocaproic acid excretion, leucine elevations, and clinical outcome.[126] Laboratory results of plasma BCAAs should be rapidly available to prevent the predicted deficiency in isoleucine and valine. When one is beginning replacement, these two amino acids may be added as free amino acids to increase their ratio to leucine in natural protein. High-energy intakes of 140 to 170 kcal/kg of body weight should be given during this period to prevent the catabolism of body protein. If osmolality of formula permits, protein at 2.5 to 3.0 g/kg should be offered. This regimen lowers the concentrations of BCAAs to near normal ranges. If deficiency of either isoleucine or valine occurs, plasma leucine concentrations will remain elevated as a function of muscle catabolism or decreased protein synthesis.

*Assessment of Nutrition Support.* Frequency of assessment is dictated by the clinical course of the patient and the response of plasma amino acids. Monitoring of therapy should employ three combined approaches.

Ion exchange chromatography should be used daily to quantitate plasma amino acid concentrations for approximately three weeks of life. The concentrations determine requirements for the individual BCAAs.

Following establishment of requirements, quantitation of plasma amino acids is used approximately every two weeks to make sure the child has not "grown out" of his prescription. Samples should be obtained at midday before the noon feeding. We have found organic acid analysis of urine to be helpful (see Fig. 63–6). Branched-chain alpha-ketoacids decrease under optimum dietary conditions. If overrestriction of energy or a specific amino acid occurs, evidence of beta-lipolysis (acetoacetic acid, β-OH-butyric acid), is found.

After hospital discharge, daily testing of urine by a parent at home with dinitrophenylhydrazine (DNPH) is a rapid screen for ketoaciduria. As a rule, "preventive" clinical evaluation of the child for cryptogenic infections before overt ketoacidosis occurs is more effective than trying to treat the child after a catabolic phase has produced its attendant ketoacidosis. If the urine DNPH results are positive, a blood sample should be collected on filter paper for assay of leucine and further analyzed by GC/MS. A physician should evaluate the child for infection or other causes for ketoacidosis. With a diet history, physician's examination, and laboratory analyses, one can usually differentiate among overrestriction, intercurrent infection, or underrestriction of diet as a cause for branched-chain α-ketoaciduria. Weekly Guthrie tests and diet records are necessary components in chronic management. Every effort should be made to maintain plasma BCAAs in the normal range. Plasma leucine concentrations greater than 600 μmol are associated with clinically significant alpha-ketoacidemia and the appearance of ataxia.[5,126]

Episodes of infection bring about catabolism of tissue protein and an increase in plasma concentrations of BCAAs. Clinical improvement is rapid if some BCAAs are administered along with an amino acid mix that provides 150 to 200 kcal/kg/day.

*Termination of Nutrition Support.* Patients with classic MSUD are unable to terminate diet. The occurrence of death in variants with intermittent maple syrup urine disease suggests the need for some form of ongoing therapy in even these relatively stable patients.[115] The branched-chain alpha-ketoacids are relatively acute neurotoxins and probably interfere with oxygen consumption and ATP production in the medullary reticular substance of the brain.[5,115]

## Isovaleric Acidemia

**Definition.** This disorder was first described by Tanaka in 1966 and was identified by the urinary excretion of isovaleric acid.[127] Subsequently, a deficiency of isovaleryl-CoA dehydrogenase (EC 1.3.99.10) was defined. This enzyme is a mitochondrial flavoprotein and uses electron transfer factor (ETF). Although deficiency of ETF is also reported, mutations in the apoenzyme are specific for isovaleryl CoA as substrate. Deficiency of isovaleryl-CoA dehydrogenase results in a block in the catabolism of leucine at the next step after branched-chain alpha-ketoacid dehydrogenase complex (see Fig. 63–4). Isovaleric acid, 3-hydroxyisovaleric acid, and the adduct isovalerylglycine accumulate in body fluids. Through gas-liquid chromatography (GC) and mass spectrometry (MS), these compounds are identified in the body fluids (Fig. 63–7).

Isovaleric acid (IVA) is responsible for the sweaty-feet odor. Because IVA is a metabolite of leucine, a defect in the enzyme that was thought to oxidize the BCAAs and straight-chain fatty acids with four to six carbons was suspected.[115] However, four major findings indicated the presence of an acyl-CoA dehydrogenase specific to isovaleryl-CoA, i.e., isovaleryl CoA dehydrogenase: (1) An oral dose of 100 mg L-leucine/kg body weight caused a 200-fold increase in serum IVA and only minimal elevations in beta-methylcrotonic acid during remission. (2) Similar oral loading tests with L-isoleucine and L-valine did not result in the accumulation of their corresponding short-chain fatty acid catabolites in the serum. (3) The ability of patients' leukocytes and cultured fibroblasts to oxidize [1-$^{14}$C] IVA to $CO_2$ in vitro was significantly impaired. (4) Other short-chain fatty acids such as isobutyric, n-butyric, 2-methylbutyric, and n-hexanoic acids failed to increase during acidotic attacks or leucine-loading tests. Subsequently, the flavin-dependent dehydrogenase, isovaleryl-CoA dehydrogenase, was identified as the enzyme responsible for the specific oxidation of isovaleryl-CoA.[115]

Further investigation revealed the presence of N-isovalerylglycine and 3-hydroxyIVA as major metabolites in the urine of individuals with isovaleric acidemia. N-isovalerylglycine (IVG) was excreted consistently during remissions and ke-

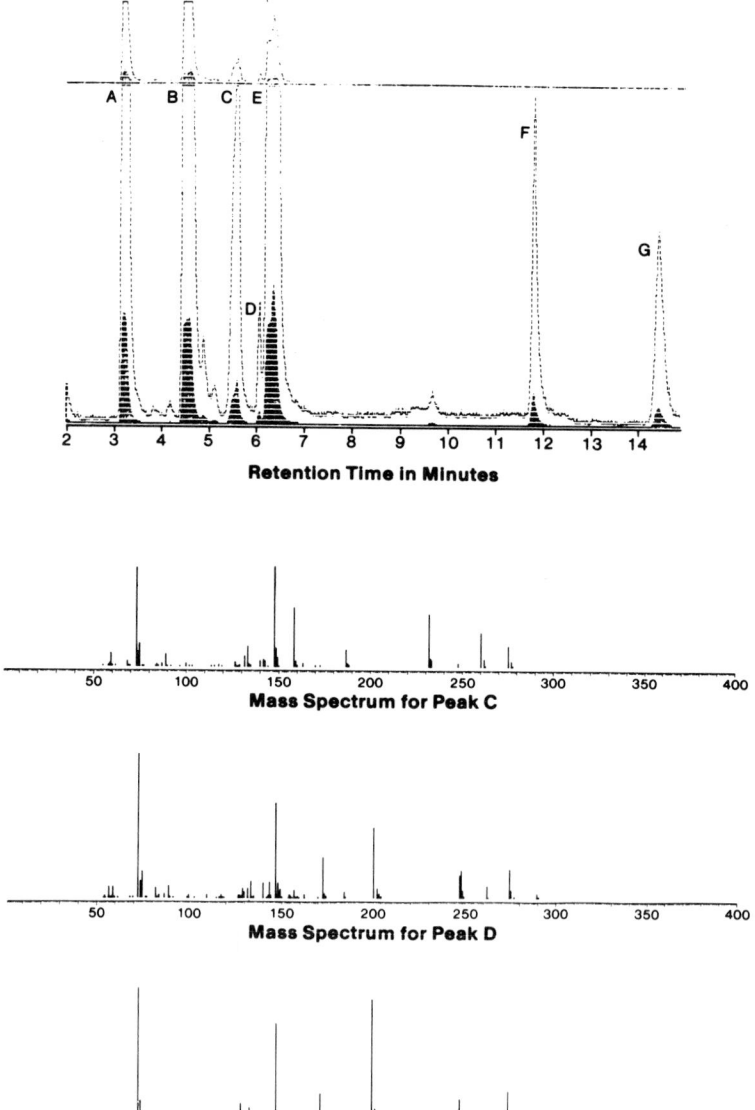

**Fig. 63–6.** Chromatogram and mass spectrum of branched-chain α-ketoacids in the urine of an untreated infant with maple syrup urine disease. Urine was oximated, extracted, derivatized, and chromatographed as described in Figure 63–3. Labeled peaks represent the following organic acids: peak A is lactic acid; peak B is 2-OH isovaleric acid; peak C is α-keto isovaleric acid (KIC); peak D is α-keto-β-methylvaleric acid (KMV); peak E is α-ketoisocaproic acid (KK); peak F is a combination of p-OH phenyllactic acid and the internal standard, pentadecanoic acid; and peak G is the external standard, tetracosane (C24). The mass spectra for peaks C, D, and E are in the lower half. Fragments of mass 275, 260, 232, 186, and 158 are characteristic of the trimethylsilyl derivative of KIV (peak C). The larger ketoacids KMV and KIC differ from KIV by a larger fragment of mass 289 and a fragment of mass 246. They differ among themselves at fragments of mass 216, 143, 129, and 110 (compare spectrum for peaks D and E). (Courtesy of R. Salvo, Division of Medical Genetics, Emory University.)

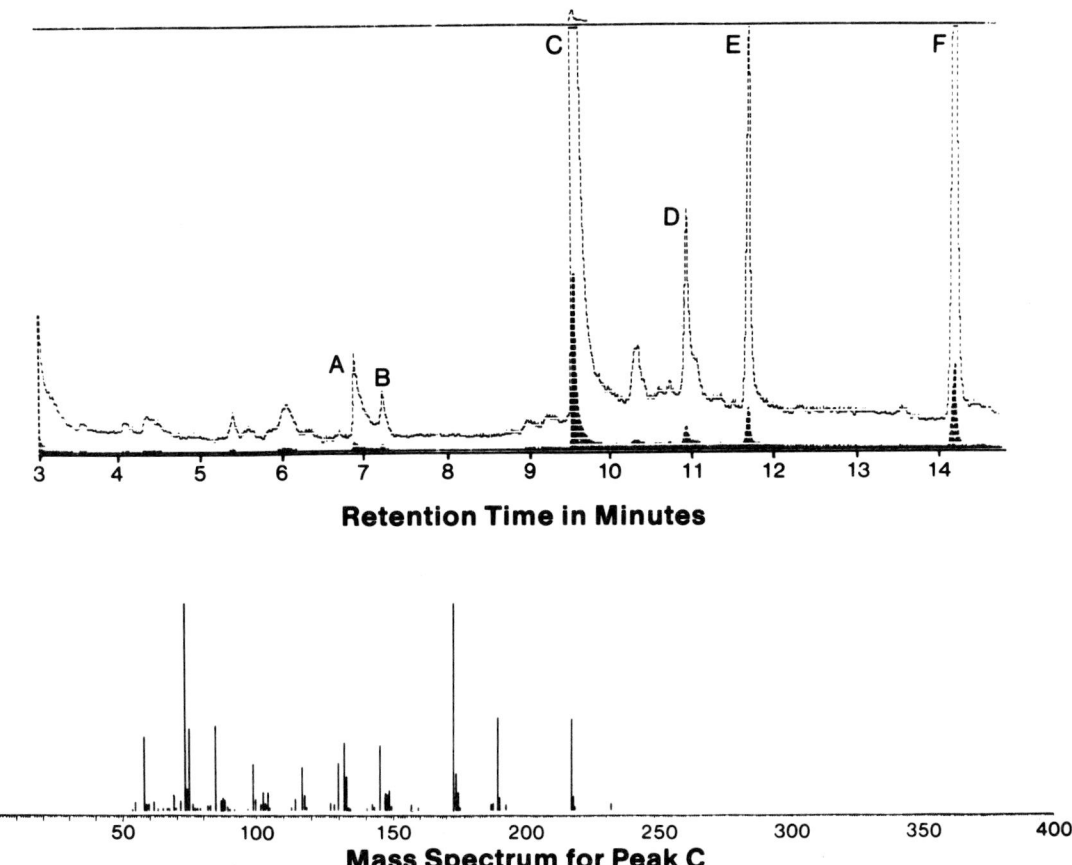

**Retention Time in Minutes**

**Mass Spectrum for Peak C**

**Fig. 63–7.** Chromatogram and mass spectrum of isovalerylglycine in the urine from a patient with isovaleric acidemia. This urine sample is from a stable nine-year-old female with isovaleric acidemia who was receiving glycine supplements (see Fig. 63–8). The sample was not oximated but was extracted, dried, and derivatized with trimethylsilane as in Figures 63–3 and 63–6. Peak A is urea; peak B is succinic acid; peak C is the monotrimethylsilyl derivative of isovalerylglycine; peak D is citric acid; peak E is the internal standard, pentadecanoic acid; peak F is the external standard, tetracosane. Below is the mass spectrum of peak C. Fragments of mass 231, 216, 189, 172, 116, 99, and 85 are characteristic of isovalerylglycine standards.

totic attacks (see Fig. 63–7). Unlike IVG, 3-hydroxyIVA is only present in significant amounts during ketotic attacks.[128] Several minor metabolites have also been identified in the urine of isovaleric acidemia patients including 4-hydroxyIVA, mesaconic acid, methylsuccinic acid, and 3-methylbutyrolactone.[129,130]

Analysis of numerous case reports of isovaleric acidemia has resulted in the classification of two different clinical presentations: the acute form and the chronic intermittent form.[115] Those patients with the acute form of isovaleric acidemia are generally normal full-term infants at birth. Within the first days of life, poor feeding, tachypnea, vomiting, and a characteristic "sweaty-feet" odor of the blood and urine are frequently noted. Diarrhea,[131] lethargy,[132] hypotonia, and tremors[133] may also be found. In some cases patients do not respond to treatment; they may be-

come cyanotic or comatose, and death often results.[131–133] The exact cause of death is frequently unknown. Severe metabolic acidosis, hyperammonemia, CNS hemorrhage, cardiac arrests, and sepsis are some probable causes. Those infants who respond to treatment and survive the neonatal period may develop appropriately and seem to progress into the chronic intermittent type of isovaleric acidemia.[115]

A second broad classification is the chronic intermittent form.[115] These babies generally are normal at birth. During late infancy they may develop episodes of vomiting, acidosis, stupor, and coma. A sweaty-feet odor is usually present, and a transient alopecia is occasionally seen. These episodes may begin as early as two weeks of age; the frequency of attacks seems to decrease with age. Urinary tract and upper respiratory infections frequently trigger these episodes, as well as excessive intake of protein and aspirin. Many children affected by the intermittent form have a strong preference for fruits and vegetables over meat and milk, whereas others consume normal quantities of protein without problems. Although several patients have developed normally, some are mildly to severely retarded.

Several patients with either the acute or chronic form of isovaleric acidemia have had moderate to severe hematologic abnormalities, including leukopenia and thrombocytopenia, with pancytopenia being the most common. This pancytopenia may be secondary to arrested maturation of hemopoietic precursors. In one instance, transfusion of packed red cells and platelets prevented further complications. A depressed hemoglobin was also seen in several patients. The occurrence of transient alopecia seems to be more common with the chronic intermittent form of the disease. Hyperammonemia (up to 814 μmol) has also been reported during acute attacks.

**Diagnosis.** Because isovalerylglycine (IVG) is excreted during both remission and ketotic attacks, measurement of urinary IVG using CG/MS is the best method of diagnosis. Normal three- to five-year-old unaffected children have no detectable urinary IVG (less than 2 mg/day). Affected children of the same age excrete 40 to 250 mg/day.[134] During ketotic episodes, urinary 3-hydroxyIVA, 4-hydroxyIVA, and methylsuccinic acids are excreted in large quantities as well.[129,130]

Diagnosis is confirmed by measuring the impaired ability of skin fibroblasts cultured from affected individuals to oxidize leucine-2-[14]C to [14]$CO_2$.[135] A more complicated assay using mitochondria and 1-[14]C-isovaleric acid has also been used.[136]

Prenatal diagnosis is available by combined organic acid analysis of amniotic fluid and enzyme assay of cultured amniotic fluid cells. A heterozygote for isovaleryl-CoA dehydrogenase deficiency has been detected prenatally.[137]

**Treatment.** During acute ketotic attacks, parenteral fluid therapy and correction of the metabolic acidosis are indicated as adjuncts to high caloric intake and glycine therapy.[115] Serum IVA levels are monitored during ketotic attacks. GC/MS analysis is the most accurate means of determining serum and urinary IVA, which is an extremely volatile substance.[138] A special method of GC/MS allows separate quantitation of the two isomers, IVA and 2-methylbutyic acid.[138] Serum IVA ranges from 0.1 to 84 mg/dl[137] depending on the patient's clinical status. A simple and rapid method of determining 4-hydroxyIVA levels in the plasma has been devised.[139] However, elevations in this metabolite lag at least 36 hours behind the

maximum plasma level of IVA,[139] which limits its use clinically. Monitoring urinary IVG provides a good parameter of nutritional therapy. Titration of IVG with free L-glycine to a stable optimum is desirable. Excess L-glycine may inhibit IVG production (Fig. 63–8). When leucine restriction is optimal and the patient is stable, higher intake (300 to 600 mg/kg/day) of glycine may be necessary during infections or if dietary leucine restriction is not followed.

*Nutrient Requirements.* A low-protein diet of 1.2 to 1.5 g/kg/day in children less than one year of age improves clinical symptoms, and many patients restrict protein by choice.[115] This amount represents only 60% of the RDA. Total protein restriction is therefore not the best mode of therapy because overrestriction of essential branched-chain amino acids (Ileu, Val) is inevitable if leucine is adequately restricted in natural food.

Leucine restriction and the use of pharmacologic doses of glycine have been reported. In six patients with isovaleric acidemia,[115] glycine therapy resulted in decreased IVA in plasma and urine. Urinary IVG simultaneously increased, often two- to threefold (see Fig. 63–5, and 63–8). Clinical improvement occurred characterized by in-

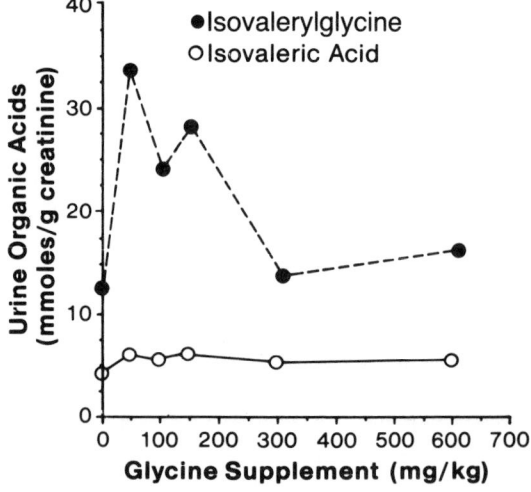

**Fig. 63–8.** Effect of oral glycine supplement on isovalerylglycine production in stable isovaleric acidemia. The oral glycine supplements indicated on the abscissa were administered at weekly intervals to the patient in Figure 63–7 while she was maintained on a constant leucine-restricted diet. Isovalerylglycine (IVG) and isovaleric acid were quantitated by gas chromatography as outlined in Figure 63–7. Symbols represent the mean of duplicate 24-hour urine samples collected over the last two days of each interval. Note the increase in IVG production at 50 to 150 mg/kg/day with decreased IVG production at 300 and 600 mg/kg/day of dietary glycine supplement. (Courtesy of M. Naglak and R. Salvo, Division of Medical Genetics, Emory University.)

creased growth, control of acidosis, and resolution of pancytopenia on glycine supplement and protein restriction over a two-week period.

Glycine used to remove isovaleric acid through an alternate pathway is a prototype for nutritional detoxification of accumulated substrates in inborn errors of metabolism (see Fig. 66–5).[140,141] The ubiquitous enzyme glycine-*N*-acylase (EC 2.3.1.13) has a broad range of substrates (Table 63–7) that accumulate in other inborn errors of metabolism and might also be amenable to this approach. The relative amounts of glycine required to optimize removal of isovaleric acid (or other substrates for the glycine-N-acylase reaction) need careful evaluation and will change with the clinical condition of the patient.

Some evidence exists for substrate inhibition of the reaction when excess glycine is added under stable conditions (see Fig. 63–7). The optimal dose of supplemental glycine was determined for a nine-year-old white female with isovaleric acidemia who was well and was maintained on an intake of leucine of 54 ± 3.6 mg/kg/day. Supplementation of glycine below or above the range of 50 to 150 mg/kg resulted in a decrease of IVG excretion by 50%. Urinary IVA excretion was consistent throughout the study. No beta-hydroxyIVA was detected in the plasma or urine. The results of this study indicated that: (1) the optimal dose of glycine for this patient under these stable clinical and nutritional conditions was 50 to 150 mg/kg; (2) an optimal dose of glycine should be quantitated for specific ages, clinical states, degree of enzyme activity, and levels of leucine intake in the treatment of isovaleric acidemia, and (3) glycine supplements above 300 mg/kg/day increased plasma and urine concentrations of glycine, but resulted in decreased IVG excretion as if this substrate were inhibiting glycine-N-acylase when concentrations of its cosubstrate, isovaleryl CoA, were controlled.

Systemic carnitine deficiency has been demonstrated in several patients with isovaleric acidemia.[142] Although plasma levels of carnitine were low in these patients, the acyl-carnitine ester, i.e., isovalerylcarnitine (IVC), was increased, especially during illness.[142,143] Relative deficiency of muscle carnitine and use of carnitine as an adduct for isovaleric acid are two reasons for considering treatment with extra L-carnitine. The relative therapeutic value of L-carnitine has been compared with that of glycine in the treatment of isovaleric acidemia in a 4½-year-black male.[143] Administration of glycine plus leucine resulted in the excretion of more isovaleryl-CoA as IVG than when leucine was administered alone. Excretion of IVG during leucine and L-carnitine administration was not above that observed with leucine administration alone. Leucine plus L-carnitine increased IVC excretion from a pretreatment level of 7 μmol/24 hours to a post-treatment level of 1,470 μmol/24 hours. Hippuric acid excretion always increased over pretreatment levels. Because hippuric acid did not increase significantly while IVC excretion did, the authors suggest a competitive formation of IVC over hippuric acid when leucine is given along with L-carnitine.[143]

## SULFUR-CONTAINING AMINO ACIDS

The biochemistry and nutritional requirements for sulfur-containing amino acids has been largely elucidated in man by studies of inherited blocks in their metabolic pathways.

### Biochemistry

Natural protein contains approximately 0.3 to 5.0% methionine. Some dietary methionine is used by the body for tissue protein synthesis, but the majority is utilized through the transsulfuration pathway to form adenosylmethionine, adenosylhomocysteine, homocysteine, cystathionine, alpha-ketobutyrate, cysteine, and their derivatives (Fig. 63–9). The first step in the transsulfuration pathway is the synthesis of S-adenosylmethionine (SAM), a reaction catalyzed by methionine adensyltransferase (EC 2.5.1.6). In this

**Table 63–7. Kinetic Constants for Glycine-N-Acylase from Bovine Liver***

| Substrate | Km | V max |
|---|---|---|
| | $(10^{-4}M)$ | *(μmol/min/mg protein)* |
| Tiglyl-CoA | 1.1 | 33.3 |
| Isovaleryl-CoA | 1.8 | 12.3 |
| Benzoyl-CoA | 0.09 | 10.4 |
| 2-Methylbutyryl-CoA | 1.1 | 8.3 |
| 3-Methylcrotonyl-CoA | 0.14 | 5.7 |
| Propionyl-CoA | 1.8 | 4.4 |
| Acetyl-CoA | 2.1 | 2.6 |

*From Bartlett, K, Gompertz, D,[140] with permission of Biochem. Med.

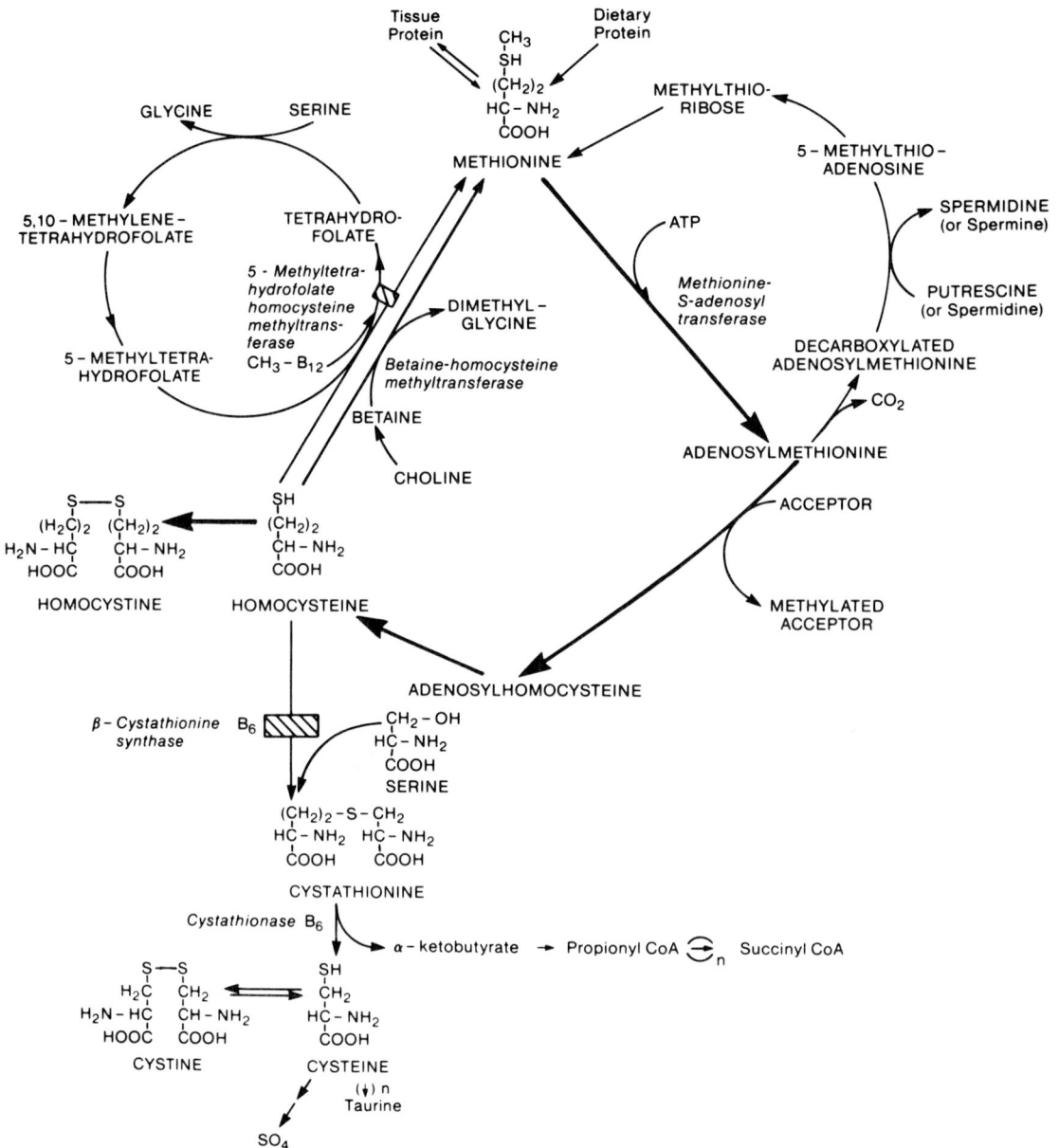

**Fig. 63–9.**  Metabolic pathways of sulfur amino acids. Hatched bars represent impaired reactions in two inherited metabolic disorders resulting in homocystinuria.

reaction, the adenosyl portion of ATP is transferred to methionine. Biologically important compounds that obtain their methyl group from SAM include: creatine, choline and phosphatidylcholines, methylated DNA and RNA, and epinephrine. Decarboxylated SAM is the source of the three carbon moieties of spermidine and spermine. S-adenosylhomocysteine is formed as an intermediary product in this pathway. S-adenosylhomocysteine is hydrolyzed to homocysteine. Homocysteine then has four possible pathways

open to it. Homocysteine reacts with serine in the presence of cystathionine beta-synthase (EC 4.2.1.22), found in liver and brain, to form cystathionine (see Fig. 63–9). Cystathionine beta-synthase requires pyridoxal phosphate as a coenzyme.

Homocysteine can also be remethylated to form methionine through two different enzymatic reactions. In one reaction, the methyl group is derived from betaine and is catalyzed by betaine-homocysteine methyltransferase (EC 2.1.1.5). The second reaction requires N5-methyltetrahydrofolate as a methyl donor and methylcobalamin (CH3B12) as coenzyme (see Fig. 63–9). The enzyme catalyzing this reaction is 5-methyltetrahydrofolate-homocysteine methyl-transferase (EC 2.1.1.13). Finkelstein and Martin used an in vitro system that approximated in vivo conditions in rat liver to measure the simultaneous product formation by the three enzymes that utilize homocysteine.[144] In this control system, 5-methyltetrahydrofolate homocysteine methyltransferase, betaine homocysteine methyltransferase, and cystathionine beta-synthase accounted for 27%, 27%, and 46%, respectively, of the homocysteine consumed.

The fourth pathway open to homocysteine is spontaneous oxidation to homocystine (see Fig. 63–9). This reaction occurs only when homocysteine is present in tissue in abnormal amounts. It is essentially irreversible because the disulfide bond of homocystine is covalent. Homocystine is not further metabolized. Cystathionine beta-synthase metabolizes most homocysteine with high affinity to cystathionine using serine as cosubstrate and pyridoxal phosphate as coenzyme. Cystathionine is then hydrolyzed to cysteine and alpha-ketobutyrate. The enzyme cystathionase (EC 4.4.1.1), which also utilizes pyridoxal phosphate as coenzyme, is required for this reaction (see Fig. 63–9). A deficiency of cystathionase results in cystathioninuria, which has no pathologic consequence. Alpha-ketobutyrate is converted to propionyl CoA, which is carboxylated to methylmalonyl CoA and isomerized to succinyl CoA, a Kreb's cycle intermediate. L-Cysteine is catabolized to pyruvate, $NH_3$, and $H_2S$.

## Homocystinuria

**Definition.** One of several genetically determined errors of methionine metabolism that produce defects in function of cystathionine beta-synthase or 5-methyltetrahydrofolate-homocysteine methyltransferase may result in homocystinuria. Impaired activity of the latter enzyme may be caused by failure to synthesize methylcobalamin from vitamin $B_{12}$ or by a deficiency in 5, 10 methylenetetrahydrofolate reductase (EC 1.1.1.68). Several different defects impair the uptake, transfer, and conversion of dietary vitamin $B_{12}$ to methylcobalamin.[15,145,145a]

The most common form of homocystinuria is due to a deficiency of cystathionine beta-synthase. The mutant enzymes are now being chemically characterized, and one deletion of 60 amino acid residues was reported.[146] Severely impaired enzyme function produces accumulation of plasma homocyst(e)ine and methionine and decreased cyst(e)ine in cells and physiologic fluids. If this biochemical circumstance is not treated early in life, skeletal changes, dislocated lenses, intravascular thromboses, osteoporosis, malar flushing and, in some patients, mental retardation will occur.

The skeletal changes and dislocated lenses are presumably due to a structural defect in collagen formation produced by homocystine interaction with aldose groups on collagen.[145] Intravascular thromboses may occur at any age and have been found in coronary, renal, carotid, and intracranial arteries. Fifty percent of untreated patients die before 20 years of age, and 95% before 50 years of age.[147] The natural history of homocystinuria due to cystathionine beta-synthase deficiency has been clarified in a large series of patients.[148] Heterozygosity for homocystinuria may predispose to the development of premature occlusive arterial disease.[149]

It is not known to what degree the mental retardation in homocystinuria is due to a metabolic sequela, such as deficient cystathionine in myelin formation, or is a result of multiple small cerebrovascular thromboses. In a series of 84 patients, one half were of average intelligence, several were university graduates, and one held a Ph.D.[147] Mental deficiency may occur with severely impaired cystathionine beta-synthase as a consequence of multiple cerebral-arteriolar obstructions if homocystinemia is not controlled by diet.

**Screening.** Cystathionine beta-synthase deficiency is inherited as an autosomal recessive disease. Accurate estimates of the incidence for homocystinuria are not available, but in limited newborn screening, figures varying from 1 in 36,000 to 1 in 330,000 have been found.[145] Five years of screening for homocystinuria in Georgia have yielded an incidence of approximately 1 in 221,000 live births (see Table 63–3). Homocystinuria occurs in many ethnic groups, but has a higher frequency in persons of Irish extraction than in other ethnic groups.[145] This finding may be a bias of ascertainment because of the original description of and continued screening for this disorder in the Irish population. Worldwide screening for homocystinuria is not yet available.

Selective screening uses the inexpensive urinary nitroprusside reaction. In this reaction, reduced homocysteine and cysteine form a stable red color with nitroprusside if present in excessive amounts. This selective screening test for sulfur amino acids should be included in the evaluation of any patient with an unknown cause for arterial thrombosis, dislocated lens, or mental retardation. The test is also positive in cystinuria and should be included as a screen for patients with nephrolithiasis.

In a large survey of patients with homocystinuria due to cystathionine beta-synthase deficiency, only 13% were $B_6$ responsive.[148] Most of these patients were "leaky mutants" who had residual cystathionine beta-synthase activity and expressed their disease in adolescence or young adulthood rather than early childhood. $B_6$ responsivity may be common to all mutations where some enzyme activity is present because the mechanism is through stabilizing enzyme turnover.[145] The more residual enzyme activity present, the more dramatic the $B_6$ response. Hypermethioninemia may not be present in the newborn if more than 15% activity of cystathionine beta-synthase is present.

**Diagnosis.** A positive screen by bacterial inhibition assay for methionine or urinary nitroprusside reaction should be followed by assay of plasma amino acids using ion exchange chromatography. With a cystathionine beta-synthase defect, homocystine, cysteine-homocysteine, and methionine are all elevated in plasma. Normal or low plasma methionine concentrations are associated with homocystinuria due to decreased remethylation pathways (see Fig. 3–9). Demonstration of significantly decreased cystathionine beta-synthase, $CH_3B$-12, or homocysteine methyltransferases is necessary to confirm the diagnosis and to implement appropriate therapy. Methionine may be elevated in the absence of homocystinemia in liver disease and in specific impairment of S-adenosylmethionine methyl transferase (EC 2.5.1.6). By contrast, in defects of homocysteine remethylation to methionine, methionine is low while homocysteine concentrations are elevated. Thus, disorders of cobalamin methylation to $CH_3$-$B_{12}$ or the two homocysteine methyltransferases will not be detected by nonselective newborn screening that only discriminates elevated blood methionine.

Management of these rare forms of homocystinuria does not include methionine-restricted diets. Rather, pharmacologic amounts of vitamin $B_{12}$, folate, or choline are added depending on the primary defect. Liver biopsy specimens, transformed lymphoblasts, or cultured skin fibroblasts express cystathionine β-synthase and are used to confirm the most common cause of homocystinuria. Prenatal diagnosis has been accomplished.[145,148] "Leaky mutants" should be suspected later in life when unexplained arterial thrombosis, mental retardation, or dislocated lenses are encountered.

**Treatment.** Objectives of nutrition support in homocystinuria vary according to the age at which diagnosis is made and the type and degree of enzymatic impairment. If homocystinuria is due to cystathionine beta-synthase deficiency expressed in the newborn, the clinical objectives are: (1) to prevent the development of skeletal and ocular abnormalities, (2) to prevent intravascular thromboses, and (3) to assure normal intellectual development.

Pharmacologic doses of pyridoxine should be tried in all patients with hypermethioninemia and homocystinemia.[148,150] Trials of 1 g of pyridoxine daily should be given to determine its effects on plasma methionine and homocysteine levels. Because enzyme stabilization is the most common mechanism of vitamin responsivity, weeks may be required for a biochemical response to occur. If the plasma methionine and homocysteine concentrations are reduced, the amount of pyridoxine should be gradually lowered until the minimum dose required to maintain biochemical normality is reached. Doses of 25 to 750 mg/day have been required for some patients.[150] Excess $B_6$ for prolonged periods may cause peripheral neuropathy[151] and liver injury;[152] consequently, if $B_6$ is not helpful, it should be discontinued. Betaine supplements (6 g daily) assist in maintaining postprandial plasma homocysteine concentrations in the near normal range in $B_6$-responsive individuals.[153]

Patients who do not respond to pyridoxine require a methionine-restricted diet supplemented with L-cysteine. L-cysteine becomes an essential amino acid in homocystinuria (see Fig. 63–9). If plasma folate concentrations are below normal owing to excess use in remethylating homocysteine to methionine, folate should be added as a supplement.

*Nutrient Requirements.* In prescribing and implementing care plans for infants and children with homocystinuria due to cystathionine beta-synthase deficiency, one must consider energy, protein, methionine, cysteine, folate, $B_6$, $B_{12}$, betaine, and fluid needs. Younger infants have a greater methionine requirement per kilogram of body weight than older infants. Suggested daily methionine intakes range from 50 mg/kg in the young infant to 5 mg/kg in the 15- to 19-year-old. Suggested beginning energy, protein, methionine, and fluid intakes for infants and children of different ages are given in Table 63–5. If the medical food provides more than 20 kcal/oz, extra fluid should be offered between feedings to prevent dehydration.[16]

Calcium cystinate, a soluble form of L-cysteine, should supplement the methionine-restricted diet at all ages. The young infant should be offered 300 mg/kg body weight. This amount may be decreased to 200 mg/kg at six months of age and 100 mg/kg at three years and thereafter. The calcium cystinate should be mixed with the chemically defined low-methionine or methionine-free formula to provide even distribution throughout the day.

*Low-Methionine and Methionine-Free Chemically Defined Medical Foods.* Several medical foods have been developed as protein sources for patients with homocystinuria.[57–61] These include Analog X Meth, Low Methionine Diet Powder, Maxamaid X Meth, Hom 1, and Hom 2. For a complete description of the Analog and Maxamaid range of products, see the section on low-phenylalanine and phenylalanine-free chemically defined medical foods. Sources and formulation of these products are given in Appendix Tables A-43b and A-43c. Composition is given in Appendix A-43d-4. Low Methionine Diet Powder, a soy protein isolate that contains carbohydrate, fat, minerals, and vitamins, is relatively high in methionine: 138 mg/100 g powder. Taurine (31 mg/100 g) is added. Hom 1 and Hom 2 are formulated from L-amino acids, minerals, and vitamins and are free of methionine, fat, chromium, and selenium (Appendix Table A-43d-4).

*Serving Lists.* Methionine may be provided for the young infant through the addition of specified amounts of evaporated milk or proprietary infant formula to the low-methionine or methionine-free medical foods. As growth and development proceed, solid foods should be added at the usual ages. Methionine requirement is small, and most foods contain moderate amounts in relation to requirement.[51–56] Because of this, the amount of solid food that can be ingested is small. To provide variety to the methionine-restricted diet, serving lists have been prepared.[107] Average methionine, cysteine, protein, and energy contents of these lists are given in Appendix Table A-43g.

*Assessment of Nutrition Support.* Following introduction of diet and stabilization, plasma methionine and cysteine concentrations should be monitored twice weekly until three months of age. Weekly monitoring is suggested until six months of age and twice monthly monitoring thereafter if blood levels are stable. Following a diet change, plasma methionine and cysteine should be measured after three days have elapsed. A three-day record prior to each blood sample is necessary to evaluate plasma methionine and cysteine. Plasma methionine should be maintained between 15 and 30 $\mu$mol in fasting plasma.[101] Little or no homocystine should be present in blood and urine. The pulses, skeletal growth and development, and ocular lenses are routinely assessed clinically.

*Results of Nutrition Support.* In a retrospective study of 629 patients with cystathionine beta-syn-thase deficiency, methionine restriction initiated neonatally prevented mental retardation, slowed the rate of lens dislocation, and reduced the incidence of seizures.[148] Pyridoxine treatment of late-detected $B_6$-responsive patients decreased the rate of thromboembolic events.

*Termination of Nutrition Support.* Most clinicians who treat individuals with homocystinuria believe that patients should be kept on diet indefinitely. Termination of diet after growth is achieved may lead to thromboembolisms and ciliary muscle laxity with lens dislocation. Where initiation or maintenance of nutrition support is not possible, acetylsalicylic acid (1 g daily) and dipyridamole (100 mg daily) increase platelet survival time and decrease thrombotic events.[154]

**Reproductive Performance.** For both men and women, fewer conceptions were reported for $B_6$-nonresponsive than for $B_6$-responsive patients. Offspring of male patients did not suffer excess losses and were generally reported to be normal. Higher rates of fetal loss occurred in presumptive heterozygous fetuses carried by cystathionine beta-synthase-deficient mothers than occurred in normal women.[148] Whether hypermethioninemia, homocysteinemia, or other metabolic variations in methionine metabolism are teratogenic is as yet unclear, but a teratogenic mechanism as defined for "maternal PKU" is possible.

## AMMONIA

Nutritional management of disorders involving ammonia fixation and urea production use all the traditional rules for treating inborn errors of metabolism; restricting toxic precursor, adding deficient product, and encouraging alternate pathways for nitrogen excretion are three essential rules to follow. Additionally, the biologic variation imparted on ammonia fixation and the urea cycle by heritable mutations has greatly increased our understanding of the normal physiology, biochemistry, and molecular biology of these complex functions.

### Biochemistry

Normally, ammonia is converted to urea in the liver through the Krebs-Henseleit cycle (Fig. 63–10). The first two enzymes of the cycle as well as N-acetylglutamate synthetase (EC 2.3.1.1) are mitochondrial. N-acetylglutamate synthetase catalyzes the conversion of acetyl-CoA plus glutamate to N-acetylglutamate, an essential cofactor for carbamylphosphate synthesis. Carbamylphosphate synthetase I (EC 6.3.4.16) catalyzes the conversion of ammonia, ATP, and bicarbonate to carbamylphosphate. Ornithine transcarbamylase (EC 2.1.3.3) carboxylates ornithine, forming citrulline.

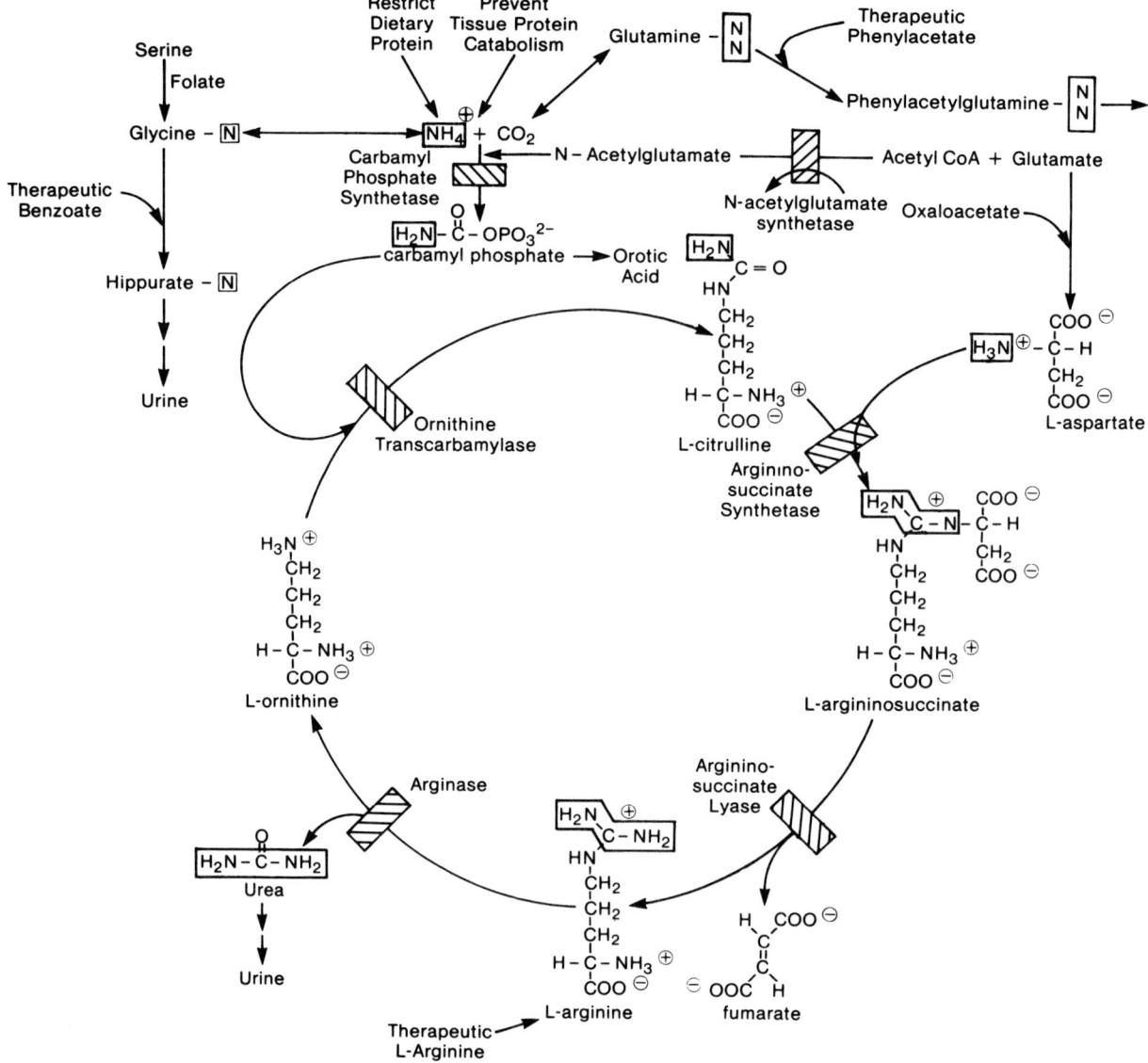

**Fig. 63–10.** Inborn errors in the urea cycle and nutritional approaches to their management. Ammonia fixation and urea production are metabolically cycled with inherited blocks producing hyperammonemia indicated by hatched bars. Important nitrogen molecules and their biochemical origins are outlined in boxes. Mitochondrial enzymes in urea synthesis are carbamylphosphate synthetase, N-acetylglutamate synthetase, and ornithine transcarbamylase. The use of benzoate and phenylacetate is indicated to provide alternate pathways for nitrogen excretion. The addition of dietary arginine is to provide urea cycle substrate distal to genetically impaired reactions. Restriction of dietary protein and addition of dietary energy to prevent catabolism are also indicated.

Citrulline is exported from mitochondria to the cytoplasm where it combines with aspartate to form argininosuccinic acid, a reaction catalyzed by argininosuccinic acid synthetase (EC 6.3.4.5). Fumarate is cleaved from argininosuccinic acid by argininosuccinic acid lyase (EC 4.3.2.1), yielding arginine. Urea is then formed by the action of arginase (EC 3.5.3.1), regenerating ornithine, which is transported back into the mitochondria.

## Urea Cycle Enzyme Deficiencies

**Definition.** Disorders of the urea cycle are a heterogeneous group of inherited defects of ureagenesis.[155] These disorders may result from impairment of one of six enzymes, three of which occur in the mitochondria and three in the cytosol (hatched bars in Figure 63–10). With the exception of ornithine transcarbamylase (OTC) deficiency, all have an autosomal recessive mode of inheritance. OTC deficiency is inherited as an X-linked dominant trait that is usually lethal in males.[155]

Hyperammonemia is a biochemical manifestation characteristic of all disorders of the urea cycle. Other biochemical characteristics of each defect follow: Carbamylphosphate synthetase I defect causes decreased plasma citrulline; OTC deficiency results in orotic aciduria and X-linked patterns of transmission; argininosuccinate synthetase deficiency is associated with increased plasma citrulline accompanied by orotic aciduria; argininosuccinate lyase deficiency causes increased argininosuccinate in plasma and urine; and arginase deficiency has increased arginine in plasma and urine. Clinical features in the newborn suggestive of urea cycle defects occur with protein ingestion. In order of severity, they include: poor feeding, vomiting, lethargy, hypotonia or spasticity, irritability, respiratory distress, convulsions, and coma. Mental retardation occurs in survivors, but successful control of hyperammonemia in the newborn may prevent this sequela.

*Variability of Expression.* Hyperammonemia and its clinical sequelae of vomiting, lethargy, and coma relate to excessive protein intake or catabolism and are observed in all the defects. However, the biochemical and phenotypic manifestations differ in the individual enzyme deficiencies. In argininosuccinate lyase deficiency, a specific hair abnormality, trichorrhexis nodosa, is evident (Fig. 63–11). This condition is related to arginine deficiency and the relatively high arginine content of normal hair protein. Hair reverts to normal with arginine supplementation (see Fig. 63—11). In patients with defects of the first four enzymes, arginine deficiency has also been associated with progressive degeneration of the central nervous system, with control of hyperammonemia through protein restriction alone.[156]

Within each enzyme defect there is a spectrum of clinical manifestations ranging from death in the newborn period to cyclical vomiting and migraine in adolescence. For example, the typical male with OTC deficiency has less than 5% activity and dies in the neonatal period. A surviving male child with a variant form of OTC deficiency shows decreased affinity for ornithine, a shift of pH optimum, and 25% of normal activity under physiologic conditions.[157]

Enzymatic evidence for genetic heterogeneity comes from kinetic studies in fibroblasts of patients with argininosuccinic acid synthetase deficiency. Enzymes from patients all showed decreased binding of citrulline and/or aspartate, but the residual argininosuccinic acid synthetase had a distinct and different curve of activity in each patient.[158] In a case of argininosuccinic acid lyase deficiency, the enzyme was defective in the liver but not in the brain and kidney, suggesting that more than one gene may be responsible for the activity of this enzyme.[159]

The genes for ornithine transcarbamylase, argininosuccinate synthetase, and arginase have all

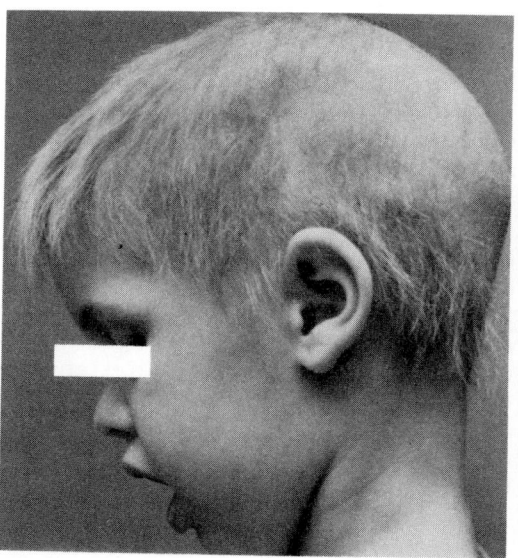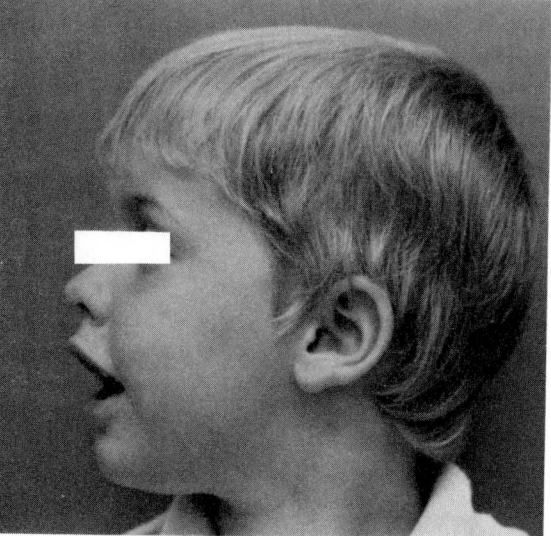

**Fig. 63–11.** Effect of arginine on hair growth in argininosuccinic aciduria. A six-year-old boy with hyperammonemia, trichorrhexis nodosa, and developmental delay was diagnosed with argininosuccinic aciduria. Before diet therapy he had diffuse brittle hair (left panel). Six months later, while receiving 350 mg/kg/day arginine, he had luxuriant blond hair and his first haircut (right panel). (Courtesy of P. Fernhoff, Division of Medical Genetics, Emory University.)

been cloned.[160] Interestingly, the cytosolic enzyme argininosuccinate synthetase has multiple pseudogenes requiring that mRNA be used from patients in northern blots to evaluate mutations leading to citrullinemia. This technique indentifies the expressed transcripts by hybridization with the cDNA probe and digestion with S-1 nuclease.[161,162] Several different types of abnormal mRNA have been defined in citrullinemia.[162] In OTC deficiency, mutations are found that produce immunologically absent mitochondrial protein in addition to variation in enzyme function. Regulation of the mechanisms involved in mitochondrial import of this nuclear-coded X-linked protein is under current intensive study.[163,164] Arginase may have differing genetic origin in kidney, liver, and brain.[165] Molecular analysis of the autosomal gene(s) is also under investigation. A syndrome known as HHH, for hyperammonemia, homocitrullinemia, and hyperornithinemia, may be caused by defective ornithine transport by mitochondria.[166]

*Expression of the Heterozygous State for OTC Deficiency.* The heterozygous state of OTC deficiency may be characterized by mild protein intolerance manifested clinically by migraine in adults and by cyclic vomiting in children.[167] A grandmother and mother of two children with OTC deficiency suffered from migrainous attacks and voluntarily avoided high-protein foods. Ammonium chloride tolerance tests were done, and within four hours both women developed nausea and headache and their plasma ammonium levels rose to three times normal.

When protein or ammonium chloride loads were administered to 15 children with migraine and cyclic vomiting, nine had abnormally high baseline plasma ammonium levels. The tests produced marked hyperammonemia in eight; six developed migraine symptoms. Of seven girls with cyclic vomiting subjected to enzyme assay, three had deficient activity of ornithine transcarbamylase.[167] Heterozygous females with OTC deficiency may be asymptomatic or as severely affected as hemizygous males.[168]

**Screening.** Nonselected screening of all newborns for urea cycle disorders is routinely conducted only in Massachusetts.[169] With the use of a bacterial auxotroph that required arginine, nine of 700,000 newborn tests were found to be homozygous-affected or heterozygous for argininosuccinate lyase deficiency.[169] Selective screening tests for disorders of the urea cycle are available.[170–174] One method for selective screening for hyperammonemia in the newborn nursery requires only one drop of blood, can be performed at the bedside, and gives results in 15 minutes.[173]

This method can be readily adopted in offices and hospitals for selective screening.

The incidence of hyperammonemia in an institutionalized mentally retarded population was studied.[174] Thirty female patients with a history of protein intolerance out of a population of 6,000 were evaluated; of 21 for whom ammonia was reported, 17 were abnormally high. Unfortunately, enzyme diagnoses were not completed and artifactual elevation of blood ammonia due to contamination with feces, nail polish, and tobacco smoke was not considered. The true incidence of disorders of ureagenesis is not known, but genetic variation may well remain undiagnosed as causes of idiopathic mental retardation.

**Diagnosis.** The presence of hyperammonemia in association with other appropriate biochemical and clinical characteristics is suggestive of a urea cycle disorder.[155,175]

The enzyme defect can be inferred from the specific metabolite in addition to ammonia that accumulates in blood and urine: orotic acid in the urine in OTC deficiency; and citrulline, argininosuccinic acid, and arginine in the plasma and urine in argininosuccinate synthetase, argininosuccinate lyase, and arginase deficiencies, respectively. Carbamylphosphate synthetase deficiency is suggested by exclusion of the other four enzymopathies. Hyperammonemia can also be caused by acute or chronic liver diseases, Reye's syndrome, asparaginase treatment, propionicacidemia, hyperlysinemia, hyperornithinemia, isovaleric acidemia, methylmalonic aciduria, and FreAmine II solution exposure in infants. Definitive diagnosis depends on biochemical and enzymatic assays in addition to adequate clinical history.[175]

**Treatment.** The treatment of inherited urea cycle enzymopathies can be divided into acute and chronic therapy.[177]

*Acute Therapy.* Peritoneal dialysis may be useful in the presence of coma in reducing plasma ammonium levels.[176] Peritoneal dialysis for seven days in a male neonate with OTC deficiency removed 50 times more ammonia than a single exchange transfusion.[178] However, peritoneal dialysis is not without difficulties and risks including *Candida* peritonitis and continued catabolism. We prefer to begin orogastric perfusion with high calories (150 kcal/kg/day) but no protein. Protein-Free Diet Powder is useful for this approach (Appendix Tables A-43b, A-43c, A-43d-5). L-arginine (350 to 500 mg/kg/day) should be added to this formulation. Sodium benzoate (300 mg/kg/day) can successfully reduce acute hyperammonemia in the neonatal period. Phenylacetic acid may also be given to form phenylacetylglutamate, which is excreted in the urine, eliminating from the body two nitrogen atoms per molecule (see Fig. 63–10).[179] A priority of newborn therapy is to "force" the neonate into an anabolic phase with high calorie feeds. Peripheral venous hyper-alimentation with 10 to 20% glucose and Intralipid (2 to 4 g/kg) may be necessary if gavage is not tolerated. As gavage feeds are increased, peripheral alimentation should be decreased. After four days of "no-protein," high-calorie arginine- and benzoate-supplemented feeds, blood ammonia should revert to near normal. Cautious addition of 1.0 to 1.5 g/kg/day of protein is then necessary.

*Chronic Therapy.* The objectives of therapy in a child with a defect of the urea cycle are to maintain plasma concentrations of ammonia as near normal as possible, but to supply protein and other essential amino acids and nutrients that will allow maximal development of intellect and optimal growth. Four major approaches are used in treatment of individuals with urea cycle defects (see Fig. 63–10). These include (1) reducing precursors of ammonia, (2) correcting arginine deficiency, (3) enhancing alternate mechanisms of waste nitrogen loss, and (4) accelerating renal excretion of accumulated intermediates.[179]

Methods used to reduce ammonia precursors include protein restriction, prevention of body protein catabolism, and use of only essential and semiessential amino acids.[177] In any situation in which intake of protein or essential amino acids is severely restricted, precursors for synthesis of carnitine (lysine, methionine), glutathione (cysteine, glutamate), and taurine (cysteine) may be limiting. Restricted methionine intake may result in a decrease in the available pool of labile methyl groups required for synthesis of important metabolic compounds.

L-arginine supplementation is required in all the urea cycle defects except arginase deficiency. To maintain normal or slightly elevated plasma arginine concentrations, 350 to 500 mg/kg of body weight daily are used.[180] L-arginine can then produce ornithine for ammonia fixation and drive the "cycle" to citrulline and argininosuccinate (see Fig. 63–10). These two amino acids are poorly absorbed by kidney and allow nitrogen loss.

Acceleration of renal excretion of accumulated intermediates in the impaired cycle is sought. Arginine supplementation increases citrulline and argininosuccinic acid excretion in argininosuccinic acid synthetase and argininosuccinic acid lyase deficiency, respectively.[177,180]

Waste nitrogen urinary loss can be enhanced by the use of sodium benzoate or phenylacetate[174] (see Fig. 63–10). Glycine conjugates with benzoate

using glycine-N-acylase and leads to the excretion of a nearly stoichiometric quantity of nitrogen as hippurate (see Fig. 63–10). Toxicity is low on 200 to 500 mg/kg/day. Folate must be administered to provide a source of one-carbon fragments for synthesis of glycine from serine in order to prevent glycine depletion.[181] Pyridoxine is necessary for transamination.

Phenylacetate increases urinary nitrogen excretion as phenylacetylglutamine[179,181] (see Fig. 63–10). Suggested dosage is 250 mg/kg body weight.

Catabolism during a febrile illness may lead to life-threatening elevations in blood ammonia. In addition to prompt diagnosis and treatment of the infection, decreased protein intake (to 0 g for one to two days), increased energy intake, and peritoneal dialysis may all be required.

In planning nutrition support of the infant or child with a defect of a urea cycle enzyme, a formal prescription should be written that includes recommended amounts of protein, energy, fluid, L-arginine, and benzoic acid for the day. The prescription for protein should be based on blood ammonia concentrations and correlated with growth.

Protein intakes suggested in Table 63–8 are based on amounts required to cover obligatory losses and growth needs[182] of infants and children fed an excellent protein source such as egg or milk. Intakes may need to be increased if the child fails to grow adequately on the recommended intake or if sodium benzoate or phenylacetate is administered.

Energy intakes recommended in Table 63–8 are somewhat greater than those for normal infants and children in order to provide ketoacid precursors from carbohydrate for synthesis of nonessential amino acids and to prevent protein degrada-

**Table 63–8.   Recommended Protein and Energy Intakes for Infants and Children with Disorders of the Urea Cycle**

| Age | Protein (g/kg) | Energy (kcal/kg) |
|---|---|---|
| <3 mo. | 1.6–1.2 | 130–145 |
| 3<6 mo. | 1.3–1.0 | 125–145 |
| 6<9 mo. | 1.3–1.0 | 120–125 |
| 9<12 mo. | 1.2–0.9 | 115–135 |
| 1<4 yr. | 1.0–0.7 | 110–120 |
| 4<7 yr. | 0.8–0.6 | 100–110 |
| 7<11 yr. | 0.7–0.5 | 80–90 |
| 11<18 yr. | 0.6–0.4 | 55–65 |
| ≥18 yr. | 0.5–0.3 | 35–50 |

tion. Carbohydrate should not provide more than 50% of the energy because of frequently elevated plasma triglyceride concentrations.

In any situation in which protein-restricted diets are fed, carnitine supplements may be necessary. If carnitine deficiency occurs, recommended amounts of supplemental L-carnitine are 50 to 100 mg/kg/day.

L-cysteine or L-methionine may be required with protein-restricted diets to provide precursors for synthesis of sulfur amino acids and taurine. If UCD 1 is used as the protein source (see next section), adequate cysteine and methionine are included. Monitoring plasma amino acids helps to prevent this type of iatrogenic deficiency.

*Medical Foods for Urea Cycle Disorders.* Nutrition support of urea cycle disorders requires restriction of nitrogen intake. This restriction is best accomplished by providing protein in the form of essential amino acids only. UCD 1, intended for the infant, is formulated from essential L-amino acids, L-cystine, L-tyrosine, sucrose, minerals, and vitamins. UCD 2 is formulated in a similar fashion, but it is free of L-cystine and L-tyrosine (Appendix Tables A-43c, A-43d-6). UCD 1 contains 55 mg L-cystine/g protein. These two products contain no fat, chromium, or selenium.

*Serving Lists.* Serving lists of natural foods are available to simplify the protein-restricted diets for professionals and families (Appendix Table A-43e).

*Assessment of Nutrition Support.* Frequency of assessment is, in part, dictated by the clinical course of the patient. Blood ammonia concentrations should be monitored routinely and maintained below 50 $\mu$mol. Plasma concentrations of amino acids should be monitored and maintained in the normal range. Plasma albumin and globulin concentrations are indices of protein status and should be evaluated frequently. Retinol-binding protein has a shorter half-life than albumin and can provide information on protein status at an earlier stage in deficiency than albumin. Caretakers should provide diet diaries and records of health status in tandem with blood for ammonia and plasma amino acids. Growth and development should be routinely assessed. If growth is not maintained, increased protein intake may be necessary.

*Results of Nutrition Support.* Results of therapy in infants with complete or near-complete enzyme deficiencies have been less than optimal, with delayed death and below-normal development. When onset is delayed, physical growth and mental development are more nearly normal with nutrition and pharmacologic support.[155,175,180] If diagnosis is anticipated and treatment begun in early infancy in affected siblings with citrullinemia or argininosuccinic acidemia, relatively normal outcome is observed even in the severe enzyme defects.

## GALACTOSE

### Biochemistry

Because lactose is the principal carbohydrate and energy source for infants and young children, galactose maintains a central metabolic role in human nutrition. Lactose is hydrolyzed in the intestine by lactase (EC 3.2.1.23) to glucose and galactose (Fig. 63–12). Prior to utilization, galactose must be converted to glucose. This conversion occurs primarily in the liver where galactose becomes glucose through three enzymatic steps. First, galactose is phosphorylated to galactose-1-phosphate by galactokinase (EC 2.7.1.6). Then the phosphorylated hexose is interchanged with the glucose moiety of uridyldiphosphoglucose by galactose-1-phosphate uridyl transferase (EC 2.7.7.10). Finally, galactose is rearranged to glucose by uridine diphosphate UDP galactose-4-epimerase (EC 5.1.3.2.) (Fig. 63–12). The glucose thus formed can be used for glycogen synthesis or phosphorylated to glucose-1-phosphate for further utilization.

### Galactosemias

**Definition.** Galactosemia may occur because of deficient functioning of any of three enzymes: galactokinase, galactose-1-phosphate uridyl transferase (gal-1-P transferase), or UDP galactose-4-epimerase (see Fig. 63–12). Patients with galactokinase deficiency have only cataracts. Galactokinase deficiency does not produce severe clinical manifestations or the accumulation of galactose-1-phosphate seen with gal-1-P transferase deficiency. At least nine variants with different degrees of function and structure have been described for mutant gal-1-P transferase.[183] This gene locus is on chromosome 9p.[155,184]

Galactosemia due to deficiency of gal-1-P transferase leads to accumulation of galactose-1-phosphate, which acts as a phosphate sink reducing intracellular phosphate for high-energy phosphate bonds. Thus, ATP, GTP, and CTP are reduced. Progressive damage to the central nervous system, liver, and renal tubule results if treatment is not instituted in the first few days of life.

Clinical symptoms of the gal-1-P transferase defect appear early in infancy. Some infants are born with cataracts and cirrhosis, which may be due to maternal lactose ingestion. Symptoms generally appear with the onset of milk feedings. Prolonged neonatal jaundice at 4 to 10 days of age is com-

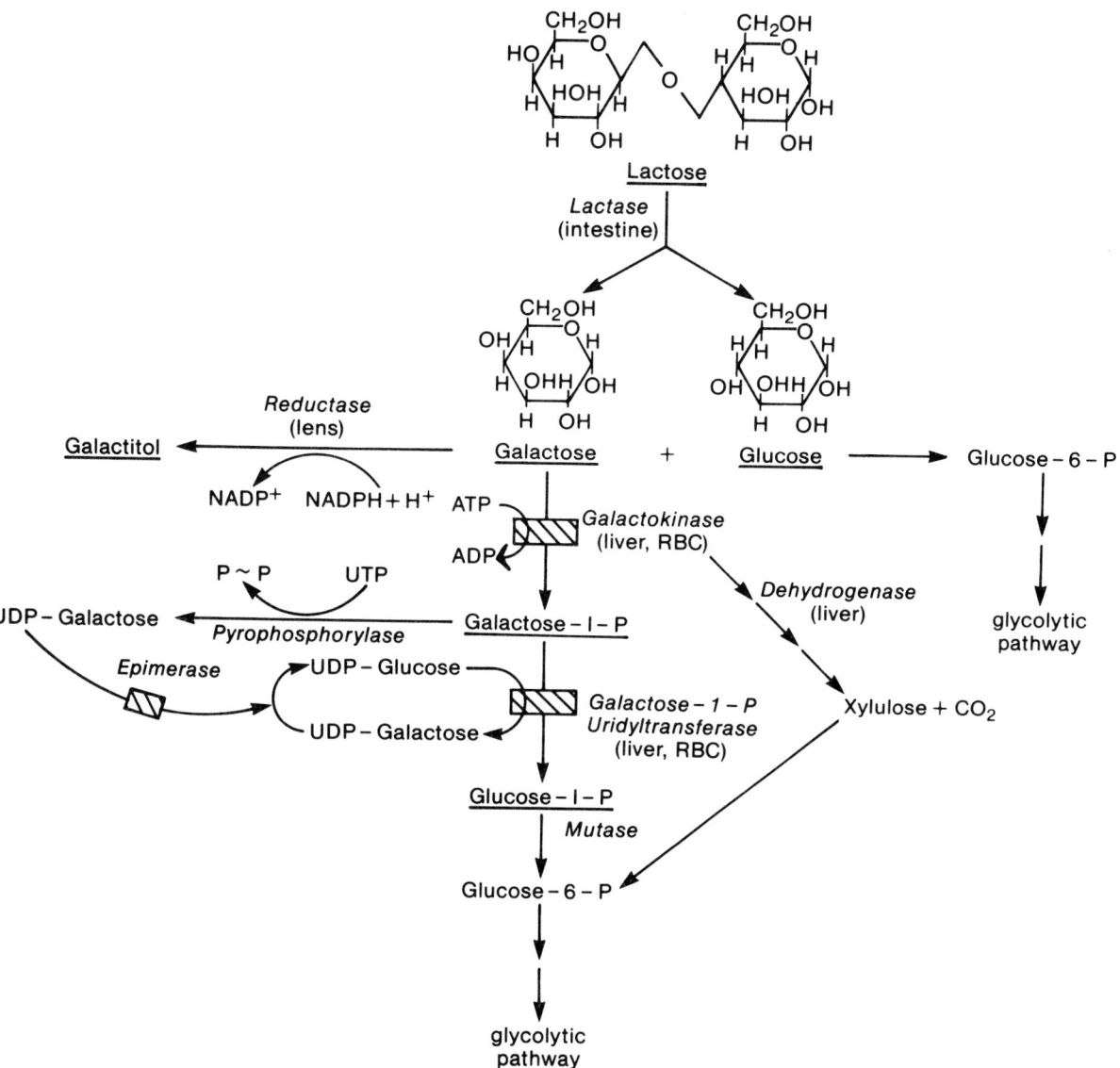

**Fig. 63–12.**   Metabolic blocks in galactose metabolism that lead to galactosemia. Genetic disorders of catalyzed reactions are indicated by hatched bars.

mon. Hyperbilirubinemia is secondary to toxic injury to liver cells by gal-1-P, delayed maturation of glucuronyl transferase,[185] mild hemolysis, and bleeding. Bleeding diatheses, *E. coli* sepsis, and shock are catastrophic events that occur during the neonatal period. Therefore, rapid screening, retrieval, diagnosis, and treatment are essential for population-based newborn screening programs if the clinical sequelae of galactosemia are to be prevented. Other relatively minor symptoms occur. Anemia from various causes is present in about 40% of untreated patients. Lethargy, hypotonia, food refusal, vomiting, and diarrhea are also common symptoms.

Retarded mental and physical growth occur in most of the untreated infants who survive. The basis for the mental retardation is unknown, but three theories include:[185] (1) an altered UDP galactose: UDP glucose ratio that may influence cellular oxidation by neural cells and myelin formation, (2) inhibition by galactose and gal-1-P of brain protein synthesis, or (3) increased levels of galactitol in the brain. Phosphatidyl inositol is an integral constituent of cell membranes, and galactitol inhibits the incorporation of inositol into essential lipids of neural cell membranes. Inhibition of synthesis of nerve cell membrane (myelin) may lead to permanently altered function. Additional effects, such as retarded physical development, may be due to food refusal, vomiting, diarrhea, renal failure, loss of galactose-derived energy, and depressed protein synthesis.

Cataracts occur in about 45% of untreated individuals. They are thought to result from the formation and accumulation of galactitol in the lens of the eye, which is impermeable to efflux. Galactitol creates an osmotic gradient that allows glutathione to efflux with consequent decreased concentrations of lens glutathione. When glutathione concentrations are decreased, glutathione peroxidase (EC 1.11.1.9) is inactivated and hydrogen peroxide accumulates to toxic levels. Hydrogen peroxide denatures lens protein, causing production of lenticular cataracts.[183]

Hepatomegaly occurs in nearly all cases of gal-1-P transferase deficiency, and cirrhosis develops in untreated patients. The hepatomegaly is associated with abnormally large amounts of gal-1-P, UDP galactose, and glycogen in the liver. Liver damage results in decreased synthesis of prothrombin and albumin.

Because of decreased albumin synthesis and proteinuria, ascites and generalized edema occur in about 36% of patients.[183] The albumin synthesized by untreated galactosemic patients contains large amounts of galactose, whereas albumin of normal individuals is free of galactose.[186] Untreated or poorly controlled patients are extremely susceptible to infection with gram-negative organisms. Immunoincompetence is probably a direct result of inhibition by gal-1-P of immune protein synthesis by lymphocytes and inactivation of leukocyte phagocytosis.

Galactose and its accumulated metabolites are toxic to the glomeruli and tubules of the kidney. Additionally, active tubular transport is impaired because of deficient ATP. Aminoaciduria is generalized.

On rare occasions, hypoglycemia occurs. Causes include defective hepatic gluconeogenesis, the inability to convert glycogen to glucose because of inhibition of phosphorylase kinase by gal-1-P, and hyperinsulinemia that may result from galactose stimulation of pancreatic beta cells and decreased hepatic extraction of insulin.[185]

**Screening.** Gal-1-P transferase deficiency is inherited via an autosomal recessive mode. Estimates of the frequency of the gal-1-P transferase defect have increased with the improvement of screening and diagnostic procedures. Five years of experience with screening over 700,000 infants for galactosemia in Georgia have yielded 1.8 in 100,000 patients with classic galactosemia and 4.0 in 100,000 patients with variant forms (see Table 63–3). Others have reported variable frequencies in United States populations between 1 in 18,000 and 1 in 70,000.[183]

The most common screening method is the Beutler fluorescent test[187] for galactosemia. This procedure consists of incubating dried blood on filter paper disks with a mixture of uridine diphosphoglucose (UDPG), phosphoglucokinase (EC 2.7.1.0), glucose-6-phosphate dehydrogenase (EC 1.1.1.49), and NADP. Erythrocytes from normal individuals contain the enzyme gal-1-P transferase and produce glucose-1-phosphate:

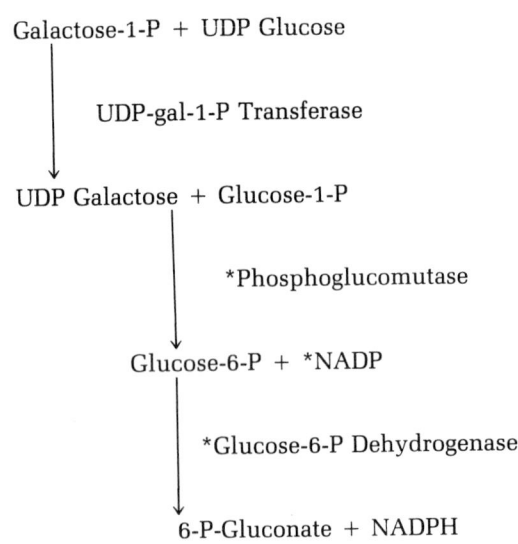

Galactose-1-P + UDP Glucose

UDP-gal-1-P Transferase

UDP Galactose + Glucose-1-P

*Phosphoglucomutase

Glucose-6-P + *NADP

*Glucose-6-P Dehydrogenase

6-P-Gluconate + NADPH

---

*Added to produce enzyme-linked NADPH by U.V. fluorescent assay.

Glucose-1-phosphate is converted to glucose-6-phosphate which, in the presence of glucose-6-dehydrogenase, reduces NAD to NADPH. Blood from patients with classic galactosemia has impaired gal-1-P transferase activity. This enzyme-linked reaction is determined by the presence or absence of produced NADPH, which is fluorescent when viewed under shortwave ultraviolet light.

Positive screening results occur if variants of gal-1-P transferase are inactivated by exposure of the blood disks to heat, as in the summer. The Duarte/galactosemia compound heterozygote is more sensitive to heat than the homozygous normal. Confirmation of a positive Beutler screening test uses erythrocyte hemolysates for quantitative enzyme activity. Quantitation of intact erythrocyte gal-1-P content in the erythrocytes of the probands and isoenzymal analysis of parental galactose-1-P uridyltransferase are necessary for final diagnosis and genetic counseling.

An alternative screening test to determine the presence of excess galactose concentrations has been developed.[7] This test depends on the fact that lysis of certain strains of *E. coli* by bacteriophage is inhibited by galactose or gal-1-P. Climatic changes should not affect this screening procedure.

**Diagnosis.** Patients with a positive Beutler and/or a positive *E. coli* bacteriophage test should have all lactose removed from their diets immediately while enzyme diagnosis and family work-up proceed. Fresh, sterile heparinized blood should be sent to a central laboratory experienced in enzyme analysis. Both patient and family should be evaluated by the center for genotype and form of impaired enzyme.

Diagnosis of galactosemia is accomplished through measurement of activity of gal-1-P transferase in erythrocytes. No activity occurs in individuals homozygous for the classic disease (G/G), whereas heterozygotes (G/N) have approximately one half normal activity (Table 63–9). Several types of gal-1-P transferase deficiency have been described based on percentage of activity in the erythrocyte and on isozyme patterns on starch gel electrophoresis (see Table 63–9). The need for therapy in patients with activity of 25% or less of gal-1-P transferase, as in compound heterozygotes for Duarte/galactosemia alleles, has not been established. However, galactose should be restricted in early life for patients with any mutant genotype if erythrocyte gal-1-P is elevated above 2 mg/dl.

Gal-1-P transferase is expressed in cultured amniotic fluid cells from the normal fetus. Thus, prenatal detection of gal-1-P transferase deficiency is possible. Amniotic fluid of a fetus with galactosemia was found to have an elevated concentration of galactitol. Assessment of the galactitol content of amniotic fluid by GC/MS provides a rapid, ancillary method for prenatal diagnosis of galactosemia.[188]

**Treatment.** Objectives of therapy in galactosemia are to ameliorate or to prevent symptoms while providing adequate energy and nutrients for normal growth and development. Treatment should begin as early in the first week of life as possible, and consists of removal of all sources of lactose and galactose from the diet.

*Nutrient Requirements.* Energy and nutrient requirements of well-controlled infants and children with galactosemia are the same as those for normal individuals of the same age, gender, and physical activity. Whether greater than normal energy and protein intakes will prevent the linear growth retardation seen in poorly controlled children is not known.

*Formulas.* Human milk contains 6 to 8% lactose, cow's milk 3 to 4% lactose, and many proprietary infant formulas 7% lactose. These milks must be replaced by a formula low in galactose (Isomil, Nutramigen, Pregestimil, or ProSobee).

Formulas containing soy protein isolate have about 14 mg galactose/L in the form of raffinose and stachyose, oligosaccharides that contain galactose. At one time it was thought that these oligosaccharides yielded free galactose on hydrolysis in the intestine. It is now known that the human intestine has no enzymes to hydrolyze these oligosaccharides.[189] Thus, they may be safely used for feeding infants and children with galactosemia. Casein hydrolysates such as Nutramigen and Pregestimil have been treated to remove lactose but contain about 160 mg galactose/L.[190]

*Solid Foods.* When solid foods (Appendix Table A-43b) are added at appropriate ages, careful reading of labels is required to ensure that neither galactose nor lactose has been added in food processing (see also Appendix Table A-34). Lactose is added to baked goods, dry mixes, ice cream, sherbets, confections, and batter mixes, among others, to improve flavor, texture, body, viscosity, and mouth feel.[191] Standards of identity for "standard name" foods that do not require ingredient lists on the label should be obtained from the Food and Drug Administration. Examples of such foods are imitation milk, white bread, and mayonnaise. Foods such as peas and organ meats that naturally contain galactose must also be excluded from the diet. Certain artificial sweeteners contain lactose as an extender. These artificial sweeteners and any products prepared with these sugar substitutes must be avoided.

Some clinical centers treating patients with ga-

**Table 63–9. Allelic Disorders of Galactose-1-Phosphate Uridyl Transferase**

| Type | Genotype | Erythrocyte UDP-Gal-1-P Transferase |
|------|----------|-------------------------------------|
| | | *(% of control)* |
| Classic | N/N | 0 |
| Chicago | C/N | 75 |
| | D/N | 75 |
| Duarte | D/D | 50 |
| | G/N | 50 |
| Duarte/Gal | D/G | 25 |
| Indiana | I/N | 0–45 |
| Negro | gt/gt (mosaic) | 0 (normal hepatic activity) |
| Rennes | R/N | 7 |

lactosemia have allowed fermented dairy products and aged cheese under the mistaken impression that all lactose has been converted to lactic acid. This is not the case,[192–196] however, and these products should be excluded from the diet. Vegetable gums such as agar, acacia (gum arabic), carrageenan, locust bean (carob), and guar are complex galactosides or galactomannans that contain mostly β-D-1→3, 1→4, and 1→6 linkages that are not digested by humans. Thus, foods containing these gums may be used in galactose-restricted diets. Only tragacanthic acid, which has a main chain of 1→4-alpha-D-galacturonopyranosyl units, may need to be excluded from the diet. One report suggested that all legumes, textured vegetable protein, spinach, and vegetable gums be excluded from the galactose-restricted diet.[196] However, no scientific data were presented to justify this recommendation.

*Drugs.* Drugs often contain lactose for a variety of purposes. Lists of sugar-free drug preparations are published that should be updated frequently and scrutinized when galactosemic children require drug therapy.

*Results of Nutrition Support.* Treatment, while lifesaving, may not result in complete freedom from the sequelae of accumulated gal-1-P. Those infants diagnosed and treated early who maintain excellent dietary control have better intellectual function than those who have poor control or are diagnosed late.[197,198] Control is defined on the basis of erythrocyte gal-1-P levels and is considered excellent if consistently below 3 mg/dl.[199] However, even with excellent control, children frequently have lower IQs than their normal siblings.[200] They may have difficulty with language,[201] abstract thinking, and visual perception. These deficits may be related to intrauterine brain damage from maternal blood galactose crossing the placenta into the vulnerable fetus.[202]

However, galactose is normally synthesized by man and is essential for membrane mucoproteins. These membranes are constantly being synthesized and degraded, producing galactose. Prevention of some gal-1-P accumulation by restriction of exogenous galactose is thus impossible. Early-onset cataracts and infertility in affected females are reported despite "good" dietary control. Galactose (i.e., milk) restriction in at-risk pregnant females is generally advised.[203]

*Assessment of Nutrition Support.* Frequent evaluation of growth, development, and erythrocyte gal-1-P concentrations is necessary to determine if the diet is being followed. Use of galactosylated hemoglobin A1 as an index of dietary control has been suggested, but is less sensitive and is an indirect test.[204]

*Diet Termination.* Although some investigators have recommended liberalization of the galactose-restricted diet at 12 to 13 years of age, this suggestion is not warranted because the damaging effects of accumulated galactitol in the lens and gal-1-P in the liver and kidney remain. Galactosemic females must continue treatment with galactose exclusion to prevent gonadal atrophy and in utero damage to the fetus.[205] Hypogonadism has been reported in female patients with gal-1-P transferase deficiency in whom nutrition support was delayed.[206–209] Males examined had normal gonadal function. Offspring of pregnant rats fed a 50% galactose diet had a striking reduction in oocyte number. The most prominent effects were noted after exposure to galactose during the premeiotic stages of oogenesis.[210,211]

## REFERENCES

1. McKusick, V.A.: Mendelian Inheritance in Man: Catalog of Autosomal Dominant, Recessive, X-Linked Phenotypes. 6th ed. Baltimore, Johns Hopkins University Press, 1983.
2. Harris, H.: The Principles of Human Biochemical

Genetics. 3rd ed. Amsterdam, North-Holland Publishing Company, 1980.

3. Naylor E.W., Flores, N.E.: Evaluation of neonatal screening for maple syrup urine disease. *In* Neonatal Screening. (Naruse, H., Irie, M., Eds.) Amsterdam, Excerpta Medica, 1983.

4. Marshall L., DiGeorge, A.: Am. J. Hum. Genet. *33*:138A, 1981.

5. Elsas, L., et al.: Metabolic consequences of inherited defects in branched chain α-ketoacid dehydrogenase: mechanisms of thiamine action. *In* Metabolism and Clinical Implications of Branched Chain Amino Acids and Ketoacids. (Walser, M., Williamson, J., Eds.) New York, Elsevier Science Publishing Co., Inc., 1981.

6. Snyderman, E.: Maple syrup urine disease. *In* Congenital Metabolic Disease: Diagnosis and Treatment (Wapnir, L.A., Ed.) New York, Marcel Dekker, Inc., 1985.

7. Elsas, L.J.: Newborn Screening. *In* Pediatrics. 17th ed. (Rudolph, A.M., Ed.) New York, Appleton-Century Crofts, 1982.

8. Elsas, L., Brown, A., Fernhoff, P.: Newborn Screening for metabolic disorders in the state of Georgia. *In* Neonatal Screening. (Naruse, H., Irie, M., Eds.) Amsterdam, Excerpta Medica, 1983.

9. Burns J.J.: Am. J. Med. *26*:740, 1959.

10. Jackson: Hosp. Pract. *15*:39, 1985.

11. Lipson, M.H., et al.: J. Clin. Invest. *66*:188, 1980.

12. Elsas L.J., Danner D.J.: Ann. N.Y. Acad. Sci. *378*:404, 1982.

13. Baumgartner, E.R., et al: Helv. Paediatr. Acta *34*:483, 1979.

14. Elsas, McCormick: *In* Vitamins and Hormones, Vol. 43. New York, Academic Press, 1987, pp. 103–144.

15. Elsas, L., McCormick: Vitamins and Hormones, Vol. 44. New York, Academic Press, In press, 1987.

15a.Belmont, Caskey: *In* Gene Transfer. (Kucherlapati, Ed.) New York, Plenum Publishing Corp., 1986.

16. Acosta, P.B.: *In* Practice of Pediatrics. (Kelly, V, Ed.) Philadelphia, J.B. Lippincott Co., 1983.

17. Chipponi, J.X., et al.: Am. J. Clin. Nutr. *35*:1112, 1982.

18. Acosta, P.B., Stepnick-Gropper, S.: J. Inherited. Metab. Dis. 9 (Suppl. 2):183, 1986.

19. Cashel, K.M., et al.: J. Hum. Nutr. *32*:264, 1978.

20. Abrams, C.A.L., et al.: JAMA. *232*:1136, 1975.

21. Coodin, F.J., et al.: Pediatrics *47*:438, 1971.

22. Seegar, W.E., Chesney: Am. J. Dis. Child. *131*:137, 1977.

23. Endres, W., et al: J. Inherited Metab. Dis. *7*:8, 1984.

24. Anderson, K., et al.: J. Inherited Metab. Dis. *9*:39, 1986.

25. Martin, S., Acosta, P.B.: J. Am. Diet. Assoc. *87*:48, 1987.

26. Krause, W., et al.: J. Clin. Invest. *75*:40, 1985.

27. Friedman, et al.: Proc. Natl. Acad. Sci. USA *70*:552, 1973.

28. Griffin, R.F., Elsas, L.J.: J. Pediatr. *86*:572, 1975.

29. Ledley, F.D., et al.: N. Engl. J. Med. *314*:1276, 1986.

30. Niederwieser, A., et al.: J. Inherited Metab. Dis. 8 (Suppl. 1):34, 1985.

31. Kaufman, S.: Raine Memorial Lecture. J. Inherited Metab. Dis. *8*(Suppl. 1):20, 1985.

31a.Curtius, et al.: J. Inherited Metab. Dis. 8 (Suppl. 1):28, 1985.

32. Dobbing, J.: The later development of the brain and its vulnerability. *In* Scientific Foundations of Paediatrics. (Davis, J.A., Dobbing, Eds.) London, Heinemann, 1981.

33. Pardridge, W.M., Choi, T.B.: Fed. Proc. *45*:2073, 1986.

34. Guthrie, R.A., Susi, A.: Pediatrics *32*:338, 1963.

35. Genetic Screening: Programs, Principles, and Research. Washington, D.C., National Academy of Sciences, 1975.

36. Fernhoff, P.M., et al.: South. Med. J. *75*:529, 1982.

37. Berry, H., et al.: Am. J. Dis. Child. *136*:111, 1982.

38. Daiger, S.P, et al.: Lancet *1*:229, 1986.

39. Jordan, M.K., et al.: Dev. Med. Child. Neurol. *27*:33, 1985.

40. Ledley, F.D., et al.: Proc. Natl. Acad. Sci. USA, in press, 1987.

41. Reichle, et al.: JAMA. *178*:939, 1961.

42. Acosta, P.B., et al.: J. Am. Diet. Assoc. *72*:164, 1978.

43. Rose: Nutr. Abstr. Rev. *27*:631, 1957.

44. Hanley, W.B., et al.: Pediatr. Res. *4*:318, 1970.

45. Acosta, P.B.: The contribution of therapy of inherited amino acid disorders to knowledge of amino acid requirements. *In* Congenital Metabolic Disease: Diagnosis and Treatment. (Wapnir, Ed.) New York, Marcel Dekker, Inc., 1985.

46. Batshaw, M.L., et al.: J. Pediatr. *99*:159, 1981.

47. Holt, L.E., Jr. et al.: Protein and Amino Acid Requirements in Early Infancy. New York, New York University Press, 1960.

48. Food and Nutrition Board. Recommended Dietary Allowances. 9th ed. Washington, D.C., National Academy of Sciences National Research Council, 1980.

49. Kindt, E., et al.: Am. J. Clin. Nutr. *37*:778, 1983.

50. Barness, L.: *In* Nelson's Textbook of Pediatrics. 12th ed. (Behrman, Vaughan, Eds.) Philadelphia, W.B. Saunders Co., 1983.

51. Douglass, J.S., et al.: Composition of Foods: Breakfast Cereals: Raw, Processed, Prepared. Agric. Handbook 8-8. Washington, D.C., U.S. Government Printing Office, 1982.

52. Gebhardt, J.E., et al.: Composition of Foods: Fruits and Juices: Raw, Processed, Prepared. Agric. Handbook 8-9. Washington, D.C., U.S. Government Printing Office, 1982.

53. Haytowitz, Matthews, R.H.: Composition of Foods: Vegetables and Vegetable Products: Raw, Processed, Prepared. Agric. Handbook 8-11. Washington, D.C., U.S. Government Printing Office, 1984.

54. Pennington, J.A.T., Church, H.N.: Bowes and Church's Food Values of Portions Commonly Used. 14th ed. New York, Harper and Row Publishers, Inc., 1985.

55. Posati, L.P.: Composition of Foods: Poultry Products: Raw, Processed, Prepared. Agric. Handbook 8-5. Washington, D.C., U.S. Government Printing Office, 1979.

56. Posati, L.P., Orr, M.L.: Composition of Foods: Dairy and Egg Products: Raw, Processed, Prepared. Agric. Handbook 8-1. Washington, D.C., U.S. Government Printing Office, 1976.

57. Mead Johnson Nutritional Division: Pediatric Products Handbook. Evansville, Mead Johnson & Co., 1986.

58. Mead Johnson Nutritional Division: Products for Dietary Management of Inborn Errors of Metabolism and Other Special Feeding Problems. Evansville, Mead Johnson & Co., 1983.

59. Polycose. Glucose Polymers. Columbus, Ohio, Ross Laboratories, 1984.

60. Scientific Department, International Division: Milupa Special Products. Friedrichsdorf/Taunus, Milupa AG, 1986.
61. Scientific Hospital Supplies, Limited: Dietitian's Checklist. Liverpool, Speirs Brakell Limited, 1985.
62. Acosta, P.B., et al.: Parents' Guide to the Child with PKU. Tallahassee, Florida State University, 1984.
63. Wannemacher, R.W.: Am. J. Clin. Nutr. 30:1269, 1977.
64. Umbarger, B., et al.: JAMA. 193:128, 1965.
65. Ingall, et al.: J. Pediatr. 65:1073A, 1964.
66. Elsas, L.J., et al.: J. Biol. Chem. 243:1846, 1968.
67. Elsas, L.J., et al.: J. Biol. Chem. 246:6452, 1971.
68. Nakagawa, I., et al.: J. Nutr. 77:61, 1962.
69. Sibinga, M.S, et al.: Dev. Med. Child. Neurol. 13:63, 1971.
70. McCaman, Robins: J. Lab. Clin. Med. 59:885, 1962.
71. Acosta, P.B., et al.: PKU—A Guide to Management. Berkeley, California State Department of Health, 1972.
72. Holm, V.A., et al.: Pediatrics 63:700, 1979.
73. Dobson, J.C., et al.: Pediatrics 60:822, 1977.
74. Acosta, P.B., et al.: Am. J. Clin. Nutr. 30:198, 1977.
75. Wong, R., et al.: J. Am. Diet. Assoc. 57:229, 1970.
76. Acosta, P.B., et al.: J. Parent. Ent. Nutr. 5:406, 1981.
77. Acosta, P.B., et al.: J. Inher. Metab. Dis. 5:107, 1982.
78. Acosta, P.B., et al.: J. Parenter. Enter. Nutr. In press, 1987.
79. Lewis, J.S., et al.: Am. J. Clin. Nutr. 26:136, 1973.
80. Lewis, J.S., et al.: Fed. Proc. 33:666A, 1974.
81. Hudson, F.P.: Arch. Dis. Child. 42:198, 1967.
82. Holtzman, N.A., et al.: N. Engl. J. Med. 293:1121, 1975.
83. Horner, F.A., et al.: N. Engl. J. Med. 266:79, 1962.
84. Seashore, M.R., et al.: Pediatrics 75:226, 1985.
85. Holtzman, N.A., et al.: N. Engl. J. Med. 314:593, 1986.
86. Krause, W., et al.: Pediatr. Res. 20:1112–1116, 1986.
87. Lenke, R.R., Levy, H.L.: N. Engl. J. Med. 303:1202, 1980.
88. Ghadimi, H., Pecora, P.: Pediatrics 33:500, 1964.
89. Okano, Y., et al.: J. Inherited Metab. Dis. 9:15, 1986.
90. Lindblad, B., et al.: Proc. Natl. Acad. Sci. USA 74:4641, 1971.
91. Sassa, S., Kappas, A.: J. Clin. Invest. 71:625, 1983.
92. Christensen, E., et al.: Clin. Chim. Acta 116:331, 1981.
93. Kvittingen, E.A., et al.: Pediatr. Res. 14:541, 1983.
94. Furukawa, N., et al.: Pediatr. Res. 18:409, 1984.
95. Goldsmith, L.A.: Tyrosinemia and related disorders. In The Metabolic Basis of Inherited Disease. 5th ed. (Stanbury, JB, et al. Eds.) New York, McGraw-Hill Co., 1983.
96. Mamunes, P., et al.: Pediatrics 57:675, 1976.
97. Gagne, R., et al.: Prenatal Diagnosis 2:185, 1982.
98. Kvittingen, E.A., et al.: Pediatr. Res. 19:334, 1985.
98a. Elsas, L.J. Personal experience.
99. Sassa, S., Granick: Proc. Natl. Acad. Sci. USA 67:517, 1970.
99a. Goetsch, C.A., Bissell, D.M.: N. Engl. J. Med. 315:235, 1986.
100. Tolbert, Watts, J.: J. Nutr. 80:111, 1963.
101. Acosta, P.B., Elsas, L.J.: Dietary Management of Inherited Metabolic Diseases: Phenylketonuria, Galactosemia, Tyrosinemia, Homocystinuria and Maple Syrup Urine Disease. Atlanta, ACELMU Publ., 1976.
102. Michals, K., et al.: J. Am. Diet. Assoc. 73:507, 1978.
103. Soirdahl, S., et al.: Pediatr. Res. 13:74, 1979.

104. Bonkowsky, H.L., et al.: Metabolism 25:405, 1976.
105. Tschudy, D.P., et al.: Metabolism 13:396, 1964.
106. Welland, F.H., et al.: Metabolism 13:232, 1964.
107. Training Manual: Microcomputers in Nutrition Support of Genetic Disease. Tallahassee, Florida State University, 1984.
108. Cohn, R.M., et al.: Am. J. Clin. Nutr. 30:209, 1977.
109. Danner, D.J., et al.: J. Clin. Invest. 75:858, 1985.
110. Litwer, S., Danner, D.J.: Biochem. Biophys. Res. Commun. 131:961, 1985.
111. Elsas, L.J., Danner, D.J.: Ann. N.Y. Acad. Sci. 378:404, 1982.
112. Danner, D.J., Elsas, L.J.: Biochem. Med. 13:7, 1975.
113. Heffelfinger, S., et al.: Am. J. Hum. Genet. 36:802, 1984.
114. Fernhoff, P.M., et al.: Pediatr. Res. 19:1011, 1985.
115. Tanaka, K., Rosenberg, L.E.: Disorders of branched chain amino acid metabolism. In The Metabolic Basis of Inherited Disease. 5th ed. (Stanbury, J.B., et al., Eds.) New York, McGraw-Hill Book Co., 1983.
116. Elsas, L.J., et al.: Metabolism 21:929, 1972.
117. Naylor, E.W., Guthrie, R.: Pediatrics 61:262, 1978.
118. Elsas, L.J., et al.: Metabolism 23:569, 1974.
119. Wendel, L.L., et al.: Eur. J. Pediatr. 138:293, 1982.
120. Clow, C.L., et al.: Pediatrics 68:856, 1981.
121. Wendel, L.L., et al.: Eur. J. Pediatr. 138:293, 1982.
122. Duran, M., Wadman, S.K.: J. Inherited Metab. Dis. 8 (Suppl. 1):70, 1985.
123. Szmelcman, S., Guggenheim, K.: Biochem. J. 100:7, 1966.
124. Hammerson, G., et al.: Monogr. Hum. Genet. 9:84, 1978.
125. DiGeorge, et al.: N. Engl. J. Med. 307:1492, 1982.
126. Snyderman, J.E., et al.: Pediatr. Res. 18:851, 1984.
127. Tanaka, K., et al.: Proc. Natl. Acad. Sci. USA 56:236, 1966.
128. Shigamatsu, Y., et al.: Pediatr. Res. 16:771, 1982.
129. Truscott, R.T.W., et al.: Clin. Chim. Acta 110:187, 1981.
130. Lehnert, W., Niederhoff, H.: Eur. J. Pediatr. 136:281, 1981.
131. Mendiola, J., et al.: Tex. Med. 80:52, 1984.
132. Wysocki, S.J., et al.: Clin. Chem. 29:1002, 1983.
133. Yoshino, M., et al.: Adv. Exp. Biol. Med. 153:141, 1982.
134. Cohn, et al.: J. Pediatr. 92:813, 1978.
135. Dubiel, et al.: J. Clin. Invest. 72:1543, 1983.
136. Ikeda, et al.: In Metabolism and Clinical Implications of Branched Chain Amino Acids and Ketoacids. (Walser, Williamson, Eds.) New York, Elsevier North Holland, Inc., 1981.
137. Blascovics, M., Donnell, G.: J. Inherited Metab. Dis. 1:9, 1978.
138. Tanaka, K., Yu: Clin. Chim. Acta 138:333, 1984.
139. Shigematsu, Y., et al.: Clin. Chim. Acta 138:333, 1984.
140. Bartlett, K., Gompertz, D.: Biochem. Med. 10:15, 1974.
141. Nandi, D.L.A., et al.: J. Biol. Chem. 254:7230, 1979.
142. Stanley, C.A., et al.: Pediatr. Res. 17:296A, 1983.
143. Roe, C.R., et al.: J. Clin. Invest. 74:2290, 1984.
144. Finkelstein, J.D., Martin J.J.: J. Biol. Chem. 259:9508, 1984.
145. Mudd, S.H., Levy, H.L.: Disorders of transsulfuration. In The Metabolic Basis of Inherited Disease. 5th ed. (Stanbury, J.B., et al. Eds.) New York, McGraw-Hill Book Co., 1983.
145a. Rosenberg, L.E.: In Advances in Human Genetics.

Vol. 6. (Harris, Hirschorn, Eds.) New York, Plenum Publishing Corp., 1976, pp. 1–69.
146. Skovby, F., et al.: Am. J. Hum. Genet. *36*:452, 1984.
147. McCusick, V.A., et al.: *In* Inherited Disorders of the Sulfur Metabolism. (Carson, N., Raine, Eds.) London, Churchill Livingstone, 1971.
148. Mudd, J.H., et al.: Am. J. Hum. Genet. *37*:1, 1985.
149. Boers, G.H.J., et al.: N. Engl. J. Med. *313*:709, 1985.
150. Fernhoff, P.M., et al.: *In* Human Nutrition: Clinical and Biochemical Aspects. (Garry, P., Ed.) Washington, D.C., American Association of Clinical Chemistry, 1980.
151. Schaumburg, et al.: N. Engl. J. Med. *309*:445, 1983.
152. Yoshida, I., et al.: J. Inherited Metab. Dis. *8*:91, 1985.
153. Wilcken, D.E.L., et al.: Metabolism *34*:1115, 1985.
154. Marcus, A.J.: N. Engl. J. Med. *309*:1515, 1983.
155. Walser, M.: Urea cycle disorders and other hereditary hyperammonemic syndromes. *In* The Metabolic Basis of Inherited Disease. 5th ed. (Stanbury, et al. Eds.) New York, McGraw-Hill Book Co., 1983.
156. Cederbaum, S., et al.: J. Pediatr. *90*:5–69, 1977.
157. Levin, et al.: Arch. Dis. Child. *44*:152, 1969.
158. Kennaway, N., et al.: Pediatr. Res. *9*:554, 1975.
159. Glick, et al.: Am. J. Hum. Genet. *28*:22, 1976.
160. Beaudet, A.: Am. J. Hum. Genet. *37*:386, 1985.
161. Su, et al.: J. Biol. Chem. *256*:11826, 1981.
162. Beaudet, A., et al.: Adv. Hum. Genet. *15*:161, 1986.
163. Horwich, et al.: Science, *224*:1068, 1984.
164. Kraus, et al.: Nucleic Acids Res. *13*:943, 1985.
165. Spector, et al.: Pediatr. Res. *17*:941, 1983.
166. Valle, D., Simell, O.: *In* The Metabolic Basis of Inherited Disease. 5th ed. (Stanbury, et al. Eds.). New York, McGraw-Hill Book Co., 1983.
167. Russell: Mt. Sinai J. Med. *40*:723, 1973.
168. Rowe, et al.: N. Engl. J. Med. *314*:541, 1986.
169. Levy, H., et al.: *In* Neonatal Screening for Inborn Errors of Metabolism. (Bickel, H., et al., Eds.) Berlin, Springer-Verlag, 1980.
170. Naylor, E.W., et al.: J. Lab. Clin. Med. *89*:987, 1977.
171. Naylor, E.W.: Pediatrics *68*:453, 1981.
172. Talbot, et al.: Pediatrics *70*:526, 1982.
173. Tada, et al.: Eur. J. Pediatr. *130*:105, 1979.
174. Rett: Wien. Med. Wochenschr. *118*:311, 1968.
175. Symposium on Disorders of the Urea Cycle: Pediatrics *68*:271, 1981.
176. Batshaw, M.L., et al.: Pediatr. Res. *13*:472, 1979.
177. Brusilow: Hosp. Pract. Oct. 15, 1985, p. 65.
178. Snyderman, S.E., et al.: Pediatrics *56*:65, 1975.
179. Bachmann, C.: Enzyme *32*:56, 1984.
180. Batshaw, M.L., et al.: Pediatrics *68*:290, 1981.
181. Msall, M., et al.: N. Engl. J. Med. *310*:1500, 1984.
182. Ad Hoc Expert Committee: Energy and Protein Requirements. Rome, Food and Agriculture Organization of the United Nations, 1973.
183. Segal, S.: Disorders of galactose metabolism. *In* The Metabolic Basis of Inherited Disease. 5th ed. (Stanbury, J.B., et al., Eds.) New York, McGraw-Hill Book Co., 1983.
184. Sparkes, et al.: Am. Hum. Genet. (London) *43*:343, 1980.
185. Sidbury: *In* Galactosemia. (Hsia, D., Ed.) Springfield, Charles C Thomas, Publishers, 1969.
186. Urbanowski, et al.: N. Engl. J. Med. *306*:84, 1982.
187. Beutler, Baluda: J. Lab. Clin. Med. *68*:137, 1966.
188. Jakobs, C., et al.: Pediatr. Res. *18*:714, 1984.
189. Gitzelman, R., Auricchio, S.: Pediatrics *36*:231, 1965.
190. Galactosemia in Infancy. Evansville, Mead Johnson, 1976.
191. Nickerson, TA: Food Tech. *32*:40, 1978.
192. Hettinga, D.H.: J. Dairy Sci. *53*:1377, 1970.
193. Gallagher, C.R.: J. Am. Diet. Assoc. *65*:418, 1974.
194. Lee, P.E., Lillibridge, C.B.: Am. J. Clin. Nutr. *29*:428, 1976.
195. Fagen, J.H.: J. Dairy Sci. *35*:779, 1952.
196. Clothier, C.M., Davidson, D.C.: Hum. Nutr. Appl. Nutr. *37A*:483, 1983.
197. Fishler, K., et al.: Pediatrics *50*:412, 1972.
198. Lee: J. Ment. Defic. Res. *16*:173, 1972.
199. Donnell, G., et al.: Pediatrics *31*:802, 1963.
200. Gitzelman, R., Steinmann, B.: Enzyme *32*:37, 1984.
201. Waisbren S.E., et al.: J. Pediatr. *102*:75, 1983.
202. Irons, M., et al.: J. Pediatr. *107*:261, 1985.
203. Fensom, et al.: Br. Med. J. *4*:386, 1974.
204. Howard, N.J., et al.: Acta Paediatr. Scand. *70*:695, 1981.
205. Komrower, G.M.: J. Inherited Metab. Dis. *5* (Suppl. 2):96, 1982.
206. Anon: Lancet *2*:1379, 1982.
207. Komrower, G.M.: Lancet *1*:190, 1983.
208. Kaufman, F.R., et al.: N. Engl. J. Med. *30*:994, 1981.
209. Kaufman, et al.: J. Inherited Metab. Dis. *9*:140, 1986.
210. Chen, Y.T., et al.: Science, *214*:1145, 1981.
211. Chen, Y.T., et al.: Pediatr. Res. *18*:345, 1984.

*Chapter* **64**

# NUTRITION AND DIET IN CANCER

Maurice E. Shils

## DIET AND NUTRITION AS MODIFYING FACTORS IN TUMOR GENESIS AND GROWTH

The major components of diet serve as the energy sources for the host and for the neoplasm it can harbor. The amino acids from the diet provide the building blocks for the proteins and peptides of normal cells and tumor cells. Minerals have structural, metabolic, and metallic coenzyme functions, and vitamins are coenzymes and regulators in many steps of intermediary metabolism in normal and malignant cells. It is no surprise, therefore, to find that experimental manipulations of diet can affect tumor development and growth. However, the complexity, variability, and unexpectedness of some of these relations and the potential for therapy impart considerable interest and importance to this subject. Attention is directed in this section to dietary influences on tumor development and growth, with brief attention to nutritional factors affecting carcinogenic action and immune responses.

## Calories and Nutrients in Spontaneous Tumor Development in Experimental Animals

**Macronutrients.** Dietary components have been manipulated to test the effects of their intake. Tannenbaum pioneered in showing the dependence of tumor formation on caloric intake in animal models.[1a,1b] In some experiments, the experimental diets were adequate in all components except for a major caloric contribution, usually carbohydrate, partially withheld from the experimental diet but present in the control diet; this approach is designated "caloric restriction." Another approach to energy deficit has involved restricting all components that are present in the control diet; this has been termed "underfeeding." In most studies of these types, the experimental animals were allowed to ingest only 50 to 70% of the intake of their fully fed controls. The development of spontaneous tumors in mice and rats was inhibited by such restriction; however, the magnitude of inhibition was influenced by tumor type, the degree of restriction, and the presence of carcinogenic agents.

Early study on spontaneous mammary tumors indicated that inclusion of fat in the diet stimulates tumor development apparently beyond the fat's caloric contribution.[1a] Boutwell et al and others demonstrated that one factor in the tumor-promoting action of fat was the more efficient use of the energy in a high-fat diet compared to an isocaloric low-fat diet.[2a,2b] In addition, saturated and polyunsaturated fats affected tumorigenesis differently, apparently because of a requirement for essential fatty acids; in rats, tumor yield increases with increasing amounts of essential fatty acids (EFA) up to a threshold of about 4% of total calories; further amounts of EFA do not increase tumor yield.[3] The differing effects of high- and low-fat diets were overcome when animals were subjected to caloric restriction.[4]

Underfeeding reduced production by the anterior pituitary gland, reducing circulating levels of prolactin, luteinizing hormone, follicle-stimulating hormone, thyrotropin, and growth hormone as compared to levels in fully fed animals.[5] Severe food restriction can increase production of ACTH and adrenocortical hormones. With endocrine-sensitive tumors, such as the spontaneous mammary tumors, the principal effect of underfeeding appears to be related to reduced estrogen and prolactin.[5]

Several long-term studies in rats confirmed the older studies and provided additional data. When a commercial diet was compared to four purified diets varying in protein (casein), carbohydrate (sucrose), or total calories administered to male rats, total tumor risk was found to be directly and exponentially related to caloric intake. Within each dietary group risk, heavier rats had greater tumor risk than lighter rats. Occurrence and malignancy of certain tumors correlated either directly or inversely with the level of protein intake. Lowest incidence, greatest delay in occurrence, absence of malignant epithelial tumors, and greatest life expectancy were observed when intakes of protein, carbohydrate, and total calories were low.[6]

When 10%, 22%, or 51% casein in isocaloric diets was fed to male rats on an ad libitum or calorie restricted basis, the highest incidence of adenomas of the anterior pituitary gland was associated with the dietary group having the highest ad libitum intake of protein. Restriction in both calories and protein depressed the incidence to the greatest extent. Among all six dietary groups, body weight of the rats in early life correlated with the tumor prevalence in later life.[6b] Short-term (7-week) restriction of food intake by rats after weaning followed by an ad libitum regimen substantially reduced long-term growth and the incidence of neoplasms, particularly of benign tumors and endocrine adenomas. Animals restricted in their food intake throughout life had appreciably lower tumor incidence (benign and malignant) than did those on the short-term restriction or those fed ad libitum.[6c]

Spontaneous lymphoproliferative disease was decreased in a certain mouse strain restricted in protein, fat, and carbohydrate.[7] Yields of spontaneous liver tumors in mice and of pituitary, mammary, and skin tumors in rats were decreased by long-term reduction (20%) in food intake.[8]

Interest in various aspects of the question of the role of energy intake on carcinogenesis has been renewed. The importance of energy intake relationships and relative contributions is particularly critical in the interpretation of epidemiologic data.[9] An entire symposium was devoted to a review of the effects of energy sources and their contributions to total energy intake and to energy expenditure in carcinogenesis.[10]

**Micronutrients.** Important exceptions exist to the preceding evidence for decreased spontaneous tumor incidence with restrictions of calories and major dietary components. Deficiencies of certain micronutrients have been associated with an increased incidence of spontaneous tumors in rats. Vitamin A deficiency has been related to the development of odontomas[11] and salivary gland tumors.[12] A cereal-based diet low in iodide has led to increased frequency of thyroid tumors and pituitary enlargement.[13] Magnesium deficiency in rats has been reported to induce an invasive thymoma.[14] Other investigators, however, have not found the resulting enlarged thymus to be invasive, although it does cause death.[15] Chronic myelogenous leukemia has also been reported in magnesium-deficient rats,[16] but independent confirmation has not been reported. Cirrhosis and hepatoma were noted to develop in rats on choline-deficient diets[17] but may have been related to the concomitant exposure to aflatoxin, the effects of which were unknown at the time of the original experiments.[18]

## FORMATION AND ACTION OF CARCINOGENS

Evidence that chemical carcinogens play a significant role in the cause of cancer in man is increasing. Hence, attention is being given to searching out any maneuver that will prevent exposure to carcinogens of susceptible cells, inhibit interaction of carcinogens and cells, or reverse such a reaction at an early phase. Such carcinogenic agents develop in the environment in many ways—through ionizing radiation, in industrial chemical processes and their end-products and effluents, in certain chemicals added to food or present as contaminants, as natural toxicants, and as products of microbial action in the intestine. The literature on actual or potential carcinogens arising from the food supply is enormous.[19-25] (Numerous original references are given in Chapters 27 and 38.)

Carcinogens can be divided into two classes based on the electrophilic hypothesis of carcinogenesis, which states that most, if not all, chemical carcinogens are metabolized to biologically reactive electrophils that exert their carcinogenic activity.[26,27] The two classes are the electrophilic and nonelectrophilic carcinogens; the latter and much smaller group includes hormones, antimetabolites, and such compounds as thioacetamide. A close relation exists between electrophilicity and mutagenesis in standard assays[27]; hence, the two classes can be described as genotoxic and nongenotoxic (epigenetic), respectively.

Electrophils, which bind DNA in target tissues, include the major categories of well-known carcinogens such as aromatic amines, polycyclic aromatic hydrocarbons, alkylated agents, and nitrosoamines. Such compounds may exist as procarcinogens, which require metabolic conversion to exert their carcinogenic activities, or as ultimate carcinogens that exist in reactive electrophilic form requiring no further metabolic change to exert their actions.

Initiation, an early and irreversible stage in the carcinogenic process, is produced by a single or very limited application of a carcinogen. Promotion is the stimulation of development from an initiated cell to a tumor. A complete carcinogen performs both functions.[27] The first precancerous changes in a cell progress through a series of qualitative and independent changes to tumor growth and development. Some dietary modifications have been shown to be capable of altering each of these stages of tumor development.[27-30]

Initiation and promotion is best illustrated by the steps by which chemical carcinogens are used to produce skin cancer.[28] Tumors are initiated by treating the skin with a carcinogen at a dose so low that tumors either will not develop or will do so only rarely during the lifetime of the treated animal. Initiation can also be accomplished by feeding or injecting any of a variety of carcinogens. The treated skin appears to contain some cells that are irreversibly altered (initiated) so that subsequent application of a second agent will elicit many tumors. The second agent, the promoter, is not an effective carcinogen when applied as an initiator.

# DIETARY AND NUTRIENT INTERACTIONS WITH CARCINOGENS

A large number of xenobiotic compounds occur in foods, particularly those of plant origin. Wattenberg pointed out that "without effective detoxication systems that rid the organism of anutrient foreign compounds, it would not be possible for species to consume herbivorous foods and survive."[29] The available detoxication systems protect not only against such dietary foreign compounds, but also against naturally occurring and synthetic toxic compounds including many drugs and toxins such as chemical carcinogens.

Certain dietary constituents—nutrients and nonnutrients (anutrients)—inhibit carcinogenesis by one of several mechanisms. The classification of Wattenberg is based on the time in the carcinogenic process during which the inhibitors are effective.[19] The categories are (1) compounds that prevent the formation of carcinogens from precursors (ascorbic acid and tocopherol have this type of action, as well as other actions); (2) compounds that prevent carcinogenic substances from reaching or reacting with critical target sites in the tissue, i.e., "blocking agents"; (3) compounds that act by suppressing the expression of neoplasia in cells previously exposed to doses of carcinogens that ordinarily would result in cancer, i.e., "suppressive agents." Some inhibitors are capable of acting at one or more times and certain compounds are differentiated into subgroups of actions within each category.[29]

Included in the blocking agent subgroups are those that inhibit the metabolic conversion of the procarcinogen to the ultimate carcinogen. The amount of conjugating enzymes can be stimulated, such as the enzyme induced by the antioxidant butylated hydroxyanisole (BHA) or by agents that increase microsomal mono-oxygenase activity, e.g., β-naphthoquinone. Such inhibitors also enhance the activity of major conjugating systems, such as glutathione (GSH)-S-transferase. The microsomal mono-oxygenase system can both activate and detoxify chemical carcinogens, depending on whether ring hydroxylation or nitrogen hydroxylation occurs.[29] Wattenberg noted that, in experimental animals, the usual reactions tend to inhibit chemical carcinogenesis; however, under certain conditions, enhancement of carcinogenicity might occur.[30]

The relationship between the type of diet with its specific dietary constituents and GSH-S-transferase activity has been studied. The enzyme activity is significantly higher in tissues of animals fed crude diets than in those fed purified diets. This high activity was produced particularly by diets containing high concentrations of cruciferous vegetables, citrus fruit oils, and green or roasted coffee beans.[29] Such crude diets or those containing added active compounds (e.g., p-methoxyphenol, 2-BHA, and coumarin) inhibited certain carcinogen-induced neoplasia in rats.[29]

Efforts to identify the chemical natures of the inducers present in natural foods disclosed that the most potent sources were vegetables of the Brassicaceae family, including brussels sprouts, cabbages, and broccoli; various indoles with inducing activity were isolated, namely indole-3 acetonitrile, indole-3 carbinol, and 3′-diindolylmethane, derived from hydrolysis of a parent compound.[31]

The activities of these drug metabolizing enzymes can be depressed by starvation, protein deficiency, fat and carbohydrate modification, and certain mineral and vitamin deficiencies.[32] Both starvation and feeding of purified diets to the animals led to total loss of the ability to hydroxylate aromatic polycyclic hydrocarbons.

Protection against a variety of chemical carcinogens has been afforded also by other inducers of microsomal enzymes; these include polycyclic hydrocarbons (which are toxic), flavones (which have little toxicity), barbiturates, and phenothiazines.[28]

The activities of microsomal oxidase enzymes in the small intestine and lung of experimental animals have been studied in relation to the effects of dietary factors. It has been suggested that the presence of these drug-metabolizing enzymes in the major portals of entry of food and air acts as an important protection against the entrance of carcinogens by these routes.[29,30]

Another form of blocking includes chemical reactions with the electrophilic ultimate carcinogen, i.e., trapping reactions by nucleophiles such as flavones[33] or methionine; these reactions are a form of detoxification. Another example of blocking is the prevention of a carcinogen's binding to DNA; when added in vitro, selenite can inhibit the binding of dimethylbenzanthracene (DMBA) to the DNA of fetal mouse cell cultures.[34] Selenium given in relatively large doses can act in vivo either as an inhibitor of initiation of mammary tumors (when given *before* and during exposure to DMBA) or as an inhibitor of promotion (when given *after* exposure for a prolonged period).[27,35] Selenium-low diets can inhibit tumor incidence but only in rats on a high-fat diet.[35]

In the 1930s, Japanese investigators observed that rats subsisting on rice developed liver cancer when given the dye DMBA. Addition of yeast or liver to the diet prevented the tumors. Riboflavin and casein together when added to the rice diet markedly reduced tumor incidence. The amelioration of cancer by these nutritional factors was observed even after the initiating effect of the dye had been operating for some time; however, once adenomatous hyperplasia of the bile ducts, cholangioma, or hepatoma was present, improvement in diet was without effect.[36] A biochemical basis for the effect of riboflavin was established by the finding that azo dye reductase (which splits DMBA) in liver requires riboflavin adenine nucleotide as a cofactor. Demethylation of DMBA by drug-metabolizing enzymes resulted in loss of carcinogenicity.[37]

The third category of inhibitors (suppressive agents) acts subsequent to exposure to carcinogens and suppresses the expression of such agents. Included in this class are nutrients such as retinoids and selenium. Other subgroups include soybean protease inhibitors[38]; inhibitors of prostaglandin synthesis such as indomethacin; a group of substances in plant materials that include benzoyl isothiocyanate (a constituent of cruciferous vegetables); and substances present in green coffee beans, cabbage, cauliflower, and orange oil—all of which inhibited mammary tumor formation following DMBA administration.[29] Part of the action of these anticarcinogens appears to be their ability to prevent the action of those tumor promoters that induced the formation of free radicals. These free radicals formed in metabolism induce single-strand breaks in DNA.[39] (The formation and quenching of free radical by selenium and vitamin E are noted in Chapters 10A and 15.) It appears that the inhibitory action of selenium on mammary carcinogenesis is not attributable to its glutathione peroxidase activity,[40] but rather to its prevention of carcinogenic action on DNA.[34]

Provision of polyunsaturated fatty acids, particularly linoleate (C18:2,ω6), enhances mammary tumorigenesis, with about 4% EFA being necessary for tumorgenesis.[41] When the EFA was in a diet containing a variety of natural foods (cereals, fish meal, and dry skim milk), the tumorgenic effect was appreciably less than when it was a purified diet containing casein and dextrose. The cyclo-oxygenase inhibitor, indomethacin, inhibited the promotional effects of linoleate-rich diet with the DMBA-induced mammary tumor model and with a transplantable DMBA-4-tumor model; this inhibition suggests strongly that the tumor promotion of the ω6 EFA is mediated, at least in part, by eicosanoids, particularly products of arachidonic acid.[42] Plant phenolic compounds in vitro inhibit both lipoxygenase and cyclo-oxygenase and are also known to prevent the induction of experimental bladder tumors.[43]

Eicosapentaenoic acid (C20:5,ω3) = (EPA) and

docosahexaenoic acid (C22:6,ω3) = (DHA) are known to inhibit arachidonic acid; thus, including ω3 fatty acids in the diet can partially decrease the overproduction of eicosanoids.[42] A number of reports have appeared indicating that relatively large amounts of commercial fish oils such as MaxEPA and menhaden oil suppress tumor development in various tumor models in mice and rats.[42]

Subcutaneous implantation of cellulose-paraffin discs impregnated with 5% 3-methylcholanthrene (which leads to virtually 100% tumor induction in susceptible strains) into mice depleted of phenylalanine-tyrosine resulted in more rapid development of tumors and death than in controls.[44] Deficiencies of isoleucine or leucine resulted in no significant differences in tumor incidence as compared to controls.

**Vitamins and Minerals.** Along with the development of experimental animal models of carcinogen-induced neoplasia in various organ systems has been active interest in the effects of excesses or deficiencies of various vitamins and minerals (particularly trace elements) on tumorigenesis.

Vitamin A has been of particular interest because of its fundamental role in epithelial cell differentiation. A basic effect of its deficiency is increased DNA synthesis and mitotic activity with resultant hyperplasia of the basal cells of epithelium. The literature provides a spectrum of tumorigenic responses involving vitamin A: vitamin A–deficient rats have been found to be more susceptible than controls to induction of colon cancer by aflatoxin $B_1$[45]; vitamin A, although initially suppressive to the effect of benzo(α)pyrene, eventually ceases to be inhibitory[46]; vitamin A status did not appreciably affect dimethylhydrazine (DMH) carcinogenesis[45]; and vitamin A deficiency appeared to protect against induction of colon cancer by N-methyl-N'-nitro-N-nitrosoguanidine.[47]

Increased susceptibility to various carcinogens has been noted in the respiratory tract[48] and bladder[49] of vitamin A–deficient rats. Vitamin A administration has been associated with inhibition of development in hamsters of carcinoma of the forestomach and cervix,[50] tracheobronchial and bronchogenic epithelium,[51] skin,[52] and breast.[38] Other investigators have obtained conflicting results.[53]

**Retinoids.** The common retinyl esters have limitations as antitumor agents in pharmacologic doses because their metabolic pathways limit availability at specific target sites (e.g., bladder epithelium) or because of their toxicity.[54] Accordingly, Sporn and associates developed synthetic analogues (included in the general term *retinoids,*

which Sporn et al. introduced) that were less toxic and had different patterns of tissue distribution, metabolism, and storage. The basic structure of the retinoid molecule has been modified to form hundreds of analogues, and certain changes can have a dramatic effect on organ distribution and activity.[54–56]

Preliminary evidence has emerged for the value of specific retinoids in preventing development and growth of specific types of epithelial cancer. Retinoic acid and certain retinoids inhibit production of skin cancer following initiation and application of the promoter 12-0-tetradecanoylphorbol-13-acetate (TPA) if the retinoid is applied within an hour or so before or after TPA.[28] This inhibitory action correlates very well with inhibition of induction of ornithine decarboxylase (ODC). On the other hand, retinoic acid can augment the tumor response to DMBA applied to mouse skin.[25] Various retinoids have been tested for their inhibitory action (chemoprevention) with a variety of carcinogens that produce cancer of the skin, mammary gland, bladder, segments of the alimentary tract, and cervix.[55,56] They have been found most effective when administered shortly after carcinogen administration, though treatment is still effective against breast and bladder cancer even after delay.[28,55]

**Carotenoids.** Since the 1981 review of Peto et al. concerning a possible anticancer role in humans of β-carotene,[57] appreciably more data have appeared. β-carotene appears to be an unusual type of lipid antioxidant in that it exhibits good free radical–trapping antioxidant behavior only at partial pressures of oxygen significantly less than that of 150 torr, the pressure of oxygen in normal air.[58] Such low-oxygen partial pressures obtain in most tissues under physiologic conditions. At higher pressures, β-carotene loses its antioxidant activity and shows an autocatalytic, pro-oxidant effect. The antioxidant effectiveness of β-carotene at low partial pressures of oxygen would complement that of vitamins E at high-oxygen concentrations.[48] β-carotene and canthaxanthin (which is not converted to vitamin A) protected hairless mice against tumor production induced by ultraviolet B irradiation and other means.[59]

**Vitamin D Metabolites.** It was noted in Chapter 13 that vitamin D metabolites induced differentiation of marrow stem cells into monocytes or macrophages and can inhibit growth of several neoplastic cell lines. $1\alpha25(OH)_2D_3$ in amounts of 0.12 to 12 nmol induced differentiation of human promyelocytic leukemia cells into mature granulocytes in vitro.[60] Calcitriol or $1\alpha25(OH)_2D_3$ increased the survival of mice inoculated with murine myeloid leukemia cells without inducing hypercalcemia.[61] Calcitriol has been reported to stimulate cancer cell replication at low "physiologic" concentrations and to inhibit replication at higher concentrations; these biphasic effects have been noted in a human breast cancer and malignant melanoma lines.[62]

**Ascorbic Acid.** The potential role of nitrosamines as carcinogenic, mutagenic, and cytotoxic agents has focused attention on the nature and sources of their precursors. Nitrite ion reacts with naturally occurring and synthetic secondary and tertiary amines to form nitroso compounds. The findings that ascorbic acid reacts very rapidly with nitrite[63] and effectively competes with amines for nitrite in vitro[64] and in vivo[65] suggested that coadministration of ascorbic acid with potentially nitrosatable drugs and nitrite-containing foods might reduce the hazards associated with ingestion of these substances.[64,67a] Ascorbic acid inhibited tumor induction in rats given nitrite with urea or amines or given N-nitroso compounds[67a,67b] and decreased the formation of nitrosoamine in food incubated in vitro under simulated gastric conditions.[68] (This subject is discussed further in considering gastric and colon cancer.)

**Zinc.** Dietary zinc deficiency increased the incidence and shortened the lag time for induction of esophageal tumors in rats given methylbenzylnitrosamine.[69] The protective roles of tocopherol and selenium have been noted above.

Examples of the opposite effect, in which increased amounts of nutrients augment carcinogens, have been noted. Addition of tryptophan or other indoles to 2-acetylaminofluorene (AAF) markedly increased the incidence of bladder tumor in rats.[70] Extra thiamin, given to rats on a grain diet containing bracken fern (which contains a thiaminase), increased the incidence of bladder tumor, though it did not affect the high incidence of intestinal tumors occurring in animals subsisting on the basic diet with AAF.[71] A single injection of streptozocin, a naturally occurring nitrosurea, when given with two injections of large doses of nicotinamide resulted in the appearance of insulin-secreting pancreatic islet cell tumors in 92% of male rats 226 to 547 days later. Streptozocin by itself caused tumors in 7% of cases; nicotinamide by itself had no effect.[72]

## EFFECTS OF DIETARY CHANGES ON ESTABLISHED TUMORS

The rationale for attempting to inhibit or to actually reverse established neoplastic growth by inducing nutritional deficiencies is based on the possibility that certain tumor cells may be more sensitive than normal cells to such depletion. An increased sensitivity may depend on quantitative or even qualitative differences in the requirement for certain nutrients, so that depletion by dietary means or the use of nutritional analogues (antimetabolites), which block metabolic pathways, will adversely affect tumor cells to a greater degree than host cells.

Caloric intake retards the establishment and growth of transplanted tumors only when the host's weight diminishes or is depressed below that of controls.[1] Similarly, protein deprivation and most other deficiencies inhibit tumor growth only when associated with poor host (carcass) growth or weight loss.[1] Zinc deficiency in rats is an exception; growth of transplanted Walker 256 tumor was significantly reduced despite only small growth differences with weight-matched controls.[73] Another report indicated a 14% weight loss of zinc-deficient tumor (mammary R3230 AC)–bearing rats compared to their nondeficient tumor-bearing controls.[74]

In magnesium deficiency, the growth of the same tumor in rats was depressed, but the host carcass was only about two thirds the weight of the nondeficient controls.[75] Variation in the proportion of dietary fat appears to have no consistent effect on transplant take and growth. When protein intakes of 0%, 18% and 30% were fed to rats for 2 weeks and Walker carcinosarcoma 256 was injected intraportally, it was noted that the greater the protein intake, the greater the number of animals demonstrating hepatic metastases and the larger the tumors present.[76] The level of protein influenced the growth of metastases rather than the "take" of tumor cells.

**Amino Acids.** When a single amino acid was omitted from the diets of rats with Walker 256 transplants, tumor growth was inhibited; however, loss of host body weight occurred as well.[77] This effect was noted for many though not all of the essential amino acids.[77] Diets restricted in phenylalanine and tyrosine inhibited the growth of transplanted S91 melanoma in mice but not of S37 sarcoma.[78] Rather similar restrictions of these amino acids had an insignificant effect on the growth of a hepatoma (BW7756) or mammary adenocarcinoma (C3HBA) in certain mouse strains.[79]

Theuer has systematically studied the effects of restriction of each essential amino acid on the growth of the transplanted BW10232 adenocarcinoma in female C57BL/J6 mice.[80] Dietary levels of tryptophan, threonine, leucine, or methionine that significantly inhibited tumor growth also depressed host weight. However, reduced dietary levels of phenylalanine, valine, or isoleucine significantly inhibited tumor weight without affecting host weight. Lysine restriction had no effect

on either weight gain or tumor growth. Phenylalanine-tyrosine deficiency resulted in more rapid
tumor growth and death in rats exposed to meth-
ylcholanthrene; (MCA) isoleucine and leucine deficiencies were not associated with any differences from controls in tumor growth.[44]

The conflicting results of phenylalanine-tyrosine and other amino acid restrictions in mice
with transplanted or induced tumors emphasize
again the fact that effective nutritional or other
manipulation with one type of tumor or carcinogen may be ineffective with another type. Attention is directed to discussion below on varying
degrees of tumor immunogenicity as one explanation of these differences.

Certain neoplastic cells in tissue culture have
been found to require L-asparagine because of a
deficiency of L-asparagine synthetase. A number
of studies have shown that the enzyme L-asparaginase (which deaminates L-asparagine to aspartic acid) has antitumor action in neoplasms of the
mouse, rat, and dog.[81] A wide variety of human
neoplasms have been treated with L-asparaginase;
at this time, acute lymphocytic leukemia appears
to be the most sensitive, with a high percentage
of remissions that were not sustained[81,82]; L-asparaginase is currently used on occasion with
other agents.

**Vitamins.** Deficiencies of folic acid,[83] pyridoxine,[84] or riboflavin[85] have each been found to result in significant inhibition of the growth of certain tumors beyond the effect of the vitamin
deficiency per se. Studies of the vitamin composition of various experimental tumors indicate
that the tumors show no specific qualitative differences from normal tissues. While a number of
tumors tend to be low in certain vitamins, values
as low or even lower are noted in some normal
tissues.

Various vitamin antimetabolites have been
tested against human neoplasms. At present, the
only clinically useful analogue is methotrexate,
which plays an important role in the treatment of
acute leukemias, metastatic choriocarcinoma, and
other malignancies. Large dosages are often given
followed by leucovorin ("citrovorum rescue") to
ameliorate damage to normal cells. Pyridoxine-
low diets, combined in some cases with 4-deoxy-
pyridoxine, had no definite antitumor effect in
patients with advanced neoplastic diseases.[86]

The inhibition by dietary means of tumorigenesis and growth involves a potentially complex
and poorly understood problem. Dietary restriction or specific deficiency leads to many changes
in the organism. For example, with endocrine-
sensitive tumors, such as spontaneous mammary
tumors, the principal growth inhibitory effect is

related to reduced estrogen or other hormone production.[5] A general phenomenon may be involved, such as that suggested by Bullough, who
postulated that growth inhibition resulting from
deficiency is secondary to a decrease in the mean
mitotic activity of the tissue.[87] When a deficiency
leads to tumor development, the converse may
occur, with increased mitotic activity of certain
cells with neoplastic potential.

## Metabolic Advantages and Influences of Malignant Cells: Response to Nutrition Support

One of the more interesting associations of tumor metabolism with nutrition concerns the ability of various experimental tumors to obtain their
energy sources and amino acids from the host,
especially in periods of deprivation.[88–90] There is
also evidence that tumors are capable of taking up
amino acids from the blood and concentrating
them to a greater extent than some other normal
tissues can. In ad libitum–fed rats with certain
transplanted tumors, the host tissues lose weight
when the tumor begins to grow rapidly; anorexia
is associated with this phase.[91] Forced feeding by
tube of such rats largely can prevent loss of host
tissue,[92,93] but with continued feeding in the absence of definitive antitumor therapy, the tumor
also grows; with no antitumor treatment, undesirable metabolic reactions occur and death ensues.[88,89]

In ad libitum studies, repletion with a complete
diet of tumor-bearing (Walker 256) animals that
were previously on a protein-depleted diet resulted in improvement in host weight, serum albumin, and the nitrogen and DNA contents of various organs, provided that the tumor burden was
less than 5% of body weight initially. Tumor
weight was double that of animals continued on
the protein-free diet, while the carcass weights of
the refed animals had increased approximately
70% over those of the protein-depleted rats.[94] In
contrast, the presence of a larger initial tumor burden (> 25% of carcass weight) significantly inhibited the ability of the host to utilize the improved diet.[94] Mice with a transplanted MCA-
induced tumor became quite anorectic (consuming 50 to 60% of initial food intake) 7 to 8 days
after the tumors became palpable. Loss of dry body
weight was due primarily to loss of lipid. Pair-
fed, nontumor bearing controls had a carcass dry
weight 16% greater and had twice as much lipid,
indicating that decreased food intake alone did
not explain all of the tissue depletion.[90]

A series of studies have reported on the effect
of intravenous feeding of small animals on host
and tumor weights and other changes following

tumor cell transplantation. Comparisons have been made of various dietary regimens including intake of an ad libitum chow diet, no food intake at all, intake of intravenous carbohydrate or amino acids as the only sources of partial calories and intake of complete total parenteral nutrition (TPN) solutions varying in their carbohydrate and fat contents.

In general, complete TPN formulas resulted in about the same or somewhat better carcass weight than did ad libitum chow diets and resulted in about the same ratio of tumor to carcass weight as did the ad libitum diet; the tumor and carcass weights were appreciably greater than in those animals that were starved or given only some carbohydrate or amino acids. Tumors studied included Morris hepatocarcinoma in ACI-N rats,[95] Walker 256 carcinosarcoma in Sprague Dawley rats,[96] and Lewis lung carcinoma in Swiss mice.[97]

Comparison of high glucose—TPN solutions with varying glucose-lipid contents and with a high-lipid TPN solution revealed no differences in these studies.[95-97] Doubling time of tumor growth was significantly less in animals given chow or casein oral diet or TPN of any glucose-lipid or high-lipid content than in the starved and semistarved animals.[95-97] These findings are in contrast to a report using rats of the Lewis-Wistar type with a nonmetastasizing transplanted mammary tumor, in which rats on the high-fat TPN maintained weight better and had a lower ratio of tumor weight to host weight than did the chow-fed controls, animals given glucose TPN, or those given mixed glucose-lipid TPN[98]; a significantly slower doubling time was noted also with the lipid TPN formula than with glucose TPN or mixed glucose-lipid TPN.[98]

The problem of overnutrition in tumor-bearing animals is emphasized by a study in which TPN was progressively increased in different groups from 33% of normal caloric intake up to 167%.[99] Host weight and tumor weight progressively increased, while protein content remained stable. Above 133%, liver fat was increased to a greater extent than in nontumor-bearing controls. At 167%, all tumor-bearing animals died (cause undetermined), whereas controls did not.

An area requiring continuing investigations concerns modifications of the composition of forced feeding formulations such as TPN. For example, a major increase in the arginine concentration of TPN solution (5.5% as against 0.66%) over an 8-day period in rats transplanted with the Yoshida sarcoma suppressed growth, prevented metastases, and enhanced phagocytosis.[100]

## Immunity and Nutritional Influences

Immune responses have important relationships to cancer. Depressed cellular immunity has been known to occur in cancer patients and, in the past, has frequently been attributed to the effects of cancer per se. However, studies done initially in children,[101] in adults,[102] and then in cancer patients[103] have shown that altered immune responses can result from malnutrition.

Undernutrition of a general or specific type can affect each aspect of the immune mechanisms of the organism (see Chap. 32). With respect to the cancer-bearing host, efforts can be made to improve immunity by improving nutritional status, by modifying concentrations of certain nutrients (i.e., lipids), or by inducing certain deficiencies in an effort to slow tumor growth sufficiently to allow immune responses to develop. Years ago, Stoerk and Emerson observed that induction of riboflavin deficiency in C3H mice at 6 to 14 days resulted in a 30 to 37% cure rate of transplanted tumors, whereas riboflavin-repleted mice all died; tumor reinoculated into "cured" mice with or without riboflavin in the diets failed to "take."[104] The authors postulated that the nutrient deficiency slowed growth sufficiently to permit immune defenses to become effective.

Worthington et al. studied the effect of restriction of dietary phenylalanine-tyrosine, isoleucine, or leucine on the immune resistance of mice to a transplanted 3-MCA-induced tumor.[105] Tumor developed rapidly, with 100% incidence in nonimmune mice on the control diet. Mice on the various deficient and control diets were immunized by inoculation of MCA tumor cells; in each case, when the tumor reached a certain size it was totally excised. Three days later, the same animals were again inoculated with tumor cells. These reinoculated animals had a much slower tumor development and lower incidence than nonimmunized controls, but the amino acid–deficient diets had neither a protective nor a deleterious influence compared to control diets with adequate amino acids.

One possible explanation for the failure of host immune defenses to destroy malignant cells is the presence of serum inhibitors ("blocking antibody"). It has been suggested that certain deficiencies could inhibit formation of blocking antibody without depressing cellular immunity.[106] Moderate reduction of the amino acids phenylalanine-cystine, isoleucine and tryptophan produced marked depression of hemagglutinin and blocking antibody responses without affecting cytotoxic cell-mediated immunity.[107] Limitation of arginine, histidine, and lysine produced only slight depression of the immune responses. Moderate restriction of leucine resulted in a paradoxical depression of cytotoxicity with little effect on serum blocking antibody.

A key issue concerns the apparent immunogenicity of tumors, either of human or animal origin. If immunogenicity is absent or minimal, nutritional influences capable of depressing or modifying immune reactions to tumor antigens will not be apparent or will be minimally effective; on the other hand, when immunogenetic response is marked, the effects of decreasing or increasing immune responses by nutritional means may be significant.

McCarrick et al. have addressed this important issue.[108] They used the fact that the C-1300 neuroblastoma (NB) derived from mice is an immunogenic tumor whereas a variant of this tumor (TBJ-NB) is nonimmunizing, is faster growing, and has a metastatic potential despite its common origin and histologic identity. Male strain A mice were randomly placed on either a complete chow diet (23.4% protein and 4.2 kcal/g) or a low-protein diet (2.5% protein, and 3.65 kcal/g). The animals were pair-fed amounts equal in caloric content. After varying periods on the diets, half of each group received an inoculation of C-1300-NB cells and the other half of each group received the TBJ-NB cells; the animals were periodically sacrificed with analyses of tumor and host characteristics.

The following results were obtained. (1) Nonimmunogenic TBJ-NB tumors grew more rapidly than C-1300-NB tumors in mice on both types of diets. (2) There were no differences in either TBJ-NB tumor size or tumor weight/carcass weight ratios in the mice on the control or the deficient diets. (3) Immunogenetic C-1300-NB tumors grew significantly better in the protein-depleted mice than they did in the well-fed mice. (4) Prior sublethal whole-body irradiation eliminated the inhibiting effect of the control diet on tumor growth in the C-1300-NB inoculated mice. It was concluded that the influence of malnutrition is most likely to be apparent with that tumor type that induces an immunologic antitumor response.

McCarrick et al. also reviewed the contradictory literature regarding the influence of nutritional repletion in experiments with various rodent tumors.[108] They pointed out that differing results in studies by various investigators using different mouse hepatomas can be explained by differences in immunogenicity of the hepatomas. They also noted that the same Walker 256 carcinosarcoma has different growth properties in different rat "strains," i.e. growth is slower in the Wistar-bred rat than in the Sprague Dawley rat, and that his-

tocompatibility difference rather than tumor antigenicity may explain differences in tumor growth in nutritional studies reported by others.

Clinical correlations of the type made by McCarrick et al. are not available because of a lack of ability to quantify human tumor immunogenicity, although, as they note, most but not all human tumors are regarded as minimally immunogenic or nonimmunogenic.[108] The entire problem of relating malnutrition to patient prognosis is complicated seriously by the contribution of tumor burden to malnutrition and its impact on metabolic functions.

What is the effect of nutritional status on immune function of the cancer-bearing host? Copeland and associates studied the effects of nutritional depletion and rehabilitation on immune competence, tumor growth, and responsiveness to antitumor therapy.[103] Their data indicate that malnutrition leads to immunosuppression, as do surgery, radiation therapy, and chemotherapy. The majority of patients who on initial testing gave a negative response to various intradermal antigens became positive (i.e., had increased cellular immunity) to skin testing following nutritional treatment with total parenteral nutrition, despite chemotherapy and surgery. Radiation therapy prevented or reversed improved immune responses. Others have also found improved immune status in cancer patients given parenteral nutrition.[109a,109b] Tumor-bearing rats with depressed cellular immunity induced by protein deficiency also responded to nutritional repletion with return of their immunity.[109c] Provision of all amino acids administered as the only source of nutrition did not reverse the depressed immunity.

Increasing clinical evidence suggests that reestablishment of cellular immunity by nutritional means, together with control of infection, plays an important role in decreasing morbidity and mortality.[110] The importance of optimum defenses against infection in the cancer patient emphasizes the need for providing adequate nutrition, completely separate from the issue of improving host resistance to tumor growth, which, as noted above, has an important relationship to tumor immunogenicity.

## EPIDEMIOLOGIC DATA ON NEOPLASIA AND DIETARY PRACTICES

From the earliest medical records to the present, physicians and laymen have postulated an association (either protective or predisposing) between diet and the development of cancer.[111] This area has proved fertile for a wide range of speculation, extending from charlatans and food faddists to epidemiologists and laboratory scientists.

Interest in this field has increased as the result of epidemiologic surveys indicating (1) marked differences in the prevalence of malignancies originating in different organ systems within a given population, (2) variations in the prevalence of malignancy in a specific organ among different populations that may or may not be geographically distant, and (3) changes in the prevalence of certain cancers associated with population migrations. Such data suggest that environmental factors are important even though they do not prove specific cause-effect relationships. The role of diet as an important environmental variable has gained increasing attention as further epidemiologic studies have associated some differences in diet composition with regional differences in prevalence of types of cancer.

Many recent general reviews of epidemiologic and experimental studies have explored the relationship among dietary and other environmental factors and cancer causation.[19–25,112–116] One of the most detailed is that of the Committee on Diet, Nutrition and Cancer of the National Research Council.[20]

Differences in the intake of a specific dietary constituent, e.g., fat or carbohydrate, among population groups must, by the nature of usual human diet composition, be associated with differences in intakes of other essential nutrients, caloric sources, and food-related factors; hence, although ascribed to a difference of a given dietary constituent, the actual changes may be and usually are complex. Such potential complexity should lead to caution and the development of more precise evidence before noncausative associations are mistakenly ascribed to "proven" etiologic factors.

Problems inherent in epidemiologic studies have been reviewed in references given above. With respect to certain human tumors, for example those arising in the gastrointestinal tract, evidence suggests that their development and clinical expression may run a course of many years. The initiating factors might not be present at the time of the survey, thereby creating uncertainty about the accuracy of retrospective data. Studies comparing migrant populations with those remaining at the point of origin would appear to permit a more objective evaluation of environmental influence, but pitfalls still persist. For example, migrants are not necessarily representative of the derivative population in a number of ways.

Nevertheless, epidemiologic studies are important, and a number of important relations have been established concerning neoplasms occurring at different sites. These studies in turn have stimulated studies in laboratory animals as well as prospective human studies, case-control studies, and the important intervention-type study. With the current poor prognosis of many human cancers, efforts to develop effective preventive measures appear most important.

## Diet and Cancer Etiologic Relations At Specific Sites

**Oral and Pharyngeal Carcinoma.** Alcohol and tobacco use are risk factors in human oral cancer.[117] The chewing of tobacco in the United States is associated with higher rates of cancer induction, as is the chewing of betel nut in countries such as India. The role of dietary factors is uncertain, with either no relation being determined[117] or with evidence that decreased intake of foods containing vitamins A and C and carotenoids is a positive risk factor after controlling for alcohol and tobacco usage.[118]

As association was noted between the occurrence of Plummer-Vinson syndrome (sideropenic anemia with epithelial lesions) and cancer of the hypopharynx in Swedish women.[119] The syndrome was believed to be secondary to iron deficiency, but vitamin deficiencies were also involved. Incidence of both the syndrome and the cancer has decreased in association with improved nutrition, improved health care, and decreasing number of pregnancies.[120]

**Esophageal Cancer.** This carcinoma has a worldwide but variable distribution. The highest rates are observed in South Central Asia (a region involving Turkey, Iran, China, and the Soviet Union) related to diets high in bread and very low in vegetables, to poor economic status, and, in some areas, possibly to opium smoking.[113,121] Aflatoxin does not appear to be involved. Other countries with a high incidence include France, India, Finland, the West Indies, and parts of Africa; it is practically unknown in the west of Africa but is very common in the eastern and southern parts.[113]

Increased use of alcohol and tobacco are major risk factors for the occurrence of esophageal cancer in certain areas (e.g., France, especially Brittany and Normandy,[122,123] and New York City[124]). The prevalence is much greater among men than among women. However, in certain areas with particularly high incidence, alcohol and tobacco appear to very weak risk factors. The poorer economic groups appear to be more affected by the malignancy. A series of surveys indicate an association with ingestion of diets low in fruits, vegetables, and dairy products.[113] In the United States, esophageal cancer, which has been considered mainly a disease of males, has been declining in whites and rising significantly in blacks of both sexes.[124a] In Japan it has been associated with the eating of wheat, dried and salted fish and pork; it has been declining since the 1970s, as has gastric cancer.[125]

A randomized double-blind intervention study in a Chinese province with a high incidence of esophageal cancer indicated that retinol (50,000 I.U.), riboflavin (200 mg), and zinc (50 mg) supplements once weekly over 13.5 months did not affect the prevalence of precancerous lesions of the esophagus.[125a]

It is apparent that the associations between some dietary factors and esophageal cancer, while present, are not specific and require more detailed investigation. It is clear that in the United States and Western Europe, efforts to control alcohol and tobacco use should have a high priority, as should efforts to improve nutrition in economically underprivileged groups.

**Gastric Cancer.** As noted by Byers and Graham,[113] the most striking feature of the distribution of gastric cancer is its strong inverse relation with industrialization (except in Japan), while within countries, an inverse relation exists between its prevalence and the socioeconomic status of affected individuals. Males tend to have much higher rates than females. Gastric cancer—50 years ago the most prevalent—is decreasing consistently in the United States (Fig. 64–1); it is now at a level at which it is not listed among the 11 major organ system sites by estimated new cases and deaths.[124a] Similar downtrends became apparent later in Europe and Japan, particularly in large city populations,[126] but their rates of gastric cancer are still five or more times that of the United States.[127]

Following migration from a high-incidence area to a low-incidence area, usually within two generations the gastric cancer rate in migrants falls to rates rather similar to the new country. Japanese males born primarily in Japan who migrated to Hawaii had an overall gastric cancer incidence of 156/100,000, while males of Japanese descent born in Hawaii had a rate of 112. White males primarily from the continental United States who migrated to Hawaii had a rate of 30.9/100,000 compared to their white counterparts born in Hawaii, who had a rate of 61.3. Japanese females had rates approximately one third of the males, and white females had rates approximately one third (Hawaiian-born) to one half (continental U.S.-born) of their male counterparts.[128] A lower gastric incidence has been noted in Eastern European immigrants to the United States, with rates remaining high in their countries of origin.[129]

A large number of case-control studies have attempted to find an association between diet and gastric cancer. Byers and Graham[113] and the National Research Council (NRC) committee[20] have reviewed these data. The former conclude, "considering all case-control and prospective studies together, it is difficult to identify any consistent pattern of foods which seems to increase risk."

**Nitrate, Nitrite, and Nitrosoamines.** Exposure to these compounds has been implicated as a causative factor in cancer, particularly gastric cancer. A current view is that neither nitrate nor nitrite are carcinogenic in themselves.[130] Any risk derives from the formation of various nitrosoamines, which in experimental laboratory animals are either active carcinogens or are converted to the active form.

Nitrate and nitrite are added to red-meat products and smoked fish to produce a reddish pink color and to inhibit outgrowth of the spores of Clostridium botulinum and the production of its toxin as well as of other pathogens. Nitrate is taken up by plants and enters the food cycle.

The NRC committee has reviewed estimates of per capita daily nitrate and nitrite intakes of the United States population and has presented its own data.[131] It estimates an intake of 75 mg/day of nitrate, with 87% coming from vegetables, 6% from fruits and juices, 2.6% from water (this can vary widely depending on source), 1.6% from cured meats, 1.6% from baked goods and cereals, 0.6% from fresh meats, and 0.2% from milk and its products. Quadrupling of intake of cured meats added 3 mg/day, while quadrupling of vegetable intake and omission of meat by vegetarians resulted in an average daily intake of 268 mg.

Average per capita intake of nitrite is much smaller with an estimate of 0.77 mg/day, with 39% derived from cured meats, 34% from baked goods and cereals, 16% from vegetables, 7.7% from fresh meats, and 1.3% each from water, fruits and juices, and milk and its products. Quadrupling the intake of cured meat would result in approximately 1.7 mg, while ingestion of a vegetarian diet would result in 0.77 mg.

Nitrogen oxides in the air may contribute significantly to the nitrate and nitrite exposure, but currently exact estimates are conjectural. Nitric oxide from the smoke from cigarettes, if inhaled and if efficiently converted to nitrate, would result in ingestion of approximately 21 mg of nitrate; low-tar cigarettes would probably contribute one half to one third as much nitric oxide.[132]

The metabolism and pharmacokinetics of nitrate and nitrite are rather complex.[133] In individuals with normal gastric acidity, approximately 5% of ingested nitrate is reduced to nitrite in the

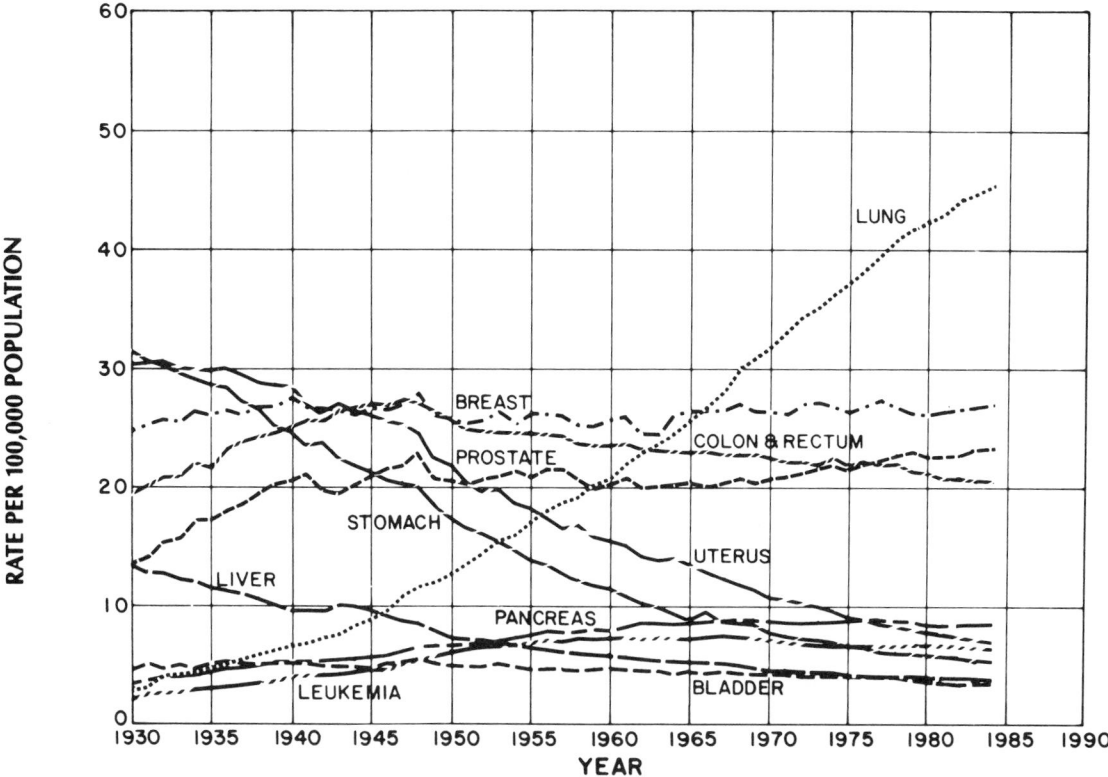

**Fig. 64–1.** Cancer death rates for 10 organ sites in the United States, 1930 to 1984. Rates are for both sexes combined, except for breast and uterus cancer (in the female population only) and for prostate cancer (in the male population). Rate for the population standardized for age on the 1970 United States population. (From Cancer Facts and Figures 1987, p. 5. New York, American Cancer Society, 1987.)

saliva (this amount varies, however, depending on the mouth flora). The nitrate and nitrite enter the stomach, where some endogenously formed nitrate enters. Normally, little or no nitrate or nitrite is absorbed in the stomach, and some nitrite may be converted to nitrate. Nitrate absorption is rapid and efficient in the upper small bowel. Absorbed nitrate travels to the salivary gland, where a proportion is secreted, the amount depending on competition with other ions. At oral doses of nitrate above a threshold (approximately 54 mg), nitrate secreted by the salivary glands is approximately 25% of that ingested; of that secreted, approximately 20% is reduced to nitrite in the saliva.

Gastric hypoacidity with pH values above pH 5 is associated with bacterial growth in the stomach, including bacteria from the oral cavity. Under such conditions and with appropriate organisms, nitrate is reduced to nitrite; this conversion can contribute an increased gastric nitrite load that can be about 90% of the total.[134] Patients with pernicious anemia have a mean nitrite concentration in their gastric juice nearly 50 times that of age-matched normal controls; this disease is as-

sociated with an increased incidence of gastric cancer.[135] Hypoacidity of gastric juice is increasingly common in older populations.[22] The chronic use of $H_2$ histamine antagonists (e.g., cimetidine) in ulcer disease raises gastric pH and has been associated with an increase in gastric bacteria.[136]

Heterotrophic bacterial nitrification was suggested to account for the apparent endogenous synthesis of nitrate and nitrite[137]; however, it is more likely that any endogenous synthesis occurs metabolically in mammalian tissues.[138]

Nitrosation usually results from reactions of compounds (e.g., nitrite) that can generate a nitrosonium ion ($NO^+$) and, less often, nitric oxide (NO). Their reactions with amines and amides may produce carcinogenic compounds including nitrosoamine and nitrosoamides. Nitrosation leading to nitrosoamine formation can occur in food prior to ingestion (as the result of food processing, cooking and preservation procedures, gamma radiation, and photolysis) or during digestion.[130,139a] Inhibitors occurring in foods naturally or in the form of additives reduce the nitrosation reactions. Ascorbic acid blocks the formation of nitrosoamines at low pH and in the absence of oxygen,[139b] and α tocopherol (unesterified) acts in a lipid setting, most effectively at low pH, reacting with nitrite.[139b] Certain phenols (e.g., propyl gallate, vanillin, tannic acid), bisulfite, and thiols such as cysteine and glutathione are also effective inhibitors.

In 1978, the U.S. Department of Agriculture published a regulation specifying the amount of nitrite that can be added to bacon (i.e., sodium nitrite at 120 mg/kg or potassium nitrite at 148 mg/kg); sodium ascorbate or erythorbate (550 mg/kg) must also be added to inhibit nitrosoamine formation.[140a] The levels of nitrite in preserved meats and fish usually decline very significantly (i.e., 90%) from processing to storage and to final preparation.[68,140b]

Exposure to these groups of compounds has been implicated as a causative agent in human cancer, particularly gastric cancer, with particular reference to the influence of N-nitroso compounds, especially nitrosoamides. This literature has been reviewed in the NRC report.[141a] It pointed out that "evidence implicating nitrate, nitrite, and N-nitroso compounds in the development of cancer is largely circumstantial." It recommended, however, that the use of nitrate salts in the curing process be discontinued in all meat and poultry products and that efforts be made to reduce its content in vegetables and drinking water.

Because nitrosoamines formed endogenously from nitrite ingested in cured meats provide only a small proportion of the total exposure of the public to nitrosoamines from all sources, and because, according to the NRC report, "the degree or protection against botulism is likely to decrease if the essential preservation uses of nitrite are substantially reduced," nitrite should continue to be used for this purpose until efficacious and safer alternatives against botulism are developed. "The speculative risk estimates made by the committee indicate that approximately 6 to 138 cases of cancer could be avoided in the United States annually if nitrite were removed from cured meats." The NRC report points out that an FDA task force estimated in 1979 that 22 deaths from botulism would result from the omission of nitrite in meat products. However, the committee did not believe that such a comparison was advisable (e.g., 22 versus 6 to 138 deaths) because these figures are rough estimates.[141b]

**Colon Cancer.** Although older vital statistics included carcinoma of the sigmoid with carcinoma of the rectum and combined nonrectal colon cancer with cancer of the small intestine, it is clear that there is site heterogeneity in the cancer frequency among populations.[142] More recent observations give specific data on occurrence in the cecum and ascending colon, transverse colon, descending colon, sigmoid colon (these sites are included in the general term "colon"), and rectum (up to 8 cm from the anus).[124a,142] Lower-risk population groups show a proportionately greater incidence of left-sided colon (rectal) cancer, and higher-risk groups show an increased incidence of cancer in the remainder of the colon. Carcinomas of the small intestine are uncommon.

When large-bowel (e.g., colon and rectal) cancers are considered together, they are second in frequency only to lung cancer and common skin cancers.[124a] Hence, major attention is paid to these cancers in terms of early diagnosis and efforts at prevention.

The overall trend in the United States is shown in Figure 64–1. In a number of countries, death rates for cancer of the large bowel have a strong negative correlation with the rate of gastric cancer and with industrialization (Japan and Finland being exceptions). Colon cancer is increasing in Japan.[143] However, in a number of countries the risk for both types is relatively low.[144] Despite the increased incidence in industrialized countries, no socioeconomic gradient has been found by intrapopulation comparisons in the United States and Western Europe. However, studies have indicated a fourfold excess risk in the upper classes in both sexes in Cali, Colombia[145] and a twofold risk in Hong Kong[146]; this excess was associated with increased intake of meat and other foods.

As with gastric cancer, the association of incidence with environment for colon cancer has been strengthened by observed changes following migration from a country of low risk to one of high risk. However, the incidence of colon cancer is the reverse of that of gastric cancer. For example, mortality from colon cancer increases progressively when comparing those Japanese born and living in Japan to those migrating to Hawaii and to those of Japanese descent born in Hawaii.[142] Similar trends have been noted in Japanese in California and in Puerto Ricans living in Puerto Rico as compared to those living in the continental United States. Contrary to the decline in gastric cancer, which does not express itself clearly until the first generation born to emigrants from the high-risk areas, the increase in large-bowel cancer is seen during the immigrant generation. This indicates a strong environmental influence expressing itself clearly in a matter of about 10 years.

The strong environmental association has led to an increasing number of epidemiologic and experimental studies of dietary and nutritional influences. Wynder[147] and others have emphasized the worldwide correlation of colon cancer incidence, fat consumption, and myocardial infarction. Others have reported positive correlations with consumption of animal protein,[148] of both animal fat and protein,[149] of meat and animal protein,[150] of meat (particularly beef),[151] and of total calories, total and saturated fat, and cholesterol but not of crude fiber or vitamin C.[152] Contrariwise, no correlation between total fat or cholesterol intake and population mortality data was found in a study in Hawaii of five ethnic groups.[152a]

Comparison of patients with colon cancer with case-control orthopedic patients indicated that at dietary extremes, a high-meat, low-vegetable diet had a risk ratio of 8 compared to a low-meat, high-vegetable diet.[153] Estimates of availability of dietary components in 38 countries in relation to male colon cancer death rates indicated a positive correlation with meat and fats, a negative correlation with dietary fiber, and no protective effect of vitamins A and C and cruciferous vegetables.[154,155]

Reports of case-control studies relative to fat intake are contradictory. Adult males in Kupio, Finland had one fourth the incidence of colon cancer of adult males in Copenhagen, Denmark, where the fat intake was the same; there were, however, specific food differences—the low-incidence group consumed more fiber and milk.[156] Fat intake was similar in a low-risk group in Kupio and high-risk group in New York, but again, food sources were different, with more meat and less dairy products and fiber consumed in New York.[157] In a case-control study, fat intake was the same in individuals with colon cancer and in their tumor-free controls, but fiber intake was reportedly higher in controls[158]; however, review of the data indicates that differences in fiber intake were not clear-cut.[159,160]

In a prospective Japanese study, no apparent relation was noted between the frequency of meat intake and colorectal cancer risk; however, in a correlational study in health centers, a strong positive correlation was found between individuals eating meat daily and mortality from colon cancer in the relevant district.[161] Colon cancer mortality was analyzed between 1911 and 1978 in two enclosed religious orders of women who ate little or no meat in adult life; mortality was not lower (nor were the deaths from breast cancer fewer) than mortality in the general English population.[162] In South Africa, the frequency of colon cancer in urban blacks is about 20% that of whites, and in Indians and "coloreds" it is about 30% of the white rate. Dietary analysis of representative noncancer subjects among these groups indicated a similar protein and fiber intake, but blacks ate

only about one half as much fat as the other three groups did. An association was found between fecal pH and colon cancer risk; namely, a more acidic pH was associated with a lower risk.[163] Colorectal cancer is much lower in Seventh-Day Adventists—who are often lacto-ovovegetarians—than in non-Adventists; Mormons also have relatively low rates, yet their meat consumption is virtually the same as the remainder of the United States population.[164,165]

Other reports on fiber raise further questions about the validity of claims for a causative relation to colon cancer. The variety of compounds (and their sources) included in the term "fiber" may be a major complicating factor. (See Chap 2*b*. For further relations of fiber to colon cancer, see Chap. 56D2.) The NRC report states in one place that the hypothesis for "a protective effect of dietary fiber" is supported[166] but in another that "the Committee found no conclusive evidence to indicate that dietary fiber (such as that present in certain fruits, vegetables, grains, and cereals) exerts a protective effect against colorectal cancer in humans."[167] A review by the Life Sciences Research Office of the Federation of American Societies for Experimental Biology noted that "numerous specific questions require additional study before a role for dietary fiber in the prevention of human colonic diverticulosis and cancer of the colon can be established."[168] In addition, it has been noted that "There is little direct evidence that increasing the intake of fibre by itself has any beneficial effect on health."[168a]

The fiber issue is further complicated by a community-based case-control study of large-bowel cancer in Adelaide, Australia. The intake of numerous nutrients as well as total energy was examined.[169] Total protein intake was the most consistent risk factor, with a two- to threefold risk for women above the baseline of case controls; in males this risk held only for old age. Total energy intake was a positive risk factor, as was total alcohol intake. Women showed a gradient of increased relative risk with increased consumption of total fat and protein at low levels of fiber consumption; however, the same increase in relative risk occurred with an increasing intake of fiber, even controlling for total energy intake.

Men showed increased risk with higher fat and protein at low consumption of fiber, but a reduced risk with increasing intake of fiber at high levels of nutrient intake. Vitamin C but not vitamin A reduced risk. Fiber from vegetables and cereal sources was considered in separate analyses. There appeared to be little relationship between consumption of both kinds of fiber and risk of colon cancer in males and little difference between colon and rectal cancer. For females, cereal fiber was associated with increased risk depending on the amount consumed; the increased risk was explained largely by its strong positive association with risk of distal colon cancer (transverse colon to sigmoid).

The NRC report concluded that "of all the dietary components it studied, the combined epidemiological and experimental evidence is most suggestive for a causal relation between fat intake and the occurrence of cancer."[170]

Many studies have been done on the relationship between serum cholesterol levels and colon cancer. In the majority of studies an inverse relation was observed.[171a–d] For example, in the Framingham Study, a cholesterol level of 190 mg/dl was suggested as a threshold below which there were elevated cancer risks.[171a] On the other hand, another study found no difference from case controls in the mean serum cholesterol levels for patients for all colon cancers, right-sided, left-sided, or rectal.[171b] Still others have found a positive association between serum cholesterol level (obtained some time prior to the diagnosis of cancer) and the risk of rectal cancer for men; when cholesterol and beta-lipoprotein levels were taken together, the association for colon and rectal cancer was significant for men but not for women.[171c] Similarly, men and women found to have colorectal adenomas (believed to be precursors of colon cancer), but no actual cancer, had significantly elevated serum cholesterol levels compared to those found to be free of adenomas.[171d]

At present, no substantiated objective evidence links colon cancer to exposure to nitrate and nitrite.[172] The speculative assumptions of 6 to 138 cancer deaths per year that may occur in the United States population as a result of consumption of nitrite in meat products have been mentioned above.

Various hypotheses have been advanced in efforts to explain possible dietary influences in terms of causative mechanisms. One is the "fiber" theory. As originally proposed, this theory postulated that a high-fiber diet results in a more rapid transit of food and other substances through the intestines and that the decreased transit time minimized opportunities for gut bacteria to produce carcinogens and also reduced the chance for carcinogen–mucosal cell interaction; therefore, populations living primarily on foods of legume and cereal origin with a relatively high-fiber content should have a low incidence of colon cancer, while those ingesting foods that have a high content of refined or nonvegetable-derived foods should have a high incidence.[173,174]

How do the postulates of the fiber hypothesis hold up in epidemiologic investigation? A western type of diet often includes a significant amount of fiber from vegetables and fruits. Although the origins of fiber are different, the amounts are not necessarily less than in a diet high in cereals and legumes. Japanese immigrants in Hawaii who changed to a western diet actually increased their total fiber intake.[175] Contrary to the early claims for decreased transit time with increased fiber intake,[173,174] other studies have noted variable changes depending on previous transit times of individuals[176]; still others have found no effect,[177] a decrease in transit time, or no change, depending on methodology used.[178]

The transit time hypothesis is also challenged by studies that noted that Hawaiian-Japanese (both Issei and nisei) had bowel transit times that were shorter than those of whites of the same age[175] and similar to Japanese in Japan, although colon cancer rates of the two Japanese populations are different.[180] There was no difference in mouth to anus transit time of food between population samples in Denmark and Finland despite a fourfold variation in colon cancer incidence.[181]

An alternative hypothesis attempting to relate diet patterns to colon cancer was based on two postulates concerning western types of diets (as compared to nonwestern types): western diets increased bile secretion, and they induced a pattern of colonic flora characterized by increased anaerobes and the presence of certain strains of Clostridia capable of dehydrogenating bile acids into actual or potential carcinogens.[182a,182b] This hypothesis has led to major epidemiologic and research efforts in a number of directions, including research into the influences of dietary differences and alterations on fecal flora patterns, bile acid metabolism, bacterial enzyme reactions, and fecal mutagens, and into the effects of carcinogens and dietary factors on colonic mucosa. (See Chaps. 27 and 56D1.) The area is one of continuing research. A recent postulate is that the ratio of lithocholic acid to deoxycholic acid in fecal extracts may be an important marker for colorectal cancer.[183]

Certain nutrients, fiber, alcohol, hormonal factors, and stool characteristics have been suggested as factors possibly contributing to colon cancer. The complexity of the situation is exemplified in the comments of Potter and McMichael, who emphasize the need for a multifactorial hypothesis.[169]

Intervention studies have been initiated in which the influence of dietary changes (including fat restriction) on biomarkers of increased susceptibility to colonic cancer and on polyp formation[184] are under investigation in human subjects.

Another intervention approach relates to a possible protective effect of dietary calcium. Oral calcium was found to reduce the proliferative effects of bile acids and fatty acids on rodent colonic mucosa.[185,186] It was suggested that the adverse effects of dietary fat in human colonic epithelium might be modified by increased calcium intake.[187] Calcium carbonate (1.25 g orally/day) was reported to reduce the proliferative epithelium of colonic crypts of subjects at high risk for familial colonic cancer, with the result that the mucosa "approached that previously observed in subjects at low risk for colonic cancer."[188] This preliminary study did not involve a double-blind controlled study, and its relation to prevention of colon cancer is not established at this time.

Of interest is the fact that increased calcium can cause a rapid terminal differentiation with formation of cornified cells and cell death in monolayers of mouse epidermal cells.[189] The role of calcitriol in cell differentiation has been mentioned above. Of possible relevance is the finding that increased extracellular calcium can block the growth-inhibitory effect of calcitriol[190a] and also modulate the hormone's effect in promoting cellular differentiation.[190b]

**Hormone-Dependent Cancers.** These include malignant lesions of the breast, endometrium, ovary, prostate, and thyroid. The relation of cancer of the thyroid to iodide deficiency is well established and will not be discussed here.

**Breast Cancer.** As with large-bowel cancer, breast cancer is more prevalent in industrialized countries (an exception being Japan). A shift in breast cancer incidence to the pattern of the host country has been shown for emigrants from various countries with relatively low rates, e.g., for Poles immigrating to the United States[191] and Australia[192] and for Japanese residing in the United States.[193,194] The trends are the reverse of the trends for gastric cancer and similar to the trends for colon cancer, in that the increases manifest themselves in the generation born after the immigration, suggesting that environmental effects play a key role. In the case of breast cancer, physiologic factors include the time of puberty and breast development. There is increasing evidence of the importance of puberty in influencing the risk of breast cancer.[195] Risk factors also include the family history of the disease, early menarche, nulliparity, and first child after age 30. Alcohol consumption has been repeatedly documented as a risk factor.[196]

A positive correlation between fat consumption and breast cancer mortality has been found in epidemiologic surveys.[197–201] Analyses of the diets of the five main ethnic groups in Hawaii indicated that the intake of total fat had a good correlation with the ethnic-specific incidence rates of breast cancer in Hawaii.[152a] A prospective study in Japan found that women who ate meat daily had higher breast cancer rates than those who did not, but this effect was noted only in women 55 years and older.[161] Case-control study results vary: a very slightly lower fat intake by *controls* as compared to cases has been noted (69 vs 73 g/day)[202]; a greater fat intake by cases than by controls was noted[203]; and no difference in frequency of meat or fat intake in cases but a slight decrease in green vegetable consumption compared to controls was noted in another study.[204] There was no statistical significance between cases and controls in Japanese women in Japan,[205] nor in Japanese women or white women in Hawaii.[205a]

Ingram reported that, beginning with the onset of World War II, a marked reduction in breast cancer mortality in England and Wales coincided with a major decrease in the intake of sugar, meat, and fat and an increase in consumption of cereals and fruits and vegetables.[206a] However, reexamination of that mortality data by others revealed that the apparent sudden decrease in breast cancer mortality was an artifact of a change in the method of selecting cause of death.[206b]

In a prospective four-year study involving almost 90,000 nurses initially 34 to 59 years of age with no previous history of cancer, there was no evidence that fat intake within the limits involved (which varied from about 32% to about 44% of total calories) was related to breast cancer development.[207] As the authors note, a reduction in fat of approximately 25% had no detectable influence; this reduction brought the fat down to approximately 30% of total calories, the level recommended by the NRC Committee on Diet, Nutrition and Cancer[20] and the National Cancer Institute (NCI).[208a] This level is significantly higher than the goal of the preventive dietary trials of the NCI, which is a long-term reduction to 20% of total calories as fat,[208b] and is higher still than the 15% goal in an adjuvant study of the NCI.[208c]

Seventh-Day Adventist women, who have a very slightly lower incidence of breast cancer than women in other population groups, have a lower mortality rate. This lower rate has been explained by earlier diagnosis; when differences in stage-at-diagnosis were accounted for, mortality figures of both Adventist vegetarians and nonvegetarians were not significantly different.[209]

Up to the time of menopause, age-specific mortality rates for female breast cancer in United States and Japanese women are fairly comparable with some comparative slowing in postmenopausal Japanese women. The two populations show marked differences in intakes of animal protein, fat, and carbohydrates.[195] Stage-specific analyses of breast cancer incidence by age among Japanese and white women in Hawaii between 1960 and 1979 indicated that postmenopausal breast cancer in the Japanese had slower average growth rates, which may explain Japanese women's better survival.[210]

Studies in two Dutch cities and Aichi prefecture, Japan among women 45 to 50 years and older with breast cancer suggest that approximately 50% of the difference in incidence are attributable to differences in body weight and height (i.e., body size).[211] Similar differences for postmenopausal women hold when cancer incidence is plotted against surface area. Overweight (excessive weight for a given height) was not deemed a risk factor. The rise in breast cancer incidence noted in Japanese-Americans in the United States can be explained by associated increasing body weight and height following migration.[212] However, other data indicate that significant overweight is a risk factor.[213a-c] For example, a large prospective study by the American Cancer Society associates women overweight by more than 40%, as compared to women of normal weight, with higher mortality for breast cancer as well as for cancers of the ovary, endometrium, gallbladder, and cervix.[213a] Several case-control studies have indicated that obesity is a risk factor for breast cancer, especially after menopause.[214-216] This increased risk may be related to adipose production of estrone.

Although a woman's family and reproductive histories with respect to breast cancer are established risk factors,[124a,207,207b] a definite positive relationship to fat intake remains to be demonstrated unequivocally in view of mounting negative data.

**Endometrial, Ovarian, and Prostate Cancers.** In international and national studies, these malignancies, like those of the breast and colon, are associated with industrialization (except in Japan), higher socioeconomic status, and high per capita intake of fat. An association has been noted between serious obesity and endometrial cancer.[213a,217,218] Though several case-control studies do not appear to relate ovarian carcinoma to obesity,[219,220] an association has been found in the American Cancer Society survey.[213a] A case-control study in white women found that the cancer patients ate foods higher in animal fat but consumed less vegetable fat; there were no differences in their coffee, alcohol, and tobacco use.[221]

Prostate cancer rates are low in Japan and increase after immigration into the United States. Several case-control studies have indicated that patients with cancer consumed more fat, protein, and vitamin A.[113] The level of consumption of green and yellow vegetables in Japan was inversely correlated with risk in one study[222]; in another study in Hawaii, no relation was detected with respect to total vitamin or ascorbic acid in men less than 70 years and a weak positive association was found for ones above 70.[222a]

Analyses of dietary histories of controls and of patients with ovarian cancer and endometrial cancer indicated that consumption of vegetables was slightly lower in the patients. The serum selenium levels in samples obtained over a 5-year period in 111 subjects prior to the development of cancer were compared with levels from controls that did not develop cancer. The risk of cancer for those in the lowest quintile of serum selenium was twice that of subjects in the highest quintile, and the association with low serum selenium levels was highest for gastrointestinal and prostate cancers.[223] While the selenium levels of patients with gastrointestinal and prostate cancer was significantly different from the selenium levels of controls, the difference in concentration was slight (6 ng/ml or 5%), and only the lowest quintile had increased cancer risk. No quantitative data are given on the distribution of serum selenium values in this group of cancer patients, which had a mean of 0.10 μg/ml. The mean ± SEM of 0.129 ± 0.002 μg/ml of all of the cancer subjects appears to be within the accepted normal range for the United States population. Relative risk was increased with lower vitamin A and E serum values.[223]

**Primary Liver Cancer.** Primary hepatocellular carcinoma (PHC or hepatoma) is one of the ten most common cancers in the world (at least 250,000 new cases occur yearly) and one of the most prevalent in developing countries.[224,225] It is common in Southeast Asia, the Western Pacific, and Sub-Saharan Africa. In many areas it is the most frequent malignancy in the male population, the case rate being approximately 500 times that observed in the United States in the 24- to 34-year age group.[226] Its case fatality rate approaches 100%.

It was noted more than 40 years ago that PHC usually occurred in livers that were affected with cirrhosis. PHC was associated with cirrhosis of the postnecrotic type, and hence with viral hepatitis (specifically hepatitis B virus [HBV]). The linkage between HBV and postnecrotic liver cirrhosis has been greatly strengthened by many relevant findings.[225] Strategies under active consideration include primary prevention with safe and effective vaccines, and injection of hepatitis B immune globulin into children born of carrier mothers within 48 hours of birth. The magnitude of the task is indicated by the estimate that there are 200 million HBV carriers in the world, a large proportion of which are infectious.

In developed countries, PHC occurs most commonly in patients with cirrhosis that is often associated with alcoholism; association exists also with both hemachromatosis and α-antitrypsin deficiency.[225] However, some studies in the United States do not support the association with alcohol.[226a]

In areas of high incidence of PHC, a correlation has been found between estimated intake of aflatoxin $B_1$, which is a potent hepatoxic carcinogenic compound in many species (see Chap. 38), and incidence of PHC.[227] Aflatoxins can be ingested as metabolites of Aspergillus flavus and closely related fungi in contaminated foods.[228] Because of the strong association of PHC with HBV, however, it is more likely that aflatoxin, if it is a causative factor at all, acts as a cocarcinogen with HBV.[225]

**Pancreatic Cancer.** Increased incidence and mortality from pancreatic cancer in individuals with diabetes mellitus has been noted in case-control cohort and correlated studies, especially in women.[229–231] However, the evidence associating this malignancy with dietary factors is limited and conflicting. Increased mortality has been associated with higher intake of sources of animal protein, fat, sugar, and coffee,[150,230,232] while incidence correlates only with increased intake of eggs.[150] Increased risk with intake of meat has been noted in cohort[233] and case-control studies[234a,234b] but only with grilled or fried meat in another study.[235] In case-control studies, increased risk has been associated with decreased vegetable intake,[234a,234b] especially intake of carrots and citrus fruits,[235] and with increased intake of margarine (but *not* butter)[235] and of white bread.[234b] The association with alcohol ingestion is contradictory, with reports of no correlation in case-control studies[230,235,236]; a negative correlation with wine[234b]; a positive correlation with beer but not with total alcohol intake in ethnic groups in Hawaii[237]; a correlation with total alcohol in a United States counties survey,[238] and a correlation with wine intake in female patients but not in males, as compared to controls.[239] Similarly, the relation to coffee intake was variable, with no relation noted,[234b,235] with increased risk only with decaffeinated coffee,[236] or increased risk with coffee generally.[236]

**Lung Cancer.** Lung cancer is now the most prevalent malignancy in the United States (other than skin cancers), with cigarette smoking as a major risk factor in the most common type (squamous cell). Because many smokers do not develop lung cancer and because not all cases and types of lung cancer are explained by smoking, other factors besides smoking and occupational carcinogen exposure have been explored as contributory or cofactors. Many studies on types of food intake and serum nutrient levels have been reported. Interpretation of data has been confused by the indiscriminate use of the term "vitamin A" in extrapolating from diet histories; both retinol and carotenoids are included in food composition tables as sources of vitamin A and some investigators failed to distinguish sources of vitamin A. An early study reported an inverse relation between risk of lung cancer and increasing "vitamin A" intake, although vitamin A intake was not measured per se.[240] It is apparent that populations subsisting primarily on cereals and vegetables with little or no animal fats or fortified margarine are ingesting little preformed vitamin A; in such populations, those individuals ingesting increased amounts of green or yellow vegetables or certain fruits are ingesting more carotenoids and not more vitamin A.

Studies for the period 1976 to 1983 uniformly reporting protection against cancer by increased intake of green-yellow vegetables, dark green leafy vegetables, and vitamin A intake have been reviewed elsewhere[20,113]; of 22 case-control studies using food frequency questionnaires, 18 reported that a high intake of vegetables and fruits (i.e., foods rich in carotene) was associated with a decreased risk of epithelial cancers in different sites.[241] In some studies of smokers in which intake of preformed vitamin A was differentiated from intake of carotene, it was apparent that carotene was the protective nutrient.[242,243]

Levels of certain nutrients have been determined in sera collected from various populations and then frozen, with chemical analyses performed later; when the data were reviewed seeking relationship to the subsequent occurrence of lung cancer, the results were contradictory. Three reports with data on small numbers of individuals noted lower levels of retinol[244]; on the other hand, 7 reports into 1986 indicated a lack of association between serum retinol levels before the diagnosis of lung cancer and lung cancer's later development.[241]

Serum β-carotene has been inversely related to the incidence of lung cancer in Hawaii,[245] Switzerland,[246] and Washington County, Maryland,[244] while one study noted no association with cancer of the lung or other sites.[247] A strong inverse relation with β-carotene was noted for the risk of squamous cell carcinoma.[244] The same study noted that mean serum vitamin E levels were lower than controls with all histologic types of lung cancer. A similar study found no association with vitamin E.[247] A positive association was noted with serum selenium,[244] in contrast to a report of no association.[223,248,249] Even if β-carotene supplements significantly reduced lung cancer deaths, the risk imposed by cigarettes would continue to be very high.[241] Nevertheless, intervention trials with β-carotene are indicated and are underway.

### Summary

In this brief overview of studies of diet and nutrition associations with cancer, the approach has been through a site-specific review considering energy and nutrients that had been given most attention in the past. The NRC committee has presented a detailed review by specific nutrients, as well as by site.[20] A summary of recent, ongoing, and projected cancer prevention trials using various nutrients has been published.[208b]

The difficulties in getting consistent, semiquantitative data by dietary histories of various types has been reviewed in Chapter 47; many epidemiologic studies have obtained less than adequate data. Byers and Graham made the interesting statement: "In our study of cancer in western New York in which we have been collecting during the last 5 years data from cases and neighborhood-matched controls regarding diet, we have expanded our dietary interviews from what was a 15-minute interview 20 years ago to a 2- to 3-hour interview which covers a wide variety of dietary items, including means of preparation and usual serving size."[113] This greater detail in diet-history taking will provide more quantitatve data on the intakes and amounts of specific foods. It will not solve questions about the accuracy of patient recall, the degree of patient variability of intake over the years, and the significant differences between actual intake of nutrients and non-nutrients in foods and the mean values of these items as listed in food tables.

The need for quantitative data of specific nutrient intakes of individuals who develop cancer compared to those who do not is a critical issue. How much (if any) of a particular nutrient is needed to protect against cancer development? Are the optimum or desirable protective amounts (if any) of a specific nutrient below, at, or above the RDA?

As a final point, I find *less* consensus now than in the past on the effect of specific foods and nutrients as specific etiologic or protective factors in cancer development in man; this disagreement results from the increasing number of conflicting reports and the realization that new and unre-

solved issues can be answered only by long-term research on human subjects.

Specific health claims made on containers of specific foods (even with the imprimatur of the National Cancer Institute thereon) are not helpful in improving public understanding of complex and unresolved health issues. Legitimating such claims weakens the Food and Drug and Cosmetic Act and key regulatory functions of the FDA designed to protect the public.[250a–c]

## NUTRITIONAL EFFECTS OF CANCER

A number of effects of cancer—either systemic or localized cancer—and of various antitumor treatments can have adverse effects on the nutritional status of the affected patient. In order for the physician to develop a rational program designed to either maintain good nutritional status or renourish the undernourished cancer patient, he must understand the underlying pathophysiologic factors. After delineation of these factors, a specific dietary regimen can then be prepared by the dietitian.

### Systemic Effects

Even though a cancer may still be localized, it may exert systemic (i.e., generalized) effects in the patient. As the tumor grows and metastasizes, these influences often become more obvious. This section reviews some of these effects (Table 64–1).

**Anorexia.** Loss of appetite can occur in a variety of situations and may be caused by intestinal obstruction, surgical intervention, sepsis, abdominal radiation, or certain drugs. In this section, anorexia is considered a systemic effect of the malignancy per se. As voluntary food intake is progressively depressed below the level necessary to meet energy and various nutritional needs, negative balances develop. When persistent and severe, the anorexia, possibly in association with other poorly understood metabolic influences, can eventually lead to cancer cachexia, or severe undernutrition and wasting of body tissues.

Although anorexia is not unique to cancer, its high incidence in certain types and its severity and persistence in a significant number of patients make it a matter of special concern. It is manifested most noticeably in patients with cancer in one or more areas of the alimentary tract, especially the liver, stomach, and pancreas and in many patients with widely disseminated tumors. As stated, it is not present with all types of tumors under certain conditions. For example, women with breast cancer are usually not anorectic, even though there may be major bone involvement, but anorexia occurs in such women when the liver becomes involved. Its onset may be insidious and

**Table 64–1.  Nutritional Problems Associated with the Presence of Neoplastic Disease**

1. Anorexia with progressive weight loss and undernutrition
2. Taste changes causing depressed or altered food intake
3. Alterations in protein, carbohydrate, and fat metabolism
4. Hypermetabolism in a variable number of patients
5. Impaired food intake and malnutrition secondary to bowel obstruction at any level
6. Malabsorption associated with:
   A. Deficiency or inactivation of pancreatic enzymes
   B. Deficiency or inactivation of bile salts
   C. Failure of food to mix with digestive enzymes (e.g., enzyme dilution; pancreaticocibal asynchrony)
   D. Fistulous bypass of small bowel
   E. Infiltration of small-bowel or lymphatics and mesentery by malignant cells
   F. Blind loop syndrome occurring with depressed gastric secretion or partial upper small-bowel obstruction leading to bacterial overgrowth
   G. Malnutrition-induced villous hypoplasia
7. Protein-losing enteropathy with various malignancies
8. Hormonal abnormalities induced by tumors
   A. Hypercalcemia induced by increased serum calcitriol and other hormones or by osteoclastic processes
   B. Osteomalacia with hypophosphatemia often associated with depressed serum calcitriol
   C. Hypoglycemia of insulin-secreting tumors
   D. Hyperglycemia, e.g., with islet glucagonoma or somatostatinoma
9. Anemia of chronic blood loss
10. Electrolyte and fluid problems with:
    A. Persistent vomiting with intestinal obstruction or intracranial tumors
    B. Intestinal fluid losses through fistulas or diarrhea
    C. Intestinal secretory abnormalities with hormone-secreting tumors (e.g., carcinoid syndrome, Zollinger-Ellison syndrome [gastrinoma], Verner-Morrison syndrome, increased calcitonin, villous adenoma)
    D. Inappropriate antidiuretic hormone secretion associated with certain tumors (e.g., lung carcinomas)
    E. Hyperadrenalism with tumors producing corticotropin or corticosteroid
11. Miscellaneous organ dysfunction with nutritional implications, e.g., intractable gastric ulcers with gastrinomas, Fanconi's syndrome with light-chain disease, coma with brain tumors

unaccompanied by manifestations of disease other than progressive weight loss. It is a dictum of medicine that the patient with an unexplained weight loss should undergo a search for a neoplasm. The initial medical evaluation usually reveals the cause.[250d]

The anorexia of malignancy appears to be a general phenomenon that is exhibited by a number of other tumor-bearing species; as in humans, it is not necessarily induced by all tumor types.

A comparison of two tumor types transplanted to rats is instructive. A Leydig cell–derived tumor (LTW) caused early anorexia and failure of growth in transplanted young rats, whereas a breast carcinosarcoma was not associated with significant anorexia; tumor and host grew almost until death.[91] In parabiosis studies, rats bearing one of these two tumors were attached to nontumor-bearing rats, with attached sham-operated rats serving as controls. After a suitable feeding and growth period, the host and tumor weights were determined in the tumor-bearing paired animals as were the weights of the paired animals with no tumors. Neither the breast cancer–bearing animals nor their parabiotic pairs lost any weight in comparison to the sham-operated rats. In contrast, the Leydig cell tumor–bearing rats lost weight (as expected), but so did their parabiotic nontumor-bearing pairs. In parabiosis experiments a small but persistent exchange of blood occurs across the pairs. This study suggested that a substance or substances derived from anorexia-inducing tumors can pass through the bloodstream to induce anorexia and weight loss in nontumor-bearing parabiotic paired rats.

A large number of substances including naturally occurring hormones act peripherally, centrally, or by both mechanisms to depress food intake in laboratory animals and man[251] (see Chap. 30). Efforts have been made to study the possible influence of certain hormones on the anorexia occurring with certain transplanted tumors. Chance et al. noted that such rats had elevated levels of unbound tryptophan in plasma, whereas brain tryptophan and serotonin levels were significantly increased[252a]; nevertheless, depletion of brain serotonin by the injection of several antiserotonin drugs did not modify the anorectic response to the Walker 256 tumor despite significant reductions of brain serotonin and hydroxyindoleacetic acid.[252b] Immunoreactive cholecystokinin in parts of the brain was reduced during MCA sarcoma–induced anorexia[253a]; however, cholecystokinin administration at various intraperitoneal dosages was not more effective in inducing hypophagia in rats with several types of tumors than it was in nontumor bearing rats.[253b]

The history of administration of insulin to non-diabetic malnourished individuals to overcome anorexia extends back to the time that insulin first became available commercially. Morrison studied the response to protamine zinc insulin injected once daily for 4 days in two different strains of rats, each with a different transplanted tumor that induced anorexia and cachexia.[254a] Insulin treatment increased the food intake 2 to 3 times that of tumor-free controls and was not associated with tumor growth acceleration. Intake was related to the amount of insulin given; blood sugar levels were not measured.

Rats with a nonmetastasizing sarcoma that induced anorexia and death were given 2 units of long-acting insulin/100 g of body weight.[254b] When insulin was given from the time that the tumors were palpable, the carcass weights of the treated animals were significantly greater than those of the untreated tumor-bearing controls; though the tumors were not larger, survival times were slightly reduced with the insulin. Those rats given insulin in the late cachectic period also had increased food intake and weight gain and no increased survival.

Administration of 2 units of insulin produced marked hypoglycemia and elevated insulin levels at 6 hours when measured in tumor-bearing rats and their controls. Others have found that with the same tumor and rat strain, 2 units of NPH insulin/100 g once daily increased food intake by the tumor-bearing animals, but only for 6 days; appetite decreased and insulin-treated rats died for unknown reasons despite continuing insulin and hypoglycemia.[254c] Carcass weight of the insulin-treated tumor-bearing animals increased and tumor weight decreased as compared to tumor-bearing controls but the differences were not statistically significant.

If these experiences with rats are applicable to anorectic cancer patients, insulin therapy is not an effective agent against anorexia, partly because hypoglycemia appears to be insulin's mechanism of action, but primarily because it does not extend survival.

Anorexia developed in Walker (256) tumor-bearing rats that were previously made hyperphagic by lesions in the ventromedial hypothalamus, thus indicating that tumor anorexia is not mediated by this mechanism.[255]

**Taste Changes.** In addition to inhibition of food intake resulting from substances that are derived from tumors directly or indirectly, other factors must be considered. One of these is altered taste that makes previously tolerated food unacceptable in whole or part. Many patients ascribe diminished appetite to taste changes. The anatomy and

physiology of taste and smell are complex and the number of drugs affecting these senses is large.[256,257] Hormonal changes including those of opioids are involved.

Excluding drug effects and antitumor treatments, researchers have attempted to determine the prevalence and types of taste alterations in cancer patients. Most studies have used the method of detecting the lowest perceptible solution concentration of sodium chloride (for salt), hydrochloric or citric acid (for sour), urea (for bitter), and sucrose (for sweet). This method has been criticized and forced-choice methods recommended to eliminate some response biases[258]; these methods are more time-consuming, however.

An early paper in this field noted that 25 of 50 patients with metastatic carcinoma of various primary sites had altered (less pleasurable) taste of food.[259] This change was associated with an elevated taste threshold for sweetness (i.e., food tasted less sweet) and a lowered taste threshold for bitterness. The likelihood of a taste abnormality's being present increased with the increasing extent of disease but not with histologic type of neoplasm. Subsequent papers have challenged the concept of a consistent pattern of altered taste. No threshold taste differences were noted between matched controls and patients with esophageal cancer[260]; others have found a higher threshold for sour (p = 0.05) and sweet (p > 0.05)[261]; a higher threshold for salt in breast cancer patents; a higher threshold for sweet in colon cancer patients[262]; or a higher threshold for bitter in various malignancies.[263]

Responses of patients with upper gastrointestinal cancers to five suprathreshold concentrations of the four basic tastes were graded on the basis of the range of intensity and hedonic reactions.[264] Intensity scores indicated no abnormalities of taste perception among patients on the basis of tumor site, type of therapy, or appetite. Hedonic reactions differed among individuals and groups. Patients on chemotherapy were less likely to express a preference for any of the sucrose concentrations; anorectic patients were most likely to prefer lower sweetness levels than nonanorectic patients, but they did ingest a greater percentage of sweet foods. Of a total of 133 patients with a large variety of malignancies, 77 (59%) reported that they had no food aversions (defined as two or more specific foods or a group of foods that became unpleasant since they learned of their cancer diagnosis).[265] Weight loss and anorexia or early satiety was reported by more patients with reported food aversion than without food aversion.

The findings on taste are inconsistent or variable both within patient groups and among reports. It behooves physicians and dietitians to ascertain the preferences and dislikes of their individual patients and develop a diet pattern based on their responses. Alterations in taste appear to be factors in anorexia that are associated with more fundamental metabolic changes initiated by tumors and influenced to some extent by psychosomatic factors.

**Learned Food Aversion.** Psychologic factors undoubtedly play a role in appetite. The fear and uncertainty engendered by the diagnosis of cancer and its uncertain outcome and the stress of diagnostic procedures are exacerbated by the physiologic and metabolic effects of various antitumor interventions. One aspect of this is so-called learned aversion; this means that dislike for a food or foods develops after exposure to this food or foods in association with unpleasant systemic reactions such as nausea or vomiting. In cancer patients, the unpleasant reactions could occur with antitumor therapy such as a chemotherapeutic drug or ionizing radiation. Investigators tested for learned food aversion in children given anticancer drugs that induced nausea or vomiting by offering the experimental group an unusually flavored ice cream shortly before drug administration; controls were not given this flavored ice cream. When tested later for aversion to the same ice cream, controls chose it three times more frequently than did the experimental group.[266] These results were extended and included adult patients also.

The possible role of learned food aversions was investigated in tumor-bearing animals using the hypothesis that tumor-bearing rats would avoid foods associated with aversive physiologic effects of the tumor itself, without any relation to treatment. Comparison was made with rats bearing one of two anorexigenic transplanted tumors in studies in which the animals were exposed persistently to one of two diets for 19 days of tumor growth; this exposure was followed by a single preference test in which the rats' intake of the previously used diet was compared with their intake of the other diet, to which they had not previously been exposed.[267] Those rats with a Leydig–cell tumor developed an aversion to their usual diet, whereas those with the Walker 256 did not. Obviously, tumor-specific factors that were not identified were involved. In a discussion of such experiments, Morrison expressed concern about the validity of learned aversions in relation to animal studies; namely, as a conditioned response, removal of the stimulus should be associated with a fairly slow extinction time. However, when an anorexigenic transplanted tumor is excised, food intake improves very quickly;

hence, aversive conditioning, if it occurs, must be interacting with physiologic impairments.[268]

**Other Metabolic Factors.** As noted above, persistent anorexia is associated with progressive wasting and a state of undernutrition (cancer cachexia). The etiologic factors leading to this state have been a source of speculation and research over many years, with periodic reviews.[88,89,269–273] Numerous metabolic alterations have been reported in laboratory animals and humans bearing malignancies. Some have been mentioned earlier in discussions of the effects of transplanted and spontaneous animal tumors; that is, the advantage of tumors in the starving or nitrogen-deprived host to retain nitrogen and undergo cell division at the expense of host tissues (the "nitrogen trap" concept),[88,89] and the observation that decreased food intake per se did not account entirely for tissue wasting by tumor-bearing rats.[90] It is clear that many aspects of metabolism are affected.

**Weight Loss.** Weight loss is a risk factor for survival;[274,275a,b] Heymsfield et al. reported that the minimum range of corrected arm muscle area of cancer patients compatible with survival is 9 to 11 cm$^2$.[276a] Weight loss in both cancer patients and those with anorexia nervosa was accounted for primarily by loss of fat and of skeletal muscle; however, the loss of visceral organ volume in cancer patients was less.[276b]

**Energy Expenditure.** Increased energy production was noted in a leukemic patient more than a century ago by Pettenkofer and Voit. Eight reports with relatively few cases published between 1922 and 1974 on the basal metabolic rate of cancer patients indicated variable results but showed that some patients, especially those with leukemia and Hodgkin's disease, had elevations.[277] More recent studies confirm the observations that metabolic rate is increased in some but not all cancer patients and varies markedly.[278–283] Resting energy expenditures in patients with gastrointestinal cancer with metastases were found to increase by only 10%.[279] Comparison of resting energy expenditure in a heterogeneous group of weight-losing cancer patients with that in noncancer patients both with and without weight loss indicated that malnourished cancer patients had energy expenditure similar to that predicted for healthy, well-nourished individuals but had greater energy expenditure than malnourished noncancer patients, and that the differences became less when both cancer and noncancer groups were very depleted.[281]

Of 200 malnourished afebrile cancer patients (44% gastrointestinal, 29% gynecological, and 29% genitourinary malignancies) with resting energy expenditure measured by indirect calorim-

etry, 33% were hypometabolic (< 90% of that predicted by the Harris-Benedict equation), 41% were
normometabolic, and 20% were hypermetabolic
(> 110 of predicted). The hypermetabolic patients
had significantly longer duration of disease.[282a]
Similar observations in 173 stable patients with
cancers of the alimentary tract who were not
undergoing therapy had a rather similar distribution of resting energy expenditure (36% hypermetabolic, 42% normometabolic and 22% hypermetabolic).[282b] Differences between metabolic
groups were not explained by differences in age,
sex, body size, nutritional status, tumor burden,
or duration of disease. Patients with pancreatic or
hepatobiliary tumors were predominantly hypometabolic; those with gastric cancer tended to be
hypermetabolic; those with esophageal or colorectal malignancies were distributed more evenly
across the metabolic groups.[282b]

Without actual measurements of energy expenditure, one cannot predict with assurance actual expenditure in the afebrile cancer patient.
Obviously, when hypermetabolism is present, the
patient with anorexia will lose more weight than
the equally anorectic patient who is normo- or
hypometabolic.

**Glucose Kinetics.** A significant number of studies in cancer patients indicate alterations in glucose metabolism in at least some cancer patients,
particularly those with an increased tumor burden
or greater extent of spread. An increased rate of
Cori cycling (i.e., glucose → lactate → glucose)
has been noted.[283a-e] Holroyde et al. noted increased cycle activity in patients with metastatic
disease and progressive weight loss,[283b] while others found no association between Cori cycle activity and extent of colon cancer or on the basis
of weight loss (> 10%);[283e] others have found no
increase in net recycling (Cori + alanine-glucose
cycles) between cancer patients and controls.[283f]

Based on a hypothesis that hydrazine modifies
futile cycling and inhibits gluconeogenesis in cancer,[283c] this drug's effect on intake and weight was
studied, with placebo controls. The subjects had
a variety of advanced cancers and were undergoing chemotherapy regimens.[283d] The claim was
made that the hydrazine-treated subjects had "an
increased caloric intake more commonly associated with weight gain" as compared to controls. . . "although caloric intake was only slightly
greater in hydrazine-treated patients." The large
percentage of drop-outs in both groups, major differences in distribution of tumor types, and paucity of data indicate the need for further observations to substantiate this claim.

Increased glucose turnover has been recorded
frequently.[283–285] Kokal et al.[283e] and Shaw and

Wolfe[285] noted that the rate was increased in those
with more extensive disease. In the former case,
Duke's C and D patients had significantly increased turnover rates compared with Duke's B
colon cancer, and there was no relation with
preillness weight loss; others have noted no relation between turnover rate and extent of weight
loss in patients with esophageal cancer.[284]

Rates of glucose and urea turnover and glucose
oxidation have been determined in normal volunteers, in a group of patients with early gastrointestinal (colon) cancer, and in those with advanced gastrointestinal malignancies (esophagus,
stomach, pancreas).[285] Basal rates of glucose turnover were similar in the first two groups (13.9 and
13.3 μmol/kg/min) but significantly higher in
those with advanced cancer (17.6 μmol/kg/min).
When glucose was infused, less suppression of
endogenous production of glucose occurred in
both cancer groups (76% and 69%) than in controls (94%). The glucose oxidation rate increased
progressively in proportion to tumor burden
(23.9% for controls, 32.8% for early tumors, and
43.0% for advanced tumors). After curative resection in the early tumor group, glucose utilization
decreased significantly. Urea turnover was significantly higher in the advanced tumor group (8.4%
μmol/kg/min) as compared to controls (5.9 μmol/
kg/min); glucose infusion significantly suppressed urea turnover·in the healthy controls but
did not induce a significant decrease in the advanced tumor group.

Increased glucose turnover indicates a need for
an increased supply if metabolism is to proceed.
Cori cycling does not appear to account completely for increased need, averaging in colon cancer patients about 14%.[283c] Glycerol has been calculated to contribute about 3% to glucose
supply.[283d] It is known that gluconeogenesis from
amino acids increases in cancer patients.[286] The
increased turnover of urea[285] and the data provided in the next section support this concept.
The increased rate of metabolism of gluconeogenic amino acids for this purpose may lead to
skeletal and visceral protein depletion.

**Protein Kinetics.** Of special concern in the wasting of cancer patients is the loss of lean body mass
and the body's apparent inability to adapt metabolically to impaired intake. A number of studies
of rates of protein flux (Q), synthesis (S), and
breakdown (C) in cancer patients (c) have been
published in the past 7 years.[287a-i] The majority of
studies have reported increases in Q, S, and C as
compared to normal individuals or other controls;[278a-g] however, two reports on children with
newly diagnosed cancer were complicated by the
presence of fever in most subjects.[278d,g]

Weight loss of some degree was common in the patients as compared to controls, and a variety of tumors were involved in a number of these studies. In one,[278e] two patients with acute leukemia with increased kinetics had a return to normal with chemotherapy. Two studies found no differences in kinetic compared to controls. Patients with stage III testicular carcinoma and on TPN had Q, S, and C that before chemotherapy were not significantly different from their healthy controls'; chemotherapy induced major declines in these rates.[287h] In the only report of which at this writing I am aware in which measurements were performed in the same patients before and after surgical resection of the malignancies, Glass et al. found no differences[287i]; some individual differences were noted at the two periods, but these could not be accounted for by tumor stage, preoperative anorexia, or preoperative weight loss. Of the 11 patients, the extent of disease was relatively restricted in most (Duke A [2 patients], B [6 patients] and C [3 patients]).

Protein kinetics were compared in 7 malnourished untreated cancer patients (mean weight loss 22%) later proven to be free of liver metastases, 11 malnourished patients with nonmalignant diseases (mean weight loss 17%), and 5 normal subjects who had been starved for 10 days.[287f] Protein turnover and synthesis were measured using primed constant infusion of $^{15}$N-glycine while the subjects received 500 kcal/day as 5% glucose. Whole-body turnover in the cancer patients was 32% higher than in the noncancer subjects and 35% higher (p < .025) than in the starved subjects. Similarly, the rate of protein synthesis was 35% (not significant) and 54% higher (p < 0.025) in the cancer patients than in the noncancer and starved subjects, respectively. Mean urinary loss with the hypocaloric glucose infusion in the cancer patients was only slightly greater than in the noncancer controls but less than in the starved individuals.

Other data suggested that tumor growth alone in cancer patients is unlikely to cause a great decrease in whole-body synthesis of protein because the rate of protein synthesis of human tumors is similar to that in the normal tissues from wich they arise.[288]

Thus, some but not all cancer patients have been noted to have protein kinetics similar to those patients in the catabolic phase of severe trauma, sepsis, or chronic infection. When the catabolic rate exceeds the synthetic rate persistently, depletion of body protein occurs in accordance with the degree of discrepancy.

**Catabolic Cell-Derived Factors.** Substances that affect metabolic changes and induce certain changes associated with a hypercatabolic state are being studied. Japanese workers reported many years ago the existence of a factor they termed "toxohormone," derived from human and laboratory animal tumor tissue, capable of causing lipid depletion, immunosuppression, and thymic involution in the host;[289] to my knowledge, this substance has never been chemically isolated and identified.

More recently, a factor termed toxohormone-L (originally identified in ascitic fluid from tumor-bearing mice and from patients with liver and ovarian cancer) caused lipid mobilization in vitro and when injected into laboratory animals with adipose tissue pads; injection of a partially purified preparation into the lateral ventricle of rats significantly suppressed food and water intake after a 5-hour lag period.[290] Despite the similarity of names, toxohormone-L differs in molecular weight and in certain metabolic actions from the other toxohormone. Additional evidence confirming the action of another lipid mobilizing factor has been reported in serum of tumor-bearing mice.[291]

Endotoxin, which induced cachexia in laboratory animals, was associated with lipoprotein-lipase deficiency and hyperlipidemia in treated animals. Similar effects resulted from injection of supernates from stimulated macrophages in vivo[292] and in in vitro culture of adipocytes.[293] The macrophage factor was termed cachectin.[293] When cachectin was added to cells before or near confluence and RNA was subsequently isolated, researchers noted that cachectin had prevented the appearance of new RNAs associated with differentiation and also prevented the accumulation of lipid; cachectin added to adipocytes resulted in loss of the stainable lipid in 80 to 90% of these cells.[294] Structurally related compounds have cytotoxic action on tumor and other cells; tumor necrosis factor (TNF) is produced by stimulated macrophages,[295] and lymphotoxin is produced by mitogen-stimulated lymphocytes.[296a] Interleukin I[296b] and TNF produce changes on injection into animals with a hypermetabolic state. The roles of such substances in the development of human cancer undernutrition will undoubtedly be explored.

**"Ectopic" Hormones.** A diffuse system of endocrine cells characterized by certain cytochemical capabilities has been termed APUD (amine precursor uptake and decarboxylation). The peptide hormones these cells secrete have a powerful influence on adjacent and distant organs. Pearse stated that the APUD cells were derived from "neuroendocrine programmed embryonic ectoblast,"[297] although this concept has been challenged. It has been suggested that differentiation of malignant cells results in a wide spectrum of ectopic peptide production[298] and is a universal capability of neoplastic cells.[299] Every known, naturally occurring hormone has been found to be produced by one or more human tumor types. Unlike the normal hormone control mechanism, ectopic hormone production is autonomous.

Metabolic, nutritional, electrolyte, and other clinical problems can result from such increased production.[300,301] Hormones with nutritional implications include gastrin, vasoactive intestinal peptide (VIP), serotonin, glucagon, insulin, vasopressin, parathyroid hormone, growth hormone, ACTH, calcitonin, somatostatin, and the vitamin D derivative, calcitriol. Insulin from insulinomas is produced by the cells that normally produce it and hence is not an ectopic hormone. Similarly, gastrin from pancreatic tumor cells can also be produced by cells normally capable of its production. Somatomedins, which are believed to account for the development of hypoglycemia in instances of hepatic carcinomas, are normally produced in the liver and act like insulin. Of the types of neoplasms producing hypoglycemia, 21% were found to be hepatic in origin, and a few were adenocarcinomas of stomach and colon.[301]

While the syndrome of inappropriate antidiuretic hormone (SIADH) has been associated with carcinoma of the lung, 12 of 28 patients with colon carcinoma were found by radioimmunoassay to have vasopressin concentrations that were above normal. Although without clinical evidence of SIADH, these patients would presumably have manifested this syndrome if water-loaded.[299] Pancreatic islet cell, carcinoid, and adenocarcinoma account for 10% of cases manifesting clinically apparent ectopic ACTH production.[301]

VIP- and serotonin-producing tumors also elaborate other hormones that have (e.g., prostaglandins, histamine, kinins) or appear not to have (e.g., pancreatic polypeptide) supplementary metabolic effects. Severe diarrhea can occur with tumors secreting serotonin (carcinoid syndrome), calcitonin, gastrin (Zollinger-Ellison syndrome), and VIP (Verner-Morrison syndrome). Zollinger-Ellison syndrome can be associated with steatorrhea induced by the inhibitory effects of decreased intestinal pH on pancreatic lipase function, as well as by epithelial damage.[302] Potassium and fluid losses in the diarrhea of Verner-Morrison syndrome may be severe.[303]

Gastrointestinal hormones have trophic effects on normal gastrointestinal mucosa and pancreas. Receptors for steroid and peptide hormones have been detected in a wide variety of human tumors.[304] Gastrin and some other hormones have been found to stimulate growth of human tumors transplanted to laboratory animals and in vitro; the possible role of such hormones in human neoplasms has been discussed.[304]

Hypercalcemia is one of the most common metabolic complications of cancer. It is steadily progressive unless treated and may be symptomatic at relatively lower calcium concentrations than is the case with hyperparathyroidism. The more common symptoms are nausea, vomiting, anorexia, lethargy, confusion, and stupor progressing to coma.

A pathogenetic classification of the hypercalcemia of cancer has been given by Mundy et al.[305] Three clinical groupings have been delineated. First are hematologic cancers (e.g., myeloma, lymphosarcoma, T-cell lymphoma, and Hodgkin's and Burkitt's lymphomas), which are associated with increased osteoclastic bone resorption (osteolytic lesions mainly) adjacent to neoplastic cells. Osteoclast-activating factor as well as calcitriol[306] are associated causative factors. The second group is bone-metastasizing solid tumors such as breast, lung, and pancreatic tumors causing increased osteoclastic bone resorption with variable osteoblastic response; bone demonstrates discrete lytic lesions with a variable sclerotic response; direct erosion by tumor cells and prostaglandins are factors. The third group is solid tumors (without metastases) of lung, renal, pancreatic, and ovarian types operating systemically with increased osteoclastic bone resorption and decreased bone formation. Increased fractional excretion of phosphate, increased nephrogenic cyclic AMP, and decreased PTH have been noted; factors implicated include PTH, prostaglandins, transforming growth factors, factors interacting with PTH receptor, and colony-stimulating activity.

**Osteomalacia.** Another effect of tumors involves reduced concentration of calcitriol in conjunction with hypophosphatemia and is demonstrated in oncogenic or oncogenous osteomalacia. An increasing number of cases have been recognized in recent years, with approximately 50 cases reported as of 1986; undoubtedly many more cases occurred before calcitriol was recognized.[307]

Most reported cases have involved malignancies of mesenchymal or bone origin (e.g., hemangiopericytoma or giant cell tumor).[308,309] In addition, hypophosphatemic osteomalacia has been noted with prostatic carcinoma, usually advanced.[310] Muscle weakness of varying degree and variable back pain have been frequent complaints with findings of hypophosphatemia, renal phosphate wasting, and decreased calcitriol; calcidiol has been normal. Serum PTH and calcium have been normal. Histologically, osteoclast activity has been markedly enhanced. Gastrointestinal malabsorption of calcium and phosphate has been observed.[310]

Where resection of the tumor has been possible, serum calcitriol and phosphate levels rose within 36 hours, with subsequent correction of the bone disease.[308,309] As of 1987, 15 cases with this type of osteomalacia have been reported primarily in patients with myelomatosis associated with adult Fanconi syndrome caused by light-chain nephropathy with proteinuria and decreased renal tubular reabsorption of phosphate, glucose, amino acids, uric acid, and bicarbonate.[311] Where eradication of the tumor is not successful, treatment with high doses of phosphate and, where indicated, of calcitriol have been effective in treating the bone problem. Calcitriol may or may not be depressed in this specific syndrome.

**Villous Changes.** Creamer suggested that malignancies external to the gastrointestinal tract induced an abnormal small-intestinal mucosa, to which he attributed some of the ill health and loss of weight in malignancy.[312] A number of papers followed that supported or denied these findings. In a more definitive study, Barry showed that malnourished patients with extra-alimentary tract malignancies often had abnormalities of mucosal cell structure, epithelial cell loss, and decreased lactose utilization; however, he found similar changes in seriously malnourished patients without cancer and suggested that such mucosal changes are the *result* of malnutrition rather than a direct effect of nongastrointestinal tract malignancies.[313] Once present, impaired mucosal function can contribute further to malnutrition by depressing the efficiency of absorption.

**Vitamin and Trace Elements.** A number of reports describe abnormalities of these nutrients, usually subnormal blood levels. Some authors tend to attribute either to diminished nutrients a role in cancer causation, or to the tumor an effect on nutrient metabolism. Rarely have the authors been able to eliminate the most likely factors leading to low serum values, i.e., depressed intake or losses in stool. It is well known that serum folate and zinc reflect recent intake and that zinc losses in diarrhea may be very high. It is also well established that serum copper is often high in cancer patients (not because of the tumor directly but because ceruloplasmin is an acute-phase protein that is often elevated in cancer patients); vitamin $B_{12}$[314] or folate[315] may be high in myeloproliferative disorders because of the increased leukocytes per se, because of increased levels of in tissues, or because of elevation of $B_{12}$-binding alpha-globulin (see also Chap. 21). Copper and manganese

in serum will rise in the presence of biliary obstruction of any cause.

### Localized Tumor Effects

In addition to the systemic effects of cancer, a number of more localized effects of various neoplasms lead to nutritional problems (Table 64–1).

**Obstruction Along the Alimentary Tract.** The most common direct effect of alimentary tract neoplasms on nutritional status relates to partial or complete obstruction at one or more sites.

It is estimated that about 20% of surgical admissions for acute abdominal conditions are associated with intestinal obstruction and that the third most common cause of obstruction is neoplasm of the bowel.[316] When obstruction occurs acutely, the patient is likely to seek medical attention immediately. However, most neoplasms obstruct slowly and progressively. It is commonly observed that a significant number of patients will defer seeking medical care until their dysphagia, anorexia, pain, nausea, vomiting, diarrhea, or anemia from chronic blood loss have persisted to the point at which weight loss and weakness are prominent. In addition to weight loss secondary to poor intake of food, problems relating to fluid, electrolyte, and acid-base balance result from persistent vomiting or diarrhea or as a consequence of malnutrition per se.

**Malabsorption.** Malabsorption occurs for various reasons.

*Blind Loop Syndrome.* This syndrome occurs secondary to partial obstruction in the upper small bowel or in the jejunal diverticuli or secondary to lack of gastric acid secretion. It is associated with bacterial overgrowth, which may result in steatorrhea and vitamin $B_{12}$ deficiency. This syndrome involves not only direct interaction of bacteria with certain nutrients but also the development of abnormalities of the intestinal epithelium to account for associated malabsorption.[317]

*Internal Fistula.* Bypass of significant portions of the small bowel can result in malabsorption; malabsorption can occur with fistulas between the stomach and colon (gastrocolic-), with fistulas between widely separated portions of the small bowel (enteroentero-), or with fistulas diverting bowel contents through the skin (enterocutaneous). The severity depends on the extent of small-bowel bypass. When diarrhea or steatorrheic stools occur rather abruptly in the patient with suspected or known abdominal tumors, particularly when there has been previous surgery or radiation, the physician should include this possibility in the differential diagnosis and workup.

*Intestinal Lymphoma or Carcinoma.* When these involve the small-bowel mesentery lymph nodes they can present as malabsorption.[318] Patients with abdominal lymphomas and malabsorption can present with abdominal pain, weight loss, anorexia, and bulky stool suggestive of steatorrhea. They may have clubbing, glossitis, angular stomatitis, and peripheral edema. Laboratory finding may include abnormal D-xylose absorption, flat glucose tolerance curves, hypoalbuminemia, and fat and $B_{12}$ malabsorption; megaloblastosis may be present, as may deficits in fat-soluble vitamins and folic acid.

The mechanisms for the development of malabsorption in patients with primary small-bowel malignancies are several. The intestinal epithelium may be abnormal, with villous atrophy and crypt hyperplasia of the involved mucosa; although the clinical diagnosis may initially be celiac disease, such patients might not respond to a gluten-free diet;[319] this observation per se does not rule out previous celiac disease.[320] Infiltration of the lamina propria and draining lymph nodes can lead to obstructions of mesenteric lymph channels and dilatation of the lymphatics within the intestinal villi; this obstruction, in turn, can lead to development of a protein-losing enteropathy with hypoalbuminemia, hypoglobulinemia, and lymphocytopenia.[321] Protein-losing enteropathy has also been described with cases of gastric carcinoma[321] and may also occur in patients with tumors outside the alimentary tract, e.g., malignant melanoma, ovarian carcinoma, and metastatic carcinoma of the lung.[322] Nutritional replacement and support in such malabsorption syndromes are useful while direct antineoplastic treatment with radiation and chemotherapy are undertaken.

A well-established association exists between pre-existing celiac disease and the development of alimentary tract malignancies, approximately half of which have been found to be malignant lymphomas.[320] The development of newer diagnostic tests has clarified the origin of the lymphomas, which recently have been classified as T-cell in origin.[323] Carcinomas also arise in patients with pre-existing celiac disease with an incidence varying from 5 to 7%,[324,325] with lymphomas occurring at an incidence of 6 to 10%.[324–327] Various hypotheses have been suggested for the malignant involvement in these patients, including the possibility that the abnormal small-bowel epithelium permits increased absorption of carcinogens, that the chronic inflammation of the lamina propria or lymphoid hyperactivity somehow plays a role, or that environmental factors such as prolonged nutritional deficiency secondary to malabsorption or the presence of intestinal organisms may induce the malignant changes.

Cooper et al. concluded that no evidence exists that a gluten-free diet provides protection against the development of either lymphoma or carcinoma of the intestinal tract.[324] However, they point out that the gluten-free diet was ingested for a short time compared to the usual diet. Others have found that the number of patients who had never received a gluten-free diet was too small to allow comparison with those who had; furthermore, all those treated with this diet had started it in adult life.[320] Determining whether a gluten-free diet will prevent malignancy will require study of a population on the gluten-free diet from early childhood.

Other workers[325] have noted that the majority of patients with celiac disease who claimed adherence to their diet were actually ingesting variable amounts of gluten. It would seem essential to insist on maintenance of a strict gluten-free diet by patients of all ages and to exercise close surveillance at all ages, with particular concern for those who present with celiac disease in middle life and in those with the disease who deteriorate without apparent reason after a stable period on the diet.

**Fluid and Electrolyte Changes.** The major causes of fluid and electrolyte disturbances in cancer patients are vomiting and diarrhea secondary to partial or complete obstruction, and fluid losses through a fistula. Losses of sodium, chloride, potassium, magnesium, and zinc can be serious.

Fluid and electrolyte imbalances are often seen in patients with widespread hepatic metastases, ascites, and liver failure, with cardiac metastases and failure, with metastatic ovarian carcinoma and ascites, with renal failure secondary to obstruction of the urinary tract by tumor or radiation fibrosis, with obstruction of lymphatic or venous drainage in major areas, and other situations listed in Table 64–1 and described above. Factitious hyperkalemia can be reported in patients with very high platelet counts as the result of release of potassium into the supernate in blood samples awaiting analysis.

**Hypoalbuminemia.** Hypoalbuminemia is frequently noted in advanced cancer cases. The depressed albumin levels are usually secondary to inability to produce sufficient albumin as a result of serious protein-calorie deficiency, as a result of the metabolic effects of tumors, or as a result of hepatic insufficiency secondary to parenchymal cell damage or replacement by tumor. Also, depressed albumin levels are often secondary to losses of albumin from the body in excess of synthetic capacity, e.g., as occurs in protein-losing enteropathy or nephrotic syndrome. Depressed albumin levels can also be secondary to dilution of albumin into abnormally large extracellular compartments (e.g., ascites and edema). Hypoalbuminemia will usually improve with appropriate nutritional therapy when malnutrition is the primary or an important contributory factor. Antitumor therapy is obviously indicated to treat the direct effects of neoplastic growth.

**Anemia.** Anemia is common and occasionally can be secondary to insufficiency of hematopoietic nutritional factors, especially if chronic blood loss without iron replacement has occurred. A normochromic normocytic anemia is not infrequently associated wth cancer and does not respond to nutritional factors. Tumor involvement of the bone marrow and bone marrow suppression because of radiation and chemotherapy are contributing factors.

**Nutrition Support Recommendations.** Reversal for any significant period of the undesirable clinical, metabolic, and nutritional changes secondary to systemic and localized effects of cancer depends primarily on complete elimination of the malignancy or on major palliation. The physician frequency faces the problem of having to correct significant malnutrition and fluid and electrolyte imbalances in those patients requiring surgical intervention or in those needing prolonged maintenance in therapeutic trials of radiation or chemotherapy. For such patients, careful attention to correction of abnormalities is indicated. As with all chronic wasting diseases, in cancer management one cannot and should not expect to restore significant amounts of tissue in a short period of time. Urgent surgery cannot and should not wait for achievement of the goal of nutritional rehabilitation. In such a situation, correction of acute or chronic vitamin and mineral deficiencies, blood loss, and electrolyte and fluid imbalances, which achievement reduces the surgical risk, can often be accomplished within a matter of days.

When surgery, radiation, or chemotherapy are indicated for the debilitated patient who faces a further significant period of little or no oral intake of food as a consequence of such treatments, use of adequate parenteral or enteral feeding to improve nutritional and metabolic status can aid survival or decrease morbidity and the period of convalescence (see Chaps. 54 and 62).

## NUTRITIONAL PROBLEMS ARISING FROM CANCER TREATMENTS

Significant nutritional problems can arise from the presence of the tumor and from specific treatments undertaken to control the neoplastic process.

## Therapy of Head and Neck Cancer

Patients with head and neck tumors, especially males, often have a history of chronic heavy alcohol intake. For this reason and because of the tumor's effects on food intake, these patients may be in a nutritionally depleted state prior to therapy.[328] Treatment frequently involves combined surgery, radiation, and chemotherapy (Table 64–2). Radiation induces loss of taste ("mouth blindness") and xerostomia (dry mouth) as the result of salivary gland damage; injury to teeth may also occur. These effects may be long-term: of 13 patients studied 1 to 7 years after radiotherapy, 9 had measurable taste losses, especially for salt and bitter; 12 had reduced salivary flow and secretion rates, with no saliva being collected in 7; 9 complained of dry mouth.[329] Surgery may include partial or total glossectomy and mandibulectomy and resection of portions of the hard or soft palate and muscles of the lower face and neck. These procedures add to the difficulties in chewing and swallowing. The possibility of the patient's aspirating on swallowing may be serious enough for him to require tube feeding or, alternatively, laryngectomy with its physical separation of the respiratory and alimentary tracts and resultant loss of normal voice.

**Nutrition Support Recommendations.** For the patient who is seriously malnourished prior to workup and therapy, nutritional intervention should be instituted early. Because surgery or radiation can interfere with placement of central catheters in the neck or subclavian areas, parenteral nutrition through a peripheral vein or through a long antecubital central line or tube feedings are routes to be considered to initiate nutritional improvement. Post-treatment attention is directed to providing attractive foods with pleasant aroma, lubricated by gravies and salad dressings and with high caloric and nutritional content to encourage better food intake. Nutritious liquid formulas by mouth if they can be swallowed, or, alternatively, by intermittent tube feeding are often helpful. Such tubes reduce the need for permanent esophagostomy or gastrostomy tubes, which can be inserted for long-term maintenance of patients unable or opposed to repeatedly placing their own tubes or opposed to persistent indwelling nasopharyngeal tubes. (See Chap. 54 for detailed discussion of enteral feeding procedures and formulations.)

For patients who are at serious risk of aspirating regurgitated food and who have an absent gag reflex (especially in the presence of significant pul-

**Table 64–2. Consequences of Cancer Treatment Predisposing to Nutrition Problems**

1. Radiation treatment
   A. Radiation of oropharyngeal area
      1) Destruction of sense of taste; xerostomia and odynophagia; loss of teeth
   B. Radiation to lower neck and mediastinum
      1) Esophagitis with dysphagia
      2) Fibrosis with esophageal stricture
   C. Radiation of abdomen and pelvis
      1) Bowel damage, acute and chronic, with diarrhea, malabsorption, stenosis and obstruction, fistulization
2. Surgical treatment
   A. Radical resection of oropharyngeal area
      1) Chewing and swallowing difficulties
   B. Esophagectomy
      1) Gastric stasis and hypochlorhydria secondary to vagotomy
      2) Steatorrhea secondary to vagotomy
      3) Diarrhea secondary to vagotomy
      4) Early satiety
      5) Regurgitation
   C. Gastrectomy (high subtotal or total)
      1) Dumping syndrome
      2) Malabsorption
      3) Achlorhydria and lack of intrinsic factor and R protein
      4) Hypoglycemia
      5) Early satiety
   D. Intestinal resection
      1) Jejunum
         a) Decreased efficiency of absorption of many nutrients
      2) Ileum
         a) Vitamin $B_{12}$ deficiency
         b) Bile salt losses with diarrhea or steatorrhea
         c) Hyperoxaluria and renal stone
         d) Calcium and magnesium depletion
         e) Fat and fat-soluble vitamin malabsorption
      3) Massive bowel resection
         a) Life-threatening malabsorption
         b) Malnutrition
         c) Metabolic acidosis
         d) Dehydration
      4) Ileostomy and colostomy
         a) Complications of salt and water balance
   E. Blind loop syndrome
      1) Vitamin $B_{12}$ malabsorption
   F. Pancreatectomy
      1) Malabsorption
      2) Diabetes mellitus
3. Drug treatment
   A. Corticosteroids
      1) Fluid and electrolyte problems
      2) Nitrogen and calcium losses
      3) Hyperglycemia
   B. Sex hormone analogues
      1) May induce nausea and vomiting
   C. Immunotherapy
      1) Interleukin-2
         a) Azotemia
         b) Hypotension
         c) Fluid retention
   D. Antimetabolites, alkylating agents, and other drugs (see Table 64–3)

monary disease), a feeding tube with its tip in the lower esophagus or stomach imposes a certain hazard. The danger of aspiration can be reduced by infusing the formula by slow drip over a number of hours using a pump to assure a regular flow rate. The hazard can be further reduced by using tubes that have been passed into the upper small bowel prior to initiation of feeding. These tubes are very well tolerated and can be left in place unless there is an important reason for their temporary removal.

## Therapy of Esophageal Carcinoma

Radiation to the lower neck and mediastinum can induce esophagitis, but this usually disappears following cessation of therapy. However, some patients may develop fibrosis with resultant esophageal stricture. Chemotherapy can induce nausea, anorexia, sore mouth, and odynophagia, further inhibiting food intake and decreasing the acceptance of tube feeding. Surgical treatment usually involves total or distal esophagectomy requiring bilateral vagotomy, proximal gastrectomy, and gastric pull-up into the chest. Esophageal anastomotic leakage can occur (see below). Easy regurgitation, rapid satiety, decreased rate of gastric emptying of solid food despite pyloroplasty, diarrhea (intermittent or continuous), and steatorrhea (mild to moderate) are common (Table 64–2).[330] The causes of diarrhea and steatorrhea are unknown.

Total vagotomy has been associated with an increase in basal serum gastrin levels in man, though postprandial gastrin output is only slightly elevated. GIP (gastrone) levels are increased in basal serum concentration and in response to glucose. The plasma pancreatic polypeptide response to insulin hypoglycemia is markedly reduced, as is its response to a meal.[331]

**Nutrition Support Recommendations.** A significant number of these patients will have lost weight as a result of decreased intake secondary to progressive dysphagia. When obstruction is not complete, instruction and attention to ingestion of adequate amounts of complete liquid formulas are often beneficial in preventing malnutrition. When serious anorexia is also present, passage of a feeding tube is possible. However, in my experience, oral or tube feeding in the period of radiation and chemotherapy is usually inadequate to meet the need, either because of interference with the feeding program or because of nausea, pain, or combinations thereof. In such instances, adequate parenteral feeding is indicated to maintain acceptable nutritional status.

An interesting example of the value of nutritional support—in this case, total parenteral nutrition—is given by Riboli et al. in their review of 16 cases of esophageal anastomotic leakages after cancer resection.[332] In the period 1978 to 1980, 8 patients with this complication underwent immediate reoperation with a new anastomosis being created; 7 of these patients died postoperatively. In the period 1980 to 1982, 8 patients with leakage were treated by total parenteral nutrition and complete fasting; 6 survived, with spontaneous healing of the leaks; 2 died of septic mediastinitis and respiratory failure.

Postoperative dietary and nutritional intervention involves providing frequent small meals to overcome easy satiety and the tendency to regurgitate, providing meals high in carbohydrate and protein, and if steatorrhea is marked, restricting large amounts of long-chain fats and substituting medium-chain triglycerides (MCT). True "dumping" does not occur in such patients eating solid food because of the normal gastric-duodenal continuity and, usually, because of a delayed gastric emptying are present despite pyloroplasty. Dumping symptoms can occur if large amounts of hyperosmolar liquid formulas are taken by mouth or given rapidly by tube. Postoperative stricture can occur and requires dilatation; the patient with stricture might require oral or tube-fed liquid formulas to assure adequate intake.

Carcinoma of the esophagogastric junction creates physiologic and nutritional problems similar to those of the patient who has had an esophagogastrectomy and reanastomosis for carcinoma of the esophagus. Because a larger portion of the proximal stomach is resected, early satiety may be more marked, and production of gastric secretions and of their $B_{12}$ binding and other factors can be reduced.

## Therapy of Gastric Cancer

Surgical treatment for gastric cancer involves either high subtotal gastrectomy with a gastrojejunal anastomosis or total gastrectomy with esophagojejunotomy. Removal of most or all of the stomach reduces or deletes its reservoir, digestive, secretory diluting, and metering functions. These modifications from the normal have both physiologic and nutritional consequences that may vary from mild to severe depending on the extent of resection, the individual patient's response, and the preventive intervention of the physician. The physiologic and nutritional problems of patients with high subtotal or total gastrectomy are different than those occurring with esophagogastrectomy (Table 64–2).

Depending on the types and amounts of foods ingested and the response of the patient, a variety of signs and symptoms that have been termed the "dumping syndrome" can occur. This syndrome together with malabsorption and hypoglycemic reactions can occur in the gastrectomized patient (see Chap. 56 A4).

**Nutrition Support Recommendations (see also Chap. 56 A4).** The dumping syndrome can be greatly minimized or prevented by provision of and adherence to a dietary regimen called the antidumping diet (Appendix Table A-31). This diet is high in protein and fat, quite low in soluble carbohydrates, and generally somewhat restricted in all carbohydrate and fluids; it is served approximately 6 times/day. Additional measures for those who continue to be symptomatic include reclining for a period immediately after eating. The use of pectin derivative has been reported to prolong gastric emptying and to decrease dumping, blood volume changes, hyperglycemia, and serum insulin.[333] Because antidumping diets tend to be high in long-chain triglycerides (LCT), steatorhea may be significant. Steatorrhea can be reduced by progressive replacement of LCT by medium-chain triglycerides (MCT), as tolerated. MCT can be used in cooking, in salad dressings, and in nourishing beverages.

When steatorrhea is present, a trial of pancreatic extract is indicated to rule out luminal pancreatic enzyme insufficiency resulting from dilution of pancreatic enzymes or a pancreatic secretory defect. Deficiencies of vitamins and minerals can be prevented or treated by oral administration in adequate amounts. Supplementary iron taken with ascorbic acid, injection of vitamin $B_{12}$ (100 μg once monthly), and use of a *complete* supplementary multi-vitamin preparation are indicated. High-potency vitamin formulations are usually not necessary. It should be recalled that some supplementary and high-potency vitamins can be lacking or low in folate. Increased amounts of vitamin D might be indicated when fat malabsorption is significant; the need can be determined by measuring the levels of 25 OH vitamin D.

Symptoms of milk intolerance, which are common in these patients, can be prevented and adequate calcium obtained by having the patient ingest milk in small amounts (e.g., small glasses) frequently during the day; by using lactaid-treated milk, which hydrolyzes lactose, or by using yogurt as tolerated; or, if these methods are unsatisfactory, by providing during the day calcium salts sufficient to provide at least 1 g of calcium, taken in divided doses with meals.

The weight loss seen so often in gastrectomized patients is not primarily the result of malabsorption; much of it is attributable to poor food intake. In addition to the food antipathy related to the occurrence of the dumping syndrome, discomfort associated with the afferent loop syndrome or chemical esophagitis secondary to bile regurgitation, psychologic depression, the effects of drugs, or unknown factors can produce weight loss. When one adds to the physiologic and nutritional problems imposed by gastrectomy the additional anorexigenic effects of postoperative chemotherapy, the resulting nutritional problems may be severe. When the most careful dietary advice and adherence to an antidumping diet do not enable the patient either to avoid the dumping syndrome or ingest a sufficient diet to maintain or gain weight, testing of intermittent slow-drip tube feedings of a complete formula is recommended. Because of the very slow entry of food by this technique, dumping is not likely to occur. Such feedings may need be given only during the period of chemotherapy, following which appetite may improve. On the other hand, some patients remain anorectic following cessation of chemotherapy even though their tumors are not a problem; in such instances nightly tube feedings should be continued.

### Therapy of Pancreatic Carcinoma

The adverse impact on nutritional status of this tumor type and its treatments have been reviewed in Chapter 56B2 (Table 64–2). Pancreatic carcinoma is a malignancy that often presents with anorexia and weight loss. Eating may aggravate pain, which is often present. Carcinoma of the pancreas can cause digestive enzyme deficiency, especially when this organ is involved extensively, particularly in the head region, or when a major portion of the duct is obstructed elsewhere. The resulting malabsorption combined with anorexia contributes to progressive weight loss. Bile insufficiency can occur with obstruction such as occurs with involvement by tumor of the ampulla of Vater, of the common duct behind the pancreatic head, or at the porta hepatis. Bile insufficiency reduces intestinal absorption of vitamin K and leads to reduction in plasma levels of the vitamin K–dependent coagulation factors.

**Pancreatoduodenectomy.** This operative procedure was described by Whipple et al. in 1935 for the surgical treatment of carcinoma of the ampulla of Vater. Other carcinomas of the periampullary region that are amenable to treatment by this operation include those of the distal common bile duct and duodenum. Some surgeons use pancreatoduodenectomy to treat carcinoma of the head of the pancreas. In the usual operative procedure the distal portion of the stomach is removed, the pancreas is transected (usually at its neck, though varying amounts or even the entire organ may be removed), and the duodenum and

a few inches of jejunum distal to the ligament of Treitz are resected. The management of the pancreatic stump has nutritional implications, because ligation of the pancreatic duct as some surgeons perform it, with oversewing of the transected end of the pancreas will lead to complete pancreatic exocrine insufficiency.[334]

The rate of postoperative complication in this procedure is significant, and such complications may result in prolonged hospitalization, with a number of problems interfering with normal food intake. Fat malabsorption occurred in 50% of patients of one study[335] and in 27% of another study[334,336] surviving after pancreatoduodenectomy in which the pancreatic stump was anastomosed to the jejunum or stomach.

**Diabetes.** Approximately 10 to 20% of patients presenting with carcinoma of the pancreas are overtly diabetic,[337] and depending on the site of the tumor, 10 to 35% have asymptomatic glycosuria or hyperglycemia.[336] Another aspect of pancreatoduodenectomy concerns the endocrine function of the postoperative remnant of the pancreas. Decreased glucose tolerance has been noted in pancreatoduodenectomized patients in whom fasting blood sugar levels were within normal limits.[338] Insufficient insulin response to a glucose load from the remnant of the pancreas appears to be a major cause of the glucose intolerance.[339]

**Total Pancreatectomy.** Total pancreatectomy has been recommended because it eliminates the danger of pancreatic fistula without significantly increasing the surgical risk and because it eliminates the possibility of failure to remove carcinoma existing more distally either because of spread or because of tumor arising multifocally.[337] This procedure poses a difficult metabolic situation with its resultant exocrine and endocrine insufficiency. Even with the optimum use of pancreatic extract, loss of fat and nitrogen in stool tend to be increased. The usual diabetic-type diet with its increased protein and fat tends to exacerbate malabsorption and diarrhea. Replacing dietary fat with glucose to decrease steatorrhea increases the requirement for insulin.

In a series of 48 totally pancreatectomized patients followed with respect to their control of diabetes, Pliam et al. found that 50% were easily managed, 8% were managed with difficulty only when there was concomitant illness, 19% had occasional hypoglycemic reactions managed with oral carbohydrate, 4% did poorly with persistent glycosuria, and 20% were found to be very difficult to manage, with ketoacidosis or hyperglycemic episodes requiring hospitalization.[340]

**Regional Pancreatectomy.** The more radical surgery of regional pancreatectomy has been developed in an effort to improve the poor survival by en bloc removal of the pancreas, adjacent tissue and primary lymph drainage.[341a,b] The type 1 procedure involves, total removal of the pancreas, pancreatic segment of portal vein, transverse mesocolon with middle colic vessels, surrounding soft tissues, regional lymph nodes, distal stomach, duodenum, spleen, gallbladder, and common bile duct, with skeletonizing of the porta hepatis, celiac axis and superior mesenteric artery, vena cava, and aorta. Involvement of the celiac axis, superior mesenteric artery, or hepatic artery is treated additionally with arterial resection and reconstruction. Because of anorexia, marked diarrhea, and severe malabsorption, usually occurring together, total parenteral nutrition has been employed in maintaining a number of these patients postoperatively and has proved to be lifesaving with progressive improvement.

**Nutrition Support Recommendations.** Postoperatively anorexia, diabetes mellitus, pancreatic insufficiency, and other types of malabsorption present serious problems to the totally pancreatectomized patient. Adequate amounts of pancreatic extract must be administered with all meals and snacks, particularly to those with moderate to severe fat or protein malabsorption.[342a] Good control of the diabetes maximizes carbohydrate utilization and minimizes fluid and sodium losses secondary to osmotic diuresis caused by glycosuria. Medium-chain triglycerides are more efficiently absorbed in the absence of pancreatic enzymes than the usual long-chain fats are. They are also absorbed more efficiently when conjugated bile salts are insufficient or when absorptive mechanisms are impaired.

Glucose oligosaccharides can also be helpful in increasing the caloric intake and absorption of pancreatically insufficient patients, since these relatively short-chain glucose polymers can be hydrolyzed to glucose by the brush-border enzyme sucrase-α-dextrinase. This white powdery material is not sweet and may be used in a variety of ways to supplement intake. When nutritional problems are severe and parenteral nutrition is not required, intermittent tube feeding may be instituted using formulas with protein hydrolysate, oligosaccharides, MCT, minerals and vitamins; such a formula does not require pancreatic extract (see Appendix Table A–40c). Slow-drip infusion improves absorption.

## Therapy of Intestinal Resection or Damage

Major resection of the small bowel because of primary gastrointestinal malignancies is relatively uncommon, as is resection of only the jejunum.

The ileum is damaged, bypassed, or removed to a varying extent in cancer patients because of involvement with metastatic disease or with fistula development or as a result of ionizing radiation. Resection of the ileum leads to certain physiologic and nutritional problems (see Chap. 56C4 and C5 and Table 64–2); however, certain aspects are discussed further here.

**Nutrition Support Recommendations.** If the ileal resection is not extensive (usually less than 100 cm), sufficient bile salts enter the large bowel to induce a brown watery diarrhea that can be quite distressing to the patient.[342b] Cholestyramine is dramatically effective in controlling this diarrhea through its mechanism of binding bile salts.[342b] It is my policy to begin with a relatively large dose (e.g., 4 g four times daily) in order to demonstrate quickly to the patient that effective control of the diarrhea is possible. Following control of diarrhea, the doses may be reduced to half or less. It is of interest that a significant proportion of patients with such "choleraic" diarrhea find that their cholestyramine can be reduced to very low doses or to intermittent doses once they are certain that it can control this problem, suggesting that this diarrhea has an important psychologic component.

The loss of bile salts with larger distal ileal resections (usually more than 100 cm) may be so great that very little of the amount of bile salt entering the normal enterohepatic circulation is reabsorbed. The synthetic capacity of the liver to synthesize sufficient new bile salts is exceeded and the concentration of bile salts in the intestinal lumen falls below the critical micellar concentration necessary for efficient fat absorption.

**Nutrition Support Recommendations.** In such a situation, the patient may be helped by the feeding of a diet restricted in LCT and by the use of MCT, which do not require bile salt absorption.[342b] The use of a water-soluble form of vitamin K and of increased amounts of the other fat-soluble vitamins as well as calcium, magnesium and zinc are indicated to prevent deficiency of these nutrients. Sufficient polyunsaturated fats (which are not provided by MCT) must be provided to assure adequate intake of essential fatty acids.

Another consequence of ileal resection is hyperoxaluria with increased incidence of renal oxalate stone formation. The normal precipitation of oxalate ion by intestinal calcium ion is prevented by the shortage of free calcium ions that results from their binding to unabsorbed fatty acids present in increased amounts in the remaining small bowel and colon. Soluble oxalate is then absorbed in the colon and appears in the urine in increased concentrations and can precipitate as the oxalate salt in the renal tubule.

Nutrition support is designed to minimize oxalate stone formation by decreasing the intake of long-chain triglycerides and increasing MCT, decreasing oxalate intake (see Appendix Table A-25), providing at least 1 g of oral calcium ion/day to precipitate oxalate, and assuring intake of sufficient magnesium to permit normal serum levels and daily urinary excretion of at least 6 meq; this amount of magnesium is desirable because urinary magnesium tends to solubilize tubular calcium, and a normal magnesium status maintains a good urinary citrate excretion. Magnesium depletion can markedly reduce urinary concentration of this calcium-complexing ion.[343] Patients may have difficulty ingesting sufficient magnesium to provide adequate magnesium levels without experiencing increased diarrhea. This problem can be overcome by reducing fat intake to reduce fecal magnesium excretion; periodic injections or IV infusions of magnesium may be necessary to achieve adequate intake (see Chap. 6). Increased intake of oral citrate may also be necessary to increase solubility of calcium ion. A high intake (> 0.5 g daily) of ascorbic acid should be avoided to minimize oxalate output. Patient compliance and need for modifications of therapy can be monitored by periodic analyses for oxalate and citrate in 24-hour urine samples.

### Radiation Enteritis

Radiation to the upper abdomen, including the stomach, frequently leads to acute nausea and vomiting. When the pelvis or lower abdomen is irradiated, diarrhea and weight loss are the most common symptoms.[344] The acute and chronic changes in the jejunum with minor and severe radiation damage have been described.[345] Radiation-induced damage is often subclinical. Though patients may not complain of gastrointestinal changes, on questioning it is apparent that these changes may have occurred; for example, of 17 patients who had no complaints, when examined in a radiotherapy follow-up clinic 12 had permanent changes in bowel habits and 16 had some evidence of malabsorption.[346] It has been estimated that about 5% of patients with radiation enteritis have lesions that require surgical intervention; these include perforation, fistula, stricture, and hemorrhage.[347] Other estimates of postradiation injury vary widely (i.e., 6.7% to 36%[348,349]), but the data must be considered approximate because of patients lost to follow-up.

The natural history of clinically established radiation enteritis has been reviewed. It is a progressive disease in which complications including malabsorption developed in about half of those surviving the initial lesion.[347] In one study, symptoms of chronic radiation enteritis became apparent in most cases within a year of treatment but sometimes not for 10 or more years. A report exists on the occurrence of radiation-induced intestinal pseudo-obstruction 30 years after radiotherapy.[350] Intestinal disaccharidases can be reduced or a blind loop syndrome can occur with bowel damage or partial obstruction. Surgical intervention requiring intestinal bypass or resection can result in additional malabsorption.[351] The combination of damage and resection can be severe enough to result in the short bowel syndrome. Enteral or parenteral nutrition might be necessary to maintain a good nutritional status (see Chap. 54).

### Colectomy

Resection of the right colon with the ileocecal valve and a portion of the distal ileum can be associated with watery diarrhea, in large part because of entry of increased amounts of bile salts into the colon as well as because of functional loss of the valve.[352] Even if the distal ileum is functionally intact, significant losses of water and sodium can occur through the ileostomy within the first 10 days. However, most patients adapt and decrease the fluid and electrolyte losses. Generally these stabilized individuals will lose 300 to 600 ml of water daily with 40 to 100 meq of sodium and 2.5 to 10 meq of potassium, emphasizing the physiologic role of the colon in absorbing water and sodium and in exchanging potassium for sodium. A small portion of patients fail to adapt; these include those with some underlying disease of the ileum. Such patients require special care to assure adequate water and electrolyte intake to meet their needs. In those who adapt well, an episode of gastroenteritis, partial intestinal obstruction, or prolonged excessive sweating cause additional losses and dehydration. With progressive salt loss, reduction of sodium concentration in the ileostomy output occurred; this was accompanied by increased potassium concentration.[353]

### Chemotherapy

**Use and Side Effects.** Chemotherapeutic agents are a major method of treatment in cancer, often used in combination with surgery, radiation therapy, or both. Use of multicombination high-dose cyclical chemotherapy is common as the result of (1) the frequent resistance of malignant cells to a single drug, (2) the realization of the need to kill the entire population of neoplastic cells in order to obtain a "cure," and (3) improved understanding of the chemical actions in DNA and RNA synthesis and other cellular processes at which various chemotherapeutic agents exert their actions.

Because these drug activities are not specific to cancer cells, side effects on the host are common, with severity and type being related to the specific agent, dosage, duration of treatment, accompanying drugs, and individual susceptibility. Because the epithelial cells of the alimentary tract have a relatively rapid turnover, it is to be expected that many of the drugs affecting cell division will have adverse effects there as well as on cells in the bone marrow; in some instances, there are major effects on renal tubules as well as on hepatic, cardiac, pulmonary, and nerve cells. Table 64–3 summarizes adverse effects on appetite and on the functions of the alimentary tract of a number of anticancer drugs in current use. Quantitation of severity is obviously important.

Nausea and vomiting tend to be marked in the usually given dosages of dactinomycin, mithramycin, mitomycin, cisplatin, dacarbazine, and others. Mucositis and stomatitis are serious with bleomycin, dactinomycin, fluorouracil, and methotrexate. Diarrhea may be marked with dactinomycin, fluorouracil, hydroxyurea, and methotrexate. The use of combinations may exacerbate symptoms. Vincristine alkaloid causes neurologic damage leading to obstipation. Abdominal pain occurs with dactinomycin, cyclophosphamide, methotrexate, and vincristine. Nephrotoxicity is frequent with asparaginase, cisplatin, gallium, and methotrexate and, to a lesser extent, with some others. Hormonal agents (not listed) such as dexamethasone, cytadren, tamoxifen citrate, and megestrol acetate can induce nausea and anorexia. Corticosteroids cause sodium and water retention and nitrogen and calcium loss. Cisplatin leads to renal wasting of magnesium with resultant hypokalemia and hypocalcemia if magnesium is not

given. Daunorubicin and doxorubicin are cardiotoxic. Bleomycin and busulfan can induce pulmonary toxicity. The immunotherapeutic agent interleukin-2 induces hypotension, fluid retention, oliguria, and azotemia.

**Dietary Influences on Toxicity.** Can the nature of the diet alter the intestinal toxicity of certain chemotherapeutic agents? This issue has been explored periodically in laboratory animals. Bounous et al. claimed that the feeding of an elemental diet (hydrolyzed protein with a major percentage of its amino acids in free form) reduced 5-fluorouracil toxicity in humans[354] and in rats.[355] However, a series of reports have indicated that various defined-formula diets—including those with intact protein, hydrolyzed protein, or free amino acids—have failed to exert a beneficial effect against this drug on intestinal function or body weight.[356–358]

Bounous et al.[359] and others[356] reported that elemental diets may actually increase the lethal effect of this drug. Rats fed a chemically defined liquid diet and injected intraperitonelly with methotrexate showed a marked increase in mortality from severe enteritis compared to those rats on a chow diet.[360] The defined diet delayed clearance of the drug from serum and intestinal tissue. The enhanced toxicity was reversible by feeding rats the chow diet within 24 hours before drug injection. A protein-depleted diet markedly increased the incidence of hemorrhagic cystitis in rats with Morris hepatoma given cyclophosphamide; protein-repleted rats were free of this complication.[361]

**Dietary Influences on Tumor Responsiveness: Experimental.** Does diet composition or nutritional status influence the antitumor effectiveness of chemotherapy? Enhanced tumor responsiveness occurred following methotrexate administra-

**Table 64–3. Alimentary Tract Effects of Cancer Chemotherapeutic Agents**

| Drug | Effect* | Drug | Effect* |
|------|---------|------|---------|
| AMSA | N,V,D,M | Fluorouracil | N,V,M |
| Asparaginase | A,N,V | Gallium nitrate | sl N,V |
| Bleomycin | N,V,D.M | Hydroxyurea | N,V,M,D |
| Busulfan | N,V | Methotrexate | A,N,U,P,M |
| Carmustine (BCNU) | A,N,V | Methyl GAG | N,V,D,E,M |
| Cyclophosphamide† | A,N,V,P | Mitomycin | N,V,D |
| Cytarabine | N,V,M | Procarbazine | A,N,U |
| Dacarbazine | N,V | Streptozocin | N,V,D |
| Dactinomycin | A,N,V,C,M,P | Vinblastine | N,V,P,O |
| Doxorubicin‡ | A,N,V,M | Vincristine | N,V,P,O |
| Daunorubicin | A,N,V,M | Vindesine (DVA) | O,sl N,V |
| Cisplatin | A,N,V | | |

*A = anorexia, N = nausea, D = diarrhea, E = esophagitis, M = mucositis, P = abdominal pain, O = obstipation, U = intestinal ulceration
†Cytoxan
‡Adriamycin

tion when rats previously protein depleted were protein repleted.[362] When methotrexate was administered to rats with transplanted mammary tumors 2 hours after initiation of various nutritional regimens, significant reduction in tumor volume occurred in those animals given TPN or parenteral amino acids as compared to those on a protein-depleted diet.[363]

**Nutritional Influences on Patient Status.** In humans, what is the influence, if any, of nutrition support in either augmenting the effectiveness or modifying the side effects of radiation therapy protocols and various chemotherapy regimens? Early retrospective and hence uncontrolled reports indicated that the undernourished cancer patient was more responsive and had fewer side effects with these treatments when given nutrition support. However, prospective studies have rather uniformly failed to find decreased toxicity or better adherence to therapeutic plan. Lowry and Brennan summarized four randomized trials of parenteral feeding in children and adults receiving radiation therapy (in some studies with chemotherapy).[273] There appeared to be no advantage in achieving the planned radiation schedule for the patients on parenteral feeding. In some cases the mortality data were documented for too short a period to be meaningful but in general indicated no difference from controls for the periods involved. Body weight was increased or better maintained with IV feeding.

The same authors summarized a number of controlled trials of intravenous feeding in cancer patients receiving various chemotherapy protocols (some also with radiation therapy).[273] The same general observations were made as with radiation; namely, while parenteral nutrition maintained the patients' weight, its provision compared to controls did not give an advantage in adherence to drug delivery scheduling or in other indicators of toxicity, infections morbidity, or reduction in requirement for blood products, transfusions, or survival. In some studies the presence of a central venous catheter was associated with an increased infection rate. The same or related controlled studies of the effect of parenteral nutrition in patients undergoing chemotherapy, radiation therapy, or both have been reviewed by Koretz, who arrived at the same conclusions.[364]

The issue of survival and the value of nutritional support merits comment. For example, improved nutrition itself can improve immune status of the debilitated individual; on the other hand, many of the drugs and radiation are immunosuppressive. In the presence of a potentially lethal malignancy, survival depends on the ultimate responsiveness of the particular neoplasm to the applied antitumor therapy. The key role of nutrition support is to improve or maintain nutrition as effectively as possible during the interval for which it is deemed necessary, i.e. in association with the clinical trial of the antitumor therapy in malnourished individuals.

Neither of the reviews mentioned above[273,364] points out that, in many of the reported studies, although parenteral nutrition was administered for only relatively short periods and often with the infusions being interrupted during outpatient periods, observations about the patients were noted over much longer periods. In other words, parenteral nutrition was often short term.[365,366] Furthermore, in some of the studies, it was apparent that some of the controls had lost so much weight that parenteral nutrition had to be instituted.

**Additional Studies of Nutritional Support.** Ascorbic acid in the high dose of 10 g daily had no advantage over a placebo in 100 patients with advanced colorectal cancer who had no previous chemotherapy.[367] The double-blind study indicated no difference in the progression of measurable disease or in survival. The same group had demonstrated earlier that this vitamin had no advantage over a placebo when given in conjunction with chemotherapy.

Investigators have reported periodically on the negative impact of certain chemotherapeutic agents or combinations on metabolism. A well-documented recent study that includes data on protein kinetics before and with chemotherapy (vinblastine, cisplatin, and bleomycin) was performed on patients with stage III testicular carcinoma.[287h] The nitrogen equilibrium present before chemotherapy changed to negative nitrogen balance; protein turnover, synthesis, and catabolism (which were initially similar to those of normal controls) decreased with the drug therapy by 23%, 34%, and 30%, respectively, despite continuing IV nutrition support.

Analysis of six randomized trials of intravenous feeding in patients with major surgery for cancer of the alimentary tract indicated that this support procedure was beneficial with respect to body weights, serum albumin, and decreased complications.[273] A randomized study of patients with gastrointestinal cancer not stratified for nutritional status indicated that 10 days of preoperative TPN was associated with significant decreases in serious postoperative complications and mortality as compared to those days without TPN.[368] Body composition studies performed initially and after 2 weeks of TPN in 17 malnourished cancer patents indicated that 8 had appreciable improvement in body cell mass and decreased extracellular mass; those patients that did not improve had advanced neoplastic disease sepsis, or both.[369] Many other studies have been performed in cancer patients before and during nutrition support. Such support was often associated with weight gain and reversal of negative nitrogen balance.[273,370]

In patients with localized esophageal cancer, both enteral and parenteral nutrition stabilized nutritional status and protein kinetics.[371] The ability of patients with untreated advanced testicular cancer to maintain normal protein kinetics (as well as nitrogen balance) on TPN has been noted.[287h] Bennegard et al. compared malnourished cancer patients with malnourished noncancer subjects before and after a period of enteral feeding; both groups responded well with weight gain and restored energy and nitrogen balance.[372] Nutrition support in malnourished children is particularly important.[365,373–375]

Evidence indicates that in at least some patients (e.g., those with advanced cancer), the weight gain tends to be primarily fat and water.[376a,376b] Balance data of minerals indicates that increased nitrogen retention and weight does not represent synthesis of expected amounts of normal lean body mass.[376a] Conflicting results have been obtained on potassium retention in cancer patients given enteral feeding,[371,372] whereas with parenteral nutrition, potassium retention tends to occur rather generally.[370] How much of the retained potassium is in new lean tissue is unknown, since the ratio of total body nitrogen to lean body mass (based on total body potassium) in cancer patients differs from the ratio in normals;[376b] others have found discordant results between total body potassium and the total body nitrogen when measured by neutron activation in patients on parenteral feedings.[377]

**Nutrition Support Recommendations.** Despite the metabolic problems, complications, and uncertainties that have been briefly mentioned here, the physician frequently must decide whether to initiate some form of nutrition support. The many and varied causes of undernutrition in these patients have been reviewed here in some detail. Because adequate nutrition support can produce the subjective and objective responses of an improved feeling of well-being, increased strength and activity, and extended life, nutrition support, where indicated, can be worth instituting as part of the overall patient care program. The following guidelines are offered:

1. For the patient with mild to moderate anorexia and taste changes, careful evaluation of food likes and dislikes and properly timed provision of attractive solid and liquid foods can make the difference between weight maintenance and loss.

2. Criteria for instituting nutrition support are progressive weight loss or the likelihood of significant weight loss if the current clinical situation persists. The specific period of active support will depend on the nature and duration of the specific antitumor therapy or therapies and on patient responsiveness.

3. Factors affecting the decision for enteral versus parenteral routes have been discussed (Chap. 54). In general, the obstructed, vomiting, or seriously ill patient who also may be leukopenic and thrombocytopenic is a candidate for parenteral nutrition through a central vein.

4. Enteral and parenteral nutrition formulations for the afebrile cancer patient are basically the same as for the mildly to moderately stressed patient wthout cancer, with due consideration for special problems related to organ failure.

5. For the seriously anorectic patient who is no longer a candidate for further antitumor therapy of any kind, who has a functioning alimentary tract, and whose quality of life is reasonably acceptable and likely to be maintained or improved by enteral feeding, this method of feeding should be used if desired by the patient.

6. For the patient with intestinal obstruction because of active abdominal disease and for whom all therapy has failed, a rapid downhill course out of a hospital is very common. This situation presents difficult emotional problems, particularly if prior use of parenteral nutrition had improved physical capacity and weight and if consideration was being given to cessation of TPN. All too frequently the physician is pressured to continue TPN in hospital or at home despite the clear statement that it has no antitumor benefit and may have its own complications. The attending physician must present the options and drawbacks of home parenteral nutrition (including financial costs); the mentally competent patient must then make the decision.

## UNPROVEN DIET AND NUTRITION CLAIMS

Cancer has its share of procedures and methods of treatment that either have never been demonstrated to be effective in scientifically acceptable clinical trials or have failed such trials. Despite this failure, a series of such methods continue to be advertised, advocated, and practiced by some individuals and groups under some beguiling phrase such as "alternative cancer therapy." The American Cancer Society maintains a file of more than 70 such unorthodox therapies.[378] Dietary and nutritional practices play a major role in most of these systems. Chapter 36 considers the issues of food fads and faddism and factors that lead individuals to embrace unproven practices.

Cancer meets four conditions that help explain the widespread and persistent appeal of unproven or disproven health claims to cancer patients and their families. First, cancer is a major disease in terms of prevalence and in its advanced forms has a relatively low and unpredictable cure rate by current medical methods; second, patients know that aggressive surgery, radiation, or chemotherapy, alone or in combinations, in the treatment of advanced disease can have serious side effects; third, physicians and others exist who will dispense one or another unproven system of treatments; and fourth, patients or their families seek out or self-administer such therapies because often they fear the effects of medically accepted treatments, have a dislike or distrust of their regular physicians, or have a general distrust of scientific medicine and of governmental regulations on drugs, health, and other matters.[379]

Descriptions of such treatments unproven or disproven have been published.[379-382] Chapter 25 reviews in some detail amygdalin ("laetrile") and "pangamic acid"—two major props of such treatments. Herbert has reviewed the subject from the viewpoints of criteria of the scientific method, the operations of quacks and their costs, and legal actions that have been undertaken to curb this problem.[383]

It is highly desirable for physicians, dietitians, and nurses who care for cancer patients to be aware of the extent of this problem, to know the details of some of the more common components of unproven systems of care, and to be willing to frankly discuss this area with patients who ask questions about such methods.

The reasons for an informed and understanding approach to patients on this issue are underscored by data collected on cancer patients by Cassileth et al.[384] Three hundred and four cancer center inpatients were interviewed, as were 356 patients with cancer (primarily outpatients) under the care of "unorthodox" practitioners; 202 (31%) of the total were on conventional (i.e., medically accepted) therapy only; 325 (49%) were on both conventional and unorthodox therapy; and 53 (8%) were on the unorthodox therapy only.

With reference to 171 patients on both therapies who received chemotherapy and/or radiation and/or surgery, it was found that an additional 10% of

patients had refused recommended chemotherapy, 9% had refused recommended radiation therapy, and 2% had refused recommended surgery. Of the 53 patients only on unorthodox therapy, 28% had refused recommended chemotherapy, 26% had refused recommended radiation therapy and 28% had refused recommended surgery. Patients on the combination of conventional and unorthodox treatment tended to be better educated than those on conventional treatment only. Of the 325 patients on the two types of therapies, 64% had sought conventional treatment first, adding alternative treatment an average of 24 months later; while 60% continued both systems of treatment, 40% had discontinued conventional care entirely after an average of 8 months. This study revealed that it was physicians (constituting 60% of unorthodox practitioners) who played a very active role in prescribing unorthodox treatments for the 378 patients receiving such therapies, particularly "metabolic," megavitamin, and "immune" treatments.

Of those patients on dual systems, 75% had informed their regular physicians of their adoption of alternative care; 39% of conventional physicians reacted with disapproval to this information, while 30% were supportive and 12% were neutral. Disapproval resulted in refusal of further physician treatment in 4% of patients. Unfortunately, no data are provided on the nature of the unorthodox treatments that led to rejection, disapproval, or approval.

In my opinion, "benign" unorthodox therapies such as a reasonable dietary variation, routine supplementary vitamins, innocuous glandular extracts, imagery, or spiritual guidance including "laying on of hands" would be acceptable in addition to medically indicated therapies. However, there is a real basis for physician concern about vigorous coffee enemas (which have been associated with deaths),[385] high-dose Laetrile by mouth, and persistent use of extreme diets deficient or excessive in one or more essential nutrients. The latter types of therapies call for an informed and calm discussion of potential dangers and an effort to discontinue or reduce their use; if the patient persists, sufficiently close follow-up is necessary to detect and act on incipient metabolic abnormalities. Support of the patient, including continuation of indicated chemotherapy, radiation, or surgery, rather than patient rejection, is the goal.

While Cassileth et al.[384] provide no data on why 40% of those on conventional therapy later discontinued it, it is possible that lack of support by the medical care team played a role. Members of the group of patients willing to use both systems of therapy are intermediate among the three groups in their attitudes about the value of medically accepted therapies. As such they tend to respond positively to informative and continuing discussions about their therapy and the need for persevering with it. A major attraction of unproven therapies is the argument that they are painless and without side effects such as hair loss, immune system depression, bone marrow depression, and infection. An understanding by the patient and family members as to why the effects of chemotherapy and radiation are worth undergoing is not likely to be obtained by a very brief, even though reassuring, statement by a physician, without any real opportunity for adequate discussion. Patients (and/or families and friends) read in the press or in "alternative therapy" group publications about statements in recognized medical publications such as that concluding that "35 years of intense effort focused largely on improving treatment must be judged a qualified failure."[386]

There is another reason why health professionals should be conversant and concerned about this issue namely, the need to inform the public, the press, and members of various legislatures about the personal and societal costs of health frauds. The failures of the health professions as well as the press and legislators are made clear in the review of the debacle with Laetrile.[387] At least 21 legislatures passed and governors approved decriminalization of this agent; such laws are still on the books in most of these states. Such legislation was a fundamental attack on the integrity of the Food, Drug, and Cosmetic Act and on the powers of the Food and Drug Administration by giving state appointees power without adequate investigational authority to approve a federally unapproved substance, thus opening the door to legalized charlatanism. It misled the public by giving the false impression that Laetrile was safe. It derogated the role of physicians as patient advocates by mis-stating health facts to the public and introducing potential mistrust between physician and patient. The obvious failure of the health professions to exert significant influence in many states should stimulate long-term educational activities at many levels to better resist the successors to krebiozen and Laetrile, whatever they may be.

## REFERENCES

1a. Tannenbaum: Cancer Res. *5*:616, 1945.
1b. Tannenbaum, Silverstone: Adv. Cancer Res. *1*:451, 1953.
2a. Boutwell, Brush, Rusch: Cancer Res. *9*:741, 1949.
2b. Boissonveault, Elson, Pariza: J. Nat. Cancer Inst. *76*:335, 1986.
3. Carroll, Khor: Prog. Biochem. Pharmacol. *10*:308, 1975.
4. Thompson, Meeken, Tagliaferro, et al.: Nutr. Cancer *7*:37, 1985.
5. Leung, Aylworth, Meites: Proc. Soc. Exp. Biol. Med. *173*:159, 1983.
6a. Ross, Bras: J. Nutr. *87*:245, 1965.
6b. Ross, Bras, Ragbeer: J. Nutr. *100*:177, 1970.
6c. Ross, Bras: J. Nutr. *103*:944, 1973.
7. Kubo, Day, Good: Proc. Nat. Acad. Sci. (USA) *81*:5831, 1984.
8. Tucker: Int. J. Cancer. *23*:803, 1979.
9. Willett, Stampfer: Am. J. Epidem. *124*:17, 1986.
10. Calories and Energy Expenditure in Carcinogenesis. Proc. Symp. 2/24–25, 1986. (Pariza, Simopoulos eds) Am. J. Clin. Nutr. *45*:149–372, 1987.
11. Orten, Burn, Smith: Proc. Soc. Exp. Biol. Med. *36*:82, 1937.
12. Rowe, Grammer, Watson, et al.: Cancer *26*:436, 1970.
13. Axelrad, Leblond: Cancer *8*:339, 1955.
14. Bois, Sandborn, Messier: Cancer Res. *29*:763, 1969.
15. Alcock, Shils, Leiberman, et al.: Cancer Res. *33*:2196, 1973.
16. Barrifora, et al.: Arch. Pathol. *86*:610, 1968.
17. Copeland, Salmon: Am. J. Pathol. *22*:1059, 1946.
18. Butler, Newberne: Cancer Res. *29*:236, 1969.
19. Doll, Peto: J. Nat. Cancer Inst. *66*:1191, 1981.
20. Committee on Diet, Nutrition and Cancer: Diet, Nutrition and Cancer. National Research Council. Washington, D.C., National Academy Press, 1982.
21. Sugimura: Cancer *49*:1970, 1982.
22. Hartman: Environ. Mutagen. *5*:111, 1983.
23. Ames: Science *221*:1256, 1983.
24. Prival: Nutr. Cancer *6*:236, 1984.
25. Huberman, Barr (eds.): The Role of Chemicals and Radiation in the Etiology of Cancer. New York, Raven Press, 1985.
26. Miller: Cancer Res. *38*:1479, 1978.
27. Poierier: Am. J. Clin. Nutr. *45*:185, 1987.
28. Boutwell: Cancer Res. (Suppl.) *43*:2465S, 1983.
29. Wattenberg: Cancer Res. (Suppl.) *43*:2448S, 1983.
30. Wattenberg: J. Natl. Cancer Inst. *60*:11, 1978: Adv. Cancer Res. *26*:197, 1978.
31. Loub, Wattenberg, Davis: J. Natl. Cancer Inst. *54*:985, 1975.
32. Campbell, Hayes: Pharmacol. Rev. *26*:171, 1974.
33. Newmark: Nutr. Cancer *6*:58, 1984.
34. Milner, Pigott, Dipple: Cancer Res. *45*:6347, 1985.
35. Ip: Fed. Proc. *44*:2573, 1985.
36. Sugiura: J. Nutr. *44*:345, 1951.
37. Conney, Miller, Miller: Cancer Res. *16*:450, 1956.
38. Yavelow, Finley, Kennedy, et al: Cancer Res. (Suppl.) *43*:2454S, 1983.
39. Birnboim: Science *215*:1247, 1982.
40. Medena, Lane, Tracey: Cancer Res. (Suppl.) *43*:2460S, 1983.
41. Ip: Am. J. Clin. Nutr. *45*:218, 1987.
42. Karmali: Am. J. Clin. Nutr. *45*:225, 1987.
43. Lands: Am. J. Clin. Nutr. *45*:235, 1987.
44. Worthington, Syrotuck, Ahmed: J. Nutr. *108*:1402, 1978.
45. Rogers, Newberne: Cancer Res. *35*:3427, 1975.
46. McCormick, Burns, Albert: J. Nat. Cancer Inst. *66*:559, 1981.
47. Reddy, et al.: Cancer Res. *35*:3426, 1975.
48. Nettesheim, Williams: Int. J. Cancer *17*:351, 1976.
49. Cohen, Wittenberg, Bryan: Cancer Res. *36*:2334, 1976.

50. Chu, Malmgren: Cancer Res. *25*:884, 1965.
51. Saffiotti, et al.: Cancer *20*:857, 1967.
52. Shamberger: J. Natl. Cancer Inst. *47*:667, 1971.
53. Smith, et al.: Cancer Res. *35*:11, 1975.
54. Sporn: Nutr. Rev. *35*:65, 1977; Fed. Proc. *35*:1332, 1976.
55. Moon, McCormick, Mehta: Cancer Res. (Suppl.) *43*:2469S, 1983.
56. Sporn, Roberts, Goodman (eds): The Retinoids. Vol 2. New York, Academic Press, 1984, pp. 327–371.
57. Peto, Doll, Buckley, et al.: Nature *290*:201, 1981.
58. Burton, Ingold: Science *224*:569, 1984.
59. Matthews-Roth: Pure Appl. Chem. *57*:717, 1985.
60. Tanaka, Abe, Miyaura, et al.: Biochem. J. *204*:713, 1982.
61. Honma, Hozumi, Abe, et al.: Proc. Nat. Acad. Sci. (USA) *80*:201, 1983.
62. Frampton, Omond, Eisman: Cancer Res. *43*:4443, 1983.
63. Dahn, Loewe, Bunton: Helv. Chim. Acta. *43*:320, 1960.
64. Mirvish, et al.: Science *177*:65, 1972.
65. Ivancovic, et al.: Z. Krebsforsch *79*:145, 1973.
66. Newberne: Science *204*:1079, 1979.
67a. Mirvish: Toxicol. Appl. Pharmacol. *31*:225, 1975.
67b. Mirvish, et al.: J. Natl. Cancer Inst. *55*:633, 1975.
68. Weisburger, Raineri: Cancer Res. *35*:3469, 1975.
69. Fong, Sivak, Newberne: J. Natl. Cancer Inst. *61*:145, 1978.
70. Dunning, Curtis, Mann: Cancer Res. *10*:454, 1959.
71. Pamukcu, Yalciner, Price, et al.: Cancer Res. *30*:2671, 1970.
72. Rakieten, et al.: Proc. Soc. Exp. Biol. Med. *137*:280, 1971.
73. DeWys, Pories, Richter, et al.: Proc. Soc. Exp. Biol. Med. *135*:17, 1970.
74. Mills, Broghamer, Higgins, et al.: J. Nutr. *114*:746, 1984.
75. Mills, Broghamer, Higgins, et al.: J. Nutr. *114*:739, 1984.
76. Fisher, Fischer: Cancer *14*:547, 1961.
77. Sugimura, Birnbaum, Winitz, et al.: Arch. Biochem. Biophys. *81*:439, 1959.
78. Demopolous: J. Natl. Cancer Inst. *37*:185, 1966.
79. Ryan, Elliott: Arch. Biochem. Biophys. *125*:797, 1968.
80. Theuer: J. Nutr. *101*:223, 1971.
81. Cooney, Handschumacher: Annu. Rev. Pharmacol. *10*:421, 1970.
82. Capizzi, Bertino, Handschumacher: Annu. Rev. Med. *21*:433, 1970.
83. Rosen, Sotobayashi, Nichol: Proc. Am. Assoc. Cancer Res. *5*:54, 1964.
84. Rosen, Hihich, Nicol: Vitam. Horm. *22*:609, 1964.
85. Morris, Robertson: J. Natl. Cancer Inst. *3*:479, 1943.
86. Gailani, Holland, Nussbaum, et al.: Cancer *21*:975, 1968.
87. Bullough: Br. J. Cancer *4*:329, 1950.
88. Mider: Annu. Rev. Med. *4*:187, 1953.
89. Henderson, LePage: Cancer Res. *19*:887, 1959.
90. Lundholm, Edstrom, Karlberg, et al.: Cancer Res. *40*:2516, 1980.
91. Mordes, Rossini: Science *213*:565, 1981.
92. Begg, Dickinson: Cancer Res. *11*:409, 1951.
93. Allison, Wannemacher, Hilf, et al.: J. Nutr. *54*:593, 1954.
94. Daly, Copeland, Dudrick, et al.: J. Surg. Res. *28*:507, 1980.
95. King, Boelhouwer, Kingsnorth, et al.: J. Parenter. Enteral. Nutr. *9*:422, 1985.
96. Hak, Raasch, Hammer et al.: J. Parenter. Enteral. Nutr. *8*:657, 1984.
97. Mahaffey, Copeland, Economides, et al.: J. Pediatr. Surg. *20*:775, 1985.
98. Buzby, Mullen, Stein: Cancer *45*:2940, 1980.
99. Popp, Wagner, Brito: Surgery *94*:300, 1983.
100. Tachibana, Hiraoka, Moriguchi, et al.: J. Parenter. Enteral. Nutr. *9*:428, 1985.
101. Suskind (ed.): Malnutrition and the Immune Response. New York, Raven Press, 1977.
102. Law, Dudrick, Abdou: Ann. Surg. *179*:168, 1974.
103. Copeland, Macfadyen, Dudrick: Ann. Surg. *184*:60, 1976.
104. Stoerk, Emerson: Proc. Soc. Exp. Biol. Med. *70*:703.
105. Worthington, Syrotuck, Admed: J. Nutr. *108*:1402, 1978.
106. Jose, Cooper, Good: Nature *231*:323, 1971.
107. Jose, Good: J. Exp. Med. *137*:1, 1973.
108. McCarrick, Ikeda, Ziegler: J. Parenter. Enteral. Nutr. *10*:21–28, 1986.
109a. Dionigi, Zonta, Dominioni, et al.: Ann. Surg. *185*:467, 1977.
109b. Serrou, Cupissol: Cancer Treatment Reports 65 (Suppl 5):*115*, 1981.
109c. Daly, Copeland, Quinn, et al.: Surg. Forum *27*:113.
110. Meakins, Pietsch, Bubenick, et al.: Ann. Surg. *186*:241, 1977.
111. Hoffman: Cancer and Diet. Baltimore, Williams & Wilkins, 1937.
112. Lowenthal (ed): Nutrition in cancer causation and prevention. Cancer Res. *43* (Suppl 5) 2386S–2519S, 1983.
113. Byers, Graham: Adv. Cancer Res. *41*:1–69, 1984.
114. Willett, McMahon: N. Engl. J. Med. *310*:633; 310:697, 1984.
115. Wynder: Cur. Concepts Nutr. *13*:171, 1984.
116. Reddy, Cohen (eds): Diet, Nutrition and Cancer. A Critical Evaluation. Vol 1. Macronutrients and Cancer. Boca Raton, Fl, CRC Press, 1986.
117. Byers, Graham: Adv. Cancer Res. *41*:42–43, 1984.
118. Marshall, Graham, Mettlin, et al.: Nutr. Cancer *3*:145, 1982.
119. Ahlbom: Acta Radiol. *18*:163, 1937.
120. Larrson, Sandstrom, and Westling: Cancer Res. *35*:3308, 1975.
121. Cook-Mozaffari, Azordegan, Day, et al.: Br. J. Cancer *39*:293, 1979.
122. Day: Cancer Res. *35*:3304, 1975.
123. Tuyns: Nutr.Cancer *5*:195, 1983.
124. Wynder, Bross: Cancer *14*:389, 1961.
124a. American Cancer Society: Cancer Facts and Figures 1987, New York, Am. Cancer Soc., 1987.
125. Nagai, Hashimoto, Yanagawa, et al.: Cancer *3*:257, 1982.
125a. Munoz, Wahrendorf, Bang, et al.: Lancet *2*:111, 1985.
126. Hirayama: Cancer Res. *35*:3460, 1975.
127. Haenzel, Correa: Cancer Res. *35*:3452, 1975.
128. Kolonel, Nomura, Hirohata, et al.: Am. J. Clin. Nutr. *34*:2478, 1981.
129. Haenzel: J. Nutr. Cancer Inst. *26*:37, 1961.
130. Committee on Nitrate and Alternative Curing Agents in Food, National Academy of Sciences: The Health Effects of Nitrate, Nitrite and N-nitroso Compounds, Natl. Acad. Press, Washington, D.C., 1981.
131. See Ref 130: Tables 5–20 and 5–21, pp 5-48, 5-49.

132. See Ref 130: pp 5-53, 5-54.
133. See Ref 130: Chapter 8.
134. See Ref 130: Table 8-2, pp 8-11.
135. Ruddell, Bone, Hill, et al.: Lancet *1*:521, 1978.
136. Ruddell, Axon, Findlay, et al.: Lancet *1*:672, 1980.
137. Tannenbaum, Fett, Young, et al.: Science *200*:1487, 1978.
138. See Ref 130: pp 8-15 to 8-17.
139a.Scanlan: Cancer Res. (Suppl. 43): 2435S, 1983.
139b.Mirvish: Cancer *58*:1842, 1986.
140a.U.S. Dept. Agriculture. Fed. Register. *43*:20992, 1978.
140b.Issenberg: Fed. Proc. *35*:1322, 1976.
141a.See Ref 130: pp 9-3 to 9-17.
141b.See Ref 130: pp 10-33, 10-34.
142. Correa, Haenzel: Adv. Cancer Res. *26*:1, 1978.
143. Hirayama: Cancer Res. *35*:3460, 1975.
144. Correa: Cancer Res. *35*:3395, 1975.
145. Haenzel, Correa: Cancer *28*:14, 1975.
146. Hill, MacLennan, Newcombe: Lancet *1*:436, 1979.
147. Wynder: Cancer Res. *35*:3388, 1975.
148. Gregor, Toman, Prusova: Gut *10*:1031, 1969.
149. Drasar, Irving: Br. J. Cancer *27*:167, 1973.
150. Armstrong, Doll: Int. J. Cancer *18*:617, 1975.
151. Berg, Howell: Cancer *34*:807, 1974.
152. Jain, Cook, Davis, et al.: Int. J. Cancer *26*:757, 1980.
152a.Kolonel, Hankin, Nomura, et al.: Cancer Res. *41*:3727, 1981.
153. Manousas, Day, Trichopoulos, et al.: Int. J. Cancer *32*:1, 1983.
154. McKeown-Eyssen, Bright-See: Nutr. Cancer *6*:160, 1984.
155. McKeown-Eyssen, Bright-See: Nutr. Cancer *7*:251, 1985.
156. Ref. omitted
157. Reddy, Hedges, Laakso, et al.: Cancer *42*:2832, 1978.
158. Modan, Barrell, Lubin, et al.: J. Nat. Cancer Inst. 55:15, 1975.
159. Shils: Nutrition and neoplasia. *In* Modern Nutrition and Health and Disease (Goodhart, Shils, eds.) 6th Ed. Philadelphia, Lea & Febiger, 1980.
160. Potter, McMichael: J. Nat. Cancer Inst. *76*:566, 1976.
161. Hirayama: Nutr. Cancer *1*:67, 1979.
162. Kinlen: Lancet *1*:946, 1982.
163. Walker, Walker, Walker: Br. J. Cancer *53*:489, 1986.
164. Enstrom: *In* Cancer Incidence in Defined Populations (Cairns, Lyon, Skolnick, eds.) Cold Spring Harbor. New York, Cold Spring Harbor Laboratory, 1980, pp 69–90.
165. Lyon, Sorenson: Am. J. Clin. Nutr. *31*:S227, 1978.
166. See Ref 20, p 17-11.
167. See Ref 20, p 1-7.
168. Talbot: Fed. Proc. *40*:2337, 1981.
168a.Editorial: Lancet *1*:782, 1987.
169. Potter, McMichael: J. Nat. Cancer Inst. *76*:557, 1986.
170. See Ref 20, p 5-21.
171a.Williams, Sorlie, Fernleib, et al.: J.A.M.A. *245*:247, 1981.
171b.Sidney, Friedman, Hiatt: Am. J. Epidemiol *124*:33, 1986.
171c.Tornberg, Holm, Carstensen, et al.: N. Engl. J. Med. *315*:1629, 1986.
171d.Mannes, Maier, Thieme, et al.: N. Engl. J. Med. *315*:1634, 1986.
172. Haenzel, Berg, Segi, et al.: J. Natl. Cancer Inst. *51*:1765, 1973.

173. Burkitt: Lancet *2*:1229, 1969.
174. Burkitt, Walker, Painter: Lancet *2*:1408, 1972.
175. Glober, Klein, Moore, et al.: Lancet *2*:80, 1974.
176. Harvey, Pomare, Heaton: Lancet *1*:1278, 1973.
177. Eastwood, Kirkpatrick, Mitchell, et al.: Br. Med. J. *4*:392, 1973.
178. Walter, Baird, Davies, et al.: Br. Med. J. *2*:536, 1975.
179. Reference omitted.
180. Glober, Kamiyama, Nomura, et al.: Lancet *2*:110, 1977.
181. International Agency for Research in Cancer: Lancet *2*:207, 1977.
182a.Aries, Crowther, Drasar et al.: Gut. *10*:334, 1969.
182b.Hill: Cancer Res. *35*:3398, 1975.
183. Owen, Dodo, Thompson, et al.: Nutr. Cancer *9*:73, 1987.
184. Lipkin: Gastroenterology *92*:1083, 1987.
185. Wargovich, Eng, Newmark, et al.: Carcinogenesis *4*:1205, 1983.
186. Wargovich, Eng, Newmark: Cancer Lett. *23*:253, 1984.
187. Newmark, Wargovich, Bruce: J. Nat. Cancer Inst. *72*:1325, 1984.
188. Lipkin, Newmark: N. Engl. J. Med. *313*:1381, 1985.
189. Hemmings, Holbrook, Yuspa: J. Cell Physiol. *116*:265, 1983.
190a.Simpson, Arnold: Endocrinology *119*:2284, 1986.
190b.Miyaura, Aye, Suda: Endocrinology *115*:1891, 1984.
191. Staszewski, Haenszel: J. Natl. Cancer Inst. *35*:291, 1965.
192. Staszewski, McCall, Stenhouse: Br. J. Cancer *25*:559, 1971.
193. Haenzel, Kurihara: J. Natl. Cancer Inst. *40*:43, 1968.
194. Dunn: Cancer Res. *35*:3240, 1975.
195. Weisburger, Cohen, Wynder: *In* Origin of Human Cancer (Hiatt, Watson, Winsten, eds.) Cold Spring Harbor, New York, Cold Spring Harbor Laboratory, 1977, pp 584-594.
196. Schatzkin, Jones, Hoover, et al.: N. Engl. J. Med. *316*:1169, 1987.
197. Lea: Lancet *2*:323, 1966.
198. Carroll, Gammal, Plunkett: Can. Med. Assoc. J. *98*:590, 1968.
199. Armstrong, Doll: Int. J. Cancer *15*:617, 1975.
200. Hems: Br. J. Cancer *37*:974, 1978.
201. Gray, Pike, Henderson: Br. J. Cancer *39*:1, 1979.
202. Miller, Kelly, Choi, et al.: Am. J. Epidemiol. *107*:499, 1978.
203. Lubin, Burns, Blot, et al.: Int. J. Cancer: *28*:685, 1981.
204. Graham, Marshall, Mettin, et al.: Am. J. Epidemiol. *116*:68, 1982.
205. Hirohata, Shigamatsu, Nomura, et al.: Natl. Cancer Inst. Monogr. *69*:187, 1985.
205a.Nomura, Hirohata, Kolonel, et al.: Natl. Cancer Inst. Monogr. *69*:191, 1985.
206a.Ingram: Nutr. Cancer *3*:75, 1981.
206b.Key, Darby, Pike: Nutr. Cancer *10*:1, 1987.
207. Willett, Stampfer, Colditz et al.: N. Eng. J. Med. *316*:22, 1987.
208a.Natl. Cancer Inst.: DHHS Publ. No (NIH) *84*:2671, 1984.
208b.DeWys, Malone, Butrum, et al.: Cancer *58*:1954, 1986.
208c.Wynder, Rose, Cohen: Cancer *58*:1804, 1986.
209. Zollinger, Phillips, Kuzma: Am. J. Epidemiol. *119*:503, 1984.

210. Ward-Hinds, Kolonel, Nomura, et al.: Br. J. Cancer *45*:118, 1982.
211. de Waard, Cornelis, Aoki, et al.: Cancer *40*:126, 1977.
212. Buell: J. Natl. Cancer Inst. *51*:1479, 1973.
213a.Garfinkel: Ann Intern. Med. *103*:1034, 1985.
213b.Dubin, Hutter, Strax, et al.: J. Natl. Cancer Inst. *73*:1273, 1984.
213c.Greenberg, Vessey, McPherson, et al.: Br. J. Cancer *51*:691, 1985.
214. Kelsey: Am. J. Epidemiol. *1*:74, 1979.
215. Mohla, Criss: The relationship of diet to cancer and hormones. *In* Nutrition and Cancer. Etiology and Treatment. (Newell, Ellison, eds.) New York, Raven Press, 1981, pp 93–110.
216. Rose, Boyar: In Ref 116, p 151.
217. Wynder, Escher, Mantel: Cancer *19*:489, 1966.
218. Elwood, Cole, Rothman, et al.: J. Natl. Cancer Inst. *59*:1055, 1977.
219. Annegers, Strom, Decker, et al.: Cancer *43*:723, 1979.
220. Hildreth, Kelsey, LiVolsi, et al.: Am. J. Epidemiol. *114*:398, 1981.
221. Cramer, Welch, Hutchison, et al.: Obstet. Gynecol. *63*:833, 1984.
222. Hirayama: Natl. Cancer Inst. Monogr. *53*:149–154, 1979.
222a.Kolonel, Hinds, Nomura, et al.: Natl. Cancer Inst. Mongr. *69*:137, 1985.
223. Willett, Polk, Morris, et al.: Lancet *2*:130, 1983.
224. World Health Organization: W.H.O. Tech. Rep. Ser. No. 691, 1983.
225. Arthur, Hall, Wright: Lancet *1*:607, 1984.
226. Higginson: Gastroenterology *57*:587, 1969.
226a.See Ref 20: pp 17–11, 17–12.
227. Munoz, Linsell: Epidemiology of primary liver cancer. *In* Epidemiology of Cancer of the Digestive Tract (Correa, Haenzel, eds.) Hague, Netherlands, Martinus Nijhoff, 1982.
228. Enwonwu: Lancet *2*:956, 1984.
229. Kessler: J. Natl. Cancer Inst. *44*:673, 1970.
230. Wynder, Mabuchi, Maruchi, et al.: J. Natl. Cancer Inst. *50*:645, 1973.
231. Armstrong, Lea, Adelstein, et al.: Br. J. Prev. Soc. Med. *30*:151, 1976.
232. Lea: Ann. R. Coll. Surg. Engl. *41*:432, 1967.
233. Hirayama: *In* Origins of Human Cancer (Hiatt, Watson, Winsten, eds). Cold Spring Harbor, New York, Cold Spring Harbor Laboratory, 1977, pp 55–75.
234a.Committee on Diet, Nutrition and Cancer: National Research Council. Ishii, Nakamura, Ozaki, et al.: cited p 17–13.
234b.Gold, Gordis, Diener et al.: Cancer *55*:460, 1985.
235. Norell, Ahlbom, Erwald, et al.: Am. J. Epidemiol. *124*:894, 1986.
236. MacMahon, Yen, Trichopolous, et al.: N. Engl. J. Med. *304*:630, 1981.
237. Hinds, Kolonel, Lee, et al.: Br. J. Cancer: *41*:929, 1980.
238. Blot, Fraumeni, Stone: Cancer *42*:373, 1978.
239. Lin and Kessler: J.A.M.A. *245*:147, 1981.
240. Bjelke: Int. J. Cancer. *15*:561, 1975.
241. Hennekens: (Editorial) N. Engl. J. Med. *315*:1288, 1986.
242. Shekelle, Lepper, Liu, et al.: Lancet *2*:1185, 1981.
243. Ziegler, Mason, Steinhagen, et al.: Am. J. Epidemiol. *123*:1080, 1986.
244. Menkes, Comstock, Vuilleumier, et al.: N. Engl. J. Med. *315*:1250, 1986.

245. Nomura, Stemmerman, Heilbrun, et al.: Cancer Res. *45*:2369, 1985.
246. Stahelin, Rosel, Buess, et al.: J. Natl. Cancer Inst. *73*:1463, 1984.
247. Willett, Polk, Underwood, et al.: N. Engl. J. Med. *310*:430, 1984.
248. Friedman, Blaner, Goodman, et al.: Am. J. Epidemiol. *123*:781, 1986.
249. Saloneu, Saloneu, Lappetaläinen, et al.: Br. Med. J. *290*:417, 1985.
250a.Forbes: Am. J. Clin. Nutr. *43*:629, 1986.
250b.N.Y. Acad. Med.: Statement and Resolution Regarding Proposed Revision of FDA Regulations Concerning Disease Related Health Claims on Labels. Bull. N.Y. Acad. Med. *63*:410, 1987.
250c.Federal Register. FDA 21 CFR Pt. 101: Food Labeling; Public Health Messages on Food Labels and Labeling. *52*:No. 149, 28843–28849, 8/4/1987.
250d.Morton, Sox, Krupp: Ann. Intern. Med. *95*:568, 1981.
251. Symposium: Neuropeptidergic Regulation of Food Intake: Fed. Proc. *43*:2888–2906, 1984.
252a.Chance, Von Meyenfeldt, Fischer: Neurosc. Behav. Rev. *7*:471, 1983.
252b.Chance, von Meyenfeldt, Fischer: Pharmacol. Biochem. Behav. *18*:115, 1983.
253a.Chance, Van Lammeren, Chen, et al.: J. Surg. Res. *36*:490, 1984.
253b.Van Lammeren, Chance, Fischer: Peptides *5*:97, 1984.
254a.Morrison: Cancer Res. *42*:3642, 1982.
254b.Moley, Morrison, Norton: Cancer Res. *45*:4925, 1985.
254c.Chance, Muggia-Sullam, Chen, et al.: J. Natl. Cancer Inst. *77*:497, 1986.
255. Baille, Millar, Pratt: Am. J. Physiol. *209*:296, 1965.
256. Schiffman: N. Engl. J. Med. *308*:1275; *308*:1337, 1983.
257. Weiner: Intl. J. Eating Disorders *4*:347, 1985.
258. Bartoshuk: Am. J. Clin. Nutr. *31*:1068, 1978.
259. DeWys, Walters: Cancer *36*:1888, 1975.
260. Kamath, Booth, Lad, et al.: Cancer *52*:386, 1983.
261. Williams, Cohen: Am. J. Clin. Nutr. *31*:122, 1978.
262. Carson, Gormican: J. Am. Diet. Assoc. *70*:361, 1977.
263. Settle, Quinn, Kare: Cited in Shamberger, J. Natl. Cancer Inst.*47*:667, 1971.
264. Trant, Serin, Douglass: Am. J. Clin. Nutr. *36*:44, 1982.
265. Nielsen, Theologides, Vickers: Am. J. Clin. Nutr. *33*:2253, 1980.
266. Bernstein: Cancer Res. (Suppl.) *42*:715S, 1982.
267. Bernstein, Fenner: Appetite J. Intake Res. *4*:79, 1983.
268. Morrison: Cancer Res. (Suppl.) *42*:720S, 1982.
269. Goodlad: *In* Mammalian Protein Metabolism. Vol. 2 (Munro, Allison, eds.) New York, Academic Press, 1964, pp. 415–444.
270. DeWys: Cancer Res. (Suppl.) *42*:721, 1982.
271. Lawson, Richmond, Nixon, et al.: Ann. Rev. Nutr. *2*:227, 1982.
272a.Wesdorp, Krause, von Myenfeldt: Br. J. Surg. *70*:352, 1983.
272b.Editorial: Cancer cachexia. Lancet *1*:833, 1984.
273. Lowry, Brennan: Intravenous feeding of the cancer patient. *In* Parenteral Nutrition (Rombeau, Caldwell, eds.) Philadelphia, W.B. Saunders, 1986.
274. Costa, Vincent, Aragon: Cancer Res. *20*:387, 1979.
275a.DeWys, Begg, Lavin, et al.: Am. J. Med. *69*:491, 1980.
275b.DeWys, Begg, Band, et al.: Cancer Treatment Repts. *65*:(Suppl. 5) 87, 1981.

276a.Heymsfield, McManus, Smith, et al.: Am. J. Clin. Nutr. *36*:680, 1982.

276b.Heymsfield, McManus: Cancer *55*:238, 1985.

277. Young: Cancer Res. *37*:2336, 1977.

278. Warmold, Lundholm, Schersten: Cancer Res. *38*:1801, 1978.

279. Macfie, Burkinshaw, Oxby, et al.: Br. J. Surg. *69*:443, 1982.

280. Edstrom, Bennegard, Eden, et al.: Arch Otolaryngol. *108*:697, 1982.

281. Lindmark, Bennegard, Eden, et al.: Gastroenterology *87*:402, 1984.

282a.Knox, Crosby, Feuer, et al.: Ann. Surg. *197*:152, 1983.

282b.Dempsey, Feuer, Knox, et al.: Cancer *53*:1265, 1984.

283a.Waterhouse: Cancer *33*:66, 1974.

283b.Holroyde, Gabuzda, Putnam, et al.: Cancer Res. *35*:3710, 1975.

283c.Gold: Oncology *22*:185, 1986.

283d.Chlebowski, Bulcavage, Grosvenor, et al.: Cancer *59*:406, 1987.

283e.Kokal, McCulloch, Wright, et al.: Ann. Surg. *198*:601, 1983.

283f.Lundholm, Edström, Karlberg, et al.: Cancer *50*:1142, 1982.

284. Burt, Gorschboth, Brennan: Cancer *49*:1092, 1982.

285. Shaw, Wolfe: Surgery *101*:181, 1987.

286. Waterhouse, Jeanprete, Keilson: Cancer Res. *39*:1966, 1979.

287a.Carmichael, Claque, Kier, et al.: Br. J. Surg. *67*:736, 1980.

287b.Norton, Stein, Brennan: Ann. Surg. *194*:123, 1981.

287c.Heber, Chlebowski, Ishibashi, et al.: Cancer Res. *42*:4815, 1982.

287d.Kien, Camitta: Cancer Res. *43*:5586, 1983.

287e.Lapidat, Nissim, Shaklai, et al.: Clin. Sci. *66*:147, 1984.

287f.Jeevanadam, Horowitz, Lowry, et al.: Lancet *1*:1423, 1984.

287g.Kien, Camitta: J. Parenter. Enteral Nutr. *11*:129, 1987.

287h.Herrmann, Garnick, Moore, et al.: Surgery *90* 381, 1984.

287i.Glass, Fern, Garlick: Clin. Sci. *64*:101, 1983.

288. Mullen, Buzby, Gertner, et al.: Surgery *87*:331, 1980.

289. Nakahara, Fukuoka: Adv. Cancer Res. *5*:157, 1958.

290. Masuno, Yoshimura, Ogawe, et al.: Eur. J. Cancer Clin. Oncol. *20*:1177, 1984.

291. Kitada, Hayes, Mead, et al.: Lipids *15*:168, 1980; J. Cell. Biochem. *20*:409, 1982.

292. Kawakami, Cerami: J. Exp. Med. *154*:631, 1981.

293. Pekala, Lane, Cerami: Proc. Natl. Acad. Sci., USA *79*:912, 1982.

294. Torti, Dieckmann, Beutler, et al.: Science *229*:867, 1985.

295. Old, Science *230*:630, 1985.

296a.Ruddle, Powell, Conta: Lymphokine Res. *2*:25, 1983.

296b.Dinarello: N. Engl. J. Med. *311*:1413, 1984.

297. Pearse: Int. Surg. *64*:5, 1979.

298. Stevens, Moore: Lancet *1*:118, 1983.

299. Odell, Wolfsen, Yoshimoto, et al.: Trans. Am. Phys. *90*:204, 1977.

300. Creutzfeldt (ed): Gastrointestinal hormones. Clinics in Gastroenterology *9*:#3, 1980. Philadelphia, W.B. Saunders.

301. Odell, Wolfsen: Annu. Rev. Med. *29*:379, 1978.

302. Shimoda, Saunders, Rubin: Gastroenterology *55*:705, 1968.

303. Fahrenkrug: Clin. Gastroenterol. *9*:633, 1980.

304. Townsend, Singh, Thompson: Gastroenterology *91*:1002, 1986.

305. Mundy, Ibbotson, D'Souza, et al.: N. Engl. J. Med. *310*:1718, 1984.

306. Stavros, Manolagas, Deftos: Editorial. Ann. Intern. Med. *100*:144, 1984.

307. Salassa, Jowsey, Arnaud: N. Engl. J. Med. *283*:65, 1970.

308. Drezner, Feinglos: J. Clin. Invest. *60*:1046, 1977.

309. Siris, Clemens, Dempster, et al.: Am. J. Med. *82*:307, 1987.

310. Lyles, Berry, Haussler, et al.: Ann. Intern. Med. *93*:275, 1980.

311. Rao, Parfitt, Villanueva, et al.: Am. J. Med. *82*:333, 1987.

312. Creamer: Br. Med. J. *2*:1435, 1964.

313. Barry: Gut *15*:562, 1974.

314. Hall, Finkler: Blood *27*:611, 1966.

315. Swendseid, Bethell, Bird: Cancer Res. *11*:864, 1951.

316. Schwartz, Storer: Manifestations of gastrointestinal disease. *In* Principles of surgery. 2nd Ed. (Schwartz, ed.) New York, McGraw Hill, 1974, p. 980.

317. Toskes, Gianelli, Jervis, et al.: Gastroenterology *68*:1193, 1975.

318. Novis, Banks, Marks, et al.: Quart. J. Med. *40*:521, 1971.

319. Isaacson, Wright: Lancet *1*:67, 1978.

320. Swinson, Slavin, Coles, et al.: Lancet *1*:111, 1983.

321. Waldman, Broder, Strober: Ann. N.Y. Acad. Sci. *230*:306, 1974.

322. Schnider, Mariolo: Dis. Month. (D.M.) *25*:7, 1979.

323. Isaacson, O'Connor, Spencer, et al.: Lancet *2*:688, 1985.

324. Cooper, Holmes, Ferguson, et al.: Medicine *59*:249, 1980.

325. Selby, Gallagher: Dig. Dis. Sci. *24*:684, 1979.

326. Brandt, Hagander, Norden, et al.: Acta. Med. Scand. *204*:467, 1978.

327. Austed, Cornes, Gough, et al.: Am. J. Digest. Dis. *12*:475, 1967.

328. Chencharick, Mossman: Cancer *51*:811, 1983.

329. Mossman, Schatzman, Chencharick: Intl. J. Radiat. Oncol. Biol. Phys. *8*:991, 1982.

330. Shils: Surg. Gynecol. Obstet. *132*:709, 1971.

331. Becker: Clin Gastroenterol *9*:755, 1980.

332. Riboli, Bertoglio, Arnulfo, et al.: J. Parenter. Enteral Nutr. *10*:82, 1986.

333. Leeds, Ebid, Ralph, et al.: Lancet *1*:1075, 1981.

334. Goldsmith, Ghosh, Hovos: Surg. Gynecol. Obstet. *132*:87, 1971.

335. Wollaeger, Comfort, Clagett, et al.: J.A.M.A. *137*:838, 1948.

336. Warren, Veidenheimer, Pratt: Surg. Clin North Am. *47*:639, 1967.

337. Brooks, Culebras: Am. J. Surg. *131*:516, 1976.

338. Christiansen, Olsen, Warming: Scand. J. Gastroenterol. (Suppl) *9*:189, 1971.

339. Miyata, Takao, Uozumi, et al: Ann. Surg. *179*:494, 1974.

340. Pliam, ReMine: Arch. Surg. *110*:506, 1975.

341a.Fortner, Kim, Cubilla, et al.: Ann. Surg. *186*:42, 1977.

341b.Fortner: Cancer *47*:1712, 1981.

342a.Perez, Newcomer, Moertel, et al.: Cancer *52*:346, 1983.
342b.Hofman, Poley: Gastroenterology *62*:918, 1972.
343. Rudman, Dedonis, Fountain, et al.: N. Engl. J. Med. *303*:657, 1980.
344. Shank: Primary Care and Cancer, April 1986, p. 49.
345. Wiernik: Gut *7*:149, 1966.
346. Neuman, Katsaris, Blendis, et al.: Lancet *2*:1471, 1973.
347. Galland, Spencer: Lancet *1*:1257, 1985.
348. DeCosse, Rhodes, Wentz, et al.: Ann. Surg. *170*:369, 1969.
349. Kwitko, Pieterse, Hecker, et al.: Austral. N.Z. J. Med. *12*:272, 1982.
350. Perino, Schuffer, Mehta, et al.: Gastroenterology *91*:994, 1986.
351. Beer, Fan, Halsted: Am. J. Clin. Nutr. *41*:85, 1985.
352. Weser, Fletcher, Urban: Gastroenterology *77*:572, 1979.
353. Gallagher, Harrison, Skyring: Gut *3*:219, 1962.
354. Bounous, Gentile, Hugon: Can. J. Surg. *14*:312, 1971.
355. Bounous, Hugon, Gentile: Can. J. Surg. *14*:298, 1971.
356. Stanford, King, Carey: J. Surg. Oncol. *9*:493, 1977.
357. Gardner, Heading: Clin. Sci. *56*:243, 1979.
358. Plumb, Gardner: J. Parenter. Enteral Nutr. *7*:351, 1983.
359. Bounous, Pageau, Regoli: Int. J. Clin. Pharmacol. Biopharmacol. *16*:265, 1978.
360. Harvey, McAnena, Mehta, et al.: J. Parenter. Enteral Nutr. *11*:119, 1987.
361. Daising, Grosfeld, Remley, et al.: J. Pediatr. Surg. *17*:721, 1982.
362. Reynolds, Daly, Rowlands, et al.: Cancer *45*:3069, 1980.
363. Torosian, Mullen, Miller, et al.: J. Parenter. Enteral Nutr. *7*:337, 1983.
364. Koretz: J. Clin. Oncol. *2*:534, 1984.

365. Ghavimi, Shils, Scott, et al.: J. Pediatr. *101*:530, 1982.
366. Samuels, Selig, Ogden, et al.: Cancer Treat. Rep. *65*:615, 1981.
367. Moertel, Fleming, Creagan, et al.: N. Engl. J. Med. *312*:127, 1985.
368. Müller, Brenner, Dienst, et al.: Lancet *1*:68, 1982.
369. Shizgal: Cancer *55*:250, 1985.
370. Brennan, Ekman: Cancer *54*:2627, 1984.
371. Burt, Stein, Brennan: J. Surg. Res. *34*:303, 1983.
372. Bennegard, Eden, Ekman, et al.: Gastroenterology *85*:92, 1983.
373. Van Eys, Copeland, Cangir, et al.: Med. Pediatr. Oncol. *8*:63, 1980.
374. Donaldson, Wesley, Ghavimi, et al.: Med. Pediatr. Oncol. *10*:129, 1982.
375. Rickard, Coates, Grosfeld, et al.: Cancer *58*:1904, 1986.
376a.Nixon, Lawson, Kutner, et al.: Cancer Res. *41*:2038, 1981.
376b.Cohn, Varsky, Vaswani, et al.: Nutr. Cancer *4*:99, 1982.
377. Jeejeebhoy, Baker, Wolman, et al.: Am. J. Clin. Nutr. *35*:1117, 1982.
378. American Cancer Society: Unproven Methods of Cancer Management. New York, American Cancer Society, 1979.
379. Shils, Hermann: Bull. N.Y. Acad. Med. *58*:323, 1982.
380. Olson: Drugs, cancer and charlatans. *In* Clinical Oncology (Horton, Hill, eds.) Philadelphia, W.B. Saunders, 1977, pp. 182–191.
381. Herbert: Nutr. Cancer *6*:196, 1984.
382. Bowman, Kushner, Dawson, et al.: J. Clin. Oncol. *2*:702, 1984.
383. Herbert: Cancer *58*:1930, 1986.
384. Cassileth, Lusk, Strouse, et al: Ann. Intern. Med. *101*:105, 1984.
385. Eisele, Reay: J.A.M.A. *244*:1608, 1980.
386. Bailar, Smith: N. Engl. J. Med. *314*:1226, 1986.
387. Lerner: Cancer *53*:815, 1984.

*Chapter* **65**

# NUTRITION AND DIET IN ALCOHOLISM

## Spencer Shaw and Charles S. Lieber

The relationship between nutrition and alcohol is complicated by many levels of interaction. Alcoholic beverages are themselves nutrients, predominantly providing energy, but in an intricate way. Ethanol affects the level of food intake by its displacement of required nutrients in the diet, its effect on appetite, and its multiple actions on almost every level of the gastrointestinal (GI) tract. The predominant metabolism of ethanol by the liver alters this organ and profoundly affects the metabolism of many nutrients. Ethanol alters the storage, mobilization, activation, and metabolism of nutrients and has a significant effect on almost every organ. Alcohol is directly toxic to many bodily tissues. Malnutrition may modify this effect. Alcoholism is also a major cause of nutritional deficiency syndromes. Nutritional therapy in the alcoholic, however, often may be a balance between maximizing recovery and avoiding iatrogenic complications. The multitude of physiologic systems affected by alcohol makes a simple approach difficult. Although much information has been gained about pathophysiology and the problems of iatrogenic complications, few well-controlled clinical studies are available.

## NUTRITIONAL VALUE OF ALCOHOLIC BEVERAGES

Alcoholic beverages may contain varying amounts of carbohydrates, trace elements, B vitamins (such as niacin and thiamin), and other congeners.[1] However, aside from their ethanol content, they provide little nutritive value. In unusual circumstances, toxic amounts of lead, cobalt, and iron may be present. Although various metabolic effects of several congeners have been postulated, none has been definitely established.

Alcoholic beverages provide mainly caloric food value, derived from their ethanol content. Average national consumption figures indicate ethanol accounts for 4.5% of calories in the average diet.[2] Ethanol liberates 7.1 kcal/g when combusted, and sometimes may be an overlooked source of calories in the diet for those attempting weight reduction. However, ethanol does not provide caloric food value equivalent to that of carbohydrate.

Isocaloric replacement of carbohydrate calories by ethanol (50% of total calories) in a balanced diet results in a decline in body weight[3] (Fig. 65–1). Furthermore, when given as supplemental calories, ethanol produces less weight gain than calorically equivalent food[3] (Figs. 65–2, 65–3). The mechanism by which this occurs is possibly related to an increase in the energy requirement of the body. Oxygen consumption is significantly higher in rats fed ethanol than in control animals fed isocaloric carbohydrate.[4] Furthermore, ethanol increases oxygen consumption in normal human subjects, and this effect is greater in alcoholics. Presumably, excess energy would be dissipated as heat. Evidence for malabsorption or maldigestion as an explanation for ethanol-induced energy losses has been lacking under conditions comparable to those pertaining to the studies depicted in Figures 65–2 and 65–3,[4] although intake of ethanol in higher amounts for more prolonged periods may affect the gastrointestinal tract.

## EFFECTS OF ETHANOL ON DIGESTION AND ABSORPTION

Acute and chronic alcohol consumption may profoundly alter digestion and gastrointestinal ab-sorption. The effects of ethanol, however, must often be differentiated from those of concurrent deficiency of nutrients such as folate. Many studies demonstrating acute effects of ethanol employ pharmacologic doses of ethanol in unphysiologic systems. The clinical relevance of such observations to the nutritional status of human alcoholics is often not established. Nevertheless, alterations in digestion and absorption caused by alcohol may produce marginal deficiencies or may potentiate deficiencies arising from other causes.

### Gastrointestinal Tract

The stomach is exposed to higher concentrations of ethanol than the lower gastrointestinal tract, which may explain the vulnerability of the stomach to acute damage from alcohol. Ethanol disrupts the gastric mucosal barrier[5] and is an accepted cause of acute gastritis. Its role in the production of gastric ulcer or chronic gastritis is controversial.[6] Acute gastritis may be accompanied by massive bleeding and thus may result in iron deficiency. In addition to direct toxic effects, alcohol may impair gastric emptying[7] and may increase acid secretion.[8] The latter effect may secondarily enhance absorption of non-heme iron[9] and may, in part, account for the tendency toward increased iron retention noted in some alcoholics.

The duodenum, like the stomach, is exposed to the highest concentrations of ethanol. Experimentally in the rat, ethanol-induced lesions in the in-

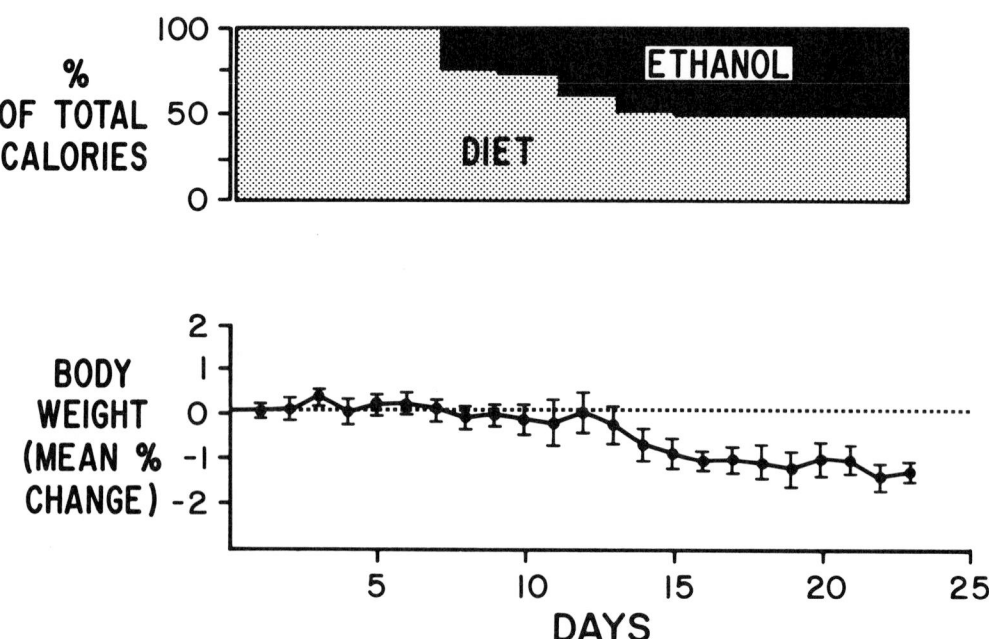

**Fig. 65–1.** Effect of the isocaloric substitution of ethanol for carbohydrate calories on body weight. Substitution of ethanol as 50% of total calories results in a decline in body weight. (From Pirola, R.C., Lieber, C.S.,[3] with permission of Pharmacology.)

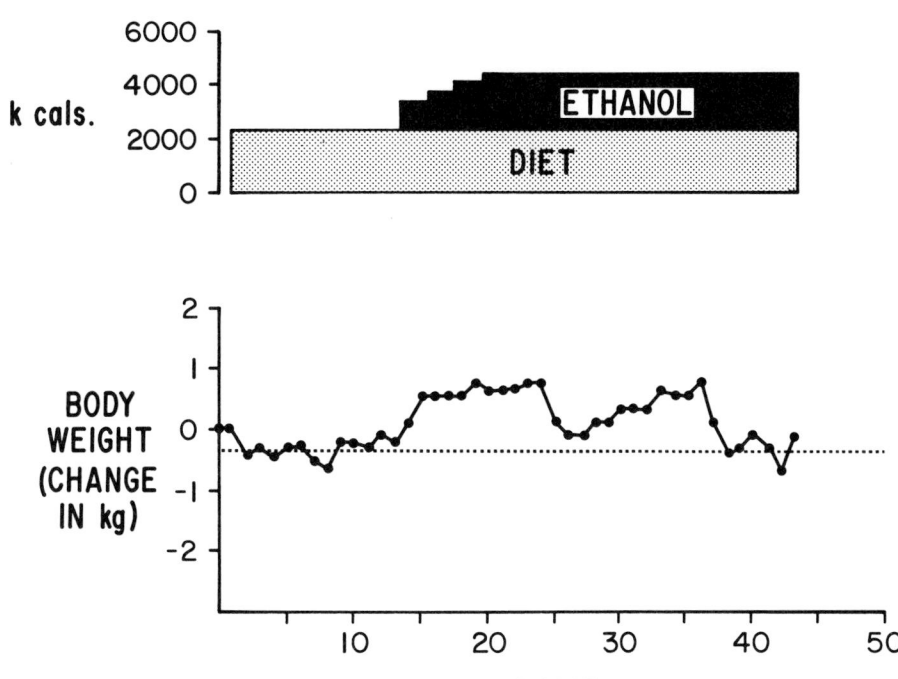

**Fig. 65–2.** Effect on body weight of the addition of alcohol-derived calories to the diet. (From Pirola, R.C., Lieber, C.S.,[3] with permission of Pharmacology.)

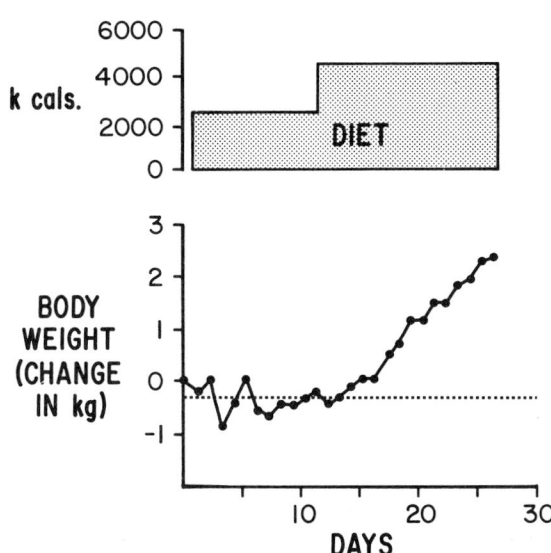

**Fig. 65–3.** Effect of nonalcohol-derived calories. Supplementary calories from ethanol produced less weight gain than calorically equivalent carbohydrate. (From Pirola, R.C., Lieber, C.S.,[3] with permission of Pharmacology.)

testine appear to be related directly to the concentration of ethanol, with the greatest damage resulting from those solutions with the highest concentrations of ethanol.[10] In man, the acute oral administration of ethanol (1 g/kg) results in endoscopic and morphologic lesions in the duodenum.[11] These lesions are patchy in nature, a condition that may explain previous failures to observe them.[12]

The morphologic effects of ethanol on the small intestine are accompanied by functional changes. Alterations in mucosal enzymes and in absorption of many nutrients have been observed.[10,13,14] Oral and intravenous alcohol produces increased type III waves (propulsive waves) in the ileum and decreased type I waves (impeding waves) in the jejunum. These changes have been proposed as possible mechanisms to explain, at least in part, the diarrhea observed in binge drinkers.[15]

Chronic ethanol consumption is associated with many alterations in intestinal function. These effects, however, must be differentiated from those resulting from nutritional deficiencies. Indeed, malnutrition may lead to intestinal malabsorption,[16,17] and folate depletion, common in alcoholics, may be especially implicated in this regard.[18–21] Impaired absorption of folate, thiamin, $B_{12}$, fat, and xylose has been described in alcoholics, with recovery after withdrawal and the institution of a nutritious diet.[19,22–25] Acute and chronic ethanol administration may impair sodium and water transport in the small intestine; this effect is potentiated by a folate-deficient diet.[26] By contrast, chronic ethanol administration with an adequate diet has been shown to result only in impairment of $B_{12}$ absorption.[27]

In well-nourished alcoholics, depressed levels of intestinal lactase and lactose intolerance have been observed,[28] with recovery following withdrawal from alcohol (Fig. 65–4). In this latter study, blacks were more susceptible to this injurious effect of ethanol than were whites (Fig. 65–5). The functional significance of the reduced lactase values was revealed by the small blood glucose rise after a lactose load (Fig. 65–6). The subjects with low intestinal lactase and small blood glucose rises had a high frequency of intolerance (Fig. 65–6). The frequency of lactase deficiency, especially among black alcoholics, must be borne in mind when diets are prescribed for alcoholics with gastritis or ulcer disease.

In alcoholics other factors may also contribute to intestinal dysfunction, such as portal hypertension,[29] therapeutic interventions as with neomycin,[30] pancreatic insufficiency, altered intestinal flora, and altered bile salts.

Despite the many levels at which alcohol may alter the upper GI tract, the incidence of related nutritional deficiencies is relatively small. Even in patients with cirrhosis, the incidence of steatorrhea is uncommon and in one series was present in only 9% of patients.[31]

## Pancreas

Acutely, ethanol causes an increase in pancreatic secretion of water and bicarbonate when given orally; this increase may be mediated by release of secretin from the duodenum.[32–34] If gastric juice is prevented from reaching the duodenum, however, intravenous or intragastric ethanol results in a decrease in pancreatic secretion.[35–37] Increased tone at the sphincter of Oddi is observed after acute ethanol administration.[38] The physiologic significance of this effect, however, is not established.

Chronic alcohol consumption may result in an increase in the protein content of pancreatic juice, with a concomitant decrease in water and electrolytes.[33] Precipitation of such protein within pancreatic ducts has been proposed as a key pathologic alteration in chronic calcific alcoholic pancreatitis. Both a high-fat, high-protein diet and, paradoxically, malnutrition have been implicated in the pathogenesis of this disorder.[39] Chronic pancreatitis may lead to pancreatic insufficiency and may contribute to steatorrhea and malabsorption. Acute pancreatitis may result in disturbances of fluid and electrolytes and diminished dietary intake. Both acute and chronic pancreatitis may cause alterations in glucose tolerance.

## Bile Salts

Steatorrhea in an alcoholic may be potentiated by alterations in bile salt metabolism. Acutely, ethanol may decrease intraluminal bile salts.[37] Chronic ethanol feeding in rats prolongs the half-

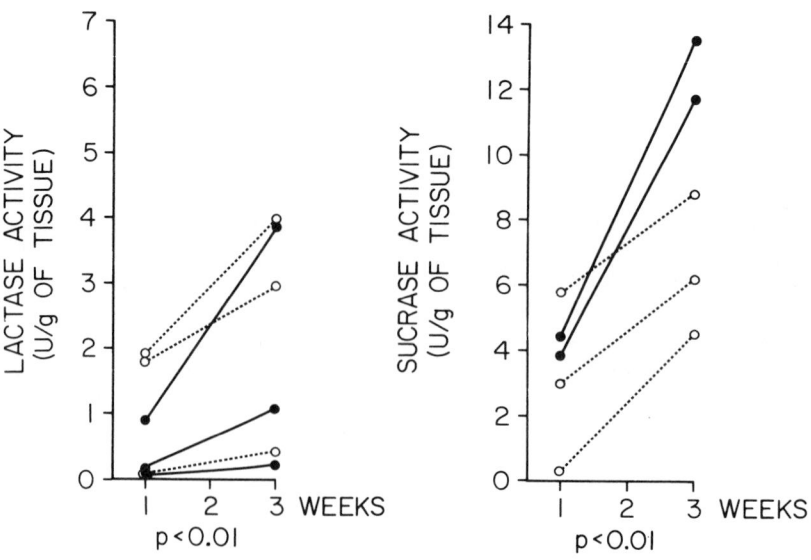

**Fig. 65–4.**   Effect of withdrawal from alcohol upon intestinal lactase. A significant increase in intestinal lactase was observed following one to three weeks of withdrawal from alcohol. A similar effect was noted for intestinal sucrase activity. (Reprinted by permission of the publisher from Perlow, W., et al., Gastroenterology *72*:680, 1977, by The American Gastroenterological Association.)

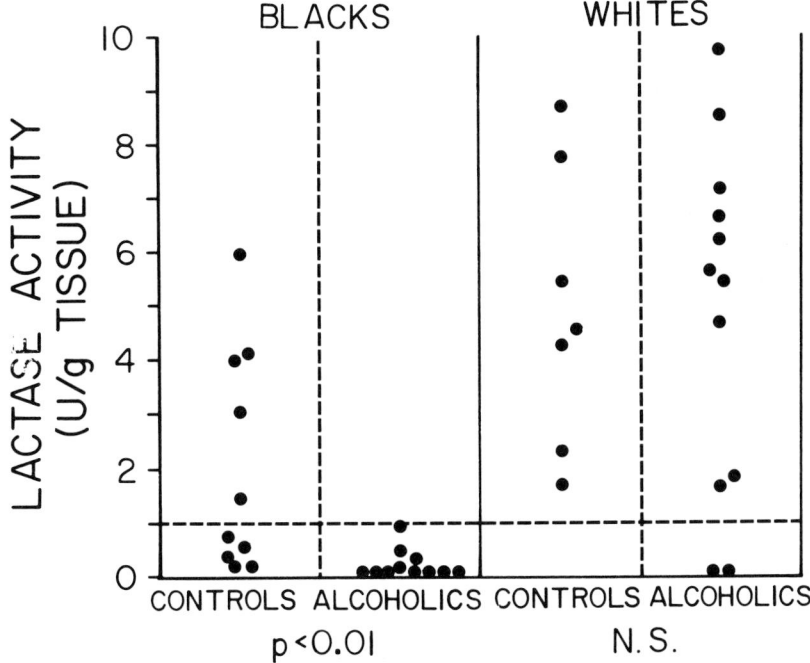

**Fig. 65–5.** The effects of chronic alcohol consumption on lowering intestinal lactase activity. Black alcoholics were found to be especially sensitive. (Reprinted by permission of the publisher from Perlow, W., et al., Gastroenterology *72*:680, 1977, by The American Gastroenterological Association.)

excretion time of cholic and chenodeoxycholic acid, increases the pool size slightly, and decreases daily excretion.[40] In patients with alcoholic cirrhosis, deoxycholate may be markedly diminished in the bile, possibly because of impaired conversion of cholate to deoxycholate by bacteria.[41] Decreased cholic acid synthesis, decreased total bile acid pools,[42] diminished concentrations of bile salts in intestinal juices, and bacterial deconjugation of bile salts by altered intestinal flora[31] may all contribute to steatorrhea in patients with cirrhosis.

The incidence of pigmented gallstones is increased in patients with cirrhosis.[43]

## ALTERATIONS OF NUTRIENT METABOLISM

### Water-Soluble Vitamins

**Overall Changes.** The alterations of the metabolism of water-soluble vitamins in the alcoholic demonstrate the many levels at which ethanol, liver disease, and other organ damage may affect nutrients. In addition to decreased intake and absorption the following have been noted: (1) decreased hepatic affinity for folate as measured by displacement studies,[44] (2) impaired activation or utilization of folate, thiamin, and $B_6$,[45–49] (3) increased hepatic clearance of pyridoxyl phosphate in cirrhosis,[50] and (4) release of B vitamins from

the perfused liver following acute addition of ethanol.[51] The clinical significance of such alteration is not, however, clearly defined. Depressed circulating levels of vitamins may be found in 40% of malnourished alcoholics, with folate and pyridoxine being most often lowered. Megaloblastic anemias related to folate or $B_6$ deficiency, and neurologic syndromes related to thiamin deficiency are the most common clinical manifestations of vitamin deficiencies in the alcoholic. The effects of marginal deficiencies on such processes as recovery from liver injury are unknown.

The water-soluble vitamins have attracted special interest because they have been proposed as both a cure for alcoholism in high doses and a cause of alcoholism when deficient.[52] However, the human studies upon which these theories were based were uncontrolled and, similarly, the animal studies used as evidence were subject to many criticisms.[53]

**Thiamin.** Thiamin metabolism in the alcoholic has been of considerable interest because of the numerous neurologic abnormalities that have been attributed completely or in part to its deficiency.

The effects of ethanol on thiamin status, however, have been a subject of controversy. The amount of alcohol consumed, the sources of dietary calories, and the degree of alcoholic liver damage may all be important variables. Even in

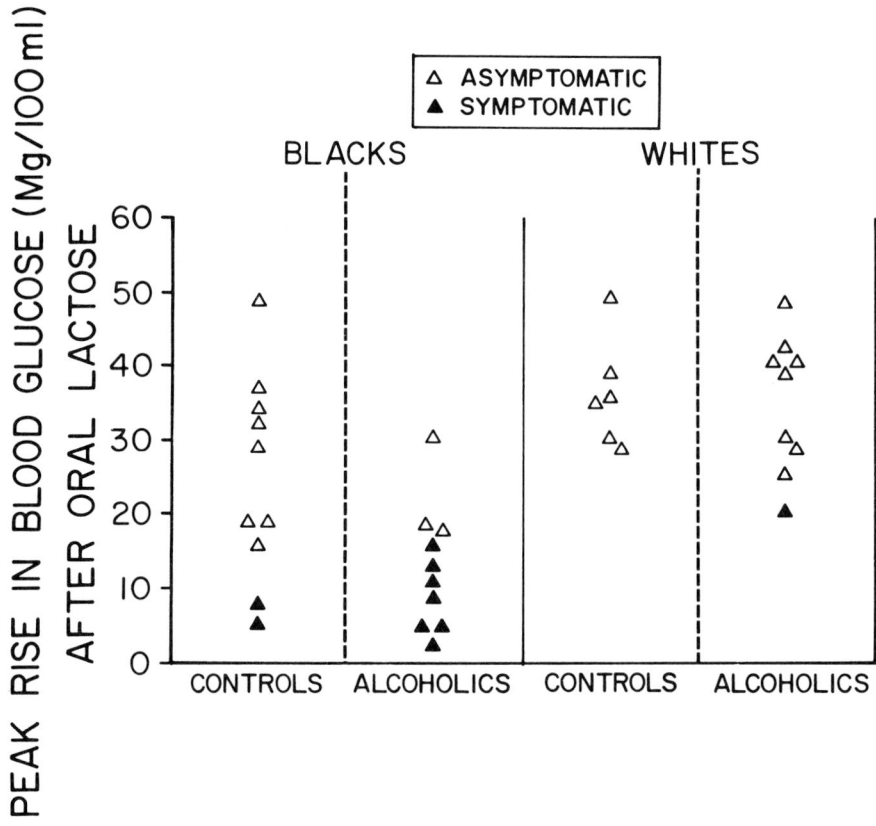

**Fig. 65–6.** Effect of lactase deficiency on rise in serum glucose after oral lactose administration. Blood glucose rose the least in subjects with the most severe lactase deficiency. There was a good correlation between symptoms and the lack of rise in glucose. (Reprinted by permission of the publisher from Perlow, W., et al., Gastroenterology *72*:682, 1977, by The American Gastroenterological Association.)

experimental models of alcohol feeding, results are conflicting: decreases in thiamin levels,[54–58] no change,[59,60] and increases have all been reported.[56] Two studies measured tissue thiamin levels after chronic alcohol feeding using the Lieber-DeCarli formula diet.[61] One study found no changes in thiamin pyrophosphate (TPP) in brain and liver[59] whereas the other found decreases in bioavailable thiamin assayed by *Ochromonas danica* in blood and liver.[57] Another study reported a decrease in transketolase activity after chronic alcohol feeding of this diet,[56] but no TPP effect was observed and the activities in brain and liver were lower than those reported with frank thiamin deficiency. The latter study, however, included an acute dose of ethanol in addition to chronic feeding prior to the measurement of enzyme activity. In one study, no change in tissue levels of bioavailable thiamin or transketolase enzymes was observed in either rodents or primates fed alcohol for up to four years along with adequate diets.[62] Furthermore, learning deficits observed with thiamin deficiency alone were not

observed after giving alcohol chronically along with adequate thiamin to rodents.

The results of this study also demonstrate the importance of thiamin deficiency in producing deficits in shuttle box avoidance learning. These results are consistent with several observations made in rodents[63] and humans[64–66] that emphasize the importance of thiamin deficiency in producing learning deficits analogous to those seen in alcoholics with Wernicke-Korsakoff syndrome. They differ from the findings of Freund and Walker who observed learning deficits in rodents after chronic alcohol feeding with diets that contained adequate thiamin.[67] In the latter studies, however, the composition of the liquid diets was not completely defined, and tissue levels of thiamin were not measured.

In many studies, alcohol was fed chronically along with diets containing excess thiamin. Ethanol in the gastrointestinal tract interferes with active but not passive transport of thiamin.[59,68,69] Thus, diets that are marginal in thiamin might be adversely affected by ethanol because at low concentrations the active transport of thiamin is most important. Furthermore, in these studies ethanol was substituted isocalorically for carbohydrates, producing a thiamin-sparing effect.[70,71] It is possible that if ethanol is consumed as additional calories it might have a greater adverse effect on thiamin balance.

In the presence of cirrhosis, activation of thiamin pyrophosphate by the liver is decreased.[72] In the presence of advanced liver damage, the storage capacity of the liver is impaired.[73] The possible significance of these facts was revealed in one study: Even in normally nourished alcoholics with well-compensated liver disease, it was found that thiamin deficiency, judged by low transketolase levels, was present in 30%.[74] Thus, one can expect that in the most severe stages of alcoholic liver damage, thiamin status may be impaired.

**Pyridoxine.** Pyridoxine has been studied extensively with respect to the effects of ethanol metabolism. Veitch found that rats fed alcohol as 36% of total calories showed a significant decrease in the hepatic content of pyridoxal phosphate when either a sufficient or insufficient dietary amount of $B_6$ was administered.[75] In isolated perfused livers, the addition of 18 mM ethanol lowered the pyridoxal phosphate content of livers and decreased the net synthesis of pyridoxal phosphate from pyridoxine in the $B_6$-deficient animals. These effects were abolished by 4-methylpyrazole, an inhibitor of alcohol dehydrogenase. Thus, the derangement in pyridoxal phosphate metabolism produced by ethanol is dependent upon its oxidation. One interpretation of these findings was that acetaldehyde may be the responsible agent, because in human erythrocytes acetaldehyde acts to enhance the enzymatic hydrolysis of pyridoxal-5-phosphate by cellular phosphatases.[76] Similar observations were made in isolated rat hepatocytes.[49] The latter study also reportedly showed that acetaldehyde can displace pyridoxal-5-phosphate from its binding protein and thereby promote its degradation.

**Vitamin $B_{12}$.** Vitamin $B_{12}$ absorption is impaired by chronic ethanol intake despite the administration of pancreatin and intrinsic factor.[27] However, in the absence of other diseases, $B_{12}$-deficiency anemia is rare among alcoholics.

**Ascorbic Acid.** In one study more than 50% of alcoholics with liver disease had depressed leukocyte ascorbic acid levels.[77] These low levels were correlated with depressed hepatic levels and impaired hepatic drug metabolism. In this study it was not ascertained whether decreased dietary intake or altered hepatic metabolism of ascorbate (such as due to peroxidation) may have been responsible for the observed changes.

**Folate.** Alcohol impairs the utilization of folate as assessed by hematologic parameters.[78] Consumption of the equivalent of 3 to 6 oz. of ethanol (95%) in volunteers produces a 50% decrease in serum levels of folate at 16 hr, followed by a rebound increase.[79] Urinary excretion of folate, however, was not enhanced under these conditions.[80] In humans, ethanol interferes with the release or formation of the principal circulating form of folate (5-methyl tetrahydrofolate).[81] In rats, Steinberg and co-workers observed that ethanol, when given acutely, shifted intracellular hepatic folate from polyglutamate toward monoglutamate, decreased serum folate, and decreased biliary folate.[81] The results were interpreted to indicate that alcohol directly inhibited the transport of folate from the hepatocyte into the bile. In studies of ethanol feeding in rats, Brown and co-workers observed that ethanol decreased hepatic uptake of folate and synthesis of pteropolyglutamate, which could lead to impaired hepatic storage.[82] Folate deficiency and related anemias are common in alcoholics and may be caused by one or more of the mechanisms just discussed.

### Fat-Soluble Vitamins

**General Changes.** The metabolism of fat-soluble vitamins may be altered in the alcoholic because of effects of alcohol, alcohol-induced tissue injury, steatorrhea, reduced dietary intake, and concomitant nutritional alterations such as those related to calcium and zinc.

**Vitamin A.** Alcoholics with cirrhosis may suffer from night blindness,[83] which is possibly related to vitamin A deficiency.[84] Studies have shown that plasma vitamin A,[85] as well as retinol-binding protein (RBP) levels,[86] are decreased in patients with alcoholic cirrhosis. These complications have usually been contributed to malnutrition, since poor dietary intake has been reported in alcoholics with[86,87] or without [87] cirrhosis. It is also possible that these complications may result from hepatic injury, because decreased plasma vitamin A and RBP levels have been reported in patients with liver disease without apparent alcohol intake.[88] These low plasma levels have been postulated to be due to defective synthesis of RBP in the liver.[88] Alcoholic cirrhosis is often associated with zinc deficiency,[85,86] which has also been postulated to decrease plasma RBP through impaired mobilization of RBP from the liver.[89]

Previous studies of hepatic vitamin A levels in various disease states involve only autopsy material, do not include biopsy data, and do not specify the alcoholism status of the subjects in the studies.[90] There are some reports of patients with alcoholic cirrhosis with evidence of a low circulating level of vitamin A,[85,86,91,92] but the actual hepatic vitamin A concentration of these subjects has not been described. Patients with alcoholic liver disease were found to have low levels of hepatic vitamin A at all stages of their disease[93] (Fig. 65–7). In such subjects with alcoholic fatty liver, hepatic vitamin A concentration was much lower than in normal livers (on the average one fifth); it was also significantly lower than in patients with chronic persistent hepatitis despite the fact that the degree of liver injury associated with the fatty liver was moderate. Furthermore, in both groups, blood levels of retinol-binding protein and prealbumin were normal and there was no evidence of deficient vitamin A intake. In patients with alcoholic hepatitis, liver levels of vitamin A were depressed even further to one tenth of normal values or less. The lowest hepatic vitamin A levels (30 times below normal) were observed in patients with cirrhosis. Thus, alcoholic liver disease is associated with severely decreased hepatic

vitamin A levels, even when liver injury is moderate (fatty liver) and when blood levels of vitamin A, RBP, and prealbumin are still unaffected. RBP, which has been considered a good index of vitamin A deficiency, and more sensitive even than dark adaptation,[94] was also normal in the subjects with alcoholic fatty liver.

The mechanism whereby alcoholic liver disease is associated with lowered hepatic vitamin A is not clear. Malnutrition, when present, could of course contribute to hepatic vitamin A depletion. However, experimental administration of ethanol with normal diets or even those enriched with vitamin A resulted in a depression of hepatic vitamin A that could not be attributed to insufficient vitamin A intake or malabsorption.[95] In contrast, vitamin A contents in the kidney and testis were increased two- to threefold in ethanol rats after nine weeks. Serum vitamin A and RBP levels were not significantly changed. In earlier experimental studies, Suschetet found no effect of chronic

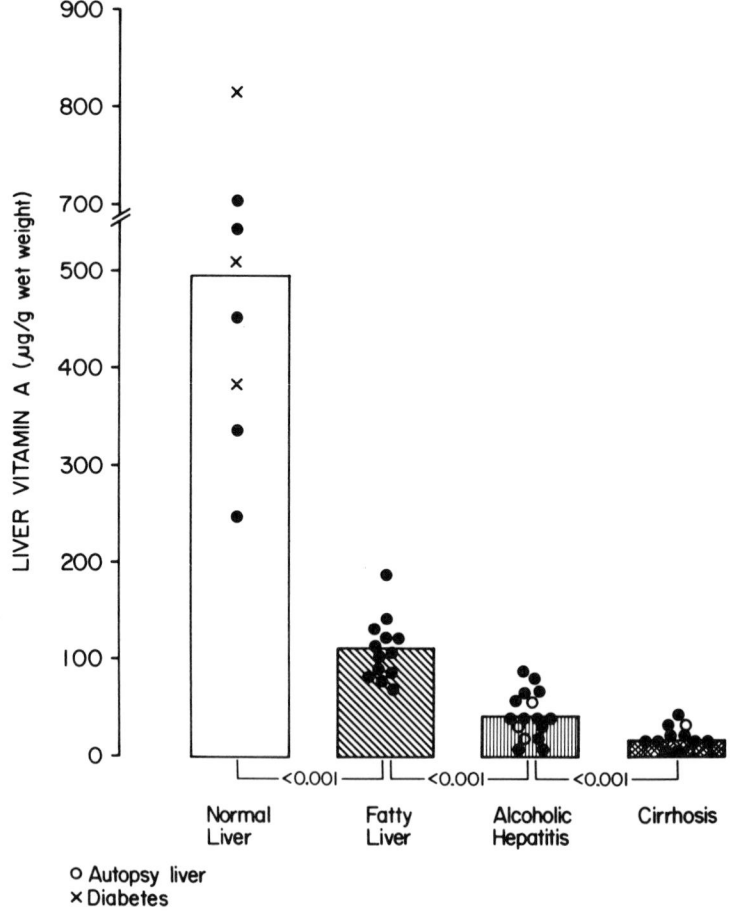

**Fig. 65–7.** Hepatic vitamin A levels in subjects with normal livers, chronic persistent hepatitis, and various stages of alcoholic injury. (From Leo, M.A., Lieber, C.S.[93]. Reprinted, by permission of the New England Journal of Medicine *37*:597–601, 1982.)

ethanol consumption on hepatic vitamin A,[96] whereas Baumann et al. noted that prolonged ethanol intake decreased hepatic vitamin A.[97] More recently, Blomstrand et al. observed a similar effect,[98] but in all three studies, ethanol was given in drinking water, and nutritionally paired controls were not assessed.

The reason for the decreased hepatic vitamin A even in the presence of adequate intake is not known. Even when dietary vitamin A intake was virtually eliminated, the difference in hepatic storage between ethanol-fed rats and controls was much greater than could be accounted for by the total vitamin A intake. Therefore, malabsorption cannot be the only reason for the depletion of hepatic vitamin A. Two possible mechanisms other than malabsorption can be considered: increased mobilization of vitamin A from the liver and increased catabolism of vitamin A in the liver or in other organs. There is experimental evidence in favor of both.[99,100] Multivesicular lysosomes (ML) in alcoholics have been observed in apparent relationship to lowered hepatic vitamin A level.[101] Additional studies are required to determine the relationship between lowered vitamin A and alterations of liver functions and structure, including the nature of the link between the lowered vitamin A and the appearance of ML, with possible involvement of a defect in lipoprotein secretion.

In view of the low vitamin A levels in the liver of patients with liver disease[93] and the symptoms of vitamin A deficiency reported in alcoholics,[94] the question of the therapeutic use of vitamin A must be raised. When manifest vitamin A deficiency is present (as corroborated by low serum vitamin A levels), such treatment might be particularly indicated.[91,92] It is noteworthy, however, that even in the presence of normal serum vitamin A, the liver levels may be severely depressed.[93] Whether vitamin A should be administered to these patients and, in the affirmative, how much should be given are still open questions. Although vitamin A deficiency might adversely affect the liver, an excess of vitamin A is also known to be hepatotoxic.[102–104] In the latter studies, the amounts used were large and exceeded greatly the dosage of vitamin A commonly used for the treatment of several clinical conditions such as xerophthalmia.[105] Among other therapeutic uses, vitamin A has been included in the treatment of alcoholics with hypogonadism and abnormal dark adaptation.[86,91] The amounts administered, which ranged from 10,000 IU/day for up to five months to 50,000 IU/day for one week, were considered safe because no adverse effects have been reported in normal individuals with these dosages. It must

be pointed out, however, that in the case of other potential hepatotoxic agents such as acetaminophen, alcoholics experienced an unusual susceptibility to the drug in terms of hepatotoxicity.[106] In addition, in rats, alcohol pretreatment potentiates the hepatotoxicity of acetaminophen.[107] Studies by Leo et al.[108] and Leo and Lieber[109] showed that similar potentiation also occurs with regard to vitamin A.

In the first study, rats were fed diets for two weeks with either normal or fivefold increased vitamin A content, both with or without ethanol.[108] Ethanol with a normal vitamin A diet produced the expected proliferation of the smooth endoplasmic reticulum and moderate mitochondrial lesions. Vitamin A supplementation by itself produced endoplasmic reticulum proliferation and slight enlargement of mitochondria. The combination of high vitamin A and ethanol resulted in more striking lesions. The blood levels of vitamin A were unaffected, whereas liver levels of vitamin A were increased by vitamin A supplementation and decreased by ethanol supplementation. As a net result, the liver vitamin A content of the high-A ethanol group was not greater than that of the normal-A control group, suggesting that a metabolite of vitamin A rather than vitamin A itself may have been responsible for the potentiation of vitamin A toxicity by ethanol. Mitochondrial toxicity reflected itself also in decreased content of various cytochromes and reduced activity of enzymes, including glutamate dehydrogenase (GDH). The activity of the latter was increased in the serum.

In the second study, nine months of vitamin A supplementation in the rat resulted in an increased number of fat-storing cells (lipocytes), and a significant correlation occurred between the latter and the vitamin A accumulation in the liver.[109] However, when vitamin A supplementation was combined with ethanol administration, both vitamin A levels in the liver and the number of fat-storing cells were decreased, with the appearance of numerous transitional cells and myofibroblasts in association with abundant collagen fibers. There was also striking hepatic inflammation and necrosis, accompanied by a rise in serum GDH and SGOT, and a decrease in retinol-binding protein and vitamin A. Thus, this study revealed that in the rat, an amount of vitamin A supplementation that normally does not produce significant liver alterations may result in hepatic inflammation, necrosis, and fibrosis when associated with alcohol consumption, even though the rat is normally refractory to ethanol-induced fibrosis.

The mechanism of the enhanced toxicity resulting from the association of moderate vitamin

A supplementation with ethanol is not known. In the rat, vitamin A in the amount used in the aforementioned study was not shown by itself to produce fibrosis, nor did ethanol treatment per se result in such an effect in rodents. It has been postulated before that toxicity of excess vitamin A may result from the overflow of vitamin A from its form associated with the RBP to an esterified form that circulates with the lipoproteins.[110,111] The latter form was not found to be increased in the studies of Leo and Lieber using much lower amounts of vitamin A supplementation.[109] It is also apparent that retinol by itself is not directly responsible for the toxicity. After chronic ethanol consumption, levels of vitamin A in the liver were in fact much lower than in the controls, yet signs of toxicity were most prominent in this group. As mentioned before, potentiation by ethanol of the toxicity of other agents, such as carbon tetrachloride and acetaminophen, is due to enhanced production of an active metabolite secondary to the induction of the microsomal system of the liver.[107,112] Since a metabolite of retinol, namely retinoic acid, can be further metabolized by liver microsomes, particularly when the latter system is "induced" by chronic ethanol consumption,[100] one can postulate that metabolites of retinoic acid, because of their increased production, might also participate in the increased toxicity. At present, however, we lack direct experimental evidence to support such a hypothesis.

In the therapeutic uses of vitamin A, the clinician might have to weigh carefully potential beneficial effects against enhanced toxicity, particularly in the case of alcoholics. Careful monitoring of patients with vitamin A is, therefore, mandatory but there are at present no readily available measurements to detect early signs of toxicity. It is noteworthy that vitamin A levels in the serum may be normal in the presence of high liver vitamin A and associated hepatotoxicity. Although increased serum levels of enzymes such as GDH and transaminase may, of course, reflect hepatotoxicity, their practical use may be limited in alcoholics by the difficulty in differentiating between an enzyme increase in the blood that reflects vitamin A toxicity and one that results from the direct hepatotoxic effects of ethanol. Similarly, measurements of vitamin A in liver biopsies may not be revealing because the actual level found may again result from two opposite changes, namely the decrease of vitamin A associated with chronic ethanol consumption and the rise of vitamin A associated with vitamin A therapy. In the absence of signs for the early detection of the toxicity of vitamin A, great caution should be exercised in the selection of the dosage of vitamin A used for the therapy of complications associated with alcoholism. In the alcoholic, the beneficial range of vitamin A supplementation may fall within a narrow therapeutic window.

**Vitamin D.** Vitamin D metabolism in conjunction with calcium metabolism is of special interest in the alcoholic. Alcoholic populations have been observed to have decreased bone density,[113] increased susceptibility to fractures,[114] and increased frequency of osteonecrosis[115] compared to other populations. Vitamin D metabolism may be affected at many levels in the alcoholic. In addition to decreased dietary intake, decreased absorption may occur because of pancreatic insufficiency and bile salt abnormalities. Similarly, calcium absorption may be impaired. Patients with alcoholic cirrhosis have decreased clearance of plasma cholecaliferol and decreased urinary glucuronide conjugates.[116] The liver is the first site of hydroxylation of vitamin $D_3$ (cholecalciferol), a process necessary for its activation; therefore, hepatocellular injury accompanied by deficient activation of dietary vitamin D was believed to explain resistance to parenteral vitamin D therapy.[116] Bjorneboe and co-workers observed decreased serum 25-OH $D_3$ levels in 58% of active alcoholics without evidence of liver disease but with normal vitamin D intakes.[117] Hepner and co-workers observed a decreased use of 25-OH $D_3$ after injection in cirrhotics but no delay in alcoholics without cirrhosis.[118] Posner and co-workers observed low levels of 25-OH vitamin D in 44% of alcoholics with cirrhosis but no alteration in the metabolism of vitamin D to 25-OH vitamin D.[119] Similarly, Luisier observed decreased serum 25-OH vitamin D in patients with Laennec's cirrhosis.[120] Thus, patients with cirrhosis frequently have low levels of 25-OH vitamin $D_3$, although the mechanism may not be caused solely by decreased activation by a damaged liver. Other postulated mechanisms of possible alterations in vitamin D metabolism include increased degradation of activated vitamin D by the cytochrome P-450 system (which may be stimulated by alcohol) and decreased storage depots of fat and muscle in debilitated patients with chronic liver disease.[117]

Baran and co-workers observed a decrease in trabecular bone in rodents after chronic alcohol feeding despite normal levels of 25-OH vitamin D, calcium, phosphorus, and testosterone.[121] They postulated that alcohol had a direct toxic effect on bone. The increased urinary losses of calcium induced by alcohol, ethanol-induced hypercorticism, and parathyroid stimulation secondary to calcium-binding proteins in cirrhosis are other mechanisms by which altered bone metabolism may contribute to clinical musculoskeletal diseases in alcoholic populations. The site or sites of the abnormalities involved and their importance, however, remain to be clarified.

**Vitamin K.** Vitamin K deficiency in the alcoholic may manifest itself as a bleeding diathesis related to failure to synthesize clotting factors in the liver. Dietary deficiency, decreased synthesis by intestinal bacteria, and malabsorption may be contributory. Deficiency states are relatively uncommon, but marginal deficiencies may be potentiated by concomitant liver injury. Vitamin K may correct a prolonged prothrombin time in such instances; failure to correct such an abnormality generally denotes severe parenchymal injury.

## WATER, MINERALS, AND ELECTROLYTES

### Sodium, Potassium, and Water

Alcoholics with chronic liver disease may have disorders of water and electrolyte metabolism. Sodium and water retention is common and presents clinically as ascites, edema, and portal hypertension. Postulated mechanisms include hypoalbuminemia, altered renal hemodynamics, endocrine abnormalities, and changes in lymph flow.[122] Rarely, dilutional hyponatremia may occur in beer drinkers because of the low sodium content of beer consumed.[123]

Increasing abdominal girth, weight gain, a dragging sensation in the abdomen, shortness of breath, and swelling of the ankles may be typical presenting symptoms of salt and water retention in patients with cirrhosis. The presence of shifting dullness, pitting edema, effusions on chest roentgenogram, and fluid on paracentesis confirm the diagnosis. Dietary regimen is adjusted according to the severity of salt and water retention. Severe symptoms and refractory cases may require rigid sodium restriction (250 mg/day). Restriction at this level is advocated even if mild hyponatremia is present, that is, if the serum sodium level is 125 to 130 meq/L.[124] Symptomatic hyponatremia with serum sodium below this level may require intervention with hypertonic saline and rigid water restriction. Fluid restriction of 1,500 to 2,000 ml/day (including all liquids taken with medications) is recommended, especially if hyponatremia is present. With less severe retention, sodium restriction of 500 to 1,000 mg/day may be attempted. Daily measurement of weight and serum electrolytes is necessary to guide therapy. Summerskill and co-workers recommend not exceeding a weight loss of 5 kg/wk by dietary or diuretic therapy.[122] In refractory patients, especially those with symptoms such as severe dyspnea, paracentesis may be necessary. Two liters per

24 hours has been recommended as a safe rate of removal. More vigorous therapy may cause acute depletion of albumin, salt, and water and may result in cardiovascular collapse. Replacement therapy with IV albumin and saline may be required during such therapy. Diuretics may be used, but with careful attention to the possible development of hypokalemia and hyponatremia. Following restriction, diuresis and improved handling of dietary sodium may result. A ceiling of 2,500 mg of Na in the diet has been suggested.[125]

Patients with chronic liver disease may have difficulty in handling fluid loads. A daily total volume of 1,500 to 2,000 ml is recommended with observation for adequate urine output, weight gain, and hyponatremia. Oliguria, azotemia, and elevated creatinine level may indicate deteriorating renal function. Patients with alcoholic liver disease are especially susceptible to acute tubular necrosis through complications such as variceal bleeding. Spontaneous renal failure of the so-called hepatorenal syndrome may also occur. A rising serum urea level caused by renal failure may present a special problem in the patient with alcoholic liver disease. Urea is secreted into the GI tract and hydrolyzed to ammonia; thus, it acts like any nitrogenous compound. With increasing levels of urea, the resultant ammonia becomes a significant problem and may worsen or precipitate hepatic coma. In this case, antibiotics may be given to prevent conversion of urea to ammonia, and enemas may decrease the total load of nitrogenous compounds absorbed. Administration of limited amounts of mixtures of essential amino acids to patients with diminished protein tolerance because of renal failure has been advocated.[122] The dietary management of acute renal failure is otherwise the same as in other etiologies.

Soler and co-workers observed low whole-body potassium levels in alcoholics with cirrhosis, usually associated with ascites and hepatic decompensation.[126] These abnormalities of potassium were difficult to correct, were only poorly correlated with the serum potassium, and often were associated with a poor prognosis. Mechanisms of low body potassium stores also include vomiting and diarrhea, hyperaldosteronism, muscle wasting, renal tubular acidosis, and diuretic therapy. Increased urinary potassium excretion has been observed during chronic alcohol consumption.[127] Depletion of potassium may be especially significant because of consequent increased renal vein ammonia and worsening of hepatic coma.

### Magnesium

The similarity of the neuromuscular excitability of hypomagnesemia and acute alcohol withdrawal has aroused considerable interest in magnesium metabolism in the alcoholic. Acute ethanol administration was observed by McCollister and co-workers to increase urinary magnesium excretion two- to threefold and did not depend upon the ethanol-induced water diuresis.[128] In experimental animals, Sargent and co-workers also observed that, given acutely, ethanol increased urinary magnesium excretion and serum magnesium; plasma levels were unaffected by chronic alcohol administration.[129] A similar increase in serum magnesium was observed by Peng and Gitelman after acute ethanol administration.[130] Hepatic soluble and mitochondrial magnesium also increased.[131] McDonald and Margen, however, observed no change in urinary magnesium during chronic alcohol feeding.[132]

Sullivan and co-workers observed low serum magnesium levels in 5 of 16 patients with cirrhosis,[133] but Lin and Jacob found low skeletal muscle magnesium levels in 7 of 10 cirrhotics and observed a poor correlation between serum magnesium and whole-body magnesium.[134] Similarly, Mendelsohn and co-workers observed decreased exchangeable magnesium in most tremulous alcoholics.[135] In this study, however, there was no correlation between magnesium blood levels and the onset of alcohol withdrawal. Furthermore, florid magnesium deficiency states in alcoholics are exceedingly rare.[136] Thus, although alcoholics may frequently have low serum or exchangeable magnesium levels, the clinical significance of such abnormalities is not established except for rare cases in which severe hypomagnesemia may be present.

## Calcium and Phosphorus

As observed in studies of vitamin D, abnormal calcium and phosphorus metabolism may be important for the increased incidence of bone abnormalities seen in the alcoholic. The effects of acute ethanol administration on serum calcium levels are conflicting. Peng and Gitelman[130] and Shah and co-workers[137] observed that a large acute dose of ethanol in the rat decreased serum calcium levels. Sargent and co-workers[129] obtained the same results in the dog. In man, however, Markkanen and Nanto observed that an intravenous infusion of ethanol increased serum calcium and phosphorus as well as urinary excretion.[138] Krawitt observed that ethanol inhibited duodenal calcium absorption in the rat independent of vitamin D.[139] Stein and co-workers observed hypophosphatemia in 50% of hospitalized alcoholics,[140] and Luisier observed decreased serum calcium and intestinal asorption of calcium in patients with Laennec's cirrhosis.[120] In the latter

study, 25-OH D was also depressed. Calcium and phosphate abnormalities may be secondary to or may potentiate deficiencies of vitamin D in the alcoholic.

Blachley and co-workers observed decreased levels of muscle phosphorus in dogs fed alcohol for 56 days and postulated a role for such depletion in the pathogenesis of alcoholic myopathy.[141] The same group observed a return of phosphorus levels toward normal with more prolonged feeding,[142] which calls into question the importance of reduced phosphate levels in the pathogenesis of myopathy observed with chronic alcohol consumption. McDonald and Margen observed increased urinary excretion of phosphorus but not of calcium during chronic alcohol consumption in man.[132]

## Iron

The question of the metabolism of iron in the alcoholic is particularly relevant because of the association of hepatic injury with excess iron. Acute alcohol administration may increase iron absorption, possibly through stimulation of gastric acid secretion, resulting in increased solubility of ferric ion in the small intestine.[9] Alcoholics may receive excessive dietary iron from beverages, such as certain wines, or through inadvertent treatment with iron-containing vitamin preparations. In addition, anemias unrelated to iron deficiency may be incorrectly treated with iron. Pancreatic insufficiency, folate deficiency, portosystemic shunting, and cirrhosis may increase iron absorption.[143]

In autopsy studies, Volini and co-workers observed increased hepatic iron in most patients with early alcoholic liver cirrhosis.[144] No relationship was found between iron absorption, serum iron concentration, percentage saturation of total iron-binding capacity, and liver iron in one study.[145] Serum ferritin was increased in nonanemic alcoholics. Measurement of the liver iron concentration may be necessary to clearly differentiate between alcoholics with significant siderosis and patients with idiopathic hemochromatosis.[145] The mechanisms responsible for the increase of iron found in the liver of alcoholic patients remain unclear. There is little or no uptake of transferrin-bound $^{52}$Fe in controls, but significant uptake is seen in alcoholics with liver disease. Increased asialotransferrins in serum due to alcohol have been postulated to play a role in producing hepatic siderosis.[146] Uptake in the alcoholic with cirrhosis is significantly less than in the patients with fatty liver disease and in patients with primary biliary cirrhosis.[147]

Iron absorption of non-heme iron is unaffected

in alcoholics with liver disease in the absence of iron deficiency anemia or ethanol in the GI tract.[148]

The potential for excess iron to produce tissue injury and the finding of increased iron stores in a significant percentage of patients with alcoholic cirrhosis make this an important area for future investigation.

Iron deficiency anemia is uncommon in alcoholics unless conditions such as GI bleeding from varices, ulcers, and gastritis, repeated phlebotomies, dietary extremes, or chronic infections are present.[149] To the contrary, as previously discussed, alcoholics have a propensity to develop increased iron stores that may potentiate tissue injury in the liver and other organs. Transfusions and iron therapy should be used with caution and only to the point of correcting deficiencies. Routine iron supplements are not indicated.

### Zinc

Zinc has been of special interest in the alcoholic because zinc is a co-factor for alcohol dehydrogenase as well as vitamin A dehydrogenases and because zinc deficiency states have been observed in alcoholic patients.

Sargent and co-workers observed no effect of acute ethanol administration on serum zinc or urinary excretion of zinc.[129] By contrast, chronic alcohol consumption increases urinary zinc excretion. In alcoholics with fatty or normal livers, Hartoma and co-workers observed increased levels of serum zinc that were positively correlated with the P-450 content of the liver as well as its capacity for drug metabolism.[150] By contrast, patients with hepatitis or cirrhosis had low levels of serum zinc. Similarly, Smith and co-workers observed low plasma levels of zinc in 40% of patients with active liver disease.[85] Furthermore, Sullivan and co-workers observed that serum zinc levels in patients with cirrhosis remained low despite administration of zinc and that these patients had hyperzincuria during the period of zinc administration.[133] Thus, hypozincemia and hyperzincuria are frequently observed in the alcoholic, but only in the presence of severe liver disease. In fact, Helwig and co-workers observed hypozincemia in only 3 of 42 subjects and no significant decreases in serum zinc levels in a group of alcoholics characterized by a low incidence of liver abnormalities.[151] By contrast, Volini and co-workers found hepatic zinc levels to be decreased in alcoholics regardless of the stage of liver disease.[145]

Zinc deficiency has been incriminated in the pathogenesis of night blindness seen in alcoholics, presumably because of its role as a cofactor of vitamin A dehydrogenase, which is needed for conversion of retinol to retinal. Russell and co-workers studied 26 patients with cirrhosis.[91] Low serum zinc levels were found in three patients with abnormal dark adaptation but not in any patients with normal dark adaptation. Most of his patients with abnormal dark adaptation responded to vitamin A, but in four who did not, two responded to zinc administration. Similar results were observed by McClain and co-workers.[86] Thus, zinc deficiency must be considered along with vitamin A deficiency in the alcoholic. Theoretical consideration and some animal data have suggested a similar importance of zinc in vitamin A metabolism in the gonad,[86] but its significance in man remains to be established.

### Copper

Hartoma and co-workers observed an increase in serum copper levels in alcoholics independent of the stage of liver disease of the hepatic capacity for drug metabolism.[150] Sullivan and co-workers observed normal levels of serum copper in 16 cirrhotic patients.[133] Volini and co-workers observed an increase in hepatic copper levels in advanced alcoholic cirrhosis.[145] The significance of any of these changes in unknown.

### Various Trace Metals

Trace elements or micronutrients have become increasingly appreciated for their potential importance in the pathogenesis of various disease states, especially in the alcoholic. Their role as cofactors for many metalloenzymes, as well as their direct toxicity to the liver in some instances, is of special importance.

Sullivan and co-workers observed decreased levels of selenium in the serum of each of 16 cirrhotics.[133] Little is known of most of the other trace metals in alcoholics. Hepatic levels of manganese and chromium are unchanged in alcoholic liver disease, nickel is consistently increased, and cobalt is decreased in advanced cirrhosis.[145] No significance has been attributed to such changes. Furthermore, acute ethanol administration has been observed to cause intracellular shifts in trace metals.[131] Thus, changes in whole liver may not be relevant to functions of particular organelles or cellular processes. Cobalt may act synergistically with ethanol to produce cardiotoxicity in alcoholics when beverages such as beer are consumed in excess. Versiek and co-workers reported increased serum molybdenum levels in patients with acute liver disease.[152] In alcoholic liver disease, levels were increased as a group, but in those patients with cirrhosis normal levels were found.

## Carbohydrates

The absorption and digestion of carbohydrates are generally regarded as normal in the alcoholic.[125] Experimentally, however, chronic alcohol administration impairs jejunal uptake and transport of carbohydrates.[153] Administration of alcohol has a priming effect on glucose-mediated insulin release[154] and causes glucose intolerance.[155] Chronic alcohol administration results in impaired glucose tolerance, elevated insulin levels, and abnormal responses to glucagon.[156] These effects have been noted in alcoholics with fatty liver as well as in those with cirrhosis. Alcohol-induced pancreatitis may result in a transient or permanent glucose intolerance because of damage to pancreatic islet cells or the secondary release of steroids and catecholamines. The many effects of alcohol on the intermediary metabolism of carbohydrates[157] may contribute to impaired gluconeogenesis and may in part explain the symptomatic hypoglycemia in human alcoholics with prolonged fasting following heavy drinking. Other mechanisms that may contribute to hypoglycemia include glycogen depletion and autonomic dysfunction.[157]

## Uric Acid

Hyperuricemia has been observed in patients following oral or intravenous administration of ethanol despite the absence of known disorders of uric acid metabolism or renal disease.[158] Following alcohol consumption, hyperuricemia may persist for several days and thus be misdiagnosed as a primary rather than secondary disorder. NADH generation during ethanol metabolism by alcohol dehydrogenase may enhance lactate production or may prevent the liver from completing the Cori cycle and utilizing lactate originating in peripheral tissues, especially lactate produced from muscle activity in alcoholic withdrawal.[159] Elevated serum lactate, which results in decreased urinary excretion of uric acid, is a major mechanism by which hyperuricemia occurs. The effect of lactate is independent of alterations in urinary pH[158] and occurs despite the administration of probenecid.[160] Alcohol-induced hyperlipemia and ketogenesis, as well as starvation-induced ketosis, may also play a role in hyperuricemia. One study in patients with gout has suggested a possible contributory role of increased urate production due to ethanol, but patients were studied on a purine-free diet with relatively low doses of ethanol.[161] The changes in serum uric acid associated with alcohol administration are sufficient to precipitate acute gouty attacks.[160] The alterations in uric acid metabolism related to alcohol-

ism may explain the clinical observation of the association between alcoholics and gout.

In advanced alcoholic liver disease, serum uric acid may actually be decreased because of low xanthine oxidase activity in the damaged liver. Short-term ethanol administration decreases the plasma clearance of caffeine (a xanthine) and increases the elimination half-life of caffeine, probably owing to an inhibition of hepatic metabolism.[162]

## Lipids

The metabolism of lipids in alcoholics is of special interest because of the frequency of fatty liver and hyperlipidemias seen in these patients. Ethanol metabolism in the liver by alcohol dehydrogenase results in excess hepatic production of NADH. Alcohol consumption also results in mitochondrial damage within the liver. These two effects may, in large part, account for the major alterations in lipid metabolism resulting from ethanol: decreased fatty acid oxidation, increased fatty acid synthesis, and increased ketogenesis.[163,164] As a result of these alterations, excess triglycerides may accumulate within the liver and produce steatosis or may be released into the blood as lipoproteins. Intestinal production of very low-density lipoproteins has been observed,[165] although the contribution of this mechanism appears to be minor.[166] The serum cholesterol may also be increased in alcoholism, a fact that may be related to an ethanol-induced increase in hepatic cholesterogenesis[40] and decreased bile salt secretion.[40]

The administration of ethanol to man results in hyperlipidemia with the major increase occurring in the serum triglycerides. This response may be greatly enhanced by a fat-containing meal.[167] Elevations in serum cholesterol and triglycerides have been directly attributed to chronic alcohol consumption.[168] A characteristic feature of alcohol-induced hyperlipemia is that all lipoprotein fractions are increased, albeit to a variable degree (Fig. 65–8). The major increase is in the very low-density liproproteins, but a small percentage of alcoholics may have chylomicrons or chylomicron-like particles even in the fasting state.[169] Furthermore, a similarly small precentage may have hypercholesterolemia due to hyperbeta-lipoproteinemia.

A marked sensitivity to the hyperlipidemic effects of alcohol may be observed in patients with type IV familial or carbohydrate-induced hyperlipemia,[170] patients with defective removal of lipids (decreased postheparin lipoprotein lipase),[171] diabetics, and patients with pancreatitis. The latter condition has been associated with an inhib-

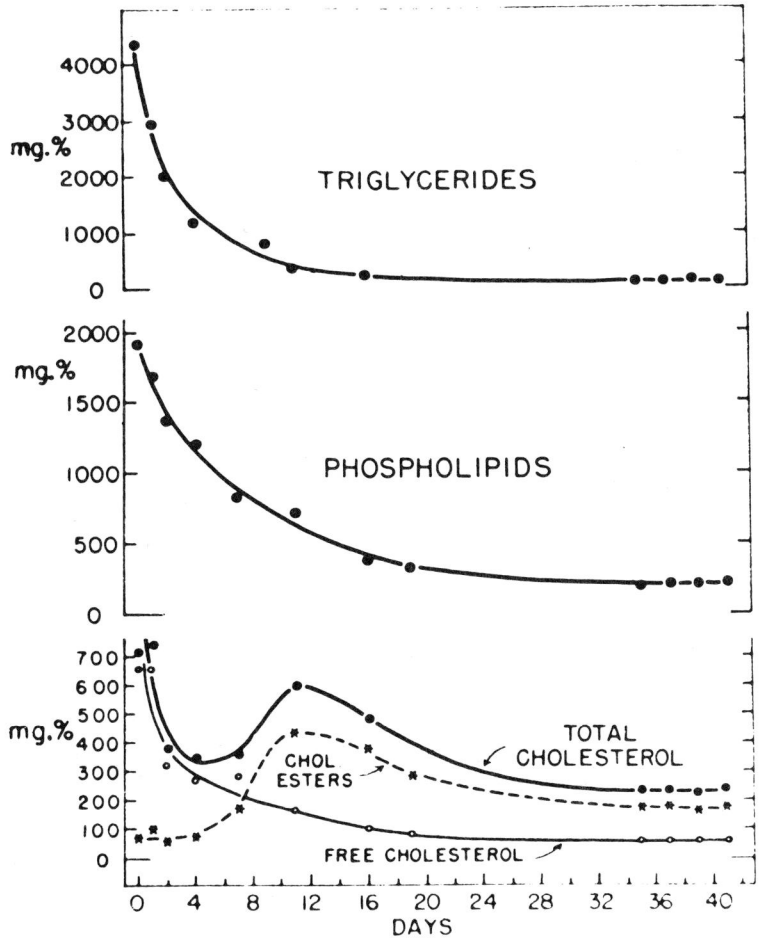

**Fig. 65—8.** Serum lipids in the alcoholic and the effect of withdrawal from ethanol. Lipid fractions decrease at varying rates. (From Losowsky, M.S., et al.,[171] with permission by Am. J. Med.)

itor of lipoprotein lipase.[172] Ethanol may thus unmask a subclinical hyperlipidemia and should be excluded as a cause of or contributor to observed hyperlipidemias. Marked hyperlipidemias may be associated with hemolysis,[173] which is transient and clears at the same time as the hyperlipidemia. Abdominal pain may occur with hyperlipidemia, and differentiation of a primary effect from associated pancreatic, GI, or hepatic disease may be difficult. The significance of alcohol-induced hyperlipidemia as a risk factor in coronary artery disease remains to be clarified. Moderate alcohol consumption appears to be associated with some protection with respect to coronary artery disease. This protective effect, however, may be reversed if the drinking pattern is variable or sporadic.[174] In patients with severe liver injury, such as cirrhosis, hypolipemia usually prevails.[175,176]

Intrahepatic fat accumulation from alcohol may be affected by dietary lipids.[177] However, low-fat diets are not practical in a clinical setting because of their unpalatability.[178]

## Protein

Acute ethanol administration has been observed to result in decreased hepatic synthesis of lipoproteins[179] and albumin.[180,181] By contrast, chronic alcohol feeding is associated with increased protein synthesis.[166] Furthermore, chronic feeding results in increased accumulation in the liver of transport protein such as albumin and transferrin.[182] This effect may be mediated by the action of ethanol (or its metabolite acetaldehyde) on hepatic microtubules.[182] The accumulation of hepatic protein is comparable in magnitude, in terms of weight, to the accumulation of lipid.

Experimentally, alcohol has a complex effect on nitrogen balance, depending upon dietary conditions. Given as supplementary calories, ethanol may be nitrogen sparing, but given as an isocaloric substitute for carbohydrate, it increases urea excretion in the urine.[183,184]

## Amino Acid Metabolism

**General Changes.** Amino acid metabolism in alcoholism is of special interest because of the relationship between amino acids and hepatic encephalopathy, the potential use of amino acids for parenteral feeding, and the role of amino acids in the synthesis of central nervous system transmitters such as serotonin. Numerous alterations in amino acid metabolism have been observed,[185,186] but the clinical relevance of most observations remains to be established. This is especially true because of the failure of many studies to control the three main variables that may affect amino acid metabolism: alcohol, nutrition, and liver injury.

Impairment of intestinal absorption of amino acids in the presence of alcohol has been noted;[13] however, increased nitrogen excretion in the stool is only rarely observed with chronic alcohol consumption. Ethanol impairs hepatic uptake of amino acids. This effect is mediated by the metabolism of ethanol.[187] However, hepatic protein and urea synthesis are increased after chronic alcohol feeding.[166,183] Therefore, the significance of the observed effects of alcohol on amino acid transport must be questioned.

Alterations of metabolism in the liver resulting from alcohol consumption and/or liver disease have been observed for almost every amino acid studied.[186] Several amino acids merit discussion in this regard.

**Methionine.** Chronic alcohol administration for 3 to 10 days to protein-deficient rats results in an increase in enzymes related to the degradation of methionine.[188] This finding is of interest because of the role of methionine as a lipotrope in rodents and because of the observation of increased alpha amino-n-butyric acid (a product of methionine catabolism) in the plasma following chronic alcohol consumption.[189]

**Tryptophan.** Tryptophan metabolism has aroused considerable interest because of its catabolism to the neurotransmitter serotonin as well as to nicotinic acid. Urinary excretion products have been measured but have yielded conflicting results regarding the effect of alcoholism on these competing pathways of catabolism.[186,190] This finding is not surprising in light of the many nutritional variables, such as pyridoxine availability, that are involved. Low levels of tryptophan have been observed in the plasma of alcoholics and may be a mechanism of depression in these patients.[191]

**Branched-Chain Amino Acids.** Branched-chain amino acids (BCAA)—valine, leucine, and isoleucine—are decreased in the plasma of patients with alcoholism and/or liver injury.[192–194] In hepatic encephalopathy related primarily to Laennec's cirrhosis, patients have depressed BCAA and normal levels with disorders such as halothane hepatitis.[195] BCAA clearance from plasma is increased in patients with cirrhosis.[196] Controlled studies conducted with animal models and patients have revealed that depressed BCAA observed in alcoholics results from dietary protein deficiency as well as advanced liver disease.[189] Furthermore, chronic alcohol feeding results in a striking increase in BCAA if dietary protein intake is maintained.[189] In addition to BCAA, chronic alcohol feeding also increases alpha amino-n-butyric acid in the plasma.[189] This amino acid has proved useful as a biochemical marker of heavy drinking.[197]

**Severe Liver Injury.** Fulminant hepatic necrosis may result in a generalized nonspecific increase in plasma amino acids.[195,198] Cirrhotics have decreased conversion of phenylalanine to tyrosine, abnormal tyrosine tolerance test, and elevated plasma levels of tyrosine, methionine, phenylalanine, tryptophan, glutamate, and aspartate.[195,199–203] Elevated plasma levels of aromatic amino acids may be associated with elevated levels of their decarboxylation products because of metabolism in the GI tract. Elevated levels of tyrosine and tyramine have been reported in hepatic encephalopathy.[202] Increased tyrosine and other aromatic amino acids and low BCAA in plasma have been implicated in the pathogenesis of hepatic encephalopathy.[201,203] Therapy related to this hypothesis is discussed in the following section.

## EFFECTS OF DIETARY FACTORS ON ETHANOL METABOLISM

Alcohol dehydrogenase (ADH) is the enzyme that figures predominantly in ethanol metabolism. Under a variety of circumstances, the level of this enzyme is rate limiting for the oxidation of ethanol.[204] The enzyme level may be affected by dietary factors that thus influence the rate of ethanol metabolism. Indeed, low-protein diets have been shown to reduce hepatic ADH levels in rats[205] and to considerably lower the rates of ethanol metabolism both in rats[205] and in man.[206]

Prolonged fasting markedly prolongs the metabolism of ethanol. In isolated rat liver cells, the rate of ethanol oxidation is approximately twice as fast in the fed state as in the fasted state. The mechanism of this alteration in rate results from decreased availability of metabolites to shuttle reducing equivalents into mitochondria needed for the metabolism of ethanol.[207]

The effects of dietary factors on the rate of ethanol metabolism may be of clinical significance. For a given alcohol intake, malnourished alcoholics may have higher and more sustained blood ethanol levels than do normal individuals.[208] This situation results in increased brain effects of ethanol and decreased effects related to ethanol metabolism.

## ALCOHOL, NUTRITION, AND ORGAN DAMAGE IN THE ALCOHOLIC

### Liver

Liver disease (fatty liver, hepatitis, and cirrhosis) is the most significant medical complication in the alcoholic in terms of morbidity and mortality. The question of the respective roles of alcohol and malnutrition in the pathogenesis of alcoholic liver disease is significant for both the prevention and the treatment of the disease.

Malnutrition has been proposed as the predominant factor producing liver injury for three reasons: (1) poor nutritional status of alcoholics seen in some hospital populations, (2) poor dietary intake by history among patients with advanced liver disease (cirrhosis), and (3) analogies between alcoholic fatty liver and the fatty liver present in kwashiorkor and following intestinal bypass for obesity. The nutritional status of alcoholics, however, is dependent upon the population studied; past stereotypes about the alcoholic may have stemmed from studies conducted primarily in skid-row alcoholics among city hospital populations. Dietary histories conducted in patients with cirrhosis[209] do not distinguish malnutrition and liver disease as cause and/or effect, since complications of cirrhosis such as ascites and encephalopathy may limit intakes. Furthermore, epidemiologic studies have failed to reveal relationships between malnutrition and cirrhosis in underdeveloped countries,[210] and liver biopsies of severely malnourished prison camp victims of World War II revealed only minimal histologic abnormalities.[211]

The role of lipotropes (such as methionine and choline) in the development of alcoholic liver disease is confusing because of inappropriate extrapolation from animal models. Primates are far less susceptible to lipotrope deficiency than are rodents[212] and, in fact, there is no evidence that a choline-deficient diet is deleterious to man. Treatment with choline of patients suffering from alcoholic liver injury has been found to be ineffective in the face of continued ethanol consumption.[213] Experimentally, massive supplementation with choline failed to prevent fatty liver produced by alcohol in volunteer subjects.[214] Furthermore, the fatty liver of choline deficiency is biochemically distinct from that observed following ethanol administration: hepatic phospholipids are increased in alcoholic fatty liver[215] but decreased in fatty liver because of choline deficiency. Even in rodents, acute or chronic alcohol administration results in liver injury despite massive supplementation with choline.[216] Thus, hepatic injury induced by choline deficiency appears to be primarily an experimental disease of animals with little or no relevance to human alcoholic liver injury.

Some experimental studies in man and rats have revealed no adverse effects of alcohol in the face of adequate nutrition[217,218] and have been used to support the arguments against the importance of alcohol itself in the pathogenesis of alcoholic liver injury. However, such studies can be criticized because of the use of dosages of alcohol much below those of heavy drinkers. By contrast, much evidence supports the direct role of alcohol in the pathogenesis of alcoholic liver injury. Epidemiologically, a direct relationship has been demonstrated between the amount of alcohol consumed and the incidence of cirrhosis during Prohibition in the United States and during the rationing of alcoholic beverages in Europe during World War II.[219,220] Lelbach has shown that the probability of developing cirrhosis is directly related to the amount and duration of ethanol consumed.[221] Menghini has observed that in sufficient quantity alcohol decreases the clearance of hepatic fat.[222] Most significantly, alcohol is directly toxic to the liver (morphologically and biochemically) in both alcoholics and nonalcoholics regardless of dietary variation in fat, protein, vitamins, and lipotropes.[19,214,215,223,224] The full spectrum of alcoholic liver disease (fatty liver and cirrhosis) has been produced in a primate model given alcohol in conjunction with an adequate diet.[225,226]

The interaction of alcohol and malnutrition with respect to liver injury remains largely unexplored. Numerous experimental studies have demonstrated such interactions,[177,227–231] but their clinical significance is unknown. In one clinical study of skid-row alcoholics with poor nutritional status, the incidence of cirrhosis was surprisingly low.[232] Furthermore, experimentally, protein deficiency prevents the development of cirrhosis following $CCL_4$ administration in rats.[233] Thus, under some circumstances it is conceivable that malnutrition may even be protective with respect to some of the effects of ethanol on the liver.

### Heart

Specific nutritional heart disease in the alcoholic may occur in the form of beriberi heart disease. Symptoms classically include those of congestive heart failure and hyperkinetic circulation. Low urinary thiamin and red cell trans-ketolase confirm the diagnosis, and other symptoms of thiamin deficiency may be present. In contrast to beriberi heart disease, alcoholic cardiomyopathy manifests itself with symptoms of congestive heart failure accompanied by a low cardiac output and peripheral vasoconstriction. The diagnosis is made essentially by exclusion. Characteristic electron microscopic changes in alcoholic cardiomyopathy have been described[234] and compared to those produced experimentally in hypomagnesemic rats.[235] This study has heightened interest in a possible nutritional etiology. However, alcoholics without evidence of heart disease or nutritional deficiency have abnormal left ventricular function when stressed.[236] Acute and chronic alcohol intake alters myocardial metabolism.[237] Acute alcohol administration sufficient to achieve blood levels of 150 mg/dl causes a rise in end diastolic pressure and decreases stroke output. Chronic alcohol administration in the face of a normal diet causes similar changes that persist for several weeks after withdrawal.[236] It is possible that alcohol and nutritional factors may, when combined, produce alcoholic cardiomyopathy. Such a case is illustrated by the cobalt-mediated cardiomyopathy in beer drinkers. The combination of small quantities of cobalt combined with large quantities of ethanol produces a fulminant cardiomyopathy in beer drinkers.[238] However, cobalt or ethanol alone taken in amounts comparable to those ingested by patients who developed cobalt beer-drinker's heart does not produce this disorder.

## Blood and Bone Marrow

Deficiencies of pyridoxine and folate may result in hematologic abnormalities in alcoholics, although the frequency and nature of the observed abnormalities are highly dependent upon the population selected. In one series of 65 patients admitted for alcoholism and not selected for hematologic problems, 40% had megaloblastic erythropoiesis secondary to folate deficiency, 30% had sideroblasts in the erythroid marrow, and a small percentage had iron deficiency anemia. A total of 75% had either anemia or bone marrow abnormalities. In middle- and upper-class alcoholics, folate levels are generally normal.[239] Small amounts of folic acid (250 μg intramuscularly and 150 μg by mouth) prevent megaloblastic changes, and 1 mg of pyridoxine per day prevents sideroblastic changes during ethanol administration. However, pharmacologic doses of folic acid do not prevent vacuolization of erythroid elements in patients fed alcohol and an adequate diet.[240] Thus,

alcohol has a direct toxic effect on the bone marrow despite adequate nutrition.

Thrombocytopenia and granulocytopenia have been described in alcoholics with varying frequency depending upon patient selection. Causes of thrombocytopenia include acute alcohol ingestion, folate deficiency, hypersplenism, infection, and disseminated intravascular coagulation. Ethanol causes a depression in circulating platelets despite the concomitant administration of a nutritious diet and vitamin supplements, including large doses of folic acid.[240] In addition, chronic alcohol administration with an adequate diet and folate supplements impairs platelet function.[241] Granulocytopenia has been reported associated with alcohol intoxication in the absence of folate deficiency, hypersplenism, or infection; there is rapid recovery after alcohol withdrawal.[242] However, in patients given alcohol chronically in the absence of nutritional deficiency, granulocytopenia does not develop.[240] Acute alcohol administration impairs leukocyte mobilization.[243]

## Nervous System

A number of neurologic disorders seen in alcoholism have been traditionally attributed to nutritional deficiencies, especially those of the B vitamins. Recently, however, the nutritional etiology of some of these disorders, especially some aspects of the Wernicke-Korsakoff syndrome, has been questioned.

Alcoholic polyneuropathy is characterized by generalized symmetrical involvement of peripheral nerves that spreads proximally. First symptoms include discomfort and fatigue in the anterior tibial muscles and paresthesias in the feet. These symptoms are usually followed by weakness in the toes and ankles, diminished ankle jerks, and decreased fine movements and vibratory sense. Finally, glove-and-stocking hypalgesia and severe weakness may result.[244] Thiamin deficiency has been most strongly implicated in etiology, but other B vitamins are mentioned as well. $B_{12}$, pyridoxine, nicotinic acid, and riboflavin deficiencies can be associated with peripheral neuropathy, and pantothenic acid deficiency may produce symptoms of peripheral nerve disease.[244]

The Wernicke-Korsakoff syndrome is the most spectacular CNS-related neurologic problem in alcoholism. Wernicke's encephalopathy is characterized by weakness of eye movements, gait disturbance, and confusion. Horizontal nystagmus, paralysis of external recti, paralysis of conjugate gaze, and ataxia of gait and stance may be observed. Korsakoff's psychosis is characterized initially by anterograde amnesia, retrograde amnesia to a lesser extent, a disordered time sense, and often confabulation in the acute stages. Cognitive deficits have also been observed.[64] Ophthalmoplegia in Wernicke's encephalopathy responds rapidly to thiamin administration, while the ataxia and confusion respond more slowly. The rapidity of response depends upon the conversion of thiamin to its active form in the liver; patients with advanced liver disease, such as cirrhosis, may therefore have a delayed response.[47]

The association of Korsakoff's psychosis with Wernicke's encephalopathy has led to their inclusion in one syndrome. However, whereas Wernicke's encephalopathy is a thiamin-responsive illness, the relationship of Korsakoff's psychosis to thiamin deficiency in terms of pathogenesis and treatment is less clearly delineated. Korsakoff's psychosis and Wernicke's encephalopathy are rarely, if ever, seen in clinical thiamin deficiency in the absence of alcoholism.[245] It has been postulated that this phenomenon may be related to the impact of alcohol on the balance of dietary calories.[245] The Wernicke-Korsakoff syndrome is characterized by symmetrical CNS lesions in periaqueductal and perivestibular areas of the diencephalon, midbrain, and cerebellum.[246] Symmetric and bilateral lesions are also observed in experimental thiamin deficiency in animals.[247] It is not surprising, therefore, that the psychosis and some aspects of the encephalopathy are only minimally or slowly responsive to thiamin treatment.[248] In addition to the structural similarity of lesions, a history of dietary deficiency in most alcoholics with memory and learning defects supports the theory that Korsakoff's psychosis is related to thiamin deficiency, or at least nutritional deficiency.[64] An abnormality of a thiamin-requiring enzyme has been observed in patients with the Wernicke-Korsakoff syndrome.[66] Clinical and pathological evidence supports the concept that Wernicke's encephalopathy and the pathologic lesions associated with it are decreasing in association with improvement in nutrition in recent years.[246] However, a study from Holland has shown an increase in the Wernicke-Korsakoff syndrome.[249] Experimentally, it is difficult to demonstrate learning deficiencies related to thiamin deficiency alone in rats,[63] while alcohol in the absence of nutritional deficiencies produces such defects.[250] Studies with a nutritionally adequate diet have revealed no deficits despite up to one year of alcohol feeding.[62] Thus, the precise interrelation of alcohol, thiamin, and Korsakoff's psychosis awaits clarification.

Nutrition amblyopia is a disorder characterized by central or centrocecal scotomata. Vitamin B deficiency has been suggested as a cause although a specific etiology is not established.[244] Similarly, the influence of nutritional factors in the pathogenesis of central pontine myelinosis, Marchiafava-Bignami syndrome, alcoholic cerebellar degeneration, and other rarer neurologic syndromes seen in alcoholics remains speculative. Cerebellar degeneration has, however, responded to thiamin.[251] Pellagra, although increasingly rare in alcoholics, may be manifested by psychosis, dementia, neuropathy, and posterior and lateral column disease. Skin changes and diarrhea may accompany the neurologic findings.

## NUTRITIONAL THERAPY

Nutritional therapy must be viewed in terms of the nutritional deficiencies requiring repletion as well as the pathologic alterations induced by alcohol. Nutritional therapy may be limited by underlying organ damage. For example, repletion of dietary protein deficiency may be limited or restricted in the presence of concomitant encephalopathy.

### Alcoholic Liver Injury

**Fatty Liver and Alcoholic Hepatitis.** Alcoholic fatty liver is the earliest and generally completely reversible stage of alcoholic liver injury. The only specific requirement is abstinence from alcohol. Patients with fatty liver may have associated deficiencies or complications that require specific therapy. Similar measures are required for alcoholic hepatitis. However, alcoholic hepatitis may require supportive measures to ensure electrolyte balance, especially if pyrexia or nausea and vomiting are present.

**Cirrhosis.** Recovery from cirrhosis is enhanced by a normal-protein, normal-fat, vitamin-enriched diet. Thus, diet remains the mainstay of the treatment of alcoholic liver disease. The components will be examined separately:

*Fat.* Low-fat diets are of theoretical interest in patients with alcoholic liver disease. However, they are generally not advocated because of the lack of palatability of such regimens, especially for a patient who is already anorectic.[178]

*Vitamins.* Several times the daily requirements of water-soluble vitamins are generally given without known harmful effects or proven efficacy. An increased requirement for folic acid has been clearly demonstrated with clinically manifested hematologic abnormalities resulting from administration of the regular daily requirement with alcohol. Abnormalities of the metabolism of other vitamins have also been observed. Therefore, it seems prudent to prevent the possibility of marginal subclinical deficiencies with supplementary vitamins. Intake of large doses of pyridoxine, however, has produced sensory neuropathy.[252]

*Protein.* Protein intake in patients with alcoholic liver injury must be adequate to prevent nitrogen wasting but not so great as to precipitate hepatic coma. Nitrogen balance studies have revealed essentially normal protein requirements in cirrhosis,[185] and some studies have even suggested increased nitrogen retention.[253] Dietary requirements for specific amino acids may be altered as evidenced by plasma levels and clearance rates. In general, patients with alcoholic liver disease have depressed plasma branched-chain amino acids,[193,194,254,255] and increased clearance of these amino acids,[196] along with increased levels of aromatic amino acids[198–201] and decreased clearance of these amino acids.[199] Amino acids may differ with respect to their ability to produce ammonia and are tolerated to a different extent in hepatic encephalopathy.[203]

*Calories.* Caloric intake should be sufficient to prevent endogenous protein breakdown. The daily caloric requirement to achieve nitrogen sparing in the alcoholic or in the presence of alcoholic liver injury is unknown,[125] but it is a reasonable practice to give an amount of calories in excess of daily requirements if feasible.

*Lipotropes.* There is no evidence that lipotropes are useful in recovery from alcoholic liver injury; in fact, they may prove harmful as an excess nitrogen load or may even cause liver toxicity.[256]

## Hepatic Encephalopathy

Hepatic encephalopathy represents a neuropsychiatric syndrome secondary to liver disease with a wide clinical spectrum ranging from personality changes to deep coma. Confusion, apathy, irritability, and personality changes may represent the earliest findings. Clinical findings include constructive apraxia, hypothermia, asterixis, and EEG changes. The etiology and pathogenesis of hepatic encephalopathy are complex. The major nutritional considerations include adjustment of exogenous and endogenous nitrogen loads and potassium and acid-base balance.

Exogenous protein load must be minimized because of the adverse effects of the resultant nitrogen load on encephalopathy. Dietary protein may be eliminated initially in the treatment of hepatic encephalopathy but must be resumed after several days to prevent endogenous catabolism. Nitrogen sparing should be maintained through intravenous glucose if caloric intake is inadequate. Because 5% dextrose (as the monohydrate) contains only 170 kcal/1,000 ml, it may be necessary to administer hypertonic glucose through a large-bore catheter, especially if fluid restriction is indicated. Hypercatabolic states, such as infections with fever, must be treated to prevent the adverse effects of protein catabolism. Patients with portacaval shunts may be especially sensitive to dietary protein.

Interest has also focused on selective abnormalities in the plasma aminogram as a possible contributor to portal-systemic encephalopathy (PSE) and as an indicator of what amino acids could be supplied in relatively greater or lesser amounts to improve nutrition and encephalopathy.[201,257] The observation that patients with PSE often have low branched-chain amino acids but elevated aromatic amino acids in their plasma generated the hypothesis that this amino acid imbalance could promote PSE. Attempts were therefore made to correct the imbalance by administering intravenously an amino acid mixture (FO80:HepatAmine) enriched with branched-chain amino acids (valine, leucine, isoleucine) but containing decreased amounts of aromatic amino acids (phenylalanine, tyrosine, tryptophan). One anecdotal report described patients with encephalopathy (due to cirrhosis, acute hepatitis, or other causes) who received HepatAmine as their protein source while other therapy for encephalopathy was continued. Encephalopathy improved in 87% of 42 patients with cirrhosis and 75% of 17 patients with hepatitis, and plasma amino acid patterns changed toward normal.[258] A multicenter, prospective controlled trial compared 4 to 14 days of treatment with intravenous HepatAmine with oral neomycin in 59 patients with acute hepatic encephalopathy.[259] The mortality rate was 17% among 30 patients treated with the amino acid mixture and 55% among 29 treated with neomycin. The latter subjects, however, received only glucose instead of the amino acid mixture. In another multicenter randomized trial by Wahren et al., intravenous branched-chain amino acid administration reduced the concentrations of aromatic amino acids but neither improved cerebral function nor decreased mortality in patients with hepatic encephalopathy.[260] Similarly, in a study by Weber and Reiser of three groups of patients with alcoholic liver disease including stable cirrhosis, acute alcoholic hepatitis without portal-systemic encephalopathy, and cirrhosis with encephalopathy, plasma amino acids did not change with improvement in PSE, and abnormalities of plasma amino acids did not prevent maintenance or attainment of positive nitrogen balance in patients with acute alcoholic hepatitis.[261]

In three patients with cirrhosis and subclinical encephalopathy given increasing amounts (20 to 100 g/day) of intravenous FO80,[262] the results showed the following: (1) Positive nitrogen balance was achieved only with 80 and 100 g FO80/day. (2) Plasma ammonia fell during negative nitrogen balance but increased during positive nitrogen balance. (3) Plasma tyrosine and cystine fell significantly (p <0.05) with all intakes of FO80. (It should be noted here that hypotyrosinemia and hypocystinemia have also been observed in some cirrhotics given parenteral nutrition with FreAmine II, a common amino acid source.[263]) (4) The abnormal branched-chain to aromatic amino acid ratio was reversed. (5) Encephalopathy did not significantly change from baseline. The authors concluded that FO80 is an inadequate nutritional formula when given as the sole protein source because it produces hypotyrosinemia and hypocystinemia. Furthermore, although the ratio of plasma branched-chain to aromatic amino acids changed, this was not accompanied by improvement in encephalopathy. Similar equivocal results were obtained in attempts at manipulating amino acids through altering dietary protein in patients with severe liver disease.

Greenberger et al. showed that not only the quantity but also the quality of the dietary protein may be important in the management of the chronic condition.[264] Vegetable-derived protein was claimed to be superior to animal protein. However, Shaw et al. found no advantage in switching from animal to vegetable protein in terms of encephalopathy or nitrogen balance.[265] In fact, vegetable protein seemed to be less well tolerated by the patient. Similar negative results were obtained by De Bruijn et al. who found that comparable changes in dietary regimen were not associated with a change in the neurologic impairment.[266] They observed, however, that with a vegetable diet the apparent nitrogen balance tended to be more positive. Uribe et al. suggested that use of a vegetable protein diet may be complicated by hypoglycemia and that patients may find such diets "voluminous."[267]

Two studies have examined the usefulness of *oral* administration of branched-chain amino acids or branched-chain enriched mixtures of amino acids in the diet. In a study by Erikson et al., patients with cirrhosis and grade 1-2 hepatic encephalopathy for six months or longer were evaluated in a randomized double-blind crossover study testing the value of supplemental branched-chain amino acids in the diet.[268] The concentration of branched-chain amino acids increased in response to the supplementation, but there was no significant change in mental status. Four of the patients studied were consuming 40 g/day of protein while others consumed between 60 and 100

g/day. Patients were given 30 g of amino acids or sucrose maltodextrin. No change was noted even after administration for as long as 22 weeks. In another study by McGhee et al., Hepatic-Aid, a BCAA-enriched mixture of amino acids, was substituted for isonitrogenous casein in the diet.[267] It was comparable to casein with respect to clinical and biochemical effects but did not cause any further improvement in hepatic encephalopathy or nitrogen balance.

A nonselective overall amino acid supplementation has been reported to be beneficial in patients with alcoholic liver disease; indeed, intravenous therapy with amino acid for four weeks seemed to be associated with lower mortality rate (p<0.02).[270] Such a beneficial effect is to be expected to the extent that amino acid supplementation corrects a deficiency without exceeding the nitrogenous tolerance of the patient.

Tolerance to dietary protein may be enhanced through concomitant administration of neomycin, lactulose, and enemas. Neomycin inhibits the action of gastrointestinal flora that convert protein and urea to ammonia and other potentially toxic nitrogenous products within the gut. Decreased renal function (as with hepatorenal syndrome) may result in oto- and nephrotoxic blood levels of neomycin. Dosage must be markedly lowered or the drug discontinued under such circumstances. Ampicillin has been found to prevent the conversion of urea to ammonia within the GI tract[271] and may prove to be a useful alternative to neomycin in these circumstances. Lactulose, also used in place of neomycin, may act through acidification of bowel contents with resultant ammonia trapping (as ammonium) or through increased motility.[272]

Hypokalemia increases renal vein ammonia via a direct effect on renal ammonia production and possibly through increased back diffusion of ammonia from alkaline urine.[273] This condition may worsen encephalopathy. Parenteral or oral potassium may be given in dosages of approximately 100 to 200 meq/day until deficits are corrected, provided that renal function is normal.

### Ascites and Edema

Dietary regimen to combat ascites and edema is adjusted according to the severity of salt and water retention. Details of management are discussed in the section on water, minerals, and electrolytes.

### Renal Disorders

Oliguria, azotemia, and elevated creatinine may indicate deteriorating renal function. Patients with alcoholic liver disease are especially susceptible to acute tubular necrosis through such complications as variceal bleeding. Spontaneous renal failure or the so-called hepatorenal syndrome may also occur. Rising serum urea caused by renal failure may present a special problem in the patient with alcoholic liver disease. Urea diffuses into the GI tract and is hydrolyzed to ammonia; thus, it acts as any nitrogenous compound. With increasing levels of urea, the resultant ammonia becomes a significant problem and may worsen or precipitate hepatic coma.[274] In this case antibiotics (see the section on encephalopathy) may be given to prevent conversion of urea to ammonia. Enemas may be required.

### Neurologic Disorders

**Peripheral Neuropathy.** In patients with peripheral neuropathy, thiamin deficiency has been most strongly implicated in etiology, but other B vitamins have a place as well. $B_{12}$, pyridoxine, nicotinic acid, and riboflavin deficiencies can be associated with peripheral neuropathy, and pantothenic acid deficiency may produce symptoms of peripheral nerve disease.[244] Peripheral neuropathy, as with other neurological disorders found in the alcoholic, is generally treated with abstinence and B-vitamin therapy. Empirically, B vitamins are given as a group rather than as a specific vitamin therapy. Although the optimal therapeutic dosage has not been established, one recommendation is 10 times the normal daily requirement for 1 week and 5 times the daily requirement thereafter.[244] Megavitamin dosages of pyridoxine may produce sensory neuropathy.[252]

**Wernicke-Korsakoff Syndrome.** In patients with the Wernicke-Korsakoff syndrome, the ophthalmoplegia responds rapidly to thiamin administration while the ataxia and confusion respond more slowly. Although 2 to 3 mg may be sufficient, usually larger doses (50 mg) are given. Rapidity of response depends upon the conversion of thiamin to its active form in the liver. Patients with advanced liver disease such as cirrhosis may, therefore, have a delayed response.[47]

**Other Central Nervous System Disorders.** Nutritional amblyopia, cerebellar degeneration, Marchiafava-Bignami syndrome, and other rare central nervous system disorders seen in the alcoholic are prudently treated with abstinence and administration of B vitamins.

### Hematologic Disorders

Iron deficiency, if present in the alcoholic, should be corrected cautiously because of the propensity of these patients, if liver disease is present, to retain iron and because of the potential injurious effects of iron excess upon the liver. Thrombocytopenia may respond simply to abstinence

from alcohol or, if caused by vitamin deficiencies such as folate deficiency, to replacement therapy.

Anemias, low serum folate, and megaloblastic marrow with or without sideroblasts may be used to diagnose folate- and pyridoxine-related hematologic abnormalities. Therapy includes abstinence and vitamin supplementation. Although smaller doses may be adequate, many times the daily requirement of folate and pyridoxine are generally administered.

### Cardiomyopathy

Thiamin repletion is the specific therapy for beriberi heart disease. Therapy of 5 to 10 mg/day is probably adequate, although generally larger amounts are administered. Empirically, however, in any alcoholic with cardiomyopathy, B vitamins are generally given as a group, with an adequate diet and abstinence from alcohol. Magnesium deficiency should be corrected if present, although this is not a common clinical problem. Congestive heart failure from alcoholic cardiomyopathy is treated with conventional salt restriction and therapy used for heart disease of other etiologies.

## NUTRITIONAL STATUS OF THE ALCOHOLIC

Alcoholism remains one of the few causes of florid nutritional deficiencies in our society. However, the stereotype of the malnourished alcoholic is based largely upon studies of inner-city and indigent populations or patients in whom malnutrition is secondary to severe liver disease. Such a stereotype is probably unfounded as it applies to the millions of alcoholics in the United States. The spread of alcoholism to various socioeconomic classes, the greater availability and enrichment of foods, and the investigation of broader populations of alcoholics have led to a modification of this view. Indeed, moderate alcohol consumption has little impact on nutrition status,[275] and no significant differences have been found among alcoholics and nonalcoholics matched for socioeconomic and health history.[276] A study of middle-class alcoholics admitted to an alcoholism treatment facility revealed dietary intake to be well within the RDA for protein, fat, carbohydrate, and most other nutrients.[277] The mean daily protein intake was 86 g/day, and 88% met or exceeded their ideal body weight. Several of the patients, however, had intakes of less than 75% of the RDA for vitamin A, thiamin, niacin, and ascorbic acid. Similarly, a study of alcoholics "free of hepatic disease" admitted to a Veterans Administration Hospital for treatment of alcoholism revealed no deficiencies of visceral protein status by biochemical, anthropometric, and nutrient intake data.[278]

Nevertheless, alcohol may interact with nutrition at many levels to produce marginal if not clinically overt deficiencies. Populations with borderline nutrition, such as the elderly, may be especially susceptible to these effects.[279] The clinical significance of such nutritional deficiencies by themselves or in conjunction with alcohol with regard to organ damage remains an interesting area for further exploration.

# REFERENCES

1. Leake, C.D., Silverman, M.: The chemistry of alcoholic beverages. *In* Biology of Alcoholism. (Kissin, B., Begleiter, H., Eds.) New York, Plenum Publishing Corp., 1974.
2. Scheig, R.: Am. J. Clin. Nutr. *23*:467–471, 1974.
3. Pirola, R.C., Lieber, C.S.: Pharmacology *7*:185–196, 1972.
4. Pirola, R.C., Lieber, C.S.: Am. J. Clin. Nutr. *19*:90–97, 1976.
5. Davenport, H.W.: Gastroenterology *56*:439–446, 1969.
6. Lorber, S.H., Dinoso, V.P., Chey, W.Y.: Disease of the gastrointestinal tract. *In* Biology of Alcoholism. (Kissin, B., Begleiter, H., Eds.) New York, Plenum Publishing Corp., 1974.
7. Barboriak, J.J., Meade, R.C.: Am. J. Clin. Nutr. *23*:1151–1153, 1970.
8. Cooke, A.R.: Gastroenterology *62*:501–502, 1972.
9. Charlton, R.W., Jacobs, P., Seftel, H., et al.: Br. Med. J. 2:1427–1429, 1964.
10. Baraona, E., Pirola, R.C., Lieber, C.S.: Gastroenterology *66*:226–234, 1974.
11. Gottfried, E.B., Korsten, M.A., Lieber, C.S.: Am. J. Gastroenterol. *70*:587–592, 1976.
12. Pirola, R.C., Bolin, M., Davis, A.E.: Am. J. Dig. Dis. *14*:239–243, 1969.
13. Israel, Y., Valenzuela, J.E., Salazar, I., et al.: J. Nutr. *98*:222–224, 1969.
14. Hillman, R.W.: *In* Biology of Alcoholism. (Kissin, B., Begleiter, H., Eds.) New York, Plenum Publishing Corp., 1974, p. 513.
15. Robles, F.A., Mezey, E., Halsted, C.H., et al.: Johns Hopkins Med. J. *135*:17–36, 1974.
16. James, W.P.T.: Lancet *1*:333–335, 1968.
17. Mayoral, L.G., Tripahty, V., Garcia, F.T., et al.: Am. J. Clin. Nutr. *20*:866–870, 1967.
18. Winawer, S.J., Sullivan, L.W., Herbert, V., et al.: N. Engl. J. Med. *272*:892–895, 1965.
19. Halsted, C.H., Robles, E.A., Mezey, E.: N. Engl. J. Med. *285*:701–706, 1971.
20. Hermos, J.A., Adams, W.M., Liu, Y.K., et al.: Ann. Intern. Med. *76*:957–965, 1972.
21. Halsted, C.H., Robles, E.A., Mezey, E.: Gastroenterology *64*:526–532, 1973.
22. Tomasulo, P.A., Kater, R.M.N., Iber, F.L.: Am. J. Clin. Nutr. *21*:1340–1344, 1968.
23. Roggin, G.M., Iber, F.L., Kater, R.M.H., et al.: Johns Hopkins Med. J. *125*:321–330, 1969.
24. Mezey, E., Jow, E., Slavin, R.E., et al.: Gastroenterology *59*:657–664, 1970.
25. Lindenbaum, J., Lieber, C.S.: Nature *224*:806–807, 1969.
26. Mekhjian, M.S., May, E.S.: Gastroenterology *72*:1280–1286, 1977.
27. Lindenbaum, J., Lieber, C.S.: Ann. NY Acad. Sci. *252*:228–234, 1975.
28. Perlow, W., Baraona, E., Lieber, C.S.: Gastroenterology *72*:680–685, 1977.
29. Losowsky, M.S., Walker, B.E.: Gastroenterology *56*:589–600, 1969.
30. Faloon, W.W.: Am. J. Clin. Nutr. *23*:645–651, 1970.
31. Linscheer, W.G.: Am. J. Clin. Nutr. *23*:488–492, 1970.
32. Walton, R., Schapiro, H., Woodward, W.A.: Surg. Forum *11*:365–371, 1960.
33. Sarles, H., Tiscornia, O.: Med. Clin. North Am. *58*:1333, 1974.
34. Straus, E., Urbach, M.J., Yalow, R.S.: N. Engl. J. Med. *293*:1031–1032, 1975.
35. Mott, C.B., Sarles, H., Tiscornia, O., et al.: Dig. Dis. Sci. *17*:902–910, 1972.
36. Bayer, M., Rudick, J., Lieber, C.S., et al.: Gastroenterology *63*:619–626, 1972.
37. Marin, G.A., Ward, N.L., Fischer, R.: Dig. Dis. Sci. *18*:825–833, 1973.
38. Pirola, R.C., Davis, A.E.: Gut *9*:557–560, 1968.
39. Sarles, H.: Gastroenterology *66*:604–616, 1974.
40. Lefevre, A.F., DeCarli, L.M, Lieber, C.S.: J. Lipid Res. *13*:48–55, 1972.
41. Knodell, R.G., Kinsey, D., Boedeker, E.C., et al.: Gastroenterology *71*:196–201, 1976.
42. Vlahcevic, S.R., Juttijudata, P., Bell, C.C., et al.: Gastroenterology *62*:1174–1183, 1972.
43. Nicholas, P., Rinaudo, P.A., Conn, H.D.: Gastroenterology *63*:112–118, 1972.
44. Cherrick, G.R., Baker, H., Frank, O., et al.: J. Lab. Clin. Med. *66*:446–451, 1965.
45. Hines, J.D.: J. Lab. Clin. Med. *74*:883–888, 1969.
46. Sullivan, L.W., Herbert, V.: J. Clin. Invest. *43*:2048–2062, 1964.
47. Cole, M., Turner, A., Frank, O., et al.: Am. J. Clin. Nutr. *22*:44–51, 1969.
48. Eichner, E.R., Hillman, R.S.: Am. J. Med. *50*:218–223, 1971.
49. Veitch, R.L., Lumeng, L., Li, T.K.: Gastroenterology *66*:868–874, 1974.
50. Mitchell, D., Wagner, C., Stone, W.J., et al.: Gastroenterology *71*:1043–1049, 1976.
51. Sorrell, M.F., Baker, H., Barak, A.J., et al.: Am. J. Clin. Nutr. *27*:743–745, 1974.
52. Williams, R.J.: Alcoholism—The Nutritional Approach. Austin, University of Texas Press, 1959.
53. Mickelsen, J.: J. Am. Diet. Assoc. *31*:570, 1955.
54. Kiessling, K.H., Tilander, K.: Q. J. Stud. Alc. *22*:535–543, 1961.
55. Kontinnen, K., Oura, E., Suomalainen, H.: Ann. Med. Exp. Penn. *45*:68–71, 1967.
56. Chan, A.W.K.: Pharmacologist *18*:237, 1976.
57. Frank, O., Baker, H.: Am. J. Clin. Nutr. *33*:221–226, 1980.
58. Abe, T., Okamoto, F., Itokawa, Y.: J. Nutr. Sci. Vitaminol. *25*:375–383, 1979.
59. Hoyumpa, A.M., Nichols, S., Henderson, G.I., et al.: Am. J. Clin. Nutr. *31*:938–945, 1978.
60. Balaghi, M., Neal, R.A.: J. Nutr. *107*:2144–2152, 1977.
61. Lieber, C.S., DeCarli, L.M.: Fed. Proc. *35*:1233–1236, 1976.
62. Shaw, S., Gorkin, B.D., Lieber, C.S.: Am. J. Clin. Nutr. *34*:856–860, 1981.
63. Vorhees, C.V., Barrett, R.J., Schenker, S.: Life Sci. *16*:1187–2000, 1975.
64. Victor, M., Adams, R.D.: Am. J. Clin. Nutr. *9*:379–387, 1961.
65. Victor, M., Adams, R.D., Collins, C.H.: The Wer-

nicke-Korsakoff Syndrome. Philadelphia, F.A. Davis Co., 1971.

66. Blass, J.P., Gibson, G.E.: N. Engl. J. Med. *297*:1367–1370, 1977.
67. Walker, D.W., Freund, G.: Physiol. Behav. *7*:773, 1971.
68. Thomson, A., Baker, M., Leevy, C.M.: Am. J. Clin. Nutr. *21*:537–538, 1968.
69. Tomasulo, P.A., Kater, R.M.H., Iber, F.L.: Am. J. Clin. Nutr. *21*:1341–1344, 1968.
70. Westerfeld, W.W., Doisy, E.A.: J. Nutr. *30*:127–136, 1945.
71. Butler, R.E., Sarrett, H.P.: J. Nutr. *35*:539–548, 1948.
72. Cole, M., Turner, A., Frank, O., et al.: Am. J. Clin. Nutr. *22*:44–51, 1969.
73. Baker, H., Frank, O., Ziffer, H., et al.: Am. J. Clin. Nutr. *14*:1–6, 1964.
74. Camilo, M.E., Morgan, M.Y., Sherlock, S.: Scand. J. Gastroenterol. *16*:273–279, 1981.
75. Veitch, R.L., Lumeng, L., Li, T.K.: J. Clin. Invest. *55*:1026–1032, 1975.
76. Lumeng, L., Li, T.K.: J. Clin. Invest. *53*:693–698, 1974.
77. Beattie, A.D., Sherlock, S.: Gut *17*:571–575, 1976.
78. Sullivan, L.W., Herbert, V.: J. Clin. Invest. *43*:2048, 1964.
79. Paine, C.J., Eichner, E.R., Dickson V.: Am. J. Med. Sci. *266*:135–138, 1973.
80. Eichner, E.R., Hillman, R.S.: J. Clin. Invest. *52*:584–591, 1973.
81. Steinberg, S.E., Campbell, C.L, Hillman, R.S.: Biochem. Pharmacol. *30*:97–98, 1981.
82. Brown, J.P., Davidson, G.E., Scott, J.M., et al.: Biochem. Pharmacol. *22*:3287, 1973.
83. Patek, A.J., Haig, C.: J. Clin. Invest. *18*:609–616, 1939.
84. Wald, G.: Science *162*:230–239, 1969.
85. Smith, J.C., Brown, E.D., White, S.C., et al.: Lancet *1*:1251–1252, 1975.
86. McClain, C.J., Van Thiel, D.H., Parker, S., et al.: Alcoholism: Clin. Exp. Res. *3*:135–140, 1979.
87. Patek, A.J., Toth, I.G., Saunders, M.G., et al.: Arch. Intern. Med. *135*:1053–1057, 1975.
88. Smith, F.R., Goodman, D.S.: J. Clin. Invest. *50*:2426–2436, 1971.
89. Smith, J.C., McDaniel, E.G., Fan, F.F., et al.: Science *181*:954–955, 1973.
90. Wolff, K.L.: Lancet *223*:617–620, 1932.
91. Russell, R.M., Morrison, S.A., Smith, F.R., et al.: Ann. Intern. Med. *88*:622–626, 1978.
92. Morbarhan, S., Russell, R.M., Underwood, B.A., et al.: Am. J. Clin. Nutr. *34*:2264–2270, 1981.
93. Leo, M.A., Lieber, C.S.: N. Engl. J. Med. *37*:597–601, 1982.
94. Vahlquist, A., Sjolund, K., Norden, A., et al.: Scand. J. Clin. Lab. Invest. *38*:301–308, 1978.
95. Sato, M., Lieber, C.S.: J. Nutr. *111*:2015—2023, 1981.
96. Suschetet, M.: J. Int. Vitaminol. Nutr. *45*:129–137, 1975.
97. Baumann, C.A., Foster, E.G., Moore, P.R.: J. Biol. Chem. *142*:597–608, 1942.
98. Blomstrand, R., Lof, A., Osling, H.: Nutr. Metab. *21*:148–151, 1977.
99. Sato, M., Lieber, C.S.: J. Nutr. *112*:1188–1196, 1982.
100. Sato, M., Lieber, C.S.: Arch. Biochem. Biophys. *213*:557–564, 1982.

101. Leo, M.A., Sato, M., Lieber, C.S.: Gastroenterology *84*:562–572, 1983.
102. Russell, R.M., Boyer, S.A., Bagheri, S.A.: N. Engl. J. Med. *291*:435–440, 1974.
103. Farrell, G.C., Bathal, P.S., Powell, L.W.: Dig. Dis. Sci. *22*:724–728, 1977.
104. Herbert, V.: Am. J. Clin. Nutr. *36*:185–186, 1982.
105. Sommer, A., Tarwotjo, I., Djunaedi, M.E., et al.: Lancet *1*:557–559, 1980.
106. Lieber, C.S.: Am. J. Gastroenterol. *74*:313–320, 1980.
107. Sato, C., Matsuda, Y., Lieber, C.S.: Gastroenterology *80*:140–148, 1981.
108. Leo, M.A., Arai, M., Sato, M., et al.: Gastroenterology *82*:194–205, 1982.
109. Leo, M.A., Lieber, C.S.: Hepatology *3*:1–11, 1983.
110. Mallia, A.K., Smith, J.E., Goodman, D.W.S.: J. Lipid Res. *16*:180–188, 1975.
111. Smith, F.R., Goodman, D.W.S.: N. Engl. J. Med. *294*:805–808, 1976.
112. Hasumura, Y., Teschke, R., Lieber, C.S.: Gastroenterology *66*:415–422, 1974.
113. Saville, P.D.: J. Bone Joint Surg. *47*:492–499, 1965.
114. Nilsson, B.E.: Acta Chir. Scand. *136*:383–387, 1970.
115. Solomon, L.: J. Bone Joint Surg. *55*:246–261, 1973.
116. Avioli, L.V., Lee, S.W., McDonald, J.E., et al.: J. Clin. Invest. *46*:983–992, 1967.
117. Bjorneboe, G.A., Johnsen, J., Bjorneboe, A., et al.: Am. J. Clin. Nutr. *44*:678–682, 1986.
118. Hepner, G.W., Roginsky, M., Moo, H.F.: Am. J. Dig. Dis. *21*:527–531, 1976.
119. Posner, D.B., Russell, R.M., Absood, S., et al.: Gastroenterology *74*:866–870, 1978.
120. Luisier, M., Vocoz, J.F., Donath, A., et al.: Schweiz. Med. Wochenschr. *107*:1529–1533, 1977.
121. Baran, D.T., Teitelbaum, S.L., Berfeld, M.A., et al.: Am. J. Physiol. *238*:507–510, 1980.
122. Summerskill, W.H.J., Barnado, D.E., Baldus, W.P.: Am. J. Clin. Nutr. *23*:499–507, 1980.
123. Hilden, T., Svendsen, T.L.: Lancet *2*:245–246, 1975.
124. Gabuzda, G.J.: Gastroenterology *58*:546–553, 1980.
125. Gabuzda, G.J.: Med. Clin. North Am. *54*:1455–1469, 1970.
126. Soler, M.G., Jain, S., James, H., et al.: Gut *17*:152–157, 1976.
127. McDonald, J.T., Margen, S.: Am. J. Clin. Nutr. *32*:817–822, 1979.
128. McCollister, R., Prasad, A.S., Doe, R.P., et al.: J. Lab. Clin. Med. *52*:928–932, 1958.
129. Sargent, W.Q., Simpson, J.R., Beard, J.D.: J. Pharmacol. Ther. *190*:507, 1974.
130. Peng, T.C., Gitelman, M.J.: Endocrinology *94*:608–612, 1974.
131. Szutowski, M.M., Lipsaka, M., Bandolet, J.P.: Polish J. Pharmacol. *28*:397–401, 1974.
132. McDonald, J.T., Margen, S.: Am. J. Clin. Nutr. *32*:823–833, 1979.
133. Sullivan, J.F., Williams, R.V., Burch, R.E.: Alcoholism: Clin. Exp. Res. *3*:235–239, 1979.
134. Lin, P., Jacob, E.: Q. J. Med. *41*:291–300, 1972.
135. Mendelson, J.H., Barnes, B., Mayman, C., et al.: Metabolism *14*:88–94, 1965.
136. Heaton, F.W., Pyrah, W., Beresford, C.L., et al: Lancet *2*:802–805, 1962.
137. Shah, J.M., Bowser, N., Hargis, G.K., et al.: Metabolism *27*:257–260, 1978.

138. Markkanen, T., Nanto, V.: Experientia *XXII*:753–754, 1966.
139. Krawitt, E.L.: J. Lab. Clin. Med. *85*:665–671, 1975.
140. Stein, J.M., Smith, W.D., Ginn, H.E.: Am. J. Med. Sci. *252*:78–83, 1966.
141. Blachley, J.D., Ferguson, E.R., Carter, N.W., et al.: Trans. Assoc. Am. Physicians *94*:110–122, 1980.
142. Ferguson, E.R., Blachley, J.D., Knochel, J.P.: Alcoholism: Clin. Exp. Res. *29*:583A, 1981.
143. Grace, N.D., Powell, L.W.: Gastroenterology *67*:1257–1268, 1974.
144. Volini, F., Huerga, J., Kent, G.: Trace metal studies in liver disease using atomic absorption spectrometry. *In* Laboratory Diagnosis of Liver Disease. (Sunderman, F.W., Sunderman, F.W., Jr., Green, W.H., Eds.) St. Louis, W.H. Green, 1968.
145. Chapman, R.W., Morgan, M.Y., Laulicht, M., et al.: Dig. Dis. Sci. *27*:909–915, 1982.
146. Regoeczi, E., Chindemi, P.A., Debanne, M.T.: Alcoholism: Clin. Exp. Res. *8*:287–292, 1984.
147. Chapman, R.W., Morgan, M.Y., Bell R., et al.: Gastroenterology *84*:143–149, 1983.
148. Chapman, R.W., Morgan, M.Y., Boss, A.M., et al.: Dig. Dis. Sci. *28*:321–327, 1983.
149. Eichner, E.R., Hillman, R.S.: Am. J. Med. *50*:218–223, 1971.
150. Hartoma, T.R., Sontaniemi, E.A., Pelkonen, O., et al.: Eur. J. Clin. Pharmacol. *12*:147–151, 1977.
151. Helwig, H.L., Hoffer, E.M., Thielen, W.C., et al.: Am. J. Clin. Pathol. *45*:156–159, 1966.
152. Versiek, J., Hoste, J., VanBallenberghe, L., et al.: J. Lab. Clin. Med. *97*:535–544, 1981.
153. Lindenbaum, J., Shea, N., Saha, S.R., et al.: Clin. Res. *20*:459, 1972.
154. Metz, R., Berger, S., Mako, M.: Diabetes *18*:517–522, 1969.
155. Phillips, G.B., Safrit, H.F.: JAMA, *217*:1513–1519, 1971.
156. Rehfeld, J.F., Juhl, E., Hilden, M.: Gastroenterology *64*:445–451, 1973.
157. Arky, R.A.: The effect of alcohol on carbohydrate metabolism. *In* Biology of Alcoholism. (Kissin, B., Begleiter, H., Eds.) New York, Plenum Publishing Corp., 1974.
158. Lieber, C.S., Jones, F., Losowsky, R.S., et al.: J. Clin. Invest *41*:1863, 1962.
159. Newcombe, D.S.: Metabolism *21*:1193–1203, 1972.
160. MacLachlan, M.J., Rodnan, C.P.: Am. J. Med. *42*:38–57, 1967.
161. Faller, J., Fox, I.H.: N. Engl. J. Med. *307*:1598–1602, 1982.
162. Mitchell, M.C., Hoyumpa, A.M., Schenker, S., et al.: J. Lab. Clin. Med. *101*:826–834, 1983.
163. Lieber, C.S.: Lipids *9*:103–107, 1974.
164. Lieber, C.S.: Ethanol and lipid disorders including fatty liver, hyperlipidemia and atherosclerosis. *In* Metabolic Aspects of Alcoholism. Lancaster, England, MTP Press, 1977, pp. 141–177.
165. Mitstillis, S.P., Ockner, R.K.: J. Lab. Clin. Med. *80*:34–46, 1972.
166. Baraona, E., Pirola, R.C., Lieber, C.S.: J. Clin. Invest. *52*:296–303, 1973.
167. Wilson, D.E., Schreibmann, P.H., Brewster, A.L., et al.: J. Lab. Clin. Med. *75*:264–274, 1974.
168. Ostrander, L.D., Lamphiear, D.E., Block, W.D., et al.: Arch. Intern. Med. *134*:451–456, 1974.
169. Chait, A., February, A.E., Mancini, M., et al.: Lancet *2*:62–64, 1972.
170. Ginsberg, H., Olefsky, J., Farquhar, J.W., et al.: Ann. Intern. Med. *80*:143–149, 1974.
171. Losowsky, M.S., Jones, D.P., Davidson, C.S., et al.: Am. J. Med. *35*:794–803, 1963.
172. Kessler, J.I., Kniffen, J.C., Janowitz, H.J.: N. Engl. J. Med. *269*:943–948, 1963.
173. Zieve, L.: Ann. Intern. Med. *48*:471–496, 1958.
174. Gruchow, M.H., Hoffman, R.G., Anderson, P.J., et al.: Atherosclerosis *43*:393–404, 1982.
175. Marzo, S., Ghirardi, P., Sandini, D., et al.: Klin. Wochenschr. *48*:949–950, 1970.
176. Guisard, D., Gonand, J.P., Laurent, J., et al.: Nutr. Metab. *13*:222–229, 1971.
177. Lieber, C.S., DeCarli, L.M.: Am. J. Clin. Nutr. *23*:474–478, 1970.
178. Crews, R.H., Faloon, W.W.: JAMA *181*:754–756, 1962.
179. Schapiro, R.H., Drummey, G.D., Shimizu, Y., et al.: J. Clin. Invest. *43*:1338–1347, 1964.
180. Rothschild, M.A., Oratz, M., Mongelli, J., et al.: J. Clin. Invest. *50*:1812–1818, 1971.
181. Jeejeebhoy, K.N., Phillips, M.J., Bruce-Robertson, A., et al.: Biochem. J. *126*:1111–1126, 1972.
182. Baraona, E., Leo, M.A., Borowsky, S.A., et al.: Science *190*:794–795, 1975.
183. Klatskin, G.: Yale J. Biol. Med. *34*:124–143, 1961.
184. Rodrigo, C., Antezana, L., Baraona, E.: J. Nutr. *101*:1307–1310, 1971.
185. Gabuzda, G.J., Shear, L.: Am. J. Clin. Nutr. *23*:479–486, 1970.
186. Lieber, C.S.: Medical Disorders of Alcoholism: Pathogenesis and Treatment. Philadelphia, W.B. Saunders, 1982.
187. Piccirillo, W., Chambers, J.W.: Res. Commun. Chem. Pathol. Pharmacol. *13*:297–308, 1976.
188. Finkelstein, J.D., Cello, J.P., Kyle, W.E.: Biochem. Biophys. Res. Commun. *61*:475–481, 1974.
189. Shaw, S., Lieber, C.S.: Gastroenterology *74*:677–682, 1978.
190. Pasquariello, G., Quadri, A., Tenconi, L.T.: Tryptophan-nicotinic acid metabolism in chronic alcoholism. *In* 6th International Congress of Gerontology, Copenhagen, 1963.
191. Branchey, L., Shaw, S., Lieber, C.S.: Life Sci. *29*:2751–2755, 1981.
192. Siegel, F.L., Roach, M.K., Pomeroy, L.R.: Proc. Natl. Acad. Sci. *51*:605, 1964.
193. Iob, V., Coon, W.W., Sloan, M.: J. Surg. Res. *7*:41–43, 1967.
194. Zinneman, H.N., Seal, U.S., Doe, P.P.: Am. J. Dig. Dis. *14*:118–126, 1969.
195. Rosen, H.M., Yoshimura, N., Hodgman, J., et al.: Gastroenterology *72*:483–487, 1977.
196. Iob, V., Coon, W.W., Sloan, M.: J. Surg. Res. *6*:233–239, 1966.
197. Shaw, S., Worner, T., Borysow, M., et al.: Alcoholism: Clin. Exp. Res. *3*:297–301, 1979.
198. Wu, A., Bollman, J.L., Butt, H.R.: J. Clin. Invest. *34*:845–849, 1955.
199. Levine, R.J., Coon, H.O.: J. Clin. Invest. *46*:2012–2020, 1967.
200. Iber, F.L., Rosen, H., Levenson, S.M., et al.: J. Lab. Clin. Med. *50*:417–425, 1957.
201. Fischer, J.E., Rosen, H.M., Ebeid, A.M., et al.: Surgery *78*:276–290, 1975.
202. Faraj, B.A., Bowen, P.A., Isaacs, J.W., et al.: N. Engl. J. Med. *294*:1360–1364, 1976.
203. Fischer, J.E., Ebeid, A.M., Rosen, H.M., et al.: Gastroenterology *70*:981, 1976.
204. Crow, K.E., Cornell, N.W., Veech, R.L.: Alcoholism: Clin. Exp. Res. *1*:43–47, 1977.

205. Bode, J.L., Goebell, H., Stähler, M.: Gesamte Exp. Med. *152*:111–124, 1970.
206. Bode, J.L., Buchwald, B., Goebell, H.: German Med. Mon. *1*:149–151, 1971.
207. Meijer, A.J., Van Woebkom, G.M., Williamson, J.R., et al.: Biochem. J. *150*:205–209, 1975.
208. Korsten, M.A., Matsuzaki, S., Feinman, L., et al.: N. Engl. J. Med. *292*:386, 1975.
209. Patek, A.L., Toth, I.G., Saunders, M.G., et al.: Arch. Intern. Med. *135*:1053–1057, 1975.
210. Davidson, C.S.: Am. J. Clin. Nutr. *23*:427–431, 1970.
211. Sherlock, S., Walshe, V.: Nature *161*:604, 1948.
212. Hoffbauer, F.W., Zaki, F.G.: Arch. Pathol. *79*:364–369, 1965.
213. Olson, R.E.: Nutrition and Alcoholism. *In* Modern Nutrition in Health and Disease. 3rd ed. (Wohl, M.G., Goodhart, R.S., Eds.). Philadelphia, Lea & Febiger, 1964, pp 779–795.
214. Rubin, E., Lieber, C.S.: N. Engl. J. Med. *178*:869–876, 1968.
215. Lieber, C.S., Jones, D.P., DeCarli, L.M.: J. Clin. Invest. *44*:1009–1020, 1965.
216. Lieber, C.S., DeCarli, L.M.: Gastroenterology *50*:316–322, 1966.
217. Hartroft, S.W., Porta, E.A.: Can. J. Physiol. Pharmacol. *46*:463–471, 1968.
218. Erenoglu, E., Edreira, J.G., Patek, A.J.: Ann. Intern. Med. *60*:814–821, 1964.
219. US Bureau of the Census: Vital Statistics Rates in the United States, 1900–1940, Washington, D.C., Government Printing Office, 1943.
220. Lederman, S.: Alcohol, Alcoholisme, Alcoholisation. Institut National d'Etudes Demographiques, Travaux et Documents, Cahier No. 41, Paris, Presses Universitaires de France, 1964.
221. Lelbach, W.K.: Acta Hepatosplenol. *14*:9–16, 1967.
222. Menghini, G.: Bull. Schweiz. Akad. Med. Wiss. *16*:36–52, 1960.
223. Rubin, E., Lieber, C.S.: Fed. Proc. *26*:1458–1462, 1967.
224. Lieber, C.S., Rubin, E.: Am. J. Med. *44*:200–211, 1968.
225. Lieber, C.S., DeCarli, L.M.: J. Med. Primatol. *3*:153–163, 1974.
226. Rubin, E., Lieber, C.S.: N. Engl. J. Med. *290*:128–134, 1974.
227. Lieber, C.S., DeCarli, L.M., Rubin, E.: Proc. Natl. Acad. Sci. *72*:437–441, 1975.
228. Lieber, C.S., Spritz, N.: J. Clin. Invest. *45*:1400–1411, 1966.
229. Klatskin, G., Krehl, W.A., Conn, H.O.: J. Exp. Med. *100*:605–614, 1966.
230. Lieber, C.S., Spritz, N., DeCarli, L.M.: J. Clin. Invest. *45*:51–62, 1966.
231. Lieber, C.S., Spritz, N., DeCarli, L.M.: J. Lipid Res. *10*:283–287, 1969.
232. Kyosola, K., Salorinne, Y.: Ann. Clin. Res. *7*:80–84, 1975.
233. Bhuyan, U.N., Nayak, N.C., Deo, M.G., et al.: Lab. Invest. *14*:184–190, 1965.
234. Hibbs, R.G., Ferrans, V.J., Black, W.L., et al.: Am. Heart J. *69*:766–771, 1965.
235. Susin, M., Herdson, P.B.: Arch. Pathol. *83*:86–92, 1967.
236. Regan, T.J., Levinson, G.E., Oldenurtel, H.A., et al.: Clin. Invest, *48*:397–403, 1969.
237. Wendt, V.E., Wu, L.A., Luni, R., et al.: Ann. Intern. Med. *62*:1068–1073, 1965.
238. Morin, Y.L., Daniel, A.: Can. Med. Assoc. J. *97*:926–931, 1967.
239. Eichner, E.R., Buchanan, B., Smith, J.W., et al.: Am. J. Med. Sci. *263*:35–42, 1972.
240. Lindenbaum, J., Lieber, C.S.: N. Engl. J. Med. *281*:333–338, 1969.
241. Haut, M.J., Cowan, D.H.: Am. J. Med. *56*:22–32, 1974.
242. Lindenbaum, J., Hargrove, R.L.: Ann. Intern. Med. *68*:526–532, 1968.
243. Brayton, R.G., Strokes, P.E., Schwartz, M.S., et al.: N. Engl. J. Med. *282*:123–128, 1970.
244. Hornabrook, P.W.: Am. J. Clin. Nutr. *9*:398, 1961.
245. Platt, B.S.: Thiamine deficiency in human beriberi and in Wernicke's encephalopathy. *In* Thiamine Deficiency: Biochemical Lesions and Their Clinical Significance. (Wolstenholme, G.E.W., Ed.) Boston, Little, Brown and Co., 1967.
246. Neubueger, K.T.: Arch. Pathol. *63*:1–6, 1957.
247. Dreyfus, P.M., Victor, M.: Am. J. Clin. Nutr. *9*:414–425, 1961.
248. Phillips, T.W., Victor, M., Adams, R.D., et al.: J. Clin. Invest. *31*:859–871, 1952.
249. Muller-Kobald, M.J.P., Endiz, C.J.: Ned. Tijdschr. Geneeskd. *119*:991–996, 1975.
250. Walker, D.W., Freund, G.: Science *182*:597–599, 1973.
251. Graham, J.R., Woodhouse, P., Read, F.S.: Lancet *2*:107, 1971.
252. Schaumburg, H., Kaplan, J., Windebank A., et al.: N. Engl. J. Med. *309*:445–448, 1983.
253. Rudman, D., Akgun, S., Galambos, J.T.: Am. J. Clin. Nutr. *23*:1203–1211, 1970.
254. Breuer, V.L., Breuer, H.: Z. Klin. Chem. Klin. Biochem. *13*:191–196, 1975.
255. Ning, M., Lowenstein, L.M., Davidson, L.S.: J. Lab. Clin. Med. *70*:554–562, 1967.
256. Lieber, C.S., Leo, M.A., Mak, K.M., et al.: Hepatology *5*:561–572, 1985.
257. Fischer, J.F.: Dig. Dis. Sci. *27*:97–102, 1982.
258. Freund, H., Dienstag, J., Lehrich, J., et al.: Ann. Surg. *196*:209–220, 1982.
259. Cerra, F.B., Cheung, N.K., Fischer, J.E., et al.: Hepatology *2*:699, 1983.
260. Wahren, J., Denis, J., Desurmont, P., et al.: Hepatology *3*:475–480, 1983.
261. Weber, F.L., Reiser, B.J.: Dig. Dis. Sci. *27*:103–110, 1982.
262. Millikan, W.J., Jr., Henderson, J.M., Warren, W.D., et al.: Ann. Surg. *197*:294–304, 1983.
263. Rudman, D., Kutner, M., Ansley, J., et al.: Gastroenterology *81*:1025–1035, 1981.
264. Greenberger, N.J., Carley, J., Schenker, S., et al.: Am. J. Dig. Dis. *22*:845–855, 1977.
265. Shaw, S., Worner, T., Lieber, C.S.: Am. J. Clin. Nutr. *38*:59–63, 1983a.
266. De Bruijn, K.M., Blendis, L.M., Zilm, D.H., et al.: Gut *24*:53–60, 1983.
267. Uribe, M., Marquez, M.A., Ramos, G.G., et al.: Dig. Dis. Sci. *27*:1109–1116, 1982.
268. Eriksson, L.S., Persson, A., Wahren, J: Gut *23*:801–806, 1981.
269. McGhee, A., Henderson, J.M., Millikan, W.J., et al.: Ann. Surg. *197*:288–293, 1983.
270. Nasrallah, S.M., Galambos, J.T.: Lancet *2*:1276–1277, 1980.
271. Meyers, S., Lieber, C.S.: Gastroenterology *70*:244–247, 1976.
272. Hubel, K.A.: Gastroenterology *65*:349, 1973.

273. Shear, L., Gabuzda, G.J.: Am. J. Clin. Nutr. *23*:614–618, 1970.
274. Lieber, C.S., Davidson, C.S.: Arch. Intern. Med. *106*:749–752, 1960.
275. Bebb, H.T., Houser, H.B., Witschi, J.C., et al.: Am. J. Clin. Nutr. *24*:1042–1047, 1971.
276. Westerfeld, W.W., Shulman, M.P.: JAMA *170*:197–200, 1959.
277. Hurt, R.D., Higgins, J.A., Nelson, R.A., et al.: Am. J. Clin. Nutr. *34*:386–392, 1981.
278. Dickson, B.J., Delaney, C.J., Walker, O., et al.: Am. J. Clin. Nutr. *37*:216–220, 1983.
279. Barboriak, J.J., Rooney, C.B., Leitschuh, T.H., et al.: J. Am. Diet. Assoc. *72*:493–495, 1981.

## SELECTED READINGS

Davidson, C.S.: Am. J. Clin. Nutr. *23*:427–436, 1970.

Gabuzda, G.J.: Med. Clin. North. Am. *54*:1455–1469, 1970.

Gabuzda, G.J., Shear, L.: Am. J. Clin. Nutr. *23*:479–486, 1970.

Leake, C.D., Silverman, M.: The chemistry of alcoholic beverages. *In* Biology of Alcoholism. (Kissin, B., Begleiter, H., Eds.) New York, Plenum Publishing Corp., 1974.

Leo, M.A., Lieber, C.S.: Alcoholism: Clin. Exp. Res. *7*:15–21, 1983.

Lieber, C.S.: Medical Disorders of Alcoholism: Pathogenesis and Treatment. Philadelphia, W.B. Saunders Co., 1982.

Lieber, C.S.: Alcohol *1*:151–157, 1984.

Lieber, C.S.: Hepatology *4*:1243–1260, 1984.

Lieber, C.S., Leo, M.A.: *In* Metabolism and Nutrition in Liver Disease. (Holm, E., Kasper, H., Eds.) Lancaster, England, MTP Press, Ltd., 1985, pp. 157–179.

Pirola, R.C., Lieber, C.S.: Pharmacology *7*:185–196, 1972.

Shaw, S., Lieber, C.S.: Alcoholism: Clin. Exp. Res. *7*:22–27, 1983.

Shaw, S., Worner, T., Lieber, C.S.: Am. J. Clin. Nutr. *38*:59–63, 1983.

*Chapter* **66**

# BEHAVIORAL DISORDERS AFFECTING FOOD INTAKE: ANOREXIA NERVOSA AND BULIMIA

Alexander R. Lucas and Diane M. Huse

Eating disorders are defined as deviations in eating patterns that lead to disease or disability, especially cachexia or obesity. They often are classified on the basis of their visible end result—that is, extreme thinness or fatness—but the variations in eating pattern also should be considered.[1] Anorexia nervosa is characterized by persistent intentional weight loss and maintenance of weight at an abnormally low level. Bulimia, which means ravenous appetite, also is the term commonly applied to a syndrome involving binge eating (rapid consumption of food in a discrete period of time, usually less than two hours), vomiting, and purging.

Historical views of anorexia nervosa, identified in the medical literature as early as 300 years ago, have been reviewed by Lucas.[2] Richard Morton first described the condition,[3] and Sir William Gull named it over a century ago.[4] There still is some confusion about the classification of anorexia nervosa. It is generally agreed that it be classified among psychogenic disorders with characteristic weight phobia. Hypothalamic dysfunction is a feature, but researchers disagree whether this dysfunction is primary or secondary to the undernutrition.[2,5,6]

Bruch emphasized that not all forms of psychogenic malnutrition should be classified as anorexia nervosa.[7] She separated those forms of undernutrition incidental to schizophrenia, depression, and certain somatic conditions. Within the remaining group of cases commonly recognized as anorexia nervosa, Bruch distinguished two categories of patients on the basis of the psychologic motivation. The patients identified as having *primary anorexia nervosa* exhibit preoccupation with body size, manifested by a relentless pursuit of thinness and a phobic avoidance of being fat, a disturbance in perception of bodily states such as hunger and satiation, and a profound sense of ineffectiveness. In *atypical anorexia nervosa*, the patient is preoccupied with the eating function itself and its distorted symbolic meaning, with thinness being only an accidental by-product. In the latter group, conversion hysteria and other psychoneurotic conflicts are recognized.

Less is known about the classification of bulimia. Russell described bulimia nervosa as a syndrome.[8] Casper reviewed the history of the syndrome as well as that of bulimia as a symptom.[9] The syndrome is thought to be common in normal-weight individuals, particularly in young women of late high school and college age.

## PATHOPHYSIOLOGY

The pathophysiologic changes seen in anorexia nervosa are similar to those observed in other states of semistarvation. For the most part, they are adaptive responses that allow the individual to survive a decreased dietary intake of energy sources. Such adaptations, however, are not without their "cost": functional impairment in other systems that limit the individual's capacity to perform normal physical and mental activities. Many of the symptoms and signs of anorexia nervosa can readily be understood within the context of "normal" adaptations to semistarvation.[10]

Starvation is associated with energy conservation, with adaptations that spare glucose and protein while favoring utilization of fat, with often dramatic shifts in fluid and electrolyte balances, and with alterations in hypothalamic-pituitary function that result especially in amenorrhea and infertility. These adaptive changes may not account for all of the decrease in energy utilization. Diminished protein synthesis and turnover probably also contribute substantially. However, the known alterations in insulin, thyroid, and catecholamine metabolism provide a framework for understanding some of the signs and symptoms experienced by semistarved patients, including the reductions in pulse rate, respiratory rate, blood pressure, oxygen consumption, carbon dioxide production, cardiac output, gut motility, and other autonomic nervous system responses.

The alterations in thyroid hormone and catecholamine metabolism may also contribute to cold intolerance, dry skin, dry hair, hypercarotenemia, hypercholesterolemia, prolongation of ankle reflexes, constipation, and other symptoms of semistarvation. A more detailed discussion of fasting diuresis and refeeding edema, energy conservation, and endocrine adaptations in fasting and semistarvation, delineated in the classic studies by Benedict and Keys et al., is published elsewhere.[10]

The hypothalamic responses to energy deprivation are also adaptive, allowing the organism to survive better than would be the case if such adaptations failed to occur. The most obvious example is the alteration in control of secretion of pituitary gonadotropins, resulting in disruption of normal cyclic patterns and producing anovulation, amenorrhea, infertility, and reduced libido. Such adaptations decrease the likelihood of becoming pregnant and also preserve the iron and protein stores that normally would be lost during menstrual flow.

Recent work has focused on the study of the hypothalamus-pituitary end-organ axis in an attempt to elucidate the neurophysiologic mechanisms underlying anorexia nervosa. Boyar and colleagues demonstrated circadian patterns of luteinizing hormone (LH) secretion in patients with anorexia nervosa, similar to those seen in prepubertal girls.[11] Information on the ability of the pituitary to secrete gonadotropins in patients with anorexia nervosa has come from the use of a single injection of luteinizing hormone–releasing hormones (LH-RH). These studies have shown im-

paired LH and follicle-stimulating hormone (FSH) response at low weight but normal response after weight gain.[12] Marshall and Kelch used low-dose injections of LH-RH every two hours to simulate the physiologic pulsations of the LH response and demonstrated the resumption of pubertal and adult LH secretion patterns in underweight anorexia nervosa patients.[13] This evidence has been used to support the hypothesis that there is hypothalamic dysfunction in anorexia nervosa.[14] However, the hypothalamic changes could be energy-conserving adaptations to protect the organism from the effects of calorie deprivation.

Another argument put forth to support the idea of "hypothalamic immaturity" is that some anorexia nervosa patients become amenorrheic before experiencing weight loss. The amenorrhea, however, can be due to any number of poorly understood mechanisms, both psychic and physiologic. In many instances, amenorrhea is a later development reflecting loss of body weight and fat. This relationship has been demonstrated in the normal population by Frisch and McArthur.[15] There is no doubt that adequate body weight and fat, subject to individual variability, are prerequisite for menstrual function. In addition, central nervous system regulatory controls originating at hypothalamic and higher centers influence this delicate endocrine mechanism. The giving up of "anorectic mental attitudes" is necessary, in addition to weight gain, in order for menstruation to resume.[16]

In bulimia, menstrual function is often maintained or may be irregular, but this subject has not been studied extensively.

## ETIOLOGY AND PATHOGENESIS

The current view is that eating disorders have multiple interacting causes. The biopsychosocial conceptualization identifies roots in three spheres: biologic, psychologic, and social. This model suggests a unique interaction of variables for each individual. An unexplained physiologic predisposition with possible genetic determinants leads to a variable degree of biologic vulnerability in persons at risk to develop eating disorders. Specific early experiences and family influences may create intrapsychic conflicts that determine the psychologic predisposition. Despite the studies by Minuchin et al. delineating certain "psychosomatic" family patterns,[17] evidence is accumulating that a considerable variety of psychodynamic patterns exists in the families of patients with anorexia nervosa.[18,19]

Social influences and expectations that exert special pressure on modern women play an important role in the development of eating disorders.[7] The biologic factors that initiate anorexia nervosa may be mediated by pubertal endocrine changes. Psychologic conflicts lead to personality and behavioral changes that promote and support dieting. The social climate, such as the cultural obsession with thinness, tends to reinforce the psychologic motivation. Each of the three factors has greater or lesser importance for particular individuals who develop the disease. Thus, some appear to have a strong innate tendency to develop the disorder, despite a supportive family environment, whereas others react particularly to conflicted family experiences, and still others react primarily to the pressures of society.[2]

Most commonly, the process of dieting begins near the time of puberty, often shortly after menstrual periods have begun. This is a time of rapid physical and psychologic change. Not infrequently, a casual comment by a friend or family member suggests that the individual is becoming fat. Often the process begins with relatively innocent dieting. The girl who develops anorexia nervosa is acutely aware of the changes in her body configuration and becomes concerned about the increasing girth of her hips and thighs. Unlike most of her peers, she persists in dieting because of her determination and eventual pleasure in achieving control over her body. At first the dieting is difficult, in the face of overpowering hunger pangs, but with persistence it becomes easier, the hunger pangs diminish, and she becomes used to smaller and smaller quantities of food at less frequent intervals. Friends and family admire her accomplishment, and she receives compliments on her willpower and slim figure. Her friends become envious of her appearance and of the clothing size that she can wear. Exercise becomes more vigorous and ritualized. As her weight diminishes, her weight goals become even lower. She becomes more and more compulsive, secretive, and idiosyncratic about her diet habits. Physical and mental signs of starvation begin to develop. The latter are often ignored or actively denied. As family and friends become worried, the individual withdraws increasingly from social interaction, becomes quiet and seclusive, immerses herself in achievement-oriented activities, persists in dieting, and becomes increasingly active. Eventually she becomes irritable and hostile toward her family. School performance may decline, despite excessive hours of studying, as she becomes distractible and preoccupied and, ultimately, depressed and apathetic.

Unsuppressible hunger (bulimia) may supervene as a reaction to chronic semistarvation. This urge may be effectively suppressed for months or even years, but may lead to rapid weight gain and obesity before stabilization at normal weight. If the bulimic individual tenaciously clings to her pursuit of thinness, she will resort to vomiting or purging through laxative and diuretic abuse in order to maintain low body weight. This practice leads to chronic anorexia and bulimia nervosa with serious consequences.

Bulimia, like anorexia nervosa, has multiple causes. Clinical presentations vary, with some patients maintaining normal weight and others remaining markedly underweight. A cycle of binge eating and purging behavior often alternates with prolonged fasting. It is becoming increasingly clear that symptoms overlap among these disorders, and considerable individual variation exists as to vulnerability, causation, and perpetuation of symptoms.[19a]

## EPIDEMIOLOGY

Anorexia nervosa most commonly begins in the second decade of life. It rarely begins earlier, but it can occur after age 20. It is 10 times more common in females than in males. Onset is most often around the time of puberty or later in adolescence, at the time of leaving home and the expectation for independent functioning. Greatest vulnerability is in individuals engaged in activities requiring visible, high-performance competition such as ballet dancing, gymnastics, and modeling. Among males, those engaged in athletic pursuits in which low weight is a consideration, such as wrestling and long-distance running, are most affected. Estimates based on psychiatric registers place the incidence of anorexia nervosa at 0.4 to 1.6 cases per 100,000 population. These figures are underestimates of the true incidence in the population.[20] In a vulnerable population of British private school teenage girls under age 18, the prevalence was 1 case per 200 girls.[21] Some evidence exists that in Sweden and Switzerland the disorder has been increasing since the 1930s.[22,23] It is thought to be more frequent in higher socioeconomic classes and virtually nonexistent in underdeveloped nations. It is rarely, if ever, identified among blacks. That this finding represents only social class differences is unlikely; it may be related to differences in biologic vulnerability.

Less is known about the frequency of the bulimia syndrome in the general population. Because it has attracted interest only recently and is not readily identifiable except through self-reports, epidemiologic studies of this condition are still rare. It is thought to be quite common in young adults, particularly college students.

## CLINICAL ASPECTS AND COMPLICATIONS

The signs and symptoms, as well as laboratory findings, in anorexia nervosa and bulimia are most easily understood in context of the stage of the illness and the diet pattern that has been followed. At the onset of the illness, and for a considerable time thereafter, there may be no observable signs other than depletion of adipose tissue, and no abnormalities on laboratory tests. The negative findings are simply confirmation that in a previously healthy individual even marked starvation is compensated for by the homeostatic mechanisms of the body. The absence of abnormal findings tends to reinforce the patient's conviction that nothing is wrong. Bulimia may lead to obesity. Occasional binge eating may be seen in normal-weight individuals without complications. Bulimia alternating with prolonged fasting, vomiting, or purging leads to serious complications. Bulimia also occurs in certain forms of morbid obesity, notably Prader-Willi syndrome.[24]

It was generally thought that patients with anorexia nervosa have similar diet patterns characterized by specific carbohydrate avoidance.[6,18,25] A study of the diet patterns in 96 patients indicated much diversity.[26] All restricted their calorie intake, but 38% maintained satisfactory quality in the selection of their diets. Of the 62% whose diets were unsatisfactory in quality, most had irregular meal patterns, and a high proportion of this group indulged in binge eating, vomiting, or fasting. Recognition of the great variability in diet preferences among anorexic patients has implications for planning individualized treatment.

Physical signs in anorexia nervosa include dry thin skin, a sallow complexion, and loss of body fat. Bradycardia, hypotension, hypothermia, and cold intolerance occur. Often there is abdominal pain and a sensation of fullness. Constipation is common. Amenorrhea is a constant feature in females; males experience an analogous loss of sexual interest. Excessive loss of scalp hair may occur and eventually fine downy hair (lanugo) may appear on the body and face.

Personality features include model behavior, compliance, perfectionism, and high academic achievement. The patient usually presents a rigid, unspontaneous demeanor and is unusually serious and polite but inhibited and brief in responses. Excessive activity occurs but may be concealed. Sleep disturbance is common. Eventually manifestations of depression appear.

Among normal-weight individuals with bulimia, binge eating generally occurs frequently, at least several times a week. Usually, the episodes tend to last less than two hours, although they may last for many hours at a time. High-calorie, easily ingested foods such as ice cream, bread products, and candy tend to be eaten during binges. Vomiting is often a part of the syndrome, and patients with the disorder may also abuse laxatives and diuretics. Personality features differ from those in patients with anorexia nervosa who restrict intake. Depressive symptoms are common and suicide attempts are not infrequent among bulimic patients. Many have impulse-control problems in other areas of their lives. Shoplifting (frequently of food) is reported, as well as other forms of stealing. The association among substance abuse, alcoholism, and bulimia is being recognized more frequently.[27]

A person with bulimia may demonstrate no physical signs until damaging eating and vomiting behaviors have appeared. Nonpainful swelling of salivary glands is suggestive of extreme variability in quantity of food intake. Erosion of dental enamel occurs with frequent vomiting, and calluses of the knuckles proclaim self-induced vomiting.

Laboratory studies are of greatest help in documenting the degree of physiologic adaptation to undernourishment, in documenting complications of anorexia nervosa and bulimia, and in identifying other illnesses resembling eating disorders. There is no laboratory profile that is diagnostic. When physical signs and laboratory findings not usually associated with anorexia nervosa, such as increased heart rate, erythrocyte sedimentation rate, or leukocyte count, are found, they should alert the physician to a possible medical complication or the presence of another disorder.[28]

The laboratory profile varies considerably from normal to severely deranged and gives only a picture of these variables at the time of the test. In an illness that may last for many years, the stage is an important consideration in evaluating the laboratory findings. Abnormalities may not be observed until the illness is advanced. Serum electrolyte values usually are in the normal range except in cases in which vomiting or laxative or diuretic abuse is a feature. The reported values may be high because of dehydration. The hematologic picture is variable because of changes in hydration. Anemia is not unusual in moderately severe cases, but may be masked by hemoconcentration.

Dietary deficiencies lead to nutritional anemias in some patients. A peculiar morphologic change of erythrocytes resembling acanthocytosis is frequently present. The erythrocyte sedimentation rate is usually low. Leukopenia with relative lymphocytosis is common. Overt vitamin deficiencies are rare.[29] Serum protein values tend to remain normal until advanced stages of starvation. The serum cholesterol level is increased in about one third of patients, and the serum carotene value may be high.[30]

Little documentation of the long-term complications exists in the literature, although various cardiovascular and renal complications can ensue. Demineralization of bone (osteoporosis) can be a long-range consequence.[30a] Kidney stones can occur. During the acute or subacute phases, gastrointestinal complications, including decreased motility and atonic gut resembling paralytic ileus, may occur. Pancreatitis has been reported but, like sialadenosis, its mechanism is not known.[31,32]

Vomiting and laxative and diuretic abuse may be accompanied by serious electrolyte imbalances, notably hypokalemia, leading to cardiac arrhythmias, muscular weakness, renal impairment, and even death.[27]

Although mortality rates of up to 21.5% have been reported, rates were less than 5% in over half of outcome studies.[33] Death from inanition is rare. It may be most often due to suicide in long-standing bulimia nervosa, but it also has been attributed to overwhelming infection and to cardiopulmonary complications.[34] Death has also been attributed to overzealous refeeding, specifically, aspiration during tube feeding, and fluid and electrolyte imbalance during intravenous therapy.[35]

## DIAGNOSIS AND DIFFERENTIAL DIAGNOSIS

The diagnosis of anorexia nervosa hinges upon the presence of significant self-induced weight loss unexplained by physical illness or other psychiatric disorder. Psychologic characteristics, including the fear of becoming fat and disturbance in the perception of one's body image, are often included among the diagnostic criteria. The criteria set forth in the report of the Pathology of Eating Group require three major features: (1) self-inflicted severe loss of weight by avoidance of foods considered to be fattening, by self-induced vomiting or abuse of purgatives, or by excessive exercise; (2) a secondary endocrine disorder of the hypothalamus-anterior pituitary-gonad axis manifested in the female by amenorrhea and in the male by a diminution of sexual interest and activity; and (3) a psychologic disorder that has as its central theme a morbid fear of being unable to control eating and becoming too fat, either specified or implied by the eating behavior.[36]

Both physical and psychiatric disorders associated with weight loss must be differentiated from anorexia nervosa. The chief physical diseases to be differentiated are gastrointestinal diseases involving malabsorption. Among psychiatric disorders, primary depression and schizophrenia can be associated with severe weight loss and resemble anorexia nervosa.

Diagnostic criteria for bulimia include the essential features of episodic binge eating accompanied by an awareness that the eating pattern is abnormal, fear of not being able to stop eating voluntarily, and depressed mood and self-deprecating thoughts after the eating binges.[37]

## SPECTRUM OF EATING DISORDERS

Many forms of eating disorder occur, ranging from extreme emaciation to super-obesity.[38] Dieters and abstainers constitute the "pure" form of anorexia nervosa. Others maintain low weight by vomiting and purging. The term "thin fat people" designates those individuals who maintain weight below their biologic set point and suffer starvation symptoms at a weight that may be average for the general population.[7] Common forms of obesity are depicted at the hyperorexic end of the continuum. Individuals with bulimia nervosa as a consequence of anorexia nervosa, as well as the large group of individuals who maintain weight within the normal range through vomiting and purging, represent the middle of the continuum. Many individuals with eating disorders change their eating patterns over time, as suggested by the arrows in Figure 66–1.

## TREATMENT: ANOREXIA NERVOSA

Most cases of anorexia nervosa can be managed by the family physician, internist, or pediatrician, but they do take much time and sincere interest on the part of the physician. Mild cases often respond to concerned counseling about adolescent growth, normal nutrition, and the consequences of starvation. Severe cases are best managed by someone particularly experienced in treating the disorder. These patients need to be followed for a long time with various combinations of support, psychologic counseling, and diet counseling. A few cases are so severe that precipitous weight loss continues despite outpatient treatment efforts, and these patients require intensive hospital treatment.

Regardless of whether the patient remains at home or is hospitalized, the general principles of treatment involve education about the physiologic and psychologic consequences of starvation, encouragement to increase food intake gradually, and emotional support for the patient and family.

**Dietary Treatment.** Treatment of anorexia nervosa involves the joint efforts of a physician and a dietitian; they meet separately with the patient

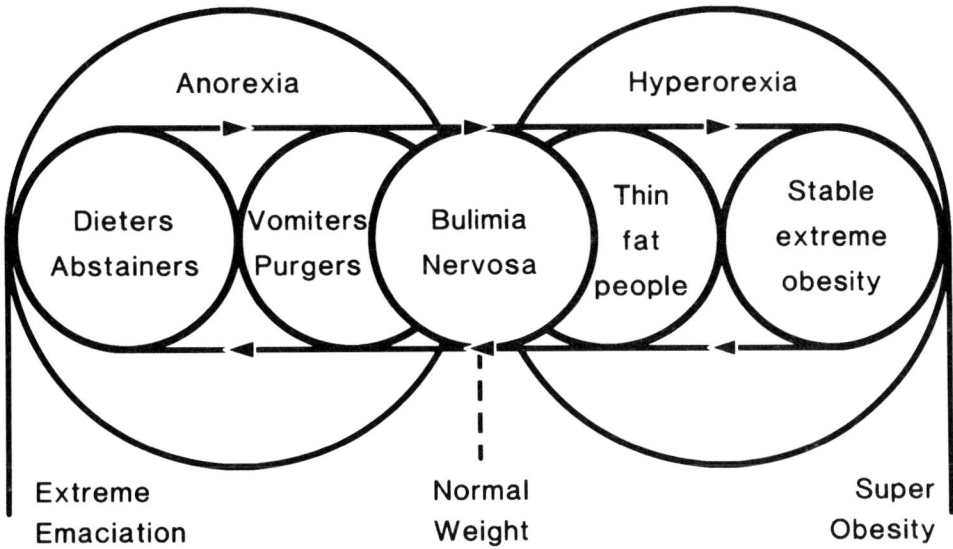

**Fig. 66–1.** Continuum of eating disorders. (Adapted from Vandereycken, W.[38])

periodically, usually once a week, after the comprehensive evaluation. The dietitian discusses specifics of diet modification in order to encourage both the resumption of normal eating patterns and the restoration of normal weight that are central to recovery from anorexia nervosa.

As in restoration of weight in other conditions involving starvation, a valid physiologic approach to treatment is to encourage the cessation of weight loss initially, to improve the nutritional state while low weight is maintained for a time, and then to encourage the gradual increase of weight through normal self-feeding. Use of artificial products or parenteral feeding is unnecessary. Contrary to the ideas espoused by some, there is no need for encouraging anorexic patients to consume above-average quantities of food. On the contrary, because of the low body weight and hypometabolic state, unusually small quantities are necessary at first (see nomogram in Appendix Table A–10). Estimated basal calorie requirements should be adjusted on the basis of the measured basal metabolic rate. The initial use of small quantities meets the psychologic needs of the patient, who is fearful of gaining weight rapidly and of becoming fat. Because some of the anorexia patients are realistically guarding against overeating, encouraging them to eat large quantities and high-calorie snacks is countertherapeutic.

Treatment involves several phases: obtaining a detailed diet history, determining the calorie content of the initial diet, designing an appropriate diet plan, planning gradual progression in the diet, considering weight gain expectations and, finally, designing a diet plan for weight maintenance. Specifics of this approach have been described in more detail elsewhere.[39]

**Specialized Outpatient Treatment.** Because of the severity of the patient's psychopathology, the intensity of conflicts within the family, or the patient's persistent resistance to weight gain, some individuals need more intense treatment. Psychotherapy may focus primarily on the patient, dealing with the particular conflicts that exist, along with supportive counseling of the parents, or it may involve more specific treatment directed toward pathologic patterns of family interaction. The dietary approach to treatment, implemented concurrently, ensures that realistic food intake is not ignored while convincing the patient that weight gain will not be excessive or too rapid.

**Hospital Treatment.** The decision regarding hospitalization is based on the severity and rapidity of weight loss, the degree of malnutrition, the severity of the psychopathology, and the extent of family problems. Hospital treatment requires a well-coordinated effort by the physician and hospital personnel. The implementation of an individualized treatment plan consistently and effectively is essential. Patients hospitalized for anorexia nervosa may be on a pediatric ward, an adolescent unit, a general medical ward, or a psychiatric unit for adolescents or adults.[40]

**Medication.** Although numerous medications have been used, they do not have an established place in the treatment of anorexia nervosa. Antipsychotic drugs and antidepressants have been used but, unless psychotic or depressive symptoms are prominent, there is no evidence that these medications will either shorten the course of anorexia nervosa or improve the chance of recovery.

### TREATMENT: BULIMIA

The understanding of treatment for bulimia is still in its early phases. Reliable medical approaches have not yet evolved. Much recent interest has centered on developing treatment approaches, including pharmacologic therapy and individual and group psychotherapeutic techniques, but their efficacy is not established.

Principles of dietary treatment used for anorexia nervosa can be adapted for patients with bulimia. This treatment should begin with a frank educational discussion about nutritional and health consequences. Encouraging regularity in diet habits can minimize the likelihood of the eating binges or long periods of fasting that contribute to the binge eating/fasting or purging cycle.

### OUTCOME

The course and outcome of anorexia nervosa are extremely variable.[25] In 64% of treated patients, weight returned to normal levels, 2% of the patients became obese, and 18% reached a level of weight that was considered to be low but adequate for physiologic function (Fig. 66–2). The range of weight, 42 to 47 kg, represents the weight threshold at which puberty is initiated and the hormonal changes leading to secondary sexual characteristics are set into motion. For many anorexic patients, the idea of weight within this range is terrifying. Fourteen percent of treated patients

remained chronically anorexic and at an inadequate weight level. In this group, menstrual function did not return. Some individuals remained chronically severely undernourished; others developed episodes of bulimia and vomiting with weight fluctuations. Two percent of treated patients died. Reviews of outcome studies have set the mean mortality rate at 6% (range, 0 to 21.5%) in different studies.[33,41]

Weight recovery is not the only or even the most important criterion for recovery, although regaining weight to a reasonable level is a necessary prerequisite to recovery. Three fourths of the patients in outcome studies were better at follow-up than at initial presentation in terms of body weight, but only one third were eating normally. Half were still consciously and purposefully avoiding high-calorie foods. Bulimia was present in 14 to 15% at follow-up, and vomiting was reported in 10 to 28%. Most continued to express a morbid attitude toward weight and shape. Outcome for menstrual function was less satisfactory than that for body weight. Only one half to three quarters were menstruating at follow-up. Psychiatric status and social adjustment were impaired in a large proportion of the patients. Economic productivity was selectivity spared: 90% were successfully employed even though social adjustment and body weight might have been poor.[33,41]

These reviews of follow-up studies confirm the impressions of the seriousness of the illness, but they also emphasize the variability of outcome.

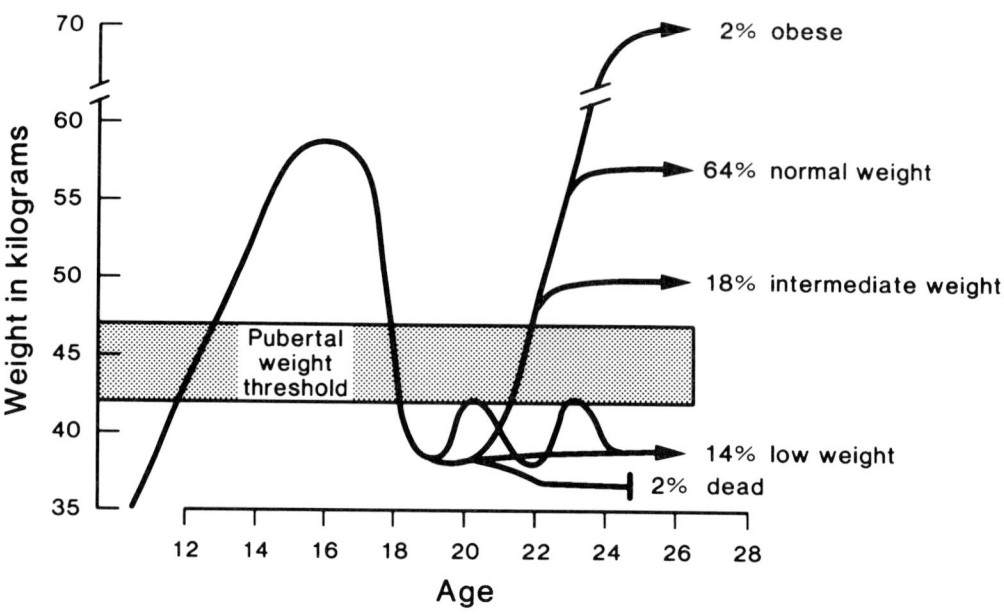

**Fig. 66–2.** Course and outcome in anorexia nervosa. (Adapted from Crisp, A.H.[25])

The nature of selection in a referral population tends to bias the studies in the direction of more severe forms of the illness. Few long-term follow-up studies have been reported, and most questions about the natural history of the illness still are unanswered. There is little documentation of the effects of treatment on outcome.

The long-range outcome of bulimia and its variants has not yet been reported. It is recognized that bulimia may be a phase in symptom evolution among some patients with an eating disorder.

## REFERENCES

1. Rau, J.H., Green, R.S.: Compr. Psychiatry *16*:223–231, 1975.
2. Lucas, A.R.: Mayo Clin. Proc. *56*:254–264, 1981.
3. Morton, R.: Phthisiologia, seu Exercitationes de Phthisi Tribus Libris Comprehensae: Totumque Opus Variis Historiis Illustratum. London, Samuel Smith, 1689.
4. Gull, W.W.: Trans. Clin. Soc. Lond. *7*:22–28, 1874.
5. Crisp, A.H.: J. Psychosom. Res. *9*:67–78, 1965.
6. Russell, G.F.M.: Anorexia nervosa: Its identity as an illness and its treatment. *In* Modern Trends in Psychological Medicine, Vol. 2. (Price, J.H., Ed.) London, Butterworth, 1970.
7. Bruch, H.: Eating Disorders: Obesity and Anorexia Nervosa. New York, Basic Books, 1973.
8. Russell, G.: Psychol. Med. *9*:429–448, 1979.
9. Casper, R.C.: Int. J. Eating Disord. *2*:3–16, 1983.
10. Lucas, A.R., Callaway, C.W.: Anorexia nervosa and bulimia. *In* Bockus Gastroenterology. 4th ed. (Beck, J.E., Ed.) Philadelphia, W.B. Saunders Co., 1984.
11. Boyar, R.M., Katz, J., Finkelstein, J.W., et al.: N. Engl. J. Med. *291*:861–865, 1974.
12. Isaacs, A.J.: Endocrinology. *In* Anorexia Nervosa. (Dally, P., Gomez, J., Eds.) London, Heinemann Medical Books, 1979.
13. Marshall, J.C., Kelch, R.P.: J. Clin. Endocrinol. Metab. *49*:712–718, 1979.
14. Weiner, H.: Int. J. Eating Disord. *2*:109–116, 1983.
15. Frisch, R.E., McArthur, J.W.: Science *185*:949–951, 1974.
16. Falk, J.R., Halmi, K.A.: Biol. Psychiatry *17*:799–806, 1982.
17. Minuchin, S., Rosman, B.L., Baker, L.: Psychosomatic Families: Anorexia Nervosa in Context. Cambridge, Harvard University Press, 1978.
18. Garfinkel, P.E., Garner, D.M.: Anorexia Nervosa: A Multidimensional Perspective. New York, Brunner/Mazel, 1982.
19. Strober, M.: An empirically derived typology of anorexia nervosa. *In* Anorexia Nervosa: Recent Developments in Research. (Darby, P., Garner, D.M., Garfinkel, P.F., Eds.) New York, Alan R. Liss, 1983.
19a. Johnson, C., Lewis, C., Hagman, J.: Psychiatr. Clin. North Am. *7*:247–273, 1984.
20. Kendell, R.E., Hall, D.J., Hailey, A., et al.: Psychol. Med. *3*:200–203, 1973.
21. Crisp, A.H., Palmer, R.L., Kalucy, R.S.: Br. J. Psychiatry *128*:549–554, 1976.
22. Theander, S.: Acta Psychiatr. Scand. [Suppl.] *214*:1–194, 1970.
23. Willi, J., Grossmann, S.: Am. J. Psychiatry *140*:564–567, 1983.
24. Holm, V.A., Sulzbacher, S., Pipes, P.L.: Prader-Willi Syndrome. Baltimore, University Park Press, 1981.
25. Crisp, A.H.: Anorexia Nervosa: Let Me Be. New York, Grune and Stratton, 1980.
26. Huse, D.M., Lucas, A.R.: Am. J. Clin. Nutr. *40*:251–254, 1984.
27. Mitchell, J.E., Pyle, R.L.: Int. J. Eating Disord. *1*:61–73, 1982.
28. Lucas, A.R.: Mayo Clin. Proc. *52*:748–750, 1977.
29. Casper, R.C., Kirschner, B., Sandstead, H.H., et al.: Am. J. Clin. Nutr. *33*:1801–1808, 1980.
30. Curran, J.M.: Ph.D. Thesis, University of Illinois, 1982.
30a. Rigotti, N.A., Nussbaum, S.R., Herzog, D.B., et al.: N. Engl. J. Med. *311*:1601–1606, 1984.
31. Nordgren, L., von Schéele, C.: Biol. Psychiatry *12*:681–686, 1977.
32. Schoettle, U.C.: J. Am. Acad. Child Psychiatry *18*:384–390, 1979.
33. Hsu, L.K.: Arch. Gen. Psychiatry *37*:1041–1046, 1980.
34. Bruch, H.: Psychosom. Med. *33*:135–144, 1971.
35. Drossman, D.A., Ontjes, D.A., Heizer, W.D.: Gastroenterology *77*:1115–1131, 1979.
36. Garrow, J.S., Crisp, A.H., Jordan, H.A., et al.: Pathology of eating group report. *In* Dahlem Workshop on Appetite and Food Intake. (Silverstone, T., Ed.) Berlin, Abakon, 1976.
37. Diagnostic and Statistical Manual of Mental Disorders. 3rd ed. Washington, D.C., American Psychiatric Association, 1980.
38. Vandereycken, W.: Uncommon eating/weight disorders related to amenorrhea, infertility and problematic pregnancy. *In* Advances in Psychosomatic Obstetrics and Gynecology. (Prill, H.J., Stauber, M., Eds.) Berlin, Springer-Verlag, 1982.
39. Huse, D.M., Lucas, A.R.: J. Am. Diet. Assoc. *83*:687–690, 1983.
40. Lucas, A.R., Duncan, J.W., Piens, V.: Am. J. Psychiatry *133*:1034–1038, 1976.
41. Schwartz, D.M., Thompson, M.G.: Am. J. Psychiatry *138*:319–323, 1981.

## SELECTED READINGS

Bruch, H.: Eating Disorders: Obesity and Anorexia Nervosa. New York, Basic Books, 1973.

Cahill, G.F., Jr., Aoki, T.T., Rossini, A.: Metabolism in obesity and anorexia nervosa. *In* Disorders of Eating and Nutrients in Treatment of Brain Diseases, Vol. 3. (Wurtman, R.J., Wurtman, J.J., Eds.) New York, Raven Press, 1979.

Garfinkel, P.E., Garner, D.M.: Anorexia Nervosa. New York, Brunner/Mazel Publishers, 1982.

Keys, A., Brožek, J., Henschel, A., et al.: The Biology of Human Starvation, Vols. 1 and 2. Minneapolis, University of Minnesota Press, 1950.

Stunkard, A.J., Stellar, E.: Eating and Its Disorders. (Association for Research in Nervous and Mental Disease.) Vol. 62. New York, Raven Press, 1984.

*Chapter* **67**

# DIET AND NUTRITION IN NEUROLOGIC DISORDERS

Pierre M. Dreyfus

Improper and inadequate nutrition that is allowed to persist over weeks and months can lead to neurologic diseases that affect the central or the peripheral nervous system, or both. Nutritional diseases of the nervous system have been carefully documented from a clinical, pathologic, and biochemical point of view since their etiology was first identified a century ago. In fact, the study of some of these diseases has been largely responsible for a number of advances in the field of modern nutrition. More specifically, the discoveries of the pathogenesis of beriberi,[1] a disease that affects the heart and the peripheral nervous system, and pellagra,[2] an affliction of the central nervous system, led to the eventual discovery of vitamins and active cofactors and an understanding of their function in metabolism. It is of interest that the successful nutritional management of beriberi antedated by some 29 years the discovery of the specific cause of the disease and the description of the deficient nutrient: thiamin. Prior to 1882, when a drastic change in the diet of the Japanese navy virtually eliminated beriberi among Japanese sailors, beriberi had occurred in epidemic proportions throughout the world. Although the disease continues to be seen in underprivileged, severely malnourished, and chronically alcoholic individuals, it no longer constitutes a major public health problem.

Nutritional disorders of the nervous system are most commonly seen as a consequence of chronic alcoholism, debilitating diseases that affect the gastrointestinal tract, starvation due to unavailability of nutrients (e.g., poverty or drought), and malnutrition caused by individual ignorance about diet and nutrition. Among the more privileged populations of the world, neurologic diseases of nutritional etiology are seen most often in patients seeking to shed excess weight by dietary, pharmacologic, or surgical means, as well as in food cultists and individuals with peculiar dietary habits. In this type of population, nutritional deficiency sufficiently severe to lead to neurologic dysfunction can also occur as the result of stress, although the dietary intake is considered to be adequate. Examples of such stressful conditions are: chronic infection, endocrine imbalance, overwhelming psychiatric disease, and pernicious vomiting; occasionally pregnancy is a culprit.

The various nutritional syndromes that affect the nervous system, all of which will be described in this chapter, may present separately in relatively pure form or together in varying combinations. Some are more common than others. Basic constitutional and genetic factors undoubtedly underlie individual responses to altered nutrition. In some individuals there are no clinical manifestations. Others experience an array of symptoms and signs referable to the central, peripheral, or autonomic nervous system. Nutritional disorders of the nervous system all share certain characteristic etiologic and pathologic attributes. The known biochemical lesions that can be demonstrated in these diseases invariably antedate the appearance of clinical manifestations and pathologic changes, which affect areas of the nervous system in a predictable, reproducible, selective, and symmetrical fashion. Most of these diseases are eminently preventable or, when they occur, can be treated by a simple dietary approach.

A number of neurologic diseases and syndromes are engendered by metabolic disturbances. In some instances the metabolic defect may be well defined whereas in others it is as yet unknown. The prevention and successful treatment of some of these disorders frequently involve nutritional manipulation consisting of the addition, elimination, or substitution of some basic nutrient or nutrients. Various chronic afflictions of the nervous system are attended by severe, life-threatening malnutrition that can be reversed with relative ease, leading to increased comfort on the part of the patient, although the course of the underlying disease remains unaltered.

The adverse consequences of diet or dietary elements on behavior, the potential neurotoxicity of certain vitamins,and the interrelationship of antiepileptic drugs and vitamins are also considered in this chapter.

Finally, the rationale behind the use of diet and vitamins as therapy for neurologic disorders that do not have a nutritional etiology, such as headache, neuralgia, and dementia, is also discussed.

## NEUROLOGIC DISORDERS CAUSED BY MALNUTRITION

The chronic ingestion of alcohol, when it is accompanied by undernutrition (in some instances, malnutrition), can lead to a number of clearly defined neurologic disorders. It is well known that during periods of heavy drinking the absorption of vitamins, their intestinal transport, tissue storage, utilization, and conversion to metabolically active forms are sharply curtailed, while at the same time the need for vitamins and essential nutrients increases. In addition, chronic alcoholism affects mineral, carbohydrate, protein, and lipid metabolism in an adverse manner. Nutritional disorders of the nervous system, although most commonly associated with chronic alcoholism, can affect malnourished, debilitated, nonalcoholic individuals who suffer from such illnesses as malabsorption syndromes, carcinomatosis, and renal disease. Considering the ever-increasing size of the chronic alcoholic population throughout the world and the magnitude of the consequent general medical problems, alcohol-induced nutritional diseases of the nervous system are relatively rare. Nutritional disorders constitute only 1 to 3% of all alcohol-related problems affecting the nervous system that come to the attention of physicians.[3]

### Wernicke-Korsakoff's Syndrome

Wernicke-Korsakoff's syndrome, although relatively rare, constitutes the most common alcoholic-nutritional affliction of the central nervous system.[4] This syndrome is not restricted to the alcoholic population; it can affect patients whose nutritional depletion is unrelated to the abusive intake of alcohol. Wernicke's encephalopathy is characterized by the acute onset of ophthalmoplegia, nystagmus, and ataxia of stance and gait. Mental symptoms, which evolve during the course of the illness, affect more than 90% of patients. At the onset of the illness, global confusion, profound disorientation, apathy, indifference, inattentiveness, drowsiness, and decreased spontaneity of speech are the characteristic presenting symptoms. On rare occasions, stupor and coma are the initial symptoms. The clinical picture of Wernicke's disease may include such superimposed symptoms of alcohol withdrawal as delirium tremens or clinical evidence of hepatic decompensation.

With improved nutrition, the clinical picture improves and patients can be more easily tested. It is then possible to demonstrate the presence of ocular palsies, nystagmus, ataxia, and peripheral neuropathy—the classic hallmarks of Wernicke's disease. These clinical signs are frequently accompanied or followed by obvious Korsakoff's psychosis, otherwise referred to as amnestic-confabulatory syndrome. This condition is characterized by spotty loss of memory, the inability to learn and form new memories, impaired conceptual or perceptual functions, and confabulation, which usually vanishes during the more chronic stage of the illness. On rare occasions, Korsakoff's psychosis may be present without the ocular signs and ataxia of Wernicke's encephalopathy.

There can be no doubt that Wernicke-Korsakoff's syndrome is caused by severe thiamin deficiency.[4] The requirements for thiamin are greatest when large amounts of glucose or alcohol are being metabolized and when metabolic demands are high. A sudden increase in brain glucose levels in a patient with marginal thiamin reserves may precipitate symptoms and signs of Wernicke-Korsakoff's syndrome.[5] Therefore, whenever glucose is being administered rapidly to a chronically malnourished and/or metabolically stressed individual, the parenteral fluids should always include a mixture of B vitamins. Since Korsakoff's psychosis that is either associated with or subsequent to the onset of Wernicke's encephalopathy is essentially irreversible, prompt therapeutic intervention is essential. The improvement of the acute neurologic signs and symptoms of Wernicke-Korsakoff's disease correlates well with erythrocyte transketolase activity, a sensitive test of the adequacy of thiamin nutriture.[6] Reduced erythrocyte transketolase activity reverts toward normal as thiamin is administered and the patient improves. For additional discussion on this syndrome, see Chapter 65.

### Nutritional Neuropathy

Nutritional neuropathy is probably the nutritional disorder of the peripheral nervous system that is most frequently encountered. In common with all nutritional disorders of the nervous system, the disease occurs in a variety of clinical settings. The characteristic clinical features of nutritional polyneuropathy,[7] as is the case with most polyneuropathies, in the early stages of the disease consist of symmetrical impairment of motor and sensory function accompanied by reduced or absent reflex activity affecting the legs to a greater extent than the arms. The distal segments of the extremities are usually more affected than are the proximal ones, and occasionally autonomic dysfunction accompanies the classic symptoms and signs of polyneuropathy. In the early stages of the disease, sensory symptoms tend to be more prominent than motor dysfunction. Patients frequently complain of paresthesias, dysesthesias, and a burning sensation. In the more advanced stages of the disease, marked motor impairment, such as foot drop, wrist drop, or complete paralysis of the legs, may be elicited. No specific clinical manifestations distinguish polyneuropathies caused by nutritional deficiency from those due to other causes.

One of the various clinical entities that have been attributed to nutritional factors is beriberi neuropathy ("dry beriberi"), which stems from a primary deficiency of thiamin. Another entity, alcoholic or nutritional neuropathy, seen predominantly in developed countries, is likely due to severe thiamin deficiency caused by abnormal vitamin metabolism, or to the inadequate intake of the vitamin in the face of a high energy intake (derived mainly from alcohol).[7] It has been demonstrated that alcohol alone may have a direct effect on neuronal metabolism. Consequently, alcoholic neuropathy is perhaps a prime example of what may be called a "toxonutritional" polyneuropathy.[8] Deficiencies of thiamin, pyridoxine,

niacin, pantothenic acid, biotin, vitamin $B_{12}$, and possibly folate are associated with disease of the peripheral nervous system. It is rare that deficiency of a single vitamin (with the exception of $B_{12}$) is identified as the sole cause of polyneuropathy. Usually the deficiency state is multifactorial, involving the lack of several vitamins and other nutrients. Whereas the peripheral nervous system may be the most susceptible to nutritional depletion, other parts of the nervous system, such as the spinal cord, optic nerve, and cerebellum, may be affected coincidentally, but to a lesser degree. In such instances, the symptoms and signs of neuropathy tend to mask those of myelopathy or cerebellar involvement. In most cases of nutritional polyneuropathy, the presence of such systemic manifestations as weight loss, seborrheic dermatitis, follicular hypokeratosis, glossitis, cheilosis, angular stomatitis, changes in the color and texture of hair, anemia, and circulatory disturbances helps in establishing the nutritional etiology of the disease.

Attempts to investigate clinically the specific etiology of nutritional polyneuropathies have encountered difficulties. The disease process is slow, with both onset and recovery being measured in terms of weeks or even months. The underlying biochemical lesion or metabolic insult usually antedates the advent of clinical signs and symptoms, abnormal physiologic parameters, and pathologic changes. By the time a patient comes to the attention of a physician, the underlying biochemical defect may already have been corrected, yet the disease continues to evolve. It is not unusual for patients to complain of severe weakness, sensory loss, or troublesome dysesthesia at the same time that electrical studies and pathologic changes suggest improvement of the underlying disease. Although electrical studies may ascertain the stage of the disease and provide some clues whether the underlying pathologic process involves primarily the axon or the myelin sheath, they cannot possibly elucidate etiologic factors.

The treatment of nutritional polyneuropathies is straightforward: provision of improved nutrition and supplemental vitamins, and removal of noxious substances.

### Nutritional Amblyopia

This remarkably uniform and stereotyped disorder of vision occurs infrequently and affects only persons who are chronically undernourished.[9] Characteristically the disease evolves slowly and subacutely with the mode of onset of symptoms being much the same in all patients. Visual impairment usually has an insidious beginning and reaches its maximum in several weeks to months. Common presenting complaints are blurred or dim vision, difficulty in reading, photophobia, and discomfort in the retrobulbar region on moving the eyes. On examination the patient is noted to have bilateral asymmetrical scotomata of varying sizes. Ophthalmoscopic changes are at first restricted to slight redness of the temporal margins of the optic discs. At a later stage of the illness minimal pallor may be observed, but frequently no abnormality is visible. Peripheral vision is intact. Although the syndrome most frequently afflicts patients who neglect their nutrition and who are habituated to alcohol or occasionally to tobacco, it has been encountered during periods of famine in undernourished populations all over the world and among civilian and military prisoners of war who have had no access to either alcohol or tobacco. On occasion, a similar syndrome may present as one of the complications of pernicious anemia as well as of other deficiency states caused by a lack of vitamin $B_{12}$.[10]

The metabolic aberration or specific vitamin deficiency responsible for the development of nutritional amblyopia has not as yet been defined. A deficiency of vitamin $B_{12}$, thiamin, riboflavin, and pyridoxine and a failure in the detoxification of the cyanide present in tobacco smoke have both been implicated in the etiology of the disease. In isolated cases, reduced serum vitamin $B_{12}$ levels, the abnormal urinary excretion of methylmalonic acid, and low levels of blood transketolase activity have been detected; none of these abnormalities is specific and to date no others have been demonstrated.[9]

Treatment with oral or parenteral B vitamins and improved nutrition is usually followed by clinical amelioration. Improvement is dependent upon the duration of the visual syndrome and its severity at the time that therapy is instituted.[9]

### Cerebellar Degeneration

Cerebellar cortical degeneration, sometimes referred to as alcoholic cerebellar degeneration, is a syndrome primarily characterized by progressive unsteadiness of stance and gait, with relative sparing of arms and cranial nerves. The disease can be set apart from all other known forms of cerebellar degeneration because of the uniformity of the clinical and pathologic manifestations.[11]

A substantial body of evidence implicates nutritional factors as the most likely causes of the disease. Although the disease is most frequently encountered in chronic alcoholic patients, it has also been reported in malnourished individuals who allegedly did not drink. Many patients with cortical cerebellar degeneration give a history of

progressive weight loss before the onset of their symptoms. Signs of malnutrition are common, and the cerebellar syndrome frequently occurs in conjunction with cirrhosis and other nutritional complications of alcoholism. It is of interest that nonalcoholic patients may develop cortical cerebellar degeneration in the setting of other diseases associated with nutritional depletion, such as pellagra, gastrointestinal cancer, and protracted vomiting.[12]

Improved nutrition and the administration of B vitamins may result in some degree of improvement of ataxia. On occasion, abstinence alone may be effective. It has been postulated that alcohol and/or some of its metabolites superimposed upon malnutrition may be responsible for the damage caused to the cerebellum.[11]

### Vitamin $B_{12}$ Deficiency

Malabsorption of vitamin $B_{12}$ from the gastrointestinal tract, such as that caused by pernicious anemia, can result in subacute degeneration of the spinal cord, optic nerves, cerebral white matter, and peripheral nerves. Most often the neurologic manifestations of vitamin $B_{12}$ deficiency are associated with the typical macrocytic anemia of pernicious anemia. On occasion, however, the latter is not present. Neurologic symptoms rarely occur as a result of vitamin $B_{12}$ deficiency secondary to fish tapeworm infestation, sprue, gastrointestinal surgery, or vegetarianism.

Progressive symmetrical paresthesia of hands and feet, weakness, spasticity and ataxia of legs, occasional confusion and dementia, and sometimes bilateral failing vision constitute the main neurologic symptoms of vitamin $B_{12}$ deficiency. The main physical findings consist of diminution or loss of position and vibratory senses (blunting of pain, temperature, and tactile sensations over the distal parts of the legs), hyperactive knee jerks, and the absence of ankle jerks and extensor plantar responses. Psychologic symptoms may range from apathy, irritability, and depression to confusion and frank dementia.

Why a deficiency of vitamin $B_{12}$ results in neurologic complications remains unknown. The neurologic manifestations of the deficiency state may occur independently of the megaloblastic anemia. Neurologic symptoms and signs may appear when the anemia has been corrected by folic acid. The biochemical lesion responsible for the neurologic manifestations of vitamin $B_{12}$ deficiency appears to involve the enzyme methylmalonyl-CoA-isomerase that normally converts methylmalonyl-CoA to succinyl-CoA, a metabolic step in the utilization of propionic acid.[13,14] The excessive urinary excretion of methylmalonic acid that results as a consequence of the deficiency state has been demonstrated in patients suffering from vitamin $B_{12}$ deficiency and neurologic complications. Detection of this substance in the urine constitutes a sensitive index of vitamin $B_{12}$ deficiency.[15] The isomerase that converts methylmalonyl-CoA to succinyl-CoA may be essential to the maintenance of the myelin sheath. Sural nerve specimens obtained from patients with pernicious anemia show abnormal fatty acid metabolism, i.e., they accumulate branched-chain and odd-chain fatty acids that are derived from labeled propionate. The presence of these abnormal fatty acids may explain, in part, the structural changes observed in central and peripheral myelin of patients.[13]

The early neurologic manifestations of vitamin $B_{12}$ deficiency are rapidly and completely reversible. Therefore, prompt initiation of therapy is of the utmost importance. The greatest degree of improvement is achieved when treatment takes place within three months of the onset of symptoms. However, variable degrees of amelioration can be obtained even 6 to 12 months after the onset of symptoms. Daily intramuscular injections of 50 μg of cyanocobalamin should be given during the first two weeks. Subsequently, 100 μg of cyanocobalamin should be given intramuscularly twice a week for two months, after which the patient should receive a minimum of 100 μg intramuscularly every month for life to prevent the possibility of a relapse that might be caused by metabolic stress.

### Pellagra

Pellagra, a disease that is characterized by dementia, dermatitis, and diarrhea, is becoming increasingly rare in the Western world as a consequence of improved nutrition, the enrichment of flour, and the increasingly common practice of vitamin supplementation. When the disease was prevalent in the United States, a large proportion of cases occurred in chronic alcoholics, among whom it can still be encountered. This is particularly true among those alcoholics who, in addition to their chronic imbibition, suffer from a combination of impaired gastrointestinal absorption and faulty nutrition. The neurologic manifestations of pellagra resemble those of an encephalopathy, occasionally accompanied by signs of peripheral nerve and spinal cord involvement. The psychologic symptoms often precede the skin changes, which characteristically develop upon exposure to sunlight. In the early stages of the disease, the patient may be depressed, apathetic, fearful, and apprehensive. Insomnia, dizziness, and headache are common. As the disease progresses, a florid psychosis characterized by confusion, delusion, disorientation, and hallucinations may develop. Later the patient may lapse into coma. Some patients exhibit spasticity of the legs and ataxic gait.[16] The neurologic symptoms and signs are promptly reversed by the administration of niacin. Both niacin (10 or 20 mg) and its precursor, tryptophan (100 to 500 mg), must be included in the daily diet.

## NEUROLOGIC DISORDERS AFFECTED BY DIET OR DIETARY ELEMENTS

### Metabolic Diseases

In several genetically determined metabolic neurologic diseases, part of the treatment consists of either the elimination of certain foods that contain nutrients known to be damaging to the nervous system and other organs or, in vitamin-dependent diseases, the supplementation of a specific vitamin because of a demonstrated enzymatic defect that can be partially overcome by pharmacologic rather than nutritional doses of the vitamin (Table 67–1). Examples of such disorders will be discussed briefly.[17]

**Wilson's Disease.** A classic example of a disease that is affected by the elimination of a nutrient is Wilson's disease (hepatolenticular degeneration),[18,19] a progressive familial illness inherited through an autosomal recessive gene. This condition is characterized by cirrhosis of the liver, neurologic signs and symptoms due to damage of the basal ganglia of the brain, and a rust-colored pigmented ring of the cornea of the eye near the scleral junction (Kayser-Fleischer ring) present in all patients with neurologic impairment. The salient symptoms and signs include progressive tremors, rigidity, dysarthria, dysphagia, drooling, dementia, and psychosis. The basic underlying biochemical defect consists of a deficiency of the copper-carrying protein, ceruloplasmin, in the blood. This genetic defect causes the increased accumulation of copper in various organs, including the liver, the nervous system, and the cornea (hence the Kayser-Fleischer ring), and the elimination of large quantities of copper in the urine. Treatment for this disease is best achieved by the exclusion from the diet of foods high in copper content, such as broccoli, oysters, cocoa, nuts, and beans. Agents that either chelate copper, such as penicillamine, or prevent its absorption from the gastrointestinal tract, such as potash, are used in conjunction with a low copper diet. The combined dietary and pharmacologic treatment leads to significant amelioration of hepatic dysfunction and of neurologic symptoms and signs.[19,20]

**Table 67–1.  Inborn Errors of Metabolism with Neurologic Manifestations**

| Disease | Defect | Dietary Treatment | Ref. |
|---|---|---|---|
| Phenylketonuria | Phenylalanine hydroxylase | Restrict phenylalanine | 26,27 |
| Maple syrup urine disease | Branched-chain ketoacid decarboxylase | 1. Restrict leucine, isoleucine, valine<br>2. Thiamin | 25,27 |
| Urea Cycle Defects | | | |
| Argininosuccinicaciduria | Argininosuccinase | | |
| Citrullinemia | Argininosuccinic synthetase | | |
| Hyperammonemia | Ornithine transcarbamylase<br>Carbamyl phosphate synthetase | Restrict protein | 25 |
| Lysine intolerance | Interference with arginase | | |
| Homocystinuria | Cystathionine synthetase | 1. Restrict methionine<br>2. Pyridoxine<br>3. Folic acid, vitamin $B_{12}$ | 25 |
| Galactosemia | Galactose-1-phosphate uridyl transferase | Lactose-free diet<br>Low-galactose diet | 25,28,29 |
| Wilson's disease | Low serum ceruloplasmin | Low-copper diet | 18,19 |
| Refsum's disease | Alpha oxidation of phytanic acid to pristanic acid | Phytol-free diet | 21,22 |

Adapted from Menkes, J.H.[25]

**Refsum's Disease (Heredopathia Atactica Polyneuritiformis).** This relatively rare autosomal recessive disease of the peripheral nervous system was first described by Refsum in 1944.[21] The illness is characterized by the onset in either late childhood or early adolescence of signs and symptoms suggestive of motor, sensory, symmetrical, areflexic neuropathy, sometimes accompanied by cerebellar ataxia, cataracts, retinitis pigmentosa, diminished hearing or deafness, cardiomyopathy, and cutaneous changes (ichthyosis). The biochemical lesion in this disease consists of a block in the alpha oxidation of phytanic acid to pristanic acid. The metabolic block causes the accumulation of a branched-chain fatty acid, phytanic acid, in the blood with increased excretion of the acid in the urine and the accumulation of abnormal lipids in peripheral nerves. Phytanic acid is derived from phytol, which is contained in a large variety of foods, such as nuts, spinach, and coffee. The ingestion of a phytol-free diet leads to decreased phytanic acid levels in the blood, followed over the course of many months by slow but steady improvement of the neurologic disorder.[22] In individuals in whom the peripheral nerve disorder is either partial or intermittent, the strict adherence to a phytol-free diet, although important, may not be crucial.

**Vitamin-Responsive Diseases.** Vitamin-responsive, or vitamin-dependent, diseases are a group of genetically determined metabolic disorders in which either a vitamin-dependent enzymatic step or a reaction involving the conversion of a vitamin to its active cofactor form is defective, causing the abnormal accumulation of metabolites, or substrates, in the blood.[17,23–25] In these diseases, blood vitamin levels are normal. The basic metabolic defect involves the structure of the apoenzyme, its coenzyme binding sites, or some aspect of coenzyme synthesis. The neurologic manifestations observed in vitamin-responsive diseases tend to be protean, ranging from mental retardation, psychiatric symptoms, and convulsive seizures to opthalmologic signs, ataxia, spasticity, and peripheral neuropathy (Table 67–2). The degree of response of these disorders to the appropriate vitamin varies considerably. In some patients marked improvement of neurologic symptoms and signs occurs following therapy with amounts exceeding nutritional or physiologic doses. In pyridoxine dependency, a disorder of neonates characterized by generalized seizures and most likely due to abnormal glutamic acid decarboxylase coenzyme binding sites, convulsions can be controlled with daily doses of pyridoxine that are 5 to 20 times greater than the recommended daily requirement.[17,23,24]

**Acquired and Hereditary Hyperammonemic Disorders.** Acute and chronic liver disease caused by either primary hepatic pathology or portacaval shunting may lead to a metabolic encephalopathy that evolves over a period of days and weeks and that proceeds to progressive mental confusion and drowsiness followed by stupor, coma, and sometimes death. On occasion these symptoms are preceded by generalized or focal seizures and asterixis (liver flap). The encephalopathy can be reversible by appropriate treatment, including dietary measures, but a fatal outcome is not infrequent. Recurring bouts of hepatic encephalopathy

**Table 67–2.   Vitamin-Responsive Diseases with Neurologic Manifestations**

| Vitamin | Disease |
|---------|---------|
| Thiamin (vitamin $B_1$) | Maple syrup urine disease<br>Pyruvate decarboxylase deficiency<br>Leigh's disease |
| Pyridoxine (vitamin $B_6$) | Neonatal convulsions<br>Homocystinuria<br>Cystathioninuria |
| Cobalamin (vitamin $B_{12}$) | Methylmalonuria<br>Homocystinuria |
| Folic acid | Homocystinuria |
| Nicotinamide | Hartnup disease |
| Biotin | Propionicacidemia<br>Methylcrotonylglycinuria |

Adapted from Mudd, S.H.[17]

may cause episodic stupor and coma or a persistent extrapyramidal movement disorder, ataxia, myelopathy, and irreversible dementia. The EEG of hepatic encephalopathy assumes a characteristic pattern consisting of triphasic delta waves at 2 Hz. These tend to correlate with the high blood ammonia levels invariably detected in well-established cases.[30]

The nutritional support of patients afflicted with acute or chronic liver disease, the prevention of hepatic encephalopathy, and the successful treatment of this devastating disorder require an understanding of its pathogenesis.

It is generally believed that hepatic encephalopathy is caused by the toxic effects on the central nervous system of ammonia that has accumulated in blood. Urea-splitting bacteria in the intestine release ammonia into the portal circulation. Under normal circumstances, this substance is effectively removed by the liver. In the presence of hepatocellular disease, or of a portalsystemic shunt, ammonia accumulates in the systemic circulation leading to brain dysfunction. Whereas blood ammonia levels correlate well with the characteristic electroencephalographic abnormality described in liver failure, they may not correlate with the patient's level of consciousness,[30,31] possibly because blood levels of ammonia do not accurately reflect tissue levels of this toxic substance. It has been postulated that the accumulation of ammonia and the adverse chain of metabolic events lead to the depletion of the neurotransmitters norepinephrine and dopamine and the accumulation of the false neurotransmitters octopamine and phenylethanolamine in the brain. The production of these false neurotransmitters is presumably caused by excessive levels of the aromatic amino acids phenylalanine, tryptophan, and methionine. In addition, hepatic dysfunction is said to lead to a reduction of serum

levels of the branched-chain amino acids valine, leucine, and isoleucine.[32,33]

The curtailment of dietary protein, whether animal or vegetable, along with an increase in carbohydrate ingestion may prevent the development of hepatic encephalopathy in patients with hepatocellular disease. Once the disease is established, the dietary treatment of hepatic encephalopathy in patients with hepatocellular disease has been the restriction of dietary protein and the removal of urea-splitting bacteria in the colon. The latter is accomplished by means of the administration of an antibiotic (neomycin) or of lactulose, which acidifies the colonic contents, or the administration of colonic enemas.[30,31]

Since dietary protein not only enhances hepatic regeneration but also maintains host resistance, a modest amount of protein is essential. Most patients with hepatic dysfunction who show evidence of encephalopathy may tolerate 35 to 40 g of protein, but even at these levels neurologic changes may occur. The administration of amino acid preparations containing increased amounts of branched-chain amino acids was reported by Fischer and associates to have a beneficial effect on the encephalopathic state in patients with portocaval shunting associated with cirrhosis. In addition to this improvement, the abnormal plasma amino acid pattern of decreased branched-chain and increased aromatic amino acids returned toward normal.[32–34] Fischer and others have suggested that this formula decreased the presence of false neurotransmitters in the brain. In addition, these investigators believe that an imbalance of amino acids noted in hepatic encephalopathy may also be noted in patients with sepsis and trauma and that administration of such branched-chain amino acid preparations has had a beneficial effect on septic encephalopathy. However, other studies comparing the effectiveness of intravenous branched-chain amino acid preparations with conservative management, such as the use of protein restriction and lactulose, have failed to show convincing evidence of the superior effect of the branched-chain amino acids on encephalopathic states despite the reversal of the abnormal plasma amino acid pattern toward normal and the development of positive nitrogen balance.[35-37] Administration of a branched-chain preparation (Hepaticaid) by tube or by mouth in a cross-over study did not ameliorate encephalopathy.[38] Another study suggesting improvement with this product was uncontrolled and was associated with simultaneous provision of ancillary anti-coma regimen.[39] Additional controlled and randomized studies are required before accepting earlier claims for the clinical usefulness of branched-chain amino acid preparations in cirrhosis-related encephalopathy. For additional discussion on this issue, see Chapter 68.

Several genetically determined disorders caused by hyperammonemia due to the failure of removal of blood urea have been recognized. In these diseases, which are inherited in an autosomal recessive manner, a deficiency of urea cycle enzymes has been detected (see Table 70–1). The clinical features of these genetic hyperammonemic disorders vary according to the degree of enzymatic defect. Symptoms may consist of mental retardation, generalized seizures, ataxia, intermittent stupor and coma, rigidity, and opisthotonos. However, some patients merely display learning disability and are otherwise normal. In general, the patient improves when the diet is restricted in protein. Of interest is the fact that some afflicted children display a natural distaste for meat.[25] (See Chap. 63.)

## Chronic Neurologic Diseases

Acute and chronic neurologic diseases of non-nutritional origin that impair consciousness of motor functions essential to adequate nutritional intake, such as paralysis or weakness of the facial muscles, the tongue, the pharynx, and the muscles of deglutition, frequently require the temporary or permanent use of a nasogastric tube or a gastrostomy for the patient's well-being. These measures make possible proper enteral nutrition and may, in fact, prove to be life-saving. In most of these disorders, nutritional support does not affect the basic pathogenesis of the disease. The use of B-complex vitamin preparations for a variety of acute and chronic neurologic diseases of cryptic origin continues to be common medical practice. To date, however, there is no objective evidence that this practice has any effect on the speed of recovery of the afflicted nervous tissue.

Specific nutritional therapy has been advocated for a number of neurologic diseases of undetermined etiology. For instance, a low-fat diet has been recommended as an effective means of reducing the incidence of exacerbations in patients suffering from multiple sclerosis. However, objective evaluation of the efficacy of this treatment modality has not yet been possible. Epidemiologic studies relating multiple sclerosis to nutritional factors have revealed a possible correlation between the incidence of the disease, the total fat intake, and the percentage of calories of animal origin consumed.[40] Multiple sclerosis tends to be more prevalent in countries where the use of animal fat is high. It has also been suggested that the administration of unsaturated fatty acids, such as linoleic or arachidonic acid, may reduce the number and the severity of multiple sclerosis attacks. This idea is based on the observation that brain and spinal cord gleaned from patients who have died of multiple sclerosis are deficient in unsaturated fatty acids and that linoleic and arachidonic acid tend to inhibit the lymphocyte-antigen interaction, the cellular mechanism that may enhance demyelination. Sensitized lymphocytes probably interact with myelin components in the affected parts of the nervous system during an attack of multiple sclerosis. That the ingestion of unsaturated fatty acids, such as linoleic acid, affects the course of multiple sclerosis remains unproved.[40]

The possibility that polyunsaturated fatty acids have an immunosuppressant effect has led to the evaluation of low-polyunsaturated-fatty-acid diets in other neurologic disorders of autoimmune-inflammatory etiology, such as Guillain-Barré syndrome, that acutely affect peripheral nerves.[41]

Although Parkinson's disease is not caused by altered nutrition, it responds favorably to a combination of specific therapy and dietary manipulation. The administration of the amino acid levodopa (L-dihydroxyphenylalanine) is known to improve the symptoms of Parkinson's disease, i.e., rigidity, bradykinesia, and tremor. Upon entry into the appropriate nerve cells of the affected parts of the brain, levodopa is converted to the deficient catecholamine, dopamine. Most of the ingested levodopa is converted to dopamine in nerve cells located in peripheral ganglia, and only 1% of the amino acid is made available to the brain. The enzymatic reaction that converts levodopa to dopamine, a vitamin-$B_6$-dependent decarboxylase, can be stimulated by excessive amounts of the vitamin, shunting even more levodopa to the periphery. As a result, the beneficial effects of levodopa may be drastically reduced when supplemental vitamin preparations containing pyridoxine are added to the daily dose of levodopa. Therefore, vitamin preparations that contain pyridoxine should be avoided. Because the amino acids contained in the standard diet tend to compete with the gastrointestial absorption of levodopa, the daily protein intake of parkinsonian patients receiving levodopa should be kept in the vicinity of 0.5 g protein/kg/day. In addition, the medication should not be ingested at the same time as foods rich in amino acids, such as meat and dairy products, are eaten.[42]

**Anticonvulsant Effect of Ketogenic Diet.** It is well established that ketosis and acidosis secondary to minimal caloric intake or starvation have an anticonvulsant effect. This knowledge has led to the successful clinical use of a diet high in fat and low in carbohydrate, the ketogenic diet, as therapy for seizure disorders in which all other forms of treatment have failed. The mechanism of action of the ketogenic diet on seizures remains unknown, but the anticonvulsant effect of the diet is maintained as long as blood ketone bodies remain elevated. Since the diet has such an impressive effect on certain seizure types (absence and myoclonic), it deserves consideration as a therapeutic mode. The diet appears to be most effective in children under the age of 10. In order to assure success, the diet must be adhered to rigidly, which presents problems in terms of acceptance and compliance. A more recently developed ketogenic diet including medium-chain triglycerides has permitted liberalization of carbohydrate and protein intake, making the diet more acceptable to the patient.[42a]

### Headache

A link between the consumption of certain foods and the occurrence of headaches, particularly of the migraine type, has been suspected since Hippocratic days.[43] Such foods as chocolate, cheese, citrus fruit, and alcoholic beverages appear to be most frequently associated with migraine headaches.[44] It is postulated that tyramine, a monoamine contained in relatively high concentrations in these foods, triggers the symptoms.[43] Tyramine is found mainly in foods and beverages that have undergone bacterial decomposition, such as cheddar and bleu cheese and certain wines.[43] It is postulated that tyramine, by virtue of sympathomimetic properties, acts either directly or indirectly through the release of norepinephrine, a powerful vasoconstrictor, on sensitive blood vessels that in turn provoke a migraine attack. Biochemical studies on the platelets of some patients suffering from migraine headaches have revealed a deficiency of phenosulfo-

transferase, an enzyme that detoxifies the phenol groups contained in certain foods by the addition of a sulfate radical.[45,46] Dietary phenylethylamine, contained in such foods as chocolate, cheese, and alcoholic beverages, may also precipitate migraine attacks in some individuals, presumably by virtue of defective phenylethylamine oxidation. A number of food additives, notably sodium nitrite and nitrate (meat preservatives used in processed meats), sodium glutamate (a flavor enhancer and a food preservative), and tartrazine (a coloring agent), have also been associated with headaches. Sodium glutamate, frequently used in certain Chinese dishes, when consumed in large quantities, may precipitate a generalized vasomotor reaction consisting of perioral numbness, flushing of the face, dizziness, and headache (Chinese restaurant syndrome) in sensitive individuals.[47,48]

Whereas nitrates and nitrites contained in such processed meats as hot dogs have been blamed for migraine attacks, one clinical study suggests that the headaches are in fact provoked by the amount of pork contained in these products, rather than by the preservatives.[49]

In general, the results of clinical investigations of the association of foods and their constituents and headaches remain controversial. Some studies seem to confirm the connection whereas others deny it, attributing "dietary-induced" headaches to psychologic factors. Until a consensus has been established, migraine sufferers should be advised to abstain whenever possible from foods thought to provoke an attack.

### Neuropathy, Neuralgia, and Dementia

Nutritional therapy consisting of vitamins and other nutrients continues to be used in neurologic disorders of unknown cause, in spite of a total lack of scientific rationale. The popularity of administering large doses of B vitamins as therapy for peripheral neuropathies, neuralgias, and dementias of uncertain etiology stems from the fact that experimentally induced deficiencies of these vitamins in animals frequently result in symptoms caused by reversible lesions of the peripheral and central nervous system. In most instances, the far-advanced lesions show demyelination and destruction of nerve fibers as well as damage to nerve cells, a frequent finding in many human neurologic diseases. These observations have led to the erroneous belief that diseases in human beings with similar clinical and pathologic attributes will improve more rapidly and more completely following the administration of vitamins in doses that frequently exceed those used to maintain adequate nutrition. In most instances, lack of knowledge, frustration on the part of the patient and the physician, and the desire to try any type of "shotgun" therapy have led to the irrational and medically unsound use of vitamins and special diets in the treatment of such neurologic disorders as neuropathies, neuralgias, and dementias.

Thiamin in huge doses is frequently used to treat peripheral neuropathy of undetermined cause. To date, there is no scientific evidence to show that the vitamin either protects peripheral nerve fibers from further damage or enhances regeneration or remyelination, except when severe thiamin deficiency has been demonstrated by appropriate laboratory tests. The same can be said for the use of large doses of vitamin $B_{12}$ in trigeminal or postherpetic neuralgia. The neuropathy, the subacute degeneration of the spinal cord, the degeneration of the optic nerve, and the dementia associated with vitamin $B_{12}$ deficiency respond dramatically to appropriate doses of the vitamin, as does the rare case of dementia caused by folate or niacin deficiency. Treatment with large doses of B vitamin complex has no effect on toxic, metabolic, familial, or traumatic neuropathies. Nor do dementias, such as Alzheimer's and Pick's disease, respond to megavitamin therapy.

## Vitamin Toxicity and Neurologic Defects

The past decade has witnessed an ever-increasing misuse of vitamins in doses that far exceed the accepted daily requirements. Along with an emphasis on weight-reduction diets, better nutrition, and improved physical and mental health, a belief has developed that vitamins will increase athletic stamina and performance and that if a small dose of a vitamin is good, a megadose must, by necessity, be better. This concept has been responsible for the overcommercialization and indiscriminate use of vitamins.[50] However, considering the large doses of vitamins consumed daily, for a variety of reasons, by an ever-increasing number of people, vitamin toxicity affecting the nervous system is relatively rare. Of all the vitamins, both water- and fat-soluble, only two—vitamin A and pyridoxine (vitamin $B_6$)—are known to produce adverse neurologic reactions when ingested in pharmacologic rather than recommended nutritional doses.

**Vitamin A.** This vitamin has been used to excess by patients suffering from acne and health food addicts. Although susceptibility to vitamin A toxicity tends to be highly variable, a dose in excess of 25,000 International Units per day (10 times the recommended daily allowance) ingested over a period of months can lead to toxic symptoms. Infants and children tend to be more susceptible.[51,52] The abusive intake of alcohol further enhances the toxicity of this vitamin.[52]

Toxicity occurs when the capacity of the retinol binding system in the plasma and cells is exceeded. The excessive vitamin A is then presented to cell membranes and organelles in unbound form. It is presumed that an excess of the vitamin leads to an increased permeability of the choroid plexus in the brain and a consequent increase in the formation of cerebrospinal fluid; hence, a clinical condition known as pseudotumor cerebri, or benign increased intracranial pressure, results. Patients complain of headache, drowsiness, blurred vision, and diplopia. They may exhibit nuchal rigidity, papilledema, and bilateral abducens weakness, all caused by increased intracranial pressure. In most cases, the classic skin changes may be noted: a desquamative scaly erythematous dermatitis with yellowish disc pigmentation of the soles of the feet, the palms of the hands, and the nasolabial folds. Once the vitamin has been withheld, recovery from toxicity occurs in two to three days. In some instances, resolution of symptoms and signs of toxicity may take several weeks.[53,54]

Vitamin A ingested in excessive amounts during the first trimester of pregnancy may be responsible for cleft palate, harelip, macroglossia, defective eye development, or hydrocephalus in the fetus.

**Vitamin $B_6$.** Excessive doses of vitamin $B_6$ have been used for general health purposes, premenstrual syndrome, carpal tunnel syndrome, schizophrenia, and childhood autism. Until recently, it was assumed that high doses of the vitamin were generally harmless. One report has shown that when pyridoxine is ingested in gram quantities per day (6 g/day) for 4 to 40 months, a severe, slowly reversible, symmetrical, distal, areflexic, sensory neuropathy may ensue.[55] Patients complain of progressive ataxia, particularly in the dark (loss of visual cues), accompanied by numbness of the feet and severe sensory dysfunction characterized by a marked decrease in joint position and vibratory sense, a decrease in the sense of touch in a distal symmetrical distribution, and a decrease in the sensation of lips and tongue. The spinal fluid examination tends to be normal. Standard electrical studies performed after the illness is well established reflect degeneration of large axons and small myelinated fibers that in turn reflect pathologic changes in the dorsal root and gasserian ganglia.[55]

## Anticonvulsant-Induced Vitamin Insufficiency

**Folate.** Patients who are being treated with anticonvulsant drugs for seizure disorders may incur a significant degree of folic acid deficiency.[56,57]

Although diphenylhydantoin appears to be the drug most frequently implicated, phenobarbital and primidone may also be involved, but to a lesser degree and frequency. These drugs are thought to affect the metabolism of folate or its metabolites because of similarities in chemical structure, because of a drug-induced impairment of absorption or of tissue transport, or because of competitive inhibition of vitamin coenzyme formation.[58] Following the long-term administration of these drugs, a fall of serum, cerebrospinal fluid, and red blood cell folate levels can be detected and, on rare occasions, a megaloblastic anemia and/or neuropsychiatric complications characterized by apathy, depression, and, eventually, dementia may occur.

The literature contains conflicting reports on the effects of folic acid on seizure control. It has been suggested that in some patients the administration of folic acid may increase the frequency of seizures and that folic acid and its derivatives may have significant convulsive properties.[60] Experimental evidence in animals suggests a possible blockade of inhibitory gamma aminobutyric acid receptors by folic acid, reducing seizure thresholds.[61]

Carefully controlled clinical studies are needed before the relationship between anticonvulsants, folate, and seizure control can be confirmed and fully understood.[62] It seems reasonable to screen the serum folate levels of patients who have received diphenylhydantoin for recurrent seizures over a prolonged period. This is particularly germane in the case of patients who demonstrate such unusual neuropsychiatric problems as dementia.

**Vitamin D.** The prolonged administration of anticonvulsant drugs, such as phenytoin, may lead to a decrease in bone mineral content. The severity of demineralization appears to be related to the dose of the drug, a deficiency of physical activity, and a lack of exposure to sunlight. However, pathologic fractures as a result of demineralization are rare.[63] The drugs interact with the vitamin and its active forms, decreasing intestinal calcium absorption and redistribution. The problem in the United States does not appear to be of sufficient clinical importance to warrant the routine vitamin D supplementation of patients treated with antiepileptic drugs; however, the possibility should be borne in mind, and vitamin D metabolites should be estimated periodically in long-term patients with poor intake or malabsorption.

**Vitamin K.** The antiepileptic drugs, phenytoin, phenobarbital, and primidone, individually or in combination, when used to treat epileptic pregnant women, can cause bleeding in the neonate by depressing the production or the release of the vitamin K-dependent clotting factors: prothrombin and factors V and VII. Vitamin K should be administered in the late stages of pregnancy to the neonate and the mother under treatment for epilepsy.[63]

## Valproic Acid and Hyperammonemia

Valproic acid, a widely used and effective anticonvulsant drug, can cause hepatic failure and hyperammonemia. The latter has been reported in the absence of laboratory evidence of hepatic dysfunction in children receiving multiple anticonvulsant drugs.[63a,-63c] In this group of patients, hyperammonemia appears to be dose-related and may occur after several years of therapy. Hyperammonemia may underlie unexplained episodes of stupor, coma, and increased seizure activity, weight loss, nausea, anorexia, and vomiting. According to some investigators, the biochemical mechanism responsible for the hyperammonemia consists of the accumulation of propionate, one of the metabolites of valproic acid, and the inhibition of carbamyl phosphate synthetase, one of the enzymes involved in the conversion of ammonia to urea.[63a] A partial inborn error of ammonia metabolism in certain children may render them more vulnerable to hyperammonemia when they are treated with valproic acid. Valproic acid therapy may cause asymptomatic hepatic dysfunction and hyperammonemia. Therefore, liver function tests, including ammonia blood levels, are indicated at periodic intervals in patients receiving this drug. It should be discontinued in the presence of abnormal liver function tests and/or hyperammonemia. In patients in whom valproic acid has proved to be the most effective anticonvulsant agent, the drug can be continued cautiously, provided the dietary intake of protein is sharply curtailed. This regimen may result in the reversal of abnormal liver function test results including hyperammonemia.[63d]

## Food Additives

The idea that food additives, such as synthetic food dyes and certain naturally occurring ingredients, adversely affect the behavior and learning of children has attracted considerable attention since it was first suggested several decades ago. Clinical data gathered to date have been extremely controversial. Investigators have claimed that strict adherence to the "Feingold diet," a diet totally devoid of additives, including dyes and antioxidants, leads to improvement or complete remission of hyperkinetic behavior and learning disability in 50 to 70% of afflicted children.[64] Furthermore, in 75% of such children, the diet has been claimed to be as effective as such stimulants as methylphenidate hydrochloride (Ritalin) and dextroamphetamine. The beneficial effect of the diet, sometimes referred to as "the Feingold effect," has been reported to occur in a matter of days to weeks, provided there is 100% adherence to the diet. The younger the child, the more rapid and complete the degree of improvement. The published accounts of the dramatic effects of the diet are either anecdotal or based mainly on essentially uncontrolled clinical trials.[64,65]

In 1982, a Consensus Development Conference was convened at the National Institutes of Health to evaluate the available information on the subject.[66] Anderson has summarized some of the conference findings as follows:[67]

> Some significant and well-controlled studies have verified the following impressions:
> 1. The Feingold type of diet may be helpful in a number of children with the attention deficit disorder with hyperkinesis (not 50% as Feingold stated).[68,69]*
> 2. The diet seemed most helpful in younger children.
> 3. Challenge with higher doses of food colors in children might produce a pharmacologic-like effect to depress learning in a specific test situation.[70]
> 4. Allergic (hypersensitivity) as well as other imreactions to foods or food additives probably have nothing to do with the effects of the diet on behavior.

Significant biochemical and neurobehavioral effects of artificial food colors have been reported by a number of research laboratories. The best-studied example is erythrosin B (FDC Red #3). This artificial coloring agent when added in vitro alters membrane conductance, changing the movement of the cations sodium and potassium across the membrane. The dye has the unique property of acting only on the sodium and potassium ATPase of brain; it is not active on the enzyme found in other tissues, such as liver and red blood cells. It is a potent noncompetitive inhibitor of dopamine uptake by nerve endings prepared from rat brain exposed to the dye for five minutes. Other studies have shown that the compound inhibits the uptake of many other neurotransmitters and precursors, an effect diluted by increasing amounts of tissue in the biochemical assay. Whether these neurochemical properties of this particular food dye can be extrapolated to hyperactive behavior and learning disorders in children remains to be shown.[71-74]

*Reference numbers in this quotation are those of this chapter, but the actual references are those of the quotation.

Well-designed clinical studies that take into consideration genetic predisposition, variability and heterogeneity, dosage, time of administration, and easily measured objective and significant clinical end points seem essential before one can establish beyond doubt that food additives have an adverse effect on behavior.

## SUMMARY

In this chapter, neurologic diseases and their relationship to nutritional and dietary factors have been discussed. In some of the disorders, improper or inadequate nutrition is implicated; therefore, dietary manipulation constitutes the main therapeutic mode. In others a combination of genetic and metabolic factors, as well as dietary factors, underlies the symptoms and signs of neurologic dysfunction that can be ameliorated by changes in the diet and/or vitamin supplementation. In some disorders, such as migraine headache and hyperactivity in children, the beneficial effects of altered nutrition remain controversial. In such neurologic diseases as dementia, in which no obvious nutritional cause has been established, dietary treatment has not been successful.

Despite significant advances over the past decades in the field of nutrition, large gaps remain in our understanding of the role of nutrition in the normal and abnormal metabolic activity of the nervous system. More sensitive and critical methods for the assessment of the nutritional status of the nervous system and for the evaluation of the dietary management of neuropsychiatric disorders are essential before more rational and effective therapeutic manipulations can be developed.

## REFERENCES

1. Williams, R.R.: Toward the Conquest of Beriberi. Cambridge, MA, Harvard University Press, 1970.
2. Terris, M.: Goldberger on Pellagra. Baton Rouge, Louisiana State University Press, 1964.
3. Victor, M., Adams, R.D.: Am. J. Clin. Nutr. 9:379–397, 1961.
4. Victor, M., Adams, R.D., Collins, G.H.: The Wernicke-Korsakoff's Syndrome. Philadelphia, F.A. Davis Co., 1971.
5. Watson, A.J.S., Walker, G.H., Tomkin, M.M.R., et al.: Ir. J. Med. Sci. 150:301–303, 1981.
6. Dreyfus, P.M.: N. Engl. J. Med. 267:596–598, 1962.
7. Victor, M.: Polyneuropathy due to nutritional deficiency and alcoholism. In Peripheral Neuropathy. (Dyck, P.J., Ed.) Philadelphia, W.B. Saunders Co., 1975.
8. Mayer, R.F., Garcia-Mullin, R.: Peripheral nerve and muscle disorders associated with alcoholism. In Biology of Alcoholism. (Kissin, B., Begleiter, H., Eds.) New York, Plenum Publishing Corp., 1972.
9. Dreyfus, P.M.: Amblyopia and other neurological disorders associated with chronic alcoholism. In Handbook of Clinical Neurology. (Vinken, P.J., Bruyn, G.W., Eds.) Amsterdam, North Holland Publishing Company, 1976.

10. Lerman, S., Feldman, A.L.: Arch. Ophthalmol. *65*:381–385, 1961.

11. Victor, M., Adams, R.D., Mancall, E.L.: Arch. Neurol. *1*:579–688, 1959.

12. Mancall, E., McEntee, W.J.: Neurology *15*:303–313, 1965.

13. Frenkel, E.P.: J. Clin. Invest. *52*:1237–1245, 1973.

14. Frenkel, E.P., Kitchens, R.L., Johnston, J.M.: J. Biol. Chem. *248*:7540–7546, 1973.

15. Dreyfus, P.M., Dube, V.: Clin. Chim. Acta *15*:525–528, 1967.

16. Jolliffe, N., Bowman, K.M., Rosenblum, L.A., et al.: JAMA *114*:307–312, 1940.

17. Mudd, S.H.: Adv. Nutr. Res. *4*:1–34, 1982.

18. Scheinberg, I.H.: Wilson's Disease. Philadelphia, W.B. Saunders Co., 1984.

19. Sternlieb, I., Scheinberg, I.H.: JAMA *189*:748–754, 1964.

20. Strickland, G.T., Blackwell, R.A., Walten, R.H.: Am. J. Med. *51*:31–40, 1971.

21. Refsum, S.: Acta Phychiatr. Scand. (Suppl.) 38, 1946.

22. Steinberg, D., Mize, C.E., Herndon, J.H., Jr., et al.: Arch. Intern. Med. *125*:75–87, 1970.

23. Rosenberg, L.E.: Curr. Concepts Nutr. *8*:55–64, 1979.

24. Dodge, P.R., Prensky, A.L., Feigin, R.D., et al.: Nutrition and the Developing Nervous System. St. Louis, C.V. Mosby Co., 1975.

25. Menkes, J.H.: Textbook of Child Neurology. 3rd ed. Philadelphia, Lea & Febiger, 1985.

26. Centerwall, W.R., Centerwall, A.S., Armon, V., et al.: Pediatrics *59*:93–101, 1961.

27. Holliday, M.A., Anderson, A.S., Barness, L.A., et al.: Pediatrics *57*:783–792, 1976.

28. Cornblath, M., Schwartz, R.: Disorders of Carbohydrate Metabolism in Infancy. 2nd ed. Philadelphia, W.B. Saunders Co., 1976.

29. Fischler, K.: Pediatrics *50*:412–419, 1972.

30. Conn, H.O.: Hosp. Pract. *8*:65–72, 1973.

31. Breen, K.J., Schenker, S.: Hepatic coma: Present concepts of pathogenesis and therapy. *In* Progress in Liver Diseases, Vol. IV. (Popper, H., Schaffner, F., Eds.) New York, Grune and Stratton, 1972.

32. Fischer, J.E., Bower, R.H.: Surg. Clin. North Am. *61*:653–660, 1981.

33. Bower, R.H., Fischer, J.E.: Nutritional management of hepatic encephalopathy. *In* Advances in Nutrition Research. (Draper, H.H., Ed.) New York, Plenum Publishing Corp., 1981.

34. Cerra, F.B., McMillen, M., Angelico, R., et al.: Surgery *94*:612–619, 1983.

35. Wahren, J., Denis, J., Desurmont, P., et al.: Hepatology *3*:475–480, 1983.

36. Rossi-Fanelli, F., Riggio, O., Cangiano, C., et al.: Dig. Dis. Sci. *27*:929–935, 1982.

37. Millikan, W.J., Jr., Henderson, J.M., Warren, W.D.: Ann. Surg. *197*:294–304, 1983.

38. McGhee, A., Henderson, J.M., Millikan, W.J., Jr., et al.: Ann. Surg. *197*:288–293, 1983.

39. Keohane, P.P., Atrill, H., Gimble, G., et al.: J. Parenter. Enter. Nutr. *7*:346–350, 1983.

40. Fields, E.J.: J.R. Soc. Med. *72*:487–488, 1979.

41. Bower, D.B., Newsholme, E.A.: Lancet, *1*:583–585, 1978.

42. Mena, I., Cotzias, G.C.: N. Engl. J. Med. *292*:181–184, 1975.

42a. Withrow, C.D.: The ketogenic diet: Mechanism of anticonvulsant action. *In* Antiepileptic Drugs. (Woodbury, D.M., Penry, J.K., Schmidt, R.P., Eds.) New York, Raven Press, 1972.

43. Kohlenberg, R.J.: Headache *22*:30–34, 1982.

44. Wilson, C.W.M., Kirker, J.G., Warnes, H., et al.: Postgrad. Med. J. *56*:617–621, 1980.

45. Littlewood, J., Glover, V., Sandler, M., et al.: Lancet *1*:983–985, 1982.

46. Glover, V., Littlewood, J., Sandler, M., et al.: Headache *23*:53–58, 1983.

47. Medina, J.L., Diamond, S.: Headache *18*:31–34, 1978.

48. Hanington, E.: J. Hum. Nut. *34*:175–180, 1980.

49. Bernstein, A.: Personal communication.

50. Rudman, D., Williams, P.J.: N. Engl. J. Med. *309*:488–489, 1983.

51. Farris, W.A., Erdman, J.W., Jr.: JAMA *247*:1317–1318, 1982.

52. Herbert, V.: Am. J. Clin. Nutr.: *36*:185–186, 1982.

53. Leo, M.A., Arai, M., Sato, M., et al.: Gastroenterology *82*:194–205, 1982.

54. Bauernfeind, J.C.: The Nutrition Foundation, New York, 1980.

55. Schaumburg, H., Kaplan, J., Windebank, A., et al.: N. Engl. J. Med. *309*:445–448, 1983.

56. Reynolds, E.H., Mattson, R.H., Gallagher, B.B.: Neurology *22*:841–844, 1972.

57. Smith, D.B., Obbens, E.A.M.T.: Antifolate-antiepileptic relationships in folic acid. *In* Neurology, Psychiatry, and Internal Medicine. (Botez, M.I., Reynolds, E.H., Eds.) New York, Raven Press, 1979.

58. Pisciotta, A.V.: Phenytoin, hematological toxicity. *In* Antiepileptic Drugs. (Woodbury, D.M., Penry, J.K., Pippenger, C.E., eds.). New York, Raven Press, 1982.

59. Reference deleted.

60. Baylis, E.M., Crowley, J.M., Preece, J.M., et al.: Lancet *1*:62–64, 1971.

61. Roberts, P.J.: Nature (London) *250*:429–430, 1974.

62. Mattson, R.H., Gallagher, B.B., Reynolds, E.H., et al.: Arch. Neurol. *29*:78–81, 1973.

63. Kutt, H., Solomon, G.E.: Antiepileptic drugs. Phenytoin: Relevent side effects. *In* Antiepileptic Drugs. (Woodbury, D.M., Penry, J.K., Schmidt, R.P., Eds.) New York, Raven Press, 1972.

63a. Coulter, D.L., Allen, R.J.: Lancet *1*:1310–1311, 1980.

63b. Rawat, S., Borkowski, W.J., Swick, H.M.: Neurology *31*:1173–1174, 1981.

63c. Murphy, J.V., Marquardt, K.: Arch. Neurol. *39*:591–592, 1982.

63d. Personal observation.

64. Feingold, B.F.: Dietary management of behavior and learning disabilities. *In* Nutrition and Behavior. (Miller, S.A., Ed.) Philadelphia, The Franklin Institute Press, 1981.

65. Feingold, B.F.: Why Your Child is Hyperactive. New York, Random House, 1975.

66. National Institutes of Health Consensus Development Conference: Defined Diets in Childhood Hyperactivity. Office for Medical Applications of Research, Bethesda, Maryland. Washington, D.C., January, 1982.

67. Anderson, J.A.: Nutr. Rev. *42*:112, 1984.

68. Harley, J.P., Ray, R.S., Tomasi, L., et al.: Pediatrics *61*:818–828, 1978.

69. Weiss, B., Williams, J.H., Margen, S.: Science *207*:1487–1488, 1980.

70. Swanson, J.M., Kinsbourne, M.: Science *207*:1485–1487, 1980.

71. Silbergeld, E.K., Anderson, S.M.: Bull. N.Y. Acad. Med. *58*:275–295, 1982.

72. Rose, T.L.: J. Appl. Behav. Anal. *11*:439–446, 1978.

73. Mailman, R.B., Ferris, R.M., Tang, F.L.M., et al.: Science *207*:535–537, 1980.

74. Dickerson, J.W., Pepler, F.: J. Hum. Nutr. *34*:167–174, 1980.

*Chapter* **68**

# NUTRITION AND DIET IN RHEUMATIC DISORDERS

Alfred J. Bollet

The field of rheumatic diseases encompasses a wide range of diseases and pathologic processes, most of which affect joint tissues, and thus cause symptoms of arthritis. The basic structure affected by these diseases is the connective tissue, and thus they are known as connective tissue diseases. An earlier name, "collagen diseases," arose when the term collagen was synonymous with connective tissue. It is reserved for a specific fibrillar protein in that tissue, and the name "collagen disease" is obsolete.

The connective tissues affected by these diseases include synovial membrane lining joint surfaces, cartilage, bone, tendons, ligaments, the interstitial tissues in all organs, and the blood vessels. Vasculitis occurs commonly in these diseases, particularly affecting arterioles and venules, but in some instances large arteries, including the aorta, are affected. By convention, arteriosclerotic vascular lesions and inflammation of large veins (phlebitis) are not considered among the connective tissue diseases.

Connective tissues all over the body can be involved, and manifestations can appear in almost any organ, but the most frequent manifestation of these diseases is arthritis. There are over 100 different diseases in the field, with a wide variety of pathologic processes, such as local or widespread inflammation, immune mechanisms, wear-and-tear processes, and inherited metabolic abnormalities. Pain is the most frequent manifestation of rheumatic diseases, and many painful syndromes are included in the spectrum of connective tissue diseases. Muscle diseases and vaguely defined painful syndromes such as "fibrositis" are common rheumatic diseases. Temporary but annoying focal connective tissue syndromes include traumatic sprains and strains, focal myositis, tendonitis, and tendon sheath abnormalities. The most frequent serious forms of arthritis are rheumatoid arthritis, osteoarthritis, gout, and systemic lupus erythematosus. This chapter concentrates primarily on nutritional considerations in those diseases.

Because therapy for most forms of arthritis is not curative, the diseases are chronic and patients are always seeking more satisfactory forms of therapy. Food faddists and other quacks prey upon patients with arthritis because of the attractiveness of nonpharmacologic approaches to therapy. The lay literature abounds in dietary "cures" for arthritis. Since many of the pathologic processes are minor and temporary, although annoying, spontaneous improvement is a frequent occurrence and usually is attributed by patients to the last method tried; if it was a diet, favorable testimonials result, providing quotations for lay publications, which rarely identify the nature of the arthritis in the patients quoted. Because the causes of arthritis are varied, any publication that fails to identify the nature of the disease treated, lumping all "arthritis" as one disaese, is without value.

## NUTRITIONAL INFLUENCES ON STRUCTURE AND METABOLISM OF CONNECTIVE TISSUE

Mature connective tissues are varied in structure and function. Hyaline cartilage is easily compressed, energy absorbing, and self-lubricating, preventing friction during joint motion. Ligaments, tendon, and bone provide support and strong attachments. Loose areolar interstitial tissue and capillary walls allow rapid movement of nutrients and wastes between cells and plasma. The cells synthesize the basic constituents of each of these forms of connective tissue and are named according to the physical characteristics of the mature tissue they form, such as osteocytes, fibrocytes, or chondrocytes. When the tissue is immature, with active synthesis of its extracellular constituents, the cells are usually referred to as "blasts," such as chondroblasts or fibroblasts.

The main fibrillar components of the connective tissues are the proteins, elastin, reticulin, and the various types of collagen. Interspersed among the fibers are the constituents of the "ground substance," including the proteoglycans, which are high-molecular-weight substances containing large, complex polysaccharides (the glycosaminoglycans). The proteoglycans can bind large amounts of water and electrolytes. A thorough description of the chemistry and metabolism of these compounds may be found elsewhere. It is worthy of emphasis, however, that the polysaccharide components are synthesized from glucose, and the rates of synthesis can be affected by the availability of this sugar or its metabolic derivatives, such as uridine diphosphoglucose. (UDPG).

The protein components of connective tissue, including the protein moieties of the proteoglycans, are affected by nutritional influences in a fashion similar to those that affect other structural proteins. The first classic connective tissue disease to be described was scurvy, since ascorbic acid is essential for synthesis of collagen. Scurvy, then, is a true "collagen disease"; weakness of the collagenous structure of small blood vessels causes the multiple small interstitial hemorrhages that occur in this disease. Collagen serves in part as a reservoir protein, providing a source of amino acids in times of negative nitrogen balance,[1] although it is not labile as muscle protein. Mobilization of collagen does occur during starvation or protein deficiency, or in states of protein catabolism, such as occurs when corticosteroids are administered.

Loss of the collagen becomes evident in the structures with the most collagen, the bone and the skin, because 50% of the collagen is in bone and 25% is in the dermis. The rest of the connective tissues contain the remaining 25% of the collagen. Mobilization of bone collagen results in thinning of the bone due to the decrease in bone matrix (osteoporosis) in starvation or other states of prolonged negative nitrogen balance.

The most frequent pathologic process affecting the connective tissue in the rheumatic diseases is inflammation. In the past it was not realized that inflammation was susceptible to nutritional influence, but now it is clear that fatty acid derivatives, the prostaglandins, play a key role in the pathogenesis of the inflammatory process. Experimental data in mice (discussed later in this chapter) have shown that dietary changes can modify the production of prostaglandins during inflammation.

The most common forms of arthritis are rheumatoid arthritis and osteoarthritis. The former is a widespread inflammation affecting small and large joints. It can begin at any age and varies greatly in severity and manifestations. Osteoarthritis, on the other hand, is a wear-and-tear process, characterized by degeneration of articular cartilage with secondary changes in underlying bone. It usually occurs in older people, mostly affecting joints that have had excessive wear for some reason, and often is limited to one or a few joints. Neither process has a major metabolic component.

Muscle wasting is a common manifestation of all types of chronic joint disease, since muscle inflammation and joint immobility due to pain occur commonly as part of the disease in all types of arthritis. Muscle atrophy, usually focal, then occurs around affected joints, but some patients with rheumatoid arthritis have fever and other systemic manifestations, leading to anorexia, weight loss, and even inanition in severe cases. In such instances, the negative nitrogen balance can contribute to the muscle wasting. Nutritional influences are of considerable importance in these patients.

## NUTRITION AND INFLAMMATION

The rheumatic diseases are characterized by inflammation, particularly in joint tissues, and immune processes. In many of the diseases antibodies are formed that react with tissue components, so-called autoantibodies, and these diseases are often referred to as "autoimmune" diseases. A variety of immune mechanisms occur in these diseases; we are beginning to recognize and understand nutritional influences on these immune phenomena,[2] which may become more important in the future.

Deposition of immune complexes is a major pathogenetic mechanism in many of these conditions. Enhanced ability to develop immune re-actions in some modern population groups may result from their improved nutritional status over that of prior generations, thus leading to the ap-parent increase in incidence of these diseases.

Inflammation is a complicated process that in-cludes activation of cascade systems of plasma proteins, resulting in release or activation of en-zymes and other factors that play a role in mo-bilization of responsive cells and tissue destruc-tion. Products of the kinin and complement systems, release of endogenous pyrogen and other mediators from cells, release of lysosomal en-zymes, appearance in the plasma of "acute phase reactants" formed in the liver, and other phenom-ena are included. Generation of a series of bio-logically active fatty acids from arachidonic acid, the prostaglandins, and leukotrienes forms an-other key component of the inflammatory process. Many of these processes can be affected by nutri-tional influences. Recent studies have focused pri-marily on the role of dietary fatty acids.

## Role of Essential Fatty Acids

Prostaglandins and leukotrienes are synthe-sized by a wide variety of cells, including leu-kocytes and platelets. These compounds are de-rived from essential fatty acids in the diet, particularly arachidonic acid. They modulate the responses of many tissues and organs, particularly those containing smooth muscle. The prostaglan-dins of the E series cause vasodilatation, hyper-emia, exudation, and increased sensitivity to painful stimuli (tenderness). Prostaglandins also mediate the interrelationships of antibody-pro-ducing cells, inhibiting the action of suppressor T cells and leading to increased antibody pro-duction, at least in vitro.[3] Dietary arachidonic acid is preferentially incorporated into the phospho-lipids of activated lymphocytes, and arachidonic acid constitutes over 20% of the total phospho-lipid fatty acid of macrophages.[4]

Diets deficient in essential fatty acids can mod-ify the response of experimental animals to in-flammatory stimuli. For example, mice on a diet deficient in essential fatty acids showed a signif-icant reduction in immune responses, both pri-mary and secondary.[5] Responses to both T-cell-dependent and T-cell-independent antigens were blunted.[6] Evidence for diminution in immune re-sponse on a diet deficient in essential fatty acids was reported in F1 hybrids of New Zealand Black and New Zealand White (NZB/NZW) mice, who developed a form of glomerulonephritis, accom-panied by antinuclear antibodies. Pathologically, this disease resembles the renal disease seen in human systemic lupus erythematosus. These rats

uniformly die before one year of age, but litter-mates kept on a diet deficient in essential fatty acids have a much lower incidence of renal dis-ease, and a considerably longer survival.[7] The rats on a diet deficient in essential fatty acids showed a decreased incidence of glomerulonephritis, de-creased subepidermal deposition of immunoglob-ulins, and decreased development of antibodies to double-stranded DNA.[7]

However, skin-graft rejection in rats deficient in polyunsaturated fatty acids is potentiated, and the incidence of induced tumors is reduced, suggest-ing that cell-mediated immune responses are aug-mented.[4,5,8] Rats on a diet deficient in essential fatty acids show reduced experimental chronic inflammation.[9,10] Adjuvant arthritis, an experi-mental form of inflammation that is widely used for screening drug effects, is suppressed in rats fed such a diet.[9] Inflammatory exudate induced experimentally in these animals is decreased in quantity, and has a lower concentration of pros-taglandins than in controls fed a normal diet.[9] In another study, a diet containing evening primrose oil comprised of 9% linoleic acid and only 0.3% arachidonic acid shifted prostaglandin synthesis toward E1 from E2. In rats on this diet, the che-motactic response of polymorphonuclear leuko-cytes is significantly impaired.

Changes in dietary fatty acids can bring about alterations of the fatty acid composition of mem-brane lipids. Feeding with diets high in omega-3 fatty acids results in such compounds substituting for the arachidonic acid in membrane lipids in man and laboratory animals. When stimuli result in prostaglandin formation, the resulting com-pounds differ from those produced from arachi-donate, which are mostly of the 2 series. The om-ega-3 fatty acid studied most extensively is eicosapentanoic acid (EPA), which is present mainly in dietary fish oils. Interest has been aroused because of reports of a decreased inci-dence of diseases characterized by thrombosis, such as myocardial infarction, in Eskimos whose diet is rich in this fatty acid.

Eicosapentanoic acid gives rise to PGE3, which is less vasodilatory and has less of an inflamma-tion-inducing effect than PGE2, and to PGI3, which has less of an antiaggregatory effect on platelets than PGI2; platelets produce throm-boxane A3, which is weakly proaggregatory com-pared to thromboxane A2. Eicosapentanoic acid is a poor substrate for the fatty acid cyclo-oxy-genase, which results in prostaglandin formation, but it is a good substrate for lipoxygenase enzymes that catalyze the biosynthesis of hydroperoxy-acids, hydroxy-acids, and leukotrienes. Leuko-triene B5 (LTB5), which results from conversion of EPA, has been shown to be at least 30 times less potent than LTB4 (which is synthesized from arachidonic acid) in causing aggregation of rat neutrophils, chemokinesis, and lysosomal enzyme release from human neutrophils, and in potentiating bradykinin-induced plasma exudation.[10a] Experimentally, supplementation of a standard rat diet with EPA caused a significant increase in the formation of LTB5 and a decrease in the synthesis of LTB4 by stimulated leukocytes, as well as a decrease in edema formation following injection of an inflammation-producing agent.[10b]

Thus, diets rich in long-chain omega-3 fatty acids (EPA) from sources such as cod liver oil or mackerel show that is is possible in man to produce a dose-related, sustained change in the spectrum of biologically active tissue prostanoids to a more favorable pattern with regard to tendency to clot formation[10c] and severity of inflammatory reaction.[10b,10d]

Most of the drugs used in the treatment of the rheumatic diseases affect synthesis of prostaglandins. Nonsteroidal anti-inflammatory drugs inhibit a key early step in the synthesis of these compounds: the cyclo-oxygenase that converts arachidonic acid to prostaglandins.[11] Phospholipase activity, which releases arachidonic acid from membrane lipids, is decreased by treatment with corticosteroids. Such approaches, diminishing prostaglandin formation, are more practical in patients at this time, but in the future dietary modifications may be found to be a safe and effective means of altering the responsiveness of the cells involved in the inflammatory process. Alterations in fatty acid content of the diet, such as supplementation with eicosapentanoic acid, could, by reducing the synthesis of prostaglandins, offer a novel and nontoxic approach to the modulation of a chronic inflammatory response.

## OTHER METABOLIC ALTERATIONS IN RHEUMATIC DISEASES

The renal involvement that occurs in some patients with systemic connective tissue disease, such as systemic lupus erythematosus, can lead to the nephrotic syndrome. Clinically this problem resembles other causes of nephrotic syndrome. Protein loss may be severe and may lead to hypoproteinemia and edema.

Some patients with arthritis have edema, partly because of salt and water retention from drug effect,[11] but also because of immobility caused by joint pain. Whatever the mechanism of the edema in these patients, salt restriction is helpful, and diuretics are also often valuable.

Salt and water retention can result in edema in patients taking nonsteroidal anti-inflammatory

drugs. These drugs can affect renal handling of sodium and water through their effect on renal prostaglandin synthesis.[11] This effect is described in the section on nutritional consequences of therapy.

Gastrointestinal abnormalities occur in some connective tissue diseases, particularly in scleroderma (progressive systemic sclerosis). Widespread gastrointestinal tract involvement can result in atrophy of the intestinal mucosa, and loss of secretory activity and absorptive surface.[12] Malabsorption, with severe nutritional consequences, may occur. Elemental diets or even parenteral nutrition may be necessary. These problems do not differ fundamentally from those seen in other causes of malabsorption, but the prognosis is usually poor.

Interference with food consumption can occur, primarily in cases of scleroderma, as a result of tightness of the skin around the mouth, or contracture of the capsules of the temporomandibular joints. Inability to open the mouth can lead to the necessity for a liquid diet. Removal of teeth has even been necessary on occasion in order to have access to the mouth with a straw.

### Obesity

Because the spine and lower extremities are weight-bearing, body weight plays a role in the strain on the joints in these areas and can contribute to the development or progression of arthritis. Osteoarthritis is the form of arthritis most likely to be affected by obesity because it is a wear-and-tear process characterized by breakdown of cartilage and bone, with secondary proliferative changes. Mechanical factors that put an extra strain on joint tissues can accelerate the development or rate of progression of this disease. Studies of dietary intake and body weight in osteoarthritis, however, have not clearly established obesity as a factor in the pathogenesis.[13] Engel reported a higher incidence of osteoarthritis in both weight-bearing and nonweight-bearing joints in obese patients,[14] but several others did not find a higher incidence in nonweight-bearing joints, such as the distal interphalangeal joints, in obese patients.[15,16] In a population survey in New Haven, Connecticut, the weight-to-height ratio correlated with the incidence of osteoarthritis.[17] A strikingly high frequency of osteoarthritis occurs in obese mice,[18] but a genetic factor was identified that did not necessarily correlate with body weight.[19]

The hip joint, which is a common site affected by both osteoarthritis and rheumatoid arthritis, has been well studied from the standpoint of the influence body weight on the progression of established arthritis.[20] In a group of 89 patients who required total hip replacement for osteoarthritis or rheumatoid arthritis, a striking correlation was found between body weight and the degree of loss of the substance of the femoral head. Another study of 25 grossly obese patients, who averaged 91 kg above their ideal weights, failed to show an increase in the frequency of osteoarthritis from that expected,[21] and the mean age of these patients was only 44.7 years, which is relatively young for a group of patients with osteoarthritis.

Obesity correlates with the finding of hyperuricemia and the development of gout.[22] Weight loss causes lowering of the plasma uric acid level in these individuals.[23]

## Arthritis Following Surgical Treatment of Obesity

Some patients with particularly severe obesity have been subjected to a surgical procedure to limit the intestinal surface available for absorption, the so-called "intestinal bypass procedure." This operation creates a blind loop of jejunum that is not involved in transport or absorption of food, giving rise to a form of "blind-loop syndrome." Such patients commonly develop arthritis, perhaps because of bacterial overgrowth in such loops leading to absorption of bacterial antigens and formation of immune complexes that reach the joints. The arthritis in these individuals has a predilection for small joints of the upper and lower extremities, and is often accompanied by a skin rash, which tends to be pustulovesicular. Bacteria are not found in the lesions, but immunoglobulins and complement components are demonstrable in vessel walls, and there are increased quantities of circulating cryoglobulins containing immunoglobulins, complement, and some immune complexes.[24]

## METABOLIC DISEASES AFFECTING CONNECTIVE TISSUE

**Gout.** The most common metabolic disorder associated with arthritis is gout. Increases in serum levels of uric acid, whatever the cause, can lead to formation of crystals of uric acid in joint tissues, producing a severe inflammatory reaction. This form of "crystal synovitis" is most often familial, especially in men. Usually there is no underlying disease, although patients with gout have a higher frequency of obesity, and some of the correlates of obesity, such as diabetes, hypertension, and ischemic heart disease, occur with higher frequency in people with gout than in the general population.[22]

Some patients with gout excrete less uric acid each day than they form from endogenous and exogenous precursors, and thus are in positive urate balance. The accumulation of urate leads to deposition of insoluble masses of crystals, particularly in cartilage, and a foreign-body granulomatous reaction around these depositions. Called tophi, these deposits can cause destruction of joint tissues, leading to chronic arthritis.

Studies of patients with gout have not revealed any significant differences in diet from control groups, with the exception of alcoholic beverage consumption. Patients with gout consumed a greater amount of beer.[25] Dietary therapy has been used in the management of patients with gout. About 15% of the urate formed each day comes from dietary sources; the remainder is an obligatory end product of tissue nucleic acid turnover. A diet markedly restricted in purine content will reduce the urinary excretion of uric acid by 200 to 400 mg per day, and will lower the serum uric acid level by about 1 mg/dl.[26]

Although severe dietary restriction is not often necessary,[26] control of obesity, reduction in alcohol intake and, when necessary, control of hypertriglyceridemia are more important aspects of the nutritional management of gout. However, it is wise for patients with gout to avoid food particularly high in purine content, such as sweetbreads, fish roe, anchovies, sardines, liver, and kidney, and to restrict intake of foods moderately high in purines, such as animal meats, seafood, beans, lentils, spinach, and peas.[26] A diet severely restricted in purine precursors is relatively unpalatable, and compliance is difficult. Fortunately it is not necessary because drugs are effective in controlling the manifestations of the disease.

Drug therapy can consist of either uricosurics, which block renal tubular reabsorption of urate, increasing excretion, or inhibitors of the enzyme xanthine oxidase, which converts hypoxanthine to xanthine, and xanthine to uric acid. Increased excretion of uric acid or inhibition of its synthesis is more effective than dietary manipulation in controlling the metabolic abnormality.

**Hyperlipidemias.** Hyperlipidemias can be associated with joint symptoms, particularly the type IIa and type IV hyperlipoproteinemias. Patients with type IA disease often have polyarthritis, Achilles tendonitis, and tenosynovitis, and thus seem to have a rheumatic disease. Because the patients usually have xanthelasma and numerous xanthomas, especially in tendons, the diagnosis is not difficult. Patients with type IV hyperlipoproteinemia commonly have mild joint pains, usually involving one or a few joints, with periodic exacerbations. The episodic nature of the symptoms provides a diagnostically helpful clue, but false positive serologic tests for rheumatoid factor in these patients may lead to confusion. Diagnosis must be made by lipoprotein electrophoresis, demonstrating elevated beta-lipoproteins and elevated serum triglycerides. Dietary therapy, including restriction of intake of carbohydrates, alcohol, and total calories, with consequent reduction in triglyceride levels, is often helpful in relieving the joint symptoms. Drug therapy is being evaluated.[27]

**Ochronosis.** An inherited metabolic disorder, ochronosis is characterized by urine that darkens on standing, owing to the presence of excessive quantities of homogentisic acid. Also called alkaptonuria, the disease is due to an inherited deficiency of the enzyme homogentisic acid oxidase. As a result, homogentisic acid increases in quantity in body fluids, and is excreted in the urine. Polymers of this acid that are deposited in cartilaginous structures, especially joint cartilage, darken with time, and black pigment is seen in cartilage as a characteristic finding. Degeneration of chondrocytes results, leading to breakdown of the cartilage matrix, a form of osteoarthritis. The abnormal cartilage becomes calcified, and thus the disease can be diagnosed by roentgenogram, as well as by the history of dark urine, and the pigmentation visible in cartilaginous structures such as the earlobes. At present no dietary therapy is useful in management of these patients.

## OTHER METABOLIC PHENOMENA IN CONNECTIVE TISSUE DISEASES

**Histidine and Sulfhydryl Groups.** The plasma of patients with rheumatoid arthritis has a lower level of free sulfhydryl groups[28] and decreased levels of histidine in the plasma compared to normal individuals.[29,30] Levels of other amino acids are in the same range as in normal people. The decrease in the level of histidine correlates with the degree of clinical activity of the rheumatoid arthritis, as measured by various parameters that reflect disease activity, such as the erythrocyte sedimentation rate, duration of morning stiffness, and titer of rheumatoid factor. The subnormal level of this amino acid in the plasma is not due to poor absorption because oral doses of histidine are absorbed as quickly in these patients as in normal individuals.[31] In view of these biochemical findings, treatment of rheumatoid arthritis with 4.5 g/day of histidine was evaluated in a double blind study. Although there was no significant improvement in the group as a whole, patients with more active and more prolonged disease did show some suggestion of benefit, compared to their status on placebo therapy,[32] but these changes were not dramatic. The only conclusion

that could be drawn from this study is that further trials of this form of therapy are warranted.

Drugs that offer significant improvement in patients with rheumatoid arthritis do not alter the abnormal plasma level of histidine with one exception. Penicillamine raises the levels of histidine and total serum sulfhydryl levels, and lowers the plasma viscosity and C-reactive protein.[33] Because penicillamine itself has free sulfhydryl (SH) groups, researchers have suggested that its mechanism of action involves those groups. This subject is controversial, however, since gold, which is given as a complex with a sulfhydryl compound, is clearly of therapeutic value in rheumatoid arthritis. It is widely believed that the gold is the therapeutic substance, but the possibility that the sulfhydryl compound accompanying the gold is the true therapeutic agent remains under consideration.[33] The amount of SH in these gold salts is not sufficient to affect the total level of SH in the serum, however. Chloroquine, another drug shown to have a disease-suppressive effect in rheumatoid arthritis, albeit a weak one, does not affect plasma levels of histidine, nor do the non-steroidal anti-inflammatory drugs (NSAIDs) or corticosteroids.

Rheumatoid factor is a characteristic finding in the plasma of patients with rheumatoid arthritis. It is an antibody to gamma globulin that has been altered in some fashion to make it antigenic. In vitro, low levels of histidine allow aggregation of gamma globulin molecules to form more readily by formation of disulfide bonds, a process that can alter the antigenicity of the protein. It has been shown that maintenance of free sulfhydryl groups in plasma is a possible protective mechanism, minimizing the tendency of the gamma globulin to become antigenic.[29] This theory is not generally accepted, however.

**Tryptophan Metabolism in Rheumatoid Arthritis.** Abnormal quantities of metabolites of tyrosine and tryptophan have been found in the urine of patients with rheumatoid arthritis and other forms of inflammatory arthritis. Degradation of tryptophan results in excretion of 3-hydroxykynurenine, xanthurenic acid, 3-hydroxyanthranilic acid, and N-methyl-nicotinamide. Increased urinary excretion of these metabolites of tryptophan has been reported in patients with rheumatoid arthritis and scleroderma, but not in a pattern that would suggest a defect at a specific enzymatic step, and the reason for these abnormalities has not been elucidated.[34] Deficiencies of vitamins involved in the metabolism of these amino acids have not been found in patients with these connective tissue diseases. Administration of pyridoxine neither benefits the patient clinically nor corrects the abnormalities in urinary excretion, but in one study pyridoxine administration caused a reversal of the increased urinary excretion of these metabolites that occurs following administration of tryptophan.[35]

There have been several reports of aggravation of rheumatoid arthritis and other systemic connective tissue diseases following oral administration of L-tyrosine, and improvement of patients on diets low in phenylalanine and tyrosine. In several patients with rheumatoid arthritis, some clinical improvement has been noted on diets low in tryptophan, with a drop in sedimentation rate; notably, these diets are low in total protein (20 g/day).[35] In a study of glomerulonephritis that develops in hybrid New Zealand Black mice (NZB/NZW), a diet low in phenylalanine and tyrosine reduced the frequency and severity of development of the renal lesions.[4]

## Metals

**Iron.** Anemia is a frequent finding in severe, uncontrolled rheumatoid arthritis, and is occasionally seen in other forms of chronic inflammatory joint disease. A low level of iron usually exists in the plasma of such patients, along with a hypochromic normocytic anemia. Total iron binding capacity of the plasma is not usually increased. Thus the clinical findings are more typical of those found in the anemia of chronic infection, or chronic inflammatory disease, rather than true iron deficiency, and bone marrow examination usually shows normal or increased iron stores in such patients.[36] Iron absorption is normal in patients with rheumatoid arthritis. Iron therapy usually does not improve the anemia in these patients unless there is a concomitant iron deficiency on the basis of blood loss, which can be demonstrated by decreased iron stores in the bone marrow.[37]

Increased amounts of iron have been demonstrated in synovial tissues of patients with rheumatoid arthritis.[38–40] These studies suggest recurrent intra-articular microhemorrhages. The rate of iron accumulation in the knee in these patients averaged 1.25 mg/day, representing bleeding of about 3.5 mg/day. No correlation was found with the serum iron, and this small amount of iron accumulation probably had no effect on the stores of iron available for marrow function.

The pathogenesis of the iron deficiency in rheumatoid arthritis and in other chronic inflammatory states probably represents a defect in reutilization of iron after red blood cell destruction, the exact cause of which is still obscure. The process is not specific for rheumatoid arthritis, and is not critical to the pathogenesis of the disease.

Only rarely does the anemia require treatment specifically directed toward it, and then there usually is another contributory factor, such as significant gastrointestinal blood loss or a superimposed, acquired, immunologically mediated hemolytic process.[41]

**Copper.** Elevated levels of both free copper and ceruloplasmin occur in the plasma of patients with rheumatoid arthritis. Both the total copper and ultrafilterable copper are elevated; no simple relationship has been found between these two levels of copper in the plasma.[42] The plasma copper levels correlate with the degree of joint inflammation. These findings have been interpreted to mean that both copper and ceruloplasmin behave as acute phase reactants in a nonspecific fashion. They are elevated in patients with a variety of inflammatory diseases without specificity.[42,43] The levels of copper decrease with therapy for the rheumatoid arthritis, as do levels of other acute phase reactants.[42]

Copper and ceruloplasmin levels are particularly elevated in female patients with rheumatoid arthritis who are receiving oral contraceptives containing estrogen, whereas normal levels are found in men and women not receiving estrogen.[42,44] Because oral contraceptives raise titers of antinuclear antibodies and rheumatoid factor, this observation is of interest.[44] The levels of total serum copper correlate inversely with the serum iron in patients with rheumatoid arthritis,[42,43] but ultrafilterable copper levels do not correlate with anything.[42] Because serum iron is decreased in this disease, as well as in other forms of chronic inflammation, this correlation is probably also nonspecific.[43]

There is a strong direct correlation between ceruloplasmin levels and antioxidant activity of the serum.[43] This phenomenon suggests a potential protective role for the increased ceruloplasmin levels in inflammatory states, since toxic oxygen radicals are formed during inflammation. Scavengers of these radicals decrease the severity of inflammation in experimental models. Ceruloplasmin may act to minimize the toxicity of such radicals.[42,43] In this context, it is notable that the wearing of copper bracelets is a folk remedy for arthritis. These bracelets usually cause some discoloration of the underlying skin, suggesting absorption of copper from the jewelry.[42]

**Zinc.** Patients with rheumatoid arthritis have lower serum levels of zinc than normal individuals or patients with other rheumatic diseases. Niedermeier and Griggs found a zinc level averaging 73 μg/dl in patients with rheumatoid arthritis, compared to a mean in controls of 115.[45] A more recent study, using atomic absorption spectrophotometry, found plasma zinc levels averaging 85.7 μg/dl in patients with rheumatoid arthritis, 99 μg/dl in controls. The decrease in plasma levels correlated with the severity of the osteoporosis observed in these patients, judging by the metacarpal index, a radiologic measurement of the width of the cortex of the second metacarpal bone. Correlation was best in women who had been treated with corticosteroids. Zinc levels correlated directly with the level of serum albumin, and inversely with the erythrocyte sedimentation rate, but did not correlate with the degree of joint tenderness.[46,47]

Low zinc levels have also been reported in patients on corticosteroid therapy, and in those who have had severe burns.[47] Zinc could be important in the genesis of manifestations of rheumatoid arthritis; zinc has been shown to stabilize lysosomal membranes, to inhibit prostaglandin synthesis, to interfere with complement action, and to impair macrophage function.[48]

In a double-blind controlled study of therapy with oral zinc sulfate in 24 patients with chronic refractory rheumatoid arthritis, significant improvement was noted in the amount of joint swelling, the duration of morning stiffness, the time needed to walk a set distance, and the overall evaluation of their status by the patients. Several other clinical trials have failed to show a beneficial effect of zinc.[49-51]

Enzymes involved in the synthesis of collagen require zinc. In zinc-deficient animals, wound healing is impaired, implying a defect in collagen synthesis. Failure of collagen synthesis is not a feature of the rheumatic diseases, however.

Most of the direct reacting zinc in the plasma is bound to histidine, and the low levels of serum histidine may be the cause or the effect of the low levels of zinc.[48] Experimentally, zinc-deficient chickens improve when given either oral zinc or histidine.[48]

At least one therapeutic agent used in patients with rheumatoid arthritis can alter zinc metabolism. Penicillamine increases both zinc absorption and urinary excretion, but a positive balance results.

**Other Trace Metals.** A deficiency of *selenium* has been reported in a patient receiving parenteral hyperalimentation, who developed muscle pain and tenderness and was unable to walk. This clinical syndrome resembles that seen in patients with myositis, the "fibrositis syndrome," and also is a component of other rheumatic diseases such as rheumatoid arthritis.

Surgical stress may have contributed to the negative balance of the metal, but it is interesting that the patient lived in an area with low selenium in the soil. This observation points to a need for further investigation of possible trace metal deficiencies that might contribute to symptoms of patients with rheumatic diseases.[52]

Cotzias studied metabolism of *manganese* and found that the turnover rate was increased in a small group of patients with rheumatoid arthritis, compared to control patients with a variety of diseases.[53] The slow turnover rates were accelerated by steroid therapy.

Manganese is a cofactor critical to the activity of some enzymes involved in glycosaminoglycan synthesis. Manganese deficiency in experimental animals results in defective synthesis of these compounds, which are key components of the extracellular material in connective tissue.[53] These findings may be relevant to disease affecting connective tissues, but there have been no clinical studies.

## Vitamins

Among the other dietary claims made regarding treatment of arthritis, "megavitamins," especially large doses of vitamins C and D, have been advocated. Vitamin D was used therapeutically for rheumatoid arthritis in the 1930s and early 1940s in uncontrolled trials. Although many physicians thought it was of benefit, and little else was available to treat these patients at that time, a great deal of toxicity occurred. Huge doses were given, often parenterally, with resulting hypercalcemia, renal calculi, and pathologic calcifications. Objective signs of improvement were few and unconvincing.[54]

**Vitamin C.** This vitamin was studied and tried in the treatment of rheumatoid arthritis in the 1940s, at a time when vitamin deficiency diseases were more common, and therapeutic use of vitamins had a major public impact. Numerous studies showed low levels of ascorbic acid in the plasma and blood cells of patients with rheumatoid arthritis, findings that have been confirmed more recently with improved methods of assay. The reason for the low levels has never been clarified. It is possible that therapy, particularly aspirin, may increase the rate of clearance of ascorbic acid, lowering blood levels secondarily. Because of these observations, therapeutic doses of ascorbic acid were tried in several studies, without evidence of clinical benefit.[55] There is no rationale for the large doses of vitamin C tried for a variety of problems in recent years, and there are no reports of controlled studies showing clinical benefit in any form of arthritis.

Ascorbic acid is essential for the synthesis of collagen, the main extracellular fiber found in connective tissue. Vitamin C deficiency is characterized by failure of synthesis of adequate quantities of collagen, accounting for the impaired wound healing and capillary fragility seen in scurvy. Decreased synthesis of collagen is not a feature of any of the rheumatic diseases. Excessive synthesis of collagen is a major aspect of the pathologic process of scleroderma (also known as progressive systemic sclerosis). Thus there is no reason to expect this form of therapy to be of benefit. On the other hand, the synthesis of collagen requires only the small amounts of ascorbic acid in the diet that have been established as the recommended daily requirements, and one should not expect benefit from intakes of larger amounts of the vitamin. In fact, deleterious effects seem more likely if collagen synthesis could be accelerated, since fibroblast proliferation and excessive collagen formation occur in many forms of arthritis. However, such harmful effects have not yet been reported.

## NUTRITIONAL EFFECTS OF THERAPY

**Gold and Zinc.** The mechanism of action of gold compounds in rheumatoid arthritis is unclear. Most research is focusing on a controlling influence on immunologic processes through an effect on either macrophages or lymphocytes. Some investigators are examining possible effects of gold on heavy metal nutrition. In patients with rheumatoid arthritis, a response to gold correlates with a decrease in the elevated plasma copper levels that occur in patients with active disease, the copper behaving in the same fashion as other "acute phase reactants." Plasma zinc levels rise more slowly as the arthritis comes under control.[33]

**Corticosteroids.** Among the therapeutic agents used in the treatment of rheumatic diseases,the one with the most metabolic effects is corticosteroid therapy. Although rarely used in the treatment of rheumatoid arthritis at present, except in very small doses, corticosteroids are used in relatively large amounts in the treatment of systemic lupus erythematosus and other serious systemic connective tissue diseases, especially those that result from immune mechanisms. The metabolic effects of corticosteroids are discussed elsewhere; only the effect on vitamin D metabolism and bone is discussed here.

The antianabolic effect of corticosteroids is well known. Inhibition of the synthetic activity of connective tissue cells is also well established, with the most important clinical manifestations seen in skin and bone, the two organs with the most abundant collagen. Osteoporosis and thin skin are thus major side effects of corticosteroid therapy, especially in the rheumatic diseases. The drugs are usually needed for long periods to treat these

chronic problems, and women, who are more susceptible to these side effects, constitute most of the patients with rheumatic diseases.

The mechanisms responsible for the altered bone metabolism when corticosteroid are administered include a direct effect on the bones, inhibiting synthesis of bone matrix, and an effect on calcium absorption in the intestine, modifying the effects of vitamin D. Collapse of vertebral bodies and increased susceptibility to femoral fractures are the most frequent serious sequelae of this phenomenon. The effect of corticosteroids on calcium results from inhibition of synthesis of the carrier protein involved in calcium absorption. As a result of the decreased calcium entering the plasma, secondary stimulation of parathyroid function occurs, contributing to the skeletal thinning.[56]

Administration of larger amounts of calcium in the diet, accompanied by increased quantities of vitamin D (10,000 to 30,000 units three times a week) or therapeutic doses of 25-hydroxy vitamin D, the metabolite of the vitamin that has the major effect on calcium transport in the intestinal mucosa, can minimize this side effect of corticosteroid therapy. There is some evidence that this approach reverses the steroid-induced bone loss, at least to some extent. (It should be noted that prevention of further progression of the bone loss would be of major clinical value, even without reversal of the bone thinning.) A prophylactic regimen including 500 to 1,000 mg of calcium daily and 50,000 units of vitamin D about two to three times a week is recommended.[56] A potential side effect of this form of therapy is the development of renal calculi. Monitoring of serum and urinary calcium, therefore, is probably wise.

**Nonsteroidal Anti-inflammatory Agents.** The most frequently used therapeutic agents in the treatment of patients with rheumatic diseases are the NSAIDs. Aspirin was the first drug in this category to be used widely and is still a mainstay of therapy for arthritis. More recently introduced NSAIDs are occasionally more effective and cause fewer gastrointestinal side effects than aspirin, although officially aspirin is still the standard of efficacy. These drugs are analgesic, anti-inflammatory, and antipyretic. A major aspect of the action of the entire group of drugs is inhibition of synthesis of prostaglandins. A consequence of the inhibition of prostaglandin synthesis in the kidney is retention of salt and water by many patients receiving these drugs. In susceptible individuals, azotemia can result, particularly in patients with antecedent kidney disease, since the prostaglandins are a major form of adaptation to altered renal perfusion.

The retention of salt and water rarely causes

serious consequences unless there are concomitant diseases such as hypertension or congestive heart failure.

## DIETS PROPOSED FOR TREATMENT OF ARTHRITIS

The lay literature abounds with suggestions of diets that will "cure" arthritis. Although published as nonfiction, often reaching bestseller lists in that category, these books should be classified as fiction. A hallmark of the group is a claim that the proposed diet is good for "arthritis" without any distinction being made among approximately 100 causes of arthritis. Clearly, in view of the diversity of the diseases in this field, no treatment can be expected to cure all forms of arthritis. A second feature of this group of publications is the use of testimonials, without mention of controlled studies. Many forms of arthritis spontaneously fluctuate in severity, and improvement can be expected from time to time in most patients. Descriptions of improvement without controlling for the frequency of these spontaneous variations make such claims impossible to evaluate and scientifically worthless. Such occurrences probably account for most of the testimonials.

A controlled study of diet was performed on 11 patients with rheumatoid arthritis. They were placed on a regimen limited in preservatives, additives, herbs, milk products, fruit, and red meat for 10 weeks, after a period of fasting, following suggestions made in a popular book (the "Dong diet"). Fifteen patients with rheumatoid arthritis who remained on their regular diets served as controls. Six patients improved on the placebo diet, and five improved on the experimental diet. Although no demonstrable effect of the elimination diet was shown, two patients elected to remain on that diet because they were convinced that it helped them.[57] It can be concluded that dietary manipulation is of value to individual patients, but no benefical regimen clearly deserves widespread adoption or the immodest claims made in lay media.

Joint pain can be a manifestation of food allergy.[58,59] Rheumatic complaints have been induced in patients with established allergic reactions to foods such as soy extracts, coffee, eggs, milk, potatoes, apples, lettuce, oranges, ethanol, beef, and pork.[59] There are also individual case reports of patients with rheumatoid arthritis who have demonstrated definite adverse reactions to specific items of food and benefit from an elimination diet. In one well-studied case, the specific food was cheese, and evidence for circulating immune complexes was found. The patient benefited from withdrawal of dairy products from the diet.[60]

When food allergy is responsible for joint complaints, or aggravation of underlying joint disease, improvement can be expected from dietary manipulation. These cases may account for some of the testimonials claiming improvement on specific diets, such as the "no nightshades diet," which eliminates potatoes, tomatoes, peppers, and related vegetables.

Experimental studies in animals demonstrating that limitation of essential fatty acid intake or decrease in intake of phenylalanine and tyrosine can modify immune responses,[4] impede the development of immune complex disease, and ameliorate the severity of experimental inflammation have been discussed previously. It is possible that carefully studied dietary manipulation can be of some benefit, at least in the inflammatory forms of arthritis, but extreme care is necessary to obtain this benefit without inducing serious nutritional deficiency syndromes. Further study of possible clinical application of these findings is warranted.

## REFERENCES

1. Bollet, A.J.: Mt. Sinai J. Med. *37*:445–449, 1970.
2. Chandra, R.K.: Lancet *1*:688–691, 1983.
3. Goodwin, J.S., Webb, D.R.: Clin. Immunol. Immunopathol. *15*:106–122, 1980.
4. Hurd, E., et al.: J. Clin. Invest. *67*:476–485, 1981.
5. Ziff, M.: Arthritis Rheum. *26*:457–471, 1983.
6. DeWille, J.W., Fraker, P.J., Romsos, D.R.: J. Nutr. *109*:1018–1027, 1979.
7. Hurd, E., Gilliam, J.N.: J. Invest. Dermatol. *77*:381–384, 1981.
8. Mertin, J., Hunt, R.: Proc. Natl. Acad. Sci. U.S.A. *73*:928–931, 1976.
9. Denko, C.W.: Agents Actions *6*:636–641, 1976.
10. Kunkel, S.L., Ogawa, H., Ward, P.A., et al.: Prog. Lipid Res. *20*:885–888, 1981.
10a.Terano, T., Salmon, J.A., Moncada, S.: Prostaglandins *27*:217–232, 1984.
10b.Terano, T., Salmon, J.A., Higgs, G.A., Moncada, S.: Biochem. Pharmacol. *35*:779–785, 1986.
10c.Fischer, S., Weber, P.C.: Biomed. Mass Spectrom. *12*:470–476, 1985.
10d.Von Schacky, C., Fisher, S., Weber, P.C.: J. Clin Investig. *76*:1626–1671, 1985.
11. Bollet, A.J.: Textbook of Rheumatology. 2nd ed. (Kelly, W.N., Harris, E.D. Jr., Ruddy, S., et al. eds.), Philadelphia, W.B. Saunders Co. In press, 1985.
12. Rodnan, G.P.: Progressive systemic sclerosis (scleroderma). *In* Arthritis and Allied Conditions. 9th ed. (McCarty, D.J., ed.) Philadelphia, Lea & Febiger, 1979.
13. Eising, L.: J. Bone Joint Surg. *45*:69–81, 1963.
14. Engel, A.: Publication *1000*:29, U.S. Public Health Service, 1968.
15. Kellgren, J.H., Lawrence, J.S.: Am. Rheum. Dis. *17*:388–397, 1958.
16. Stecher, R.M.: Ann. Rheum. Dis. *14*:1–10, 1955.
17. Acheson, R.M., Collart, A.B.: Ann. Rheum. Dis. *34*:379–387, 1975.
18. Silberberg, M., Jarrett, S.F., Silberberg, R.: Arch. Pathol. *61*:280–288, 1956.
19. Sokoloff, L., Mickelsen, O.: J. Nutr. *85*:117–121, 1965.

20. Watson, M.: Rheumatol. Rehabil. *15*:264–269, 1976.
21. Goldin, R.J., McAdam, L., Louie, J.S., et al.: Ann. Rheum. Dis. *35*:349–353, 1976.
22. Hall, A.P., Barry, P.E., Dawber, R.R., et al.: Am. J. Med. *42*:27–37, 1967.
23. Nicholls, A., Scott, J.T.: Lancet *2*:1223–1224, 1972.
24. Utsinger, P.D., Farber, N., Shapiro, R.F., et al.: Arthritis Rheum. *21*:599, 1978.
25. Gibson, T., Highton, J., Potter, C., et al.: Ann. Rheum. Dis. *39*:417–423, 1980.
26. Kelley, W.N.: Gout and related disorders of purine metabolism. *In* Textbook of Rheumatology. (Kelley, W.N., Harris, E.D. Jr., Ruddy, S., et al., eds.) Philadelphia, W.B. Saunders Co., 1981.
27. Bole, G.G.: Arthritis associated with hyperlipidemia and hypercholesterolemia. *In* Textbook of Rheumatology. (Kelley, W.N., Harris, E.D. Jr., Ruddy, S., et al., eds.) Philadelphia, W.B. Saunders Co., 1981.
28. Lorber, A., Bovy, R.A., Chang, C.C.: Metabolism *20*:446–455, 1971.
29. Gerber, D.: J. Rheumatol. *2*:384–392, 1975.
30. Gerber, D.: J. Clin. Invest. *55*:1164–1173, 1975.
31. Gerber, D.A., Tanenbaum, L., Ahrens, M.: Metabolism *25*:655–657, 1976.
32. Pinals, R.S., Harris, E., Burnett, J.B., et al.: J. Rheumatol. *4*:414–419, 1977.
33. Bird, H.A.: Ann. Rheum. Dis. *42*:474–475, 1983.
34. Houpt, J.R., Ogryzlo, M.A., Hunt, M.: Semin. Arthritis Rheum. *2*:333–353, 1973.
35. Robinson, W.: Nutrition and the rheumatic diseases. *In* Textbook of Rheumatology. (Kelley, W.N., Harris, E.D. Jr., Ruddy, S., et al., eds.), Philadelphia, W.B. Saunders, 1981.
36. Mowat, A.G.: Semin. Arthritis Rheum. *1*:195–219, 1971.
37. Boddy, K., Will, G.: Ann. Rheum. Dis. *28*:537–540, 1969.
38. Muirden, K.D., Senator, G.B.: Ann. Rheum. Dis. *27*:38–48, 1968.
39. Senator, G.B., Muirden, K.D., Balazs, N.: Ann. Rheum. Dis. *27*:49–54, 1968.
40. Bennett, R.M., et al.: Arthritis Rheum. *16*:298–304, 1973.
41. Owen, E.T., Lawson, A.A.H.: Ann. Rheum. Dis. *25*:547–552, 1966.
42. Brown, D.H., Buxhn, W.W., El-Ghobarey, A.F., et al.: An. Rheum. Dis. *38*:174–176, 1979.
43. Scudder, R., Al-Timimi, D., McMurray, W., et al.: Ann. Rheum. Dis. *37*:67–70, 1978.
44. Bajpayee, D.P.: Ann. Rheum. Dis. *34*:162–165, 1975.
45. Niedermeier, W., Griggs, J.H.: J. Chronic Dis. *23*:527–536, 1971.
46. Balogh, Z., El-Ghobarey, A.F., Fell, G.S., et al.: Ann. Rheum. Dis. *39*:329–332, 1980.
47. Kennedy, A.C., Fell, G.S., Rooney, P.J., et al.: Scand. J. Rheum. *4*:243–245, 1975.
48. Simkin, P.A.: Lancet *2*:539–542, 1976.
49. Job, C., Menkes, C.J., Delbarre, F.: Arthritis Rheum. *23*:1408–1409, 1980.
50. Mattingly, P.C., Mowat, A.G.: Ann. Rheum. Dis. *41*:456–457, 1982.
51. Mascioli, E.A., Blackburn, G.L.: *In* Texbook of Rheumatology. 2nd ed. (Kelley, W.N., Harris, E.D. Jr., Ruddy, S., et al., eds.) Philadelphia, W.B. Saunders Co., 1985.
52. Young, V.R.: N. Engl. J. Med. *304*:1228–1230, 1982.
53. Cotzias, G.C., Papavasiliou, P.S., Hughes, E.R., et al.: J. Clin. Invest. *47*:992–1001, 1968.
54. Ellman, P.: Br. J. Rheum. *1*:263–277, 1939.
55. Hall, M.G., Darling, R.C., Taylor, F.H.L.: Ann. Intern. Med. *13*:415–423, 1939.
56. Hahn, T.J., Hahn, B.H.: Arthritis Rheum. *6*:165–188, 1976.
57. Panush, R.S., Carter, R.L., Katz, P., et al.: Arthritis Rheum. *26*:462–471, 1983.
58. Bock, S.A.: Medical Times, September, 1983, pp. 27–43.
59. Mandell, M.: Medical World News *31*:16–17, 1980.
60. Parke, A.L., Hughes, G.V.R.: Br. Med. J. *282*:2027–2029, 1981.

# APPENDIX

## Abby Stolper Bloch and Maurice E. Shils

The major portion of the Appendix provides basic tabular information on nutritional standards and nutrient contents of various foods and food supplements. Specific dietary regimens supplement recommendations in the text for dietary management of disease entities. Because detailed and extensive tables of food composition are available, inclusion of this type of data has been limited. Dietary prescriptions may require modification in accordance with the clinical status and reactions of the individual patient.

There is a section on liquid formulas with detailed compositions of commercially available products and examples of special formulas for preparation by hospitals or patients at home.

### APPENDIX CONTENTS

1483

### Table A–1a.  Mean Heights and Weights and Recommended Energy Intake, U.S. Revised 1980*

| Category | Age (years) | Weight (kg) | Weight (lb) | Height (cm) | Height (in) | Energy Needs (with range) (kcal) | Energy Needs (with range) (MJ) |
|---|---|---|---|---|---|---|---|
| Infants | 0.0–0.5 | 6 | 13 | 60 | 24 | kg × 115 (95–145) | kg × .48 |
| | 0.5–1.0 | 9 | 20 | 71 | 28 | kg × 105 (80–135) | kg × .44 |
| Children | 1–3 | 13 | 29 | 90 | 35 | 1,300 (900–1,800) | 5.5 |
| | 4–6 | 20 | 44 | 112 | 44 | 1,700 (1,300–2,300) | 7.1 |
| | 7–10 | 28 | 62 | 132 | 52 | 2,400 (1,650–3,300) | 10.1 |
| Males | 11–14 | 45 | 99 | 157 | 62 | 2,700 (2,000–3,700) | 11.3 |
| | 15–18 | 66 | 145 | 176 | 69 | 2,800 (2,100–3,900) | 11.8 |
| | 19–22 | 70 | 154 | 177 | 70 | 2,900 (2,500–3,300) | 12.2 |
| | 23–50 | 70 | 154 | 178 | 70 | 2,700 (2,300–3,100) | 11.3 |
| | 51–75 | 70 | 154 | 178 | 70 | 2,400 (2,000–2,800) | 10.1 |
| | 76+ | 70 | 154 | 178 | 70 | 2,050 (1,650–2,450) | 8.6 |
| Females | 11–14 | 46 | 101 | 157 | 62 | 2,200 (1,500–3,000) | 9.2 |
| | 15–18 | 55 | 120 | 163 | 64 | 2,100 (1,200–3,000) | 8.8 |
| | 19–22 | 55 | 120 | 163 | 64 | 2,100 (1,700–2,500) | 8.8 |
| | 23–50 | 55 | 120 | 163 | 64 | 2,000 (1,600–2,400) | 8.4 |
| | 51–75 | 55 | 120 | 163 | 64 | 1,800 (1,400–2,200) | 7.6 |
| | 76+ | 55 | 120 | 163 | 64 | 1,600 (1,200–2,000) | 6.7 |
| Pregnancy | | | | | | +300 | |
| Lactation | | | | | | +500 | |

The data in this table have been assembled from the observed median heights and weights of children, together with desirable weights for adults, for the mean heights of men (178 cm) and women (163 cm) between the ages of 18 and 34 years as surveyed in the U.S. population (HEW/NCHS data).

The energy allowances for the young adults are for men and women doing light work. The allowances for the two older age groups represent mean energy needs over these age spans, allowing for a 2% decrease in basal (resting) metabolic rate per decade and a reduction in activity of 200 kcal/day for men and women between 51 and 75 years, 500 kcal for men over 75 years, and 400 kcal for women over 75 (see original text). The customary range of daily energy output is shown for adults in parentheses, and is based on a variation in energy needs of ±400 kcal at any one age (see original text and Garrow, 1978), emphasizing the range of energy intakes appropriate for any group of people.

Energy allowances for children through age 18 are based on median energy intakes of children these ages followed in longitudinal growth studies. The values in parentheses are 10th and 90th percentiles of energy intake, to indicate the range of energy consumption among children of these ages (see original text).

*From Recommended Dietary Allowances. 9th ed. Washington, D.C., National Academy of Sciences, p. 23.

## Table A–1b. Recommended Daily Dietary

| | Age | Weight | | Height | | Protein | Fat-soluble Vitamins | | |
| | | | | | | | Vitamin A | Vitamin D | Vitamin E |
| | (years) | (kg) | (lb) | (cm) | (in) | (g) | (µg R.E.)[b] | (µg)[c] | (mg α T.E.)[d] |
|---|---|---|---|---|---|---|---|---|---|
| Infants | 0.0–0.5 | 6 | 13 | 60 | 24 | kg × 2.2 | 420 | 10 | 3 |
| | 0.5–1.0 | 9 | 20 | 71 | 28 | kg × 2.0 | 400 | 10 | 4 |
| Children | 1–3 | 13 | 29 | 90 | 35 | 23 | 400 | 10 | 5 |
| | 4–6 | 20 | 44 | 112 | 44 | 30 | 500 | 10 | 6 |
| | 7–10 | 28 | 62 | 132 | 52 | 34 | 700 | 10 | 7 |
| Males | 11–14 | 45 | 99 | 157 | 62 | 45 | 1,000 | 10 | 8 |
| | 15–18 | 66 | 145 | 176 | 69 | 56 | 1,000 | 10 | 10 |
| | 19–22 | 70 | 154 | 177 | 70 | 56 | 1,000 | 7.5 | 10 |
| | 23–50 | 70 | 154 | 178 | 70 | 56 | 1,000 | 5 | 10 |
| | 51+ | 70 | 154 | 178 | 70 | 56 | 1,000 | 5 | 10 |
| Females | 11–14 | 46 | 101 | 157 | 62 | 46 | 800 | 10 | 8 |
| | 15–18 | 55 | 120 | 163 | 64 | 46 | 800 | 10 | 8 |
| | 19–22 | 55 | 120 | 163 | 64 | 44 | 800 | 7.5 | 8 |
| | 23–50 | 55 | 120 | 163 | 64 | 44 | 800 | 5 | 8 |
| | 51+ | 55 | 120 | 163 | 64 | 44 | 800 | 5 | 8 |
| Pregnant | | | | | | +30 | +200 | +5 | +2 |
| Lactating | | | | | | +20 | +400 | +5 | +3 |

[a]The allowances are intended to provide for individual variations among most normal persons living in the United States under usual environmental stresses. Diets should be based on a variety of common foods in order to provide other nutrients for which human requirements have been less well defined. See original text for detailed discussion of allowances and of nutrients not tabulated.

[b]Retinol equivalents. 1 Retinol equivalent = 1 µg retinol or 6 µg β carotene. See original text for calculation of vitamin A activity of diets as retinol equivalents.

[c]As cholecalciferol. 10 µg cholecalciferol = 400 I.U. vitamin D.

[d]α tocopherol equivalents (T.E.). 1 mg d-α-tocopherol = 1 α T.E. See original text for variation in allowances and calculation of vitamin E activity of the diet as α tocopherol equivalents.

[e]1 NE (niacin equivalent) is equal to 1 mg of niacin or 60 mg of dietary tryptophan.

## Table A–1c. Estimated Safe and Adequate Daily Dietary Intakes of

| | Age | Vitamins | | | Trace Elements[b] | |
| | (years) | Vitamin K (µg) | Biotin (µg) | Pantothenic Acid (mg) | Copper (mg) | Manganese (mg) |
|---|---|---|---|---|---|---|
| Infants | 0–0.5 | 12 | 35 | 2 | 0.5–0.7 | 0.5–0.7 |
| | 0.5–1 | 10–20 | 50 | 3 | 0.7–1.0 | 0.7–1.0 |
| Children and | 1–3 | 15–30 | 65 | 3 | 1.0–1.5 | 1.0–1.5 |
| Adolescents | 4–6 | 20–40 | 85 | 3–4 | 1.5–2.0 | 1.5–2.0 |
| | 7–10 | 30–60 | 120 | 4–5 | 2.0–2.5 | 2.0–3.0 |
| | 11+ | 50–100 | 100–200 | 4–7 | 2.0–3.0 | 2.5–5.0 |
| Adults | | 70–140 | 100–200 | 4–7 | 2.0–3.0 | 2.5–5.0 |

[a]Because there is less information on which to base allowances, these figures are not given in the main table of the RDA and are provided here in the form of ranges of recommended intakes.

[b]Since the toxic levels for many trace elements may be only several times usual intakes, the upper levels for the trace elements given in this table should not be habitually exceeded.

## Allowances,[a] U.S., Revised 1980

| | Water-soluble Vitamins | | | | | | Minerals | | | | | |
|---|---|---|---|---|---|---|---|---|---|---|---|---|
| Vita-min C (mg) | Thia-min (mg) | Ribo-flavin (mg) | Niacin (mg N.E.)[e] | Vita-min B$_6$ (mg) | Fola-cin[f] (µg) | Vita-min B$_{12}$ (µg) | Cal-cium (mg) | Phos-phorus (mg) | Mag-nesium (mg) | Iron (mg) | Zinc (mg) | Iodine (µg) |
| 35 | 0.3 | 0.4 | 6 | 0.3 | 30 | 0.5[g] | 360 | 240 | 50 | 10 | 3 | 40 |
| 35 | 0.5 | 0.6 | 8 | 0.6 | 45 | 1.5 | 540 | 360 | 70 | 15 | 5 | 50 |
| 45 | 0.7 | 0.8 | 9 | 0.9 | 100 | 2.0 | 800 | 800 | 150 | 15 | 10 | 70 |
| 45 | 0.9 | 1.0 | 11 | 1.3 | 200 | 2.5 | 800 | 800 | 200 | 10 | 10 | 90 |
| 45 | 1.2 | 1.4 | 16 | 1.6 | 300 | 3.0 | 800 | 800 | 250 | 10 | 10 | 120 |
| 50 | 1.4 | 1.6 | 18 | 1.8 | 400 | 3.0 | 1,200 | 1,200 | 350 | 18 | 15 | 150 |
| 60 | 1.4 | 1.7 | 18 | 2.0 | 400 | 3.0 | 1,200 | 1,200 | 400 | 18 | 15 | 150 |
| 60 | 1.5 | 1.7 | 19 | 2.2 | 400 | 3.0 | 800 | 800 | 350 | 10 | 15 | 150 |
| 60 | 1.4 | 1.6 | 18 | 2.2 | 400 | 3.0 | 800 | 800 | 350 | 10 | 15 | 150 |
| 60 | 1.2 | 1.4 | 16 | 2.2 | 400 | 3.0 | 800 | 800 | 350 | 10 | 15 | 150 |
| 50 | 1.1 | 1.3 | 15 | 1.8 | 400 | 3.0 | 1,200 | 1,200 | 300 | 18 | 15 | 150 |
| 60 | 1.1 | 1.3 | 14 | 2.0 | 400 | 3.0 | 1,200 | 1,200 | 300 | 18 | 15 | 150 |
| 60 | 1.1 | 1.3 | 14 | 2.0 | 400 | 3.0 | 800 | 800 | 300 | 18 | 15 | 150 |
| 60 | 1.0 | 1.2 | 13 | 2.0 | 400 | 3.0 | 800 | 800 | 300 | 18 | 15 | 150 |
| 60 | 1.0 | 1.2 | 13 | 2.0 | 400 | 3.0 | 800 | 800 | 300 | 10 | 15 | 150 |
| +20 | +0.4 | +0.3 | +2 | +0.6 | +400 | +1.0 | +400 | +400 | +150 | [h] | +5 | +25 |
| +40 | +0.5 | +0.5 | +5 | +0.5 | +100 | +1.0 | +400 | +400 | +150 | [h] | +10 | +50 |

[f]The folacin allowances refer to dietary sources as determined by *Lactobacillus casei* assay after treatment with enzymes ("conjugases") to make polyglutamyl forms of the vitamin available to the test organism.

[g]The RDA for vitamin B$_{12}$ in infants is based on average concentration of the vitamin in human milk. The allowances after weaning are based on energy intake (as recommended by the American Academy of Pediatrics) and consideration of other factors such as intestinal absorption; see original text.

[h]The increased requirement during pregnancy cannot be met by the iron content of habitual American diets nor by the existing iron stores of many women; therefore the use of 30 to 60 mg of supplemental iron is recommended. Iron needs during lactation are not substantially different from those of nonpregnant women, but continued supplementation of the mother for two to three months after parturition is advisable in order to replenish stores depleted by pregnancy.

## Additional Selected Vitamins and Minerals[a,c]

| | Trace Elements[b] | | | | Electrolytes | | |
|---|---|---|---|---|---|---|---|
| Fluoride (mg) | Chromium (mg) | Selenium (mg) | Molybdenum (mg) | | Sodium (mg) | Potassium (mg) | Chloride (mg) |
| 0.1–0.5 | 0.01–0.04 | 0.01–0.04 | 0.03–0.06 | | 115–350 | 350–925 | 275–700 |
| 0.2–1.0 | 0.02–0.06 | 0.02–0.06 | 0.04–0.08 | | 250–750 | 425–1,275 | 400–1,200 |
| 0.5–1.5 | 0.02–0.08 | 0.02–0.08 | 0.05–0.1 | | 325–975 | 550–1,650 | 500–1,500 |
| 1.0–2.5 | 0.03–0.12 | 0.03–0.12 | 0.06–0.15 | | 450–1,350 | 775–2,325 | 700–2,100 |
| 1.5–2.5 | 0.05–0.2 | 0.05–0.2 | 0.1–0.3 | | 600–1,800 | 1,000–3,000 | 925–2,775 |
| 1.5–2.5 | 0.05–0.2 | 0.05–0.2 | 0.15–0.5 | | 900–2,700 | 1,525–4,575 | 1,400–4,200 |
| 1.5–4.0 | 0.05–0.2 | 0.05–0.2 | 0.15–0.5 | | 1,100–3,300 | 1,875–5,625 | 1,700–5,100 |

[c]From Recommended Dietary Allowances. 9th ed. Washington, D.C., National Academy of Sciences 1980, p. 178.

# Table A–1d-1. Some Recommended Dietary Intakes

The Committee for the preparation of the tenth edition of the Recommended Dietary Allowances, Food and Nutrition Board, National Research Council, submitted its draft revision in 1985. It was not accepted by the National Research Council. The resulting impasse has led to a number of meetings, letters, and other comments on this issue, some of which have been published.[1-8] Members of the Committee have published, as individuals, reviews of the literature on specific nutrients; these papers include recommendations in quantitative terms as *Recommended Dietary Intakes* (RDI) for various age groups and for pregnancy and lactation. Dr. Beaton in Chapter 35 (pages 662–664) has discussed the basis for "recommended intake" with reference to the professionals who have responsibility for counseling individuals.

Although the published data cover only a relatively few nutrients and are included in a personal (rather than official committee) publication, we deemed it desirable to reproduce the data here because of the expertise of the individual authors and the potential usefulness of the figures.

## REFERENCES

1. American Institute of Nutrition: Nutr. Notes 21:1–6, 1985.
2. Guthrie, H.A.: J. Am. Diet. Assoc. 85:1646–1648, 1985.
3. Isselbacher, K.: J. Am. Diet. Assoc. 85:1648–1649, 1985.
4. Marshall, E.: Science 230:420–421, 1985.
5. Monsen, E.R., Owen, A.L.: J. Am. Diet. Assoc. 85:1649, 1985.
6. Hegsted, D.M.: J. Nutr. 116:478–481, 1986.
7. Recommended dietary allowances: Scientific issues and process for the future. A statement by the Food and Nutrition Board. J. Nutr. 116:482–488, 1986.
8. Olson, J.A.: J. Nutr. 116:1581–1584, 1986.

| Category | Age | Vitamin A* (RE) | Vitamin K† (µg) | Vitamin C‡ (mg) | Vitamin B$_{12}$§ (µg) | Folate‖ (µg/kg) | Iron# (mg) |
|---|---|---|---|---|---|---|---|
| Infants | 0–2.9 mo | 375 | 10¶ | 25 | 0.3 | 16** | φ |
| | 3–5.9 mo | 375 | 10 | 25 | 0.4 | 24** | 6.6 |
| | 6–11.9 mo | 375 | 10 | 25 | 0.5 | 32** | 8.8 |
| Children | 1–1.9 yr | 375 | 15 (1–3 yrs) | 25 | 0.7 | 3.3 | 10 |
| | 2–5.9 yr | 400 | 20 (4–6 yrs) | 25 | 1.0 | 3.3 | 10 |
| | 6–9.9 yr | 500 | 25 (7–10 yrs) | 25 | 1.5 | 3.3 | 10 |
| Males | 10–11.9 yr | 600 | 30 | 30 | 2 | 3 | 12 |
| | 12–14.9 yr | 700 | 30 | 40 | 2 | 3 | 12 |
| | 15–17.9 yr | 700 | 35 | 40 | 2 | 3 | 12 |
| | 18–70+ yr | 700 | 45 | 40 | 2 | 3 | 10 |
| Females | 10–14.9 yr | 600 | 30 | 30 | 2 | 3 | 15 |
| | 15–49.9 yr | 600 | 35 | 30 | 2 | 3 | 15 |
| | 50–70 yr | 600 | 35 | 30 | 2 | 3 | 10 |
| | 70+ yr | 600 | 35 | 30 | 2 | 3 | 10 |
| Pregnant | 0–2.9 mo | 0 | +10 | 0 | 0 | 500** | 15 + 30 add'l |
| | 3–5.9 mo | 0 | +10 | +5 | +0.5 | 500** | 15 + 30 add'l |
| | 6–9.0 mo | +200 | +10 | +10 | +0.5 | 500** | 15 + 30 add'l |
| Lactating | 0–6+ mo | +400 | +20 | +25 | +0.5 | adult dose +100 µg/d | 15 |
| | 6+ mo | +320 | +20 | +20 | +0.5 | adult dose +100 µg/d | 15 |

*Data from Olson, J.A.: Am. J. Clin. Nutr. 45:704–716, 1987. RE = retinol equivalents. One RE equals 1 µg retinol, 6 µg β-carotene, or 12 µg of other provitamin A carotenoids. Because IU are not employed in defining the RDI, the assumed distribution of carotenoids and vitamin A in the diet is no longer of key importance. Nonetheless, the present average intake, as REs, is approximately 25% provitamin A carotenoids and 75% preformed vitamin A. See Table A–1d-2 for calculation of vitamin A activity of diets as REs.

†Data from Olson, J.A.: Am. J. Clin. Nutr. 45:687–692, 1987. To convert µg of vitamin K (phylloquinone) to nmol, multiply by 2.219.

‡Data from Olson, J.A., Hodges, R.E.: Am. J. Clin. Nutr. 45:693–703, 1987. To convert mg of vitamin C to µmol, multiply by 5.679.

§Data from Herbert, V.: Am. J. Clin. Nutr. 45:671–678, 1987. To convert µg of vitamin B$_{12}$ to nmol, multiply by 1.4.

‖Data from Herbert, V.: Am. J. Clin. Nutr. 45:661–670, 1987. To convert µg of folate to nmol, multiply by 2.266.

#Data from Herbert, V.: Am. J. Clin. Nutr. 45:679–686, 1987. To convert mg of iron to nmol, multiply by 18.

¶Provided as a daily supplement or as an intramuscular injection (1 mg) at birth.

**Total per day.

φBecause of storage iron present at birth, the normal-term infant, for the first three months of life, does not require exogenous iron beyond that provided by breast milk or by formulas containing iron of bioavailability equivalent to that of breast milk.

# Table A–1d-2. Factors and Formulas Used in Interconverting Units of Vitamin A and Carotenoids*

*Factors*

1 retinol equivalent (RE)
- = 1 μg all-*trans* retinol
- = 6 μg all-*trans* β-carotene
- = 12 μg other provitamin A carotenoids
- = 3.33 $IU_a$ (i.e., the IU of vitamin A)
- = 10 $IU_c$ (i.e., the IU of provitamin A carotenoids)

1 international unit of preformed vitamin A (1 $IU_a$) = 0.3 μg of all-*trans* retinol, and

1 $IU_a$
- = 0.3 RE
- = 3 $IU_c$
- = 1.8 μg all-*trans* β-carotene
- = 3.6 μg other provitamin A carotenoids

1 IU of provitamin A carotenoids (1 $IU_c$) = 0.6 μg of all-*trans* β-carotene, and

1 $IU_c$
- = 0.1 RE
- = 0.33 $IU_a$
- = 0.1 μg all-*trans* retinol
- = 1.2 μg other provitamin A carotenoids

*Formulas*

*1)* When retinol and β-carotene are given in micrograms.

$$RE = μg \text{ retinol} + μg \text{ β-carotene}/6$$

If a diet contains 500 μg retinol and 1,800 μg β-carotene, then

$$RE = 500 + \frac{1,800}{6} = 800 \text{ RE}$$

*2)* When retinol and beta-carotene are given in IU,

$$RE = \frac{IU \text{ of retinol}}{3.33} + \frac{IU \text{ of β-carotene}}{10}$$

If a diet contains 1,667 IU retinol and 3,000 IU β-carotene, then

$$RE = \frac{1,667}{3.33} + \frac{3,000}{10} = 800 \text{ RE}$$

*Note:* The distinction between $IU_a$ and $IU_c$ is *not* made in food composition tables (see original text). In such tables, it is assumed that 1 $IU_a$ = 1 $IU_c$.

*3)* When β-carotene and other provitamin A carotenoids are given in micrograms,

$$RE = \frac{μg \text{ β-carotene}}{6} + \frac{μg \text{ other provitamin A carotenoids}}{12}$$

If a 100-g sample of sweet potato contains 2,400 μg of β-carotene and 480 μg of other provitamin A carotenoids, then

$$RE = \frac{2,400}{6} + \frac{480}{12} = 440 \text{ RE}$$

*4)* To determine the RE distribution in a food containing vitamin A derived from preformed vitamin A and from provitamin A carotenoids, but only total RE and total IU are given.

% RE as preformed vitamin A

$$= \left[ 1.5 - \frac{0.15 \text{ total IU}}{\text{total RE}} \right] \times 100$$

% RE as β-carotene $= \left[ \dfrac{0.15 \text{ total IU}}{\text{total RE}} = 0.5 \right] \times 100$

Thus, if a 100-g portion of cheese contains 300 total RE and 1,200 total IU, then

% RE as preformed vitamin A

$$= \left[ 1.5 - \frac{0.15 \times 1,200}{300} \right] \times 100 = 90\%$$

% RE as provitamin A carotenoids

$$= \left[ \frac{0.15 \times 1,200}{300} - 0.5 \right] \times 100 = 10\%$$

In the food sample, therefore, the preformed vitamin A content is 270 RE (270 μg of retinol), and the carotenoid content, expressed as β-carotene, is 30 RE (180 μg of β-carotene).

*Note:* Assumptions used from revised sections of *Handbook 8* (i.e., 8.1–8.10) are *a)* that 1 $IU_a$ = 1 $IU_c$ and *b)* that 1 RE = 1 μg retinol = 6 μg of β-carotene = 12 μg other provitamin A carotenoids.

*5)* To determine the IU distribution in a food containing vitamin A derived from preformed vitamin A and from provitamin A carotenoids, but only total RE and total IU are given,

$$IU_a = \frac{10 \text{ RE} - \text{total IU}}{2}$$

$$IU_c = \frac{(3 \times \text{total IU}) - 10 \text{ RE}}{2}$$

Thus, if a 100-g portion of cheese contains 300 total RE and 1,200 total IU, then

IU as preformed vitamin A

$$= \frac{(10 \times 300) - 1,200}{2} = 900 \text{ IU and}$$

IU as provitamin A carotenoids

$$= \frac{(3 \times 1,200) - (10 \times 300)}{2} = 300 \text{ IU}$$

*Note:* Assumptions used from revised sections of *Handbook 8* (i.e., 8.1–8.10) are *a)* that 1 $IU_a$ = 1 $IU_c$ and *b)* that 1 RE = 1 μg of retinol = 6 μg of β-carotene = 12 μg of other provitamin A carotenoids.

In some cases, small negative values for $IU_c$ are obtained when the values for total IU and total RE are given for foods containing only preformed vitamin A, particularly in fortified foods like margarine. This aberrant calculation results from the rounding of analytical values. Similarly, small negative values for $IU_a$ may result for foods containing only carotenoids. In both cases, the negative values should be taken as zero.

*From Appendix to: Olson, J.A.: Am. J. Clin. Nutr. 45:704–716, 1987 (see pp. 715–716).

**Table A–2a.   Average Energy Requirements for Various Ages, Canada, Revised 1983[a,h]**

| Age | Sex | Average Height (cm)[c] | Average Weight (kg)[c] | Requirements[b] | | | | | |
|-----|-----|------------------------|------------------------|-----------------|------|-----------|--------|----------|--------|
| | | | | kcal/kg[c,d] | MJ/kg[d] | kcal/day[e] | MJ/day[f] | kcal/cm[g] | MJ/cm[f] |
| **Months** | | | | | | | | | |
| 0–2 | Both | 55 | 4.5 | 120–100 | 0.50–0.42 | 500 | 2.0 | 9 | 0.04 |
| 3–5 | Both | 63 | 7.0 | 100–95 | 0.42–0.40 | 700 | 2.8 | 11 | 0.05 |
| 6–8 | Both | 69 | 8.5 | 95–97 | 0.40–0.41 | 800 | 3.4 | 11.5 | 0.05 |
| 9–11 | Both | 73 | 9.5 | 97–99 | 0.41 | 950 | 3.8 | 12.5 | 0.05 |
| **Years** | | | | | | | | | |
| 1 | Both | 82 | 11 | 101 | 0.42 | 1,100 | 4.8 | 13.5 | 0.06 |
| 2–3 | Both | 95 | 14 | 94 | 0.39 | 1,300 | 5.6 | 13.5 | 0.06 |
| 4–6 | Both | 107 | 18 | 100 | 0.42 | 1,800 | 7.6 | 17 | 0.07 |
| 7–9 | M | 126 | 25 | 88 | 0.37 | 2,200 | 9.2 | 17.5 | 0.07 |
| | F | 125 | 25 | 76 | 0.32 | 1,900 | 8.0 | 15 | 0.06 |
| 10–12 | M | 141 | 34 | 73 | 0.30 | 2,500 | 10.4 | 17.5 | 0.07 |
| | F | 143 | 36 | 61 | 0.25 | 2,200 | 9.2 | 15.5 | 0.06 |
| 13–15 | M | 159 | 50 | 57 | 0.24 | 2,800 | 12.0 | 17.5 | 0.07 |
| | F | 157 | 48 | 46 | 0.19 | 2,200 | 9.2 | 14 | 0.06 |
| 16–18 | M | 172 | 62 | 51 | 0.21 | 3,200 | 13.2 | 18.5 | 0.08 |
| | F | 160 | 53 | 40 | 0.17 | 2,100 | 8.8 | 13 | 0.05 |
| 19–24 | M | 175 | 71 | 42 | 0.18 | 3,000 | 12.4 | | |
| | F | 160 | 58 | 36 | 0.15 | 2,100 | 8.8 | | |
| 25–49 | M | 172 | 74 | 36 | 0.15 | 2,700 | 11.2 | | |
| | F | 160 | 59 | 32 | 0.13 | 1,900 | 8.0 | | |
| 50–74 | M | 170 | 73 | 31 | 0.13 | 2,300 | 9.6 | | |
| | F | 158 | 63 | 29 | 0.12 | 1,800 | 7.6 | | |
| 75 + | M | 168 | 69 | 29 | 0.12 | 2,000 | 8.4 | | |
| | F | 155 | 64 | 23 | 0.10 | 1,500 | 6.0 | | |

[a]See original source for references.

[b]Requirements can be expected to vary within a range of ± 30%.

[c]Figures rounded to the closest whole number when ≥10 and to the closest 0.5 when <10.

[d]First and last figures are averages at the beginning and at the end of the three-month period.

[e]Figures rounded to the nearest 50 when <1,000 and to the nearest 100 when ≥1,000.

[f]Figures included two decimals if value is <1 and 1 decimal if ≥1.

[g]Figures rounded to the nearest 0.5.

[h]Reprinted with permission from Bureau of Nutritional Sciences, Food Directorate, Health Protection Branch, Department of National Health and Welfare, Ottawa, Canada, 1983, pp. 22–23.

## Table A–2b. A Model of Energy Expenditure by a Young Adult Canadian[d]

| | *Rate of Expenditure* | | | | *Expenditure/Day* | | | | | |
| | *kcal/min* | | *KJ/min* | | *h/day* | | *kcal* | | *MJ* | |
| *Type of Activity* | *M[a]* | *F[a]* | *M* | *F* | *M* | *F* | *M* | *F* | *M* | *F* |
|---|---|---|---|---|---|---|---|---|---|---|
| Resting metabolism | 1.2 | 0.9 | 5.0 | 3.8 | 8 | 8 | 580 | 430 | 2.4 | 1.8 |
| Sitting or standing still | 1.6 | 1.2 | 6.7 | 5.0 | 10 | 11 | 960 | 792 | 4.0 | 3.3 |
| Light activity[b] | 3.2 | 2.5 | 13.4 | 10.5 | 4 | 4 | 770 | 600 | 3.2 | 2.6 |
| | (1.7–4.8) | (1.4–3.5) | (7.1–20.1) | (5.9–14.6) | | | | | | |
| Moderate activity[c] | 5.6 | 4.5 | 23.4 | 18.8 | 2 | 1 | 672 | 270 | 2.8 | 1.2 |
| | (4.9–7.4) | (3.6–5.5) | (20.5–31.0) | (15.1–23.0) | | | | | | |
| Totals | | | | | 24 | 24 | 2,982 | 2,092 | 12.4 | 8.8 |

[a]Male; female.

[b]Walking slowly; light domestic work (e.g., cooking, washing dishes, ironing, dusting, sweeping); light office or industrial work (e.g., typing, laboratory work, sewing, printing, working with light tools); sports involving light activity (e.g., golf, sailing, bowling).

[c]Walking at moderate speed; moderate domestic work (e.g., scrubbing floors, cleaning windows, polishing furniture); moderate industrial work (e.g., painting, plastering, modern farming); hobbies involving moderate activity (e.g., gardening, woodworking, dancing); sports such as tennis, cycling, skiing, swimming, skating, and jogging (the energy requirement for these activities is higher, but they represent a small fraction of the total activity).

[d]Reprinted with permission from Bureau of Nutritional Sciences, Food Directorate, Health Protection Branch, Department of National Health and Welfare, Ottawa, Canada, 1983, p. 24.

## Table A-2c. Summary Examples of Recommended Nutrient Intakes for Canadians,[a,b,l] 1983

| | | | | Fat-Soluble Vitamins | | | Water-Soluble Vitamins | | | Minerals | | | | |
|---|---|---|---|---|---|---|---|---|---|---|---|---|---|---|
| Age | Sex | Weight (kg) | Protein[c] (g/day) | Vitamin A (RE/day)[d] | Vitamin D (µg/day)[e] | Vitamin E (mg/day)[f] | Vitamin C (mg/day) | Folacin (µg/day)[g] | Vitamin $B_{12}$ (µg/day) | Calcium (mg/day) | Magnesium (mg/day) | Iron (mg/day) | Iodine (µg/day) | Zinc (mg/day) |
| **Months** | | | | | | | | | | | | | | |
| 0–2 | Both | 4.5 | 11[h] | 400 | 10 | 3 | 20 | 50 | 0.3 | 350 | 30 | 0.4[i] | 25 | 2[j] |
| 3–5 | Both | 7.0 | 14[h] | 400 | 10 | 3 | 20 | 50 | 0.3 | 350 | 40 | 5 | 35 | 3 |
| 6–8 | Both | 8.5 | 16[h] | 400 | 10 | 3 | 20 | 50 | 0.3 | 400 | 45 | 7 | 40 | 3 |
| 9–11 | Both | 9.5 | 18 | 400 | 10 | 3 | 20 | 55 | 0.3 | 400 | 50 | 7 | 45 | 3 |
| **Years** | | | | | | | | | | | | | | |
| 1 | Both | 11 | 18 | 400 | 10 | 3 | 20 | 65 | 0.3 | 500 | 55 | 6 | 55 | 4 |
| 2–3 | Both | 14 | 20 | 400 | 5 | 4 | 20 | 80 | 0.4 | 500 | 65 | 6 | 65 | 4 |
| 4–6 | Both | 18 | 25 | 500 | 5 | 5 | 25 | 90 | 0.5 | 600 | 90 | 6 | 85 | 5 |
| 7–9 | M | 25 | 31 | 700 | 2.5 | 7 | 35 | 125 | 0.8 | 700 | 110 | 7 | 110 | 6 |
| | F | 25 | 29 | 700 | 2.5 | 6 | 30 | 125 | 0.8 | 700 | 110 | 7 | 95 | 6 |
| 10–12 | M | 34 | 38 | 800 | 2.5 | 8 | 40 | 170 | 1.0 | 900 | 150 | 10 | 125 | 7 |
| | F | 36 | 39 | 800 | 2.5 | 7 | 40 | 170 | 1.0 | 1,000 | 160 | 10 | 110 | 7 |
| 13–15 | M | 50 | 49 | 900 | 2.5 | 9 | 50 | 160 | 1.5 | 1,100 | 220 | 12 | 160 | 9 |
| | F | 48 | 43 | 800 | 2.5 | 7 | 45 | 160 | 1.5 | 800 | 190 | 13 | 160 | 8 |
| 16–18 | M | 62 | 54 | 1,000 | 2.5 | 10 | 55 | 190 | 1.9 | 900 | 240 | 10 | 160 | 9 |
| | F | 53 | 47 | 800 | 2.5 | 7 | 45 | 160 | 1.9 | 700 | 220 | 14 | 160 | 8 |
| 19–24 | M | 71 | 57 | 1,000 | 2.5 | 10 | 60 | 210 | 2.0 | 800 | 240 | 8 | 160 | 9 |
| | F | 58 | 41 | 800 | 2.5 | 7 | 45 | 165 | 2.0 | 700 | 190 | 14 | 160 | 8 |
| 25–49 | M | 74 | 57 | 1,000 | 2.5 | 9 | 60 | 210 | 2.0 | 800 | 240 | 8 | 160 | 9 |
| | F | 59 | 41 | 800 | 2.5 | 6 | 45 | 165 | 2.0 | 700 | 190 | 14[k] | 160 | 8 |
| 50–74 | M | 73 | 57 | 1,000 | 2.5 | 7 | 60 | 210 | 2.0 | 800 | 240 | 8 | 160 | 9 |
| | F | 63 | 41 | 800 | 2.5 | 6 | 45 | 165 | 2.0 | 800 | 190 | 7 | 160 | 8 |
| 75+ | M | 69 | 57 | 1,000 | 2.5 | 6 | 60 | 210 | 2.0 | 800 | 240 | 8 | 160 | 9 |
| | F | 64 | 41 | 800 | 2.5 | 5 | 45 | 165 | 2.0 | 800 | 190 | 7 | 160 | 8 |

| | | | | | | | | | | | |
|---|---|---|---|---|---|---|---|---|---|---|---|
| Pregnancy (additional) | | | | | | | | | | | |
| 1st trimester | 15 | 100 | 2.5 | 2 | 0 | 305 | 1.0 | 500 | 15 | 6 | 25 | 0 |
| 2nd trimester | 20 | 100 | 2.5 | 2 | 20 | 305 | 1.0 | 500 | 20 | 6 | 25 | 1 |
| 3rd trimester | 25 | 100 | 2.5 | 2 | 20 | 305 | 1.0 | 500 | 25 | 6 | 25 | 2 |
| Lactation (additional) | 20 | 400 | 2.5 | 3 | 30 | 120 | 0.5 | 500 | 80 | 0 | 50 | 6 |

[a]Recommended intakes of energy and of certain nutrients are not listed in this table because of the nature of the variables upon which they are based. The figures for energy are estimates of average requirements for expected pattern of activity. (See Table II.1 in original.) For nutrients not shown, the following amounts are recommended: thiamin, 0.4 mg/1,000 kcal (0.48 mg/5,000 kJ); riboflavin. 0.5 mg/1,000 kcal (0.6 mg/5,000 kJ); niacin, 7.2 NE/1,000 kcal (8.6 NE/5,000 kJ); vitamin $B_6$, 15 μg, as pyridoxine, per gram of protein; phosphorus, same as calcium.

[b]Recommended intakes during periods of growth are taken as appropriate for individuals representative of the midpoint in each age group. All recommended intakes are designed to cover individual variations in essentially all of a healthy population subsisting upon a variety of common foods available in Canada.

[c]The primary units are grams per kilogram of body weight. The figures shown here are only examples; see Table V.2 in original.

[d]One retinol equivalent (RE) corresponds to the biological activity of 1 μg of retinol, 6 μg of β-carotene, or 12 μg of other carotenes.

[e]Expressed as cholecalciferol or ergocalciferol.

[f]Expressed as d-α-tocopherol equivalents, relative to which β- and γ-tocopherol and α-tocotrienol have activities of 0.5, 0.1, and 0.3 respectively.

[g]Expressed as total folate.

[h]Assumption that the protein is from breast milk or is of the same biological value as that of breast milk and that between 3 and 9 months adjustment for the quality of the protein is made.

[i]It is assumed that breast milk is the source of iron up to two months of age.

[j]Based on the assumption that breast milk is the source of zinc for the first two months.

[k]After the menopause, the recommended intake is 7 mg/day.

[l]Reprinted with permission from Bureau of Nutritional Sciences, Food Directorate, Health Protection Branch, Department of National Health and Welfare, Ottawa, Canada, 1983, pp 179–180.

## Table A–2d. Recommended Daily Amounts of Food Energy and Some Nutrients for Population Groups in the United Kingdom*

| Age Range^a (years) | Occupational Category | Energy^b MJ | Energy^b Kcal | Protein^d g | Thiamin mg | Riboflavin mg | Nicotinic Acid Equivalents mg^f | Ascorbic Acid mg | Vitamin A Retinol Equivalents μg^g | Vitamin D^h Cholecalciferol μg | Calcium mg | Iron mg |
|---|---|---|---|---|---|---|---|---|---|---|---|---|
| **Boys** | | | | | | | | | | | | |
| under 1 | | c | c | e | 0.3 | 0.4 | 5 | 20 | 450 | 7.5 | 600 | 6 |
| 1 | | 5.0 | 1,200 | 30 | 0.5 | 0.6 | 7 | 20 | 300 | 10 | 600 | 7 |
| 2 | | 5.75 | 1,400 | 35 | 0.6 | 0.7 | 8 | 20 | 300 | 10 | 600 | 7 |
| 3–4 | | 6.5 | 1,560 | 39 | 0.6 | 0.8 | 9 | 20 | 300 | 10 | 600 | 8 |
| 5–6 | | 7.25 | 1,740 | 43 | 0.7 | 0.9 | 10 | 20 | 300 | h | 600 | 10 |
| 7–8 | | 8.25 | 1,980 | 49 | 0.8 | 1.0 | 11 | 20 | 400 | h | 600 | 10 |
| 9–11 | | 9.5 | 2,280 | 57 | 0.9 | 1.2 | 14 | 25 | 575 | h | 700 | 12 |
| 12–14 | | 11.0 | 2,640 | 66 | 1.1 | 1.4 | 16 | 25 | 725 | h | 700 | 12 |
| 15–17 | | 12.0 | 2,880 | 72 | 1.2 | 1.7 | 19 | 30 | 750 | h | 600 | 12 |
| **Girls** | | | | | | | | | | | | |
| under 1 | | c | c | e | 0.3 | 0.4 | 5 | 20 | 450 | 7.5 | 600 | 6 |
| 1 | | 4.5 | 1,100 | 27 | 0.4 | 0.6 | 7 | 20 | 300 | 10 | 600 | 7 |
| 2 | | 5.5 | 1,300 | 32 | 0.5 | 0.7 | 8 | 20 | 300 | 10 | 600 | 7 |
| 3–4 | | 6.25 | 1,500 | 37 | 0.6 | 0.8 | 9 | 20 | 300 | 10 | 600 | 8 |
| 5–6 | | 7.0 | 1,680 | 42 | 0.7 | 0.9 | 10 | 20 | 300 | h | 600 | 10 |
| 7–8 | | 8.0 | 1,900 | 47 | 0.8 | 1.0 | 11 | 20 | 400 | h | 600 | 10 |
| 9–11 | | 8.5 | 2,050 | 51 | 0.8 | 1.2 | 14 | 25 | 575 | h | 700 | 12[j] |
| 12–14 | | 9.0 | 2,150 | 53 | 0.9 | 1.4 | 16 | 25 | 725 | h | 700 | 12[j] |
| 15–17 | | 9.0 | 2,150 | 53 | 0.9 | 1.7 | 19 | 30 | 750 | h | 600 | 12[j] |
| **Men** | | | | | | | | | | | | |
| 18–34 | Sedentary | 10.5 | 2,510 | 63 | 1.0 | 1.6 | 18 | 30 | 750 | h | 500 | 10 |
| | Moderately active | 12.0 | 2,900 | 72 | 1.2 | 1.6 | 18 | 30 | 750 | h | 500 | 10 |
| | Very active | 14.0 | 3,350 | 84 | 1.3 | 1.6 | 18 | 30 | 750 | h | 500 | 10 |

| | | MJ | kcal | | | | | | | | |
|---|---|---|---|---|---|---|---|---|---|---|---|
| 35–64 | Sedentary | 10.0 | 2,400 | 60 | 1.0 | 1.6 | 18 | 30 | h | 750 | 500 | 10 |
| | Moderately active | 11.5 | 2,750 | 69 | 1.1 | 1.6 | 18 | 30 | h | 750 | 500 | 10 |
| | Very active | 14.0 | 3,350 | 84 | 1.3 | 1.6 | 18 | 30 | h | 750 | 500 | 10 |
| 65–74 | Assuming a | 10.0 | 2,400 | 60 | 1.0 | 1.6 | 18 | 30 | h | 750 | 500 | 10 |
| 75+ | sedentary life | 9.0 | 2,150 | 54 | 0.9 | 1.6 | 18 | 30 | h | 750 | 500 | 10 |
| **Women** | | | | | | | | | | | | |
| 18–54 | Most occupations | 9.0 | 2,150 | 54 | 0.9 | 1.3 | 15 | 30 | h | 750 | 500 | 12[j] |
| | Very active | 10.5 | 2,500 | 62 | 1.0 | 1.3 | 15 | 30 | | 750 | 500 | 12[j] |
| 55–74 | Assuming a | 8.0 | 1,900 | 47 | 0.8 | 1.3 | 15 | 30 | h | 750 | 500 | 10 |
| 75+ | sedentary life | 7.0 | 1,680 | 42 | 0.7 | 1.3 | 15 | 30 | h | 750 | 500 | 10 |
| Pregnancy | | 10.0 | 2,400 | 60 | 1.0 | 1.6 | 18 | 60 | 10 | 750 | 1,200[i] | 13 |
| Lactation | | 11.5 | 2,750 | 69 | 1.1 | 1.8 | 21 | 60 | 10 | 1,200 | 1,200 | 15 |

[a] Since the recommendations are average amounts, the figures for each age range represent the amounts recommended at the middle of the range. Within each age range, younger children will need less, and older children more, than the amount recommended.

[b] Megajoules ($10^6$ joules). Calculated from the relation 1 kilocalorie = 4.184 kilojoules, i.e., 1 megajoule = 240 kilocalories.

[c] See Table 2 in original reference.

[d] Recommended amounts have been calculated as 10% of the recommendations for energy (paragraph 44 in original reference).

[e] See Table 2 in original reference.

[f] 1 nicotinic acid equivalent = 1 mg available nicotinic acid or 60 mg tryptophan.

[g] 1 retinol equivalent = 1 μg retinol, 6 μg β-carotene, or 12 μg other biologically active carotenoids.

[h] No dietary sources may be necessary for children and adults who are sufficiently exposed to sunlight, but during the winter children and adolescents should receive 10 μg (400 i.u.) daily by supplementation. Adults with inadequate exposure to sunlight, for example those who are housebound, may also need a supplement of 10 μg daily (paragraph 60 in original reference).

[i] For the third trimester only.

[j] This intake may not be sufficient for 10% of girls and women with large menstrual losses (paragraphs 63–70 in original reference).

Doubts have been expressed about the validity of the recommended daily amounts for folate and the figures have been withdrawn from this reprinted table. The Committee on Medical Aspects of Food Policy has decided that there is too little information at present upon which to base a practical recommendation for folate until further research has been done. A recommended daily amount for folate will be set as soon as sufficient information about folate requirements in the United Kingdom makes this possible (paragraphs 55–56 in original reference).

*Reprinted with permission from the Committee on Medical Aspects of Food Policy, Report on Health and Social Subjects—15. HMSO, for the Dept. of Health and Social Security, London, 1979 (as per Third Impression, 1985).

## Table A-2e. Japanese Recommended Dietary Allowances, Revised 1984:†
### -1. RDA for Persons with Low Activity

| Age | Energy (kcal) Men | Energy (kcal) Women | Protein (g) Men | Protein (g) Women | Energy Supplied From Fat (%) | Calcium (g) Men | Calcium (g) Women | Iron (mg) Men | Iron (mg) Women | Vitamin A (IU) Men | Vitamin A (IU) Women | Vitamin $B_1$ (mg) Men | Vitamin $B_1$ (mg) Women | Vitamin $B_2$ (mg) Men | Vitamin $B_2$ (mg) Women | Niacin (mg) Men | Niacin (mg) Women | Ascorbic Acid (mg) | Vitamin D (IU) |
|---|---|---|---|---|---|---|---|---|---|---|---|---|---|---|---|---|---|---|---|
| 0~month | 120/kg | 120/kg | 3.3 g/kg | 3.3 g/kg | 45 | 0.4 | 0.4 | 6 | 6 | 1,300 | 1,300 | 0.4 | 0.2 | 0.5 | 0.3 |  | 4 | 40 | 400 |
| 2~ | 110/kg | 110/kg | 2.5 g/kg | 2.5 g/kg | 45 | 0.4 | 0.4 | 6 | 6 | 1,300 | 1,300 | 0.5 | 0.3 | 0.7 | 0.4 |  | 6 | 40 | 400 |
| 6~ | 100/kg | 100/kg | 3.0 g/kg | 3.0 g/kg | 30~40 | 0.4 | 0.4 | 6 | 6 | 1,000 | 1,000 | 0.6 | 0.4 | 0.8 | 0.5 |  | 6 | 40 | 400 |
| 1~year | 970 | 920 | 30 | 30 | 25~30 | 0.4 | 0.4 | 7 | 7 | 1,000 | 1,000 | 0.5 | 0.4 | 0.8 | 0.5 | 6 | 6 | 40 | 400 |
| 2~ | 1,200 | 1,150 | 35 | 35 | 25~30 | 0.4 | 0.4 | 7 | 7 | 1,000 | 1,000 | 0.6 | 0.5 | 0.9 | 0.6 | 8 | 8 | 40 | 400 |
| 3~ | 1,400 | 1,350 | 40 | 40 | 25~30 | 0.4 | 0.4 | 8 | 8 | 1,000 | 1,000 | 0.6 | 0.6 | 0.9 | 0.7 | 9 | 9 | 40 | 400 |
| 4~ | 1,550 | 1,450 | 45 | 45 | 25~30 | 0.4 | 0.4 | 8 | 8 | 1,000 | 1,000 | 0.6 | 0.6 | 1.0 | 0.8 | 10 | 10 | 40 | 400 |
| 5~ | 1,600 | 1,500 | 50 | 50 | 25~30 | 0.4 | 0.4 | 8 | 8 | 1,000 | 1,000 | 0.6 | 0.6 | 1.1 | 0.8 | 11 | 10 | 40 | 400 |
| 6~ | 1,700 | 1,550 | 55 | 50 | 25~30 | 0.5 | 0.5 | 9 | 9 | 1,200 | 1,200 | 0.7 | 0.6 | 1.1 | 0.9 | 11 | 10 | 40 | 100 |
| 7~ | 1,800 | 1,650 | 60 | 55 | 25~30 | 0.5 | 0.5 | 9 | 9 | 1,200 | 1,200 | 0.7 | 0.7 | 1.2 | 0.9 | 12 | 11 | 40 | 100 |
| 8~ | 1,850 | 1,700 | 65 | 60 | 25~30 | 0.5 | 0.6 | 9 | 9 | 1,200 | 1,200 | 0.7 | 0.7 | 1.2 | 0.9 | 12 | 11 | 40 | 100 |
| 9~ | 1,950 | 1,800 | 65 | 65 | 25~30 | 0.6 | 0.7 | 10 | 10 | 1,500 | 1,500 | 0.8 | 0.7 | 1.3 | 1.0 | 13 | 12 | 40 | 100 |
| 10~ | 2,000 | 1,950 | 70 | 70 | 25~30 | 0.6 | 0.7 | 10 | 10 | 1,500 | 1,500 | 0.8 | 0.8 | 1.3 | 1.1 | 13 | 13 | 40 | 100 |
| 11~ | 2,150 | 2,100 | 75 | 75 | 25~30 | 0.7 | 0.7 | 10 | 10 | 1,500 | 1,500 | 0.9 | 0.8 | 1.4 | 1.2 | 14 | 14 | 40 | 100 |
| 12~ | 2,300 | 2,200 | 80 | 80 | 25~30 | 0.8 | 0.7 | 12 | 12 | 1,500 | 1,500 | 0.9 | 0.9 | 1.4 | 1.2 | 15 | 15 | 40 | 100 |
| 13~ | 2,450 | 2,250 | 85 | 80 | 25~30 | 0.9 | 0.7 | 12 | 12 | 1,500 | 1,500 | 1.0 | 0.9 | 1.5 | 1.2 | 16 | 15 | 40 | 100 |
| 14~ | 2,600 | 2,250 | 85 | 75 | 25~30 | 0.9 | 0.7 | 12 | 12 | 1,500 | 1,500 | 1.0 | 0.9 | 1.5 | 1.2 | 17 | 15 | 40 | 100 |
| 15~ | 2,650 | 2,200 | 85 | 70 | 25~30 | 0.8 | 0.7 | 12 | 12 | 1,500 | 1,500 | 1.1 | 0.9 | 1.5 | 1.2 | 17 | 15 | 40 | 100 |
| 16~ | 2,700 | 2,150 | 80 | 70 | 25~30 | 0.8 | 0.6 | 10 | 12 | 1,500 | 1,500 | 1.1 | 0.9 | 1.5 | 1.2 | 18 | 14 | 50 | 100 |
| 17~ | 2,700 | 2,100 | 80 | 70 | 25~30 | 0.7 | 0.6 | 10 | 12 | 1,500 | 1,500 | 1.1 | 0.8 | 1.5 | 1.2 | 18 | 14 | 50 | 100 |
| 18~ | 2,650 | 2,100 | 75 | 65 | 25~30 | 0.7 | 0.6 | 10 | 12 | 1,500 | 1,500 | 1.1 | 0.8 | 1.4 | 1.1 | 17 | 14 | 50 | 100 |
| 19~ | 2,600 | 2,050 | 75 | 60 | 25~30 | 0.7 | 0.6 | 10 | 12 | 1,500 | 1,500 | 1.0 | 0.8 | 1.4 | 1.1 | 17 | 14 | 50 | 100 |
| 20~ | 2,500 | 2,000 | 70 | 60 | 20~25 | 0.6 | 0.6 | 10 | 12* | 2,000 | 1,800 | 1.0 | 0.8 | 1.4 | 1.1 | 17 | 13 | 50 | 100 |
| 30~ | 2,450 | 1,950 | 70 | 60 | 20~25 | 0.6 | 0.6 | 10 | 12* | 2,000 | 1,800 | 1.0 | 0.8 | 1.3 | 1.1 | 16 | 13 | 50 | 100 |
| 40~ | 2,350 | 1,900 | 70 | 60 | 20~25 | 0.6 | 0.6 | 10 | 12* | 2,000 | 1,800 | 0.9 | 0.8 | 1.3 | 1.0 | 16 | 13 | 50 | 100 |
| 50~ | 2,200 | 1,850 | 70 | 60 | 20~25 | 0.6 | 0.6 | 10 | 12* | 2,000 | 1,800 | 0.9 | 0.7 | 1.2 | 1.0 | 15 | 12 | 50 | 100 |
| 60~ | 2,000 | 1,700 | 70 | 60 | 20~25 | 0.6 | 0.6 | 10 | 12* | 2,000 | 1,800 | 0.8 | 0.7 | 1.1 | 0.9 | 13 | 11 | 50 | 100 |
| 70~ | 1,800 | 1,550 | 65 | 55 | 20~25 | 0.6 | 0.6 | 10 | 10 | 2,000 | 1,800 | 0.8 | 0.7 | 1.1 | 0.9 | 13 | 11 | 50 | 100 |
| 80~ | 1,600 | 1,350 | 65 | 55 | 20~25 | 0.6 | 0.6 | 10 | 10 | 2,000 | 1,800 | 0.8 | 0.7 | 1.1 | 0.9 | 13 | 11 | 50 | 100 |

*Decrease to 10 mg after menopause.

†From Ministry of Health and Welfare, Tokyo, Japan.

## -2. RDA for Persons with Medium Activity†

| Age (year) | Energy (kcal) Men | Energy (kcal) Women | Protein (g) Men | Protein (g) Women | Energy Supplied From Fat (%) | Calcium (g) Men | Calcium (g) Women | Iron (mg) Men | Iron (mg) Women | Vitamin A (IU) Men | Vitamin A (IU) Women | Vitamin B₁ (mg) Men | Vitamin B₁ (mg) Women | Vitamin B₂ (mg) Men | Vitamin B₂ (mg) Women | Niacin (mg) Men | Niacin (mg) Women | Ascorbic Acid (mg) | Vitamin D (IU) |
|---|---|---|---|---|---|---|---|---|---|---|---|---|---|---|---|---|---|---|---|
| 15~ | 3,150 | 2,650 | 100 | 85 | | 0.8 | 0.7 | | | | | 1.3 | 1.1 | 1.7 | 1.4 | 21 | 17 | | |
| 16~ | 3,200 | 2,550 | 95 | 80 | | 0.8 | | 12 | 12 | | | 1.3 | 1.0 | 1.8 | 1.4 | 21 | 17 | | |
| 17~ | 3,200 | 2,500 | 95 | 80 | | 0.7 | | | | | | 1.3 | 1.0 | 1.8 | 1.4 | 21 | 17 | | |
| 18~ | 3,150 | 2,500 | 90 | 75 | 25~30 | 0.7 | 0.6 | | | 2,000 | 1,800 | 1.3 | 1.0 | 1.7 | 1.4 | 21 | 16 | 50 | 100 |
| 19~ | 3,100 | 2,450 | 90 | 70 | | 0.7 | | | | | | 1.2 | 1.0 | 1.7 | 1.3 | 21 | 16 | | |
| 20~ | 3,000 | 2,400 | 85 | 70 | | | | | 12* | | | 1.2 | 1.0 | 1.7 | 1.3 | 20 | 16 | | |
| 30~ | 2,900 | 2,300 | 85 | 70 | | 0.6 | | 10 | | | | 1.2 | 0.9 | 1.6 | 1.3 | 19 | 15 | | |
| 40~ | 2,800 | 2,300 | 85 | 70 | | | | | | | | 1.1 | 0.9 | 1.5 | 1.3 | 19 | 15 | | |
| 50~ | 2,650 | 2,200 | 85 | 70 | | | | | | | | 1.1 | 0.9 | 1.5 | 1.2 | 17 | 14 | | |
| 60~70 | 2,350 | 2,000 | 80 | 70 | | | | | 10 | | | 0.9 | 0.8 | 1.3 | 1.1 | 16 | 13 | | |

*Decrease to 10 mg after menopause.
†From Ministry of Health and Welfare, Tokyo, Japan.

## -3. RDA for Persons with High Activity†

| Age (year) | Energy (kcal) Men | Energy (kcal) Women | Protein (g) Men | Protein (g) Women | Energy Supplied From Fat (%) | Calcium (g) Men | Calcium (g) Women | Iron (mg) Men | Iron (mg) Women | Vitamin A (IU) Men | Vitamin A (IU) Women | Vitamin B₁ (mg) Men | Vitamin B₁ (mg) Women | Vitamin B₂ (mg) Men | Vitamin B₂ (mg) Women | Niacin (mg) Men | Niacin (mg) Women | Ascorbic Acid (mg) | Vitamin D (IU) |
|---|---|---|---|---|---|---|---|---|---|---|---|---|---|---|---|---|---|---|---|
| 15~ | 3,700 | 3,050 | 115 | 95 | | 0.8 | 0.7 | | | | | 1.5 | 1.2 | 2.0 | 1.7 | 24 | 20 | | |
| 16~ | 3,700 | 3,000 | 110 | 95 | | 0.8 | | 12 | 12 | | | 1.5 | 1.2 | 2.0 | 1.6 | 25 | 20 | | |
| 17~ | 3,700 | 2,950 | 110 | 95 | | 0.7 | | | | | | 1.5 | 1.2 | 2.0 | 1.6 | 25 | 19 | | |
| 18~ | 3,700 | 2,900 | 105 | 90 | 25~30 | 0.7 | 0.6 | | | 2,000 | 1,800 | 1.5 | 1.2 | 2.0 | 1.6 | 24 | 19 | 50 | 100 |
| 19~ | 3,600 | 2,850 | 105 | 85 | | 0.7 | | | | | | 1.5 | 1.1 | 2.0 | 1.6 | 24 | 19 | | |
| 20~ | 3,500 | 2,800 | 100 | 85 | | | | | 12* | | | 1.4 | 1.1 | 1.9 | 1.5 | 23 | 18 | | |
| 30~ | 3,400 | 2,700 | 100 | 85 | | 0.6 | | 10 | | | | 1.4 | 1.1 | 1.9 | 1.5 | 22 | 18 | | |
| 40~ | 3,250 | 2,650 | 100 | 85 | | | | | | | | 1.3 | 1.1 | 1.8 | 1.5 | 22 | 18 | | |
| 50~ | 3,100 | 2,550 | 100 | 80 | | | | | | | | 1.2 | 1.0 | 1.7 | 1.4 | 20 | 17 | | |
| 60~70 | 2,750 | 2,300 | 95 | 80 | | | | | 10 | | | 1.1 | 0.9 | 1.5 | 1.3 | 18 | 15 | | |

*Decrease to 10 mg after menopause.
†From Ministry of Health and Welfare, Tokyo, Japan.

## Table A–3a-1.  Basal Metabolic Rates of Adolescent Boys and Girls[d]

| Age (years) | Height[a] (cm) | Weight[b] (kg) | BMR[c] Total (kcal$_{th}$/day) | Total (MJ/day) | per kg (kcal$_{th}$/day) | per kg (MJ/day) |
|---|---|---|---|---|---|---|
| **Boys** | | | | | | |
| 10–11 | 140 | 32.2 | 1215 | 5.08 | 37.7 | 0.16 |
| 11–12 | 147 | 37.0 | 1300 | 5.43 | 35.1 | 0.15 |
| 12–13 | 153 | 40.9 | 1370 | 5.73 | 33.4 | 0.14 |
| 13–14 | 160 | 47.0 | 1465 | 6.12 | 31.4 | 0.13 |
| 14–15 | 166 | 52.6 | 1570 | 6.57 | 29.9 | 0.12 |
| 15–16 | 171 | 58.0 | 1665 | 6.96 | 28.7 | 0.12 |
| 16–17 | 175 | 62.7 | 1750 | 7.32 | 27.9 | 0.12 |
| 17–18 | 177 | 65.0 | 1790 | 7.48 | 27.5 | 0.12 |
| **Girls** | | | | | | |
| 10–11 | 142 | 33.7 | 1160 | 4.85 | 34.3 | 0.14 |
| 11–12 | 148 | 38.7 | 1220 | 5.10 | 31.5 | 0.13 |
| 12–13 | 155 | 44.0 | 1280 | 5.38 | 29.1 | 0.12 |
| 13–14 | 159 | 48.8 | 1340 | 5.60 | 27.5 | 0.12 |
| 14–15 | 161 | 51.4 | 1375 | 5.75 | 26.7 | 0.11 |
| 15–16 | 162 | 53.0 | 1395 | 5.83 | 26.3 | 0.11 |
| 16–17 | 163 | 54.0 | 1405 | 5.87 | 26.0 | 0.11 |
| 17–18 | 164 | 54.4 | 1410 | 5.89 | 25.9 | 0.11 |

[a]Median height for age from NCHS standards.
[b]Median weight for height and age from Baldwin's standards (Annex 2(B)).
[c]Boys: BMR = 17.5 W + 651 kcal$_{th}$/day (2.72 MJ/day). Girls: 12.2 W + 746 kcal$_{th}$/day (3.12 MJ/day).
[d]Reprinted with permission from WHO Energy and Protein Requirements, TRS No. 724, 1985, p. 94.

## Table A–3a-2.  Basal Metabolic Rate in Adult Men and Women in Relation to Height and Median Acceptable Weight for Height[a] (values given in kcal$_{th}$ with MJ in parentheses)[c]

| Height (m) | Weight[b] (kg) | 18–30 years Per kg per day | 18–30 years Per day | 30–60 years Per kg per day | 30–60 years Per day | >60 years Per kg per day | >60 years Per day |
|---|---|---|---|---|---|---|---|
| **Men** | | | | | | | |
| 1.5 | 49.5 | 29.0 (121) | 1440 (6.03) | 29.4 (123) | 1450 (6.07) | 23.3 (98) | 1150 (4.81) |
| 1.6 | 56.5 | 27.4 (115) | 1540 (6.44) | 27.2 (114) | 1530 (6.40) | 22.2 (93) | 1250 (5.23) |
| 1.7 | 63.5 | 26.0 (109) | 1650 (6.90) | 25.4 (106) | 1620 (6.78) | 21.2 (89) | 1350 (5.65) |
| 1.8 | 71.5 | 24.8 (104) | 1770 (7.41) | 23.9 (99) | 1710 (7.15) | 20.3 (85) | 1450 (6.07) |
| 1.9 | 79.5 | 23.9 (100) | 1890 (7.91) | 22.7 (95) | 1800 (7.53) | 19.6 (82) | 1560 (6.53) |
| 2.0 | 88 | 23.0 (96) | 2030 (8.49) | 21.6 (90) | 1900 (7.95) | 19.0 (80) | 1670 (6.99) |
| **Women** | | | | | | | |
| 1.4 | 41 | 26.7 (112) | 1100 (4.60) | 28.8 (120) | 1190 (4.98) | 25.0 (105) | 1030 (4.31) |
| 1.5 | 47 | 25.2 (105) | 1190 (4.98) | 26.3 (110) | 1240 (5.19) | 23.1 (97) | 1090 (4.56) |
| 1.6 | 54 | 23.9 (100) | 1290 (5.40) | 24.1 (101) | 1300 (5.44) | 21.6 (90) | 1160 (4.85) |
| 1.7 | 61 | 22.9 (96) | 1390 (5.82) | 22.4 (94) | 1360 (5.69) | 20.3 (85) | 1230 (5.15) |
| 1.8 | 68 | 22.0 (92) | 1500 (6.28) | 20.9 (87) | 1420 (5.94) | 19.3 (81) | 1310 (5.48) |

[a]BMR from equations in Table 5 of original reference rounded to 10 kcal$_{th}$.
[b]Weight taken as median acceptable weight for height; body mass index (Wt/Ht$^2$) = 22 in men, 21 in women.
[c]Reprinted with permission from WHO Energy and Protein Requirements, TRS No. 724, 1985, p. 72.

## Table A–3b. Calculated Energy Requirements of Infants from Birth to One Year[d]

| Age (months) | Intake[a] (kcal_th/kg per day) | Intake[a] (kJ/kg per day) | Calculated Energy Requirement[b] (kcal_th/kg per day) | Calculated Energy Requirement[b] (kJ/kg per day) | Median Body Weight[c] Boys (kg) | Median Body Weight[c] Girls (kg) | Total Requirement Boys (kcal_th/day) | Total Requirement Boys (kJ/day) | Total Requirement Girls (kcal_th/day) | Total Requirement Girls (kJ/day) |
|---|---|---|---|---|---|---|---|---|---|---|
| 0.5 | 118 | 494 | 124 | 519 | 3.8 | 3.6 | 470 | 1,965 | 445 | 1,860 |
| 1–2 | 114 | 477 | 116 | 485 | 4.75 | 4.35 | 550 | 2,300 | 505 | 2,115 |
| 2–3 | 107 | 448 | 109 | 456 | 5.6 | 5.05 | 610 | 2,550 | 545 | 2,280 |
| 3–4 | 101 | 423 | 103 | 431 | 6.35 | 5.7 | 655 | 2,740 | 590 | 2,470 |
| 4–5 | 96 | 402 | 99 | 414 | 7.0 | 6.35 | 695 | 2,910 | 630 | 2,635 |
| 5–6 | 93 | 389 | 96.5 | 404 | 7.55 | 6.95 | 730 | 3,055 | 670 | 2,800 |
| 6–7 | 91 | 381 | 95 | 397 | 8.05 | 7.55 | 765 | 3,220 | 720 | 3,010 |
| 7–8 | 90 | 377 | 94.5 | 395 | 8.55 | 7.95 | 810 | 3,390 | 750 | 3,140 |
| 8–9 | 90 | 377 | 95 | 397 | 9.0 | 8.4 | 855 | 3,580 | 800 | 3,350 |
| 9–10 | 91 | 381 | 99 | 414 | 9.35 | 8.75 | 925 | 3,870 | 865 | 3,620 |
| 10–11 | 93 | 389 | 100 | 418 | 9.7 | 9.05 | 970 | 4,060 | 905 | 3,790 |
| 11–12 | 97 | 406 | 104.5 | 437 | 10.05 | 9.35 | 1,050 | 4,395 | 975 | 4,080 |
| 12 | 102 | 427 | | | | | | | | |

[a]Observed intakes at ages indicated, from data of sources given in original publication. Average intake predicted from equation (age in months): 1 (kcal_th/kg) = 123 − 8.9 age + 0.59 age. See original reference.
[b]Requirement over interval indicated, calculated as predicted intake + 5%. See original reference.
[c]NCHS median weights at midpoint of month.
[d]Reprinted with permission from WHO Energy and Protein Requirements, TRS No. 724, 1985, p. 91.

## Table A–3c. Estimated Average Daily Energy Intakes and Requirements, Ages 1–10 Years[d]

| Age (years) | Boys Intake[a] (kcal_th/day) | Boys Intake[a] (MJ/day) | Boys Requirement[b] (kcal_th/day) | Boys Requirement[b] (MJ/day) |
|---|---|---|---|---|
| 1–2 | 1,140 | 4.76 | 1,200 | 5.02 |
| 2–3 | 1,340 | 5.60 | 1,410 | 5.89 |
| 3–4 | 1,490 | 6.23 | 1,560 | 6.52 |
| 4–5 | 1,610 | 6.73 | 1,690 | 7.07 |
| 5–6 | 1,720 | 7.19 | 1,810 | 7.57 |
| 6–7 | 1,810 | 7.57 | 1,900 | 7.94 |
| 7–8 | 1,895 | 7.92 | 1,990 | 8.32 |
| 8–9 | 1,970 | 8.24 | 2,070 | 8.66 |
| 9–10 | 2,045 | 8.55 | 2,150 | 8.99 |

| Age (years) | Girls Intake[a] (kcal_th/day) | Girls Intake[a] (MJ/day) | Girls Requirement[b] (kcal_th/day) | Girls Requirement[b] (MJ/day) | Requirement by Weight[c] Boys (kcal_th/kg per day) | Requirement by Weight[c] Boys (kJ/kg per day) | Requirement by Weight[c] Girls (kcal_th/kg per day) | Requirement by Weight[c] Girls (kJ/kg per day) |
|---|---|---|---|---|---|---|---|---|
| 1–2 | 1,090 | 4.56 | 1,140 | 4.76 | 104 | 435 | 108 | 452 |
| 2–3 | 1,250 | 5.23 | 1,310 | 5.48 | 104 | 410 | 102 | 427 |
| 3–4 | 1,370 | 5.73 | 1,440 | 6.02 | 99 | 414 | 95 | 397 |
| 4–5 | 1,465 | 6.12 | 1,540 | 6.44 | 95 | 397 | 92 | 385 |
| 5–6 | 1,550 | 6.48 | 1,630 | 6.81 | 92 | 385 | 88 | 368 |
| 6–7 | 1,620 | 6.77 | 1,700 | 7.11 | 88 | 368 | 83 | 347 |
| 7–8 | 1,685 | 7.05 | 1,770 | 7.40 | 83 | 347 | 76 | 318 |
| 8–9 | 1,740 | 7.28 | 1,830 | 7.65 | 77 | 322 | 69 | 268 |
| 9–10 | 1,795 | 7.51 | 1,880 | 7.86 | 72 | 301 | 62 | 259 |

[a]From data of Ferro-Luzzi and Durnin, Rome, FAO, 1981 (Document ESN: FAO/WHO/UNU/EPR/81/9).
[b]Intakes + 5%. See original reference.
[c]From NCHS median weights at midyear.
[d]Reprinted with permission from WHO Energy and Protein Requirements, TRS No. 724, 1985, pp. 94–95.

**Table A–3d.** **Calculated Average Energy Expenditure and Observed Intakes and Comparison with Recommendations of 1971 Committee for Adolescents Aged 10–18 Years**[d]

| Age (years) | Expenditure (× BMR)[a] | Expenditure (kcal_{th}/day) | (MJ/day) | Intake[b] (kcal_{th}/day) | (MJ/day) | 1971 Committee[c] Recommended Requirement (kcal_{th}/day) | (MJ/day) |
|---|---|---|---|---|---|---|---|
| Boys | | | | | | | |
| 10–11 | 1.76 | 2,140 | 8.95 | 2,110 | 8.82 | 2,500 | 10.46 |
| 11–12 | 1.73 | 2,240 | 9.37 | 2,170 | 9.07 | 2,600 | 10.87 |
| 12–13 | 1.69 | 2,310 | 9.66 | 2,200 | 9.20 | 2,700 | 11.29 |
| 13–14 | 1.67 | 2,440 | 10.20 | 2,280 | 9.53 | 2,800 | 11.71 |
| 14–15 | 1.65 | 2,590 | 10.83 | 2,340 | 9.79 | 2,900 | 12.13 |
| 15–16 | 1.62 | 2,700 | 11.29 | 2,390 | 9.99 | 3,000 | 12.55 |
| 16–17 | 1.60 | 2,800 | 11.71 | 2,440 | 10.20 | 3,050 | 12.76 |
| 17–18 | 1.60 | 2,870 | 12.0 | 2,490 | 10.41 | 3,100 | 12.97 |
| Girls | | | | | | | |
| 10–11 | 1.65 | 1,910 | 7.99 | 1,850 | 7.74 | 2,300 | 9.62 |
| 11–12 | 1.63 | 1,980 | 8.28 | 1,890 | 7.90 | 2,350 | 9.83 |
| 12–13 | 1.60 | 2,050 | 8.57 | 1,930 | 8.07 | 2,400 | 10.04 |
| 13–14 | 1.58 | 2,120 | 8.87 | 1,970 | 8.24 | 2,450 | 10.25 |
| 14–15 | 1.57 | 2,160 | 9.03 | 2,010 | 8.40 | 2,500 | 10.46 |
| 15–16 | 1.54 | 2,140 | 8.95 | 2,050 | 8.57 | 2,500 | 10.46 |
| 16–17 | 1.53 | 2,130 | 8.91 | 2,080 | 8.70 | 2,420 | 10.12 |
| 17–18 | 1.52 | 2,140 | 8.95 | 2,120 | 8.87 | 2,340 | 9.79 |

[a]Expenditure calculated as in original publication.
[b]Intakes from reference in original publication.
[c]Reference in original 1971 publication. (cf ref. d)
[d]Reprinted with permission from WHO Energy and Protein Requirements, TRS No. 724, 1985, p. 98.

**Table A–3e. Energy Expenditure Distributed Over 24 Hours and Effect of Occupation***

**65-kg Reference Man**

| Distribution of Activity | Light Activity | | Moderately Active | | Very Active | | Exceptionally Active | |
|---|---|---|---|---|---|---|---|---|
| | (kcal) | (MJ) | (kcal) | (MJ) | (kcal) | (MJ) | (kcal) | (MJ) |
| In bed (8 hours) | 500 | 2.1 | 500 | 2.1 | 500 | 2.1 | 500 | 2.1 |
| At work (8 hours) | 1,100 | 4.6 | 1,400 | 5.8 | 1,900 | 8.0 | 2,400 | 10.0 |
| Nonoccupational activities (8 hours) | 700–1,500 | 3.0–6.3 | 700–1,500 | 3.0–6.3 | 700–1,500 | 3.0–6.3 | 700–1,500 | 3.0–6.3 |
| Range of energy expenditure (24 hours) | 2,300–3,100 | 9.7–13.0 | 2,600–3,400 | 10.9–14.2 | 3,100–3,900 | 13.0–16.3 | 3,600–4,400 | 15.1–18.4 |
| Mean (24 hours) | 2,700 | 11.3 | 3,000 | 12.5 | 3,500 | 14.6 | 4,000 | 16.7 |
| Mean (per kg of body weight) | 42 | 0.17 | 46 | 0.19 | 54 | 0.23 | 62 | 0.26 |

**55-kg Reference Woman**

| Distribution of Activity | Light Activity | | Moderately Active | | Very Active | | Exceptionally Active | |
|---|---|---|---|---|---|---|---|---|
| | (kcal) | (MJ) | (kcal) | (MJ) | (kcal) | (MJ) | (kcal) | (MJ) |
| In bed (8 hours) | 420 | 1.8 | 420 | 1.8 | 420 | 1.8 | 420 | 1.8 |
| At work (8 hours) | 800 | 3.3 | 1,000 | 4.2 | 1,400 | 5.9 | 1,800 | 7.5 |
| Nonoccupational activities (8 hours) | 580–980 | 2.4–4.1 | 580–980 | 2.4–4.1 | 580–980 | 2.4–4.1 | 580–980 | 2.4–4.1 |
| Range of energy expenditure (24 hours) | 1,800–2,200 | 7.5–9.2 | 2,000–2,400 | 8.4–10.1 | 2,400–2,700 | 10.1–11.8 | 2,800–3,200 | 11.7–13.4 |
| Mean (24 hours) | 2,000 | 8.4 | 2,200 | 9.2 | 2,600 | 10.9 | 3,000 | 12.5 |
| Mean (per kg of body weight) | 36 | 0.15 | 40 | 0.17 | 47 | 0.20 | 55 | 0.23 |

*From Passmore, Nicol, and Rao: Handbook on Human Nutritional Requirements. Geneva, WHO Monogr. Ser. No. 61, 1974.

## Table A–3f. Estimates of Energy Cost of Weight Gain[b,c]

| Subjects | | Energy Cost | |
| --- | --- | --- | --- |
| | | $(kcal_{th}/g)$ | $(kJ/g)$ |
| Premature infants | | 4.9 | 20.5 |
| Premature infants | | 5.7 | 23.8 |
| Normal infants | | 5.6 | 23.4 |
| Infants recovering from malnutrition | | 5.55 | 23.2 |
| | | 4.6 | 19.2 |
| | | 3.5 | 14.6 |
| | | 4.4 | 18.4 |
| | | 7.1 | 29.7 |
| Adults, recovering from anorexia nervosa | | 6.4 | 26.7 |
| Adults, intentional overfeeding | | 8.2 | 34.3 |
| Pregnancy | Theoretical estimate[a] | 6.4 | 26.7 |

[a]Calculated as 80,000 kcal$_{th}$ (335 MJ) stored for 12.5 kg of weight gain.
[b]See original references for data sources.
[c]Reprinted with permission from WHO Energy and Protein Requirements, TRS No. 724, 1985, p. 185.

## Table A–3g.    Recommended Intakes of Nutrients—WHO, 1974*

| Age | Body Weight (kg) | Energy[1] (kcal) | Energy[1] (MJ) | Protein[1,2] (g) | Vitamin A[3,4] (µg) | Vitamin D[5,6] (µg) | Thiamin[3] (mg) | Riboflavin[3] (mg) | Niacin[3] (mg) | Folic Acid[5] (µg) | Vitamin $B_{12}$[5] (µg) | Ascorbic Acid[5] (mg) | Calcium[7] (g) | Iron[5,8] (mg) |
|---|---|---|---|---|---|---|---|---|---|---|---|---|---|---|
| Children | | | | | | | | | | | | | | |
| <1 | 7.3 | 820 | 3.4 | 14 | 300 | 10.0 | 0.3 | 0.5 | 5.4 | 60 | 0.3 | 20 | 0.5–0.6 | 5–10 |
| 1–3 | 13.4 | 1,360 | 5.7 | 16 | 250 | 10.0 | 0.5 | 0.8 | 9.0 | 100 | 0.9 | 20 | 0.4–0.5 | 5–10 |
| 4–6 | 20.2 | 1,830 | 7.6 | 20 | 300 | 10.0 | 0.7 | 1.1 | 12.1 | 100 | 1.5 | 20 | 0.4–0.5 | 5–10 |
| 7–9 | 28.1 | 2,190 | 9.2 | 25 | 400 | 2.5 | 0.9 | 1.3 | 14.5 | 100 | 1.5 | 20 | 0.4–0.5 | 5–10 |
| Male adolescents | | | | | | | | | | | | | | |
| 10–12 | 36.9 | 2,600 | 10.9 | 30 | 575 | 2.5 | 1.0 | 1.6 | 17.2 | 100 | 2.0 | 20 | 0.6–0.7 | 5–10 |
| 13–15 | 51.3 | 2,900 | 12.1 | 37 | 725 | 2.5 | 1.2 | 1.7 | 19.1 | 200 | 2.0 | 30 | 0.6–0.7 | 9–18 |
| 16–19 | 62.9 | 3,070 | 12.8 | 38 | 750 | 2.5 | 1.2 | 1.8 | 20.3 | 200 | 2.0 | 30 | 0.5–0.6 | 5–9 |
| Female adolescents | | | | | | | | | | | | | | |
| 10–12 | 38.0 | 2,350 | 9.8 | 29 | 575 | 2.5 | 0.9 | 1.4 | 15.5 | 100 | 2.0 | 20 | 0.6–0.7 | 5–10 |
| 13–15 | 49.9 | 2,490 | 10.4 | 31 | 725 | 2.5 | 1.0 | 1.5 | 16.4 | 200 | 2.0 | 30 | 0.6–0.7 | 12–24 |
| 16–19 | 54.4 | 2,310 | 9.7 | 30 | 750 | 2.5 | 0.9 | 1.4 | 15.2 | 200 | 2.0 | 30 | 0.5–0.6 | 14–28 |
| Adult man (moderately active) | 65.0 | 3,000 | 12.6 | 37 | 750 | 2.5 | 1.2 | 1.8 | 19.8 | 200 | 2.0 | 30 | 0.4–0.5 | 5–9 |
| Adult woman (moderately active) | 55.0 | 2,200 | 9.2 | 29 | 750 | 2.5 | 0.9 | 1.3 | 14.5 | 200 | 2.0 | 30 | 0.4–0.5 | 14–28 |
| Pregnancy (later half) | | +350 | +1.5 | 38 | 1,200 | 10.0 | +0.1 | +0.2 | +2.3 | 400 | 3.0 | 50 | 1.0–1.2 | (9) |
| Lactation (first 6 months) | | +550 | +2.3 | 46 | 1,200 | 10.0 | +0.2 | +0.4 | +3.7 | 300 | 2.5 | 50 | 1.0–1.2 | (9) |

[1] Energy and Protein Requirements. Report of a Joint FAO/WHO Expert Group, FAO, Rome, 1972. [2] As egg or milk protein. [3] Requirements of vitamin A, thiamin, riboflavin and niacin. Report of a Joint FAO/WHO Expert Group, FAO, Rome, 1965. [4] As retinol. [5] Requirements of ascorbic acid, vitamin D, vitamin $B_{12}$, folate and iron. Report of a Joint FAO/WHO Expert Group, FAO, Rome, 1970. [6] As cholecalciferol. [7] Calcium requirements. Report of a FAO/WHO Expert Group, FAO, Rome, 1961. [8] On each line the lower value applies when over 25% of calories in the diet come from animal foods, and the higher value when animal foods represent less than 10% of calories. [9] For women whose iron intake throughout life has been at the level recommended in this table, the daily intake of iron during pregnancy and lactation should be the same as that recommended for nonpregnant, nonlactating women of childbearing age. For women whose iron status is not satisfactory at the beginning of pregnancy, the requirement is increased, and in the extreme situation of women with no iron stores, the requirement can probably not be met without supplementation.

*From Passmore, Nicol, and Rao: Handbook on Human Nutritional Requirements. Geneva, WHO Monogr. Ser. No. 61, 1974, Table 1.

ADDENDUM: Dietary allowances, official or unofficial for many European countries, as of 1976 or earlier, appear in the Proceedings of the Second European Nutrition Conference, Munich, 1976. (Nutr. Metab., 21:210, 1977.) See also International Daily Adult Dietary Allowances (Nutr. Abst. Rev. 45:89, 1975.)

## Table A–4a.  Values for the Digestibility of Protein in Man[c,d]

| Protein Source | True Digestibility (mean ±SD) | | Digestibility Relative to Reference Proteins |
|---|---|---|---|
| Egg | 97 ± 3 | | |
| Milk, cheese | 95 + 3 | 95 | 100 |
| Meat, fish | 94 ± 3 | | |
| Maize | 85 ± 6 | | 89 |
| Rice, polished | 88 ± 4 | | 93 |
| Wheat, whole | 86 ± 5 | | 90 |
| Wheat, refined | 96 ± 4 | | 101 |
| Oatmeal | 86 ± 7 | | 90 |
| Millet | 79 | | 83 |
| Peas, mature | 88 | | 93 |
| Peanut butter | 95 | | 100 |
| Soyflour | 86 ± 7 | | 90 |
| Beans | 78 | | 82 |
| Maize + beans | 78 | | 82 |
| Maize + beans + milk | 84 | | 88 |
| Indian rice diet | 77 | | 81 |
| Indian rice diet + milk | 87 | | 92 |
| Chinese mixed diet | 96 | | 98[a] |
| Brazilian mixed diet | 78 | | 82 |
| Filipino mixed diet | 88[b] | | 93 |
| American mixed diet | 96[b] | | 101 |
| Indian rice + bean diet | 78[b] | | 82 |

[a]Relative to egg measured in the same study.
[b]Recalculated from apparent digestibility, using $F_K$ = 12 mg N/kg (see original text).
[c]See original reference for data sources.
[d]Reprinted with permission from WHO Energy and Protein Requirements, TRS No. 724, 1985, p. 119.

**Table A–4b. Daily Average Energy Requirement and Safe Level of Protein Intake for Men and Women[d]**

| Men Ages (years) | Weight (kg) | BMR/kg[a] | | Daily Energy Requirement[b] According to BMR Factor Indicated: | | | | | | | | | | Safe Level of Protein Intake[c] |
| | | (kcal_tb) | (kJ) | 1.4 BMR | | 1.6 BMR | | 1.8 BMR | | 2.0 BMR | | 2.2 BMR | | (g/day) |
| | | | | (kcal_tb) | (kJ) | (kcal_tb) | (kJ) | (kcal_tb) | (kJ) | (kcal_tb) | (kJ) | (kcal_tb) | (kJ) | |
|---|---|---|---|---|---|---|---|---|---|---|---|---|---|---|
| 18–30 | 50 | 29 | 121.3 | 2,050 | 8,500 | 2,300 | 9,700 | 2,600 | 10,900 | 2,900 | 12,100 | 3,200 | 13,300 | 37.5 |
| | 55 | 27.5 | 115.1 | 2,100 | 8,900 | 2,400 | 10,100 | 2,700 | 11,400 | 3,000 | 12,700 | 3,300 | 13,900 | 41 |
| | 60 | 26.5 | 110.8 | 2,250 | 9,300 | 2,550 | 10,600 | 2,850 | 12,000 | 3,150 | 13,300 | 3,450 | 14,600 | 45 |
| | 65 | 26 | 108.7 | 2,350 | 9,900 | 2,700 | 11,300 | 3,000 | 12,700 | 3,300 | 14,100 | 3,700 | 15,500 | 49 |
| | 70 | 25 | 104.6 | 2,450 | 10,200 | 2,800 | 11,700 | 3,150 | 13,200 | 3,500 | 14,600 | 3,850 | 16,100 | 52.5 |
| | 75 | 24.5 | 102.5 | 2,550 | 10,800 | 2,900 | 12,300 | 3,300 | 13,800 | 3,650 | 15,400 | 4,000 | 16,900 | 56 |
| | 80 | 24 | 100.4 | 2,650 | 11,200 | 3,050 | 12,900 | 3,400 | 14,500 | 3,800 | 16,100 | 4,200 | 17,700 | 60 |
| 30–60 | 50 | 29 | 121.3 | 2,050 | 8,500 | 2,350 | 9,700 | 2,650 | 10,900 | 2,900 | 12,100 | 3,200 | 13,300 | 37.5 |
| | 55 | 27.5 | 115.1 | 2,100 | 8,900 | 2,450 | 10,100 | 2,750 | 11,400 | 3,050 | 12,700 | 3,350 | 13,900 | 41 |
| | 60 | 26 | 108.7 | 2,200 | 9,100 | 2,500 | 10,400 | 2,850 | 11,700 | 3,150 | 13,000 | 3,450 | 14,300 | 45 |
| | 65 | 25 | 104.6 | 2,300 | 9,500 | 2,600 | 10,900 | 2,950 | 12,200 | 3,250 | 13,600 | 3,600 | 15,000 | 49 |
| | 70 | 24 | 100.4 | 2,350 | 9,800 | 2,700 | 11,200 | 3,050 | 12,600 | 3,400 | 14,100 | 3,700 | 15,500 | 52.5 |
| | 75 | 23.5 | 98.32 | 2,450 | 10,300 | 2,800 | 11,800 | 3,150 | 13,300 | 3,500 | 14,700 | 3,850 | 16,200 | 56 |
| | 80 | 22.5 | 94.14 | 2,550 | 10,500 | 2,900 | 12,000 | 3,250 | 13,500 | 3,600 | 15,100 | 4,000 | 16,600 | 60 |
| >60 | 50 | 23 | 96.23 | 1,650 | 6,700 | 1,850 | 7,700 | 2,100 | 8,700 | 2,300 | 9,600 | 2,550 | 10,600 | 37.5 |
| | 55 | 22.5 | 94.14 | 1,700 | 7,200 | 1,950 | 8,300 | 2,200 | 9,300 | 2,450 | 10,400 | 2,700 | 11,400 | 41 |
| | 60 | 21.5 | 89.96 | 1,800 | 7,600 | 2,100 | 8,600 | 2,350 | 9,700 | 2,600 | 10,800 | 2,850 | 11,900 | 45 |
| | 65 | 21 | 87.86 | 1,900 | 8,000 | 2,200 | 9,100 | 2,450 | 10,300 | 2,750 | 11,400 | 3,000 | 12,600 | 49 |
| | 70 | 20.5 | 85.77 | 2,000 | 8,400 | 2,300 | 9,600 | 2,600 | 10,800 | 2,850 | 12,000 | 3,150 | 13,200 | 52.5 |
| | 75 | 20 | 83.68 | 2,100 | 8,800 | 2,400 | 10,000 | 2,700 | 11,300 | 3,000 | 12,600 | 3,300 | 13,800 | 56 |
| | 80 | 19.5 | 81.59 | 2,200 | 9,100 | 2,500 | 10,400 | 2,800 | 11,800 | 3,150 | 13,100 | 3,450 | 14,400 | 60 |

# Table A-4b. (continued)

| Women Ages (years) | Weight (kg) | BMR/kg[a] kcal_bb | BMR/kg[a] (kJ) | Daily Energy Requirement[b] According to BMR Factor Indicated: 1.4 BMR (kcal_bb) | 1.4 BMR (kJ) | 1.6 BMR (kcal_bb) | 1.6 BMR (kJ) | 1.8 BMR (kcal_bb) | 1.8 BMR (kJ) | 2.0 BMR (kcal_bb) | 2.0 BMR (kJ) | 2.2 BMR (kcal_bb) | 2.2 BMR (kJ) | Safe Level of Protein Intake[c] (g/day) |
|---|---|---|---|---|---|---|---|---|---|---|---|---|---|---|
| 18–30 | 40 | 27 | 112.9 | 1,500 | 6,300 | 1,700 | 7,200 | 1,950 | 8,100 | 2,150 | 9,000 | 2,350 | 9,900 | 30 |
| | 45 | 25.5 | 106.6 | 1,600 | 6,700 | 1,850 | 7,700 | 2,100 | 8,600 | 2,300 | 9,600 | 2,550 | 10,600 | 34 |
| | 50 | 24.5 | 102.5 | 1,700 | 7,200 | 1,950 | 8,200 | 2,200 | 9,200 | 2,450 | 10,200 | 2,700 | 11,300 | 37.5 |
| | 55 | 23.5 | 98.32 | 1,850 | 7,600 | 2,100 | 8,600 | 2,350 | 9,700 | 2,600 | 10,800 | 2,850 | 11,900 | 41 |
| | 60 | 23 | 96.23 | 1,950 | 8,100 | 2,200 | 9,200 | 2,500 | 10,400 | 2,750 | 11,500 | 3,050 | 12,700 | 45 |
| | 65 | 22.5 | 94.14 | 2,050 | 8,600 | 2,300 | 9,800 | 2,600 | 11,000 | 2,900 | 12,200 | 3,200 | 13,500 | 49 |
| | 70 | 22 | 92.05 | 2,150 | 9,000 | 2,450 | 10,300 | 2,750 | 11,600 | 3,050 | 12,900 | 3,350 | 14,200 | 52.5 |
| | 75 | 21.5 | 89.96 | 2,250 | 9,400 | 2,550 | 10,800 | 2,900 | 12,100 | 3,200 | 13,500 | 3,500 | 14,800 | 56 |
| 30–60 | 40 | 29.5 | 123.4 | 1,650 | 6,900 | 1,900 | 7,900 | 2,150 | 8,900 | 2,350 | 9,900 | 2,600 | 10,900 | 30 |
| | 45 | 27.5 | 115.1 | 1,700 | 7,300 | 1,950 | 8,300 | 2,200 | 9,300 | 2,450 | 10,400 | 2,700 | 11,400 | 34 |
| | 50 | 25.5 | 106.6 | 1,800 | 7,500 | 2,050 | 8,500 | 2,300 | 9,600 | 2,550 | 10,700 | 2,800 | 11,700 | 37.5 |
| | 55 | 24 | 100.4 | 1,850 | 7,700 | 2,100 | 8,800 | 2,350 | 9,900 | 2,650 | 11,000 | 2,900 | 12,100 | 41 |
| | 60 | 22.5 | 94.14 | 1,900 | 7,900 | 2,200 | 9,000 | 2,450 | 10,200 | 2,750 | 11,300 | 3,000 | 12,400 | 45 |
| | 65 | 21.5 | 89.96 | 1,950 | 8,200 | 2,250 | 9,400 | 2,550 | 10,500 | 2,800 | 11,700 | 3,100 | 12,900 | 49 |
| | 70 | 20.5 | 85.77 | 2,050 | 8,400 | 2,300 | 9,600 | 2,600 | 10,800 | 2,900 | 12,000 | 3,200 | 13,200 | 52.5 |
| | 75 | 20 | 83.68 | 2,100 | 8,800 | 2,400 | 10,000 | 2,700 | 11,300 | 3,000 | 12,600 | 3,300 | 13,800 | 56 |
| >60 | 40 | 25.5 | 106.6 | 1,400 | 6,000 | 1,650 | 6,800 | 1,850 | 7,700 | 2,050 | 8,500 | 2,250 | 9,400 | 30 |
| | 45 | 23.5 | 98.32 | 1,500 | 6,200 | 1,700 | 7,100 | 1,900 | 8,000 | 2,150 | 8,800 | 2,350 | 9,700 | 34 |
| | 50 | 22.5 | 94.14 | 1,550 | 6,600 | 1,800 | 7,500 | 2,000 | 8,500 | 2,250 | 9,400 | 2,450 | 10,400 | 37.5 |
| | 55 | 21.5 | 89.96 | 1,650 | 6,900 | 1,900 | 7,900 | 2,100 | 8,900 | 2,350 | 9,900 | 2,600 | 10,900 | 41 |
| | 60 | 20.5 | 85.77 | 1,700 | 7,200 | 1,950 | 8,200 | 2,200 | 9,300 | 2,450 | 10,300 | 2,700 | 11,300 | 45 |
| | 65 | 19.5 | 81.59 | 1,800 | 7,400 | 2,050 | 8,500 | 2,300 | 9,500 | 2,550 | 10,600 | 2,800 | 11,700 | 49 |
| | 70 | 19 | 79.49 | 1,850 | 7,800 | 2,150 | 8,900 | 2,400 | 10,000 | 2,650 | 11,100 | 2,950 | 12,200 | 52.5 |
| | 75 | 18.5 | 77.40 | 1,950 | 8,100 | 2,200 | 9,300 | 2,500 | 10,400 | 2,750 | 11,600 | 3,050 | 12,800 | 56 |

[a] Values of BMR/kg are presented for ease of calculation by those who wish to use different BMR factors.
[b] Calculated for each weight from the equations in Table 5 (rounded values) of original publication.
[c] At 0.75 g/kg of protein with the quality and digestibility of milk or egg.
[d] Reprinted with permission from WHO Energy and Protein Requirements, TRS No. 724, 1985, p. 133–135.

## Table A–5. Height-Weight Tables: Their Sources and Development*
### Sidney Abraham

Earlier this year the Metropolitan Life Insurance Company presented their new height and weight tables that were derived from data of the Build Study, 1979.[1] Metropolitan Life had previously utilized data from life insurance mortality studies compiled in the early 1900s and late 1950s to develop desirable weight tables in 1942,[2] 1943,[3] and 1959.[4] These studies reported the prevalence of mortality among insured persons according to variations in body build (height and weight) and also presented the average weight for height of persons by age. Such studies were designed to determine which groups (those underweight or overweight) showed a proportionately higher prevalence of mortality to yield information for underwriting purposes and for warranting changes in insurance policy premiums.

### Average Weight by Height Tables and Age-Group

**Mortality Studies.** In the American life insurance industry, interest in build (height and weight) as factors that influence mortality dates back to 1885. In that year, the Union Mutual Life Insurance Company published a pamphlet containing the results of a study of the company's records on mortality in relation to build.[5] The first in-depth study on the subject was presented in 1901 by a representative of the New York Life Insurance Company at the twelfth annual meeting of the Association of Life Insurance Medical Directors of America.[6] In this presentation it was pointed out that a certain amount of overweight had previously been looked on favorably. Nonetheless, the summary of this report noted that: "First among life insurance risks [is that] the [health] hazard increases in proportion to the degree of over- or underweight, second, whereas among overweights the mortality to be expected increases with [the] increased age of [the] applicant, among underweights the mortality decreases with advancing years."

**Height-Weight Tables.** The first height-weight table based on a considerable volume of statistics and taking age into account was the "Shepherd Table." This table was prepared in 1897 and was based on 74,162 male applicants accepted for life insurance in the United States and Canada.[7]

The basic study of height and weight based on life insurance statistics, however, was made as part of the Medico-Actuarial Mortality Investigation of 1912.[8] This study and the tables derived therefrom were the basis of the height-weight tables prepared for the general population. In addition to the study of the prevalence of mortality of certain groups of the insured population, the 1912 investigation included a study of the height and weight of a sample of persons insured from 1885 to 1900. The height and weight were recorded with the subjects wearing shoes and street clothes. A total of 221,819 men residing in the United States and Canada were included in this sample. At least 40% of the weights were estimated by the medical examiners. The data as tabulated were then smoothed to provide the figures for the height-weight age tables, and the adjusted tables became the basis for height-weight tables for males in the United States at this time.

Substantially the same procedure was employed to develop height-weight tables for women, but to secure enough cases for the preparation of tables it was necessary to add 126,504 policies issued after 1900 to the 10,000 included in the 1885 to 1900 sample.

In the Medical Impairment Study of 1929,[9] height-weight data were again collected on 667,000 men and 85,000 women. The average weights of both men and women in the 1929 study were not significantly different from those observed in the Medico-Actuarial Mortality Investigation. In fact, differences were so small that it was decided not to revise the standard height-weight tables except for those individuals younger than age 15.

*From Clinical Consultations in Nutrition Support, 3:5–8, 1983. Reprinted with permission of Sidney Abraham and Clinical Consultants in Nutrition Support.

### Tables of "Ideal" or "Desirable" Weights

An article presented in 1920, "Is the 'Average' the Same as the 'Normal' for Weight and Blood Pressure?"[10] illustrates an important development in the preparation of height-weight tables. In this paper the "normal" weight group is defined as that having the lowest mortality rate. The article presented a table of "normal" weights, so defined, for medium-sized men averaging 68 inches in height, and several discussants added their tables of similarly defined normal weights for men of small, medium, and tall height. In 1922, complete height-weight tables were presented that showed this normal weight for each inch of height and for each age group.[11] In general, all such tables of normal weight indicated that the ideal weight in terms of mortality was the average weight for height at age 30.

### Metropolitan Life Develops "Ideal" Height-Weight Tables

**Desirable Weight Tables, 1942 and 1943.** The concept of a "normal" weight, represented by the average weight of men at age 30, plus an awareness of the shortcomings of height and weight alone as complete indications of obesity led to the development of "ideal" weight tables by the Metropolitan Life Insurance Company.[2,3] Although employed for many purposes, these tables were originally intended for use in health education. The basic data were derived from the standard height-weight tables of the Medico-Actuarial Study of 1912, using the average weight for each inch of height at age 30 for men and at age 25 for women. Arbitrary ranges were then developed, using the base figures as reference points. These ranges are approximately the standard deviation of average weights for a given height and include the lightest weight for persons with small frames to the heaviest weight for persons with large frames. The total was then arbitrarily divided into three overlapping ranges, and the resulting figures represented ideal weights for individuals of small, medium, and large frames. However, no definition of frame size was presented.

These tables were intended to aid people in achieving a weight below the average for their height. Before these tables were developed, only average weights for each inch of height by age and sex were available. The new approach represented a change in concept between average weight (assuming that the average value is optimal for health) and desirable weight (weight based on the criterion of longevity). The concept underlying these tables deemphasized the use of a single average at each height and refuted the popular notion that weight increments attendant with advancing age were normal and therefore not harmful.

**Desirable Weight Tables, 1959.** The next study of build in relation to mortality was made in conjunction with the Build and Bood Pressure Study of 1959.[4] This investigation was based on the combined experience of 26 life insurance companies in the United States and Canada from 1935 to 1954 and involved observation of nearly 5 million insured persons for periods up to 20 years. Only those insured persons ages 15 through 69 were included. The height and weight data were recorded with the subjects wearing street shoes and indoor clothing. More than 90% of the insured persons were reported to have been actually weighed and measured at the time of examination for life insurance. The study presented average weights for men and women for each inch of height, ranging from 62 to 76 inches for men and from 58 to 72 inches for women. To provide some indication of the sole effect of weight on mortality, persons with heart disease, cancer, or diabetes were excluded.

When the Build and Blood Pressure Study was completed, the "ideal weight" table, originally developed by the Metropolitan Life Insurance Company in 1942 and 1943, was revised to conform to the latest data. The new table, called the "desirable weight" table (*Table A–5a*) was derived directly from weights associated with lowest mortality. Ranges of "desirable weight" for individuals 25 years and older with small, medium, and large frames were given, but again, no definition of frame size was included.

## Table A–5a. Desirable Weights for Men and Women Aged 25 and Over*
### (In pounds by Height and Frame, In Indoor Clothing)

| Men *(In Shoes, One-Inch Heels)* | | | | | Women *(In Shoes, Two-Inch Heels)* | | | | |
| Height | | Small Frame | Medium Frame | Large Frame | Height | | Small Frame | Medium Frame | Large Frame |
| Feet | Inches | | | | Feet | Inches | | | |
|---|---|---|---|---|---|---|---|---|---|
| 5 | 2 | 112–120 | 118–129 | 126–141 | 4 | 10 | 92–98 | 96–107 | 104–119 |
| 5 | 3 | 115–123 | 121–133 | 129–144 | 4 | 11 | 94–101 | 98–110 | 106–122 |
| 5 | 4 | 118–126 | 124–136 | 132–148 | 5 | 0 | 96–104 | 101–113 | 109–125 |
| 5 | 5 | 121–129 | 127–139 | 135–152 | 5 | 1 | 99–107 | 104–116 | 112–128 |
| 5 | 6 | 124–133 | 130–143 | 138–156 | 5 | 2 | 102–110 | 107–119 | 115–131 |
| 5 | 7 | 128–137 | 134–147 | 142–161 | 5 | 3 | 105–113 | 110–122 | 118–134 |
| 5 | 8 | 132–141 | 138–152 | 147–166 | 5 | 4 | 108–116 | 113–126 | 121–138 |
| 5 | 9 | 136–145 | 142–156 | 151–170 | 5 | 5 | 111–119 | 116–130 | 125–142 |
| 5 | 10 | 140–150 | 146–160 | 155–174 | 5 | 6 | 114–123 | 120–135 | 129–146 |
| 5 | 11 | 144–154 | 150–165 | 159–179 | 5 | 7 | 118–127 | 124–139 | 133–150 |
| 6 | 0 | 148–158 | 154–170 | 164–184 | 5 | 8 | 122–131 | 128–143 | 137–154 |
| 6 | 1 | 152–162 | 158–175 | 168–189 | 5 | 9 | 126–135 | 132–147 | 141–158 |
| 6 | 2 | 156–167 | 162–180 | 173–194 | 5 | 10 | 130–140 | 136–151 | 145–163 |
| 6 | 3 | 160–171 | 167–185 | 178–199 | 5 | 11 | 134–144 | 140–155 | 149–168 |
| 6 | 4 | 164–175 | 172–190 | 182–204 | 6 | 0 | 138–148 | 144–159 | 153–173 |

*Data adapted from the Statistical Bulletin, Metropolitan Life Insurance Company, New York.[4]

**1983 Metropolitan Height-Weight Tables.** Data published by the Society of Actuaries and the Association of Life Insurance Medical Directors of America in the Build Study, 1979,[1] are the source for the 1983 Metropolitan Life Insurance Height-Weight Tables (*Table A–5b*). The data are from 25 life insurance companies in the United States and Canada and show the prevalence of mortality from 1954 to 1972 of approximately 4.2 million insured men and women. Almost 90% of the recorded weights submitted for the study was obtained by actually weighing the applicants. As in the 1959 Build and Blood Pressure Study, applicants with major disease conditions at the time of policy issuance were excluded from the study. The terms "ideal body weight" and "desirable body weight," used in the earlier tables were not applied to the new height and weight tables because of the various misinterpretations of their meaning.

## Table A–5b. Height-Weight Tables,* Metropolitan 1983

| Men | | | | | Women | | | | |
| Height | | Small Frame | Medium Frame | Large Frame | Height | | Small Frame | Medium Frame | Large Frame |
| Feet | Inches | | | | Feet | Inches | | | |
|---|---|---|---|---|---|---|---|---|---|
| 5 | 2 | 128–134 | 131–141 | 138–150 | 4 | 10 | 102–111 | 109–121 | 118–131 |
| 5 | 3 | 130–136 | 133–143 | 140–153 | 4 | 11 | 103–113 | 111–123 | 120–134 |
| 5 | 4 | 132–138 | 135–145 | 142–156 | 5 | 0 | 104–115 | 113–126 | 122–137 |
| 5 | 5 | 134–140 | 137–148 | 144–160 | 5 | 1 | 106–118 | 115–129 | 125–140 |
| 5 | 6 | 136–142 | 139–151 | 146–164 | 5 | 2 | 108–121 | 118–132 | 128–143 |
| 5 | 7 | 138–145 | 142–154 | 149–168 | 5 | 3 | 111–124 | 121–135 | 131–147 |
| 5 | 8 | 140–148 | 145–157 | 152–172 | 5 | 4 | 114–127 | 124–138 | 134–151 |
| 5 | 9 | 142–151 | 148–160 | 155–176 | 5 | 5 | 117–130 | 127–141 | 137–155 |
| 5 | 10 | 144–154 | 151–163 | 158–180 | 5 | 6 | 120–133 | 130–144 | 140–159 |
| 5 | 11 | 146–157 | 154–166 | 161–184 | 5 | 7 | 123–136 | 133–147 | 143–163 |
| 6 | 0 | 149–160 | 157–170 | 164–188 | 5 | 8 | 126–139 | 136–150 | 146–167 |
| 6 | 1 | 152–164 | 160–174 | 168–192 | 5 | 9 | 129–142 | 139–153 | 149–170 |
| 6 | 2 | 155–168 | 164–178 | 172–197 | 5 | 10 | 132–145 | 142–156 | 152–173 |
| 6 | 3 | 158–172 | 167–182 | 176–202 | 5 | 11 | 135–148 | 145–159 | 155–176 |
| 6 | 4 | 162–176 | 171–187 | 181–207 | 6 | 0 | 138–151 | 148–162 | 158–179 |

Weight according to frame (ages 25 to 59) for men wearing indoor clothing weighing 5 lbs., shoes with one-inch heels; for women, indoor clothing weighing 3 lbs., shoes with one-inch heels.
*Reprinted with permission from the Metropolitan Life Insurance Company, New York.

The findings from the Build Study, 1979, showed that the gap between the weights based on lowest mortality and average weights has narrowed considerably since the 1959 Build and Blood Pressure Study. Metropolitan Life considered this factor in developing the 1983 height-weight tables. Weight for height has increased in contrast to the 1959 tables, but the increased weights are still less than the average weights (see *Table A–5e* below). Additionally, the increases in weight are not uniformly distributed throughout the 1983 height-weight tables. For each frame size, the weight increases for tall men or women were not as large as those for short men or women or for those of medium height.

In conjunction with investigations based on the life insurance data previously enumerated, long-term studies such as the Framingham Heart Study[12] and the Manitoba Study[13] all indicate that the weight associated with the greatest longevity tends to be below the average weight of the population under consideration and that "slimmer is better," provided that the underweight is not associated with a medical history of significant impairment.

**Frame Size**

The 1983 Metropolitan Height-Weight Tables relate weight to body frame size. A distinction is made among persons with small, medium, and large frames. The previous Metropolitan height-weight tables also related weight to body frame size, but although the body frame sizes were statistically defined, no generally accepted method of measuring frame size was provided. Body frame size is an integral factor in considering variation in weight, assuming that persons with larger frames have larger lean body mass and therefore weigh more. In the 1983 tables, elbow breadth is now used to determine frame size in men and women (*Table A–5c*). The frame sizes were developed from elbow breadth measurements taken from the first National Health and Nutrition Examination Survey, 1971–1975,[14] and were distributed so that 50% of the population falls within the medium frame and 25% each falls within the small and large frames.

**Table A–5c.   Height and Elbow Breadth for Men and Women*,†,‡**

| Height in One-Inch Heels | Elbow Breadth |
|---|---|
| Men | |
| 5′2″–5′3″ | 2½″–2⅞″ |
| 5′4″–5′7″ | 2⅝″–2⅞″ |
| 5′8″–5′11″ | 2¾″–3″ |
| 6′0″–6′3″ | 2¾″–3⅛″ |
| 6′4″ | 2⅞″–3¼″ |
| Women | |
| 4′10″–4′11″ | 2¼″–2½″ |
| 5′0″–5′3″ | 2¼″–2½″ |
| 5′4″–5′7″ | 2⅜″–2⅝″ |
| 5′8″–5′11″ | 2⅜″–2⅝″ |
| 6′0″ | 2½″–2¾″ |

*See Table A–5e.
†See Table A–5f for data on frame size by elbow breadth from NHANES I and II.
‡Reprinted with permission from Metropolitan Life Insurance Company, New York.
Extend your arm and bend the forearm upward at a 90-degree angle. Keep fingers straight and turn the inside of your wrist toward your body. If you have a caliper, use it to measure the space between the two prominent bones on either side of your elbow. Without a caliper, place thumb and index finger of your other hand on these two bones. Measure the space between your fingers against a ruler or tape measure. Compare it with these tables that list elbow measurements for medium-frame men and women. Measurements lower than those listed indicate you have a small frame. Higher measurements indicate a larger frame.

**Summary**

Major insurance mortality studies on insured populations in the United States and Canada conducted in 1912 by the Actuarial Society of America[8] and in 1959 and 1979 by the Society of Actuaries and the Association of Life Insurance Medical Directors of America[1,4] analyzed the mortality experience among insured persons according to variations of weight by height. The studies also presented data on the distribution of weight and height. The earliest study showed that the lowest mortality by build (weight for height) was found for those somewhat overweight at younger ages and among those underweight at older ages. In later mortality studies, it was generally found that insured persons whose weight was below the average lived longer than those whose weights were above average.

Since 1942, the Metropolitan Life Insurance Company has developed weight tables from data derived from each of the three major studies. The weights in each of the tables at given heights for men and women are classified according to frame size and refer to the weights associated with lowest mortality of policyholders. The weights were those obtained when the individual was originally insured. Because it is recognized that height and weight alone are incomplete indicators of excess weight, the weight tables also considered measurements of body build. In the tables issued in the 1940s,[2,3] 1959,[4] and 1983, three groups of frame size were identified. In each frame size, weight was given as a range rather than as a single value. However, no objective method was presented to estimate frame size in the earlier two tables. In the 1983 Metropolitan Height-Weight Tables, elbow breadth, unaffected by degree of adiposity and closely representative of bony dimension, was suggested to estimate frame size in the three categories of body build.

The views herein are solely those of the author and do not necessarily represent those of the National Center for Health Statistics.

## REFERENCES

1. Build Study, 1979. Society of Actuaries and Association of Life Insurance Medical Directors of America. Philadelphia, Recording and Statistical Corporation, 1980.
2. Ideal Weight for Men. Stat. Bull. Metropol. Life Insur. Co. 23:6, 1942.
3. Ideal Weights for Women. Stat. Bull. Metropol. Life Insur. Co. 24:6, 1943.
4. New Weight Standards for Men and Women. Stat. Bull. Metropol. Life Insur. Co. 40:1, 1959.
5. Grant, F.S.: Overweights in whom the abdominal girth is greater than the chest at full inspiration. Proc. Assoc. Life Insur. Med. Dir. Am. 2:323–327, 1902.
6. Rogers, O.H.: Build as a factor influencing longevity. Proc. Assoc. Life Insur. Med. Dir. Am. 1:280–288, 1901.
7. Shepherd, G.R.: Relation of build to longevity. Proc. Assoc. Life Insur. Med. Dir. Am. 6:46–58, 1912.
8. Medico-Actuarial Mortality Investigation. New York, Actuarial Society of America, 1912.
9. Medical Impairment Study, 1929. The association of Life Insurance Medical Directors of America and the Actuarial Society of America, New York, 1931.
10. Hunter, A.: Is the 'average' the same as the 'normal' for weight and blood pressure? Trans. Actuar. Soc. Am. 21:365–370, 1920.
11. Knight, A.S.: Tables of overweight and underweight corresponding to various mortality ratios. Proc. Assoc. Life Insur. Med. Dir. Am. 9:193–199, 1922.
12. Hubert, H.B., Feinleib, M., McNamara, P.M., et al.: Obesity as an independent risk factor for cardiovascular disease: A 26-year follow-up of participants in the Framingham Heart Study. Circulation 5:968–977, 1983.
13. Rabkin, S.W., Mathewson, F.A.L., Hsu, P.H.: Relation of body weight to development of ischemic heart disease in a cohort of young North American men after a 26-year observation period: The Manitoba study. Am. J. Cardiol. 39:452–458, 1977.
14. Public Use Data Tape, NHANES I—Anthropometry, goniometry, skeletal age, bone density, and cortical thickness, ages 1–74. Tape No. 4111, National Health and Nutrition Examination Survey, 1971–1975, National Center for Health Statistics, Hyattsville, Md.

## Table A–5d. Height-Weight Tables (Metric Units), Metropolitan 1983*

The 1983 Metropolitan Height-Weight Tables are based on the 1979 Build Study.

The values are statistical computations from individuals ranging from 25 to 59 years of weights by height and body frame at which mortality has been found to be lowest or longevity the highest. Metropolitan Life does not advocate the use of the term "ideal," which has different meanings to various individuals, because the term was used originally in their 1942–1943 tables. If one wishes to use these tables in the sense that they are "ideal" in terms of lowest mortality, they are "appropriate" in that context. These tables do not provide weights related to minimizing illness, optimizing job performance, or creating the best appearance.

| | *Males* | | | | *Females* | | |
|---|---|---|---|---|---|---|---|
| *Height (cm)* | *Small Frame (kg)* | *Medium Frame (kg)* | *Large Frame (kg)* | *Height (cm)* | *Small Frame (kg)* | *Medium Frame (kg)* | *Large Frame (kg)* |
| 157.5 | 58.2–60.9 | 59.4–64.1 | 62.7–68.2 | 147.5 | 46.4–50.5 | 49.5–55.0 | 53.6–59.5 |
| 160 | 59.1–61.8 | 60.5–65.0 | 63.6–69.5 | 150 | 46.8–51.4 | 50.5–55.9 | 54.5–60.9 |
| 162.5 | 60.0–62.7 | 61.4–65.9 | 64.5–70.9 | 152.5 | 47.3–52.3 | 51.4–57.3 | 55.5–62.3 |
| 165 | 60.9–63.7 | 62.3–67.3 | 65.5–72.7 | 155 | 48.2–53.6 | 52.3–58.6 | 56.8–63.6 |
| 167.5 | 61.8–64.5 | 63.2–68.6 | 66.4–74.5 | 157.5 | 49.1–55.0 | 53.6–60.0 | 58.2–65.0 |
| 170 | 62.7–65.9 | 64.5–70.0 | 67.7–76.4 | 160 | 50.5–56.4 | 55.0–61.4 | 59.5–66.8 |
| 173 | 63.6–67.3 | 65.9–71.4 | 69.1–78.2 | 162.5 | 51.8–57.7 | 56.4–62.7 | 60.9–68.6 |
| 175 | 64.5–68.6 | 67.3–72.7 | 70.5–80.0 | 165 | 53.2–59.1 | 57.7–64.1 | 62.3–70.5 |
| 178 | 65.4–70.0 | 68.6–74.1 | 71.8–81.8 | 167.5 | 54.5–60.5 | 59.1–65.5 | 63.6–72.3 |
| 180 | 66.4–71.4 | 70.0–75.5 | 73.2–83.6 | 170 | 55.9–61.8 | 60.5–66.8 | 65.0–74.1 |
| 183 | 67.7–72.7 | 71.4–77.3 | 74.5–85.6 | 173 | 57.3–63.2 | 61.8–68.2 | 66.4–75.9 |
| 185.5 | 69.1–74.5 | 72.7–79.1 | 76.4–87.3 | 175 | 58.6–64.5 | 63.2–69.5 | 67.7–77.3 |
| 188 | 70.5–76.4 | 74.5–80.9 | 78.2–89.5 | 178 | 60.0–65.9 | 64.5–70.9 | 69.1–78.6 |
| 190.5 | 71.8–78.2 | 75.9–82.7 | 80.0–91.8 | 180 | 61.4–67.3 | 65.9–72.3 | 70.5–80.0 |
| 193 | 73.6–80.0 | 77.7–85.0 | 82.3–94.1 | 183 | 62.3–68.6 | 67.3–73.6 | 71.8–81.4 |

*Reprinted with permission from the Metropolitan Life Insurance Company, New York.

## Table A–5e. Average Weights by Height and Age Group: 1959 and 1979 Build and Blood Pressure Studies*

| Men | Height | | | | | | | | | | | | | | |
|---|---|---|---|---|---|---|---|---|---|---|---|---|---|---|---|
| | *5'2"* | *5'3"* | *5'4"* | *5'5"* | *5'6"* | *5'7"* | *5'8"* | *5'9"* | *5'10"* | *5'11"* | *6'0"* | *6'1"* | *6'2"* | *6'3"* | *6'4"* |
| **15–16 Years†** | | | | | | | | | | | | | | | |
| 1959 Study | 107 | 112 | 117 | 122 | 127 | 132 | 137 | 142 | 146 | 150 | 154 | 159 | 164 | 169 | ‡ |
| 1979 Study | 112 | 116 | 121 | 127 | 133 | 137 | 143 | 148 | 153 | 159 | 162 | 168 | 173 | 178 | 184 |
| Weight Change | +5 | +4 | +4 | +5 | +6 | +5 | +6 | +6 | +7 | +9 | +8 | +9 | +9 | +9 | — |
| **17–19 Years** | | | | | | | | | | | | | | | |
| 1959 Study | 119 | 123 | 127 | 131 | 135 | 139 | 143 | 147 | 151 | 155 | 160 | 164 | 168 | 172 | 176 |
| 1979 Study | 124 | 129 | 132 | 137 | 141 | 145 | 150 | 155 | 159 | 164 | 168 | 174 | 179 | 185 | 190 |
| Weight Change | +5 | +6 | +5 | +6 | +6 | +6 | +7 | +8 | +8 | +9 | +8 | +10 | +11 | +13 | +14 |
| **20–24 Years** | | | | | | | | | | | | | | | |
| 1959 Study | 128 | 132 | 136 | 139 | 142 | 145 | 149 | 153 | 157 | 161 | 166 | 170 | 174 | 178 | 181 |
| 1979 Study | 130 | 136 | 139 | 143 | 148 | 153 | 157 | 163 | 167 | 171 | 176 | 182 | 187 | 193 | 198 |
| Weight Change | +2 | +4 | +3 | +4 | +6 | +8 | +8 | +10 | +10 | +10 | +10 | +12 | +13 | +15 | +17 |
| **25–29 Years** | | | | | | | | | | | | | | | |
| 1959 Study | 134 | 138 | 141 | 144 | 148 | 151 | 155 | 159 | 163 | 167 | 172 | 177 | 182 | 186 | 190 |
| 1979 Study | 134 | 140 | 143 | 147 | 152 | 156 | 161 | 166 | 171 | 175 | 181 | 186 | 191 | 197 | 202 |
| Weight Change | +0 | +2 | +2 | +3 | +4 | +5 | +6 | +7 | +8 | +8 | +9 | +9 | +9 | +11 | +12 |
| **30–39 Years** | | | | | | | | | | | | | | | |
| 1959 Study | 137 | 141 | 145 | 149 | 153 | 157 | 161 | 165 | 170 | 174 | 179 | 183 | 188 | 193 | 199 |
| 1979 Study | 138 | 143 | 147 | 151 | 156 | 160 | 165 | 170 | 174 | 179 | 184 | 190 | 195 | 201 | 206 |
| Weight Change | +1 | +2 | +2 | +2 | +3 | +3 | +4 | +5 | +4 | +5 | +5 | +7 | +7 | +8 | +7 |
| **40–49 Years** | | | | | | | | | | | | | | | |
| 1959 Study | 140 | 144 | 148 | 152 | 156 | 161 | 165 | 169 | 174 | 178 | 183 | 187 | 192 | 197 | 203 |
| 1979 Study | 140 | 144 | 149 | 154 | 158 | 163 | 167 | 172 | 176 | 181 | 186 | 192 | 197 | 203 | 208 |
| Weight Change | +0 | +0 | +1 | +2 | +2 | +2 | +2 | +3 | +2 | +3 | +3 | +5 | +5 | +6 | +5 |
| **50–59 Years** | | | | | | | | | | | | | | | |
| 1959 Study | 142 | 145 | 149 | 153 | 157 | 162 | 166 | 170 | 175 | 180 | 185 | 189 | 194 | 199 | 205 |
| 1979 Study | 141 | 145 | 150 | 155 | 159 | 164 | 168 | 173 | 177 | 182 | 187 | 193 | 198 | 204 | 209 |
| Weight Change | −1 | +0 | +1 | +2 | +2 | +2 | +2 | +3 | +2 | +2 | +2 | +4 | +4 | +5 | +4 |
| **60–69 Years** | | | | | | | | | | | | | | | |
| 1959 Study | 139 | 142 | 146 | 150 | 154 | 159 | 163 | 168 | 173 | 178 | 183 | 188 | 193 | 198 | 204 |
| 1979 Study | 140 | 144 | 149 | 153 | 158 | 163 | 167 | 172 | 176 | 181 | 186 | 191 | 196 | 200 | 207 |
| Weight Change | +1 | +2 | +3 | +3 | +4 | +4 | +4 | +4 | +3 | +3 | +3 | +3 | +3 | +2 | +3 |

## Table A–5e. (continued)

| Women | 4'10" | 4'11" | 5'0" | 5'1" | 5'2" | 5'3" | 5'4" | 5'5" | 5'6" | 5'7" | 5'8" | 5'9" | 5'10" | 5'11" | 6'0" |
|---|---|---|---|---|---|---|---|---|---|---|---|---|---|---|---|
| **15–16 Years†** | | | | | | | | | | | | | | | |
| 1959 Study | 97 | 100 | 103 | 107 | 111 | 114 | 117 | 121 | 125 | 128 | 132 | 136 | ‡ | ‡ | ‡ |
| 1979 Study | 101 | 105 | 109 | 112 | 117 | 121 | 123 | 128 | 131 | 135 | 138 | 142 | 146 | 149 | 152 |
| Weight Change | +4 | +5 | +6 | +5 | +6 | +7 | +6 | +7 | +6 | +7 | +6 | +6 | — | — | — |
| **17–19 Years** | | | | | | | | | | | | | | | |
| 1959 Study | 99 | 102 | 105 | 109 | 113 | 116 | 120 | 124 | 127 | 130 | 134 | 138 | 142 | 147 | 152 |
| 1979 Study | 103 | 108 | 111 | 115 | 119 | 123 | 126 | 129 | 132 | 136 | 140 | 145 | 148 | 150 | 154 |
| Weight Change | +4 | +6 | +6 | +6 | +6 | +7 | +6 | +5 | +5 | +6 | +6 | +7 | +6 | +3 | +2 |
| **20–24 Years** | | | | | | | | | | | | | | | |
| 1959 Study | 102 | 105 | 108 | 112 | 115 | 118 | 121 | 125 | 129 | 132 | 136 | 140 | 144 | 149 | 154 |
| 1979 Study | 105 | 110 | 112 | 116 | 120 | 124 | 127 | 130 | 133 | 137 | 141 | 146 | 149 | 155 | 157 |
| Weight Change | +3 | +5 | +4 | +4 | +5 | +6 | +6 | +5 | +4 | +5 | +5 | +6 | +5 | +6 | +3 |
| **25–29 Years** | | | | | | | | | | | | | | | |
| 1959 Study | 107 | 110 | 113 | 116 | 119 | 122 | 125 | 129 | 133 | 136 | 140 | 144 | 148 | 153 | 158 |
| 1979 Study | 110 | 112 | 114 | 119 | 121 | 125 | 128 | 132 | 134 | 138 | 142 | 148 | 150 | 156 | 159 |
| Weight Change | +3 | +2 | +1 | +3 | +2 | +3 | +3 | +3 | +1 | +2 | +2 | +4 | +2 | +3 | +1 |
| **30–39 Years** | | | | | | | | | | | | | | | |
| 1959 Study | 115 | 117 | 120 | 123 | 126 | 129 | 132 | 135 | 139 | 142 | 146 | 150 | 154 | 159 | 164 |
| 1979 Study | 113 | 115 | 118 | 121 | 124 | 128 | 131 | 134 | 137 | 141 | 145 | 150 | 153 | 159 | 164 |
| Weight Change | −2 | −2 | −2 | −2 | −2 | −1 | −1 | −1 | −2 | −1 | −1 | 0 | −1 | 0 | 0 |
| **40–49 Years** | | | | | | | | | | | | | | | |
| 1959 Study | 122 | 124 | 127 | 130 | 133 | 136 | 140 | 143 | 147 | 151 | 155 | 159 | 164 | 169 | 174 |
| 1979 Study | 118 | 121 | 123 | 127 | 129 | 133 | 136 | 139 | 143 | 147 | 150 | 155 | 158 | 162 | 168 |
| Weight Change | −4 | −3 | −4 | −3 | −4 | −3 | −4 | −4 | −4 | −4 | −5 | −4 | −6 | −7 | −6 |
| **50–59 Years** | | | | | | | | | | | | | | | |
| 1959 Study | 125 | 127 | 130 | 133 | 136 | 140 | 144 | 148 | 152 | 156 | 160 | 164 | 169 | 174 | 180 |
| 1979 Study | 121 | 125 | 127 | 131 | 133 | 137 | 141 | 144 | 147 | 152 | 156 | 159 | 162 | 166 | 171 |
| Weight Change | −4 | −2 | −3 | −2 | −3 | −3 | −3 | −4 | −5 | −4 | −4 | −5 | −7 | −8 | −9 |
| **60–69 Years** | | | | | | | | | | | | | | | |
| 1959 Study | 127 | 129 | 131 | 134 | 137 | 141 | 145 | 149 | 153 | 157 | 161 | 165 | ‡ | ‡ | ‡ |
| 1979 Study | 123 | 127 | 130 | 133 | 136 | 140 | 143 | 147 | 150 | 155 | 158 | 161 | 163 | 167 | 172 |
| Weight Change | −4 | −2 | −1 | −1 | −1 | −1 | −2 | −2 | −3 | −2 | −3 | −4 | — | — | — |

*Data source: Association of Life Insurance Medical Directors of America and Society of Actuaries. Compiled by Seltzer, F.: Dietetic Currents. 10:17–22, 1983. Reprinted with permission of Ross Laboratories, Columbus, Ohio.
†Height in shoes (feet and inches) and weight in indoor clothing (pounds).
‡Average weights omitted in classes with too few cases for analysis.

## Table A–5f. Frame Size by Elbow Breadth (cm) of U.S. Male and Female Adults Derived from the Combined NHANES I and II Data Sets*

| Age | Frame Size | | |
|---|---|---|---|
| (yr) | Small | Medium | Large |
| Males | | | |
| 18–24 | ≤6.6 | >6.6 and <7.7 | ≥7.7 |
| 25–34 | ≤6.7 | >6.7 and <7.9 | ≥7.9 |
| 35–44 | ≤6.7 | >6.7 and <8.0 | ≥8.0 |
| 45–54 | ≤6.7 | >6.7 and <8.1 | ≥8.1 |
| 55–64 | ≤6.7 | >6.7 and <8.1 | ≥8.1 |
| 65–74 | ≤6.7 | >6.7 and <8.1 | ≥8.1 |
| Females | | | |
| 18–24 | ≤5.6 | >5.6 and <6.5 | ≥6.5 |
| 25–34 | ≤5.7 | >5.7 and <6.8 | ≥6.8 |
| 35–44 | ≤5.7 | >5.7 and <7.1 | ≥7.1 |
| 45–54 | ≤5.7 | >5.7 and <7.2 | ≥7.2 |
| 55–64 | ≤5.8 | >5.8 and <7.2 | ≥7.2 |
| 65–74 | ≤5.8 | >5.8 and <7.2 | ≥7.2 |

The tenth and ninetieth percentiles, respectively, represent the predicted mean ±1.282 times the SE. Similarly, the fifteenth and eighty-fifth percentiles are the predicted mean minus and plus, respectively, 1.036 times the SE of the regression equation. There were significant black-white population differences in weight and body composition when age and height were considered. However, when the comparisons were made with reference to age, height, and frame size, there were only minor interpopulation differences. For this reason, all races (white, black, and other) included in the NHANES I and II surveys were merged together for the purpose of calculating percentiles of anthropometric measurements.

*Combined NHANES I and II data sets from Frisancho, A.R.: Am. J. Clin. Nutr. 40:808–819, 1984, with permission.

# Table A–6a-1. Selected Percentiles of Weight, Triceps and Subscapular Skinfolds, and Bone-Free Upper Arm Muscle Area (AMA) for U.S. Males and Females with Small Frames (25- to 54-yr-old)†

| Ht | | n | Wt (kg) | | | | | | | Triceps (mm) | | | | | | | Subscapular (mm) | | | | | | | Bone-free AMA (cm²) | | | | | | |
|---|---|---|---|---|---|---|---|---|---|---|---|---|---|---|---|---|---|---|---|---|---|---|---|---|---|---|---|---|---|---|
| in | cm | | 5 | 10 | 15 | 50 | 85 | 90 | 95 | 5 | 10 | 15 | 50 | 85 | 90 | 95 | 5 | 10 | 15 | 50 | 85 | 90 | 95 | 5 | 10 | 15 | 50 | 85 | 90 | 95 |
| **Males** | | | | | | | | | | | | | | | | | | | | | | | | | | | | | | |
| 62 | 157 | 23 | 46* | 50* | 52* | 64 | 71* | 74* | 77* | | | | 11 | 17 | | | | | 8 | 16 | 20 | | | | | | 52 | | | |
| 63 | 160 | 43 | 48* | 51* | 53 | 61 | 70 | 75* | 79* | | | 6 | 10 | 16 | 17 | 18 | | | 7 | 12 | 25 | 29 | | | | 32 | 48 | 54 | | |
| 64 | 163 | 73 | 49* | 53 | 55 | 66 | 76 | 76 | 80* | | 5 | 5 | 11 | 17 | 18 | 21 | | 7 | 9 | 15 | 25 | 28 | 35 | | 37 | 38 | 49 | 58 | 63 | 71 |
| 65 | 165 | 112 | 52 | 58 | 66 | 66 | 77 | 81 | 84 | 4 | 5 | 6 | 11 | 18 | 18 | 20 | 7 | 8 | 8 | 14 | 26 | 26 | 32 | 31 | 35 | 37 | 47 | 60 | 63 | 71 |
| 66 | 168 | 129 | 56 | 57 | 59 | 67 | 78 | 83 | 84 | 5 | 6 | 6 | 11 | 18 | 20 | 22 | 7 | 8 | 9 | 14 | 23 | 25 | 30 | 31 | 36 | 38 | 49 | 60 | 62 | |
| 67 | 170 | 132 | 56 | 60 | 62 | 71 | 82 | 83 | 88 | 5 | 6 | 6 | 11 | 15 | 16 | 20 | 6 | 7 | 7 | 15 | 24 | 24 | | 35 | 39 | 41 | 49 | 58 | 60 | 62 |
| 68 | 173 | 107 | 56 | 59 | 62 | 71 | 79 | 82 | 85 | 5 | 6 | 6 | 10 | 17 | 17 | 20 | 7 | 8 | 9 | 13 | 24 | 30 | | 33 | 37 | 40 | 49 | 59 | 62 | 69 |
| 69 | 175 | 97 | 57* | 62 | 65 | 74 | 84 | 87 | 88* | | 6 | 6 | 11 | 17 | | | | 7 | 7 | 13 | 24 | 26 | 40 | | 36 | 40 | 58 | 61 | 63 | |
| 70 | 178 | 46 | 59* | 62* | 67 | 75 | 87 | 86* | 90* | | | 7 | 10 | 17 | | | | | 9 | 14 | 23 | | | | | 35 | 48 | 57 | | |
| 71 | 180 | 49 | 60* | 64* | 70 | 76 | 79 | 88* | 91* | | | 7 | 10 | 16 | | | | | 8 | 13 | 22 | | | | | 39 | 47 | 52 | | |
| 72 | 183 | 21 | 62* | 65* | 67* | 74 | 87* | 89* | 93* | | | | 10 | | | | | | | 14 | | | | | | | 45 | | | |
| 73 | 185 | 9 | 63* | 67* | 69* | 79* | 89* | 91* | 94* | | | | | | | | | | | | | | | | | | | | | |
| 74 | 188 | 6 | 65* | 68* | 71* | 80* | 90* | 92* | 96* | | | | | | | | | | | | | | | | | | | | | |
| **Females** | | | | | | | | | | | | | | | | | | | | | | | | | | | | | | |
| 58 | 147 | 53 | 37* | 43 | 43 | 52 | 58 | 62 | 66* | 8 | | 13 | 24 | 30 | 33 | 37 | | 10 | 12 | 23 | 34 | 38 | | | 22 | 24 | 29 | 36 | 39 | 44 |
| 59 | 150 | 108 | 42 | 43 | 44 | 53 | 63 | 69 | 72 | 8 | 11 | 14 | 21 | 29 | 33 | 36 | 6 | 9 | 10 | 17 | 29 | 32 | 34 | 17 | 20 | 22 | 28 | 38 | 39 | 43 |
| 60 | 152 | 142 | 42 | 44 | 45 | 53 | 63 | 65 | 70 | 8 | 11 | 12 | 21 | 28 | 29 | 33 | 6 | 7 | 8 | 18 | 27 | 32 | 39 | 19 | 21 | 21 | 28 | 36 | 40 | 44 |
| 61 | 155 | 218 | 44 | 46 | 47 | 54 | 64 | 66 | 72 | 11 | 12 | 14 | 21 | 28 | 31 | 34 | 7 | 7 | 9 | 16 | 28 | 32 | 36 | 20 | 21 | 23 | 28 | 38 | 39 | 42 |
| 62 | 157 | 255 | 44 | 47 | 48 | 55 | 63 | 64 | 70 | 10 | 11 | 14 | 20 | 28 | 31 | 34 | 6 | 7 | 8 | 14 | 22 | 29 | 32 | 20 | 21 | 21 | 27 | 33 | 35 | 42 |
| 63 | 160 | 239 | 46 | 48 | 49 | 55 | 65 | 68 | 79 | 10 | 11 | 13 | 20 | 27 | 29 | 36 | 6 | 7 | 7 | 13 | 27 | 27 | 31 | 20 | 21 | 22 | 27 | 33 | 35 | 37 |
| 64 | 163 | 146 | 49 | 50 | 51 | 57 | 67 | 68 | 74 | 10 | 13 | 13 | 22 | 28 | 30 | 34 | 6 | 7 | 8 | 13 | 24 | 30 | 34 | 22 | 23 | 23 | 28 | 34 | 38 | 38 |
| 65 | 165 | 113 | 50 | 52 | 53 | 60 | 70 | 72 | 80 | 12 | 13 | 14 | 19 | 29 | 31 | 34 | 7 | 7 | 8 | 15 | 26 | | 33 | 21 | 22 | 23 | 28 | 37 | 39 | 42 |
| 66 | 168 | 47 | 46* | 49* | 54 | 58 | 65 | 71* | 74* | | | 12 | 18 | 30 | | | | 8 | 9 | 12 | 25 | | | | | 23 | 27 | 35 | | 47 |
| 67 | 170 | 18 | 47* | 50* | 52* | 59 | 70* | 72* | 76* | | | | 20 | | | | | | | 13 | | | | | | | 26 | | | |
| 68 | 173 | 18 | 48* | 51* | 53* | 62 | 71* | 73* | 77* | | | | 18 | | | | | | | 15 | | | | | | | 25 | | | |
| 69 | 175 | 5 | 49* | 52* | 54* | 63* | 72* | 74* | 78* | | | | | | | | | | | | | | | | | | | | | |
| 70 | 178 | 1 | 50* | 53* | 55* | 64* | 73* | 75* | 79* | | | | | | | | | | | | | | | | | | | | | |

*Values estimated through linear regression equation.

†From Frisancho, A.R.: Am. J. Clin. Nutr. 40:808–819, 1984, with permission.

**Table A–6a-2. Selected Percentiles of Weight, Triceps and Subscapular Skinfolds, and Bone-Free Upper Arm Muscle Area (AMA) for U.S. Males and Females with Medium Frames (25- to 54-yr-old)†**

| Ht (in) | (cm) | n | Wt (kg) | | | | | | | Triceps (mm) | | | | | | | Subscapular (mm) | | | | | | | Bone-free AMA (cm²) | | | | | | |
|---|---|---|---|---|---|---|---|---|---|---|---|---|---|---|---|---|---|---|---|---|---|---|---|---|---|---|---|---|---|---|
| | | | 5 | 10 | 15 | 50 | 85 | 90 | 95 | 5 | 10 | 15 | 50 | 85 | 90 | 95 | 5 | 10 | 15 | 50 | 85 | 90 | 95 | 5 | 10 | 15 | 50 | 85 | 90 | 95 |
| **Males** | | | | | | | | | | | | | | | | | | | | | | | | | | | | | | |
| 62 | 157 | 10 | 51* | 55* | 58* | 68 | 81* | 83* | 87* | | | 6 | 15 | 18 | 20 | | | | | 13 | | | | | | | 58 | | | |
| 63 | 160 | 30 | 52* | 56* | 59* | 71 | 82* | 85* | 89* | | | | 11 | | | | | | | 18 | | | | | | | 55 | | | |
| 64 | 163 | 71 | 54* | 60 | 61 | 71 | 83 | 84 | 90* | 6 | 7 | 8 | 12 | 16 | 18 | 22 | 8 | 7 | 9 | 17 | 30 | 32 | | 40 | 43 | 47 | 56 | 67 | 69 | 71 |
| 65 | 165 | 154 | 59 | 62 | 65 | 74 | 87 | 90 | 94 | 5 | 7 | 8 | 11 | 16 | 18 | 22 | 8 | 9 | 10 | 16 | 26 | 29 | 32 | 38 | 43 | 45 | 56 | 67 | 69 | 70 |
| 66 | 168 | 212 | 58 | 61 | 65 | 75 | 85 | 87 | 93 | 5 | 6 | 7 | 11 | 16 | 18 | 22 | 7 | 7 | 9 | 16 | 25 | 27 | 33 | 39 | 42 | 44 | 55 | 69 | 72 | 78 |
| 67 | 170 | 409 | 62 | 66 | 68 | 77 | 89 | 93 | 100 | 5 | 7 | 7 | 13 | 21 | 23 | 28 | 8 | 9 | 10 | 18 | 26 | 30 | 33 | 41 | 44 | 45 | 53 | 66 | 69 | 73 |
| 68 | 173 | 478 | 60 | 64 | 66 | 78 | 89 | 92 | 97 | 5 | 5 | 7 | 11 | 18 | 20 | 24 | 7 | 8 | 9 | 16 | 25 | 28 | 31 | 38 | 41 | 44 | 55 | 67 | 71 | 76 |
| 69 | 175 | 464 | 63 | 66 | 68 | 78 | 90 | 93 | 97 | 4 | 6 | 7 | 12 | 18 | 20 | 24 | 7 | 8 | 9 | 16 | 25 | 27 | 31 | 39 | 42 | 43 | 54 | 66 | 69 | 73 |
| 70 | 178 | 419 | 64 | 66 | 70 | 81 | 90 | 93 | 97 | 5 | 6 | 7 | 12 | 18 | 20 | 23 | 7 | 8 | 9 | 15 | 24 | 27 | 30 | 37 | 41 | 44 | 55 | 65 | 68 | 72 |
| 71 | 180 | 282 | 62 | 68 | 70 | 81 | 92 | 96 | 100 | 4 | 5 | 7 | 12 | 19 | 21 | 25 | 7 | 8 | 9 | 14 | 24 | 27 | 30 | 40 | 42 | 44 | 54 | 67 | 68 | 73 |
| 72 | 183 | 231 | 68 | 71 | 74 | 84 | 97 | 100 | 104 | 5 | 7 | 7 | 12 | 20 | 22 | 26 | 7 | 8 | 9 | 15 | 26 | 30 | 32 | 39 | 44 | 44 | 56 | 65 | 67 | 74 |
| 73 | 185 | 106 | 70 | 72 | 75 | 85 | 100 | 101 | 104 | 6 | 7 | 8 | 12 | 20 | 24 | 27 | 7 | 9 | 9 | 15 | 25 | 29 | 32 | 43 | 43 | 43 | 55 | 67 | 69 | 73 |
| 74 | 188 | 50 | 68* | 76 | 77 | 88 | 100 | 100 | 104* | | 6 | 9 | 13 | 21 | 23 | | 8 | 7 | 9 | 14 | 25 | 30 | | | 43 | 43 | 55 | 62 | 63 | |
| **Females** | | | | | | | | | | | | | | | | | | | | | | | | | | | | | | |
| 58 | 147 | 40 | 41* | 46* | 50 | 63 | 77 | 75* | 79* | 15 | 19 | 20 | 25 | 40 | 40 | | 10 | 12 | 15 | 23 | 38 | | 43 | | | 24 | 35 | 42 | | 49 |
| 59 | 150 | 104 | 47 | 50 | 52 | 66 | 76 | 79 | 85 | 14 | 15 | 21 | 30 | 37 | 40 | | 8 | 10 | 13 | 29 | 38 | 39 | 41 | 23 | 24 | 26 | 33 | 43 | 45 | 49 |
| 60 | 152 | 208 | 47 | 50 | 52 | 60 | 77 | 79 | 85 | 11 | 14 | 17 | 26 | 35 | 37 | 41 | 8 | 9 | 11 | 22 | 35 | 37 | 42 | 22 | 25 | 25 | 32 | 42 | 45 | 49 |
| 61 | 155 | 465 | 47 | 49 | 51 | 61 | 73 | 78 | 86 | 12 | 14 | 15 | 25 | 34 | 36 | 42 | 7 | 9 | 10 | 19 | 32 | 36 | 42 | 21 | 24 | 25 | 31 | 42 | 45 | 51 |
| 62 | 157 | 644 | 49 | 50 | 52 | 61 | 73 | 77 | 83 | 12 | 13 | 16 | 24 | 34 | 36 | 40 | 7 | 8 | 10 | 18 | 33 | 37 | 40 | 21 | 23 | 25 | 31 | 40 | 43 | 48 |
| 63 | 160 | 685 | 49 | 51 | 53 | 62 | 77 | 80 | 88 | 12 | 14 | 15 | 24 | 33 | 35 | 38 | 7 | 8 | 10 | 18 | 31 | 34 | 38 | 22 | 23 | 25 | 32 | 41 | 43 | 50 |
| 64 | 163 | 722 | 50 | 52 | 54 | 62 | 76 | 82 | 87 | 12 | 14 | 15 | 23 | 33 | 36 | 40 | 7 | 7 | 8 | 16 | 31 | 34 | 38 | 21 | 23 | 24 | 31 | 40 | 43 | 48 |
| 65 | 165 | 628 | 52 | 54 | 55 | 63 | 75 | 80 | 89 | 12 | 14 | 15 | 22 | 31 | 34 | 38 | 7 | 7 | 8 | 15 | 29 | 33 | 38 | 21 | 23 | 24 | 31 | 40 | 43 | 49 |
| 66 | 168 | 428 | 52 | 54 | 55 | 63 | 75 | 78 | 83 | 11 | 13 | 14 | 22 | 31 | 33 | 37 | 7 | 8 | 9 | 14 | 28 | 33 | 35 | 21 | 23 | 24 | 30 | 39 | 41 | 44 |
| 67 | 170 | 257 | 54 | 56 | 57 | 65 | 79 | 82 | 88 | 12 | 13 | 15 | 21 | 29 | 30 | 35 | 7 | 8 | 8 | 15 | 28 | 32 | 37 | 22 | 24 | 25 | 30 | 40 | 43 | 48 |
| 68 | 173 | 119 | 58 | 59 | 60 | 67 | 77 | 85 | 87 | 10 | 14 | 15 | 22 | 31 | 32 | 36 | 8 | 8 | 9 | 15 | 29 | 33 | 35 | 22 | 24 | 25 | 30 | 37 | 38 | 39 |
| 69 | 175 | 59 | 49* | 58 | 60 | 68 | 79 | 82 | 87* | | 11 | 12 | 19 | 29 | 31 | | | 8 | 8 | 12 | 25 | 29 | | | 23 | 24 | 32 | 36 | 39 | |
| 70 | 178 | 15 | 50* | 54* | 57* | 70 | 80* | 83* | 87* | | | | 19 | | | | | | | 20 | | | | | | | 32 | | | |

*Value estimated through linear regression equation.
†From Frisancho A.R.: Am. J. Clin. Nutr. 40:808–819. 1984, with permission.

## Table A–6a-3. Selected Percentiles of Weight, Triceps and Subscapular Skinfolds, and Bone-Free Upper Arm Muscle Area (AMA) for U.S. Males and Females with Large Frames (25- to 54-yr-old)†

| Ht (in) | Ht (cm) | n | Wt (kg) 5 | 10 | 15 | 50 | 85 | 90 | 95 | Triceps (mm) 5 | 10 | 15 | 50 | 85 | 90 | 95 | Subscapular (mm) 5 | 10 | 15 | 50 | 85 | 90 | 95 | Bone-free AMA (cm²) 5 | 10 | 15 | 50 | 85 | 90 | 95 |
|---|---|---|---|---|---|---|---|---|---|---|---|---|---|---|---|---|---|---|---|---|---|---|---|---|---|---|---|---|---|---|
| **Males** | | | | | | | | | | | | | | | | | | | | | | | | | | | | | | |
| 62 | 157 | 1 | 57* | 62* | 66* | 82* | 99* | 103* | 108* | | | | | | | | | | | | | | | | | | | | | |
| 63 | 160 | 1 | 58* | 63* | 67* | 83* | 100* | 104* | 109* | | | | | | | | | | | | | | | | | | | | | |
| 64 | 163 | 5 | 59* | 64* | 68* | 84* | 101* | 105* | 110* | | | | | | | | | | | | | | | | | | | | | |
| 65 | 165 | 15 | 60* | 65* | 69* | 79 | 102* | 106* | 111* | | | | | | | | | | | | | | | | | | | | | |
| 66 | 168 | 37 | 60* | 65* | 75 | 84 | 103 | 106* | 112* | | | | 14 | | | | | | | 21 | | | | | | | 62 | | |
| 67 | 170 | 54 | 62* | 70 | 71 | 84 | 102 | 111 | 113* | | | 9 | 14 | 30 | | | | | 13 | 22 | 36 | 40 | | | | 48 | 58 | 73 | 78 |
| 68 | 173 | 84 | 63* | 74 | 76 | 86 | 101 | 104 | 114* | 7 | 7 | 10 | 11 | 23 | 27 | | | 8 | 11 | 20 | 36 | 35 | 38 | | 50 | 52 | 61 | 73 | 86 |
| 69 | 175 | 126 | 68 | 71 | 74 | 89 | 103 | 105 | 114 | 9 | 7 | 8 | 14 | 22 | 29 | 31 | 9 | 12 | 14 | 20 | 31 | 32 | 38 | 46 | 51 | 53 | 65 | 73 | 78 | 83 |
| 70 | 178 | 150 | 68 | 72 | 74 | 87 | 106 | 112 | 114 | 7 | 7 | 7 | 15 | 23 | 25 | 30 | 7 | 10 | 11 | 18 | 31 | 35 | 46 | 43 | 48 | 49 | 61 | 75 | 77 | 86 |
| 71 | 180 | 123 | 73 | 78 | 82 | 91 | 113 | 116 | 123 | 6 | 8 | 10 | 14 | 25 | 27 | 31 | 9 | 11 | 11 | 17 | 35 | 40 | 36 | 47 | 47 | 50 | 61 | 75 | 81 | 83 |
| 72 | 183 | 114 | 73 | 76 | 78 | 91 | 109 | 112 | 121 | 5 | 6 | 7 | 15 | 20 | 22 | 25 | 8 | 9 | 9 | 20 | 28 | 30 | 30 | 45 | 48 | 50 | 62 | 77 | 80 | 86 |
| 73 | 185 | 109 | 72 | 77 | 79 | 93 | 106 | 107 | 116 | 5 | 6 | 7 | 12 | 19 | 22 | 31 | 7 | 9 | 9 | 19 | 27 | 28 | | 47 | 49 | 50 | 61 | 79 | 83 | 86 |
| 74 | 188 | 37 | 69* | 74* | 82 | 92 | 105 | 115* | 120* | | 8 | 8 | 13 | 19 | | | | | 9 | 18 | 32 | | | | | 53 | 66 | 78 | | |
| **Females** | | | | | | | | | | | | | | | | | | | | | | | | | | | | | | |
| 58 | 147 | 6 | 56* | 63* | 67* | 86* | 105* | 110* | 117* | | | | | | | | | | | | | | | | | | | | |
| 59 | 150 | 19 | 56* | 62* | 67* | 78 | 105* | 109* | 116* | | | | 36 | | | | | | | 35 | | | | | | | 45 | | |
| 60 | 152 | 32 | 55* | 62* | 66* | 87 | 104* | 109* | 116* | | | | 38 | | | | | | | 42 | | | | | | | 44 | | |
| 61 | 155 | 92 | 54* | 64 | 66 | 81 | 105 | 111 | 115* | 16 | 17 | 26 | 36 | 48 | 50 | 50 | 13 | 17 | 17 | 35 | 48 | 53 | 55 | 26 | 29 | 33 | 41 | 62 | 74 | 72 |
| 62 | 157 | 135 | 59 | 61 | 65 | 81 | 103 | 107 | 113 | 16 | 19 | 22 | 34 | 48 | 48 | 51 | 11 | 16 | 18 | 32 | 48 | 51 | 50 | 27 | 28 | 31 | 44 | 56 | 63 | 77 |
| 63 | 160 | 162 | 58 | 63 | 67 | 83 | 105 | 109 | 119 | 18 | 20 | 22 | 34 | 46 | 48 | 49 | 10 | 14 | 16 | 32 | 44 | 48 | 50 | 26 | 30 | 32 | 43 | 60 | 65 | 63 |
| 64 | 163 | 196 | 59 | 62 | 63 | 79 | 102 | 109 | 114 | 20 | 20 | 21 | 32 | 43 | 45 | 49 | 8 | 12 | 15 | 28 | 42 | 46 | 52 | 27 | 28 | 29 | 39 | 50 | 55 | 63 |
| 65 | 165 | 242 | 59 | 61 | 63 | 81 | 103 | 109 | 114 | 17 | 21 | 18 | 31 | 43 | 46 | 48 | 7 | 9 | 14 | 29 | 42 | 48 | 45 | 23 | 28 | 29 | 39 | 56 | 59 | 67 |
| 66 | 168 | 166 | 55 | 58 | 58 | 75 | 95 | 100 | 107 | 13 | 17 | 17 | 27 | 40 | 43 | 45 | | 10 | 11 | 25 | 36 | 48 | 55 | 28 | 24 | 29 | 35 | 59 | 53 | 69 |
| 67 | 170 | 144 | 58 | 60 | 65 | 80 | 100 | 108 | 114 | 13 | 16 | 20 | 30 | 41 | 43 | 49 | | 10 | 11 | 25 | 41 | 46 | | 25 | 28 | 30 | 37 | 50 | 53 | 55 |
| 68 | 173 | 81 | 51* | 66 | 66 | 76 | 104 | 105 | 111* | 16 | 20 | 21 | 29 | 37 | 40 | 55 | | | 12 | 21 | 45 | 48 | | | | 30 | 38 | 51 | 54 | |
| 69 | 175 | 39 | 50* | 57* | 68 | 79 | 105 | 104* | 111* | | | 21 | 30 | 42 | | | | | 11 | 20 | 43 | | | | | 27 | 35 | 49 | | |
| 70 | 178 | 17 | 50* | 56* | 61* | 76 | 99* | 104* | 110* | | | | 20 | | | | | | | 16 | | | | | | | 37 | | | |

*Value estimated through linear regression equation.
†From Frisancho A.R.: Am. J. Clin. Nutr. 40:808–819, 1984, with permission.

# Table A–6a–4. Selected Percentiles of Weight, Triceps and Subscapular Skinfolds, and Bone-Free Upper Arm Muscle Area (AMA) for U.S. Males and Females with Small Frames (55- to 74-yr-old)†

| Ht (in) | Ht (cm) | n | Wt (kg) | | | | | | | Triceps (mm) | | | | | | | Subscapular (mm) | | | | | | | Bone-free AMA (cm²) | | | | | | |
|---|---|---|---|---|---|---|---|---|---|---|---|---|---|---|---|---|---|---|---|---|---|---|---|---|---|---|---|---|---|---|
| | | | 5 | 10 | 15 | 50 | 85 | 90 | 95 | 5 | 10 | 15 | 50 | 85 | 90 | 95 | 5 | 10 | 15 | 50 | 85 | 90 | 95 | 5 | 10 | 15 | 50 | 85 | 90 | 95 |
| **Males** | | | | | | | | | | | | | | | | | | | | | | | | | | | | | | |
| 62 | 157 | 47 | 45* | 49* | 56 | 61 | 68 | 73* | 77* | | | 6 | 9 | 12 | | | | | 11 | 16 | 23 | | | | | 38 | 46 | 52 | | |
| 63 | 160 | 78 | 47* | 49 | 51 | 62 | 71 | 71 | 79* | | 5 | 5 | 10 | 16 | 16 | 17 | | 6 | 6 | 12 | 21 | 22 | | | 34 | 35 | 43 | 54 | 55 | |
| 64 | 163 | 107 | 47 | 50 | 54 | 63 | 72 | 74 | 80 | 4 | 4 | 4 | 9 | 20 | 21 | 22 | 6 | 7 | 7 | 14 | 24 | 25 | 29 | 26 | 30 | 31 | 44 | 53 | 54 | 56 |
| 65 | 165 | 132 | 48 | 54 | 59 | 70 | 80 | 90 | 90 | 4 | 6 | 7 | 11 | 18 | 19 | 24 | 6 | 8 | 8 | 16 | 28 | 28 | 29 | 26 | 30 | 34 | 48 | 57 | 60 | 62 |
| 66 | 168 | 112 | 51 | 55 | 59 | 68 | 77 | 80 | 84 | 5 | 6 | 7 | 11 | 16 | 20 | 20 | 7 | 8 | 8 | 15 | 25 | 26 | 30 | 25 | 31 | 35 | 45 | 54 | 58 | 64 |
| 67 | 170 | 128 | 55 | 60 | 61 | 69 | 79 | 81 | 88 | 5 | 6 | 6 | 10 | 15 | 17 | 25 | 7 | 8 | 9 | 13 | 22 | 25 | 31 | 30 | 36 | 37 | 45 | 53 | 55 | 59 |
| 68 | 173 | 95 | 54* | 54 | 58 | 70 | 79 | 81 | 86* | | 5 | 5 | 10 | 15 | 17 | | | 7 | 7 | 13 | 21 | 27 | | | 35 | 35 | 43 | 55 | 60 | |
| 69 | 175 | 47 | 56* | 59* | 63 | 75 | 81 | 84* | 88* | | | 8 | 11 | 15 | 17 | | | | 10 | 16 | 27 | | | | | 38 | 47 | 62 | | |
| 70 | 178 | 29 | 57* | 61* | 63* | 76 | 83* | 86* | 89* | | | | 9 | | | | | | | 13 | | | | | | | 48 | | | |
| 71 | 180 | 14 | 59* | 62* | 65* | 69 | 85* | 87* | 91* | | | | | | | | | | | 10 | | | | | | | 43 | | | |
| 72 | 183 | 6 | 60* | 64* | 66* | 76* | 86* | 89* | 92* | | | | | | | | | | | | | | | | | | | | | |
| 73 | 185 | 1 | 62* | 65* | 68* | 78* | 88* | 90* | 94* | | | | | | | | | | | | | | | | | | | | | |
| 74 | 188 | 1 | 63* | 67* | 69* | 77* | 89* | 92* | 95* | | | | | | | | | | | | | | | | | | | | | |
| **Females** | | | | | | | | | | | | | | | | | | | | | | | | | | | | | | |
| 58 | 147 | 85 | 39* | 46 | 48 | 54 | 63 | 65 | 71 | 11 | 14 | 16 | 21 | 31 | 34 | | 8 | 9 | 9 | 18 | 32 | 33 | | | 22 | 23 | 29 | 40 | 42 | |
| 59 | 150 | 122 | 41 | 45 | 48 | 55 | 66 | 68 | 74 | | 13 | 15 | 21 | 30 | 31 | 33 | 7 | 7 | 9 | 19 | 29 | 30 | 33 | | 23 | 24 | 30 | 39 | 40 | 44 |
| 60 | 152 | 157 | 43 | 45 | 47 | 54 | 67 | 70 | 73 | 10 | 11 | 13 | 20 | 29 | 31 | 35 | 5 | 7 | 8 | 15 | 27 | 32 | 36 | 20 | 22 | 23 | 30 | 37 | 41 | 44 |
| 61 | 155 | 145 | 43 | 43 | 45 | 56 | 65 | 70 | 71 | 10 | 12 | 14 | 22 | 29 | 29 | 32 | 6 | 7 | 8 | 17 | 29 | 31 | 34 | 18 | 21 | 23 | 28 | 36 | 40 | 42 |
| 62 | 157 | 158 | 47 | 49 | 52 | 58 | 67 | 69 | 73 | 11 | 11 | 12 | 21 | 29 | 30 | 32 | 7 | 8 | 9 | 17 | 25 | 26 | 30 | 20 | 23 | 24 | 30 | 37 | 40 | 43 |
| 63 | 160 | 89 | 42* | 45 | 49 | 58 | 67 | 68 | 74* | | 12 | 13 | 20 | 29 | 30 | | | 6 | 7 | 14 | 25 | 27 | | | 19 | 20 | 27 | 35 | 36 | |
| 64 | 163 | 50 | 43* | 47 | 49 | 60 | 68 | 70 | 75* | | 12 | 13 | 21 | 27 | 29 | | | 6 | 7 | 18 | 24 | 25 | | | 21 | 21 | 28 | 37 | 42 | |
| 65 | 165 | 26 | 43* | 47* | 49* | 60 | 69* | 72* | 75* | | | | 18 | | | | | | | 13 | | | | | | | 28 | | | |
| 66 | 168 | 12 | 44* | 48* | 50* | 60 | 70* | 72* | 76* | | | | 23 | | | | | | | 13 | | | | | | | 33 | | | |
| 67 | 170 | 1 | 45* | 48* | 51* | 61* | 71* | 73* | 77* | | | | | | | | | | | | | | | | | | | | | |
| 68 | 173 | 1 | 45* | 49* | 51* | 61* | 71* | 74* | 77* | | | | | | | | | | | | | | | | | | | | | |
| 69 | 175 | 0 | 46* | 49* | 52* | 62* | 72* | 74* | 78* | | | | | | | | | | | | | | | | | | | | | |
| 70 | 178 | 0 | 47* | 50* | 52* | 63* | 73* | 75* | 79* | | | | | | | | | | | | | | | | | | | | | |

*Value estimated through linear regression equation.

†From Frisancho A.R.: Am. J. Clin. Nutr. 40:808–819, 1984, with permission.

## Table A–6a-5. Selected Percentiles of Weight, Triceps and Subscapular Skinfolds, and Bone-Free Upper Arm Muscle Area (AMA) for U.S. Males and Females with Medium Frames (55- to 74-yr-old)†

| Ht (in) | Ht (cm) | n | Wt (kg) 5 | 10 | 15 | 50 | 85 | 90 | 95 | Triceps (mm) 5 | 10 | 15 | 50 | 85 | 90 | 95 | Subscapular (mm) 5 | 10 | 15 | 50 | 85 | 90 | 95 | Bone-free AMA (cm²) 5 | 10 | 15 | 50 | 85 | 90 | 95 |
|---|---|---|---|---|---|---|---|---|---|---|---|---|---|---|---|---|---|---|---|---|---|---|---|---|---|---|---|---|---|---|
| **Males** | | | | | | | | | | | | | | | | | | | | | | | | | | | | | | |
| 62 | 157 | 49 | 50* | 54* | 59 | 68 | 77 | 81* | 85* | 5 | | 5 | 12 | 25 | | | | | 11 | 19 | 27 | | | | | 39 | 48 | 61 | | |
| 63 | 160 | 89 | 51* | 57 | 60 | 70 | 80 | 82 | 87* | | 7 | 7 | 11 | 20 | | 23 | | 8 | 10 | 15 | 26 | 28 | | | 36 | 38 | 50 | 60 | 63 | |
| 64 | 163 | 210 | 55 | 59 | 62 | 71 | 82 | 83 | 91 | 5 | 6 | 6 | 10 | 17 | 19 | 24 | 6 | 7 | 9 | 15 | 25 | 27 | 35 | 35 | 39 | 40 | 51 | 64 | 66 | 71 |
| 65 | 165 | 335 | 56 | 60 | 64 | 72 | 83 | 86 | 89 | 5 | 6 | 7 | 11 | 17 | 19 | 22 | 7 | 8 | 9 | 17 | 25 | 29 | 31 | 35 | 38 | 41 | 52 | 63 | 65 | 72 |
| 66 | 168 | 405 | 57 | 62 | 66 | 74 | 83 | 84 | 89 | 6 | 6 | 7 | 12 | 18 | 19 | 22 | 7 | 9 | 10 | 16 | 28 | 29 | 31 | 34 | 39 | 42 | 51 | 60 | 62 | 67 |
| 67 | 170 | 509 | 59 | 64 | 66 | 78 | 87 | 89 | 94 | 5 | 6 | 7 | 12 | 18 | 18 | 20 | 6 | 9 | 10 | 17 | 26 | 29 | 34 | 35 | 39 | 42 | 52 | 65 | 67 | 70 |
| 68 | 173 | 413 | 62 | 66 | 68 | 78 | 89 | 95 | 101 | 6 | 7 | 8 | 12 | 18 | 21 | 23 | 7 | 9 | 10 | 17 | 26 | 29 | 32 | 37 | 40 | 42 | 52 | 65 | 67 | 70 |
| 69 | 175 | 366 | 62 | 66 | 68 | 77 | 90 | 93 | 99 | 5 | 6 | 7 | 12 | 19 | 22 | 25 | 6 | 8 | 9 | 16 | 25 | 28 | 30 | 31 | 36 | 40 | 51 | 62 | 65 | 72 |
| 70 | 178 | 248 | 62 | 68 | 71 | 80 | 90 | 95 | 101 | 6 | 7 | 7 | 11 | 18 | 19 | 21 | 7 | 9 | 10 | 16 | 25 | 27 | 30 | 36 | 41 | 44 | 53 | 63 | 65 | 68 |
| 71 | 180 | 146 | 68 | 70 | 72 | 84 | 94 | 97 | 101* | 5 | 6 | 6 | 11 | 16 | 17 | 20 | 7 | 9 | 10 | 15 | 25 | 26 | 31 | 36 | 42 | 44 | 56 | 65 | 67 | 71 |
| 72 | 183 | 81 | 66* | 65 | 69 | 81 | 96 | 97 | 101* | | 6 | 8 | 13 | 19 | 19 | 20 | 7 | 8 | 10 | 16 | 28 | | | | 27 | 39 | 50 | 58 | 59 | |
| 73 | 185 | 35 | 68* | 72* | 79 | 88 | 93 | 99* | 103* | | 8 | 8 | 11 | 16 | | | | | 10 | 15 | 26 | 30 | | | | 43 | 56 | 67 | | |
| 74 | 188 | 11 | 69* | 73* | 76* | 95 | 98* | 101* | 104* | | | | 11 | | | | | | | 18 | | | | | | | 56 | | | |
| **Females** | | | | | | | | | | | | | | | | | | | | | | | | | | | | | | |
| 58 | 147 | 105 | 40 | 44 | 49 | 57 | 72 | 82 | 85 | 5 | 13 | 17 | 28 | 40 | 40 | 41 | 3 | 7 | 10 | 25 | 37 | 43 | 48 | 21 | 23 | 25 | 32 | 46 | 47 | 51 |
| 59 | 150 | 198 | 47 | 49 | 52 | 62 | 74 | 78 | 86 | 12 | 15 | 18 | 26 | 34 | 38 | 41 | 8 | 9 | 11 | 23 | 32 | 36 | 43 | 24 | 26 | 27 | 35 | 44 | 48 | 48 |
| 60 | 152 | 358 | 47 | 50 | 52 | 65 | 76 | 79 | 86 | 13 | 17 | 18 | 25 | 33 | 34 | 38 | 8 | 10 | 12 | 22 | 34 | 36 | 40 | 21 | 24 | 26 | 35 | 45 | 49 | 57 |
| 61 | 155 | 543 | 49 | 51 | 54 | 64 | 78 | 81 | 86 | 13 | 16 | 18 | 25 | 35 | 37 | 42 | 8 | 10 | 10 | 20 | 33 | 36 | 42 | 22 | 24 | 26 | 34 | 44 | 49 | 52 |
| 62 | 157 | 576 | 49 | 53 | 54 | 64 | 78 | 82 | 88 | 13 | 15 | 17 | 24 | 33 | 36 | 39 | 7 | 8 | 10 | 20 | 33 | 36 | 38 | 24 | 25 | 26 | 35 | 45 | 47 | 54 |
| 63 | 160 | 551 | 52 | 54 | 55 | 66 | 79 | 83 | 89 | 12 | 14 | 16 | 24 | 32 | 35 | 38 | 8 | 8 | 10 | 18 | 32 | 37 | 41 | 24 | 26 | 27 | 35 | 44 | 45 | 51 |
| 64 | 163 | 406 | 51 | 54 | 57 | 66 | 78 | 81 | 87 | 12 | 14 | 16 | 25 | 33 | 34 | 37 | 7 | 9 | 10 | 17 | 30 | 33 | 38 | 21 | 24 | 26 | 33 | 44 | 46 | 49 |
| 65 | 165 | 307 | 54 | 56 | 59 | 67 | 78 | 84 | 88 | 14 | 16 | 17 | 24 | 33 | 35 | 39 | 7 | 8 | 9 | 17 | 30 | 35 | 37 | 24 | 25 | 27 | 34 | 44 | 45 | 50 |
| 66 | 168 | 119 | 54 | 57 | 57 | 66 | 79 | 85 | 88 | 12 | 13 | 16 | 24 | 33 | 33 | 36 | 6 | 7 | 8 | 16 | 30 | 31 | 34 | 24 | 26 | 27 | 33 | 41 | 43 | 49 |
| 67 | 170 | 63 | 51* | 59 | 61 | 72 | 82 | 85 | 89* | | 17 | 17 | 27 | 35 | 35 | | | 9 | 10 | 19 | 35 | | | | 27 | 28 | 32 | 41 | 43 | |
| 68 | 173 | 28 | 52* | 56* | 59* | 70 | 83* | 86* | 90* | | | | 25 | | | | | | | 16 | | | | | | | 36 | | | |
| 69 | 175 | 5 | 53* | 57* | 60* | 72* | 84* | 87* | 91* | | | | | | | | | | | | | | | | | | | | | |
| 70 | 178 | 1 | 54* | 58* | 61* | 73* | 85* | 88* | 92* | | | | | | | | | | | | | | | | | | | | | |

*Value estimated through linear regression equation.

†From Frisancho, A.R.: Am. J. Clin. Nutr. 40:808–819, 1984, with permission.

## Table A–6a-6. Selected Percentiles of Weight, Triceps and Subscapular Skinfolds, and Bone-Free Upper Arm Muscle Area (AMA) for U.S. Males and Females with Large Frames (55- to 74-yr-old)†

| | | | Wt (kg) | | | | | | | Triceps (mm) | | | | | | | Subscapular (mm) | | | | | | | Bone-free AMA (cm²) | | | | | | |
|---|---|---|---|---|---|---|---|---|---|---|---|---|---|---|---|---|---|---|---|---|---|---|---|---|---|---|---|---|---|---|
| Ht in / cm | | n | 5 | 10 | 15 | 50 | 85 | 90 | 95 | 5 | 10 | 15 | 50 | 85 | 90 | 95 | 5 | 10 | 15 | 50 | 85 | 90 | 95 | 5 | 10 | 15 | 50 | 85 | 90 | 95 |
| **Males** | | | | | | | | | | | | | | | | | | | | | | | | | | | | | | |
| 62 | 157 | 7 | 54* | 59* | 63* | 77* | 91* | 95* | 100* | | | | 15 | | | | | | | 20 | | | | | | | | | | |
| 63 | 160 | 12 | 55* | 60* | 64* | 80 | 92* | 96* | 101* | | | | 21 | | | | | | | 31 | | | | | | | 57 | | | |
| 64 | 163 | 20 | 57* | 62* | 65* | 77 | 94* | 97* | 102* | | | 11 | 14 | 22 | | | | | | | | | | | | | 44 | | | |
| 65 | 165 | 36 | 58* | 63* | 73* | 79 | 89 | 98* | 103* | | | 8 | 13 | 21 | 25 | | | | 14 | 19 | 27 | | | | | 44 | 59 | 66 | | |
| 66 | 168 | 58 | 59* | 67 | 73 | 80 | 101 | 102 | 105* | | 7 | 9 | 16 | 21 | 25 | 27 | | 9 | 11 | 20 | 31 | 35 | | | 43 | 47 | 56 | 67 | 72 | 79 |
| 67 | 170 | 114 | 65 | 71 | 73 | 85 | 103 | 108 | 112 | 6 | 8 | 8 | 13 | 20 | 21 | 23 | 8 | 11 | 12 | 20 | 35 | 35 | 38 | 41 | 43 | 44 | 56 | 71 | 73 | 74 |
| 68 | 173 | 128 | 67 | 71 | 73 | 83 | 95 | 98 | 111 | 6 | 7 | 8 | 12 | 18 | 20 | 23 | 8 | 10 | 11 | 18 | 27 | 30 | 32 | | 43 | 46 | 57 | 69 | 70 | 74 |
| 69 | 175 | 131 | 65 | 70 | 74 | 84 | 96 | 98 | 105 | 6 | 6 | 6 | 14 | 22 | 25 | 31 | 7 | 11 | 11 | 20 | 27 | 30 | 33 | 40 | 45 | 45 | 58 | 70 | 72 | 79 |
| 70 | 178 | 144 | 68 | 73 | 77 | 84 | 102 | 104 | 117 | 5 | 6 | 8 | 13 | 18 | 22 | | 9 | 11 | 13 | 20 | 30 | 33 | 37 | 43 | 48 | 50 | 59 | 70 | 71 | 87 |
| 71 | 180 | 95 | 65* | 70 | 70 | 84 | 102 | 109 | 111* | | 8 | | 13 | 23 | 26 | | | 8 | 9 | 15 | 30 | 30 | | | 46 | 47 | 54 | 70 | 75 | |
| 72 | 183 | 72 | 67* | 76 | 81 | 90 | 108 | 112 | 112* | | | | 11 | | | | | 8 | 9 | 20 | 28 | 31 | | | 47 | 48 | 59 | 73 | 78 | |
| 73 | 185 | 23 | 68* | 73* | 76* | 88 | 105* | 108* | 113* | | | | 12 | | | | | | | 19 | | | | | | | 59 | | | |
| 74 | 188 | 15 | 69* | 74* | 78* | 89 | 106* | 109* | 114* | | | | | | | | | | | 15 | | | | | | | 54 | | | |
| **Females** | | | | | | | | | | | | | | | | | | | | | | | | | | | | | | |
| 58 | 147 | 14 | 53* | 59* | 63* | 92 | 95* | 99* | 104* | | | | 45 | | | | | | | 44 | | | | | | | 50 | | | |
| 59 | 150 | 26 | 54* | 59* | 63* | 78 | 95* | 99* | 105* | | | | 36 | | | | | | | 31 | | | | | | | 49 | | | |
| 60 | 152 | 72 | 54* | 65 | 69 | 78 | 87 | 88 | 105* | | 25 | 26 | 35 | 44 | 45 | 46 | 13 | 19 | 21 | 31 | 42 | 45 | 48 | 31 | 28 | 33 | 41 | 58 | 60 | 71 |
| 61 | 155 | 117 | 64 | 68 | 69 | 79 | 94 | 95 | 106 | | 22 | 24 | 33 | 40 | 44 | 46 | 13 | 16 | 19 | 29 | 40 | 43 | 53 | 28 | 32 | 34 | 44 | 59 | 61 | 76 |
| 62 | 157 | 126 | 59 | 61 | 63 | 82 | 93 | 101 | 111 | 18 | 24 | 25 | 32 | 41 | 43 | 50 | 13 | 19 | 22 | 30 | 39 | 48 | 51 | 27 | 29 | 34 | 43 | 59 | 63 | 67 |
| 63 | 160 | 154 | 61 | 65 | 67 | 80 | 100 | 102 | 118 | 19 | 24 | 25 | 33 | 41 | 43 | 45 | 10 | 15 | 16 | 29 | 41 | 45 | 55 | 28 | 32 | 33 | 41 | 56 | 62 | 78 |
| 64 | 163 | 147 | 60 | 65 | 67 | 77 | 97 | 102 | 119 | 20 | 22 | 23 | 29 | 42 | 46 | 50 | 12 | 12 | 16 | 24 | 41 | 46 | 48 | 29 | 29 | 32 | 41 | 54 | 60 | 65 |
| 65 | 165 | 117 | 60 | 66 | 69 | 80 | 98 | 102 | 111 | 18 | 22 | 23 | 30 | 43 | 44 | 46 | 8 | 9 | 12 | 26 | 42 | 46 | | | 32 | 32 | 42 | 53 | 57 | |
| 66 | 168 | 64 | 57* | 60 | 63 | 82 | 98 | 105 | 109* | 15 | 17 | 20 | 27 | 35 | 40 | | | 9 | 12 | 26 | 34 | 36 | | | 31 | 31 | 40 | 57 | 57 | |
| 67 | 170 | 40 | 58* | 64* | 68 | 80 | 105 | 104* | 109* | | 18 | 18 | 30 | 44 | | | | | 14 | 25 | 46 | | | | | 30 | 40 | 58 | | |
| 68 | 173 | 17 | 58* | 64* | 68* | 79 | 100* | 104* | 110* | | | 22 | 32 | 44 | | | | | | 21 | | | | | | | 48 | | | |
| 69 | 175 | 7 | 59* | 65* | 69* | 85* | 101* | 105* | 110* | | | 22 | 26 | | | | | | | | | | | | | | | | | |
| 70 | 178 | 2 | 60* | 65* | 69* | 85* | 101* | 105* | 111* | | | | | | | | | | | | | | | | | | | | |

*Value estimated through linear regression equation.

†From Frisancho, A.R.: Am. J. Clin. Nutr. 40:808–819, 1984, with permission.

**Table A–6a-7. Age Correction for Estimates of Weight, Triceps and Subscapular Skinfold Thicknesses, and Bone-Free Upper Arm Muscle Area (AMA)\***

| Age Group: Frame Size | Median Age | Weight | Triceps Skinfold | Subscapular Skinfold | Arm Muscle Area |
|---|---|---|---|---|---|
| | | Males | | | |
| 25–54 | | | | | |
| Small | 39 | 0.074 | 0.016 | 0.080 | 0.030 |
| Medium | 39 | 0.080 | 0.005 | 0.083 | 0.055 |
| Large | 40 | 0.000 | − 0.024 | 0.049 | 0.026 |
| 55–74 | | | | | |
| Small | 66 | − 0.329 | − 0.036 | − 0.115 | − 0.407 |
| Medium | 67 | − 0.435 | − 0.040 | − 0.125 | − 0.521 |
| Large | 67 | − 0.562 | − 0.054 | − 0.185 | − 0.644 |
| | | Females | | | |
| 25–54 | | | | | |
| Small | 37 | 0.165 | 0.166 | 0.142 | 0.087 |
| Medium | 37 | 0.234 | 0.189 | 0.214 | 0.191 |
| Large | 37 | 0.284 | 0.191 | 0.233 | 0.270 |
| 55–74 | | | | | |
| Small | 67 | − 0.027 | − 0.072 | − 0.013 | 0.036 |
| Medium | 66 | − 0.196 | − 0.210 | − 0.221 | − 0.033 |
| Large | 67 | − 0.466 | − 0.370 | − 0.515 | − 0.378 |

\*From Frisancho, A.R.: Am. J. Clin. Nutr. 40:808–819, 1984, with permission.

**Table A–6b.** **Age- and Sex-Specific Reference Values by Percentiles for Weight for Adults 18 to 74 Years of Age*·†·‡**

| Age Group (yrs) | Percentiles | | | | | | |
|---|---|---|---|---|---|---|---|
| | *5* | *10* | *25* | *50* | *75* | *90* | *95* |
| American Men | | | | | | | |
| 18–24 | 56.4 | 60.0 | 65.9 | 73.2 | 81.8 | 92.7 | 100.9 |
| 25–34 | 60.0 | 63.6 | 69.5 | 78.2 | 87.7 | 98.6 | 105.9 |
| 35–44 | 60.0 | 65.0 | 72.7 | 80.0 | 89.1 | 96.8 | 102.3 |
| 45–54 | 59.1 | 63.2 | 71.4 | 79.5 | 87.3 | 97.7 | 102.3 |
| 55–64 | 56.8 | 62.3 | 69.1 | 77.3 | 85.0 | 94.5 | 100.9 |
| 65–74 | 55.4 | 59.1 | 66.8 | 74.1 | 81.8 | 90.0 | 95.9 |
| American Women | | | | | | | |
| 18–24 | 45.4 | 48.2 | 51.8 | 58.2 | 64.5 | 74.1 | 83.2 |
| 25–34 | 46.8 | 49.5 | 54.1 | 60.0 | 69.1 | 82.3 | 91.8 |
| 35–44 | 49.5 | 51.8 | 56.4 | 63.2 | 74.1 | 88.6 | 97.7 |
| 45–54 | 49.5 | 51.8 | 57.7 | 65.9 | 74.5 | 86.8 | 96.8 |
| 55–64 | 47.3 | 50.4 | 58.2 | 65.4 | 75.1 | 86.8 | 92.3 |
| 65–74 | 47.7 | 50.9 | 57.3 | 64.5 | 74.1 | 83.2 | 86.6 |

*Anthropometric reference values based on Health and Nutrition Examination Survey (HANES I, 1971–1974). Reported by Bishop et al.: Am. J. Clin. Nutr. 34:2530–2539, 1981. The sample of 28,043 persons represented the 194 million noninstitutionalized civilians living in the 48 contiguous states of the United States at the time of the survey. Anthropometric measurements were made on the right side of the body.

†Values are in kg. Clothing worn.

‡See Tables A–6a-1 through A–6a-7 for data compiled by Frisancho, A.R.: Am. J. Clin. Nutr. 40:808–819, 1984 from NHANES I and II.

## Table A–7a. Weight of Women Aged 18 to 74 Years by Age and Height: Mean and Selected Percentiles, U.S., 1971 to 1974*·†·‡

| Age and Height | Mean | Percentile | | | | | | |
|---|---|---|---|---|---|---|---|---|
| | | 5th | 10th | 25th | 50th | 75th | 90th | 95th |
| **18–74 years** | | | | Weight in pounds | | | | |
| 57 inches | 123 | 85 | 88 | 105 | 121 | 146 | 165 | 171 |
| 58 inches | 125 | 87 | 92 | 106 | 119 | 139 | 177 | 188 |
| 59 inches | 135 | 95 | 103 | 112 | 131 | 153 | 169 | 185 |
| 60 inches | 137 | 98 | 105 | 115 | 131 | 152 | 180 | 194 |
| 61 inches | 137 | 100 | 104 | 116 | 133 | 154 | 176 | 191 |
| 62 inches | 138 | 103 | 109 | 119 | 132 | 151 | 176 | 194 |
| 63 inches | 144 | 106 | 110 | 122 | 137 | 159 | 187 | 206 |
| 64 inches | 145 | 109 | 114 | 125 | 138 | 161 | 187 | 202 |
| 65 inches | 149 | 110 | 115 | 127 | 140 | 162 | 193 | 212 |
| 66 inches | 150 | 114 | 119 | 128 | 144 | 163 | 192 | 214 |
| 67 inches | 153 | 117 | 122 | 132 | 144 | 164 | 194 | 216 |
| 68 inches | 161 | 122 | 127 | 137 | 154 | 173 | 209 | 238 |
| 69 inches | 158 | 120 | 126 | 133 | 144 | 166 | 216 | 254 |
| 70 inches | 162 | 128 | 130 | 142 | 159 | 172 | 206 | 220 |
| **18–24 years** | | | | | | | | |
| 57 inches | — | — | — | — | — | — | — | — |
| 58 inches | 118 | 87 | 90 | 106 | 112 | 131 | 155 | 157 |
| 59 inches | 118 | 95 | 98 | 107 | 112 | 132 | 145 | 162 |
| 60 inches | 123 | 93 | 96 | 107 | 115 | 132 | 154 | 179 |
| 61 inches | 124 | 97 | 101 | 109 | 118 | 132 | 150 | 182 |
| 62 inches | 124 | 97 | 99 | 109 | 119 | 133 | 150 | 166 |
| 63 inches | 132 | 101 | 106 | 114 | 129 | 142 | 162 | 188 |
| 64 inches | 133 | 104 | 108 | 116 | 130 | 142 | 165 | 179 |
| 65 inches | 135 | 104 | 110 | 119 | 130 | 143 | 162 | 190 |
| 66 inches | 140 | 112 | 114 | 121 | 131 | 154 | 174 | 190 |
| 67 inches | 143 | 112 | 115 | 129 | 138 | 151 | 164 | 187 |
| 68 inches | 142 | 117 | 119 | 127 | 140 | 150 | 161 | 168 |
| 69 inches | 136 | 104 | 119 | 130 | 134 | 142 | 152 | 170 |
| 70 inches | — | — | — | — | — | — | — | — |
| **25–34 years** | | | | | | | | |
| 57 inches | — | — | — | — | — | — | — | — |
| 58 inches | 119 | 95 | 97 | 102 | 115 | 141 | 147 | 157 |
| 59 inches | 126 | 91 | 97 | 115 | 126 | 131 | 151 | 186 |
| 60 inches | 125 | 95 | 97 | 106 | 120 | 134 | 171 | 185 |
| 61 inches | 130 | 100 | 103 | 110 | 121 | 138 | 172 | 187 |
| 62 inches | 135 | 103 | 107 | 116 | 127 | 146 | 172 | 190 |
| 63 inches | 138 | 104 | 109 | 118 | 131 | 147 | 178 | 201 |
| 64 inches | 141 | 107 | 110 | 120 | 131 | 150 | 188 | 207 |
| 65 inches | 143 | 109 | 115 | 122 | 134 | 153 | 187 | 210 |
| 66 inches | 146 | 109 | 118 | 124 | 137 | 160 | 190 | 217 |
| 67 inches | 153 | 120 | 123 | 131 | 144 | 173 | 191 | 221 |
| 68 inches | 162 | 125 | 129 | 137 | 152 | 172 | 217 | 237 |
| 69 inches | 153 | 120 | 124 | 136 | 143 | 155 | 177 | 292 |
| 70 inches | — | — | — | — | — | — | — | — |
| **35–44 years** | | | | | | | | |
| 57 inches | — | — | — | — | — | — | — | — |
| 58 inches | 128 | 94 | 95 | 107 | 118 | 141 | 182 | 216 |
| 59 inches | 136 | 97 | 102 | 117 | 132 | 147 | 171 | 209 |
| 60 inches | 135 | 104 | 109 | 116 | 124 | 149 | 173 | 193 |
| 61 inches | 134 | 101 | 106 | 113 | 128 | 147 | 164 | 180 |
| 62 inches | 142 | 108 | 111 | 121 | 134 | 150 | 181 | 199 |
| 63 inches | 146 | 109 | 114 | 124 | 136 | 164 | 195 | 205 |
| 64 inches | 148 | 111 | 114 | 125 | 138 | 166 | 195 | 210 |
| 65 inches | 155 | 118 | 123 | 131 | 147 | 174 | 201 | 219 |
| 66 inches | 157 | 118 | 121 | 130 | 145 | 167 | 214 | 239 |
| 67 inches | 155 | 123 | 124 | 130 | 146 | 162 | 205 | 235 |
| 68 inches | 171 | 123 | 125 | 145 | 160 | 179 | 240 | 268 |
| 69 inches | 180 | 139 | 143 | 152 | 167 | 184 | 230 | 300 |
| 70 inches | — | — | — | — | — | — | — | — |

## Table A–7a. (continued)

| Age and Height | Mean | Percentile | | | | | | | |
|---|---|---|---|---|---|---|---|---|
| | | *5th* | *10th* | *25th* | *50th* | *75th* | *90th* | *95th* |
| **45–54 years** | | | | | | | | |
| 57 inches | — | — | — | — | — | — | — | — |
| 58 inches | — | — | — | — | — | — | — | — |
| 59 inches | 136 | 94 | 100 | 105 | 148 | 165 | 169 | 174 |
| 60 inches | 146 | 110 | 112 | 118 | 135 | 170 | 214 | 216 |
| 61 inches | 141 | 100 | 108 | 120 | 140 | 154 | 181 | 196 |
| 62 inches | 140 | 108 | 111 | 120 | 134 | 153 | 172 | 195 |
| 63 inches | 149 | 110 | 112 | 125 | 143 | 163 | 187 | 215 |
| 64 inches | 153 | 119 | 123 | 130 | 147 | 167 | 191 | 209 |
| 65 inches | 156 | 116 | 126 | 134 | 150 | 166 | 194 | 217 |
| 66 inches | 155 | 127 | 129 | 139 | 151 | 165 | 186 | 201 |
| 67 inches | 161 | 123 | 124 | 141 | 152 | 183 | 194 | 217 |
| 68 inches | 173 | 132 | 138 | 146 | 186 | 191 | 197 | 212 |
| 69 inches | — | — | — | — | — | — | — | — |
| 70 inches | — | — | — | — | — | — | — | — |
| **55–64 years** | | | | | | | | |
| 57 inches | — | — | — | — | — | — | — | — |
| 58 inches | 122 | 70 | 86 | 101 | 119 | 126 | 181 | 200 |
| 59 inches | 143 | 110 | 112 | 127 | 141 | 161 | 167 | 179 |
| 60 inches | 142 | 103 | 105 | 122 | 145 | 161 | 177 | 188 |
| 61 inches | 148 | 100 | 110 | 128 | 148 | 166 | 183 | 190 |
| 62 inches | 146 | 106 | 116 | 128 | 139 | 164 | 187 | 199 |
| 63 inches | 154 | 109 | 118 | 132 | 147 | 176 | 203 | 223 |
| 64 inches | 151 | 109 | 117 | 129 | 147 | 169 | 191 | 208 |
| 65 inches | 162 | 110 | 119 | 141 | 151 | 171 | 200 | 225 |
| 66 inches | 155 | 90 | 100 | 127 | 151 | 175 | 209 | 223 |
| 67 inches | — | — | — | — | — | — | — | — |
| 68 inches | — | — | — | — | — | — | — | — |
| 69 inches | — | — | — | — | — | — | — | — |
| 70 inches | — | — | — | — | — | — | — | — |
| **65–74 years** | | | | | | | | |
| 57 inches | 130 | 87 | 105 | 113 | 133 | 147 | 167 | 171 |
| 58 inches | 133 | 94 | 105 | 111 | 130 | 150 | 180 | 188 |
| 59 inches | 137 | 94 | 104 | 115 | 131 | 153 | 179 | 190 |
| 60 inches | 138 | 99 | 107 | 116 | 136 | 158 | 178 | 191 |
| 61 inches | 144 | 100 | 112 | 126 | 140 | 160 | 177 | 195 |
| 62 inches | 146 | 106 | 115 | 126 | 142 | 165 | 183 | 200 |
| 63 inches | 149 | 113 | 120 | 131 | 144 | 160 | 183 | 192 |
| 64 inches | 152 | 111 | 121 | 135 | 150 | 167 | 183 | 195 |
| 65 inches | 153 | 119 | 122 | 132 | 150 | 169 | 189 | 199 |
| 66 inches | 162 | 135 | 140 | 146 | 147 | 175 | 208 | 215 |
| 67 inches | 173 | 127 | 145 | 149 | 168 | 190 | 220 | 251 |
| 68 inches | 168 | 132 | 138 | 155 | 171 | 184 | 190 | 223 |
| 69 inches | — | — | — | — | — | — | — | — |
| 70 inches | — | — | — | — | — | — | — | — |

*Examined persons were measured without shoes; clothing weight ranged from 0.20 to 0.62 pound, which was not deducted from body weight.

†See Tables A–6a-1 through A–6a-7 for data compiled by Frisancho (Am. J. Clin. Nutr. 40:808–819, 1984) from NHANES I and II.

‡From the National Center for Health Statistics, Department of Health and Human Services (NHANES I).

**Table A–7b.  Weight of Men Aged 18 to 74 Years by Age and Height: Mean and Selected Percentiles, U.S., 1971 to 1974\*·†·‡**

| Age and Height | Mean | 5th | 10th | 25th | 50th | 75th | 90th | 95th |
|---|---|---|---|---|---|---|---|---|
| | | | | | Percentile | | | |
| **18–74 years** | | | | | Weight in pounds | | | |
| 62 inches | 140 | 108 | 123 | 126 | 140 | 150 | 163 | 169 |
| 63 inches | 147 | 109 | 116 | 126 | 148 | 159 | 177 | 182 |
| 64 inches | 153 | 112 | 124 | 135 | 151 | 166 | 184 | 199 |
| 65 inches | 155 | 116 | 122 | 137 | 155 | 172 | 189 | 198 |
| 66 inches | 162 | 124 | 133 | 148 | 161 | 176 | 191 | 196 |
| 67 inches | 168 | 130 | 135 | 151 | 167 | 183 | 201 | 213 |
| 68 inches | 168 | 129 | 138 | 151 | 168 | 182 | 199 | 212 |
| 69 inches | 173 | 137 | 143 | 153 | 169 | 188 | 210 | 225 |
| 70 inches | 179 | 138 | 144 | 159 | 176 | 195 | 212 | 232 |
| 71 inches | 182 | 141 | 150 | 163 | 181 | 197 | 215 | 230 |
| 72 inches | 188 | 139 | 151 | 166 | 185 | 211 | 225 | 241 |
| 73 inches | 195 | 154 | 159 | 173 | 192 | 214 | 230 | 253 |
| 74 inches | 197 | 148 | 158 | 173 | 196 | 218 | 233 | 264 |
| 75 inches | 208 | 169 | 173 | 179 | 192 | 216 | 274 | 288 |
| 76 inches | 198 | 144 | 164 | 169 | 197 | 213 | 231 | 232 |
| **18–24 years** | | | | | | | | |
| 62 inches | — | — | — | — | — | — | — | — |
| 63 inches | — | — | — | — | — | — | — | — |
| 64 inches | 146 | 118 | 120 | 133 | 145 | 151 | 186 | 187 |
| 65 inches | 138 | 111 | 112 | 121 | 134 | 145 | 164 | 193 |
| 66 inches | 154 | 116 | 125 | 146 | 155 | 165 | 172 | 179 |
| 67 inches | 157 | 121 | 131 | 140 | 153 | 173 | 187 | 203 |
| 68 inches | 155 | 124 | 132 | 142 | 153 | 168 | 180 | 195 |
| 69 inches | 166 | 133 | 139 | 147 | 161 | 182 | 208 | 224 |
| 70 inches | 165 | 129 | 137 | 146 | 162 | 179 | 195 | 213 |
| 71 inches | 176 | 141 | 146 | 157 | 170 | 187 | 202 | 228 |
| 72 inches | 175 | 140 | 147 | 155 | 168 | 185 | 214 | 228 |
| 73 inches | 186 | 132 | 157 | 164 | 180 | 201 | 229 | 247 |
| 74 inches | 191 | 134 | 148 | 159 | 197 | 218 | 228 | 234 |
| 75 inches | — | — | — | — | — | — | — | — |
| 76 inches | — | — | — | — | — | — | — | — |
| **25–34 years** | | | | | | | | |
| 62 inches | — | — | — | — | — | — | — | — |
| 63 inches | 151 | 109 | 110 | 130 | 155 | 159 | 196 | 197 |
| 64 inches | 151 | 111 | 126 | 133 | 148 | 161 | 195 | 206 |
| 65 inches | 155 | 123 | 128 | 136 | 150 | 162 | 194 | 201 |
| 66 inches | 160 | 129 | 134 | 145 | 157 | 176 | 191 | 194 |
| 67 inches | 168 | 134 | 136 | 152 | 167 | 182 | 199 | 207 |
| 68 inches | 166 | 129 | 140 | 149 | 164 | 181 | 196 | 201 |
| 69 inches | 176 | 140 | 148 | 154 | 167 | 194 | 225 | 233 |
| 70 inches | 185 | 141 | 148 | 159 | 180 | 197 | 215 | 253 |
| 71 inches | 178 | 128 | 142 | 154 | 175 | 193 | 212 | 224 |
| 72 inches | 190 | 154 | 157 | 168 | 185 | 210 | 224 | 244 |
| 73 inches | 195 | 156 | 165 | 176 | 192 | 211 | 224 | 241 |
| 74 inches | 191 | 157 | 158 | 167 | 182 | 217 | 226 | 244 |
| 75 inches | — | — | — | — | — | — | — | — |
| 76 inches | — | — | — | — | — | — | — | — |
| **35–44 years** | | | | | | | | |
| 62 inches | — | — | — | — | — | — | — | — |
| 63 inches | — | — | — | — | — | — | — | — |
| 64 inches | 158 | 125 | 139 | 151 | 160 | 173 | 183 | 184 |
| 65 inches | 156 | 121 | 125 | 137 | 159 | 169 | 190 | 192 |
| 66 inches | 165 | 124 | 132 | 144 | 164 | 181 | 192 | 200 |
| 67 inches | 173 | 134 | 147 | 159 | 172 | 185 | 206 | 211 |
| 68 inches | 177 | 140 | 150 | 162 | 177 | 194 | 204 | 209 |
| 69 inches | 172 | 140 | 147 | 153 | 169 | 189 | 199 | 208 |
| 70 inches | 184 | 143 | 147 | 166 | 185 | 198 | 207 | 218 |
| 71 inches | 188 | 155 | 159 | 169 | 186 | 199 | 223 | 232 |
| 72 inches | 195 | 138 | 140 | 169 | 197 | 222 | 237 | 243 |
| 73 inches | 210 | 159 | 172 | 186 | 204 | 225 | 258 | 277 |
| 74 inches | — | — | — | — | — | — | — | — |
| 75 inches | — | — | — | — | — | — | — | — |
| 76 inches | — | — | — | — | — | — | — | — |

## Table A–7b. (continued)

| Age and Height | Mean | Percentile | | | | | | |
|---|---|---|---|---|---|---|---|---|
| | | 5th | 10th | 25th | 50th | 75th | 90th | 95th |
| **45–54 years** | | | | | | | | |
| 62 inches | — | — | — | — | — | — | — | — |
| 63 inches | 151 | 107 | 136 | 143 | 154 | 161 | 168 | 169 |
| 64 inches | 165 | 101 | 126 | 140 | 159 | 193 | 224 | 236 |
| 65 inches | 161 | 116 | 131 | 143 | 161 | 177 | 189 | 211 |
| 66 inches | 166 | 136 | 137 | 151 | 165 | 179 | 194 | 200 |
| 67 inches | 172 | 129 | 143 | 158 | 168 | 185 | 202 | 215 |
| 68 inches | 170 | 126 | 130 | 154 | 173 | 185 | 210 | 223 |
| 69 inches | 178 | 136 | 142 | 162 | 176 | 190 | 215 | 220 |
| 70 inches | 183 | 143 | 147 | 164 | 184 | 199 | 211 | 234 |
| 71 inches | 187 | 134 | 153 | 169 | 190 | 199 | 220 | 236 |
| 72 inches | 193 | 156 | 164 | 176 | 193 | 213 | 225 | 240 |
| 73 inches | 196 | 144 | 156 | 173 | 192 | 217 | 222 | 234 |
| 74 inches | — | — | — | — | — | — | — | — |
| 75 inches | — | — | — | — | — | — | — | — |
| 76 inches | — | — | — | — | — | — | — | — |
| **55–64 years** | | | | | | | | |
| 62 inches | — | — | — | — | — | — | — | — |
| 63 inches | — | — | — | — | — | — | — | — |
| 64 inches | 154 | 104 | 124 | 140 | 154 | 165 | 182 | 201 |
| 65 inches | 163 | 112 | 128 | 146 | 162 | 177 | 196 | 209 |
| 66 inches | 163 | 123 | 131 | 152 | 165 | 176 | 186 | 193 |
| 67 inches | 168 | 128 | 135 | 145 | 167 | 182 | 204 | 229 |
| 68 inches | 170 | 130 | 146 | 154 | 171 | 182 | 201 | 214 |
| 69 inches | 175 | 139 | 146 | 154 | 172 | 188 | 209 | 238 |
| 70 inches | 184 | 139 | 149 | 165 | 177 | 198 | 224 | 236 |
| 71 inches | 187 | 153 | 154 | 167 | 187 | 203 | 214 | 232 |
| 72 inches | 184 | 131 | 132 | 157 | 182 | 213 | 215 | 239 |
| 73 inches | 189 | 158 | 160 | 171 | 194 | 202 | 212 | 233 |
| 74 inches | — | — | — | — | — | — | — | — |
| 75 inches | — | — | — | — | — | — | — | — |
| 76 inches | — | — | — | — | — | — | — | — |
| **65–74 years** | | | | | | | | |
| 62 inches | 148 | 120 | 124 | 138 | 148 | 155 | 172 | 179 |
| 63 inches | 146 | 112 | 121 | 132 | 144 | 156 | 177 | 182 |
| 64 inches | 147 | 110 | 121 | 132 | 148 | 161 | 175 | 182 |
| 65 inches | 155 | 118 | 124 | 141 | 156 | 170 | 181 | 188 |
| 66 inches | 160 | 117 | 129 | 147 | 159 | 175 | 189 | 199 |
| 67 inches | 167 | 127 | 135 | 153 | 167 | 180 | 197 | 212 |
| 68 inches | 169 | 126 | 137 | 152 | 167 | 182 | 204 | 214 |
| 69 inches | 172 | 139 | 143 | 152 | 168 | 187 | 209 | 214 |
| 70 inches | 181 | 139 | 149 | 161 | 177 | 193 | 214 | 236 |
| 71 inches | 188 | 146 | 153 | 178 | 190 | 204 | 218 | 230 |
| 72 inches | 183 | 143 | 149 | 161 | 185 | 202 | 211 | 233 |
| 73 inches | — | — | — | — | — | — | — | — |
| 74 inches | — | — | — | — | — | — | — | — |
| 75 inches | — | — | — | — | — | — | — | — |
| 76 inches | — | — | — | — | — | — | — | — |

*Examined persons were measured without shoes; clothing weight ranged from 0.20 to 0.62 pound, which was not deducted from body weight.
†See Tables A–6a-1 through A–6a-7 for data compiled by Frisancho (Am. J. Clin. Nutr. 40:808–819, 1984) from NHANES I and II.
‡From the National Center for Health Statistics, Department of Health and Human Services.

**Table A–8. Provisional Age- and Sex-Specific Reference Values for Weight in Elderly Subjects\*·†·‡**

| Age Group (yrs) | 5% | 50% | 95% |
|---|---|---|---|
| | | Men | |
| 65 | 62.6 (138.0) | 79.5 (175.0) | 102.0 (224.9) |
| 70 | 59.7 (131.6) | 76.5 (168.7) | 99.1 (218.5) |
| 75 | 56.8 (125.2) | 73.6 (162.3) | 96.3 (212.3) |
| 80 | 53.9 (118.8) | 70.7 (155.9) | 93.4 (205.9) |
| 85 | 51.0 (112.4) | 67.8 (149.5) | 90.5 (199.5) |
| 90 | 48.1 (106.0) | 64.9 (143.1) | 87.6 (193.1) |
| | | Women | |
| 65 | 51.2 (112.9) | 66.8 (147.3) | 87.1 (192.0) |
| 70 | 49.0 (108.0) | 64.6 (142.4) | 84.9 (187.2) |
| 75 | 46.8 (103.2) | 62.4 (137.6) | 82.8 (182.5) |
| 80 | 44.7 (98.5) | 60.2 (132.7) | 80.6 (177.7) |
| 85 | 42.5 (93.7) | 58.0 (127.9) | 78.4 (172.8) |
| 90 | 40.3 (88.8) | 55.9 (123.2) | 76.2 (168.0) |

\*Data from 119 men and 150 women. The subjects were all ambulatory. Wt in kg (lbs)
†See Tables A–6a-1 through A–6a-7 for data compiled by Frisancho (Am. J. Clin. Nutr. 40:808–819, 1984) from NHANES I and II.
‡From Chumlea, W.C., Roche, A.F., Mukherjee, D.: Nutritional Assessment of the Elderly through Anthropometry. Ohio, Wright State University School of Medicine, 1984.

# Table A–9a. Physical Growth NCHS Percentiles*
## Girls: Birth to 36 Months

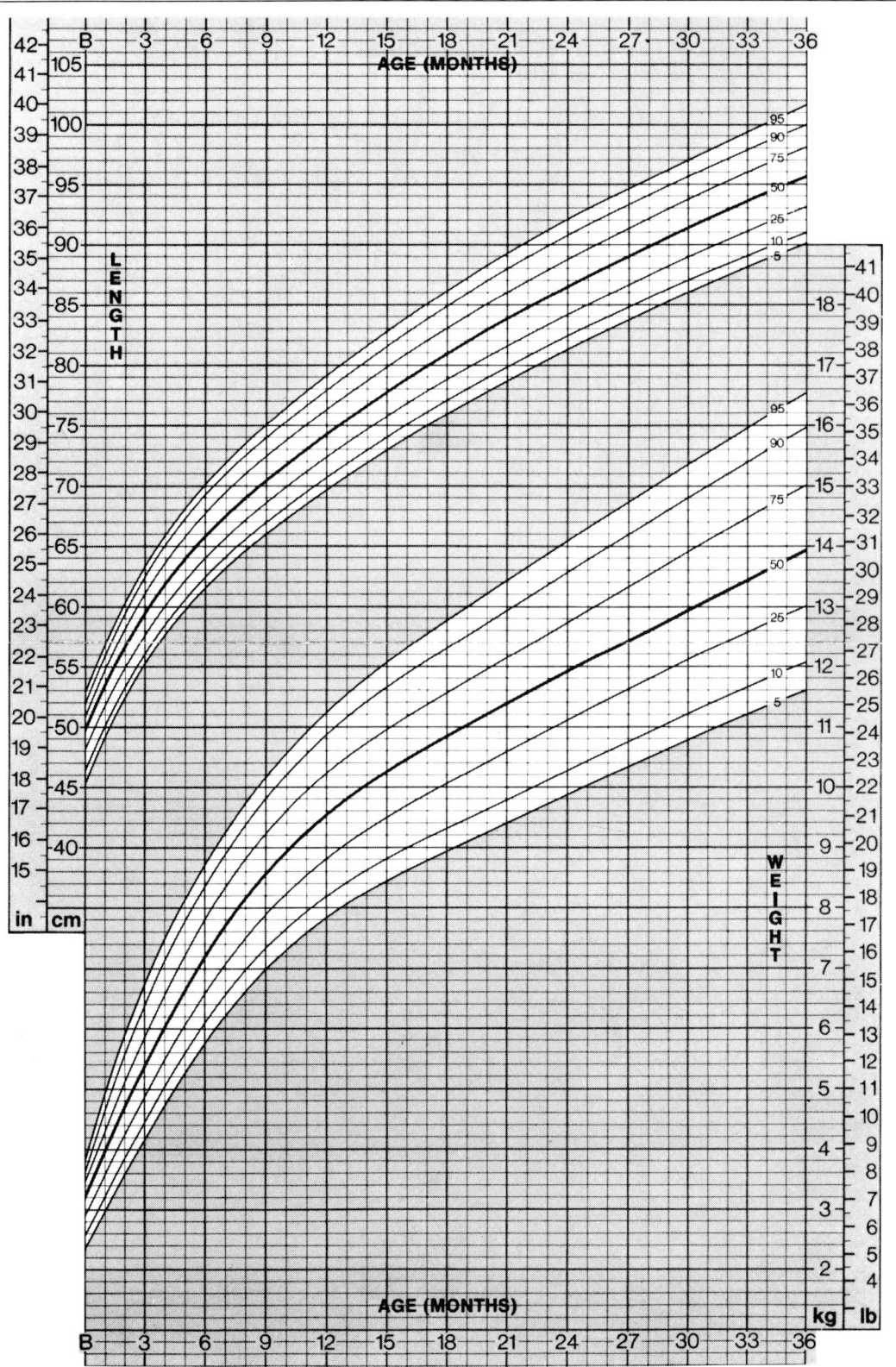

*These tables are used through the courtesy of Ross Laboratories who adapted the growth curves from the original data: National Center for Health Statistics, NCHS Growth Charts, 1976. Monthly Vital Statistics Report, Vol. 25, No. 3, Suppl. (HRA) 76–1120. Rockville, Health Resources Administration, June, 1976. Data from The Fels Research Institute, Yellow Springs, Ohio.

**Table A–9b.    Physical Growth NCHS Percentiles**
**Boys: Birth to 36 Months**

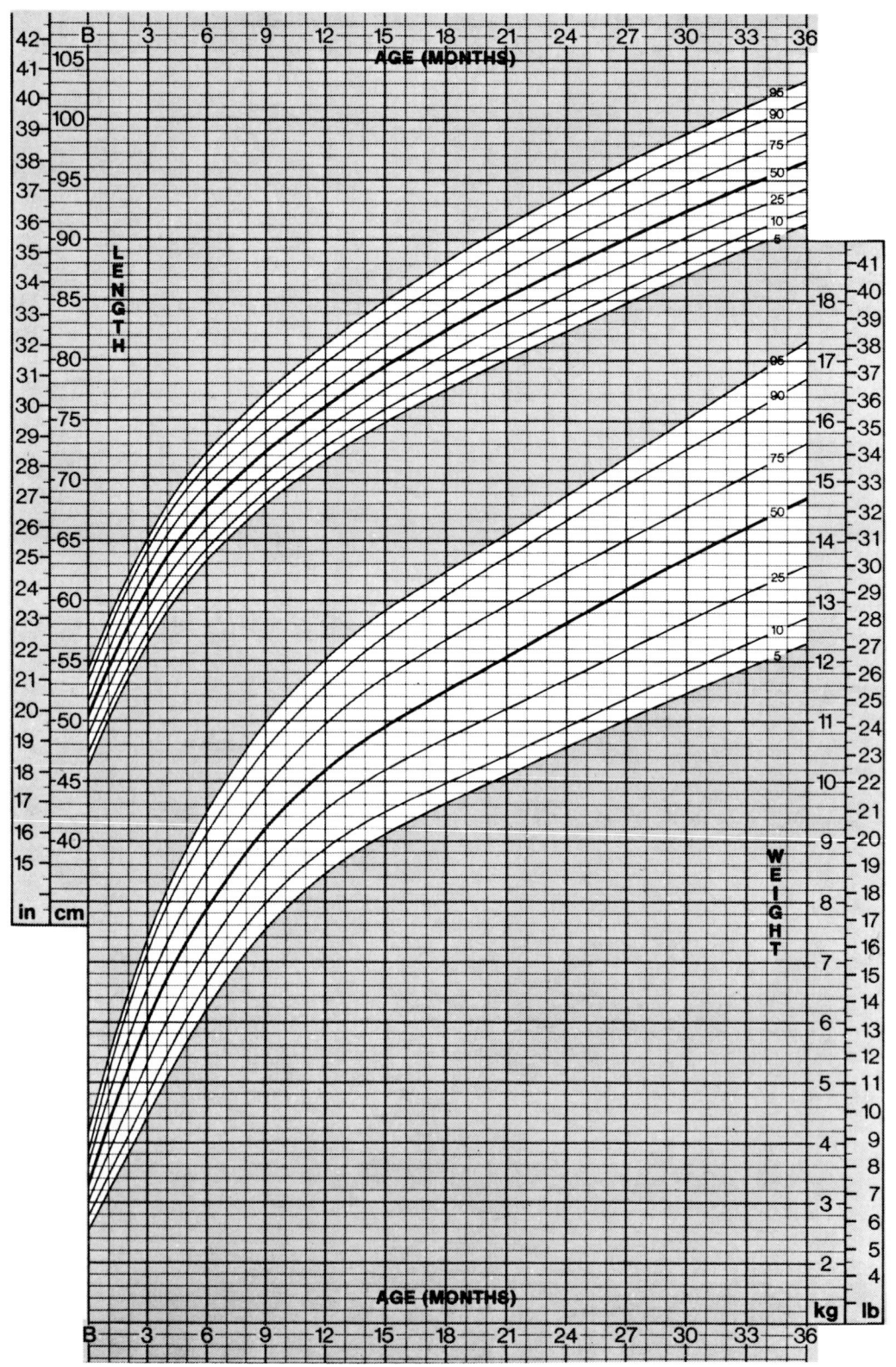

## Table A–9c. Physical Growth NCHS Percentiles
### Girls: 2 to 18 Years

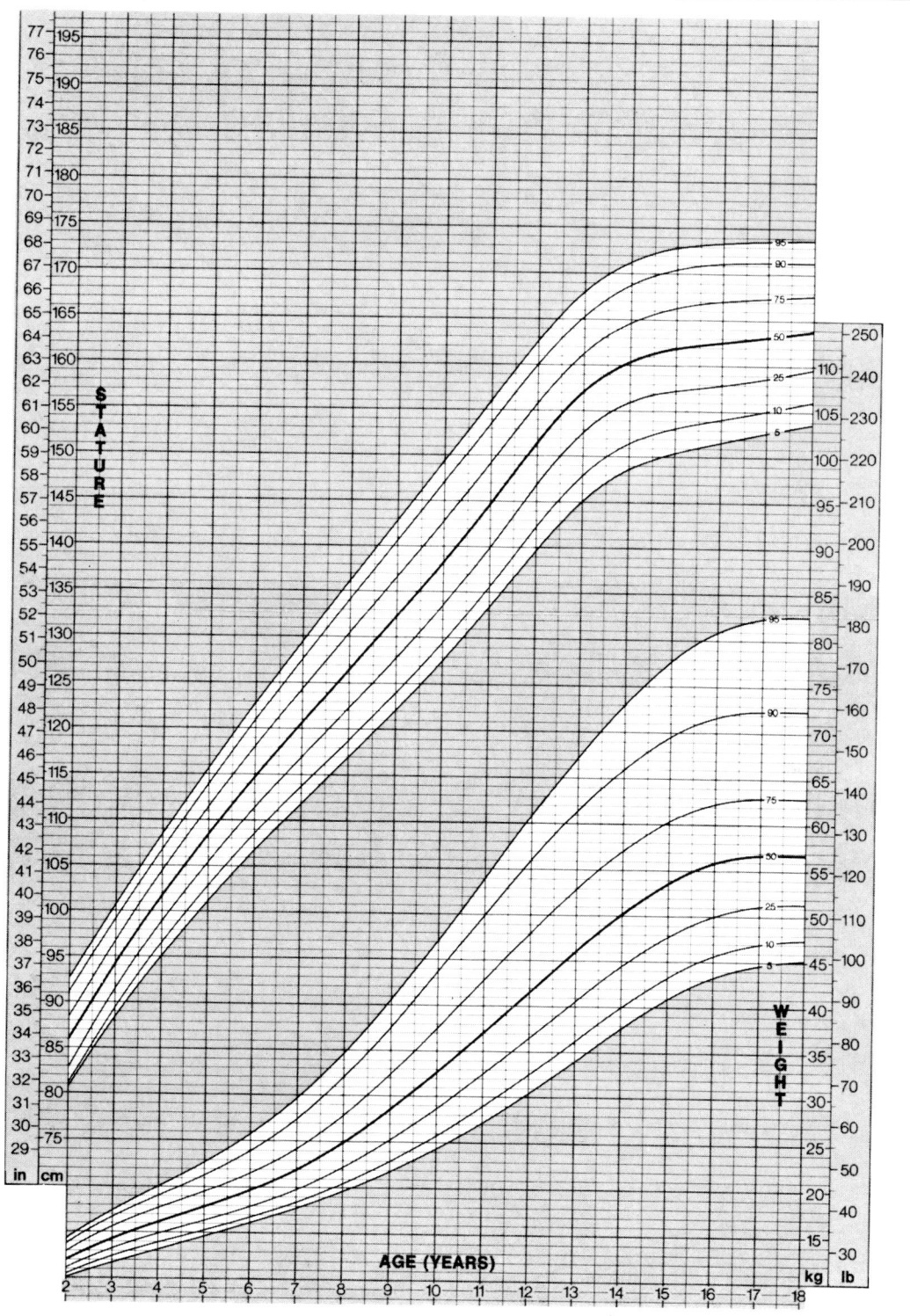

**Table A–9d.  Physical Growth NCHS Percentiles**
**Boys: 2 to 18 Years**

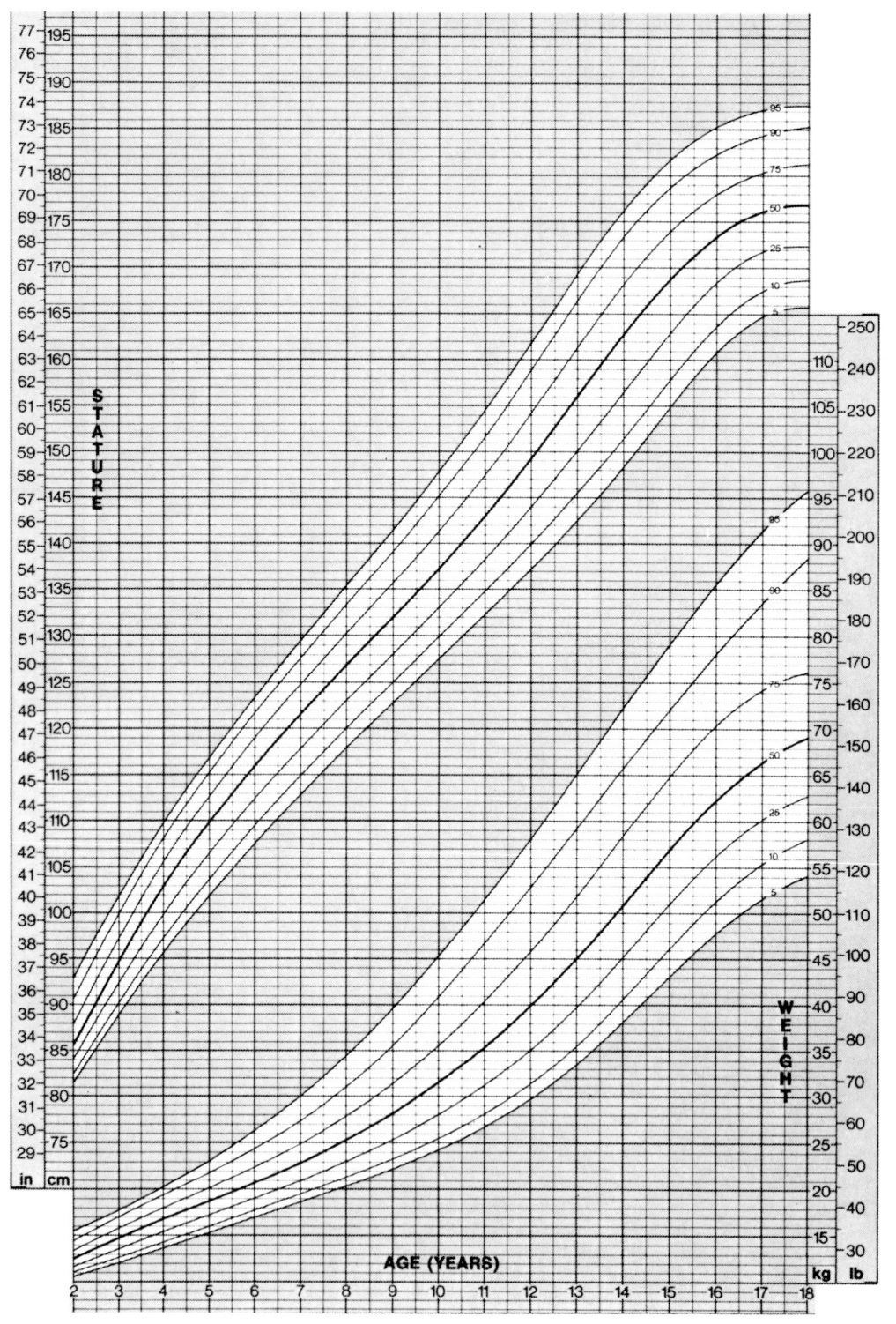

**Table A–10. Nomogram for Estimation of Caloric Requirements**

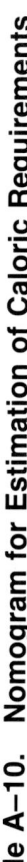

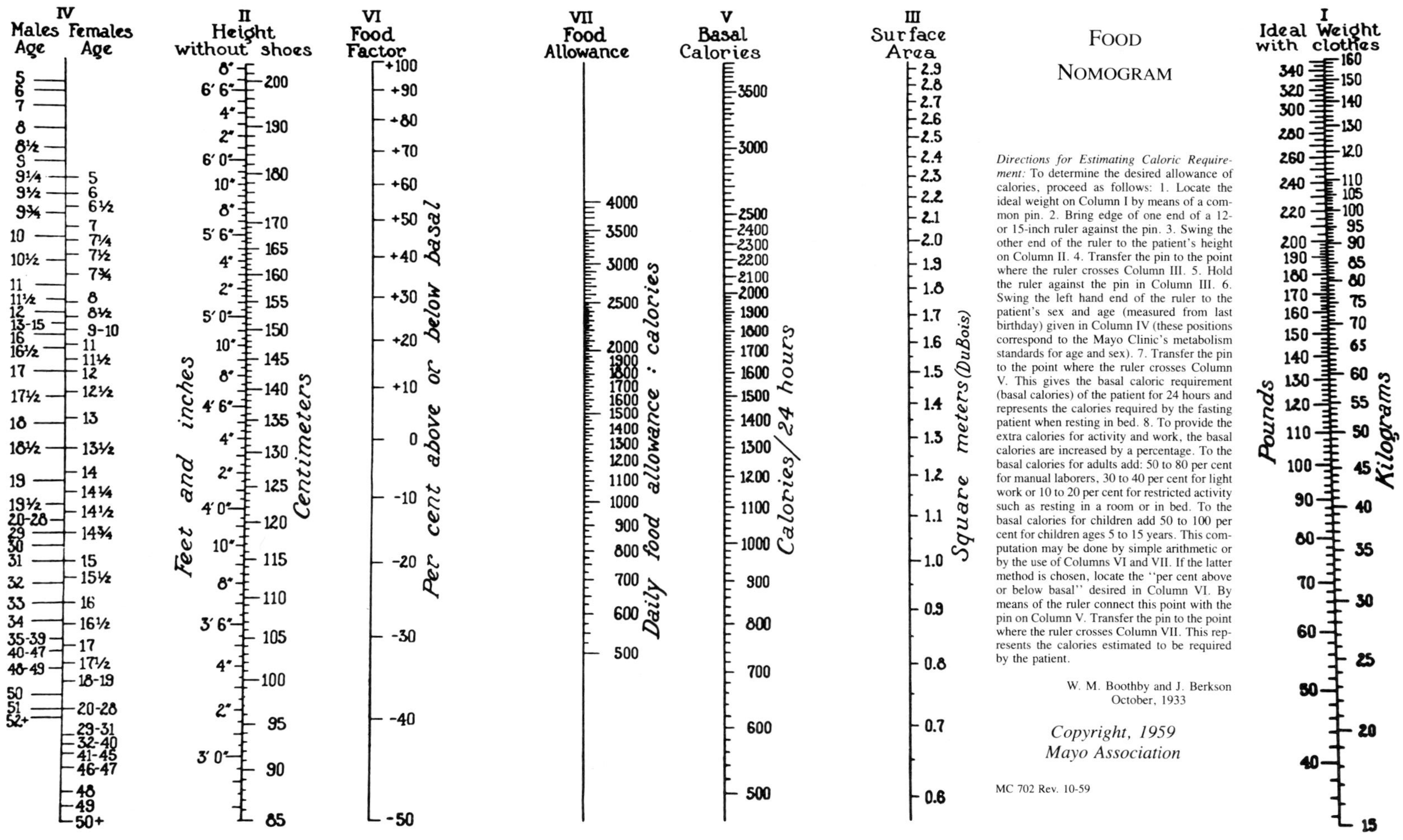

FOOD
NOMOGRAM

*Directions for Estimating Caloric Requirement:* To determine the desired allowance of calories, proceed as follows: 1. Locate the ideal weight on Column I by means of a common pin. 2. Bring edge of one end of a 12- or 15-inch ruler against the pin. 3. Swing the other end of the ruler to the patient's height on Column II. 4. Transfer the pin to the point where the ruler crosses Column III. 5. Hold the ruler against the pin in Column III. 6. Swing the left hand end of the ruler to the patient's sex and age (measured from last birthday) given in Column IV (these positions correspond to the Mayo Clinic's metabolism standards for age and sex). 7. Transfer the pin to the point where the ruler crosses Column V. This gives the basal caloric requirement (basal calories) of the patient for 24 hours and represents the calories required by the fasting patient when resting in bed. 8. To provide the extra calories for activity and work, the basal calories are increased by a percentage. To the basal calories for adults add: 50 to 80 per cent for manual laborers. 30 to 40 per cent for light work or 10 to 20 per cent for restricted activity such as resting in a room or in bed. To the basal calories for children add 50 to 100 per cent for children ages 5 to 15 years. This computation may be done by simple arithmetic or by the use of Columns VI and VII. If the latter method is chosen, locate the "per cent above or below basal" desired in Column VI. By means of the ruler connect this point with the pin on Column V. Transfer the pin to the point where the ruler crosses Column VII. This represents the calories estimated to be required by the patient.

W. M. Boothby and J. Berkson
October, 1933

*Copyright, 1959*
*Mayo Association*

MC 702 Rev. 10-59

I
Ideal Weight with clothes
*Kilograms* / *Pounds*

III
Surface Area
*Square meters (DuBois)*

V
Basal Calories
*Calories/24 hours*

VII
Food Allowance
*Daily food allowance : calories*

VI
Food Factor
*Per cent above or below basal*

II
Height without shoes
*Centimeters* / *Feet and inches*

IV
Males Females Age Age

*From Pemberton, C.M., Gastineau, C.F.: Mayo Clinic Diet Manual. 5th ed. Philadelphia, W.B. Saunders Co., 1981.

## Table A–11a. Triceps Skinfold Thickness: Females, 1 to 17 Years, United States, 1971–1974*

| Race and Age in Years | Number in Sample | Estimated Population in Thousands | Mean‡ | Standard Deviation | Percentile | | | | | | | | |
| --- | --- | --- | --- | --- | --- | --- | --- | --- | --- | --- | --- | --- | --- |
| | | | | | 5th | 10th | 15th | 25th | 50th | 75th | 85th | 90th | 95th |
| All Races† | | | | | | | | Triceps Skinfold in Millimeters | | | | | |
| 1 | 267 | 1,620 | 10.1 | 2.8 | 6.0 | 6.5 | 7.0 | 8.0 | 10.0 | 12.0 | 13.0 | 14.0 | 15.0 |
| 2 | 272 | 1,708 | 10.5 | 2.5 | 7.0 | 7.5 | 8.0 | 9.0 | 10.0 | 12.0 | 13.5 | 14.0 | 15.0 |
| 3 | 292 | 1,701 | 10.9 | 2.7 | 6.0 | 7.0 | 8.0 | 9.0 | 11.0 | 12.5 | 13.5 | 14.0 | 15.0 |
| 4 | 281 | 1,599 | 10.5 | 2.7 | 7.0 | 7.5 | 8.0 | 8.0 | 10.0 | 12.0 | 13.0 | 14.0 | 15.0 |
| 5 | 314 | 1,695 | 10.5 | 3.8 | 6.0 | 7.0 | 7.0 | 8.0 | 10.0 | 12.0 | 13.0 | 15.0 | 17.5 |
| 6 | 176 | 1,787 | 10.3 | 3.3 | 6.0 | 6.5 | 7.0 | 8.0 | 10.0 | 12.0 | 13.0 | 13.5 | 15.0 |
| 7 | 169 | 1,754 | 10.8 | 4.2 | 4.0 | 6.0 | 7.0 | 8.0 | 10.5 | 12.0 | 15.0 | 16.0 | 18.0 |
| 8 | 152 | 1,800 | 12.3 | 4.8 | 6.5 | 8.0 | 8.0 | 9.0 | 11.0 | 15.0 | 17.0 | 18.0 | 22.5 |
| 9 | 171 | 2,017 | 13.2 | 4.8 | 7.0 | 7.5 | 8.0 | 10.0 | 12.5 | 16.0 | 18.0 | 20.0 | 22.0 |
| 10 | 197 | 2,173 | 13.1 | 5.0 | 7.0 | 8.0 | 8.0 | 9.5 | 12.0 | 15.5 | 19.0 | 20.0 | 23.0 |
| 11 | 166 | 1,911 | 14.5 | 6.2 | 7.0 | 8.0 | 8.5 | 10.0 | 13.0 | 18.0 | 20.5 | 23.5 | 28.5 |
| 12 | 177 | 1,812 | 15.0 | 5.9 | 7.5 | 8.0 | 9.0 | 10.5 | 14.0 | 18.5 | 20.0 | 23.0 | 27.0 |
| 13 | 198 | 2,175 | 16.2 | 6.8 | 7.0 | 8.0 | 10.0 | 11.5 | 15.0 | 20.0 | 24.0 | 25.0 | 30.0 |
| 14 | 184 | 2,036 | 17.5 | 7.3 | 8.5 | 9.5 | 10.0 | 13.0 | 16.0 | 21.0 | 24.0 | 27.0 | 33.0 |
| 15 | 171 | 2,163 | 17.0 | 7.0 | 8.0 | 10.0 | 11.0 | 12.0 | 16.0 | 20.5 | 23.0 | 25.0 | 28.5 |
| 16 | 175 | 2,145 | 18.2 | 6.7 | 10.0 | 10.5 | 12.0 | 13.5 | 17.0 | 21.0 | 24.0 | 26.0 | 32.5 |
| 17 | 157 | 1,804 | 19.6 | 8.1 | 10.0 | 11.5 | 12.0 | 13.0 | 19.0 | 24.0 | 26.5 | 29.5 | 35.0 |
| White | | | | | | | | | | | | | |
| 1 | 189 | 1,328 | 10.2 | 2.8 | 6.0 | 7.0 | 7.0 | 8.0 | 10.0 | 12.0 | 13.0 | 13.5 | 15.5 |
| 2 | 203 | 1,434 | 10.6 | 2.6 | 7.0 | 7.5 | 8.0 | 9.0 | 10.0 | 12.0 | 13.5 | 14.0 | 15.0 |
| 3 | 211 | 1,438 | 11.1 | 2.6 | 7.0 | 8.0 | 8.5 | 9.0 | 11.0 | 13.0 | 13.5 | 14.0 | 15.0 |
| 4 | 204 | 1,339 | 10.8 | 2.6 | 7.5 | 8.0 | 8.0 | 9.0 | 10.5 | 12.0 | 13.0 | 14.5 | 16.0 |
| 5 | 224 | 1,416 | 10.7 | 3.7 | 6.0 | 7.0 | 8.0 | 8.5 | 10.0 | 12.0 | 13.0 | 15.0 | 17.5 |
| 6 | 125 | 1,445 | 10.6 | 3.3 | 6.5 | 7.0 | 7.5 | 8.0 | 10.5 | 12.0 | 13.0 | 14.0 | 16.0 |
| 7 | 122 | 1,507 | 10.9 | 4.2 | 4.0 | 6.0 | 7.0 | 8.0 | 11.0 | 12.0 | 15.0 | 15.5 | 17.5 |
| 8 | 117 | 1,507 | 12.4 | 4.7 | 7.0 | 8.0 | 8.0 | 9.0 | 11.5 | 15.0 | 16.5 | 18.0 | 22.0 |
| 9 | 129 | 1,751 | 13.6 | 4.6 | 7.5 | 8.0 | 9.0 | 10.0 | 13.0 | 16.0 | 18.0 | 20.0 | 22.0 |
| 10 | 148 | 1,855 | 13.4 | 4.8 | 7.5 | 8.0 | 8.5 | 10.0 | 12.5 | 15.5 | 19.0 | 20.0 | 23.0 |
| 11 | 122 | 1,569 | 14.9 | 6.1 | 8.0 | 8.5 | 9.0 | 10.0 | 13.0 | 17.5 | 20.5 | 24.5 | 28.5 |
| 12 | 128 | 1,506 | 15.2 | 5.6 | 8.0 | 9.0 | 10.0 | 11.0 | 14.0 | 18.5 | 20.0 | 23.0 | 26.0 |
| 13 | 153 | 1,886 | 16.2 | 6.8 | 7.0 | 8.0 | 10.0 | 11.5 | 15.0 | 20.0 | 24.0 | 25.0 | 28.5 |
| 14 | 132 | 1,731 | 17.8 | 7.3 | 9.0 | 9.5 | 10.5 | 13.0 | 16.7 | 21.0 | 24.0 | 28.5 | 33.0 |
| 15 | 125 | 1,752 | 17.7 | 6.7 | 9.0 | 10.5 | 11.0 | 13.0 | 17.0 | 21.0 | 24.0 | 25.0 | 28.5 |
| 16 | 141 | 1,933 | 18.2 | 6.6 | 10.0 | 10.5 | 12.5 | 14.0 | 17.0 | 21.0 | 24.0 | 26.0 | 32.1 |
| 17 | 117 | 1,549 | 19.8 | 8.0 | 10.0 | 12.0 | 12.5 | 13.5 | 19.0 | 24.0 | 26.5 | 29.5 | 35.0 |
| Black | | | | | | | | | | | | | |
| 1 | 73 | 257 | 10.0 | 3.0 | 5.5 | 5.5 | 7.0 | 8.0 | 10.0 | 12.0 | 13.0 | 14.0 | 15.0 |
| 2 | 66 | 261 | 10.0 | 2.3 | 7.0 | 8.0 | 8.0 | 8.0 | 10.0 | 11.0 | 12.0 | 14.0 | 15.5 |
| 3 | 78 | 245 | 9.7 | 2.9 | 6.0 | 7.0 | 7.0 | 8.0 | 10.0 | 11.0 | 12.0 | 13.0 | 14.0 |
| 4 | 73 | 246 | 8.8 | 2.7 | 5.0 | 6.0 | 7.0 | 7.0 | 8.0 | 10.5 | 12.0 | 13.0 | 14.0 |
| 5 | 88 | 265 | 9.4 | 3.9 | 5.0 | 5.0 | 6.5 | 7.0 | 8.0 | 10.0 | 12.0 | 13.5 | 17.0 |
| 6 | 50 | 336 | 9.0 | 3.1 | 5.5 | 6.0 | 6.0 | 8.0 | 8.0 | 10.0 | 11.5 | 12.0 | 13.0 |
| 7 | 46 | 241 | 10.1 | 4.0 | 5.0 | 6.0 | 7.0 | 7.5 | 9.0 | 11.0 | 17.5 | 18.0 | 18.0 |
| 8 | 35 | 293 | 11.5 | 5.1 | 5.0 | 6.5 | 7.0 | 8.0 | 10.0 | 13.5 | 18.0 | 18.0 | 23.0 |
| 9 | 41 | 247 | 10.2 | 5.1 | 5.5 | 6.0 | 6.0 | 6.5 | 8.0 | 12.0 | 18.0 | 18.0 | 20.0 |
| 10 | 48 | 303 | 11.7 | 5.6 | 6.5 | 6.5 | 7.0 | 7.5 | 10.0 | 16.0 | 18.0 | 19.0 | 24.0 |
| 11 | 42 | 315 | 12.7 | 6.4 | 4.0 | 5.0 | 6.5 | 7.5 | 10.0 | 18.0 | 22.0 | 23.0 | 23.0 |
| 12 | 47 | 284 | 13.6 | 7.6 | 5.5 | 6.0 | 6.0 | 7.5 | 12.0 | 17.0 | 22.0 | 25.0 | 30.0 |
| 13 | 44 | 287 | 16.1 | 7.0 | 7.0 | 8.5 | 10.0 | 11.0 | 14.0 | 18.0 | 24.0 | 24.0 | 33.5 |
| 14 | 50 | 265 | 15.9 | 6.7 | 8.0 | 8.0 | 9.0 | 10.5 | 14.0 | 20.5 | 24.0 | 24.5 | 24.5 |
| 15 | 46 | 411 | 14.0 | 7.6 | 6.5 | 6.5 | 8.0 | 10.0 | 12.5 | 16.0 | 16.5 | 20.0 | 32.8 |
| 16 | 33 | 203 | 18.9 | 8.0 | 8.0 | 8.0 | 10.0 | 12.0 | 19.0 | 24.0 | 24.5 | 33.0 | 33.1 |
| 17 | 39 | 239 | 16.9 | 6.6 | 7.5 | 9.0 | 11.0 | 12.0 | 14.5 | 20.0 | 24.0 | 28.0 | 31.0 |

*From the National Center for Health Statistics, Department of Health and Human Services. See also Bishop, C.W., Bowen, P.E., Ritchey, S.J.: Am. J. Clin. Nutr. 34:2530–2539, 1981.
†Includes data for races that are not shown separately.
‡Measurements made in the right arm.

## Table A–11b. Subscapular Skinfold Thickness: Females, 1 to 17 Years, United States, 1971–1974*

| Race and Age in Years | Number in Sample | Estimated Population in Thousands | Mean‡ | Standard Deviation | Percentile | | | | | | | | |
|---|---|---|---|---|---|---|---|---|---|---|---|---|---|
| | | | | | 5th | 10th | 15th | 25th | 50th | 75th | 85th | 90th | 95th |
| All Races† | | | | | Subscapular Skinfold In Millimeters | | | | | | | | |
| 1 | 267 | 1,620 | 6.2 | 1.9 | 4.0 | 4.0 | 4.0 | 5.0 | 6.0 | 8.0 | 8.0 | 9.0 | 9.0 |
| 2 | 272 | 1,708 | 6.2 | 2.4 | 4.0 | 4.0 | 4.0 | 5.0 | 6.0 | 7.0 | 8.0 | 9.0 | 10.0 |
| 3 | 292 | 1,701 | 5.8 | 2.0 | 4.0 | 4.0 | 4.0 | 4.5 | 5.5 | 6.5 | 7.0 | 8.0 | 9.0 |
| 4 | 281 | 1,599 | 5.6 | 1.9 | 3.5 | 4.0 | 4.0 | 4.5 | 5.0 | 6.0 | 7.0 | 8.0 | 9.0 |
| 5 | 314 | 1,695 | 6.2 | 3.3 | 3.5 | 4.0 | 4.0 | 4.0 | 5.0 | 6.5 | 8.0 | 9.0 | 15.0 |
| 6 | 176 | 1,787 | 6.0 | 2.8 | 3.0 | 4.0 | 4.0 | 4.5 | 5.5 | 6.5 | 7.0 | 8.0 | 10.0 |
| 7 | 169 | 1,754 | 6.2 | 3.3 | 3.0 | 4.0 | 4.0 | 4.5 | 5.0 | 7.0 | 9.0 | 10.5 | 11.5 |
| 8 | 152 | 1,800 | 7.7 | 5.5 | 3.5 | 4.0 | 4.0 | 4.5 | 5.5 | 8.0 | 12.5 | 14.5 | 19.5 |
| 9 | 171 | 2,017 | 8.5 | 5.0 | 4.0 | 4.0 | 4.5 | 5.0 | 7.0 | 10.0 | 13.0 | 17.0 | 19.0 |
| 10 | 197 | 2,173 | 8.6 | 5.1 | 4.0 | 4.5 | 5.0 | 5.5 | 6.5 | 10.0 | 13.0 | 18.0 | 20.0 |
| 11 | 166 | 1,911 | 10.1 | 6.4 | 4.0 | 5.0 | 5.0 | 6.0 | 8.0 | 13.0 | 16.0 | 19.0 | 25.5 |
| 12 | 177 | 1,812 | 11.1 | 6.8 | 5.0 | 5.0 | 5.5 | 6.0 | 9.5 | 13.0 | 16.0 | 20.0 | 25.0 |
| 13 | 198 | 2,175 | 11.9 | 7.1 | 5.0 | 6.0 | 6.0 | 7.0 | 9.5 | 15.0 | 19.0 | 23.4 | 26.0 |
| 14 | 184 | 2,036 | 13.0 | 8.0 | 5.0 | 6.0 | 6.5 | 8.0 | 10.0 | 16.0 | 19.0 | 24.0 | 28.0 |
| 15 | 171 | 2,163 | 12.2 | 7.2 | 6.0 | 6.5 | 7.0 | 7.5 | 10.0 | 14.0 | 18.0 | 20.0 | 27.0 |
| 16 | 175 | 2,145 | 13.4 | 7.8 | 6.0 | 7.0 | 7.5 | 8.0 | 10.5 | 15.0 | 21.0 | 25.5 | 29.0 |
| 17 | 157 | 1,804 | 15.6 | 9.4 | 6.5 | 7.0 | 7.5 | 9.0 | 12.5 | 20.0 | 25.5 | 27.0 | 34.1 |
| White | | | | | | | | | | | | | |
| 1 | 189 | 1,328 | 6.3 | 1.9 | 3.5 | 4.0 | 4.0 | 5.0 | 6.0 | 8.0 | 8.0 | 9.0 | 9.5 |
| 2 | 203 | 1,434 | 6.0 | 2.1 | 4.0 | 4.0 | 4.0 | 5.0 | 6.0 | 7.0 | 8.0 | 8.5 | 10.0 |
| 3 | 211 | 1,438 | 5.8 | 1.9 | 4.0 | 4.0 | 4.0 | 5.0 | 5.5 | 6.5 | 7.0 | 8.0 | 9.0 |
| 4 | 204 | 1,339 | 5.7 | 1.9 | 3.5 | 4.0 | 4.0 | 4.5 | 5.0 | 6.0 | 7.0 | 8.0 | 9.0 |
| 5 | 224 | 1,416 | 6.2 | 3.2 | 3.5 | 4.0 | 4.0 | 4.5 | 5.5 | 6.5 | 8.0 | 10.0 | 15.0 |
| 6 | 125 | 1,445 | 6.0 | 2.7 | 3.0 | 3.5 | 4.0 | 4.5 | 6.0 | 6.5 | 7.0 | 8.0 | 10.0 |
| 7 | 122 | 1,507 | 6.2 | 3.4 | 3.0 | 3.5 | 4.0 | 4.5 | 5.0 | 7.0 | 8.5 | 10.0 | 12.5 |
| 8 | 117 | 1,507 | 7.6 | 5.6 | 3.5 | 4.0 | 4.0 | 4.5 | 6.0 | 8.0 | 10.0 | 13.0 | 21.0 |
| 9 | 129 | 1,751 | 8.5 | 4.7 | 4.0 | 4.5 | 5.0 | 5.0 | 7.0 | 10.0 | 13.0 | 16.0 | 18.0 |
| 10 | 148 | 1,855 | 8.8 | 5.1 | 4.0 | 4.5 | 5.0 | 5.5 | 7.0 | 10.0 | 13.0 | 18.0 | 20.0 |
| 11 | 122 | 1,569 | 10.3 | 6.7 | 4.0 | 5.0 | 5.0 | 6.0 | 8.0 | 13.0 | 16.5 | 20.5 | 25.5 |
| 12 | 128 | 1,506 | 11.1 | 6.4 | 5.0 | 5.0 | 6.0 | 6.5 | 9.5 | 13.5 | 17.0 | 20.0 | 22.0 |
| 13 | 153 | 1,886 | 11.6 | 6.9 | 5.0 | 5.5 | 6.0 | 7.0 | 9.0 | 15.0 | 19.0 | 21.0 | 25.0 |
| 14 | 132 | 1,731 | 13.2 | 8.2 | 5.0 | 6.0 | 6.5 | 8.0 | 10.5 | 16.0 | 20.0 | 24.0 | 30.0 |
| 15 | 125 | 1,752 | 12.4 | 6.9 | 6.0 | 7.0 | 7.0 | 8.0 | 10.0 | 14.5 | 18.0 | 20.0 | 27.0 |
| 16 | 141 | 1,933 | 12.9 | 7.3 | 6.0 | 7.0 | 7.5 | 8.0 | 10.0 | 15.0 | 20.5 | 25.0 | 28.5 |
| 17 | 117 | 1,549 | 15.2 | 9.3 | 6.0 | 7.0 | 7.5 | 8.0 | 12.5 | 18.0 | 25.0 | 26.5 | 34.0 |
| Black | | | | | | | | | | | | | |
| 1 | 73 | 257 | 6.1 | 2.0 | 4.0 | 4.0 | 4.0 | 5.0 | 5.5 | 8.0 | 8.5 | 9.0 | 9.0 |
| 2 | 66 | 261 | 6.8 | 3.3 | 4.0 | 4.0 | 4.5 | 5.0 | 6.0 | 7.5 | 9.5 | 12.0 | 15.5 |
| 3 | 78 | 245 | 5.5 | 2.0 | 4.0 | 4.0 | 4.0 | 4.5 | 5.0 | 6.0 | 7.0 | 7.0 | 8.0 |
| 4 | 73 | 246 | 5.2 | 1.7 | 3.0 | 3.5 | 4.0 | 4.0 | 5.0 | 6.0 | 6.0 | 6.0 | 8.5 |
| 5 | 88 | 265 | 5.8 | 3.5 | 4.0 | 4.0 | 4.0 | 4.0 | 5.0 | 6.0 | 6.5 | 7.0 | 13.0 |
| 6 | 50 | 336 | 6.0 | 3.3 | 3.0 | 4.0 | 4.0 | 4.5 | 5.0 | 7.0 | 7.5 | 7.5 | 10.0 |
| 7 | 46 | 241 | 6.4 | 2.6 | 3.0 | 4.0 | 4.0 | 5.0 | 5.5 | 8.0 | 11.0 | 11.0 | 11.0 |
| 8 | 35 | 293 | 8.2 | 5.2 | 4.0 | 4.0 | 4.0 | 4.5 | 5.0 | 14.0 | 15.0 | 16.0 | 17.5 |
| 9 | 41 | 247 | 8.3 | 6.4 | 4.0 | 4.0 | 4.0 | 4.5 | 5.5 | 7.5 | 14.5 | 24.0 | 24.0 |
| 10 | 48 | 303 | 8.1 | 5.5 | 4.0 | 4.0 | 4.5 | 5.0 | 6.0 | 8.0 | 12.5 | 14.3 | 22.0 |
| 11 | 42 | 315 | 9.2 | 4.5 | 4.0 | 5.0 | 5.0 | 5.5 | 8.0 | 11.0 | 14.5 | 14.5 | 15.5 |
| 12 | 47 | 284 | 10.7 | 8.6 | 4.5 | 5.0 | 5.0 | 5.5 | 7.0 | 11.5 | 16.0 | 28.0 | 31.0 |
| 13 | 44 | 287 | 13.9 | 8.1 | 6.0 | 6.0 | 6.5 | 8.0 | 12.0 | 15.0 | 26.0 | 26.0 | 28.4 |
| 14 | 50 | 265 | 12.5 | 7.3 | 6.0 | 6.0 | 6.5 | 7.0 | 10.0 | 16.5 | 23.0 | 23.0 | 25.0 |
| 15 | 46 | 411 | 11.2 | 8.4 | 5.5 | 5.5 | 6.0 | 6.5 | 7.5 | 10.5 | 19.0 | 20.0 | 33.4 |
| 16 | 33 | 203 | 17.8 | 10.7 | 6.0 | 7.0 | 8.0 | 10.5 | 15.0 | 24.5 | 31.0 | 38.0 | 38.0 |
| 17 | 39 | 239 | 16.4 | 8.4 | 7.0 | 7.5 | 8.0 | 9.0 | 12.5 | 23.5 | 27.0 | 28.0 | 30.0 |

*From the National Center for Health Statistics, Department of Health and Human Services. See also Bishop, C.W., Bowen, P.E., Ritchey, S.J.: Am. J. Clin. Nutr. 34:2530–2539, 1981.
†Includes data for races that are not shown separately.
‡Measurements made in the right arm.

### Table A–11c. Triceps Skinfold Thickness: Males, 1 to 17 Years, United States, 1971–1974*

| Race and Age in Years | Number in Sample | Estimated Population in Thousands | Mean‡ | Standard Deviation | Percentile | | | | | | | | |
|---|---|---|---|---|---|---|---|---|---|---|---|---|---|
| | | | | | 5th | 10th | 15th | 25th | 50th | 75th | 85th | 90th | 95th |
| All Races† | | | | | | | | Triceps Skinfold in Millimeters | | | | | |
| 1 | 286 | 1,693 | 10.4 | 3.1 | 6.0 | 7.0 | 7.5 | 8.0 | 10.0 | 12.0 | 14.0 | 15.0 | 16.0 |
| 2 | 298 | 1,747 | 10.0 | 2.7 | 6.0 | 6.5 | 7.0 | 8.0 | 10.0 | 12.0 | 12.5 | 13.5 | 15.0 |
| 3 | 308 | 1,807 | 9.9 | 2.7 | 6.5 | 7.0 | 7.0 | 8.0 | 10.0 | 11.0 | 12.5 | 13.1 | 14.5 |
| 4 | 304 | 1,815 | 9.4 | 2.5 | 5.0 | 6.5 | 7.0 | 8.0 | 9.0 | 11.0 | 12.0 | 12.5 | 14.0 |
| 5 | 273 | 1,563 | 9.5 | 3.3 | 5.0 | 6.0 | 7.0 | 7.0 | 9.0 | 11.0 | 12.5 | 13.5 | 15.0 |
| 6 | 179 | 1,673 | 8.6 | 3.0 | 5.0 | 5.5 | 6.0 | 6.5 | 8.0 | 10.0 | 12.0 | 12.0 | 14.0 |
| 7 | 164 | 1,979 | 8.9 | 3.5 | 4.0 | 5.0 | 6.0 | 6.5 | 8.0 | 10.0 | 12.0 | 13.0 | 15.5 |
| 8 | 152 | 1,861 | 9.0 | 3.3 | 5.0 | 5.5 | 6.0 | 6.5 | 8.0 | 10.0 | 12.0 | 13.0 | 16.0 |
| 9 | 169 | 2,019 | 10.6 | 4.8 | 5.0 | 6.0 | 6.5 | 7.0 | 9.0 | 14.0 | 17.0 | 17.0 | 19.0 |
| 10 | 184 | 2,205 | 10.9 | 4.4 | 5.5 | 6.0 | 6.0 | 8.0 | 10.0 | 13.5 | 15.0 | 17.0 | 19.5 |
| 11 | 178 | 2,177 | 11.9 | 6.4 | 5.0 | 6.0 | 6.0 | 7.5 | 10.0 | 14.5 | 18.0 | 20.0 | 24.0 |
| 12 | 200 | 2,304 | 11.9 | 6.3 | 4.5 | 6.0 | 6.5 | 8.0 | 10.5 | 13.5 | 16.5 | 20.0 | 27.0 |
| 13 | 174 | 1,978 | 11.2 | 6.6 | 5.0 | 5.0 | 5.5 | 7.0 | 10.0 | 13.0 | 19.0 | 22.0 | 25.0 |
| 14 | 174 | 2,030 | 10.3 | 6.2 | 4.0 | 5.0 | 5.5 | 6.5 | 8.0 | 12.0 | 16.5 | 19.0 | 22.5 |
| 15 | 171 | 2,093 | 10.0 | 6.1 | 4.0 | 5.0 | 5.0 | 6.0 | 8.0 | 11.5 | 15.0 | 19.0 | 23.5 |
| 16 | 169 | 2,019 | 9.7 | 5.2 | 4.0 | 5.0 | 5.0 | 6.0 | 8.0 | 12.0 | 14.0 | 17.0 | 22.0 |
| 17 | 176 | 2,095 | 9.2 | 5.4 | 4.0 | 5.0 | 5.0 | 6.0 | 7.5 | 11.0 | 12.5 | 15.0 | 19.0 |
| White | | | | | | | | | | | | | |
| 1 | 211 | 1,402 | 10.7 | 3.0 | 7.0 | 7.0 | 7.5 | 8.0 | 10.0 | 12.0 | 14.0 | 15.0 | 16.5 |
| 2 | 217 | 1,461 | 9.9 | 2.6 | 6.0 | 6.5 | 7.0 | 8.0 | 10.0 | 12.0 | 12.5 | 13.0 | 14.7 |
| 3 | 226 | 1,536 | 9.9 | 2.6 | 6.5 | 7.0 | 7.0 | 8.0 | 10.0 | 11.0 | 12.5 | 13.5 | 14.5 |
| 4 | 229 | 1,547 | 9.6 | 2.4 | 6.0 | 7.0 | 7.0 | 8.0 | 10.0 | 11.0 | 12.0 | 12.5 | 14.0 |
| 5 | 207 | 1,319 | 9.8 | 3.2 | 6.0 | 6.5 | 7.0 | 7.5 | 9.0 | 11.0 | 12.5 | 13.5 | 15.0 |
| 6 | 126 | 1,343 | 8.9 | 3.1 | 5.5 | 5.6 | 6.0 | 7.0 | 9.0 | 10.0 | 12.0 | 12.5 | 14.0 |
| 7 | 125 | 1,718 | 9.1 | 3.5 | 5.0 | 6.0 | 6.0 | 7.0 | 8.0 | 10.5 | 12.0 | 13.5 | 17.0 |
| 8 | 116 | 1,644 | 9.1 | 3.3 | 5.0 | 5.5 | 6.0 | 7.0 | 8.5 | 10.5 | 12.0 | 13.0 | 16.0 |
| 9 | 117 | 1,636 | 11.1 | 4.8 | 5.5 | 6.5 | 6.5 | 7.5 | 10.0 | 14.0 | 17.0 | 17.0 | 19.0 |
| 10 | 148 | 1,909 | 11.1 | 4.2 | 5.5 | 6.0 | 7.0 | 8.0 | 10.0 | 14.0 | 15.5 | 17.0 | 19.5 |
| 11 | 132 | 1,823 | 12.5 | 6.5 | 6.0 | 6.0 | 7.0 | 8.0 | 10.0 | 15.0 | 19.0 | 20.5 | 24.5 |
| 12 | 152 | 1,970 | 12.4 | 6.1 | 6.0 | 6.0 | 7.0 | 8.5 | 11.0 | 14.0 | 18.0 | 21.0 | 27.0 |
| 13 | 129 | 1,697 | 11.7 | 6.7 | 5.0 | 5.0 | 6.0 | 7.0 | 10.0 | 14.0 | 19.0 | 22.0 | 25.5 |
| 14 | 134 | 1,730 | 10.9 | 6.4 | 4.0 | 5.0 | 6.0 | 7.0 | 9.0 | 13.0 | 18.0 | 20.0 | 24.0 |
| 15 | 124 | 1,728 | 10.2 | 6.1 | 4.0 | 5.0 | 6.0 | 6.0 | 8.0 | 12.0 | 15.0 | 19.0 | 24.0 |
| 16 | 128 | 1,752 | 10.1 | 5.2 | 4.0 | 5.0 | 5.0 | 6.5 | 9.0 | 12.5 | 15.0 | 17.0 | 22.0 |
| 17 | 139 | 1,831 | 9.3 | 5.4 | 4.5 | 5.0 | 5.5 | 6.0 | 7.5 | 11.0 | 13.0 | 15.0 | 19.0 |
| Black | | | | | | | | | | | | | |
| 1 | 72 | 280 | 9.4 | 3.4 | 4.5 | 6.0 | 7.0 | 8.0 | 8.0 | 11.0 | 12.0 | 13.0 | 15.0 |
| 2 | 77 | 267 | 10.1 | 3.2 | 4.5 | 6.0 | 6.5 | 8.0 | 10.0 | 12.0 | 14.0 | 15.0 | 15.0 |
| 3 | 72 | 212 | 9.1 | 2.6 | 6.0 | 6.5 | 6.5 | 7.0 | 9.0 | 10.5 | 12.0 | 12.0 | 13.0 |
| 4 | 74 | 260 | 8.0 | 2.6 | 5.0 | 5.0 | 5.0 | 6.5 | 7.0 | 9.0 | 10.0 | 10.5 | 15.0 |
| 5 | 64 | 226 | 7.7 | 3.4 | 4.5 | 5.0 | 5.0 | 5.0 | 7.0 | 9.0 | 10.0 | 12.0 | 15.5 |
| 6 | 52 | 321 | 7.1 | 1.8 | 4.0 | 4.0 | 5.0 | 6.0 | 7.0 | 8.0 | 9.0 | 9.0 | 9.0 |
| 7 | 38 | 253 | 7.5 | 3.2 | 4.0 | 4.0 | 4.0 | 5.0 | 6.5 | 9.0 | 11.5 | 13.0 | 15.0 |
| 8 | 33 | 203 | 7.8 | 3.4 | 4.0 | 5.0 | 5.0 | 6.0 | 6.5 | 10.0 | 11.0 | 11.0 | 12.5 |
| 9 | 52 | 383 | 8.2 | 3.9 | 3.5 | 4.0 | 4.5 | 6.0 | 7.0 | 8.0 | 12.0 | 13.0 | 18.0 |
| 10 | 33 | 251 | 9.1 | 5.3 | 5.0 | 5.0 | 6.0 | 6.0 | 7.5 | 10.0 | 13.0 | 15.0 | 20.0 |
| 11 | 43 | 313 | 8.0 | 5.0 | 4.0 | 4.0 | 5.0 | 5.0 | 6.0 | 8.5 | 11.0 | 12.0 | 15.0 |
| 12 | 47 | 316 | 9.4 | 7.0 | 4.0 | 4.0 | 4.5 | 6.0 | 7.5 | 10.7 | 11.0 | 15.0 | 24.0 |
| 13 | 45 | 281 | 8.2 | 4.4 | 4.0 | 5.0 | 5.0 | 5.0 | 7.0 | 8.5 | 11.0 | 19.0 | 19.0 |
| 14 | 39 | 282 | 6.6 | 2.6 | 3.5 | 3.5 | 3.5 | 5.0 | 6.5 | 7.0 | 8.0 | 9.0 | 12.0 |
| 15 | 43 | 310 | 8.9 | 6.1 | 4.0 | 4.5 | 5.0 | 5.0 | 6.5 | 9.0 | 10.0 | 21.0 | 21.0 |
| 16 | 41 | 267 | 7.2 | 4.8 | 4.0 | 4.0 | 4.0 | 5.0 | 6.0 | 7.5 | 8.0 | 11.0 | 15.0 |
| 17 | 35 | 235 | 8.7 | 5.8 | 3.5 | 3.5 | 5.0 | 5.0 | 7.0 | 10.5 | 12.0 | 12.0 | 23.2 |

*From the National Center for Health Statistics, Department of Health and Human Services. See also Bishop, C.W., Bowen, P.E., Ritchey, S.J.: Am. J. Clin. Nutr. 34:2530–2539, 1981.
†Includes data for races that are not shown separately.
‡Measurements made in the right arm.

## Table A–11d. Subscapular Skinfold Thickness: Males, 1 to 17 Years, United States, 1971–1974*

| Race and Age in Years | Number in Sample | Estimated Population in Thousands | Mean‡ | Standard Deviation | 5th | 10th | 15th | 25th | 50th | 75th | 85th | 90th | 95th |
|---|---|---|---|---|---|---|---|---|---|---|---|---|---|
| All Races† | | | | | | | | Subscapular Skinfold in Millimeters | | | | |
| 1 | 286 | 1,693 | 6.2 | 1.9 | 4.0 | 4.0 | 4.0 | 5.0 | 6.0 | 7.0 | 8.0 | 8.5 | 10.0 |
| 2 | 298 | 1,747 | 5.7 | 2.0 | 3.0 | 4.0 | 4.0 | 4.5 | 5.0 | 6.5 | 7.0 | 8.0 | 10.0 |
| 3 | 308 | 1,807 | 5.4 | 2.0 | 3.5 | 4.0 | 4.0 | 4.0 | 5.0 | 6.0 | 6.8 | 7.0 | 9.5 |
| 4 | 304 | 1,815 | 5.1 | 1.7 | 3.0 | 3.5 | 4.0 | 4.0 | 5.0 | 6.0 | 6.0 | 7.0 | 7.0 |
| 5 | 273 | 1,563 | 5.3 | 2.7 | 3.0 | 3.5 | 4.0 | 4.0 | 5.0 | 6.0 | 7.0 | 7.0 | 8.0 |
| 6 | 179 | 1,673 | 5.1 | 2.4 | 3.0 | 3.0 | 3.5 | 4.0 | 4.5 | 5.0 | 6.0 | 7.0 | 9.0 |
| 7 | 164 | 1,979 | 5.5 | 3.0 | 3.0 | 3.0 | 3.5 | 4.0 | 4.5 | 6.0 | 7.0 | 9.0 | 11.0 |
| 8 | 152 | 1,861 | 5.1 | 2.3 | 3.0 | 3.0 | 3.5 | 4.0 | 4.5 | 6.0 | 6.0 | 7.5 | 9.0 |
| 9 | 169 | 2,019 | 7.1 | 5.1 | 3.5 | 3.5 | 4.0 | 4.0 | 5.0 | 8.0 | 11.0 | 14.0 | 14.0 |
| 10 | 184 | 2,205 | 6.8 | 4.5 | 3.5 | 4.0 | 4.0 | 4.0 | 5.5 | 7.0 | 10.0 | 12.0 | 18.0 |
| 11 | 178 | 2,177 | 8.0 | 6.2 | 4.0 | 4.0 | 4.0 | 4.5 | 6.0 | 8.5 | 13.0 | 15.0 | 19.0 |
| 12 | 200 | 2,304 | 8.0 | 6.0 | 3.5 | 4.0 | 4.5 | 5.0 | 6.0 | 9.0 | 11.0 | 14.0 | 20.5 |
| 13 | 174 | 1,978 | 8.8 | 6.9 | 3.5 | 4.0 | 4.5 | 5.0 | 6.5 | 9.0 | 13.5 | 17.0 | 26.0 |
| 14 | 174 | 2,030 | 8.5 | 6.1 | 4.0 | 4.5 | 5.0 | 5.0 | 6.5 | 9.0 | 13.0 | 16.0 | 20.0 |
| 15 | 171 | 2,093 | 9.1 | 6.5 | 4.0 | 5.0 | 5.0 | 5.5 | 7.0 | 10.0 | 13.0 | 15.5 | 23.0 |
| 16 | 169 | 2,019 | 9.8 | 6.2 | 5.0 | 5.5 | 6.0 | 6.5 | 8.0 | 10.5 | 13.5 | 16.5 | 23.5 |
| 17 | 176 | 2,095 | 9.7 | 5.9 | 5.0 | 5.5 | 6.0 | 7.0 | 8.0 | 10.0 | 13.0 | 16.0 | 23.0 |
| White | | | | | | | | | | | | | |
| 1 | 211 | 1,402 | 6.3 | 2.0 | 4.0 | 4.0 | 4.0 | 5.0 | 6.0 | 7.0 | 8.0 | 8.5 | 10.0 |
| 2 | 217 | 1,461 | 5.6 | 1.9 | 3.0 | 3.5 | 4.0 | 4.0 | 5.0 | 6.0 | 7.0 | 7.5 | 10.0 |
| 3 | 226 | 1,536 | 5.4 | 2.0 | 3.5 | 4.0 | 4.0 | 4.0 | 5.0 | 6.0 | 6.5 | 7.0 | 10.0 |
| 4 | 229 | 1,547 | 5.2 | 1.8 | 3.0 | 4.0 | 4.0 | 4.0 | 5.0 | 6.0 | 6.0 | 7.0 | 7.0 |
| 5 | 207 | 1,319 | 5.3 | 2.7 | 3.0 | 3.5 | 4.0 | 4.0 | 5.0 | 6.0 | 7.0 | 7.0 | 8.0 |
| 6 | 126 | 1,343 | 5.1 | 2.4 | 3.0 | 3.5 | 3.5 | 4.0 | 4.5 | 5.5 | 6.0 | 7.0 | 10.0 |
| 7 | 125 | 1,718 | 5.6 | 3.1 | 3.0 | 3.0 | 3.5 | 4.0 | 5.0 | 6.0 | 7.0 | 8.0 | 11.5 |
| 8 | 116 | 1,644 | 5.1 | 2.3 | 3.0 | 3.0 | 3.0 | 4.0 | 4.5 | 6.0 | 6.0 | 7.5 | 11.0 |
| 9 | 117 | 1,636 | 7.2 | 4.7 | 3.5 | 4.0 | 4.0 | 4.0 | 5.0 | 8.5 | 11.5 | 14.0 | 14.0 |
| 10 | 148 | 1,909 | 6.8 | 4.5 | 3.0 | 4.0 | 4.0 | 4.0 | 5.5 | 7.0 | 9.5 | 12.0 | 18.0 |
| 11 | 132 | 1,823 | 8.2 | 6.4 | 3.5 | 4.0 | 4.0 | 4.5 | 6.0 | 9.0 | 14.0 | 15.0 | 20.0 |
| 12 | 152 | 1,970 | 8.1 | 5.8 | 3.5 | 4.0 | 4.0 | 5.0 | 6.0 | 9.0 | 11.5 | 14.0 | 21.0 |
| 13 | 129 | 1,697 | 9.0 | 7.1 | 3.5 | 4.0 | 4.0 | 5.0 | 6.5 | 9.0 | 14.0 | 17.0 | 27.0 |
| 14 | 134 | 1,730 | 9.0 | 6.5 | 4.0 | 5.0 | 5.0 | 5.5 | 6.5 | 9.0 | 14.0 | 16.0 | 20.0 |
| 15 | 124 | 1,728 | 8.8 | 6.4 | 4.0 | 5.0 | 5.0 | 5.5 | 7.0 | 9.0 | 13.0 | 15.0 | 22.0 |
| 16 | 128 | 1,752 | 9.9 | 6.4 | 5.0 | 5.0 | 6.0 | 6.5 | 8.0 | 11.0 | 13.5 | 17.0 | 23.5 |
| 17 | 139 | 1,831 | 9.7 | 6.1 | 5.0 | 5.5 | 6.0 | 6.5 | 8.0 | 10.0 | 13.0 | 16.0 | 23.0 |
| Black | | | | | | | | | | | | | |
| 1 | 72 | 280 | 6.0 | 1.6 | 4.0 | 4.0 | 4.0 | 5.0 | 6.0 | 7.0 | 7.5 | 8.0 | 9.0 |
| 2 | 77 | 267 | 6.5 | 2.4 | 4.0 | 4.0 | 4.0 | 5.0 | 5.5 | 7.0 | 10.0 | 11.5 | 11.5 |
| 3 | 72 | 212 | 5.3 | 1.6 | 3.5 | 4.0 | 4.0 | 4.0 | 5.0 | 6.0 | 6.5 | 6.5 | 9.0 |
| 4 | 74 | 260 | 4.8 | 1.2 | 3.0 | 3.0 | 3.5 | 4.0 | 5.0 | 5.1 | 6.0 | 6.0 | 8.0 |
| 5 | 64 | 226 | 5.1 | 2.5 | 2.5 | 3.0 | 3.0 | 4.0 | 4.5 | 5.0 | 7.0 | 7.0 | 8.5 |
| 6 | 52 | 321 | 4.9 | 2.1 | 3.0 | 3.0 | 3.5 | 4.0 | 5.0 | 5.0 | 5.5 | 7.0 | 7.0 |
| 7 | 38 | 253 | 5.2 | 2.4 | 3.0 | 3.0 | 3.0 | 3.5 | 4.0 | 6.0 | 8.0 | 10.0 | 11.0 |
| 8 | 33 | 203 | 5.5 | 2.1 | 3.5 | 3.5 | 4.0 | 4.0 | 5.0 | 6.0 | 7.5 | 9.0 | 9.0 |
| 9 | 52 | 383 | 6.6 | 6.3 | 3.0 | 3.0 | 3.0 | 4.0 | 5.0 | 6.0 | 8.0 | 8.0 | 30.0 |
| 10 | 33 | 251 | 6.7 | 3.8 | 4.0 | 4.0 | 4.0 | 4.5 | 5.0 | 7.0 | 9.0 | 12.0 | 18.5 |
| 11 | 43 | 313 | 6.7 | 4.9 | 4.0 | 4.0 | 4.0 | 5.0 | 5.5 | 6.5 | 8.0 | 8.0 | 12.5 |
| 12 | 47 | 316 | 7.4 | 6.9 | 4.0 | 4.0 | 4.5 | 4.5 | 5.0 | 7.0 | 7.0 | 17.0 | 19.0 |
| 13 | 45 | 281 | 7.6 | 5.9 | 4.0 | 4.5 | 4.5 | 5.0 | 6.0 | 7.0 | 8.0 | 18.5 | 26.0 |
| 14 | 39 | 282 | 6.1 | 2.1 | 4.0 | 4.0 | 5.0 | 5.0 | 6.0 | 7.0 | 7.0 | 7.5 | 12.0 |
| 15 | 43 | 310 | 10.6 | 6.7 | 4.0 | 5.0 | 5.5 | 7.0 | 9.0 | 12.0 | 12.0 | 24.0 | 24.0 |
| 16 | 41 | 267 | 8.5 | 4.2 | 5.5 | 5.5 | 6.5 | 6.5 | 7.0 | 9.0 | 9.5 | 10.0 | 16.0 |
| 17 | 35 | 235 | 9.6 | 5.2 | 6.0 | 6.0 | 6.0 | 7.0 | 8.0 | 10.0 | 12.0 | 16.0 | 16.0 |

*From the National Center for Health Statistics, Department of Health and Human Services. See also Bishop, C.W., Bowen, P.E., Ritchey, S.J.: Am. J. Clin. Nutr. 34:2530–2539, 1981.
†Includes data for races that are not shown separately.
‡Measurements made in the right arm.

## Table A–12a. Triceps Skinfold Thickness: Adult Women, United States, 1971–1974*·†·‡

| Race and Age in Years | Number in Sample | Estimated Population in Thousands | Mean‡ | Standard Deviation | 5th | 10th | 15th | 25th | 50th | 75th | 85th | 90th | 95th |
|---|---|---|---|---|---|---|---|---|---|---|---|---|---|
| All Races† | | | | | | | Triceps Skinfold in Millimeters | | | | | | |
| | 8,410 | 67,837 | 23.0 | 8.4 | 11.0 | 13.0 | 14.0 | 17.0 | 22.0 | 28.0 | 32.0 | 34.0 | 37.5 |
| 18–19 | 280 | 3,679 | 18.6 | 6.8 | 9.0 | 11.0 | 12.0 | 14.0 | 17.5 | 22.0 | 24.0 | 27.0 | 32.0 |
| 20–24 | 1,243 | 9,215 | 19.7 | 7.8 | 10.0 | 11.0 | 12.0 | 14.0 | 18.0 | 24.0 | 27.9 | 30.5 | 34.5 |
| 25–34 | 1,896 | 13,933 | 21.9 | 8.2 | 10.5 | 12.0 | 13.5 | 16.0 | 21.0 | 26.5 | 30.5 | 33.5 | 37.0 |
| 35–44 | 1,664 | 11,593 | 24.0 | 8.4 | 12.0 | 14.0 | 16.0 | 18.0 | 23.0 | 29.5 | 32.5 | 35.5 | 39.0 |
| 45–54 | 836 | 12,163 | 25.4 | 8.3 | 13.0 | 15.0 | 17.0 | 20.0 | 25.0 | 30.0 | 34.0 | 36.0 | 40.0 |
| 55–64 | 669 | 9,976 | 24.9 | 8.5 | 11.0 | 14.0 | 16.0 | 19.0 | 25.0 | 30.5 | 33.0 | 35.0 | 39.0 |
| 65–74 | 1,822 | 7,277 | 23.3 | 7.5 | 11.5 | 14.0 | 16.0 | 18.0 | 23.0 | 28.0 | 31.0 | 33.0 | 36.0 |
| White | | | | | | | | | | | | | |
| | 6,757 | 59,923 | 22.9 | 8.1 | 11.0 | 13.0 | 14.5 | 17.0 | 22.0 | 28.0 | 31.0 | 34.0 | 37.0 |
| 18–19 | 208 | 3,159 | 18.9 | 6.6 | 9.5 | 12.0 | 13.0 | 14.5 | 18.0 | 22.5 | 24.0 | 26.5 | 33.5 |
| 20–24 | 956 | 7,972 | 19.8 | 7.7 | 10.0 | 11.0 | 12.0 | 14.0 | 19.0 | 24.0 | 27.9 | 30.5 | 34.0 |
| 25–34 | 1,539 | 12,161 | 21.8 | 8.0 | 11.0 | 12.5 | 14.0 | 16.0 | 20.5 | 26.0 | 30.0 | 33.0 | 36.5 |
| 35–44 | 1,302 | 10,111 | 23.7 | 8.3 | 12.0 | 14.0 | 15.9 | 18.0 | 22.5 | 29.0 | 32.0 | 35.1 | 38.5 |
| 45–54 | 705 | 10,879 | 25.3 | 8.1 | 13.0 | 15.0 | 17.0 | 20.0 | 25.0 | 30.0 | 33.5 | 35.5 | 39.5 |
| 55–64 | 551 | 9,037 | 24.6 | 7.9 | 11.5 | 14.5 | 16.0 | 19.0 | 24.0 | 30.0 | 33.0 | 34.1 | 38.0 |
| 65–74 | 1,496 | 6,603 | 23.3 | 7.3 | 12.0 | 14.0 | 16.0 | 18.0 | 23.0 | 28.0 | 31.0 | 33.0 | 35.5 |
| Black | | | | | | | | | | | | | |
| | 1,557 | 7,302 | 23.7 | 10.3 | 9.0 | 11.0 | 12.0 | 15.5 | 23.0 | 30.5 | 34.0 | 36.6 | 41.0 |
| 18–19 | 70 | 504 | 16.2 | 7.3 | 8.0 | 9.0 | 9.0 | 11.5 | 14.0 | 20.0 | 25.0 | 29.0 | 32.0 |
| 20–24 | 259 | 1,073 | 19.3 | 8.7 | 9.0 | 10.0 | 11.5 | 12.5 | 17.0 | 24.5 | 28.6 | 32.0 | 36.0 |
| 25–34 | 335 | 1,646 | 22.5 | 9.6 | 8.5 | 10.0 | 12.0 | 14.0 | 22.0 | 30.0 | 32.6 | 34.1 | 40.0 |
| 35–44 | 334 | 1,318 | 25.8 | 9.2 | 11.5 | 13.0 | 16.0 | 20.0 | 25.5 | 32.0 | 35.0 | 36.5 | 41.0 |
| 45–54 | 126 | 1,237 | 26.8 | 9.8 | 12.0 | 14.0 | 17.0 | 20.0 | 26.0 | 34.0 | 37.1 | 40.0 | 42.2 |
| 55–64 | 115 | 871 | 28.2 | 12.9 | 10.0 | 11.0 | 13.0 | 19.0 | 28.0 | 34.0 | 40.0 | 45.0 | 51.5 |
| 65–74 | 318 | 652 | 23.8 | 9.0 | 7.5 | 11.5 | 15.0 | 17.5 | 24.0 | 30.0 | 32.2 | 35.5 | 40.0 |

*From the National Center for Health Statistics, Department of Health and Human Services. See also Bishop, C.W., Bowen, P.E., Ritchey, S.J.: Am. J. Clin. Nutr. 34:2530–2539, 1981.
†Includes data for races that are not shown separately. Measurements made in the right arm.
‡See Tables A–6a-1 through A–6a-7 for data compiled by Frisancho (Am. J. Clin. Nutr. 40:808–819, 1984) from NHANES I and II.

## Table A–12b. Subscapular Skinfold Thickness: Adult Women, United States, 1971–1974*·†·‡

| Race and Age in Years | Number in Sample | Estimated Population in Thousands | Mean‡ | Standard Deviation | 5th | 10th | 15th | 25th | 50th | 75th | 85th | 90th | 95th |
|---|---|---|---|---|---|---|---|---|---|---|---|---|---|
| All Races† | | | | | | | Subscapular Skinfold in Millimeters | | | | | | |
| | 8,410 | 67,837 | 18.8 | 10.2 | 6.5 | 7.5 | 8.5 | 10.5 | 16.0 | 25.2 | 30.0 | 33.2 | 38.0 |
| 18–19 | 280 | 3,679 | 14.4 | 7.7 | 6.5 | 7.0 | 7.0 | 9.0 | 12.0 | 19.0 | 22.0 | 26.0 | 30.0 |
| 20–24 | 1,243 | 9,215 | 15.4 | 8.6 | 6.0 | 7.0 | 8.0 | 9.0 | 13.0 | 19.5 | 23.0 | 27.0 | 32.1 |
| 25–34 | 1,896 | 13,933 | 17.4 | 10.1 | 6.0 | 7.0 | 8.0 | 10.0 | 14.5 | 22.5 | 29.0 | 32.1 | 38.0 |
| 35–44 | 1,664 | 11,593 | 19.6 | 10.8 | 6.5 | 8.0 | 9.0 | 11.0 | 17.0 | 26.5 | 32.0 | 34.1 | 39.1 |
| 45–54 | 836 | 12.163 | 21.2 | 10.5 | 7.0 | 8.5 | 10.0 | 12.0 | 20.0 | 28.0 | 32.5 | 35.0 | 40.0 |
| 55–64 | 669 | 9,976 | 20.9 | 10.3 | 7.0 | 8.0 | 9.5 | 12.5 | 20.0 | 28.0 | 32.0 | 34.5 | 38.0 |
| 65–74 | 1,822 | 7,277 | 19.5 | 9.3 | 7.0 | 8.0 | 10.0 | 12.0 | 18.0 | 25.0 | 30.0 | 32.5 | 37.0 |
| White | | | | | | | | | | | | | |
| | 6,757 | 59,923 | 18.2 | 9.8 | 6.5 | 7.5 | 8.0 | 10.0 | 16.0 | 25.0 | 29.4 | 32.0 | 36.5 |
| 18–19 | 208 | 3,159 | 14.2 | 7.4 | 6.5 | 7.0 | 7.0 | 8.5 | 12.0 | 19.0 | 22.0 | 26.0 | 30.0 |
| 20–24 | 956 | 7,972 | 15.1 | 8.5 | 6.0 | 7.0 | 7.5 | 9.0 | 13.0 | 19.0 | 23.0 | 27.0 | 32.0 |
| 25–34 | 1,539 | 12,161 | 16.8 | 9.8 | 6.0 | 7.0 | 8.0 | 9.5 | 14.0 | 21.5 | 27.5 | 32.0 | 37.0 |
| 35–44 | 1,302 | 10,111 | 18.8 | 10.5 | 6.5 | 7.5 | 8.5 | 10.5 | 16.0 | 25.0 | 30.0 | 34.0 | 38.0 |
| 45–54 | 705 | 10,879 | 20.4 | 10.0 | 7.0 | 8.5 | 10.0 | 12.8 | 19.0 | 27.0 | 31.5 | 34.0 | 38.0 |
| 55–64 | 551 | 9,037 | 20.2 | 9.8 | 6.5 | 8.0 | 9.0 | 12.0 | 19.0 | 27.0 | 31.0 | 34.0 | 37.0 |
| 65–74 | 1,496 | 6,603 | 19.2 | 9.1 | 7.0 | 8.0 | 10.0 | 12.0 | 18.0 | 25.0 | 29.0 | 32.0 | 36.0 |
| Black | | | | | | | | | | | | | |
| | 1,557 | 7,302 | 23.4 | 12.0 | 7.0 | 9.0 | 10.0 | 13.0 | 28.0 | 31.5 | 36.1 | 39.0 | 44.1 |
| 18–19 | 70 | 504 | 14.9 | 9.4 | 6.5 | 7.0 | 7.5 | 9.0 | 12.0 | 19.0 | 20.0 | 26.0 | 38.0 |
| 20–24 | 259 | 1,073 | 17.6 | 9.3 | 7.0 | 8.0 | 9.0 | 11.0 | 15.0 | 22.5 | 28.0 | 30.5 | 35.1 |
| 25–34 | 335 | 1,646 | 21.7 | 11.3 | 6.5 | 8.0 | 10.0 | 12.0 | 20.0 | 30.0 | 33.1 | 36.0 | 41.0 |
| 35–44 | 334 | 1,318 | 26.0 | 11.0 | 9.0 | 10.0 | 12.0 | 17.0 | 26.5 | 34.0 | 38.0 | 40.1 | 42.4 |
| 45–54 | 126 | 1,237 | 28.5 | 12.0 | 10.5 | 11.5 | 14.0 | 17.5 | 30.0 | 37.1 | 40.0 | 43.1 | 46.0 |
| 55–64 | 115 | 871 | 27.5 | 13.4 | 7.5 | 9.5 | 12.0 | 19.0 | 27.0 | 35.5 | 40.0 | 47.0 | 55.0 |
| 65–74 | 318 | 652 | 22.8 | 10.5 | 6.0 | 8.0 | 10.0 | 14.0 | 24.0 | 31.0 | 34.0 | 35.5 | 39.0 |

*From the National Center for Health Statistics, Department of Health and Human Services. See also Bishop, C.W., Bowen, P.E., Ritchey, S.J.: Am. J. Clin. Nutr. 34:2530–2539, 1981.
†Includes data for races that are not shown separately. Measurements made in the right arm.
‡See Tables A–6a-1 through A–6a-7 for data compiled by Frisancho (Am. J. Clin. Nutr. 40:808–819, 1984) from NHANES I and II.

## Table A–12c.  Triceps Skinfold Thickness: Adult Men, United States, 1971–1974*·†·‡

| Race and Age in Years | Number in Sample | Estimated Population in Thousands | Mean‡ | Standard Deviation | Percentile 5th | 10th | 15th | 25th | 50th | 75th | 85th | 90th | 95th |
|---|---|---|---|---|---|---|---|---|---|---|---|---|---|
| **All Races†** | | | | | | | | | | | | | |
| | 5,261 | 61,180 | 12.0 | 5.9 | 4.5 | 6.0 | 6.5 | 8.0 | 11.0 | 15.0 | 18.0 | 20.0 | 23.0 |
| 18–19 | 260 | 3,673 | 11.0 | 6.1 | 4.5 | 5.0 | 6.0 | 7.0 | 8.5 | 15.0 | 18.0 | 19.5 | 23.5 |
| 20–24 | 513 | 8,110 | 11.2 | 6.2 | 4.0 | 5.0 | 6.0 | 7.0 | 10.0 | 14.0 | 17.5 | 20.0 | 23.0 |
| 25–34 | 804 | 13,003 | 12.6 | 6.4 | 4.5 | 5.5 | 6.0 | 8.0 | 12.0 | 16.0 | 18.5 | 21.5 | 24.0 |
| 35–44 | 664 | 10,676 | 12.4 | 5.5 | 5.0 | 6.0 | 7.0 | 8.5 | 12.0 | 15.5 | 17.5 | 20.0 | 23.0 |
| 45–54 | 765 | 11,150 | 12.4 | 5.9 | 5.0 | 6.0 | 7.0 | 8.0 | 11.0 | 15.0 | 18.0 | 20.0 | 25.5 |
| 55–64 | 598 | 9,073 | 11.6 | 5.2 | 5.0 | 6.0 | 6.5 | 8.0 | 11.0 | 14.0 | 16.5 | 18.0 | 21.5 |
| 65–74 | 1,657 | 5,496 | 11.8 | 5.5 | 4.5 | 5.5 | 6.5 | 8.0 | 11.0 | 15.0 | 17.0 | 19.0 | 22.0 |
| **White** | | | | | | | | | | | | | |
| | 4,344 | 54,694 | 12.2 | 5.8 | 5.0 | 6.0 | 6.5 | 8.0 | 11.0 | 15.0 | 18.0 | 20.0 | 23.0 |
| 18–19 | 203 | 3,206 | 11.3 | 5.9 | 5.0 | 5.5 | 6.0 | 7.0 | 9.0 | 15.0 | 18.0 | 20.0 | 23.0 |
| 20–24 | 423 | 7,094 | 11.5 | 6.0 | 4.0 | 5.0 | 6.0 | 7.0 | 10.0 | 15.0 | 18.0 | 21.0 | 23.0 |
| 25–34 | 672 | 11,594 | 12.7 | 6.2 | 5.0 | 6.0 | 6.5 | 8.0 | 12.0 | 16.0 | 18.5 | 21.0 | 24.0 |
| 35–44 | 569 | 9,516 | 12.6 | 5.4 | 5.0 | 6.0 | 7.0 | 9.0 | 12.0 | 15.5 | 17.5 | 20.0 | 23.0 |
| 45–54 | 628 | 10,039 | 12.6 | 5.9 | 5.5 | 6.5 | 7.0 | 8.5 | 11.0 | 15.0 | 18.0 | 20.0 | 26.0 |
| 55–64 | 505 | 8,275 | 11.7 | 5.0 | 5.0 | 6.0 | 7.0 | 8.0 | 11.0 | 14.0 | 16.5 | 18.0 | 21.0 |
| 65–74 | 1,344 | 4,970 | 12.0 | 5.4 | 5.0 | 6.0 | 7.0 | 8.0 | 11.0 | 15.0 | 17.0 | 19.0 | 22.0 |
| **Black** | | | | | | | | | | | | | |
| | 847 | 5,753 | 10.6 | 7.0 | 3.5 | 4.0 | 4.5 | 6.0 | 8.5 | 13.0 | 16.0 | 20.0 | 23.0 |
| 18–19 | 52 | 404 | 8.9 | 6.7 | 2.0 | 4.0 | 5.0 | 5.1 | 7.0 | 8.0 | 12.0 | 21.0 | 24.0 |
| 20–24 | 80 | 866 | 10.0 | 7.9 | 3.0 | 4.0 | 4.0 | 6.0 | 8.0 | 11.0 | 13.0 | 18.0 | 24.0 |
| 25–34 | 119 | 1,232 | 11.8 | 8.4 | 4.0 | 4.0 | 4.0 | 5.0 | 10.0 | 15.0 | 20.0 | 22.0 | 23.0 |
| 35–44 | 87 | 1,005 | 11.3 | 6.5 | 4.0 | 4.5 | 5.0 | 7.0 | 10.0 | 14.0 | 17.0 | 18.4 | 22.0 |
| 45–54 | 130 | 1,057 | 10.0 | 5.1 | 4.0 | 4.0 | 5.0 | 6.0 | 10.0 | 12.5 | 14.0 | 16.0 | 20.0 |
| 55–64 | 85 | 703 | 10.7 | 7.2 | 3.0 | 4.0 | 4.5 | 5.0 | 8.0 | 14.0 | 20.0 | 22.0 | 26.0 |
| 65–74 | 294 | 486 | 9.7 | 5.4 | 4.0 | 4.5 | 5.0 | 6.0 | 9.0 | 12.0 | 14.0 | 15.0 | 19.5 |

*From the National Center for Health Statistics, Department of Health and Human Services. See also Bishop, C.W., Bowen, P.E., Ritchey, S.J.: Am. J. Clin. Nutr. 34:2530–2539, 1981.
†Includes data for races that are not shown separately. Measurements made in the right arm.
‡See Tables A–6a-1 through A–6a-7 for data compiled by Frisancho (Am. J. Clin. Nutr. 40:808–819, 1984) from NHANES I and II.

## Table A–12d.  Subscapular Skinfold Thickness: Adult Men, United States, 1971–1974*·†·‡

| Race and Age in Years | Number in Sample | Estimated Population in Thousands | Mean‡ | Standard Deviation | Percentile 5th | 10th | 15th | 25th | 50th | 75th | 85th | 90th | 95th |
|---|---|---|---|---|---|---|---|---|---|---|---|---|---|
| **All Races†** | | | | | | | | | | | | | |
| | 5,261 | 61,180 | 15.9 | 7.7 | 6.0 | 7.0 | 8.0 | 10.0 | 14.5 | 20.0 | 24.0 | 26.0 | 30.5 |
| 18–19 | 260 | 3,673 | 12.3 | 7.1 | 6.0 | 6.5 | 7.0 | 8.0 | 10.0 | 13.0 | 18.0 | 23.5 | 28.5 |
| 20–24 | 513 | 8,110 | 13.7 | 7.4 | 6.0 | 7.0 | 7.0 | 8.0 | 12.0 | 17.0 | 20.5 | 24.0 | 30.0 |
| 25–34 | 804 | 13,003 | 15.9 | 8.1 | 6.5 | 7.0 | 8.0 | 10.0 | 14.0 | 20.0 | 24.5 | 26.0 | 30.5 |
| 35–44 | 664 | 10,676 | 16.8 | 7.2 | 7.0 | 8.0 | 10.0 | 11.5 | 16.0 | 21.0 | 24.0 | 26.0 | 30.5 |
| 45–54 | 765 | 11,150 | 17.5 | 7.9 | 7.0 | 8.0 | 9.0 | 12.0 | 16.5 | 22.0 | 25.0 | 29.0 | 32.0 |
| 55–64 | 598 | 9,073 | 16.5 | 7.5 | 6.0 | 7.0 | 8.5 | 11.0 | 15.5 | 21.0 | 24.5 | 27.0 | 30.0 |
| 65–74 | 1,657 | 5,496 | 15.9 | 7.2 | 6.0 | 7.5 | 9.0 | 10.5 | 15.0 | 20.0 | 23.0 | 25.0 | 30.0 |
| **White** | | | | | | | | | | | | | |
| | 4,344 | 54,694 | 15.9 | 7.5 | 6.5 | 7.5 | 8.0 | 10.0 | 14.5 | 20.0 | 24.0 | 26.0 | 30.0 |
| 18–19 | 203 | 3,206 | 12.5 | 7.1 | 6.0 | 6.5 | 7.0 | 8.0 | 10.0 | 13.5 | 18.0 | 23.5 | 28.5 |
| 20–24 | 423 | 7,094 | 13.8 | 7.3 | 6.0 | 7.0 | 7.0 | 8.0 | 12.0 | 17.0 | 21.0 | 24.0 | 30.0 |
| 25–34 | 672 | 11,594 | 15.8 | 7.6 | 7.0 | 7.5 | 8.0 | 10.0 | 14.0 | 20.0 | 25.0 | 26.0 | 30.0 |
| 35–44 | 569 | 9,516 | 16.6 | 7.0 | 7.0 | 8.5 | 10.0 | 11.5 | 16.0 | 20.0 | 24.0 | 26.0 | 30.0 |
| 45–54 | 628 | 10,039 | 17.6 | 7.6 | 7.0 | 8.0 | 10.0 | 12.0 | 16.5 | 22.0 | 25.0 | 28.5 | 31.0 |
| 55–64 | 505 | 8,275 | 16.5 | 7.2 | 6.0 | 7.0 | 8.5 | 11.0 | 15.5 | 21.0 | 24.0 | 26.5 | 30.0 |
| 65–74 | 1,344 | 4,970 | 15.9 | 7.0 | 6.5 | 8.0 | 9.0 | 11.0 | 15.0 | 20.0 | 23.0 | 25.0 | 30.0 |
| **Black** | | | | | | | | | | | | | |
| | 847 | 5,753 | 16.1 | 9.9 | 6.0 | 6.5 | 7.0 | 8.5 | 14.0 | 21.9 | 25.0 | 28.0 | 35.0 |
| 18–19 | 52 | 404 | 10.9 | 7.2 | 4.0 | 5.5 | 6.0 | 7.0 | 9.0 | 11.1 | 15.0 | 23.5 | 32.0 |
| 20–24 | 80 | 866 | 13.6 | 8.6 | 5.5 | 6.0 | 7.0 | 8.0 | 11.0 | 17.0 | 19.0 | 26.0 | 30.0 |
| 25–34 | 119 | 1,232 | 16.6 | 11.8 | 6.0 | 6.5 | 7.0 | 8.0 | 11.0 | 21.5 | 25.0 | 30.5 | 42.0 |
| 35–44 | 87 | 1,005 | 18.9 | 8.4 | 7.0 | 7.0 | 8.0 | 12.0 | 19.0 | 24.0 | 25.5 | 31.0 | 33.1 |
| 45–54 | 130 | 1,057 | 16.6 | 9.7 | 6.0 | 7.0 | 7.0 | 9.0 | 13.0 | 22.0 | 26.0 | 32.0 | 35.0 |
| 55–64 | 85 | 703 | 17.0 | 10.5 | 5.0 | 5.0 | 6.5 | 10.0 | 14.5 | 23.0 | 25.0 | 28.0 | 35.0 |
| 65–74 | 294 | 486 | 15.2 | 8.6 | 6.0 | 6.0 | 7.0 | 8.0 | 13.0 | 20.0 | 23.0 | 26.0 | 33.0 |

*From the National Center for Health Statistics, Department of Health and Human Services. See also Bishop, C.W., Bowen, P.E., Ritchey, S.J.: Am. J. Clin. Nutr. 34:2530–2539, 1981.
†Includes data for races that are not shown separately. Measurements made in the right arm.
‡See Tables A–6a-1 through A–6a-7 for data compiled by Frisancho (Am. J. Clin. Nutr. 40:808–819, 1984) from NHANES I and II.

## Table A–13.  Midarm Muscle Circumference in Adults (18–74 Years), United States*·†·‡

| Age Group (yrs) | Sample Size | Estimated Population (millions) | Mean (cm) | Percentile | | | | | | |
|---|---|---|---|---|---|---|---|---|---|---|
| | | | | 5 | 10 | 25 | 50 | 75 | 90 | 95 |
| | | | | Men | | | | | | |
| 18–74 | 5,261 | 61.18 | 28.0 | 23.8 | 24.8 | 26.3 | 27.9 | 29.6 | 31.4 | 32.5 |
| 18–24 | 773 | 11.78 | 27.4 | 23.5 | 24.4 | 25.8 | 27.2 | 28.9 | 30.8 | 32.3 |
| 25–34 | 804 | 13.00 | 28.3 | 24.2 | 25.3 | 26.5 | 28.0 | 30.0 | 31.7 | 32.9 |
| 35–44 | 664 | 10.68 | 28.8 | 25.0 | 25.6 | 27.1 | 28.7 | 30.3 | 32.1 | 33.0 |
| 45–54 | 765 | 11.15 | 28.2 | 24.0 | 24.9 | 26.5 | 28.1 | 29.8 | 31.5 | 32.6 |
| 55–64 | 598 | 9.07 | 27.8 | 22.8 | 24.4 | 26.2 | 27.9 | 29.6 | 31.0 | 31.8 |
| 65–74 | 1,657 | 5.50 | 26.8 | 22.5 | 23.7 | 25.3 | 26.9 | 28.5 | 29.9 | 30.7 |
| | | | | Women | | | | | | |
| 18–74 | 8,410 | 67.84 | 22.2 | 18.4 | 19.0 | 20.2 | 21.8 | 23.6 | 25.8 | 27.4 |
| 18–24 | 1,523 | 12.89 | 20.9 | 17.7 | 18.5 | 19.4 | 20.6 | 22.1 | 23.6 | 24.9 |
| 25–34 | 1,896 | 13.93 | 21.7 | 18.3 | 18.9 | 20.0 | 21.4 | 22.9 | 24.9 | 26.6 |
| 35–44 | 1,664 | 11.59 | 22.5 | 18.5 | 19.2 | 20.6 | 22.0 | 24.0 | 26.1 | 27.4 |
| 45–54 | 836 | 12.16 | 22.7 | 18.8 | 19.5 | 20.7 | 22.2 | 24.3 | 26.6 | 27.8 |
| 55–64 | 669 | 9.98 | 22.8 | 18.6 | 19.5 | 20.8 | 22.6 | 24.4 | 26.3 | 28.1 |
| 65–74 | 1,822 | 7.28 | 22.8 | 18.6 | 19.5 | 20.8 | 22.5 | 24.4 | 26.5 | 28.1 |

*From Bishop, C.W., Bowen, P.E., Ritchey, S.J.: Am. J. Clin. Nutr. 34:2530–2539, 1981. (NHANES I 1971–74)
†Measurements were made in the right arm.
‡See Tables A–6a-1 through A–6a-7 for data compiled by Frisancho (Am. J. Clin. Nutr. 40:808–819, 1984) from NHANES I and II.

## Table A–14.  Midarm Muscle Area in Adults (18–74 Years), United States*·†·‡

| Age Group (yrs) | Sample Size | Estimated Population (millions) | Mean (cm) | Percentile | | | | | | |
|---|---|---|---|---|---|---|---|---|---|---|
| | | | | 5 | 10 | 25 | 50 | 75 | 90 | 95 |
| | | | | Men | | | | | | |
| 18–74 | 5,261 | 61.18 | 62.4 | 45.1 | 49.0 | 55.1 | 62.0 | 69.8 | 78.5 | 84.1 |
| 18–24 | 773 | 11.78 | 59.8 | 44.0 | 47.4 | 53.0 | 58.9 | 66.5 | 75.5 | 83.1 |
| 25–34 | 804 | 13.00 | 63.8 | 46.6 | 51.0 | 55.9 | 62.4 | 71.7 | 80.0 | 86.2 |
| 35–44 | 664 | 10.68 | 66.0 | 49.8 | 52.2 | 58.5 | 65.6 | 73.1 | 82.0 | 86.7 |
| 45–54 | 765 | 11.15 | 63.3 | 45.9 | 49.4 | 55.9 | 62.9 | 70.7 | 79.0 | 84.6 |
| 55–64 | 598 | 9.07 | 61.5 | 41.4 | 47.4 | 54.7 | 62.0 | 69.8 | 76.5 | 80.5 |
| 65–74 | 1,657 | 5.50 | 57.2 | 40.3 | 44.7 | 51.0 | 57.6 | 64.7 | 71.2 | 75.0 |
| | | | | Women | | | | | | |
| 18–74 | 8,410 | 67.84 | 39.2 | 27.0 | 28.7 | 32.5 | 37.8 | 44.3 | 53.0 | 59.8 |
| 18–24 | 1,523 | 12.89 | 34.8 | 24.9 | 27.2 | 30.0 | 33.8 | 38.9 | 44.3 | 49.4 |
| 25–34 | 1,896 | 13.93 | 37.5 | 26.7 | 28.4 | 31.8 | 36.5 | 41.8 | 49.4 | 56.3 |
| 35–44 | 1,664 | 11.59 | 40.3 | 27.2 | 29.4 | 33.8 | 38.5 | 45.9 | 54.2 | 59.8 |
| 45–54 | 836 | 12.16 | 41.0 | 28.1 | 30.3 | 34.1 | 39.2 | 47.0 | 56.3 | 61.5 |
| 55–64 | 669 | 9.98 | 41.4 | 27.5 | 30.3 | 34.4 | 40.7 | 47.4 | 55.1 | 62.9 |
| 65–74 | 1,822 | 7.28 | 41.4 | 27.5 | 30.3 | 34.4 | 40.3 | 47.4 | 55.9 | 62.9 |

*Calculated from Bishop, C.W., Bowen, P.E., Ritchey, S.J.: Am. J. Clin. Nutr. 34:2530–2539, 1981. (NHANES I)
†Measurements were made in the right arm.
‡See Tables A–6a-1 through A–6a-7 for data compiled by Frisancho (Am. J. Clin. Nutr. 40:808–819, 1984) from NHANES I and II.

## Table A–15. Provisional Percentiles for Triceps Skinfold Thickness in the Elderly*·†·‡

| Age Group (yrs) | 5% | 50% | 95% |
|---|---|---|---|
| Men | | | |
| 65 | 8.6 | 13.8 | 27.0 |
| 70 | 7.7 | 12.9 | 26.1 |
| 75 | 6.8 | 12.0 | 25.2 |
| 80 | 6.0 | 11.2 | 24.3 |
| 85 | 5.1 | 10.3 | 23.4 |
| 90 | 4.2 | 9.4 | 22.6 |
| Women | | | |
| 65 | 13.5 | 21.6 | 33.0 |
| 70 | 12.5 | 20.6 | 32.0 |
| 75 | 11.5 | 19.6 | 31.0 |
| 80 | 10.5 | 18.6 | 30.0 |
| 85 | 9.5 | 17.6 | 29.0 |
| 90 | 8.5 | 16.6 | 28.0 |

*Data are from 119 men and 150 women. All subjects were ambulatory, and measurements were made in the recumbent position on the left side.
†From Chumlea, W.C., Roche, A.F., Mukherjee, D.: Nutritional Assessment of the Elderly Through Anthropometry. Ohio, Wright State University School of Medicine, 1984.
‡See Tables A–6a-1 through A–6a-7 for data compiled by Frisancho (Am. J. Clin. Nutr. 40:808–819, 1984) from NHANES I and II.

## Table A–16. Provisional Percentiles for Midarm Muscle Area (cm²) in the Elderly*·†·‡

| Age Group (yrs) | 5% | 50% | 95% |
|---|---|---|---|
| Men | | | |
| 65 | 43.2 | 59.4 | 77.1 |
| 70 | 41.4 | 57.7 | 75.3 |
| 75 | 39.6 | 55.9 | 73.5 |
| 80 | 37.8 | 54.1 | 71.7 |
| 85 | 36.0 | 52.3 | 69.9 |
| 90 | 34.3 | 50.5 | 68.2 |
| Women | | | |
| 65 | 33.5 | 44.5 | 66.4 |
| 70 | 33.0 | 44.1 | 65.9 |
| 75 | 32.6 | 43.6 | 65.5 |
| 80 | 32.2 | 43.2 | 65.1 |
| 85 | 31.8 | 42.8 | 64.7 |
| 90 | 31.3 | 42.4 | 64.2 |

*Data are from 119 men and 150 women. All subjects were ambulatory, and measurements were made in the recumbent position on the left side.
†From Chumlea, W.C., Roche, A.F., Mukherjee, D.: Nutritional Assessment of the Elderly Through Anthropometry. Ohio, Wright State University School of Medicine, 1984.
‡See Tables A–6a-1 through A–6a-7 for data compiled by Frisancho (Am. J. Clin. Nutr. 40:808–819, 1984) from NHANES I and II.

## Table A–17. Equivalent Fat Content, as a Percentage of Body Weight, for a Range of Values for the Sum of Four Skinfolds*·†

| Skin Folds (mm) | Males (age in yrs) | | | | Females (age in yrs) | | | |
|---|---|---|---|---|---|---|---|---|
| | *17–29* | *30–39* | *40–49* | *50+* | *16–29* | *30–39* | *40–49* | *50+* |
| 15 | 4.8 | | | | 10.5 | | | |
| 20 | 8.1 | 12.2 | 12.2 | 12.6 | 14.1 | 17.0 | 19.8 | 21.4 |
| 25 | 10.5 | 14.2 | 15.0 | 15.6 | 16.8 | 19.4 | 22.2 | 24.0 |
| 30 | 12.9 | 16.2 | 17.7 | 18.6 | 19.5 | 21.8 | 24.5 | 26.6 |
| 35 | 14.7 | 17.7 | 19.6 | 20.8 | 21.5 | 23.7 | 26.4 | 28.5 |
| 40 | 16.4 | 19.2 | 21.4 | 22.9 | 23.4 | 25.5 | 28.2 | 30.3 |
| 45 | 17.7 | 20.4 | 23.0 | 24.7 | 25.0 | 26.9 | 29.6 | 31.9 |
| 50 | 19.0 | 21.5 | 24.6 | 26.5 | 26.5 | 28.2 | 31.0 | 33.4 |
| 55 | 20.1 | 22.5 | 25.9 | 27.9 | 27.8 | 29.4 | 32.1 | 34.6 |
| 60 | 21.2 | 23.5 | 27.1 | 29.2 | 29.1 | 30.6 | 33.2 | 35.7 |
| 65 | 22.2 | 24.3 | 28.2 | 30.4 | 30.2 | 31.6 | 34.1 | 36.7 |
| 70 | 23.1 | 25.1 | 29.3 | 31.6 | 31.2 | 32.5 | 35.0 | 37.7 |
| 75 | 24.0 | 25.9 | 30.3 | 32.7 | 32.2 | 33.4 | 35.9 | 38.7 |
| 80 | 24.8 | 26.6 | 31.2 | 33.8 | 33.1 | 34.3 | 36.7 | 39.6 |
| 85 | 25.5 | 27.2 | 32.1 | 34.8 | 34.0 | 35.1 | 37.5 | 40.4 |
| 90 | 26.2 | 27.8 | 33.0 | 35.8 | 34.8 | 35.8 | 38.3 | 41.2 |
| 95 | 26.9 | 28.4 | 33.7 | 36.6 | 35.6 | 36.5 | 39.0 | 41.9 |
| 100 | 27.6 | 29.0 | 34.4 | 37.4 | 36.4 | 37.2 | 39.7 | 42.6 |
| 105 | 28.2 | 29.6 | 35.1 | 38.2 | 37.1 | 37.9 | 40.4 | 43.3 |
| 110 | 28.8 | 30.1 | 35.8 | 39.0 | 37.8 | 38.6 | 41.0 | 43.9 |
| 115 | 29.4 | 30.6 | 36.4 | 39.7 | 38.4 | 39.1 | 41.5 | 44.5 |
| 120 | 30.0 | 31.1 | 37.0 | 40.4 | 39.0 | 39.6 | 42.0 | 45.1 |
| 125 | 31.0 | 31.5 | 37.6 | 41.1 | 39.6 | 40.1 | 42.5 | 45.7 |
| 130 | 31.5 | 31.9 | 38.2 | 41.8 | 40.2 | 40.6 | 43.0 | 46.2 |
| 135 | 32.0 | 32.3 | 38.7 | 42.4 | 40.8 | 41.1 | 43.5 | 46.7 |
| 140 | 32.5 | 32.7 | 39.2 | 43.0 | 41.3 | 41.6 | 44.0 | 47.2 |
| 145 | 32.9 | 33.1 | 39.7 | 43.6 | 41.8 | 42.1 | 44.5 | 47.7 |
| 150 | 33.3 | 33.5 | 40.2 | 44.1 | 42.3 | 42.6 | 45.0 | 48.2 |
| 155 | 33.7 | 33.9 | 40.7 | 44.6 | 42.8 | 43.1 | 45.4 | 48.7 |
| 160 | 34.1 | 34.3 | 41.2 | 45.1 | 43.3 | 43.6 | 45.8 | 49.2 |
| 165 | 34.5 | 34.6 | 41.6 | 45.6 | 43.7 | 44.0 | 46.2 | 49.6 |
| 170 | 34.9 | 34.8 | 42.0 | 46.1 | 44.1 | 44.4 | 46.6 | 50.0 |
| 175 | 35.3 | | | | | 44.8 | 47.0 | 50.4 |
| 180 | 35.6 | | | | | 45.2 | 47.4 | 50.8 |
| 185 | 35.9 | | | | | 45.6 | 47.8 | 51.2 |
| 190 | | | | | | 45.9 | 48.2 | 51.6 |
| 195 | | | | | | 46.2 | 48.5 | 52.0 |
| 200 | | | | | | 46.5 | 48.8 | 52.4 |
| 205 | | | | | | | 49.1 | 52.7 |
| 210 | | | | | | | 49.4 | 53.0 |

*Biceps, triceps, subscapular, and suprailiac of males and females of different ages.
†From Durnin, J.V.G.A., Womersley, J.: Br. J. Nutr. 32:77–97, 1974, with permission.

## Table A–18.   Beverages and Alcoholic Drinks—Calories and Selected Electrolytes

| Beverage | Calories | Sodium (mg) | Sodium (meq) | Potassium (mg) | Potassium (meq) | Phosphorus (mg) |
|---|---|---|---|---|---|---|
| Cola (avg.) | 48.1–55.0† | 0.8–4.7 (mg)† | | 0–4.4 (mg)† | | 18.1–25† |
| Diet cola (avg.) | 0.1–0.5† | 0.8–13.0 (mg)† | | 0–33.2 (mg)† | | 8.5–17.6† |
| Patio grape/orange | 52 | 11.2 | 0.5 | 4.1 | 0.1 | — |
| Mountain Dew | 49 | 8.7 | 0.4 | 2.7 | 0.1 | — |
| Teem | 41 | 8.6 | 0.4 | — | — | — |
| Root beer | 45 | 1 | 0.1 | 3.9 | 0.1 | — |
| Club soda | 0 | 21.9 | 1.0 | — | — | 0 |
| Sprite | 48 | 15.4 | 0.7 | 0.4 | — | — |
| Fanta (avg.) | 53 | 6.4 | 0.3 | 0.6 | — | — |
| Fresca | 1 | 12.1 | 0.5 | — | — | — |
| Fanta ginger ale | 42 | 9.4 | 0.4 | — | — | — |
| Slice | 45 | 3 | 0.1 | 27.6 | 0.7 | — |
| Apricot nectar | 56 | 3 | 0.1 | 114 | 2.9 | 9 |
| Apple juice | 47 | 3 | 0.1 | 119 | 3 | 7 |
| Cranberry juice | 58 | 4 | 0.2 | 24 | 0.6 | 1 |
| Grape juice, cnd | 61 | 3 | 0.1 | 132 | 3.4 | 11 |
| Grapefruit juice, unsweetened | 38 | trace | — | 153 | 3.9 | 11 |
| Orange juice, unsweetened or fresh | 45 | 1 | 0.1 | 200 | 5.1 | 17 |
| Pear nectar | 60 | 4 | 0.2 | 13 | 0.3 | 3 |
| Peach nectar | 54 | 7 | 0.3 | 40 | 1 | 6 |
| Pineapple juice, unsweetened | 56 | trace | — | 134 | 3.4 | 8 |
| Tomato juice | 20 | 200.7 | 8.7 | 227 | 5.8 | 16.5 |
| Fruit-flavored beverage | 45 | — | — | — | — | — |
| Beer, regular | 41 | 5.3 | 0.2 | 25 | 0.6 | 12.4 |
| Beer, light | 28 | 2.8 | 0.1 | 18.1 | 0.5 | 12.1 |
| Gin, rum, vodka, whiskey (86 proof) | 250 | trace | — | 3.6 | 0.1 | — |
| Table wine, 12.2% alcohol/vol. | 86 | 3.5 | 0.1 | 93.1 | 2.4 | 10.3 |
| Dessert wine, 18.5% alcohol/vol. | 137 | 3.3 | 0.1 | 76.7 | 2 | — |

Alcoholic beverages are customarily served in special glassware, the size of which tends to standardize the alcoholic content:

| | | | |
|---|---|---|---|
| 1 cordial glass | = 20 ml | 1 burgundy glass | = 120 ml |
| 1 brandy glass | = 30 ml | 1 champagne glass | = 150 ml |
| 1 jigger | = 45 ml | 1 tumbler | = 240–360 ml |
| 1 sherry glass | = 60 ml | 1 mixing glass | = 360 ml |
| 1 cocktail glass | = 90 ml | | |

*Brand name data supplied by the commercial producer of the product. Other data obtained from Composition of Foods, Fruits, and Fruit Juices: Raw, Processed, Prepared. Agriculture Handbook #8–9. Consumer Nutrition Center, Washington, USDA, 1982.
†Range.

# Table A–19. Dietary Fiber and Crude Fiber Values in Common Foods*

| | Total Dietary Fiber | Crude Fiber | Noncellulosic Polysaccharides† | Cellulose | Lignin |
|---|---|---|---|---|---|
| *CEREAL PRODUCTS* | | | *(g/100 g)* | | |
| White flour | 3.15 | 0.3 | 2.52 | 0.60 | 0.03 |
| Wholemeal flour | 9.51 | 2.3 | 6.25 | 2.46 | 0.80 |
| Bran | 44.0 | 7.8 | 32.7 | 8.05 | 3.23 |
| White bread | 2.72 | 0.2 | 2.01 | 0.71 | Tr |
| Wholemeal bread | 8.50 | 1.6 | 5.95 | 1.31 | 1.24 |
| All Bran | 26.7 | 9.1 | 17.82 | 6.01 | 2.88 |
| Cornflakes | 11.0 | 0.7 | 7.26 | 2.42 | 1.32 |
| Shredded Wheat | 12.26 | 2.3 | 8.79 | 2.63 | 0.84 |
| Swiss breakfast (mixed brands) | 7.41 | — | 5.31 | 1.36 | 0.74 |
| Weetabix | 12.72 | 1.6 | 9.18 | 2.35 | 1.19 |
| Crispbread, rye | 11.73 | 2.2 | 8.33 | 1.66 | 1.74 |
| Crispbread, wheat | 4.83 | 0.3 | 3.34 | 0.94 | 0.55 |
| Matzo | 3.85 | 0.3 | 2.72 | 0.70 | 0.43 |
| Oatcakes | 4.00 | — | 3.16 | 0.40 | 0.44 |
| Semisweet biscuits, assorted, or ladyfingers | 2.31 | 0.1 | 1.76 | 0.33 | 0.22 |
| *VEGETABLES* | | | | | |
| Broccoli tops (boiled) | 4.10 | 1.5 | 2.92 | 0.85 | 0.03 |
| Brussels sprouts (boiled) | 2.86 | 1.6 | 1.99 | 0.80 | 0.07 |
| Cabbage (boiled) | 2.83 | 0.8 | 1.76 | 0.69 | 0.38 |
| Cauliflower (boiled) | 1.80 | 1.0 | 0.67 | 1.13 | Tr |
| Lettuce (raw) | 1.53 | 0.7 | 0.47 | 1.06 | Tr |
| Onions (raw) | 2.10 | 0.6 | 1.55 | 0.55 | Tr |
| Beans, baked (canned) | 7.27 | — | 5.67 | 1.41 | 0.19 |
| Beans, runner (boiled) | 3.35 | 1.0 | 1.85 | 1.29 | 0.21 |
| Peas, frozen (raw) | 7.75 | 1.9 | 5.48 | 2.09 | 0.18 |
| Sweet corn (cooked) | 4.74 | 0.7 | 4.31 | 0.31 | 0.12 |
| (canned) (drained) | 5.69 | 0.8 | 4.97 | 0.64 | 0.08 |
| Carrots, young (boiled) | 3.70 | 1.0 | 2.22 | 1.48 | Tr |
| Parsnips (raw) | 4.90 | 2.0 | 3.77 | 1.13 | Tr |
| Swedes (raw) | 2.40 | 1.1 | 1.61 | 0.79 | Tr |
| Turnips (raw) | 2.20 | 0.9 | 1.50 | 0.70 | Tr |
| Potatoes (raw) | 3.51 | 0.5 | 2.49 | 1.02 | Tr |
| *FRUIT* | | | | | |
| Apples (flesh only) | 1.42 | 0.6 | 0.94 | 0.48 | 0.01 |
| (peel only) | 3.71 | — | 2.21 | 1.01 | 0.49 |
| Bananas | 1.75 | 0.5 | 1.12 | 0.37 | 0.26 |
| Cherries (flesh and skin) | 1.24 | 0.4 | 0.92 | 0.25 | 0.07 |
| Grapefruit (canned)‡ | 0.44 | 0.2 | 0.34 | 0.04 | 0.55 |
| Guavas (canned)‡ | 3.64 | 5.6 | 1.67 | 1.17 | 0.80 |
| Mandarin oranges (canned)‡ | 0.29 | 0.1 | 0.22 | 0.04 | 0.03 |
| Mangoes (canned)‡ and raw | 1.00 | 0.9 | 0.65 | 0.32 | 0.03 |
| Peaches (flesh and skin) | 2.28 | 0.6 | 1.46 | 0.20 | 0.62 |
| Pears (flesh only) | 2.44 | — | 1.32 | 0.67 | 0.45 |
| (peel only) | 8.59 | — | 3.72 | 2.18 | 2.67 |
| Plums (flesh and skin) | 1.52 | 0.4 | 0.99 | 0.23 | 0.30 |
| Rhubarb (raw) | 1.78 | 0.7 | 0.93 | 0.70 | 0.15 |
| Strawberries (raw) | 2.12 | 1.3 | 0.98 | 0.33 | 0.81 |
| (canned)‡ | 1.00 | 0.6 | 0.48 | 0.20 | 0.33 |
| Sultanas or raisins | 4.40 | 0.9 | 2.40 | 0.83 | 1.17 |
| *NUTS* | | | | | |
| Brazils | 7.73 | 3.1 | 3.60 | 2.17 | 1.96 |
| Peanuts | 9.30 | 2.4 | 6.40 | 1.69 | 1.21 |
| Peanut butter | 7.55 | 1.9 | 5.64 | 1.91 | Tr |
| *PRESERVES* | | | | | |
| Jam (plum, | 0.96 | 1.0 | 0.80 | 0.14 | 0.03 |
| strawberry) | 1.12 | 1.0 | 0.85 | 0.11 | 0.15 |
| Marmalade | 0.71 | 0.4 | 0.64 | 0.05 | 0.01 |
| Pickle | 1.53 | 0.5 | 0.91 | 0.50 | 0.12 |

*Compiled and submitted by D.J.A. Jenkins from data of Southgate, et al.: J. Hum. Nutr. 30:303–313, 1976, and Watt and Merrill, Handbook of the Nutritional Contents of Foods, U.S.D.A. Handbook #8, New York, Dover Publ., 1975.
†This value may include heat-induced artifacts analyzing as lignin.
‡Fruit and syrup.

## Table A–20a. Average Values for Triglycerides, Fatty Acids, and Cholesterol in Selected Foods and Oils*·†·‡

| Food Item | Total Fat (g) | SFA (g) | MFA (g) | PFA (g) | Oleic (g) | LIN-LIN (g) | P/S Ratio | CHOL (mg) |
|---|---|---|---|---|---|---|---|---|
| *MEATS* | | | | | | | | |
| Beef, approx. 6% fat, cooked | 6.40 | 2.81 | 2.77 | 0.37 | 2.34 | 0.30 | 0.1 | 65.9 |
| Beef, approx. 30% fat, cooked | 32.00 | 13.30 | 15.67 | 1.33 | 13.10 | 1.10 | 0.1 | 94.0 |
| Lamb, approx. 6.0 to 10.9% fat, cooked | 8.05 | 2.69 | 3.39 | 0.55 | 3.17 | 0.48 | 0.2 | 84.0 |
| Lamb, approx. 34 to 39% fat, cooked | 36.00 | 16.80 | 14.68 | 2.10 | 13.80 | 2.04 | 0.1 | 98.0 |
| Veal, approx. 6% fat, cooked | 6.70 | 2.97 | 2.87 | 0.47 | 2.47 | 0.38 | 0.2 | 99.0 |
| Veal, approx. 25% fat, cooked | 21.20 | 9.21 | 9.24 | 1.30 | 7.82 | 1.20 | 0.1 | 101.0 |
| Chicken, turkey, Cornish hen, light meat without skin, cooked | 3.87 | 1.15 | 1.05 | 0.92 | 0.88 | 0.68 | 0.8 | 89.0 |
| Duck, goose (domestic) without skin, cooked | 11.94 | 4.37 | 4.02 | 1.49 | 3.56 | 1.49 | 0.3 | 92.5 |
| Beef, ground, % fat unknown | 24.60 | 10.30 | 11.70 | 1.09 | 9.86 | 0.98 | 0.1 | 94.0 |
| Beef bologna | 28.36 | 11.66 | 13.28 | 1.05 | 11.72 | 1.05 | 0.1 | 56.0 |
| Pork, fresh, 22.5% to 27.4% fat, cooked | 25.13 | 9.08 | 11.52 | 2.84 | 10.59 | 2.74 | 0.3 | 82.0 |
| Frankfurter, all beef, cooked | 29.42 | 11.96 | 14.35 | 1.16 | 12.56 | 1.10 | 0.1 | 48.0 |
| Frankfurter, chicken or turkey | 17.70 | 5.89 | 5.58 | 5.00 | 5.30 | 5.00 | 0.9 | 107.0 |
| Frankfurter, beef, pork | 29.15 | 10.76 | 13.67 | 2.73 | 12.36 | 2.73 | 0.3 | 50.0 |
| Smoked pork, 22.5% to 27.4% fat, cooked | 23.48 | 8.38 | 11.03 | 2.51 | 10.15 | 2.51 | 0.3 | 67.0 |
| Salami, dry or hard pork | 33.72 | 11.89 | 16.00 | 3.74 | 14.67 | 3.55 | 0.3 | 77.2 |
| Bacon, regular, cooked | 49.24 | 17.42 | 23.69 | 5.81 | 21.96 | 5.68 | 0.3 | 85.0 |
| *FISH§* | | | | | | | | |
| Fish, 0 to 2.9% fat | 0.90 | 0.16 | 0.09 | 0.34 | 0.07 | 0.00 | 2.1 | 60.0 |
| Fish, 3.0 to 6.9% fat | 4.50 | 1.03 | 1.51 | 1.48 | 1.00 | 0.31 | 1.4 | 80.0 |
| Fish, 11.0 to 14.9% fat | 13.00 | 3.22 | 4.98 | 3.31 | 2.67 | 0.25 | 1.0 | 80.0 |
| Herring, canned, smoked, pickled | 13.60 | 4.24 | 4.74 | 3.09 | 3.73 | 0.88 | 0.7 | 97.0 |
| Salmon, pink, canned | 8.20 | 2.03 | 3.14 | 2.09 | 1.68 | 0.16 | 1.0 | 35.0 |
| Sardines, canned, drained | 11.10 | 2.82 | 2.67 | 4.00 | 1.37 | 0.34 | 1.4 | 100.0 |
| Tuna, canned, oil-packed, drained | 12.00 | 1.88 | 4.98 | 4.47 | 4.89 | 4.25 | 2.4 | 26.0 |
| Tuna, canned, water packed | 0.90 | 0.24 | 0.17 | 0.30 | 0.12 | 0.02 | 1.3 | 63.0 |
| Clams, cooked, including mussels | 2.50 | 0.48 | 0.45 | 0.53 | 0.11 | 0.06 | 1.1 | 63.0 |
| Crab, all types, cooked, fresh, frozen, or canned | 1.60 | 0.28 | 0.37 | 0.63 | 0.18 | 0.05 | 2.3 | 100.0 |
| Lobster, cooked | 3.40 | 0.40 | 0.65 | 1.25 | 0.36 | 0.91 | 3.1 | 150.0 |
| Oysters, cooked | 2.30 | 0.55 | 0.41 | 1.02 | 0.19 | 0.07 | 1.9 | 45.0 |
| Scallops, cooked | 1.40 | 0.31 | 0.14 | 0.33 | 0.05 | 0.01 | 1.1 | 53.0 |
| Shrimp, cooked | 2.40 | 0.36 | 0.51 | 0.77 | 0.32 | 0.04 | 2.1 | 150.6 |
| Caviar | 15.00 | 4.19 | 4.71 | 5.37 | 1.99 | 1.44 | 1.3 | 300.0 |
| *EGGS/DAIRY* | | | | | | | | |
| Egg, whole | 11.15 | 3.35 | 4.46 | 1.45 | 4.08 | 1.27 | 0.4 | 548.0 |
| Egg, yolk | 32.93 | 9.89 | 13.16 | 4.28 | 12.06 | 3.75 | 0.4 | 1602.0 |
| Egg, white | 0.00 | 0.00 | 0.00 | 0.00 | | | | |
| Creamer, imitation, liquid, frozen, saturated (vegetable fat) | 9.97 | 9.30 | 0.11 | 0.00 | | | 0.0 | 0.0 |
| Creamer, imitation, powdered, saturated (vegetable fat) | 35.48 | 32.52 | 0.97 | 0.01 | 0.97 | 0.01 | 0.00 | 0.0 |
| Creamer, imitation (Poly Perx) | 10.00 | 1.49 | 4.30 | 3.76 | 4.25 | 3.74 | 2.5 | 0.0 |
| Cream, half-and-half, 10–12% fat | 11.50 | 7.16 | 3.32 | 0.43 | 2.89 | 0.43 | 0.1 | 37.0 |
| Cream, light, sweet, or sour, 20% fat | 19.31 | 12.02 | 5.58 | 0.72 | 4.86 | 0.72 | 0.1 | 66.0 |
| Buttermilk, 1% fat or low-fat# | 0.88 | 0.55 | 0.25 | 0.03 | 0.22 | 0.03 | 0.1 | 4.0 |
| Milk, 1% fat# | 1.06 | 0.66 | 0.31 | 0.04 | 0.27 | 0.04 | 0.1 | 4.0 |
| Milk, 2% fat# | 1.92 | 1.20 | 0.56 | 0.07 | 0.48 | 0.07 | 0.1 | 8.0 |
| Milk, whole, 3.5 to 4% fat# | 3.34 | 2.08 | 0.96 | 0.12 | 0.92 | 0.13 | 0.1 | 14.0 |
| Cheese-Parmesan, fresh, or dry | 30.02 | 19.07 | 8.73 | 0.66 | 7.74 | 0.66 | 0.0 | 79.0 |
| cottage, low-fat | 1.93 | 1.22 | 0.55 | 0.06 | 0.45 | 0.06 | 0.1 | 8.0 |
| cottage, creamed, 4% fat | 4.51 | 2.81 | 1.30 | 0.17 | 1.20 | 0.17 | 0.1 | 15.0 |
| cream, Neufchatel, 20% fat | 23.43 | 14.80 | 6.77 | 0.65 | 5.66 | 0.65 | 0.0 | 76.0 |
| natural, 20% fat | 31.75 | 19.65 | 9.11 | 1.17 | 7.94 | 1.21 | 0.1 | 81.0 |
| Yogurt, low-fat, 1–2% fat, plain# | 1.55 | 1.00 | 0.43 | 0.04 | 0.35 | 0.04 | 0.00 | 6.0 |
| part skim, all flavors | 1.08 | 0.70 | 0.30 | 0.03 | 0.25 | 0.03 | 0.0 | 4.0 |
| whole milk, all flavors | 3.40 | 2.20 | 0.93 | 0.10 | 0.85 | 0.13 | 0.1 | 13.2 |
| Ice cream, medium-rich, 16% fat, all flavors# | 16.00 | 9.96 | 4.62 | 0.59 | 4.02 | 0.59 | 0.1 | 59.0 |
| Sherbet | 1.98 | 1.23 | 0.57 | 0.07 | 0.50 | 0.07 | 0.1 | 7.0 |
| Ice milk or soft-serve ice milk, 5% fat, all flavors# | 2.64 | 1.64 | 0.76 | 0.10 | 0.66 | 0.10 | 0.1 | 8.0 |

## Table A–20a.  (continued)

| Food Item | Total Fat (g) | SFA (g) | MFA (g) | PFA (g) | Oleic (g) | LIN-LIN (g) | P/S Ratio | CHOL (mg) |
|---|---|---|---|---|---|---|---|---|
| *(per 100-g edible portion)* | | | | | | | | |
| **FATS/OILS** | | | | | | | | |
| Oil—corn | 100.00 | 12.70 | 24.20 | 58.70 | 24.20 | 58.70 | 4.6 | 0.0 |
| sunflower | 100.00 | 10.30 | 19.50 | 65.70 | 19.50 | 65.70 | 7.0 | 0.0 |
| cottonseed | 100.00 | 25.90 | 17.80 | 51.90 | 17.00 | 52.10 | 2.0 | 0.0 |
| safflower | 100.00 | 9.10 | 12.10 | 74.50 | 11.70 | 74.50 | 8.2 | 0.0 |
| sesame | 100.00 | 14.20 | 39.70 | 41.70 | 39.30 | 41.60 | 2.9 | 0.0 |
| soybean, partially hydrogenated | 100.00 | 14.90 | 43.00 | 37.60 | 42.50 | 37.50 | 2.5 | 0.0 |
| olive | 100.00 | 13.50 | 73.70 | 8.40 | 72.50 | 8.50 | 0.6 | 0.0 |
| peanut | 100.00 | 16.90 | 46.20 | 32.00 | 44.80 | 32.00 | 1.9 | 0.0 |
| coconut# | 100.00 | 86.50 | 5.80 | 1.80 | 5.80 | 1.80 | 0.0 | 0.0 |
| palm | 100.00 | 49.30 | 37.00 | 36.60 | 9.30 | 1.60 | 0.2 | 0.0 |
| palm kernel# | 100.00 | 81.40 | 11.40 | 1.60 | 11.40 | 1.60 | 0.0 | 0.0 |
| Shortening, household, vegetable | 100.00 | 24.74 | 44.50 | 26.10 | 44.50 | 26.10 | 1.1 | 0.0 |
| Margarine (corn), 80% fat, stick or tube | 80.30 | 12.64 | 29.63 | 33.77 | 29.63 | 33.77 | 2.7 | 0.0 |
| Lard, rendered | 100.00 | 39.60 | 45.10 | 11.77 | 41.20 | 11.20 | 0.3 | 95.0 |
| Butter, salted or unsalted# | 81.11 | 50.49 | 23.43 | 3.01 | 20.40 | 3.00 | 0.1 | 219.0 |
| MCT oil# | 100.00 | 94.50 | 0.00 | 0.00 | | | | 57.1 |
| Mayonnaise, commercial, 79% fat | 79.40 | 11.80 | 22.70 | 41.30 | 22.50 | 41.30 | 3.5 | 57.1 |
| **NUTS/SEEDS** | | | | | | | | |
| Peanut butter | 51.14 | 8.52 | 24.70 | 15.40 | 23.97 | 15.40 | 1.8 | 0.0 |
| Almonds, salted | 56.53 | 5.36 | 36.71 | 11.86 | 36.03 | 11.76 | 2.2 | 0.0 |
| Cashews, salted | 48.21 | 9.53 | 28.41 | 8.15 | 27.89 | 8.14 | 0.9 | 0.0 |
| Peanuts (groundnut) | 49.19 | 6.85 | 24.49 | 15.60 | 23.81 | 15.59 | 2.3 | 0.0 |
| Walnuts, unsalted | 61.87 | 5.59 | 14.17 | 39.13 | 13.30 | 38.57 | 7.0 | 0.0 |
| Olives, black | 13.80 | 1.96 | 10.16 | 1.24 | 10.01 | 1.17 | 0.6 | 0.0 |
| Candy, fudge, chocolate, no nuts | 3.05 | 1.40 | 1.28 | 0.26 | 1.27 | 0.27 | 0.2 | 20.0 |
| **FRUITS/VEGETABLES** | | | | | | | | |
| Avocado | 15.32 | 2.44 | 9.61 | 1.96 | 8.97 | 1.95 | 0.8 | 0.0 |
| Coconut, fresh# | 33.49 | 29.70 | 1.42 | 0.37 | 1.42 | 0.37 | 0.0 | 0.0 |
| Soybeans, dry, cooked, or canned | 5.70 | 0.86 | 1.31 | 3.28 | 1.30 | 3.30 | 3.8 | 0.0 |
| Peas, blackeye, chick, dry, cooked, or canned | 2.30 | 0.24 | 0.50 | 1.05 | 0.55 | 1.13 | 4.4 | 0.0 |
| Peas, split or lentils, dry, cooked, or canned | 1.17 | 0.16 | 0.19 | 0.53 | 0.19 | 0.53 | 3.4 | 0.0 |

*The figures given are approximations since climate, species, and fodder composition cause great variations.

†Data provided by The Nutrition Coding Center, University of Minnesota. Supported by Contract No. 1-HV-6-2941-L of the National Heart, Lung and Blood Institute.

‡SFA = Saturated fatty acid; MFA = monounsaturated fatty acid; PFA = polyunsaturated fatty acid; LIN-LIN = linoleic-linolenic; P/S Ratio = polyunsaturated/saturated fatty acids; CHOL = cholesterol.

§See Table A–20b for detailed information on triglycerides, fatty acids (including Omega-3), and cholesterol in selected marine foods and oils.

#The balance of saturated fatty acids is formed by fatty acids with chain lengths <12 (butter 14%) and 12, and 14 (butter 16%, coconut and palm kernel 65–70%).

## Table A–20b. Average Values for Triglycerides, Fatty Acids, and Cholesterol of Marine Foods and Oils (including Omega-3 fatty acids)*·†

| Food Item—Raw | Total Fat (g) | SFA (g) | MFA (g) | PFA (g) | 18:3 LIN-LIN (g) | 20:5 EPA (g) | 22:6 DHA (g) | CHOL (mg) |
|---|---|---|---|---|---|---|---|---|
| Finfish | | | | | | | | |
| Anchovy | 4.8 | 1.3 | 1.2 | 1.6 | — | 0.5 | 0.9 | — |
| Bass, striped | 2.3 | 0.5 | 0.7 | 0.8 | Tr | 0.2 | 0.6 | 80 |
| Bluefish | 6.5 | 1.4 | 2.9 | 1.6 | — | 0.4 | 0.8 | 59 |
| Burbot | 0.8 | 0.2 | 0.1 | 0.3 | — | 0.1 | 0.1 | 60 |
| Carp | 5.6 | 1.1 | 2.3 | 1.4 | 0.3 | 0.2 | 0.1 | 67 |
| Cod, Atlantic | 0.7 | 0.1 | 0.1 | 0.3 | Tr | 0.1 | 0.2 | 43 |
| Eel, European | 18.8 | 3.5 | 10.9 | 1.4 | 0.7 | 0.1 | 0.1 | 108 |
| Flounder | 1.0 | 0.2 | 0.3 | 0.3 | Tr | 0.1 | 0.1 | 46 |
| Haddock | 0.7 | 0.1 | 0.1 | 0.2 | Tr | 0.1 | 0.1 | 63 |
| Hake | 1.9 | 0.5 | 0.6 | 0.5 | — | 0.1 | 0.4 | — |
| Halibut, Pacific | 2.3 | 0.3 | 0.8 | 0.7 | 0.1 | 0.1 | 0.3 | 32 |
| Herring, Atlantic‡ | 9.0 | 2.0 | 3.7 | 2.1 | 0.1 | 0.7 | 0.9 | 60 |
| Mackerel, Atlantic‡ | 13.9 | 3.6 | 5.4 | 3.7 | 0.1 | 0.9 | 1.6 | 80 |
| Perch, white | 2.5 | 0.6 | 0.9 | 0.7 | 0.1 | 0.2 | 0.1 | 80 |
| Pike, walleye | 1.2 | 0.2 | 0.3 | 0.4 | Tr | 0.1 | 0.2 | 86 |
| Pollack | 1.0 | 0.1 | 0.1 | 0.5 | — | 0.1 | 0.4 | 71 |
| Sablefish | 15.3 | 3.2 | 8.1 | 2.0 | 0.1 | 0.7 | 0.7 | 49 |
| Salmon, chinook | 10.4 | 2.5 | 4.5 | 2.1 | 0.1 | 0.8 | 0.6 | — |
| Sea bass | 1.5 | 0.4 | 0.3 | 0.5 | Tr | 0.1 | 0.3 | 41 |
| Smelt, rainbow | 2.6 | 0.5 | 0.7 | 0.9 | 0.1 | 0.3 | 0.4 | 70 |
| Snapper, red | 1.2 | 0.2 | 0.2 | 0.4 | Tr | Tr | 0.2 | — |
| Sole, European | 1.2 | 0.3 | 0.4 | 0.2 | Tr | Tr | 0.1 | 50 |
| Sturgeon, Atlantic | 6.0 | 1.2 | 1.7 | 2.1 | Tr | 1.0 | 0.5 | — |
| Swordfish | 2.1 | 0.6 | 0.8 | 0.2 | — | 0.1 | 0.1 | 39 |
| Trout, rainbow | 3.4 | 0.6 | 1.0 | 1.2 | 0.1 | 0.1 | 0.4 | 57 |
| Tuna, albacore | 4.9 | 1.2 | 1.2 | 1.8 | 0.2 | 0.3 | 1.0 | 54 |
| Whitefish, lake | 6.0 | 0.9 | 2.0 | 2.2 | 0.2 | 0.3 | 1.0 | 60 |
| Crustaceans | | | | | | | | |
| Crab, Alaska king | 0.8 | 0.1 | 0.1 | 0.3 | Tr | 0.2 | 0.1 | — |
| Crab, blue | 1.3 | 0.2 | 0.2 | 0.5 | Tr | 0.2 | 0.2 | 78 |
| Lobster, northern | 0.9 | 0.2 | 0.2 | 0.2 | — | 0.1 | 0.1 | 95 |
| Shrimp | 1.1 | 0.2 | 0.1 | 0.4 | Tr | 0.2 | 0.1 | 147 |
| Mollusks | | | | | | | | |
| Abalone, New Zealand | 1.0 | 0.2 | 0.2 | 0.2 | Tr | Tr | — | — |
| Clam, littleneck | 0.8 | 0.1 | 0.1 | 0.1 | Tr | Tr | Tr | — |
| Clam, hardshell | 0.6 | Tr | Tr | 0.1 | Tr | Tr | Tr | 31 |
| Mussel, blue | 2.2 | 0.4 | 0.5 | 0.6 | Tr | 0.2 | 0.3 | 38 |
| Octopus | 1.0 | 0.3 | 0.1 | 0.3 | — | 0.1 | 0.1 | — |
| Oyster | 2.0 | 0.4 | 0.2 | 0.7 | 0.1 | 0.3 | 0.2 | 30 |
| Scallop | 0.8 | 0.1 | 0.1 | 0.3 | Tr | 0.1 | 0.1 | 45 |
| Squid, Atlantic | 1.2 | 0.3 | 0.1 | 0.5 | Tr | 0.1 | 0.3 | — |
| Fish Oils | | | | | | | | |
| Cod liver oil | 100.0 | 17.6 | 51.2 | 25.8 | 0.7 | 9.0 | 9.5 | 570 |
| Herring oil | 100.0 | 19.2 | 60.3 | 16.1 | 0.6 | 7.1 | 4.3 | 766 |
| Menhaden oil | 100.0 | 33.6 | 32.5 | 29.5 | 1.1 | 12.7 | 7.9 | 521 |
| MaxEPA concentrated fish body oils | 100.0 | 25.4 | 28.3 | 41.1 | 0.0 | 17.8 | 11.6 | 600 |
| Salmon oil | 100.0 | 23.8 | 39.7 | 29.9 | 1.0 | 8.8 | 11.1 | 485 |

*From Provisional Table on the Content of Omega-3 Fatty Acids and Other Fat Components in Selected Foods, U.S.D.A., Human Nutrition Information Service, HNIS/PT-103, May, 1986.

†SFA = saturated fatty acid; MFA = monounsaturated fatty acid; PFA = polyunsaturated fatty acid; 18:3 LIN-LIN = linoleic-linolenic; 20:5 EPA = eicosapentaenoic acid; 22:6 DHA = docosahexaenoic acid; CHOL = cholesterol.

‡Distribution of omega fatty acids varies depending on fishing grounds.

## Table A–20c. Average Triglyceride and Fatty Acid Composition of Important Edible Nonmarine Fats*

| Food | Average Fat (%) | Average Fatty Acid Composition | | | | | | |
|------|------|------|------|------|------|------|------|------|
| | | Saturated | | | Mono- and Polyunsaturated | | | |
| | | Total† | 16:0 | 18:0 | 18:1 | 18:2 | 18:3 | 20:4 |
| Milk (cow) | 3.5 | 65† | 25 | 11 | 26 | 1–3 | 2 | tr |
| Butter | 80 | identical to milk | | | | | | |
| Lard (pig) | 100 | 42 | 28 | 13 | 46 | 6–8 | 2 | 2 |
| Pork | 35 | approx. as lard | | | | | | |
| Tallow | 100 | 53 | 29 | 20 | 42 | 2 | tr | — |
| Beef | 25 | approx. as tallow | | | | | | |
| Chicken | 15 | 30 | 25 | 4 | 42 | 21 | — | — |
| Egg | 11 | identical to chicken | | | | | | |
| Turkey | 20 | approx. as chicken | | | | | | |
| Groundnut (peanut) oil | 100 | 19‡ | 11 | 3 | 40–55‡ | 20–43‡ | | |
| Groundnut | 50 | identical | | | (variable, climate-dependent) | | | |
| Sesame oil | 100 | 15 | 9 | 5 | 39 | 40 | 1 | — |
| Sesame seed | 53 | identical to oil | | | | | | |
| Soybean oil | 100 | 15 | 11 | 4 | 23 | 51 | 7 | — |
| Soybean | 18 | identical to oil | | | | | | |
| Corn oil | 100 | 13 | 11 | 2 | 25 | 55 | tr | — |
| Corn | 4 | identical to oil | | | | | | |
| Sunflower seed oil | 100 | 12 | 6 | 4 | 24 | 60–70 | tr | — |
| Olive oil | 100 | 17 | 14 | 3 | 71 | 10 | tr | — |
| Olive | 14 | identical to oil | | | | | | |
| Cottonseed oil | 100 | 30 | 25 | 3 | 18 | 51 | tr | |
| Safflower seed oil | 100 | 10 | 7 | 3 | 15§ | 75§ | tr | |
| Palm oil | 100 | 52 | 45 | 5 | 38 | 10 | — | |
| Coconut oil | 100 | 88† | 8 | 3 | 6 | 2 | — | |
| Palm kernel oil | 100 | 80† | 7 | 2 | 14 | 1 | — | |
| Rapeseed oil (new) | 100 | 7 | 5 | 2 | 53 | 22 | 10 | |
| Rapeseed oil (old) | 100 | 4 | 3 | 1 | 11 | 13 | 9 + # | |
| Mustard seed oil | 100 | 5 | 3 | 1 | 16 | 15 | 10 + # | |
| Cashew nut | 68 | 24 | 14 | 10 | 30 | 35 | tr | |
| Walnut | 63 | 10 | 7 | 2 | 15 | 60 | 10 | |

*Data compiled and submitted by Drs. W.G. Linscheer and A.J. Vergroesen (see Chap. 3). The figures given are approximations because climate, species, and fodder composition cause great variations.

†The balance of saturated fatty acids is formed by fatty acids with chain lengths <12 (butter 14%) and 12 and 14 (butter 16%, coconut and palm kernel 65–70%).

‡Approximately 4% of C 20:0 and C 22:0, peanuts from Argentina and Virginia (USA), have relatively low C 18:1 and high C 18:2 concentrations.

§Safflower seed oil with the reverse C 18:1/18:2 composition also is available.

#Contrary to new rapeseed varieties like Canbra and LEAR, old varieties of rapeseed oil and mustard seed oil have 10% C 20:1 n-9 and 30–50% C 22:1 n-9.

## Table A–21.  Exchange Lists*·‡

The reason for dividing food into six different groups is that foods vary in their carbohydrate, protein, fat, and calorie content. Each exchange list contains foods that are alike; each choice contains about the same amount of carbohydrate, protein, fat, and calories.

The following chart shows the amount of these nutrients in one serving from each exchange list.

| Exchange List | Carbohydrate (g) | Protein (g) | Fat (g) | Calories |
|---|---|---|---|---|
| Starch/bread | 15 | 3 | trace | 80 |
| Meat (lean) | — | 7 | 3 | 55 |
| (medium-fat) | — | 7 | 5 | 75 |
| (high-fat) | — | 7 | 8 | 100 |
| Vegetable | 5 | 2 | — | 25 |
| Fruit | 15 | — | — | 60 |
| Milk (skim) | 12 | 8 | trace | 90 |
| (low-fat) | 12 | 8 | 5 | 120 |
| (whole) | 12 | 8 | 8 | 150 |
| Fat | — | — | 5 | 45 |

As you read the exchange lists, you will notice that one choice often is a larger amount of food than another choice from the same list. Because foods are so different, each food is measured or weighed so the amount of carbohydrate, protein, fat, and calories is the same in each choice.

*The exchange lists are based on material in the *Exchange Lists for Meal Planning* prepared by Committees of the American Diabetes Association, Inc. and the American Dietetic Association in cooperation with the National Institute of Arthritis, Metabolism, and Digestive Diseases and the National Heart and Lung Institutes of Health, Public Health Service, U.S. Department of Health and Human Services.
‡From the American Diabetes Assoc., 1986, with permission.

## Table A–21. (continued)

**STARCH/BREAD LIST**

Each item in this list contains about 15 g of carbohydrate, 3 g of protein, a trace of fat, and 80 calories.

Whole-grain products average about 2 g of fiber per serving. Some foods are higher in fiber. Those foods that contain 3 or more g of fiber per serving are identified with the fiber symbol.†

You can choose your starch servings from any of the items on this list. If you want to eat a starch food that is not on this list, the general rule is that:

- ½ cup of cereal, grain, or pasta is one serving
- 1 ounce of a bread product is one serving

| | |
|---|---|
| *Cereals/Grains/Pasta* | |
| Bran cereals†, flaked | ½ cup |
| Bran cereals†, concentrated (such as Bran Buds, All Bran) | ⅓ cup |
| Puffed cereal | 1½ cup |
| Grapenuts | 3 Tbsp |
| Shredded wheat | ½ cup |
| Other ready-to-eat unsweetened cereals | ¾ cup |
| Cooked cereals | ½ cup |
| Bulgur (cooked) | ½ cup |
| Grits (cooked) | ½ cup |
| Pasta (cooked) | ½ cup |
| Rice, white or brown (cooked) | ⅓ cup |
| Cornmeal (dry) | 2½ Tbsp |
| Wheat germ† | 3 Tbsp |
| *Dried Beans, Peas/Lentils* | |
| Beans† and peas† (cooked), e.g., kidney, white, split, blackeye | ⅓ cup |
| Lentils† (cooked) | ⅓ cup |
| Baked beans† | ¼ cup |
| *Starchy Vegetables* | |
| Corn† | ½ cup |
| Corn on cob†, 6″ long | 1 |
| Lima beans† | ½ cup |
| Peas, green† (canned or frozen) | ½ cup |
| Plantain† | ½ cup |
| Potato, baked | 1 small (3 oz) |
| Potato, mashed | ½ cup |
| Squash, winter† (acorn, butternut) | ¾ cup |
| Yam, sweet potato, plain | ⅓ cup |
| *Bread* | |
| Whole wheat | 1 slice (1 oz) |
| Pita, 6″ across | ½ |
| Raisin, unfrosted | 1 slice (1 oz) |
| Rye†, pumpernickel† | 1 slice (1 oz) |
| White (including French, Italian) | 1 slice (1 oz) |
| Bagel | ½ (1 oz) |
| Bread sticks, crisp, 4″ long × ½″ | 2 (⅔ oz) |
| Croutons, low-fat | 1 cup |
| English muffin | ½ |
| Plain roll, small | 1 (1 oz) |
| Frankfurter or hamburger bun | ½ (1 oz) |
| Tortilla, 6″ across | 1 |
| *Crackers/Snacks* | |
| Animal crackers | 8 |
| Graham crackers, 2½″ square | 3 |
| Matzoth | ¾ oz |
| Melba toast | 5 slices |
| Oyster crackers | 24 |
| Popcorn (popped, no fat added) | 3 cups |
| Pretzels | ¾ oz |
| Rye crisp, 2″ × 3½″ | 4 |
| Saltine-type crackers | 6 |
| Whole-wheat crackers, no fat added (crispbreads, such as Finn, Kavli, Wasa) | 2–4 slices (¾ oz) |
| *Starch Foods Prepared With Fat (Count as 1 starch/bread serving plus 1 fat serving)* | |
| Biscuit, 2½″ across | 1 |
| Chow mein noodles | ½ cup |
| Corn bread, 2″ cube | 1 (2 oz) |
| Cracker, round butter type | 6 |
| French fried potatoes, 2″ to 3½″ long | 10 (1½ oz) |
| Muffin, plain, small | 1 |
| Pancake, 4″ across | 2 |
| Waffle, 4½″ square | 1 |
| Stuffing, bread (prepared) | ¼ cup |
| Taco shell, 6″ across | 2 |
| Whole-wheat crackers, fat added (such as Triscuits) | 4–6 (1 oz) |

†3 g or more of fiber per serving.

## Table A–21. (continued)

### MEAT LIST

Each serving of meat and substitutes on this list contains varying amounts of fat and calories. The list is divided into three parts based on the amount of fat and calories: lean meat, medium-fat meat, and high-fat meat. One ounce (one meat exchange) of each of these includes:

|  | Carbohydrate (g) | Protein (g) | Fat (g) | Calories |
|---|---|---|---|---|
| Lean | 0 | 7 | 3 | 55 |
| Medium-fat | 0 | 7 | 5 | 75 |
| High-fat | 0 | 7 | 8 | 100 |

You are encouraged to use more lean and medium-fat meat, poultry, and fish in your meal plan. This will help decrease your fat intake, which may help decrease your risk for heart disease. The items from the high-fat group are high in saturated fat, cholesterol, and calories. You should limit your choices from the high-fat group to three (3) times per week. Meat and substitutes do not contribute any fiber to your meal plan. Meat and meat substitutes that have 400 mg or more of sodium are identified with a § symbol.

*Tips:*

1. Bake, roast, broil, grill, or boil these foods rather than frying them with added fat.
2. Use a nonstick pan spray or a nonstick pan to brown or fry these foods.
3. Trim off visible fat before and after cooking.
4. Do not add flour, bread crumbs, coating mixes, or fat to these foods when preparing them.
5. Weigh meat after removing bones and fat, and after cooking. Three ounces of cooked meat is about equal to 4 ounces of raw meat. Some examples of meat portions are:

    2 oz meat (2 meat exchanges) = 1 small chicken leg or thigh
    ½ cup cottage cheese or tuna

    3 oz meat (3 meat exchanges) = 1 medium pork chop
    1 small hamburger
    ½ chicken breast (1 side)
    1 unbreaded fish fillet
    cooked meat, about the size of a deck of cards

6. Restaurants usually serve prime cuts of meat, which are high in fat and calories.

## Table A–21.   (continued)

### *Lean Meat and Substitutes*
(One exchange is equal to any one of the following items)

| | | |
|---|---|---|
| Beef: | USDA Good or Choice grades of lean beef, such as round, sirloin, and flank steak, tenderloin, and chipped beef§ | 1 oz |
| Pork: | Lean pork, such as fresh ham; canned, cured, or boiled ham; Canadian bacon§, tenderloin | 1 oz |
| Veal: | All cuts are lean except for veal cutlets (ground or cubed). Examples of lean veal are chops and roasts. | 1 oz |
| Poultry: | Chicken, turkey, Cornish hen (without skin) | 1 oz |
| Fish: | All fresh and frozen fish | 1 oz |
| | Crab, lobster, scallops, shrimp, clams (fresh, or canned in water§) | 2 oz |
| | Oysters | 6 medium |
| | Tuna§ (canned in water) | ¼ cup |
| | Herring (uncreamed or smoked) | 1 oz |
| | Sardines (canned) | 2 medium |
| Wild Game: | Venison, rabbit, squirrel | 1 oz |
| | Pheasant, duck, goose (without skin) | 1 oz |
| Cheese: | Any cottage cheese | ¼ cup |
| | Grated Parmesan | 2 Tbsp |
| | Diet cheese§ with less than 55 calories per oz | 1 oz |
| Other: | 95% fat-free luncheon meat§ | 1 oz |
| | Egg whites | 3 whites |
| | Egg substitutes with less than 55 calories per ¼ cup | ¼ cup |

### *Medium-Fat Meat and Substitutes*
(One exchange is equal to any one of the following items)

| | | |
|---|---|---|
| Beef: | Most beef products fall into this category. Examples are all ground beef, roast (rib, chuck, rump), steak (cubed, Porterhouse, T-bone), and meatloaf | 1 oz |
| Pork: | Most pork products fall into this category. Examples are chops, loin roast, Boston butt, cutlets | 1 oz |
| Lamb: | Most lamb products fall into this category. Examples are chops, leg, and roast | 1 oz |
| Veal: | Cutlet (ground or cubed, unbreaded) | 1 oz |
| Poultry: | Chicken (with skin), domestic duck or goose (well-drained of fat), ground turkey | 1 oz |
| Fish: | Tuna§ (canned in oil and drained), salmon§ (canned) | ¼ cup |
| Cheese: | Skim or part-skim milk cheeses, such as | |
| | Ricotta | ¼ cup |
| | Mozzarella | 1 oz |
| | Diet cheeses§ with 56–80 calories per oz | 1 oz |
| Other: | 86% fat-free luncheon meat§ | 1 oz |
| | Egg (high in cholesterol, limit to 3 per week) | 1 |
| | Egg substitutes with 56–80 calories per ¼ cup | ¼ cup |
| | Tofu (2½″ × 2¾″ × 1″) | 4 oz |
| | Liver, heart, kidney, sweetbreads (high in cholesterol) | 1 oz |

### *High-Fat Meat and Substitutes*
Remember, these items are high in saturated fat, cholesterol, and calories, and should be used only three (3) times per week.
(One exchange is equal to any one of the following items)

| | | |
|---|---|---|
| Beef: | Most USDA Prime cuts of beef, such as ribs, corned beef§ | 1 oz |
| Pork: | Spareribs, ground pork, pork sausage§ (patty or link) | 1 oz |
| Lamb: | Patties (ground lamb) | 1 oz |
| Fish: | Any fried fish product | 1 oz |
| Cheese: | All regular cheese,§ such as American, Blue, Cheddar, Monterey, Swiss | 1 oz |
| Other: | Luncheon meat,§ such as bologna, salami, pimento loaf | 1 oz |
| | Sausage,§ such as Polish, Italian, knockwurst, smoked | 1 oz |
| | Bratwurst§ | 1 oz |
| | Frankfurter§ (turkey or chicken)†† | 1 frank (10/lb) |
| | Peanut butter (contains unsaturated fat) | 1 Tbsp |

§400 mg or more of sodium per exchange.

††Frankfurter (beef, pork or combination). Count as one high-fat meat plus one fat exchange: 1 frank (10/lb).

## Table A–21. (continued)

### VEGETABLE LIST

Each vegetable serving on this list contains about 5 g of carbohydrate, 2 g of protein, and 25 calories. Vegetables contain 2–3 g of dietary fiber. Vegetables that contain 400 mg or more of sodium per serving are identified with a § symbol.

Vegetables are a good source of vitamins and minerals. Fresh and frozen vegetables have more vitamins and less added salt. Rinsing canned vegetables will remove much of the salt.

Unless otherwise noted, the serving size for vegetables is:

- ½ cup of cooked vegetables or vegetable juice
- 1 cup of raw vegetables

| | | |
|---|---|---|
| Artichoke (½ medium) | Eggplant | Rutabaga |
| Asparagus | Greens (collard, mustard, turnip) | Sauerkraut§ |
| Beans (green, wax, Italian) | Kohlrabi | Spinach, cooked |
| Bean sprouts | Leeks | Summer squash (crookneck) |
| Beets | Mushrooms, cooked | Tomato (one large) |
| Broccoli | Okra | Tomato/vegetable juice§ |
| Brussels sprouts | Onions | Turnips |
| Cabbage, cooked | Pea pods | Water chestnuts |
| Carrots | Peppers (green) | Zucchini, cooked |
| Cauliflower | | |

Starchy vegetables such as corn, peas, and potatoes are found on the Starch/Bread list.

For free vegetables, see Free Food list.

§400 mg or more of sodium per serving.

## Table A–21.  (continued)

### FRUIT LIST

Each item on this list contains about 15 g of carbohydrate and 60 calories. Fresh, frozen, and dry fruits have about 2 g of fiber per serving. Fruits that have 3 g or more of fiber per serving have a † symbol. Fruit juices contain very little dietary fiber.

The carbohydrate and calorie content for a fruit serving are based on the usual serving of the most commonly eaten fruits. Use fresh fruits, or fruits frozen or canned without sugar added. Whole fruit is more filling than fruit juice, and may be a better choice for those who are trying to lose weight. Unless otherwise noted, the serving size for fruit is:

- ½ cup of fresh fruit or fruit juice
- ¼ cup of dried fruit

**Fresh, frozen, and unsweetened canned fruit**

| | |
|---|---|
| Apple (raw, 2″ across) | 1 apple |
| Applesauce (unsweetened) | ½ cup |
| Apricots (medium, raw) | 4 apricots |
| Apricots (canned) | ½ cup, or 4 halves |
| Banana (9″ long) | ½ banana |
| †Blackberries (raw) | ¾ cup |
| †Blueberries (raw) | ¾ cup |
| Cantaloupe (5″ across) | ⅓ melon |
| (cubes) | 1 cup |
| Cherries (large, sweet, raw) | 12 cherries |
| Cherries (canned) | ½ cup |
| Figs (raw, 2″ across) | 2 figs |
| Fruit cocktail (canned) | ½ cup |
| Grapefruit (medium) | ½ grapefruit |
| Grapefruit (segments) | ¾ cup |
| Grapes (small) | 15 grapes |
| Honeydew melon (medium) | ⅛ melon |
| (cubes) | 1 cup |
| Kiwi (large) | 1 kiwi |
| Mandarin oranges | ¾ cup |
| Mango (small) | ½ mango |
| †Nectarine (1-½″ across) | 1 nectarine |
| Orange (2-½″ across) | 1 orange |
| Papaya | 1 cup |
| Peach (2-¾″ across) | 1 peach, or ¾ cup |
| Peaches (canned) | ½ cup, or 2 halves |
| Pear | ½ large, 1 small |
| Pears (canned) | ½ cup, or 2 halves |

| | |
|---|---|
| Persimmon (medium, native) | 2 persimmons |
| Pineapple (raw) | ¾ cup |
| Pineapple (canned) | ⅓ cup |
| Plum (raw, 2″ across) | 2 plums |
| †Pomegranate | ½ pomegranate |
| †Raspberries (raw) | 1 cup |
| †Strawberries (raw, whole) | 1-¼ cup |
| †Tangerine (2-½″ across) | 2 tangerines |
| Watermelon (cubes) | 1-¼ cup |

**Dried Fruit**

| | |
|---|---|
| †Apples | 4 rings |
| †Apricots | 7 halves |
| Dates | 2-½ medium |
| †Figs | 1-½ |
| †Prunes | 3 medium |
| Raisins | 2 Tbsp |

**Fruit Juice**

| | |
|---|---|
| Apple juice/cider | ½ cup |
| Cranberry juice cocktail | ⅓ cup |
| Grapefruit juice | ½ cup |
| Grape juice | ⅓ cup |
| Orange juice | ½ cup |
| Pineapple juice | ½ cup |
| Prune juice | ⅓ cup |

†3 g or more of fiber per serving.

## MILK LIST

Each serving of milk or milk products on this list contains about 12 g of carbohydrate and 8 g of protein. The amount of fat in milk is measured in percent (%) of butterfat. The calories vary, depending on what kind of milk you choose. The list is divided into three parts based on the amount of fat and calories: skim/very low-fat milk, low-fat milk, and whole milk. One serving (one milk exchange) of each of these includes:

|  | Carbohydrate (g) | Protein (g) | Fat (g) | Calories |
|---|---|---|---|---|
| Skim/Very low-fat | 12 | 8 | trace | 90 |
| Low-fat | 12 | 8 | 5 | 120 |
| Whole | 12 | 8 | 8 | 150 |

Milk is the body's main source of calcium, the mineral needed for growth and repair of bones. Yogurt is also a good source of calcium. Yogurt and many dry or powdered milk products have different amounts of fat. If you have questions about a particular item, read the label to find out the fat and calorie content.

Milk is good to drink, but it can also be added to cereal and to other foods. Many tasty dishes such as sugar-free pudding are made with milk (see the Combination Foods list). Plain yogurt is delicious with one of your fruit servings mixed with it.

*Skim and Very Low-fat Milk*
- 1 cup skim milk
- 1 cup ½% milk
- 1 cup 1% milk
- 1 cup low-fat buttermilk
- ½ cup evaporated skim milk
- ⅓ cup dry nonfat milk
- 8-oz carton plain nonfat yogurt

*Low-Fat Milk*
- 1 cup fluid 2% milk
- 8-oz carton plain low-fat yogurt (with added nonfat milk solids)

*Whole Milk*
The whole milk group has much more fat per serving than the skim and low-fat groups. Whole milk has more than 3¼% butterfat. Try to limit your choices from the whole milk group as much as possible.
- 1 cup whole milk
- ½ cup evaporated whole milk
- 8-oz carton whole plain yogurt

## FAT LIST

Each serving on the fat list contains about 5 g of fat and 45 calories.

The foods on the fat list contain mostly fat, although some items may also contain a small amount of protein. All fats are high in calories and should be carefully measured. Everyone should modify their fat intake by eating unsaturated fats instead of saturated fats. The sodium content of these foods varies widely. Check the label for sodium information.

| *Unsaturated Fats* | | *Saturated Fats* | |
|---|---|---|---|
| Avocado | ⅛ medium | Butter | 1 tsp |
| Margarine | 1 tsp | Bacon# | 1 slice |
| Margarine, diet# | 1 Tbsp | Chitterlings | ½ oz |
| Mayonnaise | 1 tsp | Coconut, shredded | 2 Tbsp |
| Mayonnaise, reduced-calorie# | 1 Tbsp | Coffee whitener, liquid | 2 Tbsp |
| Nuts and seeds: | | Coffee whitener, powder | 4 tsp |
|   Almonds, dry roasted | 6 whole | Cream (light, coffee, table) | 2 Tbsp |
|   Cashews, dry roasted | 1 Tbsp | Cream, sour | 2 Tbsp |
|   Pecans | 2 whole | Cream (heavy, whipping) | 1 Tbsp |
|   Peanuts | 20 small, 10 large | Cream cheese | 1 Tbsp |
|   Walnuts | 2 whole | Salt pork# | ¼ oz |
|   Other nuts | 1 Tbsp | | |
|   Seeds, pine nuts, sunflower (without shells) | 1 Tbsp | | |
|   Pumpkin seeds | 2 tsp | | |
| Oil (corn, cottonseed, safflower, soybean, sunflower, olive, peanut) | 1 tsp | | |
| Olives# | 10 small, 5 large | | |
| Salad dressing, mayonnaise-type | 2 tsp | | |
| Salad dressing, mayonnaise-type, reduced-calorie | 1 Tbsp | | |
| Salad dressing (all varieties)# | 1 Tbsp | | |
| Salad dressing, reduced-calorie (two tablespoons of low-calorie is a free food.)§ | 2 Tbsp | | |

#If more than one or two servings are eaten, foods have 400 mg or more of sodium.
§400 mg or more of sodium per serving.

## FREE FOODS

A free food is any food or drink that contains 20 calories or less per serving. You can eat as much as you want of those items that have no serving size specified. You may eat two or three servings per day of those items that have a specific serving size. Be sure to spread them out through the day.

**Drinks:**
Bouillon§ or broth without fat†
Bouillon, low-sodium
Carbonated drinks, sugar-free
Carbonated water
Club soda
Cocoa powder, unsweetened (1 Tbsp)
Coffee/Tea
Drink mixes, sugar-free
Mineral water
Tonic water, sugar-free
**Nonstick pan spray**

**Fruit:**
Cranberries, unsweetened (½ cup)
Rhubarb, unsweetened (½ cup)

**Vegetables: (raw, 1 cup)**
Cabbage
Celery
Chinese cabbage†
Cucumber
Green onion
Hot peppers
Mushrooms
Radishes
Zucchini†
Salad greens:
 Endive
 Escarole
 Lettuce
 Romaine
 Spinach

**Sweet Substitutes:**
Candy, hard, sugar-free
Gelatin, sugar-free
Gum, sugar-free
Jam/jelly, sugar-free (2 tsp)
Pancake syrup, sugar-free (¼ cup)
Sugar substitutes (saccharin, Equal)
Whipped topping, low calorie

**Condiments:**
Catsup (1 Tbsp)
Horseradish
Mustard
Pickles§, dill, unsweetened
Salad dressing, low-calorie (2 Tbsp)
Taco sauce (1 Tbsp)
Vinegar

Seasonings can be very helpful in making food taste better. Be careful of how much sodium you use. Read the label and choose those seasonsing that do not contain sodium or salt.

Basil (fresh)
Celery seeds
Cinnamon
Chili powder
Chives
Curry
Dill
Flavoring extracts (e.g., vanilla,
  lemon, almond, walnut,
  peppermint, butter)

Garlic
Garlic powder
Herbs
Hot pepper sauce
Lemon
Lemon juice
Lemon pepper
Lime
Lime juice
Mint

Onion powder
Oregano
Paprika
Pepper
Pimento
Spices
Soy sauce§
Soy sauce, low-sodium
Wine, used in cooking (¼ cup)
Worcestershire sauce

†3 g or more of fiber per serving.
§400 mg or more of sodium per serving.

## COMBINATION FOODS

Much of the food we eat is mixed together in various combinations. These combination foods do not fit into only one exchange list. It can be difficult to tell what is in a certain casserole dish or baked food item. This is a list of average values for some typical combination foods. This list will help you fit these foods into your meal plan. Ask your dietitian for information about any other foods you'd like to eat. The *American Diabetes Association/American Dietetic Association Family Cookbooks* and the *American Diabetes Association Holiday Cookbook* have many recipes and further information about many foods, including combination foods. Check your library or local bookstore.

| Food | Amount | Exchanges |
|---|---|---|
| Casseroles, homemade | 1 cup (8 oz) | 2 starch, 2 medium-fat meat, 1 fat |
| Cheese pizza§ thin crust | ¼ of 15 oz or ¼ of 10″ | 2 starch, 1 medium-fat meat, 1 fat |
| Chili with beans†·§ (commercial) | 1 cup (8 oz) | 2 starch, 2 medium-fat meat, 2 fat |
| Chow mein† (without noodles or rice) | 2 cups (16 oz) | 1 starch, 2 vegetable, 2 lean meat |
| Macaroni and cheese§ | 1 cup (8 oz) | 2 starch, 1 medium-fat meat, 2 fat |
| *Soup* | | |
|   Bean† | 1 cup (8 oz) | 1 starch, 1 vegetable, 1 lean meat |
|   Chunky, all varieties | 10-¾ oz can | 1 starch, 1 vegetable, 1 medium-fat meat |
|   Cream§ (made with water) | 1 cup (8 oz) | 1 starch, 1 fat |
|   Vegetable§ or broth§ | 1 cup (8 oz) | 1 starch |
| Spaghetti and meatballs§ (canned) | 1 cup (8 oz) | 2 starch, 1 medium-fat meat, 1 fat |
| Sugar-free pudding (made with skim milk) | ½ cup | 1 starch |
| *If beans are used as a meat substitute:* | | |
| Dried beans,† peas,† lentils† | 1 cup (cooked) | 2 starch, 1 lean meat |

†3 g or more of fiber per serving
§400 mg or more of sodium per serving

## Table A–21. (continued)

### FOODS FOR OCCASIONAL USE

Moderate amounts of some foods can be used in your meal plan, in spite of their sugar or fat content, as long as you can maintain blood glucose control. The following list includes average exchange values for some of these foods. Because they are concentrated sources of carbohydrate, you will notice that the portion sizes are very small. Check with your dietitian for advice on how often and when you can eat them.

| *Food* | *Amount* | *Exchanges* |
|---|---|---|
| Angel food cake | $\frac{1}{12}$ cake | 2 starch |
| Cake, no icing | $\frac{1}{12}$ cake, or a 3″ square | 2 starch, 2 fat |
| Cookies | 2 small (1-¾″ across) | 1 starch, 1 fat |
| Frozen fruit yogurt | ⅓ cup | 1 starch |
| Gingersnaps | 3 | 1 starch |
| Granola | ¼ cup | 1 starch, 1 fat |
| Granola bars | 1 small | 1 starch, 1 fat |
| Ice cream, any flavor | ½ cup | 1 starch, 2 fat |
| Ice milk, any flavor | ½ cup | 1 starch, 1 fat |
| Sherbet, any flavor | ¼ cup | 1 starch |
| Snack chips,§ all varieties | 1 oz | 1 starch, 2 fat |
| Vanilla wafers | 6 small | 1 starch, 1 fat |

§If more than one serving is eaten, these foods have 400 mg or more of sodium

### MANAGEMENT TIPS

Some food you buy uncooked will weigh less after you cook it. This is true of most meats. Starches often swell in cooking, so a small amount of uncooked starch will become a much larger amount of cooked food. The following table shows some of the changes:

| *Food (Starch Group)* | *Uncooked* | *Cooked* |
|---|---|---|
| Oatmeal | 3 level Tbsp | ½ cup |
| Cream of wheat | 2 level Tbsp | ½ cup |
| Grits | 3 level Tbsp | ½ cup |
| Rice | 2 level Tbsp | ⅓ cup |
| Spaghetti | ¼ cup | ½ cup |
| Noodles | ⅓ cup | ½ cup |
| Macaroni | ¼ cup | ½ cup |
| Dried beans | 3 Tbsp | ⅓ cup |
| Dried peas | 3 Tbsp | ⅓ cup |
| Lentils | 2 Tbsp | ⅓ cup |
| *Food (Meat Group)* | | |
| Hamburger | 4 oz | 3 oz |
| Chicken | 1 small drumstick | 1 oz |
| | ½ breast (1 side) | 3 oz |

- Read food labels. Remember—*dietetic* does not mean *diabetic!* When you see the word "dietetic" on a food label, it means that something has been changed or replaced. It may have less salt, less fat, or less sugar. It does not mean that the food is sugar-free or calorie-free. Some dietetic foods may be useful. Those that contain 20 calories or less per serving may be eaten up to three times a day as free foods.

- Know your sweeteners. Two types of sweeteners are on the market: those with calories and those without calories. Sweeteners with calories, such as fructose, sorbitol, and mannitol, when used in large amounts, may cause cramping and diarrhea. Remember, these sweeteners do have calories that add up. Sweeteners without calories include saccharin and aspartame (Equal, Nutrasweet) and may be used in moderation.

## Table A–22.  Diets for Weight Reduction, Diabetes, and Reduced Soluble Carbohydrates (High-Polyunsaturated-Fat Diets)*

| Total Daily Intake | kcal | | | |
|---|---|---|---|---|
| | 800 | 1,200 | 1,800 | 2,400 |
| Carbohydrate (g) | 94 | 134 | 225 | 276 |
| Protein (g) | 57 | 68 | 90 | 122 |
| Fat (g) | 22 | 47 | 60 | 86 |
| Total Exchanges for One Day (see Table A–21): | | | | |
| Skim milk | 2 | 2 | 2 | 3 |
| Vegetable | 2 | 2 | 2 | 4 |
| Fruit | 3 | 4 | 5 | 5 |
| Bread | 2 | 4 | 9 | 12 |
| Meat† | 5 | 6 | 8 | 10 |
| Unsaturated fat | 1 | 5 | 7 | 10 |
| Sample Meal Pattern | Servings based on exchanges | | | |
| *Breakfast* | | | | |
| Fruit | 1 | 1 | 1 | 1 + 1 midmeal |
| Bread | 1 | 1 | 3 | 3 + 1 midmeal |
| Meat† | 0 | 0 | 2 | 2 |
| Fat, unsaturated | 1 | 1 | 2 | 3 |
| Milk, skim | ½ | 1 | 1 | 1 + 1 midmeal |
| Tea/coffee | | as desired | | |
| *Lunch* | | | | |
| Meat† | 2 | 2 | 3 | 3 |
| Vegetable | 0 | 1 | 1 | 2 |
| Bread | ½ | 1 | 3 | 3 |
| Fat, unsaturated | 0 | 2 | 2 | 3 |
| Fruit | 1 | 1 | 2 | 1 |
| Milk, skim | 1 | ½ | 0 | 1 |
| Tea/coffee | | as desired | | |
| *Dinner* | | | | |
| Meat† | 3 | 3 | 3 | 3 |
| Vegetable | 2 | 1 | 1 | 2 |
| Bread | ½ | 1 | 2 | 3 |
| Fat, unsaturated | 0 | 1 | 2 | 3 |
| Fruit | 1 | 2 | 2 | 2 |
| Milk, skim | ½ | 0 | 0 | 0 |
| Tea/coffee | | as desired | | |
| *Evening* | | | | |
| Meat† | 0 | 0 | 0 | 0 |
| Bread | 0 | 1 | 1 | 2 |
| Milk, skim | 0 | ½ | 1 | 0 |
| Fat, unsaturated | 0 | 0 | 2 | 1 |
| Tea/coffee | | as desired | | |

*This table, prepared by the authors, is based on the following dietary recommendations in *A Guide to Professionals: The Effective Application of Exchange Lists for Meal Planning,* American Diabetes Association, Inc., and The American Dietetic Association, 1977. Protein: 20% of total calories for growing children and pregnant women, minimum of 0.5 g/pound desirable body weight for other adults; carbohydrates: 50 to 70% of nonprotein calories; fat: 30 to 50% of nonprotein calories. An exception is the 800-kcal diet, which has 29% calories as protein. Reduce fat consumption to 30% of energy intake, providing equal proportions of saturated, monounsaturated, and polyunsaturated fatty acids, reduce cholesterol to 300 mg per day, increase complex carbohydrates and naturally occurring sugars to 48% of energy intake, reduce consumption of refined and processed sugars to account for 10% of total energy intake, and reduce salt consumption to 5 g per day.
†Eleven of 14 main meals per week should contain poultry (without skin), fish, lean veal, uncreamed cottage cheese, or skim milk yogurt. Remaining meals may include servings of lean beef, lamb, or pork. No more than 3 egg yolks (eating or cooking) should be taken per week.

## Table A–23a.  Sodium-Restricted Diets*

| Degree of Restriction: | | Strict† | Moderate | Mild |
|---|---|---|---|---|
| Na in mg | = | 500 | 1,000 | 2,400–4,500 |
| Na in meq | = | 21.7 | 43.4 | 104.3–195.6 |
| NaCl in g | = | 1.2 | 2.5 | 6.1–11.5 |
| *Approximate Composition* | *Unit* | | | |
| Carbohydrate | g | 291 | 327 | 339 |
| Protein | g | 84 | 147 | 111 |
| Fat | g | 65 | 84 | 96.5 |
| Calories | | 1,925 | 2,500 | 2,589.2 |
| Calcium | mg | 811 | 1,182 | 1,193 |
| Phosphorus | mg | 1,337 | 2,094 | 1,932 |
| Iron | mg | 12.7 | 19.5 | 15.8 |
| Sodium | mg (meq) | 455   (20) | 891   (44) | 2,444   (106) |
| Potassium | mg (meq) | 3,840   (98) | 4,765   (122) | 4,267   (109) |
| Vitamin A | I.U. | 6,178 | 7,222 | 7,358 |
| Thiamin | mg | 1.2 | 1.6 | 1.4 |
| Riboflavin | mg | 1.9 | 2.9 | 2.6 |
| Niacin equivalents | mg | 21.7 | 35.6 | 23.2 |
| Ascorbic acid | mg | 206 | 208 | 158 |

### General Rules:

1. Avoid the use of all salt, baking soda, and/or baking powder in cooking and for table use.
2. Avoid medicines, laxatives, and salt substitutes unless prescribed by physician.
3. Read labels carefully for sodium or salt content of packaged foods.

### Guidance on Food Selection:

| Type of Food | | Amount‡ | Foods Included | Foods Excluded |
|---|---|---|---|---|
| Milk | Strict<br>Moderate<br>Mild | ‡2 cups<br>}  3 cups | Evaporated, nonfat dry milk; skim milk; unsalted butter-milk and whole milk. ‡Additional milk must be low-sodium, fluid, or powdered. | Cultured buttermilk; condensed milk; all milk drinks prepared with malt, chocolate syrup and ice cream; yogurt; more than 2 cups of regular milk daily.<br>(*Mild*—No restriction except limit to 3 cups) |
| Other beverages | Strict<br>Moderate<br>Mild | 2–3 cups<br>}  as desired<br><br>as desired | Cocoa prepared with milk allowance; coffee, instant and regular; Postum: Sanka; tea; fresh and frozen fruitades; carbonated beverages limit to one 8-oz bottle daily. | Ginger ale; commercial chocolate syrup, fountain beverages; instant cocoa and all powdered beverage mixes; all those not listed as allowed; alcoholic beverages allowed with physician's permission.<br>(*Mild*—Only Dutch-process cocoa and alcoholic beverages without physician's permission.) |
| Soup | | 1 cup (8 oz per cup) | Unsalted broth; unsalted vegetable soup made with allowed vegetables; unsalted cream soup made from butter and milk allowance; unsalted tomato bouillon. | All canned, dehydrated, and frozen soups containing salt; bouillon cubes; consommé and other commercial meat-extract soups. |
| Meat, poultry, and fish | Strict<br>Moderate<br>Mild | 4 oz<br>10 oz<br>6 oz | Fresh, unsalted frozen or un-salted canned meats, fish, and poultry such as beef, chicken, duck, lamb, liver (beef, calves, or chicken liver allowed once every 2 weeks), pork, fresh tongue, turkey, veal; *use fresh fish only* such as bass, blue-fish, cod, flounder, halibut, oysters, perch, salmon, snapper, sole, trout, tuna; sweet-breads and salt-free peanut butter.<br>(*Mild*—Reg. tuna, salmon, shellfish) | All salted, koshered, smoked, corned, and canned (with salt) meats, fish and poultry; bacon, brains, kidneys, luncheon meats, chipped or corned beef, ham, frankfurters, anchovies, caviar, sardines, herring, regular canned tuna, salmon; shellfish; clams, crabs, lobsters, scallops, shrimps; regular peanut butter. |

## Table A–23a. (continued)

| Type of Food | | Amount‡ | Foods Included | Foods Excluded |
|---|---|---|---|---|
| Cheese | | 1 svg. (1 oz) | Unsalted cottage cheese, unsalted cream cheese, and unsalted American cheese. (*Mild*—American, cheddar, Swiss, cottage, cream) | All other cheese not listed as allowed. |
| Eggs | Strict | Limit to 1 a day | Boiled, poached, scrambled, or fried in unsalted butter. | None except in excess of amount allowed. |
| | Moderate Mild | } 2 a day | | |
| Potato or substitute | | 2 svgs. (½ cup per svg.) | Potatoes, white or sweet; macaroni; noodles; rice and spaghetti. | Potato chips and prepared potato products. |
| Bread | Strict | 4 svgs. | Unsalted bread and unsalted crackers such as melba toast and plain Passover or thin tea matzos. (*Mild*—regular bread; graham crackers; biscuits; muffins) | Regular bread; rolls; biscuits; muffins and cereal products prepared with salt or baking soda; commercial mixes; graham crackers; saltines; soda crackers; salted matzos and self-rising flour. |
| | Moderate | 6 svgs. | | |
| | Mild | 4 svgs. | | |
| Cereals | Strict Moderate | } 1 svg. (½ cup per svg.) | Unsalted slow-cooking unenriched cereals; barley; cornmeal; cornstarch; grits; tapioca; dry cereals; puffed rice; puffed and shredded wheat. | Quick-cooking and enriched cereals; dry cereals except those listed as allowed. (*Mild*—none) |
| | Mild | | | |
| Vegetables | Strict Moderate | } 3 svgs. (½ cup per svg.) | All fresh, frozen and unsalted canned vegetables except those listed under Foods Excluded; dried lima beans, lentils, split peas, and soybeans. (*Mild*—all fresh, unsalted, canned and unsalted, frozen vegetables) | Canned vegetables and vegetable juices to which salt has been added; artichokes; beets; beet greens; carrots; celery; collards; Swiss chard; dandelion greens; kale; mustard greens; sauerkraut; spinach; white turnips; frozen vegetables processed with salt such as lima beans, peas, and mixed vegetables. |
| | Mild | 4 svgs. | | |
| Fruit and fruit juice | Strict Moderate | } 3 svgs. (½ cup per svg.) | Any fruit or fruit juice fresh, frozen, or canned except those listed under Foods Excluded. Include one citrus fruit or juice daily. | Crystallized or glazed fruit; dried figs or raisins; tomato juice; all fruits to which sodium coloring, sodium flavoring, or sodium benzoate has been added. (*Mild*—none) |
| | Mild | | | |
| Butter or fat | Strict | 6 svgs. (1 tsp. per svg.) | Unsalted butter; unsalted margarine; unsalted salad and cooking fats such as corn, cottonseed, Crisco, olive oil, Spry; unsalted French and mayonnaise dressings; unsalted gravy; sweet and sour cream, limit 2 tbsps per day. (*Mod.*—3 pats may be salted, 6 tsp sweet or sour cream) (*Mild*—3 oz butter; margarine; mayonnaise; French dressing; oil; plus 3 oz cream) | Salted butter and salted margarine; all commercial salad and mayonnaise dressings; bacon and pork fat; salted meat gravy. (*Mild*—bacon, bacon fat, excess of amount allowed) |
| | Moderate | 6 svgs. | | |
| | Mild | 5 svgs. | | |

## Table A–23a.   (continued)

| Type of Food | Amount‡ | | Foods Included | Foods Excluded |
|---|---|---|---|---|
| Dessert | Strict<br>Moderate | } 1 svg. (1 svg. = ½ cup) | Fruit ice, gelatin made with fresh fruit juices; unsalted desserts made from milk and egg allowance such as custard, tapioca, cornstarch, and rice pudding; unsalted fruit crisps and unsalted fruit pies; junket except chocolate; unsalted sugar cookies.<br>‡Commercial ice cream and sherbet must be used as milk allowance. | All commercial cakes; cookies; pies; puddings; Jell-O; chocolate junket; rennet tablets; all dessert made with baking powder, salt, or soda; commercial ice cream and sherbet when not taken as milk allowance; gingersnaps; sandwich-type cookies; any dessert prepared with nuts. |
|  | Mild | 3 svgs. | (*Mild*—cake, cookies and pies) |  |
| Sweets | As desired | | Sugar, white and brown; honey; jams; jellies made without the addition of sodium benzoate; hard candy; maple syrup and gum drops. | Commercial candies and syrups; chocolate syrups; molasses; saccharin and Sucaryl. |
| Spices | As desired | | All except those listed in Foods Excluded. | Accent; dried or fresh celery leaves; celery salt; celery seed; garlic salt; horseradish prepared with salt; onion salt; salt substitutes unless recommended by physician; all seasonings with salt added. |
| Miscellaneous | As desired | | Dietetic catsup, low-sodium dietetic meat extracts and tenderizers; cream of tartar; yeast; unsalted popcorn; unsalted nuts; sodium-free baking powders if allowed by physician. | Regular catsup; chili sauce; meat extracts; meat tenderizers; meat sauces; prepared mustard; olives; pickles; relishes; soy sauce; Worcestershire sauce; salted pretzels and popcorn; chips and all *snacks* containing salt; salted nuts. |

*Adequacy:* This diet meets the 1980 Recommended Dietary Allowances of the National Research Council except for calories, which may be low for an active individual, and for iron for females. The calculations are based on the sample meal plan. Supplementation with iron and thiamin may be necessary in strict sodium regimens.

The use of water softeners may add significant amounts of sodium to the water supply.

†This strict diet can be modified to 250 mg sodium by eliminating regular milk and using only low-sodium milk and eliminating all commercial sherbets and ice cream.

‡Varying amounts of foods included relate to degrees of restriction.

## Table A–23b. Sample Meal Pattern for Strict Sodium Restriction (21.7 meq)

| *Breakfast* | *Serving Portion* | *Sample Menu* |
|---|---|---|
| Fruit | ½ cup | Orange juice |
| Cereal | ½ cup | Unsalted Wheatena |
| Egg | 1 | Soft-cooked egg |
| Bread | 2 slices | Low-sodium toast |
| Fat | 1 tsp | Unsalted butter |
| Milk | ½ cup | Milk |
| Beverage | 1 cup | Coffee |
| Sugar | 1 tbsp | Sugar |
| *Lunch* | | |
| Meat or substitute | 2 oz | Unsalted broiled chicken |
| Potato | 1 | Baked potato |
| Vegetable | ½ cup | Unsalted asparagus |
| Salad | ½ cup | Sliced tomato |
| Dressing | 1 tbsp | Unsalted French dressing |
| Dessert | ½ cup | Lime ice |
| Bread | 1 slice | Low-sodium bread |
| Fat | 1 tsp | Unsalted butter |
| Milk | ½ cup | Milk |
| Beverage | 1 cup | Coffee or tea |
| Sugar | 2 tsp | Sugar |
| *Dinner* | | |
| Soup | 1 cup | Unsalted broth |
| Meat | 2 oz | Unsalted roast beef |
| Potato | 1 | Unsalted boiled potato |
| Vegetable | ½ cup | Unsalted Brussels sprouts |
| Fruit | ½ cup | Canned apricots |
| Bread | 1 slice | Low-sodium bread |
| Fat | 1 tsp | Unsalted butter |
| Beverage | 1 cup | Coffee or tea |
| Sugar | 2 tsp | Sugar |
| *8:00 p.m.* | | |
| Milk | 1 cup | Milk |
| Fruit | ½ cup | Applesauce |

## Table A–23c. Approximate Sodium Content of Certain Food Groups that may be Calculated into Sodium-Restricted Diets*

| *Foods Containing 500 mg Na/Serving* | *Foods Containing 250 mg Na/Serving* | *Foods Containing 200 mg Na/Serving* | *Foods Containing 100 mg Na/Serving* | *Foods Containing 50 mg Na/Serving* |
|---|---|---|---|---|
| scant ¼ tsp salt | 1 oz canned tuna | 1 slice regular bakery bread or roll | ½ cup of the following unsalted vegetables: beet greens, frozen mixed peas and carrots, Swiss chard | ½ cup of the following fresh, frozen, or canned vegetables, canned without salt: |
| ¾ tsp monosodium glutamate | 2 oz canned sardines or salmon | 2 thin slices bacon, crisp and drained | | |
| ½ bouillon cube | ⅔ cup buttermilk | 3 oz canned shrimp cooked in salted water | | 1 artichoke, edible base and leaves |
| 1 cup tomato juice | ½ cup canned or regularly seasoned carrots, spinach, beets, celery, kale, or white turnips | | 1 oz fresh koshered meat | beets |
| 1 average serving ½ cup cooked rice, spaghetti, noodles, hominy, seasoned with salt | | ½ cup canned or regularly seasoned vegetables not listed elsewhere | 1 oz frozen fish fillets | carrots |
| | | | | celery |
| | | | | dandelion greens |
| ½ cup drained sauerkraut | 5 salted crackers (2-in square) | 1 day's supply of drinking water if it contains 100 mg Na/qt | | kale |
| | | | | mustard greens |
| 1 average frankfurter (1½ oz) | ¾ cup tomato juice | | | peas, black-eyed |
| | 1 day's supply of drinking water if it contains 120 mg Na/qt | ½ cup frozen peas or lima beans | | spinach |
| | | | | succotash |
| 1 day's supply of drinking water if it contains 220 mg Na/qt | | 1 oz natural cheddar cheese | | turnip greens |
| | | | | turnip, white |
| | | 1 tbsp catsup | | 1 day's supply of drinking water if it contains 40 mg Na/qt |

*From American Dietetic Association: Handbook of Clinical Dietetics. New Haven, Yale University Press, 1981, p. G8, with permission.

## Table A–24. Recommendations for Phased Dietary Modifications in the Prevention and Therapy of Hyperlipidemia*

The American Heart Association has outlined three progressive steps or phases to modify the "typical" American diet—especially to cut down on saturated fat and cholesterol.† Phase 1 describes the basic recommendations for all healthy Americans. Phase 2 contains additional changes designed for people who need to lower blood lipids (fats) further; those who have elevated blood lipid levels and/or other risk factors that require this approach. Phase 3 is for those who wish to make even further modifications, or who must meet particularly stringent requirements for lowering blood lipids.

The following table summarizes dietary goals for each of the three phases. The percentage signs refer to the percent of total calories each day. For example, if on Phase 1 a patient eats 1,500 calories a day, 450 calories (30%) would be from fats. P/S refers to a ratio of polyunsaturated to saturated fats. A P/S ratio of 1 means consumption of equal amounts of saturated and polyunsaturated fat. For example, to follow Phase 1, it is recommended that 30% of calories come from fat—10% from saturated fat and 10% from polyunsaturated fat. On the Phase 3 diet, the saturated fat should be no more than 6% and the polyunsaturated fat should be about 8% of total calories.

| Phase | 1 | 2 | 3 |
|---|---|---|---|
| Fat | 30% | 25% | 20% |
| Carbohydrate | 55% | 60% | 65% |
| Protein | 15% | 15% | 15% |
| Cholesterol‡ | 300 mg | 200–250 mg | 100 mg |
| P/S ratio | 1 | 1 | 1–2 |

‡The cholesterol content will vary depending on your body size and caloric intake.

*Phase 1:* Avoid high-saturated-fat, baked, fried items such as doughnuts, fried pies, sweet rolls, cheesecake, pie, cake, and cookies. Use low-fat crackers in place of high-fat crackers.

Use only 1% low-fat milk for drinking or food preparation. Replace cream with skim milk or nonfat milk powder. Use sherbet, frozen yogurt, or ice milk for ice cream.

Select only lean beef, lamb, and veal. Choose meats with very little marbling. Remove poultry skin. Limit amount of meat, seafood, and poultry to 7 oz or less per day.

Limit egg yolk to two per week (including those used in baking).

In place of butter, use margarine containing at least twice as much polyunsaturated fat as saturated fat. Use acceptable margarine or oil in place of shortening in recipes. Use oil or acceptable margarine for seasoning vegetables.

*Phase 2:* Select low-fat commercial products such as graham crackers, angel food cake, gingersnaps, and fig bars. Account for all fat used in baked goods as part of fat allowance.

Use only 1% low-fat milk for drinking and food preparation. Replace cream with skim milk or nonfat dry milk powder. Use low-fat cheese in place of high-fat cheese. Use sherbet, frozen yogurt, or ice milk in place of ice cream.

Increase use of fish and poultry in place of red meat. Increase use of meatless main dishes to at least three per week. Consume 6 oz or less of meat per day.

Use egg white or egg substitutes. Eliminate all egg yolks.

Use margarine containing at least twice as much polyunsaturated fat as saturated fat in place of butter. Use acceptable margarine or oil in place of shortening in recipes. Use oil or margarine for seasoning vegetables. Use air-popped popcorn.

*Phase 3:* Use safflower oil, corn oil, sunflower oil, or allowed margarine in quick breads. Use egg whites or fat-free egg substitutes for baked goods.

Use fat-free crackers. Use fruit and vegetables as snacks.

Use low-fat cheese in place of part of meat allowance. Use fruit ice or skim-milk sherbet in place of whole-milk sherbet and ice milk.

Limit meat meals to one per day (fish and poultry are preferable choices). Consume 3 oz or less of meat per day. Make all other meals meatless.

Use fat-free egg substitutes and egg whites.

Prepare homemade salad dressing using safflower, corn, or sunflower oil. Use fat-free desserts and homemade quick breads in place of high-fat desserts. Use only safflower, corn, or sunflower oil for food preparation.

*From American Heart Association: Eating for a Healthy Heart and Counseling the Patient with Hyperlipidemia. Dallas, Texas, National Center, 1986.

†From American Heart Association: A note about "Eating for a Healthy Heart." The Nutrition Committee, N.Y. City Affiliate, 1986, with permission from The American Heart Association.

ADDENDUM: The National Cholesterol Education Program recommends a "Step 1 diet" similar to the phase 1 diet above and a "Step 2 diet" providing saturated fat at <7% of calories and cholesterol at <200 mg/day. (N.Y. Times 10/6/87) (See details in NIH and AHA publications scheduled for 1988.)

## Table A–25a.   Protein, Sodium, Potassium, Phosphorus, and Magnesium Contents of Selected Common Foods*

| | Amount | Protein (g) | Potassium (meq)‡ | Sodium (meq)‡ | Phosphorus (mg) | Magnesium† (mg)‡ |
|---|---|---|---|---|---|---|
| *DAIRY PRODUCTS* | | | | | | |
| Eggs, large | 1 | 6.1 | 1.67 | 3.00 | 90.0 | 6.1 |
| Cottage cheese, salt-free, dry | 1 oz | 4.9 | 0.24 | 0.15 | 29.5 | 1.4 |
| Cream, light | 1 Tbsp | 0.4 | 0.46 | 0.26 | 12.0 | 1.3 |
| Cream, sour | 1 Tbsp | 0.4 | 0.44 | 0.26 | 10.0 | 1.7 |
| Milk, butter (fluid culture) | 1 cup | 8.1 | 9.51 | 11.17 | 219.0 | 26.8 |
| Milk, regular | 1 cup | 8.0 | 9.49 | 5.22 | 228.0 | 32.8 |
| Milk, skim | 1 cup | 8.3 | 10.41 | 5.48 | 247.0 | 27.8 |
| Milk, low-sodium | 1 cup | 7.6 | 15.80 | 0.26 | 209.0 | 12.2 |
| *BUTTER OR FAT* | | | | | | |
| Butter, sweet | 1 pat | 0.03 | 0.03 | 0.02 | 1.0 | 0.10 |
| Corn, olive, Crisco oil | 1 tsp | — | — | — | — | — |
| Margarine, salt-free | 1 pat | — | 0.03 | 0.02 | 1.0 | 0.15 |
| Mayonnaise | 1 tsp | 0.07 | 0.04 | 1.20 | 1.3 | 0.0 |
| *CEREAL* | | | | | | |
| Bran flakes, 40% | ½ cup | 1.8 | 1.75 | 4.50 | 68.5 | 24.0 |
| Corn flakes | ½ cup | 1.0 | 0.38 | 5.40 | 4.5 | 1.7 |
| Cream of rice, salt-free, cooked | 1 cup (8 oz) | 2.0 | trace | trace | 32.0 | 7.3 |
| Cream of wheat, salt-free, quick-cooking | 1 cup (8 oz) | 4.9 | trace | trace | 145.0 | 14.7 |
| Farina, salt-free, regular, cooked | 1 cup | 3.2 | 0.30 | 0.01 | 29.0 | 4.9 |
| Oatmeal, cooked | 1 cup | 4.8 | 3.74 | 0.01 | 137.0 | 57.6 |
| Puffed rice | ½ cup | 0.5 | 0.19 | trace | 7.0 | 1.9 |
| Puffed and shredded wheat | ½ cup | 1.1 | 0.65 | 0.50 | 24.0 | 19.3 |
| Rice Krispies | ½ cup | 0.9 | 0.37 | 6.15 | 14.0 | 5.0 |
| Tapioca, salt-free, dry | 1 Tbsp | 0.1 | 0.10 | 0.03 | 2.0 | 0.2 |
| *BREADS, COOKIES, CRACKERS* | | | | | | |
| Bread, regular | 1 slice | 2.2 | 0.66 | 5.50 | 24.0 | 6.3 |
| Bread, salt-free | 1 slice | 1.7 | 0.50 | 0.30 | — | 3.5 |
| Bread, whole wheat | 1 slice | 2.6 | 1.74 | 5.73 | 57.0 | 27.2 |
| Crackers, graham | 2 squares | 1.1 | 1.41 | 4.13 | 21.0 | 3.0 |
| Crackers, salt-free | 3 squares | 3.1 | 0.30 | 0.04 | — | 2.1 |
| Crackers, saltines | 1 square | 0.3 | 0.09 | 1.36 | 2.6 | 0.7 |
| English muffin, enriched | ½ | 1.5 | 0.64 | 3.82 | 30.0 | |
| Italian bread, enriched | 1 slice small | 0.9 | 0.17 | 2.56 | 8.0 | 3.6 |
| Roll, hard, enriched | ½ | 2.5 | 0.60 | 6.80 | 23.0 | 3.0 |
| Roll, soft, enriched | 1 | 2.3 | 0.69 | 6.17 | 24.0 | 5.9 |
| Vanilla wafers | 5 | 1.1 | 0.37 | 2.20 | 25.0 | 6.0 |
| *MEAT, FISH* | | | | | | |
| Boiled beef, cooked | 1 oz | 9.0 | 1.84 | 0.68 | 48.0 | 6.5 |
| Chopped beef, lean, cooked | 1 oz | 8.2 | 2.35 | 0.87 | 68.9 | 7.1 |
| Sirloin, cooked | 1 oz | 6.5 | 1.36 | 0.69 | 54.0 | 8.8 |
| Chicken, dark, cooked | 1 oz | 7.9 | 2.30 | 1.10 | 64.8 | 6.4 |
| Chicken, white, cooked | 1 oz | 8.9 | 3.00 | 0.80 | 74.9 | 7.6 |
| Lamb, cooked | 1 oz | 6.1 | 1.76 | 0.65 | 48.6 | 7.4 |
| Turkey, dark, cooked | 1 oz | 8.5 | 2.90 | 1.20 | — | 6.8 |
| Turkey, white, cooked | 1 oz | 9.3 | 3.00 | 1.00 | — | 7.9 |
| Veal, lean, cooked | 1 oz | 7.7 | 2.20 | 0.80 | 65.4 | 9.4 |
| Bluefish, cooked | 1 oz | 7.4 | — | 1.26 | 81.0 | 7.1 |
| Flat fish, raw | 1 oz | 4.7 | 2.47 | 0.95 | 55.2 | 8.5 |
| Cod, cooked | 1 oz | 8.1 | 2.94 | 1.34 | 78.0 | 9.9 |
| Halibut, cooked | 1 oz | 7.1 | 3.84 | 1.65 | 70.0 | 7.9 |
| Shrimp, raw | 1 oz | 5.1 | 1.59 | 1.72 | 47.0 | 11.9 |
| Tuna, regular, drained | 1 oz | 8.1 | 2.30 | 10.40 | 66.1 | 9.9 |
| Tuna, salt-free | 1 oz | 7.9 | 2.02 | 0.50 | 53.7 | 9.6 |
| *SWEETS* | | | | | | |
| Honey | 1 Tbsp | 0.1 | 0.28 | 0.04 | 1.0 | 0.4 |
| Ice cream, regular | ½ cup | 3.0 | 3.10 | 1.80 | 76.5 | 9.3 |
| Ice milk | ½ cup | 3.2 | 3.30 | 1.93 | 54.0 | 9.4 |
| Jams, preserves | 1 Tbsp | 0.1 | 0.50 | 0.40 | 2.0 | 1.2 |
| Sherbet (fruit ice) | ½ cup | 0.9 | 0.50 | 0.20 | 12.5 | 7.6 |
| Sugar, brown, packed | ½ cup | 0.0 | 4.41 | 0.65 | 9.5 | 20.0 |
| Sugar, white | 1 Tbsp | 0.0 | trace | trace | 0.0 | 0.0 |

## Table A–25a. (continued)

| | Amount | Protein (g) | Potassium (meq)‡ | Sodium (meq)‡ | Phosphorus (mg) | Magnesium† (mg)‡ |
|---|---|---|---|---|---|---|
| *JUICES* | | | | | | |
| Apple | 3½ oz | 0.1 | 2.59 | 0.03 | 8.87 | 3.5 |
| Apricot nectar | 3½ oz | 0.3 | 3.90 | trace | 11.95 | 7.0 |
| Cranberry | 3½ oz | 0.1 | 0.25 | 0.10 | 3.16 | 3.5 |
| Grape | 3½ oz | 0.2 | 2.96 | 0.08 | 11.85 | 10.3 |
| Grapefruit | 3½ oz | 0.5 | 4.14 | 0.03 | 14.17 | 10.3 |
| Lemon, canned | 3½ oz | 0.4 | 3.61 | 0.03 | 9.83 | 8.2 |
| Orange, canned | 3½ oz | 0.8 | 4.90 | 0.03 | 18.14 | 10.5 |
| Orange, fresh | 3½ oz | 0.7 | 5.12 | 0.03 | 16.93 | 10.9 |
| Pear nectar | 3½ oz | 0.3 | 1.00 | 0.05 | 5.20 | 3.5 |
| Pineapple | 3½ oz | 0.4 | 3.82 | 0.05 | 9.20 | 14.0 |
| Prune | 3½ oz | 0.4 | 6.00 | 0.09 | 19.92 | 14.0 |
| Tomato | 3½ oz | 0.9 | 5.82 | 8.70 | 18.10 | 11.0 |
| Tomato, salt-free | 3½ oz | 0.8 | 5.82 | 0.12 | 18.18 | 11.0 |
| *VEGETABLES* | | | | | | |
| Asparagus, cut, canned | ½ cup drained | 2.5 | 4.21 | 12.06 | 48.0 | 17.7 |
| Asparagus, low-sodium | ½ cup drained | 2.3 | 4.21 | 0.19 | 48.0 | 17.7 |
| Beans, green, canned | ½ cup drained | 1.0 | 1.64 | 6.93 | 17.0 | 8.8 |
| Beans, green, low-sodium | ½ cup drained | 1.0 | 1.64 | 0.06 | 17.0 | 8.8 |
| Beans, wax, canned | ½ cup drained | 0.9 | 1.64 | 6.93 | 16.5 | 8.8 |
| Beets, canned | ½ cup drained | 0.8 | 3.64 | 8.71 | 15.5 | 31.5 |
| Beets, low-sodium | ½ cup drained | 0.8 | 3.64 | 1.69 | 15.5 | 31.5 |
| Broccoli, cooked, no added salt | ½ cup drained | 2.4 | 5.30 | 0.34 | 48.0 | 51.0 |
| Cabbage, cooked, no added salt | ½ cup drained | 0.8 | 3.02 | 0.43 | 15.0 | 11.0 |
| Carrots, canned | ½ cup drained | 0.6 | 2.38 | 7.95 | 17.0 | 9.8 |
| Carrots, low-sodium | ½ cup drained | 0.6 | 2.38 | 1.30 | 17.0 | 9.8 |
| Carrots, raw | 1 medium | 0.8 | 6.30 | 1.47 | 26.0 | 15.0 |
| Cauliflower, cooked, no salt | ½ cup drained | 1.5 | 3.30 | 0.23 | 26.5 | 9.9 |
| Celery, raw | 1 stalk | 0.4 | 3.48 | 2.17 | 11.0 | 4.8 |
| Corn, canned | ½ cup drained | 2.1 | 2.05 | 8.45 | 40.5 | 27.2 |
| Corn, low-sodium | ½ cup drained | 2.1 | 2.05 | 0.06 | 40.5 | 27.2 |
| Cucumber, pared, raw | ½ cup drained | 0.4 | 2.87 | 0.17 | 12.5 | 10.1 |
| Peas, sweet, canned | ½ cup drained | 4.0 | 2.08 | 8.71 | 57.0 | 32.4 |
| Peas, low-sodium | ½ cup drained | 3.8 | 2.08 | 0.11 | 57.0 | 32.4 |
| Tomato, raw | 1 medium | 1.4 | 7.69 | 0.17 | 33.0 | 13.5 |
| Tomato, canned | ½ cup drained | 1.2 | 6.70 | 6.80 | 23.0 | 14.4 |
| Tomato, low-sodium | ½ cup drained | 1.2 | 6.70 | 0.15 | 23.0 | 14.4 |
| Potato, boiled | ½ cup drained | 1.5 | 5.66 | 0.06 | 32.5 | 18.0 |
| Noodles, egg enriched, cooked, with no salt | ½ cup drained | 3.3 | 0.89 | 0.06 | 47.0 | 10.4 |
| Rice, enriched, no added salt | ½ cup drained | 2.1 | 0.73 | trace | 28.5 | 9.3 |
| *FRUITS* | | | | | | |
| Apple, pared | 1 medium | 0.3 | 4.35 | 0.08 | 15.0 | 4.0 |
| Applesauce, unsweetened | ½ cup | 0.25 | 2.43 | 0.10 | 6.0 | 4.0 |
| Apricots, canned | 3 halves | 0.5 | 5.10 | 0.04 | 13.0 | 8.0 |
| Banana | 1 medium | 1.3 | 11.28 | 0.04 | 31.0 | 33.0 |
| Blueberries, fresh | ½ cup | 0.5 | 1.50 | 0.02 | 10.0 | 3.5 |
| Cherries, canned, pitted | ½ cup | 1.2 | 4.15 | 0.06 | 16.5 | 16.0 |
| Grapefruit, fresh | ½ cup | 0.45 | 3.02 | 0.04 | 14.0 | 9.5 |
| Orange, fresh | 1 medium | 1.3 | 6.74 | 0.04 | 26.0 | 13.0 |
| Peach, fresh, pared | 1 medium | 0.8 | 6.89 | 0.04 | 25.0 | 6.0 |
| Peach, canned, in syrup | ½ cup | 0.8 | 4.26 | 0.10 | 15.5 | 6.0 |
| Pear, raw | 1 medium | 1.1 | 5.46 | 0.13 | 18.0 | 9.0 |
| Pear, canned, syrup | ½ cup | 0.25 | 2.74 | 0.06 | 9.0 | 5.5 |
| Pineapple, canned | ½ cup | 0.4 | 3.14 | 0.06 | 6.5 | 17.5 |
| Strawberries, raw | ½ cup | 0.5 | 3.12 | 0.02 | 15.5 | 8.0 |

*Data taken from Watt and Merrill: Composition of Foods, Dairy and Egg Products, Raw-Processed-Prepared, U.S. Department of Agriculture Handbook No. 8-1. Washington, USDA, 1976. Nutritive Value of American Foods in Common Units, U.S. Department of Agriculture Handbook No. 456. Washington, USDA, 1975. Watt and Merrill: Composition of Foods, Raw-Processed-Prepared, U.S. Department of Agriculture Handbook No. 8. Washington, USDA, 1963.

— = Data are inadequate or variable.

†Data from Primary Nutrient Data Set for Food Consumption Surveys. U.S. Department of Agriculture, Human Nutrition Information Service, Nutrition Monitoring Division. Appreciation is expressed to Mr. Frank Hepburn and Mr. David Haytowitz for assistance in obtaining these data.

‡1 meq $K^+$ = 39.1 mg; 1 meq $Na^+$ = 23 mg; 12.0 mg $Mg^{++}$ = 1 meq.

## Table A–25b.    Restricted Protein, Sodium, and Potassium Diet (30 g protein, 20 meq potassium, 35 meq sodium)*

*Purpose:* This diet is designed for use in feeding patients with advanced renal disease where control of elevated blood urea and plasma sodium, potassium, and other minerals by dietary means is indicated. Patients needing this diet are frequently anorectic or nauseated, and the diet has been formulated to be palatable.

| Approximate Composition | Unit | Amount |
|---|---|---|
| Carbohydrate | g | 236 |
| Protein | g | 30 |
| Fat | g | 50 |
| Calories | | 1,510 |
| Calcium | mg | 217 |
| Phosphorus | mg | 460 |
| Iron | mg | 7.9 |
| Sodium | mg (meq) | 896 (35) |
| Potassium | mg (meq) | 80 (20) |
| Vitamin A | I.U. | 1,239† |
| Thiamin | mg | .55 |
| Riboflavin | mg | .57 |
| Niacin equivalents | mg | 6.3 |
| Ascorbic acid | mg | 25 |

*\*Adequacy:* This diet does not meet the 1980 RDA in any category and must be supplemented when prescribed for more than a few days by addition of (1) more carbohydrate and fat calories and calcium given orally, by tube, or intravenously, (2) a multivitamin several times a week, and (3) a low-mineral-low-protein liquid formula such as the R-#3 formula (see Table A–25c).

†Vitamin A content is maintained at RDA or lower because of the tendency of renally insufficient patients to have high serum vitamin A levels. Carrots should be eaten only once or twice a week to provide reasonable amounts of vitamin A. Patient vitamin A levels should be determined occasionally.

| Type of Food | Amount | Food Included | Food Excluded |
|---|---|---|---|
| Milk | None | None | Whole milk, skim milk, buttermilk, malted milk. |
| Other beverages§ | 2 cups | Ginger ale, root beer, Seven-up, Kool-aid (unrestricted amounts). | Cola drinks, cocoa, tea, coffee‡, Postum, Sanka. |
| Soup | None | None | All soups |
| Meat, poultry, fish | 1½ oz | Beef, chicken, lamb, pork, liver, beef heart, beef kidney, sweet-breads. Salt-free canned salmon and tuna. Codfish, clams, lobster, haddock, perch, oysters, shad, shrimp, red snapper, whitefish, whiting. Canned crabmeat. | Meat extracts. Halibut, scallops, veal. Canned sardines. All others not listed as allowed. |
| Cheese | ½ cup or ½ oz | Unsalted cottage cheese, Unsalted American cheese. | All others not listed as allowed. |
| Eggs | 1 | Any type prepared without milk (may be used as cheese substitute). | None |
| Potato substitute | 1 svg. 1 cup | Enriched white rice, macaroni, noodles, spaghetti. | All potatoes (white or sweet). Canned potatoes, potato chips. Brown rice. |
| Bread | 3 slices | Enriched white bread, saltines (5 only). | Rye bread, whole wheat bread, all those not listed as allowed. |
| Cereal | 1 svg. | Cream of wheat, hominy grits, farina; all served without milk. | All others not listed as allowed. |
| Vegetables | 2 svg. ½ cup | Cooked or raw cabbage; fresh, frozen, or salt-free canned green beans, cucumbers (6 slices), lettuce (2 leaves), salt-free canned peas, fresh or salt-free canned wax beans. | All others not listed as allowed. |

## Table A–25b.   (continued)

| | | | |
|---|---|---|---|
| Fruit | 2 svg. ½ cup | Canned or fresh applesauce, blueberries, Royal Anne cherries, peaches, pears, pineapple, grapefruit sections; fresh blackberries, raspberries, strawberries, pineapple, grapes, apple, cherries; frozen raspberries, strawberries, cranberry sauce. | All dried fruits; all others not listed as allowed. |
| Fruit juice | 2 svg. | Cranberry juice; frozen lemonade; frozen limeade. | All others not listed as allowed. |
| Butter or fat | 3 tsp | Butter, margarine, corn oil (unrestricted amounts); mayonnaise or commercial salad dressing; cream cheese. | Cream gravies; all others not listed as allowed. |
| Desserts | 1 svg. | Gelatin made with Kool-aid and sugar; dietetic gelatin (D'Zerta); lime ice. | Commercial Jell-O; all others not listed as allowed. |
| Sweets | In moderation | Gum drops, hard candy, marshmallows; white sugar syrup—1 tsp; jellies or jams. | Brown sugar, maple syrup, chocolate, molasses; all others not listed as allowed. |
| Spices | As desired | White pepper; vanilla; vinegar; peppermint extract; nutmeg; cinnamon; mace. | All others not listed as allowed. |
| Miscellaneous | | | Nuts; olives; pickles; catsup; coconut; peanut butter; bakers' yeast. |

*Sample Meal Pattern*

| Breakfast | Serving Portion | Sample Menu |
|---|---|---|
| Fruit | ½ cup | Cranberry juice |
| Cereal | ½ cup cooked | Farina |
| Bread | 1 slice | Enriched white bread |
| Fat | 1 tsp | Butter or margarine |
| Jelly | 1 tbsp | Jelly |
| Sugar | 1 tbsp | Sugar |
| Beverage | 1 cup | Coffee‡ |
| *Lunch* | | |
| Meat substitute | 1 medium | Soft-cooked egg |
| Potato substitute | ½ cup cooked | Unsalted white rice |
| Vegetable | ½ cup | Salt-free green beans |
| Dessert | ½ cup | Royal Anne cherries |
| Bread | 1 slice | Enriched white bread |
| Fat | 1 tsp | Butter or margarine |
| Beverage | 1 cup | Gingle ale |
| *Dinner* | | |
| Meat | 1½ oz | Salt-free roast beef |
| Vegetable | ½ cup | Salt-free canned waxed beans |
| Fruit | ½ cup | Applesauce |
| Bread | 1 slice | Enriched white bread |
| Fat | 1 tsp | Butter or margarine |
| Dessert | ½ cup | Lime ice |
| *8:00 p.m.* | | |
| Fruit juice | ½ cup | Frozen lemonade |

‡May be ordered at the discretion of the physician.
§Soft drinks vary in potassium and phosphate content (see Table A–18).

## Table A–25c. High-Calorie, Low-Protein, and Low-Mineral Liquid Supplement (R-#3)*,† (2,000-ml vol)

|  | *Gram* | *Household Measure* |
|---|---|---|
| Dextrose (sugar) | 240 | 1⅓ cups |
| Egg | 250 | 5 eggs |
| Cornstarch | 120 | 1 cup |
| Water | 1,284 | 5⅓ cups |
| Heavy cream | 200 | Skimpy cup |
| Chocolate syrup | 90 | 4 tbsp (to taste) |
| Corn oil | 30 | 1 oz |

*Preparation*

Dissolve in saucepan dextrose, egg, cornstarch, and about one half measured water. Mix until no lumps are visible and nothing is stuck to the bottom of the pan.

Begin to cook on low to medium heat. Do not boil. When mixture just begins to thicken, remove from the heat.

Pour cooked mixture in blender. Turn on low speed and add remaining ingredients. Place top on blender and turn to high speed for 1 to 2 minutes (until well blended).

Pour into container. Use remaining water to rinse blender. Pour into container. Mix everything thoroughly. Refrigerate.

3 to 4 glasses (3 to 4 oz each) to be taken each day. Total volume should give a 3-day supply.

*100 ml (3½ oz) provides the following:

| | | | |
|---|---|---|---|
| Calories | 151 | Mg (mg) | 3 |
| $CH_2O$ (g) | 21 | K (meq) | 1 |
| Protein (g) | 2 | Na (meq) | 1 |
| Fat (g) | 7 | | |
| Ca (mg) | 15 | | |

†From Clinical Nutrition Support Kitchen, Memorial Sloan-Kettering Cancer Center, New York.

## Table A–26. Restricted Fiber Diet*

*Purpose:* This diet is designed to reduce dietary fiber to 10 g or less, and to eliminate foods known to increase fecal weight.[1-3] It is recommended for use when there is intestinal narrowing, before and after extensive large-bowel surgery for conditions such as fistulae or extensive perineal repair,[4] or when a low-dietary-fiber diet is desirable for other reasons.

| Approximate Composition | Unit | Amount |
|---|---|---|
| Carbohydrate | g | 236 |
| Protein | g | 110 |
| Fat | g | 69 |
| Calories | | 1,997 |
| Calcium | mg | 1,066 |
| Phosphorus | mg | 1,489 |
| Iron | mg | 20.6 |
| Sodium | mg (meq) | 1,462 (64) |
| Potassium | mg (meq) | 4,117 (106) |
| Vitamin A | I.U. | 17,397 |
| Thiamin | mg | 1.4 |
| Riboflavin | mg | 2.2 |
| Niacin equivalents | mg | 31.4 |
| Ascorbic acid | mg | 102 |

*Adequacy:* This diet meets the 1980 Recommended Dietary Allowances of the National Research Council. The calculations are based on the sample meal plan. This sample plan is high in vitamin A because of the large amount of β-carotene.

When lactose intolerance is evidenced, milk should be eliminated. It may be increased as patient's tolerance improves.

Note: At present, the role of dietary fiber in diet therapy is volatile. Although current therapeutic diet recommendations are based on total dietary fiber content, ideally one should examine the physiologic effect of various types of fiber (e.g., cellulose, pectin, guar gums). At present, comprehensive tables listing food content of various types of fiber are unavailable.

| Type of Food | Amount | Food Included | Food Excluded |
|---|---|---|---|
| Milk | As desired | Whole milk, skim milk, buttermilk (note: milk should be given according to patient tolerance) | |
| Other beverages | As desired | Coffee, tea, carbonated beverages | Alcoholic beverages (unless ordered by physician) |
| Soup | As desired | Strained soups or soup made from allowed ingredients | |
| Meat, poultry, fish, or substitute | 6 oz or more | Tender or ground beef, pork, veal, lamb, chicken, turkey, chicken liver, beef liver, sweetbreads, bacon. Lean boneless fish. Canned salmon or tuna. Meats and fish should be baked, boiled, broiled, roasted, or used in cream mixtures. Serve meat and fish without spicy gravy. Pork mixtures, frankfurters, bologna, sausage, luncheon meats. Smoked, cured, canned, preserved meat or fish. Clams, oysters, shrimp, lobster. Processed smoked meats. Fried meats, fish, or fowl. Shellfish. All cheeses. Eggs | Tough fibrous meat with gristle; peanut butter, smooth or chunky |

## Table A–26. (continued)

| | | | |
|---|---|---|---|
| Potato or substitute | 2 svg. | White potato (no skin), boiled, baked, creamed, mashed, scalloped, au gratin. Pureed sweet potato. Plain macaroni, noodles, spaghetti, white rice (prepared with cream or mild cheese sauces or butter). | Potato skins |
| Bread | 4 svg. | Fresh or toasted enriched white, light rye bread, or rolls (without seeds). Saltines, soda crackers, melba toast, rusk, zwieback, milk toast | Whole wheat, cracked wheat, dark rye bread. Whole wheat crackers, graham crackers, pretzels. Pancakes, waffles, muffins, corn bread, quickbreads. All others not listed as allowed. |
| Cereal | 1 svg. | Cooked refined corn, rice, and wheat cereals. Hominy grits, farina, strained oatmeal, rolled wheat, Rice Krispies, puffed rice | Whole-grain cereals. Bran flakes, cornflakes, Ralston, Maltex, Wheatena, shredded wheat, Grapenut flakes, Wheat Chex. All other cereals not listed as allowed. |
| Vegetables | 2 svg. | Asparagus, cooked<br>Beans—green, cooked<br>  sprouts, raw<br>Beets, raw, cooked<br>Cauliflower, raw, cooked<br>Celery, raw<br>Cucumber, raw, peeled<br>Green pepper, raw<br>Kale, cooked<br>Lettuce, raw<br>Mushrooms, raw<br>Onions, raw, cooked<br>Potato, mashed, instant<br>Radishes, raw<br>Rutabagas, raw<br>Spinach, raw, with stem removed<br>Tomatoes, raw, cooked<br>Turnip greens, cooked | Beans—green, raw dried, cooked<br>  broad, raw, cooked<br>Broccoli, raw, cooked<br>Brussels sprouts, raw, cooked<br>Cabbage, raw, cooked<br>Carrots, raw, cooked<br>Corn, raw, cooked<br>Eggplant, raw, cooked<br>Peas—green, raw, cooked,<br>  dried, cooked<br>Potato, cooked or baked<br>Rice, brown, cooked<br>Squash—summer, raw, cooked<br>  winter, raw, cooked<br>  zucchini, raw, cooked<br>Yams, cooked |
| Fruit | 3 svg. | Cooked, canned, baked, or stewed fruits without skin or seeds. Royal Anne cherries. Peeled apricots, peaches, pears | Raw fruits except those listed as allowed. Fruits with seeds or skin. Raisins, dates, figs. Canned plums, berries, fruit cocktail, pineapple, and strawberries. Apples, banana |
| Fruit juice | 2 svg. | Apple, apricot, pear, peach nectar. Strained fruit juice | Fruit juices with pulp, prune juice |
| Butter or fat | 3 svg. | Butter, margarine. Smooth peanut butter. Vegetable oils or shortenings. Salad dressing made with allowed foods. Cream, avocado, bacon, gravy | Nuts, olives |
| Dessert | 1 svg. | Cookies, e.g., arrowroot, plain sugar, vanilla wafers. Plain custard, ice cream, flavored gelatin (plain, whipped, or with allowed fruit). Rennet dessert. Plain puddings. Fruit juice sponges. Snows, whips. Spanish cream, Bavarian cream. Sherbet. Cakes, e.g., angel food, sponge, plain white, or yellow, plain pound, ladyfingers | Tarts, pies, pastries, cakes, puddings that contain nuts, fruits, raisins, seeds, frosting, or coconut. Any others not listed as allowed |

## Table A–26. (continued)

| Sweets | In moderation | White sugar, brown sugar. Clear jelly. Honey, syrup, molasses. Clear, sweet dessert sauces. Hard candy, gumdrops. Chocolate syrup. | Candy containing fruit or nuts. Jam, marmalade, sugar, and candy in excess |
|---|---|---|---|
| Spices and miscellaneous | | Salt (in moderation). All spices as tolerated. White sauce (without daily milk allowance). Vinegar, condiments | Olives, pickles, popcorn, relishes |

*Sample Meal Pattern*

| *Breakfast* | *Serving Portion* | *Sample Menu* |
|---|---|---|
| Fruit | ½ cup | Strained orange juice |
| Cereal | ½ cup | Farina |
| Egg | 1 | Soft-cooked egg |
| Bread | 1 slice | Enriched white toast |
| Milk | ½ cup | Milk, whole or skimmed |
| Fat | 2 tsp | Butter or margarine |
| Sugar | 1 Tbsp | Sugar |
| Beverage | 1 cup | Coffee or tea |
| *Lunch* | | |
| Meat or substitute | 3 oz | Broiled chicken |
| Potato or substitute | ½ cup | Cooked rice |
| Vegetable | ¾ cup | Spinach |
| Bread | 1 slice | White enriched bread |
| Fat | 2 tsp | Butter or margarine |
| Fruit | ½ cup | Canned pears |
| Milk | ½ cup | Milk, whole or skimmed |
| Sugar | 2 tsp | Sugar |
| Beverage | 1 cup | Coffee or tea |
| *Dinner* | | |
| Meat or substitute | 5 oz | Roast beef |
| Potato or substitute | 1 | Baked potato (no skin) |
| Vegetable | ½ cup | Green beans |
| Bread | 1 slice | White enriched bread |
| Milk | 1 cup | Milk, whole or skimmed |
| Fat | 2 tsp | Butter or margarine |
| Dessert | ½ cup | Whole peeled apricot |
| Sugar | 2 tsp | Sugar |
| Beverage | 1 cup | Coffee or tea |
| *9:00 p.m.* | | |
| Fruit | 1 cup | Canned peaches |
| Dessert | 1 slice | Pound cake |

*Modified from Diet Manual, Memorial Sloan-Kettering Cancer Center, revised 1978. Appreciation is expressed to Carol Poduch, R.P.Dt., Toronto (Ontario) General Hospital, for helpful suggestions in the modifications of this diet.

### REFERENCES

1. Paul, A.A., Southgate, D.A.T.: McCance and Widdowson's The Composition of Foods. Amsterdam, New York, Elsevier/North-Holland Biomedical Press, 1978. 4th revised and extended edition of MRC special report 297

2. Williams, R.D., Olmstead, W.H.: The effect of cellulose, hemicellulose and lignin on the weight of the stool: A contribution to the study of laxation in man. J. Nutr. *11*:433–449, May, 1936.

3. Cummings, J.H., et al.: Colonic response to dietary fiber from carrot, cabbage, apple, bran and guar gum. Lancet, *1*(805):5–8, Jan. 7, 1978.

4. Bingham, S.: Low-residue diets: A reappraisal of their meaning. J. Hum. Nutr. 33:5–16, 1979.

## Table A–27.   High-Fiber Diet*

*Purpose:* The diet is designed to be high in dietary fiber. It is useful for decreasing intraluminal colonic pressure, increasing gastrointestinal motility, and increasing the volume and weight of material that reaches the distal colon.

| Approximate Composition | Unit | Amount |
|---|---|---|
| Carbohydrate | g | 324 |
| Protein | g | 95 |
| Fat | g | 130 |
| Calories | | 2,747 |
| Calcium | mg | 997 |
| Phosphorus | mg | 1,872 |
| Iron | mg | 13.6 |
| Sodium | mg (meq) | 2,551 (109) |
| Potassium | mg (meq) | 3,495 (90) |
| Vitamin A | I.U. | 10,622 |
| Thiamin | mg | 1.2 |
| Riboflavin | mg | 2.0 |
| Niacin equivalents | mg | 26 |
| Ascorbic acid | mg | 69 |

*Adequacy:* This diet meets the 1980 Recommended Daily Allowance of the National Research Council for men, but may be low in iron for women. The calculations are based on the sample meal plan.

*Foods to Emphasize on a Regular Diet*

| | |
|---|---|
| Meat or alternatives | Dried peas, dried beans, lentils, soy beans, nuts, seeds |
| Cereals | Oatmeal, whole-wheat cereals, bran-type cereals |
| Fruits | At least three servings daily of raw or cooked fruit, including seeds, skins, and membranes |
| Fruit juices | All kinds, especially orange and prune |
| Vegetables | At least three servings daily of all kinds, especially cabbage, celery, corn, string beans, spinach, beet greens, lettuce, escarole, mixed vegetables |
| Breads | Whole wheat, rye, cracked wheat, rusk, melba, zwieback, bran bread, and bran muffins |
| Beverages | Whole milk, buttermilk, skim milk |
| Miscellaneous | Jams, popcorn, olives, Miller's (natural) bran |

## Table A–27.  (continued)

| Breakfast | Sample Meal Pattern Serving Portion | Sample Menu |
|---|---|---|
| Fruit | ½ cup | Stewed prunes |
| Egg | 1 | Soft-cooked egg |
| Cereal | ½ cup | All Bran |
| Bread | 1 slice | Rye bread |
| Fat | 2 tsp | Margarine |
| Milk | 1 cup | Milk, whole or skimmed |
| Jam | 1 tsp | Jam |
| Sugar | 2 tsp | Sugar |
| Beverage | 1 cup | Coffee or tea |
| *Lunch* | | |
| Meat or substitute | 3 oz | Broiled chicken |
| Potato or substitute | ½ cup | Wild rice |
| Vegetable | ½ cup | Mixed vegetables |
| Salad | 1 slice | Lettuce and tomato |
| Dressing | 1 Tbsp | Russian dressing |
| Bread | 1 slice | Whole-wheat bread |
| Fat | 1 tsp | Butter or margarine |
| Milk | ½ cup | Milk, whole or skimmed |
| Dessert | 1 piece | Cherry pie |
| Sugar | 2 tsp | Sugar |
| Beverage | 1 cup | Coffee or tea |
| *Dinner* | | |
| Meat or substitute | 3 oz | Roast beef |
| Potato or substitute | 1 | Baked potato |
| Vegetable | ½ cup | Peas |
| Fruit | ½ cup | Canned fruit cup |
| Bread | 1 slice | Whole-wheat bread |
| Fat | 1 tsp | Butter or margarine |
| Salad | | Tossed greens |
| Dressing | 1 Tbsp | Thousand Island dressing |
| Milk | 1 cup | Milk, whole or skimmed |
| Sugar | 2 tsp | Sugar |
| Beverage | 1 cup | Coffee or tea |
| *9:00 p.m.* | | |
| Fruit | 1 | Fresh apple |

*Appreciation is expressed to Carol Poduch, R.P.Dt., Toronto (Ontario) General Hospital, for helpful suggestions in the modification of this diet.

# Table A–28.  High-Fiber, Low-Fat Diet*

*Purpose:* This diet is designed to be high in wheat bran to reduce intraluminal colonic pressure.[1,2] It is low in fat to inhibit the production of cholecystokinin, which is known to increase colonic motor activity.[3] The diet is recommended for use in the treatment of the irritable bowel syndrome. Certain vegetables may increase intracolonic pressure through the production of volatile fatty acids during digestion.[4] This process is possibly related to cellulose and hemicellulose content. Because there are no complete tables listing these fibers in foods, an individual approach is required in fruits and vegetables that patients may tolerate.

| Approximate Composition | Unit | Amount |
|---|---|---|
| Carbohydrate | g | 400 |
| Protein | g | 103 |
| Fat | g | 42 |
| Calories | | 2,296 |
| Calcium | mg | 1,161 |
| Phosphorus | mg | 2,254 |
| Iron | mg | 30.2 |
| Sodium | mg (meq) | 2,574 (112) |
| Potassium | mg (meq) | 4,191 (108) |
| Vitamin A | I.U. | 10,813 |
| Thiamin | mg | 2.9 |
| Riboflavin | mg | 3.0 |
| Niacin equivalents | mg | 43 |
| Ascorbic acid | mg | 156 |

*Adequacy:* This diet meets the 1980 Recommended Dietary Allowances of the National Research Council of all nutrients. The calculations are based on the sample meal plan.

| Type of Food | Amount | Food Included | Food Excluded |
|---|---|---|---|
| Milk | 2 cups | Skim milk, yogurt. Maximum of 500 ml daily of 2% partially skimmed milk, buttermilk, and yogurt | Cream; whole or chocolate milk; drinks made with whole or chocolate milk; sour cream; creamed cottage cheese |
| Breads and cereals | 10 | Bread and rolls—whole-grain, such as 100% whole wheat, bran, and those products with oats, barley, rice | Refined flour bread, rolls |
| | | Baked products—whole wheat crackers, graham wafers, whole wheat, bran, oatmeal, raisin muffins (note: omit 5 ml fat and oil for 1 muffin) | Shortbread cookies, cakes |
| | | Cereals—whole-grain cereals, bran cereals, cornflakes, brown rice | Granola, refined flour pasta, white rice |
| Wheat bran | 8 Tbsp | Wheat (Miller's) bran | |
| Meat or alternative | 6 oz | Total 150 g (6 oz) daily of lean meat, fish, or poultry that is baked, boiled, broiled, poached, roasted, or stewed. Skim milk cheese and cottage cheese; 1 egg daily | Fried meat, fish, poultry, poultry skin; fish canned in oil; sausages, frankfurters, luncheon meats, side bacon, spareribs, duck, goose; all other cheeses. Nuts and seeds |
| Vegetable | 2–3 | All except those not tolerated (must be individually determined) | Cabbage, Brussels sprouts, broccoli, lentils, legumes |
| Fruit | 2–3 | Raw or cooked fruits with skins, seeds, and membranes; dried fruit | Avocado; peel fruit |
| Soup | As desired | All made with water or skim milk; homemade soup with fat removed | Canned mushroom soup; cream soups |
| Fats | 3 tsp | Total of 3 tsp maximum butter, margarine, mayonnaise, peanut butter, salad dressing, oils | Fat in excess of 3 tsp daily |

## Table A–28. (continued)

| | | | |
|---|---|---|---|
| Dessert | As desired | Angel cake; puddings made with skim milk; gelatin desserts; sherbet | Pastries, deep-fried desserts such as doughnuts; ice cream |
| Miscellaneous beverage | As desired | Coffee, tea, Ovaltine, Postum, cocoa, fruit flavored drinks, carbonated beverages | Alcohol; chocolate drinks |
| Sweets | As desired | All sweets except those listed as excluded | Chocolate, fudge, toffee |
| Other | As desired | Herbs and spices as tolerated | Coconut; olives; sauces; gravy; coffee whitener; whipped topping; commercial snack foods |

### Sample Menu Pattern

| Breakfast | Serving Portion | Sample Menu |
|---|---|---|
| Fruit | 1 cup | ½ grapefruit |
| | | ½ cup juice |
| Cereal | ¾ cup | Bran cereal |
| Meat or substitute | 1 | Soft-boiled egg |
| Bread | 2 | Whole wheat bread |
| Milk | 1 cup | Skim milk |
| Fat | 1 tsp | Margarine |
| Sugar | 1 tsp | Sugar |
| Beverage | 1 cup | Coffee |
| Wheat bran | 2 Tbsp | Wheat bran |

| Lunch | | |
|---|---|---|
| Meat or substitute | 2 oz | Broiled chicken |
| Potato or substitute | ½ cup | Brown rice |
| Vegetable | ½ cup | Spinach |
| Bread | 1 | Whole wheat bread |
| Fat | 1 tsp | Margarine |
| Fruit | 1 | Large apple |
| Beverage | 1 cup | Carbonated beverage |
| Dessert | 1 slice | Angel cake |
| Wheat bran | 2 Tbsp | Wheat bran |

| Dinner | | |
|---|---|---|
| Meat or substitute | 3 oz | White fish |
| Potato or substitute | 1 cup | Potato |
| Vegetable | 1 cup | Green peas |
| Bread | 1 slice | Whole wheat bread |
| Fat | 1 tsp | Margarine |
| Fruit | ½ cup | Applesauce |
| Beverage | 8 oz | Carbonated beverage |
| Dessert | ½ cup | Sherbet |
| Wheat bran | 2 Tbsp | Wheat bran |

| 9 p.m. | | |
|---|---|---|
| Bread | 2 | Toast |
| Milk | 8 oz | Skim milk |
| Wheat bran | 2 Tbsp | Wheat bran |

*Modified from Diet Manual, Memorial Sloan-Kettering Cancer Center, revised 1978. Appreciation is expressed to Carol Poduch, R.P.Dt., Toronto (Ontario) General Hospital, for helpful suggestions in the modifications of the diet.

### REFERENCES

1. Manning, A.P., Heaton, K.W., Harvey, R.F.: Wheat fiber and irritable bowel syndrome. Lancet 2:417–418, 1977.
2. Taylor, I., Darby, C., Hyland, J., et al.: Changes in myoelectric activity in the irritable colon syndrome with prolonged treatment. Scand. J. Gastroenterol. 15:237–240, 1980.
3. Harvey, R.F., Read, A.E.: Effect of cholecystokinin on colonic motility and symptoms in patients with the irritable bowel syndrome. Lancet 1:1–3, 1973.
4. Williams, R.D., Olmsted, W.H.: The effect of cellulose, hemicellulose and lignin on the weight of the stool: A contribution to the study of laxation in man. J. Nutr. 2:433–449, 1936.

## Table A–29.  Soft-Textured Diet*

*Purpose:* This diet is designed to provide an adequate nutritional intake for edentulous patients, for occasional postoperative patients not yet able to take a regular diet, and for patients with mechanical or pathologic impairment of chewing and/or swallowing.

The diet is a modification of the regular diet and consists of food made soft enough to be mashed easily in the mouth and swallowed. The physiologic problems of patients to be placed on this diet should be given individual consideration and the diet varied where indicated.

| Approximate Composition | Unit | Amount |
|---|---|---|
| Carbohydrate | g | 246 |
| Protein | g | 84 |
| Fat | g | 128 |
| Calories | | 2,441 |
| Calcium | mg | 728 |
| Phosphorus | mg | 1,343 |
| Iron | mg | 11 |
| Sodium | mg (meq) | 2,630 (112) |
| Potassium | mg (meq) | 2,900 (74.3) |
| Vitamin A | I.U. | 17,372 |
| Thiamin | mg | 1.2 |
| Riboflavin | mg | 2.0 |
| Niacin equivalents | mg | 20 |
| Ascorbic acid | mg | 120 |

*Adequacy:* This diet meets all the 1980 Recommended Dietary Allowances of the National Research Council for men, but may be low in iron for women. The calculations are based on the sample meal plan.

| Type of Food | Amount | Food Included | Food Excluded |
|---|---|---|---|
| Milk | 2 cups daily | Milk, buttermilk, skim milk; cocoa | None |
| Other beverages | As desired | Tea, coffee, coffee substitutes; carbonated beverages | None |
| Soups | As desired | Broths; strained or regular cream, vegetable, frozen, or canned soups | None |
| Meat, poultry, fish | 6 oz or more daily | Any tender meat, fish, poultry, pureed or ground food if necessary | Tough, fibrous meat |
| Cheese† | | Ricotta, cottage cheese, cream cheese, American cheese, processed cheese | Hard cheese; all others not listed as allowed |
| Eggs | 1 or more daily | Soft, medium, hard-cooked poached, soft scrambled, chopped, fried | |
| Potatoes and substitute | 2 svg. or more daily | Pureed, mashed, baked potato (without skin); macaroni, rice, noodles, spaghetti | All not listed as allowed |
| Bread | 3 svg. or more daily | Enriched white, whole wheat, rye (all without seeds); soft rolls; crackers; plain muffins | Coarse bread or rolls with seeds, raisins, or nuts; hard rolls |
| Cereal | 1 svg. daily | Any cooked cereal; dry cereal if tolerated | None |
| Vegetables | 2 svg. or more daily | Pureed; baby or tender whole-cooked vegetables such as: asparagus tips, carrots, beets, squash (fresh, frozen, or canned) if tolerated. Include at least 1 svg. of green or yellow cooked vegetables daily; slice tomatoes if tolerated | All others not listed |
| Fruit | 2 svg. or more daily | Pureed, baby, or whole cooked fruits (fresh, canned, or frozen); avocado; ripe tender raw fruits such as: banana, peaches, pears, melon, plums | All raw fruits patient cannot tolerate |

## Table A–29.  (continued)

| | | | |
|---|---|---|---|
| Fruit juice | 1 svg. or more daily | All—include 1 svg. daily of citrus fruit juice: orange, grapefruit, blended. If throat is sore, apricot, apple, pear, peach and grape are the mildest juices | None |
| Butter or fat | 6 or more tsp. daily | Butter, margarine; cream; salad dressing; vegetable fats and oils; gravies | None |
| Desserts | As desired | Custards, junket, gelatin, puddings, fruit whips, ice cream, sherbet, soft cakes—all without nuts; soft fruit or cream pies; pureed or soft fruits | Any dessert containing nuts, coconut, or raisins |
| Spices | As desired | Any that are tolerated by the patient, i.e., salt, pepper, garlic, paprika, cinnamon | Any patient finds irritating |
| Miscellaneous | | White sauces; vinegar; salad dressing if tolerated | Nuts; olives; pickles; popcorn; those foods that are chemically, mechanically, or thermally irritating to the mouth and/or throat |
| Sweets | As desired | Hard candy; honey; jellies; jams; sugar; syrups; molasses; soft chocolates without nuts | All others not listed as allowed |

*Sample Meal Pattern*

| Breakfast | Serving Portion | Sample Menu |
|---|---|---|
| Fruit | ½ cup | Orange juice |
| Cereal | ½ cup | Farina |
| Egg | 1 | Soft-cooked egg |
| Bread | 1 slice | Enriched white toast |
| Fat | 2 tsp | Butter or margarine |
| Milk | ½ cup | Whole milk |
| Beverage | 1 cup | Coffee |
| Sugar | 1 Tbsp | Sugar |

| Lunch | | |
|---|---|---|
| Meat or substitute | 3 oz | Ground chicken |
| Potato or substitute | ½ cup cooked | Rice |
| Vegetable | ½ cup | Asparagus |
| Fruit | ½ cup | Canned cherries |
| Bread | 1 | Soft roll |
| Fat | 2½ tsp | Butter or margarine |
| Milk | 1 cup | Whole milk |
| Beverage | 1 cup | Tea |
| Sugar | 2 tsp | Sugar |

| Dinner | | |
|---|---|---|
| Soup | ½ cup | Cream of mushroom |
| Meat or substitute | 3 oz | Ground beef |
| Potato or subsitute | 1 | Baked potato (no skin) |
| Vegetable | ½ cup | Diced carrots |
| Dessert | ½ cup | Whole peeled apricots |
| Bread | 1 slice | Light rye bread (no seeds) |
| Fat | 2½ tsp | Butter or margarine |
| Milk | ½ cup | Whole milk |
| Beverage | 1 cup | Coffee |
| Sugar | 2 tsp | Sugar |

| 8:00 p.m. | | |
|---|---|---|
| Fruit | ½ cup | Applesauce |

*Modified from Diet Manual, Memorial Sloan-Kettering Cancer Center, revised 1978.
†Cheese is considered part of the protein allotment, e.g., a substitute for meat, poultry, fish.

## Table A–30.   Diet for Nonspecific Gastrointestinal Complaints (Bland Six-Feeding)*

*Purpose:* This diet is designed to aid in alleviating the symptoms of patients with nonspecific gastrointestinal complaints. It is designed to eliminate foods that may be irritating such as red pepper, black pepper, chili powder, caffeine, coffee, decaffeinated coffee, tea, cola, cocoa, alcohol, and excessively spicy foods. If there is a history of intolerance to milk and milk products, the amounts should be reduced to those tolerated; a special effort may be necessary to meet calcium and perhaps vitamin recommendations with advice of a physician and dietitian.

| *Approximate Composition* | *Unit* | *Amount* |
|---|---|---|
| Carbohydrate | g | 289 |
| Protein | g | 124.3 |
| Fat | g | 65.4 |
| Calories | — | 2,215 |
| Calcium | mg | 1,785 |
| Phosphorus | mg | 2,192 |
| Iron | mg | 17.6 |
| Sodium | mg (meq) | 2,297/99.9 |
| Potassium | mg (meq) | 5,670/145.4 |
| Vitamin A | I.U. | 11,345 |
| Thiamin | mg | 2.0 |
| Riboflavin | mg | 3.2 |
| Niacin equivalents | mg | 34.1 |
| Ascorbic acid | mg | 125.5 |

*Adequacy:* This diet meets the 1980 Recommended Dietary Allowances of the National Research Council for all nutrients. The calculations are based on the sample meal plan. This diet is high in calcium from milk and milk products and Vitamin A as β-carotene from vegetables.

| *Type of Food* | *Amount* | *Food Included* | *Food Excluded* |
|---|---|---|---|
| Milk | 1 qt. | Milk, buttermilk; skim milk; milk beverages | Chocolate-flavored beverages; cocoa |
| Other beverages | As desired | Postum; weak tea and Sanka if allowed by physician | Coffee; tea and Sanka if not permitted by physician; cocoa; carbonated beverages; chocolate; beer; wine; all alcoholic drinks |
| Soup | 1 svg. (½ cup) | Strained cream soup only, prepared with allowed vegetables and without meat stocks | Broth; all canned, dried, and frozen soups |
| Meat, fish, poultry | 2 svgs. (6 ozs.) | Tender beef; lamb; veal; liver; sweetbreads; chicken or turkey without skin; fish and shellfish, fresh, frozen, or canned without bones or skin; crisp bacon | Smoked, pickled, or cured meat or seafood; fried meats, poultry, fish, or seafood; pork; luncheon meats; frankfurters and sausages; clams; all those not listed as allowed |
| Cheese | As desired | Cottage, ricotta, farmer and pot cheese; cream cheese; mild cheese; cheddar cheese may be used in cooking | Sharp or spicy cheeses |
| Eggs | One | Poached, medium or hard cooked; soft scrambled in double boiler; baked omelet | Fried eggs |
| Potato or substitute | 2 svgs. | Potatoes, baked (served without skin), boiled, mashed, creamed, riced; mashed sweet potatoes or yams; white rice; macaroni, noodles, spaghetti with butter, oil, or plain tomato puree | Skin of potato; fried potatoes; whole-grain rice; potato chips; lentils |

## Table A–30.  (continued)

| | | | |
|---|---|---|---|
| Bread | 4 svgs. | White bread; white rolls without seeds; plain or toasted; soda crackers; saltines; melba toast; rusk; zwieback; milk toast | Whole wheat and rye bread; biscuits; cornbread; English muffins; rolls or muffins with seeds, raisins, coconut, or nuts; whole-grain crackers |
| Cereal | 1 svg. | Refined such as rice, cream of wheat, farina, hominy grits, cornmeal; cornflakes; Rice Krispies; puffed rice; Corn Kixs; strained oatmeal | Whole-grain cereals; bran; all those not listed as allowed |
| Vegetables | 2 svgs. Include 1 green or yellow | Soft cooked asparagus tips; beets; carrots; green or wax beans; peas; pumpkin (not spiced); spinach; winter squash; tomato or vegetable juices without added spices; pureed lima beans, tomatoes, or corn | Raw vegetables; all cooked vegetables except those listed as allowed |
| Fruit and fruit-juice | 3 svgs. | Cooked or canned without skin or seeds: apples; apricots; peaches; pears; cooked or canned Royal Anne and Bing cherries; fruit puree; ripe banana; avocado; all juices. (Include one citrus daily, taken at end of meal.) | Cooked or canned fruits with skin or seeds; canned grapefruit, orange, and pineapple; raw and frozen fruits except banana and avocado; melons; berries; dried fruits unless pureed; all those not listed as allowed |
| Butter or fat | 4 svgs. | Butter or margarine; homemade mayonnaise without mustard or spices; vegetable oils; cream | Spiced salad dressings; commercial mayonnaise |
| Dessert | 1 svg. | Plain rice, tapioca, white bread and cream pudding; blanc mange; custard; plain and flavored gelatin; junket (vanilla, banana, lemon); ice cream; sherbets and ices (eaten slowly); plain or iced cakes; sugar cookies; vanilla wafers; sponge cake; angel food cake; pound cake | Pies; pastries; cakes; cookies and desserts containing fruits as listed above, raisins, coconut, seeds, nuts, or chocolate; all those not listed as allowed |
| Sweets | Used in moderation | Sugar; sugar syrup; honey; molasses; jelly; gumdrops; marshmallows and fruit-flavored hard candy occasionally after meals; strained cranberry jelly | Chocolate; preserves; jams; rich sauces; excessive amounts of sweets |
| Spices | | Cinnamon; lemon; parsley; salt; vanilla; other spices taken only with physician's permission | Spices and condiments such as pepper; catsup; chili sauce; vinegar; mustard; garlic; horseradish; Worcestershire sauce; all others not listed as allowed |
| Miscellaneous | | Cream sauces without added spices; smooth peanut butter in moderation | Olives; pickles; Fritos; popcorn; pretzels; potato chips; nuts; very hot or very cold foods or fluids; fried foods; gravies; ice; all those not listed as allowed |

*GENERAL INSTRUCTIONS:*
1. Eat slowly.
2. Eat meals at same hour each day.
3. If possible, relax a few minutes before and after each meal.
4. Eat frequent small meals; never skip meals.
5. In-between nourishments must be included.

## Table A–30. (continued)

| Breakfast | Serving Portions | | Sample Menu |
|---|---|---|---|
| Fruit | ½ cup | | Orange juice |
| Cereal | ½ cup | | Farina, enriched |
| | | (or) | |
| Egg | 1 | | Soft-cooked egg |
| Bread | 1 slice | | White toast, enriched |
| Fat | 1 tsp. | | Butter or margarine |
| Milk | ½ cup | | Milk, lowfat |
| Beverage | 1 cup | | Postum |
| Sugar | 1 Tbsp. | | Sugar |
| *10:00 A.M.* | | | |
| Bread | 1 slice | | White toast, enriched |
| Fat | 1 tsp. | | Butter or margarine |
| Milk | ½ cup | | Milk, lowfat |
| *Lunch* | | | |
| Meat | 3 oz. | | Broiled chicken |
| Potato | 1 | | Baked potato (no skin) |
| Vegetable | ½ cup | | Acorn squash |
| Fruit | ½ cup | | Canned cherries |
| Bread | 1 slice | | White bread, enriched |
| Fat | 1 tsp. | | Butter or margarine |
| Milk | ½ cup | | Milk, lowfat |
| *3:00 P.M.* | | | |
| Fruit | ½ cup | | Applesauce |
| Milk | 1 cup | | Milk, lowfat |
| *Dinner* | | | |
| Soup | ½ cup | | Cream of mushroom |
| Meat | 4 oz. | | Roast beef |
| Potato | 1 svg. | | Boiled potato |
| Vegetable | ½ cup | | Spinach |
| Bread | 1 slice | | White bread, enriched |
| Fat | 1 tsp. | | Butter or margarine |
| Milk | ½ cup | | Milk, lowfat |
| *8:00 P.M.* | | | |
| Dessert | 1 svg. | | White cake |
| Milk | 1 cup | | Milk, lowfat |

*Modified from Diet Manual, Memorial Sloan-Kettering Cancer Center.

## Table A–31. Antidumping Diet*

*Purpose:* Following partial or total gastrectomy, symptoms of dumping may occur, but patients vary greatly in the severity and duration of symptoms. The following approach is recommended for such patients.

1. Each patient must be evaluated individually with respect to the diet that he can tolerate. Although there are wide variations, the majority with subtotal gastrectomy may be able to consume regular diets. Milk should be increased gradually as tolerance is proven.

2. To test and to prevent a dumping episode, a diet consists of six (6) equally spaced meals (restricted carbohydrate will be ordered). The carbohydrate should be in the form of starches, which are equally distributed among the six meals. Sucrose and other soluble carbohydrates are to be avoided. All fluids must be consumed 45 or 60 minutes after ingestion of solid food. Fluids should be 4 oz. or less per serving.

3. Patients with high subtotal gastrectomies may need stricter diet control. Consult your dietitian for the appropriate fat modification.

4. Increased food tolerance will encourage the patient to begin including foods that currently appear in the excluded list of this diet. If the patient continues to be asymptomatic, a normal diet may be tested and adopted if tolerated.

5. Because patients may have a malabsorption for fat, minerals, and vitamins, attention should be focused on the adequate intake of calories, protein, calcium, iron, and vitamins. If a large fat intake is associated with frequent, bulky, light-colored stools, the fat should be restricted and a physician consulted.

| *Approximate Composition* | *Unit* | *Amount* |
|---|---|---|
| Carbohydrate | g | 265 |
| Protein | g | 168 |
| Fat | g | 75 |
| Calories | — | 2,385 |
| Calcium | mg | 1,135 |
| Phosphorus | mg | 2,393 |
| Iron | mg | 22 |
| Sodium | mg (meq) | 2,008 (87.3) |
| Potassium | mg (meq) | 4,652 (104.6) |
| Vitamin A | I.U. | 12,869 |
| Thiamin | mg | 2.1 |
| Riboflavin | mg | 2.4 |
| Niacin equivalents | mg | 50 |
| Ascorbic acid | mg | 171 |

*Adequacy:* This diet meets the 1980 Recommended Dietary Allowances of the National Research Council for all nutrients. The calculations are based on the sample meal plan.

| Type of Food | Amount | Food Included | Food Excluded |
|---|---|---|---|
| Milk | 1½ cups<br>½ cup per svg. | Whole milk, buttermilk; plain yogurt (not chilled); tolerance to milk and milk products should be tested | All sweetened milk beverages; milk in all forms if not allowed by physician or if not tolerated. |
| Other beverages | See general instructions | Tea, coffee, Postum, Sanka; lemonade (without sugar or syrup—use artificial sweetener) | Sweetened fruit beverages; cocoa, chocolate; alcoholic beverages including beer; carbonated beverages |
| Soup | 1 svg.<br>¾ cup per svg. | Broth, cream soup (if milk is allowed) | All soups not listed as allowed; bouillon |
| Meat, poultry, fish | 16 oz. | All that are tolerated by patient | None if tolerated by patient |

## Table A–31. (continued)

| | | | |
|---|---|---|---|
| Cheese | 1–2 oz. | All cheeses | None |
| Eggs | 2–3 | May be prepared in any way | None |
| Potato, bread, or substitute | 6 | All except those excluded | Sweet baked goods, waffles, muffins, pancakes; bread or its equivalent in excess of specified amount; whole-grain and rye bread if not tolerated by patient |
| Cereal | 1 svg.<br>½ cup<br>4 oz. | All kinds | Sweetened cereals, whole-grain if not tolerated by patient |
| Vegetable | 2 svg.<br>½ cup per svg.<br>Include 1 green or yellow vegetable | All except those excluded | Raw vegetables if not tolerated by patient; corn and lima beans (unless substituted for bread) |
| Fruit | 2 svg. Include 1 citrus or 4 oz. citrus juice | Unsweetened cooked, fresh, or canned; all except those excluded | Fruit cooked or canned with sugar; sweetened fruit juice; raw fruit if not tolerated by patient; frozen and dried fruit |
| Butter or fat | 10 Tbsp.<br>2–3 strips | Butter, cream, margarine, oils, fats, mayonnaise, French dressing; crisp bacon | |
| Dessert | 1 svg. | Junket, custard, gelatin (made without sugar—use artificial sweetener) | Cake, cookies, pastries, pies, puddings; sherbet, ice cream, sweetened sauces, gelatin, candy |
| Miscellaneous | In moderation | Nuts, smooth peanut butter; condiments including salt; artificial sweetener | Sugar, jam, marmalade, jelly, honey, syrups, molasses, chocolate, marshmallows; snacks such as Fritos, popcorn, pretzels, potato chips; spices, condiments, pepper, catsup, chili sauce, mustard, vinegar |

*GENERAL INSTRUCTIONS:*
1. Eat regularly. Do not omit meals.
2. Eat small meals (six per day).
3. The major amount of fluids should be taken 45 to 60 minutes (or later) after each meal.
4. Eat slowly; relax before and after meals.
5. Some patients are not tolerant of milk and milk products following partial or total gastrectomies. Patient should test his tolerance by taking small amounts initially. Amounts may be increased gradually up to limit of acceptance by patient. If milk is not tolerated, a physician is to be consulted concerning other sources of calcium and perhaps a vitamin supplement.
6. As your tolerance for the diet improves, you may be able to return to three meals daily, gradually increase your carbohydrate intake, and shorten the period between the consumption of solid and liquid foods.

## Table A–31.   (continued)

|  | *Sample Meal Pattern* |  |
| --- | --- | --- |
| *8:00 a.m. Breakfast* | Serving Portion | *Sample Menu* |
| Fruit | ½ cup | Orange/grapefruit sections |
| Cereal (calcium-enriched) | 1 cup | Oatmeal |
| Yogurt | ½ cup | Low-fat yogurt |
| *9:00 a.m.* |  |  |
| Milk, skim | ½ cup | Milk, skim |
| *10:00 a.m. Mid-morning Nourishment* |  |  |
| Crackers | 4 each | Whole wheat crackers |
| Cheese | 1 oz. | Low-fat cottage cheese |
| *12:00 p.m. Lunch* |  |  |
| Meat | 5 oz. | Roast chicken breast |
| Potato | 1 cup | Rice, brown |
| Vegetable | ½ cup | Peas |
| Butter | 2 tsp. | Butter or margarine |
| Fruit | ½ cup | Unsweetened apricots (drained) |
| *1:00 p.m.* |  |  |
| Beverage | 1 cup | Tea with lemon |
| *3:00 p.m. Mid-Afternoon Nourishment* |  |  |
| Bread | 2 slices | Whole-grain bread |
| Cheese | 1 oz. | Low-fat cottage cheese |
| *6:00 p.m. Dinner* |  |  |
| Meat | 5 oz. | Roast beef |
| Potato | 1 medium | Baked potato |
| Butter or oil | 2 tsp. | Butter or margarine |
| Vegetable | ½ cup | Spinach |
| Dessert | ½ cup | Unsweetened peaches (drained) |
| *7:00 p.m.* |  |  |
| Beverage | 1 cup | Tea with lemon |
| *8:00 p.m. Evening Nourishment* |  |  |
| Bread | 2 slices | Whole-grain bread |
| Meat | 3 oz. | Tuna |
| Butter | 2 tsp. | Mayonnaise |
| *9:00 p.m.* |  |  |
| Beverage | 1 cup | Milk, skim |

*Modified from Diet Manual, Memorial Sloan-Kettering Cancer Center, revised 1978.

### Table A–32. Gluten-Free Diet (Wheat-, Rye-, Oats-, Barley-, and Buckwheat-Free)*,**

*Purpose:* This diet is designed for the treatment of patients with gluten enteropathy (i.e., nontropical sprue, celiac disease), a malabsorption syndrome caused by sensitivity to gliadin or its products. Gliadin is a protein fraction of gluten found in all grains other than rice and corn. Therefore, gluten-containing cereals are eliminated in this diet. Because wheat, rye, oats, barley, and buckwheat products are used in the manufacture of a variety of foods, beverages, and confections, deviation from this diet is permitted only with the approval of the physician.

| Approximate Composition | Unit | Amount |
|---|---|---|
| Carbohydrate | g | 297 |
| Protein | g | 98 |
| Fat | g | 107 |
| Calories | | 2,505 |
| Calcium | mg | 823 |
| Phosphorus | mg | 1,371 |
| Iron | mg | 18.1 |
| Sodium | mg (meq) | 2,757 (120) |
| Potassium | mg (meq) | 2,886 (74) |
| Vitamin A | I.U. | 9,631 |
| Thiamin | mg | 1.7 |
| Riboflavin | mg | 2.7 |
| Niacin equivalents | mg | 26.8 |
| Ascorbic acid | mg | 219 |

*Adequacy:* This diet meets the 1980 Recommended Dietary Allowances of the National Research Council. The calculations are based on the sample menu.

### GUIDELINES FOR GLUTEN-FREE DIETS

This menu pattern is designed to provide adequate nutrition while eliminating wheat, rye, oats, and barley from the diet. The fraction of gluten protein that injures the intestine of susceptible individuals is gliadin. When all sources of gliadin are removed from the diet, however, the intestine is able to regenerate and function normally.

Gluten may be present in foods as a basic ingredient (that is, listed as wheat, rye, oats, or barley), or added as a derivative when a food is processed or prepared. Thus, READING LABELS CAREFULLY IS VERY IMPORTANT. Because there is a great deal of confusion about the presence of gliadin-containing additives in foods, the last page of this instruction lists those commonly occurring additives that must always be checked as well as those that do not contain gluten. The Gluten Content of Products List contains helpful information on those commercially prepared products that have been checked for gliadin content.

Because flour and cereal products are often used in the preparation of foods, it is important to be aware of the methods of preparation used as well as the foods themselves. This is especially true when dining out.

| Food Group with Recommended Daily Intake | Foods Allowed | Food to Avoid |
|---|---|---|
| Milk—2 or more cups | Fresh, dry, evaporated, or condensed milk; cream; sour cream,† whipping cream; yogurt† | Malted milk; some commercial chocolate drinks; some nondairy creamers* |

## Table A–32. (continued)

| | | |
|---|---|---|
| Meat, fish, poultry—2 or more svgs. | All kinds of fresh meats, fish, other seafood, poultry; fish canned in oil or brine; some prepared meat products, such as frankfurters and lunch meats* | Prepared meats that contain wheat, rye, oats, or barley such as: some sausages,* frankfurters,* bologna,* luncheon meats,* chili con carne,* sandwich spreads.* Bread-containing products, such as: swiss steak, croquettes; meat loaf; tuna canned in vegetable broth,* and turkey with hydrolyzed vegetable protein injected as part of the basting solution |
| Cheeses (can be used for meat and milk groups) | All aged cheeses, such as: cheddar; Swiss Edam; Parmesan; cottage cheese,† cream cheese,† pasteurized processed cheese† | Any cheese product containing oat gum as an ingredient |
| Eggs | Plain or in cooking | Eggs in sauce made from gluten-containing ingredients (such as a regular, wheat-based white sauce) |
| Potato or other starch—1 or more svgs. | White and sweet potatoes; yams; hominy; rice; wild rice; special gluten-free noodles (Aproten) made by Henkel Corp.‡; some oriental rice and bean noodles | Regular noodles; spaghetti; macaroni; most packaged rice mixes* |
| Vegetables—2 or more svgs. | Use all plain, fresh, frozen or canned vegetables; dried peas and beans; lentils; some commercially prepared vegetables* | Creamed vegetables*; vegetables canned in sauce*; some canned baked beans*; commercially prepared vegetables and salads* |
| Fruits—2 or more svgs. | All fresh, frozen, canned, or dried fruits; all fruit juices; some canned pie fillings | Thickened or prepared fruits; some pie fillings* |
| Breads—3 or more svgs. | Specially prepared breads using only allowed flours; examples of commercially available brands: Ener-G Foods Brown Rice Bread and White Rice Bread‡ | All others containing wheat, rye, oat, and/or barley flours |
| Cereals—1 or more svgs. enriched cereal | Hot cereals made from: corn meal; cream of rice; hominy; rice; cold cereals as follows: puffed rice, Kellogg's Sugar Pops; Post's Fruity and Chocolate Pebbles; special cereals‡ | All others containing wheat, rye, oats, and/or barley; bran; graham; wheat germ; malt; kaska; bulgar; buckwheat,§ millet§ |
| Flours and thickening agents | Arrowroot starch (A)<br>Corn flour (B,C,D)‡<br>Corn meal (B,C,D)<br>Corn starch (A)<br>Potato flour (B,C,E)‡<br>Potato starch flour (B,C,E)<br>Rice bran (B)<br>Rice flours:‡ plain, brown (B,C,E), sweet (B,C,D,F)<br>Rice polish (B,C,G)‡<br>Soy flour (B,C,G)‡<br>Tapioca starch (A) | Wheat starch (manufacturer states it contains gluten); all flours containing wheat, rye, oats, and/or barley |

A = Good thickening agent
B = Good combined with other flours
C = Best combined with milk and eggs in baked product
D = Grainy-textured products
E = Drier product than with other flours
F = Moister product than with other flours
G = Adds distinct flavor to product—use with moderation

## Table A–32.   (continued)

| | | |
|---|---|---|
| Crackers and snack foods | Rice wafers*; pure corn meal tortillas; popcorn; some crackers and chips* | All others containing wheat, rye, oats and/or barley |
| Fats | Butter; margarine; vegetable oils; nuts; peanut butters; hydrogenated vegetable oils; some salad dressings*; mayonnaise* | Some commercial salad dressings* |
| Soups | Homemade broth and soups made with allowed ingredients; some commercially canned soups* | Most canned soups* and soup mixes*; bouillon |
| Desserts | Cakes, quick breads, pastries, puddings prepared with allowed ingredients. Cornstarch, tapioca, and rice puddings; gelatin desserts; custard; vanilla-flavored ice cream from: Arden, Carnation; Darigold; Foremost; Lucerne*; some pudding mixes* | Commercial cakes, cookes, pies, made with wheat, rye, oats, and/or barley; prepared mixes*; ice cream cones; puddings* |
| Beverages | Instant and ground coffee; instant tea; tea; carbonated beverages*; pure cocoa powder; unfortified wines; rums; some root beers*; vodka distilled from grapes | Ovaltine; malted milk; ale; beer; gin; #whiskeys; vodka distilled from grain |
| Sweets | Jelly; jam; honey; brown and white sugar; molasses; most syrups*; some candy*; chocolate; pure cocoa; coconut | Some commercial candies* |
| Miscellaneous | Salt; pepper; herbs; extracts; food coloring; cloves; ginger; nutmeg; cinnamon; chili powder; tomato puree and paste; olives; pickles; cider and wine vinegar; yeast; bicarbonate of soda; baking powder; cream of tartar; dry mustard; some other condiments*; monosodium glutamate (MSG) | Some curry powder*; some dry seasoning mixes*; some gravy extracts*; some meat sauces*; some catsup*; some mustard*; horseradish*; some soy sauce*; chip dips*; some chewing gum*; distilled white vinegar# |

*See Product Ingredient List for clarification.

†Check vegetable gum used.

‡See Special Products List for availability and ordering information.

§Although millet is botanically different from other gluten-containing grains, additional information is needed before this can be cleared.

#Distilled white vinegar uses grain as a starting material. Whiskies, including "corn whiskey" use wheat, rye, oats, or barley in their mash. According to chemistry professors consulted, in large-scale distillation processes, such as that occurring in the manufacture of whiskey and vinegar, it is possible that a very small amount of protein may be carried over into the distillate. The presence of such a small amount of gluten must be tested via immunoassay, an expensive and complex technique using laboratory animals to produce a gluten antibody. Currently, we are advising gluten-intolerant persons to use cider and wine vinegar in cooking and when making salad dressings or pickles. Avoid all whiskies.

Commercially prepared pickles, catsup, mustard, mayonnaise, steak sauce, and other condiments are usually made with distilled grain vinegar; however, the maximum amount of gluten that would be present in such products via the vinegar would be insignificant. Thus, moderate use of the aforementioned commercial condiments is recommended.

## Table A–32. (continued)

Always check the source of the following nebulous ingredients before using:

| Ingredient (as appears on label) | Include | Avoid |
|---|---|---|
| "Hydrolyzed vegetable protein" | Soy, corn | Mixtures of wheat, corn, and soya (soy) |
| "Flour" or "cereal products" | Rice flour, corn flour, corn meal, potato flour, soy flour | Wheat, rye, oats, or barley |
| "Vegetable protein" | Soy, corn | Wheat, rye, oats, barley |
| "Malt" or "malt flavoring" | Those derived from corn | Those derived from barley or barley malt syrup |
| "Starch" | When listed as such on a United States manufacturer's ingredient list, it is CORN STARCH | |
| "Modified starch" or "modified food starch" | Arrowroot, corn, potato, tapioca, waxy maize, maize | Wheat starch |
| "Vegetable gum" | Carob bean, locust bean, cellulose gum, guar gum, gum arabic, gum acacia, gum tragacanth, xanthan gum | Oat gum |
| "Soy sauce" or "soy sauce solids" | Those that DO NOT contain wheat, such as Chun King | Those that CONTAIN wheat |

These questionable ingredients must be cleared with the manufacturer before they are eaten. When writing the manufacturer, request information on the specific starting material(s) used in their nebulous ingredient. For example, when "modified food starch" appears as a labeling ingredient, ask for the specific type of starch used, i.e., potato starch, tapioca starch.

A combination of wheat, corn, and soya is primarily used as starting material for hydrolyzed vegetable protein, and thus is not allowed on a gluten-free diet. When wheat protein is "hydrolyzed," its large amino acid chains are broken down into smaller chains. Some protein researchers believe the sequence of amino acids found in these smaller chains contains the same toxicity as the intact gliadin subfraction of the gluten protein. Thus, HVP made from wheat is not recommended for use on a gluten-free diet.

### ADDITIONAL ADDITIVES THAT ARE GLUTEN-FREE

Adipic acid
BHA
BHT
Beta-carotene
Biotin

Calcium chloride
Calcium pantothenate
Calcium phosphate
Carboxymethylcellulose
Carrageenan
Citric acid
Corn sweetener
Corn syrup solids

Demineralized whey
Dextrose-dextrins
Dioctyl sodium sulfo succinate

Extracts

Folic acid-folacin
Fructose
Fumaric acid

Gums: acacia; arabic; carob bean; cellulose; guar; locust beans; tragacanth; xanthan

Invert sugar

Lactic acid
Lactose
Lecithin

Magnesium hydroxide
Malic acid
Microcrystallin cellulose
Mono- and diglycerides
Monosodium glutamate (MSG)

Niacin-niacinamide

Polyglycerol
Polysorbate 60; 80
Potassium citrate
Potassium iodide
Propylene glycol monostearate
Propylgallate
Pyridoxine hydrochloride

Riboflavin

Sodium acid pyrophosphate
Sodium ascorbate-ascorbic acid
Sodium benzoate
Sodium caseinate
Sodium citrate
Sodium hexametaphosphate
Sodium nitrate
Sodium silaco aluminate
Sorbitol-mannitol
Sucrose
Sulfosuccinate

Tartaric acid
Thiamin hydrochloride
Tricalcium phosphate

Vanillan
Vitamins and minerals
Vitamin A (palmitate)

Note: The above is not an exhaustive list.

## Table A–32.   (continued)

### SPECIAL PRODUCTS LIST

AlpineAire Foods
P.O. Box 926
Nevada City, CA 95959
(916) 272-1971

Excellent source for freeze-dried foods for backpacking and camping. All foods are vacuum-packed. They contain no preservatives, no added sugar, and no artificial flavors or colors. NOTE: Their "vegetable pasta" listed in Pasta Roma and "vegetable pasta stew" CONTAINS WHEAT FLOUR as its major ingredient. Mail orders accepted.

Anglo-Dietetics, Ltd.
P.O. Box 333
Wilton, CT 06897
(203) 762-2504

Write regarding complete ingredient listing of products prior to ordering. Some of their products contain wheat starch. Mail orders accepted.

Chicago Dietetic Supply, Inc.
Dept. 25
P.O. Box 529
La Grange, IL 60525
(312) 352-6900

Featherweight brand products. Primarily gluten-free (GF) flours, but also a few baked products. Write regarding complete ingredient listing prior to ordering. Some "low-gluten" products are *not* gluten-free. Mail orders accepted.

DeBoles
Garden City Park, N.Y. 11040

Corn pasta products, including ribbon noodles, macaroni, and spaghetti.

El Molino Mills
345 N. Baldwin Park Blvd.
City of Industry, CA 91746
(213) 962-7167

Produce a variety of GF cereals and flours. Available through local distributors only. No retail mail sales. Will forward name and address of distributor in your area and product ingredient information.

Ener-G Foods, Inc.
P.O. Box 24723
Seattle, WA 98124-0723
(206) 767-6660

Jolly Joan brand GF flours and flour mixes available. Will ship GF flours in bulk also. Variety of baked products including breads, cinnamon rolls, cookies, and pizza crusts. Mail orders accepted. Write for complete product information.

Fearn Soya Foods
Division of Richard Foods Corp.
4520 James Place
Melrose Park, IL 60160
(312) 345-2335

Variety of gluten-free flours, baking mixes, and other baking ingredients (Fearn brand). Mail orders accepted.

Gluten Intolerance Group
P.O. Box 23053
Seattle, WA 98102-0353
(206) 854-9606

Variety of publications dealing with celiac sprue. Sell xanthan gum for stabilization of homemade brown and white rice flour yeast bread. GIG COOKBOOK also available.

Henkel Corp.
4620 West 77th Street
Minneapolis, MN 55435
(612) 830-7831

Aproten brand GF noodle products. Various macaroni and spaghetti products available. Taste and cooking properties similar to those of wheat-containing pastas. Mail orders accepted.

Med-Diet Laboratories, Inc.
695 Hopkins Crossroad
Minnetonka, MN 55343
(612) 546-3285

Products include gluten-free dry soup mixes. Write concerning availability of other gluten-free products. Mail orders accepted.

NuVita Foods, Inc.
7624 S.W. Macadam
Portland, OR 97219
(503) 246-5433

Produce Lange's "Mello Gold" brand gluten-free flours. Mail orders accepted.

Van Brode's Milling Co.
Clinton, MA 01510

Manufacture GF cold breakfast cereals. Write for complete product listing and distribution information.

Vita-Wheat Bakery
1839 Hilton Road
Ferndale, MI 48220
(313) 543-0888

Variety of baked products for GF diet. Write for production information and ingredient lists. Mail orders accepted.

## Table A–32.   (continued)

| Breakfast | *Sample Meal Pattern*<br>Serving Portion | Sample Menu |
|---|---|---|
| Fruit | ½ cup | Orange juice |
| Cereal | 1 cup | Cream of rice |
| Egg | 1 | Soft-cooked egg |
| Bread | 1 slice | Rice bread |
| Fat | 2 tsps | Butter or margarine |
| Milk | 1 cup | Milk |
| Beverage | 1 cup | Coffee |
| Sugar | 1 Tbsp | Sugar |
| *Lunch* | | |
| Meat or substitute | 3 oz | Broiled chicken |
| Potato or substitute | 1 | Rice |
| Vegetable | ½ cup | Asparagus |
| Salad | | Sliced tomato |
| Dessert | ½ cup | Custard |
| Bread | 1 slice | Rice bread |
| Fat | 2 tsp | Butter or margarine |
| Milk | ½ cup | Milk |
| Beverage | 1 cup | Coffee |
| Sugar | 2 tsp | Sugar |
| *Dinner* | | |
| Soup | 1 cup | Bouillon, homemade |
| Meat or substitute | 3 oz | Roast beef |
| Potato or substitute | 1 | Baked potato |
| Vegetable | ½ cup | Brussels sprouts |
| Salad | ½ carrot | Carrot sticks |
| Fruit | ½ cup | Canned apricots |
| Fat | 1 tsp | Butter or margarine |
| Beverage | 1 cup | Coffee |
| Sugar | 2 tsp | Sugar |
| | ½ cup | Milk |
| *8 p.m.* | | |
| Fruit | ½ cup | Applesauce |

**Approximate composition and sample meal pattern are modified from Diet Manual, Memorial Sloan-Kettering Cancer Center, revised 1978. The Guidelines for Gluten-Free Diets were prepared by Elaine I. Hartsook, Ed. M., R.D., Gluten Intolerance Group, P.O. Box 23053, Seattle, Washington 98102-0353. A gluten-free product list and newsletters are available from Ms. Hartsook.

## Table A–33. Fat-Restricted Diets (20 and 40 g)*·†

*Purpose:* These diets are designed for patients with serious diseases of the biliary tract or pancreas or with malabsorption syndromes other than that caused by gluten sensitivity where a reduced fat intake may decrease diarrhea and nutrient losses. Medium-chain-length triglycerides (MCT) may be added to this diet in various recipes.‡ Pancreatic extract should be given where indicated.

| Approximate Composition | Unit | 20 g | 40 g |
|---|---|---|---|
| Carbohydrate | g | 391 | 369 |
| Protein | g | 91 | 98 |
| Fat | g | 21 | 42 |
| Saturated fatty acid | g | 6 | 14 |
| Unsaturated fatty acid | g | 7 | 19 |
| Calories | | 2,057 | 2,198 |
| Calcium | mg | 979 | 925 |
| Phosphorus | mg | 1,370 | 1,490 |
| Iron | mg | 14 | 16 |
| Sodium | mg (meq) | 2,744 (115) | 2,740 (115) |
| Potassium | mg (meq) | 3,272 (84) | 3,422 (88) |
| Vitamin A | I.U. | 12,000 | 13,000 |
| Thiamin | mg | 1.5 | 1.5 |
| Riboflavin | mg | 2.2 | 2.4 |
| Niacin equivalents | mg | 19 | 23 |
| Ascorbic acid | mg | 122 | 123 |

*Adequacy:* These diets meet the 1980 Recommended Dietary Allowances for adult men of the National Research Council, but may be low in iron for women. The calculations are based on the sample menu with an average weekly figure used for protein foods.

| Type of Food | Amount | Food Included | Food Excluded |
|---|---|---|---|
| Milk | 1 pt | Skim milk, fat-free buttermilk | Whole milk, cultured buttermilk, chocolate milk; yogurt |
| Other beverages | As desired | Coffee, tea, Sanka, Postum; carbonated beverages | All alcoholic beverages; Ovaltine, chocolate-flavored drinks, cocoa |
| Soup | As desired | Fat-free bouillon or broth, tomato bouillon; vegetable soup; skim milk soup | Any soup containing cream, fat, or whole milk |
| Meat, poultry, or fish | 6 oz cooked weights for 40-g diet; 2 oz for 20-g diet | All broiled, boiled, baked, or cooked without fat in a Teflon pan. All visible fat must be removed. Meat and fish may be wrapped in foil before broiling or baking in order to retain juices. Lean cuts of beef, Canadian bacon, lamb, liver, veal, white meat of chicken and turkey—remove skin before cooking; organ meats. All fish, including canned pink salmon and sardines in tomato sauce, except those listed as not allowed | Pork, ham, bacon, duck, goose, salami, pastrami, bologna, frankfurters, sausages, luncheon meats; frozen or canned meat dishes. Fish canned in oil (sardines, tuna); frozen fish sticks; fresh or frozen salmon |
| Cheese | 40-g diet: as desired; 20-g diet: additional 4 oz to replace meat portion | Fat-free cottage cheese, pot cheese, other skim-milk cheese§ | All others |

## Table A–33.  (continued)

| | | | |
|---|---|---|---|
| Eggs | 40-g diet: 1 daily; omit on 20-g diet | Medium- or hard-cooked, poached, scrambled in double boiler, cooked without fat in a Teflon pan, egg whites as desired | More than 1 daily; eggs fried in fat |
| Potato or substitute | 2–3 svg. | Baked, boiled, mashed without whole milk or fat; rice, spaghetti, macaroni; hominy | Escalloped or creamed potatoes, fried potatoes, potato chips, oven-browned potatoes; egg noodles |
| Bread | 5 svg. | White, whole wheat, rye, French, hard rolls, soft rolls, matzos, rye crisp, saltines, Uneeda biscuits, melba toast | All other breads and rolls; quickbreads, biscuits, popovers, muffins; egg matzos; butter crackers |
| Cereals | 1 svg. | All cooked and dry cereals | None |
| Vegetables | 3 or more svg. including 1 green or yellow | All fresh; frozen or canned vegetables prepared without cream sauce, fats, or oils | Creamed vegetables or vegetables prepared with fat or oil |
| Fruit and fruit juice | 4 or more svg. including citrus or tomato | All fresh, frozen, canned, and stewed except avocado and coconut; all fruit juices | Avocado and coconut |
| Butter or fats | 40-g diet: 1 tsp if tolerated; 20-g diet: omit | One of the following may be substituted for 1 tsp of butter or margarine:<br>light cream 2 Tbsp<br>heavy cream 1 Tbsp<br>French dressing 1 Tbsp<br>mayonnaise 1 tsp<br>oil 1 tsp | More than 1 tsp of butter or margarine; no gravies |
| Dessert | In moderation | Plain angel food cake, vanilla wafers, ladyfingers, arrowroot cookies, graham crackers, meringues, Jell-O, junket, cornstarch, rice and tapioca pudding made with skim milk and egg whites, water ices, fruit whips made with gelatin or egg whites | All other cakes, pies, doughnuts, cookies, puddings, pastry, ice cream, puddings made with whole milk and egg yolks, or eggs |
| Sweets | In moderation | Sugar, honey, jelly, jam, marmalade, molasses, maple syrup and sugar, sour balls, gumdrops, jelly beans, marshmallows, hard candy, and fondant | Chocolate, chocolate candy, chocolate syrup, candy made with cream, cocoa fats, and nuts |
| Spices | | Salt, paprika, herbs, mustard, nutmeg | Pepper |
| Miscellaneous | | Catsup, chili sauce, vinegar, pickles, garlic, unbuttered popcorn, white sauce made with skim milk, vanilla | Olives, nuts, peanut butter, apple butter; cream sauces, gravies; buttered popcorn, waffles, pancakes, fritters |

## Table A–33. (continued)

*Sample Meal Pattern for 20-g Fat Diet*

| Breakfast | Serving Portion | Sample Menu |
|---|---|---|
| Fruit | ½ cup | Orange juice |
| Cereal | ½ cup | Farina |
| Bread | 2 slices | White enriched toast |
| Jelly | 2 tsp | Jelly |
| Milk | ½ cup | Skim milk |
| Sugar | 1 Tbsp | Sugar |
| Beverage | 1 cup | Coffee or tea |
| *Lunch* | | |
| Meat or substitute | 3 oz | Broiled chicken (no skin) |
| Potato or substitute | ½ cup | Rice |
| Vegetable | ½ cup | Asparagus |
| Salad | 1 svg. | Lettuce and tomato |
| Dressing | | Vinegar |
| Fruit | ½ cup | Canned cherries |
| Bread | 1 | Hard roll |
| Jelly | 2 tsp | Jelly |
| Sugar | 2 tsp | Sugar |
| Milk | ½ cup | Skim milk |
| Beverage | 1 cup | Coffee or tea |
| *Dinner* | | |
| Soup | 1 cup | Bouillon (fat-free) |
| Meat or substitute | 3 oz | Baked flounder |
| Potato or substitute | 1 | Baked sweet potato |
| Vegetable | ½ cup | Brussels sprouts |
| | ½ cup | Carrot sticks |
| Fruit | ½ cup | Apricots |
| Bread | 1 slice | Rye bread |
| Milk | 1 cup | Skim milk |
| Jelly | 2 tsp | Jelly |
| Sugar | 2 tsp | Sugar |
| Beverage | 1 cup | Coffee or tea |
| *8:00 p.m.* | | |
| Fruit | 1 | Apple |

## Table A–33. (continued)

*Sample Meal Pattern for 40-g Fat Diet*

| Breakfast | Serving Portion | Sample Menu |
|---|---|---|
| Fruit | ½ cup | Orange juice |
| Cereal | ½ cup | Wheatena |
| Egg | 1 | Soft-boiled |
| Bread | 2 slices | White bread |
| Jelly | 1 Tbsp | Jelly |
| Milk, skim | 1 cup | Skim milk |
| Beverage | As desired | Coffee |
| Sugar | 1 Tbsp | Sugar |
| *Lunch* | | |
| Meat | 3 oz | Sliced white chicken |
| Potato substitute | 1 cup | Rice |
| Vegetable | 1 svg. | Carrots |
| Salad | 1 svg. | Sliced tomato |
| Bread | 2 slices | White bread |
| Fat | 1 tsp | Mayonnaise |
| Skim milk | ½ cup | Skim milk |
| Beverage | 1 cup | Tea |
| Sugar | 1 Tbsp | Sugar |
| Dessert | 1 svg. | Canned peaches |
| *Dinner* | | |
| Soup | ½ cup | Bouillon |
| Meat | 3 oz | Broiled steak |
| Potato | 1 svg. | Baked potato |
| Vegetable | 1 svg. | Steamed green beans |
| Salad | 1 svg. | Celery hearts |
| Bread | 1 svg. | Hard roll |
| Jelly | 1 Tbsp | Honey or jelly |
| Skim milk | ½ cup | Skim milk |
| Beverage | 1 cup | Coffee |
| Sugar | 1 Tbsp | Sugar |
| Dessert | 1 svg. | Raspberry Jell-O |
| *9 p.m.* | | |
| Fruit | 1 | Raw apple |

*Modified from Diet Manual, Memorial Sloan-Kettering Cancer Center, revised 1978.

†The 20-g restricted fat diet contains approximately 6 g saturated fatty acids or 27.9% of the total fat, 7 g polyunsaturated fatty acids or 34% of the total fat. The 40-g restricted diet contains 14 g saturated fatty acids or 33% of the total fat, 19 g polyunsaturated fatty acids or 44.8% of the total fat.

The 40 g can be decreased to 20 g by omitting the egg and 1 tsp fat, reducing the meat allowance from 6 oz to 3 oz, and adding 4 oz fat-free cottage cheese.

‡MCT oil may be added to this diet to increase calories as potentially absorbable fat. For information and recipes on MCT see Senior, J.R. (Ed): Medium-Chain Triglycerides. Philadelphia, University of Pennsylvania Press, 1968. Bach, A.C., and Babayan, V.K.: Medium-chain triglycerides: an update. Am. J. Clin. Nutr., *36*:Nov. 1982, pp. 950–962. Also, Portagen/MCT Oil recipe book. Mead Johnson Nutritional Division, Mead Johnson & Co. Evansville, IN., July 1983.

§The following is a partial list of some available low-fat cheeses: Caerphilly (70% fat-free), Gaperon (80% fat-free), Nökkelost (70% fat-free), Lorraine Swiss (85% fat-free), Swiss Chris (85% fat-free). Margarinost (100% cholesterol fat-free).

The following are part skimmed or low-fat: Jarlsberg, Fontina, Crem Havarti, Typo, Monterey Jack, and pure goat cheeses.

## Table A–34. Lactose Content of Selected Milk, Milk Products, and Substitutes*·†

| Product | | Lactose (approx. g/unit) |
|---|---|---|
| Milk | 1 C—244 g | 11 |
| Low-fat milk (2% fat) | 1 C—244 g | 9–13 |
| Skim milk | 1 C—244 g | 12–14 |
| Chocolate milk | 1 C—244 g | 10–12 |
| Sweetened condensed whole milk | 1 C—306 g | 35 |
| Dried whole milk | 1 C—128 g | 48 |
| Nonfat dry milk, instant | 1½ C—91 g | 46 |
| Buttermilk fluid | 1 C—245 g | 9–11 |
| Whipped cream topping | 1 Tbsp—3 g | 0.4 |
| Light cream | 1 Tbsp—15 g | 0.6 |
| Half and Half | 1 Tbsp—15 g | 0.6 |
| Low-fat yogurts‡ | 8 oz—227–258 g | 11–15 |
| Cheese: | | |
|   Blue, cream, Parmesan, Colby | 1 oz—28 g | 0.7–0.8 |
|   Camembert, Limburger | 1 oz—28 g | 0.1 |
|   Cheddar, Gouda | 1 oz—28 g | 0.4–0.6 |
| Cheese, pasteurized, processed: | | |
|   American | 1 oz—28 g | 0.5 |
|   Pimento | 1 oz—28 g | 0.5–1.7 |
|   Swiss | 1 oz—28 g | 0.4–0.6 |
| Cottage cheese | 1 C—210 g | 5–6 |
| Cottage cheese, low-fat (2% fat) | 1 C—226 g | 7–8 |
| Butter | 2 pats—10 g | 0.1 |
| Oleomargarine | 2 pats—10 g | 0 |
| Ice cream | | |
|   Vanilla, regular | 1 C—133 g | 9 |
|   French, soft | 1 C—173 g | 9 |
| Ice milk, vanilla | 1 C—131 g | 10 |
| Sherbet, orange | 1 C—193 g | 4 |
| Ice, orange | 100 g | 0 |

*From Walsh, J.D.: Am. J. Clin. Nutr. 31:592–596, 1978, with permission of the author and publisher.

†Lactaid milk and other dairy products have lactose reduced by 70%. With further treatment, these products can be 100% lactose-free.

‡Bacterial lactase in unpasteurized yogurt survives transit through the stomach allowing digestion of the lactose present in yogurt. This process enables lactase-deficient individuals to consume these dairy products in moderate amounts (from ½ to 1 pint) with fewer or no symptoms. Data from Kolars, J.C., Levitt, M.D., Aouji, M., et al.: N. Engl. J. Med. 310:1–3, 1984.

Lactase-deficient patients have been reported to experience no gastrointestinal distress after consuming pasteurized yogurt (500 g) even though the lactase activity is significantly destroyed by pasteurization. In contrast, cultured milk does result in gastrointestinal distress for lactose-intolerant individuals. Data from Savaiano, D.A., AbouElAnouar, A., Smith, D.E., et al.: Am. J. Clin. Nutr. 40:1219–1223, 1984.

## Table A–35. Oxalate Content of Selected Foods and Food Groups*

### Foods to Use: These Contain Small Amounts of Oxalate
#### 0–2 mg Oxalate per serving

| Vegetables | Fruits | Beverages | Miscellaneous |
|---|---|---|---|
| Broccoli | Avocados | Apple juice | Butter |
| Brussels sprouts | Bananas | Barley water | Cheese, cheddar |
| Cabbage | Cherries | Beer, bottled | Chicken noodle soup |
| Cauliflower | Grapes, Thompson seedless | Cider | Cornflakes |
| Chives | Mangoes | Coca-Cola | Eggs |
| Cucumbers | Melons | Grapefruit juice | Egg noodle (chow mein) |
| Lettuce | Nectarines | Lemon squash drink (lemonade) | Fish (except sardines) |
| Mushrooms | Peaches, canned | Lucozade, bottled | Jelly with allowed fruit |
| Onions |   Hiley | Milk | Lemon juice |
| Peas |   Stokes | Orange juice | Lime juice |
| Potatoes, white | Pineapples | Pepsi-Cola | Macaroni |
| Radishes | Plums, golden gage, | Pineapple juice | Margarine |
| Rice |   green gage | Sherry, dry | Meats |
| Turnips | | Wine | Oatmeal, porridge |
| | | | Oxtail soup |
| | | | Poultry |
| | | | Red plum jam |
| | | | Sweets, boiled |

### Foods to Avoid: These Contain Large Amounts of Oxalate
#### >15 mg Oxalate per serving

| Vegetables | Fruits | Beverages | Miscellaneous |
|---|---|---|---|
| Beans in tomato | Blackberries | Beer, lager | Chocolate |
|   sauce | Blueberries |   Tuborg Pilsner | Cocoa |
| Beets | Currants, red | Ovaltine (24 mg/8 oz) | Grits (white corn) |
| Celery | Gooseberries, green | Tea (132–181.2 mg/8 oz) | Peanuts |
| Chard, Swiss | Grapes, Concord | | Pecans |
| Collards | Lemon peel | | Soybean crackers |
| Dandelion | Lime peel | | Wheat germ |
|   greens | Raspberries, black | | |
| Eggplant | Rhubarb | | |
| Escarole | | | |
| Leeks | | | |
| Okra | | | |
| Parsley | | | |
| Peppers, green | | | |
| Pokeweed | | | |
| Potatoes, sweet | | | |
| Rutabagas | | | |
| Spinach | | | |
| Squash, summer | | | |

### Low-Oxalate Meal Plan
#### (40–50 mg)

| Foods | Little or No Oxalate Content <2 mg oxalate/serving Eat as desired | Moderate Oxalate Content 2–10 mg oxalate/serving Limit: two (½ cup ) servings/day | High Oxalate Content >10 mg oxalate/serving Avoid completely |
|---|---|---|---|
| Beverages/Juices | Apple juice | Coffee, any kind (8 oz. serving) | Beer: draft |
| | Beer, bottled | Cranberry juice (4 oz.) |   Stout, Guinness Draft |
| | Coca-Cola (12 oz. limit/day) | Grape juice (4 oz.) |   Lager, Tuborg Pilsner |
| | Distilled alcohol | Orange juice (4 oz.) | Juices containing berries |
| | Grapefruit juice | Tomato juice (4 oz.) | Ovaltine and other mixed |
| | Lemonade or limeade without | Nescafe powder |   beverage mixes |
| |   peel | | Tea, cocoa |
| | Wine, red, rosé | | |
| | Pepsi-Cola (12 oz. limit/day) | | |
| | Pineapple juice | | |
| | Tap water (prefered for extra | | |
| |   calcium) | | |
| Milk (2 or more cups) | Buttermilk | | |
| | Low-fat milk | | |
| | Low-fat yogurt with allowed | | |
| |   fruit | | |
| | Skim milk | | |

## Table A–35.    (continued)

| Foods | **Low-Oxalate Meal Plan (40–50 mg)** | | |
| | *Little or No Oxalate Content <2 mg oxalate/serving Eat as desired* | *Moderate Oxalate Content 2–10 mg oxalate/serving Limit: two (½ cup ) servings/day* | *High Oxalate Content >10 mg oxalate/serving Avoid completely* |
|---|---|---|---|
| Meat Group | Eggs<br>Cheese, cheddar<br>Lean lamb, beef, or pork<br>Poultry<br>Seafood | Sardines | Baked beans canned in<br>  tomato sauce<br>Peanut butter<br>Soybean curd (Tofu) |
| Vegetables | Avocados<br>Brussels sprouts<br>Cauliflower<br>Cabbage<br>Mushrooms<br>Onions<br>Peas, green<br>Potatoes (Irish)<br>Radishes | Asparagus<br>Broccoli<br>Carrots<br>Corn, sweet white, sweet yellow<br>Cucumbers, peeled<br>Green peas, canned<br>Lettuce, iceberg<br>Lima beans<br>Parsnips<br>Tomato, 1 small<br>Turnips | Beans:<br>  green, wax, dried<br>Beets:<br>  tops, root, greens<br>Celery<br>Chard, Swiss<br>Chives<br>Collards<br>Dandelion greens<br>Eggplant<br>Escarole<br>Kale<br>Leeks<br>Mustard greens<br>Okra<br>Parsley<br>Peppers, green<br>Pokeweed<br>Potatoes, sweet<br>Rutabagas<br>Spinach<br>Squash, summer<br>Watercress |
| Fruits | Avocados<br>Banana<br>Cherries, Bing<br>Grapefruit<br>Grapes, Thompson seedless<br>Mangoes<br>Melons<br>  cantaloupe<br>  casaba<br>  honeydew<br>  watermelon<br>Nectarines<br>Peaches, Hiley<br>Plums, green or Golden Age | Apples<br>Apricots<br>Cherries, edible portion<br>Currants, black<br>Oranges, edible portion<br>Peaches, Alberta<br>Pears<br>Pineapples<br>Plums, Damson<br>Prunes, Italian | Blackberries<br>Blueberries<br>Currants, red<br>Dewberries<br>Fruit cocktail<br>Gooseberries<br>Grapes, Concord<br>Lemon peel<br>Lime peel<br>Orange peel<br>Raspberries<br>Rhubarb<br>Strawberries<br>Tangerines |
| Bread/Starches | Cornflakes<br>Macaroni<br>Noodles<br>Oatmeal<br>Rice<br>Spaghetti<br>White bread | Cornbread<br>Sponge cake<br>Spaghetti, canned in tomato sauce | Fruit cake<br>Grits, white corn<br>Soybean crackers<br>Wheat germ |
| Fats & Oils | Bacon<br>Mayonnaise<br>Salad dressing<br>Vegetable oils | | Peanuts<br>Pecans |
| Miscellaneous | Jelly or preserves (made with<br>  allowed fruits)<br>Lemon, lime juice<br>Salt, pepper (1 tsp/day)<br>Soups with ingredients<br>  allowed<br>Sugar | Chicken noodle soup, dehydrated | Chocolate, cocoa<br>Pepper (in excess of 1<br>  tsp/day)<br>Vegetable soup<br>Tomato soup |

*From The Low Oxalate Diet Book. General Clinical Research Center, University of California at San Diego Medical Center and San Diego Chapter of National Foundation for Ileitis and Colitis, 1981, with permission.

## Table A–36. Diet Exchanges for a Vegetarian Diet*

List 1—*Milk Exchanges*
    Kefir                                                    1 cup (omit 2 Fat Exchanges)
    Soy milk, fortified                       1 cup (add ½ Bread Exchange)

List 2—*Vegetable Exchanges*
    Bamboo shoots                          ¾ cup
    Bean sprouts: raw or cooked
        Alfalfa                            1 cup
        Mung                             1 cup
        Soy                               1 cup
    Water chestnuts                       4

List 3—*Fruit Exchanges*
    Carrot juice                           ½ cup

List 4—*Bread Exchanges*
    Brown rice, cooked                 ⅓ cup
    Buckwheat flour, dark             3 Tbsp
    Bulgur wheat                      2 Tbsp
    Millet, cooked                      ½ cup
    Miso                                  3 Tbsp
    Oats, dry                           ¼ cup
    Pita (Syrian) bread                ½ of a 2½-oz loaf
    Rye flour                          3 Tbsp
    Wheat berries, cooked            ⅓ cup
    Wild rice, cooked                  ½ cup

List 5—*Lean Meat Exchanges†*
    Dried beans and peas            ½ cup cooked
        Black-eyed peas            (omit 1 Bread Exchange)
        Broad beans                (omit 1 Bread Exchange)
        Garbanzo                   (omit 1 Bread Exchange)
        Kidney                     (omit 1 Bread Exchange)
        Lentils                      (omit 1 Bread Exchange)
        Lima                         (omit 1 Bread Exchange)
        Mung                       (omit 1 Bread Exchange)
        Navy                        (omit 1 Bread Exchange)
        Pinto                       (omit 1 Bread Exchange)
    Soy flour                          ¼ cup (omit ½ Bread Exchange)

         *Medium-fat Meat Exchanges†*
    Cheeses:
        Camembert                  1 oz
        Edam                         1 oz
        Liederkranz                 1 oz
    Soybeans                        ⅓ cup
    Tofu                              2½″ × 2¾″ × 1″

         *High-fat Meat Exchanges†*
    Cheeses:
        Blue, Roquefort           1 oz
        Brick                       1 oz
        Gorgonzola                 1 oz
        Gouda                     1 oz
        Gruyère                  1 oz
        Limburger                1 oz
        Muenster                1 oz
        Parmesan                1 oz
        Swiss                      1 oz
    Hummus                      4 Tbsp (omit 1 Bread Exchange)
    Peanuts‡                       4 Tbsp (omit ½ Bread and 2 Fat Exchanges)
    Pignolia nuts‡               6 Tbsp (omit ½ Vegetable and 1 Fat Exchanges)
    Pumpkin seeds‡             4 Tbsp (omit ½ Bread and 1½ Fat Exchanges)
    Sesame seeds‡              4 Tbsp (omit ½ Bread and 2 Fat Exchanges)
    Sunflower seeds‡           4 Tbsp (omit ½ Bread and 2 Fat Exchanges)
List 6—*Fat Exchanges*
    Tahini                         1 tsp

## Table A–36.   (continued)

Food containing complementary proteins may be eaten together, thereby increasing protein quality. Examples of foods that may be complemented to yield high-quality protein are listed below.

| *Food* | *Complementary Protein* |
|---|---|
| Grains | Combine rice with: cheese, legumes, sesame<br>Combine wheat with: legumes, peanuts and milk, sesame, and soybean<br>Combine corn with: legumes |
| Legumes | Combine beans with: wheat, corn<br>Combine soybeans with: rice and wheat, corn and milk, wheat and sesame, peanuts and sesame, peanuts and wheat and rice |
| Nuts and seeds | Combined sesame with: beans, peanuts and soybeans, soybeans and wheat<br>Combine peanuts with: sunflower seeds |

### *Diet Patterns*

| LACTO-OVOVEGETARIAN | STRICT VEGETARIAN |
|---|---|
| Calories: 1,500 | Calories: 1,500 |
| $CH_2O$—190 g 50% | $CH_2O$—190 g 50% |
| Protein—75 g 20% | Protein—75 g 20% |
| Fat—47 g 30% | Fat—47 g 30% |

*Daily Food Allowance*

| LACTO-OVOVEGETARIAN | STRICT VEGETARIAN |
|---|---|
| 3 Skim Milk Exchanges | 3 Soybean Milk Exchanges (Note: Add ½ bread for each cup) |
| 2 Vegetable Exchanges | 2 Vegetable Exchanges |
| 4 Fruit Exchanges | 4 Fruit Exchanges |
| 7 Bread Exchanges | 7 Bread Exchanges |
| 4 Lean-meat Exchanges | 4 Lean-meat Exchanges |
| 1 Medium-fat Meat Exchange | 1 Medium-fat Meat Exchange |
| 6 Fat Exchanges | 6 Fat Exchanges |

*Meal Pattern*

*Breakfast*

| | |
|---|---|
| 1 Fruit Exchange | 1 Fruit Exchange |
| 2 Bread Exchanges | 2 Bread Exchanges |
| 1 Medium-fat Meat Exchange | 1 Medium-fat Meat Exchange |
| 2 Fat Exchanges | 2 Fat Exchanges |
| 1 Skim Milk Exchange | 1 Milk Exchange |

*Lunch*

| | |
|---|---|
| 2 Lean-meat Exchanges | 2 Lean-meat Exchanges |
| 2 Bread Exchanges | 2 Bread Exchanges |
| 1 Vegetable Exchange | 1 Vegetable Exchange |
| 2 Fruit Exchanges | 2 Fruit Exchanges |
| 2 Fat Exchanges | 2 Fat Exchanges |

*Dinner*

| | |
|---|---|
| 2 Lean-meat Exchanges | 2 Lean-meat Exchanges |
| 2 Bread Exchanges | 2 Bread Exchanges |
| 1 Vegetable Exchange | 1 Vegetable Exchange |
| 1 Fruit Exchange | 1 Fruit Exchange |
| 2 Fat Exchanges | 2 Fat Exchanges |
| 1 Skim Milk Exchange | 1 Milk Exchange |

*Bedtime Snack*

| | |
|---|---|
| 1 Skim Milk Exchange | 1 Milk Exchange |
| 1 Bread Exchange | 1 Bread Exchange |

## Table A–36. (continued)

### GUIDELINES FOR THE PROFESSIONAL

You may revise the patient's meal plan to allow more calories from carbohydrate (50 to 60%) because of the high consumption of complex carbohydrates by vegetarians.

Many vegetarians use butter instead of margarine because it is considered a natural food.

The commercial meat analogues are very high in sodium, ranging in values from 300 mg to 3,000 mg/100 g edible portion. Nutritional analyses of these products are available upon request from Loma Linda Foods, Riverside, California 92505, and Worthington Foods, Miles Laboratories, Worthington, Ohio 43085.

Some vegetarians use diet supplements such as wheat germ and brewer's yeast. Include these in the diet as follows:

Brewer's yeast, powder: 1 level Tbsp = ½ Lean-meat Exchange
Wheat germ: ¼ cup = 1 Bread Exchange

Vegetarian diets, unless fortified, could be deficient in iron. Iron absorption is enhanced by the inclusion of a vitamin C-rich food at each meal.

Vegetarian diets excluding dairy products may be inadequate in riboflavin and calcium. Two cups daily of fortified soybean milk or appropriate supplements should prevent deficiency.

For the strict vegetarian, vitamin $B_{12}$ is also required as a vitamin supplement if 2 cups of fortified soybean milk are not consumed daily.

### SUGGESTED READING FOR VEGETARIANS

1. Lappe: Diet for a Small Planet. New York, Ballantine Books, 1975.
2. Robertson, Flinders, Godfrey: Laurel's Kitchen, A Handbook for Vegetarian Cookery and Nutrition. Berkeley, Nilgiri Press, 1976.
3. National Academy of Sciences: National Research Council, Food and Nutrition Board. Committee on Nutritional Misinformation. Vegetarian Diets. Am. J. Diet Assoc., 65:121, 1974.
4. Williams: Making vegetarian diets nutritious. Am. J. Nurs., 75:12, 1975.
5. Erhard: The new vegetarians, Part 1. Vegetarianism and its medical consequences. Nutr. Today, 8:4, 1973. Part 2. The Zen macrobiotic movement and other cults based on vegetarianism. Nutr. Today, 9:20, 1974.
6. Heath, et al.: Diet Manual Utilizing a Vegetarian Diet Plan. Loma Linda. The Seventh Day Adventist Dietetic Association, 1982.
7. Smith: A guide to good eating the vegetarian way. J. Nutr. Educ., 7:109, 1975.

*Supplement to Exchange Lists for Meal Planning Vegetarian Cookery. American Diabetes Association, Washington, D.C. Area Affiliate, Inc., Food and Nutrition Committee, 1978. See Table A–11 for Standard Exchange lists.
†Meat analogs: Vegetable protein foods which closely duplicate the flavor, texture and appearance of meat—"meatless" meats. See company information in the Guidelines for the Professional given below.
‡Seeds and nuts can be considered a "High-fat Meat" exchange and a complete protein only when they are complemented.

## Table A–37. Iron, Zinc, Copper, and Selenium Content of Selected Foods (per 100 g = 3½ oz)

| | Fe* (mg) | Zn* (mg) | Cu* (mg) | Se† (µg) |
|---|---|---|---|---|
| **DAIRY PRODUCTS** | | | | |
| Cottage cheese, salt free, dry | 0.14 | 0.37 | 0.03 | 6.0 |
| Cream, light | 0.04 | 0.27 | 0.01 | |
| Cream, sour | 0.06 | 0.27 | 0.02 | |
| Eggs, large | 2.09 | 1.44 | 0.06 | 44.0 |
| Milk, butter (fluid culture) | 0.05 | 0.42 | 0.01 | |
| Milk, regular | 0.05 | 0.38 | 0.01 | 1.6 |
| Milk, skim | 0.05 | 0.39 | 0.01 | 2.7 |
| Milk, low-sodium | 0.05 | 0.38 | 0.01 | |
| **BUTTER OR FAT** | | | | |
| Butter, sweet | 0.16 | 0.05 | 0.02 | |
| Crisco | 0.00 | 0.00 | 0.00 | |
| French dressing, low-calorie | 0.40 | 0.18 | 0.01 | |
| Margarine, salt free | 0.00 | 0.00 | 0.00 | |
| Mayonnaise | 0.00 | 0.11 | 0.00 | |
| Oil, corn | 0.00 | 0.00 | 0.00 | |
| Oil, olive | 0.38 | 0.06 | 0.00 | |
| **CEREAL** | | | | |
| Bran flakes, 40% | 15.9 | 4.37 | 0.79 | 18.0 |
| Cornflakes | 6.3 | 0.28 | 0.07 | 6.3 |
| Cream of rice, salt free, cooked | 0.20 | 0.16 | 0.03 | |
| Cream of wheat, salt free, quick-cooking | 5.00 | 0.17 | 0.04 | |
| Farina, salt free, regular, cooked | 0.50 | 0.07 | 0.01 | |
| Oatmeal, cooked | 0.68 | 0.49 | 0.06 | 8.5 |
| Puffed rice | 1.06 | 1.03 | 0.17 | |
| Puffed and shredded wheat | 4.40 | 2.80 | 0.54 | |
| Rice Krispies | 6.30 | 1.70 | 0.25 | 22.0 |
| Tapioca, salt free, dry | 1.00 | 0.25 | 0.06 | |
| **BREADS, COOKIES, CRACKERS** | | | | |
| Bread, Italian, enriched | 2.80 | 0.79 | 0.20 | 56.0 |
| Bread, salt free | 2.80 | 0.30 | 0.17 | |
| Bread, regular | 2.80 | 0.74 | 0.17 | 32.0 |
| Bread, whole wheat | 3.00 | 1.78 | 0.35 | 44.0 |
| Crackers, graham | 3.50 | 0.83 | 0.30 | |
| Crackers, salt free | 4.80 | 0.56 | 0.18 | |
| Crackers, saltines | 4.80 | 0.56 | 0.18 | 8.6 |
| Muffin, English, enriched | 3.00 | 0.70 | 0.20 | 20.0 |
| Roll, hard, enriched | 2.80 | 1.13 | 0.20 | |
| Roll, soft, enriched | 2.80 | 0.72 | 0.11 | 34.0 |
| Wafers, vanilla | 2.30 | 0.31 | 0.44 | |
| **MEAT, FISH** | | | | |
| Beef, chopped, lean, cooked | 2.75 | 6.73 | 0.13 | 17.0 |
| Sirloin, cooked | 2.80 | 6.18 | 0.13 | 26.0 |
| Chicken, dark, cooked | 1.33 | 2.80 | 0.08 | 21.0 |
| Chicken, white, cooked | 1.06 | 1.23 | 0.05 | 21.0 |
| Lamb, cooked | 1.80 | 4.47 | 0.13 | 17.0 |
| Turkey, dark, cooked | 2.33 | 4.46 | 0.16 | 25.0 |
| Turkey, white, cooked | 1.35 | 2.04 | 0.04 | 25.0 |
| Veal, lean, cooked | 1.08 | 3.69 | 0.08 | 12.0 |
| Bluefish, cooked | 0.60 | 0.50 | 0.20 | |
| Flat fish, raw | 0.80 | 0.50 | 0.20 | 48.0 |
| Cod, cooked | 1.00 | 0.60 | 0.04 | |
| Halibut, cooked | 0.70 | 0.40 | 0.03 | |
| Shrimp, raw | 1.60 | 1.50 | 0.80 | 53.0 |
| Tuna, regular, drained | 1.90 | 0.40 | 0.20 | 72.0 |
| Tuna, salt free | | | | |
| **SWEETS** | | | | |
| Candy, hard sour balls | 0.20 | 0.01 | 0.02 | |
| Honey | 0.50 | 0.37 | 0.05 | |
| Ice cream, regular | 0.09 | 1.06 | 0.02 | |
| Ice milk | 0.14 | 0.42 | 0.02 | |
| Jams, preserves | 1.00 | 0.10 | 0.05 | |
| Sherbet (fruit ice) | 0.16 | 0.69 | 0.03 | |
| Sugar, brown, packed | 2.20 | 0.27 | 0.35 | |
| Sugar, white | 0.10 | 0.00 | 0.02 | |

## Table A–37.  (continued)

| | | | | |
|---|---|---|---|---|
| *JUICES* | | | | |
| Apple | 0.37 | 0.03 | 0.02 | |
| Apricot nectar | 0.38 | 0.09 | 0.07 | |
| Cranberry | | | | |
| Grape | 0.24 | 0.05 | 0.03 | |
| Grapefruit | 0.20 | 0.09 | 0.04 | |
| Lemon, canned | 0.13 | 0.06 | 0.04 | |
| Orange, canned | 0.44 | 0.07 | 0.06 | |
| Orange, fresh | 0.20 | 0.05 | 0.04 | |
| Pear nectar | 0.26 | 0.07 | 0.07 | |
| Pineapple | 0.26 | 0.11 | 0.09 | |
| Prune | 1.18 | 0.21 | 0.07 | |
| Tomato | 0.58 | 0.14 | 0.10 | |
| Tomato, salt-free | 0.58 | 0.14 | 0.10 | |
| *VEGETABLES* | | | | |
| Asparagus, cut, canned | 0.66 | 0.48 | 0.10 | |
| Asparagus, low-sodium | | | | |
| Beans, green, canned | 0.90 | 0.29 | 0.04 | |
| Beans, green, low-sodium | 0.90 | 0.29 | 0.04 | |
| Beans, wax, canned | 0.90 | 0.29 | 0.04 | |
| Beets, canned | 0.67 | 0.23 | 0.10 | |
| Beets, low-sodium | 0.62 | 0.25 | 0.06 | |
| Broccoli, cooked, no added salt | 1.15 | 0.15 | 0.07 | |
| Cabbage, cooked, no added salt | 0.39 | 0.16 | 0.03 | |
| Carrots, canned | 0.62 | 0.30 | 0.13 | 1.3 |
| Carrots, low-sodium | 0.62 | 0.30 | 0.13 | |
| Carrots, raw | 0.50 | 0.20 | 0.05 | 1.7 |
| Cauliflower, cooked, no salt | 0.42 | 0.24 | 0.09 | |
| Celery, raw | 0.48 | 0.17 | 0.04 | |
| Corn, canned | 0.42 | 0.46 | 0.05 | |
| Corn, low-sodium | 0.61 | 0.48 | 0.05 | |
| Cucumber, pared, raw | 0.35 | 0.28 | 0.05 | 6.3 |
| Peas, sweet, canned | 0.95 | 0.71 | 0.08 | |
| Peas, low-sodium | 1.11 | 0.70 | 0.11 | |
| Potatoes, boiled | 0.31 | 0.27 | 0.17 | 1.3 |
| Tomatoes, raw | 0.48 | 0.11 | 0.08 | 0.7 |
| Tomatoes, canned | 0.61 | 0.16 | 0.11 | |
| Tomatoes, low-sodium | 0.77 | 0.25 | 0.20 | |
| Noodles, egg, enriched, cooked, with no salt | 1.50 | 0.49 | 0.09 | 19.0 |
| Rice, enriched, no added salt | 1.40 | 0.41 | 0.08 | 9.0 |
| *FRUITS* | | | | |
| Apples, pared | 0.18 | 0.04 | 0.04 | 0.4 |
| Applesauce, unsweetened | 0.12 | 0.03 | 0.03 | |
| Apricots, canned | 0.39 | 0.11 | 0.08 | |
| Bananas | 0.31 | 0.16 | 0.10 | 0.9 |
| Cherries, canned, pitted | 0.36 | 0.10 | 0.15 | |
| Grapefruit, fresh | 0.09 | 0.07 | 0.05 | 1.5 |
| Oranges, fresh | 0.10 | 0.07 | 0.05 | 1.5 |
| Peaches, fresh, pared | 0.11 | 0.14 | 0.07 | |
| Peaches, canned, in syrup | 0.36 | 0.09 | 0.05 | |
| Pears, raw | 0.25 | 0.12 | 0.11 | |
| Pears, canned, in syrup | 0.28 | 0.08 | 0.05 | |
| Pineapples, canned | 0.28 | 0.10 | 0.09 | |
| Strawberries, raw | 0.38 | 0.13 | 0.05 | |

*Data from Primary Nutrient Data Set for Food Consumption Surveys, USDA, Human Nutrition Information Service, Nutrition Monitoring Division. Appreciation is expressed to Mr. Frank Hepburn and Mr. David Haytowitz for assistance in obtaining these data.
†Data adapted from Schubert, A., Holden, J.M., Wolf, W.R.: Selenium content of a core group of foods based on a critical evaluation of published analytical data. Copyright The American Dietetic Association. Reprinted by permission from J. Am. Diet. Assoc. 87:285–299, 1987.

## Table A–38.  Weights and Measures

### SYSTÈME INTERNATIONAL D'UNITÉS (SI Units)

Increasing numbers of biomedical journals and books in the United States are adopting this method of notation of the concentrations or measurements in the physical and biomedical sciences.[1,2] Conversion to SI units is occurring in stages as determined by the editors of various journals and books. SI conversion tables are extensive in clinical chemistry and have been published.[1-3]

### REFERENCES

1. Young, D.S.: Implementation of SI units for clinical laboratory data style specifications and conversion tables. Ann. Intern. Med. 106:114, 1987.
2. Lundberg, G.D., Iverson, C., Radulescu, G.: Now read this: The SI units are here. J.A.M.A. 255:2329, 1986.
3. Monsen, E.R.: The Journal adopts SI units for clinical laboratory values. J. Am. Diet. Assoc. 87:356–378, 1987.

*VOLUMES:*

| Apothecaries' Measure | Metric | Household |
|---|---|---|
| 1 fluid dram (fl dr) | 4 milliliter (ml) | 1 teaspoon (tsp) |
| 2 fl dr | 8 ml | 1 dessert spoonful |
| ½ fluid ounce (fl oz) | 15 ml | 1 tablespoon (Tbsp) (3 tsp) |
| 1 fl oz | 30 ml | 2 Tbsp (⅛ cup) |
| 1-½ fl oz | 45 ml | 1 jigger |
| 2 fl oz | 59 ml | 4 Tbsp (¼ cup) |
| 2-⅔ fl oz | 80 ml | 5-⅓ Tbsp (⅓ cup) |
| 4 fl oz | 118 ml | 8 Tbsp (½ cup) |
| 8 fl oz | 237 ml | 1 cup |
| 16 fl oz | 473 ml | 1 pint (pt) |
| 32 fl oz | 947 ml | 1 quart (qt) |
| 128 fl oz | 3,785 ml | 1 gallon (gal) |
| 3.38 fl oz | 1 deciliter (dl) (100 ml) | |
| 2.11 pt | 1 liter (L) (1,000 ml) | |

*WEIGHTS:*

| Avoirdupois | Metric |
|---|---|
| | 1 femtogram (fg) ($10^{-15}$ g) |
| | 1 picogram (pg) ($10^{-12}$ g) |
| | 1 nanogram (ng) ($10^{-9}$ g) |
| | 1 microgram ($\mu$g) ($10^{-6}$ g) |
| 1 grain (gr) | 0.065 g (65 mg) |
| 1 gram (0.035 oz) | 15.432 gr |
| 1 scruple (20 gr) | 1.296 g |
| 1 dram (dr) ( = drachm) (27.3 gr) | 1.77 g |
| 1 oz (16 dr) | 28.35 g |
| 1 lb (16 oz) | 453.59 g |
| 1 ton (2,000 lb) | 0.91 metric tons |
| 1.015 gr | 1 milligram (mg) ($10^{-3}$ g) |
| | 1 centigram (cg) ($10^{-2}$ g) |
| | 1 decigram (dg) ($10^{-1}$ g) |
| 15.4 gr (0.035 oz) | 1 gram (g) |
| 2.2 lb | 1 kilogram (kg) ($10^{3}$ g) |

## Table A–38.   (continued)

*LENGTH/AREA:*

| | *Metric* |
|---|---|
| 1 angstrom (Å) | 10 millimeter (mm) |
| 1/2500 inch (in) | 1 micron ($\mu$) ($10^{-3}$ mm) = micrometer ($\mu$m) |
| 0.039 in | 1 mm |
| 0.39 in | 1 centimeter (cm) |
| 1 in | 2.54 cm |
| 1 foot (ft) (12 in) | 30.5 cm |
| 39.4 in | 1 meter (m) |
| 1 yard (yd) (3 ft) | 0.9 m |
| 1 rod (5.5 yd) | 4.95 m |
| 1093.6 yd (0.62 mile) | 1 kilometer (km) |
| 1 mile (mi) (5,280 ft) | 1.61 km |
| 1 acre (160 square rods) | 0.4 hectare |

*TEMPERATURE CONVERSIONS:*

F to C: 5/9 (F − 32)
C to F: (9/5 × C) + 32

*ELECTROLYTE DATA:*

| *Ion* | | *Atomic Wt* (1) | *Valence* (2) | *Equivalent Wt* \* 1 ÷ 2 |
|---|---|---|---|---|
| Bicarbonate | $HCO_3^-$ | 61.0 | 1 | 61.0 |
| Calcium | $Ca^{2+}$ | 40.1 | 2 | 20.0 |
| Chloride | $Cl^-$ | 35.5 | 1 | 35.5 |
| Magnesium | $Mg^{2+}$ | 24.3 | 2 | 12.2 |
| Phosphate† | $HPO_4^{2-}$ | 96.0 | 2 | 48.0† |
| Potassium | $K^+$ | 39.1 | 1 | 39.1 |
| Sodium | $Na^+$ | 23.0 | 1 | 23.0 |
| Sulfate | $SO_4^{2-}$ | 96.1 | 2 | 48.0 |

\*Milliequivalent (meq) = Equivalent weight in milligrams (mg). To convert mg quantities of all electrolytes to meq:

$$\frac{\text{mg of electrolyte}}{\text{equivalent weight in mg}} = \text{meq}$$

To convert meq quantities of all electrolytes to mg:

$$\text{meq} \times \text{equivalent wt} = \text{mg}$$

To convert mg/dl to meq/L:

$$\frac{\text{mg/dl} \times 10}{\text{equivalent wt in mg}} = \text{meq/L}$$

To convert meq/L to mg/dl: meq/L × equivalent wt in mg × 0.1.

†At the normal pH of plasma, 20% of the total inorganic phosphate radical is combined with one equivalent of base as $BH_2PO_4$, and 80% with two equivalents of base as $B_2HPO_4$. Under these conditions, base equivalence is therefore 0.2 + (0.8 × 2) = 1.8, and the equivalent weight of 53.3 is obtained by dividing the ionic weight by 1.8 instead of by 2. For phosphorus content of phosphate solutions, 1 meq provides approximately 15 mg, and 1 mmol provides approximately 31 mg.

# Table A–39.  Amino Acid Solutions for Intravenous Use‡

| | Aminosyn 10% (Abbott)* | Aminosyn RF 5.2% (Abbott) | Aminosyn PF 7% (Abbott) | Freamine III 10% (McGaw)* | Nephramine 5.4% (McGaw) | Freamine HBC 6.9% (McGaw) | Hepatamine 8% (McGaw) | Trophamine 6% (McGaw) | Travasol 10%*,† (Travenol) | Renamine 6.5% (Travasol) | Novamine 8.5% (Kabi-Vitrum)* | Amines 5.2% (Kabi-Vitrum) | BranchAmine 4% (Travenol) |
|---|---|---|---|---|---|---|---|---|---|---|---|---|---|
| Protein equivalent (g/dl) | 10 | 5.2 | 7 | 9.6 | 5.4 | 6.13 | 7.6 | 5.8 | 10 | 6.5 | 8.5 | 5.18 | 4.0 |
| Total nitrogen (g/dl) | 1.572 | 0.786 | 1.07 | 1.53 | 0.64 | 0.97 | 1.2 | 0.93 | 1.65 | 1.0 | 1.35 | 0.66 | 0.43 |
| Osmolarity (mosm/L) | 1,000 | 475 | 586 | 950 | 435 | 620 | 785 | 525 | 1,000 | 600 | 785 | 416 | 316 |
| pH | 5.3 | 5.2 | 5.4 | 6.5 | 6.5 | 6.5 | 6.5 | 5.5 | 6.0 | 6.0 | 5.6 | 6.4 | 6.0 |
| **Essential amino acid 100 ml** | | | | | | | | | | | | | |
| L-Isoleucine | 720 | 462 | 534 | 690 | 560 | 760 | 900 | 490 | 600 | 500 | 420 | 525 | 1,380 |
| L-Leucine | 940 | 726 | 831 | 910 | 880 | 1,370 | 1,100 | 840 | 730 | 600 | 590 | 825 | 1,380 |
| L-Lysine | 720 | 535 | 475 | 730 | 640 | 410 | 610 | 490 | 580 | 450 | 673 | 600 | — |
| L-Methionine | 400 | 726 | 125 | 530 | 880 | 250 | 100 | 200 | 400 | 500 | 420 | 825 | — |
| L-Phenylalanine | 440 | 726 | 300 | 560 | 880 | 320 | 100 | 290 | 560 | 490 | 590 | 825 | — |
| L-Threonine | 520 | 330 | 360 | 400 | 400 | 200 | 450 | 250 | 420 | 380 | 420 | 375 | — |
| L-Tryptophan | 160 | 165 | 125 | 150 | 200 | 90 | 66 | 120 | 180 | 160 | 140 | 188 | — |
| L-Valine | 800 | 528 | 452 | 660 | 640 | 880 | 840 | 470 | 580 | 820 | 550 | 600 | 1,240 |
| **Nonessential amino acids 100 ml** | | | | | | | | | | | | | |
| L-Alanine | 1,280 | — | 490 | 710 | — | 400 | 770 | 320 | 2,070 | 560 | 1,200 | — | — |
| L-Arginine | 980 | 600 | 861 | 950 | — | 580 | 600 | 730 | 1,150 | 630 | 840 | 412 | — |
| L-Histidine | 300 | 429 | 220 | 280 | 250 | 160 | 240 | 290 | 480 | 420 | 500 | — | — |
| L-Proline | 860 | — | 570 | 1,120 | — | 630 | 800 | 410 | 680 | 350 | 500 | — | — |
| L-Serine | 420 | — | 347 | 590 | — | 330 | 500 | 230 | 500 | 300 | 340 | — | — |
| L-Tyrosine | 44 | — | 44 | — | — | — | — | 140 | 40 | 40 | 20 | — | — |
| L-Glycine | 1,280 | — | 270 | 1,400 | — | 330 | 900 | 220 | 1,030 | 300 | 590 | — | — |
| L-Cysteine | — | — | — | <24 | <20 | <20 | <20 | <20 | — | — | <40 | — | — |
| Glutamic acid | — | — | 576 | — | — | — | — | 300 | — | — | 420 | — | — |
| Aspartic acid | — | — | 370 | — | — | — | — | 190 | — | — | 250 | — | — |
| Taurine | — | — | 50 | — | — | — | — | 15 | — | — | — | — | — |
| Ratio of essential AA / Nonessential AA | 0.48 | 0.80 | 0.46 | 0.48 | 0.94 | 0.70 | 0.54 | 0.54 | 0.41 | 0.60 | 0.45 | 0.92 | — |
| **Electrolytes (meq/L)** | | | | | | | | | | | | | |
| Cl | — | — | — | <3 | <3 | <3 | <3 | <3 | 40 | 31 | — | — | — |
| Na | — | — | — | 10[c] | 5[d] | 10[c] | 10[c] | 10[c] | 3[e] | 3[e] | 3[e] | 3[e] | 3[e] |
| K | 5.4[a] | 5.4[a] | 3.4[b] | — | — | — | — | — | — | — | — | — | — |
| Phosphorus | — | — | — | 10 mm | — | — | 10 mm | — | — | — | — | — | — |
| Acetate | 148 | 105 | 32.5 | 89 | 44 | 57 | 62 | 56 | 87 | 60 | 88 | 50 | — |

[a] K metabisulfite 60 mg (5.4 meq K/L) as antioxidant.
[b] Na hydrosulfite (7 meq Na/L) as antioxidant.
[c] Na bisulfite 100 mg (10 meq Na/L) as antioxidant.
[d] Na bisulfite (5 meq Na/L) as antioxidant.
[e] Na bisulfite (3 meq Na/L) as antioxidant.
* Available in various concentrations (3%, 5%, 7%, 8.5%) and also with electrolytes. Novamine available as 11% solution.
† Travasol amino acid solutions in identical formulations are available in Europe, New Zealand, Australia, Taiwan under the trade name Synthamin. However, the amino acid concentrations are expressed as grams of nitrogen per liter; hence, Travasol 10% is equivalent to Synthamin 10%.
‡ Appreciation is expressed to Susan Lee, R.Ph. for preparation of this table.

**Table A–40a. Complete Diet Formulations Containing Some Natural Foods, with Varying Residue (per 1,000 kcal)\*\***

| | Biocare Shake Mix† Food Science Corp. | C.I.B.\*,† Carnation | Compleat Regular‡ Sandoz | Compleat Modified‡ Sandoz |
|---|---|---|---|---|
| Protein, g (% total kcal) | 56.1 (22%) | 55.2 (22%) | 40.0 (16%) | 40.0 (16%) |
| Source | Whey | Nonfat milk | Beef | Beef |
| | Ca caseinate | Soy protein | Nonfat milk | Ca caseinate |
| | Na caseinate | Na caseinate | | |
| Fat, g (% total kcal) | 36.3 (32%) | 29.4 (26%) | 40.0 (36%) | 34.2 (55%) |
| Source | Soy oil | Milk fat | Corn oil | Corn oil |
| | | | Beef fat | Beef fat |
| Carbohydrate, g (% total kcal) | 111.2 (44%) | 128.4 (51%) | 120.0 (48%) | 132.5 (55%) |
| Source | Sucrose | Sucrose | Hydrolyzed cereal solids | Hydrolyzed cereal solids |
| | Corn syrup solids 51.7 (21%) | Corn syrup solids 44.4 (18%) | Maltodextrins | Vegetables |
| | Lactose, 59.5 (23%) | Lactose, 84.0 (34%) | Vegetables | Peaches |
| | | | Fruits, Orange juice | Orange juice |
| | | | Lactose, 24.4 (10%) | |
| Lactose, g | 59.5 | 84.0 | 24.4 | 0 |
| Volume for 1,000 kcal (ml) | 891.0 | 880 | 935 | 935 |
| *Minerals* | | | | |
| Calcium, mg | 1,485.0 | 1,435.0 | 625.0 | 625.0 |
| Phosphorus, mg | 1,155.0 | 1,387.3 | 1,250.0 | 875.0 |
| Magnesium, mg | 391.9 | 414.7 | 250.0 | 250.0 |
| Iron, mg | 114.8 | 16.9 | 11.3 | 11.3 |
| Iodine, mcg | 123.8 | 176.2 | 93.8 | 93.8 |
| Copper, mg | 2.5 | 1.9 | 1.3 | 1.3 |
| Manganese, mg | N/A§ | N/A | 2.5 | 2.5 |
| Zinc, mg | 12.4 | 14.3 | 9.4 | 9.4 |
| Chromium, mcg | N/A | N/A | 93.8 | 93.8 |
| Selenium, mcg | N/A | N/A | 62.5 | 62.5 |
| Molybdenum, mcg | N/A | N/A | 187.5 | 187.5 |
| Sodium, meq | 39.4 | 42.6 | 51.6 | 27.2 |
| Potassium, meq | 48.0 | 70.8 | 33.6 | 33.6 |
| Chloride, meq | N/A | N/A | 22.9 | 12.3 |
| mosm/kg | N/A | 700 | 405 | 300.0 |
| Volume to provide 100% RDAs (ml)# | 1,000 | 1,060 | 1,500 | 1,500 |

## Table A–40a. (continued)

| | Meritene Liquid* Sandoz | Meritene*† Sandoz | NutriCare† Advanced Health Care | Nutrimed Robard |
|---|---|---|---|---|
| Protein, g (% total kcal) | 60.0 (24%) | 64.8 (26%) | 57.1 (23%) | 150.0 (60%) |
| Source | Concentrated skim milk | Nonfat milk | Whey | Egg white solids |
| | | | Whole milk | |
| | Na caseinate | Whole milk | | Nonfat milk |
| | | Ca caseinate | | |
| Fat, g (% total kcal) | 33.3 (30%) | 32.4 (29%) | 33.3 (30%) | 0 |
| Source | Corn oil | Milk fat | Milk fat | |
| | Mono-, diglycerides | | | |
| Carbohydrate, g (% total kcal) | 115.0 (46%) | 111.6 (45%) | 117.8 (47%) | 100.0 (40%) |
| Source | Corn syrup solids | Corn syrup solids, 14.4 (6%) | Sucrose | Sucrose, 83.3 (33%) |
| | Sucrose | Sucrose, 17.2 (7%) | Maltodextrin | Lactose, 16.7 (7%) |
| | 58.3 (23%) | | | |
| | Lactose, 56.7 (23%) | Lactose, 80.0 (32%) | Lactose | |
| Lactose, g | 56.7 | 80.0 | N/A | 16.7 |
| Volume for 1,000 kcal (ml) | 1,042 | 1,000 | 1,000 | 2,000 |
| *Minerals* | | | | |
| Calcium, mg | 1,250.0 | 2,070.0 | 1,667.9 | 2,004.0 |
| Phosphorus, mg | 1,250.0 | 1,820.0 | 1,249.5 | 1,167.0 |
| Magnesium, mg | 333.3 | 364.0 | 499.8 | 500.0 |
| Iron, mg | 15.0 | 16.0 | 22.5 | 60.1 |
| Iodine, mcg | 125.0 | 138.0 | 185.6 | 501.0 |
| Copper, mg | 1.7 | 1.8 | 2.5 | 6.7 |
| Manganese, mg | 3.3 | 3.6 | 4.6 | 13.3 |
| Zinc, mg | 12.5 | 14.0 | 18.9 | 50.0 |
| Chromium, mcg | N/A | N/A | N/A | N/A |
| Selenium, mcg | N/A | N/A | N/A | N/A |
| Molybdenum, mcg | N/A | N/A | N/A | N/A |
| Sodium, meq | 39.8 | 44.0 | 40.4 | 130.0 |
| Potassium, meq | 42.7 | 68.0 | 58.6 | 71.6 |
| Chloride, meq | 47.0 | 58.5 | N/A | N/A |
| mosm/kg | 505 | 690 | N/A | N/A |
| Volume to provide 100% RDAs (ml)# | 1,250 | 1,040 | 840 | 600 |

| | Nutrimed 420* Robard | Sustacal + Milk*,† Mead Johnson | Sustagen + Water* Mead Johnson | Vitaneed‡ Sherwood Medical |
|---|---|---|---|---|
| Protein, g (% total kcal) | 166.6 (67%) | 60.3 (24%) | 61.0 (24%) | 35.0 (14%) |
| Source | Egg white solids, Ca. Na caseinate, Nonfat milk | Nonfat milk, Whole milk | Nonfat milk, Whole milk, Ca caseinate | Beef, Na, Ca caseinate |
| Fat, g (% total kcal) | 2.4 (2%) | 24.4 (22%) | 9.1 (8%) | 40.0 (36%) |
| Source | Nonfat milk | Milk fat | Milk fat | Soy oil |
| Carbohydrate, g (% total kcal) | 76.2 (30%) | 134.4 (54%) | 171.0 (68%) | 125.0 (50%) |
| Source | Sucrose Fructose 60.3 (24%), Lactose, 15.9 (6%) | Sucrose, 36.2 (14%), Corn syrup solids, 11.8 (5%), Lactose, 85.8 (34%) | Corn syrup solids, 101.4 (40%), Sucrose, 8.0 (3%), Lactose, 61.6 (25%) | Maltodextrin, Vegetables, Peaches |
| Lactose, g | 15.9 | 85.8 | 61.6 | 0 |
| Volume for 1,000 kcal (ml) | 1,420 | 750 | 549 | 1,000 |
| *Minerals* | | | | |
| Calcium, mg | 2,380 | 1,612.4 | 1,824.0 | 500.0 |
| Phosphorus, mg | 1,475.6 | 1,334.4 | 1,368.0 | 500.0 |
| Magnesium, mg | 952.0 | 375.3 | 228.0 | 200.0 |
| Iron, mg | 42.8 | 16.7 | 10.3 | 9.0 |
| Iodine, mcg | 357.0 | 138.9 | 85.5 | 75.0 |
| Copper, mg | 4.8 | 1.9 | 1.1 | 1.0 |
| Manganese, mg | 9.5 | 2.8 | 2.9 | 2.5 |
| Zinc, mg | 35.7 | 13.9 | 11.4 | 15.0 |
| Chromium, mcg | 357.0 | N/A | N/A | N/A |
| Selenium, mcg | 357.0 | N/A | N/A | N/A |
| Molybdenum, mcg | 714.0 | N/A | N/A | N/A |
| Sodium, meq | 98.3 | 39.8 | 29.8 | 21.7 |
| Potassium, meq | 61.0 | 64.8 | 46.7 | 32.0 |
| Chloride, meq | N/A | 37.6 | 43.3 | 23.9 |
| mosm/kg | N/A | 899 | 1,100 | 375 |
| Volume to provide 100% RDAs (ml)# | 600 | 800 | 960 | 2,000 |

*Vanilla.

†Value includes whole milk.

‡With residue.

§N/A = Value not available.

#Including vitamins.

**Appreciation is expressed to Mindy Hermann-Zaidins, R.D., Memorial Sloan-Kettering Cancer Center, Clinical Nutrition Support Kitchen, for revision of this table, originally prepared by A.S. Bloch and M.E. Shils in the 6th Edition of this textbook.

**Table A–40b. Defined-Formula Diets with Intact Purified Protein, Low Residue, and No Lactose (per 1,000 kcal)\*\***

| | Enrich† Ross | Ensure* Ross | Ensure HN Ross | Ensure Plus* Ross |
|---|---|---|---|---|
| Protein, g (% total kcal) | 36.1 (14%) | 35.2 (14%) | 42.0 (17%) | 36.6 (15%) |
| Source | Na, Ca caseinate Soy protein | Na, Ca caseinate Soy protein isolate | Na, Ca caseinate Soy protein isolate | Na, Ca caseinate Soy protein isolate |
| Fat, g (% total kcal) | 33.8 (30%) | 35.2 (31%) | 33.6 (30%) | 35.5 (15%) |
| Source | Corn oil | Corn oil | Corn oil | Corn oil |
| Carbohydrate, g (% total kcal) | 147.2 (56%) | 137.2 (55%) | 133.6 (53%) | 133.2 (53%) |
| Source | Hydrolyzed cornstarch Sucrose Soy polysaccharide | Hydrolyzed cornstarch Sucrose | Hydrolyzed cornstarch Sucrose | Hydrolyzed cornstarch Sucrose |
| Lactose, g | 0 | 0 | 0 | 0 |
| Volume for 1,000 kcal (ml) | 909 | 946 | 960 | 666 |
| *Minerals* | | | | |
| Calcium, mg | 654.5 | 520.0 | 720.0 | 423.0 |
| Phosphorus, mg | 654.5 | 520.0 | 720.0 | 423.0 |
| Magnesium, mg | 260.9 | 200.0 | 288.0 | 211.0 |
| Iron, mg | 11.9 | 9.0 | 13.2 | 9.5 |
| Iodine, mcg | 100.0 | 76.0 | 108.0 | 70.4 |
| Copper, mg | 1.3 | 1.0 | 1.4 | 1.1 |
| Manganese, mg | 3.2 | 2.0 | 3.6 | 1.4 |
| Zinc, mg | 14.6 | 15.0 | 16.4 | 15.9 |
| Chromium, mcg | N/A‡ | N/A | N/A | N/A |
| Selenium, mcg | N/A | N/A | N/A | N/A |
| Molybdenum, mcg | N/A | N/A | N/A | N/A |
| Sodium, meq | 33.6 | 34.8 | 38.3 | 33.1 |
| Potassium, meq | 36.3 | 37.8 | 38.0 | 39.6 |
| Chloride, meq | 36.9 | 38.4 | 38.3 | 37.3 |
| mosm/kg | 480 | 450 | 470 | 600 |
| Volume to provide 100% RDAs (ml)§ | 1,530 | 1,892 | 1,400 | 2,000 |

| | Ensure Plus HN<br>Ross | Entralife<br>Navaco | Entrition<br>Biosearch | Fortical<br>Sherwood Medical |
|---|---|---|---|---|
| Protein, g (% total kcal)<br>Source | 41.1 (17%)<br>Na, Ca caseinate<br>Soy protein isolate | 33.2 (14%)<br>Whey<br>Isolated soy protein | 35.0 (14%)<br>Na, Ca caseinate | 40.0 (16%)<br>Na, Ca caseinate |
| Fat, g (% total kcal)<br>Source | 32.8 (30%)<br>Corn oil | 33.2 (32%)<br>Corn oil | 35.0 (32%)<br>Corn oil | 40.0 (36%)<br>Corn oil<br>Lecithin |
| Carbohydrate, g (% total kcal)<br>Source | 131.5 (53%)<br>Hydrolyzed cornstarch<br>Sucrose | 129.4 (54%)<br>Hydrolyzed cornstarch<br>Sucrose | 136.0 (54%)<br>Maltodextrin | 120.0 (48%)<br>Maltodextrin |
| Lactose, g | 0 | 0 | 0 | 0 |
| Volume for 1,000 kcal (ml) | 667 | 943 | 1,000 | 667 |
| *Minerals* | | | | |
| Calcium, mg | 695.0 | 471.6 | 500.0 | 625.0 |
| Phosphorus, mg | 695.0 | 471.6 | 500.0 | 625.0 |
| Magnesium, mg | 278.0 | 188.4 | 200.0 | 250.0 |
| Iron, mg | 12.5 | 8.4 | 9.0 | 11.2 |
| Iodine, mcg | 105.6 | 70.8 | 75.0 | 100.0 |
| Copper, mg | 1.4 | 0.8 | 1.0 | 1.5 |
| Manganese, mg | 1.4 | 2.4 | 2.0 | 2.5 |
| Zinc, mg | 10.6 | 14.0 | 7.5 | 15.0 |
| Chromium, mcg | N/A | 339.6 | N/A | N/A |
| Selenium, mcg | N/A | 45.2 | N/A | N/A |
| Molybdenum, mcg | N/A | 716.8 | N/A | N/A |
| Sodium, meq | 33.8 | 32.8 | 30.5 | 29.6 |
| Potassium, meq | 30.6 | 35.6 | 30.7 | 29.5 |
| Chloride, meq | 29.8 | 36.0 | 28.2 | 29.9 |
| mosm/kg | 650 | 450 | 300 | 410 |
| Volume to provide 100% RDAs (ml)§ | 1,420 | 2,000 | 2,000 | 1,060 |

## Table A–40b. (continued)

| | Fortison Sherwood Medical | Fortison, L.S. Sherwood Medical | Isocal Mead Johnson | Isocal HCN Mead Johnson |
|---|---|---|---|---|
| Protein, g (% total kcal) | 40.0 (16%) | 40.0 (16%) | 32.5 (13%) | 37.5 (15%) |
| Source | Na, Ca caseinate | Ca, K caseinate | Na caseinate / Soy protein isolate | Na, Ca caseinate |
| Fat, g (% total kcal) | 40.0 (36%) | 40.0 (36%) | 42.0 (37%) | 51.0 (45%) |
| Source | Corn oil / Lecithin | Corn oil / Lecithin | Soy oil, 33.6 (30%) / MCT oil, 8.4 (7%) | Soy oil, 34.0 (31%) / MCT oil, 14.5 (12%) / Lecithin, 2.5 (2%) |
| Carbohydrate, g (% total kcal) | 120.0 (48%) | 120.0 (48%) | 126.0 (50%) | 100.0 (40%) |
| Source | Maltodextrin | Maltodextrin | Glucose oligosaccharides | Corn syrup solids |
| Lactose, g | 0 | 0 | 0 | 0 |
| Volume for 1,000 kcal (ml) | 1,000 | 1,000 | 960 | 500 |
| *Minerals* | | | | |
| Calcium, mg | 625.0 | 625.0 | 600.0 | 500.0 |
| Phosphorus, mg | 625.0 | 625.0 | 500.0 | 500.0 |
| Magnesium, mg | 250.0 | 250.0 | 200.0 | 200.0 |
| Iron, mg | 11.2 | 11.2 | 9.0 | 9.0 |
| Iodine, mcg | 100.0 | 100.0 | 75.0 | 75.0 |
| Copper, mg | 1.5 | 1.5 | 1.0 | 1.5 |
| Manganese, mg | 2.5 | 2.5 | 2.5 | 1.7 |
| Zinc, mg | 15.0 | 15.0 | 10.0 | 15.0 |
| Chromium, mcg | N/A | N/A | N/A | N/A |
| Selenium, mcg | N/A | N/A | N/A | N/A |
| Molybdenum, mcg | N/A | N/A | N/A | N/A |
| Sodium, meq | 29.6 | 8.7 | 21.5 | 17.5 |
| Potassium, meq | 29.5 | 29.5 | 32.1 | 21.5 |
| Chloride, meq | 29.9 | 7.0 | 28.2 | 17.0 |
| mosm/kg | 300 | 240 | 300 | 690 |
| Volume to provide 100% RDAs (ml)§ | 1,600 | 1,600 | 1,920 | 1,000 |

| | Isolife *Navaco* | Isotein HN *Sandoz* | Magnacal *Sherwood Medical* | Newtrition *Knight Medical* |
|---|---|---|---|---|
| Protein, g (% total kcal) | 42.5 (15%) | 57.1 (23%) | 35.0 (14%) | 33.3 (13%) |
| Source | Whey (processed) Soy protein | Lactalbumin Na caseinate | Na, Ca caseinate | Na, Ca caseinate Soy protein isolate |
| Fat, g (% total kcal) | 33.6 (30%) | 28.6 (25%) | 40.0 (36%) | 37.0 (33%) |
| Source | Corn oil, 23.3 (21%) MCT oil, 10.3 (9%) | Soy oil, 21.1 (19%) MCT oil, 7.5 (6%) Mono-, diglycerides | Soy oil Mono-, diglycerides Lecithin | Corn oil |
| Carbohydrate, g (% total kcal) | 137.6 (55%) | 131.4 (53%) | 125.0 (50%) | 129.6 (53%) |
| Source | Hydrolyzed cornstarch | Maltodextrin Monosaccharides | Maltodextrin Corn syrup solids Sucrose | Maltodextrin Sucrose Glucose solids |
| Lactose, g | Trace | 0 | 0 | 0 |
| Volume for 1,000 kcal (ml) | 1,000 | 843 | 500 | 926 |
| *Minerals* | | | | |
| Calcium, mg | 520.8 | 476.2 | 500.0 | 555.5 |
| Phosphorus, mg | 520.8 | 476.2 | 500.0 | 555.5 |
| Magnesium, mg | 183.3 | 190.5 | 200.0 | 222.2 |
| Iron, mg | 10.4 | 8.6 | 9.0 | 10.0 |
| Iodine, mcg | 79.2 | 71.4 | 75.0 | 55.6 |
| Copper, mg | 1.0 | 1.0 | 1.0 | 1.1 |
| Manganese, mg | 1.0 | 1.9 | 2.5 | 1.9 |
| Zinc, mg | 7.9 | 7.1 | 15.0 | 8.3 |
| Chromium, mcg | 104.1 | 71.4 | N/A | N/A |
| Selenium, mcg | 104.1 | 71.4 | N/A | N/A |
| Molybdenum, mcg | 26.0 | 142.8 | N/A | N/A |
| Sodium, meq | 23.2 | 22.8 | 21.8 | 24.2 |
| Potassium, meq | 26.7 | 23.2 | 16.0 | 23.7 |
| Chloride, meq | 40.5 | 22.8 | 13.4 | 15.6 |
| mosm/kg | 300 | 300 | 590 | 450 |
| Volume to provide 100% RDAs (ml)§ | 1,000 | 1,770 | 1,000 | 1,667 |

## Table A–40b. (continued)

| | Newtrition High Nitrogen Knight Medical | Newtrition Isotonic Knight Medical | Nutrex Besure Nutrex | Nutrex Drink Nutrex |
|---|---|---|---|---|
| Protein, g (% total kcal) | 50.0 (20%) | 34.0 (14%) | 35.2 (14%) | 52.5 (20%) |
| Source | Na. Ca caseinate<br>Soy protein isolate | Na. Ca caseinate<br>Soy protein isolate | Na. Ca caseinate<br>Soy protein isolate | Egg white solids |
| Fat, g (% total kcal) | 33.3 (28%) | 34.0 (30%) | 35.2 (32%) | 0.7 (0.6%) |
| Source | Corn oil. 16.7 (15%)<br>MCT oil. 16.6 (13%)<br>Mono-. diglycerides | Corn oil<br>MCT oil<br>Mono-. diglycerides | Vegetable oil<br>Mono-. diglycerides<br>Lecithin | Mono-. diglycerides |
| Carbohydrate, g (% total kcal) | 133.2 (53%) | 139.6 (56%) | 137.2 (55%) | 198.8 (80%) |
| Source | Maltodextrin | Maltodextrin | Maltodextrin<br>Sucrose | Corn syrup solids<br>Sucrose |
| Lactose, g | 0 | 0 | 0 | 0 |
| Volume for 1,000 kcal (ml) | 832 | 943 | 960.0 | 1,408 |
| *Minerals* | | | | |
| Calcium, mg | 666.0 | 566.0 | 520.0 | 1,126.4 |
| Phosphorus, mg | 666.0 | 566.0 | 520.0 | 1,126.4 |
| Magnesium, mg | 266.4 | 188.7 | 200.0 | 475.9 |
| Iron, mg | 12.0 | 8.5 | 9.0 | 26.8 |
| Iodine, mcg | 99.9 | 56.6 | 76.0 | 178.8 |
| Copper, mg | 1.3 | 0.9 | 1.0 | 2.4 |
| Manganese, mg | 1.7 | 0.2 | 2.0 | 3.0 |
| Zinc, mg | 10.0 | 7.1 | 15.0 | 17.9 |
| Chromium, mcg | N/A | N/A | N/A | N/A |
| Selenium, mcg | N/A | N/A | N/A | N/A |
| Molybdenum, mcg | N/A | N/A | N/A | N/A |
| Sodium, meq | 21.7 | 24.6 | 34.8 | 36.7 |
| Potassium, meq | 21.3 | 24.2 | 37.9 | 57.8 |
| Chloride, meq | 16.4 | 18.6 | 38.3 | 24.7 |
| mosm/kg | 300 | 300 | 450 | 450 |
| Volume to provide 100% RDAs (ml)§ | 1,250 | 2,000 | 1,920 | 1,200 |

| | Nutrex Encaret Nutrex | Nutrex Protamin Nutrex | Osmolite Ross | Osmolite HN Ross |
|---|---|---|---|---|
| Protein, g (% total kcal) | 26.8 (11%) | 31.3 (12%) | 35.2 (14%) | 41.9 (17%) |
| Source | Na, Ca caseinate | Na, Ca caseinate | Na, Ca caseinate | Na, Ca caseinate |
| | Egg white solids | Soy protein | Soy protein isolate | Soy protein isolate |
| Fat, g (% total kcal) | 125.7 (23%) | 29.9 (27%) | 36.4 (31%) | 34.7 (30%) |
| Source | Soy oil | Corn oil | MCT oil, 17.2 (14%) | MCT oil, 18.3 (15%) |
| | | Lecithin | Corn oil | Corn oil, 13.5 (12%) |
| | | | Soy oil, 19.2 (17%) | Soy oil, 3.4 (3%) |
| Carbohydrate, g (% total kcal) | 162.2 (65%) | 149.8 (60%) | 137.2 (55%) | 133.0 (53%) |
| Source | Corn syrup solids | Corn syrup solids | Hydrolyzed cornstarch | Hydrolyzed cornstarch |
| | Sucrose | Sucrose | | |
| | Fiber | | | |
| Lactose, g | 0 | 0 | 0 | 0 |
| Volume for 1,000 kcal (ml) | 676 | 799 | 946 | 946 |
| *Minerals* | | | | |
| Calcium, mg | 540.8 | 666.0 | 498.1 | 714.0 |
| Phosphorus, mg | 540.8 | 666.0 | 498.1 | 714.0 |
| Magnesium, mg | 228.5 | 266.4 | 199.0 | 284.9 |
| Iron, mg | 10.3 | 12.0 | 9.0 | 12.8 |
| Iodine, mcg | 85.5 | 99.9 | 74.5 | 106.6 |
| Copper, mg | 1.1 | 1.3 | 1.0 | 1.4 |
| Manganese, mg | 2.2 | 2.5 | 2.4 | 3.6 |
| Zinc, mg | 8.6 | 10.0 | 11.2 | 16.0 |
| Chromium, mcg | N/A | N/A | N/A | N/A |
| Selenium, mcg | N/A | N/A | N/A | N/A |
| Molybdenum, mcg | N/A | N/A | N/A | N/A |
| Sodium, meq | 2.9 | 5.8 | 26.0 | 38.2 |
| Potassium, meq | 29.5 | 34.1 | 24.4 | 37.7 |
| Chloride, meq | 15.2 | 16.9 | 22.4 | 38.2 |
| mosm/kg | 460 | 450 | 300 | 300 |
| Volume to provide 100% RDAs (ml)§ | 1,200 | 1,200 | 1,887 | 1,321 |

## Table A–40b. (continued)

| | Portagen Mead Johnson | Precision HN Sandoz | Precision Isotonic Sandoz | Precision LR Sandoz |
|---|---|---|---|---|
| Protein, g (% total kcal) | 35.0 (14%) | 41.7 (17%) | 30.0 (12%) | 23.6 (10%) |
| Source | Na caseinate | Egg white solids | Egg white solids | Egg white solids |
| Fat, g (% total kcal) | 47.7 (40%) | 1.2 (1%) | 31.3 (28%) | 1.4 (1%) |
| Source | MCT oil, 41.0 (34%) Corn oil, 5.5 (5%) Lecithin, 1.3 (1%) | Soy oil | Soy oil | Soy oil |
| Carbohydrate, g (% total kcal) | 115.0 (46%) | 205.7 (82%) | 150.0 (60%) | 225.4 (89%) |
| Source | Corn syrup solids, 85.3 (34%) Sucrose, 29.1 (12%) | Maltodextrin Sucrose | Maltodextrin Sucrose | Maltodextrin Sucrose |
| Lactose, g | 0 | 0 | 0 | 0 |
| Volume for 1,000 kcal (ml) | 1,000 | 952 | 1,000 | 909 |
| *Minerals* | | | | |
| Calcium, mg | 936.0 | 333.3 | 640.0 | 527.3 |
| Phosphorus, mg | 702.0 | 333.3 | 640.0 | 527.3 |
| Magnesium. mg | 208.0 | 133.3 | 256.0 | 212.7 |
| Iron, mg | 18.7 | 6.0 | 11.5 | 9.5 |
| Iodine, mcg | 72.9 | 50.0 | 96.2 | 80.0 |
| Copper, mg | 1.6 | 0.7 | 1.3 | 1.1 |
| Manganese, mg | 1.2 | 1.3 | 2.7 | 2.2 |
| Zinc, mg | 9.4 | 5.0 | 9.6 | 8.0 |
| Chromium, mcg | N/A | 50.5 | 96.0 | 79.7 |
| Selenium, mcg | N/A | 58.1 | 64.0 | 53.2 |
| Molybdenum, mcg | N/A | 100.0 | 192.0 | 159.1 |
| Sodium, meq | 20.8 | 40.6 | 33.5 | 27.6 |
| Potassium, meq | 32.2 | 22.2 | 24.6 | 20.5 |
| Chloride, meq | 23.9 | 32.0 | 29.0 | 28.2 |
| mosm/kg | 320 | 525 | 300 | 480 |
| Volume to provide 100% RDAs (ml)§ | 960 | 2,850 | 1,560 | 1,710 |

| | Pre-Fortison Sherwood Medical | Resource Sandoz | Ross SLD Ross |
|---|---|---|---|
| Protein, g (% total kcal) | 40.0 (16%) | 34.9 (14%) | 53.6 (21%) |
| Source | Na, Ca caseinate | Na, Ca caseinate / Soy protein isolate | Egg white solids |
| Fat, g (% total kcal) | 40.0 (36%) | 34.9 (32%) | 0.7 (1%) |
| Source | Corn oil / Lecithin | Soy oil / Mono-, diglycerides | |
| Carbohydrate, g (% total kcal) | 120.0 (48%) | 135.9 (55%) | 195.6 (78%) |
| Source | Maltodextrin | Maltodextrin / Sucrose | Sucrose / Hydrolyzed cornstarch |
| Lactose, g | 0 | 0 | 0 |
| Volume for 1,000 kcal (ml) | 2,000 | 943 | 1,428 |
| *Minerals* | | | |
| Calcium, mg | 625.0 | 515.5 | 1,192.3 |
| Phosphorus, mg | 625.0 | 515.5 | 1,192.3 |
| Magnesium, mg | 500.0 | 197.8 | 478.4 |
| Iron, mg | 22.5 | 8.9 | 21.4 |
| Iodine, mcg | 200.0 | 75.0 | 178.5 |
| Copper, mg | 3.0 | 1.0 | 2.4 |
| Manganese, mg | 5.0 | 2.0 | 6.0 |
| Zinc, mg | 30.0 | 14.9 | 27.1 |
| Chromium, mcg | N/A | N/A | N/A |
| Selenium, mcg | N/A | N/A | N/A |
| Molybdenum, mcg | N/A | N/A | N/A |
| Sodium, meq | 29.6 | 34.6 | 51.7 |
| Potassium, meq | 29.5 | 37.5 | 30.5 |
| Chloride, meq | 29.9 | 37.0 | 40.2 |
| mosm/kg | 150 | 450 | 545 |
| Volume to provide 100% RDAs (ml)§ | 1,600 | 1,896 | 1,200 |

# Table A–40b. (continued)

| | Susta II† Mead Johnson | Sustacal Liquid Mead Johnson | Sustacal HC Mead Johnson | Travasorb Liquid Travenol |
|---|---|---|---|---|
| Protein, g (% total kcal) | 43.2 (17%) | 60.1 (24%) | 40.0 (16%) | 35.0 (14%) |
| Source | Na caseinate Soy protein isolate | Na, Ca caseinate Soy protein | Na, Ca caseinate | Na, Ca caseinate Soy protein isolate |
| Fat, g (% total kcal) | 33.2 (30%) | 23.1 (21%) | 37.8 (34%) | 35.0 (31%) |
| Source | Corn oil | Soy oil | Soy oil Lecithin | Corn oil Soy oil |
| Carbohydrate, g (% total kcal) | 132.0 (53%) | 137.8 (55%) | 122.2 (49%) | 136.4 (55%) |
| Source | Corn syrup solids Sucrose Soy polysaccharide | Sucrose, 97.0 (39%) Corn syrup solids, 40.8 (16%) | Corn syrup solids Sucrose | Sucrose Corn syrup solids |
| Lactose, g | 0 | 0 | 0 | 0 |
| Volume for 1,000 kcal (ml) | 960 | 980 | 667 | 1,000 |
| *Minerals* | | | | |
| Calcium, mg | 800.0 | 1,000.0 | 555.6 | 500.0 |
| Phosphorus, mg | 668.0 | 925.9 | 555.6 | 500.0 |
| Magnesium, mg | 268.0 | 375.0 | 222.3 | 200.0 |
| Iron, mg | 12.0 | 16.7 | 10.0 | 9.0 |
| Iodine, mcg | 100.0 | 138.9 | 83.3 | 75.0 |
| Copper, mg | 1.3 | 1.9 | 1.1 | 1.0 |
| Manganese, mg | 1.7 | 2.8 | 1.7 | 2.0 |
| Zinc, mg | 13.2 | 13.9 | 8.3 | 15.0 |
| Chromium, mcg | N/A | N/A | N/A | N/A |
| Selenium, mcg | N/A | N/A | N/A | N/A |
| Molybdenum, mcg | N/A | N/A | N/A | N/A |
| Sodium, meq | 29.0 | 39.8 | 24.2 | 30.4 |
| Potassium, meq | 33.8 | 51.9 | 24.7 | 30.8 |
| Chloride, meq | 37.2 | 43.5 | 23.6 | 28.4 |
| mosm/kg | N/A | 620* | 650 | 488 |
| Volume to provide 100% RDAs (ml)§ | 1,420 | 1,060 | 1,200 | 2,000 |

| | Travasorb MCT Travenol | | TwoCal HN Ross | |
|---|---|---|---|---|
| Protein, g (% total kcal) | 49.0 | (20%) | 41.8 | (17%) |
| Source | Lactalbumin | | Na, Ca caseinate | |
| Fat, g (% total kcal) | 32.9 | (31%) | 45.4 | (40%) |
| Source | MCT oil (25%) | | Corn oil | |
| | Sunflower oil (6%) | | MCT oil | |
| Carbohydrate, g (% total kcal) | 122.8 | (49%) | 108.5 | (43%) |
| Source | Corn syrup solids | | Hydrolyzed cornstarch | |
| | | | Sucrose | |
| Lactose, g | 0 | | 0 | |
| Volume for 1,000 kcal (ml) | 500 | | 500 | |
| *Minerals* | | | | |
| Calcium, mg | 500.0 | | 528.5 | |
| Phosphorus, mg | 500.0 | | 528.5 | |
| Magnesium, mg | 200.0 | | 211.5 | |
| Iron. mg | 9.0 | | 9.5 | |
| Iodine, mcg | 75.0 | | 79.5 | |
| Copper, mg | 1.0 | | 1.0 | |
| Manganese, mg | 2.0 | | 2.6 | |
| Zinc, mg | 15.0 | | 12.9 | |
| Chromium, mcg | N/A | | N/A | |
| Selenium, mcg | N/A | | N/A | |
| Molybdenum. mcg | N/A | | N/A | |
| Sodium, meq | 15.2 | | 23.0 | |
| Potassium, meq | 44.6 | | 29.8 | |
| Chloride, meq | 34.7 | | 22.0 | |
| mosm/kg | 312 | | 690 | |
| Volume to provide 100% RDAs (ml)§ | 2,000 | | 947 | |

*Vanilla.

†Contains fiber.

‡N/A = Not available.

§Including vitamins.

**Appreciation is expressed to Mindy Hermann-Zaidins. R.D.. Memorial Sloan-Kettering Cancer Center, Clinical Nutrition Support Kitchen, for revision of this table, originally prepared by A.S. Bloch and M.E. Shils in the 6th Edition of this textbook.

## Table A–40c. Defined-Formula Diets with Hydrolyzed Protein or Amino Acids, Low Residue, and No Lactose (per 1,000 kcal)**

| | Criticare HN *Mead Johnson* | Nutrex Aminex *Nutrex* | Pepti 2000 *Sherwood Medical* | Reabilan *Roussel* |
|---|---|---|---|---|
| Protein, g (% total kcal) | 36.0 (14%) | 38.2 (15%) | 40.0 (16%) | 31.5 (13%) |
| Source | Casein hydrolysate | Crystalline amino acids | Hydrolyzed lactalbumin | Wheat peptides<br>Casein peptides |
| Fat, g (% total kcal) | 3.0 (3%) | 2.8 (3%) | 10.0 (9%) | 38.9 (34%) |
| Source | Sunflower oil | Safflower oil | MCT oil, 5.0 (4%)<br>Corn oil, 5.0 (5%) | MCT oil, 15.5 (12%)<br>Oenothera biennis oil<br>Soy oil<br>Lecithin |
| Carbohydrate, g (% total kcal) | 210.0 (83%) | 205.7 (82%) | 188.8 (76%) | 131.5 (53%) |
| Source | Maltodextrin | Maltodextrin<br>Modified starch | Maltodextrin | Maltodextrin<br>Tapioca starch |
| Lactose, g | 0 | 0 | 0 | 0 |
| Volume for 1,000 kcal (ml) | 946 | 1,000 | 1,000 | 1,000 |
| *Minerals* | | | | |
| Calcium, mg | 500.0 | 499.5 | 625.0 | 498.7 |
| Phosphorus, mg | 500.0 | 499.5 | 625.0 | 498.7 |
| Magnesium, mg | 200.0 | 199.8 | 250.0 | 250.7 |
| Iron, mg | 9.0 | 9.0 | 11.3 | 10.0 |
| Iodine, mcg | 75.0 | 74.9 | 100.0 | 74.7 |
| Copper, mg | 1.0 | 1.0 | 1.5 | 1.6 |
| Manganese, mg | 2.5 | 1.0 | 2.5 | 2.0 |
| Zinc, mg | 10.0 | 10.0 | 15.0 | 10.0 |
| Chromium, mcg | N/A* | 16.6 | N/A | N/A |
| Selenium, mcg | N/A | 50.0 | N/A | 50.7 |
| Molybdenum, mcg | N/A | 50.0 | N/A | N/A |
| Sodium, meq | 26.0 | 20.0 | 29.6 | 30.4 |
| Potassium, meq | 32.0 | 20.1 | 29.5 | 32.1 |
| Chloride, meq | 28.0 | 23.1 | 29.9 | 56.3 |
| mosm/kg | 650 | 600 | 490 | 350 |
| Volume to provide 100% RDAs (ml)† | 1,892 | 2,000 | 1,600 | 2,000 |

| | Reabilan HN Roussel | Travasorb STD Travenol | Travasorb HN Travenol |
|---|---|---|---|
| Protein, g (% total kcal) | 43.6 (17%) | 30.0 (12%) | 45.0 (18%) |
| Source | Whey peptides<br>Casein peptides | Hydrolyzed lactalbumin | Hydrolyzed lactalbumin |
| Fat, g (% total kcal) | 39.0 (36%) | 13.4 (11%) | 13.4 (11%) |
| Source | MCT oil<br>Oenothera biennis oil<br>Soy oil<br>Lecithin | MCT oil. 9.0 (7%)<br>Sunflower oil. 4.4 (4%) | MCT oil. 9.0 (7%)<br>Sunflower oil. 4.4 (4%) |
| Carbohydrate, g (% total kcal) | 118.6 (47%) | 190.0 (76%) | 175.0 (70%) |
| Source | Maltodextrin<br>Tapioca starch | Glucose oligosaccharides | Glucose oligosaccharides |
| Lactose, g | 0 | 0 | 0 |
| Volume for 1,000 kcal (ml) | 750 | 1,000 | 1,000 |
| *Minerals* | | | |
| Calcium, mg | 338.0 | 500.0 | 500.0 |
| Phosphorus, mg | 376.0 | 500.0 | 500.0 |
| Magnesium, mg | 248.0 | 200.0 | 200.0 |
| Iron, mg | 10.0 | 9.0 | 9.0 |
| Iodine, mcg | 76.0 | 75.0 | 75.0 |
| Copper, mg | 1.0 | 1.0 | 1.0 |
| Manganese, mg | 2.0 | 1.3 | 1.3 |
| Zinc, mg | 10.0 | 7.5 | 7.5 |
| Chromium, mcg | 62.0 | N/A | N/A |
| Selenium, mcg | 50.0 | N/A | N/A |
| Molybdenum, mcg | N/A | N/A | N/A |
| Sodium, meq | 32.6 | 40.0 | 40.0 |
| Potassium, meq | 31.9 | 30.0 | 30.0 |
| Chloride, meq | 52.8 | 42.9 | 39.0 |
| mosm/kg | 490 | 560* | 560 |
| Volume to provide 100% RDAs (ml)† | 2,000 | 2,000 | 2,000 |

# Table A–40c. (continued)

| | Vital HN *Ross* | Vivonex *Norwich Eaton* |
|---|---|---|
| Protein, g (% total kcal) | 41.7 (17%) | 21.8 ( 9%) |
| Source | Partially hydrolyzed whey, meat, and soy | Crystalline amino acids |
| Fat, g (% total kcal) | 10.8 (8%) | 1.4 (1%) |
| Source | Safflower oil 5.9 (5%) MCT oil, 4.9 (3%) | Safflower oil |
| Carbohydrate, g (% total kcal) | 188.3 (75%) | 230.6 (90%) |
| Source | Hydrolyzed cornstarch Glucose | Glucose oligosaccharides |
| Lactose, g | 0.83 | 0 |
| Volume for 1,000 kcal (ml) | 1,000 | 1,000 |
| *Minerals* | | |
| Calcium, mg | 667.0 | 550.0 |
| Phosphorus, mg | 667.0 | 550.0 |
| Magnesium, mg | 267.0 | 222.2 |
| Iron, mg | 12.0 | 10.0 |
| Iodine, mcg | 100.0 | 83.3 |
| Copper, mg | 1.3 | 1.1 |
| Manganese, mg | 2.5 | 1.6 |
| Zinc, mg | 10.0 | 8.3 |
| Chromium, mcg | N/A | 27.8 |
| Selenium, mcg | N/A | 83.0 |
| Molybdenum, mcg | N/A | 83.0 |
| Sodium, meq | 16.7 | 20.4 |
| Potassium, meq | 29.8 | 30.0 |
| Chloride, meq | 18.8 | 20.4 |
| mosm/kg | 460 | 550 |
| Volume to provide 100% RDAs (ml)† | 1,500 | 1,800 |

|  | Vivonex HN Norwich Eaton | Vivonex T.E.N. Norwich Eaton |
|---|---|---|
| Protein, g (% total kcal) | 44.4 (17%) | 38.2 (15%) |
| Source | Crystalline amino acids | Crystalline amino acids (33% BCAA) |
| Fat, g (% total kcal) | 0.9 (1%) | 2.8 (2%) |
| Source | Safflower oil | Safflower oil |
| Carbohydrate, g (% total kcal) | 210.0 (82%) | 205.6 (82%) |
| Source | Glucose oligosaccharides | Maltodextrin Modified starch |
| Lactose, g | 0 | 0 |
| Volume for 1,000 kcal (ml) | 1,000 | 1,000 |
| *Minerals* | | |
| Calcium, mg | 330.0 | 500.0 |
| Phosphorus, mg | 330.0 | 500.0 |
| Magnesium, mg | 133.0 | 200.0 |
| Iron, mg | 6.0 | 9.0 |
| Iodine, mcg | 50.0 | 75.0 |
| Copper, mg | 0.7 | 1.0 |
| Manganese, mg | 0.9 | 0.9 |
| Zinc, mg | 5.0 | 10.0 |
| Chromium, mcg | 16.7 | 17.0 |
| Selenium, mcg | 50.0 | 50.0 |
| Molybdenum, mcg | 50.0 | 50.0 |
| Sodium, meq | 23.0 | 20.0 |
| Potassium, meq | 30.0 | 20.0 |
| Chloride, meq | 23.1 | 25.0 |
| mosm/kg | 810 | 630 |
| Volume to provide 100% RDAs (ml)† | 3,000 | 2,000 |

*N/A = Value not available.

†Including vitamins.

**Appreciation is expressed to Mindy Hermann-Zaidins, R.D., Memorial Sloan-Kettering Cancer Center, Clinical Nutrition Support Kitchen, for revision of this table, originally prepared by A.S. Bloch and M.E. Shils in the 6th Edition of this textbook.

# Table A–41. Supplementary Feedings* (per 1,000 kcal)**

| | Biocare Pudding Mix Food Sciences Corp.† | Biomed Pudding Robard‡ | Cal-Plus Henkel | Casec Mead Johnson | Citrotein Sandoz |
|---|---|---|---|---|---|
| Protein, g | 39.0 (14%) | 187.5 (75%) | 0 | 237.8 (95%) | 60.5 (24%) |
| Fat, g | 36.0 (32%) | <10.0 | 0 | 5.4 (5%) | 2.6 (2%) |
| Carbohydrate, g | 132.0 (53%) | 125.0# (25%) | 250.0 (100%) | 0 | 184.2 (74%) |
| Sodium, meq | 43.8 § | N/A | 12.77 | 17.6 | 45.8 |
| Potassium, meq | 40.51§ | N/A | 0.48 | 20.0 | 26.8 |
| Amount needed to give 1,000 kcal | 227.0 g dry weight | 322.0 g dry weight | 266.0 g dry weight | 270.3 g dry weight | 263.4 g dry weight |
| TYPE | Nutritional supplement | Protein carbohydrate source | Carbohydrate source | Protein source | Protein, vitamin, mineral supplement |

| | Controlyte Sandoz | Forta Pudding Ross | High MCT Navaco | High Protein Gelatin Delmark | Lipomul-Oral Saccharine-Free Upjohn |
|---|---|---|---|---|---|
| Protein, g | Trace | 27.2 (11%) | 0 | 119.7 (48%) | 0 |
| Fat, g | 48.0 (43%) | 38.8 (35%) | 77.4 (70%) | 1.4 (1%) | 106.5 (97%) |
| Carbohydrate, g | 143.0 (57%) | 136.0 (54%) | 66.6 (30%) | 126.7 (51%) | 8.0 (3%) |
| Sodium, meq | 0.85 | 38.3 | 12.8 | 76.5 | 0.73 |
| Potassium, meq | 0.20 | 30.7 | 36.4 | 37.9 | 0 |
| Amount needed to give 1,000 kcal | 198.0 g dry weight | 568.0 g dry weight | 163.0 g dry weight | 266.1 g dry weight | 159.7 ml liquid |
| TYPE | Low-protein, low-electrolyte calorie source | Nutritional supplement | Fat, carbohydrate source | Protein, calorie supplement | Fat source |

| | Hycal Beecham-Massengill | L.C. Navaco | Lipomul-Oral Upjohn | Lonalac Mead Johnson |
|---|---|---|---|---|
| Protein, g | 0.1 | 0 | 0 | 53.1 (21%) |
| Fat, g | 0.1 | 0 | 111.1 (100%) | 54.7 (49%) |
| Carbohydrate, g | 244.7 (100%) | 250.0 (100%) | | 75.0 (30%) |
| Sodium, meq | 1.48 | 10.0 | 1.2 | 1.7 |
| Potassium, meq | 0.07 | 2.0 | 0 | 48.10 |
| Amount needed to give 1,000 kcal | 407.0 ml liquid | 400.0 ml liquid | 166.7 ml liquid | 1,478.0 ml standard dilution or 197 g dry weight |
| TYPE | Carbohydrate source | Carbohydrate source | Fat source | Low-sodium, high-protein source |

| | Lytren<br>Mead Johnson | MCT Oil<br>Mead Johnson | Microlipid<br>Sherwood Medical | Moducal<br>Mead Johnson | Nutrex Broth<br>Nutrex |
|---|---|---|---|---|---|
| Protein, g | 0 | 0 | 0 | 0 | 30.8 (46%) |
| Fat, g | 0 | 120.5 (100%) | 111.0 (100%) | 0 | 0 |
| Carbohydrate, g | 253.0 (100%) | 0 | 0 | 250.0 (100%) | 216.0 |
| Sodium, meq | 97.2 | 0 | 0 | 7.9 | 12.17 |
| Potassium, meq | 83.3 | 0 | 0 | 0.3 | 19.48 |
| Amount needed to give 1,000 kcal | 268.0 g dry weight or 3,286 ml standard dilution | 120.5 g liquid | 222.0 ml liquid | 263.2 g dry weight | 261.3 g dry weight |
| TYPE | Calorie and electrolyte source | Medium-chain triglycerides | Fat source | Carbohydrate source | Protein, carbohydrate source |

| | Nutrex CLD<br>Nutrex | Nutrex ProMax<br>Nutrex | Nutrisource—Amino Acids<br>Sandoz | Nutrisource Amino Acids—High Branched Chain<br>Sandoz | Nutrisource Carbohydrate<br>Sandoz | Nutrisource Lipid—Long Chain Triglycerides<br>Sandoz | Nutrisource Lipid—Medium Chain Triglycerides<br>Sandoz |
|---|---|---|---|---|---|---|---|
| Protein, g | 114.3 (46%) | 178.6 (71%) | 250.0 (100%) | 250.0 (100%) | 0 | 0 | 0 |
| Fat, g | 0 | 21.4 (19%) | 0 | 0 | 0 | 111.1 (100%) | 61.0 (90% MCT) |
| Carbohydrate, g | 128.5 (51%) | 23.8 (10%) | 0 | 0 | 250.0 (100%) | 0 | 0 |
| Sodium, meq | 62.3 | 20.35 | 0 | 0 | 0.27 | 0 | 0 |
| Potassium, meq | 40.6 | 59.28 | 0 | 0 | 0.10 | 0 | 0 |
| Amount needed to give 1,000 kcal | 243.7 g dry weight | 235.7 g dry weight | 256.0 g dry weight | 256.0 g dry weight | 312.5 ml liquid | 455.2 ml liquid | 490.2 ml liquid |
| TYPE | Protein, calorie supplement | Protein source | Protein module | Protein module | Carbohydrate module | Fat module | Fat module |

# Table A–41.  (continued)

| | Nutrisource-Protein Sandoz | P.C. Navaco | Pedialyte Ross | Polycose Ross | Pro-Mix Navaco |
|---|---|---|---|---|---|
| Protein, g | 187.5 (75%) | 0 | 0 | 0 | 213.0 (85%) |
| Fat, g | 17.5 (16%) | 0 | 0 | 0 | 10.6 (10%) |
| Carbohydrate, g | 21.2 (8%) | 250.0 (100%) | 250.0 (100%) | 250.0 (100%) | 13.3 (5%) |
| Sodium, meq | 28.75 | 1.62 | 150.0 | 12.50 | 17.47 |
| Potassium, meq | 36.25 | 0 | 100.0 | 2.50 | 91.16 |
| Amount needed to give 1,000 kcal | 248.0 g dry weight | 259.1 g dry weight | 500.0 ml liquid | 263.0 g dry weight | 266.2 g dry weight |
| TYPE | Protein module | Carbohydrate source | Calorie and electrolyte source | Oligosaccharides | Protein source |

| | ProMod Ross | Propac Sherwood Medical | Sumacal Sherwood Medical | Sustacal Pudding Mead Johnson |
|---|---|---|---|---|
| Protein, g | 178.6 (71%) | 192.3 (77%) | 0 | 28.3 (11%) |
| Fat, g | 21.4 (19%) | 20.5 (18%) | 0 | 39.6 (36%) |
| Carbohydrate, g | 23.9 (10%) | 12.8 (5%) | 250.0 (100%) | 133.3 (53%) |
| Sodium, meq | 20.35 | 25.08 | 14.13 | 21.7 |
| Potassium, meq | 59.28 | 32.87 | 1.0 | 34.2 |
| Amount needed to give 1,000 kcal | 235.7 g dry weight | 250.0 g dry weight | 500.0 ml liquid | 590.6 g dry weight |
| TYPE | Protein source | Protein source | Carbohydrate source | Nutritional supplement |

*Individual items in this table may be used in appropriate amounts and combinations to prepare modular-type diets for patient needs.
†Cereal and soup available.
‡High-protein cocoa, soup, beverage, and gelatin available.
§Vanilla-flavored.
#Part polydextrose, at 1 calorie/g.
**Appreciation is expressed to Mindy Hermann-Zaidins, R.D., Memorial Sloan-Kettering Cancer Center, Clinical Nutrition Support Kitchen, for revision of this table, originally prepared by A.S. Bloch and M.E. Shils in the 6th Edition of this textbook.

**Table A–42. Defined-Formula Diets with Specific Disease-Related Claims (per 1,000 kcal)†**

| | Amin-Aid* Kendall-McGaw | Hepatic Aid II* Kendall-McGaw | Pulmocare Ross | Stresstein Sandoz |
|---|---|---|---|---|
| Protein, g (% total kcal) | 9.9 (4%) | 37.5 (15%) | 41.9 (17%) | 57.5 (23%) |
| Source | Essential amino acids plus histidine | Amino acids (high BC, lower aromatics) | Na, Ca caseinate Soy isolate | Amino acids BCAA (10%) |
| Fat, g (% total kcal) | 23.6 (21%) | 30.8 (28%) | 61.7 (56%) | 22.5 (20%) |
| Source | Partially hydrogenated soy oil Lecithin Mono-, diglycerides | Partially hydrogenated soy oil Lecithin Mono-, diglycerides | Corn oil | MCT Soy oil |
| Carbohydrate, g (% total kcal) | 186.4 (75%) | 143.2 (57%) | 70.8 (28%) | 142.5 (57%) |
| Source | Maltodextrin Sucrose | Maltodextrin Sucrose | Hydrolyzed cornstarch Sucrose | Maltodextrin |
| Lactose, g | 0 | 0 | 0 | 0 |
| Volume for 1,000 kcal (ml) | 500.0 | 607.0 | 667.0 | 830.0 |
| *Minerals* | | | | |
| Calcium, mg | negligible | negligible | 700.0 | 425.0 |
| Phosphorus, mg | " | " | 700.0 | 425.0 |
| Magnesium, mg | " | " | 282.0 | 167.5 |
| Iron, mg | " | " | 12.7 | 7.5 |
| Iodine, mcg | " | " | 107.0 | 62.5 |
| Copper, mg | " | " | 1.4 | 0.8 |
| Manganese, mg | " | " | 1.4 | 1.7 |
| Zinc, mg | " | " | 15.8 | 6.2 |
| Sodium, meq | 7.5 | 5.0 | 38.0 | 23.9 |
| Potassium, meq | negligible | negligible | 32.5 | 23.7 |
| Chloride, meq | " | " | 31.7 | 23.2 |
| mosm/kg | 850.0 | 560.0 | 490.0 | 910.0 |

## Table A–42. (continued)

| | Traumacal Mead Johnson | Travasorb Hepatic Travenol | Travasorb Renal Travenol |
|---|---|---|---|
| Protein, g (% total kcal) | 55.0 (23%) | 26.5 (11%) | 17.1 (7%) |
| Source | Ca, Na caseinate | Amino acids BCAA (6%) aromatic (2%) | Amino acids essential (4%) |
| Fat, g (% total kcal) | 45.7 (40%) | 13.2 (11%) | 13.3 (12%) |
| Source | Soy oil, 31.1 (28%) MCT oil, 14.5 (12%) | MCT, 9.5 (8%) Sunflower oil, 3.7 (3%) Lecithin | MCT, 9.3 (8%) Sunflower oil, 4.0 (4%) Lecithin |
| Carbohydrate, g (% total kcal) | 95.0 (38%) | 194.0 (78%) | 202.7 (81%) |
| Source | Corn syrup Sucrose | Glucose oligosaccharides Sucrose | Glucose oligosaccharides Sucrose |
| Lactose, g | 0 | 0 | 0 |
| Volume for 1,000 kcal (ml) | 667.0 | 928.0 | 749.0 |
| *Minerals* | | | |
| Calcium, mg | 500.0 | 352.4 | negligible |
| Phosphorus, mg | 500.0 | 437.2 | " |
| Magnesium, mg | 133.3 | 172.2 | " |
| Iron, mg | 6.0 | 8.0 | " |
| Iodine, mcg | 50.0 | 66.2 | " |
| Copper, mg | 1.0 | 0.9 | " |
| Manganese, mg | 1.7 | 1.1 | " |
| Zinc, mg | 10.0 | 6.6 | " |
| Sodium, meq | 34.78 | 17.63 | " |
| Potassium, meq | 23.93 | 26.64 | " |
| Chloride, meq | 20.05 | 17.69 | " |
| mosm/kg | 550.0 | 690.0 | 590.0 |

*Water for reconstituting will affect electrolyte concentration.
†Appreciation is expressed to Mindy Hermann-Zaidins, R.D., Memorial Sloan-Kettering Cancer Center, Clinical Nutrition Support Kitchen, for revision of this table, originally prepared by A.S. Bloch and M.E. Shils in the 6th Edition of this textbook.

**Table A–43a. Amino Acid and Protein Content of Exemplary Foods (per 100 g edible portion)***

| Food | Cystine (mg) | Isoleucine (mg) | Leucine (mg) | Methionine (mg) | Phenylalanine (mg) | Tyrosine (mg) | Valine (mg) | Protein (g) |
|---|---|---|---|---|---|---|---|---|
| **Cereals** | | | | | | | | |
| Corn grits, cooked | 32 | 56 | 215 | 34 | 73 | 61 | 47 | 1.4 |
| Cream of wheat, cooked | 34 | 67 | 115 | 28 | 82 | 48 | 73 | 1.5 |
| Oats, cooked | 64 | 118 | 197 | 43 | 141 | 92 | 151 | 2.6 |
| **Dairy Products** | | | | | | | | |
| Eggs | 289 | 759 | 1,066 | 392 | 686 | 505 | 874 | 12.1 |
| Cheese (cheddar) | 125 | 1,546 | 2,385 | 652 | 1,311 | 1,202 | 1,663 | 24.9 |
| **Milk** | | | | | | | | |
| Cow, whole | 30 | 199 | 322 | 83 | 159 | 159 | 220 | 3.3 |
| Human | 19 | 56 | 95 | 21 | 46 | 53 | 63 | 1.0 |
| **Fruits** | | | | | | | | |
| Apples, raw with skin | 3 | 8 | 12 | 2 | 5 | 4 | 9 | 0.2 |
| Apricots, raw | 3 | 41 | 77 | 6 | 52 | 29 | 47 | 1.4 |
| Bananas | 17 | 33 | 71 | 11 | 38 | 24 | 47 | 1.0 |
| Oranges, raw | 10 | 25 | 23 | 20 | 31 | 16 | 40 | 0.9 |
| Peaches, raw | 6 | 20 | 40 | 17 | 22 | 18 | 38 | 0.7 |
| Watermelons | 2 | 19 | 18 | 6 | 15 | 12 | 16 | 0.6 |
| **Meat, Fish, Poultry** | | | | | | | | |
| Beef, hamburger, lean, cooked | 391 | 1,576 | 2,467 | 748 | 1,240 | 1,081 | 1,673 | 30.1 |
| Chicken, light meat, fried | 420 | 1,732 | 2,463 | 908 | 1,303 | 1,108 | 1,628 | 32.8 |
| Fish, halibut, raw | 245 | 1,066 | 1,588 | 606 | 773 | 765 | 1,108 | 20.9 |
| **Proprietary Infant Formula** | | | | | | | | |
| Enfamil (per dl) | 17 | 90 | 154 | 29 | 58 | 66 | 91 | 1.5 |
| Similac (per dl) | 13 | 75 | 145 | 43 | 75 | 93 | 84 | 1.5 |
| **Vegetables** | | | | | | | | |
| Beans, green, cooked | 11 | 42 | 71 | 14 | 42 | 27 | 57 | 1.2 |
| lima, cooked | 83 | 438 | 535 | 68 | 336 | 219 | 425 | 6.8 |
| Broccoli, cooked | 21 | 115 | 139 | 36 | 90 | 67 | 136 | 3.0 |
| Cabbage, raw | 10 | 61 | 63 | 12 | 39 | 21 | 52 | 1.2 |
| Carrots, raw | 8 | 41 | 43 | 7 | 32 | 20 | 44 | 1.0 |
| Peas, green, cooked | 32 | 193 | 320 | 81 | 198 | 112 | 232 | 5.4 |
| Potatoes, baked | 29 | 93 | 138 | 36 | 102 | 85 | 130 | 2.3 |
| Spinach, cooked | 35 | 152 | 231 | 55 | 134 | 113 | 168 | 3.0 |
| Tomatoes, raw | 12 | 21 | 33 | 8 | 23 | 15 | 23 | 0.9 |

*From references 51 to 56 in Chapter 63, compiled by L.J. Elsas II, M.D., and P.B. Acosta, Dr. P.H. (see Chapter 63 for discussion).

## Table A–43b.   Sources and Indications for "Chemically Defined" Medical Foods for Amino Acid- or Nitrogen-Restricted Diets*

| Manufacturer | Product | Indication(s) |
|---|---|---|
| Mead Johnson Nutritional Division<br>2404 W. Pennsylvania St.<br>Evansville, IN 47221<br>(800) 457-3550 | Lofenalac<br>Low Methionine Diet Powder | PKU[a]<br>Hypermethioninemias<br>Homocystinuria (cystathionine beta-synthase deficiency) |
| | Low Phe/Tyr Diet Powder<br>Moducal | Tyrosinemias<br>Any disorder in which amino acids or N are restricted |
| | MSUD Diet Powder | MSUD[b]<br>IVA[c] (must add Ile[d] and Val[e])<br>Any disorder of BCAA[f] metabolism |
| | Phenyl-Free<br>Protein-Free Diet Powder | PKU<br>Any disorder in which amino acids or N are restricted |
| Milupa Company<br>397 Boston Post Rd.<br>Darien, CT 06820<br>(203) 656-1903 | HOM 1, HOM 2 | Hypermethioninemias<br>Homocystinuria (cystathionine beta-synthase deficiency) |
| | MSUD 1, MSUD 2 | MSUD<br>IVA (must add Ile and Val)<br>Any disorder of BCAA metabolism |
| | PKU 1, PKU 2, PKU 3<br>TYR 1, TYR 2<br>UCD 1, UCD 2 | PKU<br>Tyrosinemias<br>Defects in urea cycle enzymes |
| Ross Laboratories<br>Columbus, OH 43216<br>(614) 438-6200 | Polycose Powder | Any disorder in which amino acids or N must be restricted |
| | Analog Range<br>  MSUD<br>  X LEU<br>  X MET | MSUD<br>Any disorder of leucine metabolism<br>Homocystinuria (cystathionine beta-synthase deficiency) |
| |  X PHEN<br>  X PHEN, TYR<br>  X PHEN, TYR, MET | PKU<br>Tyrosinemias<br>Tyrosinemias with elevated plasma methionine |
| | Maxamaid Range<br>  X MET | Hypermethioninemias<br>Homocystinuria (cystathionine beta-synthase deficiency) |
| |  MSUD<br>  X PHEN<br>  X PHEN, TYR<br>  X PHEN, TYR, MET | MSUD<br>PKU<br>Tyrosinemias<br>Tyrosinemia with elevated plasma methionine |
| | Maxamum XP | PKU |

[a]Phenylketonuria
[b]Maple syrup urine disease
[c]Isovaleric acidemia
[d]Isoleucine
[e]Valine
[f]Branched-chain amino acid
*Compiled by L.J. Elsas II, M.D., and P.B. Acosta, Dr. P.H. (see Chapter 63 for discussion).

# Table A–43c. Formulation of "Chemically Defined" Medical Foods for Amino Acid- and Nitrogen-Restricted Diets*

| Product | Protein (%) | Fat (%) | Carbohydrate (%) | Minerals (%) | Vitamins (%) | Water (%) |
|---|---|---|---|---|---|---|
| *Mead Johnson Nutritional Division* | | | | | | |
| Lofenalac | 18.7 casein hydrolysate; 1.07 free L-amino acids | 18.0 corn oil | 49.2 corn syrup solids; 9.57 modified tapioca starch | 3.6 | all present | 3.8 |
| Moducal | none | none | 100 maltodextrin | 0.4 | none | 5.0 |
| MSUD Diet Powder | 10.0 free L-amino acids | 20.1 corn oil | 63.3 corn syrup solids and modified tapioca starch | 3.5 | all present | 3.3 |
| Low Methionine Diet Powder | 15.8 soy protein isolate | 28.0 corn oil and coconut oil | 51.1 corn syrup solids | 3.0 | all present | 2.1 |
| Low Phe/Tyr Diet Powder | 18.7 casein hydrolysate; 1.07 free L-amino acids | 18.0 corn oil | 59.6 corn syrup solids and modified tapioca starch | 3.6 | all present | 3.8 |
| Phenyl-Free | 20.3 L-amino acids | 6.8 corn oil and coconut oil | 66 sucrose, corn syrup solids, and modified tapioca starch | 3.8 | all present | 3.2 |
| Protein-Free Diet Powder | none | 22.5 corn oil | 71.8 corn syrup solids and modified tapioca starch | 2.7 | all present | 3.0 |
| *Milupa Company* | | | | | | |
| HOM 1/HOM 2 | 51.6/68.8 L-amino acids | none | 17.7/5.2 sucrose | 15.8/8.7 | 1.8/1.0 | 2.8/3.0 |
| MSUD 1/MSUD 2 | 40.9/54.3 L-amino acids | none | 30.5/22.5 sucrose | 15.8/8.3 | 1.8/1.0 | 2.8/3.0 |
| PKU 1/PKU 2 | 50.3/66.8 L-amino acids | none | 19.3/7.6 sucrose | 15.8/8.7 | 1.8/1.0 | 2.8/2.6 |
| PKU 3 | 68.0 L-amino acids | none | 3.4 sucrose | 11.4 | all present | 3.6 |
| TYR 1/TYR 2 | 47.4/63.0 L-amino acids | none | 22.7/12.1 sucrose | 15.8/8.7 | 1.8/1.0 | 2.8/2.6 |
| UCD 1/UCD 2 | 56.4/66.7 L-amino acids | none | 8.0/5.8 sucrose | 18.1/8.7 | 2.1/1.0 | 4.1/3.7 |
| *Ross Laboratories* | | | | | | |
| Analog Range | 13.0 L-amino acids | 20.9 | 58.0 maltodextrins 1.0 galactose | 1.37 | 0.22 | 3.00 |
| Polycose Powder | none | none | 94.0 glucose polymers | 0.38 | none | 6.00 |
| Maxamaid Range | 25.0 L-amino acids | 0 | 62.0 sucrose | 3.72 | 0.33 | 3.00 |
| Maxamum XP | 39.0 L-amino acids | 0 | 45.0 sucrose | 3.49 | 0.53 | 3.00 |

*From references 57 to 61 in Chapter 63, compiled by L.J. Elsas II, M.D. and P.B. Acosta, Dr. P.H. (see Chapter 63 for discussion).

**Table A–43d-1. Composition of "Chemically Defined" Medical Foods for Amino Acid- or Nitrogen-Restricted Diets (per 100 g of product)\*: Phenylalanine-Low or -Free Products**

| Nutrients | Analog XP | Lofenalac | Maxamaid XP | Maxamum XP | Phenyl-Free | PKU 1 | PKU 2 | PKU 3 |
|---|---|---|---|---|---|---|---|---|
| Energy (kcal) | 475 | 460 | 350 | 340 | 406 | 278 | 298 | 286 |
| Protein equivalent (g) | 13.00 | 15.0 | 25.0 | 39.0 | 20.3 | 50.3 | 66.8 | 68.0 |
| Alanine (g) | 0.61 | 0.68 | 1.08 | 1.68 | 0 | 2.40 | 3.10 | 3.10 |
| Arginine (g) | 1.08 | 0.56 | 2.33 | 3.18 | 0.69 | 2.00 | 2.70 | 2.70 |
| Aspartic acid (g) | 1.01 | 1.40 | 1.95 | 2.96 | 5.30 | 5.70 | 7.60 | 7.60 |
| Carnitine (g) | 0.010 | 8.60 | 0 | 0.02 | 0 | 0 | 0 | 0 |
| Cystine (g) | 0.40 | 0.06 | 0.75 | 1.17 | 0.35 | 1.40 | 1.80 | 1.80 |
| Glutamic acid (g) | 1.23 | 4.00 | 2.53 | 4.80 | 6.70 | 12.00 | 16.00 | 16.00 |
| Glutamine (g) | 0.12 | ? | 0.23 | 0.36 | 0 | 0 | 0 | 0 |
| Glycine (g) | 0.95 | 0.38 | 1.86 | 2.97 | 3.30 | 1.40 | 1.80 | 1.80 |
| Histidine (g) | 0.62 | 0.49 | 1.34 | 1.80 | 0.47 | 1.40 | 1.80 | 1.80 |
| Isoleucine (g) | 0.95 | 0.87 | 1.79 | 2.80 | 1.10 | 3.40 | 4.50 | 4.50 |
| Leucine (g) | 1.63 | 1.70 | 3.06 | 4.80 | 1.71 | 5.70 | 7.60 | 7.60 |
| Lysine (g) | 1.11 | 1.66 | 2.34 | 3.67 | 1.87 | 4.00 | 5.40 | 5.40 |
| Methionine (g) | 0.26 | 0.55 | 0.50 | 0.77 | 0.63 | 1.40 | 1.80 | 1.80 |
| Phenylalanine (g) | 0 | 0.075 | 0 | 0 | 20 | 0 | 0 | 0 |
| Proline (g) | 1.16 | 1.42 | 2.16 | 3.40 | 0 | 5.40 | 7.10 | 7.10 |
| Serine (g) | 0.71 | 0.94 | 1.33 | 2.10 | 0 | 3.00 | 4.00 | 4.00 |
| Taurine (g) | 0.020 | 0.027 | 0 | 0.15 | 0 | 0 | 0 | 0 |
| Threonine (g) | 0.80 | 0.79 | 1.50 | 2.35 | 0.93 | 2.70 | 3.60 | 3.60 |
| Tryptophan (g) | 0.32 | 0.20 | 0.60 | 0.94 | 0.28 | 1.00 | 1.40 | 1.40 |
| Tyrosine (g) | 1.44 | 0.80 | 2.70 | 4.24 | 0.93 | 3.40 | 4.50 | 6.00 |
| Valine (g) | 1.04 | 1.38 | 1.95 | 3.07 | 1.26 | 4.00 | 5.40 | 5.40 |
| Carbohydrate (g) | 59.0 | 60.0 | 62.0 | 45.0 | 66.0 | 19.3 | 7.6 | 3.4 |
| Fat (g) | 20.9 | 18.0 | 0 | 0 | 6.8 | 0 | 0 | 0 |

| | | | | | | | | |
|---|---|---|---|---|---|---|---|---|
| Calcium (mg) | 300 | 434 | 810 | 670 | 508 | 2,400 | 1,312 | 1,312 |
| Chloride (meq) | 8.0 | 9.2 | 12.9 | 16.0 | 26.7 | 47.1 | 28.2 | 28.2 |
| Chromium (µg) | 15 | ? | 0 | 50 | 0 | 0 | 0 | 0 |
| Copper (mg) | 0.4 | 0.4 | 2.0 | 1.4 | 0.6 | 6.7 | 2.0 | 3.6 |
| Iodine (µg) | 47 | 32 | 134 | 107 | 45 | 234 | 120 | 143 |
| Iron (mg) | 5.5 | 8.7 | 12.0 | 23.5 | 12.2 | 34.0 | 15.0 | 21.0 |
| Magnesium (mg) | 34 | 50 | 200 | 285 | 152 | 521 | 156 | 536 |
| Manganese (mg) | 0.31 | 0.14 | 1.30 | 1.7 | 1.02 | 2.40 | 0.70 | 4.8 |
| Molybdenum (µg) | 25.00 | ? | 60.0 | 110 | 0 | 107.00 | 32.00 | 476 |
| Phosphorus (mg) | 226 | 324 | 810 | 670 | 508 | 1,860 | 1,014 | 1,014 |
| Potassium (meq) | 10.2 | 12.1 | 21.5 | 17.9 | 35.1 | 59.8 | 34.1 | 34.1 |
| Selenium (µg) | 15 | ? | 0 | 50 | 6.1 | 0 | 0 | 0 |
| Sodium (meq) | 5.3 | 9.4 | 25.2 | 24.3 | 17.7 | 46.4 | 27.8 | 27.8 |
| Zinc (mg) | 3.9 | 3.6 | 13.0 | 13.6 | 7.1 | 26.0 | 7.8 | 23.8 |
| Vitamin A (µg) | 530 | 432 | 300 | 710 | 366 | 2,800 | 1,560 | 1,190 |
| D (µg) | 7.5 | 7.2 | 12.0 | 8.0 | 3.8 | 25.0 | 33.0 | 12.0 |
| E (mg) | 4.9 | 12.0 | 5.9 | 7.1 | 9.2 | 34 | 18.0 | 12.0 |
| K (µg) | 45 | 72 | 0 | 70 | 102 | 167 | 167 | 167 |
| Ascorbic acid (mg) | 41 | 37 | 135 | 90 | 53 | 234 | 80 | 100 |
| Biotin (mg) | 0.026 | 0.036 | 0.12 | 0.140 | 0.030 | 0.100 | 0.300 | 0.179 |
| $B_6$ (mg) | 0.35 | 0.29 | 1.00 | 2.1 | 0.9 | 2.20 | 1.50 | 3.2 |
| $B_{12}$ (µg) | 1.0 | 1.4 | 4.0 | 4.0 | 2.5 | 7.9 | 3.0 | 5.0 |
| Choline (mg) | 65 | 61 | 110 | 320 | 85 | 434 | 261 | 261 |
| Folate (µg) | 38 | 72 | 150 | 500 | 127 | 340 | 400 | 952 |
| Inositol (mg) | 100 | 22 | 56 | 86 | 30 | 500 | 300 | 300 |
| Niacin (mg)† | 4.5 | 5.8 | 12.0 | 13.6 | 8.1 | 54.0 | 24.0 | 18.0 |
| Pantothenic acid (mg) | 1.7 | 2.2 | 3.7 | 5.0 | 3.0 | 25.0 | 11.0 | 8.3 |
| Riboflavin (mg) | 0.60 | 0.4 | 1.20 | 1.4 | 1.0 | 4.00 | 2.00 | 1.8 |
| Thiamin (mg) | 0.40 | 0.4 | 1.08 | 1.4 | 0.6 | 2.70 | 1.40 | 1.8 |

*From references 57 to 61 in Chapter 63, compiled by L.J. Elsas II, M.D., and P.B. Acosta, Dr. P.H. (see Chapter 63 for discussion).
†Preformed niacin

**Table A–43d-2.    Composition of "Chemically Defined" Medical Foods for Amino Acid- or Nitrogen-Restricted Diets (per 100 g of product)\*: Tyrosine-Low or -Free Products**

| Nutrients | Analog X PHEN. TYR | Analog X PHEN. TYR. MET | Low Phe/Tyr Diet Powder | Maxamaid X PHEN. TYR | Maxamaid X PHEN. TYR. MET | TYR 1 | TYR 2 |
|---|---|---|---|---|---|---|---|
| Energy (kcal) | 475 | 475 | 460 | 350 | 350 | 280 | 300 |
| Protein equivalent (g) | 13.0 | 13.0 | 15.0 | 25.0 | 25.0 | 47.4 | 63.0 |
| Alanine (g) | 0.71 | 0.73 | 0.68 | 1.32 | 1.34 | 2.40 | 3.10 |
| Arginine (g) | 1.27 | 1.27 | 0.56 | 2.32 | 2.36 | 2.00 | 2.70 |
| Aspartic acid (g) | 1.00 | 1.06 | 1.40 | 1.94 | 1.97 | 5.70 | 7.60 |
| Carnitine (g) | 0.010 | 0.010 | ? | 0 | 0 | 0 | 0 |
| Cystine (g) | 0.46 | 0.48 | 0.06 | 0.86 | 0.87 | 1.40 | 1.80 |
| Glutamic acid (g) | 1.40 | 1.41 | 4.00 | 2.59 | 2.63 | 12.00 | 16.00 |
| Glutamine (g) | 0.14 | 0.14 | ? | 0.25 | 0.25 | 0 | 0 |
| Glycine (g) | 1.11 | 1.13 | 0.38 | 2.06 | 2.10 | 1.40 | 1.80 |
| Histidine (g) | 0.71 | 0.73 | 0.46 | 1.33 | 1.35 | 1.40 | 1.80 |
| Isoleucine (g) | 1.11 | 1.08 | 0.88 | 2.06 | 2.10 | 3.40 | 4.50 |
| Leucine (g) | 1.90 | 1.93 | 1.70 | 3.53 | 3.60 | 5.70 | 7.60 |
| Lysine (g) | 1.30 | 1.30 | 1.66 | 2.40 | 2.44 | 4.00 | 5.40 |
| Methionine (g) | 0.30 | 0 | 0.55 | 0.56 | 0 | 1.40 | 1.80 |
| Phenylalanine (g) | 0 | 0 | 0.075 | 0 | 0 | 0 | 0 |
| Proline (g) | 1.35 | 1.30 | 1.42 | 2.50 | 2.55 | 5.40 | 7.10 |
| Serine (g) | 0.83 | 0.87 | 0.94 | 1.54 | 1.57 | 3.00 | 4.00 |
| Taurine (g) | 0.02 | 0.02 | 0.036 | 0 | 0 | 0 | 0 |
| Threonine (g) | 0.91 | 0.95 | 0.79 | 1.73 | 1.76 | 2.70 | 3.60 |
| Tryptophan (g) | 0.37 | 0.40 | 0.20 | 0.69 | 0.70 | 1.00 | 1.40 |
| Tyrosine (g) | 0 | 0 | 0.038 | 0 | 0 | 0 | 0 |
| Valine (g) | 1.21 | 1.22 | 1.38 | 2.25 | 2.29 | 4.00 | 5.40 |
| Carbohydrate (g) | 59.0 | 59.0 | 60.0 | 62.0 | 62.0 | 22.7 | 12.1 |
| Fat (g) | 20.9 | 20.9 | 18.0 | 0 | 0 | 0 | 0 |

| | | | | | | | | |
|---|---|---|---|---|---|---|---|---|
| Calcium (mg) | 300 | 300 | 431 | 810 | 810 | 810 | 2,400 | 1,312 |
| Chloride (meq) | 8.0 | 12.9 | 9.3 | 12.9 | 12.9 | 12.9 | 47.1 | 28.2 |
| Chromium (µg) | 15 | 15 | ? | 0 | 0 | 0 | 0 | 0 |
| Copper (mg) | 0.4 | 0.4 | 0.4 | 2.0 | 2.0 | 2.0 | 6.7 | 2.0 |
| Iodine (µg) | 47 | 47 | 32 | 134 | 134 | 134 | 234 | 120 |
| Iron (mg) | 5.5 | 5.5 | 8.6 | 12.0 | 12.0 | 12.0 | 34.0 | 15.0 |
| Magnesium (mg) | 34 | 34 | 50 | 200 | 200 | 200 | 521 | 156 |
| Manganese (mg) | 0.31 | 0.31 | 0.7 | 1.30 | 1.30 | 1.30 | 2.40 | 0.70 |
| Molybdenum (µg) | 25.00 | 25.0 | ? | 60.0 | 60.0 | 60.0 | 107.00 | 32.00 |
| Phosphorus (mg) | 226 | 226 | 324 | 810 | 810 | 810 | 1,860 | 1,014 |
| Potassium (meq) | 10.2 | 10.2 | 12.0 | 21.5 | 21.5 | 21.5 | 59.8 | 34.1 |
| Selenium (µg) | 15 | 15 | ? | 0 | 0 | 0 | 0 | 0 |
| Sodium (meq) | 5.3 | 5.3 | 9.4 | 25.2 | 25.2 | 25.2 | 46.4 | 27.8 |
| Zinc (mg) | 3.9 | 3.9 | 2.9 | 13.0 | 13.0 | 13.0 | 26.0 | 7.8 |
| Vitamin A (µg) | 530 | 530 | 345 | 300 | 300 | 300 | 2,800 | 1,560 |
| D (µg) | 7.5 | 7.5 | 7.2 | 12.0 | 12.0 | 12.0 | 25.0 | 33.0 |
| E (mg) | 4.9 | 4.9 | 7.0 | 5.9 | 5.9 | 5.9 | 34.0 | 18.0 |
| K (µg) | 45 | 45 | 72 | 0 | 0 | 0 | 167 | 167 |
| Ascorbic acid (mg) | 41 | 41 | 37 | 135 | 135 | 135 | 234 | 80 |
| Biotin (mg) | 0.026 | 0.026 | 0.036 | 0.12 | 0.12 | 0.12 | 0.100 | 0.300 |
| $B_6$ (mg) | 0.35 | 0.35 | 0.3 | 1.00 | 1.00 | 1.00 | 2.20 | 1.50 |
| $B_{12}$ (µg) | 1.0 | 1.0 | 1.4 | 4.0 | 4.0 | 4.0 | 7.9 | 3.0 |
| Choline (mg) | 65 | 65 | 61 | 110 | 110 | 110 | 434 | 261 |
| Folate (µg) | 38 | 38 | 72 | 150 | 150 | 150 | 340 | 400 |
| Inositol (mg) | 100 | 100 | 22 | 56 | 56 | 56 | 500 | 300 |
| Niacin (mg)† | 4.5 | 4.5 | 5.8 | 12.0 | 12.0 | 12.0 | 54.0 | 24.0 |
| Pantothenic acid (mg) | 1.7 | 1.7 | 2.2 | 3.7 | 3.7 | 3.7 | 25.0 | 11.0 |
| Riboflavin (mg) | 0.60 | 0.60 | 0.4 | 1.20 | 1.20 | 1.20 | 4.00 | 2.00 |
| Thiamin (mg) | 0.40 | 0.40 | 0.4 | 1.1 | 1.1 | 1.1 | 2.70 | 1.40 |

*From references 57 to 61 in Chapter 63, compiled by L.J. Elsas II, M.D., and P.B. Acosta, Dr. P.H. (see Chap. 63 for discussion).

†Preformed niacin

**Table A–43d-3. Composition of "Chemically Defined" Medical Foods for Amino Acid- or Nitrogen-Restricted Diets (per 100 g of product)*: Branched-Chain Amino Acid-Free Products**

| Nutrient | Analog MSUD | Maxamaid MSUD | MSUD Diet Powder | MSUD 1 | MSUD 2 |
|---|---|---|---|---|---|
| Energy (kcal) | 475 | 350 | 466 | 286 | 307 |
| Protein equivalent (g) | 13.0 | 25.0 | 8.2 | 40.9 | 54.3 |
| Alanine (g) | 0.80 | 1.56 | 0.44 | 2.40 | 3.10 |
| Arginine (g) | 1.47 | 2.74 | 0.49 | 2.00 | 2.70 |
| Aspartic acid (g) | 1.23 | 2.29 | 1.14 | 5.70 | 7.60 |
| Carnitine (g) | 0.010 | 0 | 0.008 | 0 | 0 |
| Cystine (g) | 0.55 | 1.01 | 0.25 | 1.40 | 1.80 |
| Glutamic acid (g) | 1.65 | 3.05 | 2.10 | 12.00 | 16.00 |
| Glutamine (g) | 0.14 | 0.30 | 0 | 0 | 0 |
| Glycine (g) | 1.31 | 2.43 | 0.60 | 1.40 | 1.80 |
| Histidine (g) | 0.84 | 1.57 | 0.25 | 1.40 | 1.80 |
| Isoleucine (g) | 0 | 0 | 0 | 0 | 0 |
| Leucine (g) | 0 | 0 | 0 | 0 | 0 |
| Lysine (g) | 1.53 | 2.83 | 0.51 | 4.00 | 5.40 |
| Methionine (g) | 0.36 | 0.66 | 0.25 | 1.40 | 1.80 |
| Phenylalanine (g) | 1.00 | 1.84 | 0.55 | 2.40 | 3.20 |
| Proline (g) | 1.60 | 2.96 | 0.89 | 5.40 | 7.10 |
| Serine (g) | 0.98 | 1.82 | 0.60 | 3.00 | 4.00 |
| Taurine (g) | 0.02 | 0 | 0.028 | 0 | 0 |
| Threonine (g) | 1.10 | 2.05 | 0.55 | 2.70 | 3.60 |
| Tryptophan (g) | 0.44 | 0.82 | 0.20 | 1.00 | 1.40 |
| Tyrosine (g) | 1.00 | 1.84 | 0.65 | 2.90 | 3.90 |
| Valine (g) | 0 | 0 | 0 | 0 | 0 |
| Carbohydrate (g) | 59.0 | 62.0 | 63.3 | 30.5 | 22.5 |
| Fat (g) | 20.9 | 0 | 20.0 | 0 | 0 |

| Nutrient | | | | | |
|---|---|---|---|---|---|
| Calcium (mg) | 300 | 810 | 491 | 2,400 | 1,312 |
| Chloride (meq) | 8.0 | 12.9 | 10.5 | 47.1 | 28.2 |
| Chromium (μg) | 15 | 0 | 0 | 0 | 0 |
| Copper (mg) | 0.4 | 2.0 | 0.4 | 6.7 | 2.0 |
| Iodine (μg) | 47 | 134 | 33 | 234 | 120 |
| Iron (mg) | 5.5 | 12.0 | 9.0 | 34.0 | 15.0 |
| Magnesium (mg) | 34 | 200 | 52 | 521 | 156 |
| Manganese (mg) | 0.31 | 1.30 | 0.70 | 2.40 | 0.70 |
| Molybdenum (μg) | 25.00 | 60.0 | 0 | 107.00 | 32.00 |
| Phosphorus (mg) | 226 | 810 | 268 | 1,860 | 1,014 |
| Potassium (meq) | 10.2 | 21.5 | 12.5 | 59.8 | 34.1 |
| Selenium (μg) | 15 | 0 | 0 | 0 | 0 |
| Sodium (meq) | 5.3 | 25.2 | 9.7 | 46.4 | 27.8 |
| Zinc (mg) | 3.9 | 13.0 | 3.0 | 26.0 | 7.8 |
| Vitamin A (μg) | 530 | 300 | 357 | 2,800 | 1,560 |
| D (μg) | 7.5 | 12.0 | 7.4 | 25.0 | 33.0 |
| E (mg) | 4.9 | 5.9 | 7.0 | 34.0 | 18.0 |
| K (μg) | 45 | 0 | 74 | 167 | 167 |
| Ascorbic acid (mg) | 41 | 135 | 39 | 234 | 80 |
| Biotin (mg) | 0.026 | 0.12 | 0.040 | 0.100 | 0.300 |
| B6 (mg) | 0.35 | 1.00 | 0.30 | 2.20 | 1.50 |
| B12 (μg) | 1.0 | 4.0 | 1.50 | 7.9 | 3.0 |
| Choline (mg) | 65 | 110 | 63 | 434 | 261 |
| Folate (μg) | 38 | 150 | 74 | 340 | 400 |
| Inositol (mg) | 100 | 56 | 22 | 500 | 300 |
| Niacin (mg)† | 4.5 | 12.0 | 5.9 | 54.0 | 24.0 |
| Pantothenic acid (mg) | 1.73 | 3.7 | 2.2 | 25.0 | 11.0 |
| Riboflavin (mg) | 0.60 | 1.20 | 0.45 | 4.00 | 2.00 |
| Thiamin (mg) | 0.40 | 1.1 | 0.37 | 2.70 | 1.40 |

*From references 57 to 61 in Chapter 63, compiled by L.J. Elsas II, M.D., and P.B. Acosta, Dr. P.H. (see Chapter 63 for discussion).

†Preformed niacin

**Table A–43d-4.** Composition of "Chemically Defined" Medical Foods for Amino Acid- or Nitrogen-Restricted Diets (per 100 g of product)*: Methionine-Low or -Free Products

| Nutrient | Analog X MET | HOM 1 | HOM 2 | Low Methionine Diet Powder | Maxamaid X MET |
|---|---|---|---|---|---|
| Energy (kcal) | 475 | 277 | 296 | 518 | 350 |
| Protein equivalent (g) | 13.0 | 51.6 | 68.8 | 15.5 | 25.0 |
| Alanine (g) | 0.66 | 2.40 | 3.10 | 0.79 | 1.22 |
| Arginine (g) | 1.15 | 2.00 | 2.70 | 0.88 | 2.14 |
| Aspartic acid (g) | 0.96 | 5.70 | 7.60 | 1.76 | 1.79 |
| Carnitine (g) | 0.01 | 0 | 0 | 0 | 0 |
| Cystine (g) | 0.43 | 2.50 | 3.40 | 0.14 | 0.79 |
| Glutamic acid (g) | 1.29 | 12.00 | 16.00 | 5.10 | 2.39 |
| Glutamine (g) | 0.14 | 0 | 0 | ? | 0.23 |
| Glycine (g) | 1.02 | 1.40 | 1.80 | 0.53 | 1.90 |
| Histidine (g) | 0.66 | 1.40 | 1.80 | 0.36 | 1.22 |
| Isoleucine (g) | 1.02 | 3.40 | 4.50 | 0.73 | 1.90 |
| Leucine (g) | 1.76 | 5.70 | 7.60 | 1.20 | 3.26 |
| Lysine (g) | 1.19 | 4.00 | 5.40 | 0.95 | 2.21 |
| Methionine (g) | 0 | 0 | 0 | 0.16 | 0 |
| Phenylalanine (g) | 0.78 | 2.40 | 3.20 | 0.77 | 1.44 |
| Proline (g) | 1.24 | 5.40 | 7.10 | 2.40 | 2.31 |
| Serine (g) | 0.77 | 3.00 | 4.00 | 1.36 | 1.42 |
| Taurine (g) | 0.02 | 0 | 0 | 0.31 | 0 |
| Threonine (g) | 0.86 | 2.70 | 3.60 | 0.51 | 1.60 |
| Tryptophan (g) | 0.34 | 1.00 | 1.40 | 0.19 | 0.64 |
| Tyrosine (g) | 0.78 | 2.90 | 3.90 | 0.54 | 1.44 |
| Valine (g) | 1.12 | 4.00 | 5.40 | 0.73 | 2.08 |
| Carbohydrate (g) | 59.0 | 17.7 | 5.2 | 51.0 | 62.0 |
| Fat (g) | 20.9 | 0 | 0 | 28.0 | 0 |

| | | | | | |
|---|---|---|---|---|---|
| Calcium (mg) | 300 | 2,400 | 1,312 | 480 | 810 |
| Chloride (meq) | 8.0 | 47.1 | 28.2 | 12.0 | 12.9 |
| Chromium (µg) | 15 | 0 | 0 | ? | 0 |
| Copper (mg) | 0.4 | 6.7 | 2.0 | 0.48 | 2.0 |
| Iodine (µg) | 47 | 234 | 120 | 52 | 134 |
| Iron (mg) | 5.5 | 34.0 | 15.0 | 9.7 | 12.0 |
| Magnesium (mg) | 34 | 521 | 156 | 56 | 200 |
| Manganese (mg) | 0.31 | 2.40 | 0.70 | 0.16 | 1.30 |
| Molybdenum (µg) | 25.00 | 107.00 | 32.00 | ? | 60.0 |
| Phosphorus (mg) | 226 | 1,860 | 1,014 | 380 | 810 |
| Potassium (meq) | 10.2 | 59.8 | 34.1 | 15.4 | 21.5 |
| Selenium (µg) | 15 | 0 | 0 | ? | 0 |
| Sodium (meq) | 5.3 | 46.4 | 27.8 | 9.6 | 25.2 |
| Zinc (mg) | 3.9 | 26.0 | 7.8 | 4 | 13.0 |
| Vitamin A (µg) | 530 | 2,800 | 1,560 | 387 | 300 |
| D (µg) | 7.5 | 25.0 | 33.0 | 8 | 12.0 |
| E (mg) | 4.9 | 34.0 | 18.0 | 8 | 5.9 |
| K (µg) | 45 | 167 | 167 | 80 | 0 |
| Ascorbic acid (mg) | 41 | 234 | 80 | 42 | 135 |
| Biotin (mg) | 0.026 | 0.100 | 0.300 | 0.04 | 0.12 |
| $B_6$ (mg) | 0.35 | 2.20 | 1.50 | 0.32 | 1.00 |
| $B_{12}$ (µg) | 1.0 | 7.9 | 3.0 | 1.61 | 4.0 |
| Choline (mg) | 65 | 434 | 261 | 40 | 110 |
| Folate (µg) | 38 | 340 | 400 | 80 | 150 |
| Inositol (mg) | 100 | 500 | 300 | 24 | 56 |
| Niacin (mg)† | 4.5 | 54.0 | 24.0 | 6.4 | 12.0 |
| Pantothenic acid (mg) | 1.7 | 25.0 | 11.0 | 2.4 | 3.7 |
| Riboflavin (mg) | 0.60 | 4.00 | 2.00 | 0.48 | 1.20 |
| Thiamin (mg) | 0.40 | 2.70 | 1.40 | 0.4 | 1.08 |

*From references 57 to 61 in Chapter 63, compiled by L.J. Elsas II, M.D., and P.B. Acosta, Dr. P.H. (see Chapter 63 for discussion).
†Preformed niacin

**Table A–43d-5.** **Composition of "Chemically Defined" Medical Foods for Amino Acid- or Nitrogen-Restricted Diets (per 100 g of product)\*: Nitrogen-Free Products**

| Nutrients | Moducal | Polycose Powder | Protein-Free Diet Powder |
|---|---|---|---|
| Energy (kcal) | 380 | 380 | 490 |
| Protein equivalent (g) | 0 | 0 | 0 |
| Carbohydrate (g) | 95.0 | 94.0 | 71.8 |
| Fat (g) | 0 | 0 | 22.5 |
| Calcium (mg) | 0 | 30 | 540 |
| Chloride (meq) | 4.8 | 6.3 | 3.9 |
| Chromium (µg) | 0 | 0 | 0 |
| Copper (mg) | 0 | 0 | 0.5 |
| Iodine (µg) | 0 | 0 | 41 |
| Iron (mg) | 0 | 0 | 11.0 |
| Magnesium (mg) | 0 | 0 | 63 |
| Manganese (mg) | 0 | 0 | 0.9 |
| Molybdenum (µg) | 0 | 0 | 0 |
| Phosphorus (mg) | 0 | 5 | 300 |
| Potassium (meq) | 0.1 | 0.3 | 8.7 |
| Selenium (µg) | 0 | 0 | 0 |
| Sodium (meq) | 3.0 | 4.8 | 3.1 |
| Zinc (mg) | 0 | 0 | 3.6 |
| Vitamin A (µg) | 0 | 0 | 432 |
| D (µg) | 0 | 0 | 9.0 |
| E (mg) | 0 | 0 | 9.0 |
| K (µg) | 0 | 0 | 90 |
| Ascorbic acid (mg) | 0 | 0 | 45 |
| Biotin (mg) | 0 | 0 | 0.045 |
| $B_6$ (mg) | 0 | 0 | 0.36 |
| $B_{12}$ (µg) | 0 | 0 | 1.8 |
| Choline (mg) | 0 | 0 | 76 |
| Folate (µg) | 0 | 0 | 90 |
| Inositol (mg) | 0 | 0 | 27 |
| Niacin (mg)† | 0 | 0 | 7.2 |
| Pantothenic acid (mg) | 0 | 0 | 2.7 |
| Riboflavin (mg) | 0 | 0 | 0.5 |
| Thiamin (mg) | 0 | 0 | 0.4 |

\*From references 57 to 61 in Chapter 63, compiled by L.J. Elsas II, M.D., and P.B. Acosta, Dr. P.H. (see Chapter 63 for discussion).
†Preformed niacin

**Table A–43d-6.** **Composition of "Chemically Defined" Medical Foods for Amino Acid- or Nitrogen-Restricted Diets (per 100 g of product)\*: Products for Nitrogen-Restricted Diets**

| Nutrient | UCD 1 | UCD 2 |
|---|---|---|
| Energy (kcal) | 258 | 290 |
| Protein equivalent (g) | 56.4 | 66.7 |
| Alanine (g) | 0 | 0 |
| Arginine (g) | 0 | 0 |
| Aspartic acid (g) | 0 | 0 |
| Carnitine (g) | 0 | 0 |
| Cystine (g) | 3.10 | 0 |
| Glutamic acid (g) | 0 | 0 |
| Glutamine (g) | 0 | 0 |
| Glycine (g) | 0 | 0 |
| Histidine (g) | 3.10 | 3.60 |
| Isoleucine (g) | 7.60 | 8.90 |
| Leucine (g) | 12.80 | 15.00 |
| Lysine (g) | 9.00 | 10.70 |
| Methionine (g) | 3.10 | 7.10 |
| Phenylalanine (g) | 5.30 | 14.10 |
| Proline (g) | 0 | 0 |
| Serine (g) | 0 | 0 |
| Taurine (g) | 0 | 0 |
| Threonine (g) | 6.00 | 7.10 |
| Tryptophan (g) | 2.20 | 2.80 |
| Tyrosine (g) | 6.50 | 0 |
| Valine (g) | 9.00 | 10.70 |
| Carbohydrate (g) | 8.00 | 5.8 |
| Fat (g) | 0 | 0 |
| Calcium (mg) | 2,832 | 1,312 |
| Chloride (meq) | 55.5 | 28.2 |
| Chromium (µg) | 0 | 0 |
| Copper (mg) | 8.0 | 2.0 |
| Iodine (µg) | 274 | 120 |
| Iron (mg) | 40.0 | 15.0 |
| Magnesium (mg) | 0 | 0 |
| Manganese (mg) | 2.8 | 0.7 |
| Molybdenum (µg) | 128 | 32 |
| Phosphorus (mg) | 2,195 | 1,014 |
| Potassium (meq) | 70.6 | 34.1 |
| Selenium (µg) | 0 | 0 |
| Sodium (meq) | 54.6 | 27.8 |
| Zinc (mg) | 31.0 | 7.8 |
| Vitamin A (µg) | 3,360 | 1,560 |
| D (µg) | 30 | 33 |
| E (mg) | 41 | 18 |
| K (µg) | 200 | 167 |
| Ascorbic acid (mg) | 280 | 80 |
| Biotin (mg) | 0.12 | 0.30 |
| $B_6$ (mg) | 2.6 | 1.5 |
| $B_{12}$ (µg) | 8 | 3 |
| Choline (mg) | 512 | 261 |
| Folate (µg) | 400 | 400 |
| Inositol (mg) | 590 | 300 |
| Niacin (mg)† | 65 | 24 |
| Pantothenic acid (mg) | 30 | 11 |
| Riboflavin (mg) | 4.8 | 2.0 |
| Thiamin (mg) | 3.2 | 1.4 |

\*From references 57 to 61 in Chapter 63, compiled by L.J. Elsas II, M.D., and P.B. Acosta, Dr. P.H. (see Chapter 63 for discussion).
†Preformed niacin

## Table A–43e. Average Nutrient Content of Serving Lists for Phenylalanine and/or Tyrosine and Protein-Restricted Diets*

| Food List | Phenylalanine (mg) | Tyrosine (mg) | Methionine (mg) | Protein (g) | Carbohydrate (g) | Fat (g) | Energy (kcal) |
|---|---|---|---|---|---|---|---|
| Breads/cereals | 30 | 20 | 13 | 0.6 | 7 | 0 | 30 |
| Fats | 5 | 4 | 2 | 0.1 | 0 | 5 | 60 |
| Fruits | 15 | 10 | 8 | 0.5 | 15 | 0 | 60 |
| Vegetables | 15 | 10 | 6 | 0.5 | 2 | 0 | 10 |
| Free foods A† | 5 | 4 | 2 | 0.1 | 18 | 0 | 65 |
| Free foods B | 0 | 0 | 0 | 0 | 14 | varies | 55 |

*Compiled by L.J. Elsas II, M.D., and P.B. Acosta, Dr. P.H. (see Chapter 63 for discussion).
†Low-protein pastas and breads not included.

## Table A–43f. Average Nutrient Content of Equivalent Lists for Branched-Chain Amino Acid-Restricted Diets*

| Food List | Isoleucine (mg) | Leucine (mg) | Valine (mg) | Protein (g) | Fat (g) | Energy (kcal) |
|---|---|---|---|---|---|---|
| Breads/cereals | 18 | 35 | 25 | 0.5 | 0 | 30 |
| Fats | 7 | 10 | 7 | 0.1 | 8 | 70 |
| Fruits | 17 | 25 | 22 | 0.6 | 0 | 75 |
| Vegetables | 22 | 30 | 24 | 0.6 | 0 | 15 |
| Free foods A† | 3 | 5 | 4 | 0.1 | 0 | 50 |
| Free foods B | 0 | 0 | 0 | 0 | varies | 55 |

*Compiled by L.J. Elsas II, M.D., and P.B. Acosta, Dr. P.H.
†Low-protein pastas and breads not included.

## Table A–43g. Average Nutrient Content of Serving Lists for Methionine-Restricted Diets*

| Food List | Methionine (mg) | Cystine (mg) | Protein (g) | Fat (g) | Energy (kcal) |
|---|---|---|---|---|---|
| Breads/cereals | 20 | 20 | 1.2 | 0 | 55 |
| Fats | 2 | 0 | 0.1 | 2 | 25 |
| Fruits | 5 | 5 | 0.5 | 0 | 60 |
| Vegetables | 10 | 8 | 1.0 | 0 | 20 |
| Free foods A† | 1 | 1 | 0.2 | 0 | 50 |
| Free foods B | 0 | 0 | 0 | varies | 55 |

*Compiled by L.J. Elsas II, M.D., and P.B. Acosta, Dr. P.H. (see Chapter 63 for discussion).
†Low-protein pastas and breads not included.

## Table A–43h.  Galactose-Restricted Diet*

| Foods Allowed | Foods Excluded |
|---|---|
| *Beverages* <br> Isomil,† Nutramigen,‡ Pregestimil,‡ ProSobee,‡ carbonated drinks, fruit drinks, lactose-free products | *Beverages* <br> All untreated milk of any species and all products containing milk; whole, skim, dried, evaporated, or condensed; yogurt, cheese; aged cheese, ice cream, sherbet; malted milk; Ovaltine, hot chocolate; some cocoas and instant coffees (read labels); powdered soft drinks with lactose; curds; whey and casein; milk treated with lactobacillus acidophilus culture or lactose; imitation or filled milks; casein |
| *Breads and Cereals* <br> Breads, crackers, and rolls made without milk; Italian bread, some cooked and prepared cereals (read labels), soda crackers, pasta; contact bakeries in each geographic area for milk-free breads | *Breads and Cereals* <br> Prepared mixes, such as muffins, biscuits, waffles, pancakes; some dry cereals (read labels carefully); instant Cream of Wheat; cereals, breads, crackers, zwieback; French toast made with milk |
| *Cheeses* <br> None | *Cheeses* <br> All excluded |
| *Desserts* <br> Water and fruit ices; gelatin, angel food cake; homemade cakes, pies, cookies made from allowed ingredients; puddings made with water; sorbets | *Desserts* <br> Commercial cakes, cookies, and mixes, custard, puddings, sherbets, ice cream made with milk; any containing chocolate; pie crust made with butter or margarine |
| *Eggs* <br> All | *Eggs* <br> Omelets and soufflés containing milk |
| *Fats* <br> Margarines and dressings that do not contain milk or milk products, oils, shortening, bacon, some nondairy creamers (read labels), nut butters, nuts, lard | *Fats* <br> Margarines and dressings containing milk or milk products, butter, cream, cream cheese, peanut butter with milk solid fillers, salad dressings containing lactose, nondairy creamers containing sodium or calcium caseinate |
| *Fruits* <br> All canned, fresh, or frozen that are not processed with lactose | *Fruits* <br> Any canned or frozen processed with lactose |
| *Legumes* <br> All may be included if laboratory facilities are available for periodic testing of erythrocyte galactose-1-phosphate | *Legumes* <br> Fermented soybean products such as miso, natto, tempeh, or fermented soy sauce in which enzyme processing has been used |
| *Meat, Fish, Poultry* <br> Plain beef, chicken, fish, ham, lamb, pork, veal, strained or junior meats that do not contain milk or milk products; kosher frankfurters | *Meat, Fish, Poultry* <br> Creamed or breaded meat, fish, or fowl; sausage products, such as weiners, liver sausage, cold cuts containing nonfat milk solids; brains, liver, kidney, pancreas, sweetbreads |
| *Soups* <br> Clear soups, consommés, cream soups made with nondairy creamers free of caseinate, vegetable soups | *Soups* <br> Cream soups unless made with allowed ingredients, chowders, commercially prepared soups containing lactose |
| *Vegetables* <br> Fresh, canned, or frozen; artichokes, asparagus, beets, broccoli, cabbage, carrots, cauliflower, celery, chard, corn, cucumbers, eggplant, green beans, kale, lettuce, mustard, okra, onions, parsley, parsnips, potatoes, pumpkin, rutabagas, spinach, squash, tomatoes, white and sweet potatoes, yams; all vegetables if prepared without lactose | *Vegetables* <br> Any to which lactose is added during processing; peas; creamed, breaded, or buttered vegetables; instant potatoes, corn curls and frozen French fries if processed with lactose |
| *Miscellaneous* <br> Carob powder, popcorn, olives, pure sugar candy, jelly or marmalade, sugar, corn syrup, gravy made with water, baker's cocoa, pickles, pure seasoning and spices, molasses, beet sugar, pure monosodium glutamate, honey | *Miscellaneous* <br> Chewing gum; milk chocolate; some cocoas; toffee, peppermint; butterscotch, caramels; dietetic preparations (read labels); certain drugs and vitamin and mineral preparations; spice blends if they contain lactose; monosodium glutamate extender; artificial sweeteners containing lactose |

*Compiled by L.J. Elsas II, M.D. and P.B. Acosta, Dr. P.H. (see Chapter 63 for discussion).
†Ross Laboratories, Columbus, Ohio 43216.
‡Mead Johnson Nutritional Division, Evansville, IN 47221.

## Table A–44.  Customized Formulas for Hospital or Patient Self-Preparation Allowing Individual Variation (per 1,000 kcal)

MSKCC Blenderized Tube Feeding: A general formula for patients with normal absorption. Sodium restriction to varying degrees is achieved by omission of salt and use of low-salt vegetables. Potassium restriction is achieved by modification of orange juice. Volume per 1,000 kcal is 1,000 ml.

| | |
|---|---|
| Carrots, canned | 45 g |
| Chopped beef* | 105 g |
| Corn oil | 30 g |
| Dark Karo syrup | 90 g |
| Egg, cooked | 68 g |
| Farina, cooked | 114 g |
| Nonfat milk powder | 20 g |
| Orange juice | 180 ml |
| Salt | 1.5 g |
| Water or vegetable juice | 450 g |
| Wax beans, canned | 30 g |
| Multivitamins with iron (supplementary type) | 1 tablet/day |

DeR Oral or Tube Formula: A palatable low-residue defined formula as supplement. When this formula is used as the only source of nutrition, magnesium oxide or chloride and trace elements are added. Modifications are easily made as needed. Volume per 1,000 kcal is 800 ml.

| | |
|---|---|
| Calcium caseinate | 31 g |
| Chocolate syrup | 36 g |
| Cornstarch, cooked | 40 g |
| Dextrose, anhydrous or oligosaccharides | 80 g |
| Egg, cooked | 45 g |
| Intact protein‡ | 4.5 g |
| Oil (corn or MCT) | 27 g |
| Potassium chloride | 2.0 g |
| Water | 600 ml |
| Multivitamins with iron (supplementary type) | 1 or 2 tablets/day |
| Trace elements | † |

T-#23 Tube Formula: A formula with casein hydrolysate for use in patients with serious malabsorption, pancreatic insufficiency, inflammatory bowel disease, or intestinal fistulas. Modifications are easily made to meet special needs. Volume per 1,000 kcal is 900 ml.

| | |
|---|---|
| Alcolec§ | 1.0 g |
| Calcium lactate | 0.9 g |
| Calcium phosphate | 0.9 g** |
| DL-methionine | 0.23 g |
| DL-tryptophan | 0.23 g |
| Egg, cooked | 45 g** |
| Hydrolyzed protein# | 34 g** |
| Magnesium chloride | 12 meq** |
| Oil (corn or MCT), initially low | 23 g |
| Oligosaccharides | 169 g |
| Potassium gluconate and/or bicarbonate | 25 meq** |
| Sodium chloride and/or bicarbonate | 35 meq** |
| Trace elements | † |
| Water | 690 ml** |
| Multivitamins (supplementary type) | 2 tablets/day** |

*Pureed beef is used for small-bore tubes to avoid clogging.

‡Intact protein: e.g., Casec (Ca caseinate) Mead Johnson; Nutrisource Protein (lactalbumin) Sandoz; ProMix (whey) Navaco; ProMod (whey) Ross; Propac (whey) Sherwood Medical.

§Lecithin (emulsifying agent) if oil is used.

#Hydrolyzed protein: e.g., Hy-Case (casein hydrolysate) Humko Sheffield Chemical. A free amino acid mixture is also available, e.g., Nutrisource Amino Acids (essential and nonessential amino acids; this is much more expensive than the hydrolysate) Sandoz.

†For approximate requirements, see individual chapters on trace elements.

**To be modified upward or down depending on extent of malabsorption, gastrointestinal fluid losses, and severity of renal dysfunction.

## Table A–45. Modifications of MSKCC Blenderized Tube-Feeding Formula (A-44) for Special Clinical Conditions

MCT oil: Eliminate 60 g corn oil. Substitute 67 g MCT oil (to maintain 2,000 kcal). Various proportions of both oils may be added as indicated by patient's condition.

Low fat: Eliminate 60 g corn oil. Add 135 g sugar (to maintain 2,000 kcal). Meat must be very lean. Fat = 26 g.

Low Na: Eliminate 3.0 g salt (44 meq Na). If a severely restricted Na intake is indicated, substitute salt-free carrots, salt-free wax beans for regular. Na will be less than 10 meq.

Low protein, potassium, and sodium: The restrictions of this diet are substantial and require close clinical supervision. Modifications shoud be made as soon as the patient's condition permits. An example of such a diet follows:

| Wt. | Ingredients | Household Measures | Nutritive Analysis: 2,287 kcal* | | | |
|------|------------|------------|------------|--------|--------|------|
| 240 g | cooked enriched farina | 1 cup | protein | 17 | g | |
| 45 g | egg, boiled | 1 | fat | 95 | g | |
| 20 g | skim milk powder | 2 Tbsp | $CH_2O$ | 339 | g | |
| 45 g | carrots, salt-free | ¼ cup | | | | |
| 60 g | wax beans, salt-free | ½ cup | Ca | 363 | mg | |
| 90 g | corn oil | 3 oz | P | 329 | mg | |
| 300 g | sugar | 2 cups | Na | 176/8 | mg/meq | |
| | Water up to 2,000 ml | | K | 533/14 | mg/meq | |
| | volume or as indicated | | Fe | 2.8 | mg | plus |
| | | | Vitamin A | 7,347 | I.U. | those |
| | | | $B_1$ | 0.24 | mg | in |
| | | | $B_2$ | 0.97 | mg | multivitamin |
| | | | Niacin | 1.54 | mg | mineral |
| | | | Vitamin C | 17.9 | mg | supplement |

*Does not meet 1980 RDA except for vitamin A. When multivitamin and mineral prescriptions are given, vitamin and mineral allowances may be achieved.

# Index

Page numbers in *italics* indicate figures; page numbers followed by "t" indicate tables.

body composition in, 552
in sepsis
nutritional support in, 1333
Heat
theories of, 521-524
vital, 517-520
Height, 533-536
body composition and, 547
diurnal variation in, 538
elbow breadth and
as measure of body frame size,
1512t
energy requirements in
adolescence and, 971, 971t
estimation of
in elderly, 834
heredity's influence on, 535-536
in nutritional history assessment,
756-757, 757t
knee height and, 834, 853t
loss of
in aging, 536, 993
measurement of, 830
normative values for, 534, *534*,
*536*, *538*
Height-weight table(s), 1511t, 1514t
sources and development of, 1509-
1513
Helmholtz, Herman von, 523-524
Hemagglutinin(s). *See also* Lectin(s)
in plants, 687
Hematin
in immunity, 601
Hematopoiesis
ineffective
in folic acid or vitamin $B_{12}$
deficiency, 406
Hemicellulose(s)
chemical structure of, 53
Hemochromatosis, 217
clinical manifestations of, 217,
741
hereditary, 218-219
alcoholic cirrhosis and, 218, 219
susceptibility to infection in,
217
screening tests for, 218-219
shunt, 219-220
Hemodialysis. *See* Dialysis
Hemofiltration
continuous arteriovenous, 1263
Hemoglobin
normal values
in elderly, 994
racial differences in level, 974
Hemoglobin E trait, 210
Hemoglobin H disease, 210
Hemoglobin Lepore trait, 210
Hemoglobinuria
paroxysmal nocturnal, 209
Hemolytic anemia
in premature infants
vitamin E and, 350-351, *351*
Hemorrhage
iron loss in, 206, 208
Hemorrhagic disease of the
newborn, 335
Hemosiderin, 202, 203
Hemosiderosis

defined, 217
idiopathic pulmonary, 209
Henderson, L. J., 112
Henderson-Hasselbalch equation,
125
Hepatic coma
branched-chain amino acids in,
21-23, *23*
Hepatic encephalopathy, 1185-1189,
1463-1465
amino acid analogues for, 1189
branched-chain amino acids in,
1186, 1187t-1188t, 1442-1443,
1464-1465
dietary treatment of, 1186-1189,
1442-1443, 1464-1465
in sepsis
nutritional support for, 1333
pathogenesis of, 1185-1186, 1464
postoperative
nutritional support for, 1312
Hepatic failure. *See* Liver failure
Hepatitis
alcoholic
nutritional support in, 1183-
1184, 1441
Hepatitis B virus
liver cancer and, 1396-1397
Hepatolenticular degeneration. *See*
Wilson's disease
Hepatoma
in hemochromatosis, 217
Hepatorenal syndrome
in alcoholism, 1444
Hepatotoxin(s)
in plants, 688
Herb(s)
toxins in, 691-692
Hereditary hemorrhagic
telangiectasia
iron deficiency in, 209
Heredopathia atactica
polyneuritiformis, 1463
HHH syndrome, 1370
Hiatus hernia
fiber and, 66-67
High-density lipoprotein (HDL)
in cholesterol transport and
metabolism, 89-90, 1286
Histamine
in adverse reactions to foods,
1301, 1302t
in control of gastric secretions,
490
plasma
in food allergy diagnosis, 1303
Histamine blocker(s)
for pancreatic insufficiency, 1108
for peptic ulcer, 1100
Histamine poisoning, 642
Histidine
in amino acid supplements for
renal failure patients, 1250
in rheumatoid arthritis, 1476
HLA complex, 597
HLA-DR antigen(s), 597
Homeostasis, 109
Homocysteine
metabolism of, 1364-1365, *1364*

Homocystinuria, *1364*, 1365-1367
incidence of, 1346t, 1365
nutritional requirements in, 1347t,
1366-1367
treatment of, 1366-1367
defined-formula diets in, 1367,
1638t-1639t
natural foods in, 1367, 1643t
Hooke, Robert, 519
Hormone(s). *See also* particular
hormones
body composition and, 551
ectopic
in cancer, 1403-1404
nutrient interactions with, 570-584
Howship's lacuna, 864, *865*
Human chorionic gonadotrophin
for weight loss, 810
Humor(s)
Greek theory of, 516
"Hungry bone" syndrome, 182
Hydralazine
as vitamin antagonist, 639
presystemic clearance of
food and, 635
Hydroxyapatite
in bone, 143
β-Hydroxybutyrate
synthesis of
in prolonged fasting, 783
Hydroxyproline
synthesis of, 2
Hyperalimentation, 1023. *See also*
Enteral nutrition; Parenteral
nutrition
Hyperammonemia, 1463-1465. *See*
*also* Hepatic encephalopathy
differential diagnosis of, 1370
inherited, 1465. *See also* Urea
cycle disorder(s)
valproic acid and, 1468
Hypercalcemia, 146t, 146-147, 739-
740
drug-induced, 641
in cancer, 1404
in magnesium-deficient rats, 174,
178-179, *179*
Hypercalciuria
absorptive, 150
renal, 150
Hypercarotenosis, 304, 734
Hyperchloremia, 132t
Hypercholesterolemia. *See also*
Hyperlipidemia
cholesterol transport and
metabolism in, 90
coronary artery disease and, 1286,
*1286*, 1287
familial, 1288t
cholesterol synthesis regulation
in, 92
dietary management for infants
with, 1293
drug treatment for, 1296
in diabetes mellitus, 1209
management of, 1219
treatment of
candidates for, 1292
dietary, 1293-1294, 1294t